Guidelines

Maternity

Ambulatory (Walking) Epidural Analgesia, 364
Competency Validation for EFM, 388
How to Distinguish True Labor from False Labor, 395
Tests for Rupture of Membranes, 399
Leopold Maneuvers and Determination of the PMI of the FHR, 404
Vaginal Examination, 410
Support of Father/Partner, 420
Preparation for Birth, 421
Assisting at an Emergency Birth of a Fetus in the Vertex Position, 426
Administering Rh Immune Globulin, 502
Basal Body Temperature, 517
Cervical Mucus Characteristics, 517
Use and Care of the Diaphragm, 526
Use and Care of the Cervical Cap, 528
What to Expect After Tubal Ligation, 531
Assessing Attachment Behavior, 614
Physical Examination of the Newborn, 615
Physical Assessment of the High-Risk Infant, 698
Inserting a Gavage Feeding Tube, 709
Neonatal Skin Care, 728
Discharge Teaching for Parents of Compromised Newborns, 767

Pediatrics

Implementing Discipline, 834
Culturally Sensitive Interactions, 869
Using an Interpreter, 872
Communicating with Children, 873
Communicating with Adolescents, 874
Analyzing the Symptom: Pain, 879
Taking an Allergy History, 879
Review of Systems, 881
Measuring Triceps Skinfold Thickness, 899
Measuring Blood Pressure, 905
Effective Auscultation, 922
Feeding Children with Nonorganic Failure to Thrive, 983
Assessing Toilet Training Readiness, 999
Talking with Children Who Reveal Abuse, 1042
Recording Assessment Data in Suspected Abuse, 1046
Interviewing Adolescents, 1097
Encouraging Expression of Emotion, 1137
Situations Requiring Special Considerations, 1138
Developing Successful Parent-Professional Partnerships, 1139
Promoting Normalization, 1140
Supporting Grieving Families, 1153
Facilitating Lipreading, 1171
Admission, 1216
Nonpharmacologic Pain Management, 1220
Using EMLA, 1228
Using Buffered Lidocaine, 1229
Managing Opioid-Induced Respiratory Depression, 1230
Providing Support During ICU Admission, 1244
Selecting Nonthreatening Words or Phrases, 1256
Preoperative Checklist, 1259
Recommended Preoperative Feeding, 1259
Postoperative Care, 1262
Effective Teaching of Family Members, 1264
Skin Care, 1265
Feeding the Sick Child, 1269
Intramuscular Administration of Medication, 1292
Nasogastric, Orogastric, or Gastrostomy Medication Administration in Children, 1296
Nasogastric Tube Feedings in Children, 1312
Administration of Enemas to Children, 1315
Interpreting Peak Expiratory Flow Rates, 1349
Poison Prevention, 1439
Assessing Potential for Lead Poisoning, 1443
Treating Hypercyanotic Spells, 1473
The Diagnosis of Initial Attack of Rheumatic Fever, 1482
Prevention of Urinary Tract Infection, 1548
Preventing Atopy in Children, 1683
Reducing Stress of Burn Care Procedures, 1697
Traction Care, 1719
Identifying Latex Allergy, 1756

Nursing Care Plans

Maternity

Pregnancy—First Trimester, 144
Pregnancy—Second Trimester, 149
Pregnancy—Third Trimester, 168
Nutrition During Pregnancy, 197
Nonpharmacologic Management of Discomfort, 358
Lumbar Epidural Block During Labor, 370
EFM During Labor, 391
First Stage of Labor, 423
Second Stage of Labor, 436
Third Stage of Labor, 440
Preterm Labor, 451
Dysfunctional Labor—Secondary Inertia, 473
Postpartum Care—Vaginal Birth, 532
Puerperal Infection, 546
Stillbirth, 561
Home Care Follow-Up After Discharge, 576
Breastfeeding and Infant Nutrition, 690
High-Risk Premature Newborn, 721
Infant of Gestational Diabetic Mother, 745
Infant Undergoing Drug Withdrawal, 765
Infant with Hyperbilirubinemia, 770

Pediatrics

Child Who Is Maltreated, 1048
Child with Chronic Illness or Disability, 1147
Child Who Is Terminally Ill or Dying, 1152
Child with Mental Retardation, 1164
Child with Hearing Impairment, 1174
Child in the Hospital, 1235
Family of Ill/Hospitalized Child, 1241
Child Undergoing Surgery, 1260
Child with Acute Respiratory Infection, 1325
Child with Asthma, 1355
Child with Acute Diarrhea (Gastroenteritis), 1394
Child with Cleft Lip and/or Palate, 1423
Child with Congestive Heart Failure, 1471
Child with Congenital Heart Disease, 1480
Child with Anemia, 1504
Child with Cancer, 1526
Child with HIV Infection, 1532
Child with Nephrotic Syndrome, 1555
Child with Chronic Renal Failure, 1566
The Unconscious Child, 1584
Child with Diabetes Mellitus, 1651
Child with a Skin Disorder, 1665
Child with a Full-Thickness Burn More Than 25% BSA, 1701
Child Who Is Immobilized, 1710
Child with Cerebral Palsy, 1752

Maternal Child Nursing Care

Maternal Child Nursing Care

DONNA L. WONG, PhD, RN, PNP, CPN, FAAN

Nurse Consultant, The Children's Hospital at Saint Francis;
Adjunct Associate Professor, Department of Pediatrics,
University of Oklahoma College of Medicine—Tulsa;
Clinical Associate Professor, University of Oklahoma College of Nursing;
Adjunct Associate Professor and Consultant,
Oral Roberts University Anna Vaughn School of Nursing,
Tulsa, Oklahoma

SHANNON E. PERRY, PhD, RN, FAAN

Director and Professor, School of Nursing,
San Francisco State University,
San Francisco, California

Contributing Editor

CARYN STOERMER HESS, MS, RN

Nursing Consultant,
Englewood, Colorado

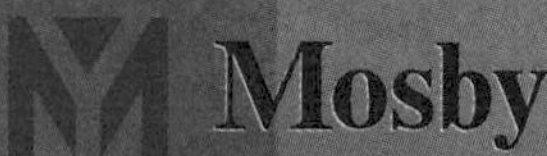

Mosby

St. Louis Baltimore Boston Carlsbad Chicago Minneapolis New York Philadelphia Portland
London Milan Sydney Tokyo Toronto

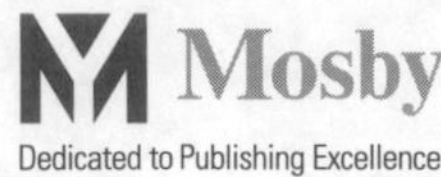

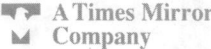

Vice President and Publisher NANCY L. COON
Executive Editor SALLY SCHREFER
Editor MICHAEL S. LEDBETTER
Developmental Editors MICHELE D. HAYDEN and LAURIE K. MUENCH
Project Manager DEBORAH L. VOGEL
Production Editor KAREN L. ALLMAN
Production Assistants MAMATA REDDY and EMILY LEVITT
Designer ELIZABETH YOUNG
Manufacturing Managers THERESA FUCHS and LINDA IERARDI

A NOTE TO THE READER:
The authors and publisher have made every attempt to check dosages and nursing content for accuracy. Because the science of pharmacology is continually advancing, our knowledge base continues to expand. Therefore we recommend that the reader always check product information for changes in dosage or administration before administering any medication. This is particularly important with new or rarely used drugs.

Printed in the United States of America
Composition by Graphic World, Inc.
Printing/binding by World Color Book Services

Mosby-Year Book, Inc.
11830 Westline Industrial Drive
St. Louis, Missouri 63146

Library of Congress Cataloging in Publication Data

Wong, Donna L.,
Maternal child nursing care / Donna L. Wong, Shannon E. Perry; contributing editor, Caryn Stoermer Hess.
p. cm.
Includes index.
ISBN 0-8151-2837-1 (alk. paper)
1. Maternity nursing. 2. Pediatric nursing. I. Perry, Shannon E. II. Hess, Caryn Stoermer. III. Title.
[DNLM: 1. Maternal–Child Nursing—methods. WY 157.3 W872m 1997]
RG951.W87 1997
610.73′62—dc21
DNLM/DLC 97-8667
for Library of Congress CIP

97 98 99 00 01 / 9 8 7 6 5 4 3 2 1

Contributors/Consultants

Elizabeth Ahmann, ScD, RN

Senior Lecturer, School of Nursing
Columbia University
New York, New York;
Consultant, Child and Family Health
Washington, D.C.;
Section Editor, *Pediatric Nursing*
Pitman, New Jersey

Kathryn R. Alden, MSN, RN, IBCLC

Clinical Assistant Professor, School of Nursing
University of North Carolina—Chapel Hill;
Lactation Consultant, Rex Home Services
Raleigh, North Carolina

Natalie Cloutman Arnold, MSN, RN, PNP

Instructor, Nursing Division
Tulsa Community College
Tulsa, Oklahoma

Debbie Fraser Askin, MN, RNC, CNS/NNP

St. Boniface General Hospital
Winnipeg, Manitoba

Jean A. Bachman, DSN, RN

Associate Professor, Barnes College of Nursing
University of Missouri—St. Louis
St. Louis, Missouri

P. Katherine Beaver, MSN, RNC, NNP

Neonatal Nurse Practitioner
Vanderbilt University Medical Center
Nashville, Tennessee

Anne M. Becker, MS, RNC

Acting Neonatal Clinical Specialist and Staff Nurse IV
Neonatal Intensive Care Nursery
Lucile Salter Packard Children's Hospital at Stanford
Palo Alto, California

Lynne Brophy, MSN, RN

Clinical Instructor, University of North Carolina—Chapel Hill;
Adult Oncology Clinical Nurse Specialist, Rex Hospital
Chapel Hill, North Carolina

Kitty Cashion, MSN, RNC

Clinical Nurse Specialist, Department of Obstetrics and Gynecology,
Division of Maternal—Fetal Medicine
College of Medicine
University of Tennessee, Memphis
Memphis, Tennessee

Nancy Friest Dahlberg, MS, RNC

Manager of Minnesota OB Homecare
Abbott Northwestern Hospital;
The OB Program, Healthspan Homecare and Hospice
Allina Health System
Minneapolis, Minnesota

Gayle Tart Davis, EdD, RN

Associate Professor, School of Nursing
University of North Carolina—Chapel Hill
Chapel Hill, North Carolina

Pamela A. DiVito-Thomas, MS, RN

Instructor
Oral Roberts University Anna Vaughn School of Nursing
Tulsa, Oklahoma

Laurie E. Doerner, MSN, RN

Instructor
Oral Roberts University Anna Vaughn School of Nursing;
Consultant, Private Practice
Pediatrics, Home Care, Infusion Therapy, and Quality Improvement
Tulsa, Oklahoma

Carol Fowler Durham, MSN, RN

Clinical Assistant Professor, School of Nursing
University of North Carolina—Chapel Hill
Chapel Hill, North Carolina

Diane Gorgal Eaton, MSN, RN

Perinatal Managed Care Specialist
Fishers, Indiana

Lienne D. Edwards, PhD, RN

Assistant Professor, Department of Family Nursing;
Director, Office of Continuing Education, College of Nursing & Health Professions
University of North Carolina at Charlotte
Charlotte, North Carolina

Jeanne O'Connor Egan, MSN, RN
Pediatric Clinical Specialist
Children's National Medical Center
Washington, D.C.

Catherine Ingram Fogel, PhD, RNC(WHNP), FAAN
Professor
University of North Carolina—Chapel Hill
Chapel Hill, North Carolina

Beverly B. Foster, PhD, RN
Associate Dean for Undergraduate Studies
University of North Carolina—Chapel Hill
Chapel Hill, North Carolina

Catherine Garner, PhD, RNC, FAAN
Research Scientist, Arizona Cancer Center
University of Arizona
Tucson, Arizona

Cynthia Garrett, MSN, RNC
Women's Health Clinical Nurse Specialist
University of North Carolina Hospitals
Chapel Hill, North Carolina

Teresa L. Hall, MS, RN
Nursing Supervisor
Hathaway Children's Services
Sylmar, California

Renee Covey Harrison, MS, RN
Assistant Professor, Nursing Division
Tulsa Community College
Tulsa, Oklahoma

Mildred G. Harvey, MSN, RNC
Consultant, Harvey, Troiano & Associates, Inc.
Houston, TX;
Clinical Nurse Specialist, Baptist Memorial Hospital
Memphis, Tennessee

Caryn Stoermer Hess, MS, RN
Nursing Consultant
Englewood, Colorado

Marilyn Hockenberry-Eaton, PhD, RN, PNP, FAAN
Director, Pediatric Nurse Practitioner Services
Texas Children's Hospital
Houston, Texas

Ellen F. Johnsen, BA, RNC
Instructor, Tulsa Training Center
Oklahoma State University
Tulsa, Oklahoma

Christina Algiere Kasprisin, MS, RN
College of Nursing
University of Vermont
Burlington, Vermont

Phyllis M. Klein, MSN, RN, C-ANP
Nurse Practitioner, Planned Parenthood
Fairfax, Virginia

Nancy E. Kline, MS, RN, CPNP
Oncology Nurse Practitioner
Texas Children's Hospital;
Instructor of Pediatrics
Baylor College of Medicine
Houston, Texas

Laura L. Kuensting, MSN(R), RN
Pediatric Clinical Nurse Specialist
Emergency Services
Christian Hospitals;
Staff Nurse
Emergency Services
Cardinal Glennon Children's Hospital
St. Louis, Missouri

Rae Langford, EdD, RN
Private Practice
Rehabilitation Nurse Consultant
Houston, Texas

Shona Swenson Lenss, BSN, RN
Attention Deficit/Hyperactivity Disorder Nurse Coordinator
Cheyenne Children's Clinic
Cheyenne, Wyoming

Sharon E. Lock, PhD, RNC
Assistant Professor
University of Virginia School of Nursing
Charlottesville, Virginia

Deitra Leonard Lowdermilk, RNC, PhD
Clinical Associate Professor, School of Nursing
University of North Carolina—Chapel Hill
Chapel Hill, North Carolina

Lynn E. Mattis, MSN, RN
Clinical Nurse Specialist
Division of Pediatric Gastroenterology/Nutrition
Department of Pediatrics
The Johns Hopkins Hospital
Baltimore, Maryland

Susan Mattson, PhD, RNC
Associate Professor, College of Nursing
Arizona State University
Scottsdale, Arizona

Mary Courtney Moore, RD, RN, PhD
Assistant Professor, Department of Molecular Physiology & Biophysics
Vanderbilt University
Nashville, Tennessee

Patricia O'Brien, MSN, RNC, PNP
Cardiovascular Clinical Nurse Specialist
Cardiovascular Program
Children's Hospital
Boston, Massachusetts

Mary L. Overfield, MN, RN, IBCLC

Partner, Lactation Consultants of North Carolina
Raleigh, North Carolina

Denise Gagnon Palmer, RN, MS

Perinatal Clinical Nurse Specialist, The Family Center
O'Connor Hospital
San Jose, California;
Assistant Clinical Professor, Department of Family Health Care Nursing
University of California at San Francisco
San Francisco, California

Kathryn A. Perry, MSN, APRN, RN,C, CNS

Clinical Nurse Specialist for Child Neurology
Children's Medical Center
Tulsa, Oklahoma

Karen A. Piotrowski, MSN, RNC

Assistant Professor of Nursing
D'Youville College
Buffalo, New York

Judith H. Poole, MN, RNC, FACCE

Perinatal Outreach Education Coordinator, Department of Obstetrics & Gynecology
Carolinas Medical Center
Charlotte, North Carolina

Kimberly J. Powell, MSN, RNC, NP

Women's Health Nurse Practitioner
University of California, San Francisco
San Francisco, California

Judy Holt Rollins, MS, RN

Consultant, Rollins & Associates, Inc.;
Coordinator, Studio G
Georgetown University Medical Center;
Adjunct Instructor
Georgetown University School of Medicine
Washington, D.C.;
Associate Editor, *Pediatric Nursing*
Pitman, New Jersey

Barbara C. Rynerson, MSN, RNC

Associate Professor, School of Nursing
University of North Carolina—Chapel Hill
Chapel Hill, North Carolina

Kathleen Rice Simpson, MSN, RNC

Perinatal Clinical Nurse Specialist
St. John's Mercy Medical Center
St. Louis, Missouri

Donna P. Smith, MS, RN

Genetic Counselor
H.A. Chapman Institute of Medical Genetics
Tulsa, Oklahoma

Sister Carol Taylor, PhD(c), MSN, RN, CSFN

Assistant Professor, Humanities;
Clinical Ethicist;
Health Care Ethicist
Holy Family College
Philadelphia, Pennsylvania

Cecilia Tiller, DSN

Assistant Professor, Department of Parent–Child Nursing
Medical College of Georgia
Augusta, Georgia

Mary Rose Tully, MPH, IBCLC

Director, Triangle Mothers' Milk Bank and Lactation Center
Wake Medical Center
Raleigh, North Carolina

Sharon W. Walters, MSN, RN, CS

Psychiatric Clinical Nurse Specialist
Harris Methodist Hospital
Fort Worth, Texas

Sara Rich Wheeler, MSN, RN

Consultant, Grief Ltd.
Covington, Indiana;
Clinical Instructor, University of Illinois Chicago
Urbana Regional Campus, College of Nursing
Urbana, Illinois

Krena Hunter White, MS, MA, RN

Assistant Professor, Nursing Division
Tulsa Community College
Tulsa, Oklahoma

Rhea P. Williams, PhD, RN

Professor
California State University—Los Angeles
Los Angeles, California

David Wilson, MS, RN,C

Instructor
Oral Roberts University Anna Vaughn School of Nursing
Tulsa, Oklahoma

Marilyn L. Winkelstein, PhD, RN

Associate Professor
University of Maryland School of Nursing
Baltimore, Maryland

Jan Lamarche Zdanuk, MSN, RNC, CNS, FNP

Family Nurse Practitioner
Fort Worth, Texas

Susan B. Zekauskas, MSN, RN, PNP

Pediatric Nurse Consultant;
Assistant Professor, Nursing Division
Tulsa Community College
Tulsa, Oklahoma

Preface

In this first edition of *Maternal Child Nursing Care,* we have worked hard to meet the increasing demands of faculty and students to teach and to learn in an environment characterized by rapid change, enormous amounts of information, fewer clinical facilities, less classroom time, and more need for community experiences.

As experienced authors and practitioners, we have combined the essential information on maternity and pediatric nursing care into one text. In this book we have condensed the size of two separate successful books by reducing duplication of material, and more importantly, we have retained the same cutting-edge, accurate, comprehensive information for which each author is known.

FEATURES

This book features a contemporary design and attractive presentation. Students will find that the logical, easy-to-follow headings and attractive design highlight important content and increase visual appeal. Hundreds of photographs and drawings throughout the text illustrate important concepts and techniques to further enhance comprehension.

To help students learn essential information quickly and efficiently, we have included numerous features that prioritize, condense, simplify, and emphasize important aspects of nursing care. In addition, this text encourages students to *think critically.*

SPECIAL FEATURES

- **Critical Thinking** boxes encourage students to consider real-life clinical situations and make appropriate clinical judgments.
- **Home Care** boxes detail important information to help prepare students and families to care for themselves in the home setting.
- **Cultural Considerations** boxes integrate concepts of culturally sensitive care throughout the text, with an emphasis on the clinical application of the information.
- **Family Focus** boxes highlight the needs or concerns of families that should be addressed when family-centered care is provided.
- **Patient Teaching** boxes teach students to help patients and families become involved in their own care with optimal outcomes.
- **Nursing Care Plans** are provided for all commonly encountered situations and disorders. The most recent NANDA-accepted nursing diagnoses and patient and family goals are included in the care plans. Rationales are added to nursing interventions for which the rationale might not be immediately evident to students.
- **Guidelines** boxes summarize important nursing interventions in an easy-to-follow format.
- **Nursing Alerts** call the reader's attention to critical information that could lead to deteriorating or emergency situations.
- **Emergency** boxes highlight important emergency procedures in a step-by-step format.
- **Atraumatic Care** boxes emphasize the importance of providing competent care while minimizing undue physical and psychologic distress for the child and family.
- **Chapter Outlines** with page numbers begin each chapter, allowing readers to quickly locate topics of interest.
- **Key Terms** are highlighted throughout each chapter to reinforce student learning.
- Hundreds of **tables** and **boxes** highlight key concepts and nursing interventions.
- **Key Points,** located at the end of each chapter, help the reader summarize major points, make connections, and synthesize information.
- A highly detailed, cross-referenced **index** allows readers to quickly access information.

TEACHING/LEARNING PACKAGE

An extensive number of ancillary products for instructors and students to use in class and clinical settings is available:

Instructor's Resource Manual and Test Bank Includes course outlines, lecture outlines, learning activities, and a 750+-question test bank.

Study Guide Includes key terms, reviews of key concepts and content, and critical thinking questions.

Overhead Transparencies Full-color transparency acetates enhance key material in the text.

Computerized Test Bank Available in IBM and Macintosh formats.

Mosby/Wong Web Site A special service that provides pediatric nursing updates, bibliographies, abstracts, announcements, additional resources, and links to other sources of pediatric Internet information. Use the address of Mosby's home page (www.mosby.com) to access this site.

Whaley & Wong's Pediatric Nursing Video Service Set of six individual videotapes featuring Donna Wong. Topics include Pediatric Assessment, Growth and Development, Medications and Injections, Family-Centered Care, Pain Assessment and Management, and Communication with Children and Families.

Donna L. Wong
Shannon E. Perry

• • •

ACKNOWLEDGMENTS

Although it is impossible to thank every individual at Mosby who has participated in the production of this text, I am grateful to Sally Schrefer and Shelly Hayden for their continued support and commitment to excellence. I'd like to extend a very special word of thanks to Caryn Hess, my friend and colleague, for her many hours of work as contributing editor on this project. Finally, as always, I thank my family—Ting and Nina—for the unselfish love, endless patience, and quiet understanding that allow me to devote such a large part of my life to my career.

Donna L. Wong

I wish to thank Michael Ledbetter, Editor; Cecily Pew and Laurie Muench, Developmental Editors; Deb Vogel, Project Manager; Karen Allman, Production Editor; and Liz Young, Designer, for their encouragement and assistance in the preparation and production of this text. I also thank Irene Bobak and Deitra Lowdermilk for their support and encouragement throughout the development of this textbook. Without their diligence and commitment to writing and editing maternity textbooks of the highest standards, I would not be in the position of co-authoring this book. I hope that we have continued their tradition of excellence. Special thanks to my husband, Bill, for his involvement in the birth and rearing of our daughter, Julie.

Shannon E. Perry

It has been a pleasure working with Sally Schrefer, Shelly Hayden, and Karen Allman of the Mosby Editorial and Production staff. I greatly appreciate their guidance and patience. Very special thanks goes to my friend and colleague, Donna Wong, who has always encouraged me in my professional endeavors. Her high standards and commitment to pediatric nursing have made this text possible. Finally, I wish to thank my family—my parents, Darold and Phyllis Stoermer, who have always loved and encouraged me; my husband, Mike; and my children, Steven, Kyle, Brian, and Kimberly, who have provided love, understanding, and patience throughout this project.

Caryn Stoermer Hess

Brief Contents

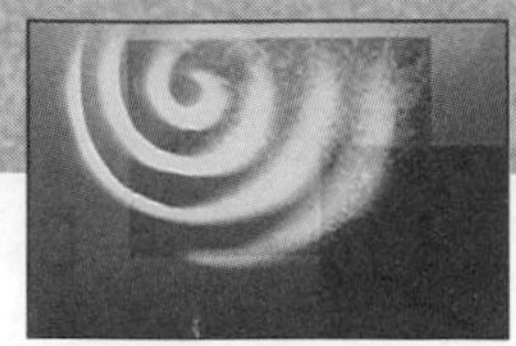

PART 1 Maternity Nursing

UNIT ONE

Introduction to Maternity Nursing

1 Contemporary Maternity Nursing, 1

2 Family and Culture, 8

3 Reproduction and Sexuality, 23

UNIT TWO

Pregnancy

4 Genetics, Conception, and Fetal Development, 51

5 Assessment for Risk Factors, 79

6 Anatomy and Physiology of Pregnancy, 103

7 Nursing Care During Pregnancy, 122

8 Maternal and Fetal Nutrition, 176

UNIT THREE

Complications of Pregnancy

9 Hypertension, Hemorrhage, and Maternal Infection, 199

10 Endocrine, Cardiovascular, and Medical-Surgical Problems During Pregnancy, 251

11 Psychosocial Problems, 296

12 Adolescent Sexuality, Pregnancy, and Parenthood, 316

UNIT FOUR

Childbirth

13 Essential Factors and Processes of Labor, 336

14 Management of Discomfort, 352

15 Fetal Assessment, 373

16 Nursing Care During Labor and Birth, 394

17 Labor and Birth at Risk, 444

UNIT FIVE

Postpartum Period

18 Maternal Physiology During the Postpartum Period, 480

19 Nursing Care During the Postpartum Period, 488

20 Postpartum Complications, 537

21 Maternal-Newborn Home Care, 565

UNIT SIX

Newborn

22 The Newborn, 591

23 Nursing Care of the Newborn, 627

24 Newborn Nutrition and Feeding, 661

25 The High-Risk Newborn, 696

26 Specific Problems of the Newborn, 724

PART 2 Pediatric Nursing

UNIT SEVEN

Children, Their Families, and the Nurse

27 Contemporary Pediatric Nursing, 783

28 Social, Cultural, and Religious Influences on Child Health Promotion, 800

29 Family Influences on Child Health Promotion, 826

30 Developmental Influences on Child Health Promotion, 844

UNIT EIGHT

Assessment of the Child and Family

31 Communication and Health Assessment of the Child and Family, 866

32 Physical and Developmental Assessment of the Child, 893

UNIT NINE

Health Promotion and Special Health Problems

33 The Infant and Family, 937

34 The Toddler and Family, 993

35 The Preschooler and Family, 1016

36 The School-Age Child and Family, 1053

37 The Adolescent and Family, 1084

UNIT TEN

Special Needs, Illness, and Hospitalization

38 Chronic Illness, Disability, and Death, 1121

39 Cognitive and Sensory Impairment, 1157

40 Family-Centered Home Care, 1186

41 Reaction to Illness and Hospitalization, 1196

42 Pediatric Nursing Interventions, 1250

UNIT ELEVEN

Health Problems of Children

43 Respiratory Dysfunction, 1321

44 Gastrointestinal Dysfunction, 1372

45 Cardiovascular Dysfunction, 1450

46 Hematologic and Immunologic Dysfunction, 1499

47 Genitourinary Dysfunction, 1542

48 Cerebral Dysfunction, 1572

49 Endocrine Dysfunction, 1624

50 Integumentary Dysfunction, 1654

51 Musculoskeletal and Articular Dysfunction, 1706

52 Neuromuscular and Muscular Dysfunction, 1746

APPENDIXES

A Standards for the Nursing Care of Women and Newborns, 1769

B Nursing Responsibilities in Implementing Intrapartum Fetal Heart Rate Monitoring, 1772

C Standard Laboratory Values: Pregnant and Nonpregnant Women, 1774

D Family APGAR Questionnaire, 1776

E Developmental/Sensory Assessment, 1778
Denver II, 1778
Denver Articulation Screening, 1780
Snellen Screening, 1782

F Growth Measurements, 1783
Height/Weight Measurements—Boys, 1783
Height/Weight Measurements—Girls, 1784
Head Circumference Charts, 1786
Percentiles for Triceps Skinfold, 1787
Percentiles for Upper Arm Circumference, 1787

G Translations of FACES Pain Rating Scale, 1788

H Pediatric Vital Signs and Parameters, 1790

I Common Laboratory Tests, 1792

Detailed Contents

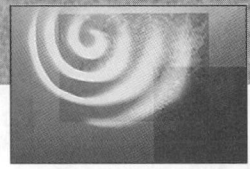

PART 1 Maternity Nursing

UNIT ONE

Introduction to Maternity Nursing

1 Contemporary Maternity Nursing, 1

Contemporary Issues and Trends, 1
- Changing health care delivery structure, 1
- Changing childbirth practices, 2
- Changing views of women, 2
- Trends in fertility and birthrate, 3
- Trends of consumer involvement, self-care, and focus on health care, 4
- Trend to high-technology care, 4
- Shift to home health care, 4
- Increase in high-risk pregnancies, 4
- Trends and issues of high costs, 4
- Access to care, 4
- Trends in nursing practice, 5

Standards of Practice, 5
- Standard of care, 5

Ethical Issues in Perinatal Nursing, 5
Research into Practice, 5

2 Family and Culture, 8

Family Function and Structure, 8
- Family function, 8
- Family structure, 8
- Family functions, 11
- Family dynamics, 12

Family Theories, 12
- Family system theory, 12
- Developmental theory, 13
- Family stress theory, 14

Key Factors in Family Health, 14
Cultural Factors Related to Family Health, 15
- Cultural context of the family, 15
- Childbearing beliefs and practices, 18
- Other factors affecting care of families, 18

3 Reproduction and Sexuality, 23

Female Reproductive System, 23
- External structures, 23
- Internal structures, 27
- Breasts, 37
- Menstrual cycle, 39

Male Reproductive System, 42
- External structures, 43
- Internal structures, 44

Sexual Response, 46
- Physiologic response to sexual stimulation, 46

Psychosocial Aspects of Sexuality, 46
Nursing Implications, 48

UNIT TWO

Pregnancy

4 Genetics, Conception, and Fetal Development, 51

Genetics, 51
- Genes and chromosomes, 51
- Cell division, 53
- Gametogenesis, 54
- Chromosomal abnormalities, 54
- Patterns of genetic transmission, 56

Conception, 58
The Embryo and Fetus, 60
- Development of the embryo, 60
- Fetal maturation, 65
- Multifetal pregnancy, 69
- Nongenetic factors influencing development, 73

Genetic Counseling, 73
- Patients seeking genetic counseling, 74
- Genetic counseling services, 74
- Management of genetic disorders, 74
- Role of the nurse in genetic counseling, 75

Preconception Care, 75
- Role of the nurse, 77

5 Assessment for Risk Factors, 79

Definition and Scope of the Problem, 79
- Maternal health problems, 79
- Fetal and neonatal health problems, 80
- Regionalization of health care services, 80

Categories of Risk Factors, 80
Biophysical Assessment, 82
- Daily fetal movement count, 82

Ultrasonography, 83
Magnetic resonance imaging, 90
Biochemical Assessment, 90
Amniocentesis, 90
Percutaneous umbilical blood sampling, 93
Chorionic villus sampling, 94
Maternal assays, 95
Electronic Fetal Monitoring, 95
Indications, 95
Fetal responses to hypoxia and asphyxia, 97
Nonstress test (fetal activity determination), 97
Contraction stress test, 98
Nursing Role in Antenatal Assessment for Risk, 100

6 Anatomy and Physiology of Pregnancy, 103

Gravidity and Parity, 103
Pregnancy Tests, 104
Adaptations to Pregnancy, 105
Signs of pregnancy, 105
Reproductive System and Breasts, 105
Hypothalamic-pituitary-ovarian axis, 105
Uterus, 106
Vagina and vulva, 110
Breasts, 111
General Body Systems, 111
Cardiovascular system, 111
Respiratory system, 114
Renal system, 115
Integumentary system, 116
Musculoskeletal system, 117
Neurologic system, 118
Gastrointestinal system, 118
Endocrine system, 119

7 Nursing Care During Pregnancy, 122

First Trimester, 122
Diagnosis of pregnancy, 123
Nursing care management, 123
Second Trimester, 146
Nursing care management, 146
Third Trimester, 157
Second-time mothers, 157
Expectant fathers/partners, 157
Nursing care management, 159
Parenthood After Age 35, 169
Older multiparous women, 169
Older nulliparous women, 169
Multifetal Pregnancy, 169
Prenatal care in multifetal pregnancies, 169
Psychosocial adjustment, 170
Prebirth Education, 170
Parent education programs, 170
Recent trends in parent education, 171
Strategies for childbirth education, 171
Options for care providers, 171
Birth setting choices, 172

8 Maternal and Fetal Nutrition, 176

Nutrient Needs During Pregnancy, 176
Energy needs, 177
Protein, 182
Water, 183
Minerals and vitamins, 184
Negative impacts on nutrition, 186
Pregnancy-induced hypertension, 187
Exercise during pregnancy, 187
Nutrient Needs During Lactation, 187
Nursing care management, 188

UNIT THREE

Complications of Pregnancy

9 Hypertension, Hemorrhage, and Maternal Infection, 199

Hypertension in Pregnancy, 199
Significance and incidence, 199
Morbidity and mortality, 199
Classification, 199
Etiology of preeclampsia, 201
Pathophysiology of preeclampsia, 201
Mild vs. severe preeclampsia, 202
HELLP syndrome, 202
Nursing care management, 204
Maternal Hemorrhagic Disorders, 216
Early pregnancy bleeding, 216
Nursing care management, 218
Late pregnancy bleeding, 224
Nursing care management, 228
Clotting disorders in pregnancy, 230
Maternal Infections, 231
Sexually transmitted disease, 232
Genital tract infections, 240
General infections, 242
Infection control, 244
Nursing care management, 244

10 Endocrine, Cardiovascular, and Medical-Surgical Problems During Pregnancy, 251

Endocrine Disorders, 251
Diabetes mellitus, 251
Nursing care management, 257
Gestational diabetes mellitus, 265
Nursing care management, 266
Hyperemesis gravidarum, 268
Nursing care management, 268
Thyroid disorders, 269
Cardiovascular Disorders, 270
Nursing care management, 271
Heart surgery during pregnancy, 276
Associated cardiovascular disorders, 276
Cardiopulmonary resuscitation of the pregnant woman, 278
Medical Disorders During Pregnancy, 279
Anemia, 279
Pulmonary Disorders, 281
Gastrointestinal disorders, 283
Integumentary disorders, 283
Neurologic disorders, 283
Autoimmune disorders, 284
Abdominal surgery during pregnancy, 285
Nursing care management, 286
Discharge planning, 287
Trauma during pregnancy, 287
Nursing care management, 287

Therapeutic and Elective Abortion, 289
Nursing care management, 289
Complications following abortion, 291
Mifepristone (RU 486), 292
Nursing considerations, 292

11 Psychosocial Problems, 296

Emotional Complications, 296
Mood disorders, 296
Schizophrenia, 298
Nursing care management, 298
Psychoactive Substance Use, 302
Legal sanctions, 302
Alcohol, 303
Marijuana, 303
Cocaine, 303
Heroin, 305
Methamphetamine, 305
Phencyclidine, 306
Nursing care management, 306
Other Addictive Substances, 309
Tobacco, 309
Caffeine, 310
Violence Against Women, 310
Dynamics of abuse, 311
Nursing care management, 311
Prevention, 313

12 Adolescent Sexuality, Pregnancy, and Parenthood, 316

Physiologic Development, 316
Cognitive Development, 317
Moral Development, 317
Psychosocial Development, 317
Adolescent Pregnancy, 317
STDs and HIV, 317
Primary Prevention of Adolescent High-Risk Sexual Behavior and Pregnancy, 318
Adolescent sexual behavior, 318
Nursing care management, 318
Secondary Prevention with Pregnant Adolescents, 321
The very young pregnant adolescent, 321
Developmental tasks of pregnancy, 321
Cultural influences, 322
Family reactions to adolescent pregnancy, 322
Adolescent fathers, 322
Nursing care management, 322
Tertiary Prevention with Adolescent Parents, 329
Adolescent parenthood, 329
Developmental tasks of parenthood, 330
The extended family, 330
Nursing care management, 330

UNIT FOUR

Childbirth

13 Essential Factors and Processes of Labor, 336

Factors Affecting Labor, 336
Passenger, 336
Passageway, 338
Powers, 343
Position of the woman in labor, 345
Process of Labor, 346
Signs preceding labor, 346
Theories of onset of labor, 346
Stages of labor, 347
Mechanism of labor, 347
Physiologic Adaptation to Labor, 349
Fetal adaptation, 349
Maternal adaptation, 349

14 Management of Discomfort, 352

Discomfort During Labor, 352
Neurologic origins, 352
Perception of pain, 352
Nonpharmacologic Management of Discomfort, 354
Childbirth preparation methods, 354
Relaxing and breathing techniques, 355
Other nonpharmacologic methods, 357
Pharmacologic Management of Discomfort, 358
Sedatives, 358
Analgesia and anesthesia, 358
Nursing care management, 367

15 Fetal Assessment, 373

Basis for monitoring, 374
The fetal response, 374
Fetal compromise, 374
Monitoring Techniques, 375
Intermittent auscultation, 375
Electronic monitoring, 376
FHR patterns, 377
Fetal blood sampling/fetal scalp stimulation: acid-base monitoring, 385
Fetal pulse oximetry, 385
Nursing care management, 386
Guidelines and standards of nursing care related to EFM, 387
Preventive measures, 388
Intrauterine resuscitation, 388
Working with the monitor, 389

16 Nursing Care During Labor and Birth, 394

First Stage of Labor, 394
Nursing care management, 394
Second Stage of Labor, 424
Nursing care management, 425
Third Stage of Labor, 436
Nursing care management, 436
Interruption in skin integrity related to childbirth, 439

17 Labor and Birth at Risk, 444

Preterm Labor and Birth, 444
Etiologic factors, 445
Nursing care management, 445
Premature Rupture of Membranes, 452
Etiologic factors, 452
Plan of care and implementation, 452
Dystocia, 452
Dysfunctional labor, 452
Alterations in pelvic structure, 453
Fetal causes, 454
Position of the woman, 456

Psychologic response, 456
Abnormal labor patterns, 456
Nursing care management, 458
Postdate Pregnancy, Labor, and Birth, 472
Maternal and fetal risks, 472
Nursing care management, 474
Obstetric Emergencies, 475
Shoulder dystocia, 475
Nursing care management, 475
Prolapsed umbilical cord, 475
Nursing care management, 475
Rupture of the uterus, 475
Nursing care management, 477
Amniotic fluid embolism, 477
Nursing care management, 477

UNIT FIVE

Postpartum Period

18 Maternal Physiology During the Postpartum Period, 480

Reproductive System and Associated Structures, 480
Uterus, 480
Endocrine System, 483
Abdomen, 483
Urinary System, 483
Gastrointestinal System, 484
Breasts, 484
Cardiovascular System, 485
Neurologic System, 486
Musculoskeletal System, 486
Integumentary System, 486
Immune System, 486

19 Nursing Care During the Postpartum Period, 488

Fourth Stage of Labor, 488
Assessment, 489
Nursing care management—physical needs, 492
Nursing care management—psychosocial needs, 502
Discharge Teaching, 512
Sexual activity, 512
Prescribed medications, 513
Routine mother and baby checkups, 513
Nursing care management—contraception, 513
Nursing care management—sterilization, 531

20 Postpartum Complications, 537

Postpartum Hemorrhage, 537
Uterine atony, 538
Lacerations of the birth canal, 538
Medical management, 539
Retained placenta, 539
Inversion of the uterus, 539
Subinvolution of the uterus, 541
Nursing care management, 541
Hemorrhagic (hypovolemic) shock, 542
Postpartum Infections, 543
Postpartum urinary tract infections, 543
Postpartum infection (sepsis), 543
Mastitis, 544
Nursing care management, 545
Sequelae of Childbirth Trauma, 546
Structural disorders of the uterus and vagina, 546
Nursing care management, 549
Loss and Grief, 550
Grief responses, 551
Anticipatory grief, 552
Tasks of mourners, 552
Nursing care management, 553
Other losses, 561
Complicated bereavement, 562

21 Maternal-Newborn Home Care, 565

The Health Care Environment that Supports Early Discharge, 565
Potential advantages of short-stay maternity care, 566
Potential disadvantages of short-stay maternity care, 566
The future of early postpartum discharge, 566
Nursing Care and Early Postpartum Discharge: Bridging Hospital and Home, 569
Critical path, 570
Nursing care management, 570
Prepatory Educational Instruction, 571
Postpartum Care, 574
Home care nursing visits, 574
The home visit, 579
Telephone follow-up, 584
Warm lines/help lines, 586
Support groups, 587
Perinatal coaching, 588
The Role of Nursing in Program Development, 589

UNIT SIX

Newborn

22 The Newborn, 591

Respiratory System, 591
Cardiovascular System, 592
Hematopoietic System, 594
Thermoregulation, 595
Fluid and Electrolyte Balance, 596
Renal System, 596
Gastrointestinal System, 597
Hepatic System, 597
Immune System, 599
Reproductive System, 599
Integumentary System, 600
Skeletal System, 602
Neuromuscular System, 603
Newborn reflexes, 603
Sensory functions, 603
Assessment, 608
Initial assessment: Apgar scoring, 608
Transitional assessment: periods of reactivity, 609
Behavioral assessment, 609
Assessment of attachment behaviors, 610
Assessment of clinical gestational age, 614
Physical Assessment, 614
General appearance, 614
Vital signs, 614
Baseline measurements of physical growth, 620
Thorax, 623
Abdomen, 624

Back and anus, 624
Genitalia, 624
Extremities, 625
Neurologic assessment, 625

23 Nursing Care of the Newborn, 627

Birth Through the First 2 Hours, 627
Nursing care management, 627
Supporting Adaptation to Extrauterine Life, 629
Body temperature, 629
Adequate oxygenation, 630
Healthy Therapeutic Interventions, 632
Eye prophylaxis, 632
Vitamin K prophylaxis, 633
2 Hours After Birth Until Discharge, 633
Nursing care management, 633
Assessment of Common Problems in the Newborn, 635
Physical injuries, 635
Physiologic problems, 636
Laboratory and Diagnostic Tests, 637
Collection of specimens, 637
Protective Environment, 642
Supporting Parents in the Care of Their Infant, 643
Social interactions, 643
Infant feeding, 645
Positioning and holding, 645
Umbilical cord care, 645
Rashes, 645
Clothing, 645
Care of the infant's linens, 646
Bathing, 646
Nursing Interventions for Therapeutic/Surgical Procedures, 649
Restraining the infant, 649
Intramuscular injection, 649
Therapy for hyperbilirubinemia, 650
Circumcision, 653
Discharge Planning and Teaching, 655
Temperature, 655
Respirations, 657
Elimination, 657
Safety, 657
Pacifiers/thumb-sucking, 657
Immunizations, 658
Infant follow-up care, 658
Home care, 658

24 Newborn Nutrition and Feeding, 661

Normal Development, 661
Physical growth, 661
Emotional development, 661
Feeding readiness, 662
Nutrient Needs, 663
Energy (calories or kcal), 663
Carbohydrate, 663
Fat, 664
Protein, 664
Fluids, 664
Vitamins and minerals, 664
Lactation, 665
Factors affecting breastfeeding practices, 665
Prenatal support for breastfeeding, 665
Unique properties of human milk, 666
Maternal benefits of lactation, 666
Overview of normal lactation, 666
Milk production, 667
Breastfeeding the baby, 668
Effects of early discharge, 674
Role of the nurse as teacher, 674
Breastfeeding support, 675
Care of the mother, 675
Expressing, pumping, and storing milk, 677
Drugs and environmental pollutants, 679
Weaning, 680
Problem-solving techniques, 680
Potentially challenging situations, 687
Nursing care management, 688
Formula Feeding, 691
Care of the bottle-feeding mother and infant, 691
Discharge Planning, 693

25 The High-Risk Newborn, 696

Classification of High-Risk Newborns, 696
Transporting High-Risk Infants, 696
Plan of Care, 697
Assessment of the high-risk newborn by systems, 697
Respiratory care, 699
Thermoregulatory care, 704
Nutritional care, 706
Developmental and emotional aspects of care, 712
Transport from a regional center ("back transport"), 718
Nursing Care of the Family, 719
Pain in Neonates, 719
Assessment of pain, 719
Management of neonatal pain, 719

26 Specific Problems of the Newborn, 724

Gestational Age and Birthweight, 724
Infant mortality and morbidity, 725
The preterm infant, 725
Nursing care management, 726
Postdate and Postmature Infants, 737
SGA, IUGR, and Dysmature Infants, 739
Common problems, 739
LGA Infants, 740
Infants of Diabetic Mothers, 741
Pathophysiology, 741
Congenital anomalies, 741
Macrosomia, 743
Birth trauma and perinatal asphyxia, 743
RDS, 744
Hypoglycemia, 744
Hypocalcemia and hypomagnesemia, 744
Cardiomyopathy, 744
Hyperbilirubinemia and polycythemia, 744
Birth Trauma, 746
Neonatal Infections, 749
Nursing care management, 750
TORCH infections, 752
Bacterial infections, 758
Fungal infections, 758
Substance Abuse, 759
Alcohol, 760
Tobacco, 761
Marijuana, 761
Cocaine, 761
Phencyclidine ("angel dust"), 761
Heroin, 761
Methadone, 762

Miscellaneous substances, 762
Nursing care management, 763
Discharge to Home for the Compromised Newborn, 766
Hyperbilirubinemia, 767
Rh incompatibility, 767
ABO incompatibility, 768
Kernicterus, 768
Congenital Anomalies, 769
Central nervous system anomalies, 770
Cardiovascular system anomalies, 772
Respiratory system anomalies, 772
Gastrointestinal system anomalies, 773
Musculoskeletal system anomalies, 775
Genitourinary system anomalies, 776
Nursing care management, 777

PART 2 Pediatric Nursing

UNIT SEVEN

Children, Their Families, and the Nurse

27 Contemporary Pediatric Nursing, 783

Health During Childhood, 783
Healthy people 2000, 783
Mortality, 783
Morbidity, 787
Evolution of child health care in the United States, 789
Pediatric Nursing, 791
Philosophy of care, 791
Role of the pediatric nurse, 793
Future trends, 796

28 Social, Cultural, and Religious Influences on Child Health Promotion, 800

Culture, 800
Social roles, 801
Subcultural influences, 801
The child and family in North America, 805
Cultural shock, 806
Cultural/Religious Influences on Health Care, 806
Susceptibility to health problems, 806
Customs and Folkways, 808
Health beliefs and practices, 811
Religious beliefs, 813
Importance of culture and religion to nurses, 813

29 Family Influences on Child Health Promotion, 826

General Concepts, 826
Definition of family, 826
Family nursing interventions, 826
Family Roles, Relationships, and Strengths, 827
Parental roles, 827
Role learning, 828
Family size and configuration, 828
Family strengths, 830
Parenting, 831
Special Parenting Situations, 835
Parenting the adopted child, 835
Parenting and divorce, 837
Single parenting, 839
Parenting in reconstituted families, 840
Parenting in dual-earner families, 840
Accommodating contemporary parenting situations, 840

30 Developmental Influences on Child Health Promotion, 844

Growth and Development, 844
Foundations of growth and development, 844
Biologic growth and physical development, 846
Physiologic changes, 848
Temperament, 849
Development of Personality and Mental Function, 850
Theoretic foundations of personality development, 850
Theoretic foundations of mental development, 852
Development of self-concept, 854
Role of Play in Development, 855
Classification of play, 855
Functions of play, 857
Toys, 858
Selected Factors that Influence Development, 858

UNIT EIGHT

Assessment of the Child and Family

31 Communication and Health Assessment of the Child and Family, 866

Communication, 866
Verbal communication, 866
Nonverbal communication—paralanguage, 867
Guidelines for Communication and Interviewing, 867
Establishing a setting for communication, 867
Communicating with Families, 868
Communicating with parents, 868
Communicating with children, 872
Communication techniques, 875
History taking, 875
Performing a health history, 875
Family Assessment, 882
Nutritional Assessment, 885

32 Physical and Developmental Assessment of the Child, 893

General Approaches Toward Examining the Child, 893
Physical Examination, 896
Growth measurements, 896
Physiologic measurements, 900
General appearance, 905
Skin, 906
Lymph nodes, 907
Head and neck, 907
Eyes, 908
Ears, 914
Nose, 918
Mouth and throat, 918
Chest, 920
Lungs, 921
Heart, 922
Abdomen, 924
Genitalia, 926
Anus, 928
Back and extremities, 928
Neurologic assessment, 930
Developmental Assessment, 931
Denver II, 931
Revised Prescreening Developmental Questionnaire (R-PDQ), 934
Developmental screening and interpretation, 934

UNIT NINE

Health Promotion and Special Health Problems

33 The Infant and Family, 937

Promoting Optimum Growth and Development, 937
Biologic development, 937
Psychosocial development, 943
Cognitive development, 943
Development of body image, 944
Social development, 944
Temperament, 948
Coping with concerns related to normal growth and development, 948
Promoting Optimum Health during Infancy, 956
Nutrition, 956
Sleep and activity, 959
Dental health, 961
Immunizations, 961
Injury prevention, 970
Anticipatory guidance—care of families, 977
Special Health Problems, 979
Feeding difficulties, 979
Failure to thrive (FTT), 980
Disorders of unknown etiology, 984
Sudden infant death syndrome (SIDS), 984
Apnea of infancy (AOI), 986
Autism, 988

34 The Toddler and Family, 993

Promoting Optimum Growth and Development, 993
Biologic development, 993
Psychosocial development, 994
Cognitive development, 995
Spiritual development, 996
Development of body image, 997
Development of sexuality, 997
Social development, 998
Coping with concerns related to normal growth and development, 999
Promoting Optimum Health During Toddlerhood, 1003
Nutrition, 1003
Sleep and activity, 1004
Dental health, 1004
Injury prevention, 1006

35 The Preschooler and Family, 1016

Promoting Optimum Growth and Development, 1016
Biologic development, 1016
Psychosocial development, 1017
Cognitive development, 1017
Moral development, 1018
Spiritual development, 1018
Development of body image, 1018
Development of sexuality, 1018
Social development, 1018
Coping with concerns related to normal growth and development, 1021
Promoting Optimum Health During the Preschool Years, 1025
Nutrition, 1025
Sleep and activity, 1026
Dental health, 1027
Injury prevention, 1027
Special Health Problems, 1028
Communicable diseases, 1028
Child Maltreatment, 1039

36 The School-Age Child and Family, 1053

Promoting Optimum Growth and Development, 1053
Biologic development, 1053
Psychosocial development, 1055
Cognitive development (Piaget), 1056
Moral development (Kohlberg), 1057
Spiritual development, 1057
Social development, 1057
Developing a self-concept, 1060
Coping with concerns related to normal growth and development, 1060
Summary of growth and development, 1063
Promoting Optimum Health During the School Years, 1063
Nutrition, 1063
Sleep and rest, 1063
Exercise and activity, 1065
Dental health, 1066
Sex education, 1068
School health, 1068
Injury prevention, 1069
Anticipatory guidance—care of families, 1069
Special Health Problems, 1072
Health problems related to sports participation, 1072
Altered growth and maturation, 1073
Tall or short stature, 1073
Sex chromosome abnormalities, 1074
Disorders with behavioral components, 1075
Attention deficit hyperactivity disorder and learning disability, 1075

Enuresis, 1077
Encopresis, 1077
Posttraumatic stress disorder, 1078
School phobia, 1078
Recurrent abdominal pain, 1079
Conversion reaction, 1079
Childhood depression, 1079
Childhood schizophrenia, 1080

37 The Adolescent and Family, 1084

Promoting Optimum Growth and Development, 1084
Biologic development, 1084
Psychosocial development, 1089
Cognitive development (Piaget), 1090
Moral development (Kohlberg), 1090
Spiritual development, 1090
Social development, 1091
Development of self-concept and body image, 1094
Promoting Optimum Health During Adolescence, 1097
Immunizations, 1098
Nutrition, 1098
Sleep and rest, 1099
Exercise and activity, 1099
Dental health, 1099
Personal care, 1099
Stress reduction, 1100
Sexuality education and guidance, 1101
Injury prevention, 1102
Anticipatory guidance—care of families, 1104
Special Health Problems, 1104
Disorders related to the reproductive system, 1104
Amenorrhea, 1104
Dysmenorrhea, 1105
Vaginitis, 1105
Disorders of the male reproductive system, 1105
Gynecomastia, 1106
Eating disorders, 1106
Obesity, 1106
Anorexia nervosa, 1109
Bulimia, 1110
Disorders with behavioral components, 1111
Smoking, 1111
Substance abuse, 1112
Suicide, 1115

UNIT TEN

Special Needs, Illness, and Hospitalization

38 Chronic Illness, Disability, and Death, 1121

Perspectives in the Care of Children with Special Needs, 1121
Scope of the problem, 1121
Changing trends in care, 1121
The Family of the Child with Special Needs, 1123
Reactions of families to a chronic illness or disability, 1123
Impact of child's chronic illness or disability on family members, 1125
Factors affecting the family's adjustment, 1128
Reactions of families to childhood death: the grief process, 1128
The Child with Special Needs, 1129
Impact of chronic illness or disability on the child, 1129
Impact of impending death on the child, 1132
Nursing care of the family and child with special needs, 1135
Nursing care of the family and child who is terminally ill or dying, 1148

39 Cognitive and Sensory Impairment, 1157

Cognitive Impairment, 1157
General concepts, 1157
Nursing care of children with cognitive impairment, 1159
Down syndrome, 1163
Fragile X syndrome, 1167
Sensory Impairment, 1168
Hearing impairment, 1168
Visual impairment, 1175
Conjunctivitis, 1181
Deaf-blind children, 1182
Retinoblastoma, 1182

40 Family-Centered Home Care, 1186

General Concepts of Home Care, 1186
Definition, 1186
Impetus for home care, 1186
Effectiveness of home care, 1187
Discharge planning and selection of a home care agency, 1187
Case management, 1187
Role of the nurse, training, and standards of care, 1188
Family-Centered Home Care, 1188
Respect for diversity, 1188
Parent-professional collaboration, 1189
The nursing process, 1190
Promotion of optimum development, self-care, and education, 1191
Safety issues in the home, 1192
Family-to-family support, 1193

41 Reaction to Illness and Hospitalization, 1196

Stressors of Hospitalization and Children's Reactions, 1196
Separation anxiety, 1196
Loss of control, 1198
Bodily injury and pain, 1200
Effects of hospitalization on the child, 1203
Nursing Care of the Child Who Is Hospitalized, 1204
Stressors and Reactions in the Family of the Child Who Is Hospitalized, 1236
Parental reactions, 1236
Sibling reactions, 1236
Altered family roles, 1236
Nursing Care of the Family, 1237
Care of the Child and Family in Special Hospital Situations, 1241

Ambulatory/outpatient setting, 1241
Isolation, 1242
Emergency admission, 1242
Intensive care unit (ICU), 1243

42 **Pediatric Nursing Interventions, 1250**

General Concepts Related to Pediatric Procedures, 1250
Informed consent, 1250
Preparation for procedures, 1252
Surgical procedures, 1257
Compliance, 1262
General Hygiene and Care, 1264
Maintaining healthy skin, 1264
Bathing, 1266
Oral hygiene, 1266
Hair care, 1267
Feeding the sick child, 1268
Controlling elevated temperatures, 1268
Family teaching and home care, 1271
Safety, 1271
Infection control, 1272
Environmental factors, 1274
Limit-setting, 1275
Transporting infants and children, 1275
Restraints, 1276
Positioning for procedures, 1278
Collection of Specimens, 1280
Urine specimens, 1280
Stool specimens, 1282
Blood specimens, 1282
Respiratory secretion/throat specimens, 1284
Administration of Medication, 1284
Preparation for safe administration, 1284
Oral administration, 1286
Intramuscular (IM) administration, 1288
Subcutaneous and intradermal administration, 1292
Intravenous (IV) administration, 1293
Nasogastric, orogastric, or gastrostomy administration, 1296
Rectal administration, 1296
Optic, otic, and nasal administration, 1297
Family teaching and home care, 1298
Procedures Related to Maintaining Fluid Balance, 1299
Measurement of intake and output (I & O), 1299
Parenteral fluid therapy, 1299
Family teaching and home care, 1302
Procedures for Maintaining Respiratory Function, 1302
Inhalation therapy, 1302
Bronchial (postural) drainage, 1305
Chest physiotherapy (CPT), 1305
Artificial ventilation, 1305
Family teaching and home care, 1310
Procedures Related to Alternative Feeding Techniques, 1311
Gavage feeding, 1311
Gastrostomy feeding, 1313
Total parenteral nutrition (TPN), 1314
Family teaching and home care, 1314
Procedures Related to Elimination, 1315
Enema, 1315
Ostomies, 1315
Family teaching and home care, 1316

UNIT ELEVEN

Health Problems of Children

43 **Respiratory Dysfunction, 1321**

Respiratory Infection, 1321
General aspects of respiratory infections, 1321
Upper Respiratory Tract Infections (URIs), 1326
Nasopharyngitis, 1326
Pharyngitis, 1327
Tonsillitis, 1328
Infectious mononucleosis, 1330
Influenza, 1331
Otitis media (OM), 1331
Croup Syndromes, 1334
Acute epiglottitis, 1334
Acute laryngitis, 1335
Acute laryngotracheobronchitis (LTB), 1335
Acute spasmodic laryngitis, 1337
Bacterial tracheitis, 1337
Infections of the Lower Airways, 1337
Bronchitis, 1337
Respiratory syncytial virus (RSV)/bronchiolitis, 1337
Pneumonias, 1339
Other Infections of the Respiratory Tract, 1341
Pertussis (whooping cough), 1341
Tuberculosis (TB), 1341
Pulmonary Dysfunction Caused by Noninfectious Irritants, 1344
Foreign body (FB) aspiration, 1344
Aspiration pneumonia, 1345
Adult respiratory distress syndrome (ARDS), 1345
Inhalation injury: smoke and carbon monoxide, 1345
Passive smoking, 1346
Long-term Respiratory Dysfunction, 1347
Asthma, 1347
Cystic fibrosis, 1356
Respiratory Emergency, 1361
Respiratory failure, 1361
Cardiopulmonary resuscitation (CPR), 1362
Airway obstruction, 1365

44 **Gastrointestinal Dysfunction, 1372**

Nutritional Disturbances, 1372
Vitamin disturbances, 1372
Mineral disturbances, 1377
Vegetarian diets, 1382
Protein and energy malnutrition (PEM), 1384
Kwashiorkor, 1384
Marasmus, 1384
Food sensitivity, 1384
Cow's milk allergy, 1385
Lactose intolerance, 1386
Gastrointestinal (GI) Dysfunction, 1386
Dehydration, 1386
Disorders of Motility, 1390
Acute diarrhea, 1390
Acute infectious diarrhea, 1393
Constipation, 1395
Hirschsprung disease, 1399
Vomiting, 1401
Gastroesophageal reflux (GFR), 1401
Intestinal Parasitic Diseases, 1403
General nursing considerations, 1403

Giardiasis, 1403
Enterobiasis (pinworms), 1405
Inflammatory Disorders, 1406
Stomatitis, 1406
Acute appendicitis, 1406
Meckel diverticulum, 1409
Inflammatory bowel disease (IBD), 1409
Peptic ulcer, 1412
Hepatic Disorders, 1414
Acute hepatitis, 1414
Cirrhosis, 1416
Biliary atresia, 1417
Structural Defects, 1418
Cleft lip (CL) and/or cleft palate (CP), 1418
Esophageal atresia (EA) and tracheoesophageal fistula (TEF), 1422
Hernias, 1425
Obstructive Disorders, 1425
Hypertrophic pyloric stenosis (HPS), 1426
Intussusception, 1429
Anorectal malformations, 1431
Malabsorption Syndromes, 1432
Celiac disease (CD), 1432
Short bowel syndrome (SBS), 1433
Ingestion of Injurious Agents, 1434
Principles of emergency treatment, 1435
Heavy metal poisoning, 1439
Lead poisoning, 1440

45 Cardiovascular Dysfunction, 1450

Cardiovascular Dysfunction, 1450
Assessment of cardiac function, 1450
Cardiac catheterization, 1451
Congenital Heart Disease, 1453
General concepts, 1453
Classification of defects, 1454
Defects with Increased Pulmonary Blood Flow, 1455
Atrial septal defect (ASD), 1456
Ventricular septal defect (VSD), 1456
Atrioventricular canal (AVC) defect, 1457
Patent ductus arteriosus (PDA), 1458
Obstructive Defects, 1455
Coarctation of the aorta (COA), 1458
Aortic stenosis (AS), 1459
Pulmonic stenosis (PS), 1460
Defects with Decreased Pulmonary Blood Flow, 1457
Tetralogy of Fallot (TOF), 1460
Tricuspid atresia, 1461
Mixed Defects, 1465
Transposition of the great arteries (TGA) or transposition of the great vessels (TGV), 1462
Total anomalous pulmonary venous connection (TAPVC), 1462
Truncus arteriosus (TA), 1463
Hypoplastic left heart syndrome (HLHS), 1464
Clinical Consequences of Congenital Heart Disease, 1465
Congestive heart failure (CHF), 1465
Hypoxemia, 1472
Nursing Care of the Family and Child with Congenital Heart Disease, 1474
Acquired Cardiovascular Disorders, 1481
Bacterial (infective) endocarditis (BE), 1481
Rheumatic fever (RF), 1482
Hyperlipidemia (hypercholesterolemia), 1483
Cardiac dysrhythmias, 1484
Vascular Dysfunction, 1486
Systemic hypertension, 1486
Kawasaki disease (KD) (mucocutaneous lymph node syndrome), 1487
Shock, 1489
Anaphylaxis, 1491
Toxic shock syndrome (TSS), 1492
Henoch-Schönlein purpura (HSP), 1493
Heart Transplantation, 1494

46 Hematologic and Immunologic Dysfunction, 1499

Hematologic and Immunologic Dysfunction, 1499
Assessment of hematologic function, 1499
Red Blood Cell (RBC) Disorders, 1499
Anemia, 1499
Iron deficiency anemia, 1503
Sickle cell anemia (SCA), 1505
B-Thalassemia (Cooley anemia), 1510
Aplastic anemia, 1511
Defects in Hemostasis, 1512
Hemophilia, 1512
Idiopathic thrombocytopenic purpura (ITP), 1515
Disseminated intravascular coagulation (DIC), 1516
Epistaxis (nosebleeding), 1516
Neoplastic Disorders, 1517
Leukemias, 1517
Lymphomas, 1528
Hodgkin disease, 1528
Non-Hodgkin lymphoma (NHL), 1530
Immunologic Deficiency Disorders, 1530
Mechanisms involved in immunity, 1530
Acquired immunodeficiency syndrome (AIDS), 1531
Severe combined immunodeficiency disease (SCID), 1533
Wiskott-Aldrich syndrome, 1534
Technologic Management of Hematologic and Immunologic Disorders, 1534
Blood transfusion therapy, 1534
Bone marrow transplantation (BMT), 1536
Apheresis, 1537

47 Genitourinary Dysfunction, 1542

Genitourinary Dysfunction, 1542
Assessment of renal function, 1542
Genitourinary Tract Disorders/Defects, 1545
Urinary tract infection (UTI), 1545
Obstructive uropathy, 1549
External defects, 1550
Glomerular Disease, 1551
Nephrotic syndrome, 1551
Acute glomerulonephritis (AGN), 1556
Miscellaneous Renal Disorders, 1558
Hemolytic-uremic syndrome (HUS), 1558
Wilms tumor, 1559
Renal Failure, 1560
Acute renal failure (ARF), 1560
Chronic renal failure (CRF), 1563
Technologic Management of Renal Failure, 1568
Dialysis, 1568
Transplantation, 1569

48 Cerebral Dysfunction, 1572

Cerebral Dysfunction, 1572
Assessment of cerebral function, 1572
Nursing Care of the Unconscious Child, 1578
Cerebral Trauma, 1585
Head injury, 1585
Near-drowning, 1593
Central Nervous System Tumors, 1594
Brain tumors, 1594
Neuroblastoma, 1599
Intracranial Infections, 1600
Bacterial meningitis, 1600
Nonbacterial (aseptic) meningitis, 1602
Encephalitis, 1603
Reye syndrome (RS), 1603
Human immunodeficiency virus (HIV) encephalopathy, 1604
Rabies, 1604
Seizure Disorders, 1605
Epilepsy, 1605
Febrile seizures, 1614
Cerebral malformations, 1615
Cranial deformities, 1615
Hydrocephalus, 1615

49 Endocrine Dysfunction, 1624

Disorders of Pituitary Function, 1624
Hypopituitarism: growth hormone (GH) deficiency, 1624
Pituitary hyperfunction, 1627
Precocious puberty, 1627
Diabetes insipidus (DI), 1628
Syndrome of inappropriate antidiuretic hormone secretion (SIADH), 1629
Disorders of Thyroid Function, 1629
Juvenile hypothyroidism, 1629
Goiter, 1630
Lymphocytic thyroiditis, 1630
Hyperthyroidism (Graves disease), 1631
Disorders of Parathyroid Function, 1633
Hypoparathyroidism, 1633
Hyperparathyroidism, 1634
Disorders of Adrenal Function, 1634
Acute adrenocortical insufficiency, 1634
Chronic adrenocortical insufficiency (Addison disease), 1635
Cushing syndrome, 1636
Congenital adrenogenital hyperplasia (CAH), 1637
Hyperaldosteronism, 1639
Pheochromocytoma, 1639
Disorders of Pancreatic Hormone Function, 1640
Diabetes mellitus (DM), 1640

50 Integumentary Dysfunction, 1654

Integumentary Dysfunction, 1654
Skin lesions, 1654
Wounds, 1655
General therapeutic management, 1660
Nursing care of the child with a skin disorder, 1662
Infections of the Skin, 1664
Bacterial infections, 1664
Viral infections, 1667
Dermatophytoses (fungal infections), 1669
Systemic mycotic (fungal) infections, 1669
Skin Disorders Related to Chemical or Physical Contacts, 1671
Contact dermatitis, 1671
Poison ivy, oak, and sumac, 1671
Drug reactions, 1672
Foreign bodies, 1672
Skin Disorders Related to Insect and Animal Contacts, 1673
Scabies, 1673
Pediculosis capitis, 1673
Arthropod bites and stings, 1674
Infections transmitted by arthropods, 1677
Animal bites, 1677
Human bites, 1678
Cat scratch disease (CSD), 1679
Miscellaneous Skin Disorders, 1679
Skin Disorders Associated with Specific Age Groups, 1679
Diaper dermatitis, 1679
Atopic dermatitis (AD) (eczema), 1682
Seborrheic dermatitis, 1685
Acne, 1685
Thermal Injury, 1687
Burns, 1687
Sunburn, 1700
Cold injury, 1703

51 Musculoskeletal and Articular Dysfunction, 1706

The Immobilized Child, 1706
Immobilization, 1706
Traumatic Injury, 1709
Soft tissue injury, 1709
Fractures, 1711
The child in a cast, 1714
The child in traction, 1716
Distraction, 1720
Amputation, 1720
Congenital Defects, 1721
Developmental dysplasia of the hip (DDH), 1721
Congenital clubfoot, 1725
Metatarsus adductus (varus), 1726
Skeletal limb deficiency, 1727
Osteogenesis imperfecta (OI), 1727
Acquired Defects, 1728
Legg-Calvé-Perthes disease, 1728
Slipped femoral capital epiphysis, 1729
Kyphosis and lordosis, 1729
Scoliosis, 1730
Infections of Bones and Joints, 1733
Osteomyelitis, 1733
Septic (suppurative, pyogenic, purulent) arthritis, 1734
Tuberculosis, 1734
Bone and Soft Tissue Tumors, 1735
General concepts: bone tumors, 1735
Osteogenic sarcoma, 1735
Ewing sarcoma, 1737
Rhabdomyosarcoma, 1737
Disorders of Joints, 1738
Juvenile rheumatoid arthritis (JRA), 1738
Systemic lupus erythematosus (SLE), 1741

52 Neuromuscular and Muscular Dysfunction, 1746

Congenital Neuromuscular or Muscular Disorders, 1746
Cerebral palsy (CP), 1746
Spina bifida (myelomeningocele), 1751
Progressive infantile spinal muscular atrophy (Werdnig-Hoffmann disease), 1759
Juvenile spinal muscular atrophy (Kugelberg-Welander disease), 1760
Muscular dystrophies (MDs), 1760
Pseudohypertrophic (Duchenne) muscular dystrophy (DMD), 1761
Acquired Neuromuscular Disorders, 1762
Guillain-Barré syndrome (GBS) (infectious polyneuritis), 1762
Tetanus, 1763
Botulism, 1764
Spinal cord injuries, 1765

APPENDIXES

A Standards for the Nursing Care of Women and Newborns, 1769

B Nursing Responsibilities in Implementing Intrapartum Fetal Heart Rate Monitoring, 1772

C Standard Laboratory Values: Pregnant and Nonpregnant Women, 1774

D Family APGAR Questionnaire, 1776

E Developmental/Sensory Assessment, 1778
Denver II, 1778
Denver Articulation Screening, 1780
Snellen Screening, 1782

F Growth Measurements, 1783
Height/Weight Measurements—Boys, 1783
Height/Weight Measurements—Girls, 1784
Head Circumference Charts, 1786
Percentiles for Triceps Skinfold, 1787
Percentiles for Upper Arm Circumference, 1787

G Translations of FACES Pain Rating Scale, 1788

H Pediatric Vital Signs and Parameters, 1790

I Common Laboratory Tests, 1792

Maternal Child Nursing Care

CHAPTER 1

Contemporary Maternity Nursing

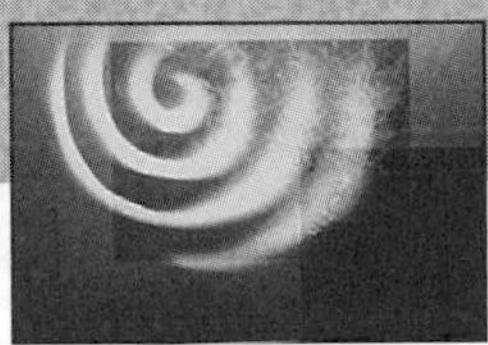

CONTEMPORARY ISSUES AND TRENDS, P. 1

Changing health care delivery structure, p. 1

Changing childbirth practices, p. 2

Changing views of women, p. 2

Trends in fertility and birthrate, p. 3

Trends of consumer involvement, self-care, and focus on health care, p. 4

Trend to high-technology care, p. 4

Shift to home health care, p. 4

Increase in high-risk pregnancies, p. 4

Trends and issues of high costs, p. 4

Access to care, p. 4

Trends in nursing practice, p. 5

STANDARDS OF PRACTICE, P. 5

Standard of care, p. 5

ETHICAL ISSUES IN PERINATAL NURSING, P. 5

RESEARCH INTO PRACTICE, P. 5

Maternity nursing focuses on the care of childbearing women and their families through all stages of pregnancy and childbirth, as well as the first 4 weeks after birth. Throughout the prenatal period, nurses, nurse practitioners, and nurse-midwives provide care for women in clinics and physicians' offices and teach classes to help families prepare for childbirth. They also care for childbearing families during labor and birth in hospitals, in birthing centers, and less often in the home. Nurses with special training may provide intensive care for high-risk neonates in special care units and for high-risk mothers in antepartal units, in critical care obstetric units, or in the home. Maternity nurses spend time teaching about pregnancy; the process of labor, birth, and recovery; and parenting skills. An investment in health promotion during childbearing can have a significant impact not only on the health of individual women and their infants, but on society as well.

The strength of a society rests on the health of its mothers and infants. In the United States, serious problems related to the health and health care of mothers and infants exist. Access to prepregnancy and pregnancy-related care for all women and the lack of reproductive health services for adolescents are major concerns (Davidson, Gibbs, and Chapin, 1991). Nurses can influence health policy by their active participation in the education of the public and state and federal legislators (Hastings, 1995).

The focus of the first portion of this book is maternity nursing. This chapter presents a general overview of issues and trends related to the health and health care of women and infants during the maternity cycle. Chapter 27 addresses issues and trends related to the health care of children.

CONTEMPORARY ISSUES AND TRENDS

Changing Health Care Delivery Structure

More than 14% of the U.S. gross domestic product was consumed by health care in 1994. To control costs, managed care has linked providers and insurers; health maintenance organizations (HMOs) were the prototypes for this system. Consolidation, mergers, and integration of hospitals occurred; these systems were designed "to provide services throughout the continuum of care" (Barter et al, 1995). The number of nurses in hospitals has declined, and unlicensed assistive personnel and multiskilled workers have been substituted. The role of the nurse is evolving from primary caregiver to leader of the interdisciplinary care team. Documentation of patient outcomes has become essential (Barter et al, 1995). Advanced practice roles will increase as nurses assume more responsibility for care of patients.

Changing Childbirth Practices

Maternity care has changed dramatically. Women can choose either a physician or a nurse-midwife as their primary care provider. In 1993, physicians attended 93.8% of all births in hospitals, and nurse-midwives attended 4.8% of all births in hospitals; 1% were out-of-hospital births (Ventura et al, 1995). Home births represented 0.6% of all births (Ventura et al, 1995). Women can give birth in a hospital labor room (rather than a delivery room), in a birthing room, in a freestanding birthing center (Ernst, 1994), or at home.

Certified nurse-midwives provide safe, quality care (Fischler and Harvey, 1995). Women who choose nurse-midwives as their primary providers participate actively in childbirth decisions and receive fewer interventions, such as epidural analgesia, for labor (Callister, 1995).

No longer are laboring mothers and their support people separated. With family-centered care, fathers, partners, grandparents, siblings, and friends may be present for labor and birth. Fathers or partners may be present for cesarean births. Newborn infants remain with the mother and may breastfeed immediately after birth. Parents participate in the care of their infants in nurseries and neonatal intensive care units (NICUs).

Nursing care is changing to *single-room maternity care*, in which a woman labors, gives birth, and recovers in the same room (labor-delivery-recovery, LDR). In some settings the entire hospital stay for a birth may occur in the same room (labor-delivery-recovery-postpartum, LDRP). Instead of having one nurse care for the baby and another nurse care for the mother, some hospitals have one nurse caring for the mother and baby as a unit (*couplet*, or *mother-baby, care*). In some hospitals, central nurseries have been eliminated, and babies "room-in" with their mothers. Many hospitals employ lactation consultants to assist mothers with breastfeeding.

Discharge of a mother and baby within 24 to 48 hours of birth is a common practice, resulting in a growing need for follow-up or home care. In some settings, discharge may occur as early as 6 hours after birth. Recent legislation ensures that mothers and babies are permitted to stay in the hospital at least 48 hours. Early discharge creates a need for focused and efficient teaching to enable the parents and infant to have a safe transition to home. Nurses may establish "warm lines" or incorporate follow-up telephone calls or home visits into their practice as they assist families needing information and reassurance.

Changing Views of Women

Women must be viewed holistically and in the context in which they live. Their physical, mental, and social needs must be considered, since these areas are interdependent and influence women's health and illness (Breslin, 1995). Even the language health care professionals use to describe women and their problems needs to be examined (Freda, 1995). For example, providers describe women who have an "incompetent cervix," who "fail to progress," or who have an "arrest" of labor, or they describe a fetus with intrauterine growth "retardation"; providers "allow" women a "trial" of labor. Caregivers might better describe women who have recurrent premature dilation of the cervix or the fetus whose intrauterine growth has been restricted (Freda, 1995). In communications with women, health care providers must move away from punitive terms associated with confinement and prison (Peterson and Cefalo, 1990).

Violence is a major factor affecting pregnant women. Violence includes battering (which may increase during pregnancy), rape or other sexual assaults, and attacks with various weapons. It is estimated that 8.3% of pregnant women are battered (Loring and Smith, 1994).

Human immunodeficiency virus (HIV) and acquired immunodeficiency syndrome (AIDS) are increasingly affecting women and children. Approximately 30% of infants born to women with HIV will also be infected with the virus (Kass, 1994). By the year 2000, AIDS will be among the top five causes of death in women of childbearing age (Covington and Collins, 1994). Limitation of reproductive choice of women infected with HIV is being discussed (Kass, 1994), and mass screening of infants and mothers is occurring (Grady, 1994).

Critical Thinking Exercises

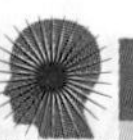

POSTPARTUM CARE

Interview three women of varying cultures in the early postpartum period.

1. **Who was with them during labor and birth? How satisfied were they with their birth experience? What contributed to their satisfaction?**
2. **Compare the birth experiences and satisfaction of the three women. What similarities and differences exist? To what do you attribute the differences?**
3. **Develop a culturally sensitive plan of care to increase satisfaction with the birth experience.**

BOX 1-1
Maternal-Infant Biostatistical Terminology

Abortus—An embryo/fetus that is removed or expelled from the uterus at 20 weeks' gestation or less, or weighing 500 g or less, or measuring 25 cm or less.

Birthrate—Number of live births in one year per 1000 population.

Fertility rate—Number of births per 1000 women between ages 15 and 44 (inclusive), calculated on a yearly basis.

Infant mortality rate—Number of deaths of infants under 1 year of age per 1000 live births.

Maternal mortality rate—Number of maternal deaths from births and complications of pregnancy, childbirth, and puerperium (the first 42 days after termination of the pregnancy) per 100,000 live births.

Neonatal mortality rate—Number of deaths of infants under 28 days of age per 1000 live births.

Perinatal mortality rate—Number of stillbirths and the number of neonatal deaths per 1000 live births.

Stillbirth—An infant who, at birth, demonstrates *no* signs of life, such as breathing, heartbeat, or voluntary muscle movements.

Trends in Fertility and Birthrate

Fertility trends and birthrates reflect women's needs for health care. Box 1-1 defines biostatistical terminology useful in analyzing maternity health care. In 1995 the **fertility rate,** the number of births to women of childbearing age (15 to 44), was 65.6 live births per 1000 women (Guyer et al, 1996). This is a slight decrease from the 66.7 rate in 1994. The highest birthrates were for women between ages 20 and 29 (Table 1-1). The **birthrate,** the number of live births per 1000 population in 1 year, was 14.8 in 1995, which is 5% lower than 1993 (Guyer et al, 1996). Almost one third of all births in the United States in 1995 were to unmarried women, with wide variation in rate among racial groups: African-American, 69.5 per 1000 and Caucasian, 25.4 per 1000 (Guyer et al, 1996). Births to unmarried women are often related to less favorable outcomes because there are typically a large number of teenagers in the unmarried group (32% in 1995). The rates of pregnancy and abortion among adolescents are higher in the United States than in any other industrialized country (Burnhill, 1994).

Number of low-birth-weight infants. Babies born weighing less than 2500 g (5 lb, 8 oz) are classified as **low birth weight (LBW),** and their risks for morbidity and mortality increase. By reducing the number of LBW infants, the health of infants improves. In 1995 the incidence of LBW was 7.3% (Guyer et al, 1996). African-American babies are more than twice as likely as Caucasian babies to be LBW and to die within the first year of life. For African-American births the incidence of LBW was 13%, whereas the rate for Caucasian births was 6.2%. Cigarette smoking is associated with LBW, prematurity, and intrauterine growth restriction (Shu et al., 1995). In 1994, 14.6% of pregnant women smoked; this proportion represented a decline from 1993 (Guyer et al, 1996).

The proportion of **preterm infants,** those born before 38 weeks of gestation, was 10.7% in 1993, a slight decline attributed to the decline in African-American preterm births from 18.9% to 18.4%. The rate of Caucasian preterm births remained at 9.1% (Ventura et al, 1994). The number of multiple births increased in 1994; most of the increase is attributed to delay in childbearing and use of fertility drugs (Guyer et al, 1996).

Infant mortality in the United States. A common indicator of the adequacy of prenatal care and the health of a nation as a whole is the **infant mortality rate** (deaths per 1000 live births). The preliminary infant mortality rate for 1995 was 7.5, the lowest ever recorded in the United States (Guyer et al, 1996). The infant mortality rate continues to be higher for African-American babies than for Caucasian babies, a gap that has widened since the mid-1970s (Kochanek and Hudson, 1995). Fig. 1-1 illustrates the trend in infant mortality over the years. Limited maternal education, young maternal age, unmarried status, poverty, and lack of prenatal care appear to be associated with higher infant mortality rates. Lack of prenatal care, poor nutrition, smoking and alcohol use, and maternal conditions such as poor health or hypertension are also important contributors to infant mortality. A shift from the current emphasis on high-technology medical interventions to a focus on improving access to preventive care for low-income families is necessary.

TABLE 1-1 Birthrate according to age—1994

AGE	RATE (/1000 WOMEN)
15-17	37.6
18-19	91.5
20-24	111.1
25-29	113.9
30-34	81.5
35-39	33.7
40-44	6.4

Data from Guyer et al: Annual summary of vital statistics—1995, *Pediatrics* 98(6):1007, 1996.

International infant mortality trends. In comparing the infant mortality rates of Canada and the United States with other industrialized nations, it is significant to note that in 1994 Canada ranked fifteenth and the United States had the twenty-first lowest rate (Guyer et al, 1996). Even though infant mortality decreased somewhat in the United States, the United States did not keep pace with other industrialized

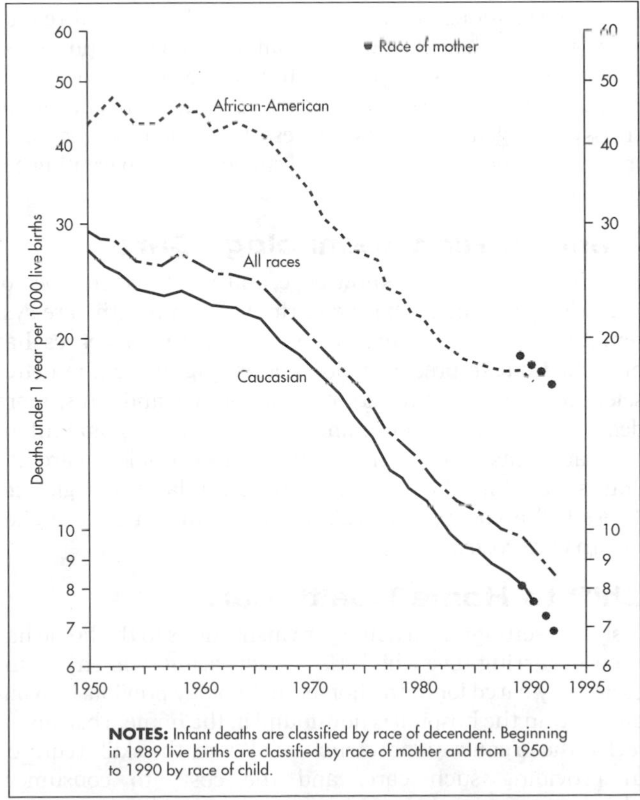

Fig. 1-1 Infant mortality rates by race: United States, 1950-1992. (From Kochanek K, Hudson B: Advance report of final mortality statistics, 1992, *Monthly Vital Stat Rep* 43(6 suppl):11, 1995.)

countries. Some suggest that the problem in the United States is rooted in economic barriers and inadequate access to prenatal care, as well as in poor financial and social benefits for childbearing women (National Commission, 1990).

Maternal mortality trends. In 1994, 270 women in the United States died from complications of pregnancy, childbirth, and the puerperium (National Center for Health Statistics, 1995). African-American women were 4 times more likely to die from these complications than were Caucasian women, at a rate of 20.5 for African-American women compared with 4.8 for Caucasian women (Mortality Patterns, 1993).

Trends of Consumer Involvement, Self-Care, and Focus on Health Care

In the 1960s, patients began to demand information about medical technology and their medical care. A movement toward self-help and assuming responsibility for wellness also occurred. No longer do patients passively accept and comply with the advice of health care providers. Patients demand information and take active roles in their health care. They make changes in health behaviors to improve pregnancy outcome (Higgins, Frank, and Brown, 1994). **Self-care** has been appealing to both patients and the health care system because of its potential to reduce health care costs.

Maternity care is especially suited to self-care because childbearing is essentially health focused, patients are usually well when they enter the system, and visits to health care providers can present the opportunity for health as well as illness interventions. Measures to improve health and reduce risks associated with poor pregnancy outcomes and illness can be addressed. Visits to health care providers provide opportunities to address topics such as nutrition education, stress management, smoking cessation, alcohol and drug treatment, improvement of social supports, and parenting education.

Trend to High-Technology Care

Advances in scientific knowledge and the large number of high-risk pregnancies have contributed to a health care system that emphasizes high-technology care. Obstetrics has branched out to preconception counseling, more and better scientific techniques to monitor the mother and fetus, more definitive tests for hypoxia and acidosis, and neonatal intensive care units (NICUs). In general, high-technology care has flourished while "health" care has been relatively neglected. These technologic advances have also contributed to higher health care costs.

Shift to Home Health Care

A shift in settings from acute care institutions to the home has been occurring. Even high-risk childbearing women are increasingly cared for in the home. Technology previously available only in the hospital is now found in the home. This has affected the organizational structure of care, the skills required in providing such care, and the costs to consumers (deLissovoy and Feustle, 1991).

Increase in High-Risk Pregnancies

High-risk pregnancies have increased, which means that a greater number of pregnant women are at risk for poor pregnancy outcomes. Escalating drug use (11% to 27% of pregnant women, depending on geographic location) has contributed to higher incidences of prematurity, LBW, congenital defects, learning disabilities, and withdrawal symptoms in infants. Alcohol use in pregnancy has been associated with miscarriages (spontaneous abortions), mental retardation, LBW, and fetal alcohol syndrome. Adequate prenatal care focusing on health and a reduction of risk factors can improve pregnancy outcomes (National Commission, 1990).

Trends and Issues of High Costs

The cost of health care is one of the fastest growing sectors of the U.S. economy. National health expenditures are 14.3% of the gross domestic product, or one seventh of the U.S. economy (Vincenzino, 1994). Perinatal care cost $27.8 billion in 1989, representing $6850 for each mother-infant pair (Long, Marquis, and Harrison, 1994). A shift in demographics, an increased emphasis on high-cost technology, and liability costs of a litigious society contribute to the high cost of care. Most researchers agree that the costs of caring for the increased number of LBW infants in NICUs have also contributed significantly to the overall health care costs, especially since 19% of all uninsured women gave birth to an infant of LBW (National Commission, 1990).

In 1991 Medicaid funded 32% of all deliveries in states reporting the data (Singh, Gold, and Frost, 1994). Nursing is making some impact on cost containment by providing midwifery care to pregnant women, but the lack of direct access to reimbursement for nurse practitioners and clinical nurse specialist services as direct care providers continues to be a problem (Ernst, 1994).

Early discharge programs are also being used to reduce costs (Brooten et al, 1994). Fullerton (1992) cautions that hospitals are adopting these programs without adequate and continual screening, without preparation for early discharge during the prenatal period, and without postpartum follow-up care and are failing to recognize that women who select early discharge are different from those forced to go home early because of limited insurance or other funding. The *safety* of shorter hospital stays must be demonstrated; it is not enough to show that they are not unsafe (U.S. Department of Health and Human Services, 1995). The American Academy of Pediatrics has published minimum criteria for early discharge of a newborn (Oh et al, 1995).

Managed care, a method of guiding care for a patient during a hospital stay, is gaining popularity as a means of controlling care costs (Marr and Reid, 1992). Managed care focuses on meeting the patient's needs while promoting efficiency and cost-effectiveness (Hicks, Stallmeyer, and Coleman, 1992). The concept of care management is applied to maternity nursing in this text. Approaches such as protocols and critical care paths are used where applicable.

Access to Care

Access to prenatal care continues to be an issue through the 1990s. The proportion of women in 1994 who began prenatal care in the first trimester was 80.2%, the highest level ever reported; 4.4% or fewer delayed care until the third trimester or had no care (Guyer et al, 1996). Older mothers (86%) sought care earlier than those under 20 years of age (59%) (Ventura et al., 1994). However, many women with

Critical Thinking Exercises 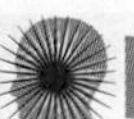

PRENATAL CARE

Not all women seek prenatal care during pregnancy. The reasons for not receiving care vary, often according to age and ethnicity. Interview three women of varying ages (younger than 20, 20 to 30, 31 to 40) who are pregnant.

1. **When did they first seek prenatal care? How often have they seen a health care provider during pregnancy? What do they see as advantages of prenatal visits? What are disadvantages or barriers to prenatal visits?**
2. **Compare the time of initiation of prenatal care among the women. Compare the advantages and disadvantages of prenatal visits. What conclusions can you draw from this information?**

access to prenatal care entered the health care system late or came only sporadically. Minority women were less likely than Caucasian women to receive early prenatal care; 82% of Caucasian women, 67% of Hispanic women, and 66% of African-American women had prenatal care in the first trimester (Ventura et al, 1995). African-American women had fewer prenatal visits than Caucasian women (LaVeist, Keith, and Gutierrez, 1995).

Barriers to access need to be removed so pregnancy outcomes can be improved. The most significant barrier to access is the inability to pay. When barriers are removed, women in the low-income bracket seek care earlier and more often (Piper, Mitchel, and Ray, 1994). Simple incentives to increase participation in prenatal care do not work (Laken and Ager, 1995). In addition to a lack of insurance and high costs, there is a lack of providers for women with low incomes, since many physicians refuse to take Medicaid patients or take only a few such patients. This presents a significant problem because one in six births are to mothers who receive Medicaid. Cited as reasons for refusal to accept Medicaid patients are low reimbursement rates and cumbersome processes for patients in obtaining reimbursement (National Commission, 1990; Scupholme, Robertson, and Kamons, 1991).

Trends in Nursing Practice

The increasing complexity of care for maternity patients has contributed to specialization of nurses working with these patients. This specialized knowledge is being gained through experience, advanced degrees, and certification programs. Nurses in advanced practice—nurse practitioners and nurse-midwives—may provide primary care throughout a woman's life, including during the pregnancy cycle.

STANDARDS OF PRACTICE

Nursing standards of practice in perinatal and women's health nursing have been described by several organizations, including the American Nurses Association (ANA), which publishes standards for maternal-child health nursing; the **Association for Women's Health, Obstetric and Neonatal Nurses (AWHONN),** which publishes standards of practice and education; and the National Association of Neonatal Nurses (NANN), which publishes standards of practice for neonatal nurses. These standards reflect current knowledge and represent levels of practice agreed on by leaders in the specialty. Because nursing practice, society, and the health care system are dynamic rather than static, standards change over time. In addition to these more formalized standards, agencies often have their own policy-and-procedure books that outline standards to be followed in that setting.

Standard of Care

In determining legal negligence, the care given is compared with the **standards of care.** If the standard was not met and harm resulted, negligence occurred. The number of legal suits in the perinatal area has typically been high. As a consequence, malpractice insurance costs have risen dramatically for physicians, nurse-midwives, and nurses (Lang and Marek, 1991; Pellegrino, Siegler, and Singer, 1991).

LEGAL TIP

Standard of Care

When you are uncertain about how to perform a procedure, consult the agency procedure book and follow the guidelines printed in the book. These guidelines are the standard of care for that agency.

ETHICAL ISSUES IN PERINATAL NURSING

Ethical concerns and debates have multiplied with increasing use of technology and scientific advances. For example, with reproductive technology, pregnancy is now possible in women who thought they would never bear children, including some who are menopausal or postmenopausal. With induced ovulation and in vitro fertilization, multiple pregnancies occur, and multifetal pregnancy reduction (selectively terminating one or more fetuses) may be considered (Lipitz, Mashiach, and Seidman, 1994). Innovations such as intrauterine fetal surgery, artificial insemination, genetic engineering, surrogate childbearing, surgery for infertility, "test tube" babies, fetal research, and treatment of very-low-birth-weight (VLBW) infants have resulted in questions about informed consent and allocation of resources. The introduction of long-acting contraceptives has created moral choices and policy dilemmas for health care providers and legislators; that is, should some women (substance abusers, women with low incomes, or women who are HIV positive) be required to take the contraceptives (Moskowitz, Jennings, and Callahan, 1995)? With the potential for great good that can come from fetal tissue transplantation, what research is ethical? What are the rights of the embryo (Robertson, 1995)? Discussion and debate about these issues will occur for many years; nurses and patients, as well as scientists, physicians, attorneys, and clergy, must be involved in the discussions. Nursing can play a constructive role in this area by providing rational, knowledgeable, and experienced voices (Pellegrino, Siegler, and Singer, 1991; Styles, 1990).

RESEARCH INTO PRACTICE

The incorporation of research findings into practice is essential to develop a science-based practice. Practicing nurses can identify problems and read research literature to identify studies that address their clinical concerns. Research utilization must increase (Gennaro, 1994). Nurses can develop protocols and procedures based on published research. Health care providers need to support researchers in their endeavors.

Key Points

- Maternity nursing focuses on women and their infants and families during the childbearing cycle.
- Nurses caring for women can play an active role in shaping health care systems to be responsive to the needs of contemporary women.
- Childbirth practices have changed to become more family-focused and to allow alternatives in care.
- Home care is an increasing and cost-effective alternative locus of care.
- The United States ranks twenty-first among industrialized nations in infant mortality.
- Ethical concerns have multiplied with increasing use of technology and scientific advances.

References

Barter M et al: The changing health care delivery structure: opportunities for nursing practice and administration, *Nurse Admin Q* 19(3):74, 1995.

Breslin E: Integrating women's health concepts in a nursing course, *Nurs Educ* 20(1):30, 1995.

Brooten D et al: A randomized trial of early hospital discharge and home follow-up of women having a cesarean birth, *Obstet Gynecol* 84(5):832, 1994.

Burnhill M: Adolescent pregnancy rates in the US, *Contemp OB GYN* 39(2):26, 1994.

Callister L: Beliefs and perceptions of childbearing women choosing different primary health care providers, *Clin Nurs Res* 4(2):168, 1995.

Covington C, Collins J: Back to the future of women's health and perinatal nursing in the 21st century, *J Obstet Gynecol Neonatal Nurs* 23(2):183, 1994.

Davidson E, Gibbs C, Chapin J: The challenge of care for the poor and underserved in the United States: an American College of Obstetricians and Gynecologists' perspective on access to care for underserved women, *Am J Dis Child* 145(5):546, 1991.

deLissovoy G, Feustle J: Advanced home health care, *Health Policy* 17:227, 1991.

Ernst E: Health care reform as an ongoing process, *J Obstet Gynecol Neonatal Nurs* 23(2):129, 1994.

Fischler N, Harvey S: Setting and provider of prenatal care: association with pregnancy outcomes among low-income women, *Health Care Women Int* 16(4):309, 1995.

Freda M: Arrest, trial, and failure, *J Obstet Gynecol Neonatal Nurs* 24(5):393, 1995.

Fullerton J: The choice of in-hospital or alternative birth environment as related to the concept of control, *J Nurs Midwifery* 27:17, 1992.

Gennaro S: Research utilization: an overview, *J Obstet Gynecol Neonatal Nurs* 23(4):313, 1994.

Grady G: HIV mass screening of infants and mothers: historical, technical, and practical issues, *Acta Paediatr Suppl* 400:39, 1994.

Guyer B et al: Annual summary of vital statistics—1995, *Pediatrics* 98(6):1007, 1996.

Hastings K: Health care reform: we need it, but do we have the national will to shape our future? *Nurse Pract* 20(1):52, 1995.

Hicks L, Stallmeyer J, Coleman J: Nursing challenges in managed care, *Nurs Econ* 10(4):265, 1992.

Higgins P, Frank B, Brown M: Changes in health behaviors made by pregnant women, *Health Care Women Int* 15:149, 1994.

Kass N: Policy, ethics, and reproductive choice: pregnancy and childbearing among HIV-infected women, *Acta Paediatr Suppl* 400:95, 1994.

Kochanek K, Hudson B: Advance report of final mortality statistics, 1992, *Monthly Vital Stat Rep* 43(suppl 6): 1, 1995.

Laken M, Ager J: Using incentives to increase participation in prenatal care, *Obstet Gynecol* 85(3):326, 1995.

Lang N, Marek K: The policy and politics of patient outcomes, *J Nurs Qual Assur* 5(2):7, 1991.

LaVeist T, Keith V, Gutierrez M: Black/white differences in prenatal care utilization: an assessment of predisposing and enabling factors, *Health Serv Res* 30(1):43, 1995.

Lipitz S, Mashiach S, Seidman D: Multifetal pregnancy reduction: the case for non-directive patient counseling, *Hum Reprod* 9(11):1978, 1994.

Long S, Marquis M, Harrison E: The costs and financing of perinatal care in the United States, *Am J Public Health* 84(9):1473, 1994.

Loring M, Smith R: Health care barriers and interventions for battered women, *Public Health Rep* 109:328, 1994.

Marr J, Reid B: Implementing managed care and case management: the neuroscience experience, *J Neurosci Nurs* 24(5):281, 1992.

Mortality patterns—1993, *MMWR* 45(8):1, 1996.

Moskowitz E, Jennings B, Callahan D: Long-acting contraceptives: ethical guidance for policymakers and health care providers, *Hastings Center Rep* 25(1):S1, 1995.

National Center for Health Statistics: *Births, marriages, divorces, and deaths for 1994*, Hyattsville, Md, 1995, US Public Health Service.

National Commission to Prevent Infant Mortality: *Troubling trends: the health of America's next generation*, Washington, DC, 1990, author.

Oh W et al: Hospital stay for healthy term newborns, *Pediatrics* 96(4):788, 1995.

Pellegrino E, Siegler M, Singer P: Future directions in clinical ethics, *J Clin Ethics* 2(1):5, 1991.

Peterson R, Cefalo R: Terms of confinement, *Obstet Gynecol* 76:308, 1990.

Piper J, Mitchel E, Ray W: Presumptive eligibility for pregnant Medicaid enrollees: its effects on prenatal care and perinatal outcome, *Am J Public Health* 84(10):1626, 1994.

Robertson J: Symbolic issues in embryo research, *Hastings Center Rep* 25(1):37, 1995.

Scupholme A, Robertson E, Kamons A: Barriers to prenatal care in a multi-clinic urban sample, *J Nurse Midwife* 36(2):111, 1991.

Shu X et al: Maternal smoking, alcohol drinking, caffeine consumption, and fetal growth: results from a prospective study, *Epidemiology* 6:115, 1995.

Singh S, Gold R, Frost J: Impact of the Medicaid eligibility expansions on coverage of deliveries, *Fam Plann Perspect* 26(1):31, 1994.

Styles M: Challenges for nursing in this new decade, *MCN Am J Maternal Child Nurs* 15(6):347, 1990.

US Department of Health and Human Services: *Maternal and newborn length of hospitalization: summary status report*, Washington, DC, 1995, DHHS.

Ventura S et al: Advance report of final natality statistics, 1992, *Monthly Vital Stat Rep* 43(suppl 1, 5): 1994.

Ventura S et al: Advance report of final mortality statistics, 1993, *Monthly Vital Stat Rep* 44(3 suppl):1, 1995.

Vincenzino J: Development in health care costs—an update, *Stat Bull* 75(1):30, 1994.

Bibliography

Alexander C, Guyer B: Adolescent pregnancy: occurrence and consequences, *Pediatr Ann* 22(2):85, 1993.

Andrews A, Patterson E: Searching for solutions to alcohol and other drug abuse during pregnancy: ethics, values and constitutional principles, *Soc Work* 40(1):55, 1995.

Barrett V, Phillips J: Reproductive health in the American workplace, *AAOHN J* 43(1):40, 1995.

Davis-Floyd R: The technocratic body: American childbirth as cultural expression, *Soc Sci Med* 38(8):1125, 1994.

Hafner-Eaton C, Pearce L: Birth choices, the law, and medicine: balancing individual freedoms and protection of the public's health, *J Health Polit Policy Law* 19(4):813, 1994.

Kuhn L et al: Maternal-infant HIV transmission and circumstances of delivery, *Am J Public Health* 84(7):1110, 1994.

Leland N et al: Variations in pregnancy outcomes by race among 10-14-year-old mothers in the United States, *Public Health Rep* 110(1):53, 1995.

Mayberry L: Intrapartal nursing care: research into practice, *J Obstet Gynecol Neonatal Nurs* 23(2):170, 1994.

Sachdev P: The abortion battle: the Canadian scene, *Med Law* 13:1, 1994.

Stewart P, Nimrod C: The need for a community-wide approach to promote healthy babies and prevent low birth weight, *Can Med Assoc J* 149(3):281, 1993.

CHAPTER 2

Family and Culture

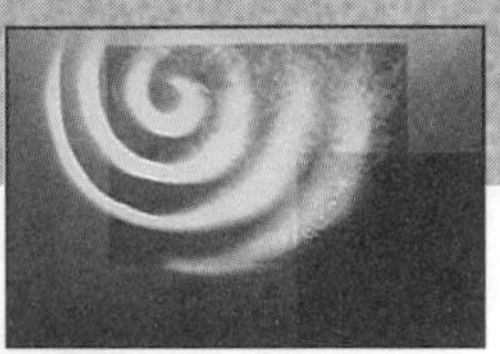

FAMILY FUNCTION AND STRUCTURE, P. 8
Family function, p. 8
Family structure, p. 8
Family functions, p. 11
Family dynamics, p. 12

FAMILY THEORIES, P. 12
Family system theory, p. 12
Developmental theory, p. 13
Family stress theory, p. 14

KEY FACTORS IN FAMILY HEALTH, P. 14

CULTURAL FACTORS RELATED TO FAMILY HEALTH, P. 15
Cultural context of the family, p. 15
Childbearing beliefs and practices, p. 18
Other factors affecting care of families, p. 19

The family is one of society's most important institutions. It represents a primary social group that influences and is influenced by other people and institutions. People recognize the family as the fundamental social unit because most people have more continuous contact with this social group than with any other. The family assumes major responsibility for the introduction and socialization of children. It transmits the fundamental cultural background of a given family to its members. Despite modern stresses and strains, the family, through its function and structure, forms a social network that acts as a potent support system for its members.

FAMILY FUNCTION AND STRUCTURE

Function refers to a special duty or performance required in the course of work or activity; it may also refer to the interactions of family members. *Structure* is a manner of organization or the arrangement of a number of parts that are interrelated in specified, recurring ways. The structure of a family may vary according to the composition of its component parts and according to its life cycle. Both structure and function are altered and modified as the needs of the family change.

Family Function

Authorities agree that families serve society in many ways. They play a vital role in the economy because they produce and consume goods and services. Furthermore, society, to maintain its continuity, must transmit its knowledge, customs, values, and beliefs to the young. When children are not an economic necessity, their primary function is to receive and to give love. Although goals for socialization and childrearing practices differ from one culture to another, in most societies the family appears to have three major objectives in relation to children: caregiving, nurturing, and training.

Family Structure

The *family structure*, or *family composition*, consists of individuals, each with a socially recognized status and position, who interact with one another on a regular, recurring basis in socially sanctioned ways. When members are gained or lost through events (e.g., marriage, divorce, birth, death, abandonment, incarceration), the family composition is altered and roles must be redefined or redistributed.

Traditionally the family structure refers to either nuclear or extended families. However, family composition has assumed new configurations in recent years, with the single-parent family and stepfamilies becoming prominent forms.

Children may belong to several different family groups during their lifetime.

Nuclear family. The **nuclear,** or **conjugal, family** consists of a husband, a wife, and their children (natural or adopted) who live in a common household. This is the reproductive unit in which the marital tie (legally or otherwise sanctioned) is the chief binding force. A strongly functional nuclear family is the prototype of human relationships and the basic unit from which more complex family forms are composed. In some instances one or more additional persons (e.g., a relative, friend, foster child, or others) may reside in the same household. Some authorities classify childless couples as nuclear families because the conjugal alliance has the theoretic potential for reproduction.

The nuclear family is more characteristic of an urban, mobile society. It is free to move where there is better financial opportunity and concomitant improvement in other areas, such as social class and prestige. It is not economically bound to a geographic area or dependent on the cooperative efforts of other members. The family members are employed on an individual basis, and economic resources are in the form of money, which allows the family to purchase goods and services from others.

Most family members maintain contact through visits, telephone calls, letters, and gift exchanges. Having no relatives readily available for advice and assistance with child care, as is common in extended families, parents in some nuclear families are more likely to turn to "experts" for child-rearing guidance.

The majority of nuclear families are associated with an extended kinship network of nuclear families living in separate households but in geographic proximity. This concept, sometimes referred to as a *modified extended family,* describes a meaningful aspect of daily existence that is reflected in frequent visiting and the exchange of services and financial aid. This family association meets the members' psychologic needs to a greater extent than do experts, friends, or organizations (Fig. 2-1). Families may reject the opportunity for social or economic advancement rather than leave such kinship associations.

Affiliative relationships. Although the nuclear family is predominantly a legally sanctioned institution, in a number of families the attachment is only *affiliative* (i.e., nonmarital) *cohabitation.* These families consist primarily of two adults but may include children. The mother and father live together, often with children from previous matings, and share family responsibilities. However, the family unit is less stable, and relationships are subject to change. Instability of the social environment in the home has been associated with juvenile delinquency, which appears to be related to the number of family constellations (changes in the adult members of the household) experienced during childhood. This is probably a reflection of repeated adjustment to a variety of authority figures with differing expectations.

Single-parent family. The **single-parent family** is not a new phenomenon. Throughout history, deaths from disease, childbirth, and wars have resulted in many one-parent families, although commonly remarriage has occurred. The contemporary single-parent family, however, has emerged partly as a consequence of women's rights movements, with more women (and men) having established separate households because of divorce, death, or desertion. In addition, a more liberal attitude in the courts has made it possible for single persons, both male and female, to adopt children, whereas previously, rigid prerequisites specified that both a father and a mother must be present in the home. Although single-parent families are usually headed by the mother, it is becoming increasingly common for fathers to be awarded custody of dependent children in divorce settlements. A significant number of single-parent families result from a single mother who wants to have a child but does not choose to have a husband. Also, unmarried mothers often choose to keep and raise their children rather than place them for adoption or marry. With the increased psychologic independence of women as a whole and the increased acceptability of single parenthood in society, more unmarried women are deliberately choosing mother-child families.

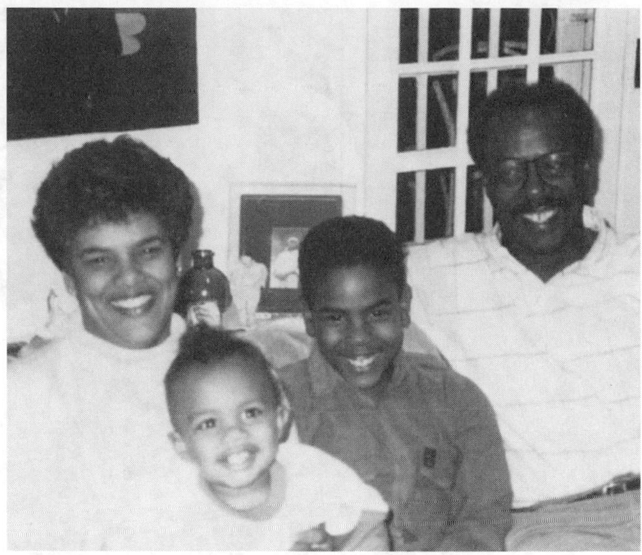

Fig. 2-1 Nuclear family.

Binuclear family. The term *binuclear family* is used to describe the situation that allows parents to continue the parenting role while terminating the spousal unit. The degree of cooperation between households and the time the child spends with each can vary. In *joint custody* the court assigns divorcing parents equal rights and responsibilities to the minor child or children. These alternate family forms are efforts on the part of those concerned to view divorce as a process of reorganization and redefinition of a family rather than as a family dissolution.

Reconstituted family. *Reconstituted families,* also referred to as *stepfamilies,* are those in which one or both the married adults have children from a previous marriage residing in the household. The term **blended families,** or *combined families,* more often refers to families composed of parents and the children each of them brings from a previous marriage. Most

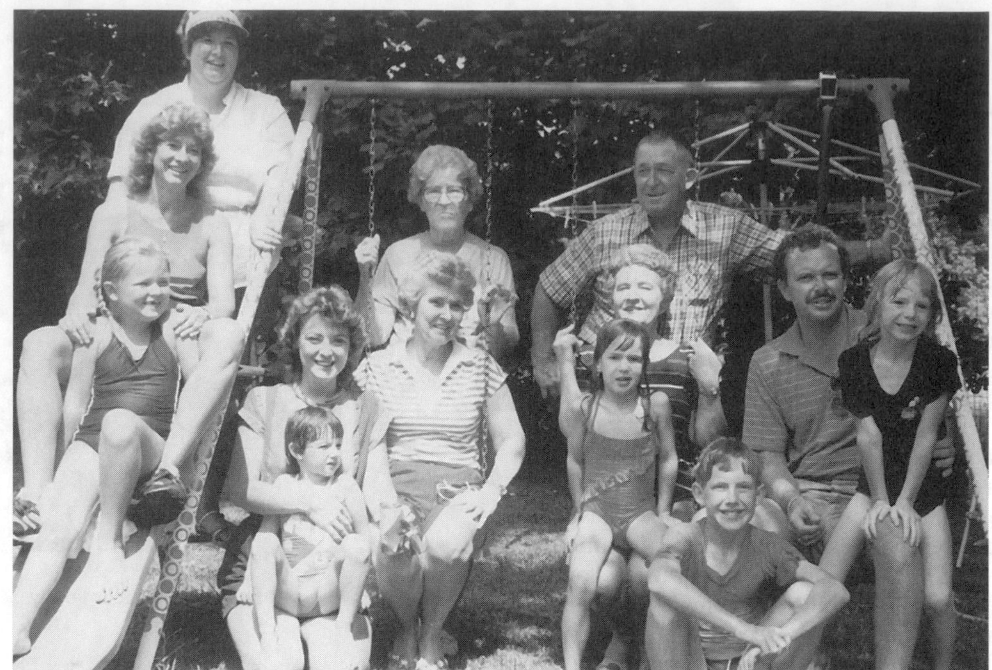

Fig. 2-2 Extended family.

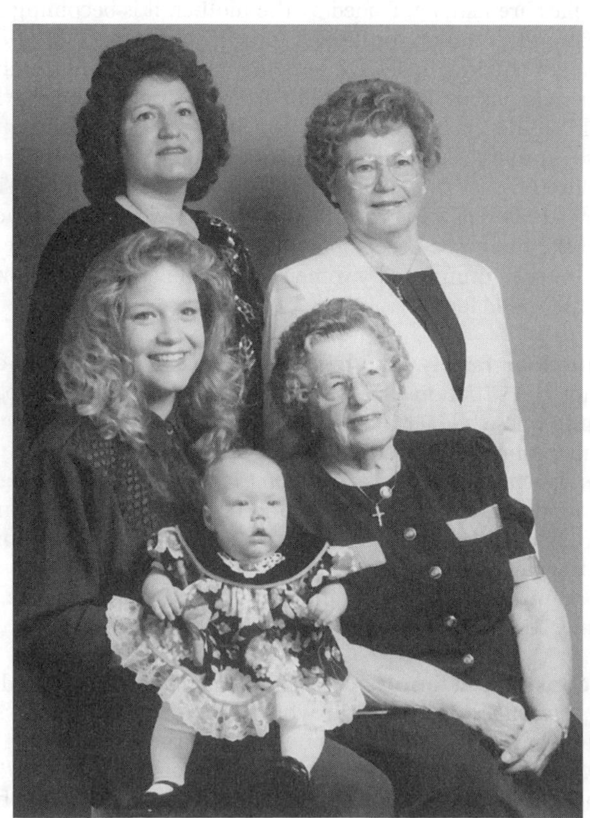

Fig. 2-3 Five generations of a family.

reconstituted families involve a mother, her children, and a stepfather.

Extended family. The **extended family** combines nuclear families into larger units through the parent-child relationship. It consists of the nuclear family plus lineal or collateral relatives. Most often it is composed of two or more residential units of three or more generations affiliated through extension of the parent-child relationship (i.e., grandparents, parents, and grandchildren) (Figs. 2-2 and 2-3).

In the extended family, childrearing is often a shared responsibility. Relatives are present and available to help young parents with household chores and child care activities. The daily lives of the children are organized around the needs and requirements of the family, with assigned tasks and obligations.

Extended family structure is more functional in areas where land is the basis of wealth and sustenance. Today the best examples of extended family units can be found among successful farmers, Native Americans, and certain recent immigrants. Extended families may form under conditions of either extreme poverty to pool resources or extreme wealth to consolidate resources.

Alternative family structures. Several other family structures exist that are much less common. The *polygamous family,* in which a spouse of either gender has more than one mate at the same time, is not legally sanctioned in the United States. In countries where it exists, polygamy is usually accorded a higher status than monogamy. It may be limited to ruling families or to high-status persons and tends to be practiced by a small segment of the population.

Another type of family structure that is relatively uncommon today is the *communal family.* The communal family emerged from a disenchantment with most contemporary life

TABLE 2-1 Stages of the family life cycle

FAMILY LIFE CYCLE STAGE	EMOTIONAL PROCESS OF TRANSITION: KEY PRINCIPLES	SECOND-ORDER CHANGES IN FAMILY STATUS REQUIRED TO PROCEED DEVELOPMENTALLY
Leaving home: single young adults	Accepting emotional and financial responsibility for self	Differentiation of self in relation to family of origin Development of intimate peer relationships Establishment of self through work and financial independence
Joining of families through marriage: new couple	Commitment to new system	Formation of marital system Realignment of relationships with extended families and friends to include spouse
Families with young children	Accepting new members into system	Adjusting marital system to make space for child(ren) Joining in childrearing, financial, and household tasks Realignment of relationships with extended family to include parenting and grandparenting roles
Families with adolescents	Increasing flexibility of family boundaries to include children's independence and grandparents' frailties	Shifting of parent-child relationships to permit adolescent to move in and out of system Refocus on midlife marital and career issues Beginning shift toward joint caring for older generation
Launching children and moving on	Accepting multitude of exits from and entries into the family system	Renegotiation of marital system as a dyad Development of adult-to-adult relationships between grown children and their parents Realignment of relationships to include in-laws and grandchildren Dealing with disabilities and death of parents (grandparents)
Families in later life	Accepting shifting of generational roles	Maintaining own and/or couple functioning and interests in face of physiologic decline; exploration of new familial and social role options Support for a more central role of middle generation Making room in the system for wisdom and experience of elderly members; supporting older generation without overfunctioning for them Dealing with loss of spouse, siblings, and other peers and preparation for own death; life review and integration

From Carter B, McGoldrick M: *The changing family life cycle: a framework for family therapy*, ed 2, Boston, 1988, Allyn & Bacon.

choices and is often seen in cults. Communal groups share common ownership of property and goods; in cooperatives there is private ownership of property, but certain goods and services are shared and exchanged cooperatively without monetary consideration. There is strong reliance on group members and material interdependence. The mother-child tie is strong during infancy and early childhood, but many parents are happy to relinquish older children to the care of others.

A **same-sex, homosexual,** or **gay/lesbian family** is one in which there is a common-law tie between two persons of the same sex who have children. Estimates of the number of children of gay or lesbian parents range from 6 to 14 million (Patterson, 1992). Although most children in gay/lesbian households are biologic from a former, legal marriage, there are other means by which homosexual adults acquire children. For example, they may be foster or adoptive parents. Lesbian mothers may conceive through artificial insemination. A gay male couple may become parents through use of a surrogate mother.

The quality of parenting and home life of gay men and lesbians, whether they are single or in a partner relationship, is equivalent to that of nongay parents (Bozett, 1984; Harris, and Turner, 1986; Turner, Scadden, and Harris, 1985). Because this family form is more common than most people may realize, it is important for the nurse to understand that gay/lesbian families are simply different from the heterosexual family form, not necessarily better or worse. The gay/lesbian family environment can be just as healthy as any other. According to reported research, children in gay/lesbian households are not more likely to be gay than children reared in heterosexual households (Bozett, 1989; Gottman, 1990; Huggins, 1989; Paul, 1986).

Nurses need to be nonjudgmental and to learn how to accept differences rather than demonstrate a homophobic prejudice that can have a detrimental effect on the nurse-family relationship. Moreover, the more knowledge of the family constellation and life-style nurses have, the greater benefit they can be to the gay or lesbian parent and the child.

Family Functions

As the family progresses through its life cycle (Table 2-1), from young adulthood to the commitment of two people to share a life, to the dissolution of the family through death or other separations, it carries out certain functions for the well-being of family members. Friedman (1992) discusses the following nine **family functions:** economic stability, status conferral, education, socialization of children, health care, religion, recreation, reproduction, and affect. These functions specify the five basic areas identified by the World

Health Organization (WHO) in 1978: biologic, economic, educational, psychologic, and sociocultural. The interdependent functions depend on the physical and mental health of family members. Each family develops common *beliefs, values,* and *sentiments* derived from their cultural perspective that are used as criteria in the choice of alternative actions.

Biologic functions include reproduction, care and rearing of children, nutrition, maintenance of health, and recreation. The ability to carry out such functions implies certain prerequisites: healthy genetic inheritance, fertility management, care during the maternity cycle, good dietary behavior, intelligent use of health services, companionship, and nurturing of family members.

Economic functions include earning enough money to carry out the other functions, developing family budgets, and ensuring the financial security of family members. To accomplish these tasks, the family must have the necessary skills, opportunities, and knowledge.

Educational functions include the teaching of skills, attitudes, and knowledge relating to the other functions. Family members must have access to resources and the necessary skills to use these resources to fulfill these functions.

The psychologic function of the family is expected to provide an environment that promotes the natural development of personality. Families should offer optimum psychologic protection and promote the ability to form relationships with people outside the family circle. These tasks require stable emotional health, common bonds of affection, and the abilities to be mutually supportive, to tolerate stress, and to cope with crises.

Sociocultural functions are associated with the socialization of children. These functions include the transfer of values relating to behavior, tradition, language, religion, and prevailing or previous social and moral attitudes. As a result, family members become conditioned to a variety of behavioral norms set by their society, which are appropriate to all stages of adult life. To do this, the family must possess "accepted standards" and be sensitive to the varying social needs of children according to their ages. A family must also accept and exemplify society's behavioral norms and be willing to explain, defend, and promote these standards. Although certain functions are relegated to or emphasized more in one phase of the family's life cycle than another (e.g., the care and socialization of children are part of the childbearing and childrearing phase of the cycle), many of the functions are continuous for the family's survival and progress.

Family Dynamics

Families work cooperatively to accomplish family functions. Through **family dynamics,** family members assume appropriate social roles. These roles are learned in the family and learned in pairs (e.g., mother-father, parent-child, brother-sister). A social role does not exist by itself; rather, it is designed to work with a role partner. Role pairing enables social interactions to take place in an orderly, predictable manner; the roles are said to be *complementary.* Some families maintain a traditional pairing of roles, whereas other families change behavior patterns to suit a change in family life-style. Rather than mother-father, brother-sister, the roles may be mother-daughter, mother-son. *Negotiation* brings these pair roles into a new alignment. Negotiation is essential to maintain family equilibrium.

Each family sets up *boundaries* between itself and society. People are extremely conscious of the difference between "family members" and "outsiders," people without kinship status. Some families isolate themselves from the outside community. Others have a wide community network to help in times of stress. Although boundaries exist for every family, family members set up *channels* through which they interact with society. These channels also ensure that the family receives its share of social resources.

Ideally the family uses its resources to provide a safe, intimate environment for the biopsychosocial development of the family members. The family provides for the *nurturing* of the newborn and the gradual *socialization* of the growing child. It serves as the source of first relationships with others. The earliest and closest relationships children form are with their parents, or parenting persons, and continue throughout a lifetime. For better or worse, parent-child relationships influence a person's self-worth and ability to form later relationships. The family influences the child's perceptions of the outside world. The family provides the growing child with an identity that possesses both a past and a sense of the future. Cultural values and rituals are passed from one generation to the next through the family (Friedman, 1992).

Through everyday interactions, the family develops and uses its own patterns of verbal and nonverbal *communication.* These patterns give insight into the emotional exchange within a family and act as reliable indicators of interpersonal functioning. Family members not only react to the communication or actions of other family members, but also interpret and define them.

Over time the family develops protocols for *problem solving,* particularly regarding important decisions such as having a baby, buying a house, or sending children to college. The criteria used in making decisions are based on *family values and attitudes* concerning the appropriateness of the behavior and the moral, social, political, and economic events of society. The *power* to make critical decisions is given to a family member through tradition or negotiation. This power is not always stated. Power reflects the family's concepts of male or female dominance and the cultural practices, social customs, and community norms. As a result, family members attain certain *statuses* or *hierarchies.* They play out these statuses by assuming various *roles.* Most families have a member who "takes charge" or "is supportive" or "can't be expected to do anything."

FAMILY THEORIES

A *family theory* can be used to describe families and how the family unit responds to events both within and outside the family. Each family theory makes certain assumptions about the family and has inherent strengths and limitations. Most nurses use a combination of theories in their work with families. A brief discussion of three family theories (system, developmental, stress) and their implications for maternal-child nursing is presented here.

Family System Theory

Family system theory is derived from general system theory, a science of "wholeness" that is characterized by interaction among the components of the system and between the system and the environment. General system theory expanded scientific thought from a simplistic view of direct cause and effect

(A causes B) to a more complex and interrelated theory (A influences B, but B also affects A). In family system theory the family is viewed as a system that continually interacts with its members and the environment. The emphasis is on the *interaction* between the members, such that a change in one family member creates a change in other members, which in turn results in a new change in the original member. Consequently, a problem or dysfunction does not lie in any one member but rather in the type of interactions used by the family. Since it is the interactions, rather than individual members, that are viewed as the source of the problem, the family becomes the patient and the focus of care. Examples of the application of family system theory to clinical problems are nonorganic failure to thrive and child abuse. According to system theory, the problem does not rest solely with the parent or child but in the type of interactions between the parent and child, as well as in a host of other factors that affect their relationship.

The family is viewed as a whole that is different from the sum of the individual members. For example, in a household of parents and one child there are not only three individuals, but also four interactive units that characterize the family system. These include three *dyads* (marital relationship, mother-child relationship, father-child relationship) and a *triangle* (the mother-father-child relationship). This concept of *nonsummativity*—"the whole is greater than the sum of its parts"—implies that when working with a family, the nurse must be aware of the relationships among family members. To effect positive change in a family, it is necessary to work with and through the several subsystems of the family.

Adaptability is characteristic of the family. When problems exist within the family, change can be effected by altering the interaction or feedback messages that perpetuate disruptive behavior. *Feedback* refers to processes within the family that help identify strengths and needs and determine how well goals are being accomplished. Positive feedback initiates change, whereas negative feedback resists change. When the family system is disrupted, change can occur at any point in the system. Although family system theorists may pursue the family history in trying to understand current family interaction and problem patterns, the emphasis is on what is occurring *now* in the family and on intervening to change that pattern. This focus allows for sometimes rapid and dramatic changes.

A major factor that influences a family's adaptability is its *boundary*, an imaginary but very real line that exists between the family and its environment. This boundary may be open or closed. An *open family* welcomes input into its system by accepting new ideas, information, resources, and opportunities. This type of family reaches out for help and uses the available support systems. In contrast, a *closed family* resists input by viewing change as threatening. The family is suspicious of any available support and strives to maintain the family system by avoiding outside influences. Knowledge of boundaries is critical when teaching or counseling families. Although open families are receptive to intervention, closed families typically resist assistance, and more effort is required to gain their trust and acceptance.

BOX 2-1

Duvall's Developmental Stages of the Family

Stage I: marriage and an independent home: the joining of families

Reestablish couple identity.
Realign relationships with extended family.
Make decisions regarding parenthood.

Stage II: families with infants

Integrate infants into family unit.
Accommodate to new parenting and grandparenting roles.
Maintain the marital bond.

Stage III: families with preschoolers

Socialize children.
Parents and children adjust to separation.

Stage IV: families with schoolchildren

Children develop peer relations.
Parents adjust to their children's peer and school influences.

Stage V: families with teenagers

Adolescents develop increasing autonomy.
Parents refocus on midlife marital and career issues.
Parents begin a shift toward concern for the older generation.

Stage VI: families as launching centers

Parents and young adults establish independent identities.
Renegotiate marital relationship.

Stage VII: middle-aged families

Reinvest in couple identity with concurrent development of independent interests.
Realign relationships to include in-laws and grandchildren.
Deal with disabilities and death of older generation.

Stage VIII: aging families

Shift from work role to leisure and semiretirement or full retirement.
Maintain couple and individual functioning while adapting to the aging process.
Prepare for own death and dealing with the loss of spouse and/or siblings and other peers.

Modified from Wright L, Leahey M: *Nurses and families: a guide to family assessment and intervention*, ed 2, Philadelphia, 1994, Davis.

Developmental Theory

Developmental theory is an outgrowth of several theories of development. Foremost among the developers is Duvall (1977), who described eight developmental tasks of the family throughout its life span (Box 2-1). The family is described as a small group, a semiclosed system of personalities that interacts with the larger cultural social system. As an interrelated system, changes do not occur in one part without a series of changes in other parts.

Developmental theory addresses family change over time by using Duvall's family life-cycle stages, based on the predictable changes in the structure, function, and roles of the family, with the age of the oldest child as the marker for stage transition. Thus the arrival of the first child marks the transition from stage I to stage II. As the first child grows and develops, the family enters subsequent stages. In every stage the family is faced with certain developmental tasks. At the same time, each member of the family must achieve individual developmental tasks as part of each family life-cycle stage.

Additions to family development theory reflect more inclusive and accurate versions of contemporary family life. New life-cycle norms have also been developed for divorced families, reconstituted families, low-income families, alcoholic families, and dual-earner families (Carter and McGoldrick, 1989). Developing norms for gay or lesbian families has been more difficult because of the absence of rituals or markers that typically delineate life-cycle stages (Slater and Mencher, 1991).

Developmental theory can be applied to nursing practice in a number of ways. For example, the nurse can assess how well new parents are accomplishing the individual and family developmental tasks associated with transition to parenthood. New applications should emerge as more is learned about developmental stages for nonnuclear and nontraditional families.

Family Stress Theory

Family stress theory, first proposed by Hill in 1949, is concerned with the ways families react to stressful events and suggests factors that promote adaptation to these events. Families encounter *stressors,* life events that affect the family unit and have the potential to produce change in the family's social system. Stressors may be predictable (e.g., parenthood) or unpredictable (e.g., illness or unemployment). These stressors are cumulative, involving simultaneous demands from work, family, and community life. Too many stressful events occurring within a relatively short period, usually 1 year, can overwhelm the family's ability to cope, thus placing the family system at risk for breakdown or its members at risk for physical and emotional health problems. When the family experiences too many stressors for it to cope adequately, a state of crisis ensues. For adaptation to occur under these circumstances, a change in family structure and/or interaction is necessary.

Family stress theory also encompasses certain capabilities the family can use to manage a crisis brought on by too many stressors. *The Typology Model of Adjustment and Adaptation* (McCubbin and McCubbin, 1989), a comprehensive family stress model, summarizes these capabilities through the following four components:

1. *Basic attributes* of the family—the family type—that explain how the family typically operates and behaves
2. *Resources* of individual family members, the family unit, and the community, including social support from extended family, friends, neighbors, and health professionals
3. *Perception* of how the family defines the situation, its impact, and their ability to manage
4. *Coping behaviors or strategies* that family members or the family unit can use to keep the family functioning as a unit; decrease an individual member's tension, anxiety, and distress; and increase understanding of the particular situation or problem.

The Typology Model of Adjustment and Adaptation helps explain why families differ in their responses to stressors. With adequate and appropriate resources, a major crisis in one family may be defined as a minor inconvenience by another.

The typology model has been further expanded to the *Resiliency Model of Family Stress Adjustment and Adaptation.* This model emphasizes family adaptation and is designed to help professionals develop strategies for intervention based on a systematic diagnosis and evaluation of the family under stress (McCubbin and McCubbin, 1993).

Incorporating systems theory, Boss (in press) offers an approach to family stress management. In her view, family stress must be studied within the larger context in which the family is living. Families mediate stress within internal and external contexts. The internal context is made up of elements that a family is able to change or control, such as family structure (i.e., boundaries, roles), psychologic defenses (i.e., perception of the event), and philosophic values and beliefs. The external context (the time and place in which a particular family finds itself) is made up of those elements over which a family has no control. These external factors include the culture of the larger society, the time in history during which the events occur to the family, the economic state of society, maturation, and genetic inheritance.

One of the expected developmental (maturational) stressor events discussed by Boss is birth. Although expected and normal, birth is a transition point and has the potential to change a family's stress level. Nurses also work with families experiencing nonnormative (unexpected or situational) stressor events such as complicated pregnancies. These events are usually highly stressful and require the interventions of nurses who understand family stress management.

Nurses can be instrumental in assisting families to change their stress level by helping them exercise their control of internal context factors. For example, the psychologic context refers to the family's perception of the stressful event. If a family's perception is based on incorrect or incomplete information, the nurse can intervene through educational strategies. Nurses can also help families experiencing stress by explaining various dimensions of the external context. For example, explaining normal infant growth and development (maturation) may reduce the stress of parenting.

KEY FACTORS IN FAMILY HEALTH

Certain factors are important in determining the quality of family health. Noteworthy among these when dealing with childbearing families are family dynamics, family socioeconomics, and family response to stress and culture. For example, family dynamics (discussed on p. 12) encompass the coordination of intrafamilial roles, the distribution of power within the family, and the decision-making process. Family dynamics also affect the use of health services.

Family socioeconomic characteristics influence the family's ability to access and use health care services. Social class affects expectations, obligations, and rewards, all of which affect the use of health services. In addition, the family acts as the primary economic unit in which incomes may be pooled, expenditure decisions are made jointly, and services are rendered internally.

Friedman (1992) considers a family's social class as the prime molder of family life-style. Social class and cultural background "exert the greatest overall influence on family life, influencing family values and practices, family behavior patterns, socialization, and world experiences families have."

The interplay among stress, perception, and resources affects the level of support afforded family members. The family's response to stress influences its members' physiologic and psychologic well-being. Cultural responses to childbearing and use of related health care services play a central role in family health. Because of the importance of culture during childbearing, this concept is discussed further.

CULTURAL FACTORS RELATED TO FAMILY HEALTH

Cultural Context of the Family

The family process within its **cultural context** is a central concern in nursing. This is especially true when the nurse is providing care to the childbearing family. Childbearing is a critical life experience and as such is often bound by traditional beliefs and practices. A culture's beliefs and practices regarding childbearing are embedded in its economic, religious, kinship, and political structures. All cultures have behavioral norms and expectations for each stage of the perinatal cycle. These norms and expectations relate to each culture's view of how people stay healthy and prevent illness. With the pluralism that exists in society and the expansion of international nursing, nurses need to focus on cultural variations in perceptions of life events and the use of health care systems. Patients have a right to expect that their health care needs, both physiologic and psychologic, will be met and that their cultural beliefs will be respected.

Culture has many definitions. Helman (1990) views culture as a set of guidelines that individuals inherit as members of a particular society and that tells people how to view the world and how to relate to other people, supernatural forces, and the natural environment. Cultural knowledge includes beliefs and values about each facet of life. These guidelines have been tested over time. They relate to food, language, religion, art, health and healing practices, kinship relationships, and all other systems of behavior.

Many subcultures may be found within each culture. *Subculture* refers to a group existing within a larger cultural system that retains its own characteristics. A subculture may be an ethnic group or a group organized in other ways. For example, in the varied culture of the United States, there are many ethnic subcultures (African-Americans, Asian-Americans, Hispanic-Americans) as well as subcultures within these groups. Nurses should also remember that the Caucasian population in the United States has diverse and multiple subcultures. Although the recent literature in the area of ethnicity and health has focused on people of color, little has been written about Caucasian ethnic communities (e.g., Italian-Americans, Polish-Americans, German-Americans) (Spector, 1991). In issues of health, illness, and major life transitions, greater differences may exist among Caucasian groups than has generally been acknowledged.

Each subculture holds rich and complex traditions, including health practices that have proved effective over time. These traditions vary from group to group. In a multicultural society, many groups can influence these traditions and practices. As cultural groups come in contact with each other, acculturation and assimilation may occur.

Acculturation refers to changes that occur in one or both groups when people from different cultures come in contact with one another. People may retain some of their own culture while adopting some of the cultural practices of the dominant society. This familiarization among cultural groups results in much overt behavioral similarity. Individuals exchange and adopt mannerisms, styles, and practices of the other group. Dress, language patterns, food choices, and health practices especially show differences among cultural groups within a society. In the United States, acculturation is generally thought to take three generations. The adult grandchild of the immigrant is usually fully Americanized (Spector, 1991). An example of acculturation is the adoption of ethnic food practices in the United States.

Assimilation, on the other hand, occurs when a cultural group loses its identity and becomes a part of the dominant culture. According to Friedman (1992), "Assimilation denotes the more complete and one-way process of one culture being absorbed into the other." Assimilation is the process by which groups "melt" into the mainstream, thus accounting for the notion of a "melting pot," a phenomenon that has been said to occur in the United States. In contrast, Spector (1991) asserts that in the United States, the "melting pot," with its dream of a common culture "has proved to be a myth and has faded; it is now time to identify and both accept and appreciate the differences among people."

Nurses must recognize that a wide range of cultural diversity exists within society. Assessment of the beliefs and practices of a group and those within the group is essential for the health care provider striving to provide culturally appropriate health care. Nurses must also be aware of factors that may prevent some providers from delivering optimum care. Understanding the concepts of ethnocentrism and cultural relativism may be helpful to nurses caring for families in a multicultural society.

Ethnocentrism "is the view that one's culture's way of doing things is the right and natural way" (Galanti, 1991). Essentially, ethnocentrism supports the notion that "my group is the best," whether it is an ethnic or a social group. For example, socialization into the profession of nursing occurs within the framework of the Western health care system. This system emphasizes the *biomedical model*, which is based primarily on the Caucasian, middle-class value system in the United States. This biomedical model represents pregnancy and childbirth as phenomena with inherent risk, most appropriately managed through specific knowledge and technology. The nurse, when encountering behavior in women who are unfamiliar with this model, may become frustrated and impatient. The women's behavior may be labeled inappropriate and in conflict with "good" health practices. Although the United States is a culturally diverse nation, the prevailing health care practices are based on beliefs held by members of the dominant culture. These practices are primarily influenced by European-Americans. If the Western health care system provides the nurse's only standard for judgment, the behavior of the nurse is called *ethnocentric*.

Cultural relativism, the opposite of ethnocentrism, involves learning about and applying the standards of another person's culture to activities within that culture. To be culturally relativistic, the nurse recognizes that people from different cultural backgrounds actually see the same objects and situations differently. For the most part, viewpoints are culturally determined.

Cultural relativism does not require nurses to *accept* the beliefs and values of another culture; rather, nurses should recognize that others' behavior may be based on a system of logic

TABLE 2-2 Traditional* cultural beliefs and practices: childbearing and parenting

PREGNANCY	CHILDBIRTH	PARENTING
Hispanic (based primarily on knowledge of Mexican-Americans)†		
Pregnancy Pregnancy desired soon after marriage Late prenatal care Expectant mother influenced strongly by mother or mother-in-law Cool air in motion considered dangerous during pregnancy Unsatisfied food cravings thought to cause a birthmark Some pica observed in the eating of ashes or dirt (not common) Milk avoided because it causes large babies and difficult births Many predictions about sex of baby May be unacceptable and frightening to have pelvic examination by male health care provider Use of herbs to treat common complaints of pregnancy Drinking chamomile tea thought to ensure effective labor	***Labor*** Use of "partera" or lay midwife preferred in some places; may prefer presence of mother rather than husband After birth of baby, mother's legs brought together to prevent air from entering uterus Loud behavior in labor ***Postpartum*** Diet may be restricted after birth; for first 2 days only boiled milk and toasted tortillas permitted (special foods to restore warmth to body) Bed rest for 3 days after birth Keep warm Delay bathing Mother's head and feet protected from cold air; bathing permitted after 14 days Mother often cared for by her own mother 40-day restriction on sexual intercourse	***Newborn*** Breastfeeding begun after third day; colostrum may be considered "filthy" or "spoiled" Olive oil or castor oil given to stimulate passage of meconium Male infant not circumcised Female infant's ears pierced Belly band used to prevent umbilical hernia Religious medal worn by mother during pregnancy; placed around infant's neck Infant protected from "evil eye" Various remedies used to treat "Mal ojo" (evil eye) and fallen fontanel (depressed fontanel)
African-American (Members of the African-American community, many of whom are descendants of slaves, have different origins. Today a number of Black Americans have immigrated from Africa, the West Indian Islands, the Dominican Republic, Haiti, and Jamaica.)		
Pregnancy Acceptance of pregnancy depends on economic status Pregnancy thought to be state of "wellness," which is often the reason for delay in seeking prenatal care, especially by lower-income African-Americans "Old wives' tales" include having a picture taken during pregnancy will cause stillbirth and reaching up will cause cord to strangle baby Craving for certain foods, including chicken, greens, clay, starch, and dirt Pregnancy may be viewed by African-American men as a sign of their virility Self-treatment for various discomforts of pregnancy, including constipation, nausea, vomiting, headache, and heartburn	***Labor*** Use of "Granny midwife" in certain parts of United States Varied emotional responses: some cry out, some display stoic behavior to avoid calling attention to selves Patient may arrive at hospital in far-advanced labor Emotional support often provided by other women, especially own mother ***Postpartum*** Vaginal bleeding seen as sign of sickness; tub baths and shampooing of hair prohibited Sassafras tea thought to have healing power Eating liver thought to cause heavier vaginal bleeding because of its high "blood" content	***Newborn*** Feeding very important: "Good" baby thought to eat well Early introduction of solid foods May breastfeed or bottle-feed; breastfeeding may be considered embarrassing Parents fearful of spoiling baby Commonly call baby by nicknames May use excessive clothing to keep baby warm Belly band used to prevent umbilical hernia Abundant use of oil on baby's scalp and skin Strong feeling of family, community, and religion

Data from Amaro, 1994; Bar-Yam, 1994; Galanti, 1991; Geissler, 1994; Mattson, 1995; Spector, 1991; and Williams, 1989.

*Variations in some beliefs and practices exist within subcultures of each group. NOTE: Most of these cultural beliefs and customs reflect the traditional culture and are not universally practiced. These lists are not intended to stereotype clients but rather to serve as guidelines while discussing meaningful cultural beliefs with a patient and her family. Examples of other cultural beliefs and practices are found throughout this text.

†Members of the Hispanic community have their origins in Spain, Cuba, Central and South America, Mexico, Puerto Rico, and other Spanish-speaking countries.

TABLE 2-2 Traditional* cultural beliefs and practices: childbearing and parenting—cont'd

PREGNANCY	CHILDBIRTH	PARENTING
Asian-Americans (Typically refers to groups from China, Korea, the Philippines, Japan, Southeast Asia [particularly Thailand], Indochina, and Vietnam)		
Pregnancy Pregnancy considered time when mother "has happiness in her body" Pregnancy seen as natural process Strong preference for female health care provider Belief in theory of hot and cold May omit soy sauce in diet to prevent dark-skinned baby Prefer soup made with ginseng root as general strength tonic Milk usually excluded from diet because it causes stomach distress Inactivity or sleeping late may cause difficult delivery	***Labor*** Mother attended by other women, especially her own mother Father does not actively participate Labor in silence Cesarean birth not welcome ***Postpartum*** Must protect self from yin (cold forces) for 30 days Ambulation limited Shower and bathing prohibited Warm room Chinese mother avoids fruits and vegetables Diet: Warm fluids Some clients are vegetarians Korean mother served seaweed soup with rice Chinese diet high in hot foods	***Newborn*** Concept of family important and valued Father is head of household; wife plays a subordinate role Birth of boy preferred May delay naming child Some groups (e.g., Vietnamese) believe colostrum is dirty; therefore they may delay breastfeeding until milk comes in
European-American (Members of the European-American [Caucasian] community have their origins in countries such as Ireland, Great Britain, Germany, Italy, and France.)		
Pregnancy Pregnancy viewed as a condition that requires medical attention to ensure health Emphasis on early prenatal care Variety of childbirth education programs available and participation encouraged Technology driven Emphasis on nutritional science Involvement of the father valued Written source of information valued	***Labor*** Birth is a public concern Technology dominated Birthing process in institutional setting valued Involvement of father expected Physician seen as head of team ***Postpartum*** Emphasis or focus on early bonding Medical interventions for dealing with discomfort Early ambulation and activity emphasized Self-care valued	***Newborn*** Increased popularity of breastfeeding Breastfeeding begins as soon as possible after childbirth ***Parenting*** Motherhood and transition to parenting seen as stressful time Nuclear family valued, although single parenting and other forms of parenting more acceptable than in the past Women often deal with multiple roles Early return to prenatal activities
Native American (Many different tribes exist within the Native-American culture; viewpoints vary according to tribal customs and beliefs.)		
Pregnancy Pregnancy considered as a normal, natural process Late prenatal care Avoid heavy lifting Herb teas encouraged	***Labor*** Prefers female attendant, although husband, mother, or father may assist with birth Birth may be attended by whole family Herbs may be used to promote uterine activity Birth may occur in squatting position ***Postpartum*** Herb teas to stop bleeding	***Newborn*** Infant not fed colostrum Use of herbs to increase flow of milk Use of cradle boards for infant Babies not handled often

different from their own. Cultural relativism affirms the uniqueness and value of every culture. Spector (1991) states that "because health care providers learn from their culture the way and the how of being healthy or ill, it behooves them to treat each patient with deference to his own cultural background."

Childbearing Beliefs and Practices

Nurses working with childbearing families in the United States and Canada care for families from different cultures and ethnic groups (Fig. 2-4). To provide a high level of care to all families, the nurse should be aware of the cultural beliefs and practices that are important to these families. Countless beliefs and practices are of a religious, cultural, or ethnic derivation and may or may not still be followed by families from diverse backgrounds.

Childbearing is one facet of health that is related to all aspects of a woman's life. Although most cultures do not regard pregnancy as an illness, it is considered to be a time of heightened susceptibility to dangerous elements. Pregnant women try to protect the fetus and pregnancy by various means. Perception of the time of greatest vulnerability varies among cultures, with some groups placing greatest emphasis on the prenatal period and others on labor and delivery or the postbirth period. Western health care culture places the greatest emphasis on the prenatal and labor and delivery periods and least on the postbirth period.

Childbearing in all cultures is complete with norms and behavioral expectations for each stage of the perinatal cycle. All relate to each culture's view of how a person maintains health and prevents illness. Some health practices reflect theories of balance and harmony among opposing forces. The intrinsic factors influencing balance and harmony include heat and cold. Other intrinsic factors are air and water, food and drink, sleep and wakefulness, movement, exercise and rest, evacuation and retention, and passions of the spirits, or emotions. Thus, for pregnant women of many cultures, maintenance of health during childbearing implies a balance and harmony in relationship with the physical, social, and spiritual environment.

Table 2-2 provides examples of some cultural beliefs and practices surrounding childbearing. Most of these cultural beliefs and customs reflect the traditional culture and are not practiced by all members of the cultural group in all parts of the United States. Variables such as degree of acculturation, educational and income levels, and amount of contact with the older generations influence the extent to which these customs are practiced. Women from these cultural-ethnic groups may adhere to some, all, or none of the practices listed.

The nurse needs to become familiar with each woman as an individual and validate the cultural beliefs, if any, that are meaningful to her. Equipped with this knowledge, the nurse supports and nurtures those beliefs that promote physical or emotional adaptation to childbearing. However, if certain beliefs are identified that might be harmful, the nurse should carefully explore those beliefs with the patient and use the beliefs in the reeducation and modification process.

Other Factors Affecting Care of Families

Several factors, including communication, space, time, and roles, are products of culture that should be considered when working with childbearing families (Giger and Davidhizar, 1995). Communication is the factor that often creates the most difficult problem for nurses working with patients from diverse cultural groups. Communication includes not only understanding the individual's language, varied dialect, and style, but also volume of speech, the meaning of touch and

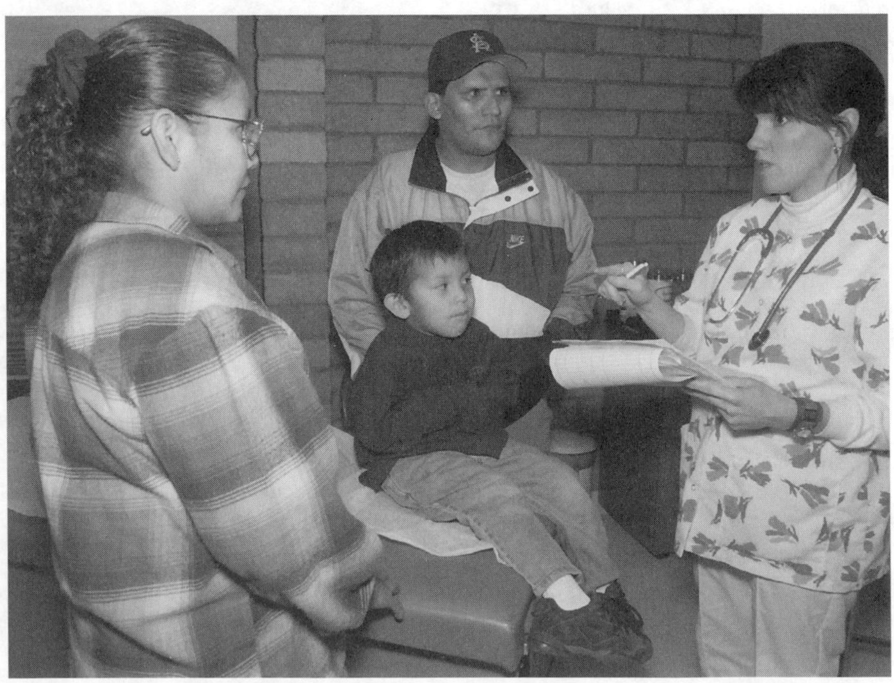

Fig. 2-4 Navajo family interacts with nurse. (Courtesy Michael S. Clement, MD, Mesa, Ariz.)

gestures, and other variables. When the patient and/or family do not speak the same language as the nurse, special approaches must be used that allow the family's health care needs to be addressed in a culturally competent manner. Such approaches include the use of interpreters. When using an interpreter, the nurse shows respect to the family by addressing questions to them and not the interpreter.

Personal space needs and feelings of territoriality are developed in a cultural setting. Although personal space is an individual matter and varies with the situation, dimensions of personal-space comfort zones vary from culture to culture. Actions such as touching the patient, placing the patient in proximity to others, taking away personal possessions, and making decisions for the patient can decrease personal security and heighten anxiety. On the other hand, when the need for distance is respected, control is maintained over personal space and personal autonomy is supported, thereby increasing the sense of security. For example, since Chinese-Americans have traditionally been a noncontact group, some members of this group may interpret closeness, increased eye contact, and touch as being offensive or impolite. Misunderstandings can be reduced by providing explanations when performing tasks that require close contact (Chang, 1995).

Nurses often use touch as an important intervention, especially in areas such as labor and delivery. The acceptance and effectiveness of these approaches must be considered in a cultural context.

As an important aspect of culture, the element of time must also be understood. People in cultural groups may be either past, present, or future oriented. Those who focus on the past strive to maintain tradition and have little motivation for formulating future goals. Some individuals who focus on the present neither save for the future nor appreciate the past. Present-oriented individuals do not necessarily adhere to a strict, time-structured schedule. Individuals with future time orientation use the present to achieve future goals.

The time orientation of the childbearing family system has important implications for nursing care. For example, bringing the infant to the clinic for follow-up examinations at a specific time may be difficult for the family who has many things happening simultaneously and who focuses on the present. On the other hand, a family with a future-oriented sense of time, for whom events are planned in advance, may be much more likely to return for the follow-up visit as scheduled. Despite the differences in time orientation, both families may be equally concerned for the well-being of their newborn.

Family roles (expectations and behaviors associated with position in the family, e.g., mother, father, grandparent) are related to social class and cultural norms. Distinct roles for men and women may be stressed. For example, the active or passive role of a man in pregnancy and childbirth is profoundly affected by culture and may have significant implications in the Western health care system. The role expectation of most health care providers that fathers will be involved may be in conflict with the expectations of patients from cultural groups such as Hispanic-Americans and Arab-Americans, who view the birthing experience as a female affair.

Critical Thinking Exercises

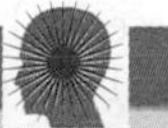

CULTURE AND VIEWS OF HEALTH

Many subcultures exist within the major cultural groups in North America. What are the major cultural groups in your geographic area? Identify two subcultures within a major cultural group (not your own) in your geographic area. Interview at least two members of each of the two subcultures identified, preferably one male and one female.

1. What do they believe will keep them healthy in pregnancy?
2. What are the roles of men and women in childbirth? Who should be present at birth?
3. What is the role of technology in the childbirth process?
4. Are there restrictions on activity and diet in the postpartum period?
5. What is the preferred method of infant feeding? How soon after birth should breastfeeding begin?
6. Are there special foods that should be eaten during pregnancy or after childbirth?
7. What will keep the baby healthy after birth?

Nursing Care Management

ASSESSMENT

To plan for the care of a family or an individual family member, the nurse may find it useful to view the family at a developmental phase in the life cycle, facing stressful life events and operating as a system. This view means that no one family member has a problem; if a problem exists, the whole family has a problem. Solutions to problems can evolve best through family participation.

Data collection process. The *process* of an assessment in planning family care is often more difficult and complicated than assessing a patient's physical health. It requires adept communication skills and the ability to establish a trusting relationship with each family member simultaneously. Families often have varying degrees of openness and privacy. All groups resent interrogation by an outsider. The reasons for obtaining information must be explained to family members in a clear, nonthreatening, and culturally appropriate manner.

Generally, family members freely give information such as address, marital status, and ages. To attain other information: (1) *observe* and note relationships, attitudes, and stress responses (who is doing what); (2) *listen* to conversation about community and family involvements or hopes and aspirations; and (3) *ask questions* in a culturally appropriate manner.

The suggestions of Stern et al. (1980) for improving communication between patients from different ethnic and cultural backgrounds and their Western health care providers are still useful. Barriers in communication exist on three levels: approach, custom, and language.

Approach includes numerous factors considered in interpersonal relationships. Americans approach most issues in health care by addressing the problem directly. For people from many cultures, such as Asians and Native Americans, engaging in small talk is vital before beginning a serious discussion. Some cultures equate commenting on flowers or pictures and having tea or a cold drink with showing respect. To begin talking to an expectant mother about the need for prenatal care before commenting on the other children, the pretty chair, or the weather could set up an atmosphere of dis-

Cultural Considerations

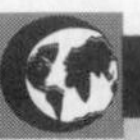

QUESTIONS TO OBTAIN CULTURAL EXPECTATIONS ABOUT CHILDBEARING

1. What do you and your family think you should do to remain healthy during pregnancy?
2. What are the things you can do or cannot do to improve your health and the health of your baby?
3. Who do you want with you during your labor?
4. What actions are important for you and your family to do after the baby's birth?
5. What do you and your family expect from the nurse(s) caring for you?
6. How will family members participate in your pregnancy, childbirth, and parenting?

trust. Women from some cultures, such as Asian-Americans and Hispanic-Americans, prefer a caregiver of the same gender. Therefore an initial encounter with a female caregiver may be critical. Showing respect and patience is essential in building trust. Native-American women may say little during interviews. They often use a low tone of voice. Note taking by the health care provider may not be welcome.

Custom includes practices and behaviors characteristic of a culture. Understanding that a cultural reason exists for all behaviors and making a sincere effort to know the person's rationale for behavior are important steps in establishing trust. Patients themselves may be the best source in helping the nurse understand cultural logic and individual differences. An assessment of health beliefs and practices is essential to achieve a holistic approach to care. For patients, adherence to a particular cultural custom provides a sense of constancy with their cultural heritage.

Language is an important factor. Stern et al. (1980) emphasize the use of clear, jargon-free English. When the family does not speak English, a bilingual nurse is ideal for assessing the family. If a bilingual nurse is not available, either a family member or a member of the same cultural group may be used as an interpreter.

The Cultural Considerations box above lists ways to elicit cultural explanations regarding childbearing.

A nurse cannot be expected to know everything about every culture and subculture and the many life-styles within each culture. To come to a better realization of why people believe as they do, people must first understand their own culture. Understanding patients' cultures, through interview, study, contact, and sincere interest, is invaluable because understanding enables nurses to give culturally appropriate nursing care.

Analysis, synthesis, and validation. After the data-gathering phase, the nurse analyzes and synthesizes the findings and makes inferences about the data. The nurse should ask the following questions: What are the significant stressors influencing this family? Do the family's beliefs reflect cultural variations? Do these beliefs promote physical or emotional well-being, or might they be harmful to the family? Is this family's immediate support system adequate for coping with the stress of childbearing and childrearing? Does family communication respect all family members in light of the individual's developmental stage?

Since inferences are subjective and based not only on the nurse's competence level but also on individual values and beliefs, the nurse needs to validate the interpretation of the data with the patient. The development of nursing diagnoses follows validation of inferences.

NURSING DIAGNOSES

Nursing diagnoses reflect the family's perception of its needs, as well as the nurse's perception. It is important to determine the family's perception of its nursing care needs rather than the perception of any one family member.

Examples of nursing diagnoses typically encountered with childbearing families include the following:

- Family coping: potential for growth
- Ineffective family coping: compromised
- Altered parenting related to
  Impaired parent-infant attachment
- Altered family processes related to
  Birth of a child with a defect
- Anxiety related to
  Expectations of parenting experience
- Social isolation related to
  Lack of interaction with peers
- Spiritual distress related to
  Conflict between ideal and personal religious practices associated with childbearing

The nurse should keep in mind that nursing diagnoses may vary with cultural groups. For example, when diagnosing "Altered parenting," the nurse must consider the family's cultural beliefs. Galanti (1991) describes the Vietnamese tradition of delaying naming the child, a tradition that Western health care providers often misinterpret as poor bonding. Traditionally, Vietnamese families decide on the baby's name in a family naming ceremony.

Once the nursing diagnoses are established, the nurse takes time to explore personal value judgments about the family that may affect and impede nursing interventions. It is also essential for nurses to validate the diagnoses to ensure that their perceptions are objective and accurate. In addition to direct validation with the family, a review of literature, an analysis of cultural norms, and discussions with other family members are also means of validation.

EXPECTED OUTCOMES

The nurse sets expected outcomes related to each diagnosis. The nurse establishes these expected outcomes with the family. Family members evaluate the expected outcomes for realism and acceptance. They establish both short-term and long-term expected outcomes. The expected outcomes are assessed to determine priority. Certain health needs require immediate attention (e.g., unexplained vaginal bleeding). Other health needs require more time to resolve (e.g., grief over birth of a child with a defect).

Working with the available data, the nursing diagnoses, and the health goals, the nurse proceeds to organize a plan for implementing the most appropriate interventions. The nurse identifies the nursing role, that is, whether the role is to teach, to provide direct care, or to refer the patient to another resource.

The nurse must be able to teach at various levels so individual family members feel understood and supported. Different strategies may be necessary for each family member. As a direct care provider, the nurse promotes activities that will lead to the family's own self-care and independence as defined by them.

PLAN OF CARE AND IMPLEMENTATION

Nurses put preventive, curative, or rehabilitative actions into practice. Then they tailor these actions to meet the individual needs of the family and its members. Nurses may also use their knowledge and skills to guide family members who will participate in the implementation. The nurse may also refer the family to appropriate internal and community support systems, as well as determine the family's willingness to use these resources.

EVALUATION

The nurse works with the family to evaluate expected outcomes using outcome criteria. These need to be stated precisely and behaviorally to measure the degree of realization. The criteria need to be realistic and flexible enough to permit modification as circumstances change.

Friedman (1992) suggests the following six questions to ask when evaluating the family nursing process:

1. Were family expectations set in relative and accurate terms?
2. Is there a consensus between the family and the health care team members of the evaluation?
3. What additional data need to be collected to evaluate progress?
4. Were the nursing diagnoses, expected outcomes, and approaches realistic and accurate?
5. If the family's behavior and perception indicate that the problem has not been satisfactorily resolved, what are the reasons?
6. Were there any unforeseen outcomes that need to be considered?

Key Points

- The family forms a social network that acts as an important support system for its members.
- Ideally, the family provides a safe, intimate environment for the biopsychosocial development of children and its adult members.
- Family system, developmental, and stress theories provide nurses with useful guides to understand family function.
- The reproductive beliefs and practices of a culture are embedded in its economic, religious, kinship, and political structures.
- The expression of parental roles and how children are viewed reflect cultural differences.
- North American culture is a pluralistic one, in which varying family forms are recognized and accepted in differing degrees.

References

Amaro H: Women in the Mexican-American community: religion, culture, and reproductive attitudes and experiences, *J Community Psychology* 16:6, 1994.

Bar-Yam N: Learning about culture: a guide for birth practitioners, *Int J Childbirth Educ* 9(2):8, 1994.

Boss P: *Family stress management*, ed 2, Newbury Park, Calif, Sage (in press).

Bozett F: Parenting concerns of gay fathers, *Top Clin Nurs* 6:60, 1984.

Bozett F: *Gay fathers: a review of the literature.* In Bozett F, editor: *Homosexuality and the family*, New York, 1989, Harrington Park.

Carter B, McGoldrick M, editors: *The changing family life cycle: a framework for family therapy*, ed 2, Boston, 1989, Allyn & Bacon.

Chang K: *Chinese Americans.* In Giger J, Davidhizar R, editors: *Transcultural nursing: assessment and intervention*, ed 2, St Louis, 1995, Mosby.

Duvall E: *Marriage and family development*, ed 5, Philadelphia, 1977, Lippincott.

Friedman M: *Family nursing theory and assessment*, New York, 1992, Appleton-Century-Crofts.

Galanti G: *Caring for patients from different cultures: case studies from American hospitals*, Philadelphia, 1991, University of Pennsylvania Press.

Geissler E: *Pocket guide to cultural assessment*, St Louis, 1994, Mosby.

Giger J, Davidhizar R, editors: *Transcultural nursing: assessment and interventions*, ed 2, St Louis, 1995, Mosby.

Gottman J: *Children of gay and lesbian parents.* In Bozett F, Sussman M, editors: *Homosexuality and family relations*, New York, 1990, Harrington Park.

Harris M, Turner P: Gay and lesbian parents, *J Homosex* 12:103, 1986.

Helman C: *Culture, health and illness*, London, 1990, Wright.

Hill R: *Families under stress*, New York, 1949, Harper & Row.

Huggins S: A comparative study of self-esteem of adolescent children of divorced lesbian mothers and divorced heterosexual mothers, *J Homosex* 18(1/2):123, 1989.

Mattson S: Culturally sensitive prenatal care for Southeastern Asians, *J Obstet Gynecol Neonatal Nurs* 24(4):335, 1995.

McCubbin M, McCubbin H: *Theoretical orientation to family stress and coping.* In Figley C, editor: *Treating families under stress*, New York, 1989, Brunner/Mazel.

McCubbin M, McCubbin H: *Families coping with illness: the resiliency model of family stress, adjustment, and adaptation.* In Danielson C, Hamel-Bissel B, Winstead-Fry P, editors: *Families, health, and illness: perspectives on coping and interventions*, St Louis, 1993, Mosby.

Patterson C: Children of lesbian and gay parents, *Child Dev* 63:1025, 1992.

Paul J: *Growing up with a gay, lesbian, or bisexual parent: an exploratory study of experiences and perceptions.* Unpublished doctoral dissertation, Berkeley, Calif, 1986, University of California at Berkeley.

Slater S, Mencher J: The lesbian family life cycle: a contextual approach, *Am J Orthopsychiatry* 61(3):372, 1991.

Spector R: *Cultural diversity in health and illness,* New York, 1991, Appleton-Century-Crofts.

Stern P et al: Culturally-induced stress during childbearing: the Filipino-American experience, *Issues Health Care Women* 2(3-4):67, 1980.

Turner P, Scadden L, Harris M: *Parenting in gay and lesbian families.* Paper presented at the First Future of Parenting Symposium, Chicago, March 1985.

Williams R: *Issues in women's health care.* In Johnson B, editor: *Psychiatric mental health nursing: adaptation and growth,* Philadelphia, 1989, Lippincott.

Wright L, Leahey M: *Nurses and families: a guide to family assessment and intervention,* ed 2, Philadelphia, 1994, Davis.

Bibliography

Callister L: Cultural meanings of childbirth, *J Obstet Gynecol Neonatal Nurs* 24(4):327, 1995.

Chalmers B, Meyer D: Companionship in the perinatal period: a cross-cultural survey of women's experiences, *J Nurse Midwife* 39(4):265, 1994.

Grace G: Families and nurses: building partnerships for growth and health, *J Obstet Gynecol Neonatal Nurs* 24(4):298, 1995.

Hutchinson M, Baqui-Aziz M: Nursing care of the childbearing Muslim family, *J Obstet Gynecol Neonatal Nurs* 23(9):767, 1994.

International Year of the Family Secretariat: The international year of the family, *Midwifery* 10:3, 1994.

Lapham S, Henley E, Kleyboecker K: Prenatal behavioral risk screening by computer among Native Americans, *Fam Med* 25:197, 1993.

Patterson J: Promoting resilience in families experiencing stress, *Pediatr Clin North Am* 42:147, 1995.

Quimby S: Women and the family of the future, *J Obstet Gynecol Neonatal Nurs* 23(2):113, 1994.

Sharts-Hopko N: Birth in the Japanese context, *J Obstet Gynecol Neonatal Nurs* 24(4):343, 1995.

Tiller C: Fathers' parenting attitudes during a child's first year, *J Obstet Gynecol Neonatal Nurs* 24(6):508, 1995.

CHAPTER 3

Reproduction and Sexuality

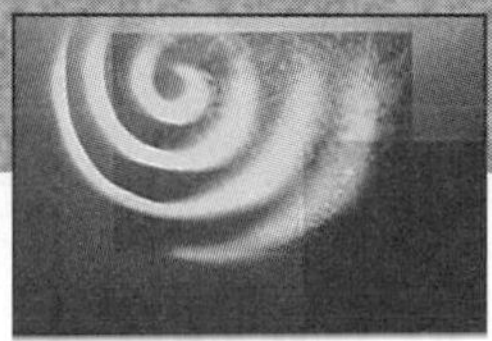

FEMALE REPRODUCTIVE SYSTEM, P. 23
External structures, p. 23
Internal structures, p. 27
Breasts, p. 37
Menstrual cycle, p. 39

MALE REPRODUCTIVE SYSTEM, P. 42
External structures, p. 43
Internal structures, p. 44

SEXUAL RESPONSE, P. 46
Physiologic response to sexual stimulation, p. 46

PSYCHOSOCIAL ASPECTS OF SEXUALITY, P. 46

NURSING IMPLICATIONS, P. 48

Nurses providing health care to women require a greater depth and breadth of knowledge of female and male anatomy and physiology than is usually taught in general courses. Knowledge of the anatomy and physiology of female and male structures involved in reproduction is basic to planning for, implementing, and evaluating nursing care of maternity patients and their families.

Although the female and male reproductive systems differ greatly in appearance, their structures are *homologous* (have the same embryonic origin) (Figs. 3-1 and 3-2). Each structure performs a vital role in continuing the human species, expressing sexuality, and generating and maintaining secondary sexual characteristics. Through hormonal influences, the genitalia, pelvis, and breasts acquire the unique adaptations necessary to childbearing. Both female and male reproductive systems consist of the following four principal components:

1. External genitalia
2. A pair of primary sex glands (gonads)
3. Ducts leading from the gonads to the body's exterior
4. Secondary (accessory) sex glands

FEMALE REPRODUCTIVE SYSTEM

The female reproductive system consists of internal organs, located in the pelvic cavity and supported by the pelvic floor, and external genitalia, located in the perineum. The internal and external reproductive structures of the woman develop and mature in response to estrogens and progesterones, starting in fetal life and continuing through puberty and the childbearing years. The reproductive structures *atrophy* (decrease in size) with age or with a decrease in ovarian hormone production. An extensive and complex innervation and a generous blood supply support the functions of these structures. The appearance of the external genitalia varies greatly from woman to woman; heredity, age, race, and the number of children a woman has borne determine the size, shape, and color of the genitalia.

External Structures

The external structures, or the *vulva,* are presented in the following order: mons pubis (mons veneris), labia majora and minora, clitoris, prepuce of clitoris, vestibule, fourchette, and perineum. Fig. 3-3 illustrates the external genitalia.

Mons pubis. The *mons pubis,* or *mons veneris,* is the rounded, soft fullness of subcutaneous fatty tissue and loose connective tissue over the symphysis pubis. It contains many sebaceous (oil) glands and develops coarse, dark, curly hair at **pubarche,** about 1 to 2 years before the onset of the menses. **Menarche** (the onset of menses) occurs on the average at age 13. Characteristics of pubic hair vary from sparse and fine among Asian women to thick, coarse, and curly among African-American women. The functions of the mons are to play a role in sensuality and to protect the symphysis pubis during coitus (sexual intercourse). As a woman ages, the amount of fatty tissue found in her body decreases and pubic hair thins.

Labia majora. The *labia majora* are two rounded, lengthwise folds of skin-covered fat and connective tissue that merge with

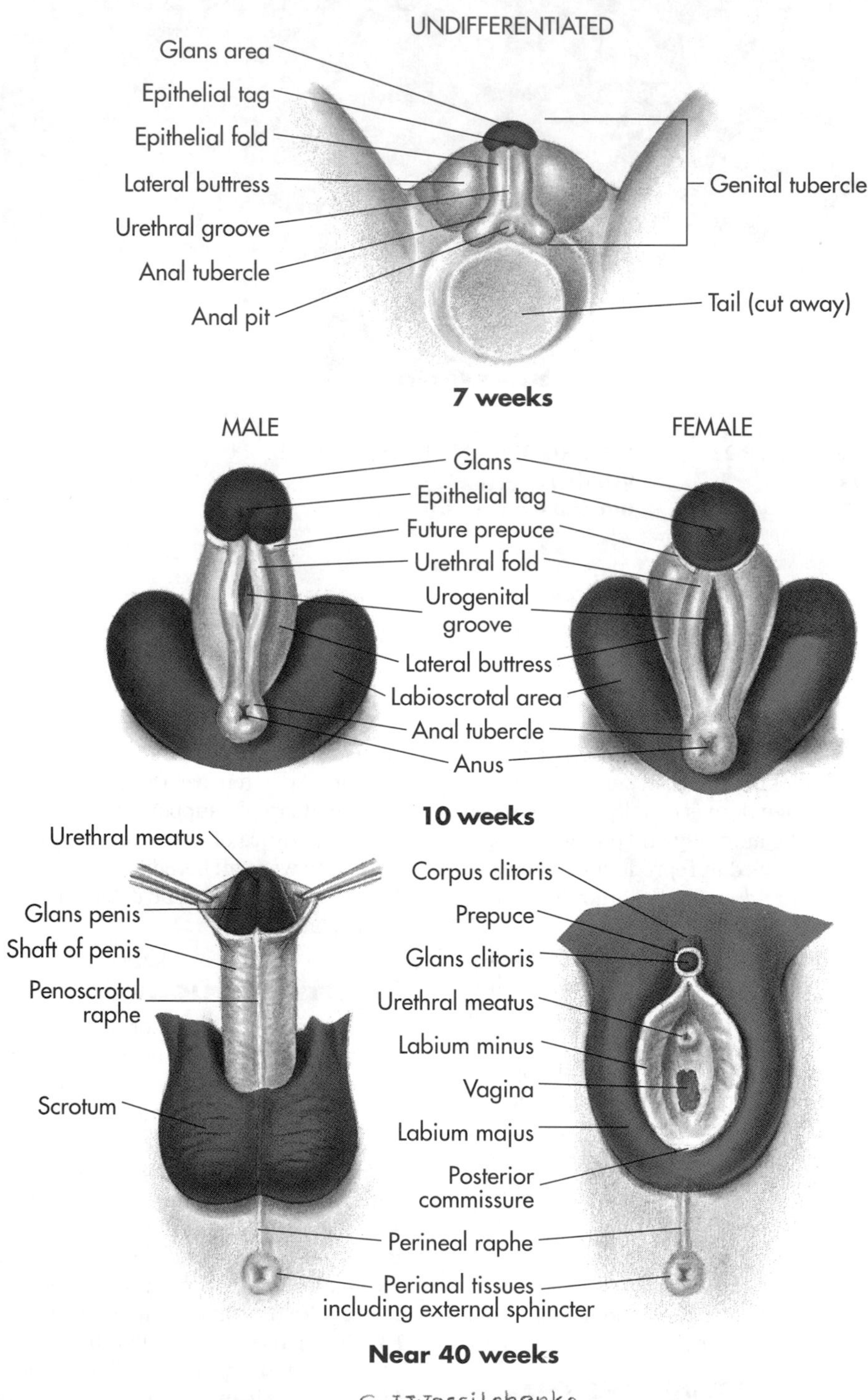
UNDIFFERENTIATED
Glans area
Epithelial tag
Epithelial fold
Lateral buttress
Urethral groove
Anal tubercle
Anal pit
Genital tubercle
Tail (cut away)
7 weeks
MALE
FEMALE
Glans
Epithelial tag
Future prepuce
Urethral fold
Urogenital groove
Lateral buttress
Labioscrotal area
Anal tubercle
Anus
10 weeks
Urethral meatus
Glans penis
Shaft of penis
Penoscrotal raphe
Scrotum
Corpus clitoris
Prepuce
Glans clitoris
Urethral meatus
Labium minus
Vagina
Labium majus
Posterior commissure
Perineal raphe
Perianal tissues including external sphincter
Near 40 weeks
G.J.Wassilchenko

Fig. 3-1 Homologues of external genitalia.

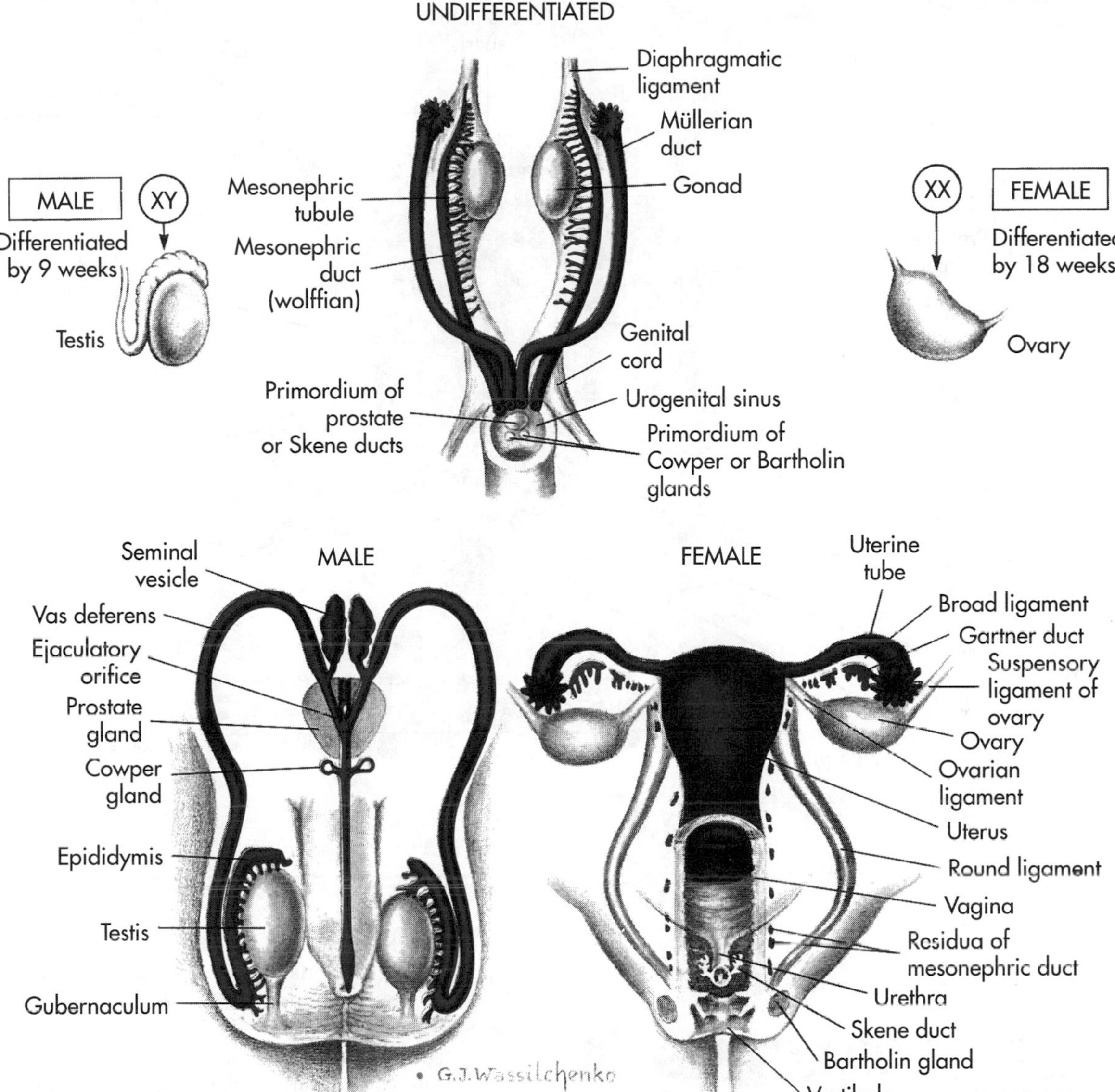

Fig. 3-2 Homologues of internal genitalia.

the mons. They extend from the mons downward around the labia minora, ending in the perineum in the midline. The labia majora protect the labia minora, urinary meatus, and vaginal introitus. In the woman who has never experienced vaginal childbirth, the labia majora lie close together in the midline, covering the underlying structures. Some labial separation and even gaping of the vaginal introitus follow childbirth and perineal or vaginal injury. Declining hormone production later in a woman's life causes the labia majora to atrophy.

On the lateral surfaces the labial skin is thick, usually pigmented darker than the surrounding tissues, and covered with coarse hair (similar to that of the mons) that thins out toward the perineum. The medial (inner) surfaces of the labia majora are smooth, thick, and without hair. They contain an abundant supply of sebaceous glands and sweat glands, are highly vascular, and contain an extensive network of nerves. The labia majora protect the inner surfaces of the vulva and enhance sexual arousal.

Labia minora. The *labia minora,* located between the labia majora, are narrow, lengthwise folds of hairless skin. The lateral and anterior aspects of the labia are usually pigmented. The medial surfaces are similar to vaginal mucosa and are pink and moist. Their rich vascularity gives them a reddish color and permits marked turgescence (swelling) of the labia minora with emotional or physical stimulation. The glands in the labia minora lubricate the vulva. A rich nerve supply makes them sensitive, enhancing their erotic function. The space between the labia minora is called the vestibule.

Clitoris. The *clitoris* is a short, cylindric, erectile organ fixed just beneath the arch of the pubis; the visible portion is about

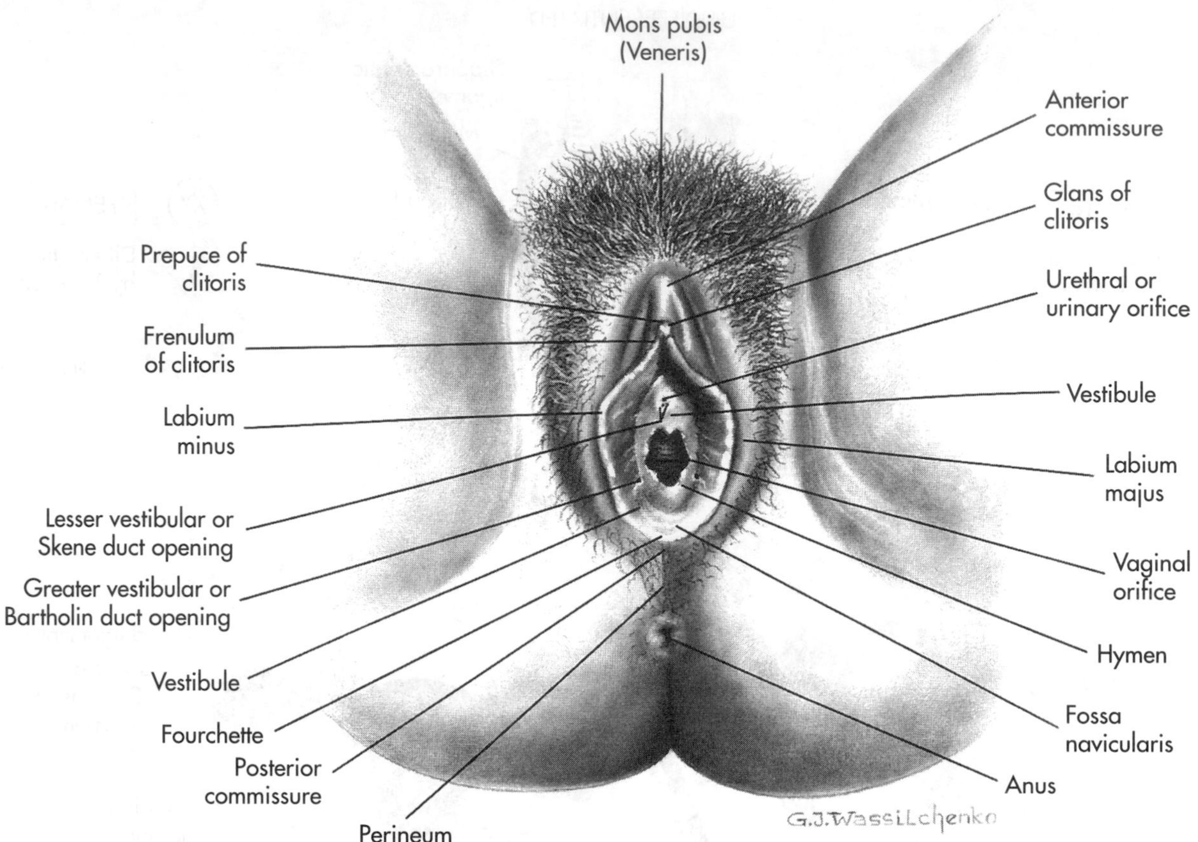

Fig. 3-3 External female genitalia.

Cultural Considerations

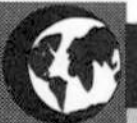

FEMALE CIRCUMCISION

Female circumcision occurs in women of many different ethnic, cultural, and religious backgrounds. Although circumcision is usually performed in childhood, some communities circumcise infants or older females.

The procedure involves removal of a portion of the clitoris but may extend to the total removal of the clitoris and labia minora. The labia majora, which are often stitched together over the urethral and vaginal openings, may also be affected.

The extent of the circumcision site affects the seriousness of complications. Common complications include bleeding, pain, local scarring, keloid or cyst formation, and infection. Impaired drainage of urine and menstrual blood may lead to chronic pelvic infections, pelvic and back pain, and chronic urinary tract infections. Some women may require surgery before vaginal examination, intercourse, or childbirth if the vaginal opening is obstructed.

Nurses are providing care to a growing number of women who have immigrated from the Middle East, Asia, and Africa, where female circumcision is more common. It is important to be sensitive to the unique needs of these patients, especially if they have concerns about maintaining or restoring the intactness of the circumcision site after childbirth.

6 × 6 mm or less in the unaroused state. The tip of the clitoral body is called the glans and is more sensitive than its shaft. When a woman is sexually aroused, the glans and shaft increase in size.

Sebaceous glands of the clitoris secrete *smegma,* a cheeselike fatty substance with a distinctive odor that serves as a *pheromone* (an organic compound that provides olfactory communication with other members of the same species to elicit a certain response, which in this case is erotic stimulation of the male human). The term *clitoris* comes from a Greek word meaning *key,* because the clitoris was seen as the key to female sexuality. Its rich vascularity and innervation make the clitoris highly sensitive to temperature, touch, and pressure sensation. Its main function is to stimulate and elevate levels of sexual tension. Some groups practice ritual removal of the clitoris during childhood (see the Cultural Considerations box to the left).

Prepuce of clitoris. Near the anterior junction the right and left labia minora separate into medial and lateral portions. The lateral portions unite above the clitoris to form its *prepuce,* a hoodlike covering; the medial portions unite below the clitoris to form its *frenulum.* Sometimes the prepuce covers the clitoris. As a result, this area has the appearance of an opening that can be mistaken for the urethral meatus if the nurse does not identify vulvar structures carefully. Attempts to insert a catheter into this sensitive area can cause considerable discomfort.

Vestibule. The *vestibule* is an oval-shaped area formed between the labia minora, clitoris, and fourchette. The vestibule contains the openings to the urethra, paraurethral (lesser vestibular or Skene) glands, the vagina, and the paravaginal (greater vestibular, vulvovaginal, or Bartholin) glands. The thin, almost mucosal surface of the vestibule is easily irritated by chemicals (e.g., feminine deodorant sprays, bubble bath salts), heat, discharges, and friction (e.g., tight jeans).

Although not a true part of the reproductive system, the *urinary (urethral) meatus* is considered here because of its closeness and relationship to the vulva. The meatus is a pink or reddened opening of varying shapes, often with slightly puckered margins. The meatus marks the terminal, or distal, part of the urethra. It is usually about 2.5 cm below the clitoris.

The *lesser vestibular* (*paraurethral* or *Skene*) *glands* are short tubular structures situated posterolaterally just inside the urethral meatus, at about the 5 and 7 o'clock positions around the meatus. They are not usually visible but produce a small amount of mucus, which functions as lubrication.

The *hymen* (Fig. 3-3) is a partial, rarely complete, elastic but tough mucosa-covered fold around the *vaginal introitus* (opening to the vagina). In virginal females the hymen may be an impediment to vaginal examination, insertion of menstrual tampons, or coitus. The hymen may be elastic and allow distention, or it may be torn easily. Occasionally the hymen covers the orifice completely, resulting in an imperforate hymen that prevents passage of menstrual flow, instrumentation (e.g., with a speculum), or coitus. A hymenotomy may be necessary in some patients. After instrumentation, use of tampons, coitus, or vaginal delivery, residual tags of the torn hymen (hymenal caruncles or carunculae myrtiformes) may be seen.

One common myth is that one can tell by the condition of the hymen whether a female is a virgin. Sexually active and even parous females may have intact hymens. For other women the hymen may be torn during strenuous physical work or exercise, masturbation, or use of tampons. Therefore the "test for virginity"—evidence of bleeding after sexual intercourse—is an unreliable criterion.

The *greater vestibular* (*vulvovaginal* or *Bartholin*) *glands* are two compound glands at the base of the labia majora, one on either side of the vaginal orifice. Several ducts, about 1.5 cm long, drain each gland. Each opens into the groove between the hymen and the labia minora. Usually the gland openings are not visible or palpable. The glands secrete a small amount of clear, viscid (sticky) mucus, especially during coitus. The alkaline pH of the mucus is supportive of sperm.

Fourchette. The *fourchette* is a thin, flat, transverse fold of tissue formed where the tapering labia majora and minora merge in the midline below the vaginal orifice.

Perineum. The **perineum** is the skin-covered muscular area between the vaginal introitus and the anus. The perineum forms the base of the perineal body (Fig. 3-15).

Internal Structures

The internal reproductive organs are discussed in the order that reflects the path of the ovum. Supportive tissues are discussed along with the internal reproductive organs they support. Internal organs include the ovaries, uterine (fallopian) tubes, uterus, and vagina. The ovaries and uterine tubes are also referred to as adnexa. A brief description of the pelvic floor and bony pelvis follows.

Ovaries. One *ovary* is located on each side of the uterus, below and behind the uterine tubes. The ovaries are held in place by two ligaments, the mesovarian portions of the uterine ***broad ligament,*** which suspend them from the lateral pelvic

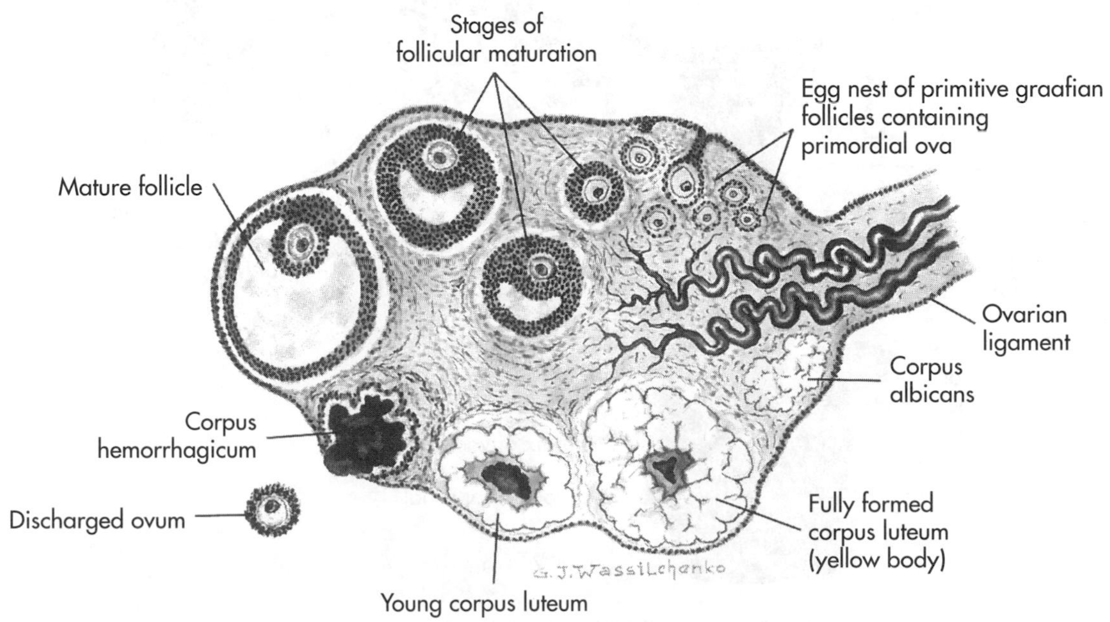

Fig. 3-4 Cross section of ovary.

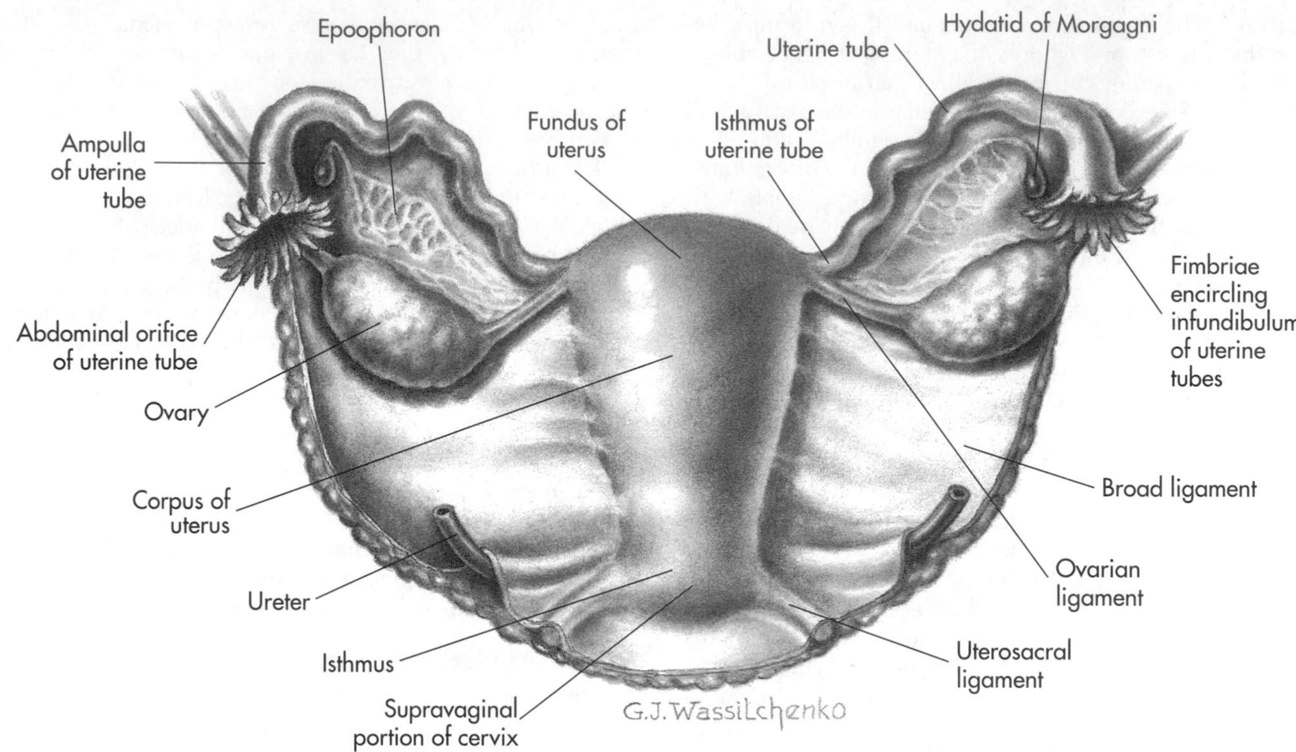

Fig. 3-5 Uterus and adnexa, posterior view.

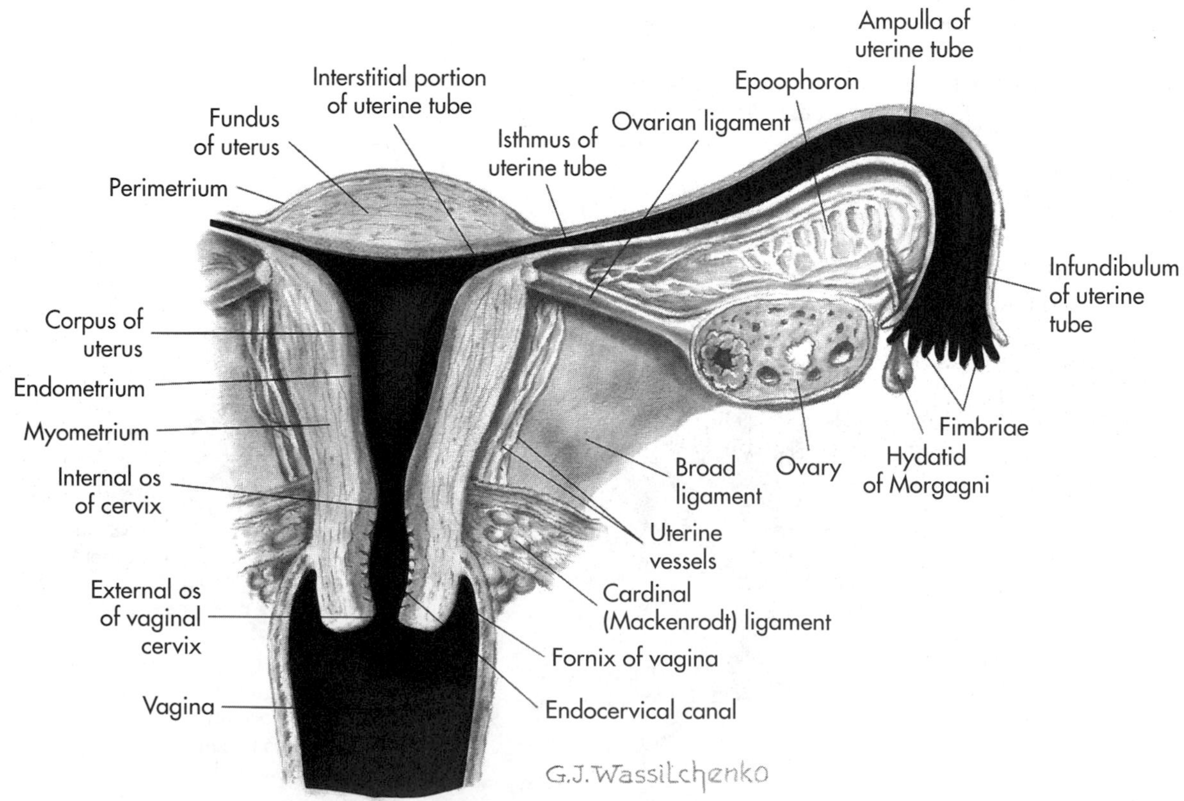

Fig. 3-6 Cross section of uterus, adnexa, and upper vagina.

side walls at about the level of the anterosuperior iliac crest, and the ***ovarian ligaments*** (Figs. 3-5 and 3-9), which anchor them to the uterus. The ovaries are movable with palpation.

The ovaries are similar in origin (homologous) to the testes in the male. Each ovary resembles a large almond in size and shape (Fig. 3-4). Each is whitish and rounded but flattened, weighs about 3 g, and measures approximately 3 × 2 × 1 cm. At the time of ovulation, ovarian size may double temporarily. The oval-shaped ovaries are firm in consistency and slightly tender. The surface of the ovary is smooth before menarche. After sexual maturity, scarring from repeated follicle rupture during ovulation roughens the nodular surface.

The two functions of the ovaries are **ovulation** and hormone production. At birth the normal female's ovaries contain countless primordial (primitive) ova. After puberty, one or more ova mature and undergo ovulation at intervals during the woman's reproductive life (generally monthly). The ovary is also the major site of production of steroid sex hormones (estrogens, progesterone, and androgens) in amounts required for normal female growth, development, and function.

Uterine tubes (fallopian tubes). The paired *uterine (fallopian) tubes* are attached to the uterine fundus (upper, rounded part of the uterus) (Figs. 3-5, 3-6, and 3-9). The tubes extend laterally, enter the free ends of the broad ligament, and curl around each ovary.

The tubes are approximately 10 cm long and 0.6 cm in diameter. Each tube has an outer coat of peritoneum; a middle, thin muscular coat; and an inner mucosa. The mucosal lining consists of columnar cells, some of which are ciliated and others of which are secretory. The mucosa is at its thinnest during the time of menstruation. Each tube, along with its mucosa, is continuous with the mucosa of the uterus and of the vagina.

The structure of the uterine tube changes along its length. Four distinctive segments can be identified (Figs. 3-5 and 3-6): (1) the infundibulum, (2) the ampulla, (3) the isthmus, and (4) the interstitial portion. The *infundibulum* is the most distal portion. Its funnel-shaped or trumpet-shaped opening is encircled with fimbriae. The fimbriae become swollen, almost erectile, at ovulation. The *ampulla* makes up the distal and middle segment of the tube. It is in the ampulla that the sperm and the ovum usually unite and **fertilization** occurs.

The *isthmus* is proximal to the ampulla. It is small and firm, similar to the round ligament. The *interstitial* (or *intramural*) portion passes through the myometrium between the fundus and the body of the uterus and has the smallest lumen (tunnel), measuring less than 1 mm in diameter. Before the fertilized ovum can pass through this lumen, it has to discard its crown of granulosa cells.

The uterine tubes provide a passageway for the ovum. The fingerlike projections (fimbriae) of the infundibulum pull the ovum into the tube with wavelike motions. The ovum is propelled along the tube, partially by the cilia but primarily by the peristaltic movements of the muscular coat, toward the uterine cavity. Peristaltic motion is influenced by estrogen and prostaglandins. Peristaltic activity of the uterine tubes and the secretory function of their mucosal lining are greatest at the time of ovulation. The columnar cells secrete a nutrient to sustain the ovum while it is in the tube.

Uterus. Between birth and puberty the *uterus* descends gradually into the true pelvis from the lower abdomen. After puberty the uterus is usually located in the midline in the true pelvis posterior to the symphysis pubis and urinary bladder and anterior to the rectum.

For most women, with the urinary bladder empty, the uterus is *anteverted* (tipped forward) and slightly anteflexed (bent forward), with the corpus (body) lying over the top of the posterior wall of the bladder. The cervix is directed downward and backward toward the tip of the sacrum so that it is usually at approximately a right angle to the plane of the vagina. For other women the uterus may be in the midposition or tipped backward (retroverted). A uterus that is bent more than usual so that the fundus (top) is closer to the cervix is called *anteflexed,* or *retroflexed* (Fig. 3-7).

A full bladder pushes the uterus back toward the rectum. A full rectum moves the uterus forward against the bladder. Uterine position also changes depending on the woman's position (e.g., lying supine, prone, on her side, or standing), her age, and pregnancy. The free mobility permits the uterus to rise slightly during the sexual response cycle (see p. 46) so the cervix is placed in a position to increase the likelihood of fertilization.

Ligaments and muscles of the pelvic floor, including the perineal body, support the uterus. A total of 10 ligaments stabilize the uterus within the pelvic cavity (Figs. 3-5, 3-6, and 3-9): four paired ligaments—broad, round, uterosacral, and cardinal (transverse or Mackenrodt); and two single ligaments—anterior (pubocervical) and posterior (rectovaginal). The posterior ligament forms the deep rectouterine pouch known as the *cul-de-sac of Douglas* (Fig. 3-8; see also Fig. 3-15).

The uterus is a flattened, hollow, muscular, thick-walled organ that resembles an upside-down pear (Fig. 3-8). In the adult woman who has never been pregnant, the uterus weighs 60 g. The uterus normally is symmetric in shape and nontender, smooth, and firm to the touch. The degree of firmness varies with several factors; for example, it is spongier during the secretory phase of the menstrual cycle, softer during pregnancy, and firmer after menopause.

The uterus has three parts (Figs. 3-5 and 3-6): the *fundus,* which is the upper, rounded prominence above the insertion of the uterine tubes; the *corpus,* or main portion, encircling the intrauterine cavity; and the *isthmus,* which is the slightly constricted portion that joins the corpus to the cervix and is known during pregnancy as the lower uterine segment.

The three functions of the uterus are cyclic menstruation with rejuvenation of the endometrium, pregnancy, and labor. These functions are essential to reproduction but not necessary for a woman's physiologic survival.

Uterine wall. The uterine wall is composed of three layers: the endometrium, the myometrium, and a partial outer layer of parietal peritoneum (Fig. 3-6).

The highly vascular *endometrium* is a lining of mucous membrane composed of three layers: a compact surface layer, a spongy middle layer of loose connective tissue, and a dense inner layer that attaches the endometrium to the myometrium. (The upper two layers are also referred to as the *functional layers,* and the inner layer is referred to as the *basal layer.*) During menstruation and after delivery, the compact

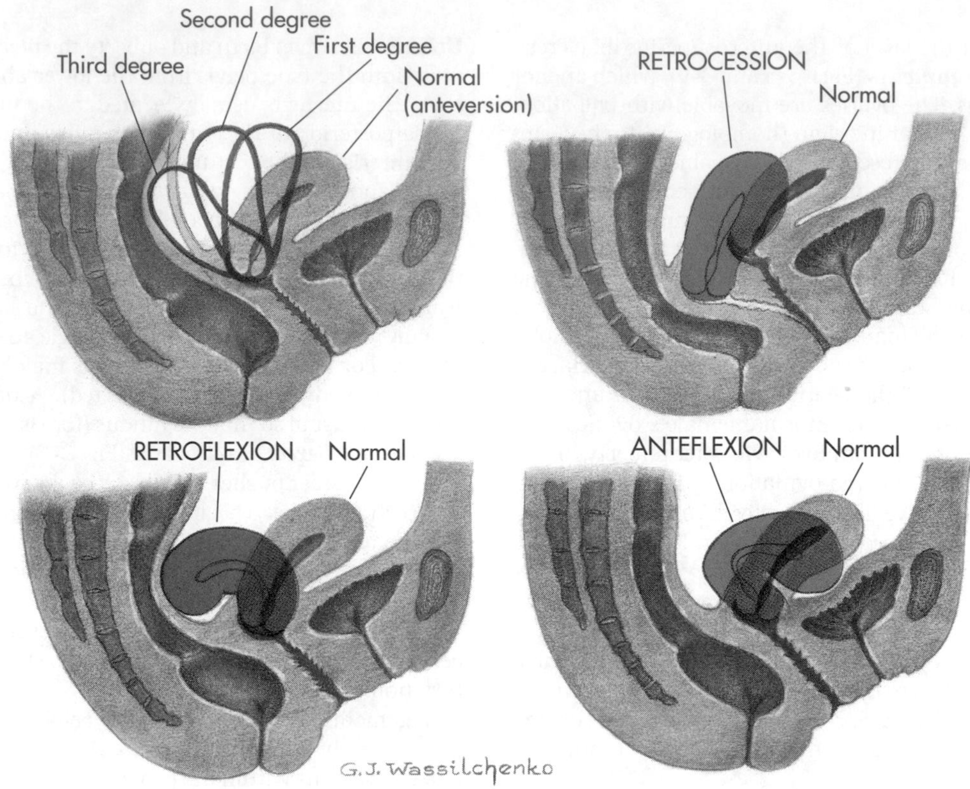

Fig. 3-7 Uterine positions.

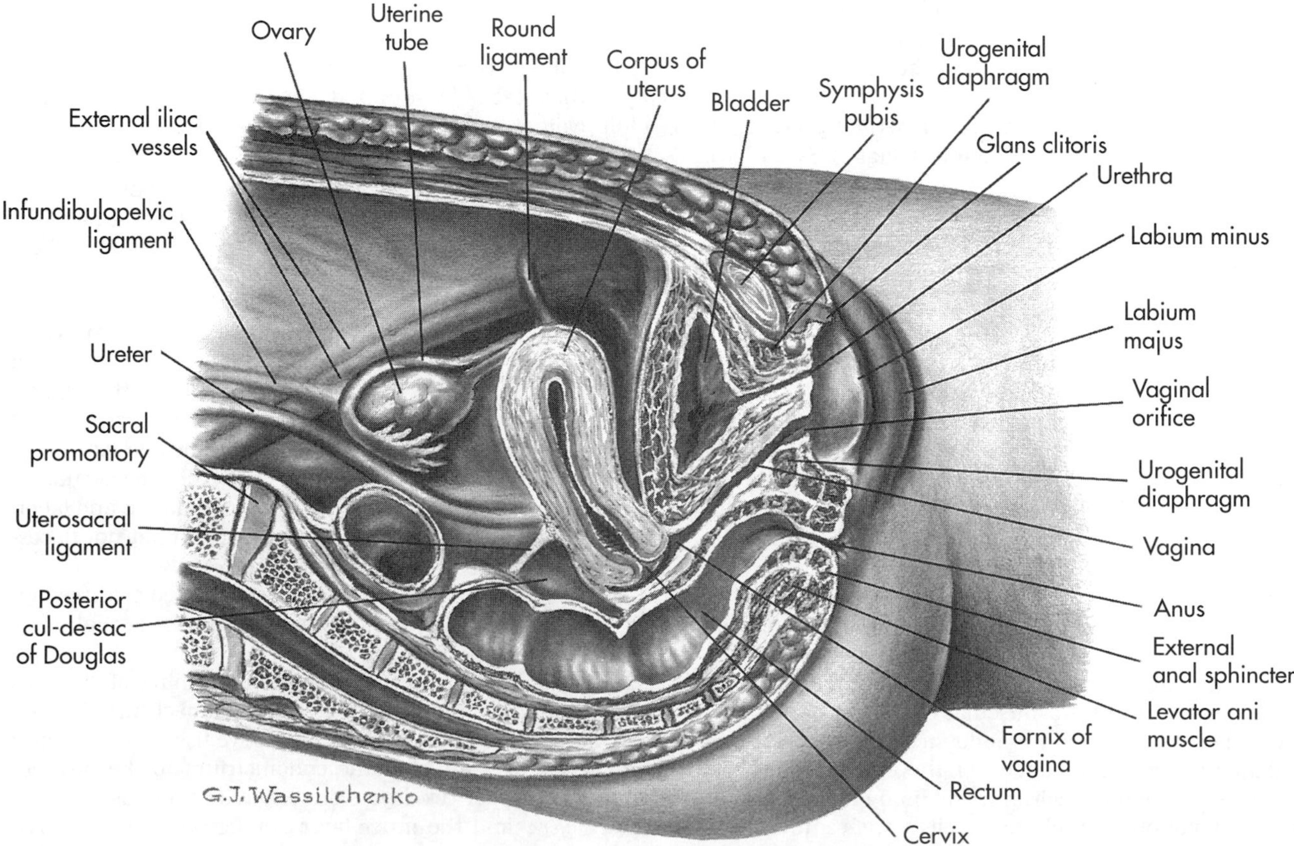

Fig. 3-8 Midsagittal view of female pelvic organs, with woman lying supine.

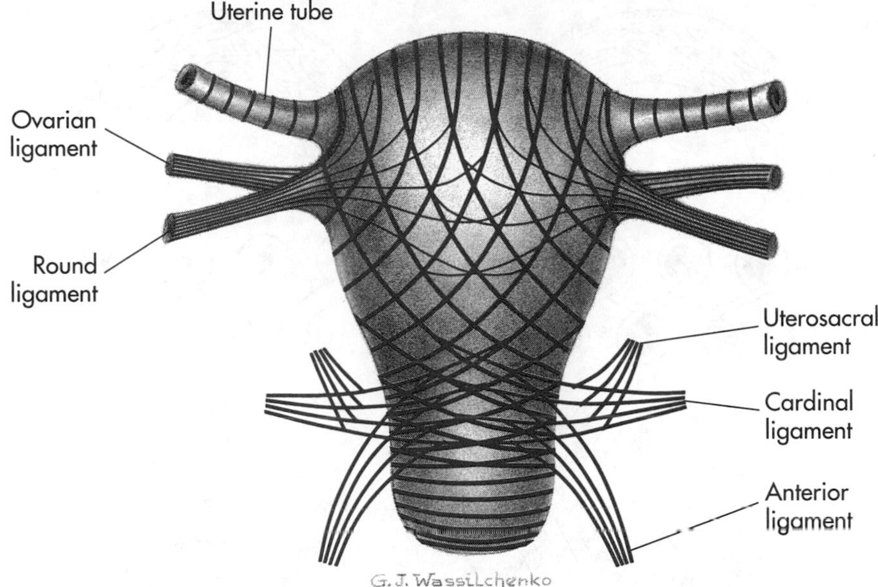

Fig. 3-9 Schematic arrangement of directions of muscle fibers. Note that uterine muscle fibers are continuous with supportive ligaments of uterus.

surface and middle spongy layers slough off. Just after menstrual flow ends, the endometrium is 0.5 mm thick; near the end of the endometrial cycle, just before menstruation begins again, it is about 5 mm thick.

Layers of smooth muscle fibers that extend in three directions (longitudinal, transverse, and oblique) make up the thick *myometrium* (Fig. 3-9). The smooth muscle fibers interlace with elastic and connective tissues and blood vessels throughout the uterine wall and blend with the dense inner layer of the endometrium. The myometrium is particularly thick in the fundus, thins out as it nears the isthmus, and is thinnest in the cervix.

Longitudinal fibers make up the *outer* myometrial layer, found mostly in the fundus, making this layer well suited for expelling the fetus during the birth process. In the thick *middle* myometrial layer the interlaced muscle fibers form a figure-eight pattern encircling large blood vessels. Contraction of the middle layer produces a hemostatic action (Fig. 3-10). Only a few circular fibers of the *inner* myometrial layer are found in the fundus. Most of the circular fibers are concentrated in the *cornua* (the place where the uterine tubes join the uterine body) and around the internal os. The sphincter action of this layer prevents the regurgitation of menstrual blood out of the uterine tubes during menstruation. This sphincter action around the internal cervical os helps retain the uterine contents during pregnancy. Injury to this sphincter can weaken the internal os and result in an internal cervical os, which opens prematurely.

Each muscle layer and its function have been described individually, but the myometrium works as a whole. The structure of the myometrium, which gives strength and elasticity, presents an example of adaptation to function:

1. To thin out, pull up, and open the cervix and to push the fetus out of the uterus, the fundus must contract with the most force.
2. Contraction of interlacing smooth muscle fibers that surround the blood vessels controls blood loss after abortion and childbirth. Because of their ability to close off (ligate) blood vessels between them, the smooth muscle fibers of the uterus are referred to as the **living ligature** (Fig. 3-10).

The *parietal peritoneum,* a serous membrane, coats all the uterine corpus except for the lower one fourth of the anterior surface, where the bladder is attached, and the cervix. Diagnostic tests and surgery involving the uterus can be performed without entering the abdominal cavity because the parietal peritoneum does not completely cover the uterine corpus.

Cervix. The lowermost portion of the uterus is the *cervix,* or neck. The attachment site of the uterine cervix to the vaginal vault divides the cervix into the longer supravaginal (above the vagina) portion (Fig. 3-5) and the shorter vaginal portion (Fig. 3-6). The length of the cervix is about 2.5 to 3 cm, of which about 1 cm protrudes into the vagina in the nonpregnant woman.

The cervix is composed primarily of fibrous connective tissue with some muscle fibers and elastic tissue. The cervix of the nulliparous woman is a rounded, almost conical, rather firm, spindle-shaped body. The narrowed opening between the uterine cavity and the endocervical canal (canal inside the cervix that connects the uterine cavity with the vagina) is the *internal os.* The narrowed opening between the endocervix and the vagina is the *external os,* a small circular opening in women who have not borne children. Childbirth changes the circular os to a small transverse opening dividing the cervix into an anterior and a posterior lip (Fig. 3-11).

When the woman is not ovulating or is not pregnant, the tip of the cervix feels firm, similar to the end of one's nose, with a dimple in the center. The dimple marks the site of the external os.

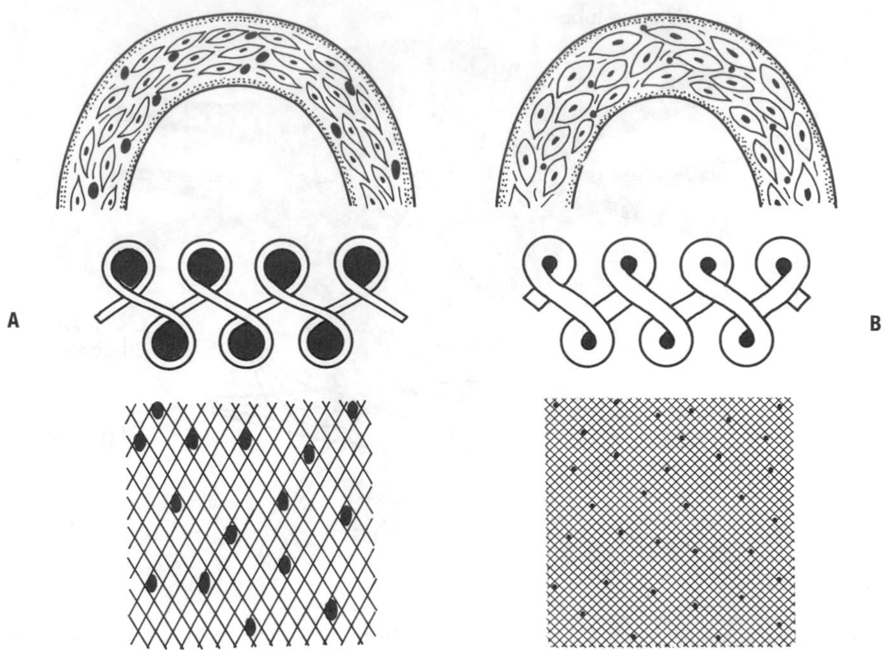

Fig. 3-10 The living ligature: interlacing smooth muscle fibers of thick middle myometrium. Color denotes blood vessels. **A,** Relaxed muscle fibers. **B,** Contracted muscle fibers ligating blood vessels.

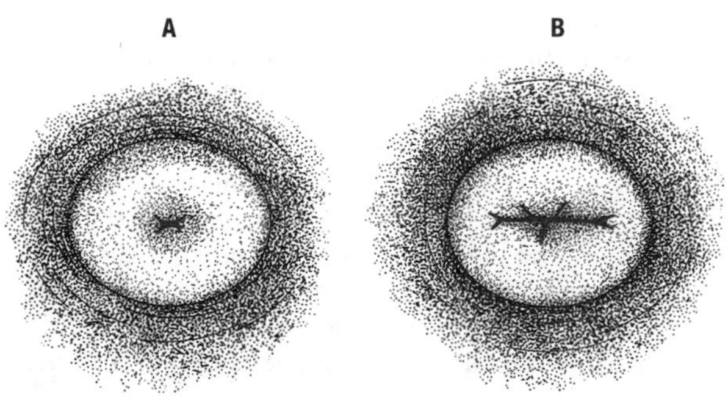

Fig. 3-11 External cervical os as seen through speculum. **A,** Nonparous cervix. **B,** Parous cervix.

The most significant characteristic of the cervix is its ability to stretch during vaginal childbirth. Several factors contribute to cervical elasticity: high connective tissue and elastic fiber content, numerous infoldings in the endocervical lining, and a 10% muscle fiber content.

Canals. The two cavities within the uterus are known as the *uterine* and *cervical canals* (Fig. 3-6). The uterine canal in the nonpregnant state is compressed by thick muscular walls so it is only a potential space, flat and triangular. The fundus forms the base of the triangle. The uterine tubes open into either end of the base. The apex of the triangle points downward and forms the internal os of the cervical canal.

The endocervical canal with its many infoldings has a surface layer of tall, columnar, mucus-producing cells. The *columnar epithelium* is beefy red, deeper, and rougher looking than the epithelial outer covering of the cervix. After menarche, *squamous epithelium* covers the outside of the cervix (ectocervix). This external covering of flat cells gives a glistening pink color to the cervix. A deeper bluish red color is seen when the woman is ovulating or pregnant. A reddened (hyperemic) cervix may indicate inflammation.

The two types of epithelium meet at the **squamocolumnar junction.** This junction line is usually just inside the external cervical os but may be found on the ectocervix in some women. The squamocolumnar junction is the most common site of neoplastic cellular changes. Therefore cells for cytologic study, the Papanicolaou (Pap) smear, are scraped from this junction.

The columnar epithelial cells produce odorless and nonirritating mucus in response to estrogen and progesterone.

Blood vessels. The abdominal aorta divides at about the level of the umbilicus and forms the two iliac arteries. Each iliac artery divides to form two arteries, the major one of which is the *hypogastric artery.* The uterine arteries branch off from the hypogastric arteries. The closeness of the uterus to the aorta ensures an ample blood supply to meet the needs of the growing uterus and conceptus.

In addition, the ovarian artery, a direct subdivision of the aorta, first supplies the ovary with the blood and then proceeds to join the uterine artery, thus adding to the blood supply (Fig. 3-12).

In the nonpregnant state the uterine blood vessels are coiled and tortuous (twisted). With advancing pregnancy and an enlarging uterus, these blood vessels straighten. The uterine veins follow along the arteries and empty into the internal iliac veins.

Innervation. The internal genitalia have a rich supply of afferent and efferent autonomic nerves, both motor and sensory.

Parasympathetic fibers from the sacral nerves are probably responsible for producing vasodilation and inhibiting

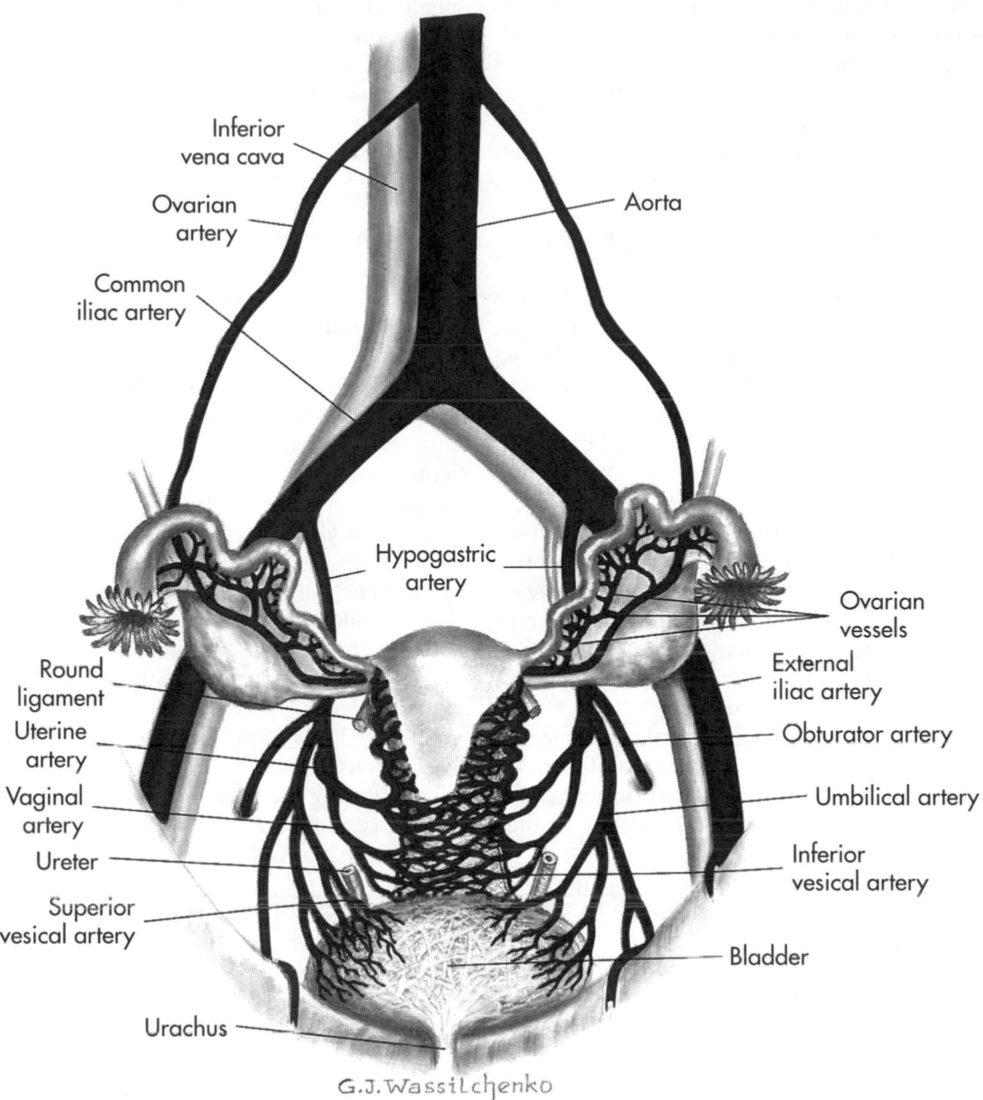

Fig. 3-12 Pelvic blood supply.

muscular contraction. Efferent sympathetic motor nerves arise from the ganglia of the fifth to tenth thoracic vertebrae (T-5 to T-10), come together over the sacrum, and reach the uterus through ganglia that lie near the base of the uterosacral ligaments. These efferent sympathetic motor nerves are believed to cause vasoconstriction and muscular contraction. The autonomic nerves just described (parasympathetic and efferent sympathetic motor) regulate the action of the uterus, but the uterus has an intrinsic motility (i.e., it can contract and relax even if the nerves to it are cut). This means that even if a woman has an accident that injures the spinal cord at or above T-5, she may still be able to have uterine contractions sufficient to give birth to an infant vaginally.

Sensory fibers carrying pain sensation from the uterus come together in the paracervical areas, proceed upward to pass just below the division (bifurcation) of the aorta, and then travel to the spinal cord at the level of T-11 and T-12. Because of this arrangement, pain that originates in the ovary or in the ureters may mimic pain that originates in the uterus, any of which may be felt in the flank and down to the inguinal and vulvar areas.

Vagina. The *vagina*, a tubular structure located in front of the rectum and behind the bladder and urethra (Fig. 3-8), extends from the introitus (the external opening in the vestibule between the labia minora of the vulva) to the cervix. When the woman is standing, the vagina slants backward and upward. It is supported mainly by its attachments to the pelvic floor musculature and fascia.

The vagina is a thin-walled, collapsible tube capable of great distention. Because of the way the cervix protrudes into the uppermost portion of the vagina, the length of the anterior wall of the vagina is only about 7.5 cm, whereas that of the posterior wall is about 9 cm. The recesses formed all around the protruding cervix are called *fornices:* right, left, anterior, and posterior. The posterior fornix is deeper than the other three (Figs. 3-6 and 3-15).

Glandular mucous membranes line the smooth muscle walls. During the reproductive years this mucosa is arranged in transverse folds called *rugae.*

The vaginal mucosa responds promptly to estrogen and progesterone stimulation. Cells are lost from the mucosa, especially during the menstrual cycle and pregnancy. Cells scraped from the vaginal mucosa can be used to estimate steroid sex hormone levels.

Vaginal fluid is derived from the lower or upper genital tract. The fluid ordinarily is slightly acidic. Interaction between vaginal lactobacilli and glycogen maintains acidity. If the pH rises above 5, the incidence of vaginal infection increases. The continuous flow of fluid from the vagina maintains relative cleanliness of the vagina. Therefore *vaginal douching in normal circumstances is neither necessary nor recommended.*

The copious blood supply to the vagina is derived from the descending branches of the uterine artery, the vaginal artery, and the internal pudendal arteries (Fig. 3-12).

The vagina is relatively insensitive. There is some innervation from the pudendal and hemorrhoidal nerves to the lowest one third of the vagina. Because of this minimal innervation and lack of special nerve endings, the vagina is the source of little sensation during sexual excitement and coitus and causes less pain during the second stage of labor than if this tissue were well supplied with nerve endings.

The *G-spot* is an area on the anterior vaginal wall beneath the urethra defined by Graefenberg as analogous to the male prostate gland. During sexual arousal it may be stimulated to the point of orgasm, with ejaculation into the urethra of fluid similar to prostatic fluid (Herbst et al, 1992).

The vagina functions as the organ for coitus, as the passageway for menstrual flow, and as the birth canal.

Pelvic floor and perineum. The pelvic diaphragm, the urogenital diaphragm or triangle, and the muscles of the external genitalia and anus comprise the pelvic floor and perineum. The perineum is sometimes defined as including all the muscles, fascia, and ligaments of the upper (pelvic) and lower (urogenital) diaphragms. The perineal body adds strength to these structures.

The *upper pelvic diaphragm,* composed of muscles and their fascia and ligaments, extends across the lowest part of the pelvic cavity like a hammock (Fig. 3-13). The largest and most significant portion of the diaphragm is formed by the pair of broad, thin *levator ani muscles,* which extend sheetlike between the ischial spines and coccyx, and the sacrum. The levator ani group of muscles is made of three muscle pairs: puborectalis, iliococcygeus, and pubococcygeus muscles. The pubococcygeus muscle is particularly significant for women. It plays a role in sexual sensory function, in bladder control, in controlling perineal relaxation during labor, and in expulsion of the fetus during birth.

The second paired muscles of the upper pelvic diaphragm are the closely joined *coccygeus muscles.* These muscles extend from the ischial spines to the coccyx and lower sacrum. The several parts of the pelvic diaphragm provide a slinglike support to abdominal and pelvic viscera.

The strength and resilience of this sling are derived from the way in which the layered parts of this sling are interwoven and interlaced. *The layers are not fixed; that is, they slide over each other.* This unique arrangement strengthens the supportive capacity of the pelvic diaphragm, allows for dilation of the vagina during the birth process and for its closure after birth, and assists with constriction of the urethra, vagina, and anal canal, which pass through the diaphragm.

The *lower pelvic diaphragm* is located in the hollow of the pubic arch and consists of the tranverse perineal muscles, which originate at the ischial tuberosities and insert into the perineal body. The strong muscle fibers provide support to the anal canal during defecation and to the lower vagina during

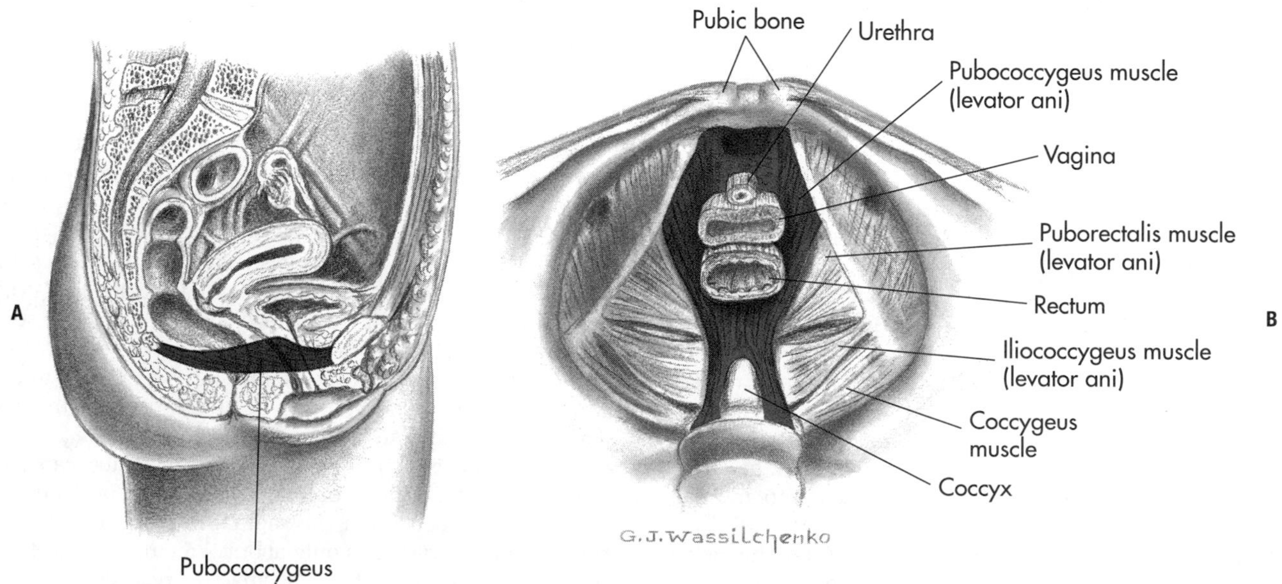

Fig. 3-13 Upper pelvic diaphragm. **A,** Pubococcygeus portion of the levator ani muscles, midsagittal view. **B,** View from above.

birth. The deep transverse perineal muscles join to form a central seam, or *raphe.* Some of their fibers encircle the urinary meatus and vaginal sphincters.

The *perineum,* or *perineal body,* located below the upper and lower pelvic diaphragm, reinforces the strength of the pelvic diaphragm and aids in constricting the urinary, vaginal, and anal openings. The *bulbocavernosus muscle* fibers originate in the perineal body and surround the vaginal opening as the muscle fibers pass forward to insert into the pubis (Fig. 3-14). The perineal body is continuous with the septum between the rectum and vagina (Fig. 3-15). This tissue is flattened and stretched as the fetus moves through the birth canal.

The *ischiocavernosus muscles* originate in the tuberosities of the ischium and continue at an angle to insert next to the bulbocavernosus muscles (Fig. 3-14). These muscle fibers contract to cause erection of the clitoris.

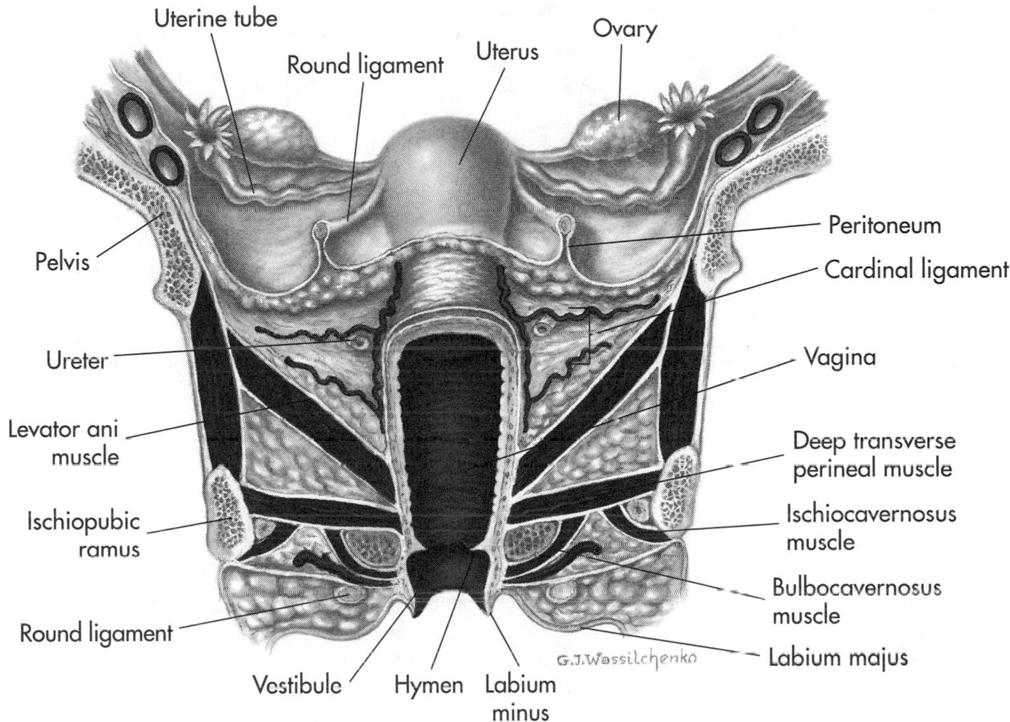

Fig. 3-14 Levator ani muscles of upper pelvic diaphragm and urogenital (lower pelvic) diaphragm, anterior view.

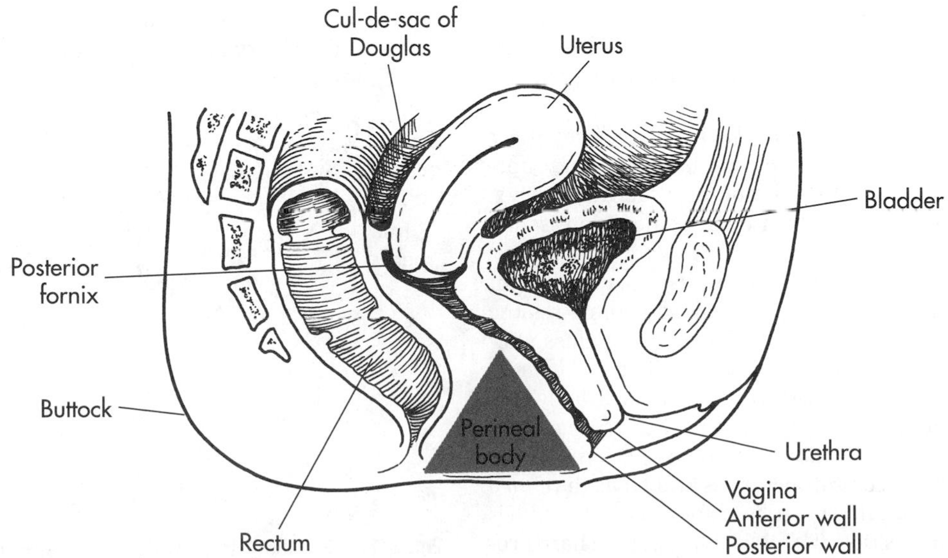

Fig. 3-15 Perineal body. Location and size relative to surrounding tissues, with woman sitting.

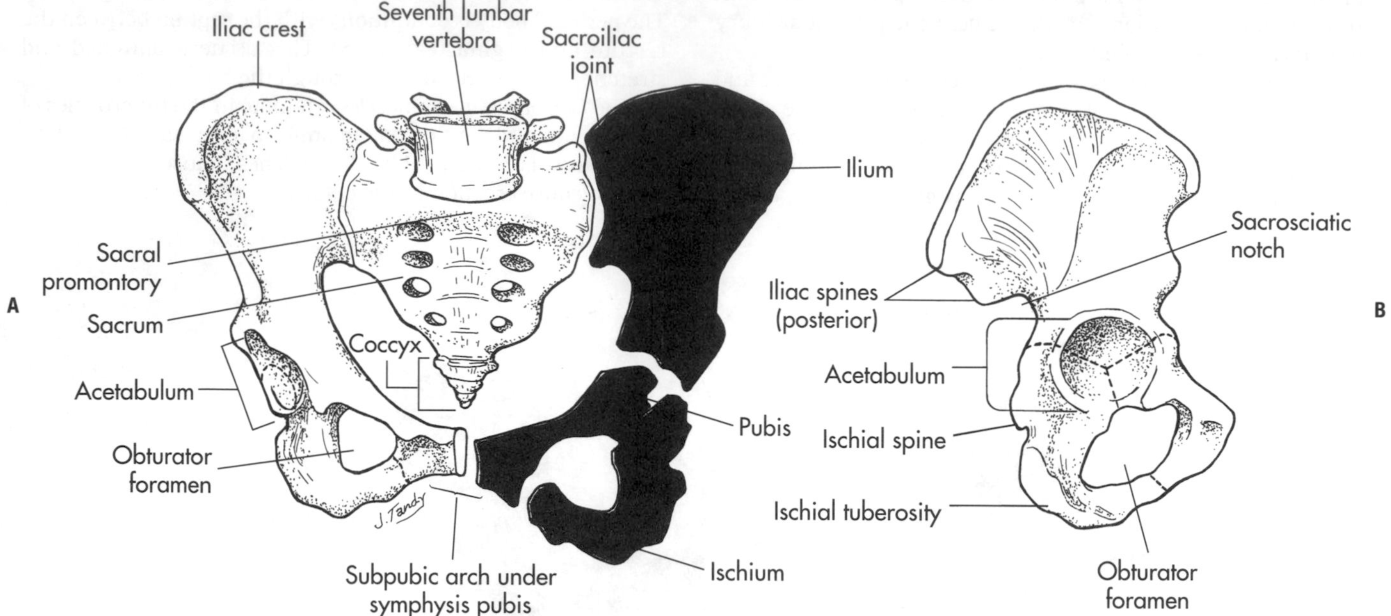

Fig. 3-16 Adult female pelvis. **A,** Anterior view. The three embryonic parts of left innominate bone are lightly shaded. **B,** External view of right innominate bone (fused).

Anal sphincter muscle fibers originate at the coccyx, separate to pass on either side of the anus, fuse, and then insert into the transverse perineal muscles.

The bulbocavernosus, transverse perineal, and anal sphincter muscle fibers can be strengthened through *Kegel exercises.*

Bony pelvis. The pelvis serves three primary purposes: (1) its bony cavity produces a protective cradle for pelvic structures; (2) its architecture is of special importance in accommodating a growing fetus throughout pregnancy and during the birth process; and (3) its strength provides stable anchorage for the attachment of supportive muscles, fascia, and ligaments.

The following structures and *landmarks of the bony pelvis* are especially important (Fig. 3-16): the iliac crest and superior, anterior iliac spine; sacral promontory; sacrum; coccyx; symphysis pubis; subpubic arch; ischial spines; and ischial tuberosities.

The pelvis (Fig. 3-16, *A*) is made of four bones: (1) the right and (2) left innominate bones, each of which comprises the right or left pubic bone, ilium, and ischium, which fuse after puberty; (3) the sacrum; and (4) the coccyx. The two *innominate bones* (hip bones) form the sides and front of the bony passage, and the sacrum and coccyx form the back.

Below the *ilium* is the *ischium,* a heavy bone terminating posteriorly in the rounded protuberances known as the *ischial tuberosities* (Fig. 3-16, *B*). The tuberosities bear the body's weight in the sitting position. The *ischial spines,* the sharp projections from the posterior border of the ischium into the pelvic cavity, may be blunt or prominent.

The *pubis,* forming the front portion of the pelvic cavity, is located beneath the mons. In the midline the two pubic bones are joined by strong ligaments and a thick cartilage to form the joint called the *symphysis pubis.* In the woman the angle formed by the subpubic arch optimally measures slightly more than 90 degrees.

The *sacrum* is formed by five fused vertebrae. The upper anterior portion of the body of the first sacral vertebra (S-1), the promontory, forms the posterior margin of the pelvic brim.

The *coccyx* (tailbone), composed of three to five fused vertebrae, articulates with the sacrum. The coccyx projects downward and forward from the lower border of the sacrum.

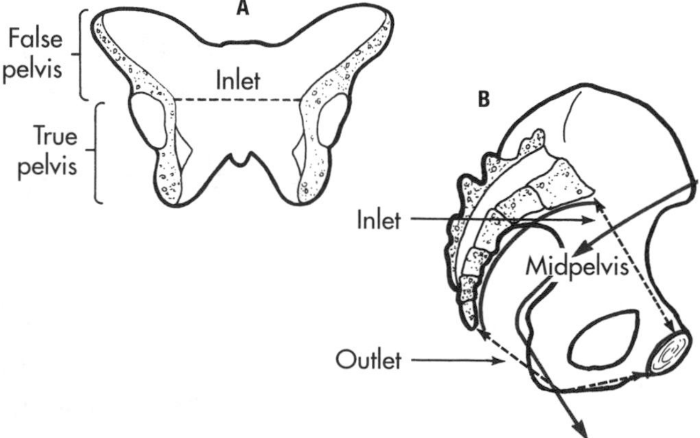

Fig. 3-17 Female pelvis. **A,** Cavity of false pelvis is shallow basin above inlet; true pelvis is deeper cavity below inlet. **B,** Cavity of true pelvis is an irregularly curved canal *(arrows).*

The pelvis is divided into two sections, the shallow upper basin, or false pelvis, and the deeper lower, or true, pelvis (Fig. 3-17, *A*). The *false pelvis* lies above the linea terminalis (brim or inlet) and varies considerably in size in different women. The *true pelvis* consists of the brim, or inlet, and the area below.

Pelvic planes include those of the *inlet*, the *midpelvis*, and the *outlet*. The cavity of the (true) midpelvis resembles an irregularly curved canal with unequal anterior and posterior surfaces (Fig. 3-17, *B*). The anterior surface is formed by the length of the symphysis. The posterior surface is formed by the length of the sacrum.

Age, sex, and race are responsible for the greatest variations in pelvic shape and size. Considerable change occurs in the pelvis during growth and development. Pelvic ossification is complete at about age 20 or slightly later. Smaller people have smaller, lighter bones than larger people.

Breasts

The *breasts* are paired mammary glands located between the second and sixth ribs (Fig. 3-18). About two thirds of the breast overlies the pectoralis major muscle, between the sternum and midaxillary line, with an extension to the axilla referred to as the *tail of Spence*. The lower one third of the breast overlies the serratus anterior muscle. The breasts are attached to the muscles by connective tissue or fascia.

The breasts of healthy mature women are approximately equal in size and shape but are often not absolutely symmetric. The size and shape vary depending on the woman's age, heredity, and nutrition. However, the contour should be smooth with no retractions, dimpling, or masses.

True glandular tissue is called *parenchyma;* supporting tissues, the fat, and fibrous connective tissue are called *stroma*. The relative amount of stroma determines the size and consistency of the breast.

Estrogen stimulates growth of the breast by inducing fat deposition in the breasts, development of stromal tissue (i.e., increase in its amount and elasticity), and growth of the extensive ductile system. Estrogen also increases the vascularity of breast tissue.

Once ovulation begins in puberty, progesterone levels increase. The increase in progesterone causes maturation of mammary gland tissue, specifically the lobules and acinar structures. During adolescence, fat deposition and growth of fibrous tissue contribute to the increase in the size of the gland. Full development of the breast is not achieved until after the end of the first pregnancy or early in the lactation period.

Each mammary gland is made of 15 to 20 *lobes*, which are divided into lobules. *Lobules* are clusters of acini. An *acinus* is a saclike terminal part of a compound gland emptying through a narrow lumen or duct. In discussions of mammary glands the correct anatomic term (acinus) is often used interchangeably with *alveolus*. The acini are lined with epithelial cells that secrete colostrum and milk. Just below the epithelium is the *myoepithelium* (*myo*, or muscle), which contracts to expel milk from the acini (Fig. 3-19).

The ducts from the clusters of acini that form the lobules merge to form larger ducts draining the lobes. Ducts from the lobes converge in a single *nipple (mammary papilla)* surrounded by an *areola*. Just as the ducts converge, they dilate to form common *lactiferous sinuses*, which are also called *ampullae*. The

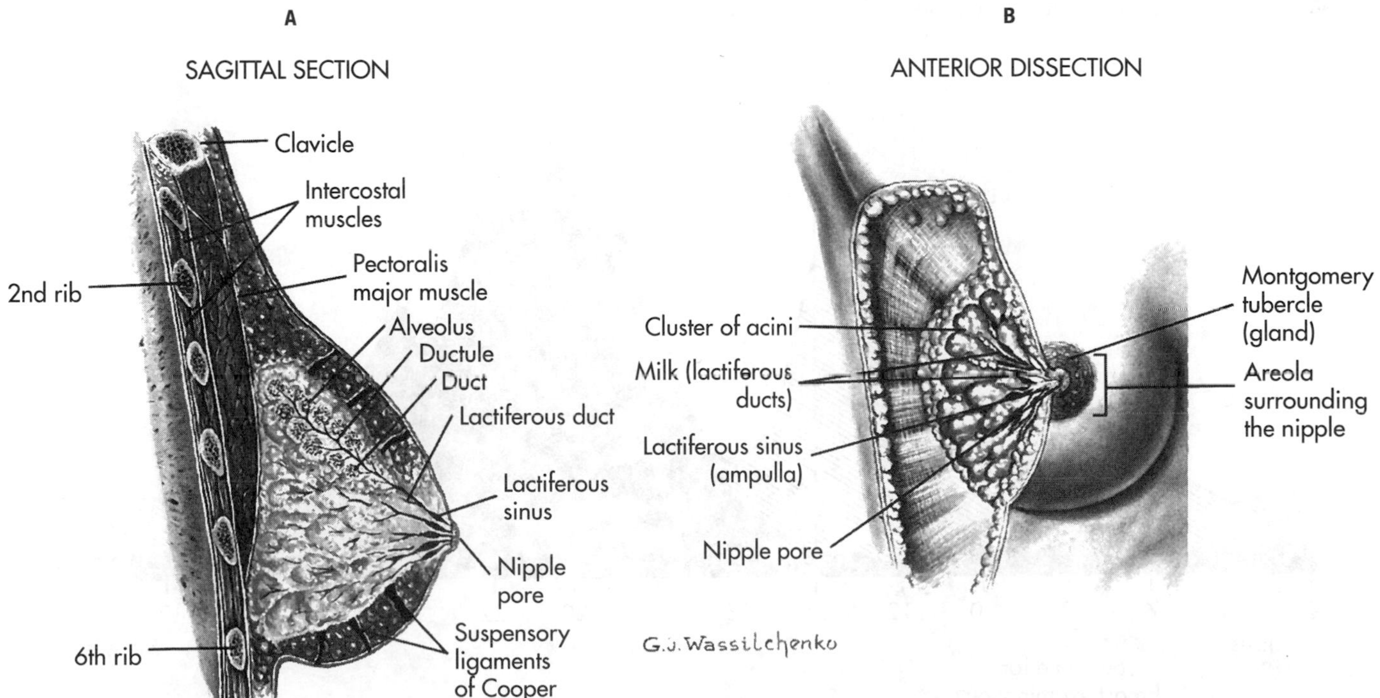

Fig. 3-18 Position and structure of mammary gland. **A**, Sagittal section. **B**, Anterior dissection. (From Seidel H et al: *Mosby's guide to physical examination*, ed 3, St Louis, 1995, Mosby.)

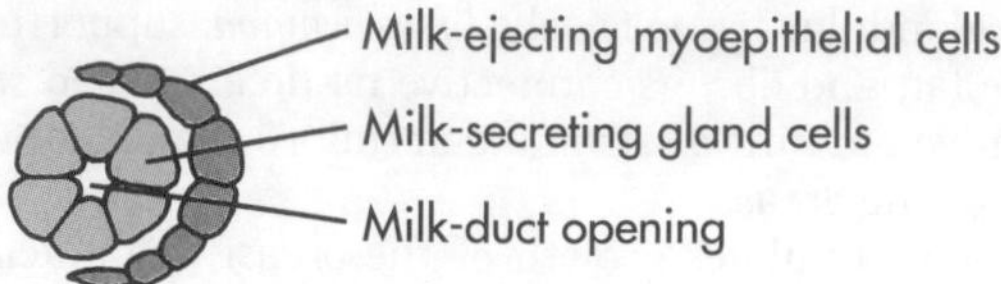

Fig. 3-19 Acinus in cross section.

lactiferous sinuses serve as milk reservoirs. Many tiny lactiferous ducts drain the ampullae and exit in the nipple.

The glandular structures and ducts are surrounded by protective fatty tissue and are separated and supported by fibrous suspensory *Cooper ligaments.* Cooper ligaments provide support to the mammary glands while permitting their mobility on the chest wall.

The round nipple is usually slightly elevated above the breast. On each breast the nipple projects slightly upward and laterally. It contains 15 to 20 openings from lactiferous ducts. The nipple is surrounded by fibromuscular tissue and covered by wrinkled skin. Except during pregnancy and lactation, there is usually no discharge from the nipple.

The nipple and surrounding areola are usually more deeply pigmented than the skin of the breast. The rough appearance of the areola is caused by sebaceous glands, *Montgomery tubercles* (Fig. 3-18), directly beneath the skin. These glands secrete a fatty substance that is thought to lubricate the nipple. Smooth muscle fibers in the areola contract to stiffen the nipple to make it easier for the breastfeeding child to grasp. Sexual stimulation can also cause the nipple to become erect.

The vascular supply to the mammary gland is abundant. In the nonpregnant state the skin may not have an obvious vascular pattern and is smooth without tightness or shininess. During pregnancy the skin of the breasts shows increased vascularity. As breast tissue increases, the skin becomes stretched and tight as the breasts become fuller.

The skin covering the breasts contains an extensive superficial lymphatic network that serves the entire chest wall and is continuous with the superficial lymphatics of the neck and abdomen. In the deeper portions of the breasts the lymphatics form a rich network as well. The primary deep lymphatic pathway drains laterally toward the axillae.

Besides their function of lactation, breasts function as organs for sexual arousal in the mature adult.

The breasts change in size and nodularity in response to cyclic ovarian changes throughout reproductive life. Increasing levels of both estrogen and progesterone in the 3 to 4 days before menstruation increase vascularity of the breasts, induce growth of the ducts and acini, and promote water retention. The epithelial cells lining the ducts proliferate in number, the ducts dilate, and the lobules distend. The acini become enlarged and secretory, and lipid (fat) is deposited within their epithelial cell lining. As a result, breast swelling, tenderness, and discomfort are common symptoms just before the onset of menstruation. After menstruation, cellular proliferation regresses, acini decrease in size, and retained water is lost.

After breasts have undergone changes numerous times in response to the ovarian cycle, the proliferation and involution (regression) are not uniform throughout the breast. In time, after repeated hormonal stimulation, small persistent areas of nodulation may develop. This normal physiologic change must be considered when breast tissue is examined. Nodules may develop just before and during menstruation, when the breast is most active. The physiologic alterations in breast size and activity reach their minimum level about 5 to 7 days after menstruation stops. Therefore breast self-examination (BSE) is best carried out during this phase of the menstrual cycle (Fig. 3-20).

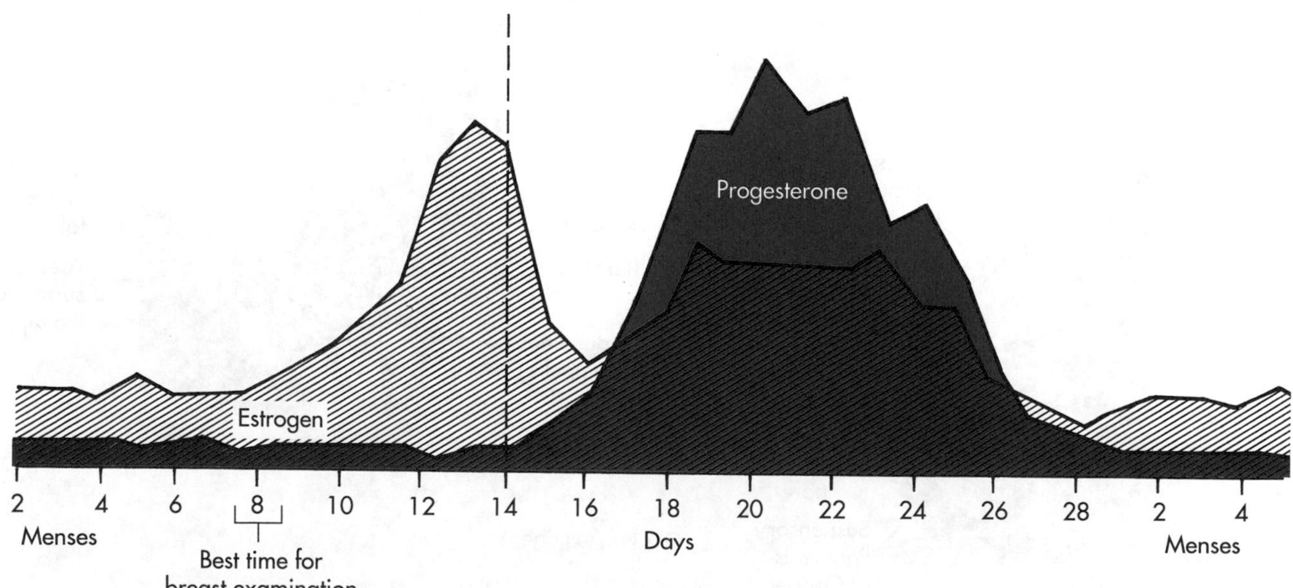

Fig. 3-20 Breast tissue changes in response to hormonal levels of menstrual cycle. BSE is done when hormonal stimulation is lowest.

Menstrual Cycle

Knowledge of the *menstrual cycle* is important for nurses providing care to women across the life span. Menstrual myths, menarche, the endometrial cycle, and hypothalamic-pituitary cycle, the ovarian cycle, other cyclic changes, and the climacterium are discussed in the following section.

Menstrual myths. Many myths have their origin in the mystery that surrounded the woman, her hidden reproductive organs, and her uniqueness in adding new members to society. As a consequence, a vast store of folklore, fancies, and superstitions has evolved. Because of their recurring nature and similar sequence, menstrual cycles were thought to be under the control of the moon. Before the discovery of ovulation in humans, it was thought that an egg was produced during menstruation only when fruitful intercourse had occurred. Not until the nineteenth century was knowledge available about the existence of the human egg, ovulation, and ovarian functioning.

As late as the second half of the twentieth century, the many behavioral changes falsely attributed to women during their menstrual cycles have been used to argue, for example, why it would be unwise for a woman to be president of the United States. Historic literature contains many references to dangers attributed to menstruating women. If a menstruating woman should walk through a farmer's fields, the crops would not grow and the flowers would wilt; if she tried to bake bread, the dough would not rise. Danger was also believed to exist for her husband, and physical contact, especially sexual intercourse, was and in some places still is prohibited. In many cultures the menstruating woman is kept in a separate menstrual hut or in separate quarters. After a ritualized "cleansing" the woman returns to her place in her family.

Menarche. Although young girls secrete small, rather constant amounts of estrogen, a marked increase occurs between 8 and 11 years of age. Moreover, increasing amounts and variations in gonadotropin and estrogen secretion develop into a cyclic pattern at least a year before *menarche,* or the first menstrual period. This occurs in most girls in North America at about age 13 (the range of onset is from ages 10 to 16).

Initially, menstrual periods are irregular, unpredictable, painless, and anovulatory in most young girls. After 1 year or more a hypothalamic-pituitary rhythm develops, and adequate cyclic estrogen is produced by the ovary to produce mature ova. Ovulatory periods tend to be regular.

In some women, ovulatory periods are associated with *dysmenorrhea* (painful uterine cramping), which may be an effect of progesterone or prostaglandins or both. This discomfort is rarely serious and is readily relieved by heat, exercise, or simple analgesics. When viewed in its proper perspective, slight cramping may be reassuring to the girl and her parents as an indication of normal ovulatory function.

Although pregnancy may occur in exceptional cases of true (constitutional) precocious puberty, most pregnancies in young girls occur well after the normally timed menarche. *All girls would benefit from knowing that pregnancy can occur at any time after the onset of menses.*

Menstruation is periodic uterine bleeding that begins approximately 14 days after ovulation. The first day of the cycle is the first day of bleeding, or *menses.* The average duration of menstrual flow is 5 days (range of 3 to 6 days), and the average blood loss is approximately 50 ml (range of 20 to 80 ml), but there is great variation.

For about 50% of women, menstrual blood does not appear to clot. The menstrual blood clots within the uterus, but the clot is liquefied before it is discharged from the uterus. Uterine discharge includes mucus and epithelial cells in addition to blood.

The menstrual cycle is a complex interplay of events that occur similtaneously in the endometrium, hypothalamus, and pituitary glands, and ovaries. The purpose of the menstrual cycle is to prepare the uterus for pregnancy. When pregnancy does not occur, menstruation follows. The woman's age, physical and emotional status, and environment influence the regularity of her menstrual cycles.

Hypothalmic-pituitary cycle. Toward the end of the normal menstrual cycle, blood levels of estrogen and progesterone fall (Figs. 3-20 and 3-21). Low blood levels of these ovarian hormones stimulate the hypothalamus to secrete gonadotropin-releasing hormone (Gn-RH). Gn-RH in turn stimulates anterior pituitary secretion of follicle stimulating hormone (FSH). FSH stimulates development of ovarian graafian follicles and their production of estrogen. Estrogen levels begin to fall, and hypothalamic Gn-RH triggers the anterior pituitary release of luteinizing hormone (LH). A marked surge of LH and a smaller peak of estrogen (day 12, Fig. 3-20) precede the expulsion of the ovum from the ovarian follicle by about 24 to 36 hours. LH peaks about the thirteenth or fourteenth day of a 28-day cycle. If fertilization and implantation of the ovum have not occurred by this time, regression of the corpus luteum follows. Therefore the levels of progesterone and estrogen decline, menstruation occurs, and the hypothalamus is once again stimulated to secrete Gn-RH. This is called the **hypothalamic-pituitary cycle** (Fig. 3-21).

Ovarian cycle. The primitive graafian follicles contain immature oocytes (primordial ova; Fig. 3-4). Before ovulation, 1 to 30 follicles begin to mature in each ovary under the influence of FSH and estrogen. The preovulatory surge of LH affects a selected follicle. Within the chosen follicle the oocyte matures, ovulation occurs, and the ovum is released. After ovulation the empty follicle begins its transformation into the corpus luteum (Fig. 3-21). This *follicular phase* (preovulatory phase) of the ovarian menstrual cycle varies in length from woman to woman. *Almost all variations in the length of the* ***ovarian cycle*** *are the result of variations in the length of the follicular phase.* On rare occasions (i.e., 1 in 100 menstrual cycles), more than one follicle is selected, and more than one oocyte matures and undergoes ovulation.

After ovulation, estrogen levels drop. For 90% of women, only a small amount of *withdrawal bleeding* occurs and it goes unnoticed. In 10% of women, sufficient bleeding occurs for it to be visible, resulting in what is known as *midcycle bleeding.*

The *luteal phase* begins immediately after ovulation and ends with the start of menstruation. This postovulatory phase of the ovarian cycle usually requires *14 days* (range of 13 to 15 days). The corpus luteum reaches its peak of functional activity 8 days after ovulation, secreting both estrogen and progesterone. Coincident with this time of peak luteal functioning, the fertilized egg is implanted in the endometrium. If no

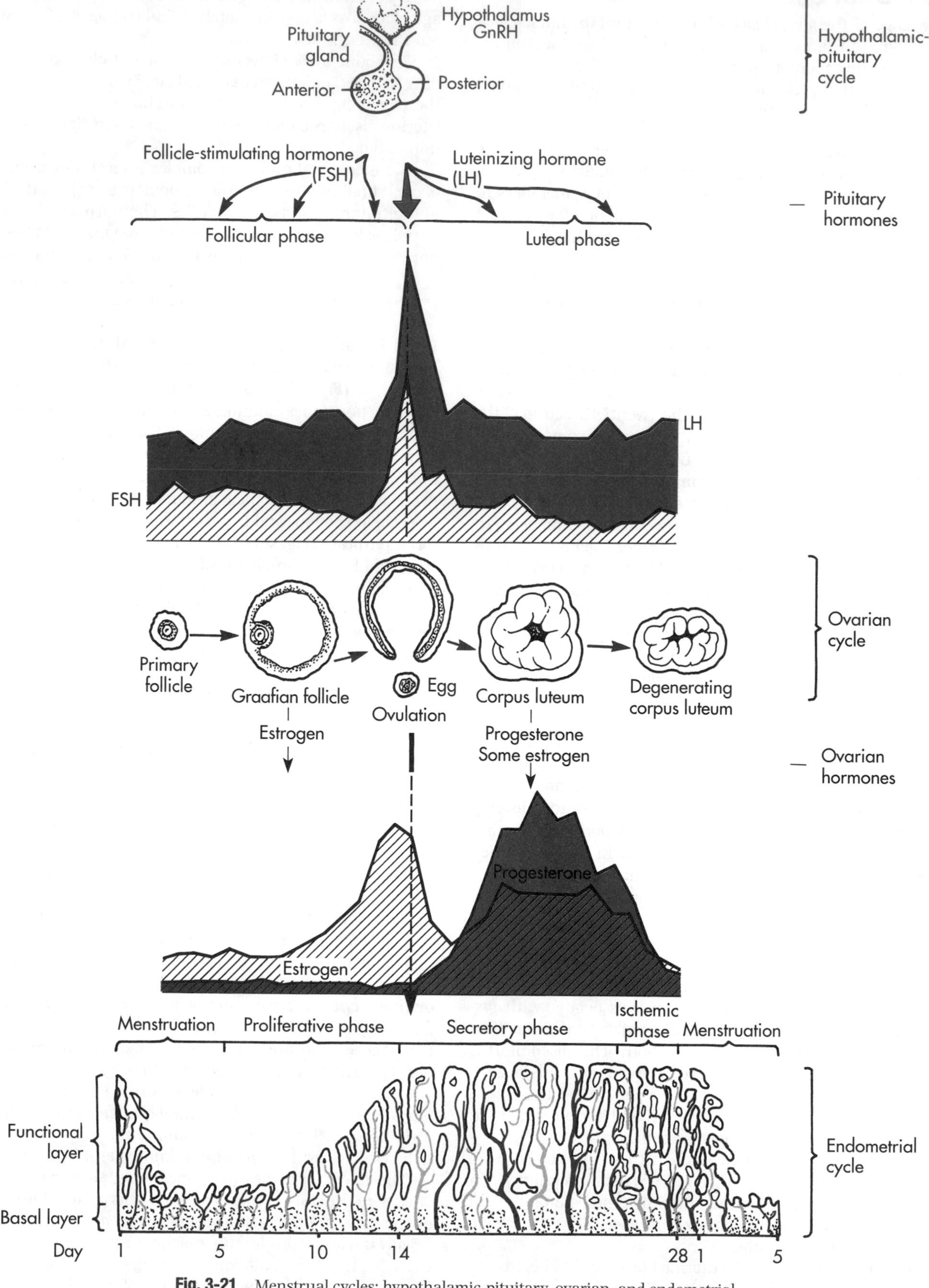

Fig. 3-21 Menstrual cycles: hypothalamic-pituitary, ovarian, and endometrial.

implantation occurs, the corpus luteum regresses, and steroid levels drop. Two weeks after ovulation, if fertilization and implantation have not occurred, the functional layer of the uterine endometrium is shed through menstruation.

Endometrial cycle. The four phases of the **endometrial cycle** are (1) the menstrual phase, (2) the proliferative phase, (3) the secretory phase, and (4) the ischemic phase (Fig. 3-21). During the *menstrual phase*, shedding of the functional two thirds of the endometrium (the compact and spongy layers) is initiated by periodic vasoconstriction of spiral arterioles in the upper layers of the endometrium. The basal layer is always retained, and regeneration begins near the end of the cycle from cells derived from the remaining glandular remnants or stromal cells in the basalis.

The *proliferative phase* is a period of rapid growth that extends from about the fifth day to the time of ovulation, which would be, for example, day 10 of a 24-day cycle, day 14 of a 28-day cycle, or day 18 of a 32-day cycle. The endometrial surface is completely restored in approximately 4 days, or slightly before bleeding ceases. From this point on, an eightfold to tenfold thickening occurs, with a leveling off of growth at ovulation. The proliferative phase depends on estrogen stimulation derived from ovarian follicles.

The *secretory phase* extends from the day of ovulation to about 3 days before the next menstrual period. After ovulation, larger amounts of progesterone are produced. An edematous, vascular, functional endometrium is now apparent.

At the end of the secretory phase the fully matured secretory endometrium reaches the thickness of heavy, soft velvet. It becomes luxuriant with blood and glandular secretions, a suitable protective and nutritive bed for a fertilized ovum, if one is available.

Implantation (nidation) of the fertilized ovum generally occurs about 7 to 10 days after ovulation. If fertilization and implantation do not occur, the corpus luteum (yellow body), which secretes estrogen and progesterone, regresses. With the rapid fall in progesterone and estrogen levels, the spiral arteries go into a spasm. During the *ischemic phase* the blood supply to the functional endometrium is blocked and necrosis develops. The functional layer separates from the basal layer, and menstrual bleeding begins, marking day 1 of the next cycle.

Other cyclic changes. When the hypothalamic-pituitary-ovarian axis functions properly, other tissues undergo predictable responses. Before ovulation the woman's basal body temperature (BBT) is lower, often below 37° C (98.6° F); after ovulation, with rising progesterone levels, her BBT rises. Changes in the cervix and cervical mucus follow a generally predictable pattern (Figs. 3-22 and 3-23). Preovulatory and postovulatory mucus is viscous (sticky), so sperm penetration is discouraged. At the time of ovulation, cervical mucus is

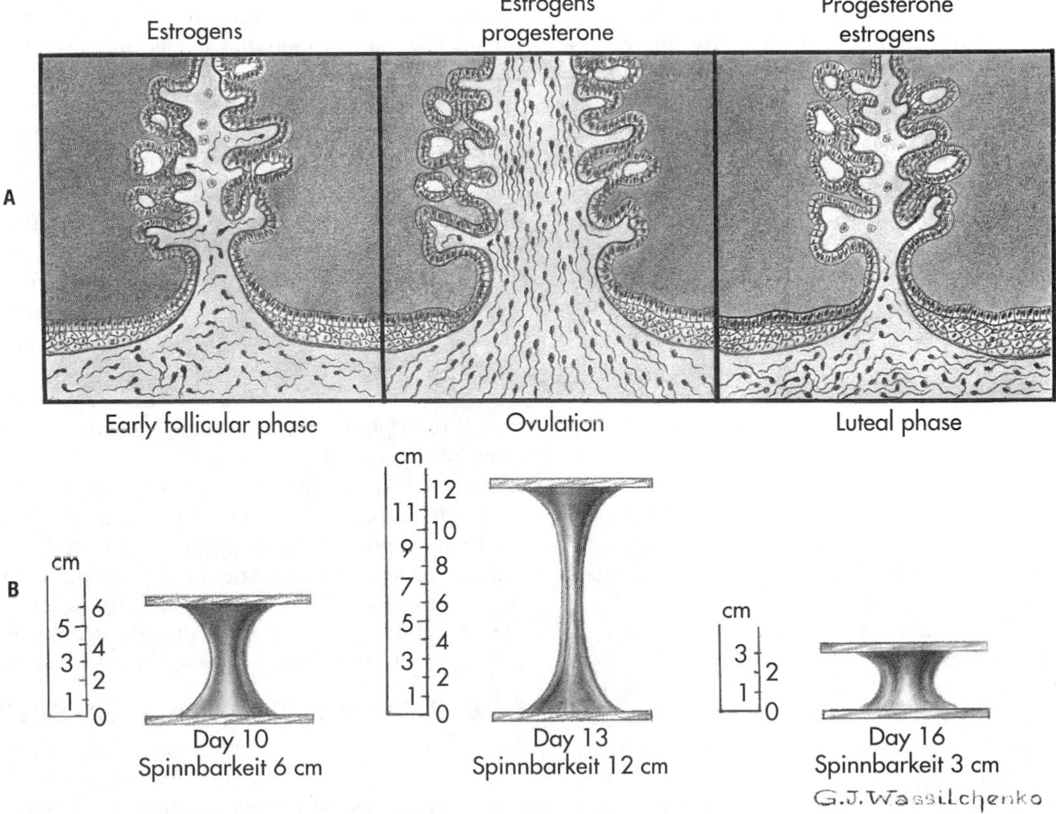

Fig. 3-22 Changes in cervix and in cervical mucus during menstrual cycle. **A,** Changes in opening of cervix that facilitates sperm migration. **B,** Characteristic stretchable quality of cervical mucus demonstrated between two glass slides.

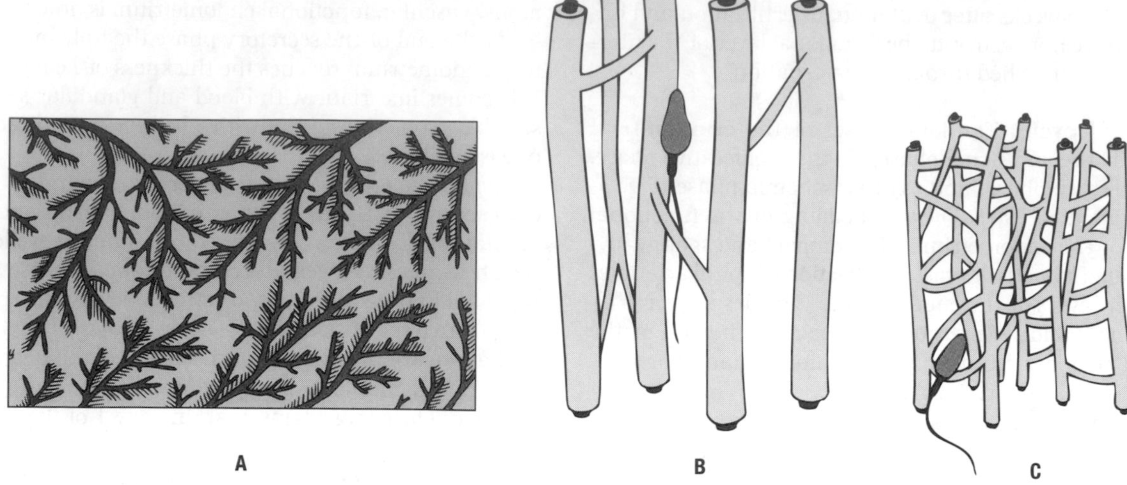

Fig. 3-23 Cervical mucus changes during menstrual cycle. **A,** Fern pattern under estrogen influence. **B,** Mucus receptive to sperm passage under estrogen influence. **C,** Mucus nonreceptive to sperm passage under progesterone influence.

thin and clear. It looks, feels, and stretches like egg white. This stretchable quality is termed *spinnbarkeit* (Fig. 3-22). Some women experience localized lower abdominal pain called *mittelschmerz* that coincides with ovulation.

These and other cyclic changes enhance fertility awareness and form the basis for the symptothermal method used for conception and contraception. The subjective and objective signs are biologic markers of the phases of the menstrual cycle (Table 3-1). Examination of women with impaired fertility includes a thorough documentation of the presence or absence of these biologic markers.

Prostaglandins. Prostaglandins (PGs) are oxygenated fatty acids now classified as hormones. The different types of PGs are distinguished by letters (PGE, PGF), numbers (PGE_2), and letters of the Greek alphabet ($PGF_{2\alpha}$).

PGs are produced in most organs of the body but most notably by the prostate and the endometrium. Therefore semen and menstrual blood are potent PG sources. PGs are metabolized quickly by most tissues. They are biologically active in minute amounts in the cardiovascular, gastrointestinal, respiratory, urogenital, and nervous systems. They also exert a marked effect on metabolism, particularly on glycolysis. PGs play an important role in many physiologic, pathologic, and pharmacologic reactions. $PGF_{2\alpha}$, PGE_1, and PGE_2 are most commonly used in reproductive medicine.

PGs affect smooth muscle contractility and modulation of hormonal activity. Indirect evidence supports effects of PGs on ovulation, fertility, changes in the cervix and cervical mucus that affect receptivity to sperm, tubal and uterine motility, sloughing of endometrium (menstruation), onset of abortion (spontaneous and induced), and onset of labor (term and preterm). After exerting their biologic actions, newly synthesized PGs are rapidly metabolized by tissues in such organs as the lungs, kidneys, and liver.

PGs may play a key role in ovulation. If PG levels do not rise along with the surge of LH, the ovum remains trapped within the graafian follicle. After ovulation, PGs may influence production of estrogen and progesterone by the corpus luteum.

The introduction of PGs into the vagina or into the uterine cavity (from ejaculated semen) increases the motility of uterine musculature, which may assist the transport of sperm through the uterus and into the oviduct. A high concentration of PGs in the semen may be necessary for normal fertility in males.

PGs produced by the woman cause regression of the corpus luteum, regression of the endometrium, and sloughing of the endometrium, which results in menstruation. PGs increase myometrial response to oxytocic stimulation, enhance uterine contractions, cause cervical dilation, and may be factors in initiating or maintaining labor. In addition, PGs may be involved in the following pathologic states: male infertility, dysmenorrhea, premenstrual syndrome, hypertensive states, preeclampsia-eclampsia, and anaphylactic shock.

Climacterium. The ***climacterium*** *(perimenopause)* is a transitional phase during which ovarian function and hormone production decline. This phase spans the years from the onset of premenopausal ovarian decline to the postmenopausal time when symptoms stop. **Menopause** (from the Latin *menis,* month, and the Greek *pausis,* to cease) refers only to the last menstrual period. However, unlike menarche, menopause can be dated with certainty only at 1 year after menstruation ceases. The average age at natural menopause is 51.4 years, with an age range of 35 to 60 years.

MALE REPRODUCTIVE SYSTEM

The male reproductive system consists of external genitalia and internal organs located in the pelvic cavity. The male's reproductive system begins to develop in response to testosterone during early fetal life. Essentially, no testosterone is produced during childhood. Resumption of testosterone production at the onset of puberty stimulates growth and maturation of reproductive structures and secondary sex charac-

TABLE 3-1 Signs and symptoms of phases of the menstrual cycle

SIGN	PREOVULATION	OVULATION	AT LEAST 2 DAYS AFTER OVULATION UP TO MENSES
Subjective signs			
Physical discomfort			
Breasts	Unreported	Unreported	Heaviness, fullness; enlarged, tender*
Abdomen	Dysmenorrhea: uterine cramping; nausea, vomiting, and diarrhea; dizziness	Intermenstrual pain (mittelschmerz) occurs 1.7 days after peak of cervical mucus and 2.5 days before increase in BBT	Premenstrual syndrome: backaches, feeling of increasing pelvic fullness
General	Increased weight, feeling of heaviness	Unreported	Headache,† acne
Affective changes‡			
Moods	Some depression may persist from premenses	Sense of well-being	Premenstrual syndrome (PMS): increased irritability, passivity, depression
Libido	Unreported	Increased sexual desire	Unreported
Energy levels	Unreported	Unreported	Spurt of energy, followed by fatigue
Objective signs			
Basal body temperature (BBT)	Individualized, often below 37° C (98.6° F)	Slight drop in BBT	Rise of about 0.2-0.4° C (3°-6° F)
Respiration	Unreported	Unreported	Hyperventilation with decrease in alveolar carbon dioxide tension
Heart rate	Unreported	Unreported	Increased slightly
Breasts	Time of least hormonal effect and smallest breast size	Increased nipple erectility, increased areolar pigmentation	Increased nodularity, enlarged
Cervix (Figs. 3-22 and 3-23)			
Mucus characteristics	"Dry" (no mucus) progressing to viscous, opaque; no ferning	Abundant, thin, clear (egg-white) mucus with spinnbarkeit (4 cm, often up to 10 cm) that dries in a fern pattern (arborization); facilitates sperm transport	Cloudy, sticky, impenetrable to sperm; dries in granular pattern (no ferning)
Mucus pH	About 7.0	7.5	Unreported
Os	Gradual, progressive widening	Open, with mucus seen spilling out	Gradual closing of os
Color of exocervix	Pink	Hyperemic (red)	Gradual return to pink
Body	Firm to touch (like tip of nose)	Soft (like earlobe)	Gradual return to firm

*Sociocultural influences may affect symptoms reported by women. Breast tenderness is rarely reported by Japanese women.
†Headaches reported with greater frequency by Nigerian women.
‡NOTE: Literature usually attributes negative premenstrual symptoms to biology, whereas good moods and rational behavior are not. When men and women are compared in activity patterns, mood changes, and symptoms, similar variability has been found in *both* men and women even though the changes in women are given more attention by society.

teristics. The size and appearance of external genitalia vary with age, heredity, race, and culture.

External Structures

The structures that make up the external genitalia are presented in the following order: mons pubis, penis, and scrotum.

At maturity, pubic hair is long, dense, coarse, and curly, forming a diamond-shaped pattern from the umbilicus to the anus. The area over the symphysis pubis is referred to as the *mons pubis.*

The *penis,* an organ of urination and copulation, consists of the shaft, or body, and the glans (Fig. 3-24). The shaft of this external male reproductive organ, which enters the vagina during coitus, is composed of three cylindric layers and erectile tissue: two lateral *corpora cavernosa* and a *corpus spongiosum,* which contains the urethra. These corpora terminate distally in the smooth, sensitive *glans penis,* which is the counterpart of the female glans clitoris.

Skin and fascia loosely envelop the penis to permit enlargement during erection. The glans is the enlarged end of the penis that contains many sensitive nerve endings and a urethral meatus at the tip (usually). The *urethra* is a common passageway for both urine and semen (Figs. 3-24 and 3-25). The *prepuce* (foreskin), an extended fold of skin, covers the glans in uncircumcised males (Fig. 3-25). In the newborn the foreskin is generally not retractable and may not be retractable for up to 2 years. It is easily retractable in the adolescent and the adult. With sexual arousal, neurocirculatory factors cause considerable increase in blood flow to the erectile tissue of the corpora, and enlargement and erection of the penis occur.

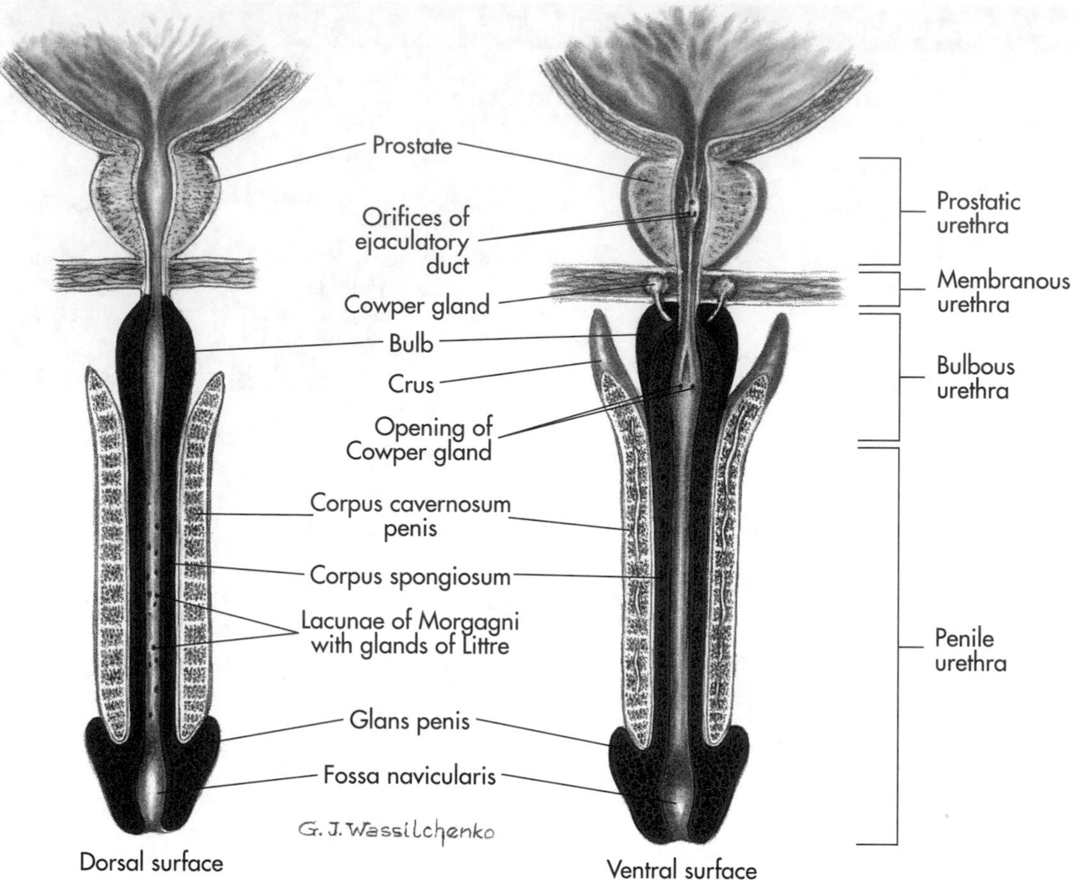

Fig. 3-24 Anatomy of urethra and penis.

The *scrotum*, a wrinkled pouch of skin, muscles, and fascia (Fig. 3-25), is divided internally by a septum, and each compartment normally contains one *testis*, *epididymis*, and *vas deferens* (seminal duct). The left side of the scrotum hangs somewhat lower (about 1 cm) than the right side. The skin is abundantly supplied with sebaceous and sweat glands and is sparsely covered with hair. Contraction and relaxation of smooth muscles under the skin result in retraction of the testes to protect them from external trauma and cold. During hot external (environmental) or internal (fever) temperature the muscles relax, lowering the testes away from the body. Conversely, cold external temperature stimulates contraction of the muscles to bring the testes close to the body.

The purpose of this mobility is to maintain the testes within an optimum temperature range for the production and viability of sperm. Hot tubs, tight underwear (jockey shorts) and pants, and long-term sitting (long-distance truck driving or cycling) present too hot an external environment or prevent testicular mobility so that spermatogenesis and sperm are jeopardized.

Internal Structures

Internal structures include testes, ducts of the testes, and accessory reproductive tract glands (Figs. 3-24 and 3-25).

Testes. The *testes* are two small oval glands located within the scrotal sac. They are suspended by attachment to scrotal tissue and the spermatic cord. Originally located in the abdomen, the testes descend through the inguinal canal by the end of the seventh lunar month of fetal life. By the ninth month, one testis or both testes may still be within the inguinal canals, with final descent into the scrotal sac occurring in the early postnatal period. The testes must be within the scrotum for spermatogenesis to occur.

The testes are similar in origin (homologous) to the ovaries in the female. Each testis is whitish, somewhat flattened from side to side and in the adult, measures about 4 or 5 cm in length. White fibrous tissue encases each testis and divides it into several lobules. Within each lobule are narrow, coiled *seminiferous tubules* about 5 to 7.5 cm long and clusters of *interstitial cells (Leydig cells)*. Spermatids attach to the germinal epithelium (Sertoli cells) within the seminiferous tubules and develop into sperm. The interstitial cells are large connective and supportive tissue (stromal) cells responsible for the production of the androgen hormone testosterone.

The two principal functions of the testes are spermatogenesis and hormone production. Primitive sex cells (spermatogonia) are present in the seminiferous tubules of the male newborn. *Spermatogenesis*, the maturation process that results in

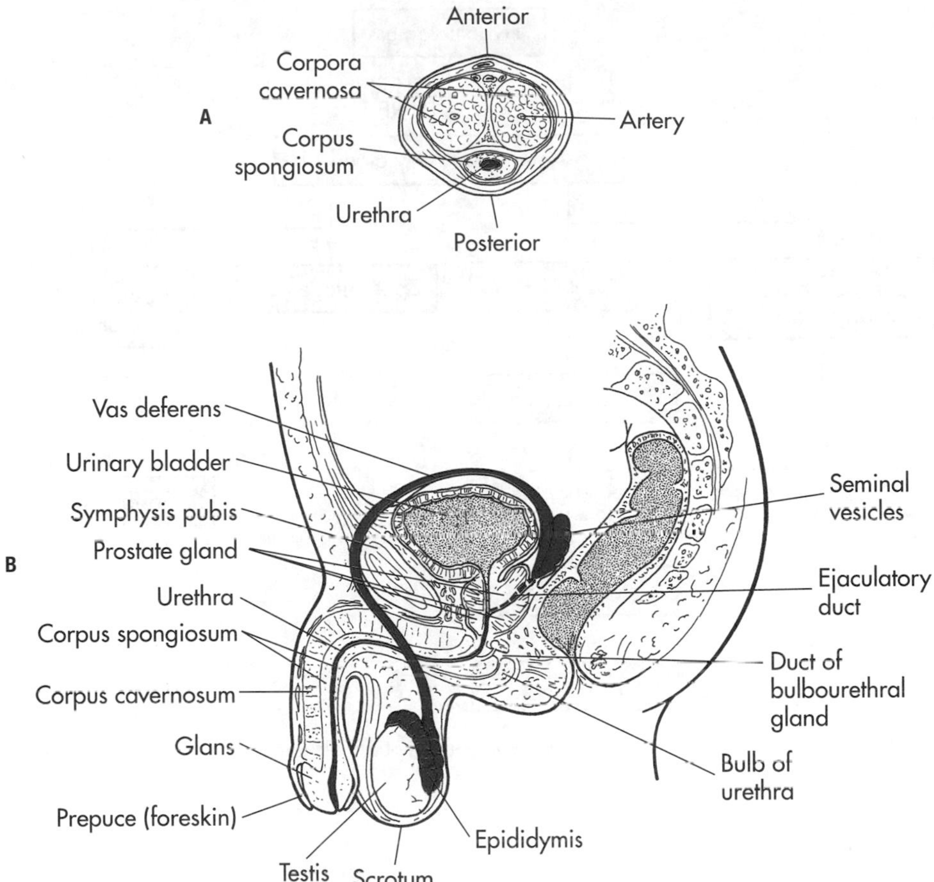

Fig. 3-25 Fascial planes of male lower genitourinary tract. **A,** Transverse section of penis. **B,** Relationship of bladder, prostate, seminal vesicles, penis, urethra, and scrotal contents.

sperm, begins during puberty and normally continues throughout a man's lifetime. The testes secrete the steroid sex hormone testosterone in the amounts that are required for normal male growth, development, and function.

Ducts (canals) of the testes. For sperm to exit the body, they must travel the full length of the duct system in succession: seminiferous tubules (mentioned earlier), epididymides (pl.), vasa deferentia (pl.), ejaculatory ducts, and the urethra. Each testis has one tightly coiled tube, about 6 m in length. This tube, the *epididymis* (Fig. 3-25), lies along the top and side of each testis. The epididymides are storage sites for maturing sperm and produce a small part of the seminal fluid (semen). Seminiferous tubules are continuous with the epididymides, which in turn connect to the vasa deferentia. When the vasa deferentia are cut or occluded for sterilization, the procedure is called a *vasectomy*.

Accessory reproductive system glands. Accessory reproductive glands secrete fluids that support the life and function of sperm. These glands include the paired *seminal vesicles*, located along the lower posterior surface of the bladder; the *prostate gland*, which surrounds the prostatic urethra; and the *bulbourethral (Cowper glands)*, located below the prostate, one at either side of the membranous urethra (Figs. 3-24 and 3-25).

Semen. Semen is the fluid ejaculated at the time of orgasm. Semen contains sperm and secretions from the seminal vesicles, prostate gland, and bulbourethral glands. An average volume per ejaculation after several days of continence (no ejaculations) is 2 to 5 ml (range: 1 to 7 ml). The volume of semen and sperm count decrease rapidly with repeated ejaculations. Semen contains constituents that provide nourishment, support and enhance sperm motility, and buffer the acidic environment of the cervical and vaginal fluids.

Semen is white to opalescent with a specific gravity of 1.028. The pH is alkaline, ranging from 7.2 to 7.8. Sperm count averages 60 million/ml, with more than 60% normal forms. About 60% of the total fluid is derived from the seminal vesicles and about 20% from the prostatic glands. Some fluid is secreted by the bulbourethral glands and probably the urethral glands.

Less than 5% of the ejaculate consists of sperm and fluid from the testes and epididymides. Since vasectomy affects only the production of this portion of the ejaculate, there is no

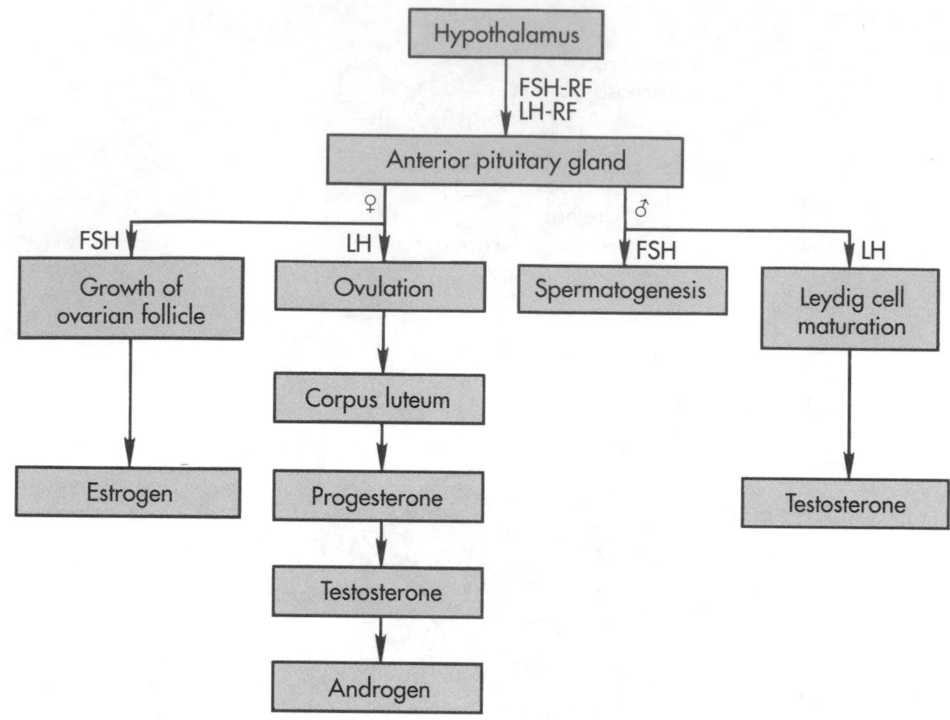

Fig. 3-26 Hypothalamic-pituitary-gonadal axis; comparison of female and male. *RF,* Releasing factor.

noticeable change in volume, even after sperm are no longer available for transport through the remaining canal system.

SEXUAL RESPONSE

The hypothalamus and anterior pituitary gland in females and males regulate the production of FSH and LH. The target tissue for these hormones is the gonad: an ovary or testis. In the female the ovary produces ova and secretes estrogen and progesterone and small amounts of testosterone; in the male the testis produces sperm and secretes testosterone. A *feedback mechanism* involving hormone secretion from the gonads, hypothalamus, and anterior pituitary aids in the control of the production of sex cells and steroid sex hormone secretion (Figs. 3-21 and 3-26).

Physiologic Response to Sexual Stimulation

Although the first outward appearance of maturing sexual development occurs at an earlier age in females than in males, both females and males achieve physical maturity at about age 17. Individuals' rates of development vary greatly. Despite anatomic and reproductive differences, women and men are more alike than different in their physiologic response to sexual excitement and orgasm. For example, the glans clitoris and the glans penis are embryonic homologues (Fig. 3-1). Little difference exists between female and male sexual response; the physical response is essentially the same whether the source of stimulation is coitus, fantasy, or mechanical/manual.

Physiologically, according to Masters and Johnson (1966), sexual response can be analyzed in terms of two processes: vasocongestion and myotonia.

Sexual stimulation results in a vasocongestive reflex dilation of penile blood vessels (erection in the male) and circumvaginal blood vessels (lubrication in the female), causing engorgement and distention of the genitalia. Venous congestion is localized primarily in the genitalia, but it also occurs to a lesser degree in the breasts and other parts of the body.

Arousal is characterized by myotonia (increased muscular tension), resulting in voluntary and involuntary rhythmic contractions. Examples of sexually stimulated myotonia are pelvic thrusting, facial grimacing, and spasms of the hands and feet (carpopedal spasms).

This **sexual response cycle** is arbitrarily divided into the following four phases: excitement, plateau, orgasm, and resolution. The four phases occur progressively, with no sharp dividing line between any two phases. Specific body changes take place in sequence. The time, intensity, and duration for cyclic completion also vary for individuals and situations. Table 3-2 compares male and female body changes during each phase of the four phases of the sexual response cycle.

PSYCHOSOCIAL ASPECTS OF SEXUALITY

Sexuality is a complex phenomenon influenced by a variety of biophysical, psychologic, sociocultural, and ethical factors. Biologic sex is determined at conception through the combination of egg and sperm. However, the development of sexuality begins in utero and extends throughout the life span.

In a culture characterized by a rapid increase in knowledge and technology, many people still are misinformed about sexuality. The following list shows some common myths about

TABLE 3-2 Four phases of sexual response

REACTIONS COMMON TO BOTH SEXES	FEMALE REACTIONS	MALE REACTIONS
Excitement phase		
Heart rate and blood pressure increase. Nipples become erect. Myotonia begins.	Clitoris increases in diameter and swells. External genitals become congested and darken. Vaginal lubrication occurs; upper two thirds of vagina lengthen and extend. Cervix and uterus pull upward. Breast size increases.	Erection of penis begins; penis increases in length and diameter. Scrotal skin becomes congested and thickens. Testes begin to increase in size and elevate toward body.
Plateau phase		
Heart rate and blood pressure continue to increase. Respirations increase. Myotonia becomes pronounced; grimacing occurs.	Clitoral head retracts under clitoral hood. Lower one third of vagina becomes engorged. Skin color changes occur; red flush may be observed across breasts, abdomen, or other surfaces.	Head of penis may enlarge slightly. Scrotum continues to grow tense and thicken. Testes continue to elevate and enlarge. Preorgasmic emission of 2 or 3 drops of fluid appears on head of penis.
Orgasmic phase		
Heart rate, blood pressure, and respirations increase to maximum levels. Involuntary muscle spasms occur. External rectal sphincter contracts.	Strong rhythmic contractions are felt in clitoris, vagina, and uterus. Sensations of warmth spread through pelvic area.	Testes elevate to maximum level. Point of "inevitability" occurs just before ejaculation with awareness of fluid in urethra. Rhythmic contractions occur in penis. Ejaculation of semen occurs.
Resolution phase		
Heart rate, blood pressure, and respirations return to normal. Nipple erection subsides. Myotonia subsides.	Engorgement in external genitalia and vagina resolves. Cervix and uterus descend to normal position. Breast size decreases. Skin flush disappears.	Fifty percent of erection is lost immediately with ejaculation; penis gradually returns to normal size. Testes and scrotum return to normal size. Refractory period (time needed for erection to occur again) varies according to age and general physical condition.

expressions of sexuality and reproduction (Stuart and Sundeen, 1995):

1. A couple must have simultaneous climaxes (orgasms) if conception is to take place.
2. A woman can become pregnant only through penile penetration or artificial insemination.
3. Urination by the woman after coitus or having sexual intercourse in a standing position will prevent pregnancy.
4. The woman determines the sex of the child.
5. Excessive masturbation is harmful.
6. Sex during menstruation is unclean and harmful.
7. Advancing age means the end of sex.
8. Oral and anal intercourse are perverted or dangerous.

Men and women tend to view sexuality differently. For example, men may think of sexuality in terms of specific numbers of activities, whereas women may focus on the meaning of a particular activity. However, no two people (man or woman) experience and express their sexuality in the same way. Sexuality is unique and individual and changes according to a person's sexual and life experiences.

Sexuality consists of at least four components: sexual response, sexual desire, view of oneself, and presentation of oneself (Bernhard, 1995). *Sexual response* refers primarily to the biophysical component of sexuality and includes the physical ability to engage in and respond to sexual activity (Table 3-2). *Sexual desire (libido)* refers to the urge (or lack thereof) for sexual activity. The intensity of sexual desire varies throughout the life span and is affected by hormonal changes (e.g., childbearing, menopause), fatigue, change of relationship with one's partner, illness and disability, and medication.

View of oneself *(gender identity)* and presentation of oneself *(sex role)* are two other important aspects of sexuality. Gender identity and sex role behaviors develop early in life (ages 2 to 4) as children identify with same-sex parents and mimic the behaviors of that parent. The feelings that children develop about themselves as sexual beings (heterosexual, homosexual, or bisexual) are related to these early experiences.

Expressions of gender identity and sex role behaviors vary with age and reflect the child's cognitive development (Piaget, 1950) and personality development (Erickson, 1959). Table 3-3 provides a review of cognitive and personality development.

TABLE 3-3 Summary of cognitive and personality development

STAGE	SIGNIFICANT OTHERS	COGNITIVE DEVELOPMENT (PIAGET)	PERSONALITY DEVELOPMENT (ERIKSON)
Infancy (birth to 18 months)	Maternal (parental) person ↓	Sensorimotor: reflex ⇄ repetition ⇄ imitation	Trust vs. mistrust
Toddlerhood (18 months to 3 years)	Parental persons and other family members ↓	Preoperational, direct experience	Autonomy vs. shame and doubt
Early childhood (3 to 6 years)	Parental persons and other family members ↓	Preoperational, direct experience	Initiative vs. guilt
Middle childhood (6 to 12 years)	Neighborhood and school ↓	Concrete thinking (not abstract)	Industry vs. inferiority
Adolescence (12 to 18 years)	Peer groups and models of leadership ↓	Formal thinking (deductive and abstract reasoning) may be limited up to 15 years	Identity vs. identity confusion, role diffusion
Early adulthood	Partners in friendship, sex, competition, and cooperation ↓	Formal thinking includes problem solving and separation of fantasy and fact	Intimacy and solidarity vs. isolation
Young and middle adulthood	Divided labor and shared household ↓	Formal thinking	Generativity vs. self-absorption, stagnation
Later adulthood (after climacterium)	Humankind, family, and friends	Formal thinking	Ego integrity vs. despair

For example, a toddler may dress up and "play mommy," whereas an adolescent may actively seek a maternal role. Selected expressions of gender identity and sex role behaviors may also give some information about gender preference: same sex, other, or both. Sexuality is dynamic; how sexuality is expressed at one moment may be different later in life.

NURSING IMPLICATIONS

The nurse is in a unique position to provide counseling and guidance to sexually maturing and sexually active individuals as well as to expectant and new parents. The role of educator is important for nurses working with families during the childbearing and childrearing years. Parents often need help with teaching their children about sex because adults are often misinformed and feel uncomfortable about many aspects of sexuality, reproduction, and body function. Accurate information about sexuality helps parents provide a supportive environment for sexual development and teach their children to be healthy, responsible sexual beings.

Parents with adolescents require additional help and information as the adolescents confront body image concerns, attempt to establish independence and mature relationships, explore sexuality, and develop socially responsible behaviors. In interactions with adolescents, nurses should provide accurate information in a private, confidential, and nonjudgmental manner and should reflect an awareness of peer and family influences and ethnocultural background.

Besides helping with childhood and adult sexuality, the nurse can help prepare patients for the sexual concerns and changes occurring with age. Many nurses have not been aware of the importance of sexuality education for older people because of the myth that the elderly are no longer interested in sex.

Sexual dysfunction problems often begin after children are born. The mother especially may become so involved with childrearing that her relationship with her partner suffers. At the same time the partner may be actively involved in career establishment, thereby leaving little energy for home life. The nurse needs to be aware of how the demands of parenting can adversely affect relationships. Simple counseling provided during these early years may prevent serious problems in later years.

The older woman in particular who has been able to move gracefully into old age and who continues to recognize herself as a sexual being is probably better able to accept the sexuality of the young. The pregnancy of a daughter then may be accepted as a continuation of her own sexuality rather than as a threat or reminder of her lost youth.

Knowledge about and comfort with one's own sexuality are important for the establishment of therapeutic relationships. A nonjudgmental nurse who recognizes personal sexual biases can contribute much to the sexual health of families. A sensitivity to alternative life-styles can help the nurse provide comprehensive care, for example, to a gay/lesbian family. Many gay/lesbian families are choosing to parent, whether through insemination, an intentional heterosexual encounter, adoption, or a previous heterosexual relationship (Deevey, 1995). Nurses can recognize potential problems and intervene, or if they are not comfortable, refer such patients to other professionals or agencies.

Box 3-1 lists questions pertinent to a sexuality screening history.

BOX 3-1
Sexual Screening History

The sexual screening history consists of at least the following five questions:

1. Are you sexually active?
   (If "No," When were you last sexually active?)
2. Do you have (or have you had) any discomfort, difficulties, or other problems during intercourse (sexual activity)*?
   (If "Yes," Do these bother you?)
3. Have you had more than one sexual partner?
   (If "Yes," How many and how long ago?)
4. Have you had any pain on urination (passing water) or unusual discharge from your genitalia?
   (If "Yes," take a history of this.)
5. Are you in a relationship in which someone physically abuses you?
   (If "Yes," explore further; inquire about safety.)

If the person has marital or emotional difficulties, ask the following:

6. How does your partner feel about your *X* (whatever the current problem is)?
7. Has *X* led to problems with how you relate to your partner or your partner relates to you, for example, emotionally and sexually?
8. If "Yes," In particular, what sexual problems have arisen or have been associated with *X*?

Modified from Ross M, Channon-Little L: *Discussing sexuality: a guide for health practitioners,* Sydney, 1991, MacLennan & Petty.
*Gay or lesbian clients may be sexually active but not have vaginal intercourse.

Critical Thinking Exercises

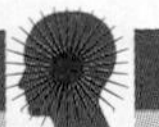

SEXUALITY EDUCATION

Age, gender, culture, religion, and life experiences affect feelings about sexuality. Therefore different content and teaching approaches are appropriate when conducting classes in reproductive anatomy and sexuality with groups of varying ages in different settings. Develop a content outline for a reproductive anatomy and sexuality education class, select appropriate teaching methods, and justify the selection of the content and teaching methods for each of the following three groups of young people:
1. Family-life class at the local junior high school
2. Young adult group from a local church
3. Group of students from a coed dormitory on the campus of a local college

Key Points

- The myometrium of the uterus is uniquely designed to expel the fetus and promote hemostasis after birth.
- Normal feedback regulation of the menstrual cycle depends on an intact hypothalamic-pituitary-gonadal mechanism.
- The female's reproductive tract structures and breasts respond predictably to changing levels of sex steroids across the life span.
- The development and maintenance of the male reproductive system throughout the life span depend on the steroid sex hormone testosterone.
- PGs play an important role in reproductive functions by their effect on smooth muscle contractility and modulation of hormones.
- Nurses need to be aware of their own feelings and values regarding sexuality before they can adequately and competently help patients meet their needs for information or refer them for further counseling.

References

Bernhard L: *Sexuality in women's lives.* In Fogel C, Woods N: *Women's health care,* Thousand Oaks, Calif, 1995, Sage.

Deevey S: *Lesbian health care.* In Fogel C, Woods N: *Women's health care,* Thousand Oaks, Calif, 1995, Sage.

Erickson E: *Identity and the life cycle: selected papers.* In *Psychological issues,* New York, 1959, International Universities Press.

Herbst A et al: *Comprehensive gynecology,* ed 2, St Louis, 1992, Mosby.

Masters W, Johnson V: *Human sexual response,* Boston, 1966, Little, Brown.

Piaget J: *The psychology of intelligence,* Boston, 1950, Routledge & Kegan Paul.

Ross M, Channon-Little L: *Discussing sexuality: a guide for health practitioners,* Sydney, 1991, MacLennon & Petty.

Stuart G, Sundeen S: *Principles and practice of psychiatric nursing,* ed 5, St Louis, 1995, Mosby.

Bibliography

Bass D: *The evolution of desire: strategies of human mating,* New York, 1994, Basic.

Butler R et al: Love and sex after 60: how to evaluate and treat the sexually-active woman, *Geriatrics* 49(11):33, 1994.

Davidson J, Moore N: Masturbation and premarital sexual intercourse among college women: making choices for sexual fulfillment, *J Sex Marital Ther* 20(3):178, 1994.

Graber J et al: The antecedents of menarcheal age: heredity, family environment, and stressful life events, *Child Dev* 66(2):346, 1995.

Holzapfel S: Aging and sexuality, *Can Fam Physician* 40:748, 1994.

Jensen L et al: Societal and parental influences on adolescent sexual behavior, *Psychol Rep* 75(2):928, 1994.

Lalonde A: Clinical management of female genital mutilation must be handled with understanding, compassion, *Can Med Assoc J* 152(6):949, 1995.

McCleary P: Female genital mutilation and childbirth: a case report, *Birth* 21(4):221, 1994.

Niswender G et al: Luteal function: the estrous cycle and early pregnancy, *Biol Reprod* 50(2):239, 1994.

Wallach E, Zacur H: *Reproductive medicine and surgery,* St Louis, 1995, Mosby.

CHAPTER 4

Genetics, Conception, and Fetal Development

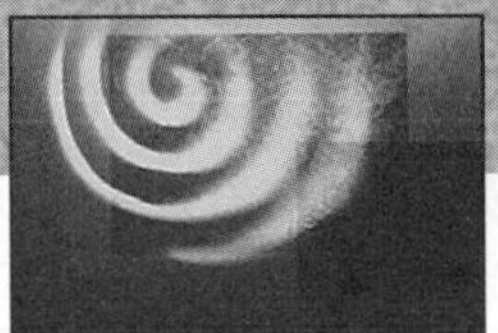

GENETICS, P. 51
Genes and chromosomes, p. 51
Cell division, p. 53
Gametogenesis, p. 54
Chromosomal abnormalities, p. 54
Patterns of genetic transmission, p. 56

CONCEPTION, P. 58

THE EMBRYO AND FETUS, P. 60
Development of the embryo, p. 60
Fetal maturation, p. 65
Multifetal pregnancy, p. 69
Nongenetic factors influencing development, p. 73

GENETIC COUNSELING, P. 73
Patients seeking genetic counseling, p. 74
Genetic counseling services, p. 74
Management of genetic disorders, p. 74
Role of the nurse in genetic counseling, p. 75

PRECONCEPTION CARE, P. 75
Role of the nurse, p. 77

This chapter presents a brief overview of the genetic basis of inheritance and the origin of common genetic disorders. The main focus of the discussion is the process of fertilization and the development of the normal embryo and fetus. The role of the nurse in genetics counseling and preconception is addressed.

GENETICS

Human development is a complicated process that depends on the systematic unraveling of instructions found in the genetic material of the egg and sperm. Development from conception to birth of a normal, healthy baby occurs without incident in most cases; occasionally, however, some anomaly in the genetic code of the embryo creates a birth defect or disorder. Parents are then left to wonder what went wrong, which parent might be "responsible," or most significantly, what are the chances of the problem recurring with the next pregnancy. The science of genetics seeks to explain the underlying causes of congenital disorders (disorders present at birth) and the patterns in which inherited disorders are passed from generation to generation. A basic understanding of genetics helps the professional nurse assist families to locate the resources (often genetics counselors) to help them cope with the questions and fears surrounding birth defects.

Genes and Chromosomes

The hereditary material carried in the nucleus of each somatic (body) cell determines an individual's physical characteristics. This material, called *deoxyribonucleic acid (DNA)*, forms threadlike strands known as **chromosomes.** Each chromosome is composed of many smaller segments of DNA referred to as **genes.** Genes or combinations of genes contain coded information that determines an individual's unique characteristics. The "code" is found in the specific linear order of the molecules that combine to form the strands of DNA. The Human Genome Project, funded by the National Institutes of Health, is involved in mapping information on the human genome (Ott, 1995). This map will facilitate study of hereditary diseases and will provide the potential for making changes at the gene level to treat or prevent hereditary diseases (Box 4-1).

All normal human somatic cells contain 46 chromosomes arranged as 23 pairs of homologous (matched) chromosomes; one chromosome of each pair is inherited from each parent. There are 22 pairs of **autosomes,** which control most traits in the body, and one pair of **sex chromosomes,** which determines sex and some other traits. The large female chromosome is called the *X;* the tiny male chromosome is the *Y.* When X and Y chromosomes are present, the embryo de-

BOX 4-1
The Human Genome Project
Jenkins J, RN, MSN and Collins F, MD, Ph D

The Human Genome Project is a federally funded, coordinated effort to assemble data on the genetic instructions found within human DNA and within DNA of several model organisms (Box 4-2) (Collins, 1995; Guyer and Collins, 1995). The ultimate goal of the project is the complete sequencing of all 3 billion base pairs of human DNA. This includes the development of genetic and physical maps that facilitate the identification of human disease genes by *positional cloning* (Table 4-1). This strategy allows the identification of disease genes without prior information about their biologic function. The focus of genetics specialists has previously been on rare genetic disorders; however, virtually every disease (except trauma) has a genetic component. Medical genetics is now poised to uncover these genetic predispositions, opening the possibility of highly sophisticated diagnostic and therapeutic strategies.

Genes that contribute to common polygenic conditions such as diabetes, hypertension, most forms of cancer, and the major mental illnesses will be identified by this approach. These gene discoveries will lead to molecular insights that will revolutionize the treatment of disease, using gene therapy or "designer drug" strategies. For many diseases, however, health care professionals will be able to predict risks but will not be able to intervene with effective treatment for some time (Scanlon and Fibison, 1995). This creates a dilemma for all health care providers. As genetic testing becomes available for risk prediction for diseases such as cancer or Alzheimer's disease, many questions will arise. How reliable is the test? What do these results mean in terms of the actual risk of developing the disease? How useful is this information? What preventive or treatment recommendations will be available based on test results? Laboratories providing genetic testing need to be monitored for quality control of genetic test results; criteria must be established to define when a test should be done only in a research setting. DNA testing, like the administration of a drug, has potential side effects and risks that need to be studied in clinical trials and managed appropriately (Andrews et al, 1994).

Until now, most physicians and nurses have not had the opportunity to incorporate genetics into their practice. An imminent challenge is to prepare providers to be able to include components of genetic risk assessment in all health care delivery, including screening, counseling, education, surveillance, and treatment, and to use this information wisely. Because of widespread concerns about misuse of information gained through genetic testing, 5% of the Human Genome Project budget is designated for research into the Ethical, Legal, and Social Implications (ELSI) Program of the project (U.S. Department of Health and Human Services, 1995). Issues of high priority for ELSI have included genetic privacy, the safety and efficacy of genetic testing, informed consent, and the potential for genetic discrimination in health insurance and employment. A recent ruling of the Equal Employment Opportunities Commmission (EEOC) renders employment discrimination on the basis of future genetic susceptibility illegal, based on the provisions of the Americans with Disabilities Act. Legislation is urgently needed to address discrimination in health insurance (Hudson et al, 1995).

All health care specialties will be required to distill this evolving body of knowledge and use the genetics information to facilitate consumer decision making. Nurses, with their long tradition of combining clinical skills and attention to the whole person, are in a critical position to lead the way.

National Center for Human Genome Research, National Institutes of Health.

BOX 4-2
Goals of the Human Genome Project

Genetic maps
Physical maps
DNA sequencing
Gene identification
Technology development
Model organisms
Informatics
Ethical, Legal, and Social Implications (ELSI) Program
Training
Technology transfer
Outreach

National Center for Human Genome Research, National Institutes of Health.

velops as a male. When two X chromosomes are present, the embryo develops as a female.

Because each gene occupies a specific chromosome location, and because chromosomes are inherited as homologous pairs, each person has two genes for every trait. In other words, if an autosome has a gene for hair color, its partner also has a gene for hair color—in the same location on the chromosome. Although both genes code for hair color, however, they may not code for the same hair color. Different genes coding for different variations of the same trait are called **alleles.** An individual with two copies of the same allele for a given trait is said to be homozygous for that trait; with two different alleles, the person is heterozygous for the trait.

Some genes are **dominant,** and their characteristics are expressed even if another allele is present on the other chromosome. Other genes are **recessive,** and their characteristics are expressed only if they are carried by both homologous chromosomes. For example, the gene for brown eyes is dominant over the gene for blue eyes. Thus a person with one gene

TABLE 4-1 Disease genes identified by positional cloning

YEAR	DISEASE	YEAR	DISEASE
1986	Chronic granulomatosus disease	1994	Aarskog-Scott syndrome
	Duchenne muscular dystrophy		Congenital adrenal hypoplasia
	Retinoblastoma		Emery-Dreifuss muscular dystrophy
1989	Cystic fibrosis		Machado-Joseph (Azorean) disease
1990	Wilms tumor	1995	Spinal muscular atrophy
	Neurofibromatosis type 1		Chondrodysplasia punctata
	Testis determining factor		Limb-girdle muscular dystrophy
	Choroideremia		Ocular albinism
1991	Fragile-X syndrome		Ataxia telangiectasia
	Familial polyposis coli		Alzheimer's disease (chromosome 14)
	Kallmann syndrome		Alzheimer's disease (chromosome 1)
	Aniridia		Hypophosphatemic rickets
1992	Myotonic dystrophy		Hereditary multiple exostoses
	Lowe syndrome		Bloom syndrome
	Norrie disease		Early-onset breast cancer (BRCA2)
1993	Menkes disease	1996	Friedreich's Ataxia
	X-linked agammaglobulinemia		Progressive Myoclonic Epilepsy
	Glycerol kinase deficiency		Treacher Collins Syndrome
	Adrenoleukodystrophy		Long QT Syndrome (Chromosome 11)
	Neurofibromatosis type 2		Barth Syndrome
	Huntington disease		Simpson-Golabi-Behmel Syndrome
	Von Hippel–Lindau disease		Werner's Syndrome
	Spinocerebellar ataxia I		X-Linked Retinitis Pigmentosa (RP3)
	Lissencephaly		Polycystic Kidney Disease, Type 2
	Wilson disease		Basal Cell Nevus Syndrome
	Tuberous sclerosis		X-Linked Myotubular Myopathy
1994	McLeod syndrome		Anhidrotic Ectodermal Dysplasia
	Polycystic kidney disease		Hemochromatosis
	Dentatorubral pallidoluysian atrophy		Chediak-Higashi Syndrome
	Fragile X "E"		Hereditary Multiple Exostoses (EXT2)
	Achondroplasia		Fanconi Anemia A
	Wiskott-Aldrich syndrome		Hermansky-Pudlak Syndrome
	Early-onset breast/ovarian cancer (BRCA1)		Spinocerebellar Ataxia 2
	Diastrophic dysplasia		CADASIL (Hereditary Stroke)

National Center for Human Genome Research, National Institutes of Health.

for brown eyes and one gene for blue eyes will have brown eyes.

When an egg and a sperm unite, the combination of alleles becomes that individual's entire genetic makeup, or **genotype,** which includes all the genes that the person carries and that can be passed to offspring. The genotype determines the person's physical appearance, or **phenotype,** but this is affected by the nature of the dominant or recessive allele. To continue the previous example, an individual with two brown-eyes alleles at the gene for eye color will have the same phenotype as one with brown-eyes and one blue-eyes allele; that is, both individuals will have brown eyes.

The pictorial analysis of the number, form, and size of an individual's chromosomes is known as a **karyotype.** A karyotype can be obtained from a blood sample specially treated and stained to make the replicating chromosomes visible under a microscope. The photographed chromosomes are cut out and arranged in a specific numeric order according to their length and shape. Fig. 4-1 illustrates the chromosomes in a body cell and a karyotype. Karyotypes can be used to determine the sex of a child and the presence of any gross chromosomal abnormalities.

Cell Division

Cells are reproduced by two different methods: mitosis and meiosis. In mitosis, the body cells replicate to yield two cells with the same genetic makeup as the parent cell. First the cell makes a copy of its DNA; then it divides, and each daughter cell receives one copy of the genetic material. The purpose of mitotic division is for growth and development or cell replacement.

Meiosis produces **gametes** (eggs and sperm). Each homologous pair of chromosomes contains one chromosome received from the mother and one from the father; thus meiosis results in cells that contain one of each of the 23 pairs of chromosomes. Because these germ cells contain 23 single chromosomes, half the genetic material of a normal somatic cell, they are said to be *haploid.* When the female gamete (egg

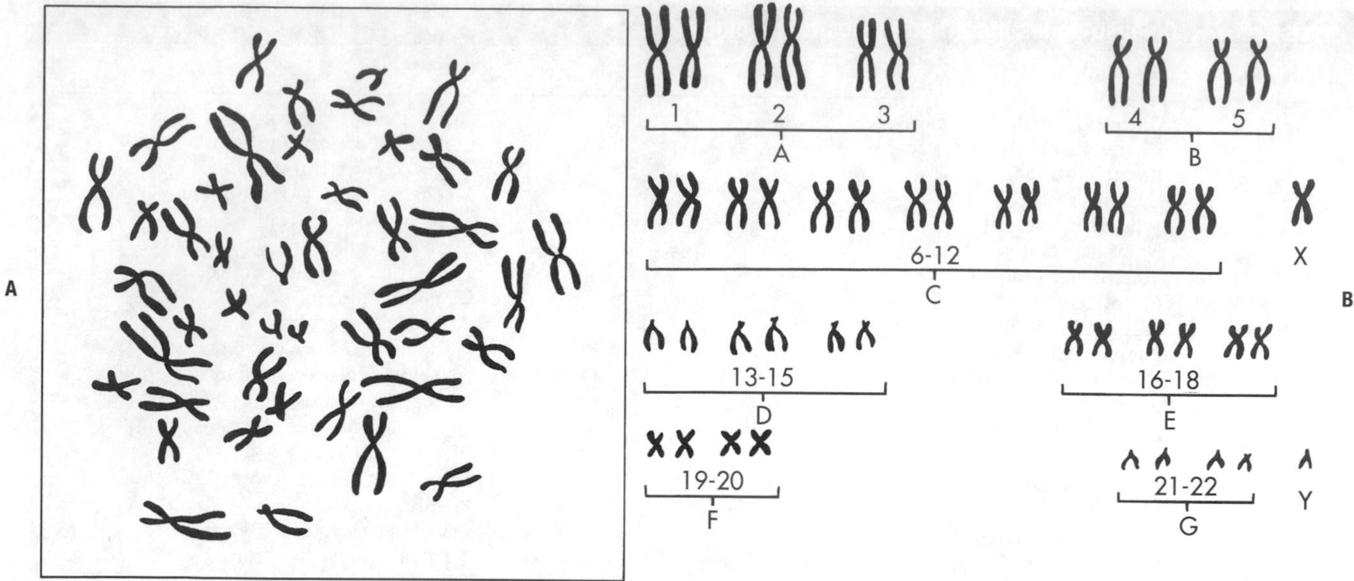

Fig. 4-1 Chromosomes during cell division. **A,** Example of photomicrograph. **B,** Chromosomes arranged in karyotype; female and male sex-determining chromosomes.

or ovum) and the male gamete (spermatozoon) unite to form the zygote, the diploid number of human chromosomes (46, or 23 pairs) is restored.

The process of DNA replication and cell division in meiosis allows different alleles for genes to be distributed at random by each parent and then rearranged on the paired chromosomes. The chromosomes then separate and proceed to different gametes. Because parents have genotypes derived from four different grandparents, many combinations of genes on each chromosome are possible. This random mixing of alleles accounts for the variation of traits seen in the offspring of the same two parents.

Gametogenesis

When a male reaches puberty, his testes begin the process of spermatogenesis. The only cells that undergo meiosis in the male are spermatocytes. The primary spermatocyte, which undergoes the first meiotic division, contains the diploid number of chromosomes. The cell has already copied its DNA before division, so four alleles for each gene are actually present. Because the copies are bound together—one allele plus its copy on each chromosome—the cell is still considered diploid.

During the first meiotic division, two haploid secondary spermatocytes are formed, each containing 22 autosomes and one sex chromosome; one contains the X chromosome (plus its copy) and the other the Y chromosome (plus its copy). During the second meiotic division the male produces two gametes with an X chromosome and two gametes with a Y chromosome, all of which will develop into viable sperm (Fig. 4-2, *A*).

Oogenesis, the process of egg (ovum) formation, begins during fetal life of the female. All the cells that may undergo meiosis in a woman's lifetime are contained in her ovaries at birth. The majority of the estimated 2 million primary oocytes (the cells that undergo the first meiotic division) degenerate spontaneously. Only 400 to 500 ova will mature during the approximately 35 years of a woman's reproductive life. The primary oocytes begin the first meiotic division (i.e., they replicate their DNA) during fetal life but remain suspended at this stage under puberty. Then, usually monthly, one primary oocyte matures and completes the first meiotic division, yielding two unequal cells: the secondary oocyte and a small polar body. Both contain 22 autosomes and one X sex chromosome (Fig. 4-2, *B*).

At ovulation the second meiotic division begins. However, the ovum does not complete the second meiotic division unless fertilization occurs. Fertilization produces a second polar body and the **zygote** (the united egg and sperm). If fertilization does not occur, the ovum degenerates (Fig. 4-2, *C*).

Chromosomal Abnormalities

Errors resulting in chromosomal abnormalities can occur in either mitosis or meiosis. These occur in either the autosomes or the sex chromosomes. Even without the presence of obvious structural malformations, small deviations in chromosomes can cause problems in fetal development.

Autosomal abnormalities. Autosomal abnormalities involve differences in the number or structure of chromosomes resulting from unequal distribution of the genetic material during gamete formation. Some of the causes and clinical effects of these genetic problems are discussed next.

Abnormalities of chromosome number. Abnormalities of chromosome number, **aneuploidy,** are most often caused by nondisjunction. Nondisjunction occurs during meiosis when a pair of chromosomes fails to separate, and one resulting cell contains both chromosomes while the other contains none. The product of the union of a normal gamete with a gamete containing an extra chromosome is a *trisomy*. The resulting individual has 47 chromosomes in each cell.

The most common trisomal abnormality is **Down syn-**

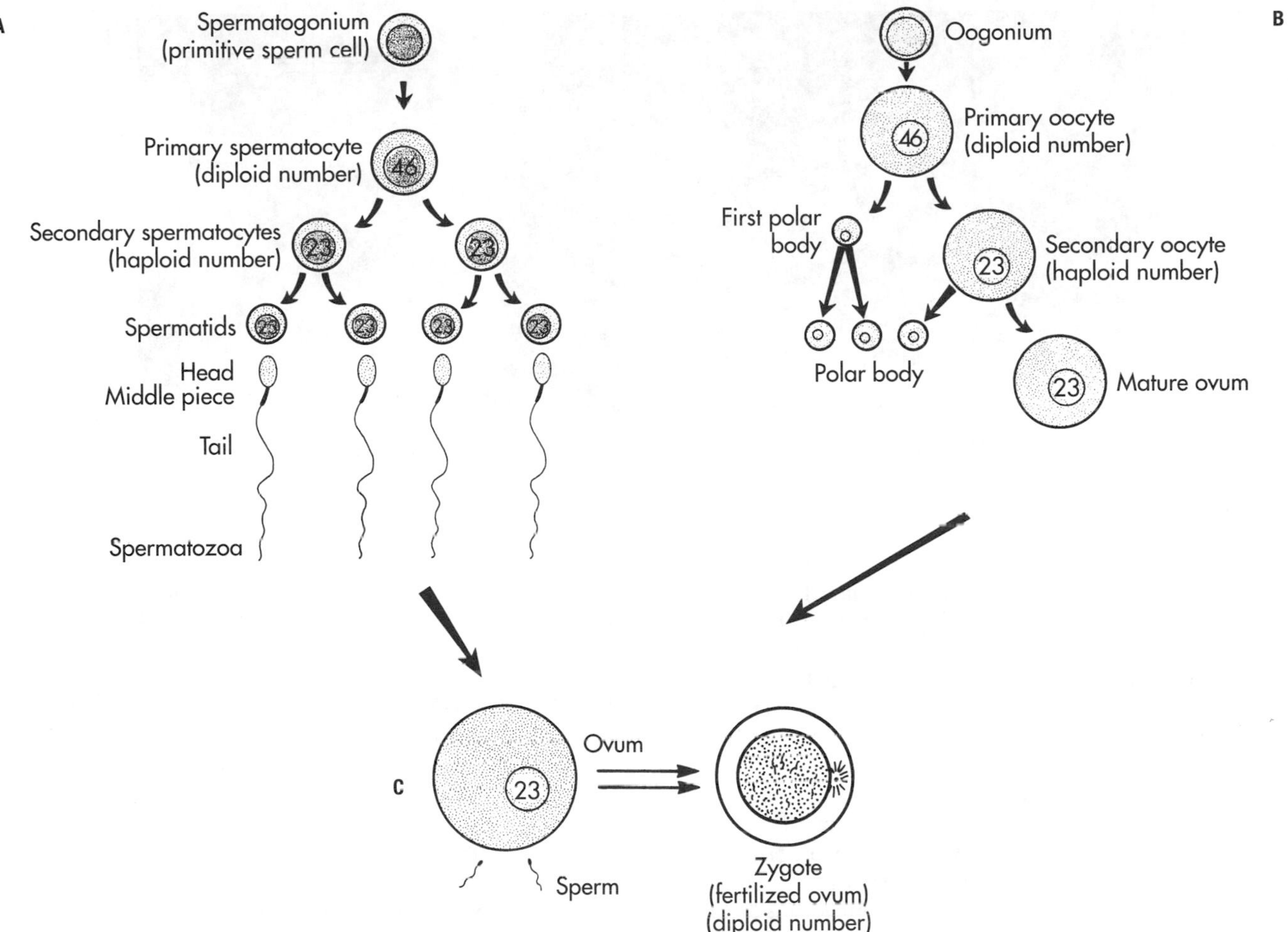

Fig. 4-2 **A**, Spermatogenesis. Gametogenesis in the male produces four mature gametes, the sperm. **B**, Oogenesis. Gametogenesis in the female produces one mature ovum and three polar bodies. Note relative difference in overall size between ovum and sperm. **C**, Fertilization results in the single-cell zygote and restoration of the diploid number of chromosomes.

drome, or trisomy 21. The affected individual has an extra chromosome 21. The clinical characteristics of Down syndrome include a broad, small skull; a flat facial profile; epicanthal folds with slanted palpebral fissures in the eyes; flat, low-set ears (Fig. 4-3, *A*); a protruding tongue; a short neck with fat pads at the nape; short, broad hands with a single transverse (simian) crease (Fig. 4-3, *B*); and hypotonic muscles with hypermobility of joints.

Individuals with Down syndrome have various degrees of mental retardation. There are increased incidences of congenital heart disease, infectious diseases, and acute childhood leukemia in individuals with Down syndrome. The incidence of Down syndrome increases with maternal or paternal age. Many affected embryos are spontaneously aborted, and some affected fetuses are stillborn.

Other autosomal trisomies that have been identified are trisomy 18 and trisomy 13. Both conditions have a very poor prognosis, with most affected children dying from cardiac or respiratory complications within 6 months of birth.

The product of the union of a normal gamete (ovum or sperm) with a gamete missing a chromosome is a **monosomy.** This individual would have only 45 chromosomes in each cell. Missing an autosomal chromosome always results in death of the embryo.

Nondisjunction can also occur during mitosis. If this occurs early in development when cell lines are forming, the individual has a mixture of cells, some with a normal number of chromosomes and others either missing a chromosome or containing an extra chromosome. This condition is known as **mosaicism.**

Mosaicism in the autosomes is most commonly seen as another form of Down syndrome. Depending on when the nondisjunction occurs during development, different body tissues will have different numbers of chromosomes. The clinical characteristics of Down syndrome may be present mildly or with varying degrees of severity, depending on the number and location of the abnormal cells. An individual with mosaic Down syndrome may have normal intelligence.

Abnormalities of chromosome structure. Abnormalities of chromosome structure involve chromosome breakage, usually resulting from one of two events: (1) translocation and (2) additions and/or deletions. Translocation occurs

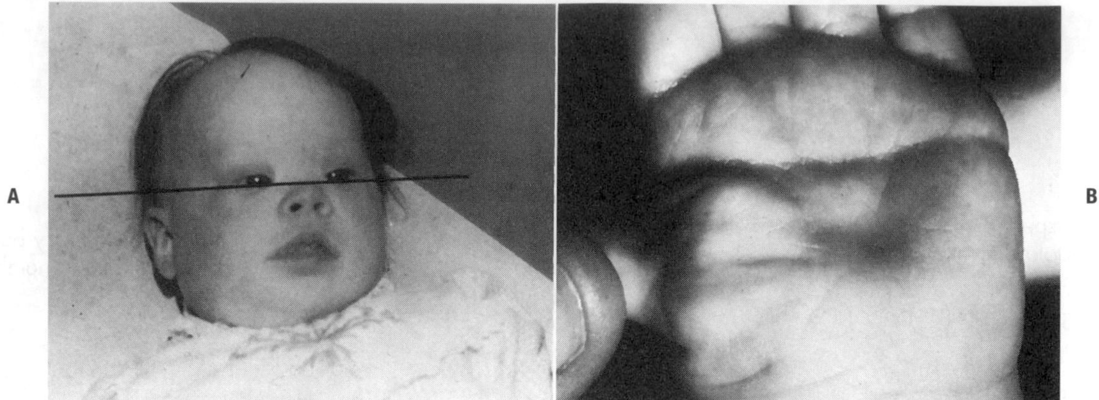

Fig. 4-3 Down syndrome (Trisomy 21). **A,** Low-set ears. **B,** Simian crease.

when genetic material is transferred from one chromosome to another different chromosome. Thus instead of two normal pairs of chromosomes, the individual has one normal chromosome of each pair and a third chromosome that is a fusion of the other two chromosomes. As long as all genetic material is retained in the cell, the individual is unaffected but is a carrier of what is known as a *balanced translocation.*

If a gamete receives the two normal chromosomes or the fused chromosome, the resulting offspring will be clinically normal. If the gamete receives one of the two normal chromosomes and the fused version, the resulting offspring will have an extra copy of one of the chromosomes. This condition is called an *unbalanced translocation* and often has serious clinical effects.

Whenever a portion of a chromosome is deleted from one chromosome and added to another, the gamete produced may have either extra copies of genes or too few copies. The clinical effects produced may be mild or severe depending on the amount of genetic material involved. Two of the more common conditions that have been described are the deletion of the short arm of chromosome 5 (cri du chat syndrome) and the deletion of the long arm of chromosome 18. Cri du chat syndrome, named after the typical mewing cry of the affected infant, causes severe mental retardation with microcephaly and unusual facial appearance. Deletion of the long arm of chromosome 18 causes severe psychomotor retardation with multiple organ malformations.

Sex chromosome abnormalities. Several sex chromosome abnormalities have been identified that are caused by nondisjunction during gametogenesis in either parent. The most common deviation in females is Turner syndrome, or monosomy X. The affected female is missing an X chromosome and exhibits juvenile external genitalia with undeveloped ovaries. She is usually short in stature with webbing of the neck. Intelligence may be impaired. Most affected embryos abort spontaneously.

The most common deviation in males is Klinefelter syndrome, or trisomy of the sex chromosomes XXY. The affected male has an extra X chromosome and exhibits poorly developed secondary sexual characteristics and small testes. He is infertile, usually tall, and effeminate. Males who are mosaic for Klinefelter syndrome may be fertile. Subnormal intelligence is usually present.

Patterns of Genetic Transmission

Heritable characteristics are those that can be passed on to offspring. The patterns by which genetic material is transmitted to the next generation are affected by the number of genes involved in the expression of the trait. Although many phenotypic characteristics result from two or more genes on different chromosomes acting together (referred to as *multifactorial inheritance*), others are controlled by a single gene *(unifactorial inheritance).*

Unlike chromosomal abnormalities, defects at the gene level cannot be determined by conventional laboratory methods such as karyotyping. Instead, genetic counselors predict the probability of the presence of an abnormal gene from the known occurrence of the trait in the individual's family and the known patterns by which the trait is inherited.

Multifactorial inheritance. Most common congenital malformations result from multifactorial inheritance, a combination of genetic and environmental factors. Examples are cleft lip, cleft palate, congenital heart disease, neural tube defects, and pyloric stenosis. Each malformation may range from mild to severe, depending on the number of genes for the defect present or the amount of environmental influence. A **neural tube defect** may range from spina bifida, a bony defect in the lumbar region of the vertebrae with little or no neurologic impairment, to anencephaly, absence of brain development, which is always fatal. Some malformations occur more often in one sex than the other. For example, pyloric stenosis and cleft lip are more common in males, and cleft palate is more common in females. Multifactorial disorders also tend to occur in families.

Unifactorial inheritance. If a single gene controls a particular trait, disorder, or defect, its pattern of inheritance is referred to as *unifactorial mendelian,* or *single-gene, inheritance.* The number of unifactorial abnormalities far exceeds the number of chromosomal abnormalities. This is understand-

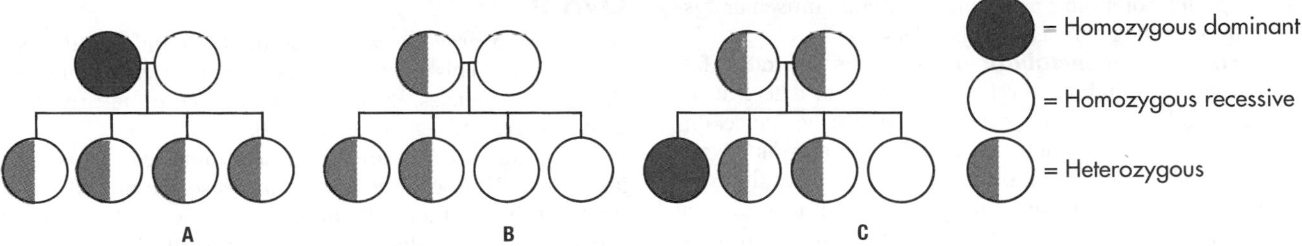

Fig. 4-4 Possible offspring in three types of matings. **A,** Homozygous-dominant parent and homozygous-recessive parent. Children all heterozygous, displaying dominant trait. **B,** Heterozygous parent and homozygous-recessive parent. Children 50% heterozygous, displaying dominant trait; 50% homozygous, displaying recessive trait. **C,** Both parents heterozygous. Children 25% homozygous, displaying dominant trait; 25% homozygous, displaying recessive trait; 50% heterozygous, displaying dominant trait.

able considering that 50,000 to 100,000 genes in the haploid number (23) of chromosomes are passed on to an offspring from each parent.

Unifactorial or single-gene disorders follow the inheritance patterns of dominance, segregation, and independent assortment described by Mendel and include autosomal dominant, autosomal recessive, and X-linked dominant and recessive modes of inheritance (Fig. 4-4).

Autosomal dominant inheritance. Autosomal dominant inheritance disorders are those in which the abnormal gene for the trait is expressed even when the other member of the pair is normal. The abnormal gene may appear as a result of a **mutation,** a spontaneous and permanent change in the normal gene structure, in which case the disorder occurs for the first time in the family. Usually an affected individual comes from multiple generations having the disorder. An affected parent who is heterozygous for the trait has a 50% chance of passing the abnormal gene to each offspring (Fig. 4-4, *B* and *C*). Males and females are equally affected.

Autosomal dominant disorders are not always expressed with the same severity of symptoms. The parent may have a minor abnormality that is not diagnosed until the birth of a more severely affected child. No way exists to predict whether an offspring will have a minor or a severe abnormality.

Examples of common autosomal dominantly inherited disorders are Marfan syndrome (disorder of connective tissue resulting in skeletal, ocular, and cardiovascular abnormalities) (Blackburn and Loper, 1992), achondroplasia (dwarfism), polydactyly (extra digits), Huntington's disease, and polycystic kidney disease.

Autosomal recessive inheritance. Autosomal recessive inheritance disorders are those in which both genes of a pair must be abnormal for the disorder to be expressed. Heterozygous individuals have only one abnormal gene and are unaffected clinically because their normal gene overshadows the abnormal gene. They are known as *carriers* of the recessive trait. Because these recessive traits are inherited by generations of the same family, an increased incidence of the disorder occurs in consanguineous matings (closely related parents). For the trait to be expressed, two carriers must each contribute the abnormal gene to the offspring (Fig. 4-4, *C*). There is a 25% chance of the trait occurring in each child. A clinically normal offspring may be a carrier of the gene. Males and females are equally affected.

Most recessive disorders tend to have severe clinical manifestations, and affected offspring do not often reproduce. If they do, all their offspring will be carriers for the disorder.

Most inborn errors of metabolism, such as phenylketonuria (PKU), galactosemia, maple syrup urine disease, Tay-Sachs disease, sickle cell anemia, and cystic fibrosis, are autosomal recessively inherited disorders.

X-linked dominant inheritance. **X-linked dominant inheritance** disorders occur in both males and heterozygous females. Because the females also have a normal gene, the effects are less severe than in affected males. Affected males transmit the abnormal gene only to their daughters on the X chromosome. Heterozygous females have a 50% chance of transmitting the abnormal gene to each offspring. An example of these extremely rare disorders is vitamin D–resistant rickets.

Fragile-X syndrome is a relatively new diagnosis. The "fragile site" on the X chromosome was identified in a central nervous system disorder affecting males and is also seen in heterozygous carrier females. Affected individuals are mentally handicapped.

X-linked recessive inheritance. Abnormal genes for **X-linked recessive inheritance** disorders are carried on the X chromosome. Females may be heterozygous or homozygous for traits carried on the X chromosome because they have two X chromosomes. Males are hemizygous because they have only one X chromosome carrying genes, with no alleles on the Y chromosome. Therefore X-linked recessive disorders are most often manifested in the male with the abnormal gene on his single X chromosome.

The male receives the defective gene from his carrier mother on her affected X chromosome. Female carriers (those heterozygous for the trait) have a 50% probability of transmitting the abnormal gene to each offspring. An affected male can pass the abnormal gene only to his daughters on the X chromosome, but not to his sons. The daughters will be carriers of the trait if they receive a normal gene on the X chromosome from their mother. They will be affected only if they receive an abnormal gene on the X chromosome from their mother as well as from their father.

Hemophilia, color blindness, and Duchenne muscular dystrophy are all X-linked recessive disorders.

Inborn errors of metabolism. Disorders of protein, fat, or carbohydrate metabolism reflecting absent or defective enzymes generally follow a recessive pattern of inheritance. Enzymes, the actions of which are genetically determined, are essential for all the physical and chemical processes that sustain body systems. Defective enzyme action interrupts the normal series of chemical reactions from the affected point onward. The result may be an accumulation of a damaging product such as phenylalanine or the absence of a necessary product such as thyroxin or melanin.

PKU is an uncommon disorder caused by autosomal recessive genes. A deficiency in the liver enzyme phenylalanine hydroxylase results in failure to metabolize the amino acid phenylalanine, allowing its metabolites to accumulate in the blood. The incidence of this disorder is 1 in every 10,000 to 20,000 births. The highest incidence is found in Caucasians from northern Europe and the United States. It is rarely seen in Jewish, African, or Japanese populations. Screening for PKU is routinely performed on all infants in the newborn nursery through a blood test.

Tay-Sachs disease, inherited as an autosomal recessive trait, results from a deficiency in hexosaminidase. It occurs primarily in Jewish families. Until 4 to 6 months of age, infants appear normal; in fact, their facial features are considered very beautiful. Then the clinical symptoms appear: apathy and regression in motor and social development and decreased vision. Death occurs between ages 3 and 4. No known treatment exists for Tay-Sachs disease.

Cystic fibrosis (mucoviscidosis or fibrocystic disease of the pancreas) is inherited as an autosomal recessive trait characterized by generalized involvement of exocrine glands. Clinical features are related to the altered viscosity of mucus-secreting glands throughout the body. It is a serious, chronic disease occurring primarily in Caucasians but can appear in those of mixed ancestry. Overall incidence is 1 per every 2000 births. It is thought that the incidence of the carrier state is 1:20 to 1:25. Advances in diagnosis and treatment have improved the prognosis so that now many affected individuals live to adulthood. Some affected women have borne children, but men generally are sterile. If the mother has cystic fibrosis and the father has no family history of the disease, offspring have a 50% chance of inheriting the gene for cystic fibrosis (MacMullen and Brucker, 1989).

Meconium ileus occurs in about 10% of newborns with cystic fibrosis. Although an initial stool may be passed from the rectum with none thereafter, usually no meconium is passed during the first 24 to 48 hours. The abdomen becomes increasingly distended, and eventually the newborn requires a laparotomy for diagnosis and treatment of the condition.

CONCEPTION

Conception, defined as the union of a single egg and sperm, marks the beginning of a pregnancy. Conception does not occur in isolation; a series of events surround it. These events include gamete (egg and sperm) formation, ovulation (release of the egg), and union of the gametes (which results in an embryo). Implantation of the embryo in the uterus is the next event in the sequence.

Ovum

As discussed previously, meiosis in the female produces an egg, or ovum. This process occurs in the ovaries, specifically in the ovarian follicles. Each month, one ovum matures with a host of surrounding supportive cells.

At ovulation the ovum is released from the ruptured ovarian follicle. High estrogen levels increase the motility of the uterine tubes so their cilia are able to capture the ovum and propel it through the tube toward the uterine cavity. The ovum cannot move by itself.

Two protective layers surround the ovum (Fig. 4-5). The first layer is a thick, acellular layer, the zona pellucida. The outer layer, the corona radiata, is composed of elongated cells.

Ova are considered fertile for about 24 hours after ovulation. If unfertilized by a sperm, the ovum degenerates and is reabsorbed.

Sperm

Ejaculation during sexual intercourse normally propels almost a teaspoon of semen containing as many as 200 to 500 million sperm into the vagina. The sperm swim with the flagellar movement of their tails. Some sperm can reach the site of fertilization within 5 minutes, but average transit time is 4 to 6 hours. Sperm remain viable within the woman's reproductive system for an average of 2 to 3 days. Most sperm are lost in the vagina, within the cervical mucus, or in the endometrium, or they enter the tube that contains no ovum.

As the sperm travel through the female reproductive tract, enzymes are produced to aid in capacitation of the sperm. Capacitation is a physiologic change that removes the protective coating from the heads of the sperm. Small perforations then form in the acrosome (a cap on the sperm) and allow enzymes (e.g., hyaluronidase) to escape. These enzymes are necessary for the sperm to penetrate the protective layers of the ovum before fertilization.

Fertilization

Fertilization takes place in the ampulla (outer third) of the uterine tube. When a sperm successfully penetrates the membrane surrounding the ovum, both sperm and ovum are enclosed within the membrane, and the membrane becomes impenetrable to other sperm; this is termed the *zona reaction*. The second meiotic division of the oocyte is completed, and the ovum nucleus becomes the female pronucleus. The head of the sperm enlarges to become the male pronucleus, and the tail degenerates. The nuclei fuse and the chromosomes combine, restoring the diploid number (46) (Fig. 4-6). Conception, the formation of the zygote (the first cell of the new individual), has been achieved.

Mitotic cellular replication, called *cleavage*, begins as the zygote travels the length of the uterine tube into the uterus. This voyage takes 3 to 4 days. Because the fertilized egg divides rapidly with no increase in size, successively smaller cells, *blastomeres*, are formed with each division. A 16-cell **morula**, a solid ball of cells, is produced within 3 days. The morula is still surrounded by the protective zona pellucida. Further development occurs as the morula floats freely within the uterus. Fluid passes through the zona pellucida into the intercellular spaces between the blastomeres. A cavity forms within the cell mass as the spaces come together, forming a structure called the *blastocyst cavity*. When the cavity be-

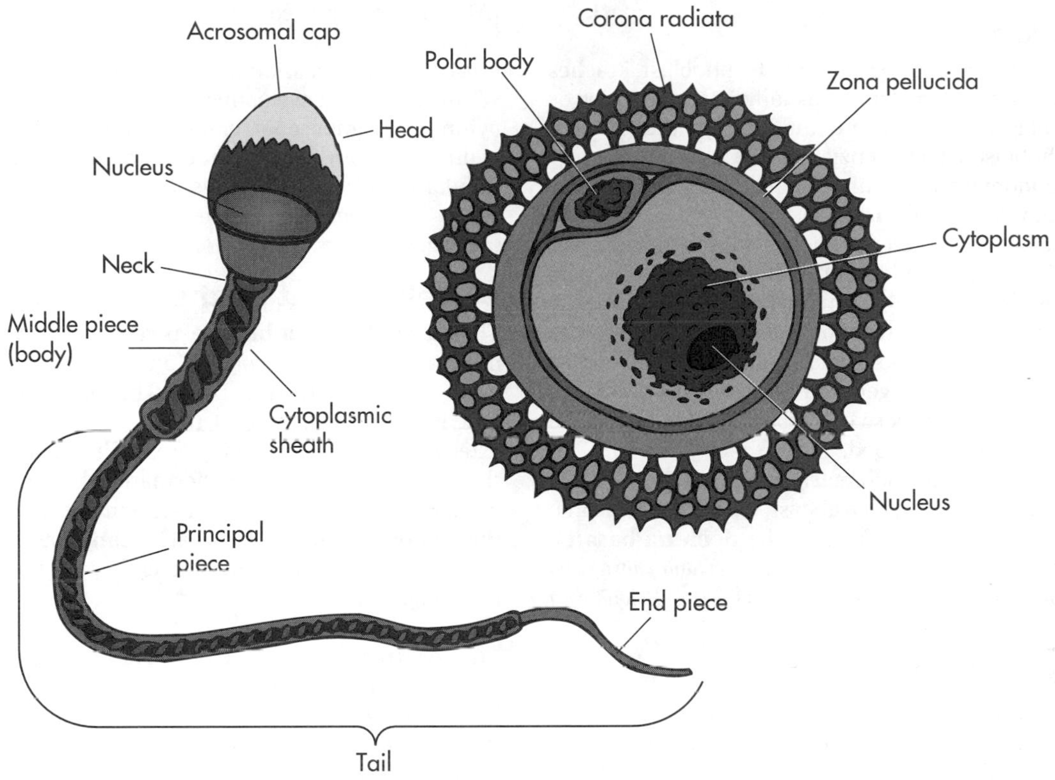

Fig. 4-5 Sperm and ovum.

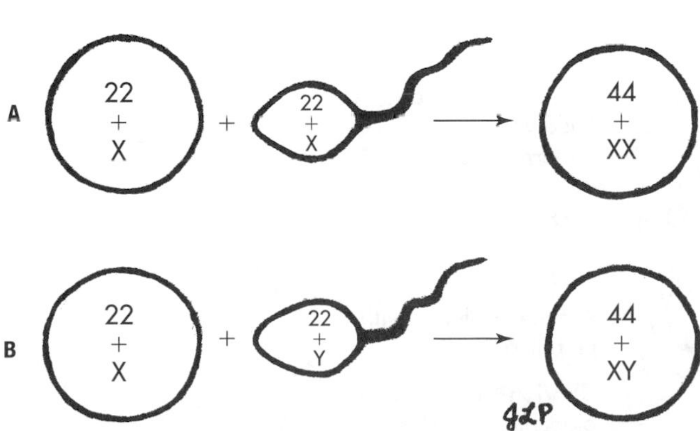

Fig. 4-6 Fertilization. **A,** Ovum fertilized by X-bearing sperm to form female zygote. **B,** Ovum fertilized by Y-bearing sperm to form male zygote.

Critical Thinking Exercises

THE ETHICS OF ADVANCES IN GENETICS

Several developments related to genetics have occurred recently. The Human Genome Project has identified a number of diseases by positional cloning. British researchers have cloned sheep. Sperm banks in the United States are storing thousands of samples of sperm. Fetal tissue is used to treat diseases.

1. What are ethical considerations related to these developments?
2. Are some of these developments ethical while others are not?
3. What considerations determine whether a development is ethical?
4. Who should decide what is ethical?

comes recognizable, the whole structure of the developing embryo is known as the **blastocyst.** The outer layer of cells surrounding the cavity is the *trophoblast.*

Implantation

The zona pellucida degenerates, and the trophoblast attaches itself to the uterine endometrium, usually in the anterior or posterior fundal region. Between 6 and 10 days after conception, the trophoblast secretes enzymes that enable it to burrow into the endometrium until the entire blastocyst is covered. This is known as **implantation.** Endometrial blood vessels erode, and some women experience slight implantation bleeding (slight spotting and bleeding during the time of the first missed menstrual period). **Chorionic villi,** fingerlike projections, develop out of the trophoblast and extend into the blood-filled spaces of the endometrium. These villi are vascular processes that obtain oxygen and nutrients from the maternal bloodstream and dispose of carbon dioxide and waste products into the maternal blood.

After implantation, the endometrium is called the *decidua.* The portion directly under the blastocyst, where the chorionic villi tap the maternal blood vessels, is the **decidua basalis.** The portion covering the blastocyst is the *decidua capsularis,* and the portion lining the rest of the uterus is the *decidua vera* (Fig. 4-7).

THE EMBRYO AND FETUS

Pregnancy lasts approximately 10 lunar months, 9 calendar months, 40 weeks, or 280 days. Length of pregnancy is computed from the first day of the last menstrual period (LMP) until the day of delivery (see discussion of Nägele's rule and adjustment for longer and shorter cycles, p. 123). However, conception occurs approximately 2 weeks after the first day of the LMP. Thus the postconceptional age of the fetus is 2 weeks less, for a total of 266 days or 38 weeks. Postconceptional age is used in the discussion of fetal development.

Intrauterine development is divided into three stages: ovum or preembryonic, embryo, and fetus. The stage of the ovum lasts from conception until day 14. This period covers cellular replication, blastocyst formation, initial development of the embryonic membranes, and establishment of the primary germ layers.

Development of the Embryo

The stage of the **embryo** lasts from day 15 until approximately 8 weeks after conception, or until the embryo measures 3 cm from crown to rump. This stage is the most critical time in the development of the organ systems and the main external features. Developing areas with rapid cell division are the most vulnerable to malformation by environmental **teratogens** (something that causes abnormal development). At the end of the eighth week, all organ systems and external structures are present, and the embryo is unmistakably human (Fig. 4-8).

Membranes. At the time of implantation, two **fetal membranes,** which will surround the developing embryo, begin to form. The *chorion* develops from the trophoblast and contains the chorionic villi on its surface. The villi burrowing into the decidua basalis increase in size and complexity as the vascu-

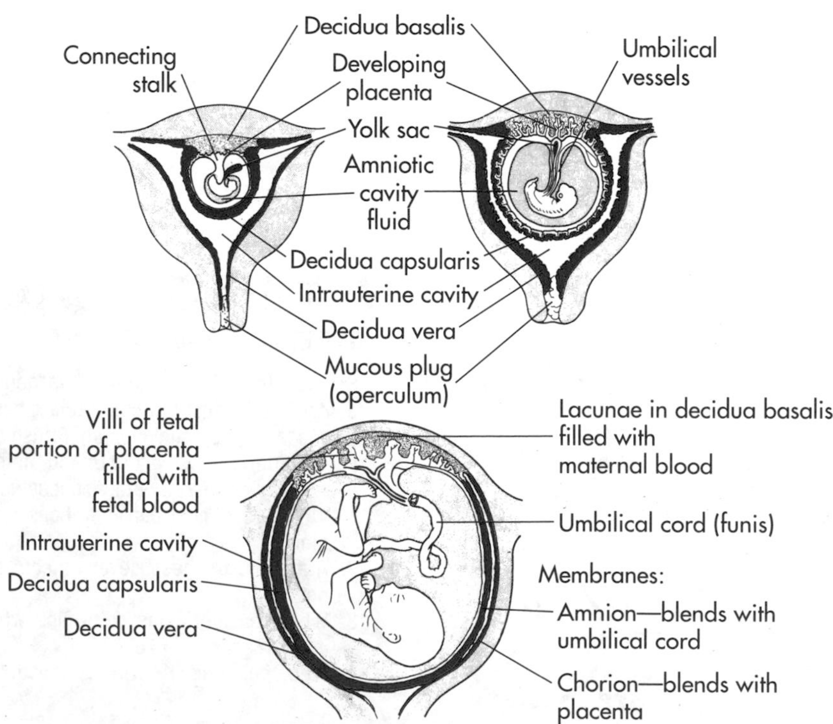

Fig. 4-7 Development of fetal membranes. Note gradual obliteration of intrauterine cavity as decidua capsularis and decidua vera meet. Also note thinning of uterine wall. Chorionic and amnionic membranes are in apposition to each other but may be peeled apart.

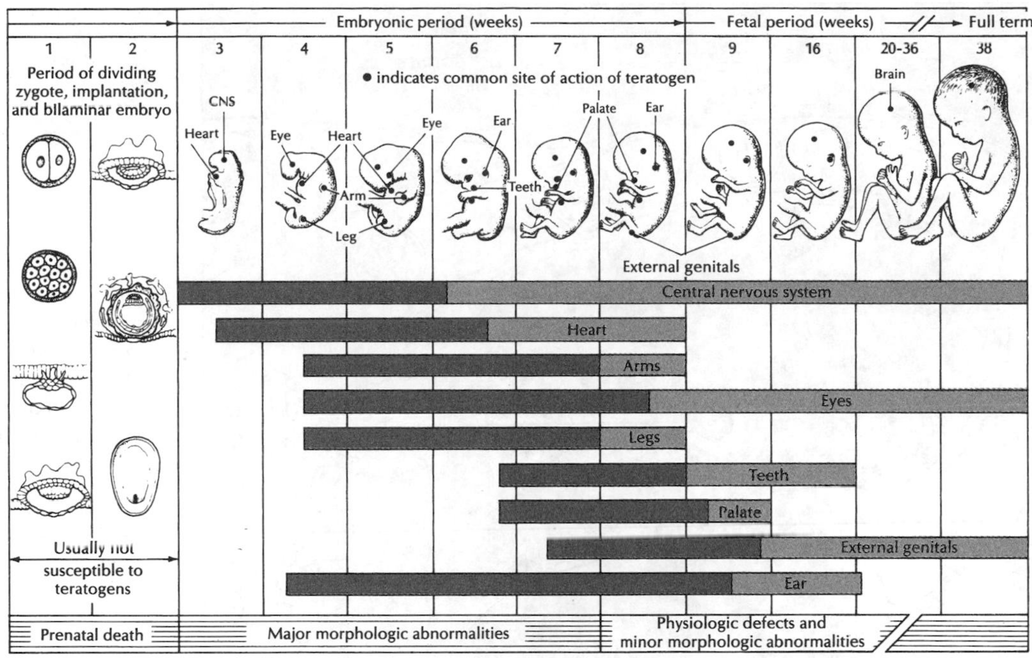

Fig. 4-8 Sensitive, or critical, periods in human development. Dark color denotes highly sensitive periods; light color indicates stages that are less sensitive to teratogens. (From Moore K: *Before we are born: basic embryology and birth defects*, ed 3, Philadelphia, 1989, Saunders.)

lar processes develop into the placenta. The chorion becomes the covering of the fetal side of the placenta. It contains the major umbilical blood vessels as they branch out over the surface of the placenta. As the embryo grows, the decidua capsularis becomes stretched. The chorionic villi on this side atrophy and degenerate, leaving a smooth chorionic membrane.

The inner cell membrane, the *amnion*, develops from the interior cells of the blastocyst. The cavity that develops between this inner cell mass and the outer layer of cells (trophoblast) is the amniotic cavity (Fig. 4-9). As it grows larger, the amnion forms on the side opposite to the developing blastocyst (Fig. 4-7). The developing embryo draws the amnion around itself, forming a fluid-filled sac. The amnion becomes the covering of the umbilical cord and covers the chorion on the fetal surface of the placenta. As the embryo grows larger, the amnion enlarges to accommodate both the embryo/fetus and its surrounding amniotic fluid. The amnion eventually comes in contact with the chorion surrounding the fetus.

Amniotic fluid. Initially the amniotic cavity derives its fluid by diffusion from the maternal blood. The amount of fluid increases weekly, so that normally 800 to 1200 ml of transparent liquid are present at term. The **amniotic fluid** volume changes constantly. The fetus swallows fluid, and fluid flows into and out of the fetal lungs. The fetus urinates into the fluid, greatly enhancing its volume.

The volume of amniotic fluid is an important factor in assessing fetal well-being (Hallak et al, 1993). Having less than 300 ml of amniotic fluid (oligohydramnios) is associated with fetal renal abnormalities. Having more than 2 L of amniotic fluid (hydramnios) is associated with gastrointestinal and other malformations.

Many functions are served by amniotic fluid for the embryo/fetus. Amniotic fluid helps maintain a constant body temperature. It serves as a source of oral fluid and as a repository for waste. It cushions the fetus from trauma by blunting and dispersing the forces. It allows freedom of movement for musculoskeletal development. It keeps the embryo from tangling with the membranes, facilitating symmetric growth of the fetus. If the embryo does intersect with the membranes, amputations of extremities or other deformities can occur from constricting amniotic bands (Reed, Claireaux, and Bain, 1989).

Amniotic fluid contains albumin, urea, uric acid, creatinine, lecithin, sphingomyelin, bilirubin, fructose, fat, leukocytes, proteins, epithelial cells, enzymes, and lanugo hair. Study of fetal cells in amniotic fluid through amniocentesis yields much information about the fetus. Genetic studies (karyotyping) provide knowledge about the sex and normality of chromosome number and structure. Other studies determine the health or maturity of the fetus.

Yolk sac. At the same time the amniotic cavity and amnion are forming, another blastocyst cavity has formed on the other side of the developing embryonic disk (Fig. 4-9). This cavity becomes surrounded by a membrane, forming the yolk sac. The yolk sac aids in transferring maternal nutrients and oxygen, which have diffused through the chorion, to the embryo. Blood vessels form to aid transport. By the third week, blood cells and plasma are manufactured in the yolk sac. At the end of the third week, the primitive heart begins to beat

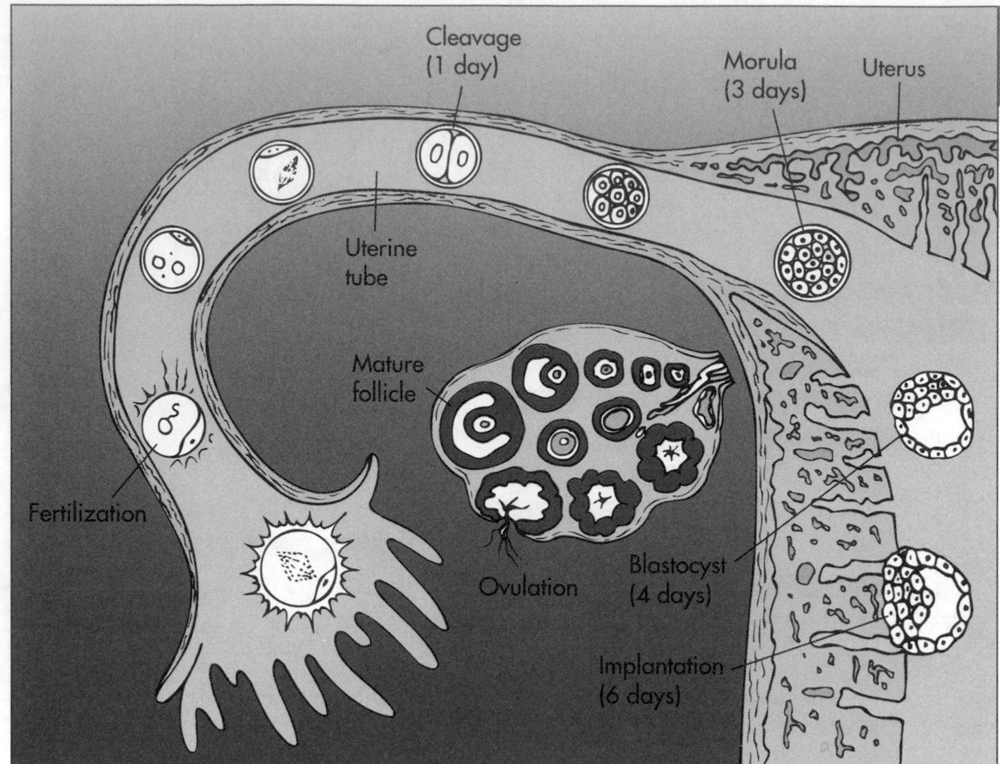

Fig. 4-9 **A,** First weeks of human development. Follicular development in ovary, ovulation, fertilization and transport of early embryo down uterine tube and into uterus, where implantation occurs. **B,** Blastocyst embedded in endometrium. Germ layers forming.

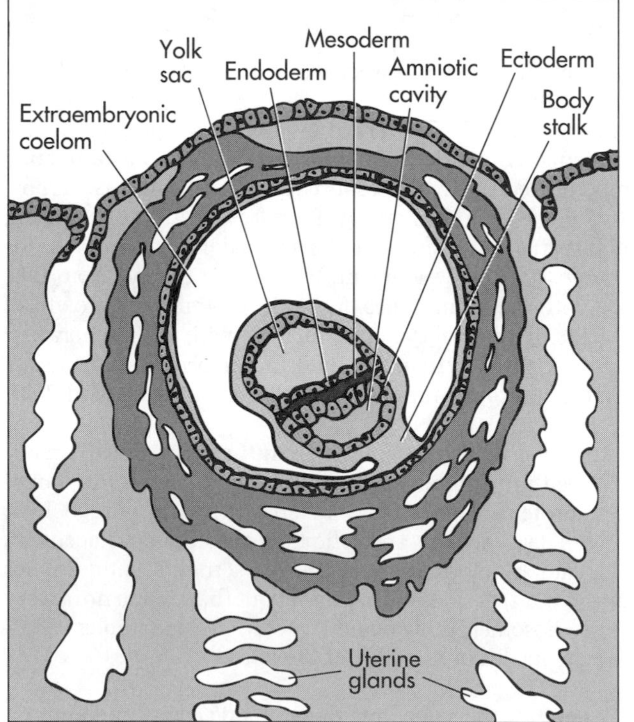

and circulate the blood through the embryo, connecting stalk, chorion, and yolk sac.

The folding in of the embryo during the fourth week results in part of the yolk sac being incorporated into the embryo's body as the primitive digestive system. Primordial germ cells arise in the yolk sac and move into the embryo. The shrinking remains of the yolk sac degenerate. By the fifth or sixth week the remnant has separated from the embryo.

Primary germ layers. During the third week after conception the embryonic disk differentiates into three primary germ layers: the ectoderm, mesoderm, and endoderm or entoderm (Fig. 4-9). All tissues and organs of the embryo develop from these three layers.

The *ectoderm,* the upper layer of the embryonic disk, gives rise to the epidermis, glands, nails and hair, the central and peripheral nervous systems, lenses of the eyes, tooth enamel, and the floor of the amniotic cavity.

The middle layer, the *mesoderm,* develops into the bones and teeth, muscles (skeletal, smooth, and cardiac), dermis and connective tissue, cardiovascular system and spleen, and urogenital system.

The lower layer, the *endoderm,* gives rise to the epithelium lining the respiratory tract and digestive tract, including the oropharynx, liver and pancreas, urethra, bladder, and vagina. The endoderm forms the roof of the yolk sac.

Umbilical cord. By day 14 after conception the embryonic disk, amniotic sac, and yolk sac are attached to the chorionic villi by the connecting stalk. During the third week the blood vessels develop to supply the embryo with maternal nutrients and oxygen. During the fifth week, after the embryo has curved inward on itself from both ends, bringing the connecting stalk to the ventral side of the embryo, the connecting stalk becomes compressed from both sides by the amnion, forming the narrower **umbilical cord** (Fig. 4-7). Two arteries carry blood from the embryo to the chorionic villi, and one vein returns blood to the embryo. One percent of umbilical cords contain only two vessels: one artery and one vein. This occurrence is sometimes associated with congenital malformations.

The cord rapidly increases in length. At term the cord ranges from 30 to 90 cm long (average 55 cm) and is 2 cm in diameter. It twists spirally on itself and loops around the embryo/fetus. A true knot is rare, but false knots occur as folds or kinks in the cord. Connective tissue called *Wharton's jelly* prevents compression of the blood vessels to ensure continued nourishment of the embryo/fetus. Compression can occur if the cord lies between the fetal head and the pelvis or is twisted around the fetal body. When the cord is wrapped around the fetal neck, it is called a *nuchal cord.*

As the placenta develops from the chorionic villi, the umbilical cord is usually located centrally. A peripheral location is less common and is known as a *battledore placenta* (Fig. 4-10, *D*). The blood vessels are arrayed out from the center to all parts of the placenta.

Placenta

Structure. During the third week after conception the trophoblast cells of the chorionic villi continue to invade the decidua basalis. As the uterine capillaries are tapped, the endometrial spiral arteries fill with maternal blood. The chorionic villi grow into the spaces with two layers of cells: the outer syncytium and the inner cytotrophoblast. A third layer develops into anchoring septa, dividing the projecting decidua

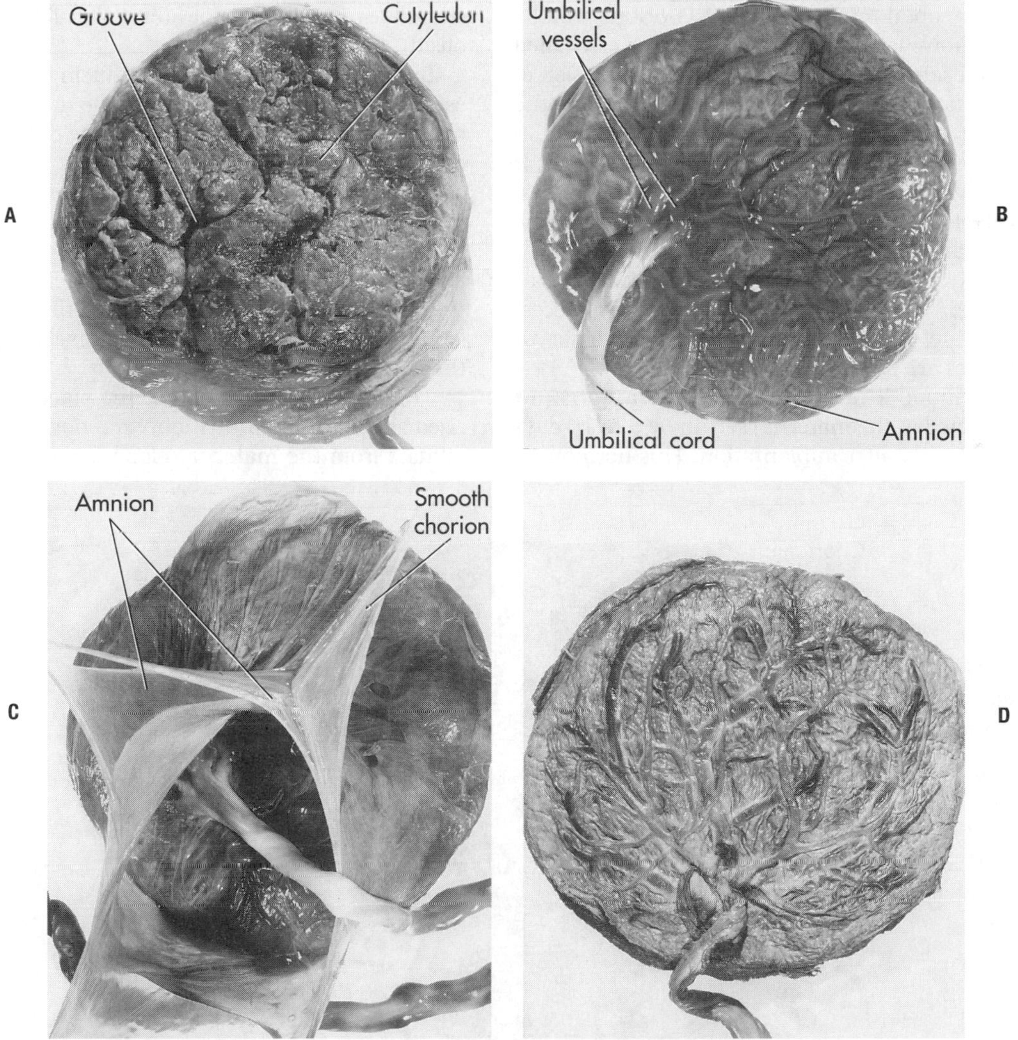

Fig. 4-10 Photographs of full-term placenta. **A,** Maternal (or uterine) surface, showing cotyledons and grooves. **B,** Fetal (or amniotic) surface, showing blood vessels running under amnion and converging to form umbilical vessels at attachment of umbilical cord. **C,** Amnion and smooth chorion are arranged to show that they are (1) fused and (2) continuous with margins of placenta. **D,** Placenta with a marginal attachment of the cord, often called a *battledore placenta* because of its resemblance to bat used in medieval game of battledore and shuttlecock. (From Moore K: *Before we were born: basic embryology and birth defects,* ed 3, Philadelphia, 1989, Saunders.)

into separate areas called *cotyledons*. In each of the 15 to 20 cotyledons, the chorionic villi branch out, and a complex system of fetal blood vessels forms. Each cotyledon is a functional unit. The whole structure is the **placenta** (Fig. 4-10).

The maternal-placental-embryonic circulation is in place by day 17, when the embryonic heart starts beating. By the end of the third week, embryonic blood is circulating between the embryo and the chorionic villi. In the intervillous spaces, maternal blood supplies oxygen and nutrients to the embryonic capillaries in the villi (Fig. 4-11). Waste products and carbon dioxide diffuse into the maternal blood.

The placenta functions as a means of metabolic exchange. Exchange is minimal at this time because the two cell layers of the villous membrane are too thick. Permeability increases as the cytotrophoblast thins and disappears by the fifth month, leaving only the single layer of syncytium between the maternal blood and the fetal capillaries. The syncytium is the functional layer of the placenta. By the eighth week, genetic testing may be done by obtaining a sample of chorionic villi by aspiration biopsy; however, limb defects have been associated with chorionic villi sampling done before 10 weeks (Hsieh et al., 1995). The structure of the placenta is complete by the twelfth week. The placenta continues to grow wider until 20 weeks, when it covers about one half of the uterine surface. It then continues to grow thicker. The branching villi continue to develop within the body of the placenta, increasing the functional surface area.

Functions. One of the early functions of the placenta is as an endocrine gland, which produces four hormones necessary to maintain the pregnancy and support the embryo/fetus. The hormones are produced in the syncytium.

The protein hormone **human chorionic gonadotropin (hCG)** can be detected in the maternal serum by 8 to 10 days after conception, shortly after implantation. This hormone is the basis for pregnancy tests. The hCG preserves the function of the ovarian corpus luteum, ensuring a continued supply of estrogen and progesterone needed to maintain the pregnancy. Spontaneous abortion occurs if the corpus luteum stops functioning before the placenta is producing sufficient estrogen and progesterone. The hCG reaches its maximum level at 50 to 70 days, then begins to decrease.

The other protein hormone produced by the placenta is human placental lactogen (hPL). This substance is similar to a growth hormone and stimulates maternal metabolism to supply needed nutrients for fetal growth. This hormone increases the resistance to insulin, facilitates glucose transport across the placental membrane, and stimulates breast development to prepare for lactation.

The placenta eventually produces more of the steroid hormone progesterone than the corpus luteum does during the first few months of pregnancy. Progesterone maintains the endometrium, decreases the contractility of the uterus, and stimulates development of breast alveoli and maternal metabolism.

By 7 weeks the placenta is producing most of the maternal estrogens, or steroid hormones. The major estrogen secreted by the placenta is estriol, whereas the ovaries produce mostly estradiol. Measuring estriol levels is a clinical assay for placental functioning. Estrogen stimulates uterine growth and uteroplacental blood flow. It causes a proliferation of the breast glandular tissue and stimulates myometrial contractility. Placental estrogen production increases greatly toward the end of pregnancy. One theory for the cause of the onset of labor is the decrease in circulating levels of progesterone and the increased levels of estrogen.

The metabolic functions of the placenta may be summarized as respiration, nutrition, excretion, and storage. Oxygen diffuses from the maternal blood across the placental mem-

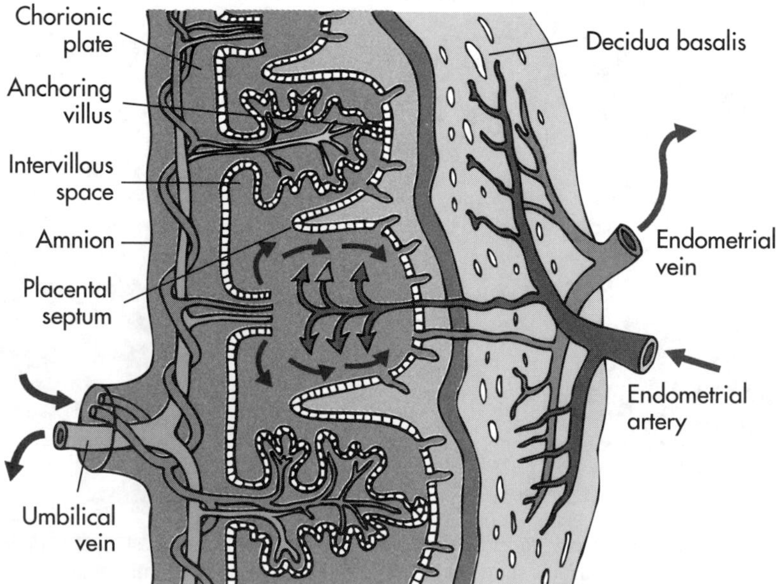

Fig. 4-11 Schematic drawing of placenta illustrating how it supplies oxygen and nutrition to embryo and removes its waste products. Deoxygenated blood leaves fetus through the umbilical arteries and enters placenta, where it is oxygenated. Oxygenated blood leaves placenta through the umbilical vein, which enters the fetus via the umbilical cord.

brane into the fetal blood, and carbon dioxide diffuses in the opposite direction. In this way the placenta functions as lungs for the fetus.

Carbohydrates, proteins, calcium, and iron are stored in the placenta for ready access to meet fetal needs. Water, inorganic salts, carbohydrates, proteins, fats, and vitamins pass from the maternal blood supply across the placental membrane into the fetal blood, supplying nutrition. Water and most electrolytes with a molecular weight less than 500 readily diffuse through the membrane. Hydrostatic and osmotic pressures aid in the flow of water and some solutions. Facilitated and active transport assist in the transfer of glucose, amino acids, calcium, iron, and substances with higher molecular weight. Amino acids and calcium are transported against the concentration gradient between the maternal blood and fetal blood.

The fetal concentration of glucose is lower than the glucose level in the maternal blood because of its rapid metabolism by the fetus. This requires transport of larger amounts of glucose from the maternal blood than would be supplied by simple diffusion alone.

Pinocytosis is a mechanism used for transferring large molecules, such as albumin and gamma globulins, across the placental membrane. This mechanism conveys the maternal immunoglobulins that render early passive immunity to the fetus.

Metabolic waste products of the fetus cross the placental membrane from the fetal blood into the maternal blood. The maternal kidneys then excrete them.

Many viruses can cross the placental membrane and infect the fetus. Some bacteria and protozoa first infect the placenta and then infect the fetus.

Drugs can also cross the placental membrane and may harm the fetus. Caffeine, alcohol, nicotine, carbon monoxide and other toxic substances in cigarette smoke, and prescription and recreational drugs (e.g., cocaine, marijuana) readily cross the placenta.

Although no direct link exists between the fetal blood in the vessels of the chorionic villi and the maternal blood in the intervillous spaces, only one cell layer separates them. Breaks in the placental membrane occasionally occur. Fetal erythrocytes then leak into the maternal circulation, and the mother may develop antibodies to the fetal red blood cells. This is often how the Rh negative mother becomes sensitized to the erythrocytes of her Rh-positive fetus.

Even though the placenta and fetus are living tissue transplants, they are not destroyed by the host mother (Cunningham, MacDonald, and Gant, 1993). The placental hormones suppress the immunologic response, or the tissue evokes no response (Willson and Carrington, 1991).

Placental function depends on the maternal blood pressure supplying the circulation. Maternal arterial blood, under pressure in the small uterine spiral arteries, spurts into the intervillous spaces (Fig. 4-11). As long as rich arterial blood continues to be supplied, pressure is exerted on the blood already in the intervillous spaces, pushing it toward drainage by the low-pressure uterine veins. At term gestation, 10% of the maternal cardiac output goes to the uterus.

If there is interference with the circulation to the placenta, the placenta cannot supply the embryo/fetus. Vasoconstriction, such as that caused by hypertension and cocaine use, diminishes uterine blood flow. Decreased maternal blood pressure or cardiac output also diminishes uterine blood flow. When a woman lies on her back with the pressure of the uterus compressing the vena cava, blood return to the right atrium is diminished (for a discussion of supine hypotension, see p. 112). Excessive maternal exercise that diverts blood to the muscles away from the uterus compromises placental circulation. Optimum circulation is achieved when the woman is lying at rest on her left side.

It is believed that *Braxton Hicks contractions* (see p. 109) enhance the movement of blood through the intervillous spaces, aiding placental circulation. However, prolonged contractions or too-short intervals between contractions during labor reduce blood flow to the placenta.

Fetal Maturation

The stage of the **fetus** lasts from 9 weeks until the pregnancy ends. Changes during the fetal period are not as dramatic, since refinement of structure and function are taking place. The fetus is less vulnerable to teratogens except for those affecting central nervous system functioning.

Viability refers to the capability of the fetus to survive outside the uterus. In the past the earliest age at which fetal survival could be expected was 28 weeks after conception. With modern technology and advancements in maternal and neonatal care, viability is now possible at 20 weeks after conception (22 weeks since LMP; fetal weight of 500 g or more). The limitations on survival outside the uterus are based on central nervous system function and oxygenation capability of the lungs.

Fetal circulatory system. The cardiovascular system is the first organ system to function in the developing human. Blood vessel and blood cell formation begin in the third week to supply the embryo with oxygen and nutrients from the mother. By the end of the third week the tubular heart begins to beat, and the primitive cardiovascular system links the embryo, connecting stalk, chorion, and yolk sac. During the fourth and fifth weeks the heart develops into the four-chambered organ. By the end of the embryonic stage the heart is developmentally complete.

The fetal lungs do not function for respiratory gas exchange, so a special circulatory pathway exists that bypasses the lungs. Oxygen-rich blood from the placenta flows rapidly through the umbilical vein into the fetal abdomen (see Fig. 22-2). When the umbilical vein reaches the liver, it divides into two branches; one circulates some oxygenated blood through the liver. Most of the blood passes through the ductus venosus into the inferior vena cava. There it mixes with the deoxygenated blood from the fetal legs and abdomen on its way to the right atrium. Most of this blood passes straight through the right atrium and through the **foramen ovale**, an opening into the left atrium. There it mixes with the small amount of blood returning deoxygenated from the fetal lungs through the pulmonary veins.

The blood flows into the left ventricle and is squeezed out into the aorta, where the arteries supplying the heart, head, neck, and arms receive the major part of the oxygen-rich blood. This pattern of supplying the highest levels of oxygen and nutrients to the head, neck, and arms enhances the

cephalocaudal (head-to-rump) development of the embryo/fetus.

Deoxygenated blood returning from the head and arms enters the right atrium through the superior vena cava. This blood is directed downward into the right ventricle, where it is squeezed into the pulmonary artery. A small amount of blood circulates through the resistant lung tissue, but the majority follows the path with less resistance through the **ductus arteriosus** into the aorta, distal to the point of exit of the arteries supplying the head and arms with oxygenated blood. The oxygen-poor blood flows through the abdominal aorta into the internal iliac arteries, where the umbilical arteries direct most of it back through the umbilical cord to the placenta. There the blood gives up its wastes and carbon dioxide in exchange for nutrients and oxygen. The blood remaining in the iliac arteries flows through the fetal abdomen and legs, ultimately returning through the inferior vena cava to the heart.

The following three special characteristics enable the fetus to obtain sufficient oxygen from the maternal blood:

1. Fetal hemoglobin carries 20% to 30% more oxygen than maternal hemoglobin.
2. The fetal hemoglobin concentration is about 50% greater than that of the mother.
3. The fetal heart rate (FHR) is 120 to 160 beats/min, making the fetal cardiac output per unit of body weight higher than that of an adult.

Hematopoietic system. Hematopoiesis, the formation of blood, occurs in the yolk sac (Fig. 4-11) beginning in the third week. Hematopoietic stem cells seed the fetal liver during the fifth week, and hematopoiesis begins there during the sixth week. This accounts for the relatively large size of the liver between the seventh and ninth weeks. Stem cells seed the fetal bone marrow, spleen and thymus, and lymph nodes between weeks 8 and 11.

The antigenic factors that determine blood type are present in the erythrocytes soon after the sixth week. For this reason the Rh-negative woman is at risk for isoimmunization in any pregnancy that lasts longer than 6 weeks after fertilization.

Respiratory system. The respiratory system begins development during embryonic life and continues through fetal life and into childhood. The development of the lungs occurs between weeks 5 and 17 with formation of the trachea, bronchi, and lung buds. Between 16 and 24 weeks the bronchi and terminal bronchioles enlarge, and vascular structures and primitive alveoli are formed. Between 24 weeks and term birth, more alveoli form. Specialized alveolar cells secrete pulmonary **surfactants** to line the interior of the alveoli. After 32 weeks, sufficient surfactant is present in developed alveoli to provide infants with a good chance of survival.

Pulmonary surfactants. The detection of the presence of pulmonary surfactants, surface-active phospholipids, in amniotic fluid has been used to determine the degree of fetal lung maturity, or the ability of the lungs to function after birth. **Lecithin (L)** is the most critical alveolar surfactant required for postnatal lung expansion. It increases in amount after the twenty-fourth week. Another pulmonary phospholipid, **sphingomyelin, (S)** remains constant in amount. Thus the measure of lecithin in relation to sphingomyelin, or the **L/S ratio** of 2:1, is used to determine fetal lung maturity. This occurs at approximately 35 weeks of gestation (Creasy and Resnik, 1994).

Certain maternal conditions alter the development of the fetal lungs. Those conditions that accelerate lung maturity generally cause decreased maternal placental blood flow. The resulting fetal hypoxia apparently stresses the fetus, increasing blood levels of corticosteroids that accelerate alveolar and surfactant development. Conditions such as maternal hypertension, placental dysfunction, infection, or corticosteroid use accelerate fetal lung maturity. Conditions such as gestational diabetes and chronic glomerulonephritis can retard fetal lung maturity.

The recent approval of the use of intrabronchial synthetic surfactant in the treatment of respiratory distress syndrome in the newborn has greatly improved the chances of survival of preterm infants (Paynton, 1991).

Fetal respiratory movements have been seen on ultrasound as early as the eleventh week. These fetal respiratory movements may aid in development of the chest wall muscles and regulate lung fluid volume. The fetal lungs produce fluid that expands the air spaces in the lungs. The fluid drains into the amniotic fluid or is swallowed by the fetus.

Before birth, secretion of lung fluid decreases. The normal birth process squeezes out approximately one third of the fluid. Infants of cesarean births do not benefit from this squeezing process; thus they have more respiratory difficulty at birth. The fluid remaining in the lungs at birth is usually reabsorbed into the infant's bloodstream within 2 hours of birth.

Renal system. The permanent kidneys form during the fifth week. Urine formation is present during the third month. Urine is excreted into the amniotic fluid and forms a major part of the amniotic fluid volume. Oligohydramnios, an abnormally small amount of amniotic fluid, is indicative of renal dysfunction. Because the placenta acts as the organ of excretion and maintains fetal water and electrolyte balance, the fetus does not need functioning kidneys while in utero. At birth, however, the kidneys are required immediately for excretory and acid-base regulatory functions.

A fetal renal malformation can be diagnosed in utero. Corrective or palliative fetal surgery may treat the malformation successfully, or plans can be made for treatment immediately after birth (Adzick and Harrison, 1994; Collins, 1994; Howell, 1994).

At term the fetus has fully developed kidneys. However, the glomerular filtration rate (GFR) is low, and the kidneys lack the ability to concentrate urine. This makes the newborn more susceptible to both overhydration and dehydration.

Most newborns void within 24 hours of birth. With the loss of the swallowed amniotic fluid and the metabolism of nutrients provided by the placenta, voidings for the first days of life are scanty until fluid intake increases.

Neurologic system. The nervous system originates from the ectoderm at 18 days after fertilization. The open neural tube forms during the fourth week. It initially closes at what will be the junction of the brain and spinal cord, leaving both ends open. The embryo folds in on itself lengthwise at this time, forming a head fold in the neural tube at this junction. The cranial end of the neural tube closes, then the caudal end closes. During week 5, different growth rates cause more flexures in the neural tube, delineating three brain areas: the forebrain, midbrain, and hindbrain.

The forebrain develops into the eyes (cranial nerve II) and cerebral hemispheres. The development of all areas of the cerebral cortex continues throughout fetal life and into childhood. The olfactory system (cranial nerve I) and thalamus also develop from the forebrain. Cranial nerves III and IV (oculomotor and trochlear) form from the midbrain. The hindbrain forms the medulla, pons, cerebellum, and the remainder of the cranial nerves. Brain waves can be recorded on an electroencephalogram (EEG) by week 8.

The spinal cord develops from the long end of the neural tube. Another ectodermal structure, the neural crest, develops into the peripheral nervous system. By the eighth week, nerve fibers traverse throughout the body. By week 11 or 12, the fetus makes respiratory movements, moves all extremities, and changes position in utero. The fetus can suck his or her thumb and swim in the amniotic fluid pool, turn somersaults, and sometimes tie a knot in the umbilical cord. Box 4-3 describes the major types of fetal movements. Sometime between 16 and 20 weeks, when the movements are strong enough to be perceived by the mother as "the baby moving," **quickening** has occurred. The perception of movement occurs earlier in the multipara than in the primipara. The mother also becomes aware of the sleeping and waking cycles of the fetus.

BOX 4-3

Major Types of Fetal Movements

General movements—These slow, gross movements involve the whole body. Their duration is from several seconds to a minute.

Startle movements—These quick (less than 1 second), generalized movements always start in the limbs and may spread to the trunk and neck.

Hiccups—These are repetitive phasic contractions of the diaphragm. A bout may last several minutes.

Fetal breathing movements—These are paradoxic movements in which the thorax moves inward and the abdomen outward with each contraction of the diaphragm.

Isolated arm or leg movements—These movements of extremities occur without movement of the trunk.

Hand-face contact—This occurs any time the moving hand makes contact with the face or mouth.

Retroflexion of the head—This is a slow to jerky backward bending of the head.

Lateral rotation of the head—This involves isolated turning of the head from side to side.

Anteflexion of the head—This is a normally slow, forward bending of the head.

Opening of mouth—This isolated movement may be accompanied by protrusion of the tongue.

Yawn—Mouth is slowly opened and rapidly closed after a few seconds.

Sucking—This burst of rhythmic jaw movements is sometimes followed by swallowing. With this movement, the fetus may be drinking amniotic fluid.

Stretch—This complex movement involves overextension of the spine, retroflexion of the head, and elevation of the arms.

From Carlson B: *Human embryology and developmental biology*, St Louis, 1994, Mosby.

Sensory awareness. Purposeful movements of the fetus have been demonstrated in response to a firm touch transmitted through the mother's abdomen. Invasive procedures to be done on a fetus require anesthesia.

Fetuses respond to sound by 24 weeks. Different types of music evoke different movements. The fetus can be soothed by the sound of the mother's voice. Acoustic stimulation can be used to evoke an FHR response (Bar-Hava and Barnhardt, 1994). The fetus does become accustomed to noises heard repeatedly.

The fetus is able to distinguish taste. By the fifth month, when the fetus is swallowing amniotic fluid, a sweetener added to the fluid causes the fetus to swallow twice as fast (Poole, 1986). The fetus also reacts to temperature changes. A cold solution placed into the amniotic fluid can cause fetal hiccups.

The fetus can see. Eyes have both rods and cones in the retina by the seventh month. A bright light shone on the mother's abdomen in late pregnancy causes abrupt fetal movements. During sleep time, rapid eye movements (REMs) have been observed similar to those occurring in children and adults while dreaming (Poole, 1986).

At term the fetal brain is approximately one-fourth the size of an adult brain. Neurologic development continues. Stressors on the fetus and neonate, such as chronic poor nutrition or hypoxia, drugs, environmental toxins, trauma, or disease, cause damage to the central nervous system long after the vulnerable embryonic time for malformations in other organ systems. Neurologic insult can result in cerebral palsy, neuromuscular impairment, mental retardation, and learning disabilities.

Gastrointestinal system. During the fourth week the embryo changes from almost straight to a C shape as both ends fold in toward the ventral surface. A portion of the yolk sac is incorporated into the body from head to tail as the primitive gut (digestive system).

The foregut produces the pharynx, part of the lower respiratory tract, the esophagus, the stomach, the first half of the duodenum, the liver, the pancreas, and the gallbladder. These structures evolve over the fifth and sixth weeks. The malformations that can occur in these areas are esophageal atresia, hypertrophic pyloric stenosis, duodenal stenosis or atresia, and biliary atresia.

The midgut becomes the distal half of the duodenum, the jejunum and ileum, the cecum and appendix, and the proximal half of the colon. The midgut loop projects into the umbilical cord between weeks 5 and 10. A malformation (omphalocele) results if the midgut fails to return to the abdominal cavity, and intestines protrude from the umbilicus. Meckel diverticulum is the most common malformation of the midgut. It occurs when a remnant of the yolk stalk that has failed to degenerate attaches to the ileum, leaving a blind sac.

The hindgut develops into the distal half of the colon, the rectum and parts of the anal canal, the urinary bladder, and the urethra. Anorectal malformations are the most commonly occurring abnormalities of the digestive system.

The fetus swallows amniotic fluid beginning in the fifth month. Gastric emptying and intestinal peristalsis occur. Fetal nutrition and elimination needs are taken care of by the placenta. As the fetus nears term, fetal waste products accumulate in the intestines as dark green to black tarry **meconium.** Normally this substance is passed through the rectum within 48 hours of birth. Sometimes with a breech birth or fetal hypoxia, meconium is passed in utero in the amniotic fluid. The failure to pass meconium after birth may indicate atresia somewhere in the digestive tract, an imperforate anus, or meconium ileus with a firm meconium plug blocking passage. Meconium ileus is seen in infants with cystic fibrosis.

The metabolic rate of the fetus is relatively low, but the infant has great growth and development needs. Beginning in week 9 the fetus synthesizes glycogen for storage in the liver. Between 26 and 30 weeks the fetus begins to lay down stores of brown fat in preparation for extrauterine cold stress. Thermoregulation in the neonate requires increased metabolism and adequate oxygenation.

The gastrointestinal system is mature by 36 weeks. Digestive enzymes, except pancreatic amylase and lipase, are present in sufficient quantity to facilitate digestion. The neonate cannot digest starches or fats efficiently. Little saliva is produced.

Hepatic system. The liver and biliary tract develop from the foregut during the fourth week of gestation. Hematopoiesis begins during the sixth week, requiring that the liver be large. The embryonic liver is prominent and occupies most of the abdominal cavity. Bile, a constituent of meconium, begins to form in the twelfth week.

Glycogen is stored in the fetal liver beginning at week 9 or 10. At term, glycogen stores are twice those of the adult. Glycogen is the major source of energy for the fetus and neonate who is stressed by in utero hypoxia or by extrauterine loss of the maternal glucose supply, by the work of breathing, or by cold stress.

Iron is stored in the fetal liver. If the maternal intake is sufficient, the fetus can store enough iron to last for 5 months after birth.

During fetal life the liver does not have to conjugate bilirubin for excretion because the unconjugated bilirubin is cleared by the placenta. Therefore the glucuronyl transferase enzyme needed for conjugation that is present in the fetal liver is less than is required after birth. This predisposes the neonate to hyperbilirubinemia.

Coagulation factors II, VII, IX, and X cannot be synthesized in the fetal liver because of the lack of vitamin K synthesis in the sterile fetal gut. This coagulation deficiency persists after birth for several days and is the rationale for the prophylactic administration of vitamin K to the newborn.

Endocrine system. The thyroid gland develops with structures in the head and neck during the third and fourth weeks. The secretion of thyroxine begins during the eighth week. Maternal thyroxine does not readily cross the placenta; therefore the fetus who does not produce thyroid hormones will be born with congenital hypothyroidism. If untreated, hypothyroidism can result in severe mental retardation. All neonates should be screened for hypothyroidism with a blood test after birth.

The adrenal cortex is formed during the sixth week and produces hormones by the eighth or ninth week. As term approaches, the fetus produces more cortisol. This is believed to aid in initiation of labor by decreasing the maternal progesterone and stimulating production of prostaglandins.

The pancreas forms from the foregut during the fifth through eighth weeks. The islets of Langerhans develop during the twelfth week. Insulin is produced by the twentieth week. In infants of mothers with uncontrolled diabetes, maternal hyperglycemia produces fetal hyperglycemia, stimulating hyperinsulinemia and islet cell hyperplasia. This results in a macrosomatic (large-sized) fetus. The hyperinsulinemia also blocks lung maturation, placing the neonate at risk for respiratory distress and hypoglycemia when the maternal glucose source is lost at delivery. Control of the maternal glucose level before and during pregnancy minimizes problems for the infant.

Reproductive system. Until the seventh week, no sex differentiation exists in the embryo. When a Y chromosome is present, testes are formed. By the end of the embryonic period, testosterone is being secreted and causes formation of the male genitalia. By week 28 the testes begin descending into the scrotum. After birth, low levels of testosterone continue to be secreted until the pubertal surge.

The female, with two X chromosomes, forms ovaries and female external genitalia. Female and male external genitalia are indistinguishable until after the ninth week. By the sixteenth week, oogenesis has been established. At birth the ovaries contain the female's lifetime supply of ova. In the female, most female hormone production is delayed until puberty. However, the fetal endometrium responds to maternal hormones, and withdrawal bleeding or vaginal discharge (pseudomenstruation) may occur at birth when these hormones are lost. The high level of maternal estrogen also stimulates mammary engorgement and secretion of fluid ("witch's milk") in newborn infants of both sexes.

Immunologic system. During the third trimester, albumin and globulin are present in the fetus. The only immunoglobulin that crosses the placenta is IgG, providing passive acquired immunity to specific bacterial toxins. The fetus produces IgM immunoglobulins by the end of the first trimester. These are produced in response to blood group antigens, gram-negative enteric organisms, and some viruses. IgA immunoglobulins are not produced by the fetus. However, colostrum, the precursor to breast milk, contains large amounts of IgA and can provide passive immunity to the neonate.

The normal term neonate can fight infection, but not as effectively as an older child. The preterm infant is at much greater risk for infection.

Musculoskeletal system. Bones and muscles develop from the mesoderm by the fourth week of embryonic development. At that time the cardiac muscle is already beating. The mesoderm next to the neural tube forms the vertebral column and ribs. The parts of the vertebral column grow toward each other to enclose the developing spinal cord. Ossification, or bone formation, begins. If there is a defect in the bony fusion, spina bifida may occur. A large defect affecting several vertebrae may allow the membranes and spinal cord to pouch out from the back, producing neurologic deficits and skeletal deformity.

The flat bones of the skull develop during the embryonic period, and ossification continues throughout childhood. At birth, connective tissue sutures exist where the bones of the skull meet. The areas where more than two bones meet, called *fontanels,* are especially prominent. The sutures and fontanels allow the bones of the skull to mold, or move during birth, enabling the head to pass through the birth canal.

The bones of the shoulders, arms, hips, and legs appear in the sixth week as a continuous skeleton with no joints. Differentiation occurs, producing separate bones and joints. Ossification will continue through childhood to allow growth. Beginning during the seventh week, muscles contract spontaneously. Arm and leg movements are visible on ultrasound, although the mother does not perceive them until the sixteenth to the twentieth week.

Integumentary system. The epidermis begins as a single layer of cells derived from the ectoderm at 4 weeks. By the seventh week, there are two layers of cells. The cells of the superficial layer are sloughed and become mixed with the sebaceous gland secretions to form the white, greasy *vernix caseosa,* the material that protects the skin of the fetus. The vernix is thick at 24 weeks but becomes scant by term.

The basal layer of the epidermis is the germinal layer, which replaces the lost cells. Until 17 weeks the skin is thin and wrinkled, with blood vessels visible underneath. The skin thickens, and all layers are present at term. After 32 weeks, as subcutaneous fat is deposited under the dermis, the skin becomes less wrinkled and red in appearance.

By 16 weeks the epidermal ridges are present on the palms of the hands, the fingers, the bottom of the feet, and the toes. This makes the handprints and footprints unique to that infant.

Hairs form from the hair bulbs in the epidermis, which project into the dermis. Cells in the hair bulb keratinize to form the hair shaft. As the cells at the base of the hair shaft proliferate, the hair grows to the surface of the epithelium. The very fine hairs, called *lanugo,* appear first at 12 weeks on the eyebrows and upper lip. By 20 weeks they cover the entire body. At this time the eyelashes, eyebrows, and scalp hair are beginning to grow. By 28 weeks the scalp hair is longer than the lanugo, which is thinning and may disappear by term gestation.

Fingernails and toenails develop from thickened epidermis at the tips of the digits beginning during the tenth week. They grow slowly. Fingernails usually reach the fingertips by 32 weeks, and toenails reach toetips by 36 weeks.

Table 4-2 summarizes embryonic and fetal development.

Multifetal Pregnancy

Twins. When two mature ova are produced in one ovarian cycle, both have the potential to be fertilized by separate sperm. This results in two zygotes, or **dizygotic twins.** (Fig. 4-12). There are always two amnions, two chorions, and two placentas that may be fused together. These dizygotic or fraternal twins may be the same sex or different sexes and are genetically no more alike than siblings born at different times. Dizygotic twinning occurs in families, more often among African-American women than Caucasian women, and least often among Asian-American women. Twinning increases in frequency with maternal age up to 35 years, with parity, and with the use of fertility drugs.

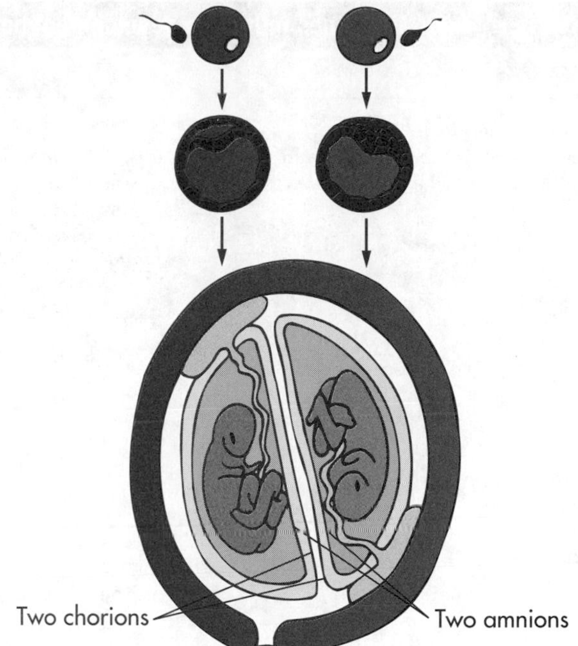

Fig. 4-12 Formation of dizygotic twins. There is fertilization of two ova, two implantations, two placentas, two chorions, and two amnions.

Identical twins develop from one fertilized ovum, which then divides, thus the term **monozygotic twins** (Fig. 4-13). They are the same sex and have the same genotype. If division occurs soon after fertilization, two embryos, two amnions, two chorions, and two placentas that may be fused will develop. Most often, division occurs between 4 and 8 days after fertilization, and there are two embryos, two amnions, one chorion, and one placenta. Rarely, division occurs after the eighth day following fertilization. In this case there are two embryos within a common amnion and a common chorion with one placenta. This often causes circulatory problems because the umbilical cords may tangle together, and one or both fetuses may die. If division occurs very late, cleavage may not be complete, and conjoined or "Siamese" twins could result.

Monozygotic twinning occurs in approximately 1 of 250 births (Cunningham, MacDonald, and Gant, 1993). There is no association with race, heredity, maternal age, or parity. Fertility drugs do increase the incidence of multiple births (Derom et al, 1987).

Other multifetal pregnancies. The occurrence of multifetal pregnancies with three or more fetuses has increased with the use of fertility drugs and in vitro fertilization. Triplets occur in about 1 of 7600 pregnancies. They can occur from the division of one zygote into two, with one of the two dividing again, producing identical triplets. Triplets can also be produced from two zygotes, one dividing into a set of identical

Text continued on p. 73.

TABLE 4-2 Milestones in human development before birth since last menstrual period (LMP)

4 WEEKS	8 WEEKS	12 WEEKS
External appearance		
Body flexed, C shaped; arm and leg buds present; head at right angles to body	Body fairly well formed; nose flat, eyes far apart; digits well formed; head elevating; tail almost disappeared; eyes, ears, nose, and mouth recognizable	Nails appearing; resembles a human; head erect but disproportionately large; skin pink, delicate
Crown-to-rump measurement; weight		
0.4 to 0.5 cm; 0.4 g	2.5 to 3 cm; 2 g	6 to 9 cm; 19 g
Gastrointestinal system		
Stomach at midline and fusiform; conspicuous liver; esophagus short; intestine a short tube	Intestinal villi developing; small intestines coil within umbilical cord; palatal folds present; liver very large	Bile secreted; palatal fusion complete; intestines have withdrawn from cord and assume characteristic positions
Musculoskeletal system		
All somites present	First indication of ossification—occiput, mandible, and humerus; fetus capable of some movement; definitive muscles of trunk, limbs, and head well represented	Some bones well outlined, ossification spreading; upper cervical to lower sacral arches and bodies ossify; smooth muscle layers indicated in hollow viscera
Circulatory system		
Heart develops, double chambers visible, begins to beat; aortic arch and major veins completed	Main blood vessels assume final plan; enucleated red cells predominate in blood	Blood forming in marrow
Respiratory system		
Primary lung buds appear	Pleural and pericardial cavities forming; branching bronchioles; nostrils closed by epithelial plugs	Lungs acquire definite shape; vocal cords appear
Renal system		
Rudimentary ureteral buds appear	Earliest secretory tubules differentiating; bladder-urethra separates from rectum	Kidney able to secrete urine; bladder expands as a sac
Nervous system		
Well-marked midbrain flexure; no hindbrain or cervical flexures; neural groove closed	Cerebral cortex begins to acquire typical cells; differentiation of cerebral cortex, meninges, ventricular foramina, cerebrospinal fluid circulation; spinal cord extends entire length of spine	Brain structural configuration almost complete; cord shows cervical and lumbar enlargements; fourth ventricle foramina (pl) developed; sucking present
Sensory organs		
Eye and ear appearing as optic vessel and otocyst	Primordial choroid plexuses develop; ventricles large relative to cortex; development progressing; eyes converging rapidly; internal ear developing	Earliest taste buds indicated; characteristic organization of eye attained
Genital system		
Genital ridge appears (fifth week)	Testes and ovaries distinguishable; external genitalia sexless but begin to differentiate	Sex recognizable; internal and external sex organs specific

Modified from Wong D: *Whaley and Wong's nursing care of infants and children,* St. Louis, 1979, Mosby.

TABLE 4-2 Milestones in human development before birth since last menstrual period (LMP)—cont'd

16 WEEKS	20 WEEKS	24 WEEKS
External appearance		
Head still dominant; face looks human; eyes, ears, and nose approach typical appearance on gross examination; arm/leg ratio proportionate; scalp hair appears	Vernix caseosa appears; lanugo appears; legs lengthen considerably; sebaceous glands appear	Body lean but fairly well proportioned; skin red and wrinkled; vernix caseosa present; sweat glands forming
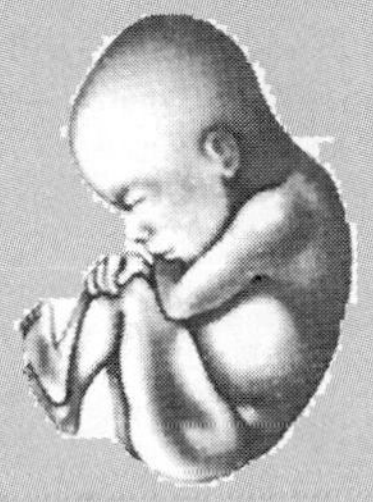	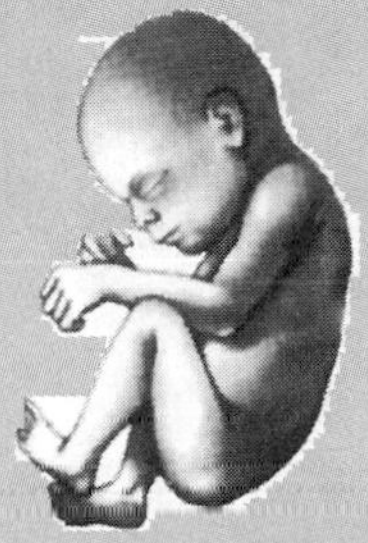	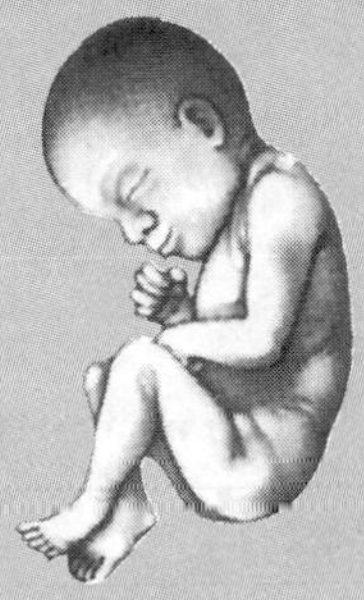
Crown-to-rump measurement; weight		
11.5 to 13.5 cm; 100 g	16 to 18.5 cm; 300 g	23 cm; 600 g
Gastrointestinal system		
Meconium in bowel; some enzyme secretion; anus open	Enamel and dentine depositing; ascending colon recognizable	
Musculoskeletal system		
Most bones distinctly indicated throughout body; joint cavities appear; muscular movements can be detected	Sternum ossifies; fetal movements strong enough for mother to feel	
Circulatory system		
Heart muscle well developed; blood formation active in spleen		Blood formation increases in bone marrow and decreases in liver
Respiratory system		
Elastic fibers appear in lungs; terminal and respiratory bronchioles appear	Nostrils reopen; primitive respiratory-like movements begin	Alveolar ducts and sacs present; lecithin begins to appear in amniotic fluid (weeks 26 to 27)
Renal system		
Kidney in position; attains typical shape and plan		
Nervous system		
Cerebral lobes delineated; cerebellum assumes some prominance	Brain grossly formed; cord myelination begins; spinal cord ends at level of first sacral vertebra (S-1)	Cerebral cortex layered typically; neuronal proliferation in cerebral cortex ends
Sensory organs		
General sense organs differentiated	Nose and ears ossify	Can hear
Genital system		
Testes in position for descent into scrotum; vagina open		Testes at inguinal ring in descent to scrotum

Continued.

TABLE 4-2 Milestones in human development before birth since last menstrual period (LMP)—cont'd

	28 WEEKS	30-31 WEEKS	36 AND 40 WEEKS
External appearance	Lean body, less wrinkled and red; nails appear	Subcutaneous fat beginning to collect; more rounded appearance; skin pink and smooth; has assumed birth position 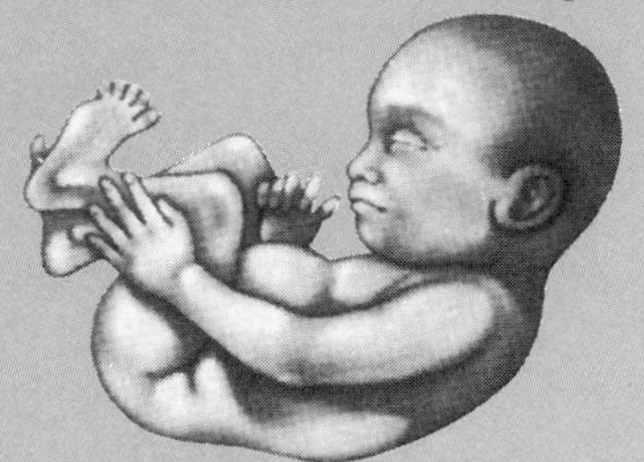	***36 weeks*** Skin pink, body rounded; general lanugo disappearing; body usually plump ***40 weeks*** Skin smooth and pink; scant vernix caseosa; moderate to profuse hair; lanugo on shoulders and upper body only; nasal and alar cartilage apparent
Crown-to-rump measurement; weight	27 cm; 1100 g	31 cm; 1800 to 2100 g	***36 weeks*** 35 cm; 2200 to 2900 g ***40 weeks*** 40 cm; 3200+ g
Musculoskeletal system	Astragalus (talus, ankle bone) ossifies; weak, fleeting movements, minimum tone	Middle fourth phalanxes ossify; permanent teeth primordia seen; can turn head to side	***36 weeks*** Distal femoral ossification centers present; sustained, definite movements; fair tone; can turn and elevate head ***40 weeks*** Active, sustained movement; good tone; may lift head
Respiratory system	Lecithin forming on alveolar surfaces	L/S ratio = 1.2:1	***36 weeks*** L/S ratio ≥ 2:1 ***40 weeks*** Pulmonary branching only two-thirds complete
Renal system			***36 weeks*** Formation of new nephrons ceases
Nervous system	Appearance of cerebral fissures, convolutions rapidly appearing; indefinite sleep-wake cycle; cry weak or absent; weak suck reflex		***36 weeks*** End of spinal cord at level of third lumbar vertebra (L-3); definite sleep-wake cycle ***40 weeks*** Myelination of brain begins; patterned sleep-wake cycle with alert periods; cries when hungry or uncomfortable; strong suck reflex
Sensory organs	Eyelids reopen; retinal layers completed, light receptive; pupils capable of reacting to light	Sense of taste present; aware of sounds outside mother's body	
Genital system		Testes descending to scrotum	***40 weeks*** Testes in scrotum; labia major well developed

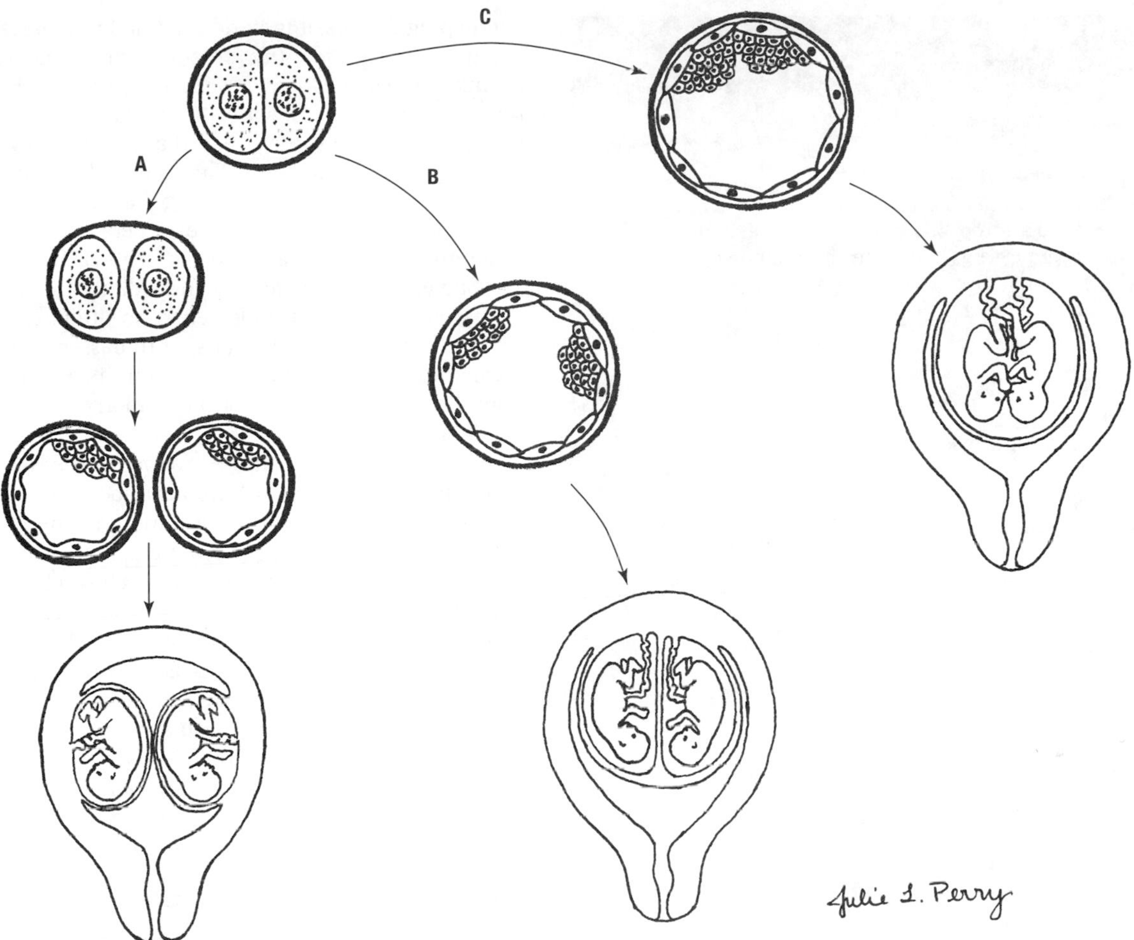

Fig. 4-13 Formation of monozygotic twins. **A,** One fertilization: blastomeres separate, resulting in two implantations, two placentas, and two sets of membranes. **B,** One blastomere with two inner cell masses, one fused placenta, one chorion, and separate amnions. **C,** One blastomere with incomplete separation of cell mass resulting in conjoined twins.

twins and the second zygote a single fraternal sibling, or from three zygotes. Quadruplets, quintuplets, sextuplets, and so on, likewise have similar possible derivations.

Nongenetic Factors Influencing Development

Not all congenital disorders are inherited. *Congenital* simply means that the condition was present at birth. Some congenital malformations may be the result of functional or structural disability. In contrast to other forms of developmental disabilities, disabilities caused by teratogens are theoretically totally preventable (Hoyme, 1990). Known human teratogens are drugs and chemicals (Brown, Bellinger, and Matthews, 1990; Thompson and Cordero, 1989), infections, exposure to radiation, and certain maternal conditions (Box 4-4). A teratogen has the greatest effect on the organs and parts of an embryo during its periods of rapid differentiation. This occurs during the embryonic period, specifically from days 15 to 60. During the first 2 weeks of development, teratogens either have no effect on the embryo or have effects so severe that they cause spontaneous abortion. Brain growth and development continue during the fetal period, and teratogens can severely affect mental development throughout gestation (Fig. 4-8).

Besides the genetic makeup and the influence of teratogens, the adequacy of maternal nutrition also influences development. The embryo and fetus must obtain the nutrients they need from the mother's diet; they cannot tap the maternal reserves. Malnutrition during pregnancy produces low-birth-weight (LBW) newborns who are susceptible to infection. Malnutrition also affects brain development during the latter half of gestation and may result in learning disabilities in the child.

GENETIC COUNSELING

Rapid expansion in the identification, understanding, and diagnosis of genetic disease has been accompanied by effective medical or surgical therapies in a small number of patients. For most genetic conditions, therapeutic or preventive measures are nonexistent or disappointingly limited. Consequently, the most useful means of reducing the incidence of these disorders is by preventing their transmission. With the

BOX 4-4
Human Teratogens

Drugs and chemicals
Alcohol
Androgens
Anticoagulants (warfarin, dicumarol)
Antithyroid drugs (propylthiouracil, iodide, methimazole)
Chemotherapeutic drugs (methotrexate, aminopterin)
Diethylstilbestrol (DES)
Isotretinoin (Accutane)
Lead
Lithium
Organic mercury
Phenytoin
Polychlorinated biphenyls (PCBs)
Streptomycin
Tetracycline
Thalidomide
Trimethadione, paramethadione
Valproic acid

Infections
Cytomegalovirus (CMV)
Rubella
Syphilis
Toxoplasmosis
Varicella

Exposure to radiation

Maternal conditions
Diabetes mellitus
Phenylketonuria (PKU)

From Reed G, Claireaux A, Bain A, editors: *Diseases of the fetus and newborn: pathology, radiology, and genetics*, St Louis, 1989, Mosby.

accumulation of knowledge about genetic disorders, the probability of recurrence in any given situation can be predicted with increased accuracy. At present the best means for reducing the number of children born with genetic defects is for health professionals to provide families with genetic information and services.

Patients Seeking Genetic Counseling

The reasons that people seek genetic counseling vary. These people may or may not be affected themselves. Those who seek counseling usually fall into the following categories:

1. People who want to know if they have or are carriers of a genetic disorder
2. People who are concerned about being at risk for giving birth to a child with a specific genetic disorder
3. People who are planning parenthood and who want to know the implications (prognosis and treatment) of a genetic disorder affecting one or both partners
4. People seeking help in making a decision about prenatal diagnosis, selective abortion, artificial insemination by donor, or adoption
5. People seeking help for a child affected with a genetic disorder

For all pregnancies, it is standard practice to assess for heritable disorders to identify potential problems (Creasy and Resnik, 1994). The interviewer inquires about the health status of family members, abnormal reproductive outcomes, history of maternal disorders (e.g., diabetes, PKU, cystic fibrosis), drug exposures, and illness (Fanaroff and Martin, 1992). Advanced maternal and paternal ages are noted. Ethnic origin should be recorded, since some disorders appear more often in some groups (Creasy and Resnik, 1994). Examples include Tay-Sachs disease in Jewish individuals of Ashkenazic or Sephardic descent, β-thalassemia in Italians and Greeks, sickle cell anemia in Africans, α-thalassemia in Southeast Asians and Filipinos, and tyrosinemia in French-Canadians from the Lac St. Jean–Chicoutimi region of Quebec (Fanaroff and Martin, 1992).

All nurses, especially those involved in the care of mothers and children, need to (1) have an understanding of genetic theory and the nature of more common genetic disorders to recognize cues that may indicate a genetically related problem, (2) be able to help families obtain counseling services, (3) augment the counseling process (Stringer, Librizzi, and Weiner, 1991), and (4) be aware of the legal and ethical issues involved (Barber, 1991). Nurses assist with preparation of patients for procedures and counseling and with diagnostic procedures and therapeutic programs. Nurses also interpret and reinforce counseling, maintain follow-up care, support the family's coping capacities, and assist family members in their problem solving. Nurses with advanced preparation in genetics and counseling may be genetic counselors.

Genetic Counseling Services

The most efficient genetic counseling services are associated with the larger universities and major medical centers where support services are available (e.g., biochemistry and cytology laboratories) and consist of a group of specialists under the leadership of a physician trained in medical genetics. Many of these regional centers maintain satellite clinics or services in outlying areas to provide contact with both consumers and health professionals. A number of specialized groups provide clinics and services for people with a specific genetic disorder, such as cystic fibrosis, muscular dystrophy, hemophilia, or diabetes. Health professionals should become familiar with people who provide genetic counseling and places where counseling services are available to patients in their area of practice (Inati, Lazar, and Haskin-Leahy, 1994).

Management of Genetic Disorders

At this time, no cures exist for genetic disorders, although remedies can be implemented to prevent or reduce the harmful effects of a few disorders. Structural defects can sometimes be modified to produce normal or near-normal function. Surgical therapy is employed for congenital heart defects and cosmetic defects such as cleft lip. Research is being conducted to devise methods to influence or change genes directly by placing substitute DNA in the cells of those with a genetic mutation, thereby preventing or curing the disease process or relieving symptoms (Crombleholme and Bianchi, 1994). Successful treatment of adenosine deaminase deficiency and cystic fibrosis has been reported (Pickler and Munro, 1995). The major thrust in therapy is modification of the internal or external environment to minimize the effects of the disorder.

Estimation of risk. The risks of recurrence of a genetic disorder are determined by the mode of inheritance. The risk of recurrence for disorders caused by a factor that segregates during cell division (genes and chromosomes) can be estimated with a high degree of accuracy by application of mendelian principles. In a dominant disorder the risk is 50%, or one in two, that a subsequent offspring will be affected; an autosomal recessive disease carries a one-in-four risk of recurrence; and an X-linked disorder is related to the child's sex, as described in the section related to X-linked inheritance. Translocation chromosomes have a high risk of recurrence.

Disorders in which a subsequent pregnancy would carry no more risk than pregnancy alone (estimated at 1 in 30) include those resulting from isolated incidences not likely to be present in another pregnancy, such as maternal infections (e.g., rubella, toxoplasmosis), maternal ingestion of drugs, most chromosomal abnormalities, and a disorder determined to be the result of a fresh mutation.

Interpretation of risk. Counselors explain the risk estimates to patients without making recommendations or decisions and avoid allowing their own biases to interfere. The counselor provides appropriate information about the nature of the disorder, the extent of the risks in the specific case, the probable consequences, and (if appropriate) alternative options available, but the final decision to become pregnant or to continue a pregnancy must be left to the family. An important nursing role is reinforcing the information the families are given and continuing to interpret this information on their level of understanding.

The most important concept that must be emphasized to families is that *each pregnancy is an independent event*. For example, in monogenic disorders in which the risk factor is one in four that the child will be affected, the risk remains the same no matter how many affected children are already in the family. Families may maintain the erroneous assumption that the presence of one affected child ensures that the next three will be free of the disorder. However, "chance has no memory." The risk is one in four for each pregnancy. On the other hand, in a family with a child who has a disorder with multifactorial causes, the risk increases with each subsequent child born with the disorder.

Role of the Nurse in Genetic Counseling

Although diagnosis and treatment of genetic disorders require medical skills and determination of risk factors for many disorders requires the expertise of a geneticist, nurses with advanced preparation are assuming an increasingly important role in counseling people about genetically transmitted or genetically influenced conditions. Nurses are usually the ones who provide follow-up care and maintain contact with the patients. They are in the best position to sustain a close relationship with families; for example, community health nurses may have already established a rapport with the families.

Follow-up care. Maintaining contact with the family after genetic counseling, testing, or therapy is one of the most important nursing responsibilities, since the success of counseling is measured by the way the family uses the information presented to them. Most counseling services try to schedule at least one postdiagnostic or postcounseling visit to assess how well the family is beginning to incorporate this new information into their lives and value systems. Follow-up visits to the counseling service or visits to the home provide additional opportunities to reexplore all aspects of the situation and to answer any questions the family may have since the previous contacts.

Referral to appropriate agencies is an essential part of the follow-up management. Many organizations and foundations, such as the Cystic Fibrosis Foundation and the Muscular Dystrophy Association, help provide services and equipment for affected children. There are also numerous parent groups with which the family can share experiences and derive mutual support from other families with similar problems. Nurses should become familiar with services available in their community that provide assistance and education to families with these special problems.

Emotional support. Probably the most important of all nursing functions is providing emotional support to the family during all aspects of the counseling process. Feelings that are generated under the real or imagined threat posed by a genetic disorder are as varied as the people being counseled. Responses may include a variety of stress reactions, such as apathy, denial, anger, hostility, fear, embarrassment, grief, and loss of self-esteem.

Factors such as religious beliefs, intellectual level, and prior attitudes toward the disorder affect the way in which families respond to counseling information. Sometimes counselors and other health personnel create barriers through their own attitudes toward a specific disorder. It is often difficult to be nonjudgmental and objective, and nurses may intentionally or unintentionally influence families in making decisions. Families may pressure the nurse to make decisions for them with questions such as, "What would you do if you were me?" Families and individuals need education, guidance, and support throughout the counseling process. They should be given the facts and possible consequences and all the assistance they need in problem solving, but the final decision regarding a course of action must be their own.

PRECONCEPTION CARE

Preconception care is as important to perinatal services as prenatal care. Preconception care is designed for health maintenance. It stresses risk assessment and healthy behaviors that promote health of the woman and her potential fetus.

The period of greatest danger for the developing fetus is 17 to 56 days after fertilization. By the end of the eighth week after conception and certainly by the end of the first trimester, major structural anomalies in the fetus are already present if they are to occur. Because many women do not realize they are pregnant, do not have their pregnancy confirmed, and do not seek prenatal care until well into the first trimester, the rapidly growing fetus may be exposed to all types of intrauterine environmental hazards during its most vulnerable developmental phase (Cefalo and Moos, 1995).

Therefore preconception care has several purposes, including the following:

- Establish life-style behaviors to maintain optimum health (e.g., eating a healthy diet; getting enough rest

BOX 4-5
Components of Preconception Care

Health promotion: general teaching

Nutrition
- Healthy diet, including folic acid
- Optimum weight

Exercise and rest
Avoidance of substance use/abuse (tobacco, alcohol, "recreational" drugs)
Use of "safer sex" practices
Attending to family and social needs

Risk factor assessment

Medical history
- Immune status (e.g., rubella)
- Family history
- Illnesses (e.g., infections)
- Genetic disorders
- Current use of medication (prescription, nonprescription)

Reproductive history
- Contraceptive
- Obstetric

Psychosocial history
- Spouse/partner and family situation, including domestic violence
- Availability of family or other support systems
- Readiness for pregnancy (e.g., age, life goals, stress)

Financial resources
Environmental (home, workplace) conditions
- Safety hazards
- Toxic chemicals
- Radiation

Interventions

Anticipatory guidance/teaching
Treatment of medical conditions and results
- Medications
- Cessation/reduction in substance use/abuse
- Immunizations (e.g., rubella, tuberculosis, hepatitis)

Nutrition, diet and weight management
Exercise
Referral for genetic counseling
Referral to and use of:
- Family planning services
- Family and social needs management

and exercise; and reducing or avoiding alcohol use, smoking, and drugs).
- Identify and treat risk factors before conception (e.g., medical conditions such as diabetes mellitus, substance abuse, and testing for immunity from infections that could cause mental retardation or other birth defects).
- Conceive a pregnancy without unnecessary risk factors (e.g., monitor the medications taken for chronic illness, health hazards in the workplace or home).
- Identify carriers of inherited diseases (e.g., Tay-Sachs disease, sickle cell disease, thalassemia).
- Prepare people psychologically for pregnancy and the responsibilities that come with parenthood.

Every woman of childbearing age should be viewed as a potential mother. Therefore identifying and treating risk fac-

BOX 4-6
Preconception Assessment

Interview

Life-style
- Nutrition
- Exercise, rest
- Substance use: alcohol, tobacco, cocaine, other
- Occupation
- Psychosocial: stress, anxiety, depression; support from partner, family, friends; domestic violence
- Financial resources

Immunization status
- Rubella
- Hepatitis B

Medications
- Over the counter, nonprescription (e.g., aspirin)
- Prescription

Medical conditions: review of systems
- Hypertension and cardiovascular disease
- Seizure disorders
- Diabetes mellitus
- Renal disease
- Tuberculosis, asthma
- Autoimmune disorders (e.g., SLE, rheumatoid arthritis)
- Allergies

Reproductive system
- Fertility problems, endometriosis
- Contraceptive history
- Obstetric history (e.g., prior pregnancies, miscarriages, child with a disorder)
- Abnormal Papanicolaou (Pap) smear results
- Results of mammogram
- Sexually transmitted diseases (STDs)
- Sexual practices

Treatment history
- Previous abdominal/reproductive surgery
- Trauma
- Transfusion

Environmental history
- Work exposures
- Home exposures

Family history, including husband/partner
- Medical conditions
- Genetic conditions (e.g., sickle cell disease, Tay-Sachs disease, cystic fibrosis, bleeding disorders, hemophilia, PKU)
- Birth defects

Physical examination

General medical with emphasis on:
- Thyroid gland
- Breasts
- Pelvic structures

Laboratory studies

General: complete blood count, urinalysis, blood type and Rh, rubella immunity, STDs (e.g., syphilis, gonorrhea, *Chlamydia*), hepatitis B surface antigen, Pap smear, cervical culture

Depending on indication:
- Purified protein derivative (PPD)
- Human immunodeficiency virus (HIV)
- Toxicology screen
- Thalassemia

tors and providing anticipatory guidance with emphasis on healthy life-styles may be the key to improving the health of the next generation (Freda, 1993). Box 4-5 outlines the components of preconception care, such as health promotion, risk assessment, and interventions as needed.

The more the health care provider knows about a woman's state of health and life-style, the better. For example, women with insulin-dependent diabetes mellitus who maintain excellent control of blood sugar at conception could reduce the risk for congenital anomalies (malformations) in the fetus (Centers for Disease Control and Prevention, 1992). Women who have an adequate intake of folic acid (0.4 mg/day) before and after conception decrease the possibility of neural tube defects (Cefalo and Moos, 1995; Werler, Shipiro, and Mitchell, 1993). Demographic information such as age and race are also important. Women under age 15 or over age 40 are at higher risk during pregnancy than women ages 16 to 39. Some ethnic groups have special risks (e.g., African-Americans and Southeast Asians are at risk for sickle cell disease; people of Jewish descent are at risk for Tay-Sachs disease).

Box 4-6 provides a preconception assessment that identifies areas to be explored.

Role of the Nurse

Prevention should be the focus of self-care. From 8% to 10% of birth defects occur as a result of environmental factors and may be amenable to nursing intervention (Pletsh, 1990). Cleanliness, ventilation, adherence to manufacturer's directions for use and disposal of materials, use of protective gear to shield against known and unknown hazards, and avoidance of exposure to radiation are examples of strategies to reduce risk.

In some instances, safer materials can be substituted for potentially hazardous ones. For example, most household cleaning needs can be met with baking soda, table salt, distilled white vinegar, lemon juice, trisodium phosphate (TSP, which does not emit fumes), a plunger, and some common sense. These substances can be used to clean drains, wash windows, degrease, prevent mold and mildew, disinfect, and scour (Dadd, 1987).

Nurses must be alert to conditions in the workplace that may affect reproductive health of workers and their partners. Stress reduction through relaxation and guided imagery and moderate exercise and rest are useful.

As private citizens, nurses must become involved in professional and political organizations to promote and support legislation to control pollution of the environment. Nurses can teach about alternative ways to clean the home and care for yards and gardens to reduce exposure to potentially harmful substances.

Evaluation of short-term results is possible to some extent. The birth of a healthy baby with no apparent disorder or disease, the uncomplicated recovery of the new mother, continued fertility, and demonstration of a life-style that supports good reproductive health are some expected outcomes when preconception and pregnancy care are effective. Long-term effects may not be known for many years or generations.

Critical Thinking Exercises

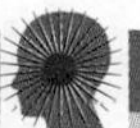

RISK OF RECURRENCE OF GENETIC DISORDERS

Estimation of the risk of recurrence of genetic disorders is often a difficult concept to understand and to explain to parents. Using the examples of Down syndrome and PKU, prepare an explanation of how these disorders are transmitted, when they can be diagnosed, and what the risk of transmission is for each pregnancy.

1. **What information do you need to provide this explanation accurately and completely?**
2. **Outline your response, keeping in mind genetics, stages of fetal development, and current diagnostic techniques.**
3. **How would your teaching materials and methods differ if you were providing this explanation to teenagers with no children rather than to parents of a child with a disorder?**

Key Points

- Genes are the basic units of heredity responsible for all human characteristics. They comprise 23 pairs of chromosomes: 22 pairs of autosomes and one pair of sex chromosomes.
- Chromosomal abnormalities of number and structure occur in both autosomes and sex chromosomes.
- Genetic disorders follow mendelian inheritance patterns of dominance, segregation, and independent assortment of normal genetic transmission.
- Multifactorial inheritance includes both genetic and environmental contributions.
- Human gestation is approximately 280 days after the LMP or 266 days after conception.
- Fertilization occurs in the uterine tube within 24 hours of ovulation. The zygote undergoes mitotic divisions, creating a 16-cell morula.
- Critical periods occur in human development during which the embryo/fetus is vulnerable to environmental teratogens.
- The best means for reducing the number of children born with genetic defects is to provide families with genetic information and services.
- Preconception care stresses healthy behaviors that promote health of the woman and her fetus.

References

Adzick N, Harrison M: Fetal surgical therapy, *Lancet* 343:897, 1994.

Andrews L et al, editors: *Assessing genetic risks: implications for health and social policy,* Washington, DC, 1994, National Academy Press (Institute of Medicine).

Barber H: Ethics, morals, and gene control, *The Female Patient* 16(10):13, 1991.

Bar-Hava I, Barnhardt Y: Fetal vibracoustic stimulation, *The Female Patient* 19(5):63, 1994.

Blackburn S, Loper D: *Maternal, fetal, and neonatal physiology: a clinical perspective,* Philadelphia, 1992, Saunders.

Brown M, Bellinger D, Matthews J: In utero lead exposure, *MCN Am J Matern Child Nurs* 15(2):94, 1990.

Cefalo R, Moos M: *Preconceptional health care,* St Louis, 1995, Mosby.

Centers for Disease Control and Prevention: Recommendation for use of folic acid to reduce number of spina bifida cases and other neural tube defects, *MMWR* 41(RR-14): 1992.

Collins F: Ahead of schedule and under budget: the Genome Project passes its fifth birthday, *Proc Natl Acad Sci USA* 92:10, 821, 1995.

Collins J: Fetal surgery: changing the outcome before birth, *J Obstet Gynecol Neonatal Nurs* 23:166, 1994.

Creasy R, Resnik J, editors: *Maternal-fetal medicine: principles and practice,* ed 3, Philadelphia, 1994, Saunders.

Crombleholme T, Bianchi D: In utero hematopoietic stem cell transplantation and gene therapy, *Semin Perinatol* 18(4):376, 1994.

Cunningham F, MacDonald P, Gant N: *Williams obstetrics,* ed 19, East Norwalk, Conn, 1993, Appleton & Lange.

Dadd D: Nontoxic cleaners for your home, *San Francisco Chronicle,* April 1, 1987, p C8.

Derom C et al: Increased monozygotic twinning rate after ovulation induction, *Lancet* 1:1237, 1987.

Fanaroff A, Martin R, editors: *Neonatal-perinatal medicine: diseases of the fetus and infant,* ed 5, St Louis, 1992, Mosby.

Freda M: Research utilization improves nursing practice, *AWHONN Voice,* 1(12):4, 1993.

Guyer M, Collins F: How is the Human Genome Project doing, and what have we learned so far? *Proc Natl Acad Sci USA* 92:10, 841, 1995.

Hallack M et al: Amniotic fluid index: gestational age-specific values for normal human pregnancy, *J Reprod Med* 38:853, 1993.

Howell L: The unborn surgical patient: a nursing frontier, *Nurs Clin North Am* 29:681, 1994.

Hoyme H: Teratogenically induced fetal anomalies, *Clin Perinatol* 17:547, 1990.

Hsieh F et al: Limb defects after chorionic villi sampling, *Obstet Gynecol* 85:84, 1995.

Hudson K et al: Genetic discrimination and health insurance: an urgent need for reform, *Science* 270:391, 1995.

Inati M, Lazar E, Haskin-Leahy L: The role of the genetic counselor in a perinatal unit, *Semin Perinatol* 18:133, 1994.

MacMullen N, Brucker M: Pregnancy made possible for women with cystic fibrosis, *MCN Am J Matern Child Nurs* 14(3):196, 1989.

Ott B: The Human Genome Project: an overview of ethical issues and public policy concerns, *Nurs Outlook,* 43(5), 1995.

Paynton A: Synthetic surfactant: giving premature infants a better chance for survival, *Nursing '91* 21(3):64, 1991.

Pickler R, Munro C: Gene therapy for inherited disorders, *J Pediatr Nurs* 10:40, 1995.

Pletsh P: Birth defect prevention: nursing interventions, *J Obstet Gynecol Neonatal Nurs* 19:482, 1990.

Poole R, editor: *The incredible machine,* Washington, DC, 1986, National Geographic Society.

Reed G, Claireaux A, Bain A, editors: *Diseases of the fetus and newborn: pathology, radiology, and genetics,* St Louis, 1989, Mosby.

Scanlon C, Fibison W: *Managing genetic information: implications for nursing practice,* Washington, DC, 1995, American Nurses Association.

Stringer M, Librizzi R, Weiner S: Establishing a prenatal genetic diagnosis: the nurse's role *MCN Am J Matern Child Nurs* 16(3):152, 1991.

Thomson E, Cordero J: The new teratogens: Accutane and other vitamin-A analogs, *MCN Am J Matern Child Nurs* 14(4):244, 1989.

US Department of Health and Human Services: *The Human Genome Project progress report fiscal years 1993-1994,* Washington, DC, 1995, National Institutes of Health.

Werler M, Shipiro S, Mitchell A: Periconceptional folic exposure and risk of occurrent neural tube defects, *JAMA* 269:1257, 1993.

Willson J et al: *Obstetrics and gynecology,* ed 9, St Louis, 1991, Mosby.

Bibliography

Anderson F et al: Attitudes of women to fetal tissue research, *J Med Ethics* 20(1):36, 1994.

Arias F: *Practical guide to high-risk pregnancy and delivery,* ed 2, St Louis, 1992, Mosby.

Forsman I: Evolution of the nursing role in genetics, *J Obstet Gynecol Neonatal Nurs* 23(6):481, 1994.

Hedrick M et al: Plug the lung until it grows (PLUG): a new method to treat congenital diaphragmatic hernia in utero, *J Pediatr Surg* 29(5):612, 1994.

Jones S: Genetic-based and assisted reproductive technology of the 21st century, *J Obstet Gynecol Neonatal Nurs* 23(2):160, 1994.

Noonan N, Senner A: Gene therapy techniques in the treatment of adenosine deaminase–deficiency severe combined immunodeficiency syndrome, *J Perinat Neonatal Nurs* 7(4):65, 1994.

Polin R, Fox W: *Fetal and neonatal physiology,* vols 1 and 2, Philadelphia, 1991, Saunders.

Snodgrass S: Cocaine babies: a result of multiple teratogenic influences, *J Child Neurol* 9(3):227, 1994.

CHAPTER 5

Assessment for Risk Factors

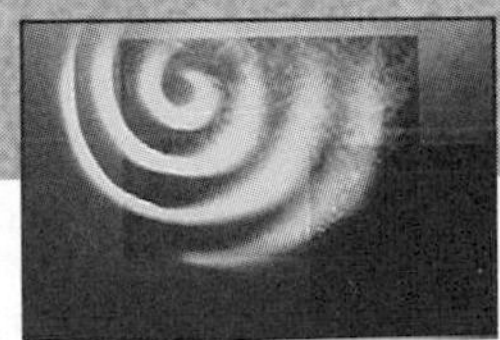

DEFINITION AND SCOPE OF THE PROBLEM, P. 79

Maternal health problems, p. 79

Fetal and neonatal health problems, p. 80

Regionalization of health care services, p. 80

CATEGORIES OF RISK FACTORS, P. 80

BIOPHYSICAL ASSESSMENT, P. 82

Daily fetal movement count, p. 82

Ultrasonography, p. 83

Magnetic resonance imaging, p. 90

BIOCHEMICAL ASSESSMENT, P. 90

Amniocentesis, p. 90

Percutaneous umbilical blood sampling, p. 93

Chorionic villus sampling, p. 94

Maternal assays, p. 95

ELECTRONIC FETAL MONITORING, P. 95

Indications, p. 95

Fetal responses to hypoxia and asphyxia, p. 97

Nonstress test (fetal activity determination), p. 97

Contraction stress test, p. 98

NURSING ROLE IN ANTENATAL ASSESSMENT FOR RISK, P. 100

Perinatal outcome depends on the early recognition and management of problems. Identification of the existence of risks, together with appropriate and timely intervention, can help prevent disabling conditions both during the neonatal period and in future developmental stages (Aumann and Baird, 1993). Emphasis is on the safe birth of normal infants who can develop to their maximum potential. Advances along many scientific fronts have provided the technology to achieve a level of perinatal health care far beyond that previously available.

Serious biologic handicaps, health problems, obstetric disorders, and social deprivation may compromise the mother and the infant in subtle or more obvious ways. Factors other than biophysical criteria contribute to risk. Homeless, single, and uninsured pregnant women who are unlikely to be able to access prenatal care early or at all are among those at risk. Psychosocial factors that involve maternal behaviors and adverse life-styles have a negative effect on the health of the mother and fetus (Fogel and Lewallen, 1995). Understanding the factors that place patients at risk will allow the nurse to provide individualized therapeutic nursing care (Kemp and Hatmaker, 1989).

DEFINITION AND SCOPE OF THE PROBLEM

A high-risk pregnancy is one in which the life or health of the mother or infant is jeopardized by a disorder coincidental with or unique to pregnancy. For the mother the high-risk status arbitrarily extends through the puerperium (30 days after childbirth). Postbirth maternal complications usually are resolved within a month of birth, but perinatal morbidity may continue for months or years.

Maternal Health Problems

Different parts of the world have different leading causes of maternal death attributable to pregnancy. In general, three major causes have persisted for the last 35 years: hypertensive disorders, infection, and hemorrhage.

In 1994, 270 women in the United States died of complications of pregnancy, childbirth, and the puerperium (National Center for Health Statistics, 1995). Women of color continue to have a maternal morbidity rate more than twice as high as Caucasian women (Atrash et al, 1990). In 1992 African-American mothers had significantly higher rates for anemia, chronic hypertension, and eclampsia compared with Caucasian mothers; the risk of a low-birth-weight (LBW, less than 2500 g) infant or preterm birth was greater for African-American than for Caucasian mothers for each of the medical risk factors associated with these outcomes. The four most commonly reported medical risk factors (anemia, diabetes, pregnancy-associated hypertension, uterine bleeding) were substantially higher for Native-American mothers than for any other racial or ethnic group (National Center for Health Statistics, 1994).

Although the number of maternal deaths overall is small, maternal mortality remains a significant problem because a high proportion of deaths are preventable, mainly through improving the access to and use of prenatal care services. Nurses can be instrumental in educating the public about the importance of obtaining early and regular care during pregnancy.

Fetal and Neonatal Health Problems

The leading causes of death in the neonatal period are congenital anomalies, disorders relating to short gestation and LBW, respiratory distress syndrome, and the effects of maternal complications. African-American women are twice as likely as Caucasian women to experience prematurity, LBW, and infant and fetal death (National Center for Health Statistics, 1994). Increased rates of survival during the neonatal period have resulted largely from the improvement in perinatal services, including the technology of neonatal intensive care units (NICUs), high-quality prenatal care, and the use of obstetric technology.

To achieve significant decline of the infant mortality rate and to eliminate racial and ethnic differences in pregnancy outcomes, a national, state, and local commitment to that goal is necessary. Reducing infant mortality requires the removal of financial, educational, sociocultural, and logistic barriers to care so pregnant women seek and receive health services.

Regionalization of Health Care Services

Mortality decreases when high-risk status is identified and intensive care applied. Follow-up studies have shown that serious residual handicaps (physical and mental) of surviving infants have been dramatically reduced when such identification and intervention exist.

It is neither feasible nor reasonable for each hospital to develop and maintain the full spectrum of medical, nursing, and other specialists; laboratory capabilities; and equipment necessary to provide optimal care for all patients. As a consequence, regionalization of health care has come into being; that is, facilities within a geographic region are organized to provide different levels of care. Ideally, a regionalized system includes primary care and three levels of facilities within the designated geographic area. The most specialized personnel and equipment are centralized in level III facilities and receive referrals from level I facilities, which provide care for patients with low-risk conditions. Level I facilities have three main functions: (1) the management of normal pregnancy, labor, and childbirth; (2) the earliest possible identification of high-risk pregnancy and high-risk neonates; and (3) the provision of stabilization care in the event of unanticipated obstetric or neonatal emergencies. Level II facilities provide care for a specified type of maternal and neonatal complications and offer a full range of maternity and neonatal care in uncomplicated cases. Staff members are specially educated and prepared for those particular complications, and appropriate equipment is available. Level III facilities, the regional centers, have the capacity to manage the most complex disorders, both maternal and neonatal. Often, pregnant women are transported to these centers before the birth of the baby to optimize the maternal/fetal/neonatal outcome. The regional centers also provide outreach educational services for medical and nursing staff within the region.

CATEGORIES OF RISK FACTORS

Traditionally, risk factors have been viewed only from the medical model: only medical, obstetric, or physiologic risk factors were considered. Today a more comprehensive approach to high-risk pregnancy is used. The factors associated with high-risk childbearing are grouped into broad categories based on threats to health and pregnancy outcome. Categories of risk include biophysical, psychosocial, sociodemographic, and environmental as follows (Box 5-1), (Fogel and Lewallen, 1995):

- *Biophysical risks* include factors that originate within the mother or fetus and affect the development or functioning of either or both.
- *Psychosocial risks* are comprised of maternal behaviors and adverse life-styles that have a negative effect on the health of the mother and/or fetus; they may include emotional distress and disturbed interpersonal relationships, as well as inadequate social support and unsafe cultural practices (see the Cultural Considerations box below).
- *Sociodemographic risks* arise from the mother and her family and place the mother-fetus unit at risk.
- *Environmental risks* include hazards of the workplace and the woman's general environment.

Risk factors are interrelated and cumulative in their effects and are shown in Fig. 5-1. Box 5-2 lists pregnancy problems and risk factors, and Box 5-3 outlines risk factors of the postpartum woman and the neonate. This chapter focuses on assessment of biophysical risks. Chapter 11 addresses psychosocial risks.

The major expected outcome of antepartum testing is the detection of potential fetal compromise. Ideally the technique used will identify fetal compromise before intrauterine asphyxia of the fetus so that the health care provider can take measures to prevent or minimize adverse perinatal outcomes. No single test can provide this information. The results of such tests must be interpreted in light of the complete clinical picture. The remainder of this chapter describes diagnostic techniques and their use in detecting fetuses at risk.

Cultural Considerations 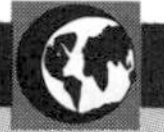

ANTEPARTUM CULTURAL ASSESSMENT

All cultures recognize pregnancy as a special transitional period, with particular customs and beliefs that dictate behavior during this time. In the antepartum period, the nurse should assess the following:

- Consideration of pregnancy as a state of illness or health
- Behavioral expectations of mother and health care provider
- Dietary prescriptions or restrictions; hot/cold balance theory; pica
- Activity restrictions or prescriptions; use of massage
- People from whom woman will usually seek advice and the appropriate time to do so; when to begin prenatal care (if at all); modesty

BOX 5-1
Categories of High-Risk Factors

BIOPHYSICAL

1. **Genetic**—may interfere with normal fetal/neonatal development, result in congenital anomalies, and/or create difficulties for the mother. Includes defective genes, transmittable inherited disorders, chromosome anomalies, multiple pregnancy, large fetal size, and ABO incompatibility.
2. **Nutritional status**—one of the most important determinants of pregnancy outcome. Fetal growth and development cannot progress normally without adequate nutrition. Includes very young age; three pregnancies in the past 2 years; tobacco, alcohol, or drug use; inadequate intake because of chronic illness or food fads; inadequate or excessive weight gain; and hematocrit less than 33%.
3. **Medical and obstetric**—medical complications of current and past pregnancies, obstetric-related illnesses, and pregnancy losses. See Box 5-2.

PSYCHOSOCIAL

1. **Smoking**—strong, consistent, causal relationship between maternal smoking and reduced birth weight. Risks include LBW infants, especially with increased age; higher neonatal mortality rates; increased spontaneous abortions; and increased incidence of premature rupture of membranes. Aggravated by low socioeconomic status, poor nutritional status, and concurrent use of alcohol.
2. **Caffeine**—not been shown to cause birth defects in humans. Heavy consumption (3 or more cups of coffee/day) has been related to a slight decrease in birth weight.
3. **Alcohol**—although exact effects of use in pregnancy have not been quantified and mode of action is largely unexplained, The conclusion is that there are specific negative reproductive effects. Includes fetal alcohol syndrome (FAS) and fetal alcohol effects (FAEs), learning disabilities, and hyperactivity.
4. **Drugs**—may adversely affect a developing fetus through several mechanisms: they may be teratogenic, cause metabolic disturbances, produce chemical effects, or cause depression and/or alteration of central nervous system function. Includes those prescribed by health care provider or bought over the counter and commonly abused drugs: heroin, cocaine, and marijuana. See Chapter 11 for more information about drug and alcohol abuse.
5. **Psychologic status**—childbearing triggers profound and complex physiologic, psychologic, and social changes; some evidence suggests a relationship between emotional distress and birth complications. Includes specific intrapsychic disturbances and addictive life styles; history of child or spouse abuse; insufficient support systems; family disruption or dissolution; maternal role changes/conflicts; noncompliance with cultural norms; unsafe cultural, ethnic, or religious practices; and situational crises.

SOCIODEMOGRAPHIC

1. **Low income**—poverty underlies many other risk factors. Includes inadequate financial resources for food and prenatal care, poor general health, and increased risk of medical complications of pregnancy; adverse environmental influences more prevalent.
2. **Lack of prenatal care**—major factor in placing woman at risk since opportunity is lost for early diagnosis and treatment of complications. May be caused by financial barriers or lack of access to care; depersonalization of the system resulting in long waits, routine visits, variability in health care personnel, and unpleasant physical surroundings; lack of understanding of need for early and continued care or cultural beliefs that do not support the need; and fear of health care providers and the system.
3. **Age**—traditionally, women at either end of the childbearing years have had a higher incidence of poor outcomes; research indicates that age may be a risk factor in some patients but not in others. Both physiologic and psychologic risks should be evaluated.

   Adolescents: more complications are seen in the very young (younger than 15 years old) and if pregnancy occurs less than 3 years after menarche. Includes anemia, pregnancy-induced hypertension (PIH), prolonged labor, contracted pelvis, and cephalopelvic disproportion; mothers under age 15 have a 60% higher mortality rate than those over age 20; long-term social implications such as lower educational attainment, lower incomes, increased dependence on government support programs, higher divorce rates, and higher parity.

   Mature mothers: risks do not arise from age alone, but rather are affected by many factors, such as number and spacing of previous pregnancies; genetic disposition of the parents; and medical history, life-style, nutrition, and prenatal care of mother. Increased risks are associated with increased likelihood of chronic diseases that adversely affect pregnancy outcomes; more invasive medical management of older women's pregnancies and labors, with resulting complications; and demographic characteristics. Specific entities more likely to be experienced by mature women include hypertension and PIH, diabetes, extended labor, cesarean delivery, placenta previa, abruptio placentae, and mortality. Her fetus is at greater risk for both LBW and macrosomia, chromosomal abnormalities, congenital malformations, and neonatal mortality.
4. **Parity**—number of previous pregnancies is a risk and is associated with age. Includes all first pregnancies and first pregnancy at either end of the childbearing age continuum; incidence of PIH and dystocia is higher in first births.
5. **Marital status**—mortality and morbidity rates are higher for nonmarital than marital births. Includes greater risk for PIH and inadequate prenatal care; more often occur in lower age-groups.
6. **Residence**—large variations in prenatal care availability and quality. Women in metropolitan areas have more prenatal visits than those in rural areas; those in rural areas have higher incidence of maternal mortality and have fewer opportunities for specialized care. Health care in an inner city may be of poorer quality than in a more affluent section, and those women are usually poorer and begin childbearing earlier and continue longer.
7. **Ethnicity**—ethnicity alone is not a major risk; race as indicator of other sociodemographic factors, however, is a risk. Non-Caucasian women are more than 3 times as likely as Caucasian women to die of pregnancy-related causes; infant mortality rates among African-Americans are more than twice as high as those among Caucasians; African-American babies have the highest rates of prematurity and LBW.

ENVIRONMENTAL

A variety of environmental substances can have an impact on fertility and fetal development, the chance of a live birth, and the child's subsequent mental and physical development. Substances include infections, radiation, chemicals such as pesticides, therapeutic drugs, illicit drugs, industrial pollutant, cigarette smoke, stress, and diet. Paternal exposure to mutagenic agents in the workplace associated with increased risk of spontaneous abortion.

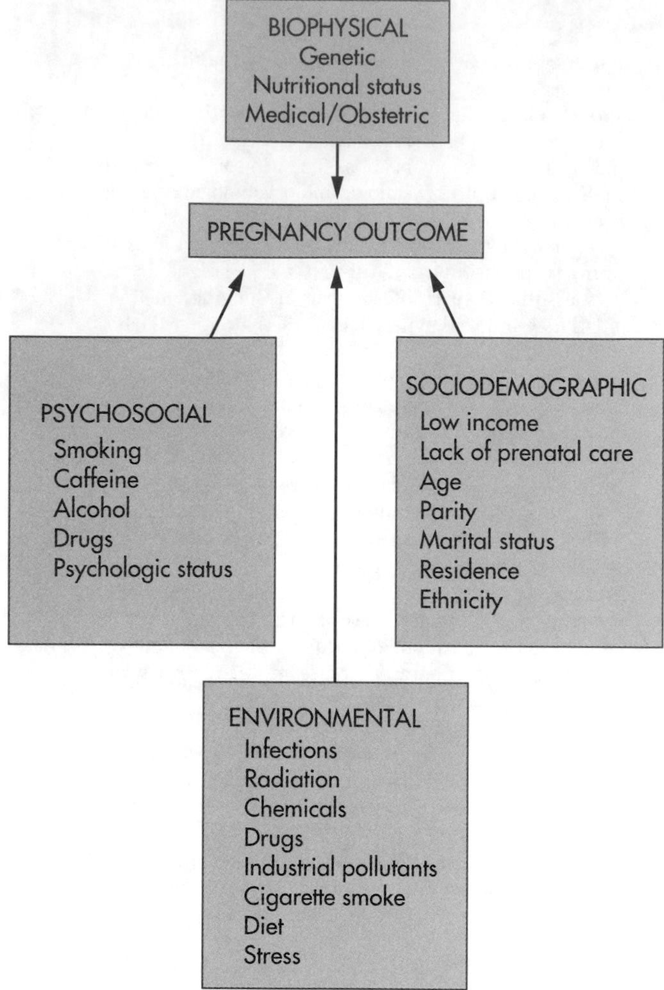

Fig. 5-1 Interrelationship of risk factors that may affect pregnancy outcome. (Modified from Fogel C, Woods D: *Health care of women,* 1981, Mosby.)

BOX 5-2
Specific Pregnancy Problems and Related Risk Factors

Preterm labor
Age below 16 or over 35
Low socioeconomic status
Maternal weight below 50 kg (110 lb)
Poor nutrition
Previous preterm birth
Incompetent cervix
Uterine anomalies
Smoking
Drug addiction and alcohol abuse
Pyelonephritis, pneumonia
Multiple gestation
Anemia
Abnormal fetal presentation
Preterm rupture of membranes
Placental abnormalities
Infection

Polyhydramnios
Diabetes mellitus
Multiple gestation
Fetal congenital anomalies
Isoimmunization (Rh or ABO)
Nonimmune hydrops
Abnormal fetal presentation

Intrauterine growth restriction (IUGR)
Multiple gestation
Poor nutrition
Maternal cyanotic heart disease
Chronic hypertension
Pregnancy-induced hypertension (PIH)
Recurrent antepartum hemorrhage
Smoking
Maternal diabetes with vascular problems
Fetal infections
Fetal cardiovascular anomalies
Drug addiction and alcohol abuse
Fetal congenital anomalies
Hemoglobinopathies

Oligohydramnios
Renal agenesis (Potter's syndrome)
Prolonged rupture of membranes
IUGR
Intrauterine fetal demise

Postterm pregnancy
Anencephaly
Placental sulfatase deficiency
Perinatal hypoxia, acidosis
Placental insufficiency

Chromosomal abnormalities
Maternal age 35 years or more at delivery
Balanced translocation (maternal and paternal)

Modified from DeCherney A, Pernoll M, editors: *Current obstetric and gynecologic diagnosis and treatment,* ed 8, East Norwalk, Conn, 1994, Appleton & Lange.

BIOPHYSICAL ASSESSMENT

Daily Fetal Movement Count

Maternal assessment of fetal activity is a simple yet valuable method for monitoring the fetal condition. **Daily fetal movement count (DFMC)** is simple to understand, is noninvasive, can be done at home, and does not interfere with most daily routines. In general the presence of fetal movements (FMs) is a reassuring sign of fetal health. Most women who experience stillbirth note a decrease in or absence of FMs (Calhoun, 1990).

Maternal awareness of FMs is reported to be at least 90% accurate, as demonstrated by simultaneous observation of the fetus by real-time ultrasound; no mothers report more FMs than are documented. Several protocols are used for counting. Except for very low daily FM or a trend toward decreased motion, the clinical value of the absolute number of FMs has not been established. The only exception is if FMs cease entirely for 12 hours (fetal alarm signal). Generally, fewer than three FMs within 1 hour warrants further evalua-

BOX 5-3
Factors that Place Postpartum Woman and Neonate at High Risk

Mother
Hemorrhage
Infection
Abnormal vital signs
Traumatic labor or birth
Psychosocial factors

Infant (for admission to NICU)
High-risk category
Infants continuing or developing signs of RDS or other respiratory distress
Asphyxiated infants (Apgar scores less than 6 at 5 minutes); resuscitation required at birth
Preterm infants; dysmature infants
Infants with cyanosis or suspected cardiovascular disease; persistent cyanosis
Infants with major congenital malformations requiring surgery; chromosomal anomalies
Infants with convulsions, sepsis, hemorrhagic diathesis, or shock
Meconium aspiration syndrome
CNS depression for longer than 24 hours
Hypoglycemia
Hypocalcemia
Hyperbilirubinemia

Moderate-risk category
Dysmaturity
Prematurity (weight between 2000 and 2500 g)
Apgar score less than 5 at 1 minute
Feeding problems
Multifetal birth
Transient tachypnea
Hypomagnesemia or hypermagnesemia
Hypoparathyroidism
Failure to gain weight
Jitteriness or hyperactivity
Cardiac anomalies not requiring immediate catheterization
Heart murmur
Anemia
CNS depression for less than 24 hours

CNS, Central nervous system; *NICU*, neonatal intensive care unit; *RDS*, respiratory distress syndrome.

tion through nonstress or contraction stress testing, **biophysical profile (BPP)**, or a combination of evaluation methods.

Ultrasonography

Sound is a waveform of energy that causes oscillation of small particles in a medium. The frequency of sound, which refers to the number of peaks or waves that traverse a given point per unit of time, is expressed in hertz (Hz). Sound with a frequency of one cycle, or one peak per second, has a frequency of 1 Hz. When directional beams of sound strike an object, an echo is returned. The time delay between the emission of the sound and the return of the echo is noted, as well as the direction from which the echo comes. From these data the object's distance and location can be calculated.

First introduced in the 1960s, diagnostic ultrasound has developed rapidly to enjoy a principle position in antepartum fetal surveillance. **Ultrasound** is sound that has a frequency higher than that of normal human hearing, that is, greater than 20,000 Hz. Diagnostic ultrasound instruments operate in a range of frequencies varying from 2 to 10 million Hz (or 2 to 10 megahertz [MHz]), still well below that used by sonar and radar.

Levels of ultrasound examination. Perinatal care providers and ultrasonographers have come to a tentative agreement on terminology describing two different levels of ultrasound. Basic screening, or level 1, examination is used most often. It can be performed by ultrasonographers or other health care professionals, including nurses who have had special training. Level 1 ultrasounds are directed toward the uses described in detail in the following sections; they are used primarily to detect fetal viability, determine the presentation of the fetus and gestational age, locate the placenta, and determine **amniotic fluid volume (AFV).** Targeted, or level 2, examinations are done if a patient is suspected of carrying an anatomically or physiologically abnormal fetus. Indications for a level 2 examination include abnormal findings on a clinical examination, especially with polyhydramnios or oligohydramnios; elevated **alpha-fetoprotein (AFP)** levels; and a history of offspring with anomalies that could be seen with ultrasound. Level 2 ultrasounds are performed by highly trained and experienced ultrasonographers.

Indications for use. Table 5-1 lists major indications for the use of obstetric sonography by trimester. During the first trimester, ultrasound examination is performed to obtain the following information: (1) number, size, and location of gestational sacs (Fig. 5-2); (2) presence or absence of fetal cardiac and body movement; (3) presence or absence of uterine abnormalities (e.g., bicornuate uterus, fibroids) or adnexal masses (e.g., ovarian cysts, ectopic pregnancy); (4) pregnancy dating (i.e., crown-rump length); and (5) presence and location of an intrauterine device (IUD).

During the second and third trimesters the following information is sought: (1) fetal viability, number, position, gestational age, growth pattern, and anomalies; (2) amniotic fluid volume; (3) placental location and maturity; (4) uterine fibroids and anomalies; and (5) adnexal masses.

Fetal heart activity. Fetal heart activity can be demonstrated as early as 6 to 7 weeks by real-time echo scanners and at 10 to 12 weeks by Doppler mode. By 9 to 10 weeks, gestational trophoblastic disease can be diagnosed (Fig. 5-3). Confirmation of fetal death can be detected by lack of heart motion, the presence of fetal scalp edema, and maceration and overlap of the cranial bones.

Gestational age. Several indicators have been established for the need of gestational dating: (1) uncertain dates for the last normal menstrual period, (2) recent discontinuation of

TABLE 5-1 Major indications for obstetric sonography

FIRST TRIMESTER	SECOND TRIMESTER	THIRD TRIMESTER

Confirm pregnancy
Confirm viability
Rule out ectopic pregnancy
Confirm gestational age†
  Birth control use
  Irregular menses
  No dates
  Postpartum pregnancy
Previous complicated pregnancy
  Cesarean birth
  Rh incompatibility
  Diabetes mellitus
  Intrauterine fetal growth restriction (IUGR)
  Clarify dates/sizes discrepancy
Large for dates—rule out:
  Leiomyomata
  Bicornuate uterus
  Adnexal mass
  Multifetal gestation
  Poor dates
  Molar pregnancy*§
Small for dates—rule out:
  Poor dates
  Missed abortion
  Blighted ovum
	Establish or confirm dates*
	If no fetal heart tones:
	  Clarify dates/size discrepancy, variability
	Large for dates—rule out:
	  Poor estimate of dates
	  Molar pregnancy
	  Multifetal gestation
	  Leiomyomata
	  Polyhydramnios
	  Congenital anomalies
	Small for dates—rule out:
	  Poor estimate of dates
	  IUGR
	  Congenital anomalies
	  Oligohydramnios
	If history of bleeding—rule out total placenta previa
	If Rh incompatibility—rule out fetal hydrops
		If no fetal heart tones:
		  Clarify dates/size discrepancy, variability
		Large for dates—rule out:
		  Macrosomia (diabetes mellitus)
		  Multifetal gestation
		  Polyhydramnios
		  Congenital anomalies
		  Poor estimate of dates‡
		Small for dates—rule out:
		  IUGR
		  Oligohydramnios
		  Congenital anomalies
		  Poor estimate of dates‡
		Determine fetal position—rule out:
		  Breech
		  Tranverse lie
		If history of bleeding—rule out:
		  Placenta previa
		  Abruptio placentae
		  Determine fetal lung maturity
		  Amniocentesis for lecithin/sphingomyelin ratio (see p. 90)
		  Placental maturity (grades 0-3)
		If Rh incompatibility—rule out fetal hydrops
		Doppler flow studies
		Biophysical profile
		Phosphatidylglycerol
		Amniotic fluid volume

Modified from Athey P, Hadlock F: *Ultrasound in obstetrics and gynecology*, ed 2, St Louis, 1985, Mosby.
*Accuracy ± 1 to 1½ weeks.
†Accuracy ± 3 days.
‡Accuracy only ± 3 weeks.
§Hydatidiform mole.

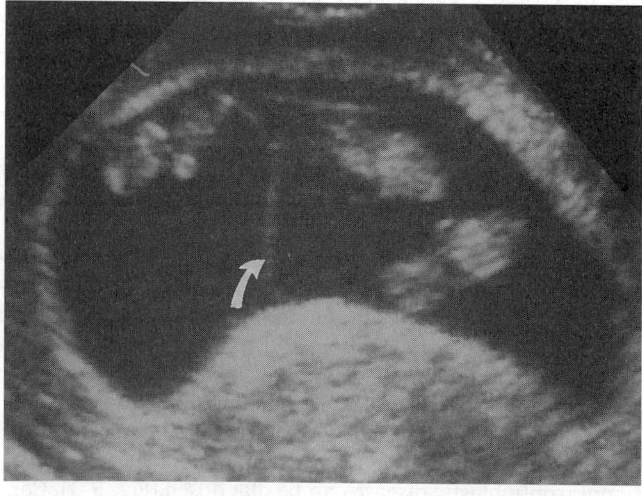

Fig. 5-2 First-trimester triplets identified at 9 weeks gestation. Transvaginal transaxial-coronal view shows three well-defined embryos. Between two of the embryos, the one on the left and the one in the middle, is a well-defined, thick dichorionic-diamniotic membrane *(curved arrow)*. (From Kurtz A, Middleton W: *Ultrasound: the requisites*, St Louis, 1996, Mosby.)

TABLE 5-2 Correlation of fetal weight and biparietal diameter (BPD)

BPD (cm)	ESTIMATED FETAL WEIGHT
8.2	2290 g (5 lb, 1 oz)
8.5	2500 g (5 lb, 8 oz)
8.8	2730 g (6 lb, 0 oz)
9.4	3180 g (7 lb, 0 oz)
10.0	3630 g (8 lb, 0 oz)
10.6	4070 g (9 lb, 0 oz)

oral contraceptives, (3) bleeding episode during the first trimester, (4) uterine size that does not agree with dates, and (5) other high-risk conditions.

During the first 18 weeks of gestation the use of ultrasound permits an extremely accurate assessment of gestational age because most normal fetuses grow at the same rate. With increased fetal age, the accuracy of gestational age estimates using ultrasound increases as more variables are measured (Chervenak and Gabbe, 1991; Manning, 1994). Four

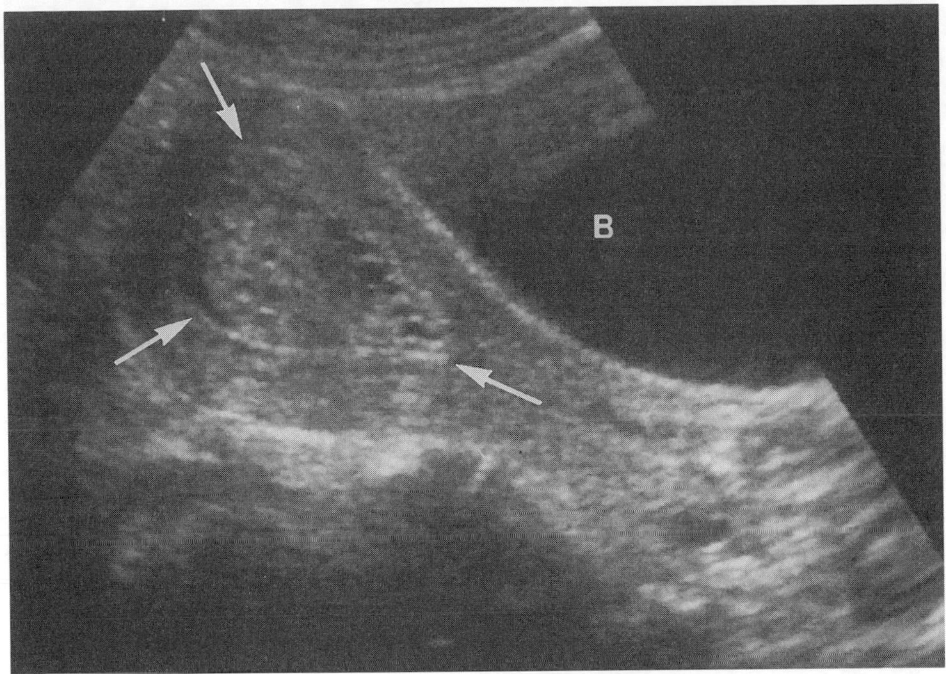

Fig. 5-3 Hydatidiform mole. This transabdominal sagittal midline image shows an enlarged first-trimester uterus. Markedly spread endometrial canal *(arrows)* is filled with hypoechoic and hyperechoic tissue. Note vesicular (grapelike) appearance. *B*, Urinary bladder. (From Kurtz A, Middleton W: *Ultrasound: the requisites*, St Louis, 1996, Mosby.)

methods of fetal age estimation are used: (1) determination of gestational sac dimensions (about 8 weeks), (2) measurement of crown-rump length (7 to 14 weeks), (3) measurement of the **biparietal diameter (BPD)** (after 12 weeks), and (4) measurement of femur length (after 12 weeks). Fetal BPD at 36 weeks should be approximately 8.7 cm. Term pregnancy and fetal maturity can be diagnosed with some confidence if the biparietal cephalometric measurement by ultrasound is greater than 9.8 cm (Figs. 5-4 and 5-5 and Table 5-2), especially when combined with appropriate femur length measurement. In later gestations the accuracy of fetal age determination is enhanced by serial measurements.

Fetal growth. Fetal growth is a result of interaction between intrinsic growth potential and environmental factors that may enhance or inhibit that growth. Conditions that serve as indicators for ultrasound assessment of fetal growth include (1) poor maternal weight gain or pattern of weight gain, (2) previous **intrauterine growth restriction (IUGR)**, (3) chronic infections, (4) ingestion of drugs (tobacco, alcohol, over-the-counter and street drugs), (5) maternal diabetes mellitus, (6) PIH or other hypertension, (6) multifetal pregnancy, and (7) other medical or surgical complications.

Serial evaluations of BPD and limb length can differentiate between inaccurate dates and true IUGR. IUGR may be symmetric (the fetus is small in all parameters) or asymmetric (head and body growth vary). Symmetric IUGR, which implies a chronic or longstanding insult, may be caused by low genetic growth potential, intrauterine infection, maternal undernutrition or heavy smoking, or chromosomal aberration. Asymmetric growth reflects an acute or late-occurring deprivation, such as placenta insufficiency resulting from hypertension, renal disease, or cardiovascular disease (Aumann and Baird, 1993; Manning, 1994).

Adjunct to amniocentesis, percutaneous umbilical blood sampling, and chorionic villus sampling. The safety of **amniocentesis** is increased when the physician knows the exact position of the fetus, placenta, and pockets of amniotic fluid. The use of ultrasound scanning has greatly reduced previous risks associated with amniocentesis, such as fetomaternal hemorrhage from a pierced placenta. **Percutaneous umbilical blood sampling (PUBS)** and **chorionic villus sampling (CVS)** are also guided by ultrasound to identify accurately the cord and chorion frondosum.

Fetal anatomy. Depending on the gestational age, the following structures may be identified: head (including ventricles and blood vessels), neck, spine, heart, stomach, small bowel, liver, kidneys, bladder, and limbs. Ultrasonography permits the confirmation of normal anatomy or the detection of major fetal malformations. The recognition of an anomaly may influence the location (e.g., delivery room vs. a labor, delivery, recovery room; a level III center vs. a level I institution) and method of birth so neonatal outcomes may be optimal. Beyond 36 weeks of gestation, more than 85% of all major anomalies can be detected by ultrasound. As a general rule, the earlier in gestation a lesion can be detected, the worse the prognostic significance (Manning, 1994).

The number of fetuses and their presentation also may be

A

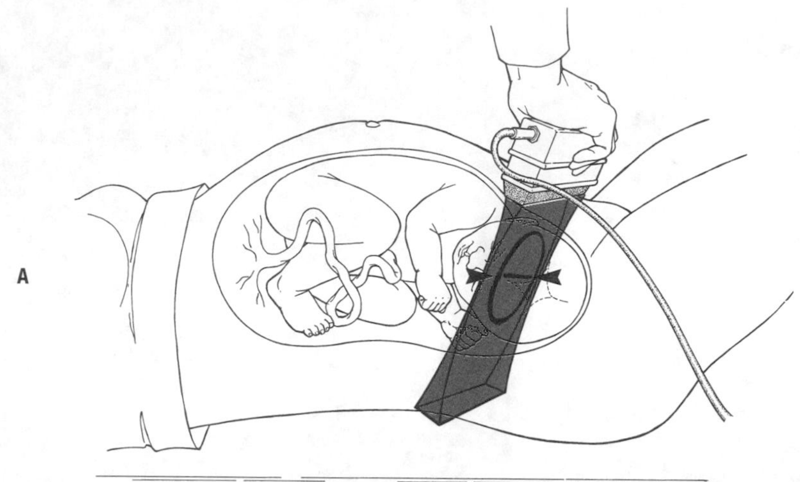

B

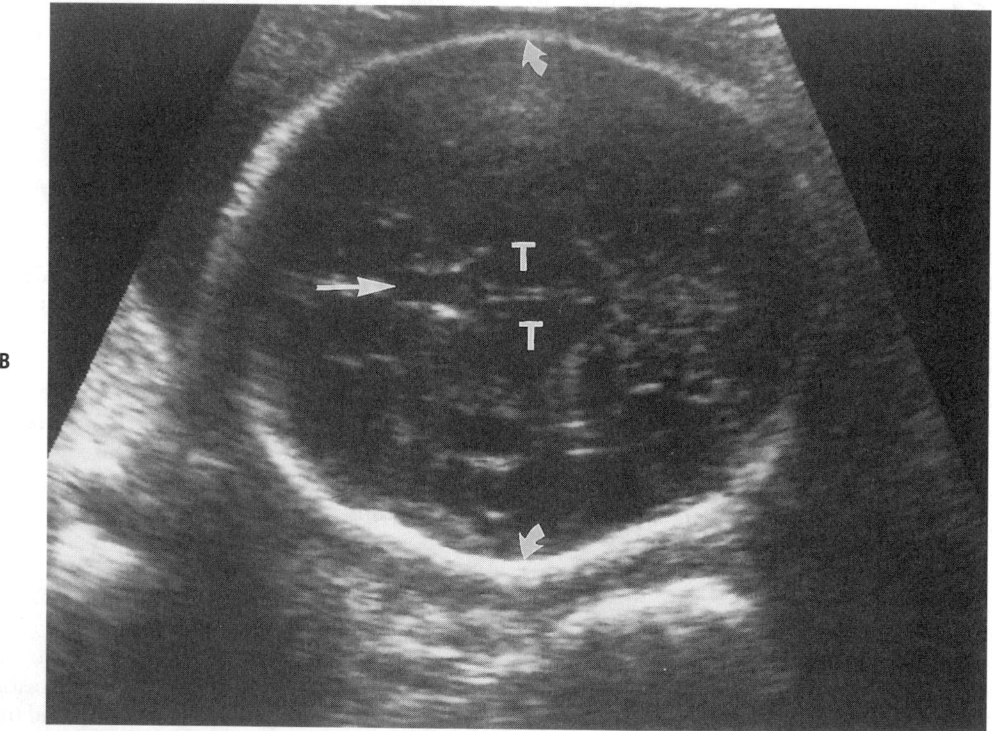

Fig. 5-4 **A,** Biparietal cephalometry by ultrasound. **B,** Transaxial image of the fetal head in the late second trimester, at the level of the thalami *(T)*. The biparietal diameter is measured from the leading edge to the leading edge *(curved arrows)*. The cavum septum pellucidum is also seen *(straight arrow)*. (**B** from Kurtz A, Middleton W: *Ultrasound: the requisites*, St Louis, 1996, Mosby.)

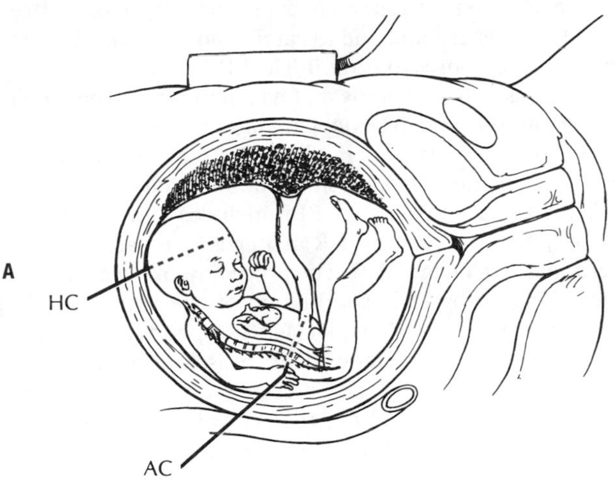

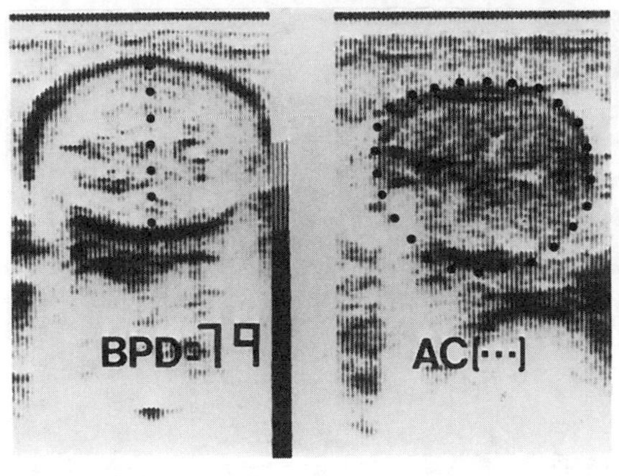

Fig. 5-5 **A**, Schematic presentation of appropriate planes of sections (*dotted lines*) for BPD, head circumference (HC), and abdominal circumference (AC). **B**, Real-time ultrasound image demonstrates typical head and body images that correspond to planes in **A**. Using these two images, one can determine BPD (7.9 cm), HC (30 cm), AC (28 cm), and estimated fetal weight (EFW) (1840 g) in this normal 32-week fetus. (From Athey P, Hadlock F: *Ultrasound in Obstetrics and gynecology*, ed 2, St Louis, 1985, Mosby.)

assessed. This knowledge assists with planning for therapy and mode of birth.

Placental position and function. The pattern of uterine and placental growth and the fullness of the maternal bladder influences the apparent location of the placenta. By 14 to 16 weeks the placenta can be clearly defined, but its relationship to the internal cervical os sometimes can be altered dramatically by changing the degree of fullness of the maternal bladder. In approximately 15% to 20% of all pregnancies in which ultrasound scanning is performed in the second trimester, the placenta seems to be overlying the os; at term the incidence of placenta previa is only 0.5%. Thus the diagnosis of placenta previa can seldom be confirmed until 27 weeks, mainly because of the elongation of the lower uterine segment as pregnancy advances.

Grading of placental maturation is another use of ultrasound (Box 5-4). The calcium deposits are also significant in postterm pregnancies in that as they increase, the available surface area that can be adequately bathed by maternal blood decreases. At exactly what point this results in fetal wastage and hypoxia cannot be pinpointed precisely; however, effects usually are observable by 42 weeks and progress thereafter (Gilbert and Harmon, 1993).

Fetal well-being. Among the many physiologic measurements of the fetus that can be performed with ultrasound scanning are the following: abnormalities of amniotic fluid volume, analysis of vascular waveforms from the fetal circulation, heart motion, **fetal breathing movements (FBMs)**, fetal urine production, and fetal limb and head movements. Assessment of these parameters yields a fairly reliable picture of fetal well-being, singly or in cohort fashion. The significance of these findings is discussed in the folowing sections.

AMNIOTIC FLUID VOLUME. Abnormalities of AFV, whether excessive or diminished, are often associated with fetal disorders. Subjective criteria for the assessment of oligohydramnios (decreased fluid) include the absence of fluid pockets throughout the uterine cavity and the impression of crowding of fetal small parts. Objective determination of decreased volume is made when the largest pocket of fluid measured in two perpendicular planes is less than 1 cm. In the case of polyhydramnios (increased fluid), subjective criteria include multiple large pockets, the impression of a floating fetus, and free movement of fetal limbs. The diagnosis may be made when the largest pocket of fluid exceeds 8 cm in two perpendicular planes (Fischer and Depp, 1995; Manning, 1994). The total volume can be evaluated by a method developed by Rutherford et al. (1987), in which the depths (in centimeters)

BOX 5-4
Placental Grading

Third-trimester grading of placental maturation can be accomplished by means of ultrasound scanning. It has been recognized that throughout gestation the placenta undergoes detectable maturational changes; a relationship has been noted between advancing placental grade and fetal pulmonary maturity. Placentas are graded on a scale of 0 to 3 (with 3 being the most mature) that is based on the identification and distribution of calcium deposits within the fetal component (Manning, 1994). Ultrasound examination can identify changes in the chorionic plate, placental substance, and basal layer of the placenta that correspond to the following grades: (1) grade 0 placentas are seen in the first and second trimester; (2) grade I placentas appear between 30 and 32 weeks and may even persist until term; (3) grade II placentas are observed at around 36 weeks and persist until term in 45% of pregnancies; and (4) grade III placentas are seen at 38 weeks and reflect the greatest maturation; however, this occurs in only a small number of placentas.

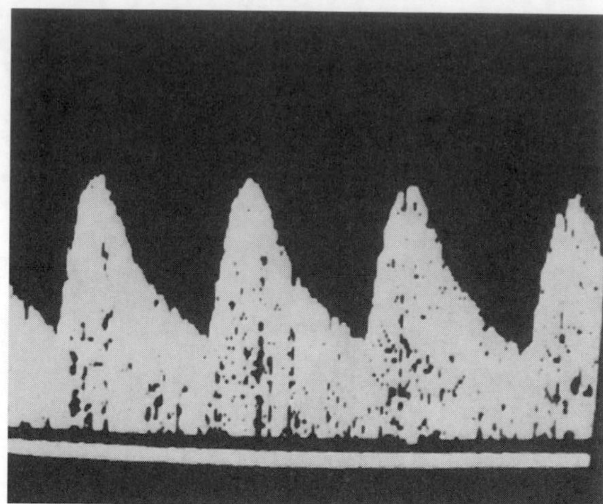

Fig. 5-6 Normal umbilical artery velocity wave forms and measurements from systole and end diastole. (From Shulman H: *Doppler ultrasound.* In Eden R, Boehm F, editors: *Assessment and care of the fetus: physiological, clinical and medicolegal principles,* Stamford, Conn, 1990, Appleton & Lange.)

of amniotic fluid in all four quadrants surrounding the maternal umbilicus are totaled, resulting in an **amniotic fluid index (AFI).** An AFI of less than 5 cm is considered to indicate oligohydramnios, 5 to 8 cm is considered borderline, and a measurement greater than 8 cm reflects polyhydramnios.

Oligohydramnios is associated with congenital anomalies (e.g., renal agenesis), IUGR, and fetal distress in labor. Polyhydramnios is found with neural tube defects, obstruction of the fetal gastrointestinal tract, multiple fetuses, and fetal hydrops (Brace, 1994; Fischer and Depp, 1995; Manning, 1994).

DOPPLER BLOOD FLOW ANALYSIS. One of the major advances in perinatal medicine is the ability to study blood flow noninvasively in the fetus and placenta using Doppler ultrasound. When a sound wave is reflected from a moving target, there is a change in frequency of the reflected wave relative to the transmitted wave. This is called the *Doppler effect.* An ultrasound beam scattered by a group of red blood cells (RBCs) is an example of this effect. The velocity of the RBCs can be determined by measuring the change in the frequency in the sound wave reflected off them (Trudinger, 1994).

Velocity waveforms from umbilical and uterine arteries, reported in systolic/diastolic (S/D) ratios, can be detected first at 15 weeks of pregnancy. Because of progressive decline in resistance in both the umbilical and the uterine artery circulation, decreasing measurement values occur as pregnancy advances. Most fetuses will achieve an S/D ratio of 3 or less by 30 weeks (Fig. 5-6). Persistent elevation of S/D ratios after 30 weeks is associated with IUGR, usually resulting from **uteroplacental insufficiency (UPI).** Abnormal velocity study results also are seen with certain chromosomal abnormalities (trisomy 13 and 18) in the fetus and lupus erythematosus in the mother (Schulman, 1990). Nicotine from maternal smoking also has been reported to increase the S/D ratio (Trudinger, 1994).

BIOPHYSICAL PROFILE. Real-time ultrasound permits detailed assessment of the physical and physiologic characteristics of the developing fetus to such an extent that it is possible to examine the fetus in detail and to catalog normal and abnormal biophysical responses to stimuli. The BPP is a noninvasive dynamic assessment of a fetus and its environment, employing ultrasonography and external fetal monitoring.

Fetal BPP scoring is a method of fetal risk surveillance based on the composite assessment of both acute and chronic markers of fetal disease. The BPP includes FBMs, FMs, fetal tone (FT), fetal heart rate (FHR) patterns by means of a **nonstress test (NST),** and AFV. The procedure may be viewed as undertaking a physical examination of the fetus, including determination of vital signs. The fetus responds to central hypoxia by alterations in movement, muscle tone, breathing, and heart rate patterns. The presence of normal fetal biophysical activities shows that the central nervous system is fully functional and that therefore the fetus is not hypoxemic (Manning and Harman, 1990).

The absence of the following three distinct biophysical variables (Table 5-3) is significant:

1. **FBMs**—initial inward movement of the thorax with descent of the diaphragm and abdominal contents, followed by a return to the original position.
2. **FMs**—single or clusters of activity involving the limbs and fetal body; isolated hand and arm movements represent normality.
3. **FT**—at least one episode of opening of the hand with finger and thumb extension with a return to closed-fist formation. In the absence of any hand movement, FT is still recorded as normal if the hand remains in the fist formation for the entire 30-minute observation.

Scoring also includes the following two other findings:

4. Qualitative **AFV**—normal is a finding of at least one pocket that measures at least 1 cm in two perpendicular planes.
5. **NST**—often performed before the BPP as a screening procedure.

Table 5-3 includes scoring and management factors. Although some clinicians advocate the use of a 3-point scoring system (0, 1, and 2), the 0 or 2 points assigned to these factors remain the more generally applied system.

The BPP provides an accurate estimate of the risk of fetal death in the immediate future. Data support the BPP as an early predictor of an acidotic fetus in the face of a nonreactive NST result and absent FBMs. In addition, when an abnormal score and oligohydramnios are encountered, labor induction is warranted (Manning and Harman, 1990). The BPP is effective as an early predictor of fetal infection in women whose membranes rupture prematurely (at fewer than 37 weeks' gestation). The change in biophysical activities precedes the clinical signs of infection and indicates the necessity for immediate birth (Gaffney, Salinger, and Vintzileos, 1990). When risk is low, as with a normal score, intervention is indicated only for obstetric or maternal factors.

Nursing role. Although a growing number of nurses perform ultrasound scans and BPPs in certain centers, most nurses are involved mainly in counseling and educating women about the procedure.

TABLE 5-3 Biophysical profile

VARIABLES	NORMAL (SCORE = 2)	ABNORMAL (SCORE = 0)
Fetal breathing movements	One or more episodes in 30 minutes, each lasting ≥30 seconds	Episodes absent or no episode of ≥30 seconds in 30 minutes
Gross body movements	Three or more discrete body/limb movements in 30 minutes (episodes of active continuous movement considered as a single movement)	Less than three episodes of body/limb movements in 30 minutes
Fetal tone	One or more episodes of active extension with return to flexion of fetal limb(s) or trunk; opening and closing of hand considered normal tone	Slow extension with return to flexion; movement of limb in full extension, or fetal movement absent
Reactive fetal heart rate	Two or more episodes of acceleration (≥15 beats/min) in 20 minutes, each lasting ≥15 seconds and associated with fetal movement	Less than two episodes of acceleration or acceleration of <15 beats/min in 20 minutes
Qualitative amniotic fluid volume	One or more pockets of fluid measuring ≥1 cm in two perpendicular planes	Pockets absent or pocket <1 cm in two perpendicular planes

SCORE	INTERPRETATION	RECOMMENDED MANAGEMENT
10	Normal infant, low risk for chronic asphyxia	Repeat testing at weekly intervals; repeat twice weekly in diabetic women and women ≥42 weeks
8	Normal infant, low risk for chronic asphyxia	Repeat testing at weekly intervals; repeat twice weekly in diabetic women and women ≥42 weeks; oligohydramnios is indication for delivery
6	Suspected chronic asphyxia	Repeat testing within 24 hours; oligohydramnios or repeat score ≤6 is indication for delivery
4	Suspected chronic asphyxia	Indications for delivery are >36 weeks and favorable cervix; if <36 weeks and lecithin/sphingomyelin ratio <2.0, repeat test in 24 hours; repeat score ≤6 or oligohydramnios is indication for delivery
2	Strong suspicion of chronic asphyxia	Extend testing time to 120 minutes; persistent score ≤4, regardless of gestational age, is indication for delivery

From Manning F et al: Fetal assessment based on fetal biophysical profile scoring: experiences in 12,620 referred high risk pregnancies, *Am J Obstet Gynecol* 151:345, 1985.

LEGAL TIP

Performance of Limited Ultrasound Examinations

Nurses who have the training and competence may perform limited ultrasound examinations if it is within the scope of practice in their state or area and if it is consistent with regulations of the agencies in which they practice. Limited ultrasound examinations include identification of fetal number, fetal presentation, fetal cardiac activity, location of the placenta, and BPP, including AFV assessment. Patients should be informed about the limited information provided by these examinations. The examinations are not meant to evaluate or identify fetal anomalies, assess fetal age, or estimate fetal weight. The obstetric health care provider is responsible for obtaining a basic or targeted examination when complete patient assessment is necessary (AWHONN, 1993).

Accurate information regarding the procedure is imperative to allay the mother's anxiety. Although ultrasound scanning has become a widely used diagnostic tool, recommendations for the procedure are based on expectations of a fetal problem and therefore may cause concern. The nurse should provide ample opportunity to answer the woman's questions and give reassurance.

For an abdominal ultrasound the woman usually is directed to come for the examination with a full bladder because it supports the uterus in position for the imaging. She is then positioned comfortably with small pillows under her head and knees. The display panel should be positioned so that the woman and her partner can observe the images on the screen if they so desire; some may not want to watch.

A transvaginal ultrasound may be performed either with the woman in a lithotomy position or with her pelvis elevated by towels, cushions, or a folded pillow. This pelvic tilt is optimal to image the pelvic structures. After a water-soluble gel is placed on the tip of the transducer to allow better sound wave transmission, a protective sheath covers the transducer. A condom, the finger of a clean rubber surgical glove, or a special probe cover provided by the manufacturer may be used. The probe is then placed in the vagina by the person conducting the examination; since a woman may be uncomfortable with this procedure, she should be permitted to insert the probe herself if she so desires. During the examination the position of the probe or the tilt of the examining table may be changed to view the complete pelvis. The procedure should not be physically painful; the woman will feel pressure as the probe is moved (see the Patient Teaching box on p. 90).

Vaginal ultrasound is well tolerated by most patients because it alleviates the need for a full bladder. It is also especially useful in obese patients, whose thick abdominal layers cannot be adequately penetrated by an abdominal approach. This technique is optimally used in the first trimester to detect ectopic pregnancies, monitor the developing embryo,

Patient Teaching

PREPARING FOR ULTRASOUND EXAMINATION

The woman should be informed that she will need to have a full bladder for an abdominal ultrasound, since this allows better imaging of the fetus. She is then positioned comfortably, with pillows under her head and knees while the test is conducted. Ultrasonic gel is applied to the abdomen and the scanner passed over it while images are reproduced. The woman and her partner can watch if they wish. The woman should not feel any discomfort.

For a transvaginal ultrasound the woman should know that she may either be in a lithotomy position or have her pelvis elevated. This position is optimal for imaging the pelvic structures. A transducer with a protective sheath covering it is introduced into the vagina. If the woman wants to insert it herself, she may be permitted to do so. The angle of the probe or the tilt of the table may be altered during the examination, but the procedure should not be painful.

help identify abnormalities, and help establish gestational age. In some instances it may be used as an adjunct to abdominal scanning to evaluate second-trimester and third-trimester pregnancies.

Safety considerations. Although no conclusive evidence indicates that humans have been harmed by diagnostic ultrasound during the 25 years it has been used, a hypothetic risk cannot be ignored. However, no biologic damage has been measured at ultrasonic intensity of less than 100 mW/cm^2, even for extended exposure times. Diagnostic ultrasonic beams all have intensities less than 10 mW/cm^2 and are applied for relatively short times. Diagnostic units also employ pulsed ultrasound with a usual duty cycle of 1/1000, which during 24 hours of continuous sampling produces only 86 seconds of ultrasonic exposure. Thus the total ultrasound exposure for the fetus depends on the number of ultrasonic examinations performed, the type of equipment used, and the amount of energy received, which depends on the duration of the procedure. It has been recommended that the length of ultrasound study and the type of equipment used be recorded. Although the possibility exists that some biologic effects may be identified in the future, current data indicate that the benefits to the patient with prudent use of diagnostic ultrasound far outweigh the possible risk (Manning, 1994).

Magnetic Resonance Imaging

Magnetic resonance imaging (MRI) is a noninvasive tool that can be used for obstetric and gynecologic diagnosis. As with computed tomography (CT), MRI provides excellent pictures of soft tissue. Unlike CT, ionizing radiation is not used; thus vascular structures within the body can be seen and evaluated without the need to inject an iodinated contrast medium, thereby eliminating any known biologic risk. As with sonography, MRI is noninvasive and can provide images in multiple planes, but interference from skeletal, fatty, or gas-filled structures is not a problem. Also, imaging of deep pelvic structures does not depend on a full bladder.

MRI can evaluate (1) fetal structure: central nervous system, thorax, abdomen, genitourinary tract, musculoskeletal system, and overall growth; (2) placenta: position, density, and evaluation of gestational trophoblastic disease; (3) amniotic fluid quantity; (4) maternal structures: uterus, cervix, adnexa, and pelvis; (5) biochemical status: pH and adenosine triphosphate (ATP) content of tissues and organs; and (6) soft tissue, metabolic, or functional malformations.

The woman is placed on a table in a supine position and slid into the bore of the main magnet that is similar in appearance to a CT scanner. Depending on the reason for the study, the entire procedure may take 20 to 60 minutes, during which time the woman must be perfectly still except for short respites. Because of the long time needed to produce MR images, it is likely that the fetus will move, which will obscure anatomic details. The only way to ensure that the fetus will not move is to administer a sedative to the mother, but this approach should be reserved for selected cases in which visualization of fetal detail is critical (Weinreb and Brown, 1990).

Although the procedure appears to have many advantages, its total safety has not been accurately determined. Thus broad use should not be encouraged until results of further study are known (Mattison and Angtuaco, 1988).

BIOCHEMICAL ASSESSMENT

Biochemical assessment involves the study of biologic components such as genes or exfoliated cells and chemical components such as the **lecithin/sphingomyelin (L/S) ratio** and bilirubin levels (Table 5-4). Specific procedures are used to obtain the specimens needed for study: amniocentesis, PUBS, CVS, and maternal assays.

Amniocentesis

Amniocentesis is performed to obtain amniotic fluid, which contains fetal cells. Under direct ultrasound visualization, a needle is inserted transabdominally into the uterus. Indications for the procedure include prenatal diagnosis of genetic disorders or congenital anomalies (neural tube defects in particular), assessment of pulmonary maturity, and diagnosis of fetal hemolytic disease. Amniotic fluid is withdrawn into a syringe, and various amniotic fluid assessments are performed. Amniocentesis is possible after week 14 of pregnancy, when the uterus becomes an abdominal organ and sufficient amniotic fluid is available for this procedure (Table 5-5 and Fig. 5-7).

Overall complications are less than 1% for both mother and fetus and include the following:

Maternal: hemorrhage, fetomaternal hemorrhage with possible maternal Rh isoimmunization, infection, labor, abruptio placentae, inadvertent damage to the intestines or bladder, amniotic fluid embolism. Because of the possibility of fetomaternal hemorrhage, it is standard practice to administer immune globulin D (RhoGAM) to the woman who is Rh negative after an amniocentesis.

Fetal: death, hemorrhage, infection (amnionitis), direct injury from the needle, abortion or preterm labor, leakage of amniotic fluid.

Many of the complications have been minimized or eliminated by performing the procedure under ultrasound guidance.

TABLE 5-4 Summary of biochemical monitoring techniques

TEST	POSSIBLE FINDINGS	CLINICAL SIGNIFICANCE
Maternal blood		
Coombs' test	Titer of 1:8 and rising	Significant Rh incompatibility
Alpha-fetoprotein	See below	
Amniotic fluid analysis		
Color	Meconium	Possible hypoxia or asphyxia
Lung profile		Fetal lung maturity
Lecithin/sphingomyelin (L/S) ratio	>2	
Phosphatidylglycerol (PG)	Present	
Creatinine	>2 mg/dl	Gestational age >36 weeks
Bilirubin (ΔOD of 450 nm)	<0.015	Gestational age >36 weeks, normal pregnancy
	High levels	Fetal hemolytic disease in Rh isoimmunized pregnancies
Lipid cells	>10%	Gestational age >35 weeks
AFP	High levels after 15 weeks' gestation	Open neural tube or other defect
Osmolality	Decline after 20 weeks' gestation	Advancing nonspecific gestational age
Genetic disorders	Dependent on cultured cells for karyotype and enzymatic activity	Counseling may be required
Sex linked		
Chromosomal		
Metabolic		

ΔOD, Change in optical density.

Genetic problems. Prenatal assessment of genetic disorders is indicated in women over age 35, those with a previous child with a chromosomal abnormality, or those with a family history of chromosomal anomalies. Inherited errors of metabolism also may be detected (e.g., Tay-Sachs disease, hemophilia, thalassemia) and other disorders for which marker genes are known.

Cells are cultured for karyotyping of chromosomes (see Chapter 4). Chromosomal aberrations appear in 1% to 2% of fetuses of women between ages 35 and 38, in 2% of women between ages 39 and 44, and in 10% of women older than age 45. Fetal cells also are assessed for sex chromatin because gender determination is important if a sex-linked disorder (occurring almost always in a male fetus) is suspected.

Biochemical analysis of enzymes produced from a cell culture can be used to detect inborn errors of metabolism. Assessment of **alpha-fetoprotein (AFP)** levels is done as a follow-up for elevated levels of maternal serum AFP. Elevated levels in the amniotic fluid help confirm the diagnosis of a open neural tube defect (e.g., spina bifida, anencephaly) or an open abdominal wall defect (e.g., omphalocele). Elevated levels result from the increased leakage of cerebrospinal fluid into the amniotic fluid through the open defect. AFP values are normally high in fetal circulation but low in amniotic fluid.

Levels also may be elevated in a normal multifetal pregnancy and with intestinal atresia, presumably caused by lack of fetal swallowing. A concurrent finding of acetylcholinesterase virtually always indicates a fetal defect (Simpson and Elias, 1994). Concurrent ultrasound examination is recommended in these patients.

Fetal maturity. Greater accuracy in estimating fetal maturity is possible through examination of amniotic fluid or its exfoliated cellular contents. Term pregnancy and fetal maturity can be demonstrated by the following laboratory studies.

Phospholipids. An **L/S ratio** greater than 2:1 indicates adequate lung maturity for extrauterine life in most cases. This is generally achieved by a gestational age of 36 weeks. A quick means of determining an approximate L/S ratio is the rapid surfactant test, also known as the *shake test* or *bubble test*. Equal parts of fresh amniotic fluid and normal saline solution are added to two parts 95% ethyl alcohol. The mixture is shaken vigorously for 30 seconds. If bubbles are still present at the meniscus 15 minutes after shaking, the fetal lung is judged to be mature.

The presence of phosphatidylglycerol, another phospholipid, also reflects fetal lung maturity. In the presence of phosphatidylglycerol, the incidence of respiratory distress syndrome (RDS) is virtually nonexistent. The turbidity of the specimen itself is believed to depend on the total amniotic fluid phospholipid concentration. Optical density (OD) 650 nm greater than 0.15 correlates extremely well with the absence of RDS (Sonek, Reiss, and Gabbe, 1990).

Bilirubin. A ΔOD (change in OD) of bilirubinoid pigments of 450 nm (less than 0.01) indicates a gestational age of greater than 36 weeks because bilirubin disappears after 36 weeks. (OD is also increased in instances of Rh incompatibility.)

Creatinine. When the creatinine (estimate of renal maturity) value is greater than 2 mg/dl, in the absence of maternal renal disease and dehydration and fetal anomaly, the gestational age is greater than 36 weeks.

Lipid cells. After fetal lipid-containing exfoliated cells are stained with Nile blue sulfate, a finding of more than 20% orange-staining cells indicates a gestational age of greater than 35 weeks; the fetus probably weighs 2500 g.

Fetal hemolytic disease. Identification and follow-up of fetal hemolytic disease in cases of isoimmunization is another indication for amniocentesis. The procedure usually is not

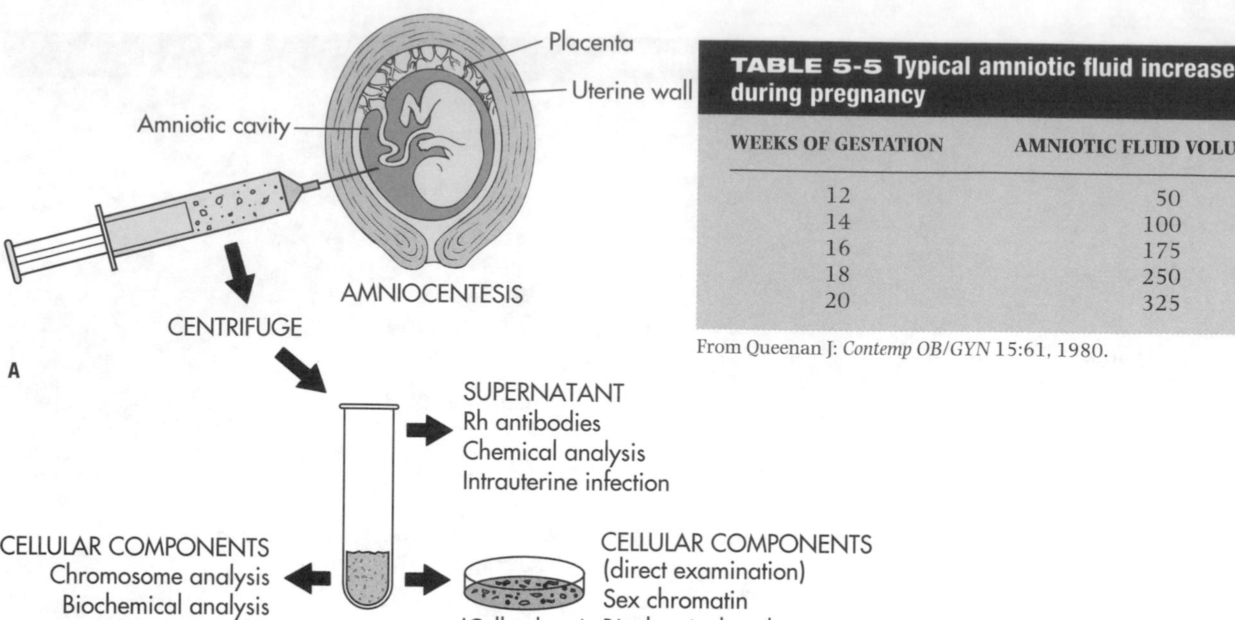

TABLE 5-5 Typical amniotic fluid increase during pregnancy

WEEKS OF GESTATION	AMNIOTIC FLUID VOLUME (ml)
12	50
14	100
16	175
18	250
20	325

From Queenan J: *Contemp OB/GYN* 15:61, 1980.

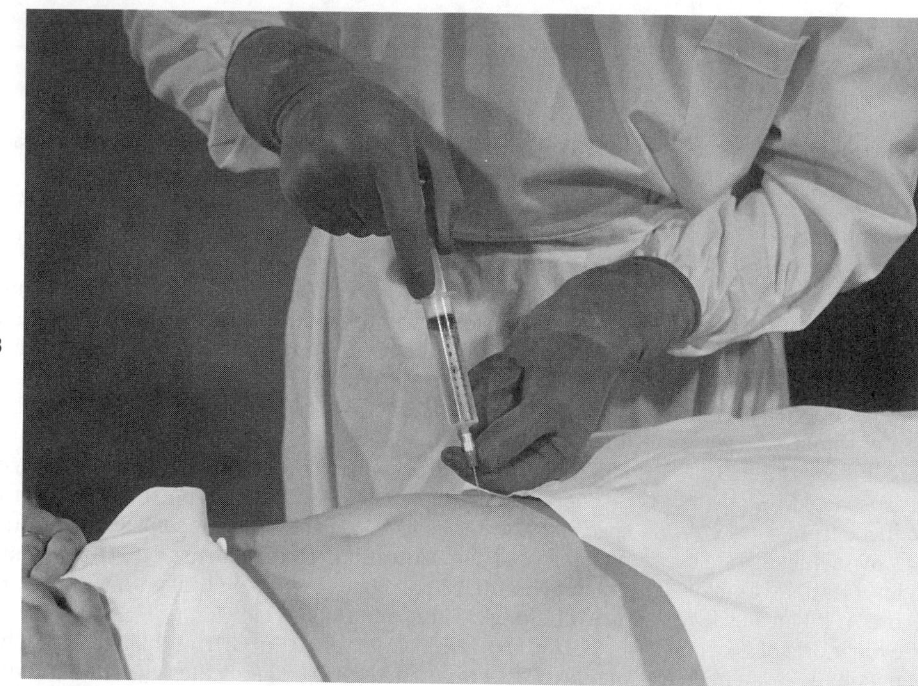

Fig. 5-7 **A,** Amniocentesis and laboratory use of amniotic fluid aspirant. **B,** Transabdominal amniocentesis.

done until the mother's antibody titer reaches 1:8 and is rising. PUBS is now the procedure of choice to evaluate and treat fetal hemolytic disease.

Apt test. The **Apt test** is used to differentiate maternal and fetal blood when vaginal bleeding occurs during pregnancy or labor. It may be performed quickly by the following method:

> Add 0.5 ml bloody fluid to 4.5 ml distilled water and shake. Add 1 ml 0.25*N* sodium hydroxide. Fetal and cord blood remains pink for 1 to 2 minutes. Maternal blood turns brown in 30 seconds.

For further confirmation of the presence of fetal blood, a Kleihauer-Betke procedure can be done in the laboratory.

Meconium. The presence of meconium in the amniotic fluid may be determined, usually by visual inspection of the sample.

Antenatal period. The presence of meconium in the amniotic fluid before early labor begins is not usually associated with an adverse fetal outcome. The finding may be the result of an acute and subsequently corrected fetal stressor, a chronic ongoing stressor, or simply the physiologic passage of meconium. Because some association has been found between meconium in amniotic fluid in the third trimester and hypertensive conditions and postmaturity, the fetus should undergo further antepartum evaluation if the birth is not imminent (Woods and Glantz, 1994).

Intrapartal period. Intrapartal **meconium-stained amniotic fluid** is an indication for more careful evaluation, such as through electronic fetal monitoring (EFM) and perhaps fetal scalp blood sampling. The presence of meconium should not be used as the sole indication for intervention (Scott et al, 1994). When membranes are ruptured and the fetal head can be touched, fetal well-being can be assessed by fetal scalp stimulation. Stimulation can be performed digitally by a vaginal examination or by applying an Allis clamp to the scalp and "wiggling" it gently. Fetal scalp stimulation can be performed by the digital method with intact membranes if the head is well applied to the cervix. Another assessment technique that can be used without the need for ruptured membranes is vibroacoustic stimulation (see discussion of non stress testing). Those fetuses whose heart rates respond with a brisk acceleration usually have a scalp blood pH greater than 7.23, which suggests fetal well-being (Harvey, 1987).

Three possible reasons exist for the passage of meconium during the intrapartal period: (1) it is a normal physiologic function that occurs with maturity (meconium passage is uncommon before weeks 23 to 24, with an increased incidence after 38 weeks); (2) it is the result of hypoxia-induced peristalsis and sphincter relaxation; and (3) it may be a sequela to umbilical cord compression–induced vagal stimulation in mature fetuses.

The following criteria have been proposed for evaluating meconium-stained amniotic fluid during the intrapartal period (Scott et al, 1994):

1. **Consistency:** "old and thin" vs. "new and thick." A new and thick consistency is more likely to be the result of fetal stress.
2. **Timing:** thick, fresh meconium passed for the first time in late labor, associated with nonremediable severe variable or late FHR decelerations, is an ominous sign. However, the presence of meconium alone is not necessarily a sign of fetal distress.
3. **Presence of other indicators:** meconium passage and nonremediable severe variable or late decelerations (especially with poor baseline variability), with or without acidosis confirmed by scalp blood sampling, are ominous signs of fetal distress.

In the presence of meconium the birth team should anticipate the need for careful suctioning of the nasopharynx at time of the birth, ideally before the first breath is taken. Suctioning at this time is effective in reducing the incidence and severity of meconium aspiration in the neonate (TePas and Cunningham, 1993).

Percutaneous Umbilical Blood Sampling

Direct access to the fetal circulation during the second and third trimesters is now possible through **PUBS,** or cordocentesis. It is the most widely used method for fetal blood sampling and transfusion (Nicolaides, Thorpe-Beeston and Noble, 1990). PUBS involves the insertion of a needle directly into

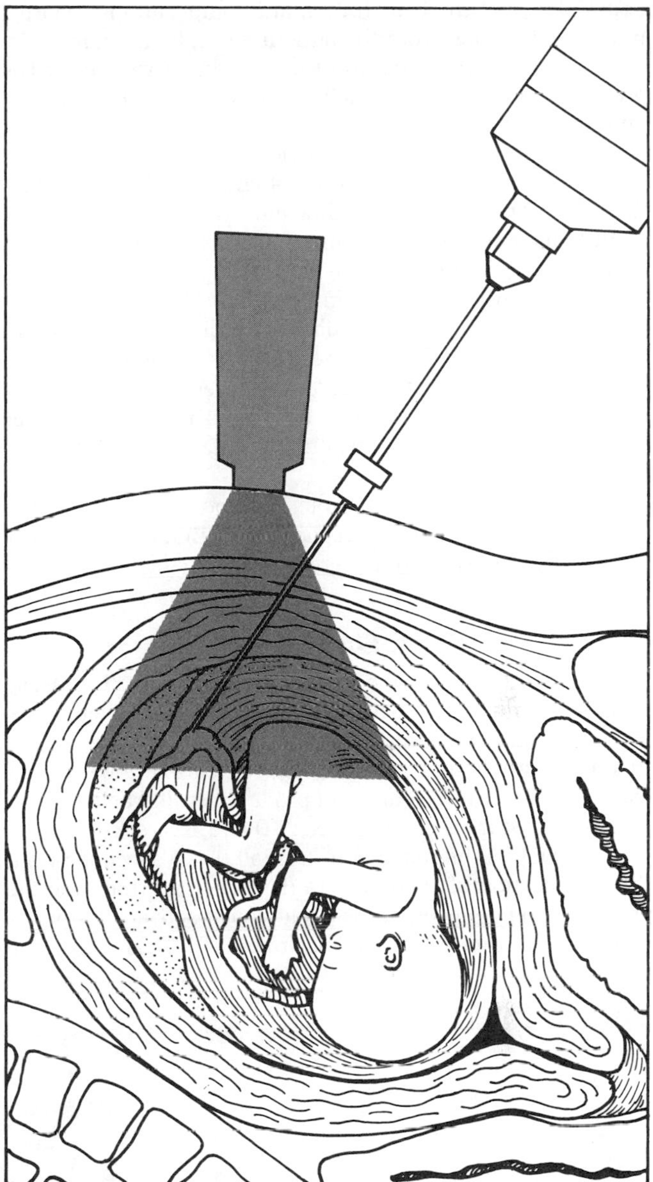

Fig. 5-8 Technique for PUBS guided by ultrasound.

the fetal umbilical vessel under ultrasound guidance. Ideally, the umbilical cord is punctured 1 to 2 cm from its placental insertion (Fig. 5-8). At this point the cord is well anchored and will not move, and the risk of maternal blood contamination (from the placenta) is slight (Ludomirski and Weiner, 1988). Generally, 1 to 4 ml of blood are removed during the puncture and immediately tested by the Kleihauer-Betke procedure to ensure fetal blood. Indications for use include prenatal diagnosis of inherited blood disorders or karyotyping of malformed fetuses, detection of fetal infection, determination of the acid-base status of fetuses with IUGR, and assessment and treatment of isoimmunization and thrombocytopenia in pregnant women (Bald et al, 1991).

In a study of more than 1600 pregnant women from 14 major North American centers, only a 1.6% mean fetal loss rate resulted from this procedure (Nicolaides, Thorpe-Beesten, and Noble, 1990). The three main complications reported were blood leakage from the puncture site, fetal bradycardia, and chorioamnionitis; none of the procedures was followed by premature rupture of the membranes (PROM) (Ludomirski and Weiner, 1988).

Since a fetal blood specimen yields a karyotype in 2 to 3 days, PUBS may be the procedure of choice when time limitations do not permit amniotic fluid cultures to be used.

In fetuses at risk for isoimmune hemolytic anemia, PUBS now permits precise identification of fetal blood type and RBC count and may avoid further interventions. If the fetus is antigen positive for maternal antibodies, a direct blood test can confirm the degree of anemia resulting from hemolysis. PUBS is now the procedure of choice for intrauterine transfusion for severely anemic fetuses; it can be done 4 to 5 weeks earlier than through the intraperitoneal route (Ludomirski and Weiner, 1988).

Follow-up includes continuous FHR monitoring for several minutes up to 1 hour and a repeat ultrasound examination 1 hour later to ensure that there was no further bleeding or hematoma formation.

Chorionic Villus Sampling

Because of its advantage of earlier diagnosis than is possible with amniocentesis, CVS has become popular for genetic studies. Although risks to the fetus exist, the greatest advantage in this technique is that genetic diagnosis can be moved to as early as the tenth week and can produce results rapidly.

The procedure is done between 10 and 12 weeks of gestation. It involves the removal of a small tissue specimen from the fetal portion of the placenta (Fig. 5-9). At that time the placenta is a heterogenous organ in which active villus proliferation is seen (Golbus and Appelman, 1990). At this stage the chorion has differentiated into two distinct structures: (1) the chorion frondosum, which overlies the basal decidua and ultimately will become the placental site, and (2) the smooth, leathery chorion laeve, from which the villi have degenerated (Wapner and Jackson, 1988). The specimen is removed either from the chorion frondosum (the preferred site) or the chorion laeve. Because chorionic villi originate in the zygote, that tissue reflects the genetic makeup of the fetus.

CVS procedures can be accomplished by either of two methods: transcervically or transabdominally. If performed transcervically, a sterile catheter is introduced into the cervix under continuous ultrasonographic guidance, and a small portion of chorionic villi is aspirated with a syringe. The aspiration cannula and obturator must be placed at the suitable site with care to avoid rupturing the amniotic sac.

If the abdominal approach is used, an 18-gauge spinal needle with stylet is inserted under sterile conditions through the abdominal wall into the chorion frondosum under ultrasound guidance. The stylet is then withdrawn, and a syringe aspirates out the chorionic tissue (Matthews and Smith, 1993) (Fig. 5-9).

Complications after the procedure, which rarely occur, include vaginal spotting or bleeding immediately afterward; spontaneous abortion (SAB), 0.3%; rupture of membranes, 0.1%; and chorioamnionitis, 0.5%. Because of the possibility of fetomaternal hemorrhage, women who are Rh negative should receive immune globulin D (RhoGAM) to avoid isoimmunization (National Institutes of Health [NIH] CVS Study Group, 1989). If CVS is done between 56 and 66 days' gestation, an increased risk of limb anomalies has been noted (Burton et al, 1992; Firth et al, 1991; Froster-Iskenius and Baird, 1989). Based on these findings, CVS may need to be restricted to 10 weeks' gestation or later. The abdominal approach does

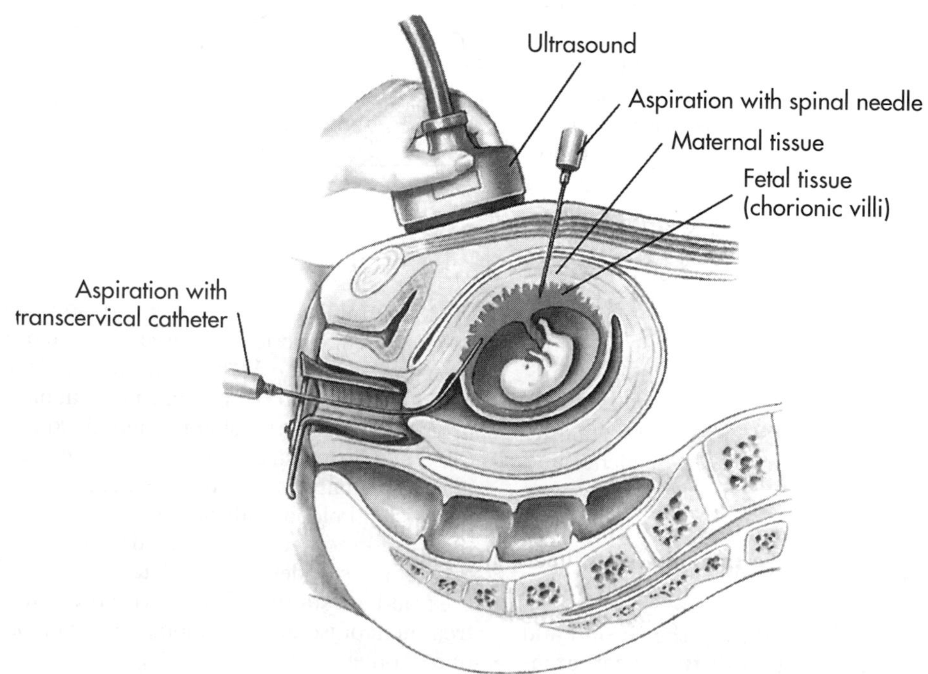

Fig. 5-9 CVS involves taking chorionic tissue for analysis of fetal problems (abdominal and transcervical methods). (Courtesy Medical and Scientific Illustration, Crozet, Va.)

BOX 5-5
Ethical Considerations Related to Fetal Rights

Amniocentesis, PUBS, and CVS are prenatal tests used for diagnosing fetal defects in pregnancy. They are invasive and carry risks to the mother and fetus. They may also involve consideration of abortion because no treatment exists for genetically affected fetuses. Thus the issue of fetal rights is a key ethical concern in prenatal testing for fetal defects.

offer the advantage of a lower risk of uterine infection and a wider window of time for safe performance.

Indications for the procedure are similar to those for amniocentesis. About 90% are performed because of advanced maternal age (over age 35) (Simpson and Elias, 1994). Other indications include biochemical and molecular assays for infections or metabolic disorders.

Box 5-5 discusses biochemical procedures and fetal rights.

Maternal Assays

Alpha-fetoprotein. A development in recent years has been the use of maternal serum AFP (MSAFP) as a screening tool for neural tube defects in pregnancy. Through this technique, approximately 80% to 85% of all open neural tube defects can be detected in pregnancy. Open abdominal wall defects may also be detected.

The cause of neural tube defects is not well understood, but it is important to note that 95% of all affected infants are born to women with no previous family history of similar anomalies. The defect occurs in 1 to 2:1000 births in most parts of the United States. After the birth of one affected child the risk of recurrence in future pregnancies is 2% to 3% (10 to 15 times) that of the general population. After two affected children the risk rises to 6% to 8% (Simpson and Elias, 1994).

AFP is produced by the fetal liver and is detectable in increasing quantities in serum of pregnant women from 14 to 34 weeks. Although amniotic fluid AFP is diagnostic, MSAFP is a screening tool only and identifies candidates for the more definitive procedures of amniocentesis and ultrasound examination. MSAFP screening can be done with reasonable reliability any time between 15 and 21 weeks' gestation (17 weeks is ideal).

Once the woman's level is determined, it is compared with normal values established by each laboratory for each week of gestation. Most use a value 2.0 to 2.5 times the normal median as abnormal (reported as *multiples of the mean*, or *MOM*). If findings are abnormal, the test should be repeated in 1 week; if two sequential MSAFP levels are elevated, the woman should be counseled regarding the significance of the findings, the nature of neural tube defects, and options for further testing.

In addition to neural tube defects, the most common reason for elevated AFPs is gestational age more advanced than assumed at the time of the test, multifetal pregnancy, unrecognized fetal demise, and severe oligohydramnios. If the fetus appears normal and of correct gestational age, an amniocentesis should be done for AFP levels (Simpson, 1991) (see the discussion of amniotic fluid AFP on p. 91).

A convincing body of evidence indicates that Down syndrome and probably other autosomal trisomies are associated with lower than normal levels of MSAFP and amniotic fluid AFP. A recent test, the **triple marker test,** is also performed at 16 to 18 weeks' gestation and is combined with maternal age to calculate a new risk. The triple marker test combines information from MSAFP, unconjugated estriol, and human chorionic gonadotropin (hCG). If a fetus has Down syndrome, it has been found that not only may the MSAFP and unconjugated estriol levels be low, but the hCG level may be elevated. With the two additional screening tests, it is estimated that 60% of fetuses with Down syndrome can be identified (Simpson, 1991; Simpson and Elias, 1994).

As with MSAFP, these tests are screening procedures only and are not diagnostic. A definitive examination of amniotic fluid for AFP and chromosomes combined with ultrasound visualization of the fetus is necessary for diagnosis.

Estriols. The steroid precursor produced by the fetal adrenals is synthesized into estriols in the placenta and is excreted by the woman's healthy kidneys. Estriol levels also may be assayed in maternal serum, the preferred method. At this time the only use of unconjugated estriols is in the triple marker test just described.

Coombs test. Coombs test for Rh incompatibility is discussed at length in Chapter 26. If the maternal Coombs titer for Rh antibodies is greater than 1:8, amniocentesis for bilirubin in amniotic fluid is indicated to determine the severity of fetal anemia from hemolysis. The Coombs titer can also detect other antibodies that may place the fetus at risk for incompatibility with maternal antigens.

Urine assessment for glycosuria, acetonuria, and proteinuria. See the Index for the pages in which these findings are discussed. See the Appendix for laboratory values. Table 5-6 presents a partial list of conditions that can be diagnosed prenatally.

ELECTRONIC FETAL MONITORING

Indications

First-trimester and second-trimester assessment is directed primarily at the diagnosis of fetal anomalies. The goal of third-trimester testing is to determine whether the intrauterine environment continues to be supportive to the fetus (Halle, 1993). The testing often is used to determine the timing of childbirth for patients at risk for uteroplacental insufficiency (the gradual decline in the delivery by the placenta of needed substances to the fetus). It has been suggested that a gradual loss of placental function occurs, in which nutritive function is lost first, leading to IUGR. Subsequently, respiratory function is compromised, resulting in fetal hypoxia (Freeman and Lagrew, 1990). Box 5-6 lists indications for both the NST or **fetal activity determination (FAD)** and the **contraction stress test (CST).**

No clinical contraindications exist for the NST. Absolute contraindications for the CST are PROM, previous classic cesarean birth, preterm labor, placenta previa, or abruptio placentae. The following are considered relative contraindications for CST: multifetal pregnancy, previous preterm labor, hydramnios, more than 36 weeks' gestation, and incompetent

TABLE 5-6 Partial list of conditions diagnosed prenatally

DISORDER	PRENATAL DIAGNOSTIC METHOD/FINDING
Chromosomal anomalies	Chromosome analysis of cultured amniotic fluid cells
Congenital defects	
Cardiac defects	Ultrasound
Central nervous system anomalies	
Anencephaly	AFP in amniotic fluid and maternal serum, ultrasound, fetoscopy, radiography
Hydrocephaly	Ultrasound, AFP, radiography
Microcephaly	Ultrasound, radiography
Spina bifida cystica	AFP, fetoscopy, ultrasound
Gastrointestinal defects	
Diaphragmatic hernia	Amniography, ultrasound
Esophageal atresia	Amniography, fetography
Gastroschisis, omphalocele	AFP, ultrasound
Meconium ileus (cystic fibrosis)	Ultrasound, radiography
Skeletal deformities (general)	Ultrasound, radiography
Osteogenesis imperfecta	Elevated amniotic fluid pyrophosphate
Fetal infections	
Cytomegalovirus	Cytomegalovirus from amniotic fluid
Rubella	Rubella virus from amniotic fluid
Syphilis	Radiography (fetal abnormalities)
Hematologic disorders	
Erythroblastosis fetalis	Amniotic fluid bilirubin, ultrasound, amniography, fetal blood sample
Sickle cell anemia	Fetal blood sample, deoxyribonucleic acid (DNA) analysis of amniotic fluid cells
Thalassemia	DNA analysis of amniotic fluid cells, fetal blood sample
Inborn errors of metabolism	Amniotic fluid analysis
Argininosuccinicaciduria (argininosuccinic lysase deficiency)	C-argininosuccinic acid in cultured cells, increased argininosuccinic acid levels
Combined immunodeficiency disease	Deficient adenosine deaminase activity in cultured cells
Congenital adrenal hyperplasia	Elevated 17α-hydroxyprogesterone, Δ^4-androstenedione, and pregnanediol levels in fluid
Congenital erythropoietic porphyria	Massive amounts of porphyrin in fluid
Cystinosis	Elevated cystine in fluid
Fabry disease	Deficient α-galactosidase activity in cultured cells
Farber disease	Deficient ceramidase activity in cultured cells
Galactosemia	Deficient galactose-1-phosphate uridyl transferase activity in cultured cells
Glutaric acidemia	Glutaric acid in fluid, deficient glutaryl-CoA dehydrogenase in cultured cells
Hunter syndrome (mucopolysaccharidosis, type II)	Deficient iduronate sulfate activity in fluid, accumulation of S-sulfate mucopolysaccharides in cultured cells
Hurler syndrome (mucopolysaccharidosis, type I)	Decreased α-L-iduronidase activity in fluid, accumulation of S-sulfate mucopolysaccharides in cultured cells
Hyperlipoproteinemid, type II	Absence of low-density lipoprotein–cell surface receptors on cultured cells
Hypophosphatasia (congenitally lethal)	Ultrasound, deficient bone and liver alkaline phosphatase isoenzyme activity in cultured cells, deficiency of total alkaline phosphatase activity in cultured cells
Krabbe disease	Deficient cerebroside β-galactosidase activity in cultured cells
Lesch-Nyhan syndrome	Deficient hypoxanthine-guanine phosphoribosyl transferase activity in cultured cells
Maple syrup urine disease	Deficient branched-chain ketoacid decarboxylase in cultured cells
Menkes syndrome (kinky-hair disease)	Increased incorporation of copper into cultured cells
Niemann-Pick disease	Deficient sphingomyelinase activity in cultured cells
Pompe disease (glycogen storage disease, type II)	Deficient α-1,4-glucosidase in cultured cells
Porphyria (acute, intermittent)	Decreased activity of uroporphyrinogen I synthetase in cultured cells
Sanfilippo syndrome	Deficient heparin sulfamidase activity in cultured cells, increased heparin sulfate in amniotic fluid
Tay-Sachs disease	Deficient β-N-acetyl-hexasaminidase A and B activity in cultured cells
Wolman disease	Deficient acid lipase activity in cultured cells

TABLE 5-6 Partial list of conditions diagnosed prenatally—cont'd

DISORDER	PRENATAL DIAGNOSTIC METHOD/FINDING
Miscellaneous conditions	
Cystic fibrosis	Reduced methylumbelliferyl-guauidinobenzoate reactive proteases in amniotic fluid
Duchenne muscular dystrophy	Elevated creatine phosphokinase levels in fetal blood
Fetal sex determination	Ultrasound (fetal outline), chromosome analysis of fluid cells, elevated testosterone levels and decreased follicle-stimulating hormone levels in amniotic fluid (male fetus)
Multifetal pregnancy	Ultrasound, radiography
Tumors and cysts	Ultrasound, radiography, amniography
Placental conditions	
Abruptio placentae	Ultrasound
Blighted ovum	Ultrasound
Ectopic pregnancy	Ultrasound
Placenta previa	Ultrasound

BOX 5-6

Indications for the Nonstress Test and the Contraction Stress Test

Maternal diabetes mellitus
Chronic hypertension
Hypertensive disorders in pregnancy
IUGR
Sickle cell disease
Maternal cyanotic heart disease
Postmaturity
History of previous stillbirth
Decreased fetal movement
Isoimmunization
Meconium-stained amniotic fluid at third-trimester amniocentesis
Hyperthyroidism
Collagen disease
Older pregnant woman
Chronic renal disease

cervix (Freeman and Lagrew, 1990). As a rule, reactive patterns with the NST or negative results with the CST are associated with favorable outcomes.

Fetal Responses to Hypoxia and Asphyxia

A number of responses occur in the fetus during hypoxia or asphyxia. Although little or no change occurs in combined cardiac output and umbilical blood flow, there is a redistribution of blood flow to certain vital organs. The series of responses (redistribution of blood flow favoring vital organs, decreased total oxygen consumption, and anaerobic glycolysis) are temporary mechanisms that enable the fetus to survive up to 30 minutes of limited oxygen supply without decompensation of vital organs. However, during more severe asphyxia or sustained hypoxemia, these responses are no longer maintained, and a decrease in the cardiac output, arterial blood pressure, and blood flow to the brain and heart then occurs (Parer, 1994). These changes may be reflected in particular FHR patterns.

Variability. Much evidence supports the clinical belief that FHR variability represents an intact nervous pathway through the cerebral cortex, midbrain, vagus nerve, and cardiac conduction system. Thus the integrity of this pathway is intact in the presence of normal FHR variability. With a 98% accuracy in predicting fetal well-being, the presence of normal variability is the most reassuring aspect of FHR monitoring. Input from various areas of the brain decreases in the presence of cerebral asphyxia, and thus variability decreases after failure of the fetal hemodynamic compensatory mechanisms to maintain cerebral oxygenation (Parer, 1994).

Nonstress Test (Fetal Activity Determination)

The NST is the most widely applied technique for antepartum evaluation of the fetus. The basis for the NST (or FAD) is that the normal fetus produces characteristic FHR patterns in response to FM. In the healthy fetus with an intact central nervous system, 90% of gross FMs are associated with FHR accelerations. This response can be blunted by hypoxia or acidosis, drugs (analgesics, barbiturates, and beta blockers), fetal sleep, and some congenital anomalies (Sonek, Reiss, and Gabbe, 1990).

Advantages. These include the ease with which the NST can be performed in an out-of-hospital setting because it is noninvasive. It also is relatively inexpensive and has no known contraindications.

Disadvantages. These center around the high false-positive rate for nonreactive findings as a result of fetal sleep cycles, medications, and fetal immaturity. There is slightly lower sensitivity to fetal compromise than with the CST or BPP.

Procedure. The woman is seated in a reclining chair (or in semi-Fowler position) to avoid supine hypotension. The FHR is recorded by Doppler transducer, and a tocotransducer is applied to detect uterine contractions or FMs. The nurse observes the strip chart for signs of fetal activity and a concurrent acceleration of FHR and monitors the woman's blood pressure. If evidence of FM is not apparent on the strip, the woman may be asked to depress a button on a hand-held event marker that is connected to the monitor when she feels FM. The FM is then noted on the strip. Because almost all accelerations are accompanied by FM, it need not be recorded with accelerations for the test to be considered reactive (Huddleston, Williams and Fabri, 1993). The test usually takes 20 to 30 minutes, but it may take longer if the fetus needs to be awakened from a sleep state.

A low-technology screening test, called the auscultated acceleration test (AAT) was developed by a nurse scientist (Paine et al, 1992). This test can be administered by a nurse with a fetoscope in 6 minutes; it has been shown to predict normal NST results more than 90% of the time.

The procedure is conducted as follows:

> Listen to the FHR with an Allen-type fetoscope for 2 minutes to establish a baseline FHR. If no acceleration of at least two beats per 5-second period occurs, stimulate fetus using a gentle 5-second shaking motion to produce FM. Repeat this shaking once more if no FM occurs in the 2 minutes after the first stimulation. Auscultation continues for an additional 2 minutes for a total of 6 minutes.

Findings on the AAT are comparable to findings on the NST, as well as to neonatal outcomes.

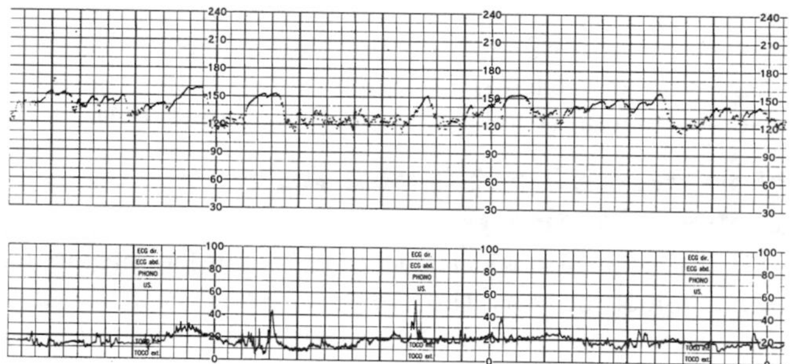

Fig. 5-10 NST. FHR accelerations with fetal movement. (From Tucker S: *Pocket guide to fetal monitoring and assessment*, ed 3, St Louis, 1996, Mosby.)

The AAT yields a better prediction of poor perinatal outcomes than does the NST; the NST, however, remains a better predictor of favorable outcomes. With modifications the AAT shows promise as a low-technology prenatal assessment method, with particular potential when perinatal risk is high and use of technology low (Paine et al, 1992).

Interpretation. Generally accepted criteria for a reactive tracing include the following:

- Two or more accelerations of 15 beats/min lasting for 15 seconds over a 20-minute period
- Normal baseline rate
- Long-term variability amplitude of 10 or more beats/min

If the test does not meet the criteria after 40 minutes, it is considered nonreactive (Fig. 5-10 and Table 5-7). Further assessments are needed with a CST or BPP.

Fetal acoustic stimulation. The **acoustic stimulation test** is another method of testing antepartum FHR response. The test takes approximately 10 minutes to complete, with the fetus monitored for 5 minutes before stimulation to obtain a baseline FHR. The sound source (usually a laryngeal stimulator) is then applied on the maternal abdomen over the fetal head. Monitoring continues for another 5 minutes, and the monitor tracing is assessed. A reactive test is achieved if there are two FHR accelerations of at least 15 beats/min for at least 15 seconds within 5 minutes of stimulus.

Fetal acoustic stimulation also may be applied during an NST if the fetus appears to be in a sleep state. Sleutel (1990) reported that nonreactive fetuses met reactive NST criteria sooner and also exhibited greater amplitude, duration, and number of accelerations after fetal acoustic stimulation. It is currently recommended that the NST be performed twice weekly or alternated weekly with CSTs for patients with diabetes or others at risk for sudden fetal death.

Contraction Stress Test

The CST is one of the first electronic methods developed for assessment of fetal well-being. Devised as a graded stress test of the fetus, its purpose is to identify the fetus in jeopardy who was stable at rest but showed evidence of compromise with the introduction of stress. Uterine contractions decrease uterine blood flow and placental perfusion. If this decrease is sufficient to produce hypoxia in the fetus, a deceleration in FHR

TABLE 5-7 Interpretation of nonstress test

RESULT	INTERPRETATION	CLINICAL SIGNIFICANCE
Reactive	Two or more accelerations of FHR of 15 beats/min lasting 15 seconds or more, associated with each FM in a 20-minute period	As long as twice-weekly NSTs remain reactive, most high-risk pregnancies are allowed to continue.
Nonreactive	Any tracing with either no FHR accelerations or accelerations <15 beats/min or lasting <15 seconds throughout any FM during testing period	Further indirect monitoring may be attempted with abdominal fetal electrocardiography (ECG) in an effort to clarify FHR pattern and quantitate variability; external monitoring should continue, and a CST or BPP should be done.
Unsatisfactory	Quality of FHR recording not adequate for interpretation	Test is repeated in 24 hours or a CST is done, depending on the clinical situation.

results, beginning at the peak of the contraction and persisting after its conclusion (late deceleration). In a healthy fetoplacental unit, uterine contractions usually do not produce late decelerations; when there is underlying uteroplacental insufficiency, contractions produce late decelerations.

Advantages. The CST provides an earlier warning of fetal compromise than does the NST, and there are fewer false-positive tests.

Disadvantages. In addition to the contraindications described earlier, CST is more time-consuming and expensive than an NST. It also is an invasive procedure if exogenous oxytocin is required.

Procedure. The woman is placed in semi-Fowler's position or sits in a reclining chair. She is monitored indirectly, and the nurse observes the strip for 10 minutes for baseline rate, long-term variability, and the possible occurrence of spontaneous contractions. Two methods of CST are the **nipple-stimulated contraction test** and the oxytocin-stimulated contraction test.

Nipple-stimulated contraction test. The nurse explains the procedure to the woman and then may apply warm, moist washcloths to both breasts for several minutes. The woman is then asked to massage one nipple for 10 minutes. Massaging the nipples causes a release of oxytocin from the posterior pituitary. An alternative approach is for her to massage the nipple for 2 minutes, rest for 2 minutes, and continue for four cycles of massage and rest. If unilateral stimulation does not achieve adequate contractions (three occurring within a 10-minute window), unilateral continuous stimulation should be tried (if the intermittent approach was used), followed by bilateral stimulation for 10 minutes. When adequate contractions are achieved or hyperstimulation occurs, stimulation should be stopped. If the stimulation and rest cycle method is

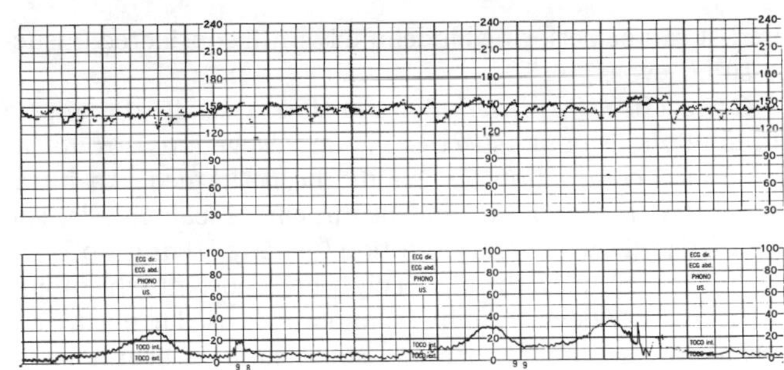

Fig. 5-11 Negative CST. (From Tucker S: *Pocket guide to fetal monitoring and assessment*, ed 3, St Louis, 1996, Mosby.)

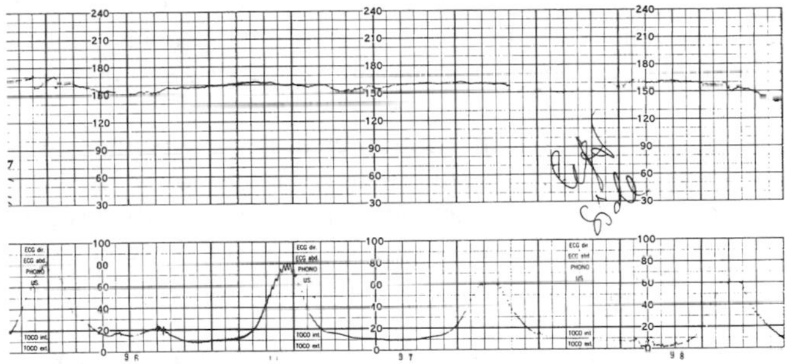

Fig. 5-12 Positive CST, compromised fetus. (From Tucker S: *Pocket guide to fetal monitoring and assessment*, ed 3, St Louis, 1996, Mosby.)

TABLE 5-8 Guide for interpretation of the contraction stress test

RESULT	INTERPRETATION	CLINICAL SIGNIFICANCE
Negative	No late decelerations, with a minimum of three uterine contractions lasting 40 to 60 seconds within a 10-minute period (Fig. 5-11)	Reassurance that fetus is likely to survive labor, should it occur within 1 week; more frequent testing may be indicated by clinical situation.
Positive	Persistent and consistent late decelerations occurring with more than half the uterine contractions (Fig. 5-12)	Management lies between use of other tools of fetal assessment (e.g., BPP) and termination of pregnancy; a positive test result indicates that fetus is at increased risk for perinatal morbidity and mortality; physician may perform an expeditious vaginal birth after a successful induction or may proceed directly to cesarean birth; decision to intervene is determined by fetal monitoring and presence of fetal heart rate reactivity.
Suspicious	Late decelerations occurring with less than half the uterine contractions once an adequate contraction pattern has been established	NST and CST should be repeated within 24 hours; if interpretable data cannot be achieved, other methods of fetal assessment must be used.*
Hyperstimulation	Late decelerations occurring with excessive uterine activity (contractions more often than every 2 minutes or lasting longer than 90 seconds) or a persistent increase in uterine tone	
Unsatisfactory	Inadequate uterine contraction pattern or tracing too poor to interpret	

*Applies to results noted as suspicious, hyperstimulation, or unsatisfactory.

used, it can be performed indefinitely until considered unsuccessful (Devoe, 1995).

Oxytocin-stimulated contraction test. If the nipple stimulation is not successful, an exogenous oxytocin-stimulated contraction test should be performed. An intravenous (IV) infusion is usually begun with a scalp needle. The oxytocin is diluted in an IV solution (usually 10 units to 1000 ml fluid) and infused through a piggyback port into the tubing of the main IV device. An infusion pump is used to ensure accurate dosage. The oxytocin infusion usually is begun at 0.5 mU/min. Most institutions have their own protocols, but the infusion usually is increased by 0.5 mU/min at 15- to 30-minute intervals until three uterine contractions of good quality are observed within a 10-minute period. The typical rate of oxytocin infusion used to elicit uterine contractions is 4 to 5 mU/min; the woman will rarely require more than 8 mU/min. The oxytocin infusion rate should probably not be increased to more than 20 mU/min; each case should be assessed individually (Devoe, 1995).

The FHR pattern is then interpreted. The oxytocin infusion is discontinued, and the maintenance IV solution infused until such time as uterine activity has returned to the preoxytocin level. The IV device is then removed and the fetal monitor discontinued.

Interpretation. If no late decelerations are observed with the contractions, the findings are considered to be negative (Fig. 5-11). Repetitive late decelerations, occurring with most contractions, render the test results positive (Fig. 5-12 and Table 5-8).

NURSING ROLE IN ANTENATAL ASSESSMENT FOR RISK

The nurse's role is that of educator and support person when the woman is undergoing such examinations as ultrasound, MRI, CVS, PUBS, and amniocentesis. In some instances the nurse may assist the physician with the procedure. In many antenatal settings, nurses perform NSTs, CSTs, BPPs, and level I ultrasounds; conduct an initial assessment; and begin necessary interventions for nonreassuring patterns. These nursing actions are accomplished after additional education and training, under guidance of established protocols, and in collaboration with physicians. Patient teaching, which is an integral component of this role, involves preparation for the procedure, intepretation of findings, and psychosocial support when needed.

All women who undergo antenatal assessments are at risk for real and potential problems. The nurse must expect the woman to be anxious. With rare exceptions, the tests are ordered because of suspected fetal compromise or deterioration of a maternal condition, or both. In the third trimester, pregnant women are most concerned about protecting themselves and their fetuses and consider themselves most vulnerable to outside influences. The label of high risk will increase this sense of vulnerability.

Most patients also exhibit a knowledge deficit in some area, whether it is related to the procedure itself, the implications of findings, or the need for further evaluation or counseling. Perinatal nurses can intervene to provide the required education. They can promote a positive parental self-image in these patients at risk.

Critical Thinking Exercises

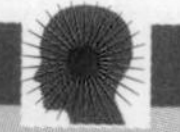

CONTRACTION STRESS TEST

Barbara has been sent from the antepartum testing center for a CST to be performed after a nonreactive NST. She is frightened and anxious about this additional test and its implications for the remainder of her pregnancy and the health of her fetus. The father of the baby is with her.

1. Explain the procedure and the rationale for doing the CST.
2. Compare and contrast the procedure and risks of noninvasive (nipple stimulation) and invasive (oxytocin by IV infusion) methods of performing the CST.
3. What is the role of the partner in the CST? Can he remain during the test? What information does he need?
4. Can the nurse provide the results of the CST to the patient? Why or why not?
5. What follow-up care is needed after the CST?

Key Points

- A high-risk pregnancy is one in which the life or well-being of the mother or infant is jeopardized by a biophysical or psychosocial disorder coincidental with or unique to pregnancy.
- Biophysical, sociodemographic, psychosocial, and environmental factors place the pregnancy and fetus/neonate at risk.
- Psychosocial perinatal warning indicators include characteristics of the parents, the child, their support systems, and family circumstances.
- Maternal and perinatal mortality for Caucasians is considerably lower than for other races in the United States.
- Evidence indicates that mortality decreases when risks are identified early and intensive care is applied.
- Diagnostic techiques include FM counts, ultrasonography, MRI, PUBS, CVS, and electronic fetal monitoring.
- Biochemical monitoring techniques involve assessment of maternal urine and blood, as well as amniotic fluid and its components.
- Reactive NSTs and negative CSTs suggest fetal well-being.

References

Association of Women's Health, Obstetric and Neonatal Nurses (AWHONN): *Nursing practice competencies and educational guidelines for limited ultrasound examination in obstetric and gynecology/infertility settings,* Washington, DC, 1993, AWHONN.

Atrash H et al: Maternal mortality in the United States, 1979-1986, *Obstet Gynecol* 76(6):1055, 1990.

Aumann G, Baird M: *Screening for the high-risk pregnancy.* In Knuppel R, Drukker J, editors: *High risk pregnancy: a team approach,* Philadelphia, 1993, Saunders.

Bald R et al: Antepartum fetal blood sampling with cordocentesis: comparison with chorionic villus sampling and amniocentesis in diagnosing karyotype anomalies, *J Reprod Med* 36:655, 1991.

Brace R: *Amniotic fluid dynamics.* In Creasy R, Resnik R, editors: *Maternal-fetal medicine: principles and practices,* ed 3, Philadelphia, 1994, Saunders.

Burton B et al: Limb anomalies associated with chorionic villus sampling, *Obstet Gynecol* 79(5 Part I):726, 1992.

Calhoun S: "Ask the experts": daily fetal movement counts, *NAACOG Newslett* 17(8):6, 1990.

Chervenak F, Gabbe S: *Obstetric ultrasound: assessment of fetal growth and anatomy.* In Gabbe S, Niebyl J, Simpson J, editors: *Obstetrics: normal and problem pregnancies,* ed 2, New York, 1991, Churchill Livingstone.

Devoe L: *Nonstress and contraction stress testing.* In Sciarra J, editor: *Gynecology and obstetrics,* vol 3, no 78, Philadelphia, 1995, Lippincott.

Firth H et al: Severe limb anomalies after chorion villus sampling at 56-66 days' gestation, *Lancet* 337(8744):762, 1991.

Fischer R, Depp R: *Amniotic fluid: physiology and assessment.* In Sciarra J, editor: *Gynecology and obstetrics,* vol 3, no 76, Philadelphia, 1995, Lippincott.

Fogel C, Lewallen L: *High-risk childbearing.* In Fogel C, Woods N, editors: *Women's health care: a comprehensive handbook,* Thousand Oaks, Calif, 1995, Sage.

Freeman R, Lagrew D Jr: *The contraction stress test.* In Eden R, Boehm F, editors: *Assessment and care of the fetus: physiological, clinical and medicolegal principles,* Stamford, Conn, 1990, Appleton & Lange.

Froster-Iskenius U, Baird P: Limb reduction defects in over one million consecutive livebirths, *Teratology* 39:127, 1989.

Gaffney S, Salinger L, Vintzileos A: The biophysical profile for fetal surveillance, *MCN Am J Matern Child Nurs* 15:356, 1990.

Gilbert E, Harmon J: *Manual of high-risk pregnancy and delivery: nursing perspectives,* St Louis, 1993, Mosby.

Golbus M, Appelman Z: *Chorionic villus sampling.* In Eden R, Boehm F, editors: *Assessment and care of the fetus: physiological, clinical and medicolegal principles,* Stamford, Conn, 1990, Appleton & Lange.

Halle J: *Diagnostic evaluation of pregnancy.* In Mattson S, Smith J, editors: *Core curriculum for maternal newborn nursing,* Philadelphia, 1993, Saunders.

Harvey C: Fetal scalp stimulation: enhancing the interpretation of fetal monitor tracings, *J Perinat Neonatal Nurs* 1:13, 1987.

Huddleston J, Williams G, Fabri E: *Antepartum assessment of the fetus.* In Knuppel R, Durkker J, editors: *High risk pregnancy: a team approach,* ed 2, Philadelphia, 1993, Saunders.

Kemp V, Hatmaker D: Stress and social support in high risk pregnancy, *Res Nurs Health* 12:331, 1989.

Ludomirski A, Weiner S: Percutaneous fetal umbilical blood sampling, *Clin Obstet Gynecol* 3:19, 1988.

Manning R: *General principles and application of ultrasound.* In Creasy R, Resnik R, editors: *Maternal-fetal medicine: principles and practices,* Philadelphia, 1994, Saunders.

Manning F, Harman C: *The fetal biophysical profile.* In Eden R, Boehm F, editors: *Assessment and care of the fetus: physiological, clinical and medicolegal principles,* Stamford, Conn, 1990, Appleton & Lange.

Matthews A, Smith A: *Genetic counseling.* In Knuppel R, Drukker J, editors: *High risk pregnancy: a team approach,* Philadelphia, 1993, Saunders.

Mattison D, Angtuaco T: Magnetic resonance imaging in prenatal diagnosis, *Clin Obstet Gynecol* 31:353, 1988.

National Center for Health Statistics: Advance report of final natality statistics, 1992, *Monthly Vital Stat Rep* 43(5 suppl), 1994.

National Center for Health Statistics: Births, marriages, divorces, and deaths for 1994, *Monthly Vital Stat Rep* 43(12):1, 1995.

National Institutes of Health (NIH) CVS Study Group: The safety and efficacy of chorionic villus sampling for early prenatal diagnosis of cytogenetic abnormalities, *N Engl J Med* 320:609, 1989.

Nicolaides K, Thorpe-Beeston J, Noble P: *Cordocentesis.* In Eden R, Boehm F, editors: *Assessment and care of the fetus: physiological, clinical and medicolegal principles,* Stamford, Conn, 1990, Appleton & Lange.

Paine L et al: A comparison of the auscultated acceleration test and the nonstress test as predictors of perinatal outcomes, *Nurs Res* 41(2):87, 1992.

Parer J: *Fetal heart rate.* In Creasy R, Resnik R, editors: *Maternal-fetal medicine: principles and practices,* ed 3, Philadelphia, 1994, Saunders.

Rutherford S et al: The four-quadrant assessment of amniotic fluid volume: an adjunct to antepartum fetal heart rate testing. I. *Obstet Gynecol* 70:353, 1987.

Schulman H: *Doppler ultrasound.* In Eden R, Boehm F, editors: *Assessment and care of the fetus: physiological, clinical and medicolegal principles,* Stamford, Conn, 1990, Appleton & Lange.

Scott J et al, editors: *Danforth's obstetrics and gynecology,* ed 7, Philadelphia, 1994, Lippincott.

Simpson J: *Genetic counseling and prenatal diagnosis.* In Gabbe S, Neibyl J, Simpson J, editors: *Obstetrics: normal and problem pregnancies,* ed 2, New York, 1991, Churchill Livingstone.

Simpson J, Elias S: *Prenatal diagnosis of genetic disorders.* In Creasy R, Resnik R, editors: *Maternal-fetal medicine: principles and practices,* Philadelphia, 1994, Saunders.

Sleutel M: Vibroacoustic stimulation and fetal heart rate in nonstress tests, *J Obstet Gynecol Neonatal Nurs* 19(3):199, 1990.

Sonek J, Reiss R, Gabbe S: *Antenatal fetal assessment.* In Iams J, Zuspan F, Quilligan E, editors: *Zuspan and Quilligan's manual of obstetrics and gynecology,* ed 2, St Louis, 1990, Mosby.

TePas K, Cunningham M: *Newborn care in the delivery room.* In Knuppel R, Drukker J, editors: *High risk pregnancy: a team approach,* ed 2, Philadelphia, 1993, Saunders.

Trudinger B: *Doppler ultrasound assessment of blood flow.* In Creasy R, Resnik R, editors: *Maternal-fetal medicine: principles and practices,* ed 2, Philadelphia, 1994, Saunders.

Wapner R, Jackson L: Chorionic villus sampling, *Clin Obstet Gynecol* 31:328, 1988.

Weinreb J, Brown C: *Magnetic resonance imaging.* In Eden R, Boehm F, editors: *Assessment and care of the fetus: physiological, clinical and medicolegal principles,* Stamford, Conn, 1990, Appleton & Lange.

Woods J, Glantz J: *Significance of amniotic fluid meconium.* In Creasy R, Resnik R, editors: *Maternal-fetal medicine: principles and practices,* ed 3, Philadelphia, 1994, Saunders.

Bibliography

Bobrowski R, Bottoms S: Unappreciated risks of elderly multipara, *Am J Obstet Gynecol* 172(6):1764, 1995.

Gregor C et al: Interpretation of biophysical profiles by nurses and physicians, *J Obstet Gynecol Neonatal Nurs* 23(5):393, 1994.

Mattson S, Smith J: *Core curriculum for maternal-newborn nursing,* Philadelphia, 1993, Saunders.

McCain G, Deatrick J: The experience of high-risk pregnancy, *J Obstet Gynecol Neonatal Nurs* 23(5):421, 1994.

McCarthy K, Narrigan D: Is there support for the use of juice to facilitate the non-stress test? *J Obstet Gynecol Neonatal Nurs* 224(4):303,1995.

Ott W: The accuracy of antenatal fetal echocardiography screening in high- and low-risk patients, *Am J Obstet Gynecol* 172(6):1741, 1995.

Sciarra J, editor: *Gynecology and obstetrics,* vol 3, Philadelphia, 1995, Lippincott.

CHAPTER 6

Anatomy and Physiology of Pregnancy

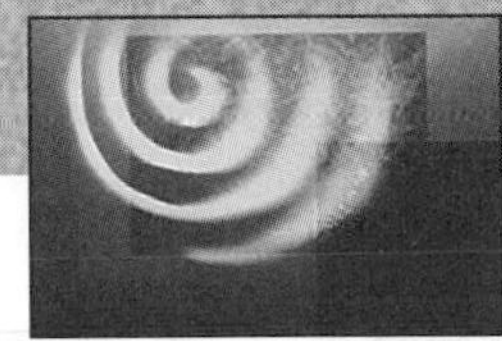

GRAVIDITY AND PARITY, P. 103
PREGNANCY TESTS, P. 104
ADAPTATIONS TO PREGNANCY, P. 105
Signs of pregnancy, p. 105
REPRODUCTIVE SYSTEM AND BREASTS, P. 105
Hypothalamic-pituitary-ovarian axis, p. 105
Uterus, p. 106
Vagina and vulva, p. 110
Breasts, p. 111
GENERAL BODY SYSTEMS, P. 111
Cardiovascular system, p. 111
Respiratory system, p. 114
Renal system, p. 115
Integumentary system, p. 116
Musculoskeletal system, p. 117
Neurologic system, p. 118
Gastrointestinal system, p. 118
Endocrine system, p. 119

The goal of maternity care is a healthy pregnancy with a physically safe and emotionally satisfying outcome for both mother and infant. Consistent health supervision and surveillance are of utmost importance. Many maternal adaptations are unfamiliar to pregnant women and their families. The knowledgeable maternity nurse can help the pregnant woman recognize the relationship between her physical status and the plan for her care. Sharing information encourages the pregnant woman to participate in her own care, depending on her interest, need to know, and readiness to learn.

GRAVIDITY AND PARITY

An understanding of the following terms to describe pregnancy and the pregnant woman is essential to the study of maternity care:

Gravida—a woman who is pregnant
Gravidity—pregnancy
Multigravida—a woman who has had two or more pregnancies
Multipara—a woman who has completed two or more pregnancies to the stage of fetal viability
Nulligravida—a woman who has never been pregnant
Nullipara—a woman who has not completed a pregnancy with a fetus or fetuses who have reached the stage of fetal viability
Parity—the number of pregnancies in which the fetus or fetuses have reached viability, not the number of fetuses (e.g., twins) born. Whether the fetus is born alive or is stillborn (fetus who shows no signs of life at birth) after viability is reached does not affect parity
Preterm—born after 20 weeks of gestation but before completion of 37 weeks of gestation
Primigravida—a woman who is pregnant for the first time
Primipara—a woman who has completed one pregnancy with a fetus or fetuses who have reached the stage of fetal viability
Term—born between the beginning of the thirty-eighth week of gestation and the end of the forty-second week of gestation
Viability—capacity to live outside the uterus, about 22 to 24 weeks since last menstrual period, or greater than 500 g.

Gravidity and parity information is obtained during history-taking interviews and may be recorded in patient records in several ways. A *two-digit system* uses abbreviations that stand for gravity and parity. For example, the abbreviation "I/0" means that a woman is pregnant for the first time (primigravida) and has not carried a pregnancy to viability (nullipara).

Another abbreviation commonly employed in maternity centers is even more detailed. It consists of five digits with hyphens for separation. The first digit represents the total number of pregnancies, including the present one (*g*ravidity); the second digit represents the total number of full-*t*erm births; the third indicates the number of *p*reterm births; the fourth identifies the number of *a*bortions (spontaneous or elective

TABLE 6-1 Gravidity and parity using five-digit (GTPAL) and two-digit systems

	FIVE-DIGIT SYSTEM					TWO-DIGIT SYSTEM
CONDITION	PREGNANCIES (GRAVIDITY, G)	TERM BIRTH (T)	PRETERM BIRTH (P)	ABORTIONS (A)	LIVING CHILDREN (L)	GRAVIDITY/ PARITY
Kathy is pregnant for the first time.	1	0	0	0	0	I/O
She carries the pregnancy to term, and the neonate survives.	1	1	0	0	1	I/I
She is pregnant again.	2	1	0	0	1	II/I
Her second pregnancy ends in abortion.	2	1	0	1	1	II/I
During her third pregnancy, she gives birth to preterm twins.	3	1	1	1	3	III/II

BOX 6-1

Using TPAL to Define Parity

T—Term birth(s)
P—Preterm birth(s)
A—Abortion(s)
L—Living children

Cultural Considerations

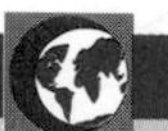

ETHNICITY AND PREGNANCY TESTING

Requests for pregnancy testing may be influenced by ethnic differences. For example, Bluestein and Levin (1992) found that African-American women request fewer pregnancy tests than Caucasian women.

termination of pregnancy before viability); and the fifth is the number of children currently *l*iving. The acronym *GTPAL* may be helpful in remembering this numeric abbreviation. For example, if a woman pregnant only once with twins gives birth at the thirty-fifth week and the babies survive, the abbreviation that represents this information is "1-0-1-0-2." During her next pregnancy the abbreviation is "2-0-1-0-2." Table 6-1 provides addtional examples.

Others prefer a four-digit system. The first digit of the five-digit system, which signifies gravidity, is dropped. The acronym *TPAL* is helpful in remembering the definition of the four digits (Box 6-1).

PREGNANCY TESTS

Early detection of pregnancy allows for early initiation of care. **Human chorionic gonadotropin (hCG)** is the biologic marker on which pregnancy tests are based. Production of hCG begins as early as the day of implantation and can be detected in the blood as early as 6 days after conception, or about 20 days since the last menstrual period (LMP) (Cunningham et al, 1993). The level of hCG increases from less than 25 mIU/ml after implantation to 12,000 to 30,000 mIU/ml at about 60 to 70 days of pregnancy and then begins to decline. The lowest level is reached between 100 to 130 days of pregnancy and remains constant until birth (Frye, 1993).

Serum and urine pregnancy tests are performed in clinics, offices, women's health centers, and laboratory settings (see the Cultural Considerations box above). Serum tests are more sensitive and can provide earlier and more accurate results than urine tests. Approximately 7 to 10 ml of venous blood is collected for serum testing. The presence of hCG can be detected as early as 6 to 9 days after ovulation (Edge and Miller, 1994; Scott et al, 1994).

Urine tests are used in most home pregnancy kits. These inexpensive tests can be purchased over the counter (OTC), and testing can be completed in a few minutes with a high degree of accuracy. Most tests require a first-voided morning urine specimen because it contains levels of hCG approximately the same as those in serum. Random urine samples usually have lower levels.

Many different tests are available, but they all depend on recognition of hCG or a beta subunit of hCG. The wide variety of tests precludes discussion of each; however, several categories of tests are described here. The nurse should read the manufacturer's directions for the test to be used.

Immunologic tests use the principle of agglutination inhibition and depend on an antigen-antibody reaction between hCG and an antiserum. Usually the antiserum is mixed with urine, and hCG-coated particles are added. If hCG is present in the urine, agglutination does not occur because the hCG neutralizes the hCG antibody, and the test is considered positive (Cunningham et al, 1993). *Latex agglutination inhibition (LAI) tests* are easy to do and give results in 2 minutes. They are accurate from 4 to 10 days after missed menses. *Hemagglutination inhibition (HAI) tests* are more sensitive than LAI tests but require 1 to 2 hours to obtain results (Barkauskas et al, 1994).

The *radioreceptor assay* is a 1-hour serum test that requires fairly sophisticated equipment to measure the ability of the blood sample to inhibit the binding of radiolabeled hCG to receptors. Radioreceptor assays are usually accurate at the time of missed menses (14 days after conception) (Pagana and Pagana, 1994).

Radioimmunoassay (RIA) pregnancy tests for the beta subunit of hCG use radioactively labeled markers, which require the testing to be done in a laboratory. Depending on the degree of sensitivity required, the test time ranges from 1 to 5 hours. RIAs are the most sensitive pregnancy tests available today (Pagana and Pagana, 1994). Pregnancy can be diagnosed 8 days after ovulation or 6 days before missed menses.

Enzyme-linked immunosorbent assays (ELISA) testing is the most popular testing procedure for pregnancy (Scott et al, 1994). It uses a specific monoclonal antibody produced by hybrid cell-line technology. An enzyme rather than a radioactive compound identifies the antigen of the substance to be measured. The enzyme induces a simple color-change reaction. The endpoint of the test can be read with either the eye or a spectrometer. ELISA testing has many advantages. The antigen-enzyme conjugate and test reagents are stable, the equipment needs are simple, and there are no nuclear waste products. As an office or home procedure, it requires minimal time and offers results in 5 minutes coupled with sensitivities as low as 25 mIU/ml of hCG in the specimen.

ELISA technology is the basis for most OTC home pregnancy tests. One-step tests for home testing are the most recent development in pregnancy tests. Virtually all OTC test kits are of this type. The woman usually applies urine to a strip and reads the results. The manufacturer provides directions for collection of the specimen (serum, plasma, or urine), care of specimen, testing procedure, and reading of results. Most companies provide a toll-free telephone number for concerns and questions about test procedures or results.

Interpreting the results of pregnancy tests requires some judgment. The type of pregnancy test and its degree of sensitivity (ability to detect low levels of a substance) and specificity (ability to discern the absence of a substance) are interpreted in conjunction with the woman's history, which includes the date of the last normal menstrual period (LNMP), usual cycle length, and results of previous pregnancy tests. It is important to know if the woman is a substance abuser. Interactions with other drugs, such as anticonvulsants and tranquilizers, can give false results. Improper collection of the specimen, hormone-producing tumors, and laboratory errors may also be responsible for false reports. When any question arises, serial testing may be the answer (Pagana and Pagana, 1994). Speed and convenience need to be weighed against sensitivity and specificity (see the Home Care box below).

ADAPTATIONS TO PREGNANCY

Maternal physiologic adaptations are attributed to the hormones of pregnancy and to mechanical pressures arising from the enlarging uterus and other tissues. These adaptations protect the woman's normal physiologic functioning, meet the metabolic demands pregnancy imposes on her body, and provide a nurturing environment for fetal development and growth. Although pregnancy is a normal phenomenon, problems can occur. The nurse needs a foundation in normal maternal physiology to accomplish the following:

1. Identify potential or actual deviation from normal adaptation to initiate remedial care.
2. Help the woman understand the anatomic and physiologic changes during pregnancy.
3. Allay the woman's (and family's) anxiety, possibly resulting from a lack of knowledge.
4. Teach the woman (and family) signs and symptoms that should be reported to the health care provider.

Along with the expected adjustments to pregnancy, some disorders also cause changes, including low hemoglobin levels, a high erythrocyte sedimentation rate, dyspnea at rest, and alterations in cardiac function and endocrine balance. These changes reflect the body's effort to protect the mother and the fetus. An understanding of these changes is necessary for anyone who participates in the care of the mother and the fetus.

Signs of Pregnancy

Some of the physiologic adaptations are recognized as **signs and symptoms of pregnancy.** The three categories are **presumptive,** those changes felt by the woman (e.g., amenorrhea, fatigue, breast changes); **probable,** those changes observed by an examiner (e.g., Hegar's sign, ballottement, pregnancy tests); and **positive,** those signs attributed only to the presence of the fetus (e.g., hearing fetal heart tones, visualizing the fetus, palpating fetal movements). Table 6-2 describes these signs of pregnancy in relation to when they might occur and other causes for their occurrence.

REPRODUCTIVE SYSTEM AND BREASTS

Hypothalamic-Pituitary-Ovarian Axis

During pregnancy, elevated levels of estrogen and progesterone (produced first by the corpus luteum in the ovary until about 14 weeks and then by the placenta) suppress secretion of follicle-stimulating hormone (FSH) and luteinizing hormone (LH) by the anterior pituitary gland. The maturation of a follicle and ovulation are thereby suppressed during pregnancy. Menstrual cycles cease. Although most women experience **amenorrhea** (absence of menses), at least 20% have some slight, painless spotting during early gestation for unexplained reasons; implantation bleeding and bleeding after intercourse related to cervical friability may account for some bleeding. A great majority of these women continue to full term and have normal infants. However, all instances of bleeding should be reported and evaluated.

After implantation the fertilized ovum and the chorionic villi produce hCG, which maintains the corpus luteum's production of estrogen and progesterone for the first 8 to 10 weeks of pregnancy until the placenta takes over their production (Scott et al, 1994).

Home Care 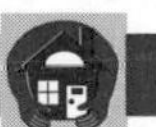

HOME PREGNANCY TESTING

- Follow manufacturer's instructions carefully. Do not omit or skip steps.
- Review manufacturer's list of drugs and other factors that could affect the test results.
- Use first-voided morning urine specimen.
- For more accurate results, wait longer than 6 to 9 days after your missed period.

TABLE 6-2 Signs of pregnancy

TIME OF OCCURRENCE (GESTATIONAL AGE)	SIGN	OTHER POSSIBLE CAUSES
	Presumptive	
3-4 weeks	Breast changes	Premenstrual changes, oral contraceptives
4 weeks	Amenorrhea	Stress, vigorous exercise, early menopause, endocrine problems, malnutrition
4-14 weeks	Nausea, vomiting	Gastrointestinal virus, food poisoning
6-12 weeks	Urinary frequency	Infection, pelvic tumors
12 weeks	Fatigue	Stress, illness
16-20 weeks	Quickening	Gas, peristalsis
	Probable	
5 weeks	Goodell's sign	Pelvic congestion
6-8 weeks	Chadwick's sign	Pelvic congestion
6-12 weeks	Hegar's sign	Pelvic congestion
4-12 weeks	Positive pregnancy test (serum)	Hydatidiform mole, choriocarcinoma
6-12 weeks	Positive pregnancy test (urine)	Pelvic infection, tumors
16 weeks	Braxton Hicks contractions	Myomas, other tumors
16-28 weeks	Ballottement	Tumors, cervical polyps
	Positive	
5-6 weeks	Visualization of fetus by ultrasound, X-ray films	No other causes
6 weeks	Fetal heart tones (FHTs) by ultrasound	
10-17 weeks	FHTs by Doppler	
17-19 weeks	FHTs by stethoscope	
19-22 weeks	Fetal movements palpated	
Late pregnancy	Visible	

Uterus

The phenomenal uterine growth in the first trimester occurs in response to the hormonal stimulus of high levels of estrogen and progesterone. Uterine enlargement results from (1) increased vascularity and dilation of blood vessels, (2) hyperplasia (production of new muscle fibers and fibroelastic tissue) and hypertrophy (enlargement of preexisting muscle fibers and fibroelastic tissue), and (3) development of the decidua (Fig. 6-1). By 7 weeks the uterus is the size of a large hen's egg; by 10 weeks it is the size of an orange (twice its nonpregnant size); and by 12 weeks it is the size of a grapefruit. Table 6-3 compares uterine measurements for the nonpregnant and pregnant uterus at 40 weeks' gestation. After the third month, uterine enlargement is primarily the result of mechanical pressure of the growing fetus (Seidel et al, 1995). In the nonpregnant woman the uterine cavity holds about 10 ml of fluid; during pregnancy its capacity increases to 5 L or more (Cunningham et al, 1993).

TABLE 6-3 Comparison of measurements for nonpregnant and pregnant uterus at 40 weeks*

MEASUREMENT	NONPREGNANT	PREGNANT (40 WEEKS)
Length	6.5 cm (2½ in)	32 cm (12½ in)
Width	4 cm (1½ in)	24 cm (9½ in)
Depth	2.5 cm (1 in)	22 cm (8½ in)
Weight	60-70 g (2½ oz)	1100-1200 g (2½ lb)
Volume	≥ 10 ml	5000 ml

*NOTE: Reports vary as to the exact values, but all authors agree on the magnitude of the growth that the uterus undergoes during pregnancy.

As the uterus increases in size, it also changes in weight, shape, and position. The muscular walls strengthen and become more elastic. At conception the uterus is shaped like an upside-down pear. During the second trimester it is spheric or globular. Later, as the fetus lengthens, the uterus becomes larger and more ovoid, and it rises out of the pelvis into the abdominal cavity.

The pregnancy may "show" after the fourteenth week, although this depends to some degree on the woman's height and weight. Abdominal enlargement may be less apparent in the primigravida with good abdominal muscle tone (Fig. 6-2). Posture also influences the type and degree of abdominal enlargement seen. In normal pregnancies the uterus enlarges at a predictable rate. This measurement is used to estimate the duration of pregnancy. Uterine enlargement is determined by measuring fundal height. Variations in the position of the fundus or the fetus, variations in the amount of amniotic fluid present, the presence of more than one fetus, and maternal obesity reduce the accuracy of this estimation of the duration of pregnancy.

As the uterus grows, it is elevated out of the pelvic area and may be palpated above the symphysis pubis sometime between the twelfth and fourteenth weeks of pregnancy (Fig. 6-3). The uterus rises gradually to the level of the umbilicus at

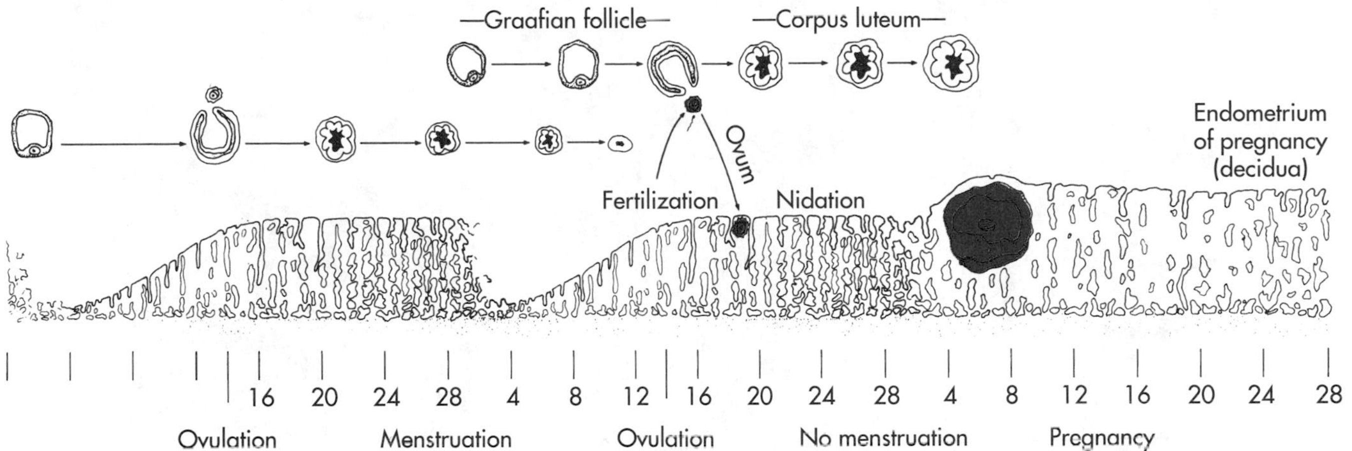

Fig. 6-1 Changes in endometrium and corpus luteum if pregnancy occurs (in days). *Nidation* refers to implantation.

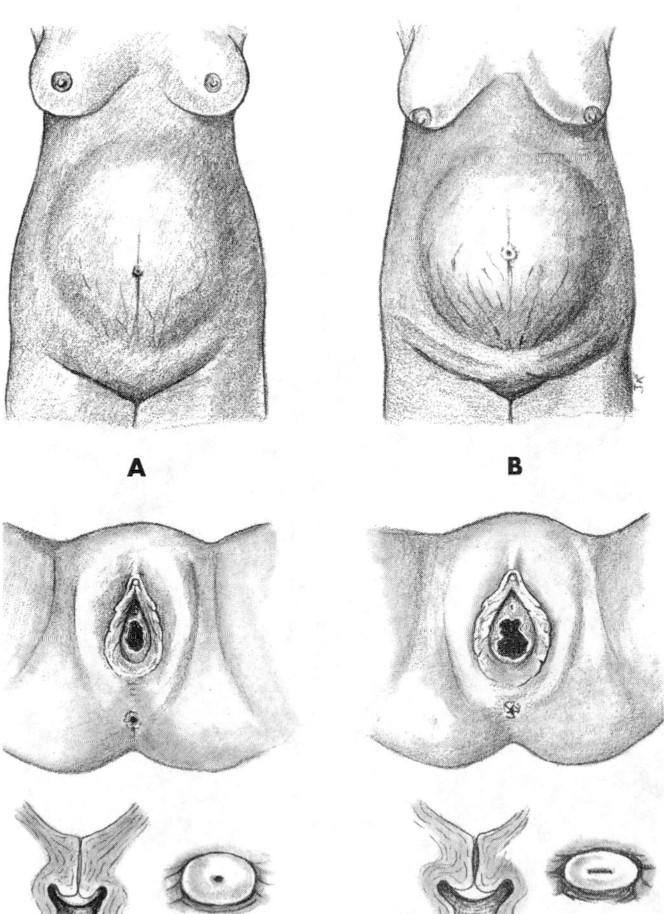

Fig. 6-2 Comparison of abdomen, vulva, and cervix in **A,** nullipara, and **B,** multipara, at same stage of pregnancy.

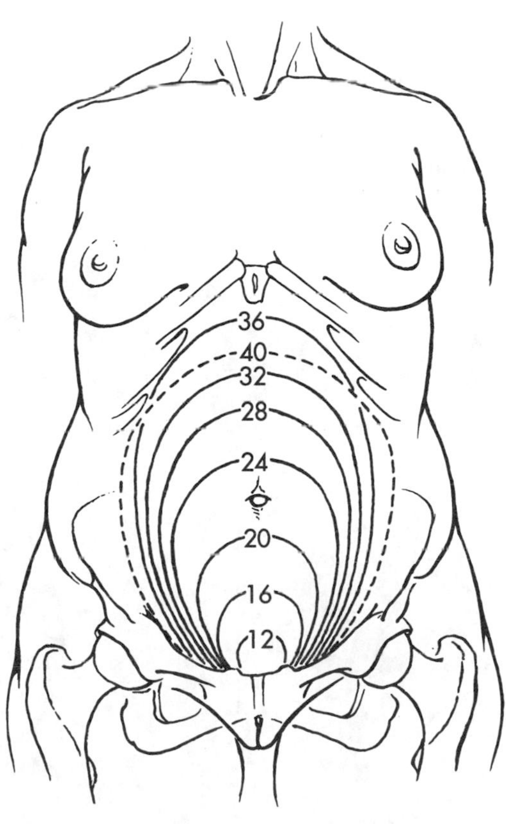

Fig. 6-3 Height of fundus by weeks of normal gestation with a single fetus. Dotted line indicates height after lightening. (From Barkauskas V et al: *Health and physical assessment,* St Louis, 1994, Mosby.)

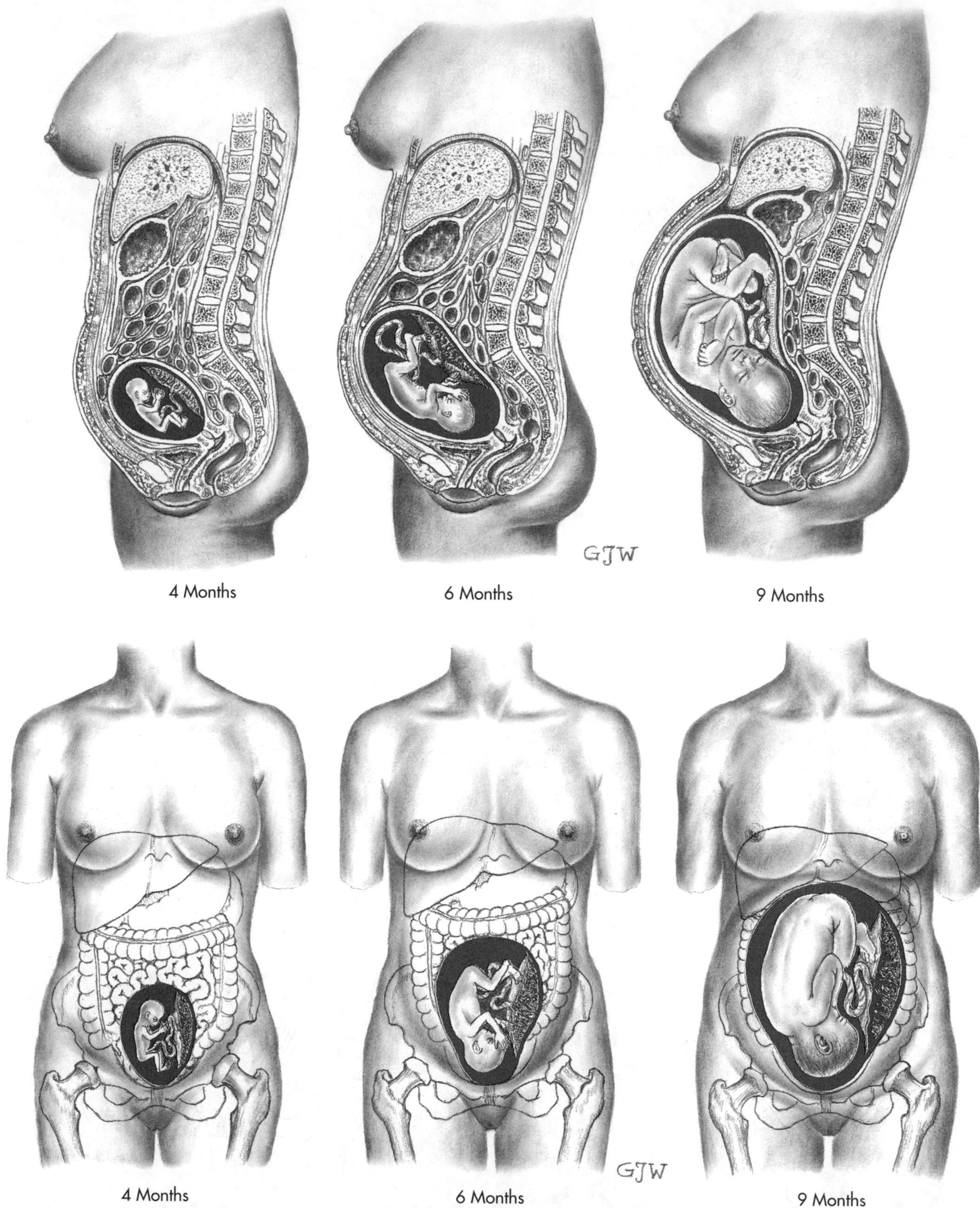

Fig. 6-4 Displacement of internal abdominal structures and diaphragm by enlarging uterus at 4, 6, and 9 months of gestation.

about 22 to 24 weeks and nearly reaches the xiphoid process at term. Between weeks 38 and 40, fundal height decreases as the fetus begins to descend and engage in the pelvis **(lightening)** (Fig. 6-3; see dotted lines). Generally, lightening occurs in the nullipara about 2 weeks before the onset of labor and at the start of labor in the multipara.

Generally the uterus is rotated to the right as it elevates, probably because of the presence of the rectosigmoid colon on the left side. However, the extensive hypertrophy (enlargement) of the round ligaments keeps the uterus in line. Eventually the growing uterus touches the anterior abdominal wall and displaces the intestines to either side of the abdomen (Fig. 6-4). When a pregnant woman stands, the major part of her uterus rests against the anterior abdominal wall and contributes to altering her center of gravity.

During the early weeks of pregnancy an increase in uterine blood flow and lymph causes pelvic congestion and edema. As a result, the uterus, cervix, and isthmus soften perceptibly and progressively, and the cervix takes on a bluish color (**Chadwick's sign,** a probable sign of pregnancy) (Scott et al, 1994).

At the seventh to eighth week the following patterns of uterine softening are noted: softening and compressibility of lower uterine segment (uterine isthmus) (**Hegar's sign;** Fig. 6-5), easy flexion of the fundus on the cervix *(McDonald's sign)*, softening and slight fullness of the fundus near the area of implantation *(Braun von Fernwald's sign)*, or a soft lateral bulge with cornual implantation *(Piskacek's sign)*. After the eighth week, general enlargement and softening of the uterine corpus and cervix are likely. These are all probable signs of pregnancy.

Some believe that the nonsteroid ovarian hormone relaxin may act along with progesterone (Cunningham et al, 1993; Scott et al, 1994). Relaxation occurs not only in the uterus but throughout various parts of the body, such as the joints, walls of blood vessels, and gastrointestinal and renal system structures.

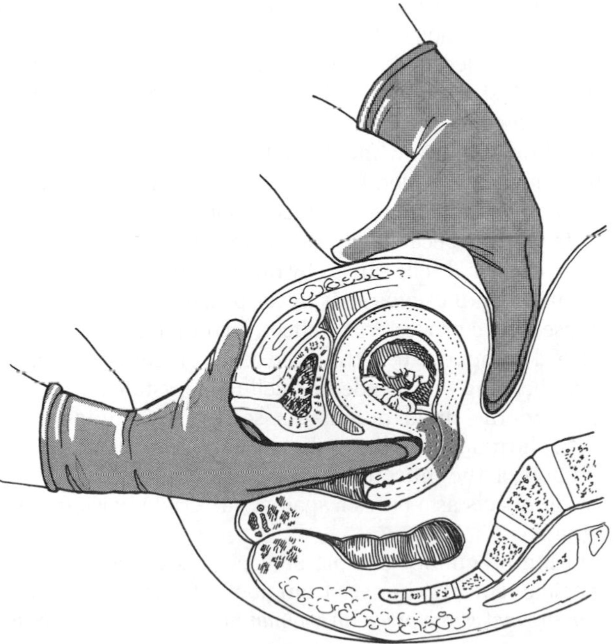

Fig. 6-5 Hegar's sign. Bimanual examination for assessing compressibility and softening of isthmus (lower uterine segment) while cervix is still firm.

Soon after the fourth month of pregnancy, uterine contractions can be felt through the abdominal wall. These contractions are referred to as **Braxton Hicks contractions,** a probable sign of pregnancy. Braxton Hicks contractions are a continuation of the irregular, painless contractions that occur intermittently throughout each menstrual cycle. The contractions are felt as uterine firmness through the abdominal wall or are evident because they raise and push the uterus forward. Contractions facilitate uterine blood flow through the intervillous spaces of the placenta and thereby promote oxygen delivery to the fetus. Although Braxton Hicks contractions are not ordinarily painful, some women do complain that they are annoying. After the twenty-eighth week, contractions become much more definite, especially in slender women. Generally these contractions cease with walking or exercise. They are rarely perceived as painful, and they do not progress in intensity, duration, and frequency as true labor contractions would.

Blood flow increases rapidly as the uterus increases in size. Although uterine blood flow increases twentyfold, the size of the conceptus grows more rapidly. Consequently, more oxygen is extracted from the uterine blood during the latter part of pregnancy (Cunningham et al, 1993). In a normal term pregnancy, one sixth of the total maternal blood volume is within the uterine vascular system. The rate of blood flow through the uterus averages 500 ml/min, and oxygen consumption of the gravid uterus averages 25 ml/min. Maternal arterial pressure, contractions of the uterus, and maternal position are three factors known to influence blood flow. Estrogens also play a role in uterine blood flow. Doppler ultrasound can be used to measure uterine blood flow velocity, especially in pregnancies at risk related to hypertension, intrauterine growth restriction (IUGR), diabetes mellitus, and multiple gestation (Scott et al, 1994).

Using an ultrasound device or a fetal stethoscope, the health care provider may hear (1) the **uterine souffle,** or bruit, a rushing or blowing sound of maternal blood flowing through uterine arteries to the placenta that is synchronous with the maternal pulse; (2) the **funic souffle,** which is synchronous with the fetal heart rate and caused by fetal blood coursing through the umbilical cord; and (3) the **fetal heart tones (FHT),** the actual heartbeat of the fetus.

Passive movement of the unengaged fetus is called **ballottement.** Ballottement can be identified generally between the sixteenth and eighteenth week. Ballottement is a technique of palpating a floating structure by bouncing it gently and feeling it rebound. The examiner's finger within the vagina taps gently upward; the fetus rises. Then the fetus sinks, and a gentle tap is felt on the finger (Fig. 6-6). Internal ballottement of a fetus within a uterus is a probable objective sign of pregnancy.

The first recognition of fetal movements, or "feeling life," by the multiparous woman may occur as early as the fourteenth to sixteenth week. The nulliparous woman may not notice these sensations until the eighteenth week or later. **Quickening,** a presumptive sign of pregnancy, is often described as a flutter and is difficult to distinguish from peristal-

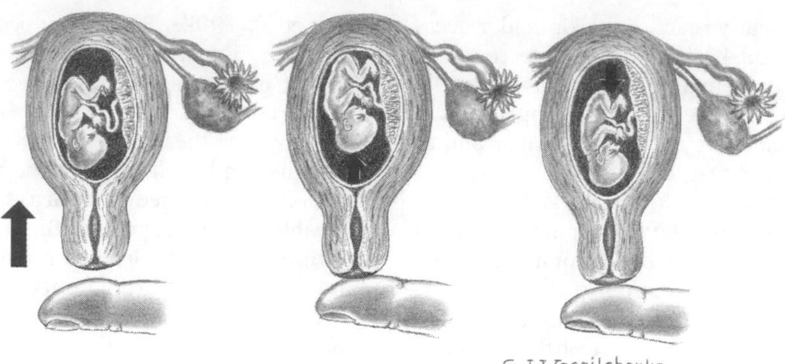

Fig. 6-6 Internal ballottement (18 weeks).

sis. Gradually, fetal movements increase in intensity and frequency. Noting the week during which quickening occurs provides a tentative clue in dating the duration of gestation.

A softening of the cervical tip may be observed about the beginning of the sixth week in a normal, unscarred cervix. This probable sign of pregnancy, **Goodell's sign,** is brought about by increased vascularity, slight hypertrophy, and hyperplasia (increase in number of cells) of the muscle and its collagen-rich connective tissue, which becomes loose, edematous, highly elastic, and increased in volume. The glands near the external os proliferate beneath the stratified squamous epithelium, giving the cervix the velvety consistency characteristic of pregnancy. The changes in the cervix as well as those of the vagina help prepare the birth canal for the fetus's passage through it (Fig. 6-7). **Friability** is increased; that is, the cervix bleeds easily when scraped or touched. Increased friability is the cause of the few drops of blood seen after coitus with deep penetration or after vaginal examination. These few drops are usually within normal limits.

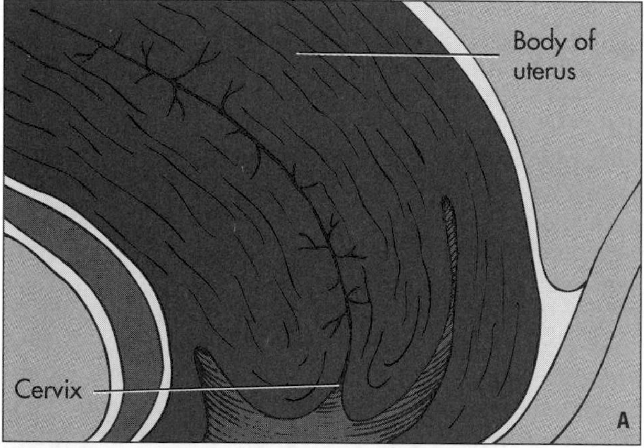

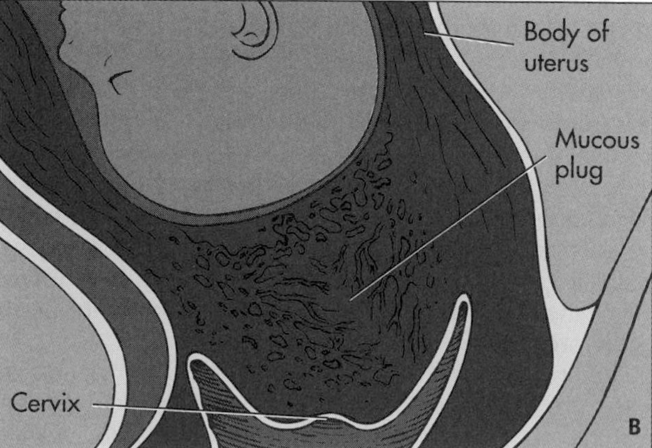

Fig. 6-7 **A**, Cervix in nonpregnant women. **B**, Changes in cervix during pregnancy.

The cervix of the nullipara is rounded. Lacerations of the cervix almost always occur during the birth process. With or without lacerations, after childbirth the cervix becomes more oval in the horizontal plane, and the external os appears as a transverse slit (Fig. 6-2).

Vagina and Vulva

Pregnancy hormones prepare the vagina for distention during labor by producing a thickened vaginal mucosa, loosened connective tissue, hypertrophied smooth muscle, and an increase in the length of the vaginal vault. Increased vascularity results in a violet-blue color of the vaginal mucosa and cervix. The deepened color, termed *Chadwick's sign* or *Jacquemier's sign,* may be evident as early as the sixth week but is easily noted at the eighth week of pregnancy.

Leukorrhea is a white or slightly gray mucoid discharge with a faint musty odor. Increased estrogen and progesterone stimulation of the cervix produces copious mucoid fluid. The fluid is whitish because of the presence of many exfoliated vaginal epithelial cells caused by normal pregnancy hyperplasia. This vaginal discharge is never pruritic or blood stained. Because of the progesterone effect, ferning (see Fig. 3-23, *A*) usually does not occur in the dried cervical mucous smear. Instead, "beading"—a beaded or cellular crystallizing pattern formed in the dried mucus—is seen (Cunningham et al, 1993). The mucus fills the endocervical canal, resulting in the formation of the mucous plug **(operculum)** (Fig. 6-7). The operculum acts as a barrier against bacterial invasion during pregnancy.

During pregnancy the pH of vaginal secretions becomes less acidic. The pH changes from about 4.0 to about 6.5. *The rise in pH makes the pregnant woman more vulnerable to vaginal infections, especially yeast infections.*

The increased vascularity of the vagina and other pelvic viscera results in a marked increase in sensitivity. The increased sensitivity may lead to a high degree of sexual inter-

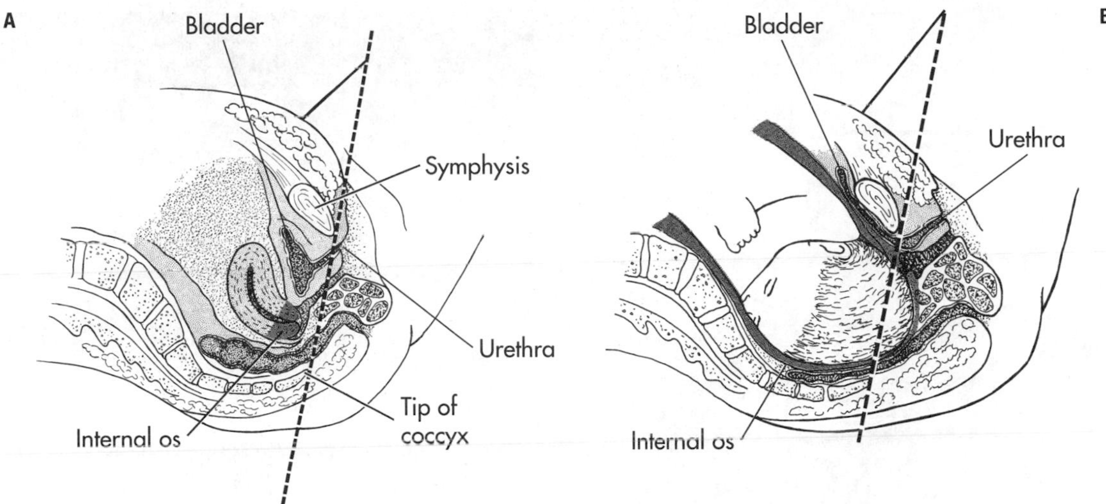

Fig. 6-8 **A,** Pelvic floor in nonpregnant women. **B,** Pelvic floor at end of pregnancy. Note marked hypertrophy and hyperplasia below the dotted line joining tip of coccyx and inferior margin of symphysis. Note elongation of bladder and urethra as a result of compression. Fat deposits are increased.

est and arousal, especially during the second trimester of pregnancy. The increased congestion plus the relaxed walls of the blood vessels and the heavy uterus may result in edema and varicosities of the vulva. The edema and varicosities usually resolve during the postpartum period.

External structures of the perineum are enlarged during pregnancy because of an increase in vasculature, hypertrophy of the perineal body, and deposition of fat (Fig. 6-8). The labia majora of the nullipara approximate and obscure the vaginal introitus; those of the parous woman separate and gape after childbirth and perineal or vaginal injury. Fig. 6-2 compares the perineum of the nullipara and the multipara in relation to the pregnant abdomen, vulva, and cervix.

Breasts

Fullness, heightened sensitivity, tingling, and heaviness of the breasts begin as early as the sixth week of gestation as a result of increased levels of estrogen and progesterone. These changes are considered presumptive signs of pregnancy because other factors can cause them to occur. Breast sensitivity varies from mild tingling to frank pain (mastodynia). Nipples and areolae become more pigmented; secondary pinkish areolae develop, extending beyond the primary areolae; and nipples become more erectile. Hypertrophy of the sebaceous (oil) glands embedded in the primary areolae, called **Montgomery tubercles** (see Fig. 3-18, *B*), may be seen around the nipples. These sebaceous glands may have a protective role in that they keep the nipples lubricated for breastfeeding. Suppleness of the nipples is jeopardized if the protective oils are washed off with soap.

The richer blood supply dilates the vessels beneath the skin. Once barely noticeable, the blood vessels now become visible, often appearing in an intertwining blue network beneath the surface of the skin. Venous congestion in the breasts is more obvious in primigravidas. Striae gravidarum (see p. 116) may appear at the outer aspects of the breasts.

During the second and third trimesters, growth of the mammary glands accounts for the progressive increase in breast size. The high levels of luteal and placental hormones in pregnancy promote proliferation of the lactiferous ducts and lobule-alveolar tissue; thus palpation of the breasts reveals a generalized, coarse nodularity. The increase in glandular tissue displaces connective tissue, and as a result the tissue becomes softer and looser. Overstretching of the fibrous, suspensory Cooper ligaments (Fig. 3-18, *A*) supporting the breasts may be reduced with a well-fitted maternity bra.

Although development of the mammary glands is functionally complete by midpregnancy, lactation is inhibited until a decrease in estrogen level occurs after the birth of the fetus and placenta. A thin, clear, viscous secretory material can be found in the acini cells by the third month of gestation. This precolostrum thickens as term approaches and is then known as **colostrum.** Colostrum, the creamy, white to yellowish to orange premilk fluid, may be expressed from the nipples as early as 16 weeks of gestation (Lawrence, 1994) (See the discussion of pituitary prolactin on p. 120).

GENERAL BODY SYSTEMS

Cardiovascular System

Maternal adjustments to pregnancy involve extensive changes in the cardiovascular system, both anatomic and physiologic. Cardiovascular adaptations protect the woman's normal physiologic functioning, meet the metabolic demands pregnancy imposes on her body, and provide for fetal developmental and growth needs.

Slight cardiac hypertrophy (enlargement) or dilation is probably secondary to increased blood volume and cardiac output. This enlargement is reversed after childbirth. As the diaphragm is displaced upward, the heart is elevated upward and rotated forward to the left (Fig. 6-9). The apical impulse, a point of maximum intensity (PMI), is shifted upward and laterally about 1 to 1.5 cm. The degree of shift depends on the duration of pregnancy and the size and position of the uterus.

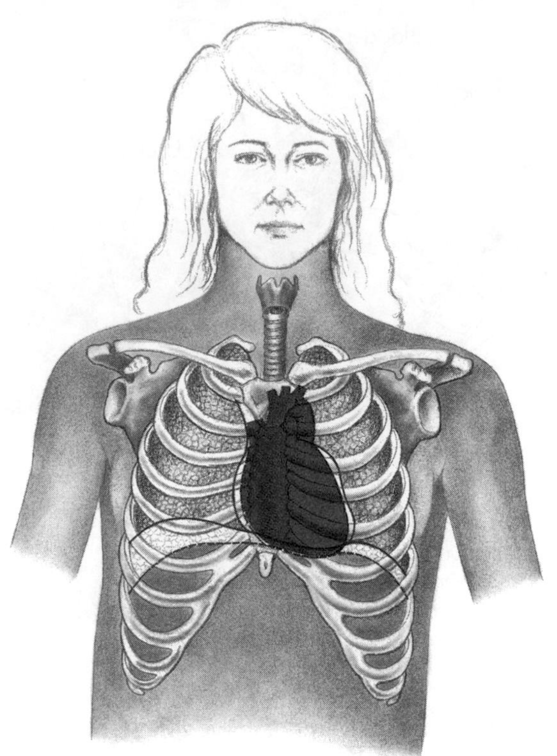

Fig. 6-9 Changes in position of heart, lungs, and thoracic cage in pregnancy: *broken line*, nonpregnant; *solid line*, change that occurs in pregnancy.

Auscultatory changes accompany the changes in heart size and position. Increases in blood volume and cardiac output also contribute to auscultatory changes common in pregnancy. More audible splitting of S_1 and S_2, and S_3 may be readily heard after 20 weeks of gestation. Additionally, grade II systolic ejection murmurs may be heard over the pulmonic area.

Between 14 and 20 weeks the pulse increases about 10 to 15 beats/min, which then persists to term. Palpitations may occur. In twin gestations the maternal heart rate may increase 40% above nonpregnant levels (Fuschino, 1992).

The cardiac rhythm may be disturbed. The pregnant woman may experience sinus dysrhythmia, premature atrial contractions, and premature ventricular systole. In the healthy woman with no underlying heart disease, no therapy is needed.

Blood pressure. Arterial blood pressure (brachial artery) varies with age, activity level, and presence of health problems. Additional factors must be considered. These factors include maternal position, maternal anxiety, and size of cuff. Maternal position affects readings. Brachial blood pressure is highest when the woman is sitting, lowest when she is lying in the lateral recumbent position, and intermediate when she is supine. Therefore the same maternal position and the same arm are used at each visit. The position and arm used are noted along with the reading.

BOX 6-2
Calculation of Mean Arterial Pressure

Blood pressure: 106/70

Formula: $\frac{\text{Systolic} + 2(\text{Diastolic})}{3}$

$\frac{106 + 2(70)}{3}$

$\frac{106 + 140}{3}$

246/3 = 82 mm Hg

Maternal anxiety can elevate readings. If an elevated reading is found, the woman is given time to rest, and the reading is repeated.

The proper size of cuff is absolutely necessary for accurate readings. The cuff should be 20% wider than the diameter of the arm around which it is wrapped: about 12 to 14 cm for average-sized individuals and about 18 to 20 cm for obese persons. Too small a cuff yields a false-high reading; too large a cuff yields a false-low reading.

In the first trimester, blood pressure usually remains the same as the prepregnancy level. During the second trimester of pregnancy, both systolic pressure and diastolic pressure decrease 5 to 10 mm Hg. The decrease in blood pressure is probably the result of peripheral vasodilation from hormonal changes during pregnancy. During the third trimester, maternal blood pressure should return to the values obtained during the first trimester.

The **mean arterial pressure (MAP)** (mean of the blood pressure in the arterial circulation) increases the diagnostic value of the findings. Normal MAP readings in the nonpregnant woman are 86.4 mm Hg ±7.5 mm Hg. MAP readings for a pregnant woman are 90.3 mm Hg ±5.8 mm Hg (Scott et al, 1994). Box 6-2 shows the calculation of a MAP.

Some degree of compression of the vena cava occurs in all women who lie on their backs during the second half of pregnancy. Some women experience a fall of more than 30 mm Hg systolic pressure. After 4 to 5 minutes a reflex bradycardia is noted, cardiac output is reduced by half, and the woman feels faint *(supine hypotension)*. Other women show an increase in blood pressure in the supine position (Cunningham et al, 1993).

Compression of the iliac veins and inferior vena cava by the uterus causes increased venous pressure and reduced blood flow in the legs, except when the woman is in the lateral position. These alterations contribute to the dependent edema, varicose veins in the legs and vulva, and hemorrhoids experienced by women in the latter part of term pregnancy.

Blood volume and composition. The degree of blood volume expansion varies considerably (Cunningham et al, 1993). Blood volume increases by approximately 1500 ml, or 40% to 50% above nonpregnancy levels. The increase is composed of 1300 ml plasma plus 450 ml red blood cells (RBCs) (Fig. 6-10). The increase in volume starts about the tenth to twelfth week, peaks at about 25% to 45% above the nonpregnant levels at the thirty-second to thirty-fourth week, then decreases slightly at the fortieth week. The volume in a multiple gestation increases above the level for a single pregnancy (Fuschino, 1992). The increased volume is a protective mechanism. It is essential for (1) the hypertrophied vascular system of the enlarged uterus, (2) adequate hydration of fetal and maternal tissues when the woman assumes an erect or supine position, and (3) fluid reserve for blood loss during the birth and the puerperium. Peripheral vasodilation maintains a normal blood pressure despite the increased blood volume in pregnancy.

During pregnancy an accelerated production of RBCs occurs (normal: 4.2 to 5.4 million/mm³). The percentage of increase depends on the amount of iron available. The RBC mass increases by 30% to 33% by term if an iron supplement is taken. The average increase is 18% in women if no supplement is taken (Bennett and Brown, 1993).

Because the plasma increase is greater than the increase of RBC production, a decrease occurs in normal hemoglobin values (12 to 16 g/dl blood) and hematocrit values (37% to 47%). This condition is referred to as **physiologic anemia.** The decrease is more noticeable during the second trimester, when rapid expansion of blood volume occurs faster than

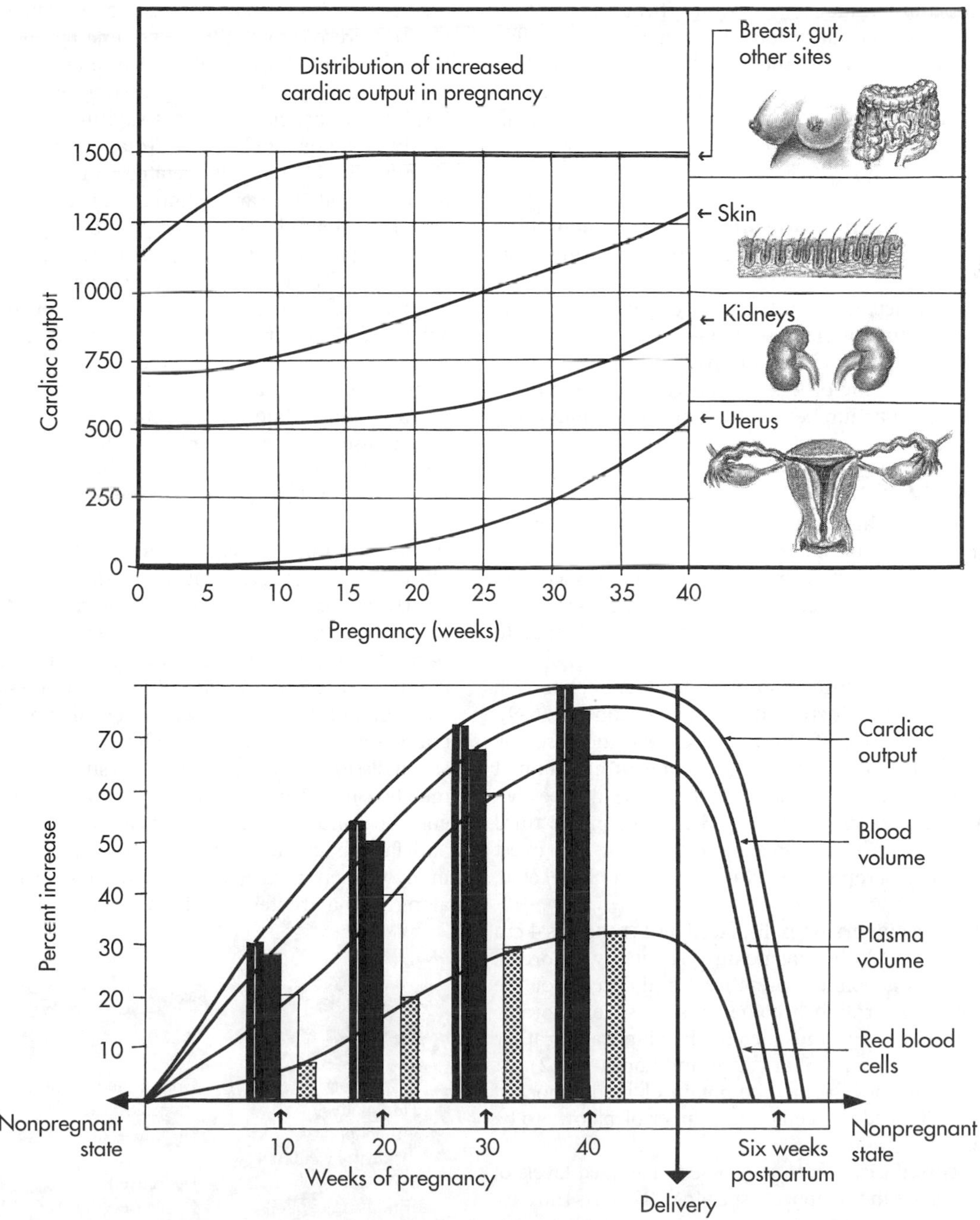

Fig. 6-10 Distribution of increased cardiac output in pregnancy.

RBC production. If the hemoglobin value drops to 10 g/dl or less or if the hematocrit drops to 35% or less, the woman is considered anemic.

The total white blood cell (WBC) count increases during the second trimester and peaks during the third trimester. This increase is primarily in the granulocytes; the lymphocyte (WBC) count stays about the same throughout pregnancy. (See the Appendix for laboratory values during pregnancy.)

Cardiac output. Cardiac output increases from 30% to 50% by the thirty-second week of pregnancy; it declines to about a 20% increase at 40 weeks. The elevated cardiac output is largely a result of increased stroke volume and in response to increased tissue demands for oxygen (nonpregnant value: 5 to 5.5 L/min; pregnant value: 6 to 7 L/min) (Scott et al, 1994) (Fig. 6-10). Cardiac output in late pregnancy is appreciably higher when the woman is in the lateral recumbant position than when she is supine. In the supine position the large, heavy uterus often impedes venous return to the heart and affects blood pressure. Cardiac output increases with any exertion, such as labor and birth.

Circulation and coagulation times. The circulation time decreases slightly by week 32. It returns to near normal near term.

A greater tendency exists for blood to coagulate (clot) during pregnancy because of increases in various clotting factors (factors VII, VIII, IX, X, and fibrinogen). Fibrinolytic activity (splitting up or dissolving of a clot) is depressed during pregnancy and the postpartum period, making the woman more vulnerable to thrombosis.

Respiratory System

Structural and ventilatory adaptations occur during pregnancy to provide for both maternal and fetal needs. Maternal oxygen requirements increase in response to the acceleration in metabolic rate and the need to add to the tissue mass in the uterus and breasts. The fetus requires oxygen and a way to eliminate carbon dioxide.

Elevated levels of estrogen cause the ligaments of the rib cage to relax, permitting increased chest expansion (Fig. 6-9). The transverse diameter of the thoracic cage increases by about 2 cm and the circumference by 6 cm (Cunningham et al, 1993). The costal angle of approximately 68 degrees before pregnancy increases to about 103 degrees in the third trimester. The lower rib cage appears to flare out. The chest may not return to its prepregnant state after birth (Seidel et al, 1995).

The level of the diaphragm is displaced by as much as 4 cm during pregnancy. With advancing pregnancy, thoracic breathing replaces abdominal breathing, and descent of the diaphragm with inspiration becomes less possible. Thoracic breathing is primarily accomplished by the diaphragm rather than by the costal muscles (Blackburn and Loper, 1992). At this stage of pregnancy, women complain of being short of breath. They may need to sleep on a number of pillows to be comfortable.

Increased vascularization in response to elevated levels of estrogen also occurs in the upper respiratory tract. As the capillaries become engorged, edema and hyperemia develop within the nose, pharynx, larynx, trachea, and bronchi. This congestion within the tissues of the respiratory tract gives rise to several conditions commonly seen during pregnancy, including nasal and sinus stuffiness, epistaxis (nosebleed), changes in the voice, and marked inflammatory response to even a mild upper respiratory infection.

Increased vascularity also swells tympanic membranes and eustachian tubes, giving rise to symptoms of impaired hearing, earaches, or a sense of fullness in the ears.

Pulmonary function changes. The pregnant woman breathes deeper (increases *tidal volume,* the volume of gas moved into or out of the respiratory tract with each breath) but increases her respiratory rate only slightly (about two breaths per minute). The increase in respiratory tidal volume associated with the normal respiratory rate results in an increase in respiratory minute volume by approximately 40% (Blackburn and Loper, 1992). Expiratory reserve volume and residual volume decrease progressively during pregnancy. The inspiratory capacity increases slightly, whereas the vital capacity remains unchanged. Total lung capacity decreases slightly. The changes are related to the elevation of the diaphragm and chest wall changes (Fuschino, 1993). Box 6-3 lists respiratory changes in pregnancy.

During pregnancy, changes in the respiratory center result in a lowered threshold for carbon dioxide. Progesterone and estrogen are presumed to be responsible for the increased sensitivity of the respiratory center to carbon dioxide. In addition, pregnant women experience increased awareness of the need to breathe; some may complain of dyspnea at rest.

Although pulmonary function is not impaired by pregnancy, diseases of the respiratory tract may be more serious during this time (Cunningham et al, 1993). One important factor may be the increased oxygen requirements.

Basal metabolic rate. The basal metabolic rate (BMR) usually rises by the fourth month of gestation. It is increased 15% to 20% by term (Worthington-Roberts and Williams, 1993). The BMR returns to nonpregnant levels by 5 to 6 days postpartum. The elevation in BMR reflects increased oxygen demands of the uterine-placental-fetal unit as well as oxygen consumption from increased maternal cardiac work. Peripheral vasodilation and acceleration of sweat gland activity assist in dissipating the excess heat resulting from the increased metabolism during pregnancy. Pregnant women may experience heat intolerance, which is annoying to some. Lassitude and fatigability after only slight exertion are described by many women in early pregnancy. These feelings may persist, along with a greater need for sleep. Lassitude and fatigability

BOX 6-3
Respiratory Changes in Pregnancy

Respiratory rate	Unchanged or slightly higher
Tidal volume	Increased 30%-40%
Vital capacity	Unchanged
Inspiratory capacity	Increased
Expiratory volume	Decreased
Total lung capacity	Decreased slightly
Oxygen consumption	Increased 15%-20%

BOX 6-4
Acid-Base Values in Arterial Blood of Pregnant Women

Carbon dioxide tension (Pco_2)	27-32 mm Hg (decreased)
Sodium bicarbonate	18-21 mEq/L (decreased)
Blood pH	Increased slightly (more alkaline)

may be caused in part by the increased metabolic activity (see the discussion of the thyroid gland later in this chapter).

Acid-base balance. By about the tenth week of pregnancy, there is a decrease of about 5 mm Hg in carbon dioxide tension, or partial pressure (Pco_2). Progesterone may be responsible for increasing the sensitivity of the respiratory center receptors so that tidal volume is increased and Pco_2 falls, the base excess (HCO_3^-, or bicarbonate) falls, and pH rises. These alterations in acid-base balance indicate that pregnancy is a state of respiratory alkalosis compensated by mild metabolic acidosis (Fuschino, 1993). Box 6-4 lists acid-base values during pregnancy.

Renal System

The kidneys are vital excretory organs. Their purpose is to maintain the body's internal environment in the relatively constant homeostatic state necessary for the efficient functioning of the body at the cellular level. The kidneys are responsible for maintaining electrolyte and acid-base balance, regulating extracellular fluid volume, excreting waste products, and conserving essential nutrients.

Anatomic changes. Changes in renal structure result from hormonal activity (estrogen and progesterone), pressure from an enlarging uterus, and an increase in blood volume. As early as the tenth week of pregnancy, the renal pelvis and the ureters dilate. Dilation of the ureters is more pronounced above the pelvic brim, in part because they are compressed between the uterus and the pelvic brim. Dilation above the pelvic brim is more marked on the right side. In most women the ureters below the pelvic brim are of normal size. The smooth-muscle walls of the ureters undergo hyperplasia and hypertrophy and relaxed muscle tone. The ureters elongate, become tortuous, and form single or double curves. In the latter part of pregnancy the right renal pelvis and ureter dilate more than on the left as a result of the displacement of the heavy uterus to the right by the sigmoid colon.

Because of these changes, a larger volume of urine is held in the pelves and ureters, and urine flow rate is slowed. Urinary stasis or stagnation has several consequences, including the following:

1. There is a lag between the time urine is formed and when it reaches the bladder. Therefore clearance test results may reflect substances contained in glomerular filtrate several hours before.
2. Stagnated urine is an excellent medium for the growth of microorganisms. In addition, the urine of pregnant women contains greater amounts of nutrients, including glucose, increasing the pH (making the urine more alkaline). Therefore during pregnancy, women are more susceptible to urinary tract infection.

Bladder irritability, nocturia, and urinary frequency and urgency (without dysuria) are commonly reported in early pregnancy. Near term, bladder symptoms may return, especially after lightening occurs.

Urinary frequency results from increased bladder sensitivity and later from compression of the bladder (Fig. 6-8). In the second trimester the bladder is pulled up out of the true pelvis into the abdomen. The urethra lengthens to 7.5 cm as the bladder is displaced upward. The pelvic congestion of pregnancy is reflected in hyperemia of the bladder and urethra. This increased vascularity causes the bladder mucosa to be traumatized and bleed easily. There may be a decrease in bladder tone, which permits distention of the bladder to approximately 1500 ml. At the same time, the bladder is compressed by the enlarging uterus, resulting in the urge to void even if the bladder contains only a small amount of urine.

Renal function changes. In normal pregnancy, renal function is altered considerably. Glomerular filtration rate (GFR) and renal plasma flow (RPF) increase early in pregnancy (Cunningham et al, 1993). The woman's kidneys must manage the increased metabolic and circulatory demands of the maternal body and also excretion of fetal waste products. Changes in renal function are caused by pregnancy hormones, an increase in blood volume, the woman's posture, physical activity, and nutritional intake.

Renal function is most efficient when the woman lies in the lateral recumbent position and least efficient when the woman assumes a supine position. A side-lying position increases renal perfusion, which increases urine output and decreases edema. When the pregnant woman is lying supine, the heavy uterus compresses the vena cava and the aorta, and cardiac output decreases. When cardiac output drops, blood flow to the brain and heart is continued at the expense of other organs, including the kidneys and uterus.

Fluid and electrolyte balance. Selective renal tubular reabsorption maintains sodium and water balance regardless of changes in dietary intake and losses through sweat, vomitus, or diarrhea. From 500 to 900 mEq of sodium is normally retained during pregnancy to meet fetal needs. The need for increased maternal intravascular and extracellular fluid volume requires additional sodium to expand fluid volume and to maintain an isotonic state. To prevent excessive sodium depletion, the maternal kidneys undergo a significant adaptation by increasing tubular reabsorption. As efficient as the renal system is, it can be overstressed by excessive dietary sodium intake or restriction or by using diuretics. *Severe hypovolemia and reduced placental perfusion are two consequences of using diuretics during pregnancy.*

The capacity of the kidneys to excrete water during the early weeks of pregnancy is more efficient than later in pregnancy. Occasionally in early pregnancy the extent of water loss may cause some women to feel thirsty. The pooling of fluid in the legs in the latter part of pregnancy decreases RPF and GFR. The diuretic response to the water load is triggered when the woman lies down, preferably on her side, and the pooled fluid reenters general circulation. This pooling of blood in the lower legs is sometimes referred to as *physiologic edema,* which requires no treatment.

Normally the kidney reabsorbs almost all the glucose and other nutrients from the plasma filtrate. In pregnant women, tubular reabsorption of glucose is impaired so *glucosuria* occurs at varying times and to varying degrees. Normal values are 0 to 20 mg/dl; that is, during any one day the urine is sometimes positive and sometimes negative. When it is positive, the amount of glucose varies from 1+ to 4+.

In nonpregnant women, blood glucose levels must be at 160 to 180 mg/dl before glucose is "spilled" into the urine (not reabsorbed). During pregnancy, glucosuria occurs when maternal glucose levels are lower than 160 mg/dl. Why glucose, as well as other nutrients such as amino acids, is wasted during pregnancy is not understood, and the exact mechanism has not been discovered. Although glucosuria may be found in normal pregnancies (1+ levels may be seen with increased anxiety states), the possibility of diabetes mellitus and gestational diabetes must be kept in mind.

Proteinuria usually does not occur in normal pregnancy except during labor or after birth (Cunningham et al, 1993). However, the increased amount of amino acids that needs to be filtered may exceed the capacity of the renal tubules to absorb them so that small amounts of protein are lost in the urine. Values of 1+ protein (dipstick assessment) or less than 300 mg/24 hr are acceptable during pregnancy (Blackburn and Loper, 1992). The amount of protein excreted is not an indication of the severity of renal disease, and an increase in protein excretion in a pregnant woman with known renal disease does not necessarily indicate a progression in her disease. However, a pregnant woman with hypertension and proteinuria must be carefully evaluated, since she may be at greater risk for an adverse pregnancy outcome. Box 6-5 lists common renal changes during pregnancy.

Integumentary System

Alterations in hormonal balance and mechanical stretching are responsible for several changes in the integumentary system during pregnancy. General changes include increases in skin thickness and subdermal fat, hyperpigmentation, hair and nail growth, accelerated sweat and sebaceous gland activity, and increased circulation and vasomotor activity. There is greater fragility of cutaneous elastic tissues, resulting in **striae gravidarum,** or "stretch marks." Cutaneous allergic responses are enhanced.

BOX 6-5
Renal Changes in Pregnancy

Bladder capacity	Increased
Glomerular filtration rate (GFR)	Increased 30%-50%
Renal plasma flow (RPF)	Increased 30%
Blood urea nitrogen (BUN)	Decreased
Creatinine	Decreased
Glucose (in urine)	Present in 20% of pregnant women

Pigmentation is caused by the anterior pituitary hormone *melanotropin,* which is increased during pregnancy. Facial melasma, also called **chloasma** or **mask of pregnancy,** is a blotchy, brownish hyperpigmentation of the skin over the malar prominences (cheeks), nose, and the forehead, especially in dark-complected expectant women. Chloasma appears in 50% to 70% of pregnant women, beginning after the sixteenth week and increasing gradually to birth. The sun intensifies this pigmentation in susceptible women. Chloasma caused by normal pregnancy usually fades after delivery. Darkening of the nipples, areolae, axillae, and vulva occurs at about the same time.

The **linea nigra** is a pigmented line extending from the symphysis pubis to the top of the fundus in the midline; this line is known as the *linea alba* before hormone-induced pigmentation. In primigravidas the extension of the linea nigra, beginning in the third month, keeps pace with the rising height of the fundus; in multigravidas the entire line often appears earlier than the third month. Not all women develop linea nigra.

Striae gravidarum, or "stretch marks" (seen over lower abdomen in Fig. 6-11), which appear in 50% to 90% of pregnant women during the second half of pregnancy, may be caused by the action of adrenocorticosteroids. Striae reflect separation within the underlying connective (collagen) tissue of the skin. These slightly depressed streaks tend to occur over areas of maximum stretch (i.e., abdomen, thighs, breasts). The stretching sometimes causes a sensation that resembles itching. Tendency to the development of striae may be familial. After birth they usually fade, although they never disappear completely. Color of striae varies depending on the pregnant woman's skin color. The striae appear pinkish on a woman with light skin and lighter than surrounding skin in dark-skinned women. In the multipara, in addition to the striae of the present pregnancy, glistening silvery lines (in light-skinned women) or purplish lines (in dark-skinned women) are commonly seen. These represent the scars of striae from previous pregnancies.

Angiomas or **telangiectasias,** are commonly referred to as *vascular spiders.* They are tiny, star-shaped or branched,

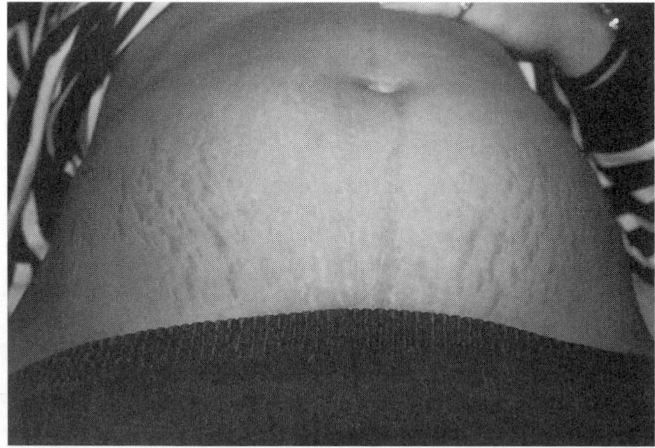

Fig. 6-11 Striae gravidarum or "stretch marks." (Courtesy Michael S. Clement, MD, Mesa, Ariz.)

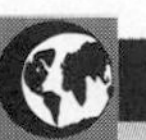

Cultural Considerations

INTEGUMENTARY CHANGES DURING PREGNANCY

Integumentary system changes such as telangiectasias and palmar erythema are seen more often in Caucasian women than in African-American women. Areolar pigmentation varies by race. African-American women have the darkest areolae, Caucasian women have the lightest, and Asian and Native-American women have intermediate pigmentation.

slightly raised, and pulsating end arterioles. The spiders, a result of elevated levels of circulating estrogen, are usually found on the neck, thorax, face, and arms. They are also described as focal networks of dilated arterioles radiating about a central core. The spiders are bluish in color and do not blanch with pressure. Vascular spiders appear during the second to fifth month of pregnancy in 65% of Caucasian women and 10% of African-American women. The spiders usually disappear after birth.

Pinkish red, diffuse mottling or well-defined blotches are seen over the palmar surfaces of the hands in about 60% of Caucasian women and 35% of African-American women during pregnancy (Cunningham et al, 1993). These color changes, called **palmar erythema,** are related primarily to increased estrogen levels (see the Cultural Considerations box above).

Gum hypertrophy may occur. An **epulis** *(gingival granuloma gravidarum)* is a red, raised nodule on the gums that bleeds easily. This lesion may develop around the third month and usually continues to enlarge as pregnancy progresses. It is usually controlled by avoiding trauma to the gums (e.g., using a soft toothbrush). An epulis usually regresses spontaneously after birth.

Nail growth may be accelerated. Some women may notice thinning and softening of the nails. Oily skin and acne vulgaris may occur during pregnancy. For other women the skin clears and looks radiant. Hirsutism, the excessive growth of hair or growth of hair in unusual places, is often reported. An increase in fine hair growth may occur. The fine hair tends to disappear after pregnancy. Growth of coarse or bristly hair does not usually disappear after pregnancy. Some women comment that their hair is thickest and most abundant during pregnancy.

Increased blood supply to the skin leads to increased perspiration. Women feel hotter during pregnancy, possibly related to a progesterone-induced increase in body temperature and vasodilation (Bennett and Brown, 1993).

Musculoskeletal System

The gradually changing body and increasing weight of the pregnant woman cause marked alterations in posture (Fig. 6-12) and walking. The great abdominal distention that gives the pelvis a forward tilt, decreased abdominal muscle tone, and increased weight bearing in late pregnancy requires a realignment of the spinal curvatures. The woman's center of gravity shifts forward. An increase in the normal lumbosacral curve (lordosis) develops, and a compensatory curvature in the cervicodorsal region (exaggerated anterior flexion of the head) is required to maintain balance. Aching, numbness, and weakness of the upper extremities may result. Large breasts and a stoop-shouldered stance further accentuate the lumbar and dorsal curves. Walking is more difficult, and the waddling gait of the pregnant woman, called "the proud walk of pregnancy" by Shakespeare, is well known. The ligamen-

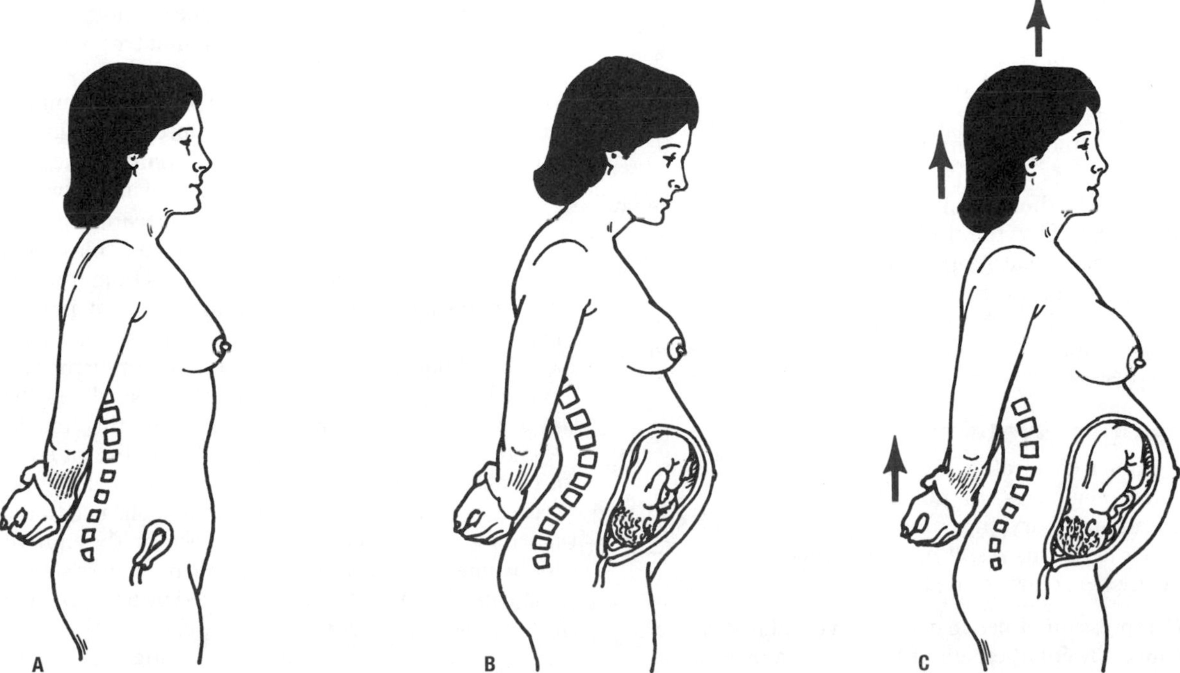

Fig. 6-12 Postural changes during pregnancy. **A,** Nonpregnant. **B,** Incorrect posture. **C,** Correct posture.

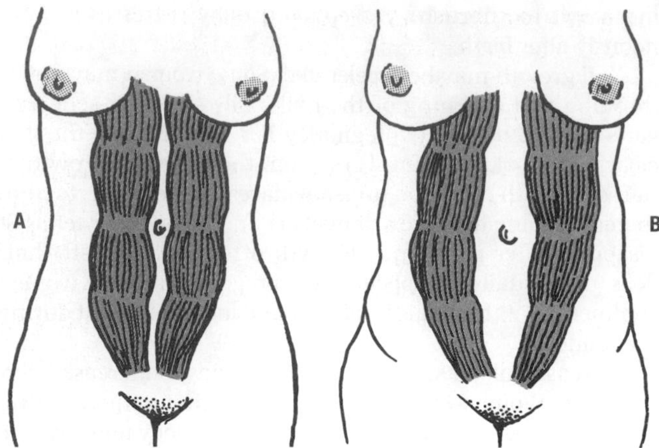

Fig. 6-13 Possible change in rectus abdominis muscles during pregnancy. **A,** Normal position in nonpregnant woman. **B,** Diastasis recti abdominis in pregnant woman.

tous and muscular structures of the middle and lower spine may be severely stressed. These and related changes often cause musculoskeletal discomfort.

The young, well-muscled woman may tolerate these changes without complaint. However, older women or those with a back disorder or a faulty sense of balance may have a considerable amount of back pain during and just after pregnancy.

Slight relaxation and increased mobility of the pelvic joints are normal during pregnancy. This is secondary to exaggerated elasticity and softening of connective and collagen tissue and is the result of increased circulating steroid sex hormones, especially estrogen. Relaxin, an ovarian hormone, assists in this relaxation and softening. These adaptations permit enlargement of pelvic dimensions to facilitate labor and birth. The degree of relaxation varies, but considerable separation of the symphysis pubis and the instability of the sacroiliac joints may cause pain and difficulty in walking. Obesity and multifetal pregnancy tend to increase the pelvic disability.

The muscles of the abdominal wall stretch and ultimately lose some tone. During the third trimester the rectus abdominis muscles may separate (Fig. 6-13), allowing abdominal contents to protrude at the midline. The umbilicus flattens or protrudes. After birth the muscles gradually regain tone. However, separation of the muscles **(diastasis recti abdominis)** may persist.

Neurologic System

Little is known regarding specific alterations in function of the neurologic system during pregnancy, aside from hypothalamic-pituitary neurohormonal changes. Specific physiologic alterations resulting from pregnancy may cause the following neurologic or neuromuscular symptoms:

1. Compression of pelvic nerves or vascular stasis caused by enlargement of the uterus may result in sensory changes in the legs.
2. Dorsolumbar lordosis may cause pain because of traction on nerves or compression of nerve roots.
3. Edema involving the peripheral nerves may result in *carpal tunnel syndrome* during the last trimester. The edema compresses the median nerve beneath the carpal ligament of the wrist. The syndrome is characterized by *paresthesia* (abnormal sensation such as burning or tingling because of a disorder of the sensory nervous system) and pain in the hand, radiating to the elbow. The dominant hand is usually affected most, although as many as 80% of women report symptoms in both hands. Symptoms usually regress after pregnancy. Some patients may require surgical treatment (Cunningham et al, 1993).
4. *Acroesthesia* (numbness and tingling of the hands) is caused by the stoop-shouldered stance (Fig. 6-12, *B*) assumed by some women during pregnancy. The condition is associated with traction on segments of the brachial plexus.
5. Tension headache is common when anxiety or uncertainty complicates gestation. However, vision problems such as refractive errors, sinusitis, or migraine may also be responsible for headaches.
6. Lightheadedness, faintness, and even syncope (fainting) are common during early pregnancy. Vasomotor instability, postural hypotension, or hypoglycemia may be responsible.
7. Hypocalcemia may cause neuromuscular problems such as muscle cramps or tetany.

Gastrointestinal System

The functioning of the gastrointestinal (GI) tract during pregnancy presents a curiously interesting picture. The appetite increases. Intestinal secretion is reduced. Liver function is altered, and absorption of nutrients is enhanced. The colon is displaced laterally upward and posteriorly. Peristaltic activity (motility) decreases. As a result, bowel sounds are diminished, and constipation, nausea, and vomiting are common. Blood flow to the pelvis increases, as does venous pressure, contributing to hemorrhoid formation in later pregnancy.

Appetite. During pregnancy the pregnant woman's appetite and food intake fluctuate. Early in pregnancy, in response to increasing levels of hCG, some pregnant women experience "morning sickness," nausea with or without vomiting that can occur throughout the day. It appears at about 4 to 6 weeks and subsides by the end of the third month (first trimester) of pregnancy. Severity varies from mild distaste for certain foods to more severe vomiting. The condition may be triggered by the sight or odor of various foods. Fatigue may also be responsible for severe nausea, but further research is needed (van Lier et al, 1993). Taste and smell may be affected as well. Appetite may be reduced during this time secondary to morning sickness or the appetite depressant effect of hCG and altered carbohydrate metabolism. Later, appetite increases in response to increasing metabolic needs. Rarely does morning sickness have harmful effects on the embryo/fetus or the woman. If the vomiting is severe or persists beyond the first trimester or if it is accompanied by fever, pain, or weight loss, medical intervention is necessary.

Women may also experience changes in their sense of taste, leading to cravings and changes in dietary intake.

Mouth. The gums are hyperemic, spongy, and swollen. They tend to bleed easily because the rising levels of estrogen cause selective increased vascularity and connective tissue proliferation (a nonspecific gingivitis). Women complain of **ptyalism** (excessive salivation). Ptyalism may be caused by the decrease in unconscious swallowing by the woman when nauseated or attributed to stimulation of salivary glands by eating starch (Cunningham et al, 1993). More information about epulis and bleeding gums can be found in the discussion of the integumentary system.

Teeth. The pregnant woman requires about 1.2 g of calcium and approximately the same amount of phosphorus every day during pregnancy. This is an increase of about 0.4 g of each of these elements over nonpregnant needs. With a well-balanced diet, these requirements are satisfied. Serious dietary deficiency, however, may deplete the mother's bony stores of these elements but does not draw on calcium in her teeth. Demineralization of teeth does not occur during pregnancy; thus the old adage, "for every child a tooth" is untrue. Gingivitis and poor dental hygiene during pregnancy (or anytime) may contribute to dental caries, which could result in the loss of a tooth.

Esophagus, stomach, and intestines. Herniation of the upper portion of the stomach *(hiatal hernia)* occurs after the seventh or eighth month of pregnancy in about 15% to 20% of pregnant women. This condition results from upward displacement of the stomach, which causes a widening of the hiatus of the diaphragm. It occurs more often in multiparas and older or obese women.

Increased estrogen production causes decreased secretion of hydrochloric acid. Therefore peptic ulcer formation or flare-up of existing peptic ulcers is uncommon during pregnancy.

Increased progesterone production causes decreased tone and motility of smooth muscles so there is esophageal regurgitation, slower emptying time of the stomach, and reverse peristalsis. As a result, the woman may experience "acid indigestion" or heartburn **(pyrosis).**

In response to increased needs during pregnancy, iron is absorbed more readily in the small intestine. In general, if an individual is deficient in iron, iron absorption is increased.

Increased progesterone (causing loss of smooth muscle tone and decreased peristalsis) results in an increase in water absorption from the colon. Constipation may result. In addition, constipation is secondary to hypoperistalsis (sluggishness of the bowel), unusual food choice, lack of fluids, decreased activity level, abdominal distention by the pregnant uterus, and displacement of intestines with some compression.

Hemorrhoids (varicose veins of the rectum and anus) may be everted or may bleed during straining at stool. Bowel habits and a characteristic type of stool are established early in life. The woman may view variations with concern and may perceive them as a disease process. A mild *ileus* (sluggishness and lack of movement) that follows birth, as well as postbirth fluid loss and perineal discomfort, contribute to continuing constipation.

Gallbladder and liver. The gallbladder is often distended because of its decreased muscle tone during pregnancy. Increased emptying time and thickening of bile secondary to prolonged retention are typical. These features, together with slight hypercholesterolemia from increased progesterone levels, may account for the development of *gallstones* during pregnancy.

Hepatic function is difficult to appraise during pregnancy. However, only minor changes in liver function develop during pregnancy. Occasionally, intrahepatic cholestasis (retention and accumulation of bile in the liver caused by factors within the liver), in response to placental steroids, occurs late in pregnancy and may result in pruritus gravidarum (severe itching) with or without jaundice. Oatmeal baths and lotions help ease the itching. Drug therapy may be needed. These distressing symptoms subside promptly after birth.

Abdominal discomfort. Intraabdominal alterations that can cause discomfort include pelvic heaviness or pressure, round ligament tension, flatulence, distention and bowel cramping, and uterine contractions. In addition to displacement of intestines, pressure from the expanding uterus increases venous pressure in the pelvic organs. Although most abdominal discomfort is a consequence of normal maternal alterations, the health care provider is constantly alert to the possibility of disorders such as bowel obstruction or an inflammatory process.

Appendicitis may be difficult to diagnose. The appendix is displaced upward and laterally, high and to the right, away from McBurney's point (see Fig. 10-5).

Endocrine System

Profound endocrine changes occur that are essential for pregnancy maintenance, normal fetal growth, and postpartum recovery.

Thyroid gland. During pregnancy an increase occurs in gland activity and hormone production. The increased activity is reflected in a moderate enlargement of the thyroid gland caused by hyperplasia of the glandular tissue and increased vascularity (Cunningham et al, 1993; Scott et al, 1994). The level of free T_4 (thyroxine) falls because of increased estrogen levels. During late pregnancy the woman may develop an iodine deficiency (Bennett and Brown, 1993). Oxygen consumption and BMR increase secondary to the metabolic activity of the products of conception.

Parathyroid gland. Pregnancy induces a slight secondary hyperparathyroidism, a reflection of increased requirements for calcium and vitamin D. When the needs for growth of the fetal skeleton are greatest, plasma parathormone levels are elevated; that is, the level peaks between 15 and 35 weeks' gestation.

Pancreas. The fetus requires significant amounts of glucose for growth and development. To meet the need for fuel, the fetus not only depletes the store of maternal glucose but also decreases the mother's ability to synthesize glucose by siphoning off her amino acids. Maternal blood glucose levels fall. Maternal insulin does not cross the placenta to the fetus. As a result, in early pregnancy the pancreas decreases its production of insulin.

As pregnancy continues, the placenta grows and produces progressively larger amounts of hormones (i.e., human placental lactogen [hPL], estrogen, progesterone). Cortisol production by the adrenals also increases. Estrogen, progesterone, hPL, and cortisol collectively decrease the mother's ability to use insulin. Cortisol stimulates increased production of insulin but also increases the mother's peripheral resistance to insulin (i.e., the tissues cannot use the insulin). Insulinase is an enzyme produced by the placenta to deactivate maternal insulin. Decreasing the mother's ability to use her own insulin is a protective mechanism that ensures an ample supply of glucose for the needs of the fetoplacental unit. The result is an added demand for insulin by the mother. The normal beta cells of the islet of Langerhans in the pancreas can meet the demand for insulin that continues to increase at a steady rate until term.

Pituitary prolactin. In pregnancy, serum prolactin begins to rise in the first trimester and increases progressively to term. It is generally believed that all the hormonal elements (estrogen, progesterone, thyroid, insulin, and free cortisol) necessary for breast growth and milk production are present in elevated concentrations during pregnancy. However, the high levels of estrogen and progesterone inhibit lactation by blocking the binding of prolactin to breast tissue until after birth (Scott et al, 1994).

Endocrine system and maternal nutrition. Progesterone and estrogen cause the deposit of fat in subcutaneous tissues over the maternal abdomen, back, and upper thighs. The fat serves as an energy reserve for both pregnancy and lactation. Estrogen promotes the enlargement of the genitals, uterus, and breasts. It also results in the growth of glandular tissues, ducts, alveoli, and nipples. Estrogen alters metabolism of nutrients by interfering with folic acid metabolism, increasing total body proteins, and promoting retention of sodium and water by kidney tubules. Estrogen may decrease secretion of hydrochloric acid and pepsin, which may be responsible for digestive upsets such as nausea.

Several other hormones affect nutrition. *Aldosterone* conserves sodium. *Thyroxine* (T_4) regulates metabolism. *Parathyroid hormone* controls calcium and magnesium metabolism. *hPL* acts as a growth hormone. *hCG* is one factor that may induce nausea and vomiting in early pregnancy.

Key Points

- The biochemical, physiologic, and anatomic adaptations that occur during pregnancy are profound and return to the nonpregnant state after birth and lactation.
- Maternal adaptations are attributed to the hormones of pregnancy and to mechanical pressures arising from the enlarging uterus and other tissues.
- The ability to recognize the beta subunit of hCG through monoclonal antibody technology has revolutionized endocrine tests for pregnancy.
- Presumptive, probable, and positive signs of pregnancy aid in the diagnosis of pregnancy; only positive signs (identification of a fetal heart tone, verification of fetal movements, and visualization of the fetus) can establish the diagnosis of pregnancy.
- Adaptations to pregnancy protect the woman's normal physiologic functioning, meet the metabolic demands pregnancy imposes, and provide for fetal developmental and growth needs.
- The rise in pH of the pregnant woman's vaginal secretions makes her more vulnerable to vaginal infections.
- Increased vascularity and sensitivity of the vagina and other pelvic viscera may lead to a high degree of sexual interest and arousal.
- Some adaptations to pregnancy result in discomforts such as fatigue, urinary frequency, nausea, and breast sensitivity.
- Balance and coordination are affected by changes in joints and the woman's center of gravity as pregnancy progresses.

References

Barkauskas V et al: *Health and physical assessment,* St Louis, 1994, Mosby.

Bennett V, Brown L: *Myles textbook for midwives,* ed 12, Edinburgh, 1993, Churchill Livingstone.

Blackburn S, Loper D: *Maternal, fetal, and neonatal physiology: a clinical perspective,* Philadelphia, 1992, Saunders.

Bluestein D, Levin J: Ethnic differences in patient requests for pregnancy testing, *J Natl Med Assoc* 84(5):403, 1992.

Cunningham F et al: *Williams obstetrics,* ed 19, East Norwalk, Conn, 1993, Appleton & Lange.

Edge V, Miller M: *Women's health care,* St Louis, 1994, Mosby.

Frye A: *Understanding diagnostic tests in the childbearing years,* ed 5, Portland, Ore, 1993, Labrys.

Fuschino W: Physiologic changes of pregnancy: impact on critical care, *Crit Care Nurs Clin North Am* 4(4):691, 1992.

Lawrence R: *Breastfeeding: a guide for the medical profession,* ed 4, St Louis, 1994, Mosby.

Pagana K, Pagana T: *Mosby's diagnostic and laboratory test reference,* ed 2, St Louis, 1994, Mosby.

Scott J et al: *Danforth's obstetrics and gynecology,* ed 7, Philadelphia, 1994, Lippincott.

Seidel H et al: *Mosby's guide to physical examination,* ed 3, St Louis, 1995, Mosby.

van Lier D et al: Nausea and fatigue during early pregnancy, *Birth* 20(4):193, 1993.

Worthington-Roberts B, Williams S: *Nutrition in pregnancy and lactation,* ed 5, St Louis, 1993, Mosby.

Bibliography

Austin D, Davis P: Valvular disease in pregnancy, *J Perinat Neonatal Nurs* 5(2):13, 1991.

Chez R: Advising pregnant women about nutrition, *Contemp OB GYN* 36(1):80, 1991.

Demystifying ovulation and pregnancy kits for your patients, *Contemp OB GYN* 38:67, 1993.

Elkayam U, Gleicher N: *Changes in cardiac findings during normal pregnancy.* In Elkayam U, Gleicher N, editors: *Cardiac problems in pregnancy,* ed 2, New York, 1990, Liss.

Fields S, Toffler W: Pregnancy testing—home and office, *West J Med* 154(3):327, 1991.

Rothman B: *Pregnancy testing.* In *Encyclopedia of childbearing: critical perspectives,* Phoenix, Ariz, 1992, Onyx.

Theunissen I, Parer J: Fluid and electrolytes in pregnancy, *Clin Obstet Gynecol* 37:3, 1994.

Wilcox A, Weinberg C, Baird D: Timing of sexual intercourse in relation to ovulation, *N Engl J Med* 333(23):1517, 1995.

CHAPTER 7

Nursing Care During Pregnancy

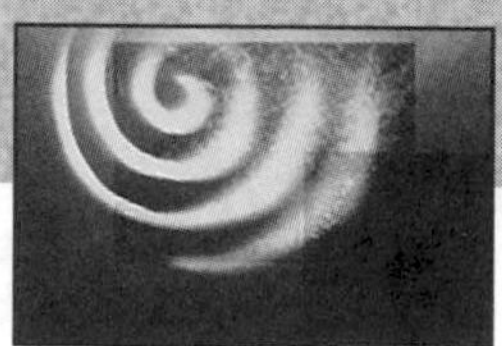

FIRST TRIMESTER, P. 122

Diagnosis of pregnancy, p. 123

Nursing care management, p.123

SECOND TRIMESTER, P. 146

Nursing care management, p. 146

THIRD TRIMESTER, P. 157

Second-time mothers, p.157

Expectant fathers/partners, p. 157

Nursing care management, p. 159

PARENTHOOD AFTER AGE 35, P. 169

Older multiparous women, p. 169

Older nulliparous women, p. 169

MULTIFETAL PREGNANCY, P. 169

Prenatal care in multifetal pregnancies, p. 169

Psychosocial adjustment, p. 170

PREBIRTH EDUCATION, P. 170

Parent education programs, p. 170

Recent trends in parent education, p. 171

Strategies for childbirth education, p. 171

Options for care providers, p. 171

Birth setting choices, p. 172

The prenatal period is a time of physical and psychologic preparation for birth and parenthood. Becoming a parent represents one of the maturational crises of people's lives, and as such it is a time of intense learning for parents and those close to them. The prenatal period provides a unique opportunity for nurses and other members of the health care team to influence family health. During this period, essentially healthy women seek regular care and guidance. The nurse's health promotion interventions can affect the well-being of the woman, her unborn child, and the rest of her family for many years to come (see the Family Focus box below).

Family Focus

PREGNANCY AND THE FAMILY

Pregnancy involves all family members, and each family member must adapt to the pregnancy in his or her own way. The process of family adaptation to pregnancy takes place within a cultural environment. Much of the research on family dynamics in pregnancy and childbirth preparation in the United States and Canada has been done with white, middle-class families. As a result, findings may not apply to subcultures, minorities, or families who do not fit the traditional American model. The terms *spouse* or *husband* or *partner* and *wife* are used consistently in the literature. The nurse may have to adapt these terms to apply to corresponding roles in many families.

Women who are happy and pleased about their pregnancies often view pregnancy as biologic fulfillment and part of their life plan. They have high self-esteem and tend to be confident about outcomes for themselves, their babies, and other family members. When pregnancy is unplanned or unwanted, acceptance of and adaptation to pregnancy are more difficult.

Regular prenatal visits, ideally beginning soon after the first missed menstrual period, offer opportunities to ensure the health of the expectant mother and her infant. This is achieved by supervising the course of pregnancy. Prenatal health supervision permits diagnosis and treatment of maternal disorders that may have preexisted or may develop during the pregnancy. It is designed to follow the growth and development of the fetus and to identify abnormalities that may interfere with the course of normal labor. The woman and her family can seek support to reduce stress and to learn parenting skills.

FIRST TRIMESTER

The woman's initial visit to the health care provider is important in setting the tone for her care. The woman needs to feel welcomed and important. This first visit may include diagnosing the pregnancy and establishing the data base, depending on the duration of gestation. If pregnancy is too early and cannot be verified, the woman's next appointment is scheduled in 2 weeks.

It is essential that professionals collaborate to provide holistic care for their patients. The case management model using care maps and critical pathways is one system that promotes comprehensive care with little or no overlap in services.

The woman's desire for pregnancy is evaluated. If the woman is pregnant and plans to carry the pregnancy to term, prenatal health supervision should begin and continue until the infant's birth. If she is pregnant and does not want to be, she is counseled about her options. If she is not pregnant and does not want to be, she is counseled about fertility management, if appropriate.

Pregnancy spans nine calendar months, 10 lunar months, or approximately 40 weeks. Pregnancy is divided into three 3-month periods, or **trimesters.** The first trimester covers weeks 1 through 13; the second, weeks 14 through 26; and the third, weeks 27 through term gestation (38 to 40 weeks). Prenatal care during each trimester focuses on different priorities of care.

Diagnosis of Pregnancy

Many women come to the first visit after having a positive home pregnancy test. However, the clinical diagnosis of pregnancy before the second missed period may be uncertain in at least 25% to 30% of women. Physical variability, lack of relaxation, obesity, or tumors, for example, may make it difficult even for the experienced obstetrician, nurse practitioner, or nurse-midwife to diagnose pregnancy. Accuracy is most important, however, because emotional, social, medical, or legal consequences of an inaccurate diagnosis, either positive or negative, can be extremely serious. A correct date for the first day of the **last menstrual period (LMP),** the date of intercourse, or the basal body temperature (BBT) record may be of great value in the accurate diagnosis of pregnancy. Reexamination in 2 to 4 weeks may be required for verifying the diagnosis. The use of sonography can assist the practitioner in verifying the pregnancy.

Great variability is possible in the subjective and objective symptoms of pregnancy. The diagnosis of pregnancy is based on signs and symptoms that are reported during history taking or found during physical examination. These signs and symptoms are classified as presumptive, probable, and positive. The **presumptive signs and symptoms** of pregnancy can be caused by conditions other than gestation. Therefore no one manifestation can be relied on for a final impression, and combinations of manifestations are not diagnostic. For example, **amenorrhea** may be caused by an endocrine disorder; lack of energy and fatigue may signify anemia or infection; and nausea or vomiting may be caused by a gastrointestinal (GI) upset or allergy.

Presumptive findings include subjective symptoms and objective signs. Subjective symptoms may include amenorrhea, nausea and vomiting **(morning sickness)**, breast changes and sensitivity, **urinary frequency,** and lack of energy or fatigue. **Quickening,** or first movement felt by the woman, may be noted between weeks 16 and 20. Objective signs include a variety of demonstrable anatomic and physiologic changes: elevation of BBT, skin changes such as **striae gravidarum** and deeper pigmentation (chloasma, linea nigra), breast changes, abdominal enlargement, and changes in the uterus and vagina.

Probable signs of pregnancy are those observed by the health care provider. When combined with presumptive signs and symptoms, they strongly suggest pregnancy. Objective signs include uterine enlargement, **Braxton Hicks contractions,** *souffle* (soft, blowing sound of blood in the arteries of the pregnant uterus and synchronous with maternal pulse), ballottement, and positive pregnancy test results.

The **positive signs** of pregnancy are demonstration of fetal heart tones distinct from heart sounds of the mother, verification of fetal movement by someone other than the mother, and visualization of the fetus with a technique such as ultrasound (Scott et al, 1994) (see the Family Focus box below).

Estimated date of birth. After pregnancy is confirmed, the woman's first question usually concerns when she will give birth. This date has traditionally been called the *estimated date of confinement (EDC)*. To promote a more positive perception of both pregnancy and birth, however, the term **estimated date of birth (EDB)** is used. Because the exact date of conception is usually unknown, many formulas or rules of thumb have been suggested for calculating the EDB. None of these rules of thumb is infallible, but Nägele's rule is reasonably accurate and is the method usually used.

Nägele's rule. **Nägele's rule** is as follows: add 7 days to the first day of the LMP, subtract 3 months, and add 1 year. For example, if the first day of the LMP was July 10, the EDB is April 17. Another method is to add 7 days to the LMP and count forward 9 months.

Nägele's rule assumes that the woman has a 28-day menstrual cycle and that the pregnancy occurred on the fourteenth day. An adjustment is in order if the cycle is longer or shorter than 28 days. If the menstrual cycle is less than 28 days, subtract that number of days from the EDB; if it is longer than 28 days, add that number of days to the EDB. On the basis of Nägele's rule, only about 4% to 10% of pregnant women will give birth spontaneously on the EDB. Most women will give birth during the period extending from 7 days before to 7 days after the EDB.

Nursing Care Management

Assessment

Ideally the woman receives continuous care for health promotion before conception and between pregnancies. The process of assessment then continues throughout the prena-

Family Focus

CONCERNS ABOUT THE FETUS

Parental concern for the health of the child seems to vary during the course of pregnancy. The first concern appears in the first trimester and relates to the possibility of spontaneous abortion. Many women delay telling others about the pregnancy until this time passes. As the child becomes more of a reality, with movement and an audible heartbeat and through ultrasound examination, parental anxiety focuses on possible defects in the child.

PRENATAL RECORD

Name		Religion	Date
Address			Telephone
Occupation	Business address		Business telephone
Husband's name	Business address		Business telephone
Husband's occupation		Referred by	

Age	Gravida	Para	Term	Premature	Abortions	Living

LMP	PMP	Quickening	EDD

Significant history

Significant findings

Date													
Wt. ( )													
BP													
Edema													
Ht. of fundus													
Position													
FH													
Urine	Sug / Pro												
Gestation													
Movement													
Initials													
RTC													

Blood group	Rh	STS	Hgb. HCT.	Pap	HBsAg

Rubella	Glucola	Alpha feto protein	GC	HIV

PPD	Chest x-ray	Vitamin supplement	Breast/bottle	Anesthesia preference	Pediatrician

Problem list

☐ Family planning information

Fig. 7-1 Prenatal history form.

Name:

Present Pregnancy			
Nausea:	Vomiting:	Other symptoms of pregnancy:	
Bleeding:	Cramping:	Pain:	Edema:
Pregnancy test Date			

Previous Pregnancies

No.	Date delivered	Feeding	Sex	Wt.	Wks. preg.	Condition		Duration of labor	Type of delivery	Remarks
						Birth	Now			
1										
2										
3										
4										
5										
6										

Past History

Menstruation onset	Frequency	Duration	Flow	Pain
Usual childhood illnesses	Rheumatic fever	Heart disease	Pulmonary disease	
Convulsions	Venereal disease	Allergies	Blood transfusion	
Injuries	Operations	Urinary disease		
Alcohol	Smoking	Drugs	Medication	

Family History

Mother	Father	Siblings	Other
Diabetes		Twins	

Physical Examination

General	Ht.	BP /	Eyes	Fundi
Ears	Mouth	Teeth	Throat	Thyroid
Chest	Breasts	Nipples	Heart	Lungs
Abdomen	Extremities			

Ext. genitalia		Perineum
Vagina		Cervix
Uterus		
Adnexa		
BI cm	DC cm	Arch
Sacrum		Spines
Post. sagittal	SS ligaments	Coccyx

____________________, MD
Signature

Fig. 7-1 cont'd. Prenatal history form.

tal period when a woman makes contact with health professionals because she suspects she is pregnant. Assessment techniques include the interview, physical examination, and laboratory tests.

Nursing ALERT

Any deviations from normal findings indicate a need for further assessments and tests.

A checklist of care needs spanning pregnancy is a valuable tool and provides the team of care providers with a communication tool to prevent gaps in care and to identify areas of repeated concern for pregnant women. When shared with pregnant women, the checklist items can provide reassurance to them and their families that their concerns are common to many pregnant women. Reading the checklist also reminds women of otherwise forgotten data. Box 7-1 provides a checklist for the first trimester.

Interview. The initial assessment interview establishes the therapeutic relationship between the nurse and the woman (see the Family Focus box below, right). It is planned, purposeful communication that focuses on specific content. Two sources are usually used in collecting data: the woman's subjective interpretation of health status and the nurse's objective observations. During the interview the nurse observes the woman's affect, posture, body language, skin color, and other physical and emotional signs. These observations provide important data in the assessment.

The initial evaluation includes a comprehensive health history emphasizing the current pregnancy, previous pregnancies, the family, a psychosocial history, a cultural history, a physical assessment, diagnostic testing, and an overall risk assessment. A prenatal history form is the best method to document the history on the initial visit (Fig. 7-1).

Reason for seeking care. The woman's description of the purpose for the request for care is quoted verbatim in the record; for example, "I think I am pregnant" or "I'm so nauseated I can't eat anything." This statement does not constitute a diagnosis, since the woman's condition needs to be confirmed by the health care provider before any care is instituted.

Nursing ALERT

Recording the chief purpose of a visit in the woman's own words alerts other personnel to the priority of need as seen by the woman.

Current pregnancy. Usually the presumptive signs of pregnancy or the results of a home pregnancy test prompt a woman to seek care. A review of symptoms she is experiencing and how she is coping with them help establish a data base to develop a plan of care.

Obstetric/gynecologic history. Data are gathered on age of menarche, menstrual history, contraceptive history, any infertility, any gynecologic anomalies (e.g., fibroids), history of any sexually transmitted diseases (STDs), sexual history, all pregnancies including the present pregnancy, and their outcomes. The date of the last Papanicolaou (Pap) smear and its result are noted. The date of the LMP is attained to establish the EDB.

Medical history. The medical history includes medical or surgical conditions that may affect the course of pregnancy or that may be affected by the pregnancy. For example, the pregnant woman who has diabetes or epilepsy will require special care. Because most women are anxious during the initial interview, reference to cues such as a Medic-Alert bracelet helps the woman explain allergies, chronic diseases, or medications being used (e.g., cortisone, insulin, anticonvulsants).

BOX 7-1

First-Trimester Checklist

- Diagnosis and expected date of birth
- Schedule and events of visits
- Counseling for self-care
  - Birthplan
  - Adaptations/discomforts
  - Breast changes
  - Urinary frequency
  - Nausea and vomiting
  - Nasal stuffiness and epistaxis
  - Gingivitis and epulis
  - Leukorrhea
  - Fatigue
  - Psychosocial responses and family dynamics
- Exercise and rest
- Relaxation
- Nutrition
- Sexuality
- Cultural variations
- Warning signs of potential complications
- Resources
- Education
- Dental evaluation
- Medical service
- Social service
- Emergency room
- Diagnostic tests
  - Specify
  - Other

Family Focus 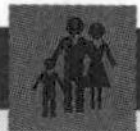

FAMILY AND THE INITIAL INTERVIEW

Often the woman is accompanied by a family member or members at her initial assessment. The nurse builds a relationship with these people as part of the social context of the patient. They also are helpful in recalling and validating information related to the patient's health. With the patient's permission, those accompanying her can be included in the initial prenatal interview. Observations and information about the woman's family are part of the interview. For example, if the woman is accompanied by small children, the nurse can inquire about her plans for child care during the forthcoming labor and birth.

Previous surgeries are described. Uterine surgery or extensive repair of the pelvic floor may necessitate cesarean birth; appendectomy rules out appendicitis as a cause of right lower quadrant pain; and spinal surgery may contraindicate spinal or epidural anesthesia. Any injury involving the pelvis is noted.

Often women who have adapted well to chronic or handicapping conditions forget to mention them because the condition is so integrated into their life-style. Special shoes or a limp may indicate a pelvic structural defect, which is an important consideration in pregnancy. The nurse who observes these special characteristics and can inquire about them sensitively obtains individualized data that will provide the basis for a comprehensive nursing care plan. Observations are vital components of the interview process because they prompt the nurse and the woman to focus on the specific needs of her and her family.

Nutritional history. This is an important component of the prenatal history. The nutritional status of a pregnant woman has a direct effect on the growth and development of the fetus. The pregnant woman is usually motivated to learn about good nutrition. A dietary assessment can reveal special diet practices, food allergies, eating behaviors, and other factors related to nutritional status (see Box 8-3).

Drug use. Past and present drug use needs to be assessed. The woman needs to be questioned about the use of both legal (over the counter [OTC], prescription, caffeine, alcohol, nicotine) and illegal (marijuana, cocaine, heroin) drug use. Many substances cross the placenta and may adversely affect the developing fetus. Periodic urine toxicology screens are often recommended during pregnancy for women who have a history of illegal drug use (Box 7-2).

Family history. The family history provides information about the woman's immediate family, including parents, siblings, and children. This helps identify familial or genetic disorders or conditions that could affect the present health status of the woman or her fetus.

Social and experiential history. Situational factors such as the family's ethnic and cultural background and socioeconomic status are determined in the social and experiential history. Perception of this pregnancy is explored. Is this pregnancy wanted or not, planned or not? Is the woman/couple pleased or displeased, accepting or nonaccepting? Is the pregnancy "hers" or "theirs"? What problems do they anticipate because of the pregnancy (e.g., financial, career, living accommodations)? The family support system is determined. What primary support is available to the woman? Are changes needed to promote adequate support for the woman? What are the existing relationships among mother, father/partner, siblings, and in-laws? What preparations are being made for the care of the woman and dependent family members during labor and for the care of the infant after birth? Is community support needed (e.g., financial, educational)? What are the woman's/couple's ideas about childbearing, expectations of infant's behavior, and outlook on life and the female role? Questions that need to be asked include the following: What will it be like to have a baby in the home? How is your life going to change by having a baby? What plans does having a baby interrupt? What is the woman's/couple's attitude toward health care, particularly during childbearing? What is expected of the health care provider, and how is the relationship between the woman/couple and nurse viewed? During interviews throughout the pregnancy, the nurse remains alert for potential parenting disorders, such as depression, lack of family support, and inadequate living conditions.

Coping mechanisms and patterns of interacting are identified. Early in the pregnancy the nurse determines the woman's/couple's knowledge of pregnancy, maternal changes, fetal growth, care of self, and care of the newborn, including feeding methods (see Family Focus box on p. 128). It is important to ask about attitudes toward unmedicated or medicated childbirth and about parental knowledge of availability of parenting skills classes. Before planning for nursing care, the nurse needs information about the woman's/couple's decision-making abilities and living habits (e.g., exercise, sleep, diet, diversional interests, personal hygiene, clothing). Common stressors in childbearing that have been identified include the baby's welfare, the labor and birth process, the behaviors of the newborn, the relationship with the baby's father, changes in body image, physical symptoms (Affonso and Mayberry, 1990), and changes in family dynamics.

BOX 7-2

Ethical Considerations Related to Screening Pregnant Women for Drug Use

Identifying pregnant women who are drug addicts by periodic urine screening during pregnancy has the potential to benefit the woman and her fetus by enabling health care providers to provide appropriate treatment. However in some instances, pregnant women have been incarcerated or otherwise punished for their addiction or for abuse of the fetus. A punitive approach is counterproductive and often leads the pregnant addict to avoid prenatal care. Health care providers must consider the possible negative effects of periodic screening when they develop prenatal screening protocols. Care should be taken to ensure that criteria for selection of women to test do not lead to bias or overrepresentation of some populations (Birchfield, Scully, and Handler, 1995).

Critical Thinking  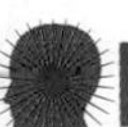

BODY CHANGES IN PREGNANCY

Anatomic and physiologic adaptations to pregnancy can cause a change in body image in a woman and her partner. The body image may change over the course of pregnancy. Interview three pregnant women (and their partners, if possible) at 16 weeks, 24 weeks, and 36 weeks of gestation.

1. How does each pregnant woman feel about changes in her body related to anatomic and physiologic adaptations?
2. How does the partner feel about the changes in the pregnant woman?
3. Which of these changes do they find pleasant?
4. Which of these changes do they find uncomfortable or troublesome?
5. What is their level of understanding of these adaptations?

Analyze your findings in relation to differences in gestation. Use your findings to develop a teaching plan for each woman. Provide rationale for your choices of topics to include.

Family Focus

MATERNAL ADAPTATION

Adaptation to the maternal role involves a complex social and cognitive learning process. Pregnancy functions as a rite of passage and indicates that maturity has been reached. Reva Rubin began studying maternal role adaptation in the 1960s. She described the **developmental tasks** of pregnancy as accepting the pregnancy, identifying the role of mother, reordering the relationships between her mother and herself and between herself and her partner, establishing a relationship with the unborn child, and preparing for the birth experience. The partner's emotional support is an important factor in the successful accomplishment of these developmental tasks. Women prepared to accept a pregnancy seek medical validation early. When pregnancy is confirmed, a woman's emotional response may range from delight to shock, disbelief, and despair. A general state of well-being predominates, but emotional lability is common. These rapid mood changes include increased irritability, explosions of tears and anger, and feelings of great joy and cheerfulness. Such changes are often attributed to hormonal changes.

Rubin described changes in pregnancy as follows. The subjective experience of time and space changes during pregnancy; early in pregnancy, nothing seems to be happening, and the woman spends much time sleeping. With quickening (feeling of fetal movement) in the second trimester, there is a reduction of time and space, both geographic and social, as the woman turns her attention inward to her pregnancy. She examines or fosters relationships with her mother and other women who have been or are pregnant. With the third trimester, there is a slower pace and a sense that time is running out as the woman's activities are curtailed. A mother's reaction to her daughter's pregnancy signifies her acceptance of the grandchild and of her daughter. If the mother is supportive, the daughter has an opportunity to discuss pregnancy and labor and her feelings of joy or ambivalence with a knowledgeable and accepting woman.

Women express two major needs within the partner relationship during pregnancy: feeling loved and valued and having the child accepted by the partner. The addition of a child changes forever the nature of the bond between partners. The partner can be a stabilizing influence, a good listener to expressions of doubts and fears, and a source of physical and emotional reassurance. The partner can also feel jealous of the unborn baby. Lesbian and unpartnered women have received little attention in the literature. Some suggest that a woman partner may be able to understand better and meet more effectively the needs of her partner for nurturing. An unpartnered woman may seek out her mother or other women friends to meet her dependence needs.

Data from Mercer R: *Becoming a mother,* New York, 1995, Springer.

The woman's **body image** is thought to be influenced by her values and personality traits. Her attitude toward her body often changes as pregnancy progresses. A positive body attitude is usually expressed during the first trimester.

Attitudes concerning the range of acceptable sexual behavior during pregnancy are explored. Questions such as the following could be asked: What has your family (partner, friends) told you about sex during pregnancy? Sexual self-concept is given more emphasis by employing questions such as, "How do you feel about the changes in your appearance? How does your partner feel about your body now? Do maternity clothes make pregnant women attractive?"

All women should be assessed for a history or risk of physical abuse, particularly since the incidence of abuse can increase during pregnancy. Although visual cues from the woman's appearance or behavior may suggest the possibility of abuse, abuse may be missed if questioning is limited to those who fit the supposed profile of the battered woman (McFarlane et al, 1992; Norton et al, 1995; Stewart and Cecutti, 1993).

Review of systems. During this portion of the interview, preexisting or concurrent problems are identified and described for all body systems and mental status. The woman is questioned about physical symptoms she has experienced, such as shortness of breath or pain. Pregnancy affects and is affected by all body systems; therefore knowledge of the present status of body systems is important in planning care. For each sign or symptom expressed, the following additional data should be obtained: body location, onset, quality, quantity, chronology, setting, aggravating or alleviating factors, and associated manifestations (onset, character, course) (Seidel et al, 1995).

Birth plan. The woman's preparation for the childbirth experience is assessed. Is she planning to attend childbirth/parent education classes (with or without her partner) during the first trimester? Is the couple considering a **birth plan**? Attendance at parent education classes and the development of a birth plan may vary with the patient's culture, usual means of coping (classes and reading material or other), and feelings about the role of the health care providers. Some women may come with a form of birth plan; for example, having experienced the birth of or preterm infant who was ill, the woman anticipating a second birth may prefer to give birth only at a tertiary care center with a neonatal intensive care unit (NICU). A highly dependent woman may allow the health care team to make decisions about birth plans, assuming that the decisions of the professionals are the wisest. A more independent, assertive woman may seek health care that is within her philosophy of care and her beliefs and knowledge, for example, home birth. She wants her wishes honored during pregnancy, labor and birth, and the postpartum period. The birth plan is also discussed in Chapter 16.

Woman with a disability. Women with serious and handicapping physical or emotional disorders—deaf, blind, depressed, physically disabled, mentally retarded, and brain-injured patients—must all be respected and the assessment approach adapted to their needs. Women who are emotionally restricted may not be able to give an effective history, but they must be respected, and the history should be obtained from them as much as is possible. Their points of view and their attitudes matter. Still, when necessary, the family, other health professionals involved in care, and the patient's record must bc queried to obtain complete information. Each woman must be fully respected and fully involved to the limit of her emotional and cognitive capacity and physical ability. Architectural accessibility must be ensured (Madorsky, 1995).

Physical examination. The initial physical examination provides the baseline for assessing subsequent changes. The examiner determines the woman's needs for basic information regarding the structure of the genital organs and provides this information, along with a demonstration of the equipment that may be used during the examination and an explanation of the procedure itself. The interaction requires an unhurried, sensitive, and gentle approach with a matter-of-fact attitude. The woman is ensured privacy for the examination without unexpected intrusions. If the woman prefers, her husband/partner may be present for the examination.

The physical examination begins with assessment of vital signs, height and weight, and blood pressure. Because the bladder must be empty before pelvic examination, the urine specimen is obtained before the examination.

Each examiner has developed a routine for proceeding with the physical examination; most choose the head-to-toe progression. Heart and lung sounds are evaluated and extremities examined. The skin is assessed for changes in pigmentation, rashes, and edema. Distribution, amount, and quality of body hair is of particular importance because the findings reflect nutritional status, endocrine function, and general emphasis on hygiene. The thyroid gland is assessed carefully, as are the breasts and abdomen. The arms and legs are assessed for swelling and varicosities. A pelvic examination is performed. The typical basic examination is usually completed without much difficulty for the healthy woman. The examiner needs to remain alert to the woman's cues that give direction to the assessment and that indicate possible problems.

Thyroid gland. The thyroid gland is the largest endocrine gland in the body and the only one accessible to direct physical examination. Assessment of thyroid function or possible dysfunction includes more than observation and palpation of the area where the thyroid gland is located. Metabolic rates and rhythms, including menstrual regularity in the woman of childbearing age, are governed by the thyroid gland. The effects of thyroid activity are widespread. Therefore observations of behavior, appearance, skin, eyes, hair, and cardiovascular status are important. Several findings require further attention (e.g., enlargement of the thyroid gland, coarse and gritty consistency, nodules).

Breasts. The physical examination includes an evaluation of the breasts, primarily to establish a data base of normal findings. However, the practitioner needs to be alert to the possibility of carcinoma at all times. Early detection of potential malignancies has been and continues to be the most important factor in the successful treatment of this disease. Because professional assessment occurs only periodically, each woman is advised to do a breast self-examination (BSE) on a monthly basis. Because of changes in breast tissue during pregnancy and lactation, BSE is not as reliable during these times. Interventions to treat inverted or flat nipples of women who plan to breastfeed are of no use (Lawrence, 1994; MAIN Trial Collaborative Group, 1994).

Abdomen. The examination of the abdomen is done carefully and systematically. The skin is assessed for general condition, color, rashes, lesions, scars, striae, dilated veins, turgor, texture, and hair distribution. Contour, symmetry, and presence of hernias are noted. Bowel sounds are auscultated. Palpation is used to assess for abdominal masses.

Pelvic examination. The woman is asked to refrain from sexual intercourse, douching, or using vaginal medications for 24 hours before a pelvic examination. (NOTE: Douching is not recommended during pregnancy or at any time.) These actions cloud the diagnosis based on secretions, cells, and odor. In addition, douching removes vaginal secretions, making insertion of the vaginal speculum more difficult.

For the examination the woman is assisted to a **lithotomy position** (Fig. 7-2). In this position she lies supine with her hips and knees flexed; her thighs are abducted and drawn upward toward her chest; her buttocks are at the edge of the table; and her feet are supported by stirrups. Some women prefer to keep their shoes or socks on, especially if the stirrups are not padded.

Critical Thinking Exercises

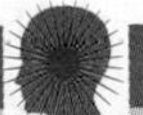

PRENATAL INTERVIEW

Pregnant women vary in perceptions of the need for medical and nursing care during pregnancy. Interview three pregnant women. If possible, select women from three cultural or ethnic groups and include both multiparous and primiparous women.

1. When did the women first consult a health care provider related to this pregnancy? Was this early or late? What were the reasons for seeking care? What were the reasons for seeking care at that time?
2. What will keep the women healthy during pregnancy? Ask the women to describe any foods/activities that the women should eat/do or avoid to protect the pregnancy.
3. Is a partner involved in this pregnancy? What was the partner's response to the diagnosis of pregnancy? If this is a second or subsequent pregnancy, did this response differ from the response to previous pregnancies?
4. What are the plans for birth? Where will the birth occur? Who will attend the birth? Will analgesia be used during labor? How soon will they go home after the birth?
5. How did responses differ among the cultural/ethnic groups and between multiparous and primiparous women?

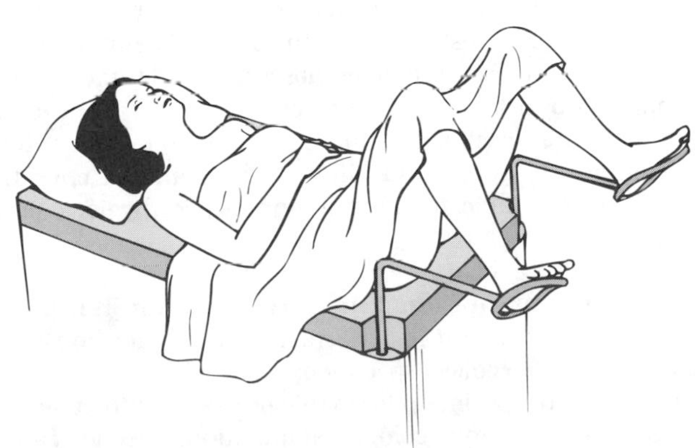

Fig. 7-2 Lithotomy position.

Many women express feelings of vulnerability when in the lithotomy position. Deep-breathing techniques and distraction may assist the woman to relax. If possible, questions should be deferred until the woman is upright and at eye level with the examiner.

Nursing ALERT

To avoid supine hypotension, the woman's upper body should be elevated.

Supine hypotension. When a woman is lying in the lithotomy position without elevation of the upper body (Fig. 7-2), the weight of abdominal contents may compress the vena cava and aorta, resulting in a drop in blood pressure **(supine hypotension)**. Pallor, breathlessness, and clammy skin are other objective signs. Nursing actions include positioning the woman on her side until her signs and symptoms subside (see the Emergency box to the right). If the woman is unable to tolerate the lithotomy position, the lateral position may be used for genital examination.

External inspection. The examiner sits at the foot of the table for the inspection of the external genitals and for the speculum examination. The woman's head is raised on a pillow, and the drape is arranged so eye-to-eye contact can be maintained.

External palpation. The examiner proceeds with the examination using palpation and inspection. The examiner wears gloves for this portion of the assessment. The woman is kept informed about the procedure. For example, the examiner says, "I am going to touch you now" before touching the genital area.

In addition to the routine assessments normally done during this part of the examination, particular attention needs to be paid to the perineum. The perineum (area between the vagina and anus) is assessed for scars from old lacerations or episiotomies and for thinning, fistulas, masses, lesions, and inflammation. The anus is assessed for hemorrhoids, hemorrhoidal tags, and integrity of the anal sphincter. Occasionally, after a vaginal birth, with lacerations that extended into the anal sphincter, the muscle may not have been correctly repaired; for example, the examiner will see a "dimple" over two ends of separated muscle, and the "wink" reflex is incomplete. If the anal sphincter was not repaired correctly, the woman may have given a history of incontinence. The anal area is also assessed for lesions, masses, abscesses, and tumors. If the woman has a history of STD, the examiner may want to obtain a culture specimen from the anal canal at this time. Throughout the genital examination the examiner notes the odor. Odor may indicate infection and/or poor hygienic practices.

Speculum examination and internal examination. A speculum examination is performed to visualize the vagina and cervix and to collect specimens.

Collection of specimens for cytologic examination is an important part of the gynecologic examination. Infection can be diagnosed through examination of specimens collected during the pelvic examination. A culture specimen for gonorrhea is obtained to screen women for gonorrheal infection that could affect the woman, her fetus, and her partner. The test is done routinely at the first prenatal visit and repeated between 20 and 28 weeks of pregnancy. A smear for *Chlamydia* and trichinosis is obtained, and an aerobic culture for bacterial vaginosis is done. If an open lesion is present at the initial pelvic examination, a viral culture specimen is obtained from the lesion and is repeated at intervals. An abnormal Pap smear result may be caused by the presence of herpes simplex virus type 2 (HSV-2) infection, or human papilloma-virus (HPV).

EMERGENCY

SUPINE HYPOTENSION

Signs/Symptoms

Pallor
Dizziness, faintness, breathlessness
Tachycardia
Nausea
Clammy (damp, cool) skin, sweating

Interventions

Position woman on her side until her signs/symptoms subside and vital signs stabilize within normal limits (WNL).

Bimanual palpation. A bimanual examination is done as it is during a routine examination. The vagina enlarges, and supporting structures are more relaxed as pregnancy advances. When the examination is performed, the tone of the pelvic musculature and need for and knowledge of Kegel exercise (see pp. 135 and 136) are assessed. Particular attention is paid to the size of the uterus, since this is an indication of the gestation of the pregnancy. Pelvic measurements are often done at this time. The nurse present during the examination can coach the woman in breathing and relaxation techniques as needed.

The examiner stands for this part of the examination. A small amount of lubricant is dropped onto the fingers of the gloved hand for the internal examination. To avoid tissue trauma and contamination, the thumb is abducted and the ring and little fingers are flexed into the palm.

The vagina is palpated for distensibility, lesions, and tenderness. The cervix is examined for position, shape, consistency, motility, and lesions. The fornix around the cervix is palpated.

The other hand is placed on the abdomen halfway between the umbilicus and symphysis pubis and exerts pressure downward toward the pelvic hand. Upward pressure from the pelvic hand traps reproductive structures for assessment by palpation. The uterus is assessed for position (see Fig. 3-7), size, shape, consistency, regularity, motility, masses, and tenderness.

Moving the abdominal hand to the right lower quadrant and the fingers of the pelvic hand in the right lateral fornix, the examiner assesses the adnexa for position, size, tenderness, and masses. The examination is repeated on her left side. Pelvic measurements are assessed.

Just before the intravaginal fingers are withdrawn, the woman is asked to tighten her vagina around the fingers as much as she can. If the muscle response is weak, the woman is assessed for her knowledge about Kegel exercise (see pp. 135 and 136).

Rectovaginal palpation. To prevent contamination of the rectum from organisms in the vagina (e.g., gonorrhea) it is best to change gloves, add fresh lubricant, and then reinsert the index finger into the vagina and the middle finger into the rectum (Fig. 7-3). Insertion is facilitated if the woman strains down. The maneuvers of the abdominovaginal examination are repeated. The rectovaginal examination permits assessment of the rectovaginal septum, the posterior surface of the uterus, and the region behind the cervix.

After the pelvic examination the woman is assisted into a sitting position and given tissues or wipes to cleanse herself and privacy to dress. The woman often returns to the examiner's office for a discussion of findings, prescriptions for therapy, and counseling.

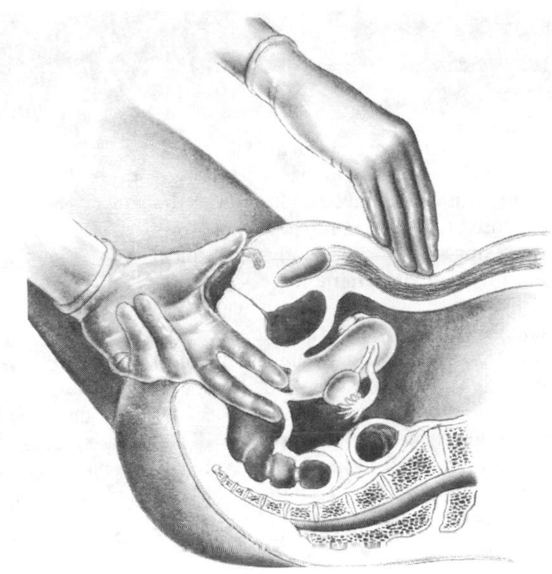

Fig. 7-3 Rectovaginal palpation. (From Seidel H et al: *Mosby's guide to physical examination*, ed 3, St Louis, 1995, Mosby.)

Laboratory tests. The data obtained from laboratory examination of specimens add important information concerning the symptoms of pregnancy and health status. Both nursing and medical diagnoses stem from such information.

Specimens are collected at the initial visit so any abnormal findings can be treated (Table 7-1). During the pelvic examination, cervical and vaginal smears for cytology and for diagnosis of infection (e.g., *Chlamydia* organisms, gonorrhea) are obtained. Blood is drawn to test for a variety of conditions: Venereal Disease Research Laboratories (VDRL) test for syphilis; complete blood cell count (CBC) with hematocrit, he-

TABLE 7-1 Laboratory tests in prenatal period

LABORATORY TEST	PURPOSE
Hemoglobin/hematocrit/WBC count, differential	Detects anemia/detects infection
Hemoglobin electrophoresis	Identifies women with hemoglobinopathies (e.g., sickle cell anemia, thalassemia)
Blood type, Rh, and irregular antibody	Identifies those fetuses at risk for developing erythroblastosis fetalis or hyperbilirubinemia in neonatal period
Rubella titer	Determines immunity to rubella
Tuberculin skin testing; chest x-ray film after 20 weeks' gestation in women with reactive tuberculin tests	Screens high-risk population for exposure to tuberculosis
Urinalysis, including microscopic examination of urinary sediment; pH, specific gravity, color, glucose, albumin, protein, RBCs, WBCs, casts, acetone; hCG	Identifies women with unsuspected diabetes mellitus, renal disease, hypertensive disease of pregnancy; infection; pregnancy
Urine culture	Identifies women with asymptomatic bacteriuria
Renal function tests: BUN, creatinine, electrolytes, creatinine clearance, total protein excretion	Evaluates level of possible renal compromise in women with a history of diabetes, hypertension, or renal disease
Pap test	Screens for cervical intraepithelial neoplasia and herpes simplex type 2
Vaginal or rectal smear for *Neisseria gonorrhoeae* (GC) *Chlamydia*, HPV, BV	Screens high-risk population for asymptomatic infection
VDRL/FTA-ABS	Identifies women with untreated syphilis
HIV antibody*, hepatitis B surface antigen, toxoplasmosis	Screens for infection
1-hour glucose tolerance	Screens for gestational diabetes; done at initial visit for women with risk factors; done at 28 weeks for all pregnant women
3-hour glucose tolerance	Screens for diabetes in women with elevated glucose level after 1-hour test; must have elevated fasting or two elevated readings for diagnosis
Cardiac evaluation: ECG, chest x-ray film, echocardiogram	Evaluates cardiac function in women with a history of hypertension or cardiac disease

WBCs, white blood cells; *RBCs*, red blood cells; *BUN*, blood urea nitrogen; *ECG*, electrocardiogram; *VDRL*, Venereal Disease Research Laboratories; *FTA-ABS*, fluorescent treponemal antibody absorption test; *hCG*, human chorionic gonadotropin; *HPV*, human papillomavirus; *HIV*, human immunodeficiency virus; *BV*, bacterial vaginosis; *GC*, gonococcus.

*With patient permission.

BOX 7-3
Ethical Considerations Related to HIV Screening

Pregnant women have an ethical obligation to seek reasonable care during pregnancy and to avoid causing harm to the fetus. Maternity nurses should be advocates for the fetus, but not at the expense of the pregnant woman.

Mandatory HIV screening involves ethical issues related to privacy invasion, discrimination, social stigma, and reproductive risks to the pregnant woman. Incidence of perinatal transmission from an HIV-positive mother to her fetus ranges from 25% to 35%. However, with maternal treatment during pregnancy with AZT, the transmission rate from the pregnant HIV-positive woman to her fetus drops to 7.9%. It is recommended that all pregnant women be tested for HIV, although testing is still voluntary. Health care providers have an obligation to make sure the pregnant woman is well informed about HIV symptoms and testing.

moglobin, and differential values; blood type and Rh factor; antibody screen (Kell, Duffy, rubella, toxoplasmosis, anti-Rh); sickle cell anemia; and level of folacin when indicated. The woman is tested for hepatitis B surface antigen (HBsAg) and hepatitis B surface antibody (HBsAb). Urine is tested for glucose (diabetes), protein (pregnancy-induced hypertension, PIH), and nitrites and leukocytes (urinary tract infection, UTI); culture and sensitivity tests are ordered as necessary. Testing for antibody to the human immunodeficiency virus (HIV) is strongly recommended for all pregnant women (Box 7-3).

Urine is tested for glucose, protein, and acetone; culture and sensitivity tests are ordered as necessary. A purified protein derivative of tuberculin (PPD) test is administered to assess for exposure to tuberculosis.

Risk factors during pregnancy may indicate the need to repeat some tests at other times. For example, exposure to tuberculosis or an STD would necessitate repeat testing.

Fetal Development

Box 7-4 and Fig. 7-4 summarize the development of the fetus at 13 weeks. Toward the end of the first trimester, before the uterus is an abdominal organ, the fetal heart tones (FHTs) can be heard with an ultrasound fetoscope or an ultrasound stethoscope (Fig. 7-5). A small amount of conduction jelly is

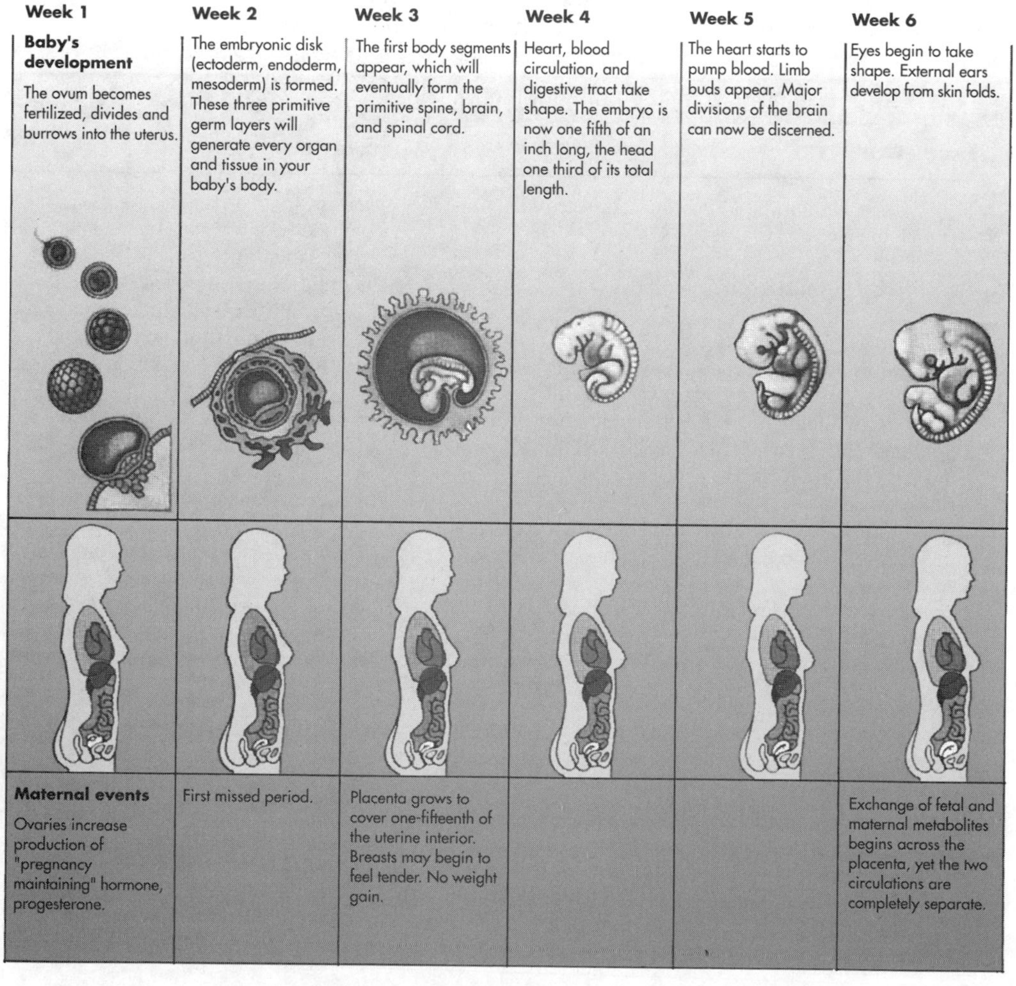

Week 1	Week 2	Week 3	Week 4	Week 5	Week 6
Baby's development The ovum becomes fertilized, divides and burrows into the uterus.	The embryonic disk (ectoderm, endoderm, mesoderm) is formed. These three primitive germ layers will generate every organ and tissue in your baby's body.	The first body segments appear, which will eventually form the primitive spine, brain, and spinal cord.	Heart, blood circulation, and digestive tract take shape. The embryo is now one fifth of an inch long, the head one third of its total length.	The heart starts to pump blood. Limb buds appear. Major divisions of the brain can now be discerned.	Eyes begin to take shape. External ears develop from skin folds.
Maternal events Ovaries increase production of "pregnancy maintaining" hormone, progesterone.	First missed period.	Placenta grows to cover one-fifteenth of the uterine interior. Breasts may begin to feel tender. No weight gain.			Exchange of fetal and maternal metabolites begins across the placenta, yet the two circulations are completely separate.

Fig. 7-4 Summary of fetal development and maternal events—first trimester. (From *Safe passage: a woman's guide to a healthier pregnancy*, Fort Washington, Pa, McNeil Consumer Products.)

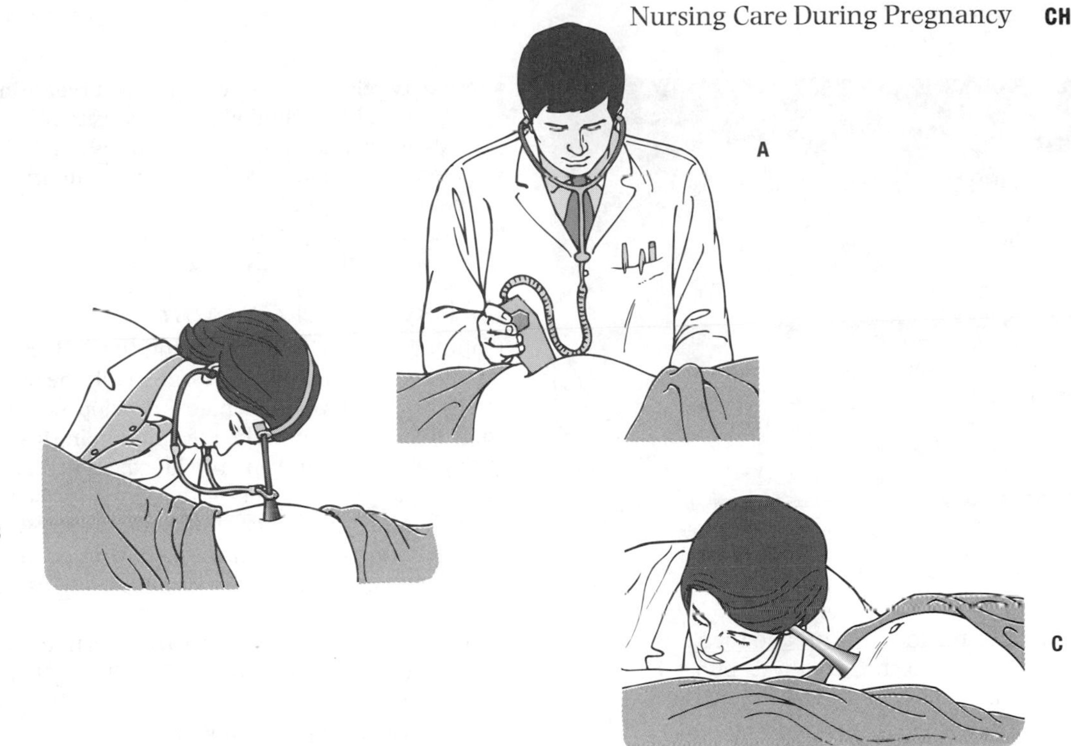

Fig. 7-5 Detecting fetal heartbeat. **A,** Fetoscope (18 to 20 weeks). **B,** Doppler ultrasound stethoscope (12 weeks). **C,** Pinard's fetoscope. NOTE: Hands should not touch stethoscope while listening.

Week 7	Week 8	Week 9	Week 10	Week 11	Week 12	Week 13
Baby's development Development is proceeding rapidly. The face is now complete with eyes, nose, lips, and tongue—even primitive milk teeth. Tiny bones and muscles appear beneath the thin skin.	The embryo is now a little more than an inch long, its tiny heart beating at about 40-80 times a minute.	Genitalia is now well defined; the baby's sex is determined. Eyelids finish forming and seal shut. The embryo has become a fetus.	The fetus assumes a more human shape as the lower body rapidly develops. Blood and bone cells form. The first movements begin.	Organs begin to function. The pancreas is producing insulin; the kidneys produce urine.	The lungs have taken shape; primitive breathing motions begin. The swallowing reflex has been mastered as the fetus sucks its thumb while floating weightlessly in the amniotic fluid.	
Maternal events No noticeable weight gain.	The placenta now covers about one third of the uterine lining.	Maternal blood volume has increased 30% to 40%.	The sensation of the first movements has been described by some women as if something were blowing bubbles through a straw in their stomachs.	2-3 lb weight gain. Possible increase in perspiration.	The placenta has reached complete functional maturity, acting as the baby's lungs, kidneys, liver, and digestive and immune systems.	

BOX 7-4
Fetal Development at 13 Weeks

Differentiation of tissues complete as period of organogenesis ends
Human appearance
Sex distinguishable
Skeleton ossifying
Tooth buds forming
Respiratory activity evident
Insulin secreted (since eighth week)
Kidneys secreting urine
Intestine returns to abdomen
Head is one third of total length
Length: 9 cm
Weight: 15 g
Fetus less susceptible to malformation from teratogenic agents after 8-10 weeks' gestation

placed on the head of the instrument, and then it is placed in the midline just anterior to the symphysis pubis. Firm pressure is needed as the scope is used. The woman and her family should be offered the opportunity to listen to the FHTs.

Signs of Potential Complications

The interview, physical examination, and laboratory tests (Table 7-1) may yield findings suggesting potential complications. When the data base is complete, a judgment is made of the woman's risk status and need for referral for specialized care or further evaluation.

During the course of pregnancy, warning signs may appear. The woman and her family need to be aware of these signs so that they can seek appropriate interventions promptly.

Nursing Diagnoses

Each woman and her family have a unique set of responses to pregnancy. To attend to these responses, the nurse begins by formulating appropriate nursing diagnoses. The following are examples of nursing diagnoses that may arise from analysis of assessment findings during the first trimester:

- Anxiety related to
  - Concern about herself
  - Physical changes with pregnancy
  - Her (or other's) feelings about pregnancy
- Pain related to
  - Early discomforts of pregnancy
- Altered family processes related to
  - Family's response to diagnosis of pregnancy
- Anxiety related to knowledge deficit regarding
  - Maternal and familial adaptations to pregnancy
  - Maternal and familial adaptations to EDB
- Altered nutrition: less than body requirements related to
  - Morning sickness
- Altered sexuality patterns, related to
  - Discomforts of early pregnancy

Expected Outcomes

Planning care for patients during the first trimester is based on the biopsychosocial assessment of the woman and her family. For each woman a plan is developed that relates specifically to her problems. The information in this chapter is general; that is, not all women will experience all problems discussed or require all facets of the care described. The nurse selects those aspects of care relevant to the woman and the woman's family based on the following patient-centered expected outcomes related to physiologic and psychosocial care:

1. The woman will demonstrate pertinent knowledge of the adaptation of the maternal body to a developing fetus as a basis for understanding the rationale and necessity for modalities of care.
2. The woman will use knowledge of self-care for nutritional needs, sexual needs, activities of daily living (ADLs), and discomforts of pregnancy.
3. The woman will identify and report symptoms that indicate deviations from normal progress.
4. The woman and her family will actively participate in her care during the first trimester of pregnancy.

Plan of Care and Implementation

The nurse-patient relationship is critical in setting the tone for further interaction. The techniques of listening with an attentive expression, touching, and using eye contact have their place, as does recognition of the woman's feelings and her right to express them. The intervention may occur in various formal or informal settings. The clinic, home visits, or telephone conversations all provide opportunities for contact and can be used effectively. Sometimes women seek information about a particular problem repeatedly. At times there may be another underlying problem that the woman is hesitant to bring up. The nurse needs to be astute in assessing unvoiced needs. The nurse can help the woman by asking for a patient-generated solution and a report of its effectiveness.

In supporting a patient, one must remember that both the nurse and the woman are contributing to the relationship. The nurse has to accept the woman's responses as a factor in

Nursing ALERT

SIGNS OF POTENTIAL COMPLICATIONS—FIRST TRIMESTER

Signs/Symptoms	Possible causes
Severe vomiting	Hyperemesis gravidarum
Chills, fever	Infection
Burning on urination	Infection
Diarrhea	Infection
Abdominal cramping, vaginal bleeding	Spontaneous abortion, miscarriage

trying to be of help. An example of one nurse-patient relationship follows:

> Mrs. Garcia had been very forthright in saying that this pregnancy was unplanned but had countered this statement with comments such as "All things happen for the best," "We always wanted the boys to have a family to turn to," and "Children bring their own love." Over time, as our relationship developed to one of mutual trust, she complained increasingly of her fear of pain, her hating to wear maternity clothes, and her having to give up helping the family. Finally I ventured to say, "Sometimes when a pregnancy is unplanned, women resent it very much and are angry about it." Her relief was evident. She said, "Oh, you don't know how angry I've been." As a result, the whole tenor of support being offered changed, and the plan was adjusted to meet her real needs.

The nurse also needs to accept that the woman must be a willing partner in a purely voluntary relationship. As such, the relationship can be refused or terminated at any time by the pregnant woman, her family, or the practitioner. When a woman refuses to do those things that are necessary to provide a safe passage for herself and the developing fetus, the practitioner may cease providing care.

Supportive care involves developing, augmenting, or changing the mechanisms used by women and families in coping with stress. An effort is made to promote active participation by the individuals in the process of solving their own problems. Women are assisted in gathering pertinent information, exploring alternative actions, making decisions as to choice of action, and assuming responsibility for the outcomes. These outcomes may be any or all of the following: living with a problem as it is, easing effects of a problem so that it can be accepted more readily, or eliminating the problem by effecting change.

At other times a successful outcome can be documented readily. A woman who early in her pregnancy had predicted a severe depressive state in the postbirth period was elated when such a state did not materialize. She remarked to the nurse who had provided support during the pregnancy and birth, "You're the best nerve medicine I've ever had!"

Education for Self-Care

Health maintenance is an important aspect of prenatal care. The patient's participation in the care ensures prompt reporting of possible problems. The patient's assumption of responsibility for health maintenance is prompted by understanding of maternal adaptations to the growth of the unborn child and a readiness to learn. Nurses provide women with the information necessary for self-care and compliance with health care measures.

The expectant mother needs an overview of the planned prenatal care and information about many other subjects. During the initial health assessment the woman may have indicated a need to learn self-care activities such as prevention of urinary tract infection, hygiene, nutrition, and Kegel exercise.

Prevention of urinary tract infection. Urinary tract infections are common in pregnancy and may be asymptomatic. Whether symptomatic or not, urinary tract infections present a risk (e.g., preterm labor) to both mother and fetus. Prevention and treatment of these infections are essential. The woman's understanding and use of good handwashing before and after urinating and wiping front to back are assessed. Before developing a plan of care, the nurse needs to determine the woman's feelings or ideas concerning cultural, ethnic, religious, or other factors affecting health practices.

Soft, absorbent toilet tissue, preferably white and unscented, should be used because harsh, scented, or printed toilet paper may cause irritation. Bubble bath or other bath oils should be avoided because these may be irritating to the urethra. Women should wear underpants and panty hose with a cotton crotch. They should avoid wearing tight-fitting slacks or jeans for long periods. A buildup of heat and moisture in the genital area may contribute to the growth of bacteria.

Some women do not have an adequate fluid and food intake. The nurse should advise the woman to drink 2 to 3 quarts (8 to 12 glasses) of liquid a day. From 8 to 10 ounces of cranberry juice may be included because cranberry juice is more acidic than other fluids and can lower the pH of the urinary tract, making it less hospitable to developing bacteria. Yogurt and acidophilic milk may also help prevent urinary tract and vaginal infections. Referral to a dietitian may be necessary.

The nurse should review with the woman healthy urination practices. Women need to maintain fluid intake to ensure frequent urination and not limit fluids to reduce frequency of urination. Women can be instructed that if urine looks dark (concentrated), they need to increase fluid intake. Blood or pain on urination should always be brought to the attention of the health care provider. Women should not ignore signals that indicate the need to urinate. Holding urine increases the time bacteria are in the bladder and allows them to multiply. Women should plan ahead in situations that require the delay of urination (e.g., long car ride). They should always urinate before going to bed at night. Bacteria also can be introduced during intercourse. Therefore women are advised to urinate before and after intercourse and then drink a large glass of water to promote additional urination. The nurse can be reasonably assured that teaching was effective if the woman does not develop a urinary tract infection. However, some women develop urinary tract infections even though they have done everything as instructed.

Kegel exercise. **Kegel exercise** (exercise for the pelvic floor) strengthens the muscles around the reproductive organs and improves muscle tone. Many women are not aware of the muscles of the pelvic floor (see Fig. 3-13) until it is pointed out that these are the muscles used during urination and sexual intercourse and can be consciously controlled. The pelvic floor muscles encircle the outlet through which the baby must pass, and it is important that they be exercised, because an exercised muscle can stretch and contract readily at birth.

To help the pelvic floor muscles return to normal functioning, Kegel exercise should be resumed immediately after giving birth. Kegel exercise can strengthen these muscles and improve muscle tone. If practiced on a regular basis, the exercise helps prevent prolapsed uterus and stress incontinence later in life (see the Patient Teaching Box on p. 136).

Additional teaching. Other subjects about which patients need information include diet, exercise, sleep, bowel habits, smoking, alcohol ingestion, drug use (both legal and illegal),

Patient Teaching

KEGEL EXERCISE

The exercise

The muscles that stop the flow of urine are the pubococcygeal muscles. Doing Kegel exercise during urination helps the woman know whether she is doing them correctly. If she can stop the stream of urine, her tone is good.

After a woman has located the correct muscles, Kegel exercise can be done in the following ways:

1. *Slow:* Tighten the muscle, hold it for the count of three, and relax it.
2. *Quick:* Tighten the muscle, and relax it as rapidly as possible.
3. *Push out, pull in:* Pull up the entire pelvic floor as though trying to suck up water into the vagina. Then bear down as if trying to push the imaginary water out. This also uses abdominal muscles.

Practice

Kegel exercise needs to be practiced several times a day to be effective. It must be done every day for the rest of the woman's life.

This exercise can be done 10 times in a row at least 3 times or more a day. Although some people recommend doing this exercise as many as 100 times in a row, this only fatigues the pelvic floor muscles.

A good time to practice is during trips to the bathroom, but additional practice at other times is even more beneficial.

and sexual relations. It is impossible to impart at one visit all the information the woman and her family may need at the time her pregnancy is diagnosed. She can be given printed information at this time, such as material prepared by her health care provider, published pamphlets, or a list of books about pregnancy for lay people. If the health care provider uses prepared material, he or she should have read the materials carefully to be certain they supply the type of information desired.

Nutritional intake is an important factor in the maintenance of maternal health during pregnancy and in the provision of adequate nutrients for embryonic/fetal development. Assessing nutritional status and providing nutritional information are part of the nurse's responsibilities in prenatal care. In some settings a dietitian conducts classes and/or interviews pregnant women regarding nutritional status and nutrition during pregnancy. Nurses can refer women to the dietitian if a need is indicated during the nursing assessment. (For detailed information concerning maternal and fetal nutritional needs and related nursing care, see Chapter 8.)

Formal classes in childbirth and parenthood education have proved successful for some women and families. "Early bird" classes provide fundamental information to meet the needs of most expectant parents during the first trimester. Allowing the expectant mother or family the opportunity to ask questions and express any anxieties or fears is also important.

Schedule for care. During the initial visit, women appreciate knowing the schedule for return prenatal visits. Most women can expect to return every 4 weeks until the twenty-eighth week of pregnancy, every 2 weeks until the thirty-sixth week of pregnancy, and then every week from week 37 until giving birth. More frequent visits may be needed to accommodate the woman's individual needs. The initial prenatal visit is usually lengthy because the assessment and examination are comprehensive.

Examination during subsequent visits is usually more focused and includes assessment and evaluation of fetal and maternal status. Blood pressure, weight, fetal heart rate (FHR), and fundal height are measured. The urine is tested for glucose and ketones at each visit. The woman is questioned about any symptoms she is having. She is given the opportunity to ask questions. This provides the nurse with the opportunity to continue patient education throughout the pregnancy. Vaginal examinations are not performed until late in the pregnancy unless there is an indication for doing them.

Signs of potential complications. One of the first responsibilities of people involved in the care of the pregnant woman is to alert her to signs and symptoms that indicate a potential complication of pregnancy. The woman needs to know how and to whom to report such warning signs (see previous Nursing Alert). When one is stressed by a disturbing symptom, it is difficult to remember specifics. Therefore the woman and her family are reassured if they receive a printed form listing the signs and symptoms that justify an investigation and the telephone numbers to call with questions or in an emergency.

Discomforts of pregnancy. Women pregnant for the first time are confronted with symptoms that would be considered abnormal in the nonpregnant state. Much of prenatal care requested by such women relates to explanations of the causes of the discomforts and what measures can be taken to relieve them. The discomforts are fairly specific to each trimester of pregnancy. Table 7-2 provides information about the physiology, prevention, and self-care of discomforts experienced during the first trimester. Nurses can provide anticipatory guidance for women. Women who understand the physical discomforts of pregnancy are less apt to become overly anxious about their health. Understanding the rationale for treatment promotes participation in their own care. Nurses need to use terminology that the woman/couple can understand.

Employment. Many women continue to work outside the home during pregnancy. Whether the expectant mother can work and for how long depends on the physical activity involved, industrial hazards, and medical or obstetric complications. A prime consideration is the avoidance of a fetotoxic environment (e.g., chemical dust particles, gases such as inhalation anesthesia). Employment of pregnant women has no negative effects of pregnancy outcomes (Henriksen et al, 1994; Messersmith-Heroman et al, 1994; Seneviratne and Fernando, 1994). Job discrimination that is based solely on pregnancy is illegal.

LEGAL TIP

Legal Considerations: Workplace Regulations

The Pregnancy Discrimination Act protects the right to work during pregnancy. Job discrimination on the basis of pregnancy is prohibited; the act requires that pregnancy or related disorders be considered like any other disability or medical

TABLE 7-2 Discomforts related to maternal adaptation during the first trimester

DISCOMFORT	PHYSIOLOGY	EDUCATION FOR SELF-CARE
Breast changes, new sensations: pain, tingling	Hypertrophy of mammary glandular tissue and increased vascularization, pigmentation, and size and prominence of nipples and areolae caused by hormone stimulation	Supportive maternity brassiere with pads to absorb discharge may be worn at night; wash with warm water and keep dry
Urgency and frequency of urination	Vascular engorgement and altered bladder function caused by hormones; bladder capacity reduced by enlarging uterus and fetal presenting part	Kegel exercise; limit fluid intake before bedtime; reassurance; wear perineal pad; refer to primary health care provider for pain or burning sensation
Languor and malaise; fatigue (usually early pregnancy)	Unexplained; may be caused by increasing levels of estrogen, progesterone, and hCG or by elevated BBT; psychologic response to pregnancy and its required physical/psychologic adaptations	Reassurance; rest as needed; well-balanced diet to prevent anemia
Nausea and vomiting; morning sickness: occurs in 50% to 75% of pregnant women, starts between first and second missed periods and lasts until about fourth missed period; may occur any time during day; expectant father may have symptoms; may be accompanied by bad taste in mouth	Cause unknown; may result from hormonal changes, possibly hCG; may be partly emotional, reflecting pride in, ambivalence about, or rejection of pregnant state	Avoid empty or overloaded stomach; maintain good posture; give stomach ample room; stop or decrease smoking; eat dry carbohydrate on awakening; remain in bed until feeling subsides, or alternate dry carbohydrate 1 hour with fluids such as hot tea, milk, or clear coffee the next hour until feeling subsides; eat five or six small meals per day; avoid fried, odorous, spicy, greasy, or gas-forming foods; consult primary care provider if intractable vomiting occurs; reassurance
Ptyalism (excessive saliva) may occur starting 2 to 3 weeks after first missed period	Possibly caused by elevated estrogen levels; may be related to reluctance to swallow because of nausea	Astringent mouthwash; chewing gum; support
Psychosocial dynamics, mood swings, mixed feelings	Hormonal and metabolic adaptations; feelings about female role, sexuality, timing of pregnancy, and resultant changes in one's life and life-style	Treatment same as prevention; both partners need reassurance and support; support significant other who can reassure woman about her attractiveness, etc.; improved communication with her partner, family, and others; refer to social worker, if needed, or supportive services (financial assistance, food stamps)

hCG, Human chorionic gonadotropin; *BBT,* basal body temperature.

condition. An applicant cannot be denied employment because of pregnancy. A pregnant worker cannot be excluded from any written or unwritten employment practice because of pregnancy or related medical conditions. Pregnant workers must be provided the same insurance benefits, sick leave, seniority credits, and reinstatement privileges awarded workers disabled by other causes.

From American College of Obstetricians and Gynecologists: *Precis V: an update in obstetrics and gynecology,* Washington, DC, 1994, ACOG.

Activities that depend on a good sense of balance should be discouraged, especially during the last half of pregnancy. Usually, excessive fatigue is the deciding factor in the termination of employment. Women in sedentary jobs need to walk around at intervals and should neither sit nor stand in one position for long periods. Activity is necessary to counter the usual sluggish, dependent circulation that potentiates development of varices and thrombophlebitis. The pregnant woman's chair should provide adequate back support. A footstool can prevent pressure on veins, relieve strain on varices, and minimize swelling of feet. Work breaks are best spent resting in the lateral side-lying position. It is recommended that employers have an area where women can lie down. Standards for maternity care and employment of mothers in industry have been recommended by the U.S. Children's Bureau to safeguard expectant mothers' interests.

Travel. Travel for low-risk pregnant women is not contraindicated. Those with high-risk pregnancies are advised to avoid long distance travel after the age of viability so as to avoid the economic and psychologic consequences of delivering a preterm infant far from home (Easa et al, 1994). Travel to areas with poor medical care, untreated water, and malaria should be avoided if possible (Bia, 1992). Many health insurance carriers do not cover birth in a foreign setting or even hospitalization for preterm labor (Barry and Bia, 1989).

If traveling for long distances, periods of activity and rest should be scheduled. While sitting, the woman can practice deep breathing, foot circling, and alternately contracting and relaxing different muscle groups. Fatigue should be avoided. Fatigue or tension, as well as altered regular personal habits and diet during arduous travel, may be detrimental.

Although travel in itself is not a cause of either abortion or preterm labor, certain precautions are recommended. A woman who does not wear automobile restraints risks injury

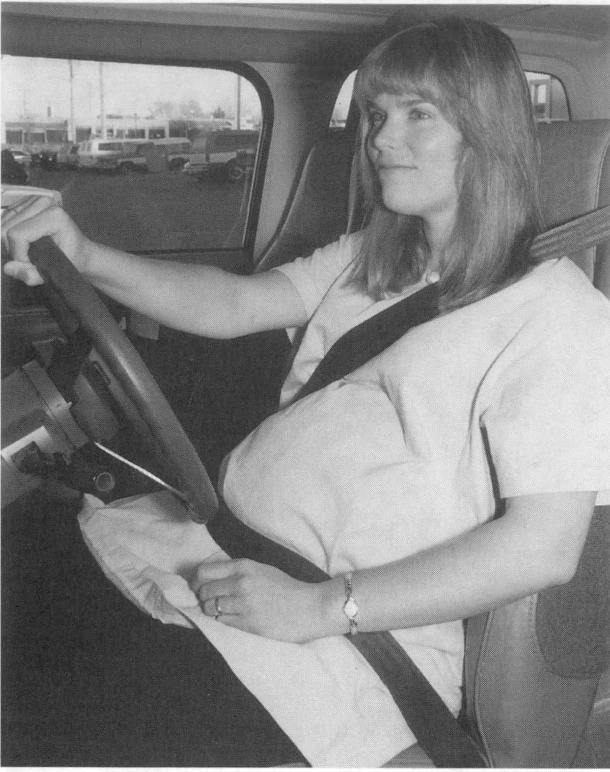

Fig. 7-6 Proper use of seat restraint and headrest. (Courtesy Michael S. Clement, MD, Mesa, Ariz.)

Patient Teaching

SAFETY DURING PREGNANCY

Maternal adaptations to pregnancy involve relaxation of joints, alteration to center of gravity, faintness, and discomforts. Problems with coordination and balance are common. Therefore the woman should follow these guidelines:

- Use good body mechanics.
- Use safety features on tools/vehicles: safety seat belts, shoulder harnesses, and headrests, goggles, helmets, as specified.
- Avoid activities requiring coordination, balance, and concentration.
- Take rest periods; reschedule daily activities to meet rest and relaxation needs.

Embryonic and fetal development is vulnerable to environmental teratogens. Many potentially dangerous chemicals are present in the home, yard, and workplace: cleaning agents, paints, sprays, herbicides, and pesticides. The soil and water supply may be unsafe. Therefore the woman should follow these guidelines:

- Read all labels for ingredients and proper use of product.
- Ensure adequate ventilation with clean air.
- Dispose of wastes appropriately.
- Wear gloves when handling chemicals.
- Change job assignments or workplace as necessary.
- Avoid high altitudes (not in pressurized aircraft), which could jeopardize oxygen intake.

to herself and her fetus. Maternal death as a result of injury is the most common cause of fetal death. The next most common cause is placental separation. Body contours change in reaction to the force of a collision. The uterus as a muscular organ can adapt its shape to that of the body. The placenta lacks the resiliency to change, and placental separation can occur. A combination lap belt and shoulder harness is the most effective automobile restraint (Fig. 7-6) (Hammond, 1990). Both shoulder and lap belts should be used. The lap belt should be worn low across the hip bones and as snug as is comfortable. The shoulder belt should be worn above the pregnant uterus and below the neck to avoid chafing. The pregnant woman should sit upright. The headrest should be used to avoid a whiplash injury.

In high-altitude regions, lowered oxygen levels may cause fetal hypoxia, especially if the pregnant woman is anemic (Barry and Bia, 1989). However, current information is limited, and there are no set recommendations.

If long-distance travel is necessary, the trip should be made by air. U.S. flight regulations do not permit pregnant women aboard during the last month without a statement from the health care provider. Most foreign airlines have a cutoff of 35 weeks' gestation.

Airline travel in large commercial jets usually poses no risk to the pregnant woman. Policies vary from airline to airline, and the pregnant woman is advised to inquire about restrictions or recommendations from her carrier (Skjenna et al, 1991). Magnetometers (metal detectors) used at airport security checkpoints are not harmful to the fetus. The 8% humidity at which cabins are maintained in commercial airlines may result in some water loss; hydration (with water) should be maintained under these conditions (Barry and Bia, 1989). Sitting in a cramped seat of an airliner for prolonged periods may increase the risk of superficial and deep thrombophlebitis. A 15-minute walk around the aircraft for every hour of travel is recommended to minimize this risk. A seat in the nonsmoking section of flights where smoking is permitted is advised to prevent elevated carboxyhemoglobin levels (see the Patient Teaching box above).

Physical activity. Many women exercise regularly and strenuously in the nonpregnant state. They are concerned about loss of physical fitness during an enforced period of decreased activity while pregnant (Culpepper, 1990; Mittelmark et al, 1991). Women who have led sedentary life-styles need to begin with physical activity of very low intensity and advance activity levels gradually (Fishbein and Phillips, 1990). A number of researchers have recommended moderate exercise during pregnancy (Culpepper, 1990; Mittelmark et al, 1991). The American College of Obstetricians and Gynecologists (ACOG, 1994b) recommends aerobic activity with a maternal heart rate no greater than 140 beats/min. Activities continued to the point of exhaustion or fatigue compromise uterine perfusion and fetoplacental oxygenation. If the woman is accustomed to jogging, she may continue; however, she should not reach the point of fatigue. Heat stress may also endanger the fetus. She should drink water during exercise to maintain hydration.

As gestation advances, the woman's center of gravity changes, her bony pelvic support loosens, her coordination usually decreases, and she notices a sensation of awkwardness. Awkwardness may cause the woman to lose balance and

Home Care

EXERCISE TIPS FOR PREGNANT WOMEN

Consult your health care provider when you know or suspect you are pregnant. Discuss your medical and obstetric history, your current regimen, and the exercises you would like to continue throughout pregnancy.

Seek help in determining an exercise routine that is well within your limit of tolerance, especially if you have not been exercising regularly.

Consider decreasing weight-bearing exercises (jogging, running) and concentrate on non-weight-bearing activities such as swimming, cycling, or stretching. If you are a runner, starting in your seventh month you may want to walk instead.

Avoid risky activities such as surfing, mountain climbing, skydiving, and racquetball. Activities requiring precise balance and coordination may be dangerous. Avoid activities that require holding your breath and bearing down (Valsalva's maneuver). Jerky, bouncy motions also should be avoided.

Exercise regularly at least three times a week, as long as you are healthy, to improve muscle tone and increase or maintain your stamina. Sporadic exercises may put undue strain on your muscles.

Limit activity to shorter intervals. Exercise for 10 to 15 minutes, rest for 2 to 3 minutes, then exercise for another 10 to 15 minutes.

Decrease your exercise level as your pregnancy progresses. The normal alterations of advancing pregnancy, such as decreased cardiac reserve and increased respiratory effort, may produce physiologic stress if you exercise strenuously for a long time.

Take your pulse every 10 to 15 minutes while you are exercising. If it is more than 140 beats/min, slow down until it returns to a maximum of 90. You should be able to converse easily while exercising. If you cannot, you need to slow down.

Avoid becoming overheated for extended periods. It is best not to exercise for more than 35 minutes, especially in hot, humid weather. As your body temperature rises, the heat is transmitted to your fetus. Prolonged or repeated fetal temperature elevation may result in birth defects, especially during the first 3 months. Your temperature should not exceed 38° C (100.4° F).

Avoid hot tubs and saunas.

Warm-up and stretching exercises prepare your joints for more strenuous exercise and lessen the likelihood of strain or injury to your joints. No exercise should be performed flat on your back after the fourth month of gestation.

A cool-down period of mild activity involving your legs after an exercise period will help bring your respiration, heart, and metabolic rates back to normal and avoid pooling of blood in the exercised muscles.

Rest for 10 minutes after exercising, lying on your left side. As the uterus grows, it puts pressure on a major vein on the right side of your abdomen, which carries blood to your heart. Lying on your left side removes the pressure and promotes return circulation from your extremities and muscles to your heart, increasing blood flow to your placenta and fetus. Care should be taken to rise gradually from the floor to avoid feeling dizzy or fainting (orthostatic hypotension).

Drink two or three 8-ounce glasses of water after you exercise to replace the body fluids you lost through perspiration. While exercising, drink water whenever you feel the need.

Increase your caloric intake to replace the calories burned during exercise and to provide the extra energy needs of pregnancy. Choose high-protein foods such as fish, cheese, eggs, and meat.

Take your time. This is not the time to be competitive or train for activities requiring long endurance.

Wear a supportive bra. Your increased breast weight may cause changes in posture and put pressure on the ulnar nerve.

Wear supportive shoes. As your uterus grows, your center of gravity shifts and you compensate by arching your back. These natural changes may make you feel off balance and more likely to fall.

Stop exercising immediately and consult your health care provider if you experience shortness of breath, dizziness, numbness, tingling, pain of any kind, more than four uterine contractions per hour, decreased fetal activity, or vaginal bleeding.

Modified from Artal R, Subak-Sharpe G: *Pregnancy and exercise,* New York, 1992, Delacorte; Fishbein E, Phillips M: How safe is exercise during pregnancy? *J Obstet Gynecol Neonatal Nurs* 19:45, 1990; ACOG: Exercise during pregnancy and the postpartum period, *Tech Bull* 189, February 1994; and Pivarnik J: Maternal exercise in pregnancy, *Sports Med* 18:215, 1994.

fall, injuring herself (ACOG, 1994b). Individually taught exercise has been shown to lower back pain in pregnant women (Ostgaard et al, 1994) (see the Home Care box above).

Exercises such as those depicted in Fig. 7-7 are taught either at prenatal classes or by the nurse in the clinic or the physician's office. The exercises promote comfort and help prepare the woman for labor. Other topics for discussion and demonstration are posture and how to lift and move objects safely to counteract the awkwardness and prevent the discomfort experienced at the start of the second trimester.

Dental health. Dental care during pregnancy is especially important. Nausea during pregnancy may lead to poor oral hygiene, and dental caries may develop. No physiologic alteration during gestation can cause dental caries. Calcium and phosphorus in the teeth are fixed in enamel. Therefore the old adage "for every child a tooth" is not true.

No scientific evidence indicates that filling teeth or even dental extraction with the use of local or nitrous oxide–oxygen anesthesia causes abortion or premature labor. Antibacterial therapy should be considered for sepsis, however, especially in pregnant women who have had rheumatic heart disease or nephritis. Emergency dental surgery is not contraindicated during pregnancy. The risks and benefits of surgery need to be explained to the mother.

Medications. Although much has been learned in recent years about fetal drug toxicity (see the Appendix), the possible teratogenicity of many drugs, both prescription and OTC, is still unknown. This is especially true for new medications and combinations of drugs. Moreover, certain subclinical errors or deficiencies in intermediate metabolism in the fetus may convert an otherwise harmless drug into a hazardous one. The greatest danger of drug-caused developmental defects in the fetus exists from the time of fertilization through the first trimester, when the woman may not realize she is pregnant.

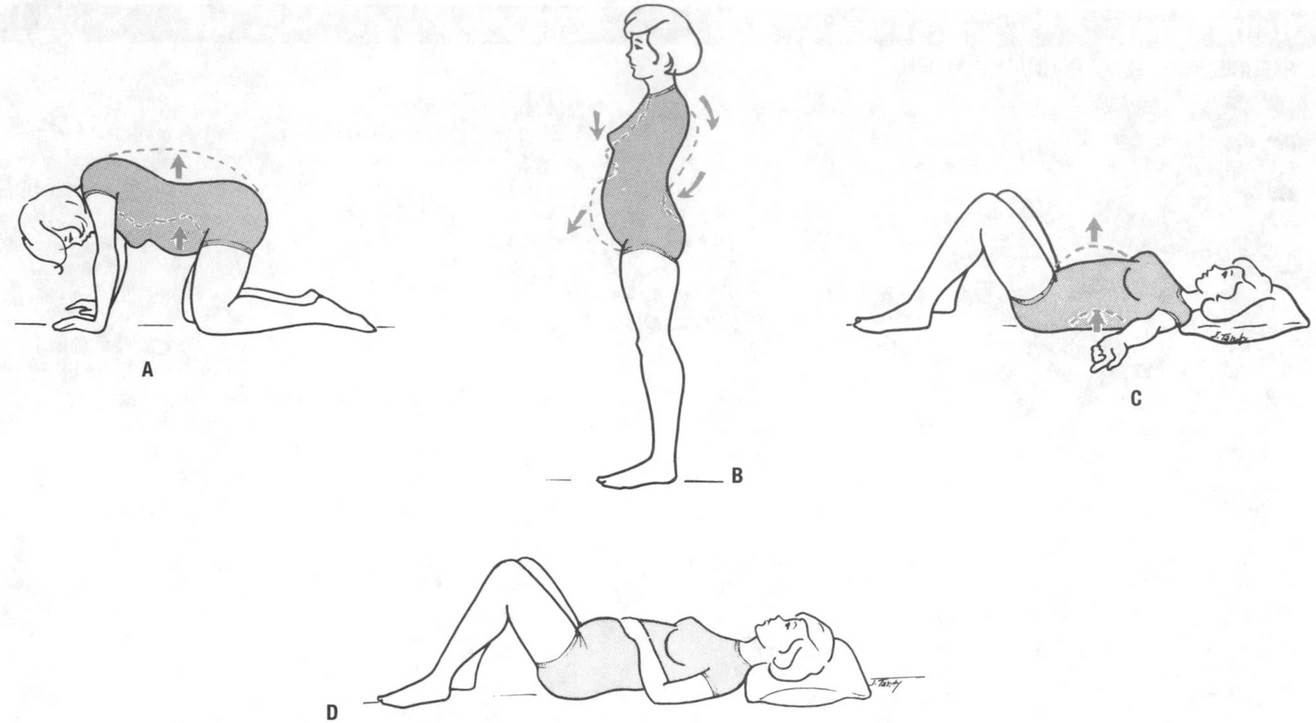

Fig. 7-7 Exercises. **A** to **C**, Pelvic rocking relieves low backache; also excellent for relief of menstrual cramps. **D**, Abdominal breathing aids relaxation and lifts abdominal wall off uterus. As pregnancy advances, a pillow or wedge is placed under one hip to prevent aortocaval compression by the enlarging uterus.

Self-treatment must be discouraged. All drugs, including OTC medications and vitamins, should be limited and a careful record kept of all therapeutic agents used (ACOG, 1994a)

Immunization. Some concern exists over the safety of various immunization techniques during pregnancy (Cunningham et al, 1993). Immunization with live or attenuated live viruses is contraindicated during pregnancy because of potential teratogenicity. Vaccines with killed viruses may be used. Live virus vaccines include measles (rubeola and rubella) (Burgess, 1990), chickenpox, mumps, and the Sabin (oral) poliomyelitis vaccine. Vaccines that may be used in pregnancy include tetanus, diphtheria, recombinant hepatitis B, and rabies.

Nursing ALERT

Rh immune globulin is administered to all Rh-negative women who have chorionic villus sampling.

Alcohol, cigarette smoke, and other substances. Alcohol consumption during pregnancy can lead to fetal alcohol syndrome or fetal alcohol effects. No safe level of alcohol consumption has yet been established. Although occasional alcoholic beverages may not be harmful to the mother or her developing embryo or fetus, complete abstinence is strongly advised. Maternal alcoholism is associated with high rates of spontaneous abortion; the risk for spontaneous abortion is dose related (three or more drinks per day) in the first trimester (Cook, Peterson, and Moore, 1990).

Cigarette smoking or continued exposure to second-hand smoke (even if the mother does not smoke) is associated with intrauterine fetal growth restriction (IUGR) and an increase in perinatal and infant morbidity and mortality. Smoking also increases the incidence of preterm labor, premature rupture of membranes (PROM), abruptio placentae, placenta previa, and fetal death resulting possibly from decreased placental perfusion. Laboratory studies indicate that smoking causes fetal hypoxia (ACOG, 1993; Cook, Peterson, and Moore, 1990; Wilcox, 1993). Exposure to nicotine has been shown to have a negative effect on the growth of the fetus (Bardy et al, 1993). All women who smoke should be strongly encouraged to quit. Pregnant women need to be advised as to the negative effects on the fetus from even second-hand smoke (ACOG, 1993; Economides and Braithwaite, 1994; Sanyal, Li, and Belanger, 1994). Early intervention may be effective in helping the woman cut down or quit smoking (Kendrick et al, 1995).

Most studies of human pregnancy report no association between caffeine consumption and birth defects or low birth weight (LBW) (Cunningham et al, 1993; Mills et al, 1993). Other effects are unknown; therefore pregnant women are advised to limit caffeine intake. Possible hazards of a commonly used artificial sweetener are discussed in Chapter 8.

Any drug or environmental agent that enters the pregnant woman's bloodstream has the potential to cross the placenta and harm the fetus (Brody et al, 1994). Marijuana, heroin, and cocaine are common examples of such substances (see Chapter 11).

Parent Education Classes

First trimester classes, or early pregnancy ("early bird") classes, provide fundamental information. Classes are developed around the following areas: (1) early fetal development, (2) physiologic and emotional changes of early pregnancy, (3) human sexuality, (4) birth settings and types of caregivers, (5) rest, exercise, and relief measures for common discomforts, (6) the nutritional needs of the mother and fetus, and (7) the development of a birth plan. Environmental and workplace hazards have become important concerns in recent years. Even though pregnancy is considered a normal process, exercises, danger signs, drugs, and self-medication are topics of interest and concern.

Throughout the series of classes there is discussion of support systems available during pregnancy and after birth. Such support systems help parents function independently and effectively. During all the classes the open expression of feelings and concerns about any aspect of pregnancy, birth, and parenting is welcomed (see the Family Focus box below).

Not all pregnant women and support people attend formal classes in preparation for childbirth. For those who do attend, extensive preparation is possible. Many do not take advantage of classes for a variety of reasons: previous experience, employment, inaccessibility because of time, cultural/ethnic/religious orientation, cost, lack of knowledge regarding choices in parent education classes, and lack of readiness. Therefore clinicians need to provide this information as needed and encourage participation.

Birth Plan

The **birth plan** is a natural evolution of the contemporary wellness-oriented life-style. It is a tool by which parents can explore their childbirth options and choose those that are most important to them. Many parents have already indicated some of their preferences by the type of health care provider and birth setting they have chosen (hospital, free-standing birth center, or home). Some pregnant women enlist the services of a health care provider only after an interview and a tour of the birth facility. Others have not given conscious thought to the conduct of their pregnancies, labors and birth, recovery, and early parenthood. These women may need help with decision making. After the confirmation of pregnancy, couples tend to focus on the reality of their situation and their emotional responses. However, it is acceptable for the nurse to initiate a discussion of a birth plan during the first and second prenatal visits. Some maternity clinics have printed material describing available options and answers to commonly asked questions. In addition, tours of the birth setting are offered by almost all facilities that provide perinatal services.

Patients' expectations must be reasonable for the resources available in the community. The nurse can provide couples with pertinent information for informed decision making, alerting them to various options and the advantages and consequences of each.

The nurse needs to assess patients' readiness to learn and to avoid overload. Some health care providers provide birth plan lists. A review and discussion of the printed list serve as a means of starting couples to think about, discuss, and identify what is personally important. Some options may only be appropriate for low-risk women; women with a high-risk pregnancy or those who develop complications during labor may have their options severely limited.

Topics for discussion and decision making may include any or all of the following:

- *Partner's participation.* Attend prenatal visits? Parent education classes? Present during labor? During birth? During cesarean birth?
- *Birth setting.* Hospital delivery room or birthing room, if available? Birthing center? Home?
- *Labor management.* Would you like to walk around during labor? Use a rocking chair? Use a shower? Jacuzzi, if available? Consider an electronic fetal monitor? Telemetry monitoring, if available? Consider stimulation of labor? Consider medication—what kind? Be interested in having music or dimmed lighting? Older children or other people present?
- *Birth.* Have you considered the various positions for birth: side lying, on hands and knees, kneeling or squatting, or using a birthing bed or delivery table? Will you be photographing, videotaping, or recording any of the labor or birth? Who would you like to be present: partner, older siblings, other family member(s), or friend(s)? What are your feelings about forceps, vacuum extraction, or episiotomies? Will your partner choose to cut the umbilical cord?

Other relevant topics might best be presented during the second trimester.

The birth plan also can serve as a tool for open communication between the pregnant woman and her partner and between them and health care providers. Early introduction to the idea of a birth plan allows the couple time to think about events or situations that could make their childbearing experience meaningful and those they would prefer to avoid. The nurse-patient interaction concerning the birth plan needs to occur in an accepting atmosphere in which patients can see themselves as unique and yet normal.

Family Focus 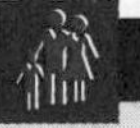

PARENT EDUCATION CLASSES

A typical preparation-for-parenthood program recognizes that expectant parents and their families have different interests and information needs as the pregnancy progresses. Consequently, the program is designed to meet the informational needs of parents at the three major stages of pregnancy and after birth: first-trimester classes, second-trimester classes, third-trimester classes, lactation classes, and postpartum ("fourth trimester") classes.

Sexual Counseling During Pregnancy

Sexual counseling includes countering misinformation, providing reassurance of normality, and suggesting alternative behaviors. The uniqueness of each couple is considered within a biopsychosocial framework (see the Patient Teaching box on p. 142).

Patient Teaching

SEXUALITY IN FIRST TRIMESTER OF PREGNANCY

- Be aware that maternal physiologic changes, such as breast enlargement, nausea, fatigue, abdominal changes, perineal enlargement, leukorrhea, pelvic vasocongestion, and orgasmic responses, may affect sexuality and sexual expression.
- Discuss responses to pregnancy with your partner.
- Keep in mind that cultural prescriptions (dos) and proscriptions (don'ts) may affect your responses.
- Although your libido may be depressed during the first trimester, it increases during the second and third trimesters.
- Discuss and explore with your partner:
  —Alternative behaviors (e.g., mutual masturbation, foot massage, cuddling)
  —Alternative positions (e.g., female superior, side lying) for sexual intercourse (see Fig. 7-8)
- Intercourse is safe as long as it is not uncomfortable. No correlation exists between intercourse and spontaneous abortion, but observe the following precautions:
  —Abstain from intercourse if you experience uterine cramping or vaginal bleeding; report event to your caregiver as soon as possible.
  —Abstain from intercourse (or any activity that results in orgasm) if you have a history of cervical incompetence, until it is corrected.
- Continue to use "safer sex" behaviors. Women at high risk for acquiring or transmitting sexually transmitted diseases are encouraged to use condoms during sexual intercourse throughout pregnancy.

Counseling couples concerning sexual adjustment during pregnancy demands assessment by nurses of their own comfort with sexuality as well as a knowledge of the physical, social, and emotional responses to sex during pregnancy (Rynerson and Lowdermilk, 1993). Not all maternity nurses are comfortable dealing with the sexual concerns of their patients. Nurses who are aware of their personal strengths and limitations in dealing with sexual content are better prepared to make referrals when necessary.

A significant number of women merely need permission to be sexual during pregnancy. Many other women need information about the physiologic changes that occur during pregnancy and to have myths associated with sex during pregnancy dispelled. Giving permission and providing information are within the purview of the maternity nurse and should be an integral component of providing health care.

Some couples must be referred for either sex therapy or family therapy. Couples with longstanding sexual dysfunction problems that are intensified by pregnancy are candidates for sex therapy. When a sexual problem is a symptom of a more serious relationship problem, the couple would benefit from family therapy.

Obtaining a history. The history provides a baseline for sexual counseling. History taking is an ongoing process. Receptivity to changes in attitudes, body image, partner relationships, and physical status are relevant topics throughout pregnancy. When changes occur, unexpected problems may develop that require intervention. The history reveals the client's knowledge of female anatomy and physiology and of attitudes about sex during pregnancy, as well as perceptions of the pregnancy, the couple's health status, and the quality of their relationship. Identification of the couple's subjective experience provides the direction and focus of sexual counseling.

Countering misinformation. Many myths and much of the misinformation related to sex and pregnancy are masked behind seemingly unrelated issues. For example, a question about the baby's ability to hear and see in utero may be related to the baby's role as an observer in lovemaking. The counselor must be extremely sensitive to questions behind the question when counseling in this highly charged emotional area.

Suggesting alternative behaviors. To date, research has not proved conclusively that coitus and orgasm are contraindicated at any time during pregnancy for the obstetrically and medically healthy woman (Cunningham et al, 1993; Scott et al, 1994). However, a history of more than one spontaneous abortion or a threatened abortion in the first trimester, impending miscarriage in the second trimester, or PROM, bleeding, or abdominal pain during the third trimester warrant precaution against coitus and orgasm (Rynerson and Lowdermilk, 1993).

Solitary and mutual masturbation and oral-genital intercourse may be used by couples as alternatives to penile-vaginal intercourse. Partners who enjoy cunnilingus may feel "turned off" by the normal increase in amount and odor of vaginal discharge during pregnancy. Couples who practice cunnilingus should be cautioned concerning the blowing of air into the vagina, particularly during the last few weeks of pregnancy, when the cervix may be slightly open. An air embolism can occur if air is forced between the uterine wall and fetal membranes and enters the maternal vascular system through the placenta.

Pictures of possible variations of coital position are often helpful. The female-superior, side-by-side, and rear-entry positions are possible alternative positions to the traditional male-superior position. The woman astride (superior position) allows her to control the angle and depth of penile penetration and protect her breasts and abdomen. The side-by-side position is the one of choice, especially during the third trimester, because it requires reduced energy and avoids pressure on the pregnant abdomen (Fig. 7-8).

Multiparous women have reported severe breast tenderness in the first trimester. A coital position that avoids direct pressure on the woman's breasts and decreased breast fondling during love play can be recommended. The woman should also be reassured that this condition is normal and temporary.

Some women complain of lower abdominal cramping and backache after orgasm during the first and third trimesters. A back rub can often relieve some of the discomfort and provide a pleasant experience. A tonic uterine contraction, often lasting up to a minute, replaces the rhythmic contractions of orgasm during the third trimester. Changes in FHR without fetal distress have been reported.

The objective of "safer sex" is prophylaxis against the acquisition and transmission of STDs (e.g., HSV, HPV, HIV.) Since these diseases may be transmitted to the woman as well

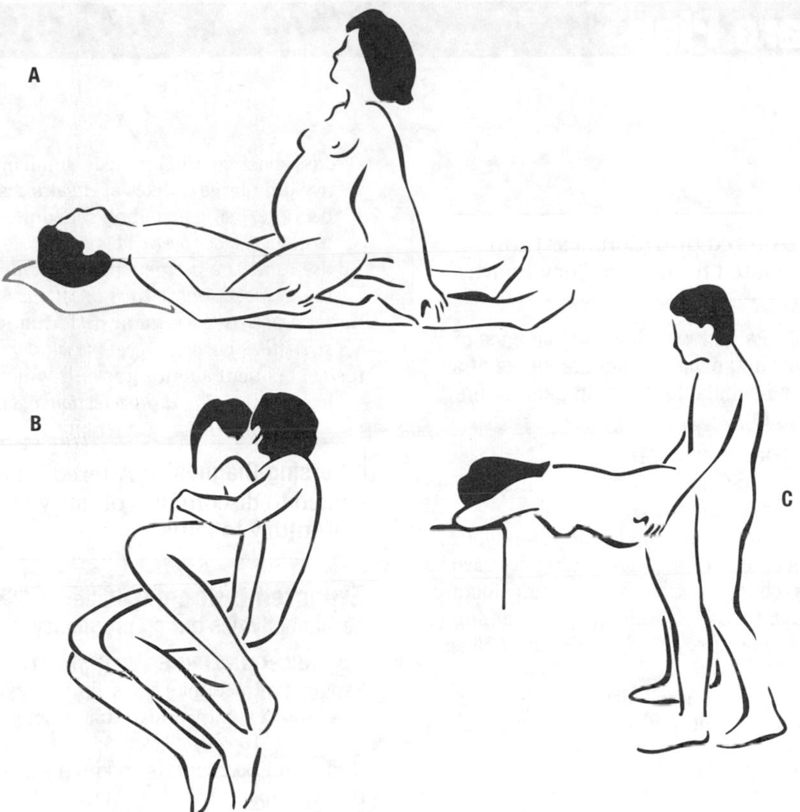

Fig. 7-8 Positions for sexual intercourse during pregnancy. **A,** Female superior; **B,** side by side; **C,** rear entry.

as to her fetus, the use of condoms is recommended throughout pregnancy if the woman is at risk for an STD.

Well-informed nurses who are comfortable with their own sexuality and the sexual counseling needs of pregnant couples can offer counseling in a valuable but often neglected area. They can establish an open environment in which couples can feel free to introduce their concerns about sexual adjustment and seek support and guidance. This is important for lesbian women and their partners as well as for women with male partners.

Cultural Variations in Prenatal Care

Prenatal care as Americans know it is a phenomenon of Western medicine. The Western biomedical model of care encourages women to seek prenatal care as early as possible in their pregnancy by visiting a physician or clinic. Visits are usually routine and follow a systematic sequence, with the initial visit followed by monthly, then semimonthly, then weekly visits. Monitoring weight and blood pressure; testing blood and urine; teaching specific information about diet, rest, and activity; and preparing for childbirth are common components of prenatal care. This model not only is unfamiliar but seems strange to many groups (Green, 1990; Kulig, 1990).

Many **cultural variations** in prenatal care exist. Even when the prenatal care described is familiar, some practices may conflict with a subculture group's beliefs and practices. Because of these and other factors, such as poor communication on the part of health care providers, lack of money, and lack of transportation, many groups do not participate in the prenatal care system (Lazarus and Philipson, 1990; Leatherman, Blackburn, and Davidhizar, 1990; Scupholme, Robertson, and Kamons, 1991). Their behavior may be misinterpreted by nurses as uncaring, lazy, or ignorant.

A concern for modesty is also a deterrent for prenatal care for many people. Exposing one's body parts, especially to a man, is a major violation of modesty. For many women, invasive procedures such as vaginal examination may be so threatening that they cannot be discussed, even with one's own husband. Thus many women prefer a female to a male health care provider (Geissler, 1994; Hutchinson and Baqi, 1994). Most women value and appreciate efforts to maintain their modesty.

For numerous cultural groups a physician is deemed appropriate only in times of illness. The services of a physician are considered inappropriate, since pregnancy is considered a normal process and the woman is in a state of health. Even when problems with pregnancy develop (according to beliefs of Western medicine), they may not be perceived as problems by the patient and may be considered normal.

Although pregnancy is considered normal by many, certain practices are expected of women of all cultures to ensure a good outcome. Cultural **prescriptions** tell women what to do, and **proscriptions** establish taboos. The purposes of these practices are to prevent maternal illness from a pregnancy-induced imbalanced state and to protect the vulnerable fetus. Prescriptions and proscriptions are related to emo-

Nursing Care Plan

PREGNANCY

First Trimester

Nursing Diagnosis: Altered nutrition: less than body requirements related to nausea, "dry heaves"

Expected Outcomes: Patient will show no evidence of nausea and/or dry heaves and exhibit adequate intake of appropriate nourishment and satisfactory weight gain for first trimester (about 1.4 kg [3 lb]).

• NURSING INTERVENTIONS/*RATIONALES*

Take a 24-hour diet history and discuss patterns of incidence *to identify probable causes of nausea.*

Discuss eliminating nausea-producing foods; eating small, frequent meals; avoiding an empty stomach; eating dry carbohydrate substances, such as crackers on awakening, followed by fluids such as hot tea or coffee within an hour; ceasing smoking; and improving posture *as ways to decrease feelings of nausea.*

Instruct patient about hyperemesis gravidarum and have her report any episode of severe vomiting *to assist in early detection of complications.*

Nursing Diagnosis: Fatigue related to physiologic/psychologic adaptations of pregnancy

Expected Outcomes: Patient will engage in normal activities of daily living (ADLs) and fulfill usual role obligations.

• NURSING INTERVENTIONS/*RATIONALES*

Identify common energy-depleting factors and energy requirements for routine ADLs and role obligations.

Discuss expected physiologic and psychologic changes that accompany pregnancy.

Teach patient to prioritize, delegate, and pace activities *to conserve energy;* to plan, schedule, and pace events (i.e., alternating activity and rest cycles) *to use energy effectively;* to maintain adequate nutrition, rest, and sleep; and to engage in stress management and a progressive physical activity program *to restore energy.*

Nursing Diagnosis: Altered patterns of urinary elimination: urinary frequency related to vascular engorgement and reduced bladder capacity

Expected Outcome: Patient will maintain or regain continence.

• NURSING INTERVENTIONS/*RATIONALES*

Identify and have patient avoid foods or beverages (e.g., coffee, citrus juice, carbonated beverages, spicy foods) *to reduce the intensity of urgency.*

Discuss spacing fluid intake in small amounts across the day, avoiding large intakes at mealtimes and intake right before bedtime, using a voiding schedule, and voiding every 2 hours *to avoid bladder overload.*

Advise to wear a perineal pad *to avoid accidents.* Change pads often *to avoid urinary tract infections.*

Instruct patient on regular performance of Kegel exercise *to strengthen pubococcygeal muscles.*

Instruct patient about signs and symptoms of urinary tract infection *to ensure early detection and treatment.*

Nursing Diagnosis: Altered sexuality patterns related to discomforts of early pregnancy and/or fear of injury to fetus

Expected Outcome: Patient will express satisfaction with sexual activities during pregnancy.

• NURSING INTERVENTIONS/*RATIONALES*

Explore (with couple) fears, doubts, expectations, and knowledge about sexuality and sexual functioning during pregnancy *to enhance coping abilities.*

Correct misperceptions and myths about sex and pregnancy.

Discuss expected changes, such as breast enlargement and tenderness, leukorrhea, nausea, fatigue, and urinary urgency, *that may affect sexual desire, expression, and function.*

Discuss alternative sexual behaviors and positions that can increase comfort during intercourse or be used as a substitute for intercourse *to maintain ongoing expressions of sexuality.*

Reinforce need for privacy, comfort, and ambiance, *which enhance a conducive environment.*

Instruct high-risk couples to use condoms during intercourse *to avoid acquiring and transmitting STDs.*

Nursing Diagnosis: Anxiety related to changes, discomforts, and/or feelings resulting from pregnancy

Expected Outcome: Patient will exhibit signs of reduced anxiety (i.e., absence of physical indicators, absence of perceived threat, absence of feelings of dread).

• NURSING INTERVENTIONS/*RATIONALES*

Identify and explore worries associated with the pregnancy.

Discuss expected changes that occur during pregnancy and strategies *for successfully coping with these changes.*

Identify successful strategies that have been used *to cope with past anxieties.*

Determine strengths and resources available *to cope with current anxiety.*

Develop a specific set of interventions *to cope with the anxiety based on data gathered.*

Nursing Care Plan

PREGNANCY

First Trimester—cont'd

Nursing Diagnosis: Knowledge deficit related to new health condition (pregnancy)

Expected Outcome: Patient will define role in health and pregnancy management.

• NURSING INTERVENTIONS/*RATIONALES*

Explore current information and expectations about pregnancy, including maternal and fetal changes, safety issues, and signs or symptoms indicative of deviation from normal progress *to identify areas of misperception and deficit.*

Devise a teaching plan *to correct misperceptions and deficits.* Include a number of readily available material and personnel resources *to accommodate learning styles and reinforce teaching.* Space the teaching plan out over a number of visits *to ensure maximum learning.*

Have patient demonstrate use of new knowledge *to reinforce correct use of information and positive adaptations in behavior.*

Nursing Diagnosis: Knowledge deficit related to self-care measures during pregnancy

Expected Outcomes: Patient will describe self-care behaviors and exhibit evidence of incorporation of behaviors.

• NURSING INTERVENTIONS/*RATIONALES*

Discuss the physiologic relationship of mother and developing fetus *to illustrate the dependence of fetus on the mother.*

Review the possible effects of ingestion/inhalation of alcohol, caffeine, tobacco, and drugs (prescription, OTC, recreational) on the fetus and discourage their use *to ensure the well-being of fetus.*

Discuss the avoidance of environmental hazards (e.g., secondhand smoke, household chemicals, occupational toxins) *to ensure the well-being of the fetus.*

Review mother's daily routine at home and at work and discuss changes in dietary habits, exercise habits, and work habits *that will assist in adapting to the changes that occur with advancing pregnancy.*

---

tional response, clothing, physical activity and rest, sexual activity, and dietary practices (see the Cultural Considerations box to the right).

Emotional response. Virtually all cultures emphasize the importance of a socially harmonious and agreeable environment. Absence of stressful relationships is important for a successful outcome for mother and baby. Harmony with other people must be fostered. Visits from extended family members may be required to demonstrate continued pleasant and noncontroversial relationships. If discord exists in any relationship with others, it is usually dealt with in culturally prescribed ways.

Imitative magic functions in proscriptions. Many Mexicans advise pregnant women not to witness an eclipse of the moon because they believe it may cause a cleft palate in the infant. Exposure to an earthquake may result in preterm delivery, miscarriage, or even a breech presentation. A pregnant woman must not ridicule someone with an affliction for fear her child might be born with the same handicap. A mother should not hate a person lest her child resemble that person, and dental work should not be done during pregnancy because it may cause a baby to have a "harelip." A widely held folk belief in many cultures is that the pregnant woman should refrain from raising her arms above her head and from tying knots so that the umbilical cord does not wrap around the baby's neck or become knotted. Other cultures believe that placing a knife under the bed of a laboring woman will "cut" her pain.

Clothing. Although most cultural groups do not prescribe specific clothing for pregnancy, modesty is an expectation for many. Some Spanish-speaking women of the Southwest wear a cord beneath the breast and knotted over the umbilicus. This cord, called a *muneco,* is thought to prevent morning sickness and ensure a safe delivery. Amulets, medals, and beads may be worn to ward off evil spirits (Spector, 1991).

Physical activity and rest. Norms that regulate physical activity of mothers during pregnancy vary tremendously. Many groups, including Native Americans and some Asian

Cultural Considerations

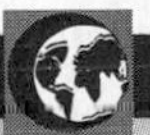

CULTURAL VARIATIONS IN PREGNANCY

The nurse taking care of pregnant women in the United States needs to be aware that women bring with them various cultural practices. The United States is made up of people with strongly held beliefs about pregnancy and childbirth. There are more than 170 Native-American groups and more than 106 ethnic groups. Each one of these groups and the individuals in the groups have beliefs and practices that will affect their care.

As part of the prenatal assessment, cultural and ethnic background needs to be explored. Asking the woman about her expectations and beliefs helps to plan care that does not conflict with proscriptions and prescriptions the pregnant woman brings with her to the pregnancy experience.

groups (Lee, 1989), encourage women to be active, to walk, and to engage in normal although not strenuous activities to ensure that the baby is healthy and not too large. Other groups, such as Filipinos, believe that any activity is dangerous, and others willingly take over work of the pregnant woman. The belief among some Filipinos is that inactivity constitutes a protection for mother and child. The mother is encouraged simply to produce the succeeding generation. Health care providers could misinterpret this behavior as laziness or noncompliance with the health regimen desired in prenatal care. Again, it is important for the nurse to find out the meaning of activity and rest for each pregnant woman.

Sexual activity. In most cultures, sexual activity is not prohibited until the end of pregnancy. Many Mexican-Americans view sexual activity as necessary to keep the birth canal lubricated (Geissler, 1994). On the other hand, Vietnamese may have definite proscriptions about sexual intercourse, requiring abstinence throughout the pregnancy, because it is thought that sexual intercourse may harm the mother and the fetus (Geissler, 1994).

Dietary practices. Nutritional information given by Western health care providers may be a source of conflict for many cultural groups. The conflict usually is not known by the health care providers unless they have an understanding of dietary beliefs and practices of the people for whom they are caring. Muslims, for example, must eat meat slaughtered in accordance with Muslim law. If this is not possible, they will accept kosher or vegetarian foods (Hutchinson and Baqi, 1994). Many cultures permit only warm foods during pregnancy (Geissler, 1994).

Evaluation

Maternal and fetal expected outcomes are evaluated according to measurable, established criteria. The clinical findings that represent normal responses are presented as goals with expected outcomes in the nursing care plan for each woman. These criteria are used as a basis for selecting appropriate nursing actions and evaluating their effectiveness (see the Nursing Care Plan on pp. 144-145).

SECOND TRIMESTER

The second trimester spans weeks 14 through 26 of pregnancy. By the second trimester the pregnancy usually has been verified. The woman and her family have had time to adjust to the pregnancy, and the initial visit and possibly a follow-up visit have been completed. For many women, discomforts common to the first trimester are resolving, but it is still too early to focus on the labor and birth.

Most women have no major problems. For them a common pattern for return visits is scheduled. Throughout the second trimester, monthly visits are sufficient; additional visits are scheduled as the need arises.

Nursing Care Management

Assessment

Interview. Follow-up visits are less intensive than the initial prenatal visit. At each visit the woman is asked for a summary of events since the previous visit. She is asked about her general emotional and physical well-being, complaints or problems, or questions she may have. Personal and family needs are identified and explored. Success or failure of self-care measures is discussed, and learning needs and readiness for learning are assessed.

Nursing ALERT

The nurse can reinforce teaching about warning signs and symptoms of potential complications by inquiring about them at each visit.

Careful, precise, and concise recording of patient responses and laboratory results contributes to the continuous supervision vital to the mother and fetus. A checklist of care needs during the second trimester of pregnancy is a valuable tool. It provides the team of care providers with a communication tool to prevent gaps and identify areas of repeated concern for patients. Box 7-5 provides a sample checklist for the second trimester.

Nursing ALERT

SIGNS OF POTENTIAL COMPLICATIONS—SECOND AND THIRD TRIMESTERS

Sign/Symptom	Possible causes
Persistent, severe vomiting	Hyperemesis gravidarum
Amniotic fluid discharge from vagina	Premature rupture of membranes (PROM)
Vaginal bleeding, severe abdominal pain	Miscarriage, placental separation
Chills, fever, burning on urination, diarrhea	Infection
Change in fetal movements: absence of fetal movements after quickening, any unusual change in pattern or amount	Fetal jeopardy or intrauterine fetal death
Uterine contractions	Preterm labor
Visual disturbances: blurring, double vision, spots	Hypertensive conditions, pregnancy-induced hypertension (PIH)
Swelling of face or fingers and over sacrum	Hypertensive conditions, PIH
Headaches: severe, frequent, or continuous	Hypertensive conditions, PIH
Muscular irritability or convulsions	Hypertensive conditions, PIH
Epigastric pain (perceived as severe stomachache)	Hypertensive conditions, PIH
Glucosuria, positive glucose tolerance test reaction	Gestational diabetes mellitus

BOX 7-5
Second-Trimester Checklist

Schedule and events of visits
Maternal assessment
  Emotional well-being
    Mood swings
    Body image changes
    Dreams
  Developmental tasks of pregnancy
    Accepted biologic fact of pregnancy
    Awareness of child as a separate being
    Increasing introspection
Fetal growth and development
Diagnostic tests
  Specify
Counseling for self-care
  Birth plan
  Adaptations/discomforts
    Skin changes
    Palpitations
    Faintness
    Gastrointestinal distress
    Varicosities
    Neuromuscular and skeletal distress
  Safety (seat belts with shoulder harness and headrest)
    Exercise and rest
    Relaxation
    Nutrition
    Alcohol and other substances
    Sexuality
    Personal hygiene
    Warning signs of potential complications
    Other

Birth plan. The nurse can answer questions and discuss concerns about the birth plan. The parents need to be reminded that no birth plan can be guaranteed, and alternative plans need to be suggested. That is, what if a cesarean birth is necessary? Does the woman want her partner to be present? Does she want to hold the baby immediately (if the baby's and mother's conditions warrant it)? Alternative plans serve to reduce disappointment. The following questions also may be asked:

- *Immediately after birth.* Do you want to hold the baby right away? To breastfeed immediately?
- *Newborn care.* What about circumcision for your baby? Will your baby be breastfed or bottle-fed?
- *Postpartum care.* What type of care do you anticipate: labor, delivery, recovery, postpartum care (LDRP), mother-baby coupling or "request" coupling (newborn cared for in nursery while mother rests)? How long does your insurance company allow you to stay in the hospital? Would you like to attend self-care classes or watch videotapes? On which subjects?

If older siblings are to be included in the labor and birth process, the possibility needs to be reviewed and cleared with the physician or nurse-midwife and the staff in the birth setting. This is done long before the EDB to avoid the stress of this type of negotiation during labor. Some facilities require that a sibling attending a birth go to preparation classes. The woman needs to specify who will be responsible for the sibling during labor and birth because this is a requirement at many facilities.

Physical examination. Physiologic changes are documented as the pregnancy progresses. This provides a basis for noting deviations from normal progress.

Nursing ALERT

Reevaluation is continuous. Each woman reacts differently to pregnancy. Careful monitoring of pregnancy and reactions to care is vital.

At each visit, temperature, pulse, and respirations are measured; blood pressure (same arm, woman sitting) is taken; weight and the determination of whether weight gain (or loss) is compatible with overall plan for weight gain are evaluated; urine is tested for protein and glucose; and presence and degree of edema are noted. These findings reflect the status of maternal adaptations. When the interview or physical examination findings are suspicious, an in-depth examination is performed.

Careful interpretation of blood pressure is important in risk-factor analysis for all pregnant women. Blood pressure is evaluated on the basis of absolute values and length of gestation and is interpreted in the light of modifying factors. PIH and *h*emolysis, *e*levated *l*iver enzyme, *l*ow *p*latelet count (HELLP) syndrome are serious complications of pregnancy and may be fatal (Sibai et al, 1995a).

Absolute values of a systolic blood pressure of 140 mm Hg or higher and a diastolic blood pressure of 90 mm Hg or greater suggest hypertension. A rise in systolic blood pressure of 30 mm Hg over baseline and/or diastolic blood pressure of 15 mm Hg over baseline are also significant regardless of whether absolute values are less than 140/90. For example, if a woman's blood pressure normally is 105/60, a change to 120/75 must be viewed as potential for hypertension. The blood pressure reaches its minimum in midpregnancy and then returns to baseline at term (Duvekot and Peeters, 1994). An increase in systolic blood pressure is a better indicator of the risk for PIH than is diastolic increase (Sibai et al, 1995b). The **roll-over test** is sometimes used to predict possible third-trimester hypertensive problems. Box 7-6 outlines the procedure for performing a roll-over test.

Laboratory tests. Routine laboratory tests during the second trimester are limited. A clean-catch urine specimen is used to detect levels of glucose (to assess for diabetes), protein (to assess for PIH), and nitrites and leukocytes (to assess for infection). Urine for culture and sensitivity, as well as blood samples, are obtained only if signs and symptoms warrant. Hematocrit (Hct) determination is done at each visit in some offices. A blood draw for alpha-fetoprotein (AFP) is done at 16 weeks. Between 20 and 28 weeks, vaginal specimens are obtained to test for gonorrhea and bacterial vaginosis.

The *multiple marker test,* or *triple screen test,* is being used to detect Down syndrome. Done at 16 to 18 weeks, it measures maternal serum alpha-fetoprotein (MSAFP), human chorionic gonadotropin (hCG), and unconjugated estriol (uE3). Ad-

BOX 7-6
Roll-Over Test

Administered at 28 to 32 weeks' gestation

Procedure:
- Position woman in left lateral recumbent position.
- Monitor blood pressure (BP) until stable, usually about 15 minutes.
- Roll woman to supine position and take B/P.
- Retake B/P in 5 minutes.

Result: increase > 20 mm Hg in diastolic B/P is considered positive.

Significance:
- If negative, chances are less than 1 in 100 that woman will develop preeclampsia.
- If positive, risk of hypertensive problem is increased; close monitoring of third trimester may be indicated.

justed values are combined to obtain a risk for Down syndrome (Heyl, Miller, and Canick, 1990). Low levels may be associated with Down syndrome and other chromosomal abnormalities (Cunningham et al, 1993). Neural tube defects are associated with a high level of MSAFP.

Fundal height. During the second trimester the uterus becomes an abdominal organ. Measurement of the height of the uterus above the symphysis pubis is used as one indicator of the progress of fetal growth. It also provides a gross estimate of the duration of pregnancy. Measurement of fundal height may aid in identification of high-risk factors: a stable or decreased fundal height may indicate intrauterine growth restriction (IUGR); an excessive increase could mean multifetal gestation or hydramnios.

A paper tape measure or a pelvimeter may be used to measure **fundal height.** To increase measurement reliability, the same person can examine the pregnant woman at each of her prenatal visits, but often multiple clinicians see the woman for prenatal visits. All clinicians who examine pregnant women should be consistent in their measurement techniques. Ideally a protocol is established for the health care setting that explicitly describes the measurement technique, including the woman's position on the examining table, the measuring device, and the method of measurement used. Conditions under which the measurements were taken can also be described, including whether the bladder was empty and whether the uterus was relaxed or contracted.

Various positions for fundal height measurement have been described in the literature. The woman can be supine, have her head elevated, have her knees flexed, or have both her head elevated and her knees flexed. Studies have shown that measurements are different in the various positions, making it even more important to standardize the fundal height measurement technique (Engstrom et al, 1993).

Placement of the tape measure can also vary. The tape can be placed in the middle of the woman's abdomen, and the measurement can be performed by measuring from the upper border of the symphysis pubis to the upper border of the fundus. The tape measure is held in contact with the skin for the entire length of the uterus (Fig. 7-9, *A*). Another measurement technique does not include the upper curve of the fundus in the measurement. One end of the tape measure is held at the upper border of the symphysis pubis with one hand; the other hand is placed at the upper border of the fundus. The tape is placed between the middle and index fingers and the measurement taken at the point the hand intercepts the tape measure (Fig. 7-9, *B*) (Engstrom and Sittler, 1993).

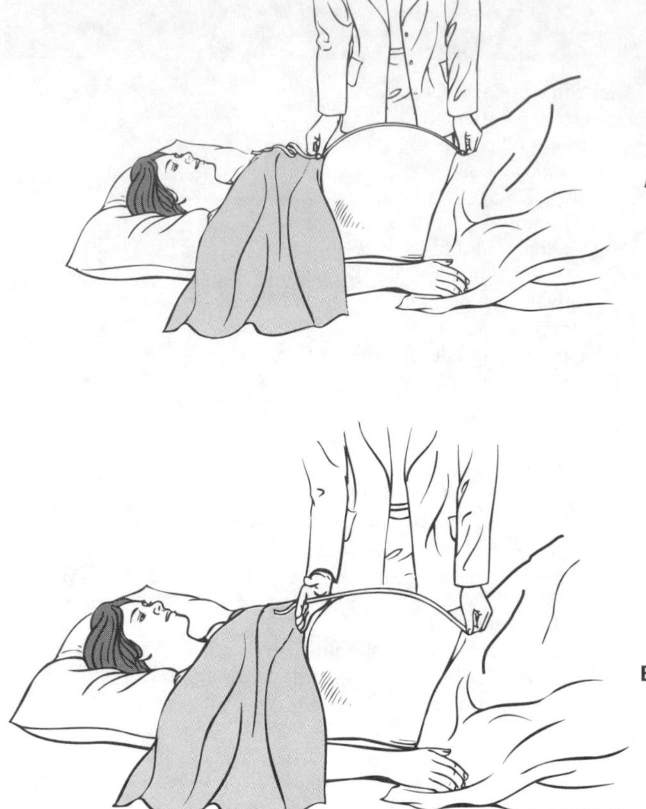

Fig. 7-9 Measurement of fundal height from symphysis that **A,** includes the upper curve of the fundus, and **B,** does not include the upper curve of the fundus. Note position of hands and measuring tape.

During the second and third trimesters (weeks 18 to 30) the height of the fundus in centimeters is approximately the same as weeks of gestation if the woman's bladder is empty (Cunningham et al, 1993).

Gestational age. In an uncomplicated pregnancy, **fetal gestational age** is estimated after determining the duration of pregnancy and the EDB. Fetal gestational age is determined from the menstrual history, contraceptive history, and pregnancy test and from the clinical evaluation, as follows:

- First uterine size estimate: date, size
- FHT first heard: date, Doppler stethoscope, fetoscope
- Date of quickening
- Current fundal height, estimated fetal weight (EFW)
- Current week of gestation
- Ultrasound: date, week of gestation, biparietal diameter (BPD)
- Reliability of dates

Nursing Care Plan

PREGNANCY

Second Trimester

Nursing Diagnosis: Joint and/or back pain related to pregnancy-related changes in pelvic structure and stress on abdominal musculature

Expected Outcome: Patient will exhibit relief of pain.

• NURSING INTERVENTIONS/*RATIONALES*

Discuss and demonstrate the use of good body mechanics while standing, stooping, and lifting and correct posture positions while standing, sitting, and reclining *to reduce strain on muscles and joints.*

Demonstrate the use of specific exercises such as the pelvic tilt and squatting *to strengthen musculature* and conscious relaxation *to relax and ease fatigue.*

Discuss external changes in routine or environment such as wearing low-heeled shoes, wearing a maternity girdle and maternity bra, and using a firm mattress and a small support pillow to the lower back *to decrease strain.*

Nursing Diagnosis: Constipation related to slowed gastrointestinal motility and intestinal tract compression from enlarging uterus

Expected Outcome: Patient will show evidence of regular bowel pattern with normal stool consistency.

• NURSING INTERVENTION/*RATIONALE*

Discuss use of dietary factors such as adequate fiber intake, adequate daily fluid intake, and regular eating schedule; use of daily aerobic exercise; use of regular defecation routines; and use of relaxation and deep-breathing techniques *to promote normal bowel function.* (Do not use stool softeners, laxatives, enemas, or other medication without first consulting a health care provider.)

Nursing Diagnosis: Pain of perineum and lower extremities related to formation of hemorrhoids and varicose veins during pregnancy

Expected Outcome: Patient will exhibit relief of aching and tenderness in legs and itching and pain in perineal area.

• NURSING INTERVENTIONS/*RATIONALES*

Discuss use of moderate exercise program and rest periods with elevation of legs and hips *to reduce edema and improve venous circulation.* (Avoid prolonged standing or sitting, straining at stool, crossing legs at knee, and wearing constrictive clothing).

Discuss use of sitz baths, tepid oatmeal baths, and astringent compresses *for temporary relief of itching and inflammation.*

Recommend use of carefully fitted support stockings *to improve venous return in lower extremities.*

Nursing Diagnosis: Knowledge deficit related to potential complications in pregnancy (e.g., miscarriage, gestational diabetes, preeclampsia, eclampsia)

Expected Outcome: Patient and significant other will delineate signs and symptoms of potential complications.

• NURSING INTERVENTIONS/*RATIONALES*

Assess what partners know about normal vs. abnormal signs and symptoms during pregnancy *to identify areas of deficit.*

Discuss signs and symptoms that serve as warning signs to potential complications *so that patient or her partner have adequate information to detect potential problems early.*

Provide written supplemental materials that include a list of warning signs and instructions about what to do if any of the listed signs occur, *so couple can reinforce and review learning and act swiftly and appropriately should a sign occur.*

Nursing Diagnosis: Altered family processes related to impending birth

Expected Outcomes: Family members will exhibit realistic expectations about impact of pregnancy and impending birth on family unit. Family members will exhibit changes in family roles and functions.

• NURSING INTERVENTIONS/RATIONALES

Encourage family members to express full range of feelings about pregnancy *to promote communication and family well-being.*

Discuss changes that will occur as pregnancy progresses and the attendant changes that may be needed in family roles and functions *to anticipate those changes.*

Have various family members delineate specific changes that they can make to support patient during pregnancy (e.g., assistance with patient's normal roles and functions) *to facilitate the needed changes.*

Explore available support systems *to provide emotional support for family as they cope with altered roles and expectations* (e.g., childbirth classes, parenting classes, counseling, social services, health care workers, friends, relatives).

Quickening ("feeling life") refers to the mother's perception of fetal movement. It usually occurs between weeks 16 and 20 of gestation.

In some centers, ultrasonography is used with all pregnancies, and a more exact estimation of gestational age can be made. Ultrasonography may be used to establish the duration of pregnancy if the woman is unable to give a precise date for her LMP or if the size of the uterus does not conform to the stated date of the LMP. In some centers, all women have a routine ultrasound done. However, the efficacy of routine sonography in low-risk pregnancies has not been documented to improve fetal outcome (Garmel and D'Alton, 1994).

Health status. The second trimester is a period of rapid growth. Box 7-7 and Fig. 7-10 summarize fetal development.

Nursing ALERT

Assessment of **fetal health status** includes consideration of fetal movement, fetal heart rate (FHR), and abnormal maternal or fetal symptoms.

BOX 7-7

Fetal Development at 26 Weeks

Viable at week 24*
Fetal movements obvious
FHR readily heard
Scalp hair, eyebrows, eyelashes, fine downy lanugo, and vernix cover skin
Eyelids still fused
Skin red, shiny, and thin
Face wrinkled, giving an "old man" appearance
Length 30 cm
Weight 600 g
Uterus at or just above level of umbilicus

*In Canada, viability is defined as 20 weeks' gestation and 500 g in weight.

The mother is instructed to note the extent and timing of fetal movements and to report immediately if the pattern changes or if movement ceases. Regular movement has been found to be a reliable indicator of fetal health (Wilailak et al, 1992).

The FHR is checked on routine visits once it has been heard (Fig. 7-5). Early in the second trimester the FHR may be heard with the Doppler stethoscope (Fig. 7-5, *B*). Before the fetus can be palpated by Leopold's maneuvers (see p. 404 and Fig. 16-4), the scope is moved around the abdomen until the FHR is heard. Each nurse develops a set pattern for searching the abdomen, for example, starting first in the midline about 2 to 3 cm above the symphysis, followed by the left lower quadrant, and so on. The FHR is counted, and the quality and rhythm are noted. Later in the second trimester the FHR can be determined with the fetoscope or Pinard's stethoscope (see Fig. 7-5, *A* and *C*). Normal rate and rhythm are other good indicators of fetal health.

Nursing ALERT

Absence of FHR, once noted, requires immediate investigation.

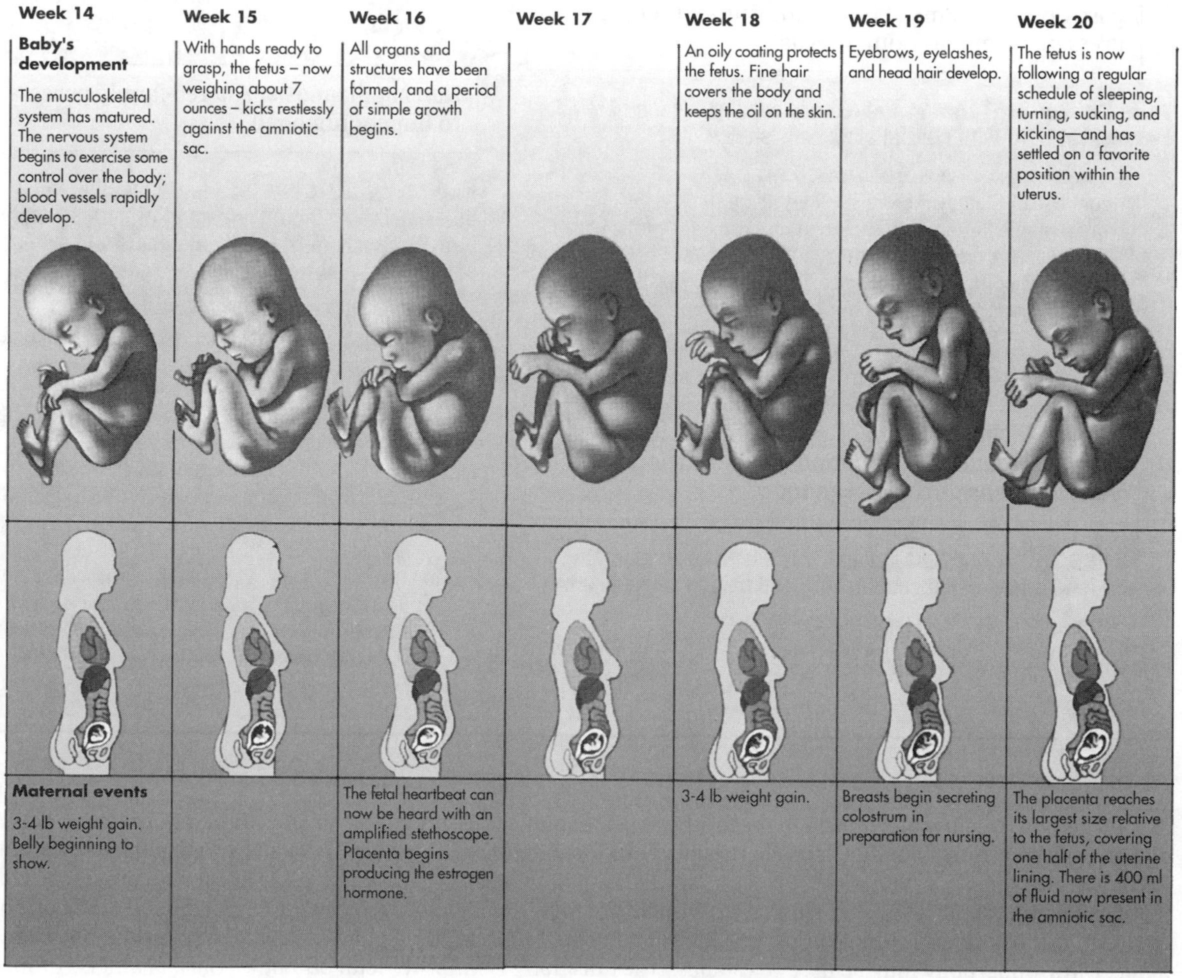

Week 14	Week 15	Week 16	Week 17	Week 18	Week 19	Week 20
Baby's development The musculoskeletal system has matured. The nervous system begins to exercise some control over the body; blood vessels rapidly develop.	With hands ready to grasp, the fetus – now weighing about 7 ounces – kicks restlessly against the amniotic sac.	All organs and structures have been formed, and a period of simple growth begins.		An oily coating protects the fetus. Fine hair covers the body and keeps the oil on the skin.	Eyebrows, eyelashes, and head hair develop.	The fetus is now following a regular schedule of sleeping, turning, sucking, and kicking—and has settled on a favorite position within the uterus.
Maternal events 3-4 lb weight gain. Belly beginning to show.		The fetal heartbeat can now be heard with an amplified stethoscope. Placenta begins producing the estrogen hormone.		3-4 lb weight gain.	Breasts begin secreting colostrum in preparation for nursing.	The placenta reaches its largest size relative to the fetus, covering one half of the uterine lining. There is 400 ml of fluid now present in the amniotic sac.

Intensive investigation of fetal health status is initiated if any maternal or fetal complications arise (e.g., maternal hypertension, IUGR, PROM, irregular or absent FHR, absence of fetal movements after quickening).

The Nursing Care Plan on p. 149 lists nursing diagnoses, outcomes, and interventions for the second trimester of pregnancy.

Nursing Diagnoses

Each individual is affected differently by pregnancy. Careful monitoring of the pregnancy and responses to care are of utmost importance. It is particularly difficult to distinguish discomforts of the second and third trimesters. Women who have given birth before tend to demonstrate some discomforts in pregnancy earlier than first-time mothers. Continuous assessment, analysis, and formulation of diagnoses are imperative. Common nursing diagnoses during the second trimester may include the following:

- Body-image disturbance related to
  - Anatomic and physiologic changes of pregnancy
- Altered health maintenance related to knowledge deficit regarding self-care measures
  - Rest and relaxation
  - Personal hygiene (increased sweating, oily skin, leukorrhea)
- Pain related to
  - Discomforts of pregnancy
- Risk for injury related to
  - Nonuse of seat and shoulder harness and headrest in automobiles
  - Exposure to harmful chemicals
- Altered family processes related to
  - Lack of understanding of second-trimester changes
  - Changing sexual relationship or partner support
- Anxiety related to
  - Discomforts of pregnancy
  - Changing family dynamics
  - Fetal well-being

Expected Outcomes

Planning care for women during the second trimester of pregnancy is guided by the nursing diagnoses. To the extent possible, the woman participates in developing an individualized plan that relates specifically to her needs. The information in this chapter is general; not all women experience all problems discussed or require all facets of care described. Expected outcomes are similar to those for the first trimester.

Expected outcomes related to physiologic care

1. The woman and her family will describe pertinent information about maternal adaptations and fetal develop-

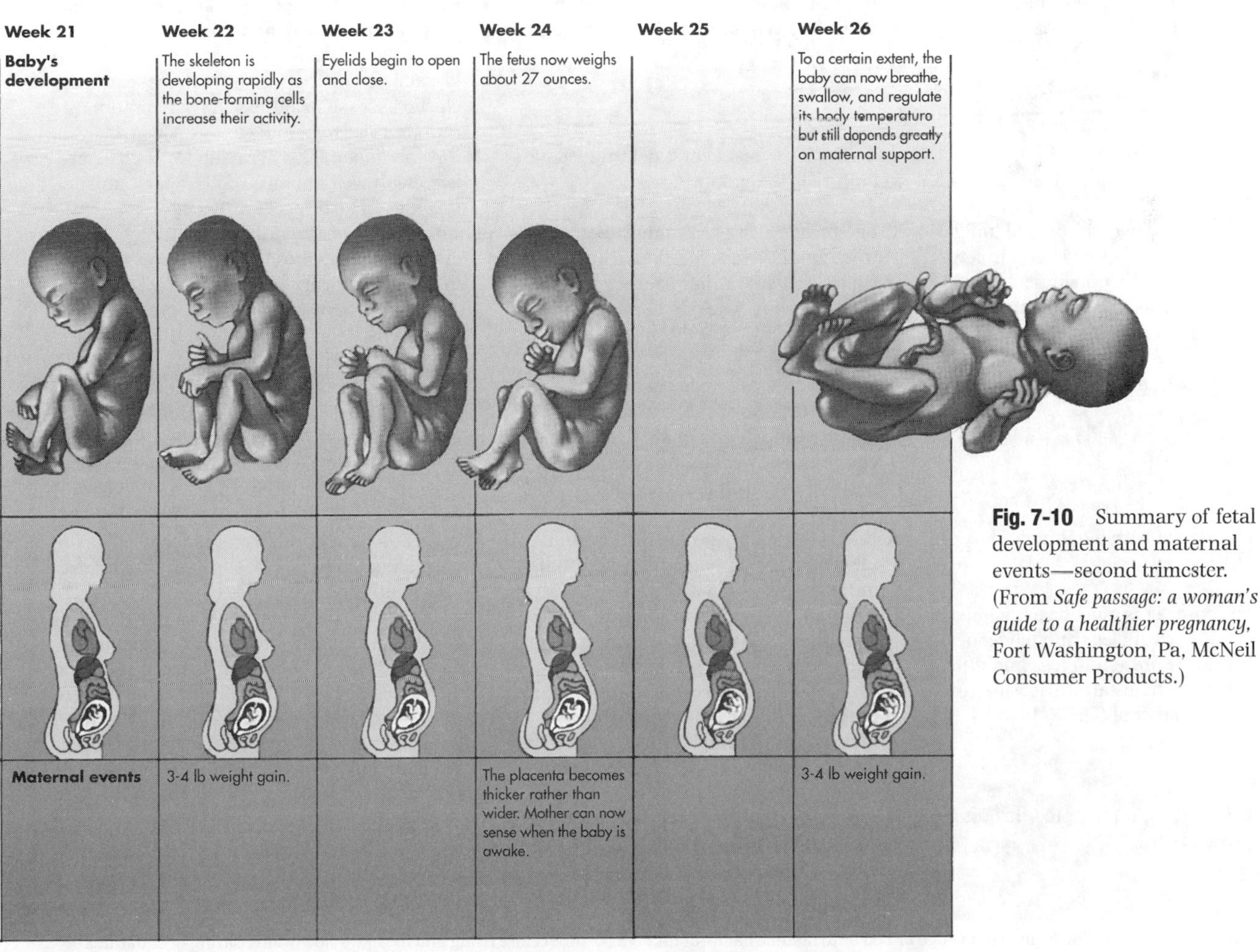

Week 21
Week 22
Week 23
Week 24
Week 25
Week 26
Baby's development
The skeleton is developing rapidly as the bone-forming cells increase their activity.
Eyelids begin to open and close.
The fetus now weighs about 27 ounces.
To a certain extent, the baby can now breathe, swallow, and regulate its body temperature but still depends greatly on maternal support.
Maternal events
3-4 lb weight gain.
The placenta becomes thicker rather than wider. Mother can now sense when the baby is awake.
3-4 lb weight gain.

Fig. 7-10 Summary of fetal development and maternal events—second trimester. (From *Safe passage: a woman's guide to a healthier pregnancy*, Fort Washington, Pa, McNeil Consumer Products.)

TABLE 7-3 Discomforts related to maternal adaptations to pregnancy in second trimester

DISCOMFORT	PHYSIOLOGY	EDUCATION FOR SELF-CARE
Pigmentation deepens, acne, oily skin	Melanocyte-stimulating hormone (from anterior pituitary)	Not preventable; usually resolved during puerperium; reassure women and their families
Spider nevi (telangiectasias) appear during trimesters 2 or 3 over neck, thorax, face, and arms	Focal networks of dilated arterioles (end arteries) from increased concentration of estrogens	Not preventable; give reassurance that they fade slowly during late puerperium; rarely disappear completely.
Palmar erythema occurs in 50% of pregnant women; may accompany spider nevi	Diffuse reddish mottling over palms and suffused skin over thenar eminences and fingertips may be caused by genetic predisposition or hyperestrogenism	Not preventable; give reassurance that condition will fade within 1 week after giving birth.
Pruritus (noninflammatory)	Unknown cause; various types as follows: Nonpapular; closely aggregated pruritic papules Increased excretory function of skin and stretching of skin possible factors	Keep fingernails short and clean; refer to health care provider for diagnosis of cause. Not preventable; symptomatic: provide Keri baths, mild sedation. Provide distraction; tepid baths with sodium bicarbonate or oatmeal added to water; lotions and oils; change of soaps or reduction in use of soap; loose clothing.
Palpitations	Unknown; should not be accompanied by persistent cardiac irregularity	Not preventable; give reassurance; refer to health care provider if accompanied by symptoms of cardiac decompensation.
Supine hypotension (vena cava syndrome), bradycardia	Posture induced by pressure of gravid uterus on ascending vena cava when woman is supine; reduces uterine-placental and renal perfusion	Assume side-lying position (see p. 155) or semi-sitting posture, with knees slightly flexed.
Faintness and rarely syncope (orthostatic hypotension) may persist throughout pregnancy	Vasomotor lability or postural hypotension from hormones; in late pregnancy may be caused by venous stasis in lower extremities	Moderate exercise, deep breathing, vigorous leg movement; avoid sudden changes in position* and warm crowded areas; move slowly and deliberately; keep environment cool; avoid hypoglycemia by eating 5 or 6 small meals per day; elastic hose; sit as necessary; if symptoms are serious, refer to health care provider.
Food cravings	Cause unknown; cravings determined by culture or geographic area	Not preventable; satisfy craving unless it interferes with well-balanced diet; report unusual cravings to health care provider.
Heartburn (pyrosis, or acid indigestion): burning sensation in lower chest or upper abdomen, occasionally with burping and regurgitation of a little sour-tasting fluid	Progesterone slows gastrointestinal (GI) tract motility and digestion, reverses peristalsis, relaxes cardiac sphincter, and delays emptying time of stomach; stomach displaced upward and compressed by enlarging uterus	Limit or avoid gas-producing or fatty foods and large meals; maintain good posture; sips of milk for temporary relief; hot tea, chewing gum; health care provider may prescribe antacid between meals; refer to health care provider for persistent symptoms.
Constipation	GI tract motility slowed because of progesterone, resulting in increased resorption of water and drying of stool; intestines compressed by enlarging uterus; predisposition to constipation because of oral iron supplementation	Six glasses of water per day; roughage in diet; moderate exercise; regular schedule for bowel movements; use relaxation techniques and deep breathing; do not take stool softener, laxatives, mineral oil, other drugs, or enemas without first consulting health care provider.
Flatulence with bloating and belching	Reduced GI motility because of hormones, allowing time for bacterial action that produces gas; swallowing air	Chew foods slowly and thoroughly; avoid gas-producing foods, fatty foods, large meals; exercise; maintain regular bowel habits.
Varicose veins: may be associated with aching legs and tenderness; may be present in legs and vulva; hemorrhoids are varicosities in perianal area (Fig. 7-11)	Hereditary predisposition; relaxation of smooth muscle walls of veins because of hormones, causing pelvic vasocongestion; condition aggravated by enlarging uterus, gravity, and bearing down for bowel movements; thrombi from leg varices rare but may be produced by hemorrhoids	Avoidance of obesity, lengthy standing or sitting, constrictive clothing, and constipation and bearing down with bowel movements; moderate exercises; rest with legs and hips elevated (Fig. 7-12); wear support stockings; thrombosed hemorrhoid may be evacuated; relieve swelling and pain with warm sitz baths, local application of astringent compresses.
Leukorrhea: often noted throughout pregnancy	Hormonally stimulated cervix becomes hypertrophic and hyperactive, producing abundant amount of mucus	Not preventable; *do not douche;* hygiene; perineal pads; reassurance; refer to health care provider if accompanied by pruritus, foul odor, or change in character or color.

*Caution woman to rise slowly and sit on edge of bed or to assume hands-and-knees posture before rising and to get up slowly after sitting or squatting.

TABLE 7-3 Discomforts related to maternal adaptations to pregnancy in second trimester—cont'd

DISCOMFORT	PHYSIOLOGY	EDUCATION FOR SELF-CARE
Headaches (through week 26)	Emotional tension (more common than vascular migraine headache); eye strain (refractory errors); vascular engorgement and congestion of sinuses from hormone stimulation	Emotional support; prenatal teaching; conscious relaxation; refer to health care provider for constant "splitting" headache, after assessing for PIH.
Carpal tunnel syndrome (involves thumb, second and third fingers, lateral side of little finger)	Compression of median nerve from changes in surrounding tissues: pain, numbness, tingling, burning; loss of skilled movements (typing); dropping of objects	Not preventable; elevation of affected arms, splinting of affected hand may help; surgery is curative.
Periodic numbness, tingling of fingers (*acrodysesthesia*) occurs in 5% of pregnant women	Brachial plexus traction syndrome from drooping of shoulders during pregnancy (occurs especially at night and early morning)	Maintain good posture; wear supportive maternity bras; reassure that condition will disappear if lifting and carrying baby does not aggravate it.
Round ligament pain (tenderness)	Stretching of ligament caused by enlarging uterus	Not preventable; reassurance, rest, good body mechanics to avoid overstretching ligament; relieve cramping by squatting or bringing knees to chest.
Joint pain, backache, and pelvic pressure; hypermobility of joints	Relaxation of symphyseal and sacroiliac joints because of hormones, resulting in unstable pelvis; exaggerated lumbar and cervicothoracic curves caused by change in center of gravity from enlarging abdomen	Good posture and body mechanics; avoid fatigue; wear low-heeled shoes; conscious relaxation; firm mattress; local heat or ice and back rubs; pelvic rock exercise; rest; reassure that condition will disappear 6 to 8 weeks after birth.

ment as a basis for understanding the management of care during the second trimester.
2. The woman will list information for self-care.
3. The woman will list symptoms that indicate deviations from normal progress and protocols for reporting them.

Expected outcomes related to psychosocial care
1. The woman and her family will be active participants in her care during the second trimester of pregnancy.
2. The woman will continue to develop a birth plan.
3. The woman will describe continued confidence in her care.

Plan of Care and Implementation

The supportive and therapeutic nurse-patient relationship grows as the nurse implements the nursing process during the second trimester. The nausea often experienced in the first trimester has resolved. Nutrition counseling is offered at each visit, and the woman is complimented on her progress, as appropriate. Women experience several new discomforts or changes as maternal adaptations continue in the second trimester. Clear separation of discomforts and changes by trimester is impossible. However, for the benefit of this discussion, they have been separated (Table 7-3).

Reinforcement and counseling about sexuality and exposure to alcohol, cigarette smoke, and other substances are provided as necessary (see Chapter 11). Alcohol abuse during pregnancy is the leading cause of mental retardation in the infant. It is also associated with an increased risk of spontaneous abortion. No determination as to what is a safe amount of alcohol consumption during pregnancy has been made; therefore it is prudent to advise pregnant women to abstain completely (ACOG, 1994a).

Women who are prepared for the possibility of experiencing emotional changes are more likely to feel reassured that they are not unusual or unnatural and that it is acceptable to talk about their reactions. As pregnancy progresses, women become more open about their feelings toward themselves and others. Active listening by the nurse can help reassure women. If psychologic disturbance is severe, referral for appropriate treatment may be necessary.

Clothing. Comfortable, loose clothing is best. Washable fabrics (e.g., absorbent cottons) are often preferred. Maternity clothes may be purchased new or found at thrift shops or garage sales in good condition because they rarely wear out. Pregnant women should avoid tight bras and belts, stretch pants, garters, tight-top knee socks, panty girdles, and other constrictive clothing. Tight clothing over the perineum encourages vaginitis and miliaria (heat rash). Impaired circulation in the legs can cause varices.

Maternity bras are constructed to accommodate the increased breast weight, chest circumference, and size of breast tail tissue (under the arm). These bras have drop-flaps over the nipples to facilitate breastfeeding. A good bra can help prevent neckache and backache.

Elastic hose have been shown to give considerable comfort and result in greater venous emptying in women with large varicose veins (Fig. 7-11) (Nillson, Austrell, and Norgren, 1992; Priollet et al, 1994). Ideally, support stockings should be put on before the woman gets out of bed in the morning. Comfortable shoes that provide firm support and promote good posture and balance are advisable. High heels and platform shoes are not recommended because of the woman's changed center of gravity and a tendency to lose her balance. In the third trimester the woman's pelvis tilts forward and her

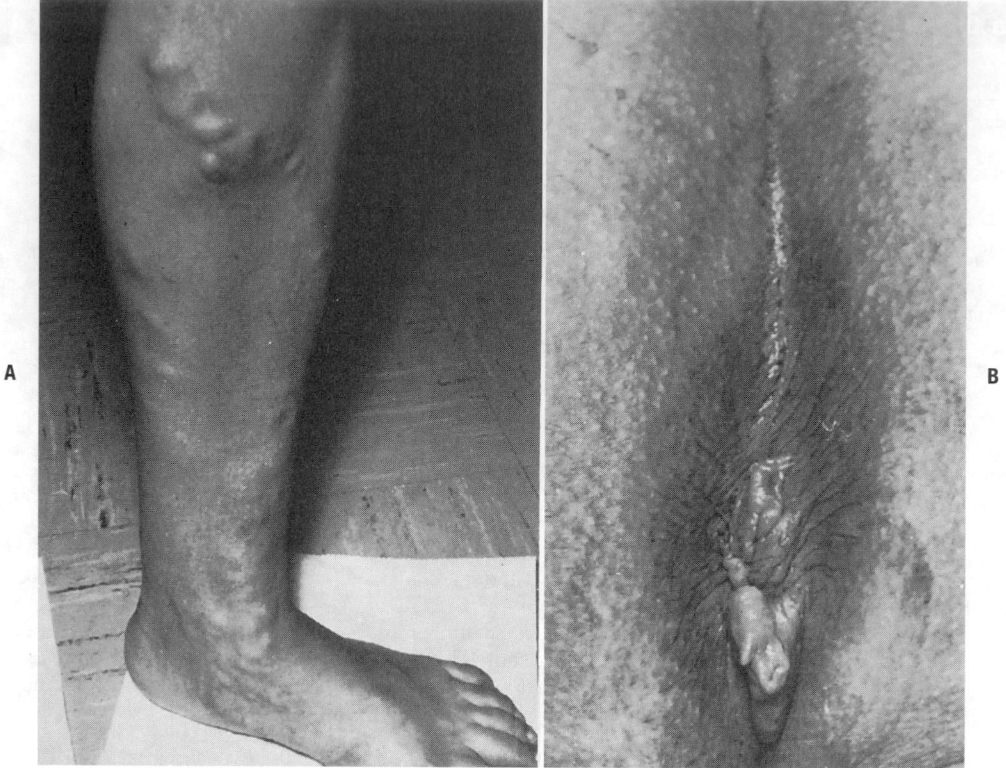

Fig. 7-11 **A,** Varicose veins of lower extremity. **B,** Varicosities of rectal area (hemorrhoids). (Courtesy Mercy Hospital and Medical Center, San Diego, Calif.)

lumbar curve increases. Leg aches and leg cramps are aggravated by nonsupportive shoes. Fig. 7-12 demonstrates a position to rest the legs and reduce swelling.

Posture and body mechanics. Many maternal adaptations predispose the woman to backache and possible injury. The pregnant woman's center of gravity changes. Pelvic joints soften and relax. Stress is placed on abdominal musculature (see Figs. 6-12 and 6-13). Poor posture and body mechanics contribute to discomfort and potential for injury. Women can acquire a kinesthetic sense for good body posture (Fig. 7-13).

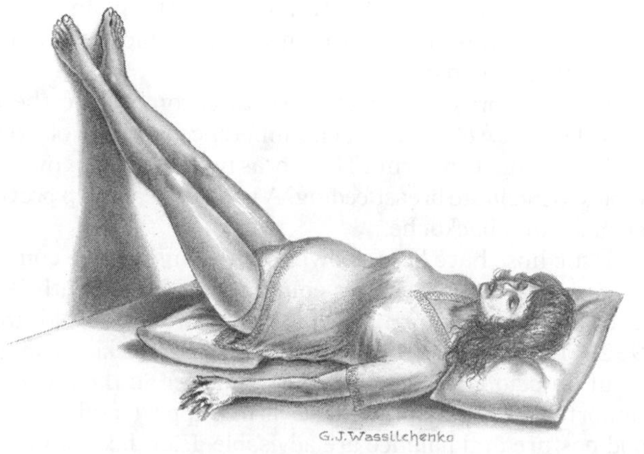

Fig. 7-12 Position for resting legs and for reducing swelling, edema and varicosities. Encourage woman with vulvar varicosities to include pillow under her hips.

In addition to fostering good posture, the activities discussed in the Patient Teaching box on p. 155 can be used.

Bathing and swimming. Tub bathing is permitted even in late pregnancy because water does not enter the vagina unless under pressure. However, tub bathing is usually contraindicated after rupture of the membranes. Baths and warm showers can be therapeutic because they relax tense tired muscles, help counter insomnia, and make the pregnant woman feel fresh. However, physical maneuverability presents a problem (increased chance of falling) late in pregnancy.

Swimming is permitted during normal pregnancy, although diving is discouraged because of possible injury.

Physical activity. Physical activity promotes a feeling of well-being in the pregnant woman. It improves circulation, assists relaxation and rest, and counteracts boredom, as it does in the nonpregnant woman. Exercise tips for pregnancy are presented in detail in the Home Care box on p. 136. Suggestions for teaching the patient Kegel exercise to strengthen the muscles around the reproductive organs and improve muscle tone are discussed on p. 136. Exercises that help relieve low back pain that often occurs during the second trimester from the increased weight of the fetus are demonstrated in Figure 7-7.

Rest and relaxation. The pregnant woman is encouraged to plan regular rest periods, particularly as pregnancy advances (Fig. 7-14). The side-lying position is recommended to promote uterine perfusion and fetoplacental oxygenation by

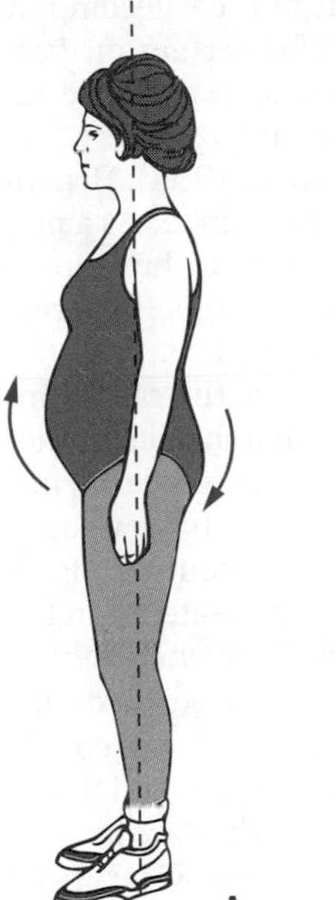

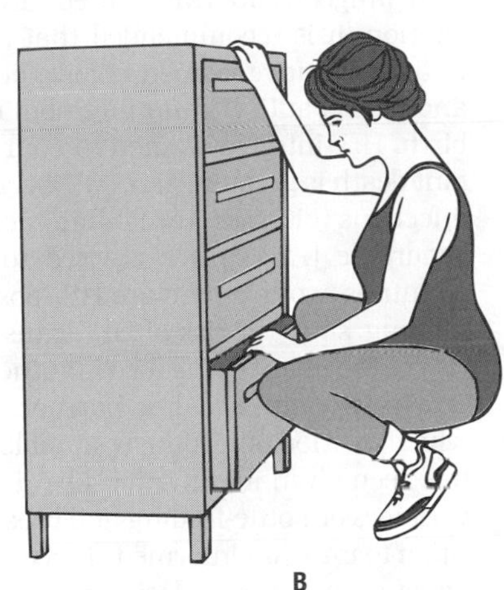

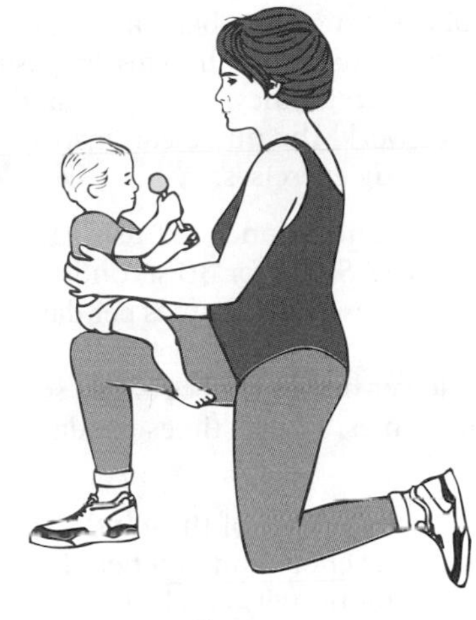

Fig. 7-13 Correct body mechanics. **A,** Standing. **B,** Squatting. **C,** Lifting.

Patient Teaching

POSTURE AND BODY MECHANICS

To prevent or relieve backache

- Perform pelvic tilt:
  —Do **pelvic tilt (rock)** on hands and knees and while sitting in straight-back chair (Fig. 7-7, *A*).
  —Do pelvic tilt (rock) in standing position against a wall or lying on floor (Fig. 7-7, *B* and *C*).
  —Perform abdominal muscle contractions during pelvic tilt while standing, lying, or sitting to help strengthen rectus abdominis muscle (Fig. 7-7, *D*).
- Use good body mechanics:
  —Use leg muscles to reach objects on or near floor. Bend at knees, not back. Knees are bent to lower body to squatting position. Feet are kept 12 to 18 inches apart for a solid base to maintain balance (Fig. 7-13, *B*).
  —Lift with legs. To lift heavy object (e.g., young child), one foot is placed slightly in front of the other and kept flat as woman lowers herself on one knee. She lifts the weight holding it close to her body and never higher than chest level. To stand up or sit down, one leg is placed slightly behind the other as she raises or lowers herself (Fig. 7-13, *C*).

To restrict lumbar curve

- Wear maternity girdle to support weak abdominal muscles.
- For prolonged standing (e.g., ironing, out-of-home employment), place one foot on low footstool or box; change positions often.
- Move car seat forward so that knees are bent and higher than hips. If needed, use small pillow to support low back area.
- Sit in chairs low enough to allow both feet on floor and preferably with knees higher than hips.

To prevent round ligament pain and strain on abdominal muscles

- Implement suggestions given in Table 7-3.

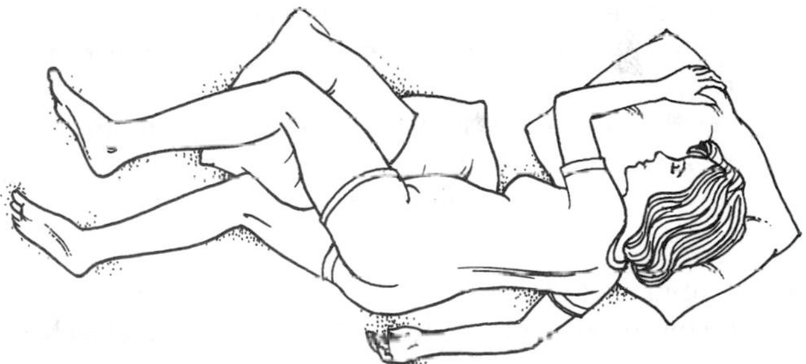

Fig. 7-14 Side-lying position for rest and relaxation. Some women prefer to support upper leg with pillows.

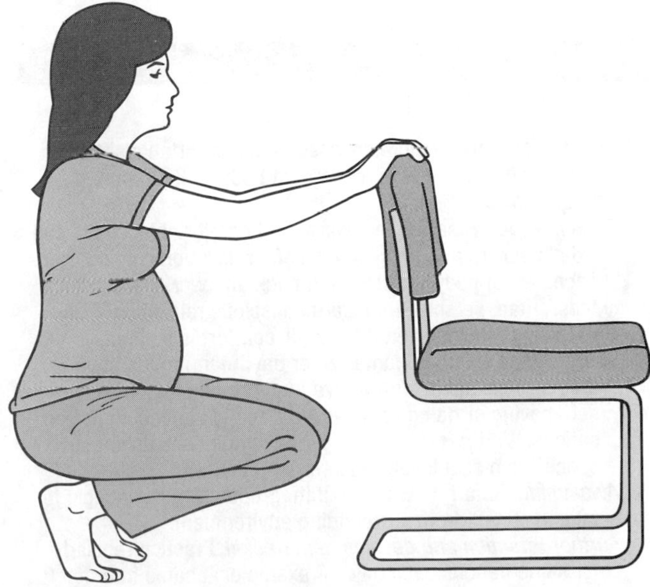

Fig. 7-15 Squatting for muscle relaxation and strengthening and for keeping leg and hip joints flexible.

eliminating pressure on the ascending vena cava and descending aorta (supine hypotension). During shorter rest periods the woman can assume the position in Fig. 7-12 to promote venous drainage from the legs and relieve leg edema and varicose veins. The mother is shown how to rise slowly from a side-lying position to avoid strain on the back and minimize the orthostatic hypotension caused by changes in position common in the latter part of pregnancy. To stretch and rest back muscles at home or at work, the nurse can instruct the woman to perform the following exercises:

Stand behind a chair. Support and balance self using the back of the chair (Fig. 7-15). Squat for 30 seconds; stand for 15 seconds. Repeat 6 times, several times per day, as needed.

While sitting in the chair, lower head to knees for 30 seconds. Raise up. Repeat 6 times, several times per day, as needed.

Conscious relaxation is the release of the mind and body from tension through conscious effort and practice. The ability to relax consciously and intentionally can be beneficial for the following reasons:

Relief of normal discomforts related to pregnancy

Reduction of stress and therefore diminished pain perception during the childbearing cycle

Heightened self-awareness and trust in own ability to control one's responses and functions

Coping with stress in everyday life situations, pregnant or not

The techniques for conscious relaxation are numerous and varied. The guidelines given in the Patient Teaching box below can be used by anyone.

Preparation for feeding newborn. Pregnant women are usually eager to discuss their plans for feeding the newborn. Breast milk is the food of choice, and breastfeeding is associated with a decreased incidence in perinatal morbidity and mortality. However, deep-seated aversion to breastfeeding by the mother or father, the mother's need for certain medications, and certain medical complications, such as active tuberculosis, newly diagnosed breast cancer, and hepatitis C, are contraindications to breastfeeding (Lawrence, 1994). Hepatitis B antigen is not transmitted through breast milk. As a precaution, it is recommended that infants born to hepatitis B antigen–positive women receive both the hepatitis B vaccine and the hepatitis B immune globulin (HBIG) immediately after birth. HIV-infected women in countries where the rate of infant death is greater than 50% because of diarrhea and other infectious diseases (excluding acquired immunodeficiency syndrome [AIDS]) are advised to breastfeed. In developed countries, women who are HIV positive are discouraged from nursing, since the risk of HIV transmission is greater than the risk of the infant dying form another cause (Lawrence, 1994).

The woman and her partner are encouraged to decide which method of feeding is suitable for them. Once the couple has been given information about the advantages and disadvantages of bottle-feeding and breastfeeding, they are in a position to make an informed choice. Health care providers need only to support their decisions.

The **pinch test** determines whether the nipple is everted or inverted (Fig. 7-16). The nurse guides the woman through this test. The woman places her thumb and forefinger on her areola and presses inward gently. This causes her nipple to stand erect or to invert. Most nipples stand erect.

In the past it was recommended that women with flat or inverted nipples do exercises to break the adhesions that cause the nipple to invert. Studies have shown that this does not work and that it may cause uterine contractions (Lawrence, 1994). The use of breast shells for women with flat or inverted nipples is still recommended (Fig. 7-17). A continuous, gentle pressure exerted around the areola pushes the nipple through a central opening in the inner shield. Breast shells should be worn during the last trimester of pregnancy for 1 to 2 hours daily. The time for wearing them should be increased gradually (Lawrence, 1994). Alexander, Grant, and Campbell (1990) found that women who wore breast shells or did nipple-rolling exercises (now contraindicated in all patients) were less likely to breastfeed than those women who had no treatment. Therefore the decision to recommend the use of breast shells to women with flat or inverted nipples must be made judiciously. Continuous support and guidance to the woman must be part of the plan.

Patient Teaching

CONSCIOUS RELAXATION

Preparation. Loosen clothing, assume a comfortable sitting or side-lying position with all parts of body well-supported with pillows.

Beginning. Allow self to feel warm and comfortable. Inhale and exhale slowly, and imagine peaceful relaxation coming over each part of body, starting with neck and working down to toes. Often, persons who learn conscious relaxation speak of feeling relaxed even if some discomfort is present.

Maintenance. Imagine (fantasize or daydream) to maintain state of relaxation. With *active imagery,* one imagines oneself moving or doing some activity and experiencing its sensations. With *passive imagery,* one imagines watching a scene, such as a lovely sunset.

Awakening. Return to wakeful state gradually. Slowly begin to take in stimuli from surrounding environment.

Further retention and development of skill. Practice regularly for some periods each day, for example, at same hour for 10 to 15 minutes each day to feel refreshed, revitalized, and invigorated.

Nursing ALERT

Breast stimulation may produce uterine activity and is not recommended for women at risk for preterm labor.

The woman is taught that nipples are cleansed with warm water to prevent blocking of the ducts with dried colostrum. Soap, ointments, alcohol, and tinctures are not used because they remove protective oils that keep nipples supple. The use of these substances may cause cracking of the nipple during early lactation (Lawrence, 1994).

The woman who plans to breastfeed should purchase a nursing bra that will accommodate the increased size required for the last few months of pregnancy, as well as for lac-

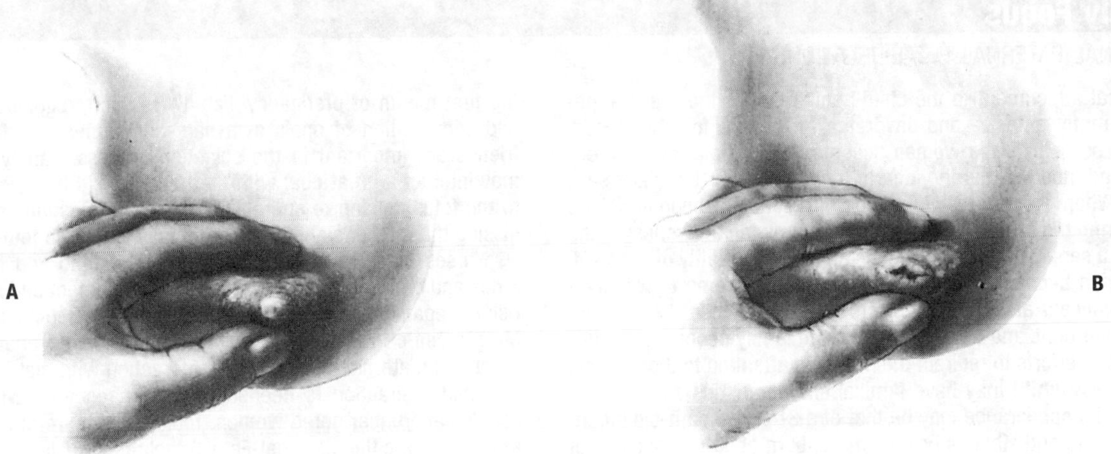

Fig. 7-16 Pinch test. **A,** Normal nipple everts with gentle pressure. **B,** Inverted or tied nipple inverts with gentle pressure. (Modified from Lawrence R: *Breastfeeding: a guide for the medical profession* ed 4, St Louis, 1994, Mosby.)

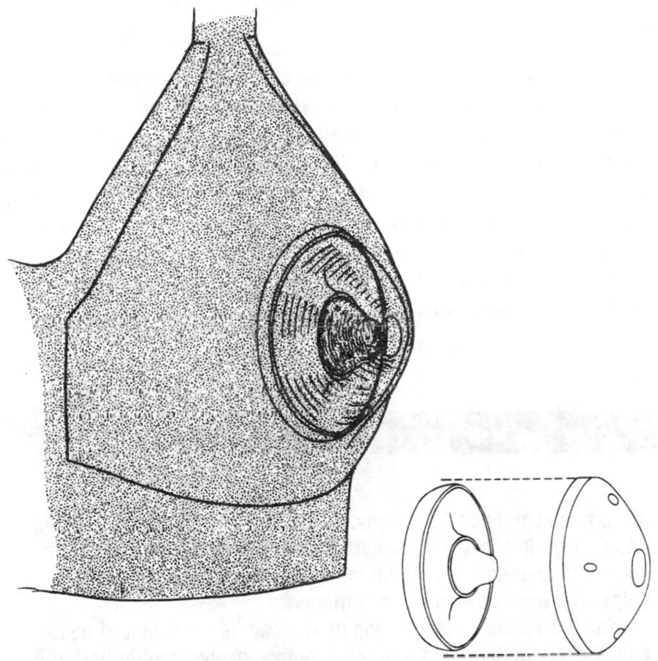

Fig. 7-17 Breast shell in place inside bra to evert nipple. (Modified from Lawrence R: *Breastfeeding: a guide for the medical profession,* ed 4, St. Louis, 1994, Mosby.)

tation. If her breasts are very heavy, or if the woman feels uncomfortable with the weight unsupported, the bra can be worn day and night.

Evaluation

Maternal and fetal expected outcomes are continuously evaluated according to measurable, established criteria. The clinical findings that represent normal responses are presented as plans and expected outcomes in the nursing care plans for each patient. These criteria are used as a basis for selecting appropriate nursing actions and evaluating their effectiveness.

THIRD TRIMESTER

The quiet period of the second trimester gives way to an active period, a trimester with more emphasis on the practical realities of expectant parenthood. Parental attachment to the fetus increases in the third trimester, a period spanning weeks 27 to 40 (see the first Family Focus box on p. 158). Mixed among the daydreams about the "coming baby" are parental anxieties that focus on possible defects in mental and physical abilities of the child. The expectant mother's attention turns to thoughts of a **safe passage** (uneventful birth process) for herself and her child (Patterson, Freese, and Goldenburg, 1990). Fears of pain and mutilation and concerns about her behavior and possible loss of control and loss of self-esteem during labor are important issues.

Physical discomforts and fetal movements often interrupt the expectant mother's rest. Dyspnea, return of urinary frequency, backache, constipation, and **varicosities** are experienced by many women in late pregnancy. Increased bulkiness and awkwardness affect the woman's ability to perform ADLs. Positions of comfort are more difficult to achieve. Increasingly, she becomes more impatient to "get this over with."

Second-Time Mothers

Mothers expecting a second child have different concerns in pregnancy than first-time mothers. They may have unresolved feelings about their first labor. They may be so focused on their first child that they are less excited and think less about the second baby than they did about the first. They are concerned about the first child's reaction to separation at the sibling's birth and are aware that a change in their relationship with the first child will occur after the new baby is born. These concerns may lead to a sense of loss and sadness. Friends and family, assured of the mother's ability to care for an infant, may offer less attention and help than they did during the first pregnancy.

Expectant Fathers/Partners

Many expectant fathers/partners become more involved with the pregnancy as pregnancy progresses (see the Family Focus

Family Focus

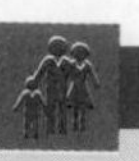

MATERNAL-PATERNAL-FETAL RELATIONSHIP

Emotional attachment to the child begins during the prenatal period. Parents fantasize and daydream to prepare for parenthood. Early in pregnancy the woman accepts the biologic fact of pregnancy and incorporates the idea of a child into her body and self-image. When the fetus is viewed on ultrasound, it becomes more real. During the second trimester there is growing awareness of the child as a separate being. When she accepts the reality of the child, the woman becomes more introspective. She seems to withdraw and to concentrate her interest on the unborn child. Her partner may feel left out, and other children in the family become more demanding in efforts to redirect the mother's attention to themselves. The **fantasy child** may have familial characteristics and superior abilities; its appearance may be that of a 3- or 4-month-old infant. Both parents and siblings believe the unborn child responds in an individualized, personal manner. Some families become involved by picking the child's name and anticipating the child's sex if it is not already known. Some families select the child's name as early as the first month of pregnancy. Family tradition, religious customs, and continuation of one's own name or names of relatives and friends are important in the selection process. Family members may interact a great deal with the unborn child by trying to listen to the fetus, talking to and playing with the fetus, and stroking or kissing the mother's abdomen, especially when the fetus moves.

Nurses must continue to seek to understand and foster attitudes and behaviors that promote early attachment and reduce the risk of negative long-term effects such as child neglect and abuse. More research relating psychologic variables to prenatal attachment and maternal-paternal-fetal interaction with maternal-paternal-child interaction is needed, including research with lesbian couples and unpartnered women. Tools to measure maternal-fetal attachment are the Maternal-Fetal Attachment Scale (MFAS) (Cranley, 1981) and the Prenatal Attachment Inventory (PAI) (Müller, 1993).

box below). Activity and energy to create and achieve characterize this phase. For men, styles of involvement differ according to their perception of the male and fathering roles within their social groups. Men begin to redefine their relationships to the fetus and to themselves as fathers. Role playing through daydreaming is common. Expectant fathers/partners have some of the same concerns as expectant mothers. Often, however, they may not share these concerns with anyone.

Some men experience emotional lability and ambivalence. Some fathers experience the **couvade** syndrome and report discomforts usually associated with women in pregnancy, such as nausea and fatigue, throughout pregnancy. *Mitleiden* (suffering along), or the experience of expectant fathers having psychomatic symptoms, has long been recognized as a phenomenon of expectant fatherhood.

If the pregnancy is unplanned or unwanted, some men find the alterations in life plans and life-styles difficult to ac-

Family Focus

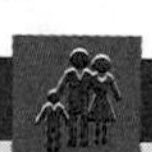

PATERNAL ADAPTATION

Expectant fathers, as with expectant mothers, have been preparing for parenthood throughout their lives. Subconsciously or consciously, most men think about having a wife and children. During courtship and early marriage, discussion of future plans may include the number, spacing, and names of their children-to-be.

In primitive societies, men enacted the ritual couvade, that is, behaved in specific ways and respected taboos associated with pregnancy and giving birth. In this way a man's new status was recognized and endorsed. His behavior acknowledged his psychosocial and biologic relationship to the mother and child.

A man's emotional responses to becoming a father, his concerns, and his informational needs change over the 9 months of pregnancy. May (1982) described three phases characterizing developmental tasks experienced by the expectant father: the announcement phase, the moratorium phase, and focusing phase.

The early period, the **announcement phase,** may last from a few hours to a few weeks. The developmental task is to accept the biologic fact of pregnancy. Men react to the confirmation of pregnancy with joy or dismay depending on whether the pregnancy is desired, unplanned, or unwanted.

The second phase, the moratorium phase, is the period of adjusting to the reality of pregnancy. This phase may be relatively short or persist until the last trimester. The developmental task is to accept the pregnancy. Men appear to put conscious thought of the pregnancy aside for a time. They become more introspective and engage in many discussions about their philosophy of life, religion, childbearing and childrearing practices, and their relationships with family members and friends.

The third phase, the focusing phase, begins in the last trimester and is characterized by the father's active involvement in both the pregnancy and his relationship with his child. The developmental task is to negotiate with his partner the role he is to play in labor and to prepare for parenthood. In this phase the man concentrates on his experience of pregnancy and begins to think of himself as a father.

The father's beliefs and feelings about the ideal mother and father and his cultural expectation of appropriate behavior during pregnancy affect his response to his partner's need for him. One man may engage in nurturing behavior. Another may feel lonely and alienated as the woman becomes physically and emotionally engrossed in the unborn child. The man may seek comfort and understanding outside the home or become interested in a new hobby or involved with his work. Some men view pregnancy as a proof of their masculinity and their dominant role. To others, pregnancy has no meaning in terms of responsibility to either mother or child. For most men, however, pregnancy is a time of preparation for the parental role, of fantasy, of great pleasure, and of intense learning.

Family Focus

SIBLING ADAPTATION TO PREGNANCY AND BIRTH

Sharing the spotlight with a new brother or sister may be the first major crisis for a child. The older child often experiences a sense of loss or feels jealous upon being "replaced" by the new baby. Some of the factors that influence the child's response are age, the parents' attitudes, the father's role, the length of separation from the mother, the hospital's visitation policy, and how the child has been prepared for the change (Mackey and Miller, 1992).

The mother with other children must devote time and energy to reorganizing her relationships with these children. She needs to prepare siblings for the child's birth and to begin the process of role transition in the family by including the children in the pregnancy and being sympathetic to older children's protests against losing their places in the family hierarchy. No child willingly gives up a familiar position.

Siblings' responses to pregnancy vary with age and dependency needs. The 1-year-old infant seems largely unaware of the process, but the 2-year-old child notices the change in mother's appearance and may comment, "Mommy's fat." The 2-year-old child's need for sameness in the environment makes the child aware of any change. Toddlers may exhibit more "clinging" behavior and revert to dependent behaviors in toilet training or eating.

By the age 3 or 4, children like to be told the story of their own beginning and accept its comparison to the present pregnancy. They like to listen to heartbeats and feel the baby moving in utero. Sometimes they worry about how the baby is being fed and what it wears. Parents often take older children with them to antepartal visits, particularly in the last few weeks. Interference with established routines can cause anger. Sharing possessions with the unborn child is often short-lived, and cribs or toys donated to the coming child are mostly reclaimed.

School-age children take a more clinical interest in their mother's pregnancy. They may want to know in more detail, "How did the baby get in there?" and "How will it get out?" Children in this age-group notice pregnant women in stores, churches, and schools and sometimes seem shy if they need to approach a pregnant woman directly. On the whole they look forward to the new baby, see themselves as "mothers" or "fathers," and enjoy buying baby supplies and readying a place for the baby. Because they still think in concrete terms and base judgments on the here and now, they respond positively to their mother's current good health and do not seem to be anxious about a future injury to her or to the unborn child. They need help to cope with any adverse change in the status of the parent or newborn, since they do not anticipate such a change.

Early and middle adolescents preoccupied with the establishment of their own sexual identity may have difficulty accepting the overwhelming evidence of the sexual activity of their parents. They reason that if they are "too young" for such activity, certainly their parents are "too old." They seem to take on a critical parental role and may ask, "What will people think?" or "How can you let yourself get so fat?" Many pregnant women with teenage children confess that their teenagers are the most difficult factor in their current pregnancy.

On the positive side, parents-to-be may be suddenly confronted by a warm, sensitive person who is able to restore the mother's self-esteem, as illustrated by the following example.

> I came home one day feeling very pregnant, tired, and heavy and dreading the idea of making dinner and being helpful—you know—the "mother bit!" Mary [age 15] was cooking some hamburger, had the table set for dinner, and even had a flower centerpiece. For some reason I just started to cry. She came to me and hugged me and said, "I think you're doing the loveliest thing in the world, having a baby." I'll always remember that—she was really my mother for the moment.

Late adolescents do not appear to be unduly disturbed. They think that they soon will be gone from home. Parents usually report they are comforting and act more as other adults than as children. One mother expecting her tenth baby remarked, "The only complaint my oldest daughter made was, 'Mother, I'm getting married in August, so don't you dare be too pregnant to come to the wedding.'"

Classes to prepare children for the birth of a new brother or sister are available in many communities (see Fig. 7-22). A general teaching plan parents can use for young children is found in the Patient Teaching box on p. 160. The general plan can be modified to fit needs of children of different ages and the needs of children who will be present during the birth.

cept. Some men engage in extramarital affairs for the first time during pregnancy. Others batter their partners (McFarlane et al, 1992).

Expectant families approaching childbirth have many needs. Siblings and grandparents need to be considered, too (see the Family Focus boxes above and on p. 160). Clearly the nurse is in a pivotal position within the health care team to assist parents with these needs during the third trimester of pregnancy. The schedule of care reflects the increased needs. Starting with week 28, visits are scheduled every 2 weeks until week 36; then they occur every week until birth.

Nursing Care Management

Assessment

During the third trimester, current family involvement in the pregnancy is assessed, for example, siblings' and grandparents' responses to the pregnancy and the coming child. In addition, the following questions are addressed:

- What anticipatory planning is in progress concerning new parenting responsibilities, sibling rivalry, recuperation from pregnancy and birth, and fertility management?
- What successes or frustrations is the mother experiencing with diet, rest and relaxation, sexuality, and emotional support?
- What is the mother's understanding of her family's needs in relation to the pregnancy and child?
- How well prepared are the parents in the event of emergency? That is, does the mother know and understand warning signs and how and to whom to report them?
- Does the mother know the signs of preterm and term labor?
- What is the mother's understanding of the labor process and expectations of herself and others during labor; does she know what to bring to the hospital or birthing center?

Patient Teaching

TIPS FOR SIBLING PREPARATION

Prenatal

1 Take your child on a prenatal visit. Let the child listen to the fetal heart beat and feel the baby move.
2 Involve the child in preparations for the baby, such as helping decorate the baby's room.
3 Move the child to a bed (if still sleeping in a crib) at least 2 months before the baby is due.
4 Read books, show videos, and/or take child to sibling preparation classes including a hospital tour.
5 Answer your child's questions about the coming birth, what babies are like, and any other question.
6 Take your child to the homes of friends who have babies so that the child has realistic expectations of what babies are like.

During the Hospital Stay

1 Have someone bring the child to the hospital to visit you and the baby (unless you plan to have the child attend the birth).
2 Don't force interactions between the child and the baby. Often the child will be more interested in seeing you and being reassured of your love.
3 Help the child explore the infant by showing how and where to touch the baby.
4 Give the child a gift (from you or you, the father, and baby).

Going Home

1 Have someone bring the child to the hospital to visit you and the baby (unless you plan to have the child attend the birth).
2 Have someone else carry the baby from the car so that you can hug the child first.

Adjustment after the Baby Is Home

1 Arrange for a special time with the child alone with each parent.
2 Don't exclude the child during infant feeding times. The child can sit with you and the baby and feed a doll or drink juice or milk with you or sit quietly with a game.
3 Prepare small gifts for the child so that when the baby gets gifts, the sibling won't feel left out. The child can also help open the baby gifts.
4 Praise the child for acting age appropriately (so that being a baby does not seem better than being older).

Family Focus

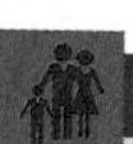

GRANDPARENT ADAPTATION TO PREGNANCY AND BIRTH

Every pregnancy affects all family relationships. For grandparents, their child's first pregnancy is undeniable evidence that they are now old enough to have a grandchild. Many think of grandparents as old, white haired, and becoming feeble of mind and body; however, some people face grandparenthood when still in their 30s or 40s. A mother-to-be announcing her pregnancy to her mother may be greeted by a negative response indicating that she is not ready to be a grandmother. Both daughter and mother may be startled and hurt by the response.

Some grandparents-to-be not only are nonsupportive but also use subtle means to decrease the self-esteem of the young parents-to-be. Mothers may talk about their terrible pregnancies; fathers may discuss the endless cost of rearing children; and mothers-in-law may describe the neglect of their sons when the concern of others is directed toward the pregnant daughters-in-law.

However, most grandparents are delighted with the prospect of a new baby in the family. It reawakens their feelings of their own youth, the excitement of giving birth, and their delight in the behavior of the parents-to-be when they were infants. They set up a memory store of first smiles, first words, and first steps that can be used later for "claiming" the newborn as a member of the family. Satisfaction comes with the realization that continuity between past and present is guaranteed.

The grandparent is the historian who transmits the history of the family and provides continuity with the present, a resource person who shares knowledge based on experience, a role model, and a support person. The grandparent's presence and support can strengthen family systems by widening the circle of support and nurturance (Barranti, 1985). Other sources of information cannot replace grandparents' unique contribution. The parent acts as negotiator in establishing the grandparent-grandchild relationship (Greene and Polivka, 1985).

Many women report that their pregnancies bridged the final gap between them and their own mothers. The estrangement that began in adolescence disappears as the now-pregnant daughter experiences joys, concerns, and anxieties similar to those her mother felt before her.

Expectant grandparenthood can be a maturational crisis for the parent of an expectant parent. To be truly family oriented, maternity care must include the grandparent in implementing the nursing process with childbearing families. Grandparents' classes represent one method of facilitating the adjustment to the grandparenting role, incorporating the grandparents into the family system, and encouraging communication between the generations (Maloni et al, 1987)

Grandparents' anxieties and concerns and their relationships with expectant parents and grandchildren should be discussed during courses for expectant parents. The expectant parents may use this opportunity to begin to resolve conflicts and perceived differences with their parents, a task that can enhance their ability to relate to their own children.

BOX 7-8
Third-Trimester Checklist

Schedule and events of visits
Counseling for self-care
- Adaptations/discomforts
  - Dyspnea
  - Insomnia
  - Psychosocial responses and family dynamics
  - Gingivitis and epulis
  - Urinary frequency
  - Perineal discomfort and pressure
  - Braxton Hicks contractions
  - Leg cramps
  - Ankle edema
- Safety (balance)
- Exercise and rest
- Relaxation
- Nutrition
- Sexuality
- Warning signs of potential complications
- Warning signs of preterm labor

Fetal growth and development
Preparation for baby
- Feeding method
- Nipple preparation

Preparation for labor
- Recognition: false vs. true
- Prenatal classes
- Control of discomfort
- Hospital tour
- Provision for other family members
- Preparation for homecoming

Diagnostic tests
- Specify

Other

- If she is having a home birth, have all the necessary supplies been obtained?
- What plans has the mother and her family made for labor?
- What anxieties are the mother or her family experiencing regarding labor or birth?
- What does the mother want to know about control of discomfort during labor?
- Is the mother (and her partner or support person) planning to attend any parent education classes?
- Does the mother have questions about fetal development and methods to assess fetal well-being?

A checklist for third-trimester assessment should be used to ensure that important areas are addressed (Box 7-8).

Signs of potential problems. The nurse is constantly on the alert for potential problems, such as the following:

- Hemorrhagic conditions
- Vaginal bleeding
- Severe abdominal pain
- Hypertensive conditions
  - Visual disturbances: blurring, double vision, or spots
  - Swelling of face or fingers and over sacrum
  - Headaches: severe, frequent, or continuous
  - Muscular irritability or convulsions
  - Epigastric pain (perceived as severe stomachache)
- Infections
  - Positive laboratory test results
  - Chills, fever
  - Burning on urination, frequency, aching back and side
  - Diarrhea
- Diabetes mellitus
- Glucosuria
- Positive glucose tolerance test reaction
- Fluid discharge from vagina
- Amniotic fluid
- Signs of preterm labor

Maternal Assessment

Interview. The initial question in the third-trimester interview is asked with the intent to identify the woman's main concern of the moment. Focusing on the woman takes advantage of her readiness to learn and affirms the caregiver's interest in her as a person.

Based on the woman's expressed needs, her status to date, and the general needs of most women in late pregnancy, the nurse's knowledge and clinical judgment guide the content and direction of the interview.

The nurse determines whether the woman attended or plans to attend classes. If so, what questions and concerns arose from the second-trimester class that need to be addressed? Does the couple plan to attend third-trimester parent-education classes? Has the birth plan been developed with realistic expectations? Is the plan feasible, flexible, and safe?

A review of physical systems is appropriate at each meeting. Any suspicious signs or symptoms are assessed in depth. Discomforts reflecting pregnancy adaptations are identified. Special inquiries are made about possible infections (e.g., genitourinary tract, respiratory tract). Knowledge of and success with self-care measures and prescribed therapy are assessed. Psychosocial responses to the pregnancy and approaching parenthood are evaluated.

Physical examination. During the third-trimester physical examination, temperature, pulse, respirations, blood pressure, and weight are assessed and noted. Suspicious signs and symptoms uncovered during the interview are evaluated. Presence, location, and degree of edema are documented carefully. Gestational age is confirmed and fundal height measured. Leopold's maneuvers are performed to determine fetal position (see p. 404). Risk assessment continues throughout the third trimester.

Laboratory tests. At each visit, urine is tested for glucose (to assess for diabetes), protein (to assess for PIH), and nitrites and leukocytes (to assess for infection). A urine culture and sensitivity test is done as necessary. Hematocrit determination by finger stick is made at each visit in some facilities. Blood tests are repeated as necessary: rapid plasma reagin (RPR) test for syphilis; Complete blood count (CBC) with hematocrit, hemoglobin, and differential values; antibody screen (Kell, Duffy, rubella, toxoplasmosis, anti-Rh, HIV); sickle cell; and level of folacin when indicated. If not done earlier in pregnancy, a glucose screen for women over age 25 is performed. Glucose challenge is usually done between 24 and 28 weeks.

Fetal Assessment

Fetal health status is evaluated at each visit. Beginning in the thirty-second week, identification of fetal presentation, position, and station (engagement), with the aid of Leopold's maneuvers (see Fig. 16-4), is done weekly. Box 7-9 and Fig. 7-18 summarize this period of rapid fetal growth.

Fundal height is measured at each visit. The method described on p. 148 is used. Uterine measurements are compared with supposed duration of pregnancy. Possible IUGR, multifetal pregnancy, or inaccuracy of the EDB may be disclosed by ultrasound.

The mother is requested to describe fetal movements. She is asked if she has warning signs to report, such as rupture of membranes or absence of or decreased fetal movement.

Nursing Diagnoses

Each woman and her family respond to and are affected by pregnancy in different ways. Careful monitoring of the pregnancy and responses to care is of the utmost importance. The following items are representative of nursing diagnoses that may be formulated in the third trimester from the data base of a low-risk pregnancy.

- Ineffective individual coping related to knowledge deficit regarding
  - Assessment for risks such as preterm labor
  - Recognizing onset of true versus false labor
  - Self-care measures
  - Emergency arrangements

BOX 7-9

Fetal Development at 40 Weeks

Nutrients and maternal immunoglobulins stored
Subcutaneous fat deposited
Dramatic storage of iron, nitrogen, and calcium
In male: testes are within well-wrinkled scrotum
In female: labia are well developed and cover vestibule
Lanugo shed, except for shoulders, generally
Body contours plump
Decreased vernix
Scalp hair 2 to 3 cm long
Cartilage in nose and ears well developed
45 to 55 cm (18 to 22 inches) in length
Weighs 3400 g ($7\frac{1}{2}$ pounds) (average)
Fundal height below xiphoid after lightening

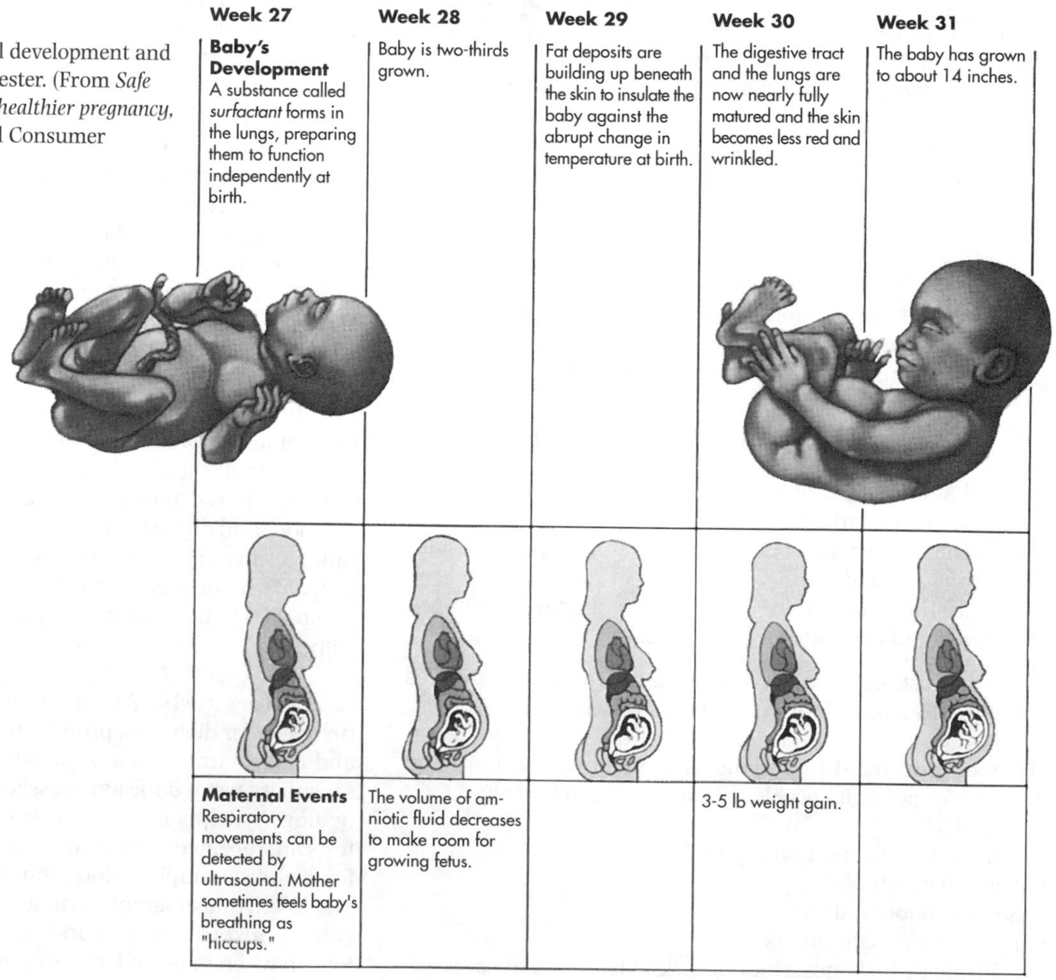

	Week 27	Week 28	Week 29	Week 30	Week 31
Baby's Development	A substance called *surfactant* forms in the lungs, preparing them to function independently at birth.	Baby is two-thirds grown.	Fat deposits are building up beneath the skin to insulate the baby against the abrupt change in temperature at birth.	The digestive tract and the lungs are now nearly fully matured and the skin becomes less red and wrinkled.	The baby has grown to about 14 inches.
Maternal Events	Respiratory movements can be detected by ultrasound. Mother sometimes feels baby's breathing as "hiccups."	The volume of amniotic fluid decreases to make room for growing fetus.		3-5 lb weight gain.	

Fig. 7-18 Summary of fetal development and maternal events—third trimester. (From *Safe passage: a woman's guide to a healthier pregnancy,* Fort Washington, Pa, McNeil Consumer Products.)

- Altered family processes related to
  Inadequate understanding of third-trimester changes and needs
  Increased concern about labor
  Insomnia or sleep deficit
- Sleep pattern disturbance related to
  Discomforts of late pregnancy
  Anxiety about approaching labor
- Activity intolerance related to
  Increased weight and change in center of gravity
  Anxiety
  Sleep disturbances

Expected Outcomes

Planning care for women and their families during the third trimester of pregnancy is given direction from identified nursing diagnoses and from a comprehensive view of the expectant family. A plan is developed mutually with the woman to the extent possible. The plan is individualized, relating specifically to the woman's and her family's needs. Expected outcomes are similar to those of the first and second trimesters.

Expected outcomes related to physiologic care

1. The woman and her family will describe pertinent information about maternal adaptations and fetal development as a basis for understanding the management of care during the third trimester.
2. The woman will list information for self-care.
3. The woman will list symptoms that indicate deviations from normal progress and protocols for reporting them.
4. The woman will list signs of preterm labor and protocols for reporting them.
5. The woman will list the differences between true and false labor.

Expected outcomes related to psychosocial care

1. The woman and her family will be active participants in her care during the third trimester of pregnancy.
2. The woman will finalize her birth plan.
3. The woman will express continued confidence in her care.

Plan of Care and Implementation

Social support. Esteem, affection, trust, concern, consideration of cultural and religious responses, and listening are components of emotional support. The woman's feelings of satisfaction with her relationships and support, as well as her feeling of competence and sense of being in control, are important issues to address in the third trimester. A discussion of parental awareness of the unborn child's responses to stimuli, such as sound, light, maternal posture, tension, and patterns of sleeping and waking can be helpful. Opportunities are also provided to discuss probable emotional tensions related to the following: childbirth experience, such as fear of pain, loss of

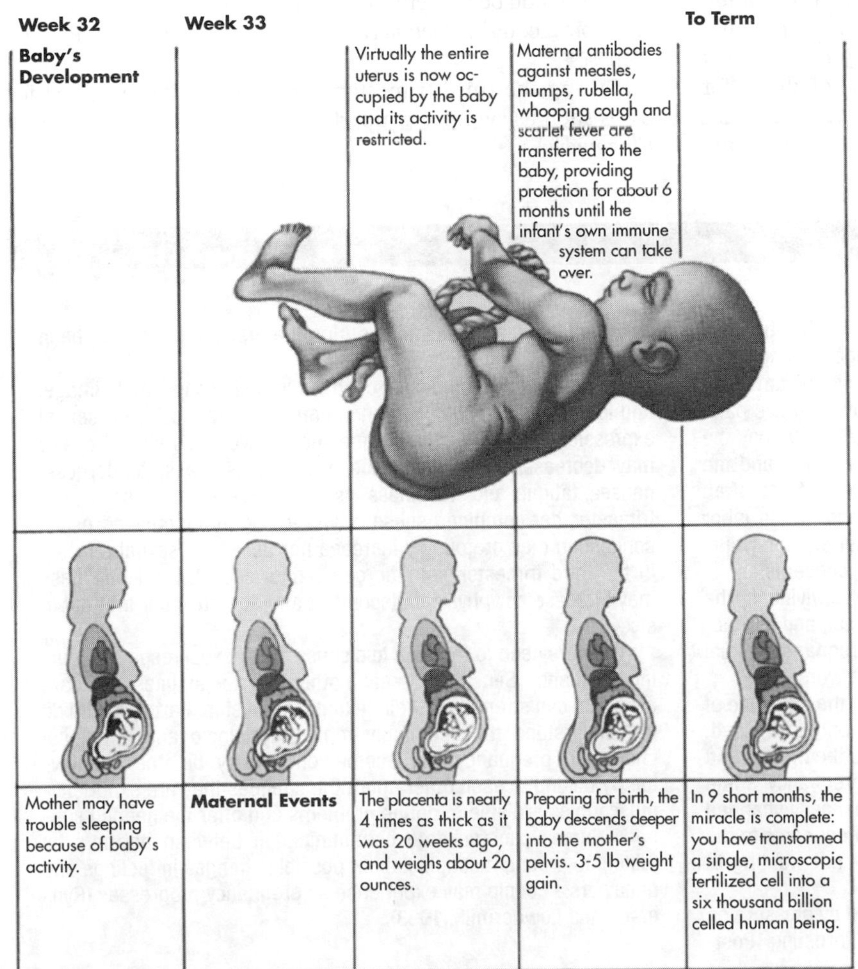
Week 32
Week 33
To Term
Baby's Development
Virtually the entire uterus is now occupied by the baby and its activity is restricted.
Maternal antibodies against measles, mumps, rubella, whooping cough and scarlet fever are transferred to the baby, providing protection for about 6 months until the infant's own immune system can take over.
Mother may have trouble sleeping because of baby's activity.
Maternal Events
The placenta is nearly 4 times as thick as it was 20 weeks ago, and weighs about 20 ounces.
Preparing for birth, the baby descends deeper into the mother's pelvis. 3-5 lb weight gain.
In 9 short months, the miracle is complete: you have transformed a single, microscopic fertilized cell into a six thousand billion celled human being.

control, and possible birth of child before reaching hospital; responsibilities and tasks of parenthood; mutual parental concerns arising from anxiety for safety of mother and unborn child; mutual parental concerns related to siblings and their acceptance of the new baby; mutual parental concerns about social and economic responsibilities; and mutual parental concerns arising from conflicts in cultural, religious, or personal value systems (Starn, 1991a; 1991b).

The father's/partner's commitment to the pregnancy, the couple's relationship, and their concerns about sexuality and sexual expression emerge as issues for many expectant parents (see the Family Focus box below). An important support measure is to validate the normality of their responses (if they fall within normal limits). Validation, feedback, and social comparison characterize appraisal support.

Providing an opportunity to discuss concerns, providing a listening ear, and validating the normality of responses will meet the expectant couple's needs in varying degrees. Nurses need to recognize that men have increased feelings of vulnerability during pregnancy. Female partners may also have these feelings. Anticipatory guidance and health promotion strategies can help partners with their concerns. Nursing intervention may directly help them with such concerns as the need to share intimate feelings or may indirectly do so through education of mothers. Health care providers can stimulate and encourage open dialogue between the couple.

During the third trimester the birth plan is finalized. When the plan is ready, it can be written out, signed by the woman and primary health care provider, and added to the prenatal record. The intent is to decrease the possibility of a conflict with staff members, for example, over the use of drugs for pain. A pleasant, relaxed atmosphere encourages expectant parents to ask questions and verbalize anxieties and fears without worrying about possible rejection. Thoughtful answers that reflect the nurse's caring can be reassuring.

Nursing ALERT

Women should not feel pressured either to attend parent education classes or to have a birth plan.

Immune system support. For women who are Rh negative, Rh sensitization is possible during pregnancy. For those who are anti-Rh immunoglobin (Rho[D]), D^U, and Coombs' test negative, Rh immunoglobulin (RhIG) is administered during pregnancy at about 28 weeks' gestation. This helps prevent the formation of antibodies by the woman to the Rh-positive cells from the fetus. RhIG is also administered at the time of the procedure to all pregnant women who have an amniocentesis.

An immunization strategy to protect newborn infants is available through the vaccination of mothers late in pregnancy. In effect, it allows for vaccination of babies before they are born. It works by passing protective antibodies from the mother to the fetus (Linder and Ohel, 1994). Hypothetically, newborns could be protected from *Haemophilus influenzae* type B, which is a potentially lethal infection that causes meningitis and pneumonia; this bacterium is a leading killer of children. Researchers are investigating whether a variety of infections could be prevented in this way: group B *Streptococcus*, whooping cough, *Pneumococcus*, *Escherichia coli*, and *Pseudomonas*.

During the third trimester, some women are retested for STDs such as syphilis, gonorrhea, group B *Streptococcus*, and *Chlamydia*.

Family Focus

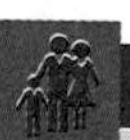

COUPLE RELATIONSHIP AND SEXUALITY

Pregnancy is a time when the couple relationship can be strengthened or stressed. In addition to the physical changes during pregnancy, the pregnant woman and her partner face significant emotional, social, and cognitive changes. Expectant fathers/male partners often experience weight gain and nausea. They may be concerned about finances, their role as fathers, sexuality, and the child's effect on the couple's relationship. Fathers/partners often worry about their role during childbirth classes and during labor and birth, as well as about the safety of their partner and baby during the birth. Female partners may have the same concerns.

Sexual expression during pregnancy is highly individual. The sexual relationship is affected by physical, emotional, and interactional factors, including myths about sex during pregnancy, sexual dysfunction problems, and physical changes in the woman.

Myths about body functions and fantasies about the influence of the fetus as a third party in lovemaking are commonly expressed. Anomalies, mental retardation, and other injuries to the mother and fetus may be attributed to sexual relations during pregnancy. Some couples fear that the woman's genitalia will be drastically changed by the birth process. Couples may not express their concerns to the health professional because of embarrassment or not wanting to appear foolish.

Discomfort during sexual activity may be caused by pressure on the woman's abdomen and deep penetration or thrusting. Postcoital cramping and backache during the first trimester have been reported.

As pregnancy progresses, changes in body shape, body image, and levels of discomfort influence both partners' desire for sexual expression. During the first trimester the woman's sexual desire may decrease, especially if she experiences breast tenderness, nausea, fatigue, and sleepiness. As she progresses into the second trimester, her combined sense of well-being and increased pelvic congestion may profoundly increase her desire for sexual release. In the third trimester, somatic complaints and physical bulkiness may increase her physical discomfort and decrease her interest in sex.

Partners need to feel free to discuss their sexual responses during pregnancy. Sensitivity to each other and a willingness to share concerns can strengthen their sexual relationship. Partners who do not understand the seemingly rapid physiologic and emotional changes of pregnancy can become confused by the other's behavior. By talking to each other about the changes they are experiencing, couples are able to define problems and offer the needed support. Nurses can facilitate communication between partners by talking to pregnant couples about possible changes in feelings and behaviors a couple may experience as pregnancy progresses (Rynerson and Lowdermilk, 1993).

Teaching for self-care. Not only are some new discomforts seen in the third trimester, but others seen previously in the first trimester (e.g., fatigue, frequency of urination) recur. Pregnant women in the older age group may experience an aggravation of varicose veins or severe backache from postural changes associated with a heavy, pendulous abdomen and relaxed joints. Such symptoms are frightening and uncomfortable.

Table 7-4 outlines the physiology, prevention, and self-care of several discomforts. Chapters 6 and 8 discuss relaxation, exercises, body mechanics, safety, employment issues, and nutrition.

Review of warning signs. The nurse needs to answer questions honestly as they arise during pregnancy. It is often difficult for the woman to know when to report signs and symptoms. The mother is encouraged to refer to a printed list of warning signs and to listen to her body. If she senses that "something is wrong," she should call her health care provider. Several signs and symptoms need to be discussed more extensively. These include vaginal bleeding, alteration in fetal movements, symptoms of PIH, rupture of membranes, and preterm labor.

If vaginal bleeding occurs in the third trimester, it is important to rule out brownish spotting occurring 48 hours after vaginal examination or sexual intercourse and a "show" of pinkish mucus. The woman should immediately telephone her primary health provider for instructions if bleeding is other than one of the preceding types.

If the woman notices cessation, noticeable lessening, or acceleration in the amount of fetal movement, she should call her physician/certified nurse-midwife (CNM) for advice. Fetal movement alterations noticed by the mother have been shown to be an accurate screen for fetal well-being (Jackson, Forouzan, and Cohen, 1991).

Appearance of edema of the hands and around the eyes,

TABLE 7-4 Discomforts related to maternal adaptation during the third trimester

PROBLEM	PHYSIOLOGY	EDUCATION FOR SELF-CARE
Shortness of breath and dyspnea in 60% of pregnant women	Expansion of diaphragm limited by enlarging uterus; diaphragm elevated about 4 cm (1½ inches); some relief after lightening	Good posture; sleep with extra pillows; avoid overloading stomach; stop smoking; refer to health care provider if symptoms worsen to rule out anemia, emphysema, and asthma.
Insomnia (later weeks of pregnancy)	Fetal movements, muscular cramping, urinary frequency, shortness of breath, or other discomforts	Reassurance; conscious relaxation; back massage or **effleurage** (Fig. 7-19); support of body parts with pillows; drink warm milk or take warm shower before retiring.
Psychosocial responses (see Chapter 11): mood swings, mixed feelings, increased anxiety	Hormonal and metabolic adaptations; feelings about impending labor, birth, and parenthood	Reassurance and support from significant other and nurse; improve communication with partner, family, and others.
Gingivitis and **epulis** (hyperemia, hypertrophy, bleeding, tenderness): condition disappears spontaneously 1 to 2 months after birth	Increased vascularity and proliferation of connective tissue from estrogen stimulation	Well-balanced diet with adequate protein and fresh fruits and vegetables; gentle brushing and good dental hygiene; avoid infection.
Urinary frequency and urgency return	Vascular engorgement and altered bladder function caused by hormones; bladder capacity reduced by enlarging uterus and fetal presenting part	Kegel exercise; limit fluid intake before bedtime; reassurance; wear perineal pad; refer to health care provider for pain or burning sensation.
Perineal discomfort and pressure	Pressure from enlarging uterus, especially when standing or walking; multifetal gestation	Rest, conscious relaxation and good posture; refer to health care provider for assessment and treatment if pain is present; rule out labor.
Braxton Hicks contractions	Intensification of uterine contractions in preparation for work of labor	Reassurance; rest; change of position; practice breathing technique when contractions are bothersome; effleurage; *rule out labor.*
Leg cramps (gastrocnemius spasm), especially when reclining	Compression of nerves supplying lower extremities because of enlarging uterus; reduced level of diffusible serum calcium or elevation of serum phosphorus; aggravating factors: fatigue, poor peripheral circulation, pointing toes when stretching legs or when walking, drinking more than 1 L (1 qt) of milk per day	Rule out blood clot by checking for Homans' sign; if clot ruled out, use massage and heat over affected muscle; dorsiflex foot until spasm relaxes (Fig. 7-20); stand on cold surface; oral supplementation with calcium carbonate or calcium lactate tablets; aluminum hydroxide gel, 30 ml, with each meal removes phosphorus by absorbing it.
Ankle edema (nonpitting) to lower extremities	Edema aggravated by prolonged standing, sitting, poor posture, lack of exercise, constrictive clothing (e.g., garters), or hot weather	Ample fluid intake for natural diuretic effect; put on support stockings before arising; rest periodically with legs and hips elevated (see Fig. 7-12) exercise moderately; refer to health care provider if generalized edema develops; *diuretics are contraindicated.*

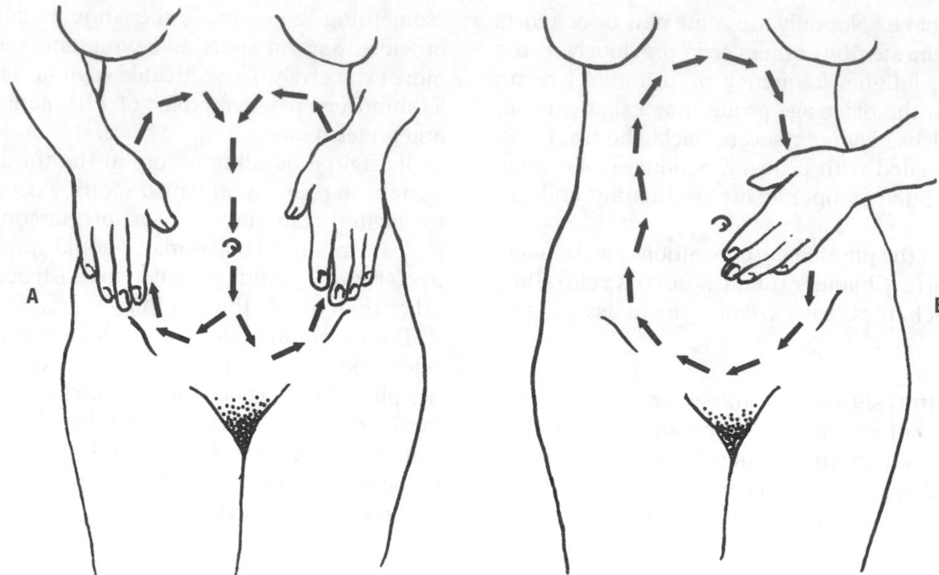

Fig. 7-19 Pattern for effleurage, a light, rhythmic stroking useful for inducing relaxation. **A,** Self-effleurage. **B,** Effleurage by another.

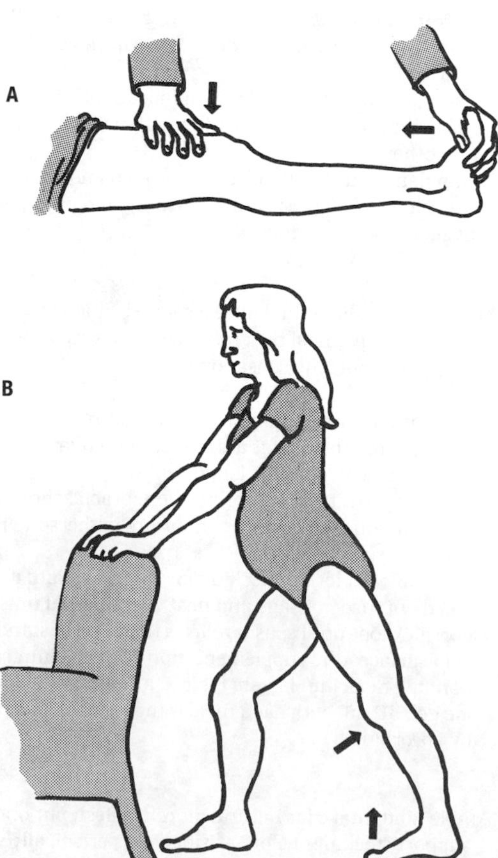

Fig. 7-20 Relief of muscle spasm (leg cramps). **A,** Another person dorsiflexes the foot with the knee extended. **B,** Woman stands and leans forward on affected leg.

severe headaches, visual changes, or feelings of jitteriness require immediate evaluation for hypertension. Severe PIH can lead to increased maternal and fetal morbidity and mortality.

A gush or trickle of clear, watery discharge that appears to come from the vagina may indicate rupture of membranes. The diagnosis usually requires a visit to the clinic or hospital for evaluation.

Recognizing preterm labor. Teaching each mother-to-be to recognize **preterm labor** is necessary (Bonovich, 1990; Hill and Lambertz, 1990). Preterm labor occurs after the twentieth week but before the thirty-seventh week of pregnancy. It is a condition in which uterine contractions cause the cervix to open earlier than normal. It could result in the birth of a preterm baby. Although certain factors may increase a woman's chances of having preterm labor, such as carrying twins or having bacterial vaginosis, the specific cause or causes are usually not known. It may be possible to prevent a preterm birth by knowing the warning signs and symptoms of preterm labor and by seeking care early if warning signs and symptoms should occur. The Patient Teaching box on p. 167 lists warning signs and symptoms of preterm labor. Fig. 7-21 shows where the signs and symptoms of preterm labor may be located.

Prebirth preparation. Not all expectant mothers and support persons attend formal classes in preparation for childbirth. For those who do attend, extensive preparation is possible. Many do not take advantage of classes for a variety of reasons: employment, inaccessibility because of time, cultural/ethnic/religious orientation, cost, lack of knowledge regarding choices in prenatal education classes, or lack of readiness. For these women, clinicians need to provide information that includes the following:

- Process of labor: admission, examination, care in labor
- Plans to get to hospital (when to go and where); care of other children

Patient Teaching

HOW TO RECOGNIZE PRETERM LABOR

Because the onset of preterm labor is subtle and often difficult to recognize, it is important to know how to feel your abdomen for uterine contractions. You can feel for contractions in the following way. While lying down, place your fingertips on the top of your uterus. A *contraction* is the periodic tightening or hardening of your uterus. If your uterus is contracting, you will actually feel your abdomen get tight or hard and then feel it relax or soften when the contraction is over.

If you think you are having any of the other signs and symptoms of preterm labor, empty your bladder, drink three or four glasses of water for hydration, lie down tilted toward your side, and place a pillow at your back for support.

Check for contractions for 1 hour. To tell how often contractions are occurring, check the minutes that elapse from the beginning of one contraction to the beginning of the next.

It is *normal* to have some uterine contractions throughout the day. They usually occur when a woman changes positions. These usually irregular and mild contractions are called Braxton Hicks contractions. They help with uterine tone and uteroplacental perfusion.

It is *not normal* to have frequent uterine contractions (every 10 minutes or more often for 1 hour).

Contractions of labor are regular, frequent, and hard. They also may be felt as a tightening of the abdomen or a backache. This type of contraction causes the cervix to efface and dilate.

Call your doctor, CNM, clinic, or labor and birth unit or go to the hospital if any of the following signs occur:

- You have uterine contractions every 10 minutes or more often for 1 hour *or*
- You have any of the other signs and symptoms for 1 hour *or*
- You have any bloody spotting or leaking of fluid from your vagina

It is often difficult to identify preterm labor. Accurate diagnosis requires assessment by the health care provider, usually in the hospital or clinic.

Post these instructions where they can be seen by everyone in your family.

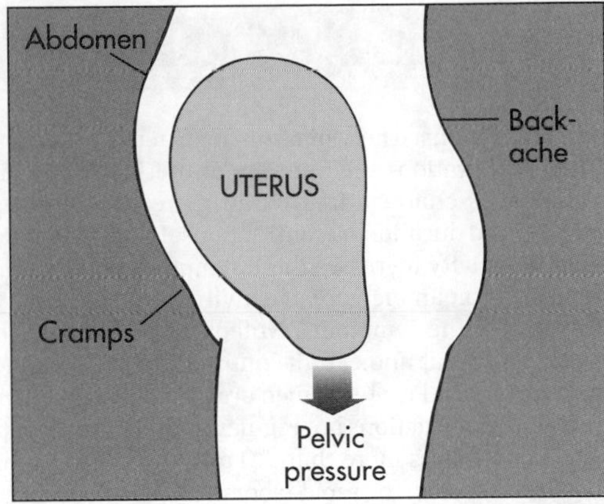

Fig. 7-21 Location of signs and symptoms of preterm labor.

- Methods to control pain (e.g., analgesia and anesthesia, breathing-relaxing techniques)
- Supplies to have in a suitcase ready for the trip to the hospital or birthing center: personal items for grooming, items for labor as desired (e.g., warm socks, focal point), supportive bra, slippers
- Responsibilities of the partner, family member, or friend who will be accompanying the woman through the labor and birth
- Emergency arrangements (e.g., precipitous birth)

A nurse needs to be ready to teach when the woman is ready to learn. One nurse described her intervention with an expectant mother as follows:

> I tried to teach her about relaxation and breathing techniques during her pregnancy, but she was not interested. When she phoned to tell me she was at the hospital in labor, she said, "What was all that stuff you were saying about breathing?" In between the next few contractions, I reviewed the crucial points.

Even if the woman/couple has attended parent-education classes, the nurse reviews preparation for childbirth. The following topics are discussed:

- Symptoms of impending labor (Box 7-10) and what information to report
- Breathing and relaxation techniques
- Involvement of significant other
- Plans to get to hospital
- Plans of labor, terminology, and what care to expect
- Preparation for baby
- Preparation of grandparents and siblings

If a hospital birth is planned, the woman is often required to preregister at the hospital of choice. Most hospitals now provide pamphlets containing information such as where to report when labor begins and policies pertaining to visitors and visiting hours. Many facilities also conduct tours.

Counseling is provided to relieve emotional tensions, which often relate directly to the childbirth experience (e.g., anxiety about pain or possible birth of the child before reaching the hospital). Nursing strategies include providing an opportunity for discussing the woman's specific fears or anxieties, helping her make definite plans concerning what she will do when labor starts, repeating instructions willingly, and having "sharing sessions" with mothers who have recently given birth. If possible, involve significant others in preparation for the birth. Arrange to have them participate in a supportive way during labor and birth. These techniques may be effective in preventing or minimizing anxiety.

Most partners of women who are approaching labor may have their anxieties decreased through intervention before the event. Fantasies can be replaced by knowledge gained through activities such as the following:

- Hospital tour to enable visualization of the labor or birthing room and waiting areas
- Demonstration of helping and supportive measures to comfort the woman during labor
- Brief review of what to expect from the woman during the labor process
- Description of what to expect of the staff during the woman's labor

BOX 7-10
Symptoms of Impending Labor

Uterine contractions. The woman is instructed to report the frequency, duration, and intensity of uterine contractions. True labor is characterized by an increase in frequency, strength, and duration of contractions. In true labor an increase in activity increases these symptoms. If the woman is in false labor, an increase in activity usually leads to a diminishing of the symptoms. Nulliparas are usually counseled to remain at home until contractions are regular and 5 minutes apart. Parous women are counseled to remain at home until contractions are regular and 10 minutes apart. If the woman lives more than 20 minutes from the hospital or has a history of rapid labors, these instructions are modified accordingly.

Rupture of the membranes.

Bloody show: The show is scant, pink, and sticky (contains mucus).

A realistic discussion of all known factors helps the father/partner problem-solve more rationally and plan for the event. Such discussions are ego strengthening because they help focus the father's/partner's energies toward more appropriate coping strategies by easing anxieties about the unknown. Today many men/partners elect to participate actively during labor and the birth of the child. However, some men/partners, because of personal or cultural reasons, neither want nor intend to participate. The important concept is that each partner agrees on the other's roles. For nurses to advocate any changes in these roles may cause confusion or feelings of guilt.

Sibling and grandparent education preparation is also available.

Evaluation

Evaluation is a continuous process as each intervention is assessed for effectiveness and an alternate intervention is used as necessary. Any change in the woman's condition or concern requires readjustment in the nursing care plan. The degree to which the expected outcomes for the mother, couple, or fetus are achieved is continuously evaluated according to the measurable established expected outcomes (See the Nursing Care Plan below).

Nursing Care Plan

PREGNANCY

Third Trimester

Nursing Diagnosis: Sleep pattern disturbance related to discomforts of late pregnancy

Expected Outcome: Patient will exhibit evidence of consistently adequate amount of restful sleep.

• NURSING INTERVENTIONS/RATIONALES

Reassure mother that insomnia is a common occurrence in late pregnancy *as validation of the normalcy of complaint.*

Discuss and demonstrate measures such as conscious relaxation, effleurage, strategic use of support pillows, and positioning *to promote and enhance sleep.*

Explore use of comfort measures such as a warm shower, whirlpool bath, and glass of warm milk *to induce relaxed state.* (Do not use medications for sleep unless specifically prescribed by physician or nurse-midwife).

Explore ways to create an environment that is optimally conducive to sleep (e.g., firm mattress, darkened room, quiet).

Nursing Diagnosis: Pain related to Braxton Hicks contractions

Expected Outcome: Patient will experience decrease in frequency and intensity of contractions.

• NURSING INTERVENTIONS/*RATIONALES*

Assess woman for frequency, strength, and regularity of contractions *to rule out preterm or true labor.*

Reassure woman that Braxton Hicks contractions are normal in pregnancy *to reduce anxiety as validation of the normalcy of complaint.*

Instruct woman to walk *to reduce contractions.*

Have woman assume left lateral lying position when at rest *to increase blood flow to uterus and decrease contractions.*

Nursing Diagnosis: Knowledge deficit related to preterm labor

Expected Outcome: Patient will delineate signs and symptoms of preterm labor.

• NURSING INTERVENTIONS/*RATIONALES*

Discuss signs and symptoms and treatment of preterm labor with woman and partner *so that adequate information is available for early detection.*

Discuss and demonstrate how to assess and time contractions *to provide needed skills to assess signs of labor.*

Provide written supplemental materials that include a list of warning signs and instructions about what to do if any of the listed signs occur *so that the couple can reinforce and review learning and act swiftly and appropriately should a sign occur.*

PARENTHOOD AFTER AGE 35

Two groups of older parents have emerged in the population of women having children late in their childbearing years. One group consists of women who have many children or who have a child during the menopausal period. The other group of older parents includes relative newcomers to maternity care. These are women who have deliberately delayed childbearing until their late 30s or early 40s.

Older Multiparous Women

Multiparous women may be those who have never used contraceptives because of personal choice or lack of knowledge concerning contraceptives, or they may be women who have used contraception successfully during the childbearing years. As menopause approaches, women in the latter group may cease to menstruate regularly, stop using contraception, and subsequently become pregnant. The older multiparous woman may think that pregnancy separates her from her peer group and that her age interferes with close associations with young mothers. Other parents welcome the unexpected infant as evidence of continuing maternal and paternal roles.

Older Nulliparous Women

The number of first-time pregnancies in women between ages 35 and 40 years has increased by 37% over the last 10 years. Women in their late 30s or even in their early 40s may be pregnant for the first time. Reasons for delaying pregnancy include advanced education, career priorities, better contraceptive measures, and infertility.

These women choose parenthood as opposed to the alternative, a child-free life-style. They often are successfully established in a career and a life-style with a partner that includes time for self-attention, establishment of a home with accumulated possessions, and freedom to travel. When questioned as to why they chose pregnancy late in life, many reply, "Because time is running out."

The dilemma of choice includes recognition that being a parent will have both positive and negative consequences (Chervenak and Kardon, 1991). Couples need to discuss the consequences of childbearing and childrearing before committing themselves to a lifelong venture. Partners in this group seem to share the preparation for parenthood, the planning for a family-centered birth, and the desire to be loving and competent parents. The reality of child care may prove difficult for these parents.

As with mothers of all ages, the mother over 35 who is accustomed to the stimulation of and contact with other adults may find the isolation with her infant difficult to accept. Anger and resentment toward the father (or infant) can result, even with "preparation" for these aspects of parenting.

First-time mothers after 35 select the right time for pregnancy; the right time is influenced by the increasing possibility of infertility or genetic defects with advancing age. Women seek information about pregnancy from books and friends. They actively seek to rule out fetal disorders and are careful in searching for the best possible maternity care. They identify sources of stress in their lives. They have concerns about having enough energy and stamina to meet the demands of parenting and their new roles and relationships.

Infertility may cause feelings of powerlessness in these couples. They have been able to plan other important events such as marriage and career changes but have no control over their ability to become parents.

If women become pregnant after treatment for infertility, they may have negative or ambivalent feelings now that they have achieved pregnancy; they may experience a multifetal pregnancy. A multifetal pregnancy may create emotional as well as physical problems. Adjusting to parenting two or more infants requires adaptability and additional resources.

During pregnancy, parents explore the possibilities and responsibilities of changing identities and new roles. They must prepare a safe and nurturing environment during pregnancy and after birth. They must integrate the child into an established family system and negotiate new roles (parent roles, sibling roles, grandparent roles) for family members.

MULTIFETAL PREGNANCY

A **multifetal pregnancy**, a pregnancy with more than one fetus, places the mother and fetuses at risk. Maternal blood volume is increased in multiple gestations, resulting in an increased strain on the maternal cardiovascular system. Anemia often develops because of a greater demand for iron by the fetuses. Marked uterine distention and increased pressure on the adjacent viscera and pelvic vasculature occur in multifetal pregnancies. Diastasis of the two rectus abdominis muscles (in the midline) may occur (see Fig. 6-13). Placenta previa develops more often in multifetal pregnancies because of the large size or placement of the placentas (Cunningham et al, 1993; Scott et al, 1994). Premature separation of the placenta may occur before the second and subsequent fetuses are born.

Twin pregnancies often end in prematurity. Spontaneous rupture of membranes before term is common. Congenital malformations are twice as common in monozygotic twins as in singletons. No increase occurs in the incidence of congenital anomalies in dizygotic twins. Two-vessel cords, that is, cords with a single umbilical artery, occur more often in twins than in singletons. This abnormality is most common in monozygotic twins. It may be associated with renal anomalies. The most serious problem for the fetus is the local shunting of blood between placentas (twin-to-twin transfusion). The recipient twin is larger. However, congenital heart failure may develop in this twin during the first 24 hours after birth. The donor twin is small, pallid, dehydrated, malnourished, and hypovolemic.

Clinical diagnosis of multifetal pregnancy is accurate in about 90% of patients. A correct diagnosis of twins is enhanced by careful assessment of the following factors (Buckley and Kulb, 1990):

- History of dizygotic twins in the female lineage
- Use of fertility drugs
- Uterine growth
- Hydramnios
- Palpation of excessive number of small or large parts
- Asynchronous fetal heartbeats or more than one fetal electrocardiographic (ECG) tracing
- Ultrasonographic evidence of more than one fetus

Prenatal Care in Multifetal Pregnancies

Prenatal care includes changes in the pattern of care and modifications in other aspects, such as weight gain and diet.

Prenatal visits by the mother with a multifetal pregnancy are scheduled at least every 2 weeks in the second trimester and weekly thereafter. Diet and weight control are supervised to allow weight gain of about 50% or more than the average woman with a singleton pregnancy (as much as 18 kg [40 pounds] above the woman's ideal nonpregnant weight). Iron and vitamin supplementation is advised.

The considerable uterine distention can cause an increase in backache. Elastic stockings or maternity tights may control leg varices. If there are risk factors for preterm birth (e.g., premature dilation of the cervix), abstinence from orgasm and nipple stimulation during the last trimester is recommended to help prevent preterm labor. Many practitioners recommend bed rest at 20 weeks when a twin pregnancy is diagnosed. This helps to avoid preterm labor in some instances. The mother needs to assume the lateral position to increase placental perfusion. If birth is delayed until after the thirty-sixth week, the risk of morbidity and mortality for the neonates decreases.

Psychosocial Adjustment

The diagnosis of a multifetal pregnancy comes as a shock to many expectant parents. They need support and education to help them cope with the changes they face. The mother needs nutrition counseling to gain more weight, counseling that maternal adaptations will probably be more uncomfortable, and information about the possibility of a preterm birth.

The degree to which parents are overwhelmed is dramatized in the following occurrence. A young couple had known they were to become parents of twins since an early sonogram revealed the presence of two gestational sacs. They had adjusted to the event and were looking forward to twins. At birth, a third baby was born. The father became irate, accused the physician of negligence in not diagnosing triplets, and threatened to sue her. This couple needed additional support during their initial adjustment period.

Additional newborns will likely strain finances, space, workload, and individual and family coping capability. Lifestyle changes may be necessary. Parents need assistance to make realistic plans for the care of the babies, for example, breastfeeding and raising them as "alike" or as separate individuals. Parents should be referred to national organizations such as Parents of Twins, Mothers of Multiples, and the La Leche League.

PREBIRTH EDUCATION

In the broadest sense the goal of childbirth education is to assist individuals and their family members to make informed decisions about pregnancy and birth. To accomplish this goal, the woman and her family need knowledge of the components of a healthy pregnancy, the process of labor and birth, and coping strategies to deal with the challenges of parenthood. Education should begin before pregnancy and continue through the postpartum period.

Some of the decisions the childbearing family must consider are the decision to have a baby, followed by choices of a care provider and type of care, the place for birth, and the type of infant feeding and care. If a woman has had a previous cesarean birth, she may consider having a vaginal birth. This section discusses these choices and the nurse's role in educating childbearing families to make informed decisions about them.

Previous pregnancy and childbirth experiences are important elements that influence current learning needs. The patient's (and support person's) age, cultural background, personal philosophy in regard to childbirth, socioeconomic status, spiritual beliefs, and learning styles all need to be assessed to develop the best plan to help the woman meet her needs.

Most parent education classes are attended by the pregnant woman and her partner, although a friend, teenage daughter, or parent may be the designated support person. Because family-centered care has supported the presence of family members at birth, classes have also evolved for grandparents and siblings to prepare them for their attendance at birth and/or the arrival of the baby (Fig. 7-22). Siblings often see a birth film and learn ways they can help welcome the baby. They also learn to cope with changes that include reduction in parental time and attention. Grandparents learn about current child care practices and how to help their adult children adapt to parenting in a supportive way.

Parent Education Programs

Expectant parents and their families have different interests and information needs as the pregnancy progresses. A typical program is designed to meet the information needs of parents at the three major stages of pregnancy and after birth.

Early pregnancy ("early bird") classes provide fundamental information. Classes are developed around the following areas: (1) early fetal development, (2) physiologic and emotional changes of pregnancy, (3) human sexuality, and (4) the nutritional needs of the mother and fetus. Environmental and workplace hazards have become important concerns in recent years. Even though pregnancy is considered a normal process, exercises, nutrition, warning signs, drugs, and self-medication are topics of interest and concern.

Midpregnancy classes emphasize the woman's participation in self-care. Classes provide information on preparation for breastfeeding and formula feeding, infant care, basic hygiene, common complaints and simple safe remedies, infant health, parenting, and updating and refining the birth plans.

Late pregnancy classes emphasize labor and birth. Different methods of coping with labor and birth have been developed and are often the basis for various prenatal classes. These include Lamaze, Bradley, and Dick-Read (see Chapter 14). The effectiveness of other methods such as hypnosis is being explored. A hospital tour is usually included.

Throughout the series of classes there is discussion of support systems that people can use during pregnancy and after birth; such support systems help parents function independently and effectively. During all the classes the open expression of feelings and concerns about any aspect of pregnancy, birth, and parenting is welcomed.

Many fathers elect to participate actively during labor and the birth of their child. As noted earlier, however, some men, through personal or cultural concepts of the father role, neither want nor intend to participate. The important concept is that the partners agree on each other's roles.

A number of women who come to the hospital in labor still have not had any prenatal care. It is the responsibility of the nurse to provide these women with the support and knowledge to successfully negotiate childbearing. A thorough assessment of immediate and long-term needs has to be done quickly. The clinician needs to provide information that includes the following:

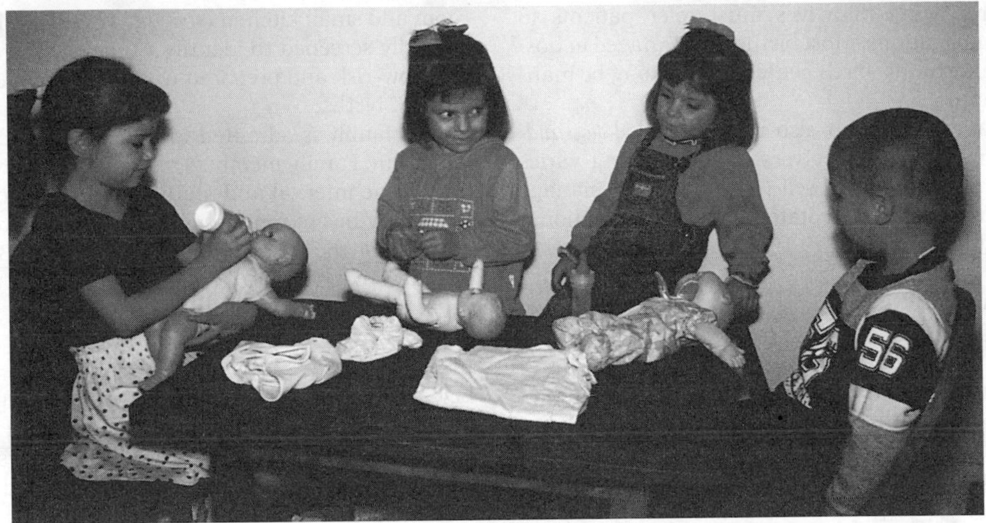

Fig. 7-22 Sibling class of preschoolers learning infant care using dolls. (Courtesy Michael S. Clement, MD, Mesa, Ariz.)

1. Process of labor: examinations, care in labor, stages of labor
2. Methods to control pain: breathing and relaxation techniques, analgesia, anesthesia
3. Responsibilities of support person

Recent Trends in Parent Education

A variety of approaches to parent education have evolved as parent educators attempt to meet learning needs. In addition to classes designed specifically for pregnant adolescents, their partners, and/or parents (Bachman, 1993), classes exist for other groups with special learning needs. These include classes for first-time mothers over 35, single women, adoptive parents, and parents of twins (Noble, 1991). Refresher classes for parents with children not only review coping techniques for labor and birth but also help couples prepare for sibling reactions and adjustments to a new baby. Cesarean birth classes are offered for couples who have a scheduled cesarean birth because of breech position or some other risk factor. Other classes focus on **vaginal birth after cesarean (VBAC),** since many women successfully give birth vaginally after previous cesarean birth (Safrin-Disler, 1990).

Because environmental influences and maternal behavior strongly affect newborn health, preconception and early pregnancy classes have been developed. These typically provide information about behaviors such as nutrition and exercise that promote improved pregnancy outcomes and about the risks of environmental hazards, smoking, alcohol, and drugs. Prenatal exercise classes during pregnancy should be based on ACOG exercise guidelines for pregnancy and the postpartum period (ACOG, 1994b) (see the Home Care box on p. 139).

Strategies for Childbirth Education

Because of the multicultural composition of the population in North America, there is great diversity in attitudes, expectations, and behaviors judged appropriate during pregnancy and early parenthood. No one approach can meet all needs. For example, classes for new immigrants are particularly effective when taught in a native language (e.g., Spanish, Tagalog, Chinese). For classes to be meaningful, parent educators must understand the value systems in other cultures and their influence on issues such as nutrition, exercise, valuing of early prenatal care, maternal weight gain, and infant feeding practices. Parent educators must establish rapport, be understood, and build on cultural practices, reinforcing the positive and promoting change only if a practice, such as pica, is directly harmful (Waxler-Morrison, Anderson, and Richardson, 1990).

Options for Care Providers

Some parents-to-be deal with decision making by developing a birth plan (see related discussion) to help them identify options and to set priorities for what they want. Often the first decision the woman makes is who will be her primary health care provider for the pregnancy and birth. This decision is doubly important because it usually affects where the birth will take place.

The nurse can provide information about the different types of health care providers and what kind of care to expect from each type. Physicians (obstetricians and family practice physicians) attend about 95% of births in the United States and Canada (National Center for Health Statistics, 1993). They see both low-risk and high-risk patients. Care often includes pharmacologic and medical management of problems as well as use of technicologic procedures. Family practice physicians may need backup by obstetricians if a specialist is needed for a problem (e.g., a cesarean birth). Most physicians manage births in a hospital setting.

Nurse-midwives are registered nurses with advanced training in care of obstetric patients. They provide care for about 4% of the births in the United States and Canada (National Center for Health Statistics, 1993). Nurse-midwives may practice with physicians or independently and with an arrangement for physician backup. They usually see low-risk obstetric patients. Care is often noninterventionist, and the woman and her family are encouraged to be active participants in the care. Nurse-midwives must refer patients to physicians for complications. Most births are managed in hospital settings or alternative birth centers; a few may be managed in a home setting.

Independent midwives, who also may be called *lay midwives,* are nonprofessional caregivers. Their training varies greatly, from formal training to self-teaching. They manage about 1% of births in the United States and Canada (National Center for Health Statistics, 1993). Patients who develop problems need to be seen by a physician. Almost all births are managed in the home setting.

Birth Setting Choices

The concept of family-centered maternity care can be implemented in any setting with careful thought. Today there are three primary options of birth settings: the hospital, an alternative birth center, and home. Women consider a variety of factors in choosing a setting for childbirth, including the preference of their health care provider, the characteristics of the birthing unit, and the preference of their third-party payer (Mackey, 1990). Approximately 98% of all births in the United States take place in a hospital setting (National Center for Health Statistics, 1993). However, the types of labor and birth services vary greatly, from the traditional labor and delivery rooms with separate postpartum and newborn units to in-hospital birthing centers where all or almost all care takes place in a single unit.

Labor, delivery, recovery, postpartum (birthing) rooms. Labor, delivery, recovery (LDR) and **labor, delivery, recovery, postpartum (LDRP)** rooms offer families a comfortable, private space for childbirth (see Fig. 16-16). There are few admission or risk criteria for the use of these rooms. Some hospitals incorporate labor support by highly trained nurses, or by monitrices. Women labor, give birth, and spend the first bonding time with their families in the LDR room. If they are not in an LDRP room, transfer to a postpartum room is usually the only room change they have to make. The woman and her family may choose this environment because it is more homelike but also because assistance is immediately available in case of emergencies.

Alternative birth centers. Alternative birth centers (ABCs) may be physically separate from or part of the traditional obstetrics department. Delivery and operating rooms and medical or NICUs are readily accessible for use if serious problems arise. Hospital ABCs, as well as free-standing birth centers, are intended to offer families an alternative to home birth, providing a compromise between hospital and home. These birth setting choices have been shown to be safe alternatives to birth in a traditional delivery setting (Alden and Harris, 1995; Eakins et al, 1989; Hutti and Johnson, 1988). In addition, they can be designed to ensure quality control and to be cost-effective, two significant issues in the delivery of health care today.

ABCs typically have homelike accommodations, including a double bed for the couple and a crib for the newborn (see Fig. 16-18, *A*). Emergency equipment and drugs are discreetly stored within cupboards, out of view but easily accessible. Private bathroom facilities are incorporated into each birth unit in the center. There may be an early labor lounge or living room and small kitchen (see Fig. 16-18, *B*). Each applicant is carefully screened to identify women with risk factors, since only low-risk and prepared women or couples are candidates for ABC births.

The family is admitted to the ABC where labor and birth will occur. Family members may remain there until discharge if the time interval and requirements for room use permit. If the family has to remain in the ABC for more than 24 hours after the birth, the demand for use of the ABC by other families may require transfer of the first family to a postpartum room in the hospital setting.

Free-standing birth centers. Although most ABCs or LDR/LDRP rooms are located in hospitals, a growing number of **free-standing birth centers** have been developed. Most free-standing birth centers are staffed by physicians who have privileges at the local hospital and by certified nurse-midwives who are prepared to attend low-risk women.

Services provided by the free-standing birth centers include those necessary for safe management during the childbearing cycle. There are some significant additions, however. Attendance at childbirth and parenting classes is required of all patients. Prenatal supervision of the woman begins in the first trimester. Her nutritional and health status must be good, and she must be experiencing a low-risk pregnancy. Patients must understand that situations may require transfer to a hospital and must have agreed to abide by those guidelines. Expectant families develop birth plans, that is, the practices and procedures they would like to include in or exclude from their childbirth experience. Developing birth plans provides a means for caregivers and parents-to-be to discuss options, preferences, and situations that might necessitate variations from their preferred birth.

Birth centers may have resources such as a lending library for parents, including books and videotapes, reference files on related topics, recycled maternity clothes and baby clothes and equipment, and supplies and reference materials for childbirth educators. The centers may also have referral files for community resources that offer services relating to childbirth and early parenting, including support groups (e.g., single parents, postbirth support group, parents of twins), genetic counseling, women's issues, and consumer action. These units, located outside the hospital, are often close to a major hospital so that quick transfer to that institution is possible if necessary. Ambulance service and emergency procedures must be readily available. Fees vary with the services provided but typically are less than or equal to those charged by local hospitals. Some base fees on the ability of the family to pay (reduced-fee sliding scale). Several third-party payers, as well as Medicaid and Civilian Health and Medical Programs of the Uniformed Forces (CHAMPUS), recognize and reimburse these centers.

Home birth. Home birth has always been popular in certain countries, such as Sweden and The Netherlands. In developing countries, hospitals or adequate lying-in facilities often are unavailable to most pregnant women, and home birth is a necessity. In North America, home births account for less than 1% of births (National Center for Health Statistics, 1993).

National groups supporting home birth are the Home Oriented Maternity Experience (HOME) and the National Association of Parents for Safe Alternatives in Childbirth (NAPSAC). These groups work to foster more humane childbearing practices at all levels, integrating the alternatives for childbirth to meet the needs of the total population. The literature on childbirth demonstrates that medically directed home birth services with skilled nurse-midwives and medical backup have excellent outcome statistics (Jones, 1991).

With a home birth the family is in control of the experience, and the birth may be more physiologically natural in familiar surroundings. The mother may be more relaxed than she would be in the hospital environment. The family can assist in and be a part of the birth, and mother-father/partner-infant (and sibling-infant) contact is immediate and sustained. Serious infection may be less likely, assuming strict aseptic principles are followed, since people generally are relatively immune to their own home bacteria (Jones, 1991).

Some disadvantages to a home birth need to be considered. Although some physicians and nurses support home births that use good medical and emergency backup systems, many regard this practice as exposing the mother and the fetus to unnecessary danger. Thus home births are not widely accepted by the medical community, making it difficult for a family to find a qualified health care provider to give prenatal care and to attend the birth. Backup emergency care by a physician in a hospital may be difficult to arrange in advance. If an emergency delivery is necessary, no effective way exists to do this rapidly in the home setting.

Factors increasing the safety of birth at home. Most health care providers agree that if home birth is the woman's choice, certain criteria must be met for a safe home birth experience. The woman should do the following (Jones, 1991):

- Be comfortable with her decision to have her baby at home.
- Be in good health. Home birth is not indicated for women with a high-risk pregnancy, such as when the woman has diabetes, heart disease, preeclampsia, or a multifetal pregnancy.
- Live no more than 10 to 15 minutes from the hospital.
- Be attended by a well-trained physician or midwife with adequate medical supplies and resuscitation equipment, including oxygen.

Key Points

- The prenatal period is a preparatory one both physically and psychologically.
- Psychosocial aspects of care may affect pregnancy, childbirth, and the adjustment of the new family.
- The pregnant woman's readiness to learn is at a high level, making this an excellent time to help her expand her self-care skills.
- Maternal physical and familial adaptations to pregnancy generate needs that the nurse can anticipate and meet.
- Detailed and carefully recorded findings from the interview, a comprehensive physical examination, and selected laboratory tests are important components of the prenatal visit.
- Even with a normal pregnancy the nurse must remain alert to hazards such as supine hypotension, warning signs and symptoms, and signs of family maladaptions.
- Each pregnant woman needs to know how to recognize and report preterm labor.
- Parent-child, sibling-child, and grandparent-child relationships are affected by pregnancy.
- Cultural prescriptions and proscriptions influence responses to pregnancy and to the health care delivery system.
- Childbirth education is a process designed to help parents make the transition from the role of expectant parents to the role and responsibilities of parents of a new baby.

References

Affonso D, Mayberry L: Common stressors reported by a group of childbearing American women, *Health Care Women Int* 11(3):331, 1990.

Alden K, Harris B: *Choices in child bearing.* In Fogel C, Woods N, editors: *Women's health care,* Thousand Oaks, Calif, 1995, Sage.

Alexander J, Grant A, Campbell M: Randomized controlled trial of breast shells and Hoffman's exercises for inverted and non-protractile nipples, *Br Med J* 304:1030, 1990.

American College of Obstetricians and Gynecologists: Smoking and reproductive health, *Tech Bull* 180, Washington, DC, May 1993, ACOG.

American College of Obstetricians and Gynecologists: *Precis V: an update in obstetrics and gynecology,* Washington, DC, 1994a, ACOG.

American College of Obstetricians and Gynecologists: Exercise during pregnancy and the postpartum period, *Tech Bull* 189, Washington, DC, February 1994b ACOG.

Bachman J: Self-described learning needs of pregnant teen participants in an innovative university/community partnership, *MCN Am J Matern Child Nurs* 21(2):65, 1993.

Bardy A et al: Objectively measured tobacco exposure during pregnancy: neonatal effects and relation to maternal smoking, *Br J Obstet Gynaecol* 100(8):721, 1993.

Barranti C: The grandparent/grandchild relationship: family resource in an era of voluntary bonds, *Fam Relat* 34:3, 1985.

Barry M, Bia F: Pregnancy and travel, *JAMA* 261:728, 1989.

Bia F: Medical considerations for the pregnant traveler, *Infect Dis Clin North Am* 6(2):371, 1992.

Birchfield M, Scully J, Handler A: Perinatal screening for illicit drugs: policies in hospitals in a large metropolitan area, *J Perinatol* 15(3):208, 1995.

Bonovich L: Recognizing the onset of labor, *J Obstet Gynecol Neonatal Nurs* 19:141, 1990.

Brody T et al: *Human pharmacology: molecular to clinical,* St Louis, 1994, Mosby.

Buckley K, Kulb N: *High risk maternity nursing manual,* Baltimore, 1990, Williams & Wilkins.

Burgess M: Rubella vaccination just before or during pregnancy, *Med J Aust* 152:507, 1990.

Chervenak J, Kardon N: Advancing maternal age: the actual risks, *Female Patient* 16:17, 1991

Cook P, Peterson R, Moore D: *Alcohol, tobacco, and other drugs may harm the unborn,* DHHS Pub No (ADM) 90-1711, Rockville, Md, 1990, Office for Substance Abuse Prevention, US Department of Health and Human Services.

Cranley M: Development of a tool for the measurement of maternal attachment during pregnancy, *Nurs Res* 30:28, 1981.

Culpepper L: *Exercise during pregnancy.* In Merkatz T, Thompson J, editors: *New perspectives on prenatal care,* New York, 1990, Elsevier.

Cunningham F et al: *Williams obstetrics,* ed 19, East Norwalk, Conn, 1993, Appleton & Lange.

Duvekot J, Peeters L: Maternal cardiovasular hemodynamic adaptation to pregnancy, *Obstet Gynecol Surv* 49(12 suppl):S1, 1994.

Eakins P et al: Obstetric outcomes at the Birth Place in Menlo Park: the first seven years, *Birth* 16:123, 1989.

Easa D et al: Unexpected preterm delivery in tourists: implications for long-distance travel during pregnancy, *J Perinatol* 14(4):264, 1994.

Economides D, Braithwaite J: Smoking, pregnancy and the fetus, *J R Soc Health* 114(4):198-201, 1994.

Engstrom J, Sittler C: Fundal height measurement. I. Technique for measuring fundal height, *J Nurse Midwife* 38(1):5, 1993.

Engstrom J et al: Fundal height measurement. III. The effect of maternal position on fundal height measurement, *J Nurse Midwife* 38(1):23, 1993.

Fishbein E, Phillips M: How safe is exercise during pregnancy? *J Obstet Gynecol Neonatal Nurs* 19:45, 1990.

Garmel S, D'Alton M: Diagnostic ultrasound in pregnancy: an overview, *Semin Perinatol* 18(3):117, 1994.

Geissler E: *Pocket guide to cultural assessment,* St Louis, 1994, Mosby.

Green N: Stressful events related to childbearing in African-American women: a pilot study, *J Nurse Midwife* 35(4):231, 1990.

Greene R, Polivka J: The meaning of grandparent day cards: an analysis of the intergenerational network, *Fam Relat* 34:2, 1985.

Hammond T: The use of automobile safety restraint systems during pregnancy, *J Obstet Gynecol Neonatal Nurs* 19:339, 1990.

Henriksen T et al: Employment during pregnancy in relation to risk factors and pregnancy outcome, *Br J Obstet Gynaecol* 101(10):858, 1994.

Heyl P, Miller W, Canick J: Maternal serum screening for aneuploid pregnancy, alphafetoprotein, hCG, and unconjugated estriol, *Obstet Gynecol* 76:1025, 1990.

Hill W, Lambertz E: Let's get rid of the term "Braxton-Hicks contractions," *Obstet Gynecol* 75:709, 1990.

Hutchinson M, Baqi A: Nursing care of the childbearing Muslim family, *J Obstet Gynecol Neonatal Nurs* 23:767, 1994.

Hutti M, Johnson J: Newborn Apgar scores of babies born in birthing rooms vs. traditional delivery rooms, *Appl Nurs Res* 1(2):68, 1988.

Jackson G, Forouzan I, Cohen A: Fetal well-being: nonimaging assessment and the biophysical profile, *Semin Roentgenol* 26(1):21, 1991.

Jones C: *Alternative birth: the complete guide,* Los Angeles, 1991, Tarcher.

Kendrick J et al: Integrating smoking cessation into routine public prenatal care: the smoking cessation in pregnancy project, *Am J Public Health* 85(2):217, 1995.

Kulig J: Childbearing beliefs among Cambodian refugee women, *West J Nurs Res* 12:108, 1990.

Lawrence R: *Breastfeeding: a guide for the medical profession,* ed 4, St Louis, 1994, Mosby.

Lazarus E, Philipson E: A longitudinal study comparing the prenatal care of Puerto Rican and white women, *Birth* 17(1):6, 1990.

Leatherman J, Blackburn D, Davidhizar R: How postpartum women explain their lack of obtaining adequate prenatal care, *J Adv Nurs* 15(3):256, 1990.

Lee R: Understanding Southeast Asian mothers-to-be, *Childbirth Educ* 8:32, 1989.

Linder N, Ohel F: In utero vaccination, *Clin Perinatol* 21:663, 1994.

Mackey M: Women's preparation for the childbirth experience, *MCN Am J Matern Child Nurs* 19(2):143, 1990.

Mackey M, Miller H: Women's views of postpartum sibling visitation, *Matern Child Nurs J* 20(1):40, 1992.

May K: Three phases of father involvement in pregnancy, *Nurs Res* 31:337, 1982.

Madorsky J: Influence of disability on pregnancy and motherhood, *West J Med* 162(2):153, 1995.

MAIN Trial Collaborative Group: Preparing for breast feeding: treatment of inverted and non-protractile nipples in pregnancy, *Midwifery* 10(4):200, 1994.

Maloni J, McIndoe J, Rubenstein G: Expectant grandparents class, *J Obstet Gynecol Neonatal Nurs* 16:26, 1987.

McFarlane J et al: Assessing for abuse during pregnancy: severity and frequency of injuries and associated entry into prenatal care, *JAMA* 267(23):3176, 1992.

Messersmith-Heroman K et al: Pregnancy outcome in military and civilian women, *Milit Med* 159(8):577, 1994.

Mills J et al: Moderate caffeine use and the risk of spontaneous abortion and intrauterine growth retardation, *JAMA* 269(5):593, 1993.

Mittelmark R et al, editors: *Exercise in pregnancy*, ed 2, Baltimore, 1991, Williams & Wilkins.

Müller M: Development of the prenatal attachment inventory, *West J Nurs Res* 15:199, 1993.

National Center for Health Statistics: Advance report of final natality statistics, 1991, *Monthly Vital Stat Rep* 42(suppl 3), 1993.

Nicholas R: High altitude sojourn in pregnancy and childhood, *Ther Umsch* 50(4):246, 1993 (German).

Nilsson L, Austrell C, Norgren L: Venous function during late pregnancy: the effect of elastic compression hosiery, *Vasa* 21(2):203, 1992.

Noble E: *Having twins: a parent's guide to pregnancy, birth, and early parenthood*, Boston, 1991, Houghton-Mifflin.

Norton L et al: Battering in pregnancy: an assessment of two screening methods, *Obstet Gynecol* 85(3):321, 1995.

Ostgaard J et al: Reduction of back and posterior pelvic pain in pregnancy, *Spine* 19(6):694, 1994.

Patterson E, Freese M, Goldenburg R: Seeking safe passage: utilizing health care during pregnancy, *Image J Nurs Sch* 22:27, 1990.

Priollet P et al: Study and treatment of varicose veins: truths and countertruths, *Ann Cardiol Angeiol Paris* 43(5):275, 1994 (French).

Rynerson B, Lowdermilk D: *Sexual intimacy in pregnancy*. In Knuppel R, Drukker J: *High-risk pregnancy: a team approach*, ed 2, Philadelphia, 1993, Saunders.

Safrin-Disler C: Vaginal birth after cesarean, *ICEA Rev* 14(3):9, 1990.

Sanyal M, Li Y, Belanger K: Metabolism of polynuclear aromatic hydrocarbon in human term placenta influenced by cigarette smoke exposure, *Reprod Toxicol* 8(5):411, 1994.

Scott J et al: *Danforth's obstetrics and gynecology*, ed 7, Philadelphia, 1994, Lippincott.

Scupholme A, Robertson E, Kamons A: Barriers to prenatal care in a multiethnic, urban sample, *J Nurse Midwife* 36(2):111, 1991.

Seidel H et al: *Mosby's guide to physical examination*, ed 3, St Louis, 1995, Mosby.

Seneviratne S, Fernando D: Influence of work on pregnancy outcome, *Int J Gynaecol Obstet* 45(1):35, 1994.

Sibai B et al: Pregnancies complicated by HELLP syndrome (hemolysis, elevated liver enzymes and low platelets): subsequent pregnancy outcome and long-term prognosis, *Am J Obstet Gynecol* 172(1, pt 1):125, 1995a.

Sibai B et al: Risk factors for preeclampsia in healthy nulliparous women: a prospective multicenter study, *Am J Obstet Gynecol* 172(2, pt 1):642, 1995b.

Skjenna O et al: Helping patients travel by air, *Can Med Assoc J* 144(3):287, 1991.

Spector R: *Cultural diversity in health and illness*, East Norwalk, Conn, 1991, Appleton & Lange.

Starn J: Childbirth classroom: labor after birth, *Childbirth Instructor* 1:27, 1991a.

Starn J: Cultural childbearing: beliefs and practices, *Int J Childbirth Educ* 6:38, 1991b.

Stewart D, Cecutti A: Physical abuse in pregnancy, *Can Med Assoc J* 149(9):1257, 1993.

Waxler-Morrison N, Anderson J, Richardson E, editors: *Cross-cultural nursing*, Vancouver, 1990, University of British Columbia Press.

Wilailak S et al: Assessment of fetal well-being: fetal movement and count versus non stress test, *Int J Gynaecol Obstet* 38(1):23, 1992.

Wilcox A: Birth weight and perinatal mortality: the effects of maternal smoking, *Am J Epidemiol* 137(10):1098, 1993.

Bibliography

Bobrowski R, Bottoms S: Underappreciated risks of the elderly multipara, *Am J Obstet Gynecol* 172(6):1764, 1995.

Chalmers B, Meyer D: Companionship in the perinatal period: a cross-cultural survey of women's experiences, *J Nurse Midwife* 39(4):265, 1994.

Conover E: Hazardous exposures during pregnancy, *J Obstet Gynecol Neonatal Nurs* 23(6):524, 1994.

Enkin M et al: Effective care in pregnancy and childbirth: a synopsis, *Birth* 22(2):101, 1995.

Roberts W et al: The irritable uterus: a risk factor for preterm birth, *Am J Obstet Gynecol* 172(1, pt 1):138, 1995.

CHAPTER 8

Maternal and Fetal Nutrition

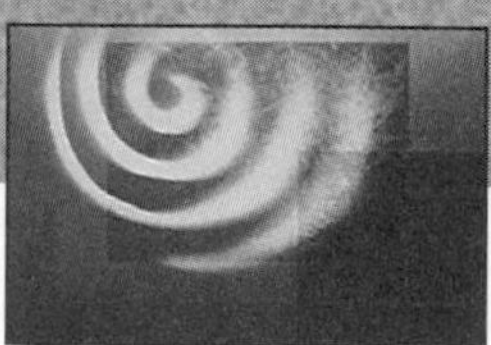

NUTRIENT NEEDS DURING PREGNANCY, P. 176

Energy needs, p. 177

Protein, p. 182

Water, p. 183

Minerals and vitamins, p. 184

Negative impacts on nutrition, p. 186

Pregnancy-induced hypertension, p. 187

Exercise during pregnancy, p. 187

NUTRIENT NEEDS DURING LACTATION, P. 187

Nursing care management, p. 188

Nutrition is one of the many factors that influence the outcome of pregnancy (Fig. 8-1). Poverty, deprived environment, limited education, unhealthy or bizarre food habits, and chronic illnesses have adverse effects on nutritional health.

The incidence of **low birth weight (LBW),** defined as a birth weight of 2500 g (5½ lb) or less, is of particular concern. LBW infants may be preterm and/or small for gestational age (SGA); in either case they are at high risk of morbidity and mortality. Currently, 75% of infant deaths in the first month of life occur among LBW infants. Rates of LBW have not declined for the past 2 decades, and in fact they have risen slightly in recent years (Guyer et al, 1995). Many factors contribute to LBW, but good maternal nutrition both before and during pregnancy is believed to be one of the most important preventive measures. It is essential that the importance of good nutrition be emphasized to all women with childbearing potential. Therefore the nurse must have a thorough understanding of nutrient needs during pregnancy, and nutrition assessment, intervention, and evaluation must be an integral part of nursing care for the pregnant woman.

NUTRIENT NEEDS DURING PREGNANCY

Pregnant women need greater amounts of some nutrients than do their nonpregnant counterparts. Nutrient needs are determined, at least in part, by the stage of gestation. During the first trimester, when the embryo/fetus is very small, needs are only slightly increased over those before pregnancy; synthesis of fetal tissues places relatively few demands on maternal nutrition. In contrast, during the second and third trimesters, as fetal growth progresses, pregnant women's need for some nutrients increases greatly; deposition of fetal stores of energy and minerals occurs in the third trimester. Factors that contribute to the increase in nutrient needs include the following:

1. *Uterine-placental-fetal unit.* Placentas of well-nourished mothers are able to provide adequate nutrients to the fetus. Placentas of poorly nourished mothers often contain fewer and smaller cells. Poorly developed placentas have a reduced ability to synthesize substances needed by the fetus, facilitate flow of needed nutrients, and inhibit passage of potentially harmful substances. Therefore it is understandable that the infant of a poorly nourished mother would be poorly nourished and SGA. Fig. 8-2 shows a possible mechanism by which maternal malnutrition may produce **intrauterine growth restriction (IUGR),** or impaired fetal growth.
2. *Maternal blood volume and constituents.* Total blood volume increases approximately 33% above normal during pregnancy. Plasma volume increases 50% in first pregnancies and more in multiparity. Red blood cell (RBC) production is stimulated during pregnancy. The number of RBCs increases gradually; the expansion of plasma volume proceeds rapidly.
3. *Maternal mammary changes.* A marked increase of the lactiferous ducts and lobular-alveolar tissue takes place.
4. *Metabolic needs.* Basal metabolic rates (BMRs), when expressed as kilocalories (kcal) per minute, are approximately 20% higher in pregnant women than in nonpregnant women. This increase includes the energy cost for tissue synthesis.

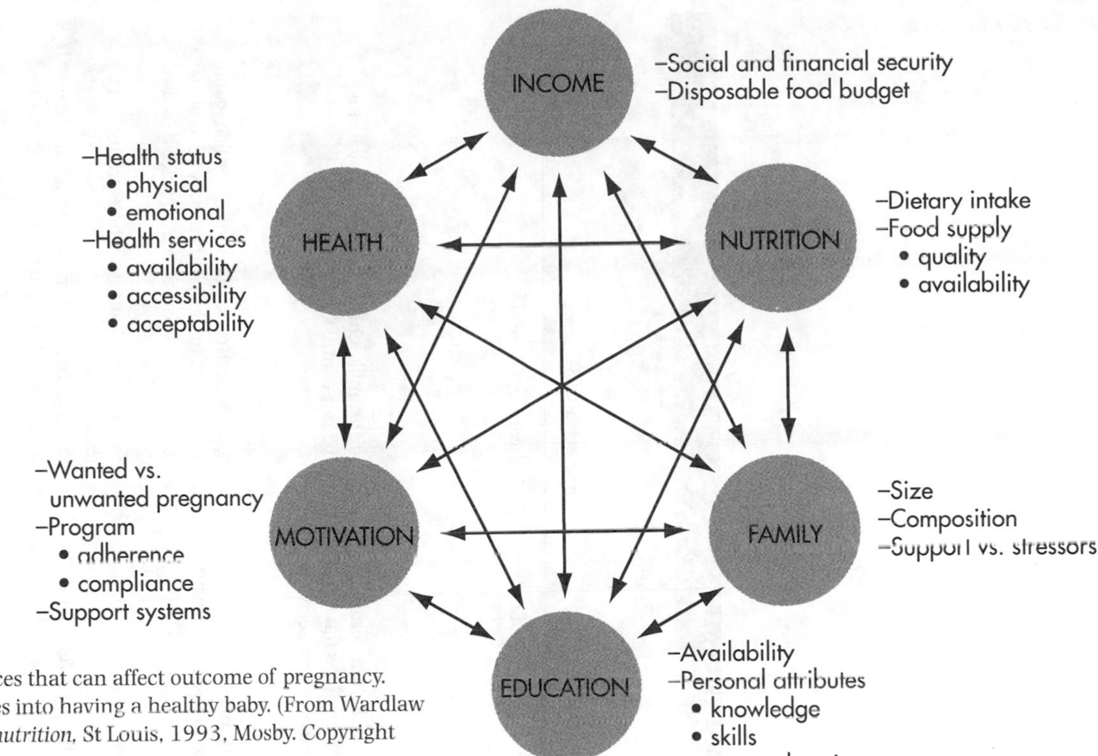

Fig. 8-1 Web of influences that can affect outcome of pregnancy. Much more than luck goes into having a healthy baby. (From Wardlaw G, Insel P: *Perspectives in nutrition*, St Louis, 1993, Mosby. Copyright McGraw-Hill.)

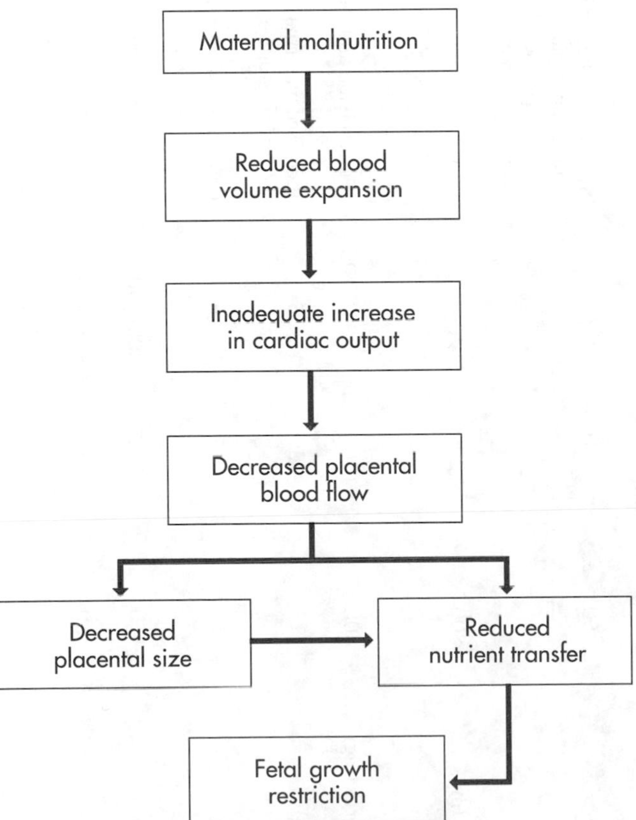

Fig. 8-2 Postulated mechanisms responsible for placental and fetal (intrauterine) growth restriction. (From Rosso P: Placental growth, development, and function in relation to maternal nutrition, *Fed Proc* 39:250, 1980.)

Recommendations for the increased intake of specific nutrients during pregnancy have been made by the National Research Council in the form of recommended daily allowances (RDAs). Table 8-1 shows RDAs for pregnancy and lactation. The RDAs were developed for use with groups of people, and it is important that these recommendations not be confused with requirements. However, they do provide a guideline to begin individualized nutrition counseling. A margin of safety has been built into these allowances to cover a wide range of individual needs. The reference woman in the typical RDA is 25 to 50 years old, weighs 58 kg (128 lb), is 164 cm (65 inches) tall, lives in a temperate climate, and is a normally active, healthy woman. Variations from this reference point need to be considered when providing individualized counseling. Age, activity level, current weight, number of fetuses, and alterations in health are examples of variations that need to be considered.

Energy Needs

Energy (kcal) needs are met by carbohydrate, fat, and protein in the diet. No specific recommendations exist for the amount of carbohydrate and fat in the diet of the pregnant woman. However, intake of these nutrients should be adequate to support the recommended weight gain. Although protein can be used to supply energy, its primary role is to provide amino acids for the synthesis of new tissues (see discussion later in chapter). The RDA for kcal during the second and third trimesters of pregnancy is 300 kcal greater than prepregnancy needs. Longitudinal assessment of weight gain during pregnancy is the best way to determine the adequacy of kcal intake; very underweight or active women may require

TABLE 8-1 Nutritional recommendations during pregnancy and lactation

NUTRIENT	RDA FOR NONPREGNANT FEMALE (25-50 YR)	RDA DURING PREGNANCY	RDA FOR LACTATION* (FIRST 6 MO/ SECOND 6 MO)	REASONS FOR INCREASED NEED	FOOD SOURCES
Calories	2200	2200 (first trimester); 2500 (second and third trimesters)	2700/2700	Increased energy needs for fetal growth and milk production	Carbohydrate, fat, protein
Protein (g)	50	60	65/62	Synthesis of the products of conception: fetus, amniotic fluid, placenta; growth of maternal tissue: uterus, breasts, RBCs, plasma proteins, secretion of milk protein during lactation	Meats, eggs, milk, cheese, legumes (dry beans and peas, peanuts), nuts, grains
Minerals					
Calcium (mg)	800	1200	1200/1200	Fetal skeleton and tooth bud formation; maintenance of maternal bone and tooth mineralization	Milk, cheese, yogurt, sardines or other fish eaten with bones left in, deep-green leafy vegetables except spinach or Swiss chard,† tofu, baked beans
Phosphorus (mg)	800	1200	1200/1200	Fetal skeleton and tooth bud formation	Milk, cheese, yogurt, meats, whole grains, nuts, legumes
Iron (mg)	15	30	15/15	Increased maternal hemoglobin formation, fetal liver iron storage	Liver, meats, whole or enriched breads and cereals, deep-green leafy vegetables, legumes, dried fruits
Zinc (mg)	12	15	19/16	Component of numerous enzyme systems; possibly important in preventing congenital malformations	Liver, shellfish, meats, whole grains, milk
Iodine (μg)	150	175	200/200	Increased maternal metabolic rate	Iodized salt, seafood, milk and milk products, commercial yeast breads and rolls
Magnesium (mg)	280	320	355/340	Involved in energy and protein metabolism, tissue growth, muscle action	Nuts, legumes, cocoa, meats, whole grains
Selenium (μg)	55	65	75/75	Antioxidant (protects cell membranes), tooth component	Organ meats, seafood, whole grains, legumes, molasses

Fat-soluble vitamins					
A (RE)‡	800	800	1300/1200	Essential for cell development, thus growth; tooth bud formation (development of enamel-forming cells in gum tissue); bone growth	Deep-green leafy vegetables, dark-yellow vegetables and fruits, chili peppers, liver, fortified margarine and butter
D (μg)§	5	10	10/10	Involved in absorption of calcium and phosphorus; improves mineralization	Fortified milk, fortified margarine, egg yolk, butter, liver, seafood
E (mg)	8	10	12/11	Antioxidant (protects cell membranes from damage), especially important for preventing hemolysis of RBCs	Vegetable oils, green leafy vegetables, whole grains, liver, nuts and seeds, cheese, fish
Water-soluble vitamins					
C (mg)	60	70	95/90	Tissue formation and integrity, formation of connective tissue, enhancement of iron absorption	Citrus fruits, strawberries, melons, broccoli, tomatoes, peppers, raw deep-green leafy vegetables
Folic acid (μg)	180	400	280/260	Increased RBC formation, prevention of macrocytic or megaloblastic anemia	Green leafy vegetables, oranges, broccoli, asparagus, artichokes, liver
Thiamin (mg)	1.1	1.5	1.6/1.6	Involved in energy metabolism	Pork, beef, liver, whole or enriched grains, legumes
Riboflavin (mg)	1.3	1.6	1.8/1.7	Involved in energy and protein metabolism	Milk, liver, enriched grains, deep-green and yellow vegetables
B_6 (pyridoxine) (mg)	1.6	2.2	2.1/2.1	Involved in protein metabolism	Meat, liver, deep-green vegetables, whole grains
B_{12} (μg)	2.0	2.2	2.6/2.6	Production of nucleic acids and proteins, especially important in formation of RBCs and prevention of megaloblastic or macrocytic anemia	Milk, egg, meat, liver, cheese
Niacin (mg)	15	17	20/20	Involved in energy metabolism	Meat, fish, poultry, liver, whole or enriched grains, peanuts

RDA, Recommended daily allowance.
*Milk production generally declines during the second 6 months of lactation as the infant's diet increasingly begins to include other foods. Thus maternal needs for many nutrients decrease.
†Spinach and chard contain calcium but also contain oxalic acid, which inhibits calcium absorption.
‡*RE*, Retinol equivalents. Replaces international units (IU). 1 RE = 5 IU.
§As cholecalciferol. 10 μg cholecalciferol = 400 IU vitamin D.

more than 300 additional kcal to sustain the desired rate of weight gain.

Weight gain. The optimal weight gain during pregnancy is not precisely known. It is known, however, that the amount of weight gained by the mother during pregnancy makes an important contribution to the course and outcome of the pregnancy. Although adequate weight gain does not necessarily indicate that the diet is nutritionally adequate, it reduces the risk of delivering an SGA or preterm infant. Desirable weight gain during pregnancy varies among individual women. The primary factor considered in making a weight gain recommendation is the appropriateness of prepregnancy weight for height, that is, whether the woman was of normal weight, underweight, or overweight before pregnancy. A commonly used method of evaluating the appropriateness of weight for height is the **body mass index (BMI).** The following formula is used to calculate BMI:

$$\text{BMI} = \text{Weight/height}^2$$

where the weight is in kilograms and height is in meters. Thus for a woman who weighed 51 kg (112 lb) before pregnancy and is 1.57 m (62 inches) tall:

$$\text{BMI} = 51/(1.57)^2, \text{ or } 20.7$$

BMI can be interpreted as falling into the following categories: less than 19.8, underweight or low; 19.8 to 26.0, normal; 26.0 to 29.0, overweight or high; and greater than 29.0, obese (Institute of Medicine, 1992). Fig. 8-3 provides an easy way of estimating and categorizing the BMI.

Women with a low BMI should gain approximately 12.5 to 18 kg (28 to 40 lb) during pregnancy (see Fig. 8-4). Women with a normal BMI should gain 11.5 to 16 kg (25 to 35 lb), and those with a high BMI should gain 7 to 11.5 kg (15 to 25 lb). Obese women should gain at least 7 kg (15 lb). Adolescents and African-American women should be encouraged to aim for the upper portion of their recommended weight gain range because their infants tend to be smaller than those of adult white women (Institute of Medicine, 1992). Adolescents who are fewer than 2 to 3 years postmenarche are believed to be at greatest nutritional risk because it is postulated that the fetus and the still-growing mother compete for nutrients. There is evidence of nutritional competition even in pregnancies of older adolescents (up to age 19), which underlines the need for especially careful nutritional teaching and follow-up during all adolescent pregnancies (Scholl and Hediger, 1993). Women shorter than 157 cm (62 inches) should have weight gain goals near the lower end of their recommended ranges to decrease the risk of mechanical complications during birth.

No recommendations have been made regarding optimal weight gain based on BMI for multifetal gestations. In twin gestations, gains of approximately 20 kg (44 lb) have been reported to be associated with the best outcomes.

Pattern of weight gain. It is important that weight gain take place throughout pregnancy. Poor weight gain early in pregnancy has been reported to increase the risk of delivering an SGA infant. Inadequate gains during the last half of pregnancy have been observed to increase the likelihood of preterm birth. These risks were found to exist even when the total gain for the pregnancy fell into the recommended range.

The optimal rate of weight gain depends on the stage of pregnancy. During the first and second trimesters, growth takes place primarily in maternal tissue, whereas during the third trimester growth occurs primarily in fetal tissues. During the first trimester there is an average total weight gain of only 1 to 2.5 kg (2 to 5 lb). Thereafter the recommended weight gain increases to approximately 0.4 kg (0.8 lb)/week for a woman of normal weight. For overweight women the recommended weekly weight gain during the second and third trimesters is 0.3 kg (0.66 lb), and for underweight women it is 0.5 kg (1.1 lb). The recommended caloric intake corresponds to this pattern of gain (Table 8-1). For the first trimester there is no increment; during the second and third trimesters an additional 300 kcal/day over the prepregnant intake is recommended. The amount of food providing 300 kcal is not great. It could be provided by one additional serving from each of the following groups: milk, yogurt, or cheese (all skim milk products); fruit; vegetable; and bread, cereal, rice, or pasta.

A chart has been developed for monitoring the progression of weight gain in normal weight, underweight, and overweight women (Fig. 8-4). Weight gain is assessed at each prenatal visit and is plotted on the chart to monitor progress toward achievement of the weight gain goal. Each pregnant woman should understand the desirable pattern and amount of weight gain. Compliance with the weight gain recommendations may be enhanced if the woman participates in establishing her own weight goal within the range recommended for her BMI.

Inadequate weight gain (less than 1 kg [2 lb]/month for normal-weight women or less than 0.5 kg [1 lb]/month for obese women during the last two trimesters) or excessive weight gain (more than 3 kg [6½ lb]/month) should be thoroughly evaluated. Possible reasons for deviations from the expected rate of weight gain include measurement or recording errors, differences in weight of clothing, time of day, and accumulation of fluids, as well as inadequate or excessive dietary intake. An exceptionally high gain is likely to be caused by an accumulation of fluids, and a gain of more than 3 kg (6½ lb) in a month, especially after the twentieth week of gestation, often heralds the development of pregnancy-induced hypertension (PIH).

Hazards of restricting adequate weight gain. An obsession with thinness and dieting permeates the North American culture. Slender, figure-conscious women may find it difficult to make the transition from guarding against weight gain before pregnancy to valuing weight gain during pregnancy. In counseling these women, the nurse can emphasize the adverse effects of maternal malnutrition (manifested by poor weight gain) on infant growth and development. This counseling includes information on the components of weight gain during pregnancy (Fig. 8-5) and the amount of this weight that will be lost at birth. Addressing the issue of how to lose weight in the postpartum period helps relieve the mother's concerns. Because lactation can help reduce maternal energy stores gradually, there is an opportunity to promote breastfeeding.

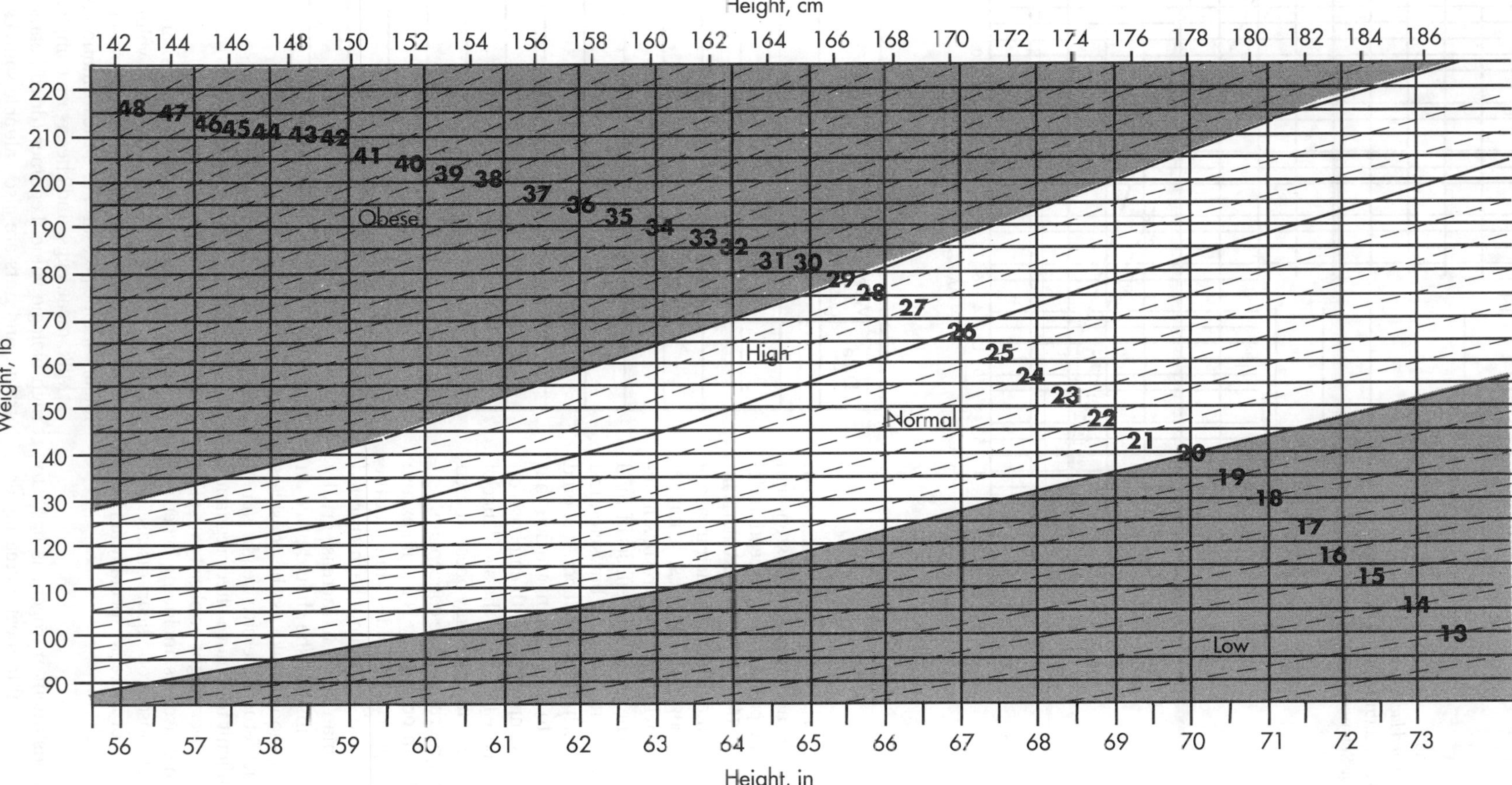

Fig. 8-3 Chart for estimating BMI category and BMI. To find BMI category (e.g., obese), find the point where height and weight intersect. To estimate BMI, read bold number on dashed line that is closest to this point. (From *Nutrition during pregnancy and lactation: an implementation guide,* Washington, DC, 1992, National Academy of Sciences.)

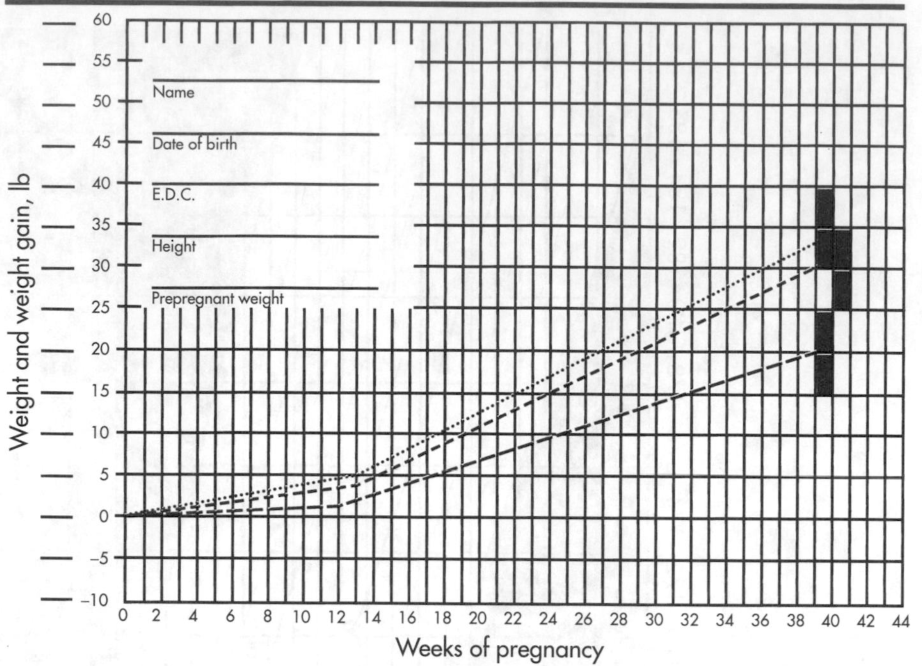

Fig. 8-4 Prenatal weight gain chart. (From *Nutrition during pregnancy and lactation: an implementation guide,* Washington, DC, 1992, National Academy of Sciences.)

Date	Weeks of gestation	Weight	Notes

B

Even obese (BMI of 26 to 29) or morbidly obese (BMI greater than 29) pregnant women need to gain at least enough weight to equal the weight of the products of conception (fetus, placenta, and amniotic fluid). If they limit their caloric intake to prevent weight gain, they may also limit their intake of other nutrients excessively. Moreover, dietary restriction results in catabolism of fat stores, which in turn results in increased production of ketones. The long-term effects of mild ketonemia during pregnancy are not known, but ketonuria has been found to be correlated with preterm labor. It should be stressed to obese women and to all pregnant women that the quality of the weight gain is important, with emphasis on the consumption of nutrient-dense foods and the avoidance of empty-calorie foods. Ideally, obese and morbidly obese women carry out a weight-reduction program before conception.

Weight gain is important, but pregnancy is not an excuse for uncontrolled dietary indulgence. The old saying that the pregnant woman is "eating for two" should not be interpreted to mean that the pregnant woman needs to increase greatly the quantity of her food intake; instead she should place an emphasis on the quality of her food intake as she considers both her needs and those of her fetus. Excessive weight gained during pregnancy may be difficult to remove after pregnancy and thus contribute to chronic overweight or obesity, an etiologic factor in a host of chronic diseases, including hypertension, diabetes mellitus, and arteriosclerotic heart disease. The woman who gains 18 kg (40 lb) or more is especially at risk.

Protein

Protein, with its essential constituent nitrogen, is basic to growth. Adequate protein is essential to meet increasing demands in pregnancy. These demands arise from the rapid growth of the fetus; the enlargement of the uterus and its supporting structures, mammary glands, and placenta; the increase in maternal circulating blood volume and the subsequent demand for increased plasma protein to maintain colloidal osmotic pressure; and the formation of amniotic fluid.

Milk, meat, eggs, and cheese are complete protein foods of high biologic value. Legumes (dried beans and peas), whole grains, and nuts are also valuable sources of protein. These protein-rich foods contribute other nutrients such as calcium, iron, and B vitamins; plant sources of protein often provide needed dietary fiber. The recommended daily food plan (Table 8-2 and Fig. 8-6) is a guide to the amounts of these foods that would supply the quantities of protein needed. Note that the RDAs provide for only a modest increase in protein intake over the prepregnant levels in adult women. Protein intake in many individuals in the United States exceeds the RDA; this means that many women may not need to increase their protein intake at all during pregnancy. Three servings of milk, yogurt, or cheese (four for adolescents) and 5 to 6 ounces (two servings) of meat, poultry, or fish supply the RDA for protein for the pregnant woman. Additional protein is provided by vegetables and breads, cereals, rice, or pasta. Inadequate protein intake is most likely to occur among pregnant adolescents, women from impoverished backgrounds, and women adhering to unusual diets such as a macrobiotic (highly restricted vegetarian) diet. High-protein supplements are not recommended because they have been associated with an increase in preterm births.

Water

Expansion of the blood volume results in increased fluid needs. Drinking 6 to 8 glasses (1500 to 2000 ml) of water, milk, and juices every 24 hours is recommended.

It is best to limit intake of caffeine-containing beverages.

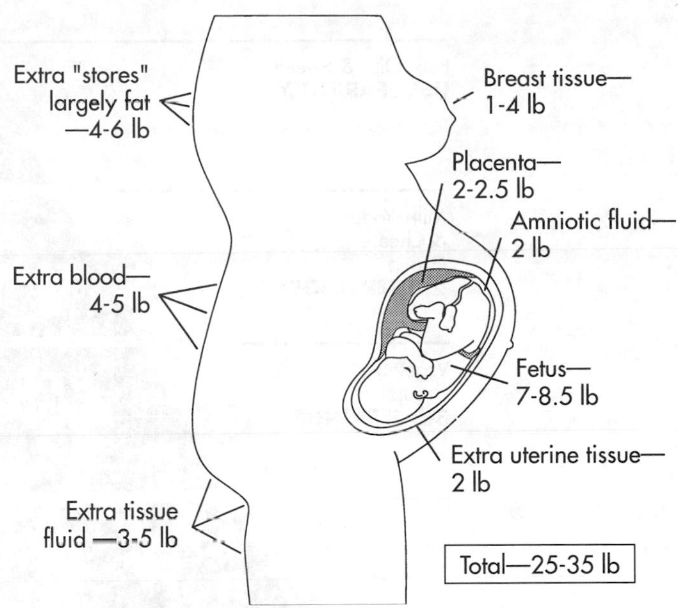

Fig 8-5 Distribution of maternal weight gain at 40 weeks. (From Worthington-Roberts B, Williams SR: *Nutrition in pregnancy and lactation*, ed 5, St Louis, 1993, Mosby. Copyright McGraw-Hill.)

TABLE 8-2 Daily food guide for pregnancy and lactation

		SUGGESTED NUMBER OF SERVINGS		
FOOD GROUP	SERVING SIZE	NONPREGNANT, NONLACTATING WOMAN	PREGNANT WOMAN	LACTATING WOMAN
Grain products				
Include whole-grain and enriched breads, cereals, pasta, and rice.	1 slice bread; ½ bun, bagel, or English muffin; 1 oz ready-to-eat cereal; ½ cup cooked grains	6-11	6-11	6-11
Vegetables				
Use dark-green leafy and deep-yellow often. Eat dry beans and peas often; count ½ cup cooked dry beans or peas as a serving of vegetables or 1 oz from meat group.	1 cup raw leafy greens; ½ cup of others	3-5	3-5	3-5
Fruits				
Include citrus fruits, strawberries, or melons frequently.	1 medium apple, orange, banana, peach, etc.; ½ cup small or diced fruit; ¾ cup juice	2-4	2-4	2-4
Milk and milk products	1 cup milk or yogurt; 1½ oz cheese	2-3	3 or more	4 or more
Meat, poultry, fish, dry beans, nuts, and eggs				
Use peanut butter or nuts rarely to avoid excessive fat intake; limit eggs to reduce cholesterol intake; trim fat from meat; remove skin from poultry.	½ cup cooked dry beans, 1 egg, or 1½ tablespoons peanut butter is equivalent to 1 oz meat	Up to 6 oz total	Up to 6 oz total	Up to 6 oz total

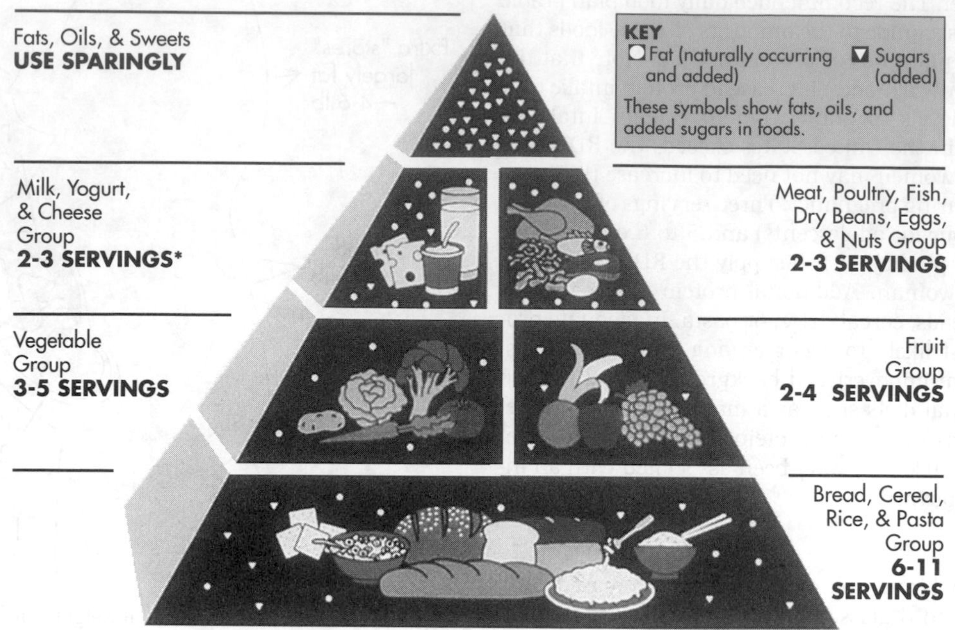

Fig. 8-6 Food Guide Pyramid: a guide to daily food choices. (Courtesy Department of Agriculture, Washington, DC.)
*3-4 for pregnant and lactating women

The effects of caffeine on the fetus are not well defined. Caffeine intake greater than 300 mg (equivalent to approximately two 6-oz cups of coffee, four 12-oz caffeine-containing soft drinks, or four to six cups of tea) a day is believed to reduce birth weight. Pregnant women would be well advised to avoid caffeine or, at a minimum, to limit their caffeine consumption to 300 mg or less until more is known about the effects of caffeine on pregnancy and the fetus (Nehlig and Debry, 1994).

The use of beverages that contain the artificial sweetener saccharin should be discouraged. Aspartame (Nutrasweet, Equal) and acesulfame K (Sweet One), two other artificial sweeteners, have not been associated with any adverse effects on the normal mother or fetus, but aspartame use should be avoided by pregnant women who are homozygous for phenylketonuria (PKU) (Position of the ADA, 1993).

Minerals and Vitamins

In general, the nutrient needs of pregnant women, with the exception of those for iron, can be met through dietary sources. Counseling about the need for a varied diet rich in vitamins and minerals should be a part of every pregnant woman's early prenatal care and should be reinforced throughout pregnancy. However, supplements of certain nutrients (listed in the following discussion) are recommended if the woman's diet is poor or if significant nutritional risk factors are present. Box 8-1 lists nutritional risk factors during pregnancy.

Iron. The changes in maternal RBC volume and mass accompanying pregnancy represent a fundamental physiologic adjustment. Full-term infants whose weight is appropriate for gestational age (AGA) are born with high hemoglobin levels of 18 to 22 g/dl and with a supply of iron stored in the liver to last 3 to 6 months. To achieve these stores, the mother must transfer approximately 300 mg of iron to the fetus during gestation. If dietary iron is not available to meet the needs of the maternal-placental-fetal unit, fetal iron reserves will not be impaired. However, maternal iron stores will be depleted and maternal RBC mass will be reduced, which may result in iron deficiency anemia in addition to the physiologic anemia of pregnancy.

The anemic woman has an impaired ability to tolerate a potential hemorrhage at birth. In addition, she may suffer from lethargy and lack of energy. The likelihood of delivering an LBW infant is increased threefold in women who are anemic early in pregnancy; women who become anemic during the third trimester have no increase in risk of LBW delivery (Scholl and Hediger, 1994). Anemia is more common among adolescents and African-American women than among adult Caucasian women (Beard, 1994). Very low maternal iron intake is associated with an increased prevalence of preterm birth (Scholl and Hediger, 1994). Diets low in iron are often low in other nutrients and calories, so it cannot be concluded that anemia and poor iron intake alone are the cause of the increased fetal risk.

The Institute of Medicine (1992) recommends that, starting by 12 weeks of gestation, all pregnant women receive a supplement providing 30 mg of ferrous iron daily. (Iron supplements may be poorly tolerated during the nausea that is prevalent in the first trimester.) If iron deficiency anemia (manifested by low levels of hematocrit or hemoglobin and serum ferritin) is present, increased dosages (60 to 120 mg daily) are required. Foods taken with an iron supplement can promote or inhibit absorption of iron from the supplement. Patient teaching regarding iron supplementation is discussed

BOX 8-1
Indicators of Nutritional Risk During Pregnancy

Adolescence
Frequent pregnancies: three or more within 2 years
Poor fetal outcome in a previous pregnancy
Poverty
Poor dietary habits with resistance to change
Use of tobacco, alcohol, or drugs
Underweight or overweight at conception
Problems with weight gain
- Any weight loss
- Weight gain less than 1 kg (2 lb)/month after first trimester
- Weight gain more than 1 kg (2 lb)/week after first trimester

Multifetal pregnancy
Low hemoglobin and/or hematocrit

on p. 196. Even though she takes an iron supplement, the woman should include good food sources of iron in her diet daily (Table 8-1). Milk and milk products contain little iron.

Calcium. Fetal calcification is responsible for most of the increase in calcium needs during pregnancy. Milk is the richest source of calcium, with 1200 mg—precisely the recommended daily amount—in 1 L (approximately 1 quart). Cottage cheese and ice cream contain less calcium than does milk, yogurt, or cheese. **Lactose intolerance** is the inability to digest milk sugar (lactose) because of the absence of the lactase enzyme in the small intestine. Lactose intolerance is relatively common in adults, particularly among African-Americans, Asians, Native Americans, and Eskimos. In these individuals, milk consumption may cause abdominal cramping, bloating, and diarrhea. Yogurt, sweet acidophilic milk, buttermilk, cheese, chocolate milk, and cocoa may be tolerated even if fresh fluid milk is not. Commercial products that contain the lactase enzyme (e.g., Lactaid) are available in pharmacies and many supermarkets. Lactase hydrolyzes, or digests, the lactose in milk, making it possible for people who are lactose-intolerant to drink milk. Large supermarkets often carry milk that has been pretreated with lactase.

In some cultures, adults rarely drink milk. For example, Puerto Ricans and other Hispanic individuals may use it only as an additive in coffee. Box 8-2 lists nondairy sources of calcium. If calcium intake appears low and the woman does not change her dietary habits in response to counseling, a supplement containing 600 mg of elemental calcium may be needed daily. Calcium supplements may also be recommended when a pregnant woman experiences leg cramps caused by an imbalance in the calcium/phosphorus ratio.

Sodium. During pregnancy there is a slight increase in the need for sodium, primarily because the body water is expanding (e.g., the expanding blood volume). Sodium is integrally involved in maintaining body water balance. Routine restriction of sodium was practiced in the past in an effort to control the peripheral edema commonly noted during pregnancy. However, moderate peripheral edema is normal in pregnancy and occurs as a response to the fluid-retaining effects of elevated levels of estrogen. Excessive emphasis on sodium restriction may make it difficult for the pregnant woman to achieve an adequate diet. Grain, milk, and meat products, which are important sources of nutrients needed in pregnancy, are significant sources of sodium. In addition, restriction of sodium intake may stress the adrenal glands and the kidney as they attempt to retain adequate sodium. In general, sodium restriction is necessary only if a maternal medical condition such as renal or liver failure or hypertension requires the restriction of sodium to control fluid retention and blood pressure.

Excessive intake of sodium is discouraged during pregnancy just as it is in nonpregnant individuals. In excess, sodium may contribute to abnormal degrees of fluid retention and edema. Table salt (sodium chloride) is the richest source of sodium. Most canned foods contain added salt unless the label specifically states otherwise. Large amounts of sodium are found in many processed foods, including meats, bakery items, mixes for casseroles or grain products, soups, and condiments. Products low in nutritive value and excessively high in sodium include pretzels, potato chips, other types of chips, pickles, catsup, prepared mustard, steak and Worcestershire sauces, some soft drinks, and bouillon. No specific RDA exists for sodium, but an intake of 2 to 3 g/day seems reasonable. This amount can usually be achieved by salting food lightly in cooking, adding no more salt at the table, and avoiding low-nutrient/high-sodium food choices.

BOX 8-2
Calcium sources for women who do not drink milk

Each of the following provides approximately the same amount of calcium as 1 cup of milk:

Fish
3 oz canned sardines
4½ oz canned salmon (if bones are eaten)

Beans and legumes
3 cups cooked dried beans
2½ cups refried beans
2 cups baked beans with molasses
1 cup tofu (calcium added in processing)

Greens
1 cup collards
1½ cups kale and turnip greens

Baked products
3 pieces cornbread
3 English muffins
4 slices French toast
2 (7-inch diameter) waffles

Fruits
11 dried figs
1⅛ cup orange juice with calcium added

Sauces
3 oz pesto sauce
5 oz cheese sauce

Zinc. The metal zinc is a constituent of numerous enzymes involved in major metabolic pathways. Zinc deficiency is associated with malformations of the central nervous system (CNS) in infants. Large intakes of iron and folate interfere with zinc absorption and decrease serum zinc levels. Because iron and folate supplements are commonly prescribed during pregnancy, pregnant women should be encouraged to consume good sources of zinc daily (see Table 8-1). Women with anemia who receive high-dose iron supplements also need supplements of the minerals zinc and copper (Institute of Medicine, 1992).

Fat-soluble vitamins. Fat-soluble vitamins—vitamins A, D, E, and K—are stored in the body tissues; with chronic overdoses these vitamins can reach toxic levels. Because of the high potential for toxicity, pregnant women are advised to take fat-soluble vitamin supplements only as prescribed. Vitamins A and D deserve special mention.

Adequate intake of vitamin A is needed to allow the fetus to store sufficient amounts of the vitamin. However, dietary sources can readily supply sufficient amounts. Congenital malformations have occurred in infants of mothers who took excessive amounts of vitamin A during pregnancy, and thus supplements are not recommended during pregnancy (Institute of Medicine, 1992). Vitamin A analogues (e.g., isotretinoin [Accutane]) prescribed for cystic acne are a special concern. Isotretinoin use during early pregnancy has been associated with heart malformations, facial abnormalities, cleft palate, hydrocephalus, deafness and blindness, and an increased risk of spontaneous abortion (ACOG, 1994). Topical agents (e.g., tretinoin [Retin-A]) do not appear to enter the circulation in any substantial amounts, but their safety in pregnancy has not been confirmed.

Vitamin D plays an important role in absorption and metabolism of calcium. The main food sources are enriched or fortified foods such as milk and ready-to-eat cereals. It is also produced in the skin by the action of ultraviolet light (in sunlight). Severe deficiency may cause neonatal hypocalcemia and tetany, as well as hypoplasia of the tooth enamel. The daily consumption of a quart of milk provides the RDA of vitamin D (and calcium) for most pregnant women. For this reason, women who do not usually drink milk should be encouraged to do so. It is advisable for women with lactose intolerance and women who refuse to include milk in the diet to take a daily supplement providing 10 μg (400 IU) of vitamin D, particularly during the winter months and in northern latitudes where sun exposure is limited (Institute of Medicine, 1992). Dark-skinned women and those who habitually wear clothing that covers most of their skin surface are also at increased risk of deficiency.

Water-soluble vitamins. Body stores of water-soluble vitamins are much smaller than those of fat-soluble vitamins; the water-soluble vitamins, in contrast to fat-soluble vitamins, are readily excreted in the urine. Therefore good sources of water-soluble vitamins must be consumed often, and toxicity with overdoses is less likely than with fat-soluble vitamins. The augmented maternal erythropoiesis of pregnancy requires substantially increased amounts of folate (folacin or folic acid), as do the rapidly growing cells in fetal and placental tissues. The birth of an infant with a neural tube defect (NTD) appears to occur more commonly among women with low levels of folate. In 1992 the U.S. Public Health Service recommended that all women who can become pregnant consume 0.4 mg of folate daily (CDC, 1992). All pregnant women should be counseled about the importance of a good diet, with the inclusion of green leafy vegetables, whole grains, and meats. A supplement of 300 μg/day is recommended for women at nutritional risk (Box 8-1). Women who have delivered infants with NTDs often receive supplemental folate during subsequent pregnancies.

Pyridoxine, or vitamin B_6, is involved in protein metabolism. Although levels of a pyridoxine-containing enzyme have been reported to be low in women with PIH, no evidence indicates that supplementation prevents or corrects the condition. No supplement is recommended routinely, but women with poor diets and those at nutritional risk (Box 8-1) may need a supplement providing 2 mg/day (Institute of Medicine, 1992).

Vitamin C, or ascorbic acid, plays an important role in tissue formation and increases the absorption of iron. The vitamin C needs of most women are readily met by a diet that includes at least one serving of citrus fruit or juice or another good source daily (Table 8-1), but smokers have an increased need. For women at nutritional risk, a supplement of 50 mg/day is recommended (Institute of Medicine, 1992). If the mother takes excessive doses of the vitamin during pregnancy, a vitamin C deficiency may develop postnatally in the infant.

Multivitamin-multimineral supplements during pregnancy. No recommendation exists for routine nutritional supplementation during pregnancy, except for iron supplementation, as described earlier. It can be difficult for women to consume adequate amounts of zinc, folate, and other nutrients, even when they consume generally good diets that follow the food guide pyramid (Keen and Zedenberg-Cherr, 1994). For this reason, many health care providers routinely prescribe a multivitamin-multimineral supplement for pregnant women.

Negative Impacts on Nutrition

Use of tobacco, alcohol, and drugs. Smoking, alcohol intake, and drug use can adversely affect the fetus. Smoking has been shown to reduce birth weight and increase the prevalence of placenta previa, abruptio placentae, and fetal and neonatal death. It is also associated with low maternal weight before pregnancy and poor weight gain during pregnancy. Women who smoke should be strongly encouraged to stop, or if this proves impossible, to reduce their use of smoking materials.

Maternal alcoholism is closely associated with spontaneous abortion. In addition, fetal alcohol syndrome (FAS), a group of characteristics that includes abnormal facies, microcephaly, impaired growth, and learning disabilities (Fig. 8-7), is seen in almost 10% of infants born to mothers with heavy prenatal alcohol use. Fetal alcohol effects (FAEs) are found in many more infants and may occur even with more moderate levels of alcohol intake (Snodgrass, 1994). At present, no safe level of alcohol intake during pregnancy is known, and abstinence is advisable.

Illegal or controlled drugs and the life-styles that com-

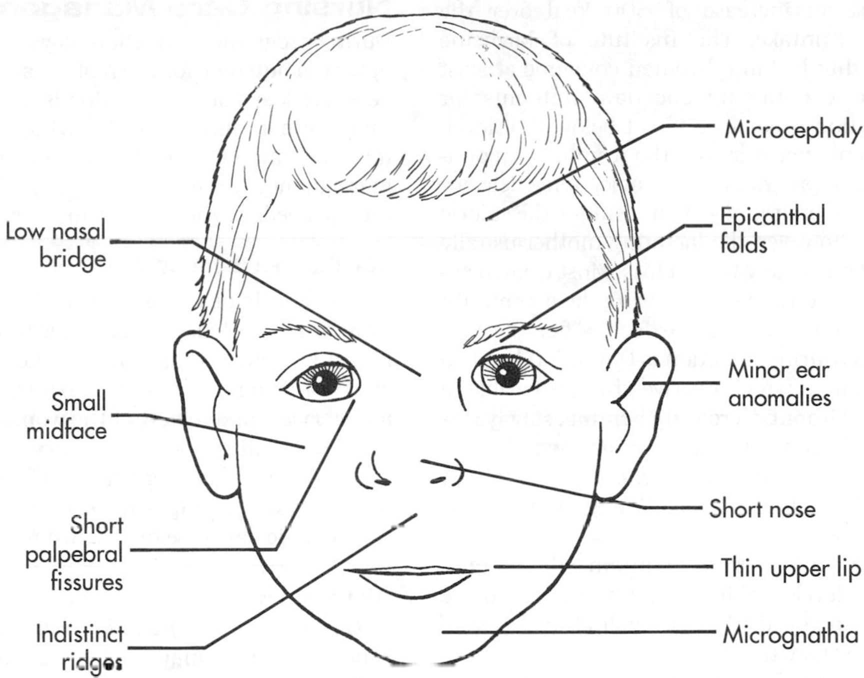

Fig 8-7 Characteristic physical effects of FAS. (From Worthington-Roberts B, Williams S: *Nutrition in pregnancy and lactation,* ed 5, St Louis, 1993, Mosby. Copyright McGraw-Hill.)

monly accompany their abuse contribute to IUGR and developmental delays (Institute of Medicine, 1992). An increased risk of complications is present in infants of women who use large amounts of cocaine or other drugs, combine the use of two or more drugs (including alcohol), come from a homeless or other deprived background, and fail to gain weight during pregnancy (Lindenberg et al, 1991; Snodgrass, 1994). Every effort should be made to convince the pregnant drug or alcohol user to cease the habit. When this proves impossible, emphasis should be placed on the importance of good nutrition, which is a key factor in preventing congenital anomalies and fetal death.

Pica. Pica, the practice of consuming nonfood substances (e.g., clay, laundry starch) or excessive amounts of foodstuffs low in nutritional value (e.g., cornstarch, ice), often is influenced by the woman's cultural background. In the United States it appears to be most common among African-American women, women from rural areas, and women with a family history of pica (Horner et al, 1991). Regular and heavy consumption of low-nutrient products may displace more nutritious foods from the diet, and the items consumed may interfere with the absorption of nutrients, especially minerals. The presence of pica, as well as details of the type and amounts of products ingested, is likely to be discovered only by the sensitive interviewer who has developed a relationship of trust with the woman. It has been proposed that pica and **food cravings** (e.g., the urge to consume ice cream, pickles, pizza) during pregnancy are caused by an innate drive to consume nutrients missing from the diet. However, research indicates that this is not likely (Worthington-Roberts and Williams, 1993).

Pregnancy-Induced Hypertension

The cause of PIH, or preeclampsia, is not known. Speculation suggests that poor intake of several nutrients, including calcium, magnesium, vitamin B_6, and protein, might contribute to the development of PIH (Newman and Fullerton, 1990; Roberts, 1994). No definite evidence indicates that nutritional deficiencies are causative factors or that nutritional supplements can help women avoid PIH. At present a diet adequate in the recommended nutrients (Table 8-1) appears to be the best means of reducing the risk of development of PIH.

Exercise During Pregnancy

Moderate exercise during pregnancy has numerous benefits, including improving muscle tone, potentially shortening the course of labor, and promoting a sense of well-being. Following careful guidelines (ACOG, 1994), most women can safely exercise throughout pregnancy. Two nutritional concepts are especially important for women who choose to exercise during pregnancy and lactation. First, fluid intake should be liberal before, during, and after exercise. Dehydration can stimulate the onset of preterm labor. Second, calorie intake should be sufficient to meet the increased needs of pregnancy and the demands of exercise.

NUTRIENT NEEDS DURING LACTATION

A varied diet chosen from all food groups (Fig. 8-6) is the best way for lactating women to receive the necessary nutrients. It is especially important that calcium intake be adequate; if it is not and if the woman does not respond to diet counseling, a supplement of 600 mg of calcium daily may be needed (Institute of Medicine, 1992).

The RDAs suggest an increase of 500 kcal over the woman's nonpregnant intake. The Institute of Medicine (1992) recommends that lactating women consume at least 1800 kcal/day because obtaining adequate nutrients for maintenance of lactation becomes difficult below that level. Because of deposition of energy stores, the woman with optimal weight gain during pregnancy is heavier after delivery than at the beginning of pregnancy. As a result of the caloric demands of lactation, however, the lactating mother usually experiences a gradual but steady weight loss. Most women experience a rapid loss of several pounds during the first month postpartum whether or not they breastfeed. After the first month the average loss during lactation is 0.5 to 1.0 kg (1 to 2 lb)/month, and a woman who is overweight may be able to lose up to 2 kg (4½ lb) without decreasing her milk supply (Institute of Medicine, 1992). On average, women who breastfeed for 12 months are 2 kg lighter at the end of the year than women who did not breastfeed (Dewey, Heinig, and Nommsen, 1993).

Fluid intake must be adequate to maintain milk production, but the mother's level of thirst is the best guide to the right amount. There is no need to consume fluids in excess of the amount needed to satisfy thirst.

Smoking and the abuse of alcohol and caffeine should be avoided during lactation. Smoking may impair milk production and also exposes the infant to the risks of passive smoking. It is speculated that the infant's psychomotor development could be affected by maternal alcohol use, and alcoholic beverages (two drinks per day) may impair the milk ejection reflex. Coffee intake may reduce the iron concentration in milk and consequently contribute to anemia in the infant. The caffeine concentration in milk is only approximately 1% of the mother's plasma level, but caffeine seems to accumulate in the infant. Some breastfed infants of mothers who drank large amounts of coffee or caffeine-containing soft drinks have been reported to be unusually active and wakeful (Lawrence, 1994).

Critical Thinking 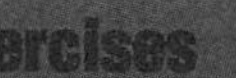 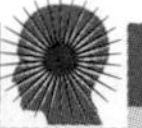

NUTRITION IN THE POSTPARTUM PERIOD

Donna is an African-American woman who works full time, pumps her breasts during her lunch break, and breastfeeds her 4-month-old daughter when she is home. Rita, who is Caucasian, also works full time and is bottle-feeding her 3-month-old son. Donna and Rita are the same height and were approximately the same weight before pregnancy; Donna gained 2.25 kg (5 lb) more than Rita did during pregnancy. Both Donna and Rita pack lunches to bring to work. Using the food guide pyramid and emphasizing the use of a variety of different foods, plan three weekday menus for Donna and Rita.

1. What other information do you need about Donna and Rita to plan appropriate menus?
2. How do the nutrient needs of Donna and Rita differ? What factors create that difference?
3. Would the menus differ if Rita weighed more than Donna?
4. How would the menus differ if Donna were a recent immigrant from Mexico? From China? An adolescent?

Nursing Care Management

During pregnancy, nutrition plays a key role in achieving an optimum outcome for the mother and her unborn baby. Motivation to learn about nutrition is usually higher during pregnancy as parents strive to "do what's right for the baby." Optimum nutrition cannot eliminate all problems that may arise in pregnancy, but it establishes a good foundation for supporting the needs of the mother and her unborn child.

Assessment

Assessment is based on a diet history (a description of the woman's usual food and beverage intake and factors affecting her nutritional status, such as medications taken and adequacy of income to allow her to purchase food) obtained from an interview and review of the woman's health records, physical examination, and laboratory analyses. Ideally a nutritional assessment is performed before conception so that any recommended changes in diet, life-style, and weight status can be undertaken before the woman becomes pregnant.

Diet history

Obstetric and gynecologic impacts on nutrition. Nutritional reserves may be depleted in the woman with high parity or frequent pregnancies, especially three or more pregnancies within 2 years. A history of preterm birth or the birth of an LBW or SGA infant may indicate inadequate dietary intake. PIH may also be a factor in poor maternal nutrition. Birth of a large-for-gestational age (LGA) infant may indicate maternal diabetes mellitus. Previous contraceptive methods also may affect reproductive health. Increased menstrual blood loss often occurs during the first 3 to 6 months that an intrauterine contraceptive device is used. Consequently the user may have low iron stores or even iron deficiency anemia. Oral contraceptive agents, on the other hand, are associated with decreased menstrual losses and increased iron stores; however, oral contraceptives may interfere with folate metabolism.

Medical history. Chronic maternal illnesses such as diabetes mellitus, renal disease, liver disease, or cystic fibrosis, as well as other malabsorptive disorders, seizure disorders, the use of anticonvulsant agents, hypertension, and PKU may affect nutritional status and dietary needs. In illnesses that result in nutritional deficits or require dietary treatment (e.g., diabetes mellitus, PKU), it is extremely important for nutritional care to begin and for optimal control of the disease condition to be achieved before conception. The registered dietitian (RD) can provide in-depth counseling for the woman who requires a therapeutic diet during pregnancy and lactation.

Usual maternal diet. The woman's usual food and beverage intake, adequacy of income and other resources to meet her nutritional needs, any dietary modifications, food allergies and intolerances, and all medications and nutrition supplements should be ascertained. In addition, the presence and severity of nutrition-related discomforts of pregnancy, such as morning sickness, constipation, and pyrosis (heartburn), should be determined (see the related discussion on pp. 195-196). The nurse should be alert to any evidence of eating disorders such as anorexia nervosa, bulimia, or frequent and rigorous dieting before or during pregnancy.

Cultural (including religious and ethnic) influences on dietary intake are extremely strong but may lessen if the woman and her family become more integrated into the dominant culture. Table 8-3 summarizes nutrition beliefs and practices of selected cultural groups. **Vegetarian diets** represent another cultural factor affecting nutritional status.

Foods basic to almost all vegetarian diets are vegetables, fruits, legumes, nuts, seeds, and grains. However, there are many variations in vegetarian diets. *Semivegetarians* (who are not truly vegetarians) include fish, poultry, eggs, and dairy products in their diets but do not eat beef or pork. This diet can be completely adequate. In addition to plant products, *lactoovovegetarians* consume both dairy products and eggs; and *lactovegetarians* consume dairy products. Iron and zinc intake may not be adequate, but these diets are otherwise nutritionally sound.

Strict vegetarians, or *vegans,* consume only plant products. Because vitamin B_{12} is found only in foods of animal origin, this diet is deficient in vitamin B_{12}. Strict vegetarians should take a supplement or use vitamin B_{12}–fortified foods (e.g., some soy milk) regularly. Vitamin B_{12} deficiency can result in megaloblastic anemia, glossitis, and neurologic deficits in the mother. Infants born to affected mothers are likely to have megaloblastic anemia and neurodevelopmental delays. Iron, calcium, zinc, and vitamin B_6 intake may be low on this diet, and some individuals have excessively low caloric intake. Protein intake should be assessed especially carefully. Plant proteins tend to be "incomplete," or lacking in one or more amino acids required for growth and maintenance of body tissues.

Eating a variety of grains, legumes (dried beans and peas), nuts, and seeds provides sufficient amounts of the essential amino acids.

The effect of food allergies and intolerances on nutritional status ranges from very important to almost nil. Lactose intolerance is of special concern during pregnancy and lactation because no other food group equals milk and milk products in calcium content. If lactose intolerance is reported, the interviewer should explore intake of other calcium sources (Table 8-1).

The assessment must include an evaluation of the woman's financial status and knowledge of sound dietary practices. The quality of the diet increases with increasing socioeconomic status and educational level. Obtaining adequate refrigeration and cooking facilities and nutritious food may be a struggle for poor women. Pregnancy rates are high among the homeless, and many homeless individuals cannot or do not take advantage of services such as food stamps (Wiecha, Dwyer, and Dunn-Strohecker, 1991).

Box 8-3 shows a simple tool that can be used for obtaining diet history information. Potential problems should be followed up with a careful interview.

Physical examination. Anthropometric (body) measurements provide both short-term and long-term indications of nutritional status and are thus essential to the assessment. At a minimum the woman's height and weight must be determined on her first entry into the health care system, and her weight must be measured at every prenatal visit thereafter (see earlier discussion of BMI).

A careful physical examination can reveal objective signs of malnutrition (Table 8-4). It is important to note, however, that some of these signs are nonspecific and that the physiologic changes of pregnancy may complicate the interpretation of physical findings. For example, lower extremity edema often occurs in caloric and protein deficiency, but it may also be a normal finding in the third trimester of pregnancy. Interpretation of physical findings is made easier by a thorough health history and by laboratory testing if indicated.

Laboratory testing. The only nutrition-related laboratory testing needed by most pregnant women is a hematocrit or hemoglobin measurement to screen for the presence of **anemia.** An individual's history or physical findings may indicate the need for additional testing, such as a complete blood cell count with a differential to identify megaloblastic or macrocytic anemia and measurement of levels of specific vitamins or minerals believed to be lacking in the diet.

Nursing Diagnoses

Nutrition-related nursing diagnoses that commonly arise from the assessment include the following

- Altered nutrition: less than body requirements related to
  - Knowledge deficit regarding nutritional needs and optimal weight gain during pregnancy
  - Inadequate income
  - Stress over an unwanted pregnancy
  - Nausea and vomiting (either mild-to-moderate effects of morning sickness or more severe effects of hyperemesis gravidarum)
  - Cultural patterns of food intake
  - Adherence to a therapeutic diet regimen
  - Concurrent use of medications
  - Drug or alcohol abuse
  - Failure to take nutritional supplements as prescribed
  - Smoking
  - Multifetal gestation
  - Adolescent pregnancy, in which increased needs of pregnancy are imposed on a girl whose own needs for growth and maturation are still high and whose eating habits are often poor
  - Poor intake and stores of iron and increase in need result in iron defiency anemia
- Altered nutrition: more than body requirements related to
  - Knowledge deficit regarding nutritional needs and optimal weight gain during pregnancy, with resultant overeating
  - Cultural patterns that foster overeating
  - A decline in activity as pregnancy progresses
  - Use of unneeded dietary supplements (particularly fat-soluble vitamins)
- Constipation related to
  - Decrease in activity with pregnancy
  - Inadequate fiber or fluid intake
  - Use of iron supplement
  - Displacement of intestines by the enlarging uterus
  - Increased progesterone levels during pregnancy, which decrease the tone and motility of intestinal musculature

Expected Outcomes

An individualized nursing care plan based on the nursing diagnoses should be developed in collaboration with the

Text continued on p. 194.

TABLE 8-3 Characteristic food patterns of some cultures

ETHNIC GROUP	MILK GROUP	PROTEIN GROUP	FRUITS AND VEGETABLES	BREADS AND CEREALS	POSSIBLE DIETARY PROBLEMS
Native American (many tribal variations; many "Americanized")	Fresh milk Evaporated milk for cooking Ice cream Cream pies	Pork, beef, lamb, rabbit Fowl, fish, eggs Legumes Sunflower seeds Nuts: walnut, acorn, pine, peanut butter Game meat	Green beans, peas Beets, turnips, squash, peppers Leafy green and other vegetables	Refined bread Whole wheat Cornmeal Rice Dry cereals "Fry" bread Tortillas	Obesity, diabetes, alcoholism, nutritional deficiencies expressed in dental problems and iron deficiency anemia Inadequate amounts of all nutrients Excessive use of sugar
Middle Eastern* (Armenian, Greek, Syrian, Turkish)	Yogurt Little butter	Lamb Nuts Dried peas, beans, lentils Sesame seeds	Peppers, tomatoes, cabbage, grape leaves, cucumbers, squash Dried apricots, raisins, dates	Cracked wheat and dark bread	Many fried meats and vegetables Lack of fresh fruits Insufficient foods from milk group High consumption of sweeteners, lamb fat, and olive oil
African-American	Milk† Ice cream Cheese: long horn, American	Pork: all cuts, plus organs, chitterlings Beef, lamb Chicken, giblets Eggs Nuts Legumes Fish, game	Leafy vegetables Green and yellow vegetables Potatoes: white, sweet Stewed fruit Bananas and other fresh fruit	Cornmeal and hominy grits Rice Biscuits, pancakes, white breads	Extensive use of frying, "smothering" in gravy, or simmering Fats: salt pork, bacon drippings, lard, gravies High consumption of sweets Insufficient citrus Vegetables often boiled for long periods with pork fat and much salt Limted amounts from milk group†
Chinese (Cantonese most prevalent)	Milk: water buffalo	Pork sausage‡ Eggs and pigeon eggs Fish Lamb, beef, goat Fowl: chicken, duck Nuts Legumes Soybean curd (tofu)	Many vegetables Radish leaves Bean/bamboo sprouts	Rice/rice flour products Cereals, noodles Wheat, corn, millet seed	Tendency of some immigrants to use large amounts of grease in cooking Limited use of milk and milk products Often low in protein, calories, or both May wash rice before cooking, removing vitamins added in fortification Soy sauce (high sodium)
Polish	Milk Sour cream Cheese Butter	Pork (preferred) Chicken	Vegetables Cabbage Roots Fruits	Dark rye	Sodium in ham, sausages, pickles High consumption of sweets Tendency to overcook vegetables Limited fruits (especially citrus), raw vegetables, and meats
Puerto Rican	Limited use of milk products Coffee with milk *(café con leche)*	Pork Poultry Eggs (Fridays) Beans *(habichuelas)*	Avocado, okra Eggplant Sweet yams Starchy vegetables and fruits *(viandas)*	Rice Cornmeal	Small amounts of pork and poultry Extensive use of fat, lard, salt pork, and olive oil Lack of milk products
Scandinavian: Danish, Finnish, Norwegian, Swedish	Cream Butter Cheeses	Wild game Reindeer Fish (fresh or dried) Eggs	Berries Dried fruit Vegetables: cole slaw, roots	Whole wheat, rye, barley, sweets (cookies, sweetbreads)	Insufficient fresh fruits and vegetables High consumption of sweets, pickled, salted meats/fish Liberal use of fat

Southeast Asian: Vietnamese, Cambodian	Generally not taken Coffee with condensed cow's milk Plain yogurt Ice cream (rare) Soybean milk	Fish (daily): fresh, dried, salted Poultry/eggs: duck, chicken Pork Beef (seldom) Dry beans Tofu	Seasonal variety: fresh or preserved Green, leafy vegetables Yams Corn	Rice: grains, flour, noodles French bread "Cellophane" (bean starch) noodles	Fresh milk products generally not consumed Poultry/eggs may be limited Meat considered "unclean" is avoided Preference for diet high in salt/pepper and rice/pork High intake of MSG and soy sauce
Jewish: Orthodox*	Milk§ Cheese§	Meat (bloodless; Kosher prepared): beef, lamb, goat, deer, poultry (all types), no pork Fish with fins and scales only No crustaceans	Wide variety	Wide variety	High intake of sodium in meat products
Filipino (Spanish-Chinese influence)	Flavored milk, milk in coffee Cheese: gouda, cheddar	Pork, beef, goat, deer, rabbit Chicken Fish Eggs, nuts, legumes	Many vegetables and fruits	Rice, cooked cereals Noodles: rice, wheat	Limited use of milk and milk products Tendency to prewash rice Tendency to have only small portions of protein foods
Italian	Cheese Some ice cream	Meat Eggs Dried beans	Leafy vegetables Potatoes Egglant, tomatoes, peppers Fruits	Pasta White breads, some whole wheat Farina Cereals	Prefer expensive imported cheeses; reluctant to substitute less expensive domestic varieties Tendency to overcook vegetables Limited use of whole grains High consumption of sweets Extensive use of olive oil Insufficient servings from milk group
Japanese (Isei, more Japanese influence; Nisei, more westernized)	Increasing amounts being used by younger generations	Pork, beef, chicken Fish Eggs Legumes: soya, red, lima beans Tofu Nuts	Many vegetables and fruits Seaweed	Rice, rice cakes Wheat noodles Refined bread, noodles	Excessive sodium: pickles, salty crisp seaweed, MSG, soy sauce Insufficient servings from milk group May use prewashed rice
Hispanic, Mexican-American	Milk Cheese Flan, ice cream	Beef, pork, lamb, chicken, tripe, hot sausage, beef intestines Fish Eggs Nuts Dry beans: pinto, chickpeas (often eaten more than once daily)	Spinach, wild greens, tomatoes, chilies, corn, cactus leaves, cabbage, avocado, potatoes Pumpkin, zapote, peaches, guava, papaya, citrus	Rice, cornmeal Sweet bread, pastries Tortilla: corn, flour Vermicelli *(fideo)*	Limited meats primarily because of cost Limited use of milk and milk products Large amounts of lard Abundant use of sugar Tendency to boil vegetables for long periods

MSG, Monosodium L-glutamate.
*Religious holidays may involve fasting, which is believed to increase the likelihood of preterm labor. Fasting requirement may be waived during pregnancy.
†Lactose intolerance relatively common in adults.
‡Lower in fat content than Western sausage.
§Milk and milk products not eaten with meat; milk may be taken before meal or 6 hours after meal; different sets of dishes and silverware are used to serve milk and meat products.

BOX 8-3
Nutrition Questionnaire

What you eat and some life-style choices you make can affect your nutrition and health now and in the future. Your nutrition can also have an important effect on your baby's health. Please answer these questions by circling the answers that apply to you.

EATING BEHAVIOR

1. Are you often bothered by any of the following? (circle all that apply):		
Nausea Vomiting Heartburn Constipation		
2. Do you skip meals at least three times a week?	No	Yes
3. Do you try to limit the amount or kind of food you eat to control your weight?	No	Yes
4. Are you on a special diet now?	No	Yes
5. Do you avoid any foods for health or religious reasons?	No	Yes

FOOD RESOURCES

1. Do you have a working stove?	No	Yes
Do you have a working refrigerator?	No	Yes
2. Do you sometimes run out of food before you are able to buy more?	No	Yes
3. Can you afford to eat the way you should?	No	Yes
4. Are you receiving any food assistance now? (circle all that apply):	No	Yes
Food stamps School breakfast School lunch		
WIC Donated food/commodities CSFP		
Food from a food pantry, soup kitchen, or food bank		
5. Do you feel you need help obtaining food?	No	Yes

FOOD AND DRINK

1. Which of these did you drink yesterday: (circle all that apply):

Soft drinks	Coffee	Tea	Fruit drinks
Orange juice	Grapefruit juice	Other juices	Milk
Kool-Aid	Beer	Wine	Alcoholic drinks
Water	Other beverages (list) ______		

2. Which of these foods did you eat yesterday? (circle all that apply):

Cheese	Pizza	Macaroni and cheese	
Yogurt	Cereal with milk		
Other foods made with cheese (e.g., tacos, enchiladas, lasagna, cheeseburgers)			
Corn	Potatoes	Sweet potatoes	Green salad
Carrots	Collard greens	Spinach	Turnip greens
Broccoli	Green beans	Green peas	Other vegetables
Apples	Bananas	Berries	Grapefruit
Melons	Oranges	Peaches	Other fruits
Meat	Fish	Chicken	Eggs
Peanut butter	Nuts	Seeds	Dried beans
Cold cuts	Hot dogs	Bacon	Sausages
Cake	Cookies	Doughnuts	Pastries
Chips	French fries		
Other deep-fried foods (e.g., fried chicken, egg rolls)			
Bread	Rolls	Rice	Cereal
Noodles	Spaghetti	Tortillas	

Were any of these whole grain?	No	Yes
3. Is the way you ate yesterday the way you usually eat?	No	Yes

LIFE-STYLE

1. Do you exercise for at least 30 minutes on a regular basis (3 times a week or more)?	No	Yes
2. Do you ever smoke cigarettes or use smokeless tobacco?	No	Yes
3. Do you ever drink beer, wine, liquor, or any other alcoholic beverages?	No	Yes

4. Which of these do you take? (circle all that apply):
Prescribed drugs or medications
Any over-the-counter products (e.g., aspirin, Tylenol, antacids, vitamins)
Street drugs (e.g., marijuana, speed, downers, crack, heroin)

Modified from Food and Nutrition Board, Institute of Medicine: *Nutrition during pregnancy and lactation: an implementation guide*, Washington, DC, 1992, National Academic Press.

TABLE 8-4 Physical assessment of nutritional status

SIGNS OF GOOD NUTRITION	SIGNS OF POOR NUTRITION
General appearance	
Alert, responsive, energetic, good endurance	Listless, apathetic, cachectic, easily fatigued, looks tired
Weight	
Normal for height, age, body build	Overweight or underweight
Posture	
Erect, arms and legs straight	Sagging shoulders, sunken chest, humped back
Muscles	
Well developed, firm, good tone, some fat under skin	Flaccid, poor tone, undeveloped, tender, "wasted" appearance
Nervous control	
Good attention span, not irritable or restless, normal reflexes, psychologic stability	Inattentive, irritable, confused, burning and tingling of hands and feet, loss of position and vibratory sense, weakness and tenderness of muscles, decrease or loss of ankle and knee reflexes
Gastrointestinal function	
Good appetite and digestion, normal regular elimination, no palpable organs or masses	Anorexia, indigestion, constipation or diarrhea, liver or spleen enlargement
Cardiovascular function	
Normal heart rate and rhythm, no murmurs, normal blood pressure for age	Rapid heart rate, enlarged heart, abnormal rhythm, elevated blood pressure
Hair	
Shiny, lustrous, firm, not easily plucked, healthy scalp	Stringy, dull, brittle, dry, thin and sparse, depigmented, can be easily plucked
Skin (general)	
Smooth, slightly moist, good color	Rough, dry, scaly, pale, pigmented, irritated, easily bruised, petechiae
Face and neck	
Skin color uniform, smooth, pink, healthy appearance; no enlargement of thyroid gland; lips not chapped or swollen	Scaly, swollen, skin dark over cheeks and under eyes, lumpiness or flakiness of skin around nose and mouth; thyroid enlarged; lips swollen, angular lesions or fissures at corners of mouth
Oral cavity	
Reddish pink mucous membranes and gums; no swelling or bleeding of gums; tongue healthy pink or deep reddish in appearance, not swollen or smooth, surface papillae present; teeth bright and clean, no cavities, no pain, no discoloration	Gums spongy, bleed easily, inflamed or receding; tongue swollen, scarlet and raw, magenta color; beefy, hyperemic, hypertrophic papillae or atrophic papillae; absent teeth or teeth with unfilled caries, worn surfaces, mottled appearance
Eyes	
Bright, clear, shiny, no sores at corners of eyelids, membranes moist and healthy pink color, no prominent blood vessels or mound of tissue (Bitot spots) on sclera, no fatigue circles beneath	Paleness of eye membranes, redness of membrane, dryness, signs of infection, Bitot spots, redness and fissuring of eyelid corners, dryness of eye membrane, dull appearance of cornea, soft cornea, blue sclerae
Extremities	
No tenderness, weakness, or swelling; nails firm and pink	Edema, tender calf, tingling, weakness; nails spoon shaped, brittle
Skeleton	
No malformations	Bowlegs, knock-knees, chest deformity at diaphragm, beaded ribs, prominent scapulae

woman. For many women with uncomplicated pregnancies the nurse can serve as the primary source of nutrition education during pregnancy. The registered dietitian, who has specialized knowledge in diet evaluation and planning, nutritional needs in illness, ethnic and cultural food practices, and translating nutrient needs into food patterns, often serves as a consultant. Pregnant women with serious nutritional problems, those with intervening illnesses such as diabetes (either preexisting or gestational), and any others requiring in-depth dietary counseling should be referred to the dietitian. The nurse, dietitian, physician, and/or nurse-midwife collaborate in helping the woman to achieve nutrition-related expected outcomes. Some common nutrition-related outcomes are that the woman will take the following actions:

1. Achieve an appropriate weight gain during pregnancy. An appropriate goal for weight gain takes into account such factors as prepregnancy weight, whether the woman is overweight/obese or underweight, and whether the pregnancy is single or multifetal
2. Consume adequate nutrients from the diet and supplements to meet estimated needs
3. Cope sucessfully with nutrition-related discomforts associated with pregnancy, such as pyrosis (heartburn), morning sickness, and constipation
4. Avoid or reduce potentially harmful practices such as smoking, alcohol consumption, and caffeine intake
5. Make an informed decision about the method of feeding her infant
6. Breastfeed her infant successfully if she chooses to do so
7. Return to prepregnancy weight (or an appropriate weight for height) within 6 months of giving birth

Plan of Care and Implementation

Nutritional care and teaching generally involve the following:

1. Acquaint the woman with nutritional needs during pregnancy and the characteristics of an adequate diet, if necessary.
2. Help the woman to individualize her diet so that she achieves an adequate intake while satisfying her personal, cultural, financial, and health needs.
3. Acquaint the woman with strategies for coping with the nutrition-related discomforts of pregnancy.
4. Help the woman use nutrition supplements appropriately.
5. Discuss with the woman the advantages and disadvantages of breastfeeding or formula-feeding her infant, and support her in her decision.
6. Consult with and make referrals to other professionals or services, as indicated.

Two programs that provide nutrition services are the food stamp program and the Special Supplement Program for Women, Infants, and Children (WIC), which provide vouchers for selected foods to pregnant and lactating women, as well as infants and children at nutritional risk. WIC foods include items such as eggs, cheese, milk, juice, and fortified cereals; these foods are chosen because they provide iron, protein, vitamin C, and other vitamins.

Adequate dietary intake. Diet teaching can take place in a one-on-one interview or in a group setting. In either case it should emphasize the importance of choosing a varied diet composed of readily available foods (rather than specialized diet supplements). Good nutrition practices and avoidance of poor practices (e.g., smoking, alcohol or drug use) are essential content for prenatal classes designed for early pregnancy.

The Food Guide Pyramid (Fig. 8-6) can be used as a guide to daily food choices during pregnancy and lactation, just as it is during other stages of the life cycle. The pyramid places the bread, cereal, rice, and pasta group at its base. This position was chosen to indicate that this group should serve as the basis for a healthful diet; 6 to 11 servings are recommended each day. Vegetables (3 to 5 servings) and fruits (2 to 4 servings) are just above the grains group. The milk, yogurt, and cheese group (2 to 3 servings for nonpregnant adults, increasing to 3 to 4 servings for pregnant and lactating women) and the meat, poultry, fish, dry beans, eggs, and nuts group (2 to 3 servings) form a narrow band near the top of the pyramid. At the apex are fats, oils, and sweets (not considered a food group), which are to be used sparingly. The importance of consuming adequate amounts from the milk, yogurt, and cheese group needs to be emphasized, especially for adolescents and women under age 25, who are still actively adding calcium to their skeletons; adolescents need at least 4 cups of milk or the equivalent daily.

Pregnancy. The pregnant woman must understand what adequate weight gain during pregnancy means, recognize the reasons for its importance, and be able to evaluate her own gain in terms of the desirable pattern. Many women, particularly those who have worked hard to control their weight before pregnancy, may find it difficult to understand why the weight gain goal is so high when a newborn infant is so small. The nurse can explain that maternal weight gain consists of increments in the weight of many tissues, not just the growing fetus (Fig. 8-5).

Dietary overindulgence, on the other hand, which may result in excessive fat stores that persist after giving birth, should be discouraged. Nevertheless, it is best not to focus unduly on weight gain, which can result in feelings of stress and guilt in the woman who does not follow the preferred pattern of gain. Box 8-4 summarizes information regarding weight gain during pregnancy.

Postpartum. The need for a varied diet with representation from all food groups continues throughout lactation. As mentioned previously, the lactating woman should be advised to consume at least 1800 kcal daily, and she should receive counseling if her diet appears to be inadequate in any nutrients. Special attention should be given to calcium, zinc, vitamin B_6, and folate intake because the RDAs for these substances remain higher than those for nonpregnant women (Table 8-1) and it may be difficult to consume enough without careful diet planning.

The woman who does not breastfeed loses weight gradually if she consumes a balanced diet that provides slightly less than her daily energy expenditure. Both lactating and nonlactating women should know that fat is the most concentrated source of calories in the diet (9 kcal/g vs. 4 kcal/g in carbohydrates and proteins), and fat calories are more efficiently converted into fat stores than are calories from carbohydrate or protein. Therefore the first step in weight reduction

BOX 8-4
Weight Gain During Pregnancy

- Progressive weight gain during pregnancy is essential for normal fetal growth and development and for deposition of maternal stores that promote successful lactation.
- Recommended weight gain during pregnancy is determined largely by prepregnancy weight for height.
- Recommended weight gains: normal-weight women, 11-16.5 kg (25-35 lb); underweight women, 12.5-18 kg (28-40 lb); overweight women, 7-11.5 kg (15-25 lb)
- Weight gain should be achieved through a balanced diet of regular foods chosen from all of the different food groups (Table 8-3).
- The pattern of weight gain is important: approximately 0.4 kg (0.9-1 lb) per week during the second and third trimesters for normal-weight women; 0.5 kg (1.1 lb) per week for underweight women; and 0.3 kg (0.67 lb) per week for overweight women.

(or controlling excessive weight gain) is to evaluate sources of fat in the diet and explore with the patient ways of reducing them. Even foods such as vegetables that are originally low in fat can become high in fat when fried or sauteed, served with excessive amounts of salad dressing, consumed with high-fat dips or sauces, or seasoned with butter or bacon drippings. A reasonable weight loss goal for nonlactating women is 0.5 to 1 kg (1 to 2 lb)/week; a loss of 1 kg (2 lb)/month is recommended for most lactating women who need to lose weight.

Daily food guide and menu planning. The daily food plan (Table 8-2 and Fig. 8-6) can be used as a guide for educating the woman regarding nutritional needs during pregnancy and lactation. This food plan is general enough to be used by individuals from a variety of cultures, including those following a vegetarian diet. One of the more helpful teaching strategies is to assist the patient to plan daily menus that follow the food plan, are affordable, have realistic preparation times, and are compatible with personal preferences and cultural practices. This activity is often especially difficult for the nurse whose socioeconomic or cultural background is different from that of the patient. Table 8-3 and some of the sources in the bibliography at the end of the chapter provide information regarding dietary practices of different ethnic and cultural groups.

Therapeutic diets. During pregnancy and lactation, modifications may need to be made in the food plan for women with special therapeutic diets. The registered dietitian instructs these women about their diets and assists them in meal planning. The nurse should understand the basic principles of the diet and be able to reinforce the diet teaching.

The nurse should be especially aware of the dietary modifications necessary for women with diabetes mellitus (either gestational or preexisting) because this disease is relatively common and because fetal deformity and death occur more often in pregnancies complicated by hyperglycemia or hypoglycemia. Every effort should be made to maintain blood glucose levels in the normal range throughout pregnancy. The woman with diabetes usually has a food plan that includes four to six meals and snacks daily, with the daily carbohydrate intake distributed fairly evenly among those meals and snacks. The complex carbohydrates—fibers and starches—should be well represented in the diet of the woman with diabetes. To maintain strict control of blood glucose, the pregnant woman with diabetes usually must monitor her own blood glucose daily. Urine glucose and ketone measurements are not sensitive enough to detect hyperglycemia accurately and provide no information about hypoglycemia. The nurse must teach the woman how to self-monitor blood glucose unless the woman has been doing so before pregnancy.

Coping with nutrition-related discomforts of pregnancy. The most common nutrition-related discomforts of pregnancy are nausea and vomiting (or "morning sickness"), constipation, and pyrosis.

Nausea and vomiting. Nausea and vomiting are most common during the first trimester. In most patients, nausea and vomiting cause only mild-to-moderate problems nutritionally, but they may cause substantial discomfort. The pregnant woman may find the following suggestions helpful:

- Eat dry, starchy foods such as dry toast, Melba toast, or crackers on awakening in the morning and at other times when nausea occurs.
- Avoid excessive amounts of fluids early in the day or when nausea is present (but compensate by drinking fluids at other times).
- Eat small amounts frequently (every 2 to 3 hours) and avoid large meals, which distend the stomach.
- Avoid skipping meals and thus becoming extremely hungry, which may worsen nausea. Have a snack such as cereal with milk, a small sandwich, or yogurt before bedtime.
- Avoid sudden movements. Arise from bed slowly.
- Decrease intake of fried and other fatty foods. Starches such as pastas, rice, and breads and low-fat protein foods (e.g., skinless broiled or baked poultry, cooked dry beans or peas, lean meats, broiled or canned fish) are good choices. Some women find that tart foods or drinks (e.g., lemonade) or salty foods (e.g., potato chips) are effective in reducing nausea (Erick, 1994).
- Fresh air may help relieve nausea. Keep the environment well ventilated (e.g., open a window), go for a walk outside, or decrease cooking odors by using an exhaust fan.
- Choose foods served at cool temperatures and foods with little aroma during periods of nausea.
- Avoid brushing teeth immediately after eating.

Box 8-5 provides a sample daily food plan, which follows these guidelines while providing an adequate diet for the pregnant woman.

Hyperemesis gravidarum, or severe and persistent vomiting causing weight loss, dehydration, and electrolyte abnormalities, occurs in up to 1% of pregnant women. Intravenous fluid and electrolyte replacement is usually necessary for women who have lost 5% of their body weight. Often this treatment is followed by improved tolerance of oral intake; therapy then consists of frequently consuming small amounts of low-fat foods. Enteral tube feeding using small-bore nasogastric tubes has been successful for some women. Because pulmonary aspiration of the feeding is a potential complica-

BOX 8-5
Food Plan for a Woman with Nausea and Vomiting During Early Pregnancy

Breakfast
Toasted oat bran bagel, plain

Midmorning
Blueberry muffin
Skim milk

Lunch
Pasta salad with tuna
Carrot sticks
Melon balls
Water

Afternoon
Vegetable juice
Rice cake

Dinner
Baked chicken with skin removed
Spinach salad
Butternut squash casserole
Skim milk

Evening/bedtime
Wheat bran cereal
Strawberries
Skim milk

BOX 8-6
Iron Supplementation

- It is difficult to consume enough iron in the diet to meet iron needs and prevent anemia during pregnancy.
- Vitamin C (in citrus fruits, tomatoes, melons, and strawberries) and heme iron (in meats, fish, and poultry) increase absorption of iron supplements. Include these in the diet often.
- Bran, tea, coffee, milk, oxalates (in spinach and Swiss chard), and egg yolks decrease iron absorption. Avoid consuming them at the same time as the supplement.
- Iron is best absorbed if it is taken when the stomach is empty; that is, it should be taken between meals with a beverage other than tea, coffee, or milk.
- Iron can be taken at bedtime if abdominal discomfort occurs when it is taken between meals.
- If an iron dose is missed, take it as soon as you remember if it is within 13 hours of the scheduled dose. Do not double the dose.
- Keep the supplement in a child-proof container and out of the reach of any children in the household.
- Stool may be black or dark green because of the iron.

tion if vomiting occurs, antiemetic medications are sometimes used in conjunction with tube feedings. Tube feedings may be used to supplement oral intake, with the volume of the tube feeding gradually decreased as oral intake improves. In some instances, total parenteral nutrition (balanced intravenous feedings of amino acids, carbohydrate, lipid, vitamins, and minerals) has been used to nourish women with hyperemesis gravidarum when nutritional status was severely imperiled (Newman, Fullerton, and Anderson, 1993).

Constipation. Improved bowel function generally results from increasing the intake of fiber (e.g., wheat bran and whole-wheat products, popcorn, raw or lightly steamed vegetables) in the diet because fiber helps to retain water within the stool, which creates a bulky stool that stimulates intestinal peristalsis. An adequate fluid intake (at least 35 ml/kg/day) helps to hydrate the fiber and increase the bulk of the stool. Making a habit of regular exercise that uses large muscle groups (walking, swimming, cycling) also helps to stimulate bowel motility.

Pyrosis. Pyrosis, or heartburn, is caused by reflux from the stomach into the esophagus. This condition can be minimized by the consumption of small, frequent meals rather than two or three larger meals daily. Because fluids increase the distention of the stomach, they should not be consumed with foods; however, the woman needs to ensure that she drinks adequate amounts between meals. Avoiding spicy foods may help alleviate the problem. Lying down immediately after eating and wearing clothing that is tight across the abdomen can contribute to the problem of reflux.

Counseling regarding iron supplementation. The nutritional supplement most commonly needed during pregnancy is iron. A variety of dietary factors can affect the completeness of absorption of an iron supplement. When bran, milk, egg yolk, coffee, tea, or oxalate-containing vegetables such as spinach and Swiss chard are consumed at the same time as iron, they inhibit iron absorption. Conversely, iron absorption is promoted by a diet rich in vitamin C sources (e.g., citrus fruits or melons) or "heme iron" (found in red meats, fish, and poultry). Iron supplements are best absorbed on an empty stomach. Thus they can be taken between meals with beverages other than milk, tea, or coffee. Some women have gastrointestinal discomfort when they take the supplement on an empty stomach; a good time for them to take the supplement is just before bedtime. Iron supplements should be kept away from any children in the household because their ingestion could result in acute iron poisoning and even death. Box 8-6 summarizes the important points of teaching about iron supplementation.

Evaluation

It is essential to set concrete measurable outcomes, to evaluate progress toward these outcomes regularly, and to revise the nursing care plan if the outcomes are not achieved.

In evaluating the adequacy of nutritional intake during pregnancy, the patient's weight gain can be compared with standardized grids showing optimal patterns (Fig. 8-4). It is helpful to remember that these grids are based on mean data and do not always account for factors such as ethnic or racial variations. To evaluate the adequacy of the woman's diet, it can be compared with the plan in Table 8-2. Again, it is essential that individual factors affecting nutritional needs and dietary intake be considered. Physical examination and laboratory testing can be used to confirm that nutritional status is adequate (see the section on assessment). For example, a hematocrit greater than 35% and a hemoglobin concentration greater than 11.5 g/dl are indicators that iron intake is adequate to prevent anemia. When weight gain is inadequate or nutritional deficits appear, the nurse must reassess the woman and her understanding of her nutritional needs, reinforce teaching as needed, and continue to reevaluate regularly (see the Nursing Care Plan below).

Nursing Care Plan

NUTRITION DURING PREGNANCY

Nursing Diagnosis: Knowledge deficit related to nutritional requirements during pregnancy

Expected Outcomes: The patient will delineate nutritional requirements and exhibit evidence of incorporating requirements into diet.

• **NURSING INTERVENTIONS/*RATIONALES***

Review basic nutritional requirements for a healthy diet using recommended dietary guidelines and the food guide pyramid *to provide knowledge baseline for discussion.*

Discuss increased nutrient needs (calories, protein, minerals, vitamins) that occur as a result of being pregnant *to increase knowledge needed for altered dietary requirements.*

Discuss the relationship between weight gain and fetal growth *to reinforce interdependence of fetus and mother.*

Calculate the appropriate total weight gain range during pregnancy using the woman's body mass index as a guide and discuss recommended rates of weight gain during the various trimesters of pregnancy *to provide concrete measures of dietary success.*

Review food preferences, cultural eating patterns or beliefs, and prepregnancy eating patterns *to enhance integration of new dietary needs.*

Discuss how to fit nutritional needs into usual dietary patterns and how to alter any identified nutritional deficits or excesses *to increase chances of success with dietary alterations.*

Discuss food aversions or cravings that may occur during pregnancy and strategies to deal with these if they are detrimental to fetus (e.g., pica) *to ensure well-being of fetus.*

Have woman keep a food diary delineating eating habits, dietary alterations, aversions, and cravings *to track eating habits and potential problem areas.*

Nursing Diagnosis: Altered nutrition: more than body requirements related to excessive intake and/or inadequate activity levels

Expected Outcome: The patient's weekly weight gain will be reduced to the appropriate rate using her body mass index and recommended weight gain ranges as guidelines.

• **NURSING INTERVENTIONS/*RATIONALES***

Review recent diet history (including food cravings) using a food diary, 24-hour recall, or food frequency approach *to ascertain food excesses contributing to excess weight gain.*

Review normal activity and exercise routines *to determine level of energy expenditure;* discuss eating patterns and reasons that lead to increased food intake (e.g., cultural beliefs or myths, increased stress, boredom) *to identify habits that contribute to excess weight gain.*

Review optimal weight gain guidelines and their rationale *to ensure that woman is knowledgeable about healthful weight gain rates.*

Set target weight gains for the remaining weeks of the pregnancy *to establish set goals.*

Discuss with the woman what changes can be made in diet, activity, and life-style *to enhance chances of meeting weight gain goals and dietary needs.* (Weight reduction diets should be avoided, since they may deprive mother and fetus of needed nutrients and lead to ketonemia.)

Nursing Diagnosis: Altered nutrition: less than body requirements related to inadequate intake of needed nutrients

Expected Outcome: The patient's weekly weight gain will be increased to the appropriate rate using her body mass index and recommended weight gain ranges as guidelines.

• **NURSING INTERVENTIONS/*RATIONALES***

Review recent diet history (including food aversions) using a food diary, 24-hour recall, or food frequency approach *to ascertain dietary inadequacies contributing to lack of sufficient weight gain.*

Review normal activity and exercise routines *to determine level of energy expenditure;* discuss eating patterns and reasons that lead to decreased food intake (e.g., morning sickness, pica, fear of becoming fat, stress, boredom) *to identify habits that contribute to inadequate weight gain.*

Review optimal weight gain guidelines and their rationale *to ensure that woman is knowledgeable about healthful weight gain rates.*

Set target weight gains for the remaining weeks of the pregnancy *to establish set goals.*

Review increased nutrient needs (calories, protein, minerals, vitamins) that occur as a result of being pregnant *to ensure woman is knowledgeable about altered dietary requirements.*

Review relationship between weight gain and fetal growth *to reinforce that adequate weight gain is needed to promote fetal well-being.*

Discuss with woman what changes can be made in diet, activity, and life-style *to enhance chances of meeting set weight gain goals and nutrient needs of mother and fetus.*

If woman has fear of being fat, if symptoms of an eating disorder are evident, or if problems in adjusting to a changing body image surface, refer woman to the appropriate mental health professional for evaluation, *since intensive treatment and follow-up may be required to ensure fetal health.*

Key Points

- A woman's nutritional status before, during, and after pregnancy contributes significantly to her and her infant's well-being.
- Many physiologic changes occurring during pregnancy influence the need for nutrients and the efficiency with which the body uses them.
- Both the total maternal weight gain and the pattern of weight gain are important determinants of the pregnancy outcome.
- The recommended weight gain during pregnancy is determined by the appropriateness of the mother's prepregnancy weight for her height.
- Nutritional risk factors include adolescent pregnancy, smoking, alcohol or drug use, multifetal gestation, poor nutritional knowledge, bizarre food habits, poverty, and frequent pregnancies.
- Iron supplementation is recommended routinely during pregnancy. Other supplements may be warranted when nutritional risk factors are present.
- The nurse and the woman are influenced by cultural and personal values and beliefs during nutrition counseling.
- Pregnancy complications that may be nutrition-related include anemia, PIH, preterm birth, and IUGR.
- Dietary adaptations can be effective interventions for some of the common discomforts of pregnancy, including nausea and vomiting, constipation, and pyrosis.

References

American College of Obstetrics and Gynecology (ACOG): Exercise during pregnancy and the postpartum period, *ACOG Tech Bull* 189, February 1994.

Beard J: Iron deficiency: assessment during pregnancy and its importance in pregnant adolescents, *Am J Clin Nutr* 59(suppl):502S, 1994.

Centers for Disease Control and Prevention (CDC): Recommendations for the use of folic acid to reduce the number of cases of spina bifida and other neural tube defects, *MMWR* 41(no RR-14):1, 1992

Dewey K, Heinig M, Nommsen L: Maternal weight-loss patterns during prolonged lactation, *Am J Clin Nutr* 58:162, 1993.

Erick M: Battling morning (noon and night) sickness: new approaches for treating an age-old problem, *J Am Diet Assoc* 94:147, 1994.

Guyer B et al: Annual summary of vital statistics—1994, *Pediatrics* 96:1029, 1995.

Horner R et al: Pica practices of pregnant women, *J Am Diet Assoc* 91:34, 1991.

Institute of Medicine: *Nutrition during pregnancy and lactation: an implementation guide*, Washington, DC, 1992, National Academy Press.

Keen K, Zedenberg-Cherr S: Should vitamin-mineral supplements be recommended for all women with child-bearing potential? *Am J Clin Nutr* 59(suppl):532S, 1994.

Lawrence R: *Breastfeeding: a guide for the medical profession*, ed 4, St Louis, 1994, Mosby.

Lindenberg C et al: A review of the literature on cocaine abuse in pregnancy, *Nurs Res* 40:69, 1991.

Nehlig A, Debry G: Consequences on the newborn of chronic maternal consumption of coffee during gestation and lactation: a review, *J Am Coll Nutr* 13:6, 1994.

Newman V, Fullerton J: Role of nutrition in the prevention of preeclampsia: review of the literature, *J Nurse Midwif* 35:282, 1990.

Newman V, Fullerton J, Anderson P: Clinical advances in the management of severe nausea and vomiting during pregnancy, *J Obstet Gynecol Neonatal Nurs* 22:483, 1993.

Position of the American Dietetic Association: Use of nutritive and nonnutritive sweeteners, *J Am Diet Assoc* 93:816, 1993.

Roberts J: Current perspectives on preeclampsia, *J Nurse Midwif* 39:70, 1994.

Scholl T, Hediger M: A review of the epidemiology of nutrition and adolescent pregnancy: maternal growth during pregnancy and its effect on the fetus, *J Am Coll Nutr* 12:101, 1993.

Scholl T, Hediger M: Anemia and iron-deficiency anemia: compilation of data on pregnancy outcome, *Am J Clin Nutr* 59(suppl):492S, 1994.

Snodgrass S: Cocaine babies: a result of multiple teratogenic influences, *J Child Neurol* 9:227, 1994.

Wiecha J, Dwyer J, Dunn-Strohecker M: Nutrition and health services needs among the homeless, *Public Health Rep* 106:364, 1991.

Worthington-Roberts B, Williams S: *Nutrition in pregnancy and lactation*, ed 5, St Louis, 1993, Mosby.

Bibliography

American College of Obstetrics and Gynecology (ACOG): Nutrition during pregnancy, *ACOG Tech Bull* 179, April 1993.

Carruth B, Skinner J: Practitioners beware: regional differences in beliefs about nutrition during pregnancy, *J Am Diet Assoc* 91:435, 1991.

Eliades D, Suitor C: *Celebrating diversity: approaching families through their food*, Arlington, Va, 1994, National Center for Education in Maternal and Child Health.

Food and Nutrition Board: *Recommended dietary allowances*, ed 10, Washington, DC, 1989, National Academy of Sciences–National Research Council.

Gizis F: Nutrition in women across the life span, *Nurs Clin North Am* 27:971, 1992.

Gutierrez Y, King J: Nutrition during teenage pregnancy, *Pediatr Ann* 22:99, 1993.

Olson C: Promoting positive nutritional practices during pregnancy and lactation, *Am J Clin Nutr* 59(suppl 2):525S, 1994.

Rees J, Worthington-Roberts B: Position of the American Dietetic Association: nutrition care for pregnant adolescents, *J Am Diet Assoc* 94:449, 1994.

CHAPTER 9

Hypertension, Hemorrhage, and Maternal Infection

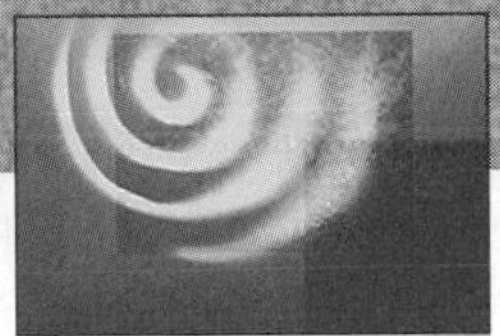

HYPERTENSION IN PREGNANCY, P. 199
Significance and incidence, p. 199
Morbidity and mortality, p. 199
Classification, p. 199
Etiology of preeclampsia, p. 201
Pathophysiology of preeclampsia, p. 201
Mild vs. severe preeclampsia, p. 202
HELLP syndrome, p. 202
Nursing care management, p. 204

MATERNAL HEMORRHAGIC DISORDERS, P. 216
Early pregnancy bleeding, p. 216
Nursing care management, p. 218
Late pregnancy bleeding, p. 224
Nursing care management, p. 228
Clotting disorders in pregnancy, p. 230

MATERNAL INFECTIONS, P. 231
Sexually transmitted disease, p. 232
Genital tract infections, p. 240
General infections, p. 242
Infection control, p. 244
Nursing care management, p. 244

Providing safe and effective care for the high-risk patient requires a joint effort from all members of the health care team, with each member contributing unique skills and talents to provide optimum outcomes for mother and infant. This chapter focuses on the three major maternal conditions that can affect the health of the woman, fetus, or newborn: hypertensive states, hemorrhage, and maternal infections.

HYPERTENSION IN PREGNANCY

Significance and Incidence

Hypertensive disorders of pregnancy greatly contribute to maternal and perinatal morbidity and mortality. It is estimated that hypertension complicates approximately 5% to 7% of all pregnancies (Gilbert and Harmon, 1993a, b). Of the women with hypertension during pregnancy, between one half and two thirds are diagnosed with preeclampsia or eclampsia (Brown, 1991). The prevalence is increased to as many as 20% to 40% of pregnancies in women with chronic renal disease or vascular disorders such as essential hypertension, diabetes mellitus, and lupus erythematosus (Fairlie and Sibai, 1993; Scott et al, 1994).

Morbidity and Mortality

Hypertension complicating pregnancy is a leading cause of maternal and infant morbidity and mortality. Preeclampsia/eclampsia may predispose the woman to potentially lethal complications such as abruptio placentae, **disseminated intravascular coagulation (DIC),** cerebral hemorrhage, cerebral vascular accident, hepatic failure, and acute renal failure (Consensus Report, 1990).

Preeclampsia contributes to intrauterine fetal death and perinatal mortality. The main causes of neonatal death from preeclampsia are placental insufficiency and abruptio placentae. Also, intrauterine growth restriction (IUGR) is common in infants of preeclamptic women (Roberts et al, 1990; Sibai, 1990a).

Eclampsia (seizures) from profound cerebral effects of pregnancy-induced hypertension is the major maternal hazard. As a rule, maternal and perinatal morbidity and mortality are highest when eclampsia presents early in gestation (before 28 weeks), maternal age is over 25 years, the woman is a multigravida, and chronic hypertension or renal disease is present. Outcomes are also more complicated in women who receive little or no prenatal care or who are transported from other health care facilities (Fairlie and Sibai, 1993). The fetus of the eclamptic woman is at increased risk from abruptio placentae, preterm birth, IUGR and acute hypoxia (Gilbert and Harmon, 1993a, b; Sibai, 1990a).

Classification

The hypertensive disorders of pregnancy refer to a variety of conditions in which maternal blood pressure is elevated with a corresponding risk to maternal and fetal well-being. Originally, hypertensive disorders of pregnancy were termed *toxemia;* however, this is inappropriate because no toxic agent or toxins have been identified. Confusion over classification continues today, causing difficulties in establishing a clinical diagnosis of the specific hypertensive disorder (Sibai and Anderson, 1991). The clinical classification is the one most frequently used today (Consensus Report, 1990).

Preeclampsia, eclampsia, and transient hypertension are gestational hypertensive disorders, often referred to as **pregnancy-induced hypertension (PIH).** Chronic hypertensive states are related to preexisting conditions.

Preeclampsia. Preeclampsia is a pregnancy-specific condition in which hypertension develops after 20 weeks of gestation in a previously normotensive woman. **Preeclampsia** is a multisystem, vasospastic disease process characterized by hemoconcentration, hypertension, and proteinuria. The diagnosis of preeclampsia has traditionally been based on the presence of hypertension with proteinuria and/or edema. However, the most significant finding is hypertension, since 20% of preeclampsia patients have no significant proteinuria before their first seizure (Willis and Blanco, 1990).

Hypertension is defined as an elevation of systolic and diastolic pressures equal to or exceeding 140/90 mm Hg. When first-trimester blood pressures are known, they serve as the woman's baseline values. Using this information, an alternative definition for hypertension is a rise in systolic pressure of 30 mm Hg or a rise in diastolic pressure of 15 mm Hg above the woman's baseline values. This latter definition is considered more sensitive to individual variations such as age, race, physiologic state, dietary habits, and heredity. The Committee on Terminology of the American College of Obstetricians and Gynecologists (ACOG) has also defined hypertension as an increase in **mean arterial pressure (MAP)** of 20 mm Hg; alternately, if prior blood pressures are unknown, a MAP of 105 mm Hg is definitive for hypertension.

The blood pressure elevation must be present on at least two occasions 4 to 6 hours apart (Fairlie and Sibai, 1993). Techniques of measurement must be standardized.

TABLE 9-1 Differentiation of mild and severe preeclampsia

	MILD PREECLAMPSIA	SEVERE PREECLAMPSIA
Maternal effects		
Blood pressure	Rise in systolic blood pressure of 30 mm Hg or more or a rise in diastolic blood pressure of ≥15 mm Hg or a reading of 140/90 mm Hg on two occasions 6 hours apart	Rise to ≥160 mm Hg systolic or 110 mm Hg diastolic on two separate occasions 6 hours apart with pregnant woman on bed rest
MAP	140/90 = 107	160/110 = 127
Weight gain	Weight gain of more than 0.5 kg (1 lb)/wk during the second and third trimesters or a sudden weight gain of 2 kg (4 to $4^1/_2$ lb)/wk at any time	Same as mild preeclampsia
Proteinuria Qualitative dipstick Quantitative 24-hour analysis	Proteinuria of 300 mg/L in a 24-hour specimen or >1 g/L in a random daytime specimen on two or more occasions 6 hours apart because protein loss is variable; with dipstick, values vary from trace to 1+	Proteinuria of 2 g/L in 24 hours or ≥2+ protein on dipstick
Edema	Dependent edema, some puffiness of eyes, face, fingers; pulmonary crackles absent	Generalized edema, noticeable puffiness of eyes, face, fingers; pulmonary crackles may be present
Reflexes	Hyperreflexia 3+; no ankle clonus	Hyperreflexia 3+ or more; ankle clonus
Urine output	Output matches intake; ≥30 ml/hr	Oliguria: <30 ml/hr or 100 ml/4 hr output
Headache	Transient	Severe
Visual problems	Absent	Blurred, photophobia, blind spots on ophthalmoscopy
Irritability/affect	Transient	Severe
Epigastric pain	Absent	Present
Serum creatinine	Normal	Elevated
Thrombocytopenia	Absent	Present
AST elevation	Minimal	Marked
Hematocrit	Increased	Increased initially, then decreased with hemolysis
Fetal effects		
Placental perfusion	Reduced	Decreased perfusion expressed as IUGR in fetus; FHR: late decelerations; oligohydramnios
Premature placental aging	Not apparent	At birth, placenta appears smaller than normal for duration of pregnancy; premature aging is apparent with numerous areas of broken syncytia; ischemic necroses (white infarcts) are numerous, and intervillous fibrin deposition (red infarcts) may be recorded

MAP, Mean arterial pressure; *AST,* aspartate aminotransferase; *IUGR,* intrauterine growth restriction; *FHR,* fetal heart rate.

Proteinuria is defined as a concentration of 0.1 g/L (greater than 2+ on dipstick) or more in at least two random urine specimens collected at least 6 hours apart. In a 24-hour specimen, proteinuria is defined as a concentration of 0.3 g/24 hours.

Edema is no longer necessary for the diagnosis of preeclampsia (Sibai and Rodriguez, 1992). If present, edema is a generalized accumulation of interstitial fluid after 12 hours of bed rest or a weight gain of more than 2 kg (4½ to 5 lb) per week. In the presence of hypertension and/or proteinuria, edema should be evaluated as a reflection of end-organ edema and possible organ hypoxia (Table 9-1).

Eclampsia. Eclampsia is the development of convulsions or coma in patients with signs and symptoms of preeclampsia, proteinuria, edema, or all of these. It is not caused by any coincidental neurologic disease such as epilepsy.

Chronic hypertension. Chronic hypertension is defined as hypertension present before the pregnancy or diagnosed before the twentieth week of gestation. Hypertension that persists longer than 6 weeks postpartum is also classified as chronic hypertension. Preconception counseling about the increased risk of superimposed preeclampsia is recommended.

Chronic hypertension with superimposed preeclampsia/eclampsia. Women with chronic hypertension may develop preeclampsia or eclampsia. The development of preeclampsia or eclampsia in the woman with chronic hypertension increases maternal and perinatal morbidity and mortality. The ACOG recommends that the diagnosis of superimposed preeclampsia be made on the basis of an increase in blood pressure together with the presence of proteinuria or generalized edema (Consensus Report, 1990).

Etiology of Preeclampsia

Preeclampsia is a condition unique to human pregnancy; signs and symptoms develop only during pregnancy and disappear quickly after birth of the fetus and placenta. The cause is unknown. No one patient profile identifies the woman who will develop preeclampsia. However, certain high-risk factors are associated with developing the disease: primigravidity, grand multigravidity, large fetus, multifetal pregnancy, and morbid obesity. Approximately 85% of preeclampsia is seen during the first pregnancy. It occurs in 14% to 20% of multifetal pregnancies and in 30% of patients with major uterine anomalies. In women with chronic hypertension or renal disease the incidence may be as high as 25% (Zuspan, 1991). Preeclampsia is a disease that progresses along a continuum from mild disease to severe preeclampsia, HELLP syndrome, or eclampsia.

Pathophysiology of Preeclampsia

The pathophysiology of preeclampsia/eclampsia is somehow related to the physiologic changes of pregnancy. Normal physiologic adaptations to pregnancy include an increase in blood plasma volume, vasodilation, decreased systemic vascular resistance (SVR), elevated cardiac output (CO), and a decreased colloid osmotic pressure (COP) (Box 9-1). In preeclampsia, circulating plasma volume decreases, resulting in hemoconcentration and an increase in maternal hematocrit. These changes lead to a decrease in maternal organ perfusion, including the uteroplacental-fetal unit. Cyclic vasospasms further decrease organ perfusion by destroying red blood cells, thereby decreasing maternal oxygen-carrying capacity.

In part, *vasospasms* are the underlying mechanism for the signs and symptoms present with preeclampsia. Vasospasms result from an increased sensitivity to circulating pressors, such as angiotensin II, and possibly an imbalance between the prostaglandins prostacyclin and thromboxane A_2 (Consensus Report, 1990; Cunningham and Lindheimer, 1992; Magness and Gant, 1994; Walsh, 1990).

Investigators have tested the ability of aspirin (a prostaglandin inhibitor) to alter the pathophysiology of preeclampsia by interfering with the production of thromboxane (Imperiale and Petrulis, 1991; Walsh, 1990). Investigation of the use of aspirin as a prophylactic treatment in the prevention of preeclampsia and its risk-benefit ratio for the mother and fetus/neonate is continuing. Other investigators are studying the use of calcium supplementation to prevent hypertension in pregnancy (Sanchez-Ramos et al, 1994).

In addition to endothelial damage (Fig. 9-1), **arterial vasospasm** may contribute to an increased capillary permeability. This increases edema and further decreases intravascular volume, predisposing the woman with preeclampsia to pulmonary edema (Dildy et al, 1991).

Easterling and Benedetti (1989) propose that preeclampsia is a hyperdynamic condition in which the characteristic findings of hypertension and proteinuria result from renal hyperperfusion. To control the large volume of blood perfusing the

BOX 9-1
Normal Physiologic Adaptations to Pregnancy

Cardiovascular

↑ Blood volume; plasma volume expansion increases to greater degree than red cell mass expansion, leading to a physiologic anemia of pregnancy
↓ Total peripheral resistance; decreases in blood pressure readings occur
↑ CO; results from increased blood volume; slight increase in heart rate to compensate for peripheral relaxation
↑ Oxygen consumption
Physiologic edema related to decreased COP and increased venous capillary hydrostatic pressure

Hematologic

↑ Clotting factors; predisposes to DIC and clotting
↓ Serum albumin results in decreases in COP; predisposes to pulmonary edema

Renal

↑ Renal plasma flow and glomerular filtration rate

Endocrine

↑ Estrogen production results in increased renin-angiotensin II–aldosterone secretion
↑ Progesterone production blocks aldosterone effect (slight decrease in Na)
↑ Vasodilator prostaglandins result in resistance to angiotensin IIC (slight decrease in blood pressure)

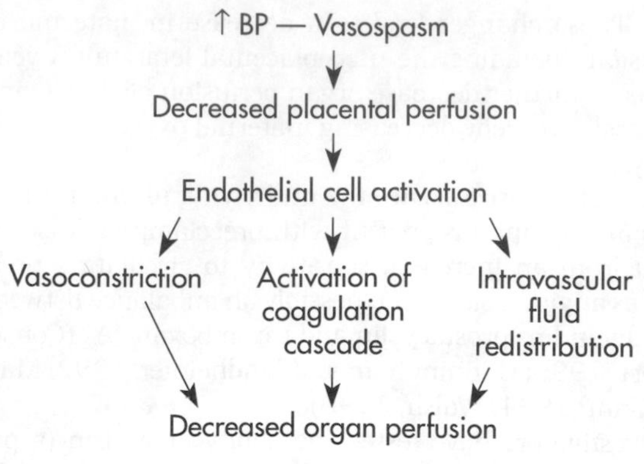

Fig. 9-1 Etiology of PIH.

kidney, renal vasospasm is initiated as a protective mechanism, but it eventually produces the proteinuria and hypertension characteristic of preeclampsia.

The relationship of the immune system to preeclampsia suggests that immunologic factors play an important role in the development of preeclampsia (Sibai, 1991a). The presence of foreign protein, the placenta, or the fetus may trigger an adverse immunologic response. This theory is supported by the increased incidence of preeclampsia/eclampsia in first-time mothers (first exposure to fetal tissue) and in women pregnant by a new partner (different genetic material) (Fig. 9-2).

Genetic predisposition may be another immunologic factor. Sibai (1991a) found a greater frequency of preeclampsia and eclampsia in daughters and granddaughters of women with a history of eclampsia, which suggests an autosomal recessive gene controlling the maternal immune response. Paternal factors also are being examined (Klonoff-Cohen et al, 1989).

A diet inadequate in all nutrients, especially protein, calcium, sodium, magnesium, and vitamins E and A, may be an etiologic factor in PIH. Proponents of this theory prescribe high-protein diets without caloric or sodium restriction to prevent and treat this disorder (Belizan et al, 1991; Newman and Fullerton, 1990). In pregnancy, especially late pregnancy when the fetus has an increased need for protein for body growth and functioning, the recommended daily allowance (RDA) for protein is increased (from 50 to 60 g/day for a singleton pregnancy). If a woman begins pregnancy with a protein deficit or if she has a multifetal pregnancy, her RDA for protein in pregnancy is even greater, and she is at risk for a deficient protein intake.

Mild vs. severe preeclampsia

As preeclampsia worsens, regardless of etiology, multiorgan system involvement is evidenced from the disease process. Renal involvement is demonstrated by changes in urine output and serum chemistries. Renal blood flow and glomerular filtration are decreased, resulting in **oliguria,** decreased urine creatinine clearance, and increases in blood urea nitrogen (BUN), serum creatinine, and serum uric acid (Dildy et al, 1991) (Table 9-1).

The pathophysiology of preeclampsia affects the central nervous system (CNS) by inducing cerebral edema and increased cerebral resistance (Dildy et al, 1991). Complications include headaches, seizures, and cerebrovascular accidents. As CNS involvement advances, the woman complains of headaches and visual disturbances (scotoma) or exhibits changes in affect and level of consciousness. A life-threatening complication is the development of eclampsia, or the onset of seizures.

Impaired placental perfusion leads to early degenerative aging of the placenta and possible IUGR of the fetus. Decreased perfusion of the liver leads to impaired function. Hepatic edema and subcapsular hemorrhage, experienced by the woman as epigastric or right upper quadrant pain, is one sign of impending eclampsia. Liver enzyme levels rise in response to liver damage. Rupture of the liver is a rare but catastrophic complication (Cunningham et al, 1993).

Debate continues whether preeclampsia contributes to or is the result of DIC or whether DIC occurs with preeclampsia (Perry and Martin, 1992; Poole, 1993, Weiner, 1991). The most common coagulation abnormality seen in preeclampsia is platelet consumption resulting in thrombocytopenia (Sibai, 1990d).

If the hypertension is difficult to bring under control, cardiac and pulmonary complications can occur. Heart failure, a common cause of maternal death attributed to preeclampsia, is rare in young, otherwise healthy women (Scott et al, 1994). Sudden circulatory collapse and shock may occur in women with a history of repeated hypertensive pregnancies. A rapid fall in systolic blood pressure by 70 mm Hg or more is most often seen a few hours after giving birth, although it may occur before or during labor.

Typically, pulmonary edema caused by preeclampsia is associated with severe generalized edema. Intravenous (IV) fluid infusion is an iatrogenic cause of fluid overload. A weak, rapid pulse, increased respiratory rate, lowered blood pressure, and pulmonary crackles suggest circulatory failure.

HELLP syndrome

HELLP syndrome (**H,** hemolysis; **EL,** elevated liver enzymes; **LP,** low platelet count) appears in only 4% to 12% of severely preeclamptic women (Gilbert and Harmon, 1993a, b). The incidence is highest among older, Caucasian, and multiparous women. Although the exact mechanism is unknown, HELLP syndrome is thought to occur secondary to changes occurring with preeclampsia (see Fig. 9-2). Arterial vasospasm, endothelial damage, and platelet aggregation with resultant tissue hypoxia are the underlying mechanisms for the pathophysiology of HELLP syndrome (Poole, 1993). The initial symptoms most often occur early in the third trimester. A circulating immunologic component may be the underlying cause. HELLP syndrome has a mortality rate of 2% to 24% (Martin et al, 1991).

For a woman to be diagnosed as having HELLP syndrome, her platelet count must be less than $100,000/mm^3$, her liver enzyme levels (specifically, (aspartate aminotransferase [AST] and alanine aminotransferase [ALT]) must be elevated and some evidence for intravascular hemolysis (schistocytes or burr cells on peripheral smear) must be present. The hemolysis that occurs accounts for the large drop in hematocrit out of proportion to the blood loss that occurs in most new mothers with HELLP syndrome during the postpartum period. A unique form of coagulopathy (not DIC) occurs with the HELLP syndrome.

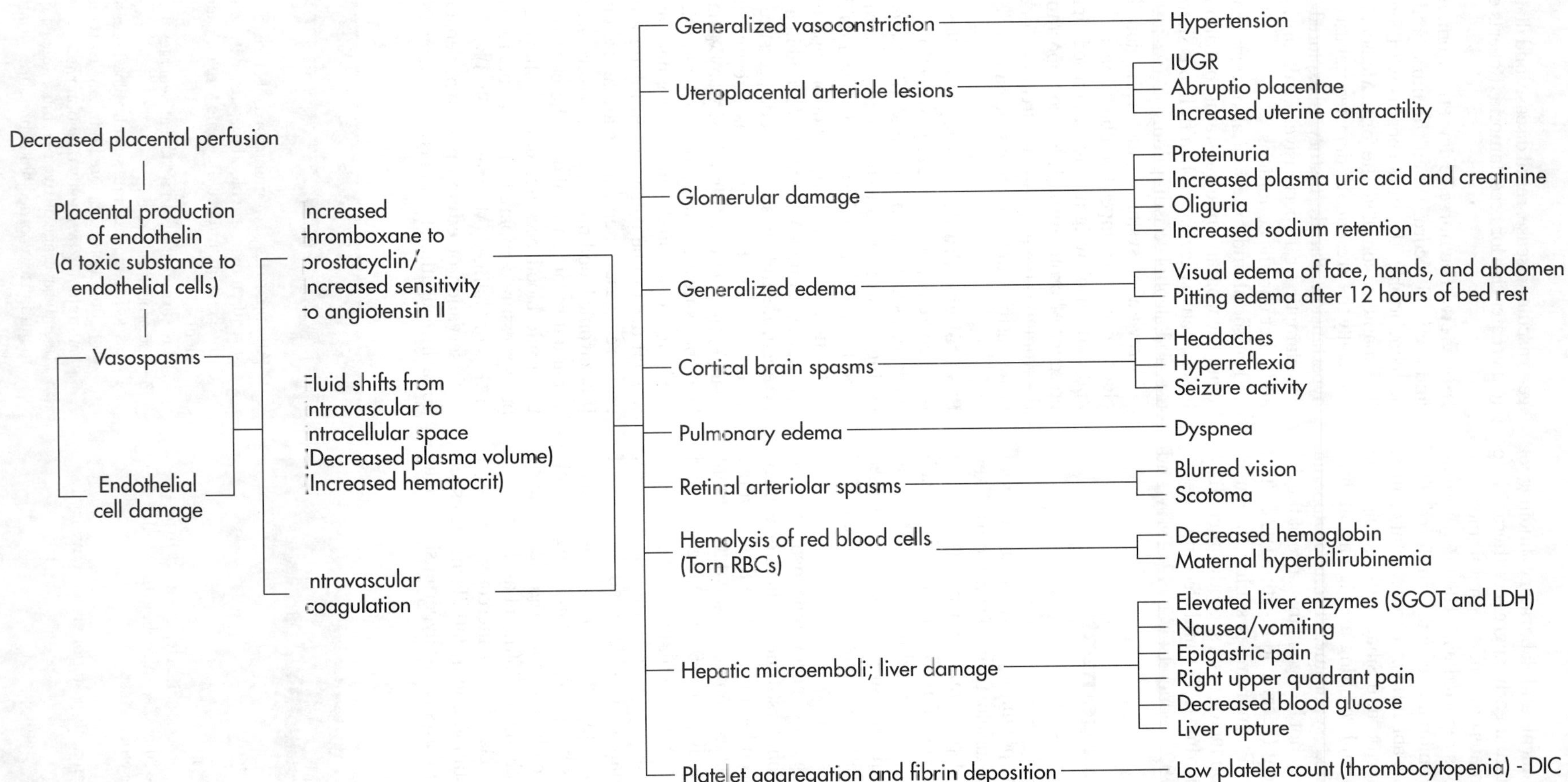

Fig. 9-2 Pathophysiology of PIH. (Modified from Gilbert E, Harmon J: *Manual of high-risk pregnancy and delivery,* St Louis, 1993, Mosby.)

Recognition of the clinical and laboratory findings of HELLP syndrome is important if early, aggressive therapy is to be initiated to prevent maternal and neonatal mortality (Sibai, 1992). Complications reported with HELLP syndrome include renal failure, pulmonary edema, ruptured liver **hematoma,** DIC syndrome, abruptio placentae, fetal demise, and perinatal asphyxia (Barton and Sibai, 1991). Epigastric pain, malaise, and nausea and vomiting are significant findings in the diagnosis of HELLP syndrome. Thrombocytopenia is a common finding but may not be a good measure of the degree of coagulopathy present (Perry and Martin, 1992). The coagulopathy seen in HELLP syndrome is similar to that in DIC, except that coagulation factor assays, prothrombin time (PT), partial thromboplastin time (PTT), and bleeding time remain normal (Guyton, 1992; Leduc et al, 1992; Perry and Martin, 1992).

Nursing Care Management

Assessment

Hypertensive disorders of pregnancy can occur without warning or with the gradual development of symptoms. A key goal is early identification of pregnant women at risk for the development of preeclampsia (Box 9-2). Therefore each woman is assessed for etiologic factors during the first prenatal visit. During each subsequent visit the woman is assessed for symptoms that suggest the onset or presence of preeclampsia.

Factors such as parity, age, and geographic location need to be taken into consideration. First-time mothers or women with a new partner have been found to be 6 to 8 times more susceptible than multiparous women are to the development of preeclampsia (Consensus Report, 1990). Daughters and sisters of preeclamptic women have a higher tendency to develop preeclampsia than do unrelated women (O'Brien, 1992). Women younger than 18 or older than 35 years of age, unmarried, and residing in the southern and western regions of the United States have a significantly higher incidence of preeclampsia. Race alone is not a significant factor for either preeclampsia or eclampsia (Saftlas et al, 1990).

Obstetric conditions associated with increased placental mass such as multifetal gestation and hydatidiform moles, as well as chronic medical disorders such as hypertension, collagen vascular disease, renal disease, and diabetes mellitus, lead to a greater risk for preeclampsia (Roberts et al, 1990).

Interview. The nurse reviews the woman's admission form and prenatal record. When the nurse and pregnant woman are comfortable, the nurse begins with the interview to clarify, expand, or complete the form. Medical history is reviewed, especially the presence of diabetes mellitus, renal disease, and hypertension. Family history is explored for occurrence of preeclamptic or hypertensive conditions, diabetes mellitus, and other chronic conditions.

The social and experiential history provides information about the woman's marital status, nutritional status, cultural beliefs, activity level, and health habits such as smoking, drug use, and alcohol consumption.

A review of systems adds to the data base for detecting blood pressure changes from baseline, abnormal weight gain and pattern of weight gain, increased signs of edema, and presence of proteinuria. It is also important to note whether the woman is having unusual, frequent, or severe headaches, visual disturbances, or epigastric pain.

Physical examination. Lack of specific reliable diagnostic tests currently hinder early detection and treatment of preeclampsia. Women with a MAP greater than 85 mm Hg during the second trimester are at greater risk for developing hypertension during the third trimester (O'Brien, 1992). Currently, no test is a good predictor of hypertensive disorders of pregnancy (Conde-Agudelo, Lodo, and Belizan, 1994).

Accurate and consistent blood pressure assessment is important for establishing a baseline and monitoring subtle changes throughout pregnancy. Many variables can influence blood pressure measurements, such as position, cuff size, arm used, and emotional state. Personnel caring for pregnant women need to be consistent in taking and recording blood pressure measurements in a standardized manner (Box 9-3). If electronic blood pressure devices are used, there should be a manual reading to validate the electronic device reading. Electronic blood pressure devices show a widening of the pulse pressure compared with manual readings; however, the MAP is unchanged (Marx et al, 1993).

Observation of **edema** plus hypertension warrants additional investigation. Edema is assessed by distribution, degree,

BOX 9-2

Risk Factors for Preeclampsia/Eclampsia

Primigravida or older multipara
Age: <18 or >35 years
Weight: <45 kg (100 lb) or obesity
Presence of chronic disease process: diabetes mellitus, hypertension, renal disease, vascular disease, collagen vascular disease (systemic lupus erythematosus)
Hydatidiform mole
Pregnancy complications: multiple gestation, large fetus, fetal hydrops
Preeclampsia in previous pregnancy
New genetic material
Antiphospholipid antibody syndrome

BOX 9-3

Blood Pressure Measurement Protocol

1. Attempt to have woman relaxed before taking blood pressure; then measure blood pressure with woman in a sitting position and use the same arm for each measurement.
2. Have arm resting on a table at heart level.
3. Use proper cuff size.
4. Assess for approximate systolic blood pressure level using palpation method before taking measurement.
5. Maintain a slow, steady deflation rate.
6. Take the average of two readings, at least 6 hours apart, to minimize recorded blood pressure variations across time.
7. Use accurate equipment.

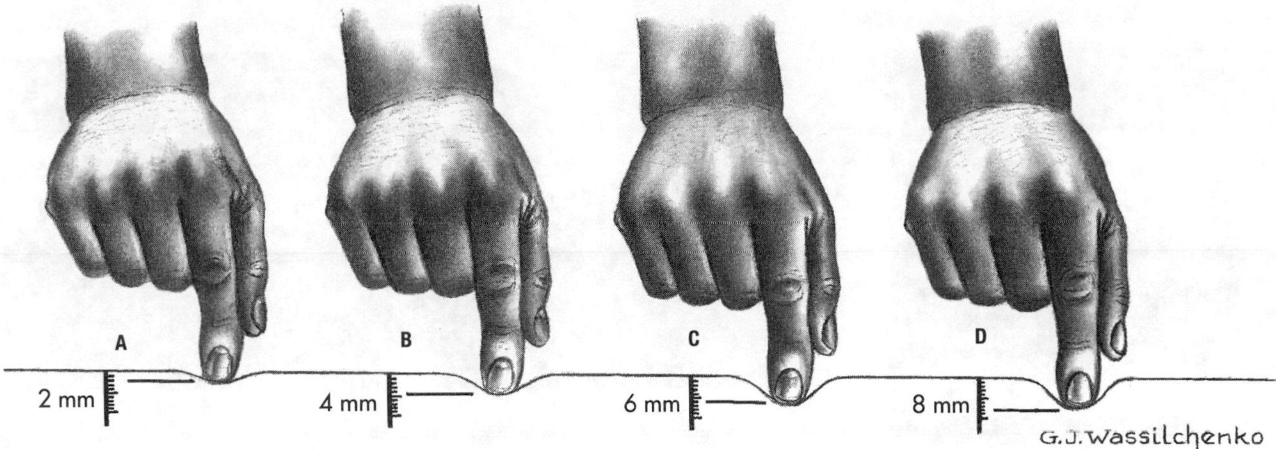

Fig. 9-3 Assessment of pitting edema. **A,** 1+; **B,** 2+; **C,** 3+; **D,** 4+.

and pitting. If periorbital or facial edema is not obvious, the pregnant woman is asked if it was present when she awoke. Edema may be described as dependent or pitting.

Dependent edema is edema of the lower or most dependent parts of the body, where hydrostatic pressure is greatest. If a person is ambulatory, this edema may first be evident in the feet and ankles. If the person is confined to bed, the edema is more likely to occur in the sacral region.

Pitting edema leaves a small depression or pit after finger pressure is applied to the swollen area. The pit is caused by movement of fluid to adjacent tissue, away from the point of pressure. Within 10 to 30 seconds the pit normally disappears. Although the amount of edema is difficult to quantitate, the method shown in Fig. 9-3 may be used to record relative degrees of edema formation.

Symptoms reflecting CNS and visual system involvement usually accompany facial edema. Although it is not a routine assessment during the prenatal period, evaluation of the fundus of the eye yields valuable data. An initial baseline finding of normal eyegrounds assists in differentiating preexisting from new disease processes. The woman may not report other symptoms such as epigastric pain or oliguria. Respirations are assessed for crackles, which may indicate pulmonary edema.

Deep tendon reflexes (DTRs) are evaluated if preeclampsia is suspected. The biceps and patellar reflexes and ankle clonus are assessed and the findings recorded (Fig. 9-4; Table 9-2).

Nursing ALERT

The evaluation of DTRs is especially important if the woman is being treated with magnesium sulfate; absence of DTRs is an early indication of impending magnesium toxicity.

To elicit the biceps reflex a downward blow is struck over the thumb, which is placed over the biceps tendon. Normal response is flexion of the arm at the elbow, or 2+ (Fig. 9-4, *A*; Table 9-2).

The **patellar reflex** is elicited with the woman's legs hanging freely over the end of the examining table, or with the woman lying on her side with the knee slightly flexed, or with both legs supported by the examiner. A blow with a percussion hammer is dealt directly to the patellar tendon, inferior to the patella. Normal response is the extension or kicking out of the leg, or 2+ (Fig. 9-4, *B* and *C*; Table 9-2).

To assess for hyperactive reflexes **(clonus)** at the ankle joint, the leg should be supported with the knee flexed. With one hand the foot is sharply dorsiflexed and the position maintained for a moment. The foot is then released (Fig. 9-4, *D* and *E*). Normal (negative clonus) response is elicited when no rhythmic oscillations (jerking) are felt while the foot is held in dorsiflexion. When the foot is released, no oscillations are seen as the foot drops to the plantar flexed position. Abnormal (positive clonus) response is recognized by rhythmic oscillations of one or more beats felt when the foot is in dorsiflexion and is seen as the foot drops to the plantar flexed position (Fig. 9-4, *F*).

An important assessment is determination of fetal status. Uteroplacental perfusion is decreased in women with preeclampsia, thereby placing the fetus in jeopardy. The fetal heart rate (FHR) is assessed for baseline rate and the presence of variability and accelerations, which indicate an intact oxygenated fetal CNS. Abnormal baseline rate, decreased or absent variability, and late decelerations are indications of fetal intolerance to its intrauterine environment. Biophysical or biochemical monitoring for fetal well-being may be ordered: fetal movement counts, nonstress testing (NST), contraction stress testing (CST), biophysical profile (BPP), and serial ultrasonography.

TABLE 9-2 Assessing deep tendon reflexes

DEGREE	GRADING
Brisk with sustained clonus	5+
Hyperactive response (brisk with transient clonus)	4+
More than normal (brisk)	3+
Normal, active	2+
Low response (sluggish or dull)	1+
No response	0

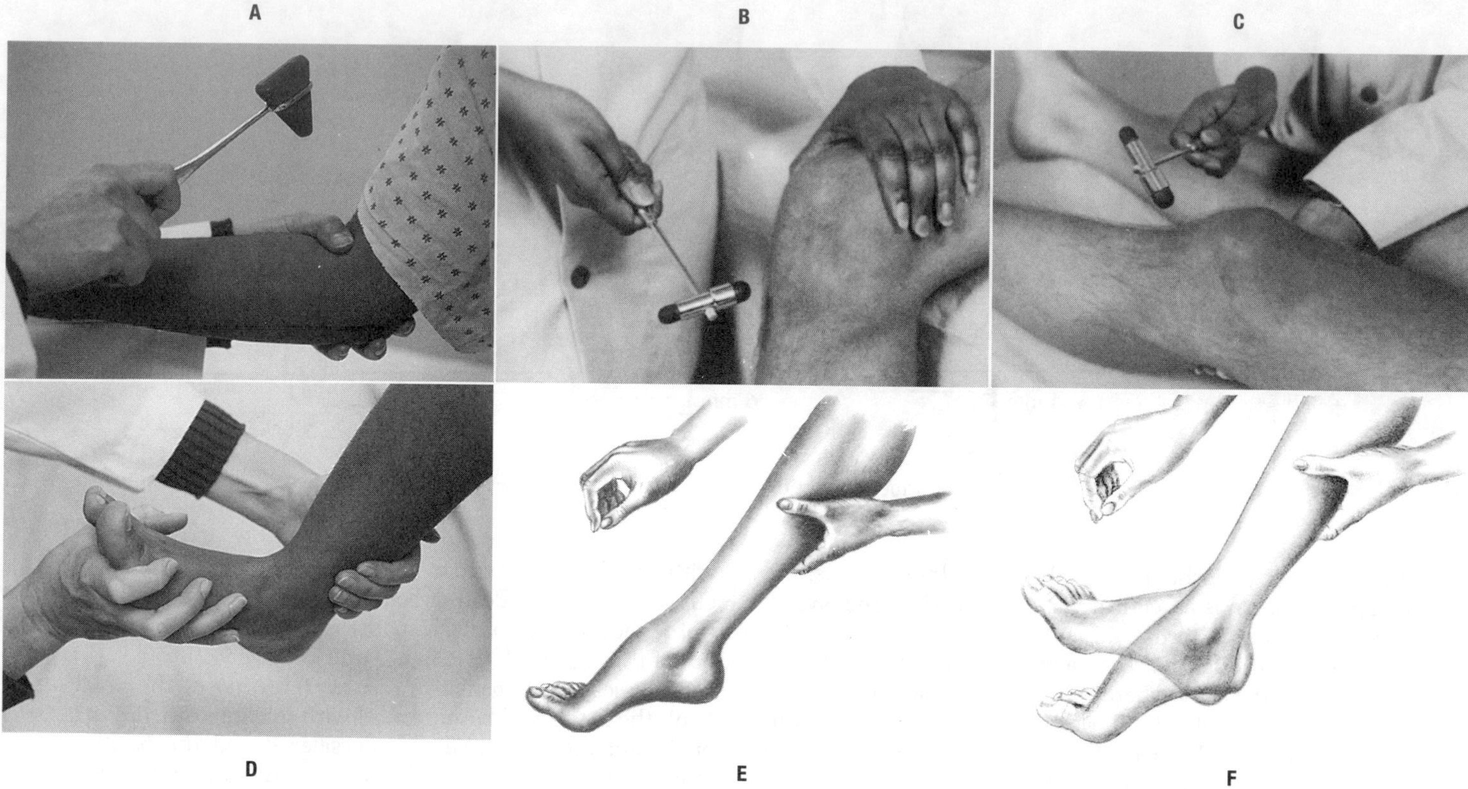

Fig. 9-4 DTRs **A,** Biceps reflex. **B,** Patellar reflex with woman's legs hanging freely over end of examining table. **C,** Patellar reflex with woman in supine position. **D,** Test for ankle clonus. **E,** Normal (negative clonus) response. **F,** Abnormal (positive clonus) response. (**A** and **D** from Seidel H et al: *Mosby's guide to physical examination,* ed 3, St Louis, 1995, Mosby; **B** and **C** from Barkauskas V et al: *Health and physical assessment,* St Louis, 1994, Mosby.)

Doppler flow velocimetry studies are used for evaluating maternal-fetal well-being (see p. 88). Uteroplacental perfusion is assessed by measuring the velocity of blood flow through the uterine or umbilical arteries, or both. A systolic/diastolic ratio greater than 3 after 26 weeks is considered abnormal, and ratios of 3.8 have been associated with preeclampsia (Fairlie, 1991; Farmakides et al, 1992).

Uterine tonicity is evaluated for signs of labor and abruptio placentae. If labor is suspected, a vaginal examination for cervical changes is indicated.

During the physical examination the pregnant woman is examined for signs of deterioration of mild preeclampsia to severe preeclampsia or eclampsia. Signs of worsening liver involvement, renal failure, worsening hypertension, cerebral involvement, and developing coagulopathies must be assessed and documented. Respirations are assessed for crackles or diminished breath sounds, which may indicate pulmonary edema. Table 9-1 summarizes warning signs of preeclampsia and the differentiation of mild from severe preeclampsia. Noninvasive assessment parameters include level of consciousness, blood pressure, hemoglobin oxygen saturation (pulse oximetry), electrocardiographic (ECG) findings, and urine output. Invasive hemodynamic monitoring may be indicated in selected patients (ACOG, 1992a).

Eclampsia usually is preceded by various premonitory symptoms and signs, including headache, severe epigastric pain, **hyperreflexia,** and hemoconcentration. However, convulsions can appear suddenly and without warning in a seemingly stable woman with only minimum blood pressure elevations (Sibai, 1992). Eclamptic seizures can result in tissue damage to the mother during the convulsion, especially if the side rails are not padded. During the convulsion the mother and fetus are not receiving oxygen. Eclamptic seizures produce a marked metabolic insult to both mother and fetus.

Laboratory tests. The nurse assists in obtaining a number of blood and urine specimens to aid in the diagnosis of preeclampsia, HELLP syndrome, or chronic hypertension. Baseline laboratory test information is useful in the early diagnosis of preeclampsia and for comparison with results obtained to evaluate progression and severity of disease. An initial blood specimen is obtained for the following tests to assess the disease process and its effect on renal and hepatic functioning:

- Complete blood count (CBC) including a platelet count
- Clotting studies (including bleeding time, PT, PTT, fibrinogen)
- Liver enzymes (lactic dehydrogenase [LDH], AST [SGOT], ALT [SGPT])
- Chemistry panel (BUN, creatinine, glucose, uric acid)
- Type and screen, possible crossmatch

The hematocrit, hemoglobin, and platelets are monitored closely for changes indicating a worsening of patient status. Since hepatic involvement is a possible complication, serum glucose levels are monitored if liver function tests indicate elevated liver enzymes. Once platelets drop below 100,000, coagulation profiles are needed to identify developing DIC (Leduc et al, 1992).

Proteinuria is determined from dipstick testing of a clean-catch or catheter urine specimen. A reading greater than +1 on two or more occasions, at least 4 hours apart, should be followed by a 24-hour urine collection (Gilbert and Harmon, 1993a). A 24-hour collection for protein and creatinine clearance is more reflective of true renal status. *Proteinuria* is defined as the excretion of 0.3 g (30 mg/dl or more in a 24-hour period. Proteinuria usually is a late sign in the course of preeclampsia (Consensus Report, 1990). Protein readings are designated as follows:

0
Trace
+1: 30 mg/dl (equivalent to 300 mg/L)
+2: 100 mg/dl
+3: 300 mg/dl
+4: Over 1000 mg (1 g)/dl

Urine output is assessed for volume of at least 30 ml/hour or 120 ml in 4 hours.

Nursing Diagnoses

Nursing diagnoses are derived by carefully analyzing the assessment findings. Common nursing diagnoses for patients with hypertensive disorders in pregnancy include the following:

- Anxiety related to
  - Preeclampsia and its effect on mother and infant
- Knowledge deficit regarding
  - Coping, Management (diet, bed rest)
- Ineffective individual and family coping related to
  - Mother's restricted activity and concern over a complicated pregnancy
  - Mother's inability to work outside the home
- Powerlessness related to
  - Inability to prevent or control condition and outcomes
- Altered tissue/organ perfusion, decreased, related to
  - Hypertension
  - Cyclic vasospasms
  - Cerebral edema
  - Hemorrhage
- Risk for injury related to signs of pulmonary edema
  - Decreased colloid osmotic pressure
  - Increased systemic vascular resistance
  - Pulmonary vascular endothelial damage
- Risk for impaired gas exchange related to
  - Magnesium sulfate therapy
  - Pulmonary edema
- Risk for decreased cardiac output related to
  - Excessive antihypertensive therapy
  - Cardiac involvement of the disease process
- Risk for injury related to signs of abruptio placentae
  - Systemic vasospasms
  - Hypertension
  - Decreased uteroplacental perfusion
  - Maternal eclamptic seizures
- Risk for injury to fetus related to
  - Uteroplacental insufficiency
  - Preterm birth
  - Abruptio placentae
  - Maternal eclamptic seizures
- Risk for injury to mother related to
  - CNS irritability secondary to cerebral edema, vasospasm, decreased renal perfusion
  - Magnesium sulfate and antihypertensive therapies

Expected Outcomes

Planning care follows medical diagnosis, choice of home or hospital management, and the woman's and family's resources. A plan is developed mutually with the woman, if possible, and should be individualized and related specifically to the needs of the patient and her family. Expected outcomes for care of patients with hypertensive disorders of pregnancy include the following:

1. The woman will recognize and immediately report abnormal signs and symptoms to prevent worsening of condition.
2. The woman will adhere to the medical regimen to minimize risk to herself and her fetus.
3. Significant other(s) will become involved and supportive in the woman's care and management of the disease to optimize emotional and physical outcomes.
4. The woman will verbalize her fears and concerns to cope with the condition and situation.
5. The woman and fetus will not suffer adverse sequelae from preeclampsia or its management.
6. The woman will not experience eclampsia and the severity of its complications.
7. The fetus will not experience distress; the newborn will be born in optimal condition with no adverse sequelae to the maternal condition and its management.
8. The woman will give birth in optimal condition with no sequelae to her condition and its management.
9. The family will be able to cope effectively with the mother's high-risk condition, its management, and outcomes.

Plan of Care and Implementation

Preeclampsia. Nursing actions are derived from medical management, health care provider directives, and nursing diagnoses.

The most effective therapy is *prevention.* Early prenatal care, identification of at-risk women during pregnancy, and recognition and reporting of physical warning signs are essential components for optimizing maternal and perinatal outcomes. The nurse's skills in assessing the woman for factors and symptoms of preeclampsia cannot be overestimated.

Nurses can do much in the advocacy role. Measures should be taken to improve public education and access to antenatal care. Counseling, referral to community resources, mobilization of support systems, nutrition counseling, and information about normal adaptation to pregnancy are essential preventive components of care. The nurse's role as educator is

Patient Teaching

PREECLAMPSIA

- The cause of pregnancy-induced hypertension is not known; symptoms are believed to occur from changes in body organ functioning.
- Vasospasm and endothelial damage lead to decreased perfusion to organs.
- Decreased perfusion to organs can result in symptoms of preeclampsia.
- An increase in blood pressure, edema, weight, and proteinuria indicates disease process is worsening.
- Decreased fetal movement may indicate fetal compromise.

Home Care

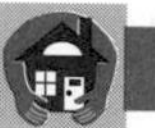

COPING WITH BED REST

- In bed, lie on your side (may alternate sides for comfort). This allows more blood to get to your uterus (womb) and baby.
- Increase your fluid intake to 8 glasses/day, and add roughage (e.g., bran, fruits, leafy vegetables) to your diet to decrease constipation.
- Include diversional activities such as puzzles, reading, and crafts to reduce boredom.
- Do gentle exercises such as circling your hands and feet or gently tensing and relaxing arm and leg muscles. This improves muscle tone, circulation, and sense of well-being.
- Encourage family participation in your care.
- Have significant others assist you with care of the house, children, etc.
- Use relaxation to help you cope with stress. Relax your body one muscle at a time or imagine some pleasant scene, word, or image. Soothing music can also help you to relax.

important in informing the woman about her condition and responsibilities in preeclampsia management, whether in the home or hospital (see the Patient Teaching box above).

Emotional and psychologic support is essential to help the woman and her family cope. Their perception of the disease process, the reasons for it, and the care received will affect their compliance with and participation in treatment. The family will need to use coping mechanisms and support systems to help them through this crisis. A plan of care for the woman with preeclampsia is superimposed on the nursing care all women need during labor and the birth process.

Home care. Interventions for preeclampsia such as bed rest and diet are considered palliative (Consensus Report, 1990). The most desired outcome for preeclampsia is preventing progression of the condition and enabling the pregnancy to continue (see the Home Care box above).

LEGAL TIP

Standard of Care for the Preeclamptic Patient at Home

Home care of the preeclamptic patient requires the same level of nursing expertise as performed the intrapartum setting. The standard of care for the preeclamptic patient at home calls for the nurse to be prepared to assess the condition, provide care, identify deviations from normal, intervene accordingly, and refer when appropriate.

Home Care

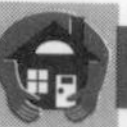

ASSESSING AND REPORTING CLINICAL SIGNS OF PREECLAMPSIA

- Report immediately any increase in your blood pressure, protein in urine, weight gain greater than 1 pound/week, or edema.
- Take your blood pressure on the same arm in a sitting position each time for consistent and accurate readings. Support arm on a table in a horizontal position at heart level.
- Use the same scale, wearing the same clothes, at the same time each day, after voiding, before breakfast, for reliable daily weights.
- Dipstick your clean-catch urine sample for assessing proteinuria; report frequency or burning on urination.
- Report to your health care provider if proteinuria is +2 or more or if you have a decrease in urine output.
- Daily assess your baby's activity. Decreased activity (three or fewer movements per hour) may indicate fetal stress.
- It is important to keep your scheduled prenatal appointments so any changes in your or the baby's condition can be detected immediately.
- Keep a daily log/diary of your assessments for your home health care nurse, or bring it with you to your next prenatal visit.

Management at home can be satisfactory if preeclampsia is mild and IUGR is not a problem. The woman's condition usually is assessed two or three times per week, either by a nurse in the home visit or by a physician in the office or high-risk clinic. Assessments may also be done by home care agencies through telephone contact.

For home care to be effective, the nurse needs to assess the home environment and the woman's ability to assume responsibility. In addition, the effects of illness, language, age, culture, beliefs, and support system need to be considered. The woman's support systems need to be mobilized and involved in planning and implementing her care. Motivation, as well as readiness and ability to learn, are essential considerations for a woman who requires instruction on self-care at home.

A knowledge of the subjective symptoms and objective signs that indicate deterioration of the condition is vital. If these symptoms occur, the woman must call her health care provider immediately (see the Home Care box above).

Bed rest in the lateral recumbent position is a standard therapy for preeclampsia and maximizes uteroplacental blood flow. It has been shown to be beneficial in decreasing blood pressure and promoting diuresis.

However, Maloni (1994) documented adverse physiologic outcomes related to complete bed rest, including cardiovascular deconditioning; diuresis with accompanying fluid, electrolyte, and weight loss; muscle atrophy; and psychologic stress. These changes begin on the first day of bed rest and continue for the duration of therapy. Risks and benefits of bed rest must be considered when developing the plan of care.

Since women with mild preeclampsia feel reasonably well, boredom from being restricted is common. Diversionary activities, visits from friends, telephone conversations, and a pleasant environment are ways to cope with boredom (see the Home Care box on p. 208). Gentle exercise (e.g., range of motion, stretching, Kegel exercise, pelvic tilts) is important in maintaining muscle tone, blood flow, regularity of bowel function, and a sense of well-being (Grohar, 1994).

Learning relaxation techniques can help to reduce stress associated with the high-risk condition and to prepare the woman for labor and the birth. Relaxation is also effective in lowering blood pressure of people with chronic hypertension.

The woman is instructed in how to take her own blood pressure and keep a record of the measurements. Women should have formal instruction in using correct, standardized techniques for obtaining accurate blood pressure measurements (see Box 9-3). Electronic devices are as accurate as mechanical ancroid units. They are easy to apply and read without need for a stethoscope or another person (Smith et al, 1990). This is particularly advantageous for women having their blood pressure monitored on an outpatient basis.

The woman is taught to weigh daily and check her urine for protein. The initial appearance of proteinuria usually indicates progressive severity of preeclampsia. An increase in weight is associated with edema formation.

Because the disease has potential adverse effects on uterine blood flow, the fetus must be evaluated regularly for hypoxia. The woman is instructed about the importance of keeping appointments for fetal monitoring tests. Explanation of the purpose of the tests and what the woman may experience during the procedures is also necessary. For home management the woman may be instructed in how to do daily fetal movement counts (see Chapter 5). Fetal activity under three counts per hour is considered serious and needs to be reported. Fetal activity decreases if hypoxia develops.

Diet and fluid recommendations are much the same as for typical pregnant women. Diets high in protein and low in salt have been suggested to prevent preeclampsia; however, the efficacy of this has not been proved (Fairlie and Sibai, 1993). Pregnant women with hypertension have less plasma volume than do normotensive women; thus sodium restriction is not recommended. Salt is needed for maintenance of blood volume and placental perfusion. The exception may be the woman with chronic hypertension successfully treated with a low-salt diet before the pregnancy. Adequate fluid intake helps to maintain optimal fluid volume and aids in renal perfusion and filtration. The nurse uses assessment data about the woman's diet and counsels her in areas of deficiency, if needed (see the Patient Teaching box above and the Nursing Care Plan on p. 210).

Although preliminary studies show that dietary calcium supplementation decreases blood pressure, insufficient data are available to recommend its use for treating hypertension (Consensus Report, 1990). The use of alcohol, smoking, and other drugs is strongly discouraged because of their harmful effects on the mother and fetus.

Patient Teaching

NUTRITION

- Eat a nutritious, balanced diet (e.g., 60 to 70 g protein, 1200 mg calcium, adequate zinc, magnesium, vitamins). Collaborate with registered dietitian for diet best suited for individual woman.
- There is no sodium restriction; however, avoid salty foods (e.g., canned foods, sodas, pretzels, potato chips, pickles, sauerkraut).
- Eat foods with roughage (e.g., whole grains, raw fruits and vegetables).
- Drink 8 to 10 glasses of water per day.
- Avoid alcohol.

Severe preeclampsia/HELLP syndrome. The woman diagnosed with severe preeclampsia/HELLP syndrome is critically ill and warrants appropriate management, usually in a tertiary care center. Management protocols are controversial among medical authorities; recommendations range from immediate birth to conservative management of the pregnancy (Dildy et al, 1991; Harvey and Burke, 1992; Sibai, 1991b). Recognition of the clinical and laboratory findings of severe preeclampsia/HELLP syndrome is important if early, aggressive therapy is to be initiated to prevent maternal and perinatal mortality. An unfavorable (uneffaced and undilated) cervix resulting from gestational age and the aggressive nature of this disorder support cesarean birth. Prolonged induction of labor could increase maternal morbidity.

Regardless of the treatment modality initiated, birth is the only definitive treatment for severe preeclampsia/HELLP syndrome. Important components of management include the administration of magnesium sulfate ($MgSO_4$) as a seizure prophylaxis and the administration of an antihypertensive agent if diastolic blood pressure is higher than 110 mm Hg. Hypoglycemia may be present in the woman with HELLP syndrome; blood sugar less than 40 mg/dl is associated with an increased maternal mortality.

Hospital care. The woman with severe preeclampsia/HELLP syndrome has multiple problems and is a tremendous challenge for the health care team. Nurses caring for this woman need an in-depth understanding of the disease process, treatment regimen, and possible complications to the mother and fetus (Table 9-1). Nursing care must focus on both the mother and the fetus.

Severe preeclampsia is diagnosed when one of the following signs and symptoms is present (Fairlie and Sibai, 1993):

1. Blood pressure $\geq$160 mm Hg systolic or $\geq$110 mm Hg diastolic (MAP $\geq$127) on two readings at least 6 hours apart.
2. Proteinuria $\geq$5 g in a 24-hour urine collection or $\geq$3+ on dipstick in at least two random clean-catch samples at least 4 hours apart
3. Oliguria $\leq$30 ml/hr or $\leq$400 ml in 24 hours
4. Cerebral or visual disturbances
5. Epigastric pain
6. Pulmonary edema or cyanosis
7. HELLP syndrome

Antepartum care focuses on stabilization and preparation for birth. Maternal and fetal surveillance, patient education regarding the disease process, and supportive measures directed toward the patient and her family are initiated. If the

Nursing Care Plan

PREECLAMPSIA

Home Care

Nursing Diagnosis: Risk for injury related to signs of preeclampsia

Expected Outcomes: Patient will: demonstrate ability to assess self and fetus for signs of worsening preeclampsia; no adverse sequelae will occur as result of preeclamptic condition.

• **NURSING INTERVENTIONS/*RATIONALES***

Review warning signs/symptoms of preeclampsia *to ensure adequate knowledge base exists for decision making.*

Assess home environment, including woman's ability to assume self-care responsibilities, support systems, language, age, culture, beliefs, and effects of illness, *to determine if home care is viable option.*

Teach woman how to do a self-assessment for clinical signs of preeclampsia (take and record blood pressure, measure urine protein, maintain daily weight log, assess edema formation, assess fetal activity) *to provide immediate evidence of a worsening condition.*

Teach woman to report any increases in blood pressure, +2 proteinuria, weight gain greater than 454 mg (1 lb) per week, presence of edema, and decreased fetal activity to her health care provider immediately *to prevent worsening of preeclamptic condition.*

Teach woman about use of bed rest, relaxation, and diet as palliative treatment options *to decrease blood pressure and promote diuresis.*

Nursing Diagnosis: Fear/anxiety related to preeclampsia and its effect on the fetus

Expected Outcome: Patient's feelings and symptoms of fear/anxiety will decrease/ease.

• **NURSING INTERVENTIONS/*RATIONALES***

Provide a calm, soothing atmosphere and teach family to provide emotional support *to facilitate coping.*

Encourage verbalization of fears *to decrease intensity of emotional response.*

Involve woman and family in the management of her preeclamptic condition *to promote a greater sense of control.*

Help woman identify and use appropriate coping strategies and support systems *to reduce fear/anxiety.*

Explore use of desensitization strategies such as progressive muscle relaxation, visual imagery, or thought stopping *to reduce fear-related emotions and related physical symptoms.*

Nursing Diagnosis: Diversional activity deficit related to imposed bed rest.

Expected Outcome: Patient will verbalize diminished feelings of boredom.

• **NURSING INTERVENTIONS/*RATIONALES***

Assist woman to explore creatively personally meaningful activities that can be pursued from the bed *to ensure activities that have meaning, purpose, and value to the individual.*

Maintain emphasis on personal choices of woman, *to promote control and minimize imposition of routines by others.*

Evaluate what support and system resources are available in the environment *to assist in providing diversional activities.*

Explore ways for woman to remain an active participant in home management and decision making *to promote control.*

Engage support of family and friends in carrying out chosen activities and making necessary environmental alterations *to ensure success.*

Teach woman about stress management and relaxation techniques *to help manage tension of confinement.*

---

woman's condition warrants and when hemodynamic monitoring is necessary, she may be placed in an obstetric critical care unit (OBCCU) or medical intensive care unit (ICU) if an obstetric CCU is not available.

Assessments include a review of the cardiovascular, pulmonary, renal, hematologic, and central nervous systems. Fetal assessments for well-being (e.g., NST, BPP, Doppler velocimetry) are important because of the potential for hypoxia related to uteroplacental insufficiency. Baseline laboratory assessments include metabolic package for liver enzyme determination, CBC with platelets, coagulation profile to assess for DIC, and electrolyte package to establish renal functioning (Farmakides et al, 1990).

The extensiveness of health assessment on admission is governed by the severity of the woman's condition. Weight is taken on admission and every day thereafter. An indwelling urinary catheter facilitates monitoring of renal function and effectiveness of therapy. If appropriate, vaginal examination reveals the status of the cervix. Abdominal palpation establishes uterine tonicity and fetal size, activity, and position. Electronic fetal monitoring is initiated to determine fetal status. The nurse's skill in implementing the techniques described can be reassuring to the woman and her family. The patient's room must be close to staff and emergency drugs, supplies, and equipment. Noise and external stimuli must be minimized. Seizure precautions are taken (Box 9-4).

Bed rest usually is ordered. The nurse's ingenuity may be called on to help the woman cope physically and psychologically with the side effects of immobility and an environment limited in stimuli and support. Thromboembolic events, which are a risk factor during normal pregnancy, pose an even greater risk with preeclampsia.

Intrapartum nursing care of the woman with severe preeclampsia or the HELLP syndrome involves maternal and fetal assessments as labor progresses. The assessment and prevention of tissue hypoxia and hemorrhage, both of which can lead to permanent compromise of vital organs, continue throughout the intrapartum and postpartum periods (Harvey and Burke, 1992).

BOX 9-4

Hospital Precautionary Measures

Environment
- Quiet
- Nonstimulating
- Lighting subdued

Seizure precautions
- Padded side rails
- Suction equipment tested and ready to use
- Oxygen administration equipment tested and ready to use

Call button within easy reach

Emergency medication tray immediately accessible
- Hydralazine and magnesium sulfate in or adjacent to woman's room
- Calcium gluconate immediately available in a well-labeled syringe

Emergency birth pack accessible

Magnesium sulfate. One of the important goals of care for the woman with severe preeclampsia/HELLP syndrome is preventing or controlling convulsions. An infusion of $MgSO_4$ is started to decrease the incidence of seizures. This is the drug of choice in the treatment of preeclampsia/eclampsia; however, seizures may develop during $MgSO_4$ therapy if the dosage is not correctly titrated according to the individual patient's clinical response (Sibai, 1990b, c; 1991b). Benefits of $MgSO_4$ therapy include an increase in uterine blood flow to protect the fetus and an increase in prostacyclin to prevent uterine vasoconstriction (Iams, Zuspan, and Quilligan, 1990) (Box 9-5).

$MgSO_4$ is administered as a secondary infusion ("piggyback") by volumetric infusion pump. An initial loading dose of 4 to 6 g in 100 ml of dextrose 5% in water (D5W) is given over 15 to 30 minutes, followed by maintenance infusion of 40 mg in 1000 ml of D5W and administered at the rate of 2 to 4 g/hour. A therapeutic serum level between 4.8 to 9.6 mg/dl is maintained by a constant infusion of at least 2 g/hour (Fairlie and Sibai, 1993). After the loading dose, there may be a transient lowering of the arterial blood pressure secondary to relaxation of smooth muscle. However, within an hour of initiating therapy, arterial blood pressures will return to pretherapy levels; *magnesium sulfate is not an antihypertensive drug. It is an anticonvulsant drug.*

Intramuscular (IM) $MgSO_4$ rarely is used because the drug absorption rate cannot be controlled, injections are painful,

BOX 9-5

Protocol for Care of Preeclamptic Patient Receiving $MgSO_4$

PATIENT/FAMILY TEACHING

Tailor information to patient's readiness to learn.

Explain technique, rationale, reactions to expect, and monitoring to anticipate.
- Technique:
  - Route and rate
  - What "piggyback" is for
- Rationale:
  - To prevent disease progression
  - To prevent seizures
- Reactions to expect:
  - Initially will feel flushed, hot, and sedated especially during the bolus infusion; then sedation will continue
- Monitoring to anticipate:
  - Maternal: blood pressure, pulse, DTRs, level of conciousness, urine output (indwelling catheter likely), presence of headache, visual disturbances, and epigastric pain
  - Fetal: Heart rate and activity

ADMINISTRATION

Position woman in side-lying position.

Prepare solution and administer with an infusion control device (pump).

Piggyback initial bolus of $MgSO_4$: 4 to 6 g in 100 ml of D5W over 20 to 30 minutes. Monitor blood pressure and pulse every 5 minutes during loading dose.

Then piggyback a solution of 40 g of $MgSO_4$ in 1000 ml of D5W or lactated Ringer's solution with an infusion control device at the ordered rate, usually 2 g/hour. Monitor blood pressure and pulse every 15 to 30 minutes depending on patient's condition.

MATERNAL/FETAL ASSESSMENTS

Monitor blood pressure, pulse, MAP, respiratory rate, FHR, and contractions every 15 to 30 minutes depending on patient's condition.

Monitor intake and output, proteinuria, DTRs, and presence of headache, visual disturbances, and epigastric pain at least hourly.

Intake is restricted to a total of 100 to 125 ml/hour, and urine output should be at least 30 ml/hour.

REPORTABLE CONDITIONS

Blood pressure: systolic >160 and/or diastolic >110 mm Hg

Respiratory rate: 12 or less.

Urine output: <30 ml/hr

Presence of headache, visual disturbances, and epigastric pain

Increasing severity of DTRs, edema, proteinuria

Any abnormal laboratory values (e.g., magnesium levels, platelet count, creatinine, uric acid, AST, ALT, PT, PTT, fibrinogen, fibrin split products)

Any other significant change in maternal/fetal status

EMERGENCY MEASURES

Keep emergency drug tray at bedside with calcium gluconate, anticonvulsant medication of choice (usually magnesium sulfate or diazepam [Valium]), and intubation equipment.

Keep side rails up and padded.

Keep lights dimmed and maintain a quiet environment.

DOCUMENTATION

All of the above

and tissue necrosis can occur. It may be used with some women who are being transported to a tertiary care center. The IM dosage is 4 to 5 g given in each buttock (1% procaine may be ordered to be added to the solution to reduce injection pain) and can be followed at 4-hour intervals with IM doses of 4 to 5 g.

$MgSO_4$ interferes with the release of acetylcholine at the synapses, decreasing neuromuscular irritability, depressing cardiac conduction, and decreasing CNS irritability (Dildy et al, 1991). Since magnesium circulates free and unbound to protein and is excreted in the urine, accurate recordings of maternal urine output must be obtained. Because $MgSO_4$ is a CNS depressant, the nurse assesses for signs and symptoms of magnesium toxicity, including loss of patellar reflexes, respiratory depression, oliguria, respiratory arrest, and cardiac arrest (see the Emergency box below). The woman's blood pressure, pulse, and respiratory status are monitored at least every 5 minutes while the IV loading dose is being administered and every 15 to 30 minutes at other times, depending on the stability of the woman's condition. It is imperative that patellar and brachial reflexes (Table 9-2 and Fig. 9-4) are assessed every hour if the woman is receiving a continuous IV infusion of $MgSO_4$. Administration is continued for at least the first 12 to 24 hours postpartum to prevent the occurrence of seizures.

Strict monitoring of IV fluid, oral intake, and urine output is important to avoid fluid overload and magnesium toxicity. $MgSO_4$ increases sodium retention and is excreted by the kidneys. Magnesium toxicity can develop very quickly and easily in women with renal involvement. Early symptoms of magnesium toxicity include nausea, a feeling of warmth, flushing, muscle weakness, decreased reflexes, and slurred speech. Maternal toxicity has been reached when respirations are fewer than 12/minute or reflex activity is absent. The drug should be discontinued immediately (Sibai, 1990b).

Urine output must be measured hourly when $MgSO_4$ is administered. The most accurate measure of urine output is with a retention catheter. The woman's urine output must total at least 120 ml every 4 hours. The nurse also must be aware of serum creatinine levels: as serum levels approach 1 mg/dl, the kidney does not excrete magnesium. If output is less than 30 ml/hour or less than 120 ml every 4 hours or if serum creatinine levels are elevated, the physician is notified. In the presence of oliguria or renal involvement the infusion of $MgSO_4$ may be reduced or discontinued.

Serum levels are obtained 4 to 6 hours after the initial loading dose. Additional serum magnesium levels are then obtained based on the woman's response and if any signs of toxicity are present.

Diuresis within 24 to 48 hours is an excellent prognostic sign. It is considered evidence that perfusion of the kidney has improved as a result of relaxation of arteriolar spasm. With improved perfusion, fluid moves from the interstitial spaces to the intravascular bed, and edema is reduced. Diuresis results in weight loss. In the presence of a large urine output (more than 200 ml/hour), the dosage of $MgSO_4$ may need to be increased.

Calcium gluconate, the antidote for $MgSO_4$, should be kept at the bedside. If toxicity occurs, 1 g (10 ml of a 10% solution) of calcium gluconate is administered by slow IV push (over at least 3 minutes) and repeated every hour until the respiratory, urinary, and neurologic depression has been alleviated.

If the woman develops eclampsia, $MgSO_4$ may be administered by slow IV push in 1 g or 2 g boluses (see the Emergency box below). For seizures unresponsive to $MgSO_4$, amobarbital sodium, 250 mg, can be administered by slow IV push over 3

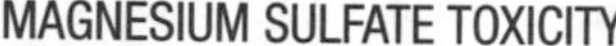

MAGNESIUM SULFATE TOXICITY

SIGNS/SYMPTOMS

Respirations <12/min
Hyporeflexia, absence of reflexes
Urine output <30 ml/hr
Toxic serum levels >9.6 mg/dl
Signs of fetal stress (e.g., fetal tachycardia or bradycardia)
Significant drop in maternal pulse or blood pressure

INTERVENTIONS

Discontinue $MgSO_4$ immediately, and change to maintenance solution.
Call for assistance and notify health care provider for immediate care.
Administer calcium gluconate as ordered (e.g., 1 g for IV injection given over 3 minutes).
Monitor return of DTRs, respiratory rate and quality, pulse rate and quality, and urine output.
Monitor $MgSO_4$ level as indicated by patient response.

EMERGENCY

ECLAMPSIA

TONIC-CLONIC CONVULSION SIGNS

Stage of invasion: 2 to 3 seconds; eyes fixed; twitching of facial muscles.
Stage of contraction: 15 to 20 seconds; eyes protrude and are bloodshot; all body muscles in tonic contraction.
Stage of convulsion: muscles relax and contract alternately (clonic). Respirations are halted and then begin again with long, deep, stertorous inhalation. Coma may ensue.

INTERVENTIONS

Keep airway patient; turn head to one side; place pillow under one shoulder or back, if possible.
Call for assistance.
Protect with side rails up and padded.
Observe and record convulsion activity.

AFTER CONVULSION/SEIZURE

Observe for postconvulsion coma and incontinence.
Use suction as needed.
Administer oxygen via face mask at 10 L/min.
Start IV fluids and monitor for potential fluid overload.
Give $MgSO_4$ or anticonvulsant drug as ordered.
Insert indwelling catheter.
Monitor blood pressure.
Monitor fetal and uterine status.
Expedite laboratory work as ordered to monitor kidney function, liver function, coagulation system, and drug levels.
Provide hygiene and a quiet environment.
Support and keep woman and family informed.
Be prepared for birth when woman is stable.

minutes (Sibai, 1990b, c). Another alternative anticonvulsant drug is diazepam (Valium). Its target tissues are the thalamus and hypothalamus, where it has a depressent effect. It is effective in the management of eclamptic convulsions refractory to $MgSO_4$ therapy. For women who have seizures unresponsive to anticonvulsant therapy, a neurologic assessment of the brain is indicated.

Because $MgSO_4$ is a tocolytic agent, its use may increase the duration of labor. The nurse must be aware that if a woman in labor is receiving $MgSO_4$, the amount of oxytocin needed to stimulate labor is higher.

$MgSO_4$ does not seem to affect FHR variability in a healthy term fetus and rarely is toxic in the healthy term newborn whose weight is within normal range for gestational age. Neonatal serum magnesium levels approximate those of the mother, and toxic levels can cause depressed respirations and hyporeflexia (Sibai, 1988). The neonate with hypermagnesemia can be treated with calcium and exchange transfusion with citrated blood or may require assisted mechanical ventilation until serum levels normalize.

Both amobarital sodium and diazepam have fetal/neonatal effects. FHR loses variability. High levels in the newborn depress sucking ability, cause hypotonia, and may result in temperature instability. The newborn's respiratory rate may be decreased. Careful surveillance of both maternal and fetal/neonatal status is warranted (see the Nursing Care Plan below).

Control of blood pressure. For the severely hypertensive woman with preeclampsia/HELLP syndrome, antihypertensive medications are ordered to lower the diastolic blood pressure. Initiation of antihypertensive therapy reduces maternal morbidity and mortality associated with left ventricular

Nursing Care Plan

PREECLAMPSIA

Hospital Care

Nursing Diagnosis: Risk for injury to mother and fetus related to CNS irritability

Expected Outcome: Patient will show diminished signs of CNS irritability (e.g., DTRs 2+, absence of clonus) and have no convulsions.

• NURSING INTERVENTIONS/*RATIONALES*

Establish baseline data (e.g., DTRs, clonus) *to use as basis for evaluating effectiveness of treatment.*

Administer IV $MgSO_4$ per physician's orders *to decrease hyperreflexia and minimize risk of convulsions.*

Monitor maternal vital signs, FHR, urine output, DTRs, IV flow rate, and serum levels of $MgSO_4$ *to assess for and prevent $MgSO_4$ toxicity (e.g., depressed respirations, oliguria, sudden drop in blood pressure, hyporeflexia, fetal distress).*

Have calcium gluconate at bedside if needed *as antidote for $MgSO_4$ toxicity.*

Maintain a quiet, darkened environment *to avoid stimuli that may precipitate seizure activity.*

Nursing Diagnosis: Altered tissue perfusion related to preeclampsia secondary to arteriole vasospasm

Expected Outcome: Patient will exhibit signs of increased vasodilation (i.e., diuresis, decreased edema, weight loss).

• NURSING INTERVENTIONS/*RATIONALES*

Establish baseline data (i.e., weight, degree of edema) *to use as basis for evaluating effectiveness of treatment.*

Administer intravenous magnesium sulfate per physician order, *which serves to relax vasospasms and increase renal perfusion.*

Place woman on bed rest in a side-lying position *to maximize uteroplacental blood flow, reduce blood pressure, and promote diuresis.*

Monitor intake and output, edema, and weight *to assess for evidence of vasodilation and increased tissue perfusion.*

Nursing Diagnosis: Risk for
- fluid volume excess related to increased sodium retention secondary to administration of $MgSO_4$
- impaired gas exchange related to pulmonary edema secondary to increased vascular resistance
- decreased cardiac output related to use of antihypertensive drugs
- injury to fetus related to ureteroplacental insufficiency secondary to use of antihypertensive medications

Expected Outcomes: Patient will exhibit signs of normal fluid volume (i.e., balanced intake and output, normal serum creatinine levels, normal breath sounds); exhibit signs of adequate oxygenation (i.e., normal respirations, fully oriented to person, time, and place); exhibit signs of normal range of cardiac output (i.e., normal pulse rate and rhythm); and exhibit signs of fetal well-being (i.e., adequate fetal movement, normal FHR).

• NURSING INTERVENTIONS/*RATIONALES*

Monitor woman for signs of fluid volume excess (increased edema, decreased urine output, elevated serum creatinine level, weight gain, dyspnea, crackles) *to prevent complications.*

Monitor woman for signs of impaired gas exchange (i.e., increased respirations, dyspnea, altered blood gases, hypoxemia) *to prevent complications.*

Monitor woman for signs of decreased cardiac output (i.e., altered pulse rate and rhythm) *to prevent complications.*

Monitor fetus for signs of difficulty (i.e., decreased fetal activity, decreased FHR) *to prevent complications.*

Record findings and report signs of increasing problems to physician *to enable timely interventions.*

failure and cerebral hemorrhage. Because a degree of maternal hypertension is necessary to maintain uteroplacental perfusion, antihypertensive therapy must not decrease the arterial pressure too low or too rapidly. Therefore the target range for the diastolic pressure is 90 to 100 mm Hg (Harvey and Burke, 1992).

IV hydralazine remains the antihypertensive of choice for the treatment of hypertension in preeclampsia (Clark et al, 1991). IV labetalol hydrochloride is also commonly used (Pickles et al, 1992). Other antihypertensive agents, such as those described in Table 9-3, may be employed (Harvey and Burke, 1992). The choice of agent depends on patient response and health care provider preference.

Eclampsia. The reported incidence of eclampsia is from 0.5% to 2% of all pregnancies. A wide range of signs and

TABLE 9-3 Pharmacologic control of hypertension in pregnancy

ACTION	TARGET TISSUE	EFFECTS: MATERNAL	EFFECTS: FETAL	NURSING ACTIONS
Hydralazine (Apresoline, Neopresol)				
Anteriolar vasodilator	Peripheral arterioles to decrease muscle tone, decreasing peripheral resistance; hypothalamus and medullary vasomotor center for minor decrease in sympathetic tone	Headache, flushing, palpitation, tachycardia, some decrease in uteroplacental blood flow, increase in heart rate and cardiac output, increase in oxygen consumption	Tachycardia: late decelerations and bradycardia if maternal diastolic pressure < 90 mm Hg	Assess for effects of medications; alert mother (family) to expected effects of medications; may be given IV bolus or by infusion; repeat no more often than every 20-30 minutes; assess blood pressure because precipitous drop can lead to shock and perhaps abruptio placentae; assess urine output; maintain bed rest in a lateral position with side rails up.
Labetalol hydrochloride (Normodyne)				
β-Blocking agent causing vasodilation without significant change in cardiac output	Peripheral arterioles (see hydralazine)	Minimal	Minimal	See hydralazine.
Methyldopa (Aldomet)				
Maintenance therapy if needed: 250 to 500 mg orally every 8 hours (α_2-receptor agonist)	Postganglionic nerve endings to cause interference with chemical neurotransmission to reduce peripheral vascular resistance, CNS to cause sedation	Sleepiness, postural hypotension, constipation; rare: drug-induced fever in 1% of women and positive Coombs' test result in 20%	After 4 months of maternal therapy, positive Coombs' test result in infant	See hydralazine.
Nifedipine (Procardia)				
Calcium channel blocker	Arterioles to reduce systemic vascular resistance via relaxation of arterial smooth muscle	Headache, flushing; possible potentiation of effects on CNS if administered concurrently with magnesium sulfate	Same as hydralazine, but less frequent	See hydralazine.
Nitroglycerin				
Potent vasodilator	Venous system	Decrease in blood pressure by decreasing cardiac output, antihypertensive effect related to maternal intravascular volume status	Stress possibly noted with MAP < 106 mm Hg, decreased FHR variability	See hydralazine; be aware of need for special IV setup; monitor blood pressure electronically; consider arterial line for more rapid assessment of BP changes.

symptoms besides convulsions are associated with eclampsia: extreme hypertension, hyperreflexia, 4+ proteinuria, generalized edema to mild hypertension without edema. The woman reports headaches with or without visual disturbances for 1 to 4 days before the onset of convulsions; proteinuria is absent in 20% of the women. Laboratory findings also vary. Hemoconcentration is evidenced by an increased hematocrit. Serum uric acid, creatinine, liver function tests, and urine creatinine clearance are elevated. DIC may be present if treatment is delayed or abruptio placentae occurs.

Immediate care. The immediate care during a convulsion is to ensure a patent airway (see the Emergency box on p. 212). Once this has been attained, adequate oxygenation must be maintained by use of supplemental oxygen. When convulsions occur, the woman is turned to her side to prevent aspiration of vomitus and supine hypotension syndrome. After the convulsion ceases, food and fluid are suctioned from the glottis or trachea. $MgSO_4$ (and amobarbital sodium for recurrent convulsions) is given as ordered (Sibai, 1990a). If an IV infusion is not in place, one is begun with a large-bore needle. Time, duration, and description of convulsions are recorded, and any urinary or fecal incontinence is noted. The fetus is monitored for adverse effects. A transient bradycardia and decreased fetal heart rate variability are common.

Aspiration is a leading cause of maternal morbidity and mortality following an eclamptic seizure. After initial stabilization and airway management, the nurse should anticipate orders for a chest x-ray film and possibly arterial blood gases (ABGs) to determine whether aspiration occurred.

A rapid assessment of uterine activity, cervical status, and fetal status is performed. During the convulsion, membranes may rupture and the cervix may dilate because the uterus becomes hypercontractile and hypertonic; birth may be imminent. If not, once the woman's seizure tendency and blood pressure are controlled, a decision should be made as to whether the birth should take place. The more serious the condition of the woman, the greater is the need to proceed to the birth, which is the definitive cure for the disease. The route of birth—induction of labor vs. cesarean birth—depends on the maternal and fetal condition. All medications and therapy are merely temporary measures (Iams, Zuspan, and Quilligan, 1990). If fetal lungs are not mature and the birth can be delayed for 48 hours, steroids such as betamethasone may be given.

Determination of central venous pressure (CVP) and pulmonary artery wedge pressure (PAWP) (Swan-Ganz catheter) may be required for accurate fluid monitoring in the presence of pulmonary edema or acute renal failure (ACOG, 1992a). Nothing by mouth (NPO) is permitted if the woman is convulsing or has symptoms of severe preeclampsia. An indwelling catheter is required for accurate measurement of hourly urine output. Blood sugar is evaluated by bedside finger stick or venous draw every 1 to 8 hours as ordered. Glucose solutions are administered as ordered. To correct hypovolemia, crystalloids (0.9% saline or Ringer's lactate solution) are infused IV at a rate that maintains a urine output of at least 30 ml/hour. Maternal response to therapy is recorded.

Medications (e.g., $MgSO_4$, antihypertensive agents) are given as directed. The woman's response is monitored and recorded, and all drugs, dosages, and times are recorded.

Laboratory tests are ordered to assess for the HELLP syndrome and to have blood typed and crossmatched. Other tests include determination of electrolytes, liver function battery, and complete hemogram and clotting profile. Blood is kept available for emergency transfusion; abruptio placentae, with accompanying hemorrhage and shock, often occurs in women with eclampsia. Other tests include determination of electrolytes, liver function battery, and complete hemogram and clotting profile, including platelets and fibrin split products (to assess for DIC).

The woman may have been incontinent of urine and stool or the membranes may have ruptured during the convulsion; she will need assistance with hygiene and a change of gown. Oral care with a soft toothbrush may be of comfort to her.

The health care provider explains procedures briefly and quietly. *The woman is never left alone.* The family is also kept informed of management, rationale, and the woman's progress.

Postpartum nursing care. After birth the symptoms of preeclampsia-eclampsia resolve quickly, usually within 48 hours. The hematopoietic and hepatic complications of HELLP syndrome may persist longer. These patients may show an abrupt decrease in platelets with a concomitant increase in LDH and AST after a trend toward normalization of values has begun. Generally, the laboratory abnormalities seen with HELLP syndrome resolve in 72 to 96 hours.

The nursing care of the woman with hypertensive disease differs from that required in a normal postpartum period in a number of respects. The following variations in the nursing process are emphasized.

Careful assessment of the woman with a hypertensive disorder continues throughout the postpartum period. Blood pressure is measured at least every 4 hours for 48 hours or more often as the woman's condition warrants. Even if no convulsions occurred before the birth, they may occur within this period. $MgSO_4$ infusion may be continued up to 48 hours after the birth. The same assessments continue until the drug is discontinued. The woman is at risk for a boggy uterus and a large lochia flow as a result of $MgSO_4$ therapy. Uterine tone and lochial flow must be monitored closely. The preeclamptic woman is hemoconcentrated and unable to tolerate excessive postpartum blood loss. Oxytocin or prostaglandin products are used to control bleeding. Ergot products (e.g., Ergotrate, Methergine) are contraindicated because they increase blood pressure. The woman is asked to report symptoms such as headaches and blurred vision. The nurse assesses affect, level of consciousness, blood pressure, pulse, and respiratory status before an analgesic is given for headache. It must be remembered that $MgSO_4$ potentiates the action of narcotics, CNS depressants, and calcium channel blockers; these drugs need to be administered with caution. The woman may need to continue antihypertensive medication if her diastolic blood pressure exceeds 100 mm Hg at discharge.

The woman's and family's responses to labor, the birth, and the newborn are monitored. Interactions and involvement in the care of the newborn are encouraged as much as the woman and her family desire. In addition, the woman and her family need opportunities to discuss their emotional response to complications. The nurse also provides information concerning the prognosis. Preeclampsia and eclampsia do not necessarily recur in subsequent pregnancies, but careful prenatal care is essential (recurrence rate is about 30%).

Critical Thinking Exercises 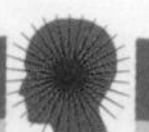

SEVERE PREECLAMPSIA

1. Marie has been diagnosed with severe preeclampsia. She is laboring in her labor, delivery, recovery, postpartum care (LDRP) room with four family members present. The family members are conversing loudly while watching a ball game on TV and taking bets. Marie states that she wants them to leave and let her rest, but she is unwilling to confront them. Role-play a nurse attempting to provide teaching to the family who resist changes in the labor plan. Ask the group to suggest different strategies.
2. Marie's blood pressure increases to 190/115. She complains of a "blinding headache," epigastric pain, and visual disturbances. On assessment the DTRs are 4+ with two beats of clonus.
   a. State the most likely diagnosis, and list in order of priority the nursing interventions to be taken.
   b. In order of priority, list the interventions during a convulsion and the specific rationale for each.
   c. Identify three medications appropriate to the care of this patient, their action, and the precautions to be used for each medication.

Evaluation

Evaluation is a continuous process. To be effective, it needs to be based on measurable criteria that reflect the expected outcomes of nursing care. Thus for severe preeclampsia/HELLP syndrome, the following conditions should be met:

1. The woman and fetus suffer no adverse sequelae from preeclampsia or its management.
2. The woman does not experience eclampsia or its complications.
3. The fetus does not experience distress.
4. The newborn is born in optimal condition with no adverse sequelae resulting from the maternal condition and its management.
5. The woman gives birth in optimal condition with no sequelae to her condition and its management.
6. The family copes effectively with the mother's high-risk condition, its management, and outcomes.

If the outcome for the mother or baby is unfavorable, the family is assisted in coping with loss and grief (see the Nursing Care Plan on p. 213).

MATERNAL HEMORRHAGIC DISORDERS

Hemorrhagic disorders in pregnancy are medical emergencies. It is estimated that 1 in 5 pregnancies are complicated by bleeding; the incidence and type of bleeding vary by trimester (Thorp, 1993). Maternal mortality has decreased significantly in recent years; however, hemorrhage remains a leading cause of maternal death (Atrash, Rowley, and Hogue, 1992; National Center for Health Statistics, 1993; Suresh and Kinch, 1991). Prompt, expert teamwork on the part of the health care providers is needed to save the lives of the mother and infant.

Blood loss during pregnancy can occur rapidly. With approximately 650 ml/minute (15% of maternal CO) of blood flow to the uterine vasculature and placenta, disruption of vascular integrity has the potential for maternal exsanguination within 8 to 10 minutes (Knuppel and Hatangadi, 1995; O'Brien, 1993; Thorp, 1993). Therefore the nurse must be alert to the signs and symptoms of hemorrhage and hypovolemic shock and be prepared to act quickly to minimize blood loss and hasten return to normal state. Supportive care for the pregnant woman and her family includes attention to physical needs, emotional well-being, and possibly grief counseling.

Early Pregnancy Bleeding

Bleeding during early pregnancy is alarming to the woman and of concern to the health care provider. The common bleeding disorders of early pregnancy include abortion, incompetent cervix, ectopic pregnancy, and hydatidiform mole.

Spontaneous abortion. Abortion is the termination of pregnancy before viability of the fetus. Viability is reached at about 20 to 24 weeks' gestation, with a fetal weight over 500 g or a crown-rump length of 18 cm. With the ever-expanding technology for neonatal care, the limits for fetal viability are becoming lower, with more aggressive management being used for an infant who has at least a chance for survival.

There are three types of abortions. A spontaneous abortion results from natural causes; a therapeutic abortion is a deliberate interruption of a pre-viable pregnancy for medical reasons; and an elective abortion is the purposeful interruption of a pre-viable pregnancy for a variety of personal reasons. This discussion includes only spontaneous abortions; for therapeutic and elective abortions, see Chapter 10.

An early spontaneous abortion, or miscarriage, is one that occurs before 12 weeks' gestation; a late abortion is one occurring between 12 and 20 weeks' gestation. The rate of spontaneous abortion is difficult to determine but may be as high as 20% (Dorfman, 1991).

Causes. The causes of early abortion may include endocrine imbalance (e.g., women with luteal phase defects or who have insulin-dependent diabetes mellitus with high blood-glucose levels in the first trimester), immunologic factors (e.g., antiphospholipid antibodies), infections (e.g., bacteriuria, *Chlamydia trachomatis*), systemic disorders (e.g., systemic lupus erythematosus), genetic factors (about 60% of early abortions display an abnormal chromosomal makeup), and cocaine use (Arias, 1993; Cunningham et al, 1993; Gilbert and Harmon, 1993b; Mills et al, 1988; Rosenak, 1990). Late spontaneous abortions usually result from maternal causes such as advancing maternal age and parity, chronic infections, incompetent cervix and other anomalies of the reproductive tract, chronic debilitating diseases, poor nutrition, and recreational drug use (Cunningham et al, 1993).

Anomalies of the reproductive tract cause second- or third-trimester pregnancy loss. Little can be done to avoid genetic causes of pregnancy loss, but prepregnancy correction of maternal disorders, immunization against infectious diseases, adequate early prenatal care, and treatment of pregnancy complications will do much to prevent abortion.

Types. The types of spontaneous abortion include threatened, inevitable, incomplete, complete, missed, and septic. Symptoms of a *threatened abortion* (Fig. 9-5, *A*) include spotting of blood and a closed cervical os. Mild uterine cramping

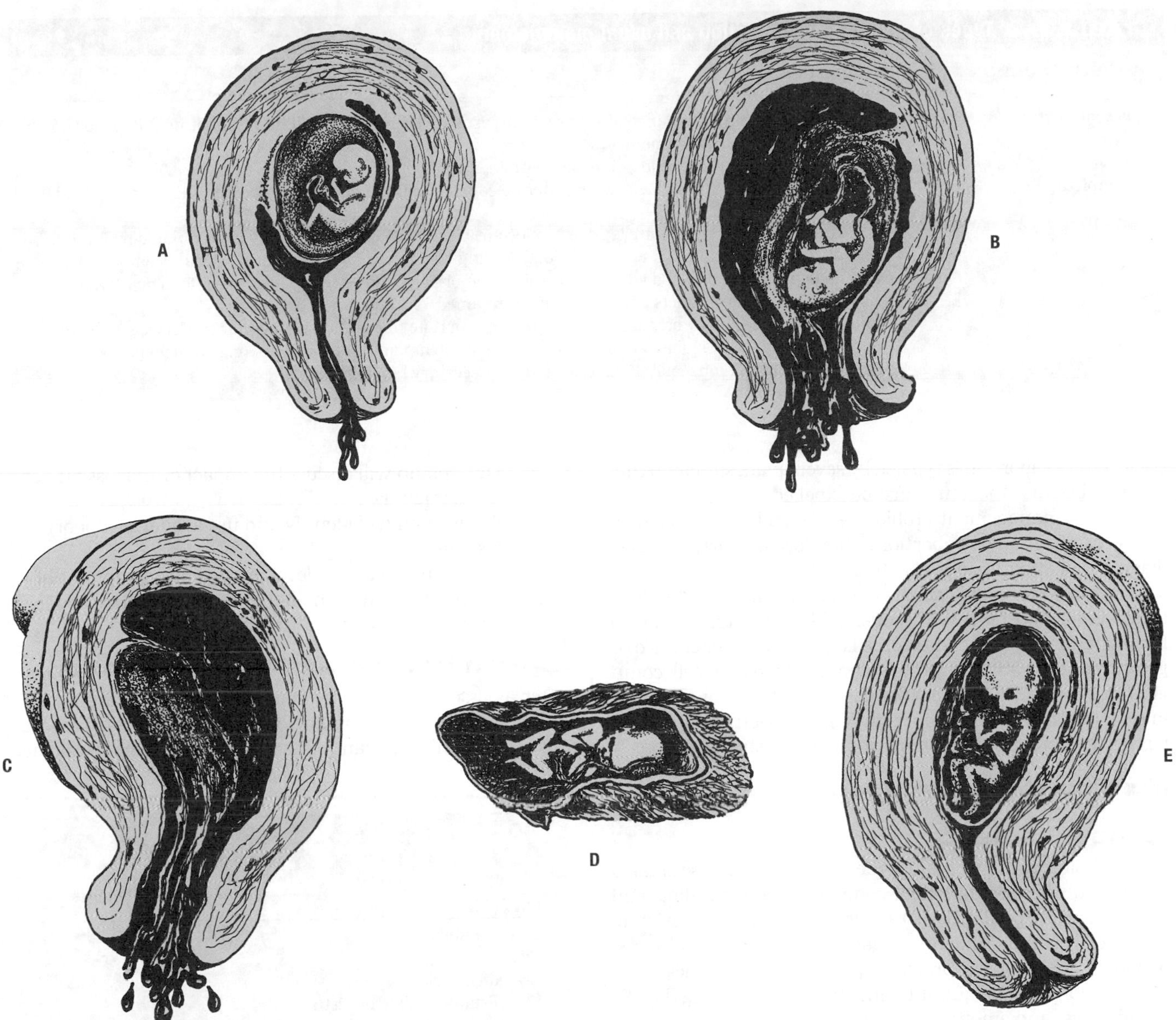

Fig. 9-5 Spontaneous abortion. **A,** Threatened. **B,** Inevitable. **C,** Incomplete. **D,** Complete. **E,** Missed.

may be present. Management includes bed rest and avoidance of stress and orgasm. Follow-up treatment is individualized.

Inevitable (Fig. 9-5, *B*) and *incomplete* (Fig. 9-5, *C*) abortions involve a moderate to heavy amount of bleeding with an open cervical os. Tissue may be present with the bleeding. Mild to severe uterine cramping may be present. Prompt termination of the pregnancy, usually by curettage, is the suggested treatment.

In a *complete abortion* (Fig. 9-5, *D*), all the fetal tissue is passed, the cervix is closed, and there may be slight bleeding. Usually no further treatment is required.

A *missed abortion* (Fig. 9-5, *E*) refers to a pregnancy in which the fetus has died but spontaneous abortion does not occur. It may be diagnosed when the uterus is smaller than expected for the duration of the pregnancy. There may be no bleeding or cramping, and the cervical os is closed. Treatment may include waiting up to 1 month for spontaneous abortion to occur with frequent monitoring of the woman's clotting factors. If spontaneous abortion does not occur, the physician will terminate the pregnancy to prevent DIC and/or sepsis in the woman.

Presenting symptoms of a *septic*, or infected, abortion include fever and abdominal tenderness. Vaginal bleeding, which may be slight to heavy, is usually malodorous. Termination of the pregnancy, antibiotic therapy, and treatment of septic shock are initiated.

Signs and symptoms. Signs and symptoms of spontaneous abortion depend on the duration of pregnancy. The woman may feel she is experiencing a heavy menstrual flow if abortion occurs before the sixth week of pregnancy. Abortion that occurs between the sixth and twelfth weeks of pregnancy will cause moderate discomfort and blood loss. After the

TABLE 9-4 Types of spontaneous abortion and usual management

TYPE OF ABORTION	MANAGEMENT
Threatened	Bed rest, sedation, and avoidance of stress and orgasm are recommended. Further treatment depends on woman's response to treatment.
Inevitable and incomplete	Prompt termination of pregnancy is accomplished, usually by dilation and curettage (D&C).
Complete	No further intervention may be needed if uterine contractions are adequate to prevent hemorrhage and if there is no infection.
Missed	If spontaneous evacuation of uterus does not occur within 1 month, pregnancy is terminated by method appropriate to duration of pregnancy. Blood clotting factors are monitored until uterus is empty. DIC and incoagulability of blood with uncontrolled hemorrhage may develop in cases of fetal death after the twelfth week if products of conception are retained for longer than 5 weeks.
Septic	Immediate termination of pregnancy by method appropriate to duration of pregnancy. Cervical culture and sensitivity (C&S) studies are done, and broad-spectrum antibiotic therapy (e.g., ampicillin) is started. Treatment for septic shock is initiated if necessary.

twelfth week, abortion is typified by severe pain, similar to that of labor, because the fetus must be expelled.

Medical management (Table 9-4) depends on the classification of spontaneous abortion. Therefore an early accurate diagnosis of spontaneous abortion is vital.

A negative or weakly positive urine pregnancy test is characteristic of abortion. With considerable or persistent blood loss, anemia is likely. If sepsis is present, temperature is greater than 100° F (38° C) and white blood cell count greater than 12,000/mm³. Endocrine studies show that human chorionic gonadotropin (hCG), estrogen, and progesterone titers are minimal or absent in established abortions.

Nursing Care Management

Assessment

On admission of the woman to the hospital, the nurse obtains a history of the woman's chief complaint, pain, bleeding, and last menstrual period (LMP) to determine the approximate length of gestation. The initial data base includes vital signs, previous pregnancies, previous pregnancy outcomes, type and location of pain, quantity and nature of bleeding (Box 9-6), allergies, and emotional status. The woman may be anxious and fearful of what may happen to her and her pregnancy.

Nursing Diagnoses

Nursing diagnoses are derived after thoughtfully analyzing assessment findings and medical management directives. Nursing diagnoses for the patient experiencing a spontaneous abortion may include the following:

- Fluid volume deficit related to
  Excessive bleeding secondary to spontaneous abortion
- Pain related to
  Uterine contractions
- Anticipatory grieving related to
  Unexpected pregnancy outcome

Expected Outcomes

The plan of care is mutually negotiated on the basis of the biophysical and psychosocial assessment of the patient. Mutually determined expected outcomes include the following:

1. The woman will discuss the impact of the loss on her and her family.
2. The woman will identify and use available support systems.
3. The woman will not develop signs and symptoms of complications (e.g., hemorrhage, infection).
4. The woman will verbalize relief from pain.

Plan of Care and Implementation

After assessing the patient, immediate nursing care focuses on stabilization of the woman. Psychosocial aspects of care focus on what this pregnancy loss means to the woman and her

BOX 9-6
Assessment of Bleeding in Pregnancy

INITIAL DATA BASE

Chief complaint
Vital signs
Gravidity, parity
LMP/Estimated date of birth (EDB)
Pregnancy history (previous and current)
Allergies
Nausea and vomiting
Pain (onset, quality, precipitating event)
Bleeding or coagulation problems
Level of consciousness
Emotional status

EARLY PREGNANCY

Confirmation of pregnancy
Bleeding (bright or dark, intermittent or continuous)
Pain (type, intensity, persistence)
Vaginal discharge

LATE PREGNANCY

EDB
Bleeding (quantity, associated pain)
Vaginal discharge
Amniotic membrane status
Uterine activity
Abdominal pain
Fetal status/viability

family. Care is patient and family centered. The nurse reinforces explanations of expected procedures, possible complications, and future implications and carries out appropriate orders. An IV line is started, laboratory work is obtained, and possibly an ultrasound test is performed. Laboratory tests include a CBC; blood typing for group, Rh factor, and cross-matching; and urinalysis. Chest x-ray films and ECG evaluation are obtained if necessary. Blood, fluid, and electrolyte imbalances are corrected as soon as possible.

If a *dilation and curettage (D&C)* is scheduled, the nurse reinforces explanations, answers any questions or concerns, and prepares the patient for surgery. D&C is a surgical procedure in which the cervix is dilated and a curette is inserted to scrape the uterine walls and remove uterine contents. General preoperative and postoperative care is appropriate for the woman requiring surgical intervention for spontaneous abortion. For late incomplete or inevitable abortions (16 to 20 weeks) and missed abortions, prostaglandins may be administered into the amniotic sac or by vaginal suppository to augment or induce labor and cause the products of conception to be expelled. IV oxytocin may also be used.

Analgesics and/or anesthetic appropriate to the procedure are used. IV administration of oxytocin, 10 U in 500 ml of infusate, may be needed to induce or augment emptying of the uterus. After evacuation of the uterus, 10 to 20 U of oxytocin in 1000 ml of infusate may be given to prevent hemorrhage.

Ergot products such as ergonovine, which contract the uterus and cervix, are contraindicated until the uterus is emptied to avoid retention of fragments or tissue. Retained fragments of fetal or placental tissue predispose to uterine relaxation and puerperal infection. Three or four doses of ergonovine, 0.2 mg orally or IM every 4 hours, may be given if the woman is normotensive. Antibiotics are given as necessary. Transfusion may be required for shock or anemia. If the woman is Rh negative and has not developed isoimmunization, she is given an intramuscular injection of $Rh_o(D)$ immune globulin within 72 hours of the abortion. The usual dose of $Rh_o(D)$ immune globulin at less than 12 weeks' gestation is 50 μg; if greater than 12 weeks', 300 μg.

Discharge teaching should emphasize the need for rest, and if significant blood loss occurred, iron supplementation may be ordered. Teaching includes information about normal physical findings, such as cramping and type/amount of bleeding, resumption of sexual activity, and family planning. Follow-up care should assess the woman's physical and emotional recovery. Referrals to local support groups or counselling are provided as necessary (see the Patient Teaching box below).

Patient Teaching

DISCHARGE TEACHING FOR WOMAN AFTER SPONTANEOUS ABORTION

- Advise woman to report any heavy, profuse, or bright red bleeding to health care provider.
- Reassure woman that a scant, dark discharge may persist for 1 to 2 weeks.
- To reduce the risk of infection, remind woman not to introduce anything into the vagina until bleeding has stopped. She should take antibiotics as prescribed.
- Acknowledge that she has experienced a loss and that time is required for recovery. She may experience mood swings and depression.
- Refer to appropriate support groups, clergy, or professional counseling.
- Attempts at pregnancy should be postponed for at least 2 months to allow her body to recover (Gilbert and Harmon, 1993b).

Evaluation

Evaluation is based on the predetermined patient-centered outcomes. The nurse can be reasonably assured that care was effective if outcomes for care have been achieved and the woman does the following:

1. Discusses the impact of the loss on her and her family
2. Identifies and uses available support systems
3. Does not develop signs and symptoms of complications
4. Verbalizes health promotion measures to decrease risk of future spontaneous abortions.

Recurrent premature dilation of cervix (incompetent cervix). Painless dilation of the cervical os without labor or contractions of the uterus may occur in the second trimester or early in the third trimester of pregnancy. Spontaneous abortion or preterm birth may result. The incidence of premature dilation of the cervix occurs in 20% or more of all second-trimester losses (Iams, Zuspan, and Quilligan, 1990).

Causes. Etiologic factors include a history of cervical lacerations during childbirth, forceful D&C, or ingestion of diethylstilbestrol (DES) by the woman's mother while pregnant with the woman. Other causes are a congenitally short cervix or uterine anomalies.

The diagnosis of recurrent **premature dilation of the cervix (incompetent cervix)** is difficult and is based on clinical history. A presumptive diagnosis can usually be made if a woman experiences appreciable cervical dilation and prolapse of the membranes through the cervix without labor. In a woman with a history of repeated spontaneous second-trimester terminations, premature cervical dilation should be suspected.

Medical management. The woman with recurrent premature dilation of the cervix may be managed conservatively with bed rest, hydration, and tocolysis (inhibition of uterine contractions) or actively by performing a cervical **cerclage.** Correction of the weakened cervix is possible by wedge trachelorrhaphy (removal of a wedge from the anterior segment of the cervix with closure) in the nonpregnant woman. During pregnancy a *McDonald cerclage,* band of homologous fascia, or nonabsorbable ribbon (Mersilene) may be placed around the cervix beneath the mucosa to constrict the internal os (Fig. 9-6). Successful continuation of the pregnancy to viability or beyond occurs in approximately 40% of women, provided the membranes remain intact and that the cervix is not more than 3 cm dilated or more than 50% effaced at the time of correction. The suture is left in place until close to term, when it is removed, and labor is allowed to begin spontaneously. This procedure must be repeated with each pregnancy.

A second method involves placement of a pursestring ligature to maintain a closed cervix. This procedure, the *Shirodkar,*

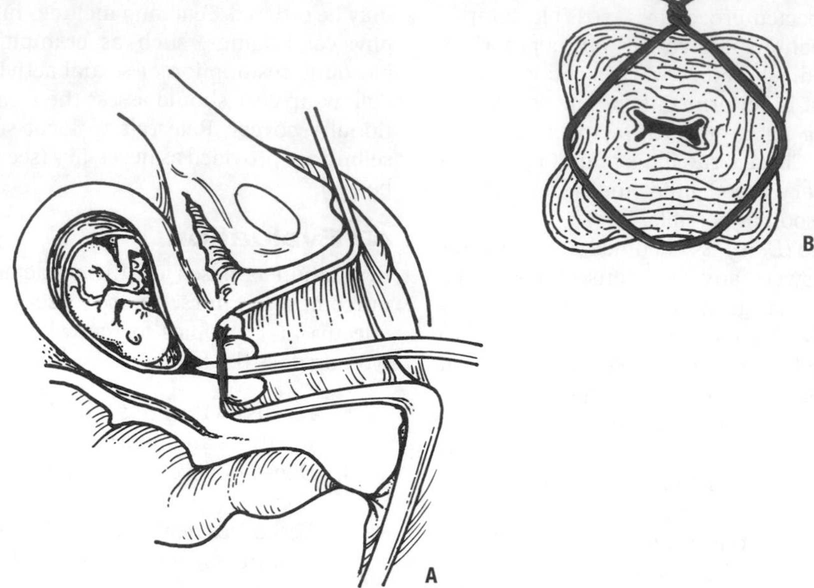

Fig. 9-6 **A**, Cerclage correction of recurrent premature dilation of cervix. **B**, Cross section of closed internal os.

allows for the suture to remain in place permanently for the woman that anticipates future pregnancies. Births are accomplished by cesarean.

Nursing care management. If recurrent premature dilation of the cervix is suspected, the assessment includes exploring the woman's feelings about her pregnancy and her understanding about early cervical dilation. It is also important to evaluate the woman's support systems. Since the diagnosis of recurrent premature dilation of the cervix usually is not made until the woman has lost one or more pregnancies, she may feel guilty or to blame for this impending loss.

Care of the woman with recurrent premature dilation of the cervix focuses on her self-concept, her ability to cope with possible pregnancy loss, and her ability to understand treatment regimens. The woman is at increased risk for premature rupture of membranes (PROM), infection, and the onset of preterm labor after surgical correction of the cervix.

If a cervical cerclage is performed, the woman is monitored postoperatively for contractions, signs of PROM, and infection. Referrals are made as appropriate for assistance once she is discharged home.

Discharge teaching focuses on signs and symptoms of preterm labor, PROM, and infection. If home uterine monitoring is used, the woman should receive her initial instructions from the home health agency before discharge.

Home care. The woman must understand the importance of bed rest at home and the need for close observation and supervision. Instruction includes the rationale for bed rest, restricting activity, and warning signs to report (Grohar, 1994; Simpson, 1992).

Tocolytics may be given to prevent uterine contractions and further dilation of the cervix. The woman must be instructed on the importance of taking oral tocolytic medication as prescribed, the expected response, and possible side effects. If home monitoring is implemented, she is taught how to apply a uterine contraction monitor and transmit the monitor tracing by telephone to the monitoring center. Nurses at the monitoring center assess the tracing for contractions, answer questions, provide emotional support and education, and report information to the woman's primary care provider (Robichaux, Stedman, Hamner, 1990).

If management of early pregnancy bleeding is unsuccessful and the fetus is born before viability, appropriate grief support should be provided. If the birth is premature, appropriate anticipatory guidance and support are necessary.

Ectopic pregnancy. Ectopic pregnancy is one in which the fertilized ovum is implanted outside the uterine cavity (Fig. 9-7). About 95% of ectopic pregnancies occur in the fallopian (uterine) tube, with most on the right side, for undetermined reasons. Other sites include the ovary, abdominal cavity, and cervix. Most extrauterine pregnancies result from abnormalities that impede or prevent the passage of the fertilized ovum through the fallopian tube (e.g., peritubal adhesions after pelvic inflammatory disease). Approximately 1 in 100 pregnancies in the United States is ectopic, and at least three fourths of these become symptomatic and are diagnosed during the first trimester. Ectopic pregnancy is a significant cause of maternal morbidity and mortality, with mortality increased 10 times more than for a vaginal birth and 50 times for an induced abortion (Cunningham et al, 1993).

Ectopic pregnancy is classified according to the site of implantation (e.g., tubal, ovarian). The uterus is the only organ capable of containing and sustaining a term pregnancy. However, the rare abdominal pregnancy, with birth by laparotomy, may result in a living infant (Fig. 9-8).

Signs and symptoms. The nurse should suspect the possibility of an ectopic pregnancy in a woman who has missed a menstrual period, has adnexal fullness and tenderness, and who has a history of pelvic infection, intrauterine device

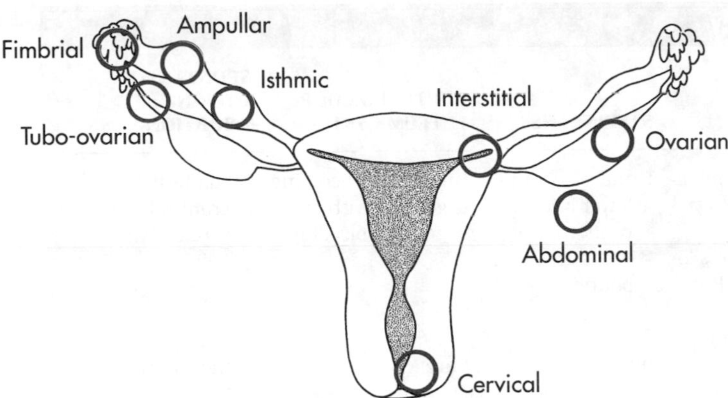

Fig. 9-7 Sites of implantation of ectopic pregnancies. Order of frequency of occurrence is ampulla, isthmus, interstitium, fimbria, tubo-ovarian ligament, ovary, abdominal cavity, and cervix (external os).

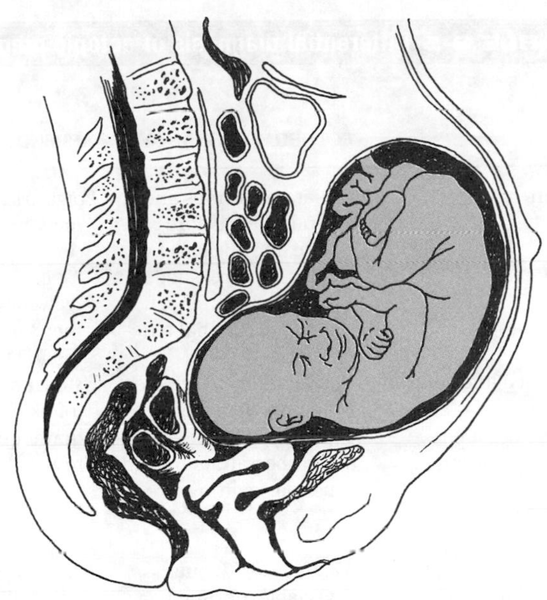

Fig. 9-8 Ectopic pregnancy, abdominal.

(IUD) use, or tubal surgery. The tenderness can progress from a dull pain to a colicky pain when the tube stretches. Pain can be unilateral, bilateral, or diffuse over the abdomen. Abnormal vaginal bleeding occurs in 50% to 80% of women. If an ectopic pregnancy ruptures, pain increases. Pain may be generalized, unilateral, or acute deep lower quadrant pain caused by blood irritating the peritoneum. Referred shoulder pain can occur related to diaphragmatic irritation caused by blood in the peritoneal cavity. The woman may exhibit signs of shock related to the amount of bleeding in the abdominal cavity and not necessarily related to obvious vaginal bleeding. Slight fever, leukocytosis, and a falling hematocrit or hemoglobin level may be noted. An ecchymotic blueness of the umbilicus (Cullen's sign), which is indicative of hematoperitoneum, may develop in a neglected, ruptured intraabdominal ectopic pregnancy.

Medical management. The use of ultrasound as an aid in the management of an ectopic pregnancy has allowed improved accuracy in the preoperative diagnosis. The differential diagnosis of ectopic pregnancy involves a consideration of numerous disorders that share many, perhaps all, of the same signs and symptoms (Table 9-5).

The major management problem in ectopic pregnancy is hemorrhage; bleeding must be quickly and effectively controlled. Blood transfusions must be available. Laparotomy is performed immediately after the diagnosis of ectopic pregnancy is made. Blood and clots are evacuated and bleeding vessels controlled.

Removal of the ectopic pregnancy through an incision into the fallopian tube or removal of a section of the tube is preferred to conserve the tube. If the tube is grossly involved, it may be removed. Ovarian pregnancy may be treated with wedge resection, but removal may be necessary depending on where the implantation occurred.

Advanced ectopic abdominal pregnancy requires laparotomy as soon as the woman is stabilized for surgery. If the placenta of a second- or third-trimester abdominal pregnancy is attached to a vital organ, such as the liver, separation and removal are usually not attempted because of risk of hemorrhage. The cord is cut flush with the placenta, and the abdomen is closed, leaving the placenta in place. Degeneration and absorption of the placenta usually occur without complication.

The diagnosis and management of ectopic pregnancy are rapidly changing as technology improves. The use of methotrexate therapy to cause regression of an ectopic pregnancy in the woman with very early (less than 6 weeks) ectopic pregnancy is being explored (Stoval and Ling, 1992).

The prognosis varies. The success of a subsequent pregnancy depends on the woman's specific reproductive history. Ectopic pregnancy recurs in approximately 10% of women, but more than 50% of women who have had an ectopic pregnancy achieve at least one normal pregnancy thereafter.

Nursing care management. A careful history with observation of a late or an actual missed period followed by slight vaginal bleeding and abdominal tenderness may identify an ectopic pregnancy. Any woman suspected of having an ectopic pregnancy should be immediately referred to a physician for a confirmative diagnosis and medical intervention. Potential nursing diagnoses pertinent to ectopic pregnancy include the following:

- Ineffective denial related to
  The possibility of a tubal pregnancy
- Decreased cardiac output, related to
  Bleeding associated with a ruptured ectopic pregnancy
- Anticipatory grieving, related to
  The loss of the pregnancy
- Pain related to
  Stretching of tube
  Rupture of tube
  Surgical treatment

Vital signs (pulse, respirations, and blood pressure) are assessed every 15 minutes or as needed, based on severity of the bleeding and the woman's condition. Laboratory tests include determination of blood type and Rh factor, CBC, and serum quantitative β-hCG values. Ultrasonography is used to con-

TABLE 9-5 Differential diagnosis of ectopic pregnancy

	ECTOPIC PREGNANCY	APPENDICITIS	SALPINGITIS	RUPTURED CORPUS LUTEUM CYST	SPONTANEOUS UTERINE ABORTION
Pain	Unilateral cramps and tenderness before rupture; may be colicky; after rupture, sudden sharp abdominopelvic pain; abdominal tenderness	Epigastric, periumbilical, then right lower quadrant pain; tenderness localizing at McBurney's point; rebound tenderness	Usually in both lower quadrants with or without rebound	Unilateral, becoming general with progressive bleeding	Mild uterine cramps to severe uterine pain
Nausea and vomiting	Occasionally before, frequently after rupture	Usual; precedes shift of pain to right lower quadrant	Infrequent	Rare	Almost never
Menstruation	Some aberration; missed period, spotting	Unrelated to menses	Hypermenorrhea or metrorrhagia or both	Period delayed, then bleeding, often with pain	Amenorrhea, then spotting, then brisk bleeding
Temperature, pulse, and blood pressure (BP)	37.2°-37.8° C; pulse variable; normal before, rapid after rupture; decreased BP after rupture	37.2°-37.8° C; pulse rapid: 90-100 beats/min;	37.2°-40° C; pulse elevated in proportion to fever	Not over 37.2° C; pulse normal unless blood loss marked, then rapid	To 37.2° C
Pelvic examination	Unilateral tenderness, especially on movement of cervix; crepitant mass on one side or in cul-de-sac	No masses; rectal tenderness high on right side	Bilateral tenderness on movement of cervix; masses only when pyosalpinx or hydrosalpinx present	Tenderness over affected ovary; no masses	Cervix slightly patulous; uterus slightly enlarged, irregularly softened: tender with infection
Laboratory findings	WBC to 15,000/μl; RBC strikingly low if blood loss large; ESR slightly elevated; pregnancy test positive in 50% of cases; culdocentesis positive for nonclotting blood	WBC: 10,000-18,000/μl (rarely normal); RBC normal; ESR slightly elevated	WBC: 15,000-30,000/μl; RBC normal; ESR greatly elevated	WBC normal to 10,000/μl: RBC normal; ESR normal	WBC: 15,000/μl

Modified from Gilbert E, Harmon J: *Manual of high-risk pregnancy and delivery*, St Louis, 1993b, Mosby.
WBC, White blood cell count; *RBC*, red blood cell count; *ESR*, erythrocyte sedimentation rate.

firm an extrauterine pregnancy. General preoperative and postoperative care is appropriate for the woman requiring surgical intervention for an ectopic pregnancy. Blood replacement may be necessary. The nurse needs to verify the woman's Rh and antibody status and administer Rh_o(D) immune globulin if appropriate.

Discharge teaching is similar to that for the woman who has had a spontaneous abortion (see the Patient Teaching box on p. 219). Additional teaching may be needed for wound care.

Hydatidiform mole. Hydatidiform mole is a gestational **trophoblastic neoplasm** (ACOG, 1993). There are two distinct types: complete—or classic—mole and partial mole.

Hydatidiform mole occurs in 1 of 1000 to 2000 pregnancies in the United States and Europe, but a much higher incidence is seen in Asia and tropical areas (Cunningham et al, 1993; Hammond and Bochus, 1994).

The etiology is unknown, although there may be an ovular defect or nutritional deficiency (e.g., carotene, protein) (Hammond and Bachus, 1994). Women at higher risk for hydatidiform mole are those who have undergone ovulation stimulation with clomiphene (Clomid) and who are in their early teens or over age 40. The risk of developing a second mole is 1% to 2%.

Types. The complete, or classic, mole results from fertilization of an egg whose nucleus has been lost or inactivated (Fig. 9-9). The mole resembles a bunch of white grapes. The hydropic (fluid-filled) vesicles grow rapidly, causing the uterus to be larger than expected for the duration of the pregnancy. Usually the complete mole contains no fetus, placenta, amniotic membranes, or fluid. Maternal blood has no placenta to receive it; therefore hemorrhage into the uterine cavity and vaginal bleeding occur. In about 20% of complete hydatidiform moles, a progression toward choriocarcinoma (a rapid-growing malignant neoplasm) occurs.

Partial mole occurs as two sperm fertilize an apparently normal ovum (Berkowitz, Goldstein, and Bernstein, 1991) (Fig. 9-10). Partial moles often have embryonic/fetal parts

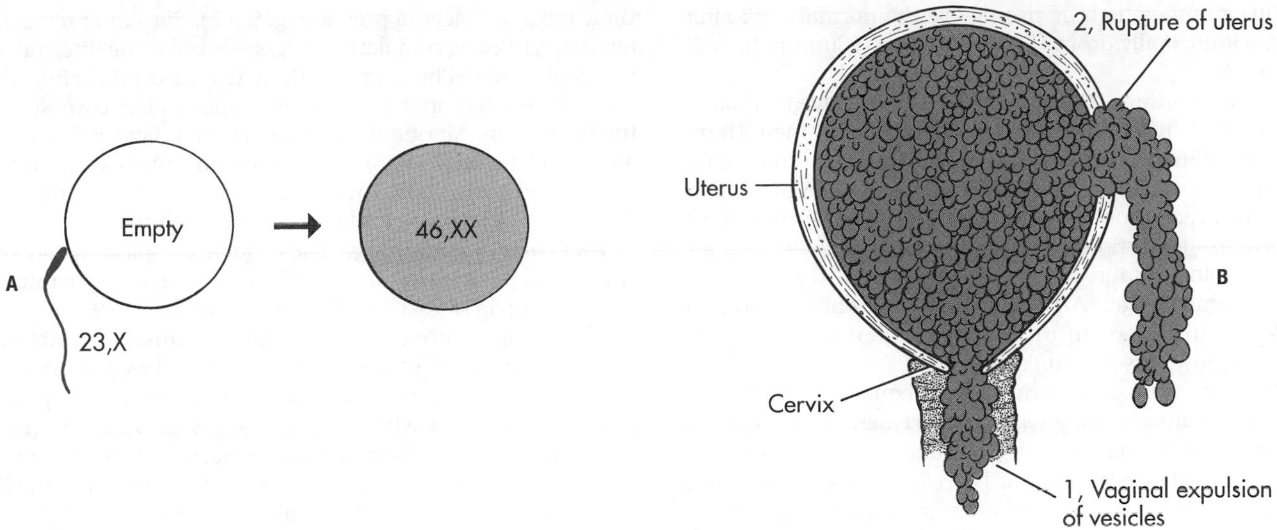

Fig. 9-9 **A,** Chromosomal origin of a complete mole. A single sperm fertilizes an "empty" ovum. Reduplication of the sperm's 23,X set gives a completely homozygous diploid 46,XX. A similar process follows fertilization of an empty ovum by two sperm with two independently drawn sets of 23,X or 23,Y; therefore karyotypes of both 46 XX and 46 XY can result. **B,** Uterine rupture with hydatidiform mole. *1,* Evacuation of mole through cervix. *2,* Rupture of uterus and spillage of mole into peritoneal cavity (rare).

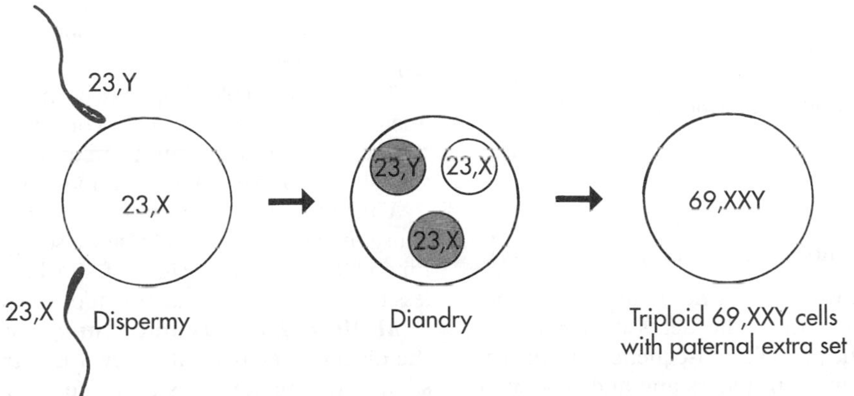

Fig. 9-10 Chromosomal origin of the triploid or partial mole. A normal ovum with a 23,X haploid set is fertilized by two sperm to give a total of 69 chromosomes. A sex configuration of XXY, XXX, or XYY, is possible.

and an amniotic sac. Congenital anomalies are usually present. The potential for malignant transformation is much less (less than 5%) than that associated with the complete hydatidiform mole (Hammond and Bachus, 1994).

Signs and symptoms. In the early stages the signs and symptoms of a complete hydatidiform mole cannot be distinguished from normal pregnancy. Later, vaginal bleeding occurs in almost 95% of patients. The vaginal discharge may be dark brown (resembling prune juice) or bright red, either scant or profuse. It may continue for only a few days or intermittently for weeks. Early in pregnancy about one half of the affected women have a uterus significantly larger than expected from the menstrual dates.

Anemia from blood loss, excessive nausea and vomiting (hyperemesis gravidarum), and abdominal cramps caused by uterine distention are relatively common findings. Preeclampsia occurs in about 15% of patients, usually between 9 and 12 gestational weeks. A partial mole causes few of these symptoms and may be mistaken for an incomplete or missed abortion.

Passage of vesicles may occur around 16 weeks' gestation. There will be no fetal movement, FHR, or palpable fetal parts. Some women exhibit signs and symptoms of hyperthyroidism. About 20% of women with hydatidiform mole may develop a trophoblastic pulmonary embolus (Berkowitz, Goldstein, and Bernstein, 1991).

Medical management. Most moles abort spontaneously. When hydropic vesicles are passed vaginally and the woman saves the specimen, the diagnosis can be established with certainty. The sonographic pattern of a molar pregnancy is characterized by a diffuse snowstorm pattern (Kulb, 1990). The hCG titer remains high or rises above the normal peak after the time it normally drops (70 to 100 days) (Cunningham et al, 1993).

Suction curettage is a safe, rapid, and effective method of evacuation of hydatidiform mole in almost all women (Hammond and Bachus, 1994). Women who want no more children may choose a primary hysterectomy as the method of choice for evacuation of hydatidiform mole and concurrent sterilization. Induction of labor with oxytocic agents or prostaglandins is not recommended because of the increased risk of hemorrhage. After evacuation, administration of Rh_o(D) immune globulin to women who are Rh negative is needed to prevent isoimmunization.

Follow-up management includes frequent physical and pelvic examinations along with measurement of serum hCG levels for at least 1 year. A rising titer and an enlarging uterus may indicate choriocarcinoma. Therefore to avoid confusion with signs of pregnancy, pregnancy should be avoided for 1 year. Oral contraceptives are usually prescribed. Cure of the malignant condition is defined as a complete absence of all clinical and hormonal evidence of disease for 5 years.

Nursing care management. Nursing diagnoses for the woman with a molar pregnancy focus on possible consequences of the disease, rationale for treatment, contraceptive counseling, and support for the grieving process. Nursing diagnoses may include the following:

- Anticipatory grieving related to
  Actual/perceived threat to self
- Fluid volume deficit related to
  Excessive bleeding secondary to evacuation of uterine contents
- Anxiety related to
  Uncertainty of disease
- Situational low self-esteem related to
  Inability to conceive a normal pregnancy

The nurse provides the woman and her family with information about the disease process, the necessity for a long course of follow-up, and the possible consequences of the disease. The nurse helps the woman understand and cope with pregnancy loss. The woman and her family are encouraged to verbalize their feelings, and information is provided about support groups or counseling resources if needed. Explanations about the importance of the need to postpone a subsequent pregnancy and contraceptive counseling are provided to emphasize the importance of consistent and reliable use of the method chosen.

Late Pregnancy Bleeding

Late pregnancy bleeding disorders include placenta previa, premature separation of placenta (abruptio placentae), and cord insertion and placental variations. Expedient assessment for and diagnosis of the cause of bleeding are essential to reduce maternal and perinatal morbidity and mortality (Fig. 9-11).

Placenta previa. In **placenta previa** the placenta is implanted in the lower uterine segment near or over the internal cervical os. The degree to which the internal cervical os is covered by the placenta has traditionally been used to classify three types of placenta previa (Fig. 9-12). Placenta previa often is described as complete, total, or central if the internal os is entirely covered by the placenta when the cervix is fully dilated. Partial placenta previa implies incomplete coverage of the internal os. Marginal placenta previa indicates that only an edge of the placenta extends to the internal os. The term *low-lying placenta* is used when the placenta is implanted in the lower uterine segment but does not reach the os.

Incidence and etiology. The incidence of placenta previa is 1 in 200 pregnancies (Scott, 1994). The recurrence rate of placenta previa is 4% to 8% (Konje and Walley, 1995).

The specific cause of placenta previa is unknown. Abnormal vascularization of the endometrium, delayed ovulation, and endometrial scarring are possible factors affecting implantation. Women who have had a low cervical cesarean birth are six times as likely to have a placenta previa. Multiple gestation may increase the woman's risk of placenta previa since there is a larger placental area (mass). Multiparity, closely spaced pregnancies, and previous placenta previa also increase the risk (Scott, 1994).

Clinical manifestations. Painless uterine bleeding, especially during the third trimester, characterizes placenta previa (Table 9-6). The first significant bleeding episode usually occurs between 29 and 30 weeks' gestation. Approximately 10% of women may go to term before bleeding occurs (Lavery, 1990). At that time, tearing and bleeding occur at the lower implantation site as the lower uterine segment stretches and thins. Rarely is the first episode life-threatening or a cause of hypovolemic shock.

The bright-red bleeding may be intermittent, may occur in gushes, or more rarely, may be continuous. It may start while the woman is resting or in the midst of any activity, including sexual intercourse, pelvic examinations, or labor.

Vital signs may be normal even with heavy blood loss because the pregnant woman can lose up to 35% of blood volume without showing signs of shock. FHR is reassuring unless there is a major detachment of the placenta.

Medical diagnosis and management. The standard for the diagnosis of placenta previa is a transabdominal ultrasound examination. It is accurate 93% to 97% of the time. Transvaginal ultrasound examination may also be used in these situations. If ultrasound scanning reveals a normally implanted placenta, a speculum examination is performed to rule out local causes of bleeding (e.g., cervicitis, polyps, carcinoma of cervix).

Management of placenta previa depends on the gestational age of the fetus and the amount of bleeding present. It includes expectant management and cesarean birth. Expectant management (e.g., bed rest) usually is implemented when the fetus is not mature. Women may be placed in the hospital on complete bed rest or managed at home (Grohar, 1994; Simpson, 1992). If a woman is bleeding, she is usually placed in the labor and birth unit, where she and the fetus can be closely monitored.

If the woman's condition stabilizes and she is at less than 36 weeks' gestation, she may remain in the hospital on bed rest with bathroom privileges and perhaps limited activity (e.g., rides in a wheelchair). Ultrasound examinations are done every 2 or 3 weeks. Fetal surveillance may include the use of an NST or BPP once or twice a week. Outpatient man-

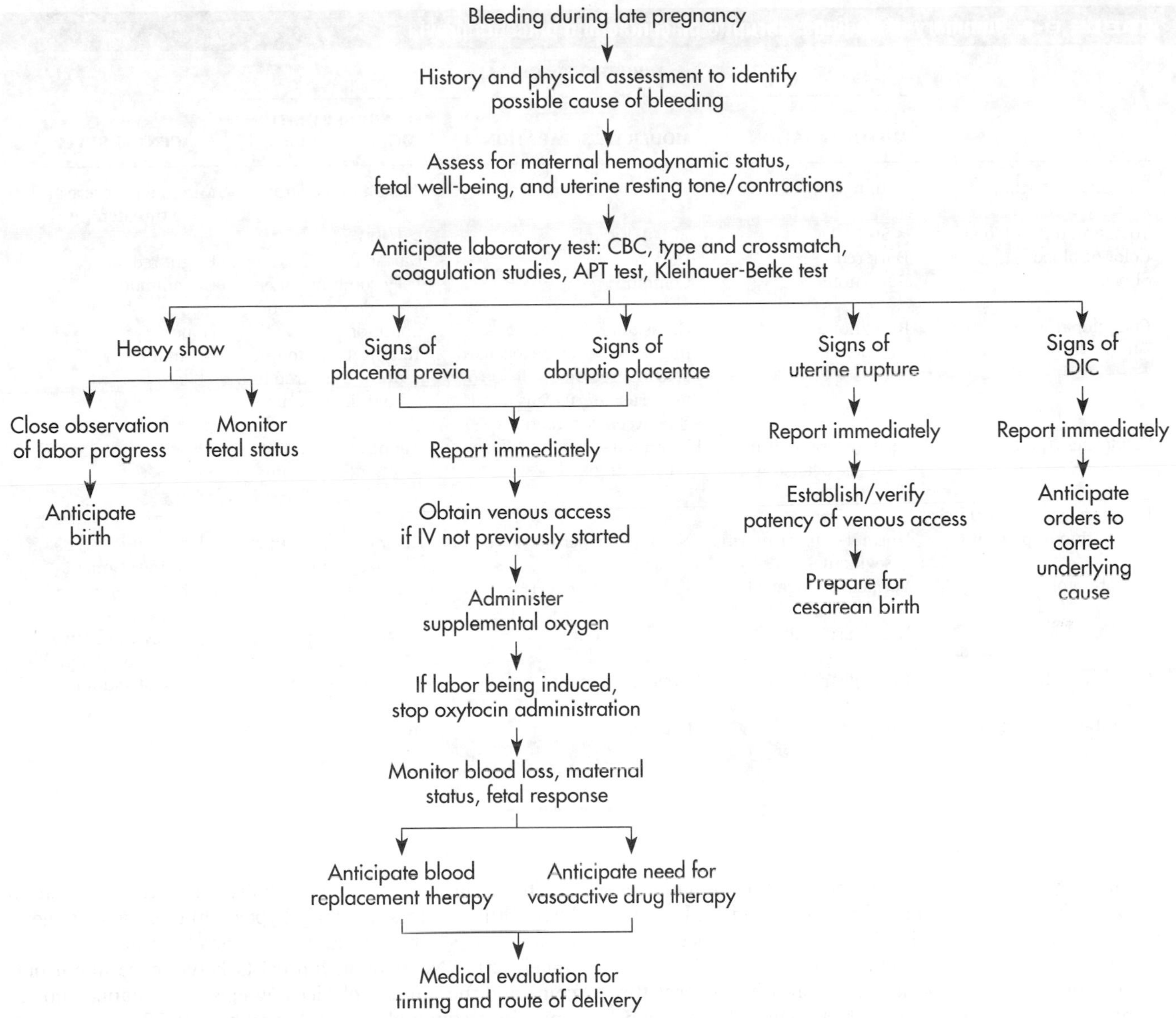

Bleeding during late pregnancy

↓

History and physical assessment to identify possible cause of bleeding

↓

Assess for maternal hemodynamic status, fetal well-being, and uterine resting tone/contractions

↓

Anticipate laboratory test: CBC, type and crossmatch, coagulation studies, APT test, Kleihauer-Betke test

↓

- Heavy show
  - Close observation of labor progress → Anticipate birth
  - Monitor fetal status
- Signs of placenta previa / Signs of abruptio placentae
  - Report immediately → Obtain venous access if IV not previously started → Administer supplemental oxygen → If labor being induced, stop oxytocin administration → Monitor blood loss, maternal status, fetal response
    - Anticipate blood replacement therapy
    - Anticipate need for vasoactive drug therapy
    - → Medical evaluation for timing and route of delivery
- Signs of uterine rupture
  - Report immediately → Establish/verify patency of venous access → Prepare for cesarean birth
- Signs of DIC
  - Report immediately → Anticipate orders to correct underlying cause

Fig. 9-11 Bleeding during late pregnancy.

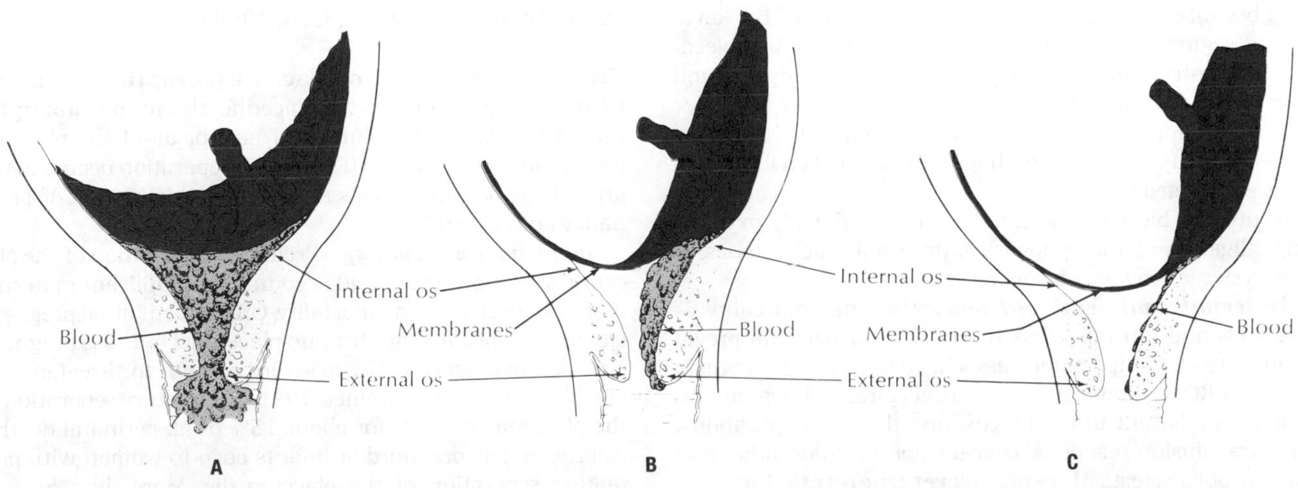

Fig. 9-12 Types of placentae previa after onset of labor. **A,** Complete or total. **B,** Incomplete or partial. **C,** Marginal or low lying.

TABLE 9-6 Summary of findings: abruptio placentae and placenta previa

	ABRUPTIO PLACENTAE			
	MILD SEPARATION	MODERATE SEPARATION	SEVERE SEPARATION (MORE THAN 66%)	PLACENTA PREVIA
Bleeding: external, vaginal	Minimal	Absent or moderate	Absent to moderate	Minimal to severe and life threatening
Total amount of blood loss	<500 ml	500-1000 ml	>1000 ml	
Color of blood	Dark red	Dark red	Dark red	Bright red
Shock	Rare; none	Common	Very common: often sudden, profound	Uncommon
Coagulopathy	Rare; none	Occasional	Common	None
Uterine tonicity	Normal	Increased—may be localized to one region or diffuse over uterus: uterus fails to relax between contractions	Tetanic, persistent uterine contraction: boardlike uterus	Normal
Tenderness (pain)	Usually absent; if present, is localized	Increased—usually diffuse over uterus	Agonizing, unremitting uterine pain	Absent
Ultrasonographic findings:				
Location of placenta	Normal—upper uterine segment	Normal—upper uterine segment	Normal—upper uterine segment	Abnormal—lower uterine segment
Station of presenting part	Variable to engaged	Variable to engaged	Variable to engaged	High—not engaged
Fetal position	Usual distribution	Usual distribution	Usual distribution	Typically transverse, breech, or oblique
Concurrent hypertensive state	Usual distribution	Typically present	Typically present	Usual distribution
Fetal status at first examination	Alive	In jeopardy	In jeopardy; dead	Alive

agement (e.g., home care) is a possibility if the woman lives close to the hospital, has available transportation, and understands the risks and the need to follow medical advice about activities (Grohar, 1994; Simpson, 1992).

If the woman is at 36 weeks' gestation or more, or if the bleeding continues or labor begins, birth will be by cesarean. Blood loss may not cease with the infant's birth. The large vascular channels in the lower uterine segment may continue to bleed because of the diminished muscle content of the lower uterine segment. The natural mechanism to control bleeding—the interlacing muscle bundles contracting around open vessels (the "living ligature"), characteristic of the upper part of the uterus—is absent in the lower part of the uterus. Therefore postpartum hemorrhage may occur even if the fundus is contracted firmly.

If uterine bleeding cannot be controlled with oxytocic drugs, ligation of the hypogastric (internal iliac) arteries or even hysterectomy may be necessary.

Maternal and fetal outcome. Maternal morbidity is about 5% and mortality less than 1% with placenta previa (Scott, 1994). Complications associated with placenta previa include PROM, preterm birth, surgery-related trauma to structures adjacent to the uterus, anesthesia complications, blood transfusion reactions, overinfusion of fluids, other placental problems (e.g., **placenta accreta, percreta, increta**), postpartum hemorrhage, anemia, and infection (see the Nursing Care Plan on p. 227).

The greatest risk of fetal mortality is the result of preterm birth. Other fetal risks include hypoxia in utero and congenital anomalies, which yield a fetal mortality rate of approximately 20%. No relationship exists between perinatal outcome and the number of bleeding episodes. Infants who are small for gestational age (SGA) and have IUGR have been associated with placenta previa and may be related to poor placental exchange or hypovolemia secondary to maternal blood loss and maternal anemia (Scott, 1994).

Premature separation of placenta (abruptio placentae). Premature separation of the placenta, also termed **abruptio placentae,** is the detachment of part or all of the placenta from its implantation site (Fig. 9-13). Separation occurs in the area of the decidua basalis after the twentieth week of pregnancy and before birth.

Incidence and etiology. Premature separation of the placenta is a serious event and accounts for significant maternal and fetal morbidity and mortality. One percent of all pregnancies are complicated by abruptio placentae; of those pregnancies, approximately 10% are severe enough to threaten fetal viability (Hunter and Weiner, 1996). Premature separation of the placenta accounts for about 15% of all perinatal deaths. Approximately one third of infants born to women with premature separation of the placenta die. More than 50% of these deaths are the result of preterm birth; many others die of intrauterine hypoxia.

Nursing Care Plan

PLACENTA PREVIA

Nursing Diagnosis: Decreased cardiac output related to bleeding secondary to placenta previa

Expected Outcomes: Patient will exhibit signs of increased blood volume and restoration of cardiac output (i.e., normal pulse and blood pressure, normal heart and breath sounds, normal skin color, tone and turgor, normal capillary refill).

• NURSING INTERVENTIONS/*RATIONALES*

Palpate uterus for tenderness and tone; assess bleeding rate, amount, color, degree of bleeding, CBC values, and coagulation profile, *to determine severity of situation.* (Do not perform vaginal examination, because it may stimulate further bleeding)

Establish baseline data for cardiac output (vital signs; heart and breath sounds; skin color, tone, turgor; capillary refill; level of consciousness; urinary output; pulse oximetry) *to use as basis for evaluating effectiveness of treatment.*

Initiate intravenous therapy and/or blood transfusions and medications per physician order *to restore vascular and blood volume and prevent organ compromise to mother and fetus.*

Place woman on bed rest *to decrease oxygen demands.*

Monitor vital signs, intake and output, hemodynamic status and laboratory values *to evaluate treatment response.*

Provide emotional support to woman and her family (i.e., explain procedures and their rationale; explain what is happening and what to expect; keep support person present) *to allay fears and provide the family with some sense of control.*

After stabilization, teach woman home management including bed rest, watching for spotting/bleeding, close follow-up with her health care provider and preparation for immediate return to hospital if needed *to prevent or stem further complications.*

Nursing Diagnosis: Risk for injury to the fetus related to decreased uterine/placental perfusion secondary to bleeding

Expected Outcome: Patient will exhibit ongoing signs of fetal well-being (i.e., adequate fetal movement, normal FHR, reactive NST, normal BPP).

• NURSING INTERVENTIONS/*RATIONALES*

Monitor fetus daily for signs of tachycardia, decreased movement, loss of reactivity on NST *to identify and treat changes in fetal status early.*

Obtain BPP per physician order *to assess for signs of chronic asphyxia.*

Maintain maternal sidelying position *to prevent compression of aorta and vena cava.*

Nursing Diagnosis: Risk for infection related to anemia and bleeding secondary to placenta previa

Expected Outcome: Patient will show no signs of intrauterine infection.

• NURSING INTERVENTIONS/*RATIONALES*

Monitor vital signs for elevated temperature, pulse, and blood pressure; monitor lab results for elevated white blood cell count, differential shift; check for uterine tenderness and malodorous vaginal discharge *to detect early signs of infection resulting from exposure of placental tissue.*

Provide/teach perineal hygiene *to decrease the risk of ascending infection.*

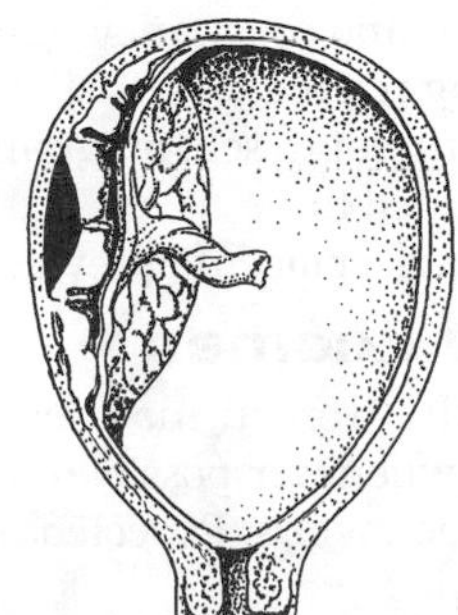
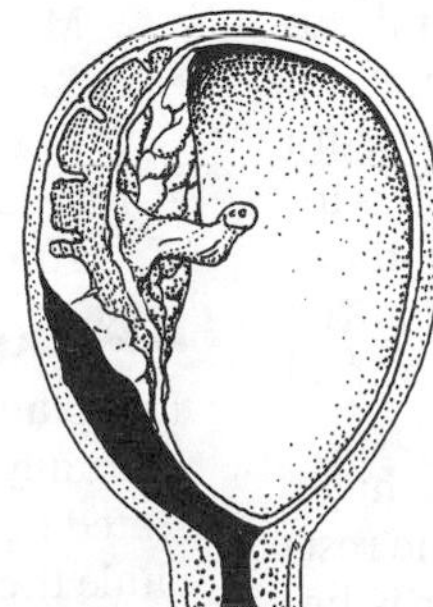
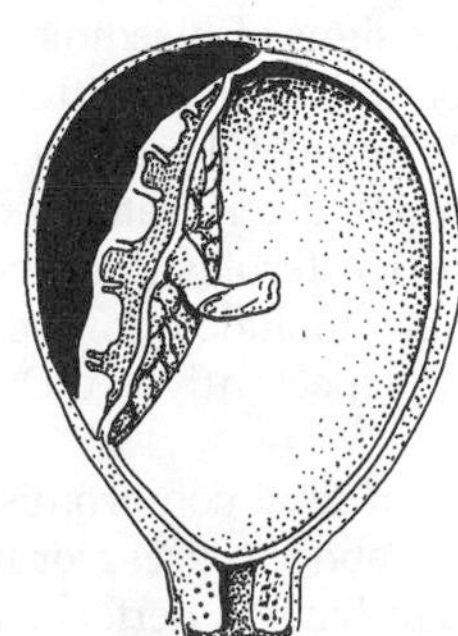

Fig. 9-13 Abruptio placentae. Premature separation of normally implanted placenta.

The risk of recurrence of abruptio placentae ranges from 10% to 30%, which yields a relative risk 30 to 40 times over that of the general population (Thorp, 1993).

Placental abruption is much more common in women with hypertension and occurs 3 times more often in women who have had more than five pregnancies. Women who smoke, use cocaine or alcohol, and ingest caffeine during their pregnancy significantly increase the incidence of abruptio placentae (Armstrong, McDonald, and Sloan, 1992; Rosenak, 1990). Women with a history of reproductive loss (abortion, preterm labor, prenatal hemorrhage, stillbirth, or neonatal death) experience premature separation of the placenta more than twice as often as do other women.

The separation may be partial or complete, or only the margin of the placenta may be involved. Bleeding from the placental site may flow out through the vagina, remain concealed (retroplacental hemorrhage) or do both (Fig. 9-13). Clinical symptoms vary with the degree of separation (Table 9-6).

Diagnosis. The diagnosis of placental abruption is based on the woman's history, physical examination, and laboratory studies. Abruptio placentae is suspected in the woman with sudden-onset, intense, usually localized uterine pain, with or without vaginal bleeding. Sonography is used to rule out placenta previa; however, it is not diagnostic for an abruption (Cunningham et al, 1993; Scott, 1994).

Significant complications accompany moderate to severe abruptio placentae. Abruption with concealed hemorrhage carries a much greater maternal hazard because the extent of hemorrhage is not recognized, and consequently blood replacement may be too little or too late (Lowe and Cunningham, 1990). Hypovolemic shock can result in renal failure and anterior pituitary necrosis (**Sheehan syndrome**). Clotting defects (e.g., DIC) may develop (McLaren, Feinstein, and Lodeiro, 1991).

A Kleihauer-Betke stain may be ordered to determine the presence of fetal-to-maternal (transplacental hemorrhage, or TPH) bleeding. Bleeding into the myometrium causes **couvelaire uterus,** with resulting myometrial tissue damage, increased tonicity, and inability of the uterus to relax between contractions. The uterus appears purplish and copper colored and is ecchymotic.

After the birth the uterus may feel firm but may not be able to contract efficiently and close off bleeding sinuses; postpartum hemorrhage should be anticipated.

Medical management. Treatment depends on maternal and fetal status. If the abruption is mild, expectant management is implemented if the fetus is younger than 36 weeks and not in distress. The woman usually is hospitalized and closely observed for signs of bleeding and labor. The fetal status is also monitored with intermittent FHR monitoring and NSTs and/or BPPs until fetal maturity is determined or until the woman's condition deteriorates and immediate birth is indicated. Use of corticosteroids to accelerate fetal lung maturity is appropriately included in the plan of care for the woman managed expectantly (ACOG, 1994; Hunter and Weiner, 1996).

In the presence of fetal compromise, severe hemorrhage, coagulopathy, poor labor progress, or increasing uterine resting tone, a cesarean birth is performed. If the mother is hemodynamically stable, a vaginal birth may be attempted when the fetus is alive and in no acute distress or if the fetus is dead. Fluid replacement must be aggressive in the presence of hemorrhage. Whole blood and Ringer's lactate are infused in quantities necessary to maintain a urine output of 30 to 60 ml/hour and a hematocrit of approximately 30% (Lowe and Cunningham, 1990).

Maternal, fetal, and neonatal outcomes. Maternal mortality approaches 1% in abruptio placentae; this condition remains a leading cause of maternal death. The mother's prognosis depends on the extent of placental detachment, overall blood loss, degree of DIC, and time between the placental "accident" and birth. Women who are Rh negative may become sensitized if the fetal Rh blood type is positive.

Perinatal mortality ranges from 25% to 35% and occurs from fetal hypoxia, preterm birth, and SGA status. Serious neurologic deficits also have been identified within the first year of life (Cunningham et al, 1993).

Nursing Care Management

Assessment

With the woman's admission to the hospital, the nurse begins with an assessment of the bleeding. Abdominal assessment reveals a soft, relaxed, nontender uterus of normal tone for placenta previa; uterine tenderness and increased tone are present with abruptio placentae. Laboratory studies include a CBC, blood type and Rh, possible type and crossmatch for packed red blood cells, and a coagulation profile.

Nursing Diagnoses

Nursing diagnoses related to the care of women with placenta previa or abruptio placentae focus on alterations in hemodynamic status, knowledge deficits, fears and anxiety of the woman, and fetal status. Potential nursing diagnoses include the following:

- Decreased cardiac output related to
  Excessive blood loss secondary to placenta previa/abruptio placentae
- Risk for fluid volume excess related to
  Fluid resuscitation
- Altered peripheral tissue perfusion related to
  Hypovolemia and shunting of blood to central circulation
- Risk for injury to fetus related to
  Decreased placental perfusion secondary to placenta previa/abruptio placentae
- Pain related to
  Bleeding between uterine wall and placenta secondary to premature separation of placenta
- Anxiety/fear related to
  Maternal condition and pregnancy outcome
- Anticipatory grieving related to:
  Actual/perceived threat to self, pregnancy, or infant
- Risk for infection related to
  Anemia, hemorrhage, placenta previa, and transfusions

Expected Outcomes

The plan of care for the woman includes patient-centered, mutually determined (whenever possible) outcomes that are stated in measureable behaviors. Expected outcomes may include the following:

1. The woman will identify and use available support systems.

2. The woman will adhere to prescribed activity limitations.
3. The woman will express relief of pain.
4. The woman will not develop complications.
5. The woman will carry her pregnancy to term or near term.
6. The woman will give birth to a healthy infant who has not undergone fetal compromise.

If the fetus dies, the woman is referred as appropriate for follow-up care (see the Nursing Care Plan on p. 227).

Plan of Care and Implementation

Nursing interventions depend on whether the woman is managed conservatively or actively. Information is given to the woman and her family about placenta previa or abruptio placentae, including causes, treatment, and expected outcomes. Vital signs and noninvasive assessments of cardiac output (Box 9-7) are obtained often to observe for signs of declining hemodynamic status. Fetal status is continuously monitored if the fetus has survived the initial insult. If placental abruption is suspected, the uterus is palpated to assess for tenderness and uterine activity. For the woman diagnosed with abruptio placentae, preparations are made for birth, remembering that an emergency cesarean birth is always a possibility.

If expectant measures are used in the management of a placenta previa, nursing care focuses on accurate assessments and appropriate referrals. The woman is instructed on the importance of bed rest and the need to report any further spotting or bleeding. Maternal vital signs are assessed as indicated based on her condition. Serial laboratory values are evaluated for the presence of falling hemoglobin/hematocrit and changes in coagulation studies. Fetal well-being is evaluated by the use of NSTs, BPPs, and ultrasonography. Any indication of fetal compromise is reported immediately to the physician.

If active management is undertaken for placenta previa, the nurse continuously assesses maternal and fetal status while preparing the woman for surgery. Maternal vital signs are assessed frequently for decreasing blood pressure, rising pulse rate, changes in level of consciousness, and oliguria. Fetal assessment is maintained by continuous electronic fetal monitoring to assess for signs of hypoxia.

Emotional support for the woman and her family is extremely important. If actively bleeding, the woman is concerned not only for her own well-being but for the well-being of her fetus. All procedures should be explained, and a support person should be present.

If the woman is discharged home after stabilization to be managed conservatively after diagnosis of placenta previa, discharge teaching focuses on the prevention of further complications. The woman will know to notify her health care provider of any further spotting or bleeding episodes and to be prepared to return to the hospital immediately (Grohar, 1994; Simpson, 1992). She must understand the importance of maintaining bed rest and the need for close follow-up monitoring.

If hospitalization or home care on bed rest is prolonged, the woman may have concerns about her work-related or family-related responsibilities or become bored with the inactivity. She should be encouraged to participate in her care and decisions about care as much as possible. Provision of diversional activities or encouragement to participate in activities she enjoys and can do while on bed rest are needed (see suggestions for activities in the Home Care box on p. 208).

Evaluation

The nurse can be reasonably assured that care was effective to the extent that the outcomes for care have been achieved. That is, the woman does the following:

1. Identifies and uses available support systems.
2. Expresses relief of pain.
3. Does not develop complications.
4. Gives birth to a healthy infant who has not experienced fetal compromise.

Cord insertion and placental variations. A **velamentous insertion of the cord** is a rare placental anomaly in which the cord vessels begin to branch at the membranes and then course onto the placenta (Fig. 9-14). *Vasa praevia* is the result of a velamentous insertion of the umbilical cord. With a vasa praevia the umbilical vein and arteries are not surrounded by Wharton's jelly and have no supportive tissue. Thus the umbilical blood vessels are at risk for laceration at any time, but this occurs most often during rupture of the membranes (Green, 1994). The sudden appearance of bright red blood at the time of rupture of membranes, spontaneous or artificial, coupled with a sudden change in the baseline FHR when no other known risk factors exist should immediately alert the nurse to the possibility of vasa praevia.

Although it occurs rarely (less than 1 in 3000 pregnancies), vasa praevia is associated with high incidence of fetal morbidity and mortality because of the potential for fetal exsanguination (Thorp, 1993). Diagnosis before birth is unusual, although examiners have reported palpating a pulsing vessel. The vasa praevia may also be noted on ultrasound examination or by direct visualization (Cunningham et al, 1993).

Battledore (marginal) insertion of the cord (Fig. 9-14, *B*) increases the risk of fetal hemorrhage, especially after marginal separation of the placenta.

BOX 9-7
Noninvasive Assessments of Cardiac Output

- Palpation of pulses (rate, quality, equality)
  - Arterial
  - Blood pressure
- Auscultation
  - Heart sounds, murmurs
  - Breath sounds
- Inspection
  - Skin color, temperature, turgor
  - Level of consciousness
  - Capillary refill
  - Urine output
  - Neck veins
  - Pulse oximetry
  - Mucous membranes
  - Presence or absence of anxiety, apprehension, restlessness, disorientation

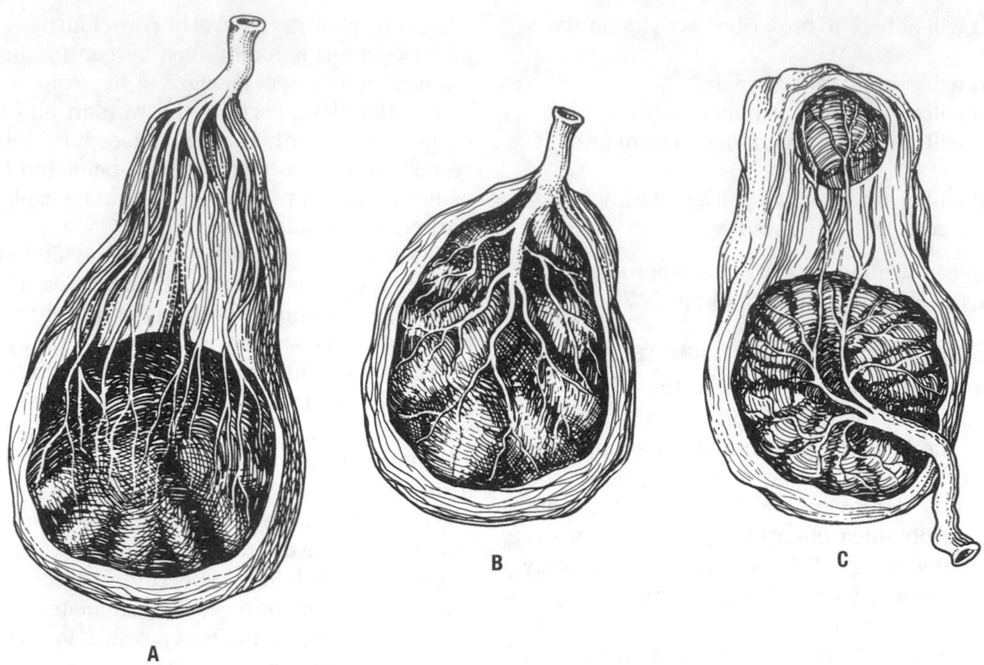

Fig. 9-14 Cord insertion and placental variations. **A,** Velamentous insertion of cord. **B,** Battledore placenta. **C,** Placenta succenturiate.

Rarely the placenta may be divided into two or more separate lobes, resulting in **succenturiate placenta** (Fig. 9-14, C). Blood vessels joining the lobes may be supported only by the fetal membranes and are therefore in danger of tearing during labor or during the birth of the baby or of the placenta. During expulsion of the placenta, one or more of the separate lobes may remain attached to the decidua basalis, preventing uterine contraction and increasing the risk of postpartum hemorrhage.

Clotting Disorders in Pregnancy

Normal clotting. Normally a delicate balance (homeostasis) is maintained between two opposing systems, the hemostatic system and the fibrinolytic system. The *hemostatic system* is involved in the life-saving process by stopping the flow of blood from injured vessels, in part through the formation of insoluble fibrin that acts as a hemostatic platelet plug. The coagulation process involves an interaction of the coagulation factors in which each factor sequentially activates the factor next in line in the so-called cascade effect sequence. The *fibrinolytic system* refers to the process by which the fibrin is split into fibrin degradation products (FDPs) and circulation is restored.

A history of abnormal bleeding, inheritance of unusual bleeding tendencies, and a report of significant aberrations of laboratory findings indicate a bleeding or clotting problem. Table 9-7 describes the tests used to determine mechanisms for the control of bleeding, that is, the function of platelets and the necessary clotting factors.

Disseminated intravascular coagulation. DIC (defibrination syndrome, defibrination coagulopathy, consumptive coagulopathy) is a pathologic form of clotting that is diffuse and consumes large amounts of clotting factors, causing widespread external and/or internal bleeding. Simply, DIC is an overactivation of the clotting cascade and the fibrinolytic system resulting in depletion of platelets and clotting factors.

The diagnosis of DIC is based on clinical findings and laboratory markers. Physical examination reveals unusual bleeding. Spontaneous bleeding from the woman's gums or nose may be noted. Petechiae may appear around the blood pressure cuff on her arm. Excessive bleeding may occur from the site of a slight trauma (e.g., venipuncture sites, IM or subcutaneous injection sites, nicks from shaving of perineum or abdomen, injury from insertion of urinary catheter). Maternal symptoms may include tachycardia and diaphoresis. Laboratory tests reveal decreased platelets, fibrinogen, proaccelerin, antihemophilic factor, and prothrombin (the factors consumed during coagulation). Other factors should be normal. Fibrinolysis is first increased but later is severely depressed. Degradation of fibrin leads to the accumulation of fibrin-split products in the blood. Fibrin-split products have anticoagulant properties and thus prolong the PT. Bleeding time is normal; coagulation time shows no clot; clot retraction time shows no clot; and PTT is increased. DIC must be distinguished from other clotting disorders before therapy is initiated.

Medical management. The primary management of DIC involves correction of the underlying cause, for example, removal of the dead fetus, treatment of existing infection or preeclampsia/eclampsia, or removal of a placental abruption. Concomitantly, treatment is directed toward support of maternal physiologic functioning. Suggested therapies may include volume replacement, blood component therapy, and optimization of oxygenation and perfusion status (Clark et al, 1991, 1994).

TABLE 9-7 Coagulation tests

TEST	COMMENTS
Activated partial thromboplastin time (PTT; measures intrinsic system): 25 to 36 seconds	Screening test of choice; very sensitive, relatively easy to perform, inexpensive; all coagulation factors except proconvertin are measured.
One-stage prothrombin time (PT; Quick's test: measures extrinsic system): 9.5 to 11.3 seconds	Test for proconvertin (factor VII), proaccelerin (V), Stuart-Prower factor (X), prothrombin (II), and fibrinogen deficiencies; it does not measure factors necessary for earlier stages of coagulation.
Thrombin time (plasma): 10 to 15 seconds	Test measures conversion of fibrinogen to fibrin and depends on concentration of fibrinogen or inhibitors such as fibrin-split-products, antithrombins, and heparin.
Platelet count: 150,000 to 300,000/mm³	*Most reliable index for DIC.*
Specific factor assays (e.g., plasma fibrinogen): 195 to 365 mg/dl	Each coagulation factor can be assessed by indirect clotting method using natural or synthetic factor-deficient substrates and compared with activity of normal plasma (100%); however, fibrinogen is only factor that can be measured directly by chemical method.
Bleeding time Template: 2 to 8 minutes Ivy: 1 to 7 minutes Duke: 1 to 3 minutes	Finger or earlobe puncture 5 mm deep and 2 mm wide (Bard-Parker blade no. 11) is made after antiseptic preparation of skin; note time of puncture: touch bleeding point gently with sterile filter paper to absorb blood every 30 seconds until bleeding stops.

Nursing Care Management. The nurse caring for the woman at risk for DIC must be aware of risk factors. Careful and thorough assessment is required, with particular attention to the signs of bleeding (e.g., petechiae, oozing from injection sites, hematuria).

Potential nursing diagnoses for the woman diagnosed with or suspected of having DIC focus on alterations in hemodynamic status, knowledge deficits, fear and anxiety of the woman, and risk for injury to the mother and fetus.

Planning care for the woman with DIC is determined primarily by the nurse and physician on the basis of the woman's biophysical assessment findings. Expected outcomes may include that the woman's hemodynamic status will be corrected, that she will receive emotional support, and that she and her fetus/newborn will have no further complications.

Nursing interventions include assessment for signs of bleeding and administration of blood and blood products. Renal failure is one consequence of DIC; therefore urine output is monitored, usually by inserting an indwelling urinary catheter. Urine output must be maintained at more than 30 ml/hour. Supportive measures include keeping the pregnant woman's right hip elevated to prevent hypotensive syndrome. Oxygen is administered by a tight-fitting rebreathing mask at 10 to 12 L/minute or per hospital protocol or physician order.

Anxiety, altered self-concept, and grief can result from perceived or actual fetal or maternal loss. The emotional needs of the woman and her family are recognized and supported.

Maternal and fetal prognosis depend on the degree and extent of the underlying disorder and the woman's response to prompt and proper treatment. Maternal risk is increased if the fetus dies in utero.

Other clotting disorders. *Autoimmune thrombocytopenic purpura (ATP)* is an autoimmune disorder in which antiplatelet antibodies decrease the life span of the platelets. Thrombocytopenia, capillary fragility, and increased bleeding time are diagnostic.

ATP may result in severe hemorrhage after cesarean birth or from cervical or vaginal lacerations. The incidence of postpartum uterine bleeding or vaginal hematomas is also increased in ATP.

Platelet transfusions are given to maintain the platelet count at 100,000/mm³. Corticosteroids are given if the diagnosis is made before or during pregnancy. Splenectomy, if needed, is deferred until after the puerperium. Neonatal thrombocytopenia, a result of the maternal disease process, occurs in about 50% of the cases and is associated with high mortality.

von Willebrand disease, a type of hemophilia, is probably the most common of all hereditary bleeding disorders (Cunningham et al, 1993). It results from a factor VIII deficiency and platelet dysfunction. It is transmitted as an incomplete autosomal dominant trait to both genders. Although von Willebrand disease is rare, it is one of the most common congenital clotting defects in American women of childbearing age. Since factor VIII increases during pregnancy, this increase may be sufficient to offset danger from hemorrhage during childbirth. However, the woman should be observed for at least 1 week postpartum. Treatment of von Willebrand disease consists of replacement of factor VIII through administration of cryoprecipitate or fresh frozen plasma.

MATERNAL INFECTIONS

Infections in pregnancy are responsible for significant morbidity and mortality. The direct financial costs of disease can be substantial. Indirect costs can be as startling and are much more difficult to measure. Some consequences of maternal infection last a lifetime, such as infertility and sterility. Psychosocial sequelae may include altered interpersonal relationships and lowered self-esteem. Other conditions, such as a congenitally acquired infection, often affect the length and quality of a child's life.

Pregnancy generally is regarded as an immunosuppressed condition. Altered immune responses in pregnancy may decrease maternal ability to fight infection. In addition, genital tract changes also may affect susceptibility. These intravaginal changes, accompanied by decreasing vaginal pH, may contribute to increased susceptibility (Brunham, Holmes, and Embree, 1990).

Education and counseling are important aspects of care for the prevention of perinatal infections. The two primary areas of risk for sexual disease transmission are sexual behaviors and lack of preventive health care behaviors. Sexual behavior risk factors include many sexual partners, high rates of acquiring new partners and changing partners, frequent contact with casual sexual partners, sexual orientation, and specific sexual practices (e.g., anal intercourse). Health care behaviors that may reduce the risk of disease transmission are the use of condoms, early examination for diagnosis and treatment, compliance with therapy, and partner referral (Adimora et al, 1994).

Additional factors may also increase the risk of sexual disease transmission. These include age younger than 20; female gender; coinfection with other sexually transmitted diseases; nonbarrier contraceptive preferences; and tobacco, alcohol, and/or illicit drug use. Alcohol and crack cocaine use are often associated with an increase in sexual disease transmission related to an increase in high-risk sexual behaviors (Adimora et al, 1994). This relationship is not well supported (Graves et al, 1995). The role of other transmission risk factors (e.g., single marital status, minority race, urban residence, low socioeconomic status) is confounding and needs further investigation (Adimora et al, 1994). Clearly the prevention of disease and reduction of maternal and neonatal sequelae continue to be challenges.

BOX 9-8
Sexually Transmitted Diseases (STDs)

BACTERIAL
Chlamydia
Gonorrhea
Syphilis
Chancroid
Lymphogranuloma venereum
Gardnerella
Shigellosis
Salmonellosis
Genital mycoplasmas
Group B streptococci

VIRAL
Human immunodeficiency virus (HIV)
Herpes simplex virus, types 1 and 2 (HSV-1, HSV-2)
Cytomegalovirus (CMV)
Hepatitis A and B viruses (HAV, HBV)
Human papillomavirus (HPV)

PROTOZOAL
Trichomoniasis
Giardiasis
Amebiasis

PARASITIC
Pediculosis
Scabies

FUNGAL
Candidiasis

Sexually Transmitted Disease

The term **sexually transmitted disease (STD)** reflects the definition as any microbe that is passed from one person to another through close, intimate contact (Spence, 1989) (Box 9-8).

Chlamydial infections. Chlamydial infections are epidemic in the United States. *Chlamydia trachomatis,* the most common sexually transmitted bacterial pathogen, is responsible for substantial morbidity, personal suffering, and heavy economic burden.

C. trachomatis is an obligatory parasitic bacterium. That is, the organisms can exist only within living cells. Therefore transmission occurs by direct sexual contact or exposure at birth. There are 15 known immunotypes of *C. trachomatis.*

Between 3 and 5 million adults are infected each year, and the number of cases of newborn conjunctivitis and pneumonia continues to grow (Webster et al, 1993). This infection is implicated in cervical dysplasia, as revealed by a Papanicolaou (Pap) smear; in ectopic pregnancy; and in sterility in the woman. In men it causes genital inflammation and damage to the prostate and sperm.

Morbidity resulting from chlamydial infections may even be higher. However, *C. trachomatis* is not a reportable STD in all states, and no comprehensive surveillance data exist (Webster et al, 1993). Difficulty in diagnosis, lack of symptomatology (especially in females), limited screening resources, and inadequate follow-up care also affect disease reporting.

Definitive laboratory diagnosis is possible with tissue culture. However, it is expensive, requires skill to perform, and requires 4 to 7 days for results. Two antigen detection methods exist: (1) a direct fluorescent antibody (DFA) test (e.g., MicroTrak) that requires a fluorescent microscope and takes 30 minutes and (2) an enzyme-linked immunosorbent assay (ELISA) test (e.g., Chlamydiazyme) that gives a color signal in 4 hours. Another viable alternative for screening populations at risk is a deoxyribonucleic acid (DNA) probe assay. A chemically luminescent DNA probe that is genetically complementary to chlamydial ribsomal ribonucleic acid (rRNA) is incorporated into the chlamydial rRNA. Studies suggest the DNA probe assay (e.g., Gen-Probe PACE 2) is a sensitive, reliable, convenient alternative to cultures and antigen detection methods (Hosein et al, 1992).

Populations at risk continue to be identified. The sexually active female under age 20 is 2 to 3 times more likely to become infected than women between ages 20 and 29. Women over 30 have the lowest rate. Women and men with multiple sexual partners are at highest risk (Evans et al, 1993; Webster et al, 1993). People who *do not* use barrier methods of birth control (condom, spermicide, diaphragm) have a higher incidence (Barnhart and Sondheimer, 1993). Lower socioeconomic status may be a risk factor, especially with regard to treatment-seeking behaviors. Sexually active men under 20 are at high risk for nongonococcal urethritis. The infection rate among homosexual men is one-third less than that of heterosexual men.

The Centers for Disease Control and Prevention (CDC) guidelines recommend screening for sexually active adolescents, women between ages 20 and 24, women who do not consistently use barrier contraceptives, and women who have new or multiple partners. All those who are presumably infected should be treated. Combination antibiotic therapy is recommended for heterosexual men and women with gonorrhea because 20% to 50% of infected individuals also harbor *C. trachomatis*. Homosexual men with gonorrhea have a low incidence of concurrent chlamydial infection. Of persons infected with *C. trachomatis*, 15% of males and 26% of females also have gonorrhea (Adimora et al, 1994).

Chlamydial infections often are asymptomatic in women, although eventual sequelae include salpingitis, ectopic pregnancy, pelvic inflammatory disease (PID), infertility, and sterility. Women may have a history of mucopurulent discharge and bleeding resulting from inflammation and erosion of cervical columnar epithelium, or they may experience breakthrough bleeding if they are taking oral contraceptives (Krettek et al, 1993). *Dysuria* (painful urination) and other urinary tract discomforts, as well as *dyspareunia* (painful intercourse), may occur.

The role of chlamydial infections in pregnancy and the perinatal period is under active study. Although infection is associated with tubal damage and ectopic pregnancy, the role of *C. trachomatis* in spontaneous abortion needs further investigation. Preterm birth, low birth weight, and postpartum endometritis also have been linked to this disease, but research data are inconclusive (Brunham, Holmes, and Embree, 1990).

Fetal or neonatal effects are common. Stillbirth and neonatal death are 10 times more common than in noninfected women. The newborn may acquire the infection by direct contact with an infected birth canal but may have no symptoms. Inclusion conjunctivitis (newborn chlamydial eye infection) initially occurs in one third of exposed newborns. Conjunctivitis appears after 3 to 4 days. Chronic follicular conjunctivitis, with conjunctival scarring and corneal neovascularization, contributes to vision sequelae. Some newborns contract chlamydial pneumonia and may exhibit symptoms of serious tachypnea, dyspnea, or apnea that require hospitalization.

Medical management. Preferred antimicrobial treatment of urethral, cervical, and rectal chlamydial infections is with doxycycline or azithromycin. All sexual partners should be tested and treated. If the woman is pregnant, erythromycin is used (CDC, 1993a). Women treated with doxycycline or azithromycin do not need to be retested unless symptoms persist; patients treated with erythromycin should be retested 3 weeks after completion of treatment. Neonatal prophylaxis is achieved with erythromycin (0.5%) ophthalmic ointment applied within 2 hours after birth; existing neonatal infections are treated with oral erythromycin syrup.

Gonorrhea. One million new cases of gonorrhea are reported each year (CDC, 1993b). Gonorrhea is caused by *Neisseria gonorrhoeae*, a diplococcus. Although gonorrhea is an STD, it also is spread by direct contact with infected lesions and indirectly by transfer from inanimate objects, or *fomites*. Self-inoculation with contaminated hands is common. Secretions on fomites, such as washcloths, towels, bed linens, and clothing, often are implicated. Risk factors include age younger than 20, early onset of sexual activity, multiple sexual partners, low socioeconomic status, urban residence, single marital status, African-American race, multiparity, and a past history of gonorrhea (Adimora et al, 1994; Evans et al, 1993).

Gonorrhea often produces only mild symptoms in women, or the diplococci may persist unsuspected in the lower genital tract. The incubation period is 2 to 5 days. Symptoms of lower urogenital tract infection include dysuria and urinary frequency, heavy green-yellow purulent discharge at the cervical os, cervical tenderness, vulvovaginitis, bartholinitis, dyspareunia, and postcoital bleeding. Swollen and painful Bartholin glands and tenderness in the lymph nodes of the groin may accompany infection. Lower abdominal pain, cervical tenderness, fever, nausea, and vomiting are accompanying symptoms. Adnexal abscess and pelvic tenderness indicate PID. PID is implicated in ectopic pregnancy or sterility. Chronic pelvic pain and low backache may be seen. Anorectal infection is diagnosed by local inflammation, burning, and pruritus. Oropharyngeal infection may be asymptomatic or result in inflammation and sore throat. Systemic infection results in gonococcemia, skin rashes, arthritis, pericarditis, and meningitis.

Gonococcal infection may be related to preterm birth, premature or prolonged rupture of membranes, and chorioamnionitis (Brunham, Holmes, and Embree, 1990). Postnatal maternal complications of untreated gonorrhea include gonococcal endometritis, acute salpingitis, dermatitis, and arthritis.

Neonatal effects include **ophthalmia neonatorum** and pneumonia. Ophthalmitis with partial or total blindness can occur. Exposed newborns also are at risk for infection elsewhere: nose, pharynx, ears, vagina, anus, and scalp electrode site. Gonorrhea in other sites may predispose the infant to bacterial sepsis. Neonatal sepsis is characterized by temperature instability, hypotonia, poor feeding, and jaundice.

Medical management. Ceftriaxone or cefixime in a single dose is recommended for treatment. Spectinomycin is the preferred alternative therapy. The CDC (1993b) suggests concomitant treatment for chlamydial infection, because coinfection is common. All recent (within 30 days) sexual partners should be treated, and condom use encouraged for oral and anogenital intercourse until repeat culture findings are negative.

Syphilis. Syphilis is caused by the spirochete *Treponema pallidum*. The incubation period is about 3 weeks, with a range of 1 to 13 weeks (Fig. 9-15). The incidence of syphilis in the United States is increasing after a period of decline and may have serious sequelae during pregnancy.

Several methods of clinical assessment of syphilis are available. Any test for antibodies may not be reactive in the presence of active infection because it takes time for the body's immune system to develop antibodies to any antigen.

Nonspecific serologic tests used for screening purposes are of two types: complement fixation (Kolmer, Wasserman) and flocculation (Kahn, rapid plasma reagin [RPR], Venereal Disease Research Laboratories [VDRL]). VDRL test results are not positive until 10 to 90 days after infection. Therefore infection may exist in the presence of a negative result from the VDRL

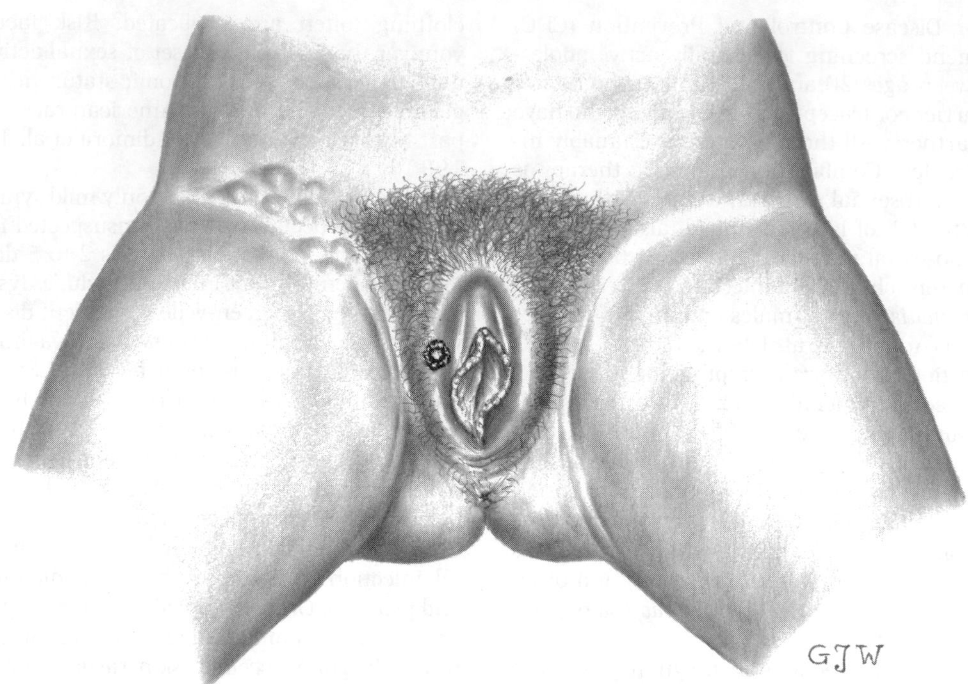

Fig. 9-15 Syphilis. Primary stage: chancre with inguinal adenopathy.

test. If the antibodies in the newborn have been acquired from the mother, titers should drop to zero by 3 months. False-positive results may occur if the newborn has an acute infection of any kind or a collagen disease. Even in the presence of a syphilitic infection, a false-negative result may occur, for example, if the mother became infected late in pregnancy. False-positive rates may be greater than 10% among IV drug abusers (Adimora et al, 1994).

Specific tests for treponemal antigen are more expensive and are used for differential diagnosis. These tests include *T. pallidum* immobilization (TPI), fluorescent treponemal antibody absorption (FTA-ABS), FTA-ABS immunoglobulin M (FTA-ABS IgM), and microhemagglutination assay for antibody to *T. pallidum* (MHA-TP). The FTA-ABS IgM is most specific for neonatal syphilis; a positive result is especially valuable in diagnosis of the condition in the symptom-free newborn. Results of the FTA-ABS IgM test may be negative, however, in the presence of active disease if infection occurred late in pregnancy and the fetus or newborn had insufficient time for an IgM response. In questionable cases the test is repeated.

Pregnancy does not alter the progression of syphilis. However, early pregnancy symptoms such as malaise and anorexia may mimic those of secondary syphilis and delay diagnosis. Syphilis probably continues to be a major cause of late abortion throughout the world, despite widespread success of diagnosis and treatment of this disease. Primary and secondary stages of untreated syphilis lead to stillbirth. Latent and tertiary stages of untreated syphilis lead to **secondary syphilis (congenital syphilis)** in the newborn.

Medical management. Benzathine penicillin G, 2.4 million U IM, is preferred for the treatment of primary and secondary syphilis. Latent syphilis infections of known or unknown duration should be treated with 7.2 million U total in three doses of 2.4 million U each at 1-week intervals. For people who are allergic to penicillin, alternate choices include tetracycline or doxycycline, erythromycin, and ceftriaxone. Tetracycline is contraindicated in pregnancy because of its effects on liver function in the mother and tooth discoloration and decreased bone growth in the fetus.

Human immunodeficiency virus/acquired immunodeficiency syndrome. Transmission of **human immunodeficiency virus (HIV)**, a retrovirus, occurs primarily through the exchange of body fluids (e.g., blood, semen, perinatal events). Although HIV is traditionally associated with homosexual populations, viral spread is currently most acute in heterosexual populations, with the largest increase among heterosexual women. Severe depression of the cellular immune system associated with HIV infection characterizes acquired immunodeficiency syndrome (AIDS). Although the populations at high risk have been well documented, *all* women should be assessed for the possibility of HIV exposure. HIV infection in women usually is reported at a later stage in the disease, with treatment initiated when the illness is more severe. The delay may partly result from the symptoms occurring differently in women than in men. Chronic vaginitis and candidiasis are common presenting problems in women. Cervical dysplasia is another complication associated with HIV infection (Angelini and Knapp, 1992).

Once HIV enters the body, seroconversion to HIV positivity usually occurs within the first 6 to 12 weeks of exposure. Although HIV seroconversion may be totally asymptomatic, it usually is accompanied by a viremic, influenza-type response.

Symptoms include fever, headache, night sweats, malaise, generalized lymphadenopathy, myalgias, nausea, diarrhea, weight loss, sore throat, and rash.

Laboratory studies may reveal leukopenia, thrombocytopenia, anemia, and an elevated erythrocyte sedimentation rate (ESR). In addition, HIV has a strong affinity for surface-marker proteins on T-lymphocytes. This affinity of HIV for T-lymphocytes leads to significant T-cell destruction. T-cell (CD4) titers less than 400 cells/mm^3 are associated with a more rapid progression to AIDS.

Pregnancy is not encouraged with positive HIV status; preconceptional counseling is recommended. Exposure to the virus has a significant impact on the woman's pregnancy, newborn feeding method, and the newborn's health status. It is hypothesized that HIV from infected women is transmitted to the fetus and newborn in the following three ways:

1. To the fetus as early as the first trimester through maternal circulation
2. To the infant during labor and birth by inoculation or ingestion of maternal blood and other infected fluids
3. To the infant through breast milk

The incidences of in utero, intrapartum, and postpartum transmission are uncertain. Rates of maternal transmission of HIV are reported as low as 10% and as high as 70%, with the most commonly reported rate being 35%. Infants born to seropositive mothers seem to be at greater risk for an HIV infection and AIDS than do infants born to seronegative mothers who later show seroconversion. Women with higher levels of viremia at more advanced stages of immunodeficiency are more likely to have negative pregnancy outcomes (Lamphear, 1994; Tinkle et al, 1992).

Prenatal period. The incidence of HIV infection in pregnant women is increasing. Physical and psychosocial health histories, physical examination, and laboratory testing must reflect this expectation if women and their newborns are to receive appropriate care. Women who fall into the high-risk category for HIV infection include the following:

1. Women and/or partners from geographic areas where HIV infection is prevalent
2. Women and/or partners who use or have used IV drugs
3. Women with persistent and recurrent STDs or a history of multiple partners
4. Women with sexual partners who are bisexual or hemophiliac
5. Women who received blood transfusions between 1978 and 1985
6. Women with clinical evidence of HIV-related infections
7. Any woman who believes she may have been exposed to HIV

HIV counseling and testing should be offered to all women at their initial entry into prenatal care. ELISA is the standard initial test for the presence of serum HIV antibody. A positive ELISA is repeated; a second positive ELISA is followed by the Western blot test, an immunoelectrophoresis procedure. False-positive ELISA results have been noted among those with autoimmune disease or a history of multiple pregnancies or blood transfusions (Tinkle et al, 1992).

BOX 9-9
Ethical Considerations and Confidentiality

Although confidentiality in the nurse-patient relationship is a basic ethical belief, sometimes the nurse is faced with a decision of whether to notify the sexual or IV needle partner who is placed at risk by the HIV-positive woman. This is an ethical dilemma involving personal and professional values regarding the issue of the patient's rights to privacy and requires careful values clarification and discussion.

Seronegativity on the first prenatal examination is not a guarantee for continued negative titers (Box 9-9). If a patient has a history of recent exposure to HIV but a negative ELISA, testing should be repeated in 3 to 4 months. After exposure to HIV, serum antibodies may take up to 12 weeks to develop. Similarly, a patient with positive ELISA and a negative Western blot needs further evaluation.

Routine prenatal tests may help identify the woman with HIV infection. Additional prenatal testing also can reveal gonorrhea, syphilis, prolonged and persistent episodes of herpes, *C. trachomatis*, hepatitis B, *Mycobacterium tuberculosis*, candidiasis (oropharyngeal or chronic vaginal infection), cytomegalovirus (CMV), and toxoplasmosis. About one half of patients with AIDS have elevated CMV titers. Because CMV inclusion disease poses a serious hazard to the fetus (Table 9-8), pregnant women are advised to avoid direct contact with HIV-infected persons with opportunistic infections.

The woman's history of vaccinations and immune status is documented. The titers for chickenpox and rubella are determined, and tuberculosis skin testing (purified protein derivative [PPD]) is done. Previous vaccination with Recombivax HB vaccine is noted because the vaccine once contained human blood products. (This vaccine is now free of association with human blood or blood products.)

Some prenatal discomforts (e.g., fatigue, anorexia, weight loss) mimic signs and symptoms of HIV infection. Differential diagnosis of *all* "pregnancy-induced" complaints and symptoms of infections is warranted. Signs of worsening HIV infection include a weight loss more than 10% of prepregnancy body weight, chronic diarrhea for longer than 1 month, and fever (intermittent or constant) for longer than 1 month.

Pharmacologic treatment for HIV infection has progressed rapidly since the discovery of the virus. The primary drug approved for treatment of HIV infection is zidovudine (AZT). Studies of pregnant women who received AZT during pregnancy (after 14 weeks, up to 34 weeks) have shown a decrease in vertical transmission rates of HIV infection from approximately 30% to 8% (CDC, 1994a, 1994b). It is recommended that all HIV-infected women be given AZT regardless of their CD4 counts (Boyer et al, 1994; CDC, 1994b). Women with CD4 counts of less than 200 cells/mm^3 should also be treated with trimethoprim prophylaxis for *Pneumocystis carcinii* pneumonia (PCP) (Acosta et al, 1992). Other opportunistic infections that persist concurrently with HIV infection are treated with medications specific to the infection; doses are commonly higher for patients with HIV/AIDS.

To support any pregnant woman's immune system, appropriate counseling is provided for optimum nutrition, sleep, rest, exercise, and stress reduction. HIV-infected women need more nutritional support and counseling about diet choices and food preparation and handling. Weight gain or maintenance in pregnancy is a challenge in these women. They are counseled regarding "safer" sex techniques. (See the Patient Teaching box in Chapter 20). Use of condoms and nonoxynol 9 spermicide is encouraged. Orogenital sex is discouraged.

As necessary, the woman is referred for drug rehabilitation. Abuse of alcohol, methamphetamines (e.g., speed, ice), marijuana, cocaine, nitrites (e.g., poppers, snappers), or other drugs compromises the body's immune system and increases the risk for AIDS and following associated conditions:

1. HIV may require the presence of an already damaged immune system before it can cause disease.
2. Alcohol and drugs interfere with many medical and alternative therapies for AIDS.
3. Alcohol and drugs affect the judgment of the user, who may become more prone to engage in activities that place persons at high risk for AIDS or increase exposure to HIV.
4. Alcohol and drug abuse causes stress, including sleep problems, which harms the functioning of the immune system.

Intrapartum period. Care of the woman in labor is not substantially altered by asymptomatic infection with HIV. The goals of nursing care are to monitor for maternal/fetal complications, provide psychosocial support, and prevent nosocomial transmission to patients and health care workers. Women with symptomatic HIV infection are more likely to experience preterm labor and birth, give birth to low-birth-weight babies, and exhibit accompanying infections, especially PCP.

External electronic fetal monitoring (EFM) is preferred if EFM is needed during labor. Inoculation of the virus into the neonate is possible if fetal scalp blood sampling is done or if a fetal scalp electrode is applied. In addition, the one who performs either of these procedures is placed at risk by accidental finger sticks.

Although the risk of transmission of HIV is considered to be low during vaginal birth, recent studies suggest that cesarean birth may decrease HIV infection in the infant (Villari et al, 1994). Cesarean birth should be based on obstetric considerations. AZT given prenatally reduces HIV antigenemia, thereby decreasing viral exposure to the infant. Immediately after vaginal or cesarean birth, infants should be wiped free of all body fluids and bathed as soon as they are stable. Adherence to infection control techniques is imperative (Craven et al, 1994).

Postpartum period. The clinical course during the postpartum period for the woman infected with HIV may be notable for infection, hemorrhage, or both (Bastin et al, 1992). Asymptomatic women may have an unremarkable postpartum course, but symptomatic, immunosuppressed women may be at increased risk for postpartum urinary tract infections, vaginitis, postpartum endometritis, and poor wound healing. HIV-related thrombocytopenias may also increase the risk of hemorrhage (Mandelbrot et al, 1994).

The cleansed newborn can be with the mother after birth, but breastfeeding is discouraged because of HIV transmission in breast milk. The World Health Organization (WHO) does not discourage breastfeeding in developing nations because of hygiene risks in the preparation and availability of formula. Standard Precautions are implemented for the mother and newborn, as they are for all patients. After discharge, the woman and her infant are referred to physicians who are experienced in the treatment of AIDS and associated conditions.

TORCH infections. *T*oxoplasmosis, *o*ther infections (e.g., hepatitis), *r*ubella virus, *c*ytomegalovirus, and *h*erpes simplex viruses, known collectively as **TORCH infections,** comprise a group of organisms capable of crossing the placenta and adversely affecting the development of the fetus. Table 9-8 outlines TORCH infections and their maternal, fetal, and newborn effects.

Toxoplasmosis. Toxoplasmosis is a protozoan infection associated with the consumption of infected raw or undercooked meat or with poor handwashing after handling infected cat litter. Pregnant women with HIV antibodies are at higher risk because toxoplasmosis is one of the common accompanying opportunistic infections. The presence of toxoplasmosis can be determined with blood studies, although laboratory diagnosis is difficult. Women in at-risk groups should have toxoplasmosis titers evaluated. Acute infection in pregnancy produces influenza-like symptoms and lymphadenopathy in some women but no symptomatology in others. Spontaneous abortion can occur.

The pharmaceutic treatment of choice for toxoplasmosis is a combination of pyrimethamine and sulfadiazine. Although pyrimethamine may be potentially harmful to the fetus, treatment of the parasitemia is essential. Some data suggest in utero improvement of fetal parasitemia with this pharmaceutic combination (Couvreur et al, 1993). If the infection is opportunistic (occurring in HIV-infected patients), leukovorin is also used. Alternating courses of this combination with spiramycin have also been suggested as experimental therapies (Matsui, 1994). Sulfa therapy should be used with caution in the third trimester to avoid neonatal kernicterus.

Other infections. The primary infection included in this category is hepatitis. *Hepatitis A virus (HAV),* or *infectious hepatitis,* is a virus spread by droplets or hands and is associated with poor handwashing after defecation. HAV is an uncommon complication of pregnancy, and perinatal transmission is rare but can occur (Watson et al, 1993). Pregnancy effects include spontaneous abortion and influenza-like symptoms such as fever, malaise, and nausea. If exposure to the fetus occurs in the first trimester and is untreated, possible effects include fetal anomalies, preterm birth, fetal or neonatal hepatitis, or intrauterine fetal death. Gamma globulin is given to mothers and exposed newborns for prophylaxis.

Hepatitis B virus (HBV) is transmitted in a manner similar to that of HIV. Routes of transmission include contaminated needles, syringes or blood products, sexual intercourse, and body fluid exchange. Routes of perinatal transmission include transplacentally and through contact with contaminated urine, feces, or vaginal secretions at birth. The presence of hepatitis B surface antigen (HBsAg) confirms diagnosis. Table 9-8 lists populations at risk for HBV.

During pregnancy, common symptoms include fever, rash, anorexia, malaise, myalgias and jaundice, right upper quadrant pain, and nausea and vomiting if the liver is acutely affected. Fetal and newborn effects include maternal-

TABLE 9-8 Maternal infections: TORCH

INFECTION	MATERNAL EFFECTS	FETAL OR NEONATAL EFFECTS	COUNSELING PREVENTION, IDENTIFICATION, AND MANAGEMENT
***T**oxoplasmosis* (protozoa)	Acute infection: similar to influenza; lymphadenopathy Mothers immune after first episode (except in immunocompromised patients)	With maternal acute infection: parasitemia Less likely to occur with maternal chronic infection Abortion likely with acute infection early in pregnancy	Use good handwashing technique. Avoid eating raw meat and exposure to litter used by infected cats; if cats in house, have toxoplasma titer checked. If titer is rising during early pregnancy, abortion may be considered an option.
***O**ther:* Hepatitis A (HAV) (infectious hepatitis) (virus)	Abortion; cause of liver failure during pregnancy Fever, malaise, nausea, abdominal discomfort	Exposure during first trimester; fetal anomalies; fetal or neonatal hepatitis; preterm birth; intrauterine fetal death	Usually spread by droplet or hand contact especially by culinary workers; gamma globulin can be given as prophylaxis for HAV.
Hepatitis B (HBV) (serum hepatitis) (virus)	May be transmitted sexually; symptoms variable: fever, rash, arthralgia, depressed appetite, dyspepsia, abdominal pain, generalized aching, malaise, weakness, jaundice, tender and enlarged liver	Infection occurs during birth. Maternal vaccination during pregnancy should present no risk for fetus; however, data are not available.	Generally passed by contaminated needles, syringes, or blood transfusions; also can be transmitted orally or by coitus, but incubation period is longer; hepatitis B immune globulin (HBIG) can be given prophylactically after exposure. HBV vaccine recommended for populations at risk and all neonates; vaccine consists of series of 3 IM doses. Infants of HBsAg-positive women should receive HBV vaccine and HBIG. Populations at risk: women from Asia, Pacific islands, Indochina, Haiti, sub-Africa, Alaska (women of Eskimo descent). Other women at risk include health care providers, IV drug users, and those sexually active with multiple partners and single partner having multiple risks.
***R**ubella* (3-day measles, German measles) (virus)	Rash, fever, mild symptoms; suboccipital lymph nodes may be swollen; some photophobia Occasionally arthritis or encephalitis Spontaneous abortion	Incidence of congenital anomalies: first month, 50%; second month, 25%, third month, 10%; fourth month, 4% Exposure during first 2 months: malformations of heart, eyes, ears, or brain; abnormal dermatoglyphics Exposure after fourth month: systemic infection, hepatosplenomegaly, intrauterine growth restriction, rash At 15-20 years of age, may experience deterioration of intellect and development or may develop epilepsy	Vaccination of pregnant women contraindicated; pregnancy should be prevented for 3 months after vaccination; pregnant women nonreactive to hemagglutinin-inhibition antigen can be safely vaccinated after the birth.
***C**ytomegalovirus* (CMV) (a herpesvirus)	Respiratory or sexually transmitted asymptomatic illness or mononucleosis-like syndrome: may have cervical discharge; no immunity develops	Fetal or neonatal death or severe, generalized disease: hemolytic anemia and jaundice; hydrocephaly or microcephaly; pneumonitis; hepatosplenomegaly, deafness	Virus may be reactivated and cause disease in utero or during birth in subsequent pregnancies; fetal infection may occur during passage through infected birth canal; disease is usually progressive through infancy and childhood.
***H**erpes genitalis* (herpes simplex virus type 2 [HSV-2]	See cytomegalovirus		

HbsAg, Hepatitis B surface antigen.

fetal transmission (approximately 90% transmission rate), sequelae of prematurity, and fetal or neonatal hepatitis.

Studies of universal screening for HBV infection in pregnant women indicate that 0.8% of women in the United States have HBsAg antibodies in pregnancy. Fewer than 50% of these women have risk factors for HBV infection. Several analyses have demonstrated the cost-effectiveness of universal screening, and the CDC (1993b) recommends that all pregnant women be screened for HBsAg at an early prenatal visit. Approximately 10% of women are chronic HBV carriers. Patients at risk who are seronegative should be given the three-dose series of HBV recombinant vaccine. Vaccination during pregnancy is not thought to pose risk to the fetus. Hepatitis B immune globulin (HBIG) vaccine may be combined with HBV vaccination to prevent infection within 14 days of HBV exposure.

Hepatitis C Virus (HCV) is another type of hepatitis commonly found in IV substance abusers and recipients of multiple blood transfusions. This viral infection is of growing concern because a few cases of perinatal transmission have been implicated, but no immunoprophylaxis is yet available. Similarly, *hepatitis D virus (HDV)* is found in IV substance abusers and patients who have received multiple transfusions; however, immunization against HBV is also protective against vertical perinatal transmission of HDV.

Rubella. Rubella, also known as *German measles* or *3-day measles,* is a viral infection transmitted by droplets. Fever, rash, and mild lymphedema usually are seen in an infected mother. Consequences for the fetus are much more serious and include spontaneous abortion, congenital anomalies (referred to as **congenital rubella syndrome**), and death. Vaccination of pregnant women is contraindicated because a rubella infection may develop after the vaccine is administered. As part of preconception counseling, rubella vaccine is given to women who are not rubella immune, and they are counseled to use contraception for at least 3 months after vaccination.

Cytomegalovirus. Maternal infection with cytomegalovirus (CMV) may begin as a mononucleosis-like syndrome. However, in most adults the onset of the disease is uncertain and asymptomatic. The virus is primarily transmitted by respiratory droplet but has also been isolated from semen, cervical/vaginal secretions, breast milk, placental tissue, urine, feces, and banked blood.

Women who show CMV infection in pregnancy (by positive viral titers) usually have chronic or recurrent infections (Brunham, Holmes, and Embree, 1990). No effective pharmacologic treatment exists for CMV; therapy focuses on symptom management.

Women at risk for infection include those who work or have children in day care centers, institutions for mentally retarded patients, or certain health care settings (e.g., nursery, dialysis, laboratories, oncology). CMV is the primary cause of congenital viral infection in the fetus and neonate and is the most common infectious cause of mental retardation. Congenital CMV infection occurs in approximately 30% to 40% of infants born to infected women (Raynor, 1993).

Herpes simplex virus. Herpes simplex virus type 1 (HSV-1) infections predominate during childhood but can also occur in adults. The virus is transmitted primarily by contact with oral secretions and causes cold sores and fever blisters. HSV-2 infections usually occur after puberty as sexual activity increases. Herpes simplex virus type 2 (HSV-2, herpes genitalis) is transmitted primarily by contact with genital secretions. Although HSV can survive for many hours on objects such as doorknobs, faucets, and toilets, scientists do not believe that human infection is likely to occur through contact with such objects. Transmission occurs through intimate contact with a person shedding the virus.

HSV interacts with epithelial or neuroepithelial cells and neurons. The incubation period from initial exposure until symptoms appear is usually 2 to 10 days. During the initial infection, HSV migrates to one or more sensory nerve ganglia, where it remains latent and dormant indefinitely. An intact immune system attacks the infection at the portal (place of entry). The primary infection involves mucocutaneous cells; recurrent infection involves stratified epithelial cells. Stressor stimuli trigger recurrent infection. Fever, another infection, emotions, menstruation, intercourse, and ultraviolet light are some common stressors.

HSV infections may involve external genitalia, the vagina, and cervix. Symptoms are more pronounced with primary infections of HSV. Painful blisters form (Fig. 9-16), rupture, and then drain, leaving shallow ulcers that crust over and disappear after 2 to 6 weeks. A vaginal discharge is seen if the cervix or vaginal mucosa is involved. The woman may have fever, malaise, anorexia, painful inguinal lymphadenopathy, dysuria, and dyspareunia.

Recurrences sometimes may be preceded by a 1 to 2-day prodrome of itching, a burning sensation in the genital area, tingling in the legs, or a slight increase in vaginal discharge. Prodromal symptoms are followed by 3 to 5 days of vesicles and ulcers. Repeated severe recurrences may result in keratitis, encephalitis, and possibly cervical carcinoma, although most recurrences tend to be milder and shorter in duration.

The pregnancy effects of primary genital herpes infection include spontaneous abortion, preterm labor, and IUGR. The main route of HSV transmission from mother to newborn is an infected birth canal; approximately 86% of isolated viral particles from exposed newborns is HSV-2. The risk of maternal-infant transmission is greater during a primary HSV-2 infection than during a recurrent episode (Adimora et al, 1994). Cesarean birth is recommended for those mothers with clinical evidence of active lesions during labor (Roberts et al, 1995). Cesarean birth should occur within 4 hours of rupture of the membranes; after 4 hours, almost all exposed newborns acquire HSV regardless of birth route (Adimora et al, 1994).

Fetal and neonatal effects are serious. Microcephaly, mental retardation, retinal dysplasia, patent ductus arteriosus, and intracranial calcification are sequelae. After intranatal infection, signs appear in 4 to 7 days. The signs include lethargy, poor feeding, jaundice, bleeding, pneumonia, convulsions, opisthotonus, bulging fontanels, and skin and mouth lesions. Neonatal infection with disseminated disease results in 82% mortality. Survivors have CNS or ocular sequelae and face recurrence in the first 5 years of life.

Acyclovir has been used since 1977 to treat life-threatening HSV infections in adults and newborns. However, data are not clear regarding safety or efficacy in pregnancy. Treatment of symptoms includes acetaminophen for fever and malaise

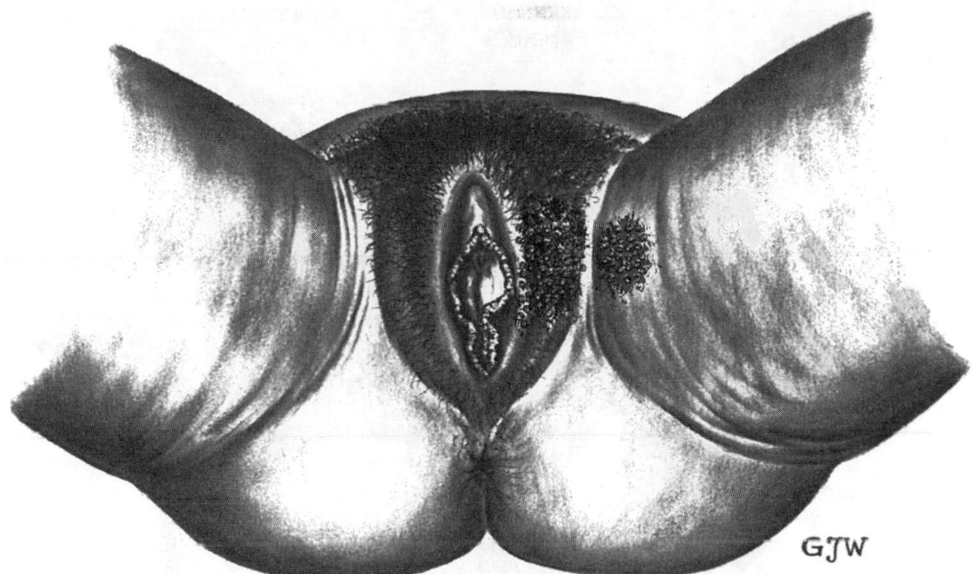

Fig. 9-16 Herpes genitalis.

and 5% lidocaine gel, local heat, or warm boric acid soaks for lesion discomfort.

Infection control measures are an important part of treatment. Thorough handwashing should be practiced by health care providers and family members. Gloves should be worn during contact with lesions or secretions. Family members with oral lesions should be discouraged from kissing the newborn. Instructions on genital hygiene and prevention of infection also should be given (see the Patient Teaching box in Chapter 20).

Many health care centers differ on isolation policies for infants of mothers with HSV infection. Infants born to mothers at risk of transmitting the infection (e.g., mothers who give birth vaginally with active lesions) may be isolated by rooming-in with the mother or by enclosure in an incubator.

Health care providers with HSV infections also should take precautions. Anyone with oral HSV lesions should wear a mask if in close contact with newborns, and anyone with skin lesions (herpetic whitlow) should not give direct care until lesions are dried and crusted.

Human papillomavirus. Condylomata acuminata, sexually transmitted lesions caused by **human papillomavirus (HPV),** is the most common viral sexually transmitted infection—3 times greater than genital herpes. More than 50 HPVs infect skin and mucosal surfaces, with HPV-6, HPV-11, HPV-16, HPV-18, and HPV-31 most often infecting the anogenital tract (Adimora et al, 1994).

Disease occurs at the entry site of the virus after an incubation period of 2 to 3 months. HPV is disseminated by skin-to-skin contact, not through body fluid exchange. Exposure to the virus is by sexual contact with an infected partner, although HPV DNA has been detected on medical instruments, underwear of infected patients, wet towels, bathing suits, and tanning salon benches (Deitch, 1995). Others at risk include those with multiple partners and smokers and oral contraceptive users, presumably related to the suppressive effects on the immune system. HPV is clinically significant because various types are associated with congenitally derived respiratory papillomatosis in children and with cervical intraepithelial neoplasia (CIN).

Condyloma acuminatum causes dry, wartlike growths on the vulva, vagina, cervix, or rectum (Fig. 9-17). These growths may be small or large, single or multiple, or have a cauliflower appearance. Chronic vaginal discharge, pruritus, or dyspareunia can occur. Diagnosis is by colposcopy and direct visualization of the growths, by biopsy, or by Pap smear.

In the immunocompetent person, condylomata acuminata may regress spontaneously. In many persons, however, the condition is difficult to treat. Available therapy is primarily cytotoxic or destructive and should be initiated with concern for patient preference. Cytotoxic agents are podofilox 0.5% solution (for self-treatment) and podophyllin (podophyllum resin). Self-treatment is less expensive, and unlike podophyllin, podofilox does not need to be washed off after application. Podophyllin, 10% to 25% in compound tincture of benzoin, is used for lesions 2 cm or less in diameter, but not in the vagina or on the cervix. Petrolatum is used to protect surrounding skin because podophyllin is caustic. The medication must be washed off after 4 hours or sooner if burning occurs, and treatment is weekly for 6 weeks. Therapy may alleviate symptoms and remove visible warts, but no cure exists for HPV. The recurrence rate is 70%. Podophyllin and podofilox are not to be used during pregnancy. The use of podophyllin during pregnancy has been associated with fetal death and preterm labor.

Destructive methods of treatment include cryotherapy with liquid nitrogen or a cryoprobe, electrocautery, surgery, and laser. The most effective destructive method is a carbon dioxide laser used with local anesthesia. Laser therapy may be used with caution in pregnancy. It is precise and sterile and is accompanied with minimum bleeding and trauma. The

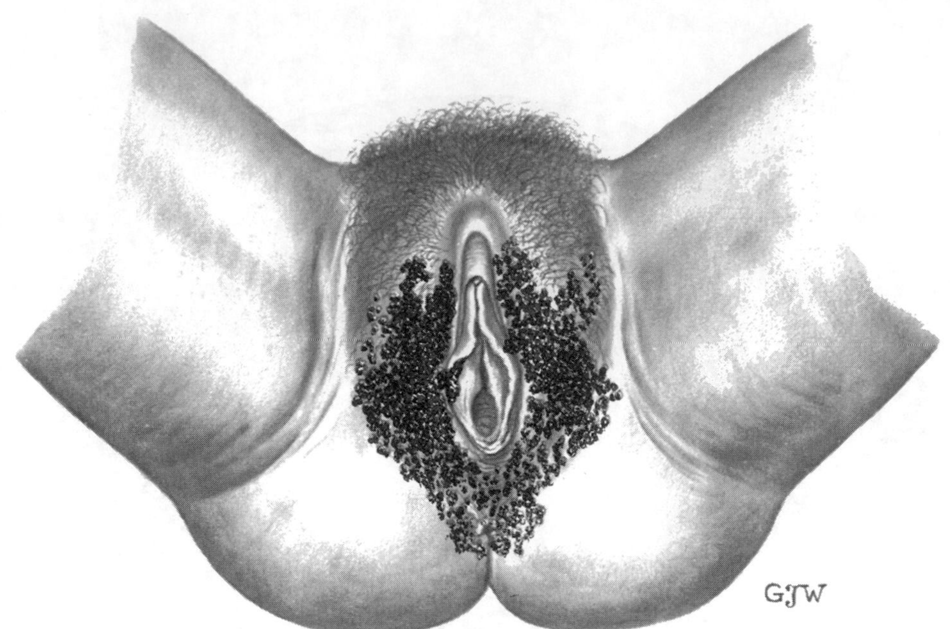

Fig. 9-17 HPV infection (condylomata acuminata).

treated area does not regain its normal pigmentation for several years, and recurrence is 25% to 100%. Instructions after laser therapy are as follows:

1. Keep area clean by irrigating with warm water twice a day (or use sitz bath).
2. Dry with electric hair dryer.
3. Apply antibacterial cream twice a day.
4. Use gauze dressing to prevent rubbing against clothing.
5. Use lidocaine gel 5% for discomfort.
6. Return to clinic as instructed.
7. Use latex condoms. Today, condoms are dense enough to prevent passage of viruses.

Trichloroacetic acid (TCA), 80% to 90% solution, is a destructive therapy that is somewhat safer to use than podophyllin. TCA can be used safely in pregnancy, but efficacy data are inconclusive. It can be self-applied with a cotton swab and does not need to be washed off. TCA is caustic to local tissues and may cause burning. Ice packs and lidocaine gel 5% may help minimize discomfort.

Pregnancy effects of HPV infection include proliferation and increased friability of lesions. Many experts recommend removal of large, outward-growing lesions during pregnancy; carbon dioxide laser treatments have been used between 30 and 32 weeks' gestation. Treatment usually is followed by vaginal birth without complications. Cesarean birth is indicated when the pelvic outlet is obstructed or when vaginal birth would result in excessive blood loss.

The primary neonatal effect of HPV infection is respiratory or laryngeal **papillomatosis.** The exact route of perinatal transmission is unknown, and disagreement exists as to the preferred mode of birth. Some infants born by cesarean have developed respiratory papillomatosis. However, the estimated risk of an infant developing papillomatosis after vaginal birth in a mother with active condyloma is 1 in 400 (Kashima, Shah, and Goodstein, 1990). The mother should make an informed decision regarding vaginal or cesarean birth.

Genital Tract Infections

Vaginal infections. The three most common vaginal infections are bacterial vaginosis, candidiasis, and trichomoniasis. Vaginal infections may be sexually transmitted.

Infections must be distinguished from normal vaginal discharge, or *leukorrhea,* which is a whitish discharge. It consists of mucus and exfoliated vaginal epithelial cells as a result of hyperplasia of the vaginal mucosa, such as occurs during pregnancy, at the time of ovulation, and before menstruation. If it is copious, it can cause discomfort from maceration.

Altered vaginal physiology during pregnancy may precipitate **vaginitis** (inflammation of the vagina). Vaginal secretions are increased, and the vagina is less acidic during pregnancy. These conditions provide an environment that promotes microbial growth.

Infectious organisms such as *Escherichia coli,* staphylococci, and streptococci change the normal acidity of the vagina. A pH of 3.5 to 4.5 is needed to support Döderlein bacillus, the vagina's main line of defense. The proximity of the urethra to the vagina predisposes the woman with vaginitis to a concurrent urethritis.

Burning, pruritus, redness, and edema of surrounding tissues are characteristic of vaginitis. These symptoms are particularly discomforting during voiding and defecating.

Objectives of management of vaginitis are to relieve discomfort, to eradicate offending organisms and thereby foster growth of Döderlein baccillus, and to prevent recurrence. During pregnancy, sitz baths and acetaminophen may be used for discomfort. Some topical creams such as hydrocortisone may relieve discomfort from tissue excoriation. Antibiotics are prescribed for treatment of specific organisms; eradication of microorganisms helps to restore vaginal acidity. Effects on the fetus from these therapies are minimal.

The most common cause of vaginal symptoms among childbearing women is *bacterial vaginosis*, also referred to as *nonspecific vaginosis*. By-products of bacterial metabolism affect vaginal pH, thus altering the flora of the vagina. The predominant microorganism is *Gardnerella vaginalis*. The homogenous vaginal discharge has an amine (fishy) odor when mixed with 10% potassium hydroxide. "Clue cells" are seen on microscopic examination of vaginal discharge.

The maternal effect of this bacterial infection is usually a mild illness. Signs and symptoms may include a milklike discharge, pruritus, burning, and pain in the vagina and around the introitus. Obstetric complications include amniotic fluid infection, PROM, preterm labor and birth, and postpartum endometritis (Andrews et al, 1995). Bacterial vaginosis also may be a risk factor for PID. Fetal and neonatal effects include septicemia and death.

Treatment of bacterial vaginosis is most effective with oral metronidazole. Topical preparations of metronidazole and clindamycin have also shown some efficacy in clinical trials. However, because of its potential teratogenic effects, oral metronidazole should not be given in the first trimester, and only single doses are approved for the second and third trimesters. The CDC (1993b) recommends the use of clindamycin cream 2% to treat the condition successfully.

Vaginal candidiasis. *Vulvovaginal candidiasis*, or candidal vaginitis, occurs throughout the world, particularly in hot, subtropical climates. Most trends suggest that the disease is increasing, in part as a result of the widespread use of antimicrobial agents. The number of healthy, symptom-free women who harbor *Candida* organisms also is increasing.

Several factors are noted, including pregnancy, use of high-estrogen oral contraceptives, and uncontrolled diabetes mellitus. Additional factors that precipitate candidiasis are steroid or immunosuppressive therapy; antibiotic therapy; immunocompromised states (e.g., AIDS); restrictive, tight, or poorly ventilated clothing; and poor genital hygiene.

Most yeastlike organisms isolated from the vagina are *Candida albicans*, a fungus normally found in the intestines. The second most common yeast is *Torulopsis glabrata*, which accounts for approximately one fourth of candidal vaginitis (Redondo-Lopez et al, 1990). The thick vaginal discharge is irritating and pruritic. Dysuria and dyspareunia are common complaints. Speculum examination usually reveals thick, white, tenacious, cheeselike patches adhering to the pale, dry, vaginal mucosa.

Maternal effects of vaginal candidiasis usually are not health-threatening, but affected mothers may be extremely uncomfortable from the pain, itching, and vaginal discharge. Pregnancy predisposes women not only to an increased rate of infection but also to increased recurrences and increased treatment failures. Treatment goals include measures to relieve symptoms and topical or vaginal antifungal agents such as clotrimazole, miconazole (available without prescription), butoconazole, and terconazole (available by prescription). Although self-medication with over-the-counter (OTC) medications is an option for treatment, pregnant women should be cautioned against this practice. Recurrent candidal vaginitis in the antepartum period may necessitate prenatal screening for other complications (e.g., AIDS, gestational diabetes).

Fetal and neonatal effects are limited to infection acquired by direct contact from the birth canal or from the contaminated hands of caregivers. However, *Candida* organisms have been isolated from the nipples of a breastfeeding mother whose infant also was infected (Johnstone and Marcinak, 1990). Oral candidiasis, or thrush, is the most commonly seen *C. albicans* infection in newborns and usually is treated with nystatin.

Trichomonas vaginalis. *Trichomonas vaginalis* is a hearty protozoan that thrives in an alkaline milieu. The role of sexual contact in the transmission of *T. vaginalis* is well documented; trichomoniasis is prevalent in approximately 30% of sexually active women (Rein and Müller, 1990).

In symptom-free persons the infection may be identified during a routine examination. *T. vaginalis* has an affinity for mucous membranes, and 75% of infected women report a vaginal discharge that may be malodorous. This profuse, frothy discharge usually is gray or yellow-green and may stream from the vagina when a speculum is inserted.

Trichomoniasis seems to have few maternal effects other than symptomatic discomfort. However, perinatal infection by *T. vaginalis* is the most common form of nonvenereal transmission of disease. Fetal and neonatal effects include fever and irritability. The preferred treatment, metronidazole (in a single 2 g dose), should be administered to pregnant women only in the second and third trimesters. Partners should also be treated.

Group B streptococci. Group B streptococcal (GBS) bacterial infections have been recognized as the leading cause of life-threatening perinatal infections in the United States (ACOG, 1992b). The transmission rate of infection from mother to infant near the time of birth ranges between 50% and 75% (Hill, 1990). Women with preterm labor or PROM are at increased risk for maternal infection as well as neonatal infection. Maternal effects include miscarriage, stillbirth, preterm birth, fever, septicemia, and puerperal infection.

Fetal and neonatal effects are also serious; GBS infections are the leading cause of neonatal sepsis and meningitis. Signs of sepsis generally are present within 72 hours after birth, and gram-positive cocci may be isolated from the umbilicus, ear, rectum, blood, and tracheal and gastric aspirates. Other neonatal effects include blindness, deafness, mental retardation, learning disabilities, and death.

Treatment of GBS infections is accomplished with penicillin, ampicillin, cephalothin, or erythromycin. Intrapartum antibiotic chemoprophylaxis for women who are GBS carriers reduces the incidence of GBS disease (ACOG, 1992b). Prophylaxis of neonates at risk for infection also is encouraged.

Urinary tract infections. Urinary tract infections (UTIs) affect about 10% of pregnant women, most of these in the prenatal period. Those who have had UTIs previously are especially prone to recurrence during pregnancy. Cervicitis, vaginitis, obstruction of the flaccid ureters, vesicoureteral reflux, and the trauma of birth predispose the pregnant woman to UTI, generally from *Escherichia coli*. Women with chronic STDs, especially gonorrhea and chlamydial infection, also are at risk. Asymptomatic bacteriuria occurs in about 5% to 15% of all pregnant women. If untreated, pyelonephritis during gestation will develop in approximately 30% of these women. Premature labor and birth may occur often as well.

Some symptoms of UTI are similar to pregnancy complaints such as urinary frequency, urgency, low back pain, suprapubic tenderness, incontinence, and incomplete bladder emptying. Other complaints help to identify UTI, including dysuria, hesitancy in starting a stream, and retention.

Urine culture and sensitivity tests should be obtained early in pregnancy, preferably at the first visit, from a clean-catch urine specimen. If infection is diagnosed, treatment with an appropriate antibiotic drug, together with increased fluid intake, urinary tract antispasmodic medication (e.g., belladonna derivatives), and frequent emptying of the bladder, is recommended. Infections caused by the colon's aerogenic organisms generally respond well to sulfisoxazole (Gantrisin) or nitrofurantoin. Treatment should be continued for 2 to 3 weeks until two negative cultures are obtained, and the infant should be observed for hyperbilirubinemia. Retreatment of the mother may be necessary if there is a recurrence.

General Infections

Many infections place the woman at risk during the childbearing cycle. Following are some maternal infections the nurse may encounter.

Coxsackievirus B. Coxsackievirus B may cause mild illness in the mother. It is responsible for death, cardiovascular anomalies, myocarditis, and meningoencephalitis in the fetus.

Varicella. Varicella (chickenpox) is highly contagious and is transmitted by direct contact with airborne virus. A maternal infection may appear as herpes zoster (shingles), especially in mothers with HIV. A severe, disseminated, epidemic type of varicella during pregnancy may be fatal for the mother (and fetus) because of necrotizing angitis (inflammation of blood and lymph vessels) and complications from varicella pneumonia.

Fetal and neonatal effects also are seen. Abortion or fetal death may occur. If maternal varicella infection occurs in the first trimester, there is about a 2% chance that the fetus will develop a pattern of defects of skin, bone, and muscle known as **congenital varicella syndrome** (Pastuszak et al, 1994). CNS effects include chorioretinitis and hydrocephalus. If maternal infection occurs within 20 days before birth, an infant should be considered possibly infectious and isolated from other infants.

Varicella-zoster immunoglobulin (VZIG) may be given prophylactically to exposed pregnant women. Some passive immunity may be delivered to the fetus through the placenta (Schuster et al, 1994). Severe varicella infections, especially if complicated by pneumonia, should be treated with IV acyclovir or vidarabine.

Influenza. Influenza is caused by a virus. Maternal effects can be serious if complicated by pneumonia. Abortion and preterm labor may result. Fetal and neonatal effects include death, preterm birth, and occasionally, anencephaly or meningomyelocele. If the woman is not pregnant, she may be given polyvalent influenza virus (attenuated live virus) vaccine.

Listeriosis. Listeriosis is caused by a gram-positive bacterium, *Listeria monocytogenes.* This organism is harbored in the vagina or cervix by 4% of pregnant women. Listeriosis may cause influenza-like symptoms. It occurs most often in summer and fall. Other symptoms include vaginitis, UTI, and enteritis. Fetal and neonatal effects are serious. This infection may result in abortion. Amnionitis or placentitis is evidenced by dirty-brown amniotic fluid. Treatment with penicillin or erythromycin usually is successful. The diagnosis of listeriosis often is obscure or delayed; thus the prognosis for the fetus or newborn generally is poor.

Lyme disease. Lyme disease is a tick-borne infection caused by the spirochete *Borrelia burgdorferi.* Infection is endemic in the Northeast, mid-Atlantic states, parts of the Midwest, and West and peaks in the late spring and summer. Most infected people develop a circular, expanding lesion (erythema chronicum migrans) at the site of the tick bite, usually on the groin, buttocks, axillae, trunk, upper part of the arms, and legs. Viremic symptoms, such as fatigue, headache, sore throat, fever, pain, and joint swelling, also may develop; some persons remain free of symptoms. Sequelae of untreated Lyme disease include chronic arthritis and neurologic and cardiac problems.

The spirochete of Lyme disease, which closely resembles that of syphilis, crosses the placenta. Maternal effects include miscarriage, preterm labor and birth, and stillbirth. Fetal and neonatal effects are not well documented because Lyme disease is still relatively new and often misdiagnosed. Congenital Lyme disease is rare (Gerber and Zalneraitis, 1994). Birth defects are common, especially cardiac and neurologic defects; however, recent data suggest maternal exposure to Lyme disease does not increase the risk of fetal death, low birth weight, preterm birth, or congenital malformations (Strobino et al, 1993). Treatment of choice for Lyme disease during pregnancy is amoxicillin or ceftriaxone.

Malaria. Malaria is caused by the protozoan *Plasmodium falciparum.* Maternal effects include chills and fever, abortion, and preterm labor. Labor may be prolonged, hazardous, and fatiguing, and it may result in cesarean birth. There is often a recurrence during the puerperium. Fetal and neonatal effects occur. There is extensive involvement of the placenta. The newborn may be SGA or stillborn if the maternal infection does not cause abortion. Infection occurs in 10% of newborns of infectious women. Quinine (chloroquine phosphate [Aralen]) given to the mother may be fetotoxic. In severe cases of malaria, however, use of appropriate medications may be an acceptable calculated risk.

Mumps. Mumps (parotitis) occurs rarely in pregnant women. In the mother, this virus may cause abortion or preterm labor. Fetal death may result. Congenital malformation such as endocardial fibroelastosis may be associated with this viral infection in survivors. Prophylaxis for epidemic parotitis is possible with administration of hyperimmune mumps gamma globulin.

Parvovirus. Parvovirus B19 is associated with a mild illness of childhood known as fifth disease or erythema infectiosum. Transmission occurs by droplets, and the primary symptoms are fever and a characteristic "slapped face" rash. Outbreaks usually occur in schools in the spring; adults who work with children are at increased risk. Maternal effects, in addition to fever and rash, include headache; malaise; and aching, swollen joints.

Fetal and neonatal effects are more serious. Parvovirus has been recently implicated as one cause of unexplained miscarriage and stillbirth. Human parvovirus infection disrupts erythropoiesis in the fetus, leading to severe anemia, cardiac failure, nonimmune hydrops fetalis (NIHF), and death. NIHF is a common result of parvovirus infection (Hadi et al, 1994; Panero et al, 1994; Yaegashi et al, 1994). No treatment exists for parvovirus infection in mothers or infants; however, fetal blood transfusions and digitalization have limited success in avoiding hydroptic sequelae in utero (Boley and Popek, 1993; Peters and Nicolaides, 1990). The need for parvovirus vaccination needs to be investigated (Jordan and Sever, 1994).

Rubeola. Rubeola, a viral infection also known as *2-week or red measles*, is uncommon because most women have been immunized or have had the disease and are immune to it. Should the woman acquire rubeola during pregnancy, fetal and neonatal effects develop. Abortion or preterm labor may occur. The newborn may be born with a rash but generally survives, usually without developmental anomalies. Prophylactic gamma globulin may prevent the disease; measles vaccination of susceptible women before (not during) pregnancy is recommended.

Tuberculosis. Tuberculosis (TB) is caused by a gram-negative, acid-fast bacillus. Pulmonary TB does not jeopardize pregnancy, although urinary and CNS TB may. Pregnancy does not affect pulmonary TB adversely; however, pulmonary TB during pregnancy is associated with prematurity, low birth weight, and perinatal death (Jana et al, 1994).

Genital infection is rare. It may be sexually transmitted or result from primary lesions in the lungs. Spontaneous abortion occurs in 20% of infected women. Many pregnancies are ectopic, or the woman has impaired fertility with genital TB. TB is gaining increased attention as one of the opportunistic infections seen commonly in people with HIV and AIDS (Margono et al, 1994; Mofenson et al, 1995). Patients with TB infections require special care to prevent respiratory droplet transmission. They are often placed on respiratory precautions in a room with negative air pressure. Care providers should be fit-tested for and wear protective face masks to protect themselves against infection. Yearly TB screening of care providers is required in many agencies to assess for exposure-related infections.

The outcome of fetal and neonatal involvement depends on the stage of TB infection of the mother. Congenital TB is rare but does occur, especially if the mother is untreated. Neonatal mortality may be as high as 30% (Machin et al, 1992).

Contraception is advocated for women with active TB; pregnancy is contraindicated until the woman has been free of the disease for $1\frac{1}{2}$ to 2 years. All pregnant women should be evaluated for TB (tine test or PPD) early in pregnancy and again later if suspicion of the disease exists. If results of the tine test or PPD are positive, a chest film may be indicated to rule out active disease. However, some practitioners recommend prophylactic treatment with isoniazid (INH) even with a negative chest film. Individuals who have been treated for TB will have a reactive TB test. Once born, the infant should have no intimate contact with the mother or others who may have the disease until contagion is no longer a problem or both mother and infant are taking medication (INH with pyroxidine, rifampin, and ethambutol).

Toxic shock syndrome. Toxic shock syndrome (TSS) is a potentially life-threatening systemic disorder that has three principal clinical manifestations: fever of sudden onset, hypotension, and rash. The erythematous macular desquamating rash is most prominent on palms and soles. The acute phase of TSS lasts about 4 to 5 days; the convalescent phase, about 1 to 2 weeks.

Diagnostic criteria for TSS include the previously mentioned signs plus the following manifestations:

1. Involvement of three or more other organ systems:

SYSTEM/AREA	MANIFESTATIONS
Gastrointestinal	Nausea, vomiting, diarrhea
Renal	Decreased urine output; pyuria
Hepatic	Jaundice; abnormal values (increased transaminase)
CNS	Altered sensorium (decreased level of consciousness); headache
Respiratory	Adult respiratory distress syndrome (ARDS)
Mucous membranes	Inflammation of vaginal, oropharyngeal, and conjunctival membranes
Muscular	Myalgia; weakness
Hematologic	Thrombocytopenia; DIC
Cardiac	Ischemic changes on ECG; decreased left ventricular contractility

2. Serologic laboratory test results for Rocky Mountain spotted fever, leptospirosis, and measles are negative. Cultures positive for *S. aureus* can be obtained from blood, urine, or stool. If the primary site of infection is tampon related, positive cultures are obtained from the vagina and cervix.

A toxin (pyrogenic exotoxin C [PEC] or enterotoxin F) secreted by strains of *S. aureus* is the causative factor in TSS. About 9% of women harbor the organism normally in their vaginas; about 1% to 5% of sexually active males have urethral cultures that are positive for *S. aureus* without having the disease. Poor perineal hygiene and lack of handwashing before touching the perineal area may increase risk. Commonly associated conditions that may predispose the person to TSS by providing a portal of entry into systemic circulation include the following:

1. Menstruation
2. Chronic vaginal infection (e.g., herpes)
3. Puerperal endometritis
4. Incisional or soft tissue abscess
5. Skin infection following a bee sting
6. IV injection of heroin
7. Use of high-absorbency tampons or barrier contraceptives (e.g., cervical cap, diaphragm)
8. Neonatal infection concurrent with maternal infection.

The population at greatest risk is women between the ages of 15 and 24 who use tampons during menstruation. The three

Patient Teaching

PREVENTION OF TOXIC SHOCK SYNDROME

GENERAL INFORMATION

- Avoid the use of tampons, cervical caps, and diaphragms during the postpartum period (6 weeks).
- Do not use any of the above if you have a history of TSS.
- Call your health care provider if you experience sudden onset of a high fever, vomiting, diarrhea, or skin rash.

TAMPON USE

- Insert only clean tampons with clean hands.
- Change tampons every 3 to 6 hours.
- Avoid use of superabsorbent tampons.
- Avoid overnight use of tampons by substituting other products such as sanitary napkins or minipads.

DIAPHRAGM OR CERVICAL CAP

- Insert clean diaphragm or cervical cap with clean hands.
- Do not use during your menstrual period.
- Remove within 6 hours after intercourse.

causes of mortality are (1) ARDS, (2) uncontrollable hypotension, and (3) DIC.

Most affected women have an uneventful recovery with no recurrence. Infection that recurs does so most often with the next menstrual cycle. Recurrence is most likely if the woman has not been treated with β-lactamase–resistant antibiotics.

Early identification of TSS is essential so that appropriate therapy can be initiated. Nursing care involves both prevention and treatment of TSS. Preventive care focuses on patient education about the relationship of TSS to the use of tampons, diaphragms, and cervical caps, (see the Patient Teaching box above). Treatment in the acute care setting may include IV fluid replacement for dehydration related to vomiting or diarrhea, administration of antibiotics, administration of transfusions for low platelet counts, and medications to treat skin rashes and hypotension (Eschenbach, 1994).

Infection Control

Infection control measures are essential to protect care providers and to prevent nosocomial infection of patients, regardless of the infectious agent. The risk of occupational transmission varies with the disease. Even if that risk is low, as it is with HIV, the possibility of any risk is significant to warrant reasonable precautions. Precautions against airborne disease transmission are available in all health care agencies. Box 9-10 describes **Standard Precautions.**

Another consideration in the prevention of occupational disease transmission is that of cross-contamination. Health care providers may develop a false sense of security about the protection that gloves provide. For example, little is gained if gloves are worn to assess a newborn and those same gloved hands are used to answer the telephone, turn on a light, or document findings on the infant's chart. Cross-contamination of surfaces is common. Proper cleaning of contaminated surfaces is essential. The following guidelines are recommended: (1) cleanse washable surfaces with a solution of sodium hypochlorite (household bleach) and water (1 cup of household bleach to 9 cups of water); health care institutions often purchase commercial products to disinfect; (2) remove all blood or other fluids before disinfection to avoid neutralizing the bleach solution. If a large spill has occurred, pour disinfectant over the spillage before removal, then disinfect as described.

Key determinants in the transmission of bloodborne pathogens include serum concentration of virus, the consistent use of Standard Precautions, and vaccination. As the serum concentration of viral pathogens increases, the rate of transmission also increases. Similarly, the numbers of hospitalized patients who test positive for HBsAg are also increasing (Lamphear, 1994). The incidence of viral infection is on the rise among health care workers; CMV is most prevalent, followed by HBV and HCV. HIV transmission in the workplace is minimal (Gerberding, 1994). Standard Precautions and vaccination offer added protection to health care workers, but data suggest adherence to Standard Precautions occurs only about half the time. In addition, although HBV vaccine is recommended for all health care workers at risk for blood and body fluid exposure, many do not complete all vaccinations in the three-dose series (Hersey and Martin, 1994).

Nursing Care Management

Assessment

Prevention, diagnosis, and treatment of maternal infections are often difficult because multiple STDs may be present at any given time. A comprehensive assessment focuses on some life-style issues that may be personal or sensitive. A culturally sensitive, nonjudgmental approach is essential for facilitating accurate data collection. Assessment includes the following key areas.

History. Factors that influence the development and management of STDs during pregnancy include a previous history of STD or PID, the number of current sexual partners, the frequency of intercourse per week, and anticipated sexual activity through the pregnancy. Life-style choices also may affect STD in the perinatal period. Mothers who are IV drug users or who have partners who use IV drugs are at risk. Other life-style factors that increase susceptibility to STDs (through suppressive effects on the immune system) include smoking, alcohol use, inadequate or poor nutrition, and high levels of fatigue or personal stress.

LEGAL TIP

Sexually Transmitted Diseases

Many STDs are also considered infectious diseases and are therefore reportable to agencies that track the incidence and prevalence of these reportable diseases. The specific infections that are reportable vary from state to state. Nurses who work in settings where infectious diseases are diagnosed may have some responsibility for reporting. It is important that nurses be aware of those diseases that are reportable in their setting and take responsibility for reporting them.

Preconception or antenatal factors that influence the development of vaginal infections or UTIs include a history of chronic UTIs or kidney infection and kidney stones; chronic

BOX 9-10
Standard Precautions

Medical history and examination cannot reliably identify all persons infected with HIV or other bloodborne pathogens. Thus blood and body fluid precautions should be used consistently for everyone. This approach should be used in the care of all persons, especially those in emergency care settings in which the risk of blood exposure is increased and the infection status of the person is usually unknown.

1. All health care workers should routinely use appropriate barrier precautions to prevent skin and mucous membrane exposure when contact with blood or other body fluids of any person is anticipated. *Latex gloves* should be worn for touching blood and body fluids, mucous membranes, or nonintact skin of all persons; for handling items or surfaces soiled with blood or body fluids; and for performing venipuncture and other vascular access procedures. Gloves should be changed after contact with each patient. *Masks and protective eyewear* or face shields should be worn during procedures that are likely to generate droplets of blood or other body fluids to prevent exposure of mucous membranes of the mouth, nose, and eyes. *Gowns or aprons* should be worn during procedures that are likely to generate splashes of blood or other body fluids.
2. Hands and other skin surfaces should be washed immediately and thoroughly if contaminated with blood or other body fluids. Hands should be washed immediately after gloves are removed.
3. All health care workers should take precautions to prevent injuries caused by needles, scalpels, and other sharp instruments or devices during procedures; when cleaning used instruments; during disposal of used needles; and when handling sharp instruments after procedures. *To prevent needle stick injuries,* needles should not be recapped, purposely bent or broken by hand, removed from disposable syringes, or otherwise manipulated by hand. After they are used, disposable syringes and needles, scalpel blades, and other sharp items should be placed immediately in puncture-resistant containers for disposal; the puncture-resistant containers should be located as close as practical to the use area.
4. Although saliva has not been implicated in HIV transmission, to minimize the need for emergency mouth-to-mouth resuscitation, mouthpieces, resuscitation bags, or other ventilation devices should be available for use in areas where the need for resuscitation is predictable.
5. Health care workers who have exudative lesions or weeping dermatitis should refrain from all direct patient care and from handling patient care equipment until the condition resolves.
6. Pregnant health care workers are not known to be at greater risk of contracting HIV infection than health care workers who are not pregnant; however, if a health care worker develops HIV infection during pregnancy, the infant is at risk of infection resulting from perinatal transmission.

PRECAUTIONS FOR INVASIVE PROCEDURES

An *invasive procedure* is defined as surgical entry into tissues, cavities, or organs or repair of major traumatic injuries (1) in an operating or birthing room, emergency department, or out-of-hospital setting, including both physicians' and dentists' offices and (2) a vaginal or cesarean birth or other invasive obstetric procedure during which bleeding may occur. The previously mentioned universal blood and body fluid precautions, combined with the following precautions, should serve as minimum precautions for all such invasive procedures.

1. All health care workers who participate in invasive procedures must routinely use appropriate barrier precautions to prevent skin and mucous membrane contact with blood and other body fluids of all patients. Gloves and surgical masks must be worn for all invasive procedures. Protective eyewear or face shields should be worn for procedures that typically result in the generation of droplets, splashing of blood or other body fluids, or the generation of bone chips. Gowns or aprons made of materials that provide an effective barrier should be worn during invasive procedures that are likely to result in the splashing of blood or other body fluids. All health care workers who perform or assist in vaginal or cesarean births should wear gloves and gowns when handling the placenta or the infant until blood and amniotic fluid have been removed from the infant's skin and should wear gloves during postnatal care of the umbilical cord.
2. If a glove is torn or a needle stick or other injury occurs, the glove should be removed and a new glove used as promptly as patient safety permits; the needle or instrument involved in the incident also should be removed from the sterile field.

conditions that impair kidney function (e.g., lupus, diabetes, sickle cell disease); chronic immunosuppressive states (e.g., steroid therapy, AIDS); poor fluid and nutritional status; failure to use condoms; and poor genital hygiene. Intrapartum events such as frequent catheterizations (especially with the use of epidural anesthesia); frequent vaginal examinations; prolonged second stage of labor; birth trauma to the vagina, cervix, bladder, and urethra; and excessive blood loss also may place the mother at greater risk for infection. Untreated or undertreated infections in the prenatal period may predispose mothers to postpartum infections. PROM and the length of time from rupture to birth also may be factors.

Physical examination. Findings on examination vary. Some infections may be asymptomatic. Vaginal discharge may or may not be present, and vesicles or sores may be unnoticed. There may be perineal edema, excoriation, erythema, and pruritus. Fever or pain may be mild and therefore dismissed. A thorough symptom assessment, coupled with a complete history and physical examination, is essential in identifying possible maternal infectious disease processes. Signs of infection may not be evident for 24 to 48 hours after the birth. A fever higher than 38° C, chills, and tachycardia are indicative of infection. Abdominal or perineal discomfort, nausea, and vomiting may also develop. Foul-smelling lochia is a sign of uterine infection; other potential sites of infection include the breasts, an episiotomy or cesarean incision, and the bladder.

Laboratory tests. Bacterial infections are easily determined from genital tract, urine, and blood studies. Viral agents also can be cultured but less successfully. An elevated white blood cell count may be of diagnostic help; other laboratory tests are useful depending on what other infectious agents are suspected. Other laboratory data to assess include hematocrit, hemoglobin, proteinuria, and BUN. Box 9-11 describes assessment for the woman suspected of having an STD.

Nursing Diagnoses

Nursing diagnoses are derived after carefully analyzing assessment findings and medical management directives. Nursing diagnoses for the patient at risk for infections include the following:

- Pain/impaired tissue integrity related to
  - Effects of infection process
  - Scratching (excoriation) of pruritic areas
  - Hygienic practices
- Knowledge deficit related to
  - Transmission/prevention of infection/reinfection
  - Safer sex behaviors
  - Management and course of infection
- Anxiety/situational low self-esteem/body image disturbance related to
  - Perceived effects on sexual relationships and family processes
  - Possible effects on pregnancy/fetus
  - Long-term sequelae to infection
- Risk for altered parenting related to
  - Fear of spread of infection to newborn
- Altered patterns of urinary elimination related to
  - Presence of edema and pain
  - Impaired urinary function
- Fear/anxiety related to
  - Possible loss of pregnancy
  - Preterm labor/birth

Critical Thinking Exercises

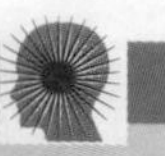

VAGINAL BLEEDING AND SEXUALLY TRANSMITTED DISEASE

You are assigned to care for a patient admitted with diagnoses of vaginal bleeding and preterm labor at 28 weeks. Vaginal speculum examination reveals bleeding from the cervical os and a thick, mucopurulent discharge. Laboratory tests show the presence of *Chlamydia trachomatis,* and intravenous antibiotics are begun. The patient is told of the findings and is upset and angry to learn that she has an STD. She is also very worried about her baby.

1. What further assessment data do you need to develop a plan of care?
2. What are some of the effects the situation may have on the patient's relationship with her partner?
3. Examine your personal reactions in light of this new information about the presence of an STD. How might these feelings affect your plan of care?
4. Formulate a plan of care, and provide rationales for your interventions.

- Altered family processes related to
  - Unexpected complication to expected postpartum recovery
  - Possible separation from newborn
  - Interruption in process of realigning relationships after addition of new family member

Expected Outcomes

A plan of care is formulated that relates specifically to the woman's physical and psychosocial needs. Goals are mutually determined with the woman. Expected outcomes include the following:

1. The woman will have her infection treated successfully.
2. The woman will experience absence or reduction of pain, relief of edema, and healing of excoriated areas.

BOX 9-11
Assessment for the Woman at Risk for Sexually Transmitted Disease

HISTORY

Chief complaint
Description of the present illness, including symptoms, self-care treatment, use of prescribed or over-the-counter medications
Sexual history, including previous history of STD, number of current sexual partners, typical frequency of sexual activity
Life-style: use of IV drugs or partner who uses IV drugs, smoking, alcohol, poor nutrition, high level of stress
General health: date of last menstrual period, date of last Pap smear, history of contraception

PHYSICAL EXAMINATION

Inspection
Palpation

LABORATORY TESTS*

Saline wet preparation (*Trichomonas*)
Potassium hydroxide wet preparation (candidiasis, *Gardnerella*)
Urinalysis
Gonorrhea culture
Cervical culture
Herpes cervical culture
Pap smear
Complete blood cell count
VDRL test
Herpes simplex virus type 1 and 2 antibodies
Western blot—HIV
Chlamydia—culture or antigen detection test

Modified from Smith L, Lauver D, Gray P: *Sexually transmitted disease.* In Fogel C, Lauver D, editors: *Sexual health promotion,* Philadelphia, 1989, Saunders.
VDRL, Veneral Disease Research Laboratories.
*Choice depends on specific STD.

3. The woman will be able to state the etiology and prevention, management, and sequelae of the infection.
4. The woman will state that she is less anxious because she does not lose the pregnancy or experience preterm labor/birth.
5. The fetus will be born free from infection and its sequelae or will experience minimal sequelae.
6. The woman and her family will verbalize acceptance of the unexpected events and positive coping measures (e.g., arrangement for home health care).

Plan of Care and Implementation

Interventions include continuous assessment for signs and symptoms of infection, assessment of pain, monitoring laboratory results, administering antimicrobial agents as ordered, initiating nonpharmacologic comfort measures, administering analgesics as ordered, and providing information to the mother and family as needed. General care, such as adequate hydration, rest, proper nutrition, and stress reduction also are implemented. Discussion of measures to avoid reinfection is essential. Topics of instruction should include proper medication administration, "safer" sex practices, and genital hygiene (see Patient Teaching boxes on pp. 545 and 546).

Evaluation

Evaluation of patient outcomes is a continuous process. To be effective, evaluation is based on patient-centered goals identified during the planning stage of nursing care. The nurse can be reasonably assured that care was effective to the extent that the expected outcomes have been met as follows:

1. The woman is free of infection, or her infection is stabilized and she does not become reinfected.
2. The woman experiences a reduction or the elimination of pain, any edema resolves, and excoriations heal.
3. The woman knows the etiology, management, and sequelae of the infection.
4. The woman reports feeling relieved that she did not lose the pregnancy or experience preterm labor/birth.
5. The fetus/neonate is born free of infection or its sequelae or experiences only minimal sequelae.

Key Points

- Hypertensive disorders during pregnancy are a leading cause of maternal and perinatal morbidity and mortality worldwide.
- The cause of preeclampsia is unknown, and there are no known reliable tests for predicting women at risk for developing preeclampsia/eclampsia.
- Preeclampsia/eclampsia is a multisystem disease, and the pathologic changes are present long before clinical manifestations, such as hypertension, are evident.
- Once preeclampsia becomes clinically evident, therapeutic interventions are palliative (e.g., bed rest, diet), and may slow the progression of the disease, allowing the pregnancy to continue, but the underlying pathology continues.
- The HELLP syndrome, which usually becomes apparent during the third trimester, is considered life-threatening.
- Magnesium sulfate, the anticonvulsant of choice for preventing eclampsia, requires careful monitoring of reflexes, respirations, and renal function; its antidote, calcium gluconate, should be at the bedside.
- Intent of emergency interventions for eclampsia is to prevent self-injury, ensure adequate oxygenation, reduce aspiration risk, and establish control with magnesium sulfate.
- Blood loss during pregnancy should always be regarded as a warning sign until ruled out by the woman's health care provider.
- Ectopic pregnancy is a significant cause of maternal morbidity and mortality even in developed countries.
- Abruptio placentae and placenta previa are differentiated by type of bleeding, uterine tonicity, and presence or absence of pain.
- Clotting disorders are associated with many obstetric complications.
- The physiologic adaptations of pregnancy mask warning signs and changes in vital signs during early shock states.
- The potential hazards of therapeutic interventions may further compromise the woman experiencing hemorrhagic disorders.
- Pregnancy confers no immunity against infection, and both mother and fetus must be considered when the pregnant woman contracts an infection.
- HIV is transmitted through blood, semen, and perinatal events.
- *Chlamydia trachomatis* is the most common sexually transmitted bacterial pathogen in the United States and is responsible for substantial morbidity, personal suffering, and heavy economic burden.
- STDs often occur in groups; what appear to be resistant infections actually may be multiple infections or reinfections.
- Abuse of alcohol and drugs compromises the body's immune system and increases the risk for AIDS and associated conditions.
- Because medical history and examination cannot reliably identify all persons with HIV or other bloodborne pathogens, blood and body fluid precautions should be used consistently for everyone.
- STDs and genital and perigenital infections are biologic events, for which all individuals have a right to expect objective, compassionate, and effective health care.

References

Acosta Y et al: HIV disease and pregnancy. II. Antepartum and intrapartum care, *J Obstet Gynecol Neonatal Nurs* 21(2):97, 1992.

Adimora A et al: *Sexually transmitted diseases*, ed 2 (companion handbook), New York, 1994, McGraw-Hill.

American College of Obstetricians and Gynecologists (ACOG): Invasive hemodynamic monitoring in obstetrics and gynecology, *ACOG Tech Bull* 175, 1992a.

American College of Obstetricians and Gynecologists (ACOG): Group B streptococcal infections in pregnancy, *ACOG Tech Bull* 170, 1992b.

American College of Obstetricians and Gynecologists (ACOG): Management of gestational trophoblastic disease, *ACOG Tech Bull* 178, 1993.

American College of Obstetricians and Gynecologists (ACOG): Antenatal corticosteroid therapy for fetal maturation, *ACOG Tech Bull* 147: 1994.

Andrews W et al: Association of post-cesarean delivery endometritis with colonization of the chorioamnion by *Ureaplasma urealyticum*, *Obstet Gynecol* 85(4):509, 1995.

Angelini D, Knapp C: *Case studies in perinatal nursing*, Gaithersburg, Md, 1992, Aspen.

Arias F: *Practical guide to high-risk pregnancy and delivery*, ed 2, St Louis, 1993, Mosby.

Armstrong B, McDonald A, Sloan M: Cigarette, alcohol and coffee consumption and spontaneous abortion, *Am J Public Health* 82:85, 1992.

Atrash H, Rowley D, Hogue C: Maternal and perinatal mortality, *Curr Opin Obstet Gynecol* 4:61, 1992.

Barnhart K, Sondheimer S: Contraception choice and sexually transmitted diseases, *Curr Opin Obstet Gynecol* 5(6):823, 1993.

Barton J, Sibai B: Care of the pregnancy complicated by HELLP syndrome, *Obstet Gynecol Clin North Am* 18(2):165, 1991.

Bastin N et al: HIV disease and pregnancy. III. Postpartum care of the HIV-positive woman and her newborn, *J Obstet Gynecol Neonatal Nurs* 21(2):105, 1992.

Belizan J et al: Calcium supplementation to prevent hypertensive disorders of pregnancy, *N Engl J Med* 325:1399, 1991.

Berkowitz R, Goldstein D, Bernstein M: Advances in management of partial molar pregnancy, *Contemp OB GYN* 38(5):33, 1991.

Boley T, Popek E: Parvovirus infection in pregnancy, *Semin Perinatol* 17(6):410, 1993.

Boyer P et al: Factors predictive of maternal-fetal transmission of HIV-1: preliminary analysis of zidovudine given during pregnancy and/or delivery, *JAMA* 271(24):1925, 1994.

Brown M: Pregnancy-induced hypertension: pathogenesis and management, *Aust NZ J Med* 21:257, 1991.

Brunham R, Holmes K, Embree J: *Sexually transmitted diseases in pregnancy*. In Holmes K et al, editors: *Sexually transmitted diseases*, ed 2, New York, 1990, McGraw-Hill.

Centers for Disease Control and Prevention (CDC): Recommendations for the prevention and management of *C. trachomatis* infections, *MMWR* 42(RR-12):1, 1993a.

Centers for Disease Control and Prevention (CDC): 1993 sexually transmitted diseases treatment guidelines, *MMWR* 42(RR-14):1, 1993b.

Centers for Disease Control and Prevention (CDC): Zidovudine for the prevention of HIV transmission from mother to infant, *MMWR* 43(16):1, 1994a.

Centers for Disease Control and Prevention (CDC): Recommendations of the US Public Health Service Task Force on the use of zidovudine to reduce perinatal transmission of human immunodeficiency virus, *MMWR* 43(RR-11):1, 1994b.

Clark S et al, editors: *Critical care obstetrics*, ed 2, Boston, 1991, Blackwell.

Clark S et al, editors: *Handbook of critical care obstetrics*, Boston, 1994, Blackwell.

Conde-Agudelo A, Lodo R, Belizan J: Evaluation of methods used in the prediction of hypertensive disorders of pregnancy, *Obstet Gynecol Surv* 49(3):210, 1994.

Couvreur J et al: In utero treatment of toxoplasmic fetopathy with the combination pyrimethamine-sulfadiazine, *Fetal Diagn Ther* 8(1):45, 1993.

Craven D et al: Human immunodeficiency virus infection in pregnancy: epidemiology and prevention of vertical transmission, *Infect Control Hosp Epidemiol* 15(1):36, 1994.

Cunningham F, Lindheimer M: Hypertension in pregnancy, *N Engl J Med* 326(14):927, 1992.

Cunningham F et al: *Williams obstetrics*, ed 19, Norwalk, Conn, 1993, Appleton & Lange.

Dildy N et al: *Complications in pregnancy-induced hypertension*. In Clark S et al, editors: *Critical care obstetrics*, ed 2, Boston, 1991, Blackwell.

Dorfman S: *Pregnancy for older parents*. In Cherry S, Merkatz I, editors: *Complications of pregnancy: medical, surgical, gynecologic, psychosocial, and perinatal*, Philadelphia, 1991, Williams & Wilkins.

Easterling T, Benedetti T: Preeclampsia: a hyperdynamic disease model, *Am J Obstet Gynecol* 160:1447, 1989.

Eschenbach D: *Pelvic infections and sexually transmitted diseases*. In Scott J et al, editors: *Danforth's obstetrics and gynecology*, ed 7, Philadelphia, 1994, Lippincott.

Evans B et al: Risk profiles for genital infection in women, *Genitourin Med* 69(4):257, 1993.

Fairlie F: Doppler flow velocimetry in hypertension in pregnancy, *Clin Perinatol* 18:749, 1991.

Fairlie F, Sibai B: *Hypertensive diseases in pregnancy*. In Reece E et al, editors: *Medicine of the fetus and mother*, Philadelphia, 1993, Lippincott.

Farmakides G et al: Pregnancy surveillance with Doppler velocimetry, *Female Patient* 15(5):49, 1990.

Farmakides G et al: Surveillance of the pregnant hypertensive patient with Doppler flow velocimetry, *Clin Obstet Gynecol* 35:387, 1992.

Gerber M, Zalneraitis E: Childhood neurologic disorders and Lyme disease during pregnancy, *Pediatr Neurol* 11(1):41, 1994.

Gerberding J: Incidence and prevalence of human immunodeficiency virus, hepatitis B virus, hepatitis C virus, and cytomegalovirus among health care personnel at risk for blood exposure: final report from a longitudinal study, *J Infect Dis* 170(6):1410, 1994.

Gilbert E, Harmon J: *Manual of high risk pregnancy and delivery*, St Louis, 1993a, Mosby.

Gilbert E, Harmon J: *Manual of high risk pregnancy and delivery*, St Louis, 1993b, Mosby.

Graves K et al: The relationship of substance use to sexual activity among young adults in the United States, *Fam Plann Perspect* 27:18, 1995.

Green J: *Placenta previa and abruptio placentae*. In Creasy R, Resnik R, editors: *Maternal-fetal medicine: principles and practice*, Philadelphia, 1994, Saunders.

Grohar J: Nursing protocols for antepartum homecare, *J Obstet Gynecol Neonatal Nurs* 23(8):687, 1994.

Guyton A: *Human physiology and mechanisms of disease*, ed 5, Philadelphia, 1992, Saunders.

Hadi H et al: Clinical significance of human parvovirus B19 infection in pregnancy, *Am J Perinatol* 11(6):398, 1994.

Hammond C, Bachus K: *Ectopic pregnancy*. In Scott J, editor: *Danforth's obstetrics and gynecology*, ed 7, Philadelphia, 1994, Lippincott.

Harvey C, Burke M: *Hypertensive disorders in pregnancy*. In Mandeville L, Troiano N, editors: *High-risk intrapartum nursing*, Philadelphia, 1992, Lippincott.

Hersey J, Martin L: Use of infection control guidelines by workers in healthcare facilities to prevent occupational transmission of HBV and HIV: results from a national survey, *Infect Control Hosp Epidemiol* 15(4, pt 1):243, 1994.

Hill H: *Group B streptococcal infections.* In Holmes K et al, editors: *Sexually transmitted diseases,* ed 2, New York, 1990, McGraw-Hill.

Hosein I et al: Detection of cervical *Chlamydia trachomatis* and *Neisseria gonorrhoeae* with deoxyribonucleic acid probe assays in obstetric patients, *Am J Obstet Gynecol* 167(3):588, 1992.

Hunter S, Weiner C: *Obstetric hemorrhage.* In Repke J, editor: *Intrapartum obstetrics,* New York, 1996, Churchill Livingstone.

Iams J, Zuspan F, Quilligan E: *Zuspan and Quilligan's manual of obstetrics and gynecology,* ed 2, St Louis, 1990, Mosby.

Imperiale T, Petrulis A: A meta-analysis of low-dose aspirin for the prevention of pregnancy-induced hypertensive disease, *JAMA* 266:260, 1991.

Jana N et al: Perinatal outcome in pregnancies complicated by pulmonary tuberculosis, *Int J Gynaecol Obstet* 44(2):119, 1994.

Johnstone H, Marcinak J: Candidiasis in the breastfeeding mother and infant, *J Obstet Gynecol Neonatal Nurs* 19:171, 1990.

Jordan E, Sever J: Fetal damage caused by parvoviral infections, *Reprod Toxicol* 8(2):161, 1994.

Kashima H, Shah K, Goodstein M: *Recurrent respiratory papillomatosis.* In Holmes K et al, editors: *Sexually transmitted diseases,* ed 2, New York, 1990, McGraw-Hill.

Klonoff-Cohen H et al: An epidemiologic study of contraception and preeclampsia, *JAMA* 262:3143, 1989.

Knuppel R, Hatangadi S: Acute hypotension related to hemorrhage in the obstetric patient, *Obstet Gynecol Clin North Am* 22(1):111, 1995.

Konje J, Walley R: *Bleeding in late pregnancy.* In James D et al, editors: *High risk pregnancy: management options,* Philadelphia, 1995, Saunders.

Krettek J et al: *Chlamydia trachomatis* in patients who used oral contraceptives and had intermenstrual spotting, *Obstet Gynecol* 81(5, pt 1):728, 1993.

Kulb N: *Abnormalities of the placenta and membranes.* In Buckley K, Kulb N, editors: *High risk maternity nursing manual,* Baltimore, 1990, Williams & Wilkins.

Lamphear B: Trends and patterns in the transmission of bloodborne pathogens to health care providers, *Epidemiol Rev* 16(2):437, 1994.

Lavery J: Placenta previa, *Clin Obstet Gynecol* 33(414), 1990.

Leduc L et al: Coagulation profile in severe preeclampsia, *Obstet Gynecol* 79:14, 1992.

Lowe T, Cunningham G: Placental abruption, *Clin Obstet Gynecol* 33(3):406, 1990.

Machin G et al: Perinatally acquired neonatal tuberculosis: report of two cases, *Pediatr Pathol* 12(5):707, 1992.

Magness R, Gant N: Control of vascular reactivity in pregnancy: the basis for therapeutic approaches to prevent pregnancy-induced hypertension, *Semin Perinatol* 18(2):45, 1994.

Maloni J: Home care of the high-risk pregnant woman requiring bed rest, *J Obstet Gynecol Neonatal Nurs* 23:696, 1994.

Mandelbrot L et al: Thrombocytopenia in pregnant women infected with human immunodeficiency virus: maternal and neonatal outcome, *Am J Obstet Gynecol* 171(1):252, 1994.

Margono F et al: Resurgence of active tuberculosis among pregnant women, *Obstet Gynecol* 83(6):911, 1994.

Martin J et al: The natural history of HELLP syndrome: patterns of disease progression and regression, *Am J Obstet Gynecol* 164:1500, 1991.

Marx G et al: Automated blood pressure measurements in laboring women: are they reliable? *Am J Obstet Gynecol* 168:796, 1993.

Matsui D: Prevention, diagnosis, and treatment of fetal toxoplasmosis, *Clin Perinatol* 21(3):675, 1994.

McLaren R, Feinstein S, Lodeiro J: Abruptio placentae with disseminated intravascular coagulation, *Female Patient* 16:22, 1991.

Mills J et al: Incidence of spontaneous abortion among normal women and insulin-dependent diabetic women whose pregnancies were identified within 21 days of conception, *N Engl J Med* 319:1617, 1988.

Mofenson L et al: *Mycobacterium tuberculosis* infection in pregnant and nonpregnant women, *Arch Intern Med* 155(10):1066, 1995.

National Center for Health Statistics: *Advance report of fetal natality statistics, 1991,* Hyattsville, Md, 1993, US Public Health Service.

Newman V, Fullerton J: Role of nutrition in the prevention of preeclampsia: review of the literature, *J Nurs Midwife* 35(5):282, 1990.

O'Brien W: The prediction of preeclampsia, *Clin Obstet Gynecol* 35:351, 1992.

O'Brien W: *Puerperal complications.* In Moore T et al, editors: *Gynecology and obstetrics: a longitudinal approach,* New York, 1993, Churchill Livingstone.

Panero C et al: Fetoneonatal hydrops from human parvovirus B19: case report, *J Perinat Med* 22(3):257, 1994.

Pastuszak A et al: Outcome after maternal varicella infection in the first 20 weeks of pregnancy, *N Engl J Med* 330(13):901, 1994.

Perry K, Martin J: Abnormal hemotasis and coagulopathy in preeclampsia and eclampsia, *Clin Obstet Gynecol* 35:338, 1992.

Peters M, Nicolaides K: Cordocentesis for the diagnosis and treatment of human fetal parvovirus infection, *Obstet Gynecol* 75:501, 1990.

Pickles C et al: Labetalol therapy for pregnancy induced hypertension, *Br J Obstet Gynaecol* 99:964, 1992.

Poole J: HELLP syndrome and coagulopathies of pregnancy, *Crit Care Nurs Clin North Am* 5:457, 1993.

Raynor B: Cytomegalovirus infection in pregnancy, *Semin Perinatol* 17(6):394, 1993.

Redondo-Lopez V et al: *Torulopsis glabrata* vaginitis: clinical aspects and susceptibility to antifungal agents, *Obstet Gynecol* 76:651, 1990.

Rein M, Müller M: Trichomonas vaginalis *and trichomoniasis.* In Holmes K et al, editors: *Sexually transmitted diseases,* ed 2, New York, 1990, McGraw-Hill.

Roberts J et al: *New developments in preeclampsia,* NIH Grant HP 24180, San Francisco, 1990, University of California.

Roberts S et al: Genital herpes during pregnancy: no lesions, no cesarean, *Obstet Gynecol* 85(2):261, 1995.

Robichaux A, Stedman C, Hamner C: Uterine activity in patients with cervical cerclage, *Obstet Gynecol* 76 (suppl 7):63, 1990.

Rosenak D: Cocaine: maternal use during pregnancy and its effect on the mother, the fetus, and the infant, *Obstet Gynecol Surv* 45:348, 1990.

Saftlas A et at: Epidemiology of preeclampsia and eclampsia in the United States, *Am J Obstet Gynecol* 163:460, 1990.

Sanchez-Ramos L et al: Prevention of pregnancy induced hypertension by calcium supplementation in angiotensin II sensitive patients, *Obstet Gynecol* 84(3):349, 1994.

Schuster V et al: Congenital varicella syndrome: studies of the virus-specific humoral and cell-mediated immune responses, *Acta Paediatr* 83(7):783, 1994.

Scott J: *Placenta previa and placental abruption.* In Scott J et al, editors: *Danforth's obstetrics and gynecology,* ed 7, Philadelphia, 1994, Lippincott.

Scott J et al, editors: *Danforth's obstetrics and gynecology,* ed 7, Philadelphia, 1994, Lippincott.

Sibai B: Pitfalls in diagnosis and management of preeclampsia, *Am J Obstet Gynecol* 159:1, 1988.

Sibai B: Eclampsia. VI. Maternal-perinatal outcome in 254 consecutive cases, *Am J Obstet Gynecol* 163:1049, 1990a.

Sibai B: Magnesium sulfate is the ideal anticonvulsant in preeclampsia/eclampsia, *Am J Obstet Gynecol* 162:1141, 1990b.

Sibai B: Preeclampsia/eclampsia: valid treatment approaches, *Contemp OB GYN* 35:84, 1990c.

Sibai B: The HELLP syndrome (hemolysis, elevated liver enzymes, and low platelets): much ado about nothing? *Am J Obstet Gynecol* 162:311, 1990d.

Sibai B: Immunologic aspects of preeclampsia, *Clin Obstet Gynecol* 34:27, 1991a.

Sibai B: Management of preeclampsia, *Clin Perinatol* 18:793, 1991b.

Sibai B: Hypertension in pregnancy, *Obstet Gynecol Clin North Am* 19(2):615, 1992.

Sibai B, Anderson G: *Hypertension.* In Gabbe S, Niebyl J, Simpson J, editors: *Obstetrics—normal and problem pregnancies,* ed 2, New York, 1991, Churchill Livingstone.

Sibai B, Rodriguez J: *Preeclampsia: diagnosis and management.* In Reece E et al, editors: *Medicine of the fetus and mother,* Philadelphia, 1992, Lippincott.

Simpson K: *Protocols for homecare management of high-risk pregnancies,* St Louis, 1992, Mosby.

Smith C et al: Reliability of compact electronic blood pressure monitors for hypertensive pregnant women, *J Reprod Med* 35:399, 1990.

Spence M: Epidemiology of sexually transmitted diseases, *Obstet Gynecol Clin North Am* 16:453, 1989.

Stoval T, Ling F: Some new approaches to ectopic pregnancy, *Contemp OB GYN* 37:35, 1992.

Strobino B et al: Lyme disease and pregnancy outcome: a prospective study of two thousand prenatal patients, *Am J Obstet Gynecol* 169(2, pt 1):367, 1993.

Suresh M, Kinch R: *Antepartum hemorrhage.* In Datta S, editor: *Anesthetic and obstetric management for high-risk pregnancy,* St Louis, 1991, Mosby.

Thorp J: *Third-trimester bleeding.* In Moore T et al, editors: *Gynecology and obstetrics: a longitudinal approach,* New York, 1993, Churchill Livingstone.

Tinkle M et al: HIV disease and pregnancy. I. Epidemiology, pathogenesis, and natural history, *J Obstet Gynecol Neonatal Nurs* 21(2):86, 1992.

Villari P et al: Cesarean section to reduce perinatal transmission of human immunodeficiency virus: a metaanalysis, *J Curr Clin Trials,* Doc No 74:2, 1994.

Walsh S: Physiology of low-dose aspirin therapy for the prevention of preeclampsia, *Semin Perinatol* 14(2):152, 1990.

Watson J et al: Vertical transmission of hepatitis A resulting in an outbreak in a neonatal intensive care unit, *J Infect Dis* 167(3):567, 1993.

Webster L et al: An evaluation of surveillance for *Chlamydia trachomatis* infection in the US, 1987-1991, *MMWR* 42(SS-3):21, 1993.

Weiner C: Preeclampsia/eclampsia syndrome and coagulation, *Clin Perinatol* 18:713, 1991.

Willis D, Blanco J: *Preeclampsia/eclampsia.* In Benrubi GI, editor: *Contemporary issues in emergency medicine: obstetric emergencies,* New York, 1990, Churchill Livingstone.

Working Group on High Blood Pressure in Pregnancy: National high blood pressure education program working group report on high blood pressure in pregnancy, *Am J Obstet Gynecol* 163:1689, 1990.

Yaegashi N et al: The frequency of human parvovirus B19 infection in nonimmune hydrops fetalis, *J Perinat Med* 22(2):159, 1994.

Zuspan F: New concepts in the understanding of hypertensive diseases during pregnancy: an overview, *Clin Perinatol* 18:653, 1991.

Bibliography

Alfirevic Z, Nielson J: Doppler ultrasonography in high risk pregnancies: systematic review with meta-analysis, *Am J Obstet Gynecol* 172:1379, 1995.

Bernstein J: Ectopic pregnancy: a nursing approach to excess risk among minority women, *J Obstet Gynecol Neonatal Nurs* 24(9):803, 1995

Creehan P: Toxic shock syndrome: an opportunity for nursing intervention, *J Obstet Gynecol Neonatal Nurs* 24(6):557, 1995.

Finch C: Human parvovirus B19 in pregnancy, *J Obstet Gynecol Neonatal Nurs* 24(6):495, 1995.

Josten E et al: Bedrest compliance for women with pregnancy problems, *Birth* 22:1, 1995.

Lindberg C: Perinatal transmission of HIV: how to counsel women, *MCN Am J Matern Child Nurs* 20(4):207, 1995.

Major C et al: Preterm premature rupture of membranes and abruptio placentae: is there an association between these pregnancy complications? *Am J Obstet Gynecol* 172:672, 1995.

McCain G, Deatrick J: The experience of high risk pregnancy, *J Obstet Gynecol Neonatal Nurs* 23:421, 1994.

Pellicano M et al: Vulvo-vaginitis and reproduction, *Clin Exp Obstet Gynecol* 22(1):51, 1995.

Poole J, Hall S, White D: *Crisis OB video series. II. Hemorrhagic disorders in pregnancy,* St Louis, 1995, Mosby.

Shermer R: Group B streptococcus during the prenatal period, *J Obstet Gynecol Neonatal Nurs* 24(6):562, 1995.

Sherwin L: Human immunodeficiency virus infection during the perinatal period: a review of literature concerning pregnant women and neonates, *J Perinatol* 15(1):54, 1995.

Sibai B et al: Risk factors for preeclampsia in healthy nulliparous women: a prospective multicenter study, *Am J Obstet Gynecol* 172:642, 1995.

Simpson K: Sepsis during pregnancy, *J Obstet Gynecol Neonatal Nurs* 24(6):550, 1995.

Stringer M, Spatz D, Donohue D: Maternal-fetal physical assessment in the home setting: role of the advanced practice nurse, *J Obstet Gynecol Neonatal Nurs* 23:720, 1994.

CHAPTER 10

Endocrine, Cardiovascular, and Medical-Surgical Problems During Pregnancy

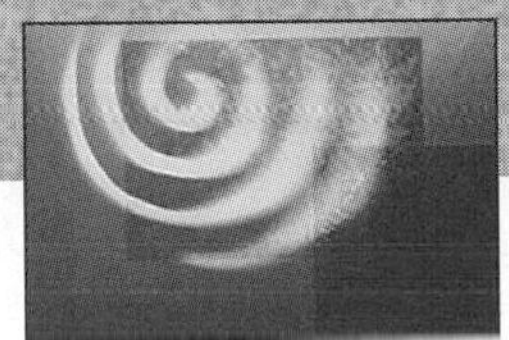

ENDOCRINE DISORDERS, P. 251

Diabetes mellitus, p. 251

Nursing care management, p. 257

Gestational diabetes mellitus, p. 265

Nursing care management, p. 266

Hyperemesis gravidarum, p. 268

Nursing care management, p. 268

Thyroid disorders, p. 269

CARDIOVASCULAR DISORDERS, P. 270

Nursing care management, p. 271

Heart surgery during pregnancy, p. 276

Associated cardiovascular disorders, p. 276

Cardiopulmonary resuscitation of the pregnant woman, p. 278

MEDICAL DISORDERS DURING PREGNANCY, P. 279

Anemia, p. 279

Pulmonary disorders, p. 281

Gastrointestinal disorders, p. 283

Integumentary disorders, p. 283

Neurologic disorders, p. 283

Autoimmune disorders, p. 284

Abdominal surgery during pregnancy, p. 285

Nursing care management, p. 286

Discharge planning, p. 287

Trauma during pregnancy, p. 287

Nursing care management, p. 287

THERAPEUTIC AND ELECTIVE ABORTION, P. 289

Nursing care management, p. 289

Complications following abortion, p. 291

Mifepristone (RU 486), p. 292

Nursing considerations, p. 292

Endocrine and metabolic disorders and other medical-surgical problems complicate many pregnancies and require careful management to promote maternal and fetal well-being and positive pregnancy outcome.

The maternity nurse is challenged to provide sound, effective care that meets the unique maternal and fetal needs prompted by these conditions. The primary objective of nursing care must be to guide and support the woman and her family in achieving optimal outcome for both the pregnant woman and the fetus. The nurse serves as teacher, counselor, and support person to assist the woman and her family in achieving the best possible outcome and to deal with the problems and disappointments that may arise.

ENDOCRINE DISORDERS

Diabetes Mellitus

Pregnancy and diabetes were incompatible before the discovery of insulin in the early 1920s. Many women of childbearing age who had diabetes were infertile or sterile, and the majority of those who became pregnant were unable to carry the pregnancy to term. Maternal and perinatal mortality was as high as 50%, with stillbirth the primary cause of perinatal death (Gabbe, 1992).

Advances in modern medicine have prompted substantial improvements in maternal and perinatal outcomes of diabetic pregnancy. In well-managed cases, the maternal and perinatal mortality rates are similar to those of the population without diabetes. However, the incidence of major congenital anomalies among infants of mothers with diabetes has not changed significantly over time. Thus experts have concluded that the key to optimal outcome of pregnancy in a woman who has diabetes is not only strict maternal glycemic control (normoglycemia) during pregnancy but also before pregnancy. Consequently, preconception counseling has become a major thrust in the management of diabetes during pregnancy.

Despite the advances in care, pregnancy complicated by diabetes is still considered to be high risk. It is most successfully managed with a multidisciplinary approach involving the obstetrician, internist or diabetologist, neonatologist, nurse, nutritionist, and social worker. Favorable outcome of pregnancy affected by diabetes requires commitment and active participation by the woman (and her family). She must comply with a schedule of frequent prenatal visits, strict adherence to dietary regimen, regular self-monitoring of blood glucose level, frequent laboratory evaluation, intensive fetal surveillance, and possible hospitalization.

Care of the pregnant woman who has diabetes requires that the nurse fully understand the normal physiologic responses to pregnancy as well as the altered metabolism of diabetes. Furthermore, the nurse must understand the relationship between pregnancy and diabetes to accurately assess the woman, plan for her care, and intervene appropriately. An awareness of the psychosocial implications of diabetes during pregnancy must guide the nurse in planning, implementing, and evaluating care of the woman and her family.

Pathogenesis of diabetes mellitus. Diabetes mellitus is a systemic disorder of carbohydrate, protein, and fat metabolism. It is characterized by **hyperglycemia** (elevated blood glucose) resulting from inadequate production of **insulin** or ineffective use of insulin at the cellular level. Insulin, produced by the beta cells in the islets of Langerhans in the pancreas, regulates blood glucose levels by enabling glucose to enter adipose and muscle cells where it is used for energy. Insulin also stimulates protein synthesis and storage of free fatty acids. When insulin is insufficient or ineffective in promoting glucose uptake by the muscle and adipose cells, glucose accumulates in the bloodstream and hyperglycemia results. Hyperglycemia causes hyperosmolarity of the blood, which attracts intracellular fluid into the vascular system, resulting in cellular dehydration and expanded blood volume. Consequently the kidneys function to excrete large volumes of urine *(polyuria)* in an attempt to regulate excess vascular volume and to excrete the unusable glucose *(glycosuria)*. Polyuria and cellular dehydration cause excessive thirst *(polydipsia)*.

The body compensates for its inability to convert carbohydrate (glucose) into energy by burning proteins (muscle) and fats. The end products of this metabolism are ketones and fatty acids, which in excess quantity produce **ketoacidosis** and *acetonuria.* Weight loss occurs because of the breakdown of fat and muscle tissue. This tissue breakdown causes a state of starvation that compels the individual to eat excessively *(polyphagia)*.

Over time, diabetes causes significant changes in both the microvascular and macrovascular circulation. These structural changes affect a variety of organ systems, primarily the heart, eyes, kidneys, and nerves. Complications resulting from diabetes include premature atherosclerosis, retinopathy, nephropathy, and neuropathy.

Although the exact cause of diabetes mellitus is uncertain, it is thought that the pancreatic beta cell damage may be the result of an interplay between genetic predisposition and environmental insult. Diabetes mellitus is not inherited, although specific genetic alterations (primarily chromosome 6) increase the potential that some individuals will experience beta cell damage and develop diabetes. The pathologic process responsible for this beta cell destruction is likely an autoimmune response to environmental factors such as viral infection, stress, or nutritional deficiencies. Early exposure to cow milk protein (during the first year) may increase the likelihood for genetically predisposed people to develop diabetes mellitus (Drash et al, 1994; Karjalainen et al, 1992).

Classification of diabetes mellitus. Although diabetes is clearly a disorder of insulin availability, it is not a single disease. Diabetes has been classified into three major types by the National Diabetes Data Group of the National Institutes of Health (ADA, 1990) (Table 10-1).

Type I: insulin-dependent diabetes mellitus. Formerly known as juvenile diabetes, type I insulin dependent diabetes mellitus (IDDM) is characterized by an absolute insulin deficiency state. Its onset is typically in people age 30 or younger. People with IDDM often experience marked alterations in blood glucose levels and are prone to ketosis.

Type II: non–insulin-dependent diabetes mellitus. Previously known as maturity-onset or adult-onset diabetes, type II non–insulin-dependent diabetes mellitus (NIDDM) occurs in all ages, but it is more common in the older overweight individual. It is associated with a lack of insulin availability or effectiveness rather than an absolute insulin deficiency. NIDDM is said to be ketosis resistant and is often controlled by diet alone.

Gestational diabetes mellitus. Glucose intolerance of variable severity with its onset or first recognition during pregnancy is considered to be **gestational diabetes mellitus (GDM).** This definition is appropriate whether insulin is used for treatment or the diabetes persists after the pregnancy. It does not exclude the possibility that the glucose intolerance preceded the pregnancy.

To identify those women with diabetes who are at greatest risk during pregnancy, a modification of White's classification (1978) can be used. This system is based on age of onset of diabetes, duration, and the severity of vascular disease (Table 10-2). Diabetes during pregnancy can also be classified according to whether the diabetes preceded the pregnancy or had its onset during gestation. **Pregestational diabetes** is the label sometimes given to type I or type II diabetes that existed before pregnancy, and gestational diabetes refers to glu-

TABLE 10-1 National Institutes of Health classification of diabetes

CLASSIFICATION	PREVIOUS NAMES	DEFINITION
Type I: IDDM	Juvenile-onset diabetes Brittle diabetes	Insulin-dependent diabetes mellitus (IDDM); pancreatic beta cells in islets of Langerhans virtually do not produce insulin
Type II: NIDDM	Adult-onset diabetes	Non–insulin-dependent diabetes mellitus (NIDDM); pancreatic beta cells in islets of Langerhans are unable to meet increased demands for insulin over time or in times of stress
Type III: GDM	Gestational diabetes	Carbohydrate intolerance that develops during pregnancy, regardless of severity

cose intolerance first recognized during the pregnancy. Although this is not a formal classification system, it is helpful in understanding the similarities and differences between the types of diabetes during pregnancy.

Metabolic changes associated with pregnancy. Normal pregnancy is characterized by complex alterations in maternal glucose metabolism, insulin production, and metabolic homeostasis. During normal pregnancy, adjustments in maternal metabolism allow for provision of adequate nutrition for both the mother and the developing fetus. Glucose, the primary fuel utilized by the fetus, is transported across the placenta through the process of carrier-mediated facilitated diffusion. This means that the glucose levels in the fetus are directly proportional to maternal levels. Although glucose crosses the placenta, insulin does not. By the tenth week of gestation the embryo/fetus secretes its own insulin at levels adequate to use the glucose obtained from the mother. Thus as maternal glucose levels rise, fetal glucose levels are increased, resulting in increased fetal insulin secretion.

During the first trimester of pregnancy, the pregnant woman's metabolic status is significantly influenced by the rising levels of estrogen and progesterone. These hormones stimulate the beta cells in the pancreas to increase insulin production, which promotes increased peripheral utilization of glucose and decreased blood glucose with fasting levels being reduced by approximately 10% (Figure 10-1, *A*). There is a concomitant increase in tissue glycogen stores and a decrease in hepatic glucose production, which further encourages lower fasting glucose levels. As a result of these normal metabolic changes of pregnancy, women with insulin-dependent diabetes are prone to hypoglycemia during the first trimester.

During the second and third trimesters, pregnancy exerts a "diabetogenic" effect on the maternal metabolic status. Because of the major hormonal changes, there is decreased tolerance to glucose, increased insulin resistance, decreased hepatic glycogen stores, and increased hepatic production of glucose. Rising levels of human placental lactogen (hPL), estrogen, progesterone, prolactin, cortisol, and insulinase increase insulin resistance through their actions as insulin antagonists. Insulin resistance is a glucose-sparing mechanism that assures an abundant supply of glucose for the fetus. Maternal insulin requirements may double or quadruple by the end of pregnancy, usually leveling off or declining slightly after 36 weeks (Figure 10-1, *B* and *C*).

At birth, expulsion of the placenta prompts an abrupt drop in levels of circulating placental hormones, cortisol, and insulinase. Maternal tissues quickly regain their prepregnancy sensitivity to insulin (Fig. 10-1, *D*). For the nonbreastfeeding mother, prepregnancy insulin-carbohydrate balance usually returns in about 7 to 10 days (Fig. 10-1, *E*). Lactation uses maternal glucose, so the breastfeeding mother's insulin requirements remain low for up to 6 to 9 months (Fig. 10-1, *E*). On completion of weaning, the mother's prepregnancy insulin requirement is reestablished (Fig. 10-1, F).

Pregestational diabetes. When a patient with recognized diabetes becomes pregnant, she is said to have pregestational diabetes; that is, the diabetes existed before conception and will continue after the pregnancy. Pregestational diabetes may be either IDDM or NIDDM, which may or may not be complicated by vascular disease, retinopathy, nephropathy, or other diabetic sequelae. Patients with NIDDM who become pregnant typically require insulin during gestation; thus the large majority of woman with pregestational diabetes are insulin-dependent during pregnancy.

The diabetogenic state of pregnancy imposed on the compromised metabolic system of the woman with pregestational diabetes has significant implications. The normal hormonal adaptations of pregnancy affect glycemic control in the patient who has pregestational diabetes. Pregnancy may also accelerate the progress of vascular complications of diabetes.

During the first trimester, while maternal blood glucose levels are normally reduced and insulin response to glucose is enhanced, glycemic control is improved. Insulin dosage for the patient whose diabetes is well under control may need to be reduced to avoid **hypoglycemia** (low blood glucose). There is an increased incidence of hypoglycemic episodes in women with IDDM during early pregnancy. Nausea, vomiting, and cravings typical of early pregnancy result in dietary fluctua-

TABLE 10-2 Modified White's classification of diabetes in pregnancy

CLASS	AGE OF ONSET		DURATION (YEARS)	VASCULAR DISEASE	TREATMENT
Gestational diabetes					
A1	During pregnancy			None	Diet alone
A2	During pregnancy			None	Insulin
Pregestational diabetes					
B	≥20	or	<10	None	Insulin
C	10-19		10-19	None	Insulin
D	≤10	or	>20	Benign (hypertension, background retinopathy)	Insulin
F	Any		Any	Nephropathy	Insulin
R	Any		Any	Proliferative retinopathy	Insulin
H	Any		Any	Cardiac disease	Insulin
T	Any		Any	Renal transplant	Insulin

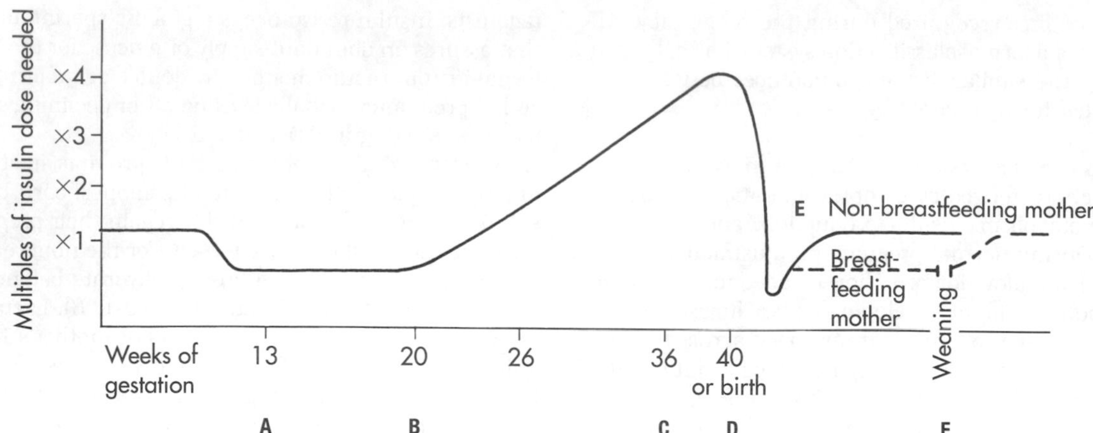

Fig. 10-1 Changing insulin needs during pregnancy. **A,** First trimester: insulin need is reduced because of increased insulin production by the pancreas and increased peripheral sensitivity to insulin; nausea, vomiting, and decreased food intake by mother as well as glucose transfer to embryo/fetus contribute to hypoglycemia. **B,** Second trimester: insulin need increases as placental hormones, cortisol, and insulinase act as insulin antagonists, decreasing insulin's effectiveness. **C,** Third trimester: insulin need may double or even quadruple, but it usually levels off after 36 weeks. **D,** Day of delivery: maternal insulin requirements drop drastically to approach prepregnancy levels. **E,** Breastfeeding mother maintains lower insulin requirements, as much as 25% less than prepregnancy; insulin need of nonbreastfeeding mother returns to prepregnancy levels in 7 to 10 days. **F,** At weaning of breastfeeding infant, mother's insulin need returns to prepregnancy levels.

tions, which influence maternal glucose levels and necessitate reduction in insulin dosage.

As insulin requirements steadily increase after the first trimester, insulin dosage must be adjusted accordingly to prevent episodes of hyperglycemia. Insulin resistance begins as early as 14 to 16 weeks and continues to rise until it levels off during the last few weeks of pregnancy.

Progression or regression of retinopathy may occur during pregnancy. Women with minimal retinopathy are unlikely to experience significant retinal changes, whereas those with moderate or severe retinopathy are likely to experience worsening of the disease during pregnancy (Chew et al, 1995; Davidorf and Chambers, 1993).

In women who have diabetes with mild to moderate renal insufficiency, pregnancy has little effect on the progression of nephropathy; detrimental effects are more often noted among women with hypertension or renal insufficiency. Women with overt nephropathy can expect progression of their disease to end-stage renal disease in approximately 10 years, regardless of pregnancy. There is an increased risk of preeclampsia, preterm labor, **intrauterine growth restriction (IUGR),** fetal distress, stillbirth, and neonatal death associated with diabetic nephropathy (Kitzmiller and Coombs, 1993; Landon and Gabbe, 1992; Reece and Homko, 1993).

In patients with insulin-dependent diabetes, the normal hemodynamic adjustments to pregnancy are impaired and result in a smaller physiologic increase in cardiac output when compared with pregnant women who are not diabetic. There is also increased risk of thromboembolic complications among pregnant women with diabetes (Meyer and Palmer, 1990). Diabetic women with coronary artery disease who become pregnant are at a significantly increased risk for mortality during pregnancy (Landon and Gabbe, 1995).

Neuropathic complications are common among patients with IDDM and NIDDM. Autonomic neuropathy such as gastroparesis (e.g., anorexia, vomiting of undigested food, belching, early satiety, weight loss) may affect diabetic control because of its effects on intake and absorption of adequate nutrition (Reece and Homko, 1993).

Preconception counseling. Preconception counseling is recommended for all women of reproductive age with diabetes and is associated with improved pregnancy outcome (Rosenn et al, 1991; Willhoite et al, 1993). Under ideal circumstances, the woman with pregestational diabetes is counseled before conception to plan the optimal time for pregnancy, to establish glycemic control before conception, and to evaluate the woman for any evidence of vascular complications of diabetes. Preconception counseling is particularly important because strict metabolic control before conception and in the early weeks of gestation is instrumental in decreasing the risk of congenital anomalies in the fetus (Kitzmiller et al, 1991; Reece and Homko, 1993) and a decreased incidence of spontaneous abortion (Rosenn et al, 1991).

The partner of the woman with diabetes should be included in the counseling process to assess the couple's level of understanding related to the effects of pregnancy on the diabetic condition and the potential complications of pregnancy as a result of diabetes. The couple should also be informed of the anticipated alterations in management of diabetes during pregnancy and the need for a multidisciplinary team approach to health care. Financial implications of diabetic pregnancy and other demands related to maternal and fetal surveillance should be discussed. Contraception is another important aspect of preconception counseling to assist the couple in effectively planning for pregnancy.

Some types of oral hypoglycemic agents (sulfonylureas such as tolbutamide) may exert teratogenic effects on the fetus and should be discontinued in the preconceptional period in women with NIDDM who had previously used them for glucose control. These women are started on insulin before pregnancy when the pregnancy is planned and as soon as the pregnancy is diagnosed when it is unplanned.

Maternal risks and complications. The pregnant woman with diabetes is at risk for the development of complications. The best predictor of pregnancy outcome for the patient with diabetes and her neonate is the degree of maternal glycemic control during pregnancy.

Poor glycemic control around the time of conception and in the early weeks of pregnancy is associated with an increased incidence of *spontaneous abortion* in women who have diabetes. Those women with good glycemic control before conception and in the first trimester appear to be no more likely than women without diabetes to experience spontaneous abortion (Combs and Kitzmiller, 1991; Greene, 1993; Rosenn et al, 1994).

Pregnancy-induced hypertension, or preeclampsia, occurs more often during diabetic pregnancy. The highest incidence occurs in women with preexisting vascular changes related to diabetes (Cunningham et al, 1993).

Hydramnios (polyhydramnios), amniotic fluid in excess of 2000 ml, occurs about 10 times more often in diabetic pregnancies than in nondiabetic pregnancies. Overdistention of the uterus caused by hydramnios increases the risk of premature rupture of membranes, preterm labor, and postpartum hemorrhage.

Infections are much more common and serious in pregnant women who are diabetic. Disorders of carbohydrate metabolism alter the body's normal resistance to infection. The inflammatory response, leukocyte function, and vaginal pH are all affected. Vaginal infections, particularly monilial vaginitis, are more common in pregnant women with diabetes. Urinary tract infections (UTIs) also are more prevalent among pregnant diabetics. Infection in the patient with diabetes is serious because it leads to increased insulin resistance and may result in ketoacidosis. These infections can precipitate preterm labor. Postpartum infection is more common among women with insulin-dependent diabetes (Stamler et al, 1990).

Ketoacidosis occurs most often during the second and third trimesters when the "diabetogenic" effect of pregnancy is the greatest. When the maternal metabolism is stressed by illness or infection, the diabetic woman is at increased risk for diabetic ketoacidosis (DKA). The use of tocolytics such as terbutaline to arrest preterm labor may contribute to the risk for hyperglycemia and subsequent DKA. Magnesium sulfate is the preferred tocolytic for women with diabetes (Foley et al, 1993; Peterson et al, 1993; Regenstein, Belluomini, and Katz, 1993). DKA may also occur because of failure to take insulin appropriately. The onset of unrecognized diabetes during pregnancy is another cause of DKA. DKA may occur with blood glucose levels barely exceeding 200 mg/dl, compared with 300 to 350 mg/dl in the nonpregnant state. In response to stress factors such as infection or illness, hyperglycemia occurs as a result of increased hepatic glucose production and decreased peripheral glucose utilization. Stress hormones that act to impair insulin action and further contribute to insulin deficiency are released. Fatty acids are mobilized from fat stores into the circulation, and as they are oxidized, ketone bodies are released into the peripheral circulation. The woman's buffering system is unable to compensate, and metabolic acidosis develops. The excessive blood glucose and ketone bodies bring about osmotic diuresis with subsequent loss of fluid and electrolytes, volume depletion, and cellular dehydration. Prompt treatment of DKA is necessary to avoid maternal coma or death. Ketoacidosis occurring at any time during pregnancy can lead to intrauterine fetal death and is also a cause of preterm labor. Perinatal mortality may be as high as 35% to 50% with maternal ketoacidosis (Chauhan and Perry, 1995; Harvey, 1992; Mintoro et al, 1993) (Table 10-3).

Although strict glycemic control is the goal of management of diabetic pregnancy, the risk of *hypoglycemia* is increased. Early in pregnancy, when hepatic production of glucose is diminished and peripheral utilization of glucose is enhanced, hypoglycemia commonly occurs, often during sleep. Later in pregnancy, hypoglycemia may also result as insulin doses are adjusted to maintain normoglycemia. Women with prepregnancy histories of severe hypoglycemia are at increased risk for severe hypoglycemia during gestation. Mild to moderate hypoglycemic episodes in pregnant women with diabetes do not appear to have significant deleterious effects on fetal well-being. The long-term fetal effects of severe maternal hypoglycemia are as yet uncertain (Langford and Bartholomew, 1992; Reece, Homko, and Wiznitzer, 1994).

Fetal/neonatal risks and complications. From the moment of conception, the infant of a mother with diabetes faces an increased risk of complications that may occur during the antenatal, intrapartal, or neonatal periods. These complications may be mild and transient, but they are often life-threatening and may result in the infant's death. Infant morbidity and mortality associated with diabetic pregnancy are significantly reduced with strict control of maternal glucose levels before and during pregnancy.

Despite the improvements in care of diabetic pregnancy, sudden and unexplained stillbirth is still a major concern. Typically this is observed in pregnancies after 36 weeks in women with vascular disease or poor glycemic control. It may also be associated with DKA, preeclampsia, hydramnios, or macrosomia (see p. 256). Although the exact cause of stillbirth is unknown, it may be related to chronic intrauterine hypoxia.

The incidence of *congenital anomalies* among infants of women with insulin-dependent diabetes is from 2 to 4 times that of the general population. Up to 50% of all perinatal deaths among infants of mothers with diabetes are the result of congenital malformations (Landon and Gabbe, 1995; Reece and Homko, 1993). The incidence of congenital malformations is related to the severity and duration of the diabetic disease process. Poor glycemic control before conception and in the early weeks of pregnancy (during the period of organogenesis) increases the risk of congenital anomalies. Hyperketonemia and hypoglycemia may also play a role in the development of congenital anomalies. Common abnormalities of the central nervous system (CNS) include caudal regression syndrome and neural tube defects such as anencephaly, hydrocephaly, microcephaly, meningocele, and meningomyelocele. Common heart anomalies are septal defects, transposition of great vessels, and coarctation of the aorta. Renal agenesis,

TABLE 10-3 Differentiation of hypoglycemia (insulin shock) and hyperglycemia (DKA)

	HYPOGLYCEMIA (INSULIN SHOCK)	HYPERGLYCEMIA (DKA)
Causes	Excess insulin Insufficient food (delayed or missed meals) Excessive exercise or work Indigestion, diarrhea, vomiting	Insufficient insulin Excess or wrong kind of food Infection, injuries, illness Emotional stress Insufficient exercise
Onset	Rapid (with regular insulin) Gradual (with modified insulin or oral hypoglycemics agents)	Slow (hours to days)
Symptoms	Hunger Sweating Nervousness Weakness Fatigue Blurred or double vision Dizziness Headache Pallor, clammy skin Shallow respirations Rapid pulse Laboratory values: Urine: negative for sugar and acetone Blood glucose: 60 mg/dl or less	Thirst Nausea or vomiting Abdominal pain Constipation Drowsiness Dim vision Increased urination Headache Flushed, dry skin Rapid breathing Weak, rapid pulse Acetone (fruity) breath odor Laboratory values: Urine: positive for sugar and acetone Blood glucose: 200 mg/dl or greater
Intervention	Check blood glucose when symptoms first appear Eat/drink carbohydrate immediately (juice, candy, etc) Repeat carbohydrate intake in 15 minutes if glucose remains low Notify health care provider if no change in glucose level If inconscious, 50% dextrose IV push, 5%-10% D/W IV drip, or glucagon Obtain blood and urine specimens for laboratory testing.	Notify health care provider Administer insulin in accordance with blood glucose levels Give intravenous (IV) fluids such as normal saline or one-half normal saline; potassium when urinary output is adequate; bicarbonate for pH <7.0 Monitor lab testing of blood and urine

hydronephrosis, hypospadias, and undescended testes are common urinary anomalies. Gastrointestinal abnormalities commonly seen are duodenal atresia, imperforate anus, and malrotation of the bowel. Single umbilical artery, ear deformities, and facial clefts also occur (Cooper et al, 1992; Greene, 1993; Kitzmiller et al, 1991; Landon and Gabbe, 1995).

Macrosomia, infant weight greater than the 90th percentile, occurs in 25% to 42% of pregnancies complicated by diabetes as compared with 8% to 14% of nondiabetic pregnancies (Jovanovic-Peterson et al, 1991). The fetal pancreas begins to secrete insulin at 10 to 14 weeks' gestation. The fetus responds to maternal hyperglycemia by secreting large amounts of insulin (hyperinsulinism). Insulin acts as a growth hormone, causing the fetus to lay down excess stores of glycogen, protein, and adipose tissue, leading to increased fetal size, or macrosomia. These infants are considered **large for gestational age (LGA).** Macrosomia is associated with dystocia, often resulting in operative vaginal delivery (episiotomy and forceps), and is responsible for the increased rate of cesarean birth among mothers with diabetes. The macrosomic infant may incur fractured clavicle, liver or spleen laceration, brachial plexus injury, facial palsy, phrenic nerve injury, or subdural hemorrhage (Landon and Gabbe, 1995; Schwartz et al, 1994). (For further discussion, see Chapter 26.)

IUGR is often seen in infants of diabetic mothers with vascular disease and results in a neonate who is **small for gestational age (SGA).** This is related to compromised uteroplacental circulation and may be worse in the presence of ketoacidosis and preeclampsia. The amount of oxygen available to the fetus is decreased as a result of maternal vascular changes. Preterm birth, common to diabetic pregnancy, may also be related to fetal hypoxia (Meyer and Palmer, 1990).

Infants of mothers with diabetes are at increased risk for respiratory distress syndrome (RDS). In past years, the incidence of respiratory distress was greater because many infants were born before term in an attempt to limit the chances of early fetal death. With advanced fetal surveillance techniques and improved maternal glycemic control, the incidence of preterm birth with resultant RDS has declined. However, there is some indication that hyperglycemia and hyperinsulinemia are instrumental in delaying pulmonary maturation in the fetus of a diabetic mother (Landon and Gabbe, 1995; Piper and Langer, 1993).

For infants of diabetic pregnancy, the transition to extrauterine life is often beset with metabolic abnormalities. Within the first 30 to 60 minutes after birth, neonatal *hypoglycemia* often occurs. This is because of the effects of fetal hyperinsulinism and rapid utilization of glucose after birth. The incidence of neonatal hypoglycemia is related to the mother's glycemic control during pregnancy as well as her glucose levels during labor and birth. *Hypocalcemia, hypomagnesemia, hyperbilirubinemia, and polycythemia* occur more often in infants of mothers with diabetes and place these neonates at increased risk (Salveson, Brudenall, and Nicolaides, 1992; Samson, 1992).

Nursing Care Management

Assessment

Interview. Whenever a pregnant woman with diabetes initiates prenatal care, thorough evaluation of her health status is completed. In addition to routine prenatal assessment, the nurse obtains a detailed history regarding the onset and course of the diabetic condition, as well as the management of diabetes and the degree of glycemic control before pregnancy. Effective management of diabetic pregnancy depends on the woman's adherence to a plan of care. For the woman to care for her diabetes on a daily basis, she must have an adequate understanding of her condition and the prescribed regimen. Thus with the initial prenatal visit, the nurse conducts a thorough assessment of the woman's knowledge regarding diabetes and pregnancy, potential maternal and fetal complications, and the plan of care. With subsequent visits, follow-up assessments are completed. Data from these assessments are used to identify the woman's specific learning needs. The support person's knowledge of diabetes is also assessed, and teaching needs are identified.

The woman's emotional status is assessed to determine how she is coping with pregnancy superimposed on preexisting diabetes. While normal pregnancy typically evokes some degree of stress and anxiety, pregnancy designated as "high risk" serves to compound anxiety and stress levels. Fear of maternal and fetal complications is a major concern. Strict adherence to the plan of care may necessitate alterations in patterns of daily living and be an additional source of stress.

The woman's support system is assessed to identify those people significant to the pregnant woman and their role in her life. It is important to assess the reactions of the family members or significant others to the pregnancy and the strict management plan, as well as their involvement in the treatment regimen. Socioeconomic factors are also reviewed. Any area of emotional stress is identified because such stress can precipitate complications (Leff, Gagne, and Jeffries, 1991; Ruggiero et al, 1990).

Physical examination. At the initial visit, a thorough physical examination is performed to assess the woman's current health status. In addition to the routine prenatal examination, specific efforts are made to assess effects of diabetes on the pregnant woman. A baseline electrocardiogram may be done to assess cardiovascular status. Evaluation for retinopathy is done, with follow-up as needed by an ophthalmologist. Blood pressure is monitored carefully throughout pregnancy because of the increased risk for pregnancy-induced hypertension. The woman's weight gain is also monitored at each visit. Fundal height is measured, and any abnormal increase in size for dates is noted because this may indicate hydramnios or fetal macrosomia. Leopold maneuvers are performed to check for fetal size and possible hydramnios.

Laboratory tests. Routine prenatal laboratory examinations are performed. In addition, baseline renal function may be assessed with a 24-hour urine specimen tested for total protein excretion and creatinine clearance. Routine urinalysis is performed on the initial prenatal visit and throughout the pregnancy to assess for the presence of urinary tract infection, which is common to diabetic pregnancy. At each visit, urine is also tested for the presence of glucose and ketones. Because of the risk of coexisting thyroid disease, thyroid function tests may also be performed (see the discussion of thyroid disorders on pp. 269-270).

For the woman with pregestational diabetes (IDDM or NIDDM), laboratory tests are done to assess glycemic control. At the initial prenatal visit, the **glycosylated hemoglobin (Hb A1c)** level may be measured. With prolonged hyperglycemia, some of the hemoglobin remains saturated with glucose for the life of the red cell. Therefore a test for glycosylated hemoglobin provides a measurement of glycemic control over time; it indicates the level of glycemic control over the previous 4 to 6 weeks. Regular measurements of glycosylated hemoglobin provide data for altering the treatment plan to promote glycemic control. Values for the measurement of Hb A_{1c}, the most commonly used index of glycosylated hemoglobin, are as follows (Pagano and Pagano, 1995):

Adult/elderly	4% to 8%
Good diabetic control	7%
Fair diabetic control	10%
Poor diabetic control	13% to 20%

Fetal surveillance. Diagnostic techniques for fetal surveillance are often performed during a pregnancy complicated by diabetes to assess fetal growth and well-being. The goals of fetal surveillance are to detect fetal compromise as early as possible and to prevent intrauterine fetal death or unnecessary preterm birth. The majority of fetal surveillance measures are concentrated in the third trimester when the risk of fetal death is greatest.

Early in pregnancy, the estimated date of birth (EDB) is determined. A baseline ultrasound is used during the first trimester to assess gestational age of the fetus. Follow-up ultrasound examinations are performed during the pregnancy, as often as every 4 to 6 weeks, to monitor fetal growth; to estimate fetal weight; and to detect hydramnios, macrosomia, and congenital anomalies.

Because diabetic pregnancies are at greater risk for neural tube defects (e.g., spina bifida, anencephaly, microcephaly), measurement of maternal serum alpha-fetoprotein (MSAFP) is performed between 16 and 18 weeks' gestation. This is often done in conjunction with a detailed ultrasound study to examine the fetus for neural tube defects.

Fetal echocardiography may be performed between 18 and 22 weeks' gestation to detect cardiac anomalies. Some practitioners repeat this fetal surveillance test at 34 weeks. Doppler studies of the umbilical artery may be performed to detect placental compromise in women with vascular disease.

Maternal evaluation of fetal movements (kick counts) is used primarily as a screening technique in fetal surveillance. Nonstress tests (NSTs) may be used weekly or more often during the third trimester to assess fetal well-being. In the presence of a nonreactive NST, a contraction stress test (CST) or fetal biophysical profile (BPP) may be used to evaluate fetal well-being (Jovanovic-Peterson and Peterson, 1992; Landon and Gabbe, 1993, 1995).

Determination of birth date and mode of delivery. In the past, preterm delivery was often elected to avoid the risk of intrauterine death. The majority of diabetic pregnancies are now allowed to progress to term (38 to 40 weeks) as long as strict glycemic control is maintained **(normoglycemia)** and all parameters of antepartum fetal surveillance remain within normal limits. In the presence of vascular disease, women may give birth before term gestation if hypertension worsens or fetal growth restriction warrants early delivery.

Many practitioners plan for elective labor induction between 38 and 40 weeks, provided maternal glucose levels are well-controlled. To confirm fetal lung maturity before birth, an amniocentesis may be performed in pregnancies of less than 39 weeks. For the pregnancy complicated by diabetes, fetal lung maturation is better predicted by the amniotic fluid **phosphatidylglycerol (PG)** than by the lecithin/sphingomyelin ratio (L/S) ratio. If the fetal lungs are still immature, birth should be postponed as long as the results of fetal assessment remain reassuring. Amniocentesis may be repeated to monitor lung maturity. Birth despite poor fetal lung maturity may be essential when testing suggests fetal compromise or if the pregnant woman develops preeclampsia, rapidly worsening retinopathy, or renal failure. The rate of cesarean births for these women is approximately 50%. Cesarean birth is usually performed when antepartum testing suggests fetal distress, the estimated fetal weight is greater than 4000 g, or the cervix fails to respond to prostaglandin ripening (Jovanovic-Peterson and Peterson, 1992; Landon and Gabbe, 1993, 1995).

Nursing Diagnoses

Each woman's experience of pregnancy complicated by diabetes is unique to her and to her family. Nursing diagnoses must be carefully formulated to reflect the actual or potential altered health-related responses that can be influenced, improved, or alleviated by nursing intervention. Examples of possible nursing diagnoses for the woman with pregestational diabetes during the antepartum, intrapartum, and postpartum periods are as follows:

Antepartum

- Knowledge deficit related to
  - Diabetic pregnancy, management, and potential effects on pregnant woman and fetus.
  - Insulin administration and its effects
  - Hypoglycemia and hyperglycemia
  - Diabetic diet
- Risk for ineffective individual or family coping related to
  - Woman's responsibility in managing her diabetes during pregnancy.
- Anxiety, fear, dysfunctional grieving, powerlessness, body-image disturbance, situational low self-esteem, spiritual distress, altered role performance, altered family processes related to
  - Stigma of being labeled "diabetic"
  - Effects of diabetes and its potential sequelae on the pregnant woman and the fetus
- Risk for noncompliance related to
  - Lack of understanding of diabetes and pregnancy and requirements of treatment plan
  - Lack of financial resources to purchase blood glucose monitoring supplies, insulin and necessary supplies, or food to follow dietary regimen
- Risk for injury to fetus related to
  - Uteroplacental insufficiency
- Risk for injury to mother related to
  - Improper insulin administration
  - Hypoglycemia and hyperglycemia
- Risk for infection related to
  - Hyperglycemia
- Altered nutrition: less or more than body requirements related to
  - Noncompliance with dietary regiment
  - Knowledge deficit regarding increased nutritional needs during pregnancy

Intrapartum

- Risk for injury related to
  - Hypoglycemia or hyperglycemia
  - Preeclampsia/eclampsia
- Altered tissue perfusion related to supine hypotension

Postpartum

- Risk for injury related to
  - Fluctuating blood glucose levels after giving birth
  - Complications of involution (hemorrhage, infection)
  - Postpartum development of preeclampsia/eclampsia
- Ineffective individual coping, altered family processes, altered parenting, related to
  - Newborn with sequelae to a diabetic pregnancy

Expected Outcomes

Planning care for the pregnant patient and her family is given direction from identified nursing diagnoses and the plan for medical management of diabetic pregnancy. The plan is individualized, relating specifically to needs identified by the health care team and to those mutually identified by the woman, her family, and the caregivers.

Expected outcomes of management of diabetic pregnancy include the following:

1. The woman and her family will demonstrate or verbalize understanding of diabetic pregnancy, the plan of care, and the importance of glycemic control.
2. The woman will comply with the plan of care.
3. The woman will achieve and maintain glycemic control.
4. The woman will demonstrate effective coping.
5. The woman will experience no complications (i.e., maternal morbidity or mortality)
6. The infant will experience no complications (i.e., perinatal morbidity or mortality)

7. The family will experience mutuality and support among its members.

Plan of Care and Implementation

As a vital member of the health care team caring for the pregnant woman with diabetes, the nurse assumes a variety of roles. Whereas normal pregnancy is a maturational crisis for most women; those pregnancies complicated by diabetes may represent a situational crisis as well because of the high-risk nature of the condition. These women require individualized, comprehensive nursing care throughout the pregnancy and in the postpartum period.

Assisting the woman with stress reduction is central to the care needed by women whose pregnancies are complicated by diabetes mellitus. Increased stress contributes to elevated blood glucose levels. Stress reduction and relaxation are taught as needed. Space, privacy, and time are provided for the woman and her family to voice their feelings and questions, as well as to problem solve among themselves. To improve the woman's motivation and understanding of diabetic management, the nurse acknowledges both positive and negative feelings about the pregnancy and diabetes. Providing care that is sensitive to individual needs and based on a collaborative relationship with the woman and family fosters their physical and emotional well-being (Leff, Gagne, and Jeffries, 1991).

Fetal surveillance techniques may identify a congenital malformation incompatible with survival. Parents need supportive care as they consider the option of early pregnancy termination. The early detection of serious fetal malformations allows for exploration of various options in planning delivery and immediate care of the newborn. The parents may also benefit from the time to prepare for the birth of a child with a congenital abnormality. Diagnostic tests for fetal malformations should be conducted under conditions that are both voluntary and informed. The risks, accuracy, and limitations of the tests should be discussed. The benefits of diagnosis and the options available when a positive diagnosis is obtained should be discussed in advance. In those instances when pregnancy loss occurs, the nurse is key in providing counseling for the woman and her family (Penha et al, 1993).

Engaging the woman as an active participant in the plan of care maintains or enhances her self-esteem and develops her self-confidence that she will be able to care for herself and her baby. Open communication with members of the health care team is encouraged to facilitate patient participation in self-care.

The nurse is most often the primary educator for the woman with diabetes and her family. Through ongoing assessment, learning needs are identified. Teaching is initiated early in pregnancy and is continued throughout the period of gestation. Adequate understanding of diabetes and pregnancy, the treatment plan, and potential complications encourages patient compliance. Euglycemia can be maintained, and maternal and fetal well-being are promoted through adherence to the plan of care.

Antepartum. Management of diabetic pregnancy is a complex process that requires the woman to be knowledgeable about the treatment regimen and the changes that may occur so she may respond appropriately. Although the woman is likely to have some knowledge and experience with the various aspects of diabetic care—diet, insulin, exercise, blood glucose monitoring—she will need assistance from the nurse to understand the effect of pregnancy on diabetes to manage her care effectively. Prenatal visits for the pregnant woman with diabetes are more frequent than for women who are not diabetic so the woman's glycemic status and pregnancy progress can be carefully monitored. Visits are scheduled every 1 to 2 weeks for the first 32 weeks, then weekly until birth.

Diet. The woman with pregestational diabetes has usually had nutritional counseling regarding the management of diabetes. Because pregnancy precipitates special nutritional concerns and needs, the woman must be educated and counseled to incorporate these changes into dietary planning. Nutritional counseling is usually provided by a registered dietician. Pregnancy is an ideal time for the diabetic to "fine-tune" her self-management skills because self-motivation is typically high. It is essential that the woman understand the importance of maintaining normal glucose levels during pregnancy.

Dietary management during diabetic pregnancy must be based on blood glucose (not urinary glucose) levels. The diet is individualized to allow for increased fetal and metabolic requirements, with consideration of such factors as prepregnancy weight and dietary habits, overall health, ethnic background, lifestyle, stage of pregnancy, knowledge of nutrition, and insulin therapy. The dietary goal is to provide weight gain consistent with a normal pregnancy, to prevent ketoacidosis, and to minimize widely-fluctuating blood glucose levels.

Energy needs are usually calculated on the basis of 30 to 35 calories per kilogram of ideal body weight, with the average diet including 2200 calories (first trimester) to 2500 calories (second and third trimesters). Total calories may be distributed among three meals and one evening snack, or more commonly, three meals and at least two snacks. Meals should be eaten on time and never skipped. Snacks must be carefully planned in accordance with insulin therapy to avoid fluctuations in blood glucose levels. A large bedtime snack of at least 25 g of carbohydrate with some protein is recommended to help prevent hypoglycemia and starvation ketosis during the night.

The ratio of carbohydrate, protein, and fat is important to meet the metabolic needs of the woman and the fetus. Ap-

Home Care

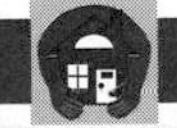

DIETARY MANAGEMENT OF DIABETIC PREGNANCY

- Follow the prescribed diet plan.
- Eat a well-balanced diet, including daily food requirements for a normal pregnancy.
- Divide daily food intake among three meals and two to four snacks, depending on individual needs.
- Eat a substantial bedtime snack to prevent a severe drop in blood glucose level during the night.
- Limit the intake of fats if weight gain occurs too rapidly.
- Take daily vitamins and iron as prescribed by the health care provider.
- Avoid foods high in refined sugar.
- Eat consistently each day; never skip meals or snacks.
- Reduce the intake of saturated fat and cholesterol.
- Eat foods high in dietary fiber.
- Avoid alcohol and caffeine.

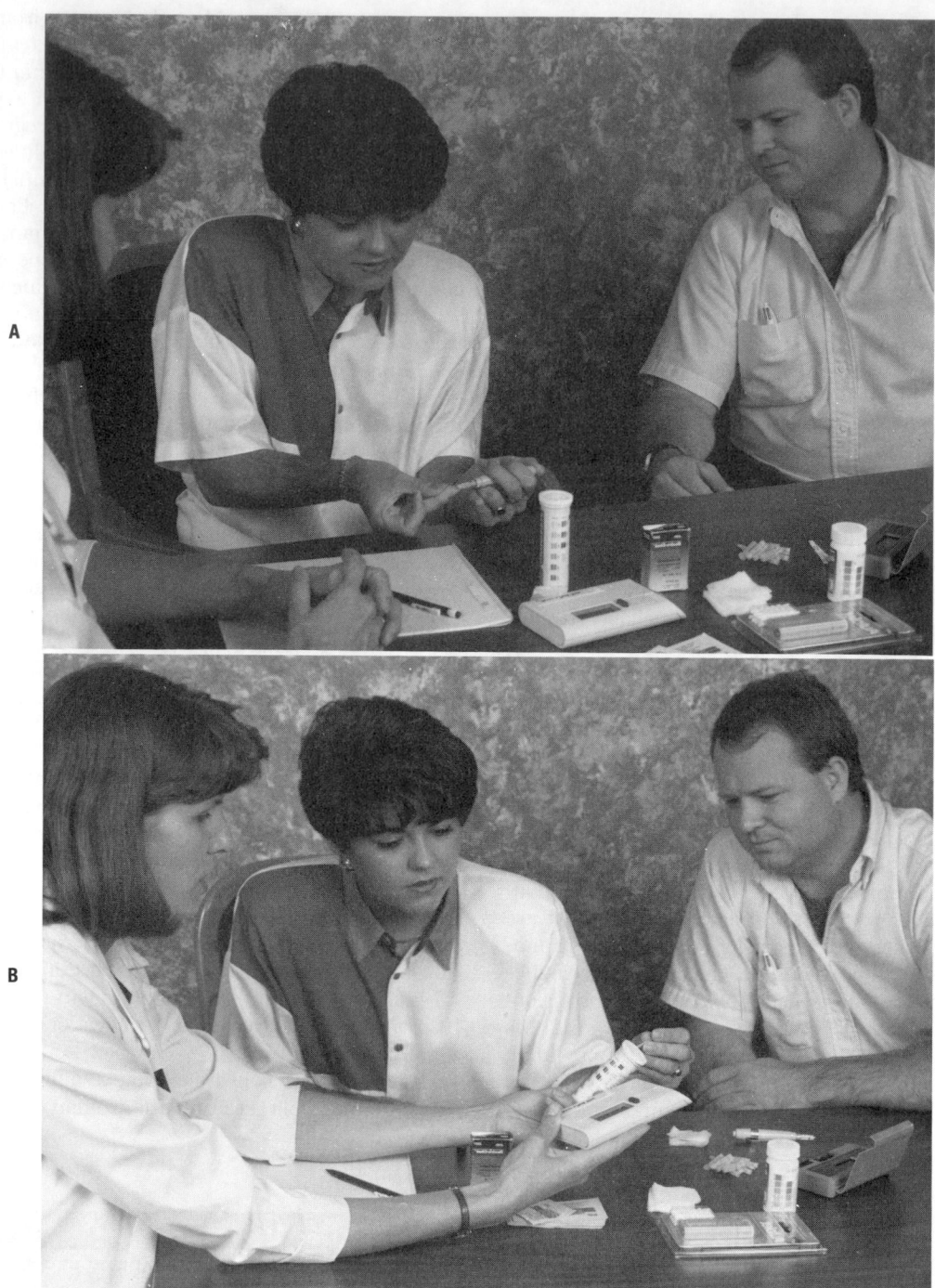

Fig. 10-2 **A,** Pregnant woman demonstrates how to collect drop of blood for glucose monitoring. **B,** Nurse assists woman and her husband in interpreting glucose values displayed by monitor. (Courtesy Jonas McKoy, University of North Carolina at Chapel Hill School of Nursing.)

proximately 50% of the total calories should be carbohydrate, with a minimum of 250 g/day. Simple carbohydrates are avoided; complex carbohydrates that are high in fiber content are recommended because the starch and protein in such foods help regulate the blood glucose level as a result of more sustained glucose release. Protein intake should constitute around 20% of the total kilocalories. Less than 30% of the daily caloric intake should come from fat, with no more than 10% from saturated fats. Vitamins and minerals are usually provided as daily supplements (Worthington-Roberts and Williams, 1993). Weight gain for most women should be 10 to 13.5 kg (22 to 30 lb) during the pregnancy, with a gain of 0.9 to 1.8 kg (2 to 4 lb) in the first trimester and .23 to .45 kg ($^1/_2$ to 1 lb) each week thereafter (Landon and Gabbe, 1995; Reece and Homko, 1993; Worthington-Roberts and Williams, 1993). (See the Home Care box on p. 259.)

Home Care

SELF-TESTING OF BLOOD GLUCOSE LEVEL

- Gather supplies, check expiration date, and read instructions on testing materials.
- Wash hands in warm water (warmth increases circulation).
- Select site on side of any finger (cleaning the site with alcohol is not necessary).
- Pierce site with lancet (be sure to rotate sites).
- Drop hand down to your side; using other hand, gently squeeze finger from hand to fingertip.
- Allow blood to drop onto reagent area of strip; be sure to cover entire reagent area.
- Follow instructions for timing and wiping of excess blood.
- At proper time, read visually or on reflectance meter.
- Record your results.
- Repeat daily according to the schedule recommended by your health care provider and as needed for signs of hypoglycemia or hyperglycemia.

From Jovanovic-Peterson L, editor: *Medical management of pregnancy complicated by diabetes,* Alexandria, Va, 1993, American Diabetes Association.

TABLE 10-4 Target blood glucose levels during pregnancy

TIME OF DAY	TARGET GLUCOSE LEVEL
Before breakfast (fasting)	60-90 mg/dl
Before lunch, dinner, bedtime	60-105 mg/dl
1 hour after meals (postprandial)	110-130 mg/dl
2 hours after meals (postprandial)	90-120 mg/dl
2:00 AM to 6:00 AM	60-120 mg/dl

From Jovanovic-Peterson L, editor: *Medical management of pregnancy complicated by diabetes,* Alexandria, Va, 1993, American Diabetes Association.

Monitoring blood glucose levels. Blood glucose testing at home with a glucose reflectance meter is the commonly accepted method for monitoring blood glucose levels and is the most important tool available to the woman to assess her degree of glycemic control (Fig 10-2). Home glucose monitoring has been credited with increasing the woman's feeling of control over self, and with decreasing or eliminating hospitalizations and consequent separation from family. It is the most accurate method of documenting the degree of glycemic control in an out-of-hospital setting and enables the woman to adjust her insulin dosage on a 24-hour basis (see the Home Care box above).

For home blood glucose monitoring to be used effectively, the woman and her family should be knowledgeable regarding proper use of the monitoring system, when to measure blood glucose levels, and the target blood glucose ranges (Table 10-4).

Blood glucose levels are routinely measured four times a day: before breakfast, lunch, and dinner, and at bedtime. Postprandial measurements, 2 hours after meals, may also be done. Some physicians recommend that at least 2 days per week a complete profile be done. This consists of eight tests per day: before meals, 2 hours after meals, at bedtime, and at 3:00 a.m. Women are also encouraged to check glucose levels at any sign of hypoglycemia or hyperglycemia. Insulin dosage, diet, and other aspects of the daily management plan are adjusted in response to blood glucose levels; thus accuracy in testing and reporting is essential.

During the second and third trimester, when insulin needs are increasing, more frequent testing is likely to be needed.

Target levels of blood glucose during pregnancy are somewhat lower than nonpregnant values. Education of the woman and her family includes the importance of achieving and maintaining lower target values than they were used to in the nonpregnant state (Table 10-4).

Insulin therapy. Adequate insulin is the primary factor in the maintenance of normoglycemia during pregnancy. Insulin requirements during pregnancy change dramatically as the pregnancy progresses, necessitating frequent adjustments in insulin dosage. In the first trimester, there is little or no change in prepregnancy insulin requirements; however, insulin dosage may need to be decreased because of hypoglycemia. During the second and third trimester, because of insulin resistance, the dosage must be increased to maintain target glucose levels. The nurse is instrumental in education and support of women who have pregestational diabetes with regard to insulin administration and adjustment of insulin dosage to maintain normoglycemia (see the Home Care box on p. 262). The total daily dose of insulin is determined based on the woman's gestational week and her body weight.

Most patients with insulin-dependent diabetes require multiple daily injections during pregnancy. Biosynthetic human insulin is recommended; a combination of intermediate-acting and regular (short-acting) insulin before breakfast and at dinner time is a common regimen. Typically, two thirds of the daily insulin dose is given in the morning before breakfast, combining NPH and regular insulin in a 2:1 ratio. The remaining one third is administered in the evening before dinner using equal doses of NPH and regular insulin (see the Home Care box on p. 262 and Table 10-5) (Jovanovic-Peterson and Peterson, 1992; Landon and Gabbe, 1995; Reece and Homko, 1993).

Although subcutaneous insulin injections are most common, continuous insulin infusion systems may be used during pregnancy. The insulin pump is designed to mimic more closely the function of the pancreas in secreting insulin by infusing regular insulin at a set basal rate and bolus doses of insulin before meals to control postmeal blood glucose levels (Fig. 10-3). The infusion tubing from the insulin pump can be left in place for several weeks without local complications. Insulin pumps are usually reserved for women whose diabetes cannot be controlled by multiple insulin injections and who are highly motivated, because meticulous blood glucose monitoring is required (Landon and Gabbe, 1995; Reece and Homko, 1993).

Urine testing. The urine is tested daily with the first morning urine. Testing should also be done if a meal is missed or delayed, when illness occurs, or when blood glucose is greater than 200 mg/dl.

Spilling a trace or small amount of ketones requires no treatment. However, if it appears repeatedly at the same time each day, some adjustment in diet may be needed. If testing

Home Care

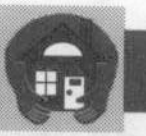

SELF-ADMINISTRATION OF INSULIN

Procedure for mixing NPH (intermediate-acting) and regular (short-acting) insulin

- Wash hands thoroughly and gather supplies. Be sure the insulin syringe corresponds to the concentration of insulin you are using.
- Check the insulin bottle to be certain it is the appropriate type and check the expiration date.
- Gently rotate (do not shake) the insulin vial to mix the insulin.
- Wipe off rubber stopper of each vial with alcohol.
- Draw back into syringe the amount of air equal to total dose.
- Inject air equal to NPH (intermediate-acting) dose into NPH vial. Remove needle from vial.
- Inject air equal to regular insulin dose into regular insulin vial.
- Invert regular insulin bottle and withdraw regular insulin dose.
- Without adding more air to NPH vial, carefully withdraw NPH dose.

Procedure for self-injection of insulin

- Select proper injection site (remember to rotate sites).
- Cleanse injection site with alcohol.
- Pinch the skin up to form a subcutaneous pocket, and holding the syringe like a pencil, puncture the skin at a 45- to 90-degree angle. If there is a great deal of fatty tissue at the site, spread the skin taut and inject the syringe at a 90-degree angle.
- Slowly inject the insulin.
- As you withdraw the needle, cover the injection site with sterile gauze and apply gentle pressure to prevent bleeding.
- Record insulin dosage and time of injection.

shows a large amount of ketones, the health care provider should be contacted immediately (Jovanovic-Peterson, 1993).

Exercise. Although exercise enhances the utilization of glucose and decreases insulin need in nonpregnant women with diabetes, there are limited data regarding exercise in the woman with pregestational diabetes. Any prescription of exercise during pregnancy for a woman with diabetes should be done by the primary health care provider and should be monitored closely to prevent complications. For those women with vasculopathy, only mild exercise is recommended because exercise causes a redistribution of blood flow, which increases the potential for ischemic injury to already compromised organs and the placenta. Also, women with vasculopathy typically depend completely on exogenous insulin and are at greater risk for wide fluctuations in blood glucose levels and ketoacidosis, which can be worsened by exercise. The best time for exercise is after meals when the blood sugar is rising. To monitor the effect of insulin on blood glucose levels, the woman can measure blood glucose before, during, and after exercise (See the Home Care box on p. 263, left).

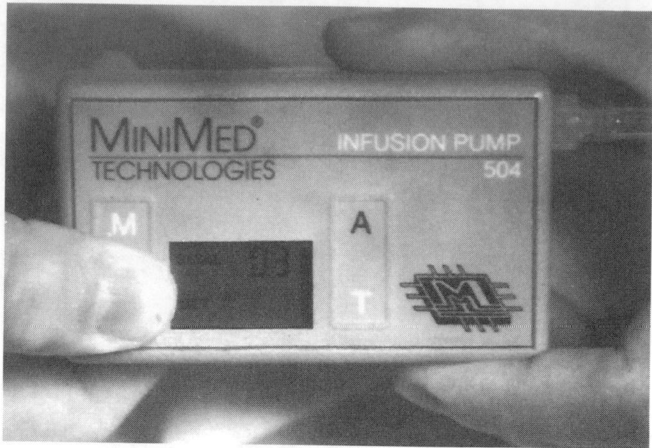

Fig. 10-3 Pregnant woman with diabetes sets basal rate on her insulin pump. (Courtesy Jonas McKoy, University of North Carolina at Chapel Hill School of Nursing.)

General care. Because the woman with diabetes is at risk for developing infections, eye problems, and neurologic changes, general skin care and foot care are discussed. A daily bath that includes good perineal care and foot care is important. For dry skin, lotions, creams, or oils can be applied. Tight clothing should be avoided. Shoes or slippers should fit properly, be worn at all times, and are best worn with socks or stockings. Feet should be inspected regularly; toenails are cut straight across, and professional help should be sought for any foot problems. Extremes of temperature are to be avoided.

Hospitalization. Despite advances in care, occasionally hospitalization may be required for regulation of insulin dosage and stabilization of glucose levels. Hospitalization offers a controlled situation to initiate and regulate insulin therapy while providing opportunity for intensive education in self-administration of insulin and regulation of blood glucose (Box 10-1).

Complications. The pregnant woman is alerted to potential complications during pregnancy and is given written instructions about the need for prompt reporting of problems such as nausea, vomiting, and infections. It is essential that the woman and her family be knowledgeable about hypo-

TABLE 10-5 Insulin administration during pregnancy: expected time of action

TYPE OF INSULIN	ONSET	PEAK	DURATION
Regular (rapid-acting)	½-1 hour	2-4 hours	5-8 hours
Intermediate acting	2-4 hours	5-10 hours	12-24 hours
Long-acting	3-4 hours	14-24 hours	24-36 hours

Home Care

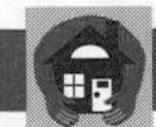

EXERCISE FOR PREGNANT WOMEN WITH PREGESTATIONAL DIABETES

- Exercise plans are individualized and should be monitored by the health care provider.
- Select exercises that are enjoyable to foster regularity.
- Exercise does not have to be vigorous to be effective.
- Avoid exercising in a warm environment.
- The best time to exercise is after meals, when blood glucose is beginning to rise.
- Monitor blood glucose levels before, during, and after exercise to determine variations in glucose levels.
- Do not administer insulin into an extremity that is to be immediately involved in exercise.

Home Care

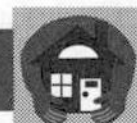

WHAT TO DO WHEN ILLNESS OCCURS:

- Be sure to take insulin even though appetite and food intake may be less than normal (insulin needs are increased with illness or infection).
- Call the health care provider and relay the following information:
  - symptoms of illness (e.g. nausea, vomiting, diarrhea)
  - fever
  - most recent blood glucose level
  - urine ketones
  - time and amount of last insulin dose
- Increase oral intake of fluids to prevent dehydration.
- Rest as much as possible.
- If unable to reach health care provider and blood glucose exceeds 200 mg/dL with urine ketones present, seek emergency treatment at the nearest health care facility. Do not attempt to self-treat for this.

BOX 10-1

Ethical Considerations Related to Pregnant Women with Medical Complications

Ethical dilemmas can occur in patient care situations involving the risk/benefit ratio of care to the mother and fetus. One issue is forced maternal bed rest or hospitalization to treat an underlying medical problem such as diabetes or cardiac disease. Traditionally, care has been provided based on the one-patient model (maternal-fetal unit), but recently the two-patient model (pregnant woman and fetus) increasingly has been used to make treatment decisions. Maternal refusal or acceptance of treatment can be ethically analyzed using these models.

glycemia and hyperglycemia, their causes, and symptoms as well as prevention and treatment measures (See the Home Care box above, right).

To prevent complications, the woman should not engage in any long-term travel without contacting her physician. Whenever she is away from home, the woman should carry along insulin, syringes, and glucose tablets. She should wear an identification bracelet at all times. It is also helpful to carry along an exchange list for dietary needs.

Labor and birth. During the intrapartum period, the woman with pregestational diabetes must be monitored closely to prevent complications related to dehydration, hypoglycemia, and hyperglycemia. Most women use large amounts of energy (calories) to accomplish the work and manage the stress of labor and birth; however, this calorie expenditure varies with the individual. Blood glucose levels and hydration must be carefully controlled during labor. An intravenous (IV) line is inserted for infusion of a maintenance fluid, such as lactated Ringer's solution or 5% dextrose/lactated Ringer's (D5LR) solution. Insulin may be administered by continuous infusion or intermittent subcutaneous injection. Determinations of blood glucose are made every hour, and fluids and insulin are adjusted to maintain blood glucose levels between 60 and 100 mg/dl. It is essential that these target glucose levels be maintained because hyperglycemia during labor can precipitate metabolic problems in the neonate, particularly hypoglycemia. Maternal hyperglycemia during labor can also lead to perinatal asphyxia and fetal/neonatal death (Palmer and Inturrisi, 1992; Reece and Homko, 1993).

During labor, continuous fetal heart monitoring is necessary. The mother should assume an upright or side-lying position during bed rest in labor to prevent supine hypotension because of a large fetus or polyhydramnios. Labor is allowed to progress, provided normal rates of cervical dilation, fetal descent, and fetal well-being are maintained. Failure to progress may indicate a macrosomic infant and cephalopelvic disproportion (CPD), which necessitates cesarean birth. The woman is observed and treated during labor for diabetic complications such as hyperglycemia, ketosis, ketoacidosis, and glycosuria. A pediatrician may be present at the birth to initiate assessment and neonatal care.

If a cesarean is the planned mode of birth, it should be scheduled in the early morning to facilitate glycemic control. The morning dose of insulin is withheld, and the woman is allowed nothing by mouth. Epidural anesthesia is recommended because hypoglycemia can be detected earlier if the woman is awake. After surgery, glucose levels are closely monitored, at least every 2 hours, and an IV solution containing 5% dextrose is infused (Landon and Gabbe, 1995).

Postpartum. In the immediate postpartum period, insulin requirements decrease substantially because the major source of insulin resistance, the placenta, has been removed. Patients with IDDM may require only one half to two thirds of the prenatal insulin dose on the first postpartum day, provided they are eating a full diet. It takes several days after delivery to reestablish carbohydrate homeostasis (Fig. 10-1). Blood glucose levels are monitored in the postpartum period, and insulin dosage is adjusted accordingly. The woman who is insulin-dependent must realize the importance of eating on time even if the baby needs feeding or other pressing demands exist. Women with NIDDM often require no insulin in the postpartum period and are able to maintain normoglycemia through diet alone or with oral hypoglycemics.

Possible postpartum complications include preeclampsia/eclampsia, hemorrhage, and infection. Hemorrhage is a possibility if the mother's uterus was overdistended (hydramnios, macrosomic fetus), or overstimulated (oxytocin induction). Infections such as monilial vaginitis are more likely to occur in a postpartum woman with diabetes.

Mothers with diabetes are encouraged to breastfeed. In addition to the advantages of maternal satisfaction and pleasure, breastfeeding has an antidiabetogenic effect. Insulin requirements may be half of prepregnancy levels because of the carbohydrate used in human milk production. Because glucose levels are lower, breastfeeding women are at increased risk for hypoglycemia, especially in the early postpartum period and after breastfeeding sessions (Neubauer et al, 1993). Insulin dosage, which is decreased during lactation, must be recalculated at the time of weaning (Benz, 1992; Lawrence, 1994) (Fig. 10-1 *E, F*).

Early breastfeeding difficulties may be experienced by the diabetic mother. Poor metabolic control may delay lactogenesis and contribute to decreased milk production (Neubauer et al, 1993). Initial contact and opportunity to breastfeed the infant may be delayed if the infant is placed in a neonatal intensive care unit (NICU) or special care nursery for observation during the first few hours after birth. Support and assistance from nursing staff and lactation specialists can facilitate the mother's early experience with breastfeeding and encourage her to continue (Ferris et al, 1993).

The new mother needs information related to family planning and contraception. While family planning is important for all women, it is essential for the woman with diabetes to

Nursing Care Plan

DIABETES

Pregestational IDDM

Nursing Diagnosis: Knowledge deficit related to interaction of new health condition (pregnancy) with preexisting condition (IDDM)

Expected Outcomes: **The patient will describe interaction of diabetes and pregnancy and potential effects on mother and fetus; follow plan of care for management of diabetes during pregnancy; and exhibit evidence of incorporation of care behaviors into daily routine.**

• **NURSING INTERVENTIONS/*RATIONALES***

Review woman's general knowledge of diabetes and prepregnancy management routines *to assess baseline knowledge and evaluate effectiveness of treatment regimens.*

Explore the woman's knowledge of effects of pregnancy on diabetes and what that means to her particular treatment regimen *to establish a teaching baseline.*

Discuss the potential sequelae of diabetes on mother and fetus, the management of a diabetic pregnancy, the need for careful adherence to the plan of care, and the importance of regular prenatal care *to ensure adequate understanding and promote compliance.*

Help woman plan any needed dietary changes *to promote adequate weight gain, maintain consistent blood glucose levels, and prevent ketoacidosis.*

Teach woman about likely insulin changes that will occur as body weight and gestational age increase and the importance of careful blood glucose monitoring *to ensure correct treatment and decrease chances of complications.*

Teach woman about importance of judicious exercise; the need for careful glucose monitoring before, during, and after exercise; and the need for close monitoring of any exercise program by a health care provider *to avoid ischemic injury to organs or placenta.*

Teach woman and significant other about potential complications and the need for prompt reporting of nausea, vomiting, infections, signs of dehydration, hypoglycemia or hyperglycemia and any wide swings in blood glucose levels *to ensure early treatment of complications and prevent potential injury to mother and fetus.*

Use multiple teaching sessions, encourage questions, clarify misconceptions, use repetition of material, provide written supplements to teaching sessions, and include significant others *to optimize teaching effectiveness.*

Help the woman individualize the knowledge and new treatment needs and integrate them into her existing management protocol *to ensure maximum treatment compliance.*

Have woman demonstrate use of new knowledge *to reinforce correct use of information and positive adaptations in behavior.*

Nursing Diagnosis: Fear/anxiety related to threat to maternal and fetal well-being

Expected Outcomes: **The patient's feelings and symptoms of fear/anxiety will decrease or abate.**

• **NURSING INTERVENTIONS/*RATIONALES***

Provide a calm, soothing atmosphere and teach family to provide emotional support *to facilitate coping.*

Encourage verbalization of fears *to decrease intensity of emotional response.*

Involve woman and family in the active management of her diabetes and pregnancy *to promote a greater sense of control.*

Encourage woman to differentiate between real and imagined threats to maternal and fetal well-being and detail what she can do to diminish the real threats *to promote a greater sense of control.*

Help woman identify and use appropriate coping strategies and support systems *to reduce fear/anxiety.*

Explore use of desensitization strategies such as progressive muscle relaxation, visual imagery, or thought stopping *to reduce fear-related emotions and related physical symptoms.*

safeguard her own health and to promote optimal outcome in any future pregnancies. The woman and her partner should be informed that the risks associated with pregnancy increase with the duration and severity of the diabetic condition and that pregnancy may contribute to vascular changes associated with diabetes. Preconception counseling is recommended because planned pregnancy and good glycemic control are instrumental in preventing congenital anomalies and spontaneous abortion in future pregnancies.

The risks and benefits of contraceptive methods are discussed with the mother and her partner before discharge from the hospital. The preferred method of contraception for the woman with insulin-dependent diabetes is a barrier method. Barrier methods such as the diaphragm or condom and spermicide pose the least risk to the diabetic woman. However, the problem with these methods is the inconsistency of use, which often leads to unplanned pregnancy (Mestman and Schmidt-Sarosi, 1993).

Use of oral contraceptives by diabetic women is controversial because of the risk of thromboembolic and vascular complications and the effect on carbohydrate metabolism. In women without vascular disease or other risk factors, low-dose oral contraceptives may be prescribed. Close monitoring of blood pressure and glucose levels is necessary to detect complications (Kjos, 1993; Landon and Gabbe, 1995).

Intrauterine devices (IUDs) are often associated with an increased risk of infection, especially during the first 4 months after insertion. However, they may be used for women with diabetes who are older or have hypertension or another vascular disease. Such individuals should be parous, in a monogamous relationship, at low risk for sexually transmitted disease, and have no history of pelvic infection. It is essential that these women recognize the signs of pelvic infection and STDs and notify their health care provider promptly if they occur (Kjos, 1993).

There is no contraindication to use of the Norplant system in diabetic women without cardiovascular complications (Jovanovic-Peterson, 1993). For the diabetic woman with significant vascular disease, effective contraception is critical to her future health and well-being. In some cases, surgical sterilization is the recommended method of contraception (Mestman and Schmidt-Sarosi, 1993).

Evaluation

Successful management of diabetic pregnancy involves a complex treatment plan and requires the woman's participation and commitment, as well as the direction and support of the health care team. Support of family and significant others is vital to the woman's physical and psychologic well-being. Effectiveness of the care plan is best measured by evaluating the degree to which the following goals have been achieved:

1. The woman and her family demonstrate/verbalize understanding of diabetic pregnancy, the plan of care, and the importance of glycemic control.
2. The woman complies with the plan of care.
3. The woman achieves and maintains glycemic control.
4. The woman demonstrates effective coping.
5. Neither the woman nor the infant experiences complications.
6. The family experiences mutuality and support among its members.

See the Nursing Care Plan on p. 264.

Gestational Diabetes Mellitus

GDM is defined as "carbohydrate intolerance of variable severity with onset or first recognition during the present pregnancy" (ADA, 1990). Gestational diabetes, most often encountered in late pregnancy, is generally characterized by mild glucose intolerance that manifests as postprandial hyperglycemia. In the majority of cases, GDM disappears at the end of the pregnancy; however, there is a high probability that it will recur in subsequent pregnancies or that NIDDM will develop later in life. Gestational diabetes occurs in 2% to 7% of all pregnant women in the United States and accounts for 90% of all cases of diabetes in pregnancy. Estimates of ethnic prevalence are variable. Caucasians seem to have the lowest risk for developing GDM, whereas African-Americans, Hispanic-Americans, South East Asians, and Native Americans appear to be at increased risk (Berkowitz et al, 1992; Dornhorst et al, 1992; Sacks et al, 1995). Classic risk factors for GDM include: (1) maternal age over 30; (2) obesity; prepregnancy weight more than 20% over ideal weight; (3) family history of NIDDM; and (4) previous obstetric history of delivery of an infant greater than 4 kg (9 lb), hydramnios, unexplained stillbirth, miscarriage, or delivery of an infant with congenital anomalies (Berkowitz et al, 1992; Jovanovic-Peterson and Peterson, 1992).

The diagnosis of gestational diabetes is usually made during the second half of pregnancy. As fetal nutrient demands rise during the late second and third trimester, maternal nutrient ingestion induces greater and more sustained levels of blood glucose. At the same time, maternal insulin resistance is also increasing as a result of the insulin antagonistic effects of the placental hormones, cortisol, and insulinase. Consequently, maternal insulin demands rise as much as threefold. The majority of pregnant women are capable of increasing insulin production to compensate for the insulin resistance and maintain normoglycemia. When the pancreas is unable to produce sufficient insulin, or if the insulin is not used effectively, gestational diabetes can result.

Some women with gestational diabetes exhibit the classic symptoms of diabetes—excessive thirst, hunger, urination, and weakness. However, because approximately 70% of gestational diabetes occurs in an asymptomatic form, universal screening of all pregnant women is essential to diagnosis and treatment. The American Diabetes Association (ADA) and the Third International Workshop-Conference on Gestational Diabetes (Metzger, 1991) recommend screening of all pregnant women between 24 and 28 weeks' gestation; those women with identified risk factors for GDM are screened earlier in pregnancy. (The American College of Obstetricians and Gynecologists [ACOG] recommends screening only for women with risk factors.) Most women with gestational diabetes show a normal fasting blood glucose level; therefore for screening/diagnostic purposes, a challenge of glucose tolerance is used. The screening tool is a 50-g **glucose tolerance test (GTT)** in which a 50-g oral glucose load is given to the woman, regardless of previous meal or time of day, followed by a plasma glucose determination 1 hour later. A glucose level of 140 mg/dl or greater is considered positive and should be followed by a 3-hour oral GTT. The 3-hour GTT is administered after an overnight fast and at least 3 days of unrestricted diet (at least 150 g carbohydrate) and physical activity. The woman is encouraged to avoid caffeine, because caffeine tends to increase glucose levels, and to abstain from smoking for 12 hours before the test. A 100-g glucose load is given, followed by measurements of plasma glucose at 1, 2, and 3 hours. The test is deemed positive for GDM if two or more of the following plasma levels are met or exceeded:

Fasting	105 mg/dl
1 hr	190 mg/dl
2 hr	165 mg/dl
3 hr	145 mg/dl

If only one of the values is elevated, the 3-hour (100 gm) GTT is repeated 1 month later. A repeat GTT is recommended at 32 to 34 weeks for those women who tested positive for the 50-g glucose test but exhibited a normal GTT if there are significant risk factors present.

Maternal and fetal risks. As with pregestational diabetes, the key to positive pregnancy outcome for both mother and fetus is strict glycemic control instituted as early as possible during gestation. Women with gestational diabetes are at increased risk for preeclampsia, UTIs, and operative birth, including cesarean birth, midforceps birth, and midvacuum extraction (Metzger, 1991; Mulford et al, 1993).

Hyperglycemia is associated with an increased risk for intrauterine fetal death and neonatal mortality. Perinatal morbidity and mortality are also higher among women who have gestational diabetes and a history of previous stillbirth, those who develop preeclampsia, and those who were diagnosed with GDM late in pregnancy. Infants of women with gestational diabetes are at significant risk for macrosomia with associated shoulder dystocia and birth trauma, neonatal hypoglycemia, hypocalcemia, polycythemia, and hyperbilirubinemia. The infant of a mother with gestational diabetes is more likely to develop obesity in childhood or later in life. There is also a greater chance that the infant will develop glucose intolerance, specifically NIDDM, in the future (Coustan, 1992; Dorner and Plagemann, 1994; Silverman et al, 1995). The woman who maintains strict glycemic control during pregnancy with normal fasting and postprandial glucose levels encounters approximately the same risk of perinatal mortality as the nondiabetic woman (Thompson et al, 1994).

Nursing Care Management

In caring for the woman diagnosed with gestational diabetes, the nursing role essentially mirrors that of pregestational diabetes. Those nurses involved in prenatal care delivery in any setting can be instrumental in the identification of those women at risk for the development of gestational diabetes.

Assessment

In the early prenatal period, a thorough history is necessary to identify any risk factors that may predispose the pregnant woman to gestational diabetes: (1) maternal age over 30, (2) prepregnancy weight more than 20% over ideal body weight, (3) family history of diabetes, and (4) previous obstetric history that includes GDM in previous pregnancy, infant weight greater than 4 kg (9 lb), congenital anomalies, hydramnios, unexplained stillbirth or miscarriage. Women who do not have diabetes with any of the risk factors for GDM are alerted to the possibility of diabetes during pregnancy and are taught to report any symptoms that may represent onset of the condition (increased thirst, hunger, or urination; weakness). The woman is instructed regarding screening measures for gestational diabetes.

With the initial prenatal interview and during subsequent visits, assessment of physical and emotional stress is important because stress is a factor known to precipitate diabetes in the individual prone to the disease. The diagnosis of gestational diabetes often represents a crisis situation to the pregnant woman and her family. Suddenly the pregnancy is labeled "high risk," which evokes fear and anxiety related to the well-being of the mother and the fetus. Whereas the woman with pregestational diabetes is usually familiar with necessary self-care skills, the woman with gestational diabetes must learn about diabetic management and master the skills on short notice. Because the diagnosis of GDM is often crisis-oriented, there may be barriers to learning and decision-making. The nurse is instrumental is assisting the pregnant woman and her family in overcoming these barriers through therapeutic communication and support, while providing the education necessary for diabetic control and self-care. Women with GDM who need insulin injections require additional support as they learn self-administration techniques (Keohane and Lacey, 1991).

Assessment of the woman's support system is an essential part of care planning. The family's reaction to the diagnosis and the necessary treatment regimen influences the woman's emotional response to the diagnosis and her compliance with the plan of care. Sources of physical and psychosocial stress are identified, with the recommendation that stress be avoided to prevent complications such as hyperglycemia (Ruggiero et al, 1990).

Nursing Diagnoses

Nursing diagnoses are identified based on assessment data and individual response to GDM. Those diagnoses appropriate for pregestational diabetes generally apply to gestational diabetes as well (See p. 258).

Expected Outcomes

Expected outcomes are formulated based on identified nursing diagnoses and the medical plan of care. The woman and her support person(s) are involved with the nurse in the mutual establishment of outcomes.

In general, the expected outcomes of care for gestational diabetes are the same as for pregestational diabetes. The major difference is that the time frame for planning may be shortened with GDM because the diagnosis is usually made later in pregnancy. Planning and implementation must necessarily occur as soon as possible after diagnosis.

Plan of Care and Implementation

Antepartum. When the diagnosis of gestational diabetes is made, treatment begins immediately, allowing little or no time for the woman and her family to adjust to the diagnosis before they are expected to implement the treatment plan. This is in contrast to the woman with pregestational diabetes who may have had years to learn about the disease and adapt to dietary modifications, self-glucose monitoring, and insulin administration. With each step of the treatment plan, it is important that the nurse and other health care providers educate the woman and her family, providing detailed and comprehensive explanations to insure understanding, participation, and compliance with the necessary interventions. Potential complications resulting from noncompliance are discussed, with emphasis placed on the need for maintenance of normoglycemia throughout the remainder of the pregnancy. It may be reassuring for the woman and her family to know that the diabetic condition typically disappears when the pregnancy is over.

Dietary modification is the mainstay of treatment for GDM. Nutritional counseling provided by a trained nutritionist is instituted as soon as possible after the diagnosis is made. The dietary program is individualized according to the woman's needs and the physician's orders. Although there are variations in dietary prescriptions, caloric intake is based on prepregnancy weight: for example, 30 cal/kg/day for women of normal weight; 24 cal/kg/day for women who are overweight; and 36 to 40 cal/kg/day for those who are underweight. A typical diet for gestational diabetes includes from 2000 to 2200 calories per day consumed in three meals and three or four snacks. The diet should contain 40% to 50% carbohydrate, composed primarily of complex carbohydrates with avoidance of simple sugars. Increased intake of soluble dietary fiber is recommended because this delays gastrointestinal absorption. Protein intake should be 20% to 25%; fats are limited to 30% to 40% and should be primarily polyunsaturated. This calorie distribution is effective in maintaining normoglycemia in 75% to 80% of women with gestational diabetes (Jovanovic-Peterson, 1993). (See the Home Care box below.)

Exercise can be an integral part of the treatment plan because it helps lower blood glucose levels and may be instrumental in eliminating the need for insulin. This is an area of controversy because some experts support exercise as an important alternative therapy for GDM (Mulford et al, 1993). It is important that the selected form of exercise does not stimulate uterine activity; arm ergometry or walking may be recommended for the woman with gestational diabetes. It is important that any exercise activity be prescribed by the health care provider, particularly for the woman with gestational diabetes who requires insulin to control glucose levels (Artal, 1992; Mulford et al, 1993; Rosas and Constantino, 1992).

Insulin is required by 10% to 25% of women with gestational diabetes to maintain normoglycemia. Once the dietary regimen is implemented, weekly determinations of fasting and postprandial glucose levels are made. Indications for the initiation of insulin therapy include a fasting plasma glucose level in excess of 105 mg/dl or a postprandial plasma level greater than 120 mg/dl. A combination of regular and NPH human insulin is administered in two or three injections per day, and the dosage is adjusted based on self-determinations of blood glucose levels (see the Home Care boxes on pp. 261 and 262) (Coustan et al, 1993; Landon and Gabbe, 1995; Langer, 1993).

The woman and her family are taught the necessary skills to manage insulin administration. In rare instances, hospitalization may be required to regulate blood glucose levels and to educate the woman about glycemic control through insulin therapy in conjunction with dietary modification.

Periodic assessment of glycosylated hemoglobin may be done to measure the degree of glycemic control. Fasting and postprandial glucose levels are usually monitored at each weekly visit. Self-monitoring of blood glucose levels is a requirement for effective insulin therapy and is usually done 4 times daily—on rising and after meals. Those patients who have gestational diabetes managed by dietary modification alone are also taught to measure blood glucose levels. Visually-read reagent strips or a glucose reflectance meter may be used for self-monitoring of blood glucose. Women with gestational diabetes are also taught to measure urine ketone levels on awakening, during illness, whenever a meal is delayed, and if blood glucose is above target values.

Women with gestational diabetes, particularly those on insulin therapy, are at risk for developing hypoglycemia and hyperglycemia. The woman and her family are taught signs and symptoms as well as causes and prevention and treatment measures (Table 10-2).

Women with gestational diabetes who maintain normal glucose levels are usually allowed to progress to term and spontaneous labor without intervention. There is no standard recommendation for fetal surveillance in gestational diabetic pregnancy. Some practitioners perform weekly NSTs or BPPs from 32 to 36 weeks. Testing begins earlier for women taking insulin and those with poor glycemic control, adverse obstetric histories, or pregnancy-induced hypertension (Coustan, 1993).

Home Care 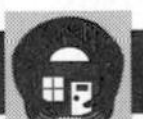

DIETARY PLANNING FOR THE WOMAN WITH GESTATIONAL DIABETES

- Avoid sugar and concentrated sweets.
- Avoid convenience foods (frozen meals, instant potatoes, canned soups, packaged stuffing).
- Eat a very small breakfast of no more than one starch or bread exchange and no fruit or juice.
- Eat small, frequent meals (every 3 hours) and include a good protein source at each meal and snack.
- Eat high fiber foods such as whole-grain breads and cereals, fresh fruits and vegetables, beans, and legumes.
- Lower fat intake.

From Jovanovic-Peterson L, editor: *Medical management of pregnancy complicated by diabetes,* Alexandria, Va, 1993, American Diabetes Association.

Intrapartum. During the labor and birth process, blood glucose levels are monitored at least every 2 hours to maintain levels at 100mg/dl or less. Glucose levels within this range decrease the severity of neonatal hypoglycemia. Intravenous fluids containing glucose are not given as a bolus to the woman with gestational diabetes, although they may be necessary as maintenance fluids.

Postpartum. Approximately 98% of woman with gestational diabetes revert to normoglycemia in the postpartum period; however, women who required insulin therapy during pregnancy are more likely to experience glucose intolerance during the early postpartum period. Four to six weeks after birth or when breastfeeding is stopped, a 75-g oral GTT is performed to assess carbohydrate intolerance. Those women with abnormal results are referred to a diabetologist for follow-up (Dacus et al, 1994; Jovanovic-Peterson and Peterson, 1992).

In planning for future pregnancies, it is important that the woman be aware that gestational diabetes is likely to recur. In addition, the woman who has experienced gestational diabetes is at risk for the development of overt diabetes. The woman is advised of the relationship between body weight and glycemic control so she can decrease her chances of developing overt diabetes in the future by controlling body weight. It is important that the woman understand the need for follow-up procedures to detect glucose intolerance, especially when considering a future pregnancy. Any woman with a history of GDM should have a random glucose level drawn at annual gynecologic examinations. Because the infant of a mother with gestational diabetes is at risk for obesity and future diabetes, regular health care for the child is essential (Howard, 1992; Jovanovic-Peterson, 1993).

Hyperemesis Gravidarum

Hyperemesis gravidarum is defined as excessive or intractable vomiting during pregnancy, leading to dehydration; nutritional deficiencies; weight loss; and fluid, electrolyte, and acid-base imbalances. The estimated incidence of hyperemesis gravidarum varies from 0.5 to 10 per 1000 births. Although most cases are mild and resolve with time, approximately 1 of every 1000 pregnant women requires hospitalization as a result of severe intractable vomiting. Hyperemesis gravidarum is generally self-limiting, but recovery is slow and frequent relapses are common. It occurs most often among primigravidas and tends to recur in subsequent pregnancies. Other predisposing factors include maternal age younger than 20, obesity, multifetal gestation, and trophoblastic disease (hydatidiform mole) (Abell and Riely, 1992; Hod et al, 1994; Singer and Brandt, 1991).

The etiology of hyperemesis gravidarum remains obscure. Several theories have been proposed as to the cause, although none of them adequately explain the disorder (Abell and Riely, 1992). Hyperemesis gravidarum may be related to high levels of estrogen or human chorionic gonadotropin and may be associated with transient hyperthyroidism during pregnancy. It may be accompanied by liver dysfunction with elevation in transaminases and bilirubin levels. Esophageal reflux, reduced gastric motility, and decreased secretion of free hydrochloric acid may contribute to the condition. Other possible causes may be vitamin B deficiencies or disturbances of carbohydrate metabolism (Goodwin, Montoro, and Mestman, 1992; Hod et al, 1994; Modigliani and Bernades, 1995).

Psychologic factors may be instrumental in the development of hyperemesis gravidarum. Ambivalence toward the pregnancy and conflicting feelings regarding prospective motherhood, body changes, and lifestyle alterations—all normal reactions to pregnancy—may contribute to episodes of vomiting, particularly if these feelings are excessive or unresolved. Women with psychologic problems whose normal reaction patterns to stress involve gastrointestinal disturbances often are affected. However, in some women, psychologic causes cannot be identified (Deuchar, 1995; Hod et al, 1994).

The effects of hyperemesis gravidarum on perinatal outcome vary with the severity of the disorder. Women who experience weight loss are more likely to have low-birth-weight (LBW) infants. There may be some relationship between hyperemesis gravidarum and the development of the CNS and skeletal anomalies in the fetus (Godsey and Newman, 1991; Hod et al, 1994).

Maternal mortality as a result of hyperemesis is rare, although in severe cases the prolonged vomiting may lead to Wernicke encephalopathy as a result of vitamin B deficiency. Symptoms of this serious complication of hyperemesis include disorientation, delusions, behavior changes, nystagmus, and uncoordinated movements. If untreated, Wernicke encephalopathy can progress to coma and death (Hod et al, 1994).

In extreme cases, persistent vomiting results in rapid weight loss and dehydration, which leads to fluid and electrolyte imbalances. Dehydration results in hypovolemia, which manifests as hypotension, tachycardia, increased hematocrit and blood urea nitrogen (BUN), and diminished urine output. Vomiting involves loss of gastric acid fluids as well as alkaline contents from deeper within the gastrointestinal tract; this can lead to the development of metabolic acidosis. Extreme maternal nutritional deprivation, or starvation, causes hypoproteinemia and hypovitaminosis. Nutritional and vitamin deficiencies may cause jaundice and bleeding from mucosal surfaces. The embryo or fetus may die, and the mother may die from irreversible metabolic alterations. Rarely, severe intractable vomiting may necessitate termination of the pregnancy by therapeutic abortion to preserve the life and health of the mother.

Conservative management of a woman experiencing hyperemesis gravidarum includes intravenous hydration, vitamin supplements, sedation, antiemetics, and in some cases psychotherapy. For more severe cases enteral or parenteral nutrition may be necessary to correct maternal nutritional deprivation (Charlin et al, 1993).

Nursing Care Management

Nursing care of the pregnant woman who is hyperemetic involves implementing the medical plan of care: initiating and monitoring intravenous therapy, administering pharmacologic agents and nutritional supplements, and monitoring the woman's response to interventions. The nurse observes the woman for any signs of complications, such as metabolic acidosis, jaundice, or hemorrhage, and alerts the physician should these occur. Accurate intake and output, including the amount of emesis, is an important aspect of nursing care. Oral hygiene while the woman is on NPO status and after episodes of vomiting helps allay associated discomforts. When the woman begins responding to therapy, limited amounts of oral fluids and bland foods such as crackers or toast are begun. The diet is progressed slowly as tolerated by the woman until she is able to consume a nutritionally sound diet. Promoting adequate rest is important for the woman with hyperemesis; the nurse can assist in coordinating treatment measures and periods of visitation to provide opportunity for rest periods. The nurse addresses the psychosocial status of the woman, recognizing that the condition is both physically and emotionally debilitating. Some women may benefit from psychotherapy such as hypnotherapy or behavior modification (Abell and Riely, 1992; Hod et al, 1994; Modigliani and Bernades, 1995; Torem, 1994).

Nursing Care Plan

HYPEREMESIS GRAVIDARUM

Nursing Diagnosis: Fluid volume deficit related to active fluid loss secondary to intractable vomiting

Expected Outcomes: The patient will exhibit signs of adequate fluid volume and electrolyte balance (i.e., normal skin turgor, moist mucous membranes, normal vital signs, stable weight; normal electrolytes, Hb and Hct, and urine specific gravity values).

• **NURSING INTERVENTIONS/*RATIONALES***

Administer intravenous fluids per physician order and monitor flow rate *to replace lost fluid and electrolytes.*

Administer antiemetics per physician order *to stop loss of fluid and electrolytes and prevent metabolic acidosis.*

Administer sedation per physician order *to relieve stress and promote rest.*

Maintain NPO status per physician order and when oral intake allowed encourage the woman's preferred liquids in increasing amounts as tolerated *to decrease vomiting and restore fluid and electrolytes.*

Provide a calm, emotionally supportive environment *to encourage rest and decrease debility.*

Maintain strict intake and output; monitor vital signs; monitor serum electrolytes, Hb and Hct, and urine specific gravity lab value; and assess skin turgor, mucous membranes, and weight *to evaluate effectiveness of interventions and prevent maternal/fetal complications.*

Nursing Diagnosis: Altered nutrition: less than body requirements related to persistent nausea and vomiting

Expected Outcomes: The patient will show no evidence of nausea or vomiting and exhibit adequate intake of appropriate nourishment and satisfactory weight gain.

• **NURSING INTERVENTIONS/*RATIONALES***

Start oral intake per physician order and as tolerated by woman beginning with small amounts of attractively served foods tailored to fit food preferences *to increase chances of successful dietary intake.*

Monitor food intake, any further episodes of nausea or vomiting, and track weight *to evaluate refeeding success.*

Refer to dietitian for development of dietary plan that meets nutritional needs of pregnancy, includes maternal eating preferences and meal scheduling *to enhance likelihood of continuing to consume needed nutrients.*

Reinforce the importance of adequate nutrition in pregnancy and assess woman's motivation to follow prescribed dietary plan *to increase likelihood of compliance.*

Nursing Diagnosis: Fear/anxiety related to threat to fetal well-being

Expected Outcomes: The patient's feelings and symptoms of fear and anxiety abate.

NURSING INTERVENTIONS/*RATIONALES*

Provide a calm, soothing atmosphere and teach family to provide emotional support *to facilitate coping.*

Encourage verbalization of fears *to decrease intensity of emotional response.*

Provide woman and family with information related to potential fetal risks and how these risks are being addressed by the health care team *to dispel anxiety stemming from the unknown.*

Involve woman and family in the active management of her diet *to promote a greater sense of control.*

Help the woman identify and use appropriate coping strategies and support systems *to reduce fear/anxiety.*

Explore use of desensitization strategies such as progressive muscle relaxation, visual imagery, or thought stopping *to reduce fear-related emotions and related physical symptoms.*

Arrange for psychologic referral as needed *to treat psychologic features of the condition and to increase coping skills.*

Usually hyperemesis gravidarum responds to therapy, and the prognosis is good. The woman is discharged home when fluid and electrolyte balance is restored and weight gain begins (see the Nursing Care Plan above).

Thyroid Disorders

Hyperthyroidism. Hyperthyroidism affects approximately 1 or 2 of every 1000 pregnancies (Burrow, 1993; Hamburger, 1992). It is most often the result of Graves disease, although other possible causes include Hashimoto thyroiditis, acute thyroiditis, toxic solitary nodules, toxic multinodular goiter, and trophoblastic disease. Typical symptoms associated with hyperthyroidism include nervousness, hyperactivity, weakness, fatigue, weight loss (or poor weight gain), diarrhea, tachycardia, shortness of breath, excessive perspiration, heat intolerance, and muscle tremors. Exophthalmos and enlargement of the thyroid gland (goiter) may also occur. Laboratory findings indicative of hyperthyroidism include elevated free thyroxine (T_4) index and increased basal metabolic rate (Kaplan, 1992; Lazarus, 1993; Molitch, 1995).

Hyperthyroidism in women may be responsible for anovulation and amenorrhea, but the disease is not a recognized cause of spontaneous abortion or fetal malformation. In women with untreated Graves disease, there is an increased risk for congenital anomalies, preterm labor, and LBW infants. Hyperemesis gravidarum is often associated with elevated thyroid hormone levels (Lazarus, 1993).

The fetus of a mother with hyperthyroidism may develop hyperthyroidism because of the transplacental passage of thyroid-stimulating immunoglobulins; fetal tachycardia as early as 25 to 30 weeks may be a symptom. Intrauterine thyrotoxicosis (hyperthyroidism) may result in growth restriction, cardiomegaly, pulmonary hypertension, craniosynostosis, prematurity, and even death (Perelman and Clemons, 1992).

The primary treatment of hyperthyroidism during pregnancy is drug therapy; the medication of choice is propylthiouracil (PTU). The usual starting dosage is 300 to 450 mg/day; the amount is gradually tapered to the smallest effective dosage to prevent unnecessary fetal hypothyroidism. PTU is usually well tolerated by the mother, with rare side effects of rash, nausea, pruritis, hepatitis, arthralgias, vasculitis, and cholestatic jaundice. The most severe side effect is agranulocytosis, which is more common with higher doses. Symptoms of agranulocytosis are fever and sore throat, which should be reported immediately to the health care provider; at the same time, the woman should cease taking PTU. Leukopenia of a transient and benign nature may occur as a result of thiouracil therapy. During therapy, thyroid activity is monitored every 2 weeks to prevent hypothyroidism and to minimize the required dosage of medication. Thiouracils readily cross the placenta and may induce fetal hypothyroidism and goiter (Lazarus, 1993; Molitch 1995). Beta-adrenergic blockers, such as propranolol may be used in severe hyperthyroidism. Long-term use is not recommended because of the potential for IUGR and altered response to anoxic stress, as well as postnatal bradycardia and hypoglycemia (Lazarus, 1993). Radioactive iodine must not be used in diagnosis or treatment of hyperthyroidism because it may compromise the fetal thyroid. If a mother on hyperthyroid medication chooses to breastfeed, she needs to be aware that physiologically significant doses of the drug are passed to the infant through the breastmilk. The infant's thyroid status should be monitored periodically so hypothyroidism can be prevented (Cunningham et al, 1993; Molitch, 1995; Sipes and Malee, 1992).

In severe cases, surgical treatment of hyperthyroidism, subtotal thyroidectomy, may be performed during the second or third trimester. Because of the increased risk of spontaneous abortion or preterm labor associated with major surgery, this treatment is usually reserved for women with severe disease, those for whom drug therapy proves toxic, and those who are unable to adhere to the prescribed medical regimen. Postoperative hypothyroidism is common, occurring in at least 20% of women with hyperthyroidism.

A serious complication of hyperthyroidism (Graves disease) is *thyroid storm,* which may occur in response to stress such as infection, birth, or surgery. A woman experiencing this emergent condition may have fever, restlessness, tachycardia, vomiting, hypotension, or stupor. Prompt treatment is essential; IV fluids and oxygen are administered along with high doses of PTU. Potassium iodide, antipyretics, dexamethasone, and beta blockers may also be given; sedation may be necessary for extreme restlessness (Molitch, 1995; Sipes and Malee, 1992).

Hypothyroidism. Hypothyroidism during pregnancy is rare because women with this condition are often infertile. Hypothyroidism is usually the result of Hashimoto thyroiditis, thyroid gland ablation by radiation, previous surgery, or antithyroid medications. Reduced thyroid function because of hypothalamic or pituitary failure is rare, with only a few reported cases (Kaplan, 1992).

Characteristic symptoms of hypothyroidism include lethargy, weakness, anorexia, weight gain, cold intolerance, mental impairment, constipation, headache, and possibly a goiter. Dry skin, thin brittle nails, alopecia, poor skin turgor, and delayed deep tendon reflexes also are common. Laboratory findings during pregnancy may reveal normal or reduced total T_4, free T_4 (thyroxine) and triiodothyronine (T_3) levels along with elevated thyroid stimulating hormone (TSH) levels (except in cases associated with hypopituitarism).

Pregnant women with hypothyroidism may be at increased risk for spontaneous abortion, preeclampsia, anemia, abruptio placentae, postpartum hemorrhage, and stillbirth. Infants born to mothers with hypothyroidism may be LBW, but for the most part are healthy, without evidence of thyroid dysfunction (Lazarus, 1993; Leung et al, 1993).

Thyroid hormone supplements are used to treat hypothyroidism. Levothyroxine (Synthroid) is most often prescribed during pregnancy, beginning with the dosage of 0.05 to 0.1 mg/day and increasing to a maximum of 0.2 mg/day over several weeks until normal levels of TSH and T_4 are reached. Women who were diagnosed with hypothyroidism before pregnancy should continue their prepregnancy doses, although it is likely the dosage will need to be adjusted as pregnancy progresses (Lazarus, 1993; Molitch, 1995).

The fetus is dependent on maternal thyroid hormones until 12 weeks' gestation, when fetal production begins. Thus maternal hypothyroidism does not cause fetal hypothyroidism. However, maternal treatment of hypothyroidism may result in increased fetal levels of thyroid hormones. Careful monitoring of the neonate's thyroid status is important to detect any abnormalities.

Postpartum thyroid dysfunction. Postpartum thyroid dysfunction (PPTD) affects from 5% to 9% of women and may be transient hyperthyroidism, transient hypothyroidism, or both. The thyroid gland, which normally enlarges during pregnancy, remains enlarged or may further increase in size during the postpartum period. The etiology of PPTD is most likely immunologic. Postpartum thyroid dysfunction usually occurs at about 6 to 12 weeks after birth with a hyperthyroid phase that lasts for 1 to 2 months, followed by a period of transient hypothyroidism. The hypothyroid state is often associated with a goiter and may last for up to 12 months. Although the majority of women progress from the hyperthyroid state to hypothyroidism, some experience resolution of hyperthyroidism without the hypothyroidism. During the hyperthyroid state, women may complain of fatigue, shoulder stiffness, nervousness, increased appetite, and sweating, although many women are asymptomatic. Symptoms during the hypothyroid state may include fatigue, weight gain, and depression. Some women diagnosed as having postpartum depression may actually have a thyroid dysfunction (Learoyd, Fung, and McGregor, 1992; Molitch, 1995).

CARDIOVASCULAR DISORDERS

During a normal pregnancy, the maternal cardiovascular system undergoes many changes that put a physiologic strain on the heart. The major cardiovascular changes that occur during a normal pregnancy that affect the patient with cardiac disease are increased intravascular volume, decreased systemic vascular resistance, cardiac output changes occurring during labor and birth, and the intravascular volume changes that occur just after childbirth. The strain is present during pregnancy and continues for a few weeks after birth. In fact, the strain is so significant the system is described as hyperdynamic during pregnancy (Harvey, 1991). The normal heart can compensate for the increased workload so pregnancy, labor, and birth are generally well tolerated, but the diseased heart is challenged hemodynamically.

If the cardiovascular changes are not well tolerated, cardiac failure can develop during pregnancy, labor, or the postpartum period (Cunningham et al, 1993). In addition, if myocardial disease develops, if valvular disease exists, or if a congenital heart defect is present, **cardiac decompensation** (inability of the heart to maintain a sufficient cardiac output) may occur.

About 1% of pregnancies are complicated by heart disease (Cunningham et al, 1993). Heart disease is the leading cause of nonobstetric maternal mortality. It ranks fourth overall as a cause of maternal death. A maternal mortality rate of 37% is expected in women who have myocardial infarctions during pregnancy (Clark, 1991). A perinatal mortality of up to 50% is anticipated with persistent cardiac decompensation.

The degree of dysfunction (disability) experienced by the woman with cardiac disease is often more important in the treatment and prognosis of cardiac disease complicating pregnancy than is the diagnosis of the valvular lesion. The New York Heart Association's (NYHA; 1964) functional classification of organic heart disease, a widely accepted standard, is as follows:

Class I: asymptomatic at normal levels of activity
Class II: symptomatic with increased activity
Class III: symptomatic with ordinary activity
Class IV: symptomatic at rest

No classification of heart disease can be considered rigid or absolute, but this one offers a basic practical guide for treatment, assuming that frequent prenatal visits, good patient cooperation, and proper obstetric care occur. Medical therapy is conducted as a team approach, including the cardiologist, obstetrical physician, and nurses. The functional classification may change over the course of the pregnancy because of the hemodynamic changes that occur in the cardiovascular system. There is a 30% to 50% increase in cardiac output compared to nonpregnancy resting values, with the majority of the increase in the first trimester and the peak in 20 to 24 weeks' gestation (Myers and Gleicher, 1992). The functional classification of the disease is determined at 3 months and again at 7 or 8 months of gestation.

Spontaneous abortion is increased, and preterm labor and birth are more prevalent in the pregnant woman with cardiac problems. In addition, IUGR is common, probably because of low oxygen pressure (Po_2) in the mother.

A cardiac diagnosis depends on the history, physical examination, x-ray findings, and if indicated, ultrasonogram results. The differential diagnosis of heart disease also involves ruling out respiratory problems, as well as other potential causes of chest pain.

Nursing Care Management

The presence of cardiac disease makes the decision to become pregnant more difficult. Planned pregnancy requires that the woman understand the peripartum risks. If the pregnancy is unplanned, the nurse needs to explore the woman's desire to continue the pregnancy in relation to the status of her cardiac condition. The nurse should review with the woman options for pregnancy termination if her cardiac status is tenuous and abortion is an acceptable alternative.

Assessment

The pregnant woman with cardiac disease requires detailed assessment to determine the potential for optimal maternal health and a viable fetus throughout the peripartum period. If she chooses to continue the pregnancy, the high-risk pregnant woman's condition may be assessed as often as weekly.

The nurse assesses for factors that would increase stress on the heart, such as anemia; infection; or a home situation that includes responsibility for the house, other children, or extended family members. The woman is observed for signs of cardiac decompensation, that is, progressive generalized edema, crackles at the base of the lungs that persist after one or two deep inspirations, or pulse irregularity (Box 10-2). Symptoms of cardiac decompensation may appear abruptly or gradually. Medical intervention must be instituted immediately to correct cardiac status. Dyspnea, chest pain, palpitations, and syncope occur commonly in pregnant women and can mask the symptoms of a developing or worsening cardiovascular disorder.

The routine assessment continues for the antepartum period, including monitoring amount and pattern of weight gain, edema, vital signs, discomforts of pregnancy, urinalysis, and blood work. The nurse documents all medications taken by the woman—including supplemental iron—and is alert to their potential side effects and interactions (Table 10-6).

The client's cultural background may affect the amount of support that she is able to receive from significant others. Family size (number of children and extended family members in the home), as well as role expectations within the family, may be dictated by cultural norms.

BOX 10-2
Signs of Potential Complications

CARDIAC DECOMPENSATION

Pregnant Woman: Subjective Symptoms

- Increasing fatigue or difficulty breathing, or both, with her usual activities
- Feeling of smothering
- Frequent cough
- Palpitations; feeling that her heart is racing
- Swelling of face, feet, legs, fingers (e.g., rings do not fit anymore)

Nurse: Objective Signs

- Irregular weak, rapid pulse (≥100 beats/min)
- Progressive, generalized edema
- Crackles at base of lungs after two inspirations and exhalations
- Orthopnea: increasing dyspnea
- Rapid respirations (≥25 breaths/min)
- Moist, frequent cough
- Increasing fatigue
- Cyanosis of lips and nail beds

TABLE 10-6 Select medications used in the treatment of the pregnant woman with cardiac disease

DRUG	CROSS PLACENTA	CONSIDERATIONS	REFERENCE SOURCES
Digitalis	Yes	■ Must consider the fetal concentration of the drug to avoid fetal toxicity (fetal toxicity exists with maternal overdose) ■ May have to increase maternal dose because of increased blood volume, but keep in therapeutic range ■ Uterine contractility can be affected, leading to preterm labor ■ Used successfully to treat fetal cardiac arrhythmias	Jackson, Clark, 1993 Gilbert, Harmon, 1993 James et al, 1994 Briggs, Garite, 1991
Procainamide	Yes	■ No teratogenic effects ■ Slow elimination from fetus, may accumulate ■ Use with caution	Jackson, Clark, 1993 James et al, 1994 Mendleson, Lang, 1995 Briggs, Garite, 1991 Kulb, 1990
Verapamil	Yes	■ Considered safe for use in pregnancy but can produce maternal hypotension with decreased uterine blood flow ■ Effects on infant not clear, use with caution	Jackson, Clark, 1993
Propranolol	Yes	■ Considered safe for use in pregnancy ■ Not teratogenic ■ Associated with fetal bradycardia, diminished uterine blood flow, IUGR, increased uterine irritability, and premature labor ■ Monitor newborn for 24-48 hours for bradycardia and hypoglycemia if woman on propranolol at the time of delivery	Jackson, Clark, 1993 James et al, 1994
Heparin	No	■ If anticoagulant therapy is needed, heparin should be used ■ Risks include maternal hemorrhage, preterm birth and stillbirth ■ Prolonged IV use may induce osteopenia in woman	James et al, 1994 Hurst, Alpert, 1994
Warfarin	Yes	■ Causes fetal anomalies and hemorrhage, mental retardation, blindness, deafness	Kulb, 1990
Furosemide	Yes	■ Fetal levels estimated to be equal to maternal levels ■ Newborns have increased diuresis, thus sodium and potassium excretion ■ No teratogenic effects ■ Uncommon to be used in first trimester ■ Monitor for decreased plasma volume, which could lead to decreased placental perfusion	Briggs, Garite, 1991
Thiazides	Yes	■ Neonatal jaundice, thrombocytopenia, fluid and electrolyte depletion	Kulb, 1990
Lidocaine	Yes	■ Safe as long as toxic levels are avoided ■ Toxic dose causes fetal CNS and cardiac toxicity	James et al, 1994
Quinidine	Yes	■ No teratogenic effects	Jackson, Clark, 1993 Mendleson, Lang, 1995 James et al, 1994
Nifedipine	Yes	■ No adverse effects on the fetus as long as the woman's blood pressure is not too low ■ Used with caution until further potential fetal toxicity has been evaluated further ■ Adverse interaction with magnesium	Fenakel et al, 1991 Briggs, Garite, 1991
Diazoxide	Yes	■ Can cause fetal and maternal hyperglycemia ■ Reserved for severe hypertension unresponsive to other medications ■ Potent relaxant of uterine smooth muscle	Wasserstrum, 1991 Barron, 1995
Nitroprusside	Yes	■ Use only in critical care unit for brief time with lowest possible therapeutic dose ■ Low dose does not appear to cause toxic cyanide levels (fetal cyanide toxicity may occur with higher doses) ■ No congenital defects have been found	Wasserstrum, 1991 Briggs, Garite, 1991 Barron, 1995

During the *intrapartum period* assessment includes the routine assessments for all women in labor as well as assessments for cardiac decompensation. The latter include measurements of the pulse and respiratory rate at least 4 times every hour during the first stage of labor and every 10 minutes during the second stage (Cunningham et al, 1993).

Nursing ALERT

The physician is alerted if the pulse rate is 100 beats/min or greater or if respirations are 25/min or greater.

Respiratory status is checked constantly for developing dyspnea, coughing, or crackles. The color and temperature of the skin are noted. Pallor, cooling, and sweating may indicate cardiac shock. The laboring woman is carefully watched for symptoms of emotional stress.

The *immediate postpartum period* is hazardous for a woman with a compromised heart. Cardiac output remains elevated for at least 48 hours after giving birth. Venous return is increased as extravascular fluid is remobilized into the vascular compartment and pressure on the inferior vena cava is reduced. Stroke volume is increased and reflex bradycardia occurs. Some health care providers favor the application of an abdominal binder or alternating tourniquets on the extremities to minimize the effects of this rapid change in the early puerperium. By 2 to 3 weeks postpartum, these changes have returned to nonpregnant levels.

Cardiac monitoring for decompensation continues through the first weeks after birth because it has been known to occur as late as the sixth postpartum week. Routine assessment as for any postpartum woman is instituted, including vital signs, lochia, uterine involution, urinary output, pain, rest, diet, and daily weight. Laboratory (e.g., hemoglobin, hematocrit, urinalysis) results are noted and reported if indicated to the physician. It is important to assess the woman's support systems, since activity will be curtailed until the cardiac system is recovered. The family's response to the birth and infant needs to be observed because the mother may not be directly involved in the infant's care for a time (e.g., prematurity of infant, health of mother).

LEGAL TIP

Cardiac and Metabolic Emergencies

The management of emergencies such as maternal cardiopulmonary distress or arrest or maternal metabolic crisis should be documented in policies, procedures, and protocols in the health care setting providing maternity care. Any independent nursing actions appropriate to the emergency should be clearly identified.

Nursing Diagnoses

The following examples are some nursing diagnoses that may be formulated. As always, individualizing diagnoses is vital.

Antepartum

- Fear related to
  - Increased peripartum risk
- Risk for ineffective individual/family coping related to
  - Woman's cardiac condition
  - Changes in relationships
- Risk for altered tissue perfusion related to
  - Hypotensive syndrome
- Risk for activity intolerance related to
  - Cardiac condition
- Knowledge deficit related to
  - Cardiac condition
  - Pregnancy and how it affects cardiac condition
  - Requirements to alter self-care activities
- Risk for self-care deficit related to
  - Activity intolerance
- Impaired home maintenance management related to
  - Mother's confinement to bed and/or limited activity level

Intrapartum

- Anxiety related to
  - Fear for infant's safety
- Fear of dying related to
  - Perceived physiologic inability to cope with the stress of labor
- Risk for impaired gas exchange related to
  - Cardiac condition
- Risk for fluid volume excess related to
  - Extravascular fluid shifts

Postpartum

- Self-care deficit related to
  - Fatigue
  - Need for bed rest
- Situational low self-esteem related to
  - Restriction placed on involvement in care of infant
- Ineffective breastfeeding related to
  - Fatigue from cardiac condition
- Risk for altered parenting related to
  - Separation as a result of prematurity
  - Fatigue from cardiac condition
- Risk for fluid volume excess related to
  - Cardiac decompensation

Expected Outcomes

The mother with cardiovascular problems faces curtailment of her activities. These restrictions can have physical and emotional implications. The community health nurse, social worker, physical or occupational therapist are some of the resource people whose services may need to be incorporated into the plan of care. Expected outcomes such as the following might be appropriate:

1. The pregnant woman (and family, if appropriate) will verbalize understanding of the disorder, management, and probable outcome.
2. The woman and her family will describe their role in management, including when and how to take medication, adjust diet, and prepare for and participate in treatment.
3. The family will cope with emotional reactions to pregnancy and an infant at risk.
4. The woman will be able to withstand the physiologic stressors of pregnancy.
5. The woman will carry her fetus to the point of viability or to term.

Plan of Care and Implementation

Therapy is focused on minimizing stress on the heart. Factors that increase the risk of cardiac decompensation are treated, and the woman is monitored closely for signs and symptoms of cardiac decompensation. The workload on the cardiovascular system is reduced by appropriate treatment of any coexisting emotional stress, hypertension, anemia, hyperthyroidism, or obesity.

Infections are treated promptly, since respiratory, urinary, and gastrointestinal tract infections can complicate the condition by accelerating heart rate and by direct spreading of organisms (e.g., *Streptococcus*) to the heart structure.

Sodium intake is restricted and accompanied by careful

monitoring for hyponatremia. The woman's intake of potassium is monitored to prevent hypokalemia, which is associated with heart and other muscular weakness and dysfunction. Anticoagulant therapy, if used, is monitored. Tests for fetal maturity and well-being and placental sufficiency may be necessary. Other therapy, which follows, is directly related to the functional classification of heart disease.

Antepartum. The pregnant woman with class I heart disease should limit stress to protect against cardiac decompensation. Additional rest, frequent evaluations and the early and effective treatment of respiratory and other infections should be stressed. Vaccines against pneumonococcal and influenza infections are recommended. Therapeutic abortion is never medically warranted.

A plan of care similar to that for class I should be followed for the pregnant woman with class II heart disease. She should avoid heavy exertion and stop any activity that causes even minor signs and symptoms of cardiac decompensation. She should be admitted to the hospital near term if signs of cardiac overload or arrhythmia develop for evaluation and treatment. Bed rest for much of each day is necessary for pregnant women with class III cardiac disease. About 30% of these women experience cardiac decompensation during pregnancy and may be hospitalized for the remainder of the pregnancy and the early puerperium. Early therapeutic abortion may be suggested, particularly if the woman has experienced a previous episode of cardiac failure. Because decompensation occurs even at rest in women with class IV cardiac disease, a major initial effort must be made to improve the cardiac status of pregnant women in this category. Early therapeutic abortion, although not without risk, may be feasible with regional anesthesia in some cases. Prophylactic antibiotic therapy may be ordered with the procedure.

Signs and symptoms of cardiac decompensation are reviewed with the pregnant woman and her family. The woman requires adequate rest. She should sleep 8 to 10 hours every day and 30 minutes after meals. Her activities are restricted; for example, if the woman is at home, she needs to limit housework, shopping, walking, and laundry to the amount recommended for the functional classification of her heart disease. Infections are treated promptly. Nutrition counseling is necessary, optimally with the woman's family present. The woman needs a diet high in iron and protein and adequate in calories to gain weight. To prevent pyrosis (heartburn), the pregnant woman is advised to assume a semi-Fowler or low Fowler position after eating. Iron supplements tend to cause constipation. She should increase her intake of fluids and fiber. A stool softener may be prescribed. It is important for the pregnant woman with cardiac disease to avoid straining during defecation. Straining or bearing down results in the *Valsalva maneuver* (forced expiration against a closed airway, which when released causes blood to rush to the heart and overload the cardiac system) (see the Home Care box above).

Cardiac medications are prescribed as needed for the pregnant woman, with attention given to fetal well-being. The hemodynamic changes that occur during pregnancy, such as increased plasma volume and increased renal clearance of drugs, can alter the amount of medication needed to establish and maintain a therapeutic drug level (Jackson and Clark, 1993). The woman's size and ethnic background must also be taken into consideration. For example, women of short stature or of Asian descent require less medication for the desired physiologic response. Therefore the nurse must monitor the pregnant woman for adverse side effects as well as the blood level of the medication in the woman's serum.

If anticoagulant therapy is required during pregnancy, heparin should be used because this large-molecule drug does not cross the placenta (James et al, 1994). Even though heparin is the anticoagulant of choice during pregnancy, it is not without risk. Heparin use can result in maternal hemorrhage, preterm birth, and stillbirth. The nurse should closely monitor the woman's blood work, including clotting factors. The woman may need to learn to self-administer heparin. She also requires specific nutritional teaching to avoid foods high in vitamin K, such as raw, deep-green and leafy vegetables, which counteract the effects of the heparin. In addition, she will require a substitute source of folic acid in her diet.

Intrapartum. Nursing care during labor and birth focuses on the promotion of cardiac function. Arterial blood gases (ABG) may be needed to assess for adequate oxygenation. A Swan-Ganz catheter may be inserted to monitor hemodynamic status accurately during labor and birth.

Anxiety is decreased or alleviated through maintaining a calm atmosphere and keeping the woman and her family informed. Uterine perfusion is facilitated by placing the woman

Home Care

WOMAN EXPERIENCING CARDIAC DECOMPENSATION

- Assess life-style patterns, emotional status, and environment of woman.
- Arrange for consultations as needed (i.e., dietitian, home care, child care, social work).
- Determine woman's and her family's understanding of her heart disease and how the disease affects her pregnancy.
- Determine stressors in woman's life. Assist woman in identifying effective coping strategies.
- Instruct woman to report signs of cardiac decompensation or congestive heart failure: generalized edema, distension of neck veins, dyspnea, pulmonary crackles, cough, palpitations, weight gain of 0.9 kg (2 lb) per day.
- Instruct woman to be watchful for signs of thromboembolism such as redness, tenderness, pain, or swelling of the legs. If such symptoms were to occur, the woman should seek medical help immediately.
- Instruct woman to avoid constipation and straining (Valsalva maneuver), by taking in adequate fluids and fiber. A stool softener may be ordered.
- Explore with woman ways to obtain needed rest throughout the day. Depending on the level of her cardiac disease, she may need to sleep 10 hours per night and rest 1/2 hour after meals (classes I and II) or rest for most of the day (class III and IV).
- Refer woman to community resources including support groups as indicated.
- Emphasize the importance of keeping her prenatal visits.

Modified from Gilbert E, Harmon J: *Manual of high risk pregnancy and delivery,* St Louis, 1993, Mosby and Grohar J: Nursing protocols for antepartum home care, *J Obstet Gynecol Neonatal Nurs* 23(8): 687, 1994.

in a side-lying position. Cardiac function is supported by keeping her head and shoulders elevated and her body parts resting on pillows. The woman is placed on a heart monitor to determine the presence of rhythm disturbances. Since pain can contribute to cardiovascular stress, discomfort is relieved with medication and supportive care. For birth the nurse assists in the administration of pharmacologic relief of discomfort. Epidural regional anesthesia provides better pain relief than narcotics and fewer alterations in hemodynamics (Cunningham et al, 1993; Gilbert and Harmon, 1993). Hypotension must be avoided.

For the woman with cardiac disease, vaginal birth is recommended if there are no obstetric problems. This is accomplished using epidural or pudendal block anesthesia with forceps for shortening the second stage of labor. Penicillin prophylaxis of nonsensitized pregnant women may be ordered to protect against bacterial endocarditis in labor and during early puerperium. Mask oxygen and pudendal block anesthesia are important. Ergot products should not be used because they tend to increase blood pressure. Diluted IV oxytocin immediately after birth may be employed to prevent hemorrhage.

Vaginal birth is accomplished with the woman in a side-lying or upright position, or if she is placed in the supine position, a pad is positioned under the hip to minimize the danger of supine hypotension. The knees are flexed, and the feet are flat on the bed. To prevent compression of popliteal veins and an increase in blood volume in the chest and trunk as a result of the efforts of gravity, stirrups are not used. Bearing down (Valsalva maneuver) must be avoided, since this reduces diastolic ventricular filling and obstructs left ventricular outflow (Scott and Branch, 1994). An episiotomy and the use of outlet forceps also decrease the work of the heart.

Beta-adrenergic agents (e.g., ritodrine, terbutaline) should not be used for tocolysis. These agents are associated with myocardial ischemia. A synthetic oxytocin *(Syntocinon)*, can be used for induction of labor. This drug does not appear to cause significant coronary artery constriction in dosage prescribed for labor induction or control of postpartum uterine atony. Cervical ripening agents containing prostaglandins are not contraindicated, but reports of use in pregnant women with cardiac disease are not available.

Postpartum. The first 24 to 48 hours postpartum are the most hemodynamically difficult. Cardiac output increases rapidly as extravascular fluid is remobilized into the vascular compartment. At the moment of birth, intraabdominal pressure is reduced drastically; pressure on veins is removed, the splanchnic vessels engorge, and blood flow to the heart is increased. When blood flow increases to the heart, a **reflex bradycardia** may result in response to the increased blood flow.

Special attention is given to the woman who is at risk for cardiac decompensation. The increased intravascular fluid can cause fluid volume excess in these women. Some physicians favor the application of an abdominal binder or alternating tourniquets on the extremities to minimize the effects of this rapid change in intraabdominal pressure. Hemorrhage and/or infection may worsen the cardiac condition. Monitoring for cardiac decompensation continues through the first week after birth because of hormonal shifts that affect hemodynamics. These shifts have been known to occur as late as the seventh postpartum day.

Care in the postpartum period is tailored to the woman's functional capacity. The woman must be protected from infection. A private room is one method to restrict traffic into her room. Positioning in bed is the same as that for the labor; that is, the head of the bed is elevated and the woman is encouraged to lie on her side. Bed rest may be ordered with or without bathroom privileges. The nurse may need to help the woman meet her grooming and hygiene needs and even help her with turning in bed, eating, and other activities. Respiratory and circulatory sequelae to immobility, as well as boredom, must be addressed. Progressive ambulation may be permitted as tolerated. The nurse assesses the woman's pulse rate, breath sounds, skin, and affect before and after walking.

Bowel and bladder elimination require special attention. Bowel movements without straining are promoted with stool softeners, diet, and fluids, plus mild analgesia and local anesthetic spray. Overdistention of the bladder is prevented, because a distended bladder can result in an atonic uterus and hemorrhage. Rapid emptying of the bladder is avoided. Rapid decompression of the bladder results in a precipitous drop in intraabdominal pressure, leading to splanchnic engorgement and generalized hypotension.

Although breastfeeding is often not advised for mothers with class III and class IV heart disease, it is not contraindicated (Lawrence, 1994). The woman can conserve her energy by breastfeeding in a resting position and by having others bring the baby to her for feedings.

Mother-child interactions warrant special planning. The interactions should not stress the mother. The mother may direct care of the infant by a designated family member. The baby can be brought regularly to the mother, held at her eye level and by her lips, and brought to her fingers so she can establish an emotional bond with her baby with a low expenditure of her energy.

Before discharge the nurse assesses the home support for the woman and infant. Preparation for discharge is carefully planned with the woman and family. Provision of help in the home for the mother by relatives, friends, and others must be addressed. If necessary, the nurse refers the family to community resources (e.g., for homemaking services). Rest and sleep periods, activity, and diet must be planned. The couple should receive information about reestablishing sexual relations and contraception (possibly sterilization of the man or the woman).

Potential hazards of a subsequent pregnancy need to be examined by the woman and her partner. If sterilization is selected as a method of contraception, the risks of surgery, especially for the woman with class III or IV heart disease need to be explained. Oral contraceptives are often contraindicated because of the risk of thromboembolism (Gilbert and Harmon, 1993). Both the woman and her partner need to be involved in the decision-making process.

Evaluation

The nurse uses the following criteria as *overall indications* for the success of therapy:

- The woman adapts to the physiologic stressors of pregnancy; for example, she is free of congestive heart failure during the postpartum period.

- The home situation is controlled, with assistance provided as necessary.
- The woman and family accept the limitations imposed on the woman by the presence of heart disease.
- The parent-child relationship is fostered by the family.
- The woman and family verbalize understanding of the disorder, management, and probable outcome.
- The woman and family describe their role in management, including when and how to take medication, adjust diet, and prepare for treatment.
- The woman and family participate in treatment.
- The woman and family cope with emotional reactions to pregnancy and an infant at risk.
- The woman is able to carry pregnancy to term or the point of viability of the fetus.

See the Nursing Care Plan for a pregnant woman with heart disease on p. 279.

Heart Surgery During Pregnancy

Operations for the correction of congenital or acquired heart disease should be performed before pregnancy if possible. Pregnancy after open heart surgery is often possible if the congenital cardiac condition was improved significantly. A woman with cardiac disease may have different signs and symptoms during pregnancy than in the nonpregnant state. When medical therapy for a pregnant woman fails, cardiac surgery should be performed (Mendelson and Lang, 1995). Early second trimester is the better time for surgery. The client, fetus, and uterus must be monitored carefully during surgery. Closed cardiac surgery, such as release of a stenotic mitral orifice, can be accomplished with little risk to mother or fetus. Open heart surgery requires extracorporeal circulation, and under these circumstances, hypoxia, fetal bradycardia, and increased uterine contractions may develop (Strickland et al, 1991). As a consequence, the risk of fetal damage or loss rises to 10% to 20%, and is thought to result from the nonpulsatile circulation created by the extracorporeal pump (Kulb, 1990).

Some women who are free of symptoms after earlier cardiac surgery have significant deterioration during pregnancy. The normal hemodynamic demands of pregnancy compromise their cardiac status. For these clients, therapeutic abortion, if acceptable to the client and her family, is advised before the hemodynamic demands fully manifest. There is an increased incidence of spontaneous abortion, stillbirth, LBW infants, and malformed fetuses born to women with valvular heart disease.

Critical Thinking Exercises

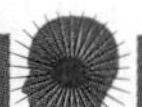

HEART DISEASE

You are assigned to a woman who has a history of class III heart disease (NYHA classification). She just learned that she is 8 weeks pregnant. She has a 2-year-old son at home and tells you that her husband, who is not present today, thinks she is healthy and that she does not need any help with household or child care activities during pregnancy.

1. Examine the options for this woman given this situation. What are the pros and cons of each?
2. Select one option. Then:
   a. Justify your choice
   b. Formulate nursing diagnoses
3. Develop a plan of care

Associated Cardiovascular Disorders

Care of the woman with cardiovascular disorders combines routine peripartum care with care specific for the cardiac diagnosis. Cardiac conditions vary in their impact on pregnancy because of acuteness or chronicity. The following discussion focuses on peripartum heart failure, hypertrophic cardiomyopathy, rheumatic heart disease, mitral valve stenosis and prolapse, Marfan syndrome, and cerebrovascular accident.

Peripartum heart failure. Peripartum heart failure (failure of the heart to maintain an adequate cardiac output to maintain adequate circulation of blood) can result from an underlying chronic hypertension, previously unrecognized mitral valve stenosis, obesity, viral myocarditis, or **idiopathic peripartum cardiomyopathy** (Cunningham et al, 1993). In addition, anemia and infection can predispose the woman to congestive heart failure.

Peripartum heart failure from an explainable cause such as an underlying heart disease usually responds well to therapy. The typical response is rapid reversal of heart failure with furosemide (Lasix) diuresis and correction of associated obstetric complications (Cunningham et al, 1993). Within days the heart size of these women returns to normal. Their long-term prognosis depends on the underlying heart disease.

Hypertrophic cardiomyopathy (HCM) is a primary disease, classified on the basis of its structural abnormality and function. In this disorder the muscle tissue of the heart walls and the septum are hypertrophied, leaving relatively small chambers. HCM usually is asymptomatic until late adolescence, early adulthood, or more rarely, middle age. Symptoms include angina, exertional dyspnea, dizziness, syncope, ventricular arrhythmias, S_4 gallop, and mild cardiomegaly. Propranolol (Inderal), a beta blocker, is given if symptoms develop (Cunningham et al, 1993). HCM is associated with sudden death, unrelated to functional status. HCM may be precipitated by physical or emotional stress, and the myocardial ischemia resulting from stress may promote ventricular fibrillation.

Peripartum cardiomyopathy comprises a syndrome of heart failure occurring during the peripartum period with no previous history of heart disease and with no specific etiologic factors. Autoimmune factors may be implicated (Cruikshank, 1994; Muller and Goldman, 1991).

The incidence of peripartum cardiomyopathy has been reported as 1 in 1500 to 1 in 4000 pregnancies (Cruikshank, 1994). It is more common in African-Americans, multiparous women age 30 and older, in twin pregnancies, and in women with preeclampsia (Mendelson and Lang, 1995). Maternal mortality has been estimated in the range of 25% to 50%, whereas infant mortality is approximately 10% (Jackson and Clark, 1993). Clinical findings are those of congestive heart failure (left ventricular failure). Symptoms include breathlessness, tachyarrhythmias, and edema, with radiologic findings of cardiomegaly. The prognosis is good if cardiomegaly does not persist after 6 months postpartum. The prognosis for women whose hearts remain enlarged after 6 months of bed rest is not as favorable. There will likely be peripartum cardiomyopathy in any future pregnancy (Jackson and Clark, 1993). Sterilization should be considered. Oral contraceptives are contraindicated because of the risk of thromboembolism.

Medical management of cardiomyopathy during pregnancy includes diuretics, potassium, anticoagulants, and digitalis. Bed rest is generally recommended, but its benefit is unclear (Jackson and Clark, 1993; Muller and Goldman, 1991).

Low sodium intake (1.5 to 2 g/day) is ordered for women with severe congestive failure. During labor, the avoidance of IV fluid overload is important. Because all women experience some rise in blood pressure at the onset of lactation, suppression of lactation is recommended to minimize stress.

The nursing care of patients with peripartum cardiomyopathies is essentially the same as for those with other types of cardiac problems. The use of the Trendelenburg position for relief of syncope has been demonstrated. The necessity for prolonged bed rest can pose social and economic hardships for the family; therefore referral to community resources for assistance may be necessary. Because sudden death is a possibility with this condition, the family needs to be trained in cardiopulmonary resuscitation. Patients need to have ready access to emergency care.

BOX 10-3

Prophylaxis of Subacute Bacterial Endocarditis

When a woman has prosthetic valves, congenital heart disease, valvular disease, cardiomyopathy or bacterial endocarditis, prophylaxis for subacute bacterial endocarditis (SBE) is given before undergoing procedures that cause significant bacteremia such as dental, urinary cystoscopy, and vaginal birth in the presence of infection (Jackson and Clark, 1993). Obstetric procedures are low risk for infective endocarditis (Barron and Lindheimer, 1995). In certain high-risk clients prophylactic antibiotics are given in uncomplicated births (vaginal and cesarean) (Jackson and Clark, 1993).

Antibiotic prophylaxis is given from 30 minutes to 1 hour before the procedure and up to 8 hours after the procedure. The standard antibiotic regimen is ampicillin 2 g IM or IV and gentamicin 1.5 mg/kg up to 80 mg (Jackson and Clark, 1993). Amoxicillin 1.5 g can be given orally for low-risk clients.

Rheumatic heart disease. Rheumatic fever usually develops suddenly, several symptom-free weeks after an inadequately treated group A beta-hemolytic streptococcal throat infection. Episodes of rheumatic fever create an autoimmune reaction in the heart tissue, leading to permanent damage of heart valves (usually the mitral valve) and the chorda tendineae cordis. This damage is referred to as **rheumatic heart disease (RHD).** RHD may be evident during acute rheumatic fever or discovered years later. Recurrences of rheumatic fever are common, each with the potential to increase the severity of heart damage. If a woman has had rheumatic fever in the past, a recurrence can occur during pregnancy. The American Heart Association recommends lifelong prophylaxis with penicillin G benzathine, even during pregnancy. For penicillin allergies, erythromycin is an acceptable alternative during pregnancy. Heart murmurs, resulting from stenosis, valvular insufficiency, or thickening of the walls of the heart, characterize RHD. Abnormal pulse rate and rhythm, as well as congestive heart failure, are common.

Mitral valve stenosis. Ninety percent of RHD in pregnancy is the result of **mitral valve stenosis** (narrowing of the opening of the mitral valve caused by stiffening of valve leaflets, obstructing blood flow from the atrium to the ventricles) (Cruikshank, 1994). As the mitral valve narrows, dyspnea worsens, occurring first on exertion and eventually at rest. A tight stenosis, plus the increase in blood volume and cardiac output of normal pregnancy may cause ventricular failure and pulmonary edema; hemoptysis may occur.

Atrial fibrillation is common because of the enlarged left atrium and can cause thromboemolism. Anticoagulants and digitalis therapy are used to treat atrial fibrillation (Cruikshank, 1994). Cardiac failure occurs for the first time during pregnancy in 25% of women with mitral valve stenosis. The care of the woman with mitral stenosis typically is managed by activity restriction, bed rest, and limitation of dietary sodium. The pregnant woman with mitral stenosis should be monitored clinically for symptoms and by echocardiograms to monitor the atrial and ventricular size as well as heart valve function. Prophylaxsis for intrapartum endocarditis and pulmonary infections is provided (Box 10-3).

Mitral valve prolapse. Mitral valve prolapse (MVP) is a common, usually benign, condition occurring in nearly 10% of women of reproductive age (Cunningham et al, 1993). The mitral valve leaflets prolapse into the left atrium during ventricular systole, allowing some backflow of blood. Midsystolic click and late systolic murmur are hallmarks of this syndrome. Most cases are asymptomatic. A few women have atypical chest pain (sharp and located in the left side of the chest) that occurs at rest, is unrelated to exercise, and does not respond to nitrates. They may have anxiety, palpitations, dyspnea on exertion, and syncope. They are usually treated with beta blockers such as propranolol (Inderal). Pregnancy and its associated hemodynamic changes may change or alleviate the murmur and click of MVP, as well as symptoms. Pregnancy usually is well tolerated unless bacterial endocarditis occurs. As with RHD, antibiotic prophylaxis is given before invasive procedures for at-risk clients and for complicated vaginal deliveries in clients with MVP (Box 10-3).

Marfan syndrome. Marfan syndrome is an autosomal dominant disorder characterized by elongation of the bones resulting in musculoskeletal disorders and general weakness of connective tissue. It is also associated with dilation of the aortic root and dissecting aneurysms (Gleicher, 1992). About 90% of individuals with this symptom have mitral valve prolapse, and 25% have aortic insufficiency. There is an increased risk of aortic dissection and rupture during pregnancy, and maternal mortality is reported at 25% to 50% (Cruikshank, 1994). Management during pregnancy includes restricted activity and beta blockers.

Cerebrovascular accident. Ischemia of the brain tissues, or *cerebrovascular accident (CVA)*, occurs from occlusion of blood vessels that normally perfuse the area. It results from a cerebral hemorrhage or an embolus. Uncontrolled hypertension during pregnancy can cause cerebral hemorrhages (Cunningham et al, 1993; Harvey, 1991). CVAs have been reported to occur in 1 in 6000 pregnancies (Simolke, Cox, and Cunningham, 1991). The extent of damage depends on the location and the extent of ischemia.

Cardiopulmonary Resuscitation of the Pregnant Woman

Trauma, pulmonary embolism, anesthesia complications, drug overdose, hypovolemia, or septic shock may result in cardiopulmonary arrest. Preexisting disorders, such as heart or pulmonary disease, hypertension, or autoimmune collagen vascular disease, increase this risk (Kulb, 1990). Some modifications of the procedure for cardiopulmonary resuscitation (CPR) (see the Emergency box below) and the Heimlich maneuver are needed (Fig. 10-4). To prevent supine hypotension, the woman is positioned on a flat firm surface, with the uterus displaced laterally (manually or with a wedge or rolled towel under her right hip). If defibrillation is needed, the paddles need to be placed one rib interspace higher than usual because the heart is displaced slightly by the enlarged uterus. If possible, the fetus should be monitored during the cardiac arrest (Elkayan and Gleicher, 1990).

Complications may be associated with CPR of a pregnant woman. These complications include laceration of the liver, rupture of the uterus, hemothorax, and hemoperitoneum (Troiano, 1989). Fetal complications also may occur. These include cardiac arrhythmia or asystole related to maternal defibrillation and medications, CNS depression related to antiarrhythmic drugs and inadequate uteroplacental perfusion, and onset of preterm labor. If the fetus dies during the resuscitative efforts, the woman should be stabilized before delivery is attempted (Kulb, 1990).

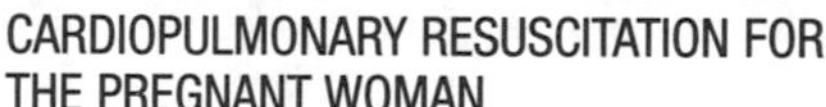

CARDIOPULMONARY RESUSCITATION FOR THE PREGNANT WOMAN

CPR

Determine unresponsiveness.
Activate emergency medical system.
Position woman on a flat firm surface with the uterus displaced laterally with a wedge (e.g., a rolled towel placed under her right hip) or manually.

Airway

Open airway with head tilt-chin lift maneuver.

Breathing

Determine breathlessness (look, listen, feel).
If the woman is not breathing, give two slow breaths.

Circulation

Determine pulselessness by feeling carotid pulse.
If there is no pulse, begin chest compressions at a rate of 80 to 100/minutes.
After four cycles of fifteen compressions and two breaths, check her pulse. If pulse is not present, then continue CPR.

Heimlich Maneuver (Fig 10-4)

If the pregnant woman is unable to speak or cough, then perform chest thrusts. Stand behind the woman and place your arms under her armpits to encircle her chest. Press backwards with quick thrusts until the foreign body is expelled.

Data from American Heart Association: *Basic life support, heart saver guide,* Dallas, 1993, AHA.

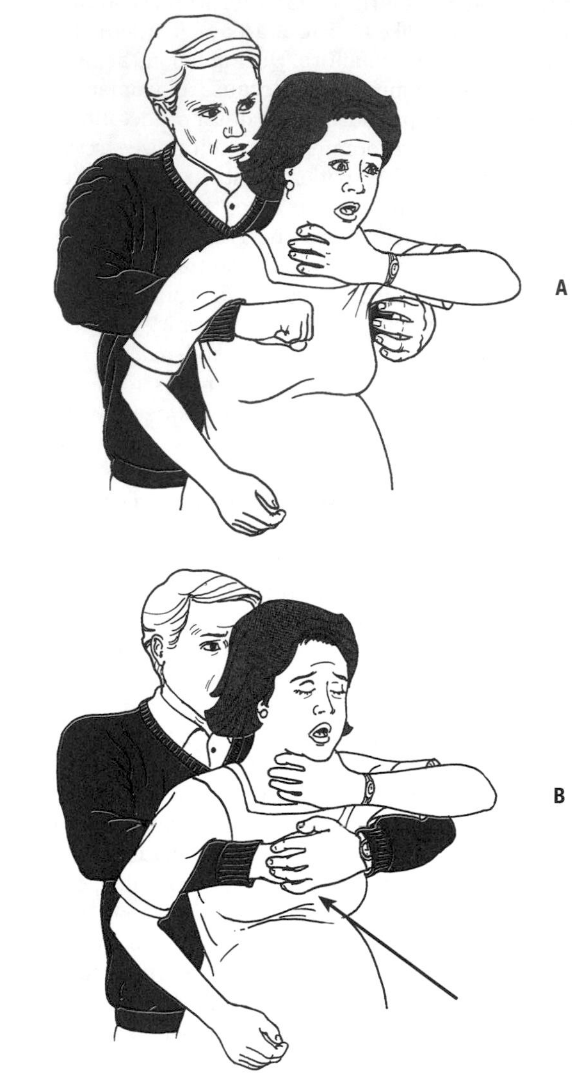

Fig. 10-4 Clearing airway obstruction in a woman in the late stages of pregnancy. **A,** Standing behind the victim, place your arms under the woman's armpits and across the chest. Place thumb side of your clenched fist against the middle of the sternum; place other hand over fist. **B,** Perform backward chest thrusts until the foreign body is expelled or woman loses consciousness. If woman becomes unconscious because of foreign body airway obstruction, place her on her back (be sure the uterus is displaced laterally, e.g., a rolled blanket under her right hip), and kneel close to the victim's side. Open the mouth with the tongue-jaw lift, perform finger sweep, attempt rescue breathing. If unable to ventilate, position hands as for chest compression. Deliver five chest thrusts firmly to remove the obstruction. Repeat the above sequence of Heimlich maneuver, finger sweep, and attempt to ventilate. Continue the above sequence until the pregnant woman's airway is clear of obstruction or help arrives to relieve you (Chandra and Hazinski, 1994). If woman is unconscious, give chest compressions as for woman without a pulse.

Nursing Care Plan

HEART DISEASE

Nursing Diagnosis: Activity intolerance related to effects of pregnant state on underlying cardiac condition

Expected Outcome: **Patient will show no evidence of cardiac decompensation (i.e., no fatigue, shortness of breath, palpitations, edema, rapid irregular pulse, crackles, rapid respirations, cyanosis of nailbeds and lips).**

• NURSING INTERVENTIONS/*RATIONALES*

Assist woman to identify factors that decrease activity tolerance and explore extent of limitations *to establish a baseline for evaluation.*

Help woman develop an individualized program of activity and rest *that maintains sufficient cardiac output.*

Teach woman to monitor physiologic response to activity (i.e., pulse rate, respiratory rate) and reduce activity that provokes fatigue and/or pain *to maintain sufficient cardiac output and prevent harm to fetus.*

Enlist significant others to assist woman in pacing activities and to provide support in performing role functions and self-care activities that are too strenuous *to increase chances of compliance with activity restrictions.*

Have woman maintain an activity log that records activities, time, duration, intensity, and physiologic response *to evaluate effectiveness of and adherence to activity program.*

Nursing Diagnosis: Risk for altered tissue perfusion related to cardiac condition secondary to increased circulatory needs during pregnancy

Expected Outcomes: **The mother will exhibit signs of hemodynamic stability (i.e., blood pressure, pulse, ABGs and white blood cell counts [WBCs] are within normal limits). The fetus will exhibit signs of well-being (i.e., fetal activity and fetal heart rate [FHR] are within normal limits).**

• NURSING INTERVENTIONS/*RATIONALES*

Monitor heart rate and rhythm, blood pressure, skin color and temperature, WBCs, Hb and Hct, ABG *to detect early signs of cardiac failure/hypoxia.*

Monitor fetal activity and FHR, perform NST as indicated *to assess fetal status and detect uteroplacental insufficiency.*

Teach woman how to detect and report early signs of cardiac decompensation *to prevent maternal/fetal complications.*

Nursing Diagnosis: Decreased cardiac output related to increased circulatory volume secondary to pregnancy and cardiac condition

Expected Outcome: **The patient will exhibit signs of adequate cardiac output (i.e., normal pulse and blood pressure, normal heart and breath sounds, normal skin color, tone and turgor, normal capillary refill, normal urine output, no evidence of edema).**

• NURSING INTERVENTIONS/*RATIONALES*

Reinforce importance for use of activity/rest cycles *to prevent cardiac complications.*

Teach woman to lie in left lateral position *to increase uterine blood flow* and to elevate legs while sitting *to promote venous return.*

Monitor intake and output and check for edema *to assess for renal complications or venous return problems.*

Monitor fetal activity and FHR, perform NST as indicated *to assess fetal status and detect uteroplacental insufficiency.*

After successful resuscitation, the woman and her fetus must receive careful monitoring. She remains at increased risk for recurrent pulmonary arrest and arrhythmias (ventricular tachycardia, supraventricular tachycardia, bradycardia). Therefore her cardiovascular, pulmonary, and neurologic status should be assessed continuously. Uterine activity and resting tone must be monitored. Fetal status and gestational age should be determined and used in the decision-making regarding continuation of the pregnancy or timing and route of delivery (Kulb, 1990). All assessment data influence both the medical and nursing plans of care (see the Nursing Care Plan above).

MEDICAL DISORDERS DURING PREGNANCY

Medical conditions may complicate pregnancy. The most common of these is anemia, especially anemia caused by iron or folic acid deficiency, sickle cell trait or disease, and thalassemia. Pulmonary, gastrointestinal, integumentary, neurologic, and autoimmune disorders also may be encountered. Pregnancy-related aspects of these conditions are addressed in the following sections.

Anemia

Anemia, the most common medical disorder of pregnancy, affects at least 20% of pregnant women. Women with anemia have a higher incidence of puerperal complications, such as infection, than do pregnant women with normal hematologic values.

Anemia results in reduction of the oxygen-carrying capacity of the blood; the heart tries to compensate by increasing the cardiac output. This effort increases the workload of the heart and stresses ventricular function. Therefore anemia that occurs with any other complication (e.g., preeclampsia) may result in congestive heart failure.

An indirect index of the oxygen-carrying capacity is the

packed red blood cell volume, or hematocrit level. The normal hematocrit range in nonpregnant women is 38% to 45%. Normal values for pregnant women with adequate iron stores may be as low as 34%. This has been explained by hydremia (dilution of blood), or the physiologic anemia of pregnancy.

At or near sea level, during the first trimester the pregnant woman is anemic when her hemoglobin level is less than 10 g/dl. In areas of high altitude, much higher values indicate anemia, for example, at 1500 m above sea level, a hemoglobin level less than 14 g/dl indicates anemia.

When a woman has anemia during pregnancy, the loss of blood at birth, even if minimal, is not well tolerated. She is at an increased risk for requiring blood transfusions. About 80% of cases of anemia in pregnancy are of the iron deficiency type (Arias, 1993). The remaining 20% of cases embrace a considerable variety of acquired and hereditary anemias, including folic acid deficiency, sickle cell anemia, and thalassemia.

Nursing care of the pregnant woman with anemia requires that the nurse be able to distinguish between the normal physiologic anemia of pregnancy and the disease states. (See the section on physiologic anemia of pregnancy, p. 113). During the prenatal visits the nurse should take a diet history and provide dietary teaching as appropriate. Pregnancy may cause increased fatigue, stress, and financial difficulties for a woman with anemia as she copes with her activities of daily living. The nurse should assess the pregnant woman's needs and provide her with appropriate resources and/or referral.

Iron deficiency anemia. Pathologic anemia of pregnancy is mainly the result of iron deficiency (James et al, 1994). Without iron therapy even pregnant women who enjoy excellent nutrition conclude pregnancy with an iron deficit. Iron for the fetus comes from the maternal serum (James et al, 1994).

Diet alone cannot replace gestational iron losses. Inadequate nutrition without therapy will certainly mean iron deficiency anemia during late pregnancy and the puerperium.

Successful iron therapy during pregnancy can be carried out in most cases with oral iron supplements (e.g., ferrous sulfate, 0.3 g, 3 times/day). It is important to teach the pregnant woman the significance of iron therapy (see Chapter 8). In addition, it is necessary to instruct the woman in dietary ways to decrease the gastrointestinal side effects of iron. Some pregnant women cannot tolerate the prescribed oral iron because of nausea and vomiting. In such cases the woman should receive parenteral iron such as an iron-dextran complex (Imferon).

Folic acid deficiency anemia. Folic acid deficiency anemia occurs in at least 2% of pregnant women in North America, an incidence much higher than that suspected even 5 years ago. Folic acid deficiency during conception and early pregnancy increases the incidence of neural tube defects, cleft lip, and cleft palate (James et al, 1994). Anemia compromises the woman's defenses, and it makes her more vulnerable to urinary tract infections and hemorrhage.

Poor diet, cooking with large volumes of water, or home canning of food (especially vegetables) may lead to folate deficiency. Malabsorption may play a part in the development of anemia caused by a lack of folic acid.

Folic acid deficiency anemia is common in multiple gestations. During pregnancy the recommended daily intake is 400 to 800 μg/day of folate.

Sickle cell hemoglobinopathy. Sickle cell hemoglobinopathy is a disease caused by the presence of abnormal hemoglobin in the blood. *Sickle cell trait* (SA hemoglobin pattern) is sickling of the red blood cells but with a normal red blood cell life span and usually causes only mild clinical symptoms. *Sickle cell anemia* (sickle cell disease) is a recessive, hereditary, familial hemolytic anemia that affects those of African-American or Mediterranean ancestry. These individuals usually have abnormal hemoglobin types (SS or SC). People with sickle cell anemia have recurrent attacks (crises) of fever and pain in the abdomen or extremities beginning in childhood. These attacks are attributed to vascular occlusion (from abnormal cells), tissue hypoxia, edema, and red blood cell destruction. Crises are associated with normochromic anemia, jaundice, reticulocytosis, positive sickle cell test, and the demonstration of abnormal hemoglobin (usually SS or SC).

Almost 10% of African-Americans in North America have the sickle cell trait, but less than 1% have sickle cell anemia. The anemia often is complicated by iron and folic acid deficiency.

Pregnancy usually results in a worsening of most aspects of the disease (Cruikshank, 1994). The anemia that occurs in normal pregnancies may aggravate sickle cell anemia and bring on more crises. Fetal loss is high, because of impaired oxygen supply and sickling, as well as infarcts in the placental circulation (James et al, 1994). Pregnant women with sickle cell anemia are prone to pyelonephritis, leg ulcers, bone abnormalities, strokes, cardiopathy, congestive heart failure, and preeclampsia. UTIs and hematuria are common. An aplastic crisis may follow serious infection. Medical therapy may include prophylactic transfusions in the mother to decrease the sickle cells and to increase the hemoglobin (Perry and Morrison, 1992). Cesarean birth is warranted only for obstetric indications. Oral contraceptives are contraindicated.

Table 10-7 identifies some potential problems faced by the woman with sickle cell disease and some preventive and maintenance interventions.

Thalassemia. Thalassemia (Mediterranean or Cooley anemia) is a relatively common anemia in which an insufficient amount of globin is produced to fill the red blood cells. Thalassemia is a hereditary disorder that involves the abnormal synthesis of the alpha or beta chains of globin. Beta thalassemia is the more common variety in the United States and is often diagnosed in individuals of Italian, Greek, southern Chinese, Mediterranean, North African, Middle Eastern, or Indo-Pakistani descent. The unbalanced synthesis of globin leads to premature red blood cell death resulting in severe anemia. Thalassemia major is the homozygous form of the disorder; thalassemia minor is the heterozygous form.

Thalassemia major complicates pregnancy. Preeclampsia is more common in women with thalassemia major. Thalassemia major may be associated with LBW infants and increased fetal wastage. Placental weight often is increased, perhaps secondary to maternal anemia. The rate of fetal distress from hypoxia is greater than in women without thalassemia major. Therefore pregnant women with thalassemia major should be monitored closely.

TABLE 10-7 Sickle cell anemia: potential problems, prevention, and maintenance

POTENTIAL PROBLEM	PREVENTION AND MAINTENANCE
1. Inadequate oxygen to meet needs of labor and prevent sickling	1. a. Monitor Hb level and HCT to maintain Hb at ≥7 g and HCT at ≥20% b. Have typed and crossmatched blood available c. Assist with transfusions d. Administer oxygen continuously during labor e. Coach for relaxation and to lessen anxiety
2. Infection resulting from anemia: urinary tract infection, pyelonephritis, pneumonia	2. a. Continue actions as under no. 1 b. Maintain adequate hydration c. Administer antibiotics, as ordered d. Maintain strict asepsis e. Encourage frequent voiding to keep bladder empty
3. Sequestration crisis caused by need for and destruction of RBCs	3. Administer folic acid supplement (15-30 mg) to decrease erythropoietic demands and reduce probability of capillary stasis
4. Crisis caused by hypoxia, hypotension, acidosis, dehydration, exertion, sudden cooling, low-grade fever	4. a. Continue actions as under no. 1 b. Avoid supine hypotension c. Maintain adequate hydration d. Maintain comfortable room temperature: use warm blankets or cool cloths as needed e. Assist with analgesia and anesthesia
5. Pseudotoxemia (hypertension, and proteinuria; *no* large weight gain); often accompanies bone pain crisis	5. a. If true PIH occurs, care is the same as for PIH b. Monitor blood pressure and urine c. Administer heparin, as ordered
6. Thromboembolism (from increased blood viscosity)	6. a. Monitor for positive Homans' sign b. Initiate bed rest if Homans' sign is positive or if reddened, warm areas, or a lump is found c. Maintain adequate hydration d. Administer heparin, as ordered e. Apply warm compresses f. Apply antiembolism stockings
7. Congestive heart failure	7. a. Assess pulse, respiratory rate every 15 min b. Auscultate for crackles frequently c. Place in semirecumbent position d. Administer oxygen and medications (e.g., digitalis, antibiotics, diuretics, analgesics) e. Prevent bearing down: reassure woman about low forceps birth under anesthesia (local or regional)
8. Pulmonary infarction (hemoptysis, cough, temperature to 40° C [102° F], friction rub)	8. Assess for this possible complication to facilitate early diagnosis
9. Postpartum hemorrhage (resulting from heparin therapy)	9. Administer ordered oxytocic medication

Hb, Hemoglobin; *HCT*, hematocrit; *PIH*, pregnancy-induced hypertension; *RBCs*, red blood cells.

Folic acid should be given to avoid folate deficiency. Regular transfusion may be necessary. Iron in any form is contraindicated. Partial exchange transfusion may be warranted in severe thalassemia. Splenectomy may be necessary if enlargement and pain occur. Women with thalassemia major may die of chronic infection or progressive hepatic or cardiac failure, the result of excessive iron deposition.

Persons with *thalassemia minor* have a mild persistent anemia, but the red blood cell level may be normal or even elevated. However, no systemic problems are caused by the anemia that is a part of the minor form of the disease. Thalassemia minor must be distinguished from iron deficiency anemia.

Pregnancy neither worsens thalassemia minor nor is compromised by the disease. The anemia will not respond to iron therapy. Prolonged parenteral iron can lead to harmful, excessive iron storage. Infants born to parents with thalassemia will inherit the disorder. Persons with thalassemia minor should have a normal life span despite a moderately reduced hemoglobin level.

Pulmonary Disorders

As pregnancy advances and the uterus moves upward in the abdominal cavity and displaces the diaphragm in the thoracic cavity, any pregnant woman may experience increased respiratory difficulty. This difficulty will be compounded by pulmonary disease.

A pregnant woman with a pulmonary disorder requires assessment, planning, and interventions specific to the disease process, in addition to the routine peripartum care. The nurse also must be alert to pulmonary complications precipitated by the pregnancy.

Bronchial asthma. Bronchial asthma is an acute respiratory illness caused by allergens, marked change in ambient temperature, or emotional tension. In many cases the actual cause may be unknown. A family history of allergy is likely in about 50% of all persons with asthma. In response to stimuli, there is widespread but reversible narrowing of the hyperreactive airways, making it difficult to breathe. The clinical manifestations are expiratory wheezing, productive cough, thick sputum, and dyspnea.

The effect of pregnancy on asthma is unpredictable. Physiologic alterations induced by pregnancy do not make the pregnant women more prone to asthmatic attacks. However, prematurity, LBW, and fetal and maternal death have been associated with asthma (Jackson and Clark, 1993).

Therapy for bronchial asthma has two objectives: (1) relief of the acute attack and (2) prevention or limitation of later attacks. In all people with asthma, known allergens should be eliminated and a comfortable home temperature maintained. Respiratory infections should be treated and mist or steam inhalation employed to aid expectoration of mucus. Bronchial asthma therapy is initiated. Acute episodes may require steroids, aminophyline, oxygen, and correction of fluid-electrolyte imbalance. Precautions specific for obstetrics include the following:

- Do not use morphine in labor because it may cause bronchospasm: meperidine (Demerol) usually will relieve bronchospasm.
- Avoid or limit the use of ephedrine and corticotropin (pressor drugs) in preeclampsia and eclampsia.
- Choose vaginal birth with use of local or regional anesthesia, whenever possible.

Adult respiratory distress syndrome. **Adult respiratory distress syndrome (ARDS),** or shock lung, occurs when the lungs are unable to maintain levels of oxygen and carbon dioxide within normal limits. Marked tachycardia, dyspnea, and cyanosis that do not respond to nasal oxygen or intermittent positive pressure breathing are the most noted signs. ARDS is not a condition specific to pregnancy; it also can result from chest trauma, drug ingestion, or pneumonia. When ARDS is associated with pregnancy, pulmonary or amniotic fluid embolism, disseminated intravascular coagulation (DIC), and aspiration pneumonia are the precipitators.

The postpartum incidence of ARDS is not affected by the means of birth but by the amount of trauma experienced during pregnancy and birth. It also may occur after spontaneous or medically induced abortion.

Laboratory reports are important in identifying the origin of acute pulmonary problems. The important observations for the nurse to note are vital signs, signs of thrombophlebitis, and hemorrhage. During the postpartum period, apprehension, distended neck veins, cyanosis, diaphoresis, and pallor provide clues. Mental confusion or disorientation also may be noted.

Temperature elevation may indicate the development of thrombophlebitis. The pulse rate increases to compensate for respiratory insufficiency of any origin. The severity of the pulmonary problem increases as the pulse rate rises. An initial rise in blood pressure occurs as cardiac output increases in an attempt to supply the tissue with oxygen. When lung damage is severe, the blood pressure drops.

Respiratory changes are the most important indicators of ARDS. The rate, depth, respiratory pattern, symmetry of chest movement, and use of accessory muscle should be noted; therefore observation of respiratory characteristics after activity is important. If there is any indication of abnormality, respirations are counted for a full minute; an error in rate of plus or minus four respirations per minute may be highly significant. On auscultation, crackles, rhonchi, wheezes, or a pleural friction rub should be reported, especially when they have occurred since an earlier normal assessment. The pregnant woman should be positioned for breathing comfort. Oxygen and emergency equipment should be available. The woman should be reassured and coached in relaxation techniques so her anxiety is lessened.

The lower extremities need to be checked for swelling, pain, inflammation, venous distention, and Homans' sign. If thrombophlebitis is suspected, the woman should be maintained on bed rest. Sudden movement or straining can dislodge a clot and lead to pulmonary embolism.

Alterations in vein distensibility have been noted, possibly because of softening of collagen induced by hormonal influences. The combination of vein distensibility and obstruction of venous blood return from the lower extremities (caused by fetal pressure on veins, especially in the last trimester) predisposes a woman to pooling of blood. Hypercoagulation and pooling may lead to thrombophlebitis. Thrombophlebitis may lead to ARDS (emboli from thromboembolism cause obstruction in the pulmonary circulation).

During pregnancy there is an increase in some of the coagulation factors. This increase in coagulation results in shortening of the partial thromboplastin time (PTT). This state predisposes the woman to an increase in rapidity of blood clotting and an increased tendency to form blood clots (hypercoagulability). Petechiae, ecchymosis, hematuria, and epistaxis are important indications of DIC. Replacement of clotting factors and heparin therapy may be required for DIC. Sources of trauma should be identified and eliminated so that outside causes of hemorrhage are avoided.

Aspiration pneumonia can be caused by changes in the gastrointestinal system during pregnancy. Progesterone relaxes smooth muscles. When the resting tone is lowered, the cardiac sphincter becomes weak and reflux of the stomach contents can easily occur. Increased intraabdominal pressure (because of fetal growth) further predisposes the mother to gastric reflux.

Food eaten as long as 24 to 48 hours before labor can be vomited and then aspirated. Aspiration of solid foods and liquids may cause bronchial obstruction leading to bronchoconstriction, which in turn can result in ARDS. Large particles can be removed by coughing, suctioning, or bronchoscopy, but liquids are harder to remove. The hydrochloric acid in the aspirated stomach contents may cause an asthmalike syndrome with necrotizing bronchitis. For this reason an antacid is given before cesarean birth as a prophylactic measure.

ARDS carries a high rate of mortality (50% to 70%) (Dorman, 1991). The prognosis is good if the woman is otherwise healthy and if ventilatory support can be maintained until the underlying disease can be treated (Cunningham et al, 1993).

Cystic fibrosis. Cystic fibrosis is a common autosomal recessive genetic disorder in which the exocrine glands produce excessive viscous secretions. Respiratory and digestive functions are impaired. Respiratory failure and early death (early 20s) are common outcomes. Improvements in diagnosis and treatment of cystic fibrosis have allowed an increasing number of women to survive to adulthood. Most women diagnosed with cystic fibrosis are infertile; however, pregnancy is not uncommon. The pregnancy is often complicated by chronic hypoxia and frequent pulmonary infections. Women with cystic fibrosis show a decrease in their residual volume during pregnancy, as do normal pregnant women. However, people with cystic fibrosis are unable to maintain vital capacity. Presumably, the pulmonary vasculature cannot accommodate the increased cardiac output of pregnancy. The results are decreased oxygen to the myocardium, decreasing cardiac output, and an increase in hypoxia. Increased maternal and perinatal mortality is related to severe pulmonary infection.

During labor, monitoring for fluid and electrolyte balance is required. The amount of sodium lost through sweat can be significant, and hypovolemia can occur. Conversely, if the woman has any degree of cor pulmonale, she must be guarded against fluid overload. Oxygen is given freely during labor. Epidural or local anesthesia is the method of choice for birth.

The infant will be heterozygous or homozygous for cystic fibrosis. Newborns with cystic fibrosis test positive for sweat chloride and may have meconium ileus. Genetic counseling and testing can identify 90% of cystic fibrosis carriers (Jackson and Clark, 1993).

Breastfeeding should be delayed until the sodium content of the mother's milk (which may be as high as 280 mmol/L) has been determined to be safe for the infant (Creasy and Resnik, 1994; Lawrence, 1994).

Gastrointestinal Disorders

Compromise of gastrointestinal function during pregnancy is of concern. Obvious physiologic alterations, such as the greatly enlarged uterus, and less apparent changes, such as hormonal differences and hypochlorhydria (deficiency of hydrochloric acid in the stomach's gastric juice), require understanding for proper diagnosis and treatment. Gallbladder disease and inflammatory bowel disease are two gastrointestinal disorders that may occur during pregnancy.

Cholelithiasis and cholecystitis. Women are four times more likely to have **cholelithiasis** (presence of gallstones in the gallbladder) than are men (Baker, 1995). Maternal adaptation significantly alters gallbladder function (Varner, 1994). Pregnancy seems to make the woman more vulnerable to gallstone formation. Decreased muscle tone allows gallbladder distention, thickening of the bile, and prolonged emptying time. Increased progesterone levels result in a slight hypercholesterolemia. However, **cholecystitis** (inflammation of the gallbladder) does not commonly occur during pregnancy. Meperidine (Demerol) or atropine alleviates ductal spasm and pain. Morphine stimulates the sphincter of Oddi and thus should be avoided (Gleicher, 1992). Generally, gallbladder surgery should be postponed until the puerperium.

Inflammatory bowel disease. Inflammatory bowel disease can be acute or chronic. Chronic inflammatory bowel disease can be classified as regional enteritis (Crohn disease) or ulcerative colitis.

Chronic inflammatory bowel diseases are prone to periods of exacerbation and remission. The cause is unknown. The clinical manifestations for this chronic disorder are liquid diarrhea, urgency of defecation, and crampy lower abdominal pain. Blood, mucus, and pus may be seen in the stool.

Treatment and therapy are the same for the pregnant woman as for the nonpregnant woman. Medications include sulfasalazine and prednisone. Folic acid and vitamin supplementation is especially important because of the problems with malabsorption and malnutrition associated with chronic inflammatory bowel disease.

The effect of inflammatory bowel disease on pregnancy is minimal unless there is marked debilitation, then spontaneous abortion, fetal death, or preterm birth may occur. In general, when pregnancy coincides with active ulcerative colitis, most women experience a severe exacerbation of the disease. When pregnancy occurs during a period of inactivity of the disorder, a flareup is unlikely.

Integumentary Disorders

Dermatologic disorders induced by pregnancy include melasma (chloasma), herpes gestationis, noninflammatory pruritus of pregnancy, vascular spiders, palmar erythema, and pregnancy granuloma (including epulides). Skin problems generally aggravated by pregnancy are acne vulgaris (acne) (in the first trimester), erythema multiforme, herpetiform dermatitis (fever blisters and genital herpes), granuloma inguinale (Donovan bodies), condylomata acuminata (genital warts), neurofibromatosis (von Recklinghausen disease), and pemphigus. Dermatologic disorders usually improved by pregnancy include acne vulgaris (in the third trimester), seborrheic dermatitis (dandruff), and psoriasis. An unpredictable course during pregnancy may be expected in atopic dermatitis, lupus erythematosus, and herpes simplex.

Elective abortion or early birth may be justified for some dermatologic conditions. These conditions include disseminated lupus erythematosus, neurofibromatosis, and herpes gestationis. Herpes gestationis (not a viral-induced disorder) is a rare blistering skin disease of pregnancy. Prednisone usually brings prompt relief and inhibits development of new lesions. The process may recur in subsequent pregnancies (Cunningham et al, 1993).

Isotretinoin (Accutane), commonly prescribed for acne, is contraindicated in pregnancy because of its high teratogenicity. Fetuses exposed to this medication are at increased risk for craniofacial, cardiac, and CNS anomalies.

Explanation, reassurance, and common sense measures should suffice for normal skin changes. In contrast, disease processes during and soon after pregnancy may be extremely difficult to diagnose and treat.

Neurologic Disorders

The pregnant woman with a neurologic disorder needs to deal with potential teratogenic effects of prescribed medications, changes of mobility during pregnancy, and impaired ability to care for the baby. The nurse should be aware of all drugs the pregnant woman is taking and the associated potential for producing congenital anomalies. As the pregnancy progresses, the woman's center of gravity shifts and causes balance and gait changes. The nurse needs to advise the woman of these expected changes and to suggest safety measures as appropriate. Family and community resources should be assessed to provide child care for the neurologically impaired woman.

Epilepsy. Epilepsy is the most common neurologic disorder accompanying pregnancy (James et al, 1994). Epilepsy may result from developmental abnormalities, injury, or have no identified cause. Epilepsy seriously complicates about 1 in 1000 gestations. Convulsive seizures may be more frequent or severe during complications of pregnancy, such as edema, alkylosis, fluid-electrolyte imbalance, cerebral hypoxia, hypoglycemia, and hypocalcemia. On the other hand, the effects of pregnancy on epilepsy are unpredictable. Seizure frequency remains the same in about 50% of women, with 25% experiencing a decrease and 25% experiencing an increase in seizure activity (Krumholz, 1992).

The differential diagnosis of epilepsy vs. eclampsia may pose a problem. Epilepsy and eclampsia can coexist. However, a history of seizures and a normal plasma uric acid level, as well as the absence of hypertension, generalized edema, or proteinuria, point to epilepsy. Electroencephalography rarely is diagnostic.

During pregnancy, risk of vaginal bleeding is doubled, and there is a threefold risk of abruptio placentae. Abnormal presentations are more common in labor and delivery, as well as the increased possibility that the fetus will experience seizures in utero (Mishell and Brenner, 1994).

Metabolic changes in pregnancy usually alter pharmacokinetics. In addition, nausea and vomiting may interfere with ingestion and absorption of medication. All anticonvulsants carry significant teratogenic risk and thus are not considered safe. The major malformations are cleft lip and cleft palate, facial abnormalities, and deformities of the extremities, as well as some neural tube defects (Kohn, 1992). Antiepileptic drugs should be monotherapy, used in the smallest therapeutic dose with the fewest side effects. Daily folic acid supplement is needed because of the depletion that occurs when taking anticonvulsants (Cartlidge, 1995).

Grand mal seizures can be controlled by intravenous sodium amobarbital or magnesium sulfate. Epilepsy is not an indication for therapeutic abortion or cesarean birth.

The neonate should be monitored for a hemorrhagic disorder because of the interference with vitamin K metabolism caused by anticonvulsants. Administration of vitamin K, 20 mEq daily by mouth to the mother for 2 weeks antepartum or 10 mg IM 4 hours before birth will prevent this complication in the newborn (Gleicher, 1992). If the pregnant woman has had to take high doses of anticonvulsants, the newborn may demonstrate sedation, respiratory depression, poor sucking, and hypotonia (Cartlidge, 1995).

Multiple sclerosis. Multiple sclerosis (MS), a patchy demyelinization of the spinal cord and CNS, may be a viral disorder. Women are affected twice as often as men, with the most common onset occurring between the ages of 20 and 40 (Cartlidge, 1995). Infertility, abortion, stillbirth, and fetal anomalies do not appear to be increased in women with MS (James et al, 1994).

MS may occasionally complicate pregnancy, but exacerbations and remissions are unrelated to the pregnant state. For this reason, medically indicated therapeutic abortion is illogical. Steroids are commonly used to treat acute exacerbations. The burden of pregnancy and subsequent child care may warrant early interruption of pregnancy and sterilization in extreme cases. Nursing care of the pregnant woman with MS is similar to the care of the normal pregnant woman. The incidence of MS in the offspring is about 3% to 5% (Rudick and Birk, 1992). During the first 3 months after birth 20% to 40% of MS patients experience a clinical relapse or worsening of the disease (Rudick and Birk, 1992).

Bell palsy. An association between idiopathic facial paralysis and pregnancy was first cited by Bell in 1830. Bell palsy occurs in about 1 in 2000 pregnancies. Incidence peaks during the third trimester and the puerperium (Cherry and Merkatz, 1991; Walling, 1993). Blinking is impaired; eye pain is often the presenting symptom (Gleicher, 1992). A causative relationship does not seem to exist between the appearance of Bell palsy and any of the complications of pregnancy.

No effects of maternal Bell palsy have been observed in infants. Maternal outcome is generally good. In most affected women, 90% or more of facial function can be expected to return (Cunningham et al, 1993; Varner, 1994). Supportive care includes prevention of injury to the exposed cornea, facial muscle massage, careful chewing and manual removal of food from inside the affected cheek, and reassurance that return of total neurologic function is likely.

Autoimmune Disorders

Autoimmune disorders comprise a large group of diseases that disrupt the function of the immune system of the body. In these types of disorders the body develops antibodies that attack its normally present antigens. Autoimmune disorders have a predilection for women in their reproductive years; therefore associations with pregnancy are not uncommon (James et al, 1994; Varner, 1994). Pregnancy may affect the disease process. Some disorders adversely affect the course of pregnancy or are detrimental to the fetus. Autoimmune disorders include rheumatoid arthritis (RA), systemic lupus erythematosus, myasthenia gravis, and immunologic thrombocytopenic purpura. Autoantibodies from rheumatoid arthritis do not cross the placenta; those of the other disorders do. The woman with immunologic thrombocytopenic purpura may give birth to a child who demonstrates thrombocytopenia. Petechiae and bleeding into the gastrointestinal and genitourinary tracts and into the brain may be evident. If the mother has myasthenia gravis, the newborn may exhibit a weak cry, sucking mechanism, and facial muscles and may have respiratory problems.

Rheumatoid arthritis. The peak prevalence of RA is between ages 35 and 45. RA affects 1 in 10,000 people in the United States and occurs 3 times more often in women than in men (Branch, 1993). All races are affected equally, but the disease is familial (Lockshin and Druzin, 1995). Spontaneous abortion is experienced by 15% to 25% of pregnant women with RA (Branch, 1993). Most women with RA find that the severity of symptoms decreases during pregnancy (Buchanan, Needs, and Brooks, 1992). For this reason many affected women attempt to become pregnant as often as possible; however, many are subfertile because of the RA. During pregnancy, women with RA experience an increase in alpha$_2$-glycoprotein. In addition, total plasma and free cortisol (especially estrogens and progesterone) show an increase. This combination apparently leads to depressed cellular immunity (Buchanan, Needs, and Brooks, 1992). Women in whom the rheumatoid factor (autoantibodies found in the synovial fluid) decreases during pregnancy report improvement in their symptoms. Researchers are now investigating the possibility of a positive effect on RA associated with the use of oral contraceptives.

Although symptoms may subside during pregnancy, they may return after giving birth. Exacerbations often recur within the first several months postpartum and return to the prepregnancy level within the first year after birth (Branch, 1993).

Management of RA during pregnancy includes an appropriate balance of rest and exercise, heat and physical therapy, salicylates and low dose steroids (Scott and Branch, 1994). Aspirin probably remains the safest and most useful antiinflammatory drug for these women. Mild hemostatic changes in the newborn, an increase in the average length of gestation, and possibly premature closure of the ductus arteriosus are attributed to maternal ingestion of large doses of aspirin (Cunningham et al, 1993).

Systemic lupus erythematosus. One of the most common serious disorders in women of childbearing age, **systemic lupus erythematosus (SLE),** is a chronic multisystem inflammatory disease that affects skin, joints, kidneys, lungs, CNS, liver, and other body organs (James et al, 1994). More than 250,000 people are known to have SLE, with an estimated 50,000 new cases per year. Although the antibody may be formed in response to a virus, a familial tendency seems to be involved.

The vague early symptoms, such as fatigue, fever, and weight loss, may be overlooked. Pericarditis is a common symptom. Eventually all organs become involved. The condition is characterized by a series of exacerbations and remissions.

If the diagnosis has been established and the woman desires a child, she is advised to wait for 2 years. At that time, if the disease has been controlled well on low doses of corticosteroids, pregnancy may be reasonably considered (Blackburn and Loper, 1992; Varner, 1994). Postpartum exacerbation may represent a rebound phenomenon as suppression of cell-mediated activity, normal during pregnancy, is terminated. Oral contraceptives are contraindicated; diaphragms and condoms are the preferred methods of fertility management if pregnancy is desired in the future. Sterilization is suggested if no more children are wanted. The outlook for persons with SLE has improved markedly in the past few years. Persons diagnosed with SLE have a 5-year survival rate of more than 90%, and more than 80% survive for 10 years or more. Infection is now a leading cause of death among persons with SLE, related to the use of immunosuppressive medications.

The effect of pregnancy on SLE seems inconsistent. The rate of spontaneous abortion is as high as 31% (Branch, 1993). Maternal complications correlate with the degree of cardiac or renal involvement (Blackburn and Loper, 1992; Varner, 1994). Renal failure, hypertension, and death are associated with diffuse proliferative lupus glomerulonephritis. When the kidneys are involved, women are subject to superimposed preeclampsia, stillbirths, preterm birth, and small-for-gestational age infants. However, if the disease is stable during pregnancy, there is only a slight risk that the disease will worsen with gestation. An exacerbation of SLE occurs during pregnancy or during postpartum in 15% to 60% of women (Branch, 1993; James et al, 1994).

Although the antibodies cross the placenta, the amount varies so that the effect on the fetus also varies. The most severely affected newborns suffer from discoid lupus, anemia, neutropenia, thrombocytopenia, and congenital complete heart block.

Myasthenia gravis. Myasthenia gravis, an autoimmune motor (muscle) end plate disorder that involves acetylcholine use, affects the motor function at the myoneural junction. Muscle weakness, particularly of the eyes, face, tongue, neck, limbs, and respiratory muscles, results. Myasthenia gravis occurs in 2 to 10 people per 100,000 and in women twice as often as in men (Branch, 1993). The peak prevalence of myasthenia gravis is about at age 25. Pregnancy may complicate the disorder, although some women experience a remission during gestation. Preterm births may be as high as 60% to 66% (Branch, 1993). The disorder is not an indication for elective abortion; an abortion does not bring about remission (Gilbert and Harmon, 1993).

Symptoms include easy fatigue, intermittent double vision, upper eyelid drooping, and facial muscle weakness (James et al, 1994). In more serious cases, upper arm weakness and breathing difficulty are seen. Infections may precipitate the onset or relapse and must be treated aggressively during pregnancy.

Women with myasthenia gravis usually tolerate labor well because of preexisting muscle relaxation. During the second stage, some women may show impairment of voluntary expulsive efforts. Meperidine is the obstetric analgesic of choice. Local anesthesia is preferred. Oxytocin may be given, but scopolamine and muscle relaxants (e.g., magnesium sulfate) are contraindicated. After birth, women must be carefully supervised, because relapses often occur during the puerperium.

All infants of mothers with myasthenia gravis should be closely monitored for muscle weakness (e.g., weak cry, respiratory distress, poor Moro reflex, difficulty in feeding). In 12% to 20% of the babies born to myasthenic mothers, transient muscle weakness occurs within the first few days after birth (Plauche, 1991; Scott and Branch, 1994). Symptoms may persist from 1 to 2 months. Of the infants who show myasthenic signs, three fourths require anticholinesterase medications. The response of the infant to the medications is usually good (Branch, 1993). With proper management, complete recovery of the infant usually occurs.

Abdominal Surgery During Pregnancy

The need for immediate abdominal surgery occurs as frequently among pregnant women as among nonpregnant women of comparable age. However, diagnosis is more difficult in the pregnant woman. An enlarged uterus and displaced internal organs may prevent adequate palpation and may alter the position of the surgical procedure (Sibai, 1992). The health care provider is confronted with both a surgical and an obstetric problem.

Laparotomy or laparoscopy may be required. Hazards of these procedures include abortion and preterm labor.

However, surgical or anesthetic intervention does not affect the incidence of congenital malformations.

Appendicitis. Acute suppurative appendicitis complicates about 1 in 1500 pregnancies (Michell and Brenner, 1994). This disorder poses the following special problems during gestation.

1. Appendicitis is more difficult to diagnose during pregnancy. The appendix is carried high and to the right, away from McBurney point, by the enlarged uterus (Fig. 10-5).
2. Appendiceal rupture and peritonitis occur two to three times more often in pregnant women than in nonpregnant women.
3. Maternal and perinatal morbidity and mortality are greatly increased when appendicitis occurs during pregnancy because of delay in diagnosis.

Most cases of acute appendicitis occur during the first 6 months of gestation, with decreasing frequency through the third trimester, labor, and puerperium. The differential diagnosis of appendicitis during pregnancy is complicated by gastrointestinal or genitourinary problems that may be confused with appendicitis. A high level of suspicion is important in the diagnosis of appendicitis.

Appendectomy before rupture is extremely important. Antibiotic therapy before rupture is of questionable value; after rupture it may be lifesaving. Therapeutic abortion is never indicated in appendicitis. Cesarean birth at or near term may be justified in association with appendectomy.

Maternal mortality increases to about 10% in the third trimester and is about 15% when appendicitis develops during labor. Perinatal mortality is approximately 10% with unruptured appendicitis but is at least 35% with peritonitis.

Intestinal obstruction. The second most common nonobstetric abdominal emergency in pregnancy is intestinal obstruction (Gleicher, 1992). Any woman with a laparotomy scar is more likely to have an intestinal obstruction (adynamic ileus) during gestation. Adhesions as a result of previous surgery or pelvic inflammatory disease, an enlarging uterus, and displacement of the intestines are etiologic factors.

Constipation, persistent cramplike, abdominal pain, vomiting, auscultatory rushes within the abdomen, and "laddering" of the intestinal shadows on x-ray films aid in the diagnosis of intestinal obstruction. Immediate surgical intervention is required for release of the obstruction.

Gynecologic problems. Ovarian cysts and twisting of ovarian cysts or adnexal tissues may occur. Pregnancy predisposes a woman to ovarian problems, especially during the first trimester. Conditions include retained or enlarged cystic corpus luteum of pregnancy, ovarian cyst, and bacterial invasion of reproductive or other intraperitoneal organs.

Laparotomy or laparoscopy may be required to discriminate between ovarian problems and early ectopic pregnancy, appendicitis, and other infectious processes.

Nursing Care Management

Fetal vital signs and activity and uterine contractility (labor may have begun) are monitored, and constant vigilance for

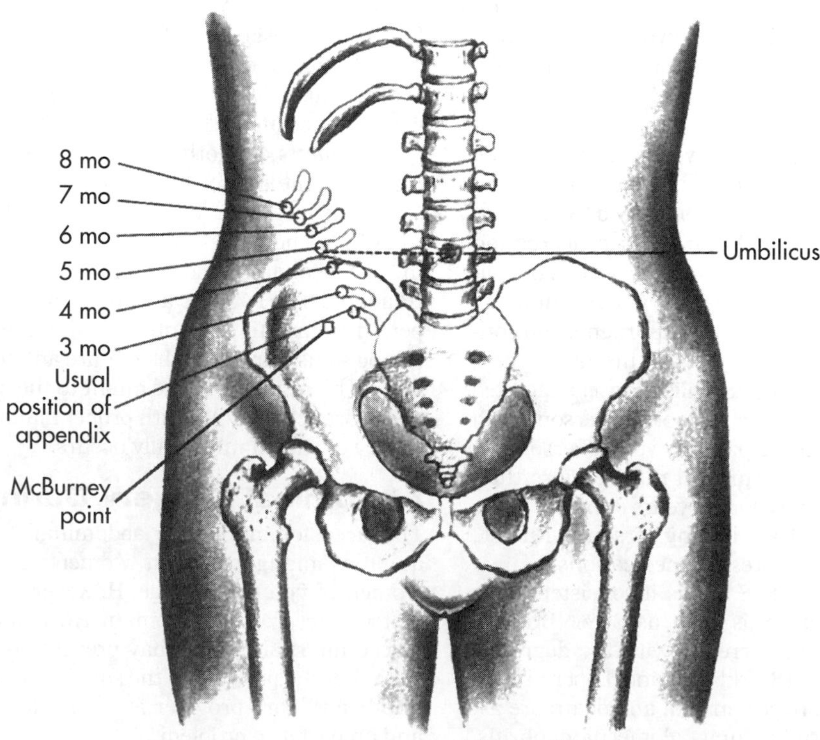

Fig. 10-5 Change in position of appendix during pregnancy.

symptoms of impending obstetric complications is maintained. The woman and her family may have heightened concerns regarding effects of the procedure and medication on fetal well-being and the course of pregnancy. The extent of preoperative assessment is determined by the immediacy of surgical intervention and the specific condition that requires surgery (Phipps, Long, and Woods, 1993).

Preoperative care for a pregnant woman differs from that of a nonpregnant woman in one significant aspect: the presence of at least one other person—the fetus. Food by mouth is restricted for several hours before a scheduled procedure or surgery. Even if she has had nothing by mouth (NPO) and especially if the surgery is unexpected the woman is in danger of vomiting and aspirating, thus special precautions are taken before anesthesia is administered (e.g., administering an antacid). Maternal ketosis and hypoglycemia rapidly occur in both the woman and fetus (Shaver, 1992). If the woman experiences a prolonged NPO status, IV fluids with dextrose should be given.

General preoperative and postoperative observations and ongoing care are the same as for any surgery. Examples of these are monitoring vital signs and fluid and electrolyte balance, providing for safety, comfort, and rest, as well as monitoring for complications. A wedge is placed under the hip during surgery to prevent compression of the vena cava. Because of the decreased respiratory excursion associated with the enlarged uterus, the pregnant woman is at greater risk of postoperative atelectasis and pulmonary complications (Shaver, 1992). The important addition to the postoperative care of the pregnant patient is that of fetal surveillance. If intrauterine pregnancy continues, monitoring of fetal heart rate and activity, as well as uterine activity, is continued.

Discharge planning. Planning for discharge begins when the pregnant woman first enters the health care system. The extent to which the preoperative expected outcomes of care can be met are reviewed, and adjustments are made accordingly. For example, if the surgery was an emergency, such as for appendicitis, there is little time for preoperative preparation. After the woman has recovered from the effects of surgery, the nurse needs to take time to encourage her to voice her fears, concerns, and questions. She may have questions regarding the effect of the surgery and anesthesia on the fetus. If she is unable to express these concerns to the surgeon, the nurse acts as patient advocate and informs the physician.

The participation of the woman and her family in discharge planning is necessary to individualize the care to fit with the available family support systems, the home situation, and the facilities. The woman may demonstrate symptoms of grief and loss, and her participation in discharge planning may be minimal. She may need assistance coping with these feelings.

The woman may need referral service to various community agencies for evaluation of the home situation, child care, home health care, and financial or other assistance. All arrangements for her return home and for convalescent care should be completed as early as possible before her expected date of discharge (Box 10-4).

Trauma During Pregnancy

The leading cause of death in women of reproductive age is trauma and not neoplasms or obstetric complications (Daddario, 1989; Troiano, 1991). Minor injury during pregnancy is common; most trauma (more than 50%) occurs during the third trimester. A change in the woman's center of gravity as well as other changes in pregnancy are responsible for syncope, loss of balance, and general clumsiness. Discomfort such as a contracting uterus or vigorous fetal movement may be distracting while the woman is driving or working.

Nursing Care Management

The woman's condition is the initial concern. The injury sustained determines the type and extent of assessment conducted. Attention is focused first on the basic ABCs: airway, breathing, and circulation. The woman's abdomen is assessed for ruptured uterus and for uterine activity. The fetus is then assessed for heart rate and activity. An individualized health assessment is performed and the woman's prenatal record is reviewed when available.

Findings from the injury must not be confused with the normal physiologic changes during pregnancy. The usual signs of organ rupture—for example, guarding, rebound tenderness, and rigidity—may only be responses to stretching of the abdominal wall. An examination of the woman in a supine position results in hypotension and a systolic value as

BOX 10-4
Discharge Teaching for Home Care

- Care of incision site
- Diet and elimination related to gastrointestinal function
- Signs and symptoms of developing complications: wound infection, thrombophlebitis, pneumonia
- Equipment needed and technique for assessing temperature
- Recommended schedule for resumption of activities of daily living
- Treatments and medications ordered
- List of resource persons and their telephone numbers
- Schedule of follow-up visits
- If birth has not occurred:
  Assessment of fetal activity (kick counts)
  Signs of preterm labor

Critical Thinking Exercises

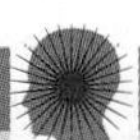

ABDOMINAL PAIN

You are assigned to admit a woman in her second trimester who is experiencing abdominal pain. She has two children at home, ages 2 and 5. Her chief complaints are fatigue, right-sided pain, and nausea.

1. **What would be your assessment questions? What physical assessments would you make? What lab values would you examine?**
2. **Given a diagnosis of appendicitis:**
   a. **What would be your nursing diagnoses? List in priority order.**
   b. **Formulate your plan of care.**
   c. **Identify home care concerns as you prepare to discharge your client.**

low as 80 mm Hg; changing her to a lateral position or simply moving the fetus raises the systolic value to more than 100 mm Hg. A silent abdomen, a sign of bowel trauma, may be a normal finding because of the decreased motility that occurs during pregnancy. Delayed emptying time of the stomach during pregnancy poses a threat of vomiting and possible aspiration if the woman has eaten within the last several hours.

During pregnancy the woman may sustain a significant blood loss (approximately a 30% reduction of circulating blood volume) without the usual signs and symptoms of hypovolemia. Pelvic blood vessels (retroperitoneal and parametrial arteries) enlarge greatly during pregnancy; thus they are more easily damaged and ruptured. The large uterus can compartmentalize and hide a hemorrhage originating in the liver and spleen. A rapid pulse may reflect only the usual increase of 10 to 15 beats/min, or it may be a sign of hypovolemia.

Laboratory and diagnostic tests are determined by the type of injury. Appropriate blood studies include tests for serum amylase and blood gases; baseline bleeding profile; and complete blood cell count, typing, and crossmatching. In normal pregnancies a white blood cell count of 18,000/mm^3 in the last trimester and 25,000/mm^3 during labor is usual; however, these same values also indicate intraabdominal hemorrhage. DIC can complicate severe trauma, placental abruption, and sepsis.

An indwelling urinary bladder catheter for drainage facilitates management of fluid therapy and aids diagnosis (Fig. 10-6). For example, difficulty in passing the catheter suggests urethral disruption, and hematuria suggests a ruptured bladder. The catheter also provides access for retrograde cystogram x-ray examination.

Intraperitoneal hemorrhage must be detected. Radiology, real-time ultrasound, and computed tomography scan are useful diagnostic modalities. The physician places a peritoneal lavage catheter for detecting intraperitoneal hemorrhage. The procedure is performed through a small incision into the peritoneum, with the woman under local anesthesia. The test

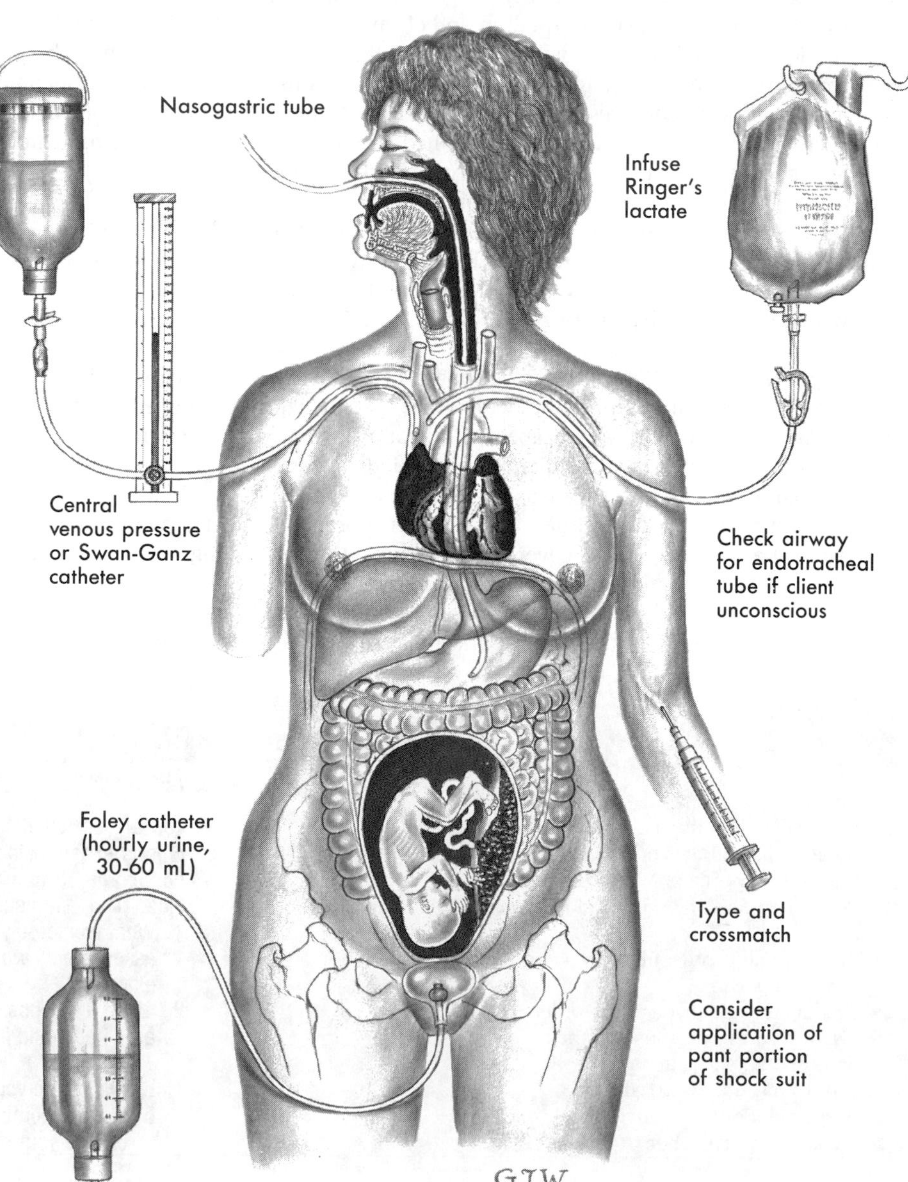

Fig. 10-6 Summary of technique used for resuscitation. Trauma care should begin in field where injury occurred, always with attention to basic ABCs: airway, breathing, and circulation.

result is positive for bleeding if the aspirate exceeds 10 ml non-clotting blood or if, after instillation of 1 L lactated Ringer's solution, bloody fluid is recovered. Radiographic studies may be necessary to guide management.

Intervention begins with prevention. The pregnant woman is counseled to discontinue activities requiring balance and coordination, to use car seat restraints appropriately, to recognize early adverse symptoms, and to seek therapy immediately. If the woman is hospitalized only for observation, she is involved in assessment for signs and symptoms of complications.

In case of minor trauma the woman is hospitalized and evaluated for the following: vaginal bleeding, uterine irritability, abdominal tenderness, abdominal pain or cramps, evidence of hypovolemia, a change in rate or absence of fetal heart tones, fetal activity, leakage of amniotic fluid, and the presence of fetal cells in maternal circulation.

Immediate trauma care consists of attention to airway, breathing, and circulation (the ABCs). While hypoxia and hypovolemia are being corrected, the woman should be transferred to a trauma center with obstetric and neonatal backup, if possible. During transfer, attendants must remember the aortocaval (supine hypotension) syndrome. The woman should be positioned on her side, or the uterus should be displaced laterally by a uterine displacer or by a pillow placed under the woman's right hip. Hypotension must be avoided to prevent compromise of cardiac output followed by decrease of blood flow to the uterus.

A nasogastric tube is inserted, if indicated because delayed gastric emptying time and increased intestinal transit time increase the risk of vomiting and aspiration. Mouth care and reassurance are used to counter any irritation caused by the tube. Fluid and electrolyte replacement is instituted and monitored. Oxygen needs are met.

Penetrating abdominal wounds, internal hemorrhage, and ruptured uterus are all indications for immediate surgical intervention. Wounds high in the abdomen have most likely penetrated a vital structure because organs such as the bowel, liver, and spleen have been displaced upward by the enlarging uterus (Fig. 10-6).

Posttraumatic uterine and fetal surveillance. When the mother's condition has been stabilized, attention is turned toward monitoring the fetus and monitoring for preterm labor and placental abruption. Usually, if these complications occur, they happen within 24 to 48 hours after the accident (Smith and Phelan, 1991). Uterine rupture can occur at the site of a previous scar or over the site of implantation, which is weakened by increased vascularity at the site. Expulsion of the uterine contents into the abdominal cavity may occur and usually is followed by massive hemorrhage.

THERAPEUTIC AND ELECTIVE ABORTION

Therapeutic abortion (TAB) is the termination of a previable pregnancy to safeguard the life or health of the mother. Indications for therapeutic abortion are as follows:

1. Preservation of the life or health of the mother (e.g., class III or IV heart disease)
2. Avoidance of the birth of an offspring with a serious developmental or hereditary disorder (e.g., Tay-Sachs disease)
3. Rape or incest

Elective abortion (EAB) is the purposeful interruption of a previable pregnancy. The indication for an elective abortion is by request of the mother but not for reasons of maternal risk or fetal disease.

Many women report more than one factor contributing to the decision to abort (Thompson and Thompson, 1990). Most women in the United States who have abortions are white and younger than age 24 (CDC, 1994). Only one fourth of abortions are obtained by married women (Wallach and Zacur, 1995). The U.S. Supreme Court set aside previous antiabortion laws in January 1973, holding that first-trimester abortion is permissible since the mortality from interruption of early gestation is now less than the mortality after normal term birth; 90% are performed at this point in pregnancy (Wallach and Zacur, 1995). Second-trimester abortion was left to the discretion of the individual states (Chavkin and Rosenfield, 1990; Rhodes, 1990, Rogers et al, 1991). Roman Catholic hospitals and some of those maintained by strict fundamentalists forbid abortion (and often sterilization) despite legal challenge.

LEGAL TIP

Abortion

Nurses need to know the laws regarding abortion in their state of practice before they offer abortion counseling or provide nursing care for a woman choosing an abortion.

Even before abortion was legalized, many abortions took place, with little-documented sequelae other than death from infection or hemorrhage or both. Although studies indicate that biologic sequelae do occur after abortion (e.g., ectopic pregnancy), rates of biologic complications tend to be low, especially if the woman aborts during the first trimester (Holt et al, 1989). Studies related to psychologic sequelae (e.g., anxiety) suggest that they are short lived (Adler et al, 1990). Sequelae are related to circumstances and support surrounding the abortion, such as the attitudes of friends, family, and health care workers. The woman facing an abortion is pregnant and may exhibit the emotional responses shared by all pregnant women, including postpartum depression.

The values and moral convictions of nurses are involved to the same extent as those of pregnant women. The conflicts and doubts of nurses can be readily communicated to women who are already anxious and overly sensitive. Health professionals need assistance to identify and come to terms with their own feelings. It is not uncommon for confusion to arise as beliefs are challenged by the reality of care (Box 10-5).

Nursing Care Management

Assessment

A thorough assessment is conducted through history, physical examination, and laboratory tests. The length of pregnancy and the condition of the woman need to be determined to select the appropriate type of abortion procedure. If the woman is Rh negative and the pregnancy is greater than 8 weeks' gestation, she is a candidate for prophylaxis against Rh

BOX 10-5
Ethical Considerations Related to Abortion

Nurses who object to abortion for ethical, religious, or other reasons may refuse to care for women having abortions except in cases where the woman's life is in danger.

isoimmunization. She will receive $Rh_0(D)$ immune globulin within 72 hours after the abortion if she is D^u negative and if Coombs test results are negative (if she is unsensitized or has not developed isoimmunization). (See Chapter 26 for a discussion of Rh isoimmunization.)

The woman's understanding of alternatives, the types of abortions, and expected recovery are assessed. Misinformation and gaps in knowledge are identified and corrected. The record is reviewed for the signed informed consent, and the patient's understanding is verified. General preoperative, operative, and postoperative assessments are performed.

Nursing Diagnoses

Analysis of data leads to the identification of the appropriate nursing diagnoses. Following are examples of nursing diagnoses for women undergoing elective abortion:

- Decisional conflict related to
  - Perceived threat to value system
- Fear related to
  - The abortion procedure
  - Potential complications
  - Implications for future pregnancies
- Anticipatory grieving related to
  - Distress at loss and/or feelings of guilt
- Risk for infection related to
  - Effects of the procedure
  - Lack of understanding of preoperative and postoperative self-care
- Pain related to
  - Effects of the procedure and/or postoperative events

Expected Outcomes

Planning is a collaborative effort among the woman, her sexual partner (as appropriate), and health care providers. Expected outcomes are established collaboratively, should be stated in patient-centered terms, and may include the following:

1. The woman will verbalize understanding of the information necessary to give informed consent.
2. The woman will experience a successful procedure, and her recovery will be uneventful.
3. The woman will verbalize that she is satisfied with the decision for elective abortion, the procedure, and the experience with the health care team.

Plan of Care and Implementation

Counseling about abortion includes help for the woman in identifying how she perceives the pregnancy; the woman needs information about choices available (i.e., having an abortion or carrying the pregnancy to term and then either keeping the child or placing the child for adoption) and information about types of abortion procedures. The expected outcome is that the woman will make an informed decision and be satisfied with her decision.

First-Trimester Abortion

Methods for performing early elective abortion include the following:

1. Menstrual extraction (vacuum extraction), or early aspiration of the endometrium in women who have not yet missed a menstrual period
2. Surgical D & C when aspiration equipment is unavailable
3. Uterine aspiration after one or two missed periods

Surgical D & C refers to cervical **dilation and curettage (D & C)** of the uterine endometrium. Curettage is the scraping of the uterine lining with a metal curette or a flexible aspiration tip to remove the products of conception implanted in the endometrium. The procedure is similar to that of uterine aspiration. Cervical trauma and uterine perforation, infection, or hemorrhage are possible, although rare, complications.

Uterine aspiration (vacuum or suction curettage) abortion is the most common procedure. The insertion of a small **laminaria** tent (cone of dried seaweed that swells as it absorbs moisture and dilates the cervix) or "seaweed stick" held in place by a vaginal tampon for 4 to 24 hours usually facilitates the purposeful interruption of a first-trimester pregnancy greater than 10 weeks' gestation by dilating the cervix atraumatically (Wallach and Zacur, 1995). On removal of the moist, expanded laminaria, the cervix will have dilated 2 or 3 times its original (dry) diameter. Rarely will further mechanical dilation of the cervix be required. The insertion of an adequate-sized aspiration cannula (8.5 to 10.5 mm) is almost always possible. Cervical laceration and bleeding are reduced by the use of laminaria. A disadvantage is the delay necessary and the need for an additional visit to the office or clinic. Prostaglandin gel may also be used to soften the cervix (Cunningham et al, 1993).

The woman comes to the clinic or physician's office the day before the abortion procedure. An antiseptic solution is used to prepare the pelvic area. A vaginal speculum is inserted, and the vaginal canal and cervix are cleansed. Injection of a local anesthetic agent into the cervix may follow. Again the area is cleansed, and the laminaria tent is inserted into the endocervical canal. Prophylactic use of an antibiotic is usually begun. Some women experience a mild cramping or have light spotting from the anesthetic injection. Discomfort can usually be controlled with mild analgesics (e.g., acetaminophen).

Aspiration abortion may be performed in the office, clinic, or in the hospital setting. If the woman chooses a hospital setting, she is admitted the day after insertion of the laminaria tent and is given preoperative sedation. The vaginal area is cleansed (shaving is not necessary). The suction procedure for accomplishing an early elective abortion (ideal time is 8 to 12 weeks since last menstrual period) usually requires less than 5 minutes and can easily be effected under paracervical block anesthesia and sedation. Independent nursing interventions have the potential to reduce pain during the procedure (Wells, 1991). During the procedure the woman is kept informed about what to expect next: for example, menstrual-like cramping and sounds of suction machine. The nurse assesses the woman's vital signs. The aspirated uterine contents must be carefully inspected to ascertain whether all fetal parts and adequate placental tissue have been evacuated. A single dose of oxytocin is used occasionally to control bleeding. The woman may remain in the health care facility for 1 to 3 hours for detection of unstable vital signs, excessive cramping, or excessive bleeding; then she is discharged. If the procedure is done in a physician's office or clinic, preoperative sedation is usually not given, and the anesthetic of choice is usually paracervical block. After the abortion the woman rests on the table until she is ready to stand. Then she remains in the waiting room until she feels she can travel. She may be discharged alone or preferably in the company of a relative or friend.

Bleeding after the operation is normally about the equivalent of a heavy menstrual period, and cramps are rarely severe. Infection such as endometritis or salpingitis occurs in about 8% of women. A D & C procedure for bleeding or sepsis caused by retained placental tissue is necessary in about 2% of women. Hakim-Elahi et al (1990) reported an overall complication rate of less than 1%. Serious depression or other psychiatric problems are rare.

Postabortal instructions differ among health care providers (e.g., use of tampons may be discouraged for 3 days or for up to 3 weeks, and resumption of sexual intercourse may be permitted within 1 week or discouraged for 3 weeks). The woman may shower daily. Instruction is given to watch for excessive bleeding (i.e., more than one large pad per hour for 4 hours), cramps, or fever and to avoid douches of any type. The woman may expect her menstrual period to resume 4 to 6 weeks from the day of the procedure. The nurse offers information about the birth control method the woman prefers, if this has not been done previously during the counseling interview that usually precedes the decision to have an abortion. The woman must be strongly encouraged to return for her follow-up visit so that complications can be detected and an acceptable contraceptive method prescribed.

Second-Trimester Abortions

There are several techniques used for second-trimester abortions.

Transabdominal intrauterine injection of hypertonic sodium chloride. The woman is admitted to the hospital for this procedure. Amniocentesis is performed. The physician determines where the needle (an 18-gauge, 7.5 cm spinal needle) will be inserted. The area is cleansed, and if desired, a local anesthetic agent is given. Approximately 200 ml of amniotic fluid is withdrawn, and a similar amount of sterile hypertonic (20% to 25%) sodium chloride solution is injected. The woman is instructed to report to the nurse when uterine contractions begin—generally, within 8 to 48 hours. In most cases augmentation with oxytocin is necessary to effect uterine evacuation in a reasonable time. Occasionally reinjection is required. In theory, labor begins because the hypertonic saline solution releases the placental uterine progesterone blockade that normally prevents the onset of labor. The same careful monitoring of uterine contractions is as necessary as for a term birth. Instruction in relaxation and breathing techniques is indicated, and an analgesic can be administered for discomfort. The assistance of a supportive person at the time of birth of the dead fetus is essential. If the woman chooses to see the fetus, emotional support should be provided. Many women are relieved to find the fetus normal and commonly inquire as to its sex. After the abortion the standard observations and postpartum care are carried out (see Chapter 19). Contraceptive counseling is given before discharge. The woman is advised to return should excessive bleeding occur.

Complications of hypertonic saline injection for second-trimester abortion may occur. Complications with the approximate rates of their occurrence include infection (10%), need for D & C to remove retained tissue (15%), failure to abort (10%), and excessive bleeding that necessitates transfusion (2%). Symptoms related to saline solution (hypernatremia) include tinnitus, tachycardia, and headache, those of water intoxication, edema, oliguria (≤200 ml/8 hours), dyspnea, thirst, and restlessness. Rarely, DIC or expulsion of the fetus through the uterine isthmus occurs.

Dilation and evacuation. Dilation and evacuation (D & E) extends the D & C and vacuum curettage up to 20 weeks of gestation (Hatcher et al, 1994). It is the predominant method of abortion used beyond the first trimester (Wallach and Zacur, 1995). The cervix requires more dilation because the products of conception are larger. Often laminaria are inserted on the 2 days preceding the procedure (i.e., two to three may be inserted on the first day; on the second day these are removed, and four to six may be inserted). This allows slow dilation of the cervix. The procedure is performed on the third day. Larger instruments are employed and additional anesthetic is required. Nursing care includes monitoring vital signs, providing emotional support, administering analgesics, and postoperative monitoring.

Injection of urea solution after amniocentesis. After the removal of about 200 ml of amniotic fluid, 200 ml of 30% solution of urea in 5% dextrose in water is introduced into the uterus by gravity drip. After 1 hour a solution of 5 units of oxytocin in 500 ml of 5% dextrose in water is started intravenously. Fetal death occurs, and expulsion of the products of conception ensues in most cases within 12 hours. Complications are less common and are less serious than with hypertonic saline solution.

Prostaglandins. Prostaglandins are now widely used for inducing second-trimester abortion (Hatcher et al, 1994). Prostaglandins can be administered in suppository form, as a gel, or by intrauterine injection. Unpleasant side effects (e.g., nausea, vomiting, and diarrhea) usually occur. Repeated doses may be needed for expulsion of the products of conception.

Abdominal hysterotomy. Hysterotomy may be chosen after more than 14 to 16 weeks of pregnancy, after failure of intrauterine injection of saline solution or prostaglandins, and when sterilization is desired. The management is comparable to that of cesarean birth; however, the risk of morbidity and mortality is much higher.

Complications Following Abortion

The most common complications after abortion include infection, retained products of conception or intrauterine blood clots, continuing pregnancy, cervical or uterine trauma, and excessive bleeding (Hatcher et al, 1994; Wallach and Zacur, 1995). Preoperative antibiotic prophylaxis has been effective in reducing the risk of infection. Women are advised to report fever, pelvic pain, and excessive bleeding. Prophylactic chlamydia and gonorrhea treatment and the use of an oral ergotrate postoperatively may reduce the incidence of infection and retained products of conception.

Mifepristone (RU 486)

Progesterone is essential for maintaining pregnancy. Mifepristone (RU 486) is a progesterone antagonist that prevents implantation of a fertilized egg. It is most effective in early gestation, during the luteal phase, within 10 days of the expected onset of what would be the first missed period after conception. It can be taken up to 5 weeks after conception. The effectiveness of mifepristone is inversely related to gestational age as determined by β-hCG levels and duration of amenorrhea (Donaldson et al, 1994). However, it is considered to be an effective and safe method for termination of early pregnancy.

Uterine bleeding begins within 4 days of administration of the first dose. Usually a period of painless, heavy bleeding is reported. Termination of pregnancy occurs for most women. For the woman in whom abortion does not occur, evacuation of the uterus by aspiration is facilitated by the softening of the uterine cervix caused by mifepristone. Some women experience slight nausea and fatigue during the period of bleeding.

Supporters of this method feel that even with known disadvantages, mifepristone offers a reasonable alternative to surgical abortion, which carries the risks of anesthesia, surgical complications, infertility, and psychologic sequelae (Henshaw et al, 1993; Norman et al, 1992; Thong and Baird, 1992; World Health Organization Task Force, 1993). Others have taken a strong stand against the use of mifepristone.

Nursing Considerations

The woman will need help exploring the meaning of the various alternatives and consequences to herself and her significant others. It is often difficult for a woman to express her true feelings (e.g., what abortion means to her now and in the future, and what support or regret her friends and peers may demonstrate). A calm, matter-of-fact approach on the part of the nurse can be helpful. Listening to what the woman has to say and encouraging her to speak are essential. Once a decision has been made, the woman must be assured of continued support. Information about what is entailed in various procedures, how much discomfort or pain can be expected, and what type of care is needed must be given. If family or friends cannot be involved, scheduling time for the nursing personnel to give the necessary support is an essential component of the care plan.

Preoperative preparation, postoperative care, and discharge planning parallel the methods used for sterilization.

Evaluation

The nurse can be reasonably assured that care was effective when the expected outcomes of care have been achieved: the woman understands all information necessary to give informed consent; the procedure is successful, recovery is uneventful, and the woman continues to be satisfied with the decision for elective abortion, the procedure, and the experience with the health care team.

Key Points

- Lack of maternal glycemic control before conception and in the first trimester of pregnancy may be responsible for fetal congenital malformations.
- Maternal insulin does not cross the placenta; the fetus begins to secrete its own insulin by the tenth week of gestation.
- Maternal insulin requirements increase as the pregnancy progresses and may quadruple by term as a result of insulin resistance created by placental hormones, insulinase, and cortisol.
- Poor glycemic control before and during pregnancy is responsible for maternal complications such as spontaneous abortion, infection, pregnancy-induced hypertension, and dystocia (difficult labor) caused by hydramnios and macrosomia.
- Home monitoring of blood glucose levels, multiple doses or constant infusion of insulin, and dietary counseling are used to create a normal intrauterine environment for fetal growth and development in the pregnancy complicated by diabetes mellitus.
- The woman with hyperemesis gravidarum is discharged home when fluid and electrolyte balance is restored and weight gain begins.
- Thyroid dysfunction during pregnancy requires close monitoring of thyroid hormone levels to regulate therapy and prevent fetal insult.
- The stress of the normal maternal adaptations to pregnancy on a heart whose functions are already taxed may cause cardiac decompensation.
- In the case of a cardiac arrest in a pregnant woman, the standard advanced cardiac life support (ACLS) guidelines should be implemented without modification.
- Anemia, the most common medical disorder of pregnancy, affects at least 20% of women.
- The chance of developing adult respiratory distress syndrome increases with the amount of trauma experienced during pregnancy or birth.
- Autoimmune disorders (e.g., systemic lupus erythematosus, myasthenia gravis) show a predilection for women in their reproductive years; therefore they may occur during pregnancy.
- Trauma during pregnancy has the potential to affect both the mother and the fetus; assessment after trauma is more difficult because of the normal physiologic changes of pregnancy.
- In the pregnant woman an enlarged uterus, displaced internal organs, and altered laboratory values may confound differential diagnosis when the need for immediate abdominal surgery occurs.
- Preoperative care for a pregnant woman differs from that for a nonpregnant woman in one significant aspect: the presence of at least one other person—the fetus.
- Elective abortion accomplished in the first trimester is 10 times safer than carrying a pregnancy to term.

References

Abell T, Riely C: Hyperemesis gravidarum, *Gastroenterol Clin North Am* 21(4):835, 1992.

Adler N et al: Psychological responses after abortion, *Science* 248(4951):41, 1990.

American Diabetes Association (ADA): Position statement: office guide to diagnosis and classification of diabetes mellitus and other categories of glucose intolerance, *Diabetes Care* 13 (suppl 1):3, 1990.

American Heart Association: *Basic life support, heart saver guide*, Dallas, 1993, The Association.

Arias F: *Practical guide to high-risk pregnancy and delivery*, St Louis, 1993, Mosby.

Artal R: Exercise and pregnancy, *Clin Sports Med* 11(2):363, 1992.

Baker A: *Liver and bilary tract disease*. In Barron W, Lindheimer M, eds: *Medical disorders during pregnancy*, St Louis, 1995, Mosby.

Barron W: *Hypertension*. In Barron W, Lindheimer M, editors: *Medical disorders during pregnancy*, St Louis, 1995, Mosby.

Barron W, Lindheimer M, editors: *Medical disorders during pregnancy*, St Louis, 1995, Mosby.

Benz, J: Antidiabetic agents and lactation, *J Hum Lact* 8(1):27, 1992.

Berkowitz, G et al: Race/ethnicity and other risk factors for gestational diabetes, *Am J Epidemiol* 135(9):965, 1992.

Blackburn S, Loper D: *Maternal, fetal and neonatal physiology: a clinical perspective*, Philadelphia, 1992, WB Saunders.

Branch D: *Autoimmune diseases in pregnancy*. In Moore T et al, editors: *Gynecology and obstetrics: a longitudinal approach*, New York, 1993, Churchill Livingstone.

Briggs G, Garlte T: *Effects on the fetus of drugs used in critical care*. In Clark S et al, editors: *Critical care obstetrics*, ed 2, Boston, 1991, Blackwell Scientific.

Buchanan W, Needs C, Brooks P: *Rheumatic diseases: the arthropathies*. In Gleicher N et al, editors: *Principles and practice of medical therapy in pregnancy*, Norwalk, Conn, 1992, Appleton & Lange.

Burrow G: Thyroid function and hyperfunction during gestation, *Endocrine Rev* 14:194, 1993.

Cartlidge N: *Neurologic disorders*. In Barron W, Lindheimer M, editors: *Medical disorders during pregnancy*, St Louis, 1995, Mosby.

Centers for Disease Control and Prevention: Abortion surveillance—pulmonary data—United States, 1991, *MMWR Morb Mortal Wkly Rep* 43: 42, 1994.

Chandra N, Hazinski M, editors: *American Heart Association textbook of basic life support for healthcare providers*, Dallas, 1994, American Heart Association.

Charlin V et al: Parenteral nutrition in hyperemesis gravidarum, *Nutrition* 9(1):29, 1993.

Chauhan S, Perry K: Management of diabetic ketoacidosis in the obstetric patient, *Obstet Gynecol Clin North Am* 22(1):143, 1995.

Chavkin W, Rosenfield A: A chill wind blows: Webster obstetrics, and the health of women, *Am J Obstet Gynecol* 163 (2):450, 1990.

Cherry S, Merkatz I: *Complications of pregnancy: medical, surgical, gynecologic, psychosocial, and perinatal*, ed 4, Baltimore, 1991, Williams & Wilkins.

Chew E, Mills J, Metzger B et al: Metabolic control and progression of retinopathy, *Diabetes Care* 18(5):631, 1995.

Clark S: *Structural cardiac disease in pregnancy*. In Clark S et al, editors: *Critical care obstetrics*, ed 2, Cambridge, Mass, 1991, Blackwell Scientific.

Combs S, Kitzmiller J: Spontaneous abortion and congenital malformations in diabetes, *Baillieres Clin Obstet Gynaecol*, 5(2):315, 1991.

Cooper M et al: Asymmetric septal hypertrophy in infants of diabetic mothers, *Am J Dis Child* 146(2):226, 1992.

Coustan D: Gestational diabetes: state of the union, *Diabetes Care* 15(5):716, 1992.

Coustan D et al: Gestational diabetes: predictors of subsequent disordered glucose metabolism, *Am J Obstet Gynecol* 168(4):139, 1993.

Creasy R, Resnik R: *Maternal-fetal medicine: principles and practice*, ed 3, Philadelphia, 1994, WB Saunders.

Cruikshank D: *Cardiovascular, pulmonary, renal and hematologic disease in pregnancy*. In Scott J et al, editors: *Danforth's obstetrics and gynecology*, ed 7, Philadelphia, 1994, JB Lippincott.

Cunningham F et al: *Williams obstetrics*, ed 19, Norwalk, Conn, 1993, Appleton & Lange.

Dacus J et al: Gestational diabetes: postpartum glucose tolerance testing, *Am J Obstet Gynecol* 171(4):927, 1994.

Daddario J: Trauma in pregnancy, *J Perinat Neonat Nurs* 3(2):14, 1989.

Davidorf F, Chambers R: Diabetic retinopathy during pregnancy, *Clin Perinatol* 20(3):57, 1993.

Deuchar N: Nausea and vomiting in pregnancy: a review of the problem with particular regard to psychological and social aspects, *Br J Obstet Gynecol* 102:6, 1995.

Donaldson K et al: RU 486: an alternative to surgical abortion, *J Obstet Gynecol Neonatal Nurs* 23(7):555, 1994.

Dorman K: *Acute pulmonary insults during pregnancy*. In Harvey C, editor: *Critical care obstetrical nursing*, Gaithersburg, M, 1991, Aspen.

Dorner G, Plagemann A: Perinatal hyperinsulinism as possible predisposing factor for diabetes mellitus, obesity, and enhanced cardiovascular risk in later life, *Horm Metab Res* 26(5):213, 1994.

Dornhurst A et al: High prevalence of gestational diabetes in women from ethnic minority groups, *Diabet Med* 9(9):820, 1992.

Drash A et al: Infant feeding practices and their possible relationship to the etiology of diabetes mellitus, *Pediatrics* 94(5):89, 1994.

Elkayan U, Gleicher N: *Changes in cardiac findings during normal pregnancy*. In Elkayan U, Gleicher N, editors: *Cardiac problems in pregnancy*, ed 2, New York, 1989, John Wiley & Sons.

Fenakel K et al: Nifedipine in the treatment of severe preeclampsia, *Obstet Gynecol* 77:331, 1991.

Ferris A et al: Perinatal lactation protocol and outcome in mothers with and without insulin-dependent diabetes mellitus, *Am J Clin Nutr* 58:43, 1993.

Foley M et al: Effect of prolonged oral terbutaline therapy on glucose tolerance in pregnancy, *Am J Obstet Gynecol* 168(1 Pt 1):100, 1993.

Gabbe S: A story of two miracles: the impact of the discovery of insulin on pregnancy in women with diabetes mellitus, *Obstet Gynecol* 79(2):295, 1992.

Gilbert E, Harmon J: *Manual of high risk pregnancy and delivery*, St Louis, 1993, Mosby.

Gleicher N, editor: *Principles and practice of medical therapy in pregnancy*, ed 2, Norwalk, Conn, 1992, Appleton and Lange.

Godsey R, Newman R: Hyperemesis gravidarum: a comparison of single and multiple admissions, *J Reprod Med* 36:287, 1991.

Goodwin T, Montoro M, Mestman J: Transient hyperthyroidism and hyperemesis gravidarum: clinical aspects, *Am J Obstet Gynecol* 167(3):148, 1992.

Greene M: Prevention and diagnosis of congenital anomalies in diabetic pregnancies, *Clin Perinatol* 20(3):533, 1993.

Grohar J: Nursing protocals for antepartum home care, *J Obstet Gynecol Neonatal Nurs* 23(8):687, 1994.

Hakim-Elahi et al: Complications of first-trimester abortion: a report of 170,000 cases, *Obstet Gynecol* 76(1):129, 1990.

Hamburger J: Diagnosis and management of Graves' disease in pregnancy, *Thyroid* 2:219, 1992.

Harvey C: *Critical care obstetrical nursing*, Gaithersburg, Md, 1991, Aspen Publishers.

Harvey M: Diabetic ketoacidosis during pregnancy, *J Perinatol Neonatal Nurs* 6(1):1, 1992.

Hatcher R et al: *Contraceptive technology: 1994-1996*, ed 15, New York, 1994, Irvington Publishers.

Henshaw R et al: Comparison of medical abortion with surgical vacuum aspiration, *BMJ* 307:714, 1993.

Hod M et al: Hyperemesis gravidarum, *J Reprod Med* 39:605, 1994.

Holt V et al: Induced abortion and the risk of subsequent ectopic pregnancy, *Am J Public Health* 79(9):1234, 1989.

Howard E: Gestational diabetes mellitus screening tests: a review of current recommendations, *J Perinatol Neonatal Nurs* 6(1):37, 1992.

Hurst, J, Alpert J: *Diagnostic atlas of the heart*, New York, 1994, Raven Press.

Jackson G, Clark S: *Cardiac and pulmonary disorders and pregnancy*. In Moore T et al, editors: *Gynecology and obstetrics: a longitudinal approach*, New York, 1993, Churchill Livingstone.

James D et al, editors: *High risk pregnancy: management options*, Philadelphia, 1994, WB Saunders.

Jovanovic-Peterson L, editor: *Medical management of pregnancy complicated by diabetes*, Alexandria, Va, 1993, American Diabetes Association.

Jovanovic-Peterson L et al: Maternal postprandial glucose levels and infant birth weight: the Diabetes in Early Pregnancy Study. The National Institute of Child Health and Human Development Diabetes in Early Pregnancy Study, *Am J Obstet Gynecol* 164: 103, 1991.

Jovanovic-Peterson L, Peterson C: Pregnancy in the diabetic woman, *Endocrinol Metab Clin North Am* 21(2):433, 1992.

Kaplan M: Assessment of thyroid function during pregnancy, *Thyroid* 2(1):57, 1992.

Karjalainen J et al: A bovine albumin peptide as a possible trigger of insulin-dependent diabetes mellitus, *N Engl J Med* 327:302, 1992.

Keohane N, Lacey L: Preparing the woman with gestational diabetes for self-care: use of a structured teaching plan by nursing staff, *J Obstet Gynecol Neonatal Nurs* 20(3):189, 1991.

Kitzmiller J, Coombs C: Maternal and perinatal implications of diabetic nephropathy, *Clin Perinatol* 20(3):561, 1993.

Kitzmiller J et al: Preconception care of diabetes: glycemic control prevents congenital anomalies, *JAMA* 265(6):731, 1991.

Kjos S: Contraception in the diabetic woman, *Clin Perinatol* 20(3):649, 1993.

Kohn N: *Neurologic diseases*. In Gleicher N, editor: *Principles and practice of medical therapy in pregnancy*, ed 2, Norwalk, Conn, 1992, Appleton & Lange.

Krumholz A: *Epilepsy in pregnancy*. In Goldstein P, Stern B, editors: *Neurological disorders of pregnancy*, Mount Kisco, NY, 1992, Futura Publishing.

Kulb N: *Cardiac disorders*. In Buckley K, Kulb N, editors: *High risk maternity nursing manual*, Baltimore, Md, 1990, Williams and Wilkins.

Landon M, Gabbe S: Diabetes mellitus and pregnancy, *Obstet Gynecol Clin North Am* 19(4):633, 1992.

Landon M, Gabbe S: Fetal surveillance in the pregnancy complicated by diabetes mellitus, *Clin Perinatol* 20(3):549, 1993.

Landon M, Gabbe S: *Diabetes mellitus*. In Barron W, Lindheimer M, editors: *Medical disorders during pregnancy*, ed 2, St Louis, 1995, Mosby.

Langer O: Management of gestational diabetes, *Clin Perinatal* 20(3):603, 1993.

Langford H, Bartholomew S: Severe hypoglycemia in diabetic pregnancy, *Va Med Q* 119(3):172, 1992.

Lawrence R: *Breastfeeding: a guide for the medical profession*, ed 4, St Louis, 1994, Mosby.

Lazarus J: Treatment of hyper- and hypothyroidism in pregnancy, *J Endocrinol Invest* 16(5):391, 1993.

Learoyd D, Fung H, McGregor A: Postpartum thyroid dysfunction, *Thyroid* 2(1):73, 1992.

Leff E, Gagne M, Jeffries S: Type I diabetes and pregnancy: are we hearing women's concerns, *MCN Am J Matern Child Nurs* 16(2):83, 1991.

Leung A et al: Perinatal outcome in hypothyroid pregnancies, *Obstet Gynecol* 81(3):349, 1993.

Lockshin M, Druzin M: *Rheumatic disease*. In Barron W, Lindheimer M, eds: *Medical disorders during pregnancy*, St Louis, 1995, Mosby.

Mendelson M, Lang R: *Pregnancy and heart disease*. In Barron W, Lindheimer M, eds: *Medical disorders during pregnancy*, St Louis, 1995, Mosby.

Mestman J, Schmidt-Sarosi C: Diabetes mellitus and fertility control: contraception management issues, *Am J Obstet Gynecol* 168(6 Pt 2):2012, 1993.

Metzger B: Summary and recommendations of the third international workshop-conference on gestational diabetes mellitus, *Diabetes* 34(suppl 2): 197, 1991.

Meyer B, Palmer S: Pregestational diabetes, *Semin Perinatol* 14(1):12, 1990.

Mintoro M et al: Outcome of pregnancy in diabetic ketoacidosis, *Am J Perinatol* 10:17, 1993.

Mishell D, Brenner P, editors: *Management of common problems in obstetrics and gynecology*, ed 3, Boston, 1994, Blackwell Scientific Publications.

Modigliani R, Bernades P: *Gastrointestinal and pancreatic diseases*. In Barron W, Lindheimer M, editors: *Medical disorders during pregnancy*, ed 2, St Louis, 1995, Mosby.

Molitch M: *Pituitary, thyroid, adrenal, and parathyroid disorders*. In Barron W, Lindheimer M, editors: *Medical disorders during pregnancy*, ed 2, St Louis, 1995, Mosby.

Mulford M et al, Alternative therapies for the management of gestational diabetes, *Clin Perinatol* 20(3):619, 1993.

Muller J, Goldman M: *Cardiovascular disease in pregnancy*. In Cherry S, Merkatz I: *Complications of pregnancy: medical, surgical, gynecologic, psychosocial, and perinatal*, ed 4, Baltimore, 1991, Williams & Wilkins.

Myers S, Gleicher N: *Physiologic changes in normal pregnancy*. In Gleicher N, editor: *Principles and practice of medical therapy in pregnancy*, ed 2, Norwalk, Conn, 1992, Appleton and Lange.

Neubauer S et al: Delayed lactogenesis in women with insulin-dependent diabetes mellitus, *Am J Clin Nutr* 58:54, 1993.

New York Heart Association (NYHA): *Diseases of the heart and blood vessels: nomenclature and criteria for diagnosis*, ed 6, Boston, 1964, Little, Brown.

Norman J et al: Medical abortion in women of less than 56 days amenorrhoea, *Br J Obstet Gynaecol* 99:601, 1992.

Pagano K, Pagano T: *Mosby's diagnostic and laboratory test reference*, ed 2, St Louis, 1995, Mosby.

Palmer D, Inturrisi M: Insulin infusion therapy in the intrapartum period, *J Perinat Neonatal Nurs*, 6(1):25, 1992.

Penha M et al: Diabetic mothers and pregnancy loss: implications for diabetes educators, *Diab Educ* 19(1):35, 1993.

Perelman A, Clemons R: The fetus in maternal hyperthyroidism, *Thyroid* 2(3):225, 1992.

Perry K, Morrison J: *Disorders of hemoglobin structure, function, and synthesis*. In Gleicher N, editor: *Principles and practice of medical therapy in pregnancy*, ed 2, Norwalk, Conn, 1992, Appleton and Lange.

Peterson A et al: Glucose intolerance as consequence of oral terbulatine treatment for preterm labor, *J Fam Pract* 36(1):25, 1993.

Phipps W et al: *Medical-surgical nursing: concepts and clinical practice*, ed 5, St Louis, 1995, Mosby.

Piper J, Langer O: Does maternal diabetes delay fetal pulmonary maturity? *Am J Obstet Gynecol* 168(3 Pt 1):783, 1993.

Plauche W: Myasthenia gravis in mothers and their newborns, *Clin Obstet Gynecol* 34:82, 1991.

Reece E, Homko C: Diabetes-related complications of pregnancy, *J Nat Med Assoc* 85(7):537, 1993.

Reece E, Homko C, Wiznitzer A: Hypoglycemia in pregnancies complicated by diabetes mellitus: maternal and fetal considerations, *Clin Obstet Gynecol* 37(1):50, 1994.

Regenstein A, Belluomini J, Katz M: Terbutaline tocolysis and glucose intolerance, *Obstet Gynecol* 81 (5 Pt 1):739, 1993.

Rhodes A: Issue update: abortion, *MCN Am J Matern Child Nurs J* 15:289, 1990.

Rogers J et al: Impact of the Minnesota parental notification law on abortion and birth, *Am J Public Health* 81(3):294, 1991.

Rosas T, Constantino N: Exercise as a treatment modality to maintain normoglycemia in gestational diabetes, *J Perinatol Neonatal Nurs* 6(1):14, 1992.

Rosenn B et al: Preconception management of insulin-dependent diabetes: improvement of pregnancy outcome, *Obstet Gynecol* 77(6):847, 1991.

Rosenn B et al: Glycemic thresholds for spontaneous abortion and con genital malformations in insulin dependent diabetes, *Obstet Gynecol* 84(4):515, 1994.

Rudick R, Birk K: *Multiple sclerosis and pregnancy.* In Goldstein P, Stern B, editors: *Neurological disorders of pregnancy,* Mount Kisco, NY, 1992, Futura Publishing.

Ruggiero L et al: Impact of social support and stress on compliance in women with gestational diabetes, *Diabetes Care* 13:441, 1990.

Sacks D et al: Toward universal criteria for gestational diabetes: the 75-gm glucose tolerance test in pregnancy, *Am J Obstet Gynecol* 172(2):607, 1995.

Salveson D, Brudenell M, Nicolaides K: Fetal polycythemia and thrombocytopenia in pregnancies complicated by maternal diabetes mellitus, *Am J Obstet Gynecol* 166(4):1287, 1992.

Samson L: Infants of diabetic mothers: current perspectives, *J Perinat Neonatal Nurs* 6(1):61, 1992.

Schwartz R et al: Hyperinsulinemia and macrosomia in the fetus of the diabetic mother, *Diabetes Care* 17(7):640, 1994.

Scott J, Branch D: *Immunologic disorders.* In Scott J ed: *Danforth's obstetrics and gynecology,* ed 7, Philadelphia, 1994, JB Lippincott.

Shaver D: *Complications of operative obstetrics.* In Gleicher N et al, editors: *Principles and practice of medical therapy in pregnancy,* Norwalk, Conn, 1992, Appleton & Lange.

Sibai B: *Surgery during pregnancy.* In Gleicher N et al, editors: *Principles and practice of medical therapy in pregnancy,* Norwalk, Conn, 1992, Appleton & Lange.

Silvermann B et al: Impaired glucose tolerance in adolescent offspring of diabetic mothers, *Diabetes Care* 18(5):611, 1995.

Simolke G, Cox S, Cunningham F: Cerebrovascular accidents complicating pregnancy and the puerperium, *Obstet Gynecol* 78:37, 1991.

Singer A, Brandt L: Pathophysiology of the GI tract during pregnancy, *Am J Gastroenterol* 86(12):1695, 1991.

Sipes A, Malee M: Endocrine disorders in pregnancy, *Obstet Gynecol Clin North Am* 19(4):655, 1992.

Smith C, Phelan J: *Trauma in pregnancy.* In Clark S, editor: *Critical care obstetrics,* Boston, 1991, Blackwell Scientific Publications.

Stamler E et al: High infectious morbidity in pregnant women with insulin-dependent diabetes: an understated complication, *Am J Obstet Gynecol* 163:1217, 1990.

Strickland R et al: Anesthesia, cardiopulmonary bypass and the pregnant client, *Mayo Clin Proc* 66:411, 1991.

Thompson D et al: Tight glucose control results in normal perinatal outcome in 150 patients with gestational diabetes, *Obstet Gynecol* 83(3):362, 1994.

Thompson J, Thompson H: *Ethical considerations in high risk pregnancies.* In Buckley K, Kulb N, editors: *High risk maternity nursing manual,* Baltimore, 1990, Williams and Wilkins.

Thong K, Baird D: Induction of abortion with mifeprisone and misoprostol in early pregnancy, *Br J of Obstet Gynaecol* 99:1004, 1992.

Torem M: Hypnotherapeutic techniques in the treatment of hyperemesis gravidarum, *Am J Clin Hypn* 37(1):1, 1994.

Troiano N: Cardiopulmonary resuscitation of the pregnant woman, *J Perinat Neonatal Nurs* 3(2):1, 1989.

Troiano N: *Trauma during pregnancy.* In Harvey C, editor: *Critical care obstetrical nursing,* Gaithersburg, Md, 1991, Aspen.

Varner M: *General medical and surgical diseases in pregnancy.* In Scott J et al, *Danforth's obstetric and gynecology,* Philadelphia, 1994, JB Lippincott.

Wallach E, Zacur H: *Reproductive medicine and surgery,* St Louis, 1995, Mosby.

Walling A: Bell's palsy in pregnancy and the puerperium, *J Fam Pract* 36:559, 1993.

Wasserstrom N: Nitroprusside in preeclampsia: circulatory distress and paradoxical bradycardia, *Hypertension* 18:79, 1991.

Wells N: Pain and distress during abortion, *Health Care Women Int,* 12(3):293, 1991.

White P: Classification of obstetrics diabetes, *Am J Obstet Gynecol* 130:228, 1978.

Willhoite M et al: The impact of preconception counseling on pregnancy outcomes: the experience of the Maine Diabetes in Pregnancy Program, *Diabetes Care* 16(2):450, 1993.

World Health Organization Task Force: Termination of pregnancy with reduced doses of mifepristone, *Br Med J* 307:532, 1993.

Worthington-Roberts B, Williams S: *Nutrition in pregnancy and lactation,* ed 5, St Louis, 1993, Mosby.

Bibliography

Avery M, Rossi M: Gestational diabetes, *J Nurs Midwife* 39(2 suppl): 9S, 1994.

Boggess K, Easterling T, Raghu G: Management and outcome of pregnant women with interstitial and restrictive lung disease, *Am J Obstet Gynecol* 173(4):1007, 1995.

Carr S et al: Precision of office-based blood glucose meters in screening for gestational diabetes, *Am J Obstet Gynecol* 173(4):1267, 1995.

Castle M et al: Listening and learning from women about mifepristone: implications for counseling and health education, *Womens Health Issues* 5(3):130, 1995.

Doshier S: What happens to the offspring of diabetic pregnancies? *MCN Am J Matern Child Nurs* 20(1):25, 1995.

Fleschler R, Sala D: Pregnancy after organ transplantation, *J Obstet Gynecol Neonatal Nurs* 24:5, 413, 1995.

Jackson J, Bash D: Management of the uncomplicated pregnant diabetic client in the ambulatory setting, *Nurse Pract* 19(12):64, 1994.

Josten E et al: Perinatal health: high-risk mothers and infants: bedrest compliance for women with pregnancy problems, *Birth* 22:1, 1995.

Kennedy B: Mitral stenosis: implications for critical care obstetric nursing, *J Obstet Gynecol Neonatal Nurs* 24(5):406, 1995.

Kuper B: Shedding new light on lupus, *Am J Nurs* 11:26, 1994.

Mitchell L: Cardiac arrest during pregnancy: maternal-fetal physiology and advanced cardiac life support for the obstetric patient, *Crit Care Nurs* 15(1):56, 1995.

Rossiter J et al: A prospective longitudinal evaluation of pregnancy in the Marfan syndrome, *Am J Obstet Gynecol* 173(5):1599, 1995.

van Stuijenberg M et al: The nutritional status and treatment of patients with hyperemesis gravidarum, *Am J Obstet Gynecol* 172:1585, 1995.

CHAPTER 11

Psychosocial Problems

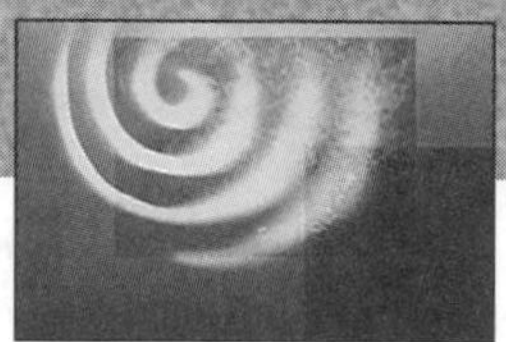

EMOTIONAL COMPLICATIONS, P. 296
Mood disorders, p. 296
Schizophrenia, p. 298
Nursing care management, p. 298

PSYCHOACTIVE SUBSTANCE USE, P. 302
Legal sanctions, p. 302
Alcohol, p. 303
Marijuana, p. 303
Cocaine, p. 303
Heroin, p. 305
Methamphetamine, p. 305
Phencyclidine, p. 306
Nursing care management, p. 306

OTHER ADDICTIVE SUBSTANCES, P. 309
Tobacco, p. 309
Caffeine, p. 310

VIOLENCE AGAINST WOMEN, P. 310
Dynamics of abuse, p. 311
Nursing care management, p. 311
Prevention, p. 313

Psychosocial conditions have implications for the health of the mother and newborn. These conditions can interfere with attachment to the newborn and family integration. Some conditions may threaten the safety and well-being of the mother and newborn. This chapter explores mental health disorders, psychoactive substance abuse disorders, tobacco and caffeine abuse, and violence against women. The nursing process with affected women and their families is emphasized.

EMOTIONAL COMPLICATIONS

Mental health problems can complicate pregnancy, childbirth, and the puerperium. Some problems predate pregnancy. For example, developmental and personality disorders generally have an onset in childhood or adolescence and usually persist into adulthood (Stuart and Sundeen, 1995). Mental retardation and autistic and disruptive behavior disorders are examples. Problems in behavioral categories include sleep and arousal disorders, schizophrenic disorders, personality disorders, and mood disorders.

Pregnancy is not a cause of psychiatric illness. However, the psychologic and physical stresses relating to pregnancy or to the new obligations of motherhood may produce an emotional crisis or be complicated by a preexisting mental illness (Affonso et al, 1993). The principal emotional disturbances complicating pregnancy and the postpartum period are mood disorders and schizophrenia. Mood disorders include depressive disorders and bipolar disorders with or without psychotic features. Schizophrenia disorders are characterized by **psychotic features** such as hallucinations, delusions, and disorganized speech or behavior. Emotional illnesses appearing during pregnancy are diagnosed by their initial features.

No one single factor has been isolated as being responsible for precipitating postpartum mental illness. Postpartum mental illness has an onset within 4 weeks of childbirth. The specifier "with postpartum onset" is applied to the current or most recent diagnosis from *The Diagnostic and Statistical Manual of Mental Disorders*, ed. 4 (DSM-IV) if the onset occurs within 4 weeks of childbirth. These DSM-IV diagnoses include major depressive, manic, or mixed episode of major depressive disorder; bipolar I disorder; bipolar II disorder; or brief psychotic disorder and schizophrenia (American Psychiatric Association, 1994). The DSM-IV is the official guide to assessment and diagnosis of psychiatric illness.

Mood Disorders

Mood disorders are defined as disorders that have as the dominant feature a disturbance in the prevailing emotional state. Although the cause of mood disorders is unknown, predisposing factors such as a family history may reveal that one or more adults have had this problem. Psychiatric complications during the course of pregnancy and a previous mental health disorder are risk factors for mood disorders in women.

Mood disorders account for approximately 50% of all pregnancy-related mental illnesses. Of these, 10% are prenatal manic or depressive states; the remainder occur during the postnatal period. However, Affonso et al (1993) reported that women's depressive symptoms may be evident during the first trimester of pregnancy—as early as 10 to 14 weeks in women who have had no prior depression. This finding disputes the myth that early pregnancy is a pleasant and happy event for everyone. Additional findings of the study included identification of depressive symptoms at 30 to 32 weeks, 1 to 2 weeks post partum, and 14 weeks post partum in women who had no depression before pregnancy (Affonso et al, 1993). Younger women seem more prone to bipolar disorders, but depression is the most common problem for women. In this chapter, the clinical manifestations of each mood disorder are discussed under each individual diagnostic category.

Postpartum symptoms of major depressive, manic, or mixed episodes do not usually differ from the symptoms of nonpostpartum mood episodes with or without psychotic features (American Psychiatric Association, 1994). Rejection of the infant, often caused by abnormal jealousy, is a prominent feature of mood disorders. The mother may be obsessed by the notion that the offspring may take her place in her partner's affections. In other instances, guilt regarding aversion to pregnancy, attempted abortion, or other personal conflicts may be the basic problem.

The mood disorders of the postpartum period can be grouped into three categories: postpartum blues, postpartum depression without psychotic features, and postpartum depression with psychotic features (previously called postpartum psychosis). Schizophrenia is discussed as a diagnostic category separate from mood disorders.

Postpartum blues. **Postpartum blues** are defined as brief episodes of labile mood and tearfulness that occur within 1 to 5 days of childbirth and last 1 to 4 days. Postpartum blues affect 50% to 80% of women who give birth (Ugarriza, 1992).

Predisposing factors for postpartum blues may include biologic changes, stress, normal responses, or social or environmental causes. Biologic theorists have studied the hormonal fluctuations associated with pregnancy and attribute some depressed mood reactions to changes in progesterone, estradiol, cortisol, and prolactin levels (Ehlert et al, 1990; Harris et al, 1989; Majewski, Ford-Rice, Falkey, 1989). Stress theory supporters propose that any stressful event (e.g., surgery) can trigger reactions such as the blues (Iles, Gath, and Kennerley, 1989). Others view the blues as a normal, physiologically based response that increases mothering instincts and protectiveness toward the infant (Majewski, Ford-Rice, and Falkey, 1989). Social and environmental issues such as strained marital and family relations, a history of premenstrual syndrome (PMS), anxiety, fear of labor, depression during pregnancy, a complicated intrapartum course, and poor social adjustment may be predisposing factors (Kennerley and Gath, 1989a; 1989b).

The clinical manifestations of postpartum blues are usually mild and transient. Diagnosing and categorizing the blues is difficult because of the lack of standardized assessment tools. The seven most common symptoms of postpartum blues are listed in Box 11-1.

BOX 11-1
Seven Most Common Symptoms of Postpartum Blues

1. Mood swings
2. Feeling low
3. Anxiety
4. Feeling overemotional
5. Tearfulness
6. Fatigue
7. Confused or muddled thinking

Postpartum depression without psychotic features. The definition of **postpartum depression** without psychotic features is intense and pervasive sadness with severe and labile mood swings. The incidence of postpartum depression without psychotic features is 10% to 15% of all childbearing women.

Predisposing factors of postpartum depression may include a history of depression or may be hormone-related or infant-related. As with postpartum blues, some researchers have identified a link between decreased postpartum depression and levels of prolactin and progesterone. Environmental and family stress issues may also be linked to postpartum depression (Gotlib et al, 1991). Women who experience depression often have fewer support systems, more stressful life events, and fewer personal resources with which to combat these events. Women with feelings of postpartum closeness to their husbands or partners report fewer depressive symptoms (Logsdon, McBride, and Birkimer, 1994). Predictive factors for postpartum depression that may assist the nurse in assessing potential problems include a previous history of mood disorder, meager or absent social support, and stressful life events (e.g., single parent, divorce, or recent death of a parent or child) (Auerbach and Jacobi, 1990; Stein et al, 1989).

The clinical manifestations of postpartum depression are severe anxiety, panic attacks, spontaneous crying long after the usual 1 to 4 days of postpartum blues, disinterest in the new infant, and insomnia that is more likely to manifest as difficulty falling asleep than as early morning awakening (American Psychiatric Association, 1994). Women may feel guilty about their depression, have negative feelings toward their infant, and be reluctant to discuss their symptoms. Alterations in maternal-infant attachment may result from postpartum depression and infant separation from the mother (American Psychiatric Association, 1994). The symptoms of postpartum depression last longer than the blues, and the mother may experience a weight change (loss or gain) and social withdrawal. In both the nonpsychotic and psychotic presentations of depression, there may be suicidal ideation, obsessional thoughts regarding violence to the child, lack of concentration, and psychomotor agitation.

Postpartum mood disorders with psychotic features. The definition of mood disorder with psychotic features is intense and pervasive sadness with severe labile mood swings and the presence of at least one of the following: delusions, hallucinations, disorganized speech, or grossly disorganized or catatonic behavior. This disorder is also called postpartum psychosis. The incidence of postpartum mood disorder with psychotic features is 1.7 cases per 1000 births. It is the least common form of postpartum mental disorders (Bright, 1994). However, once a woman has had a postpartum episode with psychotic features, the risk of recurrence with each subsequent delivery is 30% to 50% (American Psychiatric Association, 1994).

The predisposing factors of postpartum mood disorder with psychotic features are a prior history of mood disorder, especially bipolar I disorder, and a prior postpartum mood disorder. Women who do not have a history of mood disorders but who have a family history of bipolar disorders may have an increased risk of postpartum mood disorder with psychotic features (American Psychiatric Association, 1994). The clinical manifestations of postpartum mood disorder with psychotic features include delusions, hallucinations, disorganized speech, or grossly disorganized or catatonic behavior.

When delusions are present, they are often related to the newborn. The mother may think that the "newborn is possessed by the devil, has special powers, or is destined for a terrible fate" (American Psychiatric Association, 1994). Hallucinations that command the mother to kill the infant can also occur during severe episodes. Grossly disorganized behavior may manifest as disinterest in the infant or an inability to provide care.

Bipolar disorder. Bipolar disorder or "manic depressive illness" is depression with previous or current manic episodes. Manic episodes are characterized by elevated, expansive, or irritable moods. Bipolar disorder occurs in approximately 0.6% to 0.88% of the population and less often than depressive disorders (Stuart and Sundeen, 1995). Predisposing risk factors are similar to those for depression.

Clinical manifestations of a manic episode include the presence of at least three of the following to a significant degree for at least 1 week: grandiosity, decreased need for sleep, pressured speech, flight of ideas, distractibility, psychomotor agitation, and excessive involvement in pleasurable activities without regard for negative consequences (American Psychiatric Association, 1994). Even though a patient feels happy, unconcerned, and carefree, these feelings can occur without reference to reality and can include delusions of omnipotence and an inability to foresee the consequences of actions. Because patients in a manic episode are hyperactive, they may not take the time to eat or sleep, which leads to inadequate nutrition, dehydration, and sleep deprivation. Such behaviors may require prompt intervention, especially if a manic disorder occurs during pregnancy.

Critical Thinking Exercises

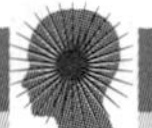

POSTPARTUM DEPRESSION

You make a home visit to a pregnant woman who started prenatal care at a county-supported clinic but missed her last two appointments. Your assessment reveals the following findings:

- Patient is tearful, feels confused, and cannot think clearly.
- Patient cannot remember when she ate last or the last time she had more than 2 hours of sleep at one time.
- Patient shows lack of concern for 18-month-old son, who is crying and has a soiled diaper.
- Patient tearfully states that she does not know if she can go on living because her husband has left her.
- Patient has a history of postpartum depression after the birth of her first baby.

For each identified problem:

1. Formulate a nursing diagnosis.
2. Prioritize the nursing diagnosis.
3. Plan patient-centered goals and expected outcomes.
4. Plan interventions and provide rationales for each.
5. List referrals and possible community resources.

Schizophrenia

Schizophrenia is defined as a "loss of ego boundaries or a gross impairment in reality testing" (American Psychiatric Association, 1994). It is a disturbance that lasts for at least six months and includes at least 1 month of two or more active-phase symptoms: delusions, hallucinations, disorganized speech, grossly disorganized or catatonic behavior, and negative symptoms. Schizophrenia appears to be not one but several distinct disorders.

The incidence of schizophrenia in the general population is a 1% lifetime risk unless an individual has a first- or second-degree relative with the disorder (Stuart and Sundeen, 1995), which equates to approximately two million people in the United States. Schizophrenia typically occurs between the late teens and mid thirties. For women, the median age of onset for the first psychotic episode is in the late twenties. Three out of four cases begin between the ages of 17 and 25, which are prime childbearing years.

Predisposing factors for schizophrenia include sociocultural, psychologic, and biologic factors. The biologic findings consistently point to structural abnormalities in the brain that have been identified in individuals with schizophrenia. Although the mechanism of transmission through the genes is not clearly defined, studies show a high incidence of schizophrenia in families. Other biologic theories suggest that symptoms of schizophrenia may be caused by changes in the structure of brain tissue (Stuart and Sundeen, 1995).

Early or prodromal clinical manifestations may include a loss of interest in social activities and work, deterioration in grooming and hygiene, and outbursts of anger. A sudden onset of delusions or hallucinations may alter a seemingly well-adjusted normal pregnancy. The symptoms indicate a woman's inability to adjust to and cope with her new obligations as a mother. The husband or significant other is totally rejected. Hostility toward the husband and medical staff is obvious. The woman may abandon reality, neglect the infant, and retreat into her own world. With prompt intervention, a good prognosis for recovery is likely for the first postpartum episode, especially if it occurs unexpectedly.

Nursing Care Management

Assessment

The nursing care plan must reflect the assessment of the clinical manifestations of the particular disorder. If predisposing factors for emotional complications are identified during the prenatal period, it is imperative to continue the assessment of emotional status at each visit. Assessment of the woman's partner, family, and infant (if post partum) is important because they may also be affected by the woman's emotional disorder.

Nursing Diagnoses

Nursing diagnoses relevant to any emotional illness that complicates pregnancy or the postpartum period may include the following:

- Risk for injury to fetus related to
  - Psychotropic medication
  - Maternal suicide
  - Untreated medical mood disorder
- Risk for injury to newborn related to
  - Unmet needs (e.g., hygiene, nutrition) and safety precautions
  - Mother's poor impulse control
- Ineffective family coping related to
  - Stigma of psychiatric diagnosis
  - Increased care needs of mother/newborn
- Impaired home maintenance management related to
  - Increased care needs of mother/newborn
- Risk for altered parenting related to
  - Inability of mother with a psychiatric illness to attach to infant
- Altered growth and development of infant related to
  - Lack of stimulation
  - Unmet needs (e.g., hygiene, nutrition) and safety precautions

Expected Outcomes

Planning focuses on the mother's dependency needs, attachment to the infant, family integration, parenting skills, care of the infant, and home maintenance management. Supervision of the mother and family in the home is a prime concern (Martell, 1990).

Expected outcomes for the woman and her family include the following:

1. The mother's psychiatric symptoms will stabilize, and she will be able to care for herself and her infant.
2. The mother's and infant's physical well-being will be maintained.
3. The mother and family will cope effectively.
4. Each family member will demonstrate continued healthy growth and development.

Plan of Care and Implementation

Prenatal and postpartum care. Emotional complications may be managed in a variety of ways and often depend on the woman's resources. If private health insurance or care through a health maintenance organization (HMO) is available, the woman may be provided with a case manager who makes frequent phone calls or home visits to provide support and manage her care. If no financial resources are available, the woman may be referred to community or state agencies for counseling and follow-up. Social workers provide invaluable assistance with referrals to community resources such as day care, foster care, homemaker services, Meals on Wheels, parenting guidance centers, mother's day out programs and telephone support groups. Community resources such as these may be used as necessary to assist with maternal dependency needs, to foster infant attachment and family integration, and to enhance parenting skills and home maintenance management.

Supervision of the mother with emotional complications is a prime concern. Sometimes it may be necessary to refer psychotic pregnant or postpartum women to an inpatient or partial day psychiatric treatment program for a brief period. A community-based approach that may include a psychiatric home health nurse for counseling and follow-up is vital for successful treatment of the emotional complications of pregnancy.

Hospitalized women present treatment challenges in three areas: psychotropic medications, legal sanctions, and management in an acute hospital setting. A brief overview of these challenges is provided in the following sections. Psychiatric texts may be consulted for specific details.

Psychotropic medications. All psychotropic medications pass through the placenta to the fetus and through breast milk to the infant. The risks of the medication are weighed against the risks of maternal agitation and potentially self-destructive behavior. Infants who were exposed to psychotropics between 8 and 10 weeks' gestation show a higher rate of congenital anomalies than infants with no such exposure (Lawrence, 1994). A higher perinatal death rate and an increased incidence of an extrapyramidal syndrome that consists of tremors, hypertonia, weakness, and poor sucking complicate the neonatal period. Medication dosages are balanced between the mother's needs and the fetal response as determined by nonstress tests (NSTs). Some medications may

BOX 11-2
Antidepressant Drugs

SELECTIVE SEROTONIN REUPTAKE INHIBITORS
Fluoxetine (Prozac)
Fluvoxamine (Luvox)
Paroxetine (Paxil)
Sertraline (Zoloft)

CYCLIC COMPOUNDS
Imipramine (Tofranil)
Desipramine (Norpramin)
Amitriptyline (Elavil)
Doxepin (Adapin, Sinequan)
Trimipramine (Surmontil)
Protriptyline (Vivactil)
Maprotiline (Ludiomil)
Amoxapine (Asendin)
Clomipramine (Anafranil)

MONOAMINE OXIDASE INHIBITORS
Phenelzine (Nardil)
Tranylcypromine (Parnate)

OTHER COMPOUNDS
Bupropion (Wellbutrin)
Venlafaxine (Effexor)
Trazodone (Desyrel and generics)
Nefazodone

BOX 11-3
Antipsychotic Drugs

Phenothiazines
Aliphatics
- Chlorpromazine (Thorazine)

Piperidines
- Mesoridazine (Serentil)
- Thioridazine (Mellaril)

Piperazines
- Fluphenazine (Prolixin, Permitil)
- Perphenazine (Trilafon)
- Trifluoperazine (Stelazine)

Thioxanthene
- Thiothixene (Navane)

Dibenzoazepines
- Loxapine (Loxitane)
- Clozapine (Clozaril)

Benzisoxazole
- Risperidone (Risperdal)

Butyrophenone
- Haloperidol (Haldol)

Indolone
- Molindone (Moban)

Diphenylbutylpiperidine
- Pimozide (Orap)

be behavioral teratogens with short- and long-term effects (Cook et al, 1990).

Postpartum blues do not usually require psychotropic medication. Postpartum depression without psychotic features may be treated with antidepressant drugs. Commonly used antidepressant drugs (Box 11-2) are often subdivided into four groups: selective serotonin reuptake inhibitors, tricyclic and related cyclic antidepressants, monoamine oxidase inhibitors (MAOIs), and other antidepressant compounds (Hyman, Arana, and Rosenbaum, 1995; Laraia and Stuart, 1995; Pastuszak et al, 1993). Antipsychotic medications may be used for acute and chronic psychotic features and schizophrenia (Box 11-3). No antipsychotic medication has been proven safe for use during pregnancy or lactation (Laraia and Stuart, 1995).

Bipolar disorder is usually treated with lithium. However, if a patient cannot tolerate the side effects of lithium or has a poor response, an anticonvulsant such as valproic acid (Depakene) or carbamazepine (Tegretol) may be prescribed for acute mania (Hyman, Arana, and Rosenbaum, 1995). Maternal shifts in fluid balance may require doubling the lithium dose to achieve a therapeutic level. Fetal lithium toxicity may cause polyhydramnios. A high incidence of fetal cardiovascular abnormalities is linked to the use of lithium during the first trimester. Fetal toxicity can result if the lithium dose is not decreased by at least 50% 1 week before birth. Regardless of the dose, the neonate may show signs of toxicity at birth: cyanosis, lethargy, low Apgar scores, and an absent Moro reflex (Krause, Ebbesen, and Lange, 1990; Lawrence, 1994).

Legal sanctions. Mental health laws that mandate psychiatric inpatient hospitalization vary from state to state. The law is usually invoked to prevent persons from harming themselves or others. If a pregnant woman has active suicidal ideations or harmful delusions about the pregnancy or fetus and is unwilling to seek treatment, legal intervention to commit the woman to an inpatient setting for assessment may be necessary.

Acute hospital management. Most treatment programs for emotional complications during pregnancy and the puerperium tend to be reactive rather than predictive. Nicholson (1990) reported that a more effective approach would be to assess postnatal depression not as an individual illness but as a normal grief reaction and a part of every postnatal profile. Interpretation by the mother of her experience may be the key to more appropriate treatment. The nurse can help mothers recognize that the childbirth experience is not always happy, positive, and a gain rather than a loss. Many mothers grieve over the loss of their former selves (figures, life-styles, jobs, sexual attractiveness) and go through upheaval and extreme stress. The nurse can help the mother acknowledge her new role and understand that depression and a grief reaction may be normal and not permanent.

The woman with depression with or without psychotic features or bipolar disorder is unable to engage in mutual interaction with the baby, which is necessary for acquaintance and subsequent attachment (bonding). If the woman wants to breastfeed, the nurse can assist with the same feeding techniques that are used for any mother. It is important to maintain and support a woman who is learning the maternal role (Auerbach and Jacobi, 1990). Within the hospital setting, the reintroduction of the baby to the mother can occur at the mother's own pace.

During these interactions, which are carefully supervised and guided, the mother's readiness for discharge and infant care is assessed. A schedule is set for increasing the hours of infant care over several days, culminating in the infant's admission to the unit for an overnight stay. The overnight stay allows the mother to experience the infant's needs and the sacrifice of sleep for the baby, a situation that is difficult for new mothers even under ideal conditions. During this time, the nurse should observe the woman for signs of bonding and attachment behaviors.

Attachment (bonding) behaviors are defined as eye-to-eye contact (en face position); physical contact (holding, touching, cuddling); talking to the baby and calling the baby by name; and initiating care as appropriate. A staff member is assigned to keep the baby in sight at all times. Indirect teaching, praise, and encouragement are designed to bolster the mother's self-esteem and self-confidence. The staff works with the father or partner at the same time as the mother.

In caring for a woman who is experiencing postpartum depression, the nurse must be aware of the effect of the depression on the family. If the mother is feeling inadequate, unable to cope with herself or the infant, withdrawn, or severely fatigued, the family is affected. Stressors are magnified and can result in isolation of the mother and family, a change in relationship with the partner, or a negative influence on parenting. The nurse must be alert for these signs of dysfunction and be prepared to help promote attachment between the mother and baby. Referral and follow-up care of the mother and family for support services and counseling are extremely important (Martell, 1990; Neuspiel et al, 1993).

Nursing Care Plan

POSTPARTUM DEPRESSION

NURSING DIAGNOSIS: Ineffective individual coping related to developing postpartum depression

Expected Outcome: **Patient will develop and maintain effective skills to cope with the demands of motherhood.**

• NURSING INTERVENTIONS/*RATIONALES*

Monitor ongoing clinical manifestations (e.g., severe anxiety, panic attacks, spontaneous crying, insomnia) *to assess depth of postpartum depression.*

Spend consistent uninterrupted periods of time talking with and actively listening to the woman *to develop a trusting and therapeutic relationship.*

Encourage open expression of feelings and emotions *to provide an atmosphere for ventilation.*

Discuss the personal meanings attached to giving birth and parenting; have the woman draw relationships between feelings and behavior *to foster a realistic assessment of the situation.*

Encourage independent behavior and decision making *to promote self-esteem and reinforce effective coping.*

Assist woman to recognize and accept responsibility for actions and set limits on manipulative behaviors *to increase a sense of responsibility and promote coping.*

Assist woman in exploring her current situation and in developing strategies for handling daily events *to develop and reinforce coping strategies.*

Help woman identify and use support systems *because effective support is essential to maintain coping skills.*

Refer woman to appropriate counseling services for *ongoing psychotherapeutic support.*

Refer woman to home health care agency if respite care of the infant is needed *to relieve stress and enhance the ability of the mother to cope.*

NURSING DIAGNOSIS: Risk for altered parenting related to inadequate maternal attachment secondary to postpartum depression

Expected Outcomes: **Contact is established with neonate, and mother is involved in care of neonate.**

• NURSING INTERVENTIONS/*RATIONALES*

Encourage touching behaviors, age-appropriate play activities, and care-taking activities by parents *to assist in developing attachment behaviors.*

Help parents perform defined touching exercises with their infant at prespecified times *to assist in the development of touching behaviors.*

Demonstrate and provide a detailed written description of the exercises *to promote understanding and use.*

Demonstrate and have parents return the demonstration of daily care-taking behaviors *to evaluate parental abilities and skills and to promote attachment.*

Teach parents about age-appropriate play activities and encourage them to have consistent playtimes with their infant *to assist in developing attachment behaviors.*

NURSING DIAGNOSIS: Risk for injury to the newborn related to neglect or poor maternal impulse control secondary to postpartum depression

Expected Outcomes: **Neonate is protected from injury; family asks for assistance when necessary.**

• NURSING INTERVENTIONS/*RATIONALES*

Assess the family home environment *to determine degree of risk to the infant's safety.*

Educate family members and support systems about early signs of neglect *to prevent abuse and injury to the infant.*

Have family call for assistance from an appropriate support service immediately if neglect is suspected *to prevent injury.*

Contact the appropriate authorities if infant safety is in question *to protect infant from harm.*

NURSING DIAGNOSIS: Risk for altered infant growth and development related to lack of stimulation/interaction secondary to maternal postpartum depression

Expected Outcome: **Growth and development milestones are reached when expected.**

• NURSING INTERVENTIONS/*RATIONALES*

Monitor infant's developmental progress (e.g., gross motor, fine motor, social, language) and growth patterns (e.g., height, weight, head circumference) at regular intervals *to evaluate developmental status and detect any deficits early to allow for amelioration.*

Assess infant for patterns of frequent restlessness, sleeplessness, agitation, unchecked crying, or resistance to cuddling and holding *to ascertain whether patterns exist that may require additional parenting skills to cope or may indicate a lack of adequate parental coping.*

If infant displays any of the previous patterns, assist parents in identifying and implementing strategies *to decrease the patterns and to help the parents cope.*

Make appropriate referrals to nutritionists, infant play groups, and occupational or physical therapists *as needed for identified growth or developmental lags.*

The onset of postpartum mood disorder with psychotic features usually is abrupt and occurs within days of childbirth. The symptoms center around the mother's relationship with the baby. The mother's response may be of an overprotective or rejecting nature. The mother may be convinced that someone is trying to take her baby and will clutch it protectively. Alternatively, she may believe that the baby is dead or defective or that the baby does not need care because God is caring for it. The mother may need assistance for alterations in patterns of sleep and rest, self-care, nutrition, fluid balance, elimination, self-esteem, and family coping. Discharge planning focuses on preparation for meeting the demands of an infant while the mother is still integrating her experience with a psychotic episode.

Schizophrenic pregnant women often experience an intensification of their disorder and are hospitalized on psychiatric or obstetric units. They require nursing care from both psychiatric and obstetric health care providers. These women may remain ambivalent toward the fetus and resist examinations and procedures. Because these women seen unaware of the signs of labor, staff members must be alert to the signs and symptoms of labor. Even though disorganization often diminishes over time, specific delusions may persist. The new mother may not be able to be close to her baby or to recognize or meet the baby's needs. In more severe cases, a mental health clinical nurse specialist or nurse practitioner can provide specialized counseling and continue to follow the mother and family after discharge from the hospital.

Evaluation

Evaluation is based on the woman's progress toward achieving the expected outcomes. The nurse can be assured that care has been effective if the physical well-being of the mother and infant is maintained, if the mother and family are able to cope effectively, and if each family member continues in a healthy growth and development pattern (see the Nursing Care Plan on p. 301).

PSYCHOACTIVE SUBSTANCE USE

The use of psychoactive (mind-altering) substances is pandemic. **Substance abuse** refers to the continued use of any drug or alcohol mind-altering agent despite the occurrence of profound individual and socially-related problems (Stuart and Sundeen, 1995). Interference with biologic integrity may be amplified during pregnancy by poor nutrition that leads to poor weight gain, anemia, and a predisposition to infection and pregnancy-induced hypertension. Poor hygiene and polydrug use, including tobacco, may compound and confuse the signs and symptoms of psychoactive substance abuse (Glantz and Woods, 1993; Little et al, 1990; Lynch and McKeon, 1990; Vaughn et al, 1993). Some drugs (e.g., morphine, heroin, diazepam) induce platelet disorders that predispose the woman to hemorrhage (Scott et al, 1994).

A pregnant woman who has been taking phencyclidine may develop an acute psychosis or be unable to attach to her infant. Expectant and new mothers who use psychoactive substances receive negative feedback from society and from health care providers who may withhold support and condemn them for endangering their unborn or newborn infant. Pregnant women who are alcohol and drug dependent often do not seek prenatal care until labor begins (Burkett, Yasin, and Palow, 1990; Cordero and Custard, 1990). Pregnant women may have little understanding of the effects of these substances on themselves, their pregnancies, or their babies. They often take the drug just before seeking admission; therefore withdrawal symptoms can be delayed for 6 to 12 hours. **Withdrawal** refers to the physiologic and cognitive changes that occur after removing the substance in the substance-dependent person.

The drug-dependent woman tends to exhibit a passive response to life and its responsibilities. She may show a high degree of depression. Substance use is a way for her to relieve psychologic distress, encourage social interaction, and blunt the feelings of loneliness and emptiness that are part of depression. Pregnancy often is not planned; it occurs as an "accidental" phenomenon. In some instances it may serve as a positive event and confirm her worth as a woman. However, after the birth the woman is faced with the parental tasks of caring for and nurturing a completely dependent infant and forming a warm, close, intimate relationship with the child.

Care of the woman who is addicted to alcohol or drugs offers a tremendous nursing challenge. The difficulty of this challenge soon becomes apparent. The woman may seek early discharge or even leave the hospital against medical advice. The demands of motherhood are being made on a person who is herself dependent and still at the stage of taking and receiving rather than giving. Most substance-dependent persons are unable to establish positive intimate relationships and often lack a meaningful support system.

Although many other substances are abused, the following discussion focuses on the use and abuse of alcohol, marijuana, cocaine, heroin, methamphetamine, tobacco, and caffeine. The care needed varies with the particular circumstances of the individual and the substance that is used. However, the nursing process is similar for all.

Legal Sanctions

Substance abuse in pregnancy, which is estimated at 2% to 11% of all births, contributes to spontaneous abortion, preterm birth, intrauterine fetal growth restriction, neonatal neurobehavioral handicaps, neonatal addiction and AIDS, and fetal and maternal death (Chasnoff, 1989; Weiss and Hansell, 1992). Increasing numbers of pregnant women who abuse substances face criminal prosecution under expanded interpretations of child abuse and drug trafficking statutes.

BOX 11-4
Ethical Considerations Related to Drug Screening

Nurses face an ethical dilemma in situations in which fetal injury can occur because of the mother's drug use. Although no specific law against drug use in pregnancy exists, it has been suggested that all pregnant women be screened routinely for illegal drug use. It has been further suggested that those women who test positive be reported to state child protective agencies, placed in jail, or placed in an inpatient psychiatric setting to protect the fetus. Fear of prosecution can prevent women from getting prenatal care and can increase the risk to the fetus.

Some states are prosecuting pregnant women for drug trafficking or child abuse because they became pregnant while addicted to drugs. Resorting to criminal charges may be counterproductive because the woman would benefit from rehabilitation more than from incarceration (Box 11-4). The problem of substance abuse in pregnancy is common and crosses all races and socioeconomic levels. However, there is bias in reporting to civil and health authorities. In one study, 80% of the women arrested for alleged substance abuse in pregnancy were women of color (Paltrow, 1990). African-American women and poor women were more likely than others to be reported. Such selective prosecution may raise charges of discrimination (Weiss and Hansell, 1992). Nurses can advocate for primary prevention programs and counseling/treatment programs for those already addicted and advocate for public policy that addresses this problem.

LEGAL TIP

Urine Drug Testing

There is no state requirement for a health care provider to test either the mother or the newborn for the presence of drugs. However, nurses need to know the policies of the states in which they practice. In some states a woman who has a positive urine drug screen test at the time of labor and birth can be referred to child protective services. If the mother is not in a drug treatment program or is assessed to be unable to provide newborn care, the infant may be placed in foster care.

Alcohol

It is estimated that 50% to 80% of all pregnant women use alcohol. Data are difficult to obtain because ethanol (alcohol) is rapidly absorbed in the small intestine and metabolized in the liver. Underreporting of alcohol use in pregnancy is a major concern of health care providers. It is estimated that 1% to 5% of pregnant women meet diagnostic criteria for alcoholism (Thorpe, 1995). Predisposing factors for alcohol abuse in pregnancy include women who smoke and who are unmarried, less educated, and younger than age 25. Alcohol abuse during pregnancy is the leading cause of fetal mental retardation in the United States (National Organization on Fetal Alcohol Syndrome, 1995). Abstinence from alcohol during pregnancy is recommended (Cefalo and Moos, 1995).

Some of the clinical manifestations of alcohol use in pregnancy are an inability to form positive relationships (which results in manipulative behavior), a low tolerance for frustration, anxiety, and expressions of guilt related to alcoholic behavior patterns. During withdrawal, central nervous system agitation is expressed as fatigue, insomnia, agitation, restlessness, and belligerence. Bruises, rashes, and other injuries may be observed. Poor physical hygiene and malnutrition are potential problems, especially in the chronic alcohol abuser (Table 11-1). Alcohol abuse in pregnancy has been associated with fetal growth restriction, altered facies, and developmental problems.

Fetal alcohol syndrome. Fetal alcohol syndrome (FAS) is a pattern of unusual facial features that includes short palpebral fissures (the distance between the inner and outer corners of the eye), a flat midface, a long or indistinct philtrum (the ridges between the nose and mouth), and a thin upper lip (Steissguth et al, 1991) (see Fig. 8-7). FAS now surpasses spina bifida and Down syndrome as the leading cause of mental retardation in the United States (National Organization on Fetal Alcohol Syndrome, 1995). The incidence is 1 in 3000 births; each year 5000 children are born in the United States with FAS, and another 50,000 children show symptoms of **fetal alcohol effect (FAE).** FAE is a lesser set of the same symptoms that constitute FAS.

Both FAS and FAE produce irreversible physical and mental damage. The economic impact is estimated at $321 million each year, with three quarters of the expense associated with the treatment and residential care of patients with mental retardation (Abel and Sokol, 1991; National Organization on Fetal Alcohol Syndrome, 1995).

FAS and FAE can be completely prevented if the woman does not drink alcohol while she is pregnant. Prevention of FAS is accomplished best with preconception counseling. Because women do not usually exaggerate their alcohol intake, a positive CAGE test (Box 11-5) would indicate a high risk for alcohol-related adverse reproductive outcomes. (See Chapter 26 for further discussion of fetal and neonatal effects.)

Marijuana

Marijuana, a substance derived from the cannabis plant, is usually rolled into cigarettes and smoked. It may also be mixed into food and eaten. It provides an intoxicating and sensory-distorting high. Marijuana smoke has the characteristics of tobacco smoke and has similar dangers (Cook et al, 1990). Marijuana readily crosses the placenta. Both cigarettes and marijuana increase carbon monoxide levels in the mother's blood, which reduces oxygen to the fetus.

Research findings regarding the effects of marijuana on pregnancy are inconsistent. That is, maternal use does not consistently increase the incidence of spontaneous abortions or stillbirths. Neonatal effects vary and may include altered sleep and arousal patterns and tremulousness. These inconsistent results may reflect variations in drug composition, maternal factors such as health or life-style, and problems of underreporting or methodologic issues (Cook et al, 1990).

Women who abuse marijuana are more likely to bear children with features suggestive of FAS. This finding supports the theory that marijuana may have a synergistic effect on alcohol and other substances (Cook et al, 1990). Marijuana rapidly passes into breast milk. Because the effects of contaminated breast milk on the newborn are unknown, breastfeeding by these mothers is not recommended. The postnatal effects of prenatal exposure to marijuana have not been identified.

Cocaine

Cocaine is a naturally occurring alkaloid obtained from the leaves of the South American cocoa plant. Cocaine is a powerful central nervous system (CNS) stimulant that works by blocking the reuptake of norepinephrine and dopamine at the nerve endings. In pregnancy, this effect results in a high level of catecholamines, which causes a hyperaroused state (Fox, 1994; Thorpe, 1995).

The increase in the use of cocaine and the even more addictive "crack" among childbearing women has been phenomenal in the past few years (Glantz and Woods, 1993; Vaughn, 1993). Crack is cocaine that is mixed with baking soda and heated until it reaches its purest form. It is sold in the form of "rocks" that are smoked in pipes. Cocaine is used in all

TABLE 11-1 Psychoactive substance effects

DRUG	PSYCHOLOGIC SIGNS	PHYSIOLOGIC SIGNS
Alcohol		
Intoxication*	Mood lability or change Impaired attention or memory Irritability Talkativeness	Slurred speech Flushed face Incoordination, unsteady gait Nystagmus
Withdrawal	Anxiety Depressed mood or irritability Maladaptive behavior	Nausea and vomiting Malaise or weakness Hyperactivity Coarse tremor of hands, tongue, eyelids Orthostatic hypotension
Cocaine ("Crack")		
Intoxication*	Psychomotor agitation Elation Grandiosity; talkativeness Hypervigilance Maladaptive behaviors	Tachycardia Pupillary dilation Hypertension Perspiration; chills Nausea; vomiting
Withdrawal	Depressed mood Disturbed sleep Increased dreaming	Fatigue Headache Convulsions (seizure)
Heroin		
Intoxication*	Euphoria, dysphoria Psychomotor retardation Apathy Maladaptive behavior Impaired attention or memory	Pupillary constriction Drowsiness Slurred speech
Withdrawal	Insomnia	Lacrimation, rhinorrhea Pupillary dilation Sweating Diarrhea Yawning Mild hypertension Tachycardia Fever
Methamphetamine ("Ice")		
Intoxication*	Hyperactivity Insomnia Restlessness Irritability Aggressiveness	Tachycardia, palpitations Tachypnea Nausea, vomiting Constipation Impotence
Withdrawal	Depression Increased sleeping Lethargy	Headache Nausea, vomiting Muscle pain Weakness
Phencyclidine (PCP)	Euphoria Psychomotor agitation Increased anxiety Emotional lability Grandiosity Sensation of slowed time Synesthesias Maladaptive behaviors	Vertical or horizontal nystagmus Hypertension Increased heart rate Numbness Decreased response to pain Ataxia; dysarthria

*State of inebriation resulting from excessive consumption of alcohol, drugs, or other toxic substances.

cultures, and its low cost and availability make it the drug of choice among the economically disadvantaged. Because crack is highly addictive, it poses new problems to health care providers, who may first see the pregnant addict in the labor and birthing area.

In the United States, it is estimated that 10% to 15% of all pregnant women use cocaine (Glantz and Woods, 1993; Lynch and McKeon, 1990). Predisposing factors and problems associated with cocaine use in pregnancy are polydrug use, poor nutrition, poverty, sexually transmitted diseases (STDs), hepatitis B infection, human immunodeficiency virus (HIV) infection, dysfunctional family systems, employment difficulties, stress, anger, poor self-esteem, and previous or present physical, emotional, and sexual abuse (Fox, 1994).

The clinical manifestations of cocaine use, such as tachycardia, pupillary dilation, and hypertension, are listed in Table 11-1. Medical complications of cocaine use in pregnancy vary from mild to severe. A variety of less serious medical problems such as lack of energy, insomnia, sinusitis, nosebleeds, sore throat, and decreased libido may be seen. More serious problems develop as general health deteriorates. The nasal septum perforates. Cardiovascular stress increases, and tachycardia, systemic hypertension, ventricular arrhythmias, sudden coronary artery spasm, and myocardial infarction develop. Cocaine-associated complications also include liver damage, intestinal ischemia, pulmonary disease with acute pulmonary edema, seizures, hemorrhagic bronchitis, headaches, and death. Needleborne diseases such as hepatitis B and acquired immunodeficiency syndrome (AIDS) are common. Needle tracks, septic phlebitis, cellulitis, and superficial abscesses are seen in intravenous drug users. Many users are poorly nourished and often have STDs (Fox, 1994). Cocaine users may mediate the effects of cocaine by a CNS depressant such as alcohol (Matera et al, 1990; Vaughn et al, 1993). Thus the woman and her fetus are exposed to the risks of both cocaine and alcohol.

Cocaine produces tachycardia and a rise in blood pressure by increasing the levels of catecholamines. During pregnancy, uterine blood vessels are maximally dilated but vasoconstrict in the presence of catecholamines. Separation of the placenta (abruption) or an acute onset of preterm labor with long, hard contractions and a precipitous birth after intravenous cocaine administration probably is secondary to acute spasm of uterine blood vessels (Chisum, 1990; Janke, 1990). Fetal effects such as an infant who is small for gestational age (SGA) and intrauterine demise are commonly seen (Chasnoff, 1989; Johnson, 1994; Mayes, Granger, and Frank, 1993).

Heroin

Heroin is a semisynthetic opioid that is related to natural opioids such as morphine. It is one of the most commonly abused drugs of this class. It is usually taken by intravenous injection but can be smoked or "snorted." The signs and symptoms of heroin use are euphoria, relaxation, pain relief, "nodding out" (apathy, detachment from reality, impaired judgment, and drowsiness), constricted pupils, nausea, constipation, slurred speech, and respiratory depression (American Psychiatric Association, 1994; Stuart and Sundeen, 1995).

The incidence of heroin use in pregnancy is unknown; however, those with a heroin dependency may use multiple drugs. Opioid dependence can begin at any age. Problems associated with opioid use are most commonly observed in the late teens and early twenties. Studies show that opioid dependence occurs in approximately 0.7% of the adult population (American Psychiatric Association, 1994). Predisposing factors include a family tendency for higher levels of psychopathology, especially an increased incidence of other substance-related disorders and antisocial personality disorders.

Medical complications of heroin include an increased risk for bloodborne pathogens such as HIV or hepatitis B. Other infections (abscesses, phlebitis, cellulitis, pneumonia, and subacute bacterial endocarditis) may occur as a result of a lack of asepsis and from sharing needles (Stuart and Sundeen, 1995). Narcotics may depress fetal movement. The most consistent perinatal effect of narcotics is interference with fetal growth and increased incidence of prematurity. A woman who is addicted to heroin is more likely to experience premature rupture of membranes and preterm labor (Ney, 1990). Because of this woman's inattention to the environment, potentially harmful events are often ignored, which leads to accidents.

Methamphetamine

The active metabolite of methamphetamine is amphetamine, a CNS stimulant known as "speed" and "meth." Closely related substances are the agents used as appetite suppressants or diet pills. The crystalline form of methamphetamine is known as "ice." When smoked, it gives a long, steady high and is more addictive than heroin. "Ice" enables a person to go without rest or food for 24 hours, only to "crash" for the next 24 hours.

Approximately 2% of the adult population experience methamphetamine abuse at some time during their lives (American Psychiatric Association, 1994). It is seen through all levels of society and is common in the 18- to 30-year-old age group.

The clinical manifestations of methamphetamine use are euphoria, abrupt awakening, increased energy, talkativeness, agitation, tachycardia, tachypnea, hyperactivity, irritability, grandiosity, diaphoresis, weight loss, insomnia, hypertension, increased temperature, ectopic heartbeat, urinary retention, constipation, dry mouth, paranoid delusions, and violent behavior. Seizures, cardiac shock, and death may occur as a result of overdose (Stuart and Sundeen, 1995). Most of the effects of amphetamines are similar to those of cocaine. Fewer maternal and neonatal complications have been attributed to this class of substances than to cocaine (American Psychiatric Association, 1994).

Methamphetamine-exposed pregnant women have higher rates of preterm births and more neonates with intrauterine growth restriction and smaller head circumferences. Neonatal behavioral patterns are altered and are characterized by abnormal sleep patterns, poor feeding, tremors, and hypertonia. These behaviors are seen if the fetus was exposed to cocaine, methamphetamine, or their combination (Cook et al, 1990). Other neonatal behaviors include state disorganization and decreased sleep. Feeding may be prolonged and accompanied by disorganized rooting and sucking. Tube feeding may be required. Withdrawal symptoms may be treated with phenobarbital or opium tincture.

Phencyclidine

Phencyclidine (PCP) is a synthetic drug known by various names (PeaCe Pill, elephant, angel dust, hog). Its use is more prevalent among ethnic minorities and in people between the ages of 18 and 40. Its effects are unpredictable and include hostility, aggressiveness, and other bizarre behaviors (Cook et al, 1990). Signs and symptoms of PCP use include confusion, disorientation, euphoria, hallucinations, paranoia, grandiosity, agitation, tendency toward violence, and antisocial behavior. Clinical manifestations include red and dry skin, dilated pupils, nystagmus, ataxia, hypertension, rigidity, and seizures (Stuart and Sundeen, 1995). The severity of these symptoms is dependent on the dose. Because some effects mimic schizophrenia, a PCP user may be admitted to a psychiatric unit.

After use, PCP persists in the brain and body fat for an extended period. It crosses the placenta and tends to be found in higher concentrations in fetal tissue than in maternal tissue. Fetal levels may be 10 times higher than maternal levels (Glantz and Woods, 1993). Because PCP tends to be used in various combinations with alcohol, cocaine, and marijuana, specific reports regarding the effects on pregnancy, the fetus, and the neonate have been limited (Cook et al, 1990; Fico and Vanderwende, 1988). The major concern with PCP is its association with polydrug abuse and the neurobehavioral effects on the neonate (Glantz and Woods, 1993).

BOX 11-5
The CAGE Questionnaire

1. Have you ever felt you ought to Cut down on your drinking?
2. Have people Annoyed you by criticizing your drinking?
3. Have you ever felt bad or Guilty about your drinking?
4. Have you ever had a drink first thing in the morning to steady your nerves or get rid of a hangover? i.e., Eye-opener.

APPLICATION:

First ask if the client uses alcohol, and if affirmative ask the CAGE questions. If negative, ask if ever and when the client stopped. A single positive response warrants investigation, 2 out of 4 suggests alcohol dependence, and 4 out of 4 is positive for alcoholism.

From Ewing J: Detecting alcoholism: the CAGE questionnaire, *JAMA* 252(14):1905, 1984.

Nursing Care Management

Assessment

The care of the substance-dependent pregnant woman is based on historic data, symptoms, physical findings, and laboratory results (Table 11-1). The social worker may assist in evaluating the woman's social, economic, and home status.

It is important for the nurse to use tact and sound judgment in the interview and to integrate screening questions for alcohol and drug abuse into the overall history of all women

BOX 11-6
The Drug Abuse Screening Test (DAST)

(*Items 4, 5, and 7 are scored in the "no" or false direction.)

1. Have you used drugs other than those required for medical reasons?
2. Have you abused prescription drugs?
3. Do you abuse more than one drug at a time?
4. Can you get through the week without using drugs (other than those required for medical reasons)?*
5. Are you always able to stop using drugs when you want to?*
6. Do you abuse drugs on a continuous basis?
7. Do you try to limit your drug use to certain situations?*
8. Have you had "blackouts" or "flashbacks" as a result of drug use?
9. Do you ever feel bad about your drug abuse?
10. Does your spouse (or parents) ever complain about your involvement with drugs?
11. Do your friends or relatives know or suspect you abuse drugs?
12. Has drug abuse ever created problems between you and your spouse?
13. Has any family member ever sought help for problems related to your drug use?
14. Have you ever lost friends because of your use of drugs?
15. Have you ever neglected your family or missed work because of your use of drugs?
16. Have you ever been in trouble at work because of drug abuse?
17. Have you ever lost a job because of drug abuse?
18. Have you gotten into fights when under the influence of drugs?
19. Have you ever been arrested because of unusual behavior while under the influence of drugs?
20. Have you ever been arrested for driving while under the influence of drugs?
21. Have you engaged in illegal activities to obtain drugs?
22. Have you ever been arrested for possession of illegal drugs?
23. Have you ever experienced withdrawal symptoms as a result of heavy drug intake?
24. Have you had medical problems as a result of your drug use (e.g., memory loss, hepatitis, convulsions, or bleeding)?
25. Have you ever gone to anyone for help for a drug problem?
26. Have you ever been in the hospital for medical problems related to your drug use?
27. Have you ever been involved in a treatment program specifically related to drug use?
28. Have you been treated as an outpatient for problems related to drug abuse?

Scoring: A score of greater than five requires further evaluation for substance abuse problems.

From Skinner H: The drug abuse screening test, *Addict Behav* 7(4):363, 1982.

at the first prenatal visit. Defensiveness on the part of the nurse will be evident to the patient and will interfere with developing trust and obtaining an accurate report of consumption (Cefalo and Moos, 1995). A concerned, nonjudgmental, and matter-of-fact approach is advisable in the hope that the woman will admit a problem if it exists.

Along with educational intervention, early recognition of alcohol or drug use through the use of a screening tool at the earliest visit is ideal. Several quick screening tools have been developed and include the Michigan Alcoholism Screening Test (MAST), the CAGE Questionnaire (Box 11-5), the T-ACE Questionnaire, and the Drug Abuse Screening Test (DAST) (Box 11-6). Scoring one "yes" answer on the CAGE Questionnaire calls for further assessment (Ewing, 1984). The CAGE Questionnaire was developed to screen for alcohol but can also be used to screen for illicit drug use by substituting the word *drug* for *alcohol*. It is not uncommon for women to abuse both alcohol and drugs.

Laboratory tests are ordered for toxicology, STDs, hepatitis B, and antibodies to HIV. Blood urea nitrogen, serum creatinine, total protein levels, albumin-to-globulin ratio, total iron-binding capacity, hemoglobin, and hematocrit values are obtained. Chest x-ray studies may be ordered for pulmonary disease. Hilar lymphadenopathy (in 95% of addicted persons), pulmonary edema, bacterial pneumonia, and foreign body emboli (from the substances used to "cut" street drugs) may be revealed.

Initial and serial ultrasound studies are used to determine gestational age because amenorrhea, which is common among drug users, precludes dating the pregnancy by the history of the last menstrual period. Because of the concern for stillbirths, increased frequency of SGA, and the potential for hypoxia, nonstress testing has been advocated (at least in the third trimester) for those pregnant women who are substance abusers (Glantz and Woods, 1993).

With the advent of early discharge, often within 12 to 24 hours after birth, assessment becomes difficult and an increasing challenge to health care professionals. Ideally the home setting should be assessed before the woman is discharged with her infant to evaluate whether or not the environment is safe and conducive to the infant's survival. The mother's ability to care for her infant after discharge should also be assessed in the home setting.

Nursing Diagnoses

The following are examples of nursing diagnoses formulated from the assessment data:

- Risk for fluid volume deficit and altered nutrition: less than body requirements related to
  - Effects of excessive use of psychoactive drugs
- Risk for injury to self, fetus, or newborn related to
  - Sensory effects of drug
- Risk for infection related to
  - Life-style
  - Dehydration and malnutrition
  - Method of administration of drug or effects of drug
- Self-care deficit, bathing/hygiene related to
  - Effects of substance abuse
- Ineffective denial related to
  - Psychodynamics of the addiction process
  - Lack of understanding of the disease process
  - Effects of a psychoactive drug or drugs on the pregnancy and the developing fetus
- Ineffective individual coping related to
  - Lack of support system
  - Low self-esteem
  - Lack of healthy mechanisms for recognition and release of anger
- Risk for violence related to
  - Maintenance of drug habit
  - Effects of substance used
  - Life-style

Expected Outcomes

Planning for care must be accomplished with recognition of the woman's life-style and habits. The ideal long-term outcome is total abstinence. However, the woman may be unable to face that level of commitment at this time. The thought of giving up the substance forever is anxiety provoking. It is rare for a substance-dependent person to stop using that substance suddenly. The goal of cutting down may be more realistic. It may also be harmful to the fetus to stop using the substance abruptly. Short-term goals are necessary. The woman must participate in the decision-making process in formulating the expected outcomes. It is particularly important that the goals be stated so that it is clear that the woman has responsibility for her behavior. The expected outcomes often are written into a contract signed by the woman and the nurse (or physician). It may be beneficial to give a copy to the woman to remind her of her commitment.

Short-term expected outcomes

1. The woman's physiologic status will be stabilized.
2. The woman will keep appointments for prenatal and postpartum care for herself and newborn care for her infant.
3. Fetal effects will be minimized; the baby will remain safe and receive appropriate care.

Long-term expected outcome

1. The woman will become involved voluntarily in long-term medical, social (e.g., Alcoholics Anonymous, withdrawal [methadone] program), psychiatric, and vocational rehabilitation.

Plan of Care and Implementation

An interdisciplinary approach is needed to plan for the care of the expectant mother. Pregnant psychoactive substance users, especially polydrug abusers, are seen in increasing numbers on maternal-newborn units (Thorpe, 1995). Hospitals are reporting an increase of three to four times as many alcohol- and drug-related births since 1985 (Fox, 1994). The needs of these mothers present special challenges to nurses. An individualized nursing care plan may be developed by the interdisciplinary team on the maternal-newborn unit. A starting point in the development of a care plan may need to be a values clarification experience. It is not uncommon for health care providers to harbor negative feelings about the behavior of psychoactive drug users. Collaboration with a mental health clinical nurse specialist/nurse practitioner will strengthen the maternal-newborn nurse's therapeutic potential with these women. Comprehensive interdisciplinary planning with nursing, medicine, social services, pastoral care, patient advocacy, case managers, human resource agencies, child protective services, foster care, outpatient treatment centers, home health agencies, and public health is essential.

The need for biologic support may be related to overdose, withdrawal, allergy, or toxicity. Physical deterioration results from the harmful effects of the alcohol or drugs, including conditions such as malnutrition, dehydration, and various infections. The acute physical condition takes priority over the woman's other health needs.

The nurse should refer the patient to a specific substance abuse counselor such as a mental health clinical nurse specialist/nurse practitioner or an outpatient/inpatient alcohol or drug treatment program. Alcohol withdrawal treatment includes the use of benzodiazepines, improvement of nutritional intake (folate and vitamins), and psychotherapy. Detoxification with disulfiram (Antabuse) is not used because of fetal teratogenicity of the drug (Lewis and Woods, 1994).

The substitution of methadone to withdraw from heroin remains controversial. If women withdraw from heroin during pregnancy, blood flow to the placenta is impaired. To prevent this occurrence, methadone is used to assist in withdrawal from heroin. Some experts advocate complete withdrawal without methadone use despite the risk of interrupted blood flow to the placenta. Others contend that the use of methadone to withdraw from heroin is good for the mother; however, for the infant methadone withdrawal may be worse than withdrawal from heroin after birth (Glantz and Woods, 1993; Stuart and Sundeen, 1995).

Interactive interventions are initiated as soon as appropri-

Nursing Care Plan

COCAINE ABUSE

Premature Labor

Nursing Diagnosis: Risk for injury to fetus related to preterm labor (PTL) secondary to cocaine use

Expected Outcome: Preterm labor will be suppressed.

• NURSING INTERVENTIONS/*RATIONALES*

Administer IV tocolytic therapy per physician order and monitor infusion *to assess effectiveness and detect any early signs of toxicity.*

Monitor maternal/fetal response to tocolytic therapy *to detect any early signs of toxicity.*

Encourage decision making about such issues as bed rest, diversion, and hygiene *to establish trust and a sense of control over the environment.*

Inform woman about effects of cocaine use on placental circulation. Refer to social worker or other mental health professional for treatment of cocaine abuse *to promote well-being of fetus.*

Prepare woman for hospital discharge by teaching about oral take-home medications and recognition of recurrent signs of PTL, encouraging continued prenatal care, and providing written resource and referral materials for emergency contacts *to enable woman to recognize breakthrough of tocolytics and seek help immediately.*

Nursing Diagnosis: Ineffective individual coping related to personal vulnerability, inadequate support systems, and pregnancy

Expected Outcome: Patient will exhibit increased responsibility in self-care and no use of cocaine during remainder of pregnancy.

• NURSING INTERVENTIONS/*RATIONALES*

Contract with woman to remain drug free for remainder of pregnancy *to ensure the well-being of the fetus.*

Discuss and help woman develop a support system network that can be used to assist her in keeping her contract (i.e., family and friends that are not involved in drug scene, medical and social services, Cocaine Anonymous) *to provide assistance to remain drug-free.*

Review the effects of cocaine, alcohol, and other toxic substances on fetus *to emphasize the importance of remaining drug free.*

Explore coping techniques that may be used to help solve problems *to enlarge coping repertoire.*

Collaborate with woman to outline needed self-care behaviors (diet, exercise) and ways that she can carry out these behaviors *so that she is actively involved in planning and deciding how to carry out needed care.*

Help woman recognize and feel good about positive personal qualities and accomplishments *to increase self-esteem.*

Set limits on any manipulative behavior and help woman to recognize and accept responsibility for her own actions *as a way to foster change.*

Nursing Diagnosis: Altered nutrition: less than body requirements related to lack of interest in food secondary to effects of cocaine use

Expected Outcome: The patient will exhibit adequate intake of appropriate nourishment and satisfactory weight gain for remainder of pregnancy.

• NURSING INTERVENTIONS/*RATIONALES*

Review the importance of diet and weight gain for mother and fetus *to assess knowledge and motivation level.*

Mutually develop a written dietary plan that incorporates likes/dislikes and includes scheduled meals *to enhance chances of use of the plan.*

ate. Interventions are directed toward reducing the stressors that apply to each individual and are identified in the nursing diagnoses. Examples of interactive interventions include group support, patient education, and individual counseling. Psychiatric nurses are skilled in intervening in denial, dependency, manipulation, and anger. Other required skills include establishing behavioral contracts and increasing self-esteem. The primary focus of care is the woman. She may already be acutely aware of the dangers to the fetus as a result of her behavior. Emphasis on the fetus's well-being instead of her own may add to her guilt, frustration, and low self-esteem.

Labor and childbirth unit nurses need to work out a standardized plan of care. Typically the woman displays poor control over her behavior and has a low threshold for pain, which is especially noticeable when she is in labor. Increased dependency needs are apparent. **Intoxication** or withdrawal signs and symptoms of the mother and fetus (Table 11-1) may challenge staff members. To prevent unsupervised drug administration, staffing should be sufficient to ensure strict surveillance of visitors. (See the Nursing Care Plan on p. 308.)

Advice regarding breastfeeding is individualized. All abused substances appear in breast milk, and some are present in greater amounts than others (Brody et al, 1994). Those substances for which breastfeeding is contraindicated include amphetamines, alcohol, cocaine, heroin, and marijuana. The baby's nutrition and safety needs are of primary importance.

Breastfeeding facilitates a closeness between the mother and child. However, during withdrawal these women have depleted energy reserves and diminished coping abilities and commonly experience severe emotional decompensation. Their condition can be aggravated by breastfeeding and caring for the infant, which can be exhausting without family support. For these reasons breastfeeding may not be chosen. For other women the need to breastfeed and care for the infant provides the impetus to break the drug dependency habit. Lactation consultants, breastfeeding educators, community support groups for new mothers, and La Leche League International are some of the resources available for additional support.

Discharge planning begins with the first contact with the woman and her family. Care is centered around the family, and whenever possible the woman and her family are involved in decision making and are encouraged to care for the infant. Mother-infant attachment is promoted. Angry or judgmental encounters between the woman and nurse are avoided; the nurse needs to respond with patience, sympathy, consistency, and at times, with firmness. The woman's strengths and positive maternal responses and feelings are supported, even when she is relinquishing her infant for adoption.

Social support systems are mobilized. Family counseling, self-help groups, transitional living programs, and community treatment programs may be involved. Home health agencies may be mobilized for supervision or guidance in postpartum self-care and infant care. Day/night care programs or halfway houses may be indicated. Some social service agencies may remove the child from the home (Neuspiel et al, 1993). Others focus on assisting troubled parents in learning to solve their problems with the child in the home. Employee assistance programs are now available in many industries, including health care agencies.

Evaluation

Evaluation is difficult because the long-range effects of substance abuse cannot be projected. Short-term positive achievements are indicators of success (e.g., the woman keeps her appointments, improves her nutrition and personal hygiene, or learns to diaper the baby). It is not reasonable to expect to see evidence of significant strides, such as complete abstinence from drugs and the assumption of mature adult behaviors within a short period. Long-term follow-up is necessary to document permanent changes.

OTHER ADDICTIVE SUBSTANCES

Tobacco

The effects of cigarette smoking on pregnancy have been known for decades. Among pregnant women, the incidence of smoking is 25% to 30% (Floyd, 1991). Smoking in pregnancy causes decreased placental perfusion and accounts for 21% to 39% of all low–birth-weight infants (Creasy and Resnik, 1994). The effect of smoking on low birth weight appears to be dose related. Smoking more than 1 pack of cigarettes daily increases by 130% the risk of delivering an infant that weighs less than 2500 g, whereas smoking less than 1 pack per day increases the risk by 53%. McDonald, Armstrong, and Sloan (1992) concluded that the odds ratio of giving birth to an SGA infant (weight <5th percentile) was 3.19 among women smoking more than 20 cigarettes daily. The difference in birth weight between the infants of smokers and nonsmokers ranges from 127 to 274 g (Abel and Sokol, 1991; Pulkkinen, 1990).

A cigarette contains more than 4000 poisonous compounds (Floyd, 1991). The oxygen-carrying capacity of hemoglobin is decreased when carbon monoxide passes through the placenta. Nicotine stimulates adrenergic release, which causes vasoconstriction and decreased uterine perfusion (Morrow, Richie, and Bull, 1988). Smokers generally have a nutrient-poor diet. Smoking interferes with the ability of the body to process essential vitamins and minerals, which results in calcium loss from the bones, decreased intestinal synthesis of vitamin B_{12}, and increased usage of vitamin C. Compensatory mechanisms are evident by decreased fetal movement, decreased beat-to-beat variability, and increased maternal and fetal heart rate after each smoking episode (Lumley and Astbury, 1989; Morrow, Richie, and Bull, 1988). The woman

BOX 11-7

Maternal Complications of Pregnancy Associated with Smoking

1. Ectopic pregnancy (Coste et al, 1991)
2. Spontaneous abortion (Armstrong, McDonald, and Sloan, 1992)
3. Premature rupture of membranes (Lumley and Astbury, 1989)
4. Preterm birth (DeHass, Harlow, and Cramer, 1991)
5. Placenta previa (Williams, 1991)
6. Abruptio placentae (Lumley and Astbury, 1989)
7. Chorioamnionitis (Dattel, 1990)

BOX 11-8
Neonatal/Pediatric Complications Associated With Maternal Smoking

1. Neurobehavioral abnormalities; learning difficulties
2. Pediatric allergies
3. Increased risk for sudden infant death syndrome (SIDS) (Floyd, 1991)
4. Increased risk for pneumonia, bronchitis, and otitis media (Floyd, 1991; Taylor, 1990)
5. Low birth weight (Lumley and Astbury, 1989)

who smokes during pregnancy is at risk for complications such as preterm birth, placenta previa, abruptio placentae, spontaneous abortion, ectopic pregnancy, premature rupture of membranes, and chorioamnionitis (Box 11-7).

Some neonatal/pediatric complications associated with maternal smoking in pregnancy are listed in Box 11-8. Breastfeeding may be contraindicated because of the nicotine in cigarettes, but this recommendation is controversial (Lawrence, 1994).

Reducing the number of cigarettes smoked per day has a positive effect on birth weight. If smoking is discontinued by the end of the first trimester, the woman has no greater risk for fetal growth abnormalities than does a nonsmoker (McDonald, Armstrong, and Sloan, 1992). Self-help educational materials to stop smoking are available through the American Cancer Society, the American Heart Association, and the American Lung Association.

Because of the evidence of complications associated with smoking in pregnancy, nurses should counsel women about these risks and encourage attempts to stop or reduce the number of cigarettes to 10 or fewer per day before or during pregnancy (McDonald, Armstrong, and Sloan, 1992). Women are often motivated during pregnancy to be successful in cutting down or quitting.

Caffeine

Caffeine-containing beverages, including coffee, tea, colas, and chocolate, are widely consumed by pregnant women. Caffeine reaches the developing fetus by crossing the placenta. The time it takes to eliminate caffeine from the body varies: it takes 3 hours in smokers, 3 to 7 hours in nonsmokers, and 10 to 20 hours in pregnant women in the third trimester. The ingestion of 600 to 1000 mg of caffeine (6 to 10 cups of caffeinated beverages) per day may lead to anxiety, restlessness, delayed sleep onset, frequent awakening, and heart palpitations. Fenster, Eskenazi, and Windham (1991) reported that consuming more than 300 mg/day of caffeine was associated with intrauterine growth restriction and low birth weight. In 1993, Mills, Holmes, and Aarons reported that there was no evidence of increased risk of spontaneous abortion, intrauterine growth restriction, or microcephaly with moderate caffeine use (<300 mg/day).

Other studies in the last decade have reported inconsistent findings regarding caffeine ingestion in pregnancy. The U.S. Food and Drug Administration advises that pregnant women should eliminate or limit their consumption of caffeine to less than 300 mg/day (e.g., 3 cups of coffee or colas). Women who consume more than 300 mg/day should be advised that their fetus could potentially suffer from decreased growth or neonatal caffeine withdrawal (McKim, 1991).

VIOLENCE AGAINST WOMEN

The frequency with which women are battered and abused and its consequent serious repercussions for women, their families, and society combine to make this one of the leading health care problems in the United States. The following is offered as a foundation for caring for the pregnant woman who may be in an abusive relationship. One in four women is physically abused, with 40% to 60% of these women experiencing battering during pregnancy (McFarlane, 1993). More teenagers than adults report abuse (Parker et al, 1993). Statistics, however, depend on reporting by the victim or by observers. Without direct and routine assessment for interpersonal violence, women do not easily disclose the violence they are experiencing. Abuse is seen as a personal stigma that must be kept concealed so that others will not think that the woman is contributing to her abuse.

The concept of domestic violence has remained confusing both because of the taboo about discussing interpersonal violence and because of the imprecise language used to identify the phenomenon. **Family violence** is a general term that is used to refer to all varieties of interpersonal violence, including child, elder, sibling, and spousal abuse. Domestic violence has referred specifically to violence between intimate adults and is sometimes erroneously called wife abuse. To more adequately identify the parties involved in the abuse, a better term might be intimate-partner abuse. This term focuses on the specific relationship, permits the wide variety of relationship configurations (e.g., heterosexual and homosexual partners, married or unmarried couples), and avoids the gender stereotyping of women as victims and men as perpetrators.

Abuse comes in many forms. Because physical assault is the easiest to measure, it is the type of abuse most discussed. In addition, emotional or psychologic abuse, characterized by intimidation and assaults on self-esteem, has immense concealed harmful effects. Although sexual abuse is receiving more attention, many women still do not identify forced sexual compliance within their marriage as rape. Social abuse occurs when a person controls and interferes with the partner's social network and contact with family or attempts to isolate the partner in other ways.

To the nurse who is inexperienced in dealing with family violence, it can be disconcerting or uncomfortable to have the patient acknowledge abuse. It is important to have a list of community resources available for abused women, including shelters, safe homes, crisis lines, and counselors. Many communities have this information available on small business cards that are easy to slip into a pocket. To find information about intimate partner abuse, the nurse may call the local battered women's organization in the closest community and ask for assistance from their staff.

The nurse must be familiar with the laws governing abuse in the state in which she practices, and she must inform the patient of these laws before she elicits the information. Awareness of the law can ensure patients' confidentiality and trust.

LEGAL TIP

Mandatory Reporting of Domestic Violence

Forty states and the District of Columbia have laws that mandate reporting by health care providers situations in which a woman has an injury that may be caused by a deadly weapon. Some states also require reports when there is reason to believe that the woman's injury may have resulted from an illegal act or an act of violence. Only six states have mandatory reporting laws specific to domestic violence or adult abuse.

Because of the wide variation from state to state in mandatory reporting, nurses must be knowledgeable about the reporting requirements of the state in which they practice.

Dynamics of Abuse

Although abuse may be physical and verbal intimidation, the underlying motive is to have power over another. Often times such power is evidenced in physical size and strength. When a woman becomes pregnant, her partner may perceive a loss of personal power in the relationship and resort to abuse as a way to restore that power. Pregnancy presents a time of transition in many ways. These changes may feel threatening and imposing.

Between 40% and 60% of battered women admit being battered during pregnancy (Parker and McFarlane, 1991); pregnancy often is the beginning or escalation of violence (Chescheir, 1992). The rate of battering in teenage pregnancies ranges from 26% to 28% (Parker, McFarlane, and Soeken, 1994). McFarlane (1993) found that 14% of Hispanic women and 19% of African-American and Caucasian women experienced episodes of abuse during pregnancy. Severity of abuse was the greatest for white women, who reported punches, kicks, cuts, contusions, burns, head and internal injuries, and use of a weapon (McFarlane, 1993). Not only is physical abuse harmful to the mother, the risk to infant health is very high.

During pregnancy, women report physical blows directed to the head, breasts, abdomen, and genitals and often report sexual assault (McFarlane, 1993). The battered pregnant woman should be treated as a high-risk obstetric patient because she is prone to anxiety, depression, alcohol and drug use, and inadequate prenatal care (Campbell et al, 1992). Battery during pregnancy results in a higher rate of low-birth-weight newborns and maternal complications of low weight gain, infections, anemia, smoking, and alcohol or drug use (Parker et al, 1994).

Battered women are reluctant to seek help for various reasons: the need to avoid the stigma associated with the nature of the family violence, the fear that they will not be believed, the fear of reprisal from their husbands and, in some states in which battering is a reportable crime, the wish to avoid involvement with police.

BOX 11-9

Indicators of Possible Abuse

1. Change in appointment pattern; either increased appointments with somatic, vague complaints or frequently missed appointments
2. Self-directed abuse, depression, attempted suicide
3. Severe anxiety, insomnia, violent nightmares
4. Alcohol or drug abuse
5. Bruises

Nursing Care Management

Patients in women's health care settings are at high risk for abuse; therefore it is important that all women entering the health care system be assessed by nurses for potential abuse (Campbell and Humphreys, 1993). Health care providers are often the first and only contact that a severely isolated woman will make with someone outside of the relationship. Failure to identify spousal abuse and to recognize the risk of serious injury or even death further endangers the lives of women and their children (Box 11-9).

While inquiring about past trauma or injuries, the nurse should ask directly if she has been injured by her husband/partner. At least the following two questions should be asked: (1) "Are you with a spouse/partner who physically, psychologically, or sexually hurts you?" and (2) "Are you afraid of your spouse/partner?" These questions give a woman permission to disclose sensitive information (Chez, 1990).

A simple abuse assessment and body map (Box 11-10 and Fig. 11-1) can help the nurse gather information in a nonthreatening and nonjudgmental way. To permit the woman to be honest without fearing reprisal later, it is important to provide privacy for this assessment and to be sure that her part-

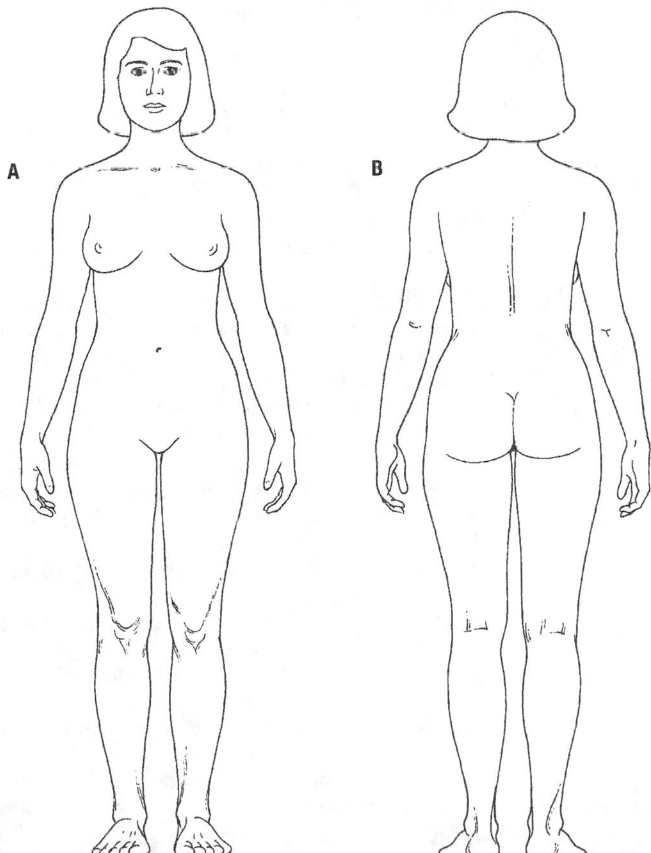

Fig. 11-1 Body maps for abuse assessment.

BOX 11-10

Abuse Assessment

These questions may help you when assessing female patients for abuse. For some women, answering "sometimes" to abuse questions is easier than *yes* or *no*.

1. Do you know where you could go or who could help you if you were abused or worried about abuse?
   Yes____ No____
   If yes, where ______________________________
2. Are you in a relationship with a man who physically hurts you?
   Yes____ No____ Sometimes____
3. Does he threaten you with abuse?
   Yes____ No____ Sometimes____

For Pregnant Patients

4. Has the man you are with hit, slapped, kicked, or otherwise physically hurt you?
   Yes____ No____ Sometimes____
5. If yes, has he hit you since you've been pregnant?
   Yes____ No____ Not Applicable____
6. If yes, did the abuse increase since you've been pregnant?
   Yes____ No____ Not Applicable____
7. Have you ever received medical treatment for any abuse injuries?
   Yes____ No____ Not Applicable____
8. If you've been abused, remembering the last time he hurt you, mark the places on the body map where he hit you.
9. Were you pregnant at the time?
   Yes____ No____ Not Applicable____

When assessing for abuse, some women may be uncomfortable with the topic and may exhibit some of the behaviors below. For some women these behaviors may be suggestive of abuse, and disclosure of battering may follow at a later date.

Actions suggestive of abuse

1. Laughing/"tittering" .... yes no
2. No eye contact (not applicable in some cultures) .... yes no
3. Crying .... yes no
4. Sighing .... yes no
5. Minimizing statements .... yes no
6. Searching/engaging eye contact (fear) .... yes no
7. Anxious body language .... yes no
   (standing to leave, dropped shoulders, depressed) .... yes no
8. Anger, defensiveness
9. Comments about emotional abuse .... yes no
10. Comments about a "friend" who is abused .... yes no

EVALUACIÓN DE ABUSO

1. ¿Sabe Ud. donde ir o quién puede ayudarle si la abusan o la maltratan o si está preocupada con la posibilidad de ser maltratada?
   Sí____ No____
   Si contesta sí, ¿adonde y con quién se iría? ______________________________
2. ¿Tiene Ud. compañia con un hombre o esposo que la maltrata fisicamente?
   Sí____ No____ A Veces____
3. ¿La ha amenazado su compañero o su esposo?
   Sí____ No____ A Veces____

Para Pacientes Embarazadas

4. ¿Ha recibido golpes en su cuerpo, su cara, o ha sido maltratada por su compañero o su esposo?
   Sí____ No____ A Veces____
5. Desde que se embarazo, ¿la ha golpeado o maltratado su compañero o su esposo?
   Sí____ No____ No Aplica____
6. Si contesta sí en la pregunta #5, conteste ahora, ¿han aumentado los maltratos?
   Sí____ No____ No Aplica____
7. ¿Ha recibido alguna vez tratamiento médico por daños o heridas causadas por el abuso o maltrato?
   Sí____ No____ No Aplica____
8. Si ha sido maltratada, por favor, marque en esta hoja los lugares donde fue golpeada la última vez.
9. ¿Estaba embarazada la última vez que fue maltratada?
   Sí____ No____ No Aplica____

ner is not present. If the woman has not experienced violence in her relationship, she will at the least be surprised by the question and at the most be educated that abuse is important enough to inquire about routinely.

Clues in the history (e.g., numerous injuries and stress-related symptoms) and evidence on physical examination of injuries such as burns or lacerations should alert the nurse to the problem. Assessment requires active listening and a detailed history of the woman's abuse and her living situation.

The nurse can respond to the woman's disclosure by acknowledging that it must be difficult for her to talk about her experiences and that she does not deserve to be treated like that. Women most fear that disclosure will result in being told that she must leave her abuser to receive further help. Such advice only alienates the woman who is socially and economically trapped in the relationship. It is least likely that she can leave the relationship while she is pregnant or has a newborn. Instead the nurse may offer resources for the woman's safety, places to call for emotional support, and counseling to help her clarify what she wants and needs (Furniss, 1993; Holtz and Furniss, 1993). The nurse can help the woman formulate a plan: What referral options (local agencies and shelters) can help her? Where can she go if she needs to leave the house immediately? Discuss a plan of action, including a prepacked bag of personal items.

The nurse's goal is to empower the woman. She needs to gain a feeling of control over her life, to set her own goals, and to make her own decisions. It is important for the nurse to communicate two messages: (1) that the nurse is deeply concerned, and (2) that the woman does not deserve to be abused.

Prevention

Nurses have the potential to make a difference in stopping the violence and preventing further injury. Educating women that abuse is a violation of their rights and facilitating their access to protective and legal services is a first step. Other measures that help discourage women from getting into abusive relationships include promoting assertiveness and self-defense courses, as well as support and self-help groups that encourage positive self-regard, confidence, and empowerment; and educational and skills development classes that enhance independence, or at least the ability to take care of one's self.

Critical Thinking Exercises 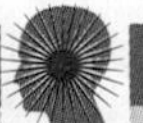

ADOLESCENT PREGNANCY—RAPE AND PSYCHOSOCIAL PROBLEMS

You are assigned to a clinic to take maternal histories at the first prenatal visit. A 16-year-old woman who comes for care gives the following history:

- She was date raped at a party 8 weeks ago. She has missed one menstrual period. Her pregnancy test was positive.
- She smokes one-half pack of cigarettes every day and drinks beer every weekend.
- She has experimented with marijuana occasionally and has tried cocaine twice in the last month.
- Her parents are divorced; she currently lives with her mother, who is unaware of the pregnancy.
- She states that she plans to keep the baby and raise it by herself. She does not have a boyfriend at this time.

For each problem you identify, do the following:

1. Formulate a nursing diagnosis.
2. Prioritize the nursing diagnosis.
3. Plan patient-centered goals and expected outcomes.
4. Plan interventions and provide rationales for each.
5. List referrals and possible community resources.

Key Points

- Psychosocial problems that may complicate childbearing can interfere with family integration and bonding with the infant.
- Involvement of the family, an interdisciplinary team approach, and community resources are required to provide long-term care for both the mother and the neonate.
- Values clarification for health care workers may be necessary to help them provide nonjudgmental care for women who abuse substances.
- Alcohol abuse during pregnancy is the leading cause of mental retardation in the United States. Alcohol-related impairments are preventable.
- Tobacco use (smoking) during pregnancy causes vasoconstriction and decreased placental perfusion, which results in maternal and neonatal complications.
- To prevent intrauterine growth restriction, low birth weight, and neonatal withdrawal, pregnant women should limit their caffeine consumption to less than 300 mg/day.
- Violence against women is a serious problem. Assessments should include questions about intimate partner abuse.

References

Abel E, Sokol R: A revised conservative estimate of the incidence of FAS and its economic impact, *Alcohol Clin Exp Res* 15:514, 1991.

Affonso D et al: Pregnancy and postpartum depressive symptoms, *J Women's Health* 2(2):157, 1993.

American Psychiatric Association: *Diagnostic and statistical manual of mental disorders*, ed 4, Washington, DC, 1994, The Association.

Armstrong B, McDonald A, Sloan M: Cigarette, alcohol and coffee consumption and spontaneous abortion, *Am J Public Health* 82:85, 1992.

Auerbach K, Jacobi A: Postpartum depression in the breastfeeding mother, *NAACOG's Clin Issues Perinatal Women Health Nurs* 1(3):375, 1990.

Bright D: Postpartum mental disorders, *Am Fam Physician* 50(3):595, 1994.

Brody T et al: *Human pharmacology, molecular to clinical*, ed 2, St Louis, 1994, Mosby.

Burkett G, Yasin S, Palow D: Perinatal implication of cocaine exposure, *J Reprod Med* 35(1):35, 1990.

Campbell J, Humphreys J: *Nursing care of survivors of family violence*, St Louis, 1993, Mosby.

Campbell J et al: Correlates of battering during pregnancy, *Res Nurs Health* 15:219, 1992.

Cefalo R, Moos M: *Preconceptional health care: a practical guide*, ed 2, St Louis, 1995, Mosby.

Chasnoff I: Cocaine, pregnancy, and the neonate, *J Women's Health* 15(3):23, 1989.

Chescheir N: Domestic violence, *Curr Pract*, 14(2):2, 1992.

Chez R: Battering during pregnancy, *Nat Perinat Assoc* 5:2, 1990.

Chisum G: Nursing interventions with the antepartum substance abuser, *J Perinat Neonat Nurs* 3:26, 1990.

Cook P et al: *Alcohol, tobacco, and other drugs may harm the unborn*, DHHS Pub No (ADM)90-1711, Rockville, Md, 1990, US Public Health Service.

Cordero L, Custard M: Effects of maternal cocaine abuse on perinatal and infant outcome, *Ohio Med* 86:410, 1990.

Coste J, Job-Spira N, Fernandez H: Increased risk of ectopic pregnancy with maternal cigarette smoking, *Am J Public Health* 81(2):199, 1991.

Creasy R, Resnik R: *Maternal fetal medicine: principles and practice*, ed 3, Philadelphia, 1994, WB Saunders.

Dattel B: Substance abuse in pregnancy, *Semin Perinatol* 14(2):179, 1990.

DeHass I, Harlow B, Cramer D: Spontaneous preterm birth: a case control study, *Am J Obstet Gynecol* 165:1290, 1991.

Ehlert U et al: Postpartum blues: salivary cortisol and psychological factors, *J Psychosom Res* 34:319, 1990.

Ewing J: Detecting alcoholism: the CAGE questionnaire, *JAMA* 252(14):1905, 1984.

Fenster L, Eskenazi B, Windham G: Caffeine consumption during pregnancy and fetal growth, *Am J Public Health* 81:458, 1991.

Fico T, Vanderwende C: Phencyclidine during pregnancy: fetal brain levels and neurobehavioral effects, *Neurotoxicol Teratol* 10:349, 1988.

Floyd R: Smoking during pregnancy: prevalence, effects and intervention strategies, *Birth* 18(1):488, 1991.

Fox C: Cocaine use in pregnancy, *J Am Board Fam Pract* 7(3):225, 1994.

Furniss K: Screening for abuse in the clinical setting, *AWHONN's Clin Issue Perinat Women Health Nurs* 4(3):402, 1993.

Glantz C, Woods J: Cocaine, heroin, and phencyclidine: obstetric perspectives, *Clinical Obstet Gynecol* 36(2):279, 1993.

Gotlib I et al: Prospective investigation of postpartum depression: factors involved in onset and recovery, *J Abnorm Psychol* 100:122, 1991.

Harris B et al: The hormonal environment of postnatal depression, *Br J Psychiatry* 154:660, 1989.

Holtz H, Furniss K: The health care provider's role in domestic violence: trends in health care, *Law Ethics* 8(2):47, 1993.

Hyman S, Arana G, Rosenbaum J: *Handbook of psychiatric drug therapy*, ed 3, Boston, 1995, Little Brown.

Iles S, Gath D, Kennerley H: Maternity blues: a comparison between postoperative women and postnatal women, *Br J Psychiatry* 155:363, 1989.

Janke J: Prenatal cocaine use: effects on perinatal outcome, *J Nurse Midwife* 35:74, 1990.

Johnson L: The legal implications of abuse of the unborn fetus, *Med Law* 13:19, 1994.

Kennerley H, Gath D: Maternity blues. I. detection and measurement by questionnaire, *Br J Psychiatry* 155:356, 1989a.

Kennerley H, Gath D: Maternity blues. III. association with obstetric, psychological, and psychiatric factors, *Br J Psychiatry* 155:367, 1989b.

Krause S, Ebbesen F, Lange A: Polyhydramnios with maternal lithium treatment, *Obstet Gynecol* 75(3):504, 1990.

Laraia M, Stuart G: *Quick psychopharmacology reference*, St Louis, 1995, Mosby.

Lawrence R: *Breastfeeding: a guide for the medical profession*, ed 4, 1994, Mosby.

Lewis D, Woods S: Fetal alcohol syndrome, *Am Fam Physician* 50(5):1025, 1994.

Little B et al: Patterns of multiple substance abuse during pregnancy: implications for mother and fetus, *South Med J* 83:507, 1990.

Logsdon M, McBride A, Birkimer J: Social support and postpartum depression, *Res Nurs Health* 17:449, 1994.

Lumley J, Astbury J: *Advice for pregnancy*. In Chalmers I, Enken M, Keirse M, editors: *Effective care in pregnancy and childbirth*, Oxford, 1989, Oxford University Press.

Lynch M, McKeon V: Cocaine use during pregnancy: research findings and clinical implications, *J Obstet Gynecol Neonat Nurs* 19:285, 1990.

Majewski M, Ford-Rice F, Falkey G: Pregnancy-induced alterations of GABA receptor sensitivity in maternal brain: an antecedent of postpartum blues? *Brain Res* 482:397, 1989.

Martell L: Postpartum depression as a family problem, *MCN Am J Matern Child Nurs* 15:90, 1990.

Matera C et al: Prevalence of use of cocaine and other substances in an obstetric population, *Am J Obstet Gynecol* 163:797, 1990.

Mayes L et al: Neurobehavioral profiles of neonates exposed to cocaine prenatally, *Pediatrics* 91(4):778, 1993.

McDonald A, Armstrong B, Sloan M: Cigarette, alcohol and coffee consumption and prematurity, *Am J Public Health* 82:87, 1992.

McFarlane J: Abuse during pregnancy: the horror and the hope, *AWHONN's Clin Issue Perinat Women's Health Nurs* 4(3):350, 1993.

McKim E: Caffeine and its effects on pregnancy and the neonate, *J Nurse Midwife* 36(4):226, 1991.

Mills J, Holmes L, Aarons J: Moderate caffeine use and the risk of spontaneous abortion and intrauterine growth retardation, *JAMA* 269:593, 1993.

Morrow R, Richie J, Bull S: Maternal cigarette smoking: the effects on umbilical and uterine blood flow velocity, *Am J Obstet Gynecol* 159(5):1069, 1988.

National Organization on Fetal Alcohol Syndrome: *Fetal alcohol syndrome fact sheet*, Washington, DC, 1995, The Organization.

Neuspiel D et al: Custody of cocaine-exposed newborns: determinants of discharge decisions, *Am J Public Health* 83(12):1726, 1993.

Ney J: The prevalence of substance abuse in patients with suspected preterm labor, *Am J Obstet Gynecol* 162:1562, 1990.

Nicolson P: Understanding postnatal depression: a mother-centered approach, *J Adv Nurs* 15(6):689, 1990.

Paltrow L: When becoming pregnant is a crime, *Criminal Justice Ethics*, 9:41, 1990.

Parker B, McFarlane J: Identifying and helping battered pregnant women, *MCN Am J Matern Child Nurs* 16:161, 1991.

Parker B, McFarlane J, Soeken K: Abuse during pregnancy: effects on maternal complications and birth weight in adult and teenage women, *Obstet Gynecol* 84(3):323, 1994.

Parker B et al: Physical and emotional abuse in pregnancy: a comparison of adult and teenage women, *Nurs Res* 42:173, 1993.

Pastuszak A et al: Pregnancy outcome following first-trimester exposure to fluoxetine (Prozac), *JAMA* 269(17):2246, 1993.

Pulkkinen P: Smoking in pregnancy with special reference to fetal growth and certain trace element distribution between mother, placenta, and fetus, *Acta Obstet Gynecol Scand* 69:543, 1990.

Scott J et al: *Obstetrics and gynecology*, ed 7, Philadelphia, 1994, JB Lippincott.

Stein A et al: Social adversity and perinatal complications: their relation to postnatal depression, *Br Med J* 2928:1073, 1989.

Steissguth A et al: Fetal alcohol syndrome in adolescents and adults, *JAMA* 265:1961, 1991.

Stuart G, Sundeen S: *Principles and practice of psychiatric nursing,* ed 5, St Louis, 1995, Mosby.

Taylor B: Prevention of pediatric pulmonary problems: the importance of maternal smoking, *Lung* 168(suppl):327, 1990.

Thorpe J: Management of drug dependency, overdose and withdrawal in the obstetric patient, *Obstet Gynecol Clin North Am* 22:4, 1995.

Ugarriza D: Postpartum affective disorders: incidence and treatment, *J Psychosoc Nursing Ment Health Serv* 30:29, 1992.

Vaughn A et al: Community-wide estimation of illicit drug use in delivering women: prevalence, demographics and associated risk factors, *Obstet Gynecol* 82(1):92, 1993.

Weiss J, Hansell M: Substance abuse during pregnancy, *Nurs Health Care* 13(9):472, 1992.

Williams M: Cigarette smoking during pregnancy in relation to placenta previa, *Am J Obstet Gynecol* 165(1):28, 1991.

Bibliography

Barton S, Harrigan R, Tse A: Prenatal cocaine exposure: implications for practice, policy development, and needs for future research, *J Perinatol* 15(1):10, 1995.

Bick C: Perceptions of nurses' caring by mothers experiencing postpartum depression, *J Obstet Gynecol Neonatal Nurs* 24(9):819, 1995.

Beck C: Screening methods for postpartum depression, *J Obstet Gynecol Neonatal Nurs* 24(4):308, 1995.

Finkelstein N: Treatment issues for alcohol- and drug-dependent pregnant and parenting women, *Health and Social Work* 19(1):7, 1994.

Kendig S: Women at risk for infection: the woman who is chemically dependent, *J Obstet Gynecol Neonatal Nurs* 24(8):776, 1995.

O'Connell K, Gerkovich M, Cook M: Mastery and sympathy in smoking cessation, *Image J Nurs Sch* 27(4):31, 1995.

CHAPTER 12

Adolescent Sexuality, Pregnancy, and Parenthood

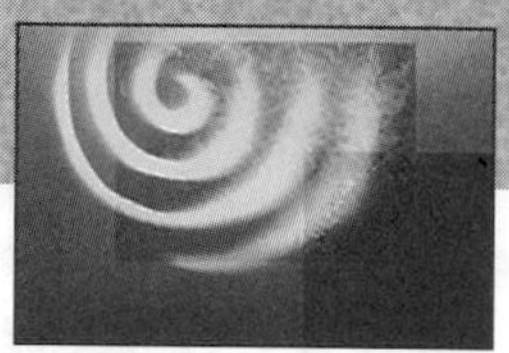

PHYSIOLOGIC DEVELOPMENT, P. 316
COGNITIVE DEVELOPMENT, P. 317
MORAL DEVELOPMENT, P. 317
PSYCHOSOCIAL DEVELOPMENT, P. 317
ADOLESCENT PREGNANCY, P. 317
STDs AND HIV, P. 317
PRIMARY PREVENTION OF ADOLESCENT HIGH-RISK SEXUAL BEHAVIOR AND PREGNANCY, P. 318
Adolescent sexual behavior, p. 318
Nursing care management, p. 318
SECONDARY PREVENTION WITH PREGNANT ADOLESCENTS, P. 321
The very young pregnant adolescent, p. 321
Developmental tasks of pregnancy, p. 321
Cultural influences, p. 322
Family reactions to adolescent pregnancy, p. 322
Adolescent fathers, p. 322
Nursing care management, p. 322
TERTIARY PREVENTION WITH ADOLESCENT PARENTS, P. 329
Adolescent parenthood, p. 329
Developmental tasks of parenthood, p. 330
The extended family, p. 330
Nursing care management, p. 330

During adolescence individuals undergo the transformation from childhood to adulthood. **Adolescence** is characterized by the onset of puberty, the establishment of independence from parents, the search for identity, and the development of cognitive processes. As adolescents undergo these changes, they may experiment with various risk-taking behaviors such as the initiation of sexual intercourse.

The proportion of teens who have had sexual intercourse by age 18 has steadily increased since 1970. More than half (56%) of the women and almost three fourths (73%) of the men in the United States have had sexual intercourse before their 18th birthday (Alan Guttmacher Institute [AGI], 1994). Teens who engage in high-risk sexual behavior, such as unprotected sexual intercourse, are at risk for pregnancy and sexually transmitted diseases (STDs), including infection with the human immunodeficiency virus (HIV). Adolescent childbearing may result in health and socioeconomic consequences for the teen mother and her baby. In addition, STDs increase the risk of pelvic inflammatory disease (PID) and future infertility. Furthermore, HIV infection is increasing among adolescents and is the sixth leading cause of death among people 15 to 24 years of age (Kochanek and Hudson, 1995).

Decreased incidences of adolescent pregnancy, STDs, and HIV infection are among the health objectives for the year 2000 (U.S. Department of Health and Human Services, 1990). Reducing high-risk sexual behavior among adolescents would contribute greatly to achieving these health objectives.

Prevention of high-risk sexual behavior and adolescent pregnancy can occur at three levels: primary, secondary, and tertiary. **Primary prevention of high-risk sexual behavior** and adolescent pregnancy refers to interventions aimed at preventing pregnancy and STDs/HIV. **Secondary prevention with pregnant adolescents** involves strategies that focus on preventing complications during pregnancy. Interventions aimed at **tertiary prevention with adolescent parents** focus on preventing complications after the infant is born (Humenick et al, 1991). This chapter reviews adolescent development and **sexuality** before exploring prevention of high-risk sexual behavior and adolescent pregnancy at each of these levels.

PHYSIOLOGIC DEVELOPMENT

Puberty begins between the ages of 9 and 14 years, when hormones from the hypothalamus trigger the secretion of hormones in the pituitary gland. Pituitary hormones increase the production of estrogen and progesterone by the ovaries. Although the sequence of events is universal, the onset of puberty is influenced by many factors, such as sex, genes, body type, nutrition, and health. The first sign of puberty is the growth spurt. This accelerated growth, which occurs approximately 2 years earlier in females than in males, continues over a 3-year period. Changes in the appearance of their bodies may make adolescents feel shy and awkward.

The development of secondary sex characteristics, such as breasts and pubic hair, has an impact on the adolescent's new body image. Primary sexual characteristics include maturation of the female ovaries and male testes, thus leading to reproductive maturity.

Maturation of the ovaries and testes is marked by menarche in girls and the first ejaculation in boys. Menarche occurs in adolescent females about 3 years after the growth spurt and occurs in about half of all girls at about age 12½ years (Forrest, 1993), but it may occur as early as age 10 years or as late as 16 years.

As the brain matures in the pubescent girl, stimulation of the hypothalamus leads to secretion of gonadotropin-releasing hormone (Gn-RH). Gn-RH stimulates the anterior pituitary to release gonadotropins, which stimulate the gonads to mature and release ova in the female and to produce sperm in the male. These physiologic changes enable the adolescent to reproduce. The first menstrual cycle is usually anovulatory, with regular ovulation not occurring for about a year.

COGNITIVE DEVELOPMENT

As the body changes, the adolescent begins to look inward and become more egocentric. Adolescent egocentrism is a stage of cognitive development in which teens consider their own experiences to be unique. Egocentric thought prompts adolescents to create imaginary audiences that allow them to think that other people are watching them. The creation of the imaginary audience explains the common feeling of self-consciousness among adolescents. The invincibility fable that "It can't happen to me" is an extension of adolescent egocentrism (Berger, 1994).

Generally, adolescents who exhibit a high degree of egocentrism have not yet mastered formal operational thought. The logical and abstract reasoning involved in formal operational thought allows adolescents to speculate, form hypotheses, and imagine possibilities (Piaget, 1969). However, Piaget maintains that maturation of the adolescent's brain and body makes formal operational thought possible, but not inevitable. Thus many adolescents continue to use concrete operational thought and cannot imagine the future consequences of their actions. Social interactions and education are essential factors in enabling an individual to attain formal operational thought (Piaget, 1969).

MORAL DEVELOPMENT

As thought processes mature, so does moral reasoning. Cognitive and psychosocial development allows adolescents to think more abstractly and to question the moral views of their parents. Social development exposes them to various ethical values. Personal experiences force adolescents to make decisions on their own and to consider moral questions more broadly than before (Berger, 1994). According to Kohlberg (1984), most young adolescents follow rules for the purpose of gaining approval from others or to be a good citizen (conventional level of morality). As late adolescents mature cognitively and gain experiences with right and wrong, they develop their own personal moral code (postconventional morality). However, Kohlberg's theory has been criticized for being biased against women, who tend to see moral dilemmas differently than men. According to Gilligan (1982), men view moral dilemmas in terms of the rights of others, whereas women are more concerned with the needs of others.

PSYCHOSOCIAL DEVELOPMENT

The primary **developmental task of adolescence** is the search for identity, both as an individual and as a member of the larger community (Berger, 1994; Erikson, 1963). The ultimate goal is identity achievement, which occurs when adolescents develop their own belief system and career goals. Although adolescents strive to achieve individuality, they have self-doubts and seek acceptance from their peers. In addition to the search for independence, adolescents also depend on their parents for financial and emotional support. Some adolescents achieve identity prematurely, a process Erikson calls *foreclosure*. Others experience identity diffusion with few commitments to goals, values, or society. Some adolescents, unable to find alternative roles, rebel and adopt a negative identity and become the opposite of what is expected of them. Some adolescents postpone career and marriage decisions (declaring a moratorium on identity formation) by attending college or serving in the military.

ADOLESCENT PREGNANCY

Over 1 million teens in the United States become pregnant annually (AGI, 1994). About 9% of sexually active girls age 14, 18% of those ages 15 to 17, and 22% of those ages 18 to 19 become pregnant every year (AGI, 1994). Of all teenage pregnancies in 1987, 35% ended in abortion and 14% ended in miscarriage. The majority of teenage births in 1987 resulted from unintended pregnancies; only 14% of births were intended (Moore, Snyder, & Glei, 1995).

The United States has the highest teenage birth rate in the industrialized world (Moore, Snyder, & Glei, 1995). In contrast, other industrialized nations have similar levels of sexually experienced adolescents with fewer teenage births and abortions than in the United States. Thus teens in other industrialized countries are using effective contraception more consistently than teens in the United States (AGI, 1994).

Motivation to avoid pregnancy is probably related to the adolescent's perception of the benefits of postponing parenthood. The adolescent's perception of the benefits are influenced by the present situation and a belief in future life options. Lower socioeconomic status offers the adolescent fewer choices. Instead of striving for high educational attainment and a professional career, adolescents of lower socioeconomic status may choose other ways to transition to adulthood. For example, sexual intercourse and having a baby may seem to be more viable alternatives than attending college.

STDs AND HIV

The incidence of STDs has risen among teens more rapidly than in the general population. Two thirds of all cases of STDs occur among persons younger than 25 years of age (Centers for Disease Control [CDC], 1993). Some STDs are more prevalent in adolescents than in older women (CDC, 1993). For example, adolescent girls 15 to 19 years old have the highest rates of gonorrhea among all women (936.4 per 100,000). The CDC estimates that 3 million teenage men and women contract STDs annually, accounting for 25% of all new cases each year (CDC, 1993).

Gonorrhea and chlamydial infection often result in PID, which can scar fallopian tubes and lead to infertility. Teenage women are at higher risk of developing PID because of young age at initiation of sexual intercourse and having more than one partner. In addition, the number of cases of acquired immunodeficiency syndrome (AIDS) among people 24 years of age and younger has increased. Heterosexual contact is the leading cause of AIDS among women 13 to 24 years old (CDC, 1993). Between October 1, 1992 and September 30, 1993, 499 cases of AIDS were reported among adolescents 13 to 19 years old. Although this accounts for only 0.4% of all AIDS cases, it is a 20% increase in this age group in 1 year. There were 3445 cases reported among young adults age 20 to 24 years (CDC, 1993). Given the long incubation period of HIV, many of the 20- to 24-year-old adults with AIDS were probably infected as teens.

Adolescent women who initiate sexual intercourse at an early age acquire multiple partners more rapidly in the first years after intercourse than young women who initiate sexual intercourse later (Kost and Forrest, 1992). About one third of teenage women report having had two to three sexual partners. The proportion of teenage women who report having four or more partners has increased from 14% in 1971 to 31% in 1988 (Kost and Forrest, 1992). Despite the media blitz about AIDS and safer sex, the average number of sexual partners has increased for adolescent males and females. In addition, teens often practice "serial monogamy" in which they are faithful to one partner until the relationship ends and then move on to a sexual relationship with another partner (AGI, 1994). However, teens are no more likely to practice serial monogamy than older unmarried women (AGI, 1994; Kost and Forrest, 1992).

Although teens are knowledgeable about AIDS (Keller et al, 1991), they continue to engage in high-risk sexual behavior. As teenage men get older they rely less on condom use and more on contraceptive methods for which the female is responsible, such as oral contraceptives (Ku, Sonenstein, and Pleck, 1993). Furthermore, once teenage women begin taking oral contraceptives, most do not use condoms consistently (Weisman et al, 1991).

Despite the rising incidence of STDs and HIV among teens, egocentric thought of adolescents leads teens to perceive themselves as being at low risk for STDs and HIV infection. This may lead to their inconsistent use of condoms and lack of communication with their partner about high-risk sexual behavior (Overby and Kegeles, 1994).

PRIMARY PREVENTION OF ADOLESCENT HIGH-RISK SEXUAL BEHAVIOR AND PREGNANCY

Adolescent Sexual Behavior

The average age for initiation of sexual intercourse is 16.2 years for females and 15.7 years for males. The proportion of Caucasian adolescent women who had ever had sexual intercourse steadily increased between 1980 and 1988, with 41.4% reporting having had premarital sexual intercourse in 1980, 43.1% in 1985, and 50.6% in 1988. The trend for adolescent African-American women was somewhat different. The proportion of African-American women having ever had sexual intercourse was 58.1% in 1980, declined to 55.4% in 1985, and increased to 58.8% in 1988 (CDC, 1991 a; 1991 b). Although African-American girls tend to initiate sexual intercourse at younger ages than do European-American girls, racial differences are beginning to narrow because of the increase in premarital sexual intercourse among Caucasian teens (AGI, 1994; Leigh et al, 1994).

In addition to racial differences, other demographic and psychosocial factors have been linked with adolescent premarital sexual intercourse. Demographic factors such as older age (Lock and Vincent, 1995; Newcomer and Baldwin, 1992), low socioeconomic status (Zabin and Hayward, 1993), single-parent family (Lock and Vincent, 1995; Young et al, 1991), and no religious affiliation (Miller and Moore, 1990) have been correlated with an increased incidence of adolescent premarital sexual intercourse. The influence of parent-adolescent communication on sexual intercourse is not clear (Perkins, 1991). Some researchers have found that parent-adolescent communication is a strong predictor of sexual intercourse, but others have found no relationship (Perkins, 1991).

Perceptions that their friends are sexually active (Lock and Vincent, 1995; National Institute of Child Health and Human Development, 1991; Yawn and Yawn, 1993) and low educational goals (Dryfoos, 1990) have also been associated with premarital sexual intercourse among adolescents. In addition, teens are more likely to engage in sexual intercourse if they engage in other risk behaviors, such as smoking and alcohol use (AGI, 1994).

The impact of self-esteem on female adolescent premarital sexual intercourse is unclear. Although low self-esteem has been emphasized as a factor associated with premarital sexual intercourse, most researchers have not found a consistent relationship (Yawn and Yawn, 1993; Zabin and Hayward, 1993).

In very young sexually experienced adolescents, sexual abuse must be suspected. In one study investigating the relationship between sexual abuse and adolescent pregnancy, researchers found that 66% of the 535 pregnant or parenting adolescent females had experienced nonvoluntary sexual intercourse (Boyer and Fine, 1992). The father of the baby is often an adult.

Nursing Care Management

When adolescent choices include engaging in sexual activity, the adolescent is at risk for various health problems. The nurse can work effectively with the sexually experienced adolescent to achieve optimal health outcomes. The nursing process can be used to accomplish this goal.

⇒ Assessment

A thorough health history interview (including menstrual, sexual, and dietary factors) with review of systems, complete physical examination (including breast and pelvic examination), and laboratory tests should be conducted. In addition, assessment of the psychosocial (e.g., sexual identity, body image, self-concept), cognitive-developmental stage, and support systems is essential. Careful assessment is needed to identify learning and care needs. The health history interview should be conducted in a quiet, private room with the adolescent fully clothed. An unhurried, nonjudgmental attitude will facilitate patient relaxation. The interview begins with nonthreatening questions.

After rapport is established with the patient, more sensitive questions may be asked. The nurse should be aware of culturally unacceptable verbal and nonverbal responses. The nurse should use direct language, such as "sexual intercourse," not "making love."

A **sexual history** is essential. It should include knowledge and use of safer sexual practices, use of contraceptives, sources of sex education, knowledge of and history of STDs, number of sexual partners, satisfaction with sexual partner, types and frequency of sexual contacts, techniques of sexual intercourse, and satisfaction with sexual intercourse.

Physical examination. A thorough physical examination is essential. The nurse should be alert for possibilities of sexual abuse in the young adolescent. Because the young adolescent has little experience with what normal body functions are, STDs may go unnoticed and unreported to health care providers for treatment. Heavy menstrual bleeding or other abnormal bleeding in adolescents may be related to abortion, trauma, endocrine diseases, infection, or other causes, such as taking oral contraceptives incorrectly or even correctly (Hilliard and Rebar, 1990).

A pelvic examination is recommended for any teenage woman who is sexually active and for those considering oral contraceptives. During puberty the vaginal epithelium is thin. Therefore it is more vulnerable to irritation and infection. Contact vaginitis can result from perfumed soap, powders, sprays, and tight jeans or other garments.

Adolescent girls are modest and are usually tense during the pelvic examination. The adolescent may consider the pelvic examination to be distasteful and anxiety provoking. It is even more threatening if sexual abuse has occurred. Before a first pelvic examination, instruction in relaxation techniques is helpful. Lidocaine ointment may be used as a lubricant. The anxious adolescent client may feel more comfortable using a mirror so she can participate in the examination. An appropriate goal is to help the adolescent feel in control and avoid embarrassment. The adolescent should be asked to decide whether her mother or partner remains in the room or leaves during the examination. If the adolescent finds the examination too painful and is truly unable to cooperate, an examination under anesthesia may be necessary (Hilliard and Rebar, 1990).

Although true breast disease is uncommon in adolescent girls, anxiety about symptoms such as swelling is common. Breast examination findings in teens commonly are hormone related and commonly occur during the hormone surge of puberty. Swelling of the breasts also may occur during pregnancy and with substance abuse. The adolescent should be reassured that breast swelling will abate spontaneously when the hormone surge regresses (Beach, 1990).

Laboratory studies. Laboratory studies for adolescents are similar to those obtained for adult women having a gynecologic examination and may include complete blood cell count, rubella antibody test, urinalysis, urine culture and sensitivity, Papanicolaou (Pap) smear, cervical culture, hemoglobin and hematocrit levels, blood typing, cultures for gonorrhea and chlamydia, and serology testing for syphilis. HIV antibody testing may also be recommended.

Nursing Diagnoses

After a review of assessment findings from the interview, physical examination, and laboratory/diagnostic tests, appropriate nursing diagnoses are formulated. Examples of nursing diagnoses that may apply include the following:

- Body-image disturbance related to
  - Puberty
- Decisional conflict related to
  - Unclear personal values or beliefs regarding premarital sexual intercourse
  - Lack of experience with sexual decision making
  - Lack of relevant information
- Health-seeking behavior: contraceptive use related to
  - Desire to avoid pregnancy
- Noncompliance: contraceptive regimen related to
  - Lack of information on correct contraceptive regimen
  - Unplanned sexual encounter
  - Side effects of contraceptives
- Health-seeking behavior: safer sexual practices related to
  - Desire to avoid sexually transmitted diseases

Expected Outcomes

A nursing care plan is based on the adolescent's health care needs. The expected outcomes for care, mutually determined by the adolescent and the nurse, are stated in patient-centered terms. Examples of possible expected outcomes include the following. The adolescent will:

1. Demonstrate acceptance of changes in body as a result of puberty (e.g., posture, grooming, dress)
2. Verbalize personal values and beliefs about premarital sexual intercourse
3. Verbalize alternatives to sexual intercourse for expressing feelings
4. Verbalize that she and her partner are practicing safer sexual behavior
5. Verbalize consequences associated with unsafe sexual practices
6. Verbalize/demonstrate correct method of using contraceptive of choice
7. Not contract an STD
8. Not become pregnant

Plan of Care and Implementation

Sexuality education. In a review of school-based **sexuality education** programs, Kirby (1992) described the evolution of sexuality education programs. Initially, sexuality education programs focused on knowledge about risks and consequences of pregnancy, values clarification, and development of decision-making and communication skills. Research indicates that these sexuality education programs did not accelerate or delay the initiation of sexual intercourse. Those who were concerned that sexuality education be value-free developed abstinence-only programs. Evaluation of abstinence-only programs has shown that they are effective in changing attitudes about premarital sexual intercourse but have had little effect on sexual behavior. Early evaluation of HIV/AIDS education programs have indicated an increase in knowledge, but few studies have measured the effect on sexual behavior (Kirby et al, 1994)

More recently, sexuality education programs have been based on theoretical models such as social learning theory. Preliminary evaluation of programs based on social learning theory suggests that they are effective in delaying sexual intercourse and reducing unprotected sexual intercourse.

Parents may not involve themselves in sexuality education for several reasons: (1) they may not have adequate information; (2) they may be uncomfortable with the topic of sex; and (3) adolescents may be uncomfortable when parents discuss sex. Some parents find it difficult to acknowledge that their "child" is a sexual person with sexual feelings and behaviors. Parental refusal to discuss sexual behavior may cause the adolescent to keep sexual activity a secret and may interfere with the adolescent's efforts to seek help. National surveys of parents reveal greater support for inclusion of comprehensive sex education in school curricula and at earlier ages for today's youth (CDC, 1991a; 1991b).

Sexuality education programs should begin before puberty (some suggest as early as kindergarten) and provide adolescents with experience in personal decision making and practice in applying the information to their lives. Programs should address how to handle peer pressure, focus on both females and males, and involve parents to enhance parent-adolescent communication and to strengthen family ties. Community institutions (e.g., churches, local lay groups, and professional groups) should also be involved to lend financial or volunteer support to the programs.

Health education at the primary prevention level includes providing information about good hygiene, prevention of STDs, and contraceptive use. Health education strategies need to be creative and developmentally, culturally, educationally, and language appropriate. Education should be appropriate for low-risk groups, high-risk groups, and parents or partners of low- or high-risk groups.

Nurses should promote school-based sexuality education for early ages. In addition, since teachers report a lack of training in sexuality education (Zabin and Hayward, 1993), nurses should take a more active role in teaching sexuality concepts in schools. Nurses can facilitate the development of peer counseling groups, with peers providing information and counseling to other adolescents.

Contraceptive use. Adolescents who are sexually active often do not use contraceptives consistently and correctly. Approximately two thirds of teens use **contraception,** usually a condom, at first intercourse (Forrest and Singh, 1990). Many demographic and psychosocial factors have been associated with adolescent contraceptive use. The older adolescents are the first time they have sexual intercourse, the more likely they are to use effective contraception (Zabin and Hayward, 1993) and to continue using it consistently (AGI, 1994). Analysis of national survey data indicates that Caucasian female adolescents are more likely to always use contraception and less likely to never use contraception than African-American female adolescents. On the other hand, African-American female adolescents are more likely than Caucasian females to use female prescription methods at first intercourse (Zabin and Hayward, 1993). These contradictory findings may be attributed to the disproportionate number of African-Americans who use family planning clinics for contraceptive counseling. In addition, the higher the socioeconomic status (SES), the more likely the adolescent is to use contraception. However, teens of lower SES visit family planning clinics and use oral contraceptives more often than those of higher SES. Teenage women are usually sexually active for several months before seeking contraceptive counseling from a health care provider.

Research indicates that those who are reliable in using contraception are more likely to have friends who use contraception (Zabin and Hayward, 1993). In addition, teenage women who are more involved with their partners may be better able to anticipate sexual activity and more likely to use reliable contraception (Zabin and Hayward, 1993).

Oral contraceptives are used more often than any other method among 15- to 19-year-old women (Peterson, 1995). Oral contraceptives do not reduce the risk of contracting STDs; however, they can reduce the risk that certain STDs, such as gonorrhea, will escalate into PID (Hatcher et al, 1994). Requirements for Title X family planning services mandate that a pelvic examination and venipuncture for hematocrit and hemoglobin be done before prescribing oral contraceptives. However, teens may delay attending family planning clinics because of this requirement (Armstrong and Stover, 1994). Research suggests that practitioners may prescribe oral contraceptives and delay the pelvic examination and laboratory work without serious complications. In one study, teens who chose to delay these procedures used condoms more often, had fewer pregnancies, and had similar STD rates compared with those who did not delay (Armstrong and Stover, 1994).

The condom is the second most common contraceptive method used (Peterson, 1995). In addition to preventing pregnancy, the latex condom and spermicide help protect against STDs. Nurses should instruct adolescents in the proper way to use condoms. Norplant (subdermal implant) and methoxyprogesterone (Depo-Provera) given intramuscularly (IM) are long-term continuous hormonal contraceptives gaining in popularity among teens.

Adolescents commonly misuse and misunderstand the rhythm method, more accurately called the fertility-awareness method. They often miscalculate the approximate midpoint between menstrual periods, abstain during what they consider to be the fertile days, and believe this makes them safe. The adolescent who wants to use this method must be taught the complex process of determining her individual fertility status so that she abstains from sexual intercourse for the full amount of time considered unsafe. This method is even less effective for adolescents who have irregular menstrual cycles (Tyre, Rothbart, and Anderson, 1990).

Teens should be taught safer sexual practices, which include using latex condoms with each sexual encounter, limiting the number of sexual partners, and communicating with sexual partners about previous high-risk sexual behavior. Teens should also be instructed in how to obtain emergency contraception (morning-after pill) if necessary.

Evaluation

The nurse can be reasonably assured that care has been effective if the expected outcomes of care have been met, that is, the adolescent:

- Demonstrates acceptance of changes in body as a result of puberty (e.g., posture, grooming, dress)
- Verbalizes personal values and beliefs about premarital sexual intercourse
- Verbalizes alternatives to sexual intercourse
- Verbalizes safer sexual practices
- Verbalizes consequences associated with unsafe sexual practices
- Verbalizes correct method of using contraceptive of choice
- Remains free of STDs
- Does not become pregnant

SECONDARY PREVENTION WITH PREGNANT ADOLESCENTS

Teenage childbearing has been associated with unfavorable consequences for mother, child, and society. After the birth of a child the adolescent mother is at high risk for low educational attainment (Klepinger, Lundberg, and Plotnick, 1995; Nord et al, 1992), low SES, and dependency on public welfare (Hayes, 1987; Zabin and Hayward, 1993). Teenage pregnancy remains the major reason female adolescents terminate their education prematurely. Leaving school early is associated with unemployment and poverty. Thus adolescent parents often fail to complete their basic education, have fewer opportunities for employment and career advancement, and have limited earning potential. More young mothers than older mothers live in families with annual incomes near the poverty level.

Payments from Aid to Families with Dependent Children (AFDC) rarely provide adequate support for the optimal development of young children. Adolescent mothers tend to have more children than they desire, and their children tend to be more closely spaced. All these factors result in limited resources that can impair optimal parenting. Children of adolescent mothers are also more likely to have problems with cognitive development (Nord et al, 1992).

Adolescent childbearing is likely to result in an increased incidence of morbidity and mortality for both the teenage mother and her infant. In an analysis of data from the National Hospital Discharge Survey, researchers found that pregnant women under 17 years old were almost 3 times more likely to develop preeclampsia than women age 30 to 34 years. In addition, women under 20 years of age were 5 times more likely to develop eclampsia than older women (Saftlas et al, 1990). Pregnancy-induced hypertension can indirectly lead to prematurity and low birth weight, since the mother often gives birth early to control the disease process. Uteroplacental insufficiency can also result from pregnancy-induced hypertension and can lead to growth restriction of the infant (Roberts, 1994).

Pregnancy puts the adolescent and her baby at risk nutritionally (Story, 1990). Poor nutritional status can lead to inadequate weight gain during pregnancy, which contributes to low birth weight in the infant (Rees et al, 1992). In addition, mothers younger than 15 years old are twice as likely to deliver preterm or low–birth-weight infants (LBW) (Nord et al, 1992). Pregnant adolescents are also at increased risk for iron deficiency anemia, which has been associated with prematurity and low birth weight (Beard, 1994; Scholl et al, 1992) (Box 12-1).

BOX 12-1
Maternal and Fetal Nutritional Risks for Pregnant Adolescents

MATERNAL
Excessive weight gain
Inadequate weight gain
Iron deficiency anemia

FETAL
Low birth weight
Preterm labor

The incidence of abandonment, abuse, separation, and divorce is 2 to 4 times higher among adolescents married in their teens than among those married in their 20s. In addition to the stress of the transition to marriage, this family instability is related to other variables, including low level of education, low level of employment, and lack of support systems.

The Very Young Pregnant Adolescent

The pregnant adolescent younger than 15 years of age is most at risk for problems in pregnancy and childbirth. The incidences of LBW infants, infant mortality, and abortion are 2 to 3 times higher in this age group than for women older than 25 years (National Center for Health Statistics, 1990).

The very young adolescent is at particular risk because she enters prenatal care later than do older adolescents and women. Late entry into prenatal care may result from late recognition of pregnancy, denial of pregnancy, or confusion about available services (Kinsman and Slap, 1992). Late presentation for care may result in inadequate time before the birth to attend to correctable problems. The very young pregnant adolescent is at higher risk for each of the confounding variables (already mentioned) associated with poor pregnancy outcomes and for those conditions associated with first pregnancy (e.g., pregnancy-induced hypertension). When prenatal care is given early and consistently and confounding variables (e.g., socioeconomic factors) are accounted for, very young pregnant adolescents are at no greater risk (nor are their infants) than older pregnant women (and their infants). The role of the nurse in reducing the risks and consequences of adolescent pregnancy is thus twofold: first, to encourage early and continued prenatal care and second, to refer the adolescent, if necessary, for appropriate social support services, which can help reverse a negative socioeconomic environment.

Developmental Tasks of Pregnancy

The pregnant adolescent faces the same **developmental tasks of pregnancy** as the pregnant adult. These tasks include the following:

- Accepting the biologic reality of pregnancy. Most adolescents do not expect to become pregnant. They may deny it until the signs are so obvious they can no longer be ignored by family members. It is common for teens to diet and wear constricting clothes to hide their condition and to succeed in concealing the pregnancy until it is quite advanced, sometimes until the birth. The level of denial in some teens and their families can be quite high.

- Accepting the reality of the unborn child. The adolescent may accept only the fantasy of having a cute, happy, healthy baby to dress up and play with like a doll. The idea of the infant's growth and development into an older child may not be a reality to the adolescent.
- Accepting the reality of parenthood. Being a parent implies being loving, concerned, and capable of providing the nurturing care an infant needs. Although there usually is the desire to be a good mother, young adolescent parents have limited life experiences, their own need to grow and develop, and little ability to cope with abstractions and to solve problems. The amount and type of support available to adolescents can significantly influence the accomplishment of these tasks.

Cultural Influences

The pregnancy rate for poor and low-income minority adolescents is high. Poverty and societal racism have a harmful effect on family and community life. Minority youth become sexually active at earlier ages and have less access to birth control information than do Caucasian adolescents. The lack of social and family support, nurturance, and supervision of the adolescent (as may occur in single-family households)—coupled with fewer opportunities to accomplish social and educational goals—places these individuals at high risk for pregnancy. The availability of social support varies across ethnic groups. In one study, African-American pregnant adolescents had fewer people in their support network than Caucasian and Hispanic-American pregnant teens. However, African-American pregnant teens identified more family members in their support network than did other teens in the study (Koniak-Griffin, Lominska, and Brecht, 1993).

In addition, cultural differences exist in adolescents' knowledge of sexuality and in their beliefs about pregnancy and pregnancy prevention. For example, in one study Native Americans believed that intrauterine devices (IUDs) were undesirable because they might mark the baby if pregnancy occurred. African-American teens considered birth control pills as well as IUDs unacceptable, whereas the beliefs and preferences of Caucasian teens varied along religious lines. Mexican-American and Central/South-American females were more likely to use effective birth control than were Puerto Rican, Cuban, and other Hispanic subjects (Durant et al, 1990).

Nurses must be aware of differences in cultural beliefs if open communication is to occur. When these beliefs are assessed and incorporated into a plan of care, more effective programs for pregnancy prevention may result and more appropriate care may be provided (Table 2-2).

Family Reactions to Adolescent Pregnancy

One of the most difficult tasks of the pregnant adolescent is telling her parents that she is pregnant. The adolescent may not talk about her pregnancy until it is obvious. Her mother usually is the first to find out and may attempt to prevent the adolescent's father from discovering his daughter's pregnancy. The usual initial reactions of grandparents-to-be to the news are shock, anger, shame, guilt, and sorrow. The nurse must assess any disharmony that is occurring in the family and assist family members in adapting to the pregnancy (or other options).

Adolescent Fathers

Teenage fathers are more likely to be children of teenage parents than are their peers who are not fathers. Consequently, they may not view pregnancy as a disruption to their young lives. In some low-income communities the capacity of adolescents to impregnate is viewed with a sense of pride and as a sign of manhood (Esman, 1990).

Adolescent fathers are more likely to be poorer and less educated than adolescent men who do not become fathers at an early age. Most adolescent fathers try to provide some support for their partners (e.g., money, gifts, transportation). They also want to be involved in the decision-making process concerning the mother's options regarding the pregnancy. However, families of the adolescent couple often exclude the adolescent father from the decision-making process because of anger about the pregnancy or because they believe that he is not capable of making a decision. However, adolescent fathers often feel that their partners do not really need them for support and thus they do not believe they are neglecting them.

Over time, contact diminishes significantly for unmarried couples, and if married, marital satisfaction tends to be low. This is true for adolescent couples from various ethnic groups. The nurse should assess the adolescent couple's relationship in planning care for the pregnant adolescent and the father of the baby.

Nursing Care Management

Many interacting biologic and social factors affect the quality of human reproduction, and these in turn are influenced by the preconceptional, maternal, and neonatal care that is made available. The adolescent and her offspring are particularly vulnerable to the risks inherent in pregnancy and parenthood. This results from circumstances characteristic of her age group, such as cognitive-developmental level, psychologic immaturity, economic dependency, delayed medical care, and lack of political power and influence. The multifaceted and complex needs of the adolescent are most effectively addressed by means of a multidisciplinary team of nurses, physicians, registered dietitians, and social workers.

Assessment

Interview. The interview for the initial prenatal visit for the pregnant adolescent is similar to that for an adult pregnant woman. A thorough health history, with a review of systems and sexual history, is warranted. Cultural considerations should also be assessed. The nurse should be aware that before pregnancy the very young adolescent usually has received care only from a pediatric health care provider and may be apprehensive about an unfamiliar health care provider. In addition to obtaining a health history from the pregnant adolescent, the nurse should elicit information about the health of the baby's father.

Nutrition assessment. Nutrition assessment is essential and includes the following components: history (medical, obstetric, life-style, psychosocial), dietary assessment, anthropometric measurements, laboratory testing, and clinical evaluation (Story, 1990). The effect of maternal age on gestational weight gain is unclear because most studies have not controlled for other factors influencing gestational weight gain, such as parity, prepregnant weight for height, ethnicity, alcohol use, and smoking (Gutierrez and King, 1993). Except for very young teens, there is little evidence that maternal age influences weight gain when other factors are controlled (Gutierrez and King, 1993).

Inadequate weight gain early in pregnancy is linked to small-for-gestational-age (SGA) infants (Scholl et al, 1993). Early weight gain may be difficult because of body image, poor prepregnancy nutritional status, and poor diet during pregnancy (Scholl et al, 1993). Late inadequate weight gain is linked to preterm birth and SGA infants (Scholl et al, 1993). Availability of nutrients to the fetus depends on whether the teenage mother continues to grow while pregnant (Scholl et al, 1993). Fetal growth restriction in teens still growing may result from competition for nutrients (Gutierrez and King, 1993; Scholl et al, 1993). If the teenage woman experienced early menarche, she may have an increased rate of growth for a longer period of time postmenarche.

Diet evaluation using a 24-hour recall provides a base for assessing the nutrients consumed by the young adolescent and can be easily obtained in any setting. The very young adolescent should also be asked about athletic participation, dance classes, and other vigorous activity that could alter her calorie requirements. The adolescent is at greater nutritional risk because of the high fat content of food served at school cafeterias and the consumption of large amounts of "fast foods." Beverage intake should also be assessed. Adolescents may inadvertently consume excessive amounts of caffeine in soft drinks and other beverages. In addition to food and beverages, life-style behaviors such as dieting, abuse of alcohol, smoking, and substance abuse affect nutritional status and should be assessed.

Information on nutritional requirements during adolescent pregnancy is limited. Nutritional needs for the young adolescent (12 to 14 years old) are higher than those of the woman whose growth has been completed. Although the recommended daily allowances (RDAs) are based on chronologic age, they provide the best available figures to use if the pregnant female is growing. A high proportion of pregnant teens, particularly low-income teens (Schneck et al, 1990), are nutritionally at risk and require nutrition intervention early and throughout their pregnancies. Adolescents' diets tend to be inadequate, particularly in iron and folic acid (Jackson and Mathur, 1991).

Health care providers should use specific, reliable procedures for obtaining and recording weight and height and should implement them consistently in classifying women according to weight for height, setting weight gain goals, and monitoring weight gain over the course of pregnancy (Institute of Medicine, 1990).

Psychosocial status. Psychosocial screening includes assessment for response to pregnancy, depression, or suicide. The nurse should also assess the adolescent's cognitive-developmental level, literacy, problem-solving ability, time orientation, body image, dependency, and peer and partner relationships.

In addition to body changes associated with puberty, the body changes associated with pregnancy may lead to a negative body image. For adult women, body changes associated with pregnancy reflect growth and survival of the infant (Richardson, 1990). Pregnant teens may be ambivalent about the pregnancy. They may deny the pregnancy, which can have a negative influence on body image and may lead to decreased nutritional intake to limit weight gain (Gong, 1990).

The pregnant adolescent should also be assessed for previous sexual abuse. Recent studies have shown that adolescent females who have been sexually abused are at increased risk for teenage pregnancy (Boyer and Fine, 1992; Stevens-Simon and Reichert, 1994). Pregnant adolescents who have been sexually abused are more likely to report substance use during pregnancy and to give birth to smaller and less mature babies (Stevens-Simon and McAnarney, 1994). Signs and symptoms of previous abuse include repeated somatic complaints (e.g., headaches, insomnia, depression), delay in seeking prenatal care, a partner who does not want to leave the patient alone with the health care provider, and missed appointments (Parker et al, 1993; Pope and Brucker, 1991). A higher proportion (22%) of adolescents are physically or sexually abused during their pregnancy than are adult pregnant women (16%) (Parker et al, 1993). Physically or sexually abused women are more likely to enter prenatal care later than women who have not been abused. Women who have been abused before pregnancy are also more likely to be abused during pregnancy (Parker et al, 1993).

Studies show significant substance abuse among pregnant adolescents (Kokotailo and Adger, 1991). Young adolescents are most likely to drink on weekends with the intent of "getting drunk." Thus the pattern of substance abuse should be assessed. Weekend binge drinking patterns are of concern in relation to fetal alcohol syndrome.

Knowledge base and perceived needs. The adolescent is assessed for her knowledge of sexuality and reproduction, prenatal development, process of labor and delivery, and pain management during labor. Basic knowledge of these factors is important to help the pregnant adolescent understand more readily the additional changes that occur during pregnancy. The nurse should refer the pregnant adolescent to childbirth classes to prepare for labor and birth. Assessment of perceived learning needs reveals valuable information that may be used as the basis for planning and intervention.

Support systems. Emotional support, particularly from the family of origin, is extremely important to the pregnant adolescent. Persons in the support system, particularly the parents, boyfriend, or husband, can significantly influence pregnancy outcome. The nurse must assess how the pregnant adolescent perceives her role and the roles and level of support from others in her support system.

Many pregnant adolescents come from socially and economically deprived families. Appropriate use of health care resources and compliance with preventive health care measures may not be part of their health value system. The nurse can assist those adolescents at risk to begin to change their own behavior so that use of the health care delivery system and its resources enhance health and well-being.

Critical Thinking Exercises

PRENATAL ASSESSMENT OF PREGNANT ADOLESCENT

Select a pregnant teenager in the prenatal setting. Follow her during her prenatal visit. Collect the following information and compare with established norms.

1. Gravida and parity
2. Last menstrual period and expected date of confinement
3. Pattern of weight gain
4. Range of blood pressure from first visit to present
5. Urine protein concentration
6. Fundal height
7. Fetal heart rate
8. Hematocrit, hemoglobin, blood type, Rh factor, and rubella titer
9. Medical problems that could have an impact on this pregnancy
10. Problems with previous pregnancies that could have an impact on this pregnancy
11. Other relevant findings

Physical examination. Physical assessment is the same as for the adult pregnant woman. Careful determination of baseline blood pressure is necessary because adolescents have lower systolic and diastolic pressures than do older women. An adolesçent could be in serious jeopardy for eclampsia with a blood pressure reading of 140/90 mm Hg.

Laboratory tests. Screenings are similar to those for the adult pregnant woman and should include hemoglobin and hematocrit levels, white blood cell and differential count, blood type, Rh factor, and antibody screen; rubella titer; serologic test for syphilis; urinalysis and urine culture; Pap smear; and vaginal or rectal smear for *Neisseria gonorrhoeae*, β-streptococcal, and chlamydial infections. A 1-hour glucose tolerance test should be obtained at 28 weeks' gestation to screen for gestational diabetes. HIV testing, tuberculin skin testing, and sickle cell screening may also be recommended for patients at risk (Van Winter and Simmons, 1990).

Nursing Diagnoses

The information gathered during the assessment, along with laboratory data, is analyzed and provides the basis for formulating nursing diagnoses. Nursing diagnoses relevant to the pregnant adolescent might include the following:

- Body-image disturbance related to
  - Pregnancy
- Post-trauma response related to
  - Physical or sexual abuse
- Altered family processes related to
  - Birth of infant to teenage mother
- Risk for altered nutrition: less than body requirements related to
  - Combined nutritional demands of teenage pregnancy and growth in the very young adolescent
  - Low socioeconomic status
- Altered growth and development related to
  - Loss of independence and disruption of peer relationships secondary to pregnancy
- Decisional conflict related to
  - Parenthood
  - Adoption
  - Abortion
- Altered health maintenance related to
  - Low socioeconomic status
  - Lack of access and availability of health care services
- Noncompliance with therapeutic regimen related to
  - Inadequate knowledge
  - Lack of social support
- Knowledge deficit: antepartum, intrapartum, postpartum, newborn care related to
  - Lack of experience

Expected Outcomes

The plan of care reflects the adolescent mother's need for increased surveillance, compliance with health care measures, and feelings of personal and social integrity. The care begins as early as possible in the prenatal period and extends through the formative period of the new family.

Whenever possible, expected outcomes for care are mutually determined. These expected outcomes may include the following. The adolescent will:

1. Demonstrate acceptance of changes in the body as a result of pregnancy (e.g., posture, grooming, dress)
2. Demonstrate clear communication with her family and will effectively resolve problems
3. Express her fears, anger, and guilt about previous sexual abuse and will identify and contact appropriate support persons/resources
4. Have adequate weight gain with hemoglobin level >11.0 g/dl
5. Seek prenatal care in the first trimester
6. Demonstrate behavior appropriate to her developmental level
7. Keep appointments for prenatal and postpartum care
8. Give birth to an infant whose birth weight is appropriate for gestational age
9. Identify and contact support systems in her community
10. Verbalize understanding of teaching related to antepartum, intrapartum, postpartum, and newborn care
11. Demonstrate appropriate self-care and newborn care

Plan of Care and Implementation

Health care professionals who work with pregnant adolescents must come to terms with their own sexuality so they can maintain a nonjudgmental approach. They should be genuinely interested in the adolescent—enthusiastic, warm, caring individuals able to view adolescents as young people worthy of respect and dignity. Nurses must be able to listen and respond with honest answers. If possible, the nurse should be available to the adolescent by telephone. An environment of trust will enable the adolescent to discuss her true feelings and enable the health care professional to determine the adolescent's real problems and set realistic goals. Knowledge of adolescent development allows the nurse to accept normal adolescent behavior rather than view it as "acting out."

Nurses must be adept in using various teaching strategies. Group discussions meet the adolescent's strong need for peer contact and acceptance. Anonymous questions and pretests can be used to identify knowledge deficits or beliefs in myths. Demonstrations by the nurse with return demonstrations by the teen facilitate assessment of the adolescent's abilities. It is important to use simple, concrete, direct language. Using correct terminology for body parts and giving direct answers to questions communicates respect. Because young adolescents have short attention spans, educational sessions should be short—15 minutes or less. In addition, stimulation of more than one of the senses by using multimethod approaches and active participation by the adolescent are helpful. For example, the use of visual models, films, charts, and role playing helps to reinforce learning and fits with the concrete cognitive style of young adolescents. Written instructional materials such as brochures and visual teaching aids should be attractive, bright in color, and contain more pictures than words. The comic book format may appeal to the very young adolescent.

Because the young adolescent is narcissistic, focusing on the needs of the fetus tends to be less successful than focusing on her own needs. Nurses must help the adolescent improve her decision-making ability, explore the risks and consequences of her actions, and assume responsibility for her behavior. Some of the techniques used to encourage growth in these areas include having the adolescent select a menu, choose appropriate types of clothing for the infant for a certain temperature, and discuss solutions to real problems. The nurse also can assist the adolescent in separating herself from her baby so that she can see the child's unique needs. Information relative to child development and to infant caregiving is basic to this goal.

Prenatal care. Risk factors, such as preeclampsia and poor nutritional status, have been linked with inadequate prenatal care (Nord et al, 1992; Roberts, 1994). In 1992 only 59% of mothers under the age of 20 years initiated prenatal care in the first trimester. In comparison, 86% of mothers age 30 to 39 years initiated prenatal care in the first trimester (Ventura et al, 1994). A study identifying barriers to prenatal care indicated that teens who received inadequate prenatal care were more likely to be confused about available services and medical coverage than teens who received better prenatal care (Kinsman and Slap, 1992). Those who received inadequate care were also more likely to think that prenatal care was unimportant, to have negative attitudes toward physicians, to have late recognition of pregnancy, and to rely on their families for prenatal advice. In addition, the teenage mothers who received inadequate prenatal care placed more importance on an "adolescent only" clinic than did other teens (Kinsman and Slap, 1992).

Attracting teens to prenatal care may improve maternal and infant outcomes (Morris et al, 1993). Teens who were referred to a special teenage clinic initiated prenatal care earlier and had more visits than teens who attended a traditional clinic (Morris et al, 1993). Although the researchers did not find differences between the two groups in health outcomes, the authors acknowledge that teenage clinics may help to build social networks and supportive relationships that may impact long-term outcomes. O'Sullivan and Jacobsen (1992)

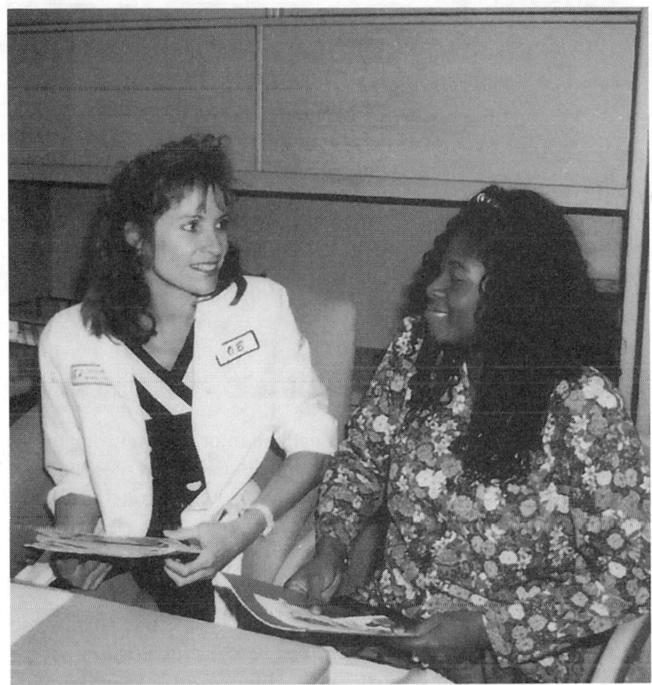
A

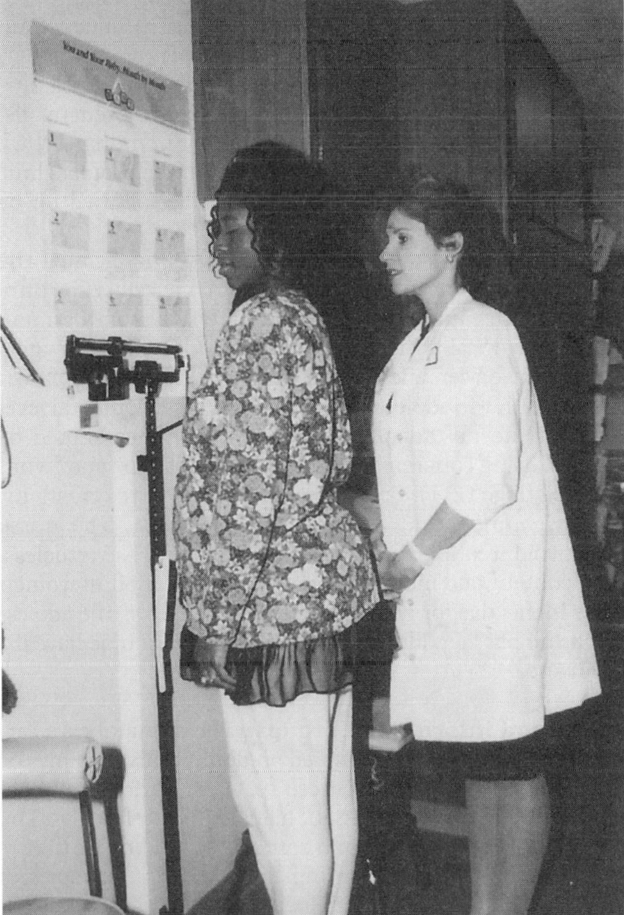
B

Fig. 12-1 Teenage expectant mothers learn about maternal adaptations to pregnancy. **A,** Expectant mother and nurse discuss prenatal concerns. **B,** Weighing in during a clinic visit. (Courtesy Marjorie Pyle, RNC, Lifecircle, Costa Mesa, Calif.)

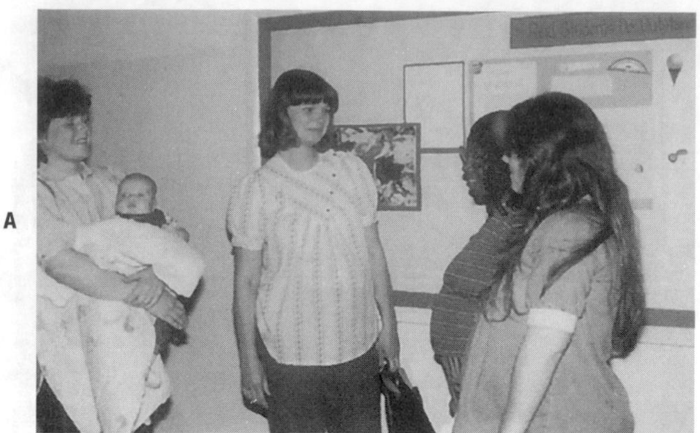

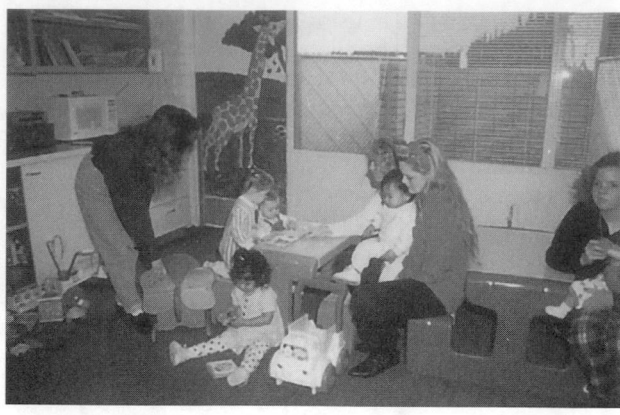

Fig. 12-2 A support and information group meeting for pregnant and parenting adolescents. **A,** Sharing experiences in prenatal clinic may decrease anxiety for teenage mothers. **B,** Teenage mothers learn child care in a day care facility. (Courtesy Marjorie Pyle, RNC, Lifecircle, Costa Mesa, Calif.)

found that teens who received rigorous follow-up with a nurse practitioner–managed program had (1) higher attendance at the scheduled 2-week visit with the infant's pediatrician, (2) infants who were fully immunized at 18 months, and (3) fewer visits to the emergency room for infant illness than teens who received routine care.

The very young adolescent is considered to be at risk during her pregnancy, and an increased number of prenatal visits should be scheduled (Van Winter and Simmons, 1990). Significant efforts should be made to encourage prompt clinic attendance; missed appointments should be followed up by telephone calls or personal contacts.

Adolescents are likely to obtain more adequate care if the prenatal site is attractive and inviting and if special efforts are made to register and retain them in care (Cartoof, Klerman, and Zazuela, 1991). Incentive programs that offer baby gifts or money have been effective. The content of prenatal classes is chosen with the adolescent's needs and developmental level in mind. Maternal adaptation during pregnancy should be discussed, using concrete examples of "what to do" and "what not to do" (Fig. 12-1). Prenatal education requires creativity, flexibility, humor, and at times, ego strength. The nurse should avoid treating the adolescent as a child. Nevertheless, typical content and methods of presentation for adult women may be ineffective for adolescents. For example, if the adolescent has no partner, films that depict a loving couple have little relevance.

Support and information groups. The prenatal care services already discussed are offered predominantly in clinics or in hospitals. In addition to these services, various self-help groups are available for pregnant teens and their families. The programs vary in structure and content, depending on the organization or agency sponsoring the program. Examples of group types include those that focus on the pregnant adolescent and her self-care, those addressing teenage parenting (which teens and their infants may attend together) (Fig. 12-2), and support groups for parents (of the pregnant adolescent) who learn how to cope and adapt to the experience (Fig. 12-3). Generally, group meetings are held on a weekly or monthly basis. Some hospitals or communities that do not currently offer such programs for adolescents may begin by designing their own or by purchasing prepackaged ones. Many of the prepackaged materials also include directions for staff training and technical assistance. For adolescents who receive little parental, partner, or peer support, as well as those who may have all these supports, such programs have proved highly effective in helping them and their families cope with the experiences associated with pregnancy and parenting.

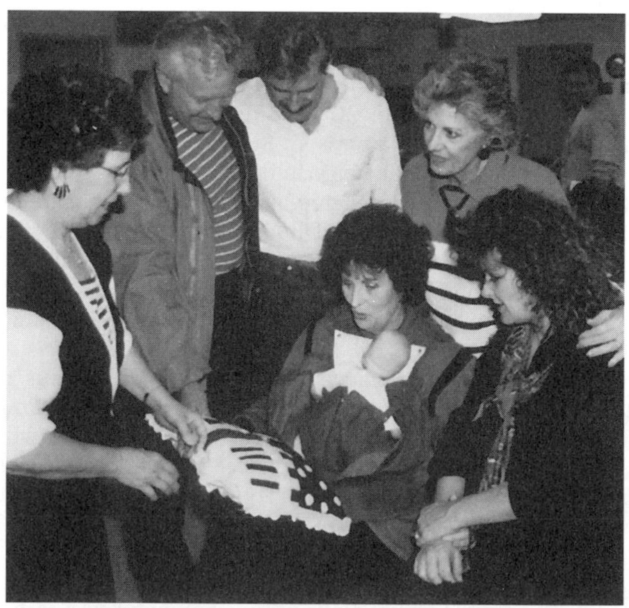

Fig. 12-3 Grandparent classes help grandparents-to-be update their knowledge and skill, such as teaching about infant stimulation (pillow is designed for infant stimulation). Grandparents discuss how best to help the adolescent with the developmental tasks of adolescence, pregnancy, and parenthood. (Courtesy Marjorie Pyle, RNC, Lifecircle, Costa Mesa, Calif.)

TABLE 12-1 Sample menus for pregnant adolescents

	DAY 1	DAY 2
Breakfast	1 cup unsweetened, ready-to-eat cereal with 1 cup 2% milk 3/4 cup orange juice	2 pancakes, 1 medium waffle, or 1 slice French toast 2 tbsp syrup 1 cup 2% milk
Snack	1 blueberry muffin 1 cup 2% milk	2 graham crackers 1 6-oz can apple juice
Lunch	1 cheeseburger (fast food) 1 banana Carrot sticks 1 cup 2% milk	3 slices pizza 1 apple Small salad 1 tbsp dressing 1 cup 2% milk
Snack	1 apple 3 tbsp peanut butter Caffeine-free soda*	1/2 cup cottage cheese dip Raw vegetables Caffeine-free soda*
Dinner	1 cup spaghetti with meat sauce Salad 2 tbsp dressing 1 roll 1/2 cup chocolate pudding 1 glass water†	3 oz baked chicken 1 cup rice 1 cup green beans 1 roll 1 ice cream sandwich 1 glass water†
Snack	1 slice angel food cake 1/2 cup fresh or frozen fruit, no sugar added Calories = 2525‡	3 cups popcorn 1 glass ginger ale Calories = 2568‡

*Sample diets should include foods that patients normally eat and, therefore, provide teaching opportunities about better choices (example: caffeinated beverage vs. caffeine-free drink).

†Encourage adequate water consumption daily—6 to 8 glasses.

‡Calorie calculations are based on the maximum allowance for growth; however, the best indication that a pregnant adolescent is eating sufficient calories is to monitor weight gain throughout pregnancy. If inadequate or excess weight gain occurs, consultation with a registered dietitian is recommended.

Nutrition counseling. The purpose of nutrition counseling is to increase the adolescent's knowledge of nutrients and ability to plan, select, and prepare optimally nutritive foods for herself and her family (Table 12-1). The nutritional needs of the mature (15 years and older) pregnant adolescent approach those of pregnant adults. Additional amounts of vitamins, minerals, and calories are needed to meet the growth needs of the pregnant adolescent and her fetus and to correct deficiencies resulting from inadequate intake of nutrients before, during, and after pregnancy. Iron supplements are needed to provide for the growing muscle mass and blood volume increase in the pregnant adolescent (Story, 1990). Most adolescent females consume at least one snack per day, with a range of one to seven. Snacks contribute more than "empty calories." Nutrients found in many of the snacks eaten by adolescent females contribute approximately half the RDA of riboflavin, vitamin C, and thiamin. Pregnant adolescents should be encouraged to eat nutritious snacks such as peanut butter crackers, cheese, fruit, and juice.

As an integral part of health care programs for pregnant adolescents, the nutrition consultant must be skillful in establishing rapport and developing a relationship that promotes effective patient counseling in the nutritional aspects of reproduction. Counseling should include setting a weight gain goal together with the pregnant adolescent, preferably at the initial prenatal examination, and explaining why weight gain is important. Additional strategies include building on cultural practices; categorizing nutrition practices as beneficial, neutral, or harmful; and reinforcing those practices that are positive and promoting change only in those that are harmful. Counseling should extend to the postpartum period to ensure a significant and lasting effect on the future of the parents and child.

Very young teens (younger than 15 years old) should gain at the upper end of recommended ranges (Gutierrez and King, 1993; Scholl et al, 1993). Weight gain should be plotted at each prenatal visit to detect erratic changes (Gutierrez and King, 1993). Erratic weight gain suggests fluid retention (Institute of Medicine [IOM], 1990). If the adolescent has an inadequate diet, vitamin and mineral supplements are recommended. Supplements should be taken between meals and at bedtime for best absorption (Gutierrez and King, 1993). Those with a recent weight loss and a body mass index (BMI) less than 19.8 should be evaluated for an eating disorder (Gutierrez and King, 1993).

Because energy expenditure for pregnant adolescents is so variable, the best assurance of adequate intake is a satisfactory weight gain. The recommended range of total weight gain and pattern of gain should be based mainly on prepregnancy weight for height. For women with a normal prepregnancy body mass index, a recommended gain at the rate of approximately 0.4 kg (1 lb) per week in the second and third trimesters of pregnancy is advised (IOM, 1990) (Table 12-2). Young adolescents and African-American women are encouraged to target their weight gain for the higher end of the appropriate range. Weight gain recommendations begin at 18 kg (40 lb) for an underweight adolescent, 16 kg (35 lb) for an adolescent of normal weight, and 11.5 kg (25 lb) for an

TABLE 12-2 Recommended weight gain for pregnant adolescents

PREPREGNANCY WEIGHT FOR HEIGHT	LB	KG
Underweight (BMI < 19.8)	35-40	16-18
Normal weight (BMI 19.8 to 26)	30-35	11.5-16
Overweight (BMI > 26)	15-25	7.0-11.5

Data from Institute of Medicine: *Nutrition during pregnancy*, Washington, DC, 1990, National Academy Press; Story M, Alton I: Nutrition and the pregnant adolescent, *Contemp Nutr* 17(5):1, 1992.

overweight adolescent. Ferrous iron (30 mg daily) is recommended for all pregnant women. If the young adolescent has an inadequate diet, she may need multivitamins and folate. If the adolescent consumes less than 600 mg calcium (698 mg in 2 cups of milk) daily, calcium supplementation (600 mg daily) is indicated (IOM, 1990). Adolescents often begin pregnancy with depleted body reserves or are still growing. Young adolescents may require higher intakes throughout their pregnancy. In general, pregnant adolescents should consume not fewer than 2000 calories per day; in many cases, higher caloric intakes are needed.

By improving her own diet and that of her family, the young mother helps build the foundation for a healthier beginning for generations to follow. Referral to the Women, Infants, and Children (WIC) Program or other food supplementation programs may ensure that nutritious food is available in the home during pregnancy and the infant's first year.

Newborn feeding. Many adolescents initially respond negatively to the idea of breastfeeding. Fear of permanent alteration in the breasts, a view of breastfeeding as "dirty," other misconceptions, and a lack of role models all contribute to the failure to choose breastfeeding as an option. Peer reactions or negative responses from the spouse or boyfriend are other factors. Thus bottle-feeding is often the feeding method chosen. The nurse may help the adolescent weigh the realities of breastfeeding, such as 24-hour commitment, against the realities of continuing her education. For successful breastfeeding the adolescent's family and school must work together. For example, the nurse may need to help the lactating adolescent arrange accommodations for pumping her breasts at school. The adolescent with a preterm infant may be encouraged to pump her breasts. All teens need much support for breastfeeding, especially after leaving the hospital. When identified counseling needs are beyond the nurse's scope, the adolescent is referred to a counselor who deals effectively with adolescents.

Labor and birth. The very young adolescent may be frightened of needles, pelvic examinations, noises from other women in labor or from equipment, and birth rooms. Single, private rooms should be provided when possible. The adolescent in labor should have the support of a knowledgeable coach, perhaps her husband, friend, parent, or nurse. Many teenage women come to labor lacking preparation; they are fearful and often alone. If they are admitted early in the first stage, teaching about relaxation with contractions, ambulation, side-lying positions, and comfort measures can be accomplished. The adolescent may be more concerned with how the baby will get out than with fetal well-being. Even though she may show an intense response to the contractions, the adolescent is trusting and will follow suggestions. Anticipatory guidance and explanation of all procedures before they are administered should always be a component of the nurse's care. Adolescents are usually responsive to staff members' sharing in their delight about the infant. For these young parents, efforts to promote parent-child attachment are particularly important.

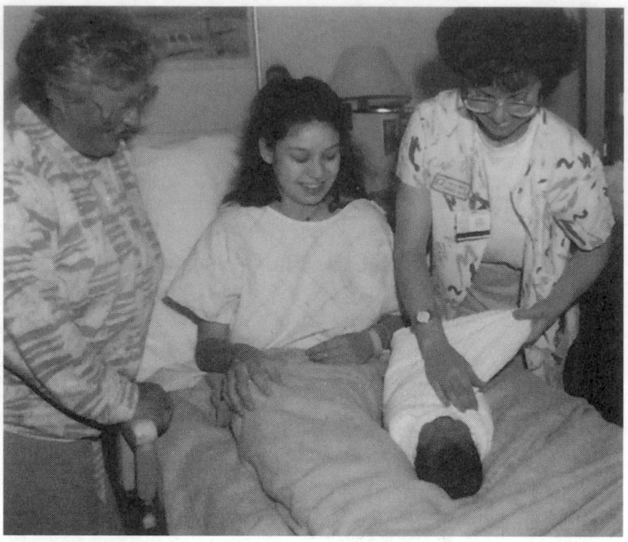

Fig. 12-4 Role modeling by the nurse and grandparent supports the adolescent's transition into parenthood. (Courtesy Marjorie Pyle, RNC, Lifecircle, Costa Mesa, Calif.)

Postpartum care. Physically the adolescent mother requires the same care as any woman who has given birth. Explicit directions for self-care and infant care are required. Most adolescents view the care of the infant as their primary area of concern. The need for continued assessment of the new mother's parenting abilities during the postbirth period is essential. In addition, continued support should be provided by involving grandparents (Fig. 12-4) or other family members through home visits and group sessions for discussion of infant care and parenting problems. Outreach programs concerned with self-care, parent-child interactions, child injuries, and instances of failure to thrive, as well as those that provide prompt and effective community intervention, prevent more serious problems.

Postpartum contraception is a high priority in very young adolescents. The risk of repeat pregnancy in adolescence is very high, and all the accompanying risks of adolescent pregnancy increase with each subsequent pregnancy. Almost universally, postpartum adolescents say they will never have sex again and therefore "need no birth control." Nevertheless, adolescents need to leave the hospital with barrier methods (foam and condoms) and the knowledge of how and when to use them. Very young adolescents may be too shy or embarrassed about touching their genitals to use a barrier method.

Critical Thinking Exercises 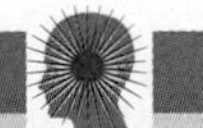

CONTRACEPTION FOR THE ADOLESCENT

A sexually experienced adolescent woman asks you which method of birth control she should use. Develop a teaching plan designed to help the adolescent make an informed decision about which contraceptive to use.

In addition, they will not likely anticipate intercourse. Adolescents may also be given a prescription of oral contraceptives with clear instructions on how to use them. Norplant may also be inserted or Depo-Provera administered before discharge. Since there is controversy about the use of hormonal contraception during lactation, breastfeeding adolescent mothers should be instructed to use spermicides and barrier methods until lactation is well established. Once lactation is established, breastfeeding adolescents can be started on progestin-only contraception (Hatcher et al, 1994). Thus the decision must be based on the individual adolescent and her life situation. Adolescent males must be considered and included in any interventions in sexuality education, family planning, and parent education.

Adoption. The adolescent will need support if she is contemplating adoption for her child. Health professionals must avoid using phrases that give negative connotations to the adoption process. Phrases such as "put up for adoption" and "give up for adoption" imply a callous, uncaring, insensitive biologic parent. Neither should the terms "real or natural parents" be used exclusively for genetic parents. The adoptive parents are the "real parents" because they care for the child. Neutral language such as "arranging for an adoption," "biologic parent" or "birth mother," and "adoptive parent" are preferred. The mother is given the option of either remaining on the postpartum floor or transferring to another unit. She is assured that she will have as much access to the baby as she desires.

Grief. Grief results from change or actual or perceived loss. The adolescent may experience grief brought on by the contemplation of adoption, giving birth to a preterm infant who may be in the intensive care unit, or the death of the infant. The nurse can help the birth mother move through the grieving process. The adolescent who gives birth to a preterm infant or one who is SGA may find it extremely difficult to reconcile this tiny, scrawny infant with her fantasized "Gerber" baby. She may experience fear over the thought of caring for the child introduced to her in the intensive care unit. The confidence and trust in her abilities gained during the prenatal period may be replaced with feelings of being overwhelmed and incompetent. The consequent alienation of mother and infant may never be overcome. Intensive teaching and continuous support programs are essential if the young mother and her vulnerable infant are not to be estranged.

Many young mothers pattern their practice on what they themselves experienced. It is vital, therefore, to determine the kind of support that those close to these young mothers are able or prepared to give and the kinds of community aid that can supplement this support. The adolescent may have conflict with dependency vs. independency issues as she performs her mothering role within the framework of her family of origin. The adolescent's family of origin also may need assistance in adapting to their new roles.

Evaluation

The nurse can be reasonably assured that care has been effective if the expected outcomes have been achieved; that is, if the adolescent:

- Demonstrates acceptance of changes in body as a result of pregnancy (e.g., posture, grooming, dress)
- Communicates clearly with her family and effectively resolves problems
- Expresses fears, anger, and guilt about previous abuse and can identify and contact appropriate support persons/resources
- Has adequate weight gain with hemoglobin level >11.0 g/dl
- Verbally acknowledges her pregnancy and seeks prenatal care in the first trimester
- Demonstrates behavior appropriate to developmental level
- Keeps appointments for prenatal and postpartum care
- Gives birth to an infant whose birth weight is appropriate for gestational age
- Identifies and contacts support systems in her community
- Verbalizes understanding of teaching related to antepartum, intrapartum, postpartum, and newborn care
- Demonstrates appropriate self-care and newborn care

TERTIARY PREVENTION WITH ADOLESCENT PARENTS

Adolescent Parenthood

The transition to parenthood may be difficult for adolescent parents. Coping with the developmental tasks of parenthood often is complicated by the unmet developmental needs and tasks of adolescence. These new parents may experience difficulty accepting a changing self-image and adjusting to new roles related to the responsibilities of infant care. They may feel different from their peers, excluded from activities, and forced prematurely to assume an adult social role. The conflict between their own desires and the demands of the infant and the low tolerance of frustration typical of adolescence further contribute to the normal psychosocial stress of childbirth.

Some differences between adolescent and adult mothers have been observed. For example, adolescents, although providing warm and attentive physical care, appear to use less verbal interaction than do older parents; in addition, they tend to be less responsive to their infants than are older mothers (Passino et al, 1993; Ruff, 1990). Psychologic aspects such as parenting attitudes and stress may play a role in how adolescents behave with their infants. East, Matthews, and Felice (1994) found that women who were teens at the time of their child's birth had little confidence in themselves as mothers and little confidence about their future relationship with their child. They also had maladaptive parenting attitudes such as valuing physical punishment, high expectations of their child's ability to nurture, and low empathy for their children's needs. The fact that teenage and adult mothers view their infants differently (e.g., teens view them as more fussy) and may respond to them inappropriately is caused by adolescents' limited knowledge of child development. For example, adolescents often expect too much of their children too soon.

Developmental Tasks of Parenthood

The **developmental tasks of parenthood** include (1) reconciling the imagined with the actual child, (2) becoming adept in caregiving activities, (3) being aware of the infant's needs, and (4) establishing oneself and one's infant as a family. Although it is biologically possible for the adolescent female to become a parent, her egocentricity and concrete thinking interfere with her ability to parent effectively. The very young adolescent is inexperienced and unprepared to recognize early signs of illness, potential danger, or household hazards. Children may be inadvertently neglected. The higher rates of infant mortality are attributed to the inexperience, lack of knowledge, and immaturity of the adolescent mother, resulting in her inability to recognize a problem and obtain necessary resources. Nevertheless, in most instances, with adequate support and developmentally appropriate teaching, effective parenting can be learned by adolescents.

Maintaining a relationship with the baby's father is beneficial for the mother and the child. Involvement of the father is related to appropriate maternal behaviors (Ruff, 1990).

The Extended Family

Childbearing in poor families often occurs without the supporting presence of the newborn's father. For very young adolescents, another member of the family may assume a significant role in the care of the infant. Commonly the baby's grandmother supports, coaches, or supervises the adolescent in her maternal role. Often the grandmother assumes the primary caretaker role if she considers the adolescent too immature or lacking in judgment to assume that role.

Nursing Care Management

Carrying the pregnancy to term and keeping the baby is one option in adolescent **sexual decision making.** Parenting ability is based on a parent's sensitivity to the infant's needs. Many factors can affect sensitivity, including stress, level of cognitive development, knowledge, infant responses, and support systems. Even though there are many books and much advice on the topic of parenting, households rarely precisely fit the descriptions of those portrayed in books. Nor are the suggestions and recommendations always appropriate. Thus parenting is a complex process that depends to a large degree on the decision-making ability of the parent within her own unique situation.

Assessment

Assessment of parenting abilities should include the following areas: the adolescent's ability to empathize with the child, her self-concept, her definition of and identification with the maternal role, her ability to problem solve and consider the child within the context of the future, and her support system. Ability to perform caregiving tasks such as feeding, stimulation, diapering, and nurturance of well and sick infants should also be assessed.

The adolescent's ability to function in a mothering role is affected by the level of stress she is experiencing. Adolescents are exposed to many stresses as they undertake the tasks and responsibilities of parenthood, a role that is best assumed by adults who are financially and educationally secure. Because stress can affect the quality of functioning, making the individual insensitive to the needs of others, the nurse should assess the type of stressors, the adolescent's reactions to the actual or perceived stress, her problem-solving ability, and her support system.

Nursing Diagnoses

Many different nursing diagnoses may evolve from the assessment data. Examples of nursing diagnoses that may apply include the following:

- Altered family processes related to
  Adaptation to teen parenthood
- Risk for altered parent/infant attachment related to
  Decreased communication with infant
- Altered role performance related to
  Lack of knowledge of maternal role
- Altered parenting related to
  Unrealistic expectations of normal infant behavior

Expected Outcomes

Mutual expected outcomes are developed on the basis of the adolescent's health care needs. Expected outcomes are stated in patient-centered terms and may include the following:

1. The adolescent's family will communicate effectively and provide support.
2. The adolescent will demonstrate appropriate interaction with her baby.
3. The adolescent will demonstrate appropriate role performance.

Plan of Care and Implementation

Because adolescents may resent the attention paid to a new baby, the nurse must demonstrate to the adolescent that she is still important. This will help establish the trust and cooperation necessary for future interaction and teaching. Before discussing topics about the care of the infant, the nurse should inquire about the adolescent and her friends, school, and social life and allow her to discuss her feelings and responses to the labor and birth process. Nurses can act as role models for adolescent parents in caring for themselves and their infants. Areas of particular importance for the mother are healthy life-styles, cleanliness, and good eating habits. The nurse's physical assessment skills can be taught to the adolescent parent so that she becomes more knowledgeable about her child's needs. Very young adolescents lack the expertise and maturity to provide 24-hour-a-day care for a child. High-risk, LBW, or preterm infants require even more care from their mothers than do term infants.

The adolescent's egocentricity makes it difficult for her to separate her own thoughts, feelings, and needs from those of the baby. She may attribute very sophisticated thought processes to the infant. It is not uncommon for the adolescent to make statements such as, "He doesn't like breast milk," "He is just crying to get attention," or "She is just doing that to make me stay home." The adolescent may try to feed her infant foods that she (the adolescent) likes—for example, pizza, soda, or potato chips—thereby placing the child in danger of choking. The nurse must attempt to demonstrate in a concrete manner the infant's limited physical and cognitive abilities. Listing specific foods that should and should not be fed to the infant is helpful.

Because adolescent mothers tend to be less sensitive and less communicative with their infants, interventions that emphasize verbal and nonverbal communication skills between mother and child are important. Because of the adolescent's own cognitive level, such intervention strategies must be concrete and specific. The neonatal behavioral assessment scale (Brazelton and Nugent, 1996) is widely used to help parents become aware of the infant's methods to communicate need and satisfaction and to see the newborn as an interactive partner. Physical self-care and infant care are essential topics that must be covered in very direct language. For some, good hygiene is a topic that must be covered in depth. Demonstrations of baby care techniques, with return demonstrations, are essential.

Because other family members may share or take on the primary caretaker role of the infant (with or without the permission of the adolescent mother), it is important to assess the adolescent's feelings about the situation and to facilitate discussion about such arrangements with the family to increase open communication and a positive experience for all involved.

Adolescent fathers. Nursing care includes the father of the child. As with the mother, the nurse must be aware of the male adolescent's cognitive-developmental levels, values, and culture.

The adolescent father, as well as the adolescent mother, is faced with immediate developmental crises: completing the developmental tasks of adolescence and making a transition to parenthood and, sometimes, to marriage. These transitions can be stressful. The nurse can initiate interaction with the adolescent father by asking the pregnant adolescent to bring the father of the baby to the clinic with her so that he may participate in the birth (Fig. 12-5). With the pregnant teen's agreement, the father may also be contacted directly. Data needed for inclusion of the young father in all aspects of the care are based on assessment of four areas: (1) the couple's relationship; (2) levels of stress, concern, and coping; (3) educational and vocational goals; and (4) the level of health education knowledge. Adolescent fathers (as all fathers) need support to discuss their emotional responses to the pregnancy. The nurse's nonjudgmental attitude is essential for open communication. The father's feelings of guilt, powerlessness, or bravado should be recognized because of their negative consequences for both parents and child. Counseling must be reality oriented. Topics such as finances, child care, parenting skills, and the father's role in the birth experience need to be discussed. Teenage fathers also require knowledge regarding reproductive physiology and birth control options.

The adolescent mother's partner, as well as her family, affects how she will deal with her pregnancy, labor and birth, and subsequent parenthood. The adolescent partner may

LEGAL TIP

Legal Issues Related To Adolescents

Emancipated minors

Minors who are married, who are in the military service, or who are living away from home and are self-supporting may be considered legally emancipated from their parents. These minors are considered mature enough to consent to their own medical care, and their parents have no legal liability to pay the bill for health care services.

Confidentiality

The Constitution protects an adolescent's right to privacy. Health care information about adolescent patients is to be kept confidential. However, parents who give consent for and pay for their children's health care are entitled to be informed about that care. They also are entitled to request and receive a copy of the adolescent's medical records. The nurse who cares for adolescents should be familiar with federal law and state statutes.

Contraception and abortion

In most states, it is legal to provide contraceptive services to minors. The role of the nurse is to determine that the minor understands the risks associated with the contraceptive as well as the associated chance of pregnancy.

Laws regarding a minor's consent to abortion are complex and vary across states. Some state statutes may require parental consent; others require parental notification before an unemancipated minor may obtain an abortion. Sterilization law also varies across states. Some states prohibit the elective sterilization of any person younger than 18 years of age. Usually the request and consent must be in writing. Federal law prohibits federal reimbursement for any sterilization of a person younger than 21 years of age (42 Code of Federal Regulations, 1989). It is each nurse's responsibility to be aware of these laws and to refer adolescent patients to legal counsel, if necessary, to ensure that their patient's rights are protected.

Retaining child custody

The adolescent mother can authorize or refuse medical treatment for her infant, regardless of her age or marital status.

Adoption

State law determines the procedures for adoption. Adoption options available to the mother include the following: agency vs. private adoption and arrangements varying from closed adoption (no sharing of any identifying information between parties and no possibility of meeting in the future) to a very open adoption (in which the birth mother may visit her child and the adoptive family regularly), as well as any combination of these options. The nurse should assess the mother's understanding of her adoption options and assist in making the appropriate referrals.

continue to be involved in an ongoing relationship with the young mother. In many instances, he plays an important role in the decisions she faces in pregnancy. He may influence her decision to continue the pregnancy, to have an abortion, to keep the child, or to place the child for adoption.

Acknowledgement of paternity is the first sign of responsibility for an absent father (Adams, Pittman, and O'Brien, 1993). Acknowledgement of paternity can be formal (legal) or informal. Legal establishment of paternity provides legal benefits for the child, such as the right to child support. Additional benefits, such as the right to Social Security benefits and veteran's benefits, are easier to obtain if paternity has been legally established. Nonfinancial benefits include access to information about family medical history and establishing legal rights to custody and visitation (Adams, Pittman, and O'Brien, 1993).

Nursing Care Plan

ADOLESCENT PREGNANCY

Nursing Diagnosis: Risk for altered growth and development related to interruption of focus on developmental tasks secondary to pregnancy

Expected Outcome: **Patient displays evidence of continuing identity formation (i.e., modifications in body image, definition of gender role, stabilizing self-esteem, projection of implications of current behavior) and desire for independence (i.e., ongoing peer relationships, detachment from parents).**

• **NURSING INTERVENTIONS/*RATIONALES***

Provide an environment conducive for interaction, including privacy and absence of parents *to encourage continued parental detachment and independence and establish trust relationship with health care provider.*

Approach teen in an adult manner, provide complete explanations of treatments and procedures, and encourage questions about options, alternatives, and fears *as she is developmentally capable of abstract thought and this encourages a sense of independence.*

Actively involve the teen in decision making and planning and impose as few restrictions as possible *to encourage independence and help her maintain a sense of control.*

Introduce teen to other teens who are pregnant or are new mothers *to establish continuing peer relationships that aid in establishing independence and provide a picture of the future.*

Accept the vacillations between childish and adult methods of coping *as part of the adolescent developmental process.*

Examine effects that impending parenthood has on life-style and have teen verbalize possible scenarios *to aid in focusing on and planning for the immediate future.*

Encourage participation of father of the baby in the pregnancy *to provide support for the teenage mother.*

Nursing Diagnosis: Risk for body image disturbance related to interaction of changes of pregnancy and adolescence

Expected Outcome: **Patient accepts and incorporates changing body into self-image.**

• **NURSING INTERVENTIONS/*RATIONALES***

Assess teen's current perceptions and feelings about body changes occurring in adolescence and pregnancy *to provide an assessment baseline and direct any needed intervention.*

Provide opportunities for teen to verbalize feelings *to explore concerns, fears, and self-doubts.*

Discuss anticipated body changes that will occur as pregnancy progresses *to prepare teen for changes and to increase feelings of control.*

Help teen to change and adapt self-care routines *to facilitate incorporation of body changes (i.e., diet, exercise, rest routines).*

Nursing Diagnosis: Risk for situational low self-esteem related to alterations in body image and role performance secondary to pregnancy and adolescence

Expected Outcome: **Patient will maintain positive self-evaluation appropriate for developmental level.**

• **NURSING INTERVENTIONS/*RATIONALES***

Assess teen's current perceptions and feelings about self *to provide assessment baseline and direct needed intervention.*

Provide opportunities for teen to verbalize feelings *to explore concerns, fears, and self-doubts.*

Have teen describe experiences that make her feel worthwhile and good about herself *to reinforce positive self-evaluation.*

Demonstrate empathy, interest in, and concern about teen *to enhance trust building.*

Listen carefully, remain nonjudgmental, and encourage and praise teen's successes *to demonstrate caring and involvement.*

Actively involve teen in all aspects of her care *to encourage feelings of independence and competence.*

Encourage teen to maintain and/or form peer relationships *as a developmentally appropriate outlet for verbalization of fears and feelings.*

Assist teen to identify additional support systems (i.e., Aid to Families with Dependent Children [AFDC], WIC, home health care, psychologic counselors, guidance counselors, and tutors) *that can assist the adolescent in adapting to motherhood and aid adolescent development.*

If teen is single, encourage her to choose one person who can attend prenatal care and prenatal classes, assist in labor and delivery, and participate in child care activities with her *to promote consistent support system.*

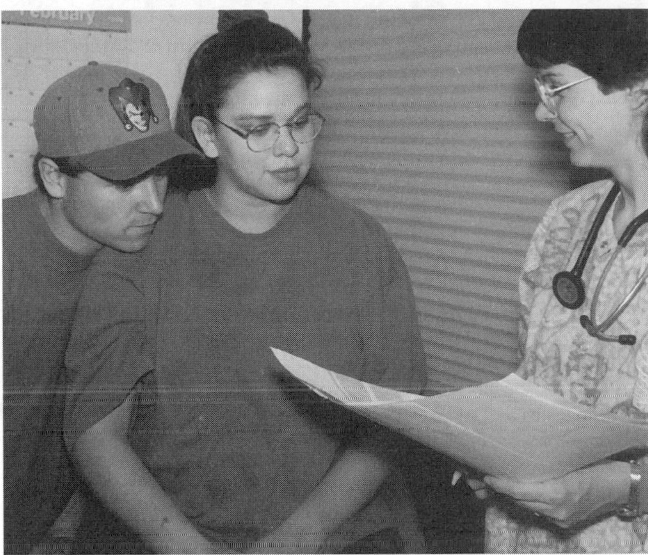

Fig. 12-5 Adolescent father with pregnant teen at a prenatal clinic visit. (Courtesy Michael S. Clement, MD, Mesa, Ariz.)

The nurse supports the young father by helping him develop realistic perceptions of his role as "father to a child." The nurse encourages his use of coping mechanisms that are not detrimental to his, his partner's, and his child's well-being. The nurse enlists support systems, parents, and professional agencies on his behalf. Encouraging mutual responsibility for birth control is a constant necessity.

The nurse must be familiar with federal and state laws regarding legal issues associated with pregnant adolescents.

Evaluation

Perinatal nurses must evaluate the care they provide to the adolescent patient to assess the effectiveness of their nursing actions. Nurses can be reasonably assured that care was effective to the extent that the expected outcomes of care have been met; that is, the adolescent's family communicates effectively and provides support, and the adolescent demonstrates appropriate interaction with her baby and appropriate role performance (see the Nursing Care Plan on p. 332).

Critical Thinking Exercises

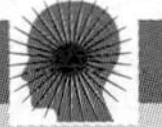

ADOLESCENT MOTHER-INFANT INTERACTION

Observe an interaction between an adolescent mother and her infant. Compare the verbal and nonverbal interaction you observe with the literature on maternal-infant interaction.

Key Points

- Adolescents see their world in far different terms than do adults; their major tasks are the development of cognitive ability and identity formation.
- Cognitive development influences sexual decision making.
- Increasingly, poverty, life-style, and risk-taking behaviors are implicated in adolescent morbidity, with associated sequelae of pregnancy and other major health problems.
- The majority of teenage pregnancies are unintended; many are the result of sexual intercourse with an adult male.
- The physiologic consequences and personal and public costs of adolescent pregnancy and parenthood are staggering.
- The adolescent's perception of pregnancy and parenthood is individual and depends on many variables.
- The developmental tasks of adolescents are interrupted by pregnancy.
- Inadequate prenatal care, poor nutrition, and poverty have been implicated in negative physiologic consequences for the adolescent mother and her fetus and newborn.
- Adolescents' reactions to perceived stress depend on the quality of their support systems, their self-esteem, and their skill in problem identification and problem solving.
- The adolescent's knowledge of child development usually is limited.
- Standard approaches to prenatal and postpartum teaching are not appropriate or appealing for most adolescents.

References

Adams G, Pittman K, O'Brien R: *Adolescent and young adult fathers: problems and solutions.* In Lawson A, Rhode D, editors: *The politics of pregnancy: adolescent sexuality and public policy,* New Haven, Ct, 1993, Yale University Press.

Alan Guttmacher Institute: *Sex and America's teenagers,* New York, 1994, The Institute.

Armstrong K, Stover M: SMART START: an option for adolescents to delay the pelvic examination and blood work in family planning clinics, *J Adolesc Health* 15(5):389, 1994.

Beach R: Breast exam: protect, reassure, educate, *Contemp OB GYN* 35:41, 1990.

Beard J: Iron deficiency: assessment during pregnancy and its importance in pregnant adolescents, *Am J Clin Nutr* 59(suppl):502S, 1994.

Berger K: *The developing person through the lifespan,* New York, 1994, Worth Publishing.

Boyer D, Fine D: Sexual abuse as a factor in adolescent pregnancy and child maltreatment, *Fam Plann Perspect* 24(1):4, 1992.

Brazelton T, Nugent J: *Neonatal behavioural scale,* ed 3, London, 1996, MacKeith Press.

Cartoof V, Klerman L, Zazueta V: The effect of source of prenatal care on care-seeking behavior and pregnancy outcomes among adolescents, *J Adolesc Health* 12:124, 1991.

Centers for Disease Control: Premarital sexual experience among adolescent women—United States, 1970-1988, *MMWR* 39(51, 52):929, 1991a.

Centers for Disease Control: *Survey: teen health and sex habits,* Atlanta, 1991b, U.S. Dept. of Health & Human Services.

Centers for Disease Control: *Division of STD/HIV Prevention annual report,* Atlanta, 1993, U.S. Dept. of Health & Human Services.

Dryfoos J: *Adolescents at risk: prevalence and prevention,* New York, 1990, Oxford University Press.

Durant R et al: Contraceptive behavior among sexually active Hispanic adolescents, *J Adolesc Health Care* 11:490, 1990.

East P, Matthews K, Felice M: Qualities of adolescent mothers' parenting, *J Adolesc Health* 15(2):163, 1994.

Erikson E: *Childhood and society,* New York, 1963, WW Norton.

Esman A: *Adolescence and culture,* New York, 1990, Columbia University Press.

Forrest J: Timing of reproductive life stages, *Obstet Gynecol* 82(1):105, 1993.

Forrest J, Singh S: The sexual and reproductive behavior of American women, 1982-1988, *Fam Plann Perspect* 22(5):206, 1990.

42 Code of Federal Regulations, 441.250-441.259, 1989.

Gilligan C: *In a different voice,* Cambridge, Mass, 1982, Harvard University Press.

Gong E: *Weight issues and management.* In Story M, editor: *Nutrition management of the pregnant adolescent,* White Plains, NY, 1990, March of Dimes.

Gutierrez Y, King J: Nutrition during teenage pregnancy, *Pediatr Ann* 22(2):99, 1993.

Hatcher R et al: *Contraceptive technology,* 16th rev ed, New York, 1994, Irvington Publishers.

Hayes C, editor: *Risking the future: adolescent sexuality, pregnancy, and childbearing,* vol I, Washington, DC, 1987, National Academy Press.

Hilliard P, Rebar R: Abnormal uterine bleeding needs a special approach, *Contemp OB GYN* 35:51, 1990.

Humenick S, Wilkerson N, Paul N, editors: *Adolescent pregnancy: nursing perspectives on prevention,* White Plains, NY, 1991, March of Dimes.

Institute of Medicine: *Nutrition during pregnancy,* Washington, DC, 1990, National Academy Press.

Jackson E, Mathur K: Adolescent pregnancy: effects of nutrients on hematocrit and birth weight, *J SC Med Assoc* 87:8, 1991.

Keller S et al: HIV-relevant sexual behavior among a healthy inner-city heterosexual adolescent population in an endemic area of HIV, *J Adolesc Health* 12(1):44, 1991.

Kinsman S, Slap G: Barriers to adolescent prenatal care, *J Adolesc Health* 13(2):146, 1992.

Kirby D: *School-based prevention programs: design, evaluation, and effectiveness.* In DiClemente R, editor: *Adolescents and AIDS: a generation in jeopardy,* Newbury Park, Calif, 1992, Sage Publications.

Kirby D et al: School-based programs to reduce sexual risk behaviors: a review of effectiveness, *Public Health Rep* 109(3):339, 1994.

Klepinger D, Lundberg S, Plotnick R: Adolescent fertility and the educational attainment of young women, *Fam Plann Perspect* 27(1):23, 1995.

Kochanek K, Hudson B: *Advance report of final mortality statistics, 1992. Monthly vital statistics report* 43(suppl 6), Hyattsville, Md, 1995, National Center for Health Statistics.

Kohlberg L: *Psychology of moral development: the nature and validity of moral stages,* San Francisco, 1984, Harper & Row.

Kokotailo P, Adger J: Substance use by pregnant adolescents, *Clin Perinatol* 18:125, 1991.

Koniak-Griffin D, Lominska S, Brecht M: Social support during adolescent pregnancy: a comparison of three ethnic groups, *J Adolesc* 16:43, 1993.

Kost K, Forrest J: American women's sexual behavior and exposure to risk of sexually transmitted diseases, *Fam Plann Perspect* 24(6):244, 1992.

Ku L, Sonenstein F, Pleck J: Young men's risk behaviors for HIV infection and sexually transmitted diseases, 1988 through 1991, *Am J Public Health* 83(11):1609, 1993.

Leigh B et al: Sexual behavior of American adolescents: results from a U.S. national survey, *J Adolesc Health* 15(2):117, 1994.

Lock S, Vincent M: Sexual decision-making among rural adolescent females, *Health Values* 19(1):47, 1995.

Miller B, Moore K: Adolescent sexual behavior, pregnancy, and parenting: research through the 1980's, *J Marriage Family* 52:1025, 1990.

Moore K, Snyder N, Glei D: *Facts at a glance,* Flint, Mich, February 1995, Charles Stewart Mott Foundation.

Morris D et al: Comparison of adolescent pregnancy outcomes by prenatal care source, *J Reprod Med* 38(5):375, 1993.

National Center for Health Statistics: *Advance report of the monthly vital statistics,* Washington, DC, 1990, U.S. Department of Health and Human Services, Public Health Service.

National Institute of Child Health and Human Development: *An evaluation and assessment of the state of the science: demographic and behavioral sciences,* Bethesda, Md, 1991, U.S. Government Printing Office.

Newcomer S, Baldwin W: Demographics of adolescent sexual behavior, contraception, pregnancy, and STD's, *J Sch Health* 62(7):265, 1992.

Nord C et al: Consequences of teenage parenting, *J Sch Health* 62(7):310, 1992.

O'Sullivan A, Jacobsen B: A randomized trial of a health care program for first time adolescent mothers and their infants, *Nurs Res* 41(4):210, 1992.

Overby K, Kegeles S: The impact of AIDS on an urban population of high-risk female minority adolescents: implications for intervention, *J Adolesc Health* 15(3):216, 1994.

Parker B et al: Physical and emotional abuse in pregnancy: a comparison of adult and teenage women, *Nurs Res* 42(3):173, 1993.

Passino A et al: Personal adjustment during pregnancy and adolescent parenting, *Adolescence* 28(109):97, 1993.

Perkins J: *Primary prevention of adolescent pregnancy.* In Humenick S, Wilkerson N, Paul N, editors: *Adolescent pregnancy: nursing perspectives on prevention,* White Plains, NY, 1991, March of Dimes.

Peterson L: *Contraceptive use in the United States: 1982-90. Advance data from vital and health statistics; no. 260,* Hyattsville, Md, 1995, National Center for Health Statistics.

Piaget J: *The intellectual development of the adolescent.* In Caplan G, Lebovici S, editors: *Adolescence: psychosocial perspectives,* New York, 1969, Basic Books.

Pope C, Brucker M: Adolescents as victims: an overview of the special impact of sexual abuse, *NAACOG's Clin Issues* 2(2):263, 1991.

Rees J et al: Weight gain in adolescents during pregnancy: rate related to birth-weight outcome, *Am J Clin Nutr* 56:868, 1992.

Richardson P: Women's experiences of body change during normal pregnancy, *Matern Child Nurs J* 19(2):93, 1990.

Roberts J: *Pregnancy-related hypertension.* In Creasy R, Resnik R, editors: *Maternal-fetal medicine: principles and practice,* Philadelphia, 1994, WB Saunders.

Ruff C: Adolescent mothering: assessing their parenting capabilities and their health education needs, *J Natl Black Nurses Assoc* 4:55, 1990.

Saftlas A et al: Epidemiology of preeclampsia and eclampsia in the United States, 1979-1986, *Am J Obstet Gynecol* 163(2):460, 1990.

Scholl T, Hediger M, Belsky D: Prenatal care and maternal health during adolescent pregnancy: a review and meta-analysis, *J Adolesc Health* 15(6):444, 1994.

Scholl T et al: Anemia vs. iron deficiency: increased risk of preterm delivery in a prospective study, *Am J Clin Nutr* 57:135, 1992.

Scholl T et al: *Growth and nutrition during adolescent pregnancy.* In Karp R, editor: *Malnourished children in the United States: caught in the cycle of poverty,* New York, 1993, Springer Publishing.

Schneck M et al: Low-income pregnant adolescents and their infants: dietary findings and health outcomes, *J Am Diet Assoc* 90:555, 1990.

Stevens-Simon C, McAnarney E: Childhood victimization: relationship to adolescent pregnancy outcome, *Child Abuse Negl* 18(7):569, 1994.

Stevens-Simon C, Reichert S: Sexual abuse, adolescent pregnancy, and child abuse: a developmental approach to an intergenerational cycle, *Arch Pediatr Adolesc Med* 148(1):23, 1994.

Story M: *Nutrition assessment of pregnant adolescents.* In Story M, editor: *Nutrition management of the pregnant adolescent,* White Plains, NY, 1990, March of Dimes.

Story M, Alton I: Nutrition and the pregnant adolescent, *Contemp Nutr* 17(5):1, 1992.

Tyre L, Rothbart B, Anderson K: Helping adolescents make the right contraceptive choice, *Contemp OB GYN* 35:37, 1990.

U.S. Department of Health and Human Services: *Healthy people 2000: national health promotion and disease prevention objectives* DHHS Publication No. PHS 91-50212, Washington, DC, 1990, U.S. Government Printing Office.

Van Winter J, Simmons P: A proposal for obstetric and pediatric management of adolescent pregnancy, *Mayo Clin Proc* 65:1061, 1990.

Ventura S, Martin J, Taffel S: *Advance report of final natality statistics, 1992: monthly vital statistics report* 43 (suppl 5), Hyattsville, Md, 1994, National Center for Health Statistics.

Weisman C et al: Consistency of condom use for disease prevention among adolescent users of oral contraceptives, *Fam Plann Perspect* 23(2):71, 1991.

Yawn B, Yawn R: Adolescent pregnancies in rural America: a review of the literature and strategies for primary prevention, *Fam Commun Health* 16(1):36, 1993.

Young E et al: The effects of family structure on the sexual behavior of adolescents, *Adolescence* 26(104):977, 1991.

Zabin L, Hayward S: *Adolescent sexual behavior and childbearing,* Newbury Park, Calif, 1993, Sage Publications.

Bibliography

Arenson J: Strengths and self-perceptions of parenting in adolescent mothers, *J Pediatr Nurs* 9(4):251, 1994.

Flanagan P et al: Communication behaviors of infants of teen mothers, *J Adolesc Health* 15(2):169, 1994.

Haskett M, Johnson C, Miller J: Individual differences in risk of child abuse by adolescent mothers: assessment in the perinatal period, *J Child Psychol Psychiatry* 35(3):461, 1994.

Jones M, Mondy L: Lessons for prevention and intervention in adolescent pregnancy: a five-year comparison of outcomes of two programs for school-aged pregnant adolescents, *J Pediatr Health Care* 8(4):152, 1994.

Lubarsky S et al: Obstetric characteristics among nulliparas under age 15, *Obstet Gynecol* 84(3):365, 1994.

Marshall E et al: Parenting and childrearing attitudes among high school students, *J Commun Health Nurs* 11(4):239, 1994.

Speiker S, Bensley L: Roles of living arrangements and grandmother social support in adolescent mothering and infant attachment, *Dev Psychol* 30(1):102, 1994.

CHAPTER 13

Essential Factors and Processes of Labor

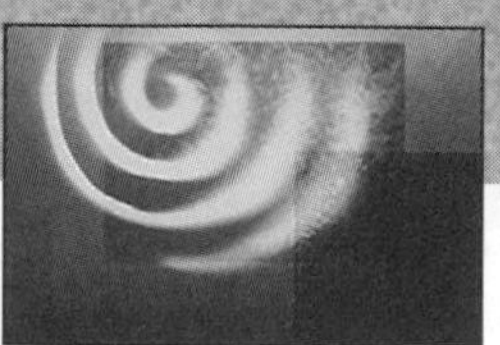

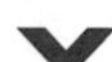

FACTORS AFFECTING LABOR, P. 336
Passenger, p. 336
Passageway, p. 338
Powers, p. 343
Position of the woman in labor, p. 345

PROCESS OF LABOR, P. 346
Signs preceding labor, p. 346
Theories of onset of labor, p. 346
Stages of labor, p. 347
Mechanism of labor, p. 347

PHYSIOLOGIC ADAPTATION TO LABOR, P. 349
Fetal adaptation, p. 349
Maternal adaptation, p. 349

During late pregnancy, the mother and the fetus prepare for the labor process. The fetus has grown and developed in preparation for extrauterine life. The mother has undergone various physiologic adaptations during pregnancy that prepare her for the process of birth and the role of motherhood. Labor and birth represent the end of pregnancy and the beginning of extrauterine life for the newborn infant.

Nurses must understand the factors affecting labor, the process involved, the normal progression of events, and the adaptations made by both the mother and fetus. Once this knowledge is mastered, nurses can apply the nursing process to each woman and her family.

FACTORS AFFECTING LABOR

Five factors affect the process of labor and birth. These are easily remembered as the five *Ps*: *p*assenger (fetus and placenta), *p*assageway (birth canal), *p*owers (contractions), *p*osition of the mother, and *p*sychologic response. The first four factors are presented here as the basis for understanding the physiologic process of labor. The fifth factor is discussed in Chapters 7, 11, and 16.

Passenger

How the *passenger*, or fetus, moves through the birth canal is a result of several interacting factors: size of the fetal head, fetal presentation, lie, attitude, and position.

Because the placenta must also pass through the birth canal, it may be considered a passenger along with the fetus. The placenta rarely impedes the process of labor in normal vaginal birth; however, some labors may be complicated by placenta previa or abruptio placentae (Chapter 9).

Size of fetal head. The fetal head, because of its size and relative rigidity, has a major effect on the birth process. The fetal skull is composed of two parietal bones, two temporal bones, the frontal bone, and the occipital bone (Fig. 13-1). These bones are united by membranous sutures: the sagittal, lambdoid, coronal, and frontal sutures. Membrane-filled spaces called **fontanels** are located where the sutures intersect. After rupture of membranes during labor, fetal presentation, position, and attitude may be palpated by fontanels and sutures during vaginal examination. Assessment of their size reveals information about the age and well-being of the newborn.

The two most important fontanels are the anterior and posterior fontanels. The larger of these, the anterior fontanel, is diamond-shaped and lies at the junction of the sagittal, coronal, and frontal sutures. It closes by 18 months after birth. The posterior fontanel lies at the junction of the sutures of the two parietal bones and the occipital bone and is triangular in shape. It closes 6 to 8 weeks after birth.

The presence of sutures and fontanels gives the skull flexibility to accommodate the infant brain, which continues to grow for some time after birth. Because the bones are not firmly united, however, slight overlapping of the bones, or **molding** of the shape of the head, occurs during labor. This capacity of the bones to slide over one another also permits adaptation to the various diameters of the maternal pelvis. Molding can be extensive, but with most newborns the head assumes its normal shape within 3 days of birth.

Although the size of the fetal shoulders may affect passage, their position can be altered relatively easily during labor so one shoulder occupies a lower level than the other. This creates a smaller shoulder diameter for negotiating the passage-

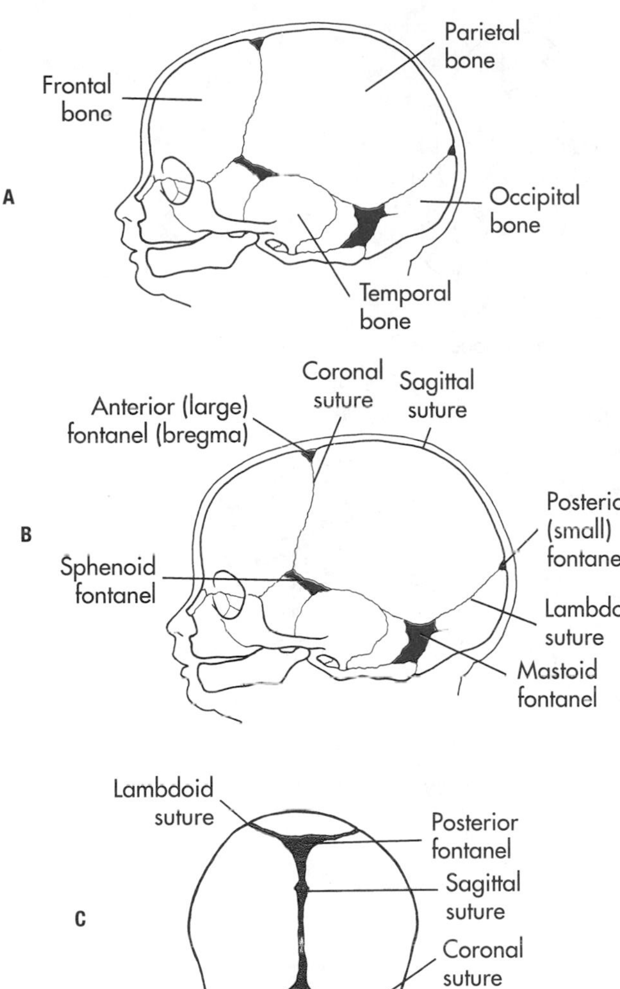

Fig. 13-1 Fetal head at term. **A,** Bones. **B** and **C,** Sutures and fontanels.

way. The circumference of the fetal hips is usually small enough not to create problems.

Fetal presentation. Presentation refers to the part of the fetus that enters the pelvic inlet first and leads through the birth canal during labor at term. The three main presentations are **cephalic** (head first), 96% (Fig. 13-2); **breech** (buttocks first), 3% (Figure 13-3, *A-C*); and shoulder, 1% (Fig. 13-3, *D*). **Presenting part** refers to that part of the fetal body first felt by the examining finger during a vaginal examination. In a cephalic presentation, the presenting part is usually the occiput; in a breech presentation, it is the sacrum; in the transverse lie, the presenting part is the scapula of the shoulder. When the presenting part is the occiput, the presentation is noted as **vertex** (Figs. 13-2; 13-4, *A;* and 13-5, *A*). Factors that determine the presenting part include fetal lie, fetal attitude, and extension or flexion or the fetus's head.

Critical Thinking Exercises

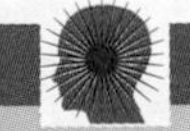

ASSESSMENT OF THE HEAD OF A NEWBORN

You are working in the newborn nursery. Select a baby and examine the head.

1. **Identify the suture lines and fontanels.**
2. **Differentiate between caput and molding if present.**
3. **Close your eyes and palpate the suture lines and fontanels. Visualize the position of the baby in relation to what you feel.**
4. **Explain how knowledge of the fetal head landmarks is used to determine the fetal position during vaginal examination during labor.**

Fetal lie. Lie is the relationship of the long axis (spine) of the fetus to the long axis (spine) of the mother. There are two lies: *longitudinal,* or vertical, in which the long axis of the fetus is parallel with the long axis of the mother; and *transverse,* or horizontal, in which the long axis of the fetus is at a right angle to that of the mother (Fig. 13-3, *D*). Longitudinal lies are either cephalic or sacral (breech) presentations, depending on the fetal structure that first enters the mother's pelvis. An oblique or unstable lie usually converts to a longitudinal or transverse lie during labor (Cunningham et al, 1993).

Fetal attitude. Attitude is the relationship of the fetal body parts to each other. The fetus assumes characteristic posture (attitude) in utero partly because of the mode of fetal growth and partly because of accommodation to the shape of the uterine cavity. Normally, the back of the fetus is markedly flexed: the head is flexed on the chest, the thighs are flexed on the abdomen, and the legs are flexed at the knees. The arms are crossed over the thorax, and the umbilical cord lies between the arms and the legs. This attitude is called *general flexion.*

Deviations from the normal attitude may cause difficulties in childbirth. For example, in a cephalic presentation the fetal head may be extended or flexed in a manner that presents a head diameter unfavorable to the limits of the maternal pelvis.

The **biparietal diameter** is the largest transverse diameter (Fig. 13-4, *B*). Of the anteroposterior diameters shown, it can be seen that the attitudes of flexion or extension allow diameters of differing sizes to enter the maternal pelvis. For example, with the head in complete flexion, the **suboccipitobregmatic diameter** (the smallest anteroposterior diameter) enters the true pelvis easily (Figs. 13-4, *A;* 13-5, *A*).

Fetal position. The presentation or presenting part indicates the portion of the fetus that overlies the pelvic inlet. **Position** is the relationship of the presenting part (occiput, sacrum, mentum [chin], or sinciput [deflexed vertex]) to the four quadrants of the mother's pelvis (Fig. 13-2). Position is described in abbreviated form determined by the first letter of each key word representing the presenting part and the quadrants of the maternal pelvis. For example, the first letter of the abbreviation for position denotes the location of the presenting part in the right *(R)* or left *(L)* side of the mother's pelvis. The middle letter stands for the specific presenting part of the

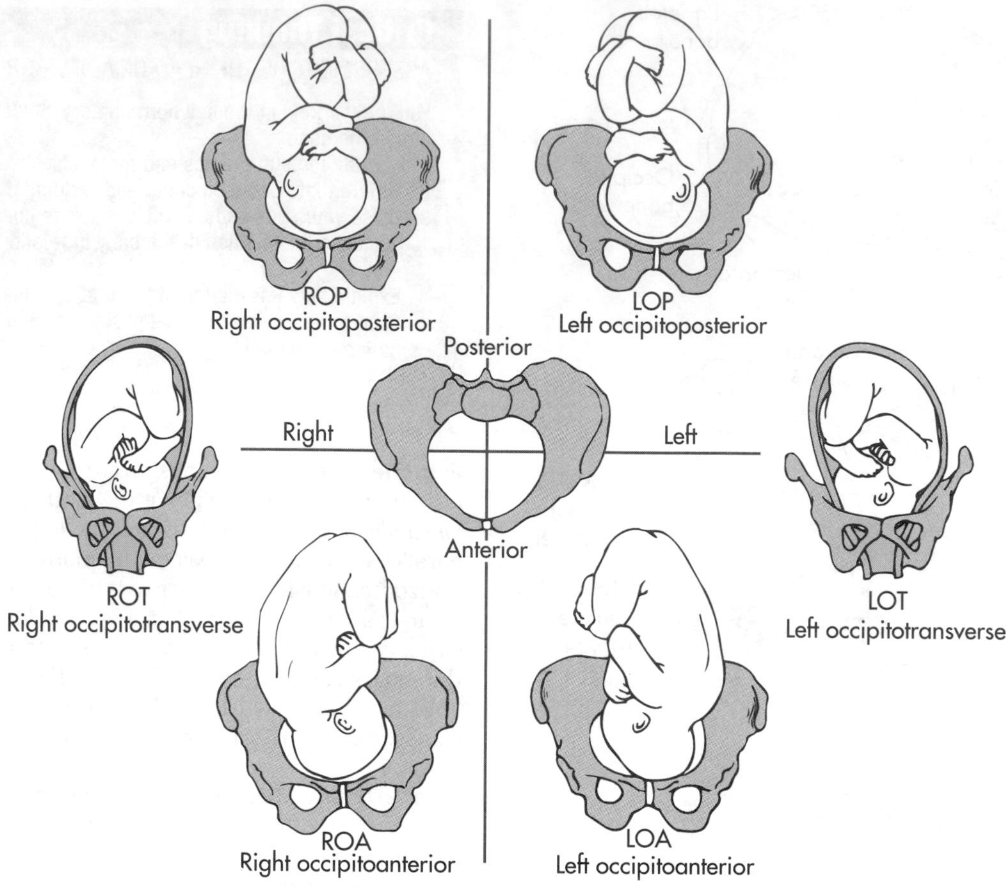

Fig. 13-2 Examples of fetal vertex (occiput) presentations in relation to front, back, or side of maternal pelvis.

fetus (*O* for occiput, *S* for sacrum, *M* for mentum [chin], and *Sc* for scapula [shoulder]). The third letter of the abbreviation stands for the location of the presenting part in relation to the anterior *(A)*, posterior *(P)*, or transverse *(T)* portion of the maternal pelvis.

The abbreviation *ROA* means that the occiput is the presenting part and is located in the right anterior quadrant of the maternal pelvis (Fig. 13-2). *LSP* means that the sacrum is the presenting part and is located in the left posterior quadrant of the maternal pelvis (Fig. 13-3).

Engagement indicates that the largest transverse diameter of the presenting part has passed through the maternal pelvic brim or inlet into the true pelvis. In a well-flexed cephalic presentation, the biparietal diameter (9.25 cm) is the widest (Fig. 13-5, *A*). Engagement can be determined by abdominal or vaginal examination.

Station is the relationship of the presenting part of the fetus to an imaginary line drawn between the maternal ischial spines. Station is expressed in terms of centimeters above or below the spines. For example, when the presenting part is 1 cm above the spines, it is noted as being minus (−)1 (Fig. 13-6). At the level of the spines, the station is referred to as zero. When the presenting part is 1 cm below the spines, the station is said to be plus (+) 1. Birth is imminent when the presenting part is at +4 to +5 cm. For accurate documentation of the rate of descent of the fetus during labor, the station of the presenting part should be determined when labor begins.

Passageway

The *passageway*, or birth canal, is composed of the mother's rigid bony pelvis and the soft tissues of the cervix, pelvic floor, vagina, and introitus (the external opening to the vagina). Although the soft tissues, particularly the muscular layers of the pelvic floor, contribute to vaginal birth of the fetus, the maternal pelvis plays a far greater role in the labor process. The fetus must successfully accommodate itself to this relatively rigid passageway. Therefore the size and shape of the pelvis must be determined before childbirth begins.

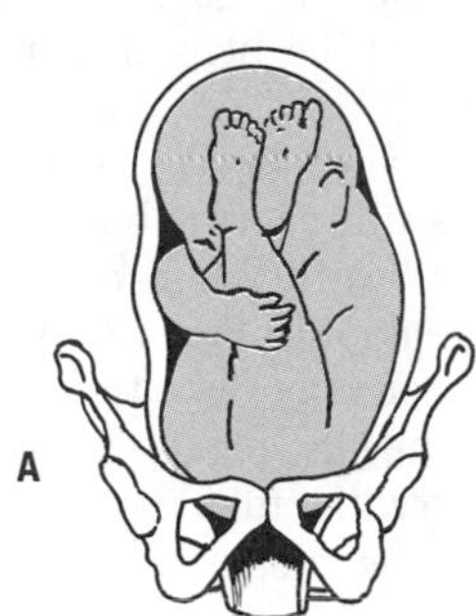

Frank breech

Lie: Longitudinal or vertical
Presentation: Breech (incomplete)
Presenting part: Sacrum
Attitude: Flexion, except for legs at knees

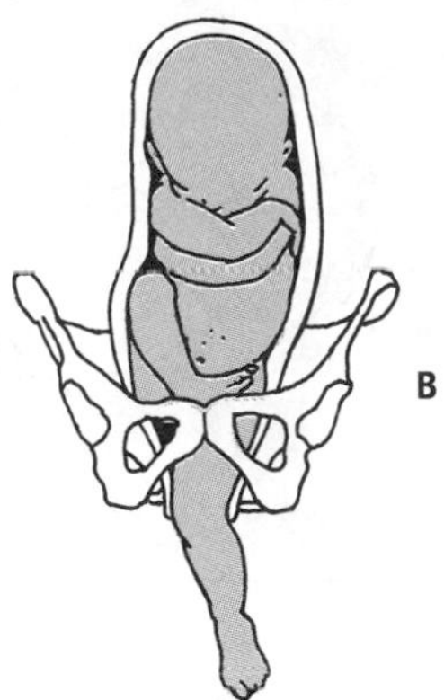

Single footling breech

Lie: Longitudinal or vertical
Presentation: Breech (incomplete)
Presenting part: Sacrum
Attitude: Flexion, except for one leg extended at hip and knee

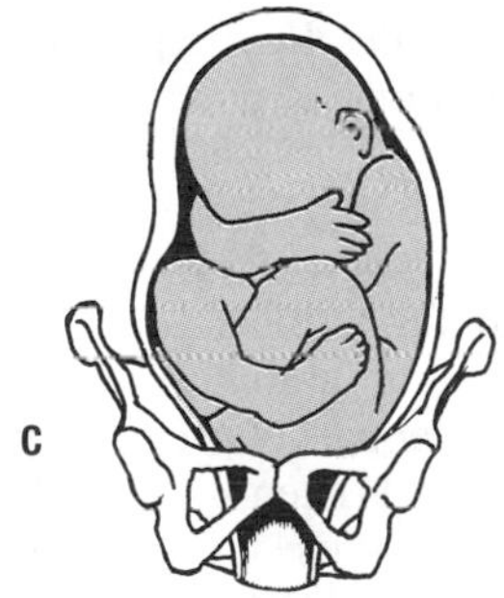

Complete breech

Lie: Longitudinal or vertical
Presentation: Breech (sacrum and feet presenting)
Presenting part: Sacrum (with feet)
Attitude: General flexion

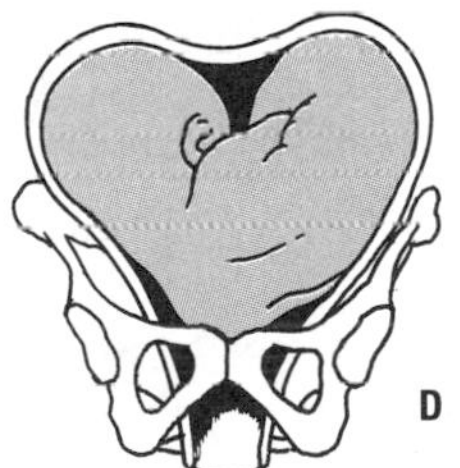

Shoulder presentation

Lie: Transverse or horizontal
Presentation: Shoulder
Presenting part: Scapula
Attitude: Flexion

Fig. 13-3 Fetal presentations. **A-C,** Breech (sacral) presentation. **D,** Shoulder presentation.

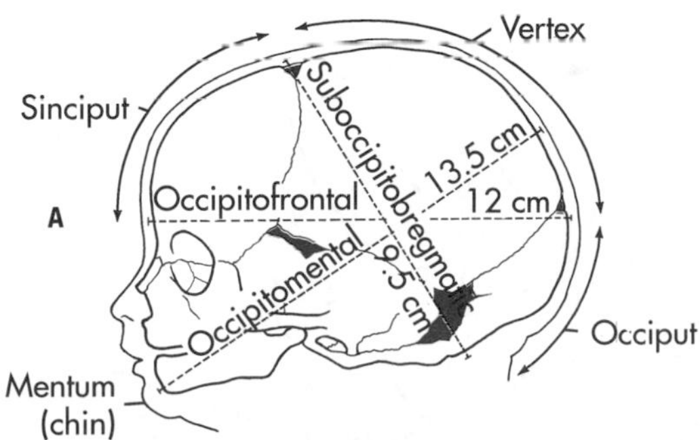

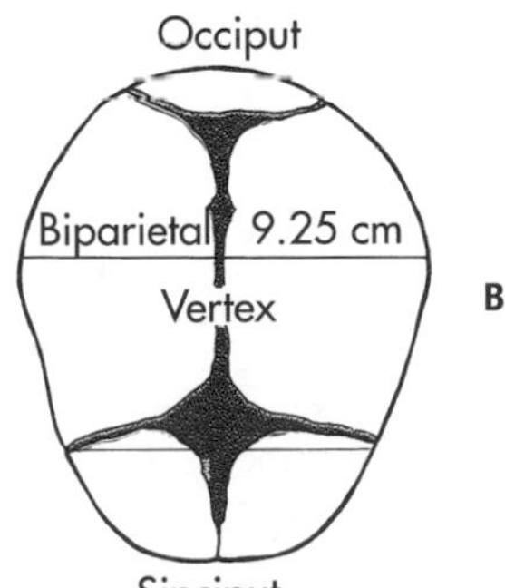

Fig. 13-4 Cephalic landmarks. **A,** Cephalic presentations: occiput, vertex, and sinciput, and cephalic diameters: suboccipitobregmatic, occipitofrontal, and occipitomental. **B,** Cephalic presentations and biparietal diameter.

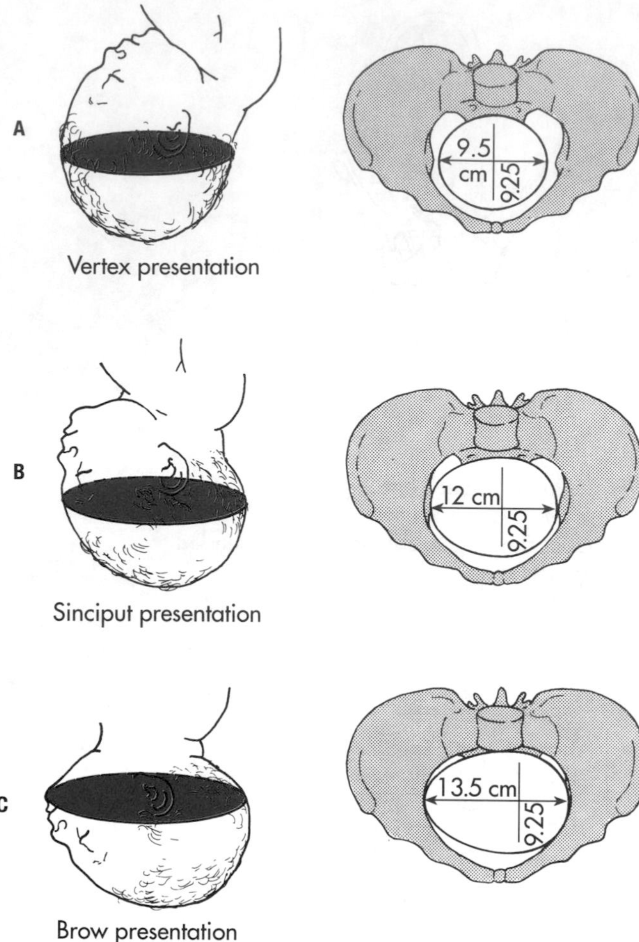

Fig. 13-5 Head entering pelvis. Biparietal diameter is indicated with an arrow (9.25 cm). **A,** Suboccipitobregmatic diameter: complete flexion of head on chest so smallest diameter enters. **B,** Occipitofrontal diameter: moderate extension (military attitude) so that large diameter enters. **C,** Occipitomental diameter: marked extension (deflection) so largest diameter, which is too large to permit head to enter pelvis, is presenting.

Bony pelvis. The anatomy of the bony pelvis is detailed in Chapter 3. The following discussion focuses on the importance of pelvic configurations as they relate to the labor process. (It may be helpful to refer back to Figs. 3-16 and 3-17.)

The bony pelvis is formed by the fusion of the ilium, ischium, pubis, and sacrum bones. The four pelvic joints are the symphysis pubis, the right and left sacroiliac joints, and the sacrococcygeal joint (Fig. 13-7). The bony pelvis is separated by the brim, or inlet, into two parts: the false pelvis and the true pelvis. The false pelvis is that part above the brim and has nothing to do with childbearing. The true pelvis is divided into three planes: the inlet or brim, the midpelvis or cavity, and the outlet.

The pelvic inlet, the upper border of the true pelvis, is formed anteriorly by the upper margins of the pubic bone; laterally by the iliopectineal lines along the innominate bones; and posteriorly by the anterior, upper margin of the sacrum and the sacral promontory.

The pelvic cavity, or midpelvis, is a curved passage with a short anterior wall and a much longer concave posterior wall. It is bounded by the posterior aspect of the symphysis pubis, the ischium, a portion of the ilium, the sacrum, and the coccyx.

The pelvic outlet is the lower border of the true pelvis. Viewed from below, it is ovoid and somewhat diamond-shaped, and it is bounded by the pubic arch anteriorly, the ischial tuberosities laterally, and the tip of the coccyx posteriorly. In the latter part of pregnancy the coccyx is movable (unless it has been broken in a fall during skiing or skating, for example, and has fused to the sacrum during healing).

The pelvic canal varies in size and shape at various levels. The diameters at the plane of the pelvic inlet, midpelvis, and outlet, plus the axis of the birth canal (Fig. 13-8) determine whether vaginal birth is possible and the manner by which the fetus may pass down the birth canal (see the discussion on the cardinal movements of the mechanism of labor, pp. 347-349).

The subpubic angle, which indicates the type of pubic

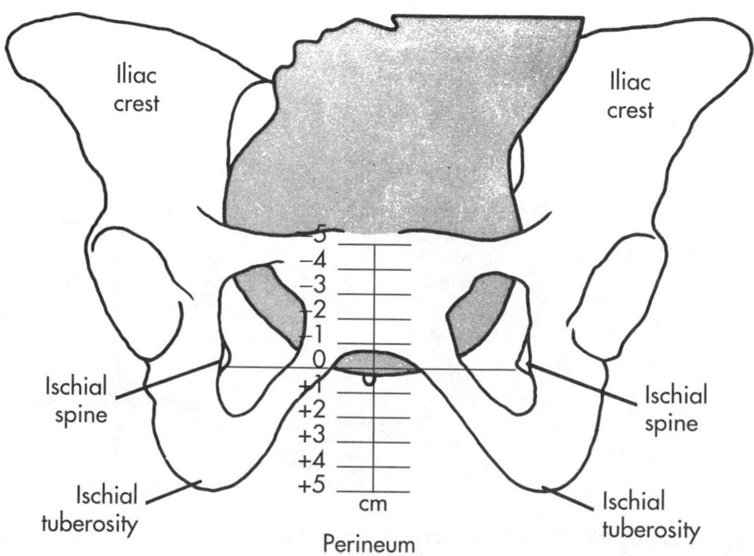

Fig. 13-6 Stations of presenting part, or degree of descent. Silhouette shows head of infant approaching station + 1. (Courtesy Ross Laboratories, Columbus, Ohio.)

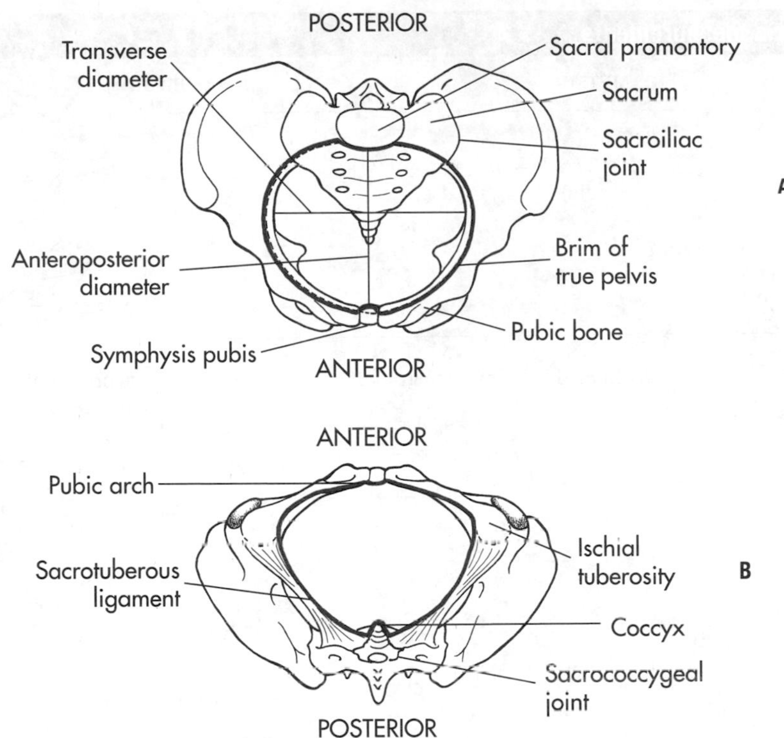

Fig. 13-7 Female pelvis. **A,** Pelvic brim from above. **B,** Pelvic outlet from below.

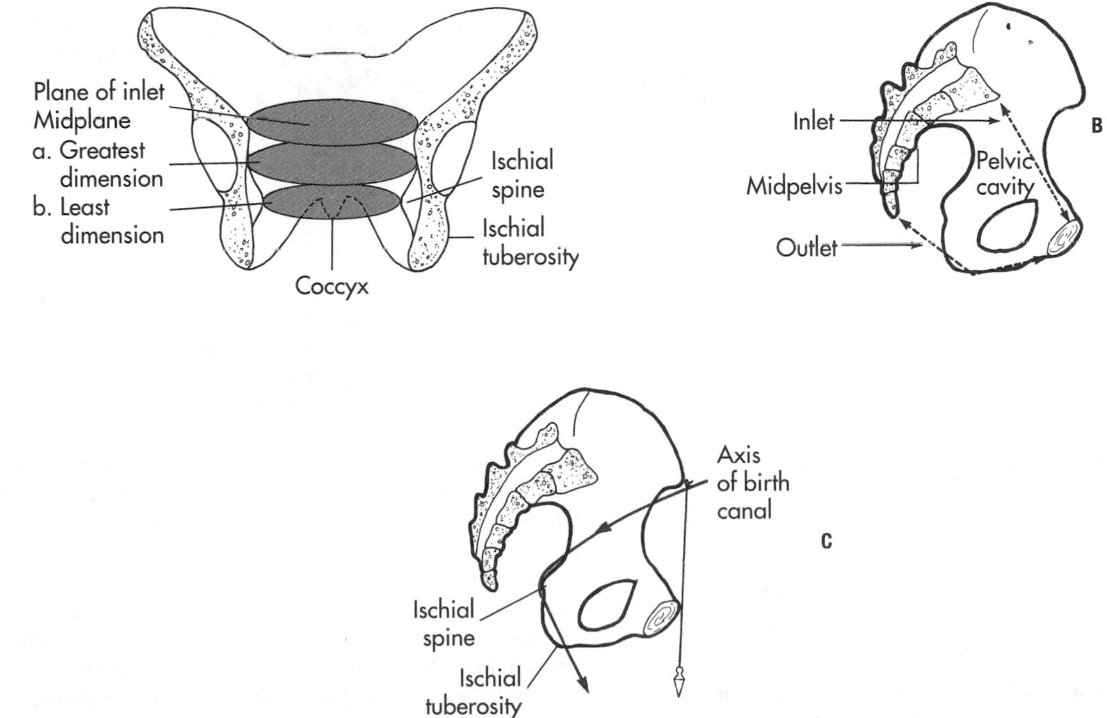

Fig. 13-8 Pelvic cavity. **A,** Inlet and midplane. Outlet not shown. **B,** Cavity of true pelvis. **C,** Note curve of sacrum and axis of birth canal.

TABLE 13-1 Obstetric measurements

PLANE	DIAMETER	MEASUREMENTS
Inlet (superior strait)	12.5 to 13 cm	
Conjugates		
Diagonal		
Obstetric: measurement that determines whether presenting part can engage or enter superior strait	1.5 to 2 cm less than diagonal (radiographic)	
True (vera) (anteroposterior)	≥11 cm (12.5 cm) (radiographic)	Length of diagonal conjugate *(solid colored line)*, obstetric conjugate *(broken colored line)*, true conjugate *(black line)*.
Midplane* Transverse diameter (interspinous diameter)	10.5 cm	Measurement of interspinous diameter. (From Malasanos et al: *Health assessment*, ed 4, St Louis, 1990, Mosby.)
Outlet† Transverse diameter (intertuberous diameter)	≥8 cm	Use of Thom's pelvimeter to measure intertuberous diameter. (From Malasanos et al: *Health assessment*, ed 4, St Louis, 1990, Mosby.)

*The midplane of the pelvis normally is its largest plane and the one of greatest diameter.
†The outlet presents the smallest plane of the pelvic canal.

arch, together with the length of the pubic rami and the intertuberous diameter, is of great importance. Because the fetus must first pass beneath the pubic arch, a narrow subpubic angle is less favorable than a rounded, wide arch. Measurement of the subpubic arch is shown in Fig. 13-9. A summary of obstetric measurements is given in Table 13-1.

The four basic types of pelvis are classified as follows:

1. Gynecoid (the classic female type)
2. Android (resembling the male pelvis)
3. Anthropoid (resembling the pelvis of anthropoid apes)
4. Platypelloid (the flat pelvis).

The **gynecoid pelvis** is the most common, with major gynecoid pelvic features present in 50% of all women. Anthropoid and android features are less common, and platypelloid pelvic features are the least common. Mixed types of pelves are more common than pure types (Cunningham et al, 1993). Examples of pelvic variations and their effects on mode of birth are given in Table 13-2.

Assessment of the bony pelvis may be performed during the first prenatal evaluation and need not be repeated if the pelvis is of adequate size and suitable shape. In the third trimester of pregnancy, the examination of the bony pelvis may be more thorough and the results more accurate because there is relaxation of the pelvic joints and ligaments. The hormones of pregnancy, especially the ovarian hormone progesterone, cause the development of considerable mobility in the pelvic joints. Widening of the joint of the symphysis pubis and instability may cause pain in any or all of the joints.

Because the examiner does not have direct access to the bony structures and because the bones are covered with vary-

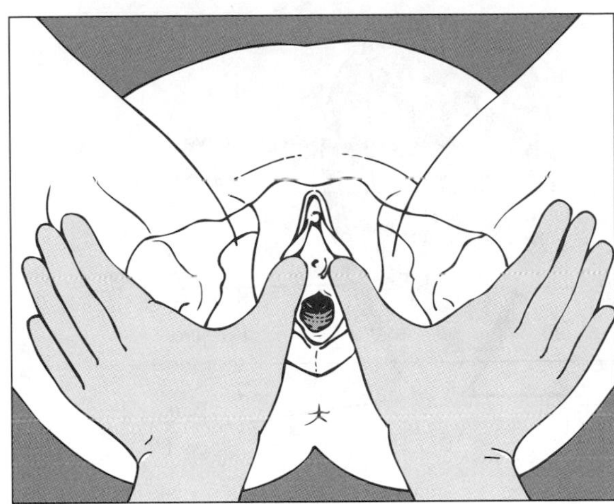

Fig. 13-9 Estimation of angle of subpubic arch. Using both thumbs, examiner externally traces descending rami down to tuberosities. (From Barkauskas V et al: *Health and physical assessment*, St Louis, 1994, Mosby.)

ing amounts of soft tissue, estimates of size and shape are approximate. Precise bony pelvis measurements can be determined by using computed tomography, ultrasound, or x-ray films. However, x-ray examination is rarely done during pregnancy because the x-rays may damage the developing fetus.

Soft tissues. The soft tissues of the passageway include the distensible lower uterine segment, cervix, pelvic floor muscles, vagina, and introitus (external opening to the vagina). Before labor begins, the uterus is composed of the uterine body (corpus) and cervix (neck). After labor has begun, uterine contractions cause the uterine body to change into a thick and muscular upper segment and a thin-walled passive muscular lower segment. A *physiologic retraction ring* separates the two segments (Fig. 13-10). The lower uterine segment gradually distends to accommodate the intrauterine contents as the wall of the upper segment becomes thick and its accommodating capacity is reduced. Contractions of the uterine body thus exert downward pressure on the fetus, pushing it against the cervix.

The cervix *effaces* (thins) and *dilates* (opens) sufficiently to allow descent of the first fetal portion into the vagina. Actually the cervix is drawn upward and over this first part as it descends.

The pelvic floor is a muscular layer that separates the pelvic cavity above from the perineal space below. This structure helps the fetus rotate anteriorly as it passes through the birth canal. As noted earlier, the soft tissues of the vagina develop throughout pregnancy until at term the vagina can dilate to accommodate the fetus and permit passage of the fetus to the external world.

Powers

Involuntary and voluntary contractions combine to expel the fetus and the placenta from the uterus. Involuntary uterine contractions, called *primary powers*, signal the beginning of labor. Once the cervix has dilated, voluntary bearing-down efforts by the woman, called *secondary powers*, augment the force of the involuntary contractions.

Primary powers. The involuntary contractions originate at certain pacemaker points in the thickened muscle layers of the upper uterine segment. From the pacemaker points, contractions move downward over the uterus in waves, separated by short rest periods. Terms used to describe these involuntary contractions include *frequency* (time between contractions—specifically, the time between the beginning of one contraction and the beginning of the next); *duration* (length of contraction); and *intensity* (strength of contraction).

TABLE 13-2 Comparison of pelvic types

	GYNECOID (50% OF WOMEN)	ANDROID (23% OF WOMEN)	ANTHROPOID (24% OF WOMEN)	PLATYPELLOID (3% OF WOMEN)
Brim	Slightly ovoid or transversely rounded	Heart shaped, angulated	Oval, wider anteroposteriorly	Flattened anteroposteriorly, wide transversely
Depth	Moderate	Deep	Deep	Shallow
Side walls	Straight	Convergent	Straight	Straight
Ischial spines	Blunt, somewhat widely separated	Prominent, narrow interspinous diameter	Prominent, often with narrow interspinous diameter	Blunt, widely separated
Sacrum	Deep, curved	Slightly curved, terminal portion often beaked	Slightly curved	Slightly curved
Subpubic arch	Wide	Narrow	Narrow	Wide
Usual mode of birth	Vaginal Spontaneous Occipitoanterior position	Cesarean Vaginal Difficult with forceps	Vaginal Forceps Spontaneous occipitoposterior or occipitoanterior position	Vaginal Spontaneous

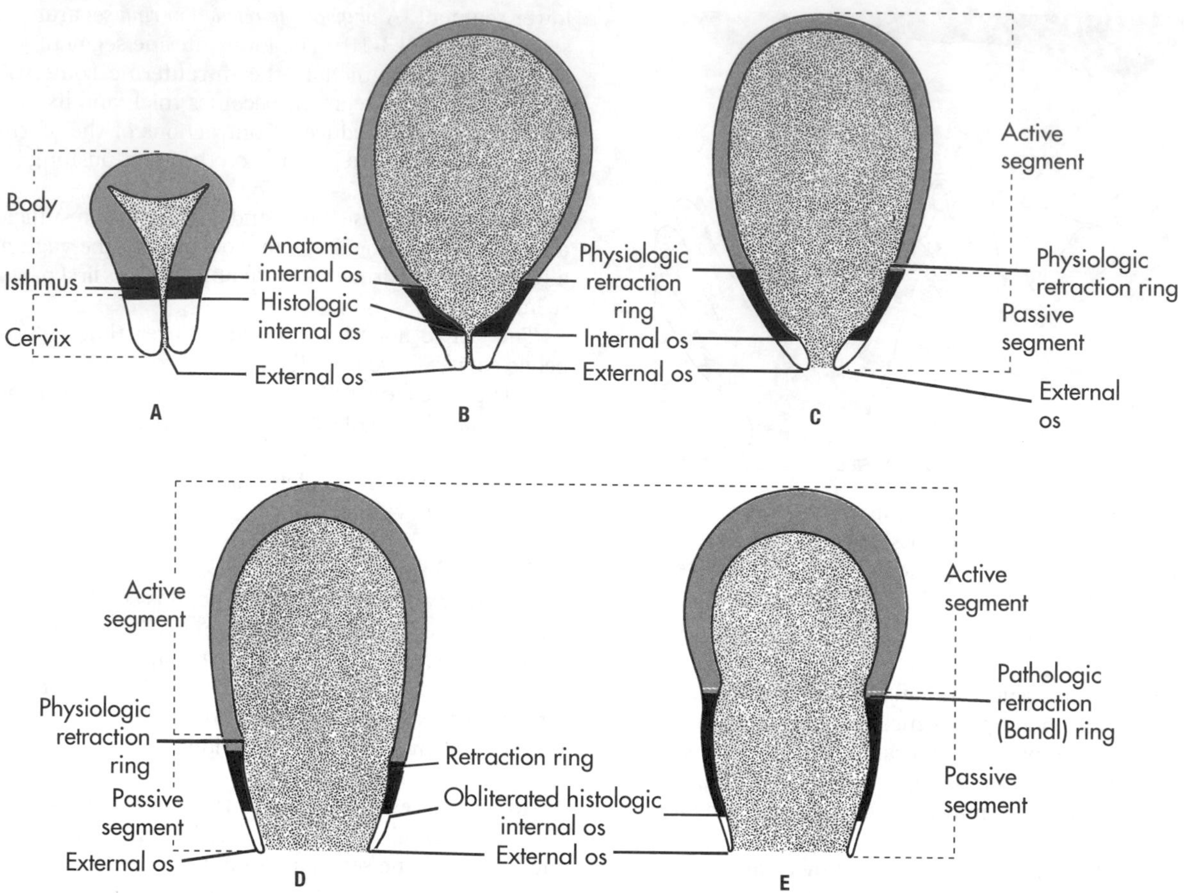

Fig. 13-10 Progressive development of segments and rings of uterus at term. Note differences in nonpregnant uterus (**A**), uterus at term (**B**), and uterus in normal labor in early first stage (**C**) and second stage (**D**). Passive segment is derived from lower uterine segment (isthmus) and cervix, and physiologic retraction ring is derived from anatomic internal os. **E,** Uterus in abnormal labor in second-stage dystocia. Pathologic retraction (Bandl) ring that forms under abnormal conditions develops from physiologic ring. (Modified from Willson J et al: *Obstetrics and gynecology,* ed 9, St Louis, 1991, Mosby.)

The primary powers are responsible for the effacement and dilation of the cervix and descent of the fetus. **Effacement** of the cervix means the shortening and thinning of the cervix during the first stage of labor. The cervix, normally 2 to 3 cm in length and about 1 cm thick, is obliterated or "taken up" by a shortening of the uterine muscle bundles during the thinning of the lower uterine segment in advancing labor. Eventually only a thin edge of the cervix can be palpated when effacement is complete. Effacement generally is advanced in first-time pregnancy at term before more than slight dilation occurs. In subsequent pregnancies, effacement and dilation of the cervix tend to progress together. Degree of effacement is expressed in percentages from 0% to 100% (e.g., a cervix is 50% effaced) (Fig. 13-11).

Dilation (or dilatation) of the cervix is the enlargement or widening of the cervical opening and the cervical canal, which occurs once labor has begun. The diameter increases from perhaps less than 1 cm to full dilation (approximately 10 cm) to allow birth of a term fetus. When the cervix is fully dilated (and completely retracted), it can no longer be palpated (Fig. 13-11). Full cervical dilation marks the end of the first stage of labor.

Dilation of the cervix occurs by the drawing upward of the musculofibrous components of the cervix with strong uterine contractions. Pressure exerted by the amniotic fluid while the membranes are intact or force applied by the presenting part also encourages cervical dilation. Scarring of the cervix as a result of prior infection or surgery may retard cervical dilation.

Mechanical stretching of the cervix (Ferguson reflex) increases uterine activity. Uterine contractions are involuntary and are usually independent from external forces. For example, uterine contractions may decrease in frequency and intensity if epidural analgesia is given early in labor, but if labor is well established, contractions are usually not affected. Also, women in labor who are paraplegic have normal uterine contractions (Cunningham et al, 1993).

Secondary powers. As soon as the presenting part reaches the pelvic floor the contractions change in character and be-

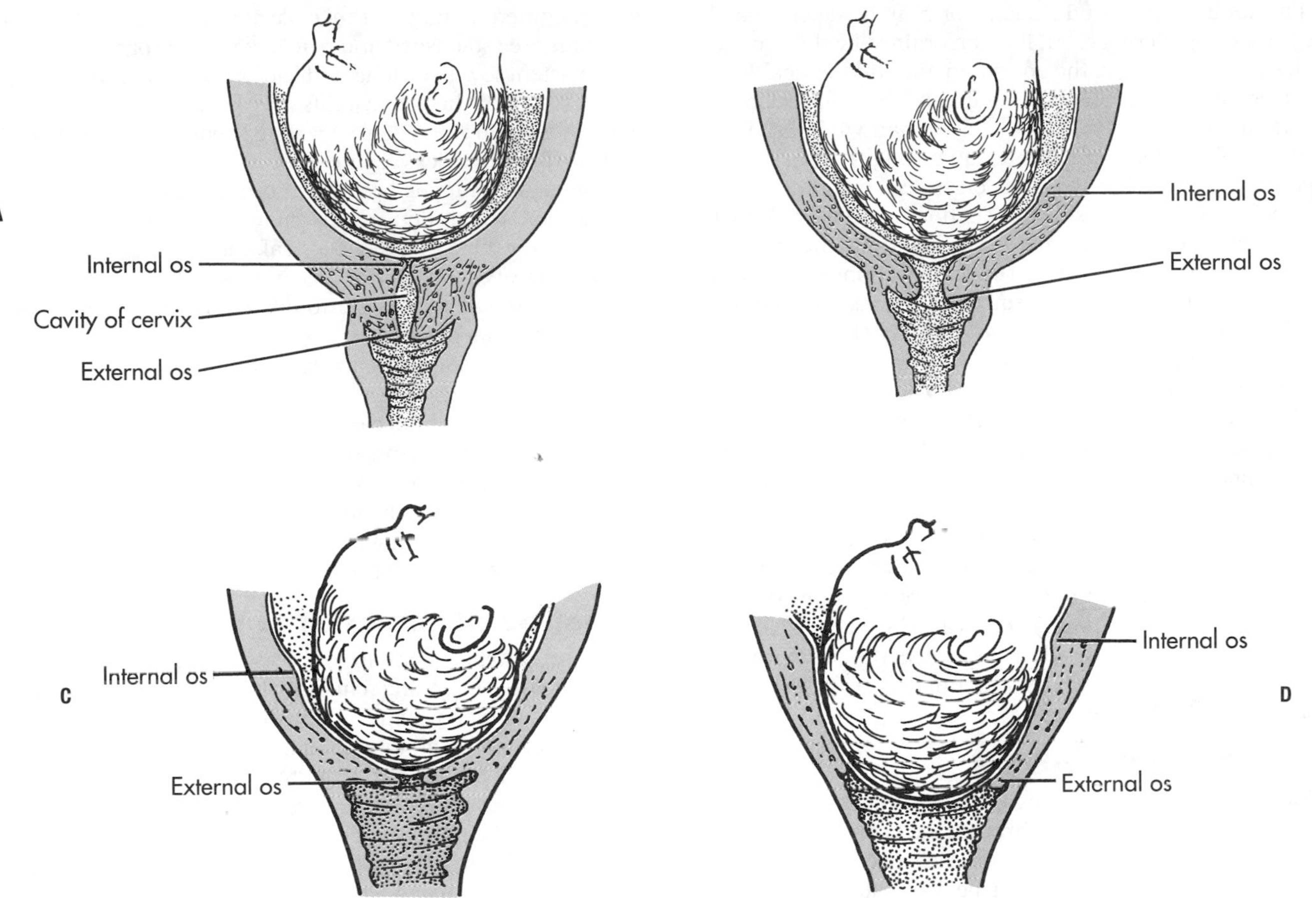

Fig. 13-11 Cervical effacement and dilation. Note how cervix is drawn up around presenting part (internal os). Membranes are intact, and head is not well applied to cervix. **A,** Before labor. **B,** Early effacement. **C,** Complete effacement (100%). Head is well applied to cervix. **D,** Complete dilation (10 cm). Some overlapping of cranial bones. Membranes still intact.

come expulsive in nature. The woman experiences an involuntary urge to push. The woman in labor uses secondary powers (bearing-down efforts) to aid in expulsion of the fetus as she contracts her diaphragm and abdominal muscles and pushes out the contents of the birth canal. Bearing down results in increased intraabdominal pressure. The pressure compresses the uterus on all sides and adds to the power of the expulsive forces. Prolonged breath holding and sustained pushing efforts may cause fetal hypoxia (Valsalva maneuver, p. 349).

The secondary forces have no effect on cervical dilation, but they are of considerable importance in the expulsion of the infant from the uterus and vagina after the cervix is fully dilated. Voluntary bearing-down efforts by the woman earlier in labor are counterproductive to cervical dilation. Straining exhausts the woman and causes cervical trauma.

Position of the Woman in Labor

Maternal position affects her anatomic and physiologic adaptations to labor. Frequent changes in position relieve fatigue, increase comfort, and improve circulation (Melzack, Belanger, and Lacroix, 1991). A woman in labor should be encouraged to find positions that are most comfortable to her.

An upright position offers a number of advantages. In an upright position (walking, sitting, kneeling, or squatting), gravity can assist in the descent of the fetus. Uterine contractions are generally stronger and more efficient in effacing and dilating the cervix, resulting in shorter labor (Andrews and Chrzanowski, 1990). In addition, assuming an upright position reduces the incidence of umbilical cord compression.

An upright position is also beneficial to the mother's cardiac output, which normally increases during labor as uterine contractions return blood to the vascular bed. Increased cardiac output improves blood flow to the uteroplacental unit and the maternal kidneys. Cardiac output is compromised if the descending aorta and ascending vena cava are compressed during labor. Compression of these major vessels may result in supine hypotension and fetal heart rate deceleration or in hypertension that decreases placental perfusion. An upright position helps reduce pressure on the maternal vessels and prevents their compression. If the woman wishes to lie down, a lateral position is most physiologic.

The "all-fours" position (hands and knees) may be used to relieve backache if the fetus is in an occipitoposterior position (Bennett and Brown, 1993).

Positioning for second-stage labor may be determined by the woman's preference, but it is constrained by the condition of the woman or fetus, the environment, and the health care provider's confidence in assisting in a birth in a specific position (Bennett and Brown, 1993). A woman who pushes in a semirecumbent position needs adequate body support to push effectively because her weight is on her sacrum, moving the coccyx forward and causing a reduction in the pelvic outlet.

In a sitting or squatting position, abdominal muscles work in greater synchrony with uterine contractions during bearing-down efforts. Kneeling or squatting moves the uterus forward and straightens the long axis of the birth canal and can facilitate the second stage of labor by increasing the pelvic outlet (Bennett and Brown, 1993).

The lateral position also is effective for assisting birth and may be an alternative for a woman who cannot abduct her hips. Support of the upper thigh may be needed during the birthing process.

There is no evidence that any of these positions for second stage-labor affect the rate of use of operative techniques (e.g., forceps delivery, vacuum extraction, cesarean birth), episiotomy, or perineal trauma. There is also no evidence that use of any of these positions adversely affects the newborn (Andrews and Chrzanowski, 1990; Bennett and Brown, 1993; Golay, Vedam and Sorger, 1993).

PROCESS OF LABOR

Labor is the process of moving the fetus, placenta, and membranes out of the uterus and through the birth canal. Various changes take place in the woman's reproductive system in the days and weeks just before labor begins. Labor itself can be discussed in terms of the mechanisms involved in the process and the stages the woman moves through.

Signs Preceding Labor

In first-time pregnancies the uterus sinks downward and forward about 2 weeks before term, when the fetus's presenting part (usually the fetal head) descends into the true pelvis. This settling is called **lightening** or "dropping" and usually happens gradually (Fig. 13-12). After lightening, women feel less congested and breathe more easily. However, there is usually more bladder pressure as a result of this shift and consequently a return of urinary frequency. In a multiparous pregnancy, lightening may not take place until after uterine contractions are established and true labor is in progress.

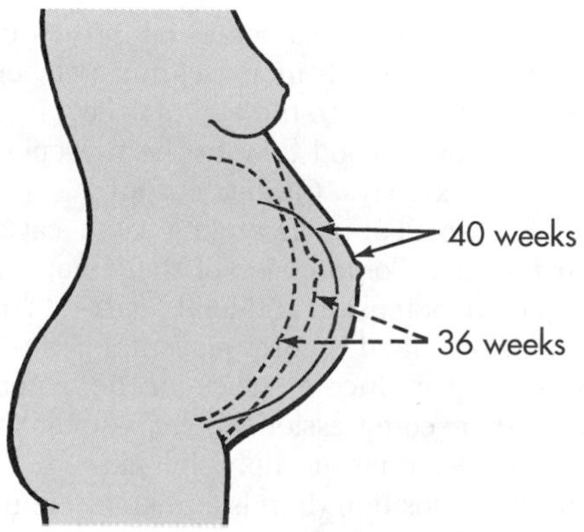

Fig. 13-12 Lightening.

Persistent low backache and sacroiliac distress as a result of relaxation of the pelvic joints may be described. Occasionally the woman may identify strong, frequent, but irregular uterine (Braxton Hicks) contractions.

The vaginal mucus becomes more profuse in response to the extreme congestion of the vaginal mucous membranes. Brownish or blood-tinged cervical mucus may be passed **(bloody show).** The cervix becomes soft (ripens) and partially effaced and may begin to dilate. The membranes may rupture spontaneously.

Two other phenomena are common in the days preceding labor: (1) loss of 0.5 to 1.5 kg (1 to 3 lb) in weight, caused by water loss resulting from electrolyte shifts that in turn are produced by changes in estrogen and progesterone levels, and (2) a surge of energy. Women speak of a burst of energy that they often use to clean the house and put everything in order. This activity has been described as the "nesting instinct." Box 13-1 lists signs that may precede labor.

Theories of Onset of Labor

The onset of true labor cannot be ascribed to a single cause. Many factors, including changes in the maternal uterus, cervix, and pituitary gland, are involved. Hormones produced by the normal fetal hypothalamus, pituitary gland, and adrenal cortex probably contribute to the onset of labor. Progressive uterine distention, increasing intrauterine pressure, and aging of the placenta seem to be associated with increasing myometrial irritability. This is a result of increased concentrations of estrogen and prostaglandins, as well as decreasing progesterone levels. The mutually coordinated effects of these factors are strong, regular, rhythmic uterine contractions. Normally, these factors working in concert result in the

BOX 13-1
Signs Preceding Labor

Lightening
Return of urinary frequency
Backache
Stronger Braxton Hicks contractions
Weight loss of 0.5 to 1.5 kg (1 to 3 lb)
Surge of energy
Increased vaginal discharge (bloody show may be present)
Cervical ripening
Rupture of membranes

Critical Thinking Exercises

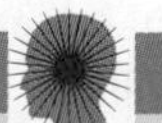

SIGNS OF LABOR

Visit a prenatal clinic. Talk to two women who are at 36 weeks' gestation or more. Ask them to tell you what they know about the signs of labor.

1. Formulate a teaching plan that will reinforce correct information and fill any gaps.
2. Implement the plan and evaluate the expected outcomes.

birth of the fetus and the expulsion of the placenta. It is still not completely understood how certain alterations trigger others and how proper checks and balances are maintained.

Stages of Labor

Labor is considered "normal" when the woman is at or near term, no complications exist, a single fetus presents by vertex, and labor is completed within 24 hours. The course of normal labor, which is remarkably constant, consists of (1) regular progression of uterine contractions, (2) effacement and progressive dilation of the cervix, and (3) progress in descent of the presenting part. *Four stages of labor* are recognized. These stages are discussed in greater detail, along with nursing care for the laboring woman and family, in Chapter 16.

The *first stage* of labor is considered to last from the onset of regular uterine contractions to full dilation of the cervix. Commonly the onset of labor is difficult to establish; the woman may be admitted to the labor floor just before birth, so the beginning of labor may be only an estimate. The first stage is much longer than the second and third combined. Great variability is the rule, however, depending on the factors discussed earlier. Full dilation may occur in less than 1 hour in some multiparous pregnancies. In first-time pregnancy, complete dilation of the cervix is seldom reached in less than 24 hours.

The first stage of labor has been divided into three phases: a *latent* phase, an *active* phase, and a *transition* phase. During the latent phase there is more progress in effacement of the cervix and little increase in descent. During the active phase and the transition phase there is more rapid dilation of the cervix and descent of the presenting part. There are no absolute values for the normal length of the first stage of labor (Willson et al, 1991). Variations may reflect differences in the patient population or in clinical practice.

The *second stage* of labor lasts from full dilation of the cervix to birth of the fetus. Labor of up to 2 hours is considered within the normal range for the second stage. Table 13-3 describes means and the limits of the first and second stages of labor based on the research of Friedman and his associates (1978).

The *third stage* of labor lasts from the birth of the fetus until the placenta is expelled. The placenta normally separates with the third or fourth strong uterine contraction after the infant has been born. It should be expelled with the next uterine contraction after placental separation. The length of time for the third stage ranges from 3 to 5 minutes, although up to 1 hour may be considered within normal limits (Bennett and Brown, 1993).

The *fourth stage* of labor arbitrarily lasts about 2 hours after the expulsion of the placenta. It is the period of immediate recovery when homeostasis is reestablished. It serves as an important period of observation for complications such as abnormal bleeding.

Mechanism of Labor

The female pelvis has varied contours and diameters at different levels, and the presenting part of the passenger is large in proportion to the passageway. For vaginal birth to occur, the fetus must adapt to the birth canal during the descent. The turns and other adjustments necessary in the human birth process are termed the **mechanism of labor** (Fig. 13-13). The seven *cardinal movements* of the mechanism of labor that occur in a vertex presentation are *engagement, descent, flexion, internal rotation, extension, external rotation (restitution)*, and finally birth by *expulsion*. Although these phases are discussed separately, a combination of movements is occurring simultaneously. For example, engagement involves both descent and flexion.

Engagement. When the biparietal diameter of the head passes the pelvic inlet, the head is said to be engaged in the pelvic inlet (Fig. 13-13, *A*). In most nulliparous pregnancies this occurs before the onset of active labor because the firmer abdominal muscles direct the presenting part into the pelvis. In multiparous pregnancies, in which the abdominal musculature is more relaxed, the head often remains freely movable above the pelvic brim until labor is established.

Descent. Descent refers to the progress of the presenting part through the pelvis. Descent depends on three forces: (1) pressure of the amniotic fluid, (2) direct pressure of the contracting fundus on the fetus, and (3) contraction of the maternal diaphragm and abdominal muscles in the second stage of labor. The effects of these forces are modified by the size and shape of the maternal pelvic planes and the size and capacity of the fetal head to mold.

The degree of descent is measured by the station of the presenting part (Fig. 13-6). There is little progress in descent

TABLE 13-3 Length of labor

STAGE OF LABOR	NULLIPARA		MULTIPARA	
	MEAN	UPPER LIMITS	MEAN	UPPER LIMITS
	HOURS		HOURS	
First stage	14.4	20	7.7	14
Latent phase	8.6		5.3	
Active phase	4.9		2.2	
Second stage	1.0	2.5*	0.2	0.8*

(Data from ACOG, 1989; Zlatnik, 1994).
*If the woman has received conduction analgesia, an extra hour is given to complete the second stage.

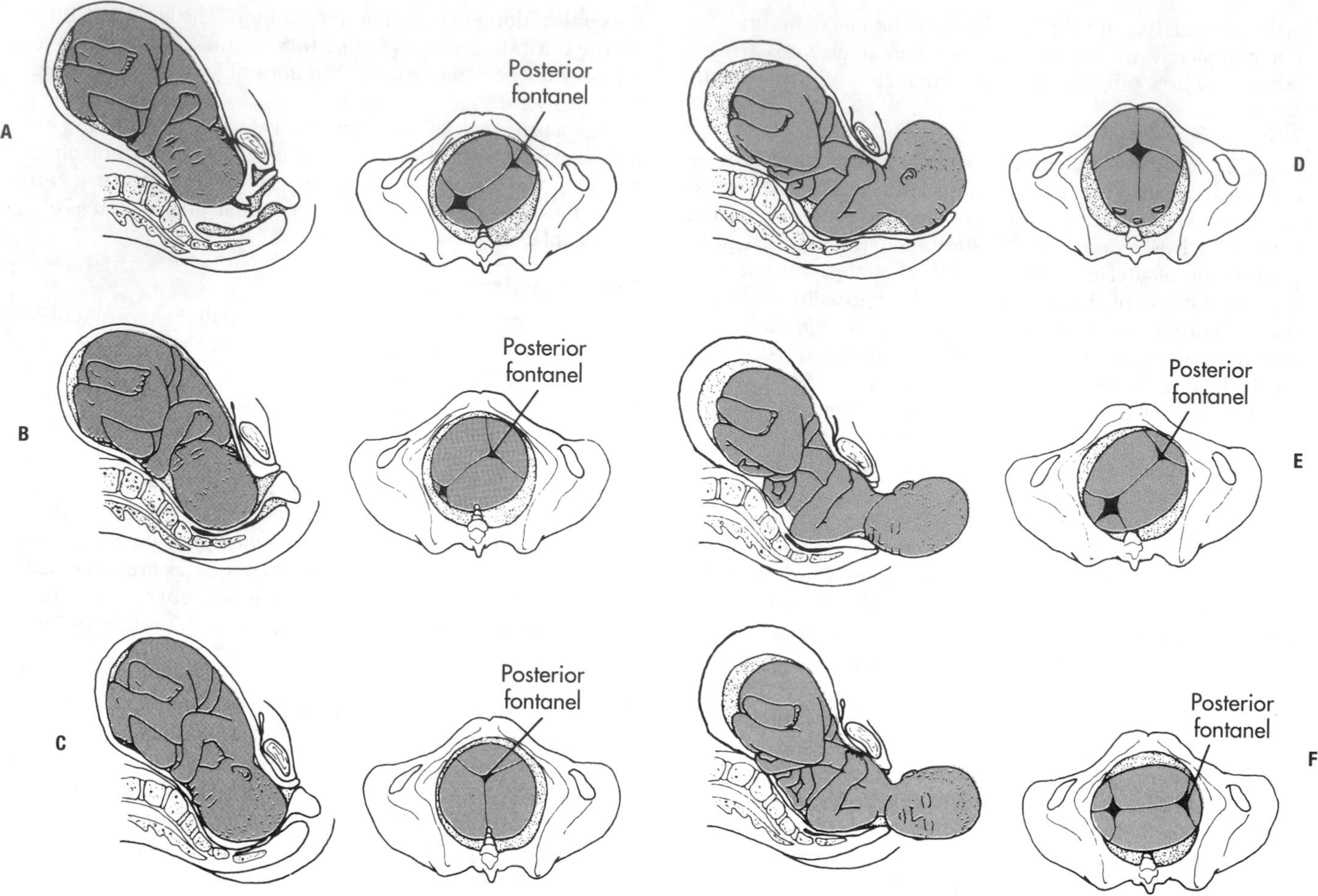

Fig. 13-13 Cardinal movements of the mechanism of labor, left occipitoanterior (LOA) presentation. **A,** Engagement and descent. **B,** Flexion. **C,** Internal rotation to occipitoanterior (OA). **D,** Extension. **E,** External rotation beginning (restitution). **F,** External rotation.

during the latent phase of the first stage of labor. Descent becomes more rapid in the active phase when the cervix has dilated to 5 to 7 cm. It is apparent especially when the membranes have ruptured.

In first-time pregnancy, this descent is slow but steady; in subsequent pregnancies the descent may be rapid. Progress in the descent of the presenting part is determined by abdominal palpation (Leopold maneuvers) and vaginal examination until the presenting part can be seen at the introitus.

Flexion. As soon as the descending head meets resistance from the cervix, pelvic wall, or pelvic floor, flexion normally occurs and the chin is brought into more intimate contact with the fetal chest (Fig. 13-13, *B*). Flexion permits the smaller suboccipitobregmatic diameter (9.5 cm) rather than the larger diameters to present to the outlet.

Internal rotation. The maternal pelvic inlet is widest in the transverse diameter. Therefore the fetal head passes the inlet into the true pelvis in the occipitotransverse position. The outlet is widest in the anteroposterior diameter, however. To exit, the fetal head must rotate. Internal rotation begins at the level of the ischial spines but is not completed until the presenting part reaches the lower pelvis. As the occiput rotates anteriorly, the face rotates posteriorly. With each contraction the fetal head is guided by the bony pelvis and the muscles of the pelvic floor. Eventually the occiput will be in the midline beneath the pubic arch. The head is almost always rotated by the time it reaches the pelvic floor (Fig. 13-13, *C*). Both the levator ani muscles and the bony pelvis are important for anterior rotation. Previous childbirth injury or regional anesthesia compromises the function of the levator sling.

Extension. When the fetal head reaches the perineum for birth, it is deflected anteriorly by the perineum. The occiput passes under the lower border of the symphysis pubis first, then the head emerges by extension: first the occiput, then the face, and finally the chin (Fig. 13-13, *D*).

Restitution and external rotation. After the head is born, it rotates briefly to the position it occupied when it was engaged in the inlet. This movement is referred to as *restitution* (Fig. 13-13, *E* and *F*). The 45-degree turn realigns the infant's head with her or his back and shoulders. The head can then be seen to rotate further. External rotation occurs as the shoulders engage and descend in maneuvers similar to those of the head. As noted earlier, the anterior shoulder descends first. When it reaches the outlet, it rotates to the midline and is delivered from under the pubic arch. The posterior shoulder is guided over the perineum until it is free of the vaginal introitus.

Expulsion. After birth of the shoulders, the head and shoulders are lifted up toward the mother's pubic bone and the trunk of the baby is born by a movement of lateral flexion in the direction of the symphysis pubis. When the baby has completely emerged, birth is complete. This is the end of the second stage of labor.

PHYSIOLOGIC ADAPTATION TO LABOR

In addition to the anatomic adaptations the mother and fetus make during the birth process, physiologic adaptations must also occur. Accurate assessment of the mother and fetus requires a knowledge of expected adaptations.

Fetal Adaptation

Several important physiologic adaptations occur. The nurse must be aware of what changes to expect in terms of fetal heart rate, fetal circulation, respiratory movements, and other behaviors.

Fetal heart rate. Fetal heart rate (FHR) monitoring provides reliable and predictive information about the condition of the fetus related to oxygenation. Stresses to the uterofetoplacental unit result in characteristic FHR patterns. It is important that the nurse have a basic understanding of the factors involved in fetal oxygenation and of the fetal responses that reflect adequate fetal oxygenation.

The average FHR at term is 140 beats/min. The normal range is 110 to 160 beats/min. Earlier in gestation the FHR is higher, with an average of approximately 160 beats/min at 20 weeks' gestation. The rate decreases progressively as the maturing fetus reaches term. However, temporary accelerations and slight early decelerations of the FHR can be expected in response to spontaneous fetal movement, vaginal examination, fundal pressure, uterine contractions, and abdominal palpation.

Fetal circulation. Fetal circulation can be affected by many factors. These factors include maternal position, uterine contractions, blood pressure, and umbilical cord blood flow. Uterine contractions during labor tend to decrease circulation through the spiral arterioles and subsequent perfusion through the intervillous space. Most healthy fetuses are well able to compensate for this stress and to exposure to increased pressure while moving passively through the birth canal during labor. Usually umbilical cord blood flow is undisturbed by uterine contractions or fetal position (Paine and Tinker, 1992).

Fetal respiration and behavior. Certain changes stimulate chemoreceptors in the aorta and carotid bodies to prepare the fetus for initiating respirations immediately after birth. These changes include items in the following list:

- 7 to 42 ml of amniotic fluid is squeezed out of the lungs (during vaginal birth).
- Fetal oxygen pressure falls (Po_2).
- Arterial carbon dioxide pressure (Pco_2) rises.
- Arterial pH falls.
- Fetal respiratory movements decrease during labor.

Maternal Adaptation

A thorough understanding of maternal adaptations to pregnancy helps the nurse anticipate and meet the woman's needs during labor. Further changes occur as the woman progresses through the stages of labor. Various body systems adapt to the process of labor, exhibiting both objective and subjective symptoms.

Cardiovascular changes. The nurse can expect some changes in the woman's cardiovascular system during labor. During each contraction, 400 ml of blood is emptied from the uterus into the maternal vascular system. This increases cardiac output by about 10% to 15% in the first stage and by about 30% to 50% in the second stage.

The nurse can anticipate changes in blood pressure. Several factors alter blood pressure in the mother. Blood flow, reduced in the uterine artery by contractions, is redirected to peripheral vessels. Peripheral resistance occurs, blood pressure rises, and the pulse rate slows. During the first stage of labor, uterine contractions increase systolic readings by about 10 mm Hg. Therefore assessing blood pressure between contractions provides more accurate data. During the second stage, contractions may increase systolic pressures by 30 mm Hg and diastolic readings by 25 mm Hg. However, both systolic and diastolic pressures remain somewhat elevated even between contractions. The woman already at risk for hypertension is then placed at increased risk for complications such as cerebral hemorrhage.

Supine hypotension occurs when the ascending vena cava and descending aorta are compressed. The laboring woman is at greater risk for supine hypotension if the uterus is particularly large because of multifetal pregnancy, hydramnios, obesity, or dehydration and hypovolemia. In addition, anxiety and pain, as well as some medications, can cause hypotension.

The woman must be encouraged to use open glottis pushing and discouraged from using the **Valsalva maneuver** (holding one's breath and tightening abdominal muscles) during the second stage. The Valsalva maneuver increases intrathoracic pressure, reduces venous return, and increases venous pressure. The cardiac output and blood pressure increase, and the pulse slows temporarily. During the Valsalva maneuver, fetal hypoxia may occur. The process is reversed when the woman takes a breath.

White blood cells (WBCs) increase, often to greater than or equal to 25,000/mm^3. Although the mechanism leading to this increase in WBCs is unknown, it may be secondary to physical or emotional stress or to tissue trauma. Labor is strenuous. Physical exercise alone can increase WBC count.

Some peripheral vascular changes occur, perhaps in response to cervical dilation or to compression of maternal vessels by the fetus passing through the birth canal. Malar flush (reddened cheeks), hot or cold feet, and eversion of hemorrhoids may result. Box 13-2 lists maternal physiologic changes during labor.

BOX 13-2
Maternal Physiologic Changes during Labor

- Cardiac output increases 10% to 15% in first stage; 30% to 50% in second stage.
- Systolic blood pressure increases during uterine contractions in first stage; systolic and diastolic pressure increase during uterine contractions in second stage.
- WBC count increases.
- Respiratory rate increases.
- Temperature may be slightly elevated.
- 1+ protein may be present in the urine.
- Gastric motility is decreased.

Respiratory changes. Respiratory system adaptations also are seen. Increased physical activity with increased oxygen consumption is reflected in an increase in the respiratory rate. *Hyperventilation* may cause respiratory alkalosis (an increase in pH), hypoxia, and hypocapnia (decrease in carbon dioxide). In the unmedicated woman in the second stage, oxygen consumption almost doubles. Anxiety also increases oxygen consumption.

Renal changes. Several renal system adaptations occur. In the second trimester, the urinary bladder becomes an abdominal organ. When filling, it is palpable above the symphysis pubis. During labor, spontaneous voiding may be difficult for various reasons: tissue edema caused by pressure from the presenting part, discomfort, sedation, and embarrassment. Proteinuria of 1+ is within normal limits inasmuch as the finding can occur in response to the breakdown of muscle tissue from the physical work of labor.

Integumentary changes. The integumentary system adaptations are evident, especially in the great distensibility in the area of the vaginal introitus (opening). The degree of distensibility varies with the individual. Despite this ability to stretch, even in the absence of episiotomy or lacerations, minute tears in the skin around the vaginal introitus do occur.

Musculoskeletal changes. The musculoskeletal system is stressed during labor. Diaphoresis, fatigue, proteinuria (1+), and perhaps an increased temperature accompany the marked increase in muscle activity. Backache and joint ache (unrelated to fetal position) occur as a result of increased joint laxity at term. The labor process itself and the woman pointing her toes can cause leg cramps.

Neurologic changes. The neurologic system reflects the stress and discomfort of labor. Sensorial changes occur as the woman moves through phases of the first stage of labor and as she moves from one stage to the next. Initially she may be euphoric. Euphoria gives way to increased seriousness, then to amnesia between contractions during the second stage, and finally to elation or fatigue after giving birth. Endogenous endorphins (morphinelike chemicals produced naturally by the body) raise the pain threshold and produce sedation. In addition, physiologic anesthesia of perineal tissues, caused by pressure of the presenting part, decreases perception of pain.

Gastrointestinal changes. Labor affects the woman's gastrointestinal system. Dry lips and mouth may result from mouth breathing, dehydration, and emotional response to labor. During labor, gastrointestinal motility and absorption are decreased and stomach emptying time is slowed. Nausea and vomiting of undigested food eaten after onset of labor are common. Nausea and belching also occur as a reflex response to full cervical dilation. The mother may state that diarrhea accompanied the onset of labor, or the nurse may palpate the presence of hard or impacted stool in the rectum.

Endocrine changes. The endocrine system is active during labor. The onset of labor may be attributed to decreasing levels of progesterone and increasing levels of estrogen, prostaglandins, and oxytocin. Metabolism increases, and blood glucose levels may decrease with the work of labor.

Key Points

- The process of labor and birth are affected by the 5 *Ps*—the passenger, passageway, powers, position of the mother, and psychologic responses.
- Because of its size and relative rigidity, the fetal head has a major effect on the birth process.
- The diameters at the plane of the pelvic inlet, midpelvis, and outlet, plus the axis of the birth canal, determine whether vaginal birth is possible and the manner by which the fetus may pass down the birth canal.
- The forces acting to expel the fetus and placenta are derived from involuntary uterine contractions during the first stage of labor, which are augmented by voluntary bearing-down efforts during the second stage.
- The first stage of labor is from the onset of regular contractions to when the cervix is fully dilated. The second stage of labor is from full dilation to the birth of the infant. The third stage of labor is from the infant's birth to the expulsion of the placenta. The fourth stage is the first 2 hours after birth.
- The cardinal movements of the mechanism of labor are engagement, descent, flexion, internal rotation, extension, restitution and external rotation, and expulsion of the baby.
- Although the reasons for the onset of labor are unknown, many factors, including changes in the maternal uterus, cervix, and pituitary gland, are thought to be involved.
- An understanding of maternal adaptations to pregnancy is fundamental to anticipating and meeting the pregnant woman's needs.
- A healthy fetus with an adequate uterofetoplacental circulation is able to compensate to the stress of uterine contractions.

References

American College of Obstetricians and Gynecologists: *Dystocia*, Tech Bull No. 137, Washington, DC, 1989, ACOG.

Andrews C, Chrzanowski M: Maternal position, labor and comfort, *Appl Nurs Res*, 3(1):7, 1990.

Bennett V, Brown L: *Myles testbook for midwives*, ed 12, Edinburgh, 1993, Churchill-Livingstone.

Cunningham F et al: *Williams obstetrics*, ed 19, Norwalk, Ct, 1993, Appleton & Lange.

Friedman E: *Labor: clinical evaluation and management*, ed 2, New York, 1978, Appleton-Century-Crofts.

Golay J, Vedam S, Sorger L: The squatting position for the second stage of labor: effects on labor and on maternal and fetal well-being, *Birth* 20(2):73, 1993.

Melzack R, Belanger E, Lacroix R: Labor pain: effect of maternal position on front and back pain, *J Pain Symptom Manage*, 6(8):476, 1991.

Paine L, Tinker D: The effect of maternal bearing-down efforts on the actual umbilical cord pH and length of second stage labor, *J Nurse Midwife* 37(1):61, 1992.

Willson J et al: *Obstetrics and gynecology*, ed 9, St Louis, 1991, Mosby.

Zlatnik F: *Normal labor and delivery*. In Scott J et al, editors: *Danforth's obstetrics and gynecology*, ed 7, Philadelphia, 1994, JB Lippincott.

Bibliography

Evans M, Dick M, Clark A: Sleep during the week before labor: relationships to labor outcomes, *Clin Nurs Res* 4(3):238, 1995.

Lowe N, Reiss R: Parturition and fetal adaptation, *J Obstet Gynecol Neonat Nurs* 25(4):339, 1996.

Mackey M: Women's evaluation of their childbirth performance, *Matern Child Nurs J* 23(2):57, 1995.

Martin E: *Intrapartum management modules*, ed 2, Baltimore, Md, 1996, Williams & Wilkins.

Tomlinson P, Bryan A, Esau A: Family centered intrapartum care: revisiting an old concept, *J Obstet Gynecol Neonat Nurs* 25(4):331, 1996.

CHAPTER 14

Management of Discomfort

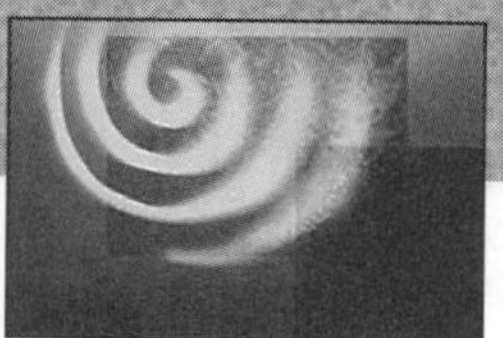

DISCOMFORT DURING LABOR, P. 352

Neurologic origins, p. 352

Perception of pain, p. 352

NONPHARMACOLOGIC MANAGEMENT OF DISCOMFORT, P. 354

Childbirth preparation methods, p. 354

Relaxing and breathing techniques, p. 355

Other nonpharmacologic methods, p. 357

PHARMACOLOGIC MANAGEMENT OF DISCOMFORT, P. 358

Sedatives, p. 358

Analgesia and anesthesia, p. 358

Nursing care management, p. 367

Pregnant women commonly worry about pain they will experience during labor and childbirth and how they will react to and deal with that pain. Interventions include a wide variety of childbirth preparation methods that help the woman or couple cope with the discomfort of labor. The interventions selected depend on the situation and the preference of both the woman and her health care provider. This chapter discusses discomfort during labor and presents nonpharmacologic and pharmacologic interventions throughout all stages of labor. This information provides the basis for understanding the nurse's role in management of discomfort during labor.

DISCOMFORT DURING LABOR

Neurologic Origins

The discomfort experienced during labor has two origins (Hughs, 1992). During the *first stage of labor,* uterine contractions cause the following two events: (1) cervical dilation and effacement, and (2) uterine ischemia (decreased blood flow and therefore local oxygen deficit) from contraction of the arteries leading to the myometrium. Pain impulses during the first stage of labor are transmitted through the spinal nerve segment (T-11 and T-12) and accessory lower thoracic and upper lumbar sympathetic nerves. These nerves originate in the uterine body and cervix.

The discomfort from cervical changes and uterine ischemia is **visceral pain.** It is located over the lower portion of the abdomen and radiates to the lumbar area of the back and down the thighs. Usually the woman experiences discomfort only during contractions and is free of pain between contractions.

During the *second stage of labor,* the stage of expulsion of the baby, the woman experiences perineal or **somatic pain.** Perineal discomfort results from stretching of perineal tissues to allow passage of the fetus and traction on the peritoneum and uterocervical supports during contractions. Discomfort also can be produced by expulsive forces or from pressure by the presenting part on the bladder, bowel, or other sensitive pelvic structures. Pain impulses during the second stage of labor are carried via S-1 through S-4 and the parasympathetic system from perineal tissues. Pain experienced during the *third stage of labor* and the so-called "afterpains" are uterine, similar to that experienced early in the first stage of labor. Areas of discomfort during labor are illustrated in Fig. 14-1.

Pain may be local, with cramping and a tearing or bursting sensation because of distention and laceration of the cervix, vagina, or perineal tissues. This discomfort is commonly perceived as an intense burning sensation as tissue stretches. Pain also may be **referred,** in which the discomfort is felt in the back, flanks, or thighs.

Perception of Pain

Although the pain threshold is remarkably similar in all people regardless of gender, social, ethnic, or cultural differences, these differences play a definite role in the individual's *perception of pain.* The effects of factors such as culture, use of counterstimuli, and distraction in coping with pain are not fully understood. The meaning of pain and the verbal and nonverbal expressions given to pain are apparently learned from interactions within the primary social group. Cultural influences may impose unrealistic expectations. For instance, Asian women believe it is shameful to scream or show pain, and they avoid verbal expression (Mattson and Smith, 1993).

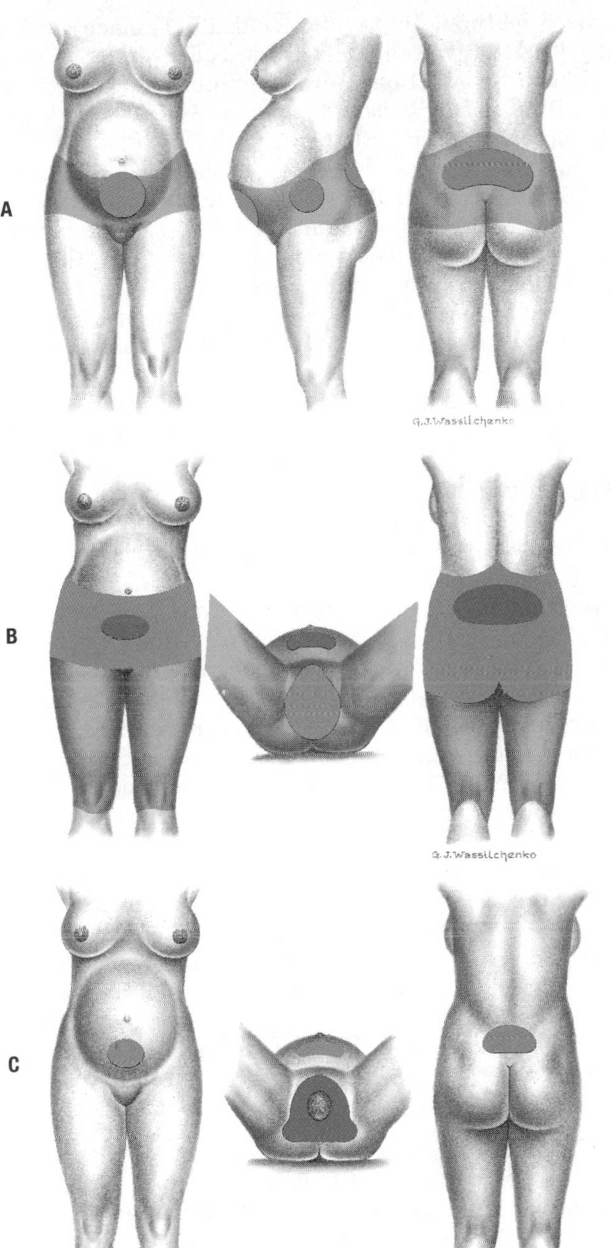

Fig. 14-1 Discomfort during labor. **A,** Distribution of labor pain during first stage. **B,** Distribution of labor pain during later phase of first stage and early phase of second stage. **C,** Distribution of labor pain during later phase of second stage and actual birth. (Gray shading indicates areas of mild discomfort; light colored shading indicates areas of moderate discomfort; dark colored areas indicate intense discomfort.)

Expression of Pain

Pain results in both psychic responses and reflex physical actions. The quality of physical pain has been described as prickling, burning, aching, throbbing, sharp, nauseating, or cramping. Pain in childbirth gives rise to symptoms that are identifiable. Increased activity of the sympathetic nervous system may occur in response to pain resulting in changes in blood pressure, pulse, respiration, and skin color. Pallor and diaphoresis may be seen (Potter and Perry, 1995). Bouts of nausea and vomiting and excessive perspiration also are commonplace.

Certain *affective expressions* of suffering are often seen. Affective changes include increasing anxiety with lessened perceptual field, writhing, crying, groaning, gesturing (hand clenching and wringing), and excessive muscular excitability throughout the body. Cultural expression of pain may vary. For example, Native-American women may endure pain quietly, whereas Hispanic women endure pain with patience but consider it acceptable to cry out (Mattson and Smith, 1993).

Pain is personalized for each individual. As pain is experienced, people develop various coping mechanisms to deal with it. Emotional tension from anxiety and fear may increase pain and perception of pain during labor (see the discussion of the Dick-Read method later in this chapter). Pain, or the possibility of pain, can induce fear in which anxiety borders on panic. Fatigue and sleep deprivation magnify pain. Parity may affect perception of labor pain because primiparous women have longer labors and thus greater fatigue, causing a vicious circle of increased pain and a more likely use of pharmacologic support (Rooks, Weatherby, and Ernst, 1992). Women with a history of substance abuse experience as much pain during labor as other women. It is usually unnecessary to withhold pain medications; however, close monitoring for complications associated with each substance is part of the nursing assessment.

At times, pain stimuli that are particularly intense can be ignored. Certain nerve cell groupings within the spinal cord, brain stem, and cerebral cortex may have the ability to modulate the pain impulse through a blocking mechanism. The **gate-control theory** is helpful in understanding the approaches used in parent education for childbirth programs or the use of hypnosis in labor. According to this theory, pain sensations travel along sensory nerve pathways to the brain, and only a limited number of sensations or messages can travel through these nerve pathways at one time. By using distraction techniques such as massage or stroking, music, and imagery, the nerve pathways for pain perception are reduced or completely blocked. These distractors are thought to work by closing down a hypothetic gate in the spinal cord, thus blocking pain signals from reaching the brain. Perception of pain stimuli is diminished.

In addition, when the woman in labor performs neuromuscular and motor skills, activity within the spinal cord itself further modifies the transmission of pain. Cognitive activities of concentration on breathing and relaxation require selective and directed cortical activity, which activates and closes the gating mechanism as well. The gate-control theory emphasizes the need for a supportive setting for birth. In such an environment the laboring woman can relax and allow the various higher mental activities to be implemented.

At other times, maternal fatigue, fetal size or position, or other factors may require the use of medications in addition to comfort measures. Labor pain may result in physiologic responses that can decrease uterine contractility and lengthen the labor. The nurse needs to understand that each woman experiences and perceives pain in her own unique way and that the pain as it is described by the woman needs to be acknowledged by the nurse. Concerns and anxieties can occur during later phases of labor and interfere with the use of the skills learned in parent education classes (Wuitchik, Hesson, and Bakel, 1990).

NONPHARMACOLOGIC MANAGEMENT OF DISCOMFORT

The alleviation of pain is important. Commonly it is not the amount of pain the woman experiences, but whether she meets her goals for herself in coping with the pain that influences her perception of the birth experience as "good" or "bad." The observant nurse looks for cues to identify the woman's desired level of control in the management of pain and its relief.

Nonpharmacologic methods for relief of discomfort are taught in many different types of prenatal preparation classes. Whether or not a woman or couple has attended these classes or read various books and magazines on the subject, the nurse can teach techniques to relieve discomfort during labor.

Childbirth Preparation Methods

Today most health care providers recommend or offer childbirth preparation classes to expectant parents. Three major methods taught in the United States are: (1) the **Dick-Read** or **natural childbirth method,** (2) the Lamaze or psychoprophylactic method, and (3) the Bradley method, or husband-coached childbirth.

Dick-Read method. Grantly Dick-Read was an English physician who published two books, *Natural Childbirth* (1933) and *Childbirth Without Fear* (1944), in which he theorized that pain in childbirth was the result of social conditioning and a fear-tension-pain syndrome. Dick-Read's work became the foundation for organized programs of childbirth preparation and teacher training throughout the United States, Canada, Great Britain, and South Africa. Nurses prepared in this method established the International Childbirth Education Association (ICEA) in 1960.

To replace fear of the unknown with understanding and confidence, Dick-Read's program includes information on labor and birth, as well as on nutrition, hygiene, and exercise. Classes include practice in three techniques: physical exercise to prepare the body for labor; conscious relaxation; and breathing patterns.

Conscious relaxation involves progressive relaxation of muscle groups in the entire body. With practice, many women are able to relax on command, both during and between contractions. Some woman actually sleep between contractions.

Breathing patterns include deep abdominal respirations for most of labor, shallow breathing toward the end of the first stage, and, until recently, breath holding for second stage of labor. Teachers of the Dick-Read method contend that the weight of the abdominal musculature of the contracting uterus increases pain. The woman is taught to force her abdominal muscles to rise as the uterus rises forward during a contraction, thus lifting the abdominal muscles off the contracting uterus.

The Dick-Read method has been adapted to ensure that labor support provided in the past by the nursing staff is now provided by the father or other support person chosen by the mother.

Lamaze method. During the 1960s the **Lamaze method** gained popularity in the United States after Marjorie Karmel introduced the **psychoprophylactic method (PPM)** in her book, *Thank You, Dr. Lamaze* (1959). The American Society for Psychoprophylaxis in Obstetrics (ASPO) was formed in 1960, and the National Association of Childbirth Education, Inc. (NACE) was formed in 1970 to promote the Lamaze method and prepare teachers in the method. In 1971 the national Council of Childbirth Education Specialists, Inc. (CCES) was founded to offer teacher-training seminars.

The Lamaze method grew out of Pavlov's work on classical conditioning. According to Lamaze, pain is a conditioned response. Women can also be conditioned not to experience pain in labor; the Lamaze method conditions women to respond to mock uterine contractions with controlled muscular relaxation and breathing patterns instead of crying out and losing control (Lamaze, 1972). Coping strategies also include concentrating on a focal point, such as a favorite picture or pattern, to keep nerve pathways occupied so they cannot respond to painful stimuli.

The woman is taught to relax uninvolved muscle groups while she contracts a specific muscle group. She applies this in labor by relaxing uninvolved muscles while her uterus contracts. Attending Lamaze-type childbirth preparation classes leads to a significantly higher level of neuromuscular control during the first stage of labor than self-preparation (Bernardini, Maloni, and Stegman, 1983). The perception of maintaining control is closely associated with satisfaction (Mackey, 1990).

Lamaze teachers believe that chest breathing lifts the diaphragm off the contracting uterus, thus giving it more room to expand. Chest-breathing patterns vary according to the intensity of the contractions and the progress of labor. Teachers also seek to eliminate fear by increasing the understanding of the way the body functions and the neurophysiology of pain. Support in labor is provided by the father or other support person or by a specially trained labor attendant called a *monitrice* or *doula.*

Bradley method. Robert Bradley, a Denver obstetrician, published *Husband-Coached Childbirth* in 1965, advocating what he calls true natural childbirth, without anesthesia or analgesia and with a husband-coach and use of labor breathing techniques. The American Academy of Husband-Coached Childbirth (AAHCC) was founded to prepare teachers and make the method available.

The **Bradley method** is based on observations of animal behavior during birth and emphasizes working in harmony with the body, using breath control, abdominal breathing, and general body relaxation (Bradley, 1981). The technique stresses environmental factors such as darkness, solitude, and quiet to make childbirth a more natural experience. Women using the Bradley method often appear to be sleeping in labor, but they are actually in a state of deep mental relaxation.

Although the father's presence during labor seems to be important to most women, the concept of the father as coach has been criticized by some (Klein et al, 1981). Some men are not comfortable with this role but can still be supportive of their wives during pregnancy and childbirth.

Comparison of childbirth methods. Most proponents of prepared childbirth agree that the major causes of pain in labor are fear and tension. All methods attempt to reduce these two factors and eliminate pain by increasing the woman's knowledge of what to expect in labor and birth, enhancing her self-confidence and sense of control, preparing a support person, and training her in physical conditioning and relaxation breathing.

There are a few fine differences in approach. For example, Bradley teachers discourage the use of medication, encouraging the woman to focus inwardly and to take direction from her own body. Lamaze teachers believe that the judicious use of pain medication can be an appropriate adjunct to relaxation techniques and stress external focusing and distraction. In reality, few instructors adhere strictly to one particular method but instead incorporate a variety of strategies aimed at increasing the woman's ability to cope with labor and minimize her need for medication.

Relaxing and Breathing Techniques

Focusing and feedback relaxation. Some women bring a favorite device for use in focusing attention. Others choose some fixed object in the labor room. As the contraction begins, they may focus on this object to reduce their perception of pain. This technique, coupled with feedback relaxation, helps the woman work with her contractions rather than against them. The coach monitors this process, giving the woman cues as to when to begin the breathing techniques (Fig. 14-2). A common feedback mechanism is for the woman and her coach to verbalize the word "relax" at the onset of each contraction and throughout it as needed. After the degree of relaxation has been assessed, relaxation techniques practiced in the prenatal period can be reviewed. The coach also keeps the woman from being disturbed by routine examinations for progress and checking of fetal heart rate. These procedures are postponed until the contraction is completed.

Breathing techniques. Different approaches to childbirth preparation stress varying techniques for using breathing as a "tool" to help the woman maintain control through contractions. In the first stage, breathing techniques can promote relaxation of abdominal muscles and thereby increase the size of the abdominal cavity. This lessens friction and discomfort between the uterus and the abdominal wall. Because the muscles of the genital area also become more relaxed, they do not interfere with descent. In the second stage, breathing is used to increase abdominal pressure and thereby assist in expelling the fetus. It also is used to relax the pudendal muscles to prevent precipitate expulsion of the fetal head.

For those couples who have prepared for labor by practicing such techniques, occasional reminders may be all that is necessary. For those who have had no preparation, instruction in simple breathing and relaxation can be given early in labor and often is surprisingly successful. Motivation is high, and learning readiness is enhanced by the reality of labor.

There are varied approaches to breathing techniques during contractions. The nurse needs to ascertain what if any information the laboring couple has before providing them with instruction. Simple patterns are more easily learned (Janke, 1992). Generally, slow abdominal breathing, approximately

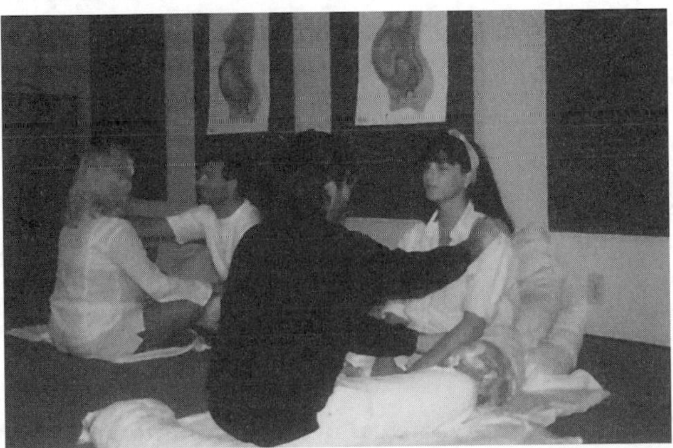

Fig. 14-2 Expectant parents learning relaxation techniques. (Courtesy Marjorie Pyle, RNC, *Lifecircle*, Costa Mesa, Calif.)

Patient Teaching

BREATHING TECHNIQUES

CLEANSING BREATH

Relaxed breath in through nose and out mouth. Used at the beginning and end of each contraction.

SLOW-PACED BREATHING (slower than normal rate)

Not less than half normal breathing rate (No. breaths/min divided by 2)

IN-2-3-4/OUT-2-3-4/IN-2-3-4/OUT-2-3-4 . . .

MODIFIED-PACED BREATHING (faster than normal rate)

Not more than twice normal breathing rate (No. breaths/min times 2); breaths should be lighter

IN-OUT/IN-OUT/IN-OUT/IN-OUT/ . . .

For more flexibility and variety, the woman may combine the slow and modified breathing by using the slow breathing for beginnings and ends of contractions and modified breathing for more intense peaks. This technique conserves energy and lessens fatigue.

PATTERNED-PACED BREATHING (SAME RATE AS MODIFIED)

Enhances concentration

a. 3:1 Patterned breathing
   IN-OUT/IN-OUT/IN-OUT/IN-BLOW
   (repeat through contraction)
b. 4:1 Patterned breathing
   IN-OUT/IN-OUT/IN-OUT/IN-OUT/IN-BLOW
   (repeat through contraction)

You may do any pattern desired, although ratios of 5:1 or higher tend to be very tiring. Some people like to do patterned breathing to a tune (Yankee Doodle, Old McDonald), to a repeated phrase (I think I can, I think I can), or in a pyramid pattern such as 1:1, 2:1, 3:1, 4:1, 5:1—5:1, 4:1, 3:1, 2:1, 1:1

c. *Coach call:* May be used when woman needs more distraction and concentration (e.g., during transition). The woman's coach signals the breathing ratio with his/her fingers or by verbal cues, changing the ratio after each "IN-BLOW."
   Example:
   IN-OUT/IN-OUT/IN-BLOW
   IN-OUT/IN-OUT/IN-OUT/IN-OUT/IN-BLOW
   IN-OUT/IN-BLOW

From Shapiro et al: *The Lamaze ready reference guide for labor and birth,* ed 2, Washington, DC, 1997, Chapter ASPO/Lamaze.

one-half the woman's normal breathing rate, is initiated when the woman can no longer walk or talk through contractions (see the Patient Teaching box on p. 355). As contractions increase in frequency and intensity, the woman may need to change to chest breathing, which is more shallow and approximately twice her normal rate of breathing.

The most difficult time to maintain control during contractions comes when the cervical dilation reaches 8 to 10 cm. This period is also called the *transition period.* Even for the woman who has prepared for labor, concentration on breathing techniques is difficult to maintain. The type used may be the 4:1 pattern: breath, breath, breath, breath, puff (as though blowing out a candle). This ratio may increase to 6:1 or 8:1. These patterns begin with the routine cleansing breath and end with a deep breath exhaled to "blow the contraction away." This type of breathing is a type of **hyperventilation.** The woman and her support person must be aware of the accompanying symptoms of the resultant *respiratory alkalosis:* lightheadedness, dizziness, tingling of fingers, or circumoral numbness. Alkalosis may be overcome by having the woman breathe into a paper bag that is held tightly around the mouth and nose. This enables her to rebreathe carbon dioxide and replace the bicarbonate ion. She can breathe into her cupped hands if no bag is available.

As the fetal head reaches the pelvic floor, the woman may experience the urge to push and may automatically begin to exert downward pressure by contracting her abdominal muscles. The traditional approach prevalent in nursing practice is to have the mother begin to push and bear down at complete dilation (10 cm) whether or not the woman feels the urge to push. This traditional view holds that pushing before full dilation is reached compresses the cervix between the fetal head and the pubic bone and that this compression may result in a nonreassuring fetal heart rate (FHR), cervical edema, or cervical laceration. It may even slow the dilation process. The woman can control the urge to push by taking panting breaths or by slowly exhaling through pursed lips. This is good practice for the type of breathing to be used as the fetal head is slowly delivered.

Another view, physiologic second-stage management of labor, asserts that the second stage is a normal physiologic event that helps women push spontaneously and give birth with minimal intervention (Cosner and deJong, 1993). McKay et al. (1990) interviewed 20 women and reported that 13 had well-defined urges to push that occurred before, at, and after complete dilation. These findings suggest that when to push should be individualized to the mother's own response rather then labor routines that dictate pushing at complete dilation.

Effleurage and sacral pressure. Effleurage and sacral pressure, or massage, are two methods that have brought relief to many women during the first stage of labor. The gate-control theory may supply the reason for the effectiveness of these measures. Firm pressure to the sacral area may assist the woman to cope with the sensations of internal pressure and pain in the lower back. **Effleurage** (see Fig. 7-20), which is a light stroking, usually of the abdomen, in rhythm with breathing during contractions, is used to distract the woman from contraction pain. The woman or her partner can perform effleurage on any area of her body. Many times the monitor belts make it difficult to perform effleurage on the abdomen; thus a thigh or the chest may be used.

Jet hydrotherapy. *Jet hydrotherapy* (whirlpool baths) is another nonpharmacologic method used for increasing comfort and relaxation during labor, although it is not universally accepted or implemented. Many new birthing units are installing baths with air jets. The buoyancy of the warm water, with or without air jets, provides support for tense muscles.

Several immediate benefits are seen. Relief from discomfort and general body relaxation reduce the woman's anxiety. Less anxiety decreases adrenalin production, which in turn allows an increase in levels of oxytocin (to stimulate labor) and endorphins (to reduce pain perception). In addition, the bubbles and gentle lapping of the water stimulate the nipples, which increases oxytocin production (hyperstimulation of the uterus has not occurred [Aderhold and Perry, 1991]). Cervical dilation of 2 to 3 cm in 30 minutes often is noted. Blood pressure readings decrease, and diuresis occurs. If the woman is experiencing "back labor" secondary to occiput posterior or transverse position, she is encouraged to assume the hands-and-knees or the side-lying position in the tub (Fig. 14-3, *A* and *C*). Because this position decreases pain and increases relaxation and the production of oxytocin, the fetus can rotate to the occiput anterior position spontaneously.

Jet hydrotherapy must be ordered by the primary health care provider. The mother's vital signs must be within normal limits, her cervix must be dilated 4 to 5 cm, and she must be in the active phase of the first stage of labor. If she is in the latent phase, her contractions may slow down. Fetal well-being must be established. Her membranes may be intact or ruptured. If ruptured, the fluid must be clear or only lightly stained with meconium (Aderhold and Perry, 1991). Heavy meconium staining necessitates an internal electrode, in which case jet hydrotherapy would be contraindicated. In a randomized trial, babies born more than 24 hours after rupture of membranes had significantly lower Apgar scores at 5 minutes in a group of bathing mothers vs. nonbathing mothers, suggesting caution for the use of jet hydrotherapy with mothers experiencing prolonged rupture of the membranes (Waldenstrom and Nilsson, 1992).

There is no set time limit, and women are often encouraged to stay in the bath as long as desired. In a randomized controlled study, most women stayed in the bath for 30 to 45 minutes, and only a few stayed longer than 60 minutes (Schorn, McAllister, and Blanco, 1993). During the bath, if the woman's temperature and FHR increase, the water is cooled down or she is asked to step out of the bath to cool down. The bath water is kept between 35.6° C to 36.7° C. The mother's temperature may remain slightly elevated for a short time after the bath. Fluids and ice chips and a cool face cloth are offered during the bath (Fig. 14-3, *A*). Maternal vital signs and labor and FHR are reassessed after the bath (Fig. 14-3, *B*).

The tub must be kept meticulously clean. Cleansing solutions vary with institutions; however, household bleach is commonly used.

Transcutaneous electrical nerve stimulation. Transcutaneous electrical nerve stimulation (TENS) may be effective because of the "placebo effect;" that is, confidence in TENS may stimulate the release of endogenous opiates (enkephalins)

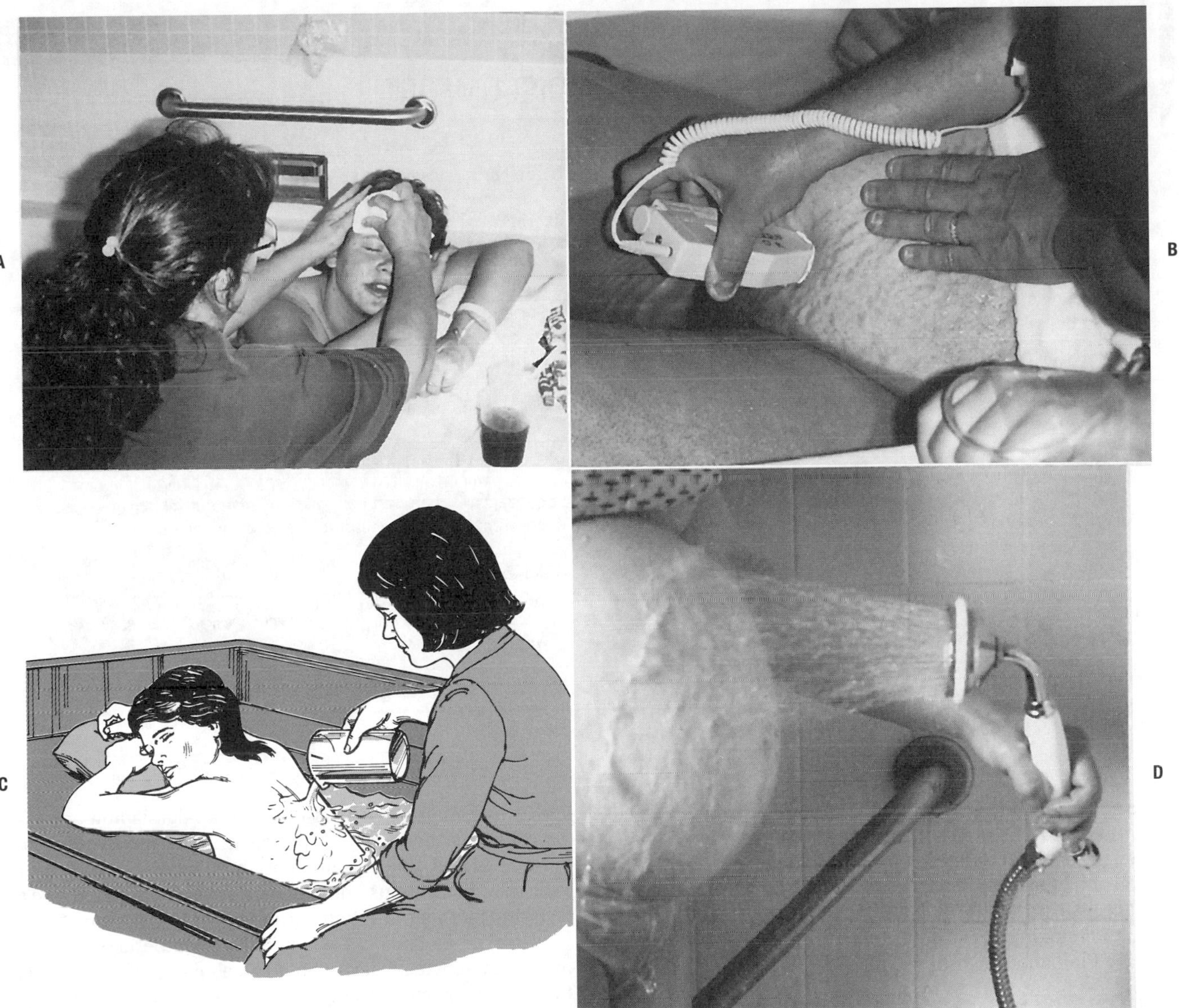

Fig. 14-3 Jet hydrotherapy during labor. **A,** Nurse provides comfort measures and ensures adequate hydration (note glass of clear fluid). **B,** Nurse assesses FHR. **C,** Woman experiencing back labor, relaxing while nurse pours warm water over her back. **D,** Use of shower as one alternative to jet hydrotherapy during labor. (**A** and **B** courtesy Kathy Aderhold, CNM, Presbyterian/St. Luke's Medical Center, Denver; **D** courtesy Kathy Harold, RN, MS, Birth Place, Barnes Hospital at Washington University Medical Center, St. Louis.)

in the woman's body and thus alleviate the discomfort (Scott et al, 1994).

Two pairs of electrodes are taped on either side of the thoracic and sacral spine. Continuous mild electrical currents are applied from a battery-operated device. During a contraction the woman increases the stimulation by turning control knobs on the device. Women describe the sensation as a tingling or buzzing and pain relief as good or very good. The use of TENS poses no risk to the mother or fetus. TENS is credited with reducing or eliminating the need for analgesia and with increasing the woman's perception of control over the experience.

The nurse assists the mother who is using TENS by explaining the device and its use, by carefully placing and securing the electrodes, and by closely evaluating its effectiveness.

Other Nonpharmacologic Methods

Various other nonpharmacologic methods for control of discomfort are practiced. Many are learned in parent education classes. These include hypnosis, acupressure, yoga, biofeedback, and therapeutic touch (Bernat et al, 1992; Kerschner and Schenck, 1991; Letts et al, 1993). Aromatherapy, the use of herbal teas or vapors, is reported to have good effects for some women (Tisserand, 1990; Valnet, 1990).

Women are encouraged to tune in to their own body cues and to incorporate natural responses. Techniques include

Nursing Care Plan

NONPHARMACOLOGIC MANAGEMENT OF DISCOMFORT

Nursing Diagnosis: Pain related to physiologic response to labor

Expected Outcomes: Woman will express decrease in intensity of discomfort and experience satisfaction with her labor and delivery performance.

• **NURSING INTERVENTIONS/*RATIONALES***

Assess whether woman and significant other have attended childbirth classes, her knowledge of labor process, and her current level of anxiety *to plan supportive strategies.*

Encourage support person to remain with woman in labor *to provide support and increase probability of response to comfort measures.*

Teach and/or review nonpharmacologic techniques available to decrease anxiety and pain during labor (i.e., focusing and feedback, breathing techniques, effleurage and sacral pressure) *to enhance chances of success in using techniques.*

Explore other techniques that the woman or significant other may have learned in childbirth classes (i.e., hypnosis, yoga, acupressure, biofeedback, therapeutic touch, aroma therapy, imaging, vocalizations) *to provide largest repertoire of coping strategies.*

Explore use of jet hydrotherapy if ordered by physician and if woman meets use criteria (i.e., vital signs within normal limits [WNL], cervix 4 to 5 cm dilated, active phase of first stage labor) *to aid relaxation and stimulate production of natural oxytocin.*

Explore use of transcutaneous nerve stimulation per physician order *to provide an increased perception of control over pain and an increase in release of endogenous opiates.*

Assist woman to change positions and to use pillows *to reduce stiffness, aid circulation, and promote comfort.*

Assess bladder for distention and encourage voiding often *to avoid bladder distention and subsequent discomfort.*

Encourage rest between contractions *to minimize fatigue.*

Keep woman and significant other informed about progress *to allay anxiety.*

Guide couple through the labor stages and phases, helping them use and modify discomfort techniques that are appropriate to each phase *to ensure greatest effectiveness of techniques employed.*

---

vocalization, or sounding, to relieve tension, imagery-assisted relaxation (IAR) (Cassidy, 1993) and visualization to guide women into positive spaces ("seeing" the vagina open up around the baby), hot compresses to the perineum, perineal massage, warm showers (Fig. 14-3, *D*) or bathing during labor, and relaxing music and subdued lighting (see the Nursing Care Plan above).

PHARMACOLOGIC MANAGEMENT OF DISCOMFORT

Sedatives

Sedatives such as barbiturates relieve anxiety and induce sleep only in prodromal or early latent labor and in the absence of pain. If the woman has pain, sedatives given without an analgesic may increase apprehension and cause the mother to become hyperactive and disoriented. Undesirable side effects include respiratory and vasomotor depression of both the mother and newborn. Because of these disadvantages, barbiturates are seldom used (Scott et al, 1994).

Analgesia and Anesthesia

The use of analgesia and anesthesia was not generally accepted as part of obstetric management until Queen Victoria used chloroform during the birth of her son in 1853. Since then much study has gone into the development of pharmacologic control of discomfort during the birth period. The goal of researchers is to develop methods that provide adequate pain relief to women without adding to maternal or fetal risk or affecting the progress of labor.

Nursing management of obstetric analgesia and anesthesia combines the nurse's expertise in maternity care with a knowledge and understanding of anatomy and physiology, as well as of medications and their desired and undesired side effects and methods of administration.

Anesthesia encompasses analgesia, amnesia, relaxation, and reflex activity. Anesthesia is the abolition of pain perception by interrupting the nerve impulses going to the brain. Loss of sensation may be partial or complete, sometimes with the loss of consciousness.

The term **analgesia** is best reserved to describe only those states in which there is alleviation of the sensation of pain or the raising of one's threshold for pain perception. With analgesia there is no loss of consciousness.

Analgesia can be induced by positive conditioning (e.g., Lamaze method, imagery, relaxation) and analgesic drugs. A basic understanding of the normal course of labor and birth and physical and psychologic preparation by the pregnant woman may reduce pain during childbirth. Especially important is good antenatal care in its broadest sense; reassurance and suggestion are beneficial. Participation in parent education classes such as those proposed by Dick-Read (1987) or psychoprophylaxis by Lamaze (1972) or Bradley (1981) can do much to alleviate distress.

The type of analgesic or anesthetic to be used is chosen in part by the stage of labor and by the method of birth (Box 14-1).

Systemic analgesia. **Systemic analgesia** remains the major method of analgesia for the woman in labor when person-

BOX 14-1
Pharmacologic Control of Discomfort by Stage of Labor and Method of Birth

FIRST STAGE
- Systemic analgesia
  - Narcotic analgesic compounds
  - Mixed narcotic agonist-antagonist compounds, analgesic potentiators
- Nerve block analgesia/anesthesia
  - Lumbar epidural analgesia
  - Paracervical block

SECOND STAGE
- Nerve block analgesia/anesthesia
  - Local infiltration anesthesia
  - Pudendal block
  - Subarachnoid (spinal) anesthesia
  - Epidural block
  - Epidural and spinal narcotics
- Inhalation analgesia/anesthesia
  - Self-administered
  - Nitrous oxide–oxygen
  - General anesthesia

VAGINAL BIRTH
- Local infiltration
- Pudendal block
- Lumbar epidural block
  - Analgesia
  - Anesthesia
- Subarachnoid block
  - Analgesia
  - Anesthesia
- Inhalation analgesia

CESAREAN BIRTH
- Subarachnoid block
  - Spinal
  - Saddle block (low spinal)
- Lumbar epidural block
  - Anesthesia
- Inhalation
  - General anesthesia

nel trained in regional analgesia are not available (Scott et al, 1994). Systemic analgesics cross the blood-brain barrier to provide central analgesic effects. They also cross the placental barrier. Effects on the fetus depend on the maternal dosage, the pharmacokinetics of the specific medication, and the route and timing of administration. Intravenous (IV) administration is often preferred over intramuscular (IM) administration because the onset of the medication's effect is faster and more reliable. Classes of analgesic medications used include narcotics, narcotic agonist-antagonist compounds, and tranquilizers such as analgesic-potentiating medications (ataractics).

Narcotic analgesic compounds. **Narcotic analgesics** such as meperidine (Demerol) and fentanyl (Sublimaze) are especially effective for the relief of severe, persistent, or recurrent pain. They have no amnesic effect. Meperidine overcomes inhibitory factors in labor and may even relax the cervix.

Meperidine is the most commonly used narcotic for women in labor (Scott et al, 1994). After IV injection, onset is rapid (30 seconds), and maximum effect is reached in 5 to 10 minutes with a duration of about 3 hours. Peak effect after IM injection of meperidine is reached in 40 to 50 minutes. In a randomized controlled study, women who received IV meperidine reported significantly lower levels of pain when compared with women who received IM meperidine (Isenor and Penny-MacGillivary, 1993). Ideally, birth should occur less than 1 or more than 4 hours after IM injection to minimize neonatal depression. Since tachycardia is a possible side effect, meperidine is used cautiously for women with cardiac disease.

Fentanyl is a potent, short-acting narcotic analgesic. After IV injection, onset of the drug effect occurs within 2 minutes and lasts about 30 to 60 minutes. Onset of the drug effect after IM injection occurs in 7 to 15 minutes, reaches its peak effect in 20 to 30 minutes, and lasts for 1 to 2 hours. Additive central nervous system (CNS) and respiratory depression occurs if fentanyl is given with alcohol, antihistamines, antidepressants, or other sedative/hypnotics.

Mixed narcotic agonist-antagonist compounds. An agonist is an agent that activates something; an antagonist is an agent that blocks something from happening. Mixed narcotic **agonist-antagonist compounds** such as butorphanol (Stadol) and nalbuphine (Nubain), in the doses used during labor, provide analgesia without causing respiratory depression of the mother or the neonate. Both IM and IV routes are used for administration. Butorphanol (1 to 3 mg IM; 0.5 to 2 mg IV) or nalbuphine (0.2 mg/kg subcutaneously (SC)/IM; 0.1 to 0.2 mg/kg IV) may be given during the first stage of labor.

Analgesic-potentiators (ataractics). Phenothiazines, so-called *tranquilizer drugs*, have the property of augmenting most of the desirable but few of the undesirable effects of analgesics or general anesthetics. These **ataractics** do not relieve pain but decrease anxiety and apprehension, as well as potentiate narcotic effects. This potentiation effect causes two drugs to work together more effectively, so the addition of an ataractic allows the narcotic dosage to be reduced. Analgesic potentiators include compounds such as promethazine (Phenergan), propiomazine (Largon), hydroxyzine (Vistaril), and promazine (Sparine).

In addition to potentiating the effects of the analgesic, the ataractic (tranquilizer) also acts as an antinauseant and antiemetic. The combination can be administered safely until the end of the first stage of labor. Usual dosages include the following: promethazine, 25 to 50 mg IM or 15 to 25 mg IV; promazine, 50 mg IM or 5 to 10 mg IV; hydroxyzine 25 to 50 mg IM. Since hydroxyzine is given only by IM injection, the onset of effect is slower and less predictable. Fetal or neonatal problems rarely develop with these dosages.

Narcotic antagonists. Narcotics such as meperidine and fentanyl can cause excessive CNS depression in the mother or newborn. **Narcotic antagonists** such as naloxone (Narcan) or the newer narcotic antagonist naltrexone (Trexan) promptly reverse the narcotic effects. In addition, the antagonist also counters the effect of stress-induced levels of endorphins. **Endorphins** are endogenous opioids secreted by the pituitary gland that act on the central and peripheral nervous systems to reduce pain. Beta-endorphin is the most potent of the endorphins. The physiologic role of endorphins is not completely understood. It is thought that endorphins increase during pregnancy and birth in humans and may increase the ability of women in labor to tolerate acute pain.

A narcotic antagonist is especially valuable if labor is more rapid than expected and birth is expected when the narcotic is at its peak effect. The antagonist may be given through the woman's IV line, or it can be administered IM into her gluteal muscle. Narcotic antagonists counteract maternal and neonatal narcotic effects. The mother needs to be told that with the administration of an antagonist the pain will return.

Nursing ALERT

Narcotic antagonists must be administered cautiously to a woman who is substance-dependent because withdrawal symptoms may occur (Box 14-2).

A narcotic antagonist can be given to the newborn. **Neonatal narcosis,** CNS depression in the newborn caused by a narcotic, may be exhibited by respiratory depression, hypotonia, lethargy, and a delay in temperature regulation. Alterations of neurologic and behavioral responses may be evident for 72 hours after birth. Meperidine may be present in the neonate's urine for up to 3 weeks. Some depression of attention and social responsiveness can be evident for up to 6 weeks (Briggs, Freeman, and Yaffe, 1986).

Nerve block analgesia and anesthesia. A variety of compounds are used in obstetrics to produce regional analgesia (some pain relief and motor block) and anesthesia (pain relief and motor block). Most of these drugs are related chemically to cocaine and carry the suffix *-caine*. This helps identify a local anesthetic.

The principal pharmacologic effect of local anesthetics is the temporary interruption of the conduction of nerve impulses, notably pain. Examples of common agents given in 0.25% to 1% solutions are lidocaine (Xylocaine), bupivacaine (Marcaine), chloroprocaine (Nesacaine), tetracaine (Pontocaine), and mepivacaine (Carbocaine).

Rarely, individuals are sensitive (allergic) to one or more local anesthetics. Sensitivity may be determined by testing with minute amounts of the medication to be used. Initially the CNS is stimulated when excessive amounts of a regional anesthetic are injected. Stimulation may be followed by depression, hypotension, and other serious adverse effects. Atropine, antihistaminic medications, oxygen, and supportive measures should bring relief.

As analgesia is established, a sympathetic blockage occurs, causing vasodilation and pooling of blood in the lower extremities. Because maternal hypotension is a secondary side effect of epidural anesthesia and is aggravated by hypovolemia, any fluid volume deficit must be corrected promptly

BOX 14-2

Signs of Potential Complications: Maternal Narcotic Withdrawal

Nausea, vomiting
Headache
Irritability
Fatigue
Perspiration, chills
Tremors, weakness, restlessness
Anxiety, apprehension, jittery feeling
Convulsions (seizures)

(Nicholson, 1990). Therefore adequate hydration for blood volume expansion is a prerequisite to epidural anesthesia. Hydration is achieved with non-n-dextrose–containing balanced salt solution (e.g., Ringer's lactate or Plasma-Lyte A). The mother receives IV hydration with 500 to 1000 ml solution within 20 minutes before the block. A vasopressor such as ephedrine and facilities for cardiopulmonary resuscitation, including oxygen and suction, must be immediately available. If maternal and fetal resuscitation is needed, left uterine displacement must be maintained to optimize venous return and therefore perfusion of the uterus.

Local infiltration anesthesia. **Local infiltration anesthesia** of perineal tissues is commonly used when an episiotomy is to be done and when time or the fetal head position does not permit a pudendal block to be administered (Scott et al, 1994). Rapid anesthesia is produced by injecting an average of 10 to 20 ml of local anesthetic with 1% lidocaine or 2% chloroprocaine into the skin and then subcutaneously into the region to be anesthetized. Epinephrine often is added to the solution to intensify the anesthesia in a limited region and to prevent excessive bleeding and systemic effects by constricting local blood vessels (Clark, Queener, and Karb, 1993). Repeated injection prolongs the anesthesia as long as needed.

Pudendal block. **Pudendal block** is useful for the second stage of labor, for episiotomy, and for birth. Although a pudendal block does not relieve pain from uterine contractions, it does relieve pain in the clitoris, the labia majora and minora, and the perineum.

Pudendal nerve block is administered 10 to 20 minutes before perineal anesthesia is needed. Vaginal and perineal pain can be eliminated by a pudendal anesthetic block (Fig. 14-4). The pudendal nerve traverses the sacrosciatic notch just medial to the tip of the ischial spine on each side. Injection of an anesthetic solution at or near these points anesthetizes the pudendal nerves peripherally. The transvaginal approach is generally used because it is less painful for the woman, has a higher success rate, and tends to cause fewer fetal complications (Scott et al, 1994). Pudendal block does not change maternal hemodynamic or respiratory functions, vital signs, or FHR. The bearing-down reflex is lessened or lost completely.

If all branches of the pudendal nerve are anesthetized, analgesia is sufficient for a spontaneous vaginal birth or for outlet (low) forceps-assisted birth. However, the anesthetic effect is insufficient to permit instrumental vaginal birth except for low forceps, and a pudendal block does not provide anal-

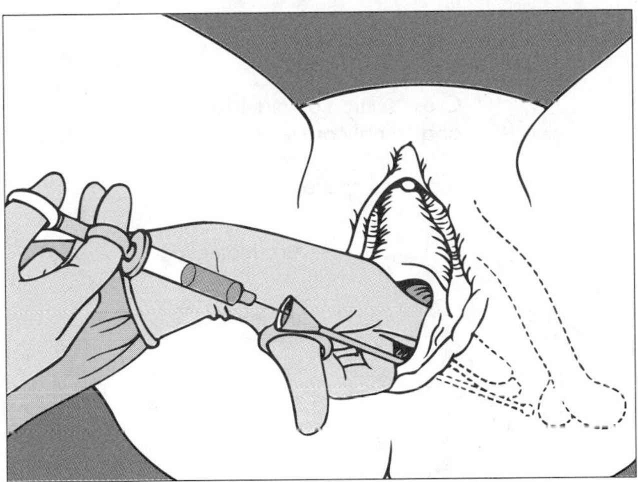

Fig. 14-4 Pudendal block. Use of needle guide ("Iowa trumpet") and Luer-Lok syringe to inject medication. (Courtesy Ross Laboratories, Columbus, Ohio.)

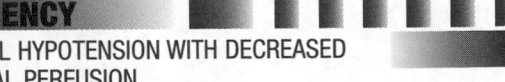

EMERGENCY

MATERNAL HYPOTENSION WITH DECREASED PLACENTAL PERFUSION

SIGNS/SYMPTOMS

- Maternal hypotension (20% drop from preblock level or less than 100 mm Hg systolic)
- Fetal bradycardia
- Decreased beat-to-beat FHR variability (Ch. 15)

INTERVENTIONS

- Turn woman to left lateral position or place pillow or wedge under right hip (see Fig. 16-3, *D*) to deflect uterus.
- Maintain IV infusion at rate specified, or increase prn per hospital protocol.
- Administer oxygen by face mask at 10-12 L/min.
- Elevate woman's legs.
- Notify physician/midwife/anesthesiologist/nurse anesthetist.
- Administer IV vasopressor (e.g., ephedrine).
- Remain with woman; continue to monitor maternal blood pressure (BP) and FHR every 5 min until stable or per primary health care provider's order.

gesia for uterine exploration or manual removal of the placenta (Scott et al, 1994).

Subarachnoid (spinal) anesthesia. In subarachnoid (spinal) block, local anesthetic is injected through the third, fourth, or fifth lumbar interspace into the subarachnoid space (Figs. 14-5 and 14-6), where the medication mixes with cerebrospinal fluid. This single-injection technique is useful for birth but not for labor. For vaginal birth, the anesthetic solution is administered during the second stage of labor when birth is imminent (e.g., fetal head is on the perineum).

For **low spinal (saddle) block anesthesia,** the injection is made with the woman in a sitting position, her legs over the side of the delivery table, and her feet supported on a stool. The nurse stands in front of her. The woman rests her chin on her chest, arches her back, and leans on the nurse for support. The nurse comforts and coaches her. This posture is thought to widen the intervertebral space for ease in inserting the spinal needle and to allow the heavy anesthetic solution to flow downward. The injection is made between contractions to avoid an unexpected high block (medication rises above T-10 with the potential of affecting the movement of the diaphragm and muscles of respiration). Once the anesthetic has been injected, the woman remains upright for a period of 30 seconds to 2 minutes (as directed by the anesthesiologist) to permit downward diffusion. Then the woman is assisted to a supine position (with wedge under one hip to prevent supine hypotension). She must remain supine with the head elevated slightly. Onset of anesthesia usually occurs within 1 to 2 minutes after injection. Duration of anesthesia is 1 to 3 hours, depending on the anesthetic used.

Marked hypotension, decreased cardiac output and placental perfusion, and respiratory inadequacy may occur during any spinal anesthesia. Therefore the woman receives hydration with IV fluids before injection of an anesthetic to decrease the potential for hypotension caused by sympathetic blockade. After injection, maternal blood pressure, pulse, respirations, and FHR must be checked and recorded every 5 to 10 minutes. If signs of serious maternal hypotension or fetal distress develop, emergency care must be given (see the Emergency box above).

Because the mother is not able to sense her contractions, she must be instructed when to bear down. If the birth occurs in a delivery room (rather than a labor-delivery-recovery room) the mother will need assistance in the transfer to a recovery bed after she has been delivered of the placenta.

Advantages of spinal anesthesia include ease of administration and absence of fetal hypoxia with maintenance of normotension. Maternal consciousness is maintained, excellent muscular relaxation is achieved, and blood loss is not excessive. Maternal alertness enables the woman to participate in the birth process. Usually no other anesthetic agents (e.g., inhalation drugs) are required. If stirrups are used for birth, care must be taken to position them properly. Spinal anesthesia may be the method of choice for women with severe respiratory problems or with liver, kidney, or metabolic disease because it decreases the stress of labor and birth on these systems.

Disadvantages of spinal anesthesia include drug reactions (e.g., allergy), rare chemical myelitis or infection, hypotension, and respiratory paralysis; cardiopulmonary resuscitation (CPR) may be needed. When a spinal anesthetic is given, the need for operative delivery (episiotomy, low forceps extraction) tends to increase because of the elimination of voluntary expulsive efforts. After birth, the incidence of bladder and uterine atony, as well as postspinal headache, is higher.

HEADACHE AFTER SPINAL (LUMBAR) PUNCTURE. Leakage of cerebrospinal fluid from the site of puncture of the *meninges* (membranous coverings of the spinal cord) is thought to be the major causative factor in postlumbar puncture (postspinal headache). Headache may be postural and occur only in the head-up or standing position. Presumably with postural changes, the diminished volume of cerebrospinal fluid creates traction on pain-sensitive CNS structures. Headache, auditory, and visual problems may persist for days or weeks.

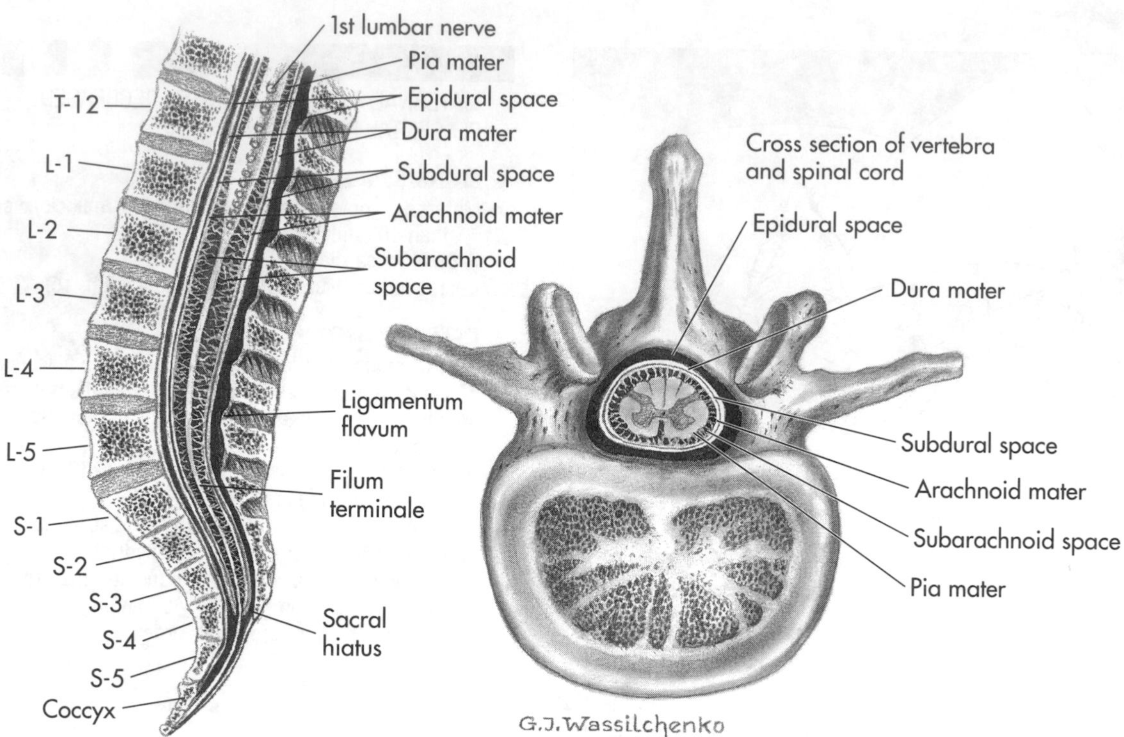

Fig. 14-5 Membranes and spaces of spinal cord; levels of sacral, lumbar, and thoracic nerves.

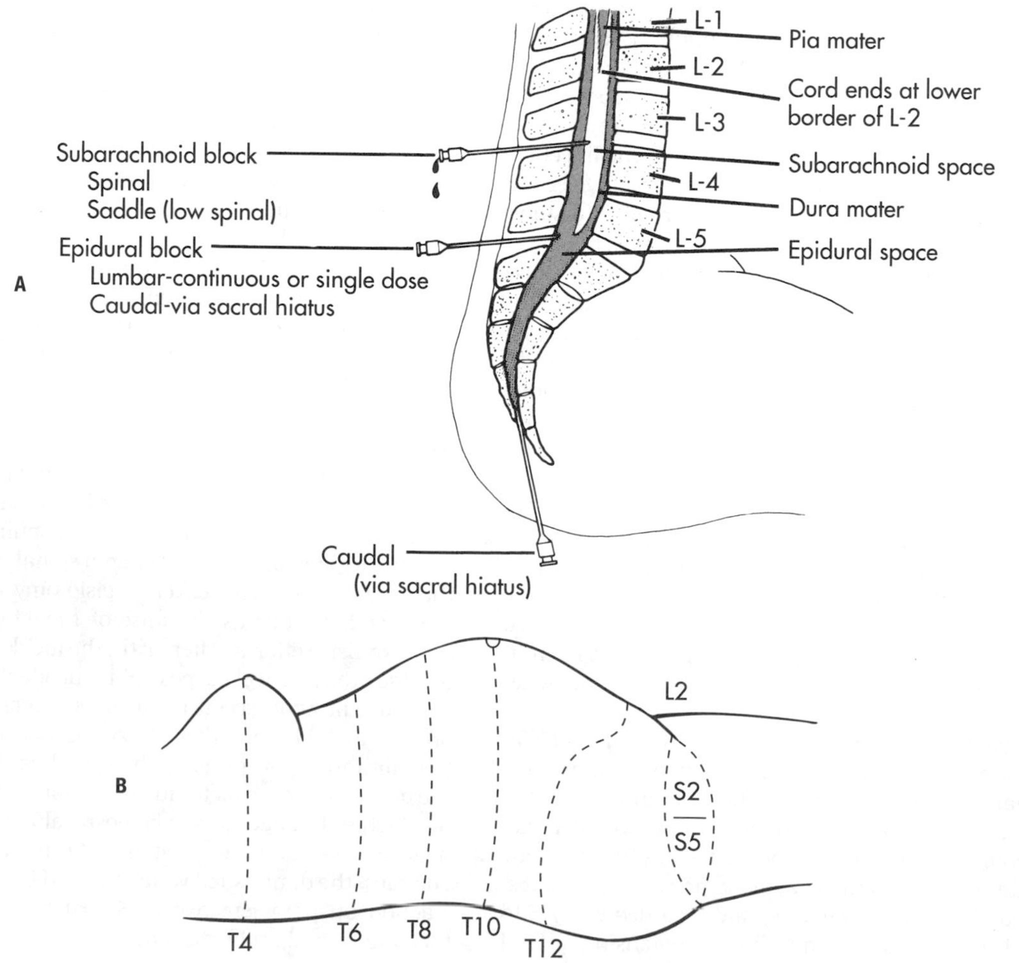

Fig. 14-6 **A,** Regional block analgesia and anesthesia in obstetrics. **B,** Sensory block levels of analgesia.

However, the likelihood of headache after lumbar puncture can be reduced if the anesthesiologist uses a small-gauge spinal needle and avoids multiple punctures of the meninges. Positioning the woman flat in bed (with only a small, flat pillow for her head) for at least 8 hours has been recommended to prevent headache after spinal anesthesia, but there is no definitive evidence that this procedure is effective. Positioning the woman on her abdomen is thought to decrease the loss of fluid through the puncture site. Hydration has been claimed to be of value, but there is no compelling evidence to support its use (Cunningham et al, 1993). Initial treatment for headache after lumbar puncture usually includes analgesics, bed rest, caffeine, and increased fluid intake (i.e., 150 ml/hr IV) (Scott et al, 1994).

An autologous **epidural blood patch** (a patch repairing a tear or a hole in the dura mater around the spinal cord) is often beneficial and may be considered if the headache does not resolve spontaneously (Scott et al, 1994). To form a patch, a few milliliters of the woman's blood without anticoagulant is injected epidurally at the site of the spinal tap (Fig. 14-7), forming a clot that covers the hole and prevents further fluid loss. Other measures that seem to provide relief are an injection of saline in larger volumes and abdominal support with a girdle or abdominal binder. For some women the headache may be improved remarkably by the third day and absent by the fifth day.

Epidural block. Relief from the pain of uterine contractions and birth (vaginal and abdominal) can be accomplished by injecting a suitable local anesthetic into the epidural (peridural) space (Figs. 14-6 and 14-8). The portal of entry into this space for obstetric analgesia and anesthesia is through either a lumbar intervertebral space or caudally through the sacral hiatus and sacral canal.

The caudal space is the lowest extent of the epidural, or peridural, space (Figs. 14-6 and 14-8). Emerging from the dural sac a few inches higher, a rich network of sacral nerves passes downward through the caudal space. A suitable anesthetic solution filling the caudal canal may eliminate the sensation of pain carried via the sacral nerves to produce anesthesia suitable for vaginal birth. Higher levels with continuous caudal technique provide both analgesia in the first and second stages of labor and anesthesia for birth. Because of analgesia early in labor, caudal epidural block is rarely used today (Writer, 1992). Specifics regarding this method are not presented here. See medical texts for this information.

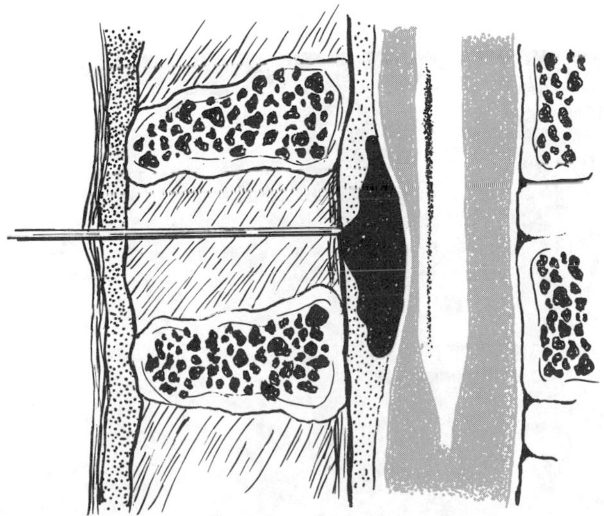

Fig. 14-7 Blood patch therapy for postspinal headache.

Complete lumbar **epidural block** for the discomfort of labor and vaginal birth requires a block from T-10 to S-5. For cesarean birth, a block is essential from at least T-8 to S-1. The diffusion of epidural anesthesia depends on the location of the catheter tip, the dose and volume of anesthetic agent used,

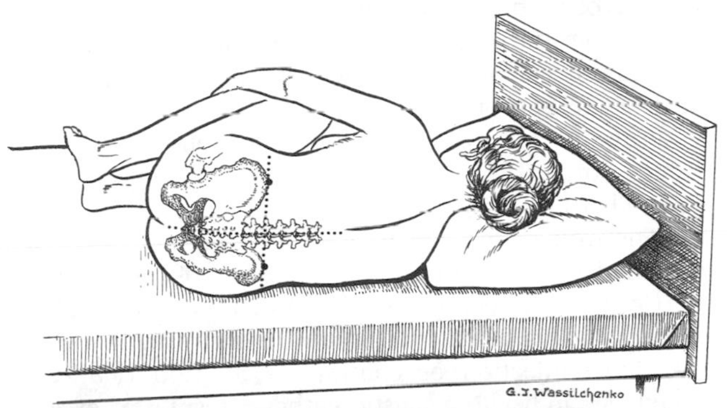

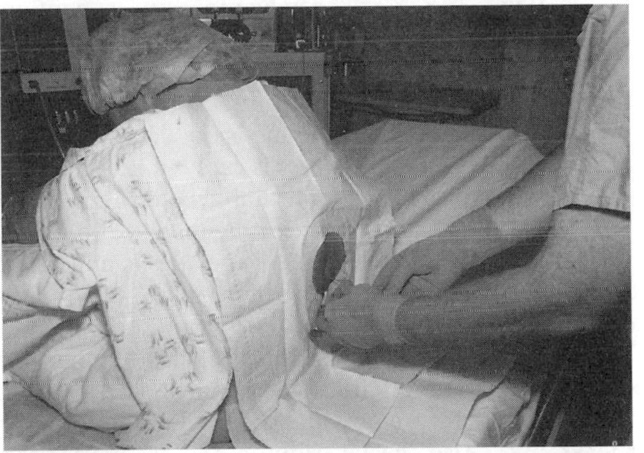

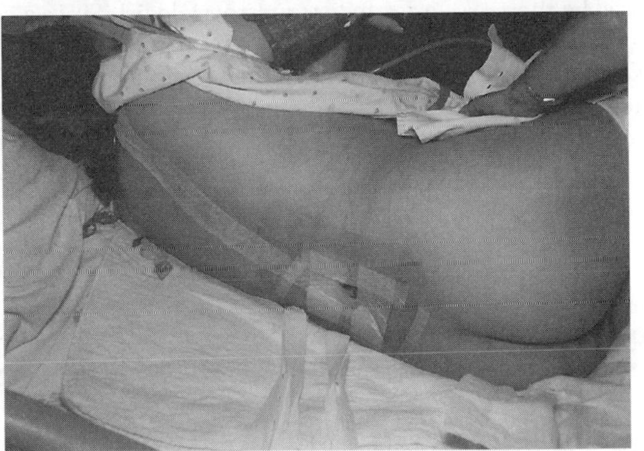

Fig. 14-8 **A,** Lateral decubitus position for epidural and subarachnoid block and anatomic landmarks to locate needle insertion site. **B,** Epidural anesthesia. Skin has been prepared with antiseptic solution (povidone-iodine; Betadine). Area is draped with sterile towels. Nurse continues to support woman. **C,** Catheter is taped to woman's back; port segment is taped near her shoulder. (**B** and **C** courtesy Michael S. Clement, MD, Mesa, Ariz.)

and the woman's position (e.g., horizontal or head-up position) (Cunningham et al, 1993).

For induction of lumbar epidural anesthesia, the woman is positioned as for a spinal injection (i.e., sitting) or in a modified Sims position (Fig. 14-8). For modified lateral Sims position, the woman is placed on her left side, shoulders parallel, legs slightly flexed, and back arched.

The woman is positioned preferably on her left side to avoid having the weight of the uterus on the ascending vena cava and descending aorta, which can impair venous return and decrease placental perfusion. Oxygen is available should hypotension occur despite maintenance of IV fluid and displacement of the maternal uterus to the left. The nurse anesthetist/anesthesiologist may need to give an injection of ephedrine (a vasopressor used to increase maternal blood pressure) and to accelerate IV fluid infusion (see the Emergency box on p. 361).

The FHR and progress in labor must be monitored carefully. The woman in labor may not be aware of changes in strength of uterine contractions or descent of the presenting part. Occasionally, depression of contractions may result, necessitating augmentation of labor with oxytocin.

A single injection or continuous infusion (via pump) through an indwelling plastic catheter results in excellent analgesia (Fig. 14-8, *C*). The advantages of a continuous block are numerous: the mother experiences excellent pain relief and remains alert and cooperative, good relaxation is achieved, airway reflexes remain intact, only partial motor paralysis develops, gastric emptying is not delayed, and blood loss is not excessive. Fetal distress is rare but may occur with rapid absorption or marked maternal hypotension. The dose, volume, and type of anesthetic can be modified to allow the mother to push, to produce perineal anesthesia, and to permit forceps or even abdominal birth if required (Cunningham et al, 1993).

The disadvantages of a continuous block for the woman include the need for an IV line, occasional dizziness, weakness of the legs, difficulty emptying the bladder, and shivering (Writer, 1992). Also special training and experience are required by the nurse anesthetist/anesthesiologist. Since a considerable amount of the drug must be used, reactions or rapid absorption of the anesthetic agent may result in maternal hypotension, convulsions, or paresthesia (Box 14-3). The incidence of operative delivery (e.g., episiotomy, use of forceps) may be increased if the woman cannot bear down effectively. Occasionally, accidental high-spinal anesthesia (and later, postspinal headache) may follow inadvertent perforation of the dural membrane when lumbar epidural anesthesia is induced.

For some women the anesthetic selected is not effective, and a second form of anesthesia is required. Establishment of effective pain relief with maximum safety takes time. Consequently, in case of rapid labor the potential for pain relief during labor and birth is not realized. For example, peridural anesthesia for women of higher parity in active labor is likely to prove not worth the bother, risk, and expense (Cunningham et al, 1993).

Epidural and spinal narcotics. There is a high concentration of narcotic receptors along the pain pathway in the spinal cord, in the brain stem, and in the thalamus. Because these receptors are highly sensitive to narcotics, a small quantity of narcotic produces marked analgesia that lasts for several hours. Medication is injected through a catheter placed in the epidural or subarachnoid space, which reaches these narcotic receptors, and pain transmission is blocked without compromising motor ability, thus the so-called "walking epidural" (see the Guidelines box below).

Administration of epidural or spinal narcotics during labor has several advantages. These narcotics do not cause maternal hypotension or affect vital signs. The woman feels contractions but not pain. Her ability to bear down during the second stage of labor is preserved because the pushing reflex is not lost and motor power remains intact.

Fentanyl may be used alone. Its effects last up to 90 minutes. When added to the local anesthetic at the time of epidural administration, it extends the duration of anesthesia. There are no cardiovascular effects. However, for most women, fentanyl does not provide adequate analgesia for second-stage labor pain, episiotomy, or birth (Cunningham et al, 1993).

The most common indication for the administration of epidural or spinal narcotics is for relief of postoperative pain. For example, women who give birth by the abdominal route receive fentanyl (Innovar) or morphine through the catheter. The catheter may then be removed, and the women are usually free of pain for 24 hours. Occasionally the catheter is left in place in case another dose is needed.

BOX 14-3
Side Effects of Epidural Anesthesia

Decreased awareness of uterine contractions
Decreased awareness of giving birth
Sensation of weakness
Sensation of numbness
Paresthesia of the lower limbs
Reduced mobility
Shivering
Bladder distension
Symptoms related to postural hypotension

Guidelines 

AMBULATORY (WALKING) EPIDURAL ANALGESIA

Patient
- No obstetric or anesthetic contraindications to ambulation
- Grossly normal leg strength
- No orthostatic hypotension
- Able to perform knee bend while standing

Nurse
- Always accompany ambulatory patients
- Assess at regular intervals

Epidurally administered morphine allows the woman to be up with surprising ease and to care for her baby. Early ambulation and freedom from pain also facilitate bladder emptying. To a woman who has had a previous cesarean birth and experienced the usual postoperative pain, the effects of this approach seem miraculous. However, the mother may not understand why she may experience pain after the narcotic effect wears off.

Side effects of morphine administered by the epidural or spinal route include nausea, vomiting, pruritus (itching), urinary retention, and delayed respiratory depression, often occurring about 12 hours after administration of the morphine. Antiemetics, antipruritics, and narcotic antagonists are used to relieve these symptoms. For example, naloxone, naltrexone promethazine, or metoclopramide (Reglan) may be administered. If these are used, the analgesic effects are obliterated and other methods of pain relief are needed. Hospital protocols should provide specific instructions for treatment of these side effects. Some health care providers believe that the risks of epidural or spinal injection are sufficient not to warrant its routine use. Respiratory depression is a serious concern; the woman's respiratory rate should be assessed and documented every hour for 24 hours or per hospital protocol.

Contraindications to subarachnoid and epidural blocks. The following contraindications to epidural analgesia apply equally to caudal and subarachnoid blocks (Scott et al, 1994):

1. *Patient refusal.*
2. *Antepartum hemorrhage.* Acute hypovolemia leads to increased sympathetic tone to maintain the blood pressure. Any anesthetic technique that blocks the sympathetic fibers can lead to significant hypotension, which can endanger the mother and baby.
3. *Anticoagulant therapy or bleeding disorder.* If a woman is receiving anticoagulant therapy or has a bleeding disorder, injury to a blood vessel may result in a hematoma. The hematoma may compress the cauda equina or the spinal cord and lead to serious CNS sequelae.
4. *Infection at the injection site.* Infection can be spread through the peridural or subarachnoid spaces if the needle traverses an infected area.
5. *Tumor at the injection site.* A tumor at the injection site is an unusual but definite contraindication.
6. *Allergy to anesthetic drug.*
7. *History of spinal injury or surgery, or CNS disease.*
8. *Marked hypotension.*

Relative contraindications to intraspinal blocks include CNS disorders, extensive back surgery, morbid obesity or anatomic abnormality in which landmarks cannot be identified, and current or prior disease of the CNS (Scott et al, 1994).

Drug effects on neonate. Debate persists concerning the effects of epidural anesthesia on the neonate's neurobehavioral responses. Findings from studies of associations between neurobehavioral outcome and epidural anesthesia are far from consistent. For example, neonatal neurobehavioral scores comparing infants born to mothers with and without epidural analgesia conflict between those showing little or no difference in the scores (Hamza, 1994), and those reporting that neonates did not score as well on neurobehavioral tests (Sepkoski et al, 1992). Today, most believe this decreased muscle tone, if present, is temporary and of no clinical significance.

Paracervical (uterosacral) block. **Paracervical block** is given to relieve pain from cervical dilation and distention of the lower uterine segment in the first stage of labor during the active (acceleration) phase. For paracervical anesthesia, a dilute local anesthetic drug (e.g., 5 ml of 1% procaine) is injected just beneath the mucosa adjacent to the outer rim of the cervix (9 and 3 o'clock positions) after the cervix is more than 5 cm dilated. A needle guide (e.g., the Iowa trumpet) is useful but not indispensable for transvaginal administration (Fig. 14-9). Relief from discomfort is noticed within approximately 5 minutes. Excellent pain relief lasts for at least 1 hour.

Anesthesia extends from the lower uterine segment and cervix to the upper third of the vagina; there is no perineal anesthesia. Although there may be a transient depression of contractions, there is little or no effect on the labor. Repeat injections may be given until the cervix is dilated to 8 cm, whereupon another method such as pudendal block may be necessary.

Paracervical-block anesthesia may cause fetal intoxication because of rapid absorption of the drug. When the anesthetic is injected into the tissues lateral to the cervix, it is picked up by the maternal circulation, which quickly involves the uterus and placenta. When overdosage occurs, the fetus may exhibit bradycardia because of the quinidine-like effect of the anesthetic on the myocardium or because of a reduction in uterine blood flow. In addition, CNS medullary depression may develop, and the neonate may show vascular collapse and apnea at birth. Hematomas can develop at the site of injection if a uterine vessel is damaged.

Because of these potential complications, paracervical block is rarely used for labor but remains an option for anesthesia during abortion or other gynecologic procedures.

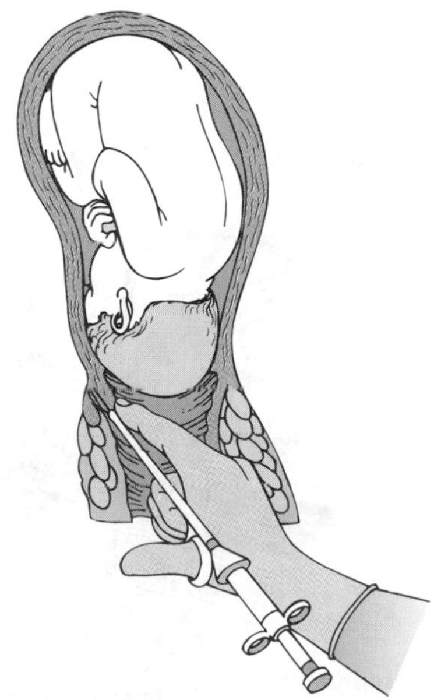

Fig. 14-9 Paracervical block. Note the position of the hand and fingers in relation to the cervix and fetal head and the shallow depth of the needle insertion. Note also that no undue pressure is applied at the vaginal fornix by the fingers or needle guide.

General anesthesia. General anesthesia rarely is indicated for uncomplicated vaginal birth. It may be necessary if there is a contraindication (including patient refusal) to nerve block analgesia/anesthesia or if fetal indications necessitate a rapid birth (vaginal or abdominal). The woman is not awake with this method, and there is danger of respiratory depression and vomiting followed by aspiration. For women with hypovolemia, general anesthesia is safer than nerve block analgesia or anesthesia. Thiopental (Pentothal) is commonly used for general anesthesia. Administered intravenously (4 mg/kg of body weight), thiopental produces rapid induction of anesthesia and does not depress the fetus (Scott et al, 1994).

If general anesthesia is being considered, the nurse gives the woman nothing by mouth and sees that an IV infusion is established. If time allows, the nurse premedicates the woman with a nonparticulate oral antacid such as sodium citrate (30 ml) to increase gastric pH and neutralize acid contents of the stomach. If there is sufficient time, some nurse anesthetists/anesthesiologists or physicians also order a histamine blocker such as cimetidine to decrease production of gastric acid and metoclopramide to increase gastric emptying (Scott et al, 1994). Before induction, a wedge should be placed under the woman's right hip to displace the uterus to the left. Uterine displacement prevents aortocaval compression, which interferes with placental perfusion. Sometimes the nurse is asked to assist with *cricoid pressure* before intubation (Fig. 14-10).

Priorities for recovery room care are to maintain an open airway and cardiopulmonary functions and to prevent postpartum hemorrhage. Routine postpartum care is organized to facilitate parent-child attachment as soon as possible and to answer the mother's questions. When appropriate, the nurse assesses the mother's readiness to see the baby and her response to the anesthesia and to the event that necessitated general anesthesia (e.g., cesarean birth when vaginal birth was anticipated).

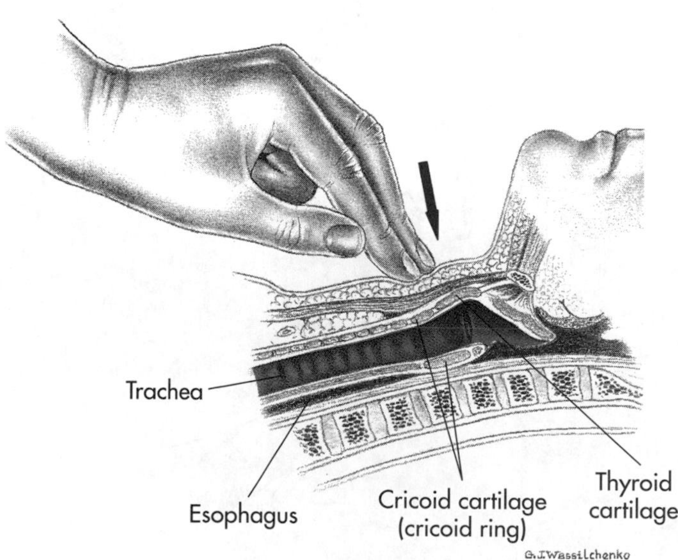

Fig. 14-10 Technique of applying pressure on cricoid cartilage to occlude esophagus; prevents pulmonary aspiration of gastric contents during anesthesia induction.

Combination anesthesia for cesarean birth. Light general anesthesia, considered by many to be ideal for cesarean birth, is achieved with a combination of thiopental, a mixture of nitrous oxide and oxygen, and succinylcholine. The woman is given 100% oxygen for 3 minutes, followed by almost simultaneous rapid administration of thiopental and succinylcholine. During intubation, cricoid pressure is maintained, often by the nurse, to prevent aspiration of vomitus (Fig. 14-10). When the woman is somnolent, a nitrous oxide-oxygen mixture is given. Excellent tolerance of this combination is widely reported.

Inhalation anesthesia. Self-administration of inhalation gases may be helpful, especially during the second stage of labor. The mother breathes subanesthetic concentrations of an inhalation anesthetic such as methoxyflurane (Penthrane). If these agents are given properly, the woman remains conscious but has profound pain relief. The gas is usually self-administered from a capsule and mask strapped to the wrist. The primary health care provider sets the desired concentration, and the woman inhales the medication during contractions. The goal of this method is for the woman to remain conscious while profound analgesia, as well as some amnesia for painful events, is achieved.

The nurse must stay with the woman and never administer the medication for her because overdose is a risk. The nurse must also monitor vital signs every 30 minutes and FHR every 15 minutes. The woman should remain conscious and not become delirious or excited. The nurse alerts the primary health care provider and removes the analgesic from the woman's hand if the mother has cardiac arrhythmia, loses consciousness, or if FHR abnormalities occur. These inhalation analgesics are rarely used in the United States today.

Other inhalation agents include halothane (Fluothane) and nitrous oxide. Halothane inhalation relaxes the uterus quickly and facilitates intrauterine manipulation, version, and extraction. The desired effect is general loss of sensitivity to touch, pain, and other stimulation.

A combination of 50% nitrous oxide and 50% oxygen may be given for analgesic effect late in the first stage and with contractions during the period of expulsion in the second stage. Administered in low concentrations, nitrous oxide relieves the mother's pain but still allows her to bear down with her contractions during the second stage of labor. Care is needed to prevent maternal and neonatal respiratory depression when nitrous oxide is used as an analgesic or anesthetic.

Anesthesia in the obese woman. Obesity affects 6% to 10% of pregnant women. Obesity is defined as an excess of body fat causing weight to be greater than 20% over ideal weight. Weight more than twice the ideal body weight is defined as morbid obesity. A study of anesthesia-related maternal mortality in Michigan between 1972 and 1989 found that obesity was a risk factor in 80% of maternal deaths (Endler et al, 1988). A retrospective study between 1978 and 1989 of morbidly obese women found that 62% gave birth by cesarean, and 48% had emergency cesarean birth (Hood and Dewan, 1993).

Maternal physiologic changes are the result of hormonal influences and mechanical effects. In obesity, the weight of fat tissue and the added metabolic demands also affect maternal physiology (Endler, 1990). Blood volume and cardiac output increase during pregnancy and obesity, expanding in proportion to the amount of fat tissue mass. During labor and vaginal birth, and in the immediate postpartum period, blood values and cardiac output reach levels 80% higher than prelabor values. The enlarged uterus and abdominal fat mass increase the possibility of aortocaval compression.

The respiratory system is also stressed (Endler, 1990). The obese woman in labor is in a precarious state of pulmonary function. Therefore oxygenation must be carefully monitored through birth and the immediate postpartum period. Monitoring by pulse oximeter has been suggested.

All pregnant women experience delayed gastric emptying time, decreased tone in the cardiac sphincter, and gastric hyperacidity. In addition, an obese woman is more likely to have a hiatal hernia and a marked increase in intragastric pressure and volume. Therefore obese women are at great risk for regurgitation and aspiration (Endler, 1990).

Management during labor should focus on efforts to minimize oxygen consumption and maximize pulmonary function. Epidural analgesia during the first stage of labor decreases demands on the metabolic and respiratory systems and improves oxygenation. This is because pain causes a rise in catecholamine levels, and this rise leads to increased cardiac output. Effective epidural analgesia slows this rise in catecholamine levels.

Intravenous narcotics may be used during the first stage of labor. However, the dosage of drugs and their effects must be monitored carefully because obese women are extremely sensitive to the respiratory depressant effects of narcotics (Endler, 1990). Epidural block during the second stage of labor provides complete pain relief and supports cardiovascular function.

If cesarean birth is necessary, epidural block is preferred over general anesthesia. Problems associated with general anesthesia include potential difficulties during intubation, hypertensive effect of laryngoscopy and intubation, and danger of aspiration and pulmonary complications. Subarachnoid block may be used if there is insufficient time for an epidural block. Uterine displacement to prevent aortocaval compression is more difficult to achieve in the obese woman. If the woman is extremely obese, elevation of the right hip on a wedge may not be sufficient to avoid compression. It may be necessary to physically lift the abdominal fat pad off the abdomen until the peritoneal cavity has been entered (Endler, 1990).

Maternal hypothermia after analgesia and anesthesia. Hypothermia is core body temperature of less than 35° C (95° F). Women are predisposed to hypothermia because of vasodilation normally occurring during pregnancy and because of the administration of analgesia and anesthesia.

Opiates and narcotics, barbiturates, tranquilizers, and antiemetics are thought to affect thermoregulation by increasing vasodilation and radiant loss; general anesthesia agents affect it by depressing thermoregulation; and epidural and spinal anesthesia affect thermoregulation by inducing peripheral dilation (Dunn et al, 1993). During labor, vaginal or cesarean birth, or immediately after birth, women may experience shivering, hypotension, and respiratory distress. Hypothermia may result in cardiovascular, pulmonary, circulatory, hematologic, neurologic, or renal complications (Dunn et al, 1993). The nurse can minimize these complications by ensuring birthing areas are warm, removing wet drapes and towels, and covering the women with warm blankets after birth and by early recognition of hypothermia. Explanation of these effects given to women and their support persons helps allay concerns.

Nursing Care Management

The choice of pain relief depends on a combination of factors, including the woman's special needs and wishes, the availability of the desired method of analgesia or anesthesia, the health care provider's preference and expertise, and the phase and stage of labor. The nurse is responsible for continuous maternal and fetal assessment and for establishing mutual goals with the woman (and her family), formulating nursing diagnosis, planning and implementing nursing care, and evaluating the effects of care based on a plan of care. Careful documentation by the nurse of all care management is essential.

Assessment

The assessment of the woman in labor, her fetus, and her labor is a joint effort of the nurse and the primary health care providers, who then consult with the woman. The needs of each woman are different. Many factors enter into the nursing assessment to determine choice of analgesia and anesthesia (see the Cultural Considerations box below). Assessment of learning needs of women in labor is also an important role for the nurse.

History. The woman's prenatal record is read for relevant information. In addition to identifying data, the woman's parity, estimated date of birth, and complications and medications during pregnancy are noted. A history of allergies is noted and displayed prominently. A history of smoking and neurologic and spinal disorders, as well as relevant psychosocial data are noted.

Cultural Considerations 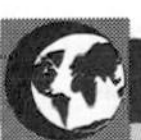

SOME CULTURAL BELIEFS ABOUT PAIN

The following are only examples of how women of different cultural backgrounds may react to pain. The nurse still needs to make assessments for each individual woman experiencing pain related to childbirth.

- Chinese women may not exhibit reactions to pain. They consider it impolite to accept something when it is first offered; therefore, pain interventions may need to be offered more than once. Accupuncture may be used for pain relief.
- Iranian women may be vocal with labor pain.
- Japanese women may be stoic with labor pain.
- Haitian women may demonstrate a high tolerance for pain.
- Southeast Asian women may endure severe pain before requesting relief.
- Mexican women may be stoic until late in labor; then they may become vocal and request pain relief.

Critical Thinking Exercises

PAIN MANAGEMENT

1. You are assigned to a Southeast Asian woman in active labor who has her fists tightly clenched and is grimacing. She is not requesting anything for pain. You are convinced that discomfort should be avoided if possible.
   a. Examine the assumptions you may have about how women of different cultures exhibit reactions to pain.
   b. Examine assumptions that both you and the patient may have about pain relief.
   c. Analyze arguments for and against use of pharmacologic agents for control of discomfort.
   d. Formulate a plan of care for pain relief in this situation, and justify your choice of interventions.
2. Talk to a woman who has experienced childbirth previously. Ask her to describe her reactions to pain, how she sought relief of pain, the atmosphere of the childbirth setting, and the attitudes of the health care providers.
   a. Analyze how the atmosphere of the setting and the attitudes of the health care providers might have influenced the woman's perception of pain.
   b. Examine the childbirth setting in which you are now assigned.

What is the atmosphere of the setting, and what are the attitudes of the health care providers regarding the expression of pain by women of a different culture?

Evaluate the impact when the nurse is from a different culture than the woman she cares for.

Interview. Interview data establish the time and type of food taken at the woman's last meal; her existing respiratory condition (cold, allergy); and unusual reactions to medications (e.g., allergy), cleansing agents, or tape. The woman is asked whether she attended parent-education or childbirth preparation classes. Her preparation and preferences for management of discomfort are noted. Her knowledge of choices for management of discomfort is assessed. The woman's perception of discomfort and her expressed need for medication add to the data base. The events since the woman's last contact with the primary health care provider are reviewed (e.g., infections, diarrhea, change in fetal behavior). If verbal and physical signs suggest substance abuse, the nurse inquires about the type of drug used, time of last use, and method of administration. Interaction with family members is noted.

Physical examination. The character and status of this labor and fetal response are assessed. The nurse notes the degree of hydration by assessing intake and output, moisture of mucous membranes, and skin turgor. Bladder distention is noted. Evidence of skin infection near sites of possible needle insertion is recorded and reported. Signs of apprehension such as fist clenching and restlessness are noted.

If the woman is in labor, maternal and fetal vital signs; uterine contractions; and cervical effacement and dilation, station, and anticipated time until birth are all considered. Length of labor and degree of fatigue are important considerations.

Laboratory tests. Laboratory tests are reviewed for anemia (hemoglobin and hematocrit), coagulopathy (bleeding disorder), and infection (white blood cell count [WBC] and differential). The prenatal record is reviewed for laboratory tests (e.g., blood, urine, amniotic fluid) related to disorders such as diabetes mellitus, cardiac disease, thyroid disease, infection, and concurrent disorders such as preeclampsia or substance abuse. Antenatal diagnostic studies (e.g., ultrasound, nonstress test, contraction stress test, amniocentesis, biophysical profile) and their findings are noted. The choice of analgesia and anesthesia varies by phase and stage of labor (Box 14-1).

Signs of potential problems. Any medication can cause an allergic reaction that may be minor or as severe as anaphylaxis. Minor reactions can be characterized by development of a rash, rhinitis, fever, asthma, and pruritus. Management of the less acute allergic response is not an emergency. The nurse should monitor the vital signs, respiratory status, cardiovascular status, platelet count, and WBC count. The woman is observed for side effects of medications, especially drowsiness; the fluid intake and output are monitored to determine fluid balance and anticipate urinary retention; and the frequency of bowel movements is monitored to assess constipation (Clark, Queener, and Karb, 1993).

Severe allergic reactions may occur suddenly and produce shock. The most dramatic form of anaphylaxis is sudden severe bronchospasm, vasospasm, severe hypotension, and death. Signs of anaphylaxis are largely caused by contraction of smooth muscles and may begin with irritability, extreme weakness, nausea, and vomiting. The reaction then proceeds to dyspnea, cyanosis, convulsions, and cardiac arrest. The acute allergic reaction—anaphylaxis—requires immediate diagnosis and treatment, usually with 1:1000 epinephrine injected subcutaneously or intramuscularly, followed by parenteral antihistamines. Supportive care addresses symptoms and is based on rapid assessment of cardiovascular and respiratory response; CPR may be necessary. The nurse must also be alert to fetal well-being; FHR decelerations are noted and reported to the primary health care provider.

Nursing Diagnoses

Nursing diagnoses vary from individual to individual. The following list includes some examples of nursing diagnoses that are relevant to control of discomfort during the birth period:

- Pain related to
  Processes of labor and birth
- Risk for altered tissue perfusion related to
  Effects of analgesia or anesthesia
  Maternal position
- Hypothermia related to
  Effects of analgesia or anesthesia
- Situational low self-esteem related to
  Negative perception of the woman's (or her family's) behavior
- Anxiety or fear related to knowledge deficit of
  Procedure for nerve block analgesia
  Expected sensation during nerve block analgesia
  Mother's role during nerve block analgesia
  Options for analgesia and anesthesia

- Risk for injury to mother related to
  Effects of analgesia and anesthesia on sensation and motor control
- Risk for injury to fetus related to
  Maternal hypotension
  Maternal position (aortocaval compression)

Expected Outcomes

The expected outcomes for nursing care related to control of discomfort include the following considerations:

1. The mother will achieve adequate pain relief without adding to maternal risk (e.g., through appropriate nonpharmacologic methods; appropriate medication; and dosage, timing, and route of administration).
2. The fetus will maintain well-being, and the neonate will adjust to extrauterine life.
3. The family/significant others will know their needs and rights in relation to the use of nonpharmacologic methods, analgesia, or anesthesia.

Plan of Care and Implementation

For each woman, a plan of care is developed that relates to her clinical and nursing problems. The plan involves the mother and family and incorporates their priorities and preferences. The nurse, in collaboration with the primary health care provider and laboring woman, selects those aspects of care relevant to the individual woman and her family.

The woman's perception of her behavior during labor is of utmost importance. If she planned a nonmedicated birth but then needs and accepts medication, her self-esteem may falter. Verbal and nonverbal acceptance of her behavior is given (as necessary) by the nurse and reinforced by discussion and reassurance the day after birth. Explanations about fetal response to maternal discomfort, the effects of maternal fatigue, and the medication itself are supportive measures. Support may be needed by family and other support persons if plans for a nonmedicated birth were altered.

Excessive stress (as yet undefined in perinatal medicine) causes increased maternal catecholamine production. Catecholamines have been linked to dysfunctional labor and fetal and neonatal distress and illness (Simkin, 1986a, b). Since women who worried about pain consistently had worse outcomes on all measures in a large prospective study, the nurse must direct attention to reduction of anxiety and stress during labor (Green, 1993). Parents may feel reassured somewhat by hearing that medication is sometimes indicated for the baby's benefit.

Informed consent. The primary health care provider and anesthesia care provider are responsible for informing women of the alternative methods of pharmacologic pain relief available in the hospital setting. The description of anesthetic techniques is essential to informed consent, even if the woman has received information about analgesia and anesthesia earlier in her pregnancy. This interview should take place just before or early in labor so the woman has time to consider alternatives. Nurses play a part in the informed consent by clarifying and describing the procedures or by acting as a patient's advocate and asking the primary health care provider for further explanations. The procedure and its advantages and disadvantages must be thoroughly explained.

LEGAL TIP

Informed Consent for Anesthesia

The Woman Receives (In An Understandable Manner):

Explanation of alternatives available for pain control
Description of anesthetic and procedure for administration
Description of the benefits, discomfort, risks, and consequences of the selected anesthetic for the mother and the fetus
Explanation of how complications can be treated
Information that the anesthetic is not always effective
Indication that she may withdraw consent at any time
Opportunity to have any questions answered
Opportunity to explain in her own words components of the consent

Consent form:

Written in woman's primary language
Woman's signature
Date of consent
Signature of anesthesia caregiver certifying the woman has received an explanation and appears to understand the explanation.

Timing of administration. Orders often are written to dispense or administer medication on the basis of the nurse's clinical judgment. These orders require clinical knowledge and expertise. It is often the nurse who alerts the primary health care provider that the woman is in need of pharmacologic relief for discomfort. Box 14-1 lists pharmacologic control by stage of labor and method of birth.

Preparation for procedures. The nurse reviews or validates the woman's choices for relief from discomfort and clarifies the information for the mother as necessary. The woman needs an explanation of the procedure and what will be asked of her (e.g., to maintain flexed position during insertion of epidural needle). The woman benefits from knowing how the medication is to be given, the degree of discomfort to expect from administration of the medication, sensations she can expect, skin preparation procedures, the time required for administration, and the interval before medication takes effect. The nurse explains the need for emptying the bladder before analgesic or anesthetic is given and for keeping the bladder empty. When an indwelling epidural catheter is threaded, the woman is informed that a momentary twinge down her leg, hip, or back may occur and that this feeling is not a sign of injury.

For paracervical and pudendal blocks a long needle is used (Figs. 14-4 and 14-9). The sight of this needle may be frightening. The woman can be reassured that only the tip of the needle will be inserted.

Administration of medication. Accuracy in the monitoring of the progress of labor is the basis for clinical judgment in the need for pharmacologic control of discomfort. Knowledge of the medications that are used during childbirth is essential. The most effective route of administration for each woman is selected. Then the medication is prepared and administered correctly.

Intravenous route. The preferred route of administration of medications such as meperidine or fentanyl is through IV tubing. The infusion of IV solution is stopped while the medication is injected into the port nearest the woman. The medication is given slowly in small doses at the *beginning* of three to five consecutive contractions. Because uterine blood vessels are constricted during contractions, the medication stays within the maternal vascular system for several seconds before the uterine blood vessels reopen. The IV infusion is restarted slowly to prevent a bolus of medication. Through this method of injection, the amount of medication crossing the placenta to the fetus is minimized. With decreased placental transfer, the mother's degree of pain relief is maximized. The IV route has the following benefits:

Onset of pain relief is more predictable.
Pain relief is obtained with small doses of the drug.
Duration of effect is more predictable.

Intramuscular route. IM injections of analgesics, although still used, are no longer the preferred route of administration for the woman in labor. Identified disadvantages of the IM route include the following:

Onset of pain relief is delayed.
Higher doses of medication are required.
Medication is released at an unpredictable rate from the muscle tissue and is available for transfer across the placenta to the fetus.

IM injections are given in the upper portion of the arm (deltoid site) if regional anesthesia is planned later in labor. This is the preferred site because the autonomic blockage from the regional (e.g., epidural) anesthesia increases blood flow to the gluteal region and accelerates absorption of the drug. The maternal plasma level of the drug necessary to bring pain relief usually is reached 45 minutes after IM injection, followed by a decline in plasma levels. The maternal drug levels (after IM injections) are unequal because of uneven distribution (maternal uptake) and metabolism. The advantage of using the IM route is quick administration.

Nerve blocks. An IV line is established before nerve blocks such as paracervical, epidural, subarachnoid spinal, and general anesthesia are introduced. Lactated Ringer's solution or Plasma-Lyte A and normal saline solution are the preferred solutions. Infusion solutions without dextrose are preferred, especially when a solution needs to be infused rapidly (e.g., in the presence of severe dehydration or to maintain blood pressure). Solutions containing dextrose raise maternal blood glucose levels rapidly. The fetus responds to high blood glucose levels by increasing insulin production; fetal or neonatal hypoglycemia may result. In addition, dextrose changes osmotic pressure so fluid is excreted from the kidneys more rapidly.

The woman needs assistance in assuming and maintaining the correct position for epidural and spinal anesthesia (see p. 363).

Safety and general care. After IV or IM injection or nerve block, the woman is protected by raised side rails and a call bell within easy reach when the nurse is not in attendance. These women must be protected from prolonged pressure on an anesthetized part (e.g., lying on one side with weight on one leg; tight bedclothes on feet). If stirrups are used, the nurse pads them, adjusts both stirrups at the same level and angle, places both of the woman's legs into them while avoiding putting pressure to the popliteal angle, and applies restraints without restricting circulation.

The nurse monitors and records the woman's response to medication, including the level of pain relief, the level of ap-

Nursing Care Plan

LUMBAR EPIDURAL BLOCK DURING LABOR

Nursing Diagnosis: Risk for maternal/fetal injury related to maternal hypotension secondary to epidural block

Expected Outcomes: The patient will show no signs of hypotension; her pulse and blood pressure will remain within normal limits; and FHR will remain within normal limits.

• **NURSING INTERVENTIONS/*RATIONALES***

Establish baseline data on maternal vital signs and fetal heart rate *to evaluate subsequent readings.*

Start intravenous infusion per physician order and monitor flow *to increase blood volume and enhance cardiac output.*

Place woman in a lateral position *to avoid aortocaval compression and support placental perfusion.*

Monitor maternal vital signs and fetal heart rate *to identify early signs of maternal hypotension and/or fetal distress.*

If hypotension occurs, elevate the woman's legs, increase infusion rate per hospital protocol, administer oxygen by face mask at 10 to 12 L/minute, notify physician or nurse anesthetist/anesthesiologist, and administer vasopressor per physician order *to quickly correct maternal hypotension and maintain placental perfusion.*

Nursing Diagnosis: Altered pattern of urinary elimination related to effects of epidural block

Expected Outcome: Patient's bladder will not show signs of distention.

• **NURSING INTERVENTIONS/*RATIONALES***

Palpate the bladder superior to the symphysis on a frequent basis *because distention may occur from increased fluid intake and inability to feel urge to void.*

Encourage frequent voiding and catheterize if necessary *to avoid bladder distention because it impedes progress of fetus down birth canal and may result in trauma to the bladder.*

prehension, the return of sensations and perception of pain, and allergic or untoward reactions (e.g., hypotension, respiratory depression, and hypothermia). The nurse continues to monitor maternal vital signs, blood pressure, strength and frequency of uterine contractions, changes in the cervix and station of the presenting part, presence of the bearing-down reflex, bladder filling, and state of hydration. Determining the fetal response after the administration of analgesia or anesthesia is vital. The woman is asked if she (or the family) has any questions. The nurse assesses the woman's and her family's understanding of the need for ensuring her safety (e.g., keeping side rails up, calling for assistance as needed).

The time between the administration of a narcotic and the baby's birth are noted. The woman's record during childbirth serves as a documented means of communication among all members of the health care team. Documentation of the events is mandatory to meet legal requirements. Precise records also serve as a reservoir for research study.

Evaluation

Evaluation is a continuous process. The nurse can be relatively assured that care was effective if expected outcomes for care are achieved: the mother has adequate pain relief without risk; the fetus and newborn maintain well-being; and family members know their needs and rights in relation to analgesia and anesthesia (see the Nursing Care Plan on p. 370).

Key Points

- The expected outcome of preparation for childbirth and parenting is "education for choice."
- Nonpharmacologic pain and stress-management strategies are valuable for managing labor discomfort.
- The type of analgesic or anesthetic to be used is chosen in part by the stage of labor and the method of birth.
- Narcotic effects can be potentiated with ataractics.
- Naloxone or naltrexone are narcotic antagonists that can reverse narcotic effects, especially respiratory depression.
- Pharmacologic control of discomfort during labor requires collaboration among the health care providers and the woman in labor.
- The nurse must understand medications, their expected effects, their potential side effects, and methods of administration.
- Placement of an IV line and maternal hydration are essential during regional nerve blocks.
- Maternal analgesia or anesthesia potentially affects neonatal neurobehavioral response.
- The use of narcotic agonist-antagonist compounds in women with preexisting narcotic dependency may cause symptoms of narcotic withdrawal.

References

Aderhold K, Perry L: Jet hydrotherapy for labor and postpartum pain relief, *MCN Am J Matern Child Nurs* 16:97, 1991.

Bernardini J, Maloni J, Stegman C: Neuromuscular control of childbirth-prepared women during the first stage of labor, *J Obstet Gynecol Neonatal Nurs* 2:105, 1983.

Bernat S et al: Biofeedback-assisted relaxation to reduce stress in labor, *J Obstet Gynecol Neonatal Nurs* 21:295, 1992.

Bradley R: *Husband-coached childbirth*, ed 3, New York, 1981, Harper & Collins.

Briggs G, Freeman R, Yaffe S: *Drugs in pregnancy and lactation*, ed 2, Baltimore, 1986, Williams & Wilkins.

Cassidy J: A picture perfect birth: guided imagery interprets the pain/anxiety cycle, *RN* 56:45, 1993.

Clark J, Queener S, Karb V: *Pharmacological basis of nursing practice*, ed 4, St Louis, 1993, Mosby.

Cosner K, deJong E: Physiologic second-stage labor, *MCN Am J Matern Child Nurs* 18:39, 1993.

Cunningham F, et al: *Williams obstetrics*, ed 19, Norwalk, Conn., 1993, Appleton & Lange.

Dick-Read G: *Natural childbirth*, London, 1933, William Heinemann.

Dick-Read G: *Childbirth without fear*, New York, 1944, Harper & Row.

Dick-Read G: *Childbirth without fear*, ed 5, New York, 1987, Harper & Collins.

Dunn P et al: Maternal hypothermia: implications for obstetric nurses, *J Obstet Gynecol Neonatal Nurs*, 23:238, 1993.

Endler G: The risk of anesthesia in obese parturients, *J Perinat* 10:175, 1990.

Endler G et al: Anesthesia-related maternal mortality in Michigan, 1972-1984, *Am J Obstet Gynecol* 159:187, 1988.

Green J: Expectations and experiences of pain in labor: findings from a large prospective study, *Birth* 20:65, 1993.

Hamza J: Effect of epidural anesthesia on the fetus and the neonate, *Cah Anesthesiol* 42(2): 265, 1994.

Hood D, Dewan D: Anesthetic and obstetric outcome in morbidly obese parturients, *Anesthesiology* 79:1210, 1993.

Hughs S: Analgesia methods during labour and delivery, *Can J Anaesth* 39:18, 1992.

Isenor L, Penny-MacGillivary T: Intravenous meperidine infusion for obstetric analgesia, *J Obstet Gynecol Neonatal Nurs* 22:349, 1993.

Janke J: Teaching breathing techniques in the 90s, *Int J Childbirth Educ* 7:33, 1992.

Karmel M: *Thank you, Dr. Lamaze*, Philadelphia, 1959, JB Lippincott.

Kershner J, Schenck V: Music therapy-assisted childbirth, *Int J Childbirth Educ* 6:32, 1991

Klein R et al: A study of father and nurse support during labor, *Birth* 8:161, 1981.

Lamaze F: *Painless childbirth*, New York, 1972, Pocket Books.

Letts P et al: The use of hypnosis in labor and delivery: a preliminary study, *J Womens Health* 2:335, 1993.

McKay S, Barrows T, Roberts J: Women's views of second-stage labor as assessed by interviews and videotapes, *Birth* 17:192 1990.

Mackey M: Women's preparation for the childbirth experience, *Matern Child Nurs J* 19:143, 1990.

Mattson S, Smith J: *Core curriculum maternal-newborn nursing,* Philadelphia, 1993, WB Saunders.
Nicholson C: Nursing considerations for the parturient who has received epidural narcotics during labor or delivery, *J Perinat Neonatal Nurs* 4:14,1990.
Potter P, Perry A: *Basic nursing: theory and practice,* ed 3, St Louis, 1995, Mosby.
Rooks J, Weatherby N, Ernst E: The national birth center study. II. Intrapartum and immediate postpartum and neonatal care, *J Nurse Midwife* 37:301, 1992.
Scott J et al: *Danforth's obstetrics and gynecology,* ed 7, Philadelphia, 1994, JB Lippincott.
Schorn M, McAllister J, Blanco J: Water immersion and the effect on labor, *J Nurse Midwife* 38:336, 1993.
Sepkoski C et al: The effects of maternal epidural anesthesia on neonatal behavior during the first month, *Dev Med Child Neurol* 34:1072, 1992.
Simkin P: Stress, pain, and catecholamines in labor. I. A review, *Birth* 13(4):227, 1986a.
Simkin P: Stress, pain, and catecholamines in labor. II. A pilot survey of new mothers, *Birth* 13(4):234, 1986b.
Tisserand M: *Aromatherapy for women,* London, 1990, Thorsons.
Valnet J: *The practice of aromatherapy,* Rochester, Vt, 1990, Healing Arts Press.
Waldenstrom U, Nilsson C: Warm tub bath after spontaneous rupture of the membranes, *Birth* 19:57, 1992.
Writer D: Epidural analgesia for labor, *Anesth Clin North Am* 10:59, 1992.
Wuitchik M, Hesson K, Bakel D: Perinatal predictors of pain and distress during labor, *Birth* 17:186, 1990.

Bibliography

Bradley L: Changing American birth through childbirth education, *Pat Educ Couns* 25(1):75, 1995.
Geissler E: *Pocket guide to cultural assessment,* St Louis, 1994, Mosby.
Gordon S, Gaines S, Hauber R: Self-administered versus nurse-administered epidural analgesia after cesarean section, *J Obstet Gynecol Neonatal Nurs* 23:99, 1994.
Manning J: Intrathecal narcotics: new approach for labor analgesia, *J Obstet Gynecol Neonatal Nures* 25(3):221, 1996.
Olden J et al: Patients' versus nurses' assessment of pain and sedation after cesarean section, *J Obstet Gynecol Neonatal Nurs* 24:137, 1995.
Youngstrom P, Baker S, Miller J: Epidurals redefined in analgesia and anesthesia: a distinction with a difference, *J Obstet Gynecol Neonatal Nurs* 25(4):350, 1996.

CHAPTER 15

Fetal Assessment

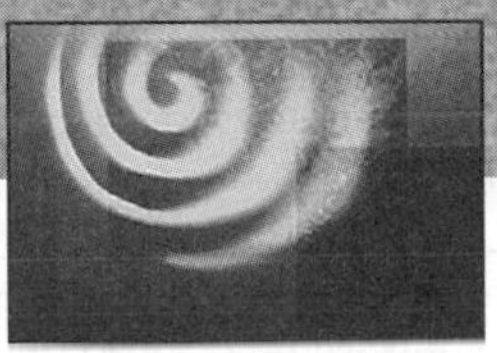

BASIS FOR MONITORING, P. 374

The fetal response, p. 374

Fetal compromise, p. 374

MONITORING TECHNIQUES, P. 375

Intermittent auscultation, p. 375

Electronic monitoring, p. 376

FHR patterns, p. 377

Fetal blood sampling/fetal scalp stimulation: acid-base monitoring, p. 385

Fetal pulse oximetry, p. 385

Nursing care management, p. 386

Guidelines and standards of nursing care related to EFM, p. 387

Preventive measures, p. 388

Intrauterine resuscitation, p. 388

Working with the monitor, p. 389

Over the last century, parents' expectations for pregnancy outcomes have changed dramatically. In the early 1900s, many women and infants did not survive the pregnancy and childbirth process. Even 50 years ago, risk of death from childbirth was significant. In 1940 the maternal mortality rate (MMR) was 364 women per 100,000 live births as compared with the current MMR of 7.8, and the infant mortality rate was 32 per 1000 live births as compared to today's rate of 7.5 (Centers for Disease Control and Prevention, Guyer et al, 1996). As childbirth moved to the hospital setting with modern technology and skilled health care providers, most pregnancies resulted in both maternal survival and the birth of a healthy infant. The fetus has evolved as a person as a result of increased prenatal education about fetal growth and development and routine use of ultrasound, during which parents are able to "see" their infant before birth. These factors have promoted the development, refinement, and use of many diagnostic procedures such as electronic monitoring of the fetus. Technologic innovations in perinatal care over the past two decades have increased health care providers' understanding of maternal-fetal physiology and anatomy, which has in turn been a driving force in fine-tuning technologic advances. Consumers are well aware of and expect to benefit personally from medical technology.

Since the 1970s, when the technology was first introduced, considerable expertise has evolved in assessing fetal hemodynamic and oxygen status as reflected by continuous **electronic fetal monitoring (EFM).** Evaluation of the fetal heart rate (FHR) remains complex because of the number of factors that must be considered and variations in the "normal" fetal response to labor. To date there is no consensus in the literature or in clinical practice on terminology to describe FHR patterns nor on objective data to determine when fetal well-being may be compromised. Current methods to describe FHR patterns are based on terminology from equipment manufacturers, researchers, and authors and can vary by region of the country, institution, and health care provider. The terminology used in this chapter is accepted by many providers; however, it is important to note that at present there is no nationally agreed-upon nomenclature for describing FHR patterns. Common terminology should be established among the members of the perinatal health care team at each institution and ideally within each perinatal network, to be sure that all members comprehend the meaning of the pattern implications, to ensure consistency in medical record documentation, and to facilitate collaboration and communication (Afriat, 1996). A nonreassuring FHR pattern is not necessarily an indication of fetal compromise; however, such a pattern requires interventions to attempt to reassure the nurse and physician of fetal well-being. A reassuring FHR pattern virtually assures the birth of a healthy, well-oxygenated newborn; however, with a nonreassuring FHR pattern, at least 50% of the time, birth of a healthy, well-oxygenated newborn will also result (Afriat, 1996). Thus, because of the low positive predictive ability of EFM and lack of consensus on objective data to determine fetal well-being, the term *fetal distress* should be avoided in documentation on the medical record.

Basic information about EFM during labor is emphasized in this chapter. Other methods of fetal surveillance (e.g., biophysical profile) are discussed in Chapter 5. Perinatal nurses caring for women in labor must be knowledgeable about methods of monitoring and the implications of various findings. Nursing responsibilities include explaining procedures to the woman and family and responding to their questions and concerns. Perinatal nurses must develop a systematic method of interpreting data from the monitor and be able to distinguish between reassuring and nonreassuring FHR patterns. They must be alert for signs of fetal compromise and be prepared to implement appropriate nursing interventions, including intrauterine resuscitation and notification of the primary health care provider. It is also important to be familiar with institutional policies related to chain of command and conflict resolution should disagreement arise between the nurse and primary health care provider about interpretation of FHR patterns. The Association of Women's Health, Obstetric, and Neonatal Nurses (AWHONN, 1993b) and the American College of Obstetricians and Gynecologists (ACOG, 1994; 1995) have developed guidelines for practice and standards of care for health care providers who care for women monitored by EFM during pregnancy and childbirth. It is the responsibility of the perinatal nurse to keep abreast of new developments in EFM technology and knowledge to ensure the best possible outcomes for mothers and newborns.

BASIS FOR MONITORING

The Fetal Response

Because labor represents a period of physiologic stress for the fetus, frequent monitoring of fetal status is an integral part of the nursing care during labor. Based on the physician's/certified nurse-midwife's (CNM's) and/or a woman's preferences, staffing ratios, and institutional protocols, fetal assessment during the intrapartum period can be either intermittent or continuous. Both methods are directed toward assessing the fetal response to uterine activity. Adequate fetal oxygenation must be maintained during labor to prevent fetal compromise and promote newborn health after birth. The fetal oxygen supply can be decreased in a number of ways:

- Reduction of blood flow through the maternal vessels as a result of maternal hypertension (chronic hypertension or pregnancy-induced hypertension), hypotension (supine maternal position, hemorrhage, or related to epidural analgesia/anesthesia), or hypovolemia (hemorrhage)
- Reduction of the oxygen content of the maternal blood as a result of hemorrhage or severe anemia
- Alterations in fetal circulation, occurring with compression of the umbilical cord (transient during uterine contractions or prolonged as a result of cord prolapse), placental separation or complete abruption, or head compression (head compression causes increased intracranial pressure and vagal nerve stimulation with a decrease in the FHR)
- Reduction in blood flow to the intervillous space in the placenta secondary to too frequent uterine contractions and an increase in resting uterine tone, known as uterine hyperstimulation (undesirable side effect of exogenous oxytocin), or secondary to deterioration of the placental vasculature from maternal disease processes such as hypertension or diabetes mellitus.

Fetal well-being during labor can be measured by the response of the FHR to uterine contractions. In general, a *reassuring FHR pattern* is characterized by a FHR baseline between 110 and 160 beats/min with average variability, and the absence of nonreassuring periodic changes. Acceleration of FHR with fetal movement is an additional reassuring sign.

A normal uterine activity pattern in labor is characterized by contractions every 2 to 5 minutes, duration of contractions less than 90 seconds, moderate to strong intensity of contractions by palpation, or less than 100 mm Hg intraamniotic pressure measured via intrauterine pressure catheter (IUPC), a period of 30 seconds or more from the end of one contraction to the beginning of the next contraction, and uterine relaxation by palpation or an average intraamniotic pressure of 15 mm Hg or less measured by IUPC between contractions.

Fetal Compromise

Fetal compromise may be suggested by a nonreassuring FHR pattern. It can be acute or chronic, depending on antepartum and intrapartum events, with the possibility of an acute insult superimposed on a chronic condition. Acute events include placental abruption, umbilical cord prolapse, uterine hyperstimulation by oxytocin, uterine rupture, and/or maternal hypotension related to supine position or epidural analgesia/anesthesia. Chronic conditions may result from maternal conditions that involve hemodynamic or vascular changes such as diabetes, hypertension, anemia, systemic lupus erythematosus, cardiac disease, and/or placenta previa.

The goals of intrapartum FHR monitoring are early detection of mild fetal hypoxemia and prevention of severe fetal hypoxia. A distinction can be made between hypoxemia and hypoxia. **Hypoxemia** is characterized by a deficiency of oxygen in the arterial blood, whereas **hypoxia** is an inadequate supply of oxygen at the cellular level. Fetal hypoxemia can deteriorate progressively to fetal hypoxia. The nurse must be thinking continually in terms of whether the FHR pattern is reassuring and whether fetal oxygenation is adequate. Discrimination must be made between reassuring FHR patterns, nonreassuring patterns generally indicative of mild fetal hypoxemia, and nonreassuring patterns that may indicate severe fetal hypoxia. Reassuring FHR patterns include the following:

- Baseline FHR in the normal range of 110 to 160 bpm with no periodic changes and average baseline variability.
- Early decelerations
- Mild variable decelerations with quick return to baseline
- Accelerations

Nonreassuring FHR patterns are as follows:

- Progressive increase or decrease in baseline FHR
- Tachycardia of 160 bpm or above
- Progressive decrease in baseline variability
- Severe variable decelerations (FHR less than 70 bpm lasting longer than 30 to 60 seconds, with rising baseline, decreasing variability, and/or slow return to baseline)
- Late decelerations of any magnitude—especially those that are repetitive and uncorrectable, with decreasing variability or a rising baseline FHR

- Absence of FHR variability
- Prolonged deceleration
- Severe bradycardia

MONITORING TECHNIQUES

Intermittent Auscultation

Intermittent (periodic) auscultation of the fetal heart is one method to assess fetal status during labor. A fetoscope or ultrasound stethoscope may be used to listen to the FHR (Fig. 15-1). NAACOG (now AWHONN) (1990) and ACOG (1995) have developed guidelines for the auscultation of FHR during labor.

Method and frequency of monitoring are based on maternal-fetal risk status. In the absence of risk factors, the standard practice is to auscultate the FHR as follows:

First stage:
—Latent phase every 60 minutes
—Active phase every 30 minutes
Second stage:
—Every 15 minutes

When risk factors are present during labor, the FHR is auscultated as follows:

First stage:
—Latent phase every 30 minutes
—Active phase every 15 minutes
Second stage:
—Every 5 minutes

Controversy continues related to the ideal method of fetal assessment during labor. Multiple research studies suggest that intermittent auscultation of the FHR at the frequencies already listed result in fetal outcomes similar to what is seen when EFM is used. The advantage of intermittent auscultation is that it is a high-touch, low-tech method of assessing fetal status during labor with fewer restrictions on maternal activity. Childbirth is a natural process. Thus most women and fetuses do well with minimal intervention and periodic assessment.

Every effort should be made to use the method of fetal assessment the woman desires, if possible. However, auscultation of the FHR according to the preceding frequency guidelines may be difficult in today's busy labor and birth units. Auscultation as the primary method of fetal assessment requires a one-to-one nurse-fetus staffing ratio (e.g., a woman with twins would require two primary nurses to meet this standard during labor if auscultation is selected). If acuity and census change so that auscultation standards can no longer be met, the nurse must notify the physician or nurse midwife that continuous EFM will be used until staffing can be arranged to meet the standards.

Auscultation is performed during a uterine contraction and for a period of 30 seconds immediately after the end of the contraction. Auscultation can reveal FHR tachycardia, bradycardia, or dysrhythmia that may occur during the brief assessment. The most important sign of fetal compromise, beat-to-beat or short-term variability of the FHR, cannot be assessed by periodic auscultation (Parer, 1994). Nonreassuring FHR patterns may not occur or be detected during the pe-

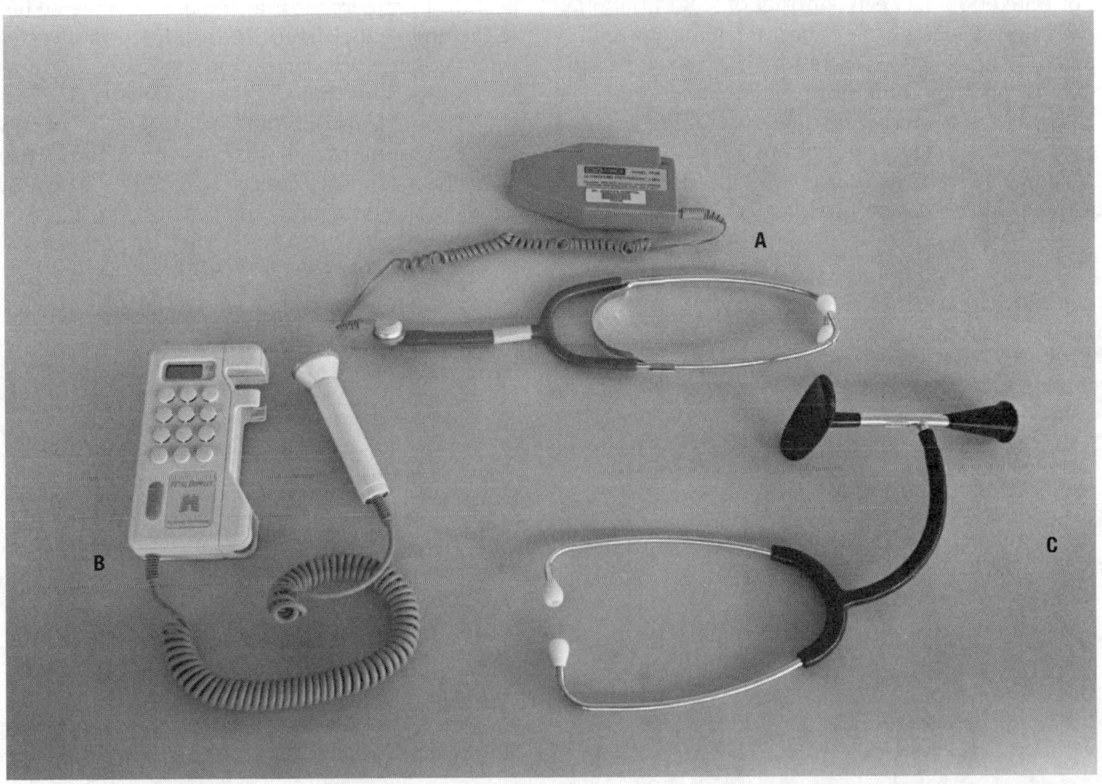

Fig. 15-1 **A,** Ultrasound fetoscope. **B,** Ultrasound stethoscope. **C,** DeLee-Hillis fetoscope. (Courtesy Michael S. Clement, MD, Mesa, Ariz.)

riods of auscultation and thus go unrecognized by the examiner (AAP/ACOG, 1992; ACOG, 1995; Freeman et al, 1991). An improved method that is more likely to aid in diagnosing fetal compromise in the high-risk pregnancy is the counting of FHR during sequential contractions and for a full 3 minutes thereafter. Persistent, postcontraction bradycardia (e.g., FHR of 100 beats/min or a persistent drop of 30 beats/min or more below baseline) or gross irregularity can indicate fetal compromise.

The woman can become anxious if the examiner cannot readily count the FHR. The inexperienced listener often takes time to locate the heartbeat and find the area of maximum intensity. The mother can be told that the nurse is "finding the spot where the sounds are loudest." If it has taken considerable time to locate the FHR, the examiner can reassure the mother by offering her an opportunity to listen, too. If the examiner cannot locate the FHR, assistance should be requested. In some cases the use of ultrasound will aid in locating the FHR. Seeing the FHR on the ultrasound screen will be reassuring for the mother if there was initial difficulty in locating the best area for auscultation.

When using intermittent auscultation, uterine activity is assessed by placing the examiner's hand over the fundus before, during, and after contractions. Contraction intensity is usually described as mild, moderate, or strong. Contraction duration is measured in seconds, from beginning to end of the contraction. Frequency of contractions is measured in minutes, from the beginning of one contraction to the beginning of the next contraction. When using palpation to assess uterine activity, it is important to maintain the examiner's hand on the fundus after the contraction is over to evaluate uterine resting tone or relaxation between contractions. Resting tone between contractions is usually described as soft or relaxed.

Accurate and complete documentation of fetal status and uterine activity is especially important when using intermittent auscultation because there is no paper tracing recording of these assessments, as occurs continuously with electronic monitoring. Labor flow records that prompt notations of all assessments are useful for comprehensive documentation.

Electronic Monitoring

There are two modes of electronic monitoring. The external mode uses transducers placed on the maternal abdomen to assess FHR and uterine activity. Newer monitors can monitor dual FHRs in twin gestations. The internal mode uses a **spiral electrode** applied to the fetal presenting part to assess the fetal electrocardiogram (ECG) and an **intrauterine pressure catheter** to assess uterine activity and intraamniotic pressure. A brief description contrasting the external and internal modes of EFM is provided in Table 15-1.

External monitoring. Separate transducers monitor the FHR and uterine contractions (Fig. 15-2). The **ultrasound transducer** acts through the reflection of high-frequency sound waves from a moving interface, in this case the fetal heart and valves. It may sometimes be difficult to reproduce a continuous and precise record of the FHR by this method because of artifacts introduced by fetal and maternal movement. The FHR is printed on specially formatted monitor paper for ease in identifying FHR baseline rate, variability, and periodic changes, and uterine activity over time. Most institutions use an EFM paper speed of 3 cm/min. Once the area of maximum intensity of FHR has been located, conduction gel is applied to the surface of the ultrasound transducer, and the transducer is then positioned over this area.

The **tocotransducer** (tocodynamometer) measures uterine activity transabdominally. A pressure-sensitive surface on the side next to the abdomen measures abdominal wall changes during uterine contractions or fetal movement. The device is placed over the fundus above the umbilicus. When monitoring the woman experiencing preterm labor, it is important to remember that the fundus may be below the level of the umbilicus. The tocotransducer can measure and record the frequency, regularity, and approximate duration of uterine contractions, but not their intensity. This method is especially valuable during the first stage of labor in women with intact membranes or for use in antepartum testing. The tocotransducer of most EFMs is designed for assessing uterine activity in the term pregnancy. Therefore if the woman is in

TABLE 15-1 External and internal modes of monitoring

EXTERNAL MODE	INTERNAL MODE
FHR	
Ultrasound transducer: High-frequency sound waves reflect mechanical action of the fetal heart. Used during the antepartum and intrapartum period.	*Spiral electrode:* This electrode converts the fetal ECG as obtained from the presenting part to the FHR via a cardiotachometer. This method can only be used when membranes are ruptured and cervix sufficiently dilated (2 to 3 cm) during the intrapartum period. Electrode penetrates into fetal presenting part by 1.5 mm and must be on securely to ensure a good signal.
Uterine activity	
Tocodynamometer: This instrument monitors frequency and duration of contractions by means of a pressure-sensing device applied to the maternal abdomen. Used during both the antepartum and intrapartum periods.	*IUPC:* This instrument monitors the frequency, duration, and intensity of contractions. There are two types of IUPCs. One is a fluid-filled system, and the other is a solid catheter. Both measure intrauterine pressure at the catheter tip and convert the pressure into millimeters of mercury on the uterine activity panel of the strip chart. Both can be used only when membranes are ruptured and the cervix sufficiently dilated (2 to 3 cm) during the intrapartum period.

A

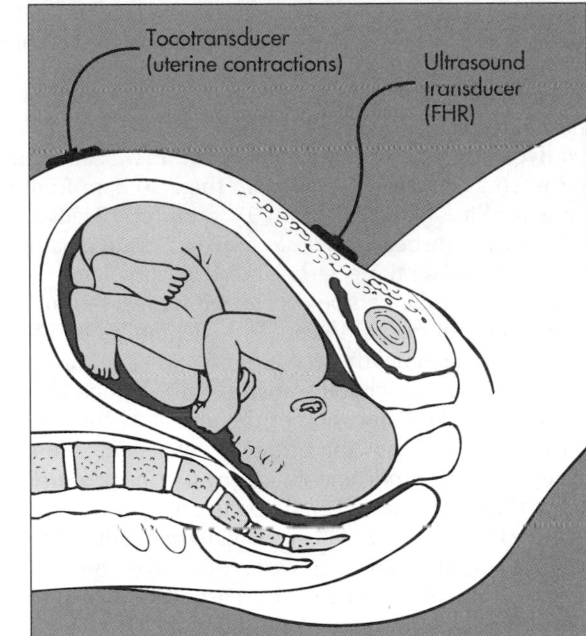

B

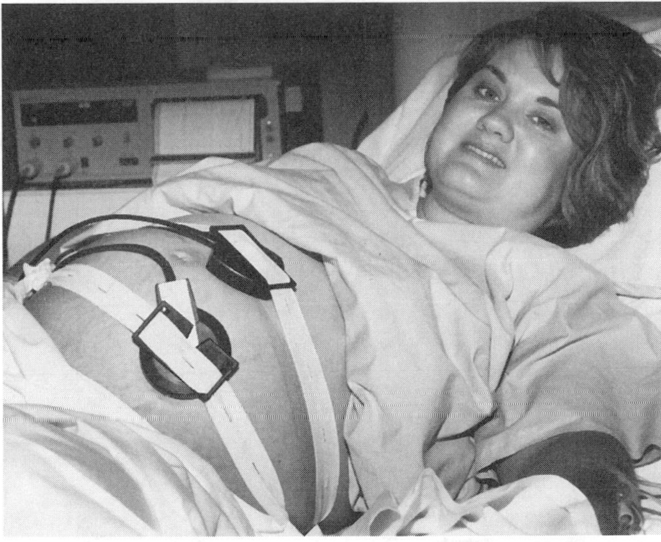

Fig. 15-2 **A,** External noninvasive fetal monitoring using tocotransducer and ultrasound transducer. **B,** Ultrasound transducer is placed below umbilicus, and tocotransducer is placed on uterine fundus. (Courtesy St John's Mercy Medical Center, St Louis, Mo.)

preterm labor, the tocotransducer may not be sensitive enough to detect preterm uterine activity (Eganhouse, 1992). When electronically monitoring the woman in preterm labor, the nurse may need to rely on the woman's indication of uterine activity and use palpation as an additional method of assessment for contraction frequency.

Internal monitoring. Continuous internal monitoring provides an accurate assessment of fetal well-being during labor (Fig. 15-3). For this type of monitoring the membranes must be ruptured, the cervix sufficiently dilated (2 to 3 cm), and the presenting part low enough for placement of the electrode. A small spiral electrode attached to the presenting part yields a continuous FHR on the fetal monitor strip. To measure uterine contractions, a pressure-sensitive catheter is introduced into the uterine cavity. As the catheter is compressed, pressure is placed on the strain gauge or pressure transducer, which is then converted into a pressure reading in millimeters of mercury of intraamniotic pressure. The average intraamniotic pressure range during a contraction is 50 to 85 mm Hg. The intrauterine pressure catheter can measure frequency, duration, and intensity of uterine contractions. The display of FHR and uterine activity on the monitor paper differs for the two modes of electronic monitoring (Fig. 15-4). Note that each small square represents 10 seconds; each larger box of six squares equals 1 minute.

Critical Thinking Exercises

EFM

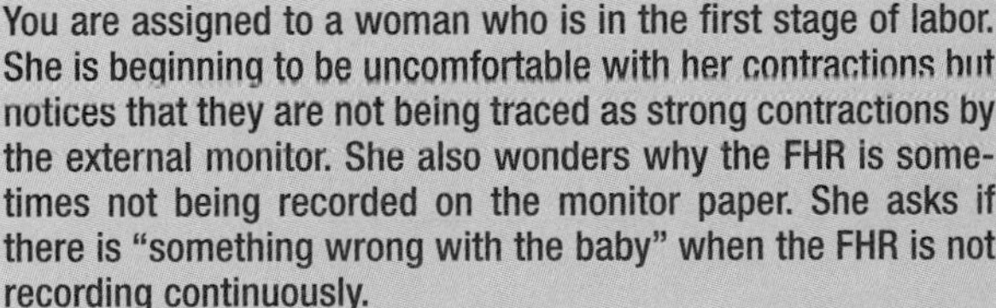

You are assigned to a woman who is in the first stage of labor. She is beginning to be uncomfortable with her contractions but notices that they are not being traced as strong contractions by the external monitor. She also wonders why the FHR is sometimes not being recorded on the monitor paper. She asks if there is "something wrong with the baby" when the FHR is not recording continuously.

1. Based on your knowledge of how the external monitor works, how would you explain the lack of continuous tracing of the FHR and the seeming inconsistency in the degree of the mother's discomfort and the appearance of contractions on the monitor paper?
2. Identify nursing diagnoses based on your analysis of the situation.
3. Develop a plan of care, including interventions that would be reassuring and supportive, and justify your choices.

FHR Patterns

Baseline FHR. The intrinsic rhythmicity of the fetal heart and the fetal autonomic nervous system control the FHR. An increase in sympathetic response results in acceleration of the FHR. An augmentation in parasympathetic response produces a slowing of the FHR. The push-pull relationship between the two divisions of the autonomic nervous system serves to balance the FHR. (This process is described in the discussion of variability in this section.)

Baseline fetal heart rate is the average rate when the woman is not in labor or is between contractions. At term this average is about 135 to 140 beats/min, a decrease from 160 beats/min early in pregnancy. The normal range at term is 110 to 160 beats/min. Ideally, the FHR should be assessed over a 10- to 20-minute period to determine baseline rate.

Tachycardia is a baseline FHR above 160 beats/min or an increase of more than 30 beats/min from the previous baseline for longer than 10 minutes. It can be considered an early

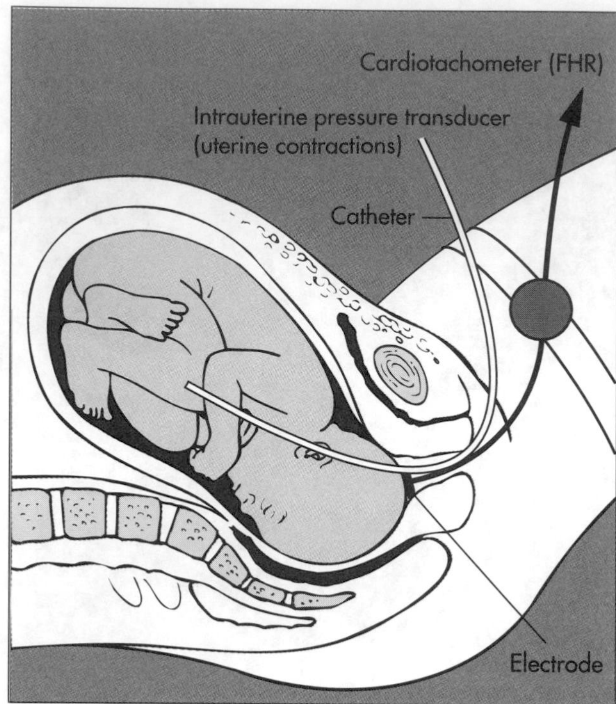

Fig. 15-3 Internal invasive fetal monitoring with intrauterine catheter and spiral electrode in place (membranes ruptured and cervix dilated).

sign of fetal hypoxemia. Causes include maternal or fetal infection, as sometimes occurs with prolonged rupture of membranes with intraamniotic infection, maternal hyperthyroidism or fetal anemia; and response to drugs such as atropine, hydroxyzine (Vistaril), ritodrine, or terbutaline.

Bradycardia is a baseline FHR below 110 beats/min in the term fetus or a decrease of more than 30 bpm from the previous baseline for longer than 10 minutes. (Bradycardia should be distinguished from prolonged deceleration patterns, which are periodic changes that are described later in this chapter.) Bradycardia can be considered a later sign of fetal hypoxemia or progression to fetal hypoxia and is also known to occur before fetal death (terminal bradycardia). Bradycardia can result from placental transfer of drugs such as anesthetics, prolonged compression of the umbilical cord, maternal hypothermia, and maternal hypotension. Maternal supine hypotensive syndrome, caused by uterine pressure (the weight of the gravid uterus) on the vena cava, decreases blood flow return to the maternal heart, which then reduces maternal cardiac output and blood pressure. These responses in the mother subsequently result in decreased blood flow to the uteroplacental unit followed by an initial increase in FHR as the fetus attempts to compensate. If blood flow is not restored quickly, a decrease in the FHR, fetal bradycardia, occurs. Table 15-2 compares tachycardia with bradycardia.

Variability of the FHR can be described as the normal irregularity of the cardiac rhythm. It is characterized by a continuous balancing interaction of the parasympathetic (cardiodeceleration) and sympathetic (cardioacceleration) divisions of the autonomic nervous system. This "push-pull" effect results in an irregular FHR, which is an indicator of fetal health. FHR variability increases gradually with gestational age of the fetus. The fetal parasympathetic division has matured sufficiently by 28 weeks' gestation to interact with

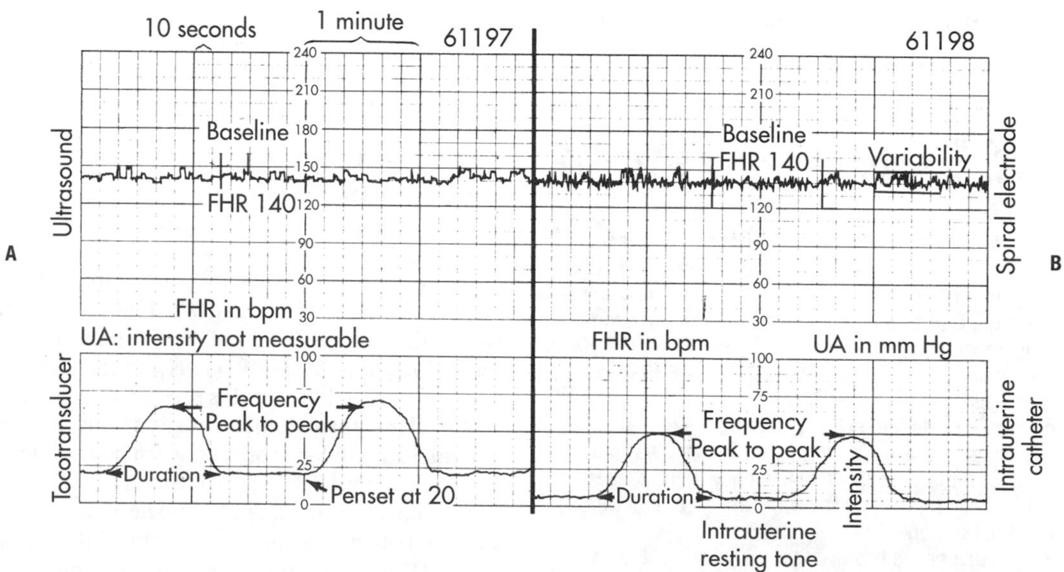

Fig. 15-4 Display of FHR and uterine activity on monitor paper. **A,** External mode with ultrasound and tocotransducer as signal source. **B,** Internal mode with spiral electrode and intrauterine catheter as signal source. (From Tucker S: *Pocket guide to fetal monitoring and assessment,* ed 3, St Louis, 1996, Mosby.)

TABLE 15-2 Tachycardia and bradycardia

TACHYCARDIA	BRADYCARDIA
Definition	
FHR above 160 beats/min lasting longer than 10 min	FHR below 110 bpm lasting longer than 10 min
Cause	
Early fetal hypoxemia Maternal fever Parasympatholytic drugs (atropine, hydroxyzine) β-sympathomimetic drugs (ritodrine, isoxsuprine) Intraamniotic infection Maternal hyperthyroidism Fetal anemia Fetal heart failure Fetal cardiac dysrhythmias	Late fetal hypoxia/hypoxemia β-adrenergic blocking drugs (propranolol; anesthetics for epidural, spinal, caudal, and pudendal blocks) Maternal hypotension Prolonged umbilical cord compression Fetal congenital heart block
Clinical significance	
Persistent tachycardia in absence of periodic changes does not appear serious in terms of neonatal outcome (especially true if tachycardia is associated with maternal fever); tachycardia is a nonreassuring sign when associated with late decelerations, severe variable decelerations, or absence of variability.	Bradycardia with average variability and absence of periodic changes is not a sign of fetal compromise if FHR remains above 80 beats/min; bradycardia caused by hypoxia is a nonreassuring sign when associated with loss of variability and late decelerations.
Nursing intervention	
Depends on cause; reduce maternal fever with antipyretics as ordered and cooling measures; oxygen at 10 to 12 L/min per face mask may be of some value; carry out physician's/CNM's orders based on alleviating cause.	Depends on cause; intervention not warranted in fetus with heart block diagnosed by ECG; oxygen at 10 to 12 L/min per face mask may be of some value; carry out physician's/CNM's orders based on alleviating cause.

the sympathetic division to produce variability of the FHR (Freeman et al, 1991).

Variability is described as being short-term or long-term. Short-term variability is the change in FHR from one heartbeat to the next. Thus even though a fetal heart may beat 140 times over the course of a minute, there are times in that minute when the heart rate is 134 or 146. Long-term variability appears as rhythmic cycles (or waves) from the baseline, and there are generally three to five cycles per minute. All monitors can present evidence of long-term variability whether the woman is monitored internally or externally. Only the internal signal source from a spiral electrode can accurately assess short-term variability (Fig. 15-5). However, most monitors in current use have an autocorrelation feature that can closely approximate short-term variability when the external signal source, the ultrasound transducer, is used.

Absence of variability, or a smooth (flat) baseline, is considered nonreassuring and a sign of potential fetal compromise. By 28 weeks' gestation, there should be evidence of FHR variability, although variability may be slightly less than in term fetuses (Freeman et al, 1991). Decreased variability can result from fetal hypoxemia and acidemia, as well as from certain drugs that depress the central nervous system (CNS), including analgesics, narcotics (meperidine [Demerol]), barbiturates (secobarbital [Seconal] and pentobarbital [Nembutal]), tranquilizers (diazepam [Valium]), ataractics (promethazine [Phenergan]), and general anesthetics. In addition, a temporary decrease in variability can occur when the fetus is in a sleep state. These sleep states do not usually last longer than 30 minutes before average variability resumes. To

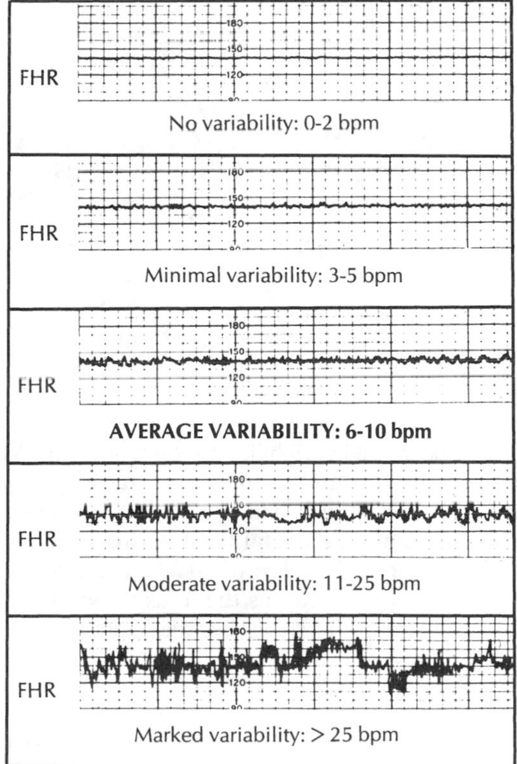

Fig. 15-5 FHR variability. Short- and long-term variability tend to increase and decrease together. *bpm*, Beats/min. (From Tucker S: *Pocket guide to fetal monitoring and assessment*, ed 3, St Louis, 1996, Mosby

TABLE 15-3 Increased and decreased variability

INCREASED VARIABILITY	DECREASED VARIABILITY
Cause	
Early mild hypoxemia Fetal stimulation caused by the following: Uterine palpation Uterine contractions Fetal activity Maternal activity	Hypoxia/acidosis CNS depressants Analgesics/narcotics Meperidine Alphaprodine (Nisentil) Morphine Pentazocine (Talwin) Barbituates Secobarbital Pentobarbital Amobarbital (Amytal) Tranquilizers (diazepam) Ataractics Promethazine (Phenergan) Propiomazine (Largon) Hydroxyzine (Vistaril) Promazine (Sparine) Parasympatholytics (atropine) General anesthetics Prematurity Fetal sleep cycles Congenital abnormalities Fetal cardiac dysrhythmias
Clinical significance	
Significance of marked variability not known; increased variability from a previous average variability is earliest FHR sign of mild hypoxemia.	Benign when associated with periodic fetal sleep states, which last 20 to 30 min; if caused by drugs, variability usually increases as drugs are excreted Decreased variability considered nonreassuring if caused by hypoxia/hypoxemia when it occurs with late decelerations; decreased variability is associated with fetal acidemia and low Apgar scores.
Nursing intervention	
Observe FHR tracing carefully for any nonreassuring patterns, including decreasing variability and late decelerations; if using external mode of monitoring, consider using internal mode (spiral electrode) for a more accurate tracing.	Depends on cause; intervention not warranted if associated with fetal sleep states or temporarily associated with CNS depressants; consider application of internal mode (spiral electrode); perform external fetal stimulation or fetal scalp stimulation during vaginal examination to attempt to elicit an acceleration of the FHR and/or return to average variability; assist physician/CNM with fetal blood sampling for pH if ordered; prepare for birth if so indicated by physician/CNM.

determine if decreased variability results from fetal sleep, the perinatal nurse can stimulate the fetus externally by placing her hands on the maternal abdomen and gently moving the fetus or by stimulating the fetal head during vaginal examination. These actions should result in a FHR acceleration and return to average variability as the fetus is awakened. Table 15-3 contrasts key differences between increased and decreased variability.

Periodic changes in FHR. Periodic changes in the FHR are referred to as accelerations or decelerations, and the latter are described as early, late, or variable, depending on their characteristics of timing, shape, and repetitiveness in relation to uterine contractions. **Accelerations** (caused by dominance of the sympathetic response) are usually encountered with breech presentations (Fig. 15-6, *A*). Pressure applied to the infant's buttocks results in accelerations, whereas pressure applied to the head results in decelerations. Accelerations may occur, however, during the second stage of labor in cephalic presentations. Accelerations (Fig. 15-6, *B*) of the FHR occurring during fetal movement are indications of fetal well-being (nonstress test).

Decelerations (caused by dominance of parasympathetic response) may be benign or nonreassuring. The three types of decelerations that are encountered during labor are early, late, and variable. FHR decelerations are described by their relation to the onset and end of a contraction and by their shape.

Early deceleration (slowing of heart rate) in response to compression of the fetal head is normal and usually does not indicate fetal compromise (Fig. 15-7, *A*). The deceleration is characterized by a uniform shape and an early onset corre-

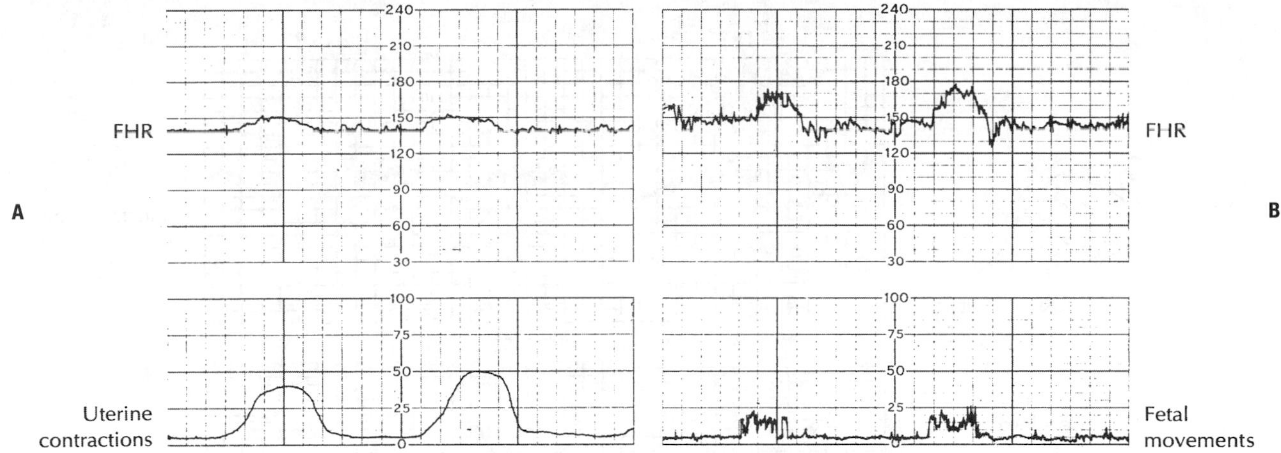

Fig. 15-6 **A,** Acceleration of FHR with uterine contractions. **B,** Acceleration of FHR with fetal movement. (From Tucker S: *Pocket guide to fetal monitoring and assessment*, ed 3, St Louis, 1996, Mosby.)

TABLE 15-4 Acceleration and early deceleration

	ACCELERATION	EARLY DECELERATION
Description	Transitory increase of FHR above baseline (see Fig. 15-6)	Transitory decrease of FHR below baseline concurrent with uterine contractions (see Fig. 15-7, *A*)
Shape	May resemble shape of uterine contraction	Uniform shape; mirror image of uterine contraction
Onset	Variable; often precedes or occurs simultaneously with uterine contraction	Early in contraction phase before peak of contraction
Recovery	Variable	By end of contraction as uterine pressure returns to its resting tone
Amplitude	Usually 15 beats/min above baseline	Usually proportional to amplitude of contraction; rarely decelerates below 100 beats/min
Baseline	Usually associated with average baseline variability	Usually associated with average baseline variability
Occurrence	Variable; may be repetitive with each contraction	Repetitious (occurs with each contraction); usually occurs between 4 to 7 cm dilation and in second stage of labor.
Cause	Spontaneous fetal movement Vaginal examination Breech presentation Occiput posterior position Uterine contractions Fundal pressure Abdominal palpation	Head compression resulting from: Uterine contractions Vaginal examination Fundal pressure Placement of internal mode of monitoring
Clinical significance	Acceleration with fetal movement signifies fetal well-being representing fetal alertness or arousal states.	Reassuring pattern not associated with fetal hypoxemia, acidemia, or low Apgar scores.
Nursing intervention	None required	None required

sponding to the rise in intraamniotic pressure as the uterus contracts. When present, it usually occurs during the first stage of labor when the cervix is dilated 4 to 7 cm. Early decelerations sometimes are seen during the second stage when the woman is pushing. Early decelerations as a response to fetal head compression can occur during vaginal examinations, as a result of fundal pressure, during placement of the internal mode for fetal monitoring, and during uterine contractions.

Early decelerations are considered to be a benign pattern; therefore interventions are not necessary. The value of identifying early decelerations is to be able to distinguish them from late or variable decelerations, which can be nonreassuring and for which interventions are appropriate. Table 15-4 contrasts accelerations of FHR with early decelerations.

Late decelerations are caused by uteroplacental insufficiency, either chronic or acute. They appear as a smooth, curvilinear, uniform heart rate pattern that closely reflects the pattern of intrauterine pressure during a contraction. However, in contrast to early decelerations, a late deceleration

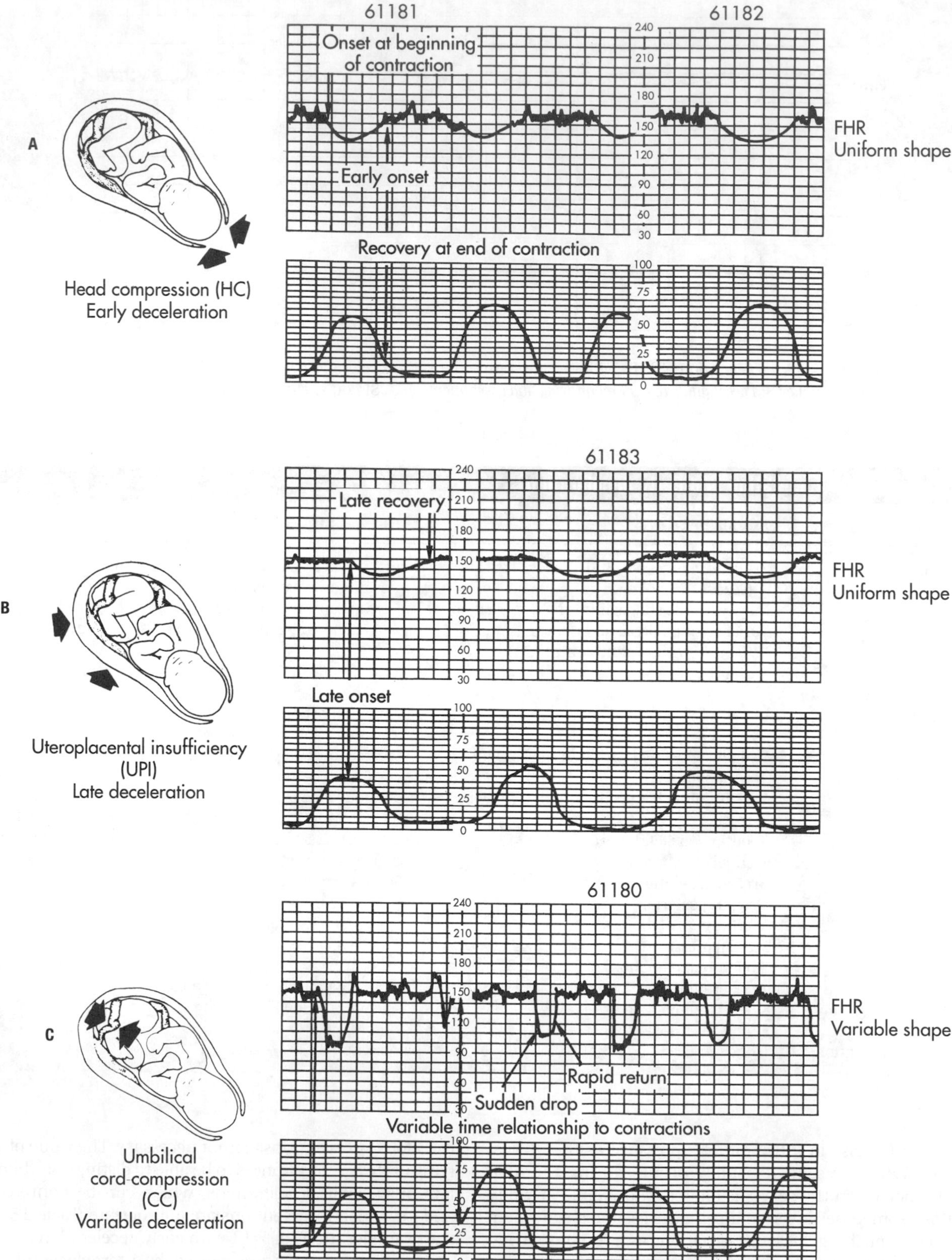

Fig. 15-7 **A,** Early decelerations caused by head compression. **B,** Late deceleration caused by uteroplacental insufficiency. **C,** Variable deceleration caused by cord compression.

begins after the contraction has been established and consistently persists into the interval after the contraction is over (Fig. 15-7, *B*). The term *late* is related to the timing or onset of the deceleration in relation to the uterine contraction. Late deceleration patterns, when persistent or recurrent, usually indicate fetal hypoxemia because of insufficient placental perfusion. Persistent and repetitive late decelerations can be associated with the progression of fetal hypoxemia to hypoxia and acidemia progressing to acidosis. They should be considered an ominous sign when they are uncorrectable, especially if they are associated with decreased variability and tachycardia. Late decelerations caused by maternal supine hypotensive syndrome are usually correctable when the woman turns to her side to displace the weight of the gravid uterus off the vena cava. Lateral positioning allows a better return of maternal blood flow to the heart, which increases cardiac output and blood pressure.

Late decelerations caused by uteroplacental insufficiency can result from uterine hyperstimulation with oxytocin, pregnancy-induced hypertension (PIH), pregnancy lasting past 42 weeks, intraamniotic infection, small-for-gestational-age (SGA) fetus, maternal diabetes, placenta previa, abruptio placentae, conduction anesthetics (producing maternal hypotension), maternal cardiac disease, and maternal anemia.

Variable decelerations, as their name implies, are variable in shape and onset and are caused by umbilical cord compression. Table 15-5 contrasts late deceleration with variable deceleration. The appearance of variable deceleration patterns is different from the early and late decelerations, which closely approximate the shape of the corresponding uterine contraction. In contrast, variable decelerations often are a U or a V shape characterized by a rapid descent and ascent to and from the nadir (or depth) of the deceleration (Fig. 15-7, *C*). Some variable decelerations are preceded and followed by brief accelerations of the FHR known as "shoulders," which are a normal physiologic response to compression of the umbilical vein and arteries.

Variable decelerations may be related to partial, brief compression of the cord. If encountered in the first stage of labor, they usually can be resolved by changing the mother's position, such as from one side to the other. Some advocate the administration of oxygen by face mask to the mother, which may be of some value for selected patients. However, the cause of variable decelerations is not related to oxygen-deficient blood, but rather to impaired delivery of blood to the fetus and return of blood to the placenta caused by cord compression. Variable decelerations most commonly are encountered during the second stage of labor as a result of umbilical cord compression during fetal descent. If repetitive variable decelerations occur during the second stage, it is important to encourage the woman not to push with every contraction, so the fetus has time to recover. Pushing with alternate contractions can sometimes be difficult if the woman does not have regional analgesia/anesthesia. Variable decelerations are associated with neonatal depression only when cord compression is severe or prolonged (i.e., tight nuchal cord, short cord, knot in cord, prolapsed cord). Neonatal depression should also be anticipated if variable decelerations have occurred with most contractions during the second stage, progressively increasing in duration and depth, with a rising FHR baseline and decreasing variability. Variable decelerations occur in about half of all labors and usually are a temporary and correctable phenomenon with maternal position change.

A nonreassuring sign is severe variable deceleration. In this sign the FHR is below 70 beats/min and lasts longer than 30 to 60 seconds. It is accompanied by any of the following: a rising baseline FHR, decreasing variability, or slow return of FHR to baseline. The return to baseline may occur with an "overshoot"; that is, the FHR goes above the baseline and then subsequently returns to baseline. As with any periodic FHR pattern, evaluation of the overall FHR characteristics, such as baseline and variability, is important in determining whether the variable decelerations are reassuring or nonreassuring.

Some primary health care providers consider treatment with **amnioinfusion** for laboring women who have oligohydramnios (insufficient amniotic fluid). In this procedure, normal saline solution is infused via the intrauterine catheter into the uterine cavity in an attempt to add fluid around the umbilical cord and thus prevent its compression during contractions (Fanaroff and Martin, 1997). The fluid can be at room temperature; however, if more than 500 ml is to be infused, it is preferable to warm the fluid to 37° C.

Controversy exists as to the benefits of prophylactic amnioinfusion for women with oligohydramnios who do not have variable FHR decelerations during labor. Recent data suggest amnioinfusion should be reserved for women who demonstrate variable FHR decelerations, rather than initiated routinely for oligohydramnios; however, more research is needed in this area (Ogundipe, Spong, and Ross, 1994). Potential iatrogenic effects of amnioinfusion include increased intraamniotic pressure, uterine overdistention, fetal hypothermia, and intraamniotic infection.

Prolonged decelerations. Prolonged decelerations are difficult to classify inasmuch as they can occur in many situations.

Generally the benign causes are pelvic examination, application of the spiral electrode, rapid fetal descent, and sustained maternal Valsalva maneuver (pp. 347,388, and 429).

Other prolonged decelerations are caused by progressive severe variable decelerations, sudden umbilical cord prolapse, hypotension produced by spinal or epidural analgesia/anesthesia, paracervical anesthesia, a tetanic contraction, and maternal hypoxia, which may occur during a seizure. When the duration of the deceleration is longer than 2 to 3 minutes, a loss of variability with rebound tachycardia usually occurs. Occasionally a period of late decelerations follows. These responses normally end spontaneously. However, when a prolonged deceleration is seen late in the course of severe variable decelerations or during a prolonged series of late decelerations, the prolonged deceleration may occur just before fetal death.

Pattern recognition. Many factors must be evaluated to determine if an FHR pattern is reassuring or nonreassuring. This includes a systematic assessment and evaluation of baseline rate, variability, accelerations, and decelerations, as well as consideration of the frequency and strength of uterine contractions. These factors must be evaluated on the basis of other obstetric information, including parity, maternal and obstetric complications, progress in labor, and analgesia or anesthesia. The estimated time interval until birth must also

TABLE 15-5 Late deceleration versus variable deceleration

	LATE DECELERATION	VARIABLE DECELERATION
Description	Transitory decrease in FHR below baseline rate in contracting phase (see Fig. 15-7, *B*)	Abrupt transitory decrease in FHR that varies in duration, intensity, and timing related to onset of contractions (Fig. 15-7, *C*)
Shape	Uniform; mirror image of uterine contraction	Variable; characterized by sudden drop in FHR in V or U shape
Onset	Late in contraction phase; after peak of contraction; low point of deceleration occurs well after peak of contraction	Variable times in contracting phase; often preceded by transitory acceleration
Recovery	Well after end of contraction	Return to baseline is rapid, sometimes with transitory acceleration or acceleration immediately preceding and following deceleration (shouldering or "overshoot"); slow return to baseline with severe variable decelerations
Deceleration	Usually proportional to amplitude of contraction; rarely decelerates below 100 beats/min	*Mild:* decelerates to any level, less than 30 sec with abrupt return to baseline *Moderate:* decelerates above 80 beats/min, any duration with abrupt return to baseline *Severe:* decelerates below 70 beats/min for greater than 30 sec, with slow return to baseline
Baseline	Often associated with loss of variability and increasing baseline rate	Mild variables usually associated with average baseline variability; moderate and severe variables often associated with decreasing variability and increasing baseline rate
Occurrence	Occurs with each contraction; proportional to strength and duration of contractions	Variable; commonly observed late in labor with fetal descent and pushing
Cause	Uteroplacental insufficiency caused by the following: Uterine hyperactivity or hypertonicity Maternal supine hypotension Epidural or spinal anesthesia Placenta previa Abruptio placentae Hypertensive disorders Postmaturity Intrauterine growth restriction Diabetes mellitus Intraamniotic infection	Umbilical cord compression caused by the following: Maternal position with cord between fetus and maternal pelvis Cord around fetal neck, arm, leg, or other body part Short cord Knot in cord Prolapsed cord
Clinical significance	Nonreassuring, worrisome pattern associated with fetal hypoxemia, acidemia, and low Apgar scores; considered ominous if persistent and uncorrected, especially when associated with fetal tachycardia and loss of variability	Variable decelerations occur in about 50% of all labors and usually are transient, correctable, and not associated with low Apgar scores; mild variable decelerations are reassuring; decelerations progressing from moderate to severe are associated with fetal acidemia, hypoxemia, and low Apgar scores; severe variable decelerations with average baseline variability just before delivery are usually well tolerated
Nursing intervention	Intrauterine resuscitation Change maternal position Correct maternal hypotension Elevate legs Increase rate of maintenance intravenous (IV) line Discontinue oxytocin if infusing Administer oxygen at 10 to 12 L/min with tight face mask Assist with birth (cesarean or vaginal assisted) if pattern cannot be corrected	Change maternal position; if decelerations do not yet meet criteria for mild variable deceleration, proceed with following measures: Discontinue oxytocin if infusing Administer oxygen at 10 to 12 L/min with tight face mask Assist with vaginal or speculum examination If cord is prolapsed, examiner will elevate fetal presenting part with cord between gloved fingers until cesarean birth is accomplished Assist with amnioinfusion if ordered Assist with birth (vaginal assisted or cesarean)

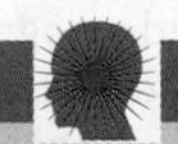

Critical Thinking Exercises

REVIEW OF FETAL MONITOR STRIPS

Review three sample or actual fetal monitor strips.

1. **Determine:**
   a. FHR: baseline, variability
   b. Periodic changes, if any
   c. Contraction interval, duration, intensity, and resting tone
2. **Corroborate your findings in clinical conference**
3. **Describe appropriate nursing actions for each of these periodic changes:**
   a. Accelerations
   b. Early decelerations
   c. Late decelerations
   d. Variable decelerations

be considered. Intervention and interruption of labor are therefore based on clinical judgment of a complex, integrated process.

Experienced perinatal nurses use a mental checklist when evaluating FHR tracings that include the following questions: What is the baseline? Is it within normal limits? Is there evidence of FHR variability? If not, does fetal stimulation elicit an acceleration and return of variability? Are there periodic patterns? If so, what are they and what are the appropriate interventions? What is the relationship between the FHR pattern and uterine activity? Do the interventions resolve the situation? Is the pattern now reassuring or are further actions needed?

The nurse's ability to interpret patterns and a comparison of nurses' and obstetricians' responses has been studied. There is not always agreement between members of the perinatal health care team when interpreting FHR patterns and deciding on a clinical course of action (Chez et al, 1990). It is important for each perinatal unit to have in place a clear procedure for quickly resolving differences between health care providers (such as a chain-of-command policy or algorithm) so maternal-fetal well-being will not be compromised. Ideally any discussion about differences in opinion takes place in private so patients and other health care providers cannot overhear. It is best to remain calm and assume both parties are interested in the same objective: an optimum maternal-fetal outcome. Using phrases such as "I have a different perspective" usually works better than saying "You are wrong" (Simpson and Chez, 1996). The discussion should be limited to the clinical situation at hand. If the situation deteriorates or one party becomes verbally abusive, a third party may be needed to mediate. The most important consideration is maternal-fetal well-being. Documentation, in concise, nonjudgmental language, of notification of each party on the chain of command, including resulting interventions until resolution of the situation, is essential.

Fetal Blood Sampling/Fetal Scalp Stimulation: Acid-Base Monitoring

It is thought that fetal acidosis occurs as a result of hypoxia. Fetal hypoxemia can progress to hypoxia; acidemia can lead to acidosis. As a part of the intrapartum fetal monitoring process, it may be useful to determine the fetal capillary pH, although the exact role of this procedure remains controversial (ACOG, 1995). When first introduced, there were high expectations that fetal scalp blood sampling would allow accurate identification of fetal compromise and reduce the cesarean birth rate for fetal distress. This procedure reached peak popularity in clinical practice in the early 1990s, but because of its invasive nature, failure to have a significant impact on decreasing cesarean birth rates, and the emerging body of knowledge related to fetal acid-base status associated with fetal scalp stimulation, the incidence of fetal blood sampling is on the decline in the United States. Knowledge of fetal acid-base status related to fetal scalp stimulation was acquired by clinical studies involving fetal scalp blood sampling. Some perinatal centers have abandoned the sampling procedure entirely with no evidence of increased cesarean birth rates or adverse perinatal outcomes (Goodwin, Milner-Masterson, and Paul, 1994).

Fetal blood sampling should be reserved for clinical situations in which noninvasive attempts to assess fetal acid-base status have been initiated, such as stimulation of the fetal scalp during a vaginal examination, external fetal stimulation, or vibroacoustic stimulation. If fetal stimulation produces a 15-beat/min acceleration of the FHR for at least 15 seconds, the nurse can be reassured that the fetus is not hypoxemic or acidemic. Because blood gas values can vary so rapidly with transient circulatory changes, the routine use of fetal blood sampling during the intrapartum period is not warranted. Some of the factors causing this variability include maternal acidemia or alkalemia, caput succedaneum, stage of labor, and time relationship of scalp sampling to uterine contraction.

The procedure is performed by a physician or nurse-midwife who obtains the sample from the fetal scalp transcervically after rupture of the membranes. The scalp is swabbed with a disinfecting solution before the puncture is made. The sample is collected and sent to the laboratory for analysis of pH, base excess or base deficit, Po_2, and Pco_2.

Fetal Pulse Oximetry

Continuous monitoring of fetal oxygen saturation by pulse oximetry is a new method of fetal assessment currently in the clinical investigation stage (Luttkus et al, 1995). Fetal pulse oximetry works in a way similar to pulse oximetry used for children and adults. During vaginal examination, in a laboring woman with ruptured membranes, a sensor is inserted next to the fetal presenting part to assess oxygen saturation. Present limitations include the intermittent loss of signal; however, when an adequate signal is obtained, information about fetal oxygen saturation is available over selected periods (Dildy et al, 1994). Previously, data related to fetal oxygenation could only be obtained through the more invasive technique of fetal scalp blood sampling. The fetal pulse oximeter has not yet been approved by the United States Food and Drug Administration (USFDA) for use in clinical practice; however, a multicenter clinical trial in the United States is currently underway. Results from European studies are promising. Improvements in equipment technology and more positive research data could lead to use of fetal pulse oximetry as an adjunct to EFM to assess fetal status in tertiary care centers.

Meconium-stained amniotic fluid. The passage of meconium from the fetal bowel before birth may indicate fetal compromise. Peristalsis of the bowel increases during hypoxia, and the contents are likely to be expelled. Although the presence of **meconium-stained amniotic fluid** is not always an indication of fetal compromise, its presence requires prompt notification of the physician or nurse-midwife. In some cases, amnioinfusion will be performed in an effort to flush out the meconium and thus decrease the risk of infant meconium aspiration syndrome; however, conflicting data continue to emerge related to the benefits of this procedure in improving neonatal outcomes (Usta et al, 1995). The nurse should be prepared at birth to assist with suctioning the newborn to prevent aspiration of meconium into the lungs. This requires gathering the appropriate equipment and notification of qualified providers who will perform tracheal suctioning.

Nursing Care Management

Care of women experiencing a low-risk labor is the same as that of women monitored by EFM or auscultation: assessment of maternal temperature, pulse, respirations, blood pressure and FHR, observation of vaginal discharge, frequent maternal position changes, care of emotional and knowledge needs, and recognition of meconium-stained amniotic fluid. Nursing students, new graduates, and nurses being cross-trained need additional education and clinical experience for the application of internal electrodes and FHR pattern recognition.

BOX 15-1

FHR Assessment Checklist

Patient's name ______________ Date/time______________

____

1. What is the baseline FHR?
   - ____ Beats per minute
   - Check one of the following as observed on the monitor strip:
   - ____ Average baseline FHR (110 to 160 beats/min)
   - ____ Tachycardia (>160 beats/min or >30 beats/min from normal/previous baseline)
   - ____ Bradycardia (<110 beats/min or <30 beats/min from normal/previous baseline)
2. What is the baseline variability?
   - ____ Average short-term variability (6 to 10 beats/min)
   - ____ Average long-term variability (3 to 5 cycles/min)
   - ____ Minimal variability
   - ____ Absence of variability
   - ____ Marked variability
3. Are there any periodic changes in FHR?
   - ____ Accelerations with fetal movement
   - ____ Repetitive accelerations with each contraction
   - ____ Early decelerations (head compression)
   - ____ Late decelerations (uteroplacental insufficiency)
   - ____ Variable decelerations (cord compression)
   - ____ Mild
   - ____ Moderate
   - ____ Severe
4. What does the uterine activity panel show?
   - ____ Frequency (peak to peak)
   - ____ Duration (beginning to end)
   - ____ Intensity (in mm Hg only with intrauterine catheter)
   - ____ Resting time at least 30 seconds
   - ____ Resting tone (<15 mm Hg pressure)

COMMENTS: ________________________________

PANEL NUMBER — WHAT CAN BE OR SHOULD HAVE BEEN DONE

Modified from Tucker S: *Pocket guide to fetal monitoring and assessment*, ed 3, St Louis, 1996, Mosby.

Assessment

Prenatal records and current labor events must be assessed to determine the degree of risk for fetal compromise. Fetal membranes must be ruptured before internal monitoring is possible. Maternal mobility and positioning needs are assessed. The laboring woman's and family's knowledge of FHR monitoring is determined.

The FHR pattern is assessed for baseline values, tachycardia, and bradycardia, variability (increased or decreased); and periodic changes (acceleration or deceleration). Decelerations are described as early, late, or variable. A checklist assists the nurse (Box 15-1). The character of amniotic fluid is assessed for amount, color, odor, and evidence of meconium passage and infection.

Nursing Diagnoses

Assessment findings are reviewed and nursing diagnoses formulated. Several nursing diagnoses are possible, including the following:

- Decreased maternal cardiac output related to
  - Supine hypotension secondary to maternal position
- Ineffective individual coping related to
  - Lack of knowledge of fetal monitoring during labor
  - Restriction of mobility or movement during EFM
- Impaired fetal gas exchange related to
  - Umbilical cord compression
  - Placental insufficiency
  - Nonrecognition of nonreassuring or ominous FHR pattern
  - Missed diagnosis because of poor tracing resulting from malposition of transducers
- Risk for fetal injury related to
  - Unrecognized hypoxemia/hypoxia or anoxia
  - Infection secondary to internal monitoring or blood sampling
- Pain related to
  - Use of belts to position transducers
  - Maternal position
  - Application of internal electrode or obtaining blood sample

Expected Outcomes

Interventions are derived from current knowledge of fetal monitoring during labor and standards for care. The woman's/family's concerns and questions are considered in planning. Expected outcomes are set for the pregnant woman and the fetus and include the following:

1. The fetus will not suffer any hypoxemic, hypoxic, or anoxic episodes.
2. Should fetal compromise occur, it will be identified promptly. Appropriate nursing interventions will be initiated, such as intrauterine resuscitation techniques and notification of the physician or nurse-midwife.

BOX 15-2
Protocol For FHR Monitoring

Patient/family teaching

Explain purpose of monitoring
Explain procedure
Provide rationale for maternal position other than supine

Care

Assist woman to a comfortable position other than supine
Change maternal position at least every 2 hours
Change placement of monitor belts every 2 hours when possible
Provide perineal care as needed when internal monitoring is implemented

Maternal/fetal assessments

Obtain a 20-minute strip by EFM on all patients admitted to labor unit

Low-risk patient:

Auscultate or assess tracing every 30 minutes in active phase of first stage
Auscultate or assess tracing every 15 minutes in second stage

High-risk patient:

Auscultate or assess tracing every 15 minutes in active phase and every 5 minutes in second stage

Auscultation—all patients:

Count baseline FHR between contractions
Assess FHR during the contraction and for at least 30 seconds after the contraction
Note presence or absence of decelerations
Assess FHR before ambulation

EFM—all patients:

Assess and interpret FHR baseline, variability (long-term for external, long-term and short-term for internal), presence or absence of decelerations and accelerations

Assessments for all patients:

Assess uterine activity for frequency, duration, intensity of contractions, and uterine resting tone
Assess FHR immediately after rupture of membranes, vaginal examinations, any invasive procedure

Reportable conditions

Presence of nonreassuring patterns
Worsening of any pattern
Presence of any fetal arrhythmias
Difficulty in obtaining adequate FHR tracing or inadequate audible FHR

Emergency measures

Implement immediately for nonreassuring patterns:

Reposition patient in lateral position to increase uteroplacental perfusion or relieve cord compression
Administer oxygen at 10 to 12 L/min or per hospital protocol via face mask
Discontinue oxytocin if infusing
Correct maternal hypovolemia by increasing IV rate per protocol or as ordered
Assess for bleeding or other cause of pattern change, such as maternal hypotension
Notify physician/certified nurse midwife
Anticipate emergency preparation for surgical intervention if nonreassuring pattern continues despite interventions

Documentation

Patient record—auscultation:

FHR baseline, rate and rhythm, presence of decelerations, and uterine activity data

Patient record—EFM:

Method of monitoring, change in method, and adjustments to equipment
FHR range, variability, presence of decelerations, and presence of accelerations
Uterine activity by palpation, external, and/or internal monitoring
Interpretation of FHR data, nursing interventions, and patient responses
Notification of physician/certified nurse midwife
Patient identification data per hospital procedure

Monitor strip:

Patient identification data
Assessments, procedures, and interventions (medications, etc.)
Notification of physician/certified nurse midwife
Significant occurrences such as sterile vaginal examination, rupture of membranes
Monitor adjustments

3. The mother and family will verbalize understanding of the need for monitoring.
4. The pregnant woman and family will recognize and avoid situations that compromise maternal/fetal circulation.
5. The pregnant woman and family will achieve the type of birth experience that is both physically safe for mother/fetus/neonate and emotionally satisfying.

Plan of Care and Implementation

It is the responsibility of the nurse providing care to women in labor to assess FHR patterns, perform independent nursing interventions, document observations and actions according to the established standard of care, and report nonreassuring patterns to the physician/certified nurse-midwife. See Box 15-2 for a sample protocol for FHR monitoring.

Guidelines and Standards of Nursing Care Related to EFM

AWHONN has established guidelines for didactic content, clinical experiences, and competency validation for FHR monitoring (1993b). The organization periodically issues statements to update practice. ACOG (1995) publishes technical bulletins to review clinical practice issues such as EFM. The Joint Commission on Accreditation of Healthcare Organizations (JCAHO) has also established guidelines for education

Guidelines

COMPETENCY VALIDATION FOR EFM

Perinatal centers with a large volume of births may have a competency validation program that is different from small institutions with nurses who may not have the opportunity to interpret many EFM strips. Experienced perinatal nurses and those new to intrapartum practice have different needs. Paper and pencil tests and skills checklists are some methods to evaluate knowledge and skills. Case study presentations, FHR strip reviews, computer-assisted instructional programs with self-assessments, peer review, medical record audits, and patient feedback are additional methods to validate competencies necessary for intrapartum nursing practice (Afriat et al, 1994).

and competency validation for nurses who work with monitoring equipment (1996). Perinatal nurses are responsible for being familiar with published educational and practice guidelines and for practicing accordingly.

In the past, much attention has been focused on EFM as a separate intrapartum nursing skill. However, knowledge of the physiologic basis of FHR monitoring, ability to interpret EFM data accurately, and initiation of appropriate interventions are integral components of intrapartum practice and should be evaluated as such (Afriat et al, 1994). The latest AWHONN (1993b) guidelines, *Didactic Content and Clinical Skills Verification for Professional Nurse Providers of Basic, High-risk and Critical-care Intrapartum Nursing,* reflect this philosophy. Both skills verification and knowledge base evaluation must be included in any program to validate intrapartum nursing competencies. No one method is superior; rather, individual unit needs and knowledge and skill level of providers should be considered (see the Guidelines box above).

Nursing liability. Nurses who care for women during the labor and birth process may be more likely to be involved in a lawsuit than nurses in less litigious nursing specialties. Prospective risk management includes a thorough related knowledge base; practice consistent with published standards, guidelines, states' nurse practice acts, and institutional protocols; careful documentation; and the establishment of collaborative provider relationships as well as good nurse-patient relationships.

LEGAL TIP

Fetal Monitoring Standards

Nurses who care for women during the childbirth process are legally responsible for correctly interpreting FHR patterns, initiating appropriate nursing interventions based on the pattern seen, and documenting the outcome of those interventions. Perinatal nurses are responsible for timely notification of the physician or nurse-midwife in the case of nonreassuring FHR patterns. Perinatal nurses are also responsible for initiating the institutional chain of command should differences in opinion arise between health care providers related to pattern interpretation and interventions.

Preventive Measures

Discouraging the Valsalva maneuver. The **Valsalva maneuver** is closed-glottis (holding one's breath) pushing. Its use during the pushing process (bearing down) may adversely affect maternal hemodynamics and fetal status (Cruttenden, 1995; Thomson, 1993; Watson, 1994). Prolonged Valsalva pushing (that lasts more than 5 to 6 seconds) can decrease maternal blood pressure and placental blood flow, alter maternal and fetal oxygenation, decrease fetal pH and Po_2, increase fetal Pco_2, increase the incidence of FHR pattern changes, and delay recovery of FHR with fetal hypoxemia (Barnett and Humenick, 1982; Blackburn and Loper, 1992; McKay and Roberts, 1985). Open-glottis (vocalization) pushing is more natural physiologically and not associated with changes in maternal blood pressure or increased fetal pH (Paine and Tinker, 1992; Thomson, 1993). Therefore during the second stage of labor, nurses should encourage the woman to keep her mouth and glottis open and to vocalize (e.g., grunt) while pushing. Nurses should *not* direct the woman to "be quiet, keep your mouth closed, hold your breath, and push."

Maternal position. Maternal hypotension and fetal hypoxemia may develop more rapidly with supine position or epidural analgesia/anesthesia (Blackburn and Loper, 1992; Fanaroff and Martin, 1997).

During the first stage of labor the supine position compromises effective uterine activity, prolongs labor, and increases the use of drugs (e.g., oxytocin) to augment labor (Roberts, 1989). Oxytocin decreases the intervals during which the uterus is relaxed and in which normal intervillous space perfusion occurs. Oxytocin also insidiously increases uterine resting tonus above the normal range of 10 to 15 mm Hg (Fanaroff and Martin, 1997). Therefore nursing care (e.g., maternal position changes) that supports a more efficient, shorter labor should be implemented. During the second stage of labor the laboring woman's involuntary pushing efforts with minimal straining are encouraged. In addition to maintaining maternal and fetal hemodynamics, this pushing pattern is associated with a shorter second stage of labor. A semi-recumbent position and spontaneous short bursts of pushing in response to involuntary bearing-down urges are most conducive to favorable outcomes (Blackburn and Loper, 1992; Cherry and Merkatz, 1991; Watson, 1994).

The nurse must coach the woman to avoid hyperventilatory breathing. Hyperventilation will result in hypoventilation between contractions. The attendant fall in Po_2 could be harmful to the fetus (Fanaroff and Martin, 1997).

Intrauterine Resuscitation

Intrauterine resuscitation refers to those interventions initiated when a nonreassuring FHR pattern is noted and which are directed primarily toward improving uterine and intervillous space blood flow and secondarily toward increasing maternal oxygenation and cardiac output (Fanaroff and Martin, 1997). Preventive interventions have been described: avoiding the supine position and encouraging maternal position changes; encouraging spontaneous short bursts of pushing in response to involuntary bearing-down urges; and open-mouth, open-glottis with vocalizing while pushing. Previously it was thought that the left lateral maternal position preferentially improved maternal cardiac output and thus enhanced blood flow to the fetus. It is now known that either right or left lateral maternal positioning works well to enhance uteroplacental blood flow (Clark et al, 1991). The key issue is to avoid positioning the laboring woman on her back to decrease risk of supine hypotension leading to decreased fetal perfusion.

Compression of the umbilical cord vessels results in variable decelerations. Amnioinfusion helps relieve pressure on the (nonprolapsed) umbilical cord. If maternal hypotension is caused by acute hemorrhage (hypovolemia), rapid infusion of blood volume expanders may be ordered. Until the infusion is established, the nurse can elevate the woman's legs. Blood pooled in the legs, especially with sympathetic blockade (e.g., epidural anesthesia), will then drain quickly into the central venous circulation and augment the effective intravascular volume (Fanaroff and Martin, 1992).

Oxytocin should always be infused as a "piggyback" connection near the indwelling needle (ACOG, 1995; AWHONN, 1993a). If FHR patterns change for any reason, oxytocin stimulation of uterine muscle activity must be discontinued. The IV line from the piggyback (containing oxytocin) is turned off, and the primary infusion line is opened.

Nurses need to prioritize interventions to maximize intrauterine resuscitation. The first priority is to open the maternal/fetal vascular systems; the second priority, to increase blood volume; and the third priority, to optimize oxygenation of the circulating blood volume. For example, to relieve acute FHR deceleration, the nurse can do the following:

- Turn woman to side-lying position
- Increase maternal blood volume by increasing the rate of the primary IV infusion or by raising the woman's legs
- Provide oxygen by face mask

Some interventions are specific to the FHR pattern seen. Nursing interventions for tachycardia and bradycardia are given in Table 15-2, and those for increased or decreased variability are shown in Table 15-3. Nursing interventions specific for FHR acceleration or early deceleration are not required (Table 15-4). Late and some types of variable FHR decelerations require aggressive intervention (Table 15-5). The decision for medical intervention or immediate vaginal or cesarean birth is made by the physician/CNM.

Working with the Monitor

Application of external EFM. The equipment is easily applied by the nurse but may need to be repositioned as the mother or fetus changes position. The woman is asked to assume a semi-sitting or lateral position. It is important that the nurse thoroughly explains to the woman and her labor support person(s) how the monitor works to assess the FHR and detect uterine activity. The importance of the nurse's role in this education has been studied. Women who felt the nurse thoroughly explained EFM before and during application of the monitor had more positive attitudes about their childbirth experience than did women who did not feel EFM was explained to them and their support persons. Women who were unsure how the monitor worked were frustrated when they had painful contractions that were not detected by the monitor. They felt they were not getting "credit" for the intensity of the contractions. Other women were worried when the EFM temporarily lost the FHR signal, causing them to think something must be wrong with their baby. The quality of the explanation of the EFM to the woman and her support person can have a significant effect on the woman's perception of the childbirth experience (Simpson, 1991). The nurse explains the procedure to the woman and labor support person(s) and performs the following steps:

- Turns on monitor; taps transducer before use to ensure sound transmission
- Places both belts under the woman's back at about waist level
- Applies a thin coat of transmission gel to the face of the diaphragm of the transducer
- Performs the first and second Leopold maneuvers to locate the fetal back (for further discussion of Leopold maneuvers, see Chapter 16 and Fig. 16-4).
- Positions the ultrasound transducer in place over the fetal heart and secures the belt
- Obtains a tracing to ensure that the transducer is picking up the FHR
- Positions the tocotransducer over the uterine fundus where it contracts; it can be in the midline or slightly to one side

BOX 15-3

Checklist for Fetal Monitoring Equipment

Preparation of monitor

1. Is the paper inserted correctly?
2. Are transducer cables plugged into the appropriate outlet of the monitor?

Ultrasound transducer

1. Has ultrasound transmission gel been applied to the transducer?
2. Was the FHR tested and noted on the monitor paper?
3. Does a signal light flash with each heartbeat?
4. Is the belt secure and snug but comfortable for the laboring woman?

Tocotransducer

1. Is the tocotransducer firmly positioned at the site of the least maternal tissue?
2. Has it been applied without gel or paste?
3. Was the pen-set knob adjusted between the 10- and 15-mm Hg marks and noted on the monitor paper?
4. Was this setting done between contractions?
5. Is the belt secure and snug but comfortable for the laboring woman?

Spiral electrode

1. Are the wires attached firmly to the posts on the leg plate?
2. Is the spiral electrode attached to the presenting part of the fetus?
3. Is the inner surface of the leg plate covered with electrode gel, if necessary?
4. Is the leg plate properly secured to the woman's thigh?

Internal catheter/strain gauge*

1. Is the length line on the catheter visible at the introitus?
2. Is it noted on the monitor paper that a calibration was done?
3. Was the uterine activity tested?

Modified from Tucker S: *Pocket guide to fetal monitoring and assessment*, ed 3, St Louis, 1996, Mosby.

*Some internal catheters are solid and do not have syringes or stopcocks.

- Tightens the belt so it is snug but not uncomfortable for the laboring woman
- Checks placement by putting one hand on the fundus and palpating for a contraction
- Adjusts the pen-set knob so that the baseline reads between 5 and 15 mm Hg on the monitor strip

In addition to knowing how to apply the monitor and interpret tracings, the nurse functions as a troubleshooter. A checklist for fetal monitoring equipment is presented in Box 15-3.

Care of mother using EFM. For quick reference, summary guidelines for the care of the woman using electronic monitoring during labor are listed in Box 15-4. It is important to remember that although the use of fetal monitoring can be reassuring to many parents, to some it can be a source of anxiety. Therefore the nurse must be particularly sensitive to and respond appropriately to the emotional, knowledge, and comfort needs of the woman as well as her family during labor.

Documentation. Clear and complete documentation is provided on the woman's monitoring strip before the initiation of

BOX 15-4

Care of Woman Using EFM

The following guidelines relate to client teaching and the functioning of the monitor:

Explain that fetal status can be continuously assessed by FHR, even during contractions.

Explain that the lower tracing on the monitor strip paper shows uterine activity; the upper tracing shows the FHR.

Reassure woman and partner that prepared childbirth techniques can be implemented without difficulty.

Explain that, during external monitoring, effleurage can be performed on sides of abdomen or upper portion of thighs.

Explain that breathing patterns based on the timing and intensity of contractions can be enhanced by the observation of uterine activity on the monitor strip paper, which shows the onset of contractions.

Note peak of contraction; knowing that contraction will not get stronger and is half over usually is helpful.

Note diminishing intensity.

Coordinate with appropriate breathing and relaxation techniques.

Reassure woman and partner that the use of internal monitoring does not restrict her movement, although she is confined to bed.*

Explain that use of external monitoring usually requires the woman's cooperation during positioning and movement.

Reassure woman and partner that use of monitoring does not imply fetal jeopardy.

Reassure her that the equipment is removed periodically to permit the applicator sites to be washed and back rubs to be given.

External monitoring (Fig 15-2)

Ultrasound transducer

Monitors FHR with high-frequency sound waves.

Tap transducer before use to ensure sound transmission.

Apply ultrasound transmission gel to maternal abdomen; clean abdomen and transducer and reapply gel q 2 hrs and prn.

Massage reddened skin areas gently and reposition belt or adhesive device q 2 hrs and prn.

Auscultate FHR with stethoscope or fetoscope if in doubt as to validity of tracing.

Position and reposition transducer prn to ensure receipt of clear, interpretable FHR data.

Tocotransducer

Monitors uterine activity via a pressure-sensing device placed on the maternal abdomen

Position and reposition qh and prn on the fundus where there is the least maternal tissue.

Keep abdominal strap snug but comfortable for the laboring woman.

Adjust pen-set between contractions to print between 10 and 15 mm Hg on monitor strip paper.

Palpate fundus every 30 to 60 minutes to assess strength of contraction; only frequency and duration of contractions can be assessed with tocotransducer.

Do not determine woman's need for analgesic based on uterine activity displayed on monitor strip.

Gently massage reddened areas under transducer and belt qh and prn.

Internal monitoring (Fig. 15-3)

Spiral electrode

Obtains fetal ECG from presenting part and converts it into FHR

Ensure that color-coded wires are appropriately attached to push post on leg plate.

Apply electrode paste to leg plate q 2 hrs and prn.

Observe FHR tracing on monitor strip for long-term and short-term variability.

Turn electrode counterclockwise to remove; never pull straight out from presenting part.

Administer perineal care after the woman voids during labor.

Intrauterine catheter

Catheter (may be fluid-filled or solid) that monitors intraamniotic pressure internally.

Flush open system catheter with sterile water before insertion and prn.

Ensure that the length line on catheter is visible at introitus.

For open system catheters, turn stopcock off to woman, then with pressure valve of strain gauge released, flush strain gauge, remove syringe, and set stylus to 0 line of chart paper; test further according to manufacturer's instructions q 3-4 hrs and prn.

For closed system catheters, set baseline rate between uterine contractions when uterus is relaxed.

Check proper functioning by tapping catheter, asking woman to cough, or applying fundal pressure; observe appropriate inflection on strip chart.

Keep catheter taped to woman's leg to prevent dislodgement.

Modified from Tucker S et al: *Patient care standards: collaborative practice planning guides*, ed 5, St Louis, 1992, Mosby.

*Portable telemetry monitors allow the FHR and uterine contraction patterns to be observed on centrally located electronic display stations. These portable units permit ambulation during electronic monitoring.

monitoring to ensure identification. This documentation is continued and updated according to institutional protocol as monitoring progresses. In some institutions, observations and interventions are noted on the monitor strip to provide a comprehensive document that depicts the course of labor and the woman's care. In other institutions, this documentation is confined to the labor flow record. Advocates of documenting on both the medical record and the EFM strip cite ease of notation directly on the strip while at the bedside and improved accuracy in documentation of critical events and interventions. Others believe charting on the EFM strip is duplicate documentation of the same information noted in the medical record and thus unnecessary additional nursing paperwork. One way to document that frequent maternal-fetal assessments at the bedside have occurred is to initial the EFM strip or depress the "mark" button during these assessments. A disadvantage of documenting on both the EFM strip and the medical record is that often the times noted for events and interventions on the EFM strip do not match what is later documented in the medical record. These discrepancies can lead to the appearance of errors. Therefore if institutional policy mandates documentation on both the monitor strip and the medical record, it is critical to make sure the times and notations of events and interventions match. No one method of documentation is right; rather, the nurse must be aware of and follow individual institutional policies and participate in changing policies as needed. Many of the aspects of care and events that can be documented on the monitor strip are listed in Box 15-5.

BOX 15-5
Documentation: Monitor Strip

Observations

Maternal vital signs
Maternal position/repositioning
Vaginal examinations and findings
Medications; anesthesia/analgesia
Voidings; emesis
Pushing/bearing down
Fetal movement
Baseline FHR, periodic changes

Adjustments

Relocation of transducers
Flushing or adjustment of catheter
Replacement of electrode
Replacement of catheter
Time lapsed while changing monitor strip paper

Interventions

Position change
Parenteral fluids
Discontinuance of oxytocin
Oxygen administration
Physician/CNM notification and response

Nursing Care Plan

EFM DURING LABOR

Nursing Diagnosis: Maternal anxiety related to lack of knowledge about use of electronic monitor

Expected outcomes: The patient will exhibit increased understanding about fetal monitoring and signs of reduced anxiety (i.e., absence of physical indicators, absence of perceived threat, and absence of feelings of dread).

• NURSING INTERVENTIONS/*RATIONALES*

Explain and demonstrate to woman and labor support partner how the electronic monitor (internal or external) works in assessing FHR and in detecting and assessing quality of uterine contractions *to remove fear of unknown and ensure that woman can work with the monitor.*

When making adjustments to the monitor, explain to the couple what is being done and why *because information increases understanding and allays anxiety.*

Explain that while a side-lying position or Fowler's position provides for optimum monitoring, position changes decrease discomfort; therefore encourage frequent changes in position (other than supine) and explain any monitoring adjustments that are being made as a result *to reduce discomfort and allay anxiety.*

Nursing Diagnosis: Risk for fetal injury related to inaccurate placement of transducers/electrodes, misinterpretation of results or failure to use other assessment techniques to monitor fetal well-being

Expected outcomes: Fetal well-being is adequately assessed, and any fetal compromise is identified immediately.

• NURSING INTERVENTIONS/RATIONALES

Carefully follow guidelines and checklist for application and initiation of monitoring *to ensure proper placement of monitoring devices and production of accurate output from monitoring device.*

Check placement throughout monitoring process *to ensure that devices remain correctly placed.*

Regularly assess and record results of EFM (FHR and variability, decelerations, accelerations, uterine activity, contractions, uterine resting tone) *to provide consistent and timely evaluation of fetal well-being and progress of labor.*

Auscultate FHR and palpate contractions on a regular basis *to provide a cross-check on the EFM output and ensure fetal well-being.*

The medical record is labeled with the following information: woman's name, identification number, date, expected date of birth (EDB); high-risk conditions such as preeclampsia or diabetes; membranes intact or ruptured; cervical dilation and station of presenting part; and the time monitor was attached and the mode used, as well as a notation that the FHR has been reviewed and evaluated on a periodic basis.

Evaluation

Evaluation is a continuous process. The nurse can assume that care was effective when the goals for care have been met. That is, the fetus does not suffer any hypoxemic or anoxemic episode, and should fetal compromise occur, it is identified promptly and appropriate interventions initiated. In addition, the mother and family understand the need for monitoring, the mother avoids situations that compromise maternal/fetal circulation, and the mother/couple achieves the type of birth experience that is both physically safe for mother/fetus/newborn and emotionally satisfying (see the Nursing Care Plan on p. 391 for the woman who is being monitored during labor).

Key Points

- Fetal well-being during labor is measured by the response of the FHR to uterine contractions.
- FHR characteristics include the baseline FHR and periodic changes in FHR.
- It is the responsibility of the nurse to assess FHR patterns, perform independent nursing interventions, and report nonreassuring patterns to the physician or nurse-midwife.
- Monitoring techniques of fetal well-being include FHR assessment and noting presence of meconium-stained fluid.
- AWHONN and ACOG have established and published standards for EFM.
- The emotional, informational, and comfort needs of the woman and her family must be addressed when the mother and her fetus are being monitored.

References

Afriat C: *Intrapartum fetal monitoring.* In Simpson K, Creehan P, editors: *AWHONN's perinatal nursing,* Philadelphia, 1996, JB Lippincott.

Afriat C et al: Electronic fetal monitoring competency—to validate or not to validate: the opinions of experts, *J Perinat Neonatal Nurs* 8(3):1, 1994.

American Academy of Pediatrics/American College of Obstetricians and Gynecologists: *Guidelines for perinatal care,* Elk Grove Village, Ill, 1992, AAP/ACOG.

American College of Obstetricians and Gynecologists: *Induction of labor,* (ACOG Technical Bull No. 217), Washington, DC, 1995, ACOG.

American College of Obstetricians and Gynecologists: *Antepartum fetal surveillance,* (ACOG Technical Bull No. 188), Washington, DC, 1994, ACOG.

American College of Obstetricians and Gynecologists: *Fetal heart rate patterns: monitoring, interpretation, and management* (ACOG Technical Bull No. 207), Washington, DC, 1995, ACOG.

Association of Women's Health, Obstetric, and Neonatal Nurses: *Cervical ripening and induction and augmentation of labor (Practice Resource),* Washington, DC, 1993a, AWHONN.

Association of Women's Health, Obstetric, and Neonatal Nurses: *Didactic content and clinical skills verification for professional nurse providers of basic, high-risk, and critical-care intrapartum nursing,* Washington, DC, 1993b, AWHONN.

Barnett M, Humenick S: Infant outcomes in relation to second stage labor pushing, *Birth* 9:221, 1982.

Blackburn S, Loper D: *Maternal, fetal and neonatal physiology: a clinical perspective,* Philadelphia, 1992, WB Saunders.

Centers for Disease Control and Prevention: Differences in maternal mortality among Black and White women—United States, 1990, *MMWR* 44(1):6, 1995.

Cherry S, Merkatz I: *Complications of pregnancy: medical, surgical, gynecologic, psychosocial, and perinatal,* Baltimore, 1991, Williams & Wilkins.

Chez B et al: Interpretations of nonstress tests by obstetric nurses, *J Obstet Gynecol Neonatal Nurs* 19:227, 1990.

Clark S et al: Position change and central hemodynamic profile during normal third trimester pregnancy and postpartum, *Am J Obstet Gynecol* 164(3):883, 1991.

Cruttenden J: To push or not to push? *Mod Midwife* 5(12):31, 1995.

Dildy G et al: Intrapartum fetal pulse oximetry: fetal oxygen saturation trends during labor and relation to delivery outcome, *Am J Obstet Gynecol* 171:679, 1994.

Eganhouse D: Nursing assessment and responsibilities in monitoring the preterm pregnancy, *J Obstet Gynecol Neonatal Nurs* 21:355, 1992.

Fanaroff A, Martin R: *Neonatal-perinatal medicine: diseases of the fetus and infant,* ed 6, St Louis, 1997, Mosby.

Freeman R, Garite T, Nageotte M: *Fetal heart rate monitoring,* Baltimore, 1991, Williams & Wilkins.

Goodwin T, Milner-Masterson L, Paul R: Elimination of fetal scalp blood sampling on a large clinical service, *Obstet Gynecol* 83:971, 1994.

Guyer B et al: Annual summary of vital statistics—1995, *Pediatrics* 98:1007, 1996.

Joint Commission on Accreditation of Healthcare Organizations: *Accreditation manual, volume I, standards,* Oakbrook Terrace, Ill, 1996, JCAHO.

Luttkus A et al: Continuous monitoring of fetal oxygen saturation by pulse oximetry, *Obstet Gynecol* 85:183, 1995.

McKay S, Roberts J: Second stage labor: what is normal? *J Obstet Gynecol Neonatal Nurs* 14:101, 1985.

NAACOG: *Fetal heart rate auscultation (OGN nursing practice resource),* Washington, DC, 1990, NAACOG.

Ogundipe O, Spong C, Ross M: Prophylactic amnioinfusion for oligohydramnios: a reevaluation, *Obstet Gynecol* 84:544, 1994.

Paine L, Tinker D: The effect of maternal bearing-down efforts on arterial umbilical cord pH and length of the second stage of labor, *J Nurse Midwife* 37(1):61, 1992.

Parer J: *Fetal heart rate.* In Creasy R, Resnik R, editors: *Maternal/fetal medicine: principles and practice,* ed 3, Philadelphia, 1994, WB Saunders.

Roberts J: *Maternal positioning during the first stage of labour.* In Chalmers I, Enkin M, Keirse M, editors: *Effective care in pregnancy and childbirth,* Oxford, 1989, Oxford University Press.

Simpson K: *Attitudes of laboring women towards continuous electronic fetal monitoring,* unpublished Master's Thesis, 1991, University of Missouri-St. Louis.

Simpson K, Chez B: *Professional and legal issues.* In Simpson K, Creehan P, editors: *AWHONN's perinatal nursing,* Philadelphia, 1996, JB Lippincott.

Thomson A: Pushing techniques in the second stage of labour, *J Adv Nurs* 18(2):171, 1993.

Tucker S: *Pocket guide to fetal monitoring and assessment,* ed 3, St Louis, 1996, Mosby.

Tucker S et al: *Patient care standards: collaborative practice planning guides,* ed 6, St Louis, 1996, Mosby.

Usta I et al: The impact of a policy of amnioinfusion for meconium-stained amniotic fluid, *Obstet Gynecol* 85(2):237, 1995.

Watson V: Maternal position in the second stage of labour, *Mod Midwife* 4(7):21, 1994.

Bibliography

Gilbert E, Harmon J: *Manual of high-risk pregnancy and delivery: nursing perspectives,* ed 3, St Louis, 1996, Mosby.

Parer J: Fetal cerebral metabolism: the influence of asphyxia and other factors, *J Perinatol* 14:376, 1994.

Paul R: Electronic fetal monitoring and later outcome: a thirty-year overview, *J Perinatol* 14:393, 1994.

Raines D: Fetal surveillance: issues and implications, *J Obstet Gynecol Neonatal Nurs* 25(7):559, 1996.

Schifrin B: Fetal heart rate patterns and the timing of fetal injury, *J Perinatol* 14:174, 1994.

Schifrin B: The ABCs of electronic fetal monitoring, *J Perinatol* 14:396, 1994.

Vintzileos A et al: Intrapartum electronic fetal heart rate monitoring versus intermittent auscultation: a meta-analysis, *Obstet Gynecol* 85, 149, 1995.

Wallerstedt C et al: Amnioinfusion: an update, *J Obstet Gynecol Neonatal Nurs* 23(7):573, 1994.

CHAPTER 16

Nursing Care During Labor and Birth

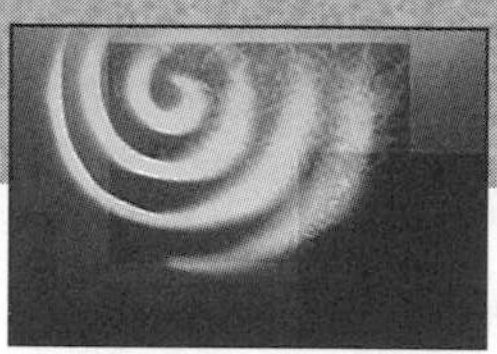

FIRST STAGE OF LABOR, P. 394
Nursing care management, p. 394

SECOND STAGE OF LABOR, P. 424
Nursing care management, p. 425

THIRD STAGE OF LABOR, P. 436
Nursing care management, p. 436
Interruption in skin integrity related to childbirth, p. 439

The labor process is an exciting and anxious time for the woman and her family. For most women, labor begins with the first uterine contraction, continues with hours of hard work during dilation and birth, and ends as the woman and her family begin the attachment process with the infant. Nursing care focuses on supporting the woman and her family throughout the labor process with the goal of ensuring the best possible outcome for all involved.

FIRST STAGE OF LABOR

The **first stage of labor** begins with the onset of regular uterine contractions and ends with complete effacement and full cervical dilation. Care begins when the woman reports one or more of the following:

- Onset of progressive, regular uterine contractions that increase in frequency, strength, and duration
- Blood-tinged vaginal discharge (bloody show)
- Fluid discharge from the vagina (spontaneous rupture of membranes)

The first stage of labor consists of three phases: the **latent phase** (up to 3 cm of dilation), the **active phase** (4 to 7 cm), and the **transition phase** (8 to 10 cm). Most nulliparous women seek entry to the hospital in the latent phase because they have not experienced labor before and are unsure of the "right" time to come in (Bonovich, 1990). Multiparous women usually do not come to the hospital until they are in the active phase. Even though no two labors are identical, women who have given birth before appear less anxious about the process unless they have had a previous negative experience.

Nursing Care Management

Assessment

Assessment begins at the first contact with the woman, whether by telephone or in person. Many women call the hospital or birthing center to receive validation that it is all right for them to come in. The manner in which the nurse communicates with the woman during this initial contact can set the tone for a positive birth experience. A caring attitude encourages the client to verbalize her questions and concerns. If possible, the nurse should have the woman's prenatal record in hand when speaking to her or admitting her for evaluation of labor. Copies of records are usually filed on the perinatal unit sometime during the third trimester.

Certain factors are assessed initially to determine if the woman is in **true labor** and should come to the hospital or be admitted (Cunningham et al, 1993) (see the Guidelines box on p. 395).

When a woman calls and there is a question about whether she is in labor (or in labor advanced enough to be admitted), the nurse should suggest that she either call her physician/certified nurse-midwife (CNM) or come to the hospital (Box 16-1, p. 398). Before the first meeting with the woman in labor, the nurse reviews the prenatal record.

When the woman arrives at the perinatal unit, assessment is the top priority (Fig. 16-1). The nurse first performs a screening assessment, using the techniques of interview and physical assessment, and obtains laboratory findings to determine the status of the woman and her fetus as well as the progress of her labor. The physician/CNM is notified, and if the woman is admitted, a detailed systems assessment is done.

Guidelines

HOW TO DISTINGUISH TRUE LABOR FROM FALSE LABOR

True labor

Contractions

- Occur regularly, becoming stronger, lasting longer, occurring closer together
- Increase in intensity with walking
- Are felt in lower back, radiating to lower portion of abdomen
- Continue despite use of comfort measures

Cervix

- Shows progressive change (softening, effacement, and dilation signaled by the appearance of bloody show)
- Moves to an increasingly anterior position
- Requires vaginal examination to detect changes

Fetus

- Presenting part usually becomes engaged in the pelvis, often referred to as the fetus "dropping" (lightening). This results in increased ease of breathing; at the same time the bladder is compressed from the downward pressure exerted by the presenting part, resulting in urinary frequency.

False labor

Contractions

- Occur irregularly or become regular only temporarily
- Often stop with walking or position change
- Are felt in the back or abdomen above the navel
- Often can be stopped with use of comfort measures

Cervix

- May be soft but there is no significant change in effacement or dilation or evidence of bloody show
- Is often in a posterior position
- Requires a vaginal examination to determine characteristics

Fetus

- Presenting part is usually not engaged in the pelvis

Admission data. Admission forms can provide guidelines for important assessment information when a woman in labor is being evaluated or admitted. Additional sources of data include the (1) prenatal record, (2) initial interview, (3) physical examination to determine baseline physiologic parameters, (4) laboratory results, (5) expressed psychosocial and cultural factors, and (6) clinical evaluation of labor status. Forms that integrate admission and labor data, as shown in Fig. 16-2, permit a more complete assessment.

Prenatal data. The admitting nurse reviews the prenatal record to identify the woman's individual needs and risks. If the woman has not had any prenatal care, certain baseline information must be obtained. If the woman experiences discomfort, the nurse asks questions between contractions when the woman can concentrate better.

It is important to know the woman's *age* so that the plan of care can be tailored to her age group. For example, a 14-year-old and a 40-year-old have different but specific needs, and their ages place them at risk for different problems. *Height and weight* relationships are important to identify the potential risk for cephalopelvic disproportion. Other factors to consider are *general health*, any current *medical conditions or allergies*, *respiratory status*, the type and time of the *last solid food* eaten, and previous *surgeries*.

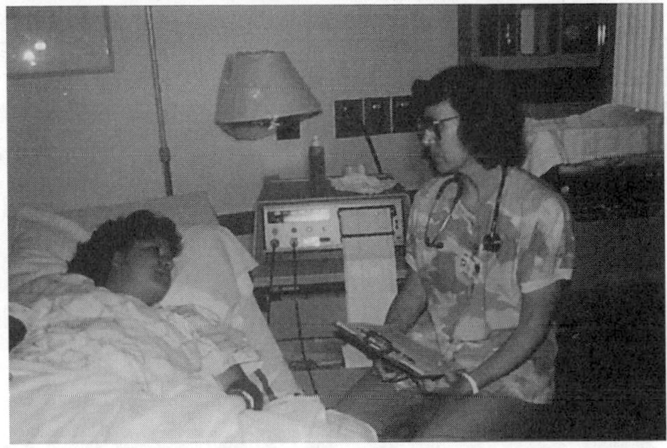

Fig. 16-1 Woman being admitted. (Courtesy Marjorie Pyle, RNC, Lifecircle, Costa Mesa, Calif.)

Past and present *obstetric and pregnancy history* is carefully assessed. The *obstetric history* includes gravidity (number of pregnancies) and parity (pregnancy outcome: term and preterm births, spontaneous and elective abortions, and number of living children). Other *obstetric problems* to consider include history of the following: vaginal bleeding, pregnancy-induced hypertension (PIH), anemia, gestational diabetes, infections (bacterial or sexually transmitted), and immunodeficiencies.

If this is not the woman's first labor and birth experience, it is important to note the characteristics of her previous experiences. This information includes the duration of previous labors, the type of anesthesia used, and the kind of birth (spontaneous vaginal or forceps-, vacuum-, or cesarean-assisted). The woman's perception of her previous labor and birth experiences should be explored, since it may influence the manner in which she approaches her current experience. Women can retain long-term memories of their childbirth experiences. Recall of labor and birth events can affect a woman's postpartum emotional adjustment, self-esteem, and ability to parent effectively (DiMatteo, 1993; Simkin, 1991).

While reviewing past births, the nurse collects data related to the condition of the babies (their weight, Apgar scores, and general health at and following birth).

It is important to confirm that the expected date of birth (EDB) is as accurate as possible. Other data in the prenatal record include patterns of maternal weight gain; physiologic measurements such as maternal vital signs (blood pressure, temperature, pulse, respiration), fundal height, baseline fetal heart rate (FHR); and laboratory test results. These tests include blood type and Rh factor, complete or partial blood count (CBC or hemoglobin and hematocrit), 50-g blood glucose test, rubella titer, serologic findings (Venereal Disease Research Laboratories [VDRL] or rapid plasma reagin [RPR]), hepatitis B surface antigen (HBsAG), group B streptococcus status, and urinalysis. Additional tests may include tuberculosis screen with purified protein derivative (PPD), human

Obstetric Admitting Record Page 1 of 2

Basic Admission Data Date ___ / ___ / ___ Time ________
□ Ambulatory □ Direct admit □ Stretcher
□ Wheelchair □ Transfer from ________

G	T	Pt	A	L	LMP / /	EDD / /	Age
						EDD By fetal assessment / /	

Race/Ethnicity ________
Occupation ________ Education ________
Marital status S M Sep D W Religion ________

MD/CNM	Tel no	Support person/Relationship	Tel no

Reasons for Admission
□ **Onset of labor**
□ Induction of labor
□ Spontaneous abortion
□ Cesarean section
□ Primary □ Repeat
(reason for primary ________)
□ VBAC
□ Tubal ligation
□ Vaginal bleeding
□ PROM
□ Preterm labor
Detail reasons for admission ________

Observation evaluation
□ Fetal status
□ Ultrasound
□ Amniocentesis
□ NST
□ CST
□ Medical complications ________
□ Obstetric complications ________

Patient Triage Data
Contractions □ **None** □ Palpation □ Tocotransducer
Frequency ________ Duration ________ Intensity ________
Began on ___ / ___ / ___ Time ________
Membranes □ **Intact** □ Bulging
□ Ruptured (Date ___ / ___ / ___ Time ________)
Fluid □ Clear □ Bloody □ Foul smelling
□ Meconium stained □ No foul odor
Vaginal bleeding □ **None** □ Normal show
□ Bleeding (describe ________)

Cervical Exam
Station ________ Effacement ________ Dilation ________ cms
Presentation
□ Vertex □ Transverse lie
□ Face/Brow □ Compound
□ Breech (type ________) □ Unknown
Medication allergy/Sensitivity □ **None**
□ Identify ________
Other allergy/Sensitivity □ **None**
□ Identify ________

Patient Care Data

Personal Effects	Disposition		
Item	With patient	With support person	Other (describe)

Illness (≤ 14 days prior to admission) □ **None**
□ Type/Treatment ________
Recent Exposure to Communicable Disease □ **None**
□ Type/Date ________ ___ / ___ / ___
Last Oral Intake
Fluids ___ / ___ / ___ Time ________
Solids ___ / ___ / ___ Time ________
Medications □ **None**

Type/Dose	Last taken	With patient No	With patient Yes	Disposition
________	________	□	□	________
________	________	□	□	________

Smoker □ No □ Yes (________ amt/day)

Alcohol/Drug use □ No □ Yes

Substances	Amt/Day	Last used
________	________	___ / ___ / ___ Time ________
________	________	___ / ___ / ___ Time ________

Plans for Birth and Hospital Stay
Support person present in L&D □ No □ Yes ________
Other family members in L&D □ No □ Yes ________
Anesthesia □ **None**
□ Local □ Epidural □ Spinal □ General
Delivery site
□ DR □ Birthing room □ LDR □ LDRP □ OR
Personal requests ________
Adoption □ No
□ Yes Contact with infant □ No □ Yes
Adoption contact ________
Feeding preference □ Breast □ Bottle
Room preference □ Private □ Semi-Private
□ Rooming-In
□ Tubal ligation Authorization signed □ Yes □ No
□ Circumcision Authorization signed □ Yes □ No

Psychosocial Data
Communication Deficit □ **None**
□ Identify ________
Other children □ No □ Yes Age/Sex ________
________, ________, ________, ________

Partner involved □ Yes □ No
Others involved □ No □ Identify ________

Admitting signature ________ Time ________

Fig. 16-2 Obstetric admitting record. (From Hollister Incorporated.)

Obstetric Admitting Record **Page 2 of 2**

Psychosocial Data (Cont'd.)

Basic needs met	Yes	No	If no, explain
Housing	□	□	
Clothing	□	□	
Food	□	□	
Transportation	□	□	

Free from apparent physical/emotional abuse □ Yes □ No

If no, explain___

Life Stress	No	Yes	If yes, explain
Living	□	□	
Working	□	□	
Serious illness	□	□	

Self-care Needs □ None □ Needs help with___

Emotional status □ Happy □ Ambivalent □ Anxious □ Depressed □ Angry

Discharge Planning Data

Discharge planning initiated □ **Yes** □ No

Discharge needs identified___

Social service referral □ No □ Yes __/__/__

Planned length of stay___days

Needs follow-up visit by RN □ No □ Yes __/__/__

Significant Prenatal Data

Prenatal Records Available on Admission

□ **Yes** □ No

Source of prenatal data___

First prenatal visit__/__/__

Attended prenatal classes □ **Yes** □ No

Infant care provider:

Lab Findings □ **None**

Blood type & Rh___

Rubella titer___

Serology___

HbSAg___

Fetal Assessment Tests □ **None**

Date	Test	Result
/		
/		
/		
/		

Maternal Problems Identified □ **None**

	Active	Resolved
1.	□	□
2.	□	□
3.	□	□

Fetal Problems Identified □ **None**

	Active	Resolved
1.	□	□
2.	□	□
3.	□	□

Physical Assessment

Detail all abnormal findings

Height		Wt pregrav/grav	
Temp	Pulse	Resp	BP

System	Normal	Abnormal
HEENT	□	□
Neurologic	□	□
Skin	□	□
Breasts	□	□
Extremities	□	□
Cardiovascular	□	□
Respiratory	□	□
Abdomen	□	□
Gastrointestinal	□	□
Urinary	□	□
Genitalia	□	□

Fetal Evaluation Data

Fundal height___cms FHR___

Estimated fetal weight___

□ Fetoscope □ Doppler □ Fetal monitor □ Other

Weeks gestation (est)

By dates___wks

By ultrasound___wks

Date__/__/__

Multiple gestation □ **No** □ Yes

Infant	Presentation	Position
1.		
2.		
3.		

Initial Problems Identified □ **None**

1.___

2.___

3.___

Specimens obtained (check all that apply)

Urine test	Time	Results	Blood test	Time	Results
□ Urinalysis			□ Hgb		
□ C + S			□ Hct		
□ Glucose			□ VDRL/RPR		
□ Albumin			□ Type/Screen		
□ Ketones			□		
□ pH			□		
□ Blood			□		

Physician/CNM___

Notified by___

Date__/__/__Time___

Admitting signature

Examiner signature

Date__/__/__Time___

Fig. 16-2, cont'd Obstetric admitting record.

BOX 16-1

Patient Care Plan Using Protocols and Nursing Standards

Patient care plan for labor **Margery Jones**
Unit No. 4587024

Date initiated: ________ Time: ________ RN: ________

Outcome standards:

1. Patient will demonstrate normal labor progress while the fetus tolerates the labor process without demonstrating nonreassuring signs. Date met: ________
2. Patient will participate as desired in decisions about her care. Date met: ________
3. Patient and her partner will verbalize knowledge of labor process and their expectations for the birth experience. Date met: ________

Initiated Date/RN	Problem	Nursing Interventions	Discontinued Date/RN
	Alteration in maternal/fetal gas exchange	Implement fetal monitoring per protocol or orders from physician/CNM (Box 15-2, p. 387)	
	Risk related to labor progress: ▪ Altered pattern of urinary elimination ▪ Tissue trauma related to birth	Provide nursing care per hospital procedure manual Implement labor care per protocol (Table 16-2) Notify physician/CNM of problems (see Signs of Potential Complications, p. 411) Provide care for vaginal birth per hospital procedure manual Provide immediate care for newborn per hospital procedure manual	
	Anxiety related to maternal/fetal status	Encourage patient and her partner to express their concerns Keep couple informed of labor progress Involve patient in decision-making regarding her care	
	Knowledge deficit about labor/procedures	Explain procedures in terms patient can understand	
	Pain associated with labor	Promote use of relaxation techniques Provide comfort measures Offer pain medications as ordered Evaluate response to pain relief measures	
	Other problems:		

immunodeficiency virus (HIV), sickle cell trait, or other genetic screening (e.g., maternal serum α-fetoprotein [MSAFP]).

Interview. The woman's chief complaint or primary reason for coming to the hospital is determined in the interview. Her primary complaint may be that her **bag of waters** (**BOW,** amniotic membranes) broke with or without contractions. The woman may have come in for an *obstetric check* (period of observation). The obstetric check is reserved for women who are unsure about onset of labor. This designation allows time on the unit for diagnosis of labor without official admission, which minimizes or avoids cost to the patient.

The woman may be scheduled for induction of labor. Induction of labor and other complications of labor, such as premature rupture of membranes, require alterations in the nursing care plan. However, even in those instances the nursing assessment remains essentially the same.

Even the experienced mother may have difficulty determining the onset of labor. The woman is asked to recall the events of the previous days. She is assessed for the prodromal signs of labor (Box 13-1, p. 344) and for the onset of regular contractions. She is asked to describe the following:

- Frequency and duration of uterine contractions.
- Location and character of discomfort from the contractions (e.g., back pain, suprapubic discomfort).
- Persistence of the contractions despite changes in maternal position and activity (e.g., walking or lying down).
- Presence and character of vaginal discharge or show.
- Status of amniotic membranes, such as gush or seepage of fluid. If there is a discharge that may be amniotic fluid, she is asked the date and time the fluid was first noted and the fluid's characteristics (e.g., amount, color, unusual odor). In many instances a sterile speculum examination and a nitrazine (pH) or fern test confirm that the membranes are ruptured (see the Guidelines box on p. 399).

These descriptions help the nurse assess the degree of progress by determining the character of the contractions and the nature of the vaginal discharge. **Bloody show** is distinguished from bleeding in that it is pink in color and feels sticky because of its mucoid nature. It is scant to begin with and increases with effacement and dilation of the cervix. A woman may report a scant brownish discharge that may be attributed to cervical trauma as a result of vaginal examination or coitus within the last 48 hours.

Guidelines

TESTS FOR RUPTURE OF MEMBRANES

Nitrazine test for pH

Explain procedure to woman/couple.

Procedure

Use **nitrazine test** paper, a dye 1-1—impregnated test paper for pH. (Differentiates amniotic fluid, which is slightly alkaline, from urine and purulent material [pus], which are acidic.)

Wearing a sterile glove lubricated with water, place a piece of test paper at the cervical os

OR

Use a sterile, cotton-tipped applicator to dip deep into vagina to pick up fluid; touch applicator to test paper. This procedure may be done during a speculum examination.

Read results:

Membranes probably intact: identifies vaginal and most body fluids that are acidic

Yellow	pH 5.0
Olive yellow	pH 5.5
Olive green	pH 6.0

Membranes probably ruptured: Identifies amniotic fluid that is alkaline

Blue-green	pH 6.5
Blue-gray	pH 7.0
Deep blue	pH 7.5

Realize that false test results are possible because of presence of bloody show, insufficient amniotic fluid, or semen.

Remove gloves and wash hands.

Chart results:

Positive or negative

Test for ferning or fern pattern

Explain procedure to woman/couple.

Wash hands, apply sterile gloves, obtain specimen of fluid (usually with sterile speculum examination).

Spread a drop of fluid from vagina on a clean glass slide with a sterile, cotton-tipped applicator.

Allow fluid to dry.

Assess slide under microscope: observe for appearance of ferning, a frondlike crystalline pattern (do not confuse with cervical mucus test, when high levels of estrogen are responsible for the ferning).

Observe for absence of ferning (alerts staff to possibility that specimen was inadequate or that specimen was urine, vaginal discharge, or blood).

Remove gloves and wash hands.

Chart results:

Positive or negative

Because of the possibility that general anesthesia may be required at a moment's notice, it is important to assess the woman's respiratory status. The nurse asks if the woman has a "cold" or related symptoms, "stuffy nose," sore throat, or cough. Allergies are rechecked, including allergies to medications routinely used, such as meperidine (Demerol) or lidocaine (Xylocaine). Some allergic responses cause swelling of mucous membranes of the respiratory system. Because vomiting and subsequent aspiration into the respiratory tract can complicate an otherwise normal labor, the nurse records the type and time of the woman's last solid food and liquid intake.

Any information not found in the prenatal record is requested during screening for admission. Pertinent data include birth plan, choice of infant feeding method, anesthesia desired, and name of pediatrician. A patient profile is obtained; this profile indicates the woman's preparation for childbirth, supportive person(s)/family desired and available, and ethnic or cultural expectations and needs.

If the woman has prepared a formal birth plan, a copy will usually be in the prenatal record. The nurse reviews it before the woman arrives in the birthing unit. If no written plan has been made, the nurse discusses the woman's wishes and preferences when she arrives and informs her of any institutional policies that might prevent granting some of the requests. The nurse also prepares the woman for the possibility that changes may be needed in her plan as labor progresses and assures her that information will be provided so that she can make informed decisions.

Requests in a birth plan may include preferences regarding presence of birth companions and others (e.g., students, male attendants, interpreters), clothing to be worn, videotaping labor and birth, activities (e.g., listening to music, hydrotherapy, walking, acceptable positions for labor and birth), interventions such as intravenous infusions (IVs) and mode of fetal monitoring, role of the father/partner, immediate handling and care of the newborn, and special customs and cultural/religious requirements. The plan should be flexible because childbirth is a dynamic process that may necessitate adaptations as labor progresses. The woman's preferences if labor deviates from the normal should also be included in the plan (Kitzinger, 1992; Moore, Hopper, and Dip, 1995; Myles, 1989). The nurse uses the birth plan information to plan individualized care for the woman's labor.

The nulliparous woman, eager for the birth of her baby, may come to the hospital in **false labor** or early in the latent phase of the first stage. It can be disheartening for the woman and her partner to find out that the contractions that feel strong and regular to her are not true labor contractions because they are not causing cervical dilation. If she lives near the hospital, she may be asked to return home to allow labor to progress in frequency and strength of contractions and/or in amount of show. The woman is encouraged to ambulate and asked to reduce her intake to either light foods and fluids or to clear liquids, depending on the preferences of her primary health care provider. The woman who lives at a considerable distance from the hospital may be admitted in early labor.

Psychosocial factors. The woman's general appearance and behavior (and that of her partner) provide valuable clues to the type of supportive care she will need. The nurse should keep in mind that general appearance and behavior may vary depending on the stage and phase of labor. Factors to assess include the following:

- *Verbal interactions.* Does the woman ask questions? Can she ask for what she needs? Does her partner do all the talking? Does she talk to her support person(s)? Does she talk freely with the nurse or respond only to questions? Verbal interactions may vary depending on stage and phase of labor.
- *Body language.* Is she relaxed or tense? What is her anxiety level? How does she react to being touched by the nurse? Support person? Does she change position or lie rigidly still? Does she avoid eye contact? Where does her partner sit? Does she look tired? How much rest has she had during the last day?
- *Perceptual ability.* Does she understand what the nurse says? Is there a language barrier? Does her anxiety level require repeated explanations? Can she repeat what she has been told or demonstrate understanding?
- *Discomfort level.* To what degree does the woman express what she is experiencing? How does she react to a contraction? Are there any nonverbal pain messages seen? Does she complain to the nurse? To her partner? Can she ask for comfort measures?

Stress in labor

Nursing ALERT

Usually women in labor have various concerns that they voice if asked, but rarely volunteer. It is therefore important for the nurse to ask the woman what she expects in order to clear up misinformation or suggest that the woman ask her physician/CNM about an issue.

The following are common concerns that women in labor have: Will my baby be all right? Will I be able to stand labor? Will my labor be long? How will I act? Will I need medication? Will it work for me? Will my partner/someone be there to support me? Do I have to have an IV, an enema, etc.?

The nurse's responsibility to the woman in labor is to answer her questions or find out the answers, to provide support to her and her family/support persons, to take care of her in partnership with those persons the woman wants as her support team, and to serve as their advocate. The nurse communicates to the woman that she is not expected to act in any particular way and that the process will end in the birth of her baby, which is the only expectation she should have. Nursing support should reflect respect for and acceptance of a woman's individuality and behaviors. The woman's views and expectations regarding the nurse's role as caregiver should be determined. The nurse/patient relationship becomes increasingly important as labor progresses (Bryanton et al, 1994).

According to McKay and Smith (1993), women equate emotional support with information giving. Nurses are perceived as supportive when they explain things in detail using positive terms and provide accurate information and specific directions. Women feel empowered when they are given information they can understand and that reflects support of their efforts. This feeling of empowerment contributes to a positive perception of the experience.

Women prepare themselves for labor in various ways. Some go to childbirth education classes, some read books and talk to friends and relatives, and some prepare elaborate birth plans of their wishes for their labor and birth. The longer the list of "wishes," the greater is the likelihood that expectations will not be met. It is the nurse's responsibility to include the desires of the woman in formulating a plan of care. The nurse can facilitate aspects of the birth plan by showing the plan to the physician or midwife and telling the woman to remind her primary health provider about what she wants in advance.

The father, coach, or significant other also experiences stress during labor. The nurse can assist and support these individuals by identifying needs and expectations and by helping him or her address these areas. What role does this person expect to play? Is he or she nervous, anxious, aggressive, or hostile? Does he or she look hungry, tired, worried, or confused? Does he or she watch television, sleep, or stay out of the room instead of paying attention to the woman? Does he or she touch the woman; what is the character of the touch? Has the couple attended childbirth classes? The nurse ascertains what role the support person intends to fulfill and whether he or she is prepared for that role. The nurse must be sensitive to needs and provide teaching and support as appropriate. Often the support this person is able to give the laboring woman is in direct proportion to the support he or she receives from the nurses and other health care providers with whom they come in contact (Nichols, 1993).

Cultural factors. It is important to note the woman's ethnic/cultural background to anticipate nursing interventions that may need to be added or deleted to individualize the plan of care. If a special request contradicts usual practices in that setting, the woman or nurse can ask her health care provider to write an order for the special request. For example, in some cultures it is traditional to take the placenta home; in others the woman is given only certain nourishments during labor (see the Cultural Considerations box below).

When assessing a woman's cultural and religious preferences, Callister (1995) suggests that the nurse ask questions

Cultural Considerations 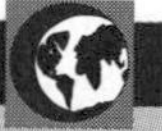

BIRTH PRACTICES IN DIFFERENT CULTURES

South Korea—Stoic response to labor pain; fathers usually not present
Japan—Natural childbirth methods practiced; may labor silently; father may be present; may eat during labor
China—Stoic response to pain; fathers not present; side-lying position preferred for labor and birth because this position is thought to reduce infant trauma
India—Natural childbirth methods preferred; fathers usually not present; female relatives usually present
Iran—Father not present; prefers female support and female caregivers
Mexico—May be stoic about discomfort until second stage, then may request pain relief; fathers and female relatives may be present
Laos—May use squatting position for birth; fathers may or may not be present; prefer female attendants

Data from Geissler E: *Pocket guide to cultural assessment,* St Louis, 1994, Mosby.

regarding (1) the value and meaning placed on the childbirth experience; (2) the view of childbirth as a wellness or illness experience, and as a private or social event; (3) practices regarding diet, medications, activity, and emotional and physical support; (4) appropriate maternal and paternal behaviors; (5) birth companions—who they should be and what they should do; and (6) views regarding the newborn and infant care immediately after birth.

Within cultures, women may learn the "right" way to behave in labor and to react to the pain experienced. These behaviors can range from total silence to moaning or screaming. A woman who moans with contractions may not be in as much physical pain as a woman who is silent but winces during contractions (Table 16-1). Some women feel it is shameful to scream or cry in pain if a man is present (D'Avanzo, 1992). If the woman's support person is her mother, she may perceive the need to "behave" more strongly than if her support person is the father of the baby. She will perceive herself as failing or succeeding on the basis of her ability to adhere to these "standards" of behavior.

The non–English-speaking woman in labor. A woman's level of anxiety in labor rises when she does not understand what is happening to her or what is being said (McKay and Smith, 1993). Some misunderstanding may occur with English-speaking women and cause some stress. The effect of misunderstanding on non–English-speaking women is much more dramatic because they often feel a complete loss of control over their situation. They can panic and withdraw or become physically abusive when someone tries to do something they perceive might harm them or their babies. Sometimes a support person is able to communicate in English. Caution must be exercised when using a support person as translator. The support person may misrepresent what the nurse or others are saying and raise the woman's stress level even more. The translator may also misrepresent what the woman is trying to say or insert his or her own beliefs or wishes. The translator may say, for example, "Her pain is not that bad—pain medications are not good for her anyway."

If there is a list of employee translators, one may be contacted for help. If no one in the hospital is able to translate, a bilingual employee or translation service can be called so a translation over the telephone can take place. For some

Critical Thinking Exercises

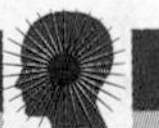

CULTURAL EXPECTATIONS IN BIRTHING

You are assigned to a laboring woman and her family who appear to be from a culture different from yours.

1. **What are your assumptions regarding their expectations?**
2. **How will you verify their perceptions and beliefs about labor and birth?**
3. **Analyze how these factors might affect the behavior of the woman, her family, and the nurse during the first stage of labor.**
4. **How would you incorporate this knowledge into your plan of care?**

TABLE 16-1 Sociocultural basis of pain experience

WOMAN IN LABOR	NURSE
Perception of meaning	
Origin: Cultural concept of and personal experience with pain; for example: Pain in childbirth is inevitable, something to be borne Pain in childbirth can be avoided completely Pain in childbirth is punishment for sin Pain in childbirth can be controlled	Origin: Cultural concept of and personal experience with pain; in addition, nurse becomes accustomed to working with certain "expected" pain trajectories; for example, in obstetrics, pain is expected to increase as labor progresses, be intermittent in character, and have an endpoint; relief can be derived from medications once labor is well established and fetus or newborn can cope with amount and elimination of medication; relief can also come from woman's knowledge, attitude, and support from family or friends
Coping mechanisms	
Woman may exhibit the following behaviors: Be traditionally vocal or nonvocal; crying out or groaning or both may be part of ritual of her response to pain Use counterstimulation to minimize pain; for example, rubbing, applying heat, using counterpressure Use relaxation, distraction, autosuggestion as pain-countering techniques Resist use of "needles" for administering pain relief	Nurse may respond by: Using self effectively; for example, tone of voice, closeness in space, and touch as media for message of interest and caring Using avoidance, belittling, or other distracting actions as protective device for self Using pharmacologic resources at hand judiciously Using comfort measures Assume responsibility for control and management of pain
Expectations of others	
Nurse may be seen as someone who will accept woman's statement of pain and act as her advocate Medical personnel may be expected to relieve woman of all pain sensations Nurse may be expected to be interested, gentle, kind, and accepting of behavior exhibited	Only certain verbal or nonverbal behaviors as responses to pain may be accepted Couple who are prepared for childbirth may be expected to refuse medication and to wish to "do everything on their own" Woman's definition of pain may not be accepted; that is, woman may wish to experience and participate in controlling pain or may not be able to accept any pain as reasonable

women a female translator may be more acceptable. The nurse can prepare a set of cards with graphics to illustrate common situations that can be used to communicate with non–English-speaking women. Even when the nurse has limited ability to communicate orally with the woman, in most instances the nurse's efforts to communicate are meaningful.

Physical examination

Nursing ALERT

A quick check (vaginal examination) may be done to rule out immiment birth before proceeding with an initial examination.

The initial examination confirms the onset of true labor. The findings serve as a baseline for assessing the woman's progress from that point. The initial physical examination includes general systems assessment, performance of Leopold maneuvers to determine fetal presentation, position, and point of maximum intensity (PMI) for auscultating the FHR, assessment of fetal staus, assessmert of uterine contractions, and vaginal examination to assess cervical effacement and dilation, fetal descent, and status of amniotic membranes and fluid. The most vital aspect of assessment is that of fetal status. Women often focus on contractions as the clearest indicator of how far advanced their labor is. However, the vaginal examination is a more valid indicator, especially for nulliparous women, for estimating the woman's phase of labor. Rupture of the membranes (ROM) significantly affects the woman's care plan. Once the membranes are ruptured, they no longer protect the intrauterine cavity and fetus from infectious organisms that can travel up the birth canal. ROM also increases the risk of umbilical cord prolapse. It is important to obtain as many related pieces of information as possible before planning and implementing care.

Complete and accurate assessment during screening provides the basis for admission and ongoing care. Minimum assessment guidelines and normal limits of maternal progress during the first stage of labor are presented in Tables 16-2 and 16-3.

Nursing ALERT

The nurse assumes much of the responsibility for making the assessment of progress. It is the nurse's responsibility to keep the physician or midwife informed about progress and any deviations from normal findings.

The assessment procedures that follow can be used as a basis for teaching women and their families. The purpose, equipment needed, and nursing actions and rationale of each procedure can be shared with the woman. All procedures are preceded by thorough handwashing. Handwashing is also important *after* the examinations are completed. Standard Precautions and precautions for invasive procedures are taken as needed (Box 16-2). The findings are explained to the woman whenever possible. Accurate documentation is done as soon as possible after interaction with the woman. Findings and the time that the procedure is performed are carefully noted and initialed on the chart and on the fetal monitoring strip (if that is agency policy).

BOX 16-2
Standard Precautions During Childbirth

Birth is a time when nurses and other health care providers are exposed to a great deal of maternal and newborn blood and body fluids. Observation of Standard Precautions is necessary if transmission of infection is to be prevented. Perinatal infections most often are transmitted through contact with body fluids. Standard Precautions as they apply to childbirth include the following:

- Wash hands before and after putting on gloves and performing procedures.
- Wear gloves (clean or sterile as appropriate) when performing procedures that require contact with the woman's genitalia and bloody show (e.g., vaginal examination, amniotomy, hygienic care of perineum, insertion of internal scalp electrode and intrauterine pressure monitor, catheterization).
- Wear cap, a mask that has a shield or protective eyewear, shoe covers, and cover gown during the birth process. Gowns should have a waterproof front and sleeves and should also be sterile for the physician/CNM who is attending the birth.
- Drape the woman as appropriate with sterile towels and sheets. Inform the woman what can be touched or not touched.
- Assist the woman's partner to put on appropriate coverings for the birth, such as cap, mask, gown, and shoe covers. Instruct the partner where to stand and what can or cannot be touched.
- Wear gloves and gown when handling the newborn immediately after birth.
- Use an appropriate method to suction the newborn's airway: mechanical wall suction or a DeLee oral suction device that keeps the newborn's mucus separate from the user's airway.

General systems assessment. A brief systems assessment is performed, including heart, lungs, and skin; presence of edema of the legs, face, hands, or sacrum; and deep tendon reflexes and clonus.

Vital signs (blood pressure, temperature, pulse, respirations) are assessed on admission, and initial values are used for comparison with future values. If blood pressure is elevated, it should be reassessed 30 minutes later, between contractions, to obtain a reading after the woman has relaxed. A correct size of cuff should be used. To avoid supine hypotension and fetal distress the woman should be encouraged to lie on her side and not in a supine position (Fig. 16-3). Her temperature is monitored for signs of infection or fluid deficit (dehydration associated with inadequate intake of fluids). The woman's intake and output should be measured every 8 hours. Urinary protein and ketone levels should be determined using a dipstick each time the woman voids.

Leopold maneuvers (abdominal palpation). After the woman is in bed, the nurse asks her to lie on her back momentarily so that *Leopold maneuvers* can be performed (see the Guidelines box on pp. 404-405 and Fig. 16-4). These maneuvers provide information about (1) the number of fetuses;

Text continued on p. 406.

TABLE 16-2 Minimum assessment of the low-risk woman during the first stage of labor*

	CERVICAL DILATION		
VARIABLES	0-3 cm (LATENT)	4-7 cm (ACTIVE)	8-10 cm (TRANSITION)
Blood pressure, pulse, respiration	q 30-60 min	q 30 min	q 15-30 min
Temperature†	q 4 hrs	q 4 hrs	q 4 hrs
Uterine activity	q 30-60 min	q 15-30 min	q 10-15 min
FHR	q 30-60 min	q 15-30 min	q 15-30 min
Vaginal show	q 30-60 min	q 30 min	q 15 min
Behavior, appearance, energy level	q 30 min	q 15 min	q 5 min

Vaginal examination‡ as necessary to identify progress of labor:

- To confirm change when symptoms indicate (e.g., increase in strength, duration, or frequency of contractions; increase in amount of bloody show; ROM; or woman feels pressure on her rectum)
- To determine whether dilation and descent are sufficient for administration of analgesic or anesthetic
- To reassess progress if labor takes longer than expected
- To determine station of presenting part

*Frequency of assessment is determined by the risk status of the maternal-fetal unit. More frequent assessment is required in high-risk situations. Frequency of assessment and method of documentation are also determined by agency policy, which is usually based on the recommended standards of medical and nursing organizations.

†If membranes have ruptured, check temperature every 2 hours; assess orally or tympanically between contractions.

‡In presence of vaginal bleeding, physician performs vaginal examination, usually under double setup, or ultrasonography.

TABLE 16-3 Maternal progress in first stage of labor within normal limits

	PHASES MARKED BY CERVICAL DILATION*		
CRITERION	0-3 cm (LATENT)	4-7 cm (ACTIVE)	8-10 cm (TRANSITION)
Duration†	About 6 to 8 hr	About 3 to 6 hr	About 20 to 40 min
Contractions			
Strength	Mild to moderate	Moderate to strong	Strong to very strong
Rhythm	Irregular	More regular	Regular
Frequency	5 to 30 min apart	3 to 5 min apart	2 to 3 min apart
Duration	30 to 45 sec	40 to 70 sec	45 to 90 sec
Descent			
Station of presenting part	Nulliparous: 0 Multiparous: 0 to −2 cm	Varies: +1 to +2 cm Varies: +1 to +2 cm	Varies: +2 to +3 cm Varies: +2 to +3 cm
Show			
Color	Brownish discharge, mucous plug, or pale pink mucus	Pink to bloody mucus	Bloody mucus
Amount	Scant	Scant to moderate	Copious
Behavior and appearance‡	Excited; thoughts center on self, labor, and baby; may be talkative or silent, calm or tense; some apprehension; pain controlled fairly well; alert, follows directions readily; open to instructions	Becomes more serious, doubtful of control of pain, more apprehensive; desires companionship and encouragement; attention more inner directed; fatigue evidenced; malar (cheeks) flush; has some difficulty following directions	Pain described as severe; backache common; frustration, fear of loss of control, and irritability surface; vague in communications; amnesia between contractions; writhing with contractions; nausea and vomiting, especially if hyperventilating; hyperesthesia; circumoral pallor, perspiration on forehead and upper lips; shaking tremor of thighs; feeling of need to defecate, pressure on anus

*In the nullipara, effacement is often complete before dilation begins; in the multipara, it occurs simultaneously with dilation. Average total duration: nullipara—10 to 16 hr; multipara—6 to 10 hr.

†Duration of each phase is influenced by such factors as parity, maternal position; and level of activity. For example, the labor of a nullipara tends to last longer, on average, than the labor of a multipara. Women who ambulate and assume upright positions or change positions frequently during labor tend to experience a shorter first stage.

‡Women who have epidural analgesia for pain relief may not demonstrate these behaviors.

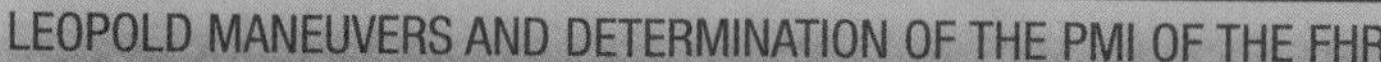

Guidelines

LEOPOLD MANEUVERS AND DETERMINATION OF THE PMI OF THE FHR

Leopold maneuvers

Wash hands.

Ask woman to empty bladder.

Position woman supine with one pillow under her head and her knees slightly flexed.

Place small rolled towel under woman's right hip to displace uterus to left of major blood vessels (avoids supine hypotension syndrome, Fig. 16-3).

If right-handed, stand on woman's right, facing her:

1. Identify fetal part that occupies the fundus. The head feels round, firm, freely movable, and palpable by ballottement; the breech feels less regular and softer. This identifies fetal lie (longitudinal or transverse) and presentation (cephalic or breech) (Fig. 16-4).
2. Using palmar surface of one hand, locate and palpate the smooth convex contour of the fetal back and the irregularities that identify the small parts (feet, hands, elbows). This assists in identifying fetal presentation (Fig. 16-4).
3. With the right hand, determine which fetal part is presenting over the inlet to the true pelvis. Gently grasp the lower pole of the uterus between the thumb and fingers, pressing in slightly (Fig. 16-4). If the head is presenting and not engaged, determine the attitude of the head (flexed or extended).
4. Turn to face the woman's feet. Using two hands, outline the fetal head (Fig. 16-4) with palmar surface of fingertips.

When presenting part has descended deeply, only a small portion of it may be outlined.

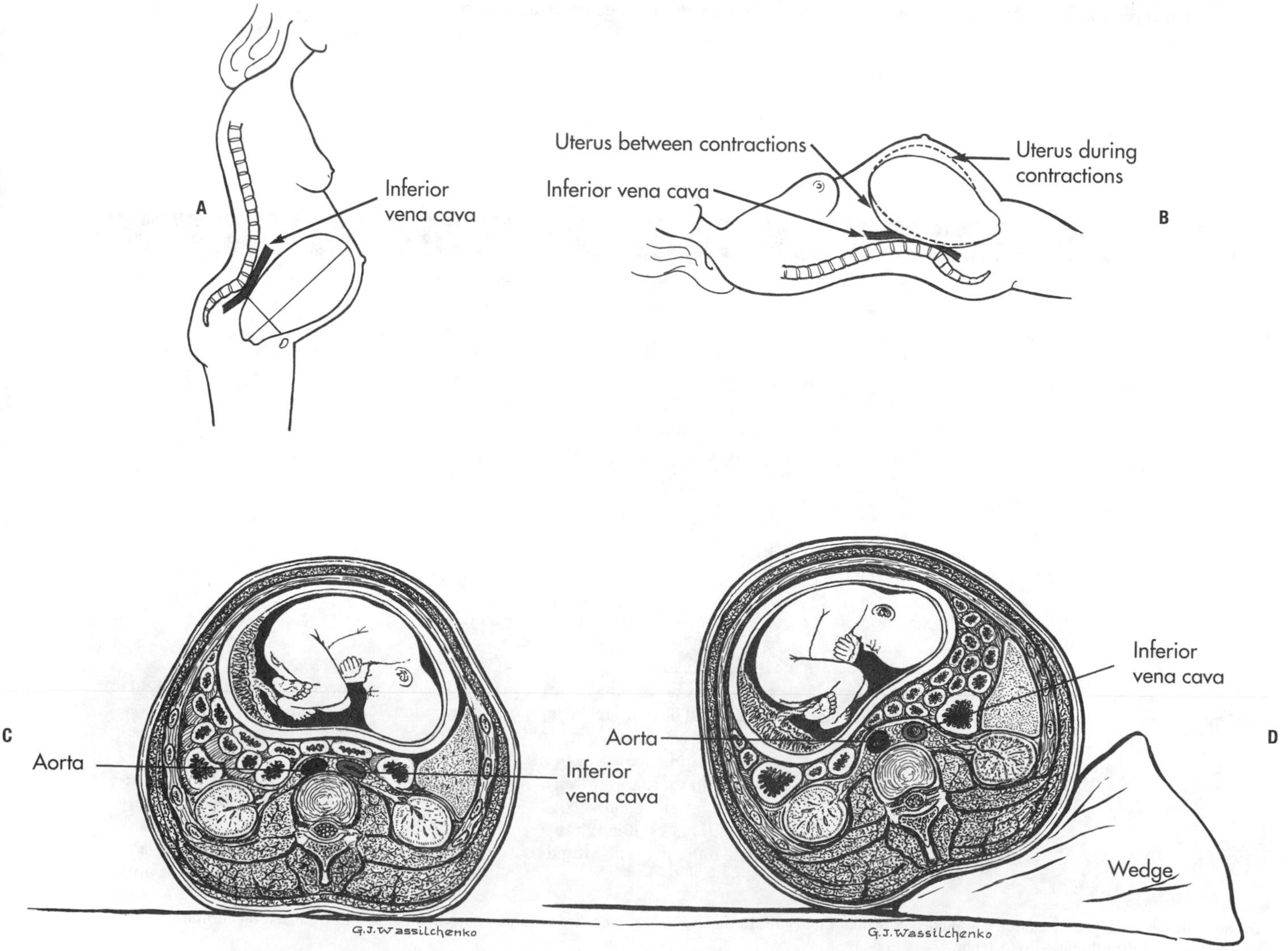

Fig. 16-3 Supine hypotension. Note relationship of gravid uterus to ascending vena cava in standing posture **(A)** and in supine posture **(B)**. **C,** Compression of aorta and inferior vena cava with woman in supine position. **D,** Relieved by use of a wedge pillow placed under woman's right side.

Guidelines

LEOPOLD MANEUVERS AND DETERMINATION OF THE PMI OF THE FHR—cont'd

Palpation of cephalic prominence assists in identifying attitude of head.

If the cephalic prominence is found on the same side as the small parts, the head must be flexed, and the vertex is presenting (Fig. 16-4). If the cephalic prominence is on the same side as the back, the presenting head is extended (Fig. 16-4).

Determination of PMI of FHR:

Wash hands.

Perform Leopold maneuvers.

Auscultate FHR (Fig. 16-4).

Chart fetal presentation, position, and lie; whether presenting part is flexed or extended, engaged or free floating. Use hospital's protocol for charting (e.g., "Vtx, LOA, floating").

Chart PMI of FHR using a two-line figure to indicate the four quadrants of the maternal abdomen, right upper quadrant (RUQ), left upper quadrant (LUQ), left lower quadrant (LLQ), and right lower quadrant (RLQ):

RUQ	LUQ
RLQ	LLQ

The umbilicus is the point where the lines cross. The PMI for the fetus in vertex presentation, in general flexion with the back on the mother's right side, commonly is found in the mother's RLQ and is recorded with an "x" or with the FHR as follows:

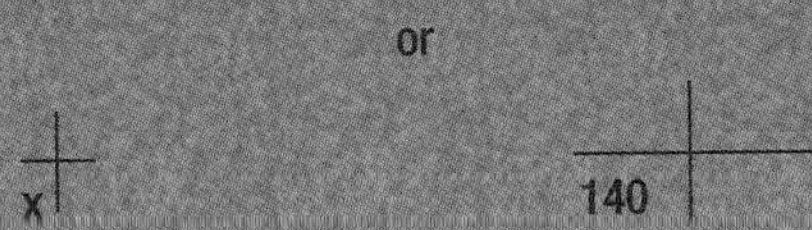

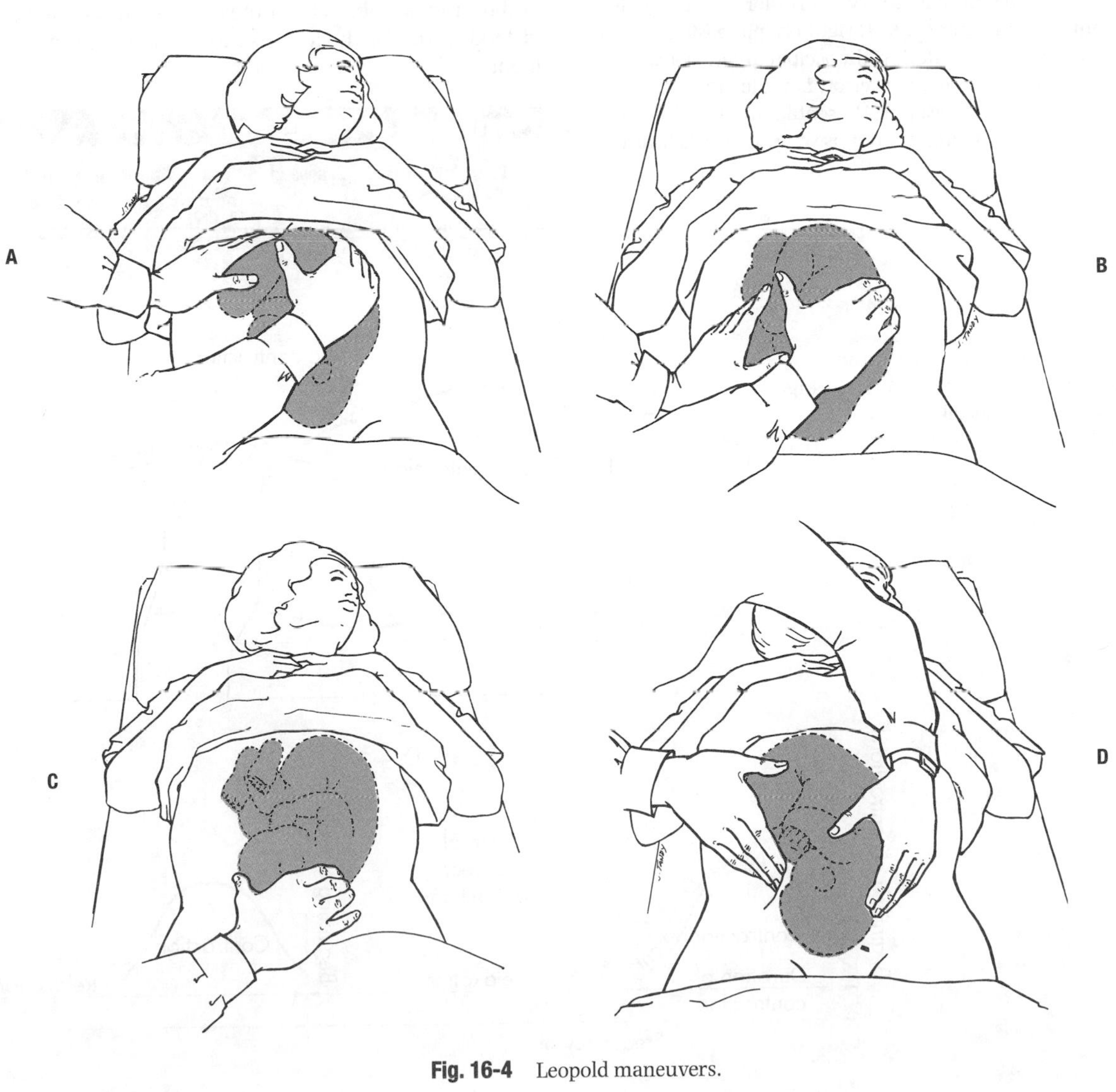

Fig. 16-4 Leopold maneuvers.

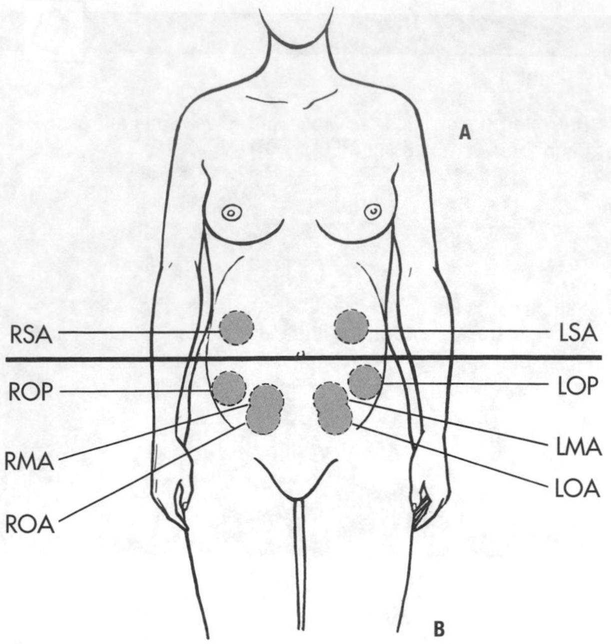

Fig. 16-5 Areas of maximum intensity of FHR for differing positions: *RSA*, right sacrum anterior; *ROP*, right occipitoposterior; *RMA*, right mentum anterior; *ROA*, right occipitoanterior; *LSA*, left sacrum anterior; *LOP*, left occipitoposterior; *LMA*, left mentum anterior; and *LOA*, left occipitoanterior. **A**, Presentation is *breech* if FHR is heard *above* umbilicus. **B**, Presentation is *vertex* if FHR is heard *below* umbilicus.

(2) the identity of the presenting part, the fetal lie, and attitude; (3) the degree of the presenting part's descent into the pelvis; and (4) the expected location of the PMI of the FHR in relation to the woman's abdomen.

Assessment of FHR and pattern. It is important for the nurse to understand the relationship between location of PMI of FHR and fetal presentation, lie, and position. Assessment of high risk for childbirth complications may be diagnosed by variations in these findings. The PMI of the FHR is the location on the maternal abdomen where the FHR is heard the loudest. This place is usually directly over the fetal back. The PMI is also an aid in determining the fetal presentation and position (Fig. 16-5). In a vertex presentation the FHR is heard *below* the mother's umbilicus in either the right or the left lower quadrant of the abdomen. In a breech presentation the FHR is heard *above* the mother's umbilicus (Fig. 16-5, *A*). As fetal descent and internal rotation occur, the FHR is heard lower and closer to the midline of the maternal abdomen. The PMI of the fetus in the right occipitoanterior (ROA) position moves to the midline just over the symphysis pubis (Fig. 16-5, *B*). Just before birth the fetal position is occipitoanterior (OA) and the fetal back is directly above the symphysis pubis. Fig. 16-5 presents diagrams of the PMI for different presentations and positions. Table 16-2 notes the recommended assessment of fetal status for the low-risk woman during the first stage of labor.

Nursing ALERT

The FHR must be assessed (1) immediately after rupture of the membranes, since this is the most common time for prolapse of the umbilical cord to occur, or (2) after any change in contraction pattern.

Fig. 16-6 Assessment of uterine contractions. **A**, Abdominal contour before and during uterine contraction. **B**, Wavelike pattern of contractile activity.

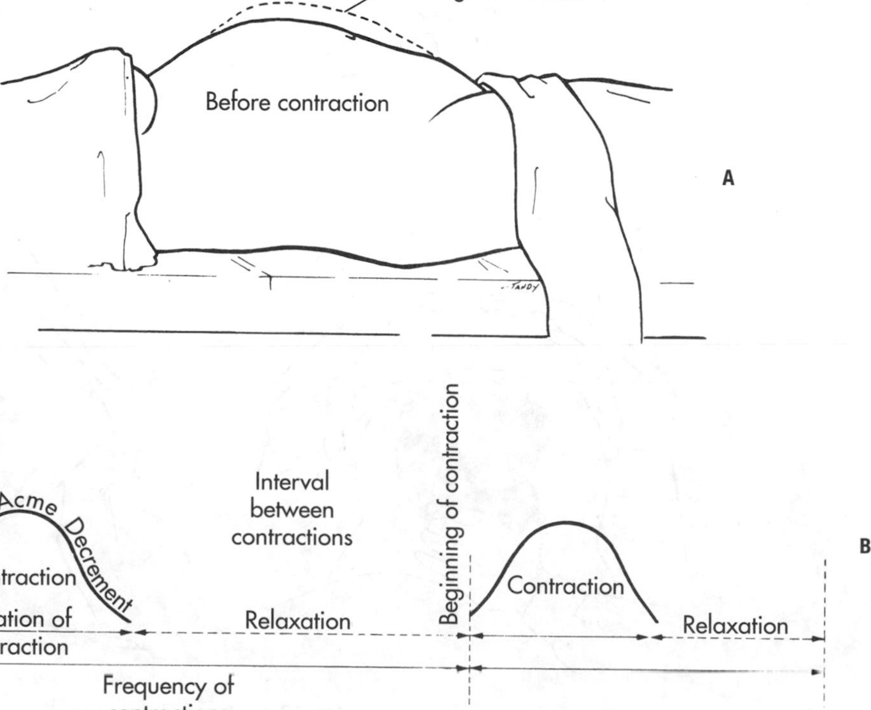

Assessment of uterine contractions. A general characteristic of effective labor is regular uterine activity; however, uterine activity is not directly related to labor progress. **Uterine contractions** are considered the primary powers that act involuntarily to expel the fetus and placenta from the uterus. Several methods are used to evaluate uterine contractions. These include the woman's subjective description, palpation and timing of the contraction by a health care provider, and electronic monitoring devices.

Each contraction exhibits a wavelike pattern. Contractions begin with a slow **increment** (the "building up" of a contraction from its onset), gradually reaching an **acme** (the peak; intrauterine pressure 50 to 75 mm Hg), and then diminishing rather rapidly to the **decrement** (the "letting down" of the contraction). An **interval** of rest follows (intrauterine pressure is 5 to 15 mm Hg), which ends when the next contraction begins. (Fig. 16-6 diagrams a typical uterine contraction.)

The following characteristics are used to describe a uterine contraction:

Frequency—how often uterine contractions occur; the period of time from the beginning of one contraction to the beginning of the next or from the peak of one contraction to the peak of the next
Intensity—the strength of a contraction at its peak
Duration—the period of time that elapses between the onset and the end of a contraction
Resting tone—the tension in the uterine muscle during the interval between contractions

The most common ways to measure uterine contractions are by palpation or by an external or internal electronic monitor. Palpation is used in the early and active phases of the first stage of labor, when the woman often is still ambulatory. At the routine time when FHR is assessed, contractions are also assessed. On admission, a 20- to 30-minute baseline monitor-

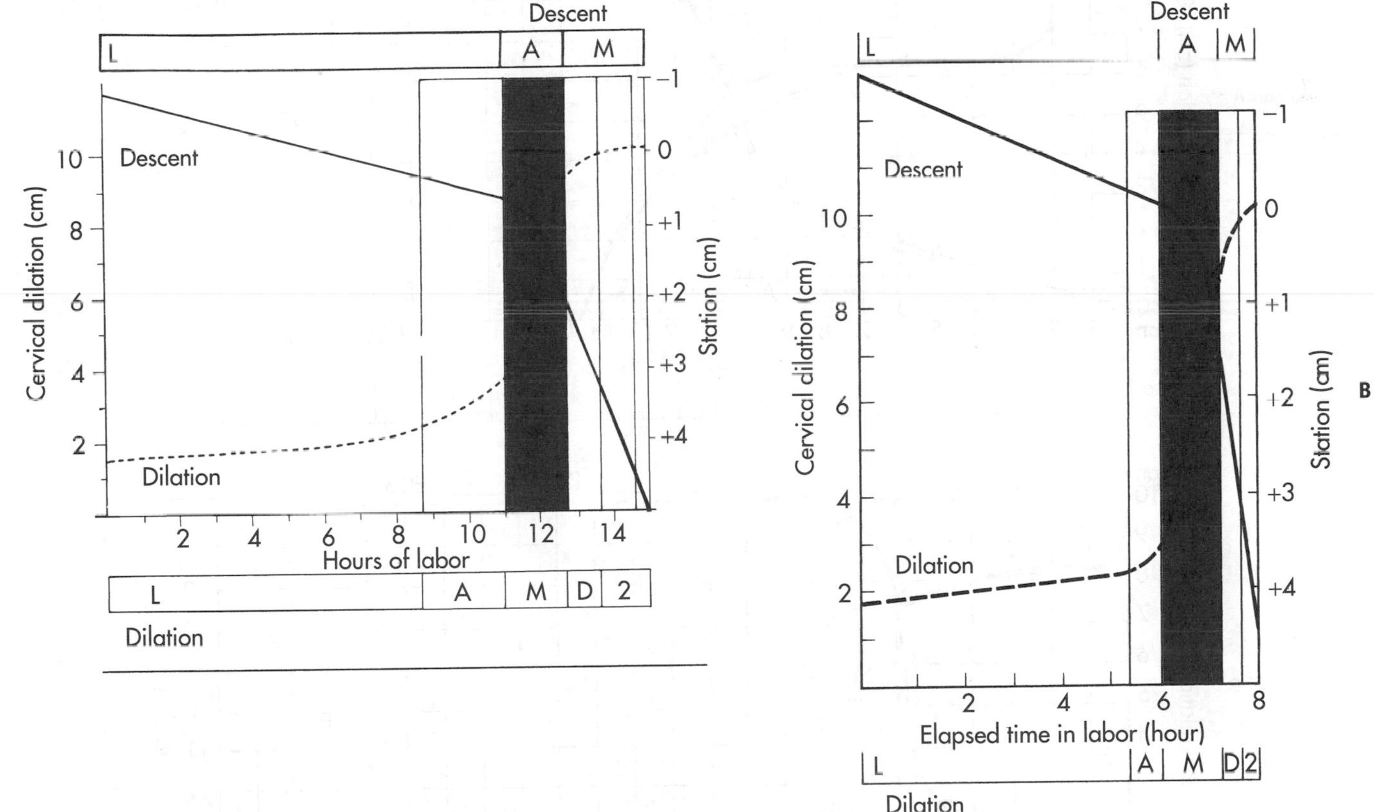

Fig. 16-7 Partogram showing relationship between cervical dilation and descent of presenting part. **A,** Nulliparous labor. **B,** Multiparous labor. The phases of cervical dilation are identified by the letters *L, A, M,* and *D.* The number *2* refers to the stage of labor. The latent phase *(L)* of the first stage of labor is that time between the onset of labor and the onset of acceleration. The active phase begins with the acceleration phase *(A)* and spans the time between the onset of the upward curve of cervical dilation and full dilation of the cervix. Freidman (1978) divides the active phase into three parts: (1) *acceleration phase (A),* (2) *phase of maximum slope (M),* and (3) *deceleration phase (D).* The dotted line denotes cervical dilation. The phases of descent are identified by the letters *L, A,* and *M,* located over the graph. The letter *L* refers to the latent phase of minimum descent. Active descent *(A)* generally begins when the cervical dilation curve reaches its phase of maximum slope. The rate of descent reaches its maximum at the beginning of the deceleration phase of cervical dilation. Maximum descent *(M)* continues in a linear manner until the perineum is reached. The solid line shows the rate of descent.

ing of uterine contractions and the FHR usually is done (Scott et al, 1994). Table 16-2 indicates continued minimum assessment times in labor, and Table 16-3 describes the expected findings as labor progresses/advances.

Frequency and duration can be determined by all three methods of uterine activity monitoring. Palpation is a less precise method of determining the intensity of uterine contractions. The following terms are used to describe what is felt on palpation; the activity in parentheses provides the novice nurse a frame of reference for the assessment:

Mild—slightly tense fundus that is easy to indent with fingertips (touching finger to lips)

Moderate—firm fundus that is difficult to indent with fingertips (touching finger to tip of nose)

Strong—rigid, boardlike fundus that is almost impossible to indent with fingertips (touching finger to forehead)

Women in labor tend to describe the pain of contractions in terms of their sensations in the lower abdomen or in the back, which may be unrelated to the firmness of the uterine fundus. Thus their report of the strength of their contractions can be less valid than that assessed by a health care provider.

External electronic monitoring provides information about the relative strength of the uterine contractions. Internal electronic monitoring with an intrauterine pressure catheter is

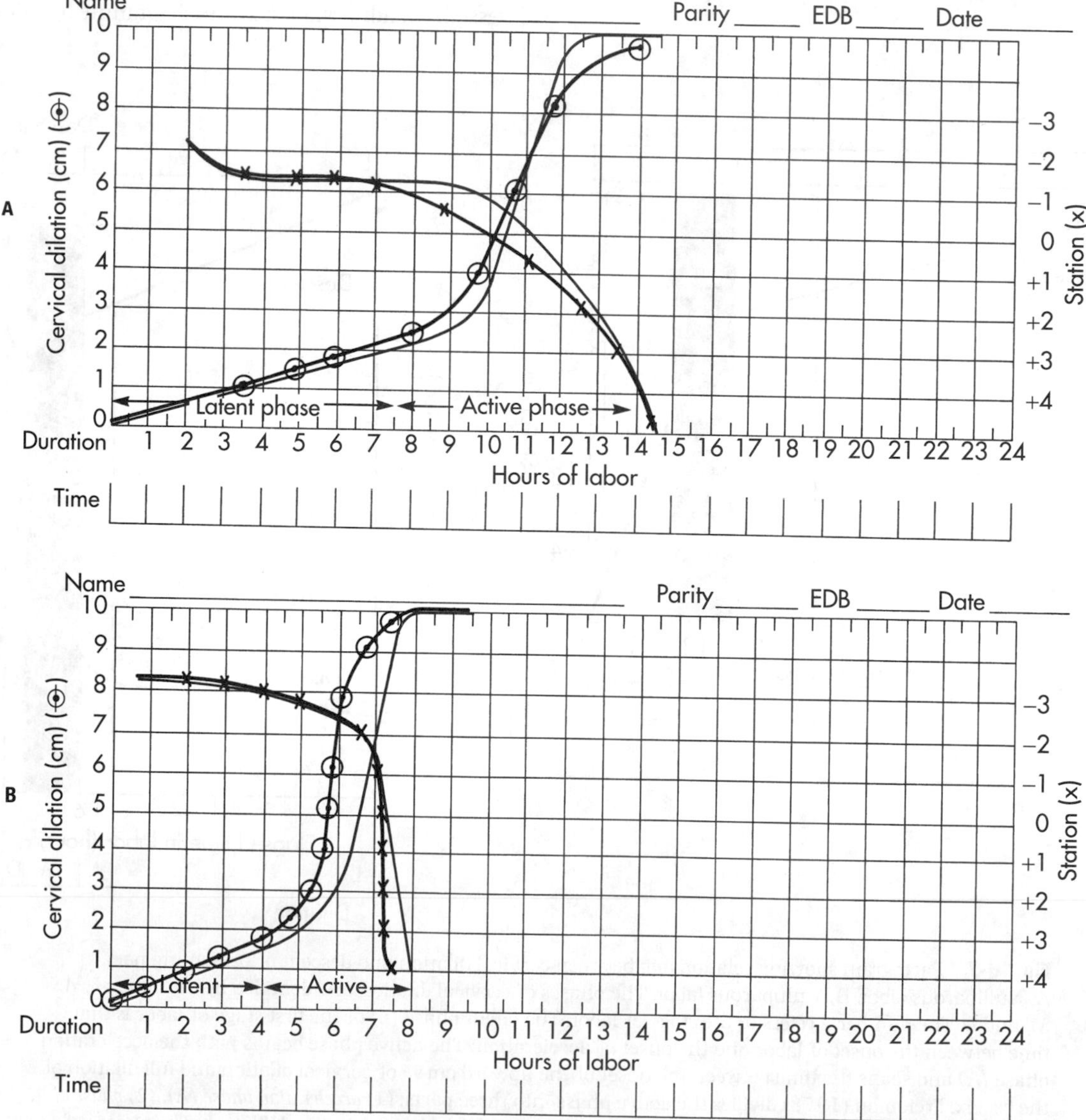

Fig. 16-8 Partogram for assessment of patterns of cervical dilation and descent. Individual woman's labor patterns *(colored)* are superimposed on prepared labor graph *(black)* for comparison. **A,** Nulliparous labor. **B,** Multiparous labor. The rate of cervical dilation is indicated by the symbol *"O"*. A line drawn through the symbols depicts the slope of the curve. Station is indicated with an *"X"*. A line drawn through the Xs reveals the pattern of descent.

the most valid method of assessing the intensity of uterine contractions.

The nurse's responsibility in monitoring uterine contractions is to ascertain whether they are powerful and frequent enough to accomplish the work of expulsion of the fetus and the placenta. If the characteristics of contractions are on either side of what is considered "acceptable" by standards, the nurse reports findings to the physician/CNM.

Cervical effacement, dilation, and fetal descent. When uterine activity is discussed, it must be related to its effect on cervical effacement and dilation and on the degree of descent of the presenting part. The effect on the fetus must also be considered. Labor progress can be effectively verified by the use of graphic charts (partograms) on which cervical dilation and station (descent) are plotted. This type of graphic charting assists an early identification of deviations from expected labor patterns. Fig. 16-7 shows the expected pattern of cervical dilation and descent for both nulliparous and multiparous women. Fig. 16-8 provides one example of a partogram; however, hospitals and birthing centers may develop their own graphs for recording assessments. Such graphs may include not only dilation and descent but also maternal vital signs, FHR, and uterine activity.

Nursing ALERT

At each assessment the nurse is responsible for documenting the findings of labor progress on the partogram and for notifying the physician or midwife should an unexpected or abnormal pattern emerge.

CERVICAL EFFACEMENT. As the cervix is retracted upward, it becomes a part of the lower uterine segment. The "taking up" of the cervix reduces the length of the cervix from about 2 cm to a few millimeters when it is 100% effaced. This upward pull on fibers of the lower uterus and downward push on the fetus presses the presenting part onto the cervix (see Fig. 16-11). As uterine contractions and retraction of the lower uterine segment continue, the cervical os dilates (opens) progressively. Effacement precedes significant cervical dilation in the first pregnancy and often accompanies dilation in subsequent pregnancies. Effacement is not recorded on the partogram.

CERVICAL DILATION. Cervical dilation is the most conclusive sign that the power of the uterine contractions is effective and labor is progressing. Thus if a cervix is long and closed, there is very little chance that birth will occur within a few hours. Once a cervix has completely dilated (10 cm) in a previous birth, as in a multiparous woman, it rarely will feel as closed as that of a nulliparous woman. The position of the cervix often is posterior in early labor, particularly in nulliparous women. The cervix moves anteriorly as labor progresses and the presenting part descends, placing pressure on the cervical rim.

STATION. *Station* refers to the relationship of the lowermost portion of the presenting part to the mother's ischial spines. In early labor the presenting part often is above the level of the ischial spines; as labor progresses, the presenting part descends. If membranes are ruptured, station is usually lower if the presenting part has accommodated into the pelvic inlet. If membranes are intact, the presenting part may be floating or engaged in the inlet. If the vertex is at 0 station or below, most often engagement of the head has occurred; that is, the biparietal diameter of the head has passed through the pelvic inlet. If the head is unusually molded or if there is an extensive formation of caput, or both, engagement might not have taken place even though the vertex is at 0 station or even lower (Cunningham et al, 1993).

VAGINAL EXAMINATION. The vaginal examination reveals whether the woman is in true labor and enables the examiner to determine whether the membranes have ruptured. It should be performed only when indicated by the status of the woman and her fetus. For example, a vaginal examination should be performed on admission, when significant change has occurred in uterine activity, on maternal perception of perineal pressure or urge to bear down, when membranes rupture, or if variable decelerations of the FHR are noted. A full explanation of the examination and support of the woman are important factors in reducing the stress and discomfort associated with the examination (Bergstrom, 1992) (see the Guidelines box on p. 410).

Laboratory and diagnostic tests. The nurse anticipates the need for urinalysis and tests for blood values and rupture of membranes.

Analysis of urine specimen. A clean-catch urine specimen is obtained to gather data about the pregnant woman's health. It is a convenient and simple procedure that can provide information about the woman's hydration status (specific gravity, color, amount), nutritional status (ketones), infection (leukocytes), or possible complications; for example, pregnancy-induced hypertension (protein). The results can be obtained quickly and will help the nurse determine appropriate interventions.

Blood tests. Blood tests vary with hospital protocol and the woman's health status. An example of minimum assessment is a hematocrit determination, in which the specimen is processed by use of a centrifuge on the perinatal unit. This can be accomplished with blood from a fingerstick or the hub of a catheter used to start an IV line. More comprehensive blood assessments such as white blood cell, red blood cell, hemoglobin, hematocrit, and platelet values are included in a CBC. A CBC may be ordered for women with a history of infection, anemia, PIH, etc.

If the woman's blood type has not been verified, blood will be drawn to establish type and Rh factor. If blood typing was done previously, the physician/CNM may choose not to repeat the test. If obvious signs of immunocompromise or substance abuse are present, other diagnostic blood tests may be ordered.

Assessment of amniotic membranes and fluid. Labor is initiated by **spontaneous rupture of membranes (SROM, SRM)** in approximately 25% of pregnant women at term. A lag period, rarely exceeding 24 hours, may precede the onset of labor. Membranes (the bag of waters) can also rupture spontaneously any time during labor. It is the nurse's responsibility to monitor FHR for several minutes immediately after **ROM,** to ascertain fetal well-being, and to document findings. Tests for assessing ROM are discussed in the Guidelines box on p. 399. **Artificial rupture of membranes** (AROM, ARM) or **amniotomy** may be done to augment or induce labor or to facilitate placement of internal monitors when fetal status requires a direct assessment method (attachment

Guidelines

VAGINAL EXAMINATION

Vaginal examinations should include the following steps:

1. The nurse assembles all the equipment needed, including single sterile glove, antiseptic solution or soluble gel, and a light source. Water should be used for lubrication during the initial examination if ROM is suspected and a nitrazine test required.
2. The nurse prepares the woman by explaining the procedure in terms of what will be done, why it is being performed, and how it will feel. The woman should be draped to prevent chilling and protect privacy, then positioned to prevent supine hypotension (Fig. 16-3). The perineum and vulva should be cleansed if needed.
3. The nurse washes her or his hands and puts on a sterile glove following aseptic technique. The nurse explains to the woman that she will feel the nurse inserting index and middle fingers into her vagina. The examination should be performed gently, with concern for the woman's comfort. The nurse should acknowledge the woman's expressions of pain or discomfort.
4. The nurse assesses the woman for the following (Fig. 16-9):
   a. Dilation and effacement of cervix
   b. Presenting part, position, station, and, if vertex, any molding of the head
   c. Status of membranes (intact, bulging, or ruptured) and characteristics of the amniotic fluid (color, clarity, odor)
   d. Presence of stool in rectum
5. The nurse helps the woman into a comfortable position and discusses the findings of the examination with the woman/couple.
6. The nurse documents all findings and reports them to the physician or midwife.

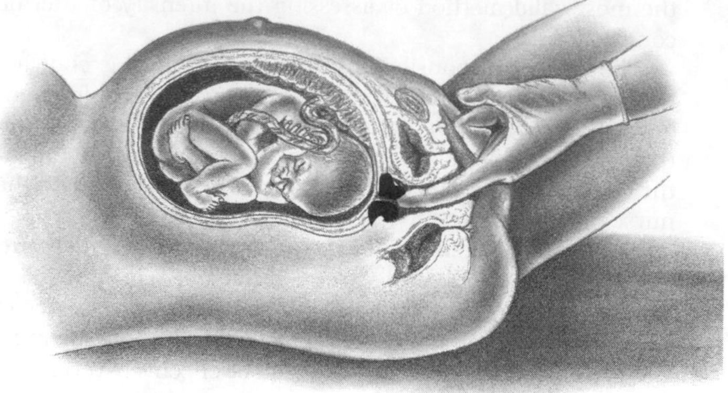

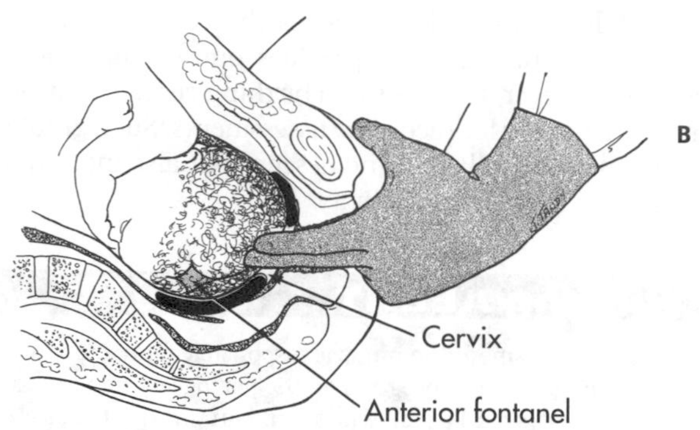

Fig. 16-9 Vaginal examination. **A,** Undilated, uneffaced cervix; membranes intact. **B,** Palpation of sagittal suture line. Cervix effaced and partially dilated.

of a cardiotachometer to the presenting part and insertion of an intrauterine pressure transducer). Amniotic fluid is assessed for the following characteristics.

COLOR. Amniotic fluid is normally pale and straw colored and may contain white particles (flecks of vernix caseosa). If the amniotic fluid is greenish brown, the fetus has probably experienced a recent hypoxic episode, causing relaxation of the anal sphincter and passage of by-products of fetal ingestion in utero called *meconium.* Yellow-stained amniotic fluid may indicate fetal hypoxia that occurred 36 hours or more before ROM, fetal hemolytic disease (Rh or ABO incompatibility), or intrauterine infection. Meconium-stained amniotic fluid may be a normal finding in a breech presentation, resulting from pressure on the fetal rectum during descent. Although meconium-stained amniotic fluid may be an ominous finding in labor, it is not always associated with fetal hypoxia and must be viewed in the context of the total clinical picture of labor (Scott et al, 1994). Amniotic fluid that is port wine colored may indicate bleeding associated with premature separation of the placenta (abruption).

VISCOSITY/ODOR. Amniotic fluid normally has a watery consistency and lacks a strong odor. If the fluid is thick, cloudy, and/or has a foul-smelling odor, infection is suspected. Large amounts of meconium can also result in amniotic fluid with a thick consistency.

AMOUNT. The expected amount of amniotic fluid is 500 to 1200 ml. Most of the amniotic fluid originates from the maternal bloodstream with additions of fetal urine. *Hydramnios* (>2000 ml of fluid) is an excessively large amount of amniotic fluid and is often associated with congenital anomalies of the fetus, resulting from the fetus's inability to drink the fluid or from fluid being trapped in the fetal body. *Oligohydramnios* (<500 ml of fluid) is an abnormally small amount of amniotic fluid and can be associated with incomplete formation or absence of the kidneys or obstruction of the urethra. If the fetus is unable to secrete and excrete urine, the volume of amniotic fluid decreases. With fetal surgery, it is now possible to correct some obstructive conditions.

INFECTION. When membranes rupture, microorganisms from the vagina can ascend into the amniotic sac. Chorioamnionitis and placentitis may develop. Even when membranes are intact, microorganisms may ascend and cause premature ROM. There is controversy regarding whether prophylactic antibiotic therapy will protect against infection (chorioamnionitis), which involves both the maternal and fetal sides of the membrane. Maternal temperature and vaginal discharge are assessed frequently (every 1 to 2 hours) for early identification of a developing infection after ROM.

The nurse's responsibility is to report findings promptly to the physician/CNM and to document findings in the labor

BOX 16-3
Signs of Potential Complications

LABOR

Intrauterine pressure >75 mm Hg (by IUPC*)
Contractions consistently lasting ≥90 sec
Contractions consistently occurring ≤2 min apart
Fetal bradycardia, tachycardia, or persistent decreased variability
Irregular FHR; suspected fetal arrhythmias
Appearance of fluid from the vagina that is meconium stained or bloody
Arrest in progress of cervical dilation/effacement and/or descent of the fetus
Maternal temperature ≥100.4° F (38° C)
Foul-smelling vaginal discharge
Persistent bright or dark red vaginal bleeding

*IUPC, Intrauterine pressure catheter.

record and on the monitor strip. If abnormal findings are obtained, continuous electronic monitoring is usually used for the duration of labor. The presence of meconium-stained amniotic fluid alerts the nurse of the necessity to observe fetal status more closely. After birth the newborn may be at high risk for alteration in respiratory status if meconium is aspirated into the lungs.

Assessment findings serve as a baseline for evaluation of the woman's progress during the first stage of labor, after she has been admitted. Although some complications of labor are anticipated, others appear only during the clinical course of labor. Knowledge of pregnancy, careful initial assessment, and follow-up of progress are necessary during normal labor as well as during a labor in which complications arise (Box 16-3).

Emergency interventions. Emergency conditions can arise with startling speed and require immediate nursing intervention. Nonreassuring FHR, inadequate uterine relaxation, vaginal bleeding, and infection are highlighted in the Emergency box on pp. 412-413. Only immediate interventions are presented. Nonreassuring FHR (see Chapter 15), inadequate uterine relaxation (see Chapter 17), and vaginal bleeding (see Chapter 9) are discussed at length in the chapters indicated. Infection does not require the same swift, emergency response; it is presented here to alert the nurse to this condition, which is potentially harmful to the fetus and mother.

Prolapse of the umbilical cord is a serious obstetric emergency that occurs most often with ROM (Fig. 16-10). This occurs in one of 400 births. Contributing factors are a long cord (>100 cm or 40 inches), malpresentation (breech), transverse lie, or unengaged presenting part.

Other predisposing factors in cord prolapse that are associated with a high presenting part are multiparity, cephalopelvic disproportion, and placenta previa.

Nursing Diagnoses

Nursing diagnoses provide direction to types of nursing actions needed to implement a plan of care. When establishing nursing diagnoses, the nurse analyzes the significance of findings collected during assessment.

Initial assessment

- Impaired verbal communication related to
  - Language barrier
- Anxiety related to
  - Knowledge deficit regarding physical examination procedures
  - Lack of previous experiences or preparation-for-parenthood classes
  - Negative experience with previous childbirth
  - Cultural differences
- Risk for injury related to
  - Inadequate prenatal care
  - Lack of prenatal testing of blood and urine
  - Inadequate forces of labor

Subsequent assessments

- Pain related to
  - Intense uterine contractions
- Fluid volume deficit related to
  - Decreased fluid intake
- Impaired physical mobility related to
  - Advanced station of fetal presenting part
  - Rupture of amniotic membranes
  - Fetal monitoring
  - Epidural anesthesia
- Altered patterns of urinary elimination related to
  - Reduced intake of oral fluids
  - Bed rest
  - Lack of privacy
  - Diminished sensation of bladder fullness
  - Epidural anesthesia/analgesia
- Risk for infection related to
  - Rupture of membranes
  - Insertion of internal monitors
  - Frequent vaginal examinations

Assessment of stress during labor

- Impaired fetal gas exchange related to
  - Maternal position
  - Hyperventilation
  - Maternal hypotension
  - Intense, frequent uterine contractions
  - Compression of umbilical cord
- Situational low maternal self-esteem related to
  - Inability to meet self-expectations
  - Loss of control during labor
- Situational low father/partner self-esteem related to
  - Unrealistic expectations regarding role as labor coach
  - Perceived ineffectiveness in meeting needs of laboring woman
- Ineffective family coping: compromised, related to
  - Knowledge deficit of comfort measures that can be used for the laboring woman

Expected Outcomes

During this important step the nurse and woman set and prioritize expected outcomes that focus on the woman/couple. Appropriate nursing and patient actions are determined to meet these expected outcomes. Planning with the woman is essential for the implementation of expected outcomes.

EMERGENCY

INTERVENTIONS FOR EMERGENCIES

Signs	*Interventions**
Nonreassuring FHR pattern	
▪ Fetal bradycardia (FHR <120 beats/min for >2 min) ▪ Fetal tachycardia (if term, FHR is >160 beats/min for >2 min) ▪ Irregular FHR, abnormal sinus rhythm with internal monitor ▪ Persistent decrease in FHR variability ▪ Late and variable deceleration patterns ▪ Absence of FHR	Notify physician/CNM† Change maternal position to side-lying Discontinue oxytocin if infusing Increase IV fluid rate if infusing Administer oxygen at 10 to 12 L/min by tight face mask Start an IV line if one is not in place
Inadequate uterine relaxation	
▪ Intrauterine pressure >75 mm Hg (by IUPC) ▪ Contractions consistently lasting >90 sec ▪ Contraction interval <2 min	Notify physician/CNM† Discontinue oxytocin (Pitocin) if infusing Change maternal position to side-lying Increase IV fluid rate if infusing Administer oxygen at 10 to 12 L/min by tight face mask Start an IV line if one is not in place Palpate and evaluate contractions Give tocolytics (terbutaline) as ordered
Vaginal bleeding	
▪ Vaginal bleeding (bright red, dark red, or in an amount exceeding that expected during normal cervical dilation) ▪ Continuous vaginal bleeding with FHR changes ▪ Pain: may or may not be present	Notify physician/CNM† Anticipate emergency (crash) cesarean delivery *Do not perform a vaginal examination*
Infection	
▪ Foul-smelling amniotic fluid ▪ Maternal temperature >100.4° F (38° C) in presence of adequate hydration (straw-colored urine) ▪ Fetal tachycardia >160 beats/min for >2 min	Notify physician/CNM† Institute cooling measures for laboring woman Start an IV line if one is not in place Assist with or perform collection of catheterized urine specimen and amniotic fluid sample and send to the laboratory for urinalysis and cultures

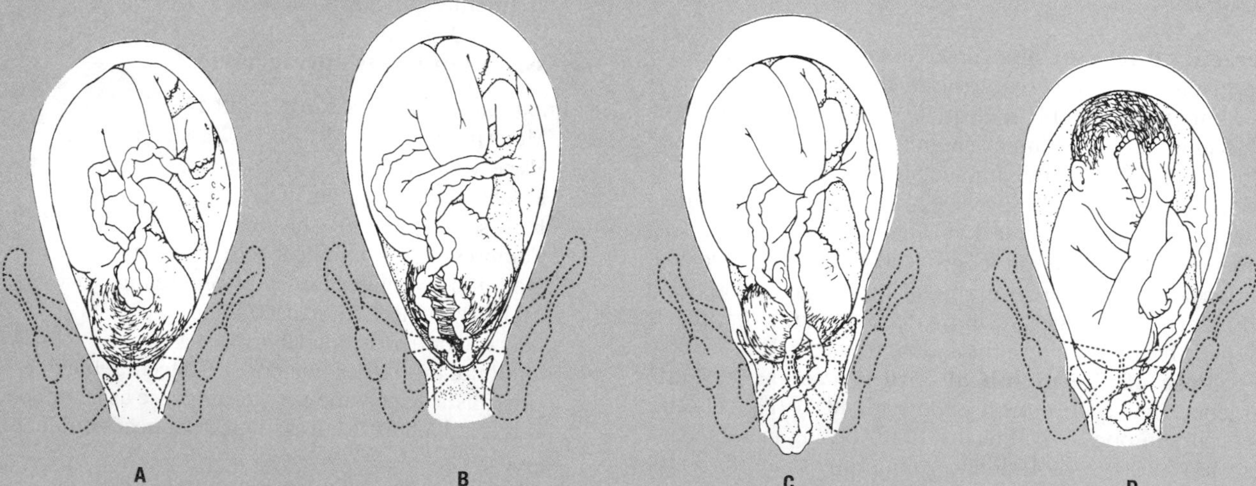

Fig. 16-10 Prolapse of umbilical cord. Note pressure of presenting part on umbilical cord, which endangers fetal circulation. **A,** Occult (hidden) prolapse of cord. **B,** Complete prolapse of cord. Note membranes are intact. **C,** Cord presenting in front of fetal head and may be seen within the vagina. **D,** Frank breech presentation with prolapsed cord.

*Since emergency situations are often frightening events, it is important for the nurse to explain to the woman and her support person(s) what is happening and how it is being managed.

†In most emergency situations, nurses take immediate action, following a protocol and standards of nursing practice. Notification of the physician/CNM can be accomplished by another person or by the nurse as soon as possible.

Signs

Prolapse of cord (Fig. 16-10)

- Fetal bradycardia with variable deceleration during uterine contraction
- Woman reports feeling the cord after membranes rupture
- Cord is seen or felt in or protruding from the vagina

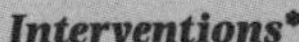

Interventions*

Call for assistance
Have someone notify the physician/CNM immediately
Glove the examining hand quickly and insert two fingers into the vagina to the cervix; with one finger on either side of the cord or both fingers to one side, exert upward pressure against the presenting part to relieve compression of the cord (Fig. 16-11, *A* and *B*); place a rolled towel under the woman's hip
Place woman into extreme Trendelenburg's or modified Sims position (Fig. 16-11, *C*) or knee-chest position (Fig. 16-11, *D*)
If the cord is protruding from the vagina, wrap it loosely in a sterile towel wet with warm sterile normal saline solution
Administer oxygen to the woman by mask, 10 to 12 L/min, until birth is accomplished
Start IV fluids or increase existing drip rate
Continue to monitor FHR by internal spiral electrode if possible

Fig. 16-11 Arrows indicate direction of pressure against presenting part to relieve compression of prolapsed umbilical cord. Pressure exerted by examiner's fingers in **A**, vertex presentation, and **B**, breech position. **C**, Gravity relieves pressure with a woman in modified Sims position with hips elevated as high as possible with pillows. **D**, Knee-chest position.

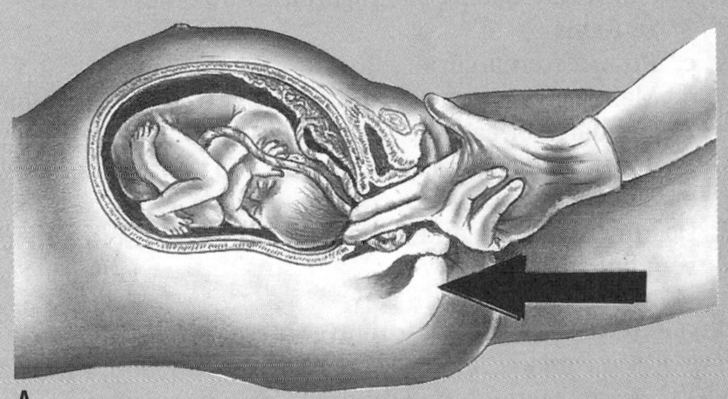

A

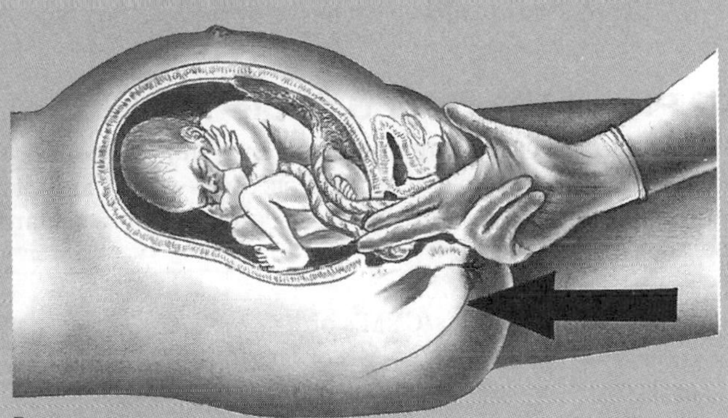

B

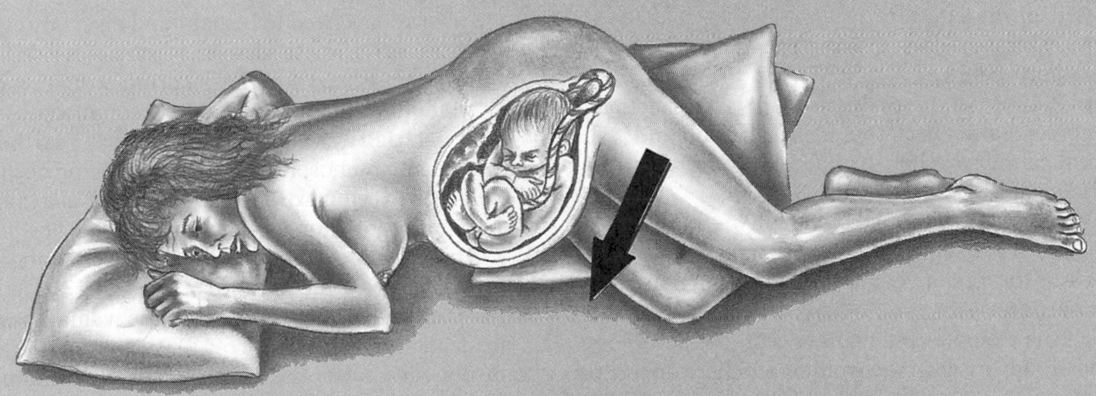

C

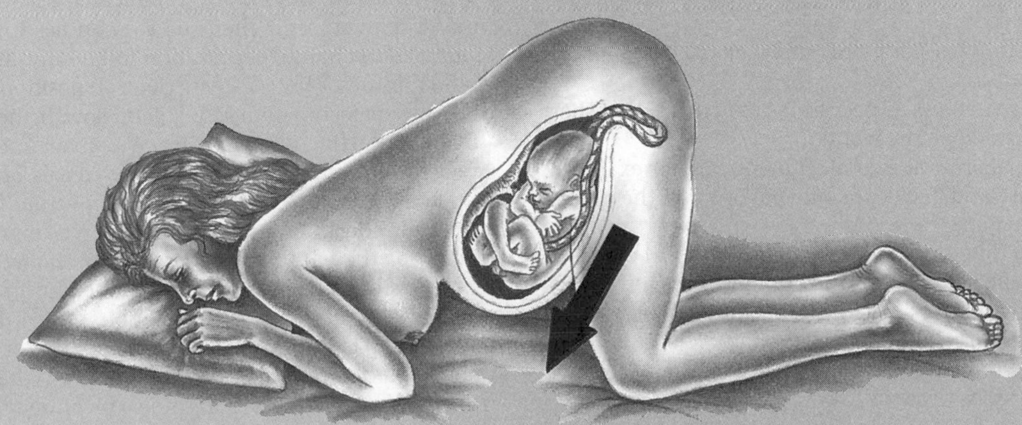

D

Throughout the first stage of labor the woman will accomplish the following:

1. Demonstrate expected progression of labor
2. Express satisfaction with the assistance of her support person(s)/family and nursing staff
3. Verbalize her desires for participation in labor and participate as tolerated throughout labor
4. Continue normal progression of labor while the FHR remains within normal range and without distress signs
5. Maintain adequate hydration status through oral and/or intravenous intake
6. Void at least every 2 hours to prevent bladder distention
7. Encourage participation of support person by verbalizing discomfort and indicating measures that help reduce discomfort and promote relaxation
8. Express satisfaction with her performance during labor

Plan of Care and Implementation

Standards of care. Standards of care guide the nurse in preparing for and implementing procedures with the expectant mother (Box 16-1). Protocols for care based on standards include the following:

1. Check the physician's/CNM's orders.
2. Assess the physician's/CNM's orders for appropriateness and correctness; for example, analgesic administration for discomfort.
3. Check labels on IV solutions, medications, and other materials used for nursing care.
4. Check the expiration date on any packs of supplies used for ordered procedures.
5. Ensure that information on the woman's identification band is correct (also check that identification band is accurate, indicating whether she has allergies, and of the appropriate color).
6. Employ an empathic approach when giving care, as follows:
   a. Use words the woman can understand when explaining procedures
   b. Respect the woman's individual needs and behaviors
   c. Establish rapport with the woman and her support person(s)/family
   d. Be kind, caring, and competent when performing necessary procedures
   e. Be aware that pain and discomfort are as the woman describes
   f. Repeat instructions as necessary and ensure that they are understood by the woman
   g. Carry out appropriate comfort measures, for example, mouth care and back care, and ensure that the support person is coping
   h. Recognize that a woman's current childbirth experience and the actions of nurses and other health care providers can have a positive or negative effect on the woman's future childbirth experiences
7. Use Standard Precautions, including precautions for invasive procedures as needed.
8. Document care according to hospital guidelines and communicate information to the physician/CNM when indicated.

LEGAL TIP

Standards of Care for Labor

1. Provide explanations to woman/family for all procedures.
2. Assess maternal and fetal status, as well as progress of labor.
   a. Continue to monitor fetal status until birth
   b. Document all assessment findings
   c. Notify physician/CNM promptly regarding assessment findings, especially those which are unexpected/abnormal
   d. Inform woman/family regarding maternal and fetal status as well as progress of labor
3. Intervene based on analysis of assessment data.
   a. Carry out all orders/protocols for care
   b. Notify physician/CNM regarding outcomes of interventions
   c. Protect woman from injury
   d. Maintain competency and currency of skills to uphold standards of care
4. Evaluate effectiveness of care given and revise care based on assessment.
5. Document all care and responses of the woman to interventions.

Physical nursing care during labor. Physical nursing care of the woman in labor is an essential function. Physical needs, nursing actions, and rationale for care are presented in Table 16-4.

Labor rooms need to be light and airy; however, the bright overhead lights are turned off when not needed. The temperature is controlled for the laboring woman's comfort. The room should be large enough to accommodate a comfortable chair for the woman's partner as well as the monitoring equipment and hospital personnel. In some hospitals, couples are urged to bring extra pillows to help make the hospital surroundings more homelike and to facilitate position changes.

Ambulation and positioning. Ambulation ad lib may be encouraged if membranes are intact, if the fetal presenting part is engaged after ROM, and if the woman has not received medication for pain (Fig. 16-12). Walking, sitting, or standing during early labor has been shown to be more comfortable than lying down (Melzack, Belanger, and Lacroix, 1991).

Ambulation may be contraindicated because of maternal and/or fetal status. When the woman lies in bed, she is encouraged to change her position frequently, at least every 30 to 60 minutes. The side-lying (lateral) position promotes optimal uteroplacental and renal blood flow. If the woman wants to lie supine, the nurse may place a pillow under one hip as a wedge to prevent pressure from the uterus on the aorta and vena cava (Fig. 16-3). Sitting is not contraindicated unless it adversely affects fetal status, which can be observed by visualization of the fetal monitor tracing. If the fetus is in the occiput posterior position, it may be helpful to encourage the woman to squat during contractions, since this position increases pelvic diameter, allowing rotation of the head to a more anterior position (Fig. 16-13, *A*). A hands-and-knees position during contractions is also recommended to facilitate

TABLE 16-4 Physical nursing care during labor

NEED	NURSING ACTIONS	RATIONALE
General hygiene		
Showers/bed baths	Assess for progress in labor	Determines appropriateness for the activity
Whirlpool bath	Supervise showers closely if woman is in true labor	Prevents injury from fall; labor may accelerate
	Suggest allowing warm water to flow over back	Aids relaxation; increases comfort
Perineum	Perform mini-prep (shave, clip hair on perineum) if ordered	Facilitates cutting and repair of episiotomy; however, may increase risk of infection
Oral hygiene	Offer toothbrush, mouthwash, or wash the teeth with an ice-cold, wet washcloth as needed	Refreshes mouth; improves morale; helps counteract dry, thirsty feeling
Hair	Brush, braid per woman's wishes	Improves morale; increases comfort
Hand washing	Offer washclothes before and after voiding and as needed	Maintains cleanliness; improves morale and comfort
Face	Offer cool washcloth	Improves morale; relief from diaphoresis
Gowns/linens	Change prn; fluff pillows	Improves morale and comfort
Fluid intake		
Oral	Offer fluids, small amounts of ice chips, or lollipops following orders of physician/certified nurse midwife (CNM)	Meets standard of care; provides hydration; provides calories; absorbs quickly and is less likely to be vomited; provides positive emotional experience
IV	Establish and maintain IV infusion as ordered	Maintains hydration; provides venous access for medications
Nothing by mouth (NPO)	Inform family of NPO and rationale	A precautionary measure if general anesthesia is a possibility; may deter vomiting and its possible sequelae
	Provide oral care	Promotes comfort; limits dryness of mouth and thirst
Elimination		
Voiding	Encourage voiding at least every 2 hours	A full bladder may impede descent of presenting part; overdistention may cause bladder atony and injury as well as postnatal voiding difficulty
Ambulatory woman	Allow ambulation to bathroom per order of physician/CNM *if:*	Reinforces normal process of urination
	The presenting part is engaged	Precautionary measure against prolapse of umbilical cord
	The membranes are not ruptured	
	The woman is not medicated	Precautionary measure against injury
Woman on bed rest	Offer bedpan	Prevents hazards of bladder distention and ambulation
	Turn on the tap water to run; pour warm water over the vulva; and give positive suggestion	Encourages voiding
	Provide privacy	Shows respect for woman
	Put up side rails on bed	Prevents injury from fall
	Place call bell within reach	
	Offer washcloth for hands	Maintains cleanliness and comfort
	Wash vulvar area	Maintains standard of care
Catheterization	Catheterize according to physician/CNM order or hospital protocols, if unable to void	Prevents hazards of bladder distention
	Insert catheter between contractions	Minimizes discomfort
	Avoid force if obstacle to insertion is noted	"Obstacle" may be caused by compression of urethra by presenting part
	If presenting part is low, introduce two fingers of free hand into introitus to apply upward pressure on presenting part while other hand inserts the catheter	Minimizes potential for injury and subsequent infection to urethra
Bowel elimination—feeling of rectal pressure	Ambulate the woman to bathroom or offer her a bedpan after careful assessment	Avoids misinterpretation of rectal pressure from the presenting part as the need to defecate

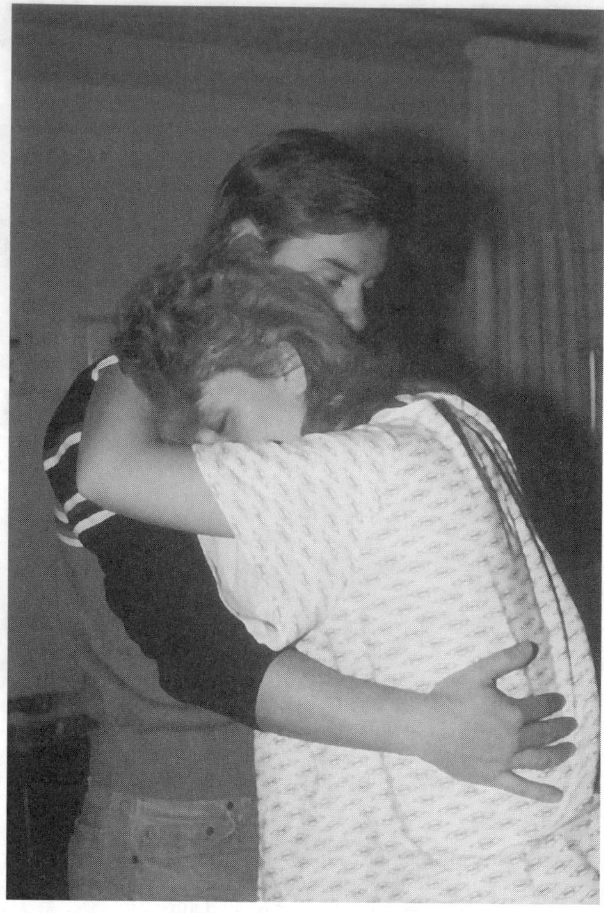

Fig. 16-12 Woman standing and leaning with partner for support. (Courtesy Marjorie Pyle, RNC, Lifecircle, Costa Mesa, Calif.)

the rotation of the fetal occiput from a posterior to an anterior position as gravity pulls the fetal back forward.

Research is being directed toward a better understanding of the physiologic and psychic effects of maternal position in labor. Fetal presentations and mechanisms of labor may be helped or hindered by maternal posture (Andrews and Chrzanowski, 1990; Biancuzzo, 1993; Liu, 1989; McKay and Roberts, 1989). Box 16-4 describes the various positions recommended for the laboring woman.

Support measures. Effective physical and emotional support provided to women during labor can result in shorter labors, reduced rates of complications and surgical/obstetric interventions (e.g., cesarean births, labor augmentations and inductions, episiotomies, forceps), and enhanced self-esteem and satisfaction (Kennell et al, 1991; Pascoe, 1993).

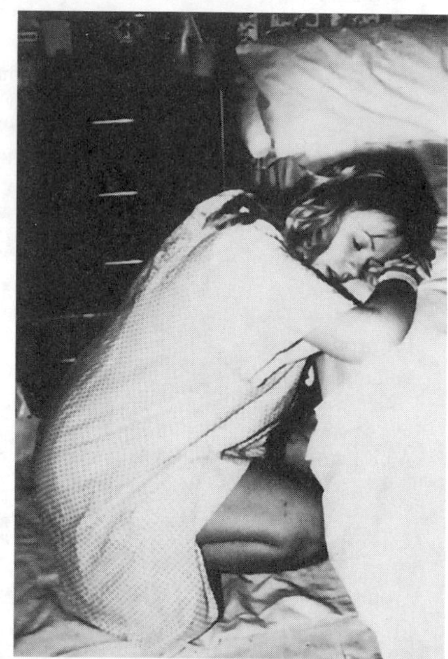

A

Fig. 16-13 Maternal positions for labor. **A,** Squatting. **B,** Woman in a knees-chest position. **C,** Woman in rocking chair using focusing and breathing with coaching from partner. (Courtesy Marjorie Pyle, RNC, Lifecircle, Costa Mesa, Calif.)

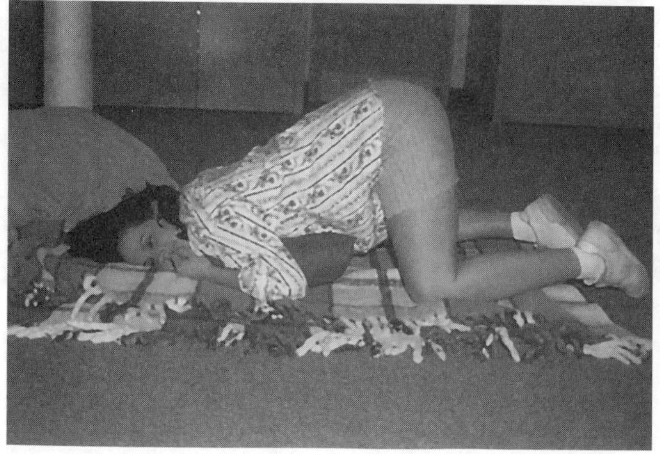

B

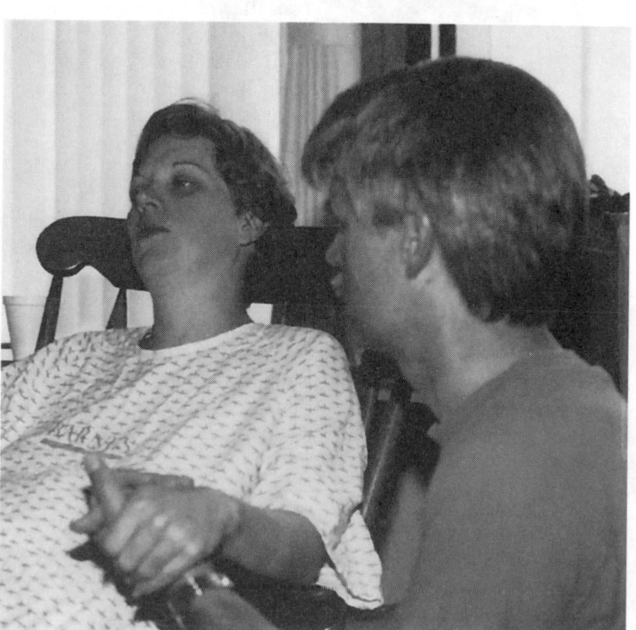

C

BOX 16-4
Some Maternal Positions During Labor and Birth*

Semi-recumbent position
- Sitting with upper body elevated to at least a 30-degree angle, place wedge/small pillow under hip to prevent vena caval compression and reduce incidence of supine hypotension
- The greater the angle of elevation, the more gravity/pressure is applied to enhance fetal descent, progress of contractions, and widening of pelvic dimensions
- Convenient for care measures and external fetal monitoring

Lateral position
- Alternate between left and right side-lying position, providing abdominal and back support as needed for comfort
- Removes pressure from the vena cava and back—enhances uteroplacental perfusion and relieves backache
- Easier to perform back massage or **counterpressure**
- Associated with less frequent, but more intense contractions
- Obtaining good external fetal monitor tracings may be more difficult
- May be used as a birthing position

Upright position
- Gravity effect enhances contraction cycle and fetal descent: fetus increases pressure on cervix; the cervix is pulled upward, facilitating effacement and dilation; impulses from cervix to pituitary gland increase, causing oxytocin to be secreted in greater amount; contractions are intensified, thereby applying more forceful downward pressure on fetus
- Fetus is aligned with pelvis and pelvic diameters are widened slightly
- Effective upright positions include:
  Ambulation
  Standing and leaning forward with support from coach (Fig. 16-12), end of bed, back of chair; relieves backache and facilitates counterpressure/back massage (Fig. 16-14, *B*)
  Sitting up in bed, chair, birthing chair (see Fig. 16-13, *C*)
  Squatting (see Fig. 16-13, *A*)

Hands-and-knees position
- Ideal position for posterior positions of the presenting part
- Assume an "all-fours" position in bed or on a covered floor
- Relieves backache characteristic of "back labor"
- Facilitates internal rotation of the fetus; increases mobility of coccyx, increases pelvic diameters; and applies the force of gravity to turn the fetal back and rotate the head

*Assess the effect of each position on the laboring woman's comfort and anxiety level, progress of labor, and FHR pattern. Alternate positions every 30 minutes to 1 hour.

Nursing ALERT

The nurse can alleviate a woman's anxiety by explaining unfamiliar terms, providing information and explanations, and preparing her for sensations and procedures that will follow.

By encouraging the woman or couple to ask questions and by providing honest, understandable answers, the nurse can play a significant role in achieving a satisfying birth experience. The learning needs a woman in labor identifies should be met by the nurse managing her care (Evans and Jeffery, 1995).

Supportive nursing care for a woman in labor includes (1) helping the woman to maintain control and participate to the extent she wishes in the birth of her infant; (2) meeting the woman's expected outcomes; (3) acting as the woman's advocate, supporting her decisions as appropriate and expressing her wishes as needed to other health care providers; (4) helping the woman conserve her energy; (5) helping control the woman's discomfort; and (5) acknowledging the woman's efforts during labor and providing positive reinforcement.

Couples who have attended childbirth education programs using the psychoprophylactic approach will know something about the labor process, coaching techniques, and comfort measures. The nurse should play a supportive role and keep the couple informed of progress. Even if the expectant parents have not attended classes, various techniques may be taught during the early phase of labor. In this case the nurse will be expected to do more of the coaching and give supportive care.

The nurse serves as a coach to the woman in the absence of other support persons or as an assistant coach to the support persons present. The nurse must have a thorough knowledge of breathing and relaxation techniques to assist the woman and her partner in coping with labor.

Comfort measures vary with the situation (Fig. 16-14). The nurse can draw on the couple's repertoire of comfort measures learned during the pregnancy. Comfort measures include maintaining a comfortable, supportive atmosphere in the labor and birth area; using touch therapeutically (e.g., warmth and counterpressure to the lower back in the case of back labor, a cool cloth to the forehead); providing nonpharmacologic management of discomfort; and administering analgesics when necessary; but, most of all, just *being there* (Table 16-5).

The woman's awareness of the soothing qualities of touch changes as labor progresses. Many women develop hyperesthesia (increased sensitivity, especially in the skin) as labor progresses. They may tell their coach to "leave me alone," or they may say, "Don't touch me." The partner who is unprepared for this normal response may feel rejected and may react by withdrawing active support. The nurse can point out that this response on the part of the woman is a positive indication that the first stage is ending and the second stage is approaching. Hyperesthesia is typical during the transition phase (Table 16-3). The woman's assertive behavior is accepted; negative comments toward the woman are unwarranted and inappropriate (Table 16-5).

Relaxation measures are often learned in childbirth classes. Guided imagery, music, and soothing massage are helpful techniques to use during labor. These techniques can

TABLE 16-5 Woman's expected responses and supportive care during labor

WOMAN	SUPPORTIVE CARE*
Dilation of cervix 0 to 3 cm (latent) (contractions 10 to 45 sec long, 3 to 30 min apart, mild to moderate)	
Mood: alert, happy, excited, mild anxiety Settles into labor room; selects focal point Rests or sleeps, if possible Uses breathing techniques Uses effleurage, focusing, and relaxation techniques	Provide encouragement, feedback for relaxation, companionship Assist to cope with contractions Encourage use of focusing techniques Help to concentrate on breathing techniques Use comfort measures Assist woman into comfortable position Inform woman of progress, explain procedures and routines Give praise Offer fluids, ice chips as ordered
Dilation of cervix 4 to 7 cm (active) (contractions 30 to 45 sec long, 3 to 5 min apart, moderate to strong)	
Mood: seriously labor oriented, concentration and energy needed for contractions, alert, more demanding Continues relaxation, focusing techniques Uses breathing techniques	Act as buffer, limit assessment techniques to between contractions Assist with contractions Encourage woman as needed to help her maintain breathing techniques Use comfort measures Assist with frequent position changes, emphasizing side-lying and upright positions Encourage voluntary relaxation of muscles of back, buttocks, thighs, and perineum; effleurage Apply counterpressure to sacrococcygeal area Encourage and praise Keep woman aware of progress Offer analgesics as ordered Check bladder, encourage woman to void Give oral care; offer fluids, ice chips as ordered
Dilation of cervix 8 to 10 cm (transition) (contractions 45 to 90 sec long, 2 to 3 min apart, strong)	
Mood: irritable, intense concentration, symptoms of transition (e.g., nausea, vomiting) Continues relaxation, needs greater concentration to do this Uses breathing techniques 4:1 breathing pattern if using psychoprophylactic techniques Panting to overcome urge to push	Stay with woman, provide constant support Assist with contractions Remind, reassure, and encourage woman to reestablish breathing pattern and concentration as needed Alert woman to begin breathing pattern before contraction becomes too intense, if she is sedated or drowsy Prompt panting respirations, if woman begins to push prematurely Use comfort measures Accept woman's inability to comply with instructions Accept irritable response to helping, such as counterpressure Support woman who has nausea and vomiting, give oral care as needed, give reassurance regarding signs of end of first stage Use relaxation techniques (effleurage and voluntary relaxation) Keep woman aware of progress

*Provided by nurses and support persons in collaboration with the nurse.

provide comfort, prevent fatigue, and conserve energy for the expulsive work of the second stage of labor. Today, many health care providers advocate the use of warm water (e.g., whirlpool bath, shower) for its soothing, relaxing effects (Aderhold and Perry, 1991; Rosenthal, 1991). Many new birthing units are installing baths with air jets. The buoyancy of the warm water, with or without air jets, provides support for tense muscles (see Fig. 14-3).

The father/partner during labor. Although females or other males may be the woman's partner during labor, this discussion focuses on the father of the baby, since he is most often the person who supports the woman during labor. The father of the baby is able to provide the comfort measures and touch that the laboring woman needs. When the woman becomes focused on her pain, sometimes the partner can persuade her to try nonpharmacologic variations of comfort measures. He usually is able to interpret the woman's needs and desires to staff members.

Throughout the last 20 years, childbirth preparation has been widely practiced. The ideal father's role was thought to be that of labor coach. Fathers were expected to actively help the woman cope with labor. This expectation may be unrealistic for all men because some men have concerns about their labor coaching abilities (Berry, 1988). Chapman (1992) reported at least three roles adopted by men during labor and

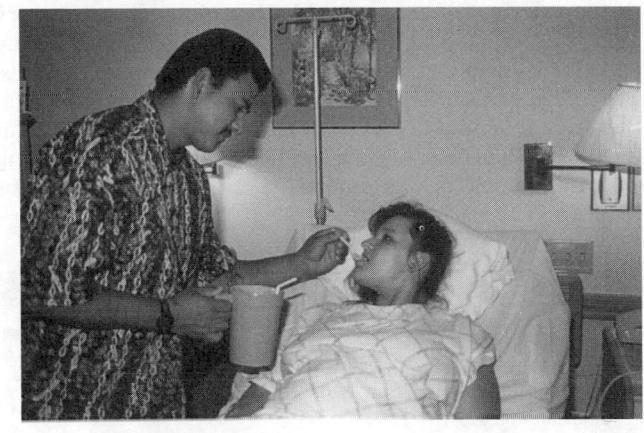

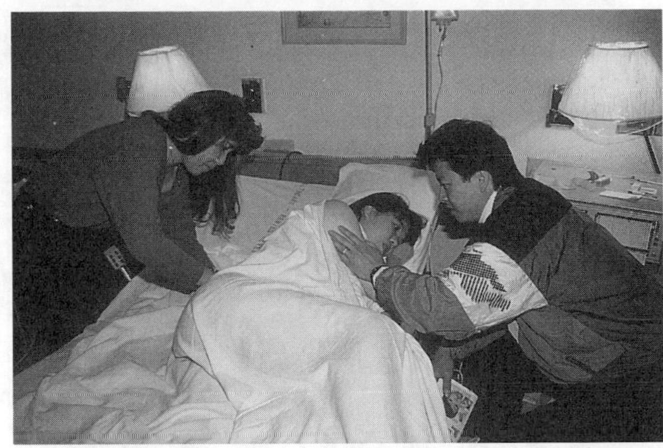

Fig. 16-14 **A,** Partner providing comfort measures. **B,** Lateral position. Support person applying sacral pressure while partner provides encouragement. (Courtesy Marjorie Pyle, RNC, Lifecircle, Costa Mesa, Calif.)

birth: coach, teammate, and witness. As the *coach,* the father actively assists the woman during and after contractions. Coaches express a strong need to be in control of themselves and of the labor experience. Women express a high desire for the father to be physically involved in labor. The father acting as the *teammate* assists the woman during labor and birth by responding to requests for physical or emotional support or both. Teammates usually adopt the follower or helper role and look to the woman or nurse to tell them what to do. Women express a strong desire to have the father present and willing to help in any way. In the role of *witness* the father acts as a companion and gives emotional and moral support. He watches the woman labor and give birth, but he often sleeps, watches television, or leaves the room for long periods of time. Witnesses believe that there is little they can do to physically help the woman and look to the nurses and other health care providers to be in charge of the experience. Women do not expect the father to do more than be present.

The degree of mutuality (level of interdependency and sharing) and understanding (the ability to know each other's needs) in a couple's relationship determines which role the father adopts. The coach and teammate roles are often adopted by men in couples with a high degree of mutuality. Men in relationships where mutuality is low tend to adopt the witness role.

Since a father/partner can participate in labor and birth in different ways, nurses need to encourage him to adopt the role most comfortable for him and for the woman, rather than an artificial role.

The father/partner will be exposed to many sights and smells he may never before have experienced. It is important to tell him what to expect and to make him comfortable about leaving the room to gather his composure should something shock him. First, of course, provision should be made for someone else to support the woman during his absence. Staff members must verbalize that the father's presence is helpful and encourage his involvement in the care of his partner to the extent of his comfort level. This is especially true when his partner has just snapped at him and told him to go away. The nurse can reassure the father that this is normal behavior for a woman in transition and that if he reenters after a few minutes, the woman will ask him why he was gone so long (Nichols, 1993).

Participation in the birth is ego building. The father can be of assistance; his presence is important. For example, a 16-year-old mother in labor with her first child thrashed about, moaning and screaming with each contraction. A nurse remained at her bedside, coaching and comforting to no avail. The adolescent father arrived and was immediately escorted into her room. The young woman continued her labor calmly and without medication through the birth.

Support of the father/partner reflects the nurse's orientation and commitment to each person, the family, and the community. Therapeutic nursing actions convey several important concepts to the father (see the Guidelines box on p. 420).

A well-informed father/partner can make a significant contribution to the health and well-being of the mother and child, their family relationship, and his self-esteem (Queenan, 1990). A significantly lower percentage of women suffer postpartum emotional upsets when their partners receive support and assistance from parent education classes, physicians, midwives, and nurses throughout the childbearing cycle.

Culture and father participation. The presence of a companion is an important source of support, encouragement, and comfort for women during childbirth. The nurse managing care for pregnant women needs to help these women identify the person(s) they wish to be their supportive companions during childbirth. The choice of birth companion is influenced by the woman's cultural and religious background and by trends occurring within the society in which she lives. For example, Western societies increasingly view the father as the ideal birth companion (Chalmers and Meyer, 1994). For European-American couples, attending childbirth classes together has become a traditional, expected activity—a rite of passage (Finn, 1994). Laotian (Hmong) husbands actively participate in the labor process often by supporting their wife's position, catching the baby as he or she emerges, cutting the cord, and burying the placenta (D'Avanzo, 1992). A Mormon woman expects her husband to be present during her labor and to lay his hands on her head in a blessing that

Guidelines

SUPPORT OF FATHER/PARTNER

The nurse can support the father/partner in the following ways:

- Regardless of the degree of involvement desired, orient him to the maternity unit, restroom, cafeteria, waiting room, nursery, visiting hours, and names and functions of personnel present. Orient him to the woman's labor room and discuss what he can do there (e.g., sleep, telephone).
- Respect his or the couple's decisions as to his degree of involvement, whether the decision is active participation in the birthing room or just being kept informed. When appropriate, provide data on which he or they can base decisions; offer freedom of choice as opposed to coercion one way or another. This is *their* experience and *their* baby.
- Indicate to him when his presence has been helpful and continue to reinforce this throughout labor.
- Offer to teach him comfort measures to the degree he wants to know them. Reassure him that he is not assuming the responsibility for observation and management of his partner's labor; rather his responsibility is to support her as she progresses.
- Communicate with him frequently regarding the woman's progress and her needs. Keep him informed of procedures to be performed, what to expect from procedures, and what is expected of him.
- Prepare him for changes in the woman's behavior and physical appearance.
- Remind him to eat; offer snacks and fluids if possible.
- Relieve him as necessary; offer blankets if he is to sleep in a chair by the bedside. Acknowledge the stress of the situation on each partner and identify normal responses. The nonjudgmental attitude of staff members helps the father and mother accept their own and each other's behavior.
- Attempt to modify or eliminate unsettling stimuli such as extra noise, extra light, and chatter.

imparts strength, comfort, and well-being for safe passage through childbirth (Callister, 1992; 1995). In some cultures the father may be available, but his presence with the mother in the labor room may not be appropriate or he may be present but resist active involvement in her care. His behavior could be misunderstood by the nursing staff as lack of concern, caring, or interest. Latina women expect their male partner to be present at their bedside during labor, to talk to them, to keep them calm, and to tell them everything is going to be okay and not to worry. The men are expected to show love and affection by telling the woman they love them, by hugging them, and by holding their hand. Latino men do not become actively involved in giving their partners care during labor by performing such activities as backrubs and helping with pushing (Khazoyan and Anderson, 1994). Lantican and Corona (1992) identify the importance of the affectional bond between Mexican-American and Filipino women and their female relatives in regard to home-related activities like childbearing. This is also true for many other cultural groups. The presence of another woman or women is highly desired for these activities. Among some cultures, if childbearing occurs in the hospital, at least one woman is desired to be present for assistance. Vietnamese and Chinese women prefer a female companion during childbirth and are very concerned about their modesty (D'Avanzo, 1992). Islamic women are very modest as well and would not accept a male presence during childbirth, including their male partner/husband (Woods, 1991). Religious beliefs of some Orthodox Jews forbid the father from touching his wife during labor or being present at the birth. While he prays, the female members of the laboring woman's family act as supportive childbirth companions (Callister, 1995).

Nursing ALERT

Because of the variation in the choice of the preferred person or persons, it is imperative for the nurse to determine from the woman and her family which persons are wanted during labor and birth.

Support of the grandparents. Especially in situations where the grandparents take the place of the father as labor coach, it is important to support them and treat them with respect. They may have a way to deal with pain based on their experience. They need to be given a chance to help if their actions will not compromise the status of the mother or the fetus. The nurse acts as a role model for parents by treating grandparents with dignity and respect, by acknowledging the value of their contributions to parental support, and by recognizing the difficulty parents have in witnessing their child's discomfort or crisis, regardless of the age of that child.

Of particular value is the availability of another person or persons to relieve the father or coach. This may be necessary to assist the woman in labor with walking, especially if IV poles are to be pushed, as well as to help the woman when she needs two tasks performed simultaneously.

Whenever possible the nurse offers the grandparents emotional support. A nurse can show support by providing liquid refreshment, even if unsolicited, and by initiating discussion with open-ended questions or statements, such as "It is sometimes hard to watch a daughter in labor. . . ." Nursing actions that provide support for the grandparents can have a therapeutic effect on all members of the family. A strong, supportive family unit is important for the optimum growth and development of its newest member.

Siblings during labor. Preparation for acceptance of the new child helps with the attachment process. Parents, brothers, sisters, and other extended family members benefit from *cognitive rehearsal* for the new addition to the family. Preparation for and participation during pregnancy and labor may help the older children accept this change. Rehearsal for the event before labor is essential. Preparation for the entire family includes the additional support person who is to be responsible for the older children throughout the childbirth process.

The age and developmental level of children influence their responses, therefore preparation is adjusted to meet each child's needs. The child younger than 2 years of age shows little interest in pregnancy and labor; for the older child the experience may reduce fears and misconceptions. Most parents have a "feel" for the maturational level and ability to cope of their children. Preparation can include a description of anticipated sights and sounds, a birth demonstration, a tour of the birthing unit, and an introduction to a real newborn (Jonquil,

1993). The children must learn that their mother will be working hard. She will not be able to talk to them during contractions. She may groan and pant at times. Labor is uncomfortable, but their mother's body is made for the job. The sights, sounds, smells, and behavior of participants will be similar to those for which fathers are prepared. Story books can be used to prepare younger children. Films for preparing older preschool and school-age children to participate in the birth experience are available.

Preparation for giving birth. The first stage of labor ends with 100% effacement and complete dilation of the cervix. For many multiparous women, birth occurs within minutes of complete dilation, perhaps only one push later. Nulliparous women usually push for 1 to 2 hours before giving birth. If the woman has epidural anesthesia, pushing can last more than 2 hours. The nurse begins preparation for birth when a multiparous woman is 6 to 8 cm dilated because progression through the last few centimeters of dilation can occur rapidly. Factors that influence the process are fetal position (e.g., occiput posterior) and size in relation to previous babies.

To prepare for birth in any setting, the birth table or case cart is usually set up during the transition phase of nulliparous women and during the active phase for multiparous women. (See Fig. 16-17 for a table setup.) A radiant warmer for the newborn is turned on when crowning begins to occur in the nulliparous woman and when the multiparous woman is 8 to 9 cm dilated. If a traditional delivery room is used, a multiparous woman is usually transferred near the end of the first stage of labor. Transfer of the nulliparous woman takes place when the presenting part begins to distend the perineum between contractions during the second stage of labor (Fig. 16-15, *A*). Transfer to the delivery room is unnecessary in labor-delivery rooms (LDRs), labor-delivery-recovery-postpartum (LDRP) rooms, and birth centers.

All nursing care and the woman's or couple's responses during this time continue to be documented to ensure continuity of care, ensure appropriate assessment of the woman's progress, and document the nursing and other care given. According to courts of law, nursing and medical care that is not

Guidelines

PREPARATION FOR BIRTH

The following are suggestions for preparation for birth. These items may vary among different facilities; therefore the protocols from each facility's procedure manual should be consulted:

1. Scrubbing facilities, scrub brushes, cuticle sticks, cleaning agent, and masks with shield or protective glasses/goggles are available.
2. The following tasks have been done:
   a. Sterile gowns and gloves for the physician/CNM, sterile drapes and towels for draping the woman, and sterile instruments and other supplies (such as bulb syringes, sutures, and anesthetic solutions) are arranged on a sterile table for convenient use.
   b. Sterile basin and water for hand washing during the birth process are readied for use.
   c. Supplies for cleansing vulva are available (sterile basin, sterile water, and cleaning solution).
   d. Birth area is warmed and free of drafts.
   e. Infant identification materials have been readied.
   f. Infant receiving blankets and heated crib are readied. Material for prophylactic care of infant's eyes and vitamin K injection are available.
3. Equipment is in working order: birth table (birthing bed or chair), overhead lights, and mirror.
4. Emergency equipment, anesthetic, laryngoscope, and supplies are available and in working order as needed for emergency situations such as control of maternal hemorrhage or fetal respiratory distress.
5. Additional supplies (anesthetics, oxytocics for injection, obstetric forceps, and vacuum extractor) are available.
6. Woman's record is up to date and ready for use in the birth area. In areas such as the labor unit, recordings are made as symptoms are noted, assessments are made, and care is given. It is imperative to have recordings complete at all times.
7. Specific orders of the physician/CNM regarding labor and birth procedures are followed.

A

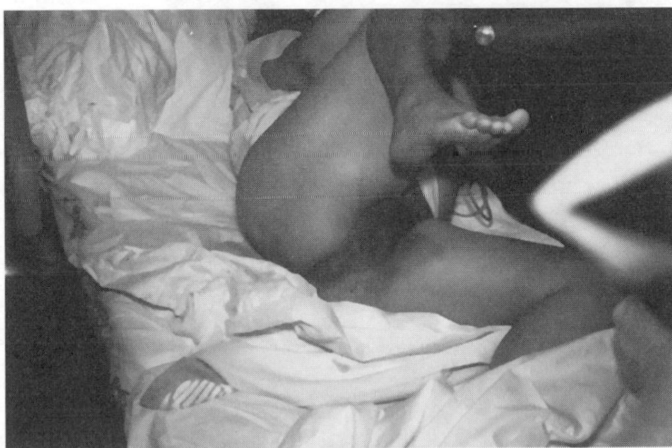

B

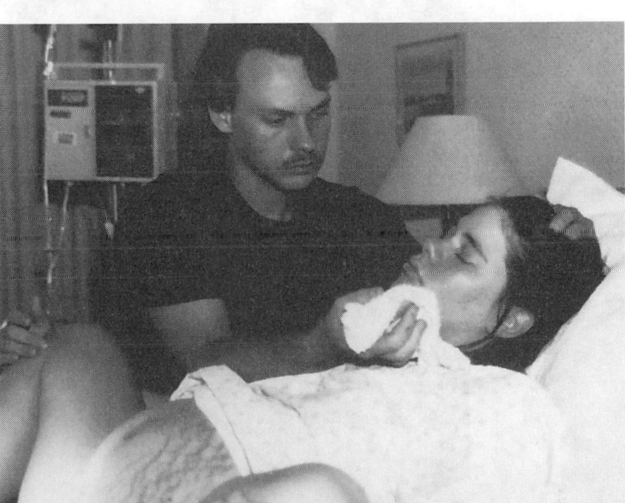

Fig. 16-15 **A**, Pushing, side-lying position, perineal bulging. **B**, Pushing, semi-sitting. Partner wiping woman's face with cool cloth between contractions. (**A**, courtesy Michael S. Clement, MD, Mesa, Ariz. **B**, courtesy Marjorie Pyle, RNC, Lifecircle, Costa Mesa, Calif.)

documented on the patient's record may not have been given (see the Guidelines box on p. 421).

The nurse estimates the time of birth and notifies the physician/CNM. Even the most experienced nurse can underestimate the time left before the birth occurs.

Nursing ALERT

Every nurse who attends a woman in labor must be prepared to perform an emergency birth if the physician/CNM is not present (see p. 426).

Significant changes have occurred in the location where birth takes place. A 1991 survey reported that more than half of all pregnant women give birth somewhere other than the traditional labor and delivery room (American College of Obstetricians and Gynecologists, 1993). The most common change in birth settings is the LDRP room, where the woman stays during her entire hospitalization (Fig. 16-16). This avoids the confusion of multiple transfers of the woman from labor room to delivery room to recovery room. Another option is the LDR room, in which the woman stays during her labor and immediate postpartum recovery period (1 to 2 hours) and

A

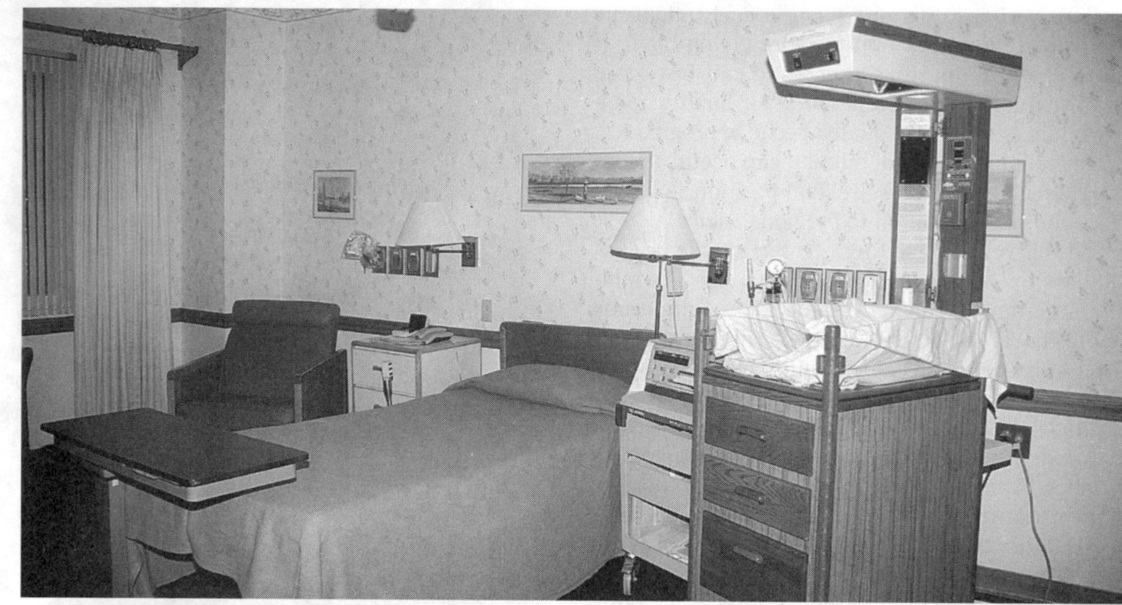

B

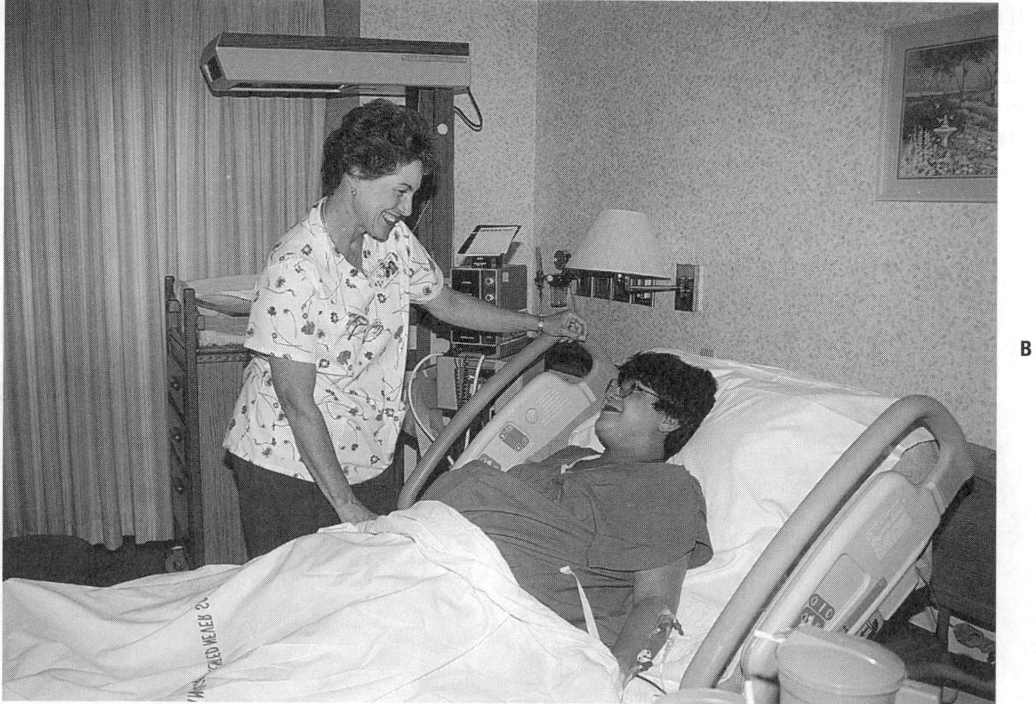

Fig. 16-16 Examples of a labor, delivery, recovery, postpartum (LDRP) room. (**A** courtesy Michael S. Clement, MD, Mesa, Ariz; **B** courtesy Marjorie Pyle, RNC, Lifecircle, Costa Mesa, Calif.)

Nursing Care Plan

FIRST STAGE OF LABOR

Nursing Diagnosis: Anxiety related to labor and the birthing process

Expected outcome: Patient exhibits decreased signs of anxiety.

• NURSING INTERVENTIONS/*RATIONALES*

Orient woman to labor and delivery suite and explain admission protocol *to allay initial feelings of anxiety.*

Assess woman's knowledge, experience, and expectations of labor; note any signs or expressions of anxiety, nervousness, or fear *to establish a baseline for intervention.*

Discuss the expected progression of labor and describe what to expect during the process *as knowledge can allay anxiety associated with the unknown.*

Actively involve woman in care decisions during labor, interpret sights and sounds of environment (monitor sights and sounds, unit activities), and share information on progression of labor (vital signs, FHR, dilation, effacement) *to increase her sense of control and allay fears.*

Actively involve significant others in care during labor *to help woman cope with the process.*

Nursing Diagnosis: Pain related to increasing frequency and intensity of contractions

Expected outcome: Patient exhibits signs of decreased discomfort.

• NURSING INTERVENTIONS/*RATIONALES*

Assess woman's level of pain and strategies that she has used to cope with pain *to establish base for intervention.*

Explain what analgesics and anesthesia are available for use during labor and delivery *to provide knowledge to help woman make decisions about pain control.*

Encourage significant other to remain as support person during labor process to assist with support and comfort measures *as measures are often more effective when delivered by a familiar person.*

Instruct woman and support person in use of specific techniques such as conscious relaxation, focused breathing, effleurage, massage, and application of sacral pressure *to increase relaxation, decrease intensity of contractions, and promote use of controlled thought and direction of energy.*

Early in labor, use diversional activities *to provide distractions.*

Encourage regular voiding to decrease chances of distention, *which can increase discomfort during contractions and impede progress of labor.*

Provide comfort measures such as frequent mouth care *to prevent dry mouth;* application of damp cloth to forehead and changing of damp gown or bed covers *to relieve discomfort associated with diaphoresis; positioning to reduce stiffness.*

Encourage conscious relaxation between contractions *to prevent fatigue, which contributes to increased pain perceptions.*

Nursing Diagnosis: Risk for fluid volume deficit related to altered intake during labor

Expected outcome: Fluid balance is maintained, and there are no signs of dehydration.

• NURSING INTERVENTIONS/*RATIONALES*

Monitor intake and output, vital signs, and electrolytes and inspect skin turgor and mucous membranes for dryness *to evaluate hydration status.*

Administer oral/parenteral fluids per physician/CNM orders *to maintain hydration.*

Monitor any emesis and administer antiemetic per physician/CNM order if necessary *to control emesis and prevent fluid loss.*

Nursing Diagnosis: Risk for infection related to rupture of membranes before or during labor

Expected outcome: Patient shows no evidence of infection.

• NURSING INTERVENTIONS/*RATIONALES*

After rupture of membranes, assess amniotic fluid for alterations in color, odor, amount, and presence of blood and meconium, *which may be indicative of intrauterine infection.*

Monitor vital signs and FHR *to evaluate for signs of infection.*

Maintain Standard Precautions, use good handwashing technique and aseptic technique when indicated, and maintain good perineal hygiene *to prevent spread of microorganisms.*

Nursing Diagnosis: Risk for altered pattern of urinary elimination related to sensory impairment secondary to labor

Expected outcome: Bladder does not show signs of distention.

• NURSING INTERVENTIONS/*RATIONALES*

Palpate the bladder superior to the symphysis on a frequent basis *as distention may occur from increased fluid intake and inability to feel urge to void.*

Encourage frequent voiding and catheterize if necessary *to avoid bladder distention as it impedes progress of fetus down birth canal and may result in trauma to the bladder.*

then tranfers to a "postpartum" room. Here she stays for the duration of her hospitalization.

Evaluation

Evaluation of progress and outcomes is a continuous activity during the first stage of labor. The nurse must carefully evaluate each interaction with the mother-to-be and her family and critically appraise how well the formulated expected outcomes for care are being met. The following results reflect effective care:

- The woman demonstrates normal labor progress while the FHR remains within normal range without signs of distress.
- She expresses satisfaction with the assistance of her support person(s) and nursing staff.
- She verbalizes her desire for participation in her care during labor and participates as tolerated throughout labor.
- She maintains adequate hydration and empties her bladder as needed.
- She indicates to her support person(s) or the nurse those measures that help to reduce her discomfort and promote relaxation.

If the evaluation process identifies that results fall short of achieving any expected outcome, further assessment, planning, and implementation is imperative to attain the appropriate quality of nursing care for the woman and her family (see the Nursing Care Plan box on p. 423).

SECOND STAGE OF LABOR

The **second stage of labor** is the stage when the infant is born. This stage begins with full cervical dilation (10 cm) and complete effacement (100%) and ends with the baby's birth. The second stage comprises three phases: *latent, descent,* and *transition.* These phases are characterized by maternal verbal and nonverbal behaviors, the status of uterine activity, the urge to bear down, and fetal descent (Table 16-6). The *latent phase* is a period of rest and relative calm. The woman is quiet and often relaxes with her eyes closed between contractions. The urge to bear down is not well established and is experienced primarily during the acme of a contraction. The *descent phase* is characterized by strong urges to bear down as the **Ferguson reflex** is activated by pressure of the presenting part on the stretch receptors of the pelvic floor. This stimulation results in release of oxytocin from the posterior pituitary gland, which causes stronger, expulsive uterine contractions. The woman becomes more focused on bearing-down efforts,

TABLE 16-6 Maternal progress in second stage of labor

CRITERION	LATENT PHASE (AVERAGE DURATION, 10 TO 30 MIN)	DESCENT PHASE (AVERAGE DURATION VARIES)*	TRANSITION PHASE (AVERAGE DURATION, 5 TO 15 MIN)
Contractions Magnitude (intensity)	Period of physiologic lull for all criteria; period of peace and rest	Significant increase	Overwhelmingly strong Expulsive
Frequency		2 to 2½ min	1 to 2 min
Duration	90 sec	90 sec	90 sec
Descent, station	0 to +2	Increases and Ferguson reflex† activated, +2 to +4	Rapid, +4 to birth
Show: color and amount		Significant increase in dark red bloody show	Fetal head visible at introitus; bloody show accompanies birth of head
Spontaneous bearing-down efforts	Slight to absent, except during acme of strongest contractions	Increased urge to bear down	Greatly increased
Vocalization	Quiet: concern over progress	Grunting sounds or expiratory vocalization; announces contractions	Grunting sounds and expiratory vocalizations continue; may scream or swear
Maternal behavior	Experiences sense of relief that transition to second stage is finished Feels fatigued and sleepy Feels a sense of accomplishment and optimism because the "worst is over" Feels in control	Senses increased urge to push Alters respiratory pattern: has short 4 to 5 sec breath holds with regular breaths in between, five to seven times per contraction Makes grunting sounds or expiratory vocalizations Frequent repositioning	Describes extreme pain Expresses feelings of powerlessness Shows decreased ability to listen or concentrate on anything but giving birth Describes **ring of fire**‡ Often shows excitement immediately after birth of head

*Duration of descent phase can vary, depending on the following: maternal parity, effectiveness of bearing-down effort, and presence of spinal anesthesia or epidural analgesia.

†Pressure of presenting part on stretch receptors of pelvic floor stimulates release of oxytocin from posterior pituitary, resulting in more intense uterine contractions.

‡Burning sensation of acute pain as vagina stretches and fetal head crowns.

Data from Aderhold and Roberts, 1991; Mahan and McKay, 1981.

which become rhythmic. She changes positions frequently to find a more comfortable pushing position. The woman frequently announces the onset of contractions and becomes more vocal as she bears down. In the *transition phase* the presenting part is on the perineum, and bearing-down efforts are most effective for birth. The woman may be more verbal about pain, may scream or swear, and may act out of control (Aderhold and Roberts, 1991). The nurse encourages the woman to listen to her body as she progresses through the phases of the second stage of labor. When a woman listens to her body to tell her when to bear down, she is using an internal locus of control and often feels more satisfied with her efforts to give birth to her baby. A sense of self-esteem and accomplishment is enhanced (Cosner and deJong, 1993).

If a woman is confined to bed in a recumbent position, the rhythmic urge to bear down is suppressed, since gravity is not being used to press the presenting part against the pelvic floor. Being moved to another room and placed on a delivery table in the lithotomy position, as has been the custom in North America for the past 30 years, also has an inhibiting effect on the urge to bear down. In most non-Western societies, labor and birth occur in the same room and women use various positions for labor, such as kneeling, sitting, standing, or squatting. In Western societies, active birth movements have developed in which women are asking for control in terms of the positions selected for childbirth and the settings where it will take place. Today, more and more births in the United States occur in birthing rooms of hospitals (LDR, LDRP) and in birthing centers. Women are using various prepared childbirth techniques (e.g., breathing, relaxation), positions, and modalities such as hydrotherapy to enhance their comfort and progress during labor and birth.

Nursing Care Management

Assessment

The only certain objective sign that the second stage of labor has begun occurs when, on vaginal examination, the examiner cannot feel the cervix, indicating that the cervix is fully dilated and effaced (Myles, 1989). Other signs that suggest the onset of the second stage include the following:

- Sudden appearance of perspiration on upper lip
- An episode of vomiting
- Increased bloody show
- Shaking of extremities
- Increased restlessness; verbalization that "I can't go on"
- Involuntary bearing-down efforts

These signs commonly appear at the time the cervix reaches full dilation (Scott et al, 1994). However, women receiving an epidural block may not exhibit signs that the second stage has begun. Other indicators for assessing progress during each phase of the second stage can be found in Table 16-6.

Assessment is continuous during the second stage of labor. Although hospital protocol determines the specific type and timing of assessments as well as the manner of documenting findings, assessments usually include the following:

- Uterine contraction frequency, strength (intensity), duration, relaxation, and fetal response
- FHR (if electrical fetal monitoring is used, variability and presence of acceleration and deceleration patterns are also assessed)
- Maternal pulse and blood pressure
- Bladder (especially in women who have epidural anesthesia, since the sensation of bladder fullness and the need to void are not perceived by the woman)
- Show; amniotic fluid
- Maternal energy level
- Emotional response of woman and partner to second stage of labor
- Fetal descent

Duration of second stage. Considerable controversy exists over the precise duration of the second stage and the time limits that should be regarded as normal. Friedman's curves (1965) for nulliparous and multiparous women are commonly used to assess the progress for the second stage (p. 408). On the basis of Friedman's data the range and average duration of the second stage of labor vary with parity, as follows:

PARITY	RANGE (MIN)	AVERAGE (MIN)
First pregnancy	25 to 75	57
Subsequent pregnancy	13 to 17	14.4

A second stage of more than 2 hours in a first pregnancy and 1½ hours in subsequent pregnancies is considered abnormal and must be reported to the physician/CNM. Using other assessment tools, FHR and pattern, the descent of the presenting part, the quality of the uterine contractions, and the fetal scalp blood pH also are considered (Mahan and McKay, 1984).

The duration of the second stage may be prolonged for the woman who has an epidural block, which causes loss of or reduction in the urge to bear down. Allowing the epidural analgesic to wear off can enhance the woman's perception of the urge to bear down, thereby increasing her expulsive efforts (Cosner and deJong, 1993).

Duration also can be affected by how and when the woman is encouraged to push. Yeates and Roberts (1984) compared the duration of the second stage when women engage in coached pushing with when they are allowed to push spontaneously as they feel the urge to bear down. Their findings are based on a small sample but suggest that spontaneous pushing may be the most effective aid in the descent and rotation of the fetus. Aderhold and Roberts (1991) found that encouraging various positions for the second stage can assist the fetus to maneuver down and out of the pelvis. The Association for Women's Health, Obstetric and Neonatal Nurses has conducted research on second-stage labor management by nurses, and preliminary findings suggest many nurses do use various positions and encourage spontaneous bearing-down efforts (Jordan, 1995).

Signs of potential problems. Prolonged second stage (see previous discussion) is reported to the physician/CNM. Signs and symptoms of impending birth (Table 16-6) may appear unexpectedly, requiring immediate action by the nurse (see the Guidelines box on p. 426).

Nursing Diagnoses

Nursing diagnoses lend direction to the nursing action(s) needed to implement care. Before establishing diagnoses the nurse analyzes the significance of the findings collected during assessment. Following are some nursing diagnoses indicating potential areas for concern during the second stage:

- Risk for injury to mother and fetus related to
  Persistent use of Valsalva maneuver
- Situational low self-esteem related to
  Knowledge deficit of normal, beneficial effects of vocalization during bearing-down efforts
  Inability to carry out plan for birth without medication
- Ineffective individual coping related to
  Coaching that contradicts woman's physiologic urge to push

Guidelines

ASSISTING AT AN EMERGENCY BIRTH OF A FETUS IN THE VERTEX PRESENTATION

1. The woman usually assumes the position most comfortable for her. A lateral position is often recommended.
2. Reassure the woman verbally. Use eye-to-eye contact and a calm, relaxed manner. If there is someone else available (e.g., the partner), that person could help support the woman in position, assist with coaching, and compliment her on her efforts.
3. Wash your hands and put gloves on, if possible.
4. Place under woman's buttocks whatever clean material is available.
5. Avoid touching the vaginal area to decrease the possibility of infection.
6. As the head begins to crown, the birth attendant should do the following:
   a. Tear the amniotic membrane (caul) if it is still intact.
   b. Instruct the woman to pant or pant-blow, thus controlling the urge to push.
   c. Place the flat side of the hand on the exposed fetal head and apply *gentle* pressure toward the vagina to prevent the head from "popping out." The mother may participate by placing her hand under yours on the emerging head. NOTE: Rapid delivery of the fetal head must be prevented because a rapid change of pressure within the molded fetal skull follows, which may result in dural or subdural tears and may cause vaginal or perineal lacerations.
7. After the birth of the head, check for an umbilical cord. If the cord is around the neck, try to slip it over the baby's head or pull *gently* to get some slack so that it can slip over the shoulders.
8. Support the fetal head as restitution (external rotation) occurs. After restitution, with one hand on each side of the baby's head, exert *gentle* pressure downward so that the anterior shoulder emerges under the symphysis pubis and acts as a fulcrum; then as *gentle* pressure is exerted in the opposite direction, the posterior shoulder, which has passed over the sacrum and coccyx, emerges.
9. Be alert! Hold the baby securely because the rest of the body may emerge quickly. The baby will be slippery!
10. Cradle the baby's head and back in one hand and the buttocks in the other. Keep the head down to drain away the mucus. If a bulb syringe is available, use it to remove mucus.
11. Dry the baby quickly to prevent rapid heat loss. Keep the baby at the same level as the mother's uterus until the end of the cord stops pulsating. NOTE: Keep the baby at the same level to prevent gravity flow of baby's blood to or from the placenta and the resultant hypovolemia or hypervolemia. Also, do not "milk" the cord.
12. Place the baby on the mother's abdomen, cover the baby (remember to keep the head warm, too) with the mother's clothing, and have her cuddle the baby. Compliment her (them) on a job well done and on the baby, if appropriate.
13. Wait for the placenta to separate; *do not* tug on the cord. NOTE: Injudicious traction may tear the cord, separate the placenta, or invert the uterus. Signs of placental separation include a slight gush of dark blood from the introitus, lengthening of the cord, and change in uterine contour from discoid to globular shape.
14. Instruct the mother to push to deliver the separated placenta. Gently ease out the placental membranes, using an up-and-down motion until membranes are removed. If the birth occurs outside the hospital setting, to minimize complications, do not cut the cord without proper clamps and a sterile cutting tool. Inspect the placenta for intactness. Place the baby on the placenta and wrap the two together for additional warmth.
15. Check the firmness of the uterus. Gently massage the fundus and demonstrate to the mother how she can massage her own fundus properly.
16. If supplies are available, clean the mother's perineal area and apply a peripad.
17. In addition to gentle massage of the fundus, the following measures can be taken to prevent or minimize **hemorrhage:**
   a. Put the baby to the breast as soon as possible. Sucking or nuzzling and licking the nipple stimulates the release of oxytocin from the posterior pituitary. NOTE: If the baby does not or cannot nurse, manually stimulate the mother's nipples.
   b. Do not allow the mother's bladder to become distended. Assess for bladder fullness and encourage her to void.
   c. Expel any clots from the mother's uterus
18. Comfort or reassure the mother and her family or friends. Keep the mother and the baby warm. Give her fluids if available and tolerated.
19. If this is a multifetal birth, identify the infants in order of birth (using letters A, B, . . .).
20. Make notations on the birth.
   a. Fetal presentation and position
   b. Presence of cord around neck (nuchal cord) or other parts and number of times cord encircles part
   c. Color, character, and amount of amniotic fluid, if ROM occurs immediately before birth
   d. Time of birth
   e. Estimated time of Apgar score (e.g., 1 and 5 minutes after birth), resuscitation efforts, and ultimate condition of baby
   f. Sex of baby
   g. Time of placental expulsion, its appearance, and completeness
   h. Maternal condition: affect, amount of bleeding, and uterine tonicity
   i. Any unusual occurrences during the birth (i.e., maternal or paternal response, verbalizations, or gestures to birth/baby)

- Pain related to
  - Bearing-down efforts and distention of the perineum
- Anxiety related to
  - Inability to control defecation with bearing-down efforts
  - Knowledge deficit regarding inexperience with perineal sensations associated with the urge to bear down
- Risk for injury to mother related to
  - Inappropriate positioning of mother's legs in stirrups
- Risk for infections related to
  - Prolonged rupture of membranes
  - Perineal incision (episiotomy)
  - Perineal lacerations
- Situational partner/father low self-esteem related to
  - Inability to support mother during final stage of labor

Expected Outcomes

Planning for the second and third stages of labor is accomplished during the first stage of labor. Previously determined expected outcomes may be modified as these stages progress.

Expected outcomes for the woman in second stage of labor may include that the woman will do the following:

1. Actively participate in the labor process
2. Sustain no injury during the labor process (nor will the fetus)
3. Obtain comfort and support from persons of choice

Plan of Care and Implementation

The nurse implements plans to constantly monitor the events of the second stage and mechanism of birth, maternal physiologic and emotional responses to the second stage, the partner's response to the second stage, and fetal response to the stress of the second stage.

The nurse continues to provide comfort measures for the mother such as positioning; mouth care; maintaining clean, dry bedding; and avoiding extraneous noise, conversation, or other distractions (e.g., laughing, talking by attending personnel in or outside the labor area). The woman is encouraged to indicate other support measures she would like.

If the mother is to be transferred to another area for birth, the nurse makes the transfer early enough to avoid rushing the patient. The birthing area is also readied for the birth. The birth table or case cart is usually set up during the transition phase for nulliparous women and during the active phase for multiparous women.

Prebirth considerations

Supplies, instruments, and equipment. The birth table is prepared, and instruments are arranged on the instrument table (Fig. 16-17). Standard procedures are followed for gloving, identifying and opening sterile packages, adding sterile supplies to the instrument table, and unwrapping and handing sterile instruments to the physician/CNM. The infant warmer and equipment are readied for the support and stabilization of the infant (Fig. 16-16, *A*) (see Box 16-2 for Standard Precautions during childbirth and Fig. 16-18 for an example of an alternative birth center).

Maternal position. The woman may want to assume various positions for childbirth. One position found to be highly effective in facilitating the descent and birth of the fetus is squatting (Andrews and Chrzanowski, 1990; Golay et al, 1993). For this position a firm surface is required, and the woman will need side support. In a birthing bed a squat bar is available to assist (Fig. 16-19). Another position is the side-lying position with the upper part of the leg held by the nurse or coach or placed on a pillow (Fig. 16-15, *A*). Some women prefer the Fowler position, which can be attained with the support of a wedged pillow or with the father/partner supporting the woman. Hands-and-knees is an effective position for birth, since it enhances placental perfusion, helps rotate a fetus from a posterior to an anterior position, and may facilitate the birth of the shoulders, especially if the fetus is large. In addition, perineal trauma may be reduced when the woman assumes this position for her birth (Biancuzzo, 1991; Gannon, 1992). When a woman uses the standing position for bearing down, her weight is borne on both femoral heads, allowing the pressure in the acetabulum to increase the transverse diameter of the pelvic outlet by up to 1 cm. This can be

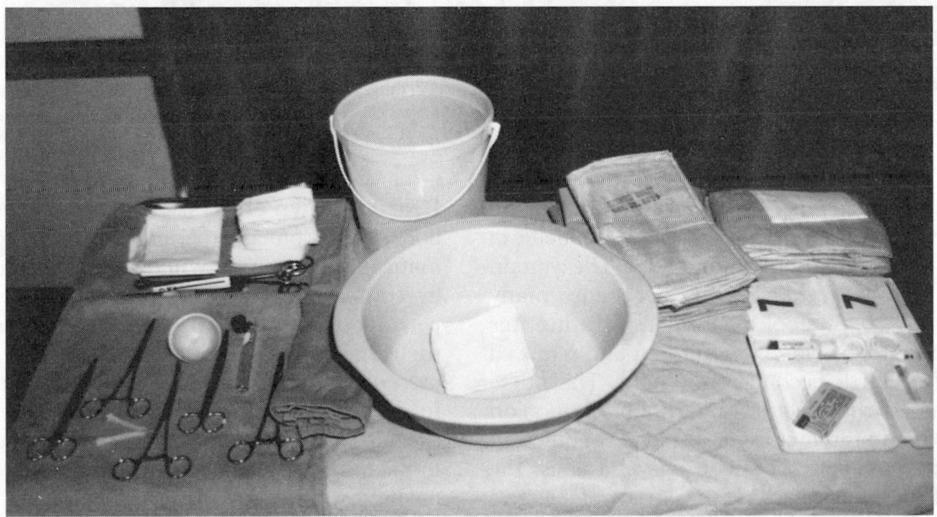

Fig. 16-17 Instrument table. (From Bobak I et al: *Maternity nursing,* ed 4, 1994, Mosby.)

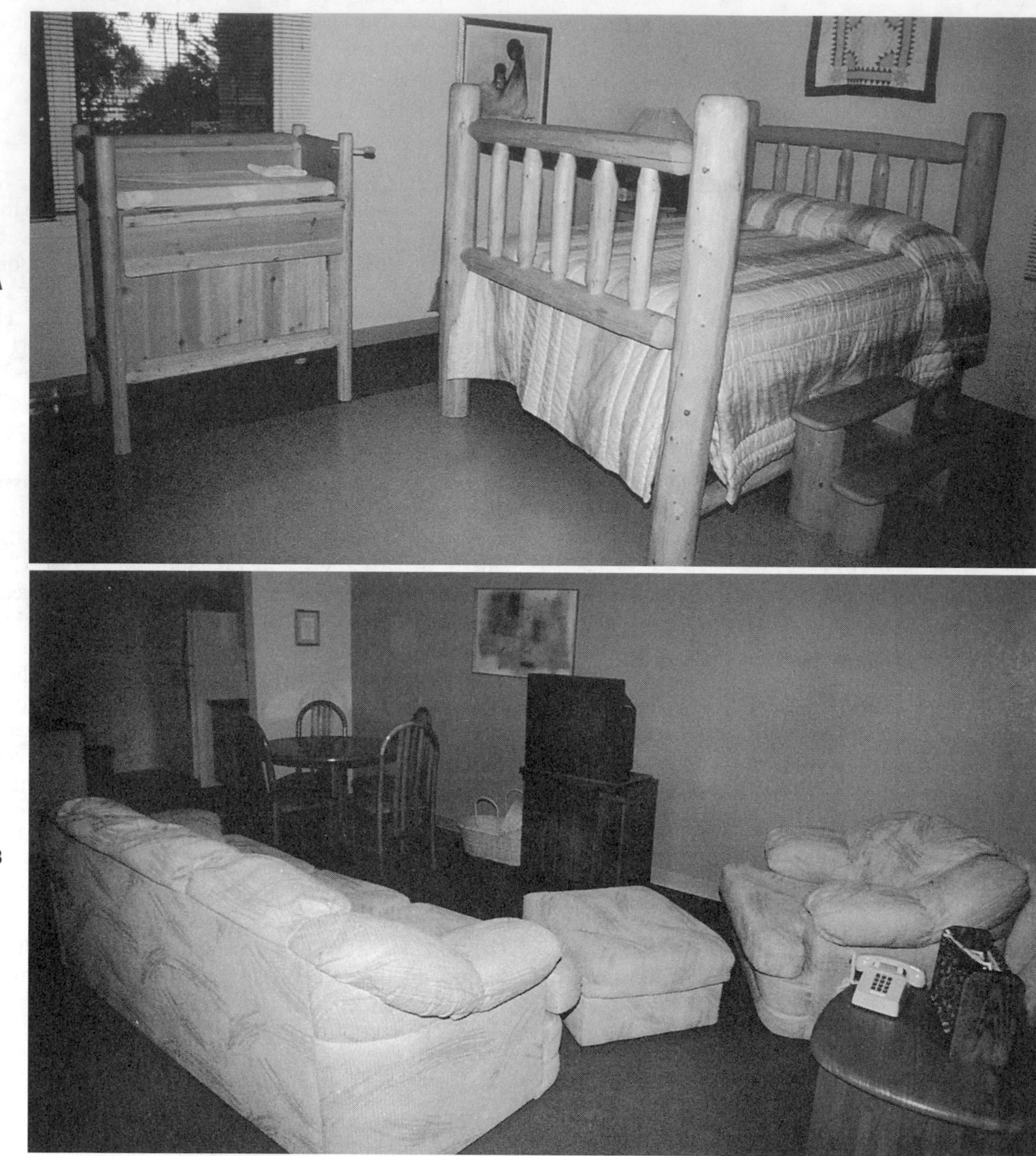

Fig. 16-18 Alternative birth center. **A,** Note double bed and crib in homelike surroundings. **B,** Lounge and kitchen. (Courtesy Michael S. Clement, MD, Mesa, Ariz.)

helpful if descent of the head is delayed as a result of failure of the occiput to rotate from the lateral (transverse diameter of pelvis) to the anterior position (Biancuzzo, 1993). The woman also may want to sit on the toilet to push because many women are concerned about stool incontinence during this stage. These women must be closely monitored and removed from the toilet before birth becomes imminent. The nurse should frequently assess the effect of maternal position(s) on fetal status. If the woman is reluctant or afraid to try different positions, the nurse must actively encourage and assist the woman to do so. Information regarding the variety of effective childbirth positions should be an essential component of prepared childbirth classes.

Bearing-down efforts. As the fetal head reaches the pelvic floor, most women experience the urge to bear down. Automatically the woman will begin to exert downward pressure by contracting her abdominal muscles while relaxing her pelvic floor. This **bearing down** is an involuntary response to the Ferguson reflex, which is activated by the pressure of the presenting part on stretch receptors of the pelvic musculature. A strong expiratory grunt *(vocalization)* may accompany the push (McKay and Roberts, 1990). When coaching women to push, the nurse encourages them to push as *they* feel like pushing rather than giving a prolonged push on command (Thomson, 1993). The nurse monitors the woman's breathing so that the woman does not hold her breath more than 5 seconds at a time. Bearing down while exhaling (open-glottis pushing) and taking breaths between bearing down efforts help maintain adequate oxygen levels for mother and fetus. Prolonged breath-holding, which is still a common practice, may trigger a **Valsalva maneuver,** which results from the woman closing the glottis (closed-glottis pushing), thereby increasing intrathoracic and cardiovascular pressure (Metzer and Therrien, 1990) (Fig. 16-20). In addition, holding the breath for more than 5 seconds diminishes the perfusion of oxygen across the placenta and results in fetal hypoxia. The nurse must remind the woman to take deep breaths to fully ventilate her lungs before and after each contraction.

Critical Thinking Exercises

UPRIGHT POSITION FOR LABOR

You are the nurse manager of a labor and birth unit in a hospital. The medical and nursing staff are reluctant to encourage laboring women to use upright positions (i.e., squatting, sitting, standing, hands and knees) to facilitate fetal descent. They state that such positions are unsafe and inconvenient. How would you respond to their concerns and convince them of the benefits of using upright positions during the second stage of labor?

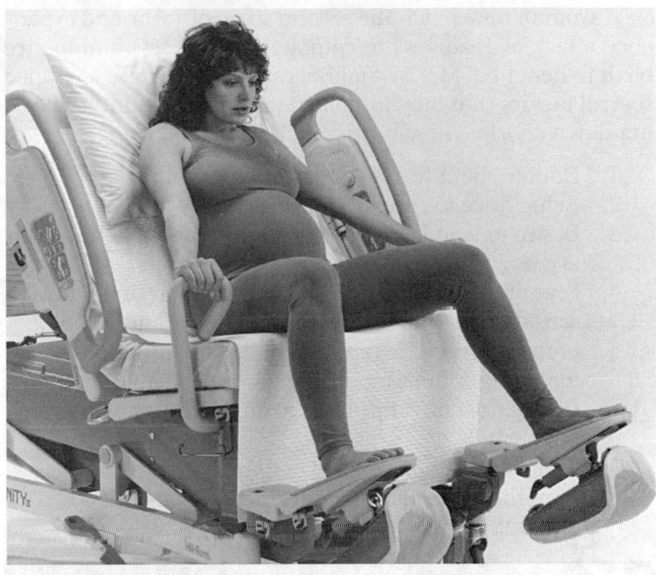

Fig. 16-19 Birthing bed. (Courtesy Hill-Rom, Batesville, Ind.)

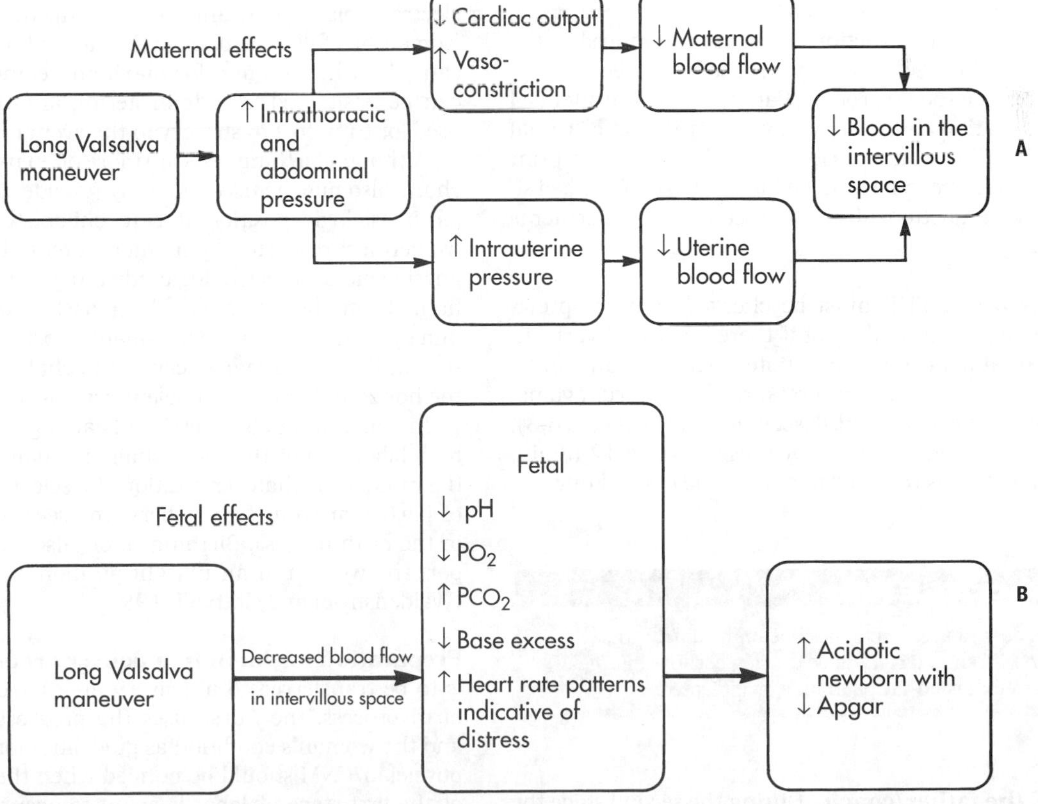

Fig. 16-20 Long Valsalva push; possible effects on mother **(A)** and on fetus **(B).** (From Barnett M, Humenick S: Infant outcome in relation to second stage labor pushing method, *Birth* 9(4):221, 1982.)

A woman may reach the second stage of labor and experience a lack of readiness to complete the process and to give birth to her child. McKay and Barrows (1991) have identified several factors that may inhibit the woman's voluntary bearing-down efforts. These factors include the following:

1. Doubts about her readiness to be a mother
2. Reluctance to care for another baby
3. Desire to wait for support person or physician/CNM to arrive
4. Fear or anxiety regarding the unfamiliar or painful sensations of the second stage of labor and pushing
5. Embarrassment regarding behaviors during pushing, including sounds made and passage of stool
6. Giving up, not wanting to go any further toward vaginal birth
7. Fear that the baby will be in danger once it emerges from the protective intrauterine environment

Nursing ALERT

Recognizing that a woman may experience a need to hold back the birth of her baby helps the nurse address the woman's individual concerns and effectively coach the woman during this stage of labor.

To ensure slow birth of the fetal head, the nurse encourages the woman to control the urge to bear down by coaching her to take panting breaths or to exhale slowly through pursed lips as the baby's head crowns. The woman needs simple, clear directions from *one* coach.

Amnesia between contractions is often pronounced in the second stage, and the woman may have to be roused to cooperate in the bearing-down process. Parents who have attended childbirth education classes may have devised a set of verbal cues for the laboring woman to follow. It is helpful if they print these on a card that can be attached to the head of the bed so that the nurse can better substitute as coach if the partner is not present.

FHR and pattern. FHR must be checked as noted previously. If the rate begins to drop or if there is a loss of variability, prompt treatment must be initiated. The woman can be turned on her side to reduce the pressure of the uterus against the ascending vena cava and descending aorta (Fig. 16-3), and oxygen can be administered by mask at 10 to 12 L/min. This is often all that is required to restore the normal rate.

Nursing ALERT

If the FHR does not return to baseline immediately, the physician/CNM should be notified quickly because medical intervention to hasten the birth may be indicated.

Support of the father/coach. During the second stage the woman needs continuous support and coaching (Tables 16-6 and 16-7). Because the coaching process can be physically and emotionally tiring for the father/coach (Jordan, 1990; Malestic, 1990; Queenan, 1990), the nurse offers nourishment, fluids, and short breaks. If birth occurs in an LDR or LDRP room, the partner may be allowed to wear street clothes or be required to wear a clean scrub outfit, cap, and mask (for the birth). The support person who attends the birth in a delivery room is given instructions regarding how and when to put on a cover gown/scrub clothes, mask, hat, and shoe covers as required. Other information for the partner includes specifying support measures for the laboring woman and pointing out areas of the room in which the partner can move freely.

Partners are encouraged to be present at the birth of their infants if this is in keeping with their cultural expectations. The psychologic closeness of the family unit is maintained, and the partner can continue the supportive care given in labor. The woman and her partner need an equal opportunity to initiate the attachment process with the baby.

Birthing beds and chairs. There is no single position for childbirth. Labor is a dynamic, interactive process among the woman and her uterus, pelvis, and voluntary muscles. Angles between the baby and the woman's pelvis constantly change as the infant turns and flexes down the birth canal. If she is able, a woman will frequently change position in labor, and she should be encouraged and assisted in this effort. The birthing bed (Fig. 16-21) can be set for different positions according to the woman's needs. The woman can squat, kneel, recline, or sit, choosing the position most comfortable for her. At the same time, there is excellent exposure for examination, electrode placement, and birth. Using the birthing bed the woman has full control of both seat and back functions and can adjust her position for maximum comfort. The bed also can be positioned for administering anesthesia and can be used for transport to surgery in the event of a cesarean birth.

Although birthing beds are more often used today, birthing chairs also may be used and may provide women with a better physiologic position during childbirth, although some women feel restricted by a chair. Potentially there is both a physiologic and psychologic advantage to the upright position. The mother can see the birth as it occurs and also maintain eye contact with the attendant. Most chairs are designed so that if an emergency occurs, the chair can be adjusted to the horizontal or the Trendelenburg position.

In some hospitals, oversized beanbag chairs are used for both labor and birth. These chairs mold around and support the mother in whatever position she selects. These chairs are of particular value for mothers who seek active involvement in the birth process. Birthing stools also can be used to support the woman in an upright position similar to squatting (Waldenstrom and Gottvall, 1991).

Preparation for birth in a delivery room. If the woman is to be transferred to a delivery area for completion of the birth process, the nurse uses the progress of fetal descent and the woman's condition as guidelines for the transfer. The physician/CNM should be notified when the transition phase of the first stage of labor is about to occur (multipara) or is occurring (nullipara) and fetal descent is progressing.

TABLE 16-7 Expected responses and support person's actions during second stage of labor

WOMAN'S RESPONSES	SUPPORT PERSON'S ACTIONS
Latent phase	
Experiences a short period of peace and rest	Encourages woman to "listen" to her body Continues support measures Suggests an upright position to encourage progression of descent if descent phase does not begin after 20 min
Descent phase	
Senses increased urgency to bear down as Ferguson reflex is activated Notes increased intensity of uterine contractions—alters respiratory pattern: short 4 to 5 sec breath-holding, five to seven times per contraction Makes grunting sounds or expiratory vocalizations	Encourages respiratory pattern of short breath-holding Stresses normality and benefits of grunting sounds and expiratory vocalization Encourages bearing-down efforts with urge to push Encourages/suggests maternal movement and position changes (upright, if descent is not occurring) Encourages woman to "listen" to her body regarding movement and position change if descent is occurring Discourages long breath-holding If birth is to occur in a delivery room, transfers woman to delivery room early to avoid rushing or, if permitted, offers her option of walking to delivery room Places woman in lateral recumbent position to slow descent if descent is too fast
Transitional phase	
Behaves in manner similar to behavior during transition in first stage (8 to 10 cm) Experiences a sense of severe pain and powerlessness Shows decreased ability to listen Concentrates on birth of baby until head is born Experiences contractions as overwhelming in intensity Reports feeling ring of fire as head crowns Maintains respiratory pattern of three to five, 5 sec breath-holding times per contraction, followed by forced expiration Eases head out with short expirations Responds with excitement and relief after head is born	Encourages slow, gentle pushing Explains that "blowing away the contraction" facilitates a slower birth of the head Provides mirror or helps woman see or touch the emerging fetal head (best to extend over two to three contractions) to help her understand the perineal sensations Coaches woman to relax mouth, throat, and neck to promote relaxation of pelvic floor Applies warm compresses to perineum to promote relaxation

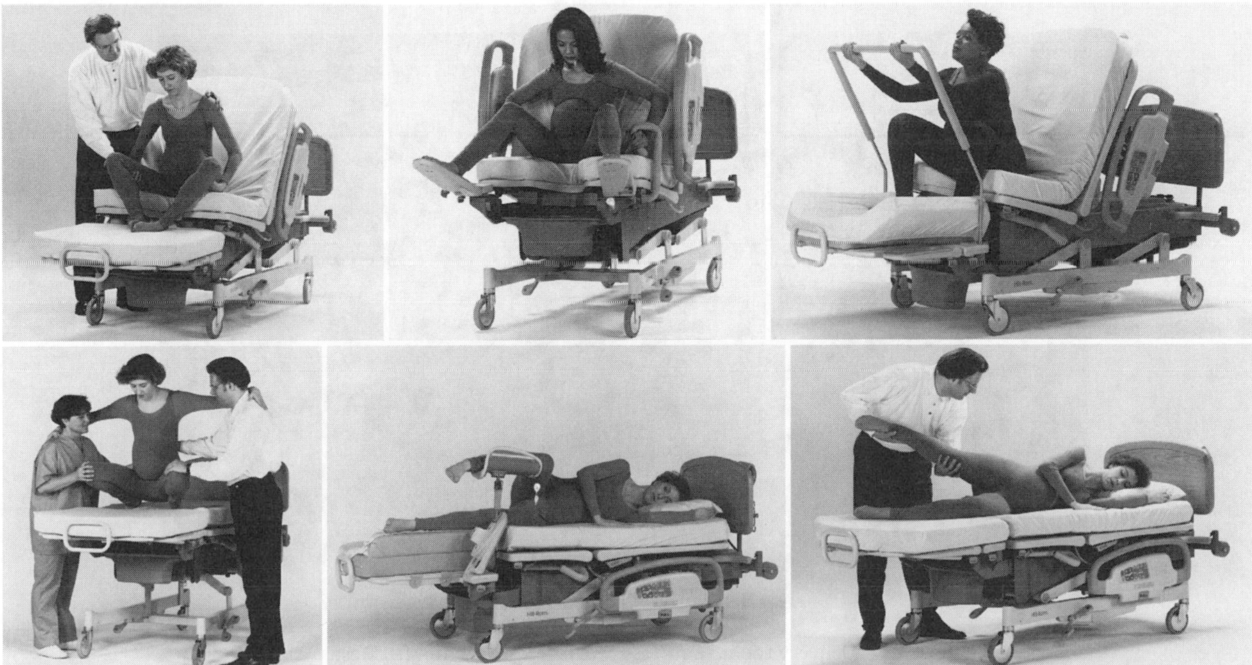

Fig. 16-21 The versatility of today's birthing bed offers mothers many options for labor and birth. (Courtesy Shapiro et al: *Lamaze ready reference guide for labor and birth*, rev ed 2, 1997, authors.)

Nursing ALERT

If *any* laboring woman states, "The baby is coming!" the baby *is* coming, and it is too late for the transfer. The baby is coming *now*, and the nurse should prepare to assist her if the physician/CNM is not yet present (see the Guidelines box on p. 426).

LEGAL TIP

Documentation

Documentation of all observations (e.g., maternal vital signs, FHR and pattern, progress of labor) and nursing interventions, including outcome of the interventions, must be done concurrently with care. The course of labor and maternal-fetal response may change without warning. It is important that all documentation be accurate and complete. Documentation is done in the labor/delivery record as well as on the monitor strip (for description of documentation on monitor strip, see p. 391).

Delivery room birth table. Delivery rooms are designed specifically to facilitate care during birth (Fig. 16-22). The birth table has many features: the entire table can be raised or lowered, and the head or foot can be raised or lowered. A wedge pillow or bolster can be inserted under the top of the mattress to raise it slightly, or the head of the table can be raised to prevent supine hypotension and facilitate pushing. The table is equipped with stirrups for supporting the legs and handle grips to aid with bearing-down efforts. If stirrups are used, the table can be "broken"; that is, the lower half of the table can be lowered and rolled back to fit under the top half.

Birth in a delivery room. If the woman must move from the labor bed to the delivery table, she will need assistance. If this is done between contractions, the woman can help, but because of her awkwardness, she cannot be rushed.

The position assumed for birth may be **Sims position** (if this is the case, the attendant will need to support the upper part of the leg), dorsal position, or lithotomy position.

The **lithotomy position** has been the position most commonly used for birth in Western cultures, although this is changing slowly. The lithotomy position makes it more convenient for the physician/CNM to deal with any complications that arise. The buttocks are brought to the edge of the table, and the legs are placed in stirrups. Care must be taken to pad the stirrups, raise and place both legs simultaneously, and adjust the shanks of the stirrups so that the calves of the legs are supported. There should be no pressure on the popliteal space. If the stirrups are not the same height, strained ligaments can develop in the woman's back as she bears down. This strain causes considerable discomfort in the postpartum period.

Once the woman is positioned for birth, the vulva and perineum are cleansed. Hospital protocols and preferences of the physician/CNM for cleansing may vary and can involve washing the area thoroughly with warm soapy water or a soapy betadine solution and then rinsing. The wash can then be followed by spraying the area with a disinfectant to prevent bacterial growth.

The circulating nurse continues to coach and encourage the woman. The nurse auscultates FHR or checks the electronic monitor tracing every 5 to 15 minutes or per protocol and informs the physician/CNM as to the rate and pattern (Tucker, 1992). The equipment for taking the blood pressure should be readied for instant use if signs of shock develop. As the woman pushes, blood pressure readings will be distorted (increased) by the increase in thoracic and abdominal pressures. A reading will be taken after birth before transferring the woman to the recovery room. An oxytocic medication (e.g., Pitocin) may be prepared for administration

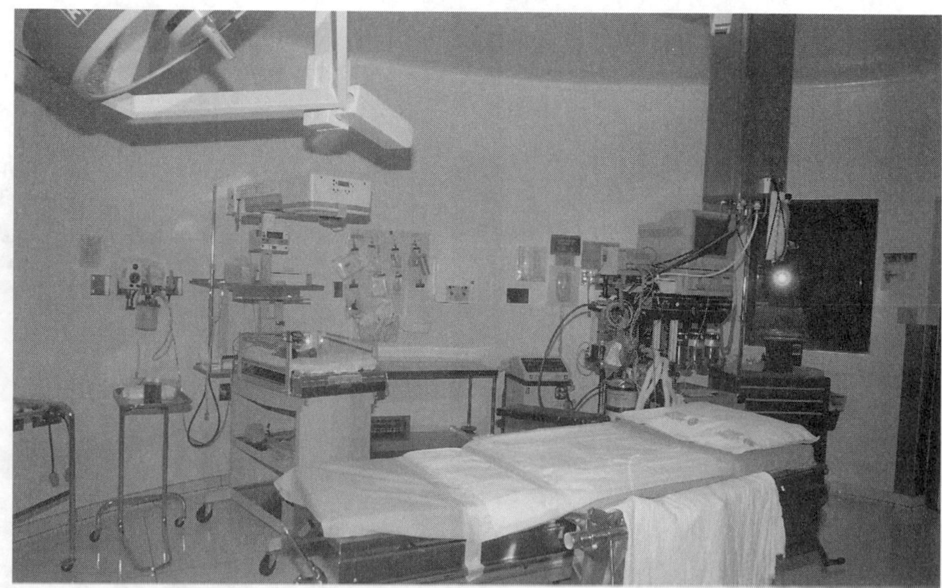

Fig. 16-22 Delivery room. (Courtesy Michael S. Clement, MD, Mesa, Ariz.)

after expulsion of the placenta. The physician/CNM puts on a cap, a mask that has a shield or protective eyewear, and shoe covers. Hands must be scrubbed and a sterile gown (with waterproof front and sleeves) and gloves put on. Nurses attending the birth may also need to wear caps, protective eyewear, masks, gowns, and gloves (Box 16-2). Then the woman may be draped with sterile towels and sheets. The partner helps the woman remember not to touch the sterile drapes.

Birth in a birthing room (LDR, LDRP) and a birthing center. In many hospitals and birthing centers, women have the opportunity to give birth without having to move to a delivery room or change beds. These settings can vary from a labor room of 60 to 80 square feet to a room the size of an operating room (300 to 350 square feet). The size of the setting dictates to a large degree who can attend the birth and what alternatives to traditional delivery room care can be offered. Women remain in these birthing rooms throughout labor, birth, recovery (LDR rooms), and perhaps the postpartum period (LDRP rooms) (Fig. 16-18). A small, back table or cart is set up with the items shown in Fig. 16-17. Position for birth varies, with possibilities such as lithotomy position with legs in stirrups, feet resting on foot rests, squat bar, or a side-lying position with leg supported by coach, nurse, or squat bar. The foot of the bed can be removed. This is done when the physician or CNM assisting with the birth specifies the need for better perineal access to perform episiotomy, for birth of a large baby, or for access to the emerging head to facilitate suctioning. Otherwise the foot of the bed is left in place and lowered slightly to form a ledge providing access for birth and a place to put the newborn infant.

Mechanism of birth: vertex presentation. The nurse's knowledge of the birth process provides a basis for the woman's preparation before and during birth. The nurse reviews with the woman or couple the cardinal movements of labor. Once the cervix is fully dilated, descent occurs. The presenting part (usually the vertex) advances with each contraction and recedes slightly as the contraction wanes; descent is constant. Descent of the presenting part elicits the Ferguson reflex as pressure from the presenting part is applied to stretch receptors of the pelvic floor, thereby producing a sensation/urge to bear down. *Bulging of the perineum* occurs during the descent phase, when the fetal presenting part is distending the perineum but is not yet visible at the introitus. The occiput generally rotates anteriorly, and with voluntary bearing-down efforts, the head appears at the introitus (Fig. 16-23). Although more and more head may be seen with each push, **crowning** occurs when the widest part of the head (the biparietal diameter) distends the vulva just before birth. Immediately before birth the perineal musculature becomes greatly distended. If an **episiotomy** (incision into the perineum to enlarge the vaginal outlet) is necessary, it is done at this time to minimize soft tissue damage (Fig. 16-24). The head is born by extension and after birth restitutes with the shoulders. Interiorly the shoulders rotate into the anteroposterior diameter of the pelvis; external rotation of the head is observed. The body is born by lateral flexion.

The three phases of a spontaneous birth of the fetus in a vertex presentation are (1) birth of the head, (2) birth of the shoulders, and (3) birth of the body and extremities.

Birth of head. The vertex first appears, followed by the forehead, face, chin, and neck. The speed of the birth of the head must be controlled, or sudden birth of the head may cause severe lacerations through the anal sphincter or even into the woman's rectum (p. 441). The birth of the head is controlled by (1) applying pressure against the rectum, drawing it downward to aid in flexing the head as the back of the neck catches under the symphysis pubis; (2) applying upward pressure from the coccygeal region (modified **Ritgen maneuver**) (Fig. 16-25) to extend the head during the actual birth, thereby protecting the musculature of the perineum; and (3) assisting the mother with voluntary control of the bearing-down efforts by coaching her to pant while letting uterine forces expel the fetus. In addition to protecting the maternal tissues, gradual birth is imperative to prevent fetal intracranial injury.

Occasionally the membranes may not be ruptured before birth. During birth of the head these membranes look like a

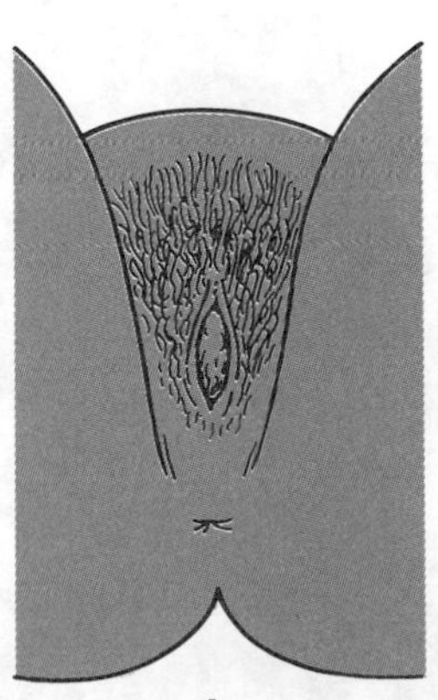

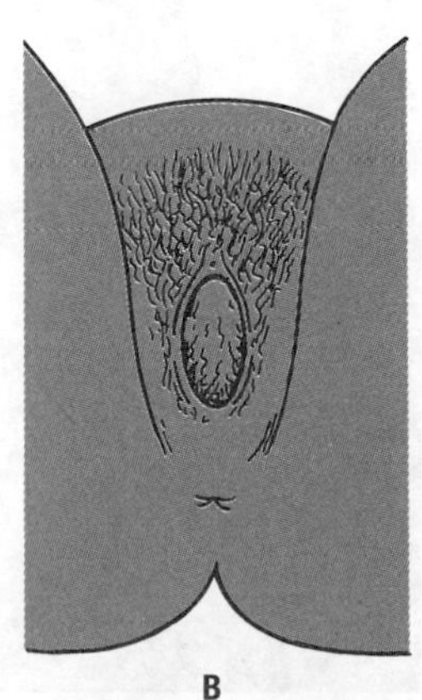

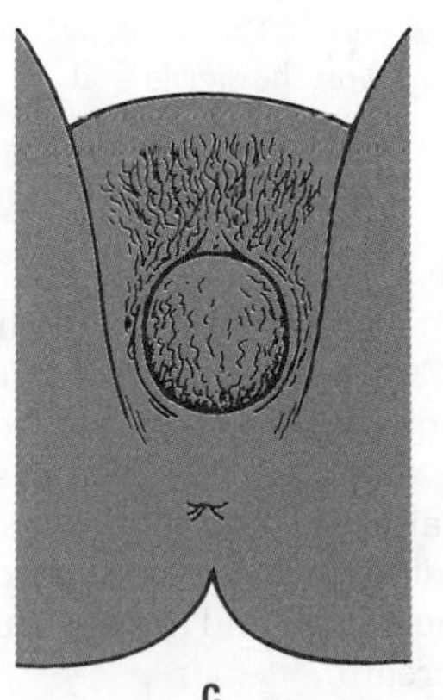

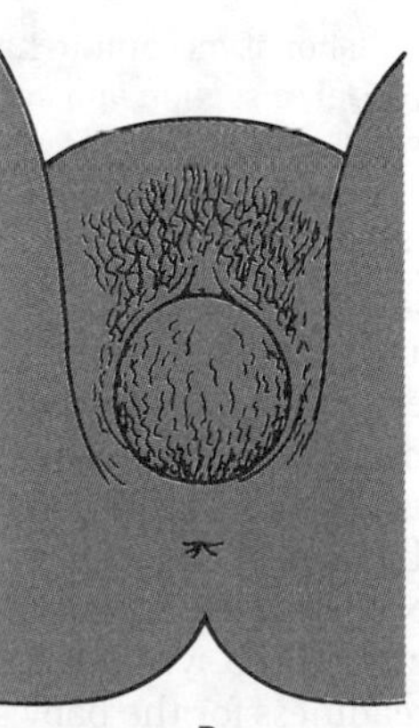

Fig. 16-23 Beginning birth with vertex presenting. **A,** Anteroposterior slit. **B,** Oval opening. **C,** Circular shape. **D,** Crowning.

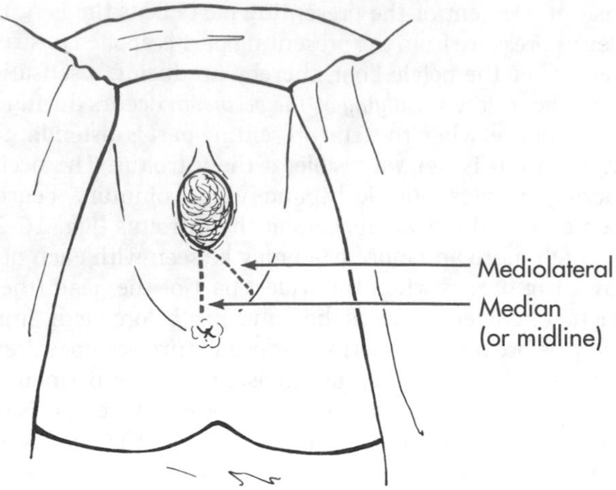

Fig. 16-24 Types of episiotomies.

hood covering the head. This hood of intact amniotic membranes covering the head during birth is known as a **caul.**

The umbilical cord often encircles the neck **(nuchal cord)** but rarely so tightly as to cause hypoxia. After the head is born, gentle palpation is used to feel for the cord. The cord should be slipped gently over the head (Fig. 16-26). If the loop is tight or if there is a second loop, the cord is clamped twice, severed between the clamps, and unwound from around the neck before the birth continues. Mucus, blood, or meconium in the nasal or oral passages may prevent the newborn from breathing. Moist gauze sponges are used to wipe the nose and mouth. A bulb syringe is inserted into the mouth and oropharynx first to aspirate contents. Next, the nares are cleared while supporting the head.

PREVENTION OF MECONIUM ASPIRATION. When the physician/CNM prepares for birth of the head, a DeLee device is connected to the suction tubing and fluids are withdrawn from the infant's mouth and nose before the first breath is taken. The care provider should refrain from using the DeLee device with oral suction to withdraw fluid from the infant unless the suction device isolates mucus from the user's airway. Instead, wall suction is recommended.

Nursing ALERT

During labor, if meconium has been present in the amniotic fluid, a DeLee suction apparatus is placed on the sterile field and wall suction is prepared.

Birth of shoulders. Before the shoulders can be born, they must engage in the pelvic inlet. Internal rotation of the shoulders occurs, accompanied by restitution and external rotation of the head so that the shoulders lie in the anteroposterior diameter of the inlet. The shoulders can then pass through the pelvic cavity. While awaiting rotation, the physician/CNM wipes the baby's face with sterile gauze squares and uses the bulb syringe to clear the mouth and nose of mucus in readiness for the baby's first breath.

The head is drawn downward and backward by the primary health care provider to help the anterior shoulder impinge beneath the arch of the symphysis and slide beneath the

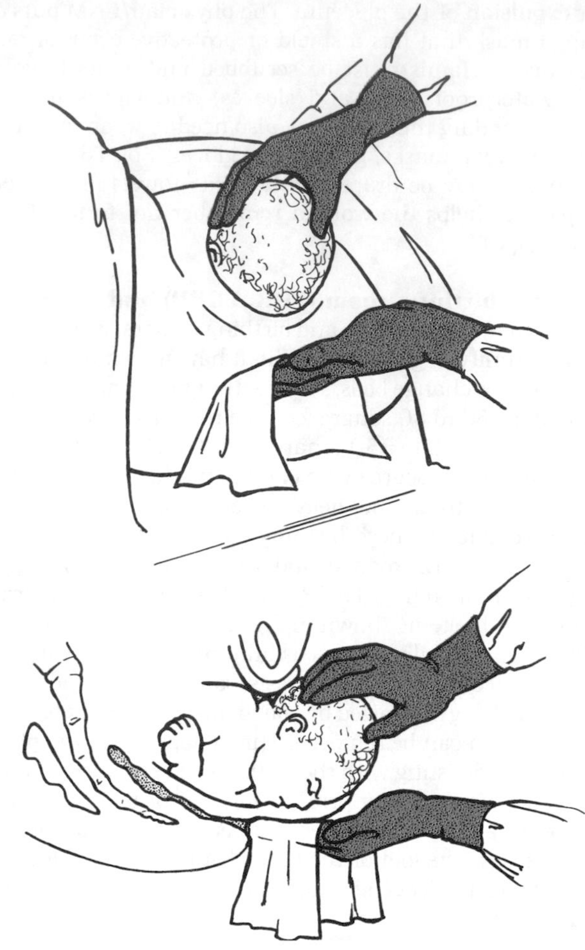

Fig. 16-25 Birth of head by modified Ritgen maneuver. Note control to prevent too-rapid birth of head.

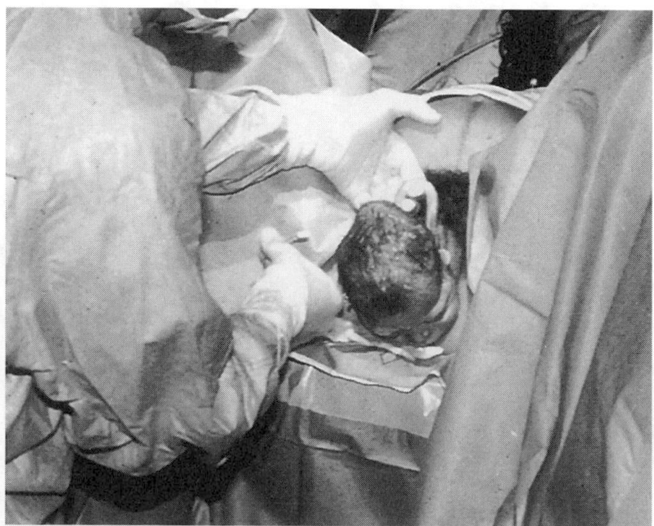

Fig. 16-26 Loosening nuchal cord (umbilical cord around neck). (Courtesy Marjorie Pyle, RNC, Lifecircle, Costa Mesa, Calif.)

pubic arch. Normally the anterior shoulder is delivered with this slight downward traction toward the perineum. The posterior shoulder distends the perineum, and, to prevent perineal trauma, the head is lifted toward the symphysis pubis, resulting in the birth of the shoulder over the perineum (Myles, 1989).

USE OF FUNDAL PRESSURE. Fundal pressure is the use of a hand and/or forearm(s) to apply gentle, steady pressure against the fundus of the uterus to facilitate the vaginal birth of the fetus. The increased use of alternative positions for pushing has decreased the use of fundal pressure. Alternative positioning assists in fetal descent. In some cases where regional or conduction anesthesia (epidural) is used, fundal pressure may be needed because of decreased maternal expulsive power. If fundal pressure is needed, a *skilled* nurse, in collaboration with the physician/CNM, performs the procedure. Fundal pressure is used most often when there is slight shoulder dystocia. In a nationwide survey, Kline-Kaye and Miller-Slade (1990) found that 84% of the respondents used fundal pressure. In some instances, nurses applied the pressure; in other instances, only physicians were responsible for fundal pressure. Few complications were noted: one respondent reported uterine rupture and nine respondents reported vaginal or cervical lacerations. Recording fundal pressure varied: 52% did not document the use of fundal pressure, 11% recorded it in the progress notes, 18% in the nursing notes, 9% in both medical and nursing notes, and 5% did not respond to the question. Nurses received no formal education in how to apply fundal pressure. No standard technique for the application of fundal pressure is available, and no current legal, professional, or regulatory standards for such application exist. Nurses with little or no knowledge or experience in application of fundal pressure may be requested to apply fundal pressure in emergency situations. Obstetric services should consider conducting an educational program on techniques of applying fundal pressure for nurses working in the labor suite. Some standardization of technique would be appropriate for individual units. Records should be kept of occurrences in which the physician/CNM believed that fundal pressure was necessary, the technique used, length of time application occurred, and outcome of the delivery. With careful record keeping, standards can be developed and the safety of women in labor enhanced.

Birth of body and extremities. Expulsion is controlled so that it occurs slowly. As lateral flexion is continued, the physician/CNM supports the weight of the baby to prevent perineal trauma. Slight rotation of the body to the right or left may be used to facilitate the birth. The time of birth is the precise time when the entire body is out of the mother. This time must be noted on the record.

In the birth of an uncompromised newborn the infant may be placed on the mother's abdomen immediately after birth and covered with a warm, dry blanket. The cord may be clamped at this time, and the physician/CNM may ask if the woman's partner would like to cut the cord. If so, the partner is given a sterile pair of scissors and instructed to cut the cord 1 inch above the clamp.

Immediate assessment and care of the newborn. Care immediately after the birth focuses on assessing and stabilizing the newborn. The nurse has primary responsibility for the infant during this period because the physician/CNM will be involved with the expulsion of the placenta and care of the mother. The nurse must be alert for any signs of distress and initiate appropriate interventions.

A brief assessment of the infant can be performed while the mother is holding him or her. The assessment includes checking the infant's airway and Apgar score. The nurse dries and then wraps the infant in a warm blanket. Further examination, identification procedures, and care can be postponed until later in the third stage of labor or early in the fourth stage.

Siblings during the second stage. Parents may wish their other children to be present during the labor and birth process. However, a young child may become frightened by the intensity of the second stage. Sights such as rupture of the membranes and sounds such as their mother's moans, screams, and grunts can be unsettling. It is not uncommon for a woman to say things during her second stage and birth that she would not say otherwise and that might scare her child, for example "I can't take any more, take this baby out of me" or "This pain is killing me, I'm going to die." The child present during birth needs someone to be close and to give explanations in a simple and calm manner. The child may want to be held.

Hospitals are more supportive of siblings' participation in the birth experience than in previous years. Organized sibling classes provide preparation for the anticipated sights, sounds, and events of the birth process, orientation to the birth environment, and impact of the addition of a new baby to the family. Jonquil (1993) uses various developmentally appropriate teaching approaches such as informal discussions, story books, play, birth demonstrations, hands-on experience with newborns, and tours of the labor unit in the sibling classes she conducts. She believes that such preparation is important for parents and children and helps to create a positive, family-oriented childbirth experience. Sibling preparation classes usually are required for a sibling to attend the birth. Although set age limits vary, most hospitals will not allow children younger than 3 years of age to attend the birth. Many hospitals deal with sibling attendance on an individual basis, taking into consideration the child's age, maturity, and preparation. Although the long-term effects on young children witnessing birth are not fully known, Jonquil (1993) has found that children who are prepared have positive experiences and long-term memories of their sibling's birth.

An alterative to sibling presence at birth is for a trusted person to remain with the sibling in the waiting area until after the birth. At that time the child can be brought into the room and see the baby held by the mother, who has become her "normal" self again.

Emergency childbirth. Even under the best of circumstances there probably will come a time when the perinatal nurse will be required to assist with the birth of an infant without medical assistance. Consider the multiparous woman who arrives at the community hospital fully dilated in the middle of the night. Since it is neither possible nor desirable to prevent an impending birth, the perinatal nurse must be able to function independently and be skilled in the safe birth of a vertex fetus (see the Guidelines box on p. 426).

Lateral Sims position for emergency childbirth. A lateral Sims posture may be the position of choice for birth when (1) the birth is progressing rapidly and there is insufficient time for slow distention of the perineum; (2) the fetal head seems too large to pass through the introitus without laceration, and episiotomy is not possible; or (3) the apparent size of the fetus is consistent with possible shoulder dystocia.

In the lateral Sims position, less stress is placed on the perineum and better visualization of the perineum is possible as the upper leg is supported by the woman's partner or the nurse (Fig. 16-15, *A*). In the event of shoulder dystocia, lateral Sims position increases the space needed for birth.

Emergency birth of preterm infant. The actual process of birthing the preterm infant does not vary from that of the term infant. However, the care of the infant after birth requires some modification as follows:

- Maintain a clear airway.
- Keep warm and minimize handling.
- Gently stimulate the preterm infant to breathe. When the infant "forgets" to breathe, rubbing the back or the soles of the feet usually is effective.
- Transport the infant to a medical facility equipped to handle preterm infants as early as possible.

Evaluation

Evaluation of outcomes is an ongoing activity. During each encounter with the woman and her family during the second stage of labor the nurse evaluates the degree to which expected outcomes are being met. For example, the woman has actively participated in the labor process, neither she nor her fetus has sustained any injury during the labor process, and she has been able to obtain comfort and support from persons of her choice. If the evaluation shows that results fall short of achieving an expected outcome, further assessment, planning, and implementation are warranted. Women should be guided in a realistic evaluation of their performance during childbirth. Women's impressions of their ability to manage during labor and birth can have an effect on future childbirth experiences (McKay, 1995). A Nursing Care Plan for a woman in the second stage of labor is provided below.

THIRD STAGE OF LABOR

The **third stage of labor** lasts from the birth of the baby until the delivery of the placenta. The goal in the management of the third stage of labor is the prompt separation and expulsion of the placenta, achieved in the easiest, safest manner.

The placenta is attached to the decidual layer of the basal plate's thin endometrium by numerous, randomized, fibrous anchor villi—much like a postage stamp is attached to a sheet of postage stamps. After the birth of the fetus, in the presence of strong uterine contractions, the placental site becomes markedly smaller. This reduced size causes the anchor villi to break and the placenta to separate from its attachments. Normally the first few strong contractions 5 to 7 minutes after the baby's birth shear the placenta from the basal plate. A placenta does not detach itself from a flaccid (relaxed) uterus because the placental site is not reduced in size.

Nursing Care Management

Assessment

Placental separation is indicated by the following signs (Fig. 16-27):

Nursing Care Plan

SECOND STAGE OF LABOR

Nursing Diagnosis: Risk for ineffective individual coping related to birthing process and fatigue of labor

Expected outcome: Woman actively participates in the birth process with no evidence of injury to her or her fetus.

• **NURSING INTERVENTIONS/*RATIONALES***

Constantly monitor events of second stage labor and birth, including physiologic responses of woman and fetus, emotional responses of woman and partner *to ensure maternal, partner, and fetal well-being.*

Provide ongoing feedback to woman and partner *to allay anxiety and enhance participation.*

Continue to provide comfort measures such as positioning; mouth care; clean, dry bedding; cool cloths on forehead; and minimizing distractions *to decrease discomfort and aid in focus on the birth process.*

Encourage woman to experiment with various positions *to assist downward movement of fetus.*

Encourage woman to bear down spontaneously on exhalation *to aid descent and rotation of fetus.*

Teach partner about importance of spontaneous bearing down *to avoid coaching to push, which may contradict or inhibit these spontaneous urges.*

Remind woman not to hold her breath while bearing down *as this may trigger a Valsalva maneuver and increase intrathoracic and cardiovascular pressure and decrease perfusion of placental oxygen, placing the fetus at risk.*

Encourage woman to vocalize as she bears down *to enhance efforts.*

Have woman take deep breaths and relax between contractions *to reduce fatigue and increase effectiveness of pushing efforts.*

If woman seems reluctant to bear down, assess possible contributing factors (i.e., doubts about readiness as a mother; desire for an absent person to be present, fear of the pain of pushing, embarrassment at passing stool while pushing, fear baby will be in danger when no longer in womb) and address specific concern *so that woman can participate in labor process effectively.*

Have mother pant as fetal head crowns *to control birth of head.*

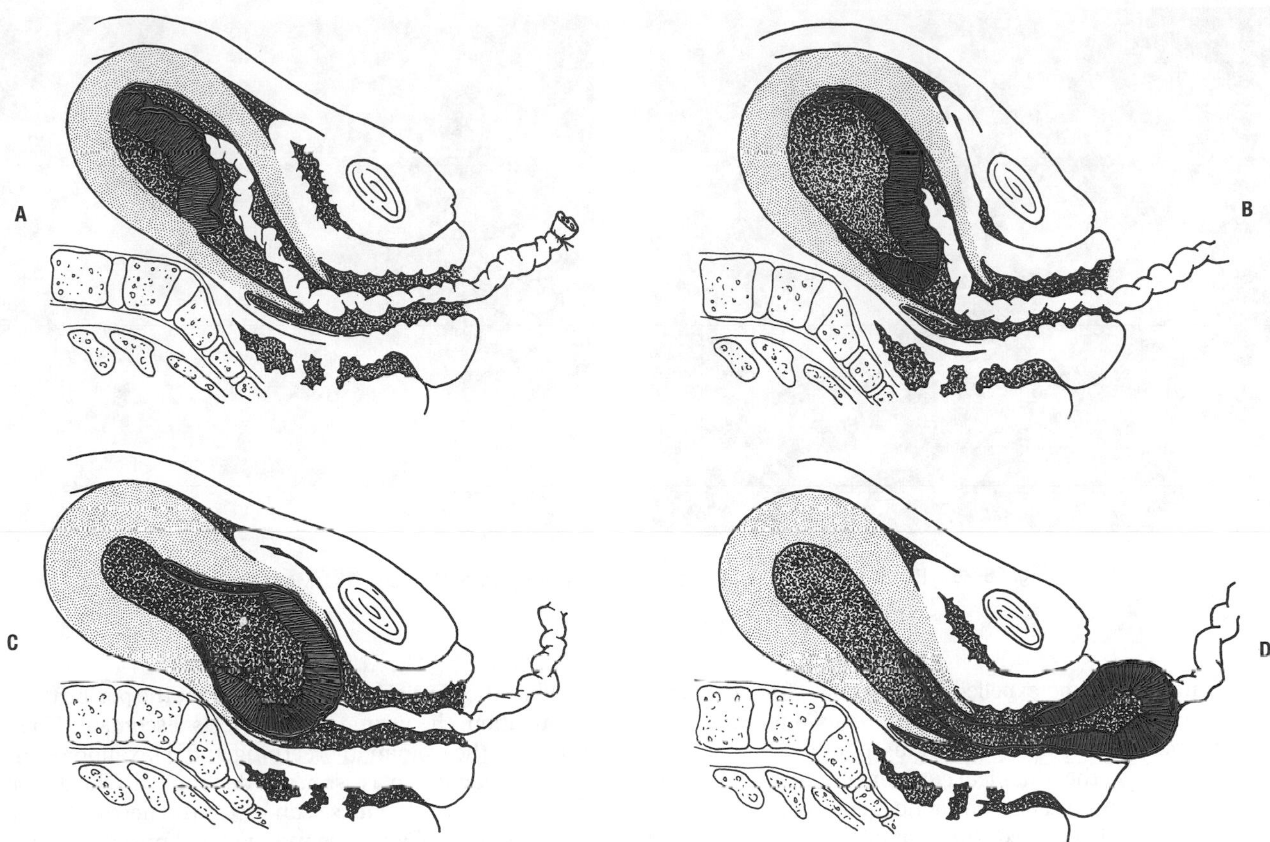

Fig. 16-27 Third stage of labor. **A,** Placenta begins the separation process in central portion with retroplacental bleeding. Uterus changes from discoid to globular shape. **B,** Placenta completes separation and enters lower uterine segment. Uterus is globular in shape. **C,** Placenta enters vagina, cord is seen to lengthen, and there may be increased bleeding. **D,** Expression (birth) of placenta and completion of third stage.

- A firmly contracting fundus
- A change in the uterus from a discoid to a globular ovoid shape as the placenta moves into the lower uterine segment
- A sudden gush of dark blood from the introitus
- Apparent lengthening of the umbilical cord as the placenta draws closer to the introitus
- A vaginal fullness (the placenta) noted on vaginal or rectal examination, or fetal membranes seen at the introitus

Whether the placenta first appears by its shiny fetal surface (Schultze mechanism) or turns to show its dark roughened maternal surface (Duncan mechanism) is of no clinical importance. After the placenta and the amniotic membranes emerge, the physician/CNM examines them for intactness to ensure that no portion remains in the uterine cavity (e.g., there are no retained fragments of the placenta or membranes) (Fig. 16-28). When indicated, parents should be consulted concerning the placenta, since some cultures have rituals regarding the handling and care of the placenta (e.g., burying the placenta near the home) after birth.

Maternal physical status. Physiologic changes after birth are profound. The cardiac output is increased rapidly as maternal circulation to the placenta ceases and the pooled blood from the lower extremities is mobilized. The pulse rate slows in response to the change in cardiac output and tends to remain slightly slower than before pregnancy for about 1 week.

Soon after the birth the woman's blood pressure usually returns to prepregnancy levels. Several factors contribute to an elevated blood pressure: the excitement of the second stage, certain medications, and the time of day (blood pressure is highest during the late afternoon). Analgesics and anesthetics may lead to hypotension in the hour after birth.

Signs of potential problems. While the physician/CNM completes the delivery of the placenta, the nurse observes the mother for signs of an altered level of consciousness (LOC) or alteration in respirations. Because of the rapid cardiovascular changes (e.g., the increased intracranial pressure during pushing and the rapid increase in cardiac output), this period represents the risk of rupture of a preexisting cerebral aneurysm and of pulmonary emboli. Another dangerous, unpredictable problem is **amniotic fluid embolism** (see Chapter 17).

Plan of Care and Implementation

To assist in the birth of the placenta, the woman is instructed to push when signs of separation have occurred. If possible,

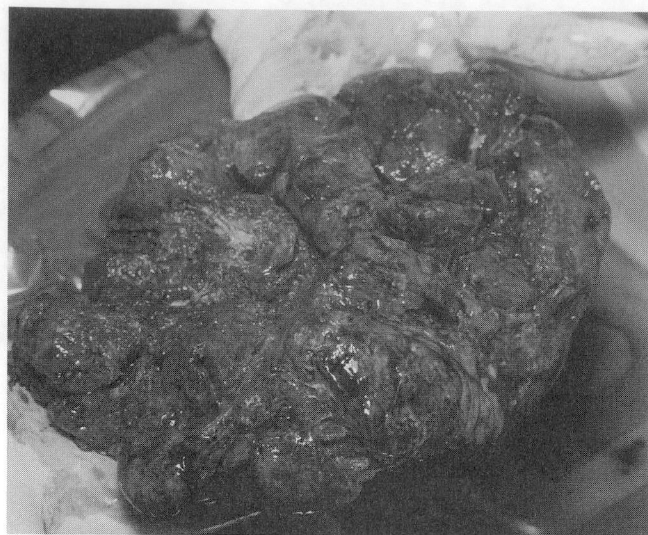
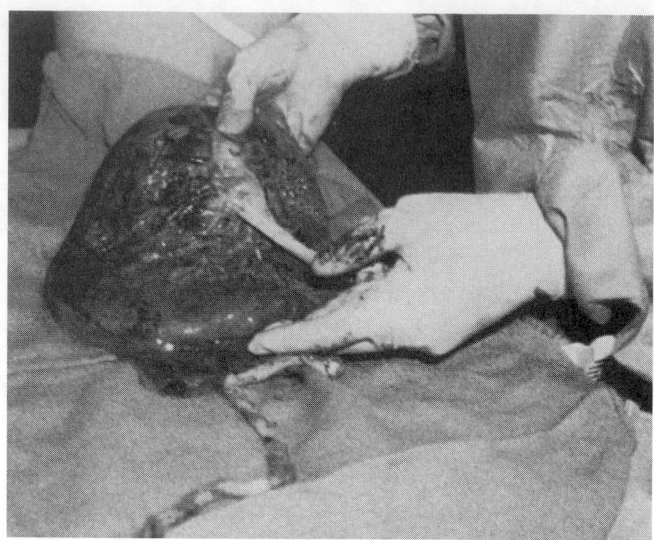

Fig. 16-28 Examination of the placenta. (Courtesy Michael S. Clement, MD, Mesa, Ariz.)

the placenta should be expelled by maternal effort during a uterine contraction, but assistance such as alternate compression and elevation of the fundus plus minimum, controlled traction on the umbilical cord may be used to facilitate delivery of the placenta and amniotic membranes. If an oxytocic medication is ordered (for example, Pitocin 10 to 20 units as an intramuscular [IM] injection or diluted in an IV solution, or methergine 0.2 mg IM injection), the nurse administers the medication in the dosage and by the route indicated after the placenta has been expelled. Oxytocics stimulate the uterus to contract, thereby helping to prevent hemorrhage after the placenta is removed. When the third stage is complete and lacerations are repaired or an episiotomy is sutured, the vulvar area is gently cleansed with warm sterile water or normal saline solution, and a sterile perineal pad is applied to the perineum.

The family during the third stage. Most parents enjoy being able to handle, hold, explore, and examine the baby immediately after birth. Both parents can assist with the thorough drying of the infant. The infant may be wrapped in a receiving blanket and placed on the woman's abdomen. If skin-to-skin contact is desired, the unwrapped infant may be placed on the woman's abdomen and then covered with a warm blanket.

Holding the newborn next to her skin helps the mother maintain the baby's body heat and provides skin contact; care must be taken to keep the head warm as well. Stockinette caps are sometimes used to cover the newborn's head. It is the nurse's responsibility to make sure the infant stays warm and is in no danger of slipping from the parent's grasp.

Many women wish to begin breast-feeding their newborns at this time to take advantage of the infant's alert state (first period of reactivity) and to stimulate the production of oxytocin, which promotes contraction of the uterus. Others wish to wait until the newborn, parents, and older siblings are together in the recovery area. In some cultures, breastfeeding is not acceptable until the milk comes in because it is believed that colostrum is unclean.

While the physician/CNM carries out the postbirth vaginal examination, the woman usually feels discomfort. The nurse can coach the woman in breathing and relaxation techniques or use distraction to assist her in dealing with the discomfort. During this time the nurse can assess the newborn's physical condition; the baby can be weighed and measured, given eye prophylaxis and vitamin K injection, given an identification bracelet, wrapped in warm blankets, and then given to the partner or back to the mother to hold. Chapter 23 provides an in-depth discussion of the care of the newborn after birth.

Parent-newborn relationships. The woman's reaction to the sight of her newborn may range from excited outbursts of laughing, talking, and even crying to apparent apathy. A polite smile and nod may acknowledge the comments of nurses and the physician/CNM. Occasionally the reaction is one of anger or indifference; the woman turns away from the baby, concentrates on her own pain, and sometimes makes hostile comments. These varied reactions can arise from pleasure, exhaustion, or deep disappointment. When evaluating parent-newborn interactions after birth, the nurse should consider the cultural characteristics of the woman and her family and the expected behaviors of that culture. Whatever the reaction and cause may be, the woman needs continuing acceptance and support from all staff. Notation regarding the parents' reaction to the newborn can be made in the recovery record. How do parents look? What do they say? What do they do? Further assessment of the parent-newborn relationship can be conducted as care is given during the period of recovery. This is especially important if warning signs (e.g., passive or hostile reactions to newborn, disappointment with sex or appearance of newborn, absence of eye contact, limited interaction of parents with each other) were noted immediately after birth. The nurse may find it helpful to discuss warning signs that may have been noted with the woman's physician/CNM. Nonverbal behaviors may vary among cultural groups, and the nurse should consider these variations when making assessments.

Siblings, who may have appeared only remotely interested

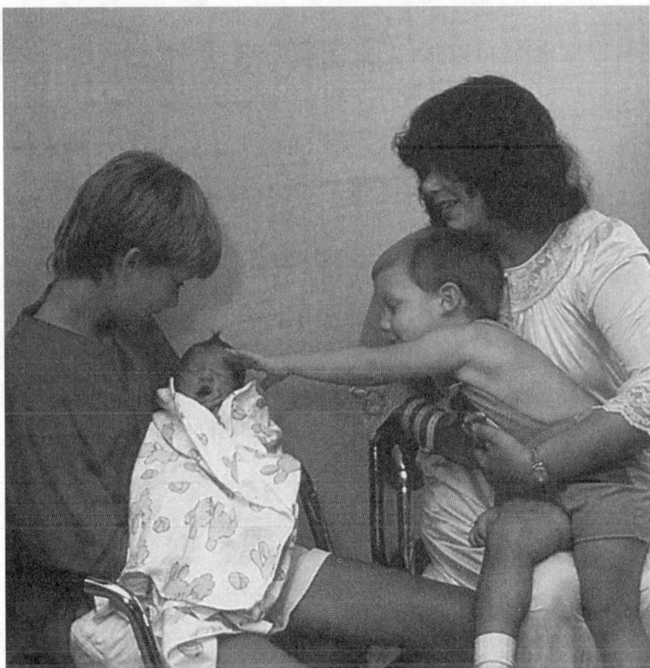

Fig. 16-29 Big brothers become acquainted with new baby sister. (From Wong D: *Whaley & Wong's nursing care of infants and children*, ed 5, St Louis, 1995, Mosby.)

in the final phases of the second stage, tend to experience renewed interest and excitement when the newborn appears and can be encouraged to hold the new family member (Fig. 16-29).

Parents are usually responsive to praise of their newborn. Many require reassurance that the dusky appearance of their baby's extremities immediately after birth is normal until circulation is well established. If appropriate, the nurse should explain the reason for the molding of the newborn's head. Information about hospital routine can be communicated. It is important, however, for nurses to recognize that the cultural background of the parents may influence expectations regarding care and handling of their newborn immediately after birth. For example, Southeast Asians believe that the head should not be touched, since it is the most sacred part of a person's body. They also believe that praise of the baby is dangerous, since jealous spirits may cause the baby harm or take it away (D'Avanzo, 1992). Hospital staff members, by their interest and concern, can do much to make this a satisfying experience for parents, family, and significant others.

Evaluation

Evaluation of outcomes is an ongoing activity. During each encounter with the new mother during the third stage of labor, the nurse evaluates the degree to which the expected outcomes are being met. For example, the woman's placenta is expelled and blood loss is less than 500 ml (<1% of body weight), the woman was prepared for the sensations she would experience and was not concerned when they occurred, and the woman, father/partner, and family initiated the process of bonding and attachment. Further assessment and collaborative care are warranted if the evaluation shows that results fall short of achieving an expected outcome (see the Nursing Care Plan on p. 440).

Interruption in Skin Integrity Related to Childbirth

Episiotomy. An episiotomy is an incision made in the perineum to enlarge the vaginal outlet. Episiotomies are performed more commonly in the United States and Canada than in Europe. The use of the side-lying position for birth is used routinely in Europe, whereas the position with legs in stirrups is more commonly used in the United States and Canada. With the side-lying position there is less tension on the perineum, and a gradual stretching of the perineum is possible. As a result there are fewer indications for the use of episiotomies.

The proponents for using the episiotomy say it serves the following purposes:

- Prevents tearing of the perineum. The clean and properly placed incision heals more properly than does a ragged tear. Some conditions that predispose a woman to perineal tearing and are therefore indications for episiotomy are a large infant, rapid labor in which there is not sufficient time for stretching of the perineum to take place, a narrow subpubic arch with a constricted outlet, and malpresentations of the fetus (e.g., the face). Research, however, does not support these claims. McGuinness et al (1991) found that women with episiotomies experienced a longer period of healing than did women without episiotomies. Midline episiotomies are also associated with a higher incidence of third- and fourth-degree lacerations (Helwig, Thorpe, and Bowes, 1993; McGuinness et al, 1991).
- Possibly minimizes prolonged and severe stretching of the muscles supporting the bladder or rectum, which may later lead to stress incontinence or to prolapse of pelvic organs (uterus, bladder, rectum). Research does not support the claim that pelvic support is protected when episiotomies are performed. Episiotomies and the third- and fourth-degree lacerations that can occur actually cut and extend into muscles, thereby prolonging recovery (Paciornik, 1990; Thorpe and Bowes, 1989).
- Reduces duration of the second stage, which may be important for maternal reasons (e.g., a hypertensive state) or fetal reasons (e.g., persistent bradycardia).
- Enlarges the vagina in case manipulation is needed for the infant's birth, for example, in a breech presentation or for application of forceps or vacuum extractor.

Those opposed to the *routine* use of episiotomies say the following:

- The perineum can be prepared for birth through use of the Kegel exercises and massage in the prenatal period. Use of Kegel exercises in the postpartum period improves and restores the tone and strength of the perineal muscles. Health practices, including good nutrition and appropriate hygienic measures, help to maintain the integrity and suppleness of the perineal tissue (Warren, 1989).
- Squatting or lateral positions during childbirth, encouraging women to push as their body tells them, and controlling the emergence of the fetal head while the woman pants increase the likelihood that the perineum will remain intact or, if lacerations occur, that they will be less severe (Golay et al, 1993; Paciornik, 1990).

Nursing Care Plan

THIRD STAGE OF LABOR

Nursing Diagnosis: Ineffective individual coping related to sense that labor process is over with emergence of neonate and lack of experience with sensations of third stage of labor

Expected outcome: Patient will actively participate in expulsion of the placenta.

• **NURSING INTERVENTIONS/*RATIONALES***

Explain to woman and labor partner what is expected in the third stage of labor *to enlist cooperation.*

Have woman maintain her position *to facilitate delivery of the placenta.*

Ask mother if she wishes to dispose of the placenta in any specific manner *to comply with certain cultural customs.*

Nursing Diagnosis: Fatigue related to energy expenditure required during labor and delivery

Expected outcome: Mother's energy levels are restored.

• **NURSING INTERVENTIONS/*RATIONALES***

Educate mother and partner about need for rest and help them plan strategies (i.e., restricting visitation, increasing role of support systems performing functions associated with daily routines) that allow specific times for rest and sleep *to ensure that woman can restore depleted energy levels in preparation for caring for a new infant.*

Monitor woman's fatigue level and the amount of rest received *to ensure restoration of energy.*

Nursing Diagnosis: Risk for fluid volume deficit related to decreased fluid intake and blood loss during delivery

Expected outcome: Fluid balance is maintained and there are no signs of dehydration.

• **NURSING INTERVENTIONS/*RATIONALES***

Monitor fluid loss (i.e., blood, urine, perspiration) and vital signs; inspect skin turgor and mucous membranes for dryness *to evaluate hydration status.*

Administer oral/parenteral fluids per physician/CNM orders *to maintain hydration.*

Monitor the fundus for firmness after placental separation *to ensure adequate contraction and prevent further blood loss.*

Administer medications per physician/CNM orders *to aid contraction of the uterus.*

- Lacerations may occur even with the use of an episiotomy; more third- and fourth-degree lacerations occur with an episiotomy (Helwig, Thorpe, and Bowes, 1993).
- Pain and discomfort from episiotomies can interfere with mother-infant interactions and the reestablishment of parental sexual intercourse.
- Episiotomies are indicated (1) if the well-being of the woman or fetus is in jeopardy, to shorten the second stage of labor; (2) if vacuum extraction or forceps are required; (3) if the infant is preterm and cerebral hemorrhage is a possibility because of capillary fragility; (4) if the infant is large (more than 4000 g [9 lb]); or (5) in most forceps and breech births (Röchner et al, 1989).

The type of episiotomy is designated by site and direction of the incision (Fig. 16-24).

Midline (median) episiotomy is most commonly used in the United States. It is effective, easily repaired, and generally the least painful. The midline episiotomy may extend through the rectal sphincter (third-degree laceration/extension) or even into the anal canal (fourth-degree laceration/extension). Primary healing and a good repair usually lead to restored sphincter tone.

Mediolateral episiotomy is employed in operative birth when posterior extension is likely. Although a fourth-degree laceration may thus be avoided, a third-degree laceration may occur. Moreover, as compared with a midline episiotomy, blood loss is greater, the repair more difficult and painful, and the mother experiences more discomfort.

Lacerations. Most acute injuries and lacerations of the perineum, vagina, uterus, and their support tissues occur during childbirth, and their management is an obstetric problem. Some injuries to the supporting tissues, whether they were acute or nonacute and whether they were repaired or not, may lead to gynecologic problems later in life (e.g., pelvic relaxation, uterine prolapse, cystocele, rectocele).

The soft tissues of the birth canal and adjacent structures suffer some damage during every birth. Damage usually is more pronounced in nulliparous women because the tissues are firmer and more resistant than in multiparous women. Perineal skin and vaginal mucosa may appear intact, obscuring numerous small lacerations in underlying muscle and its fascia. Damage to pelvic supports usually is readily apparent and thus is repaired after birth.

The individual woman's tendency to sustain lacerations varies; that is, the soft tissue in some women may be less capable of distention. Heredity may be a factor. For example, the tissue of very light-skinned (Caucasian) women, especially those with reddish hair, is not as readily distensible as that of darker-skinned women. In addition, healing may occur less efficiently in these women.

Currently, the practice in many settings is to manually support the perineum during birth and allow the perineum to tear rather than performing an episiotomy. Tears are often smaller than an episiotomy, are easily repaired, and heal quickly.

Immediate repair promotes healing and limits residual damage, plus it decreases the possibility of infection. Immediately after birth the cervix, vagina, and perineum are inspected. During the early postpartum days the nurse and physician/CNM carefully inspect the perineum and evaluate lochia and symptoms to identify any previously missed damage.

Perineal lacerations. Perineal lacerations usually occur as the fetal head is being born. The extent of the laceration is defined on the basis of depth:

First degree—Laceration extends through the skin and structures superficial to muscles.
Second degree—Laceration extends through muscles of perineal body.
Third degree—Laceration continues through anal sphincter muscle.
Fourth degree—Laceration also involves the anterior rectal wall.

Repair with absorbable suture is necessary. Third- and fourth-degree lacerations require special attention so that the woman retains fecal continence. The woman's comfort increases and healing is promoted by measures taken to ensure soft stools for a few days. Antimicrobial therapy may be used in some cases.

When the levator ani (including the iliococcygeus and pubococcygeus muscles, which form the slinglike support of the pelvic viscera) is not involved, simple perineal injuries usually heal without permanent disability regardless of whether they were repaired. However, the vaginal introitus may gape if torn or severed (episiotomy) ends of superficial perineal muscles (e.g., bulbocavernosus) are not well approximated during repair.

The ends of the torn or severed anal sphincter muscles must be repaired adequately to avoid fecal incontinence. It is easier to repair a new perineal injury to prevent sequelae than it is to correct long-term damage.

Vaginal and urethral lacerations. Vaginal lacerations often accompany perineal lacerations. Vaginal lacerations tend to extend up the lateral walls (sulci) and, if deep enough, involve the levator ani. Additional injury may occur high in the vaginal vault near the level of the ischial spines. Vaginal vault lacerations may be circular and may result from forceps rotation, especially in the presence of cephalopelvic disproportion (CPD), rapid fetal descent, and precipitous birth (Wheeler, 1991). Lacerations can occur around the urethra (periurethral) and also in the area of the clitoris. Lacerations in this very vascular area often result in profuse bleeding.

Cervical injuries. Cervical injuries occur when the cervix retracts over the advancing fetal head. These cervical lacerations occur at the lateral angles of the external os; most are shallow, and bleeding is minimal. Larger lacerations may extend to the vaginal vault or beyond the vault into the lower uterine segment; serious bleeding may occur. Extensive lacerations may follow hasty attempts to enlarge the cervical opening artificially or to deliver the fetus before full cervical dilation is achieved. Injuries to the cervix can have adverse effects on future pregnancies and childbirths.

Key Points

- The onset of labor may be difficult to determine.
- Although some complications of labor are anticipated, others are identified only as labor progresses.
- The nurse assumes much of the responsibility for assessing the progress of labor and for keeping the physician/certified nurse midwife informed about progress and deviations from expected findings.
- The fetal heart rate and pattern reveal the fetal response to the stress of the labor process.
- Meconium-staining of amniotic fluid is not always indicative of fetal distress associated with hypoxia.
- The woman's level of anxiety may rise when she does not understand what is being said to her about her labor because of the medical terminology used or because of a language barrier.
- Coaching, emotional support, and comfort measures assist the woman to use her energy constructively in relaxing and working with the contractions.
- The nurse who is aware of sociocultural aspects of helping and coping acts as an advocate/protective agent for the woman or couple during labor.
- During the second stage the woman needs continuous monitoring, support, and coaching.
- Objective signs indicate that the placenta has separated and is ready to be expelled; excessive traction (pulling) on the umbilical cord, before the placenta has separated, can result in maternal injury.
- Most parents/families enjoy being able to handle, hold, explore, and examine the baby immediately after birth.
- Nurses should observe progress in the development of parent-child relationships and be alert for warning signs that may appear during the immediate postpartum period.
- Following an emergency childbirth out of the hospital, the neonate sucking on the mother's nipple can stimulate the release of natural oxytocin from the maternal posterior pituitary gland; oxytocin stimulates the uterus to contract, thereby preventing postpartum hemorrhage.

References

Aderhold K, Perry L: Jet hydrotherapy for labor and postpartum pain relief, *MCN Am J Matern Child Nurs* 16(2):97, 1991.

Aderhold K, Roberts J: Phases of second stage labor: four descriptive care studies, *J Nurse Midwife* 36(5):267, 1991.

American College of Obstetricians and Gynecologists: More women now deliver in alternative birth sites, *ACOG Newsletter* 37(1):8, 1993.

Andrews C, Chrzanowski M: Maternal position, labor, and comfort, *Appl Nurs Res* 3(1):7, 1990.

Bergstrom L et al: "You'll feel me touching you, sweetie"; vaginal examination during the second stage of labor, *Birth* 19(1):10, 1992.

Berry L: Realistic expectations of the labor coach, *J Obstet Gynecol Neonatal Nurs* 17:354, 1988.

Biancuzzo M: Six myths of maternal posture during labor, *MCN Am J Matern Child Nurs* 18(5):264, 1993.

Biancuzzo M: The patient observer: does the hands and knees position during labor help to rotate the occiput posterior fetus? *Birth* 18(1):40, 1991.

Bonovich L: Recognizing the onset of labor, *J Obstet Gynecol Neonatal Nurs* 19(2):141, 1990.

Bryanton J, Fraser-Davey H, Sullivan P: Women's perception of nursing support during labor, *J Obstet Gynecol Neonatal Nurs* 23(8):638, 1994.

Callister L: The meaning of the childbirth experience to the Mormon woman, *J Perinatal Education* 1(1):50, 1992.

Callister L: Cultural meanings of childbirth, *J Obstet Gynecol Neonatal Nurs* 24(4):327, 1995.

Chalmers B, Meyer D: Companionship in the perinatal period: a cross-cultural survey of women's experiences, *J Nurse Midwife* 39(4):265, 1994.

Chapman L: Expectant father's roles during labor and birth, *J Obstet Gynecol Neonatal Nurs* 21(2):114, 1992.

Cosner K, deJong E: Physiologic second-stage labor, *MCN Am J Matern Child Nurs* 18(1):38, 1993.

Cunningham F, et al: *Williams obstetrics*, ed 19, Norwalk, CT, 1993, Appleton & Lange.

D'Avanzo C: Bridging the cultural gap with Southeast Asians, *MCN Am J Matern Child Nurs* 17(4):204, 1992.

DiMatteo M et al: Narratives of birth and the postpartum: analysis of the focus group responses of new mothers, *Birth* 20(4):204, 1993.

Evans S, Jeffery J: Maternal learning needs during labor and delivery, *J Obstet Gynecol Neonatal Nurs* 24(3):235, 1995.

Finn J: Culture care of Euro-American women during childbirth: using Leininger's theory, *J Transcultural Nursing* 5(2):25, 1994.

Friedman E, Sachtleben M: Station of the presenting part, *Am J Obstet Gynecol* 93:522, 1965.

Gannon J: Delivery on the hands and knees: a case study approach, *J Nurse Midwife* 37(1):48, 1992.

Gardosi J, Sylvester S, Lynch C: Alternative positions in the second stage of labour: a randomized controlled trial, *Br J Obstet Gynecol* 96:1290, 1989.

Geissler E: *Pocket guide to cultural assessment*, St Louis, 1994, Mosby.

Golay J, Vedam S, Sorger L: The squatting position for the second stage of labor: effects on labor and on maternal and fetal well-being, *Birth* 20(2):73, 1993.

Helwig J, Thorpe J, Bowes W: Does midline episiotomy increase the risk of third- and fourth-degree lacerations in operative vaginal deliveries? *Obstet Gynecol* 82:276, 1993.

Jonquil S: Preparing siblings, *Midwifery Today* 28:34, 1993.

Jordan E: *Second stage labor nursing management*, Presented at District IV AWHONN Conference, Washington, DC, October 8, 1995.

Jordan P: Laboring for relevance: expectant and new fatherhood, *Nurs Res* 39(1):11, 1990.

Kennell J et al: Continuous emotional support during labor in a US hospital: a randomized controlled trial, *JAMA* 265:2197, 1991.

Khazoyan C, Anderson N: Latina's expectations for their partners during childbirth, *MCN Am J Matern Child Nurs* 19(4):226, 1994.

Kitzinger S: Sheila Kitzinger's letter from England: birth plans, *Birth* 19(1):36, 1992.

Kline-Kaye V, Miller-Slade D: The use of fundal pressure during the second stage of labor, *J Obstet Gynecol Neonatal Nurs* 19(6):511, 1990.

Lantican S, Corona D: Comparison of the social support networks of Filipinos and Mexican American primigravidas, *Health Care Women Int* 13:329, 1992.

Liu Y: Effects of the upright position during childbirth, *Image J Nurs Sch* 21(1):14, 1989.

Luegenbiehl D et al: Standardized assessment of blood loss, *MCN Am J Matern Child Nurs* 15:241, 1990.

Luegenbiehl D: Postpartum bleeding, *NAACOG's Clinical Issues in Perinatal and Women's Health Nursing* 2(3):402, 1991.

Mackey M: Women's evaluation of their childbirth performance, *Matern Chil Nurs J* 23(2):57, 1995.

Mahan C, McKay S: Are we overmanaging second stage labor? *Contemp OB GYN* 24(12):37, 1984.

Malestic S: Fathers need help during labor, too, *RN* 53:23, 1990.

McGuinness M, Norr K, Nacion K: Comparison between different perineal outcomes on tissue healing, *J Nurse Midwife* 36(3):192, 1991.

McKay S, Barrows T: Holding back: maternal readiness to give birth, *MCN Am J Matern Child Nurs* 16(5):251, 1991.

McKay S, Roberts J: Maternal position during labor and birth: what have we learned? *Int J Childbirth Educ* 13(8):19, 1989.

McKay S, Roberts J: Obstetrics by ear. Maternal and caregiver perceptions of the meaning of maternal sounds during second stage labor, *J Nurse Midwife* 35(5):266, 1990.

McKay S, Smith S: "What are they talking about? Is something wrong?" Information sharing during the second stage of labor, *Birth* 20(3):142, 1993.

Melzak R, Belanger E, Lacroix R: Labor pain: effects of maternal position on front and back pain, *J Pain Symptom Manage* 6(8):476, 1991.

Metzer B, Therrien B: Effect of position on cardiovascular response during the Valsalva maneuver, *Nurs Res* 39(4):198, 1990.

Moore M, Hopper U, Dip G: Do birth plans empower women? Evaluation of a hospital birth plan, *Birth* 22(1):29, 1995.

Myles M: *Textbook for midwives*, ed 11, Edinburgh, 1989, Churchill Livingstone.

Nichols M: Paternal perspectives of the childbirth experience, *Matern Child Nurs J* 21(3):99, 1993.

Paciornik M: Commentary: arguments against episiotomy and in favor of squatting for birth, *Birth* 17(2):104, 1990.

Pascoe J: Social support during labor and duration of labor: a community-based study, *Public Health Nurs* 10(2):97, 1993.

Queenan J: Partners in the delivery room: a natural evolution, *Contemp OB GYN* 35(8):8, 1990.

Röchner G, Wahlberg V, Ölund A: Episiotomy and perineal trauma during childbirth, *J Adv Nurs* 14:264, 1989.

Scherer P: Supported squatting enhances the second stage of labor, *Am J Nurs* 89(10):1266, 1989.

Rosenthal M: Warm-water immersion in labor and birth, *Female Patient* 16(8):35, 1991.

Scott J et al: *Danforth's obstetrics and gynecology*, ed 7, Philadelphia, 1994, JB Lippincott.

Simkin P: Just another day in a woman's life? Women's long-term perceptions of their first birth experience. Part 1, *Birth* 18(4):203, 1991.

Thomson A: Pushing technique in the second stage of labor, *J Adv Nurs* 18:171, 1993.

Thorpe J, Bowes W: Episiotomy: can its routine use be defended, *Am J Obstet Gynecol* 160(5):1027, 1989.

Tomlinson P, Rothenberg M, Carver L: Behavioral interaction of fathers with infants and mothers in the immediate postpartum period, *J Nurs Midwife* 36:232, 1991.

Tucker S: *Pocket guide to fetal monitoring,* ed 2, St Louis, 1992, Mosby.

Waldenstrom U, Gottvall K: A randomized trial of birthing stool or conventional semirecumbent position for second stage labor, *Birth* 18(1):5, 1991.

Warren C: Making sense of . . . episiotomy, *Nurs Times* 85(44):60, 1989.

Wheeler D: Intrapartum bleeding, *NAACOGs Clin Issu Perinat Womens Health Nurs* 2(3):281, 1991.

Woods A: Nurse midwifery in rural Pakistan, *J Nurse Midwife* 36(4):249, 1991.

Yeates J, Roberts J: A comparison of two bearing-down techniques during the second stage of labor, *J Nurse Midwife* 29:3, 1984.

Bibliography

Bluff R, Halloway I: "They know best": women's perceptions of midwifery care during labour and childbirth, *Midwifery* 10:157, 1994.

Bond M, Keen-Payne R, Lucy P: The ideal nurse for the relinquishing mother: lessons from the labor room, *MCN Am J Matern Child Nurs* 20(3):156, 1995.

Buenting J: Human energy fields and birth: implications for research and practice, *Adv Nurs Sci* 15(4):53, 1993.

Greulich B et al: Twelve years and more than 30,000 nurse-midwife-attended births: the Los Angeles County and University of Southern California Women's Hospital Birth Center experience, *J Nurse Midwife* 39:185, 1994.

Mackey M, Flanders Stephan M: Women's evaluations of their labor and delivery nurses, *J Obstet Gynecol Neonatal Nurs* 23(5):413, 1994.

Martin E: *Intrapartum management modules,* ed 2, Baltimore, 1996, Williams & Wilkins.

Mayberry L: Intrapartal nursing care: research into practice, *J Obstet Gynecol Neonatal Nurs* 23(2):170, 1994.

Schorn M, McAllister J, Blanco J: Water immersion and the effect on labor, *J Nurse Midwife* 38(6):336, 1993.

Shorts Hopko N: Birth in the Japanese context, *J Obstet Gynecol Neonatal Nurs* 24(4):343, 1995.

Thilaganathan B, Meher-Homji N, Nicolaides K: Labor: an immunologically beneficial process for the neonate, *Am J Obstet Gynecol* 171:1271, 1994.

CHAPTER 17

Labor and Birth at Risk

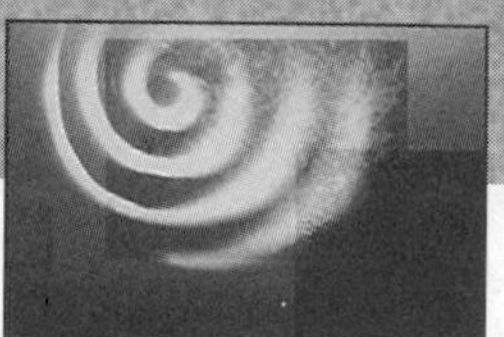

PRETERM LABOR AND BIRTH, P. 444
Etiologic factors, p. 445
Nursing care management, p. 445

PREMATURE RUPTURE OF MEMBRANES, P. 452
Etiologic factors, p. 452
Plan of care and implementation, p. 452

DYSTOCIA, P. 452
Dysfunctional labor, p. 452
Alterations in pelvic structure, p. 453
Fetal causes, p. 454
Position of the woman, p. 456
Psychologic response, p. 456
Abnormal labor patterns, p. 456
Nursing care management, p. 458

POSTDATE PREGNANCY, LABOR, AND BIRTH, P. 472
Maternal and fetal risks, p. 472
Nursing care management, p. 474

OBSTETRIC EMERGENCIES, P. 475
Shoulder dystocia, p. 475
Nursing care management, p. 475
Prolapsed umbilical cord, p. 475
Nursing care management, p. 475
Rupture of the uterus, p. 475
Nursing care management, p. 477
Amniotic fluid embolism, p. 477
Nursing care management, p. 477

When complications arise during labor and birth, perinatal morbidity and mortality increase. Some complications are anticipated, especially if the mother is identified as high risk during the antepartum period; others are unexpected or unforeseen. The woman, her family, and the obstetric team can feel devastated when things go wrong. These feelings must be recognized if nurses are to provide effective support. It is crucial for nurses to understand the normal birth process to prevent and detect deviations from normal labor and birth and to implement nursing measures when complications arise. Optimum care of the laboring woman, fetus, and family experiencing complications is possible only when the nurse and other members of the obstetric team use their knowledge and skills in a concerted effort to provide care.

This chapter focuses on labor and birth problems related to preterm labor and birth, dystocia, and postdate pregnancy and obstetric emergencies. The discussion of care of the woman experiencing preterm labor includes home and hospital assessment and management. The discussion of interventions for dystocia includes trial of labor, induction of labor, forceps-assisted birth, vacuum extraction, cesarean birth, and vaginal birth after cesarean. The discussion of the woman experiencing postdate pregnancy includes assessment strategies and management during labor and birth. Assessment and management of obstetric emergencies, including shoulder dystocia, prolapsed cord, amniotic fluid embolism, and rupture of the uterus are discussed.

PRETERM LABOR AND BIRTH

Preterm labor is defined as the onset of regular uterine contractions that cause cervical changes between 20 and 37 weeks of gestation. **Preterm birth** occurs before the end of 37 weeks of gestation. The overall incidence of preterm birth in the United States is approximately 10%. Preterm birth is responsible for 83% of infant deaths, not including those associated with congenital anomalies (Creasy, 1993).

The infant born before term does not possess the growth and development necessary for an uncomplicated adjustment to extrauterine life. His or her prospects for survival or good health may be severely compromised. For those who survive, the emotional and financial costs to families and health care systems are phenomenal. The average neonatal intensive care cost for one preterm infant is estimated to be $40,000 to $50,000. The cost for long-term care and special education for preterm infants born with severe physical and neurologic handicaps is estimated to be more than $500,000 (Blackman, 1991; Morrison, 1990).

Etiologic Factors

In approximately 50% of all preterm births, no definite cause can be identified. However, one third of all preterm labors occur after premature rupture of membranes (Gilbert and Harmon, 1993).

Risk factors for preterm labor and birth have been identified. Categories of risk include demographic risks, medical risks, current pregnancy risks, and behavioral and environmental risks (Knuppel and Drukker, 1993; Neal and Bockman, 1992; Wheeler, 1994) (Box 17-1).

In the United States, African-American women are twice as likely as Caucasian women or other non-Caucasian women (Hispanic, Native-American, Japanese) to give birth to low–birth-weight infants, many of whom are also preterm. A high risk for preterm labor is common in women who are younger than 17 or older than 35 years of age, are single, did not graduate from high school, are of low socioeconomic status, and have poor nutrition.

Women who have certain medical risks before pregnancy, especially previous preterm labor or birth or previous abortion, are at greater risk for preterm labor. Uterine anomalies, an incompetent cervix, diethylstilbestrol (DES) exposure in utero, and specific medical conditions such as hypertension and diabetes mellitus are associated with higher preterm birth rates.

Risks associated with a current pregnancy include pregnancy-induced hypertension, placental problems, anemia, spontaneous premature rupture of membranes, polyhydramnios, multifetal gestation, uterine fibroids, and fetal anomalies. Infections of the urinary tract and vagina have also been identified as risk factors (Heffner et al, 1993).

Smoking more than 10 cigarettes a day, alcohol or substance abuse, and a lack of prenatal care are among the maternal habits and activities that increase the risk of a preterm birth. Work, long commutes to work (more than 1½ hours each way), and stress also may affect the rate of preterm birth.

Uterine irritability, events that trigger uterine contractions (e.g., sexual activity, progesterone deficiency, inadequate plasma volume), and certain infections (e.g., chlamydia, group B streptococcus, *Escherichia coli*, and chorioamnionitis) may be involved in the onset of preterm labor. However, the impact of these factors is not clearly understood (Heffner et al, 1993; Main and Main, 1991; Wheeler, 1994).

BOX 17-1

Risk Factors for Preterm Labor

DEMOGRAPHIC RISKS

- Race (African-American)
- Age (<17 yr, >35 yr)
- Low socioeconomic status
- Unmarried
- Less than high school education level

MEDICAL RISKS

- Previous preterm labor or birth
- Second-trimester abortion (more than two spontaneous or therapeutic)
- Uterine anomalies
- Medical diseases (e.g., diabetes, hypertension)
- Current pregnancy risks
  - Multifetal pregnancy
  - Polyhydramnios
  - Poor weight gain
  - Placental problems (e.g., placenta previa, abruptio placentae)
  - Infections (e.g., pyelonephritis, recurrent UTIs,* chorioamnionitis
  - Incompetent cervix
  - Uterine fibroids
  - Spontaneous premature rupture of membranes
  - Fetal anomalies

BEHAVIORAL AND ENVIRONMENTAL RISKS

- Poor nutrition
- Smoking (>10 cigarettes a day)
- Alcohol and other substance abuse (especially cocaine)
- DES* exposure and other toxic exposures
- Little or no prenatal care
- Long commutes (>1½ hr each way)
- Heavy physical work

POTENTIAL RISK FACTORS

- Stress
- Uterine irritability
- Events triggering uterine contractions (e.g., orgasm)
- Cervical changes before onset of labor
- Inadequate plasma volume expansion
- Progesterone deficiency
- Infections (e.g., mycoplasma, *Chlamydia trachomatis*, group B streptococcus)

**DES*, Diethylstilbestrol; *UTIs*, urinary tract infections.

Nursing Care Management

Assessment

Obstetric management of preterm birth involves early detection of preterm labor, suppression of uterine activity, and improvement of intrapartum care of the fetus that is destined to be born early.

At their initial prenatal visit, all pregnant women are screened according to risk factors associated with preterm labor. Many risk-scoring systems have been developed to assist in identifying women who might be at high risk for preterm labor. Women need to be reassessed at each subsequent visit. Those who are considered to be high risk are followed up more closely (e.g., on a weekly basis). They receive education regarding the symptoms of preterm labor and instructions in palpating, timing, and reporting uterine contractions.

Home uterine monitoring with an ambulatory tocodynamometer (Fig. 17-1) may be implemented to detect excessive uterine contractions before they can be perceived by the woman herself. The woman records uterine activity twice a day or more often if necessary; the data are transmitted by telephone to the hospital or to a monitoring service for analysis. Appropriate therapy is instituted if labor is suspected (Hill et al, 1990). Although some studies show an association between the use of home uterine activity monitoring and a lower incidence of preterm birth, others speculate that the decrease is related to more frequent contact with health care providers (Creasy and Merkatz, 1990; Dyson et al, 1991; Hill et al, 1990). The cost of home uterine monitoring using the tocodynamometer is estimated to be $450 per day; whether this type of monitoring is cost-effective for detecting preterm

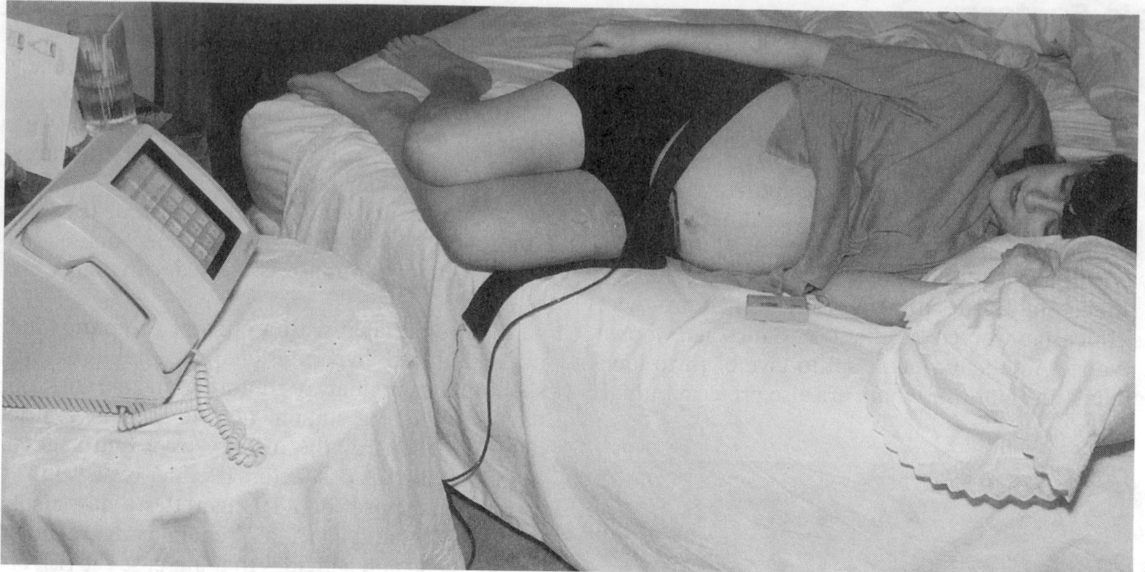

Fig. 17-1 Home uterine activity monitoring. **A,** Recording unit and transmitter. **B,** Tocodynamometer in place at center of abdomen below umbilicus. (Courtesy Michael S. Clement, MD, Mesa, Ariz.)

labor is also controversial (Wheeler, 1994). Continued study is needed.

Nursing Diagnoses

The common nursing diagnoses for the woman with preterm labor include the following:

- Knowledge deficit related to
  - Recognition of preterm labor or management of preterm labor
- Risk for maternal or fetal injury related to
  - Preterm labor and birth
  - Prescribed maternal bed rest
- Anxiety related to
  - Possible preterm birth
- Impaired physical mobility related to
  - Prescribed bed rest
- Anticipatory grieving related to
  - Potential loss of fetus
- Situational low self-esteem related to
  - Inability to carry pregnancy to term

Expected Outcomes

The nurse develops a plan of care based on whether the woman's care is managed at home or in the hospital. Common expected outcomes include the following. The woman will:

1. Demonstrate compliance with prescribed activity limitations, uterine monitoring (self-palpation or home monitoring equipment), or medication schedules
2. Not experience complications from prescribed medication management or activity restrictions
3. Carry the pregnancy to term or near-term
4. Give birth to a healthy, mature infant

Plan of Care and Implementation

Identifying preterm labor. Pregnant women should be taught to notify their health care provider if they have symptoms of preterm labor, particularly uterine contractions that occur more frequently than every 10 minutes (Box 17-2). If the woman is active, it may be helpful for her to lie on her side, drink fluids, and keep her bladder empty to increase blood flow to the uterus to correct myometrial hypoxia and to decrease uterine activity. If the woman continues to have uterine contractions after implementing these interventions for 1 hour, she usually is instructed to come to the health care provider's office or hospital for further evaluation. There the woman is positioned on her side, and an external fetal and uterine monitor is applied to assess uterine activity and fetal heart rate (FHR). Vital signs are obtained. An intravenous infusion may be started to provide additional hydration. A clean-catch or catheterized urine specimen is obtained and examined for the presence of a urinary tract infection. If substance abuse is suspected, a urine toxicology screen is obtained. A sterile speculum examination usually is performed to obtain cervical or vaginal cultures to detect the presence of an infection such as group B streptococcus, chlamydia, or gonorrhea. A cervical examination is performed to assess for dilation or effacement.

The diagnosis of preterm labor includes both uterine and cervical changes in effacement or dilation or both (Andersen and Merkatz, 1994). If uterine activity subsides and if dilation and effacement do not change from the initial examination, the woman may be discharged to home. She may be given instructions regarding activity limitations (Box 17-2) and medications for the prevention of preterm labor. If labor continues, care continues in the hospital setting until the woman's condition is stable and she can go home (on a regimen of either restricted activity or medications to prevent the recurrence of preterm labor) or until the infant is born.

BOX 17-2

Protocol for Home Management of Preterm Labor

Assessments (to be Performed Daily Unless Otherwise Specified)

Monitor uterine contractions 2-3 times per day for 30 minutes to 1 hour as instructed (by self-palpation or use of home uterine activity monitoring [HUAM] device). If HUAM is used, transmit data as instructed.

Assess for fetal activity daily by counting fetal movements as instructed. If an RN is visiting, FHR and nonstress testing may be performed as prescribed.

Review the signs and symptoms of preterm labor. Report the following occurrences to your health care provider:

- Menstrual-like cramps
- Uterine tightening
- Increase in vaginal discharge
- Low backache
- Pelvic pressure
- Rupture of membranes
- Weigh yourself, and determine your blood pressure and/or pulse as instructed.

Blood tests, urine checks, and/or cervical assessments may be performed by the visiting RN as prescribed.

Interventions

Follow instructions about limiting your activities as prescribed; for example, remain on bed rest on your side except to go to the bathroom.

Practice relaxation techniques.

Eat well-balanced meals; be sure to include roughage in your diet.

Drink 8 to 10 (8 oz) glasses of fluids every day.

Avoid or limit activities that could stimulate labor, as instructed (e.g., sexual activity that causes orgasm, breast stimulation).

Take medications as prescribed. Report side effects to your health care provider.

Keep appointments with your health care provider.

Data from Grohar J: Nursing protocols for antepartum nursing care, *J Obstet Gynecol Neonatal Nurs* 23(8):687, 1994.

Home Care 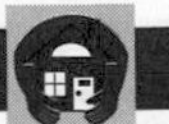

ACTIVITIES FOR CHILDREN OF WOMEN REQUIRING BED REST

- Schedule brief play periods throughout the day.
- Keep a few favorite toys in a box or basket close to the bed or couch.
- Read to the child(ren).
- Put puzzles together.
- Watch videos, play video games (a remote control for the television is ideal).
- Play cards or board games.
- Color in coloring books.
- Cut out pictures from magazines and paste on cardboard.
- Play bed basketball with a soft (sponge) ball or rolled-up sock and a trash can or empty laundry basket.

Modified from Isennock P: *Bed rest before baby: what's a mother to do?* Perry Hall, Md, 1992, Mustard Seed Publishing; Maurer L: *Confinement connection: a home support program,* Phoenix, 1992.

Home care. If the episode of preterm labor subsides and the woman is allowed to return home, she is followed in the outpatient setting with frequent visits and cervical examinations. The nurse reviews the signs and symptoms of preterm labor at each visit. Including the woman's family is essential because of the impact preterm labor has on the entire family. For example, the woman may have small children at home who need care and supervision; she may work outside the home and be forced to take a leave of absence or even lose her job. The restriction on her activities can disrupt the daily lives of all family members, causing them to assume different roles and responsibilities.

The care of the woman with preterm labor at home may or may not be supervised by a home health caregiver. The plan of care prescribed for the woman is shared with all caregivers and family members so that everyone has the information needed to assist the woman in staying motivated to comply with the plan. The woman's condition is assessed daily unless otherwise specified (Box 17-2).

Women who have their activities restricted for preterm labor must cope with the difficulties related to limited activity. The physiologic effects of bed rest include weight loss, muscle loss, decreased plasma volume, calcium loss, and increased clotting (Maloni, 1994). Psychosocial effects also occur. The need for emotional support, help with household management, time management, and child care has also been documented and may require intervention. For example, if there are children at home who need care, the nurse can suggest activities to keep the children entertained without requiring the woman to exert herself (see the Home Care box above). Boredom is a problem that the woman may face if prolonged bed rest has been prescribed. The nurse assesses the woman's interests in activities that are acceptable within her limitations. The Home Care box on p. 448 provides ideas for activities that can be performed during bed rest. Women who have preterm labor also may benefit from a referral to a high-risk support group.

Hospital care. Nursing assessments for the woman hospitalized for preterm labor are similar to those performed in the home setting, except that the nurse may be initiating the assessments and providing the interventions. These assessments may include determinations of vital signs, weight gain, lung function, FHR and fetal movement, and fundal height; urine checks for glucose, protein, and ketones; cervical examination to detect changes; uterine activity monitoring; gastrointestinal function; deep tendon reflexes; edema; and psychosocial adaptation. Prolonged hospitalization can have the same negative physiologic and psychologic effects as home care with bed rest. It is important to remember that involving the woman in as many care decisions as possible usually is beneficial to her self-esteem.

Suppression of uterine activity. Tocolytic treatment may be used to stop labor if uterine contractions persist or if cervical changes occur. **Tocolytic agents** are drugs that inhibit

Home Care

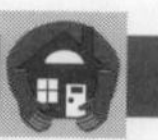

SUGGESTED ACTIVITIES FOR WOMEN REQUIRING BED REST

Set a routine for daily activities (e.g., getting dressed, moving from the bedroom to a "day bed rest place," social time, meals, self-monitoring of fetus and uterine activity).
Do passive exercises as allowed.
Review childbirth education information, or have a childbirth class at home if available.
Plan menus and grocery shopping lists.
Shop by phone.
Read books about high-risk pregnancy or other topics.
Keep a journal of the pregnancy.
Keep a calendar of the progress of the pregnancy.
Reorganize files, recipes, or the household budget.
Update address book.
Do mending, sewing.
Listen to audiotapes, watch videos, watch television.
Do crossword puzzles, jigsaw puzzles, or similar activities.
Do craft projects; make something for the baby.
Put pictures in photo albums.
Call a friend, family member, or support person each day.
For a needed lift, treat yourself to a facial, manicure, neck massage, or other special treat.

Data from Gilbert E, Harmon J: *Manual of high-risk pregnancy and delivery*, St Louis, 1993, Mosby; Isennock P: *Bed rest before baby: what's a mother to do?* Perry Hall, Md, 1992, Mustard Seed Publishing; Maloni J: Home care of the high-risk pregnant woman requiring bed rest, *J Obstet Neonatal Gynecol Nurs* 23(8):696, 1994.

EMERGENCY

PULMONARY EDEMA CAUSED BY RITODRINE THERAPY

SIGNS

Dyspnea
Crackles

INTERVENTIONS

Discontinue drug immediately.
Start oxygen via face mask.
Give intravenous diuretics as ordered.
Restrict fluids.
Notify physician.

uterine contractions. *Toko-* and *toco-* are Greek roots referring to obstetrics; *-lytic* is also Greek and means "to break down" or "to stop". The agents used include β-adrenergic drugs such as ritodrine or terbutaline and magnesium sulfate (Andersen and Merkatz, 1994).

Ritodrine. Ritodrine (Yutopar) was the first and remains the only β-sympathomimetic drug approved by the Food and Drug Administration (FDA) for use in the United States to inhibit preterm labor (Cunningham et al, 1993). Ritodrine acts on type II β-adrenergic receptors of the sympathetic nervous system, which inhibit uterine muscle activity and cause vasodilation, bronchodilation, and muscle glycogenolysis. Because β-receptor sites are present in other organs, side effects occur. The cardiovascular system is most affected, but metabolic effects also occur because receptor sites are in the liver and pancreas. Ritodrine can cause a decrease in serum potassium levels, resulting in arrhythmias. Other side effects are similar to those described for terbutaline (Box 17-3). The initial dose (50 μg/min, increased every 10 to 20 minutes until contractions stop or until a maximum dose of 350 μg/min is reached) usually is given intravenously, followed by intramuscular therapy, oral therapy, or both after the woman's condition is stabilized (Mongra and Creasy, 1995). The maintenance dose is determined by the primary health care provider and the woman's response to the medication. The oral dose ranges from 10 to 20 mg every 4 to 6 hours.

Contraindications for use include maternal diseases such as cardiovascular disease, severe preeclampsia, severe antepartum hemorrhage, chorioamnionitis, and hyperthyroidism. Fetal death and a gestational age of less than 20 weeks confirmed by ultrasound scan are two fetal-related contraindications.

Cardiopulmonary complications are possible. Some deaths in pregnant women with unrecognized preexisting cardiovascular disease have been reported with the use of ritodrine. Therefore careful assessment and monitoring are essential. Because of the possible cardiopulmonary effects, an electrocardiogram may be ordered before the first dose. A cardiac monitor for the mother may be indicated to maintain continuous assessment for *tachycardia, arrhythmia,* and *pulmonary edema* (see the Emergency box above).

Terbutaline. Terbutaline (Brethine) is another β-adrenergic agent; it is used more often than ritodrine for preterm labor. Although it has not been approved by the FDA for this use, some health care providers prefer terbutaline because of long-term clinical use with fewer serious side effects than ritodrine. Administration and contraindications are similar to those described for ritodrine, but terbutaline is more often given subcutaneously or orally.

Prolonged and continuous high-dose treatment with ritodrine or terbutaline causes desensitization of β-adrenergic receptors; preterm labor usually recurs as a result of tocolytic breakthrough. The use of subcutaneous terbutaline by pump infusion for long-term tocolysis has been reported to be effective in preventing this recurrence (Gilbert and Harmon, 1993). Pump therapy decreases desensitization by delivering a continuous low-dose infusion, with intermittent bolus doses at times when uterine activity is known to occur in the individual woman. The average daily dose by pump is 3 to 4 mg terbutaline administered subcutaneously (not including bolus doses); a daily oral dose is 30 to 60 mg over divided doses (Romero and Jones, 1994).

Women who use the terbutaline pump (Fig. 17-2) require instruction in the operation of the pump and self-injection techniques. In addition, they need to know the signs of preterm labor and how to palpate uterine contractions, recognize the warning signs and symptoms of terbutaline toxicity (Box 17-3), and follow activity precautions.

NURSING CONSIDERATIONS. Nursing interventions for women receiving ritodrine or terbutaline depend on whether the medication is administered intravenously, subcutaneously, or orally. Before intravenous therapy, the woman usually receives hydration with 500 ml isotonic crystalloid over 30 minutes. The medication is then administered via pump infusion.

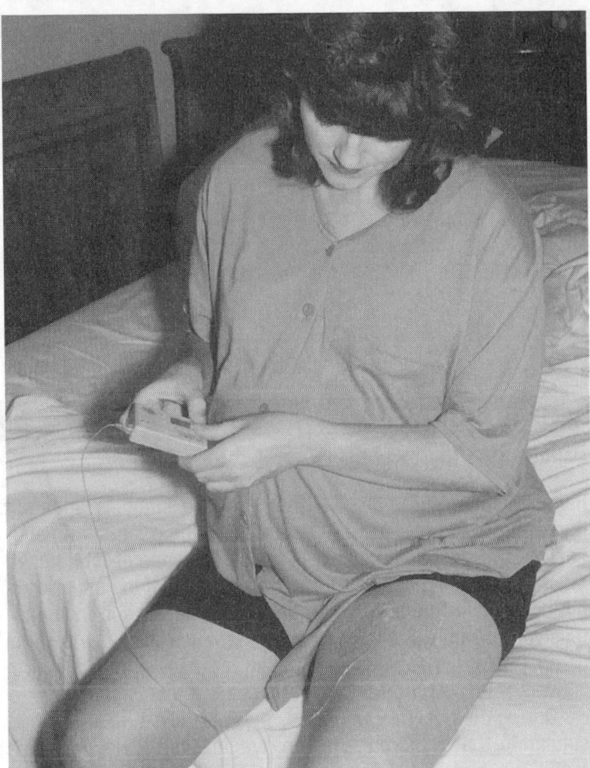

Fig. 17-2 Subcutaneous terbutaline pump attached to patient. (Courtesy Michael S. Clement, MD, Mesa, Ariz.)

BOX 17-3
Warning Signs—Side Effects of Terbutaline

MATERNAL

Central nervous system
Severe dizziness, drowsiness, headache, nervousness, restlessness

Blood pressure
Widening pulse pressure (increase in systolic, decrease in diastolic)

Heart rate
Continuous palpitations, chest pain, tachycardia ≥120 beats/min

Musculoskeletal
Severe muscle cramps and weakness

Gastrointestinal
Continuous nausea and vomiting

Respiratory
Shortness of breath, coughing, respirations >24/min, pulmonary edema (life-threatening)

Metabolic
Hyperglycemia, hypokalemia

FETAL

Tachycardia >180 beats/min
Hypoglycemia
Hyperinsulinemia

The dose is increased in increments as ordered, using the minimum amount of the medication that will stop uterine contractions. After 12 to 24 hours of successful therapy, oral therapy usually is instituted as the intravenous therapy is tapered (Gilbert and Harmon, 1993).

During intravenous therapy, the nurse monitors uterine activity and FHR continuously. FHR should not exceed 180 beats/min. Maternal vital signs, including blood pressure, are assessed per protocol; pulse should not exceed 120 beats/min. Breath sounds are assessed, and the lungs are auscultated every 8 to 12 hours. The nurse assesses the woman for other signs of medication side effects such as fluid overload, pulmonary edema, and cardiac arrhythmias. If any are noted, the medication is stopped and the primary health care provider is notified. An *antidote,* a β-blocking agent such as *propranolol (Inderal),* may be prescribed. The maximum intravenous fluid rate is 125 ml/hr. Blood samples may be drawn for laboratory analysis of glucose and potassium levels to detect hyperglycemia or hypokalemia, two common side effects of the medication. The woman is maintained on a regimen of bed rest in a side-lying position to optimize placental perfusion and to decrease pressure on the cervix. Intake and output and daily weights are monitored to detect overhydration. The woman should be told about the potential side effects of the therapy to prevent undue anxiety if they occur.

If the woman is on an oral or subcutaneous therapy regimen, maternal vital signs, FHR, fetal activity, and uterine activity are assessed per hospital routine or as ordered. If the woman's pulse is 120 beats/min or higher, the primary health care provider is usually notified before administering a dose. Medications need to be given on time every 4 to 6 hours to maintain blood levels and prevent the recurrence of uterine activity.

Magnesium sulfate. Magnesium sulfate is known to decrease uterine activity. It is used as a tocolytic agent because it is safer for the woman than ritodrine. It usually is given intravenously, but intramuscular and oral routes may be used (Andersen and Merkatz, 1994). If administered orally, magnesium oxide or gluconate is used; the main side effect is diarrhea (Creasy, 1993).

For intravenous therapy, magnesium sulfate is mixed with normal saline, and an initial 4-g dose is infused over a 20-minute period. The medication is infused via a pump at 1 to 2 g/hr and increased per protocol (usually 0.5 g/hr every 15 to 30 minutes) until the contractions stop. After 12 hours of successful therapy, oral tocolytic therapy is usually started.

NURSING CONSIDERATIONS. Nursing assessments during the intravenous administration of magnesium sulfate therapy include monitoring blood pressure, pulse, and respiratory rates; checking deep tendon reflexes; measuring intake and output; assessing level of consciousness; checking laboratory results for therapeutic levels of magnesium (4 to 8 g/dl); and checking calcium levels for hypocalcemia. Calcium gluconate

BOX 17-4
Magnesium Sulfate: Side Effects/Toxicity

Common Side Effects
Hot flushes
Nausea and vomiting
Drowsiness
Blurred vision

Signs of Toxicity
Respirations <12/min
Absent deep tendon reflexes
Severe hypotension
Urinary retention
Extreme lethargy/muscle weakness

BOX 17-5
Side Effects of Nifedipine

Headache
Fatigue
Hypotension
Dizziness
Peripheral edema
Vasodilation

should be available to reverse serious side effects (Box 17-4). Uterine activity and FHR also are monitored.

Calcium channel blockers. Calcium channel blockers prevent preterm labor by blocking the movement of calcium into the smooth muscles of the uterus, which prevents uterine contractions. Nifedipine (Procardia) is the medication usually given for preterm labor, although preterm labor is still considered an investigational use of this medication (Mongra and Creasy, 1995). The dose ranges from 10 to 20 mg orally or sublingually every 3 to 8 hours (Ferguson et al, 1990; Gilbert and Harmon, 1993). Fewer side effects are reported for nifedipine than for the β-agonists (Box 17-5). More research is needed to determine the potential benefits and risks to the woman and fetus.

Prostaglandin inhibitors. Prostaglandin antagonists (nonsteroidal inflammatory agents [naproxen, indomethacin], and salicylates) are being investigated for the treatment of preterm labor. These agents are as effective in relaxing the uterus as β-agonists. Maternal side effects are minimal but may include nausea, headache, tinnitis, and vertigo. However, concern about the potential effects on the fetus (especially premature closing of the ductus arteriosus) and bleeding continue to limit their use (Eronen et al, 1991; Mongra and Creasy, 1995). Studies suggest that the use of prostaglandin inhibitors for short periods (<48 hours) may limit fetal effects (Keirse, 1995). Investigation of prostaglandin synthesis inhibitors for preterm labor continues.

Promotion of fetal lung maturity. Respiratory distress syndrome (RDS) is common in small preterm infants with lung immaturity. The incidence and severity of RDS is reduced if glucocorticoids (e.g., betamethasone) are administered to the mother at least 24 to 48 hours before the birth. The fetus must be at less than 34 weeks of gestation. The administration must occur at least 24 hours before birth and no more than 7 days before birth.

Neither tocolytics nor steroidal therapy is universally recommended for preterm labor after premature rupture of membranes (Andersen and Merkatz, 1994). The woman who has received both tocolytics and glucocorticoids is at risk for cardiac decompensation resulting from side effects of the medications. Therefore the nurse should be vigilant in monitoring the woman for signs of cardiac decompensation (see p. 274).

Family Focus

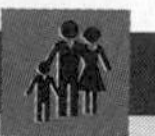

IMPACT OF PRETERM BIRTHS

Parental concern for the well-being of the infant is apparent during labor. Parents need to be aware of the interest and support of staff members. However, false assurance of fetal health must be avoided. For some parents the reality of the situation is not appreciated until they see their daughter or son in the intensive care unit. For those who experience fetal or neonatal death, the loss intensifies once the stress of labor and childbirth is over.

During the postpartum period, physical care of the mother is similar to that required after any vaginal birth. However, the family will be very anxious concerning the health and prognosis of the infant. Care of the preterm infant involves not only medical and nursing personnel but also participation of the parents. The nurse must be aware of the impact that a preterm birth may have on family dynamics. Parents must accept that the infant has special needs, and they must learn to meet these needs before discharge so that they have more realistic expectations when they are at home (Weingarten et al, 1990).

Care during preterm labor and birth. If labor cannot be stopped, the physician makes every attempt to help the woman give birth to the preterm infant safely and without trauma. If needed and if time permits, the woman is usually transferred to a center with neonatal services adequate to provide care for the preterm infant. During labor, medications such as narcotics or barbiturates that can depress the fetus are avoided. An epidural analgesic is commonly used during labor, but a pudendal block or local anesthetic may be administered for the birth. An episiotomy may be performed to shorten the second stage of labor and to reduce excessive pressure on the fragile fetal head. The route of birth is controversial, but a cesarean birth may be performed for malpresentation and maternal or fetal distress (Andersen and Merkatz, 1994). (See the Family Focus box above).

Evaluation

Evaluating the effectiveness of nursing care for women with preterm labor is based on the expected outcomes, which include the woman verbalizing an understanding of her treatment, complying with her prescribed treatment, developing no complications related to drug therapy, and giving birth at or near term to a healthy, mature infant. (See the Nursing Care Plan on p. 451).

Nursing Care Plan

PRETERM LABOR

Nursing Diagnosis: Knowledge deficit related to recognition of premature labor

Expected Outcome: Woman and significant other delineate the signs and symptoms of premature labor.

- **NURSING INTERVENTIONS/*RATIONALES***

Assess what the partners know about abnormal signs and symptoms during pregnancy *to identify areas of deficit.*

Discuss signs and symptoms that serve as warning signs of premature labor *so that the woman or her partner has adequate information to identify problems early.*

Provide written supplemental materials that include a list of warning signs and instructions regarding what to do if any of the listed signs occur *so that the couple can reinforce and review learning and act swiftly and appropriately should a sign occur.*

Discuss and demonstrate how to assess and time the contractions *to provide needed skills to assess the signs of labor.*

Nursing Diagnosis: Risk for maternal/fetal injury related to recurrence of premature labor

Expected Outcomes: Woman demonstrates ability to assess self and fetus for signs of recurring labor; maternal-fetal well-being is maintained.

- **NURSING INTERVENTIONS/*RATIONALES***

Teach woman/partner how to monitor fetal and uterine contraction activity daily *to provide immediate evidence of a worsening condition.*

Have woman/partner report rupture of membranes, vaginal bleeding, cramping, pelvic pressure, or low backache to appropriate health care resource immediately *because such symptoms are signs of labor.*

If home electronic fetal monitoring is to be used, teach woman/partner how to use the monitoring device and how to transmit the data to the health care provider via telephone *to enhance correct use of monitoring device and increase the accuracy of detection of early labor.*

Have woman monitor her weight, diet, fluid intake and vital signs on a daily basis *to evaluate for potential problems.*

Limit activities to bed rest with bathroom privileges *to decrease the likelihood of onset of labor.*

Use a side-lying position *to enhance placental perfusion.*

Abstain from sexual intercourse and nipple stimulation *because such activities may stimulate uterine contractions.*

Practice relaxation techniques *to decrease uterine tone and decrease anxiety and stress.*

Take tocolytic or other medications per physician's orders *to inhibit uterine contractions.*

Teach woman/partner about and have them report any medication side effects immediately *to prevent medication-induced complications.*

Have family arrange for alternative strategies in carrying out the woman's usual roles and functions *to decrease stress and limit temptations to increase activity.*

If small children are part of the household, encourage family to make alternative arrangements for child care *to enhance woman's compliance with the bed-rest protocol.*

Nursing Diagnosis: Fear/anxiety related to preterm labor and potentially premature neonate

Expected Outcomes: Feelings and symptoms of fear/anxiety abate.

- **NURSING INTERVENTIONS/*RATIONALES***

Provide a calm, soothing atmosphere and teach family to provide emotional support *to facilitate coping.*

Encourage verbalization of fears *to decrease intensity of emotional response.*

Involve woman and family in the home management of her condition *to promote a greater sense of control.*

Help the woman to identify and use appropriate coping strategies and support systems *to reduce fear/anxiety.*

Explore the use of desensitization strategies such as progressive muscle relaxation, visual imagery, or thought stopping *to reduce fear-related emotions and related physical symptoms.*

Nursing Diagnosis: Diversional activity deficit related to imposed bed rest

Expected Outcomes: Verbalization of diminished feelings of boredom.

- **NURSING INTERVENTIONS/*RATIONALES***

Assist woman to creatively explore personally meaningful activities that can be pursued from the bed *to ensure activities that have meaning, purpose, and value to the individual.*

Maintain emphasis on personal choices of the woman *because doing so promotes control and minimizes imposition of routines by others.*

Evaluate what support and system resources are available in the environment *to assist in providing diversional activities.*

Explore ways for the woman to remain an active participant in home management and decision making *to promote control.*

Engage support of family and friends in carrying out chosen activities and making necessary environmental alterations *to ensure success.*

Teach woman about stress management and relaxation techniques *to help manage tension of confinement.*

Critical Thinking Exercises

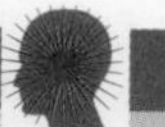

PRETERM LABOR

You are assigned to a woman who is experiencing preterm labor at 28 weeks' gestation. She has a 2-year-old-son at home. This is the woman's third admission for preterm labor during this pregnancy.

1. What impact might her history have on the nursing care she receives this time?
2. Discuss the pros and cons of home management vs. hospital management for the prevention of preterm birth for this woman.
3. On the basis of the previous discussion, develop a plan for home care for prevention of preterm birth.

Home Care

THE WOMAN WITH PREMATURE RUPTURE OF MEMBRANES

- Take your temperature at least every 4 hours during waking hours or as otherwise instructed. Report a temperature higher than 38° C (100.4° F) to your health care provider.
- Continue bed rest on your side except to go to the bathroom or as otherwise instructed.
- Assess for uterine contractions and report their occurrence if closer than 10 minutes apart.
- Do fetal movement counts daily. Report if fewer than four occur in 1 hour or if there is any other abnormal increase or decrease.
- Avoid sexual intercourse, breast stimulation, or other sexual stimulation.
- Take showers only; no tub baths.
- Use good perineal hygeine.
- Report foul-smelling vaginal discharge, an increase in amniotic fluid loss, or uterine tenderness.
- Keep all appointments with your health care provider.

PREMATURE RUPTURE OF MEMBRANES

Premature rupture of membranes (PROM) is the rupture of the amniotic sac before labor begins. PROM occurs in 2% to 18% of all pregnancies. It is the most common cause of preterm labor (Garite and Spellacy, 1994). At term, most women begin uterine contractions within 24 hours after membrane rupture; between 28 and 34 weeks of gestation, labor may not start for as long as 1 week. The earlier in pregnancy that PROM occurs, the longer the time before the onset of labor (Garite and Spellacy, 1994).

Etiologic Factors

The cause of PROM is unknown in most instances. Factors that are associated with PROM include amnionitis, placenta previa, multifetal gestation, polyhydramnios, bacterial infections, and maternal smoking (Gilbert and Harmon, 1993; Greenberg and Hankins, 1991; King, 1994). PROM may also occur after cervical cerclage or amniocentesis (Gaute and Spellacy, 1994).

Plan of Care and Implementation

If PROM is suspected, a sterile speculum examination is performed. Visualization of amniotic fluid from the cervix, a positive nitrazine test (litmus paper turns blue), or the presence of ferning (fernlike pattern in dried amniotic fluid) when the specimen is examined under a microscope indicates that the membranes are ruptured (Gilbert and Harmon, 1993).

Treatment of PROM continues to be controversial. The woman may be hospitalized until the birth of the infant or she may return home (see the Home Care box above, right). Expectant management is often used if there are no signs of infection. Expectant management includes daily assessments of maternal temperature, pulse, respirations, blood pressure, and fetal heart rate (tachycardia may be a sign of infection); palpation for uterine tenderness; assessment of vaginal discharge for color, odor, and amount; and assessment for signs of preterm labor (Grohar, 1994). Nonstress testing and ultrasound may be used to assess fetal well-being and to monitor the amniotic fluid index (see p. 88). If the woman is near term, labor may be induced.

If infection occurs, treatment with broad-spectrum antibiotics is usually initiated (Blanco, 1991). The induction of preterm labor or preterm birth by cesarean may be necessary to improve the fetal outcome.

DYSTOCIA

Dystocia is defined as long, difficult, or abnormal labor and is caused by various conditions associated with the five factors affecting labor:

1. *Dysfunctional labor,* resulting in ineffective uterine contractions or maternal bearing-down efforts (the powers)
2. *Alterations in the pelvic structure* (the passage)
3. *Fetal causes,* including abnormalities of presentation or position, anomalies, excessive size, and number of fetuses (the passenger)
4. *Maternal position* during labor and birth
5. *Psychologic responses* of the mother to labor related to past experiences, preparation, culture and heritage, and support system

These five factors are interdependent. In assessing the woman for an abnormal labor pattern, the nurse considers the interactions of these factors and how they influence labor progress. Dystocia is suspected when there is a lack of progress in the rate of cervical dilation, a lack of progress in fetal descent and expulsion, or an alteration in the characteristics of uterine contractions.

Dysfunctional Labor

Dysfunctional labor is described as abnormal uterine contractions that prevent the normal progress of cervical dilation, effacement (primary powers), or descent (secondary powers).

Hypertonic uterine dysfunction. Dysfunctional uterine contractions can be further described as being hypertonic or hypotonic. The woman who is experiencing **hypertonic**

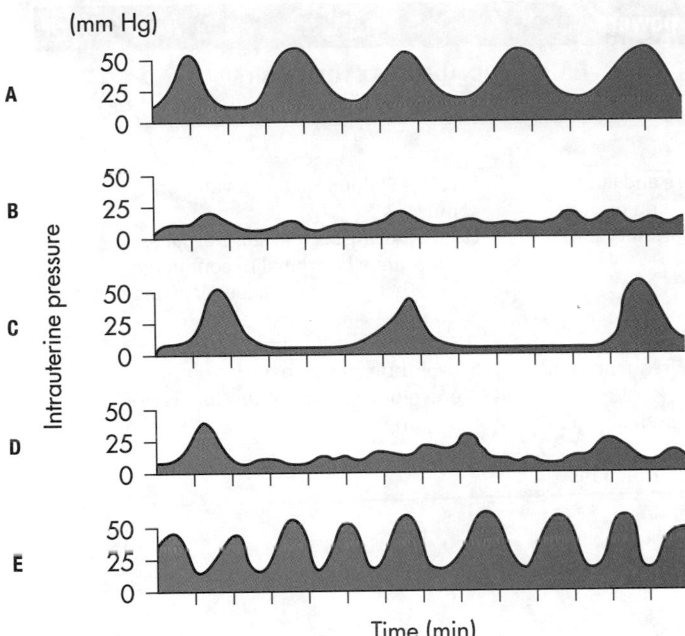

Fig. 17-3 Uterine contractility patterns in labor. **A**, Typical normal labor. **B**, Subnormal intensity, with frequency greater than needed for optimum performance. **C**, Normal contractions but too infrequent for efficient labor. **D**, Uncoordinated activity. **E**, Hypercontractility.

uterine dysfunction, or primary dysfunctional labor, often is an anxious first-time mother who is having contractions that are painful and out of proportion to their intensity and do not cause cervical dilation or effacement. These contractions usually occur in the latent stage (cervical dilation <4 cm) and usually are uncoordinated and frequent (Fig. 17-3). The force of the contraction may be in the midsection of the uterus rather than in the fundus, and the uterus may not relax completely between contractions.

Women experiencing hypertonic uterine dysfunction may be exhausted and express concern about loss of control because of the intense pain and lack of progress. Hypertonic uterine dysfunction is managed by **therapeutic rest,** which is achieved through the administration of effective analgesics such as morphine or meperidine to reduce the pain and encourage sleep. Often these women awaken with normal uterine activity.

Hypotonic uterine dysfunction. The second and more common type of uterine dysfunction is **hypotonic uterine dysfunction,** or secondary uterine inertia. The woman, who may be either in her first or a subsequent pregnancy, initially makes normal progress into the active stage of labor; the contractions then become weak and inefficient or stop altogether (Fig. 17-3, *B*). The uterus is easily indentable, even at the peak of contractions. Cephalopelvic disproportion and malpositions are common causes.

Women experiencing hypotonic uterine dysfunction may become exhausted and are at risk for infection. Medical management usually includes ruling out cephalopelvic disproportion by ultrasound or x-ray examination, followed by augmentation of labor with oxytocin (Bowes, 1989) (see p. 462).

Secondary powers. Secondary powers, or *bearing-down efforts,* are compromised by large amounts of analgesic. Anesthetics may block the bearing-down reflex and alter the effectiveness of voluntary efforts. Exhaustion from lack of sleep or a long labor and fatigue from inadequate hydration and food consumption affect the woman's voluntary efforts. Maternal position can work against the forces of gravity and decrease the strength and efficiency of the contraction. Table 17-1 summarizes dysfunctional labor.

Alterations in Pelvic Structure

Pelvic dystocia. Pelvic dystocia can occur with contractures of the pelvic diameters, which reduce the capacity of the bony pelvis, including the inlet, midpelvis, outlet, or any combination of these planes. Pelvic contractures may be caused by congenital abnormalities, maternal malnutrition, neoplasms, and lower spinal disorders. Immature pelvic size predisposes some adolescent mothers to pelvic dystocia. Pelvic deformities may result from automobile or other accidents.

Inlet contracture occurs in 1% to 2% of term births and is diagnosed when the diagonal conjugate is less than 11.5 cm. The incidence of face and shoulder presentation increases. These presentations prevent engagement and fetal descent, thereby increasing the risk of prolapse of the umbilical cord. Inlet contracture is associated with maternal rickets and a flat pelvis. Weak uterine contractions may be noted during the first stage of labor.

Midplane contracture, the most common cause of pelvic dystocia, is diagnosed when the sum of the interischial spinous and posterior sagittal diameters of the midpelvis is 13.5 cm or less. Fetal descent is arrested (transverse arrest of the fetal head) because the head cannot rotate internally. Cesarean birth is the usual management, but vacuum extraction has been used safely when the cervix has been fully dilated. Midforceps-assisted birth usually is avoided because of the increased perinatal mobidity associated with this intervention.

Outlet contracture exists when the interischial diameter is 8 cm or less. It rarely occurs without midplane contracture. Outlet contracture is associated with a long, narrow pubic arch and an android pelvis. Fetal descent is arrested. Maternal complications include extensive perineal lacerations during vaginal birth because the fetal head is pushed posteriorly.

Soft tissue dystocia. Soft tissue dystocia results from obstruction of the birth passage by an anatomic abnormality other than that of the bony pelvis. The obstruction may result from placenta previa (low-lying placenta), which partially or completely obstructs the internal os of the cervix. Other causes such as leiomyomas (uterine fibroids) in the lower uterine segment, ovarian tumors, and a full bladder or rectum may prevent the fetus from entering the pelvis. Occasionally, *cervical edema* occurs during labor when the cervix is caught between the presenting part and the symphysis or when the woman engages in bearing-down efforts prematurely, thus preventing complete dilation.

Bandl ring, a pathologic retraction ring, is associated with the prolonged rupture of membranes and protracted labor (Cunningham et al, 1993).

TABLE 17-1 Dysfunctional labor: primary and secondary powers

HYPERTONIC UTERINE DYSFUNCTION	HYPOTONIC UTERINE DYSFUNCTION	INADEQUATE VOLUNTARY EXPULSIVE FORCES
Description		
Usually occurs before 4 cm dilation; cause not known; may be related to fear and tension (primary powers) (Fig. 17-3)	Cause may be contracture and fetal malposition, overdistention of uterus (twins), or unknown (primary powers) (Fig. 17-3)	Involves abdominal and levator ani muscles Occurs during second stage of labor; cause may be related to conduction anesthetic, heavy analgesic, exhaustion
Change in pattern of progress		
Pain out of proportion to intensity of contraction Pain out of proportion to effectiveness of contraction in effacing and dilating the cervix Contractions increase in frequency Contractions uncoordinated Uterus is firm between contractions; cannot be indented	Contractions decrease in frequency and intensity Uterus easily indentable, even at peak of contraction Uterus relaxed between contractions (normal)	No voluntary urge to push or bear down or else inadequate/ineffective pushing
Potential maternal effects		
Loss of control related to intensity of pain and lack of progress Exhaustion	Infection Exhaustion Psychologic trauma	Spontaneous vaginal birth prevented
Potential fetal effects		
Fetal asphyxia with meconium aspiration	Fetal infection Fetal and neonatal death	Fetal asphyxia
Medical management		
Rule out cephalopelvic disproportion Oxytocic stimulation of labor	Analgesic (e.g., morphine, meperidine) if membranes not ruptured or cephalopelvic disproportion not present Relief of pain permits mother to rest; when she awakens, normal uterine activity may begin	Coach mother in bearing down with contractions Position mother in favorable position for pushing Low forceps or vacuum extraction if assistance for vaginal birth is needed Cesarean birth only if nonreassuring fetal status occurs

Fetal Causes

Dystocia of fetal origin may be caused by anomalies, excessive size and malpresentation, malposition, or multifetal pregnancy. Complications associated with dystocia of fetal origin include neonatal asphyxia, fetal injuries or fractures, and maternal vaginal lacerations. Although a spontaneous vaginal birth is possible, fetal dystocia often leads to the use of low forceps, vacuum extraction, or cesarean birth.

Anomalies. Gross ascites, large tumors, myelomeningocele, and hydrocephalus are fetal anomalies that can cause dystocia. These anomalies can affect the relationship between fetal anatomy and maternal pelvic capacity, resulting in failure of the fetus to descend through the birth canal.

Cephalopelvic disproportion. Cephalopelvic disproportion (CPD), also called *fetopelvic disproportion (FPD)*, is related to excessive fetal size (4000 g [8 lb, 13½ oz] or more) and occurs in approximately 5% of all term births. When CPD is present, the fetus cannot fit through the maternal pelvis to be born vaginally. Excessive fetal size, or *macrosomia*, is associated with maternal diabetes mellitus, obesity, multiparity, or the large size of one or both parents. CPD may be of maternal origin when the maternal pelvis is too small, abnormally shaped, or deformed.

Malposition. The most common fetal malposition is *persistent occipitoposterior position* (right occipitoposterior [ROP] or left occipitoposterior [LOP]) (see Fig. 13-2), which occurs in approximately 25% of all labors. Labor, especially the second stage, is prolonged; the woman complains of severe back pain from the pressure of the fetal head against her sacrum. Counterpressure to the sacral area and frequent position changes may decrease the pain. Both the hands-and-knees and the lateral position have been used to facilitate rotation of the fetus from a posterior to an anterior position (Biancuzzo, 1991).

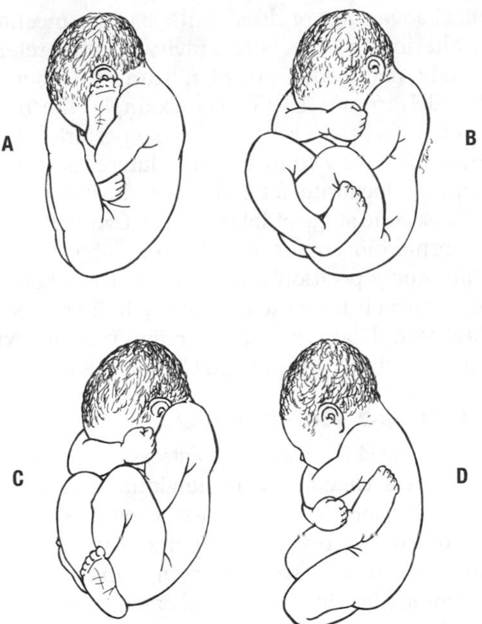

Fig. 17-4 Types of breech presentation. **A,** Frank breech. Thighs are flexed on hips; knees are extended. **B,** Complete breech. Thighs and knees are flexed. **C,** Incomplete breech. Foot extends below buttocks. **D,** Incomplete breech. Knee extends below buttocks.

Malpresentation. *Breech presentation* is the most common example of malpresentation and occurs in 3% to 4% of all births and in up to 25% of all preterm births. There are three main types of breech presentation: frank breech (thighs flexed, knees extended), complete breech (thighs and knees flexed), and incomplete breech, in which the knee or foot extends below the buttocks (Fig. 17-4). Breech presentations are associated with multifetal gestation, preterm birth, fetal and maternal anomalies, polyhydramnios, and oligohydramnios. Diagnosis is made by abdominal palpation and vaginal examination and usually is confirmed by ultrasound scan (Lydon et al, 1993).

During labor, fetal descent may be slow because the breech is not as good a dilating wedge as the fetal head; however, labor usually is not prolonged. There is a risk of prolapsed cord if the membranes rupture during early labor. The presence of meconium in amniotic fluid is not necessarily a sign of fetal distress because it results from pressure on the fetal abdominal wall as it traverses the birth canal. Fetal heart tones are best heard at or above the umbilicus. Vaginal birth is accomplished by mechanisms related to manipulation of the buttocks and lower extremities as they emerge from the birth canal (Fig. 17-5). Piper forceps sometimes are used to deliver the head (Fig. 17-10, p. 464).

Alternatives to vaginal birth of the fetus in breech presentation are external cephalic version (ECV) (in which the fetus is turned to a vertex presentation by exerting pressure on the fetus externally through the maternal abdomen) (p. 459) and cesarean birth (birth of the fetus through an abdominal incision) (p. 465).

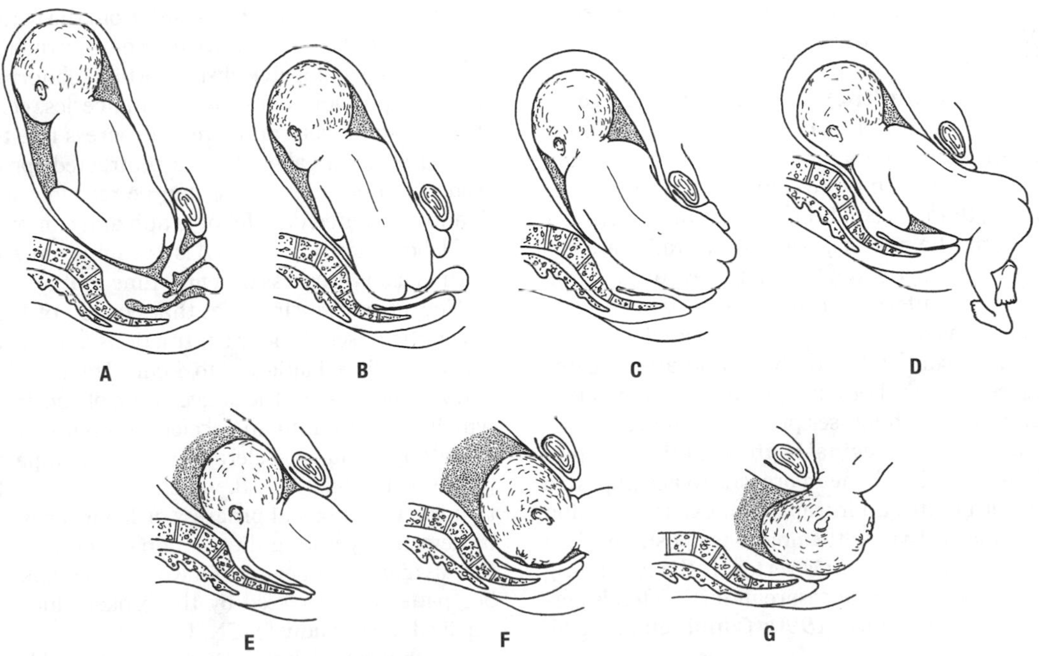

Fig. 17-5 Mechanism of labor in breech position. **A,** Breech before onset of labor. **B,** Engagement and internal rotation. **C,** Lateral flexion. **D,** External rotation or restitution. **E,** Internal rotation of shoulders and head. **F,** Face rotates to sacrum when occiput is anterior. **G,** Head is born by gradual flexion during elevation of fetal body.

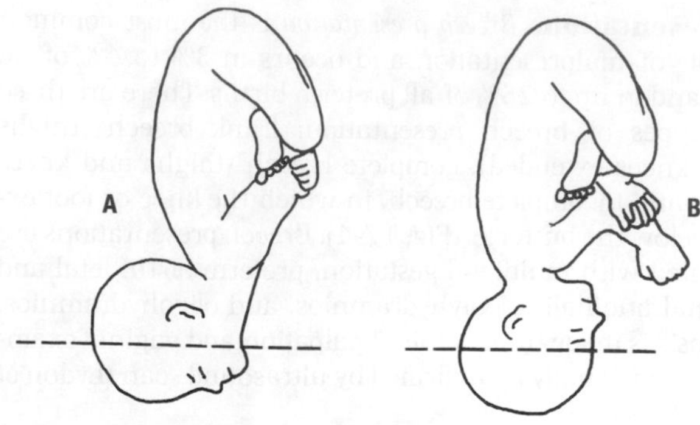

Fig. 17-6 Face **(A)** and brow **(B)** presentations.

Although opinions vary, a cesarean birth is commonly performed when the fetus is estimated to be larger than 3800 g (8 lb, 6 oz) or smaller than 1500 g (3 lb, 3 oz), if labor is ineffective, or if complications occur (Scott, 1994). Although a cesarean birth reduces the risks to the fetus, the maternal risks are increased. ECV also poses risks and is not always successful. Women with a breech presentation late in pregnancy need to be informed about the options for birth and the risks associated with each.

Face and brow presentations (Fig. 17-6) are uncommon and are associated with fetal anomalies, pelvic contractures, and cephalopelvic disproportion. Vaginal birth is possible if the fetus flexes to a vertex presentation, but forceps often are used. A cesarean birth is indicated when the presentation persists, if there is fetal distress, or if labor progress stops.

Shoulder presentations (the fetus is in a transverse lie) usually require cesarean birth, but external cephalic version may be attempted after 38 weeks' gestation (Cunningham et al, 1993).

Multifetal pregnancy. **Multifetal pregnancy** is the gestation of twins, triplets, quadruplets, or more infants. Infants of multifetal pregnancies account for 2% to 3% of all viable births and are associated with more complications, including dysfunctional labor, than are single births. The high incidence of complications and the risk of perinatal mortality are primarily related to low–birth-weight infants resulting from preterm birth and intrauterine growth restriction. In addition, fetal complications such as congenital anomalies and abnormal presentations can lead to dystocia and an increased incidence of cesarean birth. For example, in only one half of all twin pregnancies do both fetuses present in the vertex position, the most favorable for vaginal birth; one third may present as one twin in vertex and one in breech. To accomplish a vaginal birth of both twins, an intrapartum external version may be attempted for the twin in the nonvertex position when the position of the presenting twin is vertex. If the presenting twin is not in a vertex position, a cesarean birth often is performed (Adams and Chervenak, 1990; Cunningham et al, 1993).

Position of the Woman

The functional relationships between the uterine contractions, the fetus, and the mother's pelvis are altered by maternal positioning. In addition, positioning can provide either a mechanical advantage or disadvantage to the mechanisms of labor by altering the effects of gravity and the relationships among body parts that are significant to labor progress (Gilbert and Harmon, 1993). For example, the hands-and-knees position facilitates rotation from a posterior occiput position more effectively than does the lateral position. Sitting and squatting facilitate fetal descent during pushing and shorten the second stage of labor (Biancuzzo, 1993). Discouraging maternal movement or restricting labor to the recumbent or lithotomy position may compromise labor. The incidence of dystocia is increased, resulting in increased need for augmentation of labor, the use of forceps, vacuum extraction, and cesarean birth (Andrews and Chrzanowski, 1990).

Psychologic Response

Hormones released in response to stress can cause dystocia. Sources of stress vary for each individual, but pain and the absence of a support person are two recognized factors. Confinement to bed and restriction of maternal movement add a potential psychologic stress to compound the physiologic stress of immobility in the unmedicated, laboring woman. When anxiety is excessive, it can inhibit normal cervical dilation, resulting in *prolonged labor* and increased pain perception. Anxiety also causes increased levels of stress-related hormones (β-endorphin, adrenocorticotropic hormone [ACTH], cortisol, and epinephrine). These hormones act on the smooth muscles of the uterus; increased levels can cause dystocia by reducing uterine contractility (Biancuzzo, 1993).

Abnormal Labor Patterns

Abnormal labor patterns occur in 8% of all pregnancies, with the highest incidence among nulliparous women (Friedman, 1989). These patterns may result from the various causes previously described: ineffective uterine contractions, pelvic contractures, cephalopelvic disproportion, abnormal fetal presentation or position, early use of analgesics, conduction anesthesia, and anxiety and stress. Progress in either the first or second stage of labor can be protracted (prolonged) or arrested. Abnormal progress can be recognized when cervical dilation is plotted on a labor graph and compared with a normal labor curve. Fig. 17-7, *A* is a graphic representation of the normal labor progress of a first-time mother.

The *latent phase* includes that portion of the first stage between the onset of labor contractions and the acceleration in rate of cervical dilation (0 to 4 cm). The upswing in the curve denotes the onset of the active phase of the first stage of labor, which is divided into an acceleration phase, a phase of maximum slope, and a deceleration phase. Compare these normal phases with Fig. 17-7, *B*, which shows major types of deviation from the normal progress of labor. These deviations can be detected by noting the dilation of the cervix at various intervals after labor begins. If a woman exhibits an abnormal labor pattern as depicted by the broken lines, the physician/certified nurse midwife (CNM) is notified.

Six abnormal labor patterns have been identified and classified by Friedman (1989) according to cervical dilation and fetal descent. A *prolonged latent phase* is one that exceeds 20 hours in the nulliparous woman and 14 hours in the multiparous woman. The active phase of labor also can be complicated by protraction disorders (no progress). In a *protracted active phase,* the cervix dilates less than 1.2 cm/hr in the nulliparous woman and less than 1.5 cm/hr in the multiparous woman. *Arrest of the active phase* is determined when for more than 2 hours neither the nulliparous nor the multiparous woman demonstrates progress.

Descent of the presenting part also can be protracted or arrested in the active phase of labor. Active descent generally begins when cervical dilation reaches the phase of maximum slope, with the rate of descent achieving its maximum at the beginning of the deceleration phase (approximately 9 cm). A *protracted descent* pattern is one in which the rate of descent is less than 1 cm/hr in the nulliparous woman and less than 2 cm/hr in the multiparous woman. *Arrest of descent* is the lack of progress for more than 1 hour in both nulliparous and

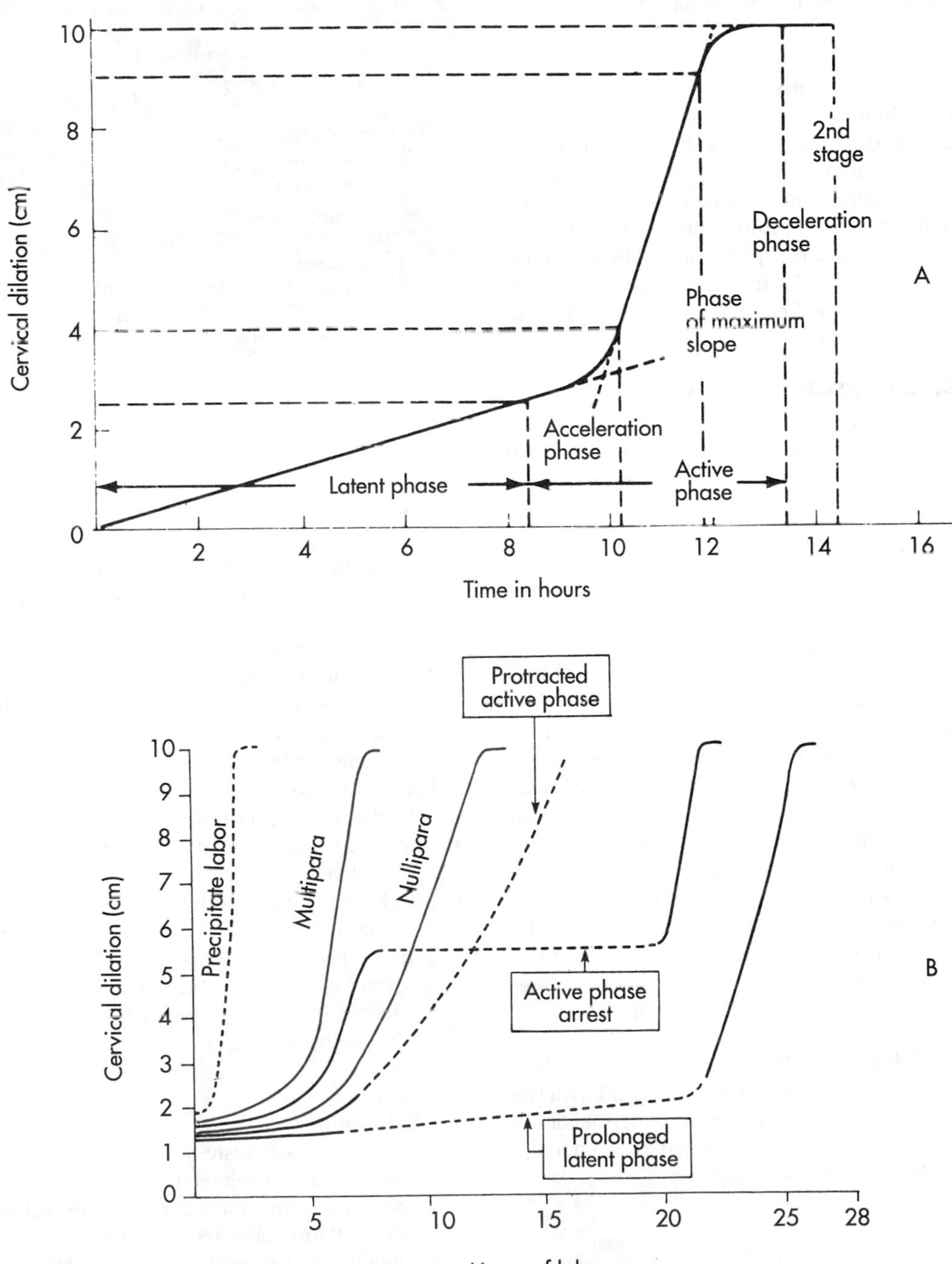

Fig. 17-7 **A,** Partogram of a normal labor. **B,** Major types of deviation from normal progress of labor may be detected by noting dilation of cervix at various intervals after labor begins. If a woman exhibits an abnormal labor pattern (as depicted by the broken lines), the physician/CNM should be notified immediately.

multiparous women. *Failure of descent* is a lack of descent of the presenting part during the deceleration phase and the second stage.

Fetal mortality increases sharply after 15 hours of the active first stage of labor. Maternal morbidity and mortality may occur as a result of uterine rupture, infection, serious dehydration, and postpartum hemorrhage. A long, difficult labor also can have an adverse psychologic effect on the mother, father, and family. Management of prolonged labor depends on the cause and can include therapeutic rest, augmentation with oxytocin, forceps birth, vacuum extraction, and cesarean birth. Table 17-2 describes labor patterns in normal and abnormal labor.

Precipitous labor. Precipitous labor is defined as labor that lasts less than 3 hours from the onset of contractions. Hypertonic uterine contractions may result in precipitous labor. Because labor is rapid, maternal and fetal complications can occur. Maternal complications include uterine rupture, lacerations of the birth canal, amniotic fluid embolism, and postpartum hemorrhage. Fetal complications include hypoxia caused by decreased periods of uterine relaxation between contractions and intracranial hemorrhage related to rapid birth (Cunningham et al, 1993).

TABLE 17-2 Labor patterns in normal and abnormal labor

NORMAL LABOR

1. Dilation: continues
   a. Latent phase: <4 cm and low slope
   b. Active phase: >5 cm or high slope
   c. Deceleration phase: ≥9 cm
2. Descent: active at ≥9 cm dilation

ABNORMAL LABOR

Pattern	Nulliparas	Multiparas
Prolonged latent phase	>20 hr	>14 hr
Protracted active phase dilation	<1.2 cm/hr	<1.5 cm/hr
Secondary arrest: no change	≥2 hr	≥2 hr
Protracted descent	<1 cm/hr	<2 cm/hr
Arrest of descent	≥1 hr	≥½ hr
Failure of descent	No change during deceleration phase and second stage	
Precipitous labor	>5 cm/hr	>10 cm/hr

Nursing Care Management

Care management of the woman at risk for problems related to abnormal labor or birth involves all members of the health care team. Nursing care is facilitated through the use of the nursing process.

Assessment

Risk assessment is a continuous process. A review of the initial interview conducted at the woman's admission to the labor unit and ongoing observations of her psychologic response to labor can reveal factors that can cause dysfunctional labor, such as anxiety or fear, the presence of a complication of pregnancy, or previous labor complications. The initial physical assessment data and ongoing assessments provide information about the frequency, duration, and intensity of uterine contractions, cervical status, FHR, presentation and station of the fetus, and status of membranes.

Fetal distress can be identified through laboratory data such as scalp pH, and potential dysfunctional labor problems related to the fetus or maternal pelvis can be identified through ultrasound. All of these assessments contribute to accurate identification of potential and actual nursing diagnoses related to dystocia and maternal-fetal compromise.

Nursing Diagnoses

Nursing diagnoses vary with the type of dystocia and with the individual needs of the woman and her family. Potential or actual nursing diagnoses that might be identified for women experiencing dystocia include the following:

- Anxiety related to
  Slowed labor progress
- Pain related to
  Dystocia
  Obstetric procedures
- Risk for fetal injury related to
  Fetal compromise
- Risk for maternal injury related to
  Interventions implemented for dystocia
- Powerlessness related to
  Loss of control
- Risk for infection related to
  Rupture of membranes, operative procedures
- Fatigue related to
  Prolonged labor
- Fear related to
  Real or potential threat to self or fetus
- Impaired tissue integrity related to
  Operative procedures
- Risk for altered parenting related to
  Unplanned cesarean birth
- Sensory/perceptual alterations related to
  Numerous interventions for dystocia
- Ineffective individual coping related to
  Disappointment
  Pain
  Fear
  Exhaustion
  Lack of support system
- Knowledge deficit related to
  Procedures, positioning, relaxation techniques
- Situational low self-esteem related to
  Inability to labor and give birth as expected
- Fluid volume excess related to
  Intravenous infusion with oxytocin
- Fluid volume deficit related to
  Nothing-by-mouth (NPO) status

Expected Outcomes

Nursing diagnoses provide direction for care. During this important step, expected outcomes are set in patient-centered terms and are prioritized. Nursing actions are selected with the woman, as appropriate, to meet the expected outcomes.

Expected outcomes for the woman who is experiencing dystocia include the following. The woman will:

1. Understand the causes and treatment of dysfunctional labor
2. Use positive patterns of coping to maintain a positive self-concept
3. Demonstrate diminished or minimal anxiety
4. Express relief of pain
5. Experience labor and birth with minimal or no complications such as infection, injury, or hemorrhage
6. Give birth to a healthy infant who has not experienced fetal distress

Plan of Care and Implementation

Nurses assume many caregiving roles when labor is complicated. Knowledge of medical management for each condition is essential to implementing the nursing process. This knowledge enables the nurse to work collaboratively with other health care providers and to meet the woman's knowledge and emotional needs. Interventions that the nurse may be assisting with or implementing include external cephalic version, trial of labor, induction/augmentation with oxytocin, amniotomy, and operative procedures such as forceps-assisted birth, vacuum extraction, and cesarean birth. The nursing role is identified with each of the procedures described.

LEGAL TIP

Standard of Care—Labor and Birth at Risk

Document all assessment, interventions, and patient responses on patient record and monitor strips according to unit protocols, procedures, and policies.

Assess whether the woman is fully informed about the procedures for which she is consenting.

Maintain safety in administering medications and treatments correctly.

Get verbal orders signed as soon as possible.

Provide care at the acceptable standard (e.g., according to hospital protocols, professional standards).

If short staffing occurs in the unit and the nurse is assigned additional patients, the nurse should document that rejecting the assignment would have placed the patient in danger as a result of abandonment.

Maternal and fetal monitoring continues according to policies, procedures, and protocols until birth, even when a decision for cesarean birth is made.

Version. Version is the turning of the fetus artificially from one presentation to another. Version may be external or internal.

External cephalic version. **External cephalic version (ECV)** is the attempt to turn the fetus from a breech or shoulder presentation to a vertex presentation for birth. ECV may be attempted in a labor and birth setting after 37 weeks' gestation. Before ECV is attempted, ultrasound scanning is used to determine the fetal position, to rule out placenta previa, and to assess the amount of amniotic fluid, the fetal age, and the presence of any anomalies. A nonstress test is performed to ensure fetal well-being. Informed consent is obtained. Contraindications to ECV include uterine anomalies, previous cesarean birth, cephalopelvic disproportion, placenta previa, multifetal gestation, and oligohydramnios (Cunningham et al, 1993).

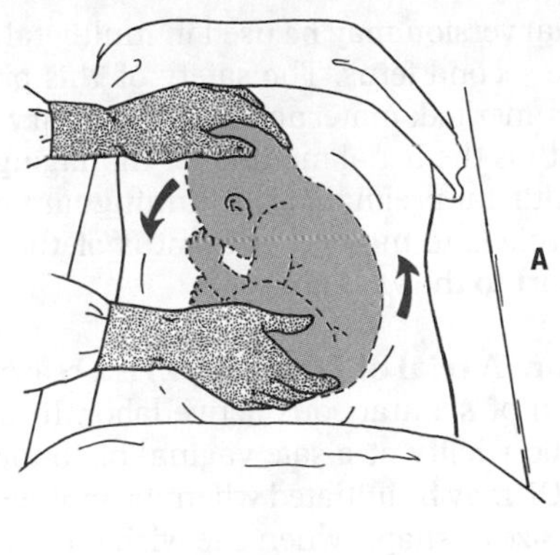

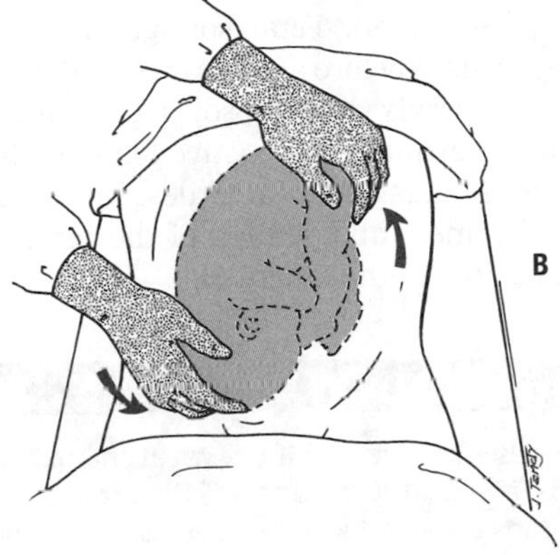

Fig. 17-8 External version of fetus from breech to vertex presentation. External version must be achieved without force. **A,** Breech is pushed up out of pelvic inlet while head is pulled toward inlet. **B,** Head is pushed toward inlet while breech is pulled upward.

ECV is accomplished by gentle, constant pressure on the abdomen accompanied by continuous fetal heart surveillance (Fig. 17-8). A tocolytic agent such as magnesium sulfate or terbutaline (p. 448) is usually given to relax the uterus and facilitate the maneuver. Ultrasound is usually used to identify potential problems such as cord entanglement and placental separation (Cunningham et al, 1993).

During an attempted ECV, the nurse continuously monitors the FHR (especially for bradycardia), checks maternal vital signs frequently, and assesses the woman's level of comfort because the procedure may cause discomfort. After the procedure is completed, the nurse continues to monitor maternal vital signs, uterine activity, and FHR and assesses for vaginal bleeding until the woman's condition is stable. Women who are Rh negative should receive Rh immune globulin because the manipulation can cause fetomaternal bleeding (Cunningham et al, 1993).

Internal version. With internal version, the fetus is turned by the physician, who inserts a hand into the uterus and changes the presentation to cephalic (head) or podalic (foot). Internal version may be used in multifetal pregnancies to deliver the second fetus. The safety of this procedure has not been documented; maternal and fetal injury are possible. Cesarean birth is the usual method for managing malpresentation in multifetal pregnancies (Cunningham et al, 1993). The nurse's role is to monitor the status of the fetus and to provide support to the woman.

Trial of labor. A **trial of labor (TOL)** is a reasonable period (4 to 6 hours) of spontaneous active labor. It allows assessment of the possibility of a safe vaginal birth for the mother and infant. TOL may be initiated when the mother's pelvis is of questionable size or shape, when she wishes to have a vaginal birth after a previous cesarean birth, and when the fetus is in an abnormal presentation. Fetal sonography or maternal pelvimetry may be used before a TOL to rule out cephalopelvic disproportion. The cervix must be soft and dilatable. During TOL, the woman is evaluated for active labor, including adequate contractions, engagement and descent of the presenting part, and effacement and dilation of the cervix. Augmentation of labor seldom is implemented.

Nursing ALERT

The nurse assesses uterine activity, cervical changes, maternal vital signs, and fetal status during TOL. If maternal or fetal complications are identified, the nurse is responsible for initiating appropriate actions, including notifying the physician/CNM and evaluating and documenting the maternal or fetal response to the interventions.

Induction of labor. **Induction of labor** is the initiation of uterine contractions before their spontaneous onset for the purpose of bringing about the birth. Induction may be indicated for a variety of medical and obstetric reasons, including pregnancy-induced hypertension, diabetes mellitus and other maternal medical problems, postdate gestation, suspected fetal jeopardy (e.g., intrauterine growth restriction), logistic factors such as history of previous rapid birth or distance of the woman's home from the hospital, and fetal death. Under such conditions the risk to the mother or fetus is less than the risk of continuing the pregnancy (Sokol, Brindley, and Dombrowski, 1994).

Both chemical and mechanical methods are used to induce labor. Intravenous oxytocin and amniotomy are the most common methods used in the United States. Prostaglandins and stripping of membranes are also used (ACOG, 1995b).

Success rates for induction of labor are higher when the cervix is favorable, or inducible. A rating system such as the **Bishop score** (Table 17-3) can be used to evaluate inducibility. For example, a score of 9 or more on this 13-point scale indicates that the cervix is soft, anterior, 50% effaced, and dilated 2 cm or more; the presenting part is engaged. Induction of labor is likely to be more successful if the score is 5 or more for nulliparas and 9 or more for multiparas.

Cervical ripening methods

CHEMICAL METHODS. Different **prostaglandins** (hormones) have been applied to the cervix before induction to induce or "ripen" (soften and thin) the cervix. A prostaglandin gel has been approved since 1993 by the FDA as a cervical ripening agent (ACOG, 1993). The gel may be administered through a catheter into the cervical canal or applied to a diaphragm that is placed next to the cervix. The intravaginal dose ranges from 1 to 5 mg; the endocervical dose is 0.5 mg (ACOG, 1993). Additional doses may be reapplied every 6 hours, with a total of two to three doses usually being sufficient. Oxytocin induction usually is not started until 6 to 12 hours later to avoid hyperstimulation (ACOG, 1995b). Side effects of prostaglandins, which include vomiting, fever, diarrhea, and hyperstimulation of the uterus, are uncommon with the low-dose gel applications (Sokol, Brindley, and Dombrowski, 1994). Prostaglandin gel is used with caution in women who have a history of asthma, glaucoma, renal disease, and cardiovascular disease (Miller and Lorkovic, 1993).

Nursing assessments after gel administration include monitoring FHR continuously for 30 minutes to 4 hours and periodically thereafter. Maternal vital signs are taken every hour for 2 hours, then every 4 hours. The woman should stay supine (with hips elevated to keep the pressure of the uterus off the vena cava) for 15 to 30 minutes to minimize leaking of the medication; the woman may then be ambulatory. If the administration is endocervical, the woman will remain at the hospital. If the administration is intravaginal and the woman shows no signs of labor, she may be allowed to go home and return the next day for oxytocin induction (Miller and Lorkovic, 1993) (see the Home Care box below).

A vaginal insert of prostaglandin (E2) is also available. After insertion, the woman should stay supine for 2 hours before ambulating. Oxytocin may be administered after 30 minutes. The insert should be removed 12 hours after insertion or with the onset of active labor.

TABLE 17-3 Bishop score

	0	1	2	3
Dilation (cm)	0	1-2	3-4	5-6
Effacement (%)	0-30	40-50	60-70	80
Station (cm)	−3	−2	−1	−1
Cervical consistency	Firm	Medium	Soft	
Cervix position	Posterior	Midline	Anterior	

Home Care

INSTRUCTIONS AFTER INTRAVAGINAL INSERTION OF PROSTAGLANDIN GEL FOR CERVICAL RIPENING

- Return to the hospital if labor begins spontaneously.
- Return to the hospital immediately if your membranes rupture or if you have vaginal bleeding, decreased fetal movement, or severe abdominal pain.
- If you do not experience labor, return for your scheduled induction.

MECHANICAL METHODS. *Hygroscopic dilators* (substances that absorb fluid from surrounding tissues and enlarge) also can be used for cervical ripening. *Laminaria tents* (natural cervical dilators made from seaweed) and synthetic dilators are inserted into the cervix. As they absorb fluid, they expand and cause cervical dilation. These dilators are left in place for 6 to 12 hours before being removed to assess cervical dilation. Fresh dilators are inserted if further treatment is necessary for cervical dilation (AWHONN, 1993).

Nursing responsibilities for women who have dilators inserted include documenting the number of dilators and sponges (used to hold the dilators in place) that have been inserted during the procedure.

Amniotomy. **Amniotomy (artificial rupture of membranes [AROM])** can be used to stimulate labor when the condition of the cervix is favorable. Labor usually begins within 12 hours of the rupture; however, if amniotomy does not stimulate labor, prolonged rupture may lead to infection. For this reason, amniotomy often is used in combination with oxytocin induction. Before the procedure, the woman is told what to expect; she also is assured that the procedure is painless for her and the fetus (Box 17-6). The membranes are ruptured with an Amnihook or other sharp instrument; the amniotic fluid is allowed to drain slowly. The fluid is assessed for color, odor, and consistency (i.e., the absence of meconium or blood). The time of rupture is recorded. The FHR is assessed before and after the procedure to detect changes that may indicate the presence of cord compression or prolapse. The woman's temperature should be checked at least every 4 hours to rule out possible infection. If the temperature is 38° C (100.4° F), the physician/CNM is notified. The nurse assesses for other signs and symptoms of infection such as maternal chills, fetal tachycardia, uterine tenderness on palpation, and foul-smelling vaginal drainage (AWHONN, 1993). Comfort measures such as frequently changing the woman's underpads should be implemented because after rupture of membranes the amniotic fluid continues to leak from the vagina until the birth.

BOX 17-6

Procedure: Assisting with an Amniotomy

Procedure

Explain to the woman what will be done.
Assess fetal heart rate as baseline data before procedure begins.
Place several underpads under the woman's buttocks to absorb the fluid.
Position the woman on a padded bed pan, fracture pan, or rolled-up towel to elevate the hips.
Assist the physician/CNM performing the procedure by providing sterile gloves and lubricant for vaginal examination.
Unwrap sterile packaging from the Amnihook or Allis forceps, and pass the instrument to the physician/CNM, who inserts it alongside the fingers to hook and tear the membranes.
Monitor FHR continuously.
Assess the color, consistency, and odor of the fluid.
Assess the woman's temperature every 4 hours.
Assess the woman for signs and symptoms of infection.

Documentation

Chart the following:
Time of rupture
Color, odor, and consistency of fluid
FHR before and after procedure
Maternal status (how the procedure was tolerated)

Oxytocin. **Oxytocin** is a hormone normally produced by the posterior pituitary gland; it stimulates uterine contractions. Oxytocin may be used either to induce the labor process or to augment a labor that is progressing slowly because of inadequate uterine contractions.

The *indications* for oxytocin induction of labor may include but are not limited to the following:

- Suspected fetal jeopardy
- Inadequate uterine contractions
- Premature rupture of membranes
- Postdate pregnancy
- Maternal medical problems (e.g., diabetic woman or woman with severe Rh isoimmunization, renal disease)
- Pregnancy-induced hypertensive diseases
- Fetal demise
- Multiparous women with a history of precipitous labor who live far away from the hospital

The management of stimulation of labor is the same regardless of indication. Because of the potential dangers associated with the use of injectable oxytocin in the prenatal and intranatal periods, the FDA has issued restrictions on its use.

Contraindications to oxytocic stimulation of labor include but are not limited to the following:

- CPD, cord presentation, abnormal lie
- Nonreassurring FHR
- Complete placenta previa or vasa previa
- Prior classic uterine incision or uterine surgery
- Active genital herpes infection
- Invasive cancer of the cervix

Oxytocin can present hazards to both the mother and the fetus. Maternal hazards include water intoxication and tumultuous labor and tetanic contractions, which may cause premature separation of the placenta, rupture of the uterus, laceration of the cervix, or postbirth hemorrhage. These complications can cause infection, disseminated intravascular coagulation, and amniotic fluid embolism. Women may become anxious or fearful if the induction is not successful because of concerns they may have about the method of birth.

Fetal hazards include fetal asphyxia and neonatal hypoxia from uterine contractions that are too frequent and too prolonged, physical injury, neonatal hyperbilirubinemia, and prematurity (if the estimated date of birth is inaccurate).

Initiation of induction or augmentation of labor with oxytocin is the responsibility of the physician/CNM, although the medication often is administered by a nurse. A written protocol for the preparation and administration of oxytocin (such as the one on p. 463) should be established by the obstetric department in each institution. The aim of induction with oxytocin has been to achieve a contraction pattern that simulates the active phase of labor as quickly as possible. Research on uterine tolerance to oxytocin has shown that lower doses given over longer time intervals are as effective as previous protocols and are less likely to cause uterine hyperstimulation and dysfunctional labor (Brodsky and Pelzar, 1991; Mercer, Pilgrim, and Sibai, 1991).

NURSING CONSIDERATIONS. After the woman has been evaluated for induction, the following recommended procedures are performed in a labor and birth setting (ACOG, 1991b; AWHONN, 1993; Davis, 1992):

- Cervical dilation and effacement are assessed.
- The woman and support person(s) are assessed regarding their understanding of the induction procedure (uterine contractions will become stronger and will occur more often and more regularly) and teaching is implemented as needed.
- A primary intravenous infusion of a physiologic electrolyte fluid is started. Intravenous medications other than oxytocin can be administered through this line.
- At least a 20-minute baseline fetal monitoring strip is recommended before the oxytocin administration.
- The woman is positioned on her side to prevent supine hypotension.
- A secondary ("piggy-back") intravenous infusion containing dilute oxytocin (usually 10 U/1000 ml) is prepared and connected to the main line close to the primary venipuncture site. No medication except oxytocin should be given through this line.
- Oxytocin should be administered through a pump delivery system to ensure an accurate dose and safe administration.
- Oxytocin is administered according to prescribed orders or protocol. Initial dosages of 0.5 to 3 mU/min, with increases of 1 to 2 mU/min, are administered at 15- to 60-minute intervals until the desired contraction pattern is achieved. That is, contractions are of 40 to 90 seconds' duration and 2 to 3 minutes apart; intensity is 40 to 90 mm Hg if intrauterine pressure is being monitored internally. In some institutions, uterine pressure is measured in Montevideo units (MVUs) (Box 17-7).
- Once the cervix is dilated to 5 to 6 cm and labor is established, the oxytocin dose can be reduced by similar decrements.
- Usually no more than 20 mU oxytocin per minute is needed to achieve progressive cervical dilation. In many cases, less than 4 mU/min is needed (Sokol, Brindley and Dombrowski, 1994).

BOX 17-7

Calculation of Montevideo Units

Montevideo units (MVUs) can be used to describe uterine intensity when an intrauterine pressure gauge is used. Subtract the baseline uterine pressure (resting tone) from the peak contraction pressure for each contraction in a 10-minute interval on the monitor tracing. Add the pressure generated by each contraction. The sum of the pressure changes for the contractions in the interval is the number of Montevideo units (average 180 to 240 MVUs).

For example, if the resting tone is 5 and if 3 contractions occurred in 10 minutes with peaks of 80, 85, and 90, the MVUs are 80 − 5 + 85 − 5 + 90 − 5 = 240 MVUs.

- The FHR, uterine resting tone, and frequency, duration, and intensity of contractions are monitored continuously (electronic fetal-maternal monitoring is suggested; internal monitoring of uterine pressure may be established).
- Maternal blood pressure and pulse are monitored when doses are changed. Institutional policies, protocol, and procedures also dictate the frequency of assessments.
- The nurse assesses intake and output to prevent water intoxication. The intravenous intake usually is limited to 1000 ml in 8 hours (125 ml/hr); urine output should be 120 ml or more in 4 hours. The nurse also assesses for the side effects of nausea, vomiting, headache, or hypotension.
- Documentation of maternal and fetal assessments is necessary in the medical record and on the fetal monitor tracing. In addition, the woman and her support persons are kept informed of her progress.

Nursing ALERT

Oxytocin is discontinued immediately and the physician/CNM notified if there is uterine hyperstimulation or nonreassuring FHR. With the latter, other nursing interventions such as administration of oxygen by face mask and positioning the woman on her side are implemented immediately (see the Emergency box on p. 463).

Augmentation. **Augmentation of labor** is the stimulation of uterine contractions after labor has started spontaneously yet progressed unsatisfactorally. Augmentation usually is implemented for hypotonic dysfunctional labor. The procedures and nursing assessments are the same as those used for oxytocin induction of labor.

Some physicians advocate *active management* of labor, which is intervention with augmentation of labor to establish efficient labor and to have the woman give birth within 12 hours of admission (ACOG, 1990). Advocates of active management indicate that early intervention (as soon as labor is not progressing at least 1 cm/hr) with aggressive use of oxytocin (e.g., increases of 6 mU/min) shortens labor and reduces the incidence of cesarean birth (ACOG, 1995c; Lopez-Zeno et al, 1992). These practices are currently under study in the United States to determine their effectiveness and impact on perinatal morbidity and mortality.

Box 17-8 summarizes the nursing responsibilities for induction of labor with oxytocin administration.

Forceps-assisted birth. A **forceps-assisted birth** is one in which an instrument with two curved blades is used to assist in the birth of the fetal head. The cephalic-like curve of the forceps commonly used is similar to the shape of the fetal head. A pelvic curve of the blades conforms to the pelvic axis. The blades are joined by a pin, screw, or groove arrangement. These locks prevent the forceps from compressing the fetal skull. Maternal indications for forceps-assisted birth include the need to shorten the second stage in dystocia (difficult labor), to correct the woman's deficient expulsive efforts (e.g., she is tired or has been given a spinal or epidural anesthetic), or to reverse a dangerous condition (e.g., cardiac decompensation).

Fetal indications include the birth of a fetus in distress, certain abnormal presentations, arrest of rotation, or delivering an aftercoming head in a breech presentation (Dennan, 1989).

Certain conditions are required for a successful forceps-assisted birth. The woman's cervix must be fully dilated to avoid lacerations and hemorrhage. The presenting part must be engaged, and a vertex presentation is desired. Membranes should be ruptured so that the position of the fetal head can be determined and a firm grasp of the forceps on the head during birth can be ensured. CPD should not be present. The woman's bladder should be emptied to avoid lacerations and injury (Sokol, Brindley, and Dombrowski, 1994).

There are different definitions of forceps applications. According to the American College of Obstetricians and Gynecologists (1991a), *outlet* forceps are appropriate when the fetal scalp is visible on the perineum without manually separating the labia (Fig. 17-9). There must be no more than a 45-degree rotation from an occiput anterior or occiput poste-

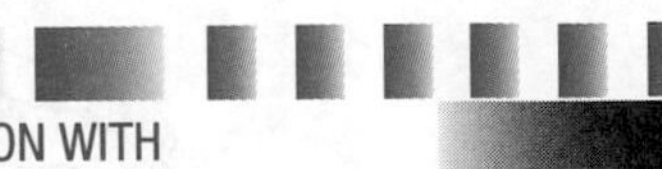

UTERINE HYPERSTIMULATION WITH OXYTOCIN

Signs

Uterine contractions >90 seconds, occurring in intervals <q2min
Uterine resting tone greater than 20 mm Hg
Nonreassuring fetal heart rate:
- Abnormal baseline
- Absent variability
- Repeated late decelerations or prolonged decelerations

Interventions

Maintain woman in sidelying position.
Turn off oxytocin; keep maintenance IV line open; increase rate.
Start oxygen via face mask per protocol or physician/CNM order.
Notify physician/CNM.
Continue monitoring FHR and uterine activity.
Document responses to actions.

BOX 17-8

Protocol for Induction of Labor with Oxytocin

Oxytocin administration

Patient/family teaching

Explain technique, rationale, and expected reactions:
- Route and rate
- What "piggyback" is for
- Reasons for use
  - Induce labor
  - Improve labor
- Reactions to expect concerning the nature of contractions. The intensity of contractions increases more rapidly, the peaks are held longer, and the contractions end more quickly. The contractions will begin to come regularly and more often.
- Monitoring to anticipate
  - Maternal: blood pressure, pulse, uterine contractions, uterine tone
  - Fetal: heart rate, activity
- Success to expect: a favorable outcome will depend on inducibility of the cervix (Bishop score of nine or more for nullipara; five or more for multipara)

Administration
- Position woman in side-lying position.
- Prepare solutions and administer according to prescribed orders with pump delivery system:
  - Infusion pump and solution is set up
  - Piggyback solution is connected to IV line
  - Solution with oxytocin is flagged with a medication label
  - Begin induction at 0.5 to 1.0 mU/min
  - Increase dose 1 to 2 mU/min at intervals of 30 to 60 minutes for up to 20 mU/min or until 300 Montevideo units are reached

When to maintain dose
- Intensity of contractions results in intrauterine pressures of 40 to 90 mm Hg (by internal monitor)
- Duration of contraction is 40 to 90 seconds
- Frequency of contractions is 2- to 3-minute intervals

Maternal/fetal assessments
- Monitor blood pressure and pulse every 30 to 60 minutes.
- Monitor contraction pattern every 15 minutes.
- Assess intake and output; limit IV intake to 1000 ml/8 hr; output should be 120 ml or more every 4 hours.
- Monitor for nausea, vomiting, headache, hypotension.
- Assess fetal status according to hospital protocol; electronic fetal monitoring is recommended.

Reportable conditions
- Uterine hyperstimulation
- Nonreassuring FHR pattern
- Suspected uterine rupture

Emergency measures

Discontinue use of oxytocin per hospital protocol:
- Turn woman on her side
- Increase primary IV rate up to 200 ml/hr unless patient has water intoxication; in presence of water intoxication, rate will be decreased to a rate that keeps the vein open
- Give woman oxygen by face mask at 8 to 10 L/min per protocol or physician order

Documentation
- Medication: type, amount, time of beginning, increasing dose, maintaining dose, and discontinuing medication in patient record and on monitoring strip
- Reactions of mother and fetus:
  - Pattern of labor
  - Progress of labor
  - FHR
  - Maternal vital signs
  - Nursing interventions and woman's response
- Notification of physician/CNM

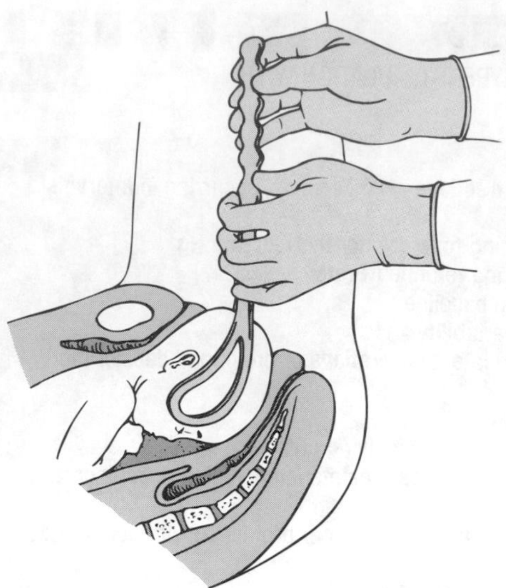

Fig. 17-9 Outlet forceps extraction of the head.

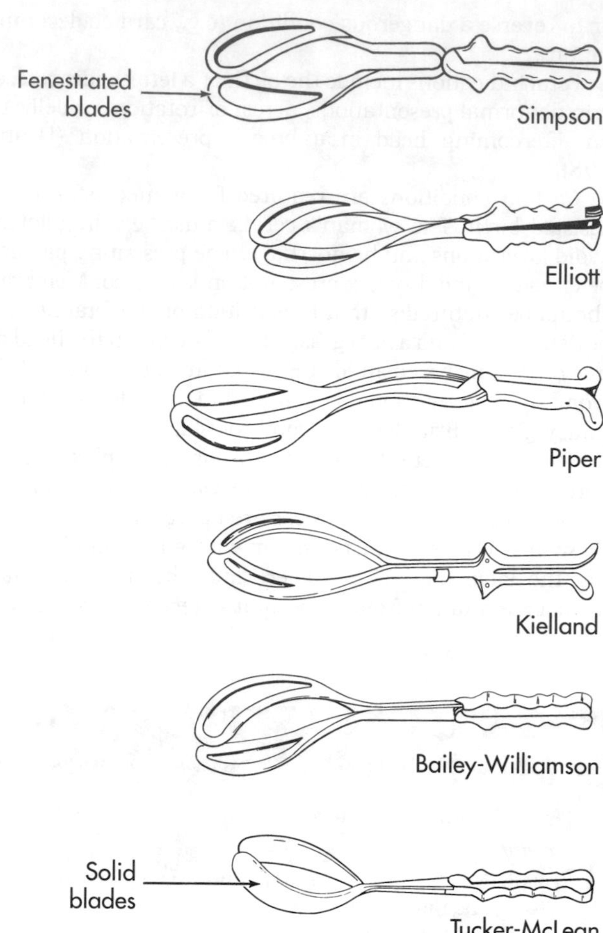

Fig. 17-10 Types of forceps. Piper forceps are used to assist delivery of the head in breech birth.

rior position. Outlet forceps are used to shorten the second stage of labor. *Low forceps* is the term used when forceps are applied to a fetal head that is at least at +2 cm station. Rotation may be more than 45 degrees. *Midforceps* are defined as forceps applied when the fetal head is engaged (no higher than station 0) but above +2 cm. There are no circumstances in which forceps should be applied to an unengaged presenting part.

Nursing considerations. The nurse obtains the type of forceps requested by the physician (Fig. 17-10). The FHR is checked, reported, and recorded *before* forceps are applied. The mother may be informed that the forceps blades fit like two tablespoons around an egg. The blades come over the baby's ears. Ordinarily traction is applied during contractions.

Nursing ALERT

After application of forceps, the FHR is rechecked, reported, and recorded *before traction* is applied. Compression of the cord between the fetal head and the forceps causes a drop in FHR. The physician would then remove and reapply the forceps.

After birth, the mother is assessed for vaginal and cervical lacerations (bleeding occurs even with a contracted uterus) and urine retention, which may result from bladder injuries. The infant should be assessed for bruising or abrasions at the site of the blade applications, facial palsy resulting from pressure of the blades on the facial nerve (cranial VII), and subdural hematoma. Newborn and postpartum caregivers should be informed that a forceps-assisted birth was performed.

Vacuum extraction. Vacuum extraction, or vacuum-assisted birth, is a birth method involving the attachment of a vacuum cup to the fetal head using negative pressure. Indications for use are similar to those for outlet forceps. Prerequisites for use include a vertex presentation, ruptured membranes, and the absence of cephalopelvic disproportion (Cunningham et al, 1993).

The woman is prepared for a vaginal birth in the lithotomy position to allow for sufficient traction. The cup is applied to the fetal head, and a caput develops inside the cup as the pressure is initiated (Fig. 17-11). Traction is applied to facilitate descent of the fetal head, and the woman is encouraged to push as suction is applied. As the head crowns, an *episiotomy* is performed if necessary; the vacuum cup is released and removed after birth of the head. If vacuum extraction is not successful, a forceps or cesarean birth is performed.

Risks to the newborn include cephalhematoma, scalp lacerations, and subdural hematoma. Maternal complications are uncommon but can include perineal, vaginal, and cervical lacerations.

Nursing considerations. The nurse's role for the woman who has given birth by use of vacuum extraction is one of support person and educator. The nurse can prepare the woman for birth and encourage her to remain active in the birth process by pushing during contractions. The FHR should be assessed frequently during the procedure. After birth, the newborn should be observed for signs of infection at the application site and cerebral irritation (e.g., poor sucking,

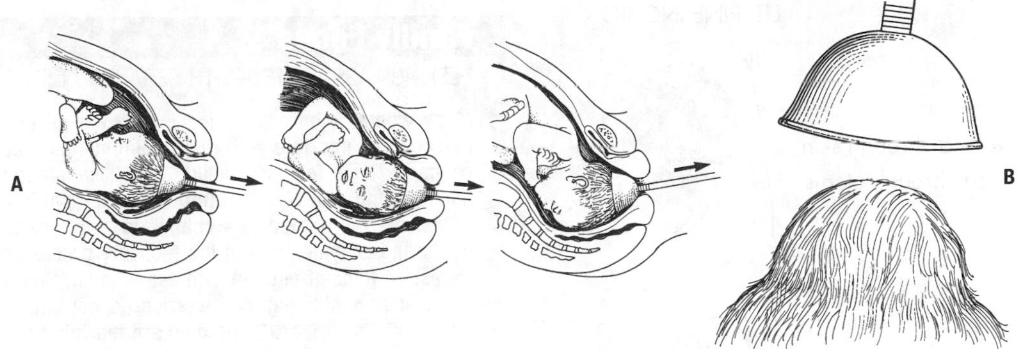

Fig. 17-11 Use of vacuum extraction to rotate the fetal head and assist with descent. **A,** Arrow indicates direction of traction on the vacuum cup. **B,** Caput succedaneum formed by the vacuum cup.

listlessness). The newborn may be at risk for cephalhematoma and neonatal jaundice as bruising resolves (Cunningham et al, 1993). The parents may need to be reassured that the caput succedaneum will begin to disappear in a few hours. Neonatal caregivers should be alerted that the birth was by vacuum extraction.

Cesarean birth. Cesarean birth is the birth of a fetus through a transabdominal incision of the uterus. Although the myth persists that Julius Caesar was born in this manner, the term is more likely derived from the Latin word *caedo* meaning "to cut." Whether a cesarean birth is planned (scheduled) or unplanned (emergency), the loss of the experience of giving birth to a child in the traditional manner may have a negative effect on a woman's self-concept. An effort is made to maintain the focus on the *birth* of a child rather than on the operative procedure. The mother experiences an abdominal rather than a vaginal birth.

The basic purpose or use of cesarean birth is to preserve the life or health of the mother and her fetus (Box 17-9). The use of cesarean birth is based on evidence of maternal or fetal stress. Maternal and fetal morbidity and mortality have decreased since the advent of antibiotics and modern surgical methods and care. However, a cesarean birth still poses threats to the health of both mother and infant. The technique of cesarean surgery has changed. Incisions are now made into the lower uterine segment rather than into the muscular body of the uterus and permit a more effective healing.

The incidence of cesarean births has increased dramatically in the last 25 years. Since the mid-1960s the cesarean birth rate has increased from less than 5% to more than 24% (Taffel, Placek, and Kosary, 1992), or approximately one fourth, of all births. Reasons cited for this increase include an increased use of electronic fetal monitoring, an increase in the number of first-time pregnancies, pregnancy at an older age, and the high incidence of repeat cesarean births (Garuffi, Strombino, and Paine, 1990; Scott, 1994). In 1992, the rate dropped slightly to 22.6% (Public Citizen Health Research Group, 1994). This decline may be attributed in part to more attempts at having a vaginal birth after giving birth by cesarean.

The type of nursing care may also influence the rate of cesarean births. A study by Radin, Harmon, and Hanson (1993) found that cesarean rates were lower for women whose nurses provided supportive care during labor.

Indications. There are few absolute indications for a cesarean birth. Today most are performed primarily for the benefit of the fetus. Four diagnostic categories are responsible for 75% to 90% of all cesarean births: dystocia, repeat cesarean, breech presentation, and fetal distress (Marieskind, 1989). Other indications for the procedure include active herpes viral infection, a prolapsed umbilical cord, medical complications such as pregnancy-induced hypertension, placental abnormalities such as placenta previa and premature separation (abruption), malpresentations such as shoulder presentation, and fetal anomalies such as hydrocephaly.

Surgical techniques. The two main types of cesarean operation are the classic and the lower segment cesarean incisions. The classic cesarean incision rarely is performed today. It may be used when rapid birth is necessary and in some cases of shoulder presentation and placenta previa. The incision is vertical into the upper body of the uterus (Fig. 17-12, *A*). The procedure is associated with a higher incidence of blood loss, infection, and uterine rupture in subsequent pregnancies than is lower segment cesarean incision. For that reason, vaginal birth after a cesarean is contraindicated with classic incisions.

BOX 17-9

Ethical Considerations Related to Forced Cesarean Birth

Refusal of a cesarean birth for fetal reasons by a woman is often described as a maternal-fetal conflict. Health care providers are ethically obliged to protect the well-being of both the mother and the fetus; it is difficult to make a decision for one without affecting the other. If a woman refuses a cesarean that is needed, health care providers need to make every effort to find out why she is refusing and provide information to persuade her to change her mind. If the woman continues to refuse surgery, then health care providers must decide if it is ethically right to get a court order for the surgery. Every effort should be made to avoid this legal step.

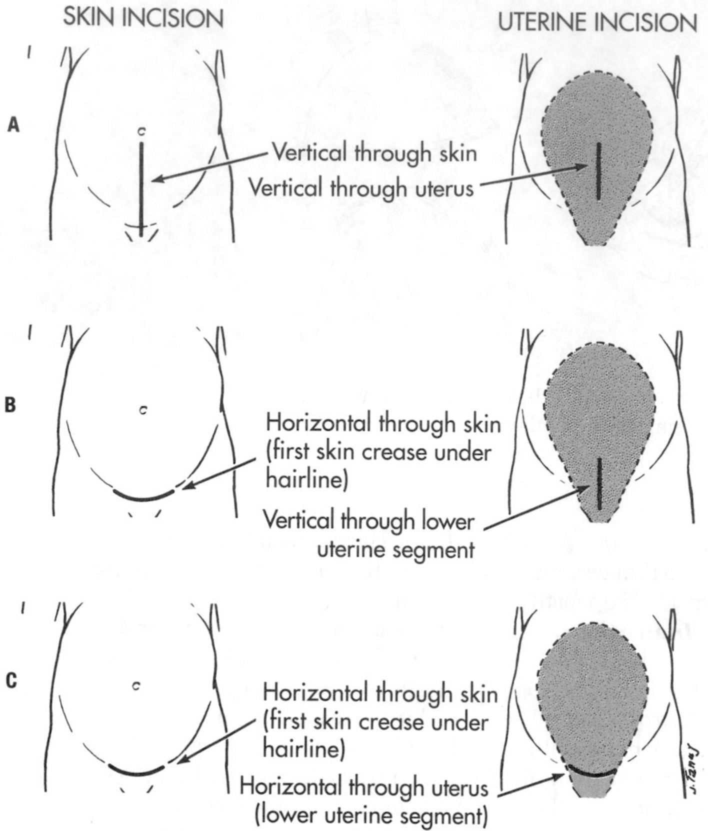

Fig. 17-12 Cesarean birth: skin and uterine incisions. **A,** Classic: vertical incisions of skin and uterus. **B,** Low cervical: horizontal incision of skin; vertical incision of uterus. **C,** Low cervical: horizontal incisions of skin and uterus.

A lower segment cesarean incision can be performed through a vertical or transverse incision (Fig. 17-12, *B* and *C*) into the uterus. The transverse incision is more popular because it is easier to perform, is associated with less blood loss and fewer postoperative infections, and is less likely to rupture in subsequent pregnancies (Cunningham et al, 1993; Scott, 1994).

Complications/risks. Cesarean births are not without complications for both the mother and fetus. Maternal complications occur in 25% to 50% of cesarean births and include aspiration, pulmonary embolism, wound infection, wound dehiscence, thrombophlebitis, hemorrhage, urinary tract infection, injuries to bladder or bowel, and complications related to anesthesia. There also is a risk that the fetus will be born prematurely if gestational age is not accurately assessed; fetal injuries can occur during the surgery (Scott, 1994). In addition, the woman is at economic risk because the cost of a cesarean birth is higher than that of a vaginal birth, and a longer recovery period may require additional expenditures. (See the Family Focus box above.)

Anesthesia. Spinal, epidural, and general anesthetics are used for cesarean births. Epidural blocks are popular because women want to be awake for and aware of the birth experience. However, the choice of anesthetic depends on several factors. The mother's medical history or present condition, such as a spinal injury or hemorrhage, may contraindicate the use of regional anesthesia. Time is another factor, especially if there is an emergency and the life of the mother or infant is at stake. In such a case a general anesthetic will most likely be used unless an epidural is in place. The woman herself is a factor. She may not know all the options or may have fears about "a needle in her back" or of being awake and feeling pain. The woman needs to be fully informed about the risks and benefits of the different types of anesthetics so that she can participate in the decision whenever there is a choice.

Family Focus

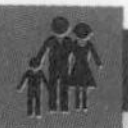

FEELINGS ASSOCIATED WITH CESAREAN BIRTH

Many women who experience a cesarean birth speak of the feelings that interfere with their maintaining an adequate self-concept. These feelings include fear, disappointment, frustration at losing control, anger (the "why me" syndrome), and loss of self-esteem related to a change in body image. Success in mothering activities and in the recovery process can do much to restore the self-esteem of these women. Some women see the scar as mutilating, and worries concerning sexual attractiveness may surface. Some men are fearful of resuming intercourse because of the fear of hurting their mates. Parents will wonder if a cesarean birth was absolutely necessary. Such feelings may surface even years later. Parents should be provided opportunities to discuss the experience to try to understand and resolve concerns.

Scheduled cesarean birth. Women face a scheduled or planned cesarean birth when labor is contraindicated (e.g., placenta previa), when birth is necessary but labor is not inducible (e.g., hypertensive states that cause a poor intrauterine environment that threatens the fetus), or when a decision is made between the physician and the woman (e.g., a repeat cesarean birth).

Women who are scheduled to have a cesarean birth have time for psychologic preparation. The psychologic response of these women may vary. Those having a repeat cesarean birth may have disturbing memories of the conditions preceding the initial surgical birth and their experiences in the postoperative recovery period. They may face with great concern the added burden of caring for an infant while recovering from a surgical operation. Others feel relieved of the uncertainty of date and time of birth and freedom from the pain of labor.

Unplanned cesarean birth. Women having unplanned or emergency cesarean births share with their families abrupt changes in their expectations for birth, postbirth care, and the care of the new baby at home. This experience may be extremely traumatic. The woman usually approaches surgery tired and discouraged after a fruitless labor. She is worried about her own and the infant's condition. She may be dehydrated and have low glycogen reserves. All preoperative procedures must be performed quickly and competently. The time for explanation of the procedures and operation is short. Because maternal and family anxiety levels are high, much of what is said is forgotten or perhaps misconstrued. After surgery, time must be spent reviewing the events preceding the operation and the operation itself to ensure that the woman understands what has happened. Fatigue is often noticeable in these women. They need much supportive care.

Prenatal preparation. Concerned professional and lay groups in the community have established councils for cesarean birth to meet the needs of these women and their families. Such groups advocate the inclusion of preparation for cesarean birth in all parenthood preparation classes. No woman can be guaranteed a vaginal birth, even if she is in good health and there is no indication of danger to the fetus before the onset of labor. Every woman needs to be aware of and prepared for this eventuality. The unknown and unexpected are ego weakening.

Childbirth educators stress the importance of emphasizing the similarities and differences between a cesarean and vaginal birth. In support of the philosophy of family-centered birth, many hospitals have policies that permit fathers and other partners to share in these births as they do in vaginal ones. Women undergoing a cesarean birth agree that the continued presence and support of their partners has helped them respond positively to the entire experience.

Preoperative care. The goal for the woman and her family is family-centered care for a cesarean birth. The *preparation* of the woman for cesarean birth is the same for either elective or emergency surgery. The primary health care provider discusses with the woman and her family the need for the cesarean birth and the prognosis for mother and infant. The anesthesiologist assesses the woman's cardiopulmonary system and presents the options for anesthesia. Informed consent is obtained for the procedure.

Maternal vital signs and blood pressure and FHR continue to be assessed per hospital routine until the operation begins. Physical preoperative preparation usually includes inserting a retention catheter to keep the bladder empty and administering prescribed preoperative medications. An abdominal-mons shave or a clipping of pubic hair may be performed. An antacid often is prescribed to neutralize gastric secretions in the event of aspiration into the woman's lungs. Intravenous fluids are started to maintain hydration and to provide an open line for the administration of blood or medications if needed. Blood and urine samples are collected and sent to the laboratory for analysis. Laboratory tests, usually ordered to establish baseline data, include a complete blood cell count and chemistry, type and crossmatching, and urinalysis.

Removal of dentures, nail polish, and jewelry may be optional depending on hospital policies. If the woman wears glasses and is going to be awake, the nurse should make sure her glasses accompany her to the operating room so she can see her infant. If the woman wears contact lenses, the nurse can find out whether they can be worn for the birth.

During preoperative preparation the support person is encouraged to remain with the woman as much as possible to provide continuing emotional support. The nurse provides essential information about the preoperative procedures. Although the nursing actions may be carried out quickly when the cesarean birth is unplanned, verbal communication, particularly explanations, is important. Silence can be frightening to the woman and her support person. The nurse's use of touch can communicate feelings of care and concern for the woman.

The nurse can assess the woman's and her partner's perceptions about the cesarean birth. For example, the woman may feel that she is a failure because she did not have a vaginal birth. As the woman expresses her feelings, the nurse may identify a risk for disturbance in self-concept during the postpartum period.

If there is time before the birth, the nurse can teach the woman about postoperative expectations, pain relief, turning, coughing, and deep breathing.

Intraoperative care. Cesarean births occur in operating rooms (ORs) in the OR suite or in labor and birth units. Once

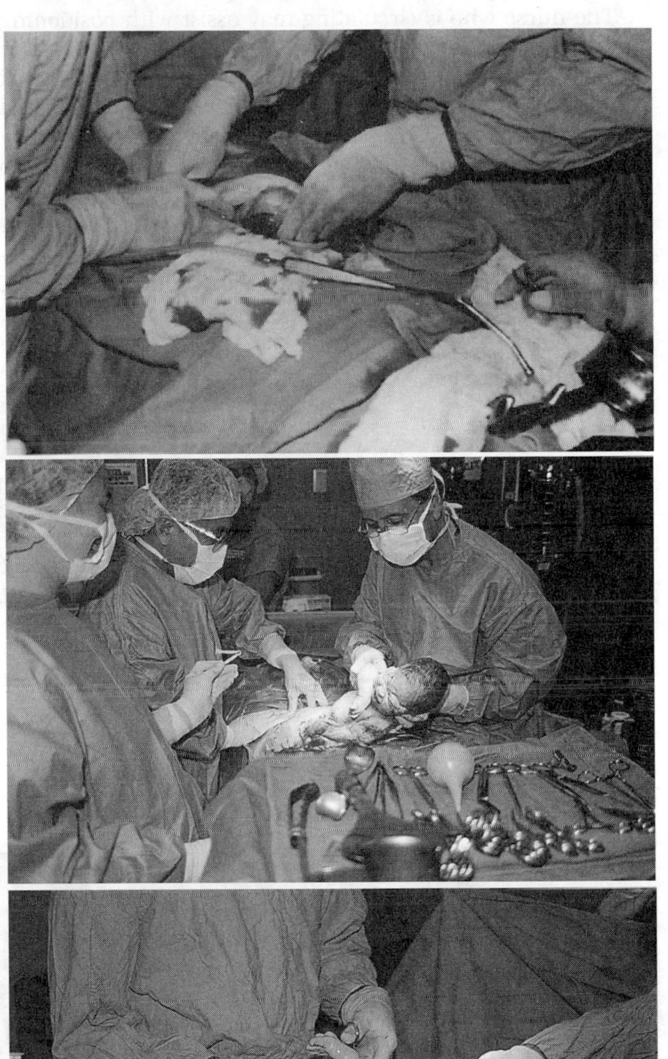

Fig. 17-13 Cesarean birth. **A,** "Bikini" incision has been made. The muscle layer is separated, the abdomen entered, the uterus has been exposed and incised; suctioning of amniotic fluid continues as head is brought up through the incision. Note small amount of bleeding. **B,** The neonate's birth through the uterine incision is complete. **C,** A quick assessment is performed. Note extreme molding of head resulting from cephalopelvic disproportion. (Courtesy Marjorie Pyle, RNC, Lifecircle, Costa Mesa, Calif.)

the woman has been taken to the operating room, her care becomes the responsibility of the obstetric team, surgeon, anesthesiologist, pediatrician, and surgical nursing staff (Fig. 17-13). In some settings, the nurse who cared for the woman in labor may scrub for or circulate during the surgery. If possible, the partner, gowned appropriately, accompanies the mother to the surgical unit and remains close to her so that continued support and comfort can be provided.

The nurse who is circulating may assist with positioning the woman on the birth (surgical) table. It is important to position her so that the uterus is displaced laterally to avoid compressing the inferior vena cava, which causes decreased placental perfusion. This position is usually accomplished by placing a wedge under the hip. A foley catheter is inserted into the bladder at this time if one is not already in place.

If the partner is not allowed or chooses not to be present, the nurse can stay in communication and give progress reports when possible. If the mother is awake during the birth, the nurse can tell her what is happening and provide support. The mother may be anxious about the sensations she is experiencing, such as cold solutions used to prepare the abdomen and pressure or pulling during the actual birth of the infant. She also may be apprehensive because of the bright lights, unfamiliar equipment, and masked and gowned personnel in the room.

When epidural anesthesia is used, the anesthetist may insert morphine into the epidural catheter after the birth of the baby. This injection provides analgesia for up to 24 hours after surgery (see pp. 364-365, 469).

Care of the infant usually is delegated to a pediatrician and/or a nurse team skilled in neonatal resuscitation, because these infants are considered to be at risk until there is evidence of physiologic stability after the birth.

A crib with resuscitation equipment is readied before surgery. Those responsible for care are expert in resuscitative techniques and in observational skills for detecting normal infant responses. If the infant's condition permits, the baby can be given to the woman's partner to hold. If the mother is

A
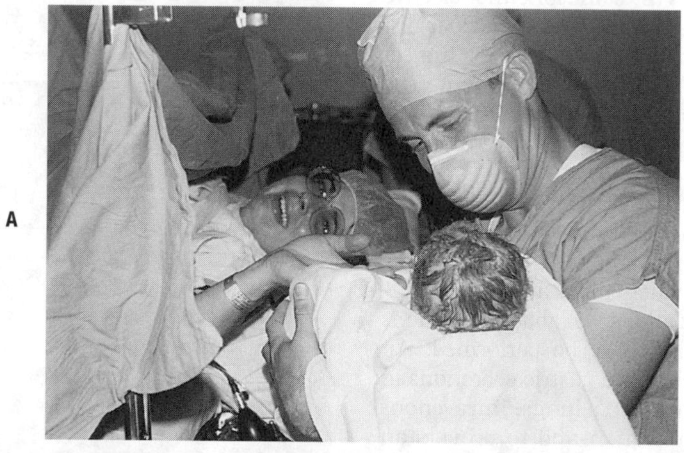

B
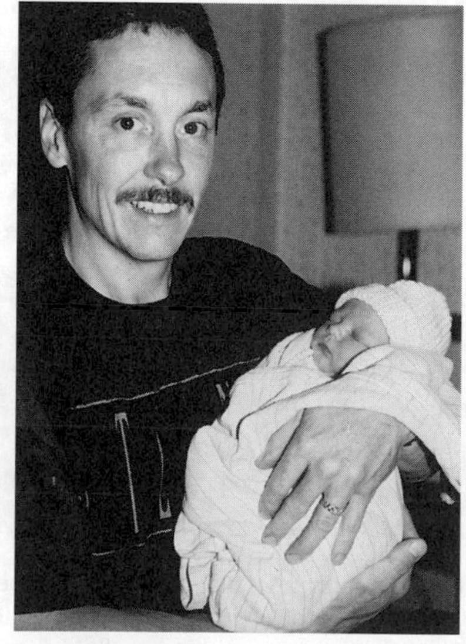

C
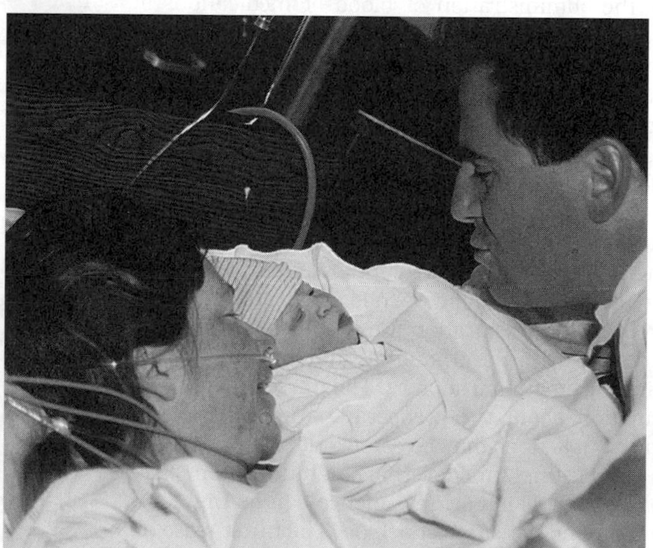

Fig. 17-14 **A,** Parents and their newborn. The physician manually removes the placenta, suctions the remaining amniotic fluid and blood from uterine cavity, and closes the uterine incision, peritoneum, muscle layer, fatty tissue, and skin while the new family is sharing some private time. **B,** The father begins bonding and attachment as mother's postoperative recovery begins. **C,** Mother-father-infant bonding is important. (**A** and **C** courtesy Marjorie Pyle, RNC, Lifecircle, Costa Mesa, Calif.)

awake, she can see and touch the baby (Fig. 17-14). The infant whose condition is compromised is transported immediately to the nursery for observation and appropriate interventions. In some institutions the partner may accompany the infant; if not, personnel keep the family informed of the infant's progress, and parent-infant contacts are initiated as soon as possible.

If the family-oriented approach is not feasible, the family is directed to the surgical or obstetric waiting room. The physician reviews with the family members the condition of the mother and child after the birth is completed. Family members may accompany the infant as he or she is transferred to the nursery, which gives the family an opportunity to see and admire the new baby.

Immediate postoperative care. The care of the woman after cesarean birth combines surgical and obstetric nursing. Once surgery is completed, the mother is transferred to a recovery room or back to her labor room. Nursing assessments in this immediate postbirth period include degree of recovery from anesthetic effects, postoperative and postbirth status, and degree of pain. A patent airway is maintained, and the woman is positioned to prevent possible aspiration. Vital signs are taken every 15 minutes for 1 to 2 hours or until stable. The condition of the incisional dressing, the fundus, and the amount of lochia are assessed, as well as intravenous intake and urine output via foley catheter. The woman is helped to turn and do deep breathing and leg exercises. Medications for pain may be administered.

If the baby is present, the mother and her partner are given some time alone to facilitate bonding and attachment with the infant. Breastfeeding can be initiated if the mother feels like trying. The woman usually is transferred to the postpartum unit after 1 to 2 hours or when her condition is stable (Box 17-10).

Postpartum care. The attitude of the nurse and other health team members can influence the woman's perception of herself after a cesarean birth. The caregivers should stress that the woman is a new mother first and a surgical patient second. This attitude helps the woman perceive herself as having the same problems and needs as other new mothers.

Physiologic concerns the first few days may be dominated by pain at the incision site and from intestinal gas and the need for pain relief. If an epidural anesthetic was used for the surgery, epidural narcotics may have been given at the time of surgery to provide pain relief for approximately 24 hours. Otherwise, pain medications usually are ordered every 3 to 4 hours, or patient-controlled analgesia (PCA) may be ordered instead. Other comfort measures such as position changes, splinting the incision with pillows, heat to the abdomen, and relaxation techniques may be implemented. Ambulation, rocking in a rocking chair, and avoiding gas-forming foods and carbonated beverages may relieve gas pains (Thomas et al, 1990). (See the Patient Teaching box above). Other physiologic concerns of women after a cesarean birth may include fatigue, activity intolerance, and incisional problems (Miovech et al, 1994).

Daily care includes perineal care, breast care, and routine hygienic care, including showering after the dressing has been removed (if showering is within the woman's cultural prescription). According to hospital policies, procedures, or protocols, the nurse assesses the vital signs, breasts, incision, fundus, and lochia. Breath sounds, bowel sounds, Homans' sign, and urinary and bowel elimination also are assessed. It is also important to note maternal affect.

Patient Teaching

POSTPARTUM PAIN RELIEF AFTER CESAREAN BIRTH

Incisional

Splint incision with a pillow when moving or coughing.
Use relaxation techniques such as music, breathing, and dim lights.
Apply a heating pad to the abdomen.

Gas

Walk as often as you can.
Do not eat or drink gas-forming foods, carbonated beverages, or whole milk.
Do not use straws for drinking fluids.
Take antiflatulent medication if prescribed.
Lie on your left side to expel gas.
Use a rocking chair.

During the postpartum period the nurse can provide care that meets the psychologic and teaching needs of mothers who have had cesarean births. The nurse can explain postpartum procedures to help the woman cooperate in her recovery from surgery. The nurse also can help the woman plan care and visits from family and friends so that adequate rest periods are provided. Information and assistance with infant care can facilitate adjustment to the mothering role. The partner can be included in infant teaching sessions and in explanations about the woman's recovery. The couple should be encouraged to express their feelings about the birth experience. Some parents are angry, frustrated, or disappointed about not having a vaginal birth. Some women express feelings of low self-esteem or negative self-image. Others express relief and gratitude that the baby is healthy and safely born. It may be helpful to have the nurse who was present during the birth visit and help fill in "gaps" about the experience. Other psychologic and life-style concerns that have been reported include depression, feeling limited in activities, and changes in family interactions (Miovech et al, 1994).

Discharge after cesarean usually occurs at a time designated by some criteria (e.g., diagnosis-related groups) and may not coincide with the woman's readiness for discharge. The nurse must provide discharge teaching in a limited time while trying to ensure that the woman is adequately prepared. The woman's information needs should be assessed. Discharge teaching includes information about diet, exercise and activity restrictions, breast care, sexual activity and contraception, medications, signs of complications (see the Patient Teaching box on p. 472), and infant care. The nurse assesses the need for continued support or counseling to facilitate the mother's emotional recovery from the birth. Referral to support groups or community agencies may be indicated.

Vaginal birth after cesarean. Indications for primary cesarean birth such as dystocia, breech presentation, or fetal distress, often are nonrecurring. Therefore a woman who has

BOX 17-10

Care Path for Cesarean Birth Without Complications
Expected Length of Stay—48 Hours

	IMMEDIATE POSTOPERATIVE CESAREAN	BY 4TH HOUR AFTER ADMISSION TO POSTPARTUM UNIT	5 HOURS TO 24 HOURS	25 HOURS TO 48 HOURS	BY DISCHARGE
Assessments					
	Recovery room/PACU admission assessment completed	PP admission assessment and care plan completed			
Vital signs	q15 min × 1 hour; q30 min × 4; WNL	q1h × 3; WNL	q4-8 h; WNL	q8h; WNL	WNL
Postpartum assessment	q15 min × 1 hour; WNL	q1h × 3; WNL	q8h; WNL	q8h; WNL	q8h; WNL
Abdominal incision	Dressing dry and intact	Dressing dry and intact	Dressing dry and intact	Dressing off or changed; incision intact	Incision intact; staples may be removed and steri-strips put in place; incision WNL
Genitourinary	Retention catheter output >30 ml/hr	Retention catheter output >30 ml/hr	Retention catheter output >30 ml/hr	Catheter discontinued; output >100 ml/void or 240 ml/8 hr	Urine output >240 ml/8 hr
Gastrointestinal		BS absent or hypoactive	Hypoactive to active BS	Active BS plus flatus	Active BS plus flatus; may or may not have BM
Musculoskeletal	Alert or easily aroused; can move legs	Alert and oriented; moving all extremities	Ambulating with help	Ambulating unassisted	Ambulating ad lib
Bonding	Evidence of parent-infant bonding; first breastfeeding if desired		Parent-infant bonding continues	Parent-infant bonding progressing	
Laboratory tests			Intrapartal CBC results on chart/computer determine Rh status and need for anti-Rh globulin; check for rubella immunity	PP HCT WNL; all lab results on chart; give anti-Rh globulin if indicated Infant will be tested for PKU after 24 hr	Give rubella vaccine if indicated
Interventions					
IV	IV continues	IV continues	IV continues	IV may be discontinued	
Diet	NPO	Ice chips; sips of clear liquids	Clear liquids	Regular diet or as tolerated	Regular diet
Perineum		Pericare by nurse	Pericare with help	Self-pericare	
Activity	Bed rest	Bed rest; change position with help	OOB × 3 with help; ADLs assisted; assisted to comfortable position to hold and feed baby	Holds baby comfortably; ambulates without assistance; ADLs unassisted	Activity ad lib
Pulmonary care	Patent airway; O_2 discontinued	TCDB q2h with splinting; incentive spirometry q1h if ordered; lungs clear	TCDB q2h while awake; lungs clear	Lungs clear	

BOX 17-10

Care Path for Cesarean Birth Without Complications Expected Length of Stay—48 Hours (cont'd)

	IMMEDIATE POSTOPERATIVE CESAREAN	BY 4TH HOUR AFTER ADMISSION TO POSTPARTUM UNIT	5 HOURS TO 24 HOURS	25 HOURS TO 48 HOURS	BY DISCHARGE
Interventions					
Medications	Oxytocin added to IV; pain control analgesics—IV or epidural narcotic	Oxytocin continued; pain control analgesics—PCA, IM, PO, epidural narcotic	Oxytocin may be discontinued; IM, PO, PCA analgesics	Stool softener, PNV; oxytocin discontinued; PO analgesics, NSAIDs, PCA discontinued	Prescription filled or given to take home
Teaching/discharge plan	Breastfeeding positioning; leg exercises	Verbalize understanding of unit routines, how to achieve rest, TCDB, involution, pain control	*Self:* comfort measures and care; reinforce TCDB and positioning; introduce teaching videos, lactation promotion or suppression *Infant:* handwashing, infant safety, positioning for feeding and burping; if breastfeeding, then positioning baby, latching on, timing, removing from breast	*Self:* diet, activity/rest, bowel/bladder function *Infant:* bonding, parent concerns, feeding, infant bath, cord care, need for car seat, newborn characteristics, circumcision, if needed; answer questions	*Self:* home care, signs of complications (infections, bleeding), normal psychologic adjustments, normal ADLs, resumption of sexual activities, contraception, identification of support system at home, self-concept issues related to cesarean birth; inform whom to call if problems; review need to keep follow-up appointment; provide information about community resources; provide copy of home care *Infant:* parents to demonstrate infant care; reinforce use of booklets for infant care; whom to call if problems; discuss immunization needs; review need to keep follow-up appointments

ADLs, Activities of daily living; *BM*, bowel movement; *BS*, bowel sounds; *CBC*, complete blood count; *HCT*, hematocrit; *IM*, intramuscular; *OOB*, out of bed; *PACU*, postanesthesia care unit; *PCA*, patient-controlled analgesia; *PKU*, phenylketonuria; *PNV*, prenatal vitamins; *PO*, by mouth; *PP*, postpartum; *NSAIDSs*, nonsteroidal antiinflammatory drugs; *TCDB*, turn, cough, deep breathe; *WNL*, within normal limits.

had a cesarean birth may subsequently become pregnant and not have any contraindications to labor and vaginal birth.

The continued practice of "once a cesarean, always a cesarean" no longer is recommended by most obstetricians. A trial of labor and **vaginal birth after cesarean (VBAC)** are now recommended as routine procedures by the American College of Obstetricians and Gynecologists (1995a) for women who have had previous cesarean birth(s) by low transverse incision. In 1992, 25.4% of women who had one previous cesarean birth had a vaginal birth with their second pregnancy (Public Citizen Health Research Group, 1994). Studies have shown that such a vaginal birth is relatively safe, with only a 0.5% risk of uterine rupture through a lower uterine segment scar (Knuppel and Drukker, 1993). Labor and a vaginal birth are not recommended if contraindications such as a previous fundal classic cesarean scar or evidence of cephalopelvic disproportion are present.

According to Scott (1994), 60% to 88% of women can give

Patient Teaching

SIGNS OF POSTOPERATIVE COMPLICATIONS AFTER DISCHARGE

Report the following signs to your health care provider:
Fever greater than 38°C (100.4°F)
Painful urination
Lochia heavier than a normal period
Wound separation
Redness or oozing at the incision site
Severe abdominal pain

Critical Thinking Exercises

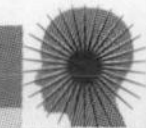

UNPLANNED CESAREAN BIRTH

You are preparing a woman for an unplanned cesarean birth for failure to progress.

1. Examine the possible reactions of the woman to this situation. How would these reactions affect the effectiveness of nursing care?
2. Examine your feelings as you think about how to prepare the woman for surgery. How would these feelings affect your care?
3. How would your preparation differ from preparing a woman for a planned cesarean?
4. Explain the differences in postpartum needs between the woman who has had a planned cesarean and the woman who has experienced an unplanned one.

birth vaginally after a trial of labor, which is recommended for women who meet the requirements for VBAC. During the antepartal period, the woman should be given information about VBAC and encouraged to choose it as an alternative to a repeat cesarean if no contraindications occur. VBAC support groups and prenatal classes can help prepare the woman psychologically for labor and vaginal birth.

This labor should occur in a hospital facility that has the equipment and personnel available to perform a cesarean within 30 minutes from the time a decision is made for cesarean birth to the beginning of the procedure. Ideally, the woman is admitted to the labor and birth unit at the onset of spontaneous labor. In the latent phase of labor, the nurse encourages normal activities such as ambulation. In the active phase of labor, FHR and uterine activity usually are monitored electronically, and intravenous access such as a heparin lock may be established. Collaboration among the woman in labor, the nurse, and other health care providers often results in a successful VBAC.

There is no evidence of contraindications for administering oxytocin to induce or augment labor or for using epidural anesthesia, but some physicians may not elect these procedures (Cunningham et al, 1993). Intravaginal prostaglandin E2 has been used safely and effectively for cervical ripening in women who are planning a VBAC (Williams et al, 1995).

Attention should be given to the woman's psychologic and physical needs during the trial of labor. Anxiety can inhibit the release of oxytocin, delaying labor progress and leading to failure and a repeat cesarean birth. The nurse can encourage the woman to use breathing and relaxation techniques and to change position to promote labor progress. The woman's partner can be encouraged to provide comfort measures and emotional support (Fawcett, Tulman, and Spedden, 1994). If a trial of labor fails, the woman will need support and encouragement to express her feelings about once again not achieving her desired outcome.

Evaluation

To evaluate the effectiveness of nursing care for a woman experiencing dystocia, the nurse reviews the expected outcomes that were met and assesses the woman's and the family's level of satisfaction with the care received. Expected outcomes include the following. The woman will:

1. Demonstrate an understanding of the causes and treatment of dysfunctional labor
2. Express decreased anxiety and fear about her condition and the status of the fetus
3. Not exhibit signs of complications such as infection, hemorrhage, and fetal distress
4. Verbalize decreased pain
5. State satisfaction with her participation in decision making about care options
6. Verbalize positive feelings about herself
7. Give birth to a healthy infant

See the Nursing Care Plan on pp. 473-474 for a woman experiencing complicated labor and cesarean birth.

POSTDATE PREGNANCY, LABOR, AND BIRTH

A **postdate birth** is the birth of an infant beyond the end of week 42 of gestation, or 294 days from the first day of the last menstrual period. The incidence of postdate pregnancy is estimated to be between 3% and 12%. The most common cause of postdate pregnancy is inaccurate dating of the pregnancy because the woman had an irregular ovulatory pattern (Spellacy, 1994).

Maternal and Fetal Risks

Maternal risks are related to the birth of an excessively large infant. The woman is at increased risk for dysfunctional labor, induction of labor, forceps-assisted birth, lacerations related to vaginal birth, and cesarean birth (Spellacy, 1994; Wood, 1994). The woman also may experience psychologic risks because she may become anxious about going past her estimated date of birth (EDB).

Fetal risks appear to be twofold. The first is related to the possibility of birth trauma and asphyxia through cephalopelvic disproportion. The second risk is believed to result from the compromising effects on the fetus of an "aging" placenta. Spellacy (1994) notes that placental function gradually decreases after 37 weeks of gestation; amniotic fluid volume declines to approximately 800 ml by 40 weeks and to approximately 250 ml by 42 weeks of gestation. Oligohydramnios is associated with fetal distress related to cord compression. If placental insufficiency is present, there is a high incidence of fetal distress during labor. Neonatal problems may include asphyxia, meconium aspiration syndrome,

Nursing Care Plan

DYSFUNCTIONAL LABOR

Secondary Inertia

Nursing Diagnosis: Risk for injury to mother and/or fetus related to oxytocin stimulation secondary to dysfunctional labor

Expected Outcomes: Maternal-fetal well-being is maintained; labor progresses and birth occurs.

• NURSING INTERVENTIONS/*RATIONALES*

Explain oxytocin protocol to woman and her labor partner *to allay apprehension and enhance participation.*

Encourage woman to void before beginning protocol *to prevent discomfort and remove a barrier to labor progress.*

Apply the electronic fetal monitor per hospital protocol and obtain a 15- to 20-minute baseline strip *to ensure adequate assessment of FHR and contractions.*

Position woman in a side-lying position and administer the oxytocin per physician order using an IV infusion pump *to stimulate uterine activity and provide adequate control of the flow rate.*

Regulate the oxytocin per protocol starting at 0.5 to 1 mU/min and advancing the dose in increments of 1 to 2 mU/minute every 15 to 60 minutes *to allow adequate evaluation of the woman's response to stimulation and to prevent hyperstimulation and fetal hypoxia.*

Maintain oxytocin dose and rate when contractions occur every 2 to 3 minutes with a duration of 40 to 90 seconds and intrauterine pressures of 40 to 90 mm Hg *to produce effective uterine stimulation without risk of hyperstimulation.*

If infusion rate is advanced to 20 mU/minute without achieving the desired contractility pattern, notify physician *because woman is at risk for hyperstimulation and water intoxication.*

Monitor maternal vital signs every 30 to 60 minutes *to assess for oxytocin-induced hypertension.*

Monitor contractility pattern and FHR pattern every 15 minutes *to assess uterine activity for possible hypertonicity or ineffective uterine response to oxytocin and to detect evidence of fetal distress.*

Monitor intake, output, and specific gravity (limit intake to 1000 ml per 8 hours; output should be at least 120 ml) *to assess for urinary retention and prevent water intoxication.*

Monitor cervical dilation, effacement, and station *to assess progress of labor.*

If hypertonicity or signs of fetal distress are detected, discontinue oxytocin immediately *to arrest the progress of hypertonicity,* turn woman on her side *to increase placental blood flow,* increase primary IV rate to 200 ml/hr (unless signs of water toxicity are present), administer oxygen per face mask *to increase the oxygen supply to the fetus,* notify physician, and continuously monitor maternal vital signs and FHRs *to provide ongoing assessment of maternal/fetal status.*

Nursing Diagnosis: Pain related to increasing frequency, regularity, intensity, and prolonged peak of contractions

Expected Outcomes: The woman exhibits signs of decreased discomfort.

• NURSING INTERVENTIONS/*RATIONALES*

Prepare woman and labor partner for the change in the nature of the contractions once the oxytocin drip is initiated *to prepare them and allow for more effective coping.*

Remind woman and labor partner that analgesics are available for use during labor *to provide knowledge to help them make decisions about pain control.*

Review the use of specific techniques such as conscious relaxation, focused breathing, effleurage, massage, and application of sacral pressure *to increase relaxation, decrease intensity of pain of contractions, and promote use of controlled thought and direction of energy.*

Provide comfort measures such as frequent mouth care *to prevent dry mouth,* application of damp cloth to forehead and changing of damp gown or bed covers *to relieve diaphoresis,* and positioning *to reduce stiffness.*

Encourage conscious relaxation between contractions *to prevent fatigue, which contributes to increased pain perceptions.*

Nursing Diagnosis: Anxiety/ineffective coping related to prolonged labor, increased pain, and fatigue

Expected Outcomes: Woman's anxiety is reduced; woman actively participates in the labor process.

NURSING INTERVENTIONS/*RATIONALES*

Provide ongoing feedback to woman and partner *to allay anxiety and enhance participation.*

Present care options when possible *to increase feelings of control.*

Continue to provide comfort measures *to maintain a posture of support and caring and to aid woman in focusing on the labor process.*

Encourage woman and partner to continue to use those mechanisms that promote effective labor (e.g., breathing, positioning) *to keep woman and partner actively involved in process.*

Nursing Diagnosis: Risk for maternal/fetal infection related to prolonged rupture of membranes or possible invasive procedures (e.g., use of fetal scalp electrodes, use of forceps, episiotomy, cesarean section)

Expected Outcomes: There is no evidence of infection.

NURSING INTERVENTIONS/*RATIONALES*

Monitor temperature *because elevation is early indicator of infection.*

Continued.

Nursing Care Plan
DYSFUNCTIONAL LABOR—cont'd

Monitor FHR/variability *because rates greater than 160 beats/minute and minimal variability may be indicative of maternal fever and infection.*
Monitor intake and output for dehydration *because signs of infection closely resemble those of dehydration, and differentiation is needed.*
Maintain Standard Precautions and use scrupulous handwashing techniques when providing care *to prevent spread of infection.*
Use strict aseptic technique when performing invasive procedures such as urinary catheterization, insertion of intravenous lines, or application of scalp electrodes *to reduce risk of nosocomial infection.*
Monitor IV sites, electrode sites, and incision sites for signs such as pain, redness, edema, heat, and drainage, *which are indicative of infection.*
Monitor urine for color, concentration, odor, clouding, casts, and sediment, *which may indicate a urinary tract infection.*
When membranes rupture, assess fluid for color, amount, and odor and for the presence of meconium stain *because alterations may be indicative of intrauterine infection.*
After membrane rupture, keep vaginal examinations to a minimum and use sterile gloves *to decrease risk of uterine infection.*
Assist woman to maintain good personal hygiene habits (e.g., wiping perineal region from front to back, keeping area dry) *to reduce introduction of bacteria.*
Monitor laboratory values (e.g., white blood cell count, cultures) *for indicators of infection.*

dysmaturity syndrome, and respiratory distress (Gilbert and Harmon, 1993). Whether or not an infant born after a postdate pregnancy has neurologic, behavioral, or intellectual developmental problems needs further investigation (Wood, 1994).

Nursing Care Management

The management of postdate pregnancy is still controversial. The induction of labor at 42 weeks is suggested by some authorities. Others allow pregnancy to proceed to 43 weeks as long as tests of fetal well-being are performed and results are normal.

LEGAL TIP

Informed Consent Regarding Care During Postdate Pregnancy

The woman with a postdate pregnancy should be informed about the risks and benefits of both treatment and nontreatment. The usual standard of practice is that antepartal surveillance (maternal assessments and tests of fetal well-being) must begin by 14 days after the EDB, no matter how it has been derived. The woman and her primary health care provider should mutually agree on a plan of care (Wood, 1994).

Antepartum assessments for postdate pregnancy may include daily fetal movement counts. Nonstress testing followed by stress tests when indicated are usually performed twice weekly. Amniotic fluid volume is usually assessed weekly. The biophysical profile may be the best indicator of fetal well-being because it combines nonstress testing with real-time ultrasound scanning to assess fetal movements, fetal breathing movements, and amniotic fluid volume (AFV). Determining the amount of AFV is critical because decreased AFV has been associated with fetal distress in postdate pregnancies (Spellacy, 1994).

Cervical checks usually are performed weekly after 40 weeks of gestation to assess whether the condition of the cervix is favorable for induction (>5 on the Bishop score) (Table 17-3). Amniocentesis or amnioscopy may be performed to detect meconium in the amniotic fluid (Spellacy, 1994).

During the postdate period the woman is encouraged to assess fetal activity daily, to assess for signs of labor, and to keep appointments with her primary health care provider (see the Home Care box below). The woman and her family should be encouraged to express their feelings about the prolonged pregnancy. Referral to a support group or other supportive resource may be needed.

If the woman's cervix is ripe, labor is usually induced with oxytocin. If her cervix is not ripe, a cervical ripening agent (e.g., prostaglandin gel) may be used before the oxytocin induction (Gilbert and Harmon, 1993).

During labor the fetus of a woman with a postdate pregnancy should be monitored electronically for a more accurate assessment of the FHR pattern. Fetal scalp pH sampling may be obtained for fetal distress or if meconium is present in the amniotic fluid. If oligohydramnios is present, amnioinfusion may be implemented to prevent cord compression or to treat a variable deceleration pattern (Gilbert and Harmon, 1993; Lake, 1992). Accurate assessment of the woman's labor pat-

Home Care

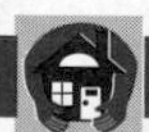

POSTDATE PREGNANCY

- Perform daily fetal movement counts.
- Assess for signs of labor.
- Call your physician/CNM if your membranes rupture.
- Keep appointments for fetal assessment tests or cervical checks.
- Come to the hospital soon after labor begins.

tern also is important because dysfunctional labor is common in this complication (Spellacy, 1994).

Emotional support is essential for the woman with a postdate pregnancy and her family. A vaginal birth is anticipated, but the couple should be prepared for a forceps-assisted birth, vacuum extraction, or cesarean birth if complications arise.

Expected outcomes include that the woman uses appropriate coping mechanisms to deal with the emotional aspects of her postdate pregnancy and that the woman and her newborn do not experience injury during the birth.

OBSTETRIC EMERGENCIES

Shoulder Dystocia

Etiologic factors. Shoulder dystocia is a rare obstetric emergency that can result in injury to the fetus or the woman during the attempt to deliver the fetus vaginally. Shoulder dystocia is a condition in which the head is born but the anterior shoulder cannot pass under the pubic arch. Fetopelvic disproportion related to excessive fetal size or maternal pelvic abnormalities may be a cause of shoulder dystocia (Willson and Carrington, 1991).

Nursing Care Management

Many maneuvers such as maternal position changes have been suggested and tried to free the anterior shoulder, but no particular maneuver has been found to be most effective (Naef and Morrison, 1994). The two most commonly described maneuvers are the application of suprapubic pressure and the McRoberts maneuver. Application of suprapubic pressure to the anterior shoulder (Fig. 17-15) may be implemented in an attempt to push it under the symphysis pubis (Naef and Morrison, 1994). The McRoberts maneuver (Fig. 17-16) is a maneuver in which the woman's legs are flexed apart with her knees on her abdomen (Piper and McDonald, 1994). This maneuver causes the sacrum to straighten, and the symphysis pubis rotates toward the mother's head; the angle of pelvic inclination is decreased, freeing the shoulder. The nurse assists the primary health care provider with implementing these maneuvers.

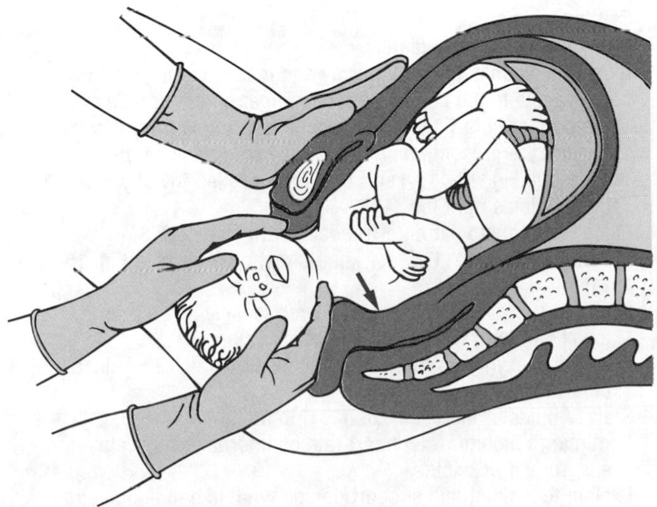

Fig. 17-15 Application of suprapubic pressure.

Having the woman move to a hands-and-knees position or a squatting position has also been used to resolve cases of shoulder dystocia (Piper and McDonald, 1994). Other alternatives require the physician/CNM to implement rotation procedures to move the shoulder and deliver the posterior arm. Fundal pressure usually is not advised (Naef and Morrison, 1994; Piper and McDonald, 1994).

Prolapsed Umbilical Cord

A **prolapsed umbilical cord** occurs when the cord lies below the presenting part of the fetus. Umbilical cord prolapse may be occult (hidden, not visible) at any time during labor whether or not membranes are ruptured (Fig. 16-10, *A* and *B*). It is most common to see frank (visible) prolapse directly after rupture of membranes (ROM), when gravity washes the cord in front of the presenting part (Fig. 16-10, *C* and *D*). Frank prolapse occurs in one of 400 births. Contributing factors are a long cord (>100 cm or 40 inches), malpresentation (breech), transverse lie, or unengaged presenting part.

When the presenting part does not fit snugly into the lower uterine segment, as in polyhydramnios or when the membranes rupture, a sudden gush of amniotic fluid may cause the cord to be displaced downward. Similarly, the cord may prolapse during AROM if the presenting part is high. A small fetus also may not fit snugly into the lower uterine segment; as a result, cord prolapse is more likely to occur.

Other predisposing factors in cord prolapse that are associated with a high presenting part are multiparity, cephalopelvic disproportion, and placenta previa. Prolapse of the cord is difficult to diagnose; however, an alert nurse or physician may make the diagnosis on vaginal examination after a sudden gush of fluid.

Nursing Care Management

Prompt recognition is important because fetal hypoxia from prolonged cord compression (occlusion of blood flow to and from the fetus for more than 5 minutes) usually results in central nervous system (CNS) damage or demise of the fetus (see the Emergency box on p. 476). Pressure on the cord is relieved by the examiner putting a sterile gloved hand into the vagina and holding the presenting part off of the umbilical cord (Fig. 16-11, *A* and *B*). The woman is assisted into a position such as a modified Sims (Fig. 16-11, *C*), Trendelenburg, or knee-chest (Fig. 16-11, *D*), where gravity keeps the presenting part off the cord. If the cervix is fully dilated, a forceps or vacuum-assisted birth can be performed for the fetus in a cephalic presentation; otherwise a cesarean birth is likely to be performed. Nonreassuring fetal status, inadequate uterine relaxation, and bleeding can also occur as a result of a prolapsed umbilical cord. Indications for immediate interventions are presented in the Emergency box on p. 476.

Rupture of the Uterus

Etiologic factors and clinical manifestations. Rupture of the uterus is a rare but very serious obstetric injury that occurs once in every 1500 to 2000 births. The most common causes of uterine rupture during pregnancy are separation of

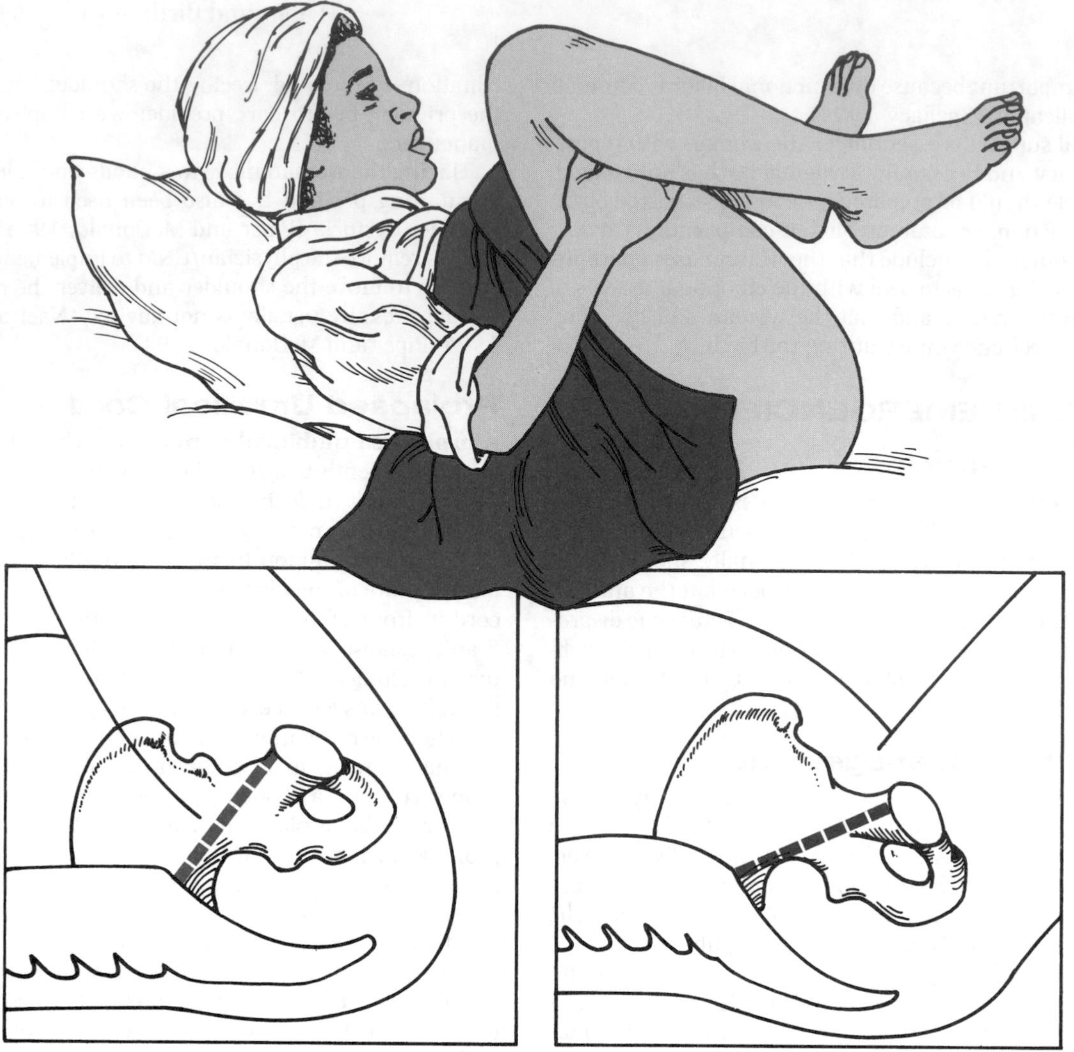

Fig. 17-16 McRoberts maneuver. (Modified from Gabbe S, Niebyl J, Simpson J: *Obstetrics, normal and problem pregnancies*, New York, 1986, Churchill Livingstone.)

EMERGENCY

PROLAPSED CORD

Signs

Fetal bradycardia with variable deceleration during uterine contraction

Woman reports feeling the cord after membranes rupture

Cord is seen in, felt in, or protruding from the vagina

Interventions

Call for assistance.

Notify physician immediately.

Glove the examining hand quickly and insert two fingers into the vagina to the cervix. With one finger on either side of the cord or both fingers to one side, exert upward pressure against the presenting part to relieve compression of the cord (see Fig. 16-11, *A* and *B*). Place a rolled towel under the woman's right hip.

Place woman into extreme Trendelenburg, modified Sims position (see Fig. 16-11, *C*), or knee-chest position (see Fig. 16-11, *D*).

If cord is protruding from vagina, wrap loosely in a sterile towel wet with warm, sterile, normal saline.

Administer oxygen to the woman by mask, 10 to 12 L/min, until birth is accomplished.

Start IV fluids or increase existing drip rate.

Continue to monitor fetal heart rate by internal fetal scalp electrode if possible.

Explain to woman and support person what is happening and how it is being managed.

the scar of a previous classical cesarean birth, uterine trauma (e.g., accidents, surgery), and congenital uterine anomaly. During labor and birth, uterine rupture may be caused by intense spontaneous uterine contractions, labor stimulation (e.g., oxytocin), an overdistended uterus, (e.g., multifetal gestation), external or internal version, and difficult forceps delivery. Uterine rupture occurs more commonly in multigravidas than primigravidas.

A uterine rupture may be classified as complete or incomplete. A complete rupture extends through the entire uterine wall into the peritoneal cavity or broad ligament. An incomplete rupture extends into the peritoneum but does not extend into the peritoneal cavity or ligament. Bleeding is usually internal. An incomplete rupture may be a partial separation of an old cesarean scar and may go unnoticed unless the woman has a subsequent cesarean birth or other uterine surgery.

Signs and symptoms vary with the extent of the rupture. In an incomplete rupture, pain may or may not be present. The fetus may or may not demonstrate nonreassuring signs such as late decelerations, decreased variability, or increased or decreased heart rate. In a complete rupture, the woman may complain of a sudden, sharp abdominal pain. If in labor, the woman's contractions will cease, and she may exhibit signs of hypovolemic shock caused by hemorrhage (e.g., hypotension; tachypnea; pallor; cool, clammy skin). The woman may complain of chest pain resulting from pulmonary embolism. If the placenta separates, the fetal heart rate will be absent. Fetal parts may be palpable through the abdomen.

Nursing Care Management

Prevention is the best treatment. Women who have had a previous classical cesarean birth are advised not to attempt a vaginal birth in subsequent pregnancies. Women at risk for uterine rupture are assessed closely during labor. Women who are induced with oxytocin are monitored for signs of uterine hyperstimulation. If hyperstimulation occurs, a tocolytic medication may be ordered to decrease the intensity of uterine contractions. After giving birth, women are assessed for excessive bleeding, especially in the presence of a firm fundus and signs of hemorrhagic shock.

If rupture occurs, medical management depends on the severity. A small rupture may be managed with a laparotomy and delivery of the infant and repair of the laceration and blood transfusions if needed. For a complete rupture, a hysterectomy and blood replacement is the usual treatment.

The nurse's role may include starting intravenous fluids, transfusing blood products, and assisting with preparation for immediate surgery. Supporting the woman's family and providing information about the treatment is important during this emergency. Mortality rates for the fetus are high (>80%) and may be as high as 50% to 75% for the woman (Cunningham et al, 1993). Providing information about (spiritual) support services or suggesting that the family contact their own support system may be warranted.

Amniotic Fluid Embolism

Etiologic factors and clinical manifestations. Amniotic fluid embolism (AFE) occurs when amniotic fluid containing particles of debris (e.g., vernix, hair, skin cells, meconium) enters the maternal circulation and obstructs pulmonary vessels, causing respiratory distress and circulatory collapse. Fluid can enter the maternal circulation any time there is an opening in the amniotic sac or maternal uterine veins and when there is enough intrauterine pressure to force the amniotic fluid into the veins (e.g., when the placenta separates or when there are rapid or strong contractions that cause the uterus to rupture or lacerate).

Amniotic fluid embolism accounts for 17% of all maternal deaths (Koonin et al, 1989). Maternal mortality occurs most often when thick meconium is present in the amniotic fluid, because it clogs the pulmonary veins more completely than other debris. Even if death does not occur immediately, serious coagulation problems (e.g., disseminated intravascular coagulopathy) usually occur.

Nursing Care Management

Medical management must be immediate. Cardiopulmonary resuscitation is often needed. The woman is usually placed on mechanical ventilation, and blood replacement is initiated. Coagulation defects are treated.

The nurse's immediate role is to assist with the resuscitation efforts. If the woman survives, she is usually moved to a critical care unit. Hemodynamic monitoring and blood replacement and coagulopathy treatment are implemented.

Support of the woman's partner/family is needed. They will likely be very anxious and distressed. Brief explanations of what is happening are important during the emergency and can be reinforced after the immediate crisis is over. If the woman dies, emotional support and involvement of the perinatal loss support team or other resource for grief counseling is needed.

Key Points

- Dystocia results from differences in the normal relationships among any of the five factors affecting labor.
- Uterine dysfunction can be described as hypertonic or hypotonic.
- The functional relationships between the uterine contractions, the fetus, and the mother's pelvis are altered by maternal positioning.
- Uterine contractility is increased by oxytocin and prostaglandin and is decreased by tocolytic agents (magnesium sulfate, β-mimetic agents, calcium channel blockers, and prostaglandin inhibitors).
- The pregnant woman and her family can be taught to treat preterm labor at home with bed rest and avoidance of activities that stimulate the uterus. Tocolytic therapy may also be implemented.
- In hospital treatment for preterm labor involves bed rest, the use of tocolytics, and pharmacologic stimulation of fetal lung maturity.
- The risk of infection is increased when premature rupture of membranes is prolonged without onset of labor.
- All expectant parents benefit from learning about operative obstetrics (e.g., use of forceps, cesarean birth) and preterm labor during the prenatal period.
- The basic purpose of a cesarean birth is to preserve the life or health of the mother and her fetus.
- Unless contraindicated, a vaginal birth is possible after a previous cesarean birth.
- Postdate pregnancy poses a risk to both the mother and the fetus.
- Obstetric emergencies (e.g., shoulder dystocia, prolapsed cord, rupture of the uterus, and amniotic fluid embolism) occur rarely but require immediate intervention.

References

Adams D, Chervenak F: Intrapartum management of twin gestation, *Clin Obstet Gynecol* 33:42, 1990.

American College of Obstetricians and Gynecologists: *Precis IV: An update in obstetrics and gynecology*, Washington, DC, 1990, ACOG.

American College of Obstetricians and Gynecologists: Technical bulletin No 152: *Operative vaginal delivery*, Washington, DC, Feb 1991, ACOG.

American College of Obstetricians and Gynecologists: *Prostaglandin E2 gel for cervical ripening*, ACOG Committee Opinion 123, Washington, DC, 1993, ACOG.

American College of Obstetricians and Gynecologists (ACOG Practice Patterns): Vaginal delivery after previous cesarean birth, Washington, DC, Aug 1995a, ACOG.

American College of Obstetricians and Gynecologists: Technical bulletin No 217: *Induction of labor*, Washington, DC, Dec, 1995b, ACOG.

American College of Obstetricians and Gynecologists: Technical bulletin No. 218: Dystocia and augmentation of labor, Washington DC, Dec 1995c, ACOG.

Andersen H, Merkatz I: *Preterm labor*. In Scott J et al: *Danforth's obstetrics and gynecology*, ed 7, Philadelphia, 1994, JB Lippincott.

Andrews C, Chrzanowski M: Maternal position, labor, and comfort, *Appl Nurs Res* 3:7, 1990.

Association of Women's Health, Obstetric, and Neonatal Nurses: *Cervical ripening and induction and augmentation of labor*, Practice Resource, Washington, DC, December 1993, AWHONN.

Biancuzzo M: The patient observer: does the hands-and-knees position during labor help to rotate the occiput posterior fetus? *Birth* 18(1):40, 1991.

Biancuzzo M: Six myths of maternal posture during labor, *MCN Am J Matern Child Nurs* 18(5):264, 1993.

Blackman J: Neonatal intensive care: is it worth it? *Pediatr Clin North Am* 38:1497, 1991.

Blanco J: Recognizing and responding to intra-amniotic infection, *Contemp OB GYN* 36(9):61, 1991.

Bowes W: *Clinical aspects of normal and abnormal labor*. In Cohen W et al, editors: *Management of labor*, ed 2, Rockville, Md, 1989, Aspen.

Brodsky P, Pelzar E: Rationale for the revision of oxytocin administration protocols, *J Obstet Gynecol Neonatal Nurs* 20(6):440, 1991.

Creasy R, Merkatz I: Prevention of preterm labor: clinical opinion, *Obstet Gynecol* 76(suppl 1):25, 1990.

Creasy R: Preterm birth prevention: where are we? *Am J Obstet Gynecol* 168:1223, 1993.

Creasy R: *Preterm labor and delivery*. In Creasy R, Resnik R: *Maternal-fetal medicine: principles and practices*, ed 3, Philadelphia, 1994, WB Saunders.

Cunningham F et al: *Williams obstetrics*, ed 19, Norwalk, Conn, 1993, Appleton & Lange.

Davis L: *Protocol for the nursing management of the patient requiring oxytocin for induction and augmentation of labor*. In Mandeville L, Troiano N, editors: *High-risk intrapartum nursing*, Philadelphia: 1992, JB Lippincott.

Dennan P: *Dennan's forceps deliveries*, ed 3, Philadelphia, 1989, FA Davis.

Dyson D et al: Prevention of preterm birth in high risk patients: the role of education and provider contact versus home uterine monitoring, *Am J Obstet Gynecol* 164:756, 1991.

Eronen M et al: The effects of indomethacin and a β-sympathomimetic agent on the fetal ductus arteriosus during treatment of premature labor: a randomized double-blind study, *Am J Obstet Gynecol* 164:141, 1991.

Fawcett J, Tulman L, Spedden J: Responses to vaginal birth after cesarean section, *J Obstet Gynecol Neonatal Nurs* 23(3):253, 1994.

Ferguson J et al: A comparison of tocolysis with nifedipine or ritodrine: analysis of efficacy and maternal, fetal, and neonatal outcome, *Am J Obstet Gynecol* 163:105, 1990.

Friedman E: *Normal and dysfunctional labor*. In Cohen W et al, editors: *Management of labor*, ed 2, Rockville, Md, 1989, Aspen.

Garuffi G, Strombino D, Paine L: Investigation of institutional differences in primary cesarean rates, *J Nurse Midwife* 35:274, 1990.

Garite T, Spellacy W: *Premature rupture of membranes*. In Scott J et al, editors: *Danforth's obstetrics and gynecology*, ed 7, Philadelphia, 1994, JB Lippincott.

Gilbert E, Harmon J: *Manual of high-risk pregnancy and delivery*, St Louis, 1993, Mosby.

Greenberg R, Hankins G: Antibiotic therapy in preterm rupture of membranes, *Clin Obstet Gynecol* 34(4):742, 1991.

Grohar J: Nursing protocols for antepartum nursing care, *J Obstet Gynecol Neonatal Nurs* 23(8):687, 1994.

Heffner L et al: Clinical and environmental predictors of preterm labor, *Obstet Gynecol* 81:750, 1993.

Hill W et al: Home uterine activity monitoring is associated with a reduction in preterm birth, *Obstet Gynecol* 76 (suppl 1):13s, 1990.

Isennock P: *Bed rest before baby: what's a mother to do?* Perry Hall, Md, 1992, Mustard Seed Publishing.

Keirse M: New perspectives for the effective treatment of preterm labor, *Am J Obstet Gynecol* 173:618, 1995.

King T: Clinical management of premature rupture of membranes, *J Nurse Midwife* 39 (suppl 2):81S, 1994.

Knuppel R, Drukker J: *High-risk pregnancy: a team approach*, ed 2, Philadelphia, 1993, WB Saunders.

Koonin L et al: Maternal mortality surveillance, United States, 1980-1985, *MMWR* 37:19, 1989.

Lopez-Zeno J et al: A controlled trial of a program for the active management of labor, *N Engl J Med* 326:450, 1992.

Lydon R et al: Accuracy of Leopold maneuvers in screening for malpresentation: a prospective study, *Birth* 20(3):132, 1993.

Main D, Main E: *Preterm birth.* In Gabbe S, Niebyl J, Simpson J, editors: *Obstetrics, normal and problem pregnancies*, ed 2, New York, 1991, Churchill Livingstone.

Maloni J: Home care of the high-risk pregnant woman requiring bed rest, *J Obstet Neonatal Gynecol Nurs* 23(8):696, 1994.

Marieskind H: Cesarean section in the United States: has it changed since 1979? *Birth* 16:196, 1989.

Maurer L: *Confinement connection: a home support program*, Phoenix, 1992.

Mercer B, Pilgrim P, Sibai B: Labor induction with continuous low-dose oxytocin infusion: a randomized trial, *Obstet Gynecol* 77:659, 1991.

Miller A, Lorkovic M: Prostaglandin E2 for cervical ripening, *MCN Am J Matern Child Nurs* 18(5):23, 1993.

Miovech S et al: Major concerns of women after cesarean delivery, *J Obstet Gynecol Neonatal Nurs* 23(1):53, 1994.

Monga M, Creasy R: Pharmacologic management of preterm labor, *Semin Perinatol* 19(1):84, 1995.

Morrison J: Preterm birth: a puzzle worth solving, *Obstet Gynecol* 76(suppl):5, 1990.

Naef R, Morrison J: Guidelines for the management of shoulder dystocia, *J Perinatol* 14(6):435, 1994.

Neal A, Bockman V: *Preterm labor and preterm premature rupture of membranes.* In Mandeville L, Troiano N, editors: *High-risk intrapartum nursing*, Philadelphia, 1992, JB Lippincott.

Piper D, McDonald P: Management of anticipated and actual shoulder dystocia: interpreting the literature, *J Nurse Midwife* 39(suppl 2):91S, 1994.

Public Citizen Health Research Group: Fewer C-sections, *USA Today*, May 19, 1994.

Radin T, Harmon J, Hanson D: Nurses' care during labor: its effects on the cesarean birth rate of healthy nulliparous women *Birth* 20(1):14, 1993.

Romero C, Jones P: Home infusion therapies for obstetric patients, *J Obstet Gynecol Neonatal Nurs* 23(8):675, 1994.

Scott J: *Cesarean section and other obstetric operations.* In Scott J et al, editors: *Danforth's obstetrics and gynecology*, ed 7, Philadelphia, 1994, JB Lippincott.

Sokol R, Brindley B, Dombrowski M: *Practical diagnosis and management of abnormal labor.* In Scott J et al, editors: *Danforth's obstetrics and gynecology*, ed 7, Philadelphia, 1994, JB Lippincott.

Spellacy W: *Postdate pregnancy.* In Scott J et al, editors: *Danforth's obstetrics and gynecology*, ed 7, Philadelphia, 1994, JB Lippincott.

Taffel S, Placek P, Kosary C: U.S. cesarean section rates 1990: an update, *Birth* 19(1):21, 1992.

Thomas L et al: The effects of rocking, diet modifications, and antiflatulent medication on postcesarean section gas pain, *J Perinat Neonatal Nurs* 4(3):12, 1990.

Weingarten C et al: Married mother's perceptions of their premature or term infants and the quality of their relationships with their husbands, *J Obstet Gynecol Neonatal Nurs* 19(1):64, 1990.

Wheeler D: Preterm birth prevention, *J Nurse Midwife* 38(suppl 2):66S, 1994.

Williams M et al: Preinduction prostaglandin E2 gel prior to induction of labor in women with a previous cesarean section, *Gynecol Obstet Invest* 40(2):89, 1995.

Willson J, Carrington E: *Obstetrics and gynecology*, ed 9, St Louis, 1991, Mosby.

Wood C: Postdate pregnancy update, *J Nurse Midwife* 39(suppl 2):110S, 1994.

Bibliography

Deutchman M, Sills D, Connor P: Perinatal outcomes: a comparison between family physicians and obstetricians, *J Am Board Fam Practice* 8(6):440, 1995.

Eganhouse D: A nursing model for a community hospital preterm birth prevention program, *J Obstet Gynecol Neonatal Nurs* 23(9):756, 1994.

Kaplan B et al: The outcome of post-term pregnancy: a comparative study, *J Perinat Med* 23(3):183, 1995.

Lucas J: The role of vacuum extraction in modern obstetrics, *Clin Obstet Gynecol* 37(4):794, 1994.

May K: Impact of maternal activity restriction for preterm labor on the expectant father, *J Obstet Gynecol Neonatal Nurs* 23(3):246, 1994.

O'Brien J: Efficacy of outpatient induction with low-dose intravaginal prostaglandin E2: a randomized, double-blind, placebo-controlled trial, *Am J Obstet Gynecol* 173(6):1855, 1995.

Olden A et al: Patients' versus nurses' assessments of pain and sedation after cesarean section, *J Obstet Gynecol Neonatal Nurs* 24(2):137, 1995.

Wing D et al: Misoprostol: an effective agent for cervical ripening and labor induction, *Am J Obstet Gynecol* 172(6):1811, 1995.

Yeomans E, Gilstrap L: The role of forceps in modern obstetrics, *Clin Obstet Gynecol* 37(4):785, 1994.

CHAPTER 18

Maternal Physiology During the Postpartum Period

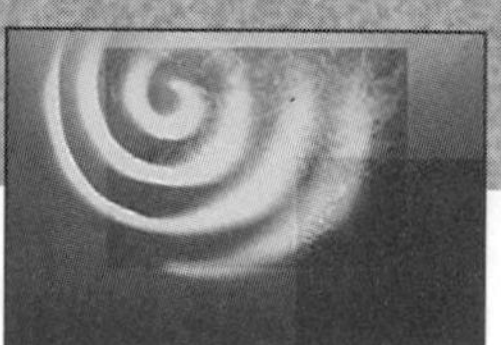

REPRODUCTIVE SYSTEM AND ASSOCIATED STRUCTURES, P. 480
Uterus, p. 480
ENDOCRINE SYSTEM, P. 483
ABDOMEN, P. 483
URINARY SYSTEM, P. 483
GASTROINTESTINAL SYSTEM, P. 484
BREASTS, P. 484
CARDIOVASCULAR SYSTEM, P. 485
NEUROLOGIC SYSTEM, P. 486
MUSCULOSKELETAL SYSTEM, P. 486
INTEGUMENTARY SYSTEM, P. 486
IMMUNE SYSTEM, P. 486

The postpartum period is the 6-week interval between the birth of the newborn and the return of the reproductive organs to their normal nonpregnant state. This period is sometimes referred to as the **puerperium**, or **fourth trimester of pregnancy.** The physiologic changes that occur during the puerperium as the processes of pregnancy are reversed are distinctive but considered normal. Many factors, including energy level, degree of psychologic and physical comfort, health of the newborn, and care and encouragement given by health professionals, contribute to the mother's well-being and response to her infant during this time. To provide care that is beneficial to the mother, her infant, and her family, the nurse must synthesize knowledge regarding maternal anatomy and physiology of the recovery period, the newborn's physical and behavioral characteristics, infant care activities, and family response to the birth of the child. This chapter focuses on anatomic and physiologic changes of the mother during the postpartum period.

REPRODUCTIVE SYSTEM AND ASSOCIATED STRUCTURES

Uterus

Involution process. The return of the uterus to a nonpregnant state following birth is known as **involution.** This process begins immediately after expulsion of the placenta with contraction of the uterine smooth muscle.

At the end of the third stage of labor the uterus is in the midline, approximately 2 cm below the level of the umbilicus, with the fundus resting on the sacral promontory. At this time, the uterus is approximately the size it was at 16 weeks of gestation (about the size of a grapefruit), and it weighs approximately 1000 g.

Within 12 hours the fundus may be approximately 1 cm above the umbilicus (Fig. 18-1). Involution progresses rapidly during the next few days. The fundus descends 1 to 2 cm every 24 hours. By the sixth postpartum day the fundus is normally halfway between the umbilicus and the symphysis pubis. The uterus should not be palpable abdominally after the ninth postpartum day.

The uterus, which at full term weighs approximately 11 times its prepregnant weight, involutes to approximately 500 g 1 week after birth and to 350 g 2 weeks after birth. One week after childbirth the uterus lies in the true pelvis once again. At 6 weeks it weighs 50 to 60 g (Fig. 18-1).

Increased estrogen and progesterone levels are responsible for the massive growth of the uterus during pregnancy. Prenatal uterine growth results from both *hyperplasia*, an increase in the number of muscle cells, and from *hypertrophy*, an enlargement of the existing cells. Postpartally, the decrease in these hormones causes autolysis, a self-destruction of excess hypertrophied tissue. However, the additional cells laid down during pregnancy remain and account for the slight increase in uterine size after each pregnancy.

Subinvolution is the failure of the uterus to return to a nonpregnant state. The most common causes of subinvolution are retained placental fragments and infection.

Contractions. Postpartum hemostasis is achieved primarily by compression of intramyometrial blood vessels as the uter-

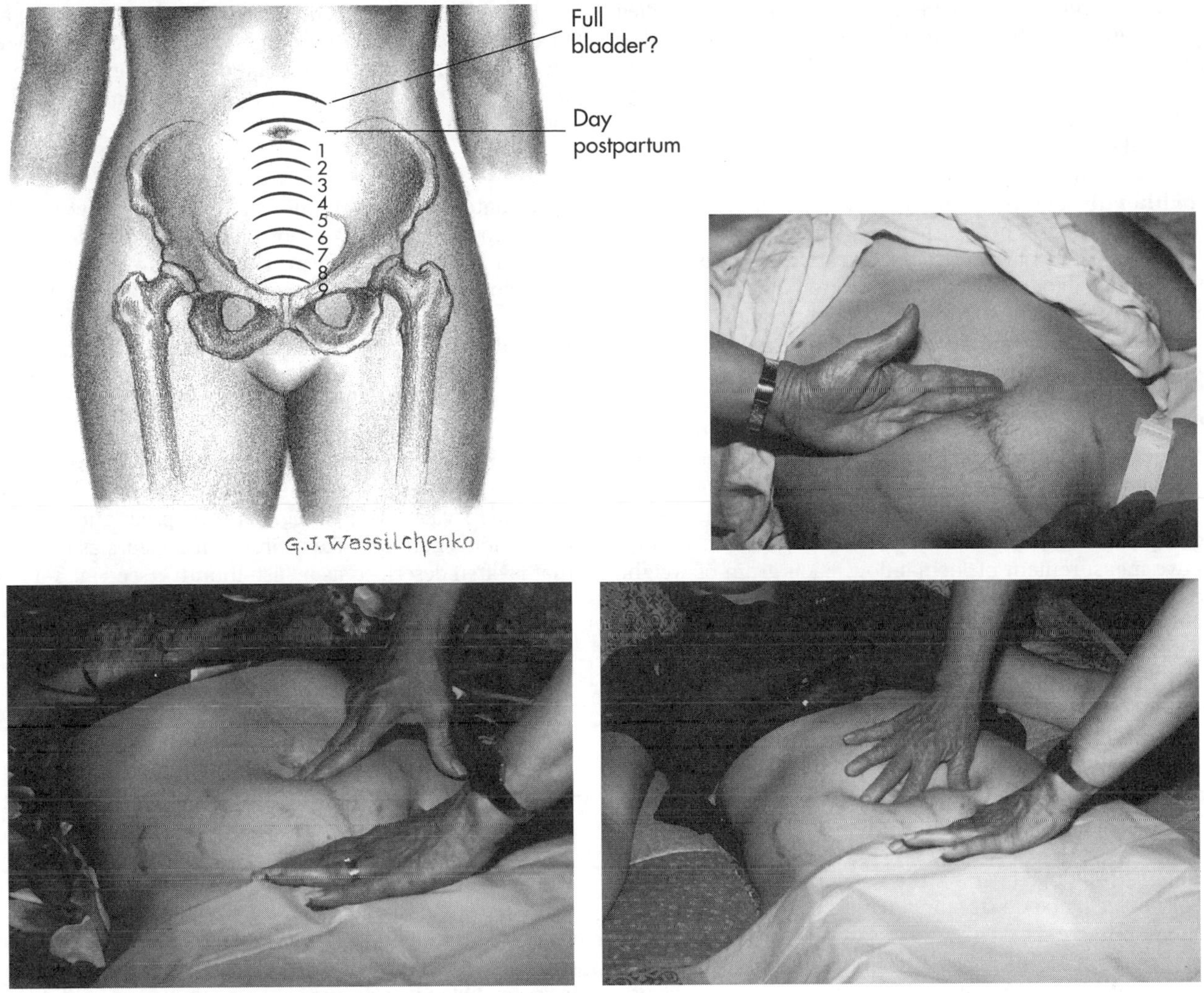

Fig. 18-1 Assessment of involution of uterus after childbirth. **A,** Normal progress, days 1 through 9. **B,** Size and position of uterus 2 hours after birth. **C,** Two days after birth. **D,** Four days after birth. (**B, C,** and **D** courtesy Marjorie Pyle, RNC, Lifecircle, Costa Mesa, Calif.).

ine muscle contracts rather than by platelet aggregation and clot formation. The hormone oxytocin is released from the pituitary gland and strengthens and coordinates these uterine contractions, which compress blood vessels and aid in hemostasis. During the first 1 to 2 postpartum hours, uterine contractions may decrease in intensity and become uncoordinated. Because it is vital that the uterus remain firm and well contracted, exogenous oxytocin (Pitocin) is usually administered intravenously or intramuscularly immediately after expulsion of the placenta. Mothers who plan to breastfeed may also be encouraged to put the baby to breast immediately after birth because suckling stimulates oxytocin release.

Afterpains. In first-time mothers, uterine tone is good, the fundus generally remains firm, and the mother does not perceive uterine cramping. Periodic relaxation and vigorous contraction are more common in subsequent pregnancies and may cause uncomfortable cramping called *afterpains,* which persist throughout the early puerperium. Afterpains are more noticeable after births in which the uterus was overdistended (e.g., large baby, multifetal gestation, polyhydramnios). Breastfeeding and exogenous oxytocic medication usually intensify these afterpains because both stimulate uterine contractions.

Placental site. Immediately after the placenta and membranes have been expelled, vascular constriction and thromboses reduce the placental site to an irregular nodular and elevated area. Upward growth of the endometrium causes sloughing of necrotic tissue and prevents the scar formation that is characteristic of normal wound healing. This unique healing process enables the endometrium to resume its usual cycle of changes and to permit implantation and placentation in future pregnancies. Endometrial regeneration is completed by the end of the third postpartum week except at the placental site. Regeneration at the placental site usually is not complete until 6 weeks after birth.

Lochia. Postchildbirth uterine discharge, commonly called *lochia,* initially is bright red and changes later to a dark red or reddish brown. It may contain small clots. For the first 2 hours after birth the amount of uterine discharge should be about that of a heavy menstrual period. After that time, the lochia flow should steadily decrease, and the color changes to yellow or white by 10 days after birth.

Lochia rubra consists mainly of blood and decidual and trophoblastic debris. The flow pales, becoming pink or brown after 3 to 4 days (lochia serosa). **Lochia serosa** consists of old blood, serum, leukocytes, and tissue debris. Approximately 10 days after childbirth the drainage becomes yellow to white (lochia alba). **Lochia alba** consists of numerous leukocytes, decidua, epithelial cells, mucus, serum, and bacteria. Lochia alba may continue for 2 to 6 weeks after the birth.

It is difficult to judge the amount of lochial flow on the basis of observation of perineal pads. Jacobson (1985) suggested one method for estimating postpartal blood loss on the basis of the amount of staining on a perineal pad (see Fig. 19-4). Weighing perineal pads before and after use provides a more objective measurement of lochial flow. Each gram of weight increase is roughly equivalent to 1 ml of blood loss. Any estimation of lochial flow is inaccurate and incomplete without consideration of the time factor. The woman who saturates a peripad in 1 hour or less is bleeding much more than the woman who saturates one peripad over an 8-hour period.

If the woman receives an oxytocic medication, the flow of lochia is usually scant until the effects of the medication wear off, regardless of the route of administration. The amount of lochia is usually less after cesarean births. Flow of lochia usually increases with ambulation and breastfeeding. After lying in bed for a prolonged period, the woman may experience a gush of pooled blood on standing, which is not to be confused with hemorrhage.

Persistence of lochia rubra early in the postpartum period suggests continued bleeding as a result of retained fragments of the placenta or membranes. Recurrence of bleeding approximately 10 days after birth indicates bleeding from the placental site, which is healing. However, after 3 to 4 weeks bleeding may be caused by infection or subinvolution. Continued lochia serosa or lochia alba may indicate endometritis, particularly if fever, pain, or tenderness is associated with the discharge. Lochia should smell like normal menstrual flow; an offensive odor usually indicates infection.

It is important to remember that all postpartal vaginal bleeding is not necessarily lochia. Common sources of vaginal bleeding after birth are unrepaired vaginal or cervical lacerations. Table 18-1 distinguishes between lochial and nonlochial bleeding.

Cervix

Immediately after birth the cervix is soft. However, by 18 hours postpartum it has shortened, developed a firm consistency, and regained its form. The cervix up to the lower uterine segment remains edematous, thin, and fragile for several days after birth. The ectocervix (portion of the cervix that protrudes into the vagina) appears bruised and has some small lacerations—optimal conditions for the development of infection. The cervical os, dilated to 10 cm during labor, closes gradually. Two fingers may still be introduced into the cervical os for the first 4 to 6 days postpartum; however, only the smallest curette may be introduced by the end of 2 weeks. The external cervical os never regains its prepregnant appearance; it is no longer shaped like a circle but appears as a jagged slit that is often described as a "fish mouth" (see Fig. 3-11). Lactation delays the production of cervical and other estrogen-influenced mucus and mucosal characteristics.

Vagina and Perineum

Postpartum estrogen deprivation is responsible for the thinness of the vaginal mucosa and the absence of rugae. The greatly distended, smooth-walled vagina gradually returns to its prepregnant size by 6 to 8 weeks after childbirth. Rugae reappear by approximately the fourth week, but they are never as prominent as they are in the nulliparous woman. Most rugae may be permanently flattened. The mucosa remains atrophic in the lactating woman, at least until menstruation begins again. Thickening of the vaginal mucosa occurs with the return of ovarian function. Estrogen deficiency is responsible for a decreased amount of vaginal lubrication and thinner vaginal mucosa. Localized dryness and coital discomfort (dyspareunia) may persist until ovarian function returns and menstruation resumes. The use of a water-soluble lubricant during intercourse is usually recommended because it is helpful in reducing discomfort.

Initially the *introitus* is erythematous and edematous, especially in the area of the episiotomy or laceration repair. Care-

Critical Thinking Exercises

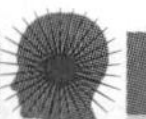

ESTIMATION OF BLOOD LOSS

Conduct an assessment of the ability to estimate blood loss.

1. Pour measured amounts of a red fluid (or expired blood from the blood bank, if possible) on perineal pads and plastic-backed underpants.
2. Ask nursing students, maternity nurses, medical students, obstetricians, anesthesiologists, and nurse anesthetists to make independent assessments of the volume.
3. Compare the results. Were profession, areas of specialization, or years of experience correlated with more accurate estimates? Were people more likely to overestimate or underestimate? Were estimates closer on perineal pads or on underpants? Were the errors in judgment large enough to cause concern about estimates of actual blood loss?

TABLE 18-1 Lochial and nonlochial bleeding

LOCHIAL BLEEDING	NONLOCHIAL BLEEDING
Lochia usually trickles from the vaginal opening. The steady flow is greater as the uterus contracts.	If the bloody discharge spurts from the vagina, there may be cervical or vaginal tears in addition to the normal lochia.
A gush of lochia may result as the uterus is massaged. If it is dark in color, it has been pooled in the relaxed vagina, and the amount soon lessens to a trickle of bright red lochia (in the early puerperium).	If the amount of bleeding continues to be excessive and bright red, a tear may be the source.

ful repair, prevention or early treatment of hematomas, and good hygiene during the first 2 weeks after birth usually result in an introitus that is barely distinguishable from that of a nulliparous woman.

Most episiotomies are visible only if the woman is lying on her side with her upper buttock raised of if she is placed in the lithotomy position. A good light source is essential for visualization of some episiotomies. The healing process of an episiotomy is the same as for any surgical incision. Signs of infection (pain, redness, warmth, swelling, or discharge) or loss of approximation (separation of the incision edges) may occur. Healing should be complete within 2 to 3 weeks.

Hemorrhoids (anal varicosities) are commonly seen (see Fig. 7-12, *B*). Internal hemorrhoids may evert while the woman is pushing during birth. Women often experience associated symptoms such as itching, discomfort, and bright red bleeding with defecation. These hemorrhoids usually decrease in size within weeks of childbirth.

Pelvic Muscular Support

The supporting structure of the uterus and vagina may be injured during childbirth and may contribute to gynecologic problems later. Supportive tissues of the pelvic floor that are torn or stretched during childbirth may require up to 6 months to regain tone. Kegel exercises, which help to strengthen perineal muscles and encourage healing, are often recommended after childbirth. (See Chapter 7 for more information.) **Pelvic relaxation** refers to the lengthening and weakening of the fascial supports of pelvic structures. These structures include the uterus, upper posterior vaginal wall, urethra, bladder, and rectum. Although relaxation can occur in any woman, it is usually a direct but delayed complication of childbirth.

ENDOCRINE SYSTEM

Placental Hormones

Great hormonal changes occur during the postpartal period. Expulsion of the placenta results in dramatic decreases of the hormones produced by that organ. Decreases in human placental lactogen (hPL), estrogens, cortisol, and the placental enzyme insulinase reverse the diabetogenic effects of pregnancy, resulting in significantly lower blood sugar levels in the immediate puerperium. Mothers with diabetes will likely require much less insulin for several days. Because these normal hormonal changes make the puerperium a transitional period for carbohydrate metabolism, the interpretation of glucose tolerance tests is more difficult during this time.

Estrogen and progesterone levels drop markedly after expulsion of the placenta and reach their lowest levels 1 week postpartum. Decreased estrogen levels are associated with breast engorgement and with the diuresis of excess extracellular fluid accumulated during pregnancy. In nonlactating women estrogen levels begin to rise by 2 weeks after birth and by postpartum day 17 are higher than in women who breastfeed (Bowes, 1991).

Pituitary Hormones and Ovarian Function

Lactating and nonlactating women differ considerably in the time of appearance of the first ovulation and the reestablishment of menstruation. The persistence of elevated serum prolactin levels in breastfeeding women appears to be responsible for suppressing ovulation. Because levels of follicle-stimulating hormone (FSH) have been shown to be identical in lactating and nonlactating women, it is thought that the ovary does not respond to FSH stimulation when increased prolactin levels are present (Bowes, 1991). Another theory is that endogenous opiate levels play an important role in regulating the hormonal levels of lactating women (Gordon et al, 1993).

Prolactin levels in blood rise progressively throughout pregnancy. In women who breastfeed, prolactin levels remain elevated into the sixth week after birth (Bowes, 1991). Serum prolactin levels are influenced by the frequency of breastfeeding, the duration of each feeding, and the degree to which supplementary feedings are used. Individual differences in the strength of an infant's sucking stimulus probably also affect prolactin levels. These variances emphasize the fact that breastfeeding is not a reliable form of birth control. In nonlactating women, prolactin levels decline after birth and reach the prepregnant range within 2 weeks.

Ovulation occurs as early as 27 days after birth in nonlactating women, with a mean time of approximately 70 to 75 days. By 2 months postpartum, most nonbreastfeeding women have resumed ovulation (Bowes, 1991; Gordon et al, 1993). Approximately 90% of nonbreastfeeding women resume menstruating by 3 months after birth (Gordon et al, 1993). In women who breastfeed, the mean length of time to ovulation is approximately 190 days (Bowes, 1991). In lactating women, both the resumption of ovulation and the return of menses are determined in large part by breastfeeding patterns (Gordon et al, 1993). The fact that 25% of breastfeeding women ovulate before their first postpartum menstrual period occurs emphasizes again the need to discuss contraceptive options early in the puerperium (Zlatnik, 1994).

The first menstrual flow after childbirth is usually heavier than normal. Within 3 to 4 cycles the amount of menstrual flow returns to the woman's prepregnant volume.

ABDOMEN

When the woman stands up during the first days after childbirth, her abdominal muscles cannot retain the abdominal contents. The abdomen protrudes and gives her a still-pregnant appearance. During the first 2 weeks after birth the abdominal wall is relaxed. Approximately 6 weeks are required before the abdominal wall almost returns to its nonpregnant state. The skin regains most of its previous elasticity, but some striae may persist. The return of muscle tone depends on previous tone, proper exercise, and the amount of adipose tissue. On occasion, with or without overdistention because of a large fetus or multiple fetuses, the abdominal wall muscles separate in a condition termed **diastasis recti abdominis** (see Fig. 6-13, *B*). The persistence of this defect may be disturbing to the woman, but surgical correction rarely is necessary. With time, the defect becomes less apparent.

URINARY SYSTEM

The hormonal changes of pregnancy (high steroid levels) contribute to an increase in renal function, whereas the diminishing steroid levels after childbirth may partly explain the reduced renal function during the puerperium. Kidney function returns to normal within 1 month after birth. Approximately 2 to 8 weeks are required for the pregnancy-induced hypotonia and dilation of the ureters and renal pelves to return to the prepregnant state (Cunningham et al, 1993). In a small percentage of women, dilation of the urinary tract may persist for 3 months. The dilation of the ureters and renal pelves increases the chance for developing a urinary tract infection.

Urine Components

The renal glycosuria induced by pregnancy disappears. Lactosuria may be expected in lactating women. The blood urea nitrogen increases during the puerperium as **autolysis** of the involuting uterus is accomplished. This breakdown of excess protein in the uterine muscle cells also results in a mild (+1) proteinuria for 1 to 2 days after childbirth in approximately 80% of women. Acetonuria may occur in women with an uncomplicated birth or after a prolonged labor with dehydration.

Postpartal Diuresis

Within 12 hours of birth, women begin to lose excess tissue fluid accumulated during pregnancy. One mechanism that reduces these retained fluids of pregnancy is the profuse **diaphoresis** that often occurs, especially at night, for the first 2 or 3 days after childbirth. Postpartal **diuresis,** caused by decreased estrogen levels, removal of increased venous pressure in the lower extremities, and loss of the remaining pregnancy-induced increase in blood volume, is another mechanism by which the body rids itself of excess fluid. Fluid loss through perspiration and increased urinary output accounts for a weight loss of approximately 2.25 kg (5 lb) during the puerperium. This elimination of excess fluid accumulated during pregnancy is sometimes referred to as *reversal of the water metabolism of pregnancy.*

Urethra and Bladder

Trauma may occur to the urethra and bladder during the birth process as the infant passes through the pelvis. The bladder wall may be hyperemic and edematous, often with small areas of hemorrhage. Clean-catch or catheterized urine specimens after the birth often reveal hematuria from bladder trauma. The urethra and urinary meatus may be edematous.

Birth-induced trauma, increased bladder capacity following childbirth, and the effects of conduction anesthesia combine to cause a decreased urge to void. In addition, pelvic soreness caused by the forces of labor, vaginal lacerations, or the episiotomy reduces or alters the voiding reflex. Decreased voiding combined with postpartal diuresis may result in bladder distention. Immediately after birth a distended bladder can lead to excessive bleeding because it prevents the uterus from firmly contracting. Later in the puerperium overdistention can make the bladder more susceptible to infection and can impede the resumption of normal voiding (Cunningham et al, 1993). If prolonged bladder overdistention occurs, further damage to the bladder wall (atony) may result. With adequate bladder emptying, bladder tone is usually restored 5 to 7 days after childbirth.

GASTROINTESTINAL SYSTEM

Appetite

The mother usually is hungry shortly after the birth and can tolerate a light diet. After full recovery from analgesia, anesthesia, and fatigue, most new mothers are hungry. Requests for double portions of food and frequent snacks are not uncommon. Lack of appetite should prompt further assessments.

Motility

Typically, decreased muscle tone and motility of the gastrointestinal tract persists for only a short time after childbirth. Excess analgesia and anesthesia may delay a return to normal tonicity and motility.

Bowel Evacuation

A spontaneous bowel evacuation may be delayed until 2 to 3 days after childbirth. This delay can be explained by decreased muscle tone in the intestines during labor and the immediate puerperium, prelabor diarrhea, lack of food, or dehydration. The mother often anticipates discomfort during the bowel movement because of perineal tenderness as a result of episiotomy, lacerations, or hemorrhoids. Regular bowel habits need to be reestablished when bowel tone returns.

BREASTS

The concentrations of hormones that stimulated breast development during pregnancy (estrogen, progesterone, human chorionic gonadotropin, prolactin, cortisol, and insulin) decrease promptly after childbirth. The time it takes for these hormones to return to prepregnancy levels is determined in part by whether the mother breastfeeds her infant.

Breastfeeding Mothers

Before lactation begins, the breasts feel soft and a yellowish fluid, **colostrum,** can be expressed from the nipples. After lactation begins, the breasts feel warm and firm. Tenderness persists for approximately 48 hours. Bluish-white milk (skim-milk appearance) or true milk can be expressed from the nipples. The nipples are examined for erectility as opposed to inversion and for signs of irritation such as cracks, blisters, or reddening. As lactation is established, a mass (lump) may be felt in the breast. Unlike the lumps associated with fibrocystic breast disease or cancer, which may be consistently palpated in the same location, a filled milk sac shifts position from day to day.

Nonbreastfeeding Mothers

In contrast to the granular feel of breasts in nonpregnant women, the breasts generally feel nodular after birth. This nodularity is bilateral and diffuse. Prolactin levels drop rapidly if the woman chooses not to breastfeed and if no antilactogenic medication is taken. Colostrum secretion and excretion persist for the first few days after childbirth. Palpation of the breast on the second or third day, as milk production begins, may reveal tissue tenderness in some women. On the third or fourth postpartum day, **engorgement** may occur. The breasts are distended (swollen), firm, tender, and warm to the touch (because of vasocongestion). Breast distention is caused primarily by the temporary congestion of veins and lymphatics rather than by an accumulation of milk. Milk can be expressed from the nipples. Axillary breast tissue (the tail of Spence) and any accessory breast or nipple tissue along the milk line may be involved. Engorgement resolves spontaneously, and discomfort decreases usually within 24 to 36 hours. If suckling is never begun (or is discontinued), lactation ceases within a few days to a week.

CARDIOVASCULAR SYSTEM

Blood Volume

Changes in blood volume depend on several variable factors such as blood loss during childbirth and mobilization and subsequent excretion of extravascular water (physiologic edema). Blood loss results in an immediate but limited decrease in total blood volume. Thereafter, normal shifts in body water result in a slow decline in blood volume. By the third to fourth week after the birth the blood volume usually has regressed to nonpregnant values.

Pregnancy-induced hypervolemia (an increase of at least 40% over nonpregnant values near term) allows most women to tolerate considerable blood loss during childbirth. Traditionally, a blood loss of more than 500 ml during the first 24 hours after birth is considered hemorrhage. In fact, however, more than half of all women giving birth vaginally and almost all giving birth by cesarean lose more than this amount. Most women can tolerate a loss of 1000 to 2000 ml without developing significant problems (Cunningham et al, 1993).

Readjustments in the maternal vasculature after childbirth are dramatic and rapid. The woman's response to blood loss during the early puerperium differs from that in a nonpregnant woman. Three postpartal physiologic changes protect the woman: (1) elimination of uteroplacental circulation reduces the size of the maternal vascular bed by 10% to 15%, (2) loss of placental endocrine function removes the stimulus for vasodilation, and (3) mobilization of extravascular water stored during pregnancy occurs. Thus hypovolemic shock usually does not occur with normal blood loss.

Cardiac Output

Pulse rate, stroke volume, and cardiac output increase throughout pregnancy. Immediately after the birth these valves remain elevated or rise even higher for 30 to 60 minutes as the blood that was shunted through the uteroplacental circuit suddenly returns to the general circulation. These values increase regardless of the type of birth or the use of conduction anesthesia (Bowes, 1991). Data regarding the exact time of return of cardiac hemodynamic levels to normal are not available, but normal cardiac output values are found when measurements are taken 8 to 10 weeks after childbirth (Bowes, 1991).

Vital Signs

Few alterations in vital signs are seen under normal circumstances. There may be a small, transient rise in both systolic and diastolic blood pressure that lasts approximately 4 days after the birth (Bowes, 1991) (Table 18-2). Respiratory function returns to nonpregnant levels by 6 months after birth. After the uterus is emptied, the diaphragm descends, the normal cardiac axis is restored, and the point of maximal impulse (PMI) and the electrocardiogram (ECG) return to nonpregnant conditions.

TABLE 18-2 Vital signs after childbirth

NORMAL FINDINGS	DEVIATIONS FROM NORMAL FINDINGS AND PROBABLE CAUSES
Temperature	
During first 24 hours may rise to 38° C (100.4° F) as a result of dehydrating effects of labor. After 24 hours the woman should be afebrile.	A diagnosis of puerperal sepsis is suggested if a rise in maternal temperature to 38° C (100.4° F) is noted after the first 24 hours after childbirth and recurs or persists for 2 days. Other possibilities are mastitis, endometritis, urinary tract infections, and other systemic infections.
Pulse	
Pulse, along with stroke volume and cardiac output, remains elevated for the first hour or so after childbirth. It then begins to decrease. By 8 to 10 weeks after childbirth the pulse has returned to a nonpregnant rate.	A rapid pulse rate or one that is increasing may indicate hypovolemia as a result of hemorrhage.
Respirations	
Respirations should fall to within the woman's normal prebirth range.	Hypoventilation may follow an unusually high subarachnoid (spinal) block.
Blood pressure	
Blood pressure is altered *slightly* if at all. Orthostatic hypotension, as indicated by feelings of faintness or dizziness immediately after standing up, can develop in the first 48 hours as a result of the splanchnic engorgement that may occur after birth.	A low or falling blood pressure may reflect hypovolemia secondary to hemorrhage. However, it is a late sign, and other symptoms of hemorrhage usually alert the staff. An increased reading may result from excessive use of vasopressor or oxytocic medications. Because pregnancy-induced hypertension (PIH) can persist into or occur first during the postpartum period, routine evaluation of blood pressure is needed. If a woman complains of headache, hypertension must be ruled out as a cause before analgesics are administered. If the blood pressure is elevated, the woman is confined to bed and the physician/nurse midwife is notified.

Blood Components

Hematocrit and hemoglobin. During the first 72 hours after childbirth, there is a greater loss of plasma volume than of blood cells. The decrease in plasma volume plus the increase in red blood cell (RBC) mass of pregnancy is associated with a rise in hematocrit and hemoglobin levels by the third to seventh day after the birth. There is no increased RBC destruction during the puerperium, but any gain in hemoglobin and hematocrit gradually disappears in accordance with the life span of the RBC. The exact time at which RBC volume returns to prepregnancy values is not known, but it is within normal limits when measured 8 weeks after childbirth (Bowes, 1991).

White blood cell count. Normal leukocytosis of pregnancy averages approximately 12,000/mm³. During the first 10 to 12 days after childbirth, values between 20,000 and 25,000/mm³ are common. Neutrophils are the most numerous white blood cells (WBCs). Leukocytosis coupled with the normal increase in erythrocyte sedimentation rate may confuse the diagnosis of acute infections during this time.

Coagulation factors. Clotting factors and fibrinogen are normally increased during pregnancy and remain elevated in the immediate puerperium. When combined with vessel damage and immobility, this hypercoagulable state causes an increased risk of **thromboembolism** (blood clots), especially after a cesarean birth. Fibrinolytic activity also increases during the first few days after childbirth (Bowes, 1991). Factors I, II, VIII, IX, and X decrease within a few days to nonpregnant levels. Fibrin split products, probably released from the placental site, can also be found in maternal blood.

Varicosities

Varicosities of the legs and around the anus (hemorrhoids) are common during pregnancy (Fig. 7-12). Varices, even the less common vulvar varices, regress (empty) rapidly immediately after childbirth. Surgical correction of varicosities is not considered during pregnancy. Total or nearly total regression of varicosities is anticipated after childbirth.

NEUROLOGIC SYSTEM

Neurologic changes during the puerperium are those that result from a reversal of maternal adaptations to pregnancy and those that result from trauma during labor and childbirth.

Pregnancy-induced neurologic discomforts abate after birth. Elimination of physiologic edema through the diuresis that follows childbirth relieves carpal tunnel syndrome by easing the compression of the median nerve. The periodic numbness and tingling of fingers that afflict 5% of pregnant women usually disappear after the birth unless lifting and carrying the baby aggravates the condition. Headaches require careful assessment. Postpartum headaches may be caused by various conditions, including pregnancy-induced hypertension (PIH), stress, and leakage of cerebrospinal fluid into the extradural space during placement of the needle for epidural or spinal anesthesia. Depending on the cause and effectiveness of the treatment, the duration of the headaches can vary from 1 to 3 days to several weeks.

Critical Thinking Exercises 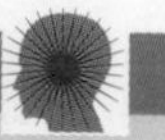

POSTPARTUM PHYSIOLOGIC CHANGES

Prepare teaching aids to explain to a patient who does not speak English the normal physiologic changes that occur during the postpartum period. How would your explanation differ if she had previously given birth to other children?

MUSCULOSKELETAL SYSTEM

Adaptations in the mother's musculoskeletal system are reversed in the puerperium. Such adaptations include those that contribute to relaxation and subsequent hypermobility of the joints and the change in the mother's center of gravity because of the enlarging uterus. Stabilization of joints is complete by 6 to 8 weeks after birth. However, although all other joints return to their normal prepregnant position before restabilization, those in the parous woman's feet do not. The new mother may notice a permanent increase in shoe size.

INTEGUMENTARY SYSTEM

Chloasma of pregnancy usually disappears at the termination of pregnancy. Hyperpigmentation of the areolae and linea nigra may not regress completely after childbirth. Some women will have permanent darker pigmentation of those areas.

Striae gravidarum (stretch marks) on the breasts, abdomen, and thighs decrease in size after delivery and turn to a pinkish white or silver tone in fair-haired women and to a brownish tone in darker-skinned women. They never completely disappear.

Vascular abnormalities such as spider angiomas (nevi), palmar erythema, and epulis generally regress in response to the rapid decline in estrogens after the end of pregnancy. For some woman, spider nevi persist indefinitely.

The abundance of fine hair seen during pregnancy usually disappears after giving birth; however, any coarse or bristly hair that appears during pregnancy usually remains. Fingernails return to their consistency and strength before pregnancy.

Diaphoresis is the most noticeable change in the integumentary system (see p. 484).

IMMUNE SYSTEM

No significant changes occur in the maternal immune system during the postpartum period. The mother's need for a rubella vaccination or for prevention of Rh isoimmunization is determined.

Key Points

- The uterus involutes rapidly after birth and returns to the true pelvis within 1 week.
- The rapid drop in estrogen and progesterone levels after expulsion of the placenta is responsible for many of the anatomic and physiologic changes in the puerperium.
- Assessment of lochia and fundal height is essential to monitoring the progress of normal involution and identifying potential problems.
- Breastfeeding is *not* a reliable form of birth control.
- Few alterations in vital signs are seen under normal circumstances after childbirth.
- Activation of blood clotting factors, immobility, and sepsis predispose the woman to thromboembolism.
- Marked diuresis, decreased bladder sensitivity, and overdistention of the bladder can lead to problems with urinary elimination.
- Postpartum physiologic changes allow the woman to tolerate considerable blood loss during childbirth.

References

Bowes W: *Postpartum care.* In Gabbe S, Niebyl J, Simpson J, editors: *Obstetrics: normal and problem pregnancies,* ed 2, New York, 1991, Churchill Livingstone.

Cunningham F et al: *Williams obstetrics,* ed 19, Norwalk, Conn, 1993, Appleton & Lange.

Gordon K et al: *Physiologic and psychologic adaptations in the puerperium.* In Moore T et al: *Gynecology and obstetrics: a longitudinal approach,* New York, 1993, Churchill Livingstone.

Jacobson H: A standard for assessing lochia volume, *MCN Am J Matern Child Nurs* 10:174, 1985.

Zlatnik F: *The normal and abnormal puerperium.* In Scott J et al: *Danforth's obstetrics and gynecology,* ed 7, Philadelphia, 1994, JB Lippincott.

Bibliography

Akins S: Postpartum hemorrhage: a 90s approach to an age-old problem, *J Nurse Midwife* 39(suppl 2): 123S, 1994.

CHAPTER 19

Nursing Care During the Postpartum Period

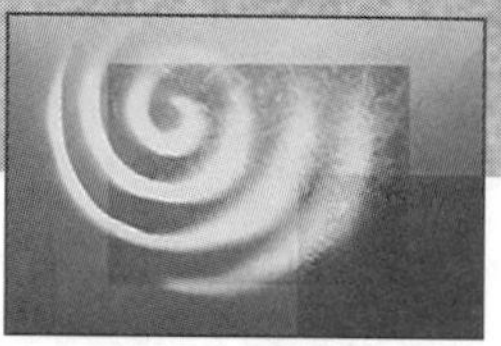

FOURTH STAGE OF LABOR, P. 488

Assessment, p. 489

Nursing care management—physical needs, p. 492

Nursing care management—psychosocial needs, p. 502

DISCHARGE TEACHING, P. 512

Sexual activity, p. 512

Prescribed medications, p. 513

Routine mother and baby checkups, p. 513

Nursing care management—contraception, p. 513

Nursing care management—sterilization, p. 531

The goal of nursing care in the immediate postpartum period is to assist women and their partners during their initial transition to parenting. The approach to the care of women after birth has changed from one modeled on sick care to one that is wellness oriented. Consequently, in the United States most women remain hospitalized no more than 1 or 2 days after giving birth, some for as few as 6 hours. Because there is so much important information to be shared with these women in a very short time, it is vital that their care be thoughtfully planned and provided. The nurse provides care that focuses on the woman's physiologic recovery, her psychologic well-being, and her ability to care for herself and her new baby. In addition, the nurse considers the needs of other family members and includes strategies in the plan of care to assist the family in adjusting to the new baby.

To provide quality care, the nurse must be knowledgeable about physical changes in the mother and psychosocial and emotional changes in the entire family. This chapter focuses on using the nursing process to meet both the mother's and the family's needs during this crucial time.

FOURTH STAGE OF LABOR

The first 1 to 2 hours after birth, sometimes referred to as the **fourth stage of labor,** are a crucial time for mother and newborn. The mother and her baby are not only recovering from the physical process of birth but are also becoming acquainted with each other and, perhaps, additional family members. During this time, maternal organs undergo their initial readjustment to the nonpregnant state and body systems begin to stabilize. Meanwhile, the newborn continues the transition from intrauterine to extrauterine existence.

Nursing ALERT

The nurse's role during the fourth stage of labor is to monitor the recovery of the new mother and infant and to identify promptly and manage any deviations in these normal processes that occur.

The fourth stage of labor is an excellent time to begin breastfeeding because the infant is in an alert state and ready to nurse. Breastfeeding at this time also aids in the contraction of the uterus and the prevention of maternal hemorrhage. Getting breastfeeding off to a good start is not just encouraging to the mother; it is physiologically vital for the infant. Colostrum loosens mucus and acts as a laxative to aid in the rapid elimination of meconium, decreasing the likelihood of hypoglycemia and the severity of hyperbilirubinemia and providing the baby with important immunologic benefits.

In most institutions the mother remains in the labor and birth area during this recovery time. In an institution using labor, delivery, and recovery (LDR) rooms, the woman will stay in the same room where she gave birth. In traditional settings, women are taken from the delivery room to a separate recovery area for observation during this time. Hospitals vary in their arrangements for care of the newborn during the

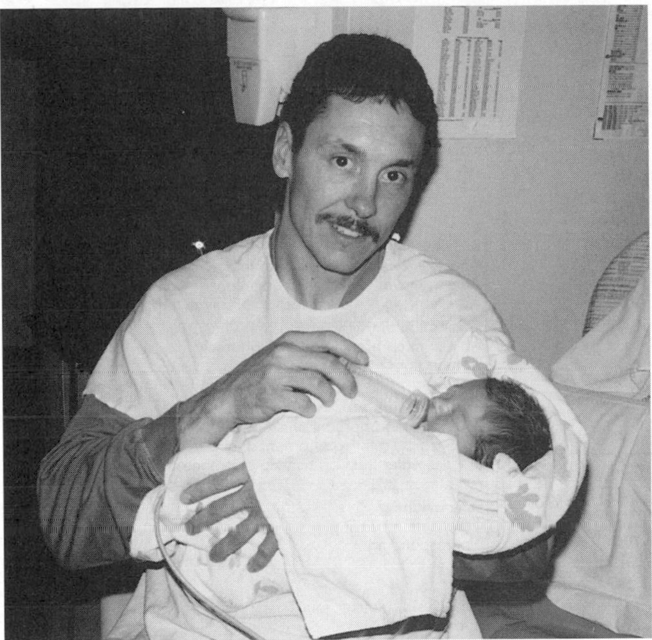

Fig. 19-1 Father gets acquainted with newborn son by feeding him a bottle.

fourth stage of labor. In some instances the baby remains at the mother's bedside and the labor/birth nurse cares for both of them. In other institutions the baby is taken to the nursery for several hours of observation after an initial bonding period with the parents (Fig. 19-1).

Assessment

If the recovery nurse has not previously cared for the new mother, assessment begins with an oral report from the nurse who attended the woman during labor and birth and a review of the prenatal, labor, and birth records. Of primary importance are conditions that could predispose the mother to hemorrhage, such as precipitous labor, large baby, grand multiparity, or induced labor. For healthy women, hemorrhage is probably the most dangerous potential complication during the fourth stage of labor.

To help the nurse provide comprehensive care, a worksheet or recovery record is suggested. Fig. 19-2 demonstrates an easy-to-use flow sheet that combines the essential immediate postpartum and anesthesia recovery assessments. During the first hour in the recovery room, physical assessment of the mother is frequent. All factors except temperature are assessed every 15 minutes for 1 hour. Temperature is assessed every 4 to 8 hours.

After the fourth 15-minute assessment, if all parameters have stabilized within the normal range, the process is usually repeated every 30 minutes during the second hour. Box 19-1 describes the physical assessment of the mother during the fourth stage of labor.

Postanesthesia recovery. The woman who has given birth by cesarean or received regional anesthesia for a vaginal birth requires special attention during the recovery period. In fact, obstetric recovery areas are held to the same standard of care

BOX 19-1
Procedure: Assessment During Fourth Stage of Labor

Before beginning the assessment, wash hands thoroughly, assemble necessary equipment, and explain the procedure to the patient.

Blood pressure

Measure per assessment schedule.

Pulse

Assess rate and regularity.

Temperature

Determine temperature.

Fundus

Put on clean examination gloves.
Position woman with knees flexed and head flat.
Just below umbilicus, cup hand, press firmly into abdomen. At the same time, stabilize the uterus at the symphysis with the opposite hand.
If fundus is firm (and bladder is empty), with uterus in midline, measure its position relative to woman's umbilicus. Lay fingers flat on abdomen under umbilicus; measure how many fingerbreadths (centimeters) fit between umbilicus and top of fundus. If the fundus is above the umbilicus, this is recorded as plus fingerbreadths or centimeters; if below, as minus fingerbreadths or centimeters.
If fundus is *not* firm, massage it gently to regain tone and expel any clots before measuring distance from umbilicus.
Place hands appropriately; massage gently only until firm.
Expel clots while keeping hands placed as in Fig. 19-3.
With upper hand, firmly apply pressure downward toward vagina; observe perineum for amount/size of expelled clots.

Bladder

Assess distention by noting location and firmness of uterine fundus and by observing and palpating bladder. Distended bladder is seen as a suprapubic rounded bulge that is dull to percussion and fluctuates like a water-filled balloon. When bladder is distended, the uterus is usually boggy, well above the umbilicus, and to the woman's right side.
Assist woman to void spontaneously. *Measure amount of urine voided.*
Catheterize as necessary.
Reassess after voiding/catheterization to make sure the bladder is not palpable and the fundus is firm and midline.

Lochia

Observe lochia on perineal pads and on linen under mother's buttocks. Determine amount and color; note size and number of clots; note odor.
Observe perineum for source of bleeding (e.g., episiotomy, lacerations).

Perineum

Ask or assist woman to turn on her side and flex upper leg on hip.
Lift upper buttock.
Observe perineum in good lighting.
Assess episiotomy for intactness, edema, bruising, redness.

Procedure: ____________________
Diagnosis: ____________________
Physician: ____________________
Anesthesia: ____________________
Anesthetist: ____________________
Armbands: ________ mother ____________ infant
Clothing: ________ c̄ family ____________ c̄ patient

Maternity Recovery Room Record

Admission note:

Par score: ADM:	DC:					Bonding	Teaching
Activity						□ appropriate	□ fundal massage
Respiration						□ inappropriate	□ TC & DB
Blood pressure						□ NA (explain)	□ breastfeeding
Conscious level							□ assistance on 1st ambulation
Color						________	
Total						________	□ ________

Homans' Sign Pos □ Neg □

Activity	
Able to move 4 extremities voluntarily or on command	2
Able to move 2 extremities voluntarily or on command	1
Able to move 0 extremities voluntarily or on command	0
Respiration	
Able to deep breathe and cough freely	2
Dyspnea or limited breathing	1
Apneic	0
Blood pressure	
BP ± mm Hg of preanesthetic level	2
BP ± 25-50 mm Hg of preanesthetic level	1
BP ± Greater than 50 mm Hg of preanesthetic level	0
Conscious level	
Fully aware	2
Arousable on calling	1
Not responding	0
Color	
Pink	2
Pale, dusky, blotchy, jaundiced, other	1
Cyanotic	0

Vital signs: Initial hour: q 15 min. then Routine: q 4 other per protocol q 1														Meds / IV / Rate	Time / Initial
	Time														
	BP														
	Pulse														
	Resp / O_2Sat														
Fundus: FB-Fingerbreadth B-Boggy FM-Firm MD-Midline	Fundus														
Lochia: CL-Clots MOD-Moderate SM-Small LG-Large	Lochia														
Bladder: D-Distended F-Foley ND-Nondistended	Bladder														
Episiotomy/Incision: NL-Normal D-Dry ABNL-Abnormal I-Intact	Epis / Inc														
q 4°	Temp														
Clear CL, Wheezing W, Diminished	Breath sounds														
q 1° / q 4°	DTR / Protein														
Admission intake total															
Admission output total														Intake total Shift 7A 3P 11P	Signature
Initials															

Discharge note | Output total Shift 7A 3P 11P

Report called to:

Anesthesia D/C:
Epidural catheter: In Out NA

IV ____cc LTC @ D/C

Fig. 19-2 An example of a maternity recovery room record. (Courtesy The Regional Medical Center at Memphis [The Med], Memphis, Tenn.)

that would be expected of any other postanesthesia recovery room. A postanesthesia recovery (PAR) score is determined for each client on arrival and updated as part of every 15-minute assessment. Components of the PAR score include activity, respirations, blood pressure, level of consciousness, and color.

Nursing ALERT

Regardless of her obstetric status, no woman can be discharged from the recovery area until she has completely recovered from the effects of anesthesia.

If the woman received general anesthesia, she should be awake and alert and oriented to time, place, and person. Her respiratory rate should be within normal limits, and her oxygen saturation levels at least 95%, as measured by a pulse oximeter. If the woman received epidural or spinal anesthesia, she should be able to raise her legs (extended at the knees, off the bed) or flex her knees, place her feet flat on the bed, and raise her buttocks well off the bed. The numb or tingling, prickly sensation should be entirely gone from her legs. Often it takes $1^1/_2$ to 2 hours for these anesthetic effects to disappear.

Transfer from the recovery area. After the initial recovery period of 1 to 2 hours has been completed, the woman may be transferred to a postpartum room in the same or another nursing unit. In labor, delivery, recovery, postpartum (LDRP) room settings the nurse who has provided care during the recovery period usually continues caring for the woman. In the LDR room or traditional setting the woman is transferred to a separate unit where the postpartum nursing staff provides her care. Women who have received general or regional anesthesia must be cleared for transfer from the recovery area by a member of the anesthesia care team. In some settings the baby will remain with the mother wherever she goes. In other institutions the baby will be taken to the nursery for several hours of observation during the mother's initial recovery period.

In preparing the transfer report the recovery nurse uses information from the admission record, the birth record, and the recovery record. Information that must be communicated to the postpartum nurse includes identity of the health care provider; gravidity and parity; age; anesthetic used; any medications given; duration of labor and time of rupture of membranes; oxytocin induction or augmentation; type of birth and repair; blood type and Rh status; state of rubella immunity; syphilis and hepatitis serology test results; intravenous (IV) infusion of any fluids; physiologic status since birth; de-

TABLE 19-1 Recovery nurse's report

ITEM	EXAMPLE OF DOCUMENTATION OF MOTHER	EXAMPLE OF DOCUMENTATION OF NEWBORN
Type of labor and birth; unusual observations, if any, of the placenta	Spontaneous or assisted (forceps) vaginal birth; vertex presentation	Spontaneous or assisted (forceps, vacuum extractor) vaginal birth in vertex presentation
Gravidity and parity, age	G1, P1, 22 years old	G1, P1, 22 years old
Anesthesia and analgesia used	None; epidural, low spinal, local	None; epidural, low spinal, or local
Condition of perineum	Episiotomy; repair of lacerations	
Events since birth	Vital signs, BP, fundus, lochia, intake and output, medications (dosage, time of administration, and results), response to newborn, observation of family interactions, including siblings, if present	Nursed at breast; took nipple well Voided × 1; meconium × 1 Eye prophylaxis Vitamin K injection Held by siblings who are happy with (or have other response to) newborn
Condition and sex of newborn; other information	Apgar at 1 and 5 min; time of birth; eye prophylaxis given; weight; whether breastfeeding or bottle feeding; if breastfeeding, whether newborn was at breast; name of pediatrician; sex of the baby	Apgar scores at 1 and 5 min Male; 3400 g (7 lb 8 oz); name of pediatrician; breastfeeding or bottle-feeding; mother's hepatitis B status
Relevant information from prenatal record	Need for rubella vaccination; presence of infections; hepatitis B status; blood type; Rh status	Unremarkable pregnancy
Miscellaneous information		
IV drip	If IV drip is infusing, rate of infusion, medications added (e.g., Pitocin), whether to keep open or discontinue after completion of bag that is hung	
Social factors	If woman is releasing baby for adoption, whether she wants to see baby, breastfeed, allow visitors, or other preferences she may have	

BP, Blood pressure

scription of fundus, lochia, bladder, and perineum; sex and weight of infant; time of birth; pediatrician; chosen method of feeding; any abnormalities noted; and assessment of initial parent-infant interaction.

This information is also documented for the nursing staff in the newborn nursery. In addition, specific information should be provided regarding the infant's Apgar scores, weight, voiding, and feeding since birth. Nursing interventions that have been completed (e.g., eye prophylaxis, vitamin K injection) also must be recorded.

Table 19-1 gives examples for documenting this information before transfer of the patient from the recovery area.

Women who give birth in birthing centers may go home within a few hours, after the woman's and infant's conditions are stable.

Nursing Care Management—Physical Needs

Assessment

A complete physical assessment, including all systems and measurement of vital signs, is performed on admission to the postpartum unit. If the woman's vital signs are within normal limits, they are likely to be assessed every 4 to 8 hours for the remainder of her hospitalization. Other components of the initial assessment include the mother's emotional status, energy level, degree of physical discomfort, hunger, and thirst. Intake and output assessments should always be included if an intravenous infusion or a urinary catheter are in place. If the woman gave birth by cesarean, her incisional dressing should also be assessed. To some degree, her knowledge level concerning self-care and infant care can also be determined at this time.

Ongoing physical assessment. The postpartum woman should be evaluated thoroughly each shift throughout hospitalization. Physical assessments include evaluation of the breasts, uterine fundus, lochia, perineum, bladder and bowel function, vital signs, and legs. Box 19-2 provides an example of a critical care path for progression of postpartum physical changes over the first 2 days. Signs of potential problems that may be identified during the assessment process are listed in Box 19-3.

Routine laboratory tests. Several laboratory tests may be performed in the immediate postpartum period. Hemoglobin and hematocrit values are often requested on the first postpartum day to assess blood loss during childbirth. In some hospitals a clean-catch or catheterized urine specimen may be obtained and sent for routine urinalysis or culture and sensitivity, especially if an indwelling urinary catheter was inserted during the intrapartum period. In addition, if the woman's rubella and Rh status are unknown, such tests should be performed and the results evaluated to determine the need for possible treatment.

Nursing Diagnoses

Although all women experience similar physiologic changes during the postpartum period, certain factors act to make each woman's experience unique. From a physiologic standpoint the length and difficulty of the labor, type of birth (vaginal or cesarean), presence of episiotomy and/or lacerations, parity, and whether she plans to breastfeed or bottle-feed are factors to be considered with each woman. After analyzing the data obtained during the assessment process, the nurse establishes nursing diagnoses that will provide a guide for planning care. Examples of nursing diagnoses commonly established for the postpartum patient include the following:

- Risk for fluid volume deficit (hemorrhage) related to
  Uterine atony after childbirth
- Risk for infection related to
  Childbirth trauma to tissues
- Urinary retention or constipation related to

BOX 19-2
Care Path: Postpartum Changes (Days 1 and 2)

Assessment	2 to 24 hours (day 1)	25 to 48 hours (day 2)
Temperature	97.1° F (36.2° C) to 100.4° F (38° C)	Within normal range
Pulse	Bradycardia: 50 to 70 beats/min	Bradycardia may persist or rate may return to normal range
Blood pressure	Within normal range	Within normal range
Energy level	Euphoric, happy, excited, or fatigued; may show need for sleep	Often tired, slow moving
Uterus	At umbilicus or just below; firm	1 cm or more below umbilicus; firm
Lochia	Rubra; moderate; few clots, if any; fleshy odor of normal menstrual flow	Rubra to serosa; moderate to scant; odor continues to be fleshy or absent
Perineum	Edematous; clean, healing, intact; episiotomy edges approximated	Edema lessening; clean, healing
Legs	Pretibial or pedal edema; Homans' sign negative	Edema lessening; Homans' sign negative
Breasts	Remain soft to palpation; colostrum can be expressed	Begin to feel firmer; occasionally feel lumpy
Appetite	Excellent; may ask for double helpings, snacks	Usually remains excellent
Elimination		
Voiding	Up to 3000 ml	Large amounts
Defecation	None expected; stool softener	None expected; stool softener
Discomfort	Generalized aching; perineal area; episiotomy, hemorrhoids, afterbirth pains	Muscle aches; perineal area; episiotomy, hemorrhoids

Postchildbirth discomfort
Childbirth trauma to tissues
- Pain related to
  - Uterine cramping (afterpains)
  - Trauma to perineum
  - Episiotomy
  - Hemorrhoids
  - Engorged breasts
- Sleep pattern disturbance related to
  - Discomforts of postpartum period
  - Long labor process
  - Infant care and hospital routine
- Risk for injury related to
  - Postpartum hemorrhage
  - Effects of anesthesia
- Knowledge deficit related to
  - Importance of voiding as deterrent to hemorrhage
- Ineffective breastfeeding related to
  - Maternal discomfort
  - Infant positioning
  - Knowledge deficit

Expected Outcomes

The nursing plan of care includes both the postpartum woman and her infant, even if the nursery nurse retains primary responsibility for the infant. In many areas, **couplet care** (also called mother and baby care or single-room maternity care) is practiced. In this approach the nurse has been educated in both mother and infant care and functions as the primary nurse for both mother and infant, even if the newborn is kept in the central nursery. This approach is a variation of rooming-in, in which the mother and child room together and the mother and nurse share in the care of the infant. The organization of the mother's care must take the newborn into consideration. The day actually revolves around the baby's feeding and care times. In couplet care, responsibility and accountability for care of both mother and infant rest with the primary nurse.

Once the nursing diagnoses are formulated, the nurse plans with the woman what nursing measures are appropriate and which are to be given priority. During her hospital stay the mother is encouraged to assume increasing responsibility for self-care and her infant's care. As the woman and her partner provide more care for herself and the baby, the nurse's role changes from one of providing direct care to one primarily of teaching, encouragement, and support.

The nursing plan of care includes assessments to detect deviations from normal physical changes, measures to relieve discomfort or pain, and safety measures to prevent injury or infection. The plan of care also includes teaching and counseling measures designed to promote the patient's feelings of competence in self-care and baby care. Family members are included in the teaching. The nurse evaluates continuously and is ready to change the plan if indicated. Almost all hospitals use standardized care plans as a base. The nurse's ability to adapt the standardized plan to specific medical and nursing diagnoses results in individualized patient care.

Expected outcomes for the postpartum period are based on the nursing diagnoses identified for the individual patient. The following are examples of common expected outcomes for physiologic needs. The woman will:

1. Saturate no more than one pad per hour during the fourth stage of labor
2. Empty her bladder either by voiding or by catheterization as necessary to keep the fundus firm and in the midline at the level of the umbilicus during the fourth stage of labor
3. Remain free of infection
4. Demonstrate normal involution and lochial characteristics
5. Remain comfortable and injury free
6. Demonstrate normal bladder and bowel patterns
7. Demonstrate knowledge of breast care, whether breastfeeding or bottle-feeding
8. Protect the health of future pregnancies and children
9. Integrate the newborn into the family

BOX 19-3
Signs of Potential Complications

PHYSIOLOGIC PROBLEMS	
Temperature	More than 38° C (100.4° F) after the first 24 hours
Pulse	Tachycardia, marked bradycardia
Blood pressure	Hypotension or hypertension
Energy level	Lethargy, extreme fatigue
Uterus	Deviated from the midline, boggy, remains above the umbilicus after 24 hours
Lochia	Heavy, foul odor; bright red bleeding that is not lochia
Perineum	Pronounced edema, not intact, signs of infection, marked discomfort
Legs	Homans sign positive; painful, reddened area; warmth on posterior aspect of calf
Breasts	Redness, heat, pain, cracked and fissured nipples, inverted nipples, palpable mass
Appetite	Lack of appetite
Elimination	Urine: inability to void, urgency, frequency, dysuria; bowel: constipation, diarrhea
Rest	Inability to rest or sleep

Plan of Care and Implementation

Nurses play many roles while implementing the nursing care plan. They provide direct physical care, teach mother and baby care, and provide anticipatory guidance and counseling. Perhaps most important, they nurture the woman by providing encouragement and support as the woman begins to assume the many tasks of motherhood. New mothers assume care at varying times, depending on their own physical and psychologic status. Nurses who take the time to "mother the mother" do much to increase feelings of self-confidence in new mothers.

The first step in providing individualized care is to confirm the woman's identity by checking her wristband. At the same time the infant's identification number is matched with the corresponding band on the mother's wrist. In some institutions the father is also given an identification band. The nurse demonstrates caring and respect by determining how the mother wishes to be addressed and then notes her preference in her record and in her nursing plan of care.

The woman and her family are oriented to their surround-

TABLE 19-2 Pharmacologic measures to stimulate uterine tone

INTERVENTION	ACTION, USES DURING PUERPERIUM	ONSET OF EFFECT, DURATION, USUAL DOSE	CONTRAINDICATIONS, PRECAUTIONS	COMMENTS
Oxytocin injection, USP (10 U/ml) (Pitocin, Syntocinon, Uteracon); oxytocic, synthetic posterior pituitary hormone	Stimulates phasic uterine muscle contraction; promotes milk ejection (let-down) reflex, facilitates flow of milk during engorgement	IV injection, 10 U; onset in 1 min IV infusion, 10 to 40 U/1000 ml 5% dextrose or physiologic electrolyte solution IM injection, 3 to 10 U; onset in 3 to 7 min; duration 30 to 60 min	Hypersensitivity; return of atony when effect wears off; may cause severe hypertension if patient is also receiving ephedrine, methoxamine, or other vasopressors	Alert: Assess for return of atony; store in cool place
Ergonovine, USP, NF (Ergotrate maleate); oxytocic, ergot alkaloid	Stimulates prolonged, nonphasic uterine contractions	Oral: 0.2 to 0.4 mg every 6 to 12 hours for 48 hours; onset in 6 to 15 min IM injection: 0.2 mg (1 ml) if nausea precludes oral preparation, onset in a few minutes Initial response: firm, tetanic contraction Subsequent response: alternating minor relaxations/contractions for 1½ hour; strong rhythmic contractions for 3 to 4 hours after injection	Severe hypertensive episodes may occur if given to hypertensive patients or those receiving vasoconstrictors; hypersensitivity; nausea, vomiting; sudden change in blood pressure or pulse; rare cases of myocardial infarction have been associated with postpartum use	Alert: Assess for changes in blood pressure, pulse; store in cool place in a light-resistant container
Methylergonovine, NF (Methergine); oxytocic, ergot alkaloid and congener of lysergic acid (LSD)	Stimulates rapid, sustained tetanic uterine contractions; used in treatment of subinvolution; has only minimum vasoconstrictive effect	Oral: 0.2 mg tab every 6 to 8 hours for maximum of 1 week; onset in 5 to 10 min IM injection 0.2 mg (1 ml) every 2 to 4 hours; onset in 2 to 5 min IV infusion (emergency only): 0.2 mg (1 ml) *slowly over 60 sec;* onset immediate	Nausea, vomiting; transient hypertension; dizziness, headache; tinnitus; diaphoresis; palpitations; temporary chest pains	Alert: Do not administer with Percodan—may result in hallucinations; assess blood pressure; store in cold place, away from light
Carboprost (Prostin/M15); oxytocic, prostaglandin	Stimulates rapid, sustained uterine contractions; used for treatment of uterine atony and uterine inversion	IM injection 1 ampule (250 μg), onset within minutes; intramyometrial injection (by physician only), ½ to 2 ampules (125 to 500 μg) diluted with 10 ml saline solution (injected transabdominally into anterior wall of uterus); onset within minutes	Severe hypertension (systolic >170 mm Hg or diastolic >100 mm Hg) and with severe symptomatic asthma Diarrhea seen with dosage above 1 ampule; systolic and diastolic blood pressure usually rises; bronchoconstriction and wheezing are concerns	Alert: Monitor blood pressure and for adverse reactions: store in refrigerator

ings. Familiarity with the unit, routines, resources, and personnel reduces one potential source of anxiety—the unknown. The mother is reassured through knowing whom and how she can call for assistance and what she can expect in the way of supplies and services. If the woman's usual daily routine before admission differs from the facility's routine, the nurse works with the woman to develop a mutually acceptable one.

Infant abduction from hospitals in the United States has increased over the past few years. The mother should be taught to check the identity of any person who comes to remove the baby from her room. Hospital personnel usually wear picture identification badges. On some units, all staff members wear matching scrubs or special badges. Other units use closed circuit television or computer monitoring systems. As a rule, the baby is never carried in a staff member's arms between the mother's room and the nursery but is always wheeled in a bassinet, which also contains baby care supplies. Patients and nurses must work together to ensure the safety of newborns in the hospital environment.

Implementation of the nursing plan of care involves putting into practice specific activities that should result in achieving the expected outcomes planned for each individual patient.

Prevention of infection. One important means of preventing infection is maintenance of a clean environment. Bed linens should be changed daily or when soiled. Disposable pads and draw sheets (if used) may need to be changed more frequently. Women should not walk about barefoot to avoid contaminating the linens when they return to bed. Supervision of the use of equipment to prevent cross-contamination is also necessary. For example, a **sitz bath** or heat lamp used in common must be scrubbed after each woman's use. Staff members are another important part of the hospital environment. Personnel must be conscientious about their handwashing techniques to prevent cross infection. Standard Precautions must be practiced. Staff members with colds, coughs, or skin infections (for example, a cold sore on the lips [herpes simplex virus type I]) must follow hospital protocol when in contact with postpartum patients.

Proper care of the episiotomy site and any perineal lacerations prevents infection in the genitourinary area and aids the healing process. Educating the woman to wipe from front to back (urethra to anus) after voiding or defecating is a simple first step. In many hospitals a squeeze bottle filled with warm water or an antiseptic solution is used after each voiding to cleanse the perineal area (Box 19-4). The woman should also be taught to change her perineal pad from front to back, each time she voids or defecates, and to wash her hands thoroughly before and after doing so.

Prevention of excessive bleeding. Postpartum hemorrhage is defined as the loss of at least 500 ml of blood within the first 24 hours after vaginal birth. Because women undergoing cesarean birth commonly lose that much, a loss of 1000 to 2000 ml of blood generally must occur before the bleeding is considered significant (Cunningham et al, 1993). A more objective criterion is a drop in hematocrit of 10%. The frequent physical assessments performed during the fourth stage of labor are designed to provide prompt identification of excessive bleeding (see the Emergency box on p. 497).

Vital signs are assessed routinely according to hospital protocol or policy to identify a decrease in blood pressure and increase in pulse rate, which are physiologic changes associated with hemorrhage and hypovolemic shock. Another routine part of the assessment is palpation of the uterus to determine its consistency (Fig 19-3). Normally the fundus (top of the uterus) is firm or may be returned to a state of firmness with intermittent gentle massage.

Nursing ALERT

If **uterine atony** (failure of the uterine muscle to contract firmly) occurs, the relaxed uterus distends with blood and clots, blood vessels in the placental site are not clamped off, and excessive bleeding results.

During each assessment, the perineal pad is checked to ensure that blood loss is not excessive.

Nursing ALERT

The nurse always checks under the mother's buttocks, as well as on the perineal pad. Blood may flow between the buttocks onto the linens under the mother while the amount on the perineal pad is slight.

A perineal pad that is soaked through from tail to tail contains approximately 68 to 80 ml of blood (Luegenbiehl et al, 1990). Finding a pad soaked in 15 minutes or observing pooling blood under the buttocks are indications of excessive blood loss that require notifying the physician/certified nurse-midwife (CNM) immediately. Blood loss is usually described subjectively as scant, light, moderate, or heavy (profuse). Fig. 19-4 shows examples of perineal pad saturation corresponding to each of these descriptions.

Although excessive blood loss in the recovery period may also be caused by vaginal or vulvar hematomas or unrepaired lacerations of the vagina or cervix, it results most often from uterine atony. Therefore the two most important interventions for preventing excessive bleeding are maintaining good uterine tone and preventing bladder distention.

Maintenance of uterine tone. A major intervention to maintain good tone is stimulation by gently massaging the uterine fundus until firm. Fundal massage may cause a temporary increase in the amount of vaginal bleeding seen as pooled blood leaves the uterus. Clots may also be expelled. Patient education is extremely important in maintaining uterine tone. Fundal massage can be a very uncomfortable procedure. Understanding the causes and dangers of uterine atony and the purpose of fundal massage can help the woman to be more cooperative. Teaching the patient to do self-fundal massage enables her to maintain some control and decreases her anxiety. Excessive force during fundal massage should be avoided because it can result in uterine prolapse. The uterus may remain boggy even with massage and expulsion of clots. If this occurs, it is important that the nurse remain with the woman and summon help. The physician/CNM should be notified immediately. Additional interventions likely to be used are administration of intravenous fluids and **oxytocic medications** (drugs that stimulate contraction of the uterine

BOX 19-4
Interventions for Episiotomy, Lacerations, and Hemorrhoids

Explain both procedure and rationale before implementation.

Cleansing

Wash perineum with mild soap and warm water or plain warm water as instructed at least once daily.
Cleanse from front to back (symphysis pubis to anal area).
Apply peripad from front to back, protecting inner surface of pad from contamination.
Wrap soiled pad and place in covered waste container.
Remind to change pad every time she voids or defecates or at least four times per day.
Wash hands thoroughly before and after changing pads.
Assess amount and character of lochia with each pad change.

Ice pack

Apply a covered ice pack to perineum
- During first 2 hours to decrease edema formation and increase comfort
- After the first 2 hours following birth to provide analgesic effect

Squeeze bottle

Demonstrate for and assist woman; explain rationale.
Fill bottle with tap water warmed to approximately 38° C (comfortably warm on the wrist). A Betadine or other solution may be used depending on the preference of the physician/certified nurse-midwife (CNM) or hospital procedure.
Instruct woman to position nozzle between her legs so that squirts of water reach perineum as she sits on toilet seat. Explain that it will take whole bottle of water over perineum.
Remind her to blot dry with toilet paper or clean wipes.
Remind her to avoid contamination from anal area.
Apply clean new pad.

Sitz bath

Built-in type:

Prepare bath by thoroughly scrubbing with cleansing agent and rinsing.
Pad with towel before filling.
Fill ⅓ to ½ full with water of correct temperature: 38° to 40.6° C or 45° C. An alternative to a warm sitz bath is a cool sitz bath. Prepare by filling with water and adding ice until the woman says the temperature is tolerable.
Encourage woman to use at least twice a day for 20 minutes.
Place call bell within easy reach.
Teach woman to enter bath by tightening gluteal muscles and keeping them tightened and then relaxing them after she is in the bath.
Place dry towels within reach.
Ensure privacy.
Check woman in 15 minutes; assess pulse as needed.

Disposable type:

Clamp tubing and fill bag with warm water.
Raise toilet seat, place bath in bowl with overflow opening directed toward back of toilet.
Place container above toilet bowl.
Attach tube into groove at front of bath.
Loosen tube clamp to regulate rate of flow; fill bath to approximately half full; continue as above for built-in sitz bath.

Dry heat

Inspect lamp for defects.
Position lamp 50 cm from perineum; use three times a day for 20-minute periods.
Teach regarding use of 40-watt bulb at home.
Provide draping over woman.
If same lamp is being used by several women, clean it carefully between uses with cleaning solution approved by the institution.

Topical applications

Apply anesthetic cream or spray if prescribed: use sparingly three to four times per day or with pad changes.
Offer witch hazel pads (Tucks) after voiding or defecating; woman pats perineum dry from front to back, then applies witch hazel pads.

smooth muscle). Table 19-2 contains information about common oxytocic medications.

LEGAL TIP
Patient Abandonment

In an emergency situation the nurse must remain with the patient and call for help. Leaving the patient can lead to a charge of patient abandonment. Abandonment also may occur if the nurse notices a change in patient status and fails to take appropriate action promptly.

Prevention of bladder distention. A full bladder causes the uterus to be displaced above the umbilicus and well to one side of midline in the abdomen. It also prevents the uterus from contracting normally. Nursing interventions focus on helping the woman to empty her bladder spontaneously as soon as possible. The first priority is to assist the woman to the bathroom or onto a bedpan if she is unable to ambulate. Having the woman listen to running water, placing her hands in warm water, or pouring water from a squeeze bottle over her perineum may stimulate voiding. Other techniques include assisting the woman into the shower or sitz bath and encouraging her to void or placing oil of peppermint in a bedpan under the woman. The vapors may relax the urinary meatus and trigger spontaneous voiding. Administering analgesics, if ordered, may be indicated because women may fear voiding because of the anticipation of pain.

If these measures are unsuccessful, a sterile catheter may be inserted to drain the urine. In the past, nurses were taught that suddenly emptying a distended bladder could result in hemorrhage, syncope, sepsis, and shock. Nursing textbooks usually recommended that no more than 750 to 1000 ml of urine be removed at one time. However, little scientific evidence exists to support this practice. Complete bladder empty-

EMERGENCY

HYPOVOLEMIC SHOCK

Signs/symptoms:

Persistent significant bleeding—perineal pad soaked within 15 minutes; may not be accompanied by a change in vital signs or maternal color or behavior
Woman states she feels weak, light-headed, "funny," "sick to my stomach," or "sees stars"
Woman begins to act anxious or exhibits air hunger
Woman's color turns ashen or grayish
Skin feels cool and clammy to touch
Increasing pulse rate
Falling blood pressure

Interventions:

Notify physician/CNM.
If uterus is atonic, massage gently and expel clots to allow uterus to contract; compress uterus manually, as needed, using two hands. Add oxytocic to IV drip, as ordered.
Give oxygen by face mask or nasal prongs at 8 to 10 L/min.
Tilt the woman to her side or elevate the right hip; elevate her legs to at least a 30-degree angle.
Provide additional or maintain existing IV of lactated Ringer's or normal saline solution to restore circulatory volume.
Administer blood or blood products as ordered.
Monitor vital signs.
Insert an indwelling urinary catheter to monitor perfusion of kidneys.
Administer emergency drugs as ordered.
Prepare for possible surgery or other emergency treatments/procedures.
Chart incident, medical and nursing interventions used, and results of treatments.

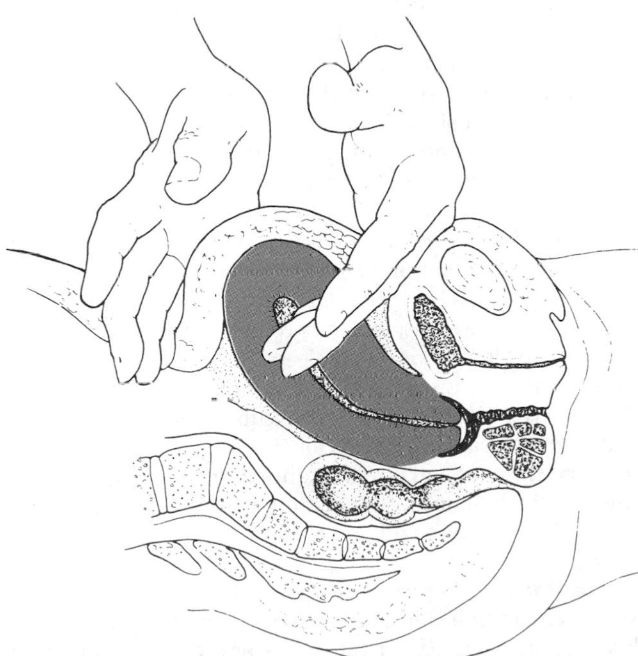

Fig. 19-3 Palpating fundus of uterus during the fourth stage of labor. Note that upper hand is cupped over fundus; lower hand dips in above symphysis pubis and supports uterus while it is massaged gently.

ing is surely more comfortable, and probably at least as safe, as serial drainage (Bristoll et al, 1989).

Evaluation of the woman's responses to intervention is an ongoing part of the nursing process. All responses to interventions should be recorded carefully. If the expected outcomes are not met or if new needs emerge, the plan of care is modified accordingly. For example, if the uterus is firm and the bladder empty, something other than uterine atony is causing the excessive bleeding. Immediately after childbirth, other causes of excessive bleeding include unrepaired vaginal or cervical lacerations and disseminated intravascular coagulation (DIC). Later in the postpartum period, subinvolution of the placental site, retained placental fragments, and infection can cause excessive uterine bleeding. Further assessment is necessary to determine the cause and correct the problem.

Promotion of comfort, rest, ambulation, and exercise

Comfort. During the fourth stage of labor many women experience intense tremors that resemble the shivering of a chill. The chilling or shivering may be related to the sudden release of pressure on pelvic nerves. According to another theory, chilling may be symptomatic of a fetus-to-mother transfusion that sometimes occurs during placental separation. The feeling of a chill may be a reaction to epinephrine (adrenaline) production during birth or to epidural anesthesia. The nurse can help the woman relax and feel comforted by providing her with warm blankets and an explanation that the tremors are commonly seen after birth and are not related to infection. Some women experience the tremors without any feeling of chill; these women also should be covered with a warm blanket. The tremors usually are self-limiting and last only a short while.

Most women experience some degree of discomfort during the postpartum period. Common causes of discomfort include afterbirth pains, episiotomy or perineal lacerations, hemorrhoids, and breast engorgement. The woman's description of the type and severity of her pain is the nurse's best guide in choosing an appropriate intervention. To confirm the location and extent of discomfort the nurse inspects and palpates areas of pain as appropriate for redness, swelling, discharge, and heat and also observes for body tension, guarded movements, and facial tension. Blood pressure, pulse, and respirations may be elevated in response to acute pain. Diaphoresis may accompany severe pain. A lack of objective signs does not nec-

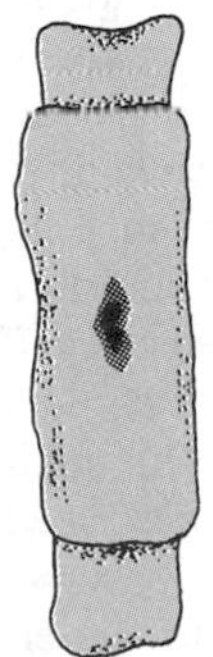
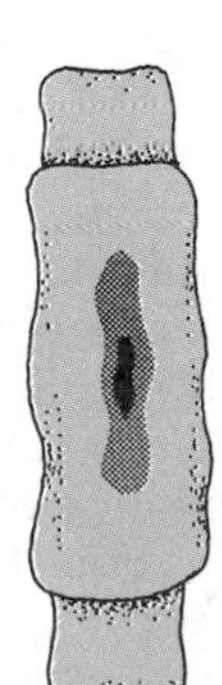
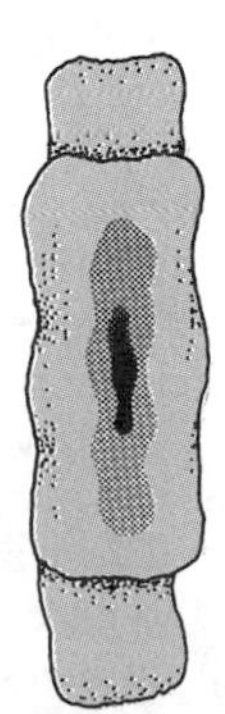
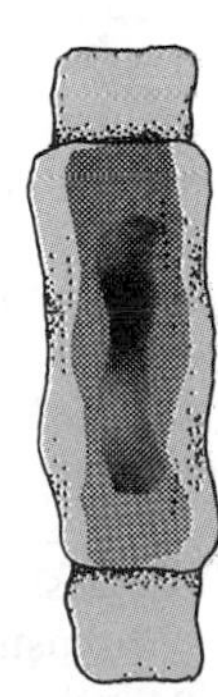

Fig. 19-4 Blood loss after birth is assessed by estimating perineal pad saturation as *(left to right)* scant, light, moderate, or heavy (profuse).

essarily mean there is no pain, because there may also be a cultural component to the expression of pain. Nursing interventions are intended to eliminate the pain sensation entirely or reduce it to a tolerable level that allows the woman to care for herself and her baby. Nurses may use both nonpharmacologic and pharmacologic interventions to promote comfort. As a rule, nonpharmacologic measures should be used first, either alone or in combination with pharmacologic interventions. Pain relief is enhanced by using more than one method or route.

NONPHARMACOLOGIC INTERVENTIONS. **Afterbirth pains** are the menstrual-like cramps experienced by many women as the uterus contracts after childbirth. Warmth, distraction, imagery, therapeutic touch, relaxation, and interaction with the infant may decrease the discomfort associated with these uterine contractions.

The episiotomy, perineal lacerations, or hemorrhoids often contribute to a new mother's discomfort. Immediately after birth, cold therapy such as ice packs are applied to the perineum directly over the episiotomy to minimize edema formation. After the first 2 hours, ice packs have little effect on minimizing edema; they are used to increase comfort by numbing the area. Disposable ice packs can be made by filling rubber examining gloves with ice chips and covering them with something clean such as a disposable wash cloth. Chemical ice packs attached to sanitary pads may also be used.

After the first 24 hours, warmth applied to the perineum increases blood flow and encourages healing. Common sources of heat include a heat lamp, a cleansing shower, a tub bath, or a sitz bath. Other simple interventions include encouraging the woman to lie on her side whenever possible and to use a pillow when sitting. Many of these interventions are also effective for hemorrhoids, especially ice packs, sitz baths, and topical applications (such as witch hazel pads). Box 19-4 gives more specific information about these interventions.

The discomfort associated with engorged breasts may be lessened by applying either ice or heat to the breasts and wearing a well-fitted support bra. Decisions about specific interventions for engorgement are based on whether the woman chooses breastfeeding or bottle-feeding (see Chapter 24).

PHARMACOLOGIC INTERVENTIONS. Most health care providers routinely order a variety of analgesics to be administered as needed, including both narcotic and nonnarcotic choices, with their dosage and time frequency ranges. Other common pharmacologic interventions include topical applications of antiseptic or anesthetic ointments or sprays. Patient-controlled analgesia (PCA) pumps and continuous epidural analgesia infusions are two newer technologies now commonly used to provide postpartum pain relief, especially after a cesarean birth. Many women want to participate in decisions about analgesia. Severe pain, however, may interfere with active participation in choosing pain relief measures. If an analgesic is to be given, the nurse must make a clinical judgment of the type, dosage, and frequency from the medications ordered. The woman is informed of the prescribed analgesic and its common side effects.

Breastfeeding mothers often have concerns about the effects of an analgesic on the infant. The timing of medications can often be adjusted to minimize infant exposure. For example, a mother may be given pain medication immediately after breastfeeding (so that the interval between medication administration and the next nursing period is as long as possible) or immediately before breastfeeding because the medication will not enter the milk already present. Although nearly all drugs present in maternal circulation are also found in breast milk, many analgesics commonly used during the postpartum period are considered relatively safe for breastfeeding mothers. The decision to administer medications of any type to a breastfeeding mother must always be made by carefully weighing the woman's need against actual or potential risks to the infant (Anderson, 1991; Briggs et al, 1994).

If acceptable pain relief has not been obtained in 1 hour and there has been no change in the initial assessment, the nurse may need to contact the physician/nurse-midwife for additional pain relief orders or further directions. Unrelieved pain results in fatigue, anxiety, and a worsening perception of the pain. It might also indicate the presence of a previously unidentified or untreated problem. Further assessment and treatment will probably be necessary to determine the cause of the pain and correct it.

Fatigue. Fatigue is common in the postpartum period (Pugh and Milligan, 1995). It involves both physiologic components associated with long labors, cesarean birth, anemia, and breastfeeding and psychologic components related to depression and anxiety. Infant behavior is also related to fatigue, with mothers of more difficult infants experiencing more fatigue (Milligan, Parks, and Lenz, 1990). Fatigue may inhibit the mother's recovery and performance as a mother (Pugh and Milligan, 1993). The side-lying position for breastfeeding minimizes fatigue in nursing mothers (Milligan, Flenniken, and Pugh, 1996).

Nursing interventions to promote rest and sleep and to minimize the expenditure of energy and decrease anxiety lessen the fatigue experienced in the postpartum period. Providing support and encouragement in initial mothering behaviors decreases the anxiety related to maternal performance. Nurses can teach mothers about the sidelying position as a means to conserve energy and rest while nursing.

Rest. Soon after giving birth, the new mother may realize that she is exhausted. A long or difficult labor may have caused her to expend so much energy that one of her first needs is for a long, restful sleep. However, the excitement and exhilaration experienced after the birth of the infant may make rest difficult. The new mother who is anxious about her ability to care for her infant or is uncomfortable may also have difficulty sleeping. The demands of the infant, the hospital environment and routines, and the presence of frequent visitors contribute to alterations in her sleep pattern.

Interventions must be planned to meet the woman's individual needs for sleep and rest. Backrubs, other comfort measures, and medication for sleep for the first few nights may be necessary. Hospital and nursing routines may also be adjusted to meet individual needs. In addition, the nurse can assist the family to limit visitors and provide a comfortable chair or bed for the partner.

Ambulation. A woman who has just given birth may need to remain in bed for a time to allow her body systems to adjust to fluid volume changes. Before assisting the woman to get out of bed for the first time, the nurse takes several factors into consideration, such as the baseline blood pressure, the amount of blood lost, and the type, amount, and timing of analgesic or anesthetic medications administered. The woman who has received regional anesthesia should remain in bed until she is able to fully move and feel sensation in her legs.

Nursing ALERT

Early and frequent ambulation is encouraged because it helps to reduce the incidence of **thromboembolism** and promote the woman's more rapid recovery of strength.

After the initial recovery period is over, the mother is encouraged to ambulate frequently.

Nursing ALERT

Having a hospital staff or family member present the first time the woman gets out of bed after childbirth is a wise idea because she may feel weak, dizzy, faint, or light-headed.

The rapid decrease in intraabdominal pressure after birth results in a dilation of blood vessels supplying the intestines, which is known as **splanchnic engorgement** and causes blood to pool in the viscera. This condition contributes to the development of orthostatic hypotension when the woman who has recently given birth stands up.

Because of the normal increase in clotting factors that occurs during pregnancy, women who must remain in bed after giving birth are at increased risk for the development of blood clots (thrombi). Prevention of clot formation is part of the nursing plan of care. If a woman remains in bed longer than 8 hours (e.g., after cesarean birth), exercise to promote circulation in the legs is indicated using the following routine:

1. Alternate flexion and extension of feet.
2. Rotate ankle in circular motion.
3. Alternate flexion and extension of legs.
4. Press back of knee to bed surface; relax.

Women with varicosities are advised to wear support hose. The woman is encouraged to walk about actively for true ambulation and is discouraged from sitting immobile in a chair. If a **thrombus** is suspected, as evidenced by a positive **Homans' sign** (complaint of pain in calf muscles when dorsiflexion of foot is forced), warmth, redness, or tenderness in the suspected leg, the physician/CNM should be notified immediately; meanwhile the woman should be confined to bed, with the affected limb elevated on pillows.

Exercise. Most women who have just given birth are extremely interested in regaining their nonpregnant figures. Postpartum exercise can begin soon after birth, although the woman should be encouraged to start with simple exercises and gradually progress to more strenuous ones. Fig. 19-5 illustrates a number of exercises appropriate for the new mother. Kegel pelvic exercises to strengthen muscle tone are extremely important, particularly after vaginal birth. To perform them, the woman alternately contracts and relaxes the muscles in her vagina, rectum, and buttocks. **Kegel exercises** (p. 135-136) help women regain the muscle tone that is often lost as pelvic tissues are stretched and torn during pregnancy and birth. Women who maintain muscle strength may benefit years later by experiencing less stress urinary incontinence (Sampselle, 1990).

Promotion of good nutrition. Restriction of food and fluid intake and the loss of fluids (blood, perspiration, or emesis) during labor cause many women to express a strong desire to eat or drink soon after giving birth. Again, the nurse considers many factors before offering food or fluids to the woman. If the woman gave birth vaginally and has recovered from the effects of the anesthetic, the vital signs are stable, the uterus is firm, and lochial flow is small to moderate, the woman can usually have sips of the liquid of her choice, followed by a regular diet. She should be cautioned to drink small amounts of fluid initially. Rapid drinking, especially of large amounts, can lead to nausea and possibly vomiting.

Heavy bleeding may signal uterine atony or retained placental fragments, either of which could require surgery. Thus the woman with heavy bleeding is given nothing by mouth (NPO) until the bleeding has been controlled. An intravenous line should be started or maintained in the woman who is kept NPO to provide fluid volume, rapid access to the vascular system if medications or blood products are required, and calorics for energy.

During their hospital stay, most women display a good appetite and eat well. They may request that family members bring to the hospital favorite foods or foods considered culturally appropriate for the postpartum period. Cultural dietary preferences must be respected. This interest in food presents an ideal opportunity for continued nutritional counseling (see Chapter 8). The woman's weight, expectations of weight loss, usual food habits, cultural preferences, laboratory findings (hemoglobin and hematocrit levels), and knowledge about nutritional needs after pregnancy should be assessed throughout this period.

Nursing interventions might include teaching about the nourishment needed to facilitate healing and increase energy. A regular diet high in protein, vitamin C, and dietary fiber, along with sufficient fluids and calories, generally is recommended for the postpartum woman to prevent constipation and promote well-being. Nutritional snacks usually are welcome. Prenatal vitamins and iron supplements often are continued.

Promotion of normal bladder and bowel patterns

Bladder. After giving birth the mother should void spontaneously within 6 to 8 hours. The first several voidings should be measured to document adequate emptying of the bladder. A volume of at least 150 ml is expected for each voiding. Some women experience difficulty in emptying the bladder, possibly a result of diminished bladder tone, edema from trauma, or fear of discomfort. Nursing interventions for inability to void and bladder distention are discussed on p. 495-496.

Bowel. Nursing interventions to promote normal bowel elimination include educating the woman about measures to avoid constipation. These interventions include ensuring adequate roughage and fluid intake and promoting exercise. Alerting the woman to side effects of medications such as narcotic analgesics (e.g., decreased gastrointestinal tract motility) may encourage her to implement measures to reduce the risk of constipation. Stool softeners or laxatives may be necessary

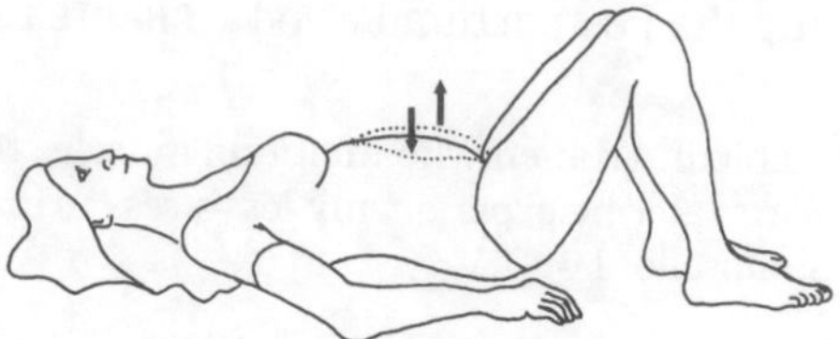

Abdominal Breathing. Lie on back with knees bent. Inhale deeply through the nose. Keep ribs as stationary as possible and allow abdomen to expand upwards. Exhale slowly but forcefully while contracting the abdominal muscles; hold for 3 to 5 seconds while exhaling. Relax.

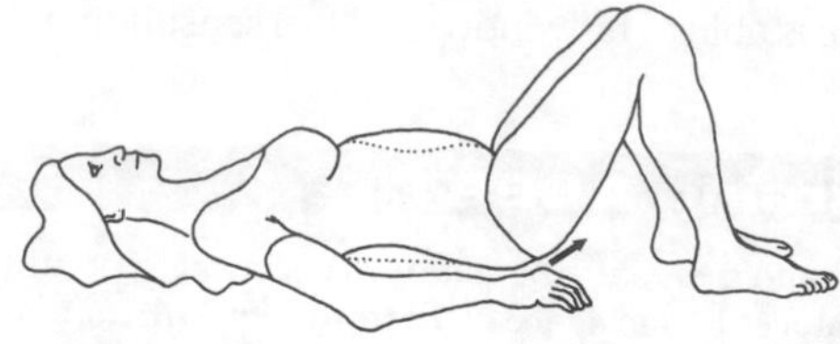

Combined Abdominal Breathing and Supine Pelvic Tilt (Pelvic Rock). Lie on back with knees bent. While inhaling deeply, roll pelvis back by flattening lower back on floor or bed. Exhale slowly but forcefully while contracting abdominal muscles and tightening buttocks. Hold for 3 to 5 seconds while exhaling. Relax.

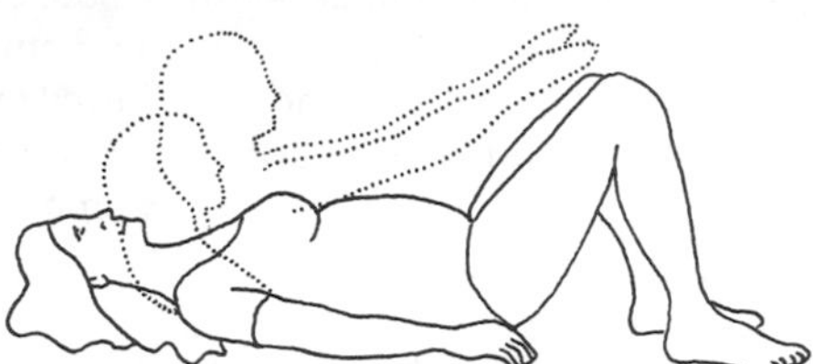

Reach for the Knees. Lie on back with knees bent. While inhaling deeply lower chin onto chest. While exhaling, raise head and shoulders slowly and smoothly and reach for knees with arms outstretched. The body should only rise as far as the back will naturally bend while waist remains on floor or bed (about 6 to 8 inches). Slowly and smoothly lower head and shoulders back to starting position. Relax.

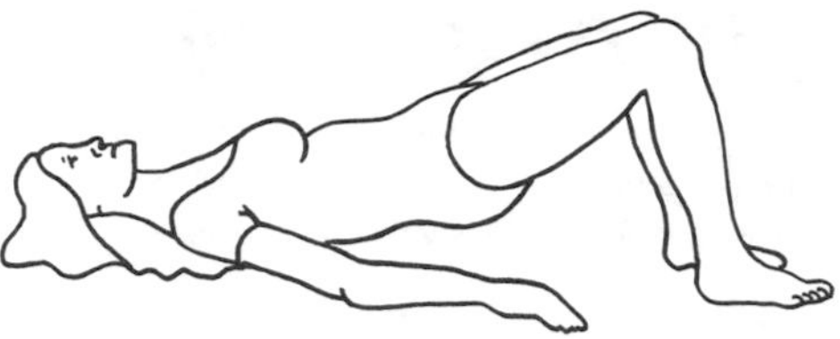

Buttocks Lift. Lie on back with arms at sides, knees bent and feet flat. Slowly raise buttocks and arch back. Return slowly to starting position.

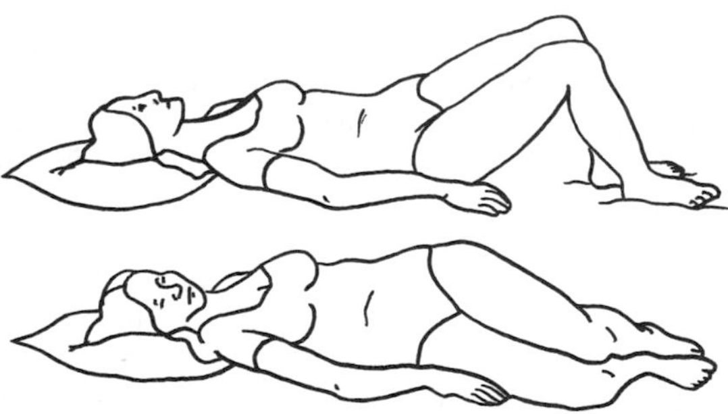

Double Knee Roll. Lie on back with knees bent. Keeping shoulders flat and feet stationary, slowly and smoothly roll knees over to the left to touch floor or bed. Maintaining a smooth motion, roll knees back over to the right until they touch floor or bed. Return to starting position and relax.

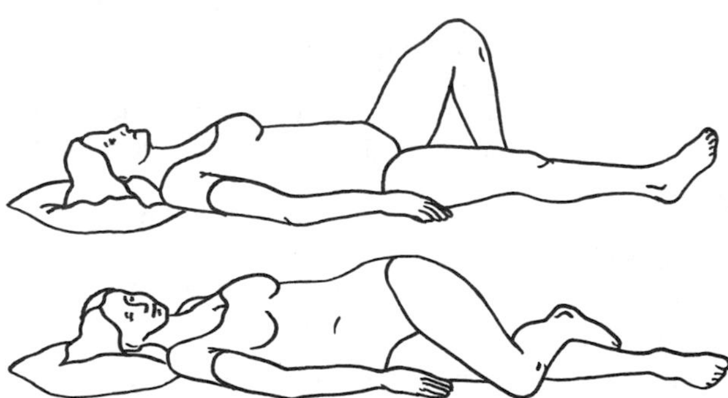

Single Knee Roll. Lie on back with right leg straight and left leg bent at the knee. Keeping shoulders flat, slowly and smoothly roll left knee over to the right to touch floor or bed and then back to starting position. Reverse position of legs. Roll right knee over to the left to touch floor or bed and return to starting position. Relax.

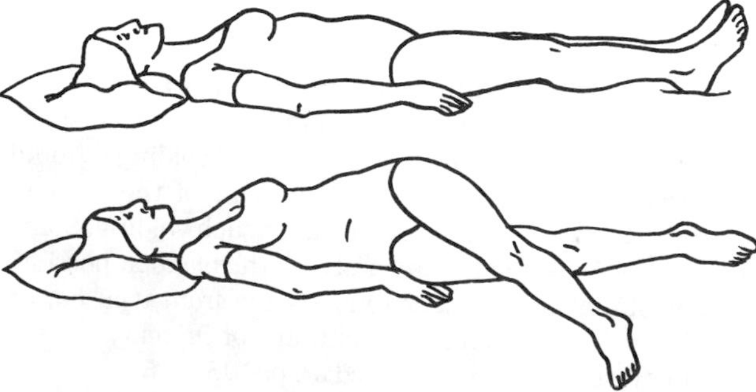

Leg Roll. Lie on back with legs straight. Keeping shoulders flat and legs straight, slowly and smoothly lift leg and roll it over to touch the right side of floor or bed and return to starting position. Repeat, rolling right leg over to touch left side of floor or bed. Relax.

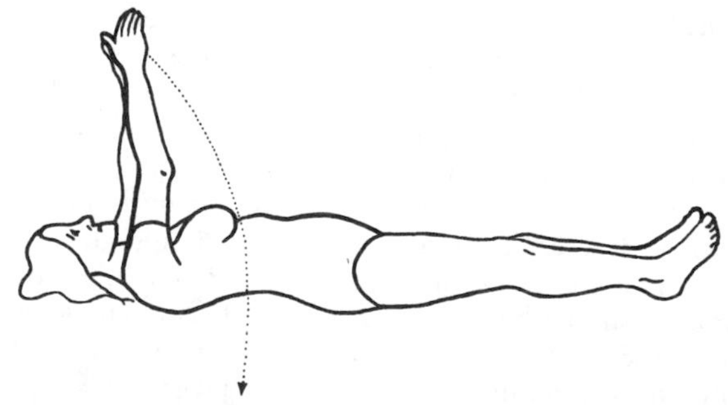

Arm Raises. Lie on back with arms extended at 90° angle from body. Raise arms so they are perpendicular and hands touch. Lower slowly.

Fig. 19-5 Postpartum exercise should begin as soon as possible. The woman should start with simple exercises and gradually progress to more strenuous ones.

during the early postpartum period. With early discharge a new mother may be home before having a bowel movement.

Some mothers experience gas pains. Ambulation or rocking in a rocking chair may stimulate passage of flatus and relief of discomfort.

Breastfeeding promotion and lactation suppression

Breastfeeding promotion. If breastfeeding was not initiated during the first 2 hours after childbirth, it should be started when the mother and infant have their first visit. Specific nursing techniques are covered in Chapter 24.

To care for the breasts, women should be taught to wash the breasts with clear water. Soap is not necessary; it may cause excessive dryness, which could result in cracked nipples. Most women, particularly those with large breasts, will be more comfortable if they wear a well-fitted nursing bra for support. A bra is also useful if breast pads are needed for leaking or when breast shields are worn for inverted nipples or nipple soreness. A bra is not necessary if the woman is comfortable without one.

Lactation suppression. Suppression of lactation is necessary when the woman has decided not to breastfeed or in the case of neonatal death. One very important nonpharmacologic intervention is wearing a well-fitted support bra or breast binder continuously for at least the first 72 hours after giving birth. Women should also avoid any breast stimulation, including running warm water over the breasts, newborn suckling, or pumping of the breasts. Few nonbreastfeeding mothers experience severe breast **engorgement** (swelling of breast tissue caused by increased blood and lymph supply to the breasts preceding lactation). If breast engorgement occurs, it can usually be managed satisfactorily with these nonpharmacologic interventions. Ice packs to the breasts are also helpful in decreasing the discomfort associated with engorgement. The woman should use a 15 minutes on, 45 minutes off schedule to prevent the rebound swelling that can occur if ice is used continuously, or she should place fresh cabbage leaves inside her bra. Cabbage leaves have been used to treat swelling in other cultures for years (Roberts, 1995). The exact mechanism of action is not known, but it is thought that naturally occurring plant estrogens or salicylates may be responsible for the effects. The leaves are replaced each time they wilt. Reduction of swelling is dramatic. A mild analgesic may also be necessary to help the mother through this uncomfortable time.

In the past an estrogen (Tace), a combination of estrogen and testosterone (Deladumone), or bromocriptine (Parlodel) was often prescribed for lactation suppression. There has been a shift away from the use of these drugs. Lactation suppression is no longer considered an indication for the use of Tace, Deladumone, or Parlodel. Seizures, strokes, and myocardial infarctions have been reported in postpartum women taking bromocriptine for lactation suppression. The exact relationship between bromocriptine use and these adverse reactions has not been established. The drug should be used with caution. Women who develop severe or progressive headaches unresponsive to usual treatment while taking bromocriptine should contact their physicians/CNMs immediately (Drug Facts and Comparisons, 1993; United States Pharmacopeial Convention, 1993).

Health promotion of future pregnancies and children. If the assessment data indicate a need, rubella vaccination and $Rh_o(D)$ immune globulin (RhoGAM) are administered during the puerperium. Failure to administer these products to women at risk of contracting rubella or developing Rh isoimmunization can seriously jeopardize the health of any future pregnancies and children.

Rubella vaccination. For women who have not had rubella (10% to 20% of all women) or women who lack immunity to the disease, a subcutaneous injection of **rubella vaccine** is recommended in the immediate postpartum period to prevent the possibility of contracting rubella in future pregnancies. Nonimmunity to rubella may be established by either of two different laboratory tests: an antibody titer or an enzyme immunoassay (EIA) test. A titer of 1:8 or less or an EIA value of <0.79 indicates nonimmunity. Seroconversion occurs in approximately 90% of women vaccinated after giving birth. The live attenuated rubella virus is not communicable in breast milk; therefore breastfeeding mothers can be vaccinated. However, because the virus is shed in urine and other body fluids, the vaccine should not be given if the mother or other household members are immunocompromised. Rubella vaccine is made from duck eggs; therefore women who have allergies to these eggs may develop a hypersensitivity reaction to the vaccine, for which they will need adrenaline. A transient arthralgia or rash is common in vaccinated women but is benign. Because it may be teratogenic, women must be told about the rubella vaccine before receiving the injection and cautioned to avoid pregnancy for 2 to 3 months after vaccination.

LEGAL TIP

Rubella Vaccination

Informed consent for rubella vaccination in the postpartum period includes information about the possible side effects and the risk of teratogenic effects. Women must understand that they must avoid pregnancy for 2 to 3 months after being vaccinated.

Prevention of Rh isoimmunization. Injection of **$Rh_o(D)$ immune globulin** (solution of gamma globulin that contains Rh antibodies) within 72 hours of childbirth prevents sensitization in the Rh-negative woman who has had a fetomaternal transfusion of Rh-positive fetal red blood cells (RBCs). $Rh_o(D)$ immune globulin promotes lysis of fetal Rh-positive RBCs circulating in the maternal bloodstream before the mother forms her own antibodies against them.

Nursing ALERT

Rh immune globulin is administered prenatally at 28 to 30 weeks' gestation to all Rh-negative, antibody (Coombs)-negative women, as well as earlier in gestation should invasive procedures such as amniocentesis be performed.

Rh immune globulin is administered postpartally to all Rh-negative, antibody (Coombs)-negative women who give birth to Rh-positive infants. Rh immune globulin is also administered after all known abortions occurring at or after 8 weeks' gestation.

The administration of 300 μg (one vial) of Rh immune

Guidelines

ADMINISTERING Rh IMMUNE GLOBULIN

Check to be sure that the identification number on the woman's hospital wristband corresponds to the identification number on the laboratory slip.

Make sure that the lot number on the laboratory slip corresponds to the lot number on the vial of Rh immune globulin.

Check the expiration date on the vial to be sure the product is usable.

Inject Rh immune globulin *intramuscularly.*

Rh immune globulin is *always* given to mothers—*never* to newborns!

Because Rh immune globulin suppresses the immune response, the woman who receives both Rh immune globulin and a rubella vaccine must be tested in 3 months to see if she has developed rubella immunity. If not, the woman will need another dose of rubella vaccine.

globulin is usually sufficient to prevent maternal sensitization. If more than 15 ml of fetal blood is present in maternal circulation, however, the dosage must be increased. A relatively inexpensive screening test, called a fetal screen, should be done initially on all Rh-negative women giving birth to infants who are Rh-positive or whose Rh status is unknown to detect the presence of fetal blood. If this screening test is positive, the **Kleihauer-Betke test,** which more accurately determines the amount of fetal blood present in maternal circulation, should be performed so that the correct dosage of Rh immune globulin can be administered.

There is some disagreement about whether Rh immune globulin should be considered a blood product. Health care providers need to discuss the most current information about this issue with women whose religious beliefs conflict with receiving blood products. In most institutions, however, precautions similar to those used for transfusing blood or blood products are taken when Rh immune globulin is administered (see the Guidelines box above.)

Evaluation

Evaluation of nursing care is ongoing and begins when the woman is admitted to the unit and ends only after discharge. If progress toward meeting the expected outcomes of care is not evident, interventions may need to be modified. As the woman's condition changes during her hospitalization, expected outcomes may need to be added or deleted. The nurse can be reasonably assured that care was effective when the expected outcomes of care have been achieved (see p. 493).

Nursing Care Management—Psychosocial Needs

Meeting the psychosocial needs of new mothers involves planning care that considers the composition and functioning of the entire family. Nurses assess the parents' reactions to the birth experience, feelings about themselves, and interactions with the new baby and other family members. Specific interventions are then planned to increase the parents' knowledge and self-confidence as they assume the care and responsibility of the new baby and integrate a new member into their existing family structure in a way that meets their cultural expectations.

Assessment

Impact of the birth experience. Many women indicate a need to examine the birth process itself and look at their own intrapartal behavior in retrospect. Their partners may express similar desires. During pregnancy the woman and her partner may have developed a specific birth plan that included a vaginal birth and very little medical intervention. If their birth experience was quite different (e.g., induction, epidural anesthesia, cesarean birth), both partners may need to mourn the loss of their expectations before they can adjust to the reality of their birth experience. Inviting them to review the events and describe how they feel helps the nurse to assess how well they understand what happened and how well they have been able to put their childbirth experience into perspective. Feelings about giving birth can affect the adaptation of both partners to parenting.

Maternal self-image. An important assessment concerns the woman's self-concept, body image, and sexuality. How this new mother feels about herself and her body during the puerperium may affect her behavior and adaptation to parenting. The woman's self-concept and body image may also affect her sexuality.

Feelings related to sexual adjustment after childbirth are often a cause of concern for new parents. Women who have recently given birth may be reluctant to resume sexual intercourse for fear of pain or may worry that coitus could damage healing perineal tissue. Because many new parents are anxious for information but reluctant to bring up the subject, postpartum nurses should matter of factly include the topic of postpartum sexuality during their routine physical assessment. While examining the episiotomy site, for example, the nurse can say, "I know you're sore right now, but it probably won't be long until you (or you and your partner) are ready to make love again. Have you thought about what that might be like? Would you like to ask me questions?" This approach assures the woman and her partner that resuming sexual activity is a legitimate concern for new parents and indicates the nurse's willingness to answer questions and share information.

Parent-infant interactions. A thorough postpartum psychosocial assessment includes evaluation of the parents' reactions to and interactions with the new baby. The psychologic state of a new mother may be euphoric and exhilarated. On the other hand, a mother who has experienced a long, difficult labor or who is in pain may be too exhausted to be interested in the baby initially. Some mothers, particularly with their firstborn, are surprised and disturbed by the passivity or disinterest they experience on seeing their long-awaited infant for the first time. The nurse can reassure the mother of the normality of these feelings. The idealized "mother love" does not necessarily appear immediately after birth. After she has had an opportunity to rest and eat, usually the new mother regains interest in the baby quickly.

Many new parents experience parenting concerns until their skills become established. Once they feel confident in their skills, the increase in self-esteem promotes a positive affective response to the child. However, some parents exhibit parenting disorders that place the child at risk. Both mother and father may experience these difficulties, although to date most research has centered on the mother (Table 19-3.) Protocols for the physical screening of high-risk pregnant women and fetuses have been developed. However, tools predicting high-risk parenting behaviors require more replication over larger samples before they can be used with precision.

Adaptive behaviors. **Adaptive behaviors** stem from the parents' realistic perception and acceptance of their newborn's needs and his or her limited abilities, immature social responses, and helplessness. Parents exhibit adaptive behaviors when they find pleasure in their infant and in the tasks done for and with him or her, when they understand their infant's emotional states and provide comfort, and when they read the infant's cues for new experiences and can sense the infant's fatigue level.

Maladaptive behaviors. Maladaptive behaviors are exhibited when parents respond inappropriately to the needs of their infant. They expect responses from the infant far in excess of the infant's ability to perform. They interpret inadequate responses as defiance or as negative judgment of parental capabilities. They obtain no pleasure from physical contact with their child. Their infants tend to be handled roughly. They are held in a manner that allows the head to dangle without support, and they are not cuddled. The par-

TABLE 19-3 Mothering behaviors*

ADAPTIVE BEHAVIORS	MALADAPTIVE BEHAVIORS
Feeding	
Offers appropriate amount and type of food to infant	Provides inadequate type or amount of food for infant
Holds infant in comfortable position during feeding	Does not hold infant or holds in uncomfortable position during feeding
Burps baby during and after feeding	Does not burp infant
Prepares food appropriately	Prepares food inappropriately
Offers food at comfortable pace for infant	Offers food at pace too rapid or slow for infant's comfort
Infant stimulation	
Provides appropriate verbal stimulation for infant during visit	Provides no, or only aggressive, verbal stimulation for infant during visit
Provides tactile stimulation for infant at times other than during feeding or moving infant away from danger	Does not provide tactile stimulation or only that of aggressive handling of infant
Provides age-appropriate toys	No evidence of age-appropriate toys
Interacts with infant in a way that provides for infant's satisfaction	Frustrates infant during interactions
Infant rest	
Provides quiet or relaxed environment for infant's rest, including scheduled rest periods	Does not provide quiet environment or consistent schedule for rest periods
Ensures that infant's needs for food, warmth, and dryness are met before sleep	Does not attend to infant's needs for food, warmth, and dryness before sleep
Perception	
Demonstrates realistic perception of infant's condition in accordance with medical and nursing diagnoses	Shows unrealistic perception of infant's condition
Has realistic expectations for infant	Demonstrates unrealistic expectations of infant
Recognizes infant's unfolding skills or behavior	Has no awareness of infant's development
Shows realistic perception of own mothering behavior	Shows unrealistic perception of own mothering behavior
Initiative	
Shows initiative in attempts to manage infant's problems, including actively seeking information about infants	Shows no initiative in attempts to meet infant's needs or to manage problems; does not follow through with plans
Recreation	
Provides positive outlets for own recreation or relaxation	Does not provide positive outlets for own recreation or relaxation
Interaction with other children	
Demonstrates positive interaction with other children in home	Demonstrates hostile-aggressive interaction with other children in home
Mothering role	
Expresses satisfaction with mothering	Expresses dissatisfaction with mothering

From Mercer R: *Parent-infant interaction.* In Sonstegard L et al, editors: *Women's health: childbearing,* vol 2, New York, 1982, Grune & Stratton.
*These describe paternal as well as maternal behaviors.

Critical Thinking Exercises

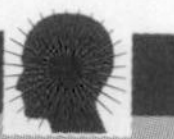

DISTURBED MOTHER-INFANT RELATIONSHIP

You admire Baby Boy Cortez' large brown eyes and button nose. Ms. Cortez, his mother, suddenly bursts into tears and says, "He looks just like Antonio, his father! I am so mad at Antonio because he told me that he didn't want this baby. I haven't seen him in months."

How would you respond to this mother? How would your response be different if:

1. **The baby had a physical anomaly?**
2. **The baby were critically ill?**
3. **The mother's behavior were warm and accepting?**

ents see the child as unattractive. The child-caring tasks of bathing and changing are viewed with disgust or annoyance. There is a lack of discrimination in responding to the infant's signals relative to hunger, fatigue, need for soothing or stimulating speech, and need for comforting body or eye contact. The parents of these infants often show excessive concern regarding the health of their child and cannot distinguish between the expected minor illnesses of childhood and serious disabilities. It appears difficult for them to accept their child as healthy and happy.

Interpretation of infant behavior. The parents' view of and response to their infant is profoundly affected by their interpretation of his or her behavior. Mothers and fathers often make value judgments about their infant's behavior and respond as though the baby had either praised or criticized them. They may see their infant as good and themselves as good parents if their infant sleeps and eats well, cries very little, and is easily consoled. In contrast, parents of babies who cry excessively, are difficult to feed, exhibit an apathetic affect, or stiffen when held may feel that the baby is bad and see themselves as failures. If parents can be helped to see newborn behavior not as bad or good but as their baby's unique way of communicating personality, needs, and desires, they will be well on the way to developing a healthy parent-child relationship.

Family structure and functioning. Another important component of the psychosocial assessment is looking at the family composition and functioning. A woman's adjustment to her role as mother is affected greatly by her relationships with her partner, her mother and other relatives, and other children. Nurses can help to ease the new mother's return home by assessing for conflicts likely to occur among family members and helping the woman to plan strategies for dealing with those problems before discharge. For example, couples may have very different ideas about parenting. Dealing with the stresses of sibling rivalry and unsolicited grandparent advice can also affect the woman's transition to motherhood. Only by asking about other nuclear and extended family members can the nurse discover potential problems in family relationships and help to plan workable solutions for them. Box 19-5 lists some signs that indicate a need for further assessment.

Impact of cultural diversity. The final component of a complete psychosocial assessment is the woman's cultural beliefs and values. Much of a woman's behavior during the postpartum period is strongly influenced by her cultural background. Nurses are likely to come into contact with women from many different countries and cultures. The nurse must remember that all cultures have developed safe and satisfying methods of caring for new mothers and babies. Only by understanding and respecting the values and beliefs of each woman can the nurse design a plan of care to meet her individual needs.

BOX 19-5 Signs of Potential Complications

PSYCHOSOCIAL NEEDS

Unable or unwilling to discuss the labor and birth experience
Refers to self as ugly and useless
Excessively preoccupied with self (body image)
Markedly depressed
Lacks a support system
Partner and/or other family members react negatively to the baby
Refuses to interact with or care for baby (e.g., does not name baby, does not want to hold or feed baby, is upset by vomiting and wet or dirty diapers)
Expresses disappointment over baby's sex
Sees baby as messy or unattractive
Baby reminds mother of family member or friend she does not like

Following is an example of one "clash of cultures." The nurse in this case was able to take this information and modify her plan of care to make it culturally congruent, and therefore more satisfying, for the woman.

> A Vietnamese woman who had been in the United States for 4 years requested rooming-in facilities after childbirth. Instead of participating in the care of her infant, she refused to do so, remained in bed, wore a woolen cap, and appeared distressed and angry. The staff were puzzled and upset by her behavior. One nurse decided to put newly learned concepts concerning cross-cultural nursing into effect. She began by praising the woman's ability to speak English and, after eliciting a smile, remarked, "Every country has developed good ways to look after mothers and babies. Would you tell me about the care in Vietnam?" There was an immediate response. The woman explained that in her country women remained in bed for 10 days after the birth and the biggest danger to their health was getting a cold. The baby was kept in the room with the mother, but either a grandmother or nurse took complete charge of the care. With this understanding, the nurse was able to develop a plan of care that was satisfactory to both the mother and the staff.

Nursing Diagnoses

After analyzing the data obtained during the assessment process, the nurse establishes nursing diagnoses to provide a guide for planning care. Examples of nursing diagnoses related to psychosocial issues that are commonly established for the postpartum patient include the following:

- Altered family processes related to
  - Unexpected birth of twins
- Impaired verbal communication related to
  - Patient's hearing impairment
  - Nurse's language not the same as patient's
- Altered parenting related to
  - Long, difficult labor
  - Postpartum pain or fatigue
  - Disappointment in sex or appearance of newborn
- Knowledge deficit related to
  - Meaning of infant behavioral cues
  - Holding, cuddling, interacting with infant
- Anxiety related to
  - Newness of parenting role, sibling rivalry, or response of grandparent
- Risk for situational low self-esteem related to
  - Lack of knowledge of infant characteristics or of care-giving skills
  - Grandparent responses
  - Using analgesics during labor
- Anxiety related to
  - Insufficient knowledge about contraception and resumption of sexual activity

Expected Outcomes

The psychosocial care plan for the postpartum woman includes all family members. The postnatal period is a crucial one for the family because it contains the potential for crisis in family adjustment. Developing a plan of care that recognizes family strengths and provides support for overcoming family weaknesses does much to help family members take on new tasks and responsibilities.

Cultural issues must also be considered when planning care. It is important that nurses not use their own cultural beliefs as a framework for care. Although the beliefs and behaviors of other cultures may be different, they can be encouraged as long as the mother wants to conform to them and she and the baby suffer no ill effects. On the other hand, the nurse should never assume that a mother wishes to participate in the behaviors practiced by a particular cultural group simply because she is a member of that culture. Many young women who are first-generation or second-generation Americans follow their cultural traditions only when other family members are present.

Non-Western cultures hold two general beliefs about the postpartum period. The first is that new mothers have a body imbalance between heat and cold. The Chinese, for example, believe that a postpartum woman's blood is weak (cold) and thickened (Ludman et al, 1989). Specific foods should be eaten and certain practices followed to restore the balance (Ahumada, 1991; D'Avanzo, 1992; Geissler, 1994; Horn, 1990; Mattson, 1995; Park and Peterson, 1991). The second general belief is that mother and baby remain in an unclean state for a period of several weeks after birth. During this time, mothers are to remain secluded, with limited activity. This period often ends with a ritual cleansing ceremony that restores purity (Geissler, 1994; Horn, 1990). Women who have immigrated to the United States or other Western nations without their extended families may not have much help at home, making it difficult for them to observe these activity restrictions (Park and Peterson, 1991). The Cultural Considerations box above lists some common cultural beliefs about the postpartum period.

Cultural Considerations

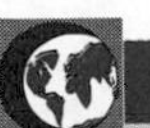

SOME CULTURAL BELIEFS ABOUT THE POSTPARTUM PERIOD AND CONTRACEPTION

Postpartum care

Chinese, Mexican, Korean, and Southeast Asian women may wish to eat only warm foods and drink hot drinks to replace blood loss and to restore the balance of hot and cold in their bodies. These women may also wish to stay warm and avoid bathing, exercising, and washing their hair for 7 to 30 days after childbirth. Self-care may not be a priority; care by family members is preferred. These women may wear abdominal binders. They may prefer not to give their babies colostrum. Other family members may care for the baby.

Haitian women may request to take the placenta home to bury or burn.

Muslim women follow strict religious laws concerning modesty and diet. A Muslim woman must keep her hair, body, arms to the wrist, and legs to the ankles covered at all times. She cannot be alone in the presence of a man other than her husband or a male relative. Observant Muslims will not eat pork or pork products. They are obligated to eat meat slaughtered according to Islamic law (halal meat), but will usually accept kosher meat, seafood, or a vegetarian diet if halal meat is not available.

Contraception

Birth control is government mandated in *China*. Most Chinese women have an IUD inserted after the birth of their first child.

Saudi Arabian women usually do not practice birth control.

Mexican women usually choose the rhythm method because most are Catholic.

(East) Indian men are encouraged to have a voluntary sterilization by vasectomy.

Muslim couples may practice contraception by mutual consent, as long as its use is not harmful to the woman. Acceptable contraceptive methods include foam and condoms, the diaphragm, and natural family planning.

As in planning care to meet physiologic needs, standardized care plans must be adapted to meet the specific needs of individual families. The nurse evaluates continuously and is ready to change the plan if necessary.

Expected psychosocial outcomes during the postpartum period are based on the nursing diagnoses identified for the individual woman and her family. Examples of common expected outcomes are included in the following list. The woman (family) will:

1. Demonstrate self-confidence in providing essential newborn care
2. Identify measures that promote a healthy personal adjustment in the postpartum period
3. Maintain healthy family functioning based on cultural norms and personal expectations

Plan of Care and Implementation

The nurse functions in the roles of teacher, encourager, and supporter rather than doer while implementing the psychosocial care plan for a postpartum patient. Implementation of the psychosocial care plan involves carrying out specific activities to achieve the expected outcome of care planned for each individual patient.

Parental attachment, bonding, and acquaintance. Parental attachment is the parents' affectional tie to the fetus and infant (Walker, 1992). Bonding is considered as a sensitive period early in the postnatal period in which parents form an emotional tie with their infant (Klaus and Kennell, 1982). Attachment and bonding are sometimes used interchangeably.

The process of attachment begins in pregnancy and continues in the postbirth period (Mercer, 1995). Attachment is developed and maintained by proximity and interaction; the parent becomes acquainted with the infant, identifies the infant as an individual, and claims the infant as a member of the family. Attachment is facilitated by feedback, that is, social, verbal and nonverbal responses, real or perceived, that indicate acceptance of one partner by the other. Attachments occur through a mutually satisfying experience. A mother commented on her son's grasp reflex, "I put my finger in his hand, and he grabbed right on. It is just a reflex, I know, but it felt good anyway" (Fig. 19-6).

An important part of attachment is acquaintance (Klaus and Kennell, 1983). Parents use eye contact (Fig. 19-7), touching, talking, and exploring as they become acquainted during the immediate postbirth period. Adoptive parents undergo the same process when they first meet their new child. During this period, families engage in identification of the new baby, or "claiming." The child is first identified in terms of "likeness" to other family members, then in terms of "differences," and finally in terms of "uniqueness." Parents make comments such as "He's the image of his father" and "His toes are shaped just like mine." Other parents may react negatively with comments such as "Be quiet, you've been enough trouble already." They may interpret the infant's normal responses as being negative toward them.

How competent parents perceive themselves to be is an important predictor for both mothers and fathers (Mercer and Ferketich, 1990). Nurses can play an important role in facilitating parental attachment by creating an environment that enhances positive parent-infant contact. They can assist the parents to be aware of infant responses and the ability to communicate. They can bolster parents' self-confidence and lend ego support as parents attempt to become competent and loving in their role. Nursing considerations for fostering maternal-infant bonding among special populations are presented in the Cultural Considerations box on p. 507.

When parents are unable or unwilling to have early contact with their infant, the delay may affect the infant's future well-being. When there is prolonged separation as a result of prematurity or illness, there is an increased percentage of neglect, abuse, and failure to thrive among these infants (Klaus and Kennell, 1982). Indifferent, neglecting patterns of maternal care are related to insecure, anxious-avoidant attachments in infants; avoidant attachments in infancy are associated with other noncompliance and antisocial behaviors in children (Shaw and Bell, 1993). Extended contact with their infant should be available for all parents, but especially for those at risk for parenting inadequacies (Box 19-6). Rooming-in or mother-baby couplet care are methods of family-centered care that promote extended contact. Fathers, siblings, and grandparents are encouraged to visit and become acquainted with the infant. Partners are encouraged to take an active role in newborn care.

Communication between parent and child. Formation of the parent-infant relationship is strengthened through the use of sensual responses or abilities by both partners in the parent-child interaction. The sensual responses and abilities used in communication between parent and child include the following: eye-to-eye contact, touch, voice, and odor. The nurse should keep in mind that there may be cultural variations in the behaviors described.

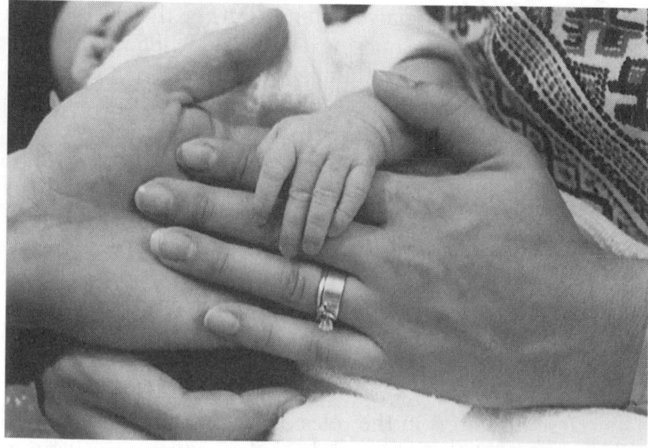

Fig. 19-6 Hands.

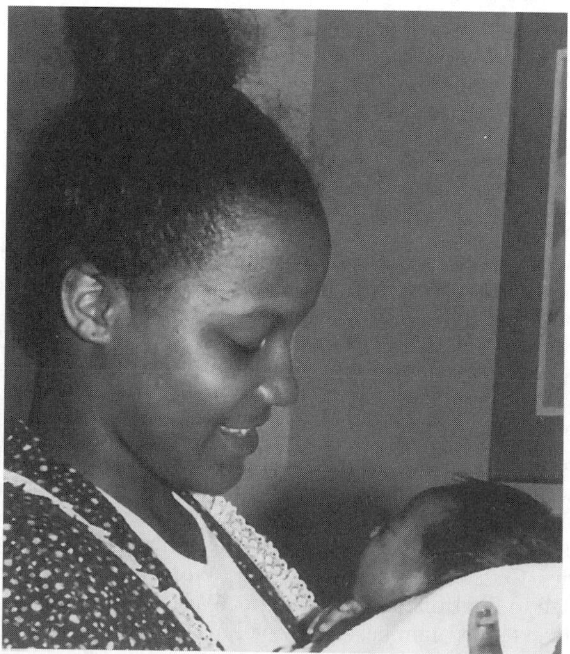

Fig. 19-7 Mother and baby make eye contact in en face position.

Eye-to-eye contact. Interest in having eye contact is demonstrated repeatedly. Parents spend considerable time stimulating their babies to open their eyes and look at them. Mothers remark that once their babies have looked at them, they feel much closer to them. In the Anglo-American culture, eye contact appears to have a cementing effect on the development of a trusting relationship and is an important factor in human relationships at all ages. In other cultures, eye-to-eye contact may be perceived differently. For example, sustained direct eye contact is considered by Mexicans to be rude, immodest, and dangerous for some. This danger may be the "mal ojo" (evil eye), resulting from excessive admiration (Geissler, 1994). As newborns become able to sustain eye contact, parents and child spend time gazing at one another, often in the en face position (a face-to-face position in which the parent's face and the infant's face are approximately 8 inches apart and on the same plane) (Fig. 19-7). Immediately after birth, lights can be dimmed so that the infant's eyes open. Instillation of prophylactic antibiotic ointment in the infant's eyes can be withheld until the infant and parents have some time together in the first hour after birth.

Touch. Touch is used extensively by parents and other caregivers as a means of becoming acquainted with the newborn. Mothers reach for their infants as soon as they are born and the cord is cut. They begin to explore their head and extremities with their fingertips, use the palm to caress the trunk, and eventually enfold the infant in their arms. They use gentle stroking and patting and rubbing to soothe the in-

Cultural Considerations

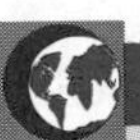

NURSING CONSIDERATIONS TO FOSTER BONDING AMONG SPECIFIC POPULATIONS

Women in economically disadvantaged situations

Low-income mothers may need to contend with stressors that distract them from developing a relationship with their babies. Inability to pay for infant supplies or child care, chaotic home situations, and worry over eligibility for social and health care services deplete these women's psychic energy.

Nurses need to conduct nonjudgmental, individual assessments of resources and social networks to avoid inaccurate and stereotypic assumptions. Nurses can help economically disadvantaged mothers access social services, such as the Women, Infants, and Children (WIC) program and Medicaid. For mothers whose home environments provide little or no support and multiple stressors, early discharge may not be optimal. Nurses can advocate for longer hospital stays for these mothers when the hospital environment is more conducive to bonding.

Economically disadvantaged mothers, especially adolescents, are not as likely to be aware of the benefits of bonding or to be knowledgeable of normal infant behaviors. These women may not be aware of maternity care options, such as rooming-in, or may be less assertive in asking for such options. The nurse needs to be a client educator and advocate, explaining the choices and the potential benefits. The nurse should ensure a supportive, encouraging environment that will help mothers engage in positive interactions with their infants. By use of the Brazelton Neonatal Behavioral Assessment Scale, the nurse can capture the mother's attention with a mother-infant interactional experience and, at the same time, increase the mother's knowledge of infant behavior. Written material can be provided after the assessment to reinforce the behavioral concepts.

Women of varying ethnic and cultural groups

Childbearing practices and rituals of other cultures may not be congruent with standard practices associated with bonding in the Anglo-American culture. For example, Chinese families traditionally use extended family members to care for the newborn so that the mother can rest and recover, especially after a cesarean birth. Some Native American, Asian, and Hispanic women do not initiate breastfeeding until their breast milk comes in. Haitian families do not name their babies until after the confinement month. Amount of eye contact varies among cultures, too. Yup'ik Eskimo mothers almost always position their babies so that eye contact can be made.

Nurses should become knowledgeable of the childbearing beliefs and practices of diverse cultural and ethnic groups. Because individual cultural variations exist within groups, nurses need to clarify with the client and family members or friends what cultural norms the client follows. Incorrect judgments may be made about mother-infant bonding if nurses do not practice culturally sensitive care.

Modified from Geissler E: *Pocket guide to cultural assessment,* St. Louis, 1994, Mosby; Symanski M: Maternal-infant bonding, *J Nurse Midwife* 37:675, 1992; Tedder J: Using the Braselton Neonatal Assessment Scale to facilitate the parent-infant relationship in a primary care setting, *Nurse Pract* 16(3):26, 1991.

BOX 19-6

Preventing Socioemotional Problems in Children Through Promotion of Attachment

Mary St. Jonn Seed

A current model using attachment theory is being tested to explore whether certain negative parental emotions expressed to an infant during the first 6 months of life are placing the child at risk for developing insecure attachments and later behavioral and emotional problems. Attachment to a significant other provides the foundation for the child's socioemotional development. Without attachment, the infant later approaches the world insecurely, without confidence and with great anxiety. Expressed Emotion (EE) is a measure of the emotional attitude expressed by an individual toward a family member with mental illness. The Camberwell Family Interview (Brown, Rutter, 1966) was developed to measure the EE constructs: hostility, criticism, overinvolvement, warmth, and positive remarks in families caring for schizophrenic adult children. Hostility/criticism and overinvolvement expressed by a family member toward the child have emerged as having the most predictive power in the relapse or recurrence of mental health symptoms. Researchers are exploring the effects of parental EE during the early development of the infant. If the EE measurement can be used to identify families at risk for developing unhealthy attachment behaviors, interventions can be designed to prevent emotional/behavioral problems in children. The early identification of a verbal indicator such as hostility and criticism expressed by a parent toward an infant could enhance the nurse's ability to detect those families at risk for poor socioemotional outcomes in their children. Nursing is in the prime position to provide early interventions that promote secure attachments in the nursery after the infant's birth and during well-baby visits in the first year of life. Research programs aimed at identifying interventions to assist parents during this important period in the development of infant attachment are imperative to prevent mental health disorders in children.

fants. Infants pat the mother's breast as they nurse. Increasing sensitivity to the infant's like or dislike of types of touch brings parents closer to their babies. Variations in touching behaviors have been noted in mothers from some cultural groups. For example, minimal touching and cuddling is a traditional Southeast Asian practice thought to protect the child from evil spirits (Galanti, 1991).

Voice. The shared response of parents and infant to each other's voice is remarkable. Parents wait tensely for the first cry. Once that cry has reassured them of the baby's health, they begin comforting behaviors. Infants respond to higher pitched voices and can distinguish their mother's voice from others soon after birth. Infants use their cries to signal hunger, pain, boredom, and tiredness. With experience, parents learn to distinguish such cries.

Odor. Parents and infants respond to each other's odor. Mothers comment on the smell of their babies when first born and have noted that each child has a unique odor; they can distinguish the smell of their own baby from other babies (Porter, Cernoch, and Perry, 1983). Infants learn rapidly to distinguish the odor of their own mother's breast milk (Stainton, 1985).

Entrainment. Newborns move in time with the structure of adult speech. They move their arms and legs in rhythm with voices. These movements are associated with culturally patterned rhythms of speech long before the infant learns to use spoken language to communicate. The shared rhythm acts to give the parent positive feedback and to establish a positive setting for effective communication.

Biorhythmicity. One of the newborn's tasks is to establish a personal rhythm or biorhythmicity. Parents help in this process by giving consistent, loving care and by using their infant's alert state to develop responsive behaviors and thereby increase social interactions and opportunities for learning.

Reciprocity and synchrony. Reciprocity is a type of body movement or behavior that provides the observer with cues. The observer/receiver interprets the cues and responds to them. Reciprocity often takes several weeks to develop with a new baby. For example, the newborn fusses and cries, the mother responds by picking up and cradling the baby, the baby becomes quiet and alert and establishes eye contact, and the mother vocalizes, sings, and coos while the child maintains eye contact. The child then averts his or her eyes and yawns; the mother decreases active response. Should the parent continue to stimulate the infant, the baby may become fussy and cry. Synchrony refers to the "fit" between the infant's cues and the parent's response. When parent and infant experience a synchronous interaction, it is mutually rewarding. It takes time for parents to correctly interpret the infant's cues. Parents may need assistance and use trial and error to develop synchrony.

Maternal adjustment. Three phases are evident as the mother adjusts to the parental role. These phases of maternal adjustment are characterized by behaviors that progress from dependent to dependent-independent to interdependent.

Dependent phase. During the first 1 to 2 days after childbirth, the mother's dependency needs predominate. To the extent that these needs are met by others, the mother is able to divert her psychologic energy to her child rather than to herself. She needs "mothering" to "mother." Rubin (1961) described this as the taking-in phase—a time when nurturing and protective care are required by the new mother. In Rubin's classic description the taking-in phase lasted 2 to 3 days. A more recent study by Ament (1990) supported Rubin's work, except women were now found to move more rapidly through the taking-in phase. For 24 hours after the birth, mature and apparently healthy women rely on others to respond to their needs for comfort, rest, nourishment, and closeness to their families and newborn.

This dependent phase is a time of great excitement, and most parents are extremely talkative. They need to verbalize their experience of pregnancy and birth. Focusing on, analyzing, and accepting these experiences help the parents move on to the next phase. Some parents are able to use staff members or other mothers as an "audience." Others are more comfortable talking with family and friends about their pregnancy and birth experience.

Because anxiety and preoccupation with her new role often narrow a mother's perceptions, information may need to be repeated. The new mother may require reminders to rest or, conversely, to ambulate enough to promote recovery. Hospital or birth center routines may not necessarily be an important priority to the new mother; she may take showers when examinations are scheduled and be involved in a telephone conversation rather than "being ready" for the baby. Regulations seem cumbersome, and sometimes mothers and their families have difficulty accepting rules that interfere with their needs to share reactions about their child.

Physical discomfort from an episiotomy, sore nipples, hemorrhoids, afterpains, and occasionally a sprained coccygeal joint can interfere with the mother's need for rest and relaxation. The selective use of comfort measures and medication depends on the nurse. Many women hesitate to ask for medication, believing that any pain they experience is normal and to be expected; few have a knowledge of how to use heat or cold to relieve local pain.

Dependent-independent phase. If the mother has received adequate nurturing in the first few hours or days, by the second or third day her desire for independent action reasserts itself. In the dependent-independent phase, the mother alternates between a need for extensive nurturing and acceptance by others and the desire to "take charge" once again. She responds enthusiastically to opportunities to learn and practice the care of the baby or, if she is an accomplished mother, to carry out or direct this care. Rubin (1961) described this phase as taking-hold, noting that it lasts approximately 10 days. Ament (1990) found that contemporary women do exhibit taking-hold behaviors sooner than the women in Rubin's study.

During this dependent-independent phase the majority of mothers are discharged home. Contemporary mothers are experiencing short hospital stays, ranging from 6 to 48 hours for low-risk uncomplicated births and 48 to 72 hours for a cesarean birth. Once home, mothers must continue to cope with physical adaptations and psychologic adjustments.

Interdependent phase. In the interdependent phase, interdependent behavior reasserts itself, and the mother and her family move forward as a system with interacting members. The relationship of the partners, although altered by the introduction of a child, resumes many of its former characteristics. A primary need is to establish a life-style that includes, but in some respects excludes, the child. The couple must share interests and activities that are adult in scope.

The couple may begin to engage in sexual intercourse by the third or fourth week after the child is born; some begin earlier, as soon as it can be accomplished without discomfort, depending on factors such as timing, amount of vaginal dryness, and whether the mother is breastfeeding. Sexual intimacy enhances the adult aspect of the family, and the adult pair shares a closeness denied to other family members. Many new fathers speak of the alienation experienced when they observe the intimate mother-child relationship, and some are frank in expressing feelings of jealousy toward the infant (Dumas, 1990). The resumption of the sexual relationship seems to bring the parents' relationship back into focus.

The interdependent phase, termed the **letting-go phase,** is often stressful for the parental pair. Interests and needs often diverge during this time. Women and their partners must resolve the effects on their relationship of their individual roles related to childrearing, homemaking, and career. Mothers (and fathers) may become more traditional in an effort to adapt during parenthood transition, with less traditional women reporting more family disorganization months into parenthood (Tomlinson and Irwin, 1993).

Little is known about postpartum maternal adjustment in the lesbian couple. Wismont and Reame (1989) discussed the literature on lesbian childbirth experience and developmental tasks. Health counselors of lesbian women reported that gay mothers expect a great deal of emotional support and nurturance from their partners. One might postulate that lesbian partners could understand this need from a female perspective and thus be more effective in meeting the mother's increased need for cuddling, holding, and fondling. However, research must be done on how pregnancy and childbirth affect the sexual relationship of lesbian couples. Some gay partners reported a deep involvement with the pregnancy as a result of the love and empathy that they share with their pregnant partners. Other gay partners expressed feelings of jealousy, ambivalence, and doubt.

Role expectations may be a significant issue for the lesbian partner, with difficulties focusing on conflicts about child care responsibilities and, more basically, "Who's Mom?" Feeling that she has no legal tie or obligation to the infant may hinder the partner's ability to form a parental role. Lesbian couples face strong social sanctions regarding their pregnancy and parenting. Their families may not have resolved the initial dismay and guilt over learning of their daughters' homosexuality. The family may disagree with the lesbian couple's decision to parent. Because family support may be limited, the couple attempts to realign with more supportive social groups, lesbian and/or heterosexual.

Paternal adjustment. First-time fathers perceive the first 4 to 10 weeks of parenthood in much the same way that mothers do; that is, as a time characterized by uncertainty, increased responsibility, disruption of sleep, and inability to control the time needed to care for the infant and reestablish the marital dyad (Dumas, 1990). Fathers express concern about (1) decreased attention from their wives relative to the marital relationship, (2) lack of wives' recognition of the fathers' desire to participate in decision making for the infant, and (3) limited time available to establish a relationship with their infants. These concerns can precipitate feelings of jealousy of the infant. Discussing feelings with their wives and becoming more involved with their infants and wives can help reduce fathers' jealous feelings. A consistent finding in the literature is that fathers who feel affection and support in the relationships with their wives or mates are more involved with infant care, and their involvement is more responsive, affectionate, and developmentally stimulating (Broom, 1994; Edwards, 1990; Nugent, 1991).

Father-infant relationship. In American culture the newborn has been found to have a powerful impact on the father. Fathers have demonstrated intense involvement with their babies (Fig. 19-8). The term used for the father's absorption, preoccupation, and interest in the infant is *engrossment.* Characteristics of engrossment include some of the sensual responses relating to touch and eye-to-eye contact that have already been discussed. The father's keen awareness of features both unique and similar to himself is another characteristic related to the father's need to claim the infant. An outstanding response is one of strong attraction to the newborn. Much time is spent "communicating" with the infant and taking delight in the infant's response to the father. Fathers feel a sense of increased self-esteem, pride, and feeling bigger, more mature, and older after seeing their baby for the first time (Fig 19-8).

Much must still be learned about the relationships between fathers and their offspring. The majority of studies on fathers of infants have focused on the amount of time fathers spend

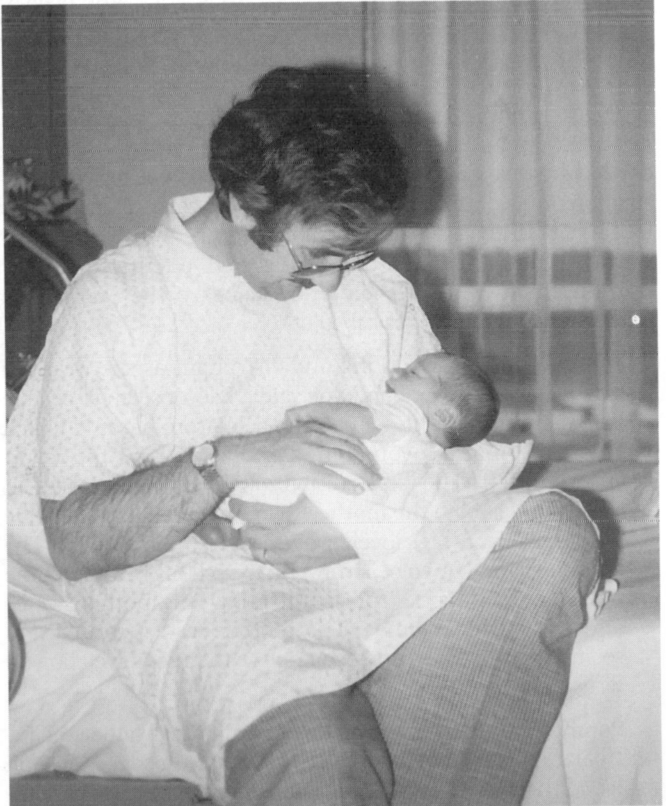

Fig. 19-8 Engrossment. Father absorbed in looking at his newborn daughter. (Courtesy Lienne Edwards, Charlotte, NC.)

and what fathers do when they are with their infants. Two consistent findings are that (1) fathers spend less time than mothers with infants, and (2) fathers' interactions with infants tend to be characterized by stimulating social play rather than caretaking.

The most influential factor on competent parenting was the one related to fathers' knowledge of infant development. Men entering parenthood with knowledge and realistic expectations about infant capabilities may be better able to cope successfully with the demands of a young infant and to develop nurturing relationships with their infants. For nurses, dissemination of information can be a highly cost-effective intervention. Successful use of videos on infant cognitive and social capabilities and on early infant care and stimulation, as well as direct parent teaching methods such as exposure to newborn assessments, has been documented (Koniak-Griffin et al, 1992; McBride, 1992; Tedder, 1991; Wolfson, Lacks, and Futteman, 1992).

Promotion of parenting skills. New parents may feel overwhelmed at the prospect of caring for a helpless, demanding newborn. Many women and men grow up with little chance to gain knowledge and experience in infant care. In our mobile society, extended family members such as aunts, uncles, and grandparents often live too far away to provide much support and assistance. Many parents hesitate to seek help from professionals, friends, or family members or feel that they have no one to call on should they wish to do so. One of the main concepts for the nurse to stress is that parenthood is a learned role. As with any other learned role, parenthood takes time to master, improves with experience, and evolves gradually and continually as the needs of the parents and child change. Parents first become acquainted with their new baby as the nurse performs a physical examination and describes any normal variations present. At this time the nurse can also discuss the baby's behavior, pointing out normal characteristics such as activity states and reflexes. Demonstrations and discussions of basic infant care skills such as feeding, bathing, and diaper changing are also included in nursing care. Through the loving and attentive manner nurses exhibit while providing physical care, they act as role models. As one nurse described it:

> I found the mother crying and distraught as she wrapped and unwrapped her baby. She said, "I don't seem to be able to do anything right." I took the baby from her and talked to him. "What are you doing to your mother? You've got her all upset!" The baby alerted to my voice and looked at me. Then I said to the mother, "Now, you talk to him." She said, "You're a big, lovely boy; don't cry so much." The baby, hearing her voice, promptly turned his head from me to look at her. I said, "You see, he knows his mother's voice and prefers it to mine." The mother was surprised and seemed very pleased and excited. We then reviewed how to wrap a baby snugly.

Parents should be given the opportunity to practice the infant care skills demonstrated by the nurse. Recognition and praise of their successes increase the parents' feelings of competence and control in their caretaking skills.

Because mothers may be discharged within 24 hours for a vaginal birth and 48 hours after giving birth by cesarean, teaching often takes place during a period when the mother may have difficulty absorbing a great deal of information. Ament (1990) suggested that the presentation of only vital highlights may be more practical during the early puerperium. Telephone warmlines to hospital, clinic, or physician's office; home visits; books; pamphlets; and videotapes are all excellent resources that can be most helpful to parents after hospital discharge. Several well-done, inexpensive videotapes on mother, baby, and child care are listed in the bibliography at the end of this chapter.

Coping strategies for new parents

Healthy personal adjustment. Because hospital stays are usually short, parents leave the protective environment of the hospital in the "honeymoon" period of parenthood. The realities of recovery and the parenting role become evident quickly, especially for those without assistance in the home. Women may misjudge the actual amount of physical and emotional energy that they possess and that care of an infant requires. They may expect to resume tasks too soon and feel discouraged when unable to do so.

Tulman and Fawcett (1991) interviewed 96 mothers of healthy, full-term infants about their recovery from childbirth when the babies were 6 months of age. Almost half the women had found the first 6 months after childbirth to be more difficult than they had expected. Perhaps providing pregnant women with more information on life-style changes after giving birth would help to ease their transition to motherhood.

Many women experience **postpartum blues,** feelings of sadness and depression sometimes called the "baby blues," in the immediate postpartum period. Symptoms begin 2 or 3 days after childbirth and usually disappear within 1 or 2 weeks. The woman experiences a letdown feeling accompanied by irritability. She may cry easily, lose her appetite, have trouble sleeping, and feel anxious. Mothers of preterm infants have been found initially to experience higher levels of anxiety and depression (Gennaro, 1988). Postpartum blues are "normal"; severe depression or outright psychosis occurs rarely. However, when symptoms do not disappear after a week or so, the family should seek professional help (see Chapter 11).

The nurse can best assist the woman and family by assuring them that this depression is both normal and temporary. Recognizing the state, helping the woman verbalize her feelings, and providing support and understanding are important nursing actions. The nurse can explain to the woman and family that the depression may be caused by hormonal changes, emotional reaction to the role transition, discomfort, or fatigue. Setting up tasks the woman can accomplish easily and successfully are interventions that can help counteract the feelings of depression. It is also important to encourage adequate rest and nutrition. Because the woman will likely continue to experience symptoms after discharge, the nurse should always include the woman's partner in all interventions to support the woman and to express concerns. Many communities now have support groups for postpartum depression. Referral to such a group may be very helpful for providing ongoing support.

Adjusting to a new family member. The birth of a baby causes enormous, permanent changes in family relationships.

Patient Teaching

COPING MECHANISMS FOR NEW FAMILIES

- Set priorities for tasks. Many tasks can be left for a later period or done by others. Be firm about not taking on extra tasks for family, friends, or community. Try not to schedule a move to a new location soon after giving birth.
- Do not become overly concerned with appearances—tidiness in the home is not as important as time spent with the family. Taking up the role of "super housekeeper" can be postponed until other adjustments are made. Sometimes new mothers become overburdened with visits from relatives eager "to take over the baby." Husbands or partners can help redirect these well-meaning people toward helping with the housework and cooking. This leaves the parent free to interact with the child.
- Get plenty of rest and sleep; rearrange schedules if necessary. Because naps may not be possible if there are other children in the family, going to bed early is recommended; let friends know when to visit.
- Do not undertake the care of another incapacitated relative at this point; such responsibilities should be undertaken by other family members.
- Arrange for some time away from the baby; enlist the help of friends, family, or others for baby-sitting. Relaxation for parents is necessary. Baby-sitting, if at all possible, must be planned and a regular schedule developed. This includes time off during the day so that you can get away from the home and its responsibilities. In some localities, churches or other agencies have developed programs attuned to the needs of mothers. The young children are cared for while the mothers take part in activities with other mothers. These activities help them establish relationships with others who also are involved in the care of young children. A mutual sharing of successes and failures in this regard helps a new mother maintain a feeling of equilibrium. At the very least you need to plan to get out of the house at least once each day. Access to a car and being able to drive are assets. Taking the baby out for a walk or shopping helps break up the daily routine.
- Make plans regarding fertility management before intercourse is resumed and the possibility of pregnancy arises.
- Be open in your communication with others. Share incidents of delight or of worry with others. Be open in your requests for assistance or support. Discussions with other mothers are helpful.
- Learn what health facilities are available, such as well-baby centers, immunization clinics, mother-infant classes (e.g., exercise, massage), and how to get in touch with the physician or nurse. If you have questions, remember that the hospital is open all day and night, and you can call the emergency or maternity department at any time.
- Prepare for returning to work. Most women are physically able to return to work by the end of the sixth week. If plans for child care were not in place before the birth, adjustments for child care must be made. Ideally a substitute parent would be one who could come to the home and provide love and care for the child. Some parents are fortunate enough to have grandparents or other relatives willing and able to fill such a role. Others must take the child to another person's home or a day care center early in the morning and pick the child up at night. The care provided by day care centers is needed by some children whose mothers must work to help support them or who are the sole support of the child. For families who require this type of service, assistance in locating such help can be obtained from the local health department and parent referrals. Unfortunately there are not enough quality places available for all children requiring day care. Arrangements for day care usually need to be made before the baby is born.
- Include the father/partner in caregiving activities.

Couples often come from very different families of origin and have conflicting expectations regarding family roles. Working through these differences in beliefs and values occurs over time as the family grows and matures. Open communication related to feelings should be encouraged between women and their partners.

Most couples have fantasized during pregnancy about how their new baby will behave. New parents can find it disconcerting to discover that their baby's behavior is not at all what they expected. Some babies cry more than expected or do not seem satisfied with their feedings. Many babies have fussy periods, often late in the afternoon or around dinner time, when they are nearly impossible to console. On the other hand, some babies are quieter and sleep more than their parents had anticipated. The Patient Teaching box above presents practical suggestions for families adjusting to life with a new baby.

Grandparents/extended family. Grandparents and other extended family members often provide much needed emotional support for new families. In addition, they can assist with housework, meals, babysitting with older children, and the new baby. Being able to verbalize experiences with others who are interested and experienced also tends to reassure the new mother. A mother, in discussing visits by the family to see the new baby, commented as follows:

> I want the family to come. You people praise him so and think he is the most wonderful baby. All my friends have their own babies and are too busy trying to get compliments for them to give us any. All babies need aunties and grandmothers!

Grandparents especially often feel the need to advise new parents on caring for the new baby. Many communities now offer grandparent classes, where grandparents can be updated on contemporary thinking. Examples of contemporary child-rearing theories with which grandparents may be unfamiliar are that one cannot spoil a newborn, that breastfeeding is superior to bottle-feeding, and that bright colors are better than pastels for the baby's room because they are more stimulating. Safer infant car seats and disposable diapers are advances that most grandparents readily appreciate.

Siblings. **Sibling rivalry** (competition between brothers and sisters) may require much parental time and attention to be handled successfully. Jealousy is usually present to some extent, even when brothers and sisters have been prepared for the new baby. Older siblings may wonder, "Why would Mommy and Daddy be getting a new baby unless the old one (me!) wasn't good enough?" Acting-out behavior, especially in preschool siblings, is common. Examples of common acting-out behaviors include whining, wetting pants or bed, asking

Home Care

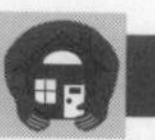

SUGGESTIONS FOR DECREASING SIBLING RIVALRY

Make changes in sleeping arrangements early enough before the birth so that the child does not feel that the new baby is taking over his or her bed.

Make arrangements for the child's care well before the birth and discuss with the child where he or she will stay and who will keep him or her.

Talk about the care that new babies require. Explain that it is okay to sometimes be angry with the baby but never okay to hurt the baby.

Spend special time with the older child. For example, Dad or another relative might take the child on an outing to the park. Mom might be able to read a story or play a game while the new baby is sleeping or feeding.

Expect babyish behavior for a while from younger children, although all children may regress for a short time. The older child needs extra love and attention, not punishment.

Do not let relatives and friends ignore the older child. For example, they might bring a small gift for the older child when giving a present to the new baby.

Let the older child help care for the new baby: sing or talk to the baby, bring Mom a diaper, help pick the clothes the baby wears home from the hospital, help select the baby's name, and help dress, feed, burp, and hold the new baby with assistance.

Do not give too many chores or expect the older child to always be ready and willing to help.

for bottle or breast, acting silly, having temper tantrums, asking if babies die, and suggesting that the baby be returned to the hospital or put in the garbage (see the Home Care box above for suggestions for decreasing sibling rivalry).

Evaluation

Evaluating nursing care in relation to psychosocial concerns can be difficult in the early postpartum period. Parental, infant, and family relationships are still undergoing rapid changes at the time most mothers are discharged home. Healthy family adjustments to the birth of a child will continue in the weeks ahead. However, the nurse can be reasonably assured that care was effective if expected outcomes for care have been met. Families should demonstrate competency in providing essential newborn care, exhibit healthy personal adjustment, and have developed plans for maintaining healthy family functioning that are congruent with their cultural norms and their personal expectations.

DISCHARGE TEACHING

Bridging the gap between hospital and home care requires sensitive and knowledgeable nursing care. Discharge planning begins at the time of admission to the unit and should be reflected in the plan of care developed for each individual patient. For example, a great deal of time during the hospital stay is usually spent in teaching about maternal and newborn care, because all women must be capable of providing basic care for themselves and their infants at the time of discharge. It is also crucial that every woman be taught to recognize the physical signs and symptoms that might indicate problems and how to obtain advice and assistance quickly if these signs appear. Box 19-5 lists several common indications of maternal physical problems in the postpartum period. Before discharge, women also need basic instruction regarding the resumption of intercourse, prescribed medications, routine mother-baby checkups, and contraception.

LEGAL TIP

Early Discharge

Whether or not the woman and her family have chosen early discharge, the nurse and the physician/CNM are held responsible if the woman is discharged before her condition has stabilized within normal limits. If complications occur, the medical and nursing staff could be sued for abandonment.

Just before the time of discharge the nurse reviews the woman's chart (audits the chart) to see that laboratory reports, medications, signatures, and other items are in order. Some hospitals have a checklist to use before the woman's discharge. The nurse verifies that any valuables kept secured during the woman's stay have been returned to her, that she has signed a receipt for them, and that the infant is ready to be discharged.

The nurse is careful not to administer any medication that would make the mother sleepy if she is the one who will be holding the baby on the way out of the hospital. In many instances the woman is seated in a wheelchair and is given the baby to hold. In other instances and depending on hospital protocol, families leave unescorted and ambulatory. The woman's possessions are gathered and taken out with her and her family; usually they are placed on some type of cart or carried by family members. *The woman's and the baby's identification bands are carefully checked.* As the woman and the baby are assisted into the car, the nurse should make sure that there is a car seat in which to secure the baby. Most states in the United States have laws requiring that babies be placed in infant car seats. The nurse is advised to know if there is such a law in the state in which he or she is practicing. Hospital policy may prohibit the nurse from placing the infant in the car seat because of liability concerns if the infant is placed in the seat incorrectly and injury occurs.

Sexual Activity

Many couples resume sexual activity before the traditional postpartum checkup 6 weeks after childbirth; sexual intercourse may resume when the bleeding has stopped. Couples may be anxious about the topic but uncomfortable and unwilling to bring it up. Health care providers often fail to mention the subject; therefore it is important that the nurse discuss the physical and psychologic effects that giving birth can have on sexual activity (see the Home Care box on p. 513). Women who are undecided about contraception at the time of discharge need information about using condoms with foam or creams until the first postpartum checkup.

Home Care

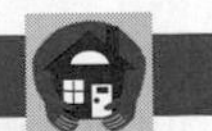

RESUMPTION OF SEXUAL INTERCOURSE

You can safely resume sexual intercourse 3 or 4 weeks after birth if bleeding has stopped and the episiotomy has healed. For the first 6 weeks to 6 months the vagina does not lubricate well because steroid depletion inhibits the vasocongestive response to sexual tension.

Your physiologic reactions to sexual stimulation for the first 3 months after birth are marked by a reduction in both rapidity and intensity of response. Vasocongestion of the labia majora and minora is delayed well into the plateau phase. The walls of the vagina are thin and pink, a condition similar to senile vaginitis. This condition results from the hormonal starvation of the involutional period. Finally, the size of the orgasmic platform and strength of the orgasmic contractions are reduced.

A water-soluble gel, cocoa butter, or a contraceptive cream or jelly might be recommended for lubrication. If some vaginal tenderness is present, your partner can be instructed to insert one or more clean, lubricated fingers into the vagina and rotate them within the vagina to help relax it and to identify possible areas of discomfort. A coital position in which the woman has control of the depth of the penile penetration also is useful. The side-by-side or female-superior position often is recommended.

The presence of the baby influences postbirth lovemaking. Parents hear every sound made by the baby; conversely you may be concerned that the baby hears every sound you make. In either case, any phase of the sexual response cycle may be interrupted by hearing the baby cry or move, leaving both of you frustrated and unsatisfied. In addition, the amount of psychologic energy you expend in child care activities may lead to fatigue.

Some women have reported sexual stimulation to plateau and orgasmic levels when nursing their babies. Although nursing mothers have a longer delay in ovarian steroid production, they often are interested in returning to sexual activity before nonnursing mothers. Nursing mothers also report higher levels of postbirth eroticism.

You should be instructed to perform Kegel exercises to strengthen your pubococcygeal muscle. This muscle is the major sphincter of the pelvis. It is associated with bowel and bladder function and with vaginal perception and response during intercourse.

Prescribed Medications

Many women have at least one medication prescribed for their use after discharge. For example, many physicians/ CNMs routinely have women continue to take their prenatal vitamins and iron during the postpartum period. It is especially important that women who are breastfeeding or who are discharged with a lower than normal hematocrit take these medications as prescribed. Women with extensive episiotomies or vaginal lacerations (third or fourth degree) are usually prescribed stool softeners to take at home. Pain relief medications (analgesics or nonsteroidal antiinflammatory drugs) may be prescribed, especially for women who had cesarean birth. The nurse should make certain that the patient knows the route, dosage, frequency, and common side effects of all ordered medications.

Critical Thinking Exercises

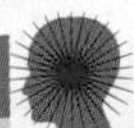

POSTPARTUM CARE

You are assigned to care for Mrs. Morgan, a 40-year-old woman who has just given birth to her first child, an 8 lb, 6 oz girl. Mrs. Morgan attended childbirth classes and intends to breastfeed her baby.

1. Formulate a plan of care for Mrs. Morgan on the basis of the information given.
2. How would your plan of care differ for a patient who:
   a. Already has two children at home?
   b. Is 16 years old and received no prenatal care?

Routine Mother and Baby Checkups

Women who have experienced uncomplicated vaginal births are still commonly scheduled for the traditional 6-week postpartum examination. Women who have had a cesarean birth are often seen in the physician's/CNM's office or clinic 2 weeks after hospital discharge. The time for the follow-up appointment should be included in the discharge instructions. If an appointment for a specific date and time was not made for the woman before leaving the hospital, she should be encouraged to call the physician's/CNM's office or clinic and schedule an appointment herself.

Parents who have not already done so need to make plans for well-child care at the time of discharge. Most offices and clinics like to see newborns for an initial examination within the first week or by 2 weeks of age. Again, if an appointment for a specific date and time was not made for the infant before leaving the hospital, the parents should be encouraged to call the office or clinic right away.

The future of postpartum care may be in the home setting because of the short hospital stay. Nurses may be making assessments and providing such care to postpartum women and their infants. Chapter 21 discusses this aspect of care in the home setting.

Nursing Care Management—Contraception

Contraception is the voluntary prevention of pregnancy and has both individual and social implications. Contraceptive options should be discussed with couples before discharge so that they can make informed decisions about fertility management before resuming sexual activity (Box 19-7). Waiting to discuss contraception at the 6-week checkup may be too late. It is possible, particularly in women who bottle-feed, for ovulation to occur as soon as 1 month after giving birth. A woman who engages in unprotected sex risks the possibility of becoming pregnant much sooner than she planned. Today, couples choosing contraception must be informed about prevention of unintended pregnancy as well as protection against sexually transmitted diseases (STDs).

A multidisciplinary approach to assisting a woman to choose an appropriate contraceptive method and to use it correctly is effective. Nurses, nurse-midwives, nurse practitioners, and other advance practice nurses and physicians have the knowledge and expertise to assist a woman in making de-

BOX 19-7
Methods of Contraception

- Methods available to people without prescription
  - Biologic periodic abstinence: natural family planning
  - Chemical barriers: spermicidal creams and gels; vaginal suppositories, and films
  - Mechanical barrier: condoms or sheaths
- Methods that require periodic medical examination and prescription
  - Hormonal therapy: estrogen or progestogen preparations or a combination of these compounds
  - Mechanical barrier: cervical uterine occlusion by diaphragms or caps
  - Intrauterine contraceptive devices
- Methods that require surgical intervention
  - Female sterilization
  - Male sterilization

cisions about contraception that will satisfy the woman's personal, social, cultural, and interpersonal needs.

Assessment

The woman's knowledge about contraception and her sexual partner's commitment to any particular method are determined. Data are required about the frequency of coitus (once every so often or several times per week), whether the woman has one sexual partner or several, the level of involvement the woman wishes to assume, and her (their) objections to any methods. The woman's level of comfort and willingness to touch her genitals and cervical mucus are assessed. Myths are identified, and religious and cultural factors are determined. The woman's verbal and nonverbal responses to hearing about the various available methods are carefully noted. An individual's reproductive life plan must be considered.*

Informed consent is a vital component in the education of the woman concerning contraception or sterilization. The nurse has the responsibility of documenting information provided and the understanding of that information by the woman. The acronym BRAIDED (NAACOG, 1991) may be useful to ensure that all elements of an informed consent are covered.

LEGAL TIP

Informed Consent

B—Benefits: information about advantages and success rates
R—Risks: information about disadvantages and failure rates
A—Alternatives: information on other methods available
I—Inquiries: opportunity to ask questions
D—Decisions: opportunity to decide or change mind
E—Explanations: information about method and how it is used
D—Documentation: information given and patient's understanding

*When contraception is begun other than immediately postpartum, a history, physical examination, and laboratory tests precede its initiation for some forms. A complete gynecologic examination is done. Menstrual, contraceptive, and obstetric histories are taken.

Nursing Diagnoses

Nursing diagnoses reflect analysis of the assessment findings. Following are examples of nursing diagnoses that may emerge:

- Risk for decisional conflict related to
  - Contraceptive alternatives
- Fear related to
  - Contraceptive method side effects
- Risk for infection related to
  - Being sexually active
  - Use of contraceptive method
- Risk for altered sexuality patterns related to
  - Fear of pain (after childbirth)
  - Fear of pregnancy
- Risk for infection related to
  - Broken skin or mucous membrane secondary to surgery, IUD insertion, hormonal implant
- Pain related to
  - Episiotomy/laceration repair
  - Postoperative recovery after sterilization
- Spiritual distress related to
  - Discrepancy between religious or cultural beliefs and choice of contraception

Expected Outcomes

Planning is a collaborative effort among the woman, her sexual partner (when appropriate), the primary health care provider, and the nurse. The expected outcomes are determined and stated in patient-centered terms and may include the following. The woman/couple will:

1. Verbalize understanding about contraceptive methods
2. State comfort and satisfaction with the method chosen
3. Achieve pregnancy when planned if further childbearing is desired
4. Experience no adverse sequelae as a result of the chosen method of contraception
5. Receive and understand all information necessary to give informed consent

Plan of Care and Implementation

Patient teaching is fundamental to initiating and maintaining any form of contraception. A care provider relationship based on trust is an important facet in patient compliance. The nurse counters myths with facts, clarifies misinformation, and fills in gaps of knowledge. The woman/couple must be fully informed of the risks, effectiveness, reversibility, and alternatives (see the Legal Tip to the left). There are various contraceptive techniques used in North America. The ideal contraceptive should be safe, easily available, economical, acceptable, simple to use, and promptly reversible. Although no means or method may ever achieve all these objectives, progress toward achieving these objectives has been made.

Contraception failure rate refers to the percentage of contraceptive users expected to experience an accidental pregnancy during the first year, even when they use a method consistently and correctly. Contraceptive effectiveness and failure rates depend on both the properties of the method and the characteristics of the user (Hatcher et al, 1994) (Box 19-8). Failure rates decrease over time either because a user gains ex-

BOX 19-8
Factors Affecting Method Effectiveness

Frequency of intercourse
Motivation to prevent pregnancy
Understanding use of the method
Compliance with method
Provision of short-term or long-term protection
Likelihood of pregnancy for the individual woman

perience with and uses a method more appropriately or because the less effective users stop using the method.

Safety of a method depends on the patient's medical history, tobacco use, and age. Barrier methods offer some protection from STDs, and oral contraceptives may lower the incidence of ovarian and endometrial cancer. "While there are risks associated with contraceptive use, the risk of death from a full-term pregnancy exceeds the risk of death from the use of any method of contraception, with the exception of the woman over age 35 who smokes and takes oral contraceptives" (NAACOG, 1991).

Methods of Contraception

The following discussion of contraceptive methods provides the nurse with information needed for patient teaching. After implementing the appropriate teaching for contraceptive use, the nurse supervises return demonstrations and practice to assess patient understanding. The woman is given written instructions and phone numbers for questions. If the woman has difficulty understanding written instructions, she (the couple) is offered graphic material and a phone number to call as necessary or an offer to return for further instruction.

Nonprescription methods. Several nonprescription methods for control of fertility (contraception) are practiced. Prescription and supervision are unnecessary for barrier methods, such as condom, foam, and spermicide or for periodic abstinence.

Two methods practiced but not recommended are douching and coitus interruptus. Douching (vaginal irrigation) after intercourse with various over-the-counter or homemade solutions can push the sperm further up the vagina and actually facilitate conception. *Coitus interruptus,* a method practiced for centuries, requires the man to withdraw his penis from the vagina before ejaculation. Extreme self-discipline is needed, and the sexual relationship may be strained. The danger of pregnancy from sperm in the preejaculatory drops is ever present. No advantages are given for this method, which has the lowest rate of effectiveness, comparable to the use of no contraceptive method (Lethbridge, 1991).

Periodic abstinence. Although **periodic abstinence,** or natural family planning (NFP), is not a method of contraception, it does prevent pregnancy by using methods that rely on avoidance of intercourse during presumed fertile days of the menstrual cycle.

Periodic abstinence methods use a combination of the following:

- Rhythm or calendar method
- Basal body temperature method
- Cervical mucus (Billings, Creighton, or ovulation) method
- Symptothermal method
- Fertility awareness method
- Predictor test for ovulation

These methods depend on the continuous observation and recording of events of the menstrual cycle. The woman or couple must be able to assess hormone-induced signs and symptoms that indicate whether she is in the fertile or infertile part of the menstrual cycle. While teaching a woman about fertility awareness, the nurse uses this opportunity for helping the woman or couple learn a great deal about their bodies.

Knowledge of the menstrual cycle is basic to the practice of NFP. To review, the human ovum can be fertilized no later than 16 to 24 hours after ovulation. Motile sperm have been recovered from the uterus and the oviducts as long as 60 hours after coitus. However, their ability to fertilize the ovum probably lasts no longer than 24 to 48 hours. Pregnancy is unlikely to occur if a couple abstains from intercourse for 4 days before and for 3 or 4 days after ovulation **(fertile period)**. More recent data suggest that the 6 days before ovulation are fertile days (Wilcox, Weinberg, and Baird, 1995). Unprotected intercourse on the other days of the cycle **(safe period)** should not result in pregnancy. However, there are two principal problems with this method: the exact time of ovulation cannot be predicted accurately, and couples may find it difficult to exercise restraint for several days before and after ovulation. Women with irregular menstrual periods have the greatest risk of failure with this form of contraception. The typical failure rate is 20% during the first year of use (Hatcher et al, 1994).

Ovulation usually occurs about 14 days before the onset of menstruation. Therefore variations in the length of menstrual cycles are usually a result of differences in the length of the preovulatory phases. The fertile period can be anticipated by the following:

- Calculating the time at which ovulation is likely to occur based on the lengths of previous menstrual cycles *(calendar method)*
- Recording the rise in BBT, a result of the thermogenic effect of progesterone *(temperature method)*
- Recognizing the changes in cervical mucus at different phases of the menstrual cycle *(ovulation, Creighton, or Billings method)*

Critical Thinking Exercises 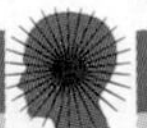
ADOLESCENT SEXUALITY

An adolescent female has approached you in your office at the local junior high school. She tells you she is having sex with several male friends but that there is no need to worry because she douches after each encounter.

1. **How would you approach your interview with this young woman?**
2. **What are your care priorities in this situation?**
3. **What legal and ethical concerns do you face?**
4. **What health care information does she urgently need?**
5. **What follow-up strategies will you use?**

- Using a predictor test for ovulation
- Using a combination of several methods

CALENDAR METHOD. Practice of the **calendar method** (*rhythm method*) is based on a count of the number of days in each cycle counting from the first day of menses (Davis, 1992). With the calendar method the fertile period is determined after accurately recording the lengths of the previous 6 to 12 menstrual cycles. The first unsafe day (beginning of the fertile period) can be determined by subtracting 18 days from the length of the shortest cycle. The last unsafe day (beginning of postovulatory safe period) can be calculated by subtracting 11 days from the length of the longest cycle. If the shortest cycle is 24 days and the longest is 30 days, application of the formula is as follows:

SHORTEST CYCLE	LONGEST CYCLE
24	30
−18	−11
6th day	19th day

To avoid conception the couple would abstain during the fertile period—days 6 through 19.

If the woman has very regular cycles of 28 days each, the formula indicates the fertile days to be as follows:

SHORTEST CYCLE	LONGEST CYCLE
28	28
−18	−11
10th day	17th day

To avoid pregnancy the couple abstains from day 10 through 17 because ovulation occurs on day 14 ± 2 days. A major drawback of the calendar method is that future events are trying to be predicted with past data. The unpredictability of the menstrual cycle is also not taken into consideration.

The method is most useful as an adjunct to the BBT or cervical mucus method. It is *not* useful in the postpartum period, during lactation, or at extremes of reproductive age when cycles are most variable (Sweezy, 1992).

BASAL BODY TEMPERATURE. The **basal body temperature (BBT)** is the lowest body temperature of a healthy person that is taken immediately after waking and before getting out of bed. The BBT usually varies from 36.2° to 36.3° C (97.2° to 97.4° F) during menses and for approximately 5 to 7 days afterward (Fig. 19-9).

If ovulation fails to occur, this pattern of lower body temperature continues throughout the cycle. Infection, fatigue, less than 3 hours of sleep per night, awakening late, and anxiety may cause temperature fluctuations, altering the expected pattern. If a new BBT thermometer is purchased, this fact is noted on the chart because the readings may vary slightly. Jet lag, alcohol taken the evening before, or sleeping in a heated waterbed must also be noted on the chart because each will affect the BBT.

About the time of ovulation a slight drop in temperature (approximately 0.05° C [0.1° F]) may be seen; after ovulation, in concert with the increasing progesterone levels of the early luteal phase of the cycle, the BBT rises slightly (approximately 0.2° to 0.4° C [0.4° to 0.8° F]) (Labbok and Queenan, 1989). The temperature remains on an elevated plateau until 2 to 4 days before menstruation. Then it drops to the low levels

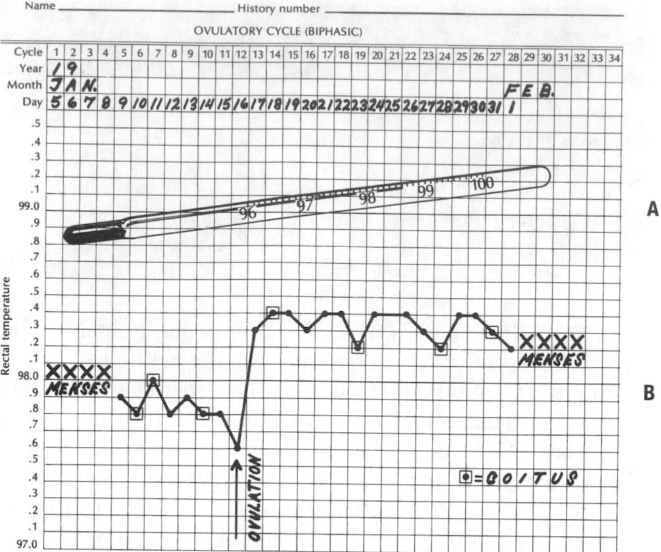

Fig. 19-9 **A,** Special thermometer for recording BBT, marked in tenths to enable person to read more easily. **B,** Basal temperature record shows drop and sharp rise at time of ovulation. Biphasic curve indicates ovulatory cycle.

recorded during the previous cycle unless pregnancy has occurred, and the temperature remains elevated.

The drop and subsequent rise in temperature are referred to as the **thermal shift.** When the entire month's temperatures are recorded on a graph, the pattern described is more apparent. It is more difficult to perceive day-to-day variations without the entire picture (see Fig. 19-9). Therefore the BBT alone is not a reliable method to predict ovulation (Labbok and Queenan, 1989). To determine if a rise in temperature is indeed the thermal shift, the woman must be aware of other signs of approaching ovulation while she continues to assess the BBT (see later discussion of symptothermal method for other indicators of ovulation).

Most counselors advise the couple who wish to prevent conception to avoid unprotected intercourse from the day of the drop in the BBT and for at least 3 days of elevated temperature (Davis, 1992). Others require the couple to abstain for the entire preovulatory period, starting with day 1 of menses until the third consecutive day of elevated BBT (Mishell, 1989) (see the Guidelines box on p. 517, left).

CERVICAL MUCUS METHOD. The **cervical mucus method** (also called the *Billings method* and the *Creighton model ovulation method*) require that the woman recognize and interpret the characteristic cyclic changes in the amount and consistency of cervical mucus (see the Guidelines box on p. 517, right). Each woman has her own unique pattern of mucus changes. The cervical mucus that accompanies ovulation is necessary for viability and motility of sperm. Without adequate cervical mucus, coitus does not result in conception. To ensure an accurate assessment of changes, the cervical mucus should be free from semen, contraceptive gels or foams, and blood or discharge from vaginal infections for at least one full cycle. Other factors that create difficulty in identifying mucus changes include douches and vaginal deodorants, being in the sexually aroused state (which thins the mucus), and

Guidelines 

BASAL BODY TEMPERATURE

Discuss BBT with the woman.
Show woman a diagram depicting the phases of the menstrual cycle.
Discuss the hormones in the woman's body that are responsible for her menstrual cycle and ovulation. Leave time for questions.
Show the woman a sample BBT graph (see Fig. 19-9) and the biphasic line seen in ovulatory cycles.
Show the woman the BBT thermometer and how it is calibrated.
Provide a demonstration.
Encourage woman to demonstrate taking and reading the thermometer and graphing the temperature while the nurse watches.
Encourage the woman to start a log to keep track of any other activity that might interfere with her true BBT.

taking medications such as antihistamines, which dry up the mucus.

Some women find this method unacceptable because they find touching their genitals uncomfortable. Whether or not a woman wants to use this method for contraception, it is to her advantage to learn to recognize mucus characteristics at ovulation. Self-evaluation of cervical mucus can be highly accurate and effective in avoiding pregnancy (Fehring et al, 1994) and can be useful diagnostically for any of the following purposes:

- To alert the couple to the reestablishment of ovulation while breastfeeding and after discontinuation of oral contraception
- To note anovulatory cycles at any time and at the commencement of menopause
- To assist couples in planning a pregnancy

SYMPTOTHERMAL METHOD. The symptothermal method combines the BBT and cervical mucus methods with awareness of secondary, cycle phase–related symptoms (see Table 3-1). Both partners take responsibility for assessments, recordings, and evaluation of their findings. Together they determine the days for abstinence. Couples who use the symptothermal method commonly report an improvement in their sexual relationship.

The couple gains fertility awareness as they learn the woman's individual psychologic and physiologic symptoms that mark the phases of her cycle. Secondary symptoms include increased libido, midcycle spotting, mittelschmerz, pelvic fullness or tenderness, and vulvar fullness. The couple, perhaps using a speculum, looks at the cervix to assess for changes indicating ovulation: that is, the os dilates slightly, the cervix softens and rises in the vagina, and cervical mucus is copious and slippery. To complete their records, the couple notes days on which coitus, changes in routine, illness, and so on have occurred (Fig. 19-10). Calendar calculations and cervical mucus changes are used to estimate the onset of the fertile period; changes in cervical mucus or the BBT are used to estimate its end.

Guidelines 

CERVICAL MUCUS CHARACTERISTICS

Setting the stage

Show charts of menstrual cycle along with changes in the cervical mucus.
Have woman practice with raw egg white.
Supply her with a BBT log and graph if she does not already have one.
Explain that the assessment of cervical mucus characteristics is best when mucus is not mixed with semen, contraceptive jellies or foams, or discharge from infections.

Content related to cervical mucus

Explain to woman (couple) how cervical mucus changes throughout the menstrual cycle.
Right before ovulation, the watery, thin, clear mucus becomes more abundant and thick. It feels like a lubricant and can be stretched 5+ cm between the thumb and forefinger; this is called **spinnbarkheit.** This characteristic indicates the period of maximum fertility. Sperm deposited in this type of mucus can survive until ovulation occurs.

Assessment technique

Stress that good handwashing is imperative to begin and end all self-assessment.
Start observation from last day of menstrual flow.
Assess cervical mucus several times a day for several cycles. Mucus can be obtained from vaginal introitus; no need to reach into vagina to cervix.
Record findings on the same record on which her BBT is en-

Effectiveness of the symptothermal method with abstinence during the fertile period ranges between 73% and 97%.

FERTILITY AWARENESS METHOD. The *fertility awareness method* is a combination of menstrual cycle charting based on observable physiologic changes and barrier contraception (Hatcher et al, 1994). During the fertile period the couple has the choice of either abstinence from genital-genital contact or the use of barrier contraception. After the fertile period the couple may enjoy freedom from contraception for the remaining nonfertile days of the menstrual cycle.

Predictor test for ovulation. The preceding discussions are about assessments that are indicative of but do not prove the occurrence and exact timing of ovulation. The **predictor test for ovulation** is a major addition to the periodic abstinence methods to help women who want to plan the time of their pregnancies and those who are trying to conceive. The predictor test for ovulation detects the sudden surge of luteinizing hormone (LH) that occurs approximately 12 to 24 hours *before* ovulation (Fehring, 1990) and is detectable in urine. Unlike BBT, the test is not affected by illness, emotional upset, or physical activity. Available for home use, a test kit contains sufficient material for several days' testing during each cycle. A positive response indicative of an LH surge is noted by color change that is easy to read. Directions for use of this home test kit vary with the manufacturer.

Chemical and mechanical contraceptive barriers. Barrier contraceptives (vaginal spermicides and condoms) are receiving great attention and increased use. These methods

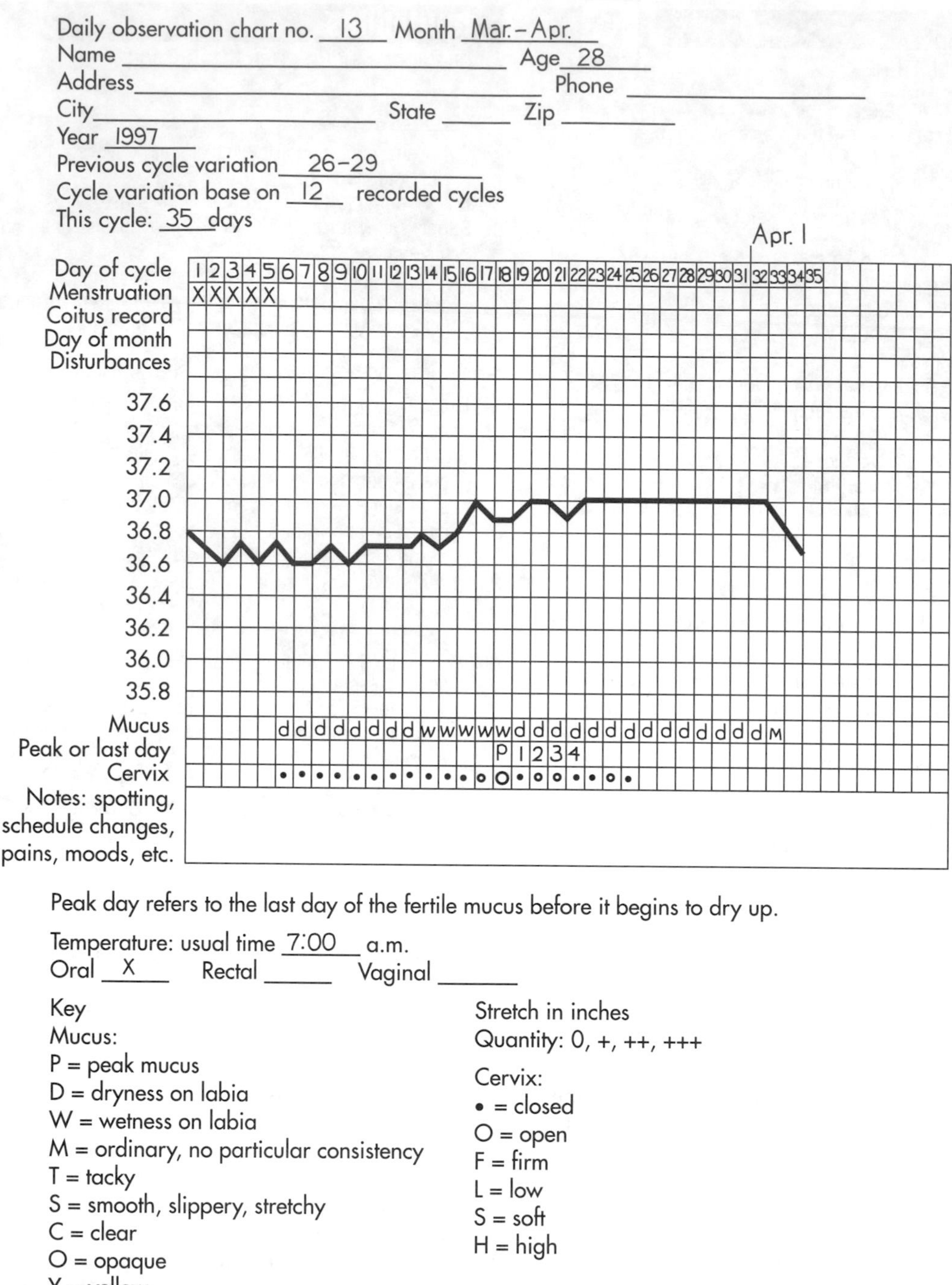

Daily observation chart no. 13 Month Mar.–Apr.
Name ______ Age 28
Address ______ Phone ______
City ______ State ______ Zip ______
Year 1997
Previous cycle variation 26–29
Cycle variation base on 12 recorded cycles
This cycle: 35 days

Apr. 1

Day of cycle: 1 2 3 4 5 6 7 8 9 10 11 12 13 14 15 16 17 18 19 20 21 22 23 24 25 26 27 28 29 30 31 32 33 34 35
Menstruation: X X X X X
Coitus record
Day of month
Disturbances
37.6
37.4
37.2
37.0
36.8
36.6
36.4
36.2
36.0
35.8
Mucus: d d d d d d d d w w w w w d d d d d d d d d d d d d d M
Peak or last day: P 1 2 3 4
Cervix: • • • • • • • • • • • • o O • o o • • o •
Notes: spotting, schedule changes, pains, moods, etc.

Peak day refers to the last day of the fertile mucus before it begins to dry up.

Temperature: usual time 7:00 a.m.
Oral X Rectal ______ Vaginal ______

Key
Mucus:
P = peak mucus
D = dryness on labia
W = wetness on labia
M = ordinary, no particular consistency
T = tacky
S = smooth, slippery, stretchy
C = clear
O = opaque
Y = yellow

Stretch in inches
Quantity: 0, +, ++, +++

Cervix:
• = closed
O = open
F = firm
L = low
S = soft
H = high

Fig. 19-10 Example of completed symptothermal method.

have an additional distinct advantage of reducing the spread of STDs (Niruthisard et al, 1992).

SPERMICIDES. A vaginal **spermicide** is a physical barrier to sperm penetration that also has a chemical action on sperm. *Nonoxynol 9* (N-9) and octoxynol 9 are the most commonly used spermicidal chemicals. Intravaginal spermicides are marketed as aerosol foams, foaming tablets, suppositories, creams, films, and gels (Fig. 19-11 and Box 19-9). Preloaded, single-dose applicators small enough to be carried in a small purse are available.

There is evidence that nonoxynol 9 plus a barrier method provides some protection against STDs (e.g., gonorrhea and chlamydia) through bacteriostatic action (Hatcher et al, 1994; Niruthisard et al, 1992). Although nonoxynol 9 has been shown to be lethal to human immunodeficiency virus (HIV) in the laboratory, effectiveness for women is still questioned (Pollack and Moore, 1994). Frequent spermicide use by women at risk for HIV infection could enhance HIV transmission if vaginal tissues are irritated. These women need to be counseled about the most up-to-date information about spermicide use and HIV. The Patient Teaching box on p. 520 provides information about spermicide use.

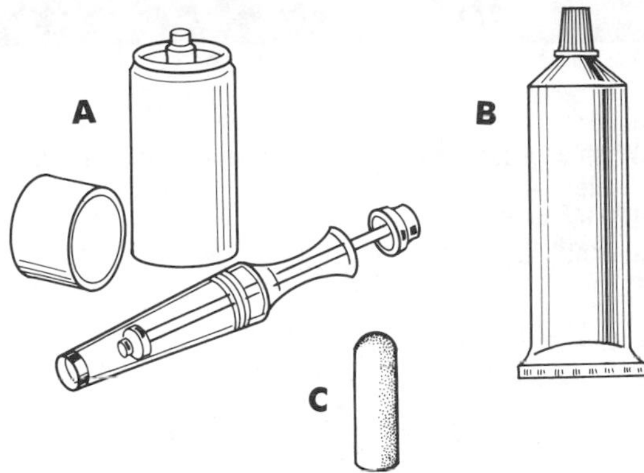

Fig. 19-11 Vaginal spermicides. **A,** Foam with applicator. **B,** Cream. **C,** Suppository.

VAGINAL SPONGE. The polyurethane vaginal sponge was approved by the Food and Drug Administration (FDA) in 1983; but is currently not manufactured in the United States. Problems with sponge removal and high failure rates may have led to this decision. It may still be sold while supplies remain and may be obtained in other countries. Water is needed to activate the spermicide (nonoxynol 9) and facilitate insertion. Spermicide is released continuously for 24 hours. A woven loop is used for retrieval from the vagina. It is recommended that at least 6 hours lapse between last intercourse and removal (Hatcher et al, 1994). Wearing the sponge for more than 24 to 30 hours is not recommended because of the rise of toxic shock syndrome (Moore, 1994). The sponge should be discarded after removal. It must not be washed and reused. Washing removes the spermicide. The mode of action is the same as that for the spermicides. Nursing actions also are similar to those for other spermicides.

VAGINAL SHEATH (FEMALE CONDOM). The vaginal sheath of natural latex rubber has flexible rings at both ends (Connell, 1994) (Fig. 19-12, *A*). This device is a combination of a diaphragm and a condom. The closed end of the pouch is inserted into the vagina and is anchored around the cervix: the open ring covers the labia. It can be applied well in advance of intercourse so that spontaneity is unaffected. Before intercourse a spermicide is added. Because it is a relatively loose sheath, it tends to heighten sensation for the man. Male condoms should not be used with female condoms. Both women and men report that intercourse with the sheath is generally about as satisfying as intercourse without the sheath. Application of this disposable barrier requires no special training. It comes in one size and is available over the counter (Greydanus and Lonchamp, 1990). This device may provide more protection against STDs than do condoms. The average 6-month failure rate is 12.5% (Moore, 1994).

MALE CONDOM. The **condom** is a thin, stretchable sheath that covers the penis (Fig. 19-12, *B*). In addition to three available sizes, four basic features differ among condoms marketed in the United States. These features are material, shape, lubricants, and spermicides. Ninety-nine percent are made of latex rubber. A functional difference in condom shape is the presence or absence of a sperm reservoir tip. To enhance vaginal stimulation, some condoms are contoured and rippled or have ribbed or roughened surfaces. Thinner construction in-

BOX 19-9
Spermicides

Mode of action

Provides a physical and chemical barrier that prevents viable sperm from entering the cervix. Effect is local within the vagina. The spermicide is placed deep in the vagina in contact with the cervix before each instance of coitus.

Failure rate

Typical failure: 21%

Advantages

- Easy to apply
- Safe
- Low cost
- Available without a prescription or previous medical examination
- Delicate vaginal mucosa is not harmed unless the woman is allergic to a particular preparation
- Aids in lubrication of the vagina
- Alternative for nursing mothers (does not interfere with lactation)
- Alternative for the premenopausal woman (to prevent masking symptoms of onset of the climacterium)
- Backup when the woman forgets her oral contraceptive
- Increases the effectiveness of condoms and other forms of contraception

STD Protection

- The barrier method containing the spermicide nonoxynol 9 provides some protection against STDs through bacteriostatic action. It is used with condoms if protection from STDs is needed.

Disadvantages

- Maximum spermicidal effectiveness usually lasts no longer than 1 hour.
- If intercourse is to be repeated, reapplication of additional spermicide must precede it.
- Some users complain it is messy and has an unpleasant fizz and taste.
- Allergic response or irritation of vaginal or penile tissue may occur.
- Possible decreased tactile sensation.

Nursing considerations/patient teaching

- The can must be shaken to distribute foam spermicide before use.
- Tablets and suppositories take from 10 to 30 minutes to dissolve.
- Douching must be avoided for at least 6 hours after coitus.
- Encourage open communication between sexual partners to discuss intravaginal contraception.
- Provide opportunity to see and handle various samples.
- Provide anatomic model to practice insertion into the vagina.
- Nurse needs to feel comfortable teaching both male and female partners.

Patient Teaching

SPERMICIDAL VAGINAL FOAM

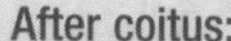

Application (10 to 15 minutes before coitus):

- Shake canister gently.
- Screw applicator to tip of canister *(A).*
- Press down until foam fills applicator.
- Unscrew applicator from canister.
- Insert applicator into vagina *(B).*
- Push plunger to release foam into vagina *(B).*
- Remove applicator from vagina.

After coitus:

- Wash applicator and plunger with mild soap and warm water.
- Dry thoroughly.
- Do not boil applicator.

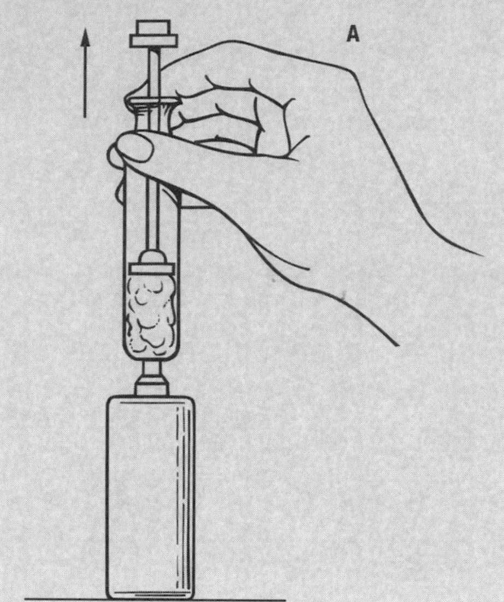

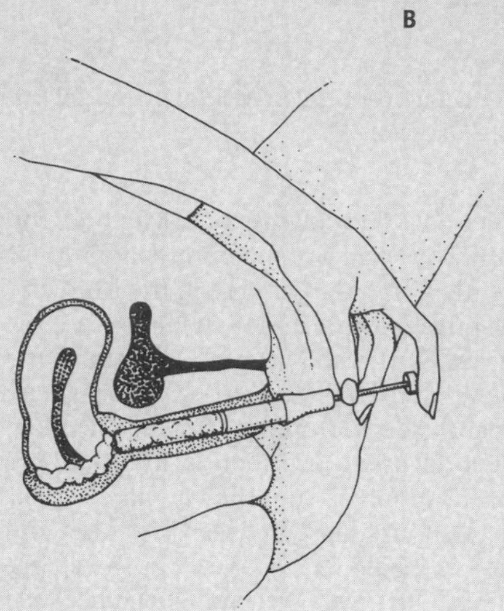

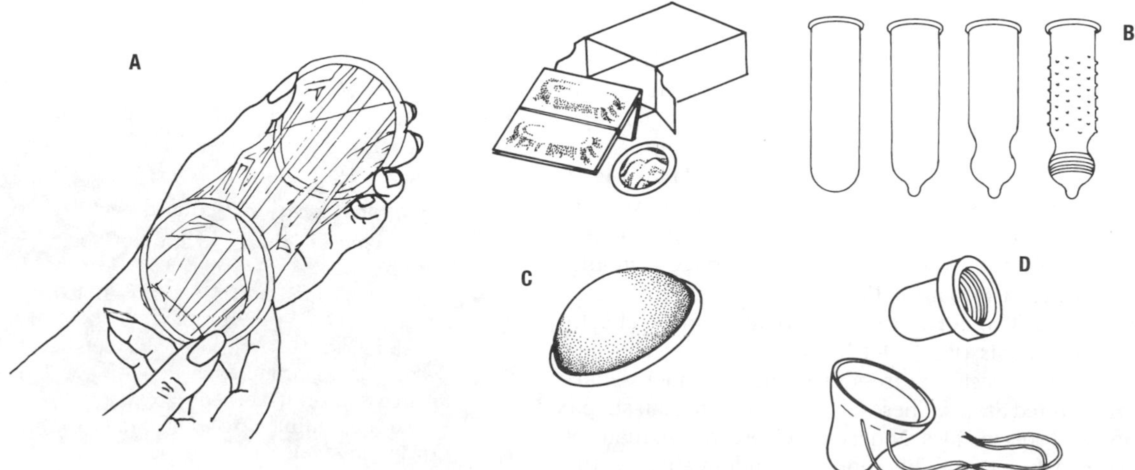

Fig. 19-12 Mechanical barriers. **A,** Vaginal sheath (female condom). **B,** Types of condoms. **C,** Diaphragm. **D,** Cervical caps.

BOX 19-10
Male Condoms

Mechanism of action

Sheath is applied over the erect penis before insertion or loss of preejaculatory drops of semen. Used correctly, condoms prevent sperm from entering the cervix. Spermicide-coated condoms cause ejaculated sperm to be immobilized rapidly, thus increasing contraceptive effectiveness.

Failure rate

- Typical users, 12%
- Correct and consistent users, 2%

Advantages

- Safe
- No side effects
- Readily available
- Premalignant changes in cervix can be prevented or ameliorated in women whose partners use condoms
- Method of male nonsurgical contraception

Disadvantages

- Must interrupt lovemaking to apply sheath
- Sensation may be altered
- If used improperly, spillage of sperm can result in pregnancy
- Occasionally condoms may tear during intercourse

STD protection

- If a condom is used throughout the act of intercourse and there is no unprotected contact with female genitals, a latex rubber condom, which is impermeable to viruses, can act as a protective measure against STDs.

Nursing considerations

- Use a new condom (check expiration date) for each act of sexual intercourse or other acts between partners that involve contact with the penis.
- Place condom after penis is erect and before intimate contact
- Place condom on head of penis (Fig. A) and unroll it all the way to the base (Fig B).
- Leave an empty space at the tip (Fig A); remove any air remaining in the tip by gently pressing air out toward the base of the penis.
- If a lubricant is desired, use water-based products such as K-Y Jelly.
- After ejaculation, carefully withdraw still erect penis, holding onto condom rim; discard.
- Store unused condoms in cool, dry place.
- Do not use condoms that are sticky, brittle, or obviously damaged.

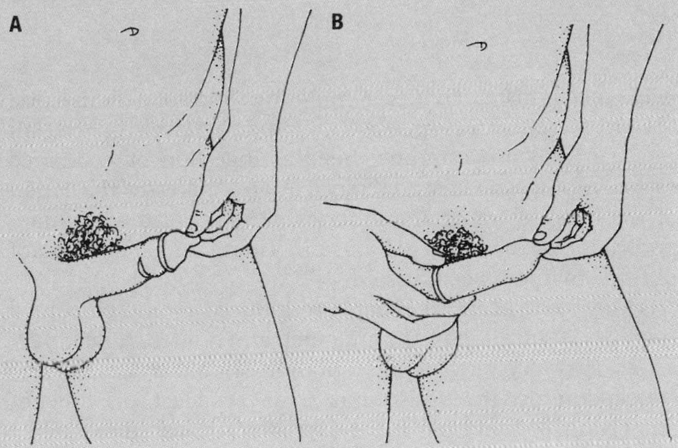

creases heat transmission and sensitivity; a variety of colors increases their acceptability and attractiveness. A wet jelly or dry powder lubricates some condoms. Since 1982, spermicide (0.5 g of nonoxynol 9) has been added to the interior or exterior surfaces of some condoms. The addition of nonoxynol 9 to latex condoms not only increases contraceptive effectiveness but also increases protection against the transmission of STDs, including HIV (Hatcher et al, 1994).

Some couples object to interrupting lovemaking to apply the sheath or complain that sensation is blunted. Occasionally, older men may have erectile problems when using condoms (Jarrett and Lethbridge, 1990). If condoms are used improperly, spillage of sperm can result in pregnancy. The sheath is applied over the erect penis before insertion or loss of preejaculatory drops of semen. Conception is possible if preejaculatory drops fall around the external vaginal opening because sperm are contained in these drops. Condom breakage during vaginal intercourse reported by users varies from 0% to 36%, with up to 6.7% of condoms bursting (Hatcher et al, 1994). The pregnancy rate with condom use is approximately 13% among typical users (Hatcher et al, 1994).

To prevent unintended pregnancy and the spread of STDs, it is essential that condoms be used correctly (Box 19-10).

Methods requiring prescription. Several methods for the control of fertility require prescription and supervision. An interview, physical examination, and occasionally laboratory tests are prerequisites for some forms of contraception. These methods of contraception include hormonal therapy, the use of diaphragms or cervical caps, and intrauterine devices.

Hormonal contraception. **Oral hormonal contraceptives** are available in several forms. General classes are described in Table 19-4. Because of the wide variety of preparations available, the woman and nurse must read the package insert for information about specific products prescribed. Guidelines issued by the FDA have standardized package insert information in an effort to increase patient compliance (Potter, 1994). In a study of package inserts, readability levels were found to be at the high school level (Swanson et al, 1990). Patient education is essential to achieve compliance.

Formulations include combined estrogen-progestin steroidal medications or progestin-only products. The formulations can be administered orally, parenterally, by implantation, or by intrauterine insertion. Combined estrogen-progestin steroidal medications are discussed first.

COMBINED ESTROGEN-PROGESTIN ORAL CONTRACEPTIVES. *Mode of action.* The normal menstrual cycle is maintained by a feed-

TABLE 19-4 Hormonal contraception

COMPOSITION	ROUTE OF ADMINISTRATION	DURATION OF EFFECT
Combination estrogen and progestin (synthetic estrogens and progestins in varying doses and formulations)	Oral	24 hours
Progestin only Norethindrone, norgestrel	Oral	24 hours
Medroxyprogesterone acetate	Intramuscular injection	3 months
Levonorgestrel	Subdermal implant	Up to 5 years
Progesterone	Intrauterine device	1 year

back mechanism. Follicle-stimulating hormone (FSH) and LH are secreted in response to fluctuating levels of ovarian estrogen and progesterone. Regular ingestion of combined estrogen-progestin steroidal medication suppresses the action of the hypothalamus and anterior pituitary leading to inappropriate secretion of FSH and LH. Therefore follicles do not mature; ovulation is inhibited.

Other contraceptive effects are induced by the combined steroids. Maturation of the endometrium is altered, making it a less favorable site for implantation should ovulation and conception occur. It also has a direct effect on the endometrium so that from 1 to 4 days after the last steroid tablet is taken the endometrium sloughs and bleeds as a result of hormone withdrawal. The **withdrawal bleeding** usually is less profuse than that of normal menstruation and may last only 2 to 3 days. Some women have no bleeding at all.

The cervical mucus remains thick as a result of the effect of the progestin. Cervical mucus under the effect of progesterone does not provide as suitable an environment for sperm penetration as does the thin, watery mucus at ovulation (Harris, 1992).

The possible role, if any, of altered tubal and uterine motility induced by the steroidal hormones is not clear. Nevertheless, combined oral hormonal contraceptives, if taken daily for 3 weeks of every 4, provide virtually absolute protection against conception (Cunningham et al, 1993).

Monophasic pills provide fixed dosages of estrogen and progestin. In phasic pills (e.g., biphasic, triphasic, and multiphasic oral contraceptives) the amount of progestin, and sometimes the amount of estrogen, varies within each cycle (Gerstman et al, 1991; Youngkin, 1993). These preparations reduce the total dosage of steroid hormones in a single cycle without sacrificing contraceptive efficacy or cycle control (Harris, 1992). The theoretic advantage is a reduction in progestin-related metabolic changes and the adverse effects attributed to those metabolic changes. The estrogen dose is also kept low, with only 30 to 40 μg of ethinyl estradiol; no tablet sold in the United States contains more than 50 μg (Facts and Comparisons, 1995).

Advantages. For motivated women it is easy to take an oral contraceptive at approximately the same time each day. Taking the pill does not relate directly to the sexual act; this fact increases its acceptability to some women. Commonly there is an improvement in sexual response once the possibility of pregnancy is not an issue. For some it is convenient to know when to expect the next "menstrual" flow.

Oral contraceptives are considered to be a safe option for older, nonsmoking women until menopause. Perimenopausal women can benefit from regular bleeding cycles, a regular hormonal pattern, and the noncontraceptive health benefits of oral contraceptives (*The Contraception Report*, 1992).

The noncontraceptive health benefits of oral contraceptives include decreased menstrual blood loss and decreased iron deficiency anemia, regulation of menorrhagia and irregular cycles, and lowered incidence of dysmenorrhea (menstrual cramps) and premenstrual syndrome (PMS). Oral contraceptives also offer protection against endometrial adenocarcinoma and possibly ovarian cancer, reduced incidence of benign breast disease, reduction of functional ovarian cysts, protection against some types of pelvic inflammatory disease (PID), and decreased risk of ectopic pregnancy.

Women taking steroidal contraceptives are examined before the medication is prescribed and yearly thereafter. The examination includes medical and family history, weight, blood pressure, general physical and pelvic examination, screening cervical cytologic analysis (Papanicolaou [Pap] smear), and hemoglobin determination. Consistent monitoring by the health care provider is also valuable in the detection of noncontraception-related disorders so that timely treatment can be initiated.

The use of oral hormonal contraceptives is initiated on one of the first 7 days of the menstrual cycle (day 1 of the cycle is the first day of menses). Other women start their use after childbirth or abortion. If contraceptives are to be started at any time other than during normal menses, or within 3 weeks after birth or abortion, another method of contraception should be used throughout the first week to avoid the risk of pregnancy (Cunningham et al, 1993). Taken exactly as directed, oral contraceptives prevent ovulation and pregnancy cannot occur; the overall effectiveness rate is almost 100%. Almost all failures (i.e., pregnancy occurs) are caused by omission of one or more pills during the regimen.

Disadvantages and side effects. Since hormonal contraceptives have come into use, the amount of estrogen and progestational agent contained in each tablet has been reduced considerably (Cunningham et al, 1993). This reduction is important because adverse effects are, to a degree, dose related.

Women must be screened for conditions that present absolute or relative contraindications to oral contraceptive use. *Absolute contraindications* include a history of thromboembolic disorders, cerebrovascular or coronary artery disease, breast cancer, estrogenic-dependent tumors, pregnancy, impaired liver function, and liver tumor. Strong *relative contraindications* include migraine headaches, hypertension, acute mononucleosis, surgery requiring immobilization for 4 weeks, age of 35 years or older and heavy smoking (more than 15 cigarettes per day), abnormal genital bleeding, diabetes mellitus, sickle cell disease, and lactation (Hatcher et al, 1994). The main causes of hospitalization and death are cardiovascular problems (e.g., myocardial infarction [heart attack], cerebrovascular accident [stroke], and thromboembolism) (Franklin, 1990).

Certain side effects of anovulatory drugs are attributable to estrogen and progestin or both. Side effects of *estrogen excess* include nausea and vomiting, dizziness, edema, leg cramps, increase in breast size, chloasma (mask of pregnancy), visual changes, hypertension, and vascular headache. Side effects of *estrogen deficiency* include early spotting (days 1 to 14), hypomenorrhea, nervousness, and atrophic vaginitis leading to painful intercourse (dyspareunia). Side effects of *progestin excess* include increased appetite, tiredness, depression, breast tenderness, vaginal yeast infection, oily skin and scalp, hirsutism, and postpill amenorrhea. Side effects of *progestin deficiency* include late spotting and breakthrough bleeding (days 15 to 21), heavy flow with clots, and decreased breast size. One of the most common side effects is bleeding irregularities (Hillard, 1989).

In the presence of side effects, especially those that are bothersome to the woman, a different product, a different drug content, or another method of contraception may be required. The "right" product for a woman contains the lowest dose of sex steroid hormones that prevents ovulation and that has the fewest and least harmful side effects. There is no way to predict the right dosage for any particular woman; trial and error is the main method for prescribing oral contraceptives, starting with the lowest possible estrogen and progestin dose.

The *changes in glucose tolerance* that occur in some women taking oral contraceptives are similar to those changes that occur during pregnancy. The dosage, type, and potency of progestin (not estrogen) produce some deterioration of glucose tolerance in normal women, as well as in those with a history of gestational diabetes (Hatcher et al, 1994).

The effectiveness of oral contraceptives is decreased when the following drugs are taken at the same time:

- Barbiturates (for sedation or seizure disorders)
- Phenytoin sodium (for seizure disorders)
- Many antibiotics such as ampicillin, tetracycline, and griseofulvin, penicillin, doxycycline, and rifampin (for tuberculosis) (Hatcher et al, 1994).

The use of oral contraceptives can also decrease the effectiveness of several drugs (e.g., oral hypoglycemics and oral anticoagulants) (Hatcher et al, 1994).

Research on the use of oral contraceptives and risk of breast cancer has been inconsistent; investigation continues on this important concern.

Women who discontinue oral contraception for a planned pregnancy commonly ask whether they should wait before attempting to conceive. Although data are controversial, studies indicate that these infants have no greater chance of being born with any type of birth defect than do infants born to women in the general population, even if conception occurred in the first month after the medication was discontinued (Mishell, 1989).

After discontinuing oral contraception there is usually a delay before ovulation and menstrual cycles recur, similar to that experienced by a new mother. However, postpill amenorrhea exceeding 6 months should be investigated.

Nursing actions. There are many different preparations of oral hormonal contraceptives. The nurse reviews the prescribing information in the package insert with the woman.

Home Care

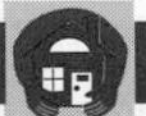

ADMINISTRATION OF ORAL CONTRACEPTIVE PILLS

- A pill should be taken at the same time every day for 21 (or 28) days.
- If one pill is missed, take it as soon as you remember it, and take the next one at the usual time.
- If you miss two or more pills in a row in the first 2 weeks of the cycle, take two for 2 days and use a backup method of contraception for the next 7 days.
- If you miss two or more pills in the third week, or three or more pills anytime: *Sunday starters* keep on taking pills until the next Sunday. Start a new pack on that day. Use a backup method of contraception for the next 7 days. *Day 1 starters* throw out the rest of the pack and start a new pack that day. Use a backup method of contraception for the next 7 days.
- *28-day pill pack:* If you miss any of the seven pills that do not have any hormones, throw out the pills you missed and keep taking one pill a day until the pack is empty. You do not need a backup method of contraception.

Modified from current "oral" contraceptive patient package inserts.

Because of the wide variations, each woman must be clear about the unique dosage regimen for the preparation prescribed for her. Directions for care after missing tablets also vary. Recent findings indicate that if two or more tablets are missed, another form of contraception must be used until the required regimen is reestablished (see the Home Care box above).

Withdrawal bleeding ("period") tends to be short and scanty when some combination pills are taken. A woman may see no fresh blood at all. Some women may have only a drop of blood or a brown smudge on their tampon or underwear. This counts as a period. This fact may explain why some women have difficulty remembering the first day of their last period.

No more than 50% to 70% of women who start taking oral contraceptives are still taking them after 1 year. It is therefore important that nurses recommend that all women choosing to use oral contraceptives also be provided with a second method of birth control and that women be instructed and comfortable with this backup method. Most women stop taking oral contraceptives for nonmedical reasons (i.e., they choose to stop), not because they develop a complication or a serious side effect.

The nurse also reviews the signs of potential complications associated with the use of oral contraceptives (Box 19-11).

Oral contraceptives do not protect a woman against STDs. A barrier method such as condoms and spermicide should also be used if protection is desired.

PROGESTIN-ONLY CONTRACEPTION. *Oral progestins (Minipill).* Progestin-only pills contain norethindrone or norgestrel and presumably impair fertility (Moore, 1994). Ovulation may occur. Progestin acts on cervical mucus to decrease sperm penetration and alters endometrial maturation to discourage implantation should conception occur. Users report a higher incidence of irregular bleeding. Progestin-only pills are slightly less effective than combined estrogen-progestin pills. Progestin-only pills are taken daily at the same time. Back-up methods are advised if two or more tablets are missed.

BOX 19-11
Signs of Potential Complications

ORAL CONTRACEPTIVES

Before oral contraceptives are prescribed and periodically throughout hormone therapy, the woman is alerted to stop taking the pill and to report any of the following symptoms to the health care provider immediately. The word *aches* helps in retention of this list:

A—Abdominal pain: may indicate a problem with the liver or gallbladder
C—Chest pain or shortness of breath: may indicate possible clot problem within lungs or heart
H—Headaches (sudden or persistent): may be caused by cardiovascular accident or hypertension
E—Eye problems: may indicate vascular accident or hypertension
S—Severe leg pain: may indicate a thromboembolic process

BOX 19-12
Ethical Considerations Concerning Enforced Contraception

The nurse may be confronted with an ethical dilemma concerning enforced contraception for a patient. There have been some judicial rulings for a woman convicted of child abuse to either obtain a Norplant device or face a jail term. Other women receiving public assistance for children may be told to get the implant or be faced with decreased or even no payments.

Some nurses may consider this punitive approach to be effective in preventing the birth of more children to unsuitable mothers; however, some individuals strongly believe that forcing women to have such procedures interferes with her constitutional rights.

Injectable progestins. Medroxyprogesterone is administered intramuscularly every 3 months. The advantages of medroxyprogesterone acetate (DMPA, Depo-Provera) include a contraceptive effectiveness comparable to combined oral contraceptives, long-lasting effects, the requirement of injections only four times a year, and lactation is not likely to be impaired (Mastroianni and Robinson, 1994). The modes of action include inhibition of ovulation and alteration in endometrial maturation and cervical mucus. The site should not be massaged following injection because doing so hastens drug absorption and shortens the period of effectiveness. Disadvantages are prolonged amenorrhea, irregular uterine bleeding, increased risk of venous thrombosis and thromboembolism, and no protection against STDs. Absolute contraindications include thrombotic problems, pregnancy, undiagnosed uterine bleeding, or a history of stroke, myocardial infarction, or breast cancer. Effectiveness approaches 100%. Because it can take up to 18 months after the last DMPA injection to regain fertility (ovulate again), women should not expect to be able to stop the injections and immediately conceive. This could be important information for couples who are trying to space children and who want to achieve pregnancy at a specific time.

Implantable progestin (Norplant). The Norplant system consists of six flexible, nonbiodegradable Silastic capsules. They contain progestin and provide up to 5 years of contraception. Insertion and removal of the capsules are minor surgical procedures involving a local anesthetic, a small incision, and no sutures. The capsules are placed subdermally in the inner aspect of the upper arm (Fig. 19-13). The progestin prevents some, but not all, ovulatory cycles and thickens cervical mucus. The effectiveness is greater than 99% over 5 years. Advantages include long-term continuous contraception, not coitus related, and reversibility. Irregular menstrual bleeding is the most common side effect (Darney et al, 1990). Other side effects, including headaches, nervousness, nausea, skin changes, and vertigo, are less common (Klaisle and Wysocki, 1992). Changes in glucose and insulin values have occurred after 6 months, especially in women who are diabetic (Konje et al, 1992).

Side effects are the most commonly reported reason for

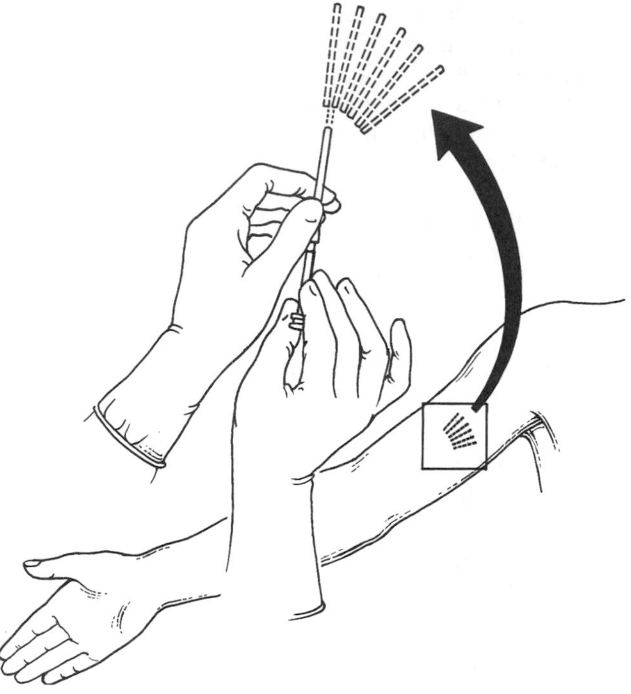

Fig. 19-13 Norplant contraceptive device.

Norplant removal. Thorough understanding of potential side effects before insertion and supportive management of side effects when they occur can result in greater user satisfaction (Hinkle, 1994). This method may be a good alternative for teenage mothers (Polaneczky et al, 1994). However, ethical concerns related to enforced contraception for vulnerable groups must be considered (Box 19-12). Implants of one and two rods, biodegradable rods, and contraceptive pellets are under investigation (Future, 1994). Because no STD protection is provided with the Norplant method, condoms should be used if protection is desired.

VAGINAL RINGS. The World Health Organization (WHO) and the Population Council are conducting research on the Silastic vaginal ring. It releases small amounts of levonorgestrel daily. Women continue to ovulate, but contraception is achieved by making cervical mucus impermeable to sperm.

The ring is designed to remain in the vagina for 3 months. Major disadvantages are irregular vaginal bleeding and irritation (Hatcher et al, 1994).

DIAPHRAGM WITH SPERMICIDE. The vaginal **diaphragm** is a shallow, dome-shaped rubber device with a flexible wire rim that covers the cervix (Fig. 19-12, *C*). There are three main styles of diaphragms available in a wide range of diameters (50 to 95 mm). Diaphragms differ in the inner construction of the circular rim. The four types of rims are flat spring, coil spring, arcing spring, and wide-seal rim. Two disposable diaphragms that contain spermicide are undergoing clinical trials (*The Contraception Report*, 1994).

The diaphragm should feel comfortable. It should be the largest size the woman can wear without her being aware of its presence. The use of a contraceptive gel or cream with the diaphragm offers both mechanical and chemical barriers to pregnancy.

The diaphragm is a mechanical barrier preventing the meeting of the sperm with the ovum. The diaphragm holds the spermicide in place against the cervix for the 6 hours it takes to destroy the sperm. The *effectiveness* of this combined method is approximately 83% to 90%. Highly motivated women may achieve rates of 99%.

Nursing actions. The woman is informed that she needs an annual gynecologic examination. The device may need to be refitted after 2 years, the loss or gain of 5 to 7 kg (10 to 15 lb) or more, and 6 weeks after giving birth or a second trimester abortion (Hawkins, Matteson, and Tabeck, 1995). Because there are various types of diaphragms on the market, the nurse uses the package insert for teaching the woman how to use and care for the diaphragm (see the Guidelines box on pp. 526-527).

Except for occasional allergic responses to the diaphragm or spermicide, there are no side effects from a well-fitted device. The diaphragm can be inserted as long as 6 hours before intercourse to increase spontaneity, but spermicide must be added each time intercourse is repeated (Hatcher et al, 1994). It must be left in place for at least 6 hours after the last intercourse. The woman who engages in intercourse infrequently may choose this barrier method. The spermicide offers additional lubrication if it is needed. A decreased incidence of vaginitis, cervicitis (including cervicitis caused by *Chlamydia trachomatis* and *Neisseria gonorrhoeae*), PID, and cervical intraepithelial neoplasia is noted among women who use contraceptive creams, foams, and gels with the diaphragm.

This method is contraindicated for the woman with relaxation of her pelvic support (uterine prolapse) or a large cystocele.

Disadvantages include the reluctance of some women to insert and remove the diaphragm. A cold diaphragm and a cold gel temporarily reduce vaginal response to sexual stimulation if insertion of the diaphragm occurs immediately before intercourse. Some women or couples object to the messiness of the spermicide. These annoyances of diaphragm use, along with failure to insert the device once foreplay has begun, are the most common reasons for failures of this method. Side effects may include irritation of tissues related to contact with spermicides. Urethritis and recurrent cystitis caused by upward pressure of the diaphragm rim against the urethra may be increased by the use of the contraceptive diaphragm.

Although reported in very small numbers, toxic shock syndrome (TSS) can occur in association with the use of the contraceptive diaphragm. The nurse should instruct the woman about ways to reduce her risk for TSS. These measures include handwashing before insertion and removal, prompt removal 6 to 8 hours after intercourse, not using the diaphragm during menses, and learning and watching for danger signs of TSS. These danger signs include a temperature of 101° F (38.4° C), diarrhea, vomiting, muscle aches, and a sunburn-like rash.

CERVICAL CAP. The Prentif cavity rim (PCR) **cervical cap** has a 1¼-inch to 1½-inch soft natural rubber dome with a firm but pliable rim (see Fig. 19-12, *D*). It fits snugly around the base of the cervix close to the junction of the cervix and vaginal fornices (Hatcher et al, 1994). The device is available in four sizes. It is recommended that the cap remain in place 8 to 12 hours after intercourse and not more than 48 hours at a time (Secor, 1992). The seal provides a physical barrier to sperm; spermicide inside the cap adds a chemical barrier.

The extended period of wear is an added convenience for women who previously used the diaphragm. Instructions for the actual insertion and use of the cervical cap closely resemble the instructions for use of the contraceptive diaphragm (see the Guidelines box on p. 528). Some of the differences are that the cervical cap can be inserted hours before sexual intercourse without a need for additional spermicide later, no additional spermicide is required for repeated acts of intercourse when the cap is used, and the cervical cap requires less spermicide than the diaphragm when initially inserted (Secor, 1992).

Some women are not good candidates for wearing the cervical cap. They include women with abnormal Pap test results, women who cannot be fitted properly with the existing cap sizes, women who find the insertion and removal of the device too difficult, women with a history of TSS, women with vaginal or cervical infections, and women who experience allergic responses to the cap or spermicide, a history of pelvic cancer, or severe cervical laceration (Secor, 1992).

Nursing actions. The nurse needs to assess the woman's understanding and skill in the use of the cervical cap (see the Guidelines box on p. 528). The angle of the uterus, the vaginal muscle tone, and the shape of the cervix may interfere with the cervical cap's ease of fitting and use. Correct fitting requires time, effort, and skill from both the woman and the clinician (Secor, 1992). The woman must check the cap's position before and after each act of intercourse.

After 3 months of use, cervical cap users had a higher rate of conversion from class I (no abnormal cells present) to class III (suspicious abnormal cells present) Pap tests when compared with diaphragm users (Mishell, 1989). These conversions may be manifestations of the human papillomavirus (HPV).

No link has been discovered between TSS and the use of the cervical cap, but such an association remains possible (Secor, 1992). The package insert recommends that another form of birth control be used during menstrual bleeding and up to at least 6 weeks postpartum. The cap should be refitted after any gynecologic surgery or birth and after major weight losses or gains. Otherwise, the size should be checked at least once a year (Secor, 1992).

Strong patient motivation is the most important criterion for successful cap use. First-year effectiveness rates are 89.7%

Guidelines

USE AND CARE OF THE DIAPHRAGM

Positions for insertion of diaphragm

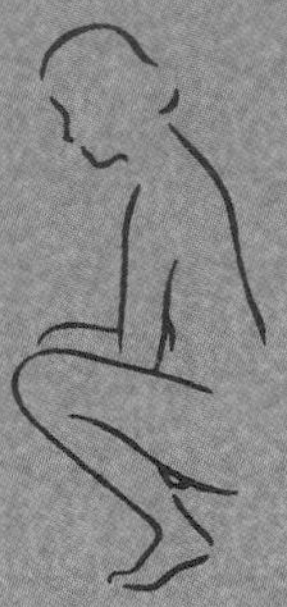

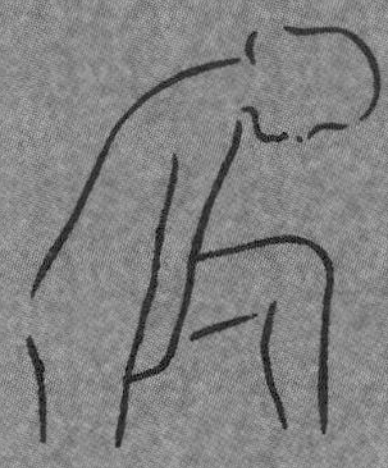

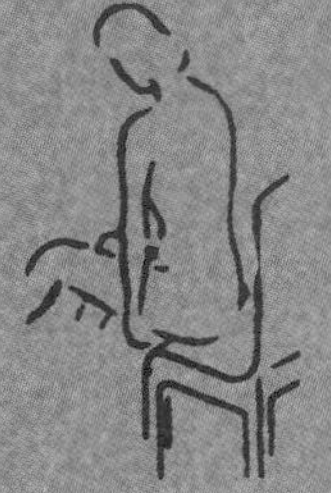

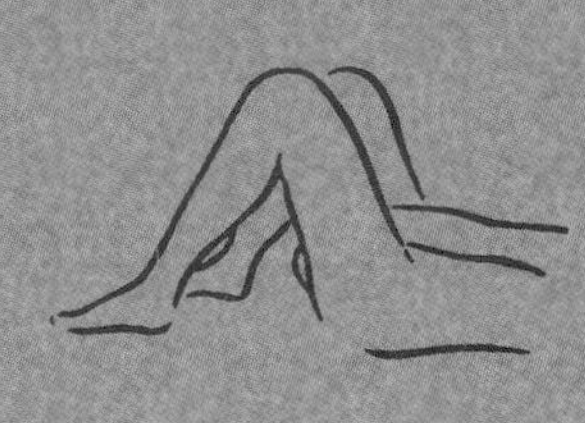

Squatting

This is the most commonly used position, and most women find this position satisfactory.

Leg up method

Another position is to raise the left foot (if right hand is used for insertion) on a low stool, and in a bending position the diaphragm is inserted.

Chair method

Another practical method for diaphragm insertion is for you to sit far forward on the edge of a chair.

Reclining

You may prefer to insert the diaphragm while in a semi-reclining position in bed.

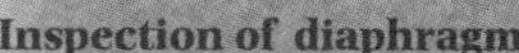

Inspection of diaphragm

Your diaphragm must be inspected carefully before each use. The best way to do this is:

Hold the diaphragm up to a light source. Carefully stretch the diaphragm at the area of the rim, on all sides, to make sure there are no holes. Remember, it is possible to puncture the diaphragm with sharp fingernails.

Another way to check for pinholes is to carefully fill the diaphragm with water. If there is any problem, it will be seen immediately.

If your diaphragm is puckered, especially near the rim, this could mean thin spots.

The diaphragm should not be used if you see any of the above; consult your health care provider.

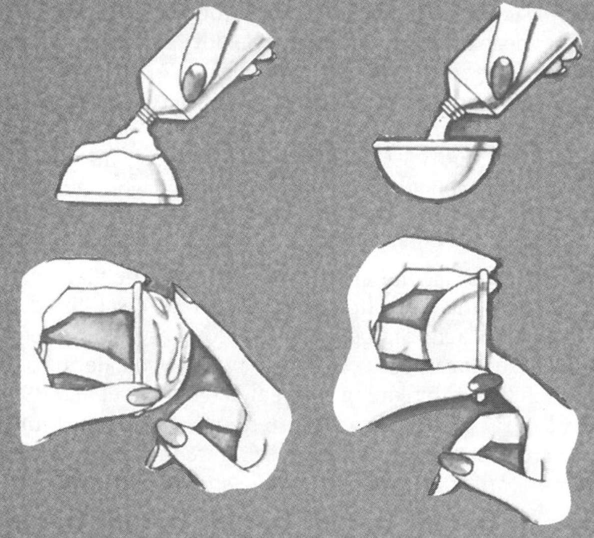

Fig. A

Preparation of diaphragm

Rinse off cornstarch. Your diaphragm must always be used with a spermicidal lubricant to be effective. Pregnancy cannot be prevented effectively by the diaphragm alone.

Always empty your bladder before inserting the diaphragm. Place about 2 teaspoonfuls of contraceptive jelly or contraceptive cream on the side of the diaphragm that will rest against the cervix (or whichever way you have been instructed). Spread it around to coat the surface and the rim. This aids in insertion and offers a more complete seal. Many women also spread some jelly or cream on the other side of the diaphragm (see Fig. A).

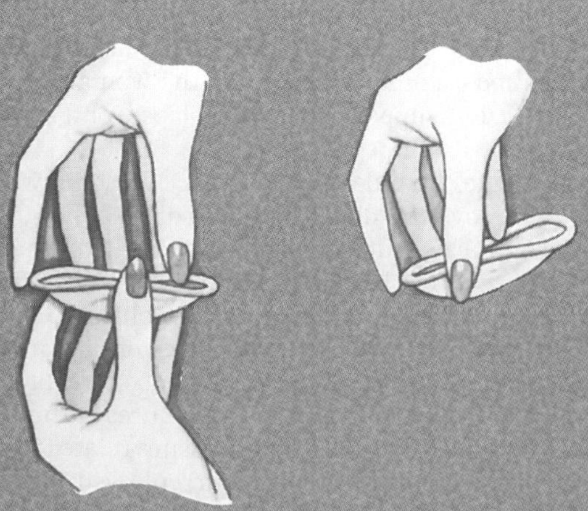

Fig. B

Insertion of diaphragm

The diaphragm can be inserted as long as 6 hours before intercourse. Hold the diaphragm between your thumb and fingers. The dome can either be up or down, as directed by your health care provider. Place your index finger on the outer rim of the compressed diaphragm (see Fig. B). Use the fingers of the other hand to spread the labia (lips of the vagina). This will assist in guiding the diaphragm into place.

Guidelines

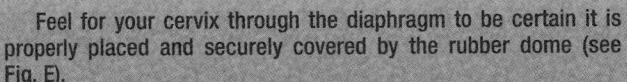

USE AND CARE OF THE DIAPHRAGM—cont'd

Insertion of diaphragm

Insert the diaphragm into the vagina. Direct it inward and downward as far as it will go to the space behind and below the cervix (see Fig. C).

Tuck the front of the rim of the diaphragm behind the pelvic bone so that the rubber hugs the front wall of the vagina (see Fig. D).

Feel for your cervix through the diaphragm to be certain it is properly placed and securely covered by the rubber dome (see Fig. E).

To clean the introducer (if one is used), wash with mild soap and warm water and rinse and dry thoroughly.

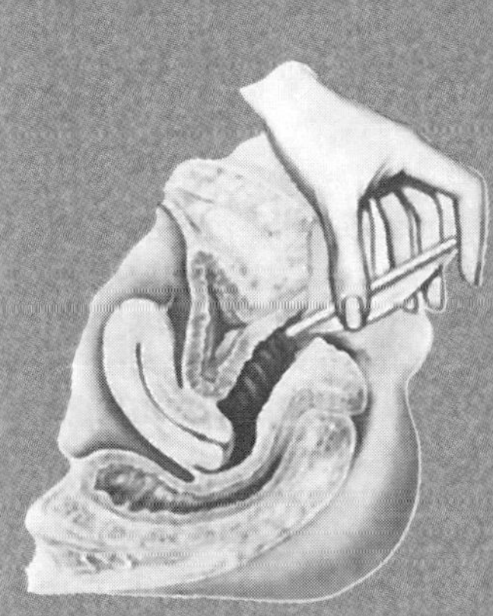

Fig. C

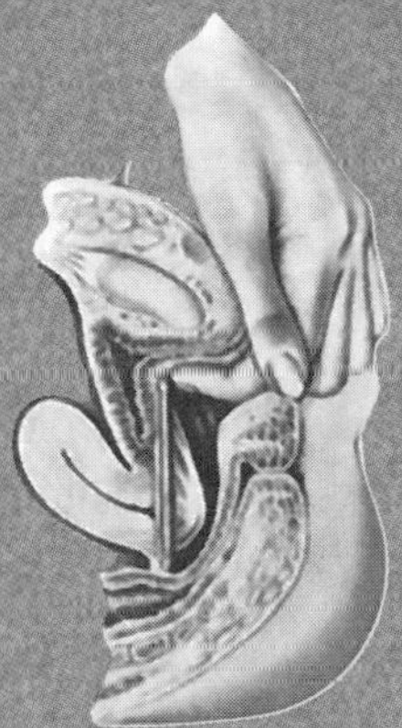

Fig. D

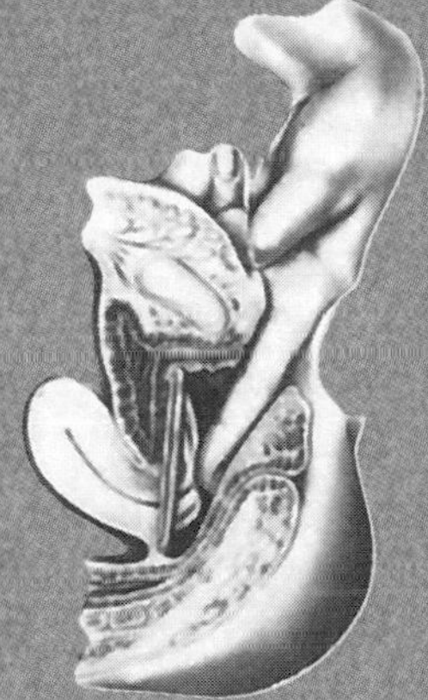

Fig. E

General information

Regardless of the time of the month, this method of contraception must be used each and every time intercourse takes place. Your diaphragm must be left in place for at least 6 hours after the last intercourse. If you remove your diaphragm before the 6-hour period, your chance of becoming pregnant could be greatly increased.

Removal of diaphragm

The only proper way to remove the diaphragm is to insert your forefinger up and over the top side of the diaphragm, and slightly to the side.

Next, turn the palm of your hand downward and backward, hooking the forefinger firmly on top of the inside of the upper rim of the diaphragm, *breaking the suction.*

Pull the diaphragm down and out. This avoids the possibility of tearing the diaphragm with the fingernails. The diaphragm *should not* be removed by trying to catch the rim from *below* the dome (see Fig. F).

Care of diaphragm

When using a vaginal diaphragm, avoid using products that may contain petroleum, such as certain body lubricants, vaginal lubricants, or vaginitic preparations. These products can weaken the rubber.

A little care means longer wear for your diaphragm. After each use the diaphragm should be washed in warm water and mild soap. Do not use detergent soaps, cold cream soaps, deodorant soaps, and soaps containing petroleum because they can weaken the rubber.

After washing, the diaphragm should be dried thoroughly. All water and moisture should be removed with your towel. The diaphragm should then be dusted with *cornstarch.* Scented talc, body powder, baby powder, and the like should not be used because they can weaken the rubber.

The diaphragm should then be placed back in the plastic case for storage. It should not be stored near a radiator or heat source or exposed to light for an extended period.

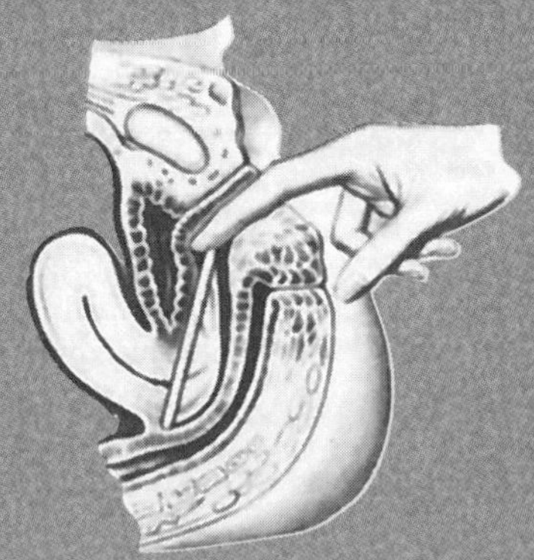

Fig. F

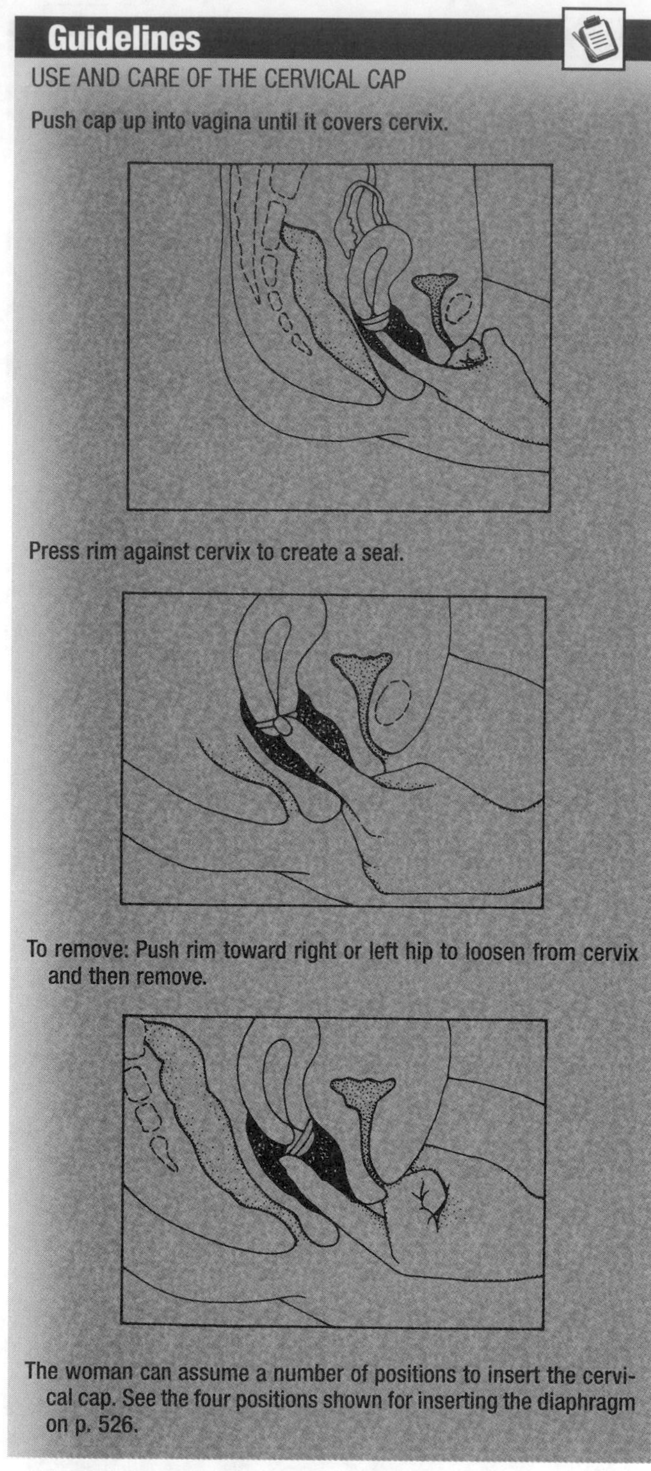

Guidelines
USE AND CARE OF THE CERVICAL CAP
Push cap up into vagina until it covers cervix.
Press rim against cervix to create a seal.
To remove: Push rim toward right or left hip to loosen from cervix and then remove.
The woman can assume a number of positions to insert the cervical cap. See the four positions shown for inserting the diaphragm on p. 526.

(Hatcher et al, 1994; Secor, 1992) and are similar to those of the diaphragm.

INTRAUTERINE DEVICES. An **intrauterine device (IUD)** is a small, T-shaped device inserted into the uterine cavity. Medicated IUDs are loaded with either copper or a progestational agent (Fig. 19-14). These chemically active substances are released continuously, for example, copper-bearing de-

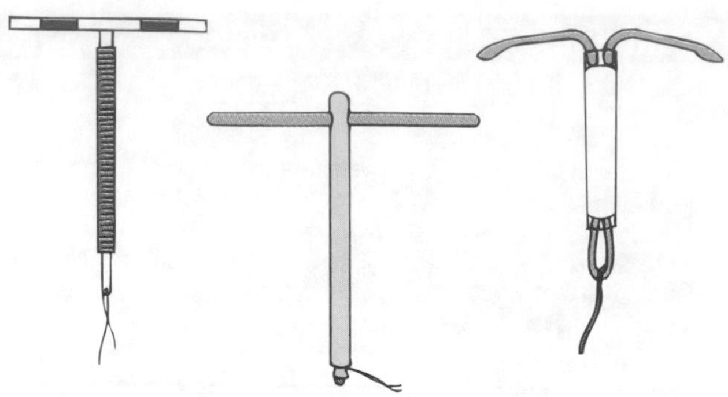

Fig. 19-14 Intrauterine devices.

vices for 4 to 8 years (at present) and progesterone devices for 1 year (*The Contraception Report,* 1992). IUDs are impregnated with barium sulfate for radiopacity. Recent evidence strongly supports a true contraceptive effect in preventing fertilization (*The Contraception Report,* 1992). The copper-bearing IUD damages sperm in transit to the uterine tubes and "interferes with the reproductive process anatomically and temporally before ova reach the uterus" (Grimes, 1989). The progesterone-bearing IUD causes progestin-related effects on cervical mucus and endometrial maturation. Because the effect is local, there is no disruption of the woman's ovulatory pattern.

The IUD offers constant contraception without the need to remember to take pills each day or engage in other manipulation before or between coital acts. If pregnancy can be excluded, an IUD may be placed at any time during the menstrual cycle. An IUD may be inserted immediately after abortion.

The absence of interference with hormonal regulation of menstrual cycles makes the IUD more appropriate than hormonal contraception for heavy smokers, women over age 35 years, women who have hypertension, or those with a history of vascular disease or familial diabetes. Contraceptive effects are reversible. When pregnancy is desired, the IUD may be removed by the health care provider.

The intrauterine progesterone contraceptive system (Progestasert) offers two important noncontraceptive progesterone-related advantages: less blood loss during menstruation and decreased primary dysmenorrhea. The mean blood loss is increased for the copper IUD. This blood loss may be clinically significant in undernourished populations.

Pregnancies that occur with IUDs in place are more likely to be ectopic. However, the risk of ectopic pregnancy is approximately the same as in women not using contraception (*Facts and Comparisons,* 1995).

The use of an IUD is contraindicated for women with a history of PID, known or suspected pregnancy, undiagnosed genital bleeding, suspected genital malignancy, or a distorted intrauterine cavity. Use of an IUD is discouraged in nulliparous women, known diabetics (because the presence of a foreign body in the uterus increases the chances of infection), and women with more than one sexual partner (the risk of infection is greater than in women in monogamous relationships).

Disadvantages of IUD use include risk of PID, especially within 3 months of insertion, and risk of bacterial vaginosis,

BOX 19-13
Signs of Potential Complications

IUDs

Signs of potential complications related to IUDs can be remembered in this manner (Hatcher et al, 1994):
P—Period late, abnormal spotting or bleeding
A—Abdominal pain, pain with intercourse
I—Infection exposure, abnormal vaginal discharge
N—Not feeling well, fever, or chills
S—String missing, shorter or longer

uterine perforation, and infection at time of insertion. The IUD offers no protection against STDs. The IUD is not recommended for teenagers but primarily for women who have had at least one child and who are involved in a stable monogamous relationship.

Nursing actions. The woman should be taught to check for the presence of the IUD thread after menstruation and at the time of ovulation as well as before coitus to rule out expulsion of the device. If pregnancy occurs with the IUD in place, the IUD should be removed immediately, if possible. Retention of the IUD during pregnancy increases the risk of septic spontaneous abortion. Some women allergic to copper develop a rash, necessitating the removal of the copper-bearing IUD. Signs of potential complications to be taught to the woman are listed in Box 19-13.

The first-year failure rate is no more than 2% in typical IUD users (Hatcher et al, 1994). The efficacy of the Copper-T 380A reportedly is greater than that of the Progestasert.

VACCINE TO BLOCK PREGNANCY. An experimental birth control vaccine for women shows promise for blocking pregnancy for 6 months without significant side effects. The vaccine was designed to spur the immune system into making antibodies that block the action of human chorionic gonadotropin, which is produced during pregnancy (*The Contraception Report*, 1994).

POSTCOITAL CONTRACEPTION. High-dose estrogen in the form of diethylstilbestrol (DES) has been used for postcoital contraception since the 1960s. It is also known as the "morning-after" pill. Because of severe immediate and long-term effects, this method is no longer recommended (Hatcher et al, 1994).

Ovral, a birth control pill containing ethinyl estradiol and norgestrel, is the most common current treatment (Narrigan, 1994). Two tablets are taken within 72 hours after intercourse and two tablets 12 hours later (Greydanus and Lonchamp, 1990). Used as a postcoital contraceptive in this manner, Ovral reduces the rate of expected pregnancy by approximately 75% (Hatcher et al, 1994). Common side effects include nausea and vomiting; antiemetics are often prescribed with this regimen. Danazol, a synthetic estrogen, is also used for emergency treatment on a similar schedule. Short-term use of progestin-only pills may be appropriate in women who cannot take estrogen. Postcoital IUD insertion has been shown to be extremely effective in preventing pregnancy (Pollack, 1992).

Turner et al (1994) found that women's knowledge of postcoital contraception was both limited and inaccurate. Patient education about contraceptive alternatives after unprotected intercourse is warranted. Postcoital contraception is most effective if administered within 12 to 24 hours of unprotected intercourse (up to 72 hours).

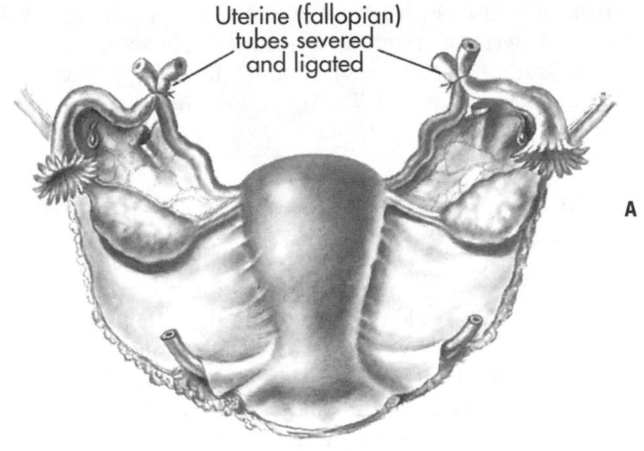

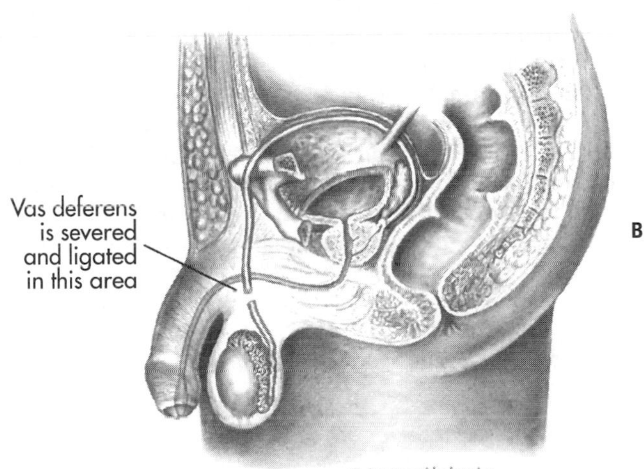

Fig. 19-15 Sterilization. **A,** Oviduct ligated and severed (tubal ligation). **B,** Sperm duct ligated and severed (vasectomy).

Sterilization. **Sterilization** refers to surgical procedures intended to render the person infertile. Most procedures involve the occlusion of the passageways for the ova and sperm (Fig. 19-15). For the female the oviducts (uterine tubes) are occluded; for the male the sperm ducts (vas deferens) are occluded. Only surgical removal of the ovaries (oophorectomy) or uterus (hysterectomy) or both will result in absolute sterility for the woman. All other operations have a small but definite failure rate; that is, pregnancy may result. Voluntary sterilization is the most prevalent method of contraception in the world (Hatcher et al, 1994). In the United States, voluntary sterilization is the most common choice of contraception for couples who are 30 years of age or older.

Laws and regulations. All states have strict regulations for informed consent. Many states in the United States permit voluntary sterilization of any mature, rational woman without reference to her marital or pregnancy status. Although the partner's consent is not required by law, the patient is encouraged to discuss the situation with the partner, and health care providers may request the partner's consent.

Sterilization of minors or mentally incompetent females is restricted by most states. The operation often requires the approval of a board of eugenicists or other court-appointed individuals.

LEGAL TIP

Female Sterilization

- If federal funds are used for sterilization, the person must be at least 21 years old on the day she signs the consent.
- The consent must be signed at least 30 days before her expected date of birth. If she gives birth less than 30 days later, the consent is still valid as long as there would have been 30 days between signing and birth had she given birth on time.
- The consent form is good for only 180 days. If a woman signs too early in pregnancy, the consent could expire before she gives birth.
- Informed consent must include an explanation of the risks, benefits, and alternatives; a statement that describes sterilization as a permanent, irreversible method of birth control; and a statement that mandates a 30-day waiting period between giving consent and the sterilization.
- Informed consent must be in the person's native language or an interpreter must be provided.
- The consent does not take the place of an operative permit for bilateral tubal ligation (BTL). In addition to the consent for sterilization, an operative permit must be signed before surgery.

Types of sterilization

FEMALE STERILIZATION. Female sterilization may be performed immediately after birth (within 24 to 48 hours), concomitantly with abortion, or as an interval procedure (during any phase of the menstrual cycle). Most sterilization procedures are performed immediately after a pregnancy, probably because of heightened motivation or increased practicality. Out-of-hospital sterilization is also safe and effective (Nisanian, 1990).

Tubal occlusion. The operation used commonly is the laparoscopic tubal fulguration (destruction of tissue by means of an electric current [electrocoagulation]). A minilaparotomy may be used for tubal ligation by cutting the tubes or removing a section (Fig. 19-16) or for the application of bands or clips. Bands (e.g., Falope ring) and clips (e.g., Hulka-Clemens) are placed around the tubes to block them (Cunningham et al, 1993). Fulguration and ligation are considered to be permanent methods. Use of the bands or clips has the theoretic advantage of possible removal and return of tubal patency. Transcervical approaches to inject occlusive material into the tubes are being investigated (Hatcher et al, 1994).

For the minilaparotomy approach the woman is admitted the morning of surgery, having received nothing by mouth since midnight. Preoperative sedation is given. The procedure may be carried out with a local anesthetic, but a regional or general anesthetic may also be used. A small vertical incision is made in the abdominal wall below the umbilicus. The woman may experience sensations of tugging but no pain, and the operation is completed within 20 minutes. She may be discharged several hours later if she has recovered from

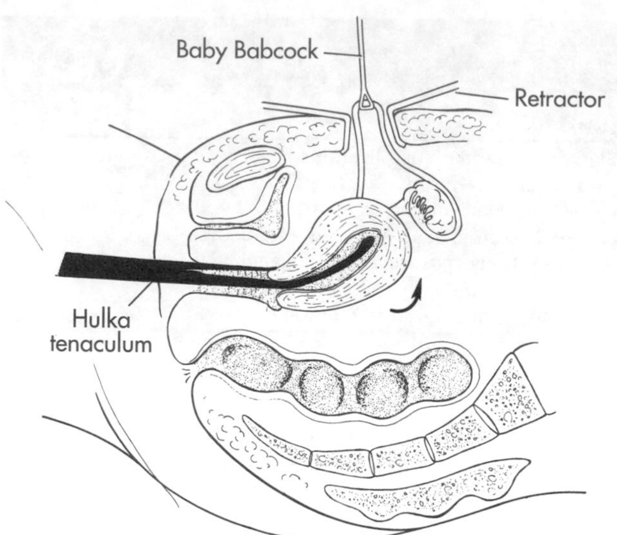

Fig. 19-16 Use of minilaparotomy to gain access to oviducts for tubal occlusion procedures. Tenaculum is used to lift uterus upward *(arrow)* toward incision.

anesthesia. Any abdominal discomfort usually can be controlled with a mild analgesic (e.g., acetaminophen). Within 10 days the scar is almost invisible (see the Guidelines box on p. 531). As occurs with any surgery, there is always a possibility of complications of anesthesia, infection, hemorrhage, and trauma to other organs. Failures, although less than 0.5%, can occur (NAACOG, 1991).

Tubal reconstruction. Restoration of tubal continuity (reanastomosis) and function is technically feasible except after laparoscopic tubal fulguration. However, sterilization reversal is costly, difficult (requiring microsurgery), and uncertain (Cunningham et al, 1993). The success rate varies with the extent of tubal destruction and removal. The incidence of successful pregnancy after reanastomosis is only approximately 15%. There is an increased risk of ectopic pregnancy. The loss of a segment of tube necessary for sperm capacitation and fertilization is the probable reason for low pregnancy rates. Women should be informed that insurance often does not cover the cost of reconstruction.

MALE STERILIZATION. Vasectomy is the easiest and most commonly used operation for male sterilization. In the United States, 500,000 men undergo vasectomy each year (Cunningham et al, 1993). Vasectomy can be carried out with local anesthesia and on an out-of-hospital basis.

In a vasectomy, small right and left incisions are made into the anterior aspect of the scrotum above and lateral to each testis over the spermatic cord (Fig. 19-15, *B*). Each vas deferens is identified and doubly ligated with fine, nonabsorbable sutures. Then each vas deferens is severed between the ligatures. Occasionally the surgeon cauterizes the cut stumps of the sperm ducts. Many surgeons bury the cut ends into scrotal fascia to lessen the chance of reunion, then close the skin incisions. Usually one nonabsorbable suture is used for closure of each skin incision. A dressing is applied.

The man is instructed in self-care to promote a safe return to routine activities. To reduce swelling and relieve discom-

Guidelines

WHAT TO EXPECT AFTER TUBAL LIGATION

You should expect no change in hormones and their influence.
Your menstrual period will be approximately the same as before the sterilization.
You may feel pain at ovulation.
The ovum disintegrates within the abdominal cavity.
It is highly unlikely that you will get pregnant.
You should not experience a change in sexual functioning; in fact, you may enjoy sexual relations more because you will not be concerned about getting pregnant.
Sterilization offers no protection against STDs; therefore you may need to use condoms.

fort, ice packs are applied to the scrotum intermittently for a few hours postoperatively. A scrotal support may be applied to decrease discomfort. Moderate inactivity for approximately 2 days is advisable because of local scrotal tenderness. The skin suture can be removed 5 to 7 days postoperatively. Sexual intercourse may be resumed as desired.

Sterility is not immediate. Some sperm will remain in the proximal portions of the sperm ducts after a vasectomy. One week to several months are required to clear the ducts of sperm (i.e., after approximately 15 ejaculations). Therefore some form of contraception is needed until the sperm count in the ejaculate on two consecutive tests is down to zero (Cunningham et al, 1993).

Vasectomy has no effect on potency (ability to achieve and maintain an erection) or volume of ejaculate. Endocrine production of testosterone continues, so secondary sex characteristics are not affected. Sperm production continues, but sperm are unable to leave the epididymis and are lysed by the immune system. Men occasionally may develop a hematoma, infection, or epididymitis (Hatcher et al, 1994). Less common are painful granulomas from accumulation of sperm.

Complications after bilateral vasectomy are uncommon and usually not serious (Giovannucci, 1992a, b). They include bleeding (usually external), suture reaction, and reaction to the anesthetic agent. Sterilization failures are rare, occurring in approximately 2 per 1000 men.

Tubal reconstruction. Microsurgery to reanastomose (restore tubal continuity) the sperm ducts can be accomplished successfully in 90% of cases (i.e., sperm in the ejaculate) (Jarow, 1987). However, the fertility (pregnancies) rate is much lower (40% to 60%). The rate of success decreases as the time since the procedure increases. The vasectomy may result in permanent changes in the testes that leave men unable to father children. The changes are those ordinarily seen only in the elderly (e.g., interstitial fibrosis [scar tissue between the seminiferous tubules]). Some men develop antibodies against their own sperm (autoimmunization). The role of antisperm antibodies in fertility after vasectomy reversal has not been completely determined.

Future trends. Contraceptive options are more limited in the United States and Canada than in some other industrialized countries. Lack of funding for research, governmental regulations, conflicting values about contraception, and high costs of liability coverage for contraception have been cited as blocks to new and improved methods.

Methods that are currently being investigated include a contraceptive vaccine, vaginal rings, transdermal patches, biodegradable implants, and sublingual tablets for delivering hormonal contraception, more reliable ovulation predictors, and reversible sterilization methods using silicone blocks and other materials (Hatcher et al, 1994).

Nursing Care Management—Sterilization

Assessment

Assessment data include the history, physical examination, and laboratory data. The nurse assesses motivation for sterilization, and alternatives are discussed. Motivation for elective sterilization includes personal preference; obstetric reasons such as multiparity; medical reasons such as hypertensive, cardiovascular, or renal disease in the woman or recurrent acute epididymitis in the man; and diagnosis of inheritable disease.

The patient's knowledge of the sterilization methods and of the chosen method is assessed. Gaps in knowledge and misinformation are noted. The record is reviewed for the signed informed consent.

Nursing Diagnoses

After analyzing the data, nursing diagnoses are identified. Examples of nursing diagnoses for the client undergoing surgical sterilization include the following:

- Decisional conflict related to
  - Alternative methods of surgical sterilization
  - Readiness for permanent termination of fertility
- Risk for infection related to
  - Broken skin or mucous membrane secondary to surgery
- Pain related to
  - Postoperative recovery
- Spiritual distress related to
  - Discrepancy between religious or cultural beliefs and choice of sterilization

Expected Outcomes

Planning is a collaborative effort among the woman and her sexual partner (if appropriate), the physician, and the nurse. Depending on the motivation for sterilization, other physicians may need to be part of the health care team. Expected outcomes are determined and stated in patient-centered terms and may include the following. The woman will:

1. Verbalize an understanding of all information necessary to give informed consent
2. Experience a successful procedure and uneventful recovery
3. Continue to be satisfied with the decision for sterilization, the procedure, and the experience with the health care team

Plan of Care and Implementation

The nurse plays an important role in assisting people with decision making so that all requirements for informed consent are met. People seek information about the various methods

Nursing Care Plan

POSTPARTUM CARE

Vaginal Birth

Nursing Diagnosis: Risk for fluid volume deficit related to uterine atony/hemorrhage

Expected Outcomes: Fundus is firm, lochia is moderate, and there is no evidence of hemorrhage.

• NURSING INTERVENTIONS/*RATIONALES*

Monitor lochia (color, amount, consistency) and count and weigh sanitary pads if lochia is heavy *to evaluate amount of bleeding.*

Monitor and palpate fundus for location and tone *to determine status of uterus and dictate further interventions because atonic uterus is most common cause of postpartum hemorrhage.*

Monitor intake and output, assess for bladder fullness, and encourage voiding *because a full bladder interferes with involution of the uterus.*

Monitor vital signs (increased pulse and respirations, decreased blood pressure) and skin temperature and color *to detect signs of hemorrhage/shock.*

Monitor postpartum hematology studies *to assess effects of blood loss.*

If fundus is boggy, apply gentle massage and assess tone response *to promote uterine contractions and increase uterine tone.* (Do not overstimulate, because doing so can cause fundal relaxation.)

Express uterine clots *to promote uterine contraction.*

Explain to the woman the process of involution and teach her to assess and massage the fundus and to report any persistant bogginess *to involve her in self-care and increase sense of self-control.*

Administer oxytoxic agents per physician/CNM order and evaluate effectiveness *to promote continuing uterine contraction.*

Administer fluids, blood, blood products, or plasma expanders as ordered *to replace lost fluid and lost blood volume.*

Nursing Diagnosis: Pain related to postpartum physiologic changes (hemorrhoids, episiotomy, breast engorgement, cracked/sore nipples)

Expected Outcome: Patient exhibits signs of decreased discomfort.

• NURSING INTERVENTIONS/*RATIONALES*

Assess location, type, and quality of pain *to direct intervention.*

Explain to the woman the source and reasons for the pain, its expected duration, and treatments *to decrease anxiety and increase sense of control.*

Administer prescribed pain medications *to provide pain relief.*

If pain is perineal (episiotomy, hemorrhoids), apply ice packs in the first 24 hours *to reduce edema and vulvar irritation and reduce discomfort;* encourage sitz baths using cool water first 24 hours *to reduce edema* and warm water thereafter *to promote circulation;* apply witch hazel compresses *to reduce edema;* teach woman to use prescribed perineal creams, sprays, or ointments *to depress response of peripheral nerves;* teach woman to tighten buttocks before sitting and to sit on flat, hard surfaces *to compress buttocks and reduce pressure on the perineum.* (Avoid donuts and soft pillows as they separate the buttocks and decrease venous blood flow, increasing pain.)

If pain is from breasts and woman is breastfeeding, encourage use of a supportive bra *to increase comfort;* ascertain that infant has latched on correctly *to prevent sore nipples;* vary infant position during feeding *to prevent sore nipples.*

If breasts are engorged, have woman use warm compresses or take a warm shower before breastfeeding *to stimulate milk flow and relieve stasis.*

If nipples are sore, have woman air-dry nipples after feeding *to toughen nipples* and apply breast creams as prescribed *to soften nipples and relieve irritation.*

If pain is from breast and woman is not breastfeeding, encourage use of a tight supportive bra or breast binder and application of ice packs *to reduce lactation and decrease heaviness.*

Nursing Diagnosis: Sleep pattern disturbance related to excitement, discomfort, and environmental interruptions

Expected Outcome: Patient sleeps for uninterrupted periods of time and feels rested after waking.

• NURSING INTERVENTIONS/*RATIONALES*

Establish woman's routine sleep patterns and compare with current sleep pattern, exploring things that interfere with sleep, *to determine scope of problem and direct interventions.*

Individualize nursing routines to fit woman's natural body rhythms (i.e., wake/sleep cycles), provide a sleep-promoting environment (i.e., darkness, quiet, adequate ventilation, appropriate room temperature), prepare for sleep using woman's usual routines (i.e., back rub, soothing music, warm milk), teach use of guided imagery and relaxation techniques *to promote optimum conditions for sleep.*

Avoid things or routines (i.e., caffeine, foods that induce heartburn, fluids, strenuous mental/physical activity) *that may interfere with sleep.*

Administer sedation or pain medication as prescribed *to enhance quality of sleep.*

Advise woman/partner to limit visitors and activities *to avoid further taxation and fatigue.*

Teach woman to use infant nap time as a time for her also to nap *to replenish energy and decrease fatigue.*

Nursing Diagnosis: Risk for infection related to altered primary defenses in the postpartum period

Expected Outcome: Patient shows no evidence of infection.

• NURSING INTERVENTIONS/*RATIONALES*

Maintain Standard Precautions and use good handwashing technique when providing care *to prevent spread of infection.*

Nursing Care Plan

POSTPARTUM CARE

Vaginal Birth—cont'd

Use strict aseptic technique when performing invasive procedures such as urinary catheterization or insertion of intravenous lines *to reduce risk of nosocomial infection.*

Monitor vital signs *because elevated temperature, pulse, respiratory rate, and blood pressure may indicate infection.*

Monitor for pallor, fatigue, malaise, chills, and loss of appetite, *which may indicate infection.*

Monitor lochia for foul smell *indicative of infection.*

Monitor IV site and episiotomy site for signs such as pain, redness, edema, heat, and drainage, *which are indicative of infection.*

Monitor urine for color, concentration, odor, clouding, casts, and sediment, *which may indicate a urinary tract infection.*

Monitor breasts for infected nipple fissures, hot engorged tissue, or obstruction of milk flow, *which are indicative of mastitis.*

Monitor laboratory values (i.e., white blood cell count, cultures) *for indicators of infection.*

Assist woman to maintain good personal hygiene habits (i.e., wiping perineal region from front to back, keeping area dry, frequent change of peripads, proper use of sitz bath, and perineal irrigation) *to reduce introduction of bacteria.*

Ensure adequate nutritional intake (high protein, iron, vitamin C) *to promote healing.*

---

of sterilization. Clinical information about the various procedures follows the evaluation section. The nurse also provides information about alternatives to sterilization (e.g., contraception).

The nurse acts as a sounding board for people who are exploring the possibility of choosing sterilization and their feelings about and motivation for this choice. The nurse records this information, which may be the basis for referral to a family planning clinic, a psychiatric social worker, or another professional health care provider.

Information must be given about what the various procedures entail, how much discomfort or pain can be expected, and what type of care is needed. Many individuals fear sterilization procedures because of the imagined effect on their sexual life. They need reassurance concerning the hormonal and psychologic basis for sexual function and the fact that uterine tube occlusion or vasectomy has no biologic sequelae on sexual adequacy (Shain et al, 1991).

Preoperative preparation. Printed instructions are usually available for patients from the physician. The physician usually performs the preoperative health assessment, which includes a psychologic assessment, physical examination, and laboratory tests. The nurse assists with the health assessment, answers questions, and confirms the patient's understanding of printed instructions (e.g., NPO after midnight). The nurse provides important emotional support throughout the process. Ambivalence and extreme fear of the procedure are reported to the physician.

Postoperative care. Postoperative care depends on the procedure performed, for example, laparoscopy or laparotomy for tubal occlusion, or vasectomy. General care includes recovery after anesthesia, vital signs, fluid-electrolyte balance (intake and output, laboratory values), prevention of or early identification of and treatment for infection or hemorrhage, control of discomfort, and assessment of emotional response to the procedure and recovery.

Discharge planning. Discharge planning depends on the type of procedure performed. In general, the client is given written instructions about observing for and reporting symptoms and signs of complications, the type of recovery to be expected, and the date and time for a follow-up appointment.

Evaluation

The nurse can be reasonably assured that care was effective if the expected outcomes of care have been achieved: the woman (couple) learns about the various methods of contraception, the couple achieves pregnancy only when it has been planned, and they experience no adverse sequelae as a result of the chosen method of contraception (see the Nursing Care Plan on pp. 532-533). If sterilization was chosen, care was effective if the patient received and understood all information necessary to give informed consent; the procedure was successful and recovery was uneventful; and the patient continues to be satisfied with the decision for sterilization, the procedure, and the experience with the health care team.

Key Points

- Postpartum care is modeled on the concept of health.
- Cultural beliefs and practices affect the patient's response to the puerperium.
- The nursing care plan includes assessments to detect deviations from normal, comfort measures to relieve discomfort or pain, and safety measures to prevent injury or infection.
- The nurse provides teaching and counseling measures designed to promote the patient's feelings of competence in self-care and baby care.
- The nurse must exhibit both clinical and decision-making skills to provide safe and effective physical care. Common nursing interventions include evaluating and treating the boggy uterus and the full urinary bladder, providing for pharmacologic and nonpharmacologic relief of pain and discomfort associated with the episiotomy or lacerations, and instituting measures to promote or suppress lactation.
- Nurses can help promote the health of the patient's future pregnancies and children by administering rubella vaccine and Rh immune globulin when indicated.
- Meeting the psychosocial needs of new mothers involves planning care that considers the composition and functioning of the entire family.
- Parenthood is a learned role. It requires time to master, improves with experience, and evolves gradually and continually as the needs of the parents and child change.
- Mothers (and partners/families) often misjudge the actual amount of physical and emotional energy required for the role transition to parenthood.
- The nurse provides anticipatory guidance that helps new mothers and their families plan ways to achieve healthy adjustments to a new family member, deal with sibling responses, and interact positively with grandparents and other extended family members.
- Attachment is the process by which parent and child come to love and accept each other.
- Attachment is strengthened through the use of sensual responses or abilities by both partners in the parent-child interaction.
- Modulation of rhythm, modification of behavioral repertoires, and mutual responsivity facilitate infant-parent adjustment.
- In adjusting to the parental role, the mother moves from a dependent state (taking in) to an interdependent state (letting go).
- There are a variety of contraceptive methods with various effectiveness rates, advantages, and disadvantages.
- Nurses must provide accurate information to couples to enable them to choose the contraceptive method(s) best suited to them.
- Effective contraceptives are available through both prescription and nonprescription sources.
- Proper concurrent use of spermicides and latex condoms provides protection against sexually transmitted diseases.
- Tubal ligations and vasectomies are sterilization methods used by increasing numbers of women and men.

Videotapes for Parents

Baby Basics (VHS, 110 minutes)
Excellent and entertaining resource on infant care in the first few months. Topics include the newborn at birth, parents caring for themselves postpartum, the first few days at home, daily care, feeding, health and safety, crying and sleeping, growth and development. (Available from Childbirth Graphics Ltd, Waco, Tex.)

Baby Talk (VHS, 60 minutes)
Excellent video on early parenting concerns and baby care. Topics include newborn appearance, sleep and awake patterns, crying and colic, illness and doctor visits, bottle feeding, and the importance of parents taking care of themselves. (Available from Childbirth Graphics Ltd, Waco, Tex.)

Hello Parents (VHS, 22 minutes)
Video that serves as a discussion starter about adapting to parenthood. Often shown in prenatal childbirth classes, the video depicts a wide variety of expectant parents and follows their transition to life with a newborn. (Available from Vida Health Communications, Cambridge, Mass.)

Hey, What About Me? (VHS, 25 minutes)
Video on sibling adjustment. Contains songs about feelings, games and lullabies, bouncing rhymes to do with the new baby, and suggestions on what the siblings can do when they feel angry or lonely. (Available from Childbirth Graphics Ltd, Waco, Tex.)

Home Before You Know It (VHS, 30 minutes)
Video covers the essentials of mother and baby care from birth to the first visit to the pediatrician. It is specifically designed to meet the educational challenges posed by today's shorter maternity stays. (Available from Vida Health Communications, Cambridge, Mass.)

References

Ahumada L: Multicultural perinatal health care, *Matern Child Health Educ Resources* 6:1, Spring 1991.

Ament L: Maternal tasks of the puerperium reidentified, *J Obstet Gynecol Neonatal Nurs* 19(4):330, 1990.

Anderson P: Therapy review: drug use during breast-feeding, *Clin Pharm* 10:594, 1991.

Briggs G et al: *Drugs in pregnancy and lactation: a reference guide to fetal and neonatal risk,* ed 4, Baltimore, 1994, Williams & Wilkins.

Bristoll S et al: The mythical danger of rapid urinary drainage, *Am J Nurs* 89(3):344, 1989.

Broom B: Impact of marital quality and psychological well-being on parental sensitivity, *Nurs Res* 43(3):138, 1994.

Brown G, Rutter M: The measurement of family activities and relationships, *Human Relations* 19:241, 1966.

Connell E: The female condom—a new contraception option, *Contemp OB GYN* 39(10):20, 1994.

Contraception choices for women over age 35: focus on benefits and risks, *The Contraception Report* 3(2):4, 1992.

Cunningham F et al: *Williams obstetrics,* ed 19, Norwalk, Conn, 1993, Appleton & Lange.

Darney P et al: Acceptance and perceptions of Norplant among users in San Francisco, USA, *Stud Fam Plann* 21(3):152, 1990.

D'Avanzo C: Bridging the cultural gap with Southeast Asians, *MCN Am J Matern Child Nurs* 17(4):204, 1992.

Davis M: Natural family planning, *NAACOG's Clin Iss Perinat Women Health Nurs* 3(2):280, 1992.

Drug facts and comparisons, ed 47, St Louis, 1993, Wolters Kluwer.

Dumas M: *A phenomenological investigation of the meaning of "being jealous" as experienced in fathers following the birth of their first child,* doctoral dissertation, Adelphi University, 1990.

Edwards L: *Paternal, infant, and social contextual characteristics as determinants of competent parental functioning by fathers with young infants,* doctoral dissertation, The University of North Carolina at Greensboro, 1990.

Facts and comparisons, Loose-Leaf Drug Information Service, St Louis, 1995, Wolters Kluwer.

Fehring R: Methods used to self-predict ovulation: a comparative study, *J Obstet Gynecol Neonatal Nurs* 19(3):233, 1990.

Fehring R et al: Use effectiveness of the Creighton Model Ovulation Method of family planning, *J Obstet Gynecol Neonatal Nurs* 23(4):303, 1994.

Franklin M: Reassessment of the metabolic effects of oral contraceptives, *J Nurse Midwife* 35(6):358, 1990.

Future methods of contraception, *The Contraception Report* 5(4):4, 1994

Galanti G: *Caring for patients from different cultures,* Philadelphia, 1991, University of Pennsylvania Press.

Geissler E: *Pocket guide to cultural assessment,* St Louis, 1994, Mosby.

Gennaro S: Postpartal anxiety and depression in mothers of term and preterm infants, *Nurs Res* 37(2):82, 1988.

Gerstman B et al: Oral contraceptive estrogen dose and the risk of deep venous thromboembolic disease, *Am J Epidemiol* 133(1):32, 1991.

Giovannucci E et al: Vasectomy and its effects of lifespan, *N Engl J Med* 326:1392, 1992a.

Giovannucci E et al: A long-term study of mortality in men who have undergone vasectomy, *N Engl J Med* 326(21):1392, 1992b.

Greydanus D, Lonchamp D: Contraception in the adolescent: preparation for the 1990s, *Med Clin North Am* 74(5):1205, 1990.

Grimes D: Whither the uterine device? *Clin Obstet Gynecol* 32(2):369, 1989.

Harris C: The birth control pill revisited, *NAACOG's Clin Iss Perinat Women Health Nurs* (2):246, 1992.

Hatcher R et al: *Contraceptive technology (1994-1996),* 16th rev ed, New York, 1994, Irvington Publishers.

Hawkins J, Matteson P, Tabeck E: *Fertility control.* In Fogel C, Woods N, editors: *Women's health care,* Thousand Oaks, Calif, 1995, Sage.

Hillard P: The patient's reaction to side effects of oral contraceptives, *Am J Obstet Gynecol* 161(5):1412, 1989.

Hinkle L: Education and counseling for Norplant users, *J Obstet Gynecol Neonatal Nurs* 23(5):387, 1994.

Horn B: Cultural concepts and postpartal care, *J Transcultural Nurs* 2(1):48, 1990.

Jarow J: Vasectomy: autoimmunity and reversal, *JAMA* 257(15):2087, 1987.

Jarrett M, Lethbridge D: The contraceptive needs of midlife women, *Nurse Pract* 15(12):34, 1990.

Klaisle C, Wysocki S: Innovations in contraception: the Norplant system, *NAACOG's Clin Issue Perinat Women Health Nurs* 3(2):267, 1992.

Klaus M, Kennell J: *Bonding: the beginnings of parent-infant attachment,* St Louis, 1983, Mosby.

Klaus M, Kennell J: *Parent-infant bonding,* ed 2, St Louis, 1982, Mosby.

Koniak-Griffin D, Verzemmnieks I, Cahill D: Using videotape instruction and feedback to improve adolescents' mothering behaviors, *J Adolesc Health* 13:570, 1992.

Konje J et al: The effect of continuous subdermal levonorgestrel (Norplant) on carbohydrate metabolism, *Am J Obstet Gynecol* 166(1):15, 1992.

Labbok M, Queenan J: The use of periodic abstinence for family planning, *Clin Obstet Gynecol* 32(2):387, 1989.

Lethbridge D: Coitus interruptus—considerations as a method of birth control, *J Obstet Gynecol Neonatal Nurs* 20(1):80, 1991.

Ludman E et al: Blood building foods in contemporary Chinese populations, *Perspect Pract* 89(8):1122, 1989.

Luegenbiehl D et al: Standardized assessment of blood loss, *MCN Am J Matern Child Nurs* 15:241, 1990.

Mastrioanni L, Robinson J: Contraception in the 1990s, *Patient Care* 28(1):107, 1994.

Mattson S: Culturally sensitive perinatal care for Southeast Asians, *J Obstet Gynecol Neonatal Nurs* 24(4):335, 1995.

McBride B: Parent education and support programs for fathers: outcome effects on paternal involvement, *Early Child Dev Care* 67:73, 1992.

Mercer R: *Parent infant interaction.* In Sonstegard L et al, editors: *Women's health: childbearing,* vol 2, New York, 1982, Grune & Stratton.

Mercer R: *Becoming a mother,* New York, 1995, Springer.

Mercer R, Ferketich S: Predictors of parental attachment during early parenthood, *J Adv Nurs* 15:268, 1990.

Milligan R, Flenniken P, Pugh L: Positioning intervention to minimize fatigue in breastfeeding women, *Appl Nurs Res* 9(2):67, 1996.

Milligan R, Parks P, Lenz E: Measuring postpartum fatigue. Paper presented at NAACOG National Research Conference: *Making a difference in women's and infants' health,* Denver, Col, July 20-21, 1990.

Mishell D: Contraception, *N Engl J Med* 320(12):777, 1989.

Moore R: *Contraception issues and options for young women: contemporary studies in women's health,* Fairlawn, NJ, 1994, MPE Communications.

NAACOG: *Contraceptive options* (OGN Practice Resource), Washington, DC, 1991, NAACOG.

Narrigan D: Postcoital contraception: has its day come? *J Nurse Midwife* 39(6):363, 1994.

Niruthisard S et al: Use of nonoxynol-9 and reduction in rate of gonococcal and chlamydial cervical infections, *Lancet* 339:1371, 1992.

Nisanian A: Outpatient minilaparotomy sterilization with local anesthesia, *J Reprod Med* 35(4):380, 1990.

Nugent J: Cultural and psychological influences on the father's role in infant development, *J Mar Fam* 53:475, 1991.

Park K, Peterson L: Beliefs, practices, and experiences of Korean women in relation to childbirth, *Health Care Women Int* 12:261, 1991.

Polaneczky M et al: The use of levonorgestrel (Norplant) for contraception in teenage mothers, *N Engl J Med* 331:1201, 1994.

Pollack A: Teen contraception in the 1990s, *J School Health* 62(7):288, 1992.

Pollack A, Moore C: New issues in spermicide use, *Contemp OB GYN* 39(4):29, 1994.

Porter R, Cernoch J, Perry S: The importance of odors in mother-infant interactions, *Maternal Child Nurs J* 12(3):147, 1983.

Potter L: Will the new OC instructions increase compliance? *Adv Nurse Pract* 2:10, 1994.

Pugh L, Milligan R: A framework for the study of childbearing fatigue, *Adv Nurs Sci* 15(4):60, 1993.

Pugh L, Milligan R: Patterns of fatigue during childbearing, *Appl Nurs Res* 8(3):140, 1995.

Roberts K: A comparison of chilled cabbage leaves and chilled gelpaks in reducing breast engorgement, *J Hum Lact* 11:17, 1995.

Rubin R: Maternal behavior, *Nurs Outlook* 9:682, 1961.

Sampselle C: Changes in pelvic muscle strength and stress urinary incontinence associated with childbirth, *J Obstet Gynecol Neonatal Nurs* 19(5):371, 1990.

Secor R: The cervical cap, *NAACOG's Clin Issue Perinat Women Health Nurs* 3(2):236, 1992.

Shain R et al: Impact of tubal sterilization and vasectomy on female marital sexuality: results of a controlled longitudinal study, *Am J Obstet Gynecol* 164(3):763, 1991.

Shaw D, Bell R: Developmental theories of parental contributors to antisocial behavior, *J Abnorm Child Psychol* 21(5):493, 1993.

Stainton M: Origins of attachment: culture and cue sensitivity, *Diss Abstracts Int* 46:3786 B (University Microfilms No. 8600606), 1985.

Swanson J et al: Readability of commercial and generic contraceptive instruction, *Image: J Nurs Sch* 22(2):96, 1990.

Sweezy S: Contraception for the postpartum woman, *NAACOG's Clin Issue Perinat Women's Health Nurs* 3(2):209, 1992.

Tedder J: Using the Brazelton neonatal assessment scale to facilitate the parent-child relationship in a primary care setting, *Nurs Pract* 16(3):26, 1991.

Tomlinson P, Irwin B: Qualitative study of women's reports of family adaptation pattern four years following transition to parenthood, *Iss Ment Health Nurs* 14:119, 1993.

Tulman L, Fawcett J: Recovery from childbirth: looking back 6 months after delivery, *Health Care Women Int* 12:341, 1991.

Turner G et al: Women's knowledge of emergency contraception, *Br J Gen Pract* 44:451, 1994.

United States Pharmacopeial Convention, Inc: *Drug information for the health care professional*, ed 13, Taunton, Mass, 1993, Rand McNally.

Youngkin E: Progestogens: a look at the "other" hormone, *Nurse Pract* 18(11):28, 1993.

Walker L: *Parent-infant nursing science: paradigms, phenomena, methods*, Philadelphia, 1992, FA Dairs.

Wilcox A, Weinberg C, Baird D: Timing of sexual intercourse in relation to ovulation: effects on the probability of conception, survival of the pregnancy, and sex of the baby, *N Engl J Med* 333(23):1517, 1995.

Wismont J, Reame N: The lesbian childbearing experience: assessing developmental tasks, *Image: J Nurs Sch* 21(3):137, 1989.

Wolfson A, Lacks P, Futteman A: Effects of parent training on infant sleep patterns, parents' stress, and perceived parental competence, *J Consult Clin Psychol* 60(1):41, 1992.

Bibliography

Beck C: Screening methods for postpartum depression, *J Obstet Gynecol Neonatal Nurs* 24(4):308, 1995.

Blegen M et al: Outcomes of hospital-based managed care: a multivariate analysis of cost and quality, *Obstet Gynecol* 86(5):809, 1995.

Callister L: Cultural meanings of childbirth, *J Obstet Gynecol Neonatal Nurs* 24(4):327, 1995.

Clark R: Infections during the postpartum period, *J Obstet Gynecol Neonatal Nurs* 24(6):542, 1995.

Coffman S: Parent and infant attachment: review of nursing research 1981-1990, *Pediatr Nurs* 18(4):421, 1992.

Freda M et al: Women's responses to depo-provera, *MCN Am J Matern-Child Nurs* 21(4):183, 1996.

Keppler A: Postpartum care center: follow-up care in a hospital-based clinic, *J Obstet Gynecol Neonatal Nurs* 24:17, 1995.

Lethbridge D: Fertility management in Taiwanese and African-American women, *J Obstet Gynecol Neonatal Nurs* 24:459, 1995.

Mapanga H, Andrews C: Influence of family and friends' basic conditioning factors and self-care agency on unmarried teenage primiparas' engagement in contraceptive practice, *J Commun Health Nurs* 12:89, 1995.

McGregor L: Short, shorter, shortest: improving the hospital stay for mothers and newborns, *MCN Am J Matern Child Nurs* 19(2):91, 1994.

Pinder P: Protocols constructed around the nursing process 2: oral contraceptives, *J Am Coll Health* 43:179, 1995.

Tiller C: Father's parenting attitudes during a child's first year, *J Obstet Gynecol Neonatal Nurs* 24(6):508, 1995.

Valaitis R, Tuff K, Swanson L: Meeting parents' postpartal needs with a telephone information line, *MCN Am J Matern Child Nurs* 21(2):90, 1996.

Walters N, Kristiansen, C: Two evaluations of combined mother-infant versus separate postnatal nursing care, *Res Nurs Health* 18:17, 1995.

CHAPTER 20

Postpartum Complications

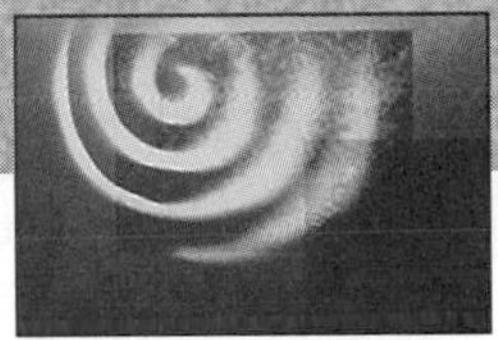

POSTPARTUM HEMORRHAGE, P. 537

Uterine atony, p. 538
Lacerations of the birth canal, p. 538
Medical management, p. 539
Retained placenta, p. 539
Inversion of the uterus, p. 539
Subinvolution of the uterus, p. 541
Nursing care management, p. 541
Hemorrhagic (hypovolemic) shock, p. 542

POSTPARTUM INFECTIONS, P. 543

Postpartum urinary tract infections, p. 543
Postpartum infection (sepsis), p. 543
Mastitis, p. 544
Nursing care management, p. 545

SEQUELAE OF CHILDBIRTH TRAUMA, P. 546

Structural disorders of the uterus and vagina, p. 546
Nursing care management, p. 549

LOSS AND GRIEF, P. 550

Grief responses, p. 551
Anticipatory grief, p. 552
Tasks of mourners, p. 552
Nursing care management, p. 553
Other losses, p. 561
Complicated bereavement, p. 562

Providing safe and effective care of the woman and family experiencing postpartum complications, sequelae of childbirth trauma, or grief related to perinatal loss requires a joint effort from all members of the health care team. This chapter focuses on the postpartum complications of hemorrhage and infection, sequelae of childbirth trauma, and loss and grief.

POSTPARTUM HEMORRHAGE

Postpartum **hemorrhage,** traditionally the loss of 500 ml of blood or more after vaginal birth, is the most common and most serious type of excessive obstetric blood loss. A more meaningful definition of postpartum hemorrhage is the loss of 1% or more of body weight, since 1 ml of blood weighs 1 g. Postpartum hemorrhage is a leading cause of maternal morbidity and mortality, accounting for approximately 10% of nonabortive maternal deaths. Approximately 8% of all births are complicated by postpartum hemorrhage (Murahata, 1991).

In defining a postpartum hemorrhage, the clinician must recognize that estimated blood loss (which is traditionally underestimated) is as important as clinical signs and symptoms (Veronikis and O'Grady, 1994). The average blood loss accompanying a spontaneous vaginal birth is approximately 500 ml; the loss is approximately 1000 ml following a cesarean birth (O'Brien, 1993). Recent reports indicate that a postpartum blood loss of up to 1000 ml is generally well tolerated by the woman, without significant changes in blood pressure and cardiac output. Therefore a more realistic definition for postpartum hemorrhage is a postpartum blood loss exceeding 1000 ml, independent of the mode of birth (Roberts, 1995). Postpartum hemorrhage may be sudden and even exsanguinating.

Nursing ALERT

Maternal exsanguination can occur within a matter of minutes (Knuppel and Hatangadi, 1995).

Moderate but persistent bleeding may continue for days or weeks. Postpartum hemorrhage may be early, within the first 24 hours after birth, or late, from 24 hours after birth until the twenty-eighth postpartum day.

Control of bleeding from the placental site is accomplished by prolonged contraction and retraction of interlacing strands of myometrium, the living ligature. A firm or contracted uterus does not normally bleed after birth unless placenta previa existed. Therefore careful assessment of uterine tone and the maintenance of uterine contractions through manual massage or oxytocic stimulation, as needed, are important parts of postpartum care.

Early postpartum hemorrhage almost invariably is caused by uterine atony, which complicates approximately 1 in 20 births (Hunter and Weiner, 1996); lacerations of the birth canal; or disseminated intravascular coagulation (DIC). *Late postpartum hemorrhage* most commonly is the result of

BOX 20-1
Risk Factors for Postpartum Hemorrhage

- Uterine atony
  - Overdistended uterus
    - Large fetus
    - Multiple fetuses
    - Polyhydramnios
    - Distention with clots
  - Anesthesia and analgesia
    - Conduction anesthesia
  - Previous history of uterine atony
  - High parity
  - Prolonged labor, oxytocin-induced labor
  - Trauma during labor and birth
    - Operative forceps birth
    - Vacuum-assisted birth
    - Cesarean birth
- Retained placental fragments
- Lacerations of the birth canal
- Ruptured uterus
- Inversion of the uterus
- Abruptio placentae
- Placenta previa
- Coagulation disorders
- Manual removal of a retained placenta
- Uterine subinvolution
- Prophylaxis for pregnancy-related complications
  - Magnesium sulfate administration during labor or postpartum
  - Aspirin therapy for antiphospholipid antibody syndrome or previous early onset, severe preeclampsia

subinvolution of the placenta site, retained placental tissue, or infection. (See Box 20-1 for predisposing factors for postpartum hemorrhage.)

It is helpful to consider the problem of excessive bleeding with reference to the stages of labor. From birth of the fetus until separation of the placenta, the character and quantity of blood passed may suggest excessive bleeding. For example, *dark blood* is probably of venous origin, perhaps from varices or superficial lacerations of the birth canal. *Bright blood* is arterial and indicates, for example, deep lacerations of the cervix. *Spurts of blood* with clots may indicate partial placental separation. *Failure of blood to clot* or remain clotted indicates coagulopathy.

The period from the separation of the placenta to its expulsion/removal is when excessive bleeding occurs as a result of incomplete placental separation. After the placenta has been expelled, persistent or excessive blood loss most commonly is a result of **atony** of the uterus (i.e., its failure to contract well or maintain its contraction) or prolapse of the uterus into the pelvis.

Complications of postpartum hemorrhage are either immediate or delayed. Hemorrhagic (hypovolemic) shock and death may occur from sudden, exsanguinating hemorrhage. Delayed complications provoked by postpartum hemorrhage include anemia, puerperal infection, and thromboembolism.

Uterine Atony

Uterine atony is marked hypotonia of the uterus. Uterine atony occurs in at least 5% of births, particularly when the woman is a grand multipara. It also can occur with polyhydramnios, when the fetus is large, or after the births of a multifetal gestation. In such conditions the uterus is overstretched and contracts poorly. Other causes of atony include traumatic birth, use of halogenated anesthesia, magnesium sulfate, rapid or prolonged labor, chorioamnionitis, and use of oxytocin for labor induction or augmentation.

Lacerations of the Birth Canal

Lacerations of the birth canal are the second major cause of postpartum hemorrhage. Continued bleeding despite efficient postpartum uterine contractions demands inspection or reinspection of the birth passage. Continuous bleeding from so-called minor sources may be just as dangerous as a sudden loss of a large amount of blood, although often it is ignored until shock develops. Birth canal lacerations may include injuries to the labia, perineum, vagina, and cervix.

Factors that influence the causes and incidence of obstetric lacerations of the lower genital tract include operative birth; uncontrolled spontaneous birth; congenital abnormalities of the maternal soft parts; contracted pelvis; size, abnormal presentation, and position of the fetus; relative size of the presenting part and the birth canal; prior scarring from infection, injury, or surgery; vulvar, perineal, and vaginal varices; and abnormalities of uterine action (e.g., precipitate birth).

Labial lacerations. Extreme vascularity in the labia and periclitoral areas often results in profuse bleeding if laceration occurs. Immediate repair, by means of fine suture on an atraumatic needle, is required.

Perineal lacerations. Lacerations of the perineum are the most common of all injuries in the lower portion of the genital tract. These are classified as first, second, third, and fourth degree (see Chapter 16). An episiotomy may extend to become either a third- or fourth-degree laceration.

Vaginal lacerations and hematomas. Prolonged pressure of the fetal head on the vaginal mucosa ultimately interferes with the circulation and may produce ischemic or pressure necrosis. Therefore the state of the tissues together with the type of birth may result in deep vaginal lacerations and predisposition to vaginal hematomas.

Vaginal hematomas occur more commonly in association with a forceps birth, an episiotomy, or in the primigravida (Ridgeway, 1995).

Nursing ALERT

During the postpartum period, if the woman complains of persistent perineal or rectal pain or a feeling of fullness in the vagina, a careful inspection of the vulva is made.

A subperitoneal hematoma may cause minimal pain, and the initial presentation may be signs of shock (Ridgeway, 1995). Once the hematoma is diagnosed, treatment or observation is begun. The initial treatment is directed toward stabilization of the patient and assessment for signs of hypovolemic shock. In general, if the hematoma is small (3 to 5 cm) and not expanding, a period of observation is appropriate.

Cold therapy (ice packs) to minimize pain and swelling and analgesics may be all that is required. If the hematoma is swelling or is larger than 5 cm, treatment consists of evacuation, ligation of the bleeding vessel if found, closure of the incision, vaginal packing if appropriate, and placement of an indwelling catheter to maintain urinary drainage (Ridgeway, 1995). Again, cold therapy, analgesia, urinary drainage, and observation are essential postoperatively.

Cervical lacerations. Cervical lacerations usually occur at the lateral angles of the external os; most are shallow, and bleeding is minimal. More extensive lacerations may extend to the vaginal vault or beyond the vault into the lower uterine segment.

Medical Management

Early recognition and diagnosis of postpartum hemorrhage is critical to the management of the woman. The first step is to evaluate the contractility of the uterus. If the uterus is hypotonic, management is directed toward increasing contractility and minimizing blood loss.

The initial management of excessive postpartum bleeding is firm massage of the uterine fundus, expression of any clots in the uterus, and rapid intravenous (IV) infusion of 20 units of oxytocin in 1000 ml Ringer's lactate or normal saline. If the uterus fails to respond to oxytocin, a dose of 0.2 mg ergonovine (Ergotrate) or methylergonovine (Methergine) may be given intramuscularly (IM) to produce sustained uterine contractions. However, use of these drugs is contraindicated in the presence of hypertension or cardiovascular disease. If first-line drugs are not effective, a derivative of prostaglandin $F_{2\alpha}$ (carboprost tromethamine) may be given IM. Most hemorrhages can be controlled after one or two injections of 0.25 mg prostaglandin $F_{2\alpha}$ IM or intramyometrially. Prostaglandin $F_{2\alpha}$ should be used cautiously in women with cardiovascular disease or reactive airway disease (asthma) (Bowes, 1994).

If bleeding persists, bimanual compression is initiated by the physician or nurse-midwife. This procedure involves inserting a fist into the vagina and pressing the knuckles against the anterior side of the uterus while placing the other hand on the abdomen, massaging the posterior uterus. Bimanual compression is also used in an acute situation until oxytocic drugs can be administered and take effect.

The woman may be moved to the delivery room or operating room for an examination to explore the uterine cavity for retained placental fragments or lacerations. If the blood being lost fails to clot, a coagulopathy (e.g., DIC) may have developed, and prompt, appropriate treatment may be lifesaving. Blood transfusion for the treatment of shock and blood replacement may be urgently needed.

If the preceding procedures are ineffective, surgical management may be the only alternative. Surgical management options include vessel ligation (uteroovarian, uterine, hypogastric), angiographic embolization, and hysterectomy (Roberts, 1995).

Retained Placenta

Nonadherent retained placenta. The normally implanted placenta separates with the first or second strong uterine contraction after birth of the infant. Placental separation occurs within 15 minutes of birth in approximately 90% of women. Within the next 15 minutes an additional 5% of women have a separated placenta. Within the third 15-minute period, only another 1% or 2% achieve placental separation. Thus if the placenta has not been recovered within 30 minutes of birth, most health care providers will attempt to remove it manually.

No supplementary anesthesia is needed for parturients who have had regional anesthesia for birth. For other women, administration of light nitrous oxide and oxygen inhalation anesthesia or IV thiopental (Pentothal) facilitates intrauterine exploration, placental separation, and recovery of the placenta.

If birth occurs early (during the fifth or sixth month), placental retention tends to occur because of poor separation.

Adherent retained placenta. Abnormal adherence of the placenta occurs for unknown reasons, but it is thought to result from zygote implantation in a zone of defective endometrium. There is no zone of separation between the placenta and the decidua. Abnormal adherence of the placenta is diagnosed in only about 1 of every 12,000 births. The mother with an abnormally attached placenta is at increased risk for postpartum hemorrhage leading to hypovolemic shock.

Unusual placental adherence may be partial or complete. The following degrees of attachment are recognized:

- *Placenta accreta*—slight penetration of myometrium by placental trophoblast
- *Placenta increta*—deep penetration by placenta
- *Placenta percreta*—perforation of uterus by placenta

At least 15% of cases of abnormally adherent placenta (all types) are associated with placenta previa (Zahn and Yeomans, 1990). The diagnosis of an abnormally adherent placenta generally is made when manual separation of a retained placenta is attempted. If the placenta does not separate readily (even a portion), immediate abdominal hysterectomy may be indicated.

Inversion of the Uterus

Inversion of the uterus (turning inside out) after birth is a potentially life-threatening complication. The incidence of uterine inversion is approximately 1 in 2000 to 2500 births (Wendel and Cox, 1995). The inversion may be partial or complete. Complete inversion of the uterus is obvious; a large, red, rounded mass (perhaps with the placenta attached) protrudes 20 to 30 cm outside the introitus. Incomplete inversion cannot be seen but must be felt; a smooth mass will be palpated through the dilated cervix, reducing the size of the uterine cavity by at least half.

Contributing factors to uterine inversion include fundal pressure and traction applied to the cord, uterine atony, leiomyomas, and abnormally adherent placental tissue. Uterine inversion occurs most often in multiparous women and with placenta accreta and increta. Although proper management of the third stage of labor prevents the majority of uterine inversions, some are unavoidable. Regardless of the precipitating factor, once an inversion occurs, prompt recognition and correction are necessary to reduce maternal morbidity and mortality.

The primary presenting signs of uterine inversion are hemorrhage, shock, and pain. Hemorrhage is the primary presenting sign in up to 94% of women with uterine inversion, with blood loss estimated to range from 800 to 1800 ml.

Up to 40% of these women may also suffer from shock (Wendel and Cox, 1995; Zahn and Yeomans, 1990).

Prevention—always the easiest, cheapest, and most effective therapy—is especially appropriate in the avoidance of puerperal uterine inversion. *One must not pull on the umbilical cord until the placenta has definitely separated.* Uterine inversion may occasionally recur in a subsequent birth.

Medical management. Uterine inversion is an emergent situation requiring immediate recognition, replacement of the uterus within the pelvic cavity, and correction of associated clinical conditions. If attempts to manually replace the uterus are not quickly successful, administration of tocolytic agents or general anesthesia may be necessary. Hemorrhagic shock can occur rapidly if the inversion is not immediately recognized.

Medical management of this condition involves all of the following interventions (Kochenour, 1991; Wendel and Cox, 1995; Zahn and Yeomans, 1990):

- Shock, which invariably is out of proportion to the blood loss, is treated. Usually, IV lactated Ringer's solution is infused; blood may also be transfused. Oxytocic agents are withheld until the uterus has been repositioned. Ergot products are strictly contraindicated because the cervix, as well as the uterus, will contract, and replacement of the uterus may be difficult.
- The fundus of the uterus is replaced. This is accomplished after the woman has received tocolytic agents or is under deep anesthesia. As soon as the uterus is repositioned, these relaxing agents are discontinued.

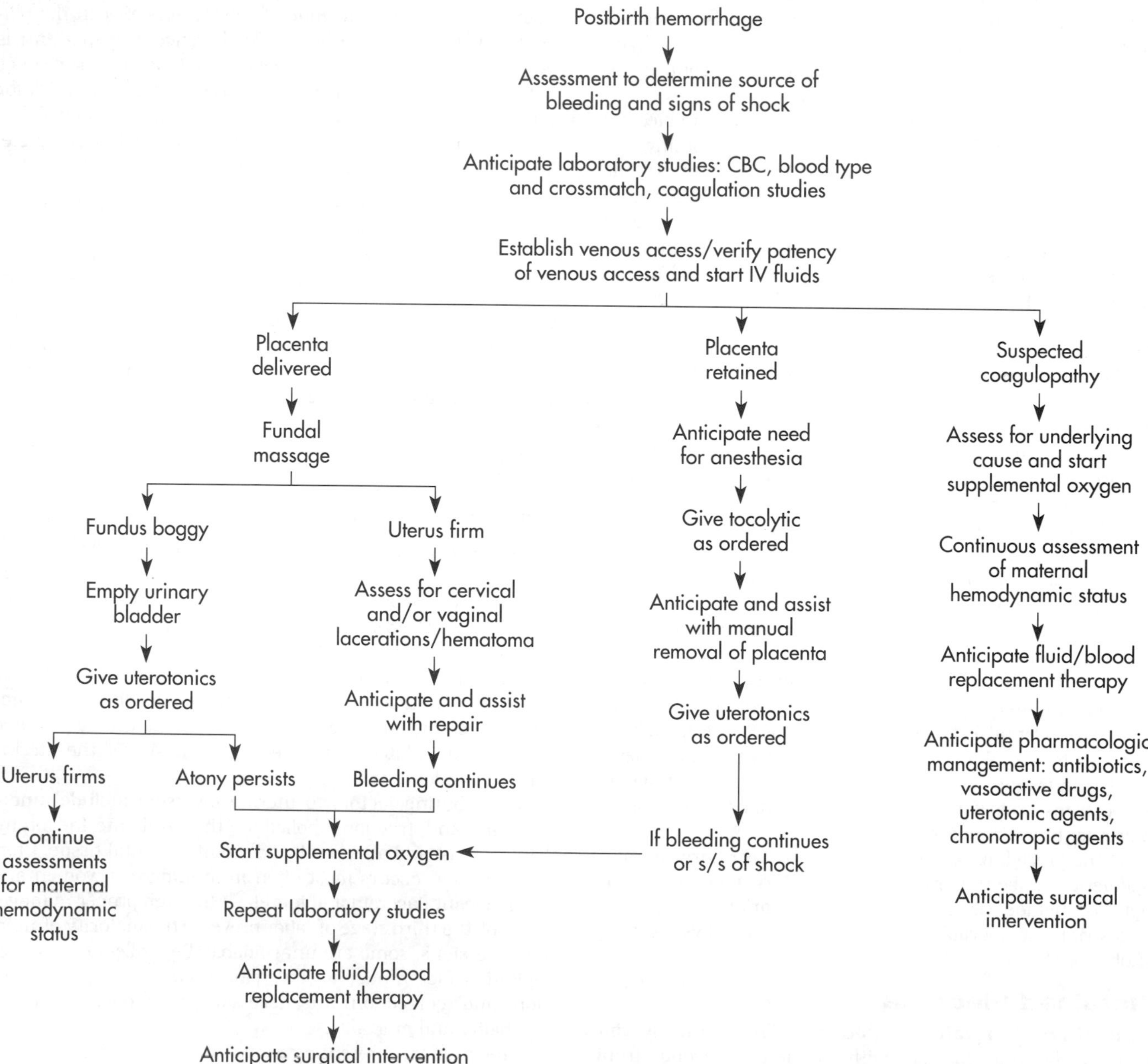

Fig. 20-1 Nursing assessments for postpartum bleeding. *CBC,* Complete blood count; *IV,* intravenous; *s/s,* signs and symptoms.

- Oxytocic agents are given after the uterus is replaced; these may include oxytocin, prostaglandin $F_{2\alpha}$ (1 to 4 mg IM or intramyometrially), and/or Prostin/15M (0.25 mg IM or intramyometrially). Bimanual compression may be effective in controlling bleeding until these drugs take effect.
- Vaginal manual replacement is successful in approximately 75% of women. Abdominal or vaginal surgery may be necessary to reposition the uterus if manual replacement is unsuccessful.
- Broad-spectrum antibiotic therapy may be initiated and a nasogastric tube inserted to prevent infection and to minimize paralytic ileus.

Subinvolution of the Uterus

Late postpartum bleeding may occur as a result of subinvolution of the uterus. Subinvolution is defined as the delayed return of the enlarged puerperal corpus to normal size and function (Cunningham et al, 1993). The causes of subinvolution include reduced circulation because of malposition, myomas, retained products of conception, infection, and gestational trophoblastic disease.

In the absence of frank bleeding, treatment is with ergonovine, 0.2 mg/4 hr for 2 or 3 days, and antibiotic therapy. With hemorrhage, dilation and curettage (D & C) to remove retained placental fragments and to debride the placental site for adequate healing generally is required, together with oxytocic agents and antibiotics.

Nursing Care Management

Assessment

Postpartum hemorrhage can progress rapidly to shock; therefore the nurse must assess the patient carefully and thoroughly (Fig. 20-1). The patient's history should be reviewed for factors that predispose the woman to postpartum hemorrhage (Box 20-1). The fundus is assessed to determine if it is firmly contracted at or near the level of the umbilicus. Bleeding should be assessed in relation to color, amount and, if possible, source. For example, the perineum is inspected for signs of lacerations and/or hematomas.

Vital signs may not be reliable indicators of shock in the immediate postpartum period because of physiologic adaptations of this period. However, frequent vital sign measurements in the first 2 hours after birth may identify trends that are related to blood loss (e.g., tachycardia, tachypnea, falling blood pressure).

Assessment should include evaluation for bladder distention because a distended bladder prevents uterine contraction. The skin is assessed for warmth and dryness; nail beds are checked for promptness of capillary refill. Laboratory studies include evaluation of hemoglobin and hematocrit levels.

Late postpartum hemorrhage may develop within several days of birth or later in the postpartum period. The patient may be at home when the symptoms occur. Discharge teaching should emphasize the signs of normal involution, as well as potential complications.

Nursing Diagnoses

Nursing diagnoses relevant to the care of the patient experiencing a postpartum hemorrhage relate to tissue perfusion, possible complications, anxiety, and knowledge deficits. Potential nursing diagnoses include the following:

- Fluid volume deficit (immediate) related to
  - Excessive blood loss secondary to uterine atony, lacerations, or uterine inversion
- Risk for infection related to
  - Excessive blood loss or exposed placental attachment site
- Risk for injury (maternal) related to
  - Attempted manual removal of retained placenta
  - Administration of blood products
  - Operative procedures
- Fear/anxiety related to
  - Threat to self
  - Knowledge deficit of procedures and operative management
- Altered parenting related to
  - Separation from infant secondary to treatment regimen
- Altered peripheral tissue perfusion related to
  - Excessive blood loss and shunting of blood to central circulation

Expected Outcomes

Expected outcomes for the woman experiencing postpartum hemorrhage may include the following. The woman will:

1. Identify and use available support systems
2. Maintain normal vital signs and laboratory values
3. Not experience complications related to excessive bleeding
4. Verbalize understanding of the condition, its management, and discharge instructions

Plan of Care and Implementation

Immediate care of the patient experiencing a postpartum hemorrhage includes assessment of vital signs and uterine consistency and administration of oxytocin or other drugs to stimulate uterine contraction. Explanations are given to the woman (and her family) regarding the rationale for procedures and the need to act quickly.

The care of the woman who has lacerations of the perineum is similar to that advocated for episiotomies (i.e., analgesia as needed for pain, and heat or cold applications as necessary).

Nursing ALERT

To avoid injury to the suture line, a woman with third- or fourth-degree lacerations is not given postpartum rectal suppositories or enemas.

The need for increased roughage in the diet and increased intake of fluids is emphasized, as well as oral stool softeners to assist the woman in reestablishing bowel habits without straining and putting stress on the suture lines.

The care of the woman experiencing an inversion of the uterus focuses on immediate stabilization of hemodynamic status. If the uterus can be replaced manually, care must be taken after the birth to avoid aggressive fundal massage.

Discharge instructions for the woman are similar to those for any postpartum patient. In addition, she should be told that she is likely to experience fatigue, even exhaustion, and needs to limit her physical activities to conserve her strength.

She may need assistance with infant care and household activities until she regains strength. Referrals for home care follow-up may be needed.

Evaluation

The nurse can be reasonably assured that care was effective to the extent that the expected outcomes have been achieved if the woman identifies and uses available support systems, maintains normal vital signs and laboratory values, does not experience complications, and verbalizes understanding of the condition, its management, and discharge instructions.

Hemorrhagic (Hypovolemic) Shock

Hemorrhage may result in **hemorrhagic or hypovolemic shock.** Shock is an emergency situation in which the perfusion of body organs may become severely compromised and death may ensue. Vigorous treatment is necessary to prevent adverse sequelae (e.g., cellular death, fluid overload, shock lung, and oxygen toxicity).

Physiologic compensatory mechanisms are activated in response to hemorrhage. The adrenal glands release catecholamines, causing arterioles and venules in the skin, lungs, gastrointestinal tract, liver, and kidneys to constrict. The available blood flow is diverted to the brain and heart and away from other organs, including the uterus. If shock is prolonged, the continued reduction in cellular oxygenation results in an accumulation of lactic acid and acidosis (from anaerobic glucose metabolism). Acidosis (lowered serum pH) causes arteriole vasodilation; venule vasoconstriction persists. A circular pattern is established; that is, decreased perfusion, increased tissue anoxia and acidosis, edema formation, and pooling of blood further decrease the perfusion. Cellular death occurs.

Medical management. Medical management of hypovolemic shock involves restoring circulating blood volume and eliminating the cause of the hemorrhage (e.g., lacerations, uterine atony, or inversion). To restore circulating blood volume, a rapid IV infusion of crystalloid solution and packed red blood cells (PRBCs) is initiated. Fresh frozen plasma (FFP) infusion may be needed if clotting factors are below normal.

Nursing Care Management

Hemorrhagic shock often occurs rapidly. As soon as a woman exhibits the signs and symptoms of shock (see the Emergency box above), the nurse summons assistance and equipment. The nurse should have standing orders to start IV fluids and know the type of infusion to use and laboratory tests to order. While waiting for the physician, the nurse ensures a patent airway, which may include airway insertion, and facilitates oxygen administration.

The nurse helps with instituting and monitoring measures to increase tissue perfusion. The nurse should be prepared to assist with placement of a central venous pressure (CVP) or Swan-Ganz catheter if needed (Clark et al, 1994).

The nurse continues to monitor, assess, and record respirations, pulse, blood pressure, skin condition, urine output, level of consciousness (LOC), and hemodynamic parameters (CVP or Swan-Ganz) to evaluate effectiveness of management.

EMERGENCY

HEMORRHAGIC SHOCK

Shock

Respirations	Rapid and shallow
Pulse	Rapid, weak, irregular
Blood pressure	Decreasing (late sign)
Skin	Cool, pale, clammy
Urine output	Decreasing
Level of consciousness	Lethargy→ coma
Mental status	Anxiety→coma
Central venous pressure	Decreased

Intervention

Summon assistance and equipment.
Start IV infusion per standing orders.
Ensure patent airway; administer oxygen.
Continue to monitor status.

Effective respiratory status is essential in that the body rids itself of excess acids by increasing the respiratory rate. Oxygen is administered, preferably by a nonrebreathing face mask, at 10 to 15 L/min. Mechanical ventilation may be needed. The pulse rate increases and becomes irregular as shock progresses in severity.

Perfusion of the skin is sacrificed in the body's attempt to maintain blood flow to the heart and brain. Therefore the condition of the skin is a valuable index to the severity of shock. The nurse assesses the degree of ischemia or cyanosis of the nail beds, eyelids, and skin inside the mouth (buccal mucosa, gums, tongue). The nurse notes the degree of coolness and clamminess of the skin to palpation.

A Foley catheter with a urometer is inserted to allow for hourly assessment of urine output. The most objective and least invasive assessment of adequate organ perfusion and oxygenation is a urine output of at least 30 ml/hr (Veronikis and O'Grady, 1994); an increased output indicates improvement in the woman's condition.

The adequacy of cerebral perfusion may be estimated by an evaluation of the woman's LOC. In early stages of decreased cerebral blood flow the woman may complain of "seeing stars," feeling dizzy, or feeling nauseated. She may become restless and orthopneic. As cerebral hypoxia increases, she may become confused and react slowly or not at all to stimuli. An improved sensorium is an indicator of improvement.

Infection is a complication of hemorrhage. Causes may include surgical procedures, multiple pelvic examinations, anemia, and loss of the white blood cell (WBC) component of the blood.

Anxiety is contagious. The nurse's calm, confident manner, coupled with brief, simple explanations, is an important aspect of care.

Fluid/blood replacement therapy. Critical to successful management of the woman experiencing a hemorrhagic complication is establishment of venous access, preferably with a large-bore Intracath. If possible, the establishment of two IV lines will facilitate fluid resuscitation. Vigorous fluid resuscitation includes the administration of crystalloids, col-

TABLE 20-1 Hazards of shock therapy

HAZARD	NURSING ACTION
Fluid overload: moist respirations, stridor, or dyspnea	Alert physician; decrease drip rate
Shock lung: tachypnea, dyspnea, anxiety, a rise in blood pressure, cyanosis, and harsh loud breaths	Alert physician; maintain ventilator between 50 and 70 mm Hg
Oxygen toxicity: muscular twitching about the face, followed by convulsions resembling grand mal seizures	Alert physician; take convulsion precautions

loids, blood, and blood components. Fluid resuscitation must be carefully monitored in that fluid overload can occur (Table 20-1). Intravascular fluid overload occurs more commonly with colloid therapy.

Transfusion therapy is used to restore oxygen-carrying capacity and intravascular volume. Packed red blood cells (PRBCs) are administered to increase vascular volume (250 to 300 ml/unit) and improve oxygen-carrying capacity. Each unit of PRBCs increases the hematocrit by 3%. Fresh frozen plasma (FFP) contains clotting factors and fibrinogen and is the only source of factors V, XI, and XII. Each unit of FFP increases intravascular volume by 250 ml and fibrinogen by 10 mg%. Each unit of platelets increases the platelet count by 5000 to 10,000 and provides limited volume expansion.

There are risks associated with administration of blood and blood components. Banked blood is cold (4° C) and has an acid pH (6.6 to 6.8), which can result in hypothermia, arrhythmias, and acidosis. In addition, banked blood can result in electrolyte imbalances caused by the electrolyte composition of the blood (sodium, 150 to 160 mEq/L; potassium, 10 to 15 mEq/L; no ionized calcium; and low levels of 2,3-diphosphoglycerate). Coagulopathies may result from massive transfusions in that banked blood is deficient in platelets and clotting factors.

Transfusion reactions may follow administration of blood or blood components. Even in an emergency, each unit should be checked per hospital protocol. Complications include hemolytic reactions, febrile reactions, allergic reactions, circulatory overloading, and air embolism. Rapid transfusion with ice-cold blood can chill the heart and cause arrhythmias or arrest.

LEGAL TIP

Standard of Care for Seizures and Bleeding Emergencies

The standard of care for obstetric emergency situations is that provision should be made for implementing independent nursing actions. Policies, procedures, and protocols for managing emergencies may include those relating to (1) seizures, (2) hemorrhage and shock, and (3) abruptio placentae.

Early recognition and appropriate management of obstetric hemorrhage are essential to prevent significant maternal and perinatal sequelae.

POSTPARTUM INFECTIONS

Postpartum Urinary Tract Infections

Postnatal urinary tract infections (UTIs) usually are caused by coliform bacteria. UTIs are common because of trauma to the base of the bladder and urethra and as a result of catheterization during or after labor.

Suprapubic or costovertebral angle pain, fever, urinary retention, hematuria, dysuria, or urinary frequency often signifies a UTI. These symptoms indicate the need for urinalysis, urine culture, bacterial sensitivity tests, and probable wide-spectrum antibiotic therapy. Substitution of a specific antibacterial drug must await an assessment of the woman's history, her response to initial therapy, and the sensitivity report.

Prompt treatment of definite UTIs is indicated. However, prophylactic therapy rarely is warranted. Most cases respond to treatment within a week. Urologic consultation is indicated if symptoms persist. Prevention of recurrence of UTI is an important part of therapy.

Postpartum Infection (Sepsis)

Postpartum infection (puerperal sepsis, or childbed fever) is any clinical infection of the genital canal that occurs within 28 days after abortion or childbirth. Infections may result from bacteria commonly found within the vagina (endogenous) or from the introduction of pathogens from outside the vagina (exogenous). An episiotomy or lacerations of the vagina or cervix may open avenues for sepsis. Even more formidable, however, may be the large placental site. Here the denuded endometrium (decidua basalis) and residual blood after birth make the uterus an ideal site for a wound infection.

Puerperal sepsis occurs after approximately 6% of births in the United States and probably is the major cause of maternal morbidity and mortality throughout the world. The most common infecting organisms are the numerous streptococcal and anaerobic organisms. *Staphylococcus aureus*, gonococci, coliform bacteria, and clostridia are less common but serious pathologic organisms that cause postpartum infection.

Commonly the infection is complicated by medical disorders such as anemia, malnutrition, and diabetes mellitus. Obstetric problems, including premature rupture of membranes (PROM), a long and exhausting labor, operative birth, hemorrhage, and retention of the products of conception, increase the likelihood and severity of puerperal sepsis.

Chorioamnionitis may be the cause or result of PROM. Chorioamnionitis may be followed by placentitis and fetal congenital pneumonia, omphalitis, or septicemia. Placentitis and chorioamnionitis may be followed by endometritis.

Endometritis, usually at the placental site, permits infection to begin. Localized infection may be followed by salpingitis, peritonitis, and pelvic abscess formation. Septicemia may develop. Secondary abscesses may arise in distant sites such as the lungs or liver. Pulmonary embolism or septic shock, often with DIC, from any serious genital infection may prove fatal. Postpartum femoral thrombophlebitis (milk leg) may result in a swollen, painful leg and, if untreated, may become septic thrombophlebitis (Fig. 20-2).

The symptoms of **puerperal infection** may be mild or severe. A temperature of 38° C (100.4° F) or more on 2 successive days, not counting the first 24 hours after birth, must be considered to have been caused by postpartum infection in the

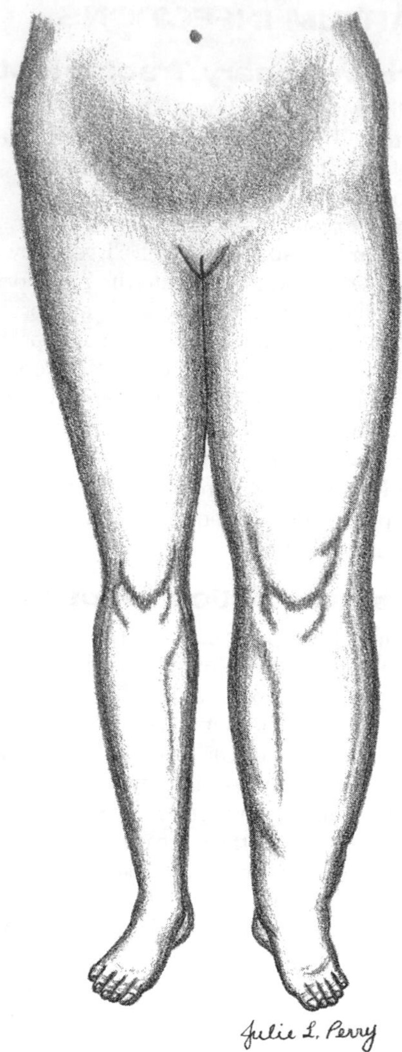

Fig. 20-2 Femoral thrombophlebitis (milk leg). (Courtesy Julie L. Perry.)

absence of convincing proof of another cause. The woman also may describe symptoms of fatigue and lethargy, lack of appetite, and chills. Perineal discomfort or lower abdominal distress, nausea, and vomiting may soon develop. Foul or profuse lochia is usually present. Intracervical or intrauterine bacterial cultures should reveal the offending pathogens within 36 to 48 hours.

The most effective and cheapest treatment of postpartum infection is prevention. Preventive measures include patient education regarding good prenatal nutrition to control anemia and intranatal hemorrhage. Good maternal perineal hygiene is emphasized. Coitus after rupture of the membranes is contraindicated. Strict adherence by all health care personnel to aseptic techniques during childbirth and the postpartum period is very important.

Infection control measures for cure and comfort are instituted. Fluid and electyrolyte balance is vital. Broad-spectrum antibiotics are administered IV until the infecting organism is identified. Then organism-specific antibiotic therapy is begun. Mother-infant contact is established on the basis of the mother's levels of fatigue and discomfort. The infant's father and other family members also may provide newborn contact. Breastfeeding may continue, depending on the prescribed antibiotic regimen.

The virulence of the organisms, the resistance of the woman, and her response to treatment affect the prognosis. Prevention, supportive therapy, and prompt massive antibiotic administration have reduced the maternal mortality in the United States to less than 0.4%.

Bacteremic shock. Critical infections, particularly those in which the causative bacteria release endotoxins, may precipitate bacteremic (septic) shock. Women with postpartum endometritis are at increased risk.

High, spiking fever and chills are pathophysiologic evidence of serious sepsis. An anxious mother may become apathetic. Body temperature often falls to slightly subnormal levels. The skin becomes cool, moist, and pale. The pulse becomes rapid and thready. Marked hypotension and peripheral cyanosis develop. Oliguria occurs.

Laboratory findings reveal marked evidence of infection. Blood cultures show bacteremia, usually consisting of enteric gram-negative bacilli. Additional studies may reflect hemoconcentration, acidosis, and coagulopathy. An electrocardiogram (ECG) may show changes indicative of myocardial insufficiency. Evidence of cardiac, pulmonary, renal, and neurologic hypoxia is notable.

Management focuses on antimicrobial therapy, as well as oxygen support to relieve tissue hypoxia, and circulatory support to prevent vascular collapse. Heart function, respiratory effort, and kidney function are closely monitored. Prompt treatment of bacteremic shock results in a good prognosis, and maternal morbidity and mortality are decreased by controlling respiratory distress, hypotension, and DIC.

Mastitis

Mastitis, or breast infection, affects approximately 1% of women soon after childbirth, most of whom are first-time mothers who are breastfeeding. Mastitis almost always is unilateral and develops well after the flow of milk has been established. The infecting organism generally is the hemolytic *Staphylococcus aureus.* An infected nipple fissure usually is the initial lesion, followed by ductal system involvement. Inflammatory edema and engorgement of the breast soon obstruct the flow of milk in the lobes. Chills, fever, malaise, and local breast tenderness are noted. Without prompt treatment, a breast abscess usually develops.

Interventions include intensive antibiotic therapy, breast support, local heat (or cold) therapy, and analgesics. Lactation is maintained (if desired) by emptying the breasts every 2 to 4 hours by manual expression or a breast pump. Most women respond to treatment, and an abscess can be prevented.

Almost all instances of acute mastitis can be avoided by proper breastfeeding to prevent cracked nipples.

Missed feedings, waiting too long between feedings, and abrupt weaning may lead to clogged milk ducts and mastitis. Cleanliness practiced by all who have contact with the newborn and new mother also reduces the incidence of mastitis.

Nursing Care Management

Assessment

History. Preconception or antenatal factors that influence the development of vaginal infections or UTIs include a history of chronic UTIs or kidney infection and kidney stones; chronic conditions that impair kidney function (e.g., lupus, diabetes, sickle cell disease); chronic immunosuppressive states (e.g., steroid therapy, acquired immunodeficiency syndrome [AIDS]); poor fluid and nutritional status; failure to use condoms; and poor genital hygiene. Intrapartum events such as frequent catheterizations (especially with the use of epidural anesthesia); frequent vaginal examinations; prolonged second stage of labor; birth trauma to the vagina, cervix, bladder, and urethra; and excessive blood loss also may place the mother at greater risk for infection. Untreated or undertreated infections in the prenatal period may predispose mothers to postpartum infections. PROM and the length of time from rupture to birth also may be factors.

Physical examination. Findings on examination vary. Some infections may be asymptomatic. Vaginal discharge may or may not be present. Fever or pain may be mild and therefore dismissed. A thorough symptom assessment, coupled with a complete history and physical examination, is essential in identifying possible maternal infectious disease processes. Signs of infection may not be evident for 24 to 48 hours after giving birth.

> **Nursing ALERT**
>
> A fever higher than 38° C (100.4° F), chills, and tachycardia are indicative of infection.

Abdominal or perineal discomfort, nausea, and vomiting may develop. Foul-smelling lochia is a sign of uterine infection; other potential sites of infection include the breasts, an episiotomy or cesarean incision, and the bladder.

Laboratory tests. Bacterial infections are easily determined from genital tract, urine, and blood studies. Viral agents also can be cultured but less successfully. An elevated WBC count may be of diagnostic help; other laboratory tests are useful depending on what other infectious agents are suspected. Other laboratory data to assess include hematocrit, hemoglobin, proteinuria, and blood urea nitrogen (BUN).

Nursing Diagnoses

Nursing diagnoses are derived after carefully analyzing assessment findings and medical management directives. Nursing diagnoses for the patient at risk for infections include the following:

- Pain/impaired tissue integrity related to
  - Effects of infection process
  - Scratching (excoriation) of pruritic areas
  - Hygienic practices
- Knowledge deficit related to
  - Transmission/prevention of infection/reinfection
  - Safer sex behaviors
  - Management and course of infection
- Anxiety/self-esteem disturbance/body-image disturbance related to
  - Perceived effects on sexual relationships and family processes
  - Long-term sequelae to infection
- Risk for altered parenting related to
  - Fear of spread of infection to newborn
- Altered patterns of urinary elimination related to
  - Presence of edema and pain
  - Impaired urinary function
- Altered family processes related to
  - Unexpected complication to expected postpartum recovery
  - Possible separation from newborn
  - Interruption in process of realigning relationships after the addition of the new family member

Expected Outcomes

A plan of care is formulated that relates specifically to the physical and psychosocial needs of the woman. Goals are mutually determined with the woman. Expected outcomes may include the following. The woman will:

1. Have her infection treated successfully
2. Be able to state the etiology and prevention, management, and sequelae of the infection
3. With her family, verbalize acceptance of the unexpected events; they verbalize positive coping measures (e.g., arrangement for home health care)

Plan of Care and Implementation

Interventions include continuously assessing for signs and symptoms of infection, assessing for pain, monitoring laboratory results, administering antimicrobial agents as ordered, initiating nonpharmacologic comfort measures, administering analgesics as ordered, and providing information to the mother and family as needed (see the Patient Teaching box below). General care such as adequate hydration, rest, proper nutrition, and stress reduction also are implemented. Discussion of measures to avoid reinfection is essential. Topics of in-

> **Patient Teaching**
>
> PREVENTION OF GENITAL TRACT INFECTIONS
>
> - Practice genital hygiene.
> - Choose underwear or hosiery with a cotton crotch.
> - Avoid tight-fitting clothing (especially tight jeans).
> - Select cloth car seat covers instead of vinyl.
> - Limit time spent in damp exercise clothes (especially swimsuits and leotards or tights).
> - Limit exposure to bath salts or bubble bath.
> - Avoid colored or scented toilet tissue.
> - If sensitive, discontinue use of feminine hygiene deodorant sprays.
> - Use condoms.
> - Void before and after intercourse.
> - Decrease dietary sugar.
> - Drink yeast-active milk and eat yogurt (with lactobacilli).
> - Avoid douching.

Patient Teaching

"SAFER" SEX

- "Safer" sex is possible only if there is no oral or genital exchange of body fluids.
- Correct use of condoms, while greatly reducing risk, is not exclusively protective.
- Use of spermicides containing nonoxynol 9 may offer additional protection.
- Select sexual partners with extreme care.
- Ask partner about history of sexually transmitted diseases.

struction should include thorough handwashing, proper medication administration, "safer" sex practices (see the Patient Teaching box above), and genital hygiene.

Evaluation

Evaluation of patient outcomes is a continuous process. To be effective, evaluation is based on patient-centered goals identified during the planning stage of nursing care. The nurse can be reasonably assured that care was effective to the extent that the following expected outcomes have been met:

1. The woman is free of infection, or her infection is stabilized and she does not become reinfected.
2. She experiences the reduction or elimination of pain.
3. The woman knows the etiology, management, and sequelae of the infection.

See the Nursing Care Plan below.

SEQUELAE OF CHILDBIRTH TRAUMA

Women are at risk for problems related to the reproductive system from the age of menarche through menopause and the older years. These problems include structural disorders of the uterus and vagina related to pelvic relaxation and are often the delayed but direct result of childbearing.

With fetopelvic disproportion, prolonged labor, or a precipitous birth, structures of the vesical and vaginal walls are stretched and may be injured. The bladder neck and urethra may be compressed between the presenting part and the pubic bones or forced downward ahead of the presenting part. Since soft tissue damage usually occurs behind an intact vaginal epithelium, there is nothing visible to repair. However, defects may also occur in women who have never been pregnant.

Structural disorders can have far-reaching effects for the woman and her family. Beyond the obvious physiologic alterations, the woman also experiences threats to her self-concept and her ability to cope. A woman's concept of herself as a sexual being can be affected by the condition and its treatments. A woman's family is also challenged by the diagnosis and treatment.

Structural Disorders of the Uterus and Vagina

Alterations in pelvic support

Uterine displacement and prolapse. Normally the round ligaments hold the uterus in anteversion, and the uterosacral ligaments pull the cervix backward and upward (see Figs. 3-5, 3-6, and 3-7). Uterine displacement is a variation of this normal placement. The most common type of displacement is posterior displacement, or *retroversion*, in which the uterus is tilted posteriorly and the cervix rotates anteriorly. Other variations include retroflexion and anteflexion (see Fig. 3-7).

By 2 months postpartum the ligaments should return to normal length, but in approximately one third of women the uterus remains retroverted. This condition is rarely symptomatic, but conception may be difficult because the cervix points

Nursing Care Plan

PUERPERAL INFECTION

Nursing Diagnosis: Infection of genital canal related to retained placental fragments

Expected Outcome: Infection is resolved with no adverse effects.

• NURSING INTERVENTIONS/*RATIONALES*

Administer and monitor broad-spectrum antibiotics per physician order *to stem invading pathogens and prevent systemic infection until specific pathogen can be identified.*

Collect intrauterine cultures per physician order for laboratory analysis *to identify specific causative organism.*

Maintain Standard Precautions and use good handwashing technique when providing care *to prevent spread of infection.*

Monitor vital signs *to assess patient's response to treatment and status of infection.*

Monitor level of fatigue and lethargy, evidence of chills, loss of appetite, nausea and vomiting, and abdominal pain, *which are indicative of extent of infection and serve as indicators of status of infection.*

Monitor lochia for foul smell and profusion *as indicators of infection state.*

Monitor laboratory values (i.e., WBC count, cultures) *for indicators of type and status of infection.*

Help patient to maintain good handwashing technique (particularly before handling her newborn) and to maintain scrupulous perineal care with frequent change and careful disposal of perineal pads *to avoid spread of infection.* Avoid use of communal sitz baths.

Ensure adequate fluid and nutritional intake *to fight infection;* administer antiemetics as needed per physician order.

Monitor intake and output and electrolyte laboratory values *to evaluate fluid and electrolyte balance.*

toward the anterior vaginal wall and away from the posterior fornix, where seminal fluid pools after coitus. Symptoms may include deep pelvic and low back pain, difficulty with elimination, exaggeration of premenstrual tension, and dyspareunia.

Uterine prolapse is a more serious type of displacement. There are varying degrees of prolapse, from mild to complete; in complete prolapse the cervix and body of the uterus protrude through the vagina and the vagina is inverted (Fig. 20-3).

Uterine displacement and prolapse can be caused by congenital or acquired weakness of the pelvic support structures (often referred to as pelvic relaxation). Although extensive damage may be noted and repaired shortly after birth, symptoms related to pelvic relaxation most often appear during the perimenopausal period, when the effects of ovarian hormones on pelvic tissues are lost and atrophic changes begin. Pelvic trauma, stress and strain, and the aging process are contributing causes. Other causes of pelvic relaxation include reproductive surgery and pelvic radiation.

CLINICAL MANIFESTATIONS. Generally, symptoms of pelvic relaxation relate to the structure involved: urethra, bladder, uterus, vagina, cul-de-sac, or rectum. The most common complaints are pulling-and-dragging sensations, pressure, protrusions, fatigue, and low backache. Symptoms may be worse after prolonged standing or deep penile penetration during intercourse. Urinary stress incontinence may be present.

Cystocele and rectocele. Cystocele and rectocele almost always accompany uterine prolapse, causing the uterus to sag even further backward and downward into the vagina. Cystocele (Fig. 20-4), protrusion of the bladder downward into the vagina, develops when supporting structures in the vesicovaginal septum are injured. Anterior wall relaxation develops gradually over time as a result of congenital defects of supports, childbearing, obesity, or advanced age. When the woman stands, the weakened anterior vaginal wall cannot support the weight of the urine in the bladder; the vesicovaginal septum is forced downward, the bladder is stretched, and its capacity is increased. With time the cystocele enlarges until it protrudes into the vagina. Complete emptying of the bladder is difficult because the cystocele sags below the bladder neck. Rectocele is the herniation of the anterior rectal wall through the relaxed or ruptured vaginal fascia and rectovaginal septum; it appears as a large bulge that may be seen through the relaxed introitus (Fig. 20-5).

CLINICAL MANIFESTATIONS. Cystoceles and rectoceles often are asymptomatic. If symptoms of cystocele are present, they may include complaints of a bearing-down sensation or that "something is in my vagina." Other symptoms include urinary frequency, retention, and/or incontinence and may include recurrent cystitis and urinary tract infections. On pelvic examination there is a bulging of the anterior wall of the vagina when the woman is asked to bear down. Unless the bladder neck and urethra are damaged, urinary continence is unaffected. Women with large cystoceles complain of having to push upward on the sagging anterior vaginal wall to be able to void.

Rectoceles may be small and produce few symptoms, but some are so large that they protrude outside of the vagina when the woman stands. Symptoms are absent when the woman is lying down. A rectocele causes a disturbance in bowel function, the sensation of "bearing down," or the sensation that the pelvic organs are falling out. With a very large rectocele it may be difficult to have a bowel movement. Each time the woman strains during bowel evacuation, the feces are forced against the thinned rectovaginal wall, stretching it more. Some women facilitate evacuation by applying digital pressure vaginally to hold up the rectal pouch.

Urinary incontinence. Many women experience uncontrollable leakage of urine as a result of vaginal childbirth injury. Conditions that disturb urinary control include stress urinary incontinence as a result of sudden increases in intraabdominal pressure (such as that caused by sneezing or coughing); urge incontinence caused by disorders of the

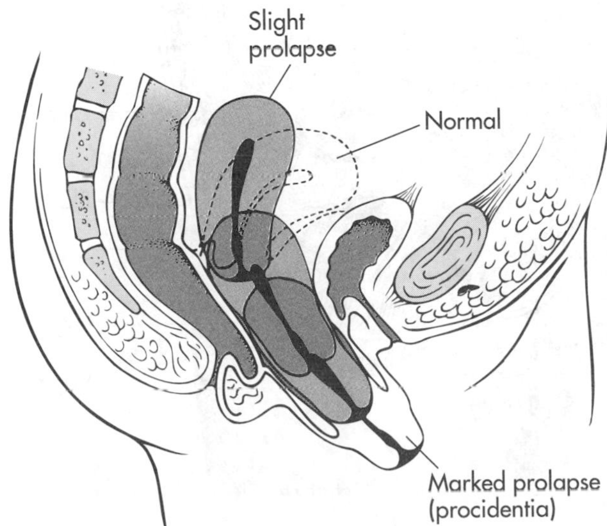

Fig. 20-3 Prolapse of uterus.

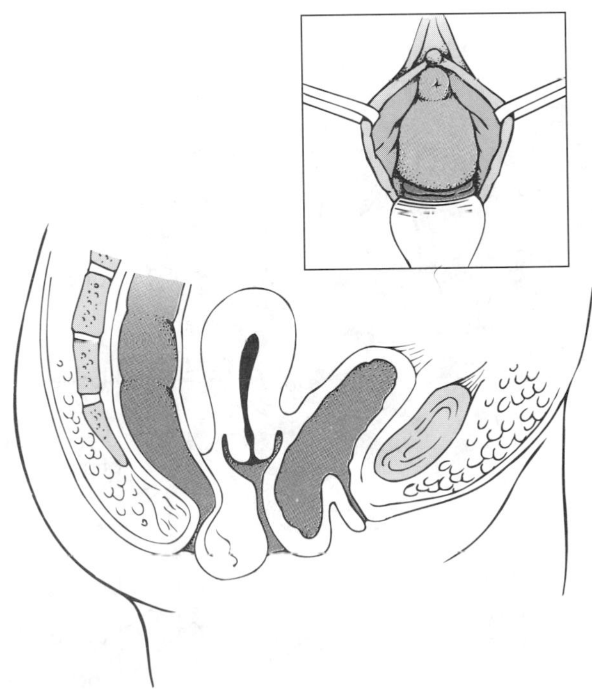

Fig. 20-4 Side and direct views of cystocele.

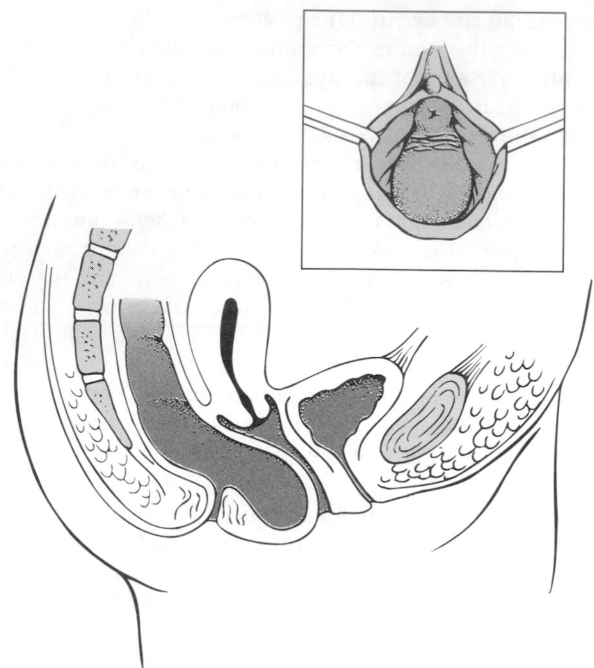

Fig. 20-5 Side and direct views of rectocele.

bladder and urethra such as urethritis and urethral stricture, trigonitis, and cystitis; neuropathies such as multiple sclerosis, diabetic neuritis, and pathologic conditions of the spinal cord; and congenital and acquired urinary tract abnormalities (Skoner, Thompson, and Caron, 1994).

Stress urinary incontinence may follow injury to bladder neck structures. A sphincter mechanism at the bladder neck compresses the upper urethra, pulls it upward behind the symphysis, and forms an acute angle at the junction of the posterior urethral wall and the base of the bladder (Fig. 20-6). To empty the bladder, the sphincter complex relaxes and the trigone contracts to open the internal urethral orifice and pull the contracting bladder wall upward, forcing urine out. The angle between the urethra and the base of the bladder is lost or increased if the supporting pubococcygeus muscle is injured; this change, coupled with a urethrocele, causes incontinence. Urine spurts out when the woman is asked to bear down or cough in the lithotomy position.

Genital fistulas. A fistula is an abnormal communication between one hollow viscus and another, or from one hollow viscus to the outside. Genital fistulas may occur between the bladder and the genital tract (e.g., vesicovaginal); between the ureter and the vagina (ureterovaginal); and between the rectum or sigmoid colon and the vagina (rectovaginal). They may be a result of a congenital anomaly, gynecologic surgery, obstetric trauma, cancer, radiation therapy, gynecologic trauma, or infection.

A *vesicovaginal fistula,* the most common urinary tract fistula, forms in the anterior vaginal wall (Fig. 20-7). It is usually a result of injury near the uterovesical junction during a radical hysterectomy for cancer. Urine is lost through the vagina, resulting in partial or complete incontinence.

A *rectovaginal fistula* is most often caused by an infection in the episiotomy site, a suture placed through the rectal wall during repair, or an unrecognized rectal injury during childbirth. Rectovaginal fistulas may also be a result of extension of cervical cancer or radiation therapy.

CLINICAL MANIFESTATIONS. Signs and symptoms of vaginal fistulas depend on the site but may include the presence of urine, flatus, or feces in the vagina; odors of urine or feces in the vagina; and irritation of vaginal tissues.

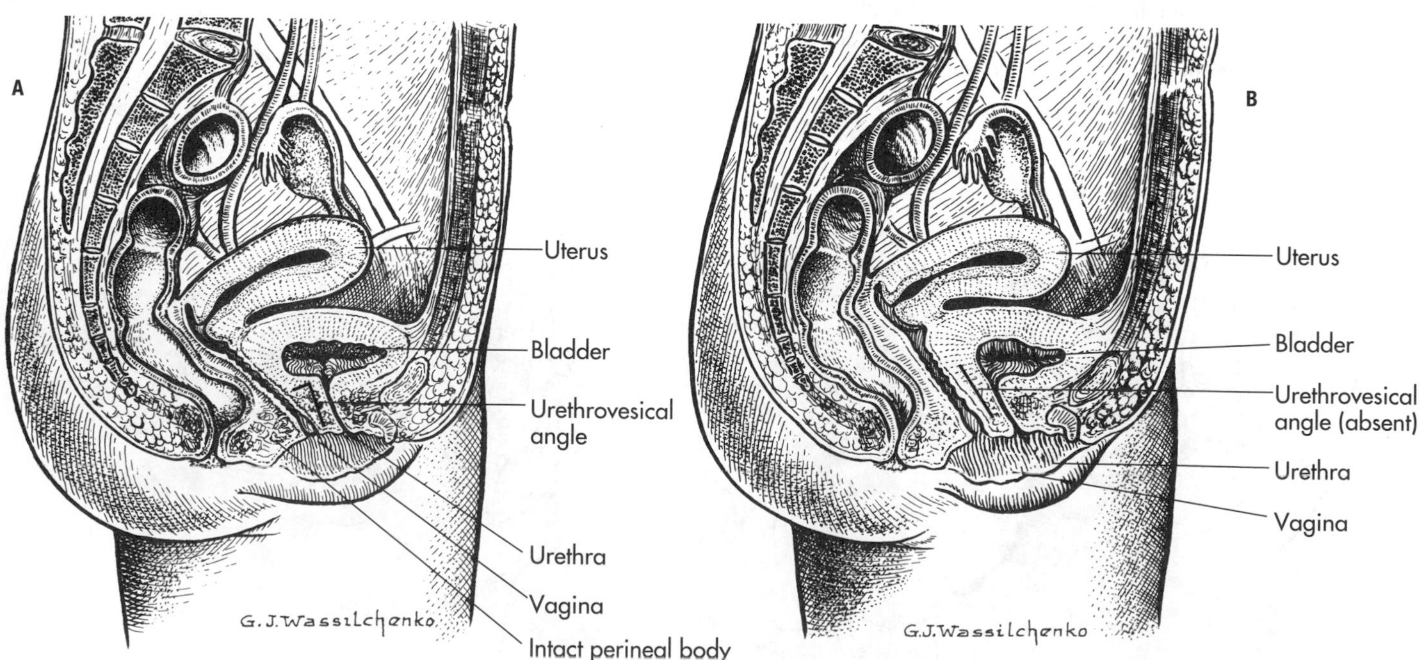

Fig. 20-6 Urethrovesical angle. **A,** Normal angle. **B,** Widening (absence) of angle.

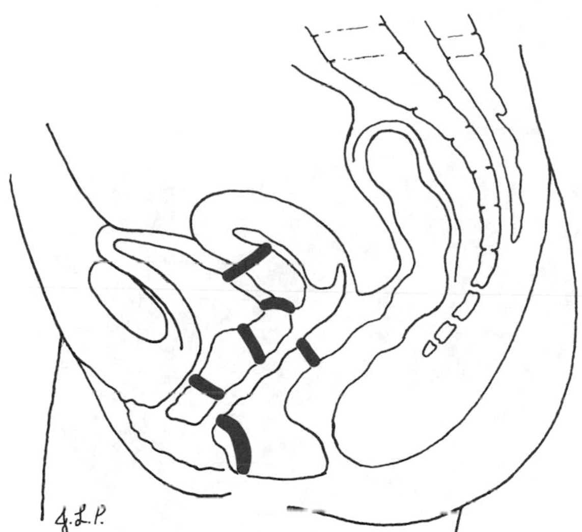

Fig. 20-7 Types of fistulas that may develop in vagina, uterus, and rectum. (Courtesy Julie L. Perry).

Nursing Care Management

Assessment

Assessment for problems related to structural disorders of the uterus and vagina focuses primarily on the genitourinary tract, the reproductive organs, bowel elimination, and psychosocial and sexual factors. A complete health history, physical examination, and laboratory tests are done to support the appropriate medical diagnosis. The nurse needs to assess the woman's knowledge of the disorder, its management, and the possible prognosis.

Nursing Diagnoses

Possible nursing diagnoses for the patient with a structural disorder of the uterus or vagina include the following:

- Knowledge deficit related to
  - Causes of structural disorders and treatment options
- Constipation or diarrhea related to
  - Anatomic changes
- Pain related to
  - Relaxation of pelvic support and/or elimination difficulties
- Ineffective individual coping related to
  - Changes in body image
- Altered family processes or interpersonal relationships related to
  - The woman's anatomic and functional changes
- Risk for injury related to
  - Lack of skill in self-care procedures
  - Lack of understanding of the rationale for the need to comply with therapy
- Social isolation, spiritual distress, body image disturbance, or self-esteem disturbance related to
  - Changes in anatomy and function
- Anxiety related to
  - Surgical procedure
  - Prognosis

Expected Outcomes

Expected outcomes are mutually negotiated and stated in patient-centered terms. Possible expected outcomes may include the following. The woman will:

1. Verbalize understanding of possible disorders related to alterations in pelvic support
2. Use good hygiene and practice measures to prevent problems related to alterations in pelvic support
3. Accept change in body functions without loss of positive body image, self-concept, and self-esteem
4. Report less anxiety related to treatment and her prognosis

Plan of Care and Implementation

Nursing interventions are directed toward educating the woman about childbirth sequelae and symptoms. The health care team works together to treat the disorders related to alterations in pelvic support and to assist the woman in management of her symptoms. If discomfort related to uterine displacement is a problem, several interventions can be implemented to treat uterine displacement. Kegel exercises can be performed several times a day to increase muscular strength (pp. 135-136). A knee-chest position performed for a few minutes several times a day can correct a mildly retroverted uterus. A pessary to support the uterus and hold it in the correct position (Fig. 20-8) may be inserted in the vagina. Usually a pessary is used only for a short time because it can lead to pressure necrosis and vaginitis. Good hygiene is important; some women can be taught to remove the pessary at night, cleanse it, and replace it in the morning. If the pessary is always left in place, regular douching with commercially prepared solutions or weak vinegar solutions (1 tablespoon to 1 quart of water) to remove increased secretions and to keep the vaginal pH at 4 to 4.5 is suggested. After a period of treatment, most women are free of symptoms and do not require the pessary. Surgical correction is rarely indicated.

Treatment for uterine prolapse depends on the degree of prolapse. Pessaries may be useful in mild prolapse. Estrogen therapy also may be used in the older woman to improve tissue tone. If these conservative treatments do not correct the problem, or if there is a significant degree of prolapse, an abdominal or vaginal hysterectomy is usually recommended.

Treatment for a cystocele includes use of a vaginal pessary or surgical repair. Pessaries may not be effective. Anterior repair (colporrhaphy) is the usual surgical procedure and is usually done for large symptomatic cystoceles. This involves a surgical shortening of pelvic muscles to provide better support for the bladder. An anterior repair is often combined with a vaginal hysterectomy.

Small rectoceles may not need treatment. The woman with mild symptoms may get relief from a high-fiber diet and adequate fluid intake, stool softeners, or mild laxatives. Vaginal pessaries usually are not effective. Large rectoceles that are causing significant symptoms are usually repaired surgically. A posterior repair (colporrhaphy) is the usual procedure. This surgery is performed vaginally and involves shortening the pelvic muscles to provide better support for the rectum. Anterior and posterior repairs may be performed at the same time and with vaginal hysterectomy.

Mild stress incontinence can be relieved by Kegel exer-

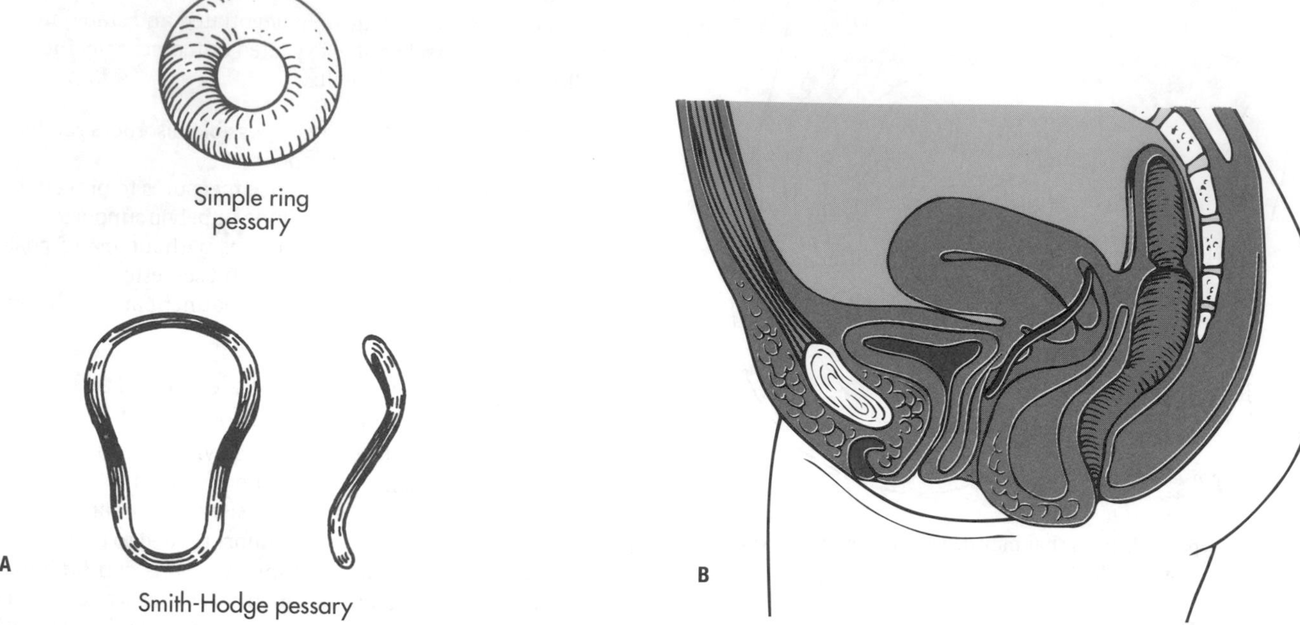

Fig. 20-8 **A**, Examples of pessaries (simple ring and Smith-Hodge). **B**, Pessary in place to hold posterior vaginal fornix and, with it, attached cervix wall backward and upward in pelvis. (**A** modified from Willson J, Carrington E: *Obstetrics and gynecology*, St Louis, 1991, Mosby).

cises. Postural changes such as crossing the legs or crossing the legs and bending over are effective for some women (Norton and Baker, 1994). Pelvic physical therapy with pelvic floor musculature retraining and functional electrical stimulation can be curative if the woman is highly motivated. A bladder neck support prosthesis inserted into the vagina may be as beneficial as surgery (Davila and Ostermann, 1994). Pessaries, diaphragms, and even tampons have been used to manage urine leakage (Marshall, 1991; Suarez, Baum, and Jacobs, 1991). Estrogen therapy may provide some relief for postmenopausal women, but surgical correction is often indicated to relieve symptoms. A transvaginal or abdominal surgical repair may be done to elevate and support the bladder neck.

Nursing care of the woman with pelvic relaxation problems or a fistula requires great sensitivity because the woman's reactions are often intense. She may become withdrawn or, conversely, hostile because of embarrassment about odors and soiling of her clothing that are beyond her control. The nurse needs to be tactful in suggesting hygienic practices that reduce odor. Commercial deodorizing douches are available, or noncommercial solutions such as diluted chlorine (1 teaspoon of chlorine household bleach to 1 quart of water) may be used. The chlorine solution is also useful for external perineal irrigation. Sitz baths and thorough washing of the genitalia with unscented, mild soap and warm water help. Sparse dusting with deodorizing powders can be useful. If a rectovaginal fistula is present, enemas given before leaving the house may provide temporary relief from oozing of fecal material until corrective surgery is performed. Irritated skin and tissues may benefit from use of a heat lamp or application of vitamin A and D ointment. Hygienic care is time consuming and may need to be repeated frequently throughout the day; protective pads or pants may need to be worn. All of these activities can be demoralizing to the woman and frustrating to her and her family.

Many of the nurse's efforts with these problems are directed toward participating in a team effort to prepare the woman for surgery. Preoperative teaching involves the primary nurse, operating room nurse, surgeon, and anesthesiologist. The nurse in the health promotion setting is usually most aware of the woman's living circumstances, physical limitations, and social problems and therefore may be best suited to coordinate continuity of care after discharge.

Evaluation

Care can be evaluated as effective if the anatomic defect is repaired and function is restored. If function cannot be fully restored through surgery, medication, or other therapy, expected outcomes are evaluated relative to self-care in compliance with the medical regimen, to the regaining or maintenance of self-esteem, and to satisfactory family and interpersonal processes.

LOSS AND GRIEF

Situational life crises can be superimposed on the experiences of childbearing. These may include infertility, premature labor/premature birth, a cesarean birth, any perception of loss of control during the birthing experience, a boy when the parents wanted a girl, the birth of a handicapped child, a maternal death, and/or fetal or neonatal death (Limbo and Wheeler, 1986a, 1986b). All of these situations have a common denominator—they are losses of what was hoped for, dreamed about, and/or planned.

From the perspective of health care providers, these crises vary in degrees. However, from the perspective of the parents, the perceived loss may be the most terrible thing that has ever happened to them. At the birth they are mourning instead of celebrating life. Those who experience a loss are bereaved. The feelings and emotions that are associated with bereavement are called **grief responses.** This section on perinatal death provides (1) a theoretic framework of mourning and grief responses on which to base nursing practice, (2) practical suggestions to help the beginning nurse know what to say and what to do in the instance of perinatal or maternal loss, and (3) suggestions to help the beginning nurse develop sensitivity to the needs of the bereaved.

The statistics on losses in the childbearing years are grim. Out of 1000 births, 180 fetuses are stillborn or die shortly after birth (Cunningham et al, 1993). Between 10% and 25% of all pregnancies end in miscarriage (spontaneous abortion)—a pregnancy that ends before 20 weeks of gestation (Cunningham et al, 1993). Each year there are approximately 30,000 stillbirths, fetuses that die in utero, and infants who die who were born after 20 weeks of gestation or who weighed at least 350 g. Neonatal death (death of babies born showing signs of life such as respiratory effort, heart rate, a pulsating cord, or muscle irritability at birth, regardless of gestational age) accounts for 25,000 deaths each year in the United States (Cunningham et al, 1993). Approximately 1.6% of all pregnancies are ectopic (i.e., occur outside of the uterus) (Goldner et al, 1993).

Grief Responses

When an individual experiences the loss of a relationship, hopes and dreams for the future end. The reestablishment of life without that particular relationship involves a process called **bereavement** or **mourning.** The subsequent feelings and emotions are grief responses. The intensity and the length of grief responses depend on the perception of the loss, one's age, religious beliefs, the changes incurred by the loss, personal ability to cope with the loss, and the presence of support systems (Sanders, 1989). Davidson (1984) described four dimensions of mourning:

1. **Shock and numbness** are experienced by parents as they express feelings of being stunned with disbelief, feelings of panic, distress, and/or anger. This experience can be interrupted by outbursts of emotion. It is difficult to make decisions during this time, and normal functioning is impeded. This phase predominates during the first 2 weeks after a loss. Parents may feel like they are in a bad dream and that they will wake up and everything will be all right.
2. **Searching and yearning** can be identified by feelings of restlessness, anger, guilt, and ambiguity. The grieving persons yearn for what might have been and search for the answer as to why the loss occurred. This phase is present at the time of the loss and peaks between 2 weeks and 4 months after the loss. They are preoccupied with thoughts about what happened, what they did or did not do to cause this terrible thing to happen, and the death itself.
3. **Disorganization** begins when the mourner turns from testing what is real to an awareness of the reality of the loss. Feelings of depression, difficulty in concentrating on work and/or in solving problems, and a general sense of not feeling well about oneself physically and emotionally exist. This phase peaks around 5 to 9 months after the death and slowly subsides. Many parents feel that they will never get over the loss and that they are losing their mind; they may feel physically ill.
4. **Reorganization** occurs when the mourner is better able to function at home and at work, with an increase in self-esteem and confidence. The mourner has the ability to cope with new challenges and has placed the loss in perspective. This phase is present when parents laugh and when they begin to enjoy the simple pleasures of life without feeling guilty. Reorganization begins to peak sometime after the first year as parents begin to move on with their lives.

Mourning is not a neat and orderly process that moves smoothly from one dimension to another. All of the dimensions of bereavement may exist at the same time, with one or more predominating at any given moment. There is much movement back and forth among the dimensions. The bereaved reveal their mourning through their language, the intensity and duration of their grief responses, and their ability to regain their life without that which was lost. The physical, emotional, and social grief responses to loss encompass many feelings and emotions (Box 20-2).

Physical grief responses associated with a perinatal loss are fatigue, headaches, tension and nervousness, insomnia,

BOX 20-2
Signs and Symptoms of Grief

Physical effects

Exhaustion/fatigue	Breathlessness/shortness of breath
Loss of appetite or increased appetite	Palpitations
Sleep problems	Aching arms
Lack of strength/muscle weakness	Restlessness
Weight loss or gain	Dry mouth
	Blurred vision
	Headaches

Emotional and/or psychologic effects

Denial	Sadness
Guilt	Sense of failure
Anger	Concentration on problems
Resentment	Failure to accept reality
Bitterness	Preoccupation with the deceased
Depression	Fluctuating mood swings
Time confusion	Decreased self-esteem
Irritability	Dreams

Social effects

Withdrawal from normal activity
Isolation (emotional and physical) from spouse, family, and/or friends

Spiritual effects

Questioning core beliefs—a spiritual crisis
Searching for the meaning of the loss
May change level of involvement in an organized religion
Anger with God (or Higher Power)
Longing for a sense of connectedness (community)

From Heath L, Gensch B, editors: *RTS counselor training manual*, ed 3, LaCrosse, Wis, 1997, Bereavement Services/RTS, Gundersen Lutheran Medical Center.

emptiness, irritability, nausea, dizziness, backaches, chest pains, heart pounding, muscle tension, numbness or tingling, and breathing that is too fast (Hardin and Urbanus, 1986; Hutti, 1986; Willis, 1991).

Emotional responses in women include crying, disappointment, preoccupation with the baby, guilt, depression, self-blame, feeling of failure, embarrassment, emotional cocooning, irritability, and anger, especially at living children (Bansen and Stevens, 1992; Hutti, 1986; Willis, 1991). Parents may blame someone for the death: God, a member of the medical profession, and/or themselves (Graham et al, 1987).

Anticipatory Grief

Anticipatory grief occurs when families have knowledge of an impending loss, such as when a baby is admitted to a neonatal intensive care unit (NICU) with problems or when a diagnosis of an anacephalic fetus is made by ultrasound examination. The fetus is still alive, but the prognosis is poor. Being able to anticipate the loss gives families an opportunity to plan, feel more in control of their situation, and be able to say good-bye in a special way. However, some individuals or family members may distance or detach themselves from the experience or the baby as a way of protecting or avoiding the pain of loss and grief.

BOX 20-3
To Jessica

The candles are lit,
but no song will be sung.
No laughter, no glee, of my little one
who would have been three.
If you only knew the plans that would be
made by your dad and me.
The cake to be baked . . .
The presents wrapped . . .
and all the funny party hats.
The pictures taken by your dad,
of course,
As loving friends fill the house.
All of this is not meant to be,
since you were taken away from me.
No birthday cake . . .
No presents unwrapped . . .
No pictures of you in your party hat.
But the candles are lit,
Never to go out,
For they burn forever in my heart.

Kathie Rataj Mayo

From La Cross, Wis, 1982, Bereavement Services/RTS, Gundersen Lutheran Medical Center.

Tasks of Mourners

Worden (1991) identified four tasks of mourners:

1. Accepting the loss
2. Working through the pain
3. Adjusting to the environment
4. Moving on

In order for the woman and her family to adapt to the loss of their baby, these tasks need to be accomplished.

Accepting the reality of the loss occurs when the woman and family come to grips with the death of the baby. Seeing, holding, touching, and/or memorialization are all ways the bereaved can perceptually confirm the baby's death. It is important for the woman and family to tell their story about the events, the experiences, and the feelings surrounding the loss to cognitively and emotionally come to terms with the death of the baby. Caregivers need to use the words "dead" and "died" rather than "lost" or "gone" to assist the bereaved in accepting the reality.

Working through the pain means the mourner must feel and express the intense emotions of grief. Not all parents/families experience the same intensity of pain. Society in general tends to minimize the death of a baby because no real social relationship with or attachment to the baby existed. Often society equates the number of years of life and visibility of a relationship to how much mourning is appropriate. However, mothers, fathers, and siblings develop images and relationships with an unborn baby, even early in pregnancy.

Families who experience perinatal loss may suppress or deny their feelings because it seems to be more socially acceptable. The nurse can be instrumental in preparing the woman and family for the reactions they may receive from others once they leave the hospital or clinic setting. A perinatal bereavement support group can help the parents work through their pain by nonjudgmental sharing of feelings. Denying the pain of grief leads to physical and emotional illness. When no physical reasons for illness can be found, complicated bereavement (p. 562) may be the source.

Being able to adjust to the environment after the loss means learning how to accommodate the changes the loss has caused. The loss of a baby means not being able to fulfill the role of mother, father, older sibling, or grandparent. Deciding what to do about the nursery and baby clothes, going back to work, parenting other children, getting pregnant again, and/or learning how to cope with insensitive family members and friends are all problems the bereaved must face.

Detachment needs to occur for the parents to adapt to their loss. Over time, the bereaved have the opportunity to change their view on how the loss has affected their lives. This change does not mean they have forgotten about their baby. It means that as the weeks and months go by, they have an opportunity to develop a new perspective, different feelings, and various ways of coping.

Moving on with life, or reorganization, means to love and live again. Once more being able to enjoy things that give pleasure, being able to nurture oneself and others, developing new interests, and reestablishing relationships are all signs of "moving on." For some women and families, the birth of a subsequent child is necessary for them to be able to move on with their lives. A bereaved parent never forgets the child, but memories become bittersweet.

Bittersweet grief (Kowalski, 1984) refers to the memories that linger after the loss has occurred (Boxes 20-3 and 20-4). This grief occurs when one is reminded of the loss. This can typically happen on birthdays, death days, and anniversaries; at school events; during changes in the seasons; and during the time of year when the loss occurred.

BOX 20-4
Bittersweet Grief

To Jessica Mayo—on her 11th Birthday
Sunday, November 18, 1990
"The child born on the Sabbath day,
is bonny and blithe and good and gay."
Sundays are special days.
. . . a day of rest, a day to play.
A day to reflect on days past.
. . . a day to thank God for all that we bless.
I bless your memory.
I wish you were here.
On your eleventh birthday, I still want to share.
. . . Your dreams of the future.
. . . Our memories past.
My baby's first cry.
My daughter's first laugh.
I was told you were an angel in heaven above.
Eleven years later, I'm an expert . . .
At long-distance love.
On your third birthday, I wrote my first poem
to you.
Eight years later, it's still true
". . . no birthday cake,
no presents unwrapped . . .
no pictures of you in your party hat.
But the candles are lit,
Never to go out
For they burn forever in my heart.
Love, Mom"

Kathie Rataj Mayo
1990

From La Cross, Wis, 1982, Bereavement Services/RTS, Gundersen Lutheran Medical Center.

Dysfunctional grieving is associated with denying the loss, expressing unresolved issues, idealizing the lost object, reliving past experiences, and maintaining a "normalcy facade" (Harris, 1984).

Fathers report restlessness, difficulty in concentrating, disorganized thoughts, feeling empty, sleep disturbances, nightmares, fatigue, weight gain, high blood pressure, diminished appetite, feelings of exhaustion, and arm pain in response to perinatal loss (Page-Leiberman and Hughes, 1990; Kimble, 1991). Fathers experience anger, sadness, unhappiness, crying, disappointment, helplessness, vulnerability, despair, and self-pity. Angry feelings of fathers are directed at God, self, peers, and unrelated events that make them feel overwhelmed with tasks (Kimble, 1991). Fathers may withdraw from others, spend time alone, and express concern for their spouse's well-being (Kimble, 1991).

Nursing Care Management

The critical intervention time is the immediate crisis period after the loss. The goal of the nurse is to provide care, support, information, and anticipatory guidance. To do this, the nurse must:

- Be knowledgeable about grief
- Anticipate what families might need and/or appreciate for future memories
- Create a nonjudgmental environment in which families can express their feelings and emotions, make decisions based on needs, and feel support for those decisions

Assessment

Families that experience loss may have many and varied feelings and responses. Some people view an early pregnancy as the union of cells; others have visions of a baby; and still others are wrapped up in the thrill of being pregnant. Assessment of family members' perceptions of the loss and their perceptions of the events surrounding the loss is crucial before intervention. This assessment is as important for families experiencing a miscarriage or ectopic pregnancy as it is for those experiencing stillbirth or neonatal loss.

Helpful questions to ask in assessing the perception of loss include the following:

- When did you find out you were pregnant?
- Who have you told about your pregnancy?
- What plans had you made for this pregnancy?
- When was your due date?

In eliciting responses, the nurse should listen for the word "baby." The language people choose to use reveals what they believe they have lost—what they will be/are grieving for. Attention should be given to verbal and nonverbal responses. The ability or inability to respond to open-ended questions provides clues that help the nurse decide which interventions to use and how much intervention is needed at any given time.

Pregnancy and birth bring about many changes in role expectations, in relationships, and in how one views oneself. The perceptions of loss that may be associated with pregnancy and birth may be any or all of the following:

- Feelings of being out of control
- Decrease in self-esteem
- Concerns about fertility or ability to bear children
- Changes in relationships with others, most specifically the father of the baby and the woman's mother
- Changes in body image
- Changes in role expectations
- Loss of the precious baby or perfect child

Listening for the words that are used by parents to describe their experiences can help the nurse formulate appropriate nursing diagnoses and a plan of care.

Nursing Diagnoses

Nursing diagnoses may include physiologic and psychosocial problems related to grieving or problems occurring in the grieving process. Possible nursing diagnoses include the following:

- Powerlessness related to
  - Hospitalization
  - Inability to care for self
  - Inability to communicate
  - Lack of knowledge
- Sleep pattern disturbance related to
  - Grieving process
  - Anticipatory grief

- Spiritual distress related to
  Loss of baby or "perfect child"
  Loss of self-esteem
- Alteration in family processes related to
  Loss of family member (i.e., baby, birth of a child with a disorder)
  Dissatisfaction over loss of control
  Inability to make decisions
  Social isolation

Expected Outcomes

Expected outcomes are set in patient-centered terms based on the mutual goals chosen by the patient and the caregiver. The expected outcomes are prioritized, and nursing actions are then selected to achieve them. Expected outcomes may include the following. The woman and her family will:

1. Be able to share their experiences and verbalize their feelings (e.g., powerlessness, loss of self-esteem) and changes in their relationships
2. Demonstrate increasing independence in participating in and making decisions regarding their plan of care
3. Be able to make decisions that reflect their religious and cultural beliefs (see the Cultural Considerations box below)
4. Be able to use family and community resources for support
5. Verbalize satisfaction with their health care professionals

When these individual expected outcomes are met, the ultimate expected outcome of positive integration of the perceived loss experience within the individual and family can, over time, be met. The overall goal of the nurse is to create a nonjudgmental atmosphere that facilitates expression of feelings and to provide anticipatory guidance, support, and information to help with decision making at the time of the loss and during any follow-up contact after hospitalization.

Cultural Considerations

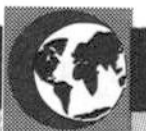

CULTURAL AND RELIGIOUS ASPECTS OF DEATH

Burial

Cremation is forbidden, discouraged, or allowed only under unusual circumstances for Baha'is, Jews, and members of the Christian and Missionary Alliance, Church of Jesus Christ of Latter-Day Saints, and Greek Orthodox Church.

Cremation is customary for Hindus and Unitarian Universalists.

Embalming

The body is not to be embalmed, unless required by state law, for Jews and Baha'is.

Sacraments

Baptism is performed only if the baby is living, for most Protestant and Roman Catholic churches.

Rituals in preparing the body for burial are performed in Judaism, Hinduism, and Islam.

Special mementos

Picture taking may be in conflict with beliefs of some cultures, such as Native American, Indian, Eskimo, Amish, Hindu, and Moslem. It would be important to offer a choice for these families. Within the culture as a whole, this may not be acceptable, but within a family it may be a desired memento.

Plan of Care and Implementation

Communicating and caring techniques. Mothers, fathers, and extended families look to the medical and nursing staff for support and understanding during the time of loss. Therapeutic communication and counseling techniques help the mother, father, and other family members express their feelings and emotions, understand their responses to the loss, and make decisions.

Nursing ALERT

Listening is the single most important communication technique nurses have in providing support, care, and understanding.

To be a good listener, the nurse should be seated comfortably in a chair positioned at a 45-degree angle approximately 2 to 4 feet from the person talking. The nurse's facial expression and demeanor should reflect concern and caring. The nurse should ask only one question at a time. Grief responses in the initial days of crisis make it difficult for individuals to concentrate on what is being asked, to think about what the question means, and to respond to the question. Leaning forward while nodding the head and saying "Uh-huh" or "Tell me more" is often encouragement enough for the bereaved person to talk about the loss. The use of silence often gives the bereaved person the opportunity to collect thoughts and to respond to questions.

The nurse should listen patiently while people tell their story of loss and grief. Asking questions that help people talk about their grief and the experiences surrounding the loss may be needed. The nurse should resist the temptation to give advice or to use clichés in offering support (Box 20-5).

Nurses need to become comfortable with their own feelings of grief and loss to effectively support and care for the bereaved. It is appropriate to express feelings with the bereaved families and to share the moment with them. It is not appropriate to be more emotional than the bereaved so that they have to comfort the nurse.

Worden (1991) identified several counseling techniques the nurse might use in helping the family share and express their grief. These include the following:

- *Actualize the loss.* Ask the bereaved questions that help them to express the experience of the loss. Use the name of their baby and view the body of the baby before speaking with family members. The following questions may help the nurse when addressing family members:
  "Tell me about your labor and birth with Lucas."
  "When did you know you were miscarrying?"
  "What was the most significant thing you remember about Jessica's funeral?"
  "Who does Angela resemble in your family?"

BOX 20-5
Responding to Grieving Families

What you can say

"I'm sad for you."
"How are you doing with all of this?"
"This must be hard for you."
"What can I do for you?"
"I'm sorry."
"I'm here, and I want to listen."

How you can help

Listen.
Touch.
Cry with the family.
Attend the funeral/memorial service.
Remember them on their baby's due date, birthday, and death day anniversaries.
Never forget.
Remember, it is *never* too late for expressing your feelings to a family about the loss of their baby.

What NOT to say

"You're young, you can have others."
"You have an angel in heaven."
"This happened for the best."
"Better for this to happen now, before you knew the baby."
"There was something wrong with the baby anyway."
Calling the baby a "fetus" or "it."

Remembrances you can give the family

Baby ring
Planter/flowers in a baby vase
Original poem
Tree or rose bush as a living memorial
Donation to a memorial fund
Needlework
Photographs
Keepsakes

From Heath L, Gensch B, editors: *RTS counselor training manual*, ed 3, La Crosse, Wis, 1997, Bereavement Services/RTS, Gundersen Lutheran Medical Center.

- *Help the survivor identify and express feelings.* Expressed grief can be overwhelming to health care professionals. Feelings of anger, guilt, and sadness are paramount in the early days and months following a loss. When the bereaved express feelings of anger, it can be helpful to identify the feeling by simply saying, "You sound angry," or "You look angry. Where is this anger coming from?" Being willing to sit down and talk about their anger can help the survivors to move past the anger and identify feelings of powerlessness and helplessness in not being able to control many aspects of the situation.

  The bereaved have many questions about their loss. "What did I do?" "What caused this to happen?" "Do you think I should have, could have done . . . ?" Part of the grief process is for the bereaved to figure out what happened, what their role was in the loss. The nurse needs to recognize that the answers to these questions must come from the bereaved. It is part of their healing. When a bereaved mother asks, "Do you think that I shouldn't have painted the baby's room? Did that cause my baby to die?" An appropriate response might be, "I understand you need to find an answer for why your baby died. What are some of the other things you've been thinking about?"

  Being with someone who is terribly sad, crying, or sobbing can be extremely difficult. The initial impulse is to touch them and/or hand them a tissue. While this action may seem supportive, it may stop or stifle the expression of emotion. The bereaved will indicate when they are ready for a tissue by beginning to wipe their eyes or nose, raising their head, and looking around or reaching for a tissue.

  Careful assessment before using touch as a therapeutic technique is important. If touch is used inappropriately, the bereaved will stiffen, pull away, look at where they were touched, or stop expressing their feelings and emotions.
- *Provide time to grieve.* Families become unaware of time frames when they first learn of and come to grips with their loss. They do not care about the change of shifts or the needs that the hospital system might have in "moving things along." When families are pushed or rushed into making decisions, they may make a decision based on the need of the health care system, not their own. Nurses need to be sensitive to the needs families might have in spending time with their baby. Providing time to see and hold their baby in private, making arrangements for their baby to be returned to them for further viewing, and delaying the processing of consent forms for autopsy or removal from the hospital are ways to give the family the opportunity to say good-bye.
- *Interpret normal feelings.* Many parents have feelings of losing control when they express the normal feelings and emotions of grief; they may feel like they are "going crazy" because of thoughts that plague them about the baby. It is essential for the nurse to reassure and educate bereaved parents about the grief process, including the physical, social, and emotional responses of individuals and families. Offering reading material on the grief process, miscarriage and/or ectopic pregnancy, responses of family and friends, talking with children, planning a special good-bye, and the differences between men and women who are grieving can satisfy some of the educational needs of bereaved families.

  After discharge, providing information/education on the grief process can be done by making follow-up phone calls to bereaved families, offering them the opportunity to talk with other bereaved parents in one-on-one support over the phone, referring them to a mutual, self-help perinatal bereavement support group, or providing a reading list of books and articles on loss, grief, and perinatal bereavement.
- *Allow for individual differences.* Grief is very personal and private. How people respond to loss and grief depends on

such things as age, gender, culture, religion, and socioeconomic status; how others around them respond to their loss; and how they coped with prior losses. Within a family, many different types of responses may occur. Typically, men want to protect their partner from further pain, and parents/grandparents want to protect their children from more hurt. The underlying feelings of powerlessness and helplessness can be hidden behind expressions of anger, resistance to ideas, overcontrol of situations, or blame. These feelings can leave the partner or grandparent feeling isolated and alone, when in fact it is the care and concern for their loved one(s) that perpetuates the expression of the feelings. The nurse can respond to these underlying feelings in the following ways:

- Recognizing what a difficult time this is for the mother, father, parent, grandparents, and/or child
- Acknowledging how hard it must be for them to feel so responsible for making sure everything (and everyone) is taken care of
- Eventually asking them about their own hopes, dreams, and subsequent feelings of loss

These communication techniques can help the nurse move the resistive person to a position of support where the person's needs can also be met.

Families need to be given the opportunity to change their mind, to express their needs to each other, and to make decisions based on their needs as individuals and as family members.

Physical comfort. Coping with loss and grief after childbirth can be an overwhelming experience for the woman and her family. Often these families request that the mother be moved off the maternity unit or be discharged to home; the thought of being on the same unit with mothers and babies is more than they can cope with. Other mothers, however, may want to remain on the maternity unit, where the staff nurses are better prepared to meet their physical and emotional needs. It should be the mother's choice as to where she wants to spend her postpartum stay.

The physical needs of a bereaved mother are the same as those of any mother who has given birth, but with an unhappy twist: the milk may come in, but there is no baby to nurse; the afterpains remind the mother of her emptiness; and gas pains feel like there is still a baby moving inside her. Many struggle with the frustration of having to go through all the pain of childbearing, only to return home with empty arms.

Hands-on interventions such as providing help with getting out of bed the first few times, bathing, answering call lights as soon as possible, and giving back massages convey caring in a tangible way. Being sensitive to the needs of the father, such as offering another meal tray, juice, and a place to sleep or perhaps the opportunity to shower in the mother's room, shows that the nurse understands the parents' needs to be together in this time of crisis.

Adequate rest, diet, and fluids must be offered to replenish the family's physical strength. Discharge instructions should be in both oral and written format. They should include the need for choosing foods based on the Food Guide Pyramid, decreasing food or fluids that contain caffeine, limiting alcohol consumption and nicotine, increasing fluids to at least a quart a day, exercising regularly, and having strategies for rest when the person is unable to sleep. Suggestions for helping the bereaved rest or sleep at night might include taking a warm bath or drinking milk before bedtime, limiting alcohol or nicotine, doing relaxation exercises or taking a nightly walk before bedtime, listening to restful music, getting a massage and, when necessary, taking a sedative. It is recommended that sedatives be used only every third night to allow the bereaved to do their needed grief work but not become sleep deprived. Sleep deprivation, poor nutrition, and inadequate fluids can be the forerunner to the development of a clinical depression that can complicate the mourning process.

Options for parents. It is sometimes difficult for the nurse to offer the bereaved information about their rights regarding options without making them feel guilty if they do not choose to exercise that right. Communicating with parents that options are their right, not their obligation, is vitally important.

Seeing and holding. One of the first options to be discussed is whether the family wants to see their baby or, in the case of miscarriage or ectopic pregnancy, the products of conception. A statement such as "Some parents have found it helpful to see their baby" (or "the products of conception") gives the parents permission to do what might seem odd or distasteful. Responses can vary greatly between someone who experiences a miscarriage or ectopic pregnancy and someone who has experienced stillbirth or **newborn death,** as well as between family members.

Parents appreciate explanations as to how their baby looks (e.g., red, peeling skin like a bad sunburn, dark discoloration similar to bruises, molding of the head that makes the head look soft and swollen, or any defects). This helps them know what to expect. The nurse should make the baby look as normal as possible. Actions such as bathing the baby, applying lotion to the baby's skin, combing the hair, placing identification bands on the arm and leg, dressing the baby in a diaper and special outfit, sprinkling powder in the baby's blanket, and wrapping the baby in a pretty blanket convey to the parents that their baby is cared for the same as any baby in the nursery.

Caring for a baby who has died can be a difficult task for the nurse. It can be even more difficult if the fetus has been dead for several days or weeks in utero. In some cases decapitation or dismemberment may have occurred. If the baby has been in the morgue, the baby can be placed underneath a warmer for 20 to 30 minutes and wrapped in a warm blanket before being brought to the parents. Cold cream rubbed over stiffened joints can help in repositioning the baby.

When bringing the baby to the parents, it is important to hold the baby close, touch a hand or cheek, use the baby's name, and talk with the parents about the special features of their child to convey that it is all right for them to do likewise. If a baby has a congenital anomaly, the nurse can have a perfect hand or foot showing.

Parents need to be offered time alone with their baby. They need to know when the nurse will return and how to call should they require anything. It is difficult to predict how much time parents will need to spend with their baby. These moments are the only ones they will have with this child.

Some parents need only a few minutes; others need hours. With the current practice of short-stay postpartum care, the nurse may need to advocate for patients who have experienced a loss to give them the time they need to grieve.

Naming the baby. Naming the baby is an important decision parents can make. Through choosing a name, the baby is made a member of their family, the loss is made more real, and it is easier for the baby to be remembered in a special way. If the sex of the baby is unable to be determined and the parents would like to name their baby, they can choose a special name for their baby, use a name already chosen for the sex they had hoped their child would be, or choose a unisex name.

Autopsy/organ donation. An autopsy can be instrumental in determining the cause of death. For some families this information is helpful in that it allows them to understand why their loss occurred, process their grief, and perhaps prevent another loss. Other parents may believe their baby has been through enough. Some religions prohibit autopsy. Organ donation can be an aid to grieving—an opportunity for the family to see something positive come out of their experience.

Bathing and dressing. When possible, families should be given the opportunity to bathe, dress, and/or anoint their baby. This can be a very symbolic ritual for many families. The skin of some babies is fragile and may crack or ooze when touched. Parents can still apply lotion with cotton balls, sprinkle powder, tie ribbons, fasten the diaper, and place amulets, medallions, rosaries, or special toys or mementos in their baby's hands or alongside their baby. They may want to do other parenting functions, such as combing hair, wrapping the baby in a blanket, placing the baby in a bassinet, or carrying their baby to the nursery. They may have special clothes for the baby at home, or they may want to purchase a special outfit for the baby.

Privacy. If at all possible, the mother should be admitted to a private room. Marking the door to the room with a special card that denotes to hospital staff that this family has experienced a loss can be helpful (Fig. 20-9).

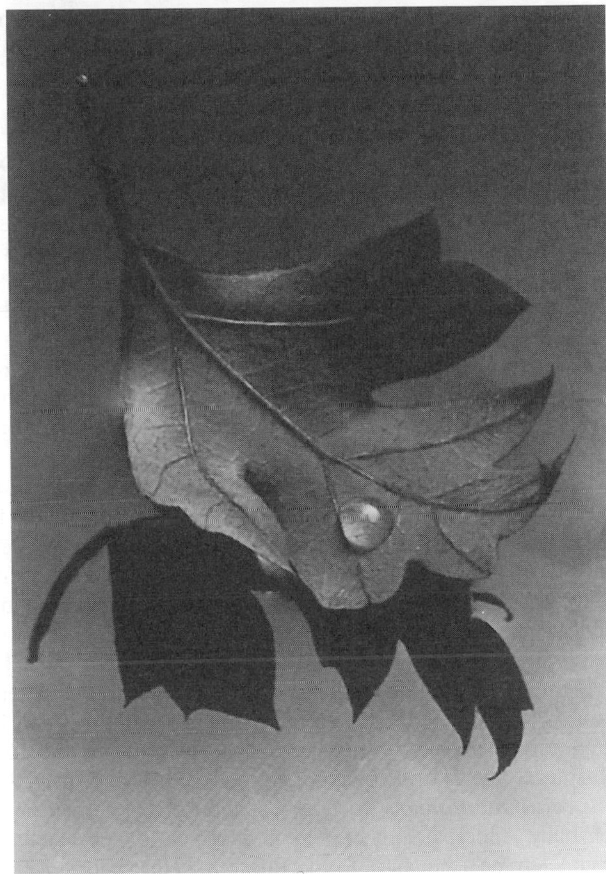

Fig. 20-9 Door card for room of mother who has experienced perinatal loss. (From Heath L, Gensch B, editors: *RTS counselor training manual*, ed 3, La Crosse, Wis, 1997, Bereavement Services/RTS, Gundersen Lutheran Medical Center.)

Visitation with other family members or friends. Families need to be offered the opportunity to have their children, grandparents, extended family members, and friends visit with them during hospitalization, as well as see and hold their baby. This affords others the opportunity to become acquainted with the baby, to understand the parents' loss, to offer their support, and to say good-bye. This experience also helps parents explain to their surviving children who their brother or sister was and what death means; it offers the children answers to their questions in a concrete manner and helps them in expressing their grief.

Religious rituals/funeral arrangements. Support from the clergy is an option that should be offered to all parents. Parents may wish to have their own pastor, priest, rabbi, or spiritual leader contacted; they may wish to see the hospital's chaplain; or they may choose neither option. A member of the clergy may offer the parents the opportunity for baptism, when appropriate. Other rituals that may be offered include a blessing, naming ceremony, anointing, ritual of the sick, memorial service, prayer, or just their physical presence as a representative of a higher being. Parents should be given information about the choices for the final disposition of their baby, regardless of gestational age. In the instance of a baby under 20 weeks of gestation, many hospitals offer to make the final disposition arrangements. Babies under 20 weeks of gestation are considered to be products of conception. Embryos, fallopian tubes removed in an ectopic pregnancy, tissue from a pregnancy obtained during a D & C, and fetuses under 20 weeks of gestation are all considered tissue. Should parents want to know what arrangements the hospital makes for their babies, the nurse should answer the parents' questions as honestly as possible. Many hospitals are currently reviewing and changing their policy on the cremation and burial of fetuses under 20 weeks of gestation to reflect more respect and dignity. In most states if a baby is over 20 weeks and 1 day of gestation or is born alive, it is the parents' responsibility to make the final arrangements for their baby.

LEGAL TIP

Live Birth

In all states there are laws that govern what constitutes a live birth. In most states a "live birth" is considered to be any product of conception expelled from a woman that shows any signs of life. Signs of life are considered to be any muscle irritability, respiratory effort, or heart rate regardless of gestational age. Nurses should be knowledgeable about their state

laws regarding what constitutes a live birth and what forms need to be completed and filed in the case of fetal death, stillbirth, or newborn death.

Final disposition of the bodies of all identifiable babies, regardless of gestational age, includes burial or cremation. Depending on the cemetery's policies, casketed babies or the ashes from cremated babies can be buried in a special place designated for babies, at the foot of a deceased relative's grave, in a plot by themselves, or in a mausoleum, or the ashes may be scattered in a designated area. Many states have regulations as to where ashes can be scattered. A local funeral director or a state vital statistics bureau should have information about rules, codes, and regulations regarding live births, burial requirements, transportation of the deceased by parents, and cremation.

In making final arrangements for their baby, parents may want a special service. They may choose to have a service in the hospital chapel, visitation at a funeral home or in their home, a funeral service, and/or a graveside service. Parents can make any of these services as special, personal, and memorable as they desire. They can choose special music, poetry, or prose written by themselves or others.

At the funeral home parents may want to hold their infant again, take pictures, dress their baby, and position their baby in the casket. All of these things are possible with a supportive funeral director who understands the needs of bereaved parents.

Special memories. Parents need tangible mementos of their baby. A lock of hair may be an important keepsake. Parents need to be asked first, for permission, before a lock of hair is cut. Hair can be removed from the nape of the baby's neck, where it is not noticeable. Parents may also bring in a baby book that had already been purchased. In addition, special memory books, cards, and information on grief and mourning are available through national perinatal bereavement organizations for purchase by parents or hospitals/clinics.

The nurse provides information about the baby's weight, length, and head circumference to the family. Footprints and handprints are taken and placed with the other information on a special card or memory/baby book. Sometimes it is difficult to obtain good handprints or footprints. Using alcohol or acetone on the palms or soles first can help the ink adhere to make the prints clearer, especially for small babies.

Any article that comes in contact or is used in caring for the baby should be saved, placed in a sealable bag, and given to the parents. Articles should not be washed or cleaned beforehand, since the parents may want to be able to keep the smell of their baby. Some examples of articles that can be given to parents are the tape measure used to measure the baby, lotions, combs, clothing, hats, blankets, pacifer, crib cards, and identification bands. Identification bands should be placed on the baby before they are given to the parents. These bands help the parents to remember the size of the baby and enable them to touch something their baby touched.

Pictures. Pictures are the most important memento a parent can have. Photographs should be taken whenever there is an identifiable baby (Fig. 20-10). It does not matter how tiny the baby is, what the baby looks like, or how long the baby has been deceased.

Pictures can be taken by an instant print camera, as well as by a 35-mm camera. Every effort should be made to make the baby appear special. Pictures should include close-ups of the baby's face, hands, and/or feet. The baby should be clothed or wrapped in a blanket with a hat or gown in some of the pictures and unclothed in other pictures. If there are any congenital anomalies, close-ups of the anomalies should also be taken. Flowers, blocks, stuffed animals, or toys can also be placed in the background to make the picture more special, like a portrait. The parents or siblings may also want to have their picture taken holding the baby. Keeping a camera nearby and taking pictures when parents are spending special time with their baby can provide wonderful memories for later on.

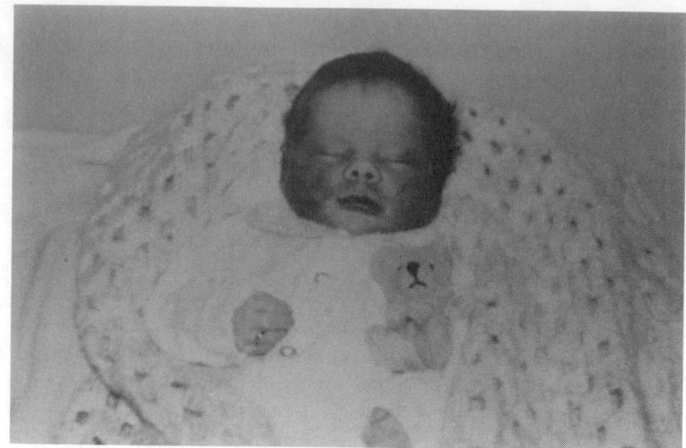

Fig. 20-10 Miranda. Full-term newborn. (From Heath L, Gensch B, editors: *RTS counselor training manual*, ed 3, La Crosse, Wis, 1997, Bereavement Services/RTS, Gundersen Lutheran Medical Center.)

Taking the baby to the morgue. Before the baby is placed in the morgue, the baby's skin should be prepared by gently putting cold cream on the eyelids, hands, and face to keep the skin from dehydrating during refrigeration. The baby should be undressed, placed on a large, smooth blanket with the hands and arms positioned at the sides, and wrapped carefully to avoid making impressions on the face.

When taking the baby to the morgue, the nurse should transport according to hospital protocol, which usually involves placing the infant in a crib. If the baby is carried, the nurse should hold the baby close, with the baby's face covered. Walking in a purposeful manner and not making any eye contact with anyone along the way should keep interested individuals from asking questions. Should the nurse be asked, a response such as "Baby's not seeing any visitors today" is appropriate.

Documentation. Many hospitals have a checklist that is used in providing care, mobilizing members of the multidisciplinary health care team, communicating options the family has chosen, and keeping track of all the details in meeting the needs of bereaved parents (Figs. 20-11 and 20-12). The checklists may or may not be a permanent part of the chart. Documentation in the nursing notes includes primary concerns, grief responses, health teaching, health care advice, and referrals of the mother or any other family members.

Follow-up after discharge. Follow-up phone calls after a loss occurs are important. The grief of the mother and her

SAMPLE

RTS Bereavement Services

CHECKLIST FOR ASSISTING PARENT(S) EXPERIENCING MISCARRIAGE/ECTOPIC PREGNANCY

RTS Counselor: ______________________ Date: ______________________

Mother's Name: ______________________ Age: ________ Due Date: ______________________

Date of Beginning of Miscarriage: ______________________ Date of Surgery: ______________________

# of Miscarriages: __________ # of Children: __________ Religion: ______________________

Address: ______________________ Occupation: ______________________

Phone Number: (   ) ______________________ Marital Status: ______________________

Father's Name: ______________________ Age: ________ Occupation: ______________________

Address: ______________________ Phone Number: (   ) ______________________

Baby's Name: ______________________ Sex: ______________________

Support people available: ______________________ Children's names: ______________________

Problem areas: ______________________ Physician: ______________________

O.K. to send written material to home address: ☐ Yes ☐ No

Date	Time	See Miscarriage Protocol RTS Manual	Comments	Initials
		Notify/Assign RTS counselor: ☐ Yes ☐ No		
		Pastoral Care: ☐ Yes ☐ No		
		Offered: ☐ Blessing ☐ Memorial Service ☐ Naming Ceremony ☐ Burial		
		Asked: "Would you like someone with you now?" ☐ Yes ☐ No		
		D&C/Surgical procedure discussed: ☐ Yes ☐ No		
		Saw baby or tissue: ☐ Mother ☐ Father		
		Touched and/or held baby: ☐ Mother ☐ Father		
		If RH negative, RhoGAM given within 72 hrs: ☐ Yes ☐ No		
		Patient's room flagged with door card: ☐ Yes ☐ No		
		Photos taken: ☐ 35 mm ☐ Polaroid ☐ Given to Parents ☐ On file		
		Footprints & handprints/weight & length: ☐ Given to Parents ☐ On file		
		Grief process discussed: ☐ Yes ☐ No		
		Incongruent grief discussed: ☐ Yes ☐ No		
		Grief packet given: ☐ Yes ☐ No		
		Info Brochure given to parents re: RTS PSG ☐ Yes ☐ No		
		Name/business card given: ☐ Yes ☐ No		
		Regular OB/Midwife notified: __________ ☐ Memo ☐ Verbally		
		Childbirth Educator notified: __________ ☐ Yes ☐ No		
		Telephone number verified: ☐ Yes ☐ No Optimal call time: __________		
		Preg & Inf Loss Card sent to RTS Secretary: ☐ Yes ☐ No		
		Given option to transfer from Maternity Unit: ☐ Yes ☐ No		
		Genetic Studies ordered: ☐ Yes ☐ No		
		Sex determination desired: (tissue in NS only) ☐ Yes ☐ No		
		Would like another parent to call: ☐ Yes ☐ No ☐ Ask Later Parent contact: __________		
		Follow-up calls: eg. ☐ 1 wk, ☐ 3 wk, ☐ 4 mo, ☐ due date/anniv date		

Forms for burial or cremation of:

a) Products of Conception - 2 copies of "Request for Return of Products of Conception to Patients" (1 copy-chart, 1 copy-lab). Obtain forms from Histology.

b) Identifiable Baby less than 20 wk or less than 350 gm - 2 copies of "Request for Return of Products of Conception to Patients" (1-chart, 1-lab). "Notice of Removal" #DOH 5043 - Responsible party for burial signs this form (either parent or a funeral director). Pink copy goes to responsible party. "Final Disposition of a Human Corpse" #DOH 5045 is required for any age identifiable baby that goes across state lines.

Note: Some cemeteries may require a "Final Disposition of a Human Corpse" report for their own record keeping.

Fig. 20-11 Checklist for assisting parent(s) experiencing miscarriage or ectopic pregnancy. (From Heath L, Gensch B, editors: *RTS counselor training manual*, ed 3, La Crosse, Wis, 1997, RTS Bereavement Services/Gundersen Lutheran Medical Center.)

SAMPLE

RTS Bereavement Services
CHECKLIST FOR ASSISTING PARENT(S)
EXPERIENCING
STILLBIRTH OR NEWBORN DEATH

Mother's Discharge Date: ______________________
Mother's Name: ______________________
Address: ______________________
Phone Number: (   ) ______________________
Father's Name: ______________________
Address: ______________________
Phone Number: (   ) ______________________
Optimal call time: ______________________
RTS Counselor: ______________________
Unit: ______________________ Ext: ________
Regular OB MD/Midwife: ______________________

Religion: ______________________
Age: _____ Gr: _____ Para: _____ L.C.: _____ Due Date: ________
Previous Loss: ______________________
Date/Time Delivered: ______________________
Date/Time Death: ______________________
Baby's Name: ______________________ Sex: ______
Children's Name(s): ______________________ Age: ______
______________________ Age: ______
______________________ Age: ______
Support People: ______________________
Attending MD &/or Pediatrician: ______________________
Notify Peds Nurse Practitioner

Date	Time		Comments	Initials
		Notify/Assign RTS counselor: ☐ Yes ☐ No		
		Pastoral Care notified: ☐ Yes ☐ No		
		Funeral Home notified: ☐ yes ☐ no Family Burial: ☐ Yes ☐ No		
		Saw baby when born and/or after delivery: ☐ Mother ☐ Father		
		Touched and/or held baby: ☐ Mother ☐ Father ☐ Siblings ☐ Grandparents ☐ Friends		
		Offered private time with their baby: ☐ Yes ☐ No		
		Baptism offered: (use seashell as vessel, give to parents) ☐ Yes ☐ No		
		Remembrance of Blessing offered: ☐ Yes ☐ No (can offer for any perinatal loss) ☐ Given to parents		
		Given option to transfer off Maternity Unit: ☐ Yes ☐ No		
		Patient's room flagged with door card: ☐ Yes ☐ No		
		Autopsy: ☐ yes ☐ no Genetic Studies: ☐ Yes ☐ No Genetic Associate notified: ☐ Yes ☐ No		
		Regular Physician/Midwife notified of death: ☐ Yes ☐ No Memo sent to Physician/Midwife: ☐ Yes ☐ No		
		Section of Fetal Monitor Strip: ☐ Given to Parents ☐ On file		
		ID Bands/Crib Cards/Tape Measure: ☐ Given to Parents ☐ On file		
		Footprints/Handprints/Weight/Length recorded on "In Memory Of" sheet: ☐ Given to Parents ☐ On file		
		Lock of hair offered (ask permission): ☐ Yes ☐ No ☐ Given to Parents ☐ On file		
		Mementos (clothing, hat, blanket, pacifier, crib cards, basin, baby ring, bear, thermometer, silk flower): ☐ Given to Parents ☐ On file		
		Complimentary birth keepsake: ☐ Given to Parents ☐ On file		
		RTS Photos taken: (clothed, unclothed, w. props, family photo) 1) Polaroid - 3 or more ☐ Given to Parents ☐ On file 2) 35 mm (6-12 pictures) ☐ Given to Parents ☐ On file 3) Medical photos ☐ Yes ☐ No		

Fig. 20-12 Checklist for assisting parent(s) experiencing stillbirth or newborn death. (From Heath L, Gensch B, editors: *RTS counselor training manual,* ed 3, La Crosse, Wis, 1997, RTS Bereavement Services/Gundersen Lutheran Medical Center).

Critical Thinking Exercises

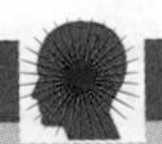

COMMUNITY RESOURCES FOR LOSS AND GRIEF

Investigate what community resources and support groups exist to assist parents who have experienced any of the following:

1. A maternal death
2. Birth of a less-than-perfect child
3. A cesarean birth
4. The death of a baby through miscarriage, stillbirth, or newborn death

family does not end with discharge but really begins once they return home, attend the funeral, and start to live their life without the baby. The calls are made to let the parents know they are still thought of and cared about. The calls are made at predictably difficult times, such as the first week at home, 1 month to 6 weeks later (parents should be invited to attend a support group at this time), 4 to 6 months after the loss, on the due date (for families who experienced a miscarriage, ectopic pregnancy, or death of a premature baby), and/or on the anniversary of the death. The calls are an opportunity for parents to ask questions, share their feelings, seek advice, and receive information to help them in processing their grief.

A grief conference is an opportunity for families to sit down with their health care providers and receive information about the baby's autopsy report or genetic studies, or just to ask questions they have had since their baby's death. Parents appreciate the opportunity to review the events of hospitalization, to go over the baby's and/or mother's chart with their primary health care provider, and to talk with those who cared for them during hospitalization. The grief conference gives health care professionals the opportunity to assess how the family is coping with their loss and to provide additional information/education on grief.

Evaluation

The evaluation of nursing care is made more difficult because of the shock and numbness of the parents during the bereavement process and the varied grief responses of the parents and other family members during hospitalization. Families need time to make decisions, the opportunity to change their minds, information on grief responses and the bereavement process, and the caring support of the nursing staff to ensure that their needs are anticipated and met. Gathering mementos and saving them until the parents are ready to have them, ensuring an opportunity for parents to spend as much time with their baby as desired, and creating precious memories are all important interventions to families who are healing after a loss. However, it is just as important to respect family systems, culture, and religious practices and to support families when they choose to do things "their way."

The evaluation of nursing care should rest on building an environment in which families can express their grief and their needs. The achievement of expected outcomes is ensured when the positive integration of the perinatal loss is expressed by the family (see the Nursing Care Plan below).

Other Losses

Perinatal diagnoses with a negative outcome. With early prenatal diagnostic tests such as ultrasonography, chorionic villi sampling, and amniocentesis, the health care team can determine the well-being of the embryo or fetus. Reasons

Nursing Care Plan

STILLBIRTH

Nursing Diagnosis: Grieving related to loss of fetus/neonate

Expected Outcome: Patient will show evidence of constructive grief process (verbalization/expression of feelings, maintenance of interpersonal relationships, use of support systems, and coping mechanisms).

• **NURSING INTERVENTIONS/*RATIONALES***

Plan time to spend with patient and significant others to sit and listen *as a way to establish trust and demonstrate concern and support.*

Allow family time to view, hold, touch, talk to, and/or bathe the dead neonate *to reinforce the reality of the event and facilitate saying good-bye.*

Secure mementos of neonate, such as footprints, handprints, and photographs for the family *to provide tangible memories of the infant.*

Encourage expression and discussion of perceptions of loss and the impact on the family *to provide ventilation and reinforcement of reality.*

Help patient and significant others to understand the grief process and to accept feelings being experienced (denial, sadness, guilt, anger, relief) as a normal part of the process *to enhance understanding and ability to cope.*

Encourage patient to make simple decisions related to primary care issues *to foster a sense of functional ability and control.*

Emphasize patient's identified strengths and provide encouragement for decisions that demonstrate effective coping skills *to help reestablish a positive self-image and reinforce ability to cope.*

Determine support sources (e.g., family, friends, church, community) and how they can help with disruptions that occur in life-style (e.g., arrangements, activities of daily living, finances, transportation) *to bolster coping and provide needed support during crisis.*

Refer patient/significant others for grief counseling if indicated *to aid in coping and to prevent complicated bereavement.*

for doing prenatal testing might be a history of chromosomal abnormality in the family; three or more miscarriages; maternal age; lack of fetal growth, movement, or heartbeat; diabetes mellitus; or other chronic illnesses.

If the fetus has a serious genetic defect that would lead to death in utero or after birth (e.g., congenital anomaly incompatible with life or genetic disorder with severe mental retardation), the choice of *medical interruption of a pregnancy, or therapeutic abortion,* may be offered. The subject of abortion is controversial and may prevent parents from sharing this decision with other family members or friends. This, of course, limits their support systems after their loss.

The decision to terminate the pregnancy paves the way to a variety of feelings, such as guilt, despair, sadness, depression, and anger (Zeanah, 1993). The nurse's role is to be a good listener. It is important to assess how these families feel about the experience and to offer options for their memories as appropriate. The healing can take place when words can be given to feelings and when needs can be met. Parents who decide to continue the pregnancy also will require emotional support.

Loss of one in a multiple birth. The death of a twin or baby in a multiple birth during pregnancy, labor, birth, or after birth requires parents to parent and grieve at the same time. It imposes a very confusing and ambivalent induction into parenthood (Swanson-Kauffman, 1988). Parents feel they cannot do anything right. They cannot parent their surviving child with all the joy and enthusiasm of new parents because their surviving child reminds them of what they have lost. They cannot grieve completely in the manner they want to because the surviving child demands their attention. These parents are at risk for altered parenting, as well as complicated bereavement. They may repress their grief to parent their surviving child(ren), or they may be overwhelmed and unable to parent the surviving child(ren).

It is important to help the parents acknowledge the birth of all the babies. They should be treated as bereaved families, and all the options discussed previously should be offered. Pictures should be taken of the babies together and separately. Parents should be offered the opportunity to hold all their babies in their arms, as well as to have private time to say good-bye to the baby who has died.

Bereaved parents should be warned that well-meaning family members or friends may say, "Well, at least you have the other baby," implying that there should be no grief because they are lucky to have one. Parents need to be able to anticipate insensitivity to their loss and be empowered to say to those people, "That is not how I feel." By simply setting a boundary on what their feelings are, they are able to acknowledge their baby who died and have an opportunity to share more about their feelings if they so choose.

Bereaved parents of twins have special problems in coping with their life without their anticipated "extra special" family, telling their surviving child about his or her twin, dealing with the possibility of that child's feelings of survivor guilt, plus deciding on how to celebrate birthdays, death days, or special holidays.

Adolescent grief. The first step for the nurse in caring for a bereaved adolescent is to acknowledge the significance of giving birth no matter what age the mother might be. Second, the nurse should make additional efforts in developing a trusting relationship in working with an adolescent. Third, the nurse should offer all of the options for saying good-bye, anticipatory guidance, support, and information to meet the adolescent's needs. It may take longer for an adolescent to process her grief because of her level of cognitive and psychoemotional maturation. Being patient, saving mementos, and giving the adolescent information on how she can contact the nurse are interventions that can help the adolescent accept the reality of the loss and process her grief.

Critical Thinking Exercises

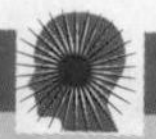

REDUCING MATERNAL MORTALITY AND COMPLICATIONS

Two of the *Healthy People 2000: National Health Promotion and Disease Prevention* objectives are to reduce the maternal mortality rate to no more than 3.3 per 100,000 live births and to reduce severe complications of pregnancy to no more than 15 per 100 deliveries. Discuss the potential impact of current health care reform initiatives in achieving these goals.

Maternal death. It is rare for a woman to die in childbirth; the incidence of maternal deaths is 7.2 per 100,000 (National Center for Health Statistics, 1994). When it does happen, families may be faced with not only mourning the death of a wife or mother but also the death of the baby, or they may be faced with parenting a baby without a surviving mother. "Death of the mother completely disrupts the family structure and often leaves the father with the care of a baby at a time when his emotional reserves are lowest" (Johnson, 1986). The same bereavement process and tasks need to be accomplished for the surviving partner, children, grandparents, other family members, and friends in order for them to heal after such a devastating loss.

The nursing care of families at this time is similar to what has already been described. Options need to be offered, memories need to be made, and mementos need to be obtained and held for the family until they are ready for them. These families are at risk for developing complicated bereavement and altered parenting of the surviving baby and other children in the family. Referral to social services to help the family mobilize support systems, as well as for counseling, can help to combat potential problems before they develop and can be beneficial not only at the time of the loss but also in the future.

The emotional toll that a maternal death takes on the nursing and medical staff must also be addressed. Guilt, anger, fear, sadness, and depression are all common responses to a maternal death. The staff may want to review the situation surrounding the events, the medical record, and their responses. This may occur in the forum of a mortality/morbidity review or a critical incident debriefing to help in coping with the feelings and emotions that result with a maternal death.

Complicated Bereavement

Working with the bereaved in the weeks and months after a loss occurs requires knowledge of how to identify **complicated bereavement.** The difficulties an individual or a family experiences may be in the grieving of the loss itself or an exacerbation of prior problems that were simply intensified during mourning. Referral to a competent therapist is part of one's professional responsibility to the family experiencing complicated bereavement.

Those who need referral include, but are not limited to, those who:

- Have symptoms of anxiety or depression that interfere with functioning in any of the three major areas of life: social/family, work, and physical health
- Have persistent thoughts of suicide that become almost constant, expression of serious suicide intent, or the development of a plan
- Are stuck in searching and yearning, which is evident by persistent anger, guilt, or obsessive thinking about the loss
- Abuse mood-altering chemicals
- Have relationship difficulties (partner, children, family, friends, co-workers)

It is the responsibility of a qualified mental health professional to distinguish between uncomplicated bereavement or an adjustment disorder with depressed mood and a major depression. However, there are certain symptoms that can signal the likelihood of major depression, something for which a person should be immediately referred:

- Loss or gain of 15% of one's body weight
- Inability to maintain or initiate basic living activities, including care of surviving children
- Persistent suicidal thoughts with or without intent or plan
- Reclusiveness

These symptoms are all indicators of depression. An individual experiencing uncomplicated bereavement who does not have a major depression feels better over time, is sad but functional, and can perform the usual activities of daily living although not with as much enthusiasm and energy as before the loss.

Finding a mental health professional with whom one can consult is imperative for the nurse doing bereavement follow-up. That person could be anyone who does therapy and is knowledgeable about bereavement and the referral process. Bereavement complications seem to be best handled by an individual therapist with knowledge of family systems or a marriage and family therapist who also does individual counseling.

Key Points

- Postpartum hemorrhage is the most common and most serious type of excessive obstetric blood loss.
- Hemorrhagic (hypovolemic) shock is an emergency situation in which the perfusion of body organs may become severely compromised and death may ensue.
- The potential hazards of therapeutic interventions may further compromise the woman with hemorrhagic disorders.
- Postpartum infection is the major cause of maternal morbidity and mortality throughout the world.
- Postpartum urinary tract infections are common because of trauma experienced during labor.
- Breast infection affects about 1% of women soon after childbirth.
- Structural disorders of the uterus and vagina related to pelvic relaxation are often the delayed but direct result of childbearing.
- An understanding of grief responses and the bereavement process is fundamental in the implementation of the nursing process.
- Therapeutic communication and counseling techniques can help families in identifying their feelings and in feeling comfortable in expressing their grief.
- Follow-up after discharge is an essential component in providing care to families who have experienced a loss.
- Nurses need to be aware of their own feelings of grief and loss to provide a nonjudgmental environment of care and support for bereaved families.

References

Bansen S, Stevens H: Women's experiences of miscarriage in early pregnancy, *J Nurse Midwife* 37(2):84, 1992.

Bowes W: *Clinical aspects of normal and abnormal labor.* In Creasy R, Resnick R, editors: *Maternal-fetal medicine: principles and practice,* Philadelphia, 1994, WB Saunders.

Clark S et al: *Handbook of critical care obstetrics,* Boston, 1994, Blackwell Scientific Publications.

Cunningham F et al: *Williams obstetrics,* ed 19, New York, 1993, Appleton & Lange.

Davidson G: *Understanding mourning,* Minneapolis, 1984, Ausburg.

Davila G, Ostermann K: The bladder neck support prosthesis: a nonsurgical approach to stress urinary incontinence in adult women, *Am J Obstet Gynecol* 171:206, 1994.

Goldner T et al: Surveillance for ectopic pregnancy—United States 1970-1989, *MMWR* 42(SS-6):76, 1993.

Graham M et al: Factors affecting psychological adjustment to fetal death, *Am J Obstet Gynecol* 157(2):254, 1987.

Hardin S, Urbanus P: Reflections on a miscarriage . . . one couple's psychological and emotional responses, *Matern Child Nurs J* 15(1):23, 1986.

Harris C: Dysfunctional grieving related to childbearing loss: a descriptive study, *Health Care Women Int* 5:401, 1984.

Hunter S, Weiner C: *Obstetric hemorrhage.* In Repke J, editor: *Intrapartum obstetrics,* New York, 1996, Churchill Livingstone.

Hutti M: An exploratory study on the miscarriage experience, *Health Care Women Int* 7:371, 1986.

Johnson S: *Nursing assessment and strategies for the family at risk: high risk parenting,* ed 2, Philadelphia, 1986, JB Lippincott.

Kimble D: Neonatal death: descriptive study of fathers' experiences, *Neonatal Network* 9(8):45, 1991.

Knuppel R, Hatangadi S: Acute hypotension related to hemorrhage in the obstetric patient, *Obstet Gynecol Clin North Am* 22(1):111, 1995.

Kochenour N: Intrapartum obstetric emergencies, *Crit Care Clin* 7(4):851, 1991.

Kowalski K: *Perinatal death: an ethnomethodological study of factors influencing perinatal bereavement,* Unpublished doctoral dissertation, Denver, 1984, University of Colorado.

Limbo R, Wheeler S: Coping with unexpected outcomes, *NAACOG Update Series* 5(3):1, 1986a.

Limbo R, Wheeler S: *When a baby dies: handbook for healing and helping,* La Crosse, Wis, 1986b, Lutheran Hospital.

Marshall S: Conservative management of stress urinary incontinence, *Urology* 28:204, 1991.

Murahata S: *Third stage of labor and postpartum hemorrhage.* In Frederickson H, Wilkins-Haug L, editors: *OB/GYN secrets,* St Louis, 1991, Mosby.

National Center for Health Statistics: *Health, United States, 1993,* Hyattsville, Md, 1994, Public Health Service.

Norton P, Baker J: Postural changes can reduce leakage in women with stress urinary incontinence, *Obstet Gynecol* 84:770, 1994.

O'Brien W: *Puerperal complications.* In Moore T et al, editors: *Gynecology and obstetrics: a longitudinal approach,* New York, 1993, Churchill Livingstone.

Page-Lieberman J, Hughes C: How fathers perceive perinatal death, *MCN Am J Matern Child Nurs,* 15:320, 1990.

Ridgeway L: Puerperal emergency: vaginal and vulvar hematomas, *Obstet Gynecol Clin North Am* 22(2):275, 1995.

Roberts W: Emergent obstetric management of postpartum hemorrhage, *Obstet Gynecol Clin North Am* 22(2):283, 1995.

Sanders C: *Grief, the mourning after: dealing with adult bereavement,* New York, 1989, Wiley Interscience.

Skoner M, Thompson W, Caron V: Factors associated with risk of stress urinary incontinence in women, *Nurs Res* 42(5):301, 1994.

Suarez G, Baum N, Jacobs J: Use of standard contraceptive diaphragm in management of stress urinary incontinence, *Urology* 28:119, 1991.

Swanson-Kauffman K: There should have been two: nursing care of parents experiencing perinatal death of a twin, *J Perinat Neonat Nurs* 2(2):78, 1988.

Veronikis D, O'Grady J: What to do—or not to do—for postpartum hemorrhage, *Contemp OB GYN* 39:11, 1994.

Wendel P, Cox S: Emergent obstetric management of uterine inversion, *Obstet Gynecol Clin North Am* 22(2):261, 1995.

Willis L: *A comparison of grief responses and physical health changes in Caucasian and African-American women following a third trimester stillbirth,* Unpublished doctoral dissertation, Columbus, 1991, The Ohio State University.

Worden W: *Grief counseling and grief therapy: handbook for the mental health practitioner,* New York, 1991, Springer.

Zahn C, Yeomans E: Postpartum hemorrhage: placenta accreta, uterine inversion and puerperal hematomas, *Clin Obstet Gynecol* 33(3):422, 1990.

Zeanah C: Do women grieve after terminating pregnancies because of fetal anomalies? A controlled study, *Obstet Gynecol* 82:270, 1993.

Bibliography

Clark R: Infections during the postpartum period, *J Obstet Gynecol Neonatal Nurs* 24(6):542, 1995.

Grabowska C: Maternal death—new figures, *Mod Midwife* 4(5):29, 1994.

Hertz E, Hebert J, Landon J: Social and environmental factors and life expectancy, infant mortality, and maternal mortality rates: results of a cross-national comparison, *Soc Sci Med* 39(1):105, 1994.

Leonard R, Parker R, O'Grady J: Postpartum hemorrhage: working with the anesthesiologist, *Contemp OB GYN* 40(4):46, 1995.

Lutz R, Kellner K: Paternal involvement after perinatal death, *J Perinatol* 14(6):743, 1994.

Poole J, Hall S, White D: *Crisis OB video series, part II, Hemorrhagic disorders in pregnancy,* St Louis, 1995, Mosby.

Primeau R, Recht C: Professional bereavement photographs: one aspect of perinatal bereavement program, *J Obstet Gynecol Neonatal Nurs* 23(1):22, 1994.

Stepanek J: A journey towards healing: coping with grief through poetry, *ACCH Advocate* 2(1):22, 1995.

Thomson A: Is the safe motherhood initiative too ambitious? *Midwifery* 11(1):1, 1995.

Wheeler S: Psychosocial needs of women during miscarriage or ectopic pregnancy, *AORN J* 60(2):221, 1994.

Willis C, Livingstone V: Infant insufficient milk syndrome associated with maternal postpartum hemorrhage, *J Hum Lact* 11(2):123, 1995.

Yancey M, Duff P: Acute hypotension related to sepsis in the obstetric patient, *Obstet Gynecol Clin North Am* 22(1):91, 1995.

CHAPTER 21

Maternal-Newborn Home Care

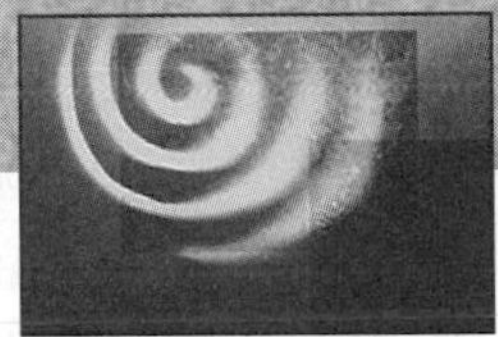

THE HEALTH CARE ENVIRONMENT THAT SUPPORTS EARLY DISCHARGE, P. 565

Potential advantages of short-stay maternity care, p. 566

Potential disadvantages of short-stay maternity care, p. 566

The future of early postpartum discharge, p. 566

NURSING CARE AND EARLY POSTPARTUM DISCHARGE: BRIDGING HOSPITAL AND HOME, P. 569

Critical path, p. 570

Nursing care management, p. 570

PREPARATORY EDUCATIONAL INSTRUCTION, P. 571

POSTPARTUM CARE, P. 574

Home care nursing visits, p. 574

The home visit, p. 579

Telephone follow-up, p. 584

Warm lines/help lines, p. 586

Support groups, p. 587

Perinatal coaching, p. 588

THE ROLE OF NURSING IN PROGRAM DEVELOPMENT, P. 589

Postpartum home care has been an area of significant growth and interest as a result of the shift in length of stay in the hospital and the need of women, newborns, and family for ongoing care in the home. **Early postpartum discharge,** shortened hospital stay, and 1-day maternity stays are terms that reflect the trend of decreasing length of stay in the hospital after a low-risk birth. This trend is affecting increasing numbers of maternity patients and the nurses who provide their care.

In years past, it was a common practice for maternity stays to be a predetermined length of time (usually counted in days) after birth. For example, 3 days after a vaginal birth and 5 days after a cesarean birth was the usual length of stay. Knowing the number of days enabled the health care team and family to plan care accordingly.

To gain perspective on how maternity hospital stays have changed over time, one can draw a quick comparison between 1950 and the 1990s. In 1950 the traditional postpartum stay after a vaginal birth was 6 days. This changed to 2 days in the early 1990s, and it is common in the mid-1990s to have the length of stay be 1 day (24 hours) after a low-risk vaginal birth.

THE HEALTH CARE ENVIRONMENT THAT SUPPORTS EARLY DISCHARGE

The latest trend is to move away from counting days (2 days, 3 days) to consideration of medical necessity and coordination of care. With predetermined medical criteria that indicate low-risk status of mothers and newborns (Box 21-1), the hospitalization can be based on medical necessity of care in an acute care setting or consideration of ongoing care in the home environment. With the approach of what is most appropriate for the individual woman and newborn, length of stay and care coordination with the health care team (physicians, inpatient nursing staff, home care staff, the multidisciplinary team) will be adjusted to deliver safe and effective care.

This is a paradigm shift away from the traditional counting days to medical necessity for the individual mother and newborn. Nursing plays a key role in all areas: prenatal, clinic, acute care, and home care for ongoing safe and effective care.

The federal government (Public Law 104-204, adopted in September, 1996) and many states have legislation requiring insurance payment for a hospital stay of 48 hours after a vaginal birth or 96 hours after a cesarean birth. Mothers and their

BOX 21-1
Criteria for Discharge

Mother

Uncomplicated pregnancy, labor, vaginal birth, and postpartum course
No evidence of premature rupture of membranes
Blood pressure, temperature stable and within normal limits
Ambulating unassisted
Voiding without difficulty
Hemoglobin >10 g
No significant vaginal bleeding
Perineum intact or no more than second-degree episiotomy or laceration repair

Infant

Term infant (38 to 42 weeks) with weight appropriate for gestational age of 2500 g (5lb, 8 oz)
Normal findings on physical assessment
Temperature, respirations, and heart rate within normal limits and stable
At least two successful feedings completed (normal sucking and swallowing)
Urination and stooling have occurred at least once
No evidence of significant jaundice in the first 24 hours after the birth
Screening tests performed according to state regulations; tests to be repeated at follow-up visit if done before the infant is 24 hours old
Initial hepatitis B vaccine given or scheduled for first follow-up visit
Laboratory data reviewed: maternal syphilis and hepatitis B status; infant or cord blood type and Coombs test results if indicated

General

No social, family, and environmental risk factors identified
Family or support person available to assist mother and infant at home
Follow-up schedule within 1 week if discharged before 48 hours after the birth
Documentation of skill of mother in feeding (breast or bottle), cord care, skin care, perineal care, infant safety (use of car seat, sleeping positions), and recognizing signs of illness and common infant problems

Modified from American Academy of Pediatrics: Hospital stay for healthy term infants, *Pediatrics* 96(1):788, 1995; Britton J, Britton H, Beebe S: Early discharge of the term newborn: a continued dilemma, *Pediatrics* 94(1):3, 1994.

families may choose to leave earlier, but this legislation is intended to provide them the option to stay if desired. Many states have included in their legislative bill that if the family chooses to leave the hospital before those hours, then insurance plans must provide coverage for one home visit by a registered nurse. Insurance companies and hospitals have been enhancing their programs to respond to this trend.

Potential Advantages of Short-Stay Maternity Care

Proponents of early postpartum discharge cite the following advantages of the practice. A shortened hospital stay may:

- Reinforce the concept of childbirth as a normal physiologic event
- Allow shorter separations of mothers and other children
- Extend a couple's sense of control and participation beyond the birth itself
- Capitalize on the security and more comfortable home environment during the stressors of early parenting
- Decrease unnecessary exposure to the pathogens in the hospital environment (Harrison, 1990)
- Allow beds on the maternity service to be used more effectively (i.e., quick turnover in patients or for someone with a complication)
- Allow more time for mother/father/partner/infant and other family members to bond (Fig. 21-1)
- Create less disruption in the daily life of the family
- Promote family/support persons active involvement in supporting the mother and parenting the newborn

Potential Disadvantages of Short-Stay Maternity Care

Opponents of early postpartum discharge cite the following disadvantages of the practice:

- Families may be or feel unprepared for the reality they face bringing the baby home
- The mother is fatigued from the labor and childbirth process
- Maternal postpartum pain/discomfort
- Decreased length of time for learning after the birth in the hospital setting
- Undetermined complications (maternal or newborn)
- Vulnerability and crisis potential that exists for both patients and families

During the immediate days and weeks of the fourth trimester, the parents experience a major life transition: recovering from the events surrounding birth, adjusting to the demands of a newborn, parenting, applying the knowledge and skill from their postdischarge instructions, shifting priorities, and realigning some roles while assuming new ones. When there are other children, an additional challenge occurs: helping them to adjust to sharing their home and parents with the newborn. The stress inherent in such profound transitions contributes tremendous crisis potential to the early postpartum experience. Table 21-1 differentiates between those patients discharged early who are at high risk for crisis and those who are at low risk.

The Future of Early Postpartum Discharge

Currently there is much debate as to the best practice for women, newborns, and their families in relationship to length of stay. When the early discharge option is supplemented by preparatory and postpartum follow-up strategies, it appears to be a safe and cost-effective alternative to traditional care (Carty and Bradley, 1990; Welt et al, 1993). Carty and Bradley (1990) conducted a randomized, controlled evaluation of early postpartum discharge. Their study randomly assigned 131 women to one of three postpartum discharge groups: 12 to 24 hours, 25 to 48 hours, and 4 days. Depending on the group assignment, the women and newborns received from one to five home visits during the first 10 days postpartum. Their findings indicated that the maternal and

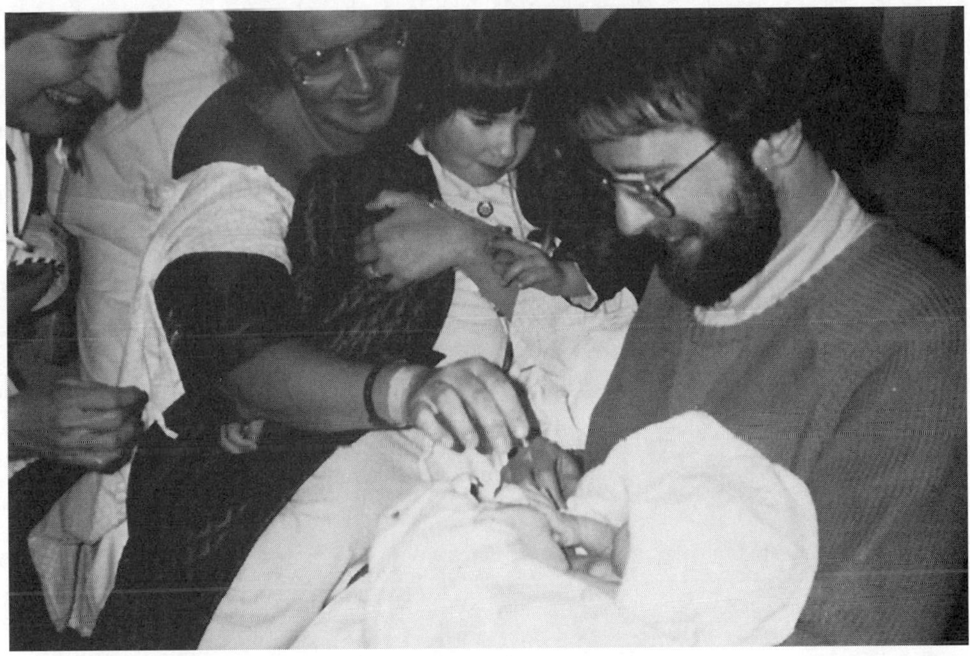

Fig. 21-1 Bonding and attachment begun early after birth is fostered in the postpartum period. Grandmother, parents, and older sibling meet the newborn. (Courtesy Marjorie Pyle, RNC, Lifecircle, Costa Mesa, Calif.)

TABLE 21-1 Postpartum clients and risk of crisis related to early discharge

PERCEPTION OF EVENT	COPING SKILLS	SUPPORT
Crisis unlikely		
Perception of uneventful, healthy pregnancy Positive labor and birth experience that met expectations Elective or desired early discharge; feels "ready" for homecoming	Effective coping/problem solving skills evident	Presence of supportive, helpful partner Helper in home for 1 to 2 weeks Readily available resources (funds, persons, agencies)
High risk for crisis		
Perception that includes unresolved negative feelings about pregnancy	Ineffective coping skills or failure to cope as a result of feeling overwhelmed by lack of preparation or lack of control	Partner or other support person physically or emotionally unavailable
Traumatic birth experience; expectations unmet; sense of failure or loss of control Physically or emotionally uncomfortable postpartum course		Lack of help at home
Concerns/worries about parenting ability, skills, maternal recovery, finances, family relations Unresolved feelings of loss Nonelective or undesired early discharge; feels unprepared for homecoming		Limited financial resources

Modified from Aguilera DC: *Crisis intervention: theory and methodology*, ed 7, St Louis, 1994, Mosby.

infant morbidity were low regardless of discharge time, although sample sizes were too small to detect significant differences in outcomes.

Similar findings were found in the study conducted by Welt et al. (1993). Of 289 early discharge families, there were 4.3% significant maternal problems and 3% significant neonatal problems identified by a nurse practitioner during a home visit in the first 72 hours. The hospital readmission rate was 1.8%.

The potential exists for early postpartum discharge programs to be compromised by the very normality of the patients. Nurses must guard against complacency in assessment of these low-risk clients. Professional nursing practice plays a key role in advocating the most appropriate care for the individual woman, newborn, and family. Care coordination throughout pregnancy is essential to assure the best possible care.

The specialty of postpartum home care has emerged as increased numbers of patients are being referred for home follow-up after a 1-day maternity stay or for follow-up after a cesarean birth. New and existing home care programs are likely

BOX 21-2

Care Path for Mother-Baby Vaginal Birth Without Complications: Expected Length of Stay—24 Hours

	Fourth Stage Labor	By 4 Hours After Birth	First Baby Visit	By 8 Hours After Birth
Assessments		PP admission assessment and care plan completed		
Vital signs	Every 15 min times 4 WNL	Every 1 hour times 3 WNL		Every 8 hours WNL
Postpartum assessment	Every 15 min times 4 WNL	Every 1 hour times 3 WNL		Every 8 hours WNL
Voiding	Empty bladder or fundus firm and not displaced	Empty bladder or fundus firm and not displaced		Empty bladder each void
Sensory	Fully alert; moving all extremities	Ambulating with help		Ambulating without help
Bonding	Evidence of parent/infant bonding at first breastfeeding		Parent/infant bonding continues	
Labs		Intrapartal CBC results on chart/computer; determine Rh status and need for anti-Rh globulin; check for rubella immunity		
Interventions				
IV	IV	May be discontinued		
Perineal	Ice pack to perineum; pericare by nurse	Self-perineal care		
Activity	Up to BR with help	Ambulates with help	Assisted to comfortable position for holding and feeding baby	Ambulates without help
Medications	Pitocin added to IV; analgesics prn	Pitocin discontinued		Stool softener; PNV
Teaching/discharge plan	Breastfeeding positioning; call for help with first ambulation	Verbalizes understanding of unit routines and how to achieve rest, pericare, involution, pain control	Handwashing, infant safety, positioning for breastfeeding, and burping; if breastfeeding, positioning baby, latching on, timing, removing from breast	Comfort measures and care related to bowel and bladder function, nutrition, lactation promotion or suppression
Sleep/rest	Assist to comfortable position	Relaxes between exams		At least one nap
Referral/consult				

PP, Postpartum; *WNL*, within normal limits; *CBC*, complete blood count; *HCT*, hematocrit; *BR*, bathroom; *prn*, as needed; *PNV*, prenatal vitamin; *Rx*, prescription.

to extend their services and service area to a greater number of patients. In addition, common problems such as maternal infection and infant hyperbilirubinemia, identified after discharge, can be treated in the home.

Favorable outcomes are ensured when preparation for early discharge and postpartum home follow-up are components of the shorter-stay alternative. Welt et al. (1993) stress the vital role the home care nurse plays in the safety and quality of the early discharge programs, which must be a routine component for all early discharge families.

NURSING CARE AND EARLY POSTPARTUM DISCHARGE: BRIDGING HOSPITAL AND HOME

The hospital-based maternity nurse assumes an invaluable role as caregiver, teacher, and patient/family advocate in settings with early postpartum discharge options. In collaboration with the physician/certified nurse-midwife (CNM), the nurse is instrumental in determining if the mother and newborn meet medical criteria and are ready for discharge. On the basis of careful assessment, the nurse plans an approach for

BOX 21-2

Care Path for Mother-Baby Vaginal Birth Without Complications: Expected Length of Stay—24 Hours, cont'd

2nd Baby Visit	By 16 Hours After Birth	3rd Baby Visit	By 24 Hours After Birth	Discharge Shift
Parent/infant bonding progressing				
	PP HCT if ordered; give anti-Rh globulin if indicated			PP HCT WNL; give rubella vaccine if indicated
	Sitz bath if ordered			Rx filled or given to take home
Bonding, parent concerns, feeding	Use of sitz bath	Infant bath, cord care, need for car seat, newborn characteristics, circumcision care if needed; answer questions; return demonstration for diaper change and feeding	Home care: signs of complications (infection, bleeding), normal psychologic adjustments, resumption of normal activities of daily living; resumption of sexual activities, contraception; identification of support system at home At least 8 hours sleep	Return demonstration infant care; reinforce use of booklets for infant and self-care; inform who should be called if problems; review need for follow-up appointment; provide information about community resources; discuss immunization needs; provide copy of home care instructions
	Assess need for referral/consults, (e.g., social work, lactation consultant)		Referral as needed before discharge	Refer to community agency as needed

meeting the needs of mother and infant during the hospitalization and provides anticipatory guidance, teaching, and referral to the home care agency for home visits to help ensure the couple's continued well-being at home.

Critical Path

Coordination of care must be incorporated throughout the pregnancy cycle.

The use of **critical path case management** for delivery of nursing care facilitates coordination of care (Zander, 1989). Critical paths are defined as shortened case management plans (Gillerman and Beckham, 1991). The schedule of care and the goals for physical recovery remain the same as those described in Chapter 19. The critical path clearly delineates what teaching/discharge planning should occur within specified times. Nurses caring for a woman after an uncomplicated vaginal birth have an average of 24 hours to prepare the postpartum mother and newborn for discharge. Therefore each nurse on each shift is expected to complete the prescribed interventions.

For example, the mother-baby care path standard after vaginal birth may include the following schedule as long as uneventful maternal or newborn recovery continues. Starting by the third hour on the postpartum unit until the end of the first 8-hour shift, the woman is assisted with ambulation; is taught about self-perineal care (including medication), hand washing, involution, and bleeding (lochia); and is given booklets and introduced to available videotapes. When the baby is with her, she learns about supporting the infant's head and extremities and proper positioning for feeding and burping. If she is breastfeeding, she also learns about rooting, latching on, and release of the nipple.

By the end of the second 8-hour shift, the woman is taught about diet, activity/rest, elimination, and medication. When her baby is with her, she is taught about bonding/attachment, usual parent concerns, normal newborn characteristics, diaper changes, cord care, frequency and timing of feedings, use of water feedings, pacifiers, and suckling patterns.

By the end of the third 8-hour shift, the woman needs a review of warning signs for which to call her health care provider. If she will need a consultation—for example, with a lactation specialist—this call is made before discharge. She is taught about safety: baby positioning, use of a car seat, the need for the baby to be attended at all times, and no bottle propping or use of microwave oven to heat baby's bottle. Sibling rivalry is discussed. Teaching is reinforced, and questions are answered. The mother is asked for return demonstrations or explanations of, for example, newborn characteristics, including crying, sneezing, diaper changes, feeding, circumcision care, and recognition of jaundice. As the woman is preparing to go home, she is reminded again of the person to call should a question arise and of the follow-up appointments.

With clearly delineated interventions for each, nurses can provide more efficient care without worry about duplication or gaps. The critical path provides clear direction to coordinating care, teaching essential information, preparing the clients for discharge, and supporting the parent toward independence (Gillerman and Beckham, 1991) (Box 21-2).

Care coordination with home care is essential. Determining which home care agency or public health/community agency will be providing the home visit is essential so the most appropriate discharge plan is made. A home care referral is completed before discharge and communicated to the family and the agency.

The critical path must be adapted to a client's special needs, for example, English as a second language or inability to read; impaired mental capacity such as retardation; substance abuse; very young chronologic age; or physical problems such as extreme fatigue, infection, or anemia. The critical path is a standard. Any deviation is noticed quickly and must be acted on. Therefore the critical path can enhance and secure quality care. It provides one method to effect the transition from hospital to home care.

Nursing Care Management

Assessment

Systematic nursing assessment of the postpartum patient and her newborn assumes significance when discharge is anticipated. Nursing assessment data may be used to help establish that criteria have been met for early discharge, thereby safeguarding mother and infant. A careful assessment enables the nurse to note normal findings and to recognize and promptly report any complications (Box 21-3). Furthermore, these assessment findings represent baseline data for continued assessment in the home by the home care nurse. These baseline data are communicated to the home care nurse on the referral form to be used by the visiting nurse.

The postpartum assessment focuses on the mother's physiologic and psychologic status, level of comfort, readiness to learn, any relevant knowledge deficit, the bonding behaviors evident, and adjustment to the transitions required for mothering. The focus of the newborn assessment is physiologic adjustment to an extrauterine environment, physical and behavioral findings, feeding ability, elimination pattern, and ability of the parents to meet the infant's needs.

Nursing Diagnoses

As women and their families anticipate postpartum discharge, they will each have unique responses. After a careful analysis of data obtained from the assessment, the nurse establishes data-based nursing diagnoses that will guide nursing actions. The following nursing diagnoses may be relevant for a woman or her family at postpartum discharge:

- Altered health maintenance related to
  Insufficient knowledge of signs of complications
- Anxiety related to
  Perceived lack of readiness for early discharge
- Ineffective breastfeeding related to
  Inadequate knowledge or insufficient support
- Ineffective family coping related to
  Disorganization and role changes of early discharge and parenting
- Fatigue related to
  Lack of opportunities to rest during hospitalization
- Risk for altered parenting related to
  Lack of knowledge/skill and unrealistic expectations

Expected Outcomes

A plan of care is formulated that relates specifically to the needs of the woman and her family. To the extent possible, the nurse involves them all in the planning and incorporates their priorities and preferences for any actions planned. Goals are set in patient-centered terms and prioritized in collaboration with the woman and her family. Expected outcomes appropriate for women/families experiencing early postpartum discharge include the following:

1. The postpartum woman will experience uncomplicated physiologic recovery.
2. The woman will experience uncomplicated psychologic adjustment to parenting.
3. The postpartum woman will verbalize an accurate knowledge base and/or demonstrate appropriate care of self and infant.
4. The woman will list available resources for home care and support and the manner in which these may be accessed.
5. The new parents will demonstrate positive interactions with each other, the newborn, and other family members.
6. The postpartum patient will be scheduled for follow-up at home.

Plan of Care and Implementation

Nurses assume both caregiving and teaching roles in preparing the woman and her family for early discharge. Discharge planning includes coordination of care with the home care agency. The nurse must verify the appropriate referral agency. Nurses who are providers of postpartum home visits extend continuity of care to families in the home setting.

Evaluation

Evaluation of patient outcomes is a continuous process. To be effective, evaluation is based on patient-centered expected outcomes identified during the planning stage of nursing care. The nurse can be reasonably assured that care was effective if the following goals have been achieved:

1. The postpartum woman has experienced uncomplicated physiologic recovery and has begun psychologic adjustment to parenting.
2. The postpartum patient verbalizes an accurate knowledge base and/or demonstrates appropriate self-care and infant care.
3. The postpartum patient lists available resources for home care and support and the manner in which these may be obtained.
4. The new parents demonstrate positive interactions with each other, the newborn, and other family members.
5. The postpartum patient has attended preparatory classes and/or is prepared for early discharge and has scheduled a follow-up visit.

If the nurse determines that patient goals are being achieved, implementation of the nursing actions continues as planned. When evaluation data suggest that expected outcomes have not been attained, the plan is revised.

PREPARATORY EDUCATIONAL INSTRUCTION

To ensure the patient's safety and well-being, a basic criterion for patient selection in short-stay maternity programs is educational preparation before discharge. Either formal classes or one-on-one instruction, both supplemented with written material, may be provided at various times throughout the pregnancy. The necessary instructions may be given initially and/or expanded during the hospital stay. Attempting to provide essential teaching only within the time constraints of a short-stay setting presents a special challenge for nurses. Postpartum teaching is complicated because the learner may be tired and uncomfortable from the demands of labor and distracted by visitors and her desire to spend time with the baby and her family. Coordination of the educational plan with the home care program is imperative to meet the needs of the new family.

The nurse recognizes that the adult's readiness to learn is associated with an acknowledgement that a problem exists or with recognition of a gap or deficit in knowledge or skill. The postpartum patient may not identify knowledge deficit as a priority concern (Pridham et al, 1991). The inexperienced mother may not realize her limitations or know what questions to ask until she is at home with the dependent newborn. The multiparous woman, not yet appreciating how unique each child is, may not realize that her existing knowledge base is insufficient. For example, one mother of an especially fussy newborn son reported that she had not learned quieting behaviors when caring for her first baby, a quiet, easily comforted daughter. Although the mother of daughters may be willing to acknowledge a need to learn how to care for the genitalia of a male newborn, she may be hesitant to reveal a knowledge deficit in other basic skills, believing it might put her previous mothering ability into question.

A **teaching plan** made jointly with the woman and her family that identifies topics to cover is essential to avoid duplication of content and to ensure that all essential information is addressed. A teaching plan coordinated with the clinic, hospital, and home care also offers consistency of the information being provided. Few things are more frustrating than hearing conflicting information, especially when the learner is pressed for time or is feeling stressed. Written and audiovisual materials can be used effectively to reinforce the oral instructions.

Teaching plans should be based on systematic assessment and joint identification of the patient's learning needs rather than on the nurse's perceptions of what constitutes essential information. Differences often exist between what nurses believe patients should know and what patients want to know. However, focusing on the informational needs common to new mothers can assist the nurse in planning with the woman the educational topics to be discussed. Mothers in short-stay perinatal programs have identified health threats to themselves and their babies, feeding, and infant care as priorities. Multiparous women are concerned about family relationships.

Once home, the postpartum woman is likely to turn to her partner and/or support person(s) as a source of information. For that reason, it is imperative to include the woman's partner or support person(s) in the instruction whenever possible. The woman may also invite the grandparents to participate because they are commonly caregivers for new families during early days at home (Fig. 21-2).

When a postpartum home visit is planned, not all the teaching is provided during the hospital stay. Some informa-

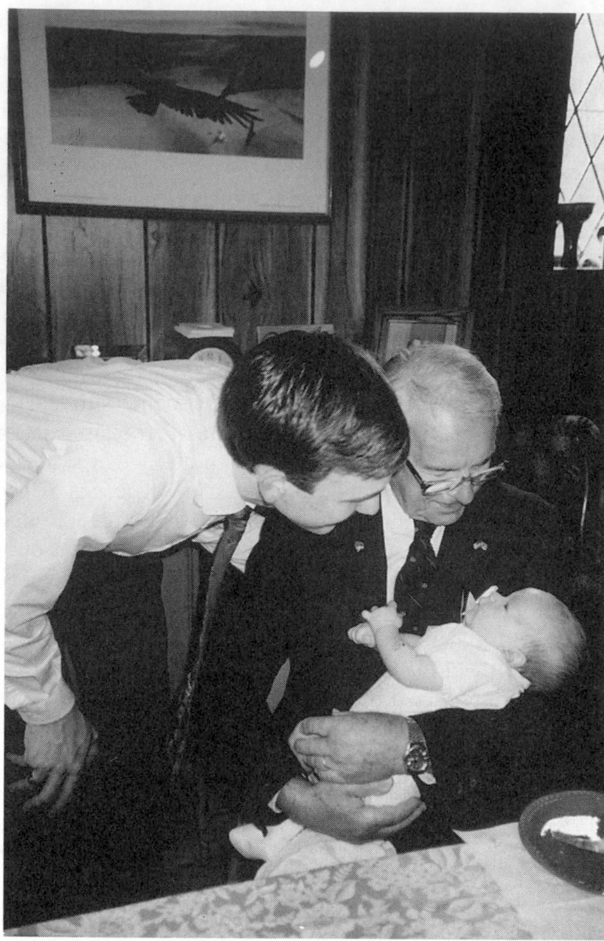

Fig. 21-2 Grandfather, son, and new grandson get acquainted. (Courtesy Eric Shultz.)

tion can be temporarily delayed until the next nurse-patient contact. The nurse can help the family anticipate what their most pressing informational needs will be between discharge and the initial follow-up contact. Together, nurse and patients can plan to meet those prioritized needs. A copy of the hospital teaching flow sheet can be included with the referral to the home care program so that the home care nurse can continue the education plan (Evans, 1991) (Fig. 21-3).

Instructions for the First Hours or Days at Home

New parents often romanticize homecoming with their newborn to the extent that they are inadequately prepared for the reality. One new mother explains, "By the time we drove an hour through traffic, my stitches were hurting and all I wanted was a warm sitz bath and some private time with Bill and the baby, in that order. Instead, a carload of visitors pulled into the driveway as we were unbuckling the baby from his car seat. I thought I would surely cry."

All couples, especially those anticipating early discharge, must be helped to anticipate what the transition from hospital to home will be like so that reality shock will not negate their joy or cause undue stress. Anticipatory guidance should focus on the immediacy of homecoming: the trip itself, providing essential infant care, ensuring rest and comfort for the mother, dealing with visitors, and enlisting help. Sometimes the most simple nursing strategies provide enormous support.

BOX 21-3
Signs of Potential Complications

POSTPARTUM (PHYSICAL) WARNING SIGNS

- Fever, with or without chills
- Foul-smelling or irritating vaginal discharge
- Excessive lochia or vaginal discharge
- Recurrence of bright red vaginal bleeding after the lochia has changed to rust color
- A swollen area on the leg that is painful, red, or hot to the touch
- Localized swelling or a painful, hot area on the breast
- A burning sensation during urination or an inability to urinate
- Pelvic or perineal pain

The Trip Home

With guidance from the nurse, the couple anticipates the actual journey home. The nurse reinforces the use of a safety-approved infant car seat, located in the back seat, with the infant facing the rear of the car. The nurse also helps the parents consider how they will respond if the baby becomes fussy during the trip. Some new mothers prefer to ride home sitting in the back seat beside the infant in the car seat. A fluffy pillow on the seat can provide comfort for a painful perineum, especially during a long trip. Before discharge the nurse may wish to administer whatever mild analgesic has been ordered for postpartum pain relief. The nurse first determines that the mother has had at least one previous dose of the medication without untoward effect.

Before the discharge, another family member may be given the task of taking all unnecessary items and any flowers or gifts home and having any prescriptions filled. This minimizes the time necessary for unloading the car or shopping, thereby increasing the availability of that person as a support after the trip home.

Dealing with Activities of Daily Life

Even the small details of daily life may become stressful, given the demands of a newborn and the discomfort or fatigue associated with birth and a busy homecoming day, or both. The nurse may intervene by suggesting that even if the plan is to use cloth diapers, the parents may wish to purchase one box of disposable diapers for those first hours at home. The nurse, offering preparatory instructions during the pregnancy, may encourage the woman to freeze extra casseroles or leftovers to be ready for use for the first few meals at home. A take-out meal can be planned if necessary to decrease one additional parental responsibility or concern during the initial hours at home.

Planning for discharge soon after an infant feeding ensures that the couple will have adequate time to get home and relatively settled before the next feeding (Fig. 21-4). Offering a sample carton of premixed bottles for the formula-fed infant prevents an immediate need for rushed preparation of for-

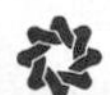

Abbott Northwestern Hospital
A HealthSpan™ Organization
SELF/FAMILY LEARNING CHECKLIST

Patient Name, Social Security #, Date of Birth

I learn best by: ☐ Group classes ☐ Individual instruction ☐ Video instruction ☐ Reading it myself

Please indicate your desired learning needs by placing a check in one of the columns next to each topic.

KEY 1 = Most important to learn before I go home
2 = I already know

(Please DATE when learning need is met.)

CARING FOR YOURSELF	1	2	DATE
Episiotomy and perineal care			
Vaginal discharge			
Hemorrhoids/Constipation			
Breast care			
Nutrition			
Activity			
Post partal exercises			
Return of menstruation			
Family planning			
Blood clots			
Post partum emotions			
Post partum warning signs			
Cesarean Birth			
Incisional care			
AFTER DISCHARGE			
When to call health care provider			
OTHER			
Working mothers			
Day care			
Sibling adjustment			
Single parent support			
Time out for parents			
Infant safety and security			
Infant As A Person Class			
New Parent Connection			

CARING FOR BABY	1	2	DATE
Diapering			
Baby bath, skin and cord care			
Circumcised/uncircumcised care			
Burping			
Bowel movements/wet diapers			
Sleeping habits			
Newborn behavior			
Jaundice			
Signs of illness			
Car seat safety			
General infant safety/poison control			
Signs/symptoms of dehydration			
Bulb syringe			
BREAST FEEDING			
Sore nipples			
Positioning			
Frequency of feedings			
Expressing/storing milk			
Engorgement			
Feeding water			
Nursing while working			
Weaning			
BOTTLE FEEDING			
Types of formula			
Preparing formula			
Frequency of feedings			

MEDICATIONS AT HOME

MEDICATIONS	STRENGTH	DOSAGE	FREQUENCY	PURPOSE/SPECIAL INSTRUCTIONS
			times per day	
			times per day	
			times per day	

RESOURCES
REFERRALS

☐ Physician Discharge Instructions ________________
☐ Home Care Agency ________________
☐ Other Referrals ________________

VALUABLES: ☐ Returned ☐ None **MEDICATIONS:** ☐ Returned ☐ None ☐ Room checked for belongings

Patient verbalized understanding of discharge information received.

PATIENT OR SUPPORT PERSON ____________ NURSE'S SIGNATURE ____________ DATE ________

SELF/FAMILY LEARNING CHECKLIST

SELF/FAMILY LEARNING CHECKLIST

Fig. 21-3 Hospital discharge teaching sheet. (Copyright Abbott-Northwestern Hospital of Allina Health System, Minneapolis and St Paul, Minn.)

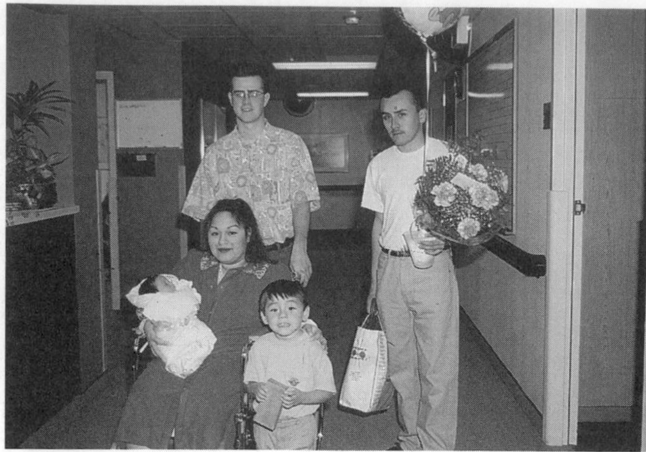

Fig. 21-4 Ready to go home. (Courtesy Marjorie Pyle, RNC, Lifecircle, Costa Mesa, Calif.)

mula. However, offering samples to nursing mothers may be perceived as discouragement of breastfeeding (Dungy et al, 1992).

Dealing with Visitors

A newborn in the family or neighborhood often seems to draw visitors like a magnet. The nurse can help the parents explore ways in which they can assert their needs in such situations. Often family/friends ask what they can do to help, and the family can respond with "Please bring us a casserole or meal," or "Could you pick up some items at the grocery store?" The couple also may want to work out some signal for alerting the partner that the new mother is becoming tired or uncomfortable and needs to have the partner invite the visitors into another part of the house. Some new mothers have found that if they remain in their robe and do not appear ready for company, visitors stay for a shorter time. New families may want to space out visitors and ask some not to visit until 3 or 4 days after being at home. A "Please Do Not Disturb" sign on the front door may be useful.

Postpartum Follow-Up Services

For postpartum families discharged early there is an obvious need for bridging hospital and home, especially early in the course of the fourth trimester when rapid physiologic and psychosocial transitions are occurring. Many types of programs have been developed to meet the needs of these families. Maternity nurses, wishing to offer continuity of care and expand their scope of practice, have joined these programs, offering various postpartum follow-up services:

- Early-discharge preparatory classes
- Telephone follow-up
- Home care programs
- Infant feeding resource centers
  - Lactation support
  - Bottle-feeding support
- Warm lines/help lines
- Parent-support groups
- Perinatal coaching

Although the services for postpartum follow-up may be offered by hospitals, maternity centers, home care agencies, public health agencies, private physicians, or entrepreneurs, it is the nursing profession that has a constant presence in each of these approaches. The goal of these services is to ensure that the mother, newborn, and family have optimal opportunity to prepare for and enjoy safe, comprehensive, quality perinatal care (Stern, 1991).

POSTPARTUM CARE

Home Care Nursing Visits

Many early discharge programs are incorporating **postpartum home visits** as a standard of care (Williams and Cooper, 1993). Home visits to maternity patients may be a service of the hospital, the private physician or clinic, a public health department, or a home care agency providing home visits. Regardless of their source, home visits are a vital component of early discharge postpartum care. Immediate follow-up contact and home visits must be available 7 days a week (see the Nursing Care Plan on p. 576-577).

The referral from the hospital to the home care agency is completed and communicated on the day of discharge (Fig. 21-5). This assures there is no delay in services for follow-up care. The hospital nurse also informs the family of the agency phone number as part of the resources to contact if needed.

On receipt of the referral, the home care agency verifies reimbursement for the home visit (unless payment for the visit is bundled with a pregnancy or labor/birth reimbursement package). This information is communicated to the family.

The day after discharge the home care agency contacts the mother to screen for maternal and newborn complications. This phone interview assists the mother and nurse in determining the most appropriate day for the home visit (Fig. 21-6).

The home visit is most commonly scheduled on the second day home from the hospital. However, the visit is based on individual family needs and may be on the first day home or the third or fourth day, depending on the individual family situation. Additional visits are planned throughout the course of the first week, as needed. A decision to extend the home visits beyond this time is made based on the family's needs and most appropriate follow-up options for the specific identified needs. A follow-up phone call after the home visit is provided by the visiting nurse/agency to give the family an opportunity to ask any questions or discuss situations that have come up since the home visit(s).

A home visit progresses more effectively if it is preplanned and well organized. The nurse reviews the hospital's discharge summary, teaching plan, and any other records, including physician's orders, that will serve to structure the interview and physical assessment and that will provide continuity in care. Before the visit the nurse obtains directions to the family's home and secures a map. Box 21-4 summarizes the protocol for a postpartum home visit.

After the visit is planned, the nurse collects necessary equipment, supplies, and instructional materials and ensures that they are clean and in working order before placing them in the visit bag. The nurse who is not known to the family identifies herself by a proper name tag, preferably with a picture for added security.

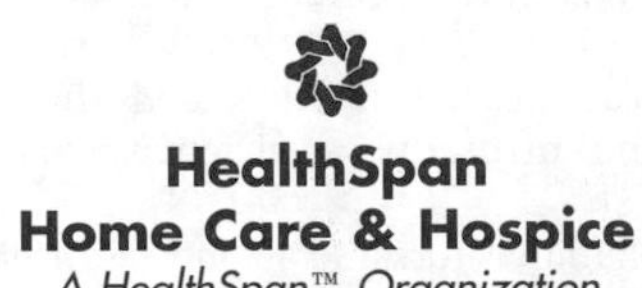

POST PARTUM HOME CARE REFERRAL

Mother's Name: ____________________
Address/phone where mother will be staying:
Address: ____________________
City: ____________________
Phone #: ____________________
Language spoken: □ English □ Other: ________
Understands English: □ Well □ Poor
□ Mother Needs Interpreter □ Hearing Impaired
Who interpreted in hospital: ____________________
Mom agrees to this referral: □ Yes □ No
Currently being seen by PHN: □ Yes □ No
Mom's M.D./Midwife: ____________________
Phone #: ____________________
Next Appt: ____________________

MOTHER:

Gravida________ T______ P______ A______ L______
Marital Status: S M W D Sep
Normal Maternal Exam: □ Yes □ No (explain below)
Epis/Incision: ____________________
Hgb pp: ____________________
Meds: ____________________
Allergies: ____________________

OTHER ISSUES:

Diabetic: ____________________
Other: ____________________
Psycho/Social Issues:
□ Parent/Child Interaction □ Adolescent Mother
□ Mental Health Status □ Drug Use/Dependency
□ Previous Losses □ Hx of Family Abuse
□ Developmentally Delayed Parents □ Limited Support System
□ Other: ____________________

Husband/Significant Other: ____________________
Baby's Name: ____________________ □ M □ F
DOB/Time: ____________________
Mother's Discharge Date/Time: ____________________
Newborn Discharge Date: (if different from mother's) ____________________
Baby's M.D. (Full Name): ____________________
Phone #: ____________________
Next Appt: ____________________

BABY:

Gestation: ____________ Weeks □ Fetal Loss
Birth Weight: ________ Discharge Weight: ________
Apgars: 1" ____________ 5" ____________
Feeding Issues: ____________________
Feedings: Breast ________ Bottle ________
Normal Infant Exam: □ Yes □ No (explain below)
Circumcised: □ Yes □ No
Cord Clamp Off: □ Yes □ No
Voidings: □ Yes □ No
Stooling: □ Yes □ No

□ Newborn screen was done in hospital—after baby 24 hours of age.

□ Newborn screen to be drawn at clinic.
□ Newborn screen to be drawn at home.
□ Lab slip sent home with family.

ADDITIONAL COMMENTS or ABNORMAL FINDINGS FOR MOTHER OR BABY: ____________________
____
____

Faxed to Home Care □ *Facesheet* □ *Referral* *Referral Completed By:* ____________________

Fig. 21-5 Referral form. (Copyright HealthSpan Home Care and Hospice of Allina Health System, St Paul, Minn.)

Nursing Care Plan

HOME CARE FOLLOW-UP AFTER DISCHARGE

Nursing Diagnosis: Risk for ineffective breastfeeding related to frustration with the process

Expected Outcomes: Woman expresses physical and psychologic comfort with the feeding process, and infant feeds successfully and appears satisfied for at least 1 hour after feeding.

• **NURSING INTERVENTIONS/*RATIONALES***

Explore woman's knowledge of breastfeeding, assess for presence of flat or inverted nipples, determine level of ambivalence and anxiety tied to breastfeeding and observe the technique being used *to evaluate the process and direct nursing interventions.*

If a problem area is identified, refer to the nursing care plan in Chapter 24 on breastfeeding.

NURSING DIAGNOSIS: Risk for infant care deficit related to lack of experience/lack of support

Expected Outcomes: Infant care routines are adequate, and infant appears healthy.

• **NURSING INTERVENTIONS/*RATIONALES***

Observe infant care routines (bathing, diapering, feeding, play) *to evaluate parental ease with care and adequacy of techniques.*

Discuss parental concerns about care issues and infant response *to assess for possible problem areas.*

Observe infant appearance (height-weight ratio, head circumference, fontanels, skin tone and turgor); assess infant's vital signs, overall tone, reflexes, and age-appropriate developmental skills *to evaluate for signs indicative of inadequate care.*

Explore available support systems for infant care *to determine adequacy of existing system.*

Help parents identify and address areas of care that need improvement *to ensure infant safety and health.*

Demonstrate troublesome care routines and have involved family members return demonstration *to facilitate improvements in care.*

Provide ongoing follow-up as needed *to ensure amelioration of identified potential and actual care deficits.*

NURSING DIAGNOSIS: Sleep pattern disturbance related to infant demands and environmental interruptions

Expected Outcome: Woman sleeps for uninterrupted periods and feels rested on waking.

• **NURSING INTERVENTIONS/*RATIONALES***

Discuss woman's routine and specify things that interfere with sleep *to determine scope of problem and direct interventions.*

Explore ways woman and significant others can make environment more conducive to sleep (i.e., privacy, darkness, quiet, back rubs, soothing music, warm milk); teach use of guided imagery and relaxation techniques *to promote optimum conditions for sleep.*

Avoid things or routines (i.e., caffeine, foods that induce heartburn, strenuous mental/physical activity) *that may interfere with sleep.*

Advise family to limit visitors and activities *to avoid further taxation and fatigue.*

Have family plan specific times to care for the newborn to allow mother time to sleep; have mother learn to use infant nap time as a time for her to nap as well as *to replenish energy and decrease fatigue.*

NURSING DIAGNOSIS: Risk for impaired home maintenance management related to addition of new family member/inadequate resources/inadequate support systems

Expected Outcome: Home exhibits signs of safe and functional environment.

• **NURSING INTERVENTIONS/*RATIONALES***

Observe the home environment (i.e., available living space and sleeping arrangements; adequacy of facilities for food preparation and storage, hygiene and toileting; overall state of repair; cleanliness; presence of safety hazards) *to determine adequacy and effective use of resources.*

Observe arrangements for the newborn, such as sleeping space, care equipment and supplies (bathing, changing, feeding, transportation) *to determine adequacy of resources.*

Explore who is responsible for cooking, cleaning, child care, and newborn care and determine whether the mother seems adequately rested *to determine adequacy of support systems.*

Collaborate with family to remedy identified safety issues immediately *to prevent physical injury.*

Identify and arrange referrals to needed social agencies (i.e., Aid to Families with Dependent Children [AFDC], Women, Infants, and Children [WIC] program, food pantries) *to ameliorate resource deficits (finances, supplies, equipment).*

Identify and arrange referrals if needed for additional support (i.e., housekeeper, child care, postpartum support groups, warm lines) *to supplement existing support systems.*

Continue home visitation as needed and provide coordination with referral services *to facilitate successful adaptation of environment.*

NURSING DIAGNOSIS: Risk for altered family processes related to inclusion of new family member

Expected Outcome: Infant is successfully assimilated into family structure.

• **NURSING INTERVENTIONS/*RATIONALES***

Explore with family the ways that the birth and neonate have changed family structure and function *to evaluate functional and role adjustment.*

Nursing Care Plan

HOME CARE FOLLOW-UP AFTER DISCHARGE—CONT'D

Observe family interaction with the newborn and note degree of bonding, evidence of sibling rivalry, and involvement in newborn care *to evaluate acceptance of newest family member.*

Assist family in reframing any perceived negative outcomes in a more positive light *to promote constructive interaction.*

Clarify identified misinformation and misperceptions *to promote clear communication.*

Assist family to explore options for solutions to identified problems *to promote effective problem resolution.*

Support family efforts as they move toward adjusting and incorporating the new member *to reinforce new functions and roles.*

If needed, make referrals to appropriate social services or community agencies *to ensure ongoing support and care.*

BOX 21-4

Protocol for Postpartum Home Visit

Previsit Interventions

1. Contact family to arrange details for home visit:
   a. Identify self, credentials, and agency role.
   b. Review purpose of home visit follow-up.
   c. Schedule convenient time for visit.
   d. Confirm address and route to family home.
2. Review and clarify appropriate data.
   a. All available assessment data for mother and infant (i.e., referral forms, hospital discharge summaries, family identified learning needs).
   b. Review records of any previous nursing contacts.
   c. Contact other professional caregivers as necessary to clarify data (i.e., obstetrician, nurse-midwife, pediatrician, referring nurse).
3. Identify community resources and teaching materials appropriate to meet needs already identified.
4. Plan the visit, and prepare bag with equipment, supplies, and materials necessary for assessments of mother and infant, actual care anticipated for mother and infant, and teaching.

In-home Interventions: Establishing a Relationship

1. Reintroduce self and establish purpose of postpartum follow-up visit for mother, infant, and family; offer family opportunity to clarify their expectations of contact.
2. Spend brief time socially interacting with family to become acquainted and establish trusting relationship.

In-home Interventions: Working With Family

1. Conduct systematic assessment of mother and newborn to determine physiologic adjustment and any existing complications.
2. Throughout visit, collect data to assess the emotional adjustment of individual family members to newborn and lifestyle changes. Note evidence of family-newborn bonding and sibling rivalry; note relationships among mother, father, children, and grandparents.
3. Determine adequacy of support system.
   a. To what extent does someone help with cooking, cleaning, and other home management tasks?
   b. To what extent is help being provided in caring for the newborn and any other children?
   c. Are support persons encouraging the new mother to care for herself and get adequate rest?
   d. Who is providing helpful information? Emotional support?
4. Throughout the visit, observe home environment for adequacy of resources:
   a. Space: privacy, safe play of children, sleeping.
   b. Overall cleanliness and state of repair.
   c. Number of steps new mother must climb.
   d. Adequacy of cooking arrangements.
   e. Adequacy of refrigeration and other food storage areas.
   f. Adequacy of bathing, toileting, and laundry facilities.
   g. Arrangements in home for newborn: sleeping, bathing, formula preparation (if needed), layette items and diapers.
5. Throughout the visit, observe home environment for overall state of repair and existence of safety hazards:
   a. Storage of medications, household cleaners, and other substances hazardous to children.
   b. Presence of peeling paint on furniture, walls, or pipes.
   c. Factors that contribute to falls, such as dim lighting, broken steps, scatter rugs.
   d. Presence of vermin.
   e. Use of crib or playpen that fails to meet safety guidelines.
   f. Existence of emergency plan in case of fire; fire alarm or extinguisher.
6. Provide care to mother and/or newborn as prescribed by their respective primary care provider or in accord with agency protocol.
7. Provide teaching on basis of previously identified needs.
8. Refer family to appropriate community agencies or resources, such as warm lines and support groups.
9. Ascertain that woman knows potential problems to watch for and whom to call if they occur.
10. Ensure that used disposable items have been handled appropriately and that reusable items are cleaned and repacked appropriately in the nurse's bag.

In-home Interventions: Ending the Visit*

1. Summarize the activities and main points of the visit.
2. Clarify future expectations, including schedule of next visit.
3. Review teaching plan, and provide major points in writing.
4. Provide information about reaching the nurse or agency if needed before the next scheduled visit.

Postvisit Interventions

1. Document the visit thoroughly, using the necessary agency forms to serve as a legal record of the visit and to allow third-party reimbursement, as possible.
2. Initiate the plan of care on which the next encounter with the patient/family will be based.
3. Communicate appropriately (by telephone, letter, progress notes, or referral form) with primary care provider, other health professionals, or referral agencies on behalf of patient/family.

*If this is the nurse's final planned encounter with the woman/family, it is important to recognize that both the women and nurse may have feelings evoked by ending a meaningful relationship and by saying goodbye. Such feelings as anger, denial, and sadness are normal in this situation. Freely expressing these feelings at the end of the relationship is encouraged. Often patients are encouraged to do so if the nurse shares such feelings first.

MINNESOTA OB HOMECARE
612-863-4478

TC **POSTPARTUM ASSESSMENT PHONE CALLS**

MOTHER'S NAME	INFANT'S NAME	
SOCIAL SECURITY #	DOB	ID #
MD	MD	

1. Are you feeling well?			
2. Do you have any concerns about your postpartum care?			
3. How many wet diapers has your baby had in the last 24 hours? (4-6)			
4. How would you describe your baby's stools?			
5. Does your baby appear jaundiced? (Describe)			
6. Do you have a clinic appointment made for your baby? When?			
INFANT FEEDING			
BOTTLE	*NURSING*		
7. How often is your baby eating?	7. How often is your baby eating?		
8. Does your baby wake to feed or do you wake him/her?	8. Does your baby wake to feed or do you wake him/her?		
9. How much formula is taken at each feeding?	9. Is your baby able to latch on without difficulty?		
10. Does your baby spit up after feeding?	10. Do you hear regular swallowing while your baby is nursing?		
	11. How long is your baby continuously sucking and swallowing when nursing? (10 minutes)		
	12. Does your baby spit up after feeding? Explain.		
	13. Does your baby fall asleep at the breast? How soon?		
	14. How do your nipples feel?		
	15. Do you feel breast feeding is going well?		
	NURSE'S SIGNATURE **DATE**		

FAXED TO: □ OB □ PEDS

□ DISCHARGED

□ VISIT SCHEDULED: DATE: ____________ □ VISIT REFUSED: REASONS: ____________

COMMENTS ____________

DISPOSITION CODES:
SC - SELF-CARE
FC - FAMILY CARE

DISCHARGE REASONS:
GM - GOALS MET
HO - HOSPITALIZATION
TR - TRANSFER TO ANOTHER AGENCY

Fig. 21-6 Telephone interview documentation record. (Copyright jointly held by Abbott Northwestern Hospital and HealthSpan Home Care and Hospice of Allina Health System, Minneapolis and St Paul, Minn.)

Safety issues. The visiting nurse may need to enter unsafe areas on occasion. Taking necessary safety precautions and avoiding dangerous visits is imperative. A confident, nonvulnerable manner is appropriate. For visits in particularly dangerous settings, nurses may wish to visit in pairs. Nurses should report to the agency by telephone at specified intervals. The same precautions and common sense that guide behavior in any potentially hazardous setting should be used on home visits. For example, the nurse should begin the day with a full tank of gas and give the agency office a list of the visits and anticipated schedule for the day. It is common for visiting nurses to have cellular phones and beepers so the nurse can make contact by phone and others are able to send messages by beeper. On visits, the nurse should park near the home or in a well-lighted area with an unobstructed route to the home's entrance. The automobile should always be locked and valuables stored out of sight. The nurse should avoid walking near groups of strangers in doorways or alleys, entering a yard with an unrestrained dog, or carrying valuables. Neither should unfamiliar shortcuts be used. If a nurse is concerned about entering a home or other building, it is best not to enter without another home care person or escort. If the nurse has an intuitive feeling that the house is unsafe, it is important to leave immediately and return later with an escort for any equipment or home care supplies.

The Home Visit

During the home visit the nurse conducts a systematic assessment of mother and newborn to determine physiologic adjustment, identify any existing complications, and answer any questions the mother has for herself and the mother/family has about the newborn or newborn care. The parents are more often ready to learn in their own home after having an opportunity to be responsible for caring for their baby (Harrison, 1990). The nurse provides education and support for the new family and links them with hospital and community resources available to them for ongoing education and support.

The first few minutes of the home visit are introductory. The nurse has an opportunity to get acquainted with the mother and her support persons and establish a trusting, professional relationship.

Although a nurse's purpose in visiting is different from that of a guest in the home, visiting nurses extend the same courtesy they would show to friends they might visit. For example, the nurse will call ahead to verify that the time scheduled for the visit is still convenient. (Not only is this common courtesy; it occasionally saves an unnecessary, sometimes costly trip.) Nurses show respect for the privacy and personal property of family members. For example, the woman is given the choice of where the interview and physical examination will be conducted to best safeguard her privacy. The nurse seeks permission before using the family's handwashing facilities, placing equipment in a particular place, or using the family telephone to call the physician/midwife.

Each home visit is unique. The home care nurse must be flexible and creative, adjusting to each family and the home environment to accomplish the home visit. If the baby is resting when the nurse arrives, it may be best for the nurse to examine the mother first and the newborn last. The nurse performs a complete maternal examination (Fig. 21-7), so it is important to support the mother's privacy. The mother may select a separate room during her physical examination. This also allows the nurse private time with the mother to ask questions and provide education on other topics such as breast care, family planning, and constipation. The assessment also focuses on the mother's emotional adjustment, including the presence of balancing factors (perception, coping, and support) that prevent crisis, and her knowledge of self- and infant care. It is important for the nurse to remember to encourage the mother to ask any questions or share concerns she may have for herself. Some families think the nurse's function is to check only on the baby and not the mother as well.

The Association of Women's Health, Obstetric, and Neonatal Nurses (AWHONN) (1994) guidelines identify the following areas that home care nurses must be prepared to address during the maternal assessment (Chapter 19):

- Evaluation of maternal adaptation
- Physical adjustment to postpartum period
  - Vital signs
  - Breasts (for both breastfeeding and formula-feeding mothers)
  - Uterine involution process
  - Perineal healing
  - Elimination: return of normal bowel and bladder function
  - Incision site, where appropriate
  - Lower extremities
  - Pain assessment
  - Sexual changes and adjustments
- Psychosocial adjustment to early motherhood
  - Self-confidence
  - Blues and/or depression
  - Specific concerns
- Health promotion activities
- Postpartum follow-up with health care provider
- List of resources

The nurse performs a complete newborn examination (Chapter 23) and throughout the examination encourages the mother/family to ask questions or express concerns they may have (Fig. 21-8). The home care nurse must verify if the newborn screen for phenylketonuria (PKU) and other inborn errors of metabolism disorders (p. 637) has been drawn. If the baby was discharged from the hospital before 24 hours of age, the newborn screen will need to be done by the home care or clinic nurse, or the family must return to the hospital laboratory. The home care nurse must clarify the plan with the family and ensure that it will be done.

AWHONN (1994) guidelines also identify the following areas that home care nurses must be prepared to address during the newborn assessment:

- Newborn examination
  - Vital signs
  - Color
  - Skin
  - Head
  - Cord condition
  - Circumcision, where applicable
  - Movement symmetry
  - Feeding patterns
  - Elimination

HealthSpan
Home Care & Hospice
A HealthSpan™ Organization
Minnesota OB Homecare

MATERNAL ASSESSMENT NOTE AND CARE PLAN

Client Name

BILLABLE ● YES ◯ NO
PAYROLL ◯ YES ● NO

Activity ID
◯ RNV 620
◯ RPV 620 (One Day Stay)

BR.
62 ●

SOCIAL SECURITY NUMBER ☐☐☐-☐☐-☐☐☐☐

TIME IN ☐☐:☐☐

MONTH DAY YEAR ☐☐-☐☐-☐☐

TIME OUT ☐☐:☐☐

Please fill in ovals completely. Write numbers centered in boxes. Use a blue or black ink pen.

PHYSICIAN NAME:	DELIVERY DATE:	HOSPITAL DISCHARGE DATE:
PHYSICIAN PLEASE NOTE:		

EXPECTED OUTCOMES:
- Client will verbalize/demonstrate knowledge of postpartum self-care and care for newborn.
- Client will demonstrate knowledge of breast and/or bottle feeding techniques and methods for problem solving.

PHYSICAL ASSESSMENT:
TPR ______ BP ______
FUNDUS ______

PERINEUM/INCISION: ◯ INTACT ◯ WITHOUT S/S OF INFECTION ◯ HEMORRHOIDS ◯ SITZ BATHS ENCOURAGED

LOCHIA: ◯ SMALL ◯ MODERATE ◯ LARGE ◯ SEROSA ◯ RUBRA ◯ NORMAL ODOR ◯ FOUL ODOR

BREASTS: ◯ NONLACTATING ◯ LACTATING ◯ REVIEWED BREAST CARE/NIPPLE CARE

FAMILY/PARENTING ADJUSTMENT: ◯ HUSBAND /S.O. SUPPORTIVE ◯ OTHERS SUPPORTIVE ◯ POSITIVE INTERACTION WITH BABY OBSERVED

PHYSICAL/EMOTIONAL — DISCUSSED:
◯ CARING FOR SELF AND BABY ◯ REST ENCOURAGED ◯ TIME FOR SELF & S.O.
◯ VERBALIZED ABILITY TO DEAL WITH PP CHANGES

ELIMINATION: ◯ HAS HAD A BM ◯ VOIDING WITHOUT DIFFICULTY

LOWER EXTREMITIES: EDEMA ◯ YES ◯ NO
◯ NEGATIVE HOMAN'S SIGN
◯ NO PAIN OR REDNESS

NUTRITION: ◯ AWARE OF DIETARY NEEDS ◯ AWARE OF FLUID NEEDS

SEXUALITY: ◯ DISCUSSED BIRTH CONTROL ◯ DISCUSSED SEXUAL ADJUSTMENT

MATERNAL TEACHING/CARE PLAN:
◯ EMERGENCY PLAN REINFORCED (I.E., POISON CONTROL, 911)
◯ HAS KNOWLEDGE OF COMMUNITY RESOURCES FOR MOTHER AND BABY (COMMUNITY PARENTING GROUPS, ETC.)
◯ BASIC HOME SAFETY ASSESSED

CLINIC VISIT SCHEDULED: ◯ NO ◯ YES ______

CONFERENCE WITH: ◯ PHYSICIAN ◯ INSURANCE ◯ OTHER ______
◯ VIA FAX

CLINICAL UPDATE:

______

NURSE'S SIGNATURE ______
FIRST MIDDLE INITIAL LAST TITLE

EMPLOYEE ID ☐☐☐☐☐☐☐☐☐☐

EMPLOYEE TYPE ☐☐

Fig. 21-7 Maternal assessment note and care plan. (Copyright jointly held by Abbott Northwestern Hospital and HealthSpan Home Care and Hospice of Allina Health System, Minneapolis and St Paul, Minn.)

HealthSpan
Home Care & Hospice
A HealthSpan™ Organization

Minnesota OB Homecare

INFANT ASSESSMENT NOTE AND CARE PLAN

Client Name

BILLABLE ◯ **YES** ◯ **NO**
PAYROLL ◯ **YES** ⬤ **NO**

Activity ID ◯ ◯ ◯
◯ RNV 620 ◯ ◯ ◯
◯ ◯ ◯ ◯
◯ ◯ ◯ ◯

BR.
62 ⬤

SOCIAL SECURITY NUMBER ☐☐☐-☐☐-☐☐☐☐

TIME IN ☐☐:☐☐

MONTH DAY YEAR ☐☐-☐☐-☐☐

TIME OUT ☐☐:☐☐

Please fill in ovals completely. Write numbers centered in boxes. Use a blue or black ink pen.

PHYSICIAN NAME:		MOTHER'S NAME:
PHYSICIAN PLEASE NOTE:		
DOB:	HOSPITAL DISCHARGE DATE:	DAYS OLD:

PHYSICAL ASSESSMENT:
TPR ______
WEIGHT: (per physician order) ______

CORD: ◯ DRYING WITHOUT REDNESS ◯ CORD CARE REVIEWED

CIRCUMCISION: ◯ CLEAN, NO S/S OF INFECTION ◯ CIRC CARE REVIEWED

SKIN CONDITION: ◯ NO RASHES ◯ NEWBORN RASH ◯ DRY

COLOR: ◯ SKIN PINK ◯ SCLERA WHITE ◯ JAUNDICE

SAFETY: ◯ SAFE ENVIRONMENT OBSERVED ◯ HAS CAR SEAT

PARENTING ASSESSMENT: ◯ BASIC NEEDS MET
◯ INFANT STIMULATION REVIEWED
◯ POSITIVE PARENT/INFANT INTERACTION OBSERVED

FEEDING: ◯ NURSING EVERY ______ HRS FOR ______ MIN, TOTAL
◯ SWALLOWING HEARD WITH NURSING
◯ BOTTLE FEEDING EVERY ______ HRS (AMT ______)
◯ CONTENT AND/OR SLEEPING BETWEEN FEEDINGS
◯ MOTHER AWARE OF DIFFERENCE BETWEEN SPITTING AND VOMITING

ELIMINATION: ◯ VOIDING ADEQUATELY [X] AMT WET DIAPERS/DAY: ______
STOOLS: ◯ GREEN ◯ MUSTARD ◯ MECONIUM

ACTIVITY: ◯ ALERT, ACTIVE PERIODS ◯ RESPONDS WELL TO STIMULI

LAB WORK: ◯ NEWBORN SCREEN DRAWN IN HOME
◯ BILIRUBIN DRAWN, RESULTS ______
◯ NONE

MATERNAL/FAMILY TEACHING — CARE PLAN:
◯ BASIC CARE SKILLS REINFORCED (TEMPING, BATHING, ETC.)
◯ ENVIRONMENT APPEARS SAFE FOR INFANT
◯ MOTHER AWARE OF S/S OF SICK BABY AND ENCOURAGED TO CALL DOCTOR WHEN IN DOUBT
◯ EMERGENCY PLAN REINFORCED (I.E., POISON CONTROL, 911)
◯ REVIEWED BABY'S GROWTH & DEVELOPMENT & SUGGESTED A LIST OF READING MATERIALS AVAILABLE IF INTERESTED
◯ REVIEWED APPROPRIATE CLOTHING FOR BABY
◯ HAS KNOWLEDGE OF COMMUNITY RESOURCES FOR MOTHER AND BABY (COMMUNITY PARENTING GROUPS, ETC.)

CLINIC VISIT SCHEDULED: ◯ NO ◯ YES ______

CONFERENCE WITH: ◯ **PHYSICIAN** ◯ **INSURANCE** ◯ **OTHER** ______
◯ **VIA FAX**

CLINICAL UPDATE:
______
______
______
______

NURSE'S SIGNATURE ______
FIRST **MIDDLE INITIAL** **LAST** **TITLE**

EMPLOYEE ID ☐☐☐☐☐☐☐☐☐☐ **EMPLOYEE TYPE** ☐☐

Fig. 21-8 Infant assessment note and care plan. (Copyright jointly held by Abbott Northwestern Hospital and HealthSpan Home Care and Hospice of Allina Health System, Minneapolis and St Paul, Minn.)

Identify problems that require interventions or referral
Perform and/or explain laboratory tests
Use technologies, when applicable

The nurse should be aware of educational materials the clinic, parent-education classes, and hospital have provided to the family for resources and instructions. The nurse can refer the family to the materials and be consistent in the education/information provided. During the home visit the nurse discusses with the parents and support persons questions and concerns about their baby and newborn care (Chapter 23).

Ideally the father or partner and/or support person(s) are present during a home visit so that the couple's adjustment to parenting can be observed. If not, the mother's perception of their adjustment can be noted. The visit also affords the nurse

Home Care

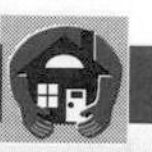

OUTCOME CRITERIA

Physiologic recovery, involution, and healing in mother

- Lists signs of problems that should be reported to primary care provider immediately
- Verbalizes understanding of normal findings
- Confirms decreasing discomfort, controlled by prescribed comfort measures
- Confirms patterns reflecting adequate rest

Breasts

- Supported by well-fitted bra
- Nontender; no signs of inflammation
- Intact nipples without cracks, fissures, or undue soreness

If breastfeeding

- Describes or demonstrates technique for placing baby on and removing baby from breast, as well as proper position to decrease stress on nipple area

If not breastfeeding

- No engorgement
- Discusses importance of not stimulating breasts

Uterus

- Fundus firm, descending below umbilicus approximately 1 cm per day

Bowels/Bladder

- Resumption of usual pattern of bowel elimination
- Hemorrhoids (if present) getting smaller; not causing undue discomfort
- Resumption of usual pattern of urinary elimination; no burning or difficulty in initiating urine flow

Lochia

- Normally progressing involution—rubra, serosa, alba in decreasing amounts—normal fleshy odor, no clots

Incision: Perineal or Abdominal

- Episiotomy (if present) well approximated without undue redness, edema, ecchymosis, discharge, or tenderness
- Cesarean incision (if present) clean, dry, well approximated; skin staples, sutures, or Steri-strips intact (if still present); evidence of normal healing

Legs

- Nontender, with negative Homans' sign bilaterally

Physiologic adaptation of infant

Temperature

- 36.5° to 37° C (97.7° to 98.6° F) by axillary route

Heart Rate

- 120 to 160 beats/min, strong, regular, normal variations with activity

Respiration

- 30 to 60 breaths/min, normal breath sounds, irregular rhythm; no retractions, or grunting; normal variations with activity

Skin

- Warm, good turgor; no rashes

Head

- Symmetric, with flat fontanels; molding or caput decreasing; no hematoma

Abdomen

- Soft, nondistended; audible bowel sounds

Color

- Consistent with racial background; no evidence of jaundice

Activity

- Alert with good muscle tone; moving all extremities equally

Umbilical Cord

- Normal atrophy noted, dry base without redness; not malodorous

Circumcision

- Bell in place (if appropriate); clean and healing; no evidence of oozing; urinary stream normal

Elimination

- Wetting a minimum of 6 to 10 diapers per day; stools consistent with feeding method in color, number, and consistency

Sleep Pattern

- Has periods of content sleep during day or night

Feeding

- Baby sucks well without excessive spitting
- Baby burps well
- Length of breastfeeding (if done) consistent with recommendations; rooting, latching on, release of nipple
- Baby sucks/swallows in sustained pattern (10 to 20 sucks), followed by a pause
- Mother identifies signs of let-down, latching on
- Mother describes the way to wake sleepy baby and keep the baby feeding
- Mother describes the way to know if baby is getting enough
- Amount of formula per feeding (if done) consistent with recommendations

an opportunity to observe interactions among those family members present within the familiarity and security of their home setting where they are in control (Hall and Carty, 1993). Observing new parents, the newborn, and other family members in this natural setting enables the nurse to elicit data about their life circumstances not accessible in any other way (Clemen-Stone, Eigsti, and McGuire, 1995). The Home Care box on p. 582 indicates criteria for evaluating the visit's outcome.

Positive feedback on parenting skills observed and newborn responses to mother and father reinforce parenting and bonding with the newborn. As the nurse holds, cuddles, and comforts the newborn, he or she is a role model to the parents and support system. Throughout the newborn examination, the nurse demonstrates and explains normal newborn behaviors and capabilities. The nurse must keep in mind the potential impact on the family of demonstrating positive parenting behaviors and skills.

Although the primary nursing interventions during a home visit involve supportive counseling, anticipatory guidance, teaching, or referral, on occasion physical care may be given. For example, on order from the physician, the nurse may remove sutures or staples from the mother's abdominal incision, change a dressing, or initiate home phototherapy for the infant (Fig. 21-9). On occasion, it may be necessary for the nurse to collect blood or urine specimens for laboratory study. For example, a clean-catch urine specimen might be needed for a mother with suspected urinary tract infection; infant blood might be collected to assess for hyperbilirubinemia or PKU follow-up. Throughout procedures of this kind and during the routine examinations of mother and newborn, Standard Precautions are followed and careful techniques used to prevent the spread of pathogens.

Ongoing support through resources offered by the hospitals and/or community groups is one way the home care nurse coordinates care for the family. Providing educational materials on community resources, public health nurse programs, and hospital postpartum groups can connect families for ongoing follow-up, education, and support. Often this information has already been introduced to the family prenatally or in the hospital, but now the family may be ready to participate in such resources. Referrals to such programs can

A

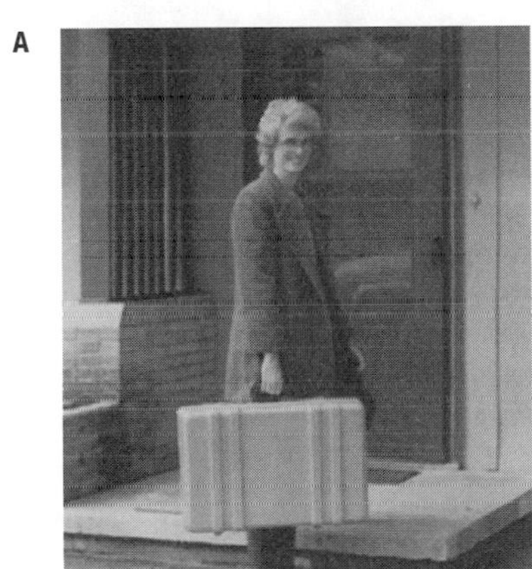

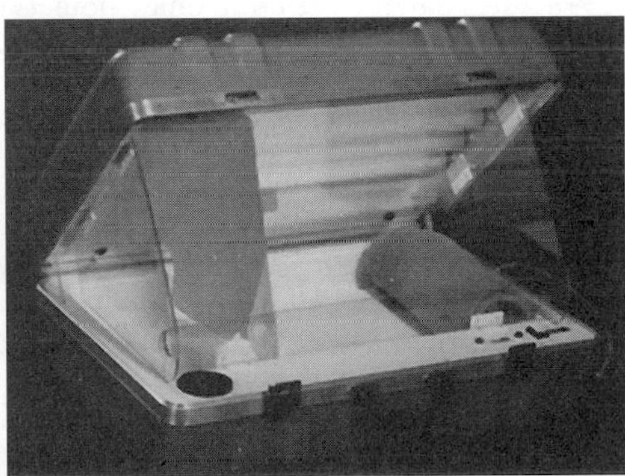

B

C

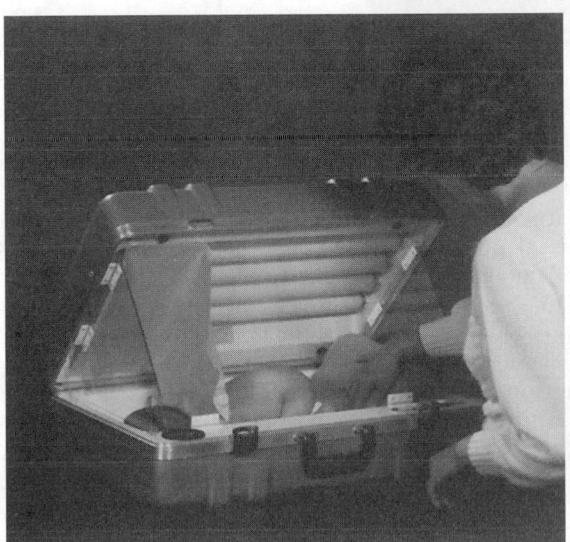

D

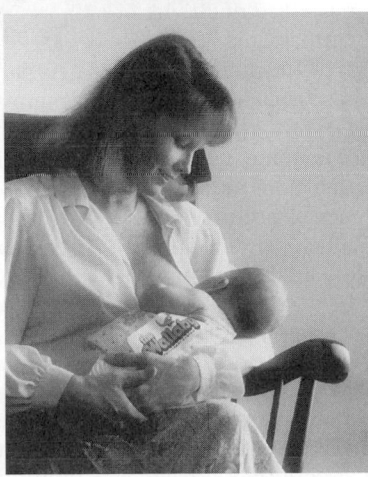

Fig. 21-9 Portable phototherapy for home use. **A,** Nurse brings portable unit to the home. **B,** Assembled unit. **C,** Infant under phototherapy with face shielded from the light. **D,** Fiberoptic method of phototherapy. Infant wrapped in covered fiberoptic panels. (**A, B, C** courtesy PEP Inc., Park Rapids, Minn; **D** courtesy Healthdyne Technology, Marietta, Georgia.)

be presented in a nonthreatening way, emphasizing the support and networking with other families in similar experiences.

One example of a community resource for new families is an infant-feeding resource center. These centers can be provided by hospitals, clinics, or entrepreneurial consultants to meet the needs of families as they breastfeed or bottle-feed their newborn/child. With early discharge, ongoing support for the breastfeeding mother is of great interest, and lactation consultants/educators have set up centers to assist families. Often the home care nurse makes a referral to a lactation consultant, pediatrician, or pediatric nurse practitioner for a mother with breastfeeding concerns that cannot be resolved during the home visit. Bottle-feeding mothers also need support and a resource center to call with their questions and concerns, and these resources can meet their needs as well. The home care nurse can assist the family to contact community resources to help with infant feeding issues.

After the home visit the visiting nurse calls the mother as a follow-up and point of discharge from home care. The purpose of the call is to address issues identified during the home visit and screen for new issues, questions, or concerns. The nurse can verify that the return appointments have been made with physician/midwife for the mother and newborn. If they have not been made, the nurse can emphasize the importance of the appointments. At this time, if there are no outstanding issues or concerns, the family can be discharged from home care. If new issues or concerns are identified, the nurse, family, and physician/midwife determine an appropriate ongoing plan of care.

Careful records that document assessment findings and all interventions, including counseling and teaching, are imperative. Such documentation is a tool of communication and care coordination with the health care team, providing ongoing care for the woman and newborn, as well as a legal record of the visit.

Advantages and limitations. A home visit has the obvious advantage of allowing the nurse to observe and interact with family members in their most natural and secure environment. Because they are at home, they are no longer anticipating how an infant will affect their lives; they are experiencing it. For that reason, family members may have questions or concerns about areas that had not been anticipated before discharge. The use of open-ended questions by the nurse, such as "What is it like being home?" "What has happened that you least expected?" "What has been your greatest joy in bringing the baby home?" and "Now that you are at home, what needs do you have?" may serve to elicit those questions or concerns.

The nurse is able to assess the adequacy of resources in the home, as well as evidence of safety in both the home and immediate surroundings. Both kinds of data are helpful in planning health teaching. Teaching that was not possible during the hospital stay can be continued on a priority basis. Learning about infant care is facilitated because the exact items to be used on a daily basis are available for demonstration and return demonstration; the mother is not required to adapt what she has learned to her own setting.

Nurses may find that the in-hospital care they provide is enhanced as a result of what they have learned during practice in homes. Furthermore, they may experience more job satisfaction as a result of extending the setting of their practice (Evans, 1991).

Critical Thinking Exercises 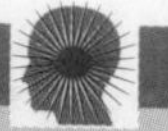

POSTPARTUM ADAPTATION

You are making a home visit to a mother and her newborn infant boy on her third postpartum day. She has two other children, both girls, ages 2 and 4 years. Assessment reveals the following findings:

- **Mother has sore, cracked nipples and reports difficulty with breastfeeding.**
- **Mother shows signs of fatigue; is not able to obtain adequate rest.**
- **Mother is uncertain about proper circumcision care.**
- **Newborn is slightly jaundiced.**
- **Newborn screen has not yet been drawn.**

For each of the identified problems:

1. **Formulate a nursing diagnosis.**
2. **Prioritize nursing diagnoses.**
3. **Plan and prioritize patient-centered expected outcomes.**
4. **Choose interventions and indicate rationale.**
5. **Indicate how you would know your interventions were effective.**
6. **Verify and justify your claims, beliefs, conclusions, decisions, and actions.**

Although telephone follow-up must, of necessity, address the mother's perceptions of her status and that of the newborn and family, home visits allow direct assessment. It is therefore more likely to facilitate identification of complicated physical or psychologic adjustment.

There are several limitations to home visits as a postpartum follow-up strategy:

- The cost of visiting families separated by great geographic distances.
- The availability of the number of nurses with expertise in caring for maternity clients and newborns in the home
- Concerns about safety in accessing families in certain areas

Telephone Follow-Up

As part of routine follow-up after discharge from the hospital, many providers are implementing one or more **postpartum telephone follow-up** calls to their patients for assessment, provision of health teaching, identification of complications to effect timely intervention, and referrals. If the family has a home care referral and visit, this follow-up is incorporated in that care. If no home care follow-up is provided, then telephone follow-up may be initiated. Telephone follow-up may be part of the services offered by the hospital, private physician/clinic, or a private agency and may be used separately or in combination with other strategies for extending postpartum care.

The nature of the telephone follow-up calls should be explained to the family before discharge from the hospital. A mutually agreeable time is scheduled for the initial call. The ideal time for a telephone call varies according to family needs. In some cases the initial call might be most appropriate

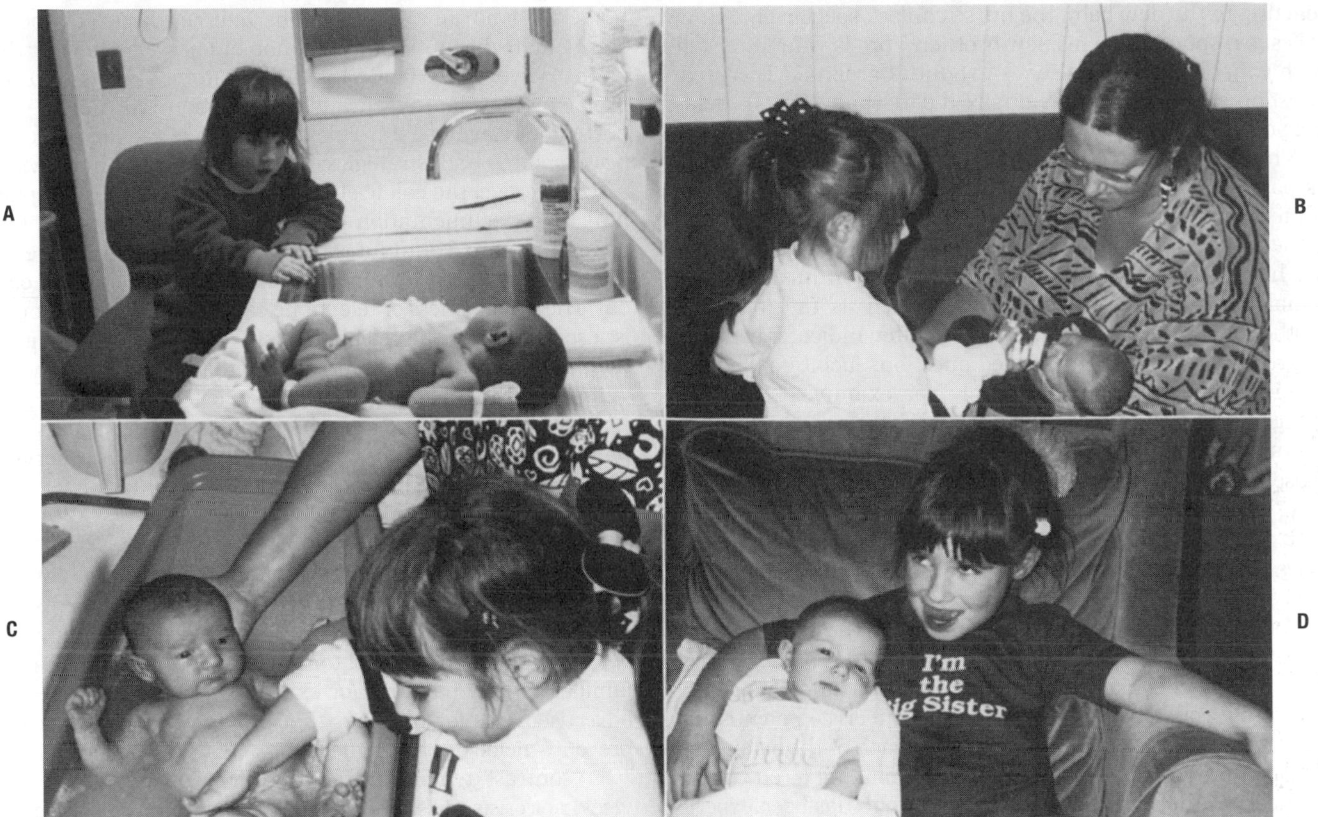

Fig. 21-10 Progress in sibling bonding and attachment. **A,** Watching during her new sister's first bath before discharge. **B,** Sibling feeds her new sister under mother's watchful eye. **C,** Sibling gives her 2-week-old sister a bath; both seem to be enjoying this time together. **D,** Sibling bonding and attachment between big sister and 1-month-old little sister. (Courtesy Nancy Mason, MD.)

within the first few hours after early discharge to ascertain that no problems have arisen since the homecoming. In other situations a follow-up call might be most appropriate the day after discharge. The timing and number of calls must be based on individual family needs.

Families also need to be able to initiate a call to the nurse when questions arise. The telephone follow-up system must be explained to the family and phone numbers provided for easy access by the family.

All therapeutic dialogue between nurse and client, including that by telephone, is purposeful and goal-directed. This is not a social call, even though there may be some small talk in reestablishing rapport between nurse and patient. During the telephone follow-up the nurse will ask questions with the following goals:

- To obtain evidence of the mother's physiologic recovery, comfort, and rest
- To determine evidence of psychologic well-being in the mother, including the presence of crisis-preventing balancing factors
- To obtain selected evidence of physiologic adaptation in the newborn
- To establish the perceived level of parental adjustment to parenthood and the stresses inherent in the early fourth trimester
- To identify learning needs of the family
- To determine the extent to which a relationship is being formed among the newborn, siblings, parents, and grandparents (Fig. 21-10)
- To explore the areas creating special concerns or challenges, as well as those placing unsettling demands on family members

In opening the conversation the nurse should provide reintroduction to family members and reinforce the reason for the telephone call. The nurse should ascertain if the call has been made at a convenient time; otherwise the effectiveness of the call is questionable. For example, a mother who has just settled a fussy baby and is attempting to relax herself will not be well served by a follow-up call at that time. Furthermore, common courtesy dictates that nurses determine if the call will create an unwelcome interruption for whatever reason. If so, a more suitable time should be mutually set.

The content of a follow-up call is planned on the basis of the discharge summary or records from the postpartum hospital stay. The use of discharge notes to guide the assessment ensures that an area of particular concern will not be overlooked. It also prompts the nurse to follow up on the basis of the woman's history. An additional advantage is in the personalization and sense of warmth and regard it communicates. For example, rather than asking how other children are reacting to the new baby, the nurse can ask specifically, "How is Leslie responding to his new brother?" or "Is your Mom still with you, or has she gone back to South Carolina?" The latter question shows more individualized care than "Who is helping you at home?"

The nurse allows the conversation to develop as naturally as possible so that the patient will not feel rushed or interrupted as rapport is established. This is particularly important if the telephoner is not the nurse who cared for the family in the health care facility. A natural progression has the additional advantage of providing cues, such as the topic the mother chooses to address first, which often indicates her area of greatest concern. Open-ended questions facilitate the telephone interaction most effectively, for example, "How are things going since you left the hospital?" "You mentioned frequent headaches since you got home. Tell me more about those." or "How are you and Peter collaborating on the baby's care?" Because specific assessment data about the mother, infant, and family are necessary, the nurse eventually guides the assessment to these areas so that the aforementioned goals for the call can be met.

An effective postpartum telephone follow-up should assess the well-being of mother and infant and the transitions each family member is making to the new life-style and changes in the family constellation. To determine the crisis potential in the family, the nurse is careful to address each of the balancing factors. Consider, for example, the nurse making a return call to check on the status of a new mother who has been experiencing sore nipples. At an earlier call, the nurse had reinforced teaching about varying the infant's position on the breast to minimize stress to the nipple and had referred the mother to a lactation consultant or La Leche League (a volunteer program that provides education and assistance for breastfeeding mothers). Today the nurse moves quickly to an assessment of the balancing factors, starting with "How have things been going since we spoke last?" Depending on the answer, the nurse may address a second factor by asking, "What have you been able to try?" After hearing the answer, the nurse might follow up by asking, "And how is that working?" The nurse would determine whether the mother has called the lactation consultant or La Leche League and how productive this intervention has been. Additional teaching or referral, possibly to the physician/CNM, may be necessary at this time.

The primary interventions available to providers extending care by telephone include patient advocacy, provision of teaching, reassurance/positive feedback, corrective feedback, supportive counseling, anticipatory guidance, and referral. Interventions are selected on the basis of a careful assessment and are provided in collaboration with the family.

Both the assessment data elicited and interventions employed during the postpartum follow-up call are recorded. This information may be faxed or copies sent to the appropriate physician/midwife for ongoing follow-up. Documentation serves both legal and reimbursement purposes.

Advantages and limitations. Telephone follow-up affords contact with the postpartum family during the vulnerable time interval during which support and intervention may be particularly effective. Most patients can be reached by telephone; according to Donaldson (1988), 92% of homes are accessible by telephone. Calls are more cost-effective than are home visits but are limited by the indirect nature of the assessment. If the mother's perception of her well-being (or that of the newborn or family) is inaccurate or falsely reported, problems may be missed and intervention will not be supported by relevant data. This disadvantage can be overcome by combining both strategies: telephone calls and home visits.

On average, the call itself lasts 15 to 20 minutes. Preplanning and documentation time can easily expand the time commitment to 30 minutes per call. Consequently, there is a potential limit to the number of calls that can be handled each day. The effectiveness of telephone calls to postpartum women is also limited by the telephone skills and listening ability of the caller and by the comfort the mother experiences in providing personal data to the faceless caller.

This service depends on the families having access to a phone. If the family does not have a phone, other services must be implemented to meet the needs of the family.

Warm Lines/Help Lines

The warm line represents another type of telephone link between the new family and concerned caregivers or experienced parent volunteers. Warm line services sometimes are best understood in contrast to "hot lines," which may be more familiar to new parents. For example, they might have seen advertisements for hot lines that provide emergency help to prevent suicide or child abuse.

In contrast, **warm lines** are helplines, or consultation services, not crisis lines. The warm line is appropriately used for less extreme concerns that may seem urgent at the time the call is placed but are not actual emergencies. Calls to warm lines commonly relate to infant feeding, prolonged crying, or sibling rivalry. One new mother called because she noticed a drop of blood on her daughter's diaper. With an explanation of the reason for the blood and that its presence was normal, she was appropriately reassured. Another mother called to talk about how it felt when her 4-year-old son screamed out, "I hate you and I hate that baby." Warm line services may extend beyond the fourth trimester. Even parents with adolescent children may profit from the helping relationship of a warm line.

Individuals who answer warm line calls must be good listeners who are empathetic and able to use techniques such as open-ended questions, restating, and reflecting to encourage the caller to communicate. The caller is given an unhurried opportunity to share feelings or concerns. It is her story, and she is allowed to tell it in her own way. Questions often are used to clarify what the caller is saying.

The caller is assessed for evidence of impending crisis: What is the situation or concern? What has already been tried in order to cope? What resources are available? Advice is not given; rather callers are helped to explore options available to them. Referrals may be made to support groups or to community agencies. When medical problems are identified, referrals are made to the appropriate physician, midwife, or nurse practitioner.

Rauen (1985), who refers to the "telephone as stethoscope," maintains that communication can be blocked when the caregiver "talks too much, makes judgmental remarks, conveys differences, takes sides, dwells on personal experiences, or assumes that the first problem mentioned is the real problem." Warm line calls always end with the caregiver summarizing the call—what concerns were identified and what resolutions have been explored. Also, the caller is invited to call again if the need arises.

Advantages and limitations. Individuals may be less hesitant to call an established warm line than to disturb their primary health care provider, especially at night, on weekends, or on holidays. The primary advantage of the warm line is quick access to a good listener, whether nurse or trained volunteer, 24 hours a day, 365 days a year. Because it is an advertised helpline, couples may feel more comfortable and less intimidated about making the call.

Inasmuch as the warm line offers round-the-clock service, there are potential difficulties in staffing; when a limited staff necessitates an answering recorder or message service, the resource is less effective. Having to leave a message negates the advantage of immediate access. Although some individuals welcome the anonymity of a faceless listener, they may be less willing to record a message.

The cost of the warm line is minimal if volunteers are used; the only costs are the telephone service itself and advertisement. The financial commitment obviously increases when any of the staff members are salaried.

For some nurses the inability to evaluate the effectiveness of their interventions is frustrating. There are generally no provisions for follow-up with the caller to determine the extent to which the problem has been resolved, if at all.

Support Groups

Humans are inherently social beings, involved on a daily basis in some kind of group, whether family members, classmates, co-workers, or friends. Often education, work, worship, and leisure time take place in groups. Thus it seems reasonable that at times of difficult transitions, people turn to groups for support. Nurses are generally familiar with the benefits of support groups for such diverse populations as the newly divorced or widowed; those with recently diagnosed acquired immunodeficiency syndrome (AIDS) or cancer; those undergoing mastectomy, colostomy, or heart attack; and those experiencing a miscarriage or early infant death.

A special group experience is sometimes sought by the woman adjusting to motherhood. On occasion, postpartum women who have met earlier in prenatal clinics or on the hospital unit may begin to associate for mutual support. Members of Lamaze classes who attend a postpartum reunion may decide to extend their relationship during the fourth trimester. Realizing the value of group support, nurses may wish to make postpartum support groups available as a strategy for bridging hospital and home.

A **postpartum support group** is a collection of individuals living the postpartum experience who are (1) striving to satisfy a personal need by belonging to a group; (2) interacting with respect to mutual goals, common interests, or common concerns; and (3) experiencing the rewards of an interdependent relationship. They perceive themselves to be members of a group; others recognize them as a group. Group behavior is governed by rules and norms that are collectively chosen, for example, "We will protect each other's confidences."

The support group setting enables parents to share and support each other in the adjustments to parenting. New parents often report surprise at the amount of fatigue they experience initially with a new infant in their lives. Schedules must be readjusted and priorities realigned to accommodate infant care and interruptions in sleep. It is not uncommon for the new mother to find it difficult to schedule time for her own shower. A father expressed his fatigue in this way, "It never ceases to amaze me that an 8-pound baby girl can wear down a 200-pound father and a 136-pound mother."

The woman must be cautioned not to overexert herself and to set priorities so that she can rest whenever possible. The group and nurse facilitator might help her explore the daily routines and ways she can best obtain rest intervals. She may need help considering her work load more realistically, asserting her need for help or support, or limiting unnecessary tasks. The woman who strives for perfection may become unduly fatigued and experience unnecessary guilt and depression.

By encouraging the woman to list all the perfect qualities she expects of herself because of her image of the ideal mother, the nurse facilitator may enable the mother to experience less guilt. The facilitator can help the new mother examine those ideal behaviors and choose to concentrate on the ones she considers most important. Together, they can explore ways of adapting to a lack of perfection, perhaps modifying those behaviors she cannot willingly let go, and asserting her need for help and support. The nurse facilitator can use this opportunity to clarify misconceptions, provide reinforcement of strengths and positive behaviors, and refer the patient to appropriate resources, such as postpartum support groups or warm lines. The nurse facilitator may provide ongoing information on normal infant growth and development and demonstrate with newborns in the class.

During successful experiences the instillation of hope provided within the group helps members believe that things can be different, perhaps better. Seeing others and themselves benefit from the group experience keeps members coming back. As they are accepted within the group and feel valued by other group members, individuals feel a bond with the group, and cohesiveness develops. Cohesion in a group also tends to reinforce the value of group membership.

Recognizing the universality of their feelings—that others feel the same way and that they are not alone or unique by virtue of their feelings or concerns—decreases anxiety and reassures members of their normality. It is comforting and offers a sense of catharsis to feel free to share feelings with others. For many women, it is a welcome relief to unburden deeply held emotions such as guilt, anger, or grief in a supportive setting where others, because of their shared emotions, are likely to be nonjudgmental.

Often in a postpartum support group an experienced mother can impart concrete information that can be valuable to other group members. For example, one new mother shared her nurse-midwife's advice about placing warm (not hot), newly brewed tea bags on sore nipples for the comfort and healing value of warmth and the tannic acid. Another shared the use she had made of her husband's socks with the foot cut out. Sliding the sock over her left arm provided enough traction to keep the wet, soapy baby from slipping off the supporting arm while she gave the infant his bath. An inexperienced mother may find herself imitating the behavior of someone in the group whom she perceives as particularly ca-

BOX 21-5

Postpartum Support Groups: Signs of Effective Functioning

- Efforts are made to make each member feel welcome, included, supported, and trusted.
- Goals are identified and/or modified so that group goals and individual goals are congruent or compatible.
- Communication is open. Expression of ideas and feelings is welcomed, even when they are not those held by others in the group.
- Being oneself is encouraged in a nonjudgmental atmosphere.
- Group members participate in group work and group leadership tasks.
- Decisions are made and problems solved with group input.
- Conflict and controversy are allowed and seen as positive events in the group's life.
- Personal growth and self-actualization are encouraged.

pable. She may imitate someone's way of positioning a baby or find herself folding her daughter's diapers differently after watching someone else's technique.

Finally, sharing oneself in a group, whether in expressing feelings or in imparting expertise, has the therapeutic value of altruism. When the woman believes that she has helped someone else, it increases her sense of esteem and self-worth. In addition to its therapeutic benefit, this factor, as well as those discussed, encourages ongoing group membership.

In addition to organizing and marketing the group, the nurse may serve in a participant/observer role in a postpartum support group. This role involves observing how the group is functioning and facilitating effective group process. In addition, the nurse might participate in the group as a resource person or content expert. Box 21-5 lists criteria by which the nurse can assess whether a postpartum support group is functioning effectively. A nurse who wishes to serve as a leader of a postpartum support group should enroll in a course in group dynamics, study the literature on group dynamics, or work initially with an experienced group leader. In planning a support group the nurse may wish to consult experts in conducting needs assessment and marketing surveys.

Advantages and limitations. There is therapeutic benefit to be gained from membership in a postpartum support group. Women find value in sharing their feelings with other women experiencing similar situations. The postpartum period is a significant time of transition for the family, and groups can meet a need for connecting and supporting the members. The presence of infants and husbands in such groups may adversely affect women in both attendance and expression of their genuine feelings, although it may be difficult for women to attend without their babies.

It may prove difficult to initiate a postpartum support group at an ideal time to meet the needs of families in transition. Although they may believe that group membership would be of value, new mothers may be too overwhelmed initially to consider seeking out such a group, much less attend one consistently. Some of the questions that must be considered by the nurse who hopes to organize and market a postpartum support group include the following:

- Will women of all ages and experiences be invited to the same group?
- Will fathers and newborns be invited or excluded?
- How can the group be marketed to benefit the new mother in the early postpartum period?
- How can ongoing commitment to the group be encouraged, given the obvious demands of this life stage?
- How can the group best be advertised?
- How can the nurse prepare most effectively for a leadership role?

Perinatal Coaching

As the name suggests, perinatal coaching occurs in the period surrounding birth and employs behaviors expected of an effective athletic coach: modeling, directing, instructing, overseeing practice, and providing cues and prompts while a learner attempts a particular skill. In this case the learners are first-time parents and the skill being coached is two-way communication between them and their newborn infant. This primary prevention model was first described by Helfer (1979) as a way of preventing child abuse and neglect by facilitating a positive parent-child relationship. Perinatal coaching offers short-term support and basic information about the newborn's amazing capacity to respond, as well as skill learning and practice in a nonthreatening environment. Parents experience less stress and more enjoyment in interaction with their newborn as a result of perinatal coaching.

Interacting with a newborn involves an ability to "speak sensory"—to use the sensory system to communicate special messages. These sensory messages occur in interaction with a child in holding, cuddling, talking or singing, touching, soothing, and rocking the infant. Such messages reach beyond the capacity of words to communicate. The ability to speak sensory does not occur naturally because new parents typically do not fully appreciate the ability of the newborn to interact with them.

Perinatal coaching can become an integral component of existing maternity care, performed by nurses or managed by nurses using experienced parents as trained volunteers. The latter approach ensures a self-perpetuating system: those who learn can subsequently volunteer for the coach's role.

Once trained, the perinatal coach will spend four 1- to 1½-hour sessions with the first-time parents, often initiating the relationship and describing the program in the final weeks of the woman's pregnancy. Box 21-6 shows a plan for typical coaching sessions. At least one follow-up session is scheduled during the mother's postpartum stay; at least one home visit is made. The four sessions provide multiple opportunities for repetition and for reinforcing learning by both positive and corrective feedback, all of which enhance skill learning. Furthermore, continued direct contact with a skillful coach offers ongoing support during the difficult transitions of the early fourth trimester. The home visit enables the perinatal coach to assess the progression of parent-infant attachment in the security of the familiar environment. It also provides an additional opportunity to determine a need for referral.

Although new parents involved in perinatal coaching programs tend to evaluate the experience favorably, there is little

BOX 21-6
The Perinatal Coaching Strategy: An Overview

Session 1: 1- to 1½-hour session with a one-on-one or small group format held in prenatal setting

Interventions

Establish rapport with individuals.
Provide overview of perinatal coaching, and offer opportunity to participate in the program.
Provide basic information about infants' sensory capabilities, wake/sleep states, reflexes, other newborn characteristics and ways of responding.
Introduce content from *The Perinatal Coaching Picture Book* and leave copy with each mother for subsequent review/reinforcement of content.

Session 2: 1- to 1½-hour private session with mother and father held in postpartum setting

Interventions

With the infant present, demonstrate and model touching, holding, looking at, rocking, talking to, and quieting behaviors.
Assist parents to identify infant's unique responses to the behaviors.
Observe as couples return the demonstration of learned skills.
Encourage couples to practice learned skills before next scheduled session.

Session 3: 1- to 1½-hour private session with mother and father held in the hospital setting or during the early days at home.

Interventions

With the infant present, observe as mother and father apply what they have learned to "speak sensory" with their newborn.
Provide reassurance by reinforcement of correctly performed skills.
Provide supportive corrective feedback of incorrectly performed skills; reteach/remodel as necessary.
Encourage continued practice.

Session 4: 1- to 1½-hour session with mother, father, and newborn in their home environment 1 to 2 weeks after discharge.

Interventions

Repeat strategies of session 3 as necessary.
Summarize and offer continued availability as social support person accessible by telephone.
Refer for additional types of assistance as necessary.

Modified from Helfer R, Wilson A: The parent-infant relationship: promoting a positive beginning through perinatal coaching, *Pediatr Clin North Am* 29:249, 1982.

empiric support for the program. Studies are needed to consider the outcome of perinatal coaching programs for diverse groups of patients, including teens and those with poor parental role models.

Advantages and limitations. Advantages of perinatal coaching include the obvious benefit of parent education and the addition of another means of social support during the transition to parenthood. It is limited by the need for trained volunteers, by the time commitment involved, and by the lack of research support.

THE ROLE OF NURSING IN PROGRAM DEVELOPMENT

There are a variety of models for delivering obstetric home follow-up services. Programs can be hospital-based, clinic-based, entrepreneurial, through home care agencies, or government-funded programs. All models of programs must be concerned with licensing and other standards; operational issues such as staffing, supplies, equipment, and reimbursement; and quality issues such as staff development, internal and external customer services, and quality improvement initiatives (Dahlberg and Koloroutis, 1994; Eaton, 1994; Goodwin, 1994).

As obstetric nurses have identified the need for postpartum home care programs, they have often been the ones to explore, promote, and develop programs to meet the families' needs. Home care gives the experienced inpatient nurse an opportunity for professional growth and diversity in practice. Nurses who participate in home care experience practice in the home setting where they function independently, adjusting to the needs and challenges of each home and family situation (Dahlberg and Koloroutis, 1994).

Key Points

- The trend for early postpartum discharge will continue as a result of consumer demand, medical necessity, and cost-containment measures.
- The short-stay option in perinatal care is safer when selection criteria are used and when home care follow-up is available.
- Early discharge classes, postpartum telephone follow-up, home visits, warm lines, and support groups, used individually or in combination, are effective means of preventing crisis and facilitating physiologic and psychologic adjustments in the postpartum period.
- Postpartum follow-up programs are most effective when planned on the basis of needs assessment and when revision is based on an evaluation of access, quality, and cost.

References

Association of Women's Health, Obstetric, and Neonatal Nurses (AWHONN): *Didactic content and clinical skills verification for professional nurse providers of perinatal home care,* Washington DC, 1994, AWHONN.

Carty E, Bradley C: A randomized, controlled evaluation of early postpartum hospital discharge, *Birth* 17(4):199, 1990.

Clemen-Stone S, Eigsti D, McGuire S: *Comprehensive family and community health nursing,* ed 4, St Louis, 1995, Mosby.

Dahlberg N, Koloroutis M: Hospital-based perinatal home-care program, *J Obstet Gynecol Neonatal Nurs* 23(8):682, 1994.

Donaldson N: Effect of telephone postpartum follow-up: a clinical trial, *Diss Abstr Int* 49:2567B (University Microfilms No DA8809495), 1988.

Dungy C et al: Effects of discharge samples on duration of breastfeeding, *Pediatrics* 90(2 pt. 1):233, 1992.

Eaton D: Perinatal home care: one entrepreneur's experience, *J Obstet Gynecol Neonatal Nurs* 23(8):726, 1994.

Evans C: Description of a home follow-up program for childbearing families, *J Obstet Gynecol Neonatal Nurs* 20:113, 1991.

Gillerman H, Beckham M: The postpartum early discharge dilemma: an innovative solution, *J Perinat Neonatal Nurs* 5:9, 1991.

Goodwin L: Essential program components for perinatal home care, *J Obstet Gynecol Neonatal Nurs* 23(8):667, 1994.

Hall W, Carty E: Managing the early discharge experience: taking control, *J Adv Nurs* 18(4):574, 1993.

Harrison L: Patient education in early postpartum discharge programs, *Am J Matern Child Nurs* 15:39, 1990.

Helfer R: *Perinatal coaching guide.* In *Pediatric basics,* No 26, Fremont, Mich, 1979, Gerber Products Co.

Pridham K et al: Early postpartum transition: progress in maternal identity and role attainment, *Res Nurs Health* 14:21, 1991.

Rauen K: The telephone as stethoscope, *MCN Am J Matern Child Nurs* 10:122, 1985.

Stern T: An early discharge program: an entrepreneurial nursing practice becomes a hospital-affiliated agency, *J Perinat Neonatal Nurs* 5:1, 1991.

Welt S et al: Feasibility of postpartum rapid hospital discharge: a study from a community hospital population, *Am J Perinatol* 10(5):384, 1993.

Williams L, Cooper M: Nurse-managed postpartum home care, *J Obstet Gynecol Neonatal Nurs* 22(1):25, 1993.

Zander K: Second generation critical paths, *Definition Center Nurs Care Manage* 4(4):1, 1989.

Bibliography

Britton J, Britton H, Beebe S: Early discharge of the term newborn: a continued dilemma, *Pediatrics* 94:3, 1994.

Brooten D: Perinatal care across the continuum: early discharge and nursing home follow-up, *J Perinat Neonatal Nurs* 9:38, 1995.

Evans C: Postpartum home care in the United States, *J Obstet Gynecol Neonatal Nurs* 24(2):180, 1995.

Keppler A: Postpartum care center: follow-up care in a hospital-based clinic, *J Obstet Gynecol Neonatal Nurs* 24(1):17, 1995.

Marrelli T: *Handbook of home health standards and documentation: guidelines for reimbursement,* ed 2, St Louis, 1996, Mosby.

Stanhope M, Lancaster J: *Community health nursing: process and practice for promoting health,* ed 4, St Louis, 1995, Mosby.

CHAPTER 22

The Newborn

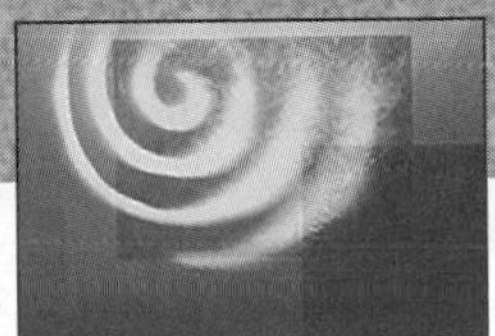

RESPIRATORY SYSTEM, P. 591
CARDIOVASCULAR SYSTEM, P. 592
HEMATOPOIETIC SYSTEM, P. 594
THERMOREGULATION, P. 595
FLUID AND ELECTROLYTE BALANCE, P. 596
RENAL SYSTEM, P. 596
GASTROINTESTINAL SYSTEM, P. 597
HEPATIC SYSTEM, P. 597
IMMUNE SYSTEM, P. 599
REPRODUCTIVE SYSTEM, P. 599
INTEGUMENTARY SYSTEM, P. 600
SKELETAL SYSTEM, P. 602
NEUROMUSCULAR SYSTEM, P. 603
Newborn reflexes, p. 603
Sensory functions, p. 603
ASSESSMENT, P. 608
Initial assessment: Apgar scoring, p. 608
Transitional assessment: periods of reactivity, p. 609
Behavioral assessment, p. 609
Assessment of attachment behaviors, p. 610
Assessment of clinical gestational age, p. 614
PHYSICAL ASSESSMENT, P. 614
General appearance, p. 614
Vital signs, p. 614
Baseline measurements of physical growth, p. 620
Thorax, p. 623
Abdomen, p. 624
Back and anus, p. 624
Genitalia, p. 624
Extremities, p. 625
Neurologic assessment, p. 625

By term gestation the fetus' various anatomic and physiologic systems have reached a level of development and functioning that permits a separate existence from the mother. At birth the newborn infant manifests behavioral competencies and a readiness for social interaction. The neonatal period, from birth through day 28, represents a time of dramatic physical change for the newborn infant. The profound biologic adaptations that occur at birth make the newborn infant's transition from intrauterine to extrauterine life possible. These adaptations set the stage for future growth and development.

RESPIRATORY SYSTEM

The most critical and immediate adjustment a newborn must make at birth is the establishment of respirations.

Initial breathing is probably the result of a reflex triggered by pressure changes, chilling, noise, light, and other sensations related to the birth process. In addition, the chemoreceptors in the aorta and carotid bodies initiate neurologic reflexes when arterial oxygen pressure (Po_2) falls, arterial carbon dioxide pressure (Pco_2) rises, and arterial pH falls. In most cases an exaggerated respiratory reaction follows within 1 minute of birth, and the infant takes the first gasping breath and cries.

The initial entry of air into the lungs is opposed by the surface tension of the fluid that filled the fetal lungs and alveoli. However, fetal lung fluid is removed by the pulmonary capillaries and lymphatic vessels. Some fluid is also removed during the normal forces of labor and delivery. As the chest emerges from the birth canal, fluid is squeezed from the lungs through the nose and mouth. After complete emergence of the neonate's chest, a brisk recoil of the thorax occurs. Air enters the upper airway to replace the lost fluid. In cesarean birth the chest is not compressed, and the newborn may have some retained lung fluid after birth.

The significance of *tactile stimulation* is questionable. Descent through the birth canal and normal handling during delivery, such as drying the skin, probably have some effect on the initiation of respiration. Slapping the neonate's heel or buttocks has no beneficial effect; it can waste precious time in the event of respiratory difficulty.

With the first breath of air the newborn begins a sequence of cardiopulmonary changes, including (1) converting from fetal to neonatal circulation, (2) emptying the lungs of fluid, and (3) establishing the characteristics of pulmonary function (Kenner, Brueggemeyer, and Gunderson, 1993). During the first hour of life, large amounts of fluid continue to be removed by the pulmonary lymphatics. Reduced pulmonary vascular resistance accommodates this flow of lung fluid; however, it is the diminished intravascular pressure that is ultimately responsible for the removal of lung fluid.

In the alveoli the surface tension of the fluid is reduced by **surfactant,** a substance produced by the alveolar epithelium that coats the alveolar surface. Acting much like a detergent, this substance reduces the surface tension of fluids that line the alveoli and respiratory passages, resulting in uniform expansion and maintenance of lung expansion at low intraalveolar pressure. Deficient surfactant production causes unequal inflation of alveoli on inspiration and collapse of alveoli on end expiration. Without surfactant, infants are unable to keep their lungs inflated and therefore exert a great deal of effort to reexpand the alveoli with each breath. Most normal term infants have adequate surfactant (Wong, 1995). Fetal pulmonary maturity can be determined by examining amniotic fluid, obtained by amniocentesis, for lecithin/sphingomyelin (L/S) ratio and other phospholipid levels. Phosphatidylglycerol appears at 35 to 36 weeks; its presence in amniotic fluid is a more predictable index of lung maturity.

Following the period of reactivity and after respirations are established, respirations are shallow and irregular, ranging from 30 to 60 breaths per minute, with short periods of apnea (less than 15 seconds). These short periods of apnea occur most often during the active (rapid eye movement [REM]) sleep cycle and decrease in frequency and duration with age. Apneic periods over 15 seconds in duration should be evaluated.

Newborn infants are preferential nose breathers. The reflex response to nasal obstruction is to open the mouth to maintain an airway. This response is not present in most infants until 3 weeks after birth. Therefore cyanosis or asphyxia may occur with nasal blockage.

The chest circumference is approximately 30 to 33 cm (12 to 13 inches) at birth. Auscultation of the chest of a newborn infant reveals loud, clear breath sounds that seem very near because little chest tissue intervenes. The ribs of the infant articulate with the spine at a horizontal rather than a downward slope; consequently the rib cage cannot expand with inspiration as readily as an adult's. Neonatal respiratory function is largely a matter of diaphragmatic contraction. The negative intrathoracic pressure is created by the descent of the diaphragm, much like negative pressure is created in the barrel of a syringe when medication is drawn up by retracting the plunger. The newborn infant's chest and abdomen rise simultaneously with inspiration. Seesaw respirations are not normal (Fig. 22-1).

CARDIOVASCULAR SYSTEM

While respiratory changes are occurring, the cardiovascular system is also undergoing many changes (Fig. 22-2). **Fetal circulation** ceases, and extrauterine circulation begins. The infant's first breath inflates the lungs, thereby reducing pulmonary vascular resistance to pulmonary blood flow. As a result there is a drop in pulmonary artery pressure. This sequence is the major mechanism by which pressure in the *right atrium* declines. The increased pulmonary blood flow returned to the left side of the heart increases the pressure in the *left atrium.* This change in pressures causes a functional closure of the shunt between the atria, the **foramen ovale.** Temporary reversal of flow through the foramen ovale may occur with crying and lead to mild cyanosis during the first few days of life.

Within the first 12 hours of extrauterine life the shunt between the pulmonary artery and the aorta, the **ductus arteriosus,** constricts in response to a decrease in circulating prostaglandin E_2 and the establishment of a high oxygen level in the arterial blood. Anatomic closure takes more time; approximately 80% of these ducts are closed by the end of the third month (Blackburn and Loper, 1992). After anatomic closure the ductus arteriosus becomes a ligament. With the clamping and severing of the cord the two umbilical arteries and one umbilical vein close immediately and within a few days become ligaments. The **ductus venosus** (vessel connecting the umbilical vein and inferior vena cava) constricts within 3 to 7 days of birth (Wong, 1995). Before birth the two ventricles act in parallel fashion (simultaneously), with shunts (foramen ovale and ductus arteriosus) adjusting any unequal outputs. After birth, however, the two ventricles act in series (one following the other), which requires that the outputs of the right and left sides of the heart be equal (Fanaroff and Martin, 1997). Table 22-1 summarizes the cardiovascular changes at birth.

Heart Rate and Sounds

The heart rate averages 140 beats/min at birth, with variations noted during sleeping and waking states. Shortly after the first cry the infant's heart rate may be as high as 175 to 180 beats/min. The range of the heart rate in the full-term infant is 80 to 100 beats/min during sleep and 120 to 160 beats/min while awake. It is not unusual to find a heart rate of 180 beats/min when the infant cries. A heart rate that is either high (faster than 160 beats/min) or low (slower than 120 beats/min) should be reevaluated within an hour or when the activity of the infant changes. After birth the heart

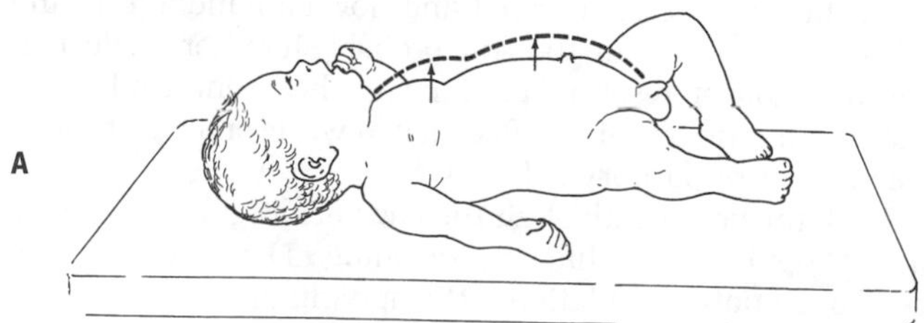

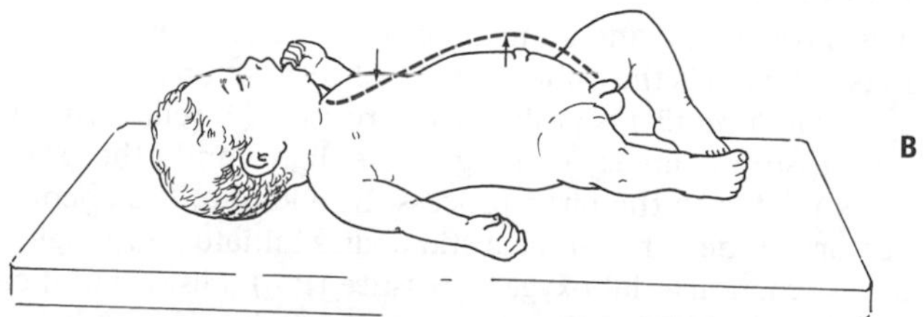

Fig. 22-1 Comparison of normal and seesaw respirations. **A,** Normal respiration. Chest and abdomen rise with inspiration. **B,** Seesaw respiration. Chest wall retracts and abdomen rises with inspiration. (Courtesy Mead Johnson & Co, Evansville, Ind.)

rate can often still be palpated by grasping the base of the umbilical cord.

The apical impulse (point of maximal impulse [PMI]) in the newborn is at the fourth intercostal space and to the left of the midclavicular line. The PMI is often visible. Heart sounds after birth reflect the series action of the heart pump. They are described as the familiar "lub, dub, lub, dub" sound. The "lub" is associated with closure of the mitral and tricuspid valves at the beginning of systole and the "dub" with closure of the aortic and pulmonic valves at the end of systole. The "lub" is the first heart sound (S_1), and the "dub" is the second heart sound (S_2). The normal cycle of the heart starts with the beginning of systole (Guyton, 1991).

Heart sounds during the neonatal period are of higher

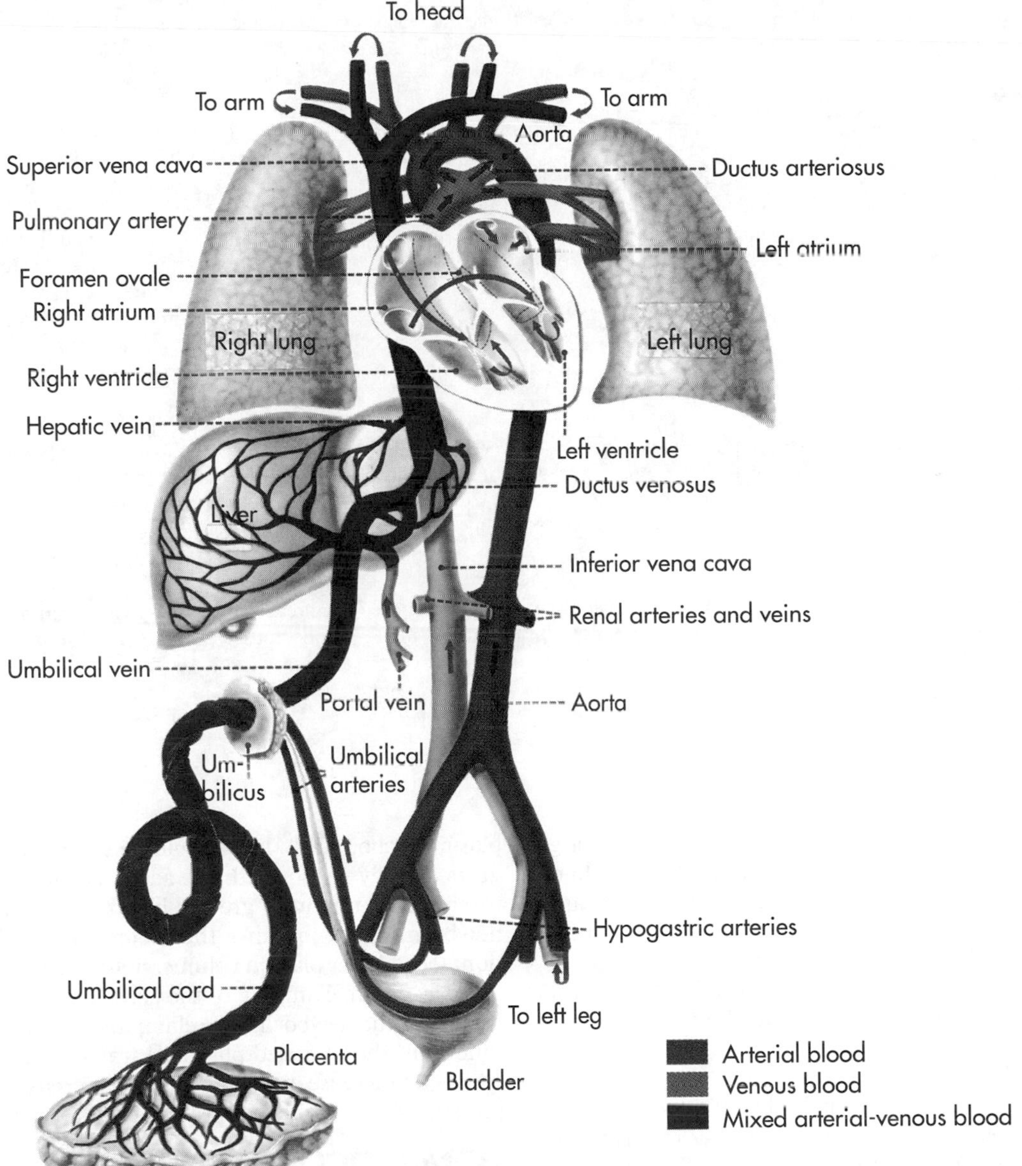

Fig. 22-2 Fetal circulation. *Before birth,* arterialized blood from the placenta flows into the fetus through the umbilical vein and passes rapidly through the liver into the inferior vena cava; from there, it flows through the foramen ovale into the left atrium, soon to appear in the aorta and arteries of the head. A portion bypasses the liver through the ductus venosus. Venous blood from the lower extremities and head passes predominantly into the right atrium, the right ventricle, and then into the descending pulmonary artery and ductus arteriosus. Thus the foramen ovale and the ductus arteriosus act as bypass channels, allowing a large part of the combined cardiac output to perfuse body tissues without flowing through the lungs. Approximately 55% of the combined ventricular output flows to the placenta; 35% perfuses body tissues; and the remaining 10% flows through the lungs. *After birth,* The foramen ovale closes; the ductus arteriosus closes and becomes a ligament; the ductus venosus closes and becomes a ligament; and the umbilical vein and arteries close and become ligaments. (Courtesy Ross Laboratories, Columbus, Ohio.)

TABLE 22-1 Cardiovascular changes at birth

PRENATAL STATUS	POSTBIRTH STATUS	ASSOCIATED FACTORS
Primary changes		
Pulmonary circulation: high pulmonary vascular resistance; increased pressure in right ventricle and pulmonary arteries	Low pulmonary vascular resistance; decreased pressure in right atrium, ventricle, and pulmonary arteries	Expansion of collapsed fetal lung with air
Systemic circulation: low pressures in left atrium, ventricle, and aorta	High systemic vascular resistance; increased pressure in left atrium, ventricle, and aorta	Loss of placental blood flow
Secondary changes		
Umbilical arteries: patent; carry blood from hypogastric arteries to placenta	Functionally closed at birth; obliteration by fibrous proliferation may take 2 to 3 months; distal portions become lateral vesicoumbilical ligaments; proximal portions remain open as superior vesicle arteries	Closure precedes that of umbilical vein; probably accomplished by smooth muscle contraction in response to thermal and mechanical stimuli and alteration in oxygen tension; mechanically severed with cord at birth
Umbilical vein: patent; carries blood from placenta to ductus venosus and liver	Closed; after obliteration it becomes *ligamentum teres hepatis*	Closure shortly after umbilical arteries; hence blood from placenta may enter neonate for short period after birth; mechanically severed with cord at birth
Ductus venosus: patent; connects umbilical vein to inferior vena cava	Closed, after obliteration it becomes *ligamentum venosum*	Loss of blood flow from umbilical vein
Ductus arteriosus: patent; shunts blood from pulmonary artery to descending aorta	Functionally closed almost immediately after birth; anatomic obliteration of lumen by fibrous proliferation requires 1 to 3 months; becomes *ligamentum arteriosum*	High systemic resistance increases aortic pressure; low pulmonary resistance reduces pulmonary arterial pressure Increased oxygen content of blood in ductus arteriosus creates vasospasm of its muscular wall
Foramen ovale: forms a valve opening that allows blood to flow directly to left atrium (shunts blood from right to left atrium)	Functionally closes at birth; constant apposition gradually leads to fusion and permanent closure within a few months or years in majority of persons	Increased pressures in left atrium together with decreased pressure in right atrium cause closure of valve over foramen

pitch, shorter duration, and greater intensity than during adult life. The first sound is typically louder and duller than the second sound, which is sharp. Most heart murmurs heard during the neonatal period have no pathologic significance, and more than half disappear by age 6 months. A persistent murmur accompanied by poor signs of transition (circumoral cyanosis, poor feeding) should be evaluated further.

Blood Pressure

The newborn infant's average systolic blood pressure is 78 mm Hg, and the average diastolic pressure is 42 mm Hg. The blood pressure varies from day to day during the first month of life. A drop in systolic blood pressure (about 15 mm Hg) the first hour of life is common. Crying and moving usually cause increases in the systolic blood pressure. Unless there is a specific indication, blood pressure is not measured in the newborn.

Blood Volume

Blood volume in the newborn ranges from 80 to 110 ml/kg during the first several days and doubles by the end of the first year. Proportionately the newborn has approximately 10% greater blood volume and nearly 20% greater red blood cell (RBC) mass than the adult. However, the newborn's blood plasma is about 20% less in volume when compared by kilogram of body weight with the adult. The infant born prematurely has a relatively greater blood volume than the term newborn. This is because the preterm infant has a proportionately greater plasma volume, not a greater RBC mass.

Early or late clamping of the cord changes circulatory dynamics of the newborn. Late clamping expands the blood volume from the so-called placental transfusion. This, in turn, causes an increase in the heart's size, increased systolic blood pressure, and a higher respiratory rate.

HEMATOPOIETIC SYSTEM

The hematopoietic system of the newborn exhibits certain variations from that of the adult. There are differences in RBCs and leukocytes and relatively few differences in platelets.

RBCs and Hemoglobin

At birth the average values of RBCs and hemoglobin are higher than those in the adult. Cord blood of the term newborn may have a hemoglobin concentration from 14 to 29 g/dl, with a mean of 17 g/dl. The hematocrit ranges from 43% to 63% (mean 55%). The RBC count is correspondingly elevated, ranging from 5.7 to 5.8 per mm^3. These values fall and reach the average levels of 11 to 17 g/dl and 4.2 to 5.2

per mm³, respectively, by the end of the first month. The blood values may be affected by delayed clamping of the cord, which results in a rise in hemoglobin, RBCs, and hematocrit. The source of the sample is another significant factor because capillary blood will yield higher values than does venous blood. The time after birth when the blood sample is obtained is significant; the slight rise in RBCs after birth is followed by a substantial drop. At birth the infant's blood contains about 80% fetal hemoglobin, but because of the shorter life span of the cells containing fetal hemoglobin, the percentage falls to 55% by 5 weeks and 5% by 20 weeks. Iron stores generally are sufficient to sustain normal RBC production for 6 months in the term infant, so the slight brief anemia is not serious.

Leukocytes

Leukocytosis, with the white blood cell (WBC) count approximately 15,000 per mm³ (range 10,000 to 30,000 per mm³), is normal at birth. The WBC count increases to about 23,000 to 24,000 per mm³ during the first day after birth. A WBC level of 11,500 per mm³ normally is maintained during the neonatal period. The initial high WBC count of the newborn decreases rapidly (see Appendix). Serious infection such as group B hemolytic streptococcus is not well tolerated by the newborn, and marked increase in the WBC count may be unlikely even in critical sepsis (infection). In many instances, sepsis is accompanied by a decline in WBCs, particularly in mature neutrophils. The activity of the bone marrow is accurately reflected by the number of circulating cells—both erythrocytes and leukocytes.

Platelets

Platelet count ranges between 200,000 and 300,000 per mm³ and is essentially the same in newborns as in adults. Factors II, VII, IX, and X, found in the liver, are decreased during the first few days of life because the newborn is unable to synthesize vitamin K. However, bleeding tendencies in the newborn are rare, and unless there has been a marked vitamin K deficiency, clotting is sufficient to prevent hemorrhage. The administration of vitamin K, 0.5 to 1 mg intramuscularly (IM), at birth enhances clotting and helps prevent bleeding (see Fig. 23-22).

Blood Groups

The infant's blood group is genetically determined and is established early in fetal life. However, during the neonatal period there is a gradual increase in the strength of the agglutinogens present in the RBC membrane. Cord blood samples may be used to identify the infant's blood type and Rh status.

THERMOREGULATION

Next to establishing respiration, heat regulation is most critical to the newborn's survival. Although the newborn's capacity for heat production is adequate, several factors predispose the newborn to excessive heat loss. First, the newborn's large surface area facilitates heat loss to the environment. The normal metabolic rate per unit weight of the newborn is about twice that of the adult, but the neonate's surface area per unit weight is about three times larger than that of the adult. Consequently, the infant produces only two thirds as much heat as an adult but loses twice as much heat per unit area. However, the large body surface area is partially compensated for by the newborn's usual position of flexion, which decreases the amount of surface area exposed to the environment.

The second factor that retards the conservation of body heat is the newborn's thin layer of subcutaneous fat. Since core body temperature is approximately 1° F higher than surface body temperature, this temperature gradient (difference) causes a heat transfer from a higher to lower temperature.

A third factor is the newborn's mechanism for producing heat. Unlike the adult, who can increase heat production through shivering, the chilled neonate cannot shiver but produces heat through **nonshivering thermogenesis.** Nonshivering thermogenesis is accomplished primarily by the metabolism of brown fat and secondarily by increased metabolic activity in the brain, heart, and liver.

Brown fat is unique to the newborn (Blackburn and Loper, 1992; Fanaroff and Martin, 1997). It has a richer vascular and nerve supply than does ordinary fat. Heat produced by intense lipid metabolic activity in brown fat can warm the neonate by increasing heat production as much as 100%. Reserves of brown fat, usually present for several weeks after birth, are rapidly depleted with cold stress. The less mature the infant, the less reserve of this essential fat is available at birth (Bliss-Holtz, 1993).

Brown fat (adipose tissue) begins to appear during gestational weeks 17 to 20. At term, brown fat accounts for 2% to 6% of the total body weight of the newborn (Thomas, 1994). It is located in superficial deposits in the interscapular region (below the nape of the neck), the axilla, posterior to the sternum, in deep deposits at the thoracic inlet, surrounding the kidneys and adrenal glands, in the perineal area, and along the vertebral column.

Heat Loss

Heat loss in the newborn occurs in four ways:

- *Convection:* the flow of heat from the body surface to cooler ambient air. For this reason, ambient temperatures are kept at 24° C and newborns are wrapped to protect them from the cold.
- *Radiation:* the loss of heat from the body surface to cooler solid surfaces not in direct contact but in relative proximity to each other. To prevent this type of loss, cribs and examining tables are placed away from outside windows.
- *Evaporation:* the loss of heat that occurs when a liquid is converted to a vapor. In the newborn, heat loss by evaporation occurs as a result of vaporization of moisture from the skin and is intensified by failure to dry the newborn directly after birth or by drying the infant too slowly after a bath.
- *Conduction:* the loss of heat from the body surface to cooler surfaces in direct contact. When admitted to the nursery, the newborn is placed in a warmed crib to minimize heat loss.

Cold Stress

Cold stress imposes metabolic and physiologic problems on all infants, regardless of gestational age and condition. The respiratory rate is increased as a response to the increased need for oxygen when the oxygen consumption increases sig-

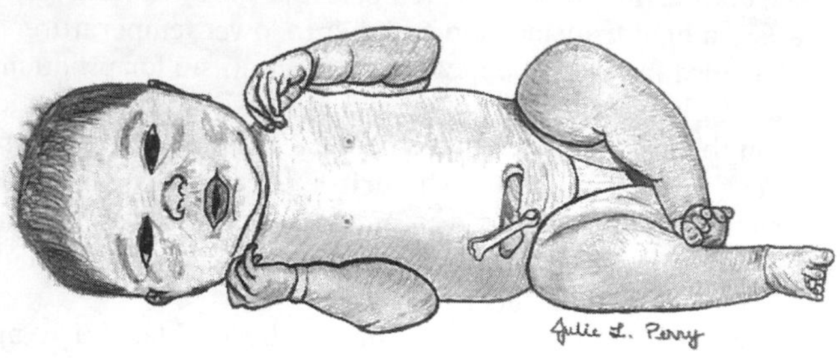

Cold → ↑O_2 consumption → ↑Respiratory rate

↓O_2 uptake by lungs ← Pulmonary vasoconstriction

↓O_2 to tissues ← Peripheral vasoconstriction

↑Anaerobic glycolysis → ↓in PO_2 and pH

Metabolic acidosis

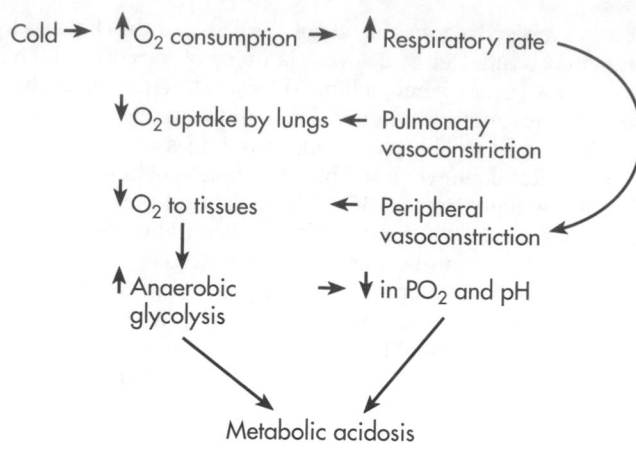

Fig. 22-3 Effects of cold stress. When an infant is stressed by cold, oxygen consumption increases and pulmonary and peripheral vasoconstriction occur, thereby decreasing oxygen uptake by the lungs and oxygen to the tissues; anaerobic glycolysis increases; and Po_2 and pH increase, leading to metabolic acidosis. (Courtesy Julie L. Perry.)

nificantly in cold stress. Oxygen consumption and energy in the cold-stressed infant are diverted from maintaining normal brain cell and cardiac function and growth to thermogenesis for survival. If the infant cannot maintain an adequate oxygen tension, vasoconstriction follows and jeopardizes pulmonary perfusion. As a consequence, arterial blood gas levels of Po_2 are decreased, and blood pH drops. These changes aggravate existing respiratory distress syndrome (RDS). Moreover, decreased pulmonary perfusion and oxygen tension may maintain or reopen the right-to-left shunt across the patent ductus arteriosus, thus decreasing the delivery of oxygenated blood to major organs such as the brain.

The basal metabolic rate is increased with cold stress. If cold stress is protracted, anaerobic glycolysis occurs, resulting in increased production of lactic acid. Metabolic acidosis develops (Fig. 22-3), and if there is a compromised respiratory function, respiratory acidosis also develops.

Hyperthermia develops more rapidly in the newborn than in the adult because of decreased ability to increase evaporative skin water losses. Although newborn infants have six times as many sweat glands per unit area as adults, these glands do not function sufficiently to allow the infant to sweat. Serious overheating of the newborn can cause dehydration, apnea, hypotension, and brain damage (Blackburn and Loper, 1992).

FLUID AND ELECTROLYTE BALANCE

Differences exist between the newborn and adult in distribution of extracellular and intracellular fluid. About 40% of the body weight of the newborn is extracellular fluid, whereas in the adult it is 20%. The rate of exchange of extracellular fluid is also different. Each day the newborn takes in and excretes roughly 600 to 700 ml of water, which is 20% of the total body fluid or 50% of the extracellular fluid. In contrast, the adult exchanges 2000 ml of water, which is 5% of the total body fluid and 14% of the extracellular fluid. The glomerular filtration rate (GFR) of a newborn is about 30% to 50% of that of the adult. This results in a decreased ability to remove nitrogenous and other waste products from the blood. However, the newborn's ingested protein is almost totally metabolized for growth.

Sodium reabsorption is decreased as a result of a lowered sodium, potassium–activated adenosine triphosphate (ATPase) activity. The decreased ability to excrete excessive sodium results in hypotonic urine compared with plasma. There is a higher concentration of sodium, phosphates, chloride, and organic acids and a lower concentration of bicarbonate ions. The infant has a higher renal threshold for glucose. The newborn can dilute urine down to 50 mOsm. Capacity to dilute urine exceeds capacity to concentrate it. There is some limitation in the ability to increase urinary volume. The newborn can concentrate urine to 600 to 700 mOsm compared with the adult's capacity of 1400 mOsm. The inability to concentrate urine is not absolute, but in terms of adult function, it is somewhat limited. Comparative laboratory values for term and preterm infants appear in the Appendix.

Loss of fluid through urine, feces, lungs, increased metabolic rate, and limited fluid intake results in a 5% to 10% loss of the birth weight. This usually occurs over the first 3 to 5 days of life.

The neonate should regain birth weight within 10 days. In addition to excretion of urine, infants lose additional water through insensible fluid loss (70% evaporates from the skin and 35% from respiratory tract). Stool water loss is estimated at 5 to 10 ml/kg/day.

RENAL SYSTEM

By the fourth month of fetal life the kidneys are formed. In utero, urine is formed in the kidneys and excreted into the amniotic fluid. At birth, small amounts (approximately 40 ml) of urine are usually present in the bladder of a full-term infant.

At term the kidneys occupy a large portion of the posterior abdominal wall. The bladder lies close to the anterior abdominal wall and is partially an abdominal, as well as a pelvic, organ. In the newborn, almost all palpable masses in the abdomen are renal in origin.

The frequency of voiding varies from 2 to 6 times during the first and second days of life and from 5 to 25 times during the subsequent 24 hours. Generally, term infants void 15 to 60 ml of urine per kilogram per day (Blackburn and Loper, 1992; Fanaroff and Martin, 1992).

Full-term infants have limited capacity to concentrate urine; therefore the specific gravity ranges from 1.005 to 1.015 (Seidel, Rosenstein, and Pathak, 1993). The ability to fully concentrate urine is attained by about 3 months of age.

After the first voiding the infant's urine may appear cloudy (because of mucus content) and have a much higher specific gravity. This decreases as fluid intake increases. Normal urine during early infancy is usually straw-colored and almost odorless. Sometimes pink-tinged uric crystal stains appear on the diaper; these stains are normal.

Because renal thresholds are low in the infant, bicarbonate concentration and buffering capacity are decreased. This may lead to acidosis and electrolyte imbalance.

GASTROINTESTINAL SYSTEM

The full-term newborn is capable of swallowing, digesting, metabolizing, absorbing proteins and simple carbohydrates, and emulsifying fats. With the exception of pancreatic amylase the characteristic enzymes and digestive juices are present even in low-birth-weight neonates.

In the adequately hydrated infant the mucous membrane of the mouth is moist and pink. The hard and soft palates are intact. Small whitish areas (Epstein pearls) may be found on the gum margins and at the juncture of the hard and soft palate. The cheeks are full because of well-developed sucking pads. These, like the labial tubercles (sucking calluses) on the upper lip, disappear around the age of 12 months, when the sucking period is over.

Even though in utero sucking motions have been recorded by ultrasound, these motions are not coordinated in any infant born who weighs less than 1500 g or is less than 32 weeks' gestation. Sucking behavior is influenced by neuromuscular maturity, maternal medications received during labor and birth, and the type of initial feeding.

A special mechanism present in healthy term newborns coordinates the breathing, sucking, and swallowing reflexes necessary for oral feeding. Peristaltic activity in the esophagus is uncoordinated in the first few days of life.

Teeth begin developing in utero with enamel formation continuing until about age 10 years. Tooth development is influenced by neonatal/infant illnesses, medications, and illnesses of, or medications taken by, the mother during pregnancy. The fluoride level in the water supply also influences tooth development. Occasionally an infant may be born with one or more teeth.

Bacteria are not present in the infant's gastrointestinal tract at birth. Soon after birth, oral and anal orifices permit entrance of bacteria and air. Generally the highest bacterial concentration is found in the lower portion of the intestine. Normal colonic bacteria are established within the first week after birth. The normal intestinal flora help synthesize vitamin K, folic acid, and biotin. Bowel sounds can usually be heard shortly after birth.

Stomach capacity varies from 30 to 90 ml, depending on the size of the infant. Emptying time for the stomach is highly variable. Several factors, such as time and volume of feedings or type and temperature of food, may affect the emptying time. The stomach empties intermittently, beginning a few minutes after the start of a feeding and ending 2 to 4 hours after feeding. The cardiac sphincter and nervous control of the stomach are immature, so some regurgitation may occur.

Digestion

The infant's ability to digest carbohydrates, fats, and proteins is regulated by the presence of certain enzymes. Most of these are functional at birth. One exception is *amylase*, produced by the salivary glands after about 3 months and by the pancreas at about 6 months of age. This enzyme is necessary to convert starch into maltose. The other exception is *lipase*, also secreted by the pancreas; it is necessary for the digestion of fat. Thus the normal newborn is capable of digesting simple carbohydrates and proteins but has a limited ability to digest fats. Parietal cell function is not fully developed, and the gastric juice is less acid than in later life (Guyton, 1991).

Further digestion and absorption of nutrients occur in the small intestine in the presence of pancreatic secretions, secretions from the liver through the common bile duct, and secretions from the duodenal portion of the small intestine.

BOX 22-1
Change in Stooling Patterns of Newborns

Meconium

Infant's first stool; composed of amniotic fluid and its constituents, intestinal secretions, shed mucosal cells, and possibly blood (ingested maternal blood or minor bleeding of alimentary tract vessels).

Passage of meconium should occur within the first 24 to 48 hours, although it may be delayed up to 7 days in very-low-birth-weight infants.

Transitional stools

Usually appear by third day after initiation of feeding; greenish brown to yellowish brown, thin, and less sticky than meconium; may contain some milk curds.

Milk stool

Usually appears by fourth day.

In *breastfed infants*, stools are yellow to golden, are pasty in consistency, and have an odor similar to that of sour milk.

In *formula-fed infants*, stools are pale yellow to light brown, are firmer in consistency, and have a more offensive odor.

Stools

At birth the lower intestine is filled with meconium. *Meconium* is formed during fetal life from the amniotic fluid and its constituents, intestinal secretions (including bilirubin), and cells (shed mucosa). Meconium is greenish black and viscous and contains occult blood. The first meconium passed is usually sterile, but within hours all meconium passed contains bacteria. About 69% of normal term infants pass meconium within 12 hours of life, 94% by 24 hours, and 99.8% in 48 hours (Blackburn and Loper, 1992). Progressive changes in the stooling pattern indicate a properly functioning gastrointestinal tract (Box 22-1).

HEPATIC SYSTEM

The liver and gallbladder are formed by the fourth week of gestation. In the newborn the liver can be palpated about 1 cm below the right costal margin because it is physiologically enlarged and occupies about 40% of the abdominal cavity. The infant's liver plays an important role in iron storage, carbohydrate metabolism, conjugation of bilirubin, and coagulation.

Iron Storage

The fetal liver (which serves as the site for production of hemoglobin after birth) begins storing iron in utero. The infant's iron store is proportional to total body hemoglobin content and length of gestation. At birth the term neonate has approximately 270 mg of iron, of which about 140 to 170 mg is hemoglobin (Blackburn and Loper, 1992).

Carbohydrate Metabolism

At birth the newborn is cut off from its maternal glucose supply and as a result experiences an initial decrease in serum glucose levels. The newborn's increased energy needs, decreased hepatic release of glucose from glycogen stores, increased RBC volume, and increased brain size may initially contribute to the rapid depletion of stored glycogen within the first 24 hours after birth. In most healthy term newborns, blood glucose levels stabilize at 50 to 60 mg/dl during the first several hours after birth, and a steady state is achieved by the fifth day of life. The initiation of feedings assists in the stabilization of the newborn's blood glucose levels (Blackburn and Loper, 1992).

Conjugation of Bilirubin

Bilirubin is a yellowish pigment that results from the breakdown of hemoglobin (Blackburn and Loper, 1992). The hemoglobin is degraded by the reticuloendothelial cells, converted to bilirubin, and released in an unconjugated form. Unconjugated or *indirect bilirubin* is relatively insoluble and is almost entirely bound to circulating albumin, a plasma protein. The term **hyperbilirubinemia** refers to an excessive accumulation of bilirubin in the blood and is characterized by *jaundice,* or *icterus,* a yellowish discoloration of the skin and other organs. Hyperbilirubinemia is a common finding in the newborn and in most instances is relatively benign. However, it can also indicate a pathologic state.

In the liver the unbound bilirubin is conjugated with glucuronide in the presence of the enzyme glucuronyl transferase. The conjugated form of bilirubin, *direct bilirubin,* is soluble and is excreted from liver cells as a constituent of bile. Along with other components of bile, direct bilirubin is excreted into the biliary tract system that carries the bile into the duodenum. Bilirubin is converted to urobilinogen and stercobilinogen within the duodenum through the action of the bacterial flora. Urobilinogen is excreted in urine and feces; stercobilinogen is excreted in the feces (Fig. 22-4). Since there are no methods for measuring indirect (unconjugated) bilirubin, it is obtained by subtracting the direct (conjugated) bilirubin from the total serum bilirubin.

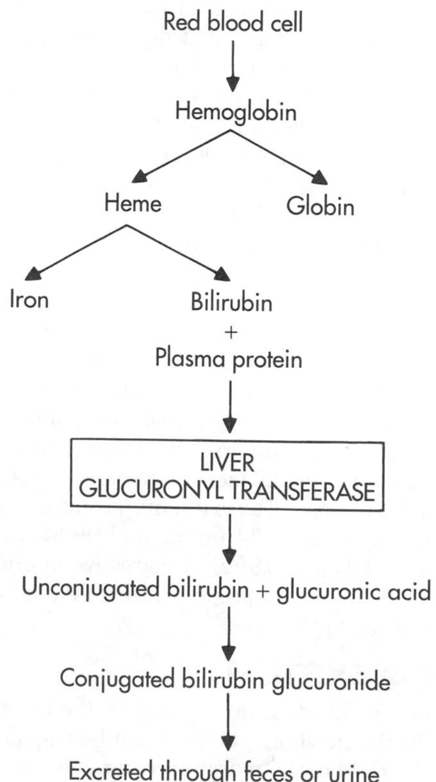

Fig. 22-4 Formation and excretion of bilirubin. (From Wong D: *Whaley & Wong's nursing care of infants and children,* ed 5, St Louis, 1995, Mosby.)

Physiologic Jaundice

The most common cause of hyperbilirubinemia is the relatively mild and self-limited **physiologic jaundice,** or *icterus neonatorum.* It is not associated with any pathologic process, as is hemolytic disease of the newborn. Although almost all newborns experience elevated bilirubin levels, only about half demonstrate observable signs of jaundice.

Physiologic jaundice fulfills the following specific criteria (Blackburn and Loper, 1992):

- The infant is otherwise well.
- In term infants, jaundice first appears after 24 hours and disappears by the end of the seventh day.
- In preterm infants, jaundice is first evident after 48 hours and disappears by the ninth or tenth day.
- Serum unconjugated bilirubin concentration usually does not exceed 12 mg/dl in term or 15 mg/dl in preterm infants.
- Hyperbilirubinemia is almost exclusively of the unconjugated variety, and conjugated (direct) bilirubin should not exceed 1 to 1.5 mg/dl.
- Daily increments of bilirubin concentration should not surpass 5 mg/dl. Bilirubin levels in excess of 12 mg/dl may indicate either an exaggeration of the physiologic handicap or the presence of a pathologic condition.

Nursing ALERT

At any serum bilirubin level the appearance of jaundice during the first day of life or persistence beyond the ages previously delineated usually indicates a pathologic process.

Jaundice may first appear in the head and then progress gradually toward the abdomen and extremities because of the neonate's circulatory pattern (cephalocaudal developmental progression); however, since it is impossible to estimate serum bilirubin levels based on the infant's clinical appearance, serum bilirubin levels are obtained to adequately establish significant levels (Tappero and Honeyfield, 1996). Noninvasive monitoring of bilirubin via cutaneous reflectance measurements *(transcutaneous bilirubinometry)* allows for repetitive estimations of bilirubin.

Feeding practices may influence the appearance and degree of physiologic jaundice. *Early feeding* tends to keep the serum bilirubin level low by stimulating intestinal activity (the gastrocolic reflex) and the passage of meconium.

Kernicterus, the most serious complication of neonatal hyperbilirubinemia, is caused by the precipitation of bilirubin in neuronal cells, resulting in their destruction. Behavioral disorders, seizures, mental retardation, delayed motor development, and sensorineural hearing loss may occur as a result of kernicterus. The exact level of serum bilirubin required to cause damage is as yet unknown. Since a number of factors (such as metabolic acidosis, hypoxemia, and hypothermia) may contribute to bilirubin neurotoxicity, serum bilirubin levels alone are not predictive of the risk for brain injury.

Jaundice in Breastfeeding Infants

Breastfeeding is associated with an increased incidence of jaundice. Two types have been identified. ***Breastfeeding-associated jaundice*** (early-onset jaundice) begins at 2 to 4 days of age and occurs in approximately 10% to 25% of breastfed newborns. The jaundice is related to the process of breastfeeding, probably from decreased caloric and fluid intake by breastfed infants before the milk supply is established, since fasting is associated with decreased hepatic clearance of bilirubin.

Breast milk jaundice (late-onset jaundice) begins at age 4 to 5 days and occurs in 2% to 3% of breastfed infants. Rising levels of bilirubin peak during the third week and then gradually diminish. Despite high levels of bilirubin that may persist for 3 to 12 weeks, these infants are well. The jaundice may be caused by a factor in the breast milk (beta-glucuronidase) that breaks down bilirubin to a lipid-soluble form, which is reabsorbed in the gut. Less frequent stooling by breastfed infants allows an extended time for reabsorption of bilirubin from stools.

Recommendations for prevention and management of early-onset jaundice in breastfed infants are to encourage frequent breastfeeding, preferably every 2 hours, and avoid supplementation. In late-onset jaundice, bilirubin levels are monitored, and breastfeeding may be discontinued for up to 24 hours when bilirubin levels reach 15 mg/dl. Breastfeeding is resumed after a decrease in the bilirubin levels occurs, which rules out other causes of hyperbilirubinemia (Lawrence, 1994).

Coagulation

Coagulation factors, which are synthesized in the liver, are activated by vitamin K. The lack of intestinal bacteria needed to synthesize vitamin K results in transient blood coagulation deficiency between the second and fifth days of life. An injection of vitamin K on the day of birth helps prevent clotting problems.

IMMUNE SYSTEM

Although nonspecific and specific body defenses are present in unborn and newborn infants, many of these defenses are not completely developed in this group. A healthy newborn does not sweat, has no tears, and is not born with "normal" skin or intestinal microbial flora. If the integrity of the skin is broken, the newborn is predisposed to tissue and blood invasion by foreign cells, such as bacteria. Infants who are preterm, small for gestational age, or postterm have different skin qualities (e.g., thin, easily torn immature skin vs. postmature cracked, peeling skin) that increase their susceptibility to invasive agents.

Full-term infants usually have passively acquired natural immunity because of the presence of maternal IgG antibodies. These antibodies are transferred from mother to infant through the placental circulation and provide short-term resistance (3 months) to the specific antigens to which the mother produced antibodies. The preterm infant may be deficient in this type of immunity, especially if born before the thirty-sixth week of gestation. Another passively acquired antibody (IgA) is present in *colostrum* and can be acquired by the newborn through breast milk. The protection provided by breastfeeding varies with the age and maturity of the infant as well as the mother's own immune system (Lawrence, 1994).

Natural barriers such as the acidity of the stomach or the production of pepsin and trypsin, which maintain sterility of the small intestine, are not fully developed until 3 to 4 weeks of age (Guyton, 1991). The membrane-protective IgA is missing from the respiratory and urinary tracts and, unless the newborn is breastfed, is absent from the gastrointestinal tract as well. The infant begins to synthesize IgG, and levels reach about 40% of adult levels by 1 year of age (Guyton, 1991). Significant amounts of IgM are produced at birth, and adult levels are reached by 9 months of age. The production of IgA, IgD, and IgE is much more gradual, and maximum levels are not attained until early childhood.

REPRODUCTIVE SYSTEM

Female

At birth the ovaries contain thousands of primitive germ cells. These represent the full complement of potential ova, since no oogonia form after delivery in term infants. The ovarian cortex, which is made up primarily of primordial follicles, forms a thicker portion of the ovary in the female newborn than in the adult. The number of ova decreases from birth of the female to sexual maturity by approximately 90%.

The infant's uterus, enlarged during pregnancy because of maternal estrogen, undergoes involution in the first weeks of life and decreases in size and weight. Hyperestrogenism (large amounts of estrogen) of pregnancy followed by a drop after birth may result in a mucoid vaginal discharge and even some slight bloody spotting (pseudomenstruation) that will disappear in 2 to 4 weeks. Vaginal tags (small additional growths to the vagina) are common findings, have no clinical significance, and do not need to be excised or treated. External genitals (labia majora and minora) are usually edematous with increased pigmentation (Fig. 22-5, *A*).

The preterm female of 30 to 36 weeks' gestation usually has a prominent clitoris that extends from the labia minora and majora. The labia majora are small and widely separated. At 36 to 40 weeks' gestation the labia majora are larger and almost cover the clitoris. In term neonates, labia majora and minora obscure the vestibule and cover the clitoris. Vernix

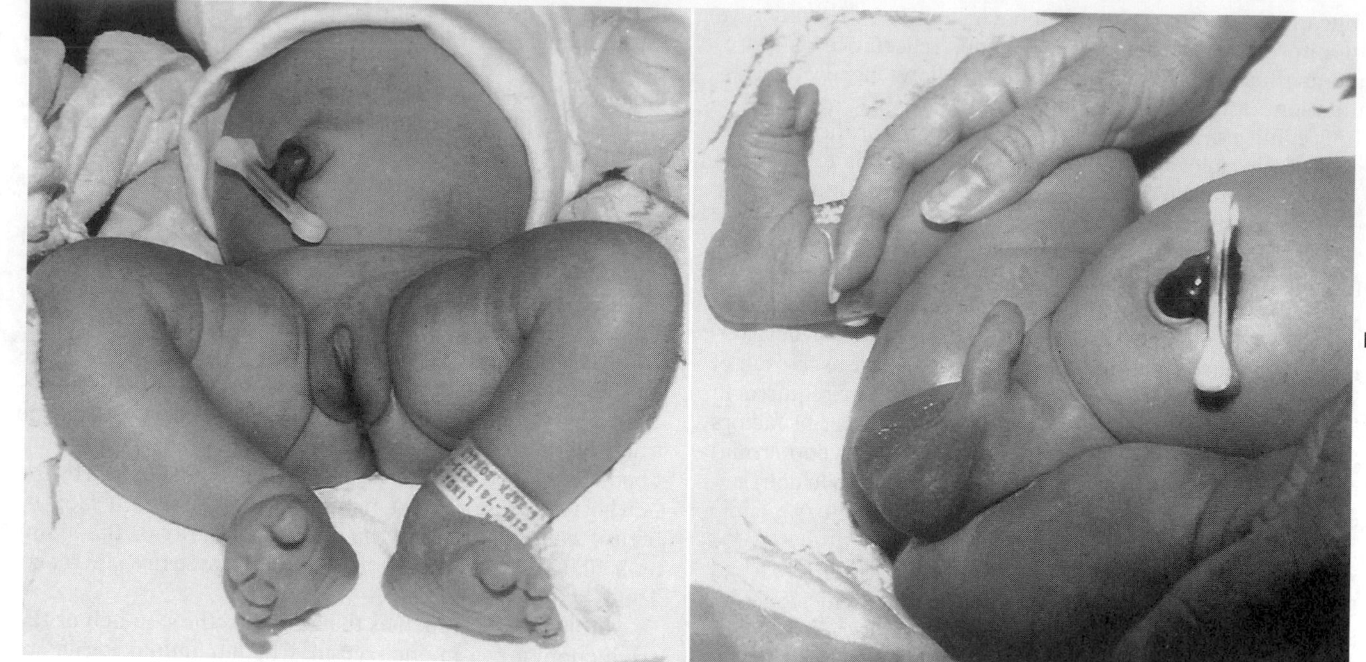

Fig. 22-5 External genitalia. **A,** Genitalia in female term infant. **B,** Genitalia in male infant (uncircumcised penis). Rugae cover scrotum, indicating term gestation. Cord has been swabbed with ethylene blue to prevent infection. (Courtesy Marjorie Pyle, RNC, Lifecircle, Costa Mesa, Calif.)

caseosa may be present in large amounts between the labia.

If the female is born in the breech position, the labia may be edematous and bruised.

Male

The testes descend into the scrotum by birth in 90% of newborn boys. Although this percentage drops with premature birth, by 1 year of age the incidence of undescended testes in all males is less than 1%.

Adhesions of the foreskin (prepuce) are almost universally present in male newborns. During prenatal development the tissue of the prepuce is continuous with the epidermis that covers the glans. Gradually the preputial space between the prepuce and glans forms. The complete separation of the two tissue areas is generally not complete at birth. For this reason the prepuce of the newborn is usually not fully retractable. Smegma, a white cheesy substance, is commonly found under the foreskin. Small, white, firm cysts called epithelial pearls may be seen at the tip of the prepuce. In the preterm male of less than 28 weeks' gestation the testes remain within the abdominal cavity and the scrotum appears high and close to the body. By 28 to 36 weeks' gestation the testes can be palpated in the inguinal canal and a few rugae appear on the scrotum. At 36 to 40 weeks' gestation the testes are palpable in the upper scrotum and rugae appear on the anterior portion. After 40 weeks the testes can be palpated in the scrotum and rugae cover the scrotal sac. The postterm neonate has deep rugae and a pendulous scrotum. The scrotum is usually more deeply pigmented than the rest of the skin (Fig. 22-5, *B*) and is especially apparent in darker-skinned infants. This pigmentation is a response to maternal estrogen. A hydrocele, caused by an accumulation of fluid around the testes, may be found. It can be transilluminated with a light and usually decreases in size without treatment. If the hydrocele is a communicating hydrocele, one in which the processus vaginalis remains open and into which peritoneal fluid may be forced by intraabdominal pressure and gravity, surgery may be indicated. A communicating hydrocele can predispose the child to herniation; therefore surgical repair is indicated if spontaneous resolution does not take place by 1 year of age (Wong, 1995).

If the male infant is born in a breech presentation, the scrotum is edematous and may be bruised. The swelling and discoloration subside within a few days.

Swelling of Breast Tissue

Swelling of the breast tissue in term infants of both sexes is caused by the hyperestrogenism of pregnancy. In a few infants a thin discharge *(witch's milk)* can be seen. This finding has no clinical significance, requires no treatment, and subsides as the maternal hormones are eliminated from the infant's body within a few days.

The nipples should be symmetrical on the chest. Breast tissue and areola size increase with gestation. The areola appears slightly elevated at 34 weeks' gestation. By 36 weeks a breast bud of 1 to 2 mm is palpable and increases to 12 mm by 42 weeks.

INTEGUMENTARY SYSTEM

All the skin structures are present at birth. The epidermis and dermis are bound loosely, are very thin, and can be easily damaged. Vernix caseosa (a cheeselike whitish substance) is present and serves as a protective skin covering. The *texture* of

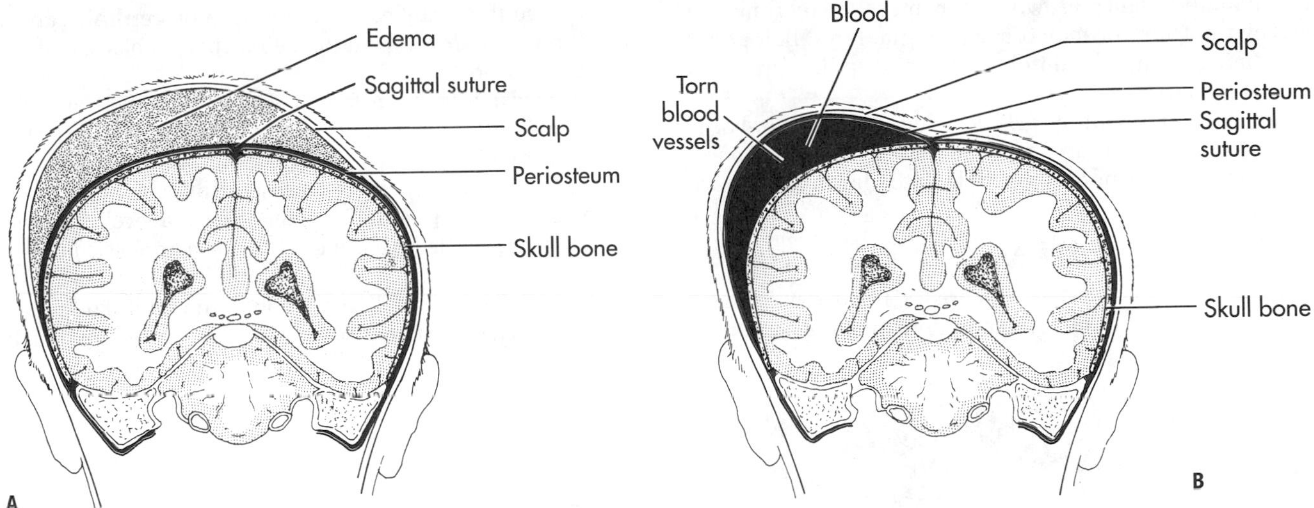

Fig. 22-6 Differences between caput succedaneum and cephalhematoma. **A,** Caput succedaneum. Edema of scalp is noted at birth and crosses suture lines. **B,** Cephalhematoma. Bleeding between periosteum and skull bone appears within first 2 days and does not cross suture lines.

the newborn's skin is velvety smooth and puffy, especially about the eyes, the legs, the dorsal aspect of the hands and feet, and the scrotum or labia. Skin *color* depends on racial and familial background and varies greatly among newborns. In general, the Caucasian infant is usually pink to red; the African-American newborn may appear as pinkish or yellowish brown. Infants of Hispanic descent may have an olive tint or a slight yellow cast to the skin. Infants of Asian descent may be a rosy or yellowish tan. The color of Native-American newborns depends on the tribe and can vary from a light pink to a dark, reddish brown. By the second or third day the skin turns to its more natural tone and is drier and flakier.

The color of the skin is observed in relation to activity, position, and temperature changes. In general, the infant becomes redder when crying and may demonstrate transient periods of cyanosis. Decreased temperature increases the degree of cyanosis because of vasoconstriction. **Mongolian spots**, darker pigmentation usually in the sacral or gluteal areas, commonly occur in newborns of darker-skinned people, i.e., African, Native-American, Asian, or Hispanic.

The hands and feet appear slightly cyanotic; this bluish discoloration, **acrocyanosis,** is caused by vasomotor instability and capillary stasis. This is normal and appears intermittently over the first 7 to 10 days, especially with exposure to cold.

Fine *lanugo* hair may be noted over the face, shoulders, and back. Actual edema of the face and *ecchymosis* (bruising) may be noted as a result of face presentation or forceps delivery.

Caput Succedaneum

Caput succedaneum is a generalized edematous area of the scalp, most commonly found on the occiput (Fig. 22-6, *A*). The sustained pressure of the presenting vertex against the cervix results in compression of local vessels and slowing of venous return. The slower venous return causes an increase in tissue fluids within the skin of the scalp, and edema develops.

This boggy edematous swelling, present at birth, extends across the suture lines of the skull and disappears spontaneously within 3 to 4 days. Often caput succedaneum and cephalhematoma occur simultaneously. Infants who are born with the assistance of vacuum extraction usually have a caput succedaneum in the area where the cup was applied.

Cephalhematoma

Cephalhematoma is a collection of blood between a skull bone and its periosteum. Therefore a cephalhematoma does not cross a cranial suture line (Fig. 22-6, *B*). Bleeding may occur with spontaneous birth from pressure against the maternal bony pelvis. Low forceps birth, as well as difficult forceps rotation and extraction, may also cause bleeding. This soft, fluctuating, irreducible fullness does not pulsate or bulge when the infant cries. It appears several hours or the day after birth. It may not become apparent until a caput succedaneum is absorbed. A cephalhematoma is usually largest on the second or third day, by which time the bleeding stops. The fullness of cephalhematoma spontaneously resolves in 3 to 6 weeks. It is not aspirated because infection may develop if the skin is punctured. As the hematoma resolves, hemolysis of RBCs occurs and jaundice may result.

Desquamation

Desquamation (peeling) of the skin of the term infant is minimal and may be localized to the extremities. The presence of peeling skin over the entire body at birth is usually an indication of postmaturity.

Sweat and Oil Glands

Sweat glands are present at birth but do not readily respond to increases in ambient or body temperature. There is some fetal sebaceous (oil) gland hyperplasia and secretion of sebum as a result of the hormonal influences of pregnancy. *Vernix caseosa* is a product of the sebaceous glands. Removal of the vernix is followed by desquamation of the epidermis in most infants (Fanaroff and Martin, 1992).

The growth phases of *hair follicles* usually occur simultaneously at birth. During the first few months the synchrony between hair loss and regrowth is disrupted, and there may be overgrowth of hair or temporary alopecia. Boys' hair grows faster than girls' hair, and in both sexes scalp hair growth is slower at the crown.

Because the amount of *melanin* is low at birth, newborns are lighter skinned than they will be as children. Consequently, infants are more susceptible to the harmful effects of direct sunlight.

SKELETAL SYSTEM

The infant's skeletal system undergoes rapid development during the first year of life. At birth there are larger amounts of cartilage than ossified bone. Because of **cephalocaudal** (head-to-rump) **development** the newborn looks somewhat out of proportion.

The head at term is one fourth of the total body length. The arms are slightly longer than the legs. In the newborn the legs are one third of the total body length but only 15% of the total body weight. As growth proceeds, the midpoint in head-to-toe measurements gradually descends from a level even with the umbilicus at birth to the level of the symphysis pubis at maturity.

The face appears small in relation to the skull. The skull is large and heavy in comparison. Cranial size and shape can be

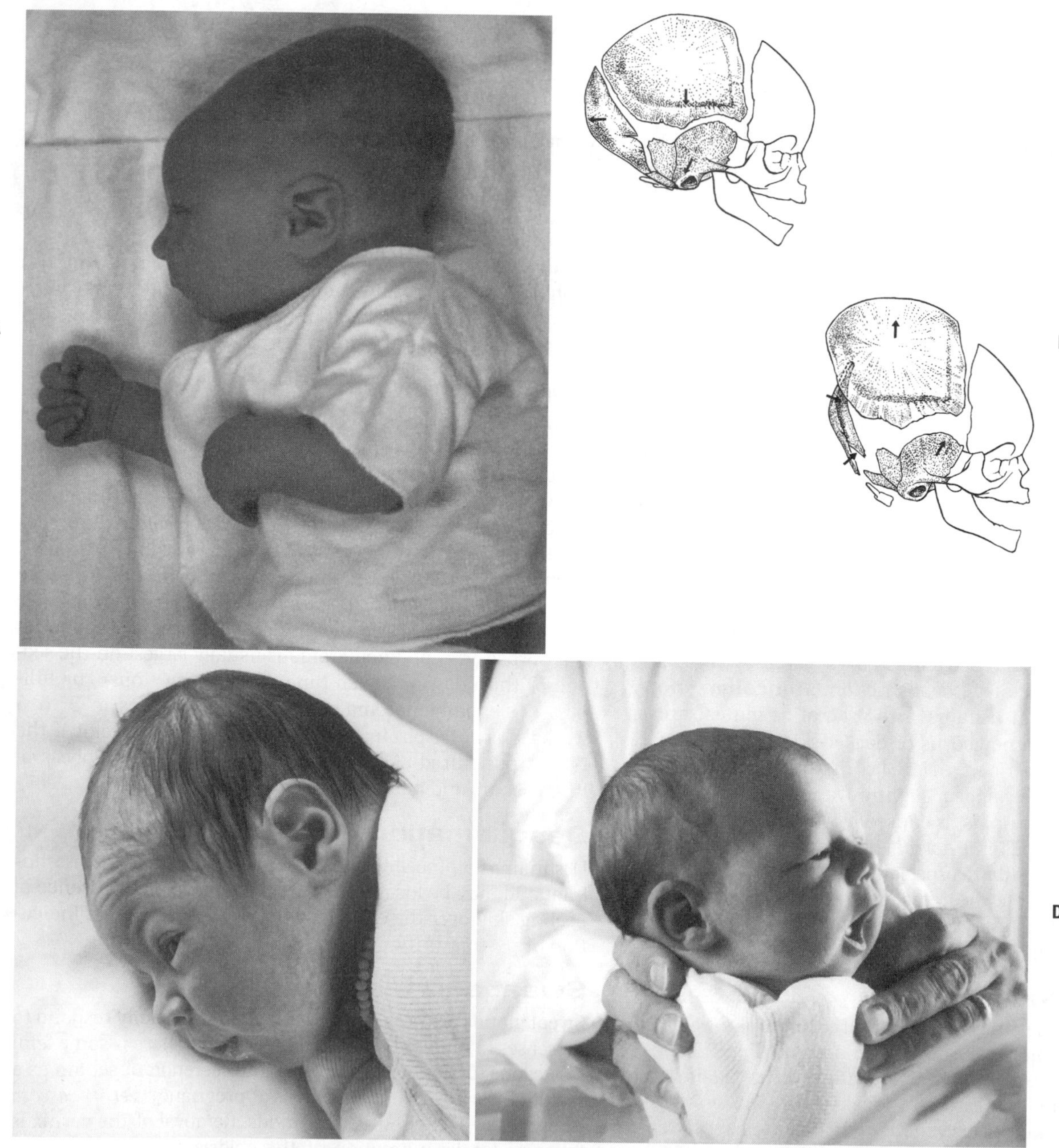

Fig. 22-7 Molding. **A,** Significant molding after vaginal birth. **B,** Schematic of bones of skull when molding is present. **C,** Some resolution of molding is seen on second or third day of life. **D,** Molding is resolved. (**A,** courtesy Kim Malloy, San Jose, Calif. **C** and **D** courtesy Marjorie Pyle, RNC, Lifecircle, Costa Mesa, Calif.)

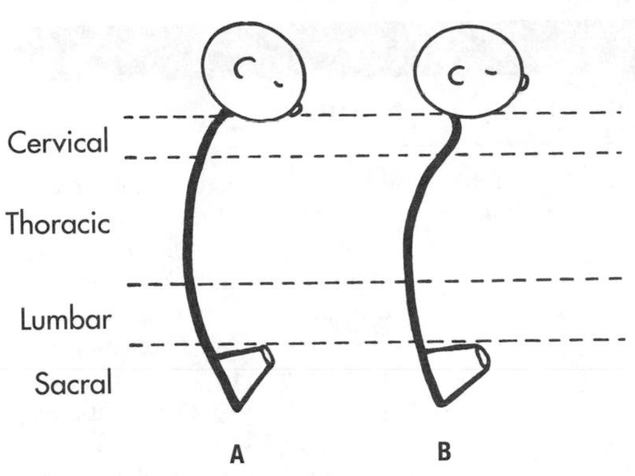

Fig. 22-8 Development of spinal curvatures. **A,** Newborn infant. **B,** Cervical secondary curvature. (From Wong D: *Whaley & Wong's nursing care of infants and children,* ed 5, St Louis, 1995, Mosby.)

distorted by molding, which is the shaping of the fetal head by overlapping of the cranial bones to facilitate movement through the birth canal during labor (Fig. 22-7). The bones in the vertebral column of the newborn form two primary curvatures, one in the thoracic region and one in the sacral region (Fig. 22-8, *A*). Both are forward, concave curvatures. As the infant gains control of his or her head, at approximately 3 months of age, a secondary curvature appears in the cervical region (Fig. 22-8, *B*).

In some newborn infants the knees show a significant separation when the ankles are held together, resulting in an appearance of bowlegs (Fig. 22-9, *A*). If the infant's presentation was breech, the knees may be extended and the infant will continue to maintain the in utero position for several weeks. What sometimes appears as a gross anomaly may simply be a result of in utero positioning. These conditions are self-limiting. The newborn is also very flat-footed with no clearly apparent arch to the foot (Fig. 22-9, *B*).

Extra digits (polydactyly) sometimes are found on the hands and feet. Alternately, fingers or toes may be fused (syndactyly). Creases can be found on the palms of the hands. The simian line, a single palmar crease, often is found in Down syndrome or in Asian infants (Fig. 4-3).

The newborn's spine appears straight and can be flexed easily. The vertebrae should appear straight and flat. The base of the spine should be free from a dimple. If a dimple is noted, further inspection is required to determine whether a sinus is present. A pilonidal dimple, especially with a sinus along with a nevus pilosis (hairy nevus), may be associated with spina bifida.

NEUROMUSCULAR SYSTEM

Unlike the skeletal system, the neuromuscular system is almost completely developed at birth.

Neuromuscular control in the newborn, although still very limited, can be noted. Infants attempt to hold their heads in line with their bodies if they are raised by their arms. Various reflexes serve to promote their safety and adequate food intake.

Spontaneous motor activity may be seen as transient tremors of the mouth and chin, especially during crying episodes, and of the extremities, notably the arms and hands. Transient tremors are normal and can be observed in nearly every newborn. These tremors should not be present when the infant is quiet and should not persist beyond 1 month of age. Persistent tremors or tremors involving the entire body may indicate a pathologic condition. Marked tonicity, clonicity, and twitching of facial muscles are possible signs of seizure activity or other neurologic and/or metabolic problems requiring evaluation.

Newborn Reflexes

The newborn infant has many primitive reflexes. The times at which these reflexes appear and disappear reflect the maturity and intactness of the developing nervous system. The most common reflexes found in the normal newborn are described in Table 22-2.

Sensory Functions

The newborn's **sensory functions** are remarkably well developed and have a significant effect on growth and development, including the attachment process.

Vision. At birth the eye is structurally incomplete. The *fovea centralis* is not yet completely differentiated from the macula.

Text continued on p. 608.

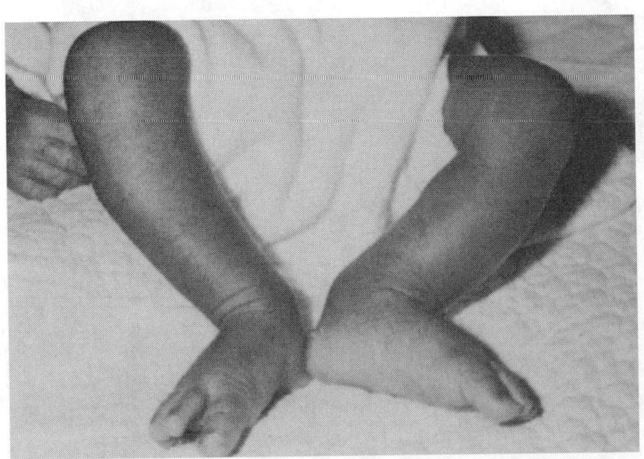

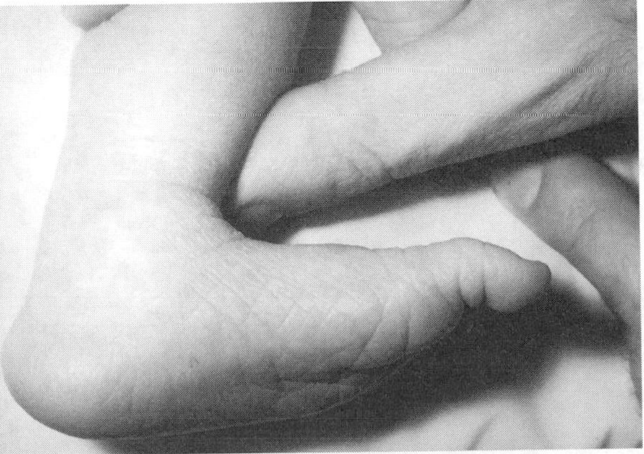

Fig. 22-9 Extremities. **A,** Bowed appearance of legs. **B,** Normal absence of arch in newborn's foot. (Courtesy Marjorie Pyle, RNC, Lifecircle, Costa Mesa, Calif.)

TABLE 22-2 Assessment of newborn's reflexes

REFLEX	ELICITING THE REFLEX	CHARACTERISTIC RESPONSE	COMMENTS
Sucking and rooting	Touch infant's lip, cheek, or corner of mouth with nipple	Infant turns head toward stimulus, opens mouth, takes hold, and sucks	Response is difficult if not impossible to elicit after infant has been fed; if response weak or absent, consider prematurity or neurologic defect Parental guidance: Avoid trying to turn head toward breast or nipple, allow infant to root: response disappears after 3 to 4* mo but may persist up to 1 yr
Swallowing	Feed infant; swallowing usually follows sucking and obtaining fluids	Swallowing is usually coordinated with sucking and usually occurs without gagging, coughing, or vomiting	If response is weak or absent, this may indicate prematurity or neurologic defect Sucking and swallowing are often uncoordinated in preterm infant
Grasp			
Palmar Plantar	Place finger in palm of hand Place finger at base of toes	Infant's fingers curl around examiner's fingers, toes curl downward	Palmar response lessens by 3 to 4 mo; parents enjoy this contact with infant; plantar response lessens by 8 mo
Extrusion	Touch or depress tip of tongue	Newborn forces tongue outward	Response disappears about fourth month of life
Glabellar (Myerson)	Tap over forehead, bridge of nose, or maxilla of newborn whose eyes are open	Newborn blinks for first four or five taps	Continued blinking with repeated taps is consistent with extrapyramidal disorder
Tonic neck or "fencing" (Fig. 22-10)	With infant falling asleep or sleeping, turn head quickly to one side	With infant facing left side, arm and leg on that side extend; opposite arm and leg flex (turn head to right, and extremities assume opposite postures)	Responses in leg are more consistent Complete response disappears by 3 to 4 mo; incomplete response may be seen until third or fourth year After 6 wk, persistent response is sign of possible cerebral palsy

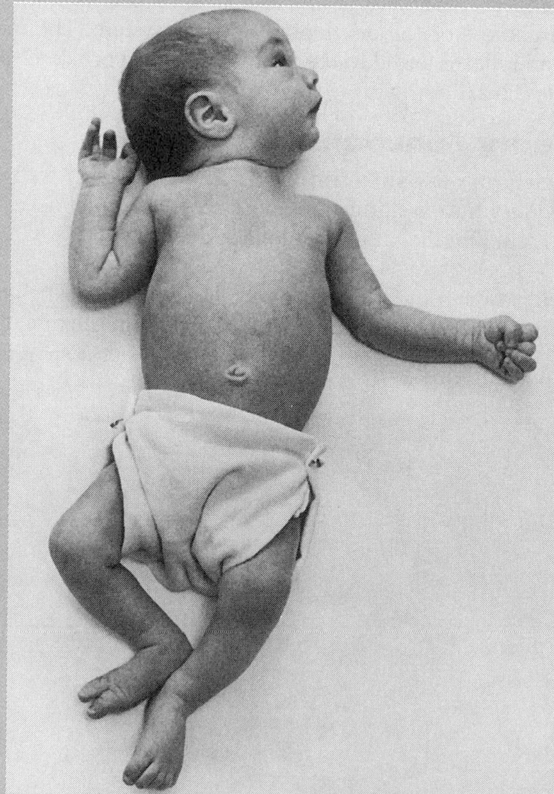

Fig. 22-10 Classic pose in spontaneous tonic neck reflex. (Courtesy Marjorie Pyle, RNC, Lifecircle, Costa Mesa, Calif.)

*All durations for persistence of reflexes are based on time elapsed after 40 weeks of gestation, that is, if this newborn was born at 36 weeks of gestation, add 1 mo to all time limits given.

TABLE 22-2 Assessment of newborn's reflexes—cont'd

REFLEX	ELICITING THE REFLEX	CHARACTERISTIC RESPONSE	COMMENTS
Moro/startle (Fig. 22-11)	Place infant on flat surface, strike surface to startle infant; best elicited if newborn is 24 to 36 hr or older	Symmetric abduction and extension of arms are seen; fingers fan out and form a C with thumb and forefinger; slight tremor may be noted; arms are adducted in embracing motion and return to relaxed flexion and movement	Response is present at birth; complete response may be seen until 8 wk of age; body jerk only is seen between 8 and 18 wk; response is absent by 6 mo if neurologic maturation is not delayed; response may be incomplete if infant is deeply asleep; give parental guidance about normal response
		Legs may follow similar pattern of response	Response is asymmetric; may connote injury to brachial plexus, clavicle, or humerus
		Preterm infant does not complete "embrace": instead, arms fall backward because of weakness	Persistent response after 6 mo indicates possible brain damage
Stepping or "walking"	Hold infant vertically, allowing one foot to touch table surface	Infant will simulate walking, alternating flexion and extension of feet: term infants walk on soles of their feet, and preterm infants walk on their toes	Response is normally present for 3 to 4 wk
Crawling	Place newborn on abdomen	Newborn makes crawling movements with arms and legs	Response should disappear about 6 wk of age
Deep tendon	Use finger instead of percussion hammer to elicit patellar, or knee jerk, reflex: newborn must be relaxed	Reflex jerk is present; even with newborn relaxed, nonselective overall reaction may occur	

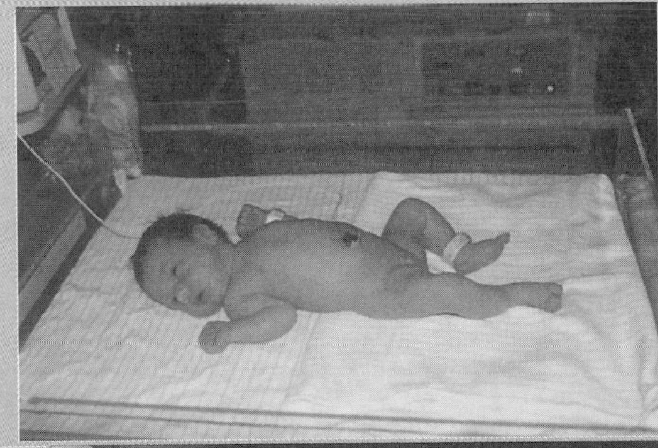

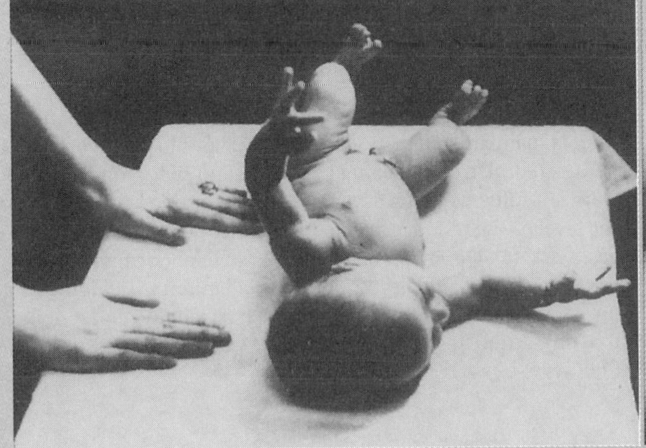

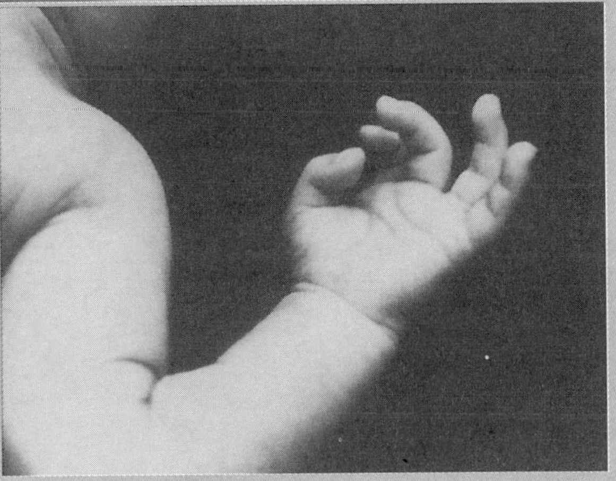

Fig. 22-11 Moro reflex. **A,** Position of rest. **B,** Moro reflex consists predominantly of abduction and extension of arms. **C,** Interesting subtlety of Moro response in newborns is C position of fingers: digits extend, except first finger and thumb, which are often semiflexed, forming shape of a C. (**A** courtesy Marjorie Pyle, RNC, Lifecircle, Costa Mesa, Calif; **B** and **C** courtesy Mead Johnson & Co, Evansville, IN.)

Continued.

TABLE 22-2 Assessment of newborn's reflexes—cont'd

REFLEX	ELICITING THE REFLEX	CHARACTERISTIC RESPONSE	COMMENTS
Crossed extension (Fig. 22-12)	Infant should be supine; extend one leg, press knee downward, stimulate bottom of foot; observe opposite leg	Opposite leg reflexes, adducts, and then extends	
Babinski sign (plantar) (Fig. 22-13)	On sole of foot, beginning at heel, stroke upward along lateral aspect of sole, then move finger across ball of foot	All toes hyperextend, with dorsiflexion of big toe—recorded as a positive sign	Absence requires neurologic evaluation; should disappear after 1 yr of age

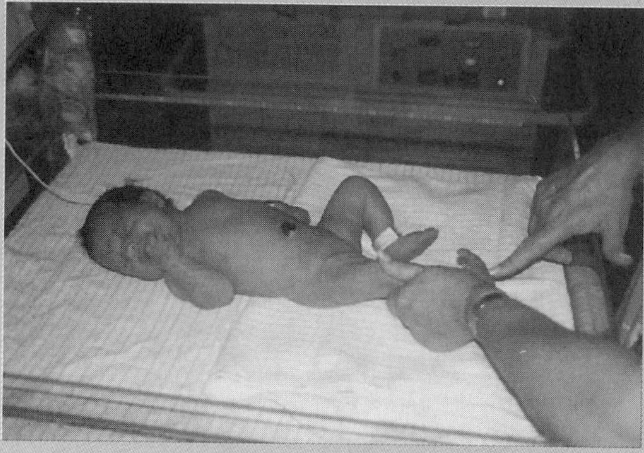

Fig. 22-12 Crossed extension reflex. With the infant in supine position, examiner extends one leg of the infant and presses the knee down. Stimulation of sole of foot of fixated limb should cause free leg to flex, adduct, and extend as if attempting to push away stimulating agent. This reflex should be present during newborn period. Absence of response suggests a spinal cord lesion; a weak response suggests peripheral nerve damage. (Courtesy Marjorie Pyle, RNC, Lifecircle, Costa Mesa, Calif.)

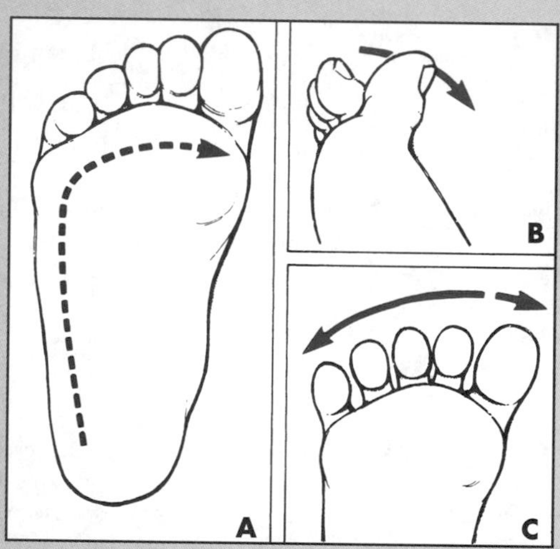

Fig. 22-13 Babinski reflex. **A,** Direction of stroke. **B,** Dorsiflexion of big toe. **C,** Fanning of toes. (From Wong D: *Whaley & Wong's nursing care of infants and children,* ed 5, St Louis, 1995, Mosby.)

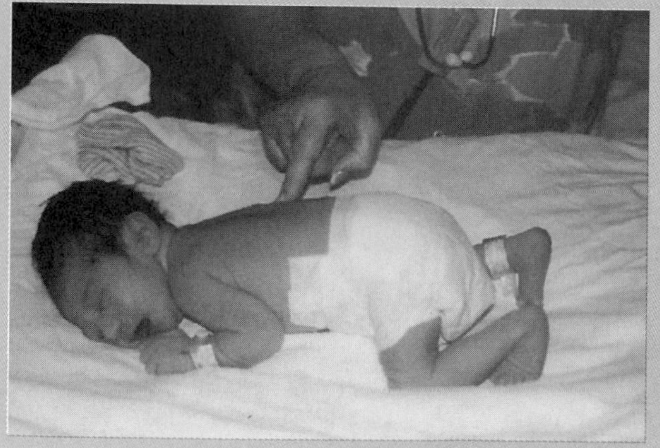

Fig. 22-14 Trunk incurvation reflex. In prone position, infant responds to linear skin stimulus (blunt end of pin or finger) along paravertebral area by flexing the trunk and swinging the pelvis toward stimulus. With transverse lesion of cord, no response below the level of the lesion is present. Complete absence of response suggests general depression or nervous system abnormality. Response may vary but should be obtainable in all infants, including preterm ones. If not seen in the first few days, it is usually apparent by age 5 to 6 days. (Courtesy Marjorie Pyle, RNC, Lifecircle, Costa Mesa, Calif.)

TABLE 22-2 Assessment of newborn's reflexes—cont'd

REFLEX	ELICITING THE REFLEX	CHARACTERISTIC RESPONSE	COMMENTS
Pull-to-sit (traction)	Pull infant up by wrists from supine position with head in midline	Head will lag until infant is in upright position, then head will be held in same plane with chest and shoulder momentarily before falling forward; infant will attempt to right head	Response depends on general muscle tone and maturity and condition of infant
Trunk incurvation (Galant) (Fig. 22-14)	Place infant prone on flat surface, run finger down back about 4 to 5 cm lateral to spine, first on one side and then down other	Trunk is flexed and pelvis is swung toward stimulated side	Response disappears by fourth week
Magnet (Fig. 22-15)	Place infant in supine position, partially flex both lower extremities and apply pressure to soles of feet	Both lower limbs should extend against examiner's pressure	
Additional newborn responses			
Yawn, stretch, burp, hiccup, sneeze	These are spontaneous behaviors	May be slightly depressed temporarily because of maternal analgesia or anesthesia, fetal hypoxia, or infection	Parental guidance: Most of these behaviors are pleasurable to parents Parents need to be assured that behaviors are normal Sneeze is usually response to lint, etc., in nose and not an indicator of a cold No treatment is needed for hiccups, sucking may help

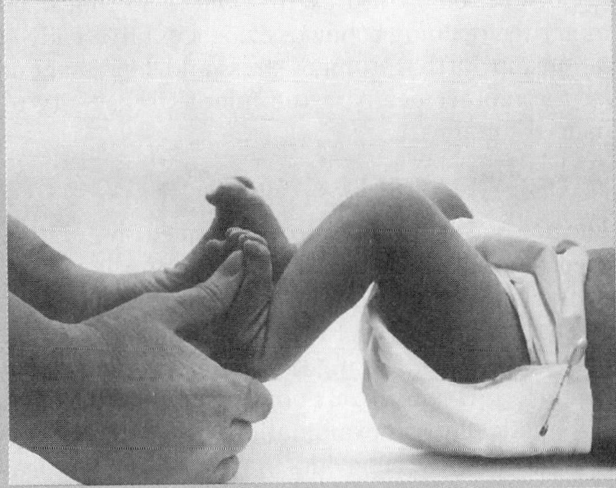

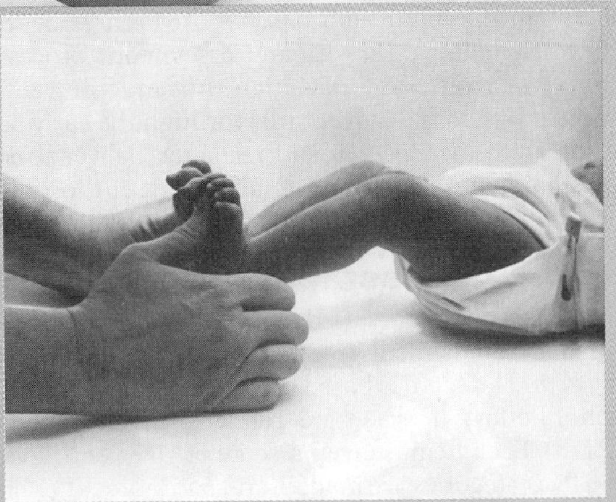

Fig. 22-15 Magnet reflex. With child in supine position and lower limbs semiflexed, light pressure is applied with fingers to both feet. Normally, while examiner's fingers maintain contact with soles of feet, the lower limbs extend. Absence of this reflex suggests damage to spinal cord or malformation. Weak reflex may be seen after breech presentation *without* extended legs or may indicate sciatic nerve stretch syndrome. Breech presentation *with* extended legs may evoke exaggerated response. (Courtesy Mead Johnson & Co., Evansville, Ind.)

The *ciliary muscles* are also immature, limiting the ability of the eyes to accommodate and fixate on an object for any length of time. The *pupils* react to light, the blink reflex is responsive to a minimal stimulus, and the corneal reflex is activated by a light touch. *Tear glands* usually do not begin to function until the infant is 2 to 4 weeks of age.

The newborn can momentarily fixate on a bright or moving object that is within 20 cm and in the midline of the visual field. In fact, the infant's ability to fixate on coordinate movement is greater during the first hour of life than during the succeeding several days. *Visual acuity* is reported to be between 20/100 and 20/400, depending on the vision measurement techniques.

The infant also demonstrates visual preferences: medium colors (yellow, green, pink) over dim or bright colors (red, orange, blue); black and white contrasting patterns, especially geometric shapes and checkerboards; large objects with medium complexity rather than small, complex objects; and reflecting objects over dull ones.

From birth onward, infants can fix their eyes and gaze intently at objects. They gaze at their parents' faces and respond to changes in them with apparent imitative effect. This ability permits parents and children to gaze into each other's eyes, and a subtle communication pattern is thereby set up. The development of eye-to-eye contact is very important for parent-infant attachment. Children of blind parents and parents who have blind children must circumvent this obstacle for the formation of a relationship.

Hearing. Once the amniotic fluid has drained from the ears, the infant probably has *auditory acuity* similar to that of an adult. The newborn is able to detect a loud sound of about 90 decibels and reacts with a startle reflex. The newborn's response to sounds of low frequency and high frequency differs; the former, such as a heartbeat, metronome, or lullaby, tends to decrease an infant's motor activity and crying, whereas the latter elicits an alerting reaction.

There is an early sensitivity to the sound of human voices and to specific speech sounds. For example, infants younger than 3 days of age can discriminate the mother's voice from that of other females (DeCasper and Fifer, 1980). As early as age 5 days, newborns can differentiate between stories repeated to them during the last trimester of pregnancy by their mother and the same stories recited after birth by a different woman (DeCasper and Spence, 1986).

The internal and middle ear structures are large at birth, but the external canal is small. The mastoid process and the bony part of the external canal have not yet developed. Consequently, the tympanic membrane and facial nerve are very close to the surface and can be easily damaged.

Smell. Newborns react to strong odors such as alcohol or vinegar by turning their heads away. Breastfed infants are able to smell breast milk and will cry for their mothers when the breasts are engorged and leaking. Infants are also able to differentiate the breast milk of their mother from the breast milk of other women by the smell (Lawrence, 1994), and maternal odors are believed to influence the attachment process.

Taste. The newborn can distinguish between tastes, and various types of solutions elicit differing gustofacial reflexes. A tasteless solution elicits no facial expression; a sweet solution elicits an eager suck and a look of satisfaction; a sour solution causes the usual puckering of the lips; and a bitter liquid produces an angry, upset expression. Newborns prefer glucose water over sterile water (Lawrence, 1994).

Critical Thinking Exercises

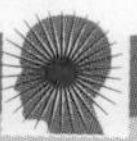

SENSORY ABILITIES AND SOCIAL RESPONSES OF THE NEONATE

Use knowledge of the newborn's sensory abilities and social responses to design a nursery (in the home) for the new baby. Focusing on these abilities, develop a list of suggestions for appropriate parent-child interactions. Discuss how this information can be used to update grandparents, knowledge of infant development (or capabilities of the infant).

Touch. The newborn perceives tactile sensation in any part of the body, although the face (especially the mouth), hands, and soles of the feet seem to be most sensitive. There is increasing documentation that touch and motion are essential to normal growth and development (Gunzenhauser, 1990). Gentle patting of the back or rubbing of the abdomen usually elicits a calming response from the infant. However, painful stimuli, such as a pinprick, elicit an angry, upset response.

The new mother uses touch (fingertip touch, soft stroking of the face, and gentle massage of the back) as one of the first interactive behaviors. Because touch between strangers is avoided in some cultures, it would seem that this automatic maternal touching behavior evidences an already intimate relationship. Birth trauma or stress and depressant drugs taken by the mother decrease the infant's sensitivity to touch or painful stimuli.

ASSESSMENT

The newborn requires thorough, skilled observation to ensure a satisfactory adjustment to extrauterine life. Physical assessment after delivery can be divided into four phases: (1) the initial assessment using the Apgar scoring system, (2) transitional assessment during the periods of reactivity, (3) assessment of gestational age, and (4) periodic assessment through systematic physical examination. In addition, the nurse must be aware of those behaviors that signal successful attachment between the infant and parents. Awareness of the expected normal findings during each assessment process helps the nurse recognize any deviation that may prevent the infant from progressing uneventfully through the early postnatal period. With increasingly shorter labor, delivery, recovery, and postpartum stays, the accomplishment of thorough newborn assessment and parent teaching has becomc a challenge.

Initial Assessment: Apgar Scoring

The most commonly used method to assess the newborn's immediate adjustment to extrauterine life is the *Apgar scoring system*. The score is based on observation of heart rate, respiratory effort, muscle tone, reflex irritability, and color (Table 22-3). Each item is given a score of 0, 1, or 2. Evaluations of all five categories are made 1 and 5 minutes after birth and are repeated until the infant's condition stabilizes. Total scores of

TABLE 22-3 Apgar scoring system

SIGN	0	1	2
Heart rate	Absent	Slow, <100	>100
Respiratory effort	Absent	Irregular, slow	Good, strong cry
Muscle tone	Limp	Some flexion of extremities	Well-flexed
Reflex irritability	No response	Grimace	Cry, sneeze
Color	Blue, pale	Body pink, extremities blue	Completely pink

0 to 3 represent severe distress, scores of 4 to 6 signify moderate difficulty, and scores of 7 to 10 indicate absence of difficulty in adjusting to extrauterine life. The Apgar score is affected by the degree of prematurity, maternal sedation or analgesia, and neuromuscular disorders.

The Apgar score reflects the general condition of the infant at 1 and 5 minutes based on the five parameters already described. The Apgar score is not a tool, however, that stands on its own to either interpret past events or predict future events linked to the infant's eventual neurologic or physical status. In addition, the Apgar score is not used to determine the newborn's need for resuscitation at birth (American Academy of Pediatrics, 1990).

Transitional Assessment: Periods of Reactivity

The newborn exhibits behavioral and physiologic characteristics that can at first appear to be signs of stress. However, during the initial 24 hours changes in heart rate, respiration, motor activity, color, mucus production, and bowel activity occur in an orderly, predictable sequence, which is normal and indicates lack of stress. Distressed infants also progress through these stages but at a slower rate.

For 6 to 8 hours after birth the newborn is in the *first period of reactivity*. During the first 30 minutes the infant is very alert, cries vigorously, may suck a fist greedily, and appears very interested in the environment. At this time the neonate's eyes are usually open, suggesting that this is an excellent opportunity for mother, father, and child to see each other. Because the newborn has a vigorous suck reflex, this is an opportune time to begin breastfeeding. The newborn usually grasps the nipple quickly, satisfying both mother and child. This is particularly important for nurses to remember, since it is likely that after this initially highly active state the infant may be quite sleepy and uninterested in sucking. Physiologically the respiratory rate can be as high as 80 breaths/min, crackles may be heard, heart rate may reach 180 beats/min, bowel sounds are active, mucus secretions are increased, and temperature may decrease slightly.

After this initial stage of alertness and activity the infant enters the *second stage* of the first reactive period, which generally lasts 2 to 4 hours. Heart and respiratory rates decrease, temperature continues to fall, mucus production decreases, and urine or stool is usually not passed. The infant is in a state of sleep and relative calm. Any attempt at stimulation usually elicits a minimal response. Because of the decrease in body temperature, undressing or bathing the infant is avoided during this time.

The *second period of reactivity* begins when the infant awakes from this deep sleep; it lasts about 2 to 5 hours and provides another excellent opportunity for child and parents to interact. The infant is again alert and responsive, heart and respiratory rates increase, the gag reflex is active, gastric and respiratory secretions are increased, and meconium is passed. This period is usually over when the amount of respiratory mucus has decreased. Following this stage is a period of stabilization of physiologic systems and a vacillating pattern of sleep and activity.

Behavioral Assessment

The healthy infant must achieve behavioral as well as biologic tasks to develop normally. Infants' behavior helps shape their environment, and their ability to react to various stimuli affects how others relate to them. The principal areas of behav-

Cultural Considerations

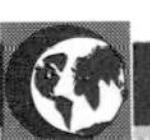

ETHNICITY AND INFANT BEHAVIOR

Researchers have found ethnic differences in infant behavior (Chitty and Winter, 1989; Freedman, 1979). Freedman (1979) found that Chinese-American infants have more self-quieting activities, fewer state changes, and more rapid responses to consoling activities than did Caucasian-American infants. A study of Navajo newborns paralleled the stereotype of the stoical impassive Native American (Freedman, 1979). Among Navajo babies, crying was rare and limb movements were reduced, and calming was almost immediate after tests for the Moro reflex. In Freedman's (1979) study, Japanese newborns were more sensitive and irritable than either the Chinese or Navajo newborns.

Asian families hold many beliefs that eating habits may result in congenital deformities. New mothers believe that cold beverages and cold food are shocking to the body and can cause problems during the postpartum period (Manio and Hall, 1987). Hispanics believe that cravings *(antojos)*, which are common in pregnancy, need to be satisfied or the newborn will have deformities often related to the wished for object. For example, the baby will have strawberry spots because the mother did not eat strawberries. Or the child may have a flat face like a tortilla because of an unsatisfied craving (Poma, 1987). A Filipino woman was told constantly by her mother-in-law that her baby's heart abnormality was caused by the mother's participating in exercise classes during pregnancy (Manio and Hall, 1987). Mexican mothers use tactile stimulation more often than vocalizations to quiet their newborns (Garcia-Coll, 1990). These studies suggest that neonatal behavior represents a behavioral phenotype, which expresses a complex relationship among genetic endowment, intrauterine environment, and maternal obstetric history (Garcia-Coll, 1990).

BOX 22-2
Clusters of Neonatal Behaviors in BNBAS

Habituation—ability to respond to and then inhibit responding to discrete stimulus (light, rattle, bell, pinprick) while asleep
Orientation—quality of alert states and ability to attend to visual and auditory stimuli while alert
Motor performance—quality of movement and tone
Range of state—measure of general arousal level or arousability of infant
Regulation of state—how infant responds when aroused
Autonomic stability—signs of stress (tremors, startles, skin color) related to homeostatic (self-regulatory) adjustment of the nervous system
Reflexes—assessment of several neonatal reflexes

ior for newborns are sleep, wakefulness, and activity, such as crying. There are ethnic differences in behavior (see the Cultural Considerations box on p. 609).

The **Brazelton Neonatal Behavioral Assessment Scale (BNBAS)** can be used to systematically assess the infant's behavior (Brazelton and Nugent, 1996). The BNBAS is an interactive examination that assesses the infant's response to 28 areas organized according to the clusters in Box 22-2. It is generally used as a research or diagnostic tool and requires special training.

The Mother's Assessment of the Behavior of her Infant (MABI) (Field et al, 1978) is based on the BNBAS and provides more parental interaction in the assessment of infant behavior.

In addition to use as initial and ongoing tools to assess neurologic and behavioral responses, the scales can be used to assess initial parent-child relationships and as a guide for parents to help them focus on their infant's individuality and to develop a deeper attachment to their child. Studies demonstrate that by showing parents the unique characteristics of their infant, a more positive perception of the infant develops, with increased interaction between infant and parent (Beal, 1989).

Patterns of sleep and activity. Newborns begin life with a systematic schedule of sleep and activity that is initially evident during the periods of reactivity. For the next 2 to 3 days, it is not unusual for infants to sleep almost constantly to recover from the exhausting birth process.

The infant's sleep comprises six distinct states; *state* refers to an interaction between the infant and the environment in which the infant's behaviors form a continuum from arousal to consciousness (Table 22-4). The cycle of these sleep states is highly variable and is based on the number of hours an infant sleeps per day, which may range anywhere from 10½ to 23 hours (average of 16½ hours). About 50% of total sleep time is spent in irregular or REM sleep. Sleep periods last 20 minutes to 6 hours with little day-night differentiation (Ferber, 1987).

Each state has its distinguishing characteristics and **state-related behaviors.** The quiet alert state is also termed the *optimum state of arousal.* During this state, infants may be observed smiling, vocalizing, or moving in synchrony (occurring

Critical Thinking Exercises 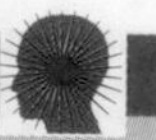
ETHNIC COMPARISONS OF NEONATES

Observe and record findings of normal newborns of at least two ethnic groups immediately after birth and in a follow-up period. Include both physiologic and behavioral data and compare findings. How can this information be used in planning care?

simultaneously) with speech. Even during the first day of life, smiling is evident in a surprising number of infants (Bamford et al, 1990). Newborns seem to watch their parents' faces carefully and respond to other people talking to them. Many infants begin a type of vocalizing by the time they are 2 weeks of age, making small, throaty, cooing noises while feeding.

The term infant uses purposeful behavior to maintain the optimum arousal state, as follows:

- Active withdrawal by increasing physical distance
- A rejecting motion of pushing away with hands and feet
- Decreasing sensitivity by falling asleep or breaking eye contact by turning head
- Use of signaling behaviors, such as fussing or crying (Brazelton and Nugent, 1996).

Use of such behaviors permits infants to quiet themselves and reinstate readiness to interact.

It is important for parents to understand these states and the methods effective in altering them. An aware infant exhibits more motor activity before feeding than after. Feeding usually terminates the state of crying when hunger is the cause. Swaddling or wrapping an infant snugly in a blanket both promotes sleep and maintains body temperature. Intermittent, vertical rocking promotes more bright-alert behavior, whereas continuous, horizontal rocking induces more drowsy behavior.

Cry. The newborn should begin extrauterine life with a strong, lusty cry. The sounds produced by crying can be described as hunger, anger, pain, and "bid for attention" cries. Discomfort (pain) sounds initially consist of gasps and cries in which the constant *H* is clearly distinguishable. The duration of crying is as highly variable in each infant as is the duration of sleep patterns. Some newborns may cry for as little as 5 minutes or as much as 2 hours or more per day.

Variations in the initial cry can indicate abnormalities. A weak, groaning cry or grunt during expiration usually indicates severe respiratory disturbances. Absent, weak, or constant crying may suggest brain damage. A high-pitched, shrill cry may be a sign of increased intracranial pressure.

Assessment of Attachment Behaviors

One of the most important areas of assessment is careful observation of those behaviors thought to indicate the formation of emotional bonds between the newborn and family, especially the mother. Although the words "bonding" and "attachment" are sometimes referred to as separate phenomena, with *bonding* representing the development of emotional ties from parent to infant and *attachment* representing the emotional ties from infant to parent, in this discussion the words are used interchangeably to denote both processes.

TABLE 22-4 States of sleep and activity

BEHAVIOR		DURATION	IMPLICATIONS FOR PARENTING
Deep sleep Closed eyes Regular breathing No movement except for sudden bodily jerks	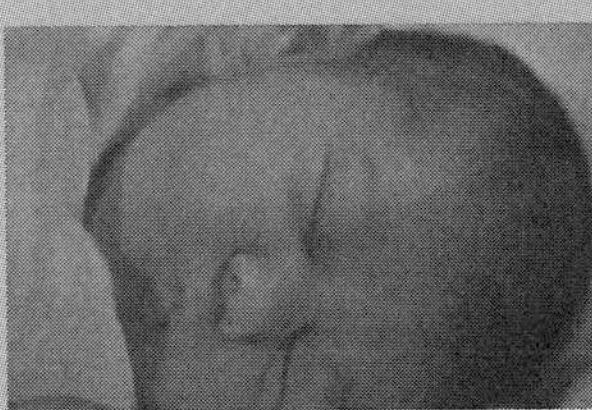	4 to 5 hrs/day, 10 to 20 mins/sleep cycle	External stimuli do not arouse infant Continue usual house noises Leave infant alone if sudden loud noise awakens infant and child cries
Light sleep Closed eyes, REM Irregular breathing Slight muscular twitching of body	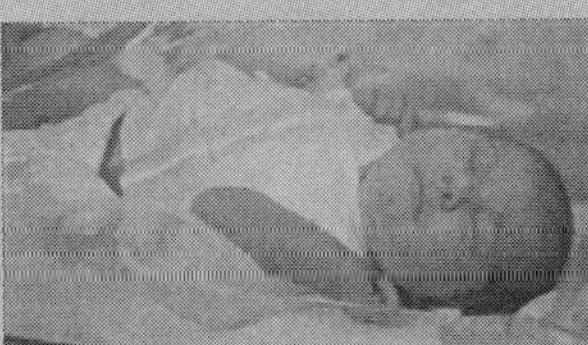	12 to 15 hrs/day, 20 to 45 mins/sleep cycle	External stimuli that did not arouse infant during regular sleep may minimally arouse child Periodic groaning or crying is usual; do not interpret as an indication of pain or discomfort
Drowsiness Eyes open and close Irregular breathing Active body movement	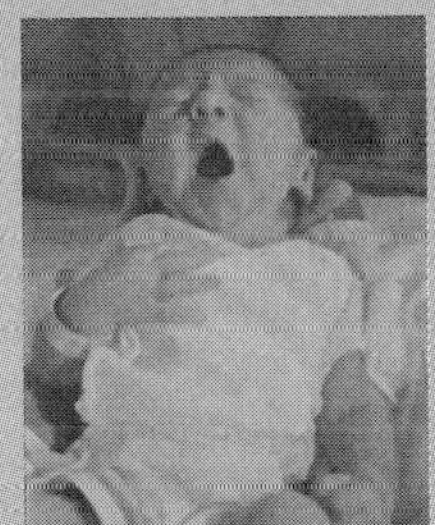	Variable	Most stimuli arouse infant Pick infant up during this time rather than leave in crib
Quiet alert Eyes open Regular breathing Very little body movement May smile or vocalize	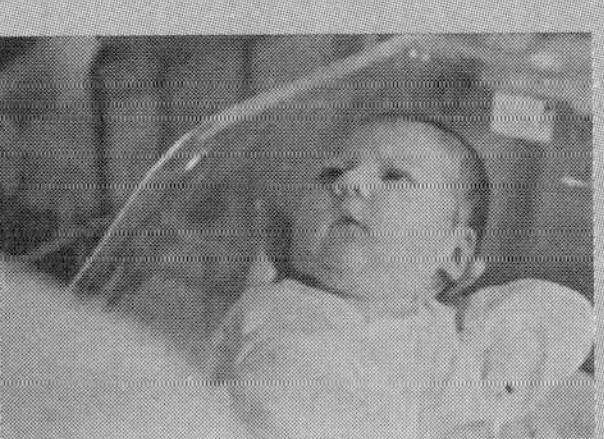	2 to 3 hrs/day	Good time to interact with infant Maintains eye contact Orients to visual stimuli
Active alert Responds to environment by active body movement and staring at close-range objects Periods of fussiness	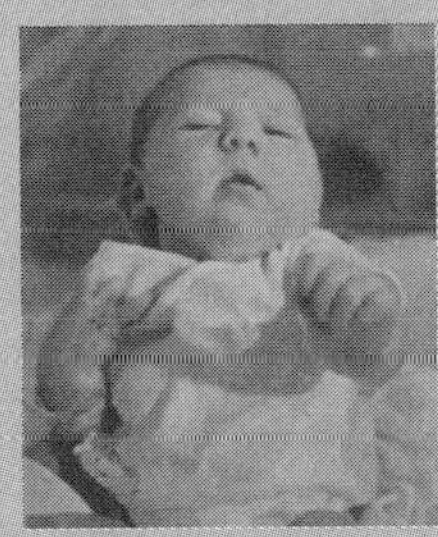	2 to 3 hrs/day	Satisfy infant's needs such as hunger Place infant in area of home where activity is continuous Place toys in crib or playpen Place objects within 17.5 to 20 cm of infant's view
Crying May begin with whimpering and slight body movement Progresses to strong, angry crying, and uncoordinated thrashing of extremities	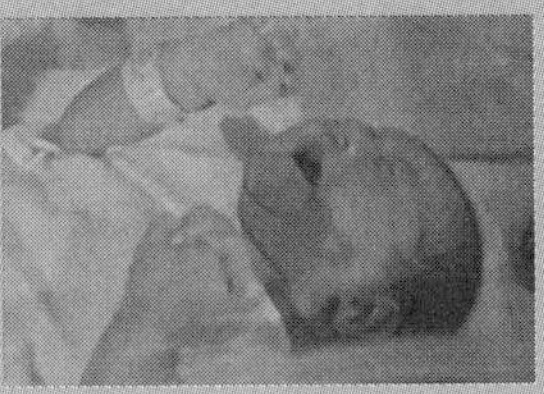	1 to 4 hrs/day	Remove intense internal or external stimuli Stimuli that were effective during alert inactivity are usually ineffective Rock and swaddle to decrease crying

Photos courtesy March of Dimes Birth Defects Foundation.

NEUROMUSCULAR MATURITY

	−1	0	1	2	3	4	5
Posture							
Square Window (wrist)	> 90°	90°	60°	45°	30°	0°	
Arm Recoil		180°	140° - 180°	110° 140°	90° - 110°	< 90°	
Popliteal Angle	180°	160°	140°	120°	100°	90°	< 90°
Scarf Sign							
Heel to Ear							

A PHYSICAL MATURITY

Skin	sticky friable transparent	gelatinous red, translucent	smooth pink, visible veins	superficial peeling &/or rash, few veins	cracking pale areas rare veins	parchment deep cracking no vessels	leathery cracked wrinkled
Lanugo	none	sparse	abundant	thinning	bald areas	mostly bald	
Plantar Surface	heel-toe 40-50 mm: -1 <40 mm: -2	>50 mm no crease	faint red marks	anterior transverse crease only	creases ant. 2/3	creases over entire sole	
Breast	imperceptible	barely perceptible	flat areola no bud	stippled areola 1-2 mm bud	raised areola 3-4 mm bud	full areola 5-10 mm bud	
Eye/Ear	lids fused loosely: -1 tightly: -2	lids open pinna flat stays folded	sl. curved pinna; soft; slow recoil	well-curved pinna; soft but ready recoil	formed & firm instant recoil	thick cartilage ear stiff	
Genitals (male)	scrotum flat, smooth	scrotum empty faint rugae	testes in upper canal rare rugae	testes descending few rugae	testes down good rugae	testes pendulous deep rugae	
Genitals (female)	clitoris prominent labia flat	prominent clitoris small labia minora	prominent clitoris enlarging minora	majora & minora equally prominent	majora large minora small	majora cover clitoris & minora	

MATURITY RATING

score	weeks
-10	20
-5	22
0	24
5	26
10	28
15	30
20	32
25	34
30	36
35	38
40	40
45	42
50	44

Fig. 22-16 Estimation of gestational age. **A,** New Ballard Scale for newborn maturity rating. Expanded scale includes extremely premature infants and has been refined to improve accuracy in more mature infants. (**A** from Ballard J et al: New Ballard Score, expanded to include extremely premature infants, *J Pediatr* 119:418, 1991.).

Unlike physical assessment of the neonate, which has concrete guidelines to follow, assessment of parent-child attachment requires much more skill in terms of observation and interviewing. The assessment process is even more challenging, with the trend toward 24-hour delivery and postpartum admissions. However, rooming-in of mother and infant and liberal visiting privileges for father, siblings, and grandparents facilitate recognition of behaviors that demonstrate positive or negative attachment. Guidelines for assessment of bonding behaviors are presented in the Guidelines box on p. 614.

Talking to the parents uncovers many variables that can affect the development of attachment and parenting. What expectations do they have for this child? In other words, how similar are their predictions of the fantasy child and their realizations about the real child? Encourage them to talk about their relationship with their own parents, since the type of parenting that parents received as a child influences their child-rearing practices. Is this a planned birth? How do they see the addition of a dependent family member affecting their life-style? What arrangements have they made in terms of such changes in life-style? What support system or significant others are available for assistance? What are their views regarding childrearing?

The labor process also significantly affects the immediate

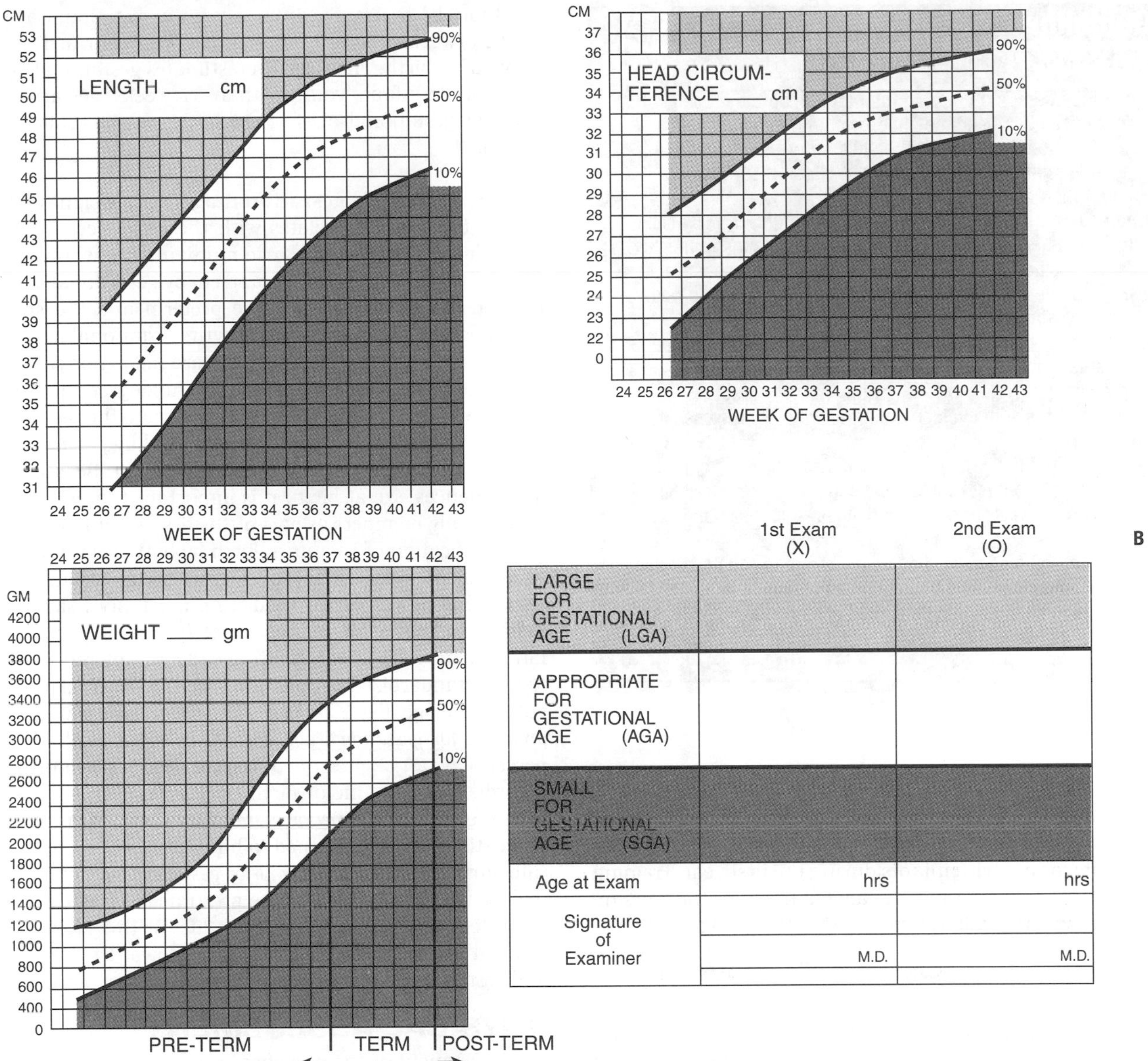

Fig. 22-16, cont'd **B,** Newborn classification based on maturity and intrauterine growth. (**B** modified from Lubchenco L, Hansman C, Boyd E: Intrauterine growth in length and head circumference as estimated from live births at gestational ages from 26 to 42 weeks, J Pediatr 37(3):403, 1966; and Battaglia F, Lubchenco L: A practical classification of newborn infants by weight and gestationl age, J Pediatr 712:159, 1967).

attachment of mothers to their newborn children. Factors such as a long labor, feeling tired or "drugged" after delivery, and problems with breastfeeding can delay the development of initial positive feelings toward the newborn (Pascoe and French, 1989).

During pregnancy, and often even before conception occurs, parents develop an image of the "ideal" or "fantasy infant." The unborn child has an imagined appearance, pattern of behavior, expected accomplishments, and predetermined effect on the life-style of the family. At birth the fantasy infant becomes the real infant. How closely the dream child resembles the real child influences the bonding process. Assessing such expectations during pregnancy and at the time of the infant's birth allows identification of discrepancies in the parents' view of the fantasy child vs. the real child.

Since attachment involves a mutually reciprocal interchange, observing the interaction between parent and infant is very important. An excellent opportunity exists during feeding. A useful instrument for systematically describing the parent's and infant's behaviors is the *Nursing Child Assessment Feeding Scale (NCAFS)* (Barnard, 1994). It consists of 76 behavioral items; 50 items describe the parent's behavior regarding sensitivity to cues, response to child's distress, social-emotional growth fosterings, and cognitive growth fostering. Twenty-six items focus on the child's behavior in terms of clarity of cues and responsiveness to parent. The results can

Guidelines

ASSESSING ATTACHMENT BEHAVIOR

When the infant is brought to the parents, do they reach out for the child and call the child by name?

Do the parents speak about the child in terms of identification—whom the infant looks like; what appears special about their child over other infants?

When parents are holding the infant, what kind of body contact is there—do parents feel at ease in changing the infant's position; are fingertips or whole hands used; are there parts of the body they avoid touching or parts of the body they investigate and scrutinize?

When the infant is awake, what kinds of stimulation do the parents provide—do they talk to the infant, to each other, or to no one; how do they look at the infant—direct visual contact, avoidance of eye contact, or looking at other people or objects?

How comfortable do the parents appear in terms of caring for the infant? Do they express any concern regarding their ability or disgust for certain activities, such as changing diapers?

What type of affection do they demonstrate to the newborn, such as smiling, stroking, kissing, or rocking?

If the infant is fussy, what kinds of comforting techniques do the parents use, such as rocking, swaddling, talking, or stroking?

also be shared with the parent to encourage discussion of feelings about the infant and to highlight behaviors of the dyad that foster successful interaction (Fuller, 1990). The NCAFS is appropriate for use with infants during the first year. Training to become a certified tester is available through the Nursing Child Assessment Satellite Training (NCAST) program.*

Assessment of Clinical Gestational Age

Assessment of gestational age is important because perinatal morbidity and mortality are related to gestational age and birth weight. A commonly used method of determining gestational age is the simplified *Assessment of Gestational Age* by Ballard, Novak, and Driver (1979) (Fig. 22-16). The Ballard scale, an abbreviated version of the *Dubowitz scale,* can be used to measure gestational ages of infants between 35 and 42 weeks (Dubowitz and Dubowitz, 1977). It assesses six external physical and six neuromuscular signs. Each sign has a number score, and the cumulative score correlates with a maturity rating of from 26 to 44 weeks of gestation.

The *New Ballard Scale,* a revision of the original scale, can be used with newborns as young as 20 weeks' gestation. The tool has the same physical and neuromuscular sections but includes −1 to −2 scores that reflect signs of extremely premature infants, such as fused eyelids; imperceptible breast tissue; sticky friable transparent skin; no lanugo; and square-window (flexion of wrist) angle greater than 90 degrees (Fig. 22-16, *A*). The examination of infants with a gestational age of 20 weeks or less should be performed at a postnatal age of less than 12 hours. For infants with a gestational age of at least 26 weeks, the examination can be performed up to 96 hours after birth. The scale overestimates gestational age by 2 to 4 days in infants younger than 37 weeks' gestation, especially at gestational ages of 32 to 37 weeks (Ballard et al, 1991).

Weight related to gestational age. The weight of the infant at birth also correlates with the incidence of perinatal morbidity and mortality. Since many infants who weigh less than 2500 g (5½ lb) are not preterm by gestational age, there is often confusion between the preterm and the small-for-gestational-age infants; fetal growth, gestational age, and fetal maturity are closely related but are not synonymous. Maturity implies functional capacity—the degree to which the neonate's organ systems are able to adapt to the requirements of extrauterine life. Therefore gestational age is more closely related to fetal maturity than is birth weight. Because heredity influences size at birth, it is important to note the size of other family members as part of the assessment process.

Classification of infants at birth by both weight and gestational age provides a more satisfactory method than weight or gestational age alone for predicting mortality risks and providing guidelines for management of the neonate. The infant's birth weight, length, and head circumference are plotted on standardized graphs that identify normal values for gestational age (Fig. 22-16, *B*). The infant whose weight is *appropriate for gestational age (AGA)* (between 10th and 90th percentile) can be presumed to have grown at a normal rate regardless of the time of birth—preterm, term, or postterm. The infant who is *large for gestational age (LGA)* (above 90th percentile) can be presumed to have grown at an accelerated rate during fetal life; the *small-for-gestational-age (SGA)* infant (below 10th percentile) can be presumed to have grown at a restricted rate during intrauterine life. Birth weight and gestational age influence mortality—the lower the birth weight and gestational age, the higher the risk of mortality.

PHYSICAL ASSESSMENT

The assessment of the newborn should progress in a systematic way from head to toe, with each system being evaluated or assessed. It may be performed in the nursery, in the labor and delivery room, in the recovery room, or at the mother's bedside (see the Guidelines box on p. 615). The following steps are included in a newborn assessment. Table 22-5 summarizes the newborn assessment.

General Appearance

The neonate's maturity level can be gauged by assessment of general appearance. Features to assess in the general survey include posture, head size, lanugo, vernix caseosa, breast tissue, sole creases, cry, and state of alertness. The normal resting position of the neonate is one of general flexion. The umbilicus is the center of the newborn's body. The neck is short, and the abdomen is rounded.

Vital Signs

Temperature. Changes in environmental temperature have the potential to disturb the body temperature. This may cause serious consequences in the newborn. Brown fat metabolism is activated in response to changes in environmental temper-

*For information contact Georgina Sumner, RN, MS, Director, NCAST, University of Washington, NCAST, WJ-10, Seattle, WA 98195; (206) 543-8528.

Guidelines

PHYSICAL EXAMINATION OF THE NEWBORN

Check that equipment and supplies are working properly and are accessible.
Provide a normothermic and nonstimulating examination area.
Undress only body area examined to prevent heat loss.
Proceed in an orderly sequence (usually head to toe) with the following exceptions:
- Observe infant's attitude and position of flexion first to avoid disturbing him/her.
- Perform all procedures that require quiet first, such as auscultating the lungs, heart, and abdomen.
- Perform disturbing procedures, such as testing reflexes, last.
- Measure head, chest, and length at same time to compare results.

Proceed quickly to avoid stressing infant.
Comfort infant during and after examination; involve parent in the following:
- Talk softly.
- Hold infant's hands against chest.
- Swaddle and hold.
- Give pacifier or gloved finger to suck.

ature that are perceived by the thermal sensors in the newborn's skin, even when the temperature of the newborn is unchanged. The newborn does not have the adult's abilities to change body posture to decrease the amount of skin surface exposed (e.g., flexion of extremities) in response to cold. When exposed to cold the newborn may cry, become restless, and increase muscular activity in an effort to generate heat. However, crying increases work load and energy is expended.

Axillary temperatures are a safe, accurate substitute for rectal temperatures (Yetman et al, 1993). The use of electronic thermometers has expedited the performance of this task and provides a reading within 1 minute. If a standard mercury thermometer is used, it should be held in place for at least 3 minutes. Taking an infant's temperature may cause the infant to cry and struggle against the placement of the thermometer in the axilla. Tympanic thermometers may be helpful in determining infants' thermal state. Before taking the temperature the examiner should take an apical heart rate and count the respiratory rate while the infant is quiet. The normal axillary temperature averages 37° C (98.6° F) with a range from 36.5° to 37.2° C (97.6° to 99° F).

Respiration. The respiratory rate varies with the state of alertness after birth. The average respiratory rate is 40 breaths/min but will vary between 30 and 60 breaths/min or may be higher than 60 breaths/min if the newborn is very active or crying. Respirations are abdominal in nature and can be counted by observing or by lightly feeling the rise and fall of the abdomen. Neonatal respirations are shallow and irregular. It is important to count the respirations for a full minute to obtain an accurate count because of normal short periods of apnea. The examiner should also observe for symmetry of chest movement.

Most term infants establish respirations spontaneously and continue to have adequate respirations. However, infants can manifest other problems through respiratory distress. Signs of respiratory distress may include nasal flaring, retractions (indrawing of tissue between ribs, below rib cage, or above sternum and clavicles), or audible grunting with expirations. Any increased use of intercostal muscles may be a sign of distress. *Seesaw respirations* instead of normal respirations are not normal and should be reported immediately (Fig. 22-1, *B*). A respiratory rate that is less than 30 or greater than 60 breaths/min, with the infant at rest, must be evaluated further. The respiratory rate of the infant may be influenced (slowed/depressed) by the analgesics or anesthetics the mother received during labor and birth. Apneic periods longer than 15 seconds must be reported to the clinician for evaluation. Even normal-appearing infants bear close observation because changes in the respiratory system can occur very rapidly.

Heart rate. Apical pulse rates should be obtained on all infants. Auscultation should be for a full minute, preferably when the infant is asleep. The infant may need to be held and comforted during assessment. Heart rate may range from 100 to 180 beats/min shortly after birth and, when the infant's condition has stabilized, from 120 to 140 beats/min.

Auscultation of the specific components of the *heart sounds* is difficult because of the rapid rate and effective transmission of respiratory sounds. However, the *first (S1)* and *second (S2) sounds* should be clear and well defined; the second sound is somewhat higher in pitch and sharper than the first. *Murmurs* are often heard in the newborn, especially over the base of the heart or at the left sternal border in the third or fourth interspace. Ordinarily they are not associated with specific cardiac defects, since they commonly represent the incomplete functional closure of fetal shunts. However, any murmur or other unusual sounds should always be recorded and reported.

Nursing ALERT

Because auscultation of neonatal breath sounds and heart tones is often difficult for the novice untrained ear, practice auscultating one parameter at a time. Close your eyes and mentally block out the extraneous sounds heard, such as room noise or neonatal movement; offer the newborn a pacifier. Auscultation of a murmur and decreased air movement in specific lung fields requires patience and practice; it may require auscultating the heart tones or breath sounds for 1 to 3 minutes each.

Weak or absent femoral pulses may indicate coarctation of the aorta or a blood clot within the vascular system. To palpate femoral pulses, the thighs are flexed on the hips, the fingers are placed along the inguinal ligament about midway between the symphysis pubis and the iliac crest, and pulses are palpated bilaterally at the same time. Femoral pulses should be equal and strong.

Blood pressure. Measurement of *blood pressure (BP)* provides useful baseline data and may indicate cardiac problems. BP is most easily and accurately assessed using oscillometry (Dinamap), although the device is less reliable when the mean arterial BP is below 40 mm Hg. It is important to use the correct size BP cuff. The average oscillometric systolic/diastolic

Text continued on p. 620.

TABLE 22-5 Summary of physical assessment of the newborn

USUAL FINDINGS	COMMON VARIATIONS/MINOR ABNORMALITIES	POTENTIAL SIGNS OF DISTRESS/ MAJOR ABNORMALITIES
General measurements		
Head circumference—33-35 cm; about 2-3 cm larger than chest circumference (Fig. 22-18, *A*) *Chest circumference*—30.5-33 cm (Fig. 22-18, *B*) *Crown-to-rump length*—31-35 cm; approximately equal to head circumference *Head-to-heel length*—48-53 cm (Fig. 22-18, *D*)	Molding after birth may decrease head circumference Head and chest circumference may be equal for first 1-2 days after birth	Head circumference <10th or >90th percentile
Birth weight—2700-4000 g (Fig. 22-17)	Loss of 10% of birth weight in first week; regained in 10-14 days	Birth weight <10th or >90th percentile
Vital signs		
Temperature		
Axillary—36.5°-37° C (97.9°-98° F)	Crying may increase body temperature slightly Radiant warmer will falsely increase axillary temperature	Hypothermia Hyperthermia
Heart rate		
Apical—120-140 beats/min	Crying will increase heart rate; sleep will decrease heart rate During first period of reactivity (6-8 hours), rate can reach 180 beats/min	Bradycardia—Resting rate below 80-100 beats/min Tachycardia—Rate above 160-180 beats/min Irregular rhythm
Respirations		
30-60 breaths/min	Crying will increase respiratory rate; sleep will decrease respiratory rate During first period of reactivity (6-8 hours), rate can reach 80 breaths/min	Tachypnea—Rate above 60 breaths/min Apnea >15 seconds
Blood pressure		
Oscillometric—65/41 mm Hg in arm and calf	Crying and activity will increase BP Placing cuff on thigh may agitate infant; thigh-blood pressure (BP) may be higher than arm or calf BP by 4-8 mm Hg	Oscillometric systolic pressure in calf 6-9 mm Hg less than in upper extremity (sign of coarctation of aorta)
General appearance		
Posture—Flexion of head and extremities, which rest on chest and abdomen	*Frank breech*—Extended legs, abducted and fully rotated thighs, flattened occiput, extended neck	Limp posture, extension of extremities
Skin		
At birth, bright red, puffy, smooth Second to third day, pink, flaky, dry Vernix caseosa Lanugo Edema around eyes, face, legs, dorsa of hands, feet, and scrotum or labia *Acrocyanosis*—Cyanosis of hands and feet *Cutis marmorata*—Transient mottling when infant is exposed to decreased temperature	Neonatal jaundice after first 24 hours Ecchymoses or petechiae caused by birth trauma *Milia*—Distended sebaceous glands that appear as tiny white papules on cheeks, chin, and nose *Miliaria or sudamina*—Distended sweat (eccrine) glands that appear as minute vesicles, especially on face *Erythema toxicum*—Pink papular rash with vesicles superimposed on thorax, back, buttocks, and abdomen; may appear in 24-48 hrs and resolve after several days *Harlequin color change*—Clearly outlined color change as infant lies on side; lower half of body becomes pink, and upper half is pale	Progressive jaundice, especially in first 24 hours Cracked or peeling skin Generalized cyanosis Pallor Mottling Grayness Plethora Hemorrhage, ecchymoses, or petechiae that persist *Sclerema*—Hard and stiff skin Poor skin turgor Rashes, pustules, or blisters *Café-au-lait spots*—Light brown spots *Nevus flammeus*—Port wine stain (Fig. 22-19, *C*) *Nevus vasculosis:* Strawberry mark (Fig. 22-16, *B*)

TABLE 22-5 Summary of physical assessment of the newborn—cont'd

USUAL FINDINGS	COMMON VARIATIONS/MINOR ABNORMALITIES	POTENTIAL SIGNS OF DISTRESS/ DISTRESS/MAJOR ABNORMALITIES
Skin—cont'd		
	Mongolian spots—Irregular areas of deep blue pigmentation, usually in sacral and gluteal regions; seen predominantly in newborns of African, Native American, Asian, or Hispanic descent *Telangiectatic nevi ("stork bites")*—Flat, deep pink localized areas usually seen in back of neck (Fig. 22-19, *A*)	
Head		
Anterior fontanel—Diamond shaped, 2.5-4.0 cm (see Fig. 8-6) *Posterior fontanel*—Triangular, 0.5-1 cm Fontanels should be flat, soft, and firm Widest part of fontanel measured from bone to bone, not suture to suture	Molding after vaginal delivery (Fig. 22-7) Third sagittal (parietal) fontanel Bulging fontanel because of crying or coughing *Caput succedaneum*—Edema of soft scalp tissue *Cephalhematoma* (uncomplicated)—Hematoma between periosteum and skull bone	Fused sutures Bulging or depressed fontanels when quiet Widened sutures and fontanels *Craniotabes*—Snapping sensation along lambdoid suture that resembles indentation of ping-pong ball
Eyes		
Lids usually edematous Color—Slate gray, dark blue, brown Absence of tears Presence of red reflex Corneal reflex in response to touch Pupillary reflex in response to light Blink reflex in response to light or touch Rudimentary fixation on objects and ability to follow to midline	Epicanthal folds in Asian infants Searching nystagmus or strabismus *Subconjunctival (scleral) hemorrhages*—Ruptured capillaries, usually at limbus	Pink color of iris Purulent discharge Upward slant in non-Asians Hypertelorism (3 cm or greater) Hypotelorism Congenital cataracts Constricted or dilated fixed pupil Absence of red reflex Absence of pupillary or corneal reflex Inability to follow object or bright light to midline Blue sclera Yellow sclera
Ears		
Position—Top of pinna on horizontal line with outer canthus of eye Startle reflex elicited by a loud, sudden noise Pinna flexible, cartilage present	Inability to visualize tympanic membrane because of filled aural canals Pinna flat against head Irregular shape or size Pits or skin tags	Low placement of ears Absence of startle reflex in response to loud noise Minor abnormalities may be signs of various syndromes, especially renal
Nose		
Nasal patency Nasal discharge—thin white mucus Sneezing	Flattened and bruised	Nonpatent canals Thick, bloody nasal discharge Flaring of nares (alae nasi) Copious nasal secretions or stuffiness (may be minor)
Mouth and throat		
Intact, high-arched palate Uvula in midline Frenulum of tongue Frenum of upper lip Sucking reflex—Strong and coordinated Rooting reflex Gag reflex Extrusion reflex Absent or minimal salivation Vigorous cry	*Natal teeth*—Teeth present at birth; benign but may be associated with congenital defects *Epstein pearls*—Small, white epithelial cysts along midline of hard palate	Cleft lip Cleft palate Large, protruding tongue or posterior displacement of tongue Profuse salivation or drooling *Candidiasis (thrush)*—White, adherent patches on tongue, palate, and buccal surfaces Inability to pass nasogastric tube Hoarse, high-pitched, weak, absent, or other abnormal cry

Continued.

TABLE 22-5 Summary of physical assessment of the newborn—cont'd

USUAL FINDINGS	COMMON VARIATIONS/MINOR ABNORMALITIES	POTENTIAL SIGNS OF DISTRESS/ MAJOR ABNORMALITIES
Neck		
Short, thick, usually surrounded by skinfolds Tonic neck reflex	*Torticollis* (wry neck)—Head held to one side with chin pointing to opposite side	Excessive skinfolds Resistant to flexion Absence of tonic neck reflex Fractured clavicle
Chest		
Anteroposterior and lateral diameters equal Slight sternal retractions evident during inspiration Xiphoid process evident Breast enlargement	Funnel chest (pectus excavatum) Pigeon chest (pectus carinatum) Supernumerary nipples Secretion of milky substance from breasts ("witch's milk")	Depressed sternum Marked retractions of chest and intercostal spaces during respiration Asymmetric chest expansion Redness and firmness around nipples Wide-spaced nipples
Lungs		
Respirations chiefly abdominal Cough reflex absent at birth, present by 1-2 days Bilateral equal bronchial breath sounds	Rate and depth of respirations may be irregular, periodic breathing Crackles shortly after birth	Inspiratory stridor Expiratory grunt Retractions Persistent irregular breathing Periodic breathing with repeated apneic spells Seesaw respirations (paradoxical) Unequal breath sounds Persistent fine crackles Wheezing Diminished breath sounds Peristaltic sounds on one side, with diminished breath sounds on same side
Heart		
Apex—Fourth to fifth intercostal space, lateral to left sternal border S_2 slightly sharper and higher in pitch than S_1	*Sinus arrhythmia*—Heart rate increases with inspiration and decreases with expiration Transient cyanosis on crying or straining	*Dextrocardia*—Heart on right side Displacement of apex, muffled Cardiomegaly Abdominal shunts Murmurs Thrills Persistent cyanosis Hyperactive precordium
Abdomen		
Cylindric in shape (Fig. 22-18, *C*) *Liver*—Palpable 2-3 cm below right costal margin *Spleen*—Tip palpable at end of first week of age *Kidneys*—Palpable 1-2 cm above umbilicus *Umbilical cord*—Bluish white at birth with two arteries and one vein *Femoral pulses*—Equal bilaterally	Umbilical hernia *Diastasis recti*—Midline gap between recti muscles *Wharton's jelly*—unusually thick umbilical cord	Abdominal distention Localized bulging Distended veins Absent bowel sounds Enlarged liver and spleen Ascites Visible peristaltic waves Scaphoid or concave abdomen Green umbilical cord Presence of only one artery in cord Urine or stool leaking from cord Palpable bladder distention following scanty voiding Absent femoral pulses Cord bleeding or hematoma
Female genitalia (Fig. 22-5)		
Labia and clitoris usually edematous Urethral meatus behind clitoris Vernix caseosa between labia Urination within 24 hrs	*Pseudomenstruation*—Blood-tinged or mucoid discharge Hymenal tag	Enlarged clitoris with urethral meatus at tip Fused labia Absence of vaginal opening Meconium from vaginal opening No urination within 24 hours Masses in labia Ambiguous genitalia

TABLE 22-5 Summary of physical assessment of the newborn—cont'd

USUAL FINDINGS	COMMON VARIATIONS/MINOR ABNORMALITIES	POTENTIAL SIGNS OF DISTRESS/MAJOR ABNORMALITIES
Male genitalia (Fig. 22-5)		
Urethral opening at tip of glans penis Testes palpable in scrotum Scrotum usually large, edematous, pendulous, and covered with rugae; usually deeply pigmented in dark-skinned ethnic groups Smegma Urination within 24 hours	Urethral opening covered by prepuce Inability to retract foreskin *Epithelial pearls*—Small, firm, white lesions at tip of prepuce Erection or priapism Testes palpable in inguinal canal Scrotum small *Hydrocele*—Fluid in scrotum	*Hypospadias*—Urethral opening on ventral surface of penis *Epispadias*—Urethral opening on dorsal surface of penis *Chordee*—Ventral curvature of penis Testes not palpable in scrotum or inguinal canal No urination within 24 hours Inguinal hernia Hypoplastic scrotum Masses in scrotum Meconium from scrotum Discoloration of testes Ambiguous genitalia
Back and rectum		
Spine intact, no openings, masses, or prominent curves Trunk incurvation reflex Anal reflex Patent anal opening Passage of meconium within 48 hours	Green liquid stools in infant under phototherapy Delayed passage of meconium in very-low-birth-weight neonates	Anal fissures or fistulas Imperforate anus Absence of anal reflex No meconium within 36 hours Pilonidal cyst or sinus Tuft of hair along spine Spina bifida (any degree)
Extremities		
Ten fingers and toes Full range of motion Nail beds pink, with transient cyanosis immediately after birth Creases on anterior two thirds of sole Sole usually flat Symmetry of extremities Equal muscle tone bilaterally, especially resistance to opposing flexion Equal bilateral brachial pulses	Partial syndactyly between second and third toes Second toe overlapping into third toe Wide gap between first (hallux) and second toes Deep crease on plantar surface of foot between first and second toes Asymmetric length of toes Dorsiflexion and shortness of hallux	*Polydactyly*—Extra digits *Syndactyly*—Fused or webbed digits *Phocomelia*—Hands or feet attached close to trunk *Hemimelia*—Absence of distal part of extremity Hyperflexibility of joints Persistent cyanosis of nail beds Yellowing of nail beds Sole covered with creases Transverse palmar (simian) crease Fractures Decreased or absent range of motion *Dislocated or subluxated hip* Limitation in hip abduction Unequal gluteal or leg folds Unequal knee height (Allis or Galeazz sign) Audible click on abduction (Ortolani sign) Asymmetry of extremities Unequal muscle tone or range of motion
Neuromuscular system		
Extremities usually maintain some degree of flexion Extension of an extremity followed by previous position of flexion Head lag while sitting, but momentary ability to hold head erect Able to turn head from side to side when prone Able to hold head in horizontal line with back when held prone	Quivering or momentary tremors	*Hypotonia*—Floppy, poor head control, extremities limp *Hypertonia*—Jittery, arms and hands tightly flexed, legs stiffly extended, startles easily Asymmetric posturing (except tonic neck reflex) *Opisthotonic posturing*—Arched back Signs of paralysis Tremors, twitches, and myoclonic jerks Marked head lag in all positions

BP is 65/41 mm Hg at 1 to 3 days of age. BP in the upper and lower extremities are compared and should be equal.

Baseline Measurements of Physical Growth

Baseline measurements must be taken and recorded to help assess the progress of the neonate. Measurements are used to determine the neonate's growth patterns. These may be recorded on growth charts.

Weight. The newborn is usually weighed shortly after birth. This may be done in the labor and birthing area or on admission to a nursery. Care must be taken to ensure the scales are balanced. The totally unclothed neonate is placed in the center of the scale, which is usually covered with a disposable pad or diaper to prevent heat loss via conduction. The nurse should place one hand over the neonate to prevent the infant from falling off the scales (Fig. 22-17). It is not uncommon for the newborn to jerk and have tremors or even cry when placed on the scales. It is common practice to weigh the infant at the same time every day and on the same scales during the hospital stay.

Birth weight of a term infant ranges from 2500 to 4000 g (5 lb, 8 oz to 8 lb, 13 oz). Neonates lose about 10% or less of

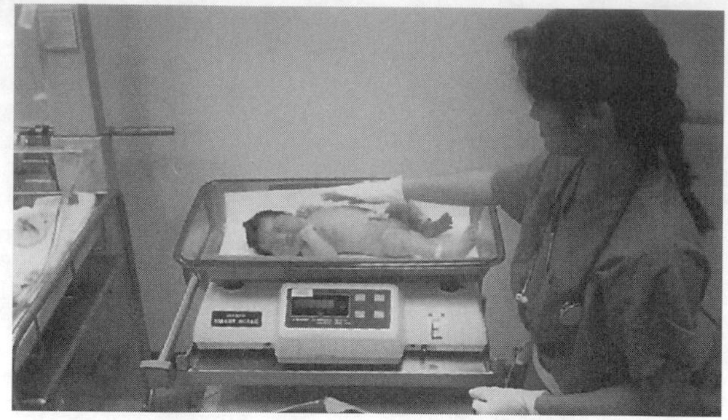

Fig. 22-17 Weighing the infant. Note that a hand is held over infant as a safety measure. The scale is covered to protect against cross infection. (Courtesy Kim Molloy, San Jose, Calif.)

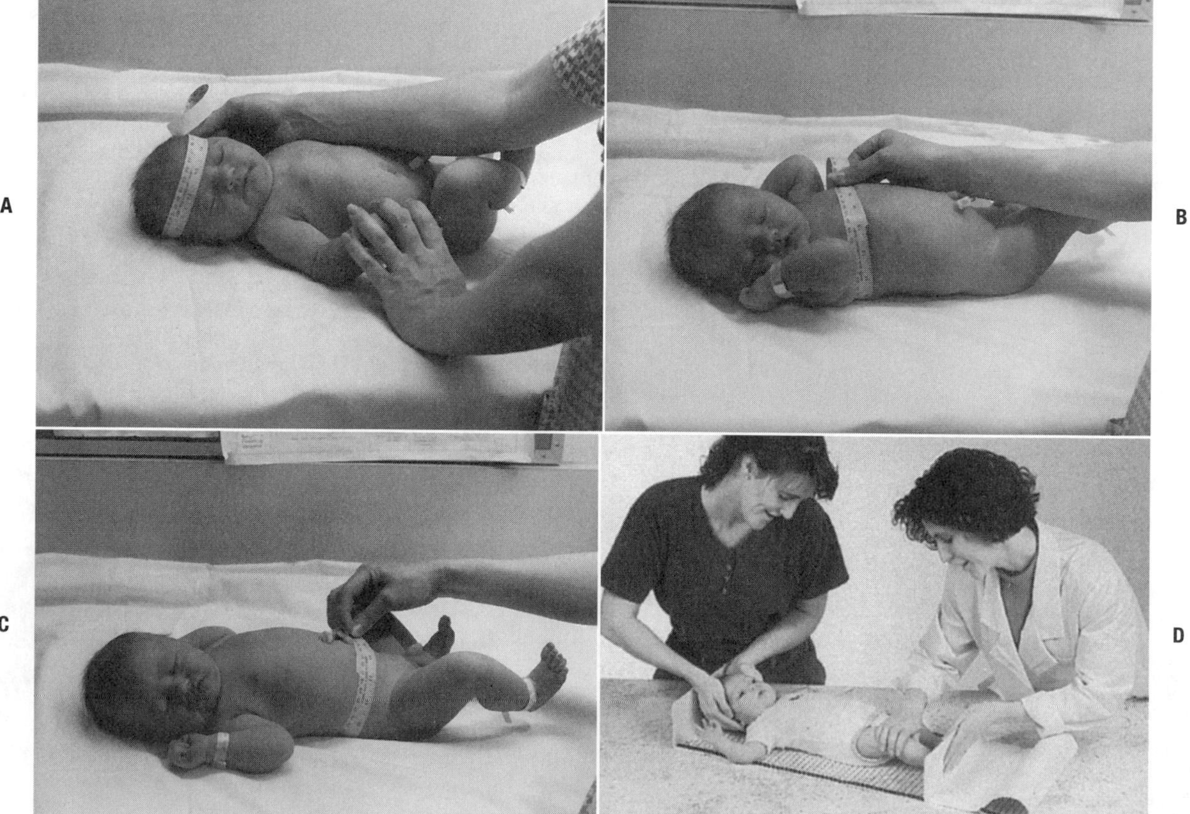

Fig. 22-18 Measurements. **A,** Circumference of head. **B,** Circumference of chest. **C,** Abdominal circumference. **D,** Length, crown to rump. To determine total length, include length of legs. If measurements are taken before the infant's initial bath, the nurse must wear gloves. (Courtesy Marjorie Pyle, RNC, Lifecircle, Costa Mesa, Calif.)

their birth weight after birth. They usually regain their birth weight by 10 to 14 days of age.

Circumferences and length. The term neonate's head circumference ranges from 32 to 36.8 cm. The head is measured at the widest part, which is the occipitofemoral diameter (Fig. 22-18, *A*).

The tape measure is placed around the head just above the infant's eyebrows. It is a good idea to remeasure the head again within 48 hours because molding may change the shape of the head and make the initial measurement inaccurate.

The chest circumference usually measures about 2 cm less than head circumference. The chest may be the same size as the head but should not exceed it. The tape is placed around the infant's chest at the nipple line (Fig. 22-18, *B*).

Abdominal circumference is measured by placing the tape around the abdomen just above the umbilicus (Fig. 22-18, *C*). Measurements vary with the size of the infant. The abdomen should be cylindrical in shape and protrude slightly. Abdominal measurements are not always taken but should be measured when there is suspicion of abdominal distention. Abdominal measurements are approximately the same as chest measurements.

In the term neonate, head-to-heel length ranges from 45 to 55 cm (18 to 22 inches). The length may be difficult to obtain because of the flexed posture of the newborn (Fig. 22-18, *D*). The examiner places the newborn on a flat surface and extends the leg until the knee is flat against the surface. Placing the head against a perpendicular surface and extending the leg may assist with this measurement. Some nurses make a pen mark on the surface of the examining table, especially if it is covered with a disposable covering, at the top of the infant's head, extend the leg, and make another mark at the infant's heel. The distance between the two marks is then measured.

Skin texture, color, and opacity. Close observation of the newborn's skin color can lead to early detection of potential problems. Any pallor, plethora (deep purplish red color from increased circulating RBCs), petechiae, cyanosis, or jaundice should be noted. The skin is examined for signs of birth injuries, such as forceps marks or lesions related to fetal monitoring. Ecchymosis or petechiae may be present on the head, neck, and face of an infant born with a nuchal cord (cord around the neck). When bruises are present, the infant's bilirubin levels may be elevated. Petechiae scattered over infant's body may indicate underlying problems such as low platelet count or infection.

Color varies with racial background, pigmentation, and physiologic changes. Acrocyanosis is characterized by bluish discoloration of the hands and feet. It is a normal condition caused by vasomotor instability and poor peripheral circulation.

The newborn's skin often appears mottled, which is a response to temperature changes. A harlequin color change may be seen. This occurs when one side of the body develops a deep red color and the other side remains pale. Harlequin color is a response to a normal vasomotor disturbance causing the blood vessels on one side of the body to constrict while those on the other side dilate.

The skin is inspected for location, size, color, and characteristics of birthmarks (Fig. 22-19).

Certain physical features vary with gestational age and usually reflect neonatal maturity. The preterm neonate has thin, translucent, ruddy skin with easily seen veins and venules (especially over the abdomen). As term gestation approaches, the skin thickens and becomes pinker; also the number of large vessels visible over the abdomen decreases. The postterm neonate typically has thick, parchment-like skin with peeling and cracking; few if any blood vessels are evident over the abdomen (NAACOG, 1991). Lanugo—soft, downy

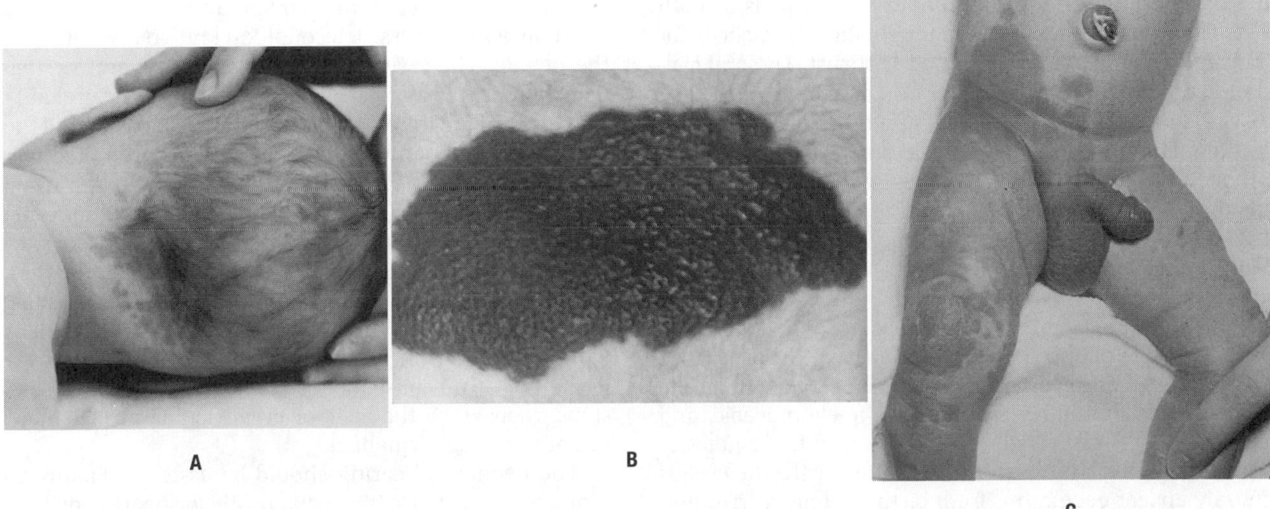

Fig. 22-19 **A,** Telangiectatic nevus (stork bite). **B,** Strawberry mark, or nevus vasculosus. **C,** Port-wine stain, or nevus flammeus. (Courtesy Mead Johnson & Co., Evansville, Ind.)

hair—appears at approximately 20 weeks' gestation. From 21 to 33 weeks, it covers the entire body. It begins to vanish from the face at 34 weeks and by 38 weeks may appear only on the shoulders. Lanugo is usually not present after 42 weeks' gestation.

Head and neck. The fontanels and suture lines are examined. The examiner palpates the suture lines to determine how much the bony edges overlap. The cranial bones commonly slide over each other during labor and delivery, causing head molding (Fig. 22-7). The anterior fontanel is diamond-shaped, located at the junction of the sagittal and coronal sutures, and measures 3 to 4 cm by 2 to 3 cm. The fontanel usually feels soft and may pulsate. The posterior fontanel is a triangular depression located at the junction of the lambdoidal and sagittal sutures. The posterior fontanel is smaller, between 0.5 and 1 cm. A third fontanel along the sagittal suture may be palpated. In most cases this represents a normal variation. African-American neonates usually have larger anterior and posterior fontanels than do Caucasian neonates.

A very large fontanel may indicate hypothyroidism. A tense or bulging fontanel may indicate increased intracranial pressure. A normal fontanel may appear slightly depressed; however, one that is severely depressed indicates dehydration. The fontanel may become fuller with crying.

The scalp should be palpated for signs of caput succedaneum or cephalhematoma. Their presence may cause the head to appear misshapen.

Hair distribution, texture, and color are other important aspects of the head examination. The amount and color of hair vary and depend on genetic factors. Unusual hair distribution may represent a minor abnormality and should be noted.

The examiner inspects the neonate's face for symmetry of features. Facial asymmetry may occur from in utero pressure, and the lopsided appearance disappears spontaneously. The mouth should appear at the midline, and its size should be appropriate for the face. Movement of the mouth should be symmetric. The lips should be sensitive to the touch; gentle stroking should trigger the sucking reflex. The chin normally is slightly receding. The term neonate has fat pads in both cheeks. The examiner touches the tongue lightly to check for the normal reaction—a forward tongue thrust. The oral cavity should not be inspected just after a feeding because the gag reflex could be stimulated, causing vomiting and subsequent aspiration. The examiner inserts the smallest gloved finger into the infant's mouth, allowing assessment of the hard and soft palates. This also stimulates the suck reflex, and intensity of the reflex can be evaluated (Tappero and Honeyfield, 1996). The neonate should have moist pink oral mucous membranes.

Eyebrows should be present and separate. Joined eyebrows across the bridge of the nose is associated with Cornelia de Lange syndrome. The eyes are examined for placement on the face; the eyelids should be of equal size, freely movable, and open adequately. Both eyeballs should be present, of equal size and shape (round), and firm. Shortly after birth, the eyelids commonly appear edematous from birth trauma or irritation caused by erythromycin instillation. In most neonates, the sclerae should be clear and white to bluish white. This iris color should be distributed evenly (Tappero and Honeyfield, 1996). Occasionally, subconjunctival hemorrhage, a result of pressure while traversing the birth canal during labor and birth, may be seen. Most neonates do not have tears; however, tears are seen occasionally.

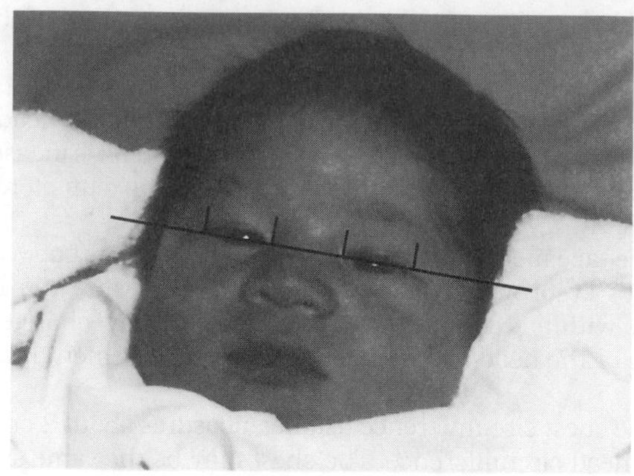

Fig. 22-20 Eyes. In pseudostrabismus, inner epicanthal folds cause the eyes to appear misaligned; however, corneal light reflexes are perfectly symmetric. Eyes are symmetric in size and shape and are well placed.

If the neonate's eyes are closed during the head-to-toe assessment, the examiner delays the eye inspection until the ophthalmic examination (which should be conducted last because it upsets the neonate). The pupils are examined with use of a penlight or flashlight and dim room lights. When exposed to light in a darkened room, the pupils should constrict equally bilaterally. If all pupil findings are normal, document them as PERRL (pupils equal, round, reactive to light). A newborn's eyes do not accommodate. To assess for the red reflex, the examiner places the penlight or ophthalmoscope directly in front of the pupil and turns on the light. When the light hits the lens, a red color is reflected from the retina to the examiner (Tappero and Honeyfield, 1996).

Movement of the eyeballs is noted. The neonate can focus momentarily and may follow to midline. Eye movements are characterized by being random and uneven. Occasionally the eyes may appear crossed, a condition known as strabismus. In the neonate, however, transient strabismus and nystagmus (constant, involuntary cyclical movement of the eyeball) may be seen until the third or fourth month; it persists until the eye muscles develop sufficiently to act in a coordinated fashion (Fig. 22-20). When the neonate's head is rotated from side to side, the eyes do not follow in response to head movements. This doll's-eye phenomenon persists for about 10 days.

The ears are inspected for symmetric shape and size. The top of the ear should align with the inner and outer canthi of the eyes (Fig. 22-21). Unilateral or bilateral periauricular papillomas (skin tags) occur fairly often. They usually are a family trait or of no consequence. Skin tags, pinpoint holes, and sinus tracts along the helix or preauricular surface may represent minor abnormalities.

The neonate's hearing should be assessed. Failure to respond to a loud noise is not diagnostic for hearing deficit. Audiology testing may be easily performed if hearing loss is suspected. The ear appears flat and shapeless until 23 weeks' gestation when incurving of the pinna (the external part of the

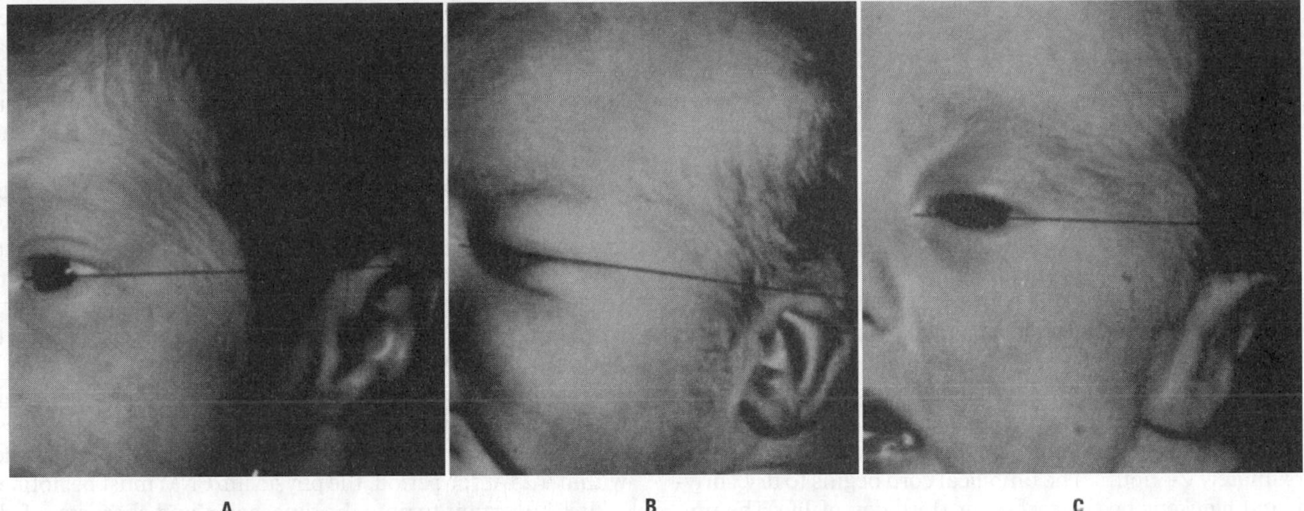

Fig. 22-21 Placement of ear on head in relation to line drawn from inner to outer canthus of eye. **A,** Normal position. **B,** Abnormally angled ear. **C,** True low-set ear. (Courtesy Mead Johnson & Co., Evansville, Ind.)

ear) begins. At 36 weeks' gestation the upper two thirds of the pinna are incurved and the pinna recoils instantly (Tappero and Honeyfield, 1996). Old blood and vernix may be in the ear canal for several days, and therefore the tympanic membrane may not be visible.

Because the neonate cannot coordinate tongue movements well, the tongue often falls backward, occluding the oral airway. Consequently, the neonate is a preferential nose breather who depends on patent nares (nostrils). To assess the nares for patency, the examiner occludes them one at a time and holds the mouth closed. The neonate should be able to breathe through the open nares. The neonate's nose is also examined for size, shape, mucous membrane integrity, and discharge. The nose should be midline on the face. The mucous membranes will appear pink and moist with no evident drainage.

The mouth should be inspected and palpated. Symmetry of the lips and lip movement, as well as the internal structure of the mouth, should be noted. Lips appear pink and moist. Some neonates are born with precocious teeth. If they are loose, they may be pulled to prevent aspiration. The hard and soft palates are inspected for cleft palate. The shape of the palate is examined. The uvula should be midline.

The tongue should be freely movable and symmetric in shape and movement. Occasionally a neonate may have a shortened frenulum ("tongue-tie"). If the tongue can extend to the alveolar ridge, usually no intervention is needed.

Small white epithelial cells—Epstein pearls—are sometimes seen on the hard palate and gums. Sucking pads can be palpated inside the cheeks. The examiner strokes the corner of the neonate's mouth to check the rooting reflex and places a finger inside the neonate's mouth to elicit the sucking reflex.

The posterior pharynx is easiest to see when the neonate is crying. Saliva usually is scant because the salivary glands are immature. The presence of excessive saliva in a neonate should alert the nurse to the possibility of tracheoesophageal fistula or esophageal atresia.

The neck should appear symmetric and without webbing; it should also be flexible enough to allow the head to move freely and equally to each side. The examiner palpates the front of the neck at the midline for the thyroid gland, as well as for the lymph nodes, which normally are not palpable (Tappero and Honeyfield, 1996).

The cardiovascular status is assessed by palpating the carotid pulses on one side at a time. They should be equal and strong bilaterally. Massage of the carotid artery should not be done because it may stimulate pressure receptors, causing reflex bradycardia (Tappero and Honeyfield, 1996).

When palpating the clavicles, the examiner moves the fingers slowly over the anterior clavicular surface. If a mass or lump is detected, the examiner then tries to move the neonate's arm gently while palpating with the other hand. A grating sensation and uneven movement of two juxtaposed bone fragments indicate a fracture, which could be from delivery trauma (Tappero and Honeyfield, 1996).

Thorax

The thoracic cavity should be cylindrical and symmetric. In the SGA or preterm neonate a smaller chest circumference is to be expected. Normally, chest wall excursion is equal bilaterally.

The ribs should be flexible and symmetric, with no palpable masses. The xiphoid process may be palpable at the bottom of the sternum. In a thin neonate, it may be visible.

Breast size. The examiner assesses breast tissue through observation and palpation. To measure breast tissue, the nipple is palpated gently with one finger or the second or third fingers placed on either side of the nipple. Measurement is taken between the two fingers to determine the amount of breast tissue.

Breast tissue and areola size increase with gestation. Increased breast tissue may indicate subcutaneous fat accumulation from accelerated intrauterine growth (as occurs in the

LGA neonate). In contrast, the SGA or postterm neonate may have decreased breast tissue from inadequate fetal growth or lost fetal weight. The nipples are inspected for spacing and number. Supernumerary nipples may appear as darkened spots just below or beside natural nipples (Tappero and Honeyfield, 1996). Any discharge is noted.

Abdomen

The abdomen should have a symmetric, slightly rounded contour. Peristaltic waves normally are not visible; however, the abdomen should move visibly during breathing. The umbilical cord remnant should appear bluish white, contain two arteries and one vein, and be free of urine leakage, a sign of a fistula from the bladder to the cord (persistent urachus).

The umbilical cord is clamped or tied at birth, and the clamp or tie is usually removed when the cord is dry, in approximately 24 hours. The umbilical cord begins to dry, shrivels, and blackens by the second or third day of life. The umbilicus should be inspected frequently for signs of infection (foul odor, redness, and/or purulent drainage), bleeding, discharge, and granuloma (small red, raw-appearing polyp where the umbilical cord separates). The cord normally falls off by 2 weeks after birth. By the time the neonate is 1 month old, the umbilicus should be healed.

Auscultation of the abdomen is performed before palpation. The examiner listens for peristaltic sounds in all four quadrants. The sounds usually are present shortly after birth. Palpation of the abdomen begins with gentle pressure, then gradually deeper pressure is used as the neonate relaxes. To promote relaxation and comfort during palpation, the neonate's legs are flexed in the fetal position. If the neonate has an asymmetric abdomen, which suggests an internal mass, great caution must be used during assessment. In many neonates, palpation may reveal a wide separation along the rectus abdominis muscles. This condition, termed *diastasis recti abdominis,* results from abdominal muscle immaturity (Tappero and Honeyfield, 1996).

Abdominal distention at birth usually indicates a serious disorder, such as intestinal obstruction or abdominal mass. Distention that occurs later may result from something simple, such as over-feeding, or may signal a gastrointestinal disorder. A scaphoid (sunken) abdomen with bowel sounds heard in the chest and signs of respiratory distress indicate a possible diaphragmatic hernia.

The amount and frequency of regurgitation ("spitting up") after feedings must be recorded. Color change, gagging, and projectile (very forceful) vomiting occur in association with esophageal or tracheoesophageal anomalies. Regurgitation during the first 1 or 2 days of life can be decreased by avoiding overfeeding, by frequently burping the infant, and by positioning the infant with the head slightly elevated.

The liver normally lies at the right costal margin. Its sharp edge should be palpated no more than 1 cm below the right costal margin; it can be felt during inspiration. The liver is a superficial organ, and deep probing is unnecessary (Tappero and Honeyfield, 1996). The spleen is on the opposite side of the abdomen. Normally the spleen is not felt. A spleen tip felt 1 cm or more below the left costal margin is an indication of disease processes seen in conjunction with hepatomegaly (Tappero and Honeyfield, 1996).

The posterior position of the kidneys makes them less accessible to palpation. If they cannot be palpated with one hand, bimanual palpation is used. In this technique the examiner places one hand behind the neonate's back while palpating the abdomen with the fingertips of the other hand. The kidney should be felt between the hands (Tappero and Honeyfield, 1996). Enlarged or cystic kidneys may be identified as masses.

Unless the bladder is distended, it should not be visible (Tappero and Honeyfield, 1996). The bladder may be palpated just above the symphysis pubis. Pressing on the bladder may induce voiding or expression of urine. The time of the first voiding should be noted.

About 17% of newborns void at the time of birth, 92% by 24 hours, and 99% within 48 hours (Fanaroff and Martin, 1992). An infant who has not voided after 24 hours should be assessed for adequacy of fluid intake, bladder distention, restlessness, and symptoms of pain. If the infant has not voided within a 24-hour period, the physician/CNM must be notified.

It is important to note the time, color, and character of the infant's first stool. A lack of passage of stool could indicate an inborn error of metabolism (e.g., cystic fibrosis) or congenital disorder (e.g., Hirschsprung disease or an imperforate anus). Stools of a newborn change in character during the first few days of life (Box 22-1).

Some infants do not digest specific formulas well. If an infant is allergic to or unable to digest a formula, the stools may become very soft with a high water content that is seen as a distinct water ring around the stool on the diaper. Forceful ejection of stool and a water ring around the stool are signs of diarrhea. Care must be taken to avoid misinterpreting transitional stools for diarrhea stools. The loss of fluid in diarrhea can rapidly lead to fluid and electrolyte imbalance.

Back and Anus

To assess the back the examiner positions the neonate prone and inspects for spinal alignment, enlargement, and masses. The back should be straight. The sacrum is examined for dimpling, a tuft of hair, or bulges. The vertebral column is palpated for enlargement and signs of pain (Kenner, Brueggemeyer, and Gunderson, 1993).

The perineum should be smooth and without dimpling or extra orifices. The anus should be midline and patent. The anal sphincter is assessed by lightly stroking the anus with a cotton-tipped applicator and observing anal constriction—a reaction called the anal wink (Mass et al, 1991). Passage of meconium indicates patency of the rectum, which should be noted.

Genitalia

The infant must be closely inspected for ambiguous genitalia and other abnormalities. Normally in a female the urethral opening is located behind the clitoris. Any deviation from this may mistakenly suggest that the clitoris is a small penis, which can occur in conditions such as adrenal hyperplasia. Nearly all females are born with hymenal tags. Absence of such could indicate vaginal agenesis. Fecal discharge from the vagina indicates a rectovaginal fistula.

The female genitalia should be assessed for signs of gestational maturity. The degree to which the labia majora and minora have come together and reduced the visual prominence of the labia minora and clitoris reflects the stage of the infant's maturity (Tappero and Honeyfield, 1996).

In the male neonate, the genitalia should be assessed for

testicular descent, scrotal size, and number of rugae (skin folds). A hydrocele is a common finding and usually decreases without intervention.

Inguinal hernias may be present and become more obvious when the infant cries. If the urinary meatus is not at the tip of the glans penis, hypospadias (urethral meatus opens on the underside of the penis) or epispadias (urethral meatus opens on the top of the penis) may be present. These problems are usually associated with other anomalies.

Extremities

The extremities are inspected for length, symmetry relative to each other and to the body as a whole, equality, muscle tone, and range of motion. Normally, the term neonate has a full range of motion, which can be tested either actively or passively. The preterm neonate has limited flexion, especially of the arms. The hands and feet are inspected for number of digits, palmar and plantar creases, and such abnormalities as webbing (Tappero and Honeyfield, 1996).

Movement of the arms should be assessed. Trauma to the brachial plexus during a difficult delivery may result in brachial palsy. The most common type of palsy involves the fifth and sixth cranial nerve roots (Duchenne-Erb paralysis). In this condition the affected arm is held in a position of tight adduction and internal rotation at the shoulder. The grasp reflex on the affected side may be intact; however, the Moro reflex will be absent on that side. With treatment, most neonates have complete recovery.

To assess leg length, the legs are extended simultaneously. They should be equal, with symmetric skin folds. The legs are inspected in both the prone and supine positions. Hip integrity is assessed using the Ortolani maneuver (Fig. 22-22). The examiner places the index and middle fingers of each hand over the greater trochanters of the hips at the same time. Downward pressure is exerted on the hips while the neonate's knees are flexed. The hips are flexed at least 70 degrees and then abducted. The motion should be smooth without any unusual clicks. Presence of a click, unequal movement, or extra skin folds is considered a positive response, indicating that the hip is dislocated.

Skeletal deformities may be congenital problems or drug induced. Clubfoot (talipes equinovarus), a deformity in which the foot turns inward and is fixed in a plantar flexion position, should be noted.

Plantar (sole) creases should be assessed immediately after birth because the drying effect of environmental exposure causes additional creases to form. The preterm neonate of 34 to 35 weeks' gestation has one or two anterior creases; at 36 to 38 weeks' gestation, creases cover the anterior two thirds of the sole. In the term neonate, creases appear over both the sole and heel. In the postterm neonate, deeper creases line the entire sole (Tappero and Honeyfield, 1996).

Neurologic Assessment

The physical assessment includes a neurologic assessment of the newborn's reflexes (Table 22-2). This provides useful information about the infant's nervous system and state of neurologic maturation. Many of the reflex behaviors are important for survival, for example, sucking and rooting. Other reflexes act as safety mechanisms, for instance, gagging, coughing, and sneezing. The assessment must be carried out as early as possible because abnormal signs present in the early neonatal period may disappear. They may reappear months or years later as abnormal functions.

Any absence of a newborn reflex could indicate major neurologic problems. Birth trauma may cause nerve damage that results in facial asymmetry and paralysis. Central nervous system depression, caused by maternal medications received during labor and delivery, also influences neuromuscular functioning.

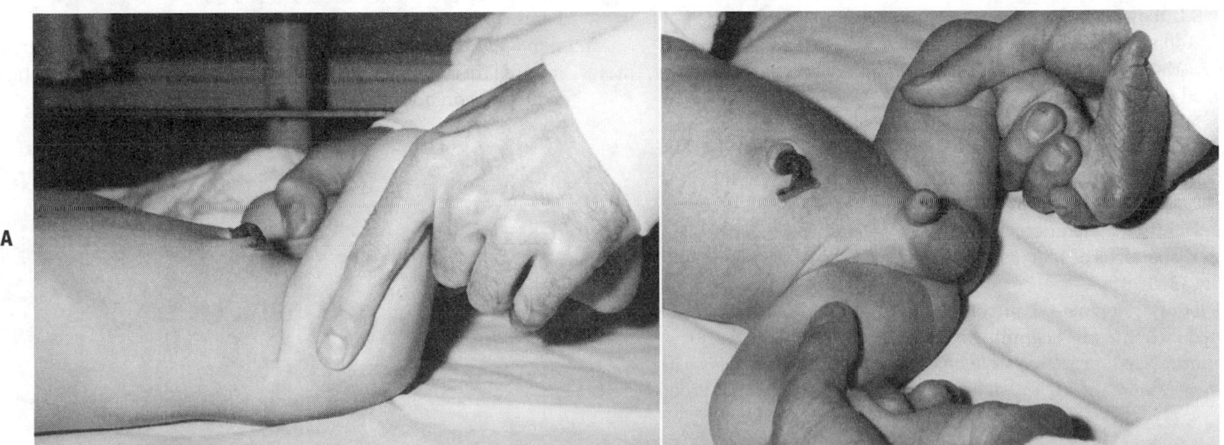

Fig. 22-22 Method of assessing for hip dysplasia or dislocation using Ortolani maneuver. **A,** Examiner's index fingers are placed over greater trochanter and thumbs over inner thigh opposite lesser trochanter. **B,** Gentle pressure is exerted to further flex thigh on hip, and thighs are rotated outward. If hip dysplasia is present, head of femur can be felt to slip forward in acetabulum and slip back when pressure is released and legs returned to their original position. A click is sometimes heard (Ortolani sign). (Courtesy Marjorie Pyle, RNC, Lifecircle, Costa Mesa, Calif.)

Key Points

- By term the infant's various anatomic and physiologic systems have reached a level of development and functioning that permits a physical existence apart from the mother and sensory capabilities that indicate a state of readiness for social interaction.
- Assessment of the newborn requires data from the prenatal, intranatal, and postnatal periods.
- The newborn assessment should proceed in a systematic manner so that each system is thoroughly evaluated.
- Many reflex behaviors are important for the newborn's survival.
- Behavioral characteristics of infants play a major role in the ultimate relationship between infants and their parents.
- Each term newborn has a predisposed capacity to handle the multitude of stimuli in the external world.
- At any serum bilirubin level the appearance of jaundice during the first day of life or persistence of jaundice beyond 7 to 8 days may indicate a pathologic process.
- Prolonged cold exposure of a newborn, even a healthy newborn, may result in acidosis and raise the level of free fatty acids, leading to cold stress.

References

American Academy of Pediatrics: *Textbook of neonatal resuscitation,* Elk Grove Village, Ill, 1990, The Academy.

Ballard J, Novak K, Driver M: A simplified score for assessment of fetal maturation of newly born infants, *J Pediatr* 95(3):769, 1979.

Ballard J et al: New Ballard Score, expanded to include extremely premature infants, *J Pediatr* 119:417, 1991.

Bamford F et al: Sleep in the first year of life, *Dev Med Child Neurol* 32:718, 1990.

Barnard K: *NCAST feeding manual,* Seattle, 1994, University of Washington.

Beal J: The effect on father-infant interaction of demonstrating the Neonatal Behavioral Assessment Scale, *Birth* 16(1):18, 1989.

Blackburn S, Loper D: *Maternal, fetal, and neonatal physiology: a clinical perspective,* Philadelphia, 1992, WB Saunders.

Bliss-Holtz J: Determination of thermoregulatory state in full-term infants, *Nurs Res* 42(4):204, 1993.

Brazelton T, Nugent J: Neonatal behavioural assessment scale, ed 3, London, 1996, MacKeith.

Chitty L, Winter R: Perinatal mortality in different ethnic groups, *Arch Dis Child* 64:1036, 1989.

DeCasper A, Fifer W: Of human bonding: newborns prefer their mother's voices, *Science* 208:1174, 1980.

DeCasper A, Spence M: Prenatal maternal speech influences newborns' perceptions of speech sounds, *Infant Behav Dev* 9:133, 1986.

Dubowitz I, Dubowitz V: *Gestational age of the newborn,* Menlo Park, Calif, 1977, Addison-Wesley.

Fanaroff A, Martin R: *Neonatal-perinatal medicine diseases of the fetus and infant,* ed 6, St Louis, 1997, Mosby.

Ferber R: Behavioral "insomnia" in the child, *Psychiatr Clin North Am* 10(4):641, 1987.

Field R et al: Mothers' assessments of the behavior of their infants, *Infant Behav Dev* 1:156, 1978.

Freedman D: Ethnic differences in babies, *Hum Nature* p 36, Jan 1979.

Fuller J: Early patterns of maternal attachment, *Health Care Women Int* 11(4):433, 1990.

Garcia-Coll C: Developmental outcome of minority infants: a process-oriented look into our beginnings, *Child Dev* 61:270, 1990.

Gunzenhauser N, editor: *Advances in touch: new implications in human development,* Skillman, NJ, 1990, Johnson & Johnson Consumer Products.

Guyton A: *Textbook of medical physiology,* ed 9, Philadelphia, 1991, WB Saunders.

Kenner C, Brueggemeyer A, Gunderson L: *Comprehensive neonatal nursing,* Philadelphia, 1993, WB Saunders.

Lawrence R: *Breastfeeding: a guide for the medical profession,* ed 4, St Louis, 1994, Mosby.

Manio E, Hall R: Asian family traditions and their influence in transcultural health care delivery, *CHC* 15:172, 1987.

Mass G et al: Routine examination in the neonatal period, *Br Med J* 302(6781):878, 1991.

Nurses Association of the American College of Obstetrics and Gynecologists (NAACOG): Physical assessment of the neonate, *OGN Nurs Pract Resource,* Washington DC, Aug 1991, NAACOG.

Pascoe J, French J: Development of positive feelings in primiparous mothers toward their normal newborns, *Clin Pediatr* 28(1):452, 1989.

Poma P: Pregnancy in Hispanic women, *J Nat Med Assoc* 79:929, 1987.

Seidel H, Rosenstein B, Pathak A: *Care of the fullterm newborn,* St Louis, 1993, Mosby.

Tappero E, Honeyfield M, editors: *Physical assessment of the newborn,* ed 2, Petaluma, Calif, 1996, NICU Ink Book Pub.

Thomas K: Thermoregulation in neonates, *Neonatal Netw* 13(2):15, 1994.

Wong D: *Whaley & Wong's nursing care of infants and children,* ed 5, St Louis, 1995, Mosby.

Yetman R et al: Comparison of temperature measurements by an aural infrared thermometer with measurements by traditional rectal and axillary techniques, *J Pediatr* 122(5):769, 1993.

Bibliography

Crockett M: Physiology of the neonatal immune system, *J Obstet Gynecol Neonatal Nurs* 24(7):627, 1995.

Bruno J: Systematic neonatal assessment and intervention, *MCN Am J Matern Child Nurs* 20(1):21, 1995.

Dodd V: Gestational age assessment, *Neonatal Netw* 15(1):27, 1996.

Medoff-Cooper B, Ray W: Neonatal sucking behaviors, *Image J Nurs Sch* 27(3):195, 1995.

CHAPTER 23

Nursing Care of the Newborn

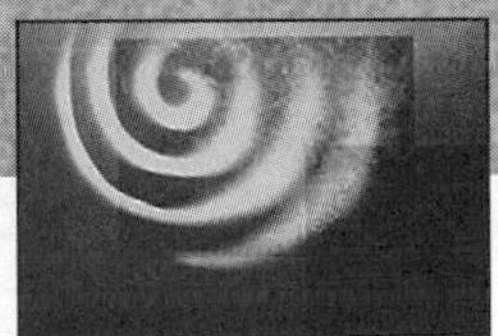

BIRTH THROUGH THE FIRST 2 HOURS, P. 627
Nursing care management, p. 627

SUPPORTING ADAPTATION TO EXTRAUTERINE LIFE, P. 629
Body temperature, p. 629
Adequate oxygenation, p. 630

HEALTHY THERAPEUTIC INTERVENTIONS, P. 632
Eye prophylaxis, p. 632
Vitamin K prophylaxis, p. 633

2 HOURS AFTER BIRTH UNTIL DISCHARGE, P. 633
Nursing care management, p. 633

ASSESSMENT OF COMMON PROBLEMS IN THE NEWBORN, P. 635
Physical injuries, p. 635
Physiologic problems, p. 636

LABORATORY AND DIAGNOSTIC TESTS, P. 637
Collection of specimens, p. 637

PROTECTIVE ENVIRONMENT, P. 642

SUPPORTING PARENTS IN THE CARE OF THEIR INFANT, P. 643
Social interactions, p. 643
Infant feeding, p. 645
Positioning and holding, p. 645
Umbilical cord care, p. 645
Rashes, p. 645
Clothing, p. 645
Care of the infant's linens, p. 646
Bathing, p. 646

NURSING INTERVENTIONS FOR THERAPEUTIC/SURGICAL PROCEDURES, P. 649
Restraining the infant, p. 649
Intramuscular injection, p. 649
Therapy for hyperbilirubinemia, p. 650
Circumcision, p. 653

DISCHARGE PLANNING AND TEACHING, P. 655
Temperature, p. 655
Respirations, p. 657
Elimination, p. 657
Safety, p. 657
Pacifiers/thumb-sucking, p. 657
Immunizations, p. 658
Infant follow-up care, p. 658
Home care, p. 658

The preceding chapter presented the numerous biologic changes the neonate makes during the transition to extrauterine life. The first 24 hours of life is critical because respiratory distress and circulatory failure can occur rapidly and with little warning (Wong, 1995).

Although most infants make the necessary biopsychosocial adjustment to extrauterine existence without undue difficulty, their well-being depends on the care they receive from others. The nursing care described in this chapter is based on careful assessment of biologic and behavioral responses and formulation of nursing diagnoses. It includes planning and implementing appropriate nursing actions and evaluating their effectiveness.

BIRTH THROUGH THE FIRST 2 HOURS

Nursing Care Management

Care begins immediately after the birth and focuses on assessing and stabilizing the condition of the newborn. The nurse has primary responsibility for the infant during this period, because the physician/midwife will be involved with delivery of the placenta and care of the mother. The nurse must be alert for any signs of distress and initiate appropriate interventions.

Assessment

Initial assessment and Apgar scoring. Before birth, the nurse who is assisting with the birth evaluates the maternal history, including labor, to identify potential problems for the neonate and alerts the nursery and/or pediatrician. The first assessment of the newborn is done immediately after birth by using the Apgar score (Table 22-2) and a brief physical assessment. The nurse, birth attendant, or pediatrician may assign the Apgar score.

Physical assessment. The nurse engages in the following activities and records findings:

1. Assesses respirations and neonate's ability to keep airway clear

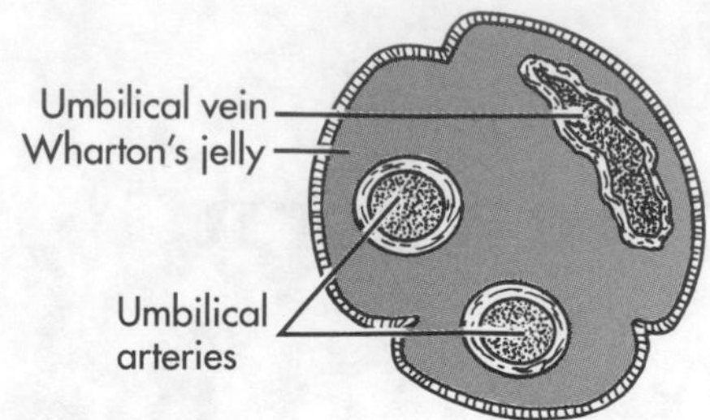

Fig. 23-1 Cross section of umbilical cord. Note collapsed appearance of thin-walled umbilical vein and contour of thicker, muscular-walled arteries.

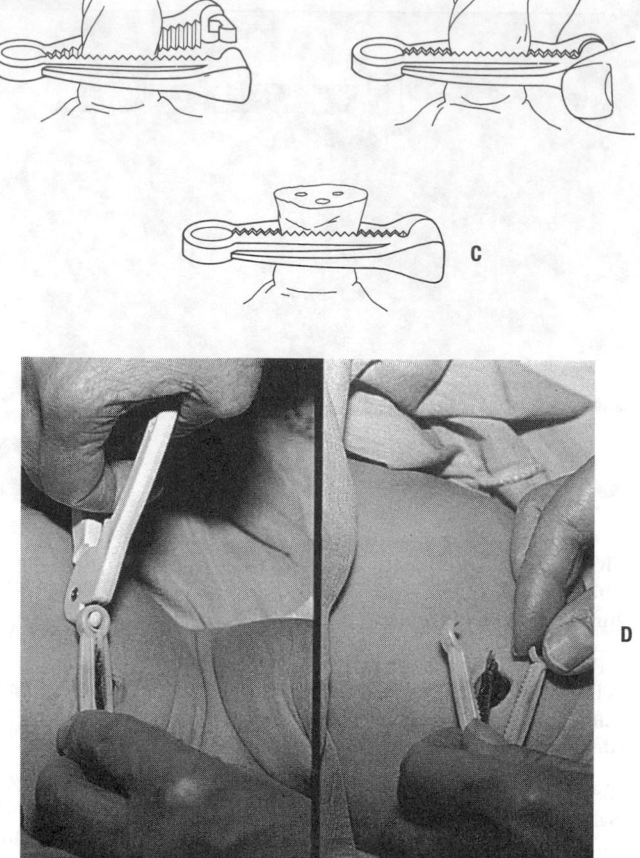

Fig. 23-2 Hollister cord clamp. **A,** Position clamp close to umbilicus. **B,** Secure cord. **C,** Cut cord. **D,** Remove clamp, using special scissors, after cord dries (about 24 hours).

2. Examines the cord for anomalies and verifies the presence of two arteries and one vein (Fig. 23-1); checks that cord clamp is in place (Fig. 23-2) or clamps the cord
3. Obtains cord blood from the placenta for analysis (Rhesus [Rh] factor, blood grouping, and hematocrit). Some hospitals do not send cord blood to the laboratory unless the mother is Rh-negative or blood type O or had no prenatal care
4. Obtains weight
5. Notes passage of meconium or urine
6. Performs initial physical examination and assessment of neonate, which includes a review of systems (Box 23-1)
   a. *External:* notes skin color, staining, peeling, or wasting (dysmaturity); considers length of nails and development of creases on soles of feet; checks for presence or absence of breast tissue; assesses nasal patency by closing one nostril at a time while observing the infant's respirations and color; notes meconium staining of cord, skin, fingernails, or amniotic fluid (may indicate fetal distress; offensive odor may indicate intrauterine infection)
   b. *Chest:* auscultates for rate and quality of heart tones and murmurs; compares and notes character of respirations and presence of crackles; notes equality of breath sounds on each side of chest by holding stethoscope in each axilla and on upper back
   c. *Abdomen:* verifies presence of a rounded abdomen and absence of anomalies
   d. *Neurologic:* checks muscle tone and reflex reaction and appraises Moro reflex; palpates anterior fontanel for fullness or bulging; notes by palpation the presence and size of the sutures and fontanels
   e. *Other observations:* notes gross structural malformations obvious at birth (described in general terms and recorded on birth record)
7. Assesses parents' response to newborn and to each other

Nursing Diagnoses

Nursing diagnoses lend direction to the nursing actions needed to implement a plan of care. Before establishing nursing diagnoses, the nurse analyzes the significance of findings collected during assessment. Following are examples of nursing diagnoses for the newborn immediately after birth:

- Ineffective airway clearance related to
  - Airway obstruction with mucus and amniotic fluid
- Ineffective thermoregulation related to
  - Environmental factors
  - Amniotic fluid moisture on the skin (evaporation)
- Altered health maintenance related to
  - Presence of congenital disorders

Expected Outcomes

During this important step, expected outcomes are set in patient-centered terms and are prioritized. Nursing actions are selected to meet these outcomes. Expected outcomes for the newborn during the immediate recovery period include the following:

1. The newborn will make the transition to extrauterine life.
2. The newborn's airway will remain clear.
3. The newborn's temperature will remain within stated normal limits.
4. The newborn will not experience bodily injury.
5. The parent-newborn's bonding process will be facilitated.

BOX 23-1
Initial Physical Assessment by Body System

CNS [ ] moves extremities, muscle tone good
[ ] symmetric features, movement
[ ] suck, rooting, Moro and grasp reflexes good
[ ] anterior fontanel soft and flat
CV [ ] heart auscultation, regular in rate and rhythm
[ ] no murmurs heard
[ ] pulses equal bilaterally
RESP [ ] lungs auscultated, clear bilaterally
[ ] respiratory rate <60 breaths/min
[ ] chest expansion symmetric
[ ] no upper airway congestion
GU [ ] male: urethral opening at tip of penis
testes descended bilaterally
female: vaginal opening apparent
GI [ ] abdomen soft, no distention
[ ] cord attached and clamped
[ ] anus patent
ENT [ ] eyes clear
[ ] palates intact
[ ] nares patent
SKIN Color [ ] pink [ ] acrocyanotic
[ ] no lesions or abrasions
[ ] birthmarks ______
[ ] caput/molding
[ ] vacuum "cap"
[ ] forceps marks
[ ] other ______
Comments: ______

Plan of Care and Implementation

Events move rapidly during this period. Assessment must be followed quickly by appropriate implementation. The physician/certified nurse midwife (CNM) may be concentrating on the progress of the third stage of labor for the mother.

The nurse responsible for the care of the newborn immediately after birth verifies that respirations have been established, dries the infant, assesses temperature, and places identical identification bracelets on the infant and the mother. In some settings, the father or partner also wears an identification bracelet. The infant may be wrapped in a warm blanket and placed in the arms of the mother, given to the partner to hold, or kept undressed under a radiant warmer. In some settings, immediately after birth the infant is placed on the mother's abdomen to allow skin to skin contact, which contributes to maintenance of the infant's optimal temperature and parental bonding (Vaughns, 1990). The infant may be admitted to a nursery or remain with the parents throughout the hospital stay.

The initial examination of the newborn can occur while the nurse is drying and wrapping the infant, or observations can be made while the infant is lying on the mother's abdomen or in her arms immediately after birth. Efforts should be directed to minimizing interference in the initial parent-infant acquaintance process. If the infant is breathing easily, has pink color, and has no life-threatening problems or congenital anomalies, then further examination can be delayed until after the parents have had an opportunity to interact with the infant.

LEGAL TIP

Infant Identification

Identical identification bands should be placed on the mother and infant (and father or partner) while they are still in the birthing room. Each time the infant is taken to the mother, the bands (number and name) should be checked to be sure that the numbers and names match.

A summary of these nursing actions and the rationale for each are given in Table 23-1.

SUPPORTING ADAPTATION TO EXTRAUTERINE LIFE

Body Temperature

If the infant does not remain with the mother during the first 1 to 2 hours after birth, the nurse places the thoroughly dried, unclothed baby under a radiant heat panel until the body temperature is stabilized. To prevent overheating, the infant should remain unclothed while under an overbed heat panel or in an isolette with a servocontrol mechanism. The servocontrol mechanism uses the desired set point temperature as the point of control. If the newborn's skin temperature fluctuates more than 1 degree from the desired set point, the heater output is increased or decreased to maintain the skin temperature at the desired level. The set point temperature on the control panel usually is maintained between 96.8° and 98.6° F (36° and 37° C). This setting should maintain the healthy term infant's skin temperature around 97.6° F (36.5° C). A **thermistor probe** (automatic sensor) is taped to the right upper quadrant of the abdomen immediately below the right costal margin, never over a bone. This will ensure detection of minor temperature changes resulting from peripheral vasoconstriction, dilation, or increased metabolism long before a change in deep body temperature develops. The other end of the probe cord is attached to the control panel. The sensor needs to be checked periodically to make sure it is securely attached to the infant's skin. The axillary temperature of the newborn is checked every hour with a thermometer. Examinations and care are performed with the newborn under the heat panel. Healthy term infants with temperatures of at least 97.6° F (36.5° C) can be bathed when the admission assessment has been completed (Penny-MacGillivray, 1996).

The nurse can help stabilize the newborn's body temperature in several ways. The ambient temperature of the nursery unit should be kept at about 75° F (24° C). The newborn is dried and wrapped in warmed blankets immediately after birth, with care to keep the head well covered while the parent is holding the newborn. The infant can also be placed directly on the mother's abdomen and covered with a warm blanket (Vaughns, 1990).

Warming infant with hypothermia. Even a healthy full-term newborn may become hypothermic. Birth in a car on the way to the hospital, a cold delivery room, or inadequate drying and wrapping immediately after birth may cause the infant's temperature to fall below neutral thermal range

TABLE 23-1 Initial nursing care of the neonate

INTERVENTION	RATIONALE
Airway	
Hold baby with head lowered (10 to 15 degrees).	Uses gravity to help remove fluids.
Suction oral pharynx with small bulb syringe as soon as head emerges.	Expedites drainage and prevents aspiration of amniotic fluid, mucus, and blood (maternal).
Suction nares next.	Prevents inspiration after stimulation of nares before mouth is clear.
Avoid deep suctioning with catheter, if possible.	May cause bradycardia or laryngospasm, or both.
Avoid suspending neonate by ankles.	Results in hyperextension of baby whose entire development occurred in flexed position.
Cord clamping	
Immediately after birth, neonate is kept at about the same level as uterus, until cord clamp is applied or until cord has stopped pulsating.	If neonate is held above level of uterus, gravity drains blood to placenta.
Without "stripping" it, cord is clamped close to umbilicus approximately 30 sec after birth if neonate appears normal and mature.	Ordinarily it is unwise to strip cord before clamping and cutting because post delivery red blood cell destruction will be increased and hyperbilirubinemia may ensue; in addition, polycythemia (increased number of red blood cells) increases blood viscosity, leading to cardiopulmonary problems.
Cord is clamped 8 to 10 cm from umbilicus if there is a possibility for exchange transfusion.	Permits access to umbilical vessels.
Assess cord for two arteries and one vein (Fig. 23-1).	Absence of one artery indicates need for further assessment.
Attachment and warmth	
Unless immediate intervention is required, dry infant and place on mother's abdomen, covering both; or wrap infant in warm blanket first.	Facilitates attachment. Assures and relaxes mother.
Caution parents to keep neonate's head covered.	Prevents cold stress.
Permit mother to breastfeed as desired.	Facilitates uterine contractions and expulsion of placenta.
Apgar score	
Appraise neonate at 1 min and again at 5 min, using Apgar scoring method (see p. 608 and Table 22-3).	Permits rapid and semiquantitative assessment of physiologic state.
Eye prophylaxis	
Instill medication per agency policy (Fig. 23-7).	Prevents infection; meets legal requirements.
Newborn weight and length	
Weigh and measure the neonate; this may be delayed until the fourth stage.	Parents usually are anxious to know and want to share data with relatives and friends.
Identification	
Identify the neonate by one of a number of techniques *before mother or baby leaves the birthing area.*	Although rare, an occasional mix-up in the identity of neonates occurs; identification and care to check both mother's and infant's ID numbers prevent unnecessary anxiety and legal complications.

(hypothermia). Warming the hypothermic baby is accomplished with care. Rapid warming may cause apneic spells and acidosis in an infant. Therefore the warming process is monitored and accomplished to progress slowly over a period of 2 to 4 hours.

Adequate Oxygenation

Establishing a patent airway is a primary objective after birth; maintaining the airway is a primary nursing objective in the nursery. Four conditions are essential for maintenance of adequate oxygenation:

- A clear airway, fundamental to adequate ventilation
- Respiratory efforts, necessary to ensure continued ventilation
- A functioning cardiopulmonary system, essential to maintain oxygenation
- Heat support, necessary because exposure to cold stress increases oxygen needs

Signs of potential complications related to abnormal newborn breathing are shown in Box 23-2.

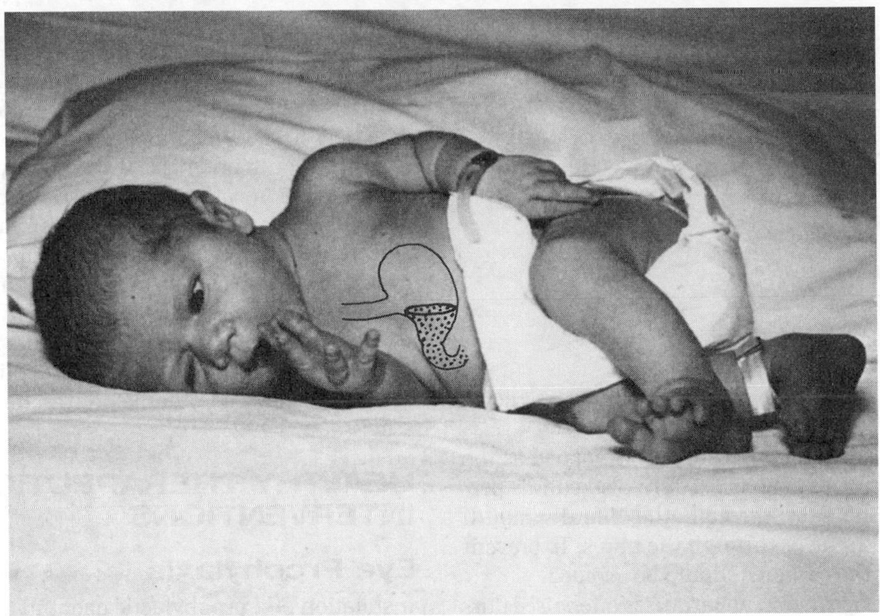

Fig. 23-3 Infant is turned to right side and supported in this position to facilitate drainage from mouth and to promote emptying of stomach contents into the small intestine.

BOX 23-2
Signs of Potential Complications

ABNORMAL NEWBORN BREATHING

1. Bradypnea: respirations < 25/min
2. Tachypnea: respirations ≥ 60/min
3. Abnormal breath sounds: crackles, rhonchi, wheezes, expiratory grunting
4. Respiratory distress: nasal flaring, retractions, labored breathing, cyanosis
5. Apnea: periodic cessation of respirations > 15-20 sec

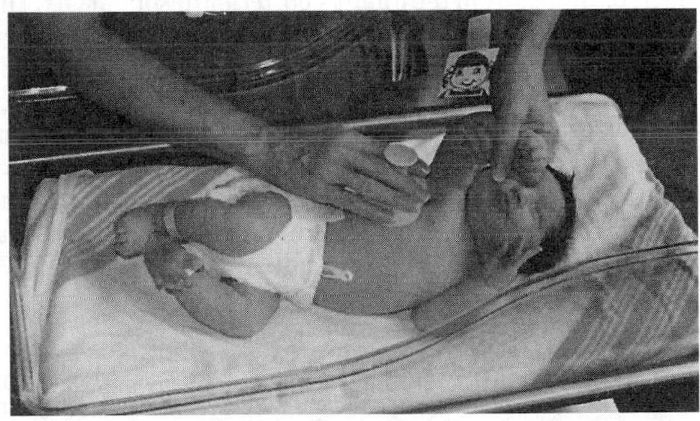

Fig. 23-4 Chest percussion. Nurse performs gentle percussion over the chest wall using a percussion cup to aid in loosening secretions before suctioning. (Courtesy Kim Molloy, San Jose, Calif.)

Maintenance of clear airway. Generally the full-term infant born vaginally has little difficulty clearing the air passages. Most secretions are drained by gravity, propelled to the oropharynx by the cough reflex, to be drained or swallowed. The infant is maintained in a side-lying position with a rolled blanket at the back to facilitate drainage (Fig. 23-3). The nurse may perform gentle percussion over the chest wall using a percussion cup to aid in loosening secretions before suctioning (Fig. 23-4). The nurse's knowledge and skill in suctioning may be critical in helping both normal and distressed infants establish or maintain adequate respirations.

Suctioning of upper airway. If the infant has excess mucus in the respiratory tract, the nurse may need to aspirate the mouth and nasal passages with a bulb syringe. The infant who is coughing and choking on the secretions should be supported with its head to the side. The mouth is suctioned first to prevent the infant from inhaling pharyngeal secretions by gasping as the nares are touched. The bulb is compressed and inserted into one side of the mouth (Fig. 23-5). The center of the infant's mouth is avoided because contact could stimulate the gag reflex. The nasal passages are suctioned one nostril at a time. The bulb syringe should always be kept in the infant's crib. The parents should be given a demonstration of how to use the bulb syringe and asked to perform a return demonstration.

A DeLee mucus-trap or a no. 5 French suction apparatus may be needed to remove secretions. The suction apparatus is

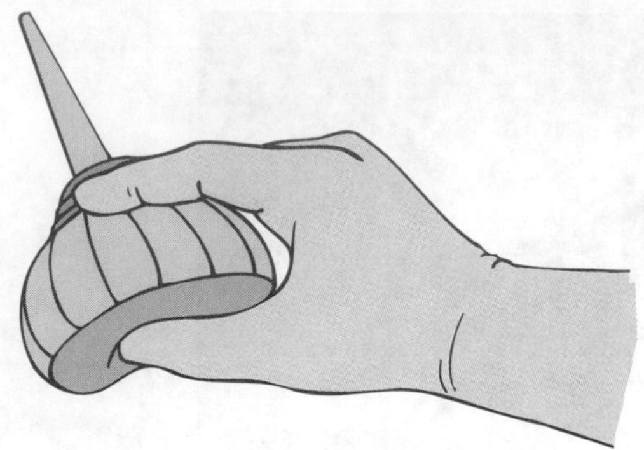

Fig. 23-5 Bulb syringe. Bulb must be compressed before insertion.

attached to wall suction, and gentle suction is applied as the tube is rotated and removed. The procedure also can be performed by inserting the tube through the infant's mouth along the base of the tongue or through the nares. To prevent tissue trauma, forcing the catheter should be avoided.

The DeLee mucus-trap suction apparatus is often used during the birth process. The DeLee suction method provides safe mechanical suctioning of neonates while preventing the transmission of bacteria, viruses, and other infectious material from the newborn to the user (Fig. 23-6).

Deeper suctioning may be necessary to remove excessive or tenacious mucus from the infant's posterior nasopharynx. The suction catheter procedure is also followed for deep suctioning. Proper tube insertion and suctioning 5 seconds or less per tube insertion will help prevent laryngospasms and oxygen depletion. If wall suction is used, the pressure should be adjusted to less than 80 mm Hg. After the catheter is properly placed, suction is created by placing one's thumb over the control, as the catheter is carefully rotated and gently withdrawn. Allow time between suctioning for adequate ventilation.

Often simple repositioning of the infant and suctioning of the mouth and nose with the bulb syringe correct the situation. The nurse listens to respirations and lung sounds with a stethoscope to determine the presence of crackles and wheezes. If the lungs are clear, the bulb syringe is used to clear the mouth and nose. If the bulb syringe does not provide relief, a suction catheter may be needed to remove mucus obstructing the nasopharynx and oropharynx. It is unusual for a newborn to experience complete airway obstruction caused by anything other than mucus, which, in most instances, is removed by either suctioning or gravity.

All personnel working with infants must have current infant CPR certification. Many institutions offer infant CPR courses to new parents before discharge (Donaher-Wagner and Braun, 1992).

HEALTHY THERAPEUTIC INTERVENTIONS

Eye Prophylaxis

Instillation of a prophylactic agent in the eyes of all neonates is mandatory in the United States (Fig. 23-7). It is a precaution against **ophthalmia neonatorum,** inflammation of the eyes from gonorrheal or chlamydial infection contracted by the newborn during passage through the mother's birth canal. In some Canadian institutions the parents may sign a form refusing eye prophylaxis. In the United States, if the family objects to this treatment, the primary care practitioner will request that the parents sign an informed refusal form, and their objection will be noted in the neonate's record. The agent used for prophylaxis varies according to hospital protocols. Usual agents include forms of erythromycin and tetracycline. Canadian hospitals have not recommended the use of silver nitrate since 1986. Its use in the United States is minimal because silver nitrate does not protect against chlamydial

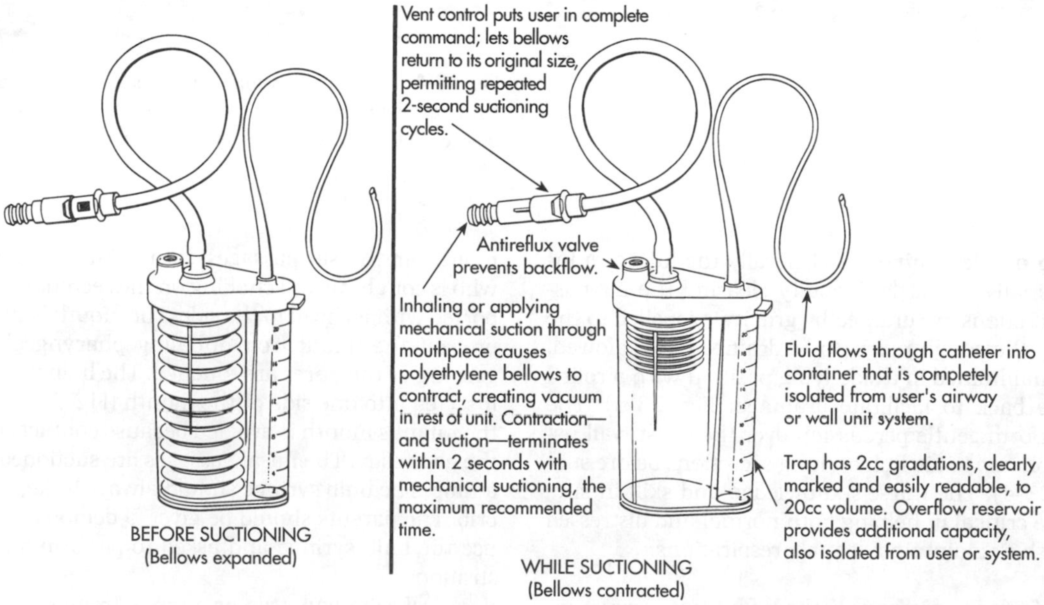
Vent control puts user in complete command; lets bellows return to its original size, permitting repeated 2-second suctioning cycles.
Antireflux valve prevents backflow.
Inhaling or applying mechanical suction through mouthpiece causes polyethylene bellows to contract, creating vacuum in rest of unit. Contraction—and suction—terminates within 2 seconds with mechanical suctioning, the maximum recommended time.
Fluid flows through catheter into container that is completely isolated from user's airway or wall unit system.
Trap has 2cc gradations, clearly marked and easily readable, to 20cc volume. Overflow reservoir provides additional capacity, also isolated from user or system.
BEFORE SUCTIONING
(Bellows expanded)
WHILE SUCTIONING
(Bellows contracted)

Fig. 23-6 DeLee suction equipment with catheter and mucus-trap. (Courtesy Busse Hospital Disposables, PO Box 011067, Hauppauge, NY 11788-0920.)

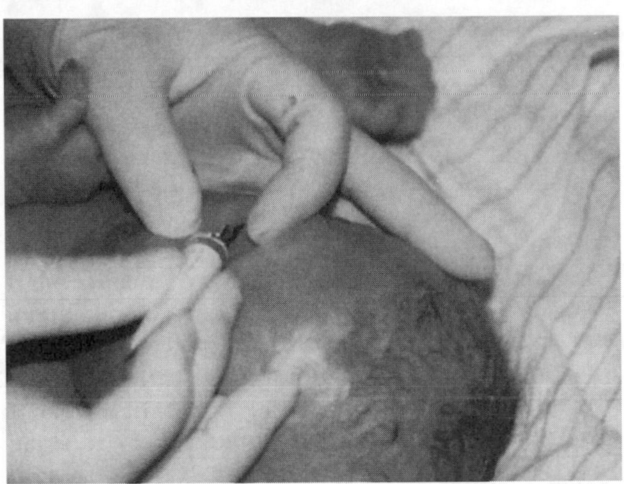

Fig. 23-7 Instillation of medication into eye of newborn. Thumb and forefinger are used to open the eye; medication is placed in the lower conjunctiva from the inner to the outer canthus. (Courtesy Marjorie Pyle, RNC, Lifecircle, Costa Mesa, Calif.)

infection and can cause chemical conjunctivitis. In some institutions instillation of eye prophylaxis is delayed until an hour or so after birth. This facilitates eye contact and enhances attachment and bonding. The Centers for Disease Control and Prevention specify that a delay of up to 2 hours is safe.

Vitamin K Prophylaxis

Administering vitamin K intramuscularly is routine in the newborn period. A single intramuscular dose of 0.5 to 1 mg of vitamin K soon after birth is given to prevent clotting problems. Vitamin K is produced in the gastrointestinal tract by bacteria; since most newborns initially have a sterile bowel, vitamin K is not produced in sufficient quantities to promote and maintain adequate blood clotting. For the administration procedure see Intramuscular Injection, p. 650.

Evaluation

Evaluation of nursing care and outcomes is an ongoing activity in the care of both mother and baby. During the third and fourth stages of labor, the nurse evaluates the degree to which expected outcomes for care are achieved. That is, the newborn's airway remains clear, temperature remains within normal limits, the infant does not experience an injury, and the parent-newborn bonding process is facilitated. If the evaluation shows that results fall short of achieving any outcome, further assessment, planning, and implementation are warranted.

2 HOURS AFTER BIRTH UNTIL DISCHARGE

Nursing Care Management

The admission to the nursery may be delayed or may never actually occur. Depending upon the routine of the hospital, the infant often remains in the labor area and is transferred to the nursery/postpartum unit with the mother. Many hospitals have adopted variations of **single-room maternity care (SRMC).** One nurse provides care for both the mother and the newborn. SRMC allows the infant to remain with the parents after the birth. Many of the procedures, such as assessment of weight and measurement, instillation of eye medications, intramuscular (IM) administration of vitamin K, and physical assessment, may be carried out in the labor and birth unit. Nurses who work in an SRMC unit; labor, delivery, recovery room (LDR); or labor, delivery, recovery, postpartum room (LDRP) are educated and competent to provide intrapartal, neonatal, and postpartum nursing care.

Regardless of the physical organization for care, many hospitals have a small holding nursery, which is available for procedures or on request of the mother who wishes her infant to be placed there. This arrangement promotes parent-infant bonding while still allowing the new parents some time to be alone.

Assessment

Even with modifications in nursery placement, the routine procedures and admission processes are still necessary. All these procedures can be carried out in any LDR, LDRP, SRMC, or separate nursery setting. The gestational age assessment should optimally be done 2 to 12 hours after birth. A complete physical assessment is also done within 2 to 8 hours of birth.

When an infant is transferred to the nursery, the infant's identification is verified by the nurse receiving the infant. The nurse places the baby in a warm environment and begins the admission process.

Some maternal conditions can affect gestational assessment. An infant who has experienced oxygen deprivation during labor may have poor muscle tone. Infants with respiratory distress tend to be flaccid and assume a "frogleg" posture. An infant who appears large, such as an infant of a diabetic mother, may respond in the same way as a premature infant.

A nurse working with infants has a responsibility to assess the health of the newborn and provide appropriate care. An eight-point check system (Ragan and Weinfield, 1989) has been developed to assist with assessing the newborn. The memory device, "Very active children need excellent comforting care always," for the acronym *VACNECCA* (vital signs, activity, color, nutrition, elimination, cord, circumcision, and attachment), facilitates a quick, thorough assessment. Such assessments should occur on every shift, be compared to the norm, and be recorded. Deviations from the norm may require intervention and notification of the physician/CNM.

Physical examination. Reviewing the maternal history and prenatal and intrapartal records provides information to help identify potential problems. Knowing the type of analgesia and anesthesia the mother received in labor is helpful. Pertinent information from the mother's prenatal record and her labor and birth record may be recorded on a form similar to the one in Fig. 23-8. The nurse can use these data to plan care for the newborn.

The parents' presence during this examination encourages prompt discussion of parental concerns and actively involves the parents in the health care of their child from birth. Also, parental interactions with the child can be observed. This aids

Neonatal Health History

Date ______ Infant ______
Date of birth ______ Sex ______
Time of birth ______ Age (in hours) now ______

Prenatal data
Maternal age ______ Blood type and Rh ______
Indirect Coombs' ______ EDB via dates ______

Previous obstetric history
Parity (explain all items) ______
Previous pregnancies:
Date ______ Gestational age ____ Sex ____ Weight ______ Birth ______ Complications ______

Complications of this pregnancy
Preeclampsia ______ Hypertension ______
Diabetes (class) ______ Bleeding ______
Viral/bacterial infection ______
Environmental teratogens ______
Drug use ______
Over-the-counter ______ Alcohol ______
Prescription ______ Cocaine ______
Heroin ______ Methadone ______
Other ______

Results of fetal testing
AFP assay ______
Ultrasound ______ Amniocentesis ______
NST ______ BPS ______

Intrapartum data
Onset of contractions ______
Rupture of membranes (ROM) ______ When? ______
Bloody ______ Meconium stained ______ Foul smell ______
Abnormalities of maternal vital signs ______
Medications during labor ______
Anesthesia/analgesia ______ Time last administered ______
Fetal monitoring (external/internal) ______
Fetal distress ______ Fetal pH ______
Length of stages of labor: 1st ______ 2nd ______ 3rd ______

Delivery
Time ______ Route ______
Reason for operative delivery ______

Resuscitation
Apgar score: 1 minute ______ 5 minute ______
Suction ______ Whiffs of O_2 ______
Positive pressure ______ via mask/endotracheal tube ______
Length ______
Time of first spontaneous breath ______
Medications ______

Other
Voided in delivery room ______ Stool ______
Breastfed ______ Bonding time ______
Observations of bonding behavior ______

In nursery
Time of transfer to nursery if applicable ______
First temperature ______ Placed in warmer/Isolette ______
Eye prophylaxis ______
Vitamin K ______ Time ______ Location ______

Fig. 23-8 Neonatal health history. (From Dickason E et al: *Maternal-infant nursing care,* ed 2, St Louis, 1994, Mosby.)

in early identification of learning needs and diagnosis of concerns in parent-child relationships.

The area used for the examination should be well lighted, warm, and free from drafts. The infant is undressed as needed and placed on a firm, flat surface. The infant may need to be picked up and cuddled at times for reassurance. The examination is carried out in a systematic manner as described in Chapter 22.

Data are recorded as descriptive notes or are summarized on standard forms. Identifying data are entered first: name, hospital number, birth date, weight, length, chest and head circumferences, race, sex, mother's and infant's blood type and Rh factor, Coombs' test results, and time of examination.

ASSESSMENT OF COMMON PROBLEMS IN THE NEWBORN

Physical Injuries

Birth trauma. *Birth trauma* includes any physical injury sustained by a newborn during labor and birth. Many injuries are minor and readily resolved in the neonatal period without treatment. Other traumas require some degree of intervention. Several factors predispose an infant to birth trauma (Fanaroff and Martin, 1997). *Maternal factors* include uterine dysfunction that leads to prolonged or precipitous labor, preterm or postterm labor, and cephalopelvic disproportion. Injury may result from dystocia caused by fetal macrosomia, multifetal gestation, abnormal or difficult presentation, and congenital anomalies. *Intrapartum events* that can result in minor scalp lacerations include the use of intrapartum fetal heart rate (FHR) monitoring and fetal scalp sampling. *Obstetric birth techniques* can also cause injury. Forceps birth, vacuum extraction, external version and extraction, and cesarean birth are all potential contributory factors.

Soft tissue injuries. *Caput succedaneum* and *cephalhematoma* are described in Chapter 22 (see Fig. 22-6).

Subconjunctival and retinal hemorrhages result from rupture of capillaries caused by increased pressure during birth. The hemorrhages clear within 5 days after birth and usually present no further problems. Parents need explanation and reassurance that these injuries are harmless.

Erythema, ecchymoses, petechiae, abrasions, lacerations, and edema of buttocks and extremities may be present. Localized discoloration may appear over presenting parts and may result from application of forceps or the vacuum extractor. Ecchymoses and edema may appear anywhere on the body. Petechiae, or pinpoint hemorrhagic areas, acquired during birth may extend over the upper trunk and face. These lesions are benign if they disappear within 2-3 days of birth and no new lesions appear. Ecchymoses and petechiae may be signs of a more serious disorder, such as *thrombocytopenia.* To differentiate hemorrhagic areas from skin rashes and discolorations, blanch the skin with two fingers. Petechiae and ecchymoses do not blanch because extravasated blood remains within the tissues.

Trauma secondary to dystocia occurs over the presenting fetal part. Forceps injury and bruising from the vacuum cup occur at the site of application of the instruments. Forceps injury commonly has a linear configuration across both sides of the face outlining the blades of the forceps. The affected areas are kept clean to minimize risk of infection. The increased use of the vacuum extractor and use of padded forceps blades may significantly reduce the incidence of these lesions (Fanaroff and Martin, 1997).

Accidental lacerations may be inflicted with a scalpel during cesarean birth. These cuts may occur on any part of the body but are most often found on the scalp, buttocks, and thighs. During vaginal deliveries scalp lacerations may occur with an episiotomy. Usually they are superficial, needing only to be kept clean. Butterfly adhesive strips will hold together the edges of more serious lacerations. Rarely are sutures needed.

Skeletal injuries. Fracture of the *clavicle,* or collarbone, is the most common birth injury. It is often associated with difficult vertex or breech birth of infants of greater than average size. *Crepitus* (the crackling sound produced by the rubbing together of fractured bone fragments) is often heard and/or felt (especially if the infant is in a prone position) on further examination, and radiographs usually reveal a complete fracture with overriding of the fragments.

A newborn with a fractured clavicle may have no symptoms, but suspect a fracture if the infant has limited use of the affected arm, malposition of the arm, an asymmetric Moro reflex, or focal swelling or tenderness or if the infant cries in pain when the arm is moved. Eliciting the scarf sign (extending arm across chest toward opposite shoulder) for assessment of gestational age is contraindicated if a fractured clavicle is suspected. Often no intervention may be prescribed other than proper body alignment, careful dressing and undressing of the infant, and handling and carrying that support the affected bone. For example, if the infant has a fractured clavicle, it is important to support the upper and lower back rather than pull the infant up from under the arms. Occasionally, for immobilization and relief of pain, the arm on the side of the fractured clavicle may be fixed on the body by pinning the sleeve to the shirt or by application of a triangular sling.

The *humerus* and *femur* are other bones that may be fractured during a difficult birth. Fractures in newborns generally heal rapidly. Immobilization is accomplished with slings, splints, swaddling, and other orthotic devices.

The infant's immature, flexible skull can withstand a great deal of molding before fracture results. Unless a blood vessel is involved, linear fractures heal without special treatment. These fractures account for 70% of all fractures in this age group. Depressed skull fractures may occur without laceration of either the skin or the dural membrane. These fractures may occur during difficult births from pressure of the head on the bony pelvis or from injudicious application of forceps.

Developmental dysplasia of the hip is often a hereditary disorder and occurs more commonly in girls because of the structure of the pelvis. In this condition, the acetabulum is abnormally shallow. The head of the femur becomes dislocated upward and backward to lie on the dorsal aspect of the ilium. The pressure of the displaced femoral head may form a false acetabulum on the ilium. A stretched joint capsule results, and ossification of the femoral head is delayed.

Before dislocation occurs, reduced movement, splinting of the affected hip, limited abduction, and asymmetry of the hip may be noted. After dislocation, all of these signs are present,

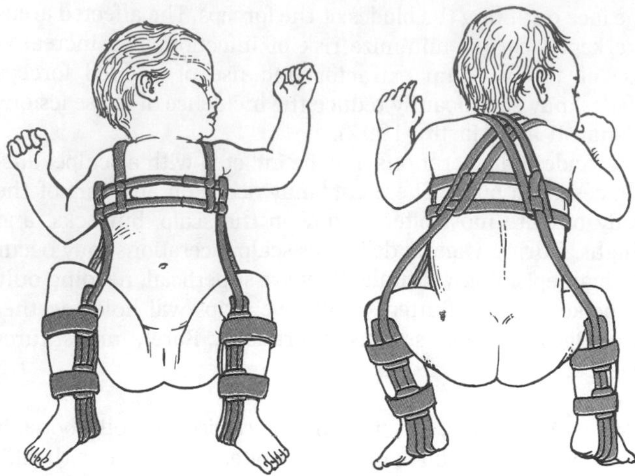

Fig. 23-9 Treatment for developmental dysplasia of the hip by application of a Pavlik harness. 1. Position the infant in a relaxed supine position. 2. The shoulder straps on the chest halter should cross in the back to prevent slippage down the shoulders. 3. The buckles for the anterior (flexor) stirrup straps should be placed at the anterior line. 4. The buckles for the posterior (abduction) stirrup straps should be placed over the scapula. 5. The self-adhesive (Velcro) straps for the proximal part of the leg should be placed just below the popliteal fossa. 6. Place the feet into the stirrups and secure the straps. 7. The posterior straps should already be attached and should not need to be unfastened when the harness is removed. 8. Secure the straps attached to the stirrups to the anterior buckles, positioning the hips at 90-degree flexion and 70-degree abduction.

together with external rotation and shortening of the leg. A clicking sound may be heard on gentle forced abduction of the leg (Ortolani sign, Fig. 22-17), and a bulge of the femoral head is felt or seen. The deformity cannot always be seen on x-ray examination in early infancy.

Treatment involves pressing the femoral head into the acetabulum to form an adequate socket before ossification is complete. A Pavlik harness is often used in treatment of developmental dysplasia of the hip (Fig. 23-9). A hip spica cast may be applied to maintain abduction, extension, and internal rotation, usually with the infant in a "frog-leg" position.

Parents need support in handling an infant with skeletal injuries because they are often fearful of hurting their newborn. Parents are encouraged to practice handling, changing, and feeding the injured newborn under the guidance of the nursing staff. This increases the parents' knowledge and confidence, in addition to facilitating attachment. A plan for follow-up therapy is developed with the parents so that the times and arrangements for therapy are convenient for them.

Physiologic Problems

Physiologic jaundice. Approximately 50% to 80% of all full-term newborns become visibly jaundiced (yellowish in color) during the first 3 days of life. Serum bilirubin levels less than 5 mg/dl usually are not reflected in visible skin jaundice. **Physiologic jaundice** is characterized by a progressive increase in serum levels of total bilirubin to a mean peak of 6 mg/dl by 72 hours of age, followed by a decline to 2 to 3 mg/dl by day 5, usually not exceeding 12 mg/dl in formula-fed newborns. These serum values are within the normal physiologic limitations of the healthy term newborn who was not exposed to perinatal complications (such as prolonged hypoxia). There is little agreement concerning the implementation of **phototherapy** and the total serum bilirubin level; the overall health status of the newborn in relation to the pattern of serum bilirubin levels must be carefully evaluated before therapy is initiated.

Every newborn is assessed for jaundice. The *blanch test* assists in the differentiation of cutaneous jaundice in infants of all races. To do the test, pressure is applied with a finger over a bony area (e.g., nose, forehead, sternum) for several seconds to empty all the capillaries in that spot. If jaundice is present, the blanched area will look yellow before the capillaries refill. The conjunctiva and buccal mucosa are assessed, especially in darker-skinned infants. It is preferable to assess for jaundice in natural light, because distortion of color from artificial lighting and reflection from nursery walls is possible.

Jaundice is reported first to be noticeable in the head and then progress gradually toward the abdomen and extremities because of the newborn infant's circulatory pattern (cephalocaudal developmental progression). Since the degree of jaundice cannot be objectively measured by visual assessment alone, serum bilirubin levels are used to assess hyperbilirubinemia. A transcutaneous bilirubin meter may be helpful to spot check certain infants with jaundice.

Nursing ALERT

Evidence of jaundice that appears before the infant is 24 hours of age is an indication for assessing bilirubin levels.

Hypoglycemia. Hypoglycemia is present when the infant's blood glucose concentration is significantly lower than that of the majority of infants of the same age and weight. Therefore the determination of an abnormally low blood glucose level varies. In the full-term newborn, hypoglycemia may be defined as plasma glucose concentrations of less than 40 mg/dl in the first 24 hours and 40 to 50 mg/dl thereafter (Cornblath and Schwartz, 1993).

Signs of hypoglycemia include jitteriness; irregular respiratory effort; cyanosis; apnea; weak, high-pitched cry; feeding difficulty; lethargy; twitching; eye rolling; and seizures. The signs may be transient but recurrent.

Blood sugar level may also be determined with a reagent strip (Dextrostix or Chemstrip-BG), which may be read either manually or with a glucose reflectance meter. Although simple procedures, the tests are very sensitive and must be performed correctly to prevent false readings. The American Academy of Pediatrics (1993a) does not recommend universal screening for hypoglycemia in full-term neonates.

Hypoglycemia in the otherwise well, low-risk term infant may be resolved by feeding the infant. Occasionally administration of intravenous glucose is required.

Hypocalcemia. Hypocalcemia (less than 7 mg/dl) may occur in newborns of diabetic mothers or with perinatal asphyxia, trauma, low birth weight (LBW), and preterm birth. Early-onset hypocalcemia occurs within the first 72 hours after birth. Signs of hypocalcemia include jitteriness, edema, apnea, intermittent cyanosis, and abdominal distention.

In most instances, early-onset hypocalcemia is self-limiting and resolves within 1 to 3 days. Treatment includes early feeding and, occasionally, administration of calcium supplements.

Jitteriness is a symptom of both hypoglycemia and hypocalcemia. Hypocalcemia must be considered if therapy for hypoglycemia is ineffective. In many newborns, jitteriness remains despite therapy and cannot be explained by either hypoglycemia or hypocalcemia (Fanaroff and Martin, 1997).

BOX 23-3
Standard Laboratory Values in a Term Newborn

Hemoglobin	14.5 to 22.5 g/dl
Hematocrit	44% to 72%
Glucose	40 to 60 mg/dl
Bilirubin, direct	0 to 1 mg/dl
Blood gases	
Arterial	pH 7.31 to 7.45
	Pco_2 33 to 48 mm Hg
	Po_2 50 to 70 mm Hg
Venous	pH 7.28 to 7.42
	Pco_2 38 to 52 mm Hg
	Po_2 20 to 49 mm Hg

LABORATORY AND DIAGNOSTIC TESTS

Blood glucose levels and urinalysis are commonly performed on newborns. Other tests may be performed as needed, including bilirubin levels, newborn screening tests (e.g., phenylketonuria [PKU], thyroid [T4], and galactosemia), hematocrits, and drug tests. See Box 23-3 for standard laboratory values in a term newborn. Some states require newborns to be tested for up to nine disorders. Information about which tests are required in a state can be obtained at state health departments. About 30 states test for sickle cell anemia and some states now test for cystic fibrosis (March of Dimes, 1994). Table 23-2 discusses some of the major disorders for which infants are checked.

Collection of Specimens

Ongoing evaluation of a newborn often requires obtaining blood and urine specimens. The following procedures are used: heel stick, venipuncture, collection of urine and specimen.

Heel stick. Many blood specimens are drawn by laboratory technicians. However, nurses may be required to perform heel sticks to obtain blood for glucose monitoring and to measure hematocrit levels. The same technique is needed to complete the PKU form or to test for galactosemia and hypothyroidism or other inborn errors of metabolism (Table 23-2).

Before the sample is taken, it is helpful to warm the heel. Application of heat for 5 to 10 minutes helps dilate the vessels in the area. A cloth soaked with warm water and wrapped loosely around the foot provides effective warming (Fig. 23-10, *A*). Second- and third-degree thermal burns have been reported from inappropriate heel warming techniques. Wrap-

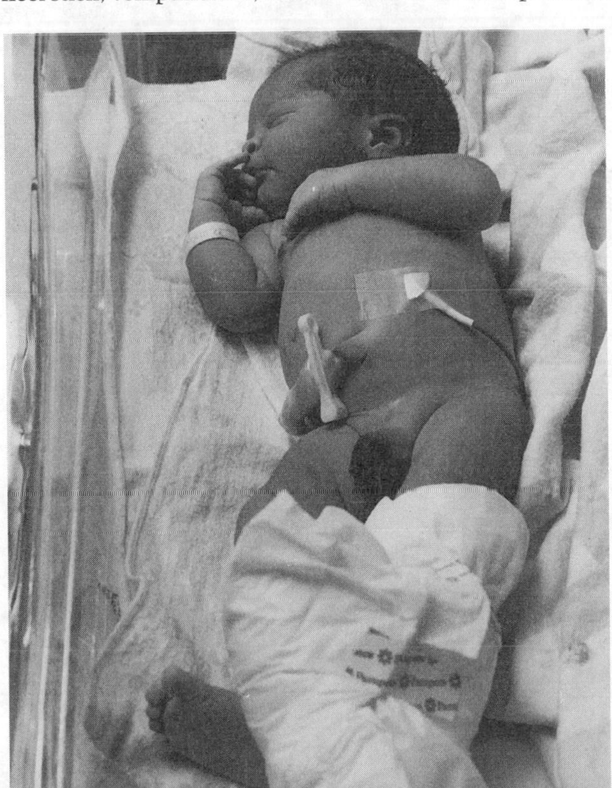

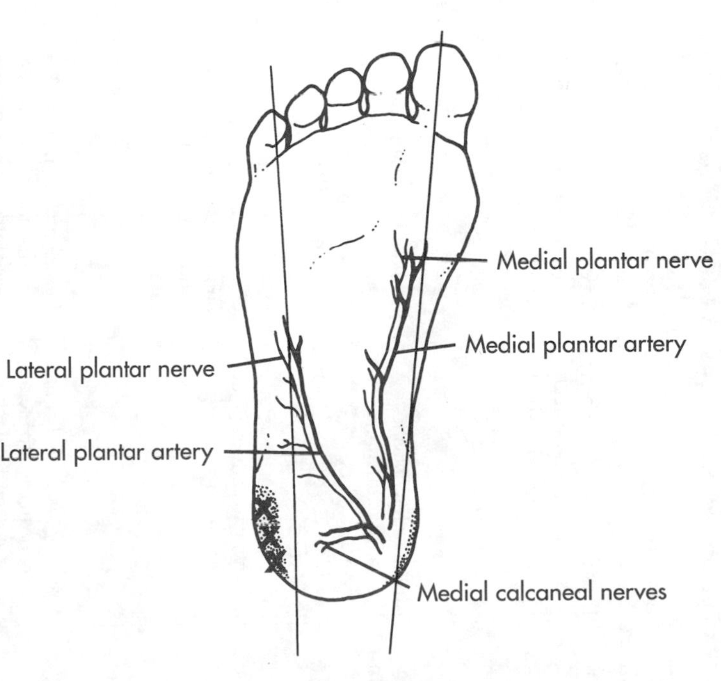

Fig. 23-10 Heel stick. **A,** Newborn with foot wrapped for warmth to increase blood flow to extremity before heel stick. **B,** Puncture sites (*x*) on infant's foot for heel stick samples of capillary blood. (Courtesy Marjorie Pyle, RNC, Lifecircle, Costa Mesa, Calif.)

TABLE 23-2 Newborn screening summary

DISORDER	BASIC DEFECT	SYMPTOMS	+ SCREENING INCIDENCE	CRITERIA	TREATMENT	FOLLOW-UP NEEDS
PKU (classic)	Lack of enzyme to properly convert the amino acid phenylalanine to tyrosine.	Severe mental retardation, eczema, seizures, behavior disorders, decreased pigmentation, distinctive "mousey" odor.	1:10,000 to 1:15,000 More common in whites	Elevated phe	Low phenylalanine diet; possible tyrosine supplementation	Lifelong dietary management; careful monitoring of hyperphe variants; careful management and preconception counseling and intervention for PKU women in the reproductive years.
Congenital hypothyroidism (primary)	Absent or hypoplastic gland; dysfunctional gland.	Mental and motor retardation, short stature, coarse, dry skin and hair, hoarse cry, constipation.	Overall 1:4000 with ethnic variation 1:12,000 African-American 1:1000 Indian	Low T_4, elevated TSH	Replacement of L-thyroxine	Maintain L-thyroxine levels in upper half of normal range; periodic bone age to monitor growth.
Galactosemia (transferase deficiency)	Absent or low activity of enzyme to convert galactose into glucose.	Neonatal death from severe dehydration, sepsis or liver abnormality; mental retardation, jaundice, blindness, cataracts.	1:10,000 to 1:90,000	Elevated galactose; low or absent fluorescence	Eliminate galactose and lactose from the diet; soy formulas in infancy; lactose-free solid foods.	Provide early monitoring for speech and neurologic problems; educate parents about hidden sources of lactose; monitor females for secondary ovarian failure; avoid medications with lactose fillers.
Maple syrup urine disease (MSUD)	Absent or low activity of enzyme needed to metabolize leucine, isoleucine, and valine.	Acidosis; hypertonicity and seizures, vomiting, drowsiness, apnea, coma; infant death or severe mental retardation and neurologic impairment; behavior disorders.	1:90,000 to 1:200,000	Elevated leucine	Diet low in leucine, isoleucine, and valine; thiamine supplement if responsive.	Educate family and friends regarding strict dietary regimen; social and education evaluation; behavior counseling; neurologic monitoring; prompt treatment of illness to minimize acidosis.
Homocystinuria	Deficiency of enzyme cytothianine synthase, which is needed for homocystine metabolism	Mental retardation, seizures, behavior disorders, early onset thromboses, dislocated lenses, tall lanky body habitus.	1:200,000	Elevated methionine	Methionine-restricted diet; cystine supplement; B_6 supplement if responsive.	Maintain lifelong low methionine diet; monitor for thrombosis (check pulses, etc); ophthalmologic care; educational and psychological evaluation; avoid unnecessary surgery.
Congenital adrenal hyperplasia (CAH)	Defect in the enzyme-21-hydroxylase	Hyponatremia, hypokalemia, hypoglycemia, dehydration and early death; ambiguous genitalia in females; progressive virilization in both sexes.	1:15,000 to 1:30,000 Native Eskimos	Elevated 17-hydroxy progesterone; abnormal electrolytes	Replace corticosteroids; plastic surgery to correct ambiguous genitalia.	Maintain adequate corticosteroids; elevate doses or give injectable doses in times of stress; periodic bone age to monitor adequate treatment; maintain pediatric endocrinology follow-up appointments.
Biotinidase deficiency	Low activity of the enzyme biotinidase; biotin deficiency	Mental retardation, seizures, ataxia, skin rash, hearing loss, alopecia, optic nerve atrophy, coma, and death.	1:60,000 to 1:100,000	Deficient or absent activity of biotinidase on calorimetric assay.	10 mg biotin daily	Monitor compliance; periodic follow-up and evaluation.

From Wright L, Brown A, Davidson-Mundt A: Newborn screening: the miracle and the challenge, *J Pediatr Nurs* 7:26, 1992. Used with permission.

ping the foot in a plastic wrap or with a plastic-covered diaper prevents dissipation of heat and can cause thermal burns (NAACOG, 1992). Disposable heel warmers are available from a variety of companies and should be used with care to prevent skin burns.

Nurses should wear gloves when collecting any specimen. The nurse cleanses the area with alcohol, restrains the infant's foot with the free hand, and punctures the selected site with a small sterile lance or "Tenderfoot" puncture device.

The most serious complication of infant heel stick is necrotizing osteochondritis from lancet penetration of the bone. To prevent this, the penetration should be no deeper than 2.4 mm and should be made at the outer aspect of the heel (Wong, 1995). To identify the appropriate puncture sites, the nurse draws an imaginary line from between the fourth and fifth toes that runs parallel to the lateral aspect of the heel, or a line running from the great toe that runs parallel to the medial aspect of the heel (Fig. 23-10, *B*). Repeated trauma to the walking surface of the heel can cause fibrosis and scarring that may lead to problems with walking (Reiner, Meltes, and Hayes, 1990; Wong, 1995).

After the specimen has been collected, pressure is applied with a dry gauze square. Reapplying alcohol will cause the site to continue to bleed. The nurse ensures proper disposal of equipment used, reviews the laboratory slip for correct identification, and checks the specimen for adequate labeling and routing.

A heel stick is traumatic for the infant and causes pain. Pain pathways are present and functional in the infant. After heel sticks infants have been observed to withdraw their feet when they are touched. To reassure the infant and promote feelings of safety, cuddle and comfort the neonate when the procedure is complete. Rocking the infant or giving a pacifier is also an effective comforting measure (Campos, 1994).

Venipuncture. Venous blood samples can be drawn from antecubital, saphenous, superficial wrist, and, rarely, scalp veins. If an intravenous (IV) site is used to obtain a blood specimen, it is important to consider the type of infusion fluid.

When venipuncture is required, positioning of the needle is extremely important. Although regular venipuncture nee-

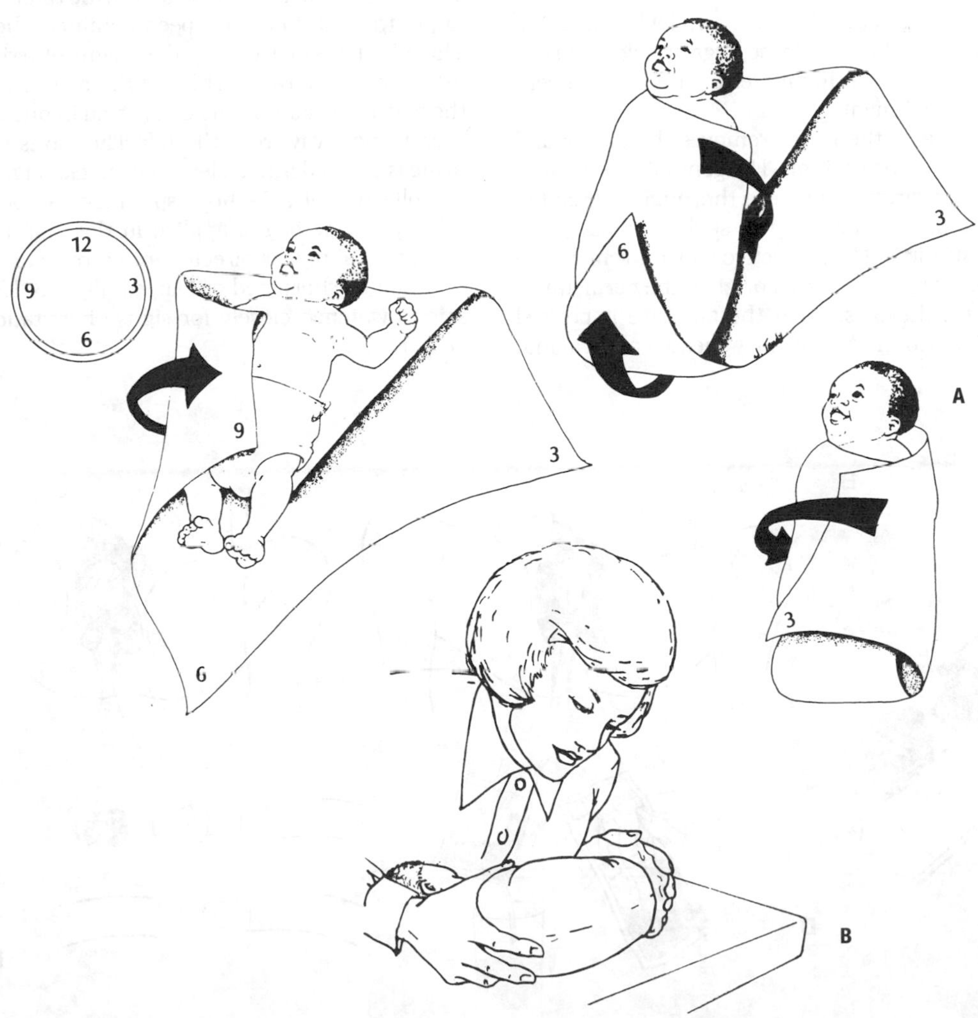

Fig. 23-11 Methods of infant restraint. **A,** Mummy technique to restrain infant. **B,** Position for lumbar puncture.

dles may be used, some individuals prefer butterfly needles. It is necessary to be very patient during the procedure because small veins yield slow blood return and the small needle must remain in place longer. The mummy restraint commonly is used to help secure the infant (Fig. 23-11).

Every effort should be made to keep the infant comfortable during the procedure. For blood gas and serum glucose studies the blood sample tubes are packed in ice to reduce blood cell metabolism and are taken immediately to the laboratory for analysis. Pressure must be maintained over an arterial puncture for at least 5 minutes to prevent bleeding and hematoma from the site.

For an hour after any venipuncture, the nurse should observe the infant often for evidence of bleeding or hematoma at the puncture site. The infant's tolerance of the procedure should be noted and recorded. The infant should be cuddled and comforted (e.g., rocked, given pacifier) when the procedure is completed.

Obtaining urine specimen. Examination of urine is a valuable laboratory tool for infant assessment. The way in which the specimen is collected may influence the results. The urine sample should be fresh and examined within 1 hour of collection.

A variety of urine collection bags are available, including the Hollister U-Bag (Fig. 23-12). These bags are clear plastic, single-use bags with self-adhering material around the opening at the point of attachment.

To prepare the infant, the nurse removes the diaper and places the infant in a supine position. The genitalia, perineum, and surrounding skin are washed and thoroughly dried because the adhesive of the bag will not stick to moist, powdered, or oily skin surfaces. The protective paper is removed to expose the adhesive (Fig. 23-12, *A*). For girls, the perineum is stretched to flatten skin folds. Then the adhesive is pressed firmly to the skin all around the urinary meatus and vagina.

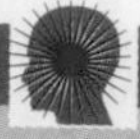

Critical Thinking Exercises

PERFORMING PROCEDURES

Select one emergency procedure and one daily care procedure. Describe what supplies and equipment are needed and how you would perform the procedure yourself and/or teach it to new parents. Justify your decisions and actions.

(NOTE: Start with the narrow portion of the butterfly-shaped adhesive patch.) The nurse must be sure to start at the bridge of skin separating the rectum from the vagina and work upward (Fig. 23-12, *B*). For boys, the penis and scrotum are tucked through the opening of the collector before the nurse removes the protective paper from the adhesive. The bag is fitted over the penis, the protective paper removed, and the flaps pressed firmly to the perineum, making sure the entire adhesive coating is firmly attached to skin with no puckering of adhesive (Fig. 23-12, *C*). This helps ensure a leak-proof seal and decreases the chance of contamination from stool. The diaper is carefully replaced. The bag is checked often. Cutting a slit in the diaper and pulling the bag through the slit may also help prevent leaking.

When a sufficient amount of urine (amount varies according to the test done) has been obtained, the bag is removed. The infant's skin is observed for signs of irritation. The specimen can be aspirated with a syringe or drained directly from the bag. For draining, the bag is held in one hand and tilted to keep urine away from the tab. The tab is removed, and the urine is drained into a clean receptacle (Fig. 23-12, *D*).

Collection of a 24-hour specimen can be a challenge. The 24-hour urine bag is applied in the manner just described, and the drainage is directed into a receptacle. The collection tube can be shortened or capped (Fig. 23-12, E). The infant's skin is watched closely for signs of irritation and lack of a proper seal.

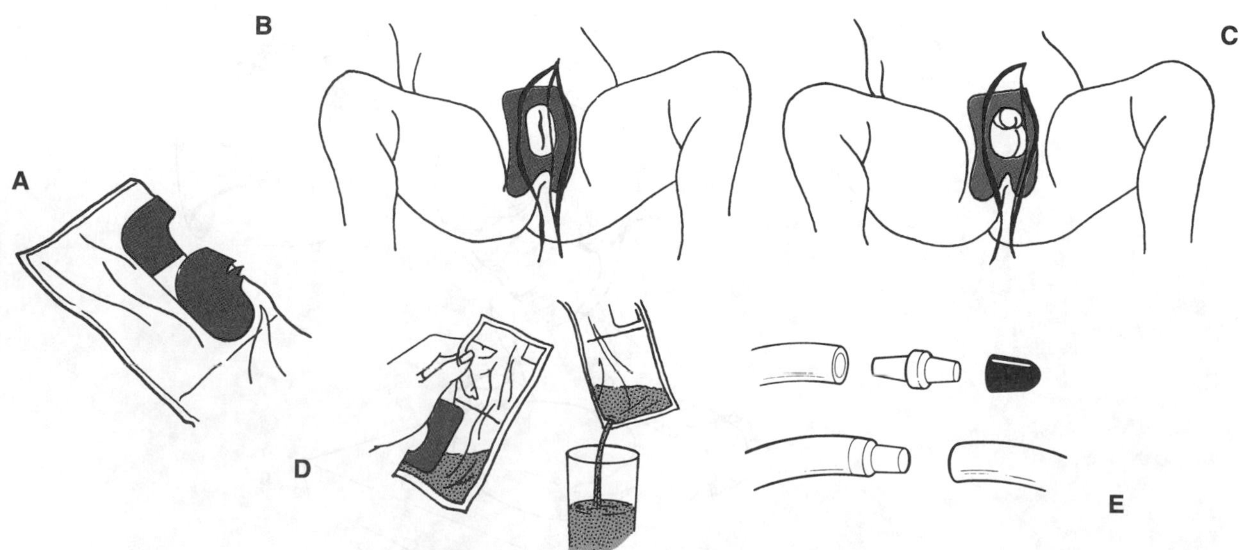

Fig. 23-12 Urine collection bag. **A,** Protective paper is being removed from the adhesive surface. **B,** Applied to girl. **C,** Applied to boy. **D,** Cut to drain urine. **E,** Collection tube. (Courtesy Hollister, Inc, Chicago, Ill.)

Nursing Care Plan

NORMAL NEWBORN

Nursing Diagnosis: Risk for ineffective airway clearance related to excess mucus/improper positioning

Expected Outcomes: Infant's airway remains patent; breathing is regular and unlabored.

• NURSING INTERVENTIONS/*RATIONALES*

Suction mouth and nasopharynx with bulb syringe as needed; clean nares of crusted secretions *to clear airway and prevent aspiration.*

Position neonate on right side after feeding *to prevent aspiration* and on back or side when sleeping *to prevent suffocation.*

Keep diapers, clothing, and covers loose enough *to allow for maximum lung expansion.*

Teach parents how to hold, suction, and position the infant with return demonstration *to ensure parental skill at airway clearance and maintenance.*

Teach parents that gagging, coughing, and sneezing are normal infant responses *that aid the infant in clearing airways.*

Teach parents feeding techniques that prevent overfeeding and distention of abdomen and teach them to burp infant frequently *to prevent regurgitation and aspiration.*

Nursing Diagnosis: Risk for ineffective thermoregulation related to immature regulatory system/changes in environment

Expected Outcome: Infant temperature remains at optimum level 36.5° C to 37.2° C (97.7° to 98.9° F).

• NURSING INTERVENTIONS/*RATIONALES*

Keep infant adequately covered with clothing and blankets (Do not overdress) *to ensure sufficient warmth to maintain temperature.*

Maintain room temperature between 75° and 78° F (24° C to 25.6° C) with 40% to 50% humidity *to optimize environment.*

Keep infant away from drafts, fans, air-conditioning vents; avoid temperature extremes and rapid changes in temperature *to prevent temperature alteration.*

Use warm water for bathing in room with stable temperature, wrap in towel, and dry immediately after bath *to prevent chilling.*

Nursing Diagnosis: Risk for infection related to immature immunologic defenses/environmental exposure

Expected Outcome: No evidence of infection of eyes, respiratory system, genital area, umbilical cord.

• NURSING INTERVENTIONS/*RATIONALES*

Have all care providers use good handwashing technique before and after handling the infant *to prevent spread of infection.*

Keep eyes and eyelashes clean and free of mucus; provide prescribed eye prophylaxis *to prevent infection.*

Keep genital areas clean and dry using proper cleansing techniques *to prevent skin irritation, cross-contamination, and infection.*

Keep umbilical stump clean and dry and place diapers below the stump *to minimize infection.*

If present, keep circumcision site clean, glans dressed with sterile petrolatum, and diaper applied loosely *to prevent trauma and infection and to promote healing.*

Monitor eyes, respiratory system, skin, genitalia, umbilical cord, circumcision site for signs of infection; monitor vital signs; monitor ordered laboratory values *to detect infection early to promote rapid treatment and healing.*

Administer topical, oral, and parenteral antibiotics per physician order *to eradicate pathogens.*

Teach parents to avoid smoke-filled environments, people with respiratory infections, substances that can induce aspiration pneumonia such as baby powder *to protect infant from respiratory compromise.*

Teach parents to avoid prolonged public outings, touching and holding by large numbers of people, people with infectious diseases, contaminated food sources *to reduce potential sources of infection.*

Nursing Diagnosis: Risk for trauma related to physical helplessness

Expected Outcome: Infant remains free of physical injury.

• NURSING INTERVENTIONS/*RATIONALES*

Employ appropriate methods of handling, holding *to prevent injury* (i.e., protect head, avoid picking up by extremities), and transporting infant (i.e., use appropriate car seat with proper technique).

Monitor environment *to prevent injury* (i.e., avoid use of pointed or sharp objects around infant, supervise infant and sibling/pet interactions, supervise infant on raised surfaces with no sides).

Modify environment *to prevent injury* (i.e., place potentially harmful objects out of reach; keep caretaker and infant fingernails trimmed, avoid jewelry that may scratch infant, check width of slats in infant crib, keep crib rails up when infant is in crib).

For some types of urine testing, urine can be aspirated directly from the diaper by means of a syringe without a needle. If the diaper has absorbent gelling material that traps urine, a small gauze or cotton balls are placed inside the diaper and the urine is aspirated from them (Wong, 1995).

Nursing Diagnoses

Analysis of the significance of assessment findings leads to the establishment of nursing diagnoses. Possible nursing diagnoses for the newborn are as follows:

- Ineffective breathing pattern related to
  Obstructed airway
- Impaired gas exchange related to
  Hypothermia (cold stress)
- Risk for ineffective thermoregulation related to
  Heat loss to environment
- Risk for infection related to
  Environmental factors
- Pain related to
  Circumcision
  Heel sticks, venipuncture

Possible nursing diagnoses for the parent(s) are as follows:

- Family coping, potential for growth related to
  Knowledge of newborn's social capabilities
  Knowledge of newborn's dependency needs
  Knowledge of biologic characteristics of the newborn
- Situational low self-esteem related to
  Misinterpretation of newborn's responses

The Nursing Care Plan on p. 641 provides examples of nursing diagnoses derived from specific assessment findings.

Expected Outcomes

Plans for care of the newborn reflect the rapid growth and development during the neonatal period. Changes in biologic and behavioral states are measured in minutes and hours after birth. The neonatal period extends up to the 28th day after birth. By that time the rate of growth changes has slowed enough so that the child's appearance and needs can be referred to in terms of weeks and months.

The focus of care changes between birth and 28 days. During the first 2 hours of life the main focus is on the infant's physiologic adaptation. By the end of the neonatal period the infant's socialization needs assume equal importance with physiologic needs.

The care given the neonate during the *first 2 hours of life* is part of the care given parents and newborns in the fourth stage of labor (p. 488). Care related to *nutritional needs* of infants, including techniques of feeding, is presented in Chapter 24. *Parent-child interactions* are discussed in Chapters 19 and 22.

The information in this section pertains to the maintenance of vital functions, the daily care of infants, and the forms of general therapy carried out routinely in the newborn period. Parental education before discharge from the hospital and at the well-baby visit is outlined.

The expected outcomes for newborn care relate to the infant and to the caregiver. The *expected outcomes for the infant* include the following:

1. The infant will maintain an effective breathing pattern.
2. The infant will maintain effective thermoregulation.
3. The infant will remain free from infection.
4. The infant will establish adequate elimination patterns.
5. The infant will experience minimal pain related to circumcision, heel stick, or other pain-causing procedure.

Expected outcomes for the parents include the following:

1. The parent(s) will attain knowledge, skill, and confidence relevant to child care activities.
2. The parent(s) will state understanding of biologic and behavioral characteristics of the newborn.
3. The parent(s) will have opportunities to intensify relationships with the newborn.
4. The parent(s) will begin to integrate the infant into the family.
5. The parent(s) will demonstrate behavior/life-style changes to reduce potential for development of problems.

PROTECTIVE ENVIRONMENT

The provision of a **protective environment** is basic to the care of the newborn. The construction, maintenance, and operation of nurseries in accredited hospitals are monitored by national professional organizations such as the American Academy of Pediatrics, the Centers for Disease Control and Prevention, the American College of Obstetricians and Gynecologists, and local or state governing bodies. In addition, hospital personnel develop their own policies and procedures directed to protecting the newborns under their care. Prescribed standards cover areas such as the following:

1. *Environmental factors*—provision of adequate lighting, elimination of potential fire hazards, safety of electric appliances, adequate ventilation, controlled temperature (warm and free of drafts) and humidity (lower than 50%).
2. *Measures to control infection*—adequate floor space to permit positioning bassinets at least 60 cm apart, hand-washing facilities, area for cleaning and storing equipment and supplies.

   Personnel are restricted to those directly involved in the care of mothers and infants, thereby reducing the opportunities for the introduction of pathogenic organisms. Personnel are instructed to use good hand-washing techniques. The most important single measure in the prevention of neonatal infection is hand washing between handling different infants.

   Health care workers must wear gloves when touching mucous membranes or nonintact skin of all patients. In addition, masks, eye coverings, and gowns must be used when indicated. Health care personnel must wear gloves when handling the infant until blood and amniotic fluid have been removed from the infant's skin, when drawing blood (e.g., heel stick), when caring for a fresh wound (e.g., circumcision), and during diaper changes.

Visitors and health care providers such as nurses, physicians, parents, brothers and sisters, department supervisors, electricians, and housekeepers are expected to wash their hands before having contact with infants or equipment. Cover gowns have not been proved to be necessary to prevent infection (Rush et al, 1990).

Individuals with infectious conditions are excluded from contact or must take special precautions when working with newborns. This includes persons with upper respiratory tract infections, gastrointestinal tract infections, and infectious skin conditions. Most agencies have now coupled this day-to-day self-screening of personnel with yearly health examinations.

3. *Safety factors*—Security measures have been implemented in many agencies in response to kidnapings from nurseries. Identical identification bracelets are placed on infants and their mothers. Infants are footprinted and/or have identification pictures taken after birth before they leave the mother's side. Personnel wear picture identification badges or other badges that identify them as newborn personnel. Infant tracking systems may be installed in mother-baby units that will set off an alarm if a baby is left alone or is with unauthorized personnel. Mothers are instructed to be certain they know the identity of anyone who cares for the infant and never to release the infant to anyone who is not wearing the appropriate identification.

SUPPORTING PARENTS IN THE CARE OF THEIR INFANT

The sensitivity of the caregiver to the social responses of the infant is basic to the development of a mutually satisfying parent-child relationship. Sensitivity increases over time as parents' awareness of their infant's social capabilities becomes more acute (see the Cultural Considerations box below).

Social Interactions

The activities of daily care during the neonatal period offer the best times for infant and family interactions. While caring for their baby, mother and father can talk to the infant, can ca-

Cultural Considerations 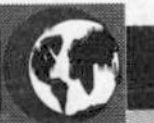

SOME CULTURAL BELIEFS ABOUT NEWBORNS

Mexican women may wish to place belly bands or coins over the infant's navel.
Muslim (Saudi Arabia) women may wish to say a prayer in the newborn's ear at the time of birth. Some groups still practice female circumcision.
Iranian male infants are usually circumcised.
Southeast Asians usually do not circumcise males. The infant should not be complimented because such compliments are believed to cause the infant to be captured by evil spirits.
A male Indian infant may be valued more than a female infant.
Haitian infants are usually not named until they are 1 month old.

Family Focus 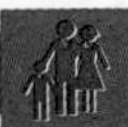

FAMILY RELATIONSHIPS AND SOCIAL SUPPORT

The family's ethnic and cultural background is important in determining the health status, genetic or familial risk factors present, and social support available to the woman throughout pregnancy and in the postpartum period. Family relationships, including husband-wife roles, vary among individuals and groups. The husband may be the decision-maker, and his consent may be necessary before the woman agrees to prenatal treatment. Female rather than male family members may be involved in the pregnancy and birth. Mothers and mothers-in-law may be present and supportive during pregnancy, birth, and the early postnatal period to provide advice and care. In such instances, they need to be included in teaching sessions. Community and church support may be available. Assessment of family and community resources is an essential component of care.

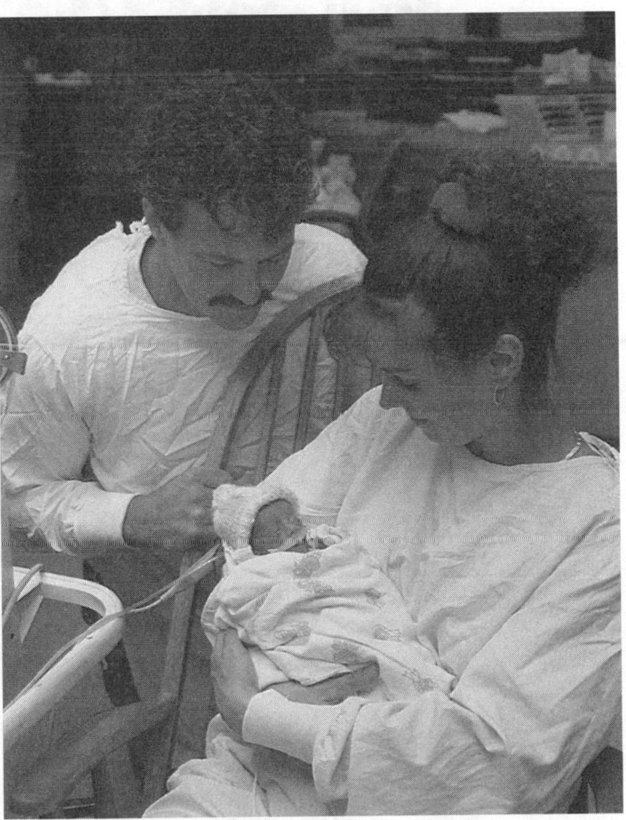

Fig. 23-13 Mother-father-baby interaction. (From Wong D: *Whaley & Wong's nursing care of infants and children,* ed. 5, St Louis, 1995, Mosby.)

ress and cuddle the child, and may use infant massage. In Fig. 23-13, mother, father, and infant engage in arousal, imitation of facial expression, and smiling. Older children's contact with a newborn needs to be supervised for strength of hugs, exploring of eyes and nose, and attempts to feed the baby. Parents often keep baby books that record their infant's progress.

Caregiving activities for the newborn are shared by the nurse and the parents. The nurse acts as teacher and support person. As soon as the mother feels physically able, she is encouraged to participate in her child's care. The mother's need for knowledge and the factors that may hinder her learning are determined through questioning and observation. The content taught and teaching aids used should reflect the mother's level of understanding. Films and tapes can be valu-

Infant care teaching record

INFANT CARE	DATE	INITIALS	TEACHING/ LEARNING CODE
Using/reading thermometer			
Temperature regulation			
Cord care*			
Dressing, wrapping, comforting*			
Voiding/stool			
Diapering*			
Bulb syringe*			
Car seat			
Circumcision			
Newborn screening			
Birth certificate			
INFANT FEEDING			
Frequency of feeding			
Positions for feeding			
Burping*			
INFANT FEEDING - BREAST			
Length of feedings			
Colostrum/when milk comes in			
Breaking suction*			
Milk supply			
Engorgement			
Hand expression			
Breast pump and milk storage			
INFANT FEEDING - BOTTLE			
Amount of feedings			
Formula preparation and storage			
Warming formula			
Don't use honey†			

Teaching/learning code:

VT = videotape
D = demonstration
VU = verbalizes understanding
NA = not applicable
V = verbal instruction
R = return demonstration
P = printed material given

*Return demonstration required before discharged at 24 hours.
†Honey contains botulism spores. Children under the age of 12 months should not be given honey.

Fig. 23-14 Infant care teaching record.

Critical Thinking Exercises

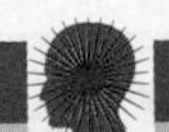

INFANT CARE CLASS

Prepare and conduct one 20-minute class in infant care for parents. Before class, prepare a written teaching plan that includes assessment of learning needs; a teaching-learning diagnosis; a plan with prioritized patient-centered goals; content and teaching methods with rationale; and evaluative criteria. After the class, critique the total experience. What insights have you achieved?

able timesavers in teaching. Most hospitals provide parents with written instructions for infant care. The care given the infant is supervised, and the parents are encouraged to ask questions. The infant care teaching record such as the one provided in Fig. 23-14 serves as a guideline for teaching parents. See the related Family Focus box on p. 643.

Infant Feeding

The infant may be put to the mother's breast shortly after birth or at least within 4 hours of birth. If the infant is to be bottle-fed, a nurse may offer a few sips of sterile water to be certain that the infant's sucking and swallowing reflexes are intact and that there are no anomalies such as a tracheoesophageal fistula before the mother feeds the baby. Most infants are on *demand feeding schedules* and are allowed to feed when they awaken. Ordinarily feedings are encouraged every 3 to 4 hours during the day and only when the infant awakens during the night in the first few days after birth. Breastfed babies will nurse more often than bottle-fed babies since human breast milk is digested faster than formulas made from cow's milk. Water supplements are usually not recommended. For a thorough discussion of infant feeding, see Chapter 24.

The nurse should assess the infant's tongue in relation to mobility and ability to suck. Ankyloglossia, or tongue-tie, an excessively tight lingual frenulum that restricts tongue movement and ability to latch on effectively to the breast, take milk from a bottle appropriately, or swallow, should be further evaluated. At times, a laser frenulectomy or a Z-plasty under general anesthesia is necessary (Godley, 1994; Pediatric Surgery Update, 1996). Simple clipping of the frenulum is no longer recommended.

Positioning and Holding

After feeding, positioning the infant on the right side promotes gastric emptying into the small intestine (Fig. 23-3). Placing the infant in the crib in a side-lying position also permits drainage of mucus from the mouth and applies no pressure to the sensitive circumcised penis. The American Academy of Pediatrics advises against the use of the prone position in the first few months of life and suggests that side lying or back lying is preferable. The prone position has been associated with an increased incidence of sudden infant death syndrome (SIDS) (Guntheroth and Spiers, 1992). Parents can be referred to "Back to Sleep," P.O. Box 29111, Washington, DC 20040; 1-800-505-CRIB for further information about infant position for sleep.

Anatomically the infant's shape—barrel chest and flat, curveless spine—makes it easy for the child to roll and startle. A folded or rolled blanket against the spine will prevent rolling to the supine position and will promote a feeling of security. Care must be taken to prevent the infant from rolling off unguarded flat surfaces. The parent or nurse who must turn away from the infant even for a moment keeps one hand securely on the infant.

The infant is held securely with support for the head because newborns are unable to maintain an erect head posture for more than a few moments. Fig. 23-15 illustrates various positions for holding an infant with adequate support.

Umbilical Cord Care

The goals of care are promotion of drying and prevention and early detection of hemorrhage or infection. If bleeding from the blood vessels of the cord is noted, the nurse checks the clamp and applies a second clamp next to the first one.

Hospital protocol directs the time and technique for routine cord care. The nurse cleanses the cord and skin area around the base of the cord with the prescribed preparation (e.g., erythromycin solution, triple-blue dye, or alcohol) and checks daily for signs of infection. The cord clamp may be removed after 24 hours when the cord is dry (Fig. 23-2, *D*).

Rashes

Diaper rash. The warm, moist atmosphere created in the diaper area provides an optimal environment for candidal growth. The dermatitis appears in the perianal area, inguinal folds, and lower abdomen. The affected area is intensely erythematous with a sharply demarcated, scalloped edge, often with numerous satellite lesions that extend beyond the larger legion. The usual source of infection is through the gastrointestinal tract when organisms are swallowed from the birth canal during delivery. It may also appear 2 to 3 days after an oral infection.

Therapy consists of applications of an anticandidal ointment, such as nystatin or clotrimazole, with each diaper change. Sometimes the infant also is given an oral antifungal preparation to eliminate any gastrointestinal source of infection.

Immediately washing and drying the wet and soiled area and changing the diaper after voiding or stooling prevent and help treat diaper rash. Parents can be taught that placing the infant in a warm room with the buttocks exposed to air or even filtered sunlight can help dry up diaper rash. Warmth can also be achieved with a 25-watt bulb placed 45 cm from the affected area for brief periods (15 minutes) several times a day. Disposable diapers and plastic pants should be avoided until healing occurs.

Other rashes. A rash on the face may result from the infant's scratching (excoriation) or from rubbing the face against the sheets, particularly if regurgitated stomach contents are not washed off promptly. Newborn rash, erythema toxicum, is a common finding (see Chapter 22).

Clothing

Parents commonly ask how warmly they should dress their infant. A simple rule of thumb is to dress the child as they dress themselves, adding or subtracting clothes and wraps for the child as necessary. A shirt or diaper may be sufficient clothing for the young infant. A cap or bonnet is needed to protect the scalp and minimize heat loss if the weather is cool or to protect against sunburn and shade the eyes if it is sunny and hot. Wrapping the infant snugly in a blanket maintains

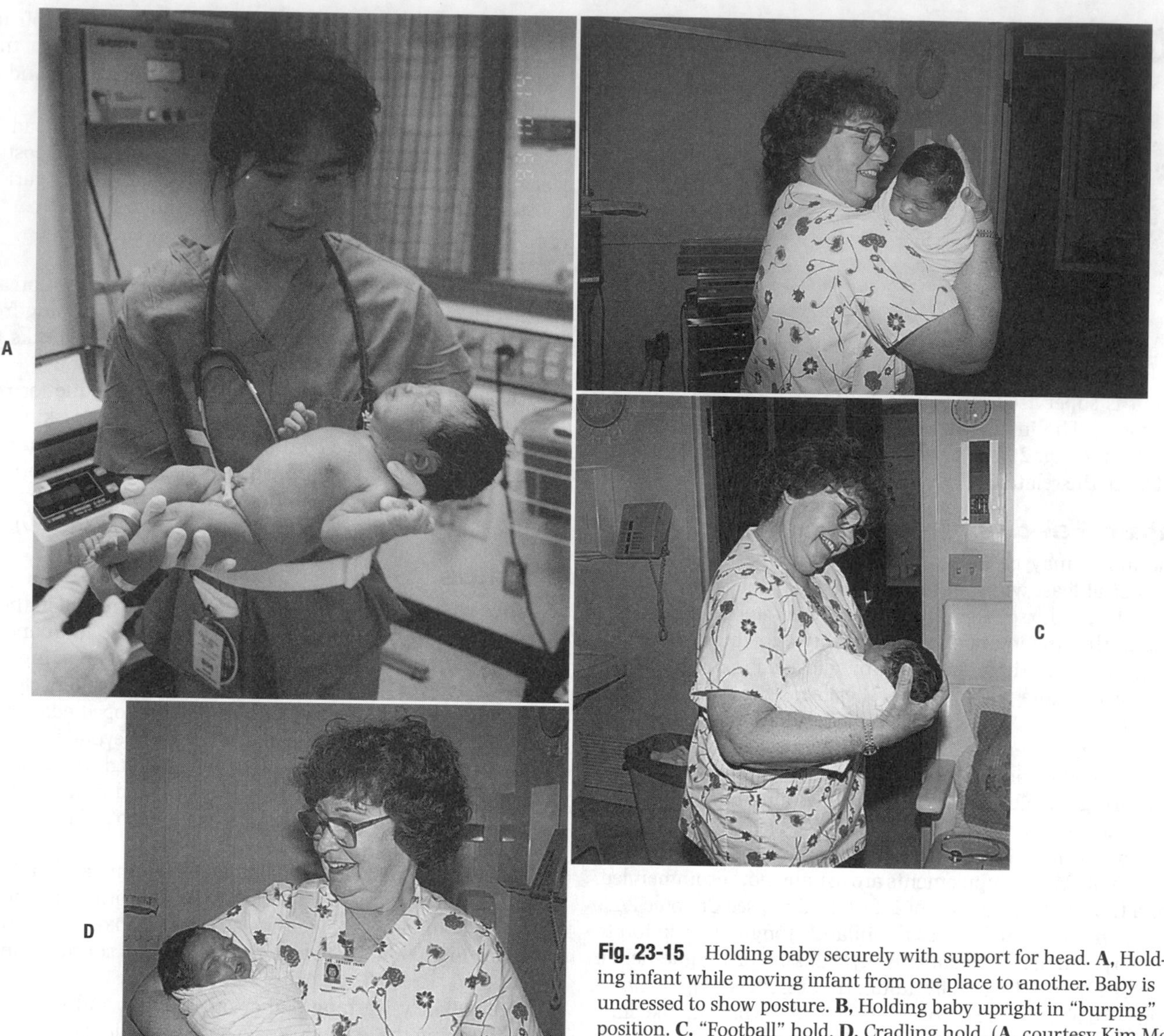

Fig. 23-15 Holding baby securely with support for head. **A,** Holding infant while moving infant from one place to another. Baby is undressed to show posture. **B,** Holding baby upright in "burping" position. **C,** "Football" hold. **D,** Cradling hold. (**A,** courtesy Kim Molloy, San Jose, Calif; **B, C, D** courtesy Marjorie Pyle, RNC, Lifecircle, Costa Mesa, Calif.)

body temperature and promotes a feeling of security. Overdressing in warm temperatures can cause discomfort as can underdressing in cold weather.

Care of the Infant's Linens

Care of the infant's clothes and bedding is directed toward minimizing cross-infection and removing residues from soap, feces, or urine that may irritate the infant's skin. In the hospital, clothing and bedding may be washed separately from other linens. Some hospitals use disposable shirts and diapers. At home the baby's clothes should be washed separately, with a mild detergent or soap and hot water. A double rinse usually removes traces of the potentially irritating cleansing agent or acid residue from the urine or stool.

Bathing

Bathing serves a number of purposes. It provides opportunities for (1) completely cleansing the infant, (2) observing the infant's condition, (3) promoting comfort, and (4) socializing of the parent-child-family. The initial bath is given when the infant's skin temperature reaches 36.5° C (97.6° F) or the core temperature is 37° C (98.6° F) (Penny-MacGillivray, 1996). Until the initial bath is completed, personnel must wear gloves when handling the newborn. In some hospitals the infant is given the initial bath with mild soap to remove blood and amniotic fluid. After the initial bath, cleansing of the genitals as necessary is deemed sufficient for the first 3 to 4 days. Bathing with warm water is sufficient for the first week. Then a mild soap may be used (NAACOG, 1992). A

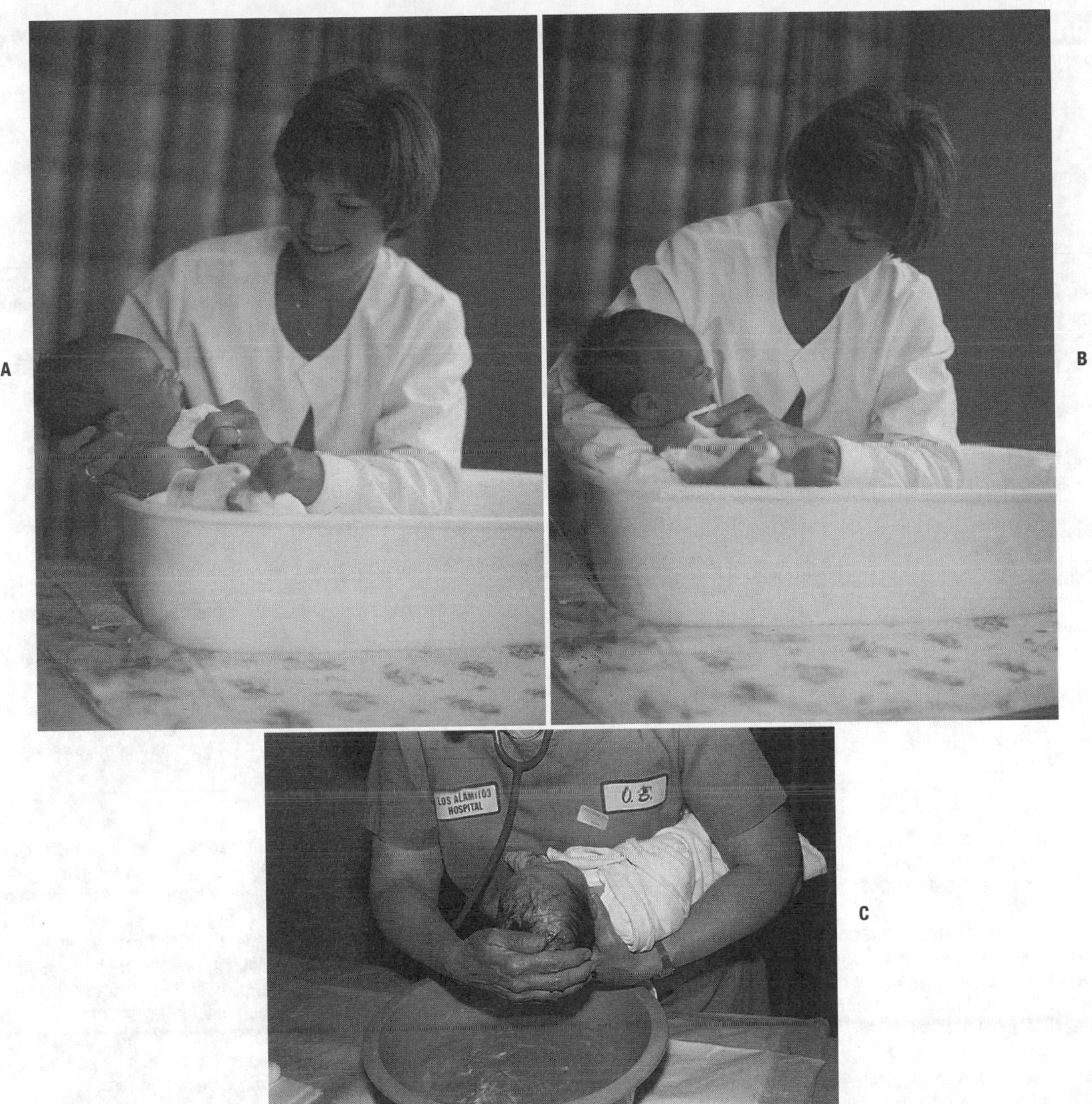

Fig. 23-16 Two methods of supporting infant during tub bath. **A,** Using hand to support neck and head. **B,** Using arm to support neck and head. **C,** Washing hair with baby wrapped to prevent heat loss from wet scalp. (**A, B** from Wong D: *Whaley & Wong's nursing care of infants and children*, ed 5, St Louis, 1995, Mosby; **C** courtesy Marjorie Pyle, RNC, Lifecircle, Costa Mesa, Calif)

newborn may not need a bath everyday. Creases under the neck and arms and in the diaper area need attention. The nurse does not need to wear gloves during the bath demonstration (Fig. 23-16).

One of the most important considerations in skin cleansing is a preservation of the skin's **acid mantle,** which is formed from the uppermost horny layer of the epidermis, sweat, superficial fat, metabolic products, and external substances such as amniotic fluid, microorganisms, and cosmetics. At birth, the skin pH is less acidic than that of older infants and adults. Within 4 days, the pH of the newborn's skin surface falls to within the bacteriostatic range ($pH < 5$) (NAACOG, 1992). Consequently, only plain warm water should be used for the bath (NAACOG, 1992). Alkaline soaps (such as Ivory), oils, powder, and lotions are not used because they alter the acid mantle, thus providing a medium for bacterial growth. The sponging technique is generally used. However, bathing the newborn by immersion has been found to cause less heat loss and less crying but is not advised until the umbilical cord falls off and has healed completely (about 10 days to 2 weeks) (see the Home Care boxes on pp. 648 and 649).

Home Care

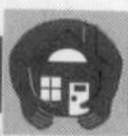

SPONGE BATHING

Fitting baths into family's schedule

Give a bath at any time convenient to you but not immediately after a feeding period because the increased handling may cause regurgitation of the feeding.

Preventing heat loss

The temperature of the room should be 24° C (75° F), and the bathing area should be free of drafts.

Control heat loss during the bath period to conserve the infant's energy. Bathing the infant quickly, exposing only a portion of the body at a time, and thoroughly drying are all parts of the bathing technique.

Gathering supplies and clothing before starting

Clothing suitable for wearing indoors: diaper, shirt; stretch suit or nightgown optional

Unscented, mild soap

Pins, if needed for diaper, closed and placed well out of baby's reach

Cotton balls

Towels for drying infant and a clean washcloth

Receiving blanket

Tub for water

Bathing the baby

Take infant to bathing area when all supplies are ready. *Never leave the infant alone on bath table or in bath water, not even for a second!* If you have to leave, take the infant with you or put back into crib.

Test temperature of the water. It should feel pleasantly warm to the inner wrist 36.7° C to 37.3° C (about 98° to 99° F).

Do not hold infant under running water—water temperature may change, and infant may be scalded or chilled rapidly.

Wash infant's head before unwrapping and undressing to prevent heat loss.

Cleanse the eyes from the inner canthus outward, using separate parts of a clean washcloth for each eye. For the first 2 to 3 days a discharge may result from the reaction of the conjunctiva to the substance (erythromycin) used as a prophylactic measure against infection. Any discharge should be considered abnormal and reported to the health care provider.

Wash the *scalp* with water and mild soap, rinse well, and dry thoroughly. Scalp desquamation, called cradle cap, often can be prevented by removing any scales with a fine-toothed comb or brush after washing. If condition persists, the health care provider may prescribe an ointment to massage into the scalp.

Creases under the chin and arms and in the groin may need daily cleansing. The crease under the chin may be exposed by elevating the infant's shoulders 5 cm and letting the head drop back.

Cleanse *ears* and *nose* with twists made of moistened cotton or a corner of the washcloth.

Do not use cotton-tipped swabs as these may cause injury.

Undress baby and wash body and arms and legs. Pat dry gently. Baby may be tub bathed after the cord drops off and umbilicus and circumcised penis are completely healed.

Preventing skin trauma

The fragile skin can be injured by too vigorous cleansing.

If stool or other debris has dried and caked on the skin, soak the area to remove it. Do not attempt to rub it off, because abrasion may result. Gentleness, patting dry rather than rubbing, and use of a mild soap without perfumes or coloring are recommended. Chemicals in the coloring and perfume can cause rashes in sensitive skin.

Care of the cord

Use a cotton swab. Dip swab in solution the physician/CNM has ordered and cleanse around base of the cord, where it joins the skin. Notify the physician/CNM of any odor, discharge, or skin inflammation around the cord. The clamp is removed when the cord is dry (about 24 hours; see Fig. 23-2). The diaper should not cover the cord. A wet or soiled diaper will slow or prevent drying of the cord and foster infection. When the cord drops off after a week to 10 days, small drops of blood may be seen when the baby cries. This will heal itself. It is not dangerous.

Care of hands and feet

Wash and dry between the fingers and toes.

Do not cut fingernails and toenails immediately after birth. The nails have to grow out far enough from the skin so that the skin is not cut by mistake. If the baby scratches himself or herself, apply loosely fitted mitts over each of the baby's hands. Do so as a last resort, however, because it interferes with the baby's ability for self-consolation. When the nails have grown, the *fingernails* and *toenails* can be cut more easily with manicure scissors (preferably scissors with rounded tips) when the infant is asleep. Nails should be kept short.

Cleansing genitalia

Cleanse the *genitals* of infants daily and after voiding and defecating. For girls, cleansing of the genitalia may be done by separating the labia and gently washing from the pubic area to the anus. For uncircumcised boys, gently pull back (retract) the foreskin. Stop when resistance is felt. Wash the tip (glans) with soap and warm water and replace the foreskin. The foreskin must be returned to its original position to prevent constriction and swelling. In most newborns the inner layer of the foreskin adheres to the glans and the foreskin cannot be retracted. By the age of 3 years, in 90% of boys the foreskin can be retracted easily without pain or trauma. For others, the foreskin is not retractable until the teens. As soon as the foreskin is partly retractable, and the child is old enough, he can be taught self-care.

Dressing the infant

When dressing the child, bunch up the shirt in both hands and expand the neck opening before placing the opening over the face; then slip the shirt over the rest of the head. Do not pull shirts roughly over the face or catch fingers in shirt sleeves.

If cloth diapers are used, absorbency can be increased by positioning the bulk of the diaper in the front for a boy and in the back for a girl. This will help absorb urine so that skin is protected. The diaper between the infant's legs should not be bulky because it can cause outward displacement of the hips. A soaker pad can be placed under the infant as a protection for the blanket. The continued use of plastic or rubber pants may lead to diaper rash.

Store infant's towels, washcloths, and supplies apart from the family's for 2 to 4 months to prevent infection.

Home Care

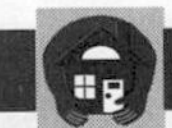

TUB BATHING

See guidelines for sponge bathing.
Place liner on bottom of tub to prevent infant from slipping.
Add 3 inches of comfortably warm water (36.7° to 37.3 C [98° to 99° F]—pleasantly warm to your inner wrist).
Wash face and shampoo hair as for sponge bath. Undress baby. Lower infant slowly into water.
Hold baby securely with fingers under the baby's armpit, with your thumb around the shoulder. The other hand supports the baby's bottom and legs.

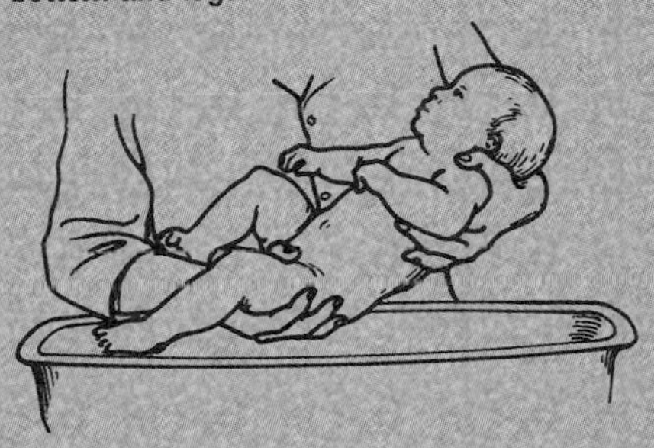

Wash the front of the baby.
Go from front to back between the legs. Rinse with the wet washcloth.

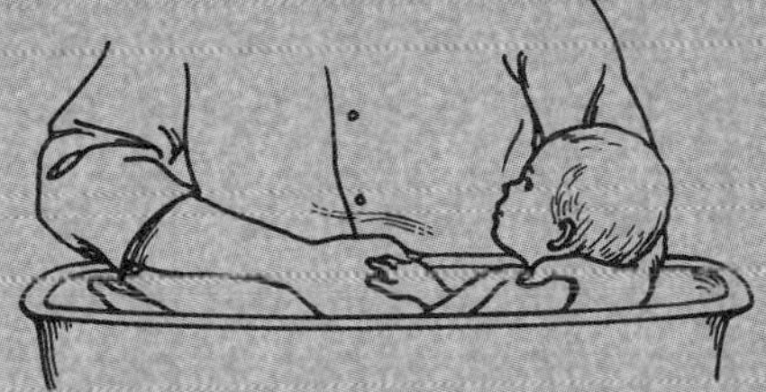

Wash the baby's back with your free hand lathered with soap. Rinse well with the wet washcloth.

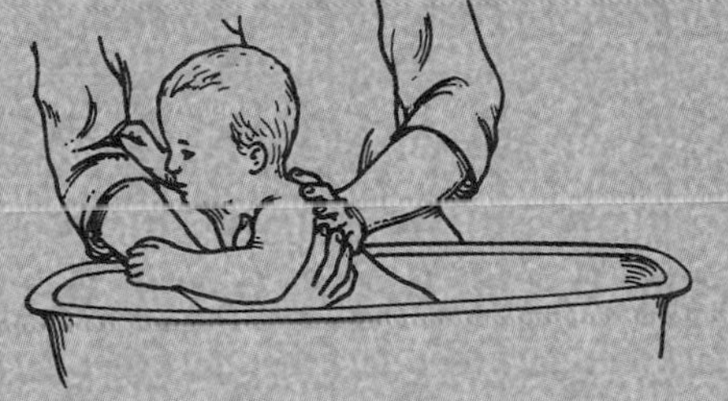

Remove infant from the water and gently pat dry.

NURSING INTERVENTIONS FOR THERAPEUTIC/SURGICAL PROCEDURES

Restraining the Infant

Reasons for restraining an infant include (1) protecting the infant from injury; (2) facilitating examinations; and (3) limiting discomfort during tests, procedures, and specimen collections. The use of restraints should only be a temporary measure; the infant should never be left unattended while any type of restraint is implemented. Institutional guidelines for the use of restraints should be carefully followed and properly documented.

Mummy technique. The mummy technique is used with the stronger, more vigorous newborn. It may be used during examinations, treatments, or specimen collections that involve the head and neck.

Equipment includes a blanket and one or two large safety pins (Fig. 23-11, *A*). The procedure is as follows:

1. Spread blanket on flat surface (e.g., a crib).
2. Fold over one corner (12 o'clock position).
3. Place newborn on blanket so that neck is at fold.
4. Fold corner at 9 o'clock position over right shoulder; tuck this corner securely under infant's left side.
5. Place corner at 6 o'clock position up over feet and either tuck it under infant's left side or, if long enough, fold it over blanket, crossing it under infant's chin.
6. Swing corner of 3 o'clock position snugly over infant and fold under infant's right side. Pin this corner into place. When tucked tightly, a pin is not always necessary.

Blanket support. Although the blanket support is not a true restraint, it controls the infant's position and movement. The blanket may be rolled and placed at the infant's sides or folded. A blanket support has the following advantages:

1. It provides comfort and security by stabilizing the infant's position.
2. It prevents the infant from rolling against the isolette or crib wall, where the child may lose heat by convection.

Temporary restraint. The nurse may restrain the infant by using the hands and body. Fig. 23-11, *B*, illustrates restraint of the infant in position for lumbar puncture.

Intramuscular Injection

Hepatitis B vaccination (Hep B) is recommended for all infants. Infants at highest risk of contracting hepatitis B are those born of women who come from Asia, Africa, South America, the South Pacific, and Southern and Eastern Europe. If the infant is born to an infected mother or to a mother who is a chronic carrier, hepatitis vaccine and hepatitis B immune globulin (HBIG) should be given within 12 hours of birth. The hepatitis vaccine is given in one site and the HBIG in another site. For infants born to healthy women, the first dose of the vaccine may be given at birth or at 1 or 2 months of age. Parental consent should be obtained before administering these medications.

In most cases a 25-gauge, 5/8-inch needle should be used for the vitamin K and hepatitis vaccine injections.

Selection of the site for injection is important. Injections must be placed in muscles large enough to accommodate the medication, yet major nerves and blood vessels must be avoided. The muscles of newborns may not tolerate more than 0.5 ml per intramuscular (IM) injection. The preferred site for newborns is the vastus lateralis (Fig. 23-17). The vastus lateralis muscle is one of the largest muscles and is well developed in the newborn. The dorsogluteal muscle is very small, poorly developed, and dangerously close to the sciatic nerve, which occupies a larger proportion of space in infants than in older children. Therefore it is not recommended as an injection site until the child has been walking for at least 1 year.

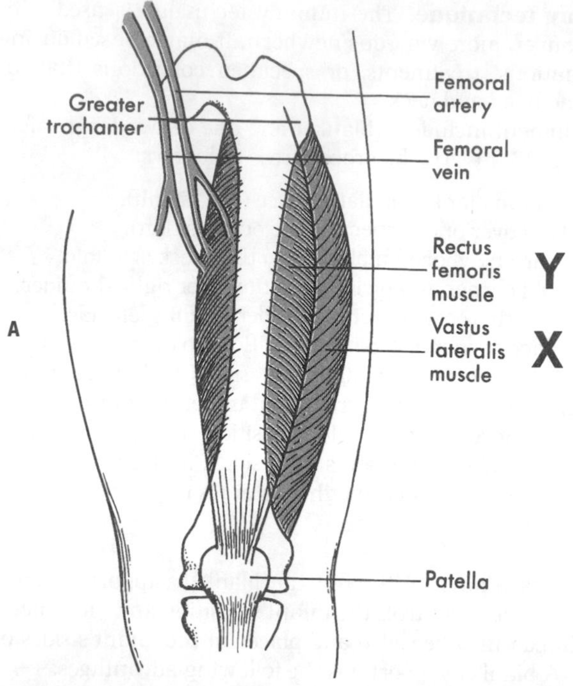

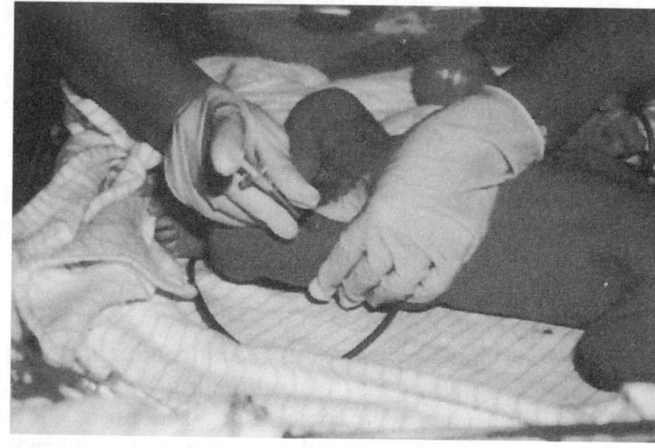

Fig. 23-17 Intramuscular injection sites. **A,** Acceptable intramuscular injection sites for children: *X,* preferred injection site; *Y,* alternative injection site. **B,** Infant's leg stabilized for intramuscular injection. Nurse is wearing gloves to give injection. (**A** from Wong D: *Whaley & Wong's nursing care of infants and children,* ed 5, St Louis, 1995, Mosby. **B** courtesy Marjorie Pyle, RNC, Lifecircle, Costa Mesa, Calif.)

The neonate's leg should be stabilized. Gloves are worn for the injection. It may be necessary to ask someone to hold the leg while the injection is being given. The nurse cleanses the injection site with alcohol and then pinches up the infant's muscle with the thumb and forefinger. The needle is inserted into the vastus lateralis at a 90-degree angle. The muscle is released and the plunger of the syringe is withdrawn. If no blood is aspirated, the medication is injected. If blood is aspirated, the needle is withdrawn and the injection is given in another site. The needle is withdrawn quickly and the site massaged with a gauze wipe. It is not uncommon for blood to ooze from the injection site. It is not necessary to cover the site with an adhesive bandage.

BOX 23-4
Effects of Phototherapy

Phototherapy causes reversible isomerization of unconjugated bilirubin in the skin (Valman, 1989). During phototherapy, infants form a substance called *lumirubin,* a water-soluble product. Lumirubin is formed slowly and excreted rapidly in both urine and feces. Because infants excrete lumirubin efficiently, increasing the formation of lumirubin improves the effectiveness of phototherapy in the treatment of neonatal jaundice.

Traditional phototherapy consists of a light source (e.g., four special blue and four daylight bulbs) that will most effectively accomplish the isomerization process. The light source is placed about 40 to 50 cm from the newborn in an incubator. The fluorescent bulbs currently used (daylight, cool light, blue, and special blue bulbs) have different distribution points on the light spectrum and different peaks of maximal emission. The generally accepted light range for maximum absorption by bilirubin is 400 to 500 nanometers. Blue or special blue lights are considered to be more specific and effective. Blue lights can make the detection of cyanosis in the infant difficult and may strain the nursery staff's eyes (NAACOG, 1986). The side effects of phototherapy do not appear to produce any long-term effects.

Bronze baby syndrome has occurred in some newborns receiving phototherapy. The serum, urine, and skin turn bronze (brown-black). The cause is unclear. Almost all newborns recover from bronze baby syndrome without sequelae.

The nurse should always remember to comfort the infant after an injection. Equipment should be properly discarded. It is important to record medication, date and time, amount, route, site of injection, and infant's tolerance of injection.

Therapy for Hyperbilirubinemia

The best therapy for **hyperbilirubinemia** is prevention. Because bilirubin is excreted in meconium, early feeding may help prevent jaundice by stimulating passage of meconium. The goal of hyperbilirubinemia treatment is to help the newborn's body reduce serum levels of unconjugated bilirubin. The term infant may have trouble conjugating the increased amount of bilirubin derived from disintegrating red blood cells. Thus the serum levels of unconjugated bilirubin rise beyond normal limits (hyperbilirubinemia) (see Chapter 22). If untreated, the levels can continue to rise and the risk of kernicterus increases in certain infants at higher risk.

There are two principal methods for reducing serum bilirubin levels: phototherapy and exchange blood transfusion. Exchange transfusion is used to treat infants whose levels of bilirubin cannot be controlled by phototherapy (Box 23-4). A number of pharmacologic agents have been used with varying results to treat hyperbilirubinemia.

The pharmacologic management of hyperbilirubinemia with phenobarbital has centered primarily on the infant with hemolytic disease and is most effective when given to the mother several days before giving birth. Phenobarbital promotes hepatic glucuronyl transferase synthesis (increasing bilirubin conjugation and hepatic clearance of the pigment in bile) and protein synthesis, which may increase albumin for more bilirubin binding sites. The use of phenobarbital in either the antenatal or the postnatal period, however, has not proved to be as effective as other treatments in reducing bilirubin. Bilirubin production in the newborn can be decreased by inhibiting heme oxygenase, an enzyme needed for heme breakdown (to biliverdin), with metalloporphyrins, especially tin-protoporphyrin and tin-mesoporphyrin. Hemeoxygenase inhibitors provide a preventive approach to hyperbilirubinemia but are not widely used.

Phototherapy. During phototherapy the infant is placed, unclothed, approximately 45-50 cm under a bank of lights for several hours or days until the serum bilirubin level drops to within acceptable range. The decision to discontinue therapy is based on a definite downward trend in total serum bilirubin values. After therapy has been terminated, the infant should be retested in several hours to ascertain whether a rebound of bilirubin level occurs.

Several precautions need to be taken while the infant is under phototherapy. The infant's eyes must be protected by an opaque mask to prevent overexposure to the light. The eye shield should be the correct size to cover the eyes completely but not occlude the nares. Before the mask is applied, the infant's eyes should be closed gently to prevent excoriation of the corneas. The mask should be removed during infant feedings so that the eyes can be checked and the infant can receive visual contact with the parents (Fig. 23-18).

Often a "string bikini" made from a disposable face mask is used instead of a diaper. This allows optimal skin exposure, yet sufficient protection to the genitals and bedding. Before the application, the metal strip must be removed from the mask to prevent burning the infant. Lotions and ointments also should be avoided because they absorb heat and can cause burns.

Phototherapy may cause the infant to sleep for longer than the usual 4-hour periods. The infant is kept on a regular feeding schedule. The number and consistency of stools are monitored. Bilirubin breakdown increases gastric motility, which

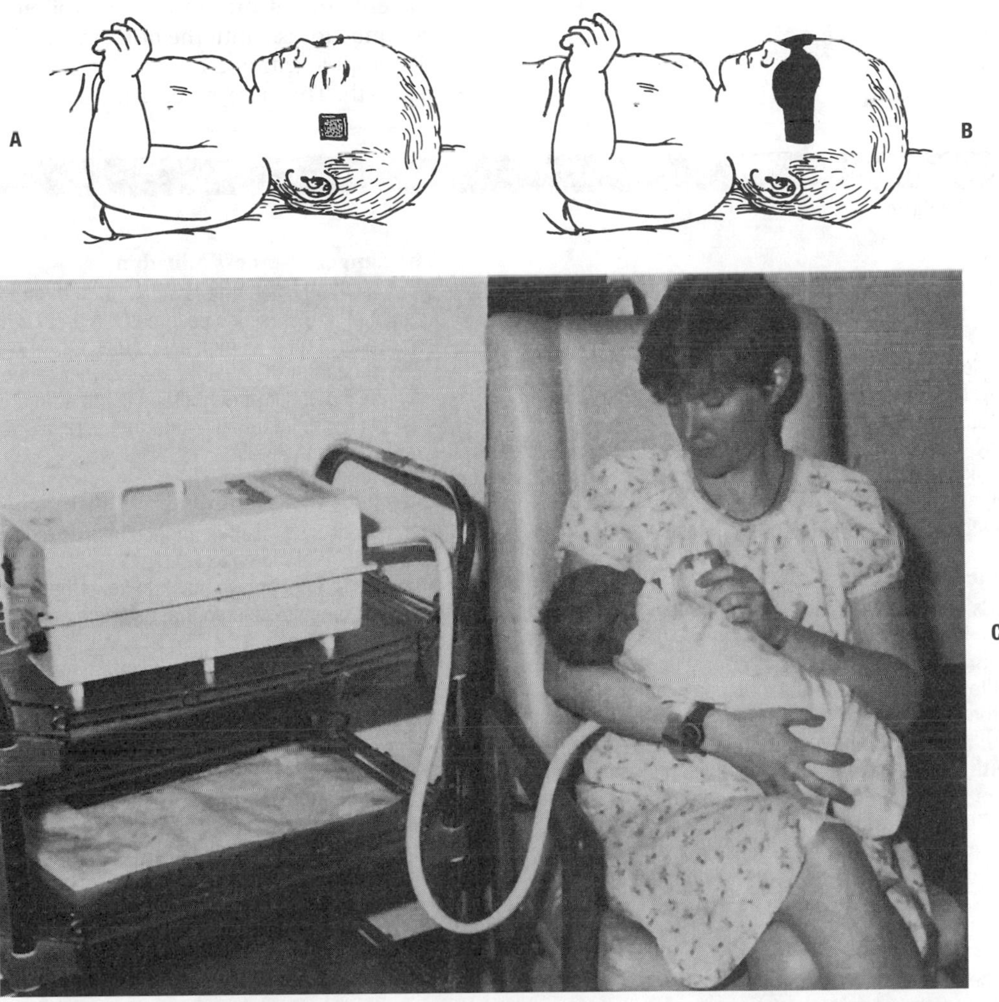

Fig. 23-18 Eye patches for newborn receiving phototherapy. **A,** Small self-adhesive (Velcro) patch stuck to both sides of head. **B,** Eye cover sticks to Velcro patch, which reduces movement of eye cover and facilitates removal for feedings. **C,** Fiberoptic phototherapy blanket permits baby to be fed, held, and changed without the need for eye patches. (**C** from Rosefeld W, Twist P, Concepcion L: A new device for phototherapy treatment of jaundiced infants, *J Perinatology* (3):243, 1990.)

Family Focus

PHOTOTHERAPY AND PARENT-INFANT INTERACTION

The traditional use of phototherapy has evoked concerns regarding a number of psychobehavioral issues, including parent-infant separation, potential social isolation, decreased sensorineural stimulation, altered biologic rhythms, altered feeding patterns, and activity changes. Parental anxiety is greatly increased, particularly at the sight of the newborn blindfolded and under special lights. The interruption of breastfeeding for phototherapy is a potential deterrent to successful maternal-infant attachment and interaction. Because research has demonstrated that bilirubin catabolism occurs primarily within the first few hours of the initiation of phototherapy, there is increased support for the removal of the infant from treatment for feeding and holding. Intermittent phototherapy may be just as effective as continuous therapy when used correctly. The benefits of stopping phototherapy for parental feeding and holding outweigh concerns related to the clearance of bilirubin (Blackburn and Loper, 1992).

results in loose stools that can cause skin excoriation and breakdown. The infant's buttocks are cleaned after each stool to help maintain skin integrity.

During phototherapy, the infant's temperature may become elevated and require monitoring. The lights increase the rate of insensible water loss (NAACOG, 1992). Therefore fluid loss and dehydration can also occur. The infant is turned every 2 hours to expose all body surfaces to the lights. Accurate charting of nursing interventions and the infant's reaction to phototherapy is necessary.

An alternative device for phototherapy consisting of a fiberoptic panel attached to an illuminator is as safe and effective as traditional phototherapy (Rosenfeld, Twist, and Concepcion, 1990). This fiberoptic blanket, which wraps light around the newborn's torso, delivers continuous phototherapy. The newborn can remain in the mother's room in an open crib or in her arms during treatment without the need for eye patches (Fig. 23-18, *C*) (Murphy and Oellrich, 1990; Rosenfeld et al, 1990). The blanket may also be used for home phototherapy (see the Family Focus box to the left).

Parent education. Serum levels of bilirubin in the newborn continue to rise until the fifth day of life. Many parents leave the hospital within 24 hours and some as early as 2 hours after birth. Therefore parents must be able to assess the new-

Patient Teaching

HYPERBILIRUBINEMIA

Definitions

Hyperbilirubinemia—above-normal levels of bilirubin in the blood
Bilirubin—end product of RBCs when they mature and break down
RBCs—red blood cells
Jaundice—yellow skin tone, whites of eyes, and mucous membranes caused by circulating bilirubin
Phototherapy—use of fluorescent light to break down the bilirubin in the skin into substances that can be excreted in the feces (stool) and urine
Bililites—fluorescent lights used for phototherapy

How jaundice happens

- When RBCs break down, they release bilirubin. Bilirubin circulates in the blood. The bilirubin combines with another substance in the liver. The substance that results moves through the blood to the kidneys and the intestines, where it is eliminated in the urine and the stool. The bilirubin gives the yellow color to urine and the brown color to the stool.
- Before birth, babies have more RBCs in each ounce of blood than adults have. The RBCs of the unborn infant have a shorter life span (70 to 90 days) than RBCs formed after birth (120 days). When the RBCs of a fetus break down, the bilirubin produced by this is carried by the fetus's blood, through the placenta, and to the mother's liver to be excreted.
- After birth, the infant's liver must get rid of the bilirubin. Even though a baby's liver functions well, it may not be able to get rid of all the bilirubin produced by breakdown of RBCs. Bilirubin seeps out of the blood and into the tissues, coloring them yellow (jaundice). The blood level of bilirubin rises quickly up to the fifth day, and then it goes down; the jaundice usually clears up by the end of the first week.

The danger of excess bilirubin

Some newborns seem to have extra bilirubin to excrete. The amount in the tissues becomes too great when the blood level is high. Bilirubin at high levels may cause damage to the brain. Consequently, the health care provider requests that the infant be placed under phototherapy lights or in a bili-blanket. This will help the infant eliminate the extra bilirubin and prevent damage to the brain.

Caring for the infant under lights for phototherapy

The newborn is placed in an incubator to keep it warm and to enable the nurse to observe it.
The infant wears an eye mask to keep the light out of the eyes.
The baby is undressed so that as much light as possible can reach the skin.
The newborn wears a "string bikini," which is made out of a paper diaper or a face mask, as a small diaper.
The baby's temperature is taken often to note any changes and to prevent the infant from becoming too hot or too cold.
The newborn is taken out from under the lights for feedings and cuddling unless a bili-blanket is being used.
The nurse obtains blood tests to check the amount of bilirubin still in the newborn's blood and updates the parents about the results.

After the newborn goes home

The parents should be encouraged to ask any questions that they have. The nurse gives them a telephone number to call at any hour with questions.

born's degree of jaundice. They should have written instructions that include the contact person to whom they should report the infant's condition. Some hospitals have a nurse make a home visit to evaluate the infant's responses. Determination of bilirubin levels may be necessary after discharge from the hospital. The home care nurse may draw the blood for the specimen, or the parents may take the baby to a laboratory for the determination. (See the Patient Teaching box on p. 652 for parental guidelines concerning hyperbilirubinemia).

Circumcision

Circumcision is commonly performed in the United States. In 1975 the American Academy of Pediatrics (AAP) released a report that supported not circumcising infants (Wiswell, 1990). However, in 1989 they revised their opinion. According to the Task Force on Circumcision (1989), a properly performed newborn circumcision prevents **phimosis** (a rare condition that can interfere with or impede flow of urine and predispose males to infection between the foreskin and glans penis) and may reduce the incidence of urinary tract infections. American men who are circumcised have a lower incidence of penile cancer. However, there is still conflicting evidence regarding the association between circumcision and sexually transmitted diseases (STDs) (Wiswell, 1990). Newborn circumcision has potential medical benefits and advantages as well as disadvantages and risks. Therefore the decision for the elective surgery is left to the parents.

Circumcision is a matter of personal parental choice. The parents' decision to have their newborn circumcised is usually based on one or more of the following factors: hygiene, religious conviction, tradition, culture, or social norms. Some people do not like to touch their infant's genitals. For these parents, circumcision may be the wisest choice. Regardless of the reason for the decision, it should be made only after parents have the available facts and sufficient time to review their options.

Expectant parents need to begin learning about circumcision during the prenatal period. However, circumcision often is not discussed with the parents before labor. In many instances it is during admission to the hospital or birth unit that the mother confronts the decision regarding circumcision. The stress of the intrapartal period makes this a difficult time for parental decision making, although consenting to their boy's circumcision is ultimately the parents' personal choice. The mother may be asked to sign a circumcision permit form during this admission procedure, although usually this request is made after the birth. Some hospitals require parents to sign a different form stating they do not wish their male infant to be circumcised if that is their desire.

Procedure. In circumcision the prepuce (foreskin) of the glans is removed. The operation is performed in the hospital before the infant's discharge. The circumcision of a Jewish male is performed on the eighth day after birth and is done at home unless the infant is unwell (see the Cultural Considerations box above). The procedure is not usually performed immediately after birth because of the danger of cold stress. Immediately after birth clotting factors drop somewhat and return to prebirth levels by the end of the first week. Therefore performing the circumcision after the baby is a week old is logical from a physiologic standpoint.

Cultural Considerations 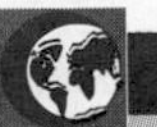

CIRCUMCISION

In the Jewish culture circumcision is performed during a highly significant ceremony called a *berith*, or *brit*, which takes place on the eighth day of life. A specially trained professional known as a *mohel* stretches the prepuce over the glans, pulling it through a slit in a shield (usually a Mogen clamp) and cutting it with a knife. The traditional technique is not sterile, and bleeding is controlled by tight bandaging around the penis (Cohen et al, 1992). The infant may be given some sweet wine before the procedure. Blankets instead of straps are usually used to restrain the infant to a board, and the parents are present (Trochtenberg, 1990).

Female circumcision (mutilation) is also practiced, particularly in Africa, the Middle East, and Southeast Asia—and among immigrants from these countries to the United States, Australia, Canada, and Europe. In the most extensive operation (excision or infibulation), the clitoris, labia minora, and medial aspects of labia majora are removed. The remaining labia majora are sewn closed, except for a small opening for urine and menses (McCleary, 1994). Anesthesia is used very rarely. In African and Asian cultures, female circumcision is used to prove virginity and to reduce sexual pleasure, thus promoting fidelity. It is estimated that 85 million to 115 million women and girls worldwide have suffered female genital mutilation, with an additional 2 million incidences occurring each year. The International Council of Nurses and the World Health Organization condemn all forms of female genital mutilation (Female genital mutilation, 1994; Female genital mutilation, 1996).

Feedings are usually withheld up to 4 hours before the circumcision to prevent vomiting and aspiration. For the circumcision procedure the infant is positioned on a plastic restraint form so that his movements are restricted (Fig. 23-19). The penis is cleansed with soap and water or other prep solution such as povidone iodine. The infant is draped to provide warmth and a sterile field. The sterile equipment is readied for use.

Some procedures require no special equipment or appliances (Fig. 23-20). However, numerous instruments have been designed for circumcision. The Yellen clamp (Fig. 23-21) may make this an almost bloodless operation. The procedure takes only a few minutes. After it is completed, a small petrolatum gauze dressing or a generous amount of petrolatum may be applied to the penis for the first day to prevent the diaper from adhering. If a bell (Plastibell) is used, it applies constant direct pressure to prevent hemorrhage. It also protects against infection, sticking to the diaper, and pain with urination. The bell is fitted over the glans, the suture is tied around the rim of the bell, and excess prepuce is cut away. The plastic rim remains in place for about a week until it falls off, after healing has taken place (Fig. 23-22). Petrolatum is not needed when the bell is used.

Discomfort. Circumcision is painful; the pain is manifested by both physiologic and behavioral changes in the infant. Local anesthesia may reduce the physiologic response to the pain. Dorsal penile nerve blocks may reduce pain and stress during newborn circumcision. In the Jewish ritual the newborn is given a few drops of wine to relax him in preparation

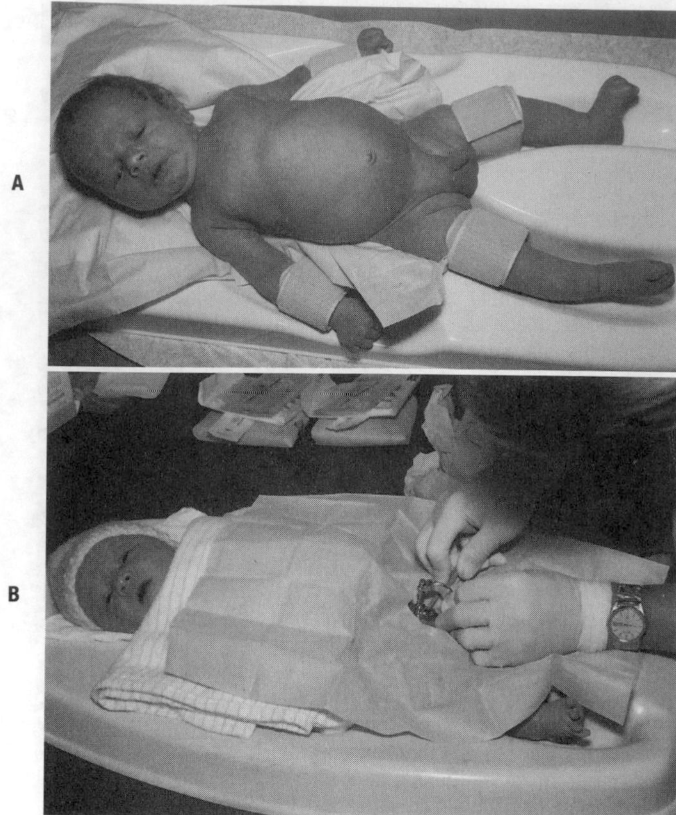

Fig. 23-19 Circumcision. **A,** Proper positioning of infant in Circumstraint. **B,** Physician performing circumcision. Baby is covered to prevent cold stress. (Courtesy Michael S. Clement, MD, Mesa, Ariz.)

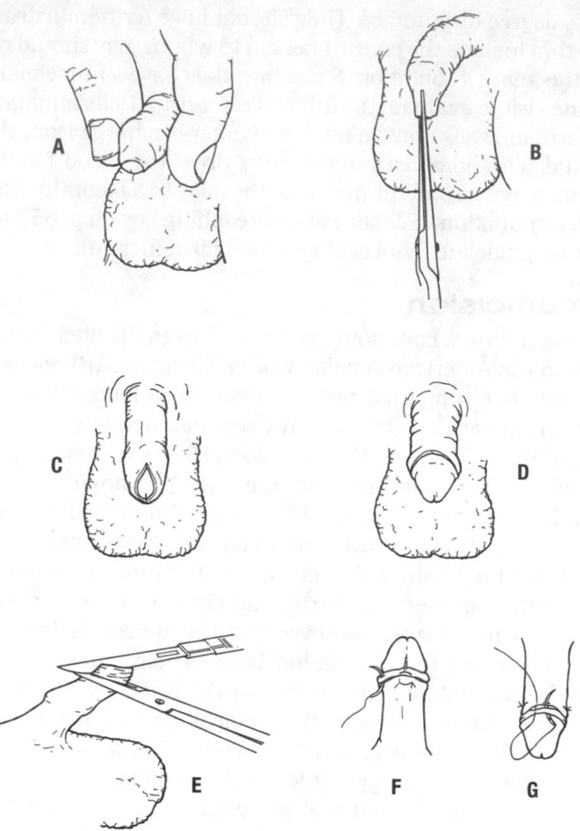

Fig. 23-20 Technique of circumcision. **A** to **D,** Prepuce is stripped and slit to facilitate its retraction behind glans penis. **E,** Prepuce is now clamped and excessive prepuce cut off. **F** and **G,** Suture material used is plain 00 or 000 catgut in very small needle; some physicians prefer silk.

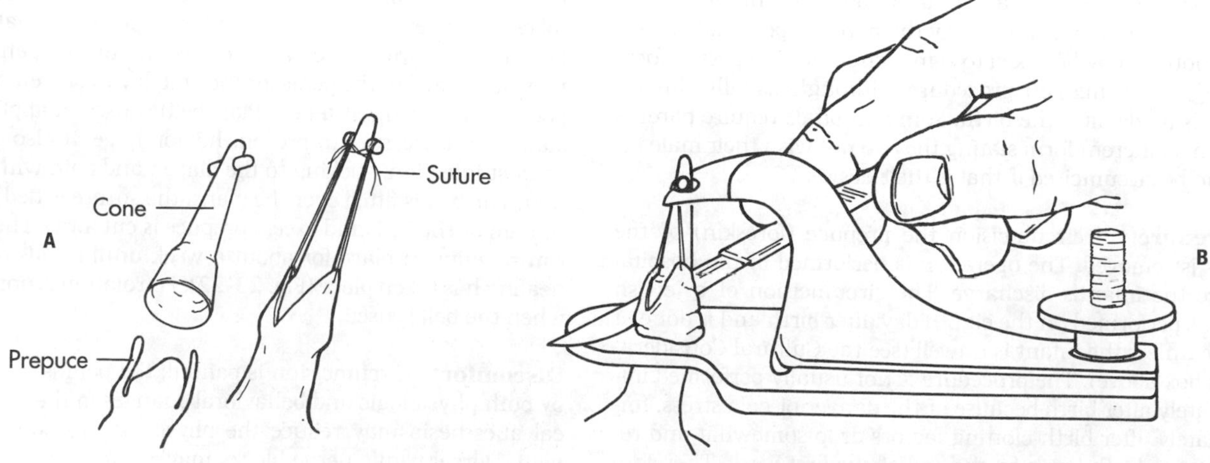

Fig. 23-21 Circumcision with Yellen clamp. **A,** Prepuce is drawn over cone. **B,** Yellen clamp is applied, hemostasis occurs, then prepuce (over cone) is cut away.

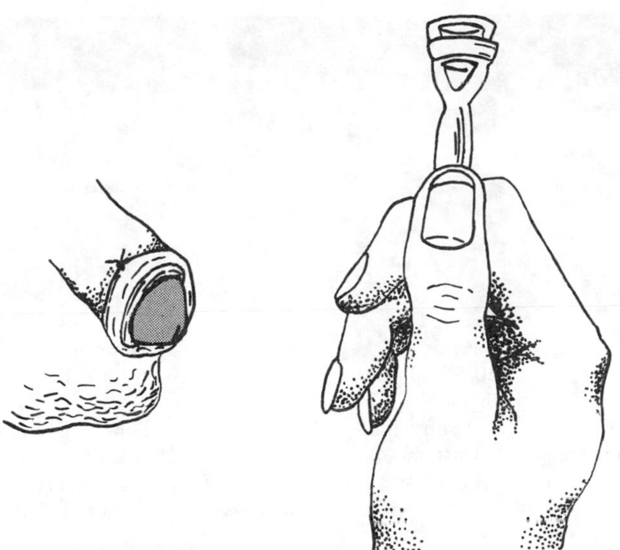

Fig. 23-22 Circumcision using the Plastibell.

for the surgery. Reported use of local anesthesia such as eutectic mixture of local anesthetics (EMLA) for circumcision is limited and needs further study. Pain may not end when the operation is over because the wound requires as long as a week to heal.

Nursing ALERT

When in doubt about pain in infants, base your decision on the following rule: Whatever is painful to an adult or child is painful to an infant, unless proved otherwise.

If the infant has undergone this surgery without anesthesia, he is comforted until he is quieted (Marchette et al, 1991). Then he is returned to his mother. These infants usually are fussy for about 2 to 3 hours and may refuse a feeding. It is not uncommon for the infant to have a loose green stool after the circumcision.

Care of the newly circumcised penis. The nurse observes the infant for bleeding and voiding. If bleeding is noted from the circumcision, the nurse applies gentle pressure to the site of bleeding with a folded sterile 4 × 4-inch gauze pad or sprinkles on powdered gel foam. If bleeding is not easily controlled, a blood vessel may need to be surgically ligated. Constant gentle pressure should be applied until bleeding stops or a physician arrives. The penis is checked hourly for bleeding for 12 hours. If the parents take the baby home before the end of 12 hours, they are taught the actions described. Before the infant's discharge, the nurse checks to see that the parents have the physician's telephone number.

Nursing actions are planned and implemented to prevent infection. Prepackaged wipes for cleaning the diaper area should be avoided because they contain alcohol. The nurse washes the penis gently with water to remove urine and feces and reapplies, if required, fresh petrolatum around the glans after each diaper change. The glans penis, normally dark red in appearance during healing, becomes covered with a yellow exudate in 24 hours. This is part of normal healing, not an infective process. No attempt is made to remove the exudate, which persists for 2 to 3 days. Parents should be taught to fanfold the diaper so that it does not press on the circumcised area. They should be encouraged to change the diaper at least every 4 hours to prevent it from sticking to the penis.

DISCHARGE PLANNING AND TEACHING

For the new parent, child care activities can cause much anxiety. Support from nursing staff members in the mother's beginning efforts can be an important factor in her seeking and accepting help in the future. Whether or not this is the couple's first baby, or whether they attended parenthood preparation classes, parents appreciate anticipatory guidance in the care of their child. The nurse should avoid covering all content at once because the parents can be overwhelmed and become anxious. With today's early discharge, teaching all the content can become a problem. Many institutions have developed home visitation programs that take the necessary teaching to the new parents (see Chapter 21), but the hospital nurse still provides most of the information for essential newborn care. In the inpatient setting, priorities of care must be established and a systematic teaching plan for infant care devised. One way to achieve this end is to use critical path case management for delivery of nursing care (Zander, 1989). The care path clearly delineates what teaching/discharge planning should occur within specified times. This ensures that essential topics are addressed and that repetition is prevented. The infant must meet criteria for early discharge (see Box 21-1). A care path may also be developed for the changes expected in the infant over the first several days. Box 23-5 is an example of a care path for infant adaptation to extrauterine life. When variations from the care path occur, further assessment and intervention may be necessary.

To set priorities for teaching, the nurse follows parental cues. Knowledge deficits should be identified before beginning to teach. Normal growth and development and the changing needs of the infant (e.g., for stimulation, exercise, and social contacts) as well as the following topics should be included during discharge planning with parents.

Temperature

The following topics should be reviewed:

1. The causes of elevation in body temperature (such as overwrapping, cold stress with resultant vasoconstriction, minimum response to infection), and the body's response to extremes in environmental temperature.
2. Symptoms to be reported, such as high or low temperatures with accompanying fussiness, stuffy nose, lethargy, irritability, poor feeding, and crying.
3. Ways to encourage normal body temperature, such as giving a tepid tub bath, dressing the infant appropriately for the temperature of the air, and protecting the infant from direct exposure to sunlight.
4. Use of warm wraps in cold weather or extra blankets.
5. Technique to take the baby's axillary temperature.

BOX 23-5
Care Path for Neonatal Adaptation to Extrauterine Life

	Day 1	Day 2	Day 3	Day 4	Day 7	Day 14
Weight		Loss of 5%-10% of birthweight	Gain of 150-300 g/day			Birth weight regained
Temperature	Stabilized at 98.6° F (37° C)					
Feedings						
Volume	*Formula* 15-60 ml *Breast* Softening of at least one breast at each feeding	*Formula* 60-90 ml *Breast* Softening of at least one breast at each feeding	*Formula* 60-90 ml *Breast* Softening of at least one breast at each feeding	*Formula* 60-90 ml *Breast* Softening of at least one breast at each feeding	*Formula* 60-90 ml *Breast* Softening of at least one breast at each feeding	*Formula* 60-90 ml *Breast* Softening of at least one breast at each feeding
Frequency	*Formula* 6-10 times/24 hrs *Breast* 8-12 times/24 hrs	*Formula* 6-10 times/24 hrs *Breast* 8-12 times/24 hrs	*Formula* 6-10 times/24 hrs *Breast* 8-12 times/24 hrs	*Formula* 6-10 times/24 hrs *Breast* 8-12 times/24 hrs	*Formula* 6-10 times/24 hrs *Breast* 8-12 times/24 hrs	*Formula* 6-10 times/24 hrs *Breast* 8-12 times/24 hrs
Voiding	At least 1 time in first 24 hrs	2-6 times/24 hrs	6-10 times/24 hrs			6-10 times/24 hrs
Stools		Meconium; at least 1 time in first 48 hrs	Transitional stool; 1-5/day	Yellow stool; 1-5/day		Yellow stool; 1-2/day
Sleep	16-20 hrs/24 hrs					16-20 hrs/24 hrs
Umbilical cord	Moist; clamped	Dry; clamp removed				Cord off
Circumcision	Red; sore	Yellow exudate covering glans	Healing	Healing		Healed
Color	Pink; acrocyanosis	Pink; slight jaundice	Peak of jaundice		Pink	
Bilirubin level	0-6 mg/dl	≤8 mg/dl	≤12 mg/dl		2 mg/dl	
Laboratory tests	Glucose when required; hematocrit (HCT)	PKU, T_4; galactose				Repeat PKU, if needed
Medications	Eye prophylaxis and vitamin K within 2 hrs of birth; hepatitis B vaccine(HBV) within 12 hrs of birth					

Respirations

Review the following points:

1. Normal variations in the rate and rhythm.
2. Reflexes such as sneezing to clear the air passage.
3. Need to protect the infant from the following:
   a. People with upper respiratory tract infections.
   b. Pollution from a smoke-filled environment (secondhand smoke).
   c. Suffocation from loose bedding, water beds, and bean bag chairs; drowning (in bath water); entrapment under excessive bedding; anything tied around the infant's neck; poorly constructed playpens, bassinets, or cribs.
   d. Sleep position—on side or back when put to sleep
   e. Aspiration pneumonia: a commonly aspirated substance is baby powder, which usually is a mixture of talc (hydrous magnesium silicate) and other silicates (Wong, 1995). Parents are advised of the danger of baby powder and discouraged from using it. If they prefer to use a powder, a corn starch preparation can be substituted. Whenever a powder is used, it should be placed in the caregiver's hand and then applied to the skin, never sprinkled directly onto the skin. The container is kept closed and immediately stored in a safe place, especially away from curious toddlers, who often imitate caregiving activities and may shake it onto the infant.
4. Symptoms of the common cold: nasal congestion, coughing, sneezing, difficulty in swallowing or breathing, low-grade fever. Advise the parents on measures to help the infant, for example:
   a. Feeding smaller amounts more frequently to prevent overtiring the infant
   b. Holding the baby in an upright position to feed
   c. For sleeping, raising the infant's head and chest by raising the mattress 30 degrees (do not use pillow)
   d. Avoiding drafts; not overdressing the baby
   e. Using only medications prescribed by a physician
   f. Covering the upper lip with a light film of petrolatum to minimize excoriation from nasal secretions

Elimination

A review includes the following reminders:

1. Changes to be expected in the color of the stool (meconium to transitional to soft yellow/golden yellow) and the number of bowel evacuations, plus the odor of stools for breastfed or bottle-fed infants (see Chapter 22)
2. Color of normal urine and number of voidings (6 to 10) to expect each day

Safety

The following measures are reviewed:

1. Protecting the infant from trauma, for example, keeping objects such as pins and scissors closed and well out of the baby's reach.
2. When infant clothes are purchased, the type of closing used should be considered: fire-retardant clothing without front buttons is appropriate.
3. Protecting the infant from falls by teaching parents to hold the infant securely (Fig. 23-15), to use safety straps in infant seats and carriers, to keep the sides up on the crib, never to leave the infant alone on changing tables or beds or in the bath, and to place pillows around the infant when on an adult bed.
4. Preventing overheating or chilling.
5. Using care in transporting infants, particularly in automobiles (Fig. 23-23). The use of approved car seats for infants is a law in 33 states.
6. Supervising brothers' and sisters' attention to the new baby.
7. Being prepared for accidental ingestion of poisonous substances by having syrup of ipecac on hand and having the telephone number of the poison control center near the telephone.

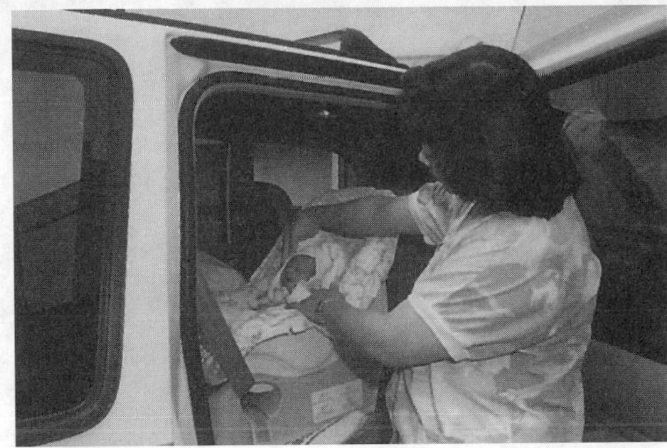

Fig. 23-23 Rearward-facing shell car seat in rear seat of car. Infant is placed in car seat when going home from hospital. (Courtesy Marjorie Pyle, RNC, Lifecircle, Costa Mesa, Calif.)

Pacifiers/Thumb-Sucking

Sucking is the infant's chief pleasure and may not be satisfied by breastfeeding or formula-feeding (Wong, 1995). It is such a strong need that infants who are deprived of sucking, such as those with cleft lip repair, will suck on the tongue. Some newborns are born with sucking pads on their fingers that developed from in utero sucking activity. Several benefits of nonnutritive sucking have been documented, such as increased weight gain in premature infants and decreased crying (Treloar, 1994).

Problems arise when parents are concerned about sucking of fingers, thumb, or pacifier and attempt to restrain this natural tendency. Before giving advice, nurses investigate the parents' feelings and base guidance on this information. For example, breastfeeding mothers may request that pacifiers not be given to their infants, and some parents may see no problem with the use of a finger but may find the use of a pacifier objectionable. In general, there is no need to restrain either unless thumb-sucking persists past 4 years of age or past the time when the permanent teeth erupt. Parents are advised to consult their pediatrician and pediatric nurse practitioner about this topic.

To decrease dependence on nonnutritive sucking, sucking pleasure can be increased by prolonging feeding time. A

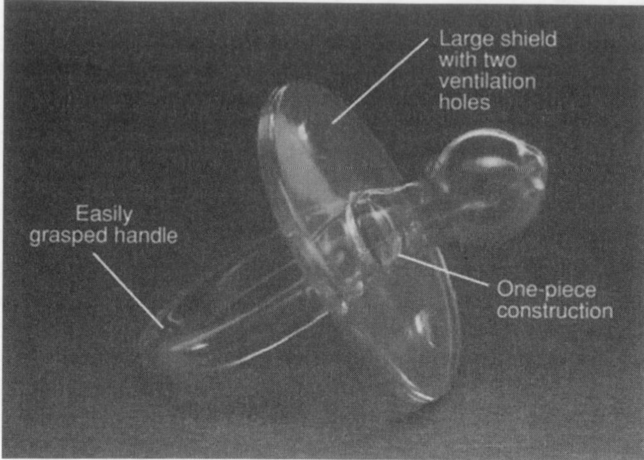

Fig. 23-24 Design of safe pacifier. (From Wong D: *Whaley & Wong's nursing care of infants and children*, ed 5, St Louis, 1995, Mosby.)

TABLE 23-3 Immunizations

IMMUNIZATION	AGE OF ORIGINAL IMMUNIZATION
DTP (diphtheria-tetanus-pertussis)	2, 4, 6 months
HibCV (*Haemophilus influenzae* B conjugate vaccine)	2, 4, 6 months (HIBTITER vaccine) 2,4 months (PedvaxHIB vaccine)
Hib and DTP	2, 4, 6 months
TOPV (trivalent oral poliovirus vaccine)*	2, 4 months
MMR (measles-mumps-rubella)	15 months (12 months if community outbreak)
Hepatitis B	Before hospital discharge, 1-2 months, 6-18 months
Tuberculin skin test (not an immunization but a test)	12-15 months

*The first two polio immunizations should be the inactivated polio vaccine (IPV); the last two doses in the series of four should be the oral polio vaccine (OPV). These doses are based on the recommendation of the Centers for Disease Control and Prevention (Pediatric Alert, 1995).

small-holed, firm nipple causes stronger sucking and slower feeding from a bottle. Also the parent's excessive use of the pacifier to calm the child should be explored. It is not unusual for parents to place a pacifier in the infant's mouth as soon as crying begins, thus reinforcing a pattern of distress relief (Wong, 1995). If the child uses a pacifier, safety considerations in purchasing one must be stressed. A homemade or poorly designed pacifier can be dangerous because the entire object may be aspirated if it is small or a portion may become lodged in the pharynx. Improvised pacifiers, such as those commonly made in hospitals from a padded nipple, also present dangers. The nipple may separate from the plastic collar and be aspirated. In addition, parents may continue to offer this pacifier to the infant at home. Safe pacifiers should be of one-piece construction, have a shield or flange that is large enough to prevent entry into the mouth, and have a handle that can be grasped (Fig. 23-24).

Immunizations

The schedule for immunizations should be reviewed (Table 23-3). The ability to protect against antigens by formation of antibodies develops sequentially. The infant must be developmentally capable of responding to antigens. A form of passive immunity is provided by colostrum and breast milk. It is specific for microbial agents present in the mother's own gastrointestinal tract. As fresh colonization occurs in the newborn, these antibodies limit bacterial growth in the gastrointestinal tract and protect against overgrowth.

This information helps health care professionals plan for the use of poliomyelitis vaccine in breastfed infants. According to Korones (1995), for its effectiveness, oral polio vaccine depends on multiplication in the intestinal tract. There is conflicting evidence that the vaccine fails to immunize babies receiving maternal breast milk with high antibody titers to poliovirus, because vaccine virus is inactivated in the gut by secretory immunoglobulin A (IgA) from breast milk (Lawrence, 1994). The Centers for Disease Control and Prevention now recommend that the first two polio immunizations be given with the inactivated poliovirus vaccine (IPV), which is believed to be less likely to cause polio than the oral (OPV) form. The last two doses in the series of four are recommended to be the OPV (Pediatric Alert, 1995). The other injections, diphtheria-tetanus-pertussis (DTP), oral poliovirus vaccine (OPV), hepatitis B, rubella, measles, and mumps, do not appear to be affected by breastfeeding and should be given at the regular recommended schedule (Lawrence, 1994).

Infant Follow-Up Care

Parents should plan for infant health follow-up care at 2 to 4 weeks of age, then every 2 months until 6 to 7 months of age, then every 3 months until 18 months, at 2 years, at 3 years, at preschool, and every 2 years thereafter. With managed care and early postpartum discharge, some institutions and their health insurance providers are encouraging either a home health visit within the first 5 to 6 days after birth or a brief outpatient visit to monitor serum bilirubin levels and breastfeeding.

The newborn's record provides a source of documented communication among all members of the health care team. The record contains accurate and complete recordings of the history, physical examination, laboratory test results, sequential observations, expected outcomes, interventions, and newborn's responses. Documentation of the parents' health education, counseling, and responses to information is included. The record should be readily accessible to health care professionals caring for the infant and family.

Home Care

With shorter hospital stays, the focus and place of infant care are changing. Home care may be provided by a nurse as part of the follow-up of patients or through a visiting nurse or community health nurse referral. Home care of the infant is discussed in Chapter 21.

Evaluation

The nurse can be reasonably assured that care was effective to the degree that the expected outcomes for care have been achieved. For the infant, outcomes include the following:

1. Maintenance of effective breathing patterns and thermoregulation
2. Freedom from infection
3. Necessary nutrition for growth
4. Adequate elimination patterns
5. Minimal pain related to heel stick, circumcision, or other pain-causing procedure

The mother/parent has achieved the following outcomes:

1. Attained knowledge, skill, and confidence relevant to child care activities
2. Can state understanding of biologic and behavioral characteristics of the newborn
3. Has taken the opportunity to intensify relationships with the newborn
4. Has begun to intergrate infant into the family
5. Has demonstrated behavioral/life-style changes to reduce potential for development of problems

Key Points

- Assessment of the newborn requires data from the prenatal, intrapartal, and postnatal periods.
- Knowledge of biologic and behavioral characteristics is essential for guiding assessment and interpreting data.
- Providing a protective environment is a key role for the nurse that includes such actions as careful identification procedures, restraining techniques, measures to prevent infection, and support of physiologic functions.
- Maintenance of adequate ventilation includes ensuring an adequate airway and body temperature.
- Parent education is a major role for the nurse and includes involving parents in all phases of the nursing process.
- Circumcision is an elective surgical procedure.
- Whether or not this is the couple's first baby, parents appreciate anticipatory guidance in the care of their child.

References

AAP releases circumcision statement, *Pediatr Nurs* 15(2):203, 1989.

American Academy of Pediatrics Committee on the Fetus and Newborn: Routine evaluation of blood pressure, hematocrit, and glucose in the newborn, *Pediatrics* 92(3):474, 1993.

Ankyloglossia, *Pediatr Surg Update* 6(1):1, 1996.

Blackburn S, Loper D: *Maternal, fetal, and neonatal physiology: a clinical perspective*, Philadelphia, 1992, WB Saunders.

Campos R: Rocking and pacifiers: two comforting interventions for heel stick pain, *Res Nurs Health* 17:331, 1994.

Cohen H et al: Postcircumcision urinary tract infection, *Clin Pediatr* 31(6):322, 1992.

Cornblath M, Schwartz R: Hypoglycemia in the neonate, *J Pediatr Endocrinol* 6(2):113, 1993.

Donaher-Wagner B, Braun D: Infant cardiopulmonary resuscitation for expectant and new parents, *MCN Am J Matern Child Nurs* 17:27, 1992.

Fanaroff A, Martin R: *Neonatal-perinatal medicine: diseases of the fetus and infant*, ed 6, St. Louis, 1997, Mosby.

Female genital mutilation, *AAP News* 10(2):3, 1994.

Female genital mutilation, (news): *J Psychosoc Nurs Ment Health Serv* 34(5):10, 1996.

Godley F: Frenuloplasty with a buccal mucosal graft, *Laryngoscope* 104(3):378, 1994.

Guntheroth W, Spiers P: Sleeping prone and the risk of sudden infant death syndrome, *JAMA* 267(17):2359, 1992.

Korones S: *High-risk newborn infants: the basis for intensive care*, ed 5, St. Louis, 1995, Mosby.

Lawrence R: *Breastfeeding: a guide for the medical profession*, ed 4, St. Louis, 1994, Mosby.

March of Dimes: *Public health information sheet: newborn screening tests*, White Plains, NY, 1994, March of Dimes.

Marchette L et al: Pain reduction interventions during neonatal circumcision, *Nurs Res* 40:241, 1991.

McCleary P: Female genital mutilation and childbirth: a case report, *Birth* 21(4):221, 1994.

Murphy M, Oellrich G: A new method of phototherapy: nursing perspectives, *J Perinatol* 10:249, 1990.

NAACOG: Neonatal skin care, *OGN Nurs Pract Resource* Jan. 1992.

Pediatric Alert: Switching from oral inactivated polio vaccine, *Pediatr Alert* 20(25):145, 1995.

Penny-MacGillivray T: A newborn's first bath: when? *J Obstet Gynecol Neonat Nurs* 25:481, 1996.

Ragan J, Weinfield A: VACNECCA: an eight-point check for neonatal assessment, *J Pract Nurs* p. 39, June, 1989.

Reiner C, Meltes S, Hayes J: Optimal sites and depths for skin puncture of infants and children as assessed from anatomical measurements, *Clin Chem* 36(3):547, 1990.

Rosenfeld W, Twist P, Concepcion L: A new device for phototherapy treatment of jaundiced infants, *J Perinatol* 10:243, 1990.

Rush J et al: A randomized trial of nursery ritual: wearing cover gowns to care for healthy newborns, *Birth* 17(1):25, 1990.

Task Force on Circumcision: Report of the task force on circumcision, *Pediatrics* 84(4):388, 1989.

Treloar D: The effect of nonnutritive sucking on oxygenation in healthy, crying full-term infants, *Appl Nur Res* 7:52, 1994.

Trochtenberg D: Neonatal circumcision, *N Engl J Med* 323(17):1206, 1990 (letter to the editor).

Valman H: Jaundice in the newborn, *Br Med J* 299:1272, 1989.

Vaughns B: Early maternal-infant contact and neonatal thermoregulation, *Neonat Netw* 8(5):19, 1990.

Wiswell T: Routine neonatal circumcision: a reappraisal, *Am Fam Physician* 41(3):859, 1990.

Wong D: *Whaley and Wong's nursing care of infants and children*, ed 5, St. Louis, 1995, Mosby.

Zander K: Second generation critical paths, *Definition* 4(4):1, 1989.

Bibliography

Corff K, Seideman R, Venkataraman P et al: Facilitated tucking: a nonpharmacologic comfort measure for pain in preterm neonates, *J Obstet Gynecol Neonat Nurs* 24(2):143, 1995.

Kemp J, Nelson V, Thach B: Physical properties of bedding that may increase risk of sudden infant death syndrome in prone-sleeping infants, *Pediatr Res* 36:7, 1994.

Klaus M, Kennell J, Klaus P: *Bonding: building the foundation of secure attachment and independence,* Menlo Park, Calif, 1995, Addison-Wesley.

Letko M: Understanding the apgar score, *J Obstet Gynecol Neonat Nurs* 25(4):299, 1996.

Page J: The newborn with ambiguous genitalia, *Neonat Netw* 13(5):15, 1994.

Stevens B, Johnston C: Physiological responses of premature infants to a painful stimulus, *Nurs Res* 43:226, 1994.

Weiss M, Poeltler D, Gocka I: Infrared tympanic thermometry for neonatal temperature assessment, *J Obstet Gynecol Neonat Nurs* 23(9):798, 1994.

CHAPTER 24

Newborn Nutrition and Feeding

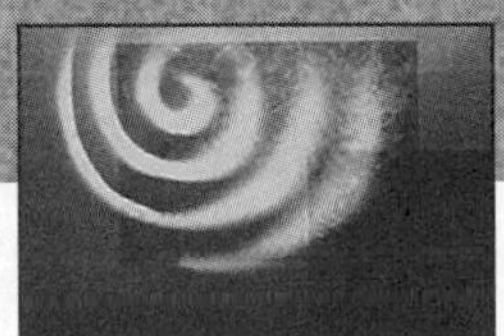

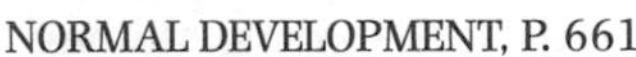

NORMAL DEVELOPMENT, P. 661

Physical growth, p. 661

Emotional development, p. 661

Feeding readiness, p. 662

NUTRIENT NEEDS, P. 663

Energy (calories or kcal), p. 663

Carbohydrate, p. 663

Fat, p. 664

Protein, p. 664

Fluids, p. 664

Vitamins and minerals, p. 664

LACTATION, P. 665

Factors affecting breastfeeding practices, p. 665

Prenatal support for breastfeeding, p. 665

Unique properties of human milk, p. 666

Maternal benefits of lactation, p. 666

Overview of normal lactation, p. 666

Milk production, p. 667

Breastfeeding the baby, p. 668

Effects of early discharge, p. 674

Role of the nurse as teacher, p. 674

Breastfeeding support, p. 675

Care of the mother, p. 675

Expressing, pumping, and storing milk, p. 677

Drugs and environmental pollutants, p. 679

Weaning, p. 680

Problem-solving techniques, p. 680

Potentially challenging situations, p. 687

Nursing care management, p. 688

FORMULA FEEDING, P. 691

Care of the bottle-feeding mother and infant, p. 691

DISCHARGE PLANNING, P. 693

Good nutrition in infancy fosters optimal growth and development. It can also establish a basis for developing lasting good eating habits. Health supervision of infants requires knowledge of their nutritional needs. This chapter focuses primarily on meeting nutritional needs for normal growth and development from birth to 6 months of age. Both breastfeeding and formula-feeding are addressed.

NORMAL DEVELOPMENT

Physical Growth

Discussion of a child's growth pattern may be a starting point for effective communication with parents regarding proper nutrition for their child. Most newborns experience a 5% to 7% weight loss during the first few days of life. Full-term infants usually regain this weight within 10 to 14 days and then continue to gain about an ounce per day until they have doubled their birth weight by age 5 months.

Typically an infant's length increases about 50% during the first year. Doubling of birth length usually does not occur until about 4 years of age. During the first year, head circumference also increases rapidly in conjunction with brain growth.

To assist in the clinical evaluation of physical growth of children in the United States, growth standards, or norms, have been developed for height or length, body weight, and head circumference. Measurements below the 5th percentile or above the 95th percentile may indicate problems with growth. Measurements between these extremes indicate that growth is within normal limits by current standards.

Emotional Development

Babies cry to communicate hunger, thirst, pain, boredom, and need for human contact. When an infant's needs are met, a sense of trust develops between the baby and the parent. The infant begins to develop a sense of competence in his or her ability to communicate. Babies learn to trust the people who answer their cries for help.

There is a special closeness that usually develops quickly between a breastfeeding mother and her baby. Mothers describe this unique relationship as reciprocal—the baby's enjoyment at the breast is matched by the mother's satisfaction at being able to nourish, nurture, and comfort her infant. Mothers feel a sense of accomplishment seeing their babies grow and develop on their milk. Also, by being able to quickly provide the opportunity to cuddle close and suck at the breast both for nourishment and comfort, the mother is able to foster a sense of well-being in her baby that can last a lifetime (Fig. 24-1).

When expecting their first baby, some men wonder what

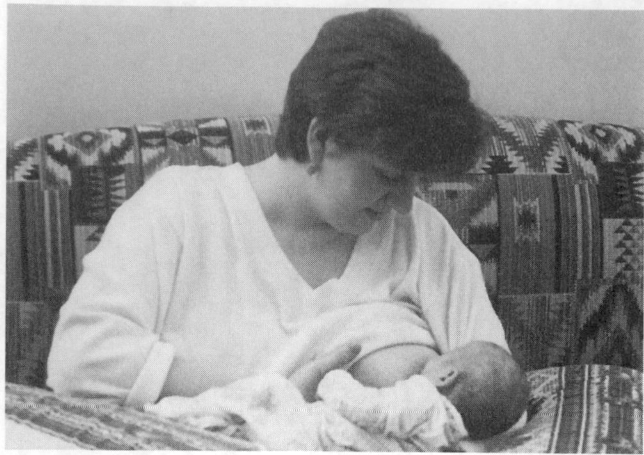

Fig. 24-1 Mother and baby enjoying breastfeeding.

the father's role in caring for the breastfed newborn might be. They fear that they will feel left out and have very little to do for the baby. The nurse can allay those fears by mentioning the many ways to interact with a baby. Fathers need to know that if they come when the baby cries—whether or not they actually feed the baby—the baby will quickly stop crying as soon as they appear. Some babies like to rest on dad's chest while the father reads or watches television. In the first few days, many babies must be awakened for feeding by a back rub. After each feeding the baby needs burping. Babies like to be held and go for walks. Newborns respond to being played with and need this type of stimulation for good development. There are also diaper changes and baths, but because fathers may feel apprehensive about these tasks before they have any experience with them, they may need instruction and encouragement.

Feeding Readiness

Feeding ability is largely determined by the maturation of the central nervous system. In the term infant, the **rooting reflex** (trying to suck on whatever touches the face), *sucking reflex*, and *swallowing reflex* are present at birth (Chapter 22). There is also an *extrusion reflex* at birth that automatically leads an infant to push the tongue out of the mouth. The healthy newborn is skilled at sucking fingers and has been doing so for several weeks. Because the placenta has provided all nourishment in utero, the newborn has no knowledge of the connection between sucking and feeding. However, infants placed on their mothers' abdomens at birth will move to seek the nipple and suck contentedly (Widstrom, Ransjo-Arvidsson, and Christensson, 1993). Early experiences with breastfeeding teach the baby to associate sucking with the good feeling of being full. The bottle-fed baby can enjoy being held while getting acquainted with the mother. The tactile stimulation of being held and cuddled makes feedings an important time for social interaction.

Most newborns express hunger by vigorous and sustained crying; however, some infants withdraw into sleep when they are uncomfortable. These babies can learn to recognize and express their hunger if they are picked up and fed each time they exhibit **feeding readiness cues** in the early weeks of life. Babies display several cues even during light sleep:

- Bringing hand to mouth
- Rooting
- Mouthing
- Sucking motions

The optimal time to begin a feeding is when the baby exhibits some of these cues rather than waiting until the baby is crying and distraught.

Newborns can focus their eyes on a point about 8 inches away from themselves. When a baby is at the mother's breast for feeding, there is a natural distance of about 8 inches between the baby's eyes and the mother's face. This allows the baby to have eye-to-eye contact with the mother. When a baby is bottle-fed, this interaction can be mimicked by holding the baby in a cradled position facing the caregiver.

In the first 3 days after birth, babies normally consume minimal volumes. **Colostrum** (early milk) is very concentrated and high in protein, uniquely suited to providing nutrition during this transition to life outside the womb. Although infant formulas are not similarly adjusted, most bottle-fed infants consume only small amounts of formula at each feeding. As the baby adjusts to extrauterine life and the digestive tract is cleared of meconium, the baby rapidly increases the volume of intake from about 10 to 15 ml per feeding in the first 24 hours to 60 to 90 ml or more per feeding thereafter.

At birth and for several months thereafter, the secretions of the infant gastrointestinal tract contain enzymes especially suited to the digestion of human milk. The ability to handle foods other than milk depends on the physiologic development of the infant. The capacities for salivary, gastric, pancreatic, and intestinal digestion increase with age. This progression indicates that the natural time for introduction of solid foods is around 6 months of age (Table 24-1). It is also at this time that the extrusion reflex becomes less pronounced.

Kidney function of the full-term newborn is not completely mature. Well-developed glomeruli satisfactorily filter the blood presented to the kidneys, but the tubules, which are functionally less mature, are somewhat limited in their ability to reabsorb water and some solutes. Therefore it is important that the kidneys not be presented with an excess renal solute load. Infants should not be fed foods with added salt.

The primary source for nutrition during the first year of life should be either breast milk or formula. Introduction of solid foods before the infant is 4 to 6 months of age may increase the infant's risk of developing allergies. Additionally, regular feeding of solid foods before this age can lead to overfeeding and decreased intake of breast milk or formula. Early introduction of solids has also been tied to early cessation of breastfeeding (Grossman et al, 1990). Even after 6 months of age the baby should be offered milk first and then the solids for an additional 2 to 3 months.

Some parents mistakenly believe that eating solid foods enables the infant to sleep through the night; however, sleep is determined by each individual's waking and sleeping pattern, not by the amount of food consumed. It is not true that early feeding of solid foods helps a baby sleep through the night.

The schedule for introducing solid foods and the types of foods to offer are discussed during the well-baby checkups at 4 to 6 months. New foods should be offered one at a time so that

TABLE 24-1 Digestion in infancy: birth to 6 months

LOCATION	FUNCTION OF ENZYME OR OTHER FACTOR	COMMENTS/IMPLICATIONS FOR FEEDING
Human milk	Lipase hydrolyzes triglycerides into free fatty acids and glycerol.	Functions in the small bowel because it must be activated by bile salts. Helps to compensate for the low pancreatic lipase activity at birth.
Mouth	Some salivary amylase is available at birth for starch digestion.	Insufficient to compensate for low pancreatic amylase levels.
	Lingual lipase released by serous glands hydrolyzes triglycerides.	Activity continues in the stomach, making an important contribution to milk fat digestion in the infant.
Stomach	Hydrochloric acid (HCl) and pepsin denature protein and begin hydrolysis.	Protein digestion begins. HCl output is low at birth but reaches adult levels by 6 months of age. Pepsin levels do not equal the adult's until 2 years.
	Gastric lipase hydrolyzes triglycerides.	Along with lingual lipase, serves as an important compensatory mechanism for low pancreatic lipase levels.
Pancreas/intestine	Trypsin, chymotrypsin, the carboxypeptidases, and elastase from the pancreas hydrolyze proteins into peptides and amino acids. Dipeptidases and tripeptidases in the intestinal brush border further digest the peptides.	Although pancreatic proteolytic enzyme release is lower than that in the adult, during the first month the infant can digest at least 80% of the protein ingested.
	Bile salts emulsify dietary fats, increasing the surface area available to pancreatic lipase activity.	Bile salt and pancreatic lipase levels are low at birth, but the activity of other lipases enables the newborn to digest 90% to 95% of dietary fat.
	Pancreatic amylase hydrolyzes starches.	Activity in term neonates is approximately 10% that of the adults. Activity increases by the end of 6 months, but maximal activity is not achieved until 2 years of age. Starch digestion may be incomplete in the young infant.
	Disaccharidases (lactase, sucrase, maltase) in the intestinal brush border hydrolyze specific disaccharides (lactose, sucrose, and maltose, respectively) to their component monosaccharides, in which form they can be absorbed.	Levels of these disaccharidases are higher at birth than they are in adults. Thus the neonate is well prepared to digest the carbohydrate in human milk, as well as the carbohydrates commonly used in preparation of formulas.

Modified from Tsang R, Nichols B, editors: *Nutrition during infancy*, Philadelphia, 1988, Hanley & Belfus.

any reaction (gas, colic, diarrhea, vomiting, diaper rash, or other skin rash) can be relieved by stopping the suspected food. Common allergens to be avoided for small babies include cow milk, egg whites, oranges, and strawberries. The nurse should counsel the mother to wait until the infant is at least 1 year old before offering these foods, especially if there is a family history of allergies. Honey should not be used on pacifiers or fed to infants under 12 months of age. It can contain spores of *Clostridium botulinum* that are not destroyed by heat during the processing of the honey. If ingested by an infant, these spores germinate, release the toxin that causes infant botulism, and, in some cases, prove fatal (Spika et al, 1989).

NUTRIENT NEEDS

Energy (Calories or kcal)

The energy requirements of the infant can be considered in terms of three areas: (1) the basal energy requirement that sustains organ metabolic function, (2) the energy needed for physical activity and digestion of food, and (3) the energy needed for growth. During the first 4 months of life, 50% to 60% of the infant's energy is expended for basal metabolism, 25% to 40% for growth, and approximately 10% to 15% for activity and other needs.

The recommended daily allowance (RDA) for energy for the first year is approximately 108 kcal/kg (49 kcal/lb) for the first 6 months and 98 kcal/kg (44.5 kcal/lb) for the second half of the year (Hendricks and Walker, 1990). Human milk supplies approximately 67 kcal/dl (20 kcal/oz); thus 720 ml (24 oz) supplies about 480 kcal/day, sufficient for an infant weighing approximately 4.2 kg ($9\frac{1}{4}$ lb). Infant formulas have been designed to approximate human milk and meet the same caloric needs.

Carbohydrate

Since newborns have only small hepatic glycogen stores, carbohydrates should provide at least 40% to 45% of total calories in the diet. Moreover, newborns may have limited ability for gluconeogenesis (formation of glucose from amino acids and other substrates) and ketogenesis (formation of ketone bodies from fat), which are mechanisms that provide alternative energy sources.

As the primary carbohydrate in human milk, lactose is the most abundant carbohydrate in the diet of infants until they reach 6 months of age. Lactose provides calories in an easily available form. Its slow breakdown and absorption probably increase calcium absorption. In cow milk–based formulas, corn syrup solids or glucose polymers are added to provide sufficient carbohydrates and supplement the lactose in the cow milk.

Fat

For infants to acquire adequate calories from the limited amount of human milk or formula they are able to consume, at least 15% of the calories provided must come from fat (triglycerides). The fat must be easily digestible. Fat in human milk is easier to digest and absorb than that in cow milk because of the arrangement of the fatty acids on the glycerol molecule and because of the presence of the enzyme lipase.

Cow milk is used in most infant formulas, but the milk fat is removed and a fat source such as corn oil, which can be digested and absorbed by the infant, is added. If whole milk or evaporated milk without added carbohydrate is fed to infants, fecal loss of fat and therefore loss of energy may be excessive because the milk moves through the infant's intestines too quickly for adequate absorption. This can lead to poor weight gain.

In addition to the energy contributions made by fat, there are essential fatty acids (EFAs) that are required for growth and tissue maintenance. EFAs are components of cell membranes and precursors of some hormones. Inadequate intake of EFAs results in eczema and growth failure. The lack of EFAs in skim and low-fat milk is another reason infants should not be fed these products.

Protein

The protein requirement is greater per unit of body weight in the newborn than at any other time of life. The RDA for protein during the first 6 months is 2.2 g/kg.

The protein content of human milk, lower than that of unmodified cow milk, is ideal for the newborn. Human milk contains far more lactalbumin in relation to casein than does cow milk; lactalbumin is more easily digested than casein. In addition, the amino acid composition of human milk is suited to the newborn infant's metabolic capabilities. For example, phenylalanine and methionine levels are low, and cystine and taurine levels are high. The protein in some commercial formulas is modified to increase the amount of lactalbumin, or whey, protein and to decrease the relative proportion of casein to more closely approximate human milk.

Fluids

The fluid requirement for normal infants is about 105 ml/kg/24 hr. Approximately 100 ml/24 hr of fluids are necessary for secretion of urine. This need is easily met by the infant who is breastfeeding or consuming properly prepared formula.

Neither breastfed nor formula-fed infants need to be given water, even those living in very hot climates (Lawrence, 1994). Indeed, being given water may decrease caloric consumption at a time when infants need to be growing rapidly. Water intoxication can result from feeding excessive amounts of water to infants (Naylor et al, 1992; Newman, 1992). Symptoms of water intoxication include hyponatremia, weakness, restlessness, nausea, vomiting, diarrhea, polyuria or oliguria, and convulsions.

Vitamins and Minerals

Human milk is the standard for determining vitamin and mineral requirements for the infant. Commercially prepared vitamins and minerals have been added to formulas to approximate the levels in human milk. In contrast, unmodified cow milk is much higher in mineral content than is human milk, which is one important reason why it is unsuitable for the feeding of human infants.

Vitamin C is present in human milk and is added to commercial formulas to provide sufficient amounts for the infant.

Most infants produce sufficient vitamin D because of their exposure to sunlight. It is estimated that a total of 30 minutes' exposure to sunlight per week wearing only a diaper, or 2 hours fully clothed without a hat, is sufficient to maintain adequate levels of this essential nutrient. Lack of sufficient vitamin D can lead to rickets. Supplementation may be recommended for preterm infants and dark-skinned children in cold climates, but it is unnecessary for the typical infant.

Vitamin K is required for blood coagulation and is produced by intestinal bacteria. However, the gut is sterile at birth, and time is required for intestinal flora to become established and produce vitamin K. Hemorrhagic disease of the newborn may result from low vitamin K levels. Excessive bruising, petechiae, prolonged bleeding from blood-sampling sites or circumcision, and intracranial hemorrhage may occur in affected infants. Therefore vitamin K is routinely administered by injection at birth to avoid such problems until the baby's gut can produce vitamin K.

In human milk the ratio of calcium to phosphorus is 2:1, which is optimal for bone mineralization. As a result, breastfed term infants receive ample calcium (28 mg/100 ml). Cow milk is very rich in calcium, but the calcium/phosphorus ratio is low. Because of the imbalance, hypocalcemia, tetany, and seizures often develop in young infants fed unmodified cow milk. The calcium/phosphorus ratio in commercial formulas is midway between human and cow milk.

Milk of all types is low in iron. However, iron from human milk is better absorbed (50%) than that from cow milk (10%), iron-fortified formula, or infant cereals (5%). Moreover, the fetus has deposited iron stores to draw on for the first few months of life. Therefore the infant who is totally breastfed normally maintains adequate hemoglobin levels for the first 6 months of life. After that time, iron-containing foods should be included in the diet. Formula-fed infants (and infants who are initially breastfed but then are weaned from the breast) should receive an iron-fortified formula until 12 months of age. Even though only a small percentage of the iron is absorbed from formulas, fortified formulas contain so much iron that the amount absorbed is usually sufficient.

Fluoride levels in human and commercial formulas are low. This mineral is involved in tooth development, which is ongoing during early infancy. A reduction in dental caries is seen in children who receive adequate fluoride. However, fluorosis (spotting) of the permanent teeth has resulted from too early or inappropriate supplementation. Thus a supplement is recommended only for those infants not receiving fluoridated water after 6 months of age (American Academy of Pediatrics, 1995).

In the United States, it is rare to find vitamin or mineral deficiencies among mothers and babies as long as the infant is breastfeeding or receiving a commercially prepared infant formula.

LACTATION

Factors Affecting Breastfeeding Practices

Cultural beliefs must be considered when planning any care. The nurse should be aware that there are many regional, ethnic, and racial cultures, which all can have significant impact on the choice to breastfeed and how to breastfeed.

Several investigators have examined various factors that have been associated with differences in breastfeeding rates among various demographic groups. These factors include support of the partner, the mother's concern about pain, fear of infant dependency, and misconceptions about the effect on appearance of the breast and the effect on sexuality (Freed, Fraley, and Schanler, 1992). Also, some cultural groups believe that colostrum is harmful, and these women delay breastfeeding until the breasts feel heavy.

In the United States, there was a steady increase in the rate of breastfeeding from a low of 25% in 1970 to a peak at 62% in 1982. The rate began to decline, and by 1989 it was only 52%. The breastfeeding rate at 6 months declined even more—from 27% in 1982 to 18% in 1989. The decline occurred across all socioeconomic strata (Ryan et al, 1991).

There are several theories that may explain these trends. In the 1980s the proportion of births to adolescents rose significantly, as did the proportion of births to unmarried and poor women (Centers for Disease Control, 1991). Both of these groups have historically been less likely to breastfeed in the United States. Also, more mothers of children under 1 year of age were in the work force than ever before. Full-time employment outside the home is significantly associated with decreased breastfeeding rates measured at 6 months (Gielen et al, 1991). Furthermore, mothers who are in the work force when their babies are less than 1 year of age include significant numbers of women who typically breastfeed: married women over 25 with some college education who are Caucasian and live in the Mountain or Pacific regions. Yet, it is important to note that there is the same rate of decline among women staying home with their children as among women returning to the work force (Ryan and Martinez, 1989). This suggests that factors other than employment must be contributing to the decline in breastfeeding initiation rates.

The low incidence of breastfeeding among women who participate in the federally funded Women, Infants, and Children's Nutrition Program (WIC) suggests possible programmatic barriers beyond the demographic barriers inherent in the population served by WIC. The primary thrust of the WIC program has been breastfeeding promotion. Generally there has been a lack of knowledgeable assistance with breastfeeding problems for this population. However, some WIC offices have implemented breastfeeding assistance programs, which have dramatically increased or even doubled breastfeeding initiation and duration rates (Valois, 1994). Since the advertising for infant formulas in many WIC settings has given a mixed message regarding the merits of breastfeeding, (MacGowan et al, 1991), a federal regulation passed in 1994 now prohibits WIC from displaying any formula company advertising.

Hospital policies that have been developed around a formula-feeding paradigm may have the most detrimental influence on breastfeeding duration. The formula-feeding paradigm rapidly evolved with the move of childbirth to the hospital setting. Among the many practices that interfere with breastfeeding are early separation of mother and infant; "test feeding" with sterile water; imposing a regimented feeding schedule; measuring feedings by ounces or minutes; keeping infants in a central nursery where early feeding cues are often overlooked; and assuming that assisting with breastfeeding is not a part of normal newborn care (Tully, 1994).

Feeding with sterile water has been done traditionally to assess the newborn for signs of tracheoesophageal fistula or esophageal atresia. However, there is no reason that this assessment cannot be done at the first breastfeeding. Colostrum has been present in the breast since the fourth month of pregnancy, and many babies suck and swallow vigorously at the initial feeding. The nurse who is with the mother and baby would observe signs of aspiration if there were a problem. If aspiration did occur, the baby's respiratory system would more readily absorb physiologic colostrum than water.

Giving a newborn a bottle may also interfere with learning to breastfeed easily because the process of sucking from a bottle is so different from breastfeeding. While breastfeeding, the baby is in control of milk flow; with a bottle, milk flows even when the baby is not sucking or ready to swallow. Infants learn to put the tongue against the rubber nipple hole to slow down the rapid flow of fluid. When infants try to use these same tongue movements during breastfeeding, they may push the human nipple out of the mouth and not be able to grasp the breast properly. The relatively inflexible rubber nipple also prevents the tongue from moving with its usual rhythmic action (Lawrence, 1989).

Additionally, the distribution of formula samples is strongly entrenched in many hospitals despite the fact that receiving these samples is associated with decreased incidence of breastfeeding as early as 3 weeks postpartum (Snell et al, 1992). Also, the use of formula company educational materials, note pads, staff name tags, infant crib tags, and mugs endorses formula-feeding, not breastfeeding.

Prenatal Support for Breastfeeding

Many parents have never seen a mother breastfeed her infant, and it is difficult to choose that with which one is unfamiliar. The nurse must ensure that prenatal classes present breastfeeding as the naturally expected way to feed an infant. Classes should also provide practical information and demonstration so that mothers know how to breastfeed. This can be more persuasive than any list of advantages. The breastfeeding mother who comes to a prenatal class can serve as a natural role model and answer expectant parents' questions. Videotapes and posters can also be useful in portraying breastfeeding as the norm for our culture.

LEGAL TIP

Informed Decision About Infant Feeding

To make an **informed decision** about feeding, parents must be given facts about the nutritional and immunologic needs of the newborn that are met with human milk, the potential benefits to the mother's health, and the risks of infant formula. The nurse must provide this information in a nonjudgmental way and then respect the parents' decision. Some health care professionals try to avoid this responsibility with the rationalization that they want to avoid making parents feel guilty. However, legally, the nurse is required to give complete information and to document that she has done so.

Unique Properties of Human Milk

Human milk provides many factors that are uniquely suited to the human infant and enhance growth and development. There are antibacterial and antiviral properties, immunoglobulins, and antiallergy factors in human milk that protect the infant against many infections and diseases. Mother's milk also contains growth factors, digestive enzymes, and proteins that foster the maturation process begun in utero (Table 24-2).

Maternal Benefits of Lactation

Because lactation is the last step in the pregnancy cycle, many mothers feel a sense of natural completion when they breastfeed. They enjoy a special sense of closeness with the baby. Often women have an enhanced sense of well-being while breastfeeding that is thought to result from the hormones necessary for lactation. The woman who breastfeeds her baby also experiences faster uterine involution, which decreases her risk of hemorrhage and speeds her body's return to a prepregnant state. The lactational amenorrhea that accompanies breastfeeding for most women protects the mother's iron stores. Absorption of many minerals appears to be enhanced so that bone density is not decreased by lactation (Hayslip et al, 1989). Studies suggest that the greater the length of time a woman breastfeeds, the less risk she has of developing premenopausal breast cancer (Layde, 1989).

Overview of Normal Lactation

Lactation is part of the normal human reproductive cycle. Successful lactation depends on the following:

- Functional breast tissue
- **Lactogenesis** (initiation of milk production)
- Effective removal of milk from the breast

Breast enlargement and tenderness during early pregnancy signal a proliferation of **milk glands,** which contain alveoli (clusters of milk-producing cells), milk ductules, and myoepithelial cells (milk-ejecting cells). The alveoli begin to produce colostrum around the sixteenth week of gestation.

After birth the baby's sucking and the mother's emotional response to her baby stimulate the hypothalamus to promote release of **oxytocin,** one of the two primary hormones of lactation, from the posterior pituitary (Table 24-3). Oxytocin triggers the myoepithelial cells surrounding the alveoli to contract, ejecting the colostrum and later milk into the milk ducts, then down into the **lactiferous sinuses** under the areola and out the nipple. This process is the **milk ejection reflex (MER),** often called the **let-down reflex.** There are several let-downs during each feeding.

Immediately after the baby is born the breasts may feel quite firm or heavy. During labor, oxytocin causes uterine contractions and triggers repeated let-downs. Some mothers even leak colostrum. From the first feeding the baby who is latched on correctly can be heard to swallow.

After the mother gives birth, there is a precipitous fall in

TABLE 24-2 Immune benefits of breast milk at a glance

COMPONENT	ACTION
White blood cells	
B lymphocytes	Give rise to antibodies targeted against specific microbes.
Macrophages	Kill microbes outright in the baby's gut, produce lysozyme, and activate other components of the immune system.
Neutrophils	May act as phagocytes, ingesting bacteria in baby's digestive system.
T lymphocytes	Kill infected cells directly or send out chemical messages to mobilize other defenses. They proliferate in the presence of organisms that cause serious illness in infants. They also manufacture compounds that can strengthen a child's own immune response.
Molecules	
Antibodies of secretory IgA class	Bind to microbes in baby's digestive tract and thereby prevent them from passing through walls of the gut into body's tissues.
B_{12}-binding protein	Reduces amount of vitamin B_{12}, which bacteria need in order to grow.
Bifidus factor	Promotes growth of *Lactobacillus bifidus,* a harmless bacterium, in baby's gut. Growth of such nonpathogenic bacteria helps to crowd out dangerous varieties.
Fatty acids	Disrupt membranes surrounding certain viruses and destroy them.
Fibronectin	Increases antimicrobial activity of macrophages: helps to repair tissues that have been damaged by immune reactions in baby's gut.
Gamma-interferon	Enhances antimicrobial activity of immune cells.
Hormones and growth factors	Stimulate baby's digestive tract to mature more quickly. Once the initially "leaky" membranes lining the gut mature, infants become less vulnerable to microorganisms.
Lactoferrin	Binds to iron, a mineral many bacteria need to survive. By reducing the available amount of iron, lactoferrin thwarts growth of pathogenic bacteria.
Lysozyme	Kills bacteria by disrupting their cell walls.
Mucins	Adhere to bacteria and viruses, thus keeping such microorganisms from attaching to mucosal surfaces.
Oligosaccharides	Bind to microorganisms and bar them from attaching to mucosal surfaces.

From Newman J: How breast milk protects newborns, *Sci Am* 273:76, 1995.

TABLE 24-3 Hormones of milk production

HORMONE	ACTION	SIGNIFICANCE	SIGNS
Oxytocin	Triggers milk ejection reflex (MER) and uterine contractions	▪ Empties milk glands ▪ If milk glands are not emptied, action of prolactin is inhibited	▪ Baby swallows rapidly ▪ Opposite breast may leak ▪ Mother experiences increased lochia flow and/or uterine cramping
Prolactin	Triggers milk production in emptied milk glands	▪ Milk glands fill with milk for each feeding ▪ Without release of prolactin, milk glands cannot transition to lactogenesis stage II and begin production of mature milk	▪ Mother feels relaxed and sleepy ▪ Baby relaxes while sucking and is content between feedings ▪ Milk changes from colostrum to mature milk ▪ Baby has adequate urine and stool output

progesterone, which allows release of **prolactin,** the other primary maternal hormone necessary for lactation. Prolactin is released by the anterior pituitary gland in response to the infant's suck. It triggers milk production in emptied milk glands. Back pressure from incomplete emptying of the breasts over several feedings can decrease milk production. This is the mechanism that inhibits milk production for the mother who is not breastfeeding. Therefore at each feeding it is important for the baby to breastfeed long enough on the first breast to thoroughly soften it, even if the baby does not take the second breast. By alternating sides, at the next feeding the baby will empty the second side.

Composition of mature milk changes during each feeding. Initially there is a release of bluish white foremilk that is skim milk (about 60% of the volume), which is followed by whole milk (about 35%). The hindmilk, or cream (about 5%), is usually let down 10 to 20 minutes into the feeding, although for a few women it occurs sooner. It is important to breastfeed long enough on one breast to supply a balanced feeding. Foremilk provides primarily lactose, protein, and water-soluble vitamins, and hindmilk contains the denser calories from fat necessary for optimal growth and contentment between feedings.

Typically, a mother produces 720 to 900 ml of milk every 24 hours by the time her baby is 2 weeks old. As the baby grows, the amount of milk needed to support the growth increases. At fairly predictable times (about 10 days, 6 weeks, 3 months, and 4 to 6 months), the baby will fuss to nurse more often than usual for about 48 hours. These times are referred to as **growth spurts.** More frequent emptying of the breasts increases milk production, and then the baby will be getting more milk each time, be more satisfied, and spread out the feedings again.

During the early weeks a well-nourished breastfed baby will have at least two bowel movements every 24 hours. Some babies stool with every feeding. The baby's bowel movements should change from black meconium to a watery, mustard-yellow stool with small white curds by the time the baby is 4 days old. As the baby gets older, the frequency of stooling decreases. Some older breastfed babies may go several days without a bowel movement. No intervention is necessary; the stool remains soft and the infant is not constipated.

Milk Production

Each female breast is composed of about 18 groups of milk glands and ducts embedded in fat and connective tissue and is well-supplied with blood vessels, lymphatic tissue, and nerves (Fig. 24-2). The size of the breast is not an indication of its capacity to make milk. The visible breast serves primarily as a storage area for milk, which is produced in the glands located in the chest wall and extending up under the arm. Regardless of breast size, milk is produced at the rate it is removed.

Stimulation of the nipple causes the pituitary gland to secrete oxytocin. This hormone is responsible for the let-down reflex during which the milk-ejecting cells contract and force the colostrum, and later the milk, from the milk-producing cells into the milk ducts, which widen to form the lactiferous

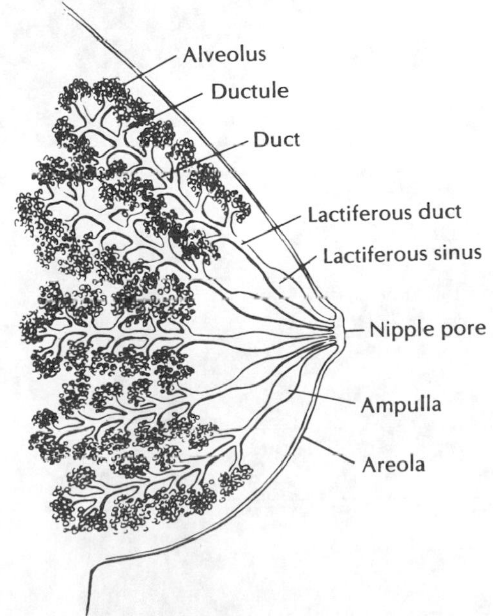

Fig. 24-2 Detailed structural features of the human breast. (From Worthington-Roberts B, Williams S: *Nutrition in pregnancy and lactation,* ed 5, St Louis, 1993, Mosby. © McGraw-Hill.)

sinuses behind the nipple. Milk pools in these lactiferous sinuses, which are located under the **areola.** The lactiferous sinuses narrow to form the many openings in the nipple through which the milk flows.

Because milk is produced in much the same way as saliva, the breast is never completely empty. As soon as milk is removed from the alveoli, synthesis resumes. Conversely, when milk is left in the breasts, milk production is limited. This explains why milk production is described as a **supply-meets-demand system.** This self-regulating mechanism allows mothers to meet the needs of their growing infants, to breastfeed multiple infants, and also to wean.

Typically, when the baby cries or brushes against the breast, the nipple becomes erect. Although there are classic breast and nipple shapes, each woman's breasts and nipples are unique. Some women's nipples remain soft and may not protrude even with stimulation. About 15% of women have at least one **inverted nipple** (Fig. 24-3). Babies can learn to breastfeed with any nipple. However, this difference in shapes and sizes makes it important that the baby not be offered bottles or pacifiers to suck until breastfeeding is well established.

Although nearly every woman can lactate, it has been estimated that 2% to 5% of women have insufficient glandular development and are not able to exclusively breastfeed (Neifert, Seacat, and Jobe, 1985). Typically these women experienced few breast changes during either puberty or early pregnancy. Women with insufficient milk production to support optimal infant growth can still breastfeed their babies while providing additional nutrition through supplementation. The baby's weight gain determines how much supplementation is needed.

Lactogenesis begins early in pregnancy. This early proliferation of milk glands and production of colostrum is referred to as lactogenesis stage I. Colostrum is a translucent yellow substance ideally suited to the needs of the newborn. It is high in protein and rich in antibodies and other infection-fighting properties. It acts as a laxative to clear the meconium that fills the gastrointestinal tract at birth and facilitates loosening of mucus. With the natural drop in progesterone and estrogen during the week after birth, the production of colostrum undergoes a transition to the production of mature milk. This is referred to as the milk "coming in," or lactogenesis stage II. If either hormone remains elevated because of a retained placental fragment or introduction of these hormones as birth control, production of mature milk may be inhibited (Box 24-1).

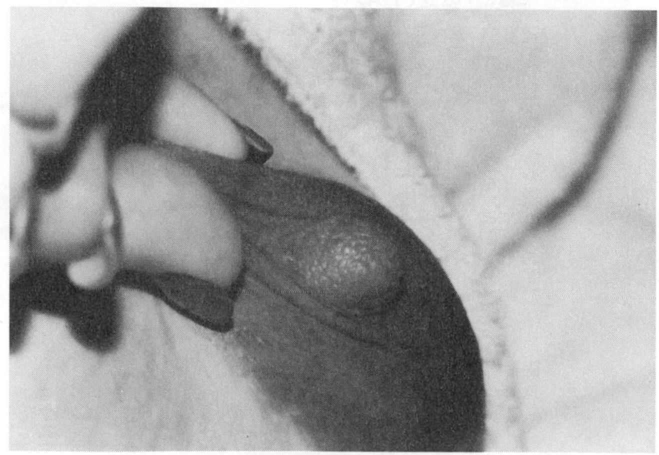

Fig. 24-3 An inverted nipple retracts when the areola is compressed, **A,** but may protrude if held at an angle, **B.** (Courtesy of Kay Hoover, IBCLC, Morton, Penn.)

Breastfeeding the Baby

Before beginning a feeding the baby should be alert and ready to suck. Once alert, the baby should be held in a comfortable position to facilitate feeding. The mother should hold the

BOX 24-1
Measuring Breast Milk Maturation

The Maturation Index of Colostrum and Milk (MICAM) uses filter paper chromatography to measure rate of breast milk maturation in individual mothers. Breast milk changes from colostrum to mature milk at different rates among women. Frequency and length of early feedings are associated with milk maturation. The MICAM can be used clinically to reassure women that their milk is maturing. The MICAM has five patterns—type 1 to type 5—that correspond with the composition of breast milk from colostrum to mature milk. The assessment is made by dropping two to three drops of milk on a piece of Whatman filter paper #1 that is placed on a ring. It takes approximately 30 minutes for the paper to dry. It is read when the paper is dry.

Early colostrum—hard, shiny, and ranges in color from very pale to bright yellow.
Late colostrum—similar to early colostrum; has a thin, translucent outer ring.
Early transitional milk—three rings; center ring yellow and 50% or more of the total area; middle ring white; outer ring translucent; spreads to a larger area than colostrum.
Late transitional milk—same three rings as transitional milk but with different proportions; yellow in the center is less than 50% of area.
Mature milk—three rings, but it is hard to see the center ring, which is almost the same color as the middle ring.

Data from Humenick S: The clinical significance of breast milk maturation rates, *Birth* 14(4):174, 1987; Humenick S et al: The maturation index of colostrum and milk (MICAM): a measurement of breast milk maturation, *J Nurs Measurement* 2(2):169, 1994.

baby's back and shoulders firmly in the palm of her hand, but not push on the back of the head. The baby's arms should be separated with one on either side of the mother's breasts. The baby's head and body must be in straight alignment. The baby should not have to turn the head or strain the neck to reach the nipple. The nurse should place firm pillows, folded blankets, or towels under the mother's arm to bring the baby's lips level with the mother's nipple. The baby's hips should be elevated nearly as high as the head. After a few weeks, most mothers find the extra support is not necessary.

Positioning. There are several positions for breastfeeding a baby. The mother should find a position that is comfortable for her (see the Patient Teaching box on pp. 670-671). She may need to use a pillow to support her back and put her feet up. Not all positions suit all mothers and babies. Once the baby has learned to latch on easily, most mothers prefer the classic cradle hold and lying-down positions.

For initial feedings the football hold usually facilitates the best latch-on. The baby is positioned so the mother can see the mouth easily. It is also preferred by most women who have had cesarean births. The across-the-lap hold gives the mother good control of the baby and allows more precise attachment for some babies. It is also helpful for nursing very small babies or for mothers with very small or very large breasts. Most mothers appreciate learning to breastfeed lying down so they can rest during feedings. Cradling provides optimal comfort for most mothers after the baby has learned to latch on easily and feed efficiently.

Latch-on. Most women find that supporting the breast in one hand with the fingers underneath and thumb on top at the back edge of the areola allows the baby to **latch on** correctly (Fig. 24-4). Most mothers need to support the breast during feedings at least for the first few weeks until the baby can stay latched on easily.

When the mother lightly touches the baby's lower lip and the tip of the tongue with her nipple, the baby responds by opening the mouth. The baby should be pulled quickly onto the breast once the mouth is open wide and the tongue is down. The baby's tongue reflexively comes out to pull the breast into the mouth. It is important to *bring the baby to the breast and not the breast to the baby* because if the breast is pushed into the baby's mouth, the baby usually closes too soon and does not latch on correctly. The amount of the areola in the baby's mouth depends on the sizes of the nipple, the areola, and the baby's mouth.

When latched on correctly, the baby's suck compresses the breast against the roof of the mouth with the tongue and creates a vacuum in the intraoral cavity at the back of the mouth, where the nipple is (see the Patient Teaching box on pp. 670-671). If the mother experiences pain after the first few sucks or does not feel a firm tugging on the nipple, the nurse should help her evaluate the baby's position to ensure that the baby's body is in straight alignment, with the back and hips well supported and no pressure on the back of the baby's head.

If the baby has difficulty keeping the tongue out over the lower gum ridge and each suck is painful, the nurse can place her index finger gently but firmly on the baby's lower jaw, which will stabilize it so the tongue stays in place. If this is helpful, the nurse can show the mother how to do it using the index finger on the hand supporting the breast. Most babies learn to latch on correctly after only a few feedings with assistance because having the nipple in the correct position is rewarding for the baby and the milk flows more quickly.

If the pain persists with better positioning and the jaw stabilized, the baby should be carefully removed from the breast and latched on again. To remove the baby from the breast without causing nipple trauma, the mother should break the suction by pushing a finger between the baby's gums and keeping it there to prevent a reflexive bite as the baby is taken off the breast (Fig. 24-5).

Once the baby is properly latched on, the mother and the nurse can observe the following:

- The cheeks are rounded, not sucked in or dimpled.
- The jaw glides smoothly as the baby sucks and swallows, and the baby's arms are relaxed.
- The mother feels a firm tug on her nipple, but no pinching or biting sensation.

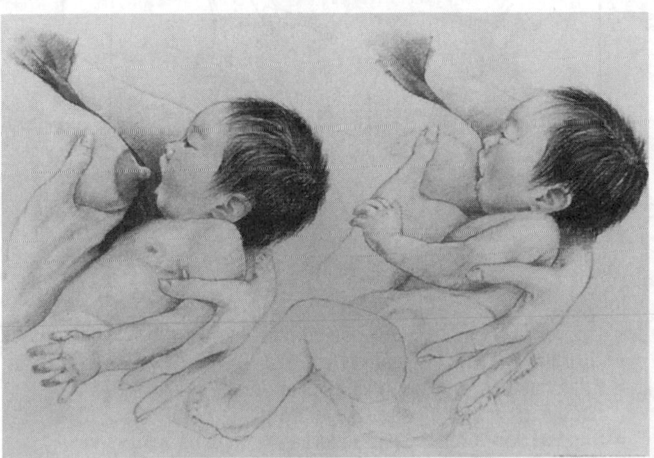

Fig. 24-4 Latching on. (Courtesy Karen Martin, Childbirth Graphics, Waco, Tex.)

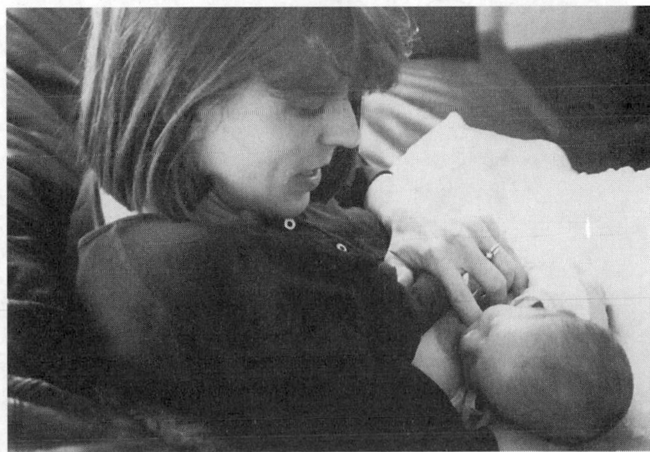

Fig. 24-5 Removing the infant from the breast.

Patient Teaching

BREASTFEEDING

How to hold your baby for feedings

- Sit or lie down comfortably with your back supported.
- Make sure your baby has one arm on either side of your breast, as you pull the baby close.
- Use firm pillows or folded blankets under the baby to keep the baby supported during the feeding. As your baby gets older, you probably will not need the extra support.
- Support the baby's back and shoulders firmly. Do not push on the back of the baby's head.
- Once the baby's mouth is open wide, pull your baby quickly onto your breast.

Four common breastfeeding positions

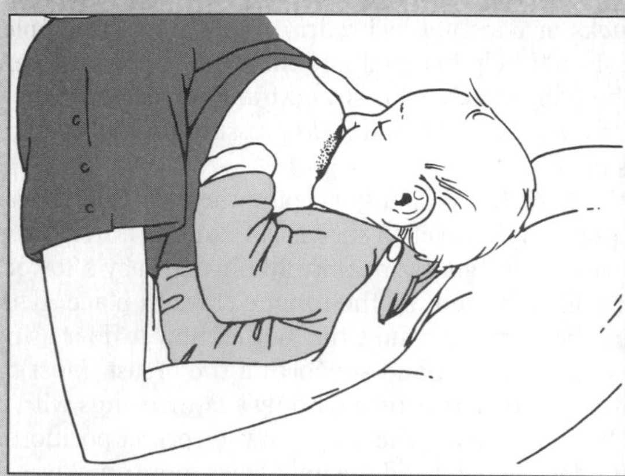

Football

- Hold the baby's back and shoulders in the palm of your hand.
- Tuck the baby up under your arm, keeping the baby's ear, shoulder, and hip in a straight line.
- Support the breast. Once the baby's mouth is open wide, pull the baby quickly to you.
- Continue to hold your breast until the baby feeds easily.

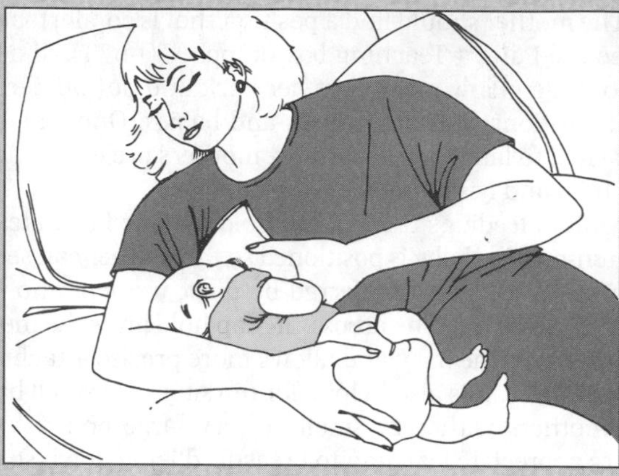

Lying down

- Lie on your side with a pillow at your back, and lay the baby so you are facing each other.
- To start, prop yourself up on your elbow and support your breast with that hand.
- Pull the baby close to you, lining up the baby's mouth with your nipple.
- Once the baby is feeding well, lie back down. Hold your breast with the opposite hand.

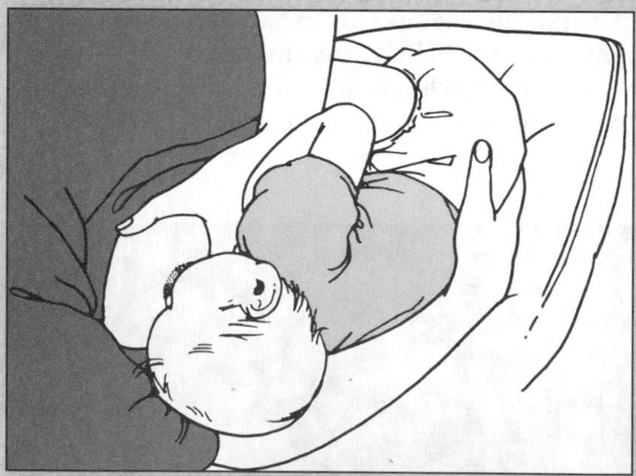

Cradling

- Cradle the baby in the arm closest to the breast, with the baby's head in the crook of your arm.
- Have your baby's body facing you, tummy to tummy.
- Use your opposite hand to support the breast.

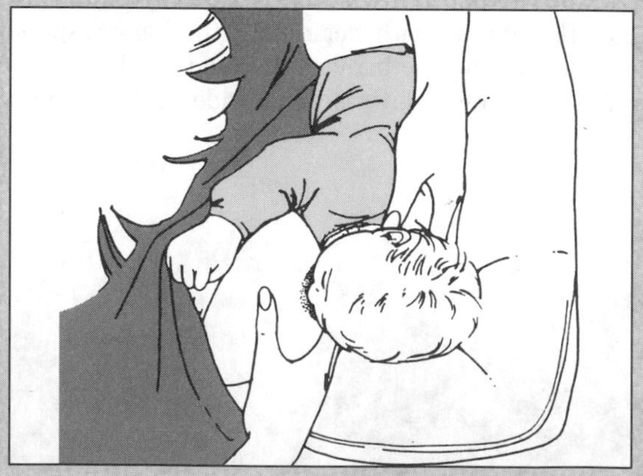

Across the Lap

- Lay your baby on firm pillows across your lap.
- Turn the baby facing you.
- Reach across your lap to support the baby's neck and shoulders with the palm of your hand.
- Support your breast from underneath to guide it into the baby's mouth.

Patient Teaching

BREASTFEEDING—cont'd

Latching-on

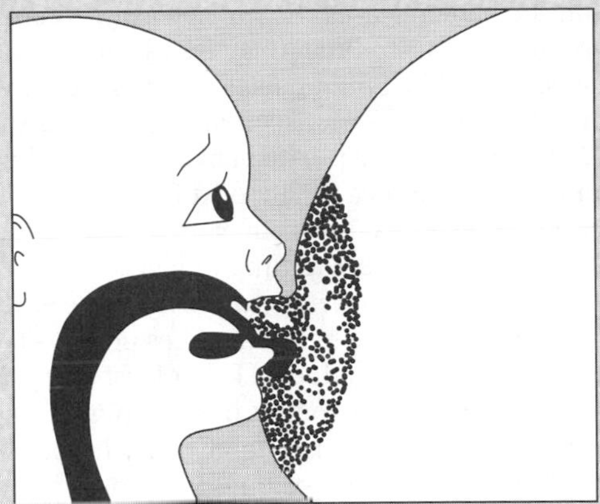

Incorrect
tongue position

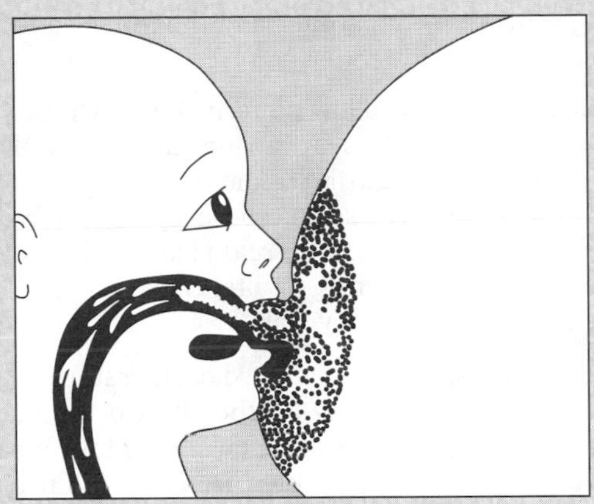

Correct
tongue position

- Hold your breast in one hand with your fingers underneath and the thumb on top.
- Have your hand back from the areola (the dark skin around the nipple).
- Line up the baby's lips with your nipple.
- Touch the lips with your nipple until the baby's mouth opens and tongue is down.
- Pull the baby quickly onto the breast.
- If nursing hurts after the first few sucks, take the baby off and start over. Make sure the baby's mouth is open wide and the tongue is down before pulling the baby close.

Breastfeeding is going well when . . .

- Your newborn is feeding about eight times in 24 hours for 30 to 40 minutes at each feeding. Some newborns need to eat more frequently until they learn to breastfeed efficiently. Other babies gain weight well feeding less often.
- At least one breast softens well at each feeding.
- You feel a tug, but not pain, when the baby sucks.
- The baby's arms and shoulders are relaxed during the feeding.
- The baby has bursts of 10 or more sucks and swallows at the beginning of each feeding.
- As your breast softens, the baby slows down to two to three sucks and swallows at a time.
- Your baby is content when you finish breastfeeding.
- By the time the baby is 4 days old, you should see at least six wet diapers and two bowel movements every 24 hours.

Let-down. The baby's mouth on the breast triggers a release of oxytocin, which causes the milk to let down. Some mothers have a tingling sensation in the breast or nipple; however, most women do not feel their milk let down. There are other reassuring signs that the mother and the nurse can identify, as follows:

- The baby's suck/swallow pattern changes from a rapid shallow suck to a deeper drawing suck and swallow.
- The breasts soften during feedings.
- The mother feels relaxed, even sleepy, during feedings.
- The mother experiences increased lochia flow and/or uterine cramping during or after the feeding.
- The opposite breast may leak.

In some cultures, and often in medical literature, there is a great deal of emphasis placed on the effect of the mother's emotions on her let-down, yet women successfully breastfeed during many adverse circumstances, from severe illness of the infant to wartime conditions. It is very rare for the milk ejection reflex not to occur automatically.

In some women the let-down reflex is inhibited by nicotine. The mother who smokes should only do so *after* feedings. It is also important for the nurse to encourage the mother to protect the baby from the effects of second-hand smoke. Smoking cessation programs can be recommended.

Typical feedings. During a typical feeding a baby begins with short, shallow sucks followed by several bursts of 10 or more long, drawing sucks and swallows when the first milk ejection reflex, or let-down, occurs. As the breast softens and the flow of milk slows, the baby will have shorter bursts of suck/swallows. The nurse should identify swallowing with the mother. If swallowing cannot be identified, it is important to reevaluate how the baby is latched on. For example, if the nipple is not centered in the mouth, is under the tongue, or is pinched at the front of the baby's mouth, milk will not flow even though the baby is sucking.

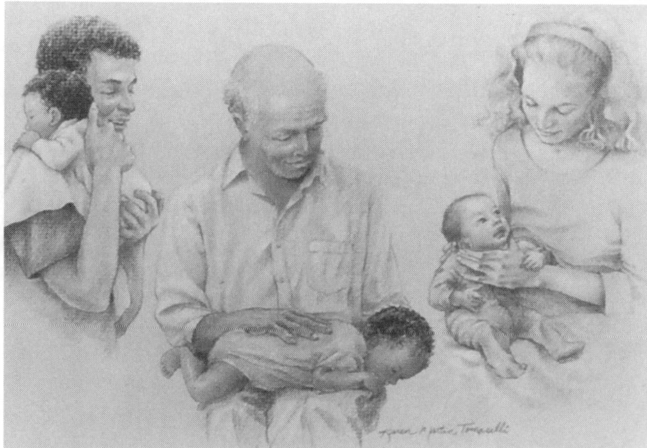

Fig. 24-6 Positions for burping infant: on the shoulder *(left)*, across the lap *(center)*, sitting *(right)*. (Note position of hand on the jaw to support the head.) (Courtesy Karen Martin, Childbirth Graphics, Waco, Tex.)

As the feeding progresses, the mother will begin to feel relaxed or even drowsy. With each suck, she will feel a firm tug on her nipple, but not chafing or pinching. The baby should stay on the first breast until it is thoroughly softened or lightened and the baby releases the nipple easily. After giving the baby an opportunity to burp (Fig. 24-6), the mother should offer the second side. Some babies need to feed only on one breast per feeding to feel satisfied and gain weight well, and not all babies need to burp. The baby who is still hungry will feed from the second breast. The next feeding should start on the breast that feels heavier or fuller.

Most newborns who are feeding well need about eight feedings per 24 hours to gain weight appropriately (see the Patient Teaching box below). The baby who does not awaken spontaneously should be wakened to be fed at least every third hour during the day and every fourth hour at night until an adequate weight gain pattern is established. The most accurate way to determine timing of feedings is to count the time from the beginning of one to the beginning of the next. Once the baby is gaining weight appropriately, the baby can determine the timing of feedings. This is often referred to as **demand feeding.** As the baby gets older, feedings will naturally be spaced farther apart.

Many babies feed more often at certain times of the day and sleep longer at others. It is important for parents to realize that every cry may not be a hunger cry. If the parents think the baby should still be full, they can first try other forms of comfort, such as diaper changing, burping, and holding, before offering a feeding. Some babies suck their own fingers or hands for comfort between feedings. This nonnutritive sucking does not necessarily mean they are hungry.

Patient Teaching

TIMING AND FREQUENCY OF FEEDINGS FOR THE BREASTFED BABY

- Put your baby near your breast skin-to-skin with you as soon after birth as possible. Be patient; it usually takes babies 1 to 2 hours before they find the nipple and latch on to feed.
- Breastfeed your baby at least every third hour during the day and once at night—more often if the baby is acting hungry. Time feedings from beginning to beginning. You may need to wake your baby for some feedings until the baby is gaining weight.
- Your baby may need several minutes to wake up enough to feed well. It may make it easier for the baby to wake up if you pick the baby up when you first notice mouthing or rooting behavior.
- Newborns need about eight feedings in 24 hours.
- Feed the baby on the first breast until it feels softer or lighter. Then try burping and offering the second breast. If the baby is not interested, start on that side at the next feeding.
- Most babies feed for about 30 minutes, but there is no set time for a feeding to last. If the feeding is lasting much longer than 40 minutes, you may need to help the baby latch on more effectively or suck more efficiently.
- As babies get older, the feeding time may shorten and the baby may not feed as often.

Since each baby takes in milk at his or her own pace and each mother's milk ejection reflex is unique, the timing of **milk transfer** is different for each mother-baby pair. Therefore telling a mother to feed her baby for a specific number of minutes is inappropriate. The length of time necessary for a feeding varies widely—some infants require approximately 5 minutes, others need closer to 45 minutes to get a complete feeding. The average time is about 30 minutes, however, which explains the traditional recommendation of 15 minutes on each breast. With such a wide range of normal feeding patterns, it is easy to see why measuring feedings by minutes at the breast could lead to either underfeeding or overfeeding. The softening or lightening of the mother's breast, the baby's decreased rate of suck/swallows, and his or her level of contentment are better markers to help a mother judge when her baby has finished a feeding. The nurse should instruct the mother in how to safely position her baby for sleep (Box 24-2).

If a baby seems to be feeding effectively and is having adequate urine output but not gaining weight well, the mother may be switching to the second breast too soon. Although the foremilk is important because it contains protein, lactose, and water-soluble vitamins, simply keeping the baby on the first breast until it is soft will ensure that the baby also receives the more calorie-dense, high-fat hindmilk, which usually results in increased weight gain.

The "colicky" infant who is having gas pains and crying inconsolably may also be having explosive stools. The gas and explosive stools may be caused by the increased lactose load that results from being overfed on the skim milk produced at the start of the feeding on each breast. Arbitrarily switching to the second breast before the baby has finished the first side may cause consumption of more lactose than the infant's system can handle. This induces a temporary lactose intolerance. Many babies thought to have colic have been cured by the simple change of finishing the first breast first at each feeding.

The practice of switching to the second breast after an arbitrary amount of time can also cause a mother to overproduce milk. Her breasts respond to the additional let-downs triggered by the repeated latch-ons. A mother who has problems with leaking between feedings may find that having her baby finish the first breast first at each feeding cures her leaking problem while giving her a happier baby.

Some babies must be awakened for feedings (see the Patient Teaching box to the right), especially in the early neonatal period. They must be taught to associate sucking and feeding with taking care of the new, unpleasant feeling of hunger. The nurse should tell the parents that a sleeping baby may be a hungry baby who is withdrawing to shut out hunger, just as babies do in situations with loud noise, bright lights, or other discomfort they cannot change. It is important for the nurse to demonstrate how to wake a sleepy baby. Often just changing the diaper works well. Unwrapping, massaging, and talking within about 8 inches of the baby's face may also help to bring the infant to an alert state. If the baby is making rooting or mouthing motions, it is not necessary for the baby's eyes to be open before beginning the feeding.

If an infant continues to **shut down** (not respond to stimulation and withdraw into sleep) after several attempts at awakening, the baby may need 10 to 15 minutes of just resting on the mother's chest before being able to respond. However, the feeding should only be delayed, not omitted.

Once the baby latches on, if the nipple has not been drawn far enough into the mouth to continue stimulating the sucking reflex, the baby may shut down again. Often massaging the baby's back or chest, or lifting the breast to reposition the nipple in the mouth, will trigger more sucking. Stroking the top of the baby's head from the crown toward the face or massaging the feet can also encourage a baby to continue sucking. Mucus in the mouth and throat may interfere with the baby's sucking. Suctioning out the baby's mouth before offering the breast again may be effective.

Some babies wake up crying frantically and cannot focus on feeding until they have been calmed (see the Patient Teaching box on p. 674). The nurse can encourage the mother to hold the baby close while talking soothingly and giving the baby a clean finger on which to suck. The baby may need a clean diaper or other comfort measures. Dripping a little water on the baby's lower lip and tongue may help the baby latch on for a feeding.

After the baby is latched on, it is important not to pull the nipple out of the baby's mouth when trying to create a breathing space. If the mother is worried about the baby's breathing,

BOX 24-2
Positioning for Sleep

The nurse should instruct the parents that the most current recommendation from the American Academy of Pediatrics is to place the baby in a side-lying or supine position for sleep, even after feedings (see Chapter 23). These positioning guidelines were developed in light of the most current research, which identifies the three most important factors in prevention of sudden infant death syndrome (SIDS) as being breastfed, avoiding exposure to second-hand smoke, and not sleeping in a prone position (Kattwinkel, 1994).

Patient Teaching

WAKING A SLEEPY BABY

1. Unwrap the baby down to a shirt and diaper.
2. Change the baby's diaper.
3. Pick up the baby and talk softly within 6 to 8 inches of the baby's face.
4. Massage the baby's whole trunk front and back using firm finger strokes in a walking motion up and down the spine and chest. Massage the arms and legs.
5. Tease the tip of the baby's tongue, and touch the lower lip until the baby begins thrusting the tongue. Then place a clean finger on the tongue, nail side down, and move it around to trigger a suck.
6. If the baby still does not start to suck, work the finger up and down to stimulate the roof of the mouth and the back of the tongue.
7. If the baby gags or tosses the head around, calm the baby and gently try again.
8. Once the baby begins to suck vigorously on the finger, regardless of whether or not the eyes are open, bring the baby to the breast.

Patient Teaching

CALMING AN UPSET NEWBORN

- Hold the baby close while talking soothingly. Do not jiggle or bounce the baby.
- Place a clean finger on the tongue, nail side down, to start the baby sucking and calming down.
- If the baby does not start to suck, work the finger up and down to stimulate the roof of the mouth and the back of the tongue to trigger sucking. Dripping a little water on the baby's tongue may also help.
- Have the mother hold her baby against her bare chest (with a blanket over both of them, if needed). The skin-to-skin contact and warmth is often calming, and the baby may be willing to suck on the mother's finger.
- The baby may need 10 to 15 minutes of rest before being ready for feeding.

she can raise the baby's hips slightly, which changes the angle of the baby's head. She will be able to see that the baby's nose is free. She can also lift the breast slightly with her hand while pushing more of the breast into the baby's mouth with her thumb. The nurse can reassure the mother that if the baby's nose were completely blocked, the baby would reflexively bite and pull back to breathe.

Because newborns are learning the connection between sucking, getting full, and feeling satisfied, it is best to avoid pacifiers at first. Some infants have nonnutritive sucking needs between feedings; however, it is important to wait to introduce a pacifier until the infant has become proficient at breastfeeding, usually a few weeks. Using a pacifier may interfere with a baby learning to suck efficiently for feeding.

Offering a bottle after breastfeeding "just to make sure the baby is getting enough" is normally unnecessary and should be avoided. This practice can contribute both to **nipple confusion** (difficulty knowing how to latch on to the breast at the next feeding) and to low milk supply because the baby becomes overly full and does not breastfeed often enough. Supplementation interrupts the supply-meets-demand milk production cycle. The parents may misinterpret the baby's taking a bottle to mean that the mother is not making sufficient milk. Since introducing the bottle nipple to the baby's mouth triggers the suck/swallow reflex, the baby usually swallows the milk. The message to the mother is that her milk is not sufficient for her baby's needs. In reality, if the baby is encouraged to continue sucking more efficiently and longer while breastfeeding, the baby will get the milk he or she needs and supplementation is not necessary.

Breastfeeding and taking a bottle require very different skills. The swallowing/breathing pattern when a baby is at the breast is distinct from that when a baby is bottle-feeding. The use of the tongue, cheeks, and lips is also very different. Whereas some babies can go easily from one to the other, others find such a transition difficult. Since it is not possible to identify which infants will have a problem, it is safer to simply suggest that all parents wait until their newborns have mastered breastfeeding skills before considering introducing any bottle-feeding, usually 4 to 6 weeks. While some parents combine breastfeeding and bottle-feeding, many babies never use bottles and wean directly to a cup when they are older.

Effects of Early Discharge

As hospital stays become shorter, responsibility for care of the breastfeeding mother and baby is shifting radically. Traditionally the hospital nurse assisted the mother not only with initial latch-on techniques, but also with establishing a feeding routine, waking a sleepy baby, and treating sore nipples and any engorgement or jaundice. Today the mother and baby are usually discharged before the transition from colostrum to mature milk even occurs and before the baby has fed often enough to have learned the connection between the discomfort of hunger and feeding and feeling good. The mother's body and the baby's needs are changing rapidly. Therefore the nurse must prepare the mother to recognize and knowledgeably meet her baby's needs independently during the critical first days and to know when to ask for help.

Although the mother is still recovering physically from giving birth and adjusting psychologically to motherhood, she may have little respite from the responsibility of running a household and serving as the primary caretaker of older children. At the same time, she is assuming the care of a new baby and may have no family or community resources for support and assistance. Some mothers have difficulty balancing employment, volunteer responsibilities, and social commitments. Because of these conflicting roles, mothers sometimes find it overwhelming to be proactive in caring for their newborns. Giving priority to initiating feedings when the baby is sleeping or taking time to encourage sufficient feeding with a drowsy infant may seem impossible to a mother when she is pulled by so many demands.

Role of the Nurse as Teacher

In the immediate postpartum period, most women are still taking in the birth experience and cannot absorb much other new information. For this reason, listening to the mother can guide the nurse in her approach to presenting information. The woman who is still retelling her birth experience may be better able to follow instructions for frequent daytime feedings if they are presented in terms of her needs for rest at night. In contrast, the mother who is taking hold of her new role and changing her focus to the baby will wake her baby for feedings because she is meeting the baby's needs.

Good nursing care and teaching during the early postpartum period can minimize several problems for both mother and baby. The mother who is assisted to breastfeed immediately after birth and frequently thereafter in a way that facilitates her infant's feeding efficiently will have fewer problems with engorgement and sore nipples. Her infant will be much less likely to become jaundiced, develop hypoglycemia, or lose more than 7% of birth weight.

Two practices that optimize teaching opportunities are listening carefully to the parents' concerns and keeping the baby in the mother's room (rooming-in or mother-baby care). For example, teaching mothers to recognize early feeding cues can be done only if the baby is with the mother. Regular feedings are facilitated when the nurse goes to the mother's room to offer assistance with waking or positioning the baby. Observing and asking questions about each feeding to determine that the baby has latched on correctly and that the mother is experiencing effective milk transfer teaches parents the significant signs they will use to determine that feedings are going well. The most meaningful teaching the nurse can do is to empower parents with knowledge. When the nurse incorporates explanations into each encounter, the parents have many opportunities to ask questions.

Demonstration is a more powerful teaching tool than a lecture. Rather than trying to present a list of information as the mother is preparing to leave, the nurse should role model appropriate infant care throughout the hospital stay. The parents may find it difficult to act on instructions to feed the baby every third hour or to feed long enough to ensure adequate intake if they were not assisted to do so consistently in the hospital. By the time of discharge the mother should have a working understanding of how to care for her baby and herself. If every feeding is charted only after the nurse asks the mother about signs that feeding is going well (see the Patient Teaching box on p. 671), the mother will have been taught what to consider as important markers that feeding is going well and when to call for help.

Breastfeeding Support

Much of the responsibility for feeding education and support rests with the nurse who is seeing the baby after hospital discharge or with a **lactation consultant** who works for the hospital or in the community. Lactation consultants come from many educational backgrounds, including nursing, nutrition, physical and occupational therapy, home economics, psychology, social work, education, or the basic sciences. A lactation consultant has postbaccalaureate education, training, and clinical experience working with breastfeeding mothers. An International Board-Certified Lactation Consultant (IBCLC) has met defined academic and clinical experience criteria and passed the certifying examination given by the International Board of Certified Lactation Consultant Examiners (IBLCE). The lactation consultants' professional organization is the International Lactation Consultants Association (ILCA). Membership is open to anyone interested in breastfeeding. Nurses who work with breastfeeding families will find the publication of the association, *The Journal of Human Lactation*, to be very informative.

Some parents worry if they need assistance with breastfeeding. Having heard that breastfeeding is "natural," they have expectations that it will be totally automatic. The nurse can explain that breastfeeding is a learned skill, much like riding a bicycle or learning to read, and may take some time and help at first. Once reassured that other babies have needed similar help, they can focus on learning the skills involved and stop worrying that there must be something wrong if their baby does not immediately breastfeed easily. Some mothers see private lactation consultants or call on community breastfeeding support groups. Health care providers who are knowledgeable about breastfeeding convey a sense of confidence to the parents and help them find workable answers to questions as they arise. The choice to breastfeed is reaffirmed when the members of the health care team comment on how well the baby is growing. The nurse has a responsibility to help the parents identify the specific breastfeeding resources available to them. Many parents will find reading material or videos helpful. Several educational materials and sources are listed in Box 24-3.

BOX 24-3
Educational Materials for Parents

"Back to Sleep," P.O. Box 2911, Washington, DC 20040

Brazelton T: *Infants and mothers: differences in development*, NY, 1986, Dell Publishing. (Book)

Childbirth Graphics: A good resource for books and pamphlets. (1-800-299-3366)

Eiger M, Olds S: *The complete book of breastfeeding*, NY, 1987, Bantam Books. (Book)

Grams M: *Breastfeeding success for working mothers*, Sheridan, Wyo, 1985, Achievement Press. (Book)

Huggins K: *The nursing mother's companion*, rev ed, Boston, 1990, The Harvard Common Press. (Book)

La Leche League: *The womanly art of breastfeeding*, ed 6, Franklin Park, Ill, 1987, La Leche League International. (Book; they also publish pamphlets)

Pryor K: *Nursing your baby*, NY, 1991, Pocket Books. (Book)

Tully M, Overfield M: *Breastfeeding: a special relationship*, Raleigh, NC, 1991, Eagle Video Productions. (1-800-869-7892; video with handout)

Woessner C, Lauwers J, Bernard B: *Breastfeeding today*, Garden City Park, NY, 1987, Avery Publishing Group. (Book)

Care of the Mother

Diet. The mother's milk automatically contains everything the baby needs, except in rare cases of maternal nutrient deficiencies. For example, vegetarian mothers who include no animal products in their diet (vegans) require a vitamin B_{12} supplement during lactation, just as they do during pregnancy (Specker et al, 1988). For most women, only 200 to 500 extra calories per day need to be added to provide adequate nutrients for the infant while protecting the mother's body stores (Riordan and Auerbach, 1993). Daily food choices should include sources of water-soluble nutrients such as vitamins C and B_6. Although a perfect diet is the ideal, the mother's body makes milk by taking from her body stores whatever is not supplied by her diet. Breast milk cannot be "weak" or inadequate. A malnourished woman may make less volume of milk, but what is produced provides excellent nutrition for her infant.

There are no specific foods or drinks that all breastfeeding mothers must have or must avoid. Although dairy products are good sources of calcium and phosphorus, the mother does not have to drink milk to make milk. However, the mother who cannot obtain adequate amounts of calcium in her diet does need a supplement. The nurse should caution the mother against "natural" sources, such as dolomite (crushed oyster shells), because such preparations are often contaminated with lead. Vegetarian mothers commonly are knowledgeable about good nutrition because they have learned how to combine nonmeat food sources to ensure adequate protein intake.

The breastfeeding mother should drink to thirst but cannot increase her milk supply by drinking extra fluids (Dusdieker et al, 1990). The mother may wish to keep a drink within reach during feedings because she will often become thirsty. If she is not consuming sufficient amounts of fluid, she will notice that her urine is concentrated. If she does not drink enough over several days, she may become constipated. These problems occur because the mother's body is meeting the needs of the baby first. Typically, women find that they are drinking as much as 2 to 3 liters of fluid each day. Many women also find that they can consume caffeine-containing drinks in moderation with no effect on their infant.

Although many individuals may be convinced that they have found a *galactagogue* (food or drink that will increase milk supply), research has not shown that any exist. Herbal teas may be suggested to the breastfeeding mother, but the nurse should warn her that many herbs are medicinal and may go through her milk to accumulate at toxic levels in the infant (Lawrence, 1994). Beer or wine used to be recommended as an aid to lactation. These substances are high in the B vitamin complex, and it may be that the individual whose milk supply appeared to increase was, in fact, deficient in these vitamins.

Weight loss. Because it takes energy to produce milk, many mothers experience a gradual weight loss while breastfeeding as fat stores deposited during pregnancy are used. For the mother who is overweight, this fact can present an added incentive for breastfeeding. The mother who wants to diet while lactating should avoid losing large amounts of weight quickly because fat-soluble environmental contaminants to which she has been exposed are stored in her body's fat reserves and may be released into her milk. Additionally, some mothers find that their milk supply decreases when caloric intake is severely restricted. Most mothers find that they can lose about 2 pounds (1 kg) per week without affecting their milk supply.

The underweight mother may worry that her milk will not be rich enough for her baby to grow well. Research has shown that even women who have been undernourished their entire lives are able to exclusively breastfeed for many months and their infants thrive. Mothers with less than 20% body fat do not produce less milk, but they require more food (Butte, 1984).

Exercise. Worldwide, the majority of women breastfeed and work very hard physically; therefore there is no reason for a breastfeeding woman to restrict her physical activity level. Women continue activities such as hiking, jogging, swimming, and aerobics with no detrimental effect on milk supply or composition (Dewey et al, 1994). The nurse can also reassure the mother that there is no scientific evidence to suggest that strenuous activity is harmful to the lactating breasts. Most women find they are more comfortable if they breastfeed just before engaging in strenuous activity so their breasts are as empty as possible. Wearing a well-designed, supportive bra may also be helpful.

Breast care. The breastfeeding mother's normal routine bathing is all that is required to keep her breasts clean. Although she should avoid soaping her breasts directly, the small amount of soap that runs down while washing her face and neck is of no concern.

Breast cream should not be used routinely because it may block the naturally occurring oil from the Montgomery glands on the areola. Some breast creams also contain alcohol, which may cause irritation or dryness. The use of vitamin E oil or cream is not recommended. It is a fat-soluble vitamin, and there is a potential risk of the baby's building up a toxic level of vitamin E. In addition, some people are allergic to it.

Research on moist wound healing suggests that purified hypoallergenic lanolin may help heal a sore nipple. However, the oils in lanolin and other breast creams can foster the growth of yeast. Therefore it should be determined that the soreness is not caused by a monilial infection (see the discussion of sore nipples on p. 683) before any breast cream is used.

Bras. If a mother needs breast support, she will be uncomfortable unless she wears a bra because the Cooper's ligament that supports the breast will stretch and be painful. The amount of breast sagging that a woman experiences depends more on her genetics than on her feeding method or use of breast support. If she is comfortable without a bra, there is no reason to wear one.

If a woman prefers to wear a bra, it must be comfortable and provide nonbinding support. The nurse can recommend that when buying a new bra, the mother test the ease with which the bra fasteners provide one-handed access to the breasts. She should look at her breasts as she removes the bra to see if there are red pressure areas where the bra fits too tightly. She may not need to purchase a new bra, but only a bra extender—a piece that adds to the length of the fastener at the back of the bra. Some mothers prefer the support of underwire bras. There is no reason to avoid them unless the mother develops plugged ducts when she wears them. A mother should breastfeed at least once each day without her bra to allow complete emptying of all milk ducts.

Leaking. Some breastfeeding mothers find that their breasts leak between feedings. Using breast pads (available as either washable or disposable) inside a bra and wearing layered tops or those with printed designs will help camouflage the leaking. The nurse should warn the mother against using plastic-lined pads because they trap moisture and may lead to sore nipples. To stop the let-down reflex the mother can become aware of any sensation such as a tingling that might serve as a warning that her milk is letting down. Pressing straight back on her nipples usually stops the let-down. In public the mother can fold her arms across her chest to apply pressure obtrusively.

Some mothers who use both breasts at each feeding may actually cause an overabundant milk supply and therefore leak. The nurse can suggest that the mother breastfeed on the first breast until it is quite soft before offering the baby the second breast. Should the second breast be too full at the end of the feeding, the mother can hand-express or pump just enough to feel comfortable. After 2 to 3 days the mother will find that she is not leaking because her milk supply has decreased to match the baby's needs.

Breast self-examination. Only 1% to 2% of breast cancer is diagnosed during pregnancy or lactation, but a breastfeeding woman should certainly do breast self-examination (BSE). The woman who is not menstruating should simply choose a convenient date on which to do her examination every month. She must become familiar with the normal lumpiness of her lactating breasts. Any lump that matches in location in both breasts is almost always breast tissue. Lumps that increase and decrease in size are milk glands or ducts. Because lactating breast tissue is very dense, mammography during lactation is of limited diagnostic value. Should a lump be discovered, a biopsy can usually be done without interrupting breastfeeding.

Effect of menstruation. Menstruation has no effect on breastfeeding. There are no hormonal effects on the infant, although some babies may seem fussy for the first day. The quality of milk is not affected (Lawrence, 1994).

Sexual sensations. Some women experience rhythmic uterine contractions during breastfeeding. Such sensations are not unusual, since uterine contractions and milk ejection are both triggered by oxytocin; however, they may be disturbing to some mothers who perceive them as similar to orgasm.

Breastfeeding as contraception. When considering large populations, exclusive breastfeeding (baby is receiving no bottle feedings or solid food) does decrease the birth rate. Breastfeeding delays the return of ovulation after childbirth for varying lengths of time for different women. However, an individual woman cannot rely on breastfeeding alone for birth control. Predicting the return of fertility is difficult because the woman may ovulate before she menstruates. Therefore use of the lactational amenorrhea (LAM) method of natural child spacing requires knowledge of reliable methods for determining ovulation, such as basal body temperature, presence of cervical mucus, and the cervical position (Lethbridge, 1989).

Effects of hormonal contraceptives. Studies have shown that some women experience a reduction in milk supply when using hormonal contraceptives, including pills, injectables, or implants. None of these contraceptives have been approved for use by lactating women before 6 weeks postpartum because of concern about the possible effects on infants less than 6 weeks of age. Additionally, since lactation is initiated by the sudden drop in progesterone and estrogen levels after the separation of the placenta, the use of any hormonal method of birth control before 6 weeks postpartum may interfere with the establishment of a full milk supply.

After 6 weeks, theoretically, progestin-only birth control pills should have the least effect on milk supply. Some mothers even take combination pills, which contain estrogen, with no decrease in milk supply. However, either type presents a potential risk for decreasing milk production. The effect is reversed if the pills are discontinued. Because initiating any hormonal method of contraception, even after 6 weeks postpartum, may cause a precipitous drop in milk supply within days, the baby whose mother has started taking birth control pills should have weight checks weekly for a few weeks to ensure continued appropriate growth.

Barrier methods of contraception do not interfere with milk supply. However, many women choose to use birth control pills because they associate all barrier methods of contraception with a lack of spontaneity in lovemaking. The nurse can suggest that the mother incorporate a diaphragm or cervical cap as an automatic part of her evening routine (for example, inserting it after brushing her teeth). The spontaneity is restored, and the woman may find using such a barrier method to be quite satisfactory.

Theoretically, progestin-only medroxyprogesterone (Depo-Provera) and levonorgestrel implants (Norplant System) should not have an effect on milk production; however, some women report an immediate reduction in milk supply. Before getting an irreversible injection of medroxyprogesterone or having to request removal of the levonorgestrel implant, a mother could take the progestin-only pill for a few months to monitor the effect of the drug on her milk supply. If her milk production is unaffected, she will probably have no reduction in supply from medroxyprogesterone or levonorgestrel implant.

Breastfeeding during pregnancy. Some mothers continue breastfeeding through a subsequent pregnancy. As long as there is no known risk for preterm labor, there is no contraindication to continuing to breastfeed. The mother must pay careful attention to her nutrition. Most women have no problems; however, a few mothers experience a decrease in milk supply or have problems with sore nipples and may choose to wean. Once the new baby is born, the breasts begin producing colostrum again.

When a mother is breastfeeding both an older child and a newborn, a practice called *tandem nursing*, the nurse should remind her to always feed the new baby first. This ensures that the newborn is receiving adequate nutrition. The supply-meets-demand principle works just as with breastfeeding multiple babies.

Expressing, Pumping, and Storing Milk

Milk can be expressed by hand or with a pump. Massaging the breasts before pumping can help to trigger the let-down reflex. Massage should start at the chest wall and move toward the nipple, with gentle but deep pressure. The mother should be told the importance of pumping sufficiently to soften her breasts to maintain her milk supply. Milk contains the hormone precursors for prolactin-inhibiting factor, which reduces milk production; therefore leaving the breasts full over time begins to decrease production. Since pumping and hand expression are rarely as efficient as a baby in removing milk from the breast, milk supply should never be assessed by volume pumped.

Hand expression. To manually express milk the mother places one hand on her breast at the edge of the areola (Fig. 24-7). With the thumb above and fingers below, she presses in toward her chest and gently compresses the breast while rolling her thumb and fingers forward. These motions are repeated rhythmically until the milk begins to flow. While the milk is flowing easily, the mother simply maintains a steady, light pressure. Her thumb and fingers should not pinch the breast or slip down to the nipple. The hand should be rotated to reach all sections of each breast. She should return to the first breast after expressing the second breast and then repeat until all readily available milk is expressed.

Pumps. There are many types of breast pumps (Figs. 24-8 and 24-9). Some are more effective than others, and they vary in price. Manual pumps are the least expensive and may be the most appropriate where portability and quietness of oper-

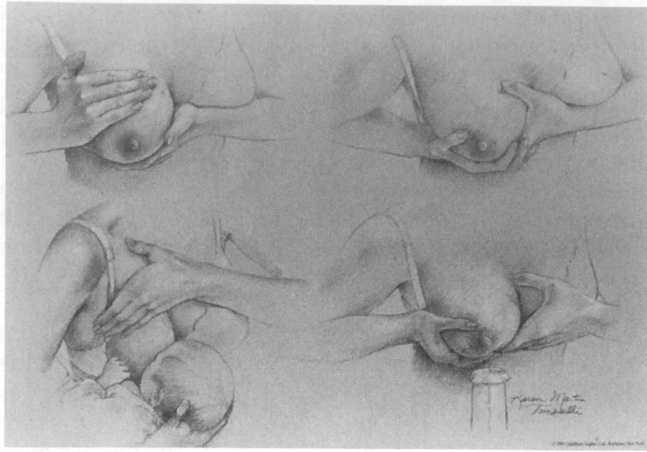

Fig. 24-7 Breast massage *(left)* and hand expression *(right)*. (Courtesy Karen Martin, Childbirth Graphics, Waco, Tex.)

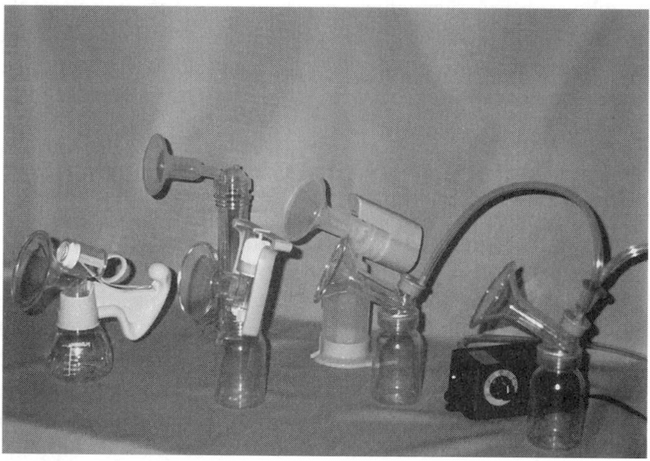

Fig. 24-8 A variety of hand pumps are available. Prices vary.

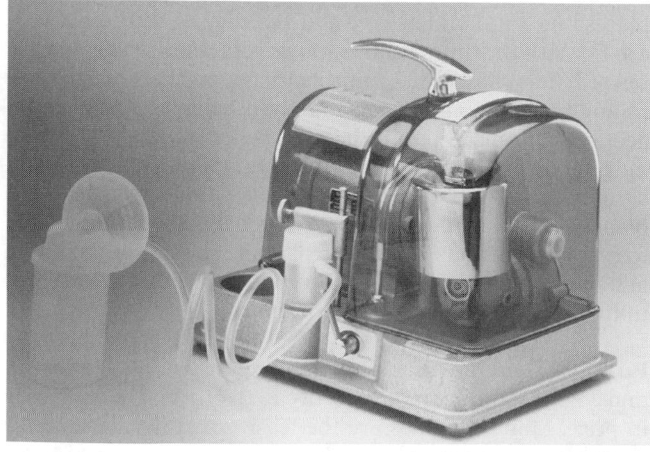

Fig. 24-9 A hospital-grade electric breast pump.

ation are critical, or when a mother is pumping only for an occasional bottle.

The battery-operated and small electric pumps have either a button to press or a small hole that the mother alternately covers and uncovers with her finger to intermittently release the vacuum. This mimics the sucking action of her infant. The nurse should instruct the mother that it is important to keep the sucking action intermittent, like the baby's suck, or it may hurt and she will obtain very little milk. A small battery-operated pump may be a good choice when the mother is going to be in a situation where access to electricity is a problem; however, using electricity is less expensive when that is an option.

Hospital-grade electrical pumps can be rented rather than purchased. They provide automatic cycling and are usually the most efficient pumps. When a mother must pump for all, or even most, of her baby's feedings (e.g., when the baby is premature or critically ill), it is imperative that she use one of these pumps to establish an optimal milk supply.

Pumping. There is no best way to approach pumping. Some mothers find it easiest to pump when they first wake up; others prefer to pump just before going to sleep. Some mothers pump whenever it seems convenient and may pour several pumpings together to make one bottle. Many women get the most milk if they pump one breast at the same time as the baby is feeding on the other side. Switching sides during pumping triggers additional let-downs, and massaging also increases the amount of milk obtained. If a mother consistently pumps at the same time each day, she will increase her supply at that time. Bilateral pumping takes less time than pumping one breast at a time but does not increase the amount of milk obtained (Fig. 24-10) (Groh-Wargo et al, 1995). The nurse can remind the mother that when she is pumping after or between feedings, she will get only the milk the baby has not taken and should not expect to get as much milk as she would when the baby is missing a feeding.

Milk storage. Milk can be stored in any clean glass or plastic container. Many parents use disposable bottle liners because they are inexpensive and take up less room in the freezer than bottles. It is suggested that the milk be double bagged, so that if the outer bag is punctured, the milk is still protected. The bags can be closed with small rubber bands or twist ties (twist ties may cause holes in neighboring bags during storage, if care is not taken when placing the bags in the freezer).

If milk must be transported, it should be kept cold. If the milk will be used within 48 hours, it can be stored in the refrigerator. If it is to be stored longer than 2 days or has not been used in that time, it should be frozen. It can be stored in a freezer at 0° C for up to 6 months, but it should be kept in the middle of the freezer, toward the back, not in the door or on the floor of the freezer where it can be subjected to wide temperature changes when the freezer is opened or during the automatic defrosting cycle. In a freezer at −20° C, it can be stored for 2 years. The nurse should instruct the mother to date her milk, so the oldest can be used first.

Milk thaws quickly when the container is placed in a bowl of warm water. The cream that rises to the top mixes back into the milk when it is gently shaken. The milk may be in layers if

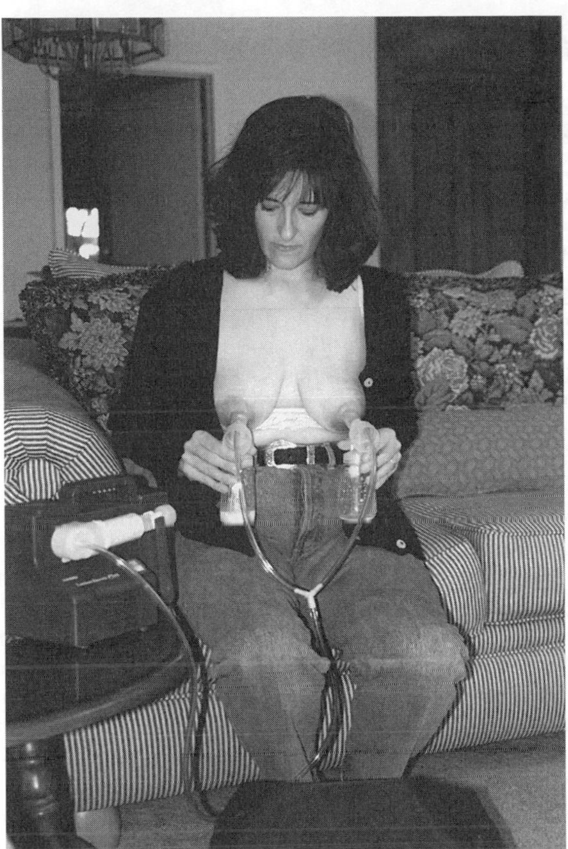

Fig. 24-10 Bilateral pumping. Mother attends graduate school and pumps between classes while away from her infant. (Courtesy Kim Molloy, San Jose, Calif.)

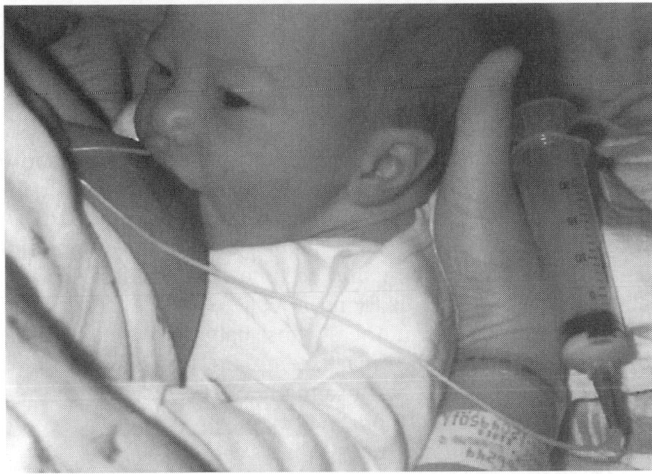

Fig. 24-11 A mother using a nursing supplementer made from a large syringe with a shortened No. 5 French gavage feeding tube attached.

it has taken several pumpings to get enough milk for one bottle. The milk may be different colors—orange, if the mother has eaten a lot of carrots; green, if she has had a big spinach salad; or even pink from beets. This does not mean that it is spoiled. The smell of milk that is spoiled is easily detected. Milk can be given to the baby in a bottle, a cup, or with a spoon.

Breast milk should not be refrozen. It should never be thawed or heated in a microwave oven because microwaving can cause encapsulated boiling bubbles in the center of the liquid that may not be detected when checking the first few drops. These hot bubbles have burned babies' palates and throats badly enough to require reconstructive surgery (Lawrence, 1994).

Being away from the baby. Many mothers successfully combine employment, attending school, or extensive volunteer commitments with breastfeeding their babies. The effect of missing feedings on a mother's milk supply varies on an individual basis. Some women's bodies adjust and only produce milk at those times of day when the mother is with the baby. Other mothers must pump while away or their supply is rapidly diminished. Still others use some formula when they miss a feeding and only pump if they become uncomfortable.

Some babies breastfeed more at night to compensate for their decreased access to their mothers during the day. As the baby gets older, the parents may prefer that the baby be fed solid foods when the mother is gone so that less pumped milk is needed.

Relactating and lactating for an adopted baby. Some mothers decide to breastfeed when they find that their infants cannot tolerate any type of formula. Other women stop breastfeeding but later decide to begin again. A few women wish to lactate for an adopted baby. Lactation can sometimes be induced simply by sucking stimulation.

The nurse should encourage the mother to have a realistic goal of feeling close to her baby rather than a possibly unrealistic expectation of providing full nutrition. The maximum breast stimulation possible should be provided by the infant sucking at the breast. Some mothers use electric breast pumps before receiving an adopted infant. Some women can restore or initiate lactation, but others find their goal elusive, no matter how hard they try.

Regardless of volume of milk actually produced, a mother can use a nursing supplementer to provide adequate nourishment at her breast (Fig. 24-11). The Lact-Aid Nursing Trainer and the Medela Supplemental Nursing System are two supplementers that are commercially available. The baby is latched onto the mother's breast with the end of the soft tubing alongside the nipple. As the infant sucks, the mother's nipple is stimulated. The baby receives whatever milk is in the breast, and supplemental nutrition comes from the formula in the nursing supplementer.

Drugs and Environmental Pollutants

Many compounds can enter human milk from the bloodstream of the lactating mother, just as they cross the placenta during pregnancy. Those which may be of concern include caffeine, alcohol, nicotine, other drugs, and environmental pollutants. Whether or not a substance appears in milk depends on many factors, including solubility in fat, degree of ionization, degree of protein binding, and active vs. passive transport. A common way of quantifying the amount of exposure for the infant is to look at the ratio of the amount of a substance found in the mother's milk to the amount found in her plasma (milk-to-plasma ratio).

Only 1% of the caffeine ingested by the mother passes into her milk. The milk-to-plasma ratio is very low. However, an infant's immature system cannot eliminate the caffeine as effectively as can an adult's. A few babies are sensitive to even a small amount of caffeine and become very irritable and unable to sleep. Caffeine is found in coffee, tea, chocolate, and many soft drinks. For mothers whose babies are sensitive, it is best to limit these while breastfeeding. Caution should also be used with herbal teas because many of these drinks contain natural substances with pharmacologic properties that could be harmful to an infant (Lawrence, 1994).

Alcoholic beverages are a common part of the daily diet in many cultures. However, since the milk-to-plasma ratio of alcohol can be greater than 1, breastfeeding after excessive consumption can have a serious effect on the infant. Frequent or excessive consumption of alcohol may also affect the milk ejection reflex (Lawrence, 1994). The level of alcohol in milk decreases over time, unlike many other drugs that stay in the milk until it is removed from the breasts. Therefore if a mother wishes to have an alcoholic drink, she should minimize her infant's exposure by having only one drink and consuming it right after a feeding. The mother who is pumping for a preterm or sick infant should be cautioned to avoid alcohol until her baby is healthy.

Nicotine can cause a decrease in milk supply over time by interfering with the milk ejection reflex and limiting breast emptying. This can cause decreased weight gain and may make the baby fussy. The nurse should inform the mother that avoiding smoking just before or during a feeding should minimize this effect and protect the baby from the effects of second-hand smoke.

Most medications do not cause problems for the infant, but breastfeeding mothers should be cautioned about taking any but essential ones. The American Academy of Pediatrics (AAP) Committee on Drugs (AAP, 1994), lists a few medications that are absolutely contraindicated for breastfeeding women. They include all drugs of abuse and the following:

- Bromocriptine—a lactation suppressant
- Cyclophosphamide—an immunosuppressant
- Cyclosporine, doxorubicin, and methotrexate—anticancer drugs
- Lithium—used to treat bipolar disorder
- Ergotamine—used to treat migraine headaches
- Phenindione—an anticoagulant not used in the United States

The AAP guidelines state that the use of certain radioactive diagnostic agents require a temporary cessation of breastfeeding. The nurse must instruct the mother to pump her breasts and discard the pumped milk until the drug has cleared her body.

In some situations a breastfeeding mother may be concerned about her exposure to environmental pollutants. However, unless she were involved in an industrial accident or exposed to a major spill, it is rare that the mother's exposure would preclude breastfeeding.

Weaning

Weaning a baby can be an almost effortless process when it is accomplished gradually. There is no discomfort for mother or infant, and the amount of milk being produced generally decreases. Many babies wean directly from the breast to a cup. With infant-led weaning, the baby moves at his or her own pace in omitting breastfeedings. Increased drinking from a cup and eating solid foods slowly substitute for breastfeeding.

With mother-led weaning the mother decides which feedings to drop. If the infant is less than 6 months old, she will probably offer a bottle. Depending on the speed with which the mother desires to wean, she can wait several days or weeks before dropping another feeding. Frequently the feeding before bedtime is the last feeding eliminated. If the infant is less than a year old, the bottle or cup should contain formula, not whole cow milk.

Some rare situations require a mother to stop breastfeeding abruptly. Should this occur, the mother often becomes painfully engorged. A mild analgesic may help. Her discomfort can be diminished by wearing a supportive bra, using ice packs and/or cabbage leaves on her breasts to decrease swelling, and pumping as necessary to remain reasonably comfortable, while keeping the breasts full enough to begin diminishing milk production.

The mother can still provide skin-to-skin contact while feeding from a bottle. The baby's additional sucking needs can be met by sucking on a parent's finger, nail side to the tongue, while being cuddled.

If a breastfeeding baby dies, the mother may not think about needing to care for her breasts. However, the nurse should assist her to pump with a hospital-grade pump so that she stays reasonably comfortable. The milk supply usually diminishes within a few days to the point that she no longer needs to pump.

Problem-Solving Techniques

Engorgement. Primary **engorgement** is a common response of the breasts to the sudden change in hormones and the presence of increased volume of milk. It usually occurs on the third to fifth day postpartum. The breasts are tender, swollen, hot, and hard and may even be shiny and red (Fig. 24-12). The swelling can extend into the axilla. Some mothers may have an elevated temperature and a headache.

The nurse can teach the mother to treat engorgement aggressively by feeding about every 2 hours, softening at least one breast at each feeding, and pumping to soften the second breast. Since back pressure on full milk glands inhibits milk production, in the first several days, frequent emptying of the breasts is essential to establishing an adequate milk supply. The nurse should reassure the mother that engorgement is not excessive milk supply, but a result of the swelling of breast tissue in response to hormone changes. Some mothers may be concerned that they will be exacerbating the problem by pumping; however, it would require several days of frequent pumping to increase milk production.

With treatment, engorgement can usually be limited to 12 to 24 hours (Tully and Overfield, 1989). Use of an anti-inflammatory pain reliever decreases swelling, pain, and

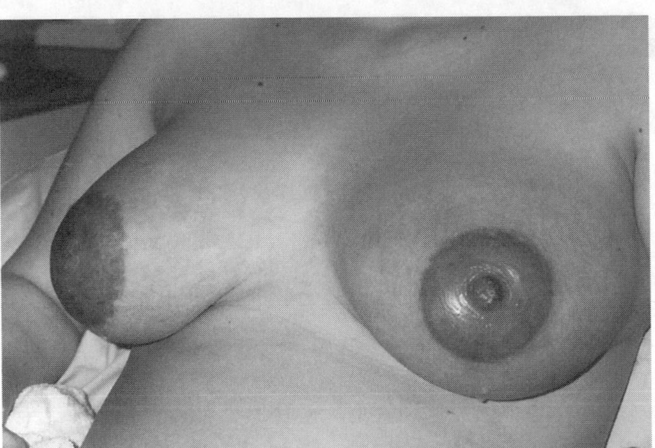

Fig. 24-12 Primary engorgement may occur during the first week postpartum.

fever. Using ice packs or raw cabbage leaves on the breasts relieves both pain and swelling and can soften the areola enough to allow the baby to latch on effectively (Roberts, 1995). The decreased swelling reduces the pressure on the ducts and allows the milk to flow. If the areola is not softened sufficiently, the nurse should assist the mother to remove enough milk to soften the areola using a hospital-grade electric pump. Ice or cabbage leaves can be applied between feedings in a 15 minutes on, 45 minutes off rotation until the mother is comfortable. Cabbage leaves should be changed when they begin to wilt.

Cabbage leaves have been used to treat swelling in other cultures for years (Roberts, 1995). Only recently have studies been undertaken in the United States to prove the efficacy of this treatment. Although the exact mechanism of action for cabbage in treating engorgement has not been identified, it is thought that continuous application might decrease milk supply. The non-breastfeeding mother may find it effective to keep cabbage leaves on her breasts continuously for several hours until the swelling has decreased.

Traditionally, heat has been used to treat engorgement because it was thought that engorgement was caused by lack of let-down. However, the primary problem is not a lack of let-down, but rather the swelling of the breast tissue that pinches the ducts shut and prevents milk flow. Since heat increases blood flow, application of heat to an already congested area is usually counterproductive. However, for an occasional mother, standing in a warm shower starts milk leaking and softens the breasts enough for the baby to latch on.

The nurse may need to reassure the mother who does not experience engorgement that her milk supply is established. Other signs of the presence of mature milk include more noticeable softening of the breasts during feeding, change in the color of the milk from yellow to white, louder swallowing sounds as the baby feeds, change in the baby's stools from meconium to breast milk stools, and at least two stools every 24 hours by the time the baby is 96 hours old (Box 24-4).

BOX 24-4
Signs of Presence of Mature Milk

- More dramatic softening of the breast as the baby nurses
- Change in color from yellow colostrum to whiter milk
- Louder sounds as the baby swallows larger volumes of milk with each suck
- Change from meconium stools to yellow breast milk stools
- At least two breast milk stools every 24 hours by the time the baby is 96 hours old

Jaundice. Jaundice in the newborn often causes considerable concern for health care providers and anxiety for parents. It can be a symptom of illness and must be monitored; however, in the 3- to 5-day old healthy term infant, some degree of hyperbilirubinemia is common and rarely a problem. This is frequently referred to as **physiologic jaundice** because the increased bilirubin level is a result of the normal breakdown of excess red blood cells. The fetus requires extra red blood cells for adequate transport of oxygen, but these cells are not needed after birth. Also, the meconium of the term infant contains about 450 mg of bilirubin, which will be reabsorbed if the meconium is not excreted within the first 2 to 3 days (Lawrence, 1994). Since the baby is usually at home before the third day, the nurse should teach the parents to recognize and report signs of jaundice, including yellow coloration of the skin and sclera, to the baby's health care provider.

Hyperbilirubinemia is often a sign of poor feeding (Table 24-4). If an infant latches on ineffectively or does not feed often enough or long enough, the baby may become jaundiced. Therefore the nurse should assist the mother to ensure that the baby has regular effective feedings, which encourage stooling and can prevent or reduce jaundice. The nurse may need to teach the parents how to wake the sleepy baby for feedings. Because bilirubin is bound by the protein albumin in milk and 98% of it is eliminated via the intestines, adequate feeding is critical. Feeding a baby water can contribute to elevated blood levels of bilirubin because only approximately 2% of bilirubin is excreted via the kidneys and water may decrease the amount of milk the baby can take.

Some researchers suggest that an enzyme in some mothers' milk may cause elevated bilirubin levels and refer to it as "late-onset breast milk jaundice." However, such a substance has never been identified.

Often when a breastfeeding baby is jaundiced, there are three other areas to investigate:

1. Lack of caloric intake, which causes the baby to be either lethargic and difficult to rouse or very irritable and frantically sucking
2. Inefficient latch-on, which causes the mother to have very sore nipples or to report she has never felt the baby suck
3. Breast engorgement, which makes correct latch-on and effective feeding difficult

These problems are often interrelated. The nurse who can intervene early with feeding assistance may be able to de-

TABLE 24-4 Comparison of major types of unconjugated hyperbilirubinemia

	PHYSIOLOGIC JAUNDICE	BREASTFEEDING ASSOCIATED JAUNDICE (EARLY ONSET)	BREAST MILK JAUNDICE (LATE ONSET)	HEMOLYTIC DISEASE
Cause	Immature hepatic function plus increased bilirubin load from red blood cell (RBC) hemolysis	Poor milk intake related to fewer calories consumed by infant before mother's milk is well established; enterohepatic shunting	Possible factors in breast milk that prevent bilirubin conjugation Less frequent stooling	Blood antigen incompatibility causes hemolysis of large numbers of RBCs Liver unable to conjugate and excrete excess bilirubin from hemolysis
Onset	After 24 hours (preterm infants, prolonged)	Third to fourth day	Fourth to fifth day	During first 24 hrs (levels increase faster than 5 mg/dl/day)
Peak	72 to 90 hours	Second to third day	Tenth to fifteenth day	Variable
Duration	Declines on fifth to seventh day		May remain jaundiced for 3 to 4 weeks	
Therapy	Phototherapy of bilirubin levels increase significantly (rise in bilirubin greater than 5 mg/dl/day)	Frequent (10 to 12 times/day) breastfeeding Phototherapy for bilirubin 17 to 22 mg/dl in healthy term infants	Increase frequency of breastfeeding; use no supplementation such as glucose water; cessation of breastfeeding no longer recommended Temporary discontinuation of breastfeeding for up to 24 hrs; if bilirubin levels decrease, breastfeeding can resume May include home phototherapy with uninterrupted breastfeeding	***Postnatal***—Phototherapy; if severe, exchange transfusion ***Prenatal***—Transfusion (fetus) Prevent sensitization (Rh incompatibility) of Rh-negative mother with RhoGAM

crease the severity of jaundice. The most effective treatment for physiologic jaundice is simply to increase the baby's milk intake. This can usually be done by ensuring correct latch-on during more frequent feedings of greater duration. Many babies require stimulation to continue sustained sucking during early feedings. Bottle-feeding or bottle supplements after breastfeeding for 24 to 48 hours are often suggested to increase intake until the bilirubin level begins to drop. However, introducing bottle nipples to a baby this young may cause nipple confusion. To minimize the risk that the baby will have difficulty continuing to breast feed, supplemental feedings can be given while the baby is latched onto the breast using a nursing supplementer (Fig. 24-11). If it is easy for the mother to pump, she can use her own milk rather than formula. If she is engorged or if the baby is not breastfeeding but rather getting formula, the nurse should assist the mother to use a hospital-grade electric pump regularly and encourage her to store the extra milk for later use.

In a few babies, elevated bilirubin levels indicate pathologic jaundice, which may result from a blood group incompatibility, an Rh factor problem, severe bruising, prematurity, or a physical anomaly. Interrupting breastfeeding is not effective treatment for these problems. Although frequent, regular feedings are important for these babies, phototherapy is often necessary as well, and occasionally these babies require exchange transfusions.

Phototherapy can be administered with a bili-blanket and/or bilirubin lights. Use of the bili-blanket allows the baby to be held and fed frequently without interrupting phototherapy. Traditional bilirubin lights require the baby to be positioned in a bed under a lamp and do not facilitate frequent feedings. If a baby is under lights and on a bili-blanket, the blanket can be left on during the feedings to maximize the effect of the therapy.

Anything out of the ordinary, especially if it requires treatment, can make new parents anxious. The nurse can reassure the parents that jaundice, except in rare cases, results from the infant's adjustment to extrauterine life. Once that adjustment has taken place, the problem does not recur. Although the feeding process may be contributing to elevated bilirubin level, the parents need to know that it is not the mother's milk that is causing the jaundice. Interrupting breastfeeding to treat jaundice has been linked to significantly shorter breastfeeding duration and to mothers seeing their children as medically vulnerable, even as preschoolers (Kemper, Forsyth, and McCarthy, 1989, 1990). The nurse who facilitates effective breastfeeding at early feedings may help to avoid such outcomes.

TABLE 24-5 Causes of sore nipples

PROBLEMS WITH	ONSET	APPEARANCE	PAINFUL SENSATION
Latch-on	Early	Abraded tip/bruised areola	At start of feeding
Suck	Early	Bruised/abraded	With sucking
Monilial infection	Early/late	"Healthy pink" or fragile	Burning, biting, and pain between feedings
Teething	Late	Abraded, but not fragile	Biting or scraping
Short frenulum	Early	Abraded	With sucking/more on bottom of nipple

Sore nipples. Sore nipples can be caused by improper suck, incorrect latch-on, or a monilial infection (Table 24-5). When a baby is latched on and sucking correctly, the mother's nipples will not be abraded, cracked, or bleeding. For the first few days the nipples may be a little tender with the initial sucks at each feeding, but the mother should quickly become comfortable as the milk flows and acts as a lubricant. The mother can make the initial sucking less painful if she moistens the nipple and areola with her milk or water before beginning the feeding.

If the mother is in pain after the first few sucks, the nurse should help her evaluate the baby's position to ensure that the baby's body is in straight alignment, with the back and hips well supported and no pressure on the back of the baby's head. If this repositioning does not help, the mother should carefully remove the baby and start the latch-on again. Once the baby's mouth is wide open, the baby should be pulled quickly to the breast. Often sore nipples are caused by attempting to push the nipple into the baby's mouth, which causes the baby to close too soon and pinch the nipple. This positions the nipple where it will be abraded by the tongue with each suck and prevents good milk transfer (see the Patient Teaching box on p. 671). Limiting time at the breast does not prevent sore nipples. The problem is normally not the length of the feeding. It is the incorrect latch-on or suck, which can usually be corrected. Once the baby is latching on and sucking correctly, sore nipples heal within just a few days, even though the baby is breastfeeding regularly.

Usually just drying the milk and saliva mixture off the nipple after feedings will facilitate healing of sore nipples. Some women find it helpful to wear breast shells (Fig. 24-13) inside the bra to keep clothing off the nipples as they heal. Breast shells also keep inverted nipples protruding between feedings, which keeps them drier.

Several additional measures can be helpful. The mother can gently rub a drop of expressed milk into the sore area. The tannic acid in brewed tea is thought to promote healing. The mother can blot a steeped, cool tea bag on the sore area after feedings.

Although using a flexible nipple shield during feedings has been marketed as a treatment for sore nipples and for latch-on difficulties, it does not protect the nipples and can present a real danger to the infant. In most cases when the nipple is covered by a shield the baby cannot get far enough back on the breast to adequately compress the lactiferous sinuses and start the milk flowing. A nipple shield can also chafe the mother's nipple as the baby sucks. If the baby sucks on just

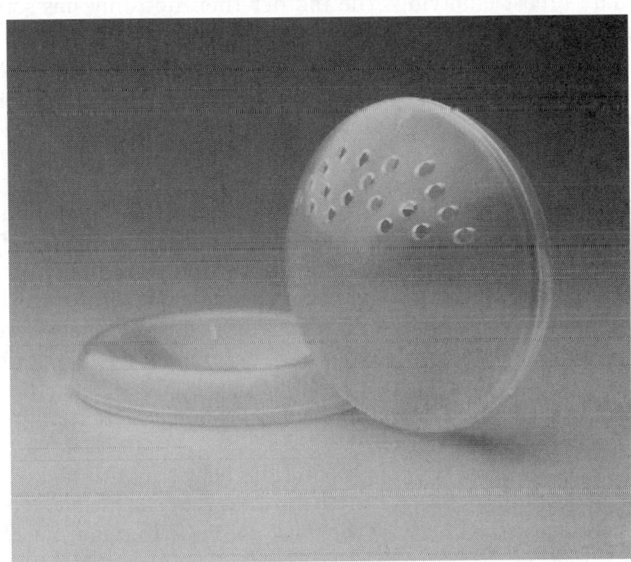

Fig. 24-13 Breast shells can be used to protect a sore nipple from clothing or to put pressure at the base of an inverted nipple to try to evert it. (Courtesy Ameda Egnell Corporation, Cary, Ill.)

BOX 24-5
Hazards of Nipple Shields

CAUTION: Nipple shields can be dangerous. There have been cases of infants breastfeeding with a shield from birth and never getting a full feeding. The shield functions as a pacifier, meeting only the baby's sucking need. Some of these babies cry because of hunger, but some of them withdraw from the pain into sleep and appear content. These babies can become dehydrated.

The nurse should discourage the use of a nipple shield and inform the mother of the risks. If a mother is already using one, the baby's urine output, number of bowel movements, and weight must be carefully monitored. The nurse should work closely with the mother during feedings to assist her in training the baby to latch on without the shield as quickly as possible (see discussion of latch-on on p. 669).

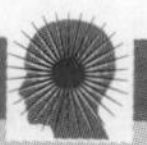

Critical Thinking Exercises

SORE NIPPLES IN BREASTFEEDING MOTHER

Role play how you could determine whether a mother's telephone call for help with sore nipples requires teaching about positioning and correct latch-on or if she might have a monilial infection on her nipples. What specific questions would you ask?

the tip of the shield, it may pinch the nipple and prevent adequate breast emptying. The mother then not only has sore nipples, but she also develops swollen breasts and her baby still has not learned how to latch on properly. The baby may use the shield as a pacifier, go to sleep without eating, and be at risk for dehydration, jaundice, and hypoglycemia (Box 24-5).

Monilial infections. If the nipples do not look abraded but the mother finds every suck painful and the pain continues after feedings, she may have a **monilial infection** on her nipples. This is caused by the same organisms as oral thrush, vaginal yeast infections, and yeast skin rashes. The baby may have a yeast diaper rash and also be experiencing pain during feedings from thrush in the mouth. Some babies shorten their feedings because of the pain, starting feeding and then pulling off crying several times.

Both the mother's nipples and the baby's mouth must be treated simultaneously, even if the infant has no visible signs of oral thrush. Otherwise they will continue to reinfect each other at every feeding. The nurse should explain to the mother that the antifungal medication is to be swabbed on the inside of the baby's mouth and rubbed on her dry nipples after feedings. To ensure that the infection is cleared, treatment should continue for at least 4 days past the last signs of pain or thrush. Careful handwashing also helps to prevent further spread of the yeast to other dark moist areas of the body.

Plugged milk duct. Occasionally a mother notices that one area of her breast is swollen and tender and does not empty or soften when she is breastfeeding or pumping. If she has no flu-like symptoms, this is probably a **plugged milk duct** (Table 24-6). Plugged milk ducts occur when some milk forms a small curd or plug in the end of the duct at the nipple. This may be caused by dry skin blocking the duct or occasionally because tight clothing (such as a bra) has put pressure on the milk duct, restricting milk flow through several feedings. Careful inspection of the tip of the nipple after the baby has breastfed usually reveals a small white "pearl" or blister, which is the curd of milk that is blocking the milk flow. Soaking the nipple in warm water for a few minutes before feeding may soften the skin and allow the plug to be released during the feeding. Massaging while breastfeeding or pumping may also help. Plugged milk ducts do not cause mastitis, but milk stasis may increase the mother's susceptibility to a breast infection.

Mastitis. A breast infection or **mastitis** is usually, but not always, first manifested by a swollen, tender breast and sudden onset of flu-like symptoms, including aching joints, fever, and severe headache. The nurse should be alert to concerns expressed by a breastfeeding mother that she feels as if she "has

TABLE 24-6 Causes of painful breasts

CAUSE	ONSET	LOCATION	SYMPTOMS	TREATMENT
Primary engorgement	First week postpartum	Bilateral	▪ Generalized breast swelling ▪ Possible fever ▪ Possible severe headache ▪ Generally feels well	▪ Frequent feeding and pumping ▪ Ice packs and/or cabbage leaves for 15 min on, 45 min off (if ice is painful, try heat) ▪ Antiinflammatory drug for fever and pain
Plugged duct	Anytime during lactation	▪ Unilateral ▪ Small white plug may be visible in tip of nipple	▪ Localized swelling and tenderness in a limited area of the breast ▪ No fever ▪ Generally feels well	▪ Soaking nipple in warm water for about 5 min before feeding or pumping ▪ Frequent feeding or pumping ▪ Massaging *behind*, not on, the swollen area during feeding or pumping
Mastitis	Anytime during lactation	▪ Typically unilateral	▪ Localized swelling with redness ▪ Usually severe localized pain ▪ Usually fever ▪ Severe flu-like symptoms ▪ May feel depressed	▪ Frequent feeding or pumping ▪ Antibiotic therapy ▪ Heat to affected area ▪ Antiinflammatory drug for fever and pain ▪ Rest and fluids (treat as any other systemic infection)

the flu" and is worried that her baby might get sick. The mother should contact her primary health care provider because she will need antibiotic treatment for the mastitis. The nurse should instruct the mother to rest and breastfeed frequently to ensure adequate emptying of the affected breast. Hot compresses on the sore breast may facilitate milk flow and be comforting for the mother. Research has shown that women who continue to breastfeed recover more quickly from mastitis than those who interrupt breastfeeding (Devereux, 1970). The most common cause of mastitis is the organism *Staphylococcus aureus,* which comes from the baby's mouth and therefore is not harmful to the baby.

Slow weight gain. Normally newborns lose about 7% of their birth weight as they eliminate amniotic fluid and meconium in the first 3 to 5 days. Then typical weight gain is 4 to 7 ounces/week (56 to 196 g) or $^3/_4$ to 1 ounce/day (21 to 28 g). The infant who continues to lose weight after 5 days, who does not regain birth weight by 2 weeks, or whose weight is below the tenth percentile after 1 month requires close supervision by a health care provider.

The nurse should talk with the parents to identify factors that may be contributing to the baby's slow weight gain, such as the following:

- How many feedings does the baby have in 24 hours? How long does a typical feeding last?
- Is at least one breast thoroughly softened at each feeding?
- Does the baby's suck cause a firm tugging on the breast?
- Does the baby have long sustained bursts of at least 10 to 15 sucks and swallows?
- Is the baby relaxed while feeding?
- How many wet diapers and bowel movements does the infant have each day?

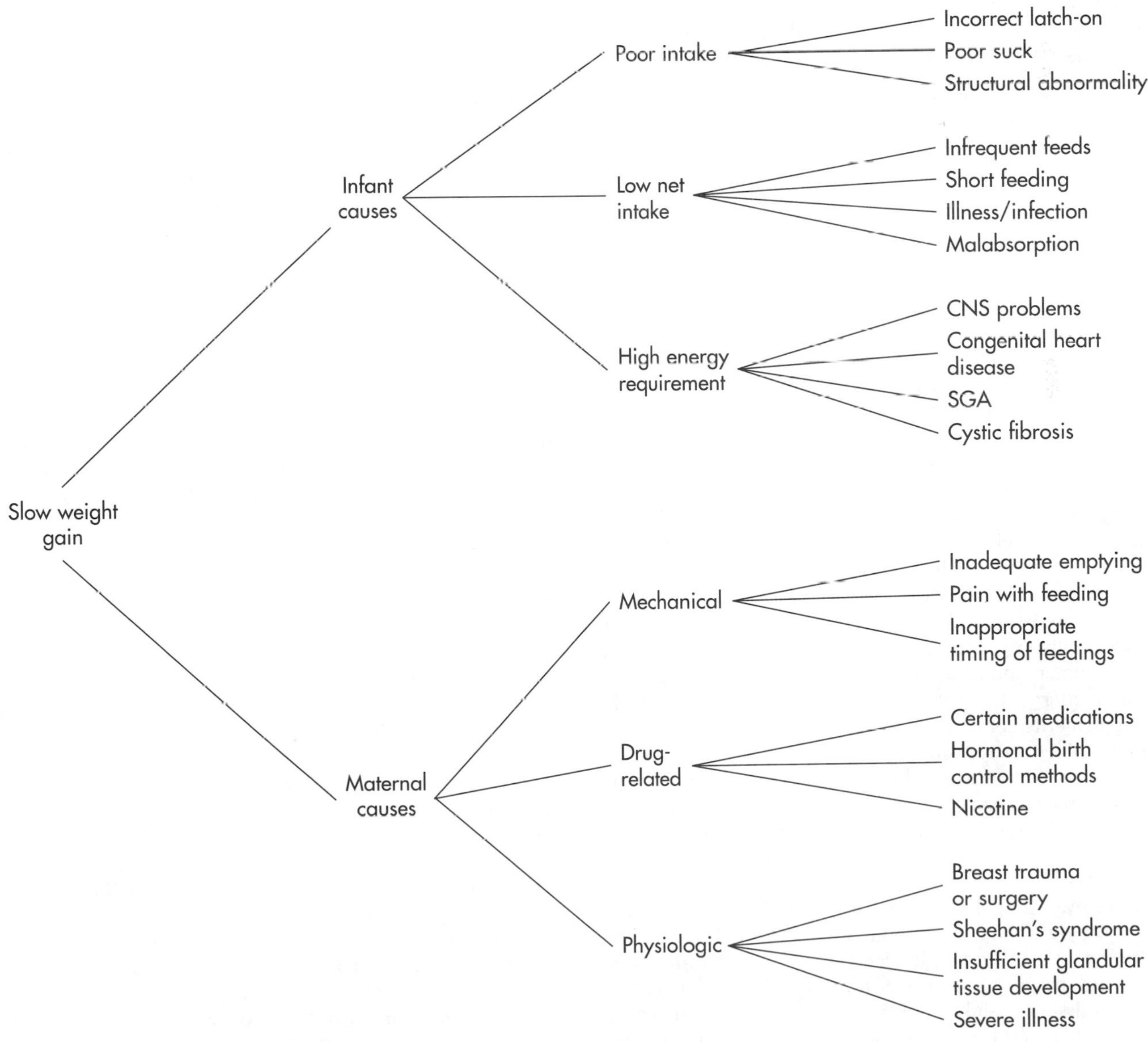

Fig. 24-14 Triaging slow weight gain. (© 1995 Lactation Consultants of North Carolina. Used with permission.)

Patient Teaching

ALTERNATE BREAST MASSAGE

- Observe when the baby stops sucking.
- Begin to massage your breast from the chest wall toward the nipple, moving more milk into the baby's mouth.
- As the baby begins sucking again, stop massaging.
- Continue to alternate massaging with the baby's sucking throughout the feeding.
- After several days the baby usually feeds more vigorously without requiring the breast massage.

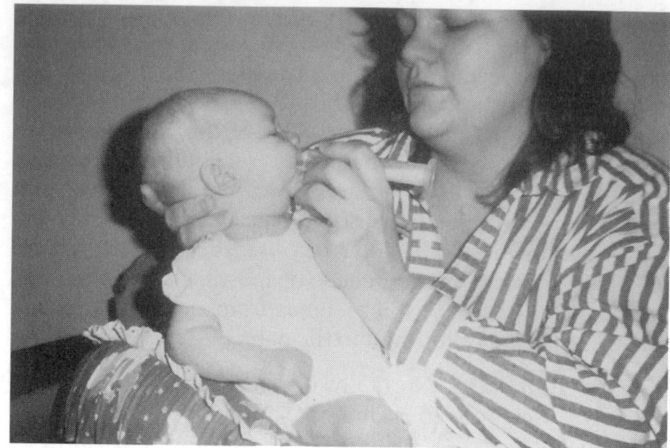

Fig. 24-15 Feeding can be done with a liquid-medicine spoon.

- For the newborn, have the stools changed from meconium to typical breast milk stools?
- Has the mother started taking birth control pills, had levonorgestrel implants (Norplant) inserted, or been given an injection of medroxyprogesterone (Depo Provera)?
- Is the mother using a nipple shield during feedings?
- Is the baby given a pacifier between feedings?

Usually the answer to a slow weight gain problem is improving feeding technique (Fig. 24-14). Fitting in an extra feeding each day can add needed calories easily. Sometimes the answer is in better positioning to facilitate a more efficient suck. Parents need to know how to wake a sleepy baby and keep the baby sucking vigorously throughout feedings. **Alternate breast massage** (see the Patient Teaching box above) may make additional milk available to the baby more quickly and keep the baby sucking (Bowles, Stutte, and Hensley, 1988).

The baby who is calorie-deprived from inadequate feeding may not have enough energy to feed well. When a baby needs supplementation, the extra breast milk or formula can be given with a spoon or cup (Fig. 24-15), with a nursing supplementer (Fig. 24-11), or with a bottle. A bottle should be avoided unless it is obvious that the baby will have no trouble latching onto the breast again. If it appears that the baby is not latching on well consistently, a spoon or cup may be an effective way to teach the baby to stick out the tongue to begin a feeding. A nursing supplementer has the advantage of improving breast stimulation, teaching the baby to breastfeed, and accomplishing feeding all at once. Normally, after a few days of supplementation, the baby begins gaining weight and has more energy. Once the baby is breastfeeding adequately, the supplements are usually not necessary.

Some babies are thriving but are at or below the tenth percentile for height and weight. The baby whose length and head circumference are increasing and who appears alert, responsive, and vigorous may be a healthy but slow-gaining baby.

Fussy baby. The baby who is fussy may be hungry. If the baby is crying to be fed more often than every 2 to 3 hours, feedings may need to last longer and/or the baby may need help to suck more effectively (see the discussion of latch-on on p. 669 and slow weight gain, p. 685). The typical newborn must be fed at least every third hour for at least eight feedings in 24 hours.

A newborn may cry as soon as positioned for feeding. A bruised head or a previously unnoticed broken clavicle may be the reason, and a change in the way the baby is held may make the baby more comfortable. Some babies stiffen and scream when anything goes near the mouth. It may be that extensive suctioning was done at birth and the baby needs some experience with being held that does not involve pain before learning how to breastfeed. The nurse can teach the parents to do kangaroo care (Anderson, 1989) by placing the baby, wearing only a diaper, on the mother's or father's bare chest (Anderson, 1989). A blanket can be placed over both of them if needed. Just cuddling quietly and relaxing together may be the most effective way to get the baby ready to learn to feed.

The newborn who is frustrated because the nipple does not stay far enough back in the mouth may cry and fuss at the breast. The baby may start feeding with well-organized suck/swallows and then, after just a few sucks, pull off the breast and scream. When the breast is firm, the baby can feel it contacting the suck/swallow trigger point at the juncture of the hard and soft palates. As the milk begins to flow and the breast softens, the breast may slip out of position in the baby's mouth. The mother of a baby like this should be shown how to support the breast to keep the nipple in place and position the baby on the breast.

Babies breastfeed and grow well when mothers eat quite varied diets. Usually if a mother continues to eat her customary diet, her breastfed infant will adapt to the flavors in her milk. Occasionally a baby experiences extreme gastrointestinal distress—cramping and gas pains. If the mother thinks back to what she has eaten during the 8 to 24 hours previous to the baby's fussing, she can often discover the cause. While for one baby, apple juice causes pain, for another it may be cabbage or beans; in yet another, it may be onions. No one person needs to avoid all these foods. The nurse should encourage the breastfeeding mother to eat her normal diet, avoiding only those foods that give her or the baby's father gas or cramping. Normally only one or two foods bother any individual baby. Some mothers find that giving the baby a dose of liquid simethicone (which is available over the counter) before each feeding makes the baby more comfortable for a while. However, persistent crying or refusing to breastfeed can also be a sign of illness, and the mother should be cautioned to call her baby's health care provider if she thinks her baby is ill.

Repeated episodes of extreme fussiness at the same time each day (colic) are often a reaction to vitamins (either the mother's or the baby's vitamin or fluoride drops). It is easy to stop these for a few days to discover if they are the source of the baby's discomfort. The healthy breastfeeding baby and mother do not require vitamin supplementation (Institute of Medicine, 1991).

For a very few babies an allergic response to cow milk products ingested by the mother is the reason for inconsolable fussiness, vomiting, or other symptoms. The baby is reacting to the cow milk protein in the mother's milk. The mother must eliminate all sources of cow milk from her diet until the baby is older. She will need a source of supplemental calcium. The nurse should alert the parents to the danger of feeding their baby any cow milk–based formula.

Some breastfed babies become fussy in response to an occasional feeding of formula, but it does not appear to affect them until the next feeding. When a baby sucks, peristaltic waves begin to move the contents of the intestines. After eliminating the large casein curd formed from the cow milk formula, the baby is content again.

The baby who has been content and then suddenly starts and continues to cry may be in pain. Ear infections, sore throat, monilial infections, etc. may go unnoticed at first. The nurse should instruct the parents that any baby who does not feed well for two feedings should be examined by a health care provider for signs of illness.

Potentially Challenging Situations

Breastfeeding twins. Caring for twins takes some planning, but breastfeeding means that feedings are always ready instantly, no one has to wash bottles and fix formula, and for some mothers, both babies can be fed at once. The mother with twins will need extra nourishment (200 to 500 kcal/day for each baby).

Each baby feeds from one breast per feeding, usually for about 20 to 30 minutes. Some mothers assign each baby a breast, whereas others switch either on a schedule or randomly. The mother may find it easiest to use a modified demand feeding schedule. She can feed the first baby who wakes up and then wake the second baby for feeding.

During the early weeks the parents may find it helpful to keep a record of feeding times and which breast was used first by which baby. If one twin nurses more vigorously than the other, that baby should alternate breasts to equalize breast stimulation.

If the mother wants to feed simultaneously, she may wish to experiment with positions (Fig. 24-16). One baby can be held in the football hold and the other in the cradle hold, or the babies can each be in a cradling position. Each baby can be supported on firm pillows while in the football hold. At first, some mothers may require assistance to get the babies off the breasts using this position.

Mothers with diabetes. Mothers with diabetes are encouraged to breastfeed, not only because of the advantages for the infant, but also because of its antidiabetogenic effect for the mother. Breastfeeding decreases the insulin requirement for most insulin-dependent women (Davies et al, 1989). During lactation the mother with diabetes can often eat more food and take less insulin. The insulin dosage must be readjusted as the baby weans (see Fig. 10-1). Some women who have diabetes have an increased risk of sore nipples caused by monilial infections.

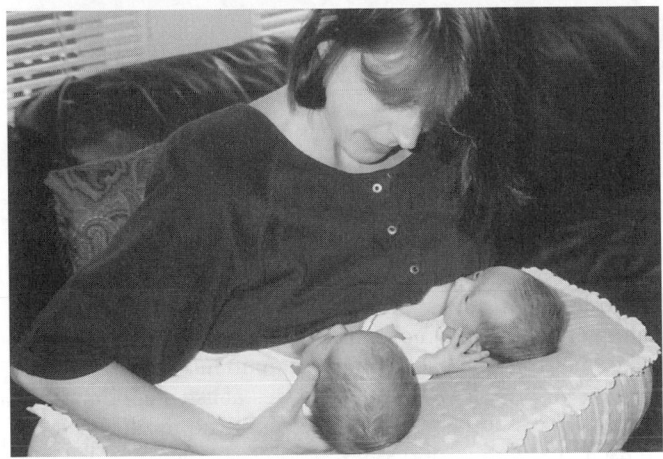

Fig. 24-16 Mothers of twins often breastfeed both babies at the same time.

Premature or sick infant. Research shows that human milk is optimal for feeding sick and preterm infants. The anti-infective, growth-promoting, and immunologic factors in human milk are significant for the baby's recovery and decrease the incidence of such diseases as neonatal necrotizing enterocolitis (Lucas and Morley, 1990). Also, preterm infants who are fed human milk even for just the first month have significantly higher IQs at school age (Lucas et al, 1992) and a decreased rate of infections (Narayanan, Prakash, and Gujral, 1981).

Often parents feel quite helpless when their infant is sick or preterm. In reflecting on the experience of having a baby who was hospitalized, many parents say that providing the mother's milk was very important to them—it was the only role they had in the early care of their infant (Kavanaugh et al, 1995).

Pumping for the preterm or sick infant. The mother who is pumping for a premature or sick baby may have difficulty getting more than a few drops at each pumping for the first 2 to 3 days. The nurse can reassure her that the baby will require very small volumes of milk at first. Many mothers find that they need to switch the pump back to each breast several times to thoroughly soften the breasts each time, at least in the beginning.

Research has shown that to establish an optimal milk supply, a mother must pump a minimum of 100 minutes during 24 hours (Hopkinson, Schanler, and Garza, 1988). This usually translates to five times a day for 10 minutes on each breast or until each breast is softened and the milk has stopped flowing. There are double pumping kits that allow the mother to pump both breasts at once (Fig. 24-10). This can save time for the mother; however, it may not be easy or efficient until the mother has some experience with pumping.

Some women always prefer to single pump. Even if the baby is only taking a small amount of her milk, the mother should pump until her breasts are softened to establish her milk production.

The nurse can help the mother plan her pumpings around visits to the baby and her other responsibilities. If the mother pumps to empty her breasts well before bed, she can probably sleep at least 6 hours before waking to pump again. Regularly emptying the breasts enough to soften them is important for establishing a milk supply. After the first few days the mother may be pumping several ounces each time while her baby is taking only a teaspoon of milk per feeding. The nurse can reassure her that the baby will catch up to her supply and that keeping the breasts well emptied will establish an optimal milk supply. Once the baby is breastfeeding, the mother can decrease her supply, if necessary. Doing so earlier may decrease the milk supply too much.

When a baby is hospitalized and being fed primarily pumped milk, the recommendations for storage and handling of the milk are more restrictive (Arnold, 1994). Milk should be stored in sterile, rigid plastic or glass containers because much of the IgA, an important immunoglobulin, is destroyed when milk is stored in soft plastic bags, including bottle liners. This is not an issue when milk is being stored for the baby who is breastfeeding most of the time and is certainly never a reason to discard any pumped milk for the hospitalized baby. Mother's own milk for her baby is ideal in virtually all circumstances.

Pumping milk for the baby who cannot breastfeed or can only breastfeed once or twice a day requires a hospital-grade electric breast pump. The mother's hospital care and discharge planning should include assistance with using and arranging to rent an appropriate pump, instructions in how to use it, how to optimize milk production, and how to store and transport the milk (Arnold, 1994).

Research has shown that breastfeeding is less physiologically stressful to small preterm babies than bottle-feeding. Although the baby may require some assistance to get started, many preterm babies can breastfeed before they can tolerate bottle-feeding (Meier, 1988).

Milk banking. A small number of infants cannot be breastfed but also cannot survive except on human milk. For those infants, banked donor milk is critically important. Because of the antiinfective and growth-promoting properties of human milk as well as its superior nutrition, donor milk is used in many neonatal intensive care units for preterm or sick infants when the mother's own milk is not available. Donor milk is also being used therapeutically in some instances for medical conditions such as transplant recipients who are immune compromised.

The Human Milk Banking Association of North America (HMBANA) established guidelines, which are reviewed annually, for the operation of donor human milk banks (Arnold and Tully, 1996). Donor milk banks collect, screen, process, and distribute milk donated by breastfeeding mothers who are feeding their own infants and pumping a few extra ounces each day for the milk bank. All donors are screened both by interview and serologically for communicable diseases. Milk is stored frozen until it is heat processed to kill potential pathogens, then it is refrozen for storage until it is dispensed for use. The heat processing adds a level of protection for the recipient that is not available in the case of any other donor tissue or organ. Milk is dispensed only on prescription. There is a per-ounce fee charged by the bank for processing; however, HMBANA guidelines prohibit payment to donors.

Nursing Care Management

The nurse should realize the possible impact of caregivers on the sense of competence and success that parents feel. Those caring for the mother can convey positive expectations by their attitude and choice of words. For example, referring to colostrum as "early milk," which is a valuable first food, rather than commenting that the mother's milk is "not in yet," creates a positive feeling for parents. It can be encouraging for a new mother to have a knowledgeable health care professional help her identify feeding-readiness cues and observe the baby feeding. Pointing out what the baby is doing correctly and suggesting changes is an effective way to teach.

Assessment

Infant. The infant is assessed for age/development, readiness for feeding, weight, feeding skills, elimination patterns, and overall behavior. Important factors to evaluate include the following:

- Maturity level—full-term or preterm; gestational age
- Traumatic birth—a bruised head, deep suctioning, a broken clavicle
- Other problems—complications such as infection, maternal medications during labor, a difficult pregnancy
- Sucking ability—suck can be partially evaluated by placing a gloved finger in the baby's mouth, with the finger pad touching the palate. The tongue should cushion the joint of the finger and come out to cover the lower gum ridge while making a stroking motion.
- Birth defects—examples include cleft lip/palate, cardiac anomalies, Down syndrome, cystic fibrosis; some may affect feeding or weight gain
- Behavior at the breast—infant's response, presence of feeding skills
- Predictable sleep/wake cycle
- Consolability

The baby must be assessed by direct observation while actually feeding at the breast. The baby who sucks well on a finger may not be able to coordinate the suck/swallow/breathe sequence necessary for effective feeding.

Assessment

Mother. The mother is assessed for physical ability to feed a newborn, psychologic readiness, knowledge of the infant's capabilities and needs, knowledge and skill in feeding methods, and self-care.

Important factors to consider include the following:

- Familiarity with infants—normal reflexes, basis for realistic expectations for feeding, sleeping, elimination, fussiness, etc.
- Feelings about breastfeeding this baby—mother says she feels too young, old, nervous, etc.; has had a previous breastfeeding experience—positive or negative; she has "always known" she would breastfeed; or she is "just trying"

- Physical features—development of breast tissue, carpal tunnel syndrome, visual or hearing impairments, breast surgery that may affect the ducts, mastectomy, chronic illness, disability that may require assistance with feeding
- Techniques—positioning and latching on
- Knowledge—using the supply-meets-demand basis for managing milk supply, growth spurts, etc.; realistic activity level; care if engorged; caution with drugs

Each of these areas can be assessed through interviews, discussion, and direct observation.

Signs of potential problems. The nurse should intervene to ensure effective feedings for the baby who:

- Does not relax while feeding but keeps fists by face
- Fusses to breastfeed within an hour of feeding
- Is too sleepy to feed well
- Does not sustain at least 10 suck/swallows in a row through several bursts of sucking
- Has fewer than six wet diapers in 24 hours by the fourth day
- Does not have at least two bowel movements each 24 hours by the fourth day
- Is still passing meconium on the fourth day
- Begins to develop jaundice

The nurse should also assist with feedings for the mother who:

- Has breasts that do not get softer or lighter with feedings
- Develops sore, cracked, or bleeding nipples
- Becomes engorged
- Does not feel a firm tug on her breast with each suck
- Does not experience increased lochia flow or uterine cramping during or after feedings
- Does not feel relaxed or drowsy during feedings
- Does not know how to judge if the baby is feeding well
- Had a cesarean birth or has a disability

Nursing Diagnoses

When the nurse has analyzed pertinent information and discussed with the parents her observation of the infant while breastfeeding, nursing diagnoses can be made regarding the infant's nutrition status. Examples of different nursing diagnoses include the following:

- Effective breastfeeding related to mother's
  - Appropriate response to infant feeding readiness cues
  - Ability to facilitate efficient breastfeeding
  - Ability to identify her physiologic signs of correct latch-on
- Risk for ineffective breastfeeding pattern related to lack of skill in
  - Positioning the baby
  - Latching the baby onto the breast
  - Facilitating sustained sucking
- Risk for ineffective breastfeeding pattern related to lack of knowledge of
  - How to wake a sleepy newborn for effective feeding
  - Appropriate length and frequency for feedings
  - Appropriate infant behavior during effective feeding

The Nursing Care Plan on p. 690 presents additional examples of nursing diagnoses based on assessment findings.

Expected Outcomes

While planning care, the nurse must consider many factors, including the following:

- The infant's ability to feed
  - Full-term or preterm
  - Any anomalies
  - Quality of suck
  - Baby's physical condition
- The mother's ability to feed
  - Mother's physical condition, including disabilities
  - Medications
  - The mother's knowledge of breastfeeding skills
- The mother's wishes and expectations regarding breastfeeding for this baby
- The mother's previous breastfeeding experience
  - Expectations resulting from that experience
  - Problems
- The mother's support system
  - Who are her sources of support
  - Does her family have questions
  - Is there anyone knowledgable to provide breastfeeding assistance
- Mother's living situation
  - Responsibilities
  - Job
  - Financial resources
- Relevant cultural influences
  - Ethnic beliefs or practices
  - Peer influences
- Access to health care
  - Geographic
  - Financial
- Availability of appropriate educational materials
  - Native language
  - Literacy level
  - Accuracy and usefulness
- Community resources
  - Breastfeeding support groups
  - Telephone hot/warm line
  - Library

The expected outcomes or goals include that the infant will:

1. Receive the necessary nutrients to grow well
2. Have minimal physiologic stress associated with digestion, metabolism, and excretion
3. Respond to the parents' caregiving in a positive manner (i.e., quieting when they try to comfort, waking and feeding appropriately, and having reasonable periods of contentment each day)

The expected outcomes for the mother include that she will:

1. Receive knowledge that can be used for sound feeding practices

Nursing Care Plan

BREASTFEEDING AND INFANT NUTRITION

Nursing Diagnosis: Risk for ineffective breastfeeding related to limited maternal experience

Expected Outcomes: **Infant is latched on correctly as evidenced by maternal comfort, signs of oxytocin and prolactin release, and sufficient milk transfer. Mother feels confident about signs of sufficient milk transfer, her own comfort, and a feeding plan after discharge.**

• **NURSING INTERVENTIONS/*RATIONALES***

Explore the mother's knowledge about breastfeeding, her questions, and her assessment of feedings since birth and compare it to the infant's feeding chart and appearance *to establish baseline to direct intervention.*

If the mother seems ambivalent about breastfeeding, explore her questions and the problems she is experiencing, assist her in solving the problems, and provide her with accurate information *to assist her in decision making and to decrease her anxiety, which could interfere with her ability to learn.*

If the woman is very anxious, spread teaching over several sessions, give her ongoing feedback during several feedings, coach her (possibly with a family member) to get her baby situated and latched on independent of your assistance, and provide her with written material she can review as needed *to ensure that she has a chance to express all of her needs and to feel competent after hospital discharge.*

Teach specific techniques that make feeding easier (i.e., how to wake a sleepy baby, how to position the baby at the breast, how to get the baby latched on without pain, how to recognize the milk transfer, how to keep the baby sucking, alternate breast massage during feeding, how to recognize when the baby is finished) *to increase her confidence in her ability to care for her baby and decrease potential for inadequate feeding.*

Teach the mother to recognize release of oxytocin and prolactin (i.e., uterine contractions and increased lochia flow, drowsiness and thirst during feedings, baby's changing suck/swallow pattern) and why they are important *to increase her confidence in her body's ability to produce milk.*

Teach the mother how to minimize and cope with engorgement if it should occur (i.e., regular 3-hour feeding schedule during the first week, thorough softening of one breast before switching to the second side, cabbage leaves or ice packs on swollen breasts before feeding, and pumping as necessary to soften breasts and provide comfort) *to minimize anxiety about engorgement and to ensure that the infant can continue to latch on successfully.*

Teach breast and nipple care (i.e., bras are necessary only if they provide comfort; dry the nipples before closing bra flaps; avoid soap on the areola and nipple; and how to heal sore or abraded nipples) *to ensure maternal comfort.*

Teach the mother what to expect in the first 2 weeks of breastfeeding (i.e., normal infant changes such as increased appetite and alertness, signs the baby is getting enough milk, why to avoid a pacifier until the baby is clearly showing signs of sufficient intake, and normal breast changes) *to establish milk supply and to increase her confidence that she can care for her baby.*

Supplement teaching with appropriate videos and other audiovisual aids, written material including how to get help after discharge, and demonstration/return demonstration as necessary *to increase maternal confidence and enhance learning.*

---

2. Become skilled and appropriately comfortable with breastfeeding
3. Receive positive feedback from the baby and develop a sense of closeness to the child as a result of breastfeeding

Plan of Care and Implementation

As the nurse defines expected outcomes, it is important to use as a framework the mother's and the partner's, wishes, expectations, and previous experiences. The outcomes and plan of care should be developed with the mother. It is most helpful if the nurse has a realistic understanding of the situation in which the mother will be living and makes suggestions based on that reality.

For example, although high goals for a mother's health may suggest a perfect diet, reality is that few new mothers are going to have one. Putting too much emphasis on ideal nutrition may make a mother feel that she cannot possibly breastfeed because she cannot follow the proposed diet. Similarly, suggesting that a new mother needs a stress-free life and plenty of rest to make milk is not only unrealistic, it is not valid. New parents do worry about their babies, and babies normally wake up at night to be fed. The nurse can help the mother put well-meant, but unfounded, advice in perspective for her situation and needs.

Evaluation

Signs that breastfeeding is going well must be elicited from both the mother and the infant. The infant who is obtaining the necessary nutrients will exhibit a steady increase in weight, an appropriate elimination pattern, good skin and muscle tone, vigorous feeding behavior, and satisfaction. The satisfied newborn sleeps, cries in moderation, and is interested in socializing.

The nurse can be reasonably assured that care was effective to the degree that the following outcomes were achieved:

1. The infant received the necessary nutrients to grow well.
2. The infant experienced minimal physiologic stress associated with digestion, metabolism, and excretion.
3. The infant responded to the parents' caregiving in a positive manner (i.e., quieting when comforted, wak-

ing and feeding at appropriate times, and having reasonable periods of contentment each day).

The expected outcomes for the mother include the following:

1. The mother verbalized understanding of sound feeding practices.
2. The mother demonstrated skill and expressed an appropriate level of comfort with breastfeeding.
3. The mother reported feeling a sense of positive feedback from the baby's responses to her efforts to calm, wake, or feed.

FORMULA FEEDING

The decision to feed a baby infant formula may be the result of the mother's or partner's personal preference, the influence of other significant family members, or simply a lack of familiarity with breastfeeding. Occasionally there is no other option: the mother may have extensive breast scarring or had a bilateral mastectomy; the mother may be taking medications that preclude breastfeeding; or the baby may be adopted. Some mothers do induce lactation for an adopted baby (see the discussion of induced lactation on p. 679). Rarely, an infant may have galactosemia and must be fed a lactose-free formula.

In the United States, formula feeding is also suggested if the mother is human immunodeficiency virus (HIV) positive. In third-world countries where the risks of dying from diarrhea and dehydration are high because of unsafe water supplies, the mother who is HIV positive is advised to breastfeed her infant.

Care of the Bottle-Feeding Mother and Infant

Inexperienced mothers who are formula-feeding their infants usually need teaching, counseling, and support. They may need assistance with the feeding process and with any problems they may experience. Some mothers who are formula-feeding express concerns that the baby will suffer as a result of their decision. Emphasis on the beneficial use of feeding times for close contact and socializing with the infant can help relieve some of this concern.

Breast care. The mother who is not breastfeeding may find it necessary to use a supportive bra, ice packs, and a mild analgesic to relieve discomfort caused by engorgement. Nipple and breast stimulation should be avoided. Cabbage leaves placed inside the bra have been found to reduce swelling as effectively as ice packs. Ice packs should be left on for about 15 to 20 minutes out of an hour. If they are left on constantly, they can cause rebound swelling. For maximum effectiveness the cabbage leaves should be changed when they wilt, usually about every hour. The drug bromocriptine (Parlodel) is sometimes prescribed as a lactation suppressant for non-breast-feeding women; however, because of the rare but serious side effects some women have experienced, such as strokes, it is no longer recommended by the manufacturer for this purpose.

Feeding patterns. Typically a newborn will drink 10 to 15 ml of formula at a feeding at first. Intake gradually increases during the first week of life. Most babies are drinking 3 to 5 ounces at a feeding by the end of the second week or sooner. Generally a baby who weighs less than 10 pounds (4.5 kg) will take about 840 ml of formula in 24 hours after the newborn period. A baby who weighs more than 10 pounds (4.5 kg) will take about 960 ml in 24 hours.

During the daytime the newborn infant should be fed at least every third hour, even if that requires waking the baby for the feedings. If the baby is fussy earlier and other comfort measures, such as holding or diaper changing, do not help, the baby may be hungry and should be fed. At night the infant with adequate weight gain can be allowed to sleep and be fed only on awakening. Night feedings should be businesslike so that the baby learns that night feedings are not play time. Most newborns need six to eight feedings in 24 hours, and the number of feedings decreases as the infant matures. Usually by 3 to 4 weeks after birth a fairly predictable feeding pattern has developed. Scheduling feedings arbitrarily at predetermined intervals may not meet a baby's needs, but initiating feedings at convenient times often moves the baby's feedings to times that work for the family.

Managing feedings. Formula can be fed at room temperature or warmed. If it is warmed, the formula's temperature should be tested before it is given to the baby.

Nursing ALERT

No foods to be given to a baby should be warmed in a microwave oven. Boiling areas may develop despite efforts to shake adequately. These areas can seriously burn the baby's mouth.

Positioning. Babies need to be held for feedings. The mother should be encouraged to cradle her infant in her arms closely and securely. Feedings provide a good time for her to talk, sing, or simply enjoy a peaceful relaxation with her baby (Fig. 24-17).

Most infants swallow air when fed from a bottle and should be given a chance to burp several times through a feeding. Swallowed air can cause excessive spitting up or gas. The bottle should be tipped so that milk fills the nipple during feedings.

A bottle should never be propped, nor should the infant be left alone during a feeding because of the risk of choking and aspiration. It would also deprive the infant of important social interaction during feedings.

Nursing ALERT

Putting a baby to bed with a bottle can cause *nursing bottle caries*, decay of the first teeth as a result of continuous contact with milk or juice.

Overfeeding. The mother should be taught to recognize the cues that her infant has had enough to eat so that she can avoid overfeeding. Overfeeding can make the baby uncomfortable, cause spitting up, and contribute to obesity. After the newborn period the infant who falls asleep, turns aside the head, or ceases to suck usually is signaling that he or she is full. Formula left in the bottle should be discarded after the feeding because the baby's saliva has mixed with the milk.

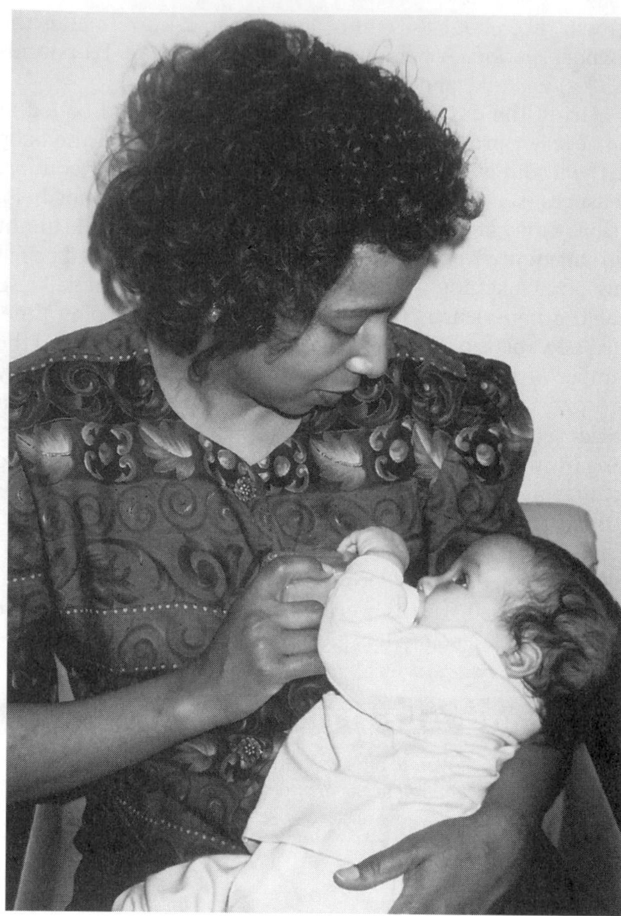

Fig. 24-17 Feeding is a time for holding the baby close and socializing with the baby.

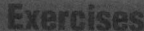

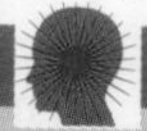

Critical Thinking Exercises

BOTTLE-FEEDING MOTHER—SLOW WEIGHT GAIN

A mother brings her baby in for a 1-month well-baby examination. She mentions to you that her mother-in-law told her the baby looks "skinny," so she has been putting less water in the formula to increase the caloric intake of each feeding. Identify assessment data that must be collected to deal with this situation. Develop a plan of care for an infant whose weight gain is (1) within normal limits or (2) less than recommended.

Growth spurts. Mothers usually notice increases in the infant's appetite between 10 days and 2 weeks; between 6 and 9 weeks; and between 3 and 6 months. These appetite spurts correspond to growth spurts. The amount of formula at each feeding should be increased by about 30 ml to meet the baby's needs.

Commercial formulas. Because human milk is uniquely designed to meet the needs of the human infant, it is used as the standard for all infant feedings. Infants who are not breastfed should be given commercial formulas. Low-income families usually are eligible for services through the WIC program, which will provide iron-fortified infant formula.

Bovine milk (cow milk) is used as the basis of most formulas. Some infants have an allergic reaction to cow milk formula. They may experience diarrhea, rash, colic, vomiting, and in extreme cases, failure to thrive. Some of these infants may be helped by switching to a soy milk formula; however, some are allergic to soy protein. If hypersensitivity to cow milk protein is suspected, a hydrolyzed casein formula may be effective. However, these special formulas are very expensive. Some women may be able to begin breastfeeding (see the discussion of relactation on p. 679) or in life-threatening cases, they may obtain human milk through a milk bank, at least temporarily.

The following list summarizes the modifications used in preparing cow-milk–based commercial formulas:

1. Butterfat is removed, and vegetable oils are added to ensure adequate fat absorption and to provide essential fatty acids.
2. Protein is heated to produce a softer curd that is more easily digested by the infant.
3. Protein and mineral concentrations are decreased to more nearly resemble those in human milk.
4. Carbohydrates are added to provide sufficient calories.

Commercial formulas are available in three forms: powder, concentrate, and ready-to-feed. All forms are equivalent in nutritional content, but there may be a considerable difference in price. Parents can weigh the considerations of convenience and cost carefully and choose the form that best suits their needs. Powdered formulas are least expensive and are convenient because they are lightweight and require no refrigeration before mixing with water. Concentrated liquid formulas must be prepared with water. Each can is sufficient to make 26 ounces and must be refrigerated after opening. Ready-to-use formula is most expensive. It comes in 8- and 32-ounce cans and is also sold in individual disposable bottles.

Formula preparation. Recent recommendations for labeling commercial infant formulas require that the directions for preparation and use of the formula include pictures and symbols for nonreading individuals. In addition, manufacturers are translating the directions from English into other languages, such as Spanish, French, Vietnamese, Chinese, and Arabic, to prevent misunderstanding and errors in formula preparation. It is important to impress on families that the proportions must not be altered—neither diluted to extend the amount of formula nor concentrated to provide more calories.

Although manufacturers of commercial formulas include directions for preparing their products, the nurse should review formula preparation with the mother. It is especially important that formula be mixed properly. The newborn's kidneys are immature, and overly concentrated formula may provide protein and minerals that exceed the kidney's excretory ability. In contrast, if the formula is diluted too much, the infant will not consume sufficient calories and will not grow well.

Sterilization of formula rarely is recommended when families have access to a safe public water supply. Instead, formula is prepared with attention to cleanliness. When water from a private well is used, parents should be advised to contact the health department to have a chemical and bacteriologic analysis of the water done before using the water in formula preparation. The presence of nitrates, excess fluoride, or bacteria may be harmful to the infant.

Evaporated milk. Although evaporated milk is concentrated and less expensive than commercial formula, mixing evaporated milk and water to feed a baby is no longer recommended because evaporated milk does not provide adequate nutrition for an infant.

Unmodified cow milk. Unmodified cow milk is not suited to the nutritional needs of the human infant in the first year of life (Table 24-1). Specific concerns include its excessive amounts of calcium, phosphorus, and other minerals; imbalance of calcium and phosphorus; excessive protein content; poorly absorbed fat; and low iron concentration. In addition, its use is apt to cause gastrointestinal blood loss in the infant through microscopic hemorrhage (Zeigler et al, 1990). This blood loss, as well as the low levels of iron in the milk, increases the likelihood of iron deficiency anemia. Anemia in the infant may have serious and long-lasting consequences. Some evidence suggests that infants who have been severely anemic, even when corrected with iron therapy, have learning delays that may persist throughout the preschool years (Oski, 1990).

Vitamin and mineral supplementation. Commercial iron-fortified formula supplies all the nutrients needed by the infant for the first 6 months of life. After 6 months the only mineral supplementation required is 0.25 mg of fluoride per day if the local water supply is not fluoridated or if the infant is given ready-to-feed formula, which eliminates the use of fluoridated tap water (AAP, 1995).

Weaning. The baby gradually learns to use a cup, and the parents find that they are preparing fewer bottles. Commonly the feeding before bedtime is the last one to remain by bottle. Babies have a strong need to suck, and the baby who has had the bottle taken away too early will compensate with nonnutritive sucking on his or her fingers, thumb, a pacifier, or even his or her own tongue. Weaning from a bottle should be a gradual process because the baby has learned to rely on the comfort that sucking provides. This comfort helps a baby cope with other events, such as toilet training, getting a new baby-sitter, moving, or the birth of a sibling (for a discussion of nursing bottle caries, see p. 691).

DISCHARGE PLANNING

Parents, whether they are breastfeeding or bottle-feeding, need varying levels of support and encouragement as they adjust to their new roles and master the skills necessary for child care. Within a few days, many babies have a fussy period each day. Most infants are alert for several hours and like social interaction. The typical newborn needs to be fed about eight times in 24 hours for about 30 minutes each time. Even with realistic expectations, many parents find these sudden demands overwhelming. For some parents the size and growth of an infant may be seen as a measure of parenting ability. Generalized anxiety about the baby can become focused on feeding. The positive feedback that comes from seeing the baby grow and thrive fosters feelings of confidence for many parents.

Nurses may be in an ideal position to provide the support the mother needs. Sometimes just knowing what is normal for a specific age can be helpful. The nurse can also give new parents phone numbers for follow-up and tell them that most new parents have feeding and other baby care questions. If the mother has questions or experiences problems, she should feel free to contact the hospital nursery, her pediatrician, or a clinic for assistance.

With early hospital discharges, most health care providers schedule a weight check during the first week of life. The nurse can confirm that this appointment has been made before the parents leave the hospital. Some hospitals and health care groups offer baby hotlines, and a few even provide a home visit. The new mother should be given information and encouraged to contact community support groups for parenting, breastfeeding, mothers of twins, etc.

A properly coordinated health care delivery system for infants and children may include various health care professionals. These professionals can be found in departments of public health and often in private physicians' offices. The nurse can make parents aware of services available from many sources, such as a lactation consultant, a nutritionist, a psychologist, a social worker, a physical therapist, or a speech pathologist.

Key Points

- Human milk is the most appropriate food for infants and provides protection from many infections and diseases even into adulthood.
- The size of the breast is not indicative of its functional capacity.
- Limiting feeding time at the breast will restrict infant intake and may contribute to engorgement, but it will not prevent sore nipples.
- There are objective, measurable signs—both maternal and infant—that effective milk transfer has taken place during breastfeeding.
- All babies should be held for feedings.
- Infants do not have the physiologic capacity to digest solid food before 4 to 6 months of age.
- Whole or skim cow milk is not appropriate for feeding the baby under 12 months of age.
- The typical newborn requires a minimum of eight feedings per 24 hours in the early weeks.
- Babies may need to be awakened for some feedings until a pattern of appropriate weight gain is established.
- Demand feeding means that the mother responds to the baby's requests for feeding in addition to ensuring that the newborn is fed at least every third hour during the day.
- Volume of milk produced is determined by volume of milk removed from the breast; breastfeeding operates on a supply-meets-demand principle.

References

American Academy of Pediatrics, Committee on Nutrition: Fluoride supplementation for children: interim policy recommendations, *Pediatrics* 95:777, 1995.

American Academy of Pediatrics (AAP): The transfer of drugs and other chemicals into human breast milk, *Pediatrics* 93:137, 1994.

Anderson G: Skin-to-skin: kangaroo care in Western Europe, *Am J Nurs* 89:662, 1989.

Arnold L: *Recommendations for collection, storage, and handling of a mother's milk for her own infant in the hospital setting,* West Hartford, Conn, 1994, Human Milk Banking Association of North America.

Arnold L, Tully M: *Guidelines for the establishment and operation of a donor human milk bank,* ed 6, West Hartford, Conn, 1996, Human Milk Banking Association of North America.

Bowles B, Stutte P, Hensley J: Alternate massage in breastfeeding, *Genesis* 9:5, 1988.

Butte N et al: Effect of maternal nutrition, diet, and body composition in lactation performance, *Am J Clin Nutr* 39:296, 1984.

Centers for Disease Control: Trends in fertility and infant and maternal health—US 1980-88, *MMWR* 40:381, 1991.

Davies H et al: Insulin requirements of diabetic women who breastfeed, *Br Med J* 298:1357, 1989.

Devereux W: Acute puerperal mastitis, *Am J Obstet Gynecol* 108:78, 1970.

Dewey K et al: A randomized study of the effects of aerobic exercise by lactating women on breast-milk volume and composition, *N Engl J Med* 330:449, 1994.

Dusdieker L et al: Prolonged maternal fluid supplementation in breastfeeding, *Pediatrics* 86:737, 1990.

Feher S et al: Increasing breast milk production for premature infants with a relaxation/imagery audiotape, *Pediatrics* 83:57, 1989.

Freed G, Fraley J, Schanler R: Attitudes of expectant fathers regarding breastfeeding, *Pediatrics* 90:224, 1992.

Gielen A et al: Maternal employment during the early postpartum period: effects on initiation and continuation of breast-feeding, *Pediatrics* 87:298, 1991.

Groh-Wagner S et al: The utility of a bilateral breast pumping system for mothers of premature infants, *Neonat Netw* 14(8):31, 1995.

Grossman L et al: The effect of postpartum lactation counseling on the duration of breast-feeding in low-income women, *Am J Dis Child* 144:471, 1990.

Gupta A, Gupta P: Metoclopramide as a lactogogue, *Clin Pediatr Phila* 24:269, 1985.

Hayslip G et al: The effect of lactation on bone mineral content in healthy postpartum women, *Obstet Gynecol* 73:588, 1989.

Hendricks K, Walker W: *Pediatric nutrition,* ed 2, Philadelphia, 1990, BC Decker.

Hopkinson J, Schanler J, Garza C: Milk production by mothers of premature infants, *Pediatrics* 81:815, 1988.

Institute of Medicine: *Nutrition during lactation,* Washington, DC, 1991, National Academy Press.

Kattwinkel J et al: Infant sleep position and sudden infant death syndrome (SIDS) in the United States, *Pediatrics* 93:820, 1994.

Kavanaugh K et al: Getting enough: mothers' concerns about breastfeeding a preterm infant after discharge, *J Obstet Gynecol Neonatal Nurs* 24:23, 1995.

Kemper K, Forsyth B, McCarthy P: Jaundice, terminating breast-feeding, and the vulnerable child, *Pediatrics* 84:773, 1989.

Kemper K, Forsyth B, McCarthy P: Persistent perceptions of vulnerability following neonatal jaundice, *Am J Dis Child* 144:238, 1990.

Lawrence R: Breast-feeding, *Pediatr Rev* 11:163, 1989.

Lawrence R: *Breastfeeding: a guide for the medical profession,* ed 4, St Louis, 1994, Mosby.

Layde P: The independent associations of parity, age at first full term pregnancy, and duration of breastfeeding with the risk of breast cancer, *J Clin Epidemiol* 42:963, 1989.

Lethbridge D: The use of breastfeeding as a contraceptive, *J Obstet Gynecol Neonatal Nurs* 18:31, 1989.

Lucas A, Morley R: Breast milk and necrotising enterocolitis, *Lancet* 336:1519, 1990.

Lucas A et al: Breast milk and subsequent intelligence quotient in children born preterm, *Lancet* 339:261, 1992.

MacGowan R et al: Breast-feeding among women attending women, infants, and children clinics in Georgia, 1987, *Pediatrics* 87:361, 1991.

Meier P: Bottle and breast feeding: effects of transcutaneous oxygen pressure and temperature in preterm infants, *Nurs Res* 37:36, 1988.

Narayanan I, Prakash K, Gujral V: The value of human milk in the prevention of infection in the high-risk low-birth weight infants, *J Pediatr* 99:496, 1981.

Naylor A et al: Oral water intoxication, *Am J Dis Child* 146:893, 1992.

Neifert M, Seacat J, Jobe W: Lactation failure due to insufficient glandular development of the breast, *Pediatrics* 76:823, 1985.

Newman J: Water intoxication: a problem of bottle-feeding, *Am J Dis Child* 146:1131, 1992.

Oski F: Whole cow milk feeding between 6 and 12 months of age? Go back to 1976, *Pediatr Rev* 12:187, 1990.

Riordan J, Auerbach K: *Breastfeeding and human lactation,* Boston, 1993, Jones & Bartlett.

Roberts K: A comparison of chilled cabbage leaves and chilled gelpaks in reducing breast engorgement, *J Hum Lact* 11:17, 1995.

Ryan A, Martinez G: Breast-feeding and the working mother: a profile, *Pediatrics* 83:524, 1989.

Ryan A et al: Recent declines in breast-feeding in the United States, 1984 through 1989, *Pediatrics* 88:719, 1991.

Snell B et al: The association of formula samples given at hospital discharge with the early duration of breastfeeding, *J Hum Lact* 8:67, 1992.

Specker B et al: Increased urinary methylmalonic acid excretion in breast-fed infants of vegetarian mothers and identification of an acceptable dietary source of vitamin B_{12}, *Am J Clin Nutr* 47:89, 1988.

Spika J et al: Risk factors for infant botulism in the United States? *Am J Dis Child* 143:828, 1989.

Tully M: *Low breastfeeding rates: is limited physician knowledge of clinical skills a contributing factor?* Unpublished master's paper, 1994, University of North Carolina at Chapel Hill, School of Public Health.

Tully M, Overfield M: *Breastfeeding counseling guide,* ed 2, Raleigh, 1989, Lactation Consultants of North Carolina.

Valois R: Breastfeeding rates among WIC recipients in Wake County, North Carolina receiving EFNEP breastfeeding support visits, personal communication, 1994.

Widstrom A, Ransjo-Arvidsson A, Christensson K: *Breastfeeding is the baby's choice,* Richmond, VA, 1993, BGK Enterprises Production (out of production).

Zeigler E et al: Cow milk feeding in infancy: further observations on blood loss from the gastrointestinal tract, *J Pediatr* 116:11, 1990.

Bibliography

Bucho B et al: Comfort measures in breastfeeding, primiparous women, *J Obstet Gynecol Neonatal Nurs* 23(1):46, 1994.

Dewey K et al: Growth of breast-fed and formula-fed infants from 0 to 18 months: the DARLING study, *Pediatrics* 89:1035, 1992.

Ellis D, Livingstone V, Hewat R: Assisting the breastfeeding mother: a problem-solving process, *J Hum Lact* 9:89, 1993.

Freed G et al: National assessment of physicians' breastfeeding knowledge, attitudes, training and experience, *JAMA* 273:472, 1995.

Newman J: How breast milk protects newborns, *Sci Am* 273:76, 1995.

Orlando S: The immunologic significance of breast milk, *J Obstet Gynecol Neonatal Nurs* 24(7):678, 1995.

Rogan W, Gladen B: Breastfeeding and cognitive development, *Early Hum Dev* 31:181, 1993.

Ziemer M, Pigeon J: Skin changes and pain in the nipple during the first week of lactation, *J Obstet Gynecol Neonatal Nurs* 22:247, 1993.

CHAPTER 25

The High-Risk Newborn

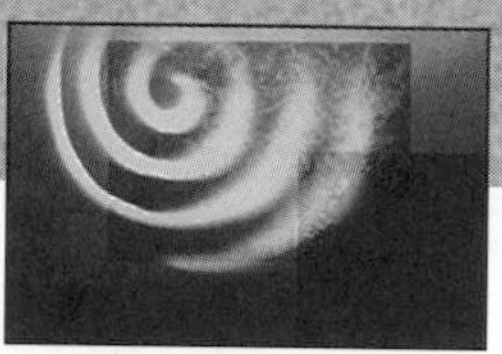

CLASSIFICATION OF HIGH-RISK NEWBORNS, P. 696

TRANSPORTING HIGH-RISK INFANTS, P. 696

PLAN OF CARE, P. 697

Assessment of the high-risk newborn by systems, p. 697

Respiratory care, p. 699

Thermoregulatory care, p. 704

Nutritional care, p. 706

Developmental and emotional aspects of care, p. 712

TRANSPORT FROM A REGIONAL CENTER ("BACK TRANSPORT"), P. 718

NURSING CARE OF THE FAMILY, P. 719

PAIN IN NEONATES, P. 719

Assessment of pain, p. 719

Management of neonatal pain, p. 719

A challenge for the nurse is the birth of an infant at risk because of conditions or circumstances that are superimposed on the normal course of events associated with birth and the adjustment to extrauterine existence. The infant may be considered high risk because of gestational age, pathophysiologic problems, or congenital anomalies.

Low-birth-weight newborns constitute the largest subgroup of high-risk infants. Of these infants, one third are small for gestational age (SGA) and two thirds are premature but appropriate for gestational age (AGA). SGA newborns also may be premature.

The more common problems related to physiologic status are closely associated with the state of maturity of the infant and usually involve chemical disturbances (e.g., hypoglycemia, hypocalcemia) and consequences of immature organs and systems (e.g., hyperbilirubinemia, respiratory distress, hypothermia). Congenital anomalies include such conditions as esophageal atresia, anencephaly, omphalocele, and heart defects.

At times, the nurse is able to anticipate such problems as when a woman is admitted in premature labor or a congenital anomaly is diagnosed by ultrasound before birth. At other times, birth of a high-risk infant is unanticipated. In either case, personnel and equipment necessary for immediate care of the infant must be available.

The outcome expectations, planning, and implementation of the nursing process for the high-risk infant should focus on maintaining the infant's physiologic systems and keeping the family adequately informed of the treatment being provided for their infant by the multidisciplinary team. The care given also focuses on family dynamics and includes an evaluation of the way in which the family is accepting the infant as a unique and individual family member.

The discussion in this chapter focuses on neonatal factors that place the newborn at risk.

A Nursing Care Plan for a high-risk infant is presented on pp. 720-721.

CLASSIFICATION OF HIGH-RISK NEWBORNS

High-risk infants are most often classified according to birth weight, gestational age, and predominant pathophysiologic problems (Box 25-1). Intrauterine growth rates are not the same for all infants, and other factors (e.g., heredity, placental insufficiency, and maternal disease) influence intrauterine growth and birth weight. The classification system in the box encompasses birth weight, gestational age, and neonatal outcome. The lowest perinatal mortality is found in the full-term infant who weighs between 3000 and 4000 g (Fanaroff, Martin, 1997).

TRANSPORTING HIGH-RISK INFANTS

The optimum site for the care of compromised neonates is in a newborn intensive care unit where specialized personnel and equipment are available. Hospitals that are not equipped to care for a high-risk mother or neonate must arrange for transfer to a specialized perinatal or regional tertiary care center. (See Chapter 5 for a description of regionalization of perinatal care.) All health care providers involved in the birth

BOX 25-1
Classification of High-Risk Infants

Classification according to size

Low-birth-weight (LBW) infant—An infant whose birth weight is less than 2500 g regardless of gestational age

Very-very-low-birth-weight (VVLBW) or extremely-low-birth-weight (ELBW) infant—An infant whose birth weight is less than 1000 g

Very-low-birth-weight (VLBW) infant—An infant whose birth weight is less than 1500 g

Moderately-low-birth-weight (MLBW)—An infant whose birth weight is 1501 to 2500 g

Appropriate-for-gestational-age (AGA) infant—An infant whose weight falls between the 10th and 90th percentiles on intrauterine growth curves

Small-for-date (SFD) or small-for-gestational-age (SGA) infant—An infant whose rate of intrauterine growth was slowed and whose birth weight falls below the 10th percentile on intrauterine growth curves

Intrauterine growth restriction (IUGR)—Found in infants whose intrauterine growth is restricted (sometimes used as a more descriptive term for the SGA infant)

Large-for-gestational-age (LGA) infant—An infant whose birth weight is above the 90th percentile on intrauterine growth charts

Classification according to gestational age

Premature (preterm) infant—An infant born before completion of 37 weeks of gestation, regardless of birth weight

Full-term infant—An infant born between the beginning of the 38 weeks and the completion of the 42 weeks of gestation, regardless of birth weight

Postmature (postterm) infant—An infant born after 42 weeks of gestational age, regardless of birth weight

Classification according to mortality

Live birth—Birth in which the neonate manifests any heartbeat, breathes, or displays voluntary movement, regardless of gestational age

Fetal death—Death of the fetus after 20 weeks of gestation and before birth, with absence of any signs of life after birth

Neonatal death—Death that occurs in the first 27 days of life; early neonatal death occurs in the first week of life; late neonatal death occurs at 7 to 27 days

Perinatal mortality—Describes the total number of fetal and early neonatal deaths per 1000 live births

Postnatal death—Death that occurs at 28 days to 1 year

of newborns should be familiar with the transport system within their own community. When possible, maternal transports (i.e., transport of pregnant women) are preferable to neonatal transports (transport of newborns). Transfer of the mother before birth has two distinct advantages: (1) neonatal morbidity and mortality decrease, and (2) the mother and infant are not separated at birth. With maternal transport, the infant does not experience the stresses of transport; rather, the infant is born at a regional center that is staffed and equipped to address the special needs of the high-risk newborn.

Arrangements for transport to an intensive care facility are made as soon as the high-risk infant is identified. Each hospital that delivers infants should be able to provide for appropriate neonatal stabilization and arrange for transport to a tertiary care facility. The infant must be kept warm and adequately oxygenated (including intubation if indicated), have vital signs and oxygen saturation monitored, and, when indicated, receive an intravenous infusion. The infant is transported in a specially designed incubator unit containing a complete life-support system and other emergency equipment that can be carried by ambulance, van, or helicopter.

The transport team may consist of one or more of the highly trained persons from the neonatal intensive care unit (NICU): a neonatologist (or a fellow in neonatology), a respiratory therapist, and one or more nurses. The professional assigned to accompany the infant must be constantly alert to every change in the infant's condition and be able to intervene appropriately.

The birth of any high-risk infant can cause profound parental stress. Parents can grieve the loss of the ideal infant. They are fearful of the possible eventual outcomes for the infant. They must also deal with the technologic world surrounding their infant, and amid all the equipment, it is sometimes difficult for them to perceive the infant and respond to its needs. Parents of high-risk infants who have been transported to regional centers therefore need special support. Many intensive care units provide the family with a handbook or pictures of the tertiary care unit to help them understand what is going on around them (Prukop, 1994).

Critical Thinking Exercises

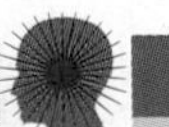

COMPARING NORMAL AND HIGH-RISK NEONATES

Observe a neonatal nurse for 1 clinical day in an intermediate care nursery, after you have spent an observation day in either a nursery for term newborns or a maternal-newborn unit, so that you could become familiar with basic newborn behaviors and care.

1. Compare the different feeding methods in the two units. Discuss with the nurse the various feeding policies and the unit's plan to implement full breastfeedings or bottle feedings for several infants.
2. Assess an infant requiring oxygen support during a nipple feeding. Why would a premature infant require oxygen support during nipple feedings but not during gavage feedings?
3. Talk with the parents of one of the infants. How do they describe their infant now and how did they perceive their infant during the acute phase of illness? Would this make a difference in the way in which you provide discharge information to the parents at admission, after the acute phase, or 2 days before discharge?

PLAN OF CARE

Assessment of the High-Risk Newborn by Systems

Assessment by systems provides a point-in-time evaluation of the infant's condition, as well as a baseline for evaluation of any change in the infant's condition. The equipment necessary for this assessment includes a stethoscope, tape measure, thermometer, blood pressure device, and *clean, warm hands.* Gloves should be worn if the infant has not had an initial bath. The assessment should be performed in a warm, safe, and comfortable environment using a systematic approach as described in Chapter 23 and in the Guidelines box below.

Blood examinations are a necessary part of the ongoing assessment and monitoring of the high-risk newborn's progress. The tests most often performed are blood glucose, bilirubin, calcium, hematocrit, and blood gases. Samples may be obtained from the heel, by venipuncture, by arterial puncture, or by an indwelling catheter in an umbilical vein, umbilical artery, or peripheral artery.

Wrapping the foot in a warm, damp washcloth or disposable diaper is a simple way to create adequate vasodilation for a heel stick. Commercial warm packs are also available but should be used with extreme caution in extremely-low-birth-weight (ELBW) and very-low-birth-weight (VLBW) infants to prevent burns.

When numerous blood samples must be drawn, it is important to maintain an accurate record of the amount of blood being removed, especially in ELBW and VLBW infants, who cannot afford to have their blood supply depleted during the acute phase of their illness. To monitor arterial blood gas

Guidelines

PHYSICAL ASSESSMENT OF THE HIGH-RISK INFANT

General Assessment

Using electronic scale, weigh daily, or more often if ordered.
Measure length and head circumference periodically.
Describe general body shape and size, posture at rest, ease of breathing, presence and location of edema.
Describe any apparent deformities.
Describe any signs of distress: poor color, mouth open, head bobbing, grimace, furrowed brow.

Respiratory Assessment

Describe shape of chest (barrel, concave), symmetry, presence of incisions, chest tubes, or other deviations.
Describe use of accessory muscles: nasal flaring or substernal, intercostal, or subclavicular retractions.
Determine respiratory rate and regularity.
Auscultate and describe breath sounds: stridor, crackles, wheezing, wet diminished sounds, areas of absence of sound, grunting, diminished air entry, equality of breath sounds.
Determine whether suctioning is needed.
Describe cry if not intubated.
Describe ambient oxygen and method of delivery; if intubated, describe size of tube, type of ventilator and settings, and method of securing tube.
Determine oxygen saturation by pulse oximetry and partial pressure of oxygen and carbon dioxide by transcutaneous oxygen ($tcPo_2$) and transcutaneous carbon dioxide ($tcPco_2$).

Cardiovascular Assessment

Determine heart rate and rhythm.
Describe heart sounds, including any murmurs.
Determine the point of maximum intensity (PMI), the point where the heartbeat sounds loudest and palpates strongest (a change in the point of maximum intensity may indicate a mediastinal shift).
Describe infant's color (may be of cardiac, respiratory, or hematopoietic origin): cyanosis, pallor, plethora, jaundice, mottling.
Assess color of nail beds, mucous membranes, lips.
Determine blood pressure. Indicate extremity used and cuff size; check each extremity at least once.
Describe peripheral pulses, capillary refill (<2 to 3 sec), peripheral perfusion (mottling).
Describe monitors, their parameters, and whether alarms are in "on" position.

Gastrointestinal Assessment

Determine presence of abdominal distention: increase in circumference, shiny skin, evidence of abdominal wall erythema, visible peristalsis, visible loops of bowel, status of umbilicus.
Determine any signs of regurgitation, and time related to feeding; character and amount of residual if gavage fed; if nasogastric tube in place, describe type of suction, drainage (color, consistency, pH, guaiac).
Describe amount, color, consistency, and odor of any emesis.
Palpate liver margin.
Describe amount, color, and consistency of stools; check for occult blood and/or reducing substances if ordered or indicated by appearance of stool.
Describe bowel sounds: presence or absence (must be present if feeding).

Genitourinary Assessment

Describe any abnormalities of genitalia.
Describe amount (as determined by weight), color, pH, labstick findings, and specific gravity of urine (to screen for adequacy of hydration).
Check weight (the most accurate measure for assessment of hydration).

Neurologic-Musculoskeletal Assessment

Describe infant's movements: random, purposeful, jittery, twitching, spontaneous, elicited; level of activity with stimulation; evaluate based on gestational age.
Describe infant's position or attitude: flexed, extended.
Describe reflexes observed: Moro, sucking, Babinski, plantar reflex, and other expected reflexes.
Determine level of response and consolability.
Determine changes in head circumference (if indicated); size and tension of fontanels, suture lines.
Determine pupillary responses in infant >32 weeks of gestation.

Temperature

Determine skin and axillary temperature.
Determine relationship to environmental temperature.

Skin Assessment

Describe any discoloration, reddened area, signs of irritation, blisters, abrasions, or denuded areas, especially where monitoring equipment, infusions, or other apparatus come in contact with skin; also check and note ***any*** skin preparation used (e.g., povidone-iodine tape).
Determine texture and turgor of skin: dry, smooth, flaky, peeling, etc.
Describe any rash, skin lesion, or birthmarks.
Determine whether intravenous infusion catheter or needle is in place and observe for signs of infiltration.
Describe parenteral infusion lines: location, type (arterial, venous, peripheral, umbilical, central, peripheral central venous); type of infusion (medication, saline, dextrose, electrolyte, lipids, total parenteral nutrition); type of infusion pump and rate of flow; type of needle (butterfly, catheter); appearance of insertion site.

levels without repeated arterial punctures, pulse oximetry, transcutaneous oxygen ($tcPo_2$), and/or carbon dioxide ($tcPco_2$) are used.

Safety measures. The proliferation of equipment technology over the past few years has increased the dangers associated with its use, especially performance malfunction and electrical hazards. Malfunction includes such things as inaccurate monitor function, erratic delivery rates in infusion devices, and low or high suction in pumps. Electrical hazards are related to defective equipment, wiring, or grounding, or improper use of equipment.

One of the most effective means for ensuring the safety of infant and staff is the nurse's knowledge, alertness, and education regarding the function of equipment. Electronic monitoring devices are checked to ensure the alarms are not turned off, which negates their effectiveness. It is important to check equipment for all correct component parts, to remove from use and report equipment that is not performing according to specifications, and to obey the basic rules of electrical safety—handle equipment with care, be alert to signs of trouble, and follow electrical safety guidelines.

Respiratory Care

The primary objective in the care of infants is to establish and maintain respiration. Many high-risk infants require supplemental oxygen and assisted ventilation. Infants with or without these supportive treatments are positioned to maximize oxygenation. Oxygen therapy is provided on the basis of the infant's requirements and illness.

Health care providers must be skilled in the resuscitation of newborns. In addition, the resuscitation of newborns requires teamwork and the availability of the proper equipment in the birthing room. Box 25-2 includes a list of neonatal resuscitation supplies and equipment.

High-risk neonates are placed in a controlled thermal environment and monitored for heart rate, respiratory activity, and temperature. Monitoring devices are equipped with an alarm system that indicates when the vital signs are above or below preset limits. However, it is essential to check the infant's heartbeat and respirations, and compare them with the monitor reading.

BOX 25-2

Neonatal Resuscitation Supplies and Equipment

Suction equipment

Bulb syringe
Mechanical suction
5- (or 6-), 8-, 10-French suction catheters
8-French feeding tube and 20-ml syringe
Meconium aspirator

Bag-and-mask equipment

Infant resuscitation bag with a pressure-release valve or pressure gauge; the bag must be capable of delivering 90% to 100% oxygen
Face masks—newborn and premature sizes (cushioned-rim masks preferred)
Oral airways—newborn and premature sizes
Oxygen source with intact flowmeter and tubing

Intubation equipment

No. 0 (premature) and No. 1 (term newborn) laryngoscope with straight blades
Extra bulbs and batteries for laryngoscope
2.5-, 3.0-, 3.5-, and 4.0-mm endotracheal tubes
Stylet
Scissors
Gloves

Medications

1:10,000 epinephrine; 3- or 10-ml ampules
0.4-mg/ml naloxone hydrochloride in 1-ml ampules or 1.0 mg/ml in 2-ml ampules
Volume expander—one or more
  Normal saline
  Ringer's lactate
  Albumin (5%)/saline solution
Sodium bicarbonate 4.2% (5 mEq/10 ml) in 10-ml ampules
250 ml of 10% dextrose
30 ml of sterile water
30 ml of normal saline

Other equipment and supplies

Radiant warmer
Stethoscope
Blood pressure monitor with transducer (desirable)
$^1/_2$- or $^3/_4$-in wide adhesive tape
1-, 3-, 5-, 10-, 20-, and 50-ml syringes
25-, 21-, and 18-gauge needles
Alcohol sponges
Umbilical artery catheterization tray
Umbilical tape
$3^1/_2$-, 5-French umbilical catheters
Three-way stopcocks
5-French feeding tube
Cardiotachometer with ECG oscilloscope (desirable)
Pressure transducer and monitor (desirable)

Data from American Heart Association/American Academy of Pediatrics: *Textbook of neonatal resuscitation*, Dallas, 1994, American Heart Association.

Nursing Care Management

Assessment

Pink color, adequate tissue perfusion, and respiratory patterns are quickly established in nonstressed newborns, and they are soon vigorous and show appropriate muscle tone. However, infants with a potential for respiratory depression at birth because of asphyxia, prematurity, or congenital malformations may exhibit cyanosis, decreased tissue perfusion, retractions, nasal flaring, or a combination of these problems.

Hypoxemia. In utero the normal fetus is exposed to lower oxygen levels than at any other period of life. The fetus thrives with a Pao_2 (oxygen tension in the arterial system) of 20 mm Hg to low 30 mm Hg (Fanaroff and Martin, 1997). At birth the exposure of the newborn to room air, which has an Fio_2 of about 21%, increases the infant's arterial oxygen saturation levels to between 80% and 100%.

Respiratory difficulty often follows a progressive pattern. Infants normally breathe between 30 to 60 breaths/min, relying significantly on their abdominal muscles to accomplish this (Hagedorn, Gardner, and Abman, 1993). However, the respiratory rate may increase without a change in rhythm. Early signs of respiratory distress include **flaring of the nares** and an expiratory grunt. Depending on the cause, **retractions** may begin as intercostal, subcostal, or suprasternal retractions. Increasing respiratory effort, for example, seesaw breathing patterns, retractions, flaring of the nares, expiratory **grunting** and apneic spells, indicates deepening distress.

Substernal retractions become more pronounced as the diaphragm works hard in an attempt to fill collapsed air sacs. Fine inspiratory crackles can be heard over both lungs, and there is an audible expiratory grunt. This grunting, a useful mechanism observed in the earlier stages of respiratory distress, serves to increase end-expiratory pressure in the lungs, thus maintaining alveolar expansion and allowing gas exchange for an additional brief period. Flaring of the nares is also a sign that accompanies tachypnea, grunting, and retractions in respiratory distress. Central cyanosis (a bluish discoloration of oral mucous membranes and generalized body cyanosis) is a late and serious sign of respiratory distress. Initially cyanosis may be abolished by supplemental oxygen. The use of pulse oximetry and arterial blood gas sampling obviates the necessity for dependence on color to determine oxygen requirements.

Periodic breathing is a respiratory pattern commonly seen in premature infants. Such infants exhibit 5- to 10-second respiratory pauses followed by 10 to 15 seconds of compensatory rapid respirations. Such periodic breathing should not be confused with **apnea,** which is a 15- to 20-second cessation of respiration. Physiologic indicators associated with apnea include cyanosis, pallor, hypotonia, or bradycardia (below 80 beats per minute). Causes of apnea include prematurity, infection, impaired oxygenation, thermal instability, maternal metabolic disorders, drugs, gastroesophageal reflux, and intracranial abnormalities (Holditch-Davis, Edwards, and Wigger, 1994; Martin, Fanaroff, and Klaus, 1993).

Respiratory distress may gradually decrease over 12 to 24 hours, with eventual recovery, or it may increase in severity. In distressed infants, cyanosis becomes more marked despite increases in ambient oxygen concentration. Often there is pallor caused by peripheral vasoconstriction, but it is often masked by cyanosis. The infant becomes flaccid and unresponsive and begins to display frequent apneic episodes. Chest auscultation reveals diminished breath sounds. The chances of recovery without assisted ventilation are then very small. Severe respiratory distress syndrome (RDS) is often associated with a shocklike state, as manifested by diminished cardiac inflow and low arterial blood pressure. The ELBW or VLBW infant, as a result of extreme pulmonary immaturity, decreased glycogen stores, and lack of accessory muscles, may have severe RDS at birth, therefore bypassing the aforementioned steps in the development of RDS.

Assessment tools. Important assessment tools include chest x-ray studies and laboratory tests. Since the cause of the respiratory distress cannot be determined by physical assessment alone, radiographic studies may reveal an underlying pathophysiologic cause such as a small pneumothorax (Wong, 1995). Blood gas results can reveal whether there is hypoxia or a metabolic imbalance, and such data can help the nurse evaluate the infant's overall status.

An accurate and timely blood pressure reading can assist in making an early diagnosis of cardiopulmonary disease and

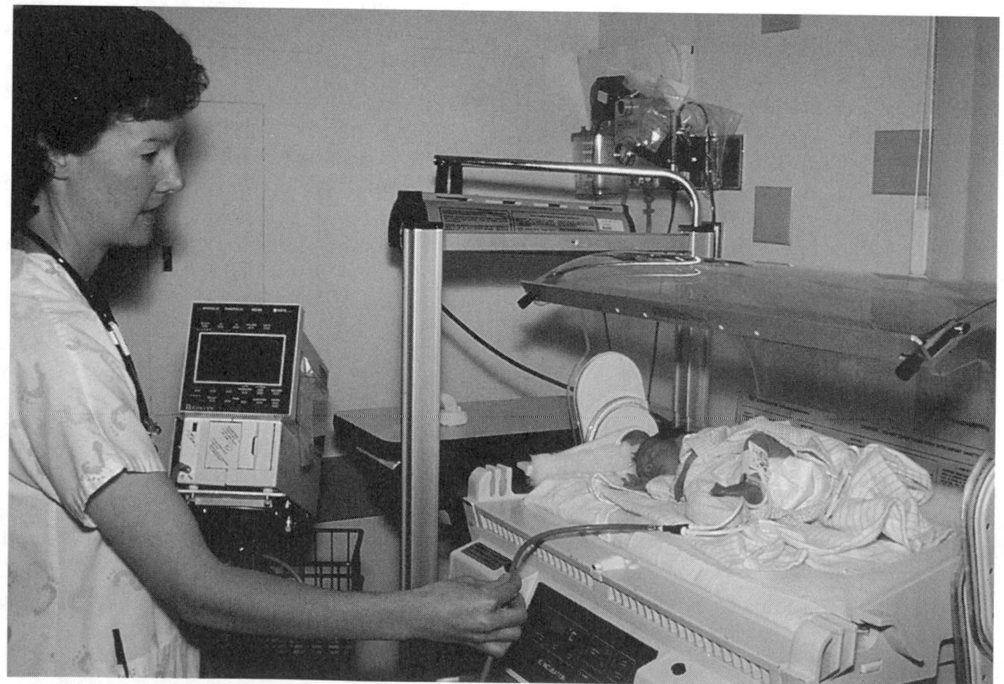

Fig. 25-1 Preparing to assess a newborn's blood pressure. Note stethoscopes for auscultation and electronic equipment. Blood pressure cuff should cover no more than 75% of the upper arm. (Courtesy Michael S. Clement, MD, Mesa, Ariz.)

in monitoring the effects of fluid therapy. Blood pressure readings can be obtained by the Doppler method or by an electronic monitor (Fig. 25-1). The monitor displays the systolic and diastolic values and the mean blood pressure (the reading midway between the diastolic and systolic pressures). An appropriate size of blood pressure cuff must be used (for example, 5 cm [2 in] wide, 15 cm [6 in] long) because an excessively wide cuff results in a falsely low reading and an excessively narrow cuff gives a falsely elevated reading. Smaller cuffs in keeping with the infant's arm size are required for premature infants. The normal systolic pressure for infants from 28 to 32 weeks' gestation is 52 mm Hg; that for term infants is up to 63 mm Hg, with a diastolic pressure of 26 to 36 mm Hg (Endo and Nishioka, 1993; Wong, 1995).

Other physiologic information, including the heart rate, respirations, and oxygen saturation, can be continuously monitored from a biometrics console using appropriate electrode attachments. To monitor heart and respiratory rates, cardiorespiratory electrodes are attached to the infant's trunk according to the manufacturer's instructions. Lead I, II, or III positions are common positions for the electrodes (Wong, 1995).

The placement of electrodes is a continual nursing problem because of the lack of flat areas on the neonate's chest and the limited space for alternating sites, the size of the electrodes, and irritation from the paste or tape. Electrodes for cardiac monitors can often be applied to the back or the upper arms to provide relief for chest areas; nonadhesive limb electrodes eliminate possible skin irritation from tape. Hydrogel electrodes are gentler to the skin and are easily removed by lifting an edge from the skin and moistening with plain water to release the adhesive. If the same electrode is reapplied to the skin, the hydrogel should be rinsed with plain water to remove accumulated sodium from perspiration, which can eventually irritate the skin. It is important to follow the manufacturer's directions for care and handling of electrodes to avoid mal function or burns to sensitive skin.

Invasive techniques such as umbilical artery catheterization and peripheral arterial puncture may be used for assessing acutely ill infants or for obtaining frequent, highly accurate results for the multidisciplinary team so that they can determine treatment options.

The **pulse oximeter** is a noninvasive monitor that measures the amount of oxygen carried by hemoglobin and can continuously assess the infant's oxygen level. A sensor, applied to any part of the infant's hand or foot, detects the amount of light (from the light source on the pulse oximeter) that passes through a vascular bed (Hagedorn, Gardner, and Abman, 1993). The monitor reads the amount of light absorbed by the oxygen-carrying hemoglobin and converts this into the saturation value. Phototherapy lights or sensor placement distal to a blood pressure cuff on an extremity may affect the reading.

Transcutaneous oxygen pressure monitoring (tcPO2) is a noninvasive means of monitoring oxygen tension for up to 4 hours at a time. The monitor probe is warmed from 42° to 45° C (107.6° to 113° F) before it is applied to stimulate faster oxygen diffusion through the skin, which may yield more accurate results. The electrodes are applied according to the manufacturer's instructions. Optimal sites are hairless and greaseless sites where an air-tight contact on the skin is possible. To prevent skin breakdown under the electrodes, the sites should also be in non–pressure-bearing areas (Hagedorn, Gardner, and Abman, 1993). In addition, infants should not be placed on top of the electrode because this compresses the capillary bed and causes poor tissue perfusion, which affects the correlation of the electrodes (Martin, Fanaroff, and Klaus, 1993).

Nursing Diagnoses

Some nursing diagnoses applicable to infants who have respiratory distress include the following:

- Impaired gas exchange related to
  - Pulmonary immaturity
- Ineffective airway clearance related to
  - Meconium aspiration
  - Respiratory infection (pneumonia)
  - Pulmonary immaturity or congenital disorder
  - Respiratory depression secondary to maternal sedation/analgesia
- Ineffective breathing pattern related to
  - Immaturity
  - Cold stress
- Ineffective thermoregulation related to
  - Physiologic immaturity
  - Large surface area to body mass ratio
  - Congenital disorder
- Altered nutrition, less than body requirements related to
  - Physiologic immaturity
  - Respiratory disorder
  - Congenital disorder
- Risk for altered parenting related to
  - Infant's physical condition at birth
  - Separation from infant

Expected Outcomes

The expected outcomes for an infant with respiratory problems include that the infant will do the following:

1. Maintain adequate gas exchange
2. Maintain a clear airway
3. Maintain an effective respiratory pattern

The expected outcomes for parents include that they will do the following:

1. Verbalize an understanding of the multidisciplinary team's basic plan of care for the infant
2. Demonstrate willingness to interact with infant through touch and verbal communication

Plan of Care and Implementation

Oxygen administration. Clinical criteria for identifying the need for oxygen administration include increased respiratory effort, respiratory distress with apnea, tachycardia, bradycardia, or central cyanosis with or without hypotonia. Additionally, the need for oxygen should be substantiated by biochemical data (arterial oxygen pressure [Pao_2] of less than 60 mm Hg or an oxygen saturation range of 89% to 92%). Continuous monitoring can reveal significant oxygen level changes, and steps can be taken to improve oxygenation and saturation as soon as possible.

BOX 25-3

Means of Administering Supplemental Oxygen

Hood therapy

Oxygen is piped into a clear plastic hood cover sized to fit over the head and neck of the infant (Fig. 25-2). Infant is protected from fluctuations in oxygen level that can occur when porthole of incubator is opened. Infant's vision may be altered by fine mist created by delivery of humidified oxygen. Nurse checks oxygen level every 1 to 2 hours and adjusts level as necessary based on infant's condition.

Nasal cannula

Nasal prongs are used when infant requires only low-flow oxygen. Infant receives an adequate, continuous flow of oxygen. Allows easier feedings and psychosocial interactions (Ludington-Hoe et al, 1994). Infant has unobstructed vision, can be positioned, held, and breastfed. Nurse checks nasal prongs regularly to ensure that they are not partially obstructed by milk or secretions. Nasal cannula can be used for home oxygen therapy.

Continuous positive airway pressure (CPAP)

CPAP infuses oxygen or air under a preset pressure (Fig. 25-3) by means of nasal prongs, a face mask, or an endotracheal tube. The pressure increases the alveolar volume by preventing the alveoli from collapsing on expiration. CPAP increases the functional residual capacity, improves the diffusion time of pulmonary gases, including oxygen, and can decrease pulmonary shunting. It can cause vascular shunting in the pulmonary beds, which can lead to persistent pulmonary hypertension and severe respiratory distress.

Mechanical ventilation

Mechanical ventilation is indicated when blood gas values reveal severe hypoxemia or severe hypercapnia (Fig. 25-4). Ventilator settings are determined by the infant's particular needs. The ventilator is set to provide a predetermined amount of oxygen to the infant during spontaneous respirations and to provide mechanical ventilation in the absence of spontaneous respirations. (A summary of common ventilator terminology is given in Box 25-4.)

Extracorporeal membrane therapy oxygenation (ECMO)

Infants with severe pulmonary dysfunction who are at more than 34 weeks gestation may be candidates for ECMO. ECMO uses cardiopulmonary bypass to oxygenate the infant's blood outside the body through a membrane oxygenator that serves as an artificial lung while the infant's lungs heal. Because of the massive systemic anticoagulation therapy required in the pump tubing and the increased risk for hemorrhage, the criteria for its use are very strict and the use of this therapy is limited. The risk for intraventricular hemorrhage in premature infants is high. ECMO has been used successfully in treatment of acute lung diseases including meconium aspiration syndrome and persistent pulmonary hypertension.

BOX 25-4

Definitions of Ventilator Terminology

Peak inspiratory pressure (PIP)

The peak level of pressure on inspiration. High pressures may cause overdistention,which can cause complications such as a pneumothorax.

Positive end-expiratory pressure (PEEP)

Creates mechanical continuous positive airway pressure (CPAP.) The therapeutic range is 3 to 8 cm H_2O (Wong, 1995).

Rate

The frequency with which the ventilator delivers the specified volume of gases (oxygen and air) to the infant. This provides the minimal number of breaths per minute needed for adequate oxygenation.

Inspiration/expiration ratio (I:E)

The amount of time during each breath spent on inspiration vs. expiration.

Mean airway pressure (MAP)

The amount of pressure exerted on the airway throughout the respiratory cycle. The average pressure is constant on high-frequency ventilators but varies during inspiratory and expiratory cycles on the conventional mode of ventilation.

Data from Hagedorn M, Gardner S, Abman S: *Respiratory distress.* In Merenstein G, Gardner S, editors: *Handbook of neonatal intensive care,* ed 3, St Louis, 1993, Mosby.

Oxygen administered to an infant is warmed and humidified to prevent cold stress and drying of the respiratory mucosa. During the administration of oxygen, the concentration, volume, temperature, and humidity of the gas are carefully controlled and monitored. Delivery of oxygen for more than a few minutes requires the use of special equipment (hood, nasal cannula, positive-pressure mask, or endotracheal tube [Box 25-3]) because the concentration of free-flow oxygen cannot be monitored accurately (Bloom and Cropley, 1994). In addition, free-flow oxygen into an incubator should not be used because the concentration fluctuates dramatically every time the doors or portholes are opened. The indiscriminant use of oxygen may be hazardous to the neonate. Possible complications of oxygen therapy include the retinopathy of prematurity and bronchopulmonary dysplasia.

Infants who need oxygen should have their respiratory status assessed accurately every 1 to 2 hrs, which should include a continuous pulse oximetry reading. Arterial or venous blood gases are drawn as the newborn's status warrants, with deterioration and/or improvement, and with changes in therapeutic interventions.

The interventions implemented are then determined on the basis of the findings yielded by the clinical assessment, including telemetry (pulse oximetry) and laboratory tests (Hagedorn, Gardner, and Abman, 1993; Wong, 1995). The interventions ordered are those that can directly manage the underlying disease process, and range from hood oxygen administration to ventilator therapy.

Respiratory assistance is withdrawn slowly as the infant's status improves. The infant is ready to be weaned from respiratory assistance once the arterial blood gas and oxygen saturation levels are maintained within normal limits. A spontaneous, adequate respiratory effort must be present, and the

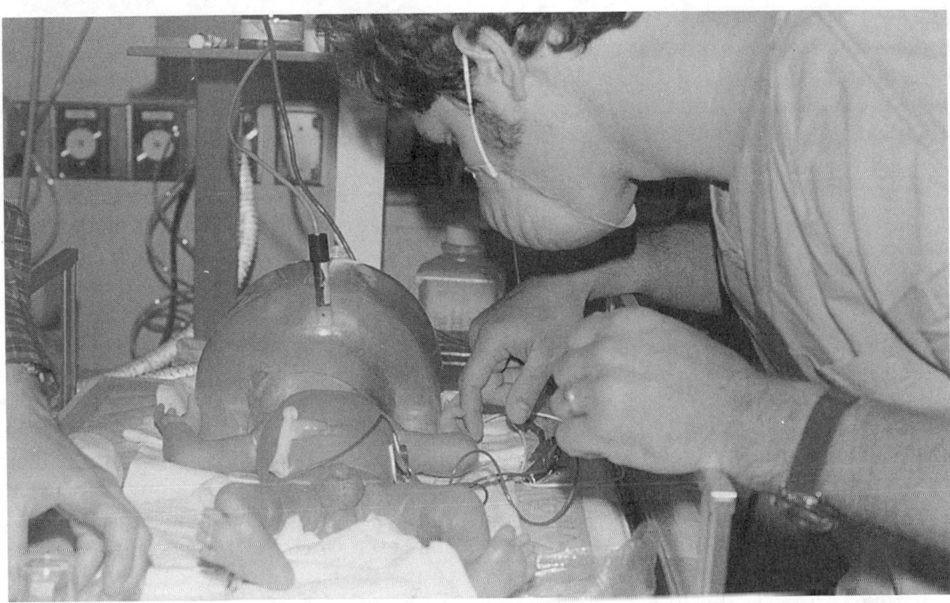

Fig. 25-2 Father interacting with his baby by touch. Note use of oxygen hood and overbed warmer. Infant's head is turned away to decrease visual stimulation. (Courtesy Marjorie Pyle, RNC, Lifecircle, Costa Mesa, Calif.)

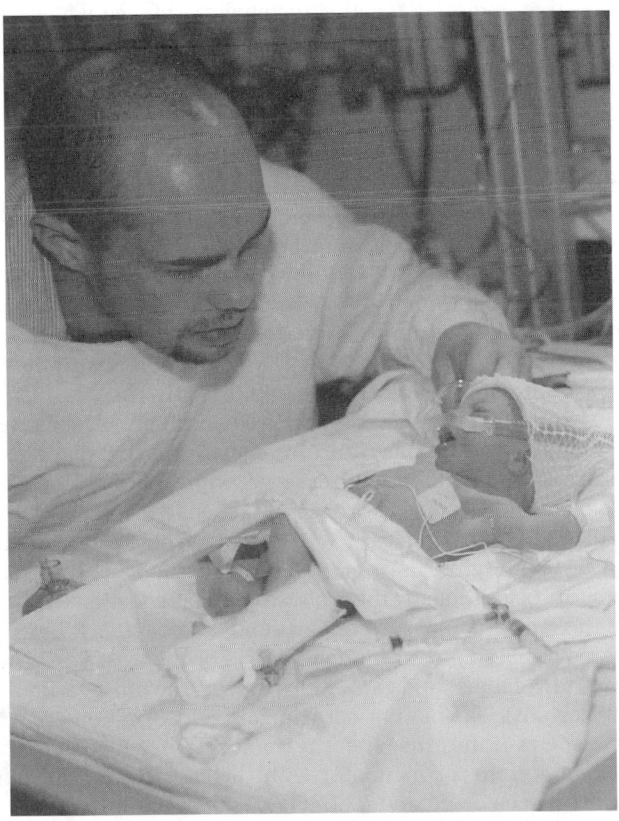

Fig. 25-3 Father interacting with his infant by touch and eye contact. Note nasal CPAP tube, double stockinette cap, pectin-based electrocardiogram lead pads, and right wrist oximeter probe. Arms are restrained to prevent infant from dislodging the CPAP tube. (Courtesy family of Daniel Jonathan Cragin and Dale Ikuta, photographer, San Jose, Calif.)

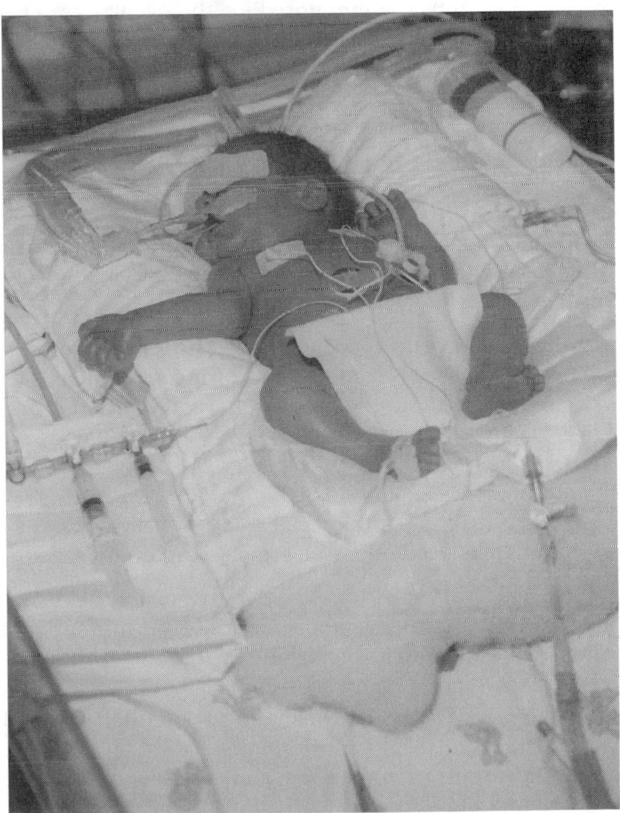

Fig. 25-4 Ventilator-dependent infant. Note phototherapy mask over eyes, pectin-based electrocardiogram lead pads, temperature probe on abdomen, umbilical line, urinary catheter drainage system, and right foot oximeter probe. (Courtesy Dale Ikuta, photographer, San Jose, Calif.)

infant must also show improved muscle tone during increased activity. Weaning is done in a stepwise and gradual manner. This may consist of the infant being extubated, placed on continuous positive airway pressure (CPAP), and then weaned to oxygen by means of a hood or nasal cannula. Throughout the weaning process the infant's oxygen levels are monitored by pulse oximetry and blood gas levels.

The parents need to be given consistent information and to be reassured about the infant's respiratory progress. Decisions regarding the nature of continued interventions should be included in a multidisciplinary plan of care, and the therapy should be frequently explained to the family. Daily or even hourly updates are imperative, especially if unexpected complications arise.

Surfactant administration. Surfactant can be administered as an adjunct to oxygen and ventilation therapy. Before 34 weeks' gestation, most infants do not produce enough surfactant to survive extrauterine life (Hagedorn, Gardner, and Abman, 1993). As a result, lung compliance is decreased and not enough gas exchange occurs as the lungs become atelectatic and require greater pressures to expand. By administering artificial surfactant, respiratory compliance is improved until the infant can generate enough surfactant on its own. Exogenous surfactant is manufactured from human, porcine, or bovine amniotic fluid and is given in several doses through an endotracheal tube (Wong, 1995). As with any drug therapy, the infant must be monitored for the occurrence of potential side effects such as a patent ductus arteriosus and pulmonary hemorrhage. Use of this drug has been associated with a significantly reduced length of time on ventilators and oxygen therapy, and an increased survival rate in premature infants (Mauskopf et al, 1995).

Evaluation

The nurse can be reasonably assured that the respiratory care of the infant was effective if the following expected outcomes for care have been met:

1. Respiratory efforts provide adequate gas exchange, and the airway remains clear during spontaneous respiration without the need for assisted ventilation or oxygen
2. All causes of the infant's respiratory problems have been identified and treated
3. The nutritional intake is adequate to provide for the metabolic needs of tissue repair, maintenance, and growth

The nurse can be reasonably assured that nursing interventions were effective in supporting the parents if the following expected outcomes have been met:

4. The parents perceive the infant as potentially normal (if this is medically substantiated)
5. The parents begin bonding and attachment to the infant

Thermoregulatory Care

After, or concurrent with, the establishment of respiration, the most crucial need of high-risk infants is the application of external warmth. To delay or prevent the effects of cold stress, infants are placed in a heated environment immediately after birth; they remain there until they are able to maintain thermal stability (balance heat production and conservation with heat dissipation). This is especially important for the preterm infant, whose ability to prevent heat loss and subsequently produce sufficient heat is inadequate.

Since overheating produces an increase in oxygen and calorie consumption, the infant is also jeopardized if he or she becomes hyperthermic. A **neutral thermal environment** is one that permits the infant to maintain a normal core temperature, with minimum oxygen consumption and calorie expenditure.

When the thermal receptors in the infant's skin are stimulated by cold, the infant attempts to minimize the loss and increase heat production. In healthy term infants this is accomplished by vasoconstriction of the peripheral blood vessels and flexion of the extremities, the latter decreasing the exposed skin surface. Heat is also generated by increasing physical activity (e.g., crying, becoming hyperactive) or metabolism (Thomas, 1994). The infant's face is particularly sensitive to cold; even when the infant's body is warm, cooling of the face causes the basal metabolic rate to rise.

Infants depend on brown fat deposits for the generation of additional heat, unlike adults who shiver to increase metabolic rate (Thomas, 1994). Although brown adipose tissue is present as early as 26 weeks' gestation, there may not be enough for adequate thermoregulation to occur until the infant is closer to term. The amount of oxygen needed for the metabolism of this adipose tissue is up to three times more than that required for the metabolism of regular tissue (Wong, 1995). In a heat-losing environment, therefore, not only can the healthy term infant's stores of substrate, such as glycogen and fat, be quickly depleted, but this can lead rapidly to acidosis and respiratory failure.

The premature or otherwise compromised infant is even more susceptible to heat loss and its attendant complications. In addition, low-birth-weight infants may be unable to increase their metabolic rate because of impaired gas exchange, caloric intake restrictions, or poor thermoregulation. Transepidermal water loss is greater because of skin immaturity in very premature infants (those at less than 28 weeks' gestation) (Endo and Nishioka, 1993) and can contribute to temperature instability.

Maintaining the thermoneutral environment is facilitated by monitoring the temperature from an overhead radiant heat source or an incubator with a servocontrol mechanism. The temperature-monitoring probe is attached to the infant's skin in the right upper quadrant of the abdomen below the right or left costal margin. However, the nurse should assess the skin integrity before placing the probe so that complications caused by the tape and pressure are prevented. Poor sites for probe placement are bony prominences (one of the least vasoreactive body regions) and extremities (one of the most vasoreactive regions). The plan of care must include rotation and reassessment of the probe site. The nurse sets the set point of the radiant warmer or incubator with the servocontrol mechanism between 36.5° and 37.0° C (97.6° to 99.0° F).

Nursing ALERT

When using a servocontrolled incubator, evaluate trends of increased or decreased ambient air temperature in response to fluctuations in the infant's body temperature to rule out sepsis or other dysfunction.

Nursing Care Management

The infant's body and extremities are assessed by touch because the skin temperature usually is the first to decrease. The infant is also assessed for physiologic signs of cold stress. Mature infants respond to cold by increasing their physical activity and crying. Immature or stressed infants may initially respond by increasing their respiratory rate. Generalized cyanosis, skin mottling and prolonged capillary refill may also be evidence of cold stress. Significantly compromised neonates may be lethargic and show increasingly severe spells of apnea and bradycardia (Klaus, Martin, and Fanaroff, 1993).

Because the signs and symptoms of temperature instability resemble those of a neonatal infection, however, an infant showing some of these signs and symptoms must also be assessed for infection. Results of laboratory tests such as a complete blood count (CBC) and measurement of the C-reactive protein (CRP) level can be used to determine whether such an infant has sepsis (Bailey and Goldfarb, 1993). An immature-to-mature neutrophil ratio that exceeds 0.20 and a CRP level of more than 1.0 mg/dl indicates the existence of an infection.

The preferred route for determining an infant's temperature is the axillary one. In the cold-stressed term neonate, the metabolism of brown fat in the axillary area may cause the readings to be falsely high. This is not the case in severely premature infants who have minimal brown fat, however. The rectal route is contraindicated because rectal perforation can occur if the thermometer is inserted the 5 cm (2 in) needed for an accurate reading to be obtained (Blake and Murray, 1993; Wong, 1995). Inguinal or tympanic routes may also be used. (Bliss-Holtz, 1993; Wells et al, 1995).

Nursing diagnoses related to thermoregulation include the following:

- Ineffective thermoregulation related to
  - Physiologic immaturity
  - Poorly controlled environment (temperature or location of room, equipment, warmer, or incubator)
  - Infection
- Risk for apnea, hypoglycemia, or acidosis related to
  - Cold stress
  - Infection

Nursing care. Nursing care is implemented to prevent or minimize temperature instability, especially cold stress. The first action a nurse takes in the birth room is to quickly dry the infant with a prewarmed, absorbent blanket, taking particular care to dry and cover the infant's head, which constitutes 21% of the infant's total body surface area. To prevent evaporative heat loss, the damp blanket is removed and the infant is then wrapped in a clean, dry one (Wong, 1995). To help maintain the newborn's temperature when the infant's condition permits, the infant can be placed in skin-to-skin contact with a parent. The parent's temperature will increase in response to a decrease in the infant's temperature during skin-to-skin contact, a phenomenon known as *thermal synchrony.* In this way the parent's body can serve as an external heat source for the infant (Ludington-Hoe et al, 1994).

When assessments or interventions are necessary, the unwrapped infant is placed in a prewarmed incubator with a servocontrol mechanism, under a radiant warmer, or on a warm surface. The use of prewarmed and properly functioning equipment helps prevent conduction heat loss. A double-walled incubator, a plastic tent, or bubble paper can also be used to help protect the infant from drafts while under a radiant heat source (Figs. 25-5 and 25-6). The portholes on the incubator are kept closed, except during direct care of the infant and parent-infant interactions. Warmers and incubators are placed away from windows, fans, and air-conditioning units, which are sources of drafts, heat, and cold (Klaus, Martin, and Fanaroff, 1993).

All surfaces and materials that the infant comes in contact with must be warm, including the nurse's hands and the stethoscope. Oxygen and air are also warmed before they are administered to the neonate. The infant's head may be kept covered with a hooded blanket or a cap. Stockinette caps should be at least double layered to adequately prevent heat loss (Klaus, Martin, and Fanaroff, 1993).

The infant's axillary temperature is assessed periodically and compared with that on the display panel. Both the axillary and display panel temperature readings are documented. The skin probe is reapplied if it becomes wet or detached.

Any temperature that is above or below the normal range is reported. In addition, the nurse should modify the environment by adjusting clothes, blankets, and thermostat settings to restore the desired body temperature.

Warming the hypothermic infant. Rapid changes in body temperature may cause apnea and acidosis in the neonate. Therefore the warming of a hypothermic infant should occur over a 2- to 4-hour period (Klaus, Martin, and Fanaroff, 1993). To accomplish this, the infant is placed either under a radiant warmer or in an incubator with a servocontrol mechanism. To ensure an optimal response during warming, the servocontrol thermostat should be increased incrementally by 0.3° C (1° F) more than each skin temperature measured. When the skin temperature reaches at least 36.5° C (97.6° F), the servocontrol thermostat is then reset to maintain a thermoneutral environment.

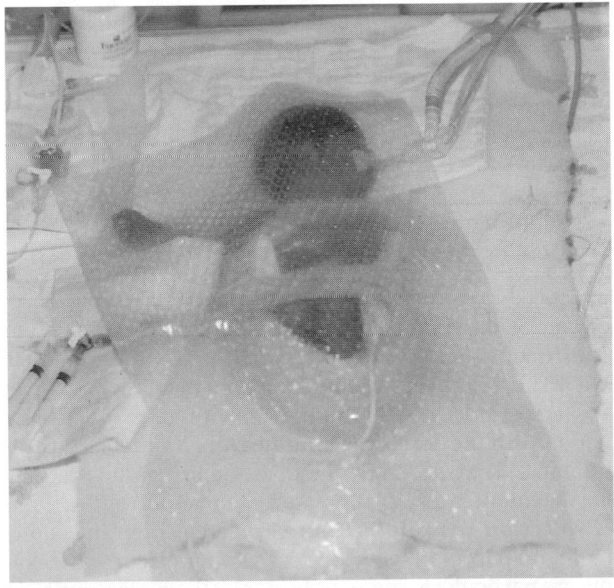

Fig. 25-5 Infant under bubble paper to ensure a draft-free environment and to prevent insensible water loss. Note nest made around infant's body to position and comfort the infant. (Courtesy Dale Ikuta, photographer, San Jose, Calif.)

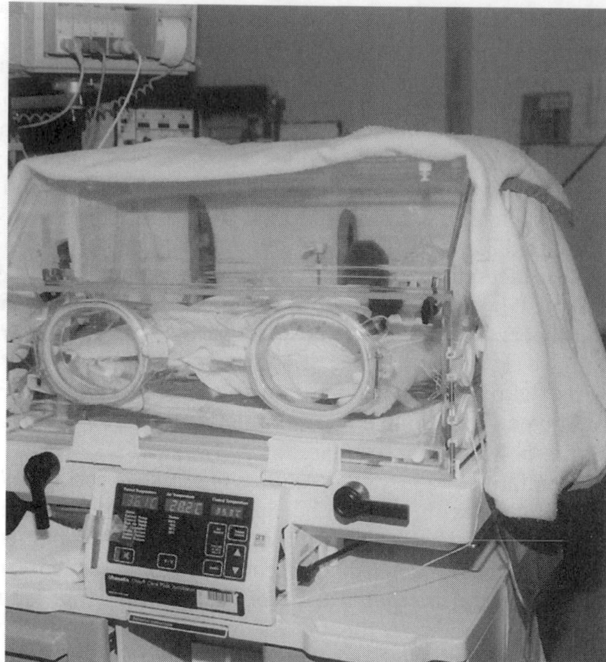

Fig. 25-6 Infant swaddled in double-walled incubator with a blanket for a light shield. (Courtesy Dale Ikuta, photographer, San Jose, Calif.)

Weaning the infant from the incubator. To wean the infant from the incubator, the incubator heat is decreased slowly over at least several hours. Infants weighing more than 1500 g who show stable self-regulation of their temperature are candidates for weaning (Gelhar et al, 1994). The nurse carries out the following measures to wean the infant from the incubator:

- Dresses the infant in a diaper, shirt, and double-thickness cap
- Lowers the incubator temperature by no more than 0.5 degree per each 2-hour period
- Records the temperature of both the infant and incubator
- Assesses the infant's responses to the changes every 15 minutes until four stable readings are obtained
- Monitors the infant's temperature and other vital signs

This procedure is repeated until the incubator temperature is the same as the room temperature and the infant's skin temperature consistently remains above 36.5° C (97.6° F) (Meier, 1994). The infant is placed in an open bassinet when the axillary temperature is stable, after which it is reassessed in conjunction with the delivery of routine care. If necessary, the infant may be returned to the incubator and weaning repeated once the infant is able to regulate its temperature.

Protection from infection. Protection from infection is an integral part of all newborn care, but preterm and sick infants are particularly susceptible to infectious organisms. Frequent and meticulous handwashing between handling of different infants and their equipment by all persons who come in contact with them is the foundation of a preventive program.

Nursing ALERT

The increased use of gloves for Standard Precautions does not eliminate the need for careful handwashing between handling neonates and between areas considered "dirty" (i.e., diapers) and "clean" (bottle feeding, intravenous drug administration).

Personnel with known infectious disorders are barred from the unit until they are no longer infectious. Standard precautions as a method of infection control are instituted in all nursery areas to protect the infants and staff. In some areas special clothing furnished by the institution is worn by everyone working in the unit. Fresh scrub dresses or suits are put on before entering the unit and are changed any time they become contaminated.

The sources of infection rise in direct relationship to the number of persons and pieces of equipment coming in contact with the infants. Equipment used in the care of infants is cleaned on a regular basis as per the manufacturer's recommendations or institutional protocol; this includes cleaning of cribs, mattresses, incubators, radiant warmers, cardiorespiratory monitors, pulse oximeters, and Dinamap monitors after use with one infant and before use with another. Since organisms thrive best in water, plumbing and humidifying equipment are particularly hazardous. Disposable equipment used for water-related therapies, such as nebulizers and plastic oxygen tubing, is changed regularly.

Nutritional Care

Effectively meeting the infant's individualized nutritional requirements promotes growth and healing. To ensure adequate nutrition, the nurse monitors the infant's total nutritional intake, including proper amounts of carbohydrates, proteins, and fats. Both breast milk and current commercial formulas provide the correct proportions of nutrients (Lien, 1994; Wong, 1995), although breast milk is the optimal source for most infants.

It is not always possible to provide enteral (by the gastrointestinal route) nourishment to a compromised infant, however. Such infants may be too ill or weak to breastfeed or bottle feed because of respiratory distress, sepsis, or prematurity (Blackburn and VandenBerg, 1993; Price and Kalhan, 1993). Early enteral feeding of the distressed neonate is also avoided to prevent bowel necrosis. In such cases, nutrition is provided parenterally. Those infants who require parenteral nutrition may have one or more of the following problems (Schanler, Shulman and Prestridge, 1994; Townsend, Johnson, and Hay, 1993):

- Lack of a coordinated suck-and-swallow reflex.
- Inability to suck because of a congenital anomaly.
- Respiratory distress requiring aggressive oxygen and/or ventilator support.
- A potential for necrotizing enterocolitis.

Nursing Care Management

The infant's tolerance of the feedings or parenteral nutrition is assessed by noting any weight gain or loss and types of elimination. Oral feedings are provided when the infant is able to coordinate sucking, swallowing, and breathing without physiologic compromise. The documentation of oral feedings includes the following:

- Type of feeding (breast or bottle)
- Evaluation of feeding
  - Strength and duration of suck
  - Length of time on each breast
  - Amount of formula taken (record number of calories per 30 ml of formula or per any special formula concentration) and time required for the feeding
- Vomiting or regurgitation with estimated volume
- Presence of cyanosis (circumoral or general)
- Presence of abdominal distention
- Effect on respirations

If instituting feeding by a gavage or a gastrostomy tube, the amount of residual food in the stomach (undigested or partially digested breast milk or formula) is first assessed by aspirating the stomach contents. The color, amount, character of any vomitus or regurgitation, time in relation to feeding, and presence of mucus are recorded. Daily weights, the volume of fluid consumed, and the caloric consumption are all assessed in infants receiving enteral and/or parenteral nutrition.

Types of nourishment. The types of formulas used, the mode and volume of feeding, and the feeding schedule of the infant are determined on the basis of the findings yielded by the assessment of the following variables:

- Initially, the birth weight, then the current weight of the compromised infant
- Pattern of weight gain or loss (infants weighing less than 1500 g require more energy for growth and thermoregulation and may gain weight poorly with either breastfeedings or bottle feedings)
- Presence or absence of suck-and-swallow reflex in all infants less than 35 weeks' gestation (Lefrak-Okikawa, and Meier, 1993)
- Demonstrated behavioral readiness to take oral feedings (Cagan, 1995)
- Physical condition, including presence or absence of bowel sounds, abdominal distention, or bloody stools, as well as presence and degree of respiratory distress or apneic episodes (Price and Kalhan, 1993)
- Residual from previous feeding, if being gavage fed
- Renal function, including urinary output and laboratory values (nitrogen balance, electrolyte balance, glucose level). Premature infants are especially susceptible to altered renal function (Schanler, Shulman, and Prestridge, 1994)

The infant's ability to tolerate the solute and fluid load is also assessed. Complications, including feeding intolerance and metabolic imbalances, may arise from inappropriate nutritional intake and the nurse should assess the infant for these (Price and Kalhan, 1993).

Weight and fluid loss or gain. For many reasons, the caloric, nutrient, and fluid requirements of compromised infants are greater than those of the term, normal newborn. One reason is that premature or dysmature newborns often have limited stores of nutrients and fluids. In addition, symptomatic or asymptomatic hypoglycemia (Box 25-5), electrolyte imbalances, or other metabolic disturbances can develop in an infant whose nutritional intake is poor. Such hypoglycemia may cause serious damage to glucose-dependent brain cells. Weight gain or loss in such infants is therefore monitored carefully to detect any need for a change in the therapy.

BOX 25-5
Clinical Signs Often Associated with Neonatal Hypoglycemia*

Apneic spells
Cardiac arrest
Cardiac failure
Cyanotic spells
High-pitched or weak cry
Hypothermia
Irritability
Lethargy or stupor
Limpness
Refusal to feed
Seizures
Tremors or jitteriness

From Fanaroff A, Martin R, editors: *Neonatal-perinatal medicine: diseases of the fetus and infant*, ed 6, St Louis, 1997, Mosby.
*The clinical sign should be alleviated with concomitant correction of the glucose level.

The infant's weight is measured and recorded daily, and the rate of weight loss or gain is calculated. Further depletion of weight and metabolic stores can occur as a result of one or a combination of the following factors:

- Increased respirations or respiratory effort
- Patent ductus arteriosus
- Hypothermic environment
- Insensible fluid loss caused by evaporation (with radiant heat or phototherapy)
- Vomiting, diarrhea, and dysfunctional absorption from the gastrointestinal tract
- Growth demands (a premature infant's growth rate approximates that of fetal growth during the last trimester and is at least two times faster than a term infant's growth rate after birth)
- Inability of the renal system to concentrate urine and maintain an adequate rate of urea excretion, as well as by an infant's inadequate response to antidiuretic hormone

The high-risk newborn is predisposed to have weight and fluid losses because of the greater amount of fluid needed to meet the demands of the increased cellular metabolic processes (resulting from stress, repair, or growth). The body weight of premature infants weighing less than 1500 g consists of 83% to 89% water, compared with the term infant's water content of 75% (Price and Kalhan, 1993). Most of this water is in the extracellular fluid compartment. Even with the early institution of fluid and nutrition intake, the premature infant's weight and fluid losses seem exaggerated. Inadequate fluid intake, resulting from either delayed administration or insufficient volume, can further cause weight and fluid losses and electrolyte disturbances in the premature infant.

Insensible water loss (IWL) is an evaporative loss that occurs largely through the skin. Approximately 30% of this

IWL comes from the respiratory tract. The total IWL in a normal infant ranges anywhere from 30 to 60 ml/kg/24 hr (Blake and Murray, 1993). This quantity can increase to up to 300% per day, depending on the infant's gestational age and skin integrity. The effects of radiant warmers, incubators, phototherapy, and other factors can augment the IWL. Some of this loss can be prevented by humidifying the oxygen administered to such compromised infants.

During the first week of extrauterine life, the premature infant can lose up to 15% of its birth weight. In contrast, a weight loss of up to only 10% is acceptable in a term, AGA infant (Price and Kalhan, 1993). After the initial week, a premature infant's loss or gain during each 24-hour period should not exceed 2% of the previous day's weight.

A method of calculating a weight gain or loss is presented in Box 25-6. If the calculations reveal a weight loss, the nurse should investigate the infant's environment to try to identify potential causes. These include increased stooling or voiding, increased evaporative losses, inadequate volume or incorrect fluid administration, and problems with malabsorption.

Interventions to correct these problems include adjusting the incubator temperature, monitoring and adjusting the volume and type of fluids being administered, assessing the urine output, including the specific gravity, and assessing the blood glucose levels. The glucose determinations are used to assess urine osmolarity, and hence renal function. High glucose levels (greater than 125 mg/dl) can stimulate an excessive osmotic diuresis (Wong, 1995).

If excessive weight gain occurs, the nurse assesses the infant to make sure overfeeding or fluid retention is not occurring. The nurse reports and records these findings and continues to assess the infant's fluid status, urine output, and blood glucose levels. The interventions implemented are determined by the infant's specific disorder and nutritional needs.

Elimination patterns. The infant's elimination patterns are also assessed. This includes the frequency of urination, as well as the amount, color, pH, and specific gravity of the urine. The assessment of the infant's bowel movements includes the frequency of stooling and the character of the stool, as well as whether there is constipation, diarrhea, or loss of fats (steatorrhea). All of these findings are documented. The nurse may request guaiac tests to assess for blood in the stool, tests to detect stool-reducing substances, and a pH determination to assess for malabsorption (Townsend, Johnson, and Hay, 1993; Wong, 1995). Infants with abdominal distention are assessed carefully to rule out the presence of hypomotility or obstructions of the gastrointestinal tract. Examples of nursing diagnoses pertaining to nutrition and elimination include the following:

- Altered nutrition, less than body requirements, related to
  - Physiologic dysmaturity
  - Immaturity
- Fluid volume deficit or overload related to
  - Immaturity or neonatal disorder
- Ineffective breathing pattern related to
  - Abdominal distention

BOX 25-6
Calculation of a Weight Loss or Gain

Example 1

Day 4 1750 g
Day 5 1730 g
20-g loss

$$\frac{20}{1750} = \frac{X\%}{100\%}$$

1750X = 2000

$1750\overline{)2000.0}$ = 1.1

X = 1.1% weight loss

Example 2

Day 4 1750 g
Day 5 1790 g
40-g gain

$$\frac{40}{1750} = \frac{X\%}{100\%}$$

1750X = 4000

$1750\overline{)4000.00}$ = 2.3

X = 2.3% weight gain

Nursing Care. Nourishment by the oral route is preferred for the infant who has adequate strength and gastrointestinal function. Breast milk may be fed by breast, bottle, intermittent gavage, or by continuous flow using a pump and feeding tube (inserted into the stomach or jejunum). Formula may be fed by the latter three routes, or by a supplementor (see Fig. 24-10). Throughout the feeding, the nurse assesses the newborn's tolerance to the procedure. When the infant breastfeeds, the nurse assists the mother by providing support and help, as necessary.

The needs of the high-risk infant must be considered when determining the type and frequency of the feedings. Many high-risk infants cannot suck well enough to breastfeed or bottle feed until they have recovered from their initial illness or matured physically (greater than 32 weeks' gestational age). Mothers of high-risk infants are encouraged to continue pumping breast milk, especially if theirs is a very premature infant who may not breastfeed for many weeks (Janke, 1994; Townsend, Johnson, and Hay, 1993). Because of the significant breastfeeding attrition rates among these mothers, they need support and encouragement every few days to continue pumping while their infant is not yet able to nurse. If there is no available breast milk (from the mother), commercial formula is used. The calories, protein, and mineral content of commercial formulas vary (see Chapter 24). The type of nipple selected ("preemie," regular, orthodontic) depends on the infant's ability to suck from the specific type of nipple. The nurse also considers the energy the infant needs to expend in the process.

Overfeeding of the high-risk infant should be avoided because this can lead to distention, with apnea, vomiting, and possibly aspiration of the feeding. The residual gastric aspirate is measured to determine whether overfeeding is occurring. Residuals of less than a quarter of a feeding can be refed to the infant to prevent the loss of gastric electrolytes. Feeding is stopped if the residual is greater than a quarter of the feeding and is not resumed until the infant can be assessed for a possible feeding intolerance (Townsend, Johnson, and Hay, 1993). The nurse also monitors the infant's abdominal girth when distention is obvious.

Gavage feeding. **Gavage feeding** is a method of providing nourishment to the infant who is compromised by respiratory distress, the infant who is too immature to have a coordinated suck-and-swallow reflex, or the infant who is easily fatigued by sucking. In gavage feeding, breast milk or formula is given to the infant through a nasogastric or orogastric tube. This spares the infant the work of sucking.

Gavage feeding can be done either with an intermittently placed tube or continuously through an indwelling feeding tube. Infants who cannot tolerate large bolus feedings are given continuous feedings. Breast milk or formula can be supplied intermittently using a syringe with gravity-controlled flow, or can be given continuously using an infusion pump. The volume of the continuous feedings is recorded hourly and the residual gastric aspirate measured every 4 hours. The type of fluid instilled is recorded with every syringe change.

The orogastric route for gavage feedings is preferred, because most infants are preferential nose breathers. However, some infants do not tolerate oral tube placement. A small nasogastric feeding tube can be placed in older infants who would otherwise gag or vomit or in ones who are learning to suck (Townsend, Johnson, and Hay, 1993). To insert the tube the nurse should follow the sequence given in the Guidelines box below.

To begin the feeding, the nurse connects the barrel of a syringe to the gavage tube. While crimping the feeding tube, the nurse pours the specified amount of breast milk or formula

Guidelines

INSERTING A GAVAGE FEEDING TUBE

1. Measure the length of the gavage tube:
   a. From the tip of the nose.
   b. To the lobe of the ear, and
   c. Down to the upper abdomen (Fig. 25-7, *A*).
2. Mark the tube with a piece of tape on the centimeter mark (average 16 to 18 cm), then
   a. Lubricate the tip of the tube with sterile water, and
   b. Insert gently (to avoid tissue trauma) through the mouth or nare (Fig. 25-7, *B*).
   c. Guide the tube down the esophagus until the predetermined mark is reached.
3. Correct placement of the tube can be checked before instilling any fluid by either:
   a. Injecting a small amount of air (1 to 3 ml) into the tube, while simultaneously listening for sounds of gurgling, or by using a stethoscope placed over the stomach area.
   b. Pulling back on the plunger to aspirate stomach contents to check for previous feeding or mucus. Lack of fluid is not necessarily evidence of improper placement.
4. Tape the tube in place and also tape it to the cheek to prevent accidental dislodgement and incorrect positioning (Fig. 25-7, *C*).
   a. Assess the infant's skin integrity before taping the tube.
   b. Edematous or very premature infants need to have a pectin barrier placed under the tape to prevent abrasions (Kuller and Lund, 1993).
5. Tube placement must be assessed before each feeding.
   a. Placement of the tube in the trachea will cause the infant to gag, cough, or become cyanotic (Townsend, Johnson, and Hay, 1993).
   b. Aspiration of respiratory secretions may be mistaken for stomach contents (Metheny et al, 1994).
   c. Check the length of the tube, because it is possible to hear air entering the stomach even if the tube is positioned above the gastroesophageal (cardiac) sphincter (Wong, 1995).

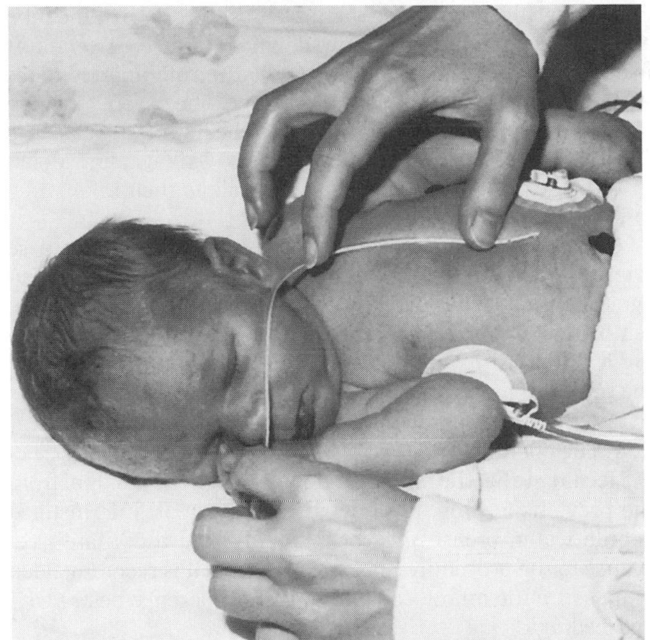

A

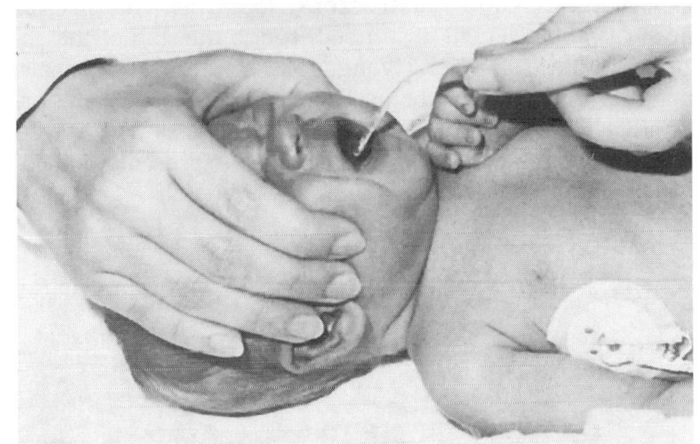

B

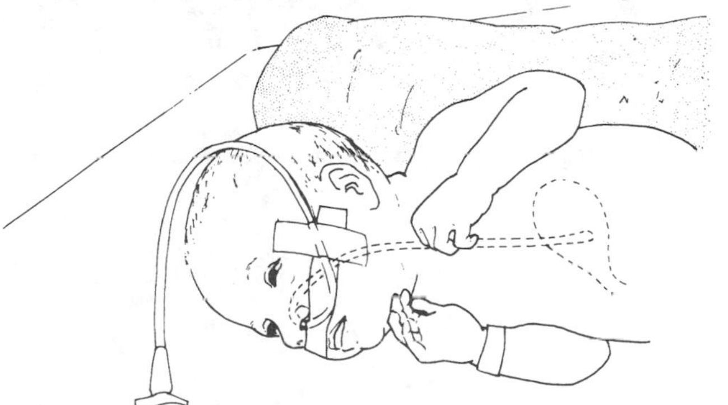

C

Fig. 25-7 Gavage feeding. **A,** Measurement of gavage feeding tube from tip of nose to earlobe and to midpoint between end of xiphoid process and umbilicus. Tape may be used to mark the correct length on the tube. **B,** Insertion of gavage tube using orogastric route. **C,** Indwelling gavage tube nasogastric route. After feeding, infant is propped on right side for 1 hour to facilitate emptying of stomach into small intestine. Note rolled towel for support.

into the syringe. The nurse then releases the crimp in the tube and allows the feeding to flow down by gravity. The infant usually tolerates the feeding better if the rate approximates that of an oral feeding (about 1 ml/min). The parent or nurse can swaddle or hold the infant to help the infant associate the feeding with positive interactions (Lefrak-Okikawa and Meier, 1993). The parents are encouraged to talk to their infant during the feedings.

Once the prescribed volume has been delivered, the nurse crimps or pinches the tube and removes the syringe. The gavage tube is capped (or the nurse continues to pinch it) while removing it in one steady motion. Capping the tube (or pinching it off) prevents breast milk or formula from leaking from the tube and being aspirated during removal of the tube.

After the feeding the infant is positioned to prevent aspiration. The documentation of the procedure includes the size of the feeding tube, the amount and quality of the residual from the previous feeding, the type and quantity of fluid instilled (sterile water, breast milk, or formula), and the infant's response to the procedure. In some instances it is recommended to measure the infant's abdominal circumference before gavage feedings.

Gastrostomy feedings. Infants with certain congenital malformations require **gastrostomy feedings.** This involves the surgical placement of a tube through the skin of the abdomen into the stomach (Wong, 1995). After the site heals, the nurse initiates small bolus feedings per the physician's orders (Fig. 25-8). Feedings by gravity are done slowly over 20 to 30 minutes. Special care must be taken to prevent rapid bolusing of the fluid because this may lead to bloating, gastrointestinal reflux into the esophagus, or respiratory compromise. Meticulous skin care at the tube insertion site is necessary to prevent skin breakdown or infection. In addition, intake and output are monitored scrupulously because these infants are prone to diarrhea until regular feedings are established.

Feeding the newborn with a cleft lip or palate. Feeding the infant with a cleft lip or palate poses a special challenge to nurses and families. These defects reduce the infant's ability to suck, which interferes with compression of the areola or nipple, and usually makes both breastfeeding and bottlefeeding difficult, time consuming, and laborious. Such infants may have other anomalies, such as a cyanotic heart lesion, which may also affect feedings. Aspiration is one of the major concerns in the feeding of infants with a cleft lip or palate. Liquid taken into the mouth has a tendency to escape by means of the cleft through the nose. For these reasons, feeding is best accomplished with the infant's head in an upright position (Wong, 1995). The infant must be fed slowly and burped more often to prevent excessive retention of the air taken in with swallowing.

The type of feeding equipment used and the rate of feeding depends on the particular infant. Regular nipples often do not work for these infants because they do not allow the infant to generate the suction required. Special nipples or other feeding devices that circumvent these problems are available. These nipples work either by covering the defect or by carrying the fluid beyond the defect (Fig. 25-9). Occasionally, gavage feedings may be needed to supplement the oral feedings in these

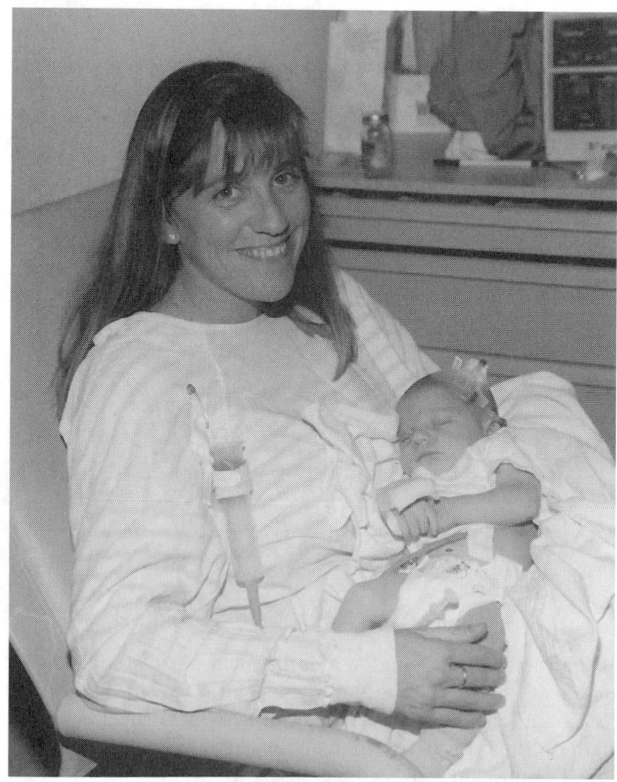

Fig. 25-8 Mother feeding infant by gastrostomy tube. Note peripheral scalp IV and armboard for peripheral TPN. (Courtesy Dale Ikuta, photographer, San Jose, Calif.)

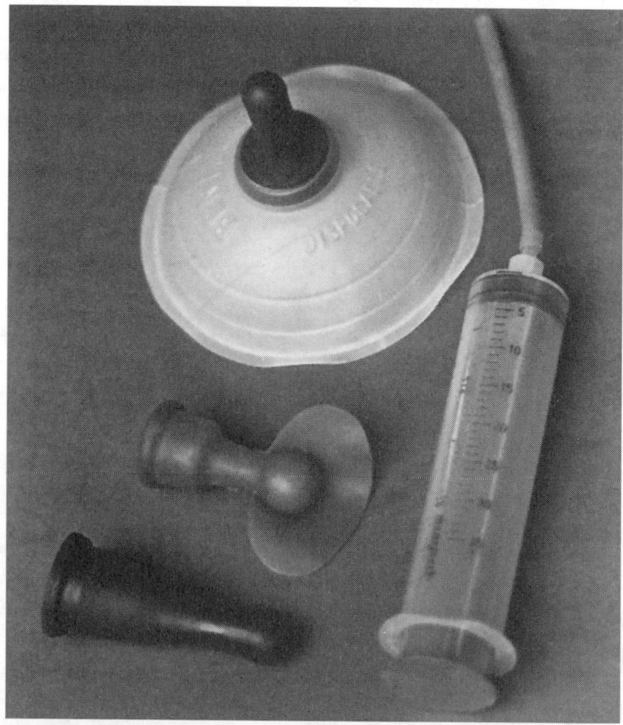

Fig. 25-9 Some devices used to feed infant with cleft palate. Clockwise, Lamb's nipple, flanged nipple, special nurser, and syringe with rubber tubing (Breck feeder). (From Wong D: *Whaley & Wong's essentials of pediatric nursing*, ed 5, St Louis, 1997, Mosby.)

infants. It has been demonstrated that such infants, when appropriate sucking, swallowing and breathing are present, tolerate breastfeeding better than bottle feeding.

Surgical repair of the cleft lip usually is performed soon after birth. Infants with no other anomalies may nipple-feed for several days before the initial repair. This promotes parent-infant attachment. The palate may be repaired some months later.

Parenteral fluids. It is not uncommon for high-risk infants to receive supplemental parenteral fluids to supply additional calories, electrolytes, and/or water.

Parenteral fluids may be given to the neonate through several routes depending on the nature of the illness, the duration and type of fluid therapy, and institutional (or NICU) preference. Common routes of fluid infusion include peripheral, peripherally inserted central venous, surgically inserted central venous or arterial, and, at times, umbilical venous or umbilical arterial catheterization. The preferred sites for intravenous (IV) infusions in neonates are peripheral veins on the dorsal surfaces of hands or feet. Alternative sites are scalp veins and antecubital veins.

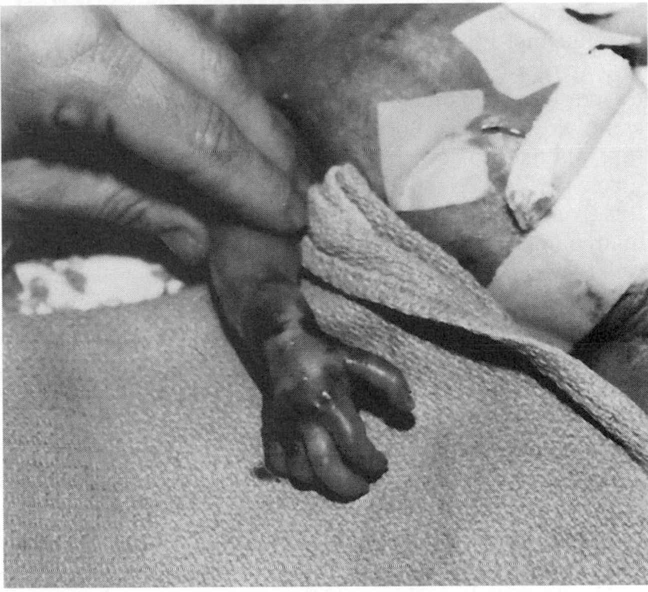

Fig. 25-10 Intravenous infiltration in small infants can cause severe ischemia.

Nursing ALERT

Nurses should be constantly alert for signs of infiltration (e.g., redness, edema, or color change of tissue, blanching at site) (Fig. 25-10) and for signs of overhydration (weight gain over 30 g/24 hr, periorbital edema, tachypnea, tachycardia, and moist crackles on lung auscultation).

Feeding with supplemental parenteral fluids is indicated for infants who are unable to obtain sufficient fluids or calories by enteral feeding. Some of these infants are dependent on **total parenteral nutrition (TPN)** for extensive periods. The nurse assesses and documents the following in infants receiving parenteral fluids or TPN:

- The type and infusion rate of the solution.
- The functional status of the infusion equipment, including the tubing and infusion pump.
- The infusion site for possible complications (phlebitis, infiltration, dislodgment).
- The caloric intake.
- The infant's responses to therapy.

The physician orders TPN per the hospital protocol. These orders must specify the electrolytes and nutrients desired, as well as the volume and rate of infusion. The amounts of calories, protein, and fat are determined on the basis of the individual infant's energy needs (Price and Kalhan, 1993).

While caring for the infant receiving parenteral fluids or TPN, the nurse secures and protects the insertion site. In addition to observing the principles of asepsis, the nurse must also observe the principles of neonatal skin care (Kuller and Lund, 1993). The nurse should also inspect the infusion site for signs of infiltration and reposition the infant frequently to maintain body alignment and protect the site. Parents of such infants need to be given explanations about TPN and the way in which the intravenous equipment and solutions affect their infant.

Advancing infant feedings. Feedings are advanced as assessment data and the infant's ability to tolerate the feedings warrant it. Documentation of a premature infant's sucking patterns can also be used to determine its readiness to nipple feed (Medoff-Cooper, Verklan, and Carlson, 1993). Feedings are advanced from passive (parenteral and gavage) to active (nipple and breastfeeding). Infants with a cleft lip or palate who have a gastrostomy are often changed to nipple feedings once the problem is repaired surgically. At each step, the nurse must carefully assess the infant's response to prevent overstressing the infant.

The infant receiving nutrition parenterally is gradually weaned off of this nutrition. To do this the nourishment given by continuous or intermittent gavage feedings is increased while the parenteral fluids are decreased. For all high-risk infants, feedings are advanced slowly and cautiously because, if feedings are advanced too rapidly, the infant may experience vomiting (with an attendant risk of aspiration), diarrhea, abdominal distention, and apneic episodes. Rapid advancement of feedings may also cause fluid retention with cardiac compromise or a pronounced diuresis with hyponatremia.

If the infant needs additional calories, a commercial human milk fortifier can be added to the gavaged breast milk or the number of calories per 30 ml of commercial formula can be increased. Soy and elemental formulas are used only for infants with very special dietary needs, such as allergies to cow's milk or chronic malabsorption (Townsend, Johnson, and Hay, 1993). Calories in breast milk can be lost if the cream separates and adheres to the tubing during continuous infusion (Brennan-Behm et al, 1994). This problem is decreased if microbore tubing is used for both continuous and intermittent gavage feedings.

The infant receiving gavage feedings progresses to bottle-feeding or breast milk feedings. To do this, the gavage feedings are decreased as the infant's ability to suckle breast milk or formula improves. Often during this transition the infant is fed by both nipple and gavage feeding to ensure the intake of both the prescribed volume of food and nutrients. However, an increased respiratory effort is a documented problem in premature infants who have a gavage tube that is left in place during nipple feedings (Shiao et al, 1995), so nurses must watch for this. The parents need support during this transition because many families measure their parenting competence by how well they can feed their child (Green, 1994).

As the time of discharge nears, the appropriate method of feeding, as well as the assessments pertaining to the method (e.g., tolerance of feedings, status of gavage tube placement), are reviewed with the parents. The parents should be encouraged to interact with the infant by talking and making eye contact with the infant during the feeding. This interaction is encouraged to stimulate the psychosocial development of the infant and to facilitate bonding and attachment (Haut, Peddicord, and O'Brien, 1994; Oehler, Hannan, and Catlett, 1993).

Nonnutritive sucking. If the infant is nourished by the gavage or the parenteral route, **nonnutritive sucking** is encouraged (Fig. 25-11) for several reasons. One is that allowing the infant to suckle on a pacifier during gavage or between oral feedings may improve oxygenation. In addition, such nonnutritive sucking may lead to a decreased energy expenditure with less restlessness and promote faster attachment to the nipple when oral feedings are initiated (Lefrak-Okikawa and Meier, 1993; Pickler and Frankel, 1995). Mothers of premature infants should also be encouraged to let their premature infants start sucking at the breast during kangaroo care because some infant's suck-and-swallow reflexes may be coordinated as early as 32 weeks' gestation.

Infants with intrauterine growth restriction may have an age-appropriate sucking reflex but require thermoregulatory support, making it difficult to breastfeed. These infants may also benefit from nonnutritive sucking at the breast for short periods.

Research findings indicate that a decrease in the incidence of necrotizing enterocolitis (NEC) correlates with the use of nonnutritive sucking during gavage feedings (Pickler and Terrell, 1994). The authors hypothesize that nonnutritive sucking has this effect because it makes the gastrointestinal tract less susceptible to the factors that precipitate NEC by promoting gastric motility and thus increasing the release of gastric enzymes. The improvement in the infant's behavioral organization brought about by nonnutritive sucking also appears to play a role in this.

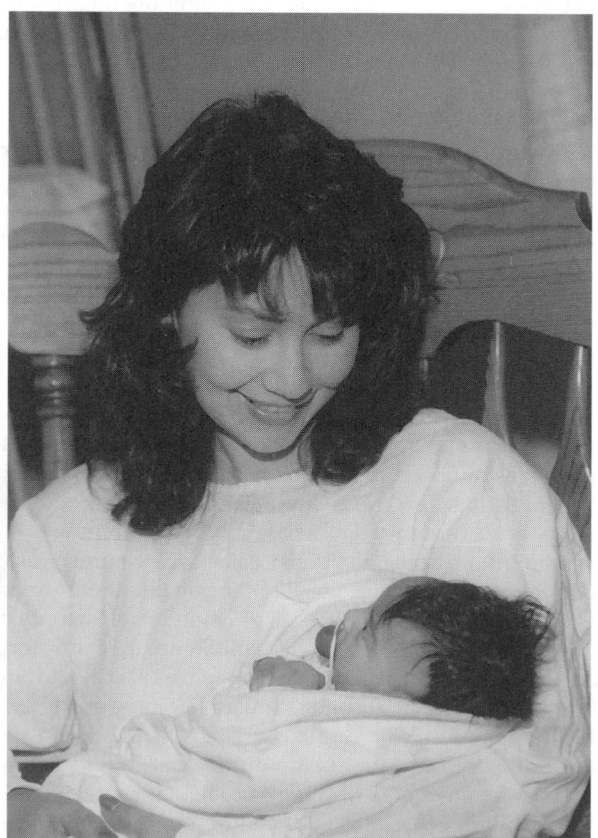

Fig. 25-11 Mother interacting with her infant during nonnutritive sucking. (Courtesy Dale Ikuta, photographer, San Jose, Calif.)

Developmental and Emotional Aspects of Care

All infants and their families have developmental and emotional needs. However, the events in the high-risk infant's life are distinctly different from those of the healthy term infant, and each challenge faced by the infant also affects the family. Whenever an infant shows increased physical distress (oxygen desaturation), the family members are affected in turn by such things as the resulting potential for more medical procedures or a longer hospital stay. The size of premature infants often distresses families, who cannot relate as well to other care issues of their infant, such as routine diaper changes because they are focused on how tiny and fragile the infant appears.

Besides these factors, the infant's vision may be altered by respiratory equipment or a phototherapy mask, making it difficult for the infant to interact with caregivers and family members. The infant may also be unable to establish diurnal and nocturnal rhythms because of the continuous exposure to overhead lighting. In addition, sedation or pain medications may affect the way in which the infant perceives the environment.

Critical Thinking Exercises 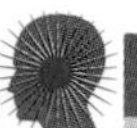

DEVELOPMENT OF HIGH-RISK INFANT

Choose either of the following:

1. Assess the developmental maturity of a 32-week gestation infant. Compare your findings with those from the assessment of a term infant. What type of feeding would each infant be given (route, frequency, and quantity)? What advice would you give the premature infant's mother about breastfeeding?
2. Observe the way in which a high-risk infant interacts with nursing staff and family members. Are the interactions the same with both? What time-out signal does the infant display when distressed? Discuss the implications of nursing care for the neonate and family on the basis of your findings.

Infants in intensive care units are exposed to high levels of auditory input from the various machine alarms, and this can have adverse effects (Fig. 25-12). For example, continuous noise levels of 45 to 85 decibels (db) are common in intensive care units. An incubator alone produces a constant noise level of 60 to 80 db (Haubrich, 1993), and each new piece of life-support equipment used adds another 20 db to the background noise (Strauch, Brandt, and Edwards-Beckett, 1993). The infant's hearing may be damaged if it is exposed to a constant decibel level of 90 db or frequent decibel swings to higher than 110 db.

An additional concern in the care of high-risk infants is that environmental hazards can be potentiated by some drugs used for infant therapy. Diuretics, especially furosemide (Lasix), antibiotics (Gentamicin), and antimalarial agents can potentiate noise-induced hearing loss (Haubrich, 1993). Therefore routine hearing screening should be performed in all infants before discharge, with universal screening completed by no later than the third month of life (National Institutes of Health, 1993).

Parents of high-risk infants must learn their new infant's special characteristics and needs under the close supervision of the nursery staff while their infant copes with its illness or physical deformities. At times they may become confused or frustrated as their infant's condition improves one day and regresses the next. Other parents may have to cope with the death of their infant. Constant support from all staff members from admission through discharge can help families get through this highly stressful and emotional time.

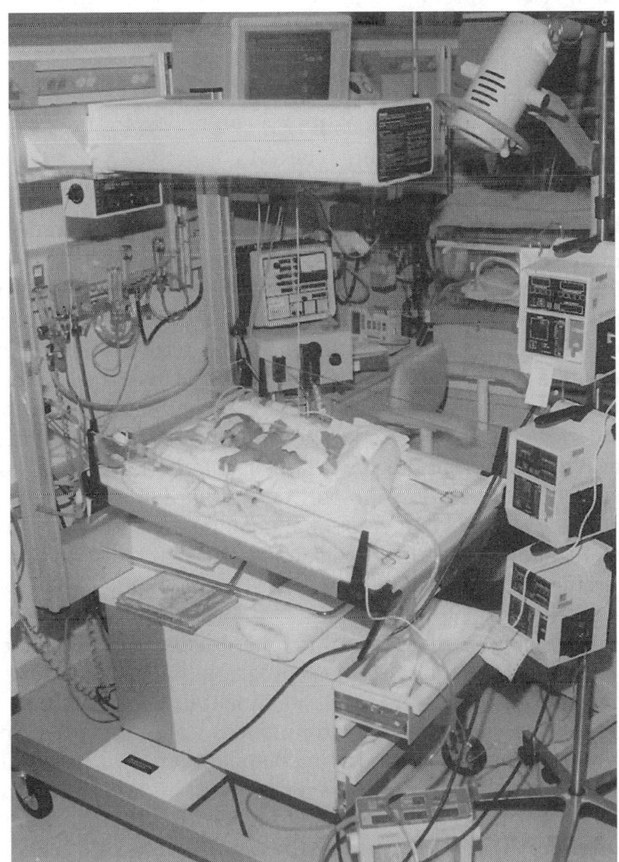

Fig. 25-12 Significant environmental stimulation. Note bed, wall oxygen attachments, monitor ventilator, incubator, pumps, and urometer, all of which have alarm systems. (Courtesy Dale Ikuta, photographer, San Jose, Calif.)

Parents may also benefit from referral to a support group. There they will be able to interact with other parents experiencing similar challenges. Support and innovative solutions to caregiving challenges can be shared among these parents.

Nursing Care Management

The creation of an environment conducive to meeting the developmental and emotional needs of the high-risk infant is limited only by human creativity. However, in a technologic environment, the nursing focus should be on the infant first and the equipment second, even though this environment may also affect the infant. The entire family's relationship with the infant must always be considered. For this reason it is essential that the effects of environmental stressors and technologic equipment on the family's perception of their infant be assessed.

Infant communication. Infants communicate their needs and ability to tolerate sensory stimulation through physiologic responses. The nurses and parents of these high-risk infants must therefore be alert to such cues. Although full-term infants may thrive on stimulation, this same stimulation in high-risk infants can instead provoke physical symptoms of stress and anxiety (Blackburn and VandenBerg, 1993; Gardner et al, 1993). Armed with a knowledge of normal gestational age responses, and by assessing such infants often, the nurse can recognize the developmental and emotional needs of even the tiniest infant. Four developmental assessment tools that can be used to identify the appropriate interventions for a particular infant are described in Box 25-7.

BOX 25-7
Four Developmental Assessment Tools

Dubowitz
A gestational age scoring system that uses for its basis the neurologic responses and physical characteristics at birth.

Ballard
A scoring system adapted from the Dubowitz examination, with the neurologic portion done on a calm infant. An adjusted Ballard assessment may be used on infants who are at more than 20 weeks' gestation.

Brazelton Neonatal Behavioral Assessment Scale (NBAS)
An assessment of a term infant's behavioral state, including motor capacity, state regulation, and interactive abilities.

Assessment of Preterm Infant Behavior (APIB)
An adaptation of the Brazelton assessment that focuses on the behavioral organization and development of premature infants from birth as early as 23 weeks' gestation to 44 weeks' postconceptional age.

Data from Blackburn S, VandenBerg K: *Assessment and management of neonatal neurobehavioral development.* In Kenner C, Brueggemeyer A, Gunderson L, editors: *Comprehensive neonatal nursing. A physiologic perspective,* Philadelphia, 1993, WB Saunders; Pittard W: *Classification of the low-birth-weight infant.* In Klaus M, Fanaroff A, editors: *Care of the high-risk neonate,* ed 4, Philadelphia, 1993, WB Saunders.

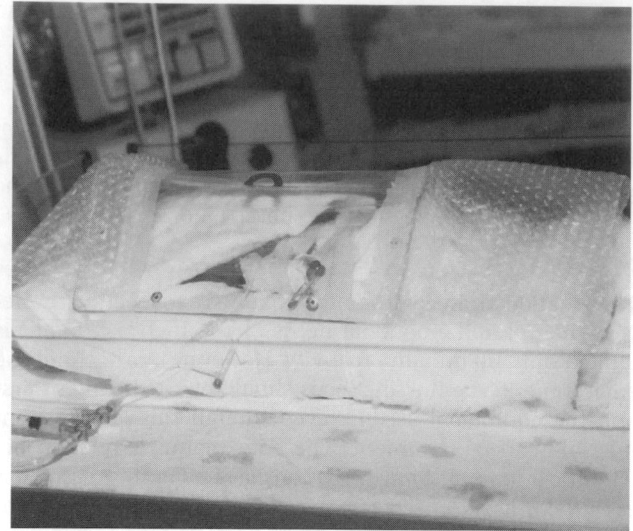

Fig. 25-13 A premature infant relaxing. (Courtesy Dale Ikuta, photographer, San Jose, Calif.)

Problems with noxious stimuli and barriers to normal contact may cause anxiety and tension. Clues to overstimulation include averting the gaze, hiccuping, gagging, or regurgitating food. Term infants exhibit a startle reflex and premature infants move all their limbs in an uncoordinated fashion in response to noxious stimuli. An irregular respiratory rate or an increased heart rate may develop in severely distressed infants, and they may then be unable to regain a calm state.

A relaxed infant state is indicated by stabilization of vital signs, closed eyes, and a relaxed posture. Nonintubated infants may make soothing verbal sounds when they are relaxed. Infants requiring artificial ventilation cannot cry audibly, and often show their distress through posturing, then relax once their needs are met (Fig. 25-13). Pinyard (1994) recommends evaluating an infant's cry as part of a developmental assessment, because specific cry sounds have been correlated with certain behavioral responses. As high-risk infants heal and mature, they increasingly respond to stimuli in a self-regulated manner rather than with a dissociated response. Infants who do not show increased self-regulation should be evaluated for a neurologic problem.

Environmental hazards. Research studies evaluating the effect of radiation, ultraviolet light, microwaves, and other environmental agents on infants are needed. There is concern that even the radiation emitted during x-ray examination of the chest film may be hazardous to the infant's entire body (Wong, 1995). Therefore the infant's genitalia and infants in adjacent incubators need to be protected from such radiation exposure by lead barriers.

Air, blood, water, and physical environment contaminants pose risks to all infants. The American Nurses Association (ANA) has published a series of position statements on many of these risks, including tuberculosis, the human immunodeficiency virus, and lead (ANA, 1991-1994). All staff and family members must observe good handwashing techniques using Standard Precautions to prevent undue exposure of the infants to harmful organisms. The institution's pipe system should be tested for lead contamination because infants are at high risk for suffering neurologic injury with blood levels even as low as 10 μg/dl (Wong, 1995). Infants may also passively acquire many substances, including lead, through breast milk. Making parents aware of the hazards of secondhand tobacco smoke should also be part of all discharge teaching. The dangers of passive exposure to tobacco smoke are borne out by the fact that there is a 35% increase in the incidence of respiratory symptoms and illnesses in the children of parents who smoke in the home. Nurses recognition of substance abuse by family members can help them assess its effect on the infant.

The gases and water supplies in nurseries may contain microorganisms that may or may not be removed even by appropriate filters. Therefore the effectiveness of any filtering system must be confirmed by laboratory testing. A related concern is that infants treated with antibiotics may be colonized by antibiotic-resistant microorganisms originating from the water supply, resulting in suprainfections (Bailey and Goldfarb, 1993).

Examples of nursing diagnoses pertaining to infant development and stimulation include the following:

- Ineffective coping related to
  - Immaturity
  - Environmental stress
  - Physiologic distress

Examples of nursing diagnoses pertaining to a family's grief include the following:

- Anticipatory grieving related to
  - Malformed infant
  - Infant's impending death
- Ineffective family coping related to
  - Potential or real loss of an infant

Nursing care. All plans for the infant and family should be interdisciplinary and set forth the expected outcomes for all aspects of developmental and emotional care. When planning a developmental program for the high-risk infant, the nurse must assess the infant's readiness to advance each time a new stimulus or therapy is added. Interventions to decrease excessive stimulation should be determined on an individual basis, and the family should be taught several ways to interact effectively and appropriately with their infant (Blackburn and VandenBerg, 1993). An important task for families is to both meet the physical and emotional demands of caring for their infant and cope with the accompanying stress. In addition, parents need to take care of themselves and any other children (Nichols, 1993).

Developmental care. A neonatal individualized developmental care and assessment program (NIDCAP) routinely integrates aspects of neurodevelopmental theory with caregivers' observations, environmental interventions, and parental support (Blackburn and VandenBerg, 1993; Gardner et al, 1993). Routine reassessment is built into the program's design. Developmental care may consist of such simple measures as placing a waterbed on the top of the infant's mattress or kangaroo (skin-to-skin) holding. The simplest calming technique is to contain the infant's extremities close to the flexed body using both hands. The care of the infant is organized to allow extended periods of undisturbed rest and sleep.

Data from studies examining the effects of high-intensity

lighting suggest that there is a link between exposure to background nursery light and the occurrence of retinopathy of prematurity. More significantly, infants exposed to a diurnal light pattern show better neuromuscular integration (Blackburn and VandenBerg, 1993). For this reason, there should be routine periods of diminished lighting in neonatal units to provide infants with a more normal environment. A folded blanket can also be arranged over the incubator to shield the infant from bright overhead lights.

In the nursery, conversation and noise are minimized. This includes setting items gently on the incubator (e.g., formula bottles, charts, and other equipment) and not slamming the porthole doors. A "do not disturb" sign can be placed on the incubator as a reminder. The volume of mechanical alarms and overhead paging systems should also be monitored. The institution of a quiet hour on each shift is one way to reduce the amount of noise and stimulation infants are exposed to on a busy unit.

Infants acquire a sense of trust as they learn the feel, sound, and smell of their parents (Gardner et al, 1993). High-risk infants must also learn to trust their caregivers to obtain comfort. However, because caregivers in the nursery may also inflict pain as part of the care they must give, some high-risk infants may not learn to trust as readily as a healthy infant. For this reason it is important for both the parents and caregivers of such infants to employ comforting interventions such as removing painful stimuli, stopping hunger, and changing wet or soiled clothing to foster trust (Green, 1994).

When the infant is ready for stimulation, the nurse has many options. All infants can tolerate being held, even if only for short periods. Additional ways for the nurse or parents to stimulate infants include cuddling, rocking, singing, or talking to the infant (Fig. 25-11). These activities are beneficial, especially during feedings. Stroking the infant's skin during medical therapy can provide tactile stimulation. The caregiver responds to the infant's cues by offering reassurance, providing for nonnutritive sucking, stroking the infant's back, and talking to the infant. Infant massage may be beneficial (see the Patient Teaching Box on pp. 716-717).

Mobiles and decals that can be changed frequently may also be placed within the infant's visual range to stimulate the infant visually. Wind-up musical toys provide rhythmic distractions as long as they are not too loud. If the infant is receiving phototherapy, the protective eye patches are removed periodically (e.g., during feeding) so that the infant can see the caregiver's face for short, comforting sessions.

Kangaroo care. **Kangaroo care** (skin-to-skin holding) helps premature infants directly interact with their parents. In this technique the infant, dressed only in a diaper, is placed directly onto the parent's bare chest and then covered with the parent's clothing or a warmed blanket (Fig. 25-14). In this way, the parent's body temperature also functions as an external heat source that enhances the infant's temperature regulation (Gale, Franck, and Lund, 1993). Even ventilator-dependent infants weighing under 1 kg have been found to benefit from this measure, although they usually tolerate it for only 30 minutes or less at a time.

Kangaroo holding originated in Bogota, Colombia, where radiant warmers and incubators were in short supply. Although such care has its roots in economic hardships, it stems from a deep respect for natural processes. Infants and parents

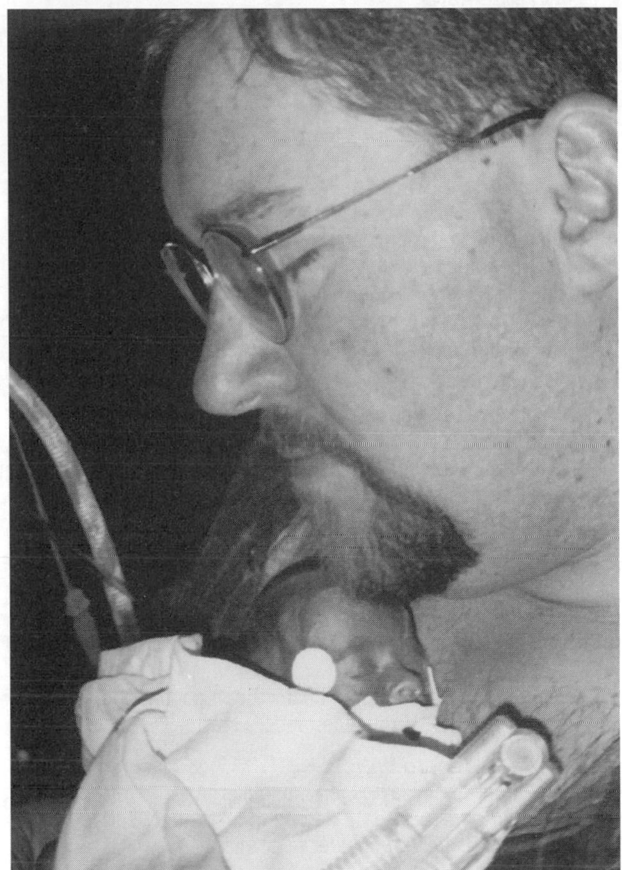

Fig. 25-14 The kangaroo method. Infant snuggled in his father's shirt in skin-to-skin contact. (Courtesy Mary Rose Tully, Raleigh, NC)

who participate in such kangaroo care have been observed to have dramatically better outcomes (Affonso et al, 1993). The mothers report increased breast milk output and fewer feelings of helplessness related to their experiences in the neonatal intensive care unit. The infants maintain their temperatures and oxygenation levels and experience fewer episodes of crying, apnea, and periodic respirations. They have also been observed to be alert and quiet longer and to have slightly higher heart rates. A further benefit of kangaroo care is that the hospital stays for these infants are shorter than those of infants treated with the traditional radiant warmer or incubator (Legault and Goulet, 1995; Ludington-Hoe et al, 1994).

Positioning. The positioning of infants plays an important role in the effectiveness of care. For example, positioning an infant in a nest or with rolls is very beneficial in reducing stress. It does so by providing defined boundaries, which helps the infant acquire organizational skills (Becker et al, 1993). In addition, it promotes the proper body alignment that is necessary to prevent developmental problems that may prevent walking as the child matures. Positioning the infant in a side-lying fetal position or prone with both legs tucked up close to the abdomen gives the infant a sense of security. Teaching parents the various ways to position the infant, and in an organized and composed manner, supports their sense of autonomy and provides them with the skills necessary for as-

Patient Teaching

INFANT MASSAGE

"When from the wearying ware of life
I seek release,
I look into my baby's face,
And there find peace."
—***Martha F. Crow***

Benefits to you, the parent:
Helps you recognize infant's cues
Soothes baby and reduces effects of stress caused by potentially overwhelming new environment
Provides baby with regular nurturing attention
Deepens attachment between parent and child
Provides fun and feels good.

Appropriate materials:
Assemble two to three pillows, two towels, a change of diapers and clothes
Purchase cold-pressed vegetable oil: almond, apricot kernel, sunflower, safflower, or coconut oil; powder.
CAUTION: Do not use mineral oil (leaches vitamins D, E, and K from skin) and scented oils or any product if baby has developed rashes from it.

To provide conducive environment:
Choose place that is warm, quiet, dimly lit, out of mainstream of activity.
Choose time when parent and baby are in good mood; use relaxation methods first if needed before starting.

To avoid injury to baby:
Handle infant gently; avoid jerking, pulling.
Place infant on lap or sit on floor with infant between legs.
Avoid creating cloud of powder near infant's face.

Head

Do not use oil on head and face.
Caution parents against jabbing or poking.
Demonstrate technique, using gentle pressure as thumbs are moved outward.
Smile at baby.

- Do gentle head "tapping" around base of neck and skull. (LeBoyer, 1981; Scheider, 1982).
- Once eyes are closed, place thumbs together over bridge of nose and move thumbs outward, gently over eyes; repeat over bridge of nose and outward over checks; repeat over lips and move thumbs outward in a "smile."
- With two fingers of each hand starting at forehead, make small circles around face at hairline and under chin.
- Gently massage each ear between thumb and forefinger; do one ear at a time.

Chest

Apply 1-2 tablespoons vegetable oil over hands.

- Do "open book" over infant's stomach. Starting with both hands flat over chest, make heart-shaped pattern down sides and over groin three or four times. Use this pattern:

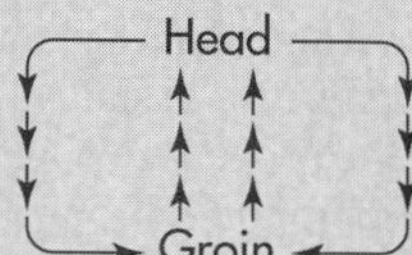

- Place hands together over abdomen, press in gently, and push outward to sides; hold baby under buttocks while thumbs are on abdomen.
- Do "butterfly." Place one hand on infant's shoulder, pull downward to opposite groin; repeat with other hand.
Repeat each technique three or four times.

To avoid stressing baby:
Watch for infant's cues to end massage; fussing, squirming, turning away.
Talk to infant, sing, hum, smile.
Limit massage to 20 minutes.

To perform massage:
Read Schneider or LeBoyer reference, and follow pictures, because not all the techniques can appear here.*

To perform techniques:
Greet infant: "Hi, I love you."

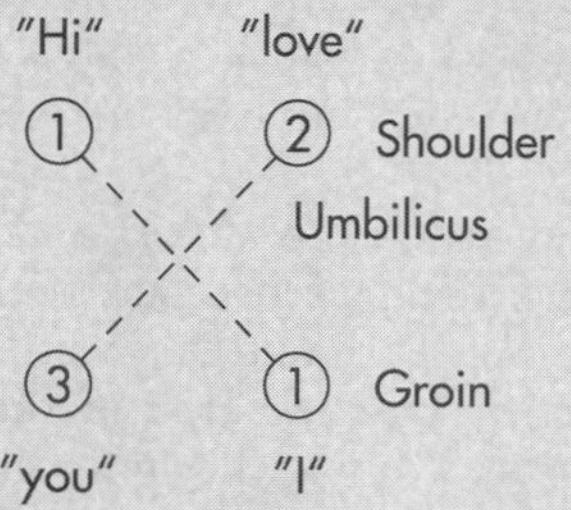

Stomach

- Do waterwheel: with outside edge of one hand, start at umbilicus and move hand downward to groin; alternate hands like a water wheel.

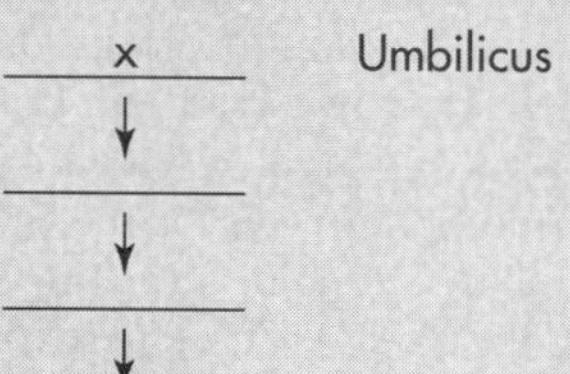

This technique is good for helping the baby with gas.

- Place thumbs together in center of abdomen, then pull out to sides.
- Perform "I love you" using this pattern

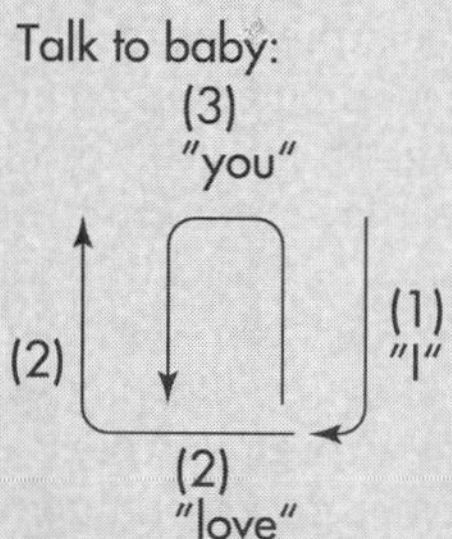

- Perform "walking": tap with fingers of both hands simultaneously, over infant's abdomen.

Arms

- Perform "Indian (Swedish) milking": hold one hand at wrist, encircle wrist with other hand and "milk" downward.
Repeat with other arm.
- Perform rolling: between palms of both hands, roll infant's arm back and forth; repeat with other arm.

*Each bullet starts a new technique.

Patient Teaching

INFANT MASSAGE—cont'd

Hands

- Make little circles in palms of each hand; then gently pull on each finger.

Legs and Feet

- Push on bottom of foot with both thumbs, making small circles; pull on each toe; roll leg between both hands; press on dorsal surface of foot to gently plantarflex foot.

Back

Carefully turn infant back onto abdomen.

- Perform "butterfly" technique making an "X" over baby's back down to the buttocks, starting at the shoulders. Use one hand at a time.
- Make small circles over baby's back with fingers of both hands simultaneously; start at shoulders and move down to buttocks.
- Perform "milking" with one hand, starting at shoulders, moving to feet. Use other hand to support infant.

Ending

- "Comb" infant's back with fingers of both hands simultaneously, starting at shoulders, moving to feet. Gradually lighten pressure so that last "combing" is barely touching skin.

Variations

Teach older child who can perform massage on doll with mother.

Learn technique during prenatal period by practicing on maternal abdomen.

sessing their infant's cues after discharge (Oehler, Hannan, and Catlett, 1993). Discharge planning should include information about the importance of placing the infant on the side or back for sleep to help decrease the risk of sudden infant death syndrome (SIDS).

Parents are often concerned about the head molding that occurs in premature infants. Chan, Kelley, and Khan (1993) investigated the effectiveness of a water mattress placed under the infant's head in preventing this phenomenon but concluded that such relief of pressure on the baby's head would not completely alter the outcome. There needs to be further research on the effectiveness of positioning in alleviating this problem.

Anticipatory grief. Families experience **anticipatory grief** when they are told of the impending death of their infant (Nichols, 1993). Parents who have an infant with a debilitating disease (with or without a congenital deformity), but that may not necessarily threaten the life of the child, may also experience anticipatory grief. An alteration in relationships, a change in life-style, and a very real threat to their hopes and dreams for the future may affect the day-to-day interaction of the family with their infant and the staff (Loizeaux, 1993; Mehren, 1991). Nurses should help facilitate the family's grieving process. If the nurse observes that a family member's day-to-day interactions with the infant change, the nurse should assess the situation and request psychosocial support or intervention by a chaplain or social worker, if necessary.

Loss of an infant. Parents who know their infant is going to die experience a very difficult time. Before the infant's death, the parents need to direct their attention, energy, and caregiving activities toward the dying infant. However, some parents find it difficult to visit their infant even for short periods once a terminal prognosis has been given. Grandparents also grieve but often are unsure how to comfort their own child (the infant's parent) during the period of impending death. Health care professionals can help by involving the family in the infant's care, providing privacy, answering questions, and preparing them for the inevitability of the death.

Adding to the problem is the fact that intensive care nurseries consist of multiple-bed rooms, making a family's grief a very public event. A designated private family room with technical support available allows the entire grieving family to have time to make their initial farewells out of the public eye (Nichols, 1993). The staff must also be prepared for the expression of a variety of grief reactions ranging from anger to copious weeping.

There may not be time for parents to anticipate the loss (Nichols, 1993). Such parents may experience a delayed grief response. Contributing to this is the fact that at the time of death parents are being asked to make decisions immediately regarding organ donation, autopsy, and funeral arrangements—things they might never have had to think of before. Because of their unpreparedness, they may react by simply refusing to discuss these issues.

Certain special circumstances also affect the parents' responses (Harrigan et al, 1993). For instance, if one or more of the infants of a multifetal pregnancy die, even if at least one is expected to live, parents may act as if all the infants are alive or dead. One reason for their denial of the infant's death may be that it causes them to lose the special status society accords the parents of twins or triplets. For weeks such parents may continue to speak of all of their children in the present tense to family and friends who have not seen the infants. Parents of infants who die after transport to another facility may also find it difficult to accept the event as a reality. The nursing staff must therefore provide every opportunity for the parents to see their infant and grieve for it. Nichols (1993) recommends that even unusual requests should be honored, when possible, since this may help the person work through the grief process.

The physical and emotional trauma felt by the families of infants who have died may have a debilitating effect and prolong their grief (Klaus and Kennell, 1993). They may desire to avoid the terrible acknowledgment that their infant is dead. This can cause them to suffer a low-level clinical depression that can be more pronounced if the mother has endured additional crises related to the pregnancy and postpartum period. The death of an infant is also made more difficult to accept by the fact that it violates one of the basic laws of nature—that parents should precede their children in death. Follow-up of the family after any death is therefore important to determine the family's well-being and their need for referral and support.

Parents of infants who have died face other issues as well, such as how to continue to function in the role of parent. Coping with one's grief while parenting and explaining the death to surviving children can be extremely difficult for bereaved parents (Loizeaux, 1993; Mehren, 1991). However, the physical, emotional, and social responses to grief that parents experience gradually diminish as they become more involved in the events of everyday life.

The nursing staff also experiences grief (Downey et al, 1995). Many primary staff nurses find themselves grieving as if an infant were their own because they often have been the primary caregiver for weeks, even months. Managers and other staff members must acknowledge this grief. Talking about the infant or attending the funeral may help the affected staff members resolve their feelings about the infant's death.

Discharge planning. Discharge planning for the high-risk infant begins at the time of admission. Throughout the infant's hospitalization, the discharge planning coordinator gathers information from all of the health care team members. This information is used to determine the infant's and family's readiness for discharge (Green, 1994). Nurses are very influential members of the planning team because as the direct caregivers throughout the infant's hospitalization they have a firsthand knowledge of the infant and the family.

As the home care needs of the infant's parents are assessed, steps are taken to eliminate any knowledge deficits. Information is provided about infant care, especially as it pertains to the particular infant's home needs (e.g., the administration of oxygen, gastrostomy feedings). Parent education includes having them give return demonstrations of their infant care skills to show whether they are becoming increasingly independent in the provision of this care. Parents should also obtain an age-appropriate car seat before the discharge of their infant. Instruction in infant cardiopulmonary resuscitation should be offered to all parents before discharge.

Referrals for appropriate resources also need to be made. Social service involvement is especially important for young or psychosocially high-risk parents (e.g., substance abusers or those with a mental illness). Social services can also provide parents with information about financial assistance (Aid to Families with Dependent Children, Medicaid, Crippled Children's Program, Social Security Disability). As our understanding of genetics increases, appropriate counseling, referral, and follow-up will become more important (Scanlon and Fibison, 1995).

Infants with developmental disabilities, or those infants who may be at risk for further problems (premature infants), are referred to appropriate community programs. Many community resources that give assistance with special educational and medical needs have been mandated by Federal Public Law #102-119 (Jenkins, Covington, and Plotnick, 1994). Such services range from family counseling to physical therapy. Some hospitals also offer infant stimulation and development programs for the parents of high-risk infants. Nursing is recognized by this law as one of the 10 qualified disciplines that can provide these services.

Referrals are made for home health assistance, as appropriate (some medical plans cover these services). These health care providers can perform actual nursing functions, as well as provide some relief from the emotional burden of caring for an infant with medical problems. Special attention should be given to parents' feelings of uncertainty, anxiety, and overwhelming frustration. Parents often experience these emotions during the planning for an infant's home care, especially if the infant has had a severe or prolonged illness (Catlett, Miles, and Holditch-Davis, 1994).

As the home care of medically fragile clients is expanded to the pediatric population, early teaching and planning become a necessity. Golberg, Gardner, and Gibson (1994) cite an example of a health care maintenance organization that saved more than a million dollars in hospital charges by having a ventilator-dependent client live at home. More facilities are investigating such home care options as one way to provide long-term care for the high-risk infant.

TRANSPORT FROM A REGIONAL CENTER ("BACK TRANSPORT")

Infants may need to be transferred back to the referring facility. Often premature infants who require thermoregulation and gavage feedings can be cared for in community hospitals closer to the parents' home. This allows parents to visit their infant more easily and to work with their personal health care provider on the long-range expected outcomes for the infant. Specialized incubators make these trips possible (Fig. 25-15). However, parents may express mixed feelings about such return transports and may be reluctant to adapt to a different facility and group of caregivers. To minimize some of these concerns, Kunley and Freston (1993) recommend giving the parents very clear information about return transports during the initial discharge planning.

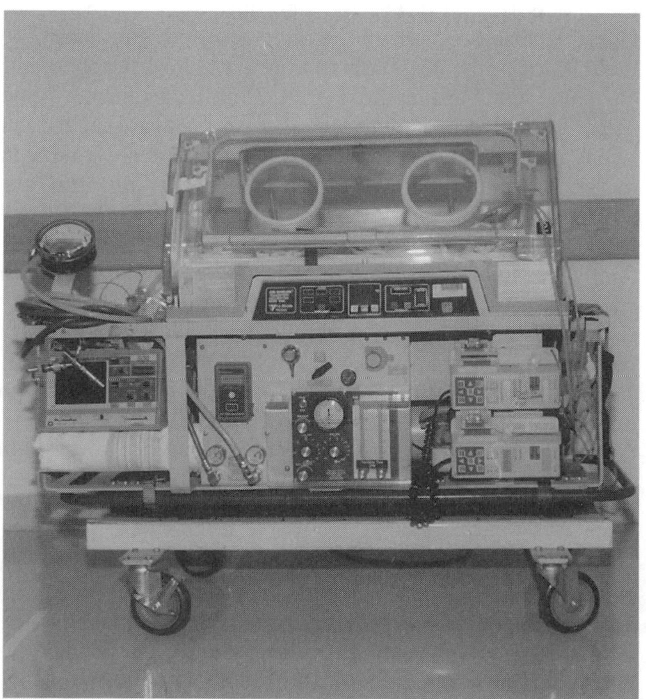

Fig. 25-15 A total life support system for transport of high-risk newborns. (Courtesy Dale Ikuta, photographer, San Jose, Calif.)

Although at the time of discharge parents may not recognize the need for information on the various resources available to help them in the care of their infant, they can be given such lists of agencies and telephone numbers for later use. Providing them with a client-specific directory covering special programs, social support, community, and funding resources can help them make the transition to the home care of their infants. As the nurse continually reinforces the idea that the infant will go home, this prompts the parents to plan for the days ahead and therefore be ready to take their infant home when the time comes.

NURSING CARE OF THE FAMILY

With the birth of a high-risk newborn, parents must readjust their expectations. They need to grieve for the loss of the "perfect" baby they had anticipated, and they may have difficulty becoming attached to their infant. Misinterpretation of their emotional cues by the health care professional can further damage this process.

Socioeconomic and cultural differences can influence parental behavior and needs. In some cultures the husband must make all decisions and attempts by health care providers to include the mother can undermine the integrity of the family. Other cultures do not name their infant until 31 days after birth, which could be misinterpreted as a lack of attachment. Non–English-speaking parents often encounter the additional difficulty of a language barrier with the health care providers.

Parents need to see and touch their baby as soon as possible. They also need consistent information regarding their infant's condition. All members of the health care team must coordinate communication so that the parents hear the same message from several sources. Other interventions to assist the parents depend, in part, on the infant's condition. Parents of preterm infants can quite possibly look forward to a "normal" child, whereas parents of infants with significant birth defects probably cannot. Normalizing the parents' interactions with their sick infant helps them accomplish the difficult task of parental attachment in the face of overwhelming grief.

The newborn's successful transition to extrauterine life, and the development of a parent-newborn relationship assures the nurse that the expected outcomes have been achieved (see the Nursing Care Plan on pp. 720-721).

PAIN IN NEONATES

Pain has physiologic and psychologic components. Because of the psychological component of pain and diffuse total body response to pain by the neonate, many health care providers believe that infants, especially premature infants, do not experience pain (Franck and Gregory, 1993). However, the central nervous system is well-developed as early as 24 weeks. The peripheral and spinal structure that transmit pain information is present and functional between the first and second trimester.

The physiologic response to pain in the neonate can be life-threatening. Pain response can decrease tidal volume, increase demands on cardiovascular system, increase metabolism and neuroendocrine imbalance. Hormonal-metabolic response to pain in a term infant has a greater magnitude and shorter duration than in adults. The premature infant has decreased lipid stores and immature enzyme activity, which results in an increase in tissue breakdown. The newborn's sympathetic response to pain is less mature and thus less predictable than an adult's (Franck and Gregory, 1993).

Assessment of Pain

Pain can be assessed in behavioral, physiologic/autonomic, and metabolic categories (Franck and Gregory, 1993).

Behavioral. The most common behavioral sign of pain is a high-pitched cry with shrill qualities (Lynam, 1995). A "cry face" is characteristic for an infant experiencing pain. Other facial features exhibited during a pain stimulus include eye squeeze, brow contraction, deepened nasolabial furrows, taut and quivering tongue, and open mouth. The infant will flex and adduct the upper body and lower limbs in an attempt to withdraw from the painful stimulus. The premature infant has a lower threshold for initiation of this flex response. Critically ill infants may become flaccid with pain stimuli (Franck and Gregory, 1993).

Physiologic/autonomic responses. Significant changes in heart rate, blood pressure (increased or decreased), intracranial pressure, vagal tone, respiratory rate, and oxygen saturation occur during noxious stimulation (Franck and Gregory, 1993; Lynam, 1995). Using physiologic parameters in assessment eliminate the subjective element associated with assessment of behavioral responses.

Metabolic. Infants release epinephrine, norepinephrine, glucagon, corticosterone, cortisol, 11-deoxycorticosterone, lactate, pyruvate, and glucose in response to pain (Franck and Gregory, 1993; Lynam, 1995).

Management of Neonatal Pain

The goals of management of neonatal pain are to (1) minimize intensity, duration, and physiologic cost of the pain, and (2) maximize the neonate's ability to cope and recover from the pain (Franck and Gregory, 1993). There are two strategies for management of pain in the neonate: nonpharmacologic and pharmacologic.

Nonpharmacologic management. Containment, also known as swaddling, has been effective in reducing excessive, immature motor responses. A blanket may also provide comfort through other senses such as thermal, tactile, and proprioceptive (Franck and Gregory, 1993; Lynam, 1995). Nonnutritive sucking (NNS) is the most common comfort measure employed by nurses. The effectiveness of NNS on the pain response is limited and confined to certain procedures (Lynam, 1995). Distraction with visual, oral, auditory or tactile stimulation may be helpful in term or older infants (Franck and Gregory, 1993).

Pharmacologic management. Pharmacologic agents have been routine for adults during painful procedures. These same agents are now becoming routine for neonates to alleviate pain with procedures. Local anesthesia may be used for circumcision and has become routine during certain invasive procedures such as chest tube insertion. Topical anesthesia has been used for lumbar puncture, venipuncture, and heel sticks (Franck, 1993). Opioids have been used as preproce-

Nursing Care Plan

HIGH-RISK PREMATURE NEWBORN

Nursing Diagnosis: Ineffective breathing pattern related to pulmonary and neuromuscular immaturity, decreased energy, fatigue

Expected Outcome: Infant exhibits adequate oxygenation (i.e., arterial blood gases and acid-base within normal limits (WNL), oxygen saturations 92% or greater, respiratory rate and pattern WNL, breath sounds clear, absence of grunting, nasal flaring, minimal retractions, skin color WNL).

• NURSING INTERVENTIONS/*RATIONALES*

Position neonate prone or supine avoiding neck hyperextension *to promote optimum air exchange.* Use a side-lying position after feeding or in cases of excessive mucus production *to avoid aspiration.* (Avoid Trendelenburg position *as it can cause increased intracranial pressure and reduce lung capacity)*

Suction nasopharynx, trachea and endotracheal tube as indicated *to remove mucus.* (Avoid oversuctioning as it can cause bronchospasm, bradycardia, hypoxia and predispose neonate to intraventricular hemorrhage).

Administer percussion, vibration, and postural drainage as prescribed *to facilitate drainage of secretions.*

Administer oxygen and monitor neonatal response *to maintain oxygen saturation.*

Maintain a neutral thermal environment *to conserve oxygen* use.

Monitor arterial blood gases, acid-base balance, oxygen saturation, respiratory rate and pattern, breath sounds, airway patency; observe for grunting, nasal flaring, retractions, cyanosis *to detect signs of respiratory distress.*

Nursing Diagnosis: Ineffective thermoregulation related to immature temperature regulation and minimal subcutaneous fat stores

Expected Outcome: Infant exhibits maintenance of stable body temperature within normal range for postconceptional age (36.5° to 37.2°C [97.6° to 99° F]).

• NURSING INTERVENTIONS/*RATIONALES*

Place neonate in a prewarmed radiant warmer *to maintain stable temperature.*

Place temperature probe on neonatal abdomen *to control heat levels in radiant warmer.*

Take axillary temperature periodically *to monitor temperature and cross check functioning of warmer unit.*

Avoid infant exposure to cool air and drafts, cold scales, cold stethoscopes, cold examination tables, prolonged bathing *that predispose the infant to heat loss.*

Monitor probe frequently *as detachment can cause overheating or warmer-induced hyperthermia.*

Transfer infant to a servocontrolled open warmer bed or incubator *when temperature has stabilized.*

Nursing Diagnosis: Risk for infection related to immature immune system

Expected Outcome: Infant exhibits no evidence of nosocomial infection.

• NURSING INTERVENTIONS/*RATIONALES*

Institute scrupulous hand washing techniques before and after handling neonate, ensure all supplies and/or equipment are clean before use, ensure strict aseptic technique with invasive procedures *to minimize exposure to infective organisms.*

Prevent contact with persons who have communicable infections and instruct parents in infection control procedures *to minimize infection risk.*

Administer prescribed antibiotics *to provide coverage for infection during sepsis workup.*

Continuously monitor vital signs for stability *as instability, hypothermia or prolonged temperature elevations serve as indicators for infection.*

Nursing Diagnosis: Risk for nutrition alteration less than body requirements related to inability to ingest nutrients secondary to immaturity

Expected Outcome: Infant receives adequate amount of nutrients with sufficient caloric intake to maintain positive nitrogen balance; demonstrates steady weight gain.

• NURSING INTERVENTIONS/*RATIONALES*

Administer parenteral fluid/total parenteral nutrition as prescribed *to provide adequate nutrition and fluid intake.*

Monitor for signs of intolerance to TPN, *which can interfere with effective replenishment of nutrients.*

Periodically assess readiness to orally feed (i.e., strong suck, swallow and gag reflexes) *to provide appropriate transition for TPN to oral feeding as soon as neonate is ready.*

Advance volume and concentration of formula when orally feeding per unit protocol *to avoid overfeeding and feeding intolerance.*

If mother desires to breast feed when neonate is stable, demonstrate how to express milk *to establish and maintain lactation until infant can breastfeed.*

Nursing Diagnosis: Risk for fluid volume deficit/excess related to immature physiology

Expected Outcome: Infant exhibits evidence of fluid homeostasis.

• NURSING INTERVENTIONS/*RATIONALES*

Administer parenteral fluids as prescribed and regulate carefully to maintain fluid balance. (Avoid hypertonic fluids such as undiluted medications, concentrated glucose as they can cause excess solute load on immature kidneys).

Implement strategies (use of plastic covers and increase of ambient humidity) *that minimize insensible water loss.*

Monitor hydration status (i.e., skin turgor, blood pressure, edema, weight, mucous membranes, fontanels, urine specific gravity, electrolytes) and intake and output *to evaluate for evidence of dehydration or overhydration.*

Nursing Care Plan

HIGH-RISK PREMATURE NEWBORN—cont'd

Nursing Diagnosis: Risk for impaired skin integrity related to immature skin structure, immobility, invasive procedures

Expected Outcome: Infant's skin remains intact with no evidence of irritation or injury.

• **NURSING INTERVENTIONS/*RATIONALES***

Cleanse skin as needed with plain warm water and apply moisturizing agents to skin *to prevent dryness and reduce friction across skin surface.*

When performing procedures: minimize use of tape and apply a skin barrier between tape and skin; use transparent elastic film for securing central and peripheral lines; use limb electrodes for monitoring or attach with hydrogel and rotate electrodes frequently; remove adhesives with soap and water rather than alcohol or acetone based adhesive removers *to minimize skin damage.*

Monitor use of thermal devices such as warmers or heating pads carefully *to prevent burns.*

Monitor skin closely for evidence of redness, rash, irritation, bruising, breakdown, ischemia, infiltration *to detect and treat potential complications early.*

Nursing Diagnosis: Risk for injury related to increased intracranial pressure and intraventricular hemorrhage secondary to immature central nervous system

Expected Outcome: Infant will exhibit normal intracranial pressure (ICP) with no evidence of intraventricular hemorrhage.

• **NURSING INTERVENTIONS/*RATIONALES***

Institute minimum stimulation protocol (i.e., minimal handling, cluster care techniques, avoidance of sudden head movements to one side, undisturbed sleep periods, light variations to simulate day and night, limit personnel and equipment noise in environment) *to decrease stress responses, which can increase ICP.*

Institute ordered pharmacologic and nonpharmacologic pain control methods *to manage pain and reduce physical stress.*

Avoid hypertonic solutions and medications *as they increase cerebral blood flow.*

Elevate head of bed 15 to 20 degrees *to decrease ICP.*

Monitor vital signs *for evidence of ICP.*

Recognize signs of overstimulation (i.e., flaccidity, yawning, irritability, crying, staring, active averting) *so stimulation can be stopped to allow rest.*

Nursing Diagnosis: Altered parenting related to separation and interruption of parent/infant attachment secondary to premature birth

Expected Outcome: Parents establish contact with neonate; demonstrate competent parenting skills and willingness to care for neonate.

• **NURSING INTERVENTIONS/*RATIONALES***

Before parents first visit to the NICU, prepare them by explaining what the neonate will look like, what the equipment will look like and its function *to diminish fear and decrease sense of shock.*

Keep parents informed about infant's condition (improvements and setbacks) and important aspects of infant's care; encourage and answer parental questions; actively listen to parent concerns *to establish trust, open communication and caring atmosphere to aid in coping.*

Encourage parents to visit the NICU often; to name the infant; to touch, hold or caress infant as physical condition permits; to be actively involved in infant's care; to bring personal items (i.e., clothing, stuffed animals or pictures of family) *to allow for formation of emotional bond.*

Reinforce parent involvement and praise care endeavors *to increase self-confidence in their contribution.*

Encourage parents to bring other siblings to visit; explain to the siblings what they are seeing; encourage siblings to draw pictures or write letters for the infant and place in or near infant crib *to promote family involvement, help ease sibling fears, and let them contribute to infant care.*

Refer parents to social services as needed *to ensure comprehensive care.*

---

dural analgesia. If the infant is not ventilated, the use of opioids is of concern related to the potential for respiratory depression (Franck, 1993; Franck and Gregory, 1993).

Anesthesia is used for prolonged surgical procedures. The American Academy of Pediatrics recommends the same guidelines for safe administration of anesthesia to critically ill infants as for unstable adult patients (Franck, 1993). During the immediate postoperative period, pain control is crucial. Low-dose continuous infusion or intermittent bolus of narcotic analgesia is given to infants. Morphine has different pharmacokinetics in the premature infant than adults. This drug has a longer half-life and delayed clearance. Other effects seen with morphine and meperidine include decreased intestinal motility, abdominal distention, and hypotension in dehydrated patients. Fentanyl has similar effects as morphine and meperidine including significant respiratory depression (Franck and Gregory, 1993). Sufentanil (Sufenta) is 10 times more potent than fentanyl and is used for neonates having cardiac surgery. Alfentanil (Alfenta) is short-acting and has been used for short procedures (Franck and Gregory, 1993). Methadone has been used for postoperative pain and treatment of neonatal abstinence syndrome. Fifty to 100 mg/kg methadone relieves pain in neonates for 6 to 10 hours (Franck and Gregory, 1993).

Acetaminophen (Tylenol) is useful for mild to moderate pain in infants and children. The use of acetaminophen in neonates is limited because it is administered only rectally (Franck and Gregory, 1993).

Key Points

- The identification of maternal and fetal risk factors in the intrapartum period is vital for planning adequate care of high-risk infants.
- High-risk infants have special problems resulting from immaturity, alterations in the functioning of systems, or metabolic imbalances.
- The nurse often is the pivotal link affecting the functional or dysfunctional survival of an infant with respiratory distress.
- For the infant receiving supplemental oxygen, periodic laboratory measurements and close clinical observation are essential so that appropriate adjustments can be made in the infant's care to minimize the risk of both hyperoxic and hypoxic insults.
- A thermoneutral environment is essential for maintaining metabolic homeostasis.
- The extent to which an infant's nutritional needs are met has a direct bearing on the infant's immediate and long-range well-being.
- Parents need to be familiar with their infant's developmental plan of care and the way in which they can participate in it.
- The aim of transporting high-risk infants to regional centers is to ensure that they have access to the required level of care.
- Parents may need support and help accepting, caring for, and taking home infants who have been compromised at birth or during the first days of life.
- Parents need assistance with coping with real or anticipated loss and grief.

References

Affonso D et al: Reconciliation and healing for mothers through skin-to-skin contact provided in an American tertiary level intensive care nursery, *Neonatal Netw* 12(3):25, 1993.

American Nurses Association Position Statement: *Availability of equipment and safety procedures to prevent transmission of blood-borne diseases*, Washington, DC, 1991, American Nurses Association.

American Nurses Association Position Statement: *AIDS/HIV and women*, Washington, DC, 1992a, American Nurses Association.

American Nurses Association Position Statement: *HIV infection and nursing students*, Washington, DC, 1992b, American Nurses Association.

American Nurses Association Position Statement: *AIDS/HIV disease and socio-culturally diverse populations*, Washington, DC, 1993a, American Nurses Association.

American Nurses Association Position Statement: *Tuberculosis and public health nursing*, Washington, DC, 1993b, American Nurses Association.

American Nurses Association Position Statement: *Lead poisoning and screening*, Washington, DC, 1994, American Nurses Association.

Bailey J, Goldfarb J: *Neonatal infections*. In Klaus M, Fanaroff A, editors: *Care of the high-risk neonate*, ed 4, Philadelphia, 1993, WB Saunders.

Becker P et al: Effects of developmental care on behavioral organization in very-low-birth-weight infants, *Nurs Res* 42(4):214, 1993.

Blackburn S, VandenBerg K: *Assessment and management of neonatal neurobehavioral development*. In Kenner C, Brueggemeyer A, Gunderson L, editors: *Comprehensive neonatal nursing: a physiologic perspective*, Philadelphia, 1993, WB Saunders.

Blake W, Murray J: *Heat balance*. In Merenstein G, Gardner S, editors: *Handbook of neonatal intensive care*, ed 3, St Louis, 1993, Mosby.

Bliss-Holtz J: Determination of thermoregulatory state in full term infants, *Nurs Res* 42(4):204, 1993.

Bloom R, Cropley C: *Textbook of neonatal resuscitation*, Elk Grove, Ill, 1994, American Heart Association.

Brennan-Behm M et al: Caloric loss from expressed mother's milk during continuous gavage infusion, *Neonat Netw* 13(2):27, 1994.

Cagan J: Feeding behavior in preterm infants [abstract]. *Neonat Netw* 14(2):82, 1995.

Catlett A, Miles M, Holditch-Davis D: Maternal perceptions of illness severity in premature infants, *Neonat Netw* 13(2):43, 1994.

Chan J, Kelley M, Khan J: The effects of a pressure relief mattress on postnatal head molding in very low birth weight infants, *Neonat Netw* 12(5):19, 1993.

Downey V et al: Dying babies and associated stress in NICU nurses, *Neonat Netw* 14(1):41, 1995.

Endo A, Nishioka E: *Neonatal assessment*. In Kenner C, Brueggemeyer A, Gunderson L, editors: *Comprehensive neonatal nursing. A physiologic perspective*, Philadelphia, 1993, WB Saunders.

Fanaroff A, Martin R: *Neonatal-perinatal medicine: diseases of the fetus and infant*, ed 6, St Louis, 1997, Mosby.

Franck L: *Identification, management, and prevention of pain in the neonate*. In Kenner C, Brueggemeyer A, Gunderson, L: *Comprehensive neonatal nursing: a physiologic perspective*, Philadelphia, 1993, WB Saunders.

Franck L, Gregory G: *Clinical evaluation and treatment of infant pain in the neonatal intensive care unit*. In Schechter M, Berde C, Yaster M, editors: *Pain in infants, children, and adolescents*, Baltimore, 1993, Williams and Wilkins.

Gale C, Franck L, Lund C: Skin-to-skin (kangaroo) holding of the intubated premature infant, *Neonat Netw* 12(6):49, 1993.

Gardner S et al: *The neonate and the environment: impact on development*. In Merenstein G, Gardner S, editors: *Handbook of neonatal intensive care*, ed 3, St Louis, 1993, Mosby.

Gelhar D et al: Research from the research utilization project: environmental temperatures, *J Obstet Gynecol Neonatal Nurs* 23(4):341, 1994.

Golberg A, Gardner G, Gibson L: Home care: the next frontier of pediatric practice, *J Pediatr* 125(5):686, 1994.

Green M, editor: *Bright futures, guidelines for health supervision of infants, children and adolescents*, Arlington, Va, 1994, National Center for Education in Maternal and Child Health.

Hagedorn M, Gardner S, Abman S: *Respiratory distress*. In Merenstein G, Gardner S, editors: *Handbook of neonatal intensive care*, ed 3, St Louis, 1993, Mosby.

Harrigan R et al: Perinatal grief: response to the loss of an infant, *Neonat Netw* 12(5):25, 1993.

Haubrich K: *Assessment and management of auditory dysfunction*. In Kenner C, Brueggemeyer A, Gunderson L, editors: *Comprehensive neonatal nursing: a physiologic perspective*, Philadelphia, 1993, WB Saunders.

Haut C, Peddicord K, O'Brien E: Supporting parental bonding in the NICU: a care plan for nurses. *Neonat Netw* 13(8):19, 1994.

Holditch-Davis D, Edwards L, Wigger M: Pathologic apnea and brief respiratory pauses in preterm infants: relation to sleep state, *Nurs Res* 43(5):293, 1994.

Janke J: Development of the breast-feeding attrition tool, *Nurs Res* 43(2):100, 1994.

Jenkins J, Covington C, Plotnick J: Early childhood intervention: the law, *MCN Am J Matern Child Nurs* 19(3):135, 1994.

Klaus M, Kennell J: *Care of the parents.* In Klaus M, Fanaroff A, editors: *Care of the high-risk neonate,* ed 4, Philadelphia, 1993, WB Saunders.

Klaus M, Martin R, Fanaroff A: *The physical environment.* In Klaus M, Fanaroff A, editors: *Care of the high-risk neonate,* ed 4, Philadelphia, 1993, WB Saunders.

Kuller J, Lund C: *Assessment and management of integumentary dysfunction.* In Kenner C, Brueggemeyer A, Gunderson I, editors: *Comprehensive neonatal nursing: a physiologic perspective,* Philadelphia, 1993, WB Saunders.

Kunley J, Freston M: Back transport: exploration of parents' feelings, *Neonat Netw* 12(1):49, 1993.

LeBoyer F: *Loving hands,* New York, 1981, Alfred A Knopf.

Lefrak-Okikawa L, Meier P: *Nutrition: physiologic basis of metabolism and management of enteral and parenteral nutrition.* In Kenner C, Brueggemeyer A, Gunderson L, editors: *Comprehensive neonatal nursing: a physiologic perspective,* Philadelphia, 1993, WB Saunders.

Legault M, Goulet C: Comparison of kangaroo and traditional methods of removing preterm infants from incubators, *J Obstet Gynecol Neonatal Nurs* 24(6):501, 1995.

Lien E: The role of fatty acid composition and positional distribution in fat absorption in infants, *J Pediatr* 125(5):S62, 1994.

Loizeaux W: *Anna. A daughter's life,* New York, 1993, Arcade Publishing.

Ludington-Hoe S et al: Kangaroo care: research results, practice implications and guidelines. *Neonat Netw* 13(1):19, 1994.

Lynam L: Research utilization: nonpharmacological management of pain in neonates, *Neonat Netw,* 14 (5): 59, 1995.

Martin R, Fanaroff A, Klaus M: *Respiratory problems.* In Klaus M, Fanaroff A, editors: *Care of the high-risk neonate,* ed 4, Philadelphia, 1993, WB Saunders.

Mauskopf J et al: Synthetic surfactant for rescue treatment of respiratory distress syndrome in premature infants weighing from 700 to 1350 grams: impact on hospital resource use and charges, *J Pediatr* 126(1):94, 1995.

Medoff-Cooper B, Verklan T, Carlson S: The development of sucking patterns and physiologic correlates in very-low-birth-weight infants, *Nurs Res* 42(2):100, 1993.

Mehren E: *Born too soon,* New York, 1991, Doubleday.

Meier P: Transition of the preterm infant to an open crib: process of the project group, *J Obstet Gynecol Neonatal Nurs* 23(4):321, 1994.

Metheny N et al: Characteristics of aspirates from feeding tubes as a method for predicting tube location, *Nurs Res* 43(5):282, 1994.

National Institutes of Health: Early identification of hearing impairment in infants and young children, *NIH Consensus Statement* 11(1), 1993.

Nichols J: *Bereavement: a state of having suffered a loss.* In Kenner C, Brueggemeyer A, Gunderson L, editors: *Comprehensive neonatal nursing. A physiologic perspective,* Philadelphia, 1993, WB Saunders.

Oehler J, Hannan T, Catlett A: Maternal views of preterm infant's responsiveness to social interaction, *Neonat Netw* 12(6):67, 1993.

Pickler R, Frankel H: The effect of non-nutritive sucking on preterm infants' behavioral organization and feeding performance [abstract], *Neonat Netw* 14(2):83, 1995.

Pickler R, Terrell R: Nonnutritive sucking and necrotizing enterocolitis, *Neonat Netw* 13(8):15, 1994.

Pinyard B: Infant cries: physiology and assessment, *Neonat Netw* 13(4):15, 1994.

Pittard W: *Classification of the low-birth-weight infant.* In Klaus M, Fanaroff A, editors: *Care of the high-risk neonate,* ed 4, Philadelphia, 1993, WB Saunders.

Price P, Kalhan S: *Nutrition and selected disorders of the gastrointestinal tract.* In Klaus M, Fanaroff A, editors: *Care of the high-risk neonate,* ed 4, Philadelphia, 1993, WB Saunders.

Prukop S, editor: *Lucile Salter Packard Children's Hospital at Stanford NICU Parent Handbook,* Palo Alto, Calif, 1994, Mead Johnson Nutritionals.

Scanlon C, Fibison W: *Managing genetic information: implications for nursing practice,* Washington, DC, 1995, American Nurses Association.

Schanler R, Shulman R, Prestridge L: Parenteral nutrient needs of very low birth weight infants, *J Pediatr* 125(6):961, 1994.

Schneider V: Infant massage: handbook for loving parents, New York, 1982, Bantam Books.

Shiao S et al: Nasogastric tube placement: effects on breathing and sucking in very-low-birth-weight infants, *Nurs Res* 44(2):82, 1995.

Strauch C, Brandt S, Edwards-Beckett J: Implementation of a quiet hour: effect on noise level and infant sleep state, *Neonat Netw* 12(2):31, 1993.

Thomas K: Back to basics: Thermoregulation in neonates, *Neonat Netw* 13(2):13, 1994.

Townsend S, Johnson C, Hay W: *Enteral nutrition.* In Merenstein G, Gardner S, editors: *Handbook of neonatal intensive care,* ed 3, St Louis, 1993, Mosby.

Wells N et al: Does tympanic temperature measure up? *MCN Am J Matern Child Nurs* 20(2):95, 1995.

Wong D, editor: *Whaley & Wong's nursing care of infants and children,* ed 5, St Louis, 1995, Mosby.

Bibliography

Chathas M, Paton J: Parenteral nutrition for hospitalized infants: 20th century advances in venous access, *J Obstet Gynecol Neonatal Nurs* 24(5):441, 1995.

Cleary J et al: Improved oxygenation during synchronized intermittent mandatory ventilation in neonates with respiratory distress syndrome: a randomized study, *J Pediatr* 126(3):407, 1995.

Cox C, Wolfson M, Shaffer T: Liquid ventilation: a comprehensive review, *Neonat Netw* 15(3):31, 1996.

Deming L: Planning earlier discharge from the NICU, *J Case Management* 2(4):13, 1996.

Gonzales I et al: Effect of enteral feeding tolerance in preterm infants, *Neonat Netw* 14(3):39, 1995.

Maroney D: Realities of a premature infant's first year: helping parents cope, *J Perinatol* 15(5):418, 1995.

Martin G: Less neonatal intensive care: a new focus, *J Perinatol* 15(1):1, 1995.

Miles M, Calson J, Funk S: Sources of support reported by mothers and fathers of infants hospitalized in a neonatal intensive care unit, *Neonat Netw* 15(3):45, 1996.

Stevens B, Franck L: Special needs of preterm infants in the management of pain and discomfort, *J Obstet Gynecol Neonatal Nurs* 24(9):856, 1995.

Symington A et al: Indwelling versus intermittent feeding tubes in premature neonate, *J Obstet Gynecol Neonatal Nurs* 24(4):321, 1995.

CHAPTER 26

Specific Problems of the Newborn

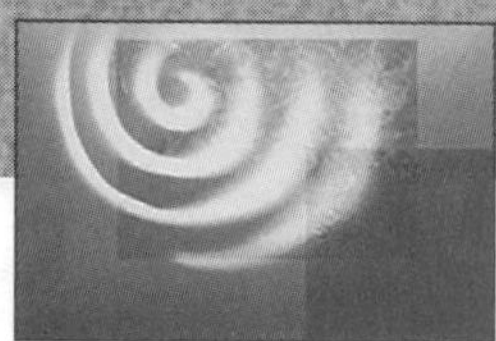

GESTATIONAL AGE AND BIRTHWEIGHT, P. 724

Infant mortality and morbidity, p. 725

The preterm infant, p. 725

Nursing care management, p. 726

POSTDATE AND POSTMATURE INFANTS, P. 737

SGA, IUGR, AND DYSMATURE INFANTS, P. 739

Common problems, p. 739

LGA INFANTS, P. 740

INFANTS OF DIABETIC MOTHERS, P. 741

Pathophysiology, p. 741

Congenital anomalies, p. 741

Macrosomia, p. 743

Birth trauma and perinatal asphyxia, p. 743

RDS, p. 744

Hypoglycemia, p. 744

Hypocalcemia and hypomagnesemia, p. 744

Cardiomyopathy, p. 744

Hyperbilirubinemia and polycythemia, p. 744

BIRTH TRAUMA, P. 746

NEONATAL INFECTIONS, P. 749

Nursing care management, p. 750

TORCH infections, p. 752

Bacterial infections, p. 758

Fungal infections, p. 758

SUBSTANCE ABUSE, P. 759

Alcohol, p. 760

Tobacco, p. 761

Marijuana, p. 761

Cocaine, p. 761

Phencyclidine ("angel dust"), p. 761

Heroin, p. 761

Methadone, p. 762

Miscellaneous substances, p. 762

Nursing care management, p. 763

DISCHARGE TO HOME FOR THE COMPROMISED NEWBORN, P. 766

HYPERBILIRUBINEMIA, P. 767

Rh incompatibility, p. 767

ABO incompatibility, p. 768

Kernicterus, p. 768

CONGENITAL ANOMALIES, P. 769

Central nervous system anomalies, p. 770

Cardiovascular system anomalies, p. 772

Respiratory system anomalies, p. 772

Gastrointestinal system anomalies, p. 773

Musculoskeletal system anomalies, p. 775

Genitourinary system anomalies, p. 776

Nursing care management, p. 777

Nurses must be prepared to provide immediate and emergency care to newborns who are born with or develop problems during the newborn period. Nurses assist in the stabilization of the infant before transporting the infant to a regional intensive care nursery. They deal with parents who are trying to cope with the birth of a baby who does not meet their expected ideal. In this chapter, some of the problems encountered during the newborn period are discussed, and nursing care of compromised infants is described.

GESTATIONAL AGE AND BIRTHWEIGHT

Modern technology and good nursing care have contributed significantly to improved health and overall survival of infants at risk because of gestational age or birth weight. However, the survival of infants born significantly before term has resulted in the development of conditions that may alter their future. These conditions include necrotizing enterocolitis (NEC), bronchopulmonary dysplasia (BPD), periventricular-intraventricular hemorrhage (PV-IVH), and retinopathy of prematurity (ROP).

The cause of preterm and **postterm** birth is largely unknown; however, the incidence of preterm birth is highest among low socioeconomic groups. This is likely a result of the lack of comprehensive prenatal health care. Other factors found to be associated with preterm birth include preeclampsia, maternal infection, multifetal pregnancy, incompetent cervix, and placental accidents.

Both **term** and preterm infants may also be classified according to birthweight; inherent therein are certain factors that place them at risk for altered development. The **large-for-gestational age (LGA)** infant has a birthweight above the ninetieth percentile and is presumed to have grown at an accelerated rate during fetal life. The **small-for-gestational**

age (SGA) infant has a birthweight below the tenth percentile and is presumed to have grown at a slower rate during fetal life.

Common causes of LGA newborns include glucose intolerance of pregnancy, true maternal diabetes mellitus, maternal overnutrition, parity, and heredity. SGA newborns may be affected by maternal smoking, hypertensive states, undernutrition, anemia, or nephritis. In addition, the birth of an SGA newborn may be associated with multifetal gestation, a discordant twin pregnancy, or congenital anomalies. High altitude, rubella, or intrauterine infection may predispose a woman to the birth of an SGA newborn. Fetal malnutrition, **intrauterine growth restriction (IUGR)** and chronic fetal distress are other processes that may result in the birth of SGA infants.

Infant Mortality and Morbidity

Preterm birth is responsible for almost two thirds of infant deaths. The infant born before term does not possess the growth and development necessary for uncomplicated adjustment to extrauterine life, and prospects for survival or good health may be severely compromised. Infants weighing more than 2500 g (5½ lb) and born after 37 weeks of pregnancy have the best prospects of survival. There is a dramatic reduction in mortality in infants, regardless of weight, who are born after week 36 of gestation. The prognosis for **low-birth-weight (LBW)** infants weighing more than 1800 g (4 lb) is more favorable than for those weighing 1500 to 1800 g (3 to 4 lb). Mortality is less than 5% if the pregnancy has progressed to 35 weeks and the fetus weighs more than 2000 g (4½ lb).

Children and adults who were LBW infants are more likely to have major problems such as cerebral palsy, mental retardation, and sensory and cognitive disabilities and are at risk for a diminished ability to successfully adapt socially, psychologically, and physically to an increasingly complex environment (Fanaroff and Martin, 1997). In addition to the potential alterations in life-style, the fiscal impact of LBW infants on our society is estimated to be in the billions of dollars each year (Box 26-1).

The Preterm Infant

The preterm infant is at risk because of immaturity of organ systems and lack of reserves. The morbidity and mortality rates for preterm infants are higher by three to four times than those of older gestational age infants of comparable weight. The potential problems and care needs of preterm infants weighing 2000 g differ from those of term, postterm, or postmature infants of equal weight.

Preterm infants are at a distinct disadvantage when they face the transition from intrauterine to extrauterine life. The

BOX 26-1

Ethical Considerations Related to Resuscitation of Extremely Premature Infants

There are many different opinions about resuscitation of extremely preterm infants weighing less than 600 g. Ethical issues that nurses are confronted with include the following:

- Whether or not to resuscitate?
- Who should decide?
- Is the cost of resuscitation justified?
- Do the benefits of technology outweigh the burdens in relation to the quality of life?

All individuals involved (health care providers and parents) should be involved in discussions that lead to resolution of these controversial issues.

BOX 26-2

Differences in Borderline, Moderately, and Extremely Premature Infants

Borderline premature infant

36 to 37 weeks' gestation
2500 to 3250 g
16% of all live births
Usually normal
Problems
- Temperature instability
- Feeding difficulties
- Jaundice
- Respiratory distress possible

Appearance
- Fewer creases on feet
- Smaller breasts
- Fuzzy hair
- Lanugo
- Vernix
- Less developed genitalia

Moderately premature infant

31 to 35 weeks' gestation
1500 to 2500 g
6% to 7% of all live births
Problems
- Temperature instability
- Glucose regulation
- Fluid balance
- Respiratory distress
- Jaundice
- Anemia
- Infections
- Feeding difficulties

Appearance
- As for borderline premature infant, but exaggerated
- Skin is thinner, more vascular

Extremely premature infants

23 to 30 weeks' gestation
400 to 1400 g
0.8% of all live births, but almost all neonatal deaths and neurologic deficits not attributable to birth defects or birth trauma
Problems
- As for moderately premature infant, but exaggerated

Appearance
- Tiny, no fat, extremely thin skin
- Eyes may be fused

degree of disadvantage depends primarily on their level of maturity (Box 26-2). Physiologic disorders and anomalies affect the infants' response to treatment as well. In general, the closer infants are to the normal term infant in gestational age and birth weight, the easier will be their adjustment to the external environment.

Nursing Care Management

Assessment

Potential problems of the preterm newborn. In assessing the preterm infant, the nurse follows a systematic approach. The response of the preterm infant to extrauterine life is different from that of the term infant. Understanding the physiologic basis of these differences helps the nurse assess these infants, determine the response of the preterm infant, and anticipate which potential problems are most likely to occur.

Respiratory function. As with the term infant, initial assessment begins with respiratory function, observing the infant's ability to make the pulmonary transition from intrauterine to extrauterine life. The preterm infant is likely to have difficulty making this transition because of numerous deficits in the respiratory system:

- Decreased number of functional alveoli
- Deficient surfactant levels
- Smaller lumen in the respiratory system
- Greater collapsibility or obstruction of respiratory passages
- Insufficient calcification of the bony thorax
- Immature and friable capillaries in the lungs
- Greater distance between functional alveoli and capillary bed to allow gas exchange

In combination, these deficits severely hinder the infant's respiratory efforts and result in respiratory distress and/or apnea. The nurse must be prepared to provide oxygen and ventilation, as necessary (Merenstein and Gardner, 1993).

Cardiovascular function. After respiratory assessment the nurse assesses the cardiovascular system and its ability to provide perfusion to essential tissues and organs. Evaluation of heart rates and rhythm, color, blood pressure, capillary refill (perfusion), pulses (brachial and femoral), oxygen saturation, and acid base status provides information concerning cardiovascular status.

The nurse must be prepared to intervene if symptoms of hypovolemia, shock, or both, are present. These symptoms include decreased blood pressure, slow capillary refill (>3 seconds), and continued respiratory distress despite provision of oxygen and ventilation.

Maintaining body temperature. As a result of numerous factors the preterm infant is susceptible to temperature instability. Heat loss is great because of the large surface area in relation to body weight. Other factors that place the preterm infant at risk for temperature instability include the following:

- Minimal insulating subcutaneous fat
- Limited stores of *brown fat* (an internal source for generation of heat present in normal term infants)
- Decreased or absent reflex control of skin capillaries (shiver response)
- Inadequate muscle mass activity (therefore the preterm infant is unable to produce his or her own heat)
- Friable (easily damaged) capillaries
- Immature temperature regulation center in the brain
- Extended rather than flexed position

The goal of thermoregulation is a neutral thermal environment (NTE). The NTE is the environmental temperature at which oxygen consumption is minimal but adequate to maintain the body temperature (Cloherty and Stark, 1991). With the knowledge of the four mechanisms of heat transfer (convection, conduction, radiation, evaporation), the nurse can ensure an environment that prevents temperature instability in the preterm infant. A regulated, external heat source and periodic assessments of temperature are essential.

Nursing ALERT

When using a servocontrolled incubator, evaluate trends of increased or decreased ambient air temperature in response to fluctuations in the infant's body temperature to rule out sepsis or other dysfunction.

Central nervous system function. The preterm infant's central nervous system (CNS) is susceptible to injury from various sources:

- Birth trauma with damage to immature structures
- Bleeding from fragile capillaries
- Impaired coagulation process, including prolonged prothrombin time
- Recurrent anoxic episodes.
- Predisposition to **hypoglycemia**

Research data suggest that the developing nervous system can reorganize neural connections after injury. Certain neurologic signs appear to have predictive power for later abnormal neurologic functions. These signs include hypotonia, decreased level of activity, weak cry for greater than 24 hours, and inability to suck and swallow (Fanaroff and Martin, 1997). Ongoing assessment and documentation of these neurologic signs is needed for discharge teaching, predictive value, and follow-up recommendations.

Maintaining adequate nutrition. Maintenance of adequate nutrition in the preterm infant is complicated by problems of intake and of metabolism. With regard to intake, the preterm infant has the following disadvantages: weak or absent suck, swallow, and gag reflexes; a small stomach capacity; and weak abdominal muscles. The preterm infant's metabolic functions are weakened by a limited store of nutrients, a decreased ability to digest proteins or absorb nutrients, and immature enzyme systems.

The nurse provides ongoing assessment of the infant's ability to take in and digest nutrients. Nourishment may need to be provided to the preterm infant by means other than the oral route (e.g., gavage or parenterally).

Nursing ALERT

Nurses must be alert to signs of both overhydration and underhydration, such as weight changes, electrolytes, output measurements, urine specific gravity, and evidence of edema.

Maintaining renal function. The preterm infant's immature renal system is unable (1) to adequately excrete metabolites and drugs, (2) to concentrate the urine, and (3) to maintain balances in acid-base, fluids, or electrolytes (Gomella et al, 1994). The nurse assesses intake and output, as well as specific gravity; monitors laboratory values for acid-base and electrolyte balance; and observes for symptoms of drug toxicity.

Maintaining hematologic status. Compared with the term infant, the preterm infant is predisposed to hematologic problems as a result of the following factors:

- Increased capillary friability
- Increased tendency to bleed (prolonged prothrombin time and partial thromboplastin time)
- Slowed production of red blood cells as a result of rapid decrease in erythropoiesis after birth
- Loss of blood from frequent laboratory tests
- Decreased red blood cell (RBC) survival related to relatively larger size of the RBC and increased permeability to sodium and potassium.

The nurse assesses for any evidence of bleeding from puncture sites, gastrointestinal tract, or skin and anemia (pale color of skin, increased apnea and bradycardia, tachycardia, and slowed weight gain) (Merenstein and Gardner, 1993).

Resisting infection. The preterm infant is at increased risk for infection because of a shortage of stored maternal immunoglobulins, an impaired ability to make antibodies, and a compromised integumentary system (thin skin and fragile capillaries). The preterm infant exhibits various nonspecific signs and symptoms of infection, including temperature instability (hypothermia or hyperthermia), lethargy, irritability, poor perfusion, color change, jaundice, feeding intolerance, vomiting, diarrhea, respiratory distress, apnea, hypotension, glucose instability, and metabolic acidosis (Gomella et al, 1994). The nurse must be diligent in assessing preterm infants for early identification and treatment of sepsis. As with all aspects of care, strict handwashing is the single most important element to prevent iatrogenic infections.

Nursing ALERT

Poor feeding behaviors such as apnea, bradycardia, cyanosis, pallor, and decreased oxygen saturation in any infant who has previously fed well may indicate an underlying illness.

Skin care. The skin of preterm infants is characteristically immature relative to that of full-term infants. Because of its increased sensitivity and fragility, no alkaline-based soap is used that might destroy the "acid mantle" of the skin. The increased permeability of the skin facilitates absorption of ingredients. All skin products (e.g., alcohol or povidone-iodine) are used with caution, and the skin is rinsed with water afterward, since these substances may cause severe irritation and chemical burns in LBW infants.

The skin is easily excoriated and denuded; therefore care must be taken to avoid damage to the delicate structure. The total skin is less thick than that of full-term infants and has fewer elastic fibers; also, there is less cohesion between the thinner skin layers. Adhesives used after heel sticks or to secure monitoring equipment or intravenous infusions may excoriate the skin or adhere to the skin surface so firmly that the skin can be separated from understructures and pulled away with the tape. The use of skin barriers protects healthy skin and helps excoriated skin heal.

It is unsafe to use scissors to remove dressings or tape from the extremities of very small and immature infants because it is easy to snip off tiny extremities or nick loosely attached skin. Solvents used to remove tape are avoided because they tend to dry and burn the delicate skin. See the guidelines for skin care in the Guidelines box on p. 728.

During skin assessment of preterm infants, nurses are also alert to the subtle signs that indicate zinc deficiency, a common problem in these infants. Breakdown usually occurs in the areas around the mouth, buttocks, fingers, and toes, In **very low birth weight (VLBW)** infants it may also occur in the creases of the neck, wrists, ankles, and around wounds. Zinc deficiency is most likely to appear in infants with sepsis, those experiencing nasogastric losses, or those who have had surgery. Any suspicious lesions are reported to the physician so that zinc supplements can be prescribed.

Growth and development potential. Although it is impossible to predict with complete accuracy the growth and development potential of each preterm newborn, some findings support an anticipated favorable outcome. The growth and development landmarks are corrected for gestational age until approximately 2.5 years (Avery et al, 1994).

The age of a preterm newborn is corrected by adding the gestational age and the postnatal age. For example, if an infant was born at 32 weeks' gestation 4 weeks ago, the infant is considered to be 36 weeks of age. The child's corrected age 6 months after the birth date is 4 months. Responses are evaluated against the norm expected for a 4-month-old infant.

The preterm infant experiences catch-up body growth during the first 2 to 3 years of life with maximum growth rates occurring between 36 and 40 weeks' postconceptional age (Avery et al, 1994; Fanaroff and Martin, 1997). Head growth is the first parameter to experience catch-up growth, followed by gain in weight and height (Avery et al, 1994).

Favorable findings that support the prediction of a growth and development pattern within the norm include certain measurable factors. At discharge from the hospital, which usually occurs between 37 and 40 weeks after the woman's last menstrual period (LMP), the infant exhibits the following characteristics:

- The baby can raise the head when prone and hold the head parallel with the body when tested for head lag response. (When the infant is pulled up by the hands, the infant's head lags, but then the head and chest will be in line as the upright position is reached. This alignment will be held momentarily before the head falls forward [pull-to-sit or traction reflex]).
- The infant cries with vigor when hungry.
- The infant shows appropriate amount and pattern of weight gain according to a growth grid.
- The infant's neurologic responses are appropriate for corrected age.
- The retinas appear normal.

At 39 to 40 weeks corrected age, the infant can focus on

Guidelines

NEONATAL SKIN CARE

General skin care

Cleanse skin with plain warm water. Use bland, nonalkaline soaps or cleansers only when necessary, such as for removal of stool.

Provide daily cleansing of eye, oral, and diaper areas and any areas of skin breakdown.

Apply moisturizing agents to skin after cleansing with warm water to retain moisture and rehydrate skin. Cleanse skin gently of any old oil or cream before applying a new layer, except in diaper area.

When safflower oil is applied, some essential fatty acids may be absorbed in addition to softening skin as a moisturizer.

Use pressure-relieving or reducing mattress to prevent pressure areas.

Use of adhesives on skin

Use minimal tape/adhesive. Evaluate need for all tape/adhesive used. Chart amount and placement of all tape used.

Use a protective, pectin-based or hydrocolloid skin barrier between skin and all tape/adhesives. Place on all areas where tape/adhesives are used, such as for securing chest tubes, nasogastric tubes, dressings, extremities to intravenous (IV) board, monitor leads, endotracheal tubes, and temperature probe (cut "keyhole" for temperature probe in barrier or place circular patch of skin barrier over probe).

Place pectin-based or hydrocolloid skin barriers directly over excoriated skin. Leave barrier undisturbed until it begins to peel off. With wet, oozing excoriations, dust site with a small amount of stoma powder (as used in ostomy care), brush excess away, and apply skin barrier. Hold barrier in place for several minutes to allow barrier to soften and mold to the skin surface.

Use transparent elastic film dressings to secure and protect central lines and peripheral arterial line insertion sites, as well as over open skin lesions. Leave dressing in place until it begins to peel off, usually within 5 to 7 days.

Alternate electrode placement and avoid standard adhesive, gelled electrode. Use limb electrodes rather than standard chest electrodes or use hydrogel or synthetic karaya gel electrodes. Assess skin thoroughly underneath electrodes. Remove and rotate electrodes minimally every 24 hours or more frequently if skin injury is noted.

Remove adhesives with warm water-soaked gauze or a small amount of bland, diluted soap, rather than alcohol or adhesive removers. To remove a skin barrier, slowly and gently peel away from skin, holding barrier in one hand and supporting skin underneath with other hand. If needed, soak off with warm water. Do not use bonding agents such as tincture of benzoin or commercial swabs.

Avoid using scissors to remove tape or dressings to prevent cutting skin or amputating digits.

Use of substances on skin

Evaluate all substances that come in contact with infant's skin.

Avoid or limit use of the following substances that have potential for percutaneous absorption and systemic effects:

Adhesive removers	Isopropyl alcohol
Boric acid	Neomycin ointment
Chlorhexidene	Povidone iodine
Chlorophenol	Salicylic acid
Epinephrine	Steroids
Estrogen	Tincture of benzoin
Hexachlorophene	Silver sulfadiazine cream
Hydrogen peroxide	

If any of the above agents are used, chart amount and frequency of application.

Before using any topical agent, analyze components of preparation and:

- Use sparingly and only when necessary.
- Confine use to smallest possible area.
- Whenever possible and appropriate, wash off with water.
- Monitor infant carefully for signs of toxicity and systemic effects.

Use of thermal devices

Avoid heat lamps because of increased potential for burns. If needed, measure actual temperature of exposed skin every 15 minutes.

When using heating pads (Aqua-K pads):

- Change infant's position every 15 minutes initially and then every 1 to 2 hours.
- Preset temperature of heating pads <40°C (104°F).

When using preheated transcutaneous electrodes:

- Avoid use on infants <1000 g.
- Set at lowest possible temperature (<44°C [111.2°F]) and secure with plastic wrap.
- Use pulse oximetry rather than transcutaneous monitoring whenever possible.

When prewarming heels before phlebotomy, avoid temperatures >40°C.

Warm ambient humidity, direct away from infant, use aerosolized sterile water, and maintain ambient temperature so as not to exceed 40°C.

Document use of all heating devices.

Use of fluid therapy/hemodynamic monitoring

Be certain fingers or toes are visible whenever extremity is used for IV or arterial line.

Secure catheter or needle with transparent dressing/tape to promote easy visualization of site.

Assess site hourly for signs of ischemia, infiltration, and inadequate perfusion (check capillary refill).

Check that any restraints (e.g., armboards) are secured safely and not restricting circulation or movement (check for pressure areas).

Modified from Malloy M, Perez-Woods R: Neonatal skin care: prevention of skin breakdown, *Pediatr Nurs* 17(1):41, 1991.

the examiner's or parent's face and is able to follow with her or his eyes.

At the corrected ages of 6 and 12 months the infant is assessed again for age-appropriate responses. The infant who continues to be a poor eater; is irritable; displays sensory, perceptual, intellectual, or motor deviations in development; and displays or develops hypertonia or hypotonia may be at risk for developmental delay.

These behaviors must be interpreted with caution; the infant requires reevaluation by an interdisciplinary team at frequent intervals. Parents need continued support and attention should these signs appear. Minor behavioral deviations also are identified so that the parents can be assisted in their understanding and acceptance of the child. Deviations such as clumsiness, varying degrees of incoordination, slowness in reading and writing, and similar problems may be distressing to the child, parents, and other family members.

Parental adaptation to preterm infant. Parents who experience the preterm birth of their infant have a different experience from parents giving birth to a full-term infant. Because of this difference, parental attachment and adaptation to the parental role also are different.

Parental tasks. Parents face a number of psychologic tasks before effective relationships and parenting patterns can evolve. These tasks include the following:

- *Anticipatory grief over the potential loss of an infant.* The parent grieves in preparation for the infant's possible death, although the parent clings to the hope that the child will survive. This begins during labor and lasts until the infant dies or shows evidence of surviving.
- *Acceptance by the mother of her failure to give birth to a healthy, full-term infant.* Grief and depression typify this phase, which persists until the infant is out of danger and is expected to survive.
- *Resumption of the process of relating to the infant.* As the baby begins to improve—gains weight, feeds by nipple, and is weaned from the incubator—the parent can begin the process of developing attachment to the infant that was interrupted by the infant's precarious condition at birth.
- *Learning how this baby differs in special needs and growth patterns.* Another parental task is to learn, understand, and accept this infant's caregiving needs and growth and development expectations.
- *Adjusting the home environment to the needs of the new infant.* Limitation of visitors is encouraged to reduce the risk of exposure to pathogens. The environmental temperature may need to be altered to optimize conditions for the infant. The need to avoid irritants such as cigarette smoke may necessitate life-style changes. Grandparents and siblings also react to the birth of the preterm infant. Parents must reconcile the grief of grandparents and the bewilderment and anger of brothers and sisters at the disproportionate amount of parental time absorbed by the newborn.

Parental responses. Parents may cope by taking each day as it comes, recognizing and accepting the lessened responses of their infant and noting the gradual progress in their child's condition. Other parents pull away from emotional attachment to the infant; they postpone becoming attached until the infant is in better health.

Parents have been observed to progress through stages as they spend more time with their infants. In the first stage they maintain an *en face* position, stroking and touching their infant (Fig. 26-1). In the second stage they assume some child care activities—feeding, bathing, diapering the infant. In the third stage the infant becomes a person and is seen as a whole child (Schraeder, 1980). Sosa and Grua (1982) reported a personal communication with Brazelton in which he correlated parental behaviors with the previously noted three stages. In the first stage, parents ask about chemical data, such as "What is his bilirubin today?" In the second stage, they note their baby yawning, sneezing, hiccoughing—reflexes that mark their infant as human. At this time the infant is still not "claimed." In later stages, they note their infant's responses to them and begin to feel that "this child is mine" and part of their family. Parents take on the role of advocate for their child.

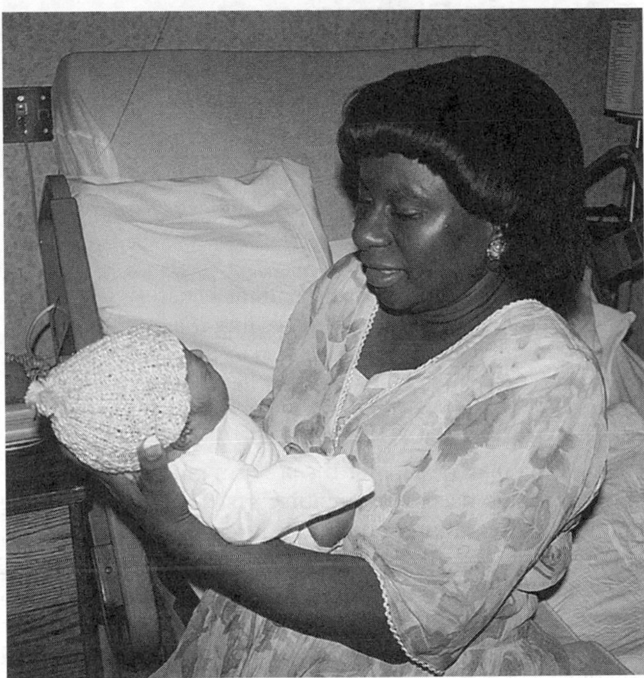

Fig. 26-1 Mother and baby make eye contact in en face position. (Courtesy Marjorie Pyle, RNC, Lifecircle, Costa Mesa, CA.)

Infant responsiveness. The preterm infant's behavior is difficult to interpret because the infant cannot provide positive reciprocal cues that encourage continued interaction with parents (Lindsay et al, 1993). The quiet alert state is less evident and is unpredictable. Field (1979) noted that if a mother concentrated her interactions on imitation of the infant's behavior, the preterm infant was increasingly attentive and interested. Too active an involvement in child care tended to result in the infant's becoming disinterested and glancing away (gaze aversion).

Parenting disorders. The incidence of physical and emotional abuse is significantly greater toward the infant who, because of preterm birth or illness, was separated from the mother for a period of time after birth. Physical abuse includes varying degrees of poor nutrition and poor hygiene. Emotional abuse ranges from subtle to outright dislike of the child. There may be preferential treatment for brothers and sisters, nagging, extremely high expectations of the child, and other types of overt or covert negative parental responses.

Factors surrounding the birth may predispose parents to subconsciously or overtly reject the child. These factors might include parental pain and anxiety, a heavy financial burden for the infant's care, unresolved anticipatory grief, threat to self-esteem, or unwanted pregnancy. The goal of health professionals is early identification and reduction of the incidence of child abuse and neglect.

Nursing Diagnoses

To formulate nursing diagnoses, the nurse analyzes data obtained from continuous monitoring of the infant and from observation of and discussions with the parents. The diagnoses may be physical, cognitive, or psychologic, for example:

- Ineffective breathing pattern related to
  Inadequate chest expansion, secondary to infant's position
- Parental anxiety related to
  Knowledge deficit regarding infant's cues
  Knowledge deficit regarding feeding the infant
- Situational low self-esteem related to
  Parent's feelings of inadequacy in caring for the infant

Expected Outcomes

The nursing plan of care for the preterm infant is dictated by the physiologic needs of immature systems, often involving emergency treatments and procedures. During this time, nursing care is a critical element in the infant's chances for survival. In addition to meeting the infant's physical needs, nursing care is planned in conjunction with parents to promote parent-infant attachment and interaction. Expected outcomes are presented in patient-centered terms.

The infant will achieve the following:

1. Maintain physiologic functioning
2. Maintain adequate nutrition
3. Experience no or minimal hematologic problems
4. Remain free of infection
5. Not develop retinal problems
6. Experience no trauma to immature musculoskeletal system
7. Experience attachment to parents

The parents will achieve the following:

1. Perceive the child as potentially normal (if this is medically substantiated)
2. Provide care comfortably
3. Experience pride and satisfaction in the care of the infant
4. Organize their time and energies to meet the love, attention, and care needs of the other members of the family as well as their own

Plan of Care and Implementation

The best environment for fetal growth and development is in the uterus of a healthy, well-nourished woman for 38 to 42 weeks. The extrauterine environment of the preterm newborn must approximate a healthy intrauterine environment for the normal sequence of growth and development to continue. The provision of such an environment is the basis for care of the preterm infant. Medical and nursing personnel and respiratory therapists work as a team to provide the intensive care needed. The nurse acts as a constant presence in the infant's support system.

Nursing actions are based on knowledge of the physiologic problems imposed on the preterm infant and on the infant's need to conserve energy for repair, maintenance, and growth. Nursing care is centered on the continuous assessment and analysis of physiologic status. Nurses fulfill many roles in providing the intensive and extended care that these infants require. Nurses continuously gather data regarding the infant's physiologic status. They make decisions and initiate therapies based on their interpretation of these data. In addition, nurses are the support persons and teachers during the first phase of the parents' adjustment to the birth of the preterm infant.

The nurse uses many technologic support systems to monitor body responses and maintain body function in the infant. Gentle touch, concern for the traumatic effects of harsh lighting, and control of machinery noise are interwoven with the technical skill of the nurse in the intensive care nursery.

Physical care. The preterm infant's environmental support consists of the following:

- Incubator or overhead heat panel. In VLBW infants a plastic bubble cover may be placed over the infant to control body temperature (NTE).
- Oxygen administration, depending on infant's cardiopulmonary and circulatory status.
- Electronic monitors as needed for observation of respiratory and cardiac functions.
- Flotation mattress and props (bolsters, rolled linens) for positioning infant to facilitate physiologic functioning and to maintain skin integrity and correct body alignment.
- Protection from noise (see discussion of infant stimulation in next section).

Metabolic support consists of measures such as the following:

- Parenteral fluids to assist in supporting nutrition, normal arterial blood gas (ABG) levels, and acid-base homeostasis
- Parenteral fluids to facilitate antibiotic therapy if sepsis is a concern
- Blood specimen analyses to monitor ABG levels, pH, blood glucose level, and sepsis.

Infant stimulation. Although preterm infants respond differently to infant stimulation than do term infants, they continue to benefit from touch as long as it is adjusted to the developmental and tolerance level of the particular infant. Both procedural and social stimulation can be used to provide the least amount of distress to the infant. For example, cycled lighting has beneficial effects on preterm infants (Blackburn and Patteson, 1991). This study suggests that decreasing the light in the room may facilitate rest and help conserve energy in preterm infants. When the lights are dimmed, activity and noise from staff members are also decreased. Nurses can provide an environment that helps preterm infants develop neurobehavioral organization. This allows the infant to conserve energy and respond more appropriately to parents. These infants need tactile stimulation provided with slow, sure motions. In changing the infant's position the nurse supports the head and holds the infant's limbs close to the body. This type of supportive movement provides stimulation while reducing motor disorganization. At 34 to 36 weeks' gestational age, the infant responds to visual and auditory stimuli when in an alert state. At 36 to 40 weeks' gestational age, infants are much more capable of tolerating stimulation from caregivers and parents. Caregivers and parents can use varied approaches to soothe the distressed infant. These include talking to the infant, controlling the infant's arms across the chest with the palm of the caregiver's hand, swaddling the infant to reduce the self-distressing effects of startle reflexes, holding and rocking the infant in an upright position, and offering a pacifier (Merenstein and Gardner, 1993).

Infant feeding. The preterm infant may be fed by breast, bottle, or gavage. Infants may be put to breast for practice feeds as soon as medically stable. For the infant who requires gavage feeding, **nonnutritive sucking** of a pacifier during the gavage procedure may facilitate earlier transition to nipple feeding. In addition, these infants may have a better weight gain, experience fewer complications, and be discharged sooner (Gill et al, 1988).

The following criteria are used for initiating nipple feedings (Merenstein and Gardner, 1993):

- Coordinated sucking, swallowing, and breathing
- Adequate gag reflex (usually established by 34 to 36 weeks' gestational age)
- Respiratory function that allows unlabored sucking (specific parameters will vary with each infant; usually respiratory rate <60 breaths per minute)
- Steady weight gain

Parent/education: cardiopulmonary resuscitation. Sudden infant death syndrome (SIDS) is more likely to develop in preterm infants than in term infants. Instruction in cardiopulmonary resuscitation (CPR) is essential for parents of all infants, although especially for parents of infants at risk for life-threatening events. Risk factors include prematurity, low Apgar scores, multiple birth, and apnea and/or bradycardia. Before taking the infant home, parents must be able to administer CPR. All parents should be encouraged to obtain instruction in CPR at their local Red Cross or other community agency. The telephone number to be dialed in case of emergency should be posted near the phone (see the Home Care box to the right).

Support of parents. The nurse as support person and teacher shapes the environment and makes caregiving more responsive to the needs of parents and child. Nurses are instrumental in helping parents learn who their infant is and to recognize behavioral cues in his or her development.

As soon as possible the parents should see and touch the infant so they can begin to acknowledge the reality of the birth and reaffirm the infant's true appearance and condition. They will need encouragement to begin working through the psychologic tasks imposed by the preterm birth. A nurse and/or physician should be present during the parent's first visit to see the infant for the following reasons:

- To help the parent "see" the infant rather than focus on the equipment. The significance and function of the apparatus that surrounds the infant should be explained.
- To explain the characteristics normal for an infant of the baby's gestational age. In this way, parents do not compare the child with a full-term healthy infant.
- To encourage the parent to express feelings about the pregnancy, labor, and birth and the experience of having a preterm infant.
- To assess the parent's perceptions of the infant and determine the appropriate time for the parent to become actively involved in care.

Home Care

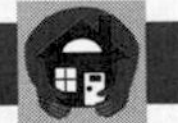

BACK TO SLEEP CAMPAIGN

The leading cause of death for infants 1 month to 1 year of age is sudden infant death syndrome (SIDS). Sleeping in the prone position is associated with SIDS. The Back to Sleep campaign is designed to promote having healthy infants sleep on a firm surface, on the back or side, with no pillows or compressible objects in bed with them. Home health nurses can promote the campaign among new parents. When SIDS occurs, home health nurses can counsel bereaved parents. Assessment and identification of grief patterns, both normal and complicated, can enable nurses to assist families and provide information about community resources. Telephone counseling and home visits are useful means of providing support to these families.

References

Buckalew P, Esposito L: The role of home health nurse in sudden infant death syndrome, *J Home Health Care Pract* 7(3):36, 1995.

Goldman M: Sudden infant death syndrome: Back to Sleep campaign, *Caring* 13(12):52, 1994.

Hirschfeld J: The "Back-to-Sleep" campaign against SIDS, *Am Fam Physician* 51(3):611, 1995.

Resources

National Institutes of Health
Back to Sleep
P.O. Box 29111
Washington, DC20040
1-800-505-CRIB

Sudden Infant Death Syndrome Clearinghouse
8201 Greensboro Dr., Suite 600
McLean, VA 22102
(703) 821-8955

American Sudden Infant Death Syndrome (SIDS) Institute
275 Carpenter Dr., Suite 100
Atlanta, GA 30328
(800) 232-SIDS (In Georgia, [800] 847-SIDS)

The Sudden Infant Death Syndrome Alliance
10500 Little Patuxent Parkway, Suite 420
Columbia, MD 21044
(301) 964-8000 or (800) 221-SIDS

Parents who have negative feelings about the pregnancy or the infant at risk need support. These parents may benefit from referral to support groups or counseling. Their feelings can be acknowledged as valid, including the burden they are experiencing financially and emotionally and their understandable feelings toward the infant. (See preceding discussion on parenting disorders.)

Soon after the birth the parents are given the opportunity to meet the infant in the *en face* position, to touch the infant, and to see his or her favorable characteristics. As soon as possible, depending primarily on her physical condition, the mother is encouraged to visit the nursery as desired and help with the infant's care. When she cannot be present physically, staff members devise appropriate methods to keep the family in frequent touch with the newborn, such as daily phone calls, notes from the infant, or photographs.

Some hospitals have instituted a support group for parents of infants in intensive care nurseries. These groups encourage parents experiencing anxiety and grief to share their feelings. An experienced neonatal intensive care unit (NICU) parent often makes contact with a new member and provides additional support. The volunteer parents provide support for the new NICU parent through hospital visits, phone contact, and home visits (Lindsay et al, 1993). Incorporating these actions into the infant's care plan acknowledges and supports nature's design by engaging and maintaining a bond between the mother and infant. This ensures the infant the continued care needed for physical and emotional survival at the optimum level.

Many NICU's use volunteers in varying capacities. After orientation, volunteers can perform various tasks, such as holding infants, stocking bedside cabinets, assembling parent packets, and in some nurseries, feeding infants.

Early discharge of some preterm infants is possible. Criteria for early discharge require the infant to be stable physiologically, be receiving adequate nutrition, and have a stable body temperature. The caregivers must exhibit physical, emotional, and educational readiness. Ideally, the environment is adequate for the infant. The caregivers must demonstrate ability in temperature taking, understanding of reportable signs and symptoms, and dietary needs (Brooten, 1995). The nurse's assessment, counseling, and teaching skills are invaluable for the success of home follow-up of infants after early hospital discharge.

Evaluation

The nurse can be reasonably assured that care was effective if the following outcomes are achieved regarding the physical aspects of care:

- Respirations are initiated and maintained.
- Body temperature is maintained.
- The infant is adequately nourished.
- CNS insult is prevented or minimized.
- Infection is prevented.
- Renal function is supported.
- Hematologic problems are prevented or minimized.
- Musculoskeletal problems are prevented or minimized.
- Retinal damage is prevented or minimized.

The nurse can be reasonably sure that care was effective if the following outcomes are achieved regarding psychosocial aspects of care:

- The mother retains a positive self-concept as a woman, mother, and sexual being.
- The mother, father/partner, and family perceive the child as potentially normal (if this is medically substantiated); provide the child with realistic care comfortably; and experience pride and satisfaction in the care of the child.
- The parents are able to organize their time and energy to meet the needs for love, attention, and care of all family members, including themselves.

A Nursing Care Plan for a preterm infant is on p. 720.

Gestational age assesment. Postnatal examination to assign gestational age that incorporates physical and neurologic criteria remains a standard assessment in all newborns in well-baby and intensive care nurseries. Ideally these tests should be performed between 2 and 8 hours after birth, with peak reliability between 30 and 48 hours of age (Ballard et al, 1979). For the first hour the infant is recovering from the stress of birth, and this is reflected in muscle movements; for example, the arm recoil is slower in a fatigued infant. After 48 hours, some responses change significantly. The plantar creases on the soles of the feet appear to increase in number and become visible as the skin loses fluid and dries.

There are four gestational age assessment methods that are used in nurseries. These methods include the Dubowitz, Ballard, and New Ballard assessment tools and assessment of the anterior vascular capsule of the lens.

The classic gestational age assessment tool, developed by Dubowitz, Dubowitz, and Goldberg in 1970, included 10 neurologic and 11 physical or "external" criteria. The decision to use neurologic and external criteria was based on the knowledge that both areas varied with gestational age (Dubowitz and Dubowitz, 1977).

Ballard et al. (1979) developed a simplified version for gestational age assessment (see Fig. 22-12). This tool used six neuromuscular criteria and six physical criteria and has been reported to overestimate preterm infants by 2 weeks and underestimate postdate infants (Avery et al, 1994; Sanders et al, 1991).

Ballard et al. (1991) have further expanded the tool for greater accuracy with the extremely premature infant (see Fig. 22-12). This assessment tool has been incorporated into most NICUs.

Examination of the anterior vascular capsule of the lens has been used to determine gestational age. This method uses direct ophthalmoscopy of the lens (Hittner et al, 1977). The hyaloid system and the tunica vasculosa lentis are an embryologic vascular system that invades the eye beginning at approximately 27 weeks and atrophies after 34 weeks (Trotter, 1993). In infants less than 27 weeks' gestation the corneas are too hazy to visualize the lens vessels. The lens vessels in infants older than 34 weeks' gestation are minimal. Therefore the use of the anterior vascular capsule of the lens for gestational age assessment is limited to the period between 27 and 34 weeks and by the capability of the observer (Hittner et al, 1977).

An accurate assessment of gestational age is critical to assist the nurse in identifying potential problems a preterm newborn is likely to experience (Fig. 26-2).

Complications associated with prematurity

Respiratory distress syndrome. **Respiratory distress syndrome (RDS)** is a lung disorder resulting from a lack of pulmonary surfactant, which leads to progressive atelectasis, loss of functional residual capacity, and ventilation-perfusion imbalance with an uneven distribution of ventilation. Surfactant deficiency may result from insufficient production, ab-

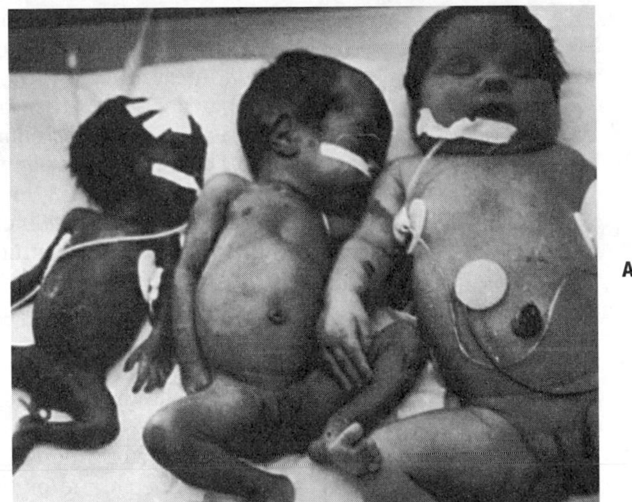
A

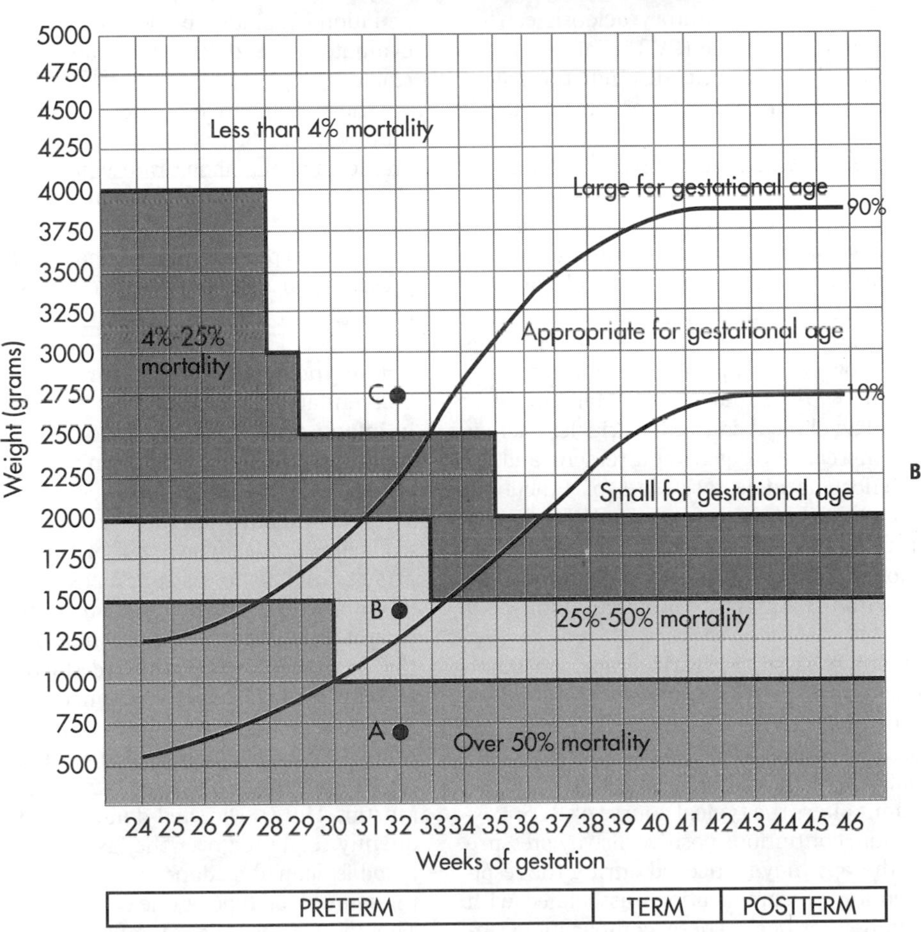

B

Fig. 26-2 Three babies of same gestational age, with weights of 600, 1400, and 2750 g, respectively, from left to right. Their weights are plotted at points *A*, *B*, and *C*. (**A**, from Korones S: *High-risk newborn infants: the basis for intensive nursing care*, ed 4, St Louis, 1986, Mosby; **B**, courtesy Mead Johnson & Co, Evansville, Ind; modified from Battaglia F, Lubchenco L: *J Pediatr* 71:59, 1967.)

BOX 26-3
Clinical Signs of RDS

Tachypnea
Grunting
Flaring
Retracting
Cyanosis
Increased work of breathing
Hypercarbia
Respiratory or mixed acidosis
Hypotension and shock

normal composition and function, disruption of surfactant production, or a combination of the aforementioned conditions. This sequence is further compromised by weak respiratory muscles and an overly compliant chest wall. Lung capacity is compromised by the presence of proteinaceous material and epithelial debris in the airways. Decreased oxygenation, cyanosis, and metabolic and/or respiratory acidosis can increase pulmonary vascular resistance (PVR). This increased PVR can lead to right-to-left shunting through the patent ductus arteriosus and foramen ovale (Avery et al, 1994; Gomella et al, 1994).

Clinical symptoms of RDS include tachypnea, grunting, nasal flaring, intercostal, supraclavicular, or subcostal retractions, and cyanosis with increasing oxygen requirement (Box 26-3). These respiratory symptoms usually present immediately after birth or within 6 hours of birth. Physical examination reveals crackles, poor air exchange, pallor, use of accessory muscles, and occasionally apnea. Radiographic findings include uniform reticulogranular appearance and air bronchograms (Avery et al, 1994; Fanaroff and Martin, 1997; Gomella et al, 1994). The clinical course is variable. There is usually a pattern of increased oxygen requirement and increased respiratory effort as atelectasis, loss of functional residual capacity, and ventilation-perfusion imbalance progress. RDS is a self-limiting disease with respiratory symptoms abating after 72 hours. The disappearance of respiratory symptoms coincides with the surfactant production in type II cells of the alveoli.

The treatment for RDS is supportive therapy. Adequate ventilation and oxygenation must be established and maintained in an attempt to prevent ventilation-perfusion mismatch and/or atelectasis. Administration of exogenous surfactant may be initiated at birth or shortly after birth. The use of exogenous surfactant alters the typical course of RDS. Positive pressure ventilation, continuous positive airway pressure (CPAP), and oxygen therapy may be needed during the respiratory illness. Prevention of complications associated with mechanical ventilation is critical. These complications include pulmonary interstitial emphysema (PIE), pneumothorax, pneumomediastinum, pneumopericardium, and bronchopulmonary dysplasia.

Positioning the infant on the abdomen with legs tucked up and arms flexed helps achieve better ventilation. Building a nest of blanket rolls or diapers around the infant decreases heat loss (there will be less surface area to lose heat from), lowers oxygen and glucose consumption (a quiet, warm infant has a lower metabolic rate), and presumably promotes comfort (the boundaries replicate the contained space of the intrauterine environment).

The infant needs periods of rest to recover from the stresses of RDS, but this condition necessitates repeated noxious interventions. Multiple examinations, obtaining blood for blood gas and other laboratory values, suctioning the endotracheal tube, and administration of medications and perhaps blood products all interfere with this rest. *Care clustering* is used to provide uninterrupted periods of rest. This term describes the organization of nursing and medical care to allow the infant periods of uninterrupted rest. Mortality and morbidity with RDS are attributed to the immature organ systems and complications associated with treatment of the disease (Avery et al, 1994; Fanaroff and Martin, 1997; Gomella et al, 1994).

Acid-base balance is evaluated by monitoring ABGs. Frequent blood sampling requires arterial access by umbilical artery catheterization (UAC) or a peripheral arterial line. Pulse oximetry and/or transcutaneous carbon dioxide and oxygen monitors document trends in ventilation and oxygenation. Capillary blood gas (CBG) levels may be used to evaluate pH and P_{CO_2} in infants whose condition is more stable.

The maintenance of an NTE continues to be critical for infants with RDS. Infants with hypoxemia are unable to increase their metabolic rate when stressed by cold (Fanaroff and Martin, 1997) (see Chapter 22 on consequences of cold stress).

Neonatal pneumonia may have a clinical and radiographic presentation similar to that of RDS, with radiodense lung fields and air bronchograms. Fluid in the minor fissure may also be noted with neonatal pneumonia. Therefore sepsis evaluation, including blood culture, complete blood count with differential, and occasionally a lumbar puncture, is indicated in infants with RDS who have risk factors for sepsis. Broad-spectrum antibiotics are begun while cultures are being evaluated (Avery et al, 1994; Cloherty and Stark, 1991).

Fluid and nutrition must be maintained for the infant critically ill with RDS. The use of parenteral nutrition can provide protein and fats to assist in a positive nitrogen balance. Daily monitoring of electrolytes, urine output, specific gravity, and weight assists in the evaluation of hydration status (Cloherty and Stark, 1991; Fanaroff and Martin, 1997).

Blood transfusions may be necessary because of the need for frequent blood sampling. A venous hematocrit of more than 40% is usually needed by the critically ill infant to maintain adequate oxygen-carrying capacity (Fanaroff and Martin, 1997). Directed-donor blood has become more frequently requested over the last several years. Directed-donor blood is defined as donor blood obtained from a person with the same blood type or one compatible with that of the infant. The donor is usually a family member or close friend of the family. Notification of the potential for blood transfusion on admission may be necessary to allow for the processing of directed-donor blood. Reassurance for the family that stringent testing occurs with all blood products may alleviate some anxiety. Some religions prohibit the use of blood transfusions. It is critical to have a complete history from the family, including religious preference. Other strategies for maintaining hematocrit may be needed in these instances.

Bronchopulmonary dysplasia. **Bronchopulmonary dysplasia (BPD)** is a chronic pulmonary condition in infants who have experienced respiratory failure, oxygen dependence for longer than 28 days and continued beyond 36 weeks' postconceptual age, abnormal radiographic findings with areas of overinflation and areas of atelectasis, and respiratory symptoms (Avery et al, 1994; Lund, 1990). The etiology of BPD is multifactorial and includes pulmonary immaturity, surfactant deficiency, lung injury and stretch, barotrauma, oxygen exposure, inflammation, and genetic predisposition (Gomella et al, 1994; Knoppert and Mackanjee, 1994; Lund, 1990). The incidence of BPD in infants weighing less than 1500 g who require mechanical ventilation for RDS ranges from 5% to 38% (Fanaroff and Martin, 1997; Lund, 1990).

Clinical symptoms include tachypnea, retractions, nasal flaring, increased work of breathing, and tachycardia. Auscultation of lung fields reveals crackles, decreased air movement, and occasionally expiratory wheezing (Gomella et al, 1994).

Treatment for BPD includes oxygen, nutrition, fluid restriction, and medications (diuretics, corticosteroids, bronchodilators). The key for BPD is prevention (Gomella et al, 1994).

The prognosis for infants with BPD depends on the degree of pulmonary dysfunction. Most deaths occur within the first year of life and result from cardiorespiratory failure, sepsis, or respiratory infection, or occur as a sudden, unexplained death (Gomella et al, 1994).

Retinopathy of prematurity. **Retinopathy of prematurity (ROP)** is a disorder of developing retinal vessels in premature infants. The incidence of ROP increases with decreasing gestational age, with a 65.8% occurrence in infants weighing less than 1251 g. The normal retinal vessels begin to form in utero at approximately 16 weeks' gestation in response to an unknown stimulus. The retinal vessels continue to develop until reaching maturity at approximately 42 to 43 weeks after conception. Once the retina is completely vascularized, the retinal vessels are not susceptible to ROP. The mechanism of injury in ROP is unclear. Possible mechanisms of injury are early vasoconstriction in response to hyperoxia, which causes decreased blood flow, vasoproliferation, and an increased number of gap junctions between spindle cells exposed to hyperoxia, resulting in developmental arrest (Cloherty and Stark, 1991; Gomella et al, 1994).

The International Classification of ROP includes the following:

Stage 1—A thin line of demarcation between the vascularized area of the retina and the avascular area

Stage II—This line becomes a ridge protruding into the vitreous

Stage III—Extraretinal fibrovascular proliferation is evident with the ridge

Stage IV—Scarring and fibrosis occurs as neovascularization extends into the vitreous; this extension of new vessels produces traction on the retina, resulting in retinal detachment

Stage IVA—Partial retinal detachment with macula remaining intact; disease occurs when the vessels around the ridge become dilated and tortuous.

Stage IVB—Partial retinal detachment with macular damage

Stage V—Total retinal detachment (Gomella et al, 1994; Korones and Bada-Ellzey, 1993)

ROP is a complex multicausal disease of preterm birth. All premature infants less than 35 weeks' gestation or weighing less than 1800 g with oxygen exposure and all infants less than 30 weeks' gestation and/or less than 1500 g need an indirect ophthalmoscopy examination at 4 to 6 weeks of age. Reexamination should occur every 1 to 2 weeks until retinal vascularization is complete (Cloherty and Stark, 1991; Gomella et al, 1994; Korones and Bada-Ellzey, 1993).

The key to management of ROP is prevention and early detection of premature birth. Circumferential cryopexy, laser photocoagulation, vitamin E, and decreased light intensity are used in the treatment of ROP with varying results (Fanaroff and Martin, 1997; Gomella et al, 1994).

Patent ductus arteriosus. Patent ductus arteriosus (PDA) is a common complication of prematurity in which the fetal ductus arteriosus fails to constrict after birth or reopens after constriction has occurred. The ductus arteriosus is a muscular contractile structure connecting the left pulmonary artery and the dorsal aorta and should functionally close by 12 to 24 hours of life. Ductal construction is promoted by increased oxygenation, levels of circulating prostaglandins, and muscle mass. Other factors that promote ductal closure include catecholamines, low pH, bradykinin, and acetylcholine (Korones and Bada-Ellzey, 1993). The incidence of PDA in premature infants weighing less than 1500 g is 40% to 60%, with an increased percentage occurring in premature infants weighing less than 1000 g (Gomella et al, 1994).

The clinical presentation for an infant with a PDA includes systolic murmur, active precordium, bounding peripheral pulses, tachycardia, tachypnea, crackles, and hepatomegaly. The systolic murmur is heard best at the second or third intercostal space at the upper left sternal border. An active precordium results from increased left ventricular stroke volume. A widened pulse pressure may result in increased peripheral pulses (Gomella et al, 1994).

Radiographic studies with PDA reveal cardiac enlargement and pulmonary edema. ABG findings reveal hypercarbia and metabolic acidosis. Echocardiography demonstrates PDA and can quantitate the amount of blood shunting across the PDA (Avery et al, 1994; Gomella et al, 1994).

The PDA can be managed medically or surgically. Medical management involves ventilatory support, fluid restriction, diuretics, and indomethacin. Indomethacin is a prostaglandin synthetase inhibitor that produces constriction of the PDA in approximately 85% of infants (Avery et al, 1994). Ventilatory support is adjusted based on ABG levels. Fluid restriction is implemented to decrease cardiovascular volume overload in association with diuretics (Gomella et al, 1994). Surgical ligation is done when PDA is clinically significant and medical management is contraindicated or has failed (Gomella et al, 1994).

Nursing care of the infant with PDA focuses on supportive care. The infant needs an NTE, adequate oxygenation, meticulous fluid balance, and parental support.

Periventricular-intraventricular hemorrhage. Periventricular-intraventricular hemorrhage (PV-IVH) is one of

BOX 26-4
Classifications of PV-IVH

Small hemorrhage
Grade I
Isolated germinal matrix hemorrhage
Grade II
Intraventricular hemorrhage with normal ventricular size

Moderate hemorrhage
Grade III
Intraventricular hemorrhage with acute ventricular dilation

Severe hemorrhage
Grade IV
Intraventricular hemorrhage with parenchymal hemorrhage

the most common types of brain injury encountered in the neonatal period and among the most severe in both short-term and long-term outcomes. The incidence of PV-IVH is 50% to 70% in infants weighing less than 1000 g (Dietch, 1993; Fanaroff and Martin, 1997).

The pathogenesis of PV-IVH includes intravascular factors (fluctuating or increasing cerebral blood flow, increases in cerebral venous pressures, and coagulopathy), vascular factors, extravascular factors, and nursery care (Dietch, 1993). PV-IVH events occur within the first week of life, with 50% occurring in the first 24 hours, 90% in the first 72 hours, and 95% in the first week (Gomella et al, 1994; Volpe, 1992).

Classification of PV-IVH uses a grading system of I to IV, with grade I being the least severe and grade IV the most severe. The categories are further delineated as small, moderate, and severe hemorrhage (Fanaroff and Martin, 1997) (Box 26-4).

Long-term neurodevelopmental outcome is determined by the severity of the PV-IVH. In studies comparing infants with small PV-IVH to similar infants without PV-IVH, the incidence of handicaps in both groups increased threefold in the moderate PV-IVH category and sevenfold in the severe PV-IVH category (Fanaroff and Martin, 1997).

Necrotizing enterocolitis. Necrotizing enterocolitis (NEC) is an acute inflammatory disease of the gastrointestinal mucosa, commonly complicated by perforation. This often fatal disease occurs in about 2% to 5% of newborns in intensive care nurseries. Although the cause of NEC is unknown, the following factors contribute to its development: immaturity, hypoxemia (postbirth), high-solute feedings, excessive amounts of feedings, perinatal asphyxia (commonly in utero), polycythemia and hyperviscosity syndromes, exchange transfusions, and bacterial or viral gastrointestinal infection (Box 26-5) (Gomella et al, 1994).

Recent research suggests that reversal of perinatal asphyxia (p. 739) within 30 minutes may prevent gastrointestinal tract insult and thus prevent the initiation of NEC pathophysiology. After 30 minutes, the distribution of cardiac output tends to be directed more toward the heart and brain and away from the abdominal organs. Therefore prompt birth of the intrauterine-asphyxiated fetus or ventilation of the asphyxiated newborn may be beneficial to the gastrointestinal tract as well as to other organs.

BOX 26-5
Proposed Risk Factors for NEC

Asphyxia
Respiratory distress syndrome
Umbilical artery catheter
Exchange transfusion
Early enteral feedings
PDA
Congenital heart disease
Polycythemia
Anemia
Shock

The onset of NEC in the full-term infant usually is between 4 and 10 days. In the preterm infant the onset may be delayed up to 30 days. Signs of developing NEC are nonspecific, which is characteristic of many neonatal disease processes. Some generalized signs include decreased activity, hypotonia, pallor, recurrent apnea and bradycardia, decreased oxygen saturation, respiratory distress, metabolic acidosis, oliguria, hypotension, decreased perfusion, temperature instability, and cyanosis. Gastrointestinal symptoms include abdominal distention, increasing or bile-stained residuals, vomiting (bile and/or blood), grossly bloody stools, abdominal tenderness, and erythema of the abdominal wall (Korones and Bada-Ellzey, 1993).

Prevention of NEC and its complications by early detection is an important part of the nursing care of high-risk infants. Nurses are in a unique position to assess the infant's behavioral cues and feeding behavior and alert clinicians to the subtle signs that may signal the onset of NEC.

Nursing ALERT

Observe for indications of early development of NEC by checking the abdomen frequently for distention (measuring abdominal girth, measuring residual gastric contents before feedings, and listening for the presence of bowel sounds) and performing all routine assessments for high-risk neonates.

Diagnosis of NEC is confirmed by radiographic examination that reveals bowel loop distention, pneumatosis intestinalis, pneumoperitoneum, and/or portal air. Laboratory evaluation includes a complete blood cell count with differential, coagulation studies, ABG levels, serum electrolyte levels, and blood culture (Korones and Bada-Ellzey, 1993). The abnormal radiograph results from the bacteria associated with NEC causing an ileus. Pneumatosis intestinalis, pneumoperitoneum, and portal air are products of the gas produced by the bacteria invading the wall of the intestines and escaping into the peritoneum and portal system when perforation occurs. The white blood cell (WBC) count on the complete blood count reveals an increased or decreased WBC level. The platelet count and coagulation studies may be abnormal, with thrombocytopenia and disseminated intravascular coagulation (DIC). The electrolyte levels may be abnormal, with leaking capillary beds and fluid shifts resulting from the infection.

Treatment is supportive. Oral or tube feedings are discontinued to rest the gastrointestinal tract. An orogastric tube is placed and attached to low suction to provide gastric decompression. Parenteral therapy (often by total parenteral nutrition [TPN]) is begun. NEC is an infectious disease; therefore control of infection is imperative, with an emphasis on careful handwashing before and after patient contact. Antibiotic therapy may be instituted, and surgery is performed when perforation or clinical deterioration occurs. Therapy may be prolonged and recovery delayed by adhesions, complications of bowel resection, short gut syndrome (especially if the ileocecal valve is removed), and intolerance of oral feedings.

Multidimensional evaluation of the care given to preterm infants and their families is required. In some families the infant dies despite all medical and nursing knowledge and skill. In other families the sequelae of preterm birth result in infants who will face disability throughout their lives. For these families, evaluation criteria concern loss, grief, and self-concept (see Chapter 25). For many other infants and their families the immediate threat to their well-being is overcome by intensive neonatal care.

The nurse can be reasonably assured that care was effective if the following expected outcomes regarding the physical aspects of care are achieved:

- Respirations are initiated and maintained.
- Body temperature is maintained.
- The infant is adequately nourished.
- CNS trauma is prevented or minimized.
- Infection is prevented.

POSTDATE AND POSTMATURE INFANTS

Postdate infants are those whose gestation is prolonged beyond 42 weeks, regardless of birth weight. These infants may be LGA or SGA, but most often their weight is **appropriate for gestational age (AGA).** Commonly these infants have little vernix caseosa other than in the skin creases, and that may be stained yellow or green (caused by intrauterine release of meconium). The cause of prolonged pregnancy is unknown. Certain groups are more likely to have gestations longer than 42 weeks, including first-time mothers, multiparous women (four or more children), and women with a history of a postdate pregnancy.

Postmaturity implies progressive placental insufficiency, resulting in a dysmature newborn. It is important to note that not all postdate infants are **postmature.** In the SGA postdate infant, fetal malnutrition and hypoxia occur as a result of deteriorating metabolic exchange in the aging placenta. The depletion of subcutaneous fat produces the wasted appearance of the dysmature infant.

Perinatal mortality is significantly higher in the postdate fetus and neonate. During labor and birth, increased oxygen demands of the postmature fetus cannot be met. Insufficient gas exchange by the postmature placenta causes an increased incidence of intrauterine hypoxia, which may result in the passage of meconium in utero and a greater risk for meconium aspiration syndrome. Of all the deaths of postdate newborns, half occur during labor and birth, about one third occur before the onset of labor, and one sixth occur in the newborn period.

Nursing Care Management

Assessment

Maternal assessment. For safe birth of the fetus, it becomes important to determine whether prolonged pregnancy actually has developed and whether there is any evidence of fetal jeopardy. Data for determining fetal gestational age are obtained from several sources and correlated.

Verification of the LMP is important to the diagnosis of prolonged pregnancy. A correlation of the LMP with the estimated duration of pregnancy at two of the earliest obstetric examinations may lead to substantiation or recalculation of the estimated date of birth (EDB). If the uterus is larger than expected for dates, hydramnios or multifetal pregnancy may be the cause. If the dates seem correct but the size of the fetus is disparate, IUGR may be the cause.

The woman's medical status is reappraised. Women with diabetes and women who have glucose intolerance of pregnancy (gestational diabetes) have large babies, and this may confuse the estimate of gestational age. Amniocentesis to ascertain lung maturity is advised in these situations.

Two serial ultrasound examinations and measurement of the fetal biparietal diameter should be accomplished. Ultrasound examination is the most accurate when performed during the first 12 weeks of gestation. A second ultrasound examination at approximately 20 weeks can provide supporting evidence for the gestation when coupled with information from the LMP and first trimester ultrasound. Fetal monitoring includes fetal activity determination, weekly estimate of fetal weight, nonstress test (NST) or oxytocin challenge test (OCT), and biophysical profile (BPP) (see Chapter 5).

Newborn assessment. Most postterm and postmature infants are oversized but otherwise normal, with advanced development and bone age. A postmature infant will have some but not necessarily all of the following physical characteristics:

- Generally has normal skull, but reduced dimensions of rest of body make skull look inordinately large
- Dry, cracked skin (desquamation), parchmentlike at birth
- Nails of hard consistency extending beyond fingertips
- Profuse scalp hair
- Subcutaneous fat layers depleted, leaving skin loose and giving an "old person" appearance
- Long and thin body contour
- Absent vernix
- Often meconium staining (golden yellow to green) of skin, nails, and cord
- May have an alert, wide-eyed appearance symptomatic of chronic intrauterine hypoxia

Persistent pulmonary hypertension of the newborn (PPHN). This term is applied to the combination of pulmonary hypertension, right-to-left shunting, and a structurally normal heart. PPHN may present either as a single entity or as the main component of meconium aspiration syndrome, congenital diaphragmatic hernia, RDS, hyperviscosity syndrome, or neonatal pneumonia or sepsis. PPHN is also called *persistent fetal circulation (PFC)* because the syndrome includes reversion to fetal pathways for blood flow.

A brief review of fetal blood flow can help visualize the problems with PPHN (Fig. 22-2 illustrates fetal circulation). In utero, oxygen-rich blood leaves the placenta via the umbilical vein, goes through the ductus venosus, and enters the inferior vena cava. From here, it empties into the right atrium and is mostly shunted across the foraman ovale to the left atrium, effectively bypassing the lungs. This blood enters the left ventricle, leaves via the aorta, and preferentially perfuses the carotid and coronary arteries. Thus the heart and brain receive the most oxygenated blood. Blood drains from the brain into the superior vena cava, reenters the right atrium, proceeds to the right ventricle, and exits via the main pulmonary artery. The lungs are a high-pressure circuit, needing only enough perfusion for growth and nutrition. The ductus arteriosus (connecting the main pulmonary artery and the aorta) is the path of least resistance for the blood leaving the right side of the fetal heart, shunting most of the cardiac output away from the lungs and toward the systemic system. This *right-to-left shunting* is the key to fetal circulation.

After birth, both the foraman ovale and the ductus arteriosus close in response to various biochemical processes, pressure changes within the heart, and dilation of the pulmonary vessels. This dilation allows virtually all of the cardiac output to enter the lungs, become oxygenated, and provide oxygen-rich blood to the tissues for normal metabolism. Any process that interferes with this transition from fetal to neonatal circulation may precipitate PPHN. PPHN characteristically proceeds into a downward spiral of exacerbating hypoxia and pulmonary vasoconstriction. Prompt recognition and aggressive intervention are required to reverse this process.

The infant with PPHN is typically born at term or postterm and presents with tachycardia and cyanosis. Management depends on the underlying etiology of the persistent pulmonary hypertension. The development of extracorporeal membrane oxygenation (ECMO) has improved the survival of these infants. This process is similar to the heart-lung bypass used in intracardiac surgery. Large catheters are placed in the carotid artery and jugular vein, blood is siphoned off, oxygenated, and then returned to the body. This process rests the lungs, allowing time for healing and vasodilation. This treatment is a maximum intervention, used after conventional treatments have failed. Salvaging the carotid artery is possible with vascular microsurgery after decannulation.

Another mode of treatment for PPHN and other respiratory disorders of the newborn is high-frequency ventilation, a group of assisted ventilation methods that deliver small volumes of gas at high frequencies and limit the development of high airway pressure, thus reducing barotrauma (Fanaroff and Martin, 1997). Innovative treatment modalities such as inhaled nitric oxide and liquid ventilation bear promising results in limited clinical trials for the treatment of PPHN (Greenspan, 1993; Roberts et al, 1992).

Meconium aspiration syndrome. Intrauterine passage of meconium is a common indication of fetal stress. Stress, such as fetal asphyxia, may cause increased intestinal peristalsis, combined with relaxation of the external anal sphincter, and passage of meconium in utero (Gomella et al, 1994). Continued intrauterine stress or the stress of birth causes the fetus to make gasping respiratory efforts in utero or during labor and delivery that draw the meconium-stained fluid into the respiratory passage (Gomella et al, 1994). This process results in **meconium aspiration.** This sticky, tarlike stool clings to the walls of alveoli and impairs respiratory function. Meconium aspiration causes physical obstruction of the airways and hinders gas exchange. Meconium fosters the growth of virulent pathogens within the respiratory tract because it is a good medium for bacterial growth (Merenstein and Gardner, 1993). Symptoms of respiratory distress syndrome are common after meconium aspiration.

The presence of a team skilled in neonatal resuscitation is required at the birth of any infant with meconium-stained amniotic fluid. The mouth and nares of the infant should be suctioned on the perineum before the infant's first breath. It is imperative that tactile stimulation in these infants be avoided until after tracheal suctioning to prevent further aspiration of meconium into the bronchi. With thick or particulate meconium the infant is intubated at birth and suctioned to remove any meconium visualized below the vocal cords. Appropriate management of the airway at birth can largely prevent meconium aspiration syndrome (MAS).

If meconium is not removed from the airway at birth, it can migrate down to the terminal airways, causing mechanical obstruction. Meconium aspiration can cause a chemical pneumonitis. These infants may develop PPHN, further complicating their management.

Nursing Diagnoses

The postmature infant's size and condition will determine whether the nursing diagnoses suitable for the "normal" newborn or those formulated for the preterm infant are appropriate. Examples include the following:

- Ineffective airway clearance related to
  Meconium aspiration syndrome
- Risk for hypothermia related to
  Depleted stores of subcutaneous fat
- Risk for injury (permanent disability) related to
  Birth trauma
  Chronic intrauterine hypoxia
- Risk for injury secondary to hypoglycemia related to
  Depleted glycogen stores

Expected Outcomes

Physiologic problems of postmaturity are reflected in the plan of care. Immediate outcomes are as follows:

1. The newborn will initiate and maintain respirations.
2. The newborn will experience no CNS trauma or infection.
3. Any birth trauma present will be identified and treated promptly without sequelae.

The long-term expected outcome is that the infant will not experience adverse effects of postmaturity.

Plan of Care and Implementation

Immediate care is similar to that given to the preterm infant. Procedures to support physiologic function (e.g., respiration, body temperature, nutrition) are discussed in Chapter 23. Potential complications experienced by postmature infants include polycythemia, hypoglycemia, and meconium aspiration (Avery et al, 1994).

Evaluation

The nurse can be assured that care was effective when the short-term outcomes for care have been achieved. These outcomes include that the newborn initiated and maintained respirations and experienced no CNS trauma or infection; if there was birth trauma, it was identified and treated promptly without sequelae. Evaluation of the degree to which the long-term outcomes are achieved is delayed beyond the period of infancy.

SGA, IUGR, AND DYSMATURE INFANTS

Infants whose birth weight falls below the tenth percentile expected at term or is two standard deviations below the mean for gestational age, for reasons other than heredity, are considered at high risk, with an increase of four to eight times in perinatal mortality (Gomella et al, 1994).

Various conditions can affect and impede growth in the developing fetus. The cause, severity, and gestational age at which the insult occurs determine how fetal growth is affected and what problems will be present in the newborn. Conditions occurring in the first trimester that affect all aspects of fetal growth (infections, teratogens, and chromosomal abnormalities), or extrinsic conditions early in pregnancy result in symmetric IUGR (head circumference, length, and weight are all less than 10%). Conditions causing symmetric growth retardation result in a short, SGA infant, usually with a smaller head circumference and reduced brain capacity (Gomella et al, 1994).

Growth restriction in later stages of pregnancy, as a result of maternal or placental factors, results in asymmetric growth restriction (with respect to gestational age, weight will be less than the tenth percentile whereas length and head circumference will be greater than the tenth percentile). Asymmetric growth restriction occurs as a result of maternal, fetal, and placental conditions (Box 26-6) (Korones and Bada-Ellzey, 1993). Infants with asymmetric IUGR have the potential for normal growth and development. Abnormal fetal size may indicate an adaptive response, with diminished fetal weight-sparing brain growth (Fanaroff and Martin, 1997).

BOX 26-6
Prenatal Factors Associated With IUGR

Maternal
Socioeconomic factors
Preeclampsia
Advanced diabetes
Malnutrition
Cigarette smoking
Alcohol consumption
Narcotic addiction
High altitude residence

Fetal
Multiple fetuses
Congenital anomalies (chromosomal and nonchromosomal)
Chronic infection (rubella and cytomegalovirus)

Placental
Placental insufficiency
Arteriovenous anastomosis

From Korones S, Bada-Ellzey H: *Neonatal decision making,* St Louis, 1993, Mosby.

Common Problems

Perinatal asphyxia. Commonly, IUGR infants have been exposed to chronic hypoxia for varying periods before labor and birth. Labor is a stressor to the normal fetus; it is an even greater stressor for the growth-restricted fetus. The chronically hypoxic infant is severely compromised by even a normal labor and has difficulty compensating after birth. The alert, wide-eyed appearance of the newborn is attributed to prolonged prenatal hypoxia. Appropriate management and resuscitation are essential for the depressed infant.

The birth of SGA babies with perinatal asphyxia may be associated with a maternal history of heavy cigarette smoking; preeclampsia; low socioeconomic status; multifetal gestation; gestational infections such as rubella, cytomegalovirus, and toxoplasmosis; advanced diabetes mellitus; and cardiac problems. When a woman with this background arrives in labor, the nursing staff must be alert to and prepared for possible perinatal asphyxia. Sequelae to perinatal asphyxia include meconium aspiration syndrome and hypoglycemia.

Meconium aspiration. See the discussion on p. 738.

Hypoglycemia. Stressed infants are at risk for the development of hypoglycemia (Merenstein and Gardner, 1993). Stress may include perinatal asphyxia and IUGR. Definitions of hypoglycemia vary for the term and the preterm infant. Within the first 3 days of life, hypoglycemia is defined as a blood glucose level of less than 40 mg/dl in the term infant or less than 30 mg/dl in the preterm infant. Symptoms of hypoglycemia include poor feeding, hypothermia, and diaphoresis. CNS symptoms can include tremors and jitteriness, weak cry, lethargy, floppy posture, seizures, or coma. Diagnosis is confirmed by laboratory blood glucose determinations or with reagent strips such as Chemstrip-BG or Dextrostix (Merenstein and Gardner, 1993).

Heat loss. As a result of a number of factors, SGA infants require particular attention to maintain thermoneutrality. These infants have less muscle mass, less brown fat (an internal fuel source for the generation of heat found in large amounts in normal term infants), less heat-preserving subcutaneous fat, and little ability to control skin capillaries. Nursing considerations focus on maintenance of thermoneutrality to support recovery from perinatal asphyxia; cold stress jeopardizes recovery from asphyxia (Merenstein and Gardner, 1993).

Nursing Care Management

Assessment

The following physical findings are characteristic of the SGA neonate:

- Generally has normal skull, but reduced dimensions of rest of body make skull look inordinately large

- Reduced subcutaneous fat
- Loose and dry skin
- Diminished muscle mass, especially over buttocks and cheeks
- Sunken abdomen (scaphoid) as opposed to being normally well rounded
- Thin, yellowish, dry, and dull-appearing umbilical cord (normal cord is gray, glistening, round, and moist)
- Sparse scalp hair
- Wide skull sutures (inadequate bone growth)

SGA infants are likely to experience perinatal asphyxia, MAS, hypoglycemia, and heat loss.

Nursing Diagnoses

Analysis of assessment findings determines suitable nursing diagnoses, such as the following examples:

- Impaired gas exchange related to
  Meconium aspiration
- Risk for injury related to
  Hypoglycemia
- Ineffective thermoregulation related to
  Reduced subcutaneous fat
  Increased surface area in relation to body weight (mass)
  Diminished muscle mass
- Risk for altered parenting related to
  Physical appearance and condition at birth

Expected Outcomes

The nursing care plan for the SGA infant is similar to that for the preterm infant. Expected outcomes are established with patients and, whenever possible, are stated in client-centered terms.

The infant will have the following outcomes:

1. Maintain physiologic functioning
2. Maintain adequate gas exchange
3. Maintain blood glucose levels within normal range and experience no episodes of hypoglycemia
4. Maintain effective thermoregulation
5. Begin bonding and attachment to parents

The parents will have the following outcomes:

1. Perceive the infant as potentially normal (if this is medically substantiated)
2. Provide care comfortably
3. Experience pride and satisfaction in the care of the infant
4. Organize their time and energies to meet the love, attention, and care needs of the other members of the family as well as their own
5. Begin bonding and attachment to the infant

Plan of Care and Implementation

Care of the SGA infant is based on the clinical problems present. The nursing care related to those problems is the same as for the preterm infant (see Implementation, p. 730). Gas exchange is supported by maintaining a clear airway (for discussion of suctioning, see pp. 631-632) and preventing cold stress (for discussion of oxygen administration and ventilation, see pp. 701-704). Hypoglycemia is treated with oral feedings (e.g., breast, formula, dextrose solution) per hospital protocol. Parenteral infusions may be necessary. An external heat source is used until the infant's temperature is stabilized (p. 705). Nursing support of parents is similar to that given to parents of preterm infants (p. 729).

Evaluation

The nurse can be reasonably assured that care was effective when the outcomes have been achieved. Specifically, the infant maintained physiologic functioning, adequate gas exchange, blood glucose levels within normal range, and normal temperature, and began bonding and attachment to the parent(s). The parents perceive the infant as potentially normal (if this is medically supported), provide care comfortably, experience pride and satisfaction in the care of the infant, organize their time and energies to meet the love, attention, and care needs of the other members of the family as well as their own, and have begun bonding and attachment to the infant.

LGA INFANTS

The LGA, or oversized, infant traditionally has been one who weighs 4000 g (8 lb 13 oz) or more at birth. An infant is considered LGA despite gestation when weight is plotted at above the 90th percentile on growth charts or two standard deviations above the mean weight for gestational age (Gomella et al, 1994; Korones and Bada-Ellzey, 1993). About 10% of newborns are of this weight, and about 0.4% to 0.9% weigh 4500 g (9 lb 15 oz) or more (Korones and Bada-Ellzey, 1993). Most of these newborns have other proportionately larger measurements. Many are born well after the EDB. Better maternal health and nutrition probably are responsible for this greater growth during recent generations as well as genetic disposition: large mothers have large babies. Certain fetal disorders result in LGA infants. These include transposition of the great vessels and Beckwith-Wiedemann syndrome (Korones and Bada-Ellzey, 1993).

Maternal pelvic diameters have not kept pace with better maternal health and nutrition resulting in larger babies; thus fetopelvic disproportion often occurs, particularly in obese women, women who gain 16 kg (35 lb) or more during gestation, and women with undiagnosed and/or uncontrolled diabetes, who are prone to have large babies. Birth trauma, especially associated with breech or shoulder presentation, is a serious hazard for the oversized neonate. Asphyxia, CNS injury, or both may occur.

A biparietal diameter greater than 10 cm verified by fetometry (ultrasound or x-ray examination), a uterine fundal measurement greater than 42 cm in the absence of hydramnios, and only average or smaller interior pelvic diameters are common findings when LGA infants are born. All pregnancies of longer than 42 weeks' gestation must be carefully evaluated. All large fetuses are monitored during a trial of labor, and preparation is made for a cesarean birth if nonreassuring fetal status or poor progress of labor occurs. LGA newborns may be preterm, term, or postdate; children of diabetic (or prediabetic) mothers; or postmature. Each of these categories has special concerns. Regardless of coexisting potential problems, the oversized infant is at risk by virtue of size alone.

Any one or a combination of injuries discussed in nursing actions for LGA infants may occur in normal- or small-sized infants. In addition to the large size of the infant, factors that predispose to birth trauma include the following:

- Preterm labor and birth
- Length of labor
- Size and shape of maternal pelvis
- Fetal presentation, attitude, and lie

Assessment

The nurse assesses the LGA infant for hypoglycemia and trauma from vaginal or cesarean birth.

Nursing Diagnoses

The nursing diagnoses are based on the type of condition the newborn has experienced. Diagnoses are individualized and may include any of the following:

- Risk for injury related to
  - Hypoglycemia
  - Cephalopelvic disproportion and vaginal birth
  - Operative birth (e.g., forceps- or vacuum-assisted birth; cesarean birth)
- Risk for altered parenting related to
  - Difficult labor and birth
  - Physical appearance and condition at birth
  - Permanent sequelae from birth trauma (e.g., Duchenne-Erb's palsy)

Expected Outcomes

Planning for care depends on the LGA infant's condition. Expected outcomes include the following:

1. The neonate will remain euglycemic.
2. The neonate will experience no birth trauma, and, if present, it will be identified and managed in a timely manner.
3. The parents will begin the bonding and attachment process.

Plan of Care and Implementation

Blood glucose levels are monitored, and hypoglycemia is corrected. Specific birth injuries are treated appropriately.

Evaluation

The nurse can be reasonably assured the outcomes for care of the LGA infant were achieved if hypoglycemia is treated and blood glucose levels are within normal limits, if birth trauma is managed with minimal or no sequelae, and if parents begin the bonding and attachment process.

INFANTS OF DIABETIC MOTHERS

No single physiologic or biochemical event can explain the diverse clinical manifestations seen in the **infants of diabetic mothers (IDMs)** or infants of gestational diabetic mothers (IGDMs). A better understanding of maternal and fetal metabolism, resulting in stricter control of maternal diabetes and improved obstetric and neonatal intensive care, has led to a decrease in perinatal mortality in diabetic pregnancy from more than 10% to less than 4% in the last 25 years (Fanaroff and Martin, 1997). However, maternal diabetes continues to play a significant role in neonatal morbidity and mortality.

All infants born to mothers with diabetes are at some risk for complications. The degree of risk is affected by the severity and duration of maternal disease. Problems seen in IDMs include congenital anomalies, macrosomia, birth trauma and perinatal asphyxia, RDS, hypoglycemia, hypocalcemia and hypomagnesemia, cardiomyopathy, hyperbilirubinemia, and polycythemia.

Pathophysiology

The mechanisms responsible for the problems seen in IDMs are not fully understood. In early pregnancy, fluctuations in blood glucose levels and episodes of ketoacidosis are believed to cause congenital anomalies. Later in pregnancy, when the mother's pancreas cannot release sufficient insulin to meet increased demands, maternal hyperglycemia results. The high levels of glucose cross the placenta and stimulate the fetal pancreas to release insulin. The combination of the increased supply of maternal glucose and other nutrients, the inability of maternal insulin to cross the placenta, and increased fetal insulin results in excessive fetal growth called macrosomia (see later discussion).

Hyperinsulinemia accounts for many of the problems the fetus or infant develops. In addition to fluctuating glucose levels, maternal vascular involvement or superimposed maternal infection adversely affects the fetus. Normally, maternal blood has a more alkaline pH than does carbon dioxide–rich fetal blood. This phenomenon encourages the exchange of oxygen and carbon dioxide across the placental membrane. When the maternal blood is more acidotic than the fetal blood, such as during ketoacidosis, little carbon dioxide or oxygen exchange occurs at the level of the placenta. The mortality for the unborn baby resulting from an episode of maternal ketoacidosis may be as high as 50% or more (Fanaroff and Martin, 1997).

Some neonatal conditions—macrosomia, hypoglycemia, hypocalcemia, hyperbilirubinemia, and perhaps fetal lung immaturity—may be eliminated or the incidence decreased by maintaining control over maternal glucose levels within narrow limits (Creasy and Resnik, 1994). Good control is defined as the maintenance of maternal blood glucose levels between 100 and 120 mg/dl.

Nursing Care Management

Assessment

The IDM is examined carefully at birth for macrosomia and for evidence of congenital anomalies, birth trauma, cardiomyopathy or asphyxia. Blood glucose, calcium and magnesium levels are measured as indicated, as low levels of these substances are common in IDMs. Respirations are monitored to detect developing RDS and skin color and blood values assessed for hyperbilirubinemia and polycythemia.

Congenital Anomalies

Congenital anomalies occur in about 7% to 10% of IDMs. Their incidence is two to four times that for infants born to mothers without diabetes (Ogata, 1994). The incidence is greatest among SGA newborns. The most frequently occurring anomalies involve the cardiac, musculoskeletal, and central nervous systems.

The incidence of congenital heart lesions in these infants is five times higher than that in the general population. Coarc-

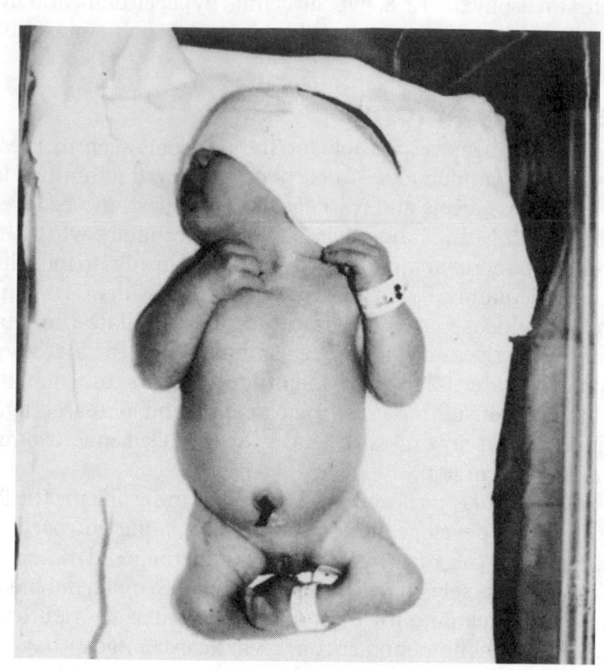

Fig. 26-3 IDM with caudal regression syndrome (sacral agenesis). (From Fanaroff A, Martin R, editors: *Neonatal-perinatal medicine: diseases of the fetus and infant,* ed 6, St Louis, 1997, Mosby.)

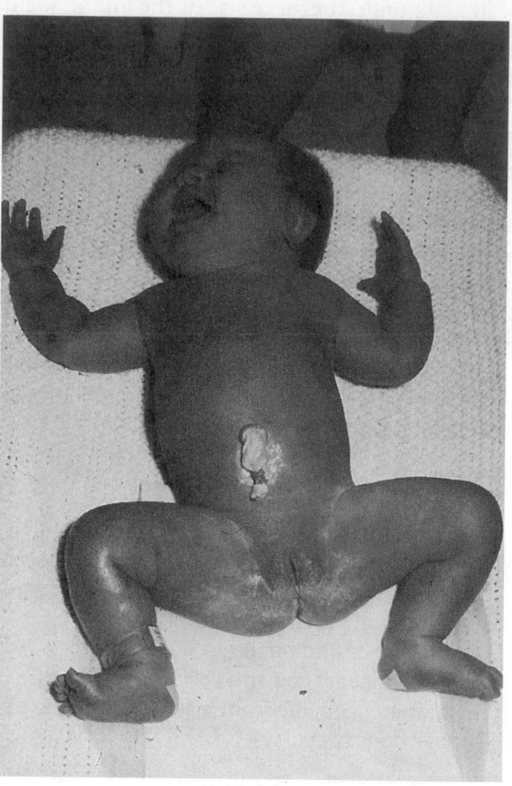

Fig. 26-4 IDM with plethora and edema. (From O'Doherty N: *Micro atlas of the newborn,* Nutley, NJ, 1980, Hoffmann-La Roche, Inc.)

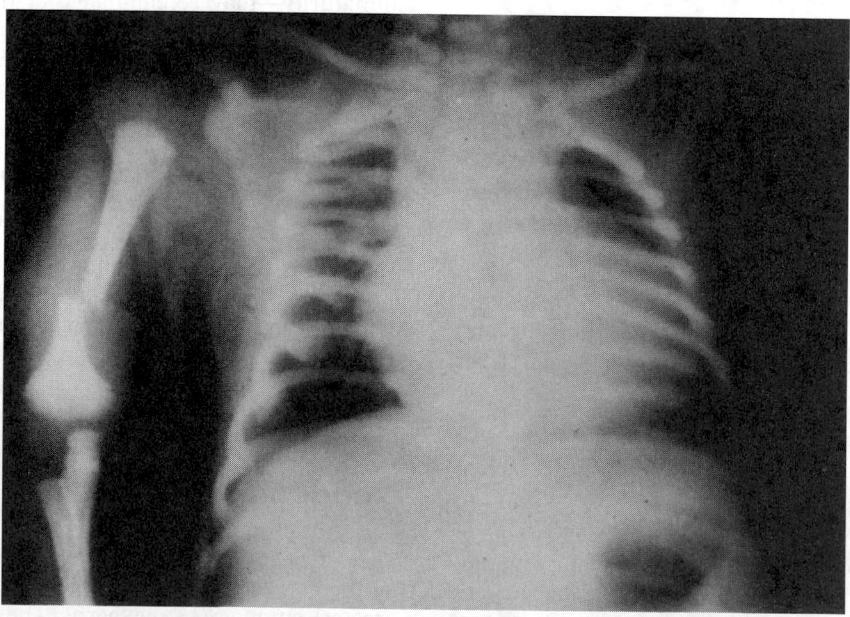

Fig. 26-5 Chest roentgenogram of a vaginally born, full-term infant (4.7 kg) of a diabetic mother. The infant had cardiomegaly, hepatomegaly, congested lung fields, and fractures of the right humerus and left clavicle. (From Fanaroff A, Martin R, editors: *Neonatal-perinatal medicine: diseases of the fetus and infant,* ed 6, St Louis, 1997, Mosby.)

tation of the aorta, transposition of the great vessels, and atrial or ventricular septal defects are the most common lesions encountered in the IDM.

CNS anomalies include anencephaly, encephalocele, meningomyelocele, and hydrocephalus. The musculoskeletal system may be affected by *caudal regression syndrome* (*sacral agenesis*, with weakness or deformities of the lower extremities, malformation and fixation of the hip joints, and shortening or deformity of the femurs) (Fig. 26-3). Hypertrichosis on the pinnae (excessive hair growth on the external ear) has been added to the list of characteristic clinical features (Fanaroff and Martin, 1997). Other defects noted in this population include gastrointestinal atresia and urinary tract malformations.

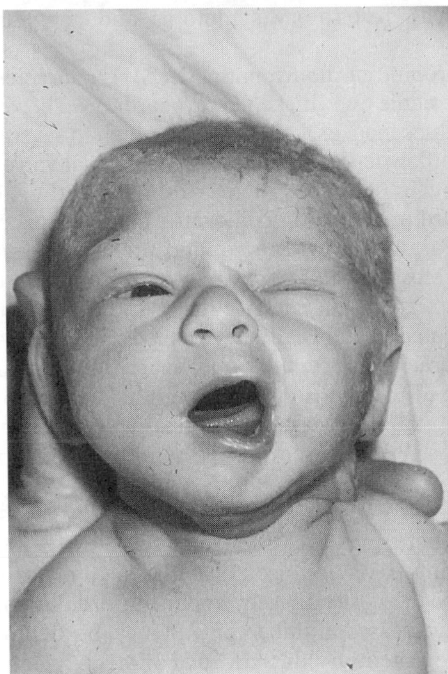

Fig. 26-6 Facial paralysis 15 minutes after forceps delivery. Absence of movement on affected side is especially noticeable when infant cries. (From O'Doherty N: *Micro atlas of the newborn*, Nutley, NJ, 1980, Hoffmann-La Roche, Inc.)

Macrosomia

Despite improvements in the control of maternal blood sugar levels, the incidence of **macrosomia** in the insulin-dependent diabetic is 20% to 30% (Ogata, 1994). At birth the typical LGA infant has a round, cherubic ("tomato" or cushingoid) face, chubby body, and a plethoric or flushed complexion (Fig. 26-4). The infant has enlarged internal organs (hepatosplenomegaly, splanchnomegaly, cardiomegaly) (Fig. 26-5) and increased body fat, especially around the shoulders. The placenta and umbilical cord are larger than average. The brain is the only organ that is not enlarged. IDMs may be LGA but physiologically immature.

The excessive shoulder size in these infants often leads to dystocia, particularly because the head may be smaller in proportion to the shoulders than in a nonmacrosomic infant. Macrosomic infants, who may be born vaginally or by cesarean birth after a trial of labor, may incur birth trauma.

Birth Trauma and Perinatal Asphyxia

Birth injury (resulting from macrosomia or method of birth) and perinatal asphyxia occur in 20% of IGDMs and 35% of

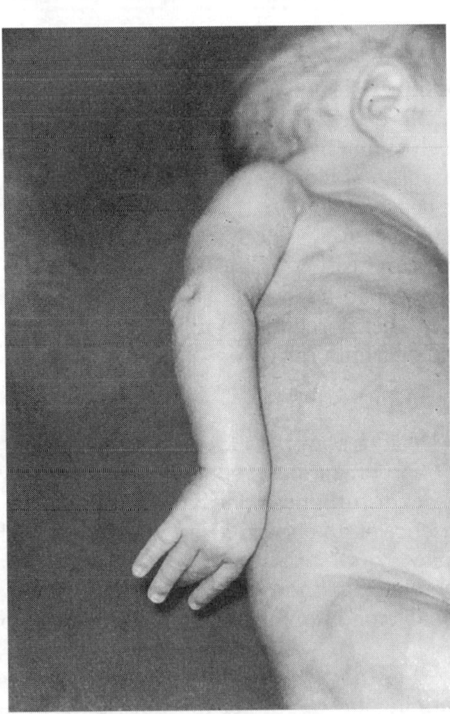

Fig. 26-7 Duchenne-Erb paralysis in newborn infant. The Moro reflex was absent in right upper extremity. Recovery was complete. (From O'Doherty N: *Micro atlas of the newborn*, Nutley, NJ, 1980, Hoffmann-La Roche, Inc.)

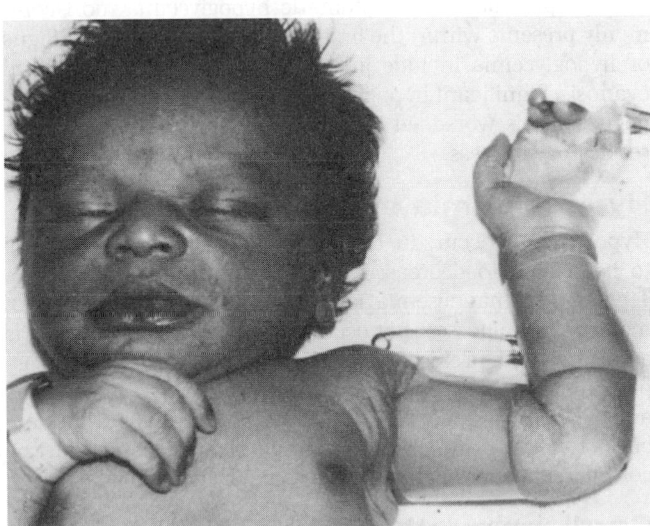

Fig. 26-8 Recommended corrective positioning for treatment of Duchenne-Erb paralysis. Notice abduction and external rotation at shoulder, flexion at elbow, supination of forearm, and slight dorsiflexion at wrist. (From Behrman R, editor: *Neonatology: diseases of the fetus and infant*, St Louis, 1973, Mosby.)

IDMs. Examples of birth trauma include cephalhematoma; paralysis of the facial nerve (seventh cranial nerve) (Fig. 26-6); fracture of the clavicle or humerus; brachial plexus paralysis, usually Duchenne-Erb (right upper arm) palsy (Figs. 26-7 and 26-8); and phrenic nerve paralysis, invariably associated with diaphragmatic paralysis.

RDS

IDMs or IGDMs are four to six times more likely than normal infants to develop RDS. With improved maternal glucose control, this risk has been substantially reduced. Some studies have found no increased risk of RDS in matched controlled studies of IDM and non-IDM infants (Mimouni et al, 1987), whereas others have shown a continued delay in lung maturation in the presence of maternal diabetes (Piper and Langer, 1993).

In the fetus exposed to high levels of maternal glucose, synthesis of surfactant may be delayed because of the high fetal serum level of insulin (Philip, 1987). Fetal lung maturity, as evidenced by a lecithin/sphingomyelin (L/S) ratio of 2:1, is not reassuring if the mother has diabetes mellitus or gestation-induced diabetes mellitus. For the infants of such mothers, an L/S ratio of 3:1 or more or the presence of *phosphatidylglycerol* in the amniotic fluid is more indicative of adequate lung maturity.

Hypoglycemia

Hypoglycemia (blood glucose levels less than 40 mg/dl in term infants) affects many IDMs. After constant exposure to high circulating levels of glucose, hyperplasia of the fetal pancreas occurs, resulting in hyperinsulinemia. Disruption of the fetal glucose supply occurs with the clamping of the umbilical cord, and the neonate's blood glucose level falls rapidly in the presence of fetal hyperinsulinism. Hypoglycemia is most common in the macrosomic infant, but blood glucose levels should be monitored in all infants of known or suspected diabetic mothers.

Asymptomatic or symptomatic hypoglycemia most commonly presents within the first 1 to 3 hours after birth. Signs of hypoglycemia include jitteriness, apnea, tachypnea, and cyanosis. Significant hypoglycemia may result in seizures. Hypoglycemia is worsened by the presence of hypothermia or respiratory distress.

Hypocalcemia and Hypomagnesemia

Hypocalcemia occurs in 10% to 20% of IDMs and is believed to be related to decreased levels of parathormone (Ogata, 1994). Hypomagnesemia is believed to develop because of maternal renal losses that occur in diabetes. Hypocalcemia is associated with preterm birth, birth trauma, and perinatal asphyxia. Signs of hypocalcemia, a prevalent finding in IDMs and IGDMs, are similar to those of hypoglycemia, but they occur between 24 and 36 hours of age. Hypocalcemia must be considered if therapy for hypoglycemia is ineffective.

Cardiomyopathy

All IDMs need careful observation for cardiomyopathy because an increased heart size is often found in this client population. Two types of cardiomyopathy can occur. Clinicians must be alert to identify correctly the type of lesion so that appropriate therapy is instituted. Both types of lesions are associated with respiratory symptoms and congestive heart failure.

Hypertrophic cardiomyopathy (HCM) is characterized by a hypercontractile and thickened myocardium. The ventricular walls are thickened, as is the septum, which in severe cases results in outflow tract obstructions. The mitral valve is poorly functioning. In nonhypertrophic cardiomyopathy (non-HCM) the myocardium is poorly contractile and overstretched. The ventricles are increased in size, and there is no outflow obstruction. Most infants are asymptomatic, but severe outflow obstruction may cause left ventricular heart failure. HCM may be treated with a β-adrenergic blocker (such as propranolol to decrease contractility and heart rate). A cardiotonic agent is used to treat non-HCM (such as digoxin to increase contractility and decrease heart rate). The abnormality usually resolves in 3 to 12 months (Fanaroff and Martin, 1997).

Hyperbilirubinemia and Polycythemia

Hyperbilirubinemia develops in 20% to 25% of IDMs (Ogata, 1994). Many IDMs are also polycythemic. Polycythemia increases blood viscosity, thereby impairing circulation. In addition, this increased number of RBCs to be hemolyzed increases the potential bilirubin load that the neonate must clear. The excessive RBCs are produced in extramedullary foci (liver and spleen) in addition to the usual sites in bone marrow. Therefore both liver function and bilirubin clearance may be adversely affected. Bruising associated with birth of a macrosomic infant will contribute further to high bilirubin levels. See also the discussion of hyperbilirubinema on p. 767.

Nursing Diagnoses

Following are examples of relevant nursing diagnoses.

Newborn

- Risk for injury related to
  - Metabolic effects of maternal condition
  - Hypoglycemia, hypocalcemia, hyperbilirubinemia, hyperviscosity of blood
  - Birth trauma
- Risk for ineffective gas exchange related to
  - Lung immaturity
  - Cardiomyopathy
- Ineffective thermoregulation related to
  - Physiologic immaturity

Parents/family

- Anxiety, fear, or powerlessness related to
  - Uncertainty regarding neonate's prognosis
- Self-esteem disturbance related to
  - Experience of an abnormal pregnancy and high-risk neonate
- Anxiety related to knowledge deficit related to
  - Neonate's condition, management, and prognosis

Expected Outcomes

Ideally, planning for the IDM begins during the antenatal period. Pediatric staff members are present at the birth. For each child an individualized plan of care is developed.

Expected outcomes for the infant include:

1. The infant will not develop respiratory distress.

2. The infant will maintain blood glucose levels within normal limits.
3. The infant will maintain temperature stability.

Expected outcomes for the family may include:

1. The family will understand the effects of diabetes mellitus or the birth injury.
2. The family will willingly comply with management.
3. If the newborn exhibits a disorder or dies, the family will exhibit appropriate grief reactions.

Plan of Care and Implementation

Implementation of care depends on the neonate's particular problems. General care of the compromised newborn is addressed in Chapter 25. If the maternal blood glucose level was well controlled throughout the pregnancy, the infant may require only monitoring. Because euglycemia is not always possible, the nurse must promptly recognize and treat any consequences of maternal diabetes that arise.

Evaluation

The nurse can be assured that care has been effective if the expected outcomes are achieved. Specifically, the newborn has a birth without trauma or injury and a neonatal period without sequelae of trauma or pregnancy complicated by maternal diabetes; the family has an understanding of diabetes or any birth injury and they willingly comply with management; and if the newborn exhibits a disorder or dies, the family initiates the grieving process (see the Nursing Care Plan below).

Nursing Care Plan

INFANT OF GESTATIONAL DIABETIC MOTHER

Nursing Diagnosis: Risk for injury related to hypoglycemia, hypocalcemia, polycythemia, hyperbilirubinemia secondary to maternal gestational diabetes

Expected Outcomes: Patient will exhibit blood glucose, serum calcium, hematocrit and serum bilirubin levels that are within normal limits.

• NURSING INTERVENTIONS/*RATIONALES*

Monitor blood glucose levels (less than 40 mg/dl indicative of hypoglycemia); serum calcium levels (less than 7 mg/dl indicative of hypocalcemia); serum bilirubin levels (over 15 mg/dl indicative of hyperbilirubinemia) *to assess and detect early onset to prevent complications.*

Observe for signs of hypoglycemia (i.e., jitteriness, twitching, lethargy, apathy, convulsions, cyanosis, sweating, eye rolling, refusal to eat); hypocalcemia (i.e., jitters, apnea, high pitched cry, abdominal distension); polycythemia (plethora), hyperbilirubinemia (i.e., jaundice) *to assess and detect signs of onset to prevent complications.*

Early feeding of infant, glucose supplements as prescribed *to prevent or treat early hypoglycemia;* increased milk feedings/calcium supplements per physician order *to prevent or treat early hypocalcemia;* early and frequent feedings *to reduce hematocrit and enhance excretion of bilirubin in stool;* phototherapy *for bilirubin over 18 to 20 mg/dl.*

Reduce environmental factors (i.e., stimuli such as jarring or shaking, cold stress, and respiratory distress), *which can predispose infant to hypoglycemia or precipitate a seizure.*

Nursing Diagnosis: Risk for impaired gas exchange related to lung immaturity/cardiomyopathy secondary to maternal gestational diabetes

Expected Outcomes: Patient will exhibit signs of adequate oxygen supply (respiratory rate, rhythm, and amplitude, blood gas levels within normal limits).

• NURSING INTERVENTIONS/*RATIONALES*

Monitor infant vital signs, blood gas levels per order, patency of airway *to evaluate pulmonary and circulatory status.*

Avoid activities that may lower body temperature and lead to cold stress, *which can induce respiratory distress.*

Suction as needed *to keep airway patent and prevent aspiration.*

Position infant on side *to facilitate mucus drainage.*

Have resuscitation equipment and oxygen available *for quick treatment of respiratory distress.*

Nursing Diagnosis: Risk for ineffective thermoregulation related to physiologic immaturity; potential for infection related to immature immunologic defenses/environmental exposure

See the Nursing Care Plan for the normal newborn in Chapter 23, p. 641.

Nursing Diagnosis: Anxiety (risk for powerlessness, situational low self-esteem, ineffective coping) related to neonate's condition, management, and prognosis

Expected Outcome: Parents demonstrate understanding of prognosis and therapy for infant.

• NURSING INTERVENTIONS/*RATIONALES*

Explain potential effects of maternal diabetic condition on newborn *to relieve fear of unknown and support ability to cope.*

Encourage open communication (i.e., inform parents of ongoing condition, procedures, and treatment; answer questions; correct misperceptions; actively listen to parental concerns) *to provide support and help provide sense of control.*

Encourage parents to interact with infant and to become involved in care routines *to foster emotional connection.*

BIRTH TRAUMA

Birth trauma (injury) is physical injury sustained by a neonate during labor and birth.

In theory, most birth injuries may be avoidable, especially if careful assessment of risk factors and appropriate planning of birth occur. The use of ultrasonography allows antepartum diagnosis of macrosomia, hydrocephalus, and unusual presentations. Elective cesarean birth can be chosen for some pregnancies to prevent significant birth injury (Merenstein and Gardner, 1993). A small percentage of significant birth injuries are unavoidable despite skilled and competent obstetric care, as in especially difficult or prolonged labor or when the infant is in an abnormal presentation (Fanaroff and Martin, 1997). The same injury might be caused in several ways. For example, a cephalhematoma could result from an obstetric technique such as forceps birth or vacuum extraction or from pressure of the fetal skull against the maternal pelvis.

Many injuries are minor and resolve readily in the neonatal period without treatment. Other trauma requires some degree of intervention. A few are serious enough to be fatal. The nurse's contributions to the welfare of the newborn begin with early observation and accurate recording. The prompt reporting of signs that indicate deviations from normal permits early initiation of appropriate therapy. Table 26-1 provides an overview of neurologic birth injuries and the sites in which they occur.

TABLE 26-1 Types of birth injuries

SITE OF INJURY	TYPE OF INJURY
Scalp	Caput succedaneum Subgaleal hemorrhage Cephalhematoma
Skull	Linear fracture Depressed fracture Occipital osteodiastasis
Intracranial	Epidural hematoma Subdural hematoma (laceration of falx, tentorium, or superficial veins) Subarachnoid hemorrhage Cerebral contusion Cerebellar contusion Intracerebellar hematoma
Spinal cord (cervical)	Vertebral artery injury Intraspinal hemorrhage Spinal cord transection or injury
Plexus	Duchenne-Erb palsy Klumpke paralysis Total (mixed) brachial plexus injury Horner syndrome Diaphragmatic paralysis Lumbosacral plexus injury
Cranial and peripheral nerve	Radial nerve palsy Medial nerve palsy Sciatic nerve palsy Laryngeal nerve palsy Diaphragmatic paralysis Facial nerve palsy

From Minarcik C, Beachy P: *Neurologic disorders.* In Merenstein G, Gardner S, editors: *Handbook of neonatal intensive care,* ed 3, St Louis, 1993, Mosby.

Nursing Care Management

Assessment

During the initial physical examination, the nurse assesses for soft tissue, neurologic, and skeletal injuries.

Nursing Diagnoses

The nursing diagnoses depend on the particular injury incurred. Thus the following list represents examples only.

Infant

- Impaired physical mobility related to
  Brachial plexus injury
- Impaired gas exchange related to
  Diaphragmatic paralysis (partial or complete)
- Pain related to
  Injury
- Injury related to
  Bruising, cephalhematoma, hyperbilirubinemia

Parents and family

- Anxiety related to knowledge deficit regarding
  Injury
  Cause of injury
  Management and therapy
  Prognosis
- Anticipatory grieving related to
  Possible sequelae of the birth injury

Expected Outcomes

Meeting the unique needs of the birth-injured newborn requires constant vigilance. Expected outcomes are established and prioritized. Nursing actions are selected in terms of the particular disorder and individual needs of the infant and family. The overall outcomes for care of infants with birth trauma include the following:

1. The newborn will suffer minimal or no sequelae of trauma.
2. The infant will receive prompt and appropriate treatment.
3. The parents will initiate and maintain a positive parent-child relationship.
4. The parents' and family's educational needs regarding the injury and its management will be met.

Plan of Care and Implementation

Soft tissue injuries. *Caput succedaneum* is a localized edematous swelling of the scalp that is not confined within the suture lines of the skull. The swelling persists for a few days after birth and then disappears without treatment. It is most often seen after vertex vaginal births and has no pathologic significance (see Fig. 22-6, *A*).

Cephalhematoma is a collection of blood from ruptured blood vessels between the periosteum and the surface of the skull. Because blood collects beneath the periosteum, it does not cross the cranial suture lines (see Fig. 22-6, *B*). The swelling may appear unilaterally or bilaterally, usually is minimal or absent at birth, increases over the first 3 days of life, and disappears gradually in 2 to 3 weeks. Occasionally, hyperbilirubinemia may result from breakdown of the accumulated blood.

Subconjunctival (scleral) and retinal hemorrhages result from rupture of capillaries caused by increased intracranial pressure (ICP) during birth. They clear within 5 days after birth and usually present no problems. However, parents need reassurance about their presence.

Erythema, ecchymoses, petechiae, abrasions, lacerations, and edema of buttocks and extremities may be present. Localized discoloration may appear over presenting or dependent parts. Ecchymoses and edema may appear anywhere on the body and on the presenting body part from the application of forceps. They also may result from manipulation of the infant's body during birth.

Bruises over the face may be the result of face presentation (Fig. 26-9). In a breech presentation, bruising and swelling may be seen over the buttocks or genitalia (Fig. 26-10). The skin over the entire head may be ecchymotic and covered with petechiae caused by a tight nuchal cord. Petechiae, or pinpoint hemorrhagic areas, acquired during birth may extend over the upper portion of the trunk and face. These lesions are benign if they disappear within 2 days of birth and no new lesions appear. Ecchymoses and petechiae may be signs of a more serious disorder, such as thrombocytopenia. If they do not disappear spontaneously in 2 days, the physician is notified. To differentiate hemorrhagic areas from skin rashes and discolorations such as mongolian spots, the nurse blanches the skin with two fingers. Because extravasated blood remains within the tissues, petechiae and ecchymoses do not blanch.

Forceps injury occurs at the site of application of the instrument. Forceps injury typically has a linear configuration across both sides of the face, outlining the placement of the forceps. The affected areas are kept clean to minimize the risk of secondary infection. These injuries usually resolve spontaneously within several days with no specific therapy. The increased use of padded forceps blades and vacuum-assisted birth may reduce the incidence of these lesions (Fanaroff and Martin, 1997).

Accidental lacerations may be inflicted with a scalpel during cesarean birth or with scissors during an episiotomy. These cuts may occur on any part of the body but most often are found on the scalp, buttocks, and thighs. Usually they are superficial, needing only to be kept clean. Butterfly adhesive strips will hold the edges of more serious lacerations together. Rarely, sutures are needed.

Skeletal injuries. The newborn's immature, flexible skull can withstand a great degree of deformation (molding) before fracture results. Considerable force is required to fracture the newborn's skull. Two types of skull fractures typically are identified in the newborn: linear fractures and depressed fractures. The location of the fracture and involvement of underlying structures determine its significance.

If an artery lying in a groove on the undersurface of the skull is torn as a result of the fracture, increased ICP will ensue. Unless a blood vessel is involved, linear fractures (which account for 70% of all fractures for this age group) heal without special treatment. The soft skull may become indented without laceration of either the skin or the dural membrane. These depressed fractures, or "ping-pong ball" indentations, may occur during difficult births from pressure of the head on the bony pelvis (Fig. 26-11). They also can occur as a result of injudicious application of forceps.

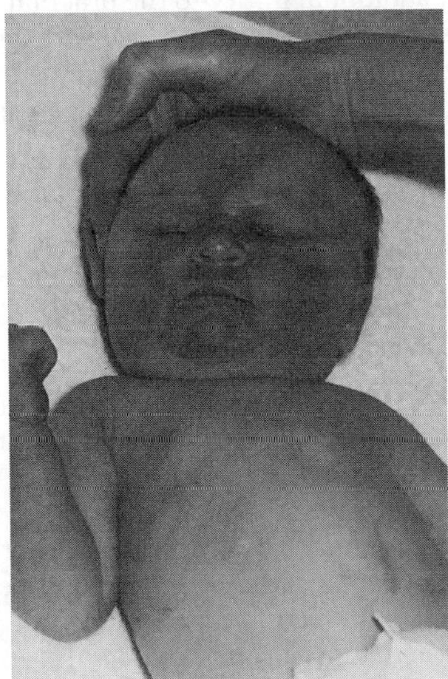

Fig. 26-9 Marked bruising of the entire face of an infant born vaginally after face presentation. Less severe ecchymoses were present on the extremities. Phototherapy was required for treatment of jaundice resulting from the breakdown of accumulated blood. (From O'Doherty N: *Micro atlas of the newborn*, Nutley, NJ, 1980, Hoffmann-La Roche, Inc.)

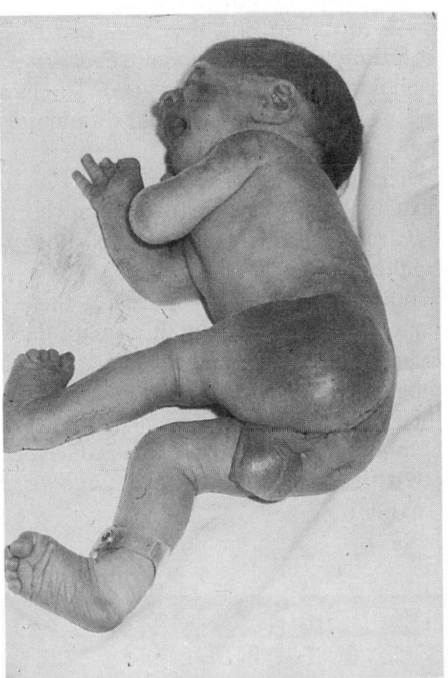

Fig. 26-10 Swelling of the genitals and bruising of the buttocks after a breech birth. Note extension of lower extremities typical of a breech birth. (From O'Doherty N: *Micro atlas of the newborn*, Nutley, NJ, 1980, Hoffmann-La Roche, Inc.)

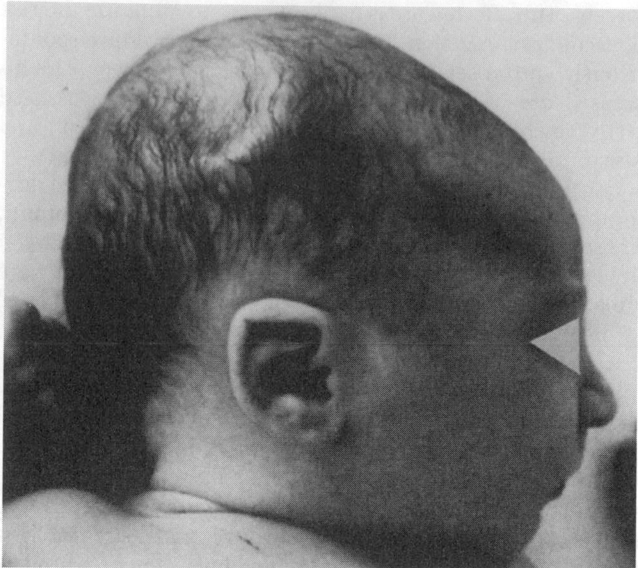

Fig. 26-11 Depressed skull fracture in a full-term male born after rapid (1-hour) labor. The infant was delivered by occiput-anterior position after rotation from occiput-posterior position. (From Fanaroff A, Martin R, editors: *Neonatal-perinatal medicine: diseases of the fetus and infant,* ed 6, St Louis, 1997, Mosby.)

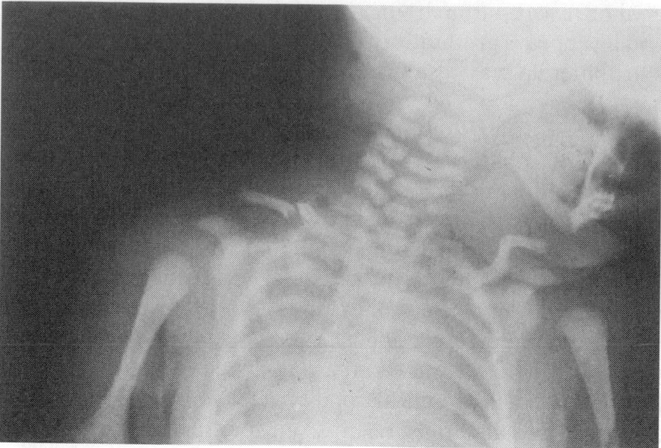

Fig. 26-12 Fractured clavicle after shoulder dystocia. (From O'Doherty N: *Micro atlas of the newborn,* Nutley, NJ, 1980, Hoffmann-La Roche, Inc.)

The clavicle is the bone most often fractured during birth. Generally the break is in the middle third of the bone (Fig. 26-12). Dystocia, particularly shoulder impaction, may be the predisposing problem. Limitation of motion of the arm, crepitus over the bone, and the absence of the Moro reflex on the affected side are diagnostic. Except for use of gentle rather than vigorous handling, no accepted treatment for fractured clavicle exists, and the prognosis is good. The figure-of-eight bandage appropriate for the older child should not be used for the newborn.

The humerus and femur are other bones that may be fractured during a difficult birth. Fractures in newborns generally heal rapidly. Immobilization is accomplished with slings, splints, swaddling, and other devices.

The parents need support in handling these infants because they often are fearful of hurting them. Parents are encouraged to practice handling, changing, and feeding the affected neonate under the guidance of nursery personnel. This increases their confidence and knowledge and facilitates attachment. A plan for follow-up therapy is developed with the parents so that the times and arrangements for therapy are acceptable to them.

Critical Thinking Exercise

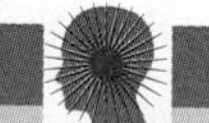

PARENTS' RESPONSE TO BIRTH INJURY

Role-play the interactions of a nurse with the parents who are angry because their infant suffered a birth injury. What do you expect the parents to say? To whom will they direct their anger? How will you respond? Who might help in this situation?

Peripheral nervous system injuries. *Duchenne-Erb paralysis* (brachial paralysis of the upper portion of the arm) is the most common type of paralysis associated with a difficult birth, occurring at rates of 0.5 to 1.9 per 1000 live births (Merenstein and Gardner, 1993) (Fig. 26-7). Injury to the upper plexus results from stretching or pulling the head away from the shoulder during a difficult birth. Typical symptoms are a flaccid arm with the elbow extended and the hand rotated inward, absence of the Moro reflex on the affected side, sensory loss over the lateral aspect of the arm, and an intact grasp reflex.

Treatment is by intermittent immobilization, proper positioning, and range of motion (ROM) exercises. Gentle manipulation and ROM exercises are delayed until about the tenth day to prevent additional injury to the brachial plexus.

Immobilization may be accomplished with a brace or splint or by pinning the infant's sleeve to the mattress. The infant should be positioned for 2 or 3 hours at a time as follows (Fig. 26-8):

- Abduct the arm 90 degrees.
- Externally rotate the shoulder.
- Flex the elbow 90 degrees.
- Supinate the wrist with the palm directed slightly toward the face.

Damage to the lower plexus, *Klumpke paralysis,* is less common. With lower arm paralysis the wrist and hand are flaccid, the grasp reflex is absent, deep tendon reflexes are present, and dependent edema and cyanosis may be apparent (in the affected hand). Treatment consists of placing the hand in a neutral position, padding the fist, and gently exercising the wrist and fingers. Full recovery is expected in 85% to 95% of infants (Merenstein and Gardner, 1993).

Facial palsy or *paralysis* (Fig. 26-6) generally is caused by pressure on the facial nerve during birth. The face on the affected side is flattened and unresponsive to the grimace that accompanies crying or stimulation, and the eye remains open. Moreover, the forehead will not wrinkle. Often the condition is transitory, resolving within hours or days of birth. Permanent paralysis is rare.

Treatment involves assistance with feeding, prevention of damage to the cornea of the open eye, and supportive care of the parents. Usually the infant's face appears distorted, especially when crying. Feeding may be prolonged, with the milk flowing out the newborn's mouth around the nipple on the affected side. The mother needs understanding and sympathetic encouragement while learning how to feed and care for the infant, as well as how to hold and cuddle the baby.

Phrenic nerve injury almost always occurs as a component of brachial plexus injury rather than as an isolated problem. Injury to the phrenic nerve results in diaphragmatic paralysis. Cyanosis and irregular thoracic respirations, with no abdominal movement on inspiration, are characteristic of paralysis of the diaphragm. Babies with diaphragmatic paralysis usually require mechanical ventilatory support, at least for the first few days after birth. Other treatments include diaphragmatic pacing or surgical correction.

Central nervous system injuries. All types of *intracranial hemorrhage (ICH)* occur in newborns. ICH as a result of birth trauma is more likely to occur in the full-term, large infant. The frequency and degree of severity of ICH are different in the newborn than in older children or adults. In the newborn, more than one type of hemorrhage can and does frequently occur (Fanaroff and Martin, 1997; Wong, 1995).

Subdural hemorrhages (hematomas), life-threatening collections of blood in the subdural space, most often are produced by the stretching and tearing of the large veins in the tentorium of the cerebellum, the dural membrane that separates the cerebrum from the cerebellum. When this type of bleeding occurs, the typical history includes a nulliparous mother, with the total labor and birth occurring in less than 2 or 3 hours, a difficult birth involving high or midforceps application, or an LGA infant. Subdural hematoma occurs infrequently today because of improvements in obstetric care. However, it is especially serious because of its inaccessibility to aspiration by subdural tap (Fanaroff and Martin, 1995; Wong, 1997).

Subarachnoid hemorrhage, the most common type of ICH, occurs in term infants as a result of trauma and in preterm infants as a result of hypoxia. Small hemorrhages are the most common. Bleeding is of venous origin, and underlying contusion also may occur (Wong, 1995).

The clinical presentation of hemorrhage in the full-term infant can vary considerably. In many infants, signs are absent, and hemorrhaging is diagnosed only because of abnormal findings on lumbar puncture, for example, RBCs in the cerebrospinal fluid (CSF). The initial clinical manifestations of neonatal subarachnoid hemorrhage may be the early onset of alternating depression and irritability, with refractory seizures (Fanaroff and Martin, 1997). Occasionally the infant appears normal initially and then has seizures on the second or third day of life, followed by no apparent sequelae.

Intracerebellar hemorrhage, although infrequent, may occur in LBW infants in association with perinatal trauma and asphyxia. At present the exact causes are not fully understood. The clinical picture is characterized by severe progressive apnea, a falling hematocrit level, and death (Fanaroff and Martin, 1997).

In general, nursing care of an infant with ICH is supportive and includes monitoring of ventilatory and intravenous therapy, observation and management of seizures, and prevention of increased ICP. Minimal handling to promote rest and reduce stress should guide nursing care (Wong, 1995).

Spinal cord injuries almost always result from breech births, especially difficult ones in which version and extraction are used. Brow and face presentations, dystocia, preterm birth, maternal nulliparity, and precipitous birth have also been identified as predisposing factors in these types of injuries. Stretching of the spinal cord, usually by forceful longitudinal traction on the trunk while the head is still firmly engaged in the pelvis, is the most common mechanism of injury. This injury is rarely seen today because cesarean birth is often used for breech presentation (Fanaroff and Martin, 1997).

Clinical manifestations depend on the severity and location of the injury. High cervical cord injuries are more likely to cause stillbirths or rapid death of the neonate. Lower lesions cause an acute spinal cord syndrome. Common signs of spinal shock include flaccid extremities, diaphragmatic breathing, paralyzed abdominal movements, atonic anal sphincter, and distended bladder. Therapy is supportive and usually unsatisfactory. Infants who survive present a therapeutic challenge that requires combined treatment from many health care providers, including the pediatrician, neurologist, neurosurgeon, urologist, orthopedist, nurse, physical therapist, and occupational therapist. Parents must understand fully the implications of severe injury to the spinal cord and the overwhelming implications it presents for the family (Fanaroff and Martin, 1997; Merenstein and Gardner, 1993).

Evaluation

The nurse can be assured that care has been effective if the outcomes for care have been achieved. Specifically, the injury receives prompt and appropriate therapy, and the newborn suffers no or minimal sequelae of trauma. In addition, the parents initiate and maintain a positive parent-child relationship, and the educational needs of parents and family regarding the injury and its management are met.

NEONATAL INFECTIONS

Sepsis (the presence of microorganisms or their toxins in the blood or other tissues) continues to be one of the most significant causes of neonatal morbidity and mortality. The newborn infant is uniquely susceptible to infection. Maternal immunoglobulin M (IgM) does not cross the placenta. Immunoglobulin A (IgA) and IgM require time to reach optimum levels after birth. Phagocytosis is less efficient. Serum complement levels are inadequate; serum complement (C1 through C6) is involved in immunologic reactions, some of which kill or lyse bacteria and enhance phagocytosis. Dysmaturity seen with IUGR and preterm and postdate birth further compromise the neonate's immune system.

Table 26-2 outlines risk factors for neonatal sepsis. Special precautions for preventing infection, as well as prompt recognition when it occurs, are necessary for optimum newborn care. Neonatal infections may be acquired in utero, during birth, during resuscitation, and nosocomially (Fanaroff and Martin, 1997).

Prenatal acquisition of infection occurs by organisms placentally transferred directly into the fetal circulatory system and from infected amniotic fluid, such as with herpes simplex virus (HSV), cytomegalovirus (CMV), and rubella. Microor-

TABLE 26-2 Risk factors for neonatal sepsis

SOURCE	RISK FACTORS
Maternal	Low socioeconomic status Poor prenatal care Poor nutrition Substance abuse
Intrapartum	Premature rupture of fetal membranes Maternal fever Chorioamnionitis Prolonged labor Premature labor Maternal urinary tract infection
Neonatal	Twin gestation Male Birth asphyxia Meconium aspiration Congenital anomalies of skin or mucous membranes Galactosemia Absence of spleen Low birth weight or prematurity Malnourishment Prolonged hospitalization

ganisms ascend from the vagina and pass through the cervix. The membranes become infected and may rupture. Infection of the fetal skin and respiratory or gastrointestinal tract may result.

During birth, contact with an infected birth canal can result in generalized or local infection. The upper airway and gastrointestinal tract are again the principal pathways for generalized infections. The conjunctiva and oral cavity are the usual sites of local infection.

Postnatal infection may be acquired during resuscitation or through the introduction of foreign objects such as indwelling catheters or endotracheal tubes. Nursery-acquired infections may be transferred to the infant by the hands of the parents or health care personnel or spread from contaminated equipment. The umbilicus is a receptive site for cutaneous infection leading to sepsis (Fanaroff and Martin, 1997).

Viral infections may cause abortion, stillbirth, intrauterine infection, congenital malformations, and acute disease. These pathogens also may cause chronic infection, with subtle manifestations that may be recognized only after a prolonged period. It is important to recognize the manifestations of infections in the neonatal period, not only to treat the acute infection and to prevent nosocomial infections in other infants, but also to anticipate effects on the infant's subsequent growth and development.

Fungal infections are of greatest concern in the immunocompromised or premature infant. Occasionally, fungal infections such as thrush are found in otherwise healthy term infants.

Septicemia refers to a generalized infection in the bloodstream. *Pneumonia*, the most common form of neonatal infection, is one of the leading causes of perinatal death (Fanaroff and Martin, 1997). *Bacterial meningitis* affects 1 in 2500 liveborn infants. *Gastroenteritis* is sporadic, depending on epidemic outbreaks. *Local infections* such as conjunctivitis and omphalitis occur frequently, but incidence rates are unavailable. Infection continues to be a significant factor in fetal and neonatal morbidity and mortality.

Nursing Care Management

Assessment

The prenatal record is reviewed for risk factors associated with infection and signs and symptoms suggestive of it. Maternal vaginal or perineal infection may be transmitted directly to the infant during passage through the birth canal. Psychosocial history and history of sexually transmitted diseases (STDs) may indicate possible human immunodeficiency virus (HIV), hepatitis B virus (HBV), or CMV infection.

The perinatal events also are reviewed. Premature rupture of membranes (PROM) may be caused by maternal or intrauterine infection. Ascending infection may occur after prolonged PROM, prolonged labor, or intrauterine fetal monitoring. A maternal history of fever during labor or the presence of foul-smelling amniotic fluid may also indicate the presence of infection. Antibiotic therapy initiated during labor should be noted. Resuscitation that requires intubation and deep suctioning may result in infection. The neonate's gestational age, maturity, birth weight, and sex all affect the incidence of infection. Sepsis occurs about twice as often and results in a higher mortality in male than in female infants. The neonate is assessed for respiratory distress, skin abscesses, rashes, and other indications of infection.

During the postnatal period the time of onset of suspicious signs is noted. Onset within the first 48 hours of life is more often associated with prenatal or perinatal predisposing factors. Onset after 2 or 3 days more frequently reflects disease acquired at or subsequent to birth (Fanaroff and Martin, 1997).

The earliest clinical signs of neonatal sepsis are characterized by a lack of specificity. The nonspecific signs include lethargy, poor feeding, poor weight gain, or irritability. The nurse or parent may simply note that the infant is just not doing as well as before. Differential diagnosis may be difficult because signs of sepsis are similar to signs of noninfectious neonatal problems such as anemia or hypoglycemia. Additional clinical and laboratory information and appropriate cultures supplement the findings described. Table 26-3 outlines signs of sepsis.

Laboratory studies are performed. Specimens for cultures include blood, CSF, stool, and urine. Increased direct (conjugated) bilirubin levels may be found, especially if the infecting microorganism is gram negative. Complete blood cell count with differential is performed to determine the presence of anemia and increased or decreased WBC count (the latter is an ominous sign). C-reactive protein may or may not be elevated.

Vigilant assessment continues during and after treatment. The newborn continues to be assessed for sequelae to septicemia. Before the advent of antibiotics, 90% of newborns with sepsis died. Antibiotic therapy decreased mortality to between 13% and 45%, depending on the causative organism.

Sequelae to septicemia include meningitis, DIC, and septic shock.

Septic shock results when the toxins are released into the bloodstream. The most common sign is a drop in blood pressure, a vital sign often overlooked in the care of the neonate.

TABLE 26-3 Signs of sepsis*

SYSTEM	SIGNS
Respiratory	Apnea, bradycardia
	Tachypnea
	Grunting, nasal flaring
	Retractions
	Decreased oxygen saturation
	Acidosis
Cardiovascular	Decreased cardiac output
	Tachycardia
	Hypotension
	Decreased perfusion
Central nervous	Temperature instability
	Lethargy
	Hypotonia
	Irritability, seizures
Gastrointestinal	Feeding intolerance
	Abdominal distention
	Vomiting, diarrhea
Integumentary	Jaundice
	Pallor
	Petechiae

*Laboratory findings include neutropenia, increased bands, hypoglycemia or hyperglycemia, metabolic acidosis, and thrombocytopenia.

Other signs are rapid, irregular respirations and pulse (similar to septicemia in general).

Nursing Diagnoses

Any number of nursing diagnoses are possible, depending on the infant's gestational age and birth weight, the organ systems involved, and the nature of the infection. Following are examples of nursing diagnoses related to neonatal infections.

Newborn

- Infection related to
  - Maternal vaginal (or other) infection
  - Resuscitation or ventilation therapy
  - Indwelling umbilical catheters, TPN, parenteral fluids
  - Intrauterine electronic fetal monitoring
  - Dysmaturity, IUGR, gestational age
- Ineffective thermoregulation related to
  - Infection
- Impaired tissue integrity related to
  - Multiple supportive measures (for example, biometric monitoring, TPN, inhalation therapy)
- Pain related to
  - Multiple supportive measures

Parents and family

- Anxiety, fear, or anticipatory grieving related to
  - Uncertainty about infant's prognosis
  - Poor prognosis
- Risk for altered parent-infant attachment related to
  - Separation of parent and newborn
  - Feelings of inadequacy in caring for infant
  - Inability to breastfeed
- Powerlessness or spiritual distress related to
  - Perinatal events or newborn's condition

Expected Outcomes

Planning begins with the development of standards for preventive measures in nurseries and protocols for the diagnosis and treatment of infections. Individual assessment findings are used to plan care for each infant. Parents and family are encouraged to participate in planning. Expected outcomes include the following:

1. The newborn will remain free of sepsis.
2. The newborn's early signs of sepsis will be recognized, and appropriate therapy will be instituted.
3. If therapy is necessary, the newborn will suffer no harmful sequelae.
4. Parents will begin bonding and attachment to newborn.
5. Parents will maintain self-esteem.
6. Staff members will establish caring relationship with parents to foster their trust and to encourage continuing, active, positive interactions of family with members of health care system.

Plan of Care and Implementation

Preventive measures. Virtually all controlled clinical trials have demonstrated that effective handwashing is responsible for the prevention of nosocomial infection in nursery units (Fanaroff and Martin, 1997). Nursing is directly or indirectly responsible for minimizing or eliminating environmental sources of infectious agents in the nursery. Measures to be taken include Standard Precautions, careful and thorough cleaning, frequent replacement of used equipment (for example, changing intravenous tubing per hospital protocol, cleaning resuscitation and ventilation equipment), and disposal of excrement and linens in an appropriate manner. Overcrowding must be avoided in nurseries.

Instillation of antibiotic into newborns' eyes 1 to 2 hours after birth is done to prevent infection. The skin, its secretions, and normal flora are natural defenses that protect against invading pathogens. Warm water may be used to remove blood and meconium from the neonate's face, head, and body. A mild nonmedicated soap (in single-use container or in a small bar reserved for a single newborn) can be used with careful water rinsing. The vernix caseosa is left in place if it is not easily removed with rinsing. No single method of cord care has been shown to prevent colonization and subsequent disease. Alcohol, triple dye, or an antimicrobial agent are typically used. Nurses need to follow agency protocols for cord care.

Curative measures. Breastfeeding or feeding the newborn breast milk from the mother is encouraged. Protective mechanisms exist in breast milk. Colostrum contains IgA, which offers protection against infection in the gastrointestinal tract. Human milk contains iron-binding protein that exerts a bacteriostatic effect on *Escherichia coli.* Human milk also contains macrophages and lymphocytes. The vulnerability of infants to common mucosal pathogens such as respiratory syncytial virus (RSV) may be reduced by passive transfer of maternal immunity in the colostrum and breast milk.

Administering medications, taking precautions when performing treatments, and following isolation procedures are also interventions to be considered when a newborn has an infection.

Monitoring the intravenous infusion rate and administering antibiotics are the nurse's responsibility. It is important to administer the prescribed dose of antibiotic within 1 hour after it is prepared to avoid loss of drug stability. If the intravenous fluid the infant is receiving contains electrolytes, vitamins, or other medications, the nurse should check with the hospital pharmacy before adding antibiotics. The antibiotic (or other medication) may be deactivated or may form a precipitate when combined with other substances. In that case a piggyback solution of the prescribed fluid is attached with a three-way stopcock at the infusion site.

Nursing ALERT

Nurses should be constantly alert for signs of infiltration (such as redness, edema, or color change of tissue, blanching at site) and for signs of overhydration (weight gain over 30 g/24 hr, periorbital edema, tachypnea, tachycardia, and moist crackles on lung auscultation).

Care must be taken in suctioning secretions from any newborn's oropharynx or trachea. These secretions may be infected.

Isolation procedures are implemented according to hospital policy as indicated. Isolation protocols are changing rapidly, and the nurse is urged to participate in continuing education and in-service programs to remain up to date.

Rehabilitative measures. Rehabilitative measures vary with the individual needs of the neonate. Some neonates need to be weaned from ventilatory support systems. Those who suffer sequelae such as mental retardation and epilepsy require a knowledgeable family and supportive community resources. Some children require corrective care for problems with dentition, vision, and hearing.

Evaluation

The nurse can be reasonably assured that care was effective if the following outcomes for care are achieved: the newborn remains free of sepsis; the newborn's early signs of sepsis are recognized and appropriately treated; if therapy is necessary, the newborn suffers no harmful sequelae; parents begin bonding and attachment to the newborn and maintain self-esteem; and staff members establish a caring relationship with parents to foster their trust and to encourage continuing, active, positive interactions of family with members of the health care team.

TORCH Infections

The occurrence of certain maternal infections during early pregnancy is known to be associated with various congenital malformations and disorders (see Chap. 9). The most common and best understood infections are represented by the acronym **TORCH,** for *t*oxoplasmosis, *o*ther (gonorrhea, syphilis, varicella, parvovirus, HBV, and HIV), *r*ubella, *c*ytomegalovirus, and *h*erpes simplex virus (HSV) (Box 26-7). HSV may result in a severe, often fatal systemic illness in neonates. Survivors of herpetic infection may have residual neurologic defects and chorioretinitis. The other congenital infections also may result in encephalopathy with various anomalies, including microcephaly, chorioretinitis, intracranial calcifications, microphthalmos, and cataracts. To a certain extent the varied clinical manifestations of these infections overlap, but a specific diagnosis can be made by the clustering of clinical findings, as well as specific antibody studies (Fanaroff and Martin, 1997).

BOX 26-7
TORCH Infections Affecting Newborns

T Toxoplasmosis
O Other: gonorrhea, syphilis, varicella, HBV, HIV, parvovirus
R Rubella
C CMV infections or CMID
H HSV infection

Toxoplasmosis. Toxoplasmosis is a multisystem disease caused by the protozoan *Toxoplasma gondii.* Cats who hunt infected birds and mice harbor the parasite and excrete the infective oocysts in their feces. Human infection follows hand-to-mouth contact, such as after disposal of cat litter or after handling or ingesting raw meat from cattle or sheep that grazed in contaminated fields.

About 30% of women who contract toxoplasmosis during gestation transmit the disease to their offspring. Fetal infection occurs in 0.07% to 0.13% of all pregnancies (Samson, 1988). The diagnosis of toxoplasmosis in the neonate is supported by elevated levels of cord blood serum IgM.

More than 70% of affected infants are free of symptoms. The clinical features of toxoplasmosis resemble cytomegalic inclusion disease (CMID) in the infant. Both diseases are responsible for serious perinatal mortality and morbidity: 10% to 15% die, 85% have severe psychomotor problems or mental retardation by age 2 to 4 years, and 50% have visual problems by age 1 year.

Severe toxoplasmosis is associated with preterm birth, growth restriction, microcephaly or hydrocephaly, microphthalmos, chorioretinitis, CNS calcification, thrombocytopenia, jaundice, and fever. Petechiae or a maculopapular rash may also be evident. Some clinical manifestations do not develop until later in life. The affected infant may be treated with pyrimethamine, as well as oral sulfadiazine, but folic acid supplement will be required to prevent anemia.

Gonorrhea. The incidence of gonococcal infection in pregnant women has ranged from 2.5% to 7.3% in recent studies (Fanaroff and Martin, 1997). With this high incidence, it is not surprising that neonatal infection with *Neisseria gonorrhoeae* occurs frequently. After rupture of membranes, ascending infection can result in orogastric contamination of the fetus. The organism also may invade mucosal surfaces such as the conjunctiva (ophthalmia neonatorum), rectal mucosa, and pharynx. Contamination may occur as the infant passes through the birth canal, or it may occur postnatally from an infected adult. Neonatal gonococcal-arthritis, septicemia, meningitis, vaginitis, and scalp abscesses can also develop.

Eye prophylaxis (for example, with 0.5% erythromycin ointment or 1% silver nitrate) is administered at or shortly after birth to prevent ophthalmia neonatorum. The infant with a mild infection often recovers completely with appropriate treatment, such as neonatal ceftriazone. Occasionally, infants die of overwhelming infection in the early neonatal period.

Syphilis. Congenital and neonatal syphilis have reemerged in recent years as significant health problems. It is estimated that for every 100 women diagnosed with primary or secondary disease, 2 to 5 infants will contract congenital syphilis. If syphilis during pregnancy is untreated, 40% to 50% of neonates born to these women will have symptomatic congenital syphilis. Treatment failure can occur, particularly when treatment is given in the third trimester; therefore infants born to women treated after 20 weeks' gestation should be investigated for congenital syphilis (Ault and Faro, 1993).

Fetal infestation with the spirochete *Treponema pallidum* is blocked by Langhans' layer in the chorion until this layer begins to atrophy between 16 and 18 weeks' gestation. If spirochetemia is untreated, it will result in fetal death by midtrimester abortion or stillbirth in one in four cases. All neonates in whom the infection occurs before 7 months' gestation are affected. Only 60% are affected if the infection occurs late in pregnancy. If maternal infection is treated adequately before the eighteenth week, neonates seldom demonstrate signs of the disease. Although treatment after the eighteenth week may cure fetal spirochetemia, pathologic changes may not be prevented completely.

Because the fetus becomes infected after the period of organogenesis (first trimester), maldevelopment of organs does not result. Congenital syphilis may stimulate preterm labor, but no evidence indicates that it causes IUGR. Stigmas of congenital syphilis (Fig. 26-13) may include inflammatory and destructive changes in the placenta; in organs such as the liver, spleen, kidneys, adrenal glands; and in bone covering and marrow. Disorders of the CNS, teeth, and cornea may not become evident until several months after birth.

The most severely affected infants may be hydropic (edematous) and anemic, with enlarged liver and spleen. Hepatosplenomegaly probably results from extramedullary hematopoietic activity stimulated by the severe anemia.

In some infants, signs of congenital syphilis do not appear

A

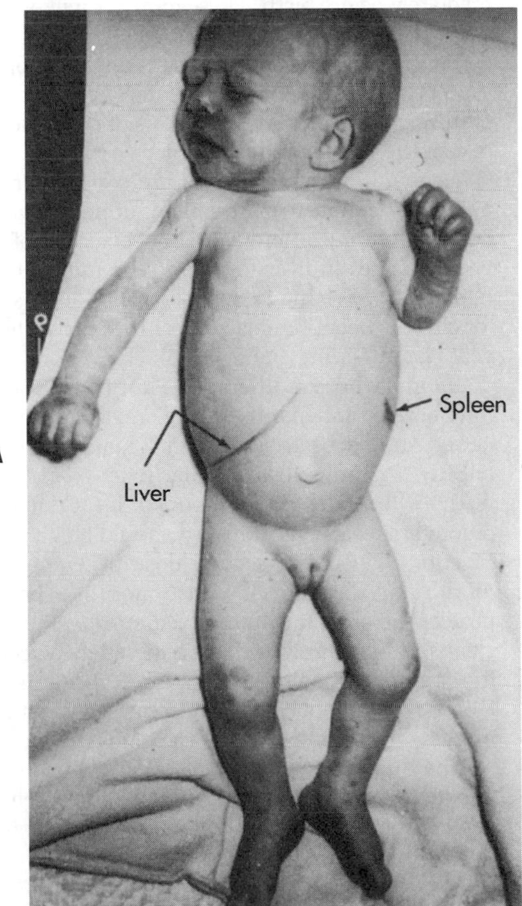

B

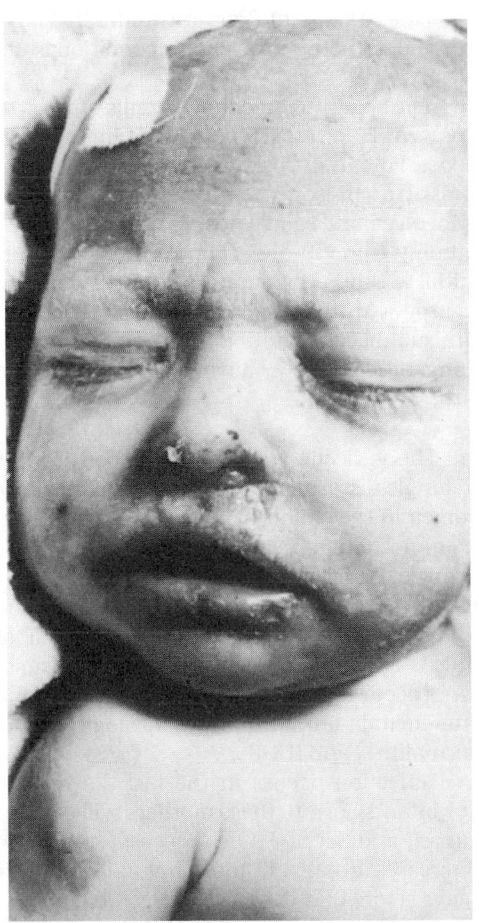

Fig. 26-13 Early congenital syphilis apparent at birth, which corresponds to secondary syphilis in the adult. (Late congenital syphilis, corresponding to tertiary syphilis, becomes apparent after 2 years of age.) **A,** Cutaneous lesions of congenital syphilis. Lines drawn on body indicate hepatosplenomegaly. No destruction of bridge of nose (common finding in congenital syphilis) is noted on this infant. **B,** Rhinitis (snuffles) resulting in rhagades and excoriation of upper lip. Red-colored rash is around mouth and on chin. (From Shirkey H, editor: *Pediatric therapy*, ed 6, St Louis, 1980, Mosby.)

until late in the neonatal period. In these newborns, early signs, such as poor feeding, slight hyperthermia, and snuffles, may be nonspecific. *Snuffles* refers to the copious, clear, serosanguineous mucous discharge from the obstructed nose. A mucopurulent discharge indicates secondary infection, usually by streptococci or staphylococci.

By the end of the first week of life, a copper-colored maculopapular dermal rash appears in untreated newborn cases. The rash is characteristically first noticeable on the palms of the hands, soles of the feet, the diaper area, and around the mouth and anus. The maculopapular lesions may become vesicular and confluent and extend over the trunk and extremities. Condylomata (elevated wartlike lesions) may be seen around the anus. Rough, cracked, mucocutaneous lesions of the lips heal to form circumoral radiating scars known as *rhagades.* If the mother was adequately treated before giving birth and serologic testing of the infant does not show syphilis, generally the infant is not treated with antibiotics. In this case the infant is checked for antibody titer (received from the mother via the placenta) every 2 weeks for 3 months, at which time the test result should be negative. Some physicians recommend antibiotic therapy for asymptomatic or inconclusive cases.

Penicillin is the usual treatment (Paryani et al, 1994). After 12 hours of antibiotic therapy, the child's condition is not considered contagious.

Even adequate treatment of congenital syphilis after birth does not always prevent late (5 to 15 years after initial infection) complications. Potential complications include neurosyphilis, deafness, Hutchinson's teeth (notched incisors), saber shins, joint involvement, saddle nose (depressed bridge), gummas (soft, gummy tumors) over the skin and other organs, and interstitial keratitis (inflammation of the cornea). The failure of therapy with the persistence of spirochetes in the eyes is not unusual because antibiotics penetrate ocular tissue poorly. Congenital syphilis during early childhood rarely causes death.

Varicella zoster. The varicella zoster virus responsible for chickenpox and shingles is a member of the herpes family. About 95% of women in the childbearing years are immune; therefore the risk of infection in pregnancy is low (1 to 7 cases per 10,000 pregnancies) (Freij and Sever, 1994).

Varicella transmission to the fetus may occur across the placenta when the disease is contracted in the first half of pregnancy, but this is relatively infrequent. When transmission to the fetus does occur in the early part of pregnancy, the effects on the fetus include limb atrophy, neurologic abnormalities, eye abnormalities, and IUGR.

When maternal infection occurs in the last 3 weeks of pregnancy, 25% of infants born to these mothers will develop clinical varicella (Freij and Sever, 1994). The severity of the infant's illness increases greatly if maternal infection occurred within 5 days before or 2 days after birth. The mortality in severe illness is 30% (Freij and Sever, 1994).

Seroimmune pregnant women exposed to active chickenpox can be given varicella zoster immune globulin (VZIG), which does not reduce the incidence of infection but should decrease the effects of the virus on the fetus. The immunoglobulin must be given within 72 hours of exposure to be effective.

Infants born to mothers who develop chickenpox between 5 days before birth and 48 hours after should be given VZIG at birth because of the risk of severe disease. Vidarabine or acyclovir can be used to treat infants with generalized involvement and pneumonia (Lott et al, 1994).

Term infants exposed to chickenpox after birth will have a mild or no infection if they are born to immune mothers. Those born to nonimmune mothers may develop chickenpox, but the course is not usually severe. Experts are divided as to whether this group of infants should receive VZIG. Infants less than 28 weeks are at risk regardless of their mother's status and likely benefit from VZIG if exposed to chickenpox.

Hepatitis B. HBV infection during pregnancy is not associated with an increase in malformations, stillbirths, or IUGR; however, about a 32% increase in risk exists for preterm birth (Fanaroff and Martin, 1997). The transmission rate of HBV to the newborn is as high as 90% (Pastorek, 1993). Transmission occurs transplacentally, serum to serum, and by contact with contaminated urine, feces, saliva, semen, or vaginal secretions during birth. Infants are most frequently infected during birth or in the first few days of life. The rate of transmission is highest when the mother contracts the virus immediately before birth. These mothers will be positive for hepatitis B surface antigen (HBsAg). Transmission may occur through breast milk, but antigens also develop in formula-fed infants at the same or higher rate. Diagnosis is made by viral culture of amniotic fluid as well as the presence of HBsAg and IgM in the cord or baby's serum.

Neonatal and fetal effects are serious. Preterm birth exposes the neonate to the problems of prematurity. Infants may be symptom free at birth or show evidence of acute hepatitis with changes in liver function. The mortality for full-blown hepatitis is 75%. Infants who become carriers are at high risk for chronic hepatitis, cirrhosis of the liver, or liver cancer even years later (Fanaroff and Martin, 1997).

Infants whose mothers have antibodies for HBsAg or who have developed hepatitis during pregnancy or the postpartum period should be treated with hepatitis B immunoglobulin (HBIG), 0.5 ml intramuscularly, as soon as possible after birth—within the first 12 hours of life. Concurrently, but at a different site, the vaccine also should be given (Fanaroff and Martin, 1997). The second dose of vaccine is given at 1 month and the third dose at 6 months. The vaccine should protect the child for up to 9 years. After the infant has been cleansed thoroughly and has received the vaccine, breastfeeding may be initiated. Vaccination for infants not exposed to HBV is recommended before discharge; breastfeeding for these infants may begin before the vaccine is given.

The Public Health Service defines women at high risk for hepatitis B as those who are Indochinese refugees, of Asian descent, or born in Haiti or South Africa; women with a history of liver disease; women who have occupational exposure to HBV, such as laboratory technologists, nurses, and physicians; and women who work with mentally retarded individuals. Intravenous drug abusers, prostitutes, and household contacts of hepatitis B carriers also are at high risk (Merenstein and Gardner, 1993).

The Centers for Disease Control (CDC) recommends that all pregnant women be screened for HBsAg at an early prenatal visit (Fanaroff and Martin, 1997).

Human immunodeficiency virus—acquired immunodeficiency syndrome. Maternal infection with the retrovirus HIV is discussed in Chapter 9. The focus of this discussion is the neonate at risk for infection with HIV. Although the transmission rate of HIV infections has been reported by some authors to be as high as 50% to 60% in infants born to mothers infected with HIV, most researchers cite a transmission rate of 20% to 35% (Bastin et al, 1992; Lindberg, 1995; Merenstein and Gardner, 1993). Pediatric acquired immunodeficiency syndrome (AIDS) accounts for 1.5% of reported AIDS cases in the United States, and 89% of these children are the offspring of HIV-infected mothers (Shannon, 1995). The incidence is likely to increase. The blood supply in the US and Canada is now screened for HIV, thus decreasing the chance of transmission by this route. However, the number of women of childbearing age infected with HIV is increasing.

Transmission of HIV from the mother to the infant occurs transplacentally at various gestational ages, perinatally through maternal blood and secretions, and postnatally through breast milk (Fanaroff and Martin, 1997; Shannon, 1995).

Routine screening and counseling of all pregnant women have been a source of controversy but have been recommended by several groups, including the American Academy of Pediatrics (Frenkel and Gaur, 1994; Provisional Committee on Pediatric AIDS, 1995). This has become especially important in light of findings that indicate that the administration of zidovudine to HIV-infected pregnant women and their infants significantly reduces the perinatal transmission of HIV (Connor et al, 1994).

Diagnosis. The diagnosis of HIV infection in the neonate is problematic (Rogers et al, 1991). Pregnant women infected with HIV produce IgG antibodies, which cross the placenta to the fetus. Therefore cord blood is positive for antibody when tested by enzyme-linked immunosorbent assay (ELISA) or Western blot techniques. Because of their physiologically depressed immune response, infants generally produce a less vigorous and more limited antibody response to HIV infection.

Virtually every baby born to a mother who is seropositive for HIV will have HIV antibody at birth; however, only 13% to 40% are actually infected (Connor and McSherry, 1994). Uninfected infants lose this maternal antibody during the first 8 to 15 months of life. Most infected infants begin to develop their own antibody and remain seropositive (Fanaroff and Martin, 1997). Many tests are used to diagnose HIV infection in infants and children (Bryant and Ratner, 1992), but improvements in sensitivity and reliability of tests are needed (Lindberg, 1995; Rogers et al, 1991).

Typically the HIV-infected neonate is asymptomatic at birth and bears no obvious physical stigma. The occurrence of an *opportunistic infection* (caused by an organism that does not usually cause disease) in the neonate may alert the caregiver to the presence of HIV infection or assist in the confirmation of the diagnosis of HIV infection. The average age of onset for an opportunistic infection is 3 to 6 months of age (Provisional Committee on Pediatric AIDS, 1995). In pediatrics the presence of lymphoid interstitial pneumonitis is now considered a criterion for diagnosis (Fanaroff and Martin, 1997). The presence of oral candidiasis (thrush) that does not respond to treatment with topical antifungal agents carries a high index of suspicion for HIV infection (Frenkel and Gaur, 1994).

Before 1 year of age, infected infants usually manifest some symptoms similar to those seen in adults, including lymphadenopathy, hepatosplenomegaly, chronic diarrhea, interstitial pneumonitis, and persistent thrush. In addition, infants fail to thrive and have developmental delays, recurrent severe bacterial infections, and occasionally recurrent enlargement of the parotid glands. *Pneumocystis carinii* pneumonia has occurred in 62% and Kaposi's sarcoma in 5% of affected infants. Viral infection caused by CMV and Epstein-Barr virus is frequently observed in children with AIDS. Bacterial sepsis also may be an initial manifestation (Fanaroff and Martin, 1997).

The average survival time between testing positive for HIV infection and death for infants is 9 months, with a 70% to 85% death rate by 2 years of age (Shannon, 1995). The disease progression has been slower and the mortality lower in infants with a later onset than with those diagnosed at birth.

Management begins by implementing Standard Precautions and precautions for invasive procedures to prevent further transmission of HIV (Craven et al, 1994; Fanaroff and Martin, 1997). Measures should also be undertaken to protect the infant from further exposure to maternal blood and body fluids. The infant's skin should be cleansed with soap and water and alcohol before invasive procedures such as vitamin K administration or heel punctures. Umbilical cord stumps are cleaned meticulously every day until healing is complete. Isolation is not required, and the infant can usually be cared for in the normal nursery. The use of gloves is not required for care activities such as dressing or feeding the infant (Benson, 1994).

Therapy for the symptomatic infant includes antimicrobial medications specific for the infections encountered and corticosteroids in the presence of lymphoid interstitial pneumonitis. Prophylaxis for PCP should be administered according to the guidelines set out by the U.S. Public Health Service (Centers for Disease Control and Prevention, 1993a). Pediatric data are not available, but it has been recommended that asymptomatic infants receive zidovudine (ZDV; formerly azidothymidine, AZT) according to their lymphocyte counts (Connor and McSherry, 1994). In industrialized countries it is generally recommended that mothers with HIV infections not breastfeed; however, the World Health Organization (WHO) does not discourage women with HIV in developing countries from breastfeeding.

Some parents opt to place the infected infants in foster homes despite the low risk for transmission among members of the same household. Social services are required in these cases. If the parent chooses to keep the infant, home health care is arranged. For more information and updated information, parents are offered the following resource: the National AIDS hotline, 1-800-342-AIDS.

The family must be counseled about vaccinations. Children with symptomatic or asymptomatic HIV infection should receive all routine vaccines except oral poliovirus vaccine. The family should be advised that household contacts should not receive oral polio vaccine (OPV) because the virus can be transmitted to the immunocompromised child. Inactivated poliomyelitis vaccine (IPV) can be given (Wong, 1995).

Rubella infection. *Congenital rubella infection* is a major concern. Since vaccination was begun in 1969, congenital rubella cases have been reduced dramatically.

More than two thirds of infected infants show no apparent involvement at birth, but consequences develop years later. Central and peripheral hearing defects, the most common result, appear to be progressive after birth. The major teratogenic effects of rubella involve the cardiovascular system (pulmonary artery hypoplasia, patent ductus arteriosus, and coarctation of the aortic isthmus) and cataract formation. Multiple other abnormalities typically occur, including intrauterine and postnatal growth restriction, thrombocytopenia (Fig. 26-14), dermal erythropoiesis, interstitial pneumonia, bony radiolucencies, retinopathy, and hepatosplenomegaly. Severe infections may result in fetal death. Delayed effects of infection manifest as thyroid dysfunction, diabetes mellitus, growth hormone deficiency, and progressive rubella panencephalopathy (Fanaroff and Martin, 1997).

The risk of a congenitally infected infant varies with the gestational age of the fetus when maternal infection occurs. Anomalies are most severe if the mother contracts the virus during the first trimester.

The rubella virus has been cultured in infants for up to 18 months after their birth. These infants are a serious source of infection to susceptible individuals, particularly women in the childbearing years. Extended pediatric isolation is mandatory until the noncontagious stage of rubella has been reached. (The infant should be isolated until pharyngeal mucus and urine are free of virus.)

Cytomegalovirus infection. Maternal CMID during pregnancy may result in abortion, stillbirth, or congenital or neonatal CMID in a live-born infant. It is the most common cause of congenital viral infections in humans, occurring in 1% of all newborns (Fanaroff and Martin, 1997). Most (90% to 95%) of the affected infants are asymptomatic at birth; however, hearing loss and learning disabilities have been reported in previously asymptomatic infants (Kenner and Lott, 1994).

The neonate with classic, full-blown CMID displays IUGR and has microcephaly. The neonate also has a rash, jaundice, and hepatosplenomegaly (Fig. 26-15). Anemia, thrombocytopenia, and hyperbilirubinemia are to be expected. Intracranial, periventricular calcification often is noted on x-ray films. Inclusion bodies ("owl's eye" figures) in cells sedimented from freshly voided urine or in liver biopsy specimens are typical.

Elevated levels of cord blood IgM are suggestive of disease. The virus may be isolated from urine or saliva of the newborn. Differential diagnosis includes other causes of jaundice, syphilis (positive Venereal Disease Research Laboratories [VDRL] findings), toxoplasmosis (positive Sabin-Feldman dye test result), hemolytic disease of the newborn (positive **Coombs'** test reaction), or coxsackievirus infection (positive culture).

Despite the extensive, endemic nature of the disease in women and men and its potential for havoc in perinatal life, critically affected newborns are born only occasionally. Milder forms of the disease often result when the fetus is affected late in pregnancy. CMV can be transmitted through breast milk while the mother is experiencing acute CMV syndrome. CMV infections acquired after birth are often asymptomatic and have no sequelae. Exceptions to this occur in preterm infants, in whom postnatal acquisition of CMV can result in pneumonia, hepatitis, thrombocytopenia, and long-term neurologic sequelae.

Antenatally infected infants who are asymptomatic at birth are at risk for late sequelae. Hearing loss may not be apparent until after the first year of life. Chorioretinitis, microcephaly, mental retardation, and neuromuscular deficits may occur by 2 years of age. Some children are at risk for a defect in tooth enamel, resulting in severe caries.

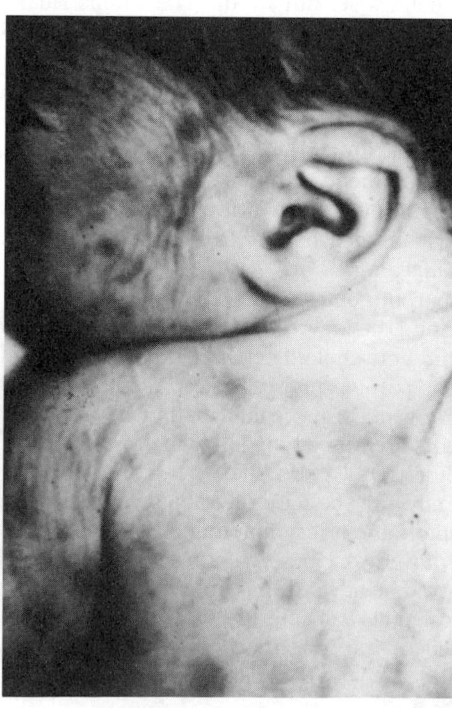

Fig. 26-14 Newborn with congenital rubella syndrome showing multiple purpuric lesions over face. (Courtesy Donald C. Anderson, Baylor College of Medicine, Houston, Tex.)

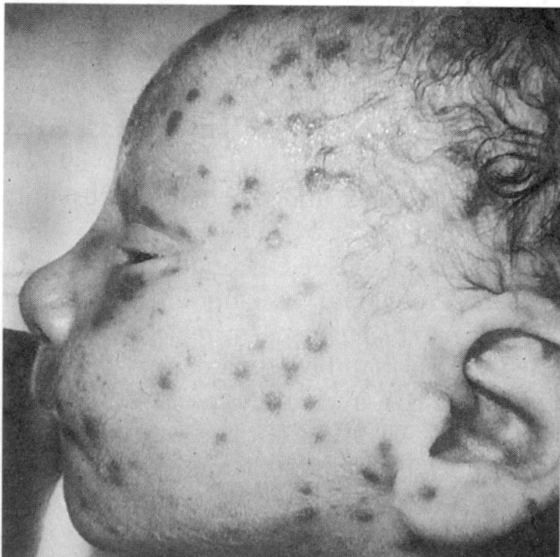

Fig. 26-15 Neonatal CMV infection. Typical rash seen in a severely affected infant. Note the small head size. (Courtesy David A. Clarke, Philadelphia.)

Herpes simplex virus. HSV infections among newborns are being diagnosed more frequently. HSV infection is estimated to occur in as many as 1 in 2000 to 1 in 5000 births (Fanaroff and Martin, 1997).

The neonate may acquire the virus by any of four modes of transmission:

- Transplacental infection
- Ascending infection by way of the birth canal
- Direct contamination during passage through an infected birth canal
- Direct transmission from infected personnel or family

Transplacental transmission of HSV infection to the neonate may occur during maternal viremia. However, an ascending transcervical infection first involves the intact fetal membranes, causing chorioamnionitis. This infection then is likely to be the cause of rupture of membranes rather than the sequela to their rupture. Transcervical infection can be accelerated by fetal monitoring scalp electrodes. The electrodes break the fetal skin barrier and increase the risk of infection; however, most infants show no evidence of infection in utero.

Congenital infection is rare and characterized by in utero destruction of normally formed organs. Affected infants are growth restricted. They have severe psychomotor restriction, with intracranial calcifications, microcephaly, hypertonicity, and seizures. They suffer eye involvement, including microphthalmos, cataracts, chorioretinitis, blindness, and retinal dysplasia. Some infants have patent ductus arteriosus, limb anomalies, and recurrent skin vesicles, with a short life expectancy.

Most infants are infected directly during passage through the birth canal. The risk of infection during vaginal birth in the presence of genital herpes has not been clearly delineated. It may be as high as 40% to 60%, with active primary infection at term. Primary maternal infections after 32 weeks' gestation carry a higher risk for the fetus and newborn than do recurrent infections (Fanaroff and Martin, 1997). The transmission rate of chronic vaginal herpes from the pregnant woman to her newborn is low, 8% or less (Toltzis, 1991). Passive intrauterine immunity to herpes may be responsible.

Postnatal acquisition of the virus and spread within a nursery have been documented by DNA analysis. Both mother and father, as well as maternal breast lesions, have been implicated in neonatal infections. There also is concern regarding symptomatic and asymptomatic shedding among hospital personnel. Nursery personnel with cold sores should practice strict handwashing and wear a mask, but no evidence indicates they should be removed from the nursery unless they have a herpetic whitlow (primary HSV infection of the terminal segment of a finger) (Fanaroff and Martin, 1997).

Clinically, neonatal HSV infections are classified as disseminated infection, encephalitis, or localized infection of the skin, eye, or mouth (Fig. 26-16). Clinical manifestations include skin vesicles in about 50% of infants (Fig. 26-17). Death results from progression of CNS involvement, respiratory distress and pneumonitis, shock, DIC, and bleeding. Overall, the mortality without antiviral therapy is 82%.

Gloves should be worn when caregivers are in contact with these infants. The neonate's eyes, oral cavity, and skin are inspected carefully for the presence of any lesions. Cultures are obtained from the mouth, eyes, and any possible lesions. Circumcision, if performed, is delayed until the infant is ready to be discharged. The infant may be discharged with the mother if the infant's cultures are negative for the virus. As long as no suspicious lesions are on the mother's breasts, breastfeeding is

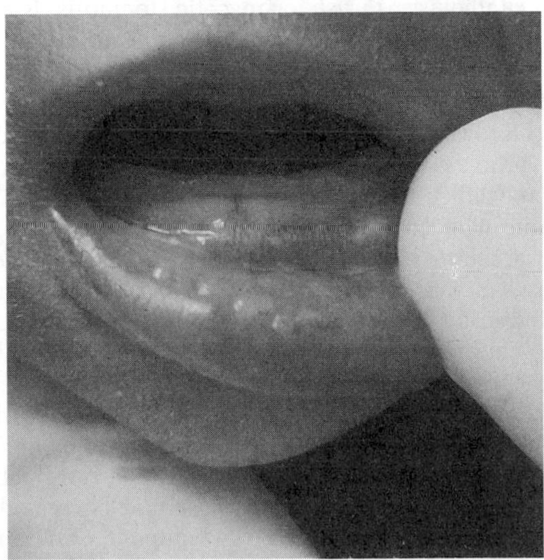

Fig. 26-16 Neonatal HSV oral lesions. (Courtesy David A. Clarke, Philadelphia.)

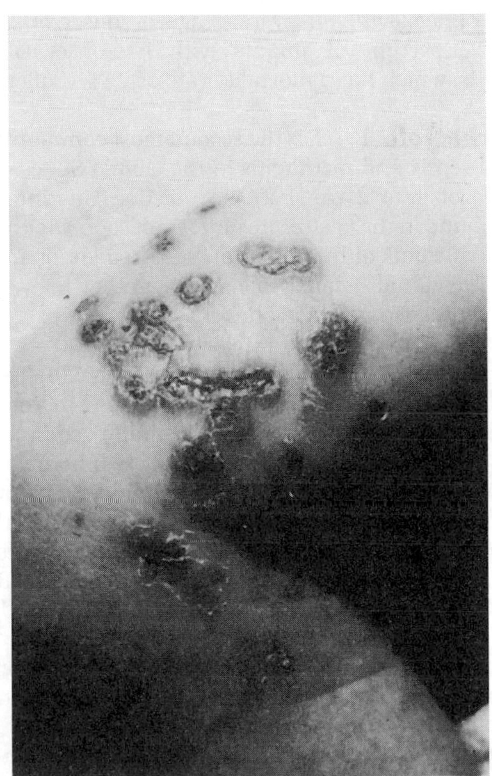

Fig. 26-17 Neonatal herpes simplex virus (HSV) skin infection. (From Fanaroff A, Martin R, editors: *Neonatal-perinatal medicine: diseases of the fetus and infant,* ed 6, St Louis, 1997, Mosby.)

allowed. For the infant at risk, prophylactic topical eye ointment (vidarabine) is administered for 5 days to prevent keratoconjunctivitis. No current recommendations exist for prophylactic systemic therapy; each case should be considered individually. Blood, urine, and CSF specimens should be cultured when indicated clinically. If herpetic lesions first occur after 6 weeks of life, the risk of dissemination and severe illness is very low (Fanaroff and Martin, 1997).

Therapy includes general supportive measures, as well as treatment with vidarabine or acyclovir. Acyclovir is the most frequently used drug. It is considered safe because only viral replication is inhibited, although long-term sequelae are not yet known. Acyclovir is easier to administer and is more effective than vidarabine for herpes encephalitis. The current recommended dose of acyclovir is 10 mg/kg/day intravenously every 8 hours for at least 14 days. Continuing therapy may be required in recurrences. Ophthalmic ointment should be administered simultaneously (Fanaroff and Martin, 1997).

Bacterial Infections

Group B streptococcus. The most common cause of neonatal sepsis and meningitis in the United States is the group B β-*hemolytic streptococcus* (GBS) (Guerina, 1991). Early-onset GBS infection in the neonate most often presents within 24 hours of birth and is most common in premature infants (Lott et al, 1994). Transplacental or vertical transmission to the fetus results in a respiratory illness that initially mimics the symptoms of severe respiratory distress. The infant rapidly deteriorates and often develops septic shock, which has a mortality rate of 30% to 50% (Fuller, 1992).

Late-onset GBS infection presents between 1 week and 3 months of age with an average age of onset of 24 days. Eighty-five percent of infants with late-onset GBS have meningitis, which has a mortality rate of 25% (Fuller, 1992).

Escherichia coli. *E. coli* is the second most common cause of neonatal sepsis and meningitis in the United States, with an incidence of 1 to 2 per 1000 live births (Guerina, 1991). *E. coli* is found in the gastrointestinal tract soon after birth and makes up the bulk of human fecal flora. In addition to meningitis, *E. coli* can also cause infections in other body systems, including the urinary tract.

Tuberculosis. The incidence of tuberculosis (TB), caused by *Mycobacterium tuberculosis*, is once again increasing in Canada and the United States. Congenitally acquired TB, although rare, can cause otitis media, pneumonia, hepatosplenomegaly, enlarged lymph glands, or disseminated disease. After delivery, exposed infants contract TB through droplets expelled by infected individuals, which results in pneumonia and necrosis of lung tissue. Untreated TB of the neonate is almost always fatal (Smith and Teele, 1990).

Listeriosis. *Listeria monocytogenes* is a bacterium capable of producing significant intrapartum illness. Prenatal infection causes chorioamnionitis or endometritis and should be suspected in cases of meconium-stained amniotic fluid in infants less than 37 weeks' gestation. With disseminated fetal infection, microabscesses have been reported in the liver, lungs, and adrenal glands of stillborn infants. Live-born infants demonstrate granulomas on the skin and posterior pharyngeal wall. Listeriosis can also present as meningitis in a late-onset infection (Bortolussi and Seelinger, 1990).

***Chlamydia* infection.** *Chlamydia trachomatis* is an intracellular bacterium that causes neonatal conjunctivitis and pneumonia. The conjunctivitis (congestion and edema), with minimal discharge, develops 5 days to 2 weeks after birth. Inclusion conjunctivitis is usually self-limiting, but if untreated, chronic follicular conjunctivitis, with conjunctival scarring and corneal neovascularization, has been reported (Hess, 1993).

The neonate is treated with oral erythromycin for 2 to 3 weeks. Silver nitrate is not effective against *C. trachomatis*, but erythromycin or tetracycline ointment may prevent ophthalmic infection (Fanaroff and Martin, 1997). Eye prophylaxis is not sufficient to prevent the development of chlamydial pneumonia; therefore infants at risk should also be treated with systemic antibiotics such as oral erythromycin syrup.

Fungal Infections

Candidiasis. *Candida* infections, formerly known as moniliasis, may occur in the newborn. *C. albicans*, the organism usually responsible, may cause disease in any organ system. It is a yeastlike fungus (producing yeast cells and spores) that can be acquired from a maternal vaginal infection during birth, by person-to-person transmission, or from contaminated hands, bottles, nipples, or other articles. It usually is a benign disorder in the neonate, often confined to the oral and diaper regions (Wong, 1995).

Candidal diaper dermatitis appears on the perianal area, inguinal folds, and lower portion of the abdomen. The affected area is intensely erythematous, with a sharply demarcated, scalloped edge, frequently with numerous satellite lesions that extend beyond the larger lesion. The source of the infection is through the gastrointestinal tract. Treatment is with applications of an anticandidal ointment, such as nystatin (Mycostatin) or miconazole 2% (Monistat), with each diaper change. The infant also may be given an oral antifungal preparation to eliminate any gastrointestinal source of infection (Wong, 1995).

Oral candidiasis (*thrush*, or mycotic stomatitis) is characterized by the appearance of white plaques on the oral mucosa, gums, and tongue. The white patches are easily differentiated from milk curds; the patches cannot be removed and tend to bleed when touched. In most cases the infant does not seem to be in discomfort from the infection. A few infants may have some difficulty swallowing.

Infants who are sick, debilitated, or receiving antibiotic therapy are more susceptible to thrush. Those with conditions such as cleft lip or palate, neoplasms, and hyperparathyroidism seem to be more vulnerable to mycotic infection.

The objectives of management are to eradicate the causative organism, to control exposure to *C. albicans*, and to improve the infant's resistance. Interventions include maintenance of scrupulous cleanliness to prevent reinfection (nursing personnel, parents, others). Good handwashing technique is always essential. Clean surfaces should be provided for neonates. Proper cleanliness of the equipment and environment is ensured. If the infant is breastfeeding, the mother is also treated with topical nystatin.

Medications are administered as ordered. Nystatin is in-

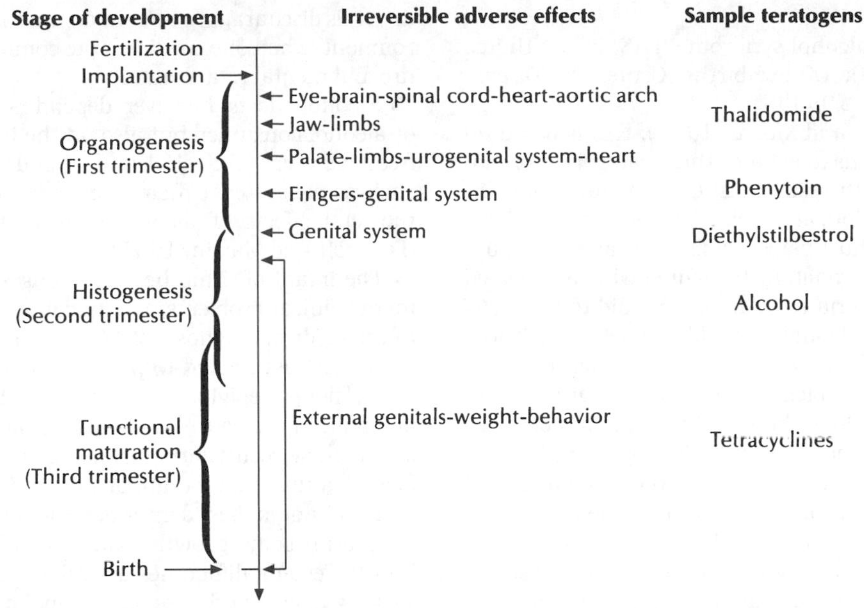

Fig. 26-18 Critical periods in human embryogenesis. (From Fanaroff A, Martin R, editors: *Neonatal-perinatal medicine: diseases of the fetus and infant*, ed 6, St Louis, 1997, Mosby.)

TABLE 26-4 Summary of neonatal effects of commonly abused substances

SUBSTANCE	NEONATAL EFFECTS
Alcohol	FAS: craniofacial anomalies, including short eyelid opening, flat midface, flat upper lip groove, thin upper lip: microcephaly, hyperactivity, developmental delays, attention deficits FAEs: milder forms of FAS; cardiac anomalies
Cocaine	Prematurity, SGA, microcephaly, poor feeding, irregular sleep pattern, diarrhea, visual attention problems, hyperactivity, difficult to console, hypersensitivity to noise and external stimuli, irritability, developmental delays, congenital anomalies such as prune belly syndrome (distended, flabby, wrinkled abdomen caused by lack of abdominal muscles)
Heroin	LBW, SGA, neonatal abstinence syndrome (see Table 26-6)
Amphetamines	SGA, prematurity, poor weight gain, lethargy
Tobacco	Prematurity, LBW, increased risk for sudden infant death syndrome (SIDS), increased risk for bronchitis, pneumonia, developmental delays
Marijuana	Possible neonatal tremors, possible LBW

stilled into the newborn's mouth with a medicine dropper after the infant is given sterile water to wash out any residual milk. Nystatin may also be swabbed over mucosa, gums, or tongue. Less frequently, an aqueous solution of gentian violet (1% to 2%) is applied with a swab to oral mucosa, gums, and tongue. The nurse should guard against staining the skin, clothes, and equipment and should warn parents about the purple staining of the baby's mouth.

SUBSTANCE ABUSE

Certain maternal behaviors result in perinatal risk. Maternal habits hazardous to the fetus and neonate include drug addiction, smoking, and alcohol abuse. Occasional withdrawal reactions have been reported in neonates of mothers who use to excess such drugs as barbiturates, alcohol, or amphetamines. Serious reactions are seen in neonates whose mothers abuse psychoactive drugs or are treated with methadone. Almost 50% of pregnancies of women addicted to opioids result in LBW infants who are not necessarily preterm. Alcohol is a teratogen. Maternal ethanol abuse during gestation creates a readily identifiable fetal alcohol syndrome.

The adverse effects of exposure of the fetus to drugs are varied and include transient behavioral changes such as fetal breathing movements or irreversible effects such as fetal death, IUGR, structural malformations, or mental retardation. Critical determinants of the effect of the drug on the fetus include the specific drug, the dosage, the route of administration, the genotype of the mother or fetus, and the timing of the drug exposure. Fig. 26-18 shows critical periods in human embryogenesis and the teratogenic effects of drugs. Table 26-4 summarizes the effects of commonly abused substances on the fetus and neonate.

Alcohol

The incidence of fetal alcohol syndrome (FAS) in the United States is about 2 per 10,000 live births (Centers for Disease Control and Prevention, 1993b).

According to Weiner and Morse (1991), FAS is based on minimum criteria of signs in each of three categories: prenatal and postnatal growth restriction; CNS malfunctions, including mental retardation; and facial features such as microcephaly, small eyes or short palpebral fissures, and a thin upper lip. Infants exposed prenatally to alcohol who are affected but do not meet the criteria for FAS may be said to have *fetal alcohol effects (FAEs)* or alcohol-related birth defects (ARBDs) (Coles, 1993). These effects run the gamut from learning disabilities and behavioral problems to speech or language problems and hyperactivity. Often these problems are not detected until the child goes to school and learning problems become evident. FAEs can be seen with other disorders, such as fetal hydantoin syndrome, so a careful history is needed.

Predictable abnormal patterns of fetal and neonatal morphogenesis are attributed to severe, chronic alcoholism in women who continue to drink heavily during pregnancy. The pattern of growth deficiency begun in prenatal life persists after birth, especially in the linear growth rate, rate of weight gain, and growth of head circumferences.

Ocular structural anomalies are common findings (Fig. 26-19). Limb anomalies and various cardiocirculatory anomalies, especially ventricular septal defects, pose problems for the child. Table 26-5 outlines physical findings in FAS. Mental retardation (IQ of 79 or below at 7 years of age), hyperactivity, and fine motor dysfunction (poor hand-to-mouth coordination, weak grasp) add to the handicapping problems that maternal alcoholism can impose. Genital abnormalities are seen in daughters of alcohol-addicted mothers. Two thirds of newborns with FAS are girls; the cause of this altered fetal sex ratio is unknown. Severe and chronic alcoholism (ethanol toxicity), not maternal malnutrition, is responsible for the severity and consistency of postnatal performance problems (Fanaroff and Martin, 1997). High alcohol levels are lethal to the developing embryo. Lower levels cause brain and other malformations. Long-term prognosis (no studies are available as yet) is discouraging even in an optimum psychosocial environment, when one considers the combination of growth failure and mental retardation.

Alcohol effects, however, depend not only on the amount of alcohol consumed but also on the interaction of quantity, frequency, type of alcohol, and other drug abuse. Other drugs, such as cigarettes, caffeine, and marijuana, may potentiate the fetal effects of alcohol consumption during gestation (Fanaroff and Martin, 1997).

The infant of a mother who abuses alcohol is faced with many clinical problems. Identification of the problems leads to the medical diagnosis of FAS. The infant may suffer respiratory distress related to preterm birth, neurologic damage, and a "floppy" epiglottis and small trachea. Tracheoepiglottal anomalies may cause cardiopulmonary arrest. Other disorders include recurrent otitis media and hearing loss. Craniofacial features may be important in diagnosing craniofacial and oral anomalies, dental development abnormalities, and long-term body growth patterns (Hudson and Hussain, 1990). Feeding difficulties are related to preterm birth, poor sucking ability, and possible cleft palate. The infant may exhibit brain dysfunction, microcephaly, and grand mal seizures.

Long-term effects into childhood may include impaired visuomotor perception and performance, lowered IQ scores, and delayed receptive and expressive language (Hill, Hegemier, and Tennyson, 1990), as well as reduced capacity to process and store factual data (Becker, Warr-Leeper, and Leeper, 1990). It is now recognized as one of the leading causes of mental retardation in the United States. Although the distinctive facial features of the infant tend to become less evident, the mental capacities never become normal (Streissguth et al, 1991).

Nursing care involves many of the same strategies used for

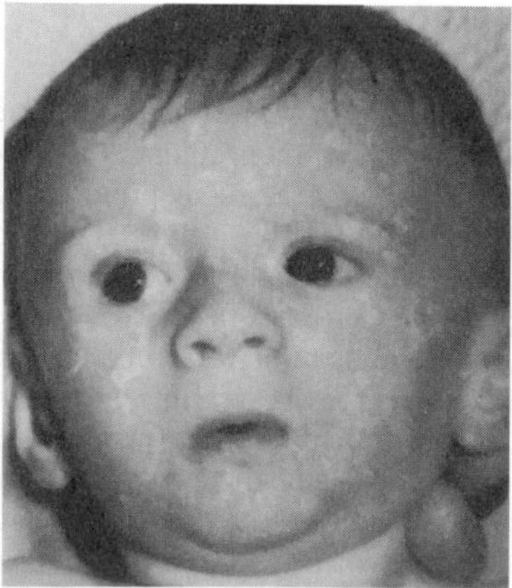

Fig. 26-19 Fetal alcohol syndrome. (Courtesy Dr. Charles Linder, Medical College of Georgia. From Goodman R, Gorlin R: *Atlas of the face in genetic disorders*, ed 2, St Louis, 1977, Mosby.)

TABLE 26-5 Features of FAS

AFFECTED PART	CHARACTERISTICS
Eyes	Epicanthal folds, strabismus, ptosis, hypoplastic retinal vessels
Mouth	Poor suck, cleft lip, cleft palate, small teeth
Ears	Deafness
Skeleton	Radioulnar synostosis, fusion of cervical vertebrae, restricted bone growth
Heart	Atrial and ventricular septal defects, tetralogy of Fallot, patent ductus arteriosus
Kidney	Renal hypoplasia, hydronephrosis, urogenital sinus
Liver	Extrahepatic biliary atresia, hepatic fibrosis
Immune system	Increased infections: otitis media, upper respiratory infections, immune deficiencies
Tumors	Nonspecific neoplasms
Skin	Abnormal palmar creases, irregular hair, whorls

From Weiner L, Moore B: *FAS: clinical perspectives and prevention.* In Chasnoff I, editor: *Drugs, alcohol, pregnancy and parenting*, Boston, 1991, Kluewer.

the care of preterm infants. Special efforts are made to involve the parents in their child's care and to encourage opportunities for parent-child attachment (see the Nursing Care Plan on p. 765).

Infants placed in a warm, caring environment with understanding caregivers who can deal with the infant's hyperirritability can be helped to lead a more normal existence than their condition might warrant (Barbour, 1989). These caregivers provide extensive cuddling and human contact and can deal with the eating problems that typically lead to a diagnosis of failure to thrive. However, these infants may not go home to such an environment. Often the family is dysfunctional.

Tobacco

Cigarette smoking in pregnancy has been found to be associated with birth weight deficits of up to 250 g for a full-term neonate (Fanaroff and Martin, 1997). Maternal cigarette smoking is implicated in 21% to 39% of LBW infants. Passive exposure to second-hand smoke by a pregnant woman may also result in the birth of an LBW infant. Also, if pregnant smokers drink five or more cups of coffee and one or more drinks of alcohol per day, the risk of IUGR is increased considerably (Fried, 1993).

The rate of spontaneous abortion and preterm birth is increased in the smoking population. When other variables have been controlled for, no association has been found between maternal smoking and congenital anomalies (Fried, 1993). Nicotine and cotinine, the two pharmacologically active substances in tobacco, are found in higher concentrations in infants whose mothers smoke. These substances can be secreted in breast milk for up to 2 hours after the mother has smoked. Cigarette smoke contains more than 2000 compounds, including carbon monoxide, dioxin, cyanide, and cadmium. Long-term studies show residual effects beyond the neonatal period (Floyd et al, 1993). Deficits in growth, in intellectual and emotional development, and in behavior have been documented. These include poor auditory responsiveness, increased fine motor tremors, hypertonicity, and decreased verbal comprehension.

Pregnant women must be aware of the harmful effects of smoking on their unborn baby's health. These include IUGR, spontaneous abortions, PROM, placenta previa, and SIDS (Feng, 1993). Increasing concern surrounds second-hand smoke and its potential effects on infants and siblings. Mothers and all others need to refrain from smoking near the infant. Several studies have reported a positive association between maternal smoking and SIDS (Floyd et al, 1993; Zuckerman, 1991). It is not clear whether this association reflects in utero exposure, passive exposure postnatally, or both.

Marijuana

Marijuana crosses the placenta. Its use during pregnancy may result in a shortened gestation and a higher incidence of IUGR (Day, Cottreau, and Richardson, 1993). Some investigators have found a higher incidence of meconium staining (Fanaroff and Martin, 1997). Some association has been reported between the use of marijuana and a decrease in infant birth weight and length and the occurrence of congenital anomalies; however, the findings have been inconsistent (Zuckerman, 1991). A longitudinal study by Fried (1993) followed infants of marijuana users for 2 years and found no association between marijuana use and cognitive abilities at 12, 24, or 36 months, but at 48 months found memory and verbal measures of cognitive ability affected in the infants of heavy marijuana users. Compounding the issue of the effects of marijuana is multidrug use, especially among adolescents, thus combining the harmful effects of marijuana, tobacco, alcohol, and cocaine. Long-term follow-up studies on exposed infants are needed.

Cocaine

Cocaine crosses the placenta and is found in breast milk. Approximately 20% to 30% of cocaine-exposed infants have resulting physical abnormalities (Chasnoff, 1992).

Antenatal effects of maternal cocaine ingestion include infarctions to developing organs, resulting in defects such as hydronephrosis, hypospadias, prune belly syndrome (distended flabby abdomen and renal anomalies), congenital heart disease, skull defects, ileal atresia, and limb reduction. Infants born to cocaine-abusing mothers show a high rate of perinatal morbidity, IUGR, preterm birth, and cerebral hemorrhage or infarction (Chasnoff, 1992; Kennard, 1990).

Cocaine-dependent neonates do not experience a process of withdrawal seen in narcotic exposed infants but rather suffer from neurotoxic effects of the drug. Signs of exposure have some of the same characteristics as heroin withdrawal but can be quite varied. There may be an increased risk for SIDS (Plessinger and Woods, 1993). Box 26-8 summarizes neonatal effects of maternal cocaine use.

Phencyclidine ("Angel Dust")

Phencyclidine (PCP) increases the risk of injury to the pregnant woman and therefore also to her passively dependent fetus. The user may be unaware that she is ingesting PCP because it frequently is misrepresented as another drug of abuse or mixed with other drugs (Carroll, 1990).

PCP crosses the placenta and is found in breast milk. Literature about the effects on infants is limited. Infants exposed to PCP may exhibit abnormal motor behavior such as irritability, jitteriness, and hypertonicity (Glantz and Woods, 1993).

Heroin

Heroin crosses the placenta and frequently results in IUGR. Heroin may have a direct growth-inhibiting effect on the fetus, but the exact mechanisms of growth inhibition is not clear. There is an increased rate of stillbirths but not of congenital anomalies. Most medical complications attributed to heroin ingestion result from prematurity (Finnegan, 1991).

Maternal detoxification in the first trimester carries an increased risk of spontaneous abortion. Detoxification is not recommended after the thirty-second week because of possible withdrawal-induced fetal distress (Glantz and Woods, 1993).

Heroin withdrawal occurs in 50% to 75% of infants born to addicted mothers, usually within the first 24 to 48 hours of life. The signs depend on the length of maternal addiction, the amount of drug taken, and the time of injection before birth. The infant whose mother is taking methadone may not demonstrate signs of withdrawal until a week or so after birth. The symptoms of infants whose mothers used heroin or methadone are similar in nature. Initially the infant may be

BOX 26-8

Neonatal Effects of Maternal Cocaine Use

Physical		Behavioral
Decreased gestational age	Fever	Irritability
Decreased birth weight	Tachypnea	Tremors
Decreased length	Congenital heart disease	Poor feeding
Decreased head circumference	Skull defects	Frantic fist sucking
Prematurity	Hypertension	Abnormal sleep patterns
Intrauterine growth restriction	Cerebral infarction	Sneezing
Anemia	Absent digits	Yawning
Ileal atresia	Vomiting	High-pitched cry
Prune belly syndrome	Diarrhea	Increased startles
Cryptorchidism		Disorganized behavior
Hypospadias		Lability
Hydronephrosis		Poor visual processing
Hypertonia		Decreased spontaneous activity
Seizures		Dull alert periods
Tachycardia		Difficult to console

From Kennard M: Cocaine use during pregnancy: fetal and neonatal effects, *J Perinat Neonatal Nurs* 3(4):58, 1990.

depressed. The withdrawal syndrome may manifest as a combination of any of the following signs. The infants may be jittery and hyperactive. Usually the infant's cry is shrill and persistent. The infant may yawn or sneeze frequently. The tendon reflexes are increased, but the Moro reflex is decreased. The neonate may exhibit poor feeding and sucking, tachypnea, vomiting, diarrhea, hypothermia or hyperthermia, and sweating. In addition, an abnormal sleep cycle, with absence of quiet sleep and disturbance of active sleep, has been described in these infants (Fanaroff and Martin, 1997).

If withdrawal is not treated, vomiting, diarrhea, dehydration, apnea, and convulsions may develop. Death may follow. Therapy is individualized. Dehydration and electrolyte imbalance are prevented or treated. Usually one of the following drugs is ordered: phenobarbital, paregoric (compound tincture of opium), or diazepam, singly or in combination.

The long-term effect on these infants is now being studied. The risk of SIDS is 5 to 10 times higher for infants with significant withdrawal problems than for infants in the general population.

Methadone

Methadone, a synthetic opiate, has been the therapy of choice for heroin addiction since 1965. It does cross the placenta. An increasing number of infants have been born to methadone-maintained mothers, who seem to have better prenatal care and a somewhat better life-style than those taking heroin (Fanaroff and Martin, 1997).

Some question exists concerning the benefits of methadone therapy during pregnancy because of its effect on the fetus. In one study (Levine and Rebarber, 1995), nonstress tests performed on women receiving methadone were found to be significantly less reactive than nonstress tests reported in the general population of pregnant women. These findings question the benefits of methadone treatment for pregnant heroin abusers and the related ethical issues. Methadone withdrawal occurs in about 80% to 95% of infants born to these women.

Methadone withdrawal resembles heroin withdrawal but tends to be more severe and prolonged. In addition, the incidence of seizures is higher. Seizures usually occur between days 7 and 10. These infants exhibit a disturbed sleep pattern similar to that seen in heroin withdrawal. They have a higher birth weight than those infants in heroin withdrawal, usually AGA. No increased incidence of congenital anomalies is seen.

Late-onset withdrawal occurs at age 2 to 4 weeks and may continue for weeks or months. A higher incidence of SIDS also has been reported in these infants. This factor is important for perinatal nurses who coordinate follow-up care for the infant and education for the mother or other caregiver. Community health nurses must know about the potential for withdrawal symptoms to occur.

Therapy for methadone withdrawal is similar to that for heroin withdrawal. The few available follow-up studies of these infants reveal a high incidence of hyperactivity, learning and behavior disorders, and poor social adjustment (Fanaroff and Martin, 1997).

Miscellaneous Substances

The fetal and neonatal effects of maternal use of methamphetamines in pregnancy are not well known. The effects appear to be dose related. LBW, preterm birth, and perinatal mortality may be consequences of higher doses used throughout pregnancy. Infants may be drowsy and jittery and may experience respiratory distress soon after birth (Evans, 1991). Lethargy may continue for several months, along with frequent infections and poor weight gain. Emotional disturbances and delays in gross and fine motor coordination may be seen during early childhood.

Phenobarbital crosses the placenta readily and is subsequently found in high levels in the fetal liver and brain. Because of its slow metabolic rate, when withdrawal does occur, onset is generally 2 to 14 days after birth and duration is about 2 to 4 months. Irritability, crying, hiccoughs, and sleepiness mark the initial response. During the second stage the infant is extremely hungry, regurgitates and gags frequently, and demonstrates episodic irritability, sweating, and a disturbed sleep pattern.

Treatment consists of swaddling, frequent feedings, and protection from noxious external stimuli. If no improvement occurs with these methods, the neonate should be given phenobarbital and then slowly withdrawn from this drug after control of symptoms (Fanaroff and Martin, 1997).

Caffeine has not been implicated as a teratogen in humans. Fenster, Eskenazi, and Windham (1991) reported that caffeine consumption greater than 300 mg a day was associated with IUGR and LBW. Mills et al. (1993) reported no adverse effects in the fetus with consumption of less than 300 mg of caffeine a day.

Planning for care of the newborn presents a challenge to the health care team. Parents are included in the planning for the newborn's care and are also encouraged to plan for their own care. A multidisciplinary approach is needed that includes home health or community resource personnel (e.g., regulatory agencies such as child protective services).

Expected outcomes are stated in patient-centered terms and include the following:

1. The newborn will suffer no adverse sequelae to drug withdrawal.
2. The infant's malformations and dysfunction will be identified and appropriate curative and rehabilitative measures instituted.
3. Parents will accept the newborn's condition and participate in the newborn's management.

Nursing Care Management

Assessment of the newborn requires a review of the mother's prenatal record. A medical and social history of drug abuse and detoxification is noted. The infant may have IUGR or be preterm with LBW.

The woman who is addicted to narcotics may have infections that compound the risk to the infant, including hepatitis, septicemia, and STDs, including AIDS (Niebyl, 1988).

The nurse often is the first to observe the signs of drug dependence in the infant. The nurse's observations help the physician differentiate between drug dependence and other conditions, such as tracheoesophageal fistula, CNS disorder, sepsis, hypoglycemia, and electrolyte imbalance.

The infant is assessed by means of the guidelines discussed in Chapter 22. The infant's gestational age and maturity are noted. In utero exposure to some drugs results in observable malformations or dysmorphism (abnormality of shape). Neonatal behavior may arouse suspicion. *Neonatal abstinence syndrome* is the term given to the group of signs and symptoms associated with drug withdrawal in the neonate (Table 26-6). Fig. 26-20 provides an example of a scoring system for assessing withdrawal symptoms. Because many women are multidrug users, the newborn initially may exhibit a confusing complex of signs.

Urine or meconium screening may be used to identify substances abused by the mother. Initially costly and of limited availability, tests of meconium collected on the first or second day of life have been shown to be both sensitive and reliable in detecting the metabolites of several street drugs, including cocaine (Bibb et al, 1995) (Box 26-9).

Nursing diagnoses, which depend on the assessment findings, are tailored to the individual needs of the neonate and the family. Following are examples of nursing diagnoses:

Neonate

- Risk for infection related to
  - Maternal risk behaviors
  - PROM
- Altered growth and development related to
  - Effects of maternal substance abuse
- Sleep pattern disturbance related to
  - Drug withdrawal
- Disorganized infant behavior related to
  - Effects of maternal substance abuse

Parents

- Altered parenting related to
  - Continuation of substance abuse or detoxification program
  - Guilt about infant's condition
  - Inability to cope with care needs of a special infant
- Anxiety related to knowledge deficit regarding
  - Care needs of an affected infant
- Violence: self-directed or directed toward infant related to
  - Drug-dependent life-style

Nursing care. Planning for care of the infant born to a substance-abusing mother presents a challenge to the health care team. Parents are included in the planning for the newborn's care and also are encouraged to plan for their own care. A multidisciplinary approach is needed that includes home

TABLE 26-6 Signs of neonatal abstinence syndrome

SYSTEM	SIGNS
Gastrointestinal	Poor feeding, vomiting, regurgitation, diarrhea, excessive sucking
Central nervous	Irritability, tremors, shrill cry, incessant crying, hyperactivity, little sleep, excoriations on knees and face, convulsions
Metabolic, vasomotor, respiratory	Nasal congestion, tachypnea, sweating, frequent yawning, increased respiratory rate >60/min, fever >37.2° C (99° F)

BOX 26-9
Ethical Considerations Related to Neonatal Drug Screening

Testing of neonatal urine or meconium for the presence of drug metabolites is a sensitive and reliable means of identifying neonates at risk for withdrawal symptoms. Controversy arises over whether universal drug screening should be instituted and whether informed consent is needed for screening neonates.

Ethical issues include the cost versus benefit of universal testing and the rights of parents versus the medical need to diagnose withdrawal.

NEONATAL ABSTINENCE SCORING SYSTEM

SYSTEM	SIGNS AND SYMPTOMS	SCORE	AM	PM	Daily Weight: COMMENTS
CENTRAL NERVOUS SYSTEM DISTURBANCES	Excessive High Pitched (Or other) Cry Continuous High Pitched (Or other) Cry	2 3			
	Sleeps < 1 Hour After Feeding Sleeps < 2 Hours After Feeding Sleeps < 3 Hours After Feeding	3 2 1			
	Hyperactive Moro Reflex Markedly Hyperactive Moro Reflex	2 3			
	Mild Tremors Disturbed Moderate-Severe Tremors Disturbed	1 2			
	Mild Tremors Undisturbed Moderate-Severe Tremors Undisturbed	3 4			
	Increased Muscle Tone	2			
	Excoriation (Specific Area)	1			
	Myoclonic Jerks	3			
	Generalized Convulsions	5			
METABOLIC/VASOMOTOR/RESPIRATORY DISTURBANCES	Sweating	1			
	Fever <101 (99-100.8° F/37.2-38.2° C) Fever >101 (38.4° C. and Higher)	1 2			
	Frequent Yawning (> 3-4 Times/Interval)	1			
	Mottling	1			
	Nasal Stuffiness	1			
	Sneezing (> 3-4 Times/Interval)	1			
	Nasal Flaring	2			
	Respiratory Rate > 60/min Respiratory Rate > 60/min with Retractions	1 2			
GASTRO-INTESTINAL DISTURBANCES	Excessive Sucking	1			
	Poor Feeding	2			
	Regurgitation Projectile Vomiting	2 3			
	Loose Stools Watery Stools	2 3			
	TOTAL SCORE				
	INITIALS OF SCORER				

Fig. 26-20 Neonatal abstinence scoring (NAS) system, developed by L. Finnegan. (From Nelson N: *Current therapy in neonatal-perinatal medicine,* ed 2, St Louis, 1990, Mosby.)

health or community resource personnel (for example, regulatory agencies such as child protective services).

Education and social support to prevent the abuse of drugs provide the ideal approach. However, given the scope of the drug abuse problem, total prevention is unrealistic.

Nursing care of the drug-dependent neonate involves supportive therapy for fluid and electrolyte balance, nutrition, infection control, and respiratory care. Swaddling, holding, reducing stimuli, and feeding as necessary may be helpful in easing withdrawal (see the Nursing Care Plan below). Specific suggestions for providing care to infants experiencing withdrawal are listed in the Patient Teaching box on p. 766.

Pharmacologic treatment is usually based on the severity of withdrawal symptoms, as determined by an assessment tool such as the one shown in Fig. 26-20. When indicated, medications are given as ordered. The dosage of phenobarbital is as follows: 20 mg/kg loading dose followed by 10 mg/kg every 12 hours until symptoms are under control; 2 mg is then given orally four times a day for 3 or 4 days as ordered. The dose is reduced by one third every 2 days for about 2 weeks, at which time treatment is discontinued. Paregoric may be ordered in a dosage of 0.8 ml/kg/day in six divided doses initially with increments of 0.4 ml/kg/day until symptom control is achieved. The dose is then decreased by 10% per day.

Drug dependence in the neonate is physiologic, not psy-

Nursing Care Plan

INFANT UNDERGOING DRUG WITHDRAWAL

Nursing Diagnosis: Risk for injury related to hyperactivity, seizures secondary to passive narcotic addiction resulting from maternal substance abuse during pregnancy

Expected Outcome: Patient exhibits no signs of seizure activity.

• **NURSING INTERVENTIONS/*RATIONALES***

Administer phenobarbital, diazepam per physician order *to decrease CNS irritability and control seizure activity.*

Decrease environmental stimuli *that may trigger irritability and hyperactive behaviors.*

Plan care activities carefully *to allow for minimum stimulation.*

Wrap infant snugly and hold infant tightly *to reduce self-stimulation behaviors and protect skin from abrasions.*

If infant is cocaine addicted, position to avoid eye contact, swaddle infant, use vertical rocking techniques, use a pacifier *to counter poor organizational response to stimuli and depressed interactive behaviors.*

Monitor activity level, note the relationship between activity level and external stimulation, and stop external stimulation *if it causes activity increase.*

Nursing Diagnosis: Altered nutrition, less than body requirements related to CNS irritability, poor suck reflex, vomiting, and diarrhea

Expected Outcome: Patient exhibits ingestion and retention of adequate nutrients and appropriate weight gain.

• **NURSING INTERVENTIONS/*RATIONALES***

Feed in frequent small amounts, elevate head during and after feeding, burp well *to diminish vomiting and aspiration.*

Experiment with various nipples *to find one most effective in compensating for poor suck reflex.*

Monitor weight daily and maintain strict intake and output *to evaluate success of feeding.*

If intake is insufficient, feed by oral gavage per physician order *to ensure ingestion of needed nutrients.*

Have suction available as required *to reduce chances of aspiration.*

Nursing Diagnosis: Risk for fluid volume deficit related to diarrhea and vomiting

Expected Outcome: Patient exhibits evidence of fluid homeostasis.

• **NURSING INTERVENTIONS/*RATIONALES***

Administer oral and parenteral fluids per physician order and regulate *to maintain fluid balance.*

Monitor hydration status (i.e., skin turgor, weight, mucous membranes, fontanels, urine specific gravity, electrolytes) and intake and output *to evaluate for evidence of dehydration.*

Nursing Diagnosis: Ineffective maternal coping, anxiety, powerlessness related to drug use, infant distress during withdrawal, and single parent status

Expected Outcome: Woman will accept newborn's condition and participate in care activities, showing evidence of maternal-infant bonding process.

• **NURSING INTERVENTIONS/*RATIONALES***

Explain effects of maternal drug use on newborn and the withdrawal process *to provide understanding and reality concerning effects of drug use.*

Encourage open communication (i.e., inform mother of ongoing condition, procedures, and treatment; answer questions; correct misperceptions; actively listen to her concerns) *to provide a sense of respect, support, and encourage a sense of control.*

Encourage mother to interact with infant and to become involved in care routines *to foster emotional connection.*

Explain how to do care procedures, how to avoid excess stimulation, how to hold and rock infant *to enhance mother's care abilities and her sense of confidence and control.*

If the mother is addicted to cocaine, explain infant's inability to interact, gaze aversion, arching back, and lack of response to cuddling *to enhance understanding of infant behaviors.*

Make appropriate referrals to social agencies for treatment of maternal drug addiction, infant development programs, and other needed support services *to ensure adequate resources for care of self and infant.*

Patient Teaching

CARE OF INFANT EXPERIENCING WITHDRAWAL

- Place the infant in a side-lying position with the spine and legs flexed.
- Position the infant's hands in midline with the arms at the side.
- Carry the infant in a flexed position.
- When interacting with the infant, introduce one stimulus at a time when the infant is in a quiet, alert state. Watch for time-out or distress signals (gaze aversion, yawning, sneezing, hiccoughs, arching, mottled color).
- When the infant is distressed, swaddle in a flexed position and rock in a slow, rhythmic fashion.
- Put the infant in a sitting position with chin tucked down for feeding.

TABLE 26-7 Drugs of abuse contraindicated during breastfeeding*

DRUG	REPORTED EFFECT OR REASONS FOR CONCERN
Amphetamine†	Irritability, poor sleeping pattern
Cocaine	Cocaine intoxication
Heroin	Tremors, restlessness, vomiting, poor feeding
Marijuana	Only one report in literature; no effect mentioned; at risk for inhaling smoke
Nicotine (smoking)	Shock, vomiting, diarrhea, rapid heart rate, restlessness; decreased milk production
Phencyclidine	Potent hallucinogen

Modified from American Academy of Pediatrics: Drug and chemical transfer, *Pediatrics* 93:138, 1994; also in Lawrence R: *Breastfeeding*, ed 4, St Louis, 1994, Mosby.

*The Committee on Drugs strongly believes that nursing mothers should not ingest any compounds listed here. Not only are they hazardous to the nursing infant, but they are also detrimental to the physical and emotional health of the mother. This list is obviously not complete; no drug of abuse should be ingested by nursing mothers even though adverse reports are not in the literature.

†Drug is concentrated in human milk.

chologic. Thus a predisposition to dependence later in life is not believed to be a factor. However, the psychosocial environment in which the infant may be raised can create a tendency to addiction.

The mother requires considerable support. Her need for and abuse of drugs result in a decreased capacity to cope. The infant's withdrawal signs and decreased consolability stress her coping abilities even further. Home health care, treatment for addiction, and education are important considerations. Sensitive exploration of the woman's options for the care of her infant and herself and for future fertility management may help her see that she has choices. This approach helps communicate respect for the new mother as a person who can make responsible decisions.

The issue of breastfeeding in this population is difficult. Although breast milk remains the optimum source of nutrition for these infants, care must be taken to avoid exposing the infant to additional drugs through the breast milk. The American Academy of Pediatrics has compiled a list of drugs contraindicated in breastfeeding (Table 26-7).

DISCHARGE TO HOME FOR THE HIGH-RISK NEWBORN

Discharge planning for the high-risk newborn begins on admission. The admission history should include important information regarding the family of the infant that can affect discharge. Who makes up the immediate family? Does the mother have others who depend on her for support? How are they being taken care of during this period?

Questions about the home environment should be asked as soon as possible. Is there gas or electric heating in the home, or is the family dependent on a fireplace or wood-burning stove? Is there access to a telephone for emergencies? Is there a home at all, or is the family living in a shelter? Problems posed by these questions require the intervention of social services and can take a long time to resolve.

Successful discharge of high-risk infants to their homes or community hospital requires a multidisciplinary approach. Medical, nursing, and social services are crucial to the smooth transition of these infants and their families to the community and home. If the infant is transported back to the community hospital that referred either the mother before birth or the infant after birth, interfacility communication is essential to continuity of care.

Discharge to home, whether from the regional center or the community hospital setting, requires parental competence. Discharge teaching begins as soon as the infant is stable and the parents wish to become involved in the care. Discharge teaching must include normal newborn care as well as specific information pertinent to the medical condition of the infant. Discharge teaching for the high-risk newborn is extensive, requires time, and cannot be adequately accomplished on the day of discharge. Important considerations in the discharge teaching of the parents of high-risk newborns are listed in the Guidelines box on p. 767.

Discharge to home for high-risk infants does not mean they can be treated like normal newborns. Follow-up by a pediatrician or nurse practitioner familiar with the complications common to the high-risk newborn is essential. Further follow-up of specific complications by qualified specialists and referral to high-risk centers for developmental interventions can help ensure the best outcome possible for these fragile infants.

Final evaluation may not be possible. Short-term expected outcomes include the following examples:

1. The newborn suffers no adverse sequelae to drug withdrawal.
2. The infant's malformations and dysfunction are identified, and appropriate curative and rehabilitative measures are instituted.
3. The parents come to terms with the newborn's condition and management.

Guidelines

DISCHARGE TEACHING FOR PARENTS OF HIGH-RISK NEWBORNS

Discharge teaching includes (but is not limited to) the following:

- Helping parents understand their baby's condition
- Infant/child car safety
- Safety measures in the home
- Feeding
- Elimination
- Bathing
- Cord care
- Taking the baby's temperature
- Medication administration
- Cardiopulmonary resuscitation (CPR) for infants
- Impact of environmental factors (maintaining thermoregulation at home)
- Teaching related to the infant's specific condition (signs and symptoms of deterioration, etc.)
- Developmental concerns related to their infant
- Follow-up appointments/consultations

However, both the infant and the parent have long-term needs. The extent to which expected outcomes have been achieved may not be known for years.

HYPERBILIRUBINEMIA

Hyperbilirubinemia is a condition in which the bilirubin level in the blood is increased. It is characterized by a yellow discoloration of the skin, mucous membranes, sclera, and various organs. This yellow discoloration is referred to as **jaundice,** or *icterus.* Jaundice is caused primarily by the accumulation in the skin of unconjugated bilirubin, a breakdown product of hemoglobin forming after its release from hemolyzed RBCs. Physiologic jaundice, discussed in Chapter 22, is the most common finding in newborns and is usually benign. The challenge in the care of neonates with hyperbilirubinemia is to distinguish physiologic jaundice from a serious clinical pathologic condition.

Following are the findings that support a diagnosis of pathologic jaundice and that, if encountered in an infant, warrant further investigation (Fanaroff and Martin, 1997):

- Serum bilirubin concentrations of greater than 4 mg/dl in cord blood
- Clinical jaundice evident within 24 hours of birth
- Total serum bilirubin levels increasing by more than 5 mg/dl in 24 hours or increasing at a rate of 0.5 mg/dl or greater over a 4- to 8-hour period
- A serum bilirubin level in a full-term newborn that exceeds 13 to 15 mg/dl at any time or clinical jaundice lasting more than 10 days
- A serum bilirubin level in a preterm newborn that exceeds 10 mg/dl at any time. Any case of visible jaundice, even if serum bilirubin levels are as low as 5 mg/dl, should be carefully monitored, especially if this lasts more than 14 to 21 days

Various etiologic factors cause hyperbilirubinemia. The main focus of this section is isoimmune hemolytic disease of the newborn secondary to Rh or ABO incompatibility.

Rh Incompatibility

There are several forms of the Rh antigen, with the D antigen the most significant one because it causes the most antibody production in a person who is Rh negative. Rh incompatibility, or **iso-immunization,** occurs when an Rh-negative mother has an Rh-positive fetus who inherits the dominant Rh-positive gene from the father. If the mother is Rh negative and the father is Rh positive and homozygous for the Rh factor, all the offspring will be Rh positive. If the father is heterozygous for the factor, there is a 50% chance that each infant born of the union will be Rh positive and a 50% chance that each will be born Rh negative. An Rh-negative fetus is in no danger because it has the same Rh factor as the mother. An Rh-negative fetus with an Rh-positive mother is also in no danger. It is only the Rh-positive offspring of an Rh-negative mother who is at risk. From 10% to 15% of all Caucasian couples and about 5% of African-American couples have Rh incompatibility. It is rare in Asian couples. The incidence of Rh sensitization and resulting hemolytic disease of the newborn have decreased dramatically since the development of Rh_0 (D) immune globulin in 1968. However, hemolytic disease of the fetus or newborn resulting from isoimmunization still occurs in 1.5% of all pregnancies (Vomund and Witter, 1994).

Nursing ALERT

RhIG is administered intramuscularly, not intravenously, only to Rh-negative women with a negative Coombs' test—never to the infant or father.

The pathogenesis of Rh incompatibility is as follows. Hematopoiesis in the fetus, or the formation of blood cells, begins as early as the eighth week of gestation, and, in up to 40% of pregnancies, these cells pass through the placenta into the maternal circulation. Whenever the fetus is Rh positive and the mother Rh negative, the mother forms antibodies against the fetal blood cells—first IgM antibodies that are too large to pass through the placenta and then, later, IgG antibodies that can cross the placenta. The process of antibody formation is called *maternal sensitization.* Once in the fetal circulation, the antibodies attack the fetal blood cells, causing lysis of the blood cells. Usually women become sensitized in their first pregnancy with an Rh positive fetus, but lysis of the fetal blood cells does not occur. During subsequent pregnancies, antibodies form in response to repeated contact with the antigen from the fetal blood, such as during placental separation, which allows the transfer of fetal blood to the maternal circulation.

Severe Rh incompatibility results in marked fetal hemolytic anemia because the fetal erythrocytes are destroyed by maternal Rh-positive antibodies. Although the placenta usually clears the bilirubin generated by the RBC breakdown, in extreme cases fetal bilirubin levels increase. This results in fetal jaundice, also known as *icterus gravis.*

The fetus compensates for the anemia by producing large numbers of immature erythrocytes to replace those hemolyzed, thus the name for this condition—**erythroblastosis fetalis.** In the most severe form of this disease, **hydrops fetalis,** the fetus has marked anemia, together with cardiac decompensation, cardiomegaly, and hepatosplenomegaly. Hypoxia results from the severe anemia. In addition, because of the decreased intravascular oncotic pressure involved, fluid leaks out of the intravascular space, resulting in generalized edema as well as effusions into the peritoneal (ascites), pericardial, and pleural (hydrothorax) spaces. The placenta is often edematous, which, along with the edematous fetus, can cause the uterus to rupture.

Intrauterine or early neonatal death may occur as a result of hydrops fetalis, although intrauterine exchange transfusions and early birth of the fetus may avert this. **Intrauterine transfusion** involves the infusion of Rh-negative, type O blood into the umbilical vein or the peritoneal cavity of the fetus, where it is absorbed by the lymphatics and enters the fetal circulation. Such transfusions are administered as needed until birth. This is a risky procedure, however, and is reserved for use in seriously affected fetuses in whom the hazards of transfusion are judged to be less than the complications of prematurity, should premature birth prove necessary (Fanaroff and Martin, 1997).

ABO Incompatibility

ABO incompatibility is more common than Rh incompatibility but causes less severe problems in the affected infant. It occurs if the fetal blood type is A, B, or AB and the maternal type is O. It rarely occurs in infants with type B blood born to mothers with type A blood. The incompatibility arises because naturally occurring anti-A and anti-B antibodies are transferred across the placenta to the fetus. Unlike the situation that pertains to Rh incompatibility (discussed in previous section), first-born infants may be affected because mothers with type O blood already have anti-A and anti-B antibodies in their blood. Such a newborn may show a weakly positive result to a direct Coombs' test. The cord bilirubin level usually is less than 4 mg/dl, and any resulting hyperbilirubinemia usually can be treated with phototherapy. Exchange transfusions are required only occasionally. Although ABO incompatibility is a frequent cause of hyperbilirubinemia, it rarely precipitates significant anemia resulting from the hemolysis of RBCs.

Kernicterus

The goal of the care given the infant with hyperbilirubinemia is the prevention of kernicterus. **Kernicterus,** or bilirubin encephalopathy, is caused by the deposition of bilirubin in the brain, especially within the basal ganglia, cerebellum, and hippocampus. This deposition can occur because unconjugated bilirubin is highly lipid soluble, making it capable of crossing the blood-brain barrier if it is not bound to protein. It results in the yellowish staining of the brain tissue and the necrosis of neurons and occurs if the concentration of unconjugated bilirubin reaches toxic levels. Kernicterus, which can develop in newborns who show no apparent signs of clinical jaundice, is generally considered to be directly related to the total serum bilirubin level, although these levels alone do not predict the risk of brain injury.

There is currently no quantitative total serum bilirubin level at which kernicterus is known to occur in either the term or preterm infant. Since the goal of phototherapy is to prevent bilirubin toxicity, quantitative total serum bilirubin levels have been proposed for treatment but are commonly recognized as being treatment guidelines and not predictive of pathology. Furthermore, it is imperative that the infant's overall clinical status be evaluated rather than serum bilirubin levels alone. Infants experiencing hypoxia, infection, hypercarbia, and dehydration are at higher risk for developing kernicterus because of the subsequent alteration in the blood-brain barrier, which permits the entry of both bound and unbound bilirubin (Blackburn, 1995). There is concern that sick preterm infants are at higher risk for developing kernicterus at lower bilirubin levels, thus the recommendation that phototherapy be initiated earlier (5 to 8 mg/dl in infants weighing less than 1500 g; 8 to 12 mg/dl in infants weighing 1500 to 1999 g) in sick and preterm newborns (Maisels 1994). Others recommend the initiation of phototherapy in healthy term infants as follows:

AGE (hr)*	TOTAL SERUM BILIRUBIN LEVEL (mg/dl)
25 to 48	>15
49 to 72	>18
>72	>20

Kernicterus has been associated with acute and long-term symptoms of neurologic damage; it is never present at birth. The clinical manifestations typically appear between 2 and 6 days after birth and go through several phases as the disease progresses, generally beginning after the bilirubin level has peaked. About half of the affected infants survive, although they often suffer permanent neurologic sequelae, such as choreoathetoid cerebral palsy or ataxia, sensorineural hearing loss, perceptual problems, mental retardation, or an attention deficit disorder.

There have been recent reports of several cases of kernicterus in infants of mothers who were discharged early after birth. The follow-up of infants who are discharged early is therefore imperative.

Nursing Care Management

Assessment

The blood type and Rh factor of the pregnant woman are determined prenatally. A thorough inventory is obtained in the Rh-negative pregnant woman to assess for the existence of events that could have caused her to develop antibodies to the Rh factor. Such events include (1) previous pregnancy with an Rh-positve fetus, (2) transfusion with Rh-positve blood, which causes immediate sensitization, (3) spontaneous or elective abortions after 8 or more gestational weeks, (4) amniocentesis performed for any reason, (5) premature separation of the placenta, and (6) trauma. If any of these events have occurred, the woman's record is checked to determine whether she has received Rh_o (D) immune globulin, such as Rhogam.

An indirect Coombs' test should be done at the first prenatal visit of an Rh-negative woman with a fetus who may be Rh-positve to determine whether she has antibodies to the Rh

*Adapted from American Academy of Pediatrics, Provisional Committee for Quality Improvement and Subcommittee on Hyperbilirubinemia: Practice parameter: management of hyperbilirubinemia in the healthy term newborn. *Pediatrics* 94(4):558,1994.

antigen. In this test the maternal blood serum is mixed with Rh-positive red blood cells. If the Rh-positve red blood cells agglutinate or clump, this indicates that maternal antibodies are present. The dilution of the specimen of blood at which clumping occurs determines the titer, or level, of maternal antibodies. This titer indicates the degree of maternal sensitization. If the titer reaches 1:16, amniocentesis is performed to permit delta optical density (delta OD) analysis to confirm Rh incompatibility.

The indirect Coombs' test is repeated at 28 weeks and, if the result remains negative, indicating that sensitization has not occurred, the woman is given an intramuscular injection of Rh_o (D) immune globulin. If the test result is positive, showing that sensitization has occurred, it is then repeated at frequent intervals to monitor the maternal antibody titer, as just described.

Nursing Diagnoses

The following are examples of nursing diagnoses pertinent to newborns at risk because of hyperbilirubinemia:

- Risk for injury to neurons and cells in the kidney, pancreas, and intestine related to
  Hyperbilirubinemia
- Impaired gas exchange related to
  Hemolytic anemia
- Risk for fluid volume deficit related to
  Phototherapy
- Risk for parental anxiety related to
  Hyperbilirubinemia, its management, and potential sequelae
- Risk for impaired skin integrity related to
  Increased stooling while undergoing phototherapy

Expected Outcomes

Expected outcomes for care are stated in patient-centered terms, as in the following:

1. The infant's prenatal and perinatal risk factors will be identified, and intervention will be implemented when appropriate.
2. The infant will not develop hyperbilirubinemia or its sequela, kernicterus.
3. The infant will have minimal or no sequelae from hyperbilirubinemia and its treatment
4. The infant's serum bilirubin levels will return to normal
5. The infant's parents will demonstrate an understanding of the infant's condition, the therapies, and the possible sequelae of the condition

Plan of Care and Implementation

The neonate's cord blood is sent to the laboratory to determine the infant's blood type and Rh status. A direct Coombs' test is performed on this cord blood to determine whether there are maternal antibodies in the fetal blood.

Phototherapy is used to reduce the serum bilirubin levels, particularly if the jaundice is physiologic rather than pathologic. Phototherapy using bili-lights or a phototherapy blanket is carried out in the normal newborn nursery (see Chapter 23 and Fig. 23-19).

> **Nursing ALERT**
>
> While blood is drawn, the bilirubin lights are turned off, and the blood is transported in a covered tube to avoid a false reading from bilirubin destruction in the test tube.

Exchange transfusions are needed less frequently today because of the decrease in the incidence of hemolytic disease in newborns resulting from isoimmunization. Other factors must always be considered as well, particularly the clinical condition of the infant, because the risks of treatment must be weighed against the risks of the outcome if the infant is not treated (Klaus and Fanaroff, 1993).

Exchange transfusion is accomplished by alternately removing a small amount of the infant's blood and replacing it with an equal amount of donor blood. If the infant has Rh incompatibility, type O Rh-negative blood is used for transfusion, so the maternal antibodies still present in the infant do not hemolyze the transfused blood. Depending on the infant's size, maturity, and condition, amounts of 5 to 15 ml of the infant's blood are removed at one time and replaced with donor blood.

Evaluation

The nurse can be reasonably assured that care was effective if the following outcomes were achieved:

- The infant's prenatal and perinatal risk factors were identified and intervention was implemented when appropriate.
- The infant did not develop hyperbilirubinemia or kernicterus.
- The infant had minimal or no sequelae from hyperbilirubinemia or its treatment.
- The infant's serum bilirubin levels returned to normal.
- The infant's parents demonstrated an understanding of the infant's condition, the therapies, and the possible sequelae of the condition (see the Nursing Care Plan box on p. 770).

CONGENITAL ANOMALIES

The desired and expected outcome of every wanted pregnancy is a normal, functioning infant with a good intellectual potential. Fulfillment of this hope depends on numerous hereditary and environmental factors. Probably all human characteristics have a genetic component, including those that produce symptoms or physical abnormalities that impair the fitness of the person. Some disorders or diseases occur through the influence of a single gene or the combined action of many genes inherited from the parents; others result from the action of the intrauterine environment. Many defects appear to occur as the result of multifactorial inheritance, which is the interaction of multiple genes with environmental factors that affect the embryonic development of the affected system. Examples of these include neural tube defects, congenital heart defects, congenital hip dysplasia, and cleft lip or palate. A disease or disorder that is transmitted from generation to generation is termed *genetic* or *hereditary*. A

Nursing Care Plan

INFANT WITH HYPERBILIRUBINEMIA

Nursing Diagnosis: Risk for injury related to hemolytic disease and treatment effects

Expected Outcome: **Bilirubin levels decrease with treatment, there is no evidence of harmful effects from phototherapy (i.e., no eye irritation, dehydration, temperature instability, or skin breakdown), and there are no complications from exchange transfusions.**

• **NURSING INTERVENTIONS/*RATIONALES***

Initiate early feedings *to enhance excretion of bilirubin in stools.*

Observe skin and mucous membranes for signs of jaundice, *indicative of rising bilirubin levels;* monitor serum bilirubin levels *to determine rate of rise and treatment response.*

Note time of jaundice onset *to help distinguish physiologic from other causes of jaundice.*

Observe for signs of hypoxia, hypothermia, hypoglycemia, and metabolic acidosis, *which occur as a result of hyperbilirubinemia and increase the risk of brain damage.*

Initiate phototherapy per physician order *to decrease bilirubin levels.*

During phototherapy, shield infant's eyes *to prevent damage to corneas and retinas;* keep infant nude and change positions frequently *for maximum body surface exposure;* cleanse skin frequently *to prevent irritation;* maintain adequate fluid intake *to prevent dehydration;* monitor body temperature *to prevent hyperthermia.*

Before exchange transfusion, keep infant NPO (2 to 4 hours) *to prevent aspiration;* check donor blood for compatibility *to prevent transfusion reaction;* have resuscitation equipment (oxygen, ambu bag, endotracheal tubes, laryngoscope) at bedside *in preparation for emergency action.*

Assist physician with exchange transfusion procedure; track amounts of blood withdrawn and transfused *to maintain balanced blood volume;* maintain body temperature *to avoid hypothermia and cold stress;* monitor vital signs and observe for rash *for indicators of transfusion reaction.*

After transfusion, continue to monitor vital signs *for transfusion reaction or other complications;* check umbilical cord *for bleeding or signs of infection.*

Nursing Diagnosis: Risk for knowledge deficit related to administration of home phototherapy

Expected Outcome: **Family demonstrates ability to provide home therapy.**

• **NURSING INTERVENTIONS/*RATIONALES***

Explore family's willingness to try home phototherapy *to evaluate feasibility of home therapy option.*

Explore family's understanding of jaundice and proposed therapy *to establish baseline for teaching.*

Teach family with demonstration–return demonstration, allowing for several practice sessions and supplement with written materials with pictorial representations *to ensure safe and optimum results.*

Include the following in your instructions: placement of lamp or fiberoptic unit; proper eye care and patching; proper skin care; proper positioning under lamp; provision of increased fluid intake; monitoring of time under lamp; monitoring of vital signs, skin, eyes, feeding patterns, stooling and voiding patterns; observe for complications.

Stress importance of obtaining the prescribed bilirubin tests on schedule *as a way of tracking success of therapy.*

Give parents a contact if they have any questions while carrying out therapy *to offer ongoing support and increase parent comfort.*

---

congenital disorder is one that is present at birth and can be caused by genetic or environmental factors, or both.

Congenital defects occur in 3% to 4% of all live births (Wardinsky, 1994), but this number increases if one includes the congenital defects that are diagnosed later in childhood. In addition, the incidence of congenital malformations in fetuses that are aborted is higher than that in infants who are born alive, thus also adding to the overall incidence. Major congenital defects are the leading cause of death in infants younger than 1 year of age in the United States and account for 20% of neonatal deaths. Although there has been a decrease in the incidences of other causes of neonatal mortality, the death rate associated with most congenital anomalies has essentially remained stable since 1932. For example, although the incidence of congenital heart defects (CHDs) has increased, probably because of better diagnostic capabilities, the death rate in such children has remained at approximately 1.5 per 10,000 children (Hoekelman et al, 1992).

The seriousness of congenital anomalies in terms of their effect on society is reflected in the more than 6 million hospital days and $200 billion a year required for the care and treatment of these neonates. Ways of preventing and detecting these anomalies are being improved continuously, as are techniques for the care of the fetus with certain anomalies. However, the promotion of the availability of these services to populations at risk challenges the community health care systems. An interdisciplinary team approach is vital for providing holistic care: the surgical treatment, rehabilitation, and education of the child, as well as psychosocial and financial assistance for the parents. Parental disappointment and disillusion, along with any negative feelings the nurse may have regarding the infant's disorder, add to the complexity of the nursing care needed for these infants.

Central Nervous System Anomalies

Most congenital anomalies of the CNS result from defects in the closure of the neural tube during fetal development. Although the cause of **neural tube defects** is unknown, they are thought to stem from the interaction of many genes that may be influenced by factors in the fetal environment, such as exposure to potato blight or organic solvents. There is growing evidence that a maternal folic acid deficit has a direct bearing on failure of the neural tube to close, therefore in 1993 the American Academy of Pediatrics issued recommendations that folic acid be administered to women of childbearing age (Rowe et al, 1995).

Some neural tube defects can be diagnosed prenatally by ultrasound studies and the finding of elevated levels of alphafetoprotein in the amniotic fluid and maternal serum.

Encephalocele and anencephaly. Encephalocele and anencephaly are abnormalities resulting from failure of the anterior end of the neural tube to close. An *encephalocele* is a herniation of the brain and meninges through the skull. Treatment consists of surgical repair and shunting to relieve hydrocephalus, unless a major brain malformation is present. Some of these infants will have some degree of cognitive deficit. **Anencephaly** is the absence of both cerebral hemispheres and of the overlying skull. It is a condition that is incompatible with life; many of the infants are stillborn or die within a few days of birth. Warmth, fluids, and comfort measures are supplied until the infant eventually dies of respiratory failure.

Spina bifida. Spina bifida, the most common defect of the CNS, results from failure of the neural tube to close at some point. There are two categories of spina bifida: spina bifida occulta and spina bifida cystica. Spina bifida occulta is a malformation in which the posterior portion of the laminas fails to close but the spinal cord or meninges do not herniate or protrude through the defect (Fig. 26-21). It is usually asymptomatic and may not be diagnosed unless there are associated problems. Spina bifida cystica includes meningocele and myelomeningocele. A *meningocele* is an external sac that contains meninges and CSF and that protrudes through a defect in the vertebral column. A **myelomeningocele** is similar, except that it also contains nerves; therefore the infant has motor and sensory deficits below the lesion. In the United States, myelomeningocele occurs in approximately 1 in 1000 live births (Romanczuk and Brown, 1994).

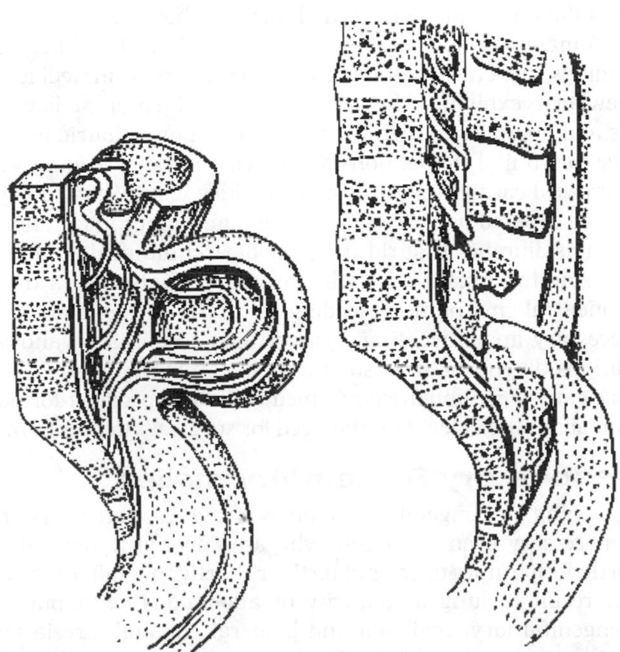

Fig. 26-21 **A,** Myelomeningocele. Note absence of vertebral arches. **B,** Dermal sinus tract with dermoid cyst, often associated with spina bifida occulta.

A myelomeningocele, which is visible at birth and most often in the lumbosacral area, is usually covered with a very fragile, thin membrane (Fig. 26-21). The sac can tear easily, allowing CSF to leak out, as well as providing an entry for infectious agents into the CNS. Myelomeningocele usually is associated with an Arnold-Chiari malformation, which results from the improper development and downward displacement of part of the brain into the cervical spinal canal. This in turn results in the development of hydrocephalus, which affects about 90% of children with myelomeningocele, although it may not be present at birth. The long-term prognosis in an affected infant can be determined to a large extent at birth, with the degree of neurologic dysfunction related to the level of the lesion, which determines the nerves involved.

A major preoperative nursing intervention for a neonate with a myelomeningocele is to protect the protruding sac from injury to prevent its rupture and resultant risk of CNS infection. Such infants should be positioned in a side-lying or prone position to prevent pressure on the sac until surgical repair is done. If the infant is allowed to be held, the nurse or parent must be careful to keep the defect from being injured. The sac should be covered with a sterile, moist, nonadherent dressing and sterile technique used in its care. The skin around the defect must be cleansed and dried carefully to prevent breakdown, which would establish a portal of entry for infectious agents. Because a lack of normal innervation may prevent the bladder from emptying completely, the nurse should use Credé's method at regular intervals to express urine from the bladder.

Nursing ALERT

Observe for early signs of infection, such as elevated temperature (axillary), irritability, lethargy, and nuchal rigidity, and for signs of increased ICP, which might indicate developing hydrocephalus.

Surgical repair is often done in the neonatal period, preferably within the first 24 hours. Very early closure can prevent CNS infection and trauma to the exposed nerves. It can also prevent stretching of other nerve roots, which can occur as the sac continues to enlarge after birth. Surgical shunt procedures to prevent increasing hydrocephalus may be needed. Other problems, such as infection, are treated as they occur.

Congenital hydrocephalus. Hydrocephalus is a condition in which the ventricles of the brain are enlarged as a result of an imbalance between the production and absorption of the CSF. It is almost always caused by interference with the circulation and absorption of CSF. Congenital hydrocephalus usually arises as a result of a malformation in the brain or an intrauterine infection. It occurs in approximately 3 to 4 per 1000 live births (Shiminski-Maher and Disabato, 1994).

About one third of all cases of congenital hydrocephalus result from stenosis of the aqueduct of Sylvius in the brain. Hydrocephalus frequently occurs in conjunction with a myelomeningocele, which blocks the flow of CSF.

An infant with congenital hydrocephalus initially has a bulging anterior fontanel and a head circumference that increases at an abnormal rate, resulting from the increase in CSF pressure. Enlargement of the forehead with depressed eyes that are rotated downward, causing a "setting sun" sign, occurs as the condition worsens. If the surgical shunting of excess CSF from the brain is not done soon after birth, the resulting increasing ICP will lead to irreversible neurologic damage, as evidenced by palpably widening sutures and fontanels, lethargy, poor feeding, vomiting, irritability, opisthotonos, and a high-pitched, shrill cry.

Nursing actions appropriate to the needs of a newborn with hydrocephalus include careful documentation of the ongoing observations. Measurement of the head circumference and other neurologic assessments are done frequently. If the infant's head is large, the placement of a flotation mattress or foam pad under the infant and frequent position changes are necessary to prevent skin breakdown resulting from the pressure. Chapter 48 contains a more detailed description of the evaluation and management of the child with hydrocephalus.

Microcephaly. **Microcephaly** refers to a small brain in a generally normally formed head. It can be an autosomal-recessive disorder or caused by a chromosomal abnormality; exposure of the woman to x-rays; or rubella, cytomegalovirus, or other maternal infections. Microcephalic infants require supportive nursing care and medical observation to determine the extent of the psychomotor retardation that almost always accompanies this abnormality. There is no treatment. Parents need support to learn to care for a child with such cognitive impairment.

Cardiovascular System Anomalies

CHDs are anatomic abnormalities in the heart that are present at birth, although they may not be diagnosed immediately. Some type of pediatric cardiovascular problem is present in 10 of every 1000 live births (Hoffman, 1995). Ventricular septal defects, constituting more than 20% of all CHDs, are the most common type that is usually acyanotic. Tetralogy of Fallot, constituting 10% of all CHDs, is the most common type resulting in cyanosis. After prematurity, CHDs are the next major cause of death in the first year of life.

The etiology of CHDs is unknown in more than 90% of the cases. Maternal factors that are associated with a higher incidence of CHD include maternal rubella, alcoholism, diabetes, poor nutrition, or age over 40 years. The maternal ingestion of folic acid antagonists, anticonvulsants, progesterone, estrogen, lithium, or coumadin, or the use of the acne medication Accutane (isotretinoin), is thought to be involved in the cause of heart defects, as is radiation exposure.

Genetic factors are implicated in the pathogenesis of CHD. As a general rule, these defects are thought to be multifactorial in origin, involving both genetic and environmental influences; however, a familial occurrence of virtually all forms of CHD has been noted.

Chromosomal abnormalities may also be associated with CHDs. For example, 40% of children with trisomy 21, or Down syndrome, have a cardiac defect. All children who have trisomy 18, the second most common chromosomal abnormality, have cardiac anomalies, and most die within a week of birth. See Chapter 45 for a discussion of classifications of CHDs.

Severe CHDs are often evident immediately after birth, especially defects that cause cyanosis such as transposition of the great vessels. Infants with these anomalies are transferred directly to special care nurseries or pediatric units.

If symptoms are present at birth, they may be obvious with the first cry, which may be weak and muffled or loud and breathless. Affected newborns may be cyanotic and unrelieved by oxygen treatment, with the cyanosis increasing whenever the child is in the supine position or cries. The bluish gray, dusky color of cyanotic infants may be mild, moderate, or severe. Other infants may be acyanotic and pale, with or without mottling on exertion, which includes crying, feeding, or stooling.

The affected newborn's activity level varies from restlessness to lethargy, and possibly unresponsiveness, except to pain. Persistent bradycardia (resting heart rate of less than 80 to 100 beats/min) or tachycardia (rate exceeding 160 to 180 beats/min) may be noted (Wong, 1995). The cardiac rhythm may be abnormal, and murmurs may be heard. Signs of congestive heart failure, diminished cardiac output, and decreased tissue perfusion may be evident. Diaphoresis, uncommon in the normal newborn, may be present in the infant with heart failure.

Because the cardiac and respiratory systems function together, cardiac disease may be manifested by respiratory signs and symptoms. The respiratory rate should be determined when the newborn is in a resting state. Abnormal findings may include tachypnea, which is a rate of 60 breaths/min or more; retractions with nasal flaring; grunting occurring with or without exertion; and dyspnea, which may worsen when the infant is supine or exerting himself or herself.

A major role of the nurse is to assess infants for abnormal findings, which, if observed, must be reported immediately. Newborns exhibiting these symptoms require prompt diagnosis and appropriate therapy in a neonatal or pediatric intensive care unit. Interventions planned if a nursing diagnosis of decreased cardiac output is made include administering oxygen as ordered as well as cardiotonic and other medications such as diuretics that rid the body of accumulated fluid, decreasing the work load of the heart by maintaining a thermoneutral environment, feeding using the gavage method if necessary, and preventing crying if this precipitates cyanosis. Various diagnostic tests such as echocardiography and cardiac catheterization are performed to obtain specific information about the defect and the need for surgical intervention.

Respiratory System Anomalies

Screening for congenital anomalies of the respiratory system is necessary even in infants who are apparently normal at birth. Respiratory distress at birth or shortly thereafter may be the result of lung immaturity or anomalous development. Congenital laryngeal web and bilateral choanal atresia are readily apparent at birth. Respiratory distress caused by diaphragmatic hernia and tracheoesophageal fistula may appear immediately or be delayed, depending on the severity of the defect.

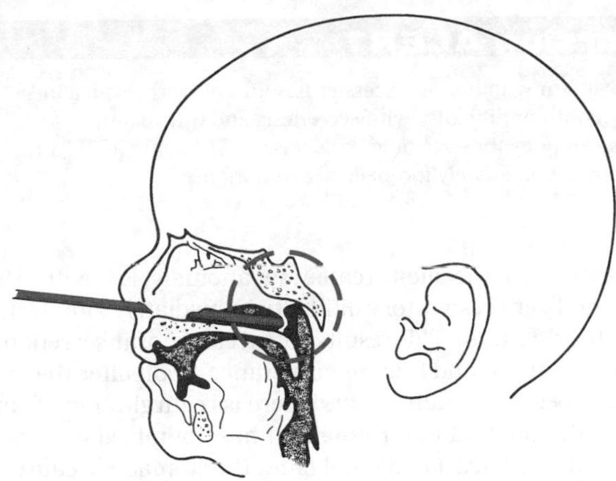

Fig. 26-22 Choanal atresia. Posterior nares are obstructed by membrane or bone either bilaterally or unilaterally. Infant becomes cyanotic at rest. With crying, newborn's color improves. Nasal discharge is present. Snorting respirations often are observed with increased respiratory effort. Newborn may be unable to breathe and eat at same time. Diagnosis is made by noting inability to pass small feeding tube through one or both nares. (Courtesy Ross Laboratories, Columbus, Ohio)

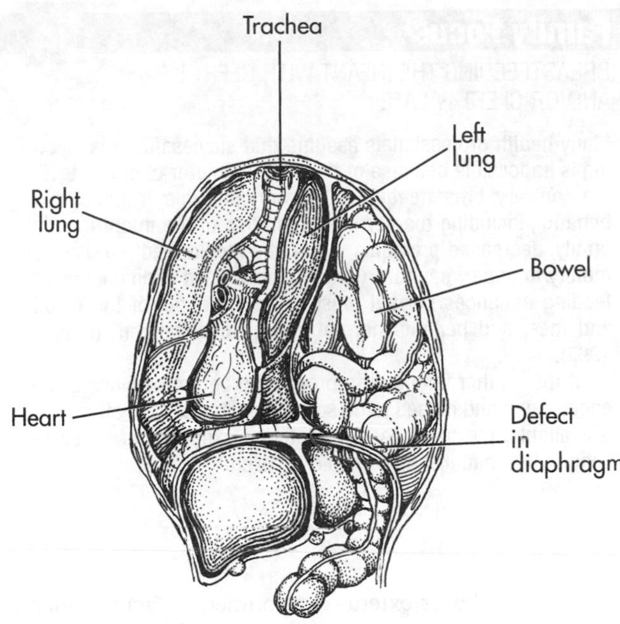

Fig. 26-23 Diaphragmatic hernia. (Courtesy Ross Laboratories, Columbus, Ohio)

Laryngeal web and choanal atresia. A laryngeal web, which is uncommon, results from the incomplete separation of the two sides of the larynx and is most often between the vocal cords. **Choanal atresia** (Fig. 26-22) is the most common congenital anomaly of the nose; it is a bony or membranous septum located between the nose and the pharynx. Inability to pass a suction catheter through the nose into the pharynx usually leads to its detection. Nearly half of the infants with choanal atresia have other anomalies. Infants with either a laryngeal web or choanal atresia require emergency surgery.

Diaphragmatic hernia. Diaphragmatic hernia results from a defect in the formation of the diaphragm, allowing the abdominal organs to be displaced into the chronic cavity. It occurs in approximately 1 in 3000 live births (Guzzetta et al, 1994); however, if stillbirths resulting from this defect are included, the incidence increases to 1 in 2000. Herniation of the abdominal viscera into the thoracic cavity may cause severe respiratory distress and represent a neonatal emergency (Fig. 26-23). The defect and herniation may be minimal and easily repaired, or the defect may be so extensive that the viscera present in the thoracic cavity during embryonic life have prevented the normal development of pulmonary tissue. The defect is usually on the left because that is the side of the diaphragm that fuses last.

Most congenital diaphragmatic hernias are discovered prenatally on ultrasound studies and may be repaired by fetal surgery in some research institutions. At birth, most affected infants have severe respiratory distress, and respiratory assessment reveals worsening distress as the bowel fills with air. Typically the breath sounds are diminished and bowel sounds are heard in the chest. Heart sounds may be heard on the right side of the chest because the heart has been displaced there by the abdominal contents. Physical examination reveals a flat or scaphoid abdomen and a prominent ipsilateral chest. Diagnosis can be made on the basis of the x-ray study finding of loops of intestine in the thoracic cavity and the absence of intestine in the abdominal cavity.

Nursing ALERT

Any newborn infant with a scaphoid abdomen, moderate to severe respiratory distress, decreased breath sounds unilaterally, and a history of polyhydramnios should be suspected of having a CDH. Ventilation should not be given with bag and mask to prevent further intestinal air and subsequent respiratory compromise.

The prognosis depends largely on the degree of pulmonary development and the success of diaphragmatic closure, but the prognosis in severe cases is guarded. The overall survival for infants who are symptomatic within the first few hours of life is about 50%, although it has improved recently with the advent of ECMO.

Gastrointestinal System Anomalies

Anomalies in the gastrointestinal system can occur anywhere along the gastrointestinal tract, from the mouth to the anus. Some anomalies, such as cleft lip, omphalocele, and gastroschisis, are apparent at birth. Others, including cleft palate, esophageal atresia, pyloric stenosis, intestinal obstructions, and imperforate anus become apparent as the infant is further assessed or becomes symptomatic.

Cleft lip and palate. Cleft lip or palate is a commonly occurring congenital midline fissure, or opening, in the lip or palate resulting from failure of the primary palate to fuse (see Fig. 44-4). One or both deformities may occur. Multiple ge-

Family Focus

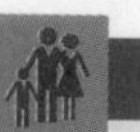

BREASTFEEDING THE INFANT WITH CLEFT LIP AND/OR CLEFT PALATE

Many health professionals assume that successful breastfeeding is impossible because of the cleft lip and/or cleft palate. On the contrary, breastfeeding is not only possible, it has several benefits, including the normal integration of the infant into the family, decreased problems with otitis media, and passive immunity to upper respiratory tract infections. In addition, breastfeeding enhances normal muscular movements of the mouth and face, and benefits normal speech development (Danner, 1992).

If the mother intended to breastfeed before delivery, she is encouraged and helped to do so as soon as possible after birth. If available, the services of a lactation expert or of La Leche League International, Inc. should be used.

netic and, to a lesser extent, environmental factors, such as maternal infection, radiation exposure, alcohol ingestion, and treatment with medications such as corticosteroids, some tranquilizers, and anticonvulsants, appear to be involved in their development. Pathophysiology, evaluation, and treatment are addressed in Chapter 44.

Feeding is difficult because the cleft lip renders the newborn unable to maintain a seal around a nipple; the cleft palate renders the infant unable to form a vacuum to maintain suction when feeding. In addition, the inability to suck and swallow normally allows milk to pool in the nasopharynx, which increases the likelihood of aspiration. Furthermore, as the infant attempts to suck, milk often comes out through the cleft and out of the nares.

Breastfeeding can be successful in some infants (Danner, 1992) (see the Family Focus box above). There are also special nipples, bottles, and appliances available to aid in feeding. In general, parents of infants with these defects need a great deal of education and support as they learn to feed their baby, to prevent what should be a normal part of infant care from becoming a very frustrating experience.

Parents of infants with a cleft lip or palate need much support, particularly in the case of a cleft lip because this is both a cosmetic and functional defect. Recognizing that this may interfere with normal parent-infant bonding in the neonatal period, the nurse must assess for this and intervene appropriately.

Esophageal atresia and tracheoesophageal fistula. Esophageal atresia (EA) and tracheoesophageal fistula (TEF), the most life-threatening anomalies of the esophagus, often occur together, although they can also occur singly. EA is a congenital anomaly in which the esophagus ends in a blind pouch or narrows into a thin cord, thus failing to form a continuous passageway to the stomach (see Fig. 44-6). TEF is an abnormal connection between the esophagus and trachea. Hydramnios is a common finding in pregnancy, particularly if the fetus has a EA without TEF. Variations of the anomalies are possible, depending on the presence or absence of a TEF, the site of the fistula, and the location and degree of the esophageal obstruction (see Fig. 44-6).

Nursing ALERT

Any infant who has an excessive amount of frothy saliva in the mouth or difficulty with secretions and unexplained episodes of cyanosis should be suspected of having a TEF and referred immediately for medical evaluation.

Infants with the life-threatening anomaly EA with TEF show significant respiratory difficulty immediately after birth. EA with or without TEF results in excessive oral secretions, abundant mucus, and feeding intolerance. Soon after the first feeding is begun in such infants, there is regurgitation of unaltered formula, that is, formula that has not mixed with gastric secretions, since it could not enter the stomach because of the EA. Respiratory distress can result from aspiration or from the acute gastric distention produced by the TEF. Choking, coughing, and cyanosis occur after even a small amount of fluid is taken by mouth.

Nursing interventions are supportive until surgery is performed. Any infant with excessive oral secretions and respiratory distress should not be fed orally until further evaluation is carried out. Surgical correction done in one stage, if possible, consists of ligating the fistula and anastomosing the two segments of the esophagus. The prognosis for a normal life is good, however, with an overall survival rate of 85% to 90%; the chances for survival in those infants in a good-risk category exceed 95%. See Chapter 44 for further discussion of surgical treatment and nursing care.

Omphalocele and gastroschisis. An **omphalocele** is a covered defect of the umbilical ring into which varying amounts of the abdominal organs may herniate (Fig. 26-24). Although it is covered with a peritoneal sac, the sac may rupture during or after birth.

Gastroschisis is the herniation of the bowel through a defect in the abdominal wall to the right of the umbilical cord. No membrane covers the contents, as occurs with an omphalocele. Unlike infants with omphalocele, these infants rarely have associated anomalies. Omphalocele occurs in approximately 1 in 5000 live births; the incidence of gastroschisis is much less than that of omphalocele (Rowe et al, 1995).

The preoperative nursing care for infants with both defects is similar. It is vital to protect the exposed viscera, which cause problems with thermoregulation and fluid and electrolyte balance. Before closure is performed, the exposed viscera are covered with moistened saline gauze and plastic wrap. Antibiotics, fluid and electrolyte replacement, gastric decompression, and thermoregulation are needed for physiologic support. If complete closure is impossible because of the small size of the defect and the large amount of viscera to be replaced, a Silastic silo pouch (Dow Corning, Midland, Mich.) is created to protect the contents as they are gradually placed back into the abdominal cavity. The defect is closed surgically after the reduction of contents is complete. Gastric decompression is necessary preoperatively to prevent aspiration pneumonia and to allow as much bowel as possible to be placed into the abdomen during surgery. Surgery is usually performed soon after birth. With surgical treatment and nutritional support, the survival rate is greater than 90% in such infants (Rowe et al, 1995).

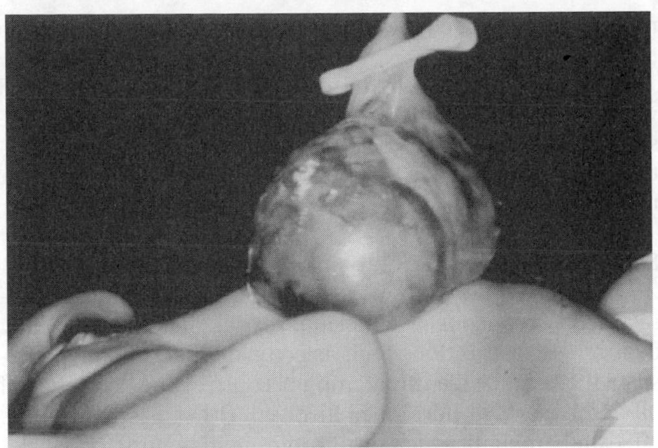

Fig. 26-24 Omphalocele containing liver. (Courtesy John R. Campbell, University of Oregon Health Sciences Center, Portland, Ore.)

Gastrointestinal obstruction. Congenital intestinal obstruction occurs in between 1 in 400 and 1 in 5000 live births (Rowe et al, 1995). Such an obstruction can occur anywhere in the gastrointestinal track and occur in the form of atresia, which is a complete obliteration of the passage; partial obstruction, in which the symptoms may vary in severity and sometimes not be detected in the neonatal period; or malrotation of the intestine, which leads to twisting of the intestine (volvulus) and obstruction. Meconium ileus is an obstruction caused by impacted meconium and is the earliest symptom of cystic fibrosis, a life-threatening chronic illness. Infants presenting with this type of obstruction should be tested for cystic fibrosis. EA, discussed previously, is a type of gastrointestinal obstruction.

In infants with an intestinal obstruction, surgery consists of resecting the obstructed area of bowel and anastomosing the nonaffected bowel. In recent years the survival rate for these infants has risen to 85% to 90% as a result of better treatments, better neonatal intensive care, and a better understanding of the total problem.

Imperforate anus. Imperforate anus is a term used to describe a wide range of congenital disorders involving the anus and rectum (see Fig. 44-9). These anomalies are relatively common, with an incidence of approximately 1 in 500 live births (Wong, 1995). Occurring more in male than in female infants, they result from the failure of anorectal development in weeks 7 and 8 of gestational life. Such infants have no anal opening, and frequently there is also a fistula from the rectum to the peritoneum or genitourinary system. The anomalies can be further classified according to the location of the defect into a "high" or "low" type, which determines the treatments necessary, as well as the prognosis. Infants with high anomalies require a colostomy in the neonatal period, with corrective surgery done in stages over time. Low anomalies may involve stenotic areas, or there may be a thin translucent membrane covering the anal opening. Treatment for such a membrane is excision followed by daily dilation, which parents are taught to do. See Chapter 44 for further discussion of surgical treatment.

Musculoskeletal System Anomalies

Developmental dysplasia of the hip. Developmental dysplasia of the hip consists of disorders that result from the abnormal development of one or all of the components of the hip joint, resulting in instability of the hip. This causes one or both of the femoral heads to be displaced from the hip socket, or acetabulum. The dislocated femoral head does not exert pressure on the acetabulum, causing delayed development of the femoral head and failure of the acetabulum to form normally. The etiology is considered to be multifactorial, with genetic factors involved, and females are more often affected than males. Risk factors for the defect include breech presentation, a positive family history, the birth order (firstborn), and prenatal maternal oligohydramnios with fetal compression and deformation. The effect of maternal hormones during pregnancy may foster hip joint capsule laxity, especially in the female. The defect occurs in approximately 1.5 to 2 per 1000 live births (Speers and Speers, 1992). The examiner tests for an unstable or actually dislocated femoral head by abducting the hips and feeling for a click when the femoral head passes back into the acetabulum (see Figs. 22-22 and 51-13).

Early detection, often by the nurse during a routine newborn assessment, allows for early treatment, which is more effective than later treatment and can prevent complications. Treatment involves the use of a Pavlik harness, a device that keeps the hips and knees flexed, the hips abducted, and the femoral head in the acetabulum (see Figs. 23 9 and 51-14). Worn continuously for 3 to 6 months, it promotes the development of muscle and cartilage, resulting in a stable hip. Although the harness is effective up to 90% of the time, traction, casting, and even surgery may be necessary to stabilize the hip. See Chapter 51 for more detailed discussion of developmental dysplasia of the hip.

Clubfoot. Clubfoot is a congenital deformity in which portions of the foot and ankle are twisted out of normal position. There are varying degrees of severity and various combinations of abnormal positions. The most common, seen in approximately 95% of infants with clubfoot, is talipes equinovarus. In this abnormality the foot points downward and inward, the ankle is inverted, and the Achilles tendon is shortened. Unless treated, further stiffening occurs, and bony changes result.

Clubfoot is one of the most common congenital anomalies, occurring in approximately 1 per 700 to 1 per 1000 live births, with two times more males than females affected (Wong, 1995). Treatment begins soon after birth. This consists of manipulation and frequent serial casting, which is necessary because of the rapid growth of the infant. If this is ineffective, surgical correction is necessary.

Because these infants are often placed in a cast before they are discharged, the nurse must teach the parents the way to care for an infant in a cast, including protecting the cast and assessing the toes for neurovascular compromise. This is particularly important because of the growth of the child, which could cause the child to outgrow the cast. See Chapter 51 for a discussion of the correction of this anomaly.

Polydactyly. Extra digits on the hands or feet occur occasionally. In some instances, polydactyly is hereditary. If there is little or no bone involvement, the extra digit is tied with silk suture soon after birth. The finger falls off within a few days, leaving a small scar. When there is bone involvement, surgical repair is indicated.

Genitourinary System Anomalies

Hypospadias and epispadias. Hypospadias constitutes a range of penile anomalies associated with an abnormally located urinary meatus. The meatus can open below the glans penis or anywhere along the ventral surface of the penis, the scrotum, or the peritoneum. It is the most common anomaly of the penis, affecting approximately 1 in 300 to 500 male infants (Rowe et al, 1995). It is classified according to the location of the meatus and the presence or absence of chordee, which is a ventral curvature of the penis.

Mild cases of hypospadias are often repaired for cosmetic reasons and involve a single surgical procedure. In more severe cases, several operations are required to reconstruct the urethral opening and correct the chordee, thereby straightening the penis. The goals are to improve the appearance of the genitalia and make it possible for the child to be able to urinate in a standing position and have a sexually adequate organ. These infants are not circumcised because the foreskin may be needed during surgical repair.

Epispadias is rare, occurring in approximately 1 in 100,000 live births (Kaplan, 1994). The urethral opening is located along the dorsal surface of the penis, and the severity ranges from a mild to a severe anomaly that is associated with exstrophy of the bladder. Surgical correction is necessary, and affected male infants should not be circumcised.

Exstrophy of the bladder. The most common bladder anomaly is exstrophy (Fig. 26-25), which often occurs in conjunction with epispadias. It is rare, occurring only in about 1 in 25,000 live births and twice as frequently in females (Kaplan, 1994). It results from the abnormal development of the bladder, abdominal wall, and the symphysis pubis that causes the bladder, urethra, and ureteral orifices to all be exposed. The bladder is visible in the suprypubic area as a red mass with numerous folds, with urine draining from it onto the infant's skin.

Immediately after birth the exposed bladder is covered with a sterile, nonadherent dressing to protect it until closure can be performed. It is recommended that reconstructive surgery be started in the neonatal period, although it may be delayed.

Sexual ambiguity. Sexual ambiguity in the newborn (Fig. 26-26) often is discovered by the nurse during a physical assessment. Erroneous or abnormal sexual differentiation may be a genetic aberration, such as congenital adrenal hypoplasia, which can be life threatening because of the deficiency of all adrenocortical hormones involved. Other possible causes of sexual ambiguity include chromosomal abnormalities, defective sex hormone synthesis in males, and the placental transfer of masculinizing agents to female fetuses. Gender assignment should be done very cautiously, integrating a multidisciplinary approach to avoid further traumatizing the parents and family. The data on which this is based may be gathered from the following sources: maternal and family history, including the ingestion of steroids during pregnancy and relatives with ambiguous genitalia or who died during the neonatal period; physical examination; chromosomal analysis (results are available in 2 to 3 days); endoscopy, ultrasonography, and radiographic contrast studies; biochemical tests, such as analysis of urinary steroid excretion, which helps detect several of the adrenal cortical syndromes; and, in some instances, laparotomy or gonad biopsy (Wong, 1995). Therapeutic intervention, including any surgery, should be started as soon as possible to prevent long-term psychosocial problems. Parents need much support as they learn to deal with this very challenging situation.

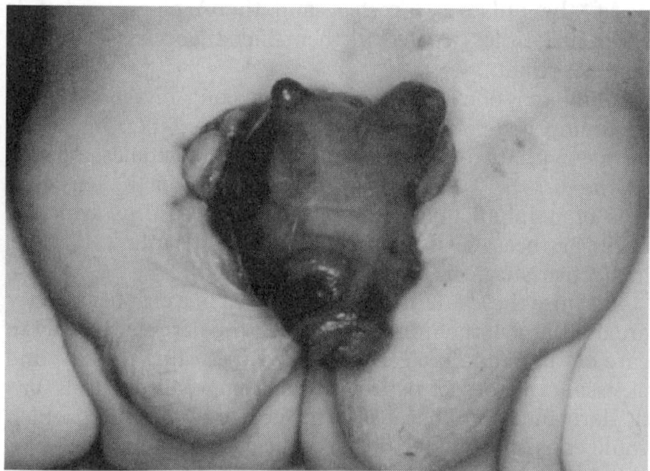

Fig. 26-25 Exstrophy of bladder. (Courtesy Edward S. Tank, MD, Division of Urology, University of Oregon Health Sciences Center, Portland, Ore.)

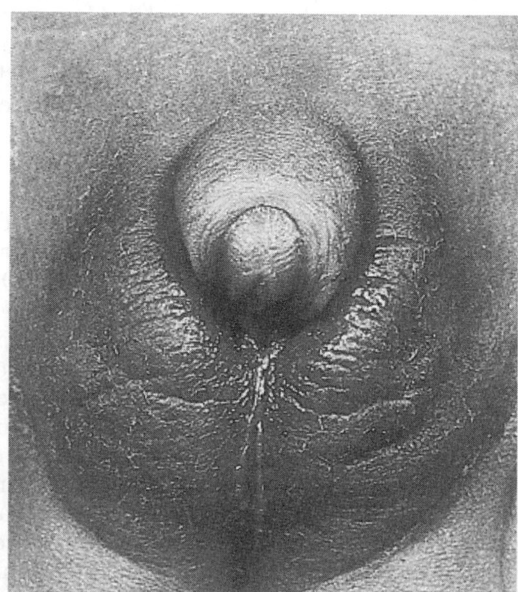

Fig. 26-26 Ambiguous external genitalia (that is, structure could be an enlarged clitoral hood and clitoris or a malformed penis). (Courtesy Edward S. Tank, MD, Division of Urology, University of Oregon Health Sciences Center, Portland, Ore.)

Teratoma. A **teratoma** is an embryonal tumor that may be solid, cystic, or mixed. It is composed of at least two and usually three types of embryonal tissue: ectoderm, mesoderm, and endoderm. A teratoma in the newborn may occur in the skull, mediastinum, abdomen, or sacral area, with more than half located in the sacrococcygeal area; 80% of all teratomas are benign. They are uncommon, occurring in approximately 1 in 35,000 live births (Rowe et al, 1995). The treatment of choice for such neonates is complete surgical resection. Most such sacrococcygeal tumors are benign, and no additional therapy is needed after complete resection done in the neonatal period. If the tumor is not surgically resected before the infant is 1 to 2 months old, the likelihood of the teratoma becoming malignant increases rapidly.

Nursing Care Management

Prenatal diagnosis. Refined testing procedures have become available to monitor the development of the fetus. Prenatal diagnostic techniques such as amniocentesis, ultrasonography, alpha-fetoprotein measurements, chorionic villus sampling, percutaneous umbilical cord blood sampling, and gene probes contribute information to the data base (see Chapter 7). Although they represent a valuable adjunct to prenatal care, these tests are not 100% accurate in detecting congenital defects (Brambati et al, 1991; Zacharias, 1990). Furthermore, not all congenital disorders are or can be anticipated. The history and medical information in the prenatal record is reviewed for factors that are associated with congenital disorders. These factors include various medical, surgical, and social conditions and their treatments (see Chapters 10 and 11), maternal infection (see Chapter 9), maternal endocrine and metabolic disorders (see Chapter 10), and infection and drug dependence in the newborn).

Perinatal diagnosis. Many congenital anomalies require intervention soon after birth. By careful observations in the birth room or nursery, the nurse can identify most of these conditions. An excessive amount of amniotic fluid, **hydramnios,** is commonly associated with congenital anomalies in the newborn, and such infants should be examined closely at the earliest possible time.

Oligohydramnios, which is an insufficient amount of amniotic fluid, is associated primarily with anomalies of the urinary tract that prevent normal micturition in utero. It is most often associated with renal agenesis or dysplasia and obstructive lesions in the lower urinary tract. Anomalies of the ears sometimes occur with renal abnormalities. Bilateral renal agenesis, resulting in oligohydramnios, commonly presents as Potter's syndrome, which is characterized by atypical facial appearance consisting of a flat nose, recessed chin, epicanthal folds, and low-set abnormal ears; limb abnormalities; pulmonary hypoplasia; and fetal growth restriction. These conditions may be diagnosed prenatally.

Postnatal diagnosis. Apgar scoring and a brief assessment are completed for all neonates after birth. Any deviations from normal are reported to the physician or midwife immediately. A thorough assessment of all body systems follows, with identification of both visible anomalies and those that might not be visible.

Some infants have multiple congenital anomalies. A recognized pattern of malformations is referred to as a *syndrome.* The most common is Down syndrome (Table 26-8 and Fig. 26-27), with the diagnosis confirmed early in the neonatal period.

Diagnostic procedures for the detection of genetic disorders are performed after birth at any time from the postnatal period through adulthood. There are many tests for various disorders; only the most frequently used ones are discussed here.

Biochemical tests. The most widespread use of postnatal testing for genetic disease is the routine screening of newborns for inborn errors of metabolism such as phenylketonuria (PKU), galactosemia, and hypothyroidism, which is mandatory in most states in the United States. An **inborn error of metabolism** is the term applied to a large group of disorders caused by a metabolic defect that results from the absence of or change in a protein, usually an enzyme, and mediated by the action of a certain gene. These defects can involve any substrate produced from protein, carbohydrate, or fat metabolism. Inborn errors of metabolism are recessive disorders, and, for this reason, for them to occur, a person must receive a defective gene from each parent. The parents usually are unaffected because their normal dominant gene directs the synthesis of sufficient protein to meet their metabolic needs under normal circumstances. With the advent of new biochemical techniques, it is now possible to detect the abnormal gene responsible for causing an increasing number of these disorders.

PKU results from a deficiency of the enzyme phenylalanine dehydrogenase (see Chapter 4). The test for PKU is not reliable, however, until the newborn has ingested an ample amount of the amino acid phenylalanine, a constituent of both human and cow milk. The nurse must document the initial ingestion of milk and perform the test at least 24 hours after that time.

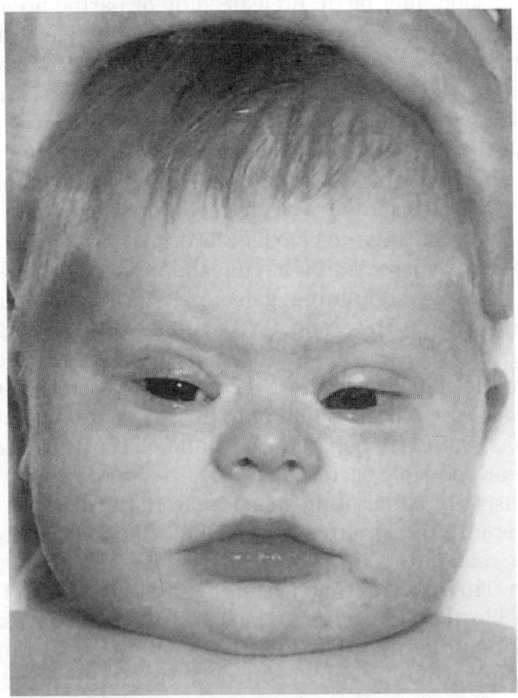

Fig. 26-27 Clinical features of Down syndrome. (From Zitelli B: *Atlas of Pediatric diagnosis,* ed 2, London, 1991, Mosby-Wolfe, Ltd.)

TABLE 26-8 Common autosomal aberrations

SYNDROME	CHROMOSOMAL ABNORMALITY AND NOMENCLATURE	AVERAGE INCIDENCE* (LIVE BIRTHS)	MAJOR CLINICAL MANIFESTATIONS
Cri-du-chat	Deletion of short arm of a B (no. 5) chromosome—46,XY,5p	1:50,000	Distinctive weak, high-pitched mew-like cry resembling the cry of a cat; small head; hypertelorism; failure to thrive; severe mental retardation
Trisomy 12 (Patau)	Trisomy of a group D (no. 13) chromosome—47,XY,13+	1:4000 to 1:15,000	Multiple anomalies, including cleft lip and palate (frequently bilateral); ear malformations; microphthalmia; polydactyly; eye defects; mental retardation; early death
Trisomy 18 (Edwards)	Trisomy of a group E (no. 18) chromosome—47,XY,18+	1:3500 to 1:8000	Deformed and low-set ears; micrognathia; rocker-bottom feet; overlapping (index over third) fingers; prominent occiput; hypertelorism; failure to thrive and early death; mental retardation
Trisomy 21 (Down)	Trisomy of a group G (no. 21) chromosome—47,XY,21+ (trisomy); 46XY,D—G–, (Dq-Gq)+ (translocation); 46,XY/47,XY,21+ (mosaic)	1:70†	Brachycephaly with flat occiput; inner epicanthal folds; small ears, nose, and mouth with protruding tongue; muscular hypotonia; broad, short hands with stubby fingers and simian palmar crease; broad, stubby feet with wide space between big and second toes; mental retardation; variable life expectancy

*Data from Nora I, Fraser F: *Medical genetics: principles and practice*, ed 3, Philadelphia, 1989, Lea & Febiger; D'Alton M, DeCherney A: Prenatal diagnosis, *N Engl J Med* 328:114, 1993.

†Risk related to maternal age: 30 years, 1/952; 35 years, 1/385; 40 years, 1/106; 45 years, 1/30; 49 years, 1/11.

If the infant is found to have PKU, a diet low in phenylalanine is begun soon after birth. Breastfeeding or partial breastfeeding may be possible for some infants if the phenylalanine levels are monitored carefully and remain within acceptable limits (Lawrence, 1994). Many affected children have some intellectual impairment.

Galactosemia, caused by a deficiency of the enzyme galactose-1-phosphate uridyltransferase, results in the inability to convert galactose to glucose. Galactosemia can also be detected by measuring the blood levels of galactose in the urine of newborns suspected of having the disease who have ingested formula containing galactose. Early symptoms are vomiting, weight loss, and CNS symptoms, including poor feeding, drowsiness, and seizures. If the disorder goes untreated, the galactose levels will continue to increase and the affected infant will show failure to thrive, mental retardation, cataracts, jaundice, hepatomegaly, and cirrhosis of the liver, with death possibly occurring in the first month of life. Therapy consists of eliminating galactose from the diet.

In recent years, many states in the United States have begun to mandate routine newborn screening for hypothyroidism. This involves the measurement of thyroxine (T_4) in a drop of blood obtained from a heel stick at 2 to 5 days of age. At this time the normally expected increase in T_4 would be lacking in newborns with hypothyroidism. Cretinism develops in untreated affected people. The same blood sample can be used to test for all three of these metabolic disorders—PKU, galactosemia, and hypothyroidism.

Cytologic studies. Abnormalities can occur in either the autosomes or the sex chromosomes. Chromosomal disorders often can be diagnosed on the basis of the clinical manifestations alone. However, an infant may have a clinical appearance that is only suggestive of a problem. Cytologic studies then need to be done to confirm or rule out a suspected diagnosis.

Disorders in the number or structure of chromosomes can be diagnosed by a karyotype (see Fig. 4-1), which is a photographic enlargement of the chromosomes arranged by their numbered pairs.

Abnormalities of the sex chromosomes make up about half of all the chromosomal abnormalities occurring in the newborn. The most common test for sex chromosome abnormalities is the buccal smear, using cells scraped from the mucosa inside the mouth. When prepared and stained, these show the number of inactive X chromosomes, also known as an *X-chromatin mass* or *Barr body*. Each cell, whether male or female, has one genetically active X chromosome. Therefore a normal female has one active X chromosome and one Barr body, which is on the inactive X chromosome. A normal male has no Barr bodies because he has only one genetically active X chromosome.

Dermatoglyphics. Dermatoglyphics is the study of the patterns formed by the ridges in the skin on the hands and feet. These patterns, formed early in development, are strongly correlated with the effects of chromosomes. Many disorders that affect multiple body systems also affect these dermal ridges. The addition or deletion of genetic material produces alterations in the loops, swirls, and arches of the finger and toe prints, in the palm lines, and in the flexion creases on the palms of the hands and soles of the feet. Characteristic dermatoglyphic patterns have been noted for almost all the chromosomal abnormalities, such as Down syndrome. The characteristic dermatoglyphic feature in a child with Turner syndrome is the large size of the dermal patterns on the fingers and toes. Certain fingerprint patterns may also be found in those people who have cardiac valvular problems later in life. As other techniques for chromosomal analysis have been developed, however, dermatoglyphics has decreased in importance in the assessment of clients with possible chromosomal abnormalities.

The nursing diagnoses formulated for an infant born with a congenital anomaly depend on the anomaly the infant has. For example, the diagnoses in an infant born with a CHD causing cyanosis will relate to inadequate oxygenation of body tissues, such as "activity intolerance related to imbalance between oxygen supply and demand." General nursing diagnoses pertain to the care of neonates with congenital abnormalities. These need to be adapted to the individual infant, and include the following:

Newborn

- Risk for injury or death related to
  Presence of a congenital disorder
- Risk for infection related to
  Anomaly or its treatment
- Risk for impaired gas exchange, nutrition, or mobility related to
  Congenital anomaly
- Risk for altered growth and development related to
  Inborn error of metabolism

Parents/Family

- Dysfunctional grieving or spiritual distress related to
  Birth of a child with a defect
- Risk for ineffective individual or family coping related to
  Birth of a child with a defect
- Knowledge deficit related to
  Cause of disorder, its management, alternative courses of action, community resources, prognosis, and the care needed by the child after discharge
- Anxiety related to
  Uncertainty regarding prognosis or ability to care for child
- Risk for altered parenting related to
  Birth of a child with a disorder or defect

Interventions: newborn. A collaborative health team approach that includes specialists (for example, orthodontists, physical therapists, geneticists) and community service representatives is needed in the care of infants with some disorders. Surgical intervention in the neonatal period may be necessary for the infant requiring either immediate correction or a palliative procedure to relieve the symptoms of the anomaly until definitive correction can be done. However, the complications induced by the stress of surgery may upset the delicate metabolic balance in a neonate already attempting to adapt to its extrauterine environment. This is compounded by the fact that there is only a limited amount of nutrient reserves normally present in the neonate and these reserves are already being drawn on by the energy-expending processes involved in rapid growth. Any surgical procedures performed during this time of growth place additional demands on these reserves. There is also a higher morbidity and mortality in neonates than in older children or adults undergoing similar procedures (Rowe et al, 1995). However, despite these problems unique to neonates, advances in surgical techniques, anesthesia, and the nursing care given in intensive care nurseries have together been responsible for lessening the risk of surgery in neonates.

The health care team must be highly skilled to meet the needs of these infants. These needs are similar to those of the compromised infant. In addition to stabilization of the infant's condition, other preoperative interventions, such as orogastric tube placement for abdominal decompression, pain management, and the maintenance of fluid and electrolyte balance, are implemented to manage specific problems.

Postoperatively, the infant is returned to the intensive care nursery, where close monitoring is maintained. The infant's respiratory efforts are supported; this often requires suctioning and usually mechanical ventilation. Constant surveillance is necessary to detect any respiratory complications resulting from the anesthesia. A pulse oximeter is attached to measure the oxygen saturation in hemoglobin, which closely correlates with arterial oxygen saturation. Oxygen is provided as needed. An indwelling gastric catheter attached to intermittent suction is placed to remove gastric secretions, thereby preventing aspiration and the abdomen from becoming distended. The infant's fluid, electrolyte, and acid-base status are monitored and adjusted as needed. Urinary output is monitored and should equal 1 to 2 ml/kg/hr. Other nursing interventions are focused on caring for the surgical site, maintaining thermoregulation, pain management, and promoting comfort.

Interventions: parents and family. While the infant is receiving optimal care, the parents also have needs that must be met as they deal with the crisis of having an infant with an abnormal condition. Their reactions are carefully assessed and are likely to be those typical of a grief response. Facilitating their understanding of the information given them about their infant's condition is a vital nursing intervention. A newly diagnosed disorder often implies the need for the implementation of a therapeutic regimen. For example, the disorder may be an inborn error of metabolism, such as PKU, which requires consistent and rigid adherence to a diet. The family may need help with securing the required formula and receiving counseling from the clinical dietitian. The importance of maintaining the diet, keeping an adequate supply of special preparations, and avoiding the use of unauthorized substitutions must be impressed on the family.

Referral to appropriate agencies is another essential component of the follow-up management, and the nurse should make the parents aware of all possible sources of aid, including pertinent literature, parent groups, and national organizations. Many organizations and foundations, such as the Cystic Fibrosis Foundation and the Muscular Dystrophy Association, provide services and equipment for affected children. There are also numerous parent groups the family can

Critical Thinking Exercises

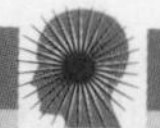

BIRTH OF A CHILD WITH A CONGENITAL ANOMALY

You have been assigned to care for Emilie, an 18-year-old single mother who has just given birth to a son, John, who has a cleft lip and palate. You are bringing the baby to the mother for the first time.

1. Identify your feelings about the infant and his physical defect.
2. Anticipate how the mother is likely to react to this encounter.
3. Rehearse how you will describe the infant to his mother.
4. Describe the surgical treatment of the defects.
5. Describe care necessary for John, including feeding and preoperative and postoperative care.

join where they can share experiences and derive mutual support in coping with problems similar to those of other group members. Nurses must be familiar with the services available in their community that provide assistance and education to families with these special problems.

A major nursing function is providing emotional support to the family during all aspects of the care of the child born with a defect or disorder (Stringer et al, 1991). The feelings stemming from the real or imagined threat posed by a congenital anomaly are as varied as the people being counseled. Responses may include apathy, denial, anger, hostility, fear, embarrassment, grief, and loss of self-esteem (see Chapter 20).

Parents benefit from seeing before-and-after pictures of other babies born with the same defect. Coupled with other verbal and nonverbal supportive care, this visual reassurance may be effective in allaying their concerns.

Families need much information, guidance, and support as they make decisions regarding the care of their infant. Once they have been given the facts and possible consequences and all the assistance they need in problem solving, the final decision regarding a course of action must be their own. It is then incumbent on health care providers to support the decision of the family.

The nurse can be reasonably assured that care for the infant was effective if the congenital disorder was treated, infection was avoided, impairments in gas exchange, nutrition, or mobility were treated, and growth and development of the child was within normal limits or the child was able to adapt effectively to any impairments. The care for the parents was effective if knowledge deficits related to the condition, its treatment, and community resources available were removed, the family grieved appropriately for the loss of their idealized child, the family was able to cope with the care of an infant with a defect, anxiety regarding prognosis and ability to care for the infant was decreased, and the parents attached emotionally to the infant.

Key Points

- A small percentage of significant birth injuries may occur despite skilled and competent obstetric care.
- Metabolic abnormalities of diabetes mellitus in pregnancy adversely affect embryonic and fetal development.
- Infection in the newborn may be acquired in utero, during birth, during resuscitation, and from within the nursery.
- Preterm infants are at risk for problems related to the immaturity of organ systems.
- Hyperbilirubinemia has a variety of etiologic factors, including maternal-fetal Rh and ABO incompatibility.
- The nurse often first observes signs of newborn drug withdrawal and acquires information from the maternal history.
- Major congenital defects are now the leading cause of death in term neonates born to mothers who had good perinatal care.
- The curative and rehabilitative problems of a child with a congenital disorder are often complex, requiring a multidisciplinary approach to care.
- Parents need special instruction (e.g., CPR, oxygen therapy, suctioning) before they take a high-risk infant home.

References

Ault K, Faro S: Viruses, bacteria and protozoa in pregnancy: a sample of each, *Clin Obstet Gynecol* 36(4):878, 1993.

Avery G, Fletcher M, MacDonald M: *Neonatology: pathophysiology and management of the newborn*, ed 4, Philadelphia, 1994, Lippincott.

Ballard J, Novak K, Driver M: A simplified score for assessment of fetal maturity of newly born infants, *J Pediatr* 95(5):769, 1979.

Ballard J et al: New Ballard score, expanded to include extremely premature infants, *J Pediatr* 119(3):417, 1991.

Barbour: B Is fetal alcohol syndrome completely irreversible? *MCN Am J Matern Child Nurs* 14:44, 1989.

Bastin N et al: HIV disease and pregnancy: postpartum care of the HIV positive woman and her newborn, *J Obstet Gynecol Neonatal Nurs* 21(2):105, 1992.

Becker M, Warr-Leeper G, Leeper I: Fetal alcohol syndrome: a description of oral motor, articulatory, short-term memory, grammatical, and semantic abilities, *J Commun Disord* 23:97, 1990.

Benson M: Management of infants born to women infected with human immunodeficiency virus, *J Perinat Neonatal Nurs* 7(4):79, 1994.

Bibb K et al: Drug screening in mothers using meconium samples, paired urine samples and interviews, *J Perinatol* 15(3):199, 1995.

Blackburn S: Hyperbilirubinemia and neonatal jaundice, *Neonat Netw* 14(7):15, 1995.

Blackburn S, Patteson D: Effects of cycled light on activity state and cardiorespiratory function in preterm infants, *J Perinat Neonatal Nurs* 4:47, 1991.

Bortolussi R, Seelinger H: *Listeriosis.* In Remington J, Klein J: *Infectious diseases of the fetus and newborn infant,* Philadelphia, 1990, Saunders.

Brambati B et al: Genetic diagnosis before the eighth gestational week, *Obstet Gynecol* 77:318, 1991.

Brooten D: Perinatal care across the continuum: early discharge and nursing home follow-up, *J Perinat Neonatal Nurs* 9(1):38, 1995.

Bryant M, Ratner L: Biology and molecular biology of human immunodeficiency virus, *Pediatr Infect Dis J* 11(5):390, 1992.

Carroll M: PCP and hallucinogens, *Adv Alcohol Substance Abuse* 9:167, 1990.

Centers for Disease Control and Prevention: 1993 Sexually transmitted diseases treatment guidelines, *MMWR* 42(RR-14):1, 1993a.

Centers for Disease Control and Prevention: Fetal alcohol syndrome in the United States—1979-1992, *MMWR* 42(17):339, 1993b.

Chasnoff I: Cocaine, pregnancy and the growing child, *Curr Probl Pediatr* 22(7):302, 1992.

Cloherty J, Stark A: *Manual of neonatal care,* ed 3, Boston, 1991, Little, Brown.

Coles C: Impact of prenatal alcohol exposure on the newborn and the child, *Clin Obstet Gynecol* 36(2):255, 1993.

Connor E, McSherry G: Treatment of HIV infection in infancy, *Clin Perinatol* 21(1):163, 1994.

Connor E et al: Reduction of maternal-infant transmission of human immunodeficiency virus type I with zidovudine treatment, *N Engl J Med* 331:1173, 1994.

Craven D et al: Human immunodeficiency virus infection in pregnancy: epidemiology and prevention of vertical transmission, *Infect Control Hosp Epidemiol* 15(1):36, 1994.

Creasy R, Resnik R: *Maternal-fetal medicine: principles and practice,* ed 3, Philadelphia, 1994, Saunders.

Danner S: Breastfeeding the infant with a cleft palate, *NAACOG Clin Issues Perinat Womens Health Nurs* 3:634, 1992.

Day N, Cottreau C, Richardson G: Epidemiology of alcohol, marijuana and cocaine use, *Clin Obstet Gynecol* 36(2):232, 1993.

Dietch J: Periventricular-intraventricular hemorrhage in the very low birth weight infant, *Neonat Netw* 12(1):7, 1993.

Dubowitz L, Dubowitz V: *Gestational age of the newborn,* Reading, Mass, 1977, Addison-Wesley.

Dubowitz L, Dubowitz V, Goldberg C: Gestational age of the newborn, *J Pediatr* 77(1):1, 1970.

Evans A: *Perinatal chemical use.* In Niswander K, Evans A, editors: *Manual of obstetrics,* ed 4, Boston, 1991, Little, Brown.

Fanaroff A, Martin R: *Neonatal-perinatal medicine: diseases of the fetus and infant,* ed 6, St Louis, 1997, Mosby.

Feng T: Substance abuse in pregnancy, *Curr Opin Obstet Gynecol* 5:16, 1993.

Fenster L, Eskenazi B, Windham G: Caffeine consumption during pregnancy and fetal growth, *Am J Public Health* 81:458, 1991.

Field T: *Interaction patterns of preterm and term infants.* In Field T, editor: *Infants born at risk,* Jamaica, NY, 1979, Spectrum Publications.

Finnegan L: *Drug addiction and pregnancy: the newborn.* In Chasnoff I, editor: *Drugs, alcohol, pregnancy and parenting,* Boston, 1991, Kluwer.

Floyd R et al: A review of smoking in pregnancy: effect on pregnancy outcome and cessation efforts, *Ann Rev Public Health* 14:379, 1993.

Freij B, Sever I: *Chronic infection.* In Avery G, Fletcher M, MacDonald M: *Neonatology: pathophysiology and management of the newborn,* ed 4, Philadelphia, 1994, Lippincott.

Frenkel L, Gaur S: Perinatal HIV infection and AIDS, *Clin Perinatol* 21(1):95, 1994.

Fried P: Prenatal exposure to tobacco and marijuana: effects during pregnancy, infancy and early childhood, *Clin Obstet Gynecol* 36(2):319, 1993.

Fuller R: Group B streptococcal infection in the newborn, *Crit Care Clin North Am* 4(3):487, 1992.

Gill N et al: Effect of nonnutritive sucking on behavioral state in preterm infants before feeding, *Nurs Res* 37(6):347, 1988.

Glantz J, Woods J: Cocaine, heroin and phencyclidine: obstetric perspectives, *Clin Obstet Gynecol* 36(2):279, 1993.

Gomella T, Cunningham M, Eyal F: *Neonatology: management, procedure, on-call problems, diseases and drugs,* ed 3, Norwalk, Conn, 1994, Appleton & Lange.

Greenspan J: Liquid ventilation: a developing technology, *Neonat Netw* 12(4):23, 1993.

Guerina N: *Bacterial and fungal infections.* In Cloherty J, Cloherty A, editors: *Manual of neonatal care,* ed 3, Boston, 1991, Little, Brown.

Guzzetta P et al: *General surgery.* In Avery G et al, editors: *Neonatology: pathophysiology and management of the newborn,* Philadelphia, 1994, Lippincott.

Hess D: *Chlamydia* in the neonate, *Neonat Netw* 12(3):9, 1993.

Hill R, Hegemier S, Tennyson L: The fetal alcohol syndrome: a multi-handicapped child, *Neurotoxicology* 10:585, 1990.

Hittner H, Hirsch N, Rudolph A: Assessment of gestational age by examination of the anterior vascular capsule of the lens, *J Pediatr* 91(3):455, 1977.

Hoekelman R et al: *Primary pediatric care,* St Louis, 1992, Mosby.

Hoffman J: Incidence of congenital heart disease. I. Postnatal incidence, *Pediatr Cardiol* 16:103, 1995.

Hudson I, Hussain K: Craniofacial and oral manifestations of fetal alcohol syndrome, *Plast Reconstr Surg* 85:505, 1990.

Kaplan G: *Structural abnormalities of the genitourinary system.* In Avery G et al, editors: *Neonatology: pathophysiology and management of the newborn,* Philadelphia, 1994, Lippincott.

Kennard M: Cocaine use during pregnancy: fetal and neonatal effects, *J Perinat Neonatal Nurs* 3(4):53, 1990.

Kenner C, Lott J: *Types of microorganisms.* In Lott J, editor: *Neonatal infection: assessment, diagnosis and management,* Petaluma, Calif, 1994, NICU Ink.

Klaus M, Fanaroff A: *Care of the high-risk neonate,* Philadelphia, 1993, WB Saunders.

Knoppert D, Mackanjee H: Current strategies in the management of bronchopulmonary dysplasia: the role of corticosteroids, *Neonat Netw* 13(3):53, 1994.

Korones S, Bada-Ellzey H: *Neonatal decision making,* St Louis, 1993, Mosby.

Lawrence R: *Breastfeeding: a guide for the medical profession,* ed 4, St Louis, 1994, Mosby.

Levine A, Rebarber A: Methadone maintenance, treatment and the nonstress test, *J Perinatol* 15(3):229, 1995.

Lindberg C: Perinatal transmission of HIV: how to counsel women, *MCN Am J Matern Child Nurs* 20(4):207, 1995.

Lindsay J et al: Creative caring in the NICU: parent-to-parent support, *Neonat Netw* 12(4):37, 1993.

Lott J et al: *Assessment and management of immunologic dysfunction.* In Kenner C, Brueggemeyer A, Gunderson L: *Comprehensive neonatal nursing,* Philadelphia, 1994, Saunders.

Lund C, editor: *Bronchopulmonary dysplasia: strategies for total patient care,* Petaluma, Calif, 1990, NICU Ink.

Maisels M: *Jaundice.* In Avery G, Fletcher M, MacDonald M, editors: *Neonatology: pathophysiology and management of the newborn,* ed 4, Philadelphia, 1994, Lippincott.

Merenstein G, Gardner S: *Handbook of neonatal intensive care,* ed 3, St Louis, 1993, Mosby.

Mills J et al: Moderate caffeine use and the risk of spontaneous abortion and intrauterine growth retardation, *JAMA* 269(5):593, 1993.

Mimouni F et al: Respiratory distress syndrome in infants of diabetic mothers in the 1980's: no direct adverse effect of maternal diabetes with modern management, *Obstet Gynecol* 69:191, 1987.

Niebyl J: *Drug use in pregnancy,* ed 2, Philadelphia, 1988, Lea & Febiger.

Ogata E: *Carbohydrate homeostasis.* In Avery G, Fletcher M, MacDonald M, editors: *Pathophysiology and management of the newborn,* Philadelphia, 1994, Lippincott.

Paryani S et al: Treatment of asymptomatic congenital syphilis: benzathine versus procaine penicillin G therapy, *J Pediatr* 125(3):471, 1994.

Pastorek J: The ABC's of hepatitis in pregnancy, *Clin Obstet Gynecol* 36(4):843, 1993.

Philip A: *Neonatology: a practical guide,* ed 3, Philadelphia, 1987, Saunders.

Piper I, Langer O: Does maternal diabetes delay fetal pulmonary maturity? *Am J Obstet Gynecol* 168(3):783, 1993.

Plessinger M, Woods J: Maternal, placental and fetal pathophysiology of cocaine exposure during pregnancy, *Clin Obstet Gynecol* 36(2):267, 1993.

Provisional Committee on Pediatric AIDS: Perinatal human immunodeficiency virus testing, *Pediatrics* 95(2):303, 1995.

Roberts J et al: Inhaled nitric oxide in persistent pulmonary hypertension of the newborn, *Lancet* 340:818, 1992.

Rogers M et al: *Advances and problems in the diagnosis of HIV infection in infants.* In Pizzo P, Wilfert C, editors: *Pediatric AIDS: the challenge of HIV infection in infants, children, and adolescents,* Baltimore, 1991, Williams & Wilkins.

Romanczuk A, Brown J: Folic acid will reduce risk of neural tube defects, *MCN Am J Matern Child Nurs* 19:331, 1994.

Rowe M et al: *Essentials of pediatric surgery,* St Louis, 1995, Mosby.

Samson L: Perinatal viral infections and neonates, *J Perinat Neonatal Nurs* 1(4):56, 1988.

Sanders M et al: Gestational age assessment in preterm neonates weighing less than 1500 grams, *Pediatrics* 88(3):542, 1991.

Schraeder B: Attachment and parenting despite lengthy intensive care, *MCN Am J Matern Child Nurs* 5:37, 1980.

Shannon L: Clinical perspectives and future trends of HIV infection in the newborn and child, *Neonat Netw* 14(3):21, 1995.

Shiminski-Maher T, Disabato, J: Current trends in the diagnosis and management of hydrocephalus in children, *J Pediatr Nurs* 9:74, 1994.

Smith M, Teele D: *Tuberculosis.* In Remington J, Klein J: *Infectious diseases of the fetus and newborn infant,* Philadelphia, 1990, Saunders.

Sosa R, Grua P: Perinatal responses to normal and premature birth experiences, *J Calif Perinat Assoc* 2:36, 1982.

Speers A, Speers M: Care of the infant in a Pavlik harness, *Pediatr Nurs* 18:229, 1992.

Streissguth A et al: Fetal alcohol syndrome in adolescents and adults, *JAMA* 265:1961, 1991.

Stringer M et al: Establishing a prenatal genetic diagnosis: the nurse's role, *MCN Am J Matern Child Nurs* 16:152, 1991.

Toltzis P: Current issues in neonatal herpes simplex virus infection, *Clin Perinatol* 18(2):193, 1991.

Trotter C: *Gestational age assessment.* In Tappero E, Honeyfield M: *Physical assessment of the newborn,* Petaluma, Calif, 1993, NICU Ink.

Volpe J: *Intraventricular hemorrhage in the premature infant: morphologic characteristics.* In Polin R, Fox W, editors: *Fetal and neonatal physiology,* vol 2, Philadelphia, 1992, Saunders.

Vomund S, Witter S: Advanced techniques for the treatment of severe isoimmunization, *MCN Am J Matern Child Nurs* 19:18, 1994.

Wardinsky T: Visual clues to diagnosis of birth defects and genetic disease, *J Pediatr Health Care* 8:63, 1994.

Weiner L, Morse B: *FAS: clinical perspectives and prevention.* In Chasnoff I, editor: *Drugs, alcohol, pregnancy and parenting,* Boston, 1991, Kluwer.

Wong D: *Whaley and Wong's nursing care of infants and children,* ed 5, St Louis, 1995, Mosby.

Zacharias J: The new genetics, *J Obstet Gynecol Neonatal Nurs* 19:122, 1990.

Zuckerman B: *Marijuana and cigarette smoke.* In Chasnoff I, editor: *Drugs, alcohol, pregnancy and parenting,* Boston, 1991, Kluwer.

Bibliography

Cavaliere T: Pharmacologic treatment of neonatal sepsis: antimicrobial agents and immunotherapy, *J Obstet Gynecol Neonatal Nurs* 24(7):647, 1995.

Corff K et al: Facilitated tucking: a nonpharmacologic comfort measure for pain in preterm neonates, *J Obstet Gynecol Neonatal Nurs* 24(2):143, 1995.

Cronin C et al: The impact of very low-birth weight infants on the family is long lasting: a maternal control study, *Arch Pediatr Adolesc Med* 149:151, 1995.

Lynam L: Research utilization: nonpharmacological management of pain in neonates, *Neonat Netw* 14(5):59, 1995.

McFarlane J, Parker B, Soekin K: Physical abuse, smoking and substance use during pregnancy: prevalance, relationships, and effects on birth weight, *J Obstet Gynecol Neonatal Nurs* 25(4):313, 1996.

Stevens B, Franck L: Special needs of preterm infants in the management of pain and discomfort, *J Obstet Gynecol Neonatal Nurs* 24(9):856, 1995.

Thompson D, Cohen D: Nursing management of the infant with a congenital malignancy, *J Obstet Gynecol Neonatal Nurs* 25(1):32, 1996.

CHAPTER 27

Contemporary Pediatric Nursing

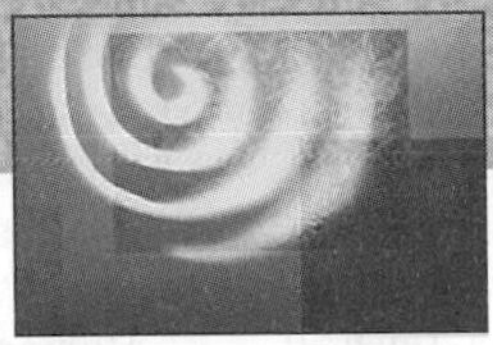

HEALTH DURING CHILDHOOD, P. 783
***Healthy people 2000*, p. 783**
Mortality, p. 783
Morbidity, p. 787
Evolution of child health care in the United States, p. 789
PEDIATRIC NURSING, P. 791
Philosophy of care, p. 791
Role of the pediatric nurse, p. 793
Future trends, p. 796

Health During Childhood

Health is a complex phenomenon. As defined by the World Health Organization (WHO), it is "a state of complete physical, mental, and social well-being and not merely the absence of disease." Despite this broad definition, however, health is traditionally assessed by observing **mortality (death)** and **morbidity (illness)** over a period of time. Therefore the *presence* of disease becomes a prime indicator of health.

Information concerning mortality and morbidity is of importance to nurses. Such data yield significant information about (1) the causes of death and illness, (2) high-risk age groups for certain disorders or hazards, (3) advances in treatment and prevention, and (4) specific areas of health counseling. Nurses who are aware of such information can better guide their planning and delivery of care.

HEALTHY PEOPLE 2000

Although the health of people, including children, in the United States has improved dramatically during the twentieth century, there remains cause for concern. There is a growing awareness that many of the serious domestic problems such as acquired immunodeficiency syndrome (AIDS), drug abuse, violence, and unwanted pregnancies have a direct effect on the health of the nation. Most importantly, the solutions to these problems do not lie in better or more innovative medical treatment but in *prevention.*

In 1990 *Healthy People 2000* (1991) was issued. It sets the following three broad goals for public health over the 1990s: (1) increase the span of healthy life for Americans, (2) reduce health disparities among Americans, and (3) achieve access to preventive services for all Americans.

Three broad approaches—health promotion, health protection, and preventive services—are employed to achieve the 22 priority areas, which contain approximately 300 measurable objectives. Selected objectives pertaining to pediatrics include improving nutritional and infant health, reducing unintentional injuries, improving oral health, reducing and controlling human immunodeficiency virus (HIV) infection, preventing sexually transmitted diseases, increasing immunization and preventing infectious diseases, and improving clinical preventive services by reducing barriers to health care (Mason and McGinnis, 1990). All health professionals, especially nurses, in any practice setting should be aware of the priority areas and work toward improving the health of U.S. children. Since the main intervention is prevention, many of the strategies nurses use, such as counseling, education, and screening, can be implemented *independently* to help achieve these goals.

MORTALITY

Figures describing rates of occurrence for events such as death in children are often referred to as **vital statistics. Mortality statistics** describe the incidence or number of individuals who have died over a specific period of time. They are usually presented as rates per 100,000 because of their lower frequency of occurrence. Such rates are calculated from a sample of death certificates.

Nursing ALERT

Because of the complexity of compiling such data, statistics may vary in different reports and should be interpreted cautiously. For example, figures may be **estimated** (from previously collected data), **provisional** (from temporary current data), or **final** (from complete provisional data). Final statistics are often published 2 or more years after data collection.

Infant Mortality

The infant mortality rate is the number of deaths per 1000 live births during the first year of life. It may be further divided into neonatal mortality (<28 days of life) and postneonatal mortality (28 days to 11 months). In the United States, there has been a dramatic decrease in infant mortality. At the beginning of the twentieth century the rate was about 200 infant deaths per 1000 live births. In 1994 the number dropped to 7.9 deaths per 1000 live births, the lowest rate ever recorded in the United States. This decrease has resulted primarily from improvements in perinatal care, such as treatment of respiratory distress syndrome and fewer deaths from sudden infant death syndrome (SIDS).

From a worldwide perspective, the United States lags significantly behind other developed countries. In 1992, it ranked last among the 22 countries with the lowest infant death rates, with Japan having the lowest rate. This is far behind neighboring countries such as Canada, which ranked sixth. The rank of the United States has fallen over several years. Although the reason is unknown, a major difference between the United States and the other 21 countries is that they all have a national health program (Wegman, 1994).

Birth weight is considered the major determinant of neonatal death in technologically developed countries and is closely related to gestational age (Wilcox and Skjaerven, 1992). The relationship between birth weight (and gestational age) and mortality shows that the lower the birth weight, the higher the mortality. The relatively high incidence of low birth weight (LBW) (<2500 g) in the United States is considered a key factor in its higher neonatal mortality rates when compared with other countries. Access to and use of high-quality prenatal care is the single most promising preventive strategy to decrease early delivery and infant mortality (Naeye, 1993). Other factors that increase the risk of infant mortality include African-American race, male gender, short or long gestation, birth order (all but second), maternal age (younger or older), and lower level of maternal education (Schoendorf et al, 1992).

Although there has been a steady and significant decline in infant mortality, the number of deaths occurring in the first year of life is still proportionately high when compared with death rates at other ages (Table 27-1). This is also true of other countries such as Canada (Table 27-2). In the United States and Canada the death rate for infants under 1 year of age is greater than the rates for individuals ages 1 through 54 years. It is not until age 55 and over that the death rate begins to exceed the rate for infants.

During the first half of the 1900s, neonatal mortality rates had not shown the remarkable reduction observed in postneonatal infant mortality. In the early 1960s attention focused on perinatal health care in an effort to decrease the number of neonatal deaths. As a result, neonatal mortality declined from 20 per 1000 live births in 1950 to 5 per 1000 live births in 1994 (Guyer et al, 1995).

As Table 27-3 demonstrates, most of the 10 leading causes of death during infancy continue to occur during the perinatal period. The first four causes—congenital anomalies, SIDS, disorders related to short gestation and unspecified LBW, and respiratory distress syndrome—accounted for about half of all deaths of infants under 1 year of age in 1992.

Although a number of perinatal problems have benefited from improved treatment, congenital anomalies continue to be a leading cause of infant mortality, accounting for over 20% of those deaths. The incidence of the majority of birth defects has remained substantially the same. Some, such as heart defects, have been rising, but the increase is the result of improved methods of detection, not increased births of af-

TABLE 27-1 Death rates by age, United States, 1994 (estimated rates per 100,000)

AGE (YEARS)	RATE	AGE (YEARS)	RATE
Under 1	811.1	45-54	452.3
1-4	44.5	55-64	1139.0
5-14	22.7	65-74	2590.9
15-24	99.6	75-84	5909.7
25-34	141.0	85 and over	15,312.6
35-44	239.5		

From Singh GK et al: Annual summary of births, marriages, divorces, and deaths: United States, 1994, *Monthly Vital Statistic Reports,* 43(13):6, Hyattsville, Md, 1995, National Center for Health Statistics.

TABLE 27-2 Death rates for children, Canada, 1988 (rates per 100,000)

	RATE		
AGE (YEARS)	TOTAL	MALE	FEMALE
Under 1	717.9	801.6	630.0
1-4	41.4	45.9	36.2
5-9	21.7	26.8	16.4
10-14	24.6	31.0	17.8
15-19	70.8	103.4	36.3
20-24	90.5	138.8	41.1

Data from Canadian Center for Health Information: *Statistics Canada,* 1988.

TABLE 27-3 Leading causes of death in infants under 1 year of age, United States, 1992 (rate per 100,000 live births)

RANK	CAUSES OF DEATH	RATE
1	Congenital anomalies	183.2
2	Sudden infant death syndrome	120.3
3	Disorders relating to short gestation and unspecified low birthweight	99.3
4	Respiratory distress syndrome	50.8
5	Newborn affected by maternal complications of pregnancy	35.9
6	Newborn affected by complications of placenta, cord, and membranes	24.4
7	Infections specific to the perinatal period	22.2
8	Accidents and adverse effects	20.1
9	Intrauterine hypoxia and birth asphyxia	15.1
10	Pneumonia and influenza	14.8

From Kochanek KD, Hudson BL: Advance report of final mortality statistics, 1992, *Monthly Vital Statistic Reports,* 43(6):65, Hyattsville, Md, 1995, National Center for Health Statistics.

fected infants (Khoury and Erickson, 1992). Two defects—anencephaly and spina bifida—are expected to decrease as much as 50% with the current recommendation of folic acid supplementation for all women of childbearing age (see Spina Bifida [Myelomeningocele], Chapter 52). Most birth defects are significantly associated with LBW; therefore prevention of congenital anomalies depends to a large extent on reducing the number of LBW infants (Mili et al, 1991).

When infant death rates are categorized according to race, a disturbing difference is seen. The infant mortality for whites is considerably lower than for all other races in the United States, with African-Americans having twice the rate for Caucasians. Although the infant mortality of both groups has declined, the gap has remained fairly constant. Unfortunately, data on minority groups are less readily available. For example, the Hispanic infant mortality rate may not represent all Hispanic subgroups, such as Cubans, who have more favorable statistics regarding prenatal care and LBW newborns. (Kochanck and Hudson, 1995).

One encouraging note is that the gap in mortality rates between all non-Caucasian races has been narrowing. Since the Indian Health Service assumed responsibility for the health of Native Americans, infant mortality for Native Americans has declined from 62.7 deaths per 1000 live births in the 1950s to 9.8 in the mid 1980s. This improvement, however, is primarily a result of declines in neonatal mortality. The postneonatal death rates for Native Americans remains more than twice as high as in the Caucasian race. This suggests that Native-American infants leave the hospital healthy but go to unsafe environments, which decreases their chances of survival past the first year (Nakamura et al, 1991).

Childhood Mortality

For children under 1 year of age, death rates have always been less than those for infants, as Table 27-4 shows. Children ages 5 to 14 years have the lowest rate of death. However, a sharp rise occurs during later adolescence, primarily from injuries, homicide, and suicide—all potentially preventable conditions that in 1992 were responsible for about 80% of deaths in teenagers and young adults 15 to 24 years old (Kochanek and Hudson, 1995). A general trend in racial differences that occurs in infant mortality is also apparent in childhood deaths for all ages and for both genders. Caucasians have fewer deaths for all ages, and for both Caucasian and African-Americans, male deaths outnumber female deaths.

There is a dramatic change in the causes of death after 1 year of age, with injuries being the leading cause during childhood, adolescence, and young adulthood. In addition, violent deaths have been steadily increasing among young people ages 10 to 25 years, especially African-Americans and males (Rachuba, Stanton and Howard, 1995). Homicide is the second leading cause of death in the 15- to 24-year age group. Children 12 years of age and older tend to be killed by non-family members (acquaintances and gangs, typically of the same race) and most often by firearms. Suicide, a form of self-violence, is the third leading cause of death among teenagers and young adults 15 to 24 years old. Caucasian males in this age group are especially at risk (see Suicide, Chapter 37).

The causes of increased violence against children and self-inflicted violence are not fully understood. In young children the increase in homicide may represent more accurate identification of child abuse. In all cases the problem of child homicides is an extremely complex one, involving numerous social, economic, and other influences. Prevention lies in a better understanding of the social and psychologic factors that lead to the high rates of homicide and suicide. Nurses need to be especially aware of young people who are depressed, repeatedly in trouble with the criminal justice system, or associated with groups known to be violent. Prevention requires identification of these youngsters, as well as therapeutic intervention by qualified professionals.

The major declines in death rates during childhood have been in deaths related to gastrointestinal diseases, infectious diseases, perinatal conditions, neoplasms, and injuries. The absence of infectious diseases as a leading cause of death is testimony to the role antibacterial agents and immunizations have played in the declining mortality rates. More effective treatment of severe infections has resulted in other disorders becoming more prominent in the list of leading killers. (Most notable among these are the neoplasms, although fewer children die from cancer than ever before. See Leukemias, Chapter 46.) However, infectious disease may again play a prominent role in childhood mortality. Of particular concern is the increasing incidence of HIV infection in children. In 1992, HIV infection ranked as the seventh

TABLE 27-4 Leading causes of death in children at selected age intervals, United States, 1992, (rates per 100,000)

RANK	AGES 1-4	RATE	AGES 5-14	RATE	AGES 15-24	RATE
	All causes	43.6	All causes	22.5	All causes	95.6
1	Injuries	15.9	Injuries	9.3	Injuries	37.8
2	Congenital anomalies	5.5	Cancer	3.0	Homicide	22.2
3	Cancer	3.1	Homicide	1.6	Suicide	13.0
4	Homicide	2.8	Congenital anomalies	1.2	Cancer	5.0
5	Heart disease	1.8	Heart disease	0.8	Heart disease	2.7
	HIV infection (7)*	1.0			HIV infection (6)*	1.6

From Kochanek KD, Hudson BL: Advance report of final mortality statistics, 1992, *Monthly Vital Statistic Reports* 43(6):23, Hyattsville, Md, 1995, National Center for Health Statistics.

*HIV (Human immunodeficiency virus); rank in parenthesis

leading cause of death for ages 1 to 14 years, and sixth for ages 15 to 24 years. Although HIV infection was the seventh leading cause of death for ages 1 to 4, the number of deaths resulting from this cause was relatively small—161 deaths, or 2% of deaths from all causes for that age group. During 1994, 1768 cases of AIDS were reported in adolescents. Of these, 64% were exposed to HIV primarily through transfusions of clotting factor for hemophilia/coagulation disorder (*Child Health,* 1995).

Injuries—the leading killer. Injuries cause more deaths and disabilities in children than do all causes of disease combined. As children grow older, the percentage of deaths from injuries increases (Table 27-5). Injuries have not shown the dramatic declines seen in other areas of childhood mortality. Injury has traditionally been regarded as an unavoidable accident or a behavioral problem, rather than a health problem. The term *accident* suggests a chaotic, random event that is "luck" or "chance"; the term *injury* is preferred because it connotes a sense of responsibility and control.

In addition, injury control, including research, has not received high priority or sufficient financial support. Research on injuries has not been based on a theoretic framework, as has been done with diseases. There is a need to view injuries and their prevention in terms of **host,** the affected person, **environment,** the time and place, and **agent,** the object that is the direct cause.

The pattern of deaths caused by unintentional injuries, especially from motor vehicles, drowning, and burns, is remarkably consistent in most Western societies such as Canada. However, the United States far exceeds other countries in the number of violent deaths. The leading causes of deaths from injuries for each age-group according to gender are presented in Table 27-5. Fortunately, prevention strategies such as use of car restraints, bicycle helmets, and smoke detectors have resulted in a significant decrease in fatalities for children ages 1 to 19 years (*Child Health,* 1995). Currently, all states in the United States have enacted legislation requiring young children to be properly restrained in motor vehicles.

Despite safety efforts, the overwhelming cause of death in children over 1 year of age is motor vehicle (MV)–related fatalities, including occupant, pedestrian, bicycle, and motorcycle deaths (Fig. 27-1). The majority of deaths from injuries occur in males. Even though the *percentage* of infants dying from MV injuries is small compared with the total number of deaths in that age group, children under 1 year of age still have a high death rate from MV occupant deaths, primarily from failure to be properly restrained.

When deaths from injuries are compared according to gender and age, the causes of death differ. The developmental stage of the child partially determines the types of injuries that are most likely to occur at a specific age. Children ages 1 to 4 years are equally likely to die as an occupant or as a pedestrian in MV injuries. However, children ages 5 to 9 years

TABLE 27-5 Mortality from leading types of injuries, United States, 1990 (rates per 100,000 population in each age-group)

	AGE (YEARS)			
TYPE OF ACCIDENT	UNDER 1	1-4	5-14	15-24
Males				
All causes	1083.1	52.4	28.5	147.4
Accidents (all types)	25.2	20.8	13.5	65.9
Motor vehicle	5.0 (2)*	6.9 (1)	7.0 (1)	49.5 (1)
Drowning†	2.2 (5)	5.0 (2)	2.1 (2)	4.4 (2)
Fires and burns	2.9 (4)	4.4 (3)	1.0 (3)	1.1 (5)
Firearms	—	—	1.0 (4)	2.4 (3)
Ingestion of food/object	4.6 (3)	0.8 (4)	—	—
Mechanical suffocation	6.7 (1)	0.6 (5)	—	—
Poisoning	—	—	—	1.5 (4)
Accidents as a percent of all deaths	2.3%	40%	47%	45%
Females				
All causes	855.5	41.0	19.3	49.0
Accidents (all types)	21.8	13.7	7.2	20.8
Motor vehicle	4.9 (2)	5.6 (1)	4.7 (1)	17.9 (1)
Drowning†	1.7 (5)	2.6 (3)	0.7 (3)	0.4 (4)
Fires and burns	2.7 (4)	2.9 (2)	0.8 (2)	0.5 (3)
Firearms	—	—	0.1 (4)	0.2 (5)
Ingestion of food/object	3.0 (3)	0.5 (4)	—	—
Mechanical suffocation	5.4 (1)	0.3 (5)	—	—
Poisoning	—	—	—	0.6 (2)
Accidents as percent of all deaths	2.5%	34%	37%	42%

Modified from National Center for Health Statistics, Public Health Service, U.S. Department of Health and Human Services: *Accident facts,* Chicago, 1993, National Safety Council.

*Indicates rank among the leading types of accidents.

†Exclusive of deaths in water transportation.

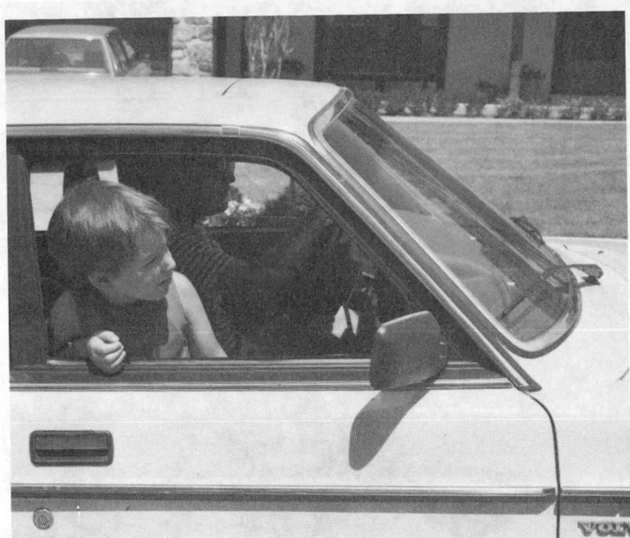

Fig. 27-1 Motor-vehicle injuries are the leading cause of death in children over age 1 year. The majority of the fatalities involve occupants who are unrestrained.

are more likely to die from pedestrian crashes, whereas adolescents are more likely to die from occupant crashes. Children ages 10 to 14 are at greatest risk of bicycling fatalities. The majority of bicycling deaths are from head injuries. Helmets can reduce the risk of head injury by 85%, but a minority of children wear them (American Academy of Pediatrics, 1995).

Drowning and burns are the second and third leading causes of death in boys ages 1 to 14, but the order is reversed in girls (Fig. 27-2). Drowning continues to be a significant cause of death in older teenagers. In addition, firearms are a major cause of death in males but not in females (Fig. 27-3). During infancy, aspiration or suffocation often ranks as the leading cause of death but is infrequent in older children (Fig. 27-4). More than half of all poisonings occur in children under 2 years of age (Fig. 27-5). By age 4 to 5 years, nonintentional poisonings are uncommon. Another increase occurs in the 15- to 24-year age group, where it is the fourth leading cause of death from injury. Poisoning in this age-group is typically intentional and usually represents death from suicide (especially in females) or drug abuse. Deaths from falls are primarily seen in children ages 1 to 14 years.

Analyzing deaths from specific types of injuries by age and gender is useful in identifying high-risk groups. When comparing deaths from injuries with other causes of childhood mortality, it is clear that preventing injuries offers the greatest promise for improving survival. Recent data indicate that advanced physical development imposes additional risks for 5-to-8 year olds. Nurses certainly play a major role in providing anticipatory guidance to parents and older children regarding hazards during each age period (Christoffel et al, 1996). Injury prevention is discussed in each chapter on health promotion of the various age-groups.

MORBIDITY

The prevalence of a specific illness in the population at a particular time is known as **morbidity statistics.** These are generally presented as rates per 1000 population because of their greater frequency of occurrence. Unlike mortality statistics, morbidity is difficult to define and may denote acute illness, chronic disease, or disability. Unlike death rates, which are updated annually, morbidity statistics are revised much less often and do not necessarily represent the general population.

A

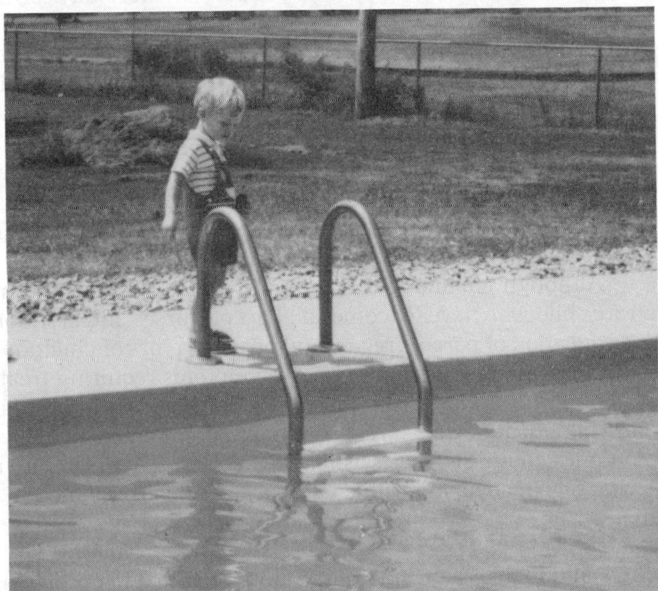

B

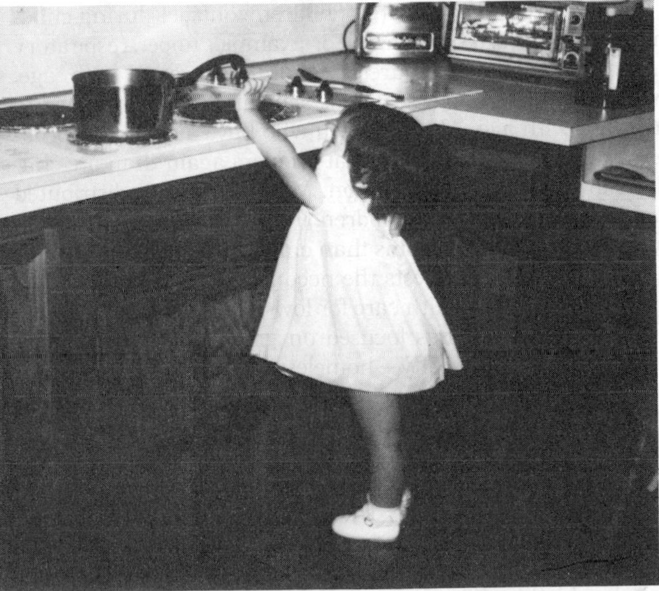

Fig. 27-2 **A,** Drowning is the second leading cause of death from injury in boys and the third in girls ages 1 to 14 years. It remains the second leading cause of death from injury for both genders ages 15 to 24 years. **B,** Burns are the second leading cause of death from injury in girls and the third in boys ages 1 to 14 years.

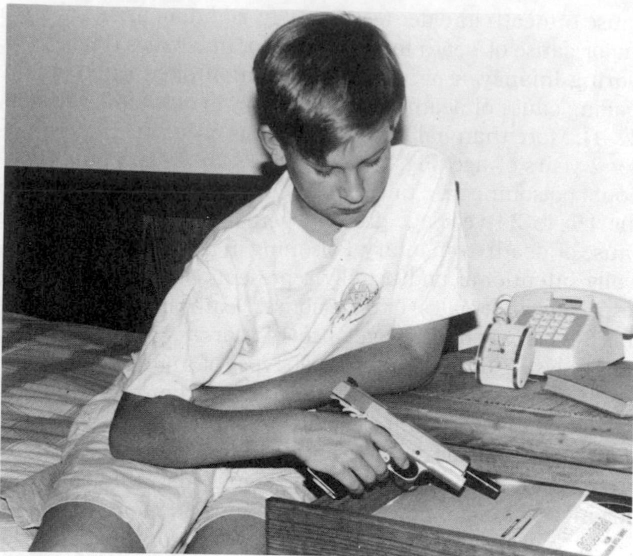

Fig. 27-3 Improper use of firearms is the fourth leading cause of death from injury in boys and girls ages 5 to 14 years and the third leading cause of death from injury in boys ages 15 to 24 years.

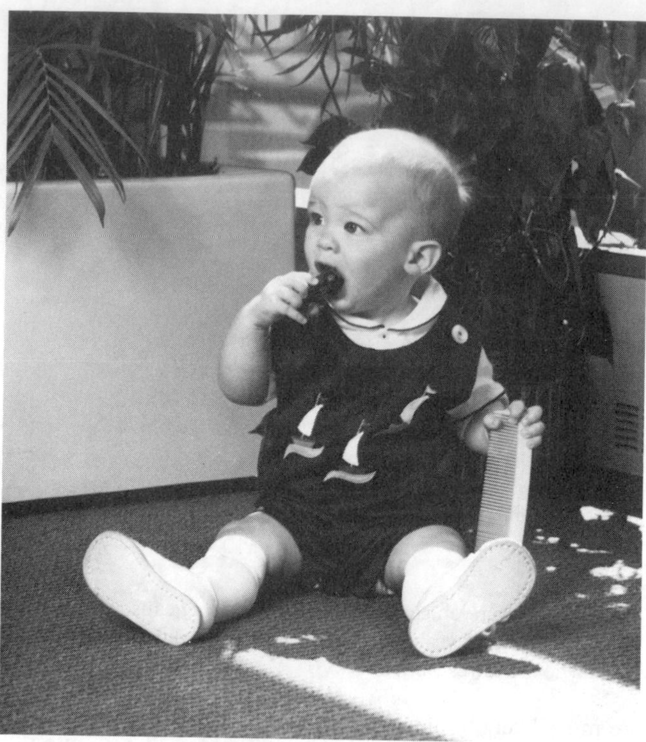

Fig. 27-4 Aspiration/suffocation is often the leading cause of death from injury in infants, especially boys.

The following discussion is intended to present an overview of illness in children from a variety of perspectives.

Childhood Morbidity

Acute illness may be defined as symptoms severe enough to limit activity or require medical attention. Respiratory illness accounts for about 50% of all acute conditions; about 11% are caused by infections and parasitic disease, and 15% are caused by injuries. The chief illness of childhood is the common cold (Pless, 1992).

The types of diseases that children contract during childhood vary according to age. For example, upper respiratory tract infection and enuresis tend to decrease with age, whereas other disorders such as acne and headaches tend to increase with age. Also, children who have any type of problem are more likely to have that problem again than are children in the general population. Morbidity is not distributed randomly in children. Children from poor families tend to have more health problems than children from nonpoor families. This finding suggests the need for heightened efforts to improve access to health care for low-income children.

Recent concern has focused on groups of children who have increased morbidity—homeless children, children living in poverty, LBW children, children with chronic illnesses, foreign-born adopted children, and children in day care centers. A number of different factors account for these at-risk groups. A major cause is limited access to health care, especially for the homeless, the poverty stricken, and those with chronic health problems. Other reasons include improved survival of children with chronic health problems, particularly infants of very low birth weight (VLBW). Children affected by certain at-risk environments such as country of origin (for adopted children) and day care centers are more likely to have a variety of medical conditions, especially infections (American Academy of Pediatrics, 1991).

Injury-related morbidity is also significant. Almost 16 million children are seen in emergency rooms for their injuries—600,000 children are hospitalized, and about 30,000 youngsters have permanent disability from injuries each year (Division of Injury Control, 1990).

Probably the most important aspect of morbidity is the degree of disability it produces. *Disability* can be measured in days off from school or days confined to bed. It can be the result of an acute or chronic disorder. On an average, a child loses 5.3 days per year because of injury or illness. Of all children under 17 years of age, over 95% are not disabled in any way. About 2% have mild disability, another 2% have moderate disability, and 0.2% are severely disabled (Pless, 1992). (The incidence of chronic conditions is discussed in Chapter 38.)

Although childhood is a time of relative health, it is the rare child who never becomes ill. Part of nurses' intervention is education of parents regarding the usual types of childhood illnesses and recognition of those symptoms requiring treatment. Future progress in decreasing childhood morbidity, as in childhood mortality, rests more on parent education than on miraculous discoveries such as antibiotics. Nurses play a vital role in advancing child care through health promotion.

The New Morbidity

In addition to disease and injury, children face other problems that can significantly affect their health. These include behavioral, social (family), and educational problems that are sometimes referred to as the new morbidity. Estimates on the incidence of these problems vary, but they represent at least 5% and as much as 25% to 30% of health problems in specific age

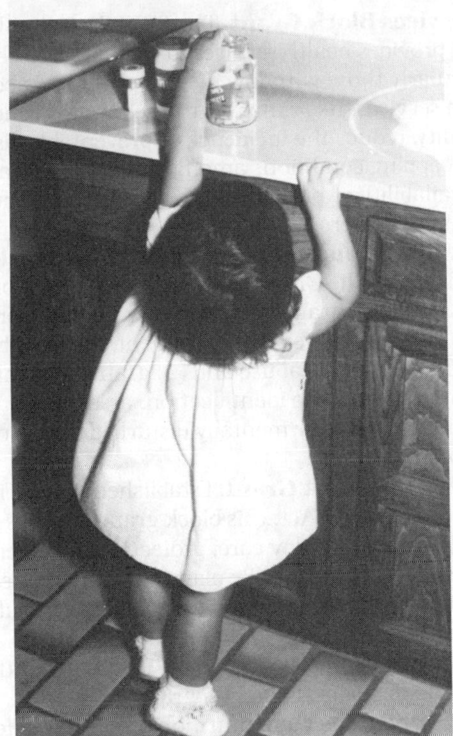

Fig. 27-5 Poisoning causes a considerable number of injuries in children under 4 years of age but is the fourth leading cause of death from injury (usually from suicide) in young people ages 15 to 24 years.

groups, social classes, and medical facilities. Although no conclusive characteristics have been identified for children with new-morbidity problems, some findings are significant in terms of defining a high-risk group. This group includes children (1) from the lowest socioeconomic strata, (2) ages 7 to 14 years, (3) of male gender, (4) from one-parent families, (5) with a presenting complaint of a chronic physical disorder, (6) with reading skills below grade level, and (7) with higher rates of school absenteeism (Gortmaker et al, 1990). As new "epidemics" such as violence, poverty, technology-dependent children, drug-addicted infants, and HIV continue to emerge, nurses will need to continue professional education efforts to effectively manage children's psychosocial problems (American Academy of Pediatrics, 1993).

EVOLUTION OF CHILD HEALTH CARE IN THE UNITED STATES

Children in colonial America were born into a world with many hazards to their health and survival. Epidemics were common, and no control or treatment was known. Physicians were few, and only a small number had any formal training. Midwives also were untrained, basing their practice on past experiences. Books providing information on child care and feeding were scarce and, when available, were useful only to a minority of literate parents.

Medical care by physicians was limited to wealthy families who lived in or could travel to more developed cities. Children who lived on farms were mainly cared for by another family member or by a competent neighbor. Traveling medicine men, with their various forms of quackery, were common. African-American slave children had only as much care as their owner was able or willing to provide. Native American children were treated for disease according to the tradition of each tribe, which was often a mixture of medicine, magic, and religion. With the colonization of America the tribes were exposed to many new, often fatal, diseases.

Statistics on childhood mortality during the colonial period are largely unavailable. Epidemic diseases were prevalent, however, and included smallpox, measles, mumps, chickenpox, influenza, diphtheria, yellow fever, cholera, and whooping cough, but the disease that surpassed all others as a cause of childhood death was dysentery. Sometimes entire families succumbed to this illness. Other diseases that were major contributors to childhood illness were the "slow epidemics" of tuberculosis, nutritional diseases, and injuries (Schmidt, 1976).

Although scientific knowledge was accumulating, especially from work done in Europe, there were no organized efforts in the United States to apply that knowledge to the care of the sick. It was not until the Industrial Revolution was well under way in the nineteenth century that the consequences of childhood illness and injury and the effects of child labor, poverty, and neglect became more widely recognized. The end of the nineteenth century is often regarded as the dark ages of pediatrics, and the first half of the twentieth century as the dawn of improved health care for children (Cone, 1976).

The study of pediatrics began in the last half of the 1800s, particularly under the influence of a Prussian-born physician, *Abraham Jacobi* (1830-1919), who is referred to as the *Father of Pediatrics.* Along with several other physicians, he was a pioneer in the scientific and clinical investigation of childhood diseases. One outstanding achievement was the establishment of "milk stations," where mothers could bring sick children for treatment and learn the importance of pure milk and its proper preparation.

The crusade for pure milk helped bring the dairy industry under legal control and led to the establishment of infant welfare stations. The remarkable decline in infant mortality since 1900 has been achieved through prevention and health-promoting measures such as improved sanitation and pasteurization of milk. Before these regulations existed, the unsanitary milk supply was a chief source of infantile diarrhea and bovine tuberculosis.

At about the same time, increasing concern developed for the social welfare of children, especially those who were homeless or employed as factory laborers. The work of one such reformer, *Lillian Wald* (1867-1940), had far-reaching effects on child health and nursing. She founded the Henry Street Settlement in New York City, which eventually provided nursing service, social work, and an organized program of social, cultural, and educational activities. Wald is regarded as the founder of public health or community nursing. She was instrumental in establishing the role of the first full-time school nurse, *Lina Rogers.* Soon other nurses were employed to teach parents and children about the prevention or need for treatment of minor skin conditions, malnutrition, and other impairments or illnesses identified in the school. An outgrowth of nursing involvement in school health was the development of pediatric courses and specialized clinical experience in schools of nursing.

As more causes of disease were identified, there was an emphasis on isolation and asepsis. In the early 1900s children with contagious diseases were isolated from adult patients. Parents were prohibited from visiting because they might transmit disease to and from the home. Even toys and personal articles of clothing were kept from the child. It was not until the 1940s and the famous work of Spitz and Robertson on institutionalized children that the effects of isolation and maternal deprivation were recognized. This brought forth a surge of interest in the psychologic health of children and resulted in changes for hospitalized children, such as rooming-in, sibling visitations, child life (play) programs, prehospitalization preparation, parent education, and hospital schooling.

Influenced by social reformers such as Lillian Wald, national leaders began to take action to improve children's living conditions. By 1909 President Theodore Roosevelt called the first *White House Conference on Children.* It focused on care of dependent children and attempted to address the deplorable working conditions of youngsters. As a result of this conference, the *U.S. Children's Bureau* was established in 1912. This marked the beginning of a period of studies of economic and social factors related to infant mortality, maternal deaths, and maternal and infant care in rural areas, all of which created the basis for stimulating better standards of care for mothers and children. This helped lead to the first Maternity and Infancy Act (Sheppard-Towner Act) in 1921, which provided grants to states to develop a Division of Maternal and Child Health (MCH) as a unit of the health department.

With the passage of *Title V of the Social Security Act (SSA)* in 1935, a federal-state partnership was established under the administration of the Children's Bureau. Title V included federal grants-in-aid to states, matched by state funds, for three types of work: *maternal and child health, Crippled Children's Services (CCS),* and *child welfare services.* The first programs provided by Title V were prenatal, postnatal, and child health clinics and training of personnel. The early emphasis of the CCS was on orthopedic care. With the recognition that a child's ability to function could also be limited by a chronic illness, state CCS programs became involved with children with developmental, behavioral, and educational problems and more recently with home care of children with complex medical conditions. This broadened concept was officially reflected in the 1985 passage of legislation that changed the name of the CCS to the *Program for Children with Special Health Needs (CSHN).*

Numerous other federal programs have been developed. Some that have had a major impact on maternal and child health include the following:

Medicaid. In 1965, Medicaid was created under Title XIX of the Social Security Act to reduce financial barriers to health care for the poor. It is the largest maternal-child health program. A major project under Medicaid is the Child Health Assessment Program (CHAP), which provides services for a large number of pregnant women and children. Not all poor children are eligible for Medicaid; financial eligibility varies considerably from state to state.

Aid to Families with Dependent Children (AFDC). AFDC was established by the Social Security Act of 1935 as a cash grant program to enable states to aid needy children without fathers.

MCH Services Block Grant. The MCH Services Block Grant provides health services to mothers and children, particularly those with low income or limited access to health services. Its primary purposes are to reduce infant mortality, reduce the incidence of preventable disease and handicapping conditions among children, and increase the availability of prenatal, delivery, and postpartum care to eligible mothers.

Alcohol, Drug Abuse, and Mental Health Block Grant. Established by the Omnibus Budget Reconciliation Act of 1981, the block grant provides funds to states for (1) projects to support prevention, treatment, and rehabilitation related to substance abuse and (2) grants to community health centers for the identification, assessment, and treatment of severely mentally disturbed children and adolescents.

Social Services Block Grant. Established under Title XX of the Social Security Act, this block grant provides states with funds for child day care, protective and emergency services, counseling, family planning, home-based services, information and referral, and adoption and foster care services.

Women, Infants, and Children (WIC). In 1974 the WIC Special Supplemental Food Program was started. It provides nutritious food and nutrition education to low-income, pregnant, postpartum, and lactating women and to infants and children up to age 5 years. Other nutrition programs include Food Stamps, National School Lunch Program, School Breakfast Program, and Child Care Food Program, which provides financial assistance for nutritious meals to children in day care centers, family and group day care homes, and Head Start centers.

Education for All Handicapped Children Act (P.L. 94-142). In 1975 P.L. 94-142 was passed to provide a free, appropriate public education to all handicapped children from ages 3 to 21 and to provide for those supportive services (speech, counseling, and so on) that ensure the benefit of special education.

Education of the Handicapped Act Amendments of 1986 (P.L. 99-457). In 1986 P.L. 99-457 was passed to allow for the provision of federal funding to states to develop and implement a statewide, comprehensive, coordinated, and multidisciplinary program of early intervention services for handicapped infants and toddlers and their families.

Family and Medical Leave Act (FMLA). Signed into law in 1993 FMLA allows eligible employees to take up to 12 weeks of unpaid leave from their jobs every year to care for newborn or newly adopted children; to care for children, parents, or spouses who have serious health conditions; or to recover from their own serious health conditions. After the leave, the law entitles employees to return to their previous jobs or to equivalent jobs with the same pay, benefits, and other conditions.

Despite the number of federal and state programs available to assist children and families, there are serious barriers to health care in the United States, including (1) **financial barriers,** such as not having insurance or having insurance that does not cover certain services; (2) **system barriers,** such as having to travel great distances for health care or state-to-state variations in Medicaid benefits; and (3) **knowledge barriers,** such as not knowing about the need or value of prenatal or child health supervision or being unaware of the services that are available. The current thrust in health care initiative is to improve children's and families' access to health care.

One of the most drastic changes in health care delivery has been the establishment of a prospective payment system based on *diagnosis-related groups (DRGs)*. The DRG categories allow pretreatment (prospective) billing for almost all U.S. hospitals reimbursed by Medicare. With hospitals now financially responsible when Medicare patients exceed the allotted admission stay, more patients are being discharged early. This has created an immense need for home care and other sources of community-based services. The exact impact DRGs will have on pediatric care is uncertain, but because health care cost containment is a national priority, it is inevitable that some form of prospective payment will affect children. Nurses need to be aware of the changing economics and prepared to meet the challenges, especially those related to the movement of care to **health maintenance organizations (HMOs).**

Pediatric Nursing

PHILOSOPHY OF CARE

Nursing of infants and children is consistent with the **definition of nursing** as "the diagnosis and treatment of human responses to actual or potential health problems." The definition incorporates the four essential features of contemporary nursing practice:

1. Attention to the full range of human experiences and responses to health and illness without restriction to a problem-focused orientation
2. Integration of objective data with knowledge gained from an understanding of the patient or group's subjective experience
3. Application of scientific knowledge to the processes of diagnosis and treatment
4. Provision of a caring relationship that facilitates health and healing (American Nurses Association, 1995)

Its goal is to promote the highest possible state of health in each child within the family system. To accomplish this goal, this section focuses on key philosophies of care that guide nursing practice regardless of the child's condition.

Family-Centered Care

The philosophy of **family-centered care** recognizes the family as the constant in a child's life and that service systems and personnel must support, respect, encourage, and enhance the strength and competence of the family (Johnson, McGonigel, and Kaufmann, 1989). Families are supported in their natural caregiving and decision-making roles by building on their unique strengths as individuals and families. Patterns of living at home and in the community are promoted. The needs of all family members, not just the child's, are considered (Box 27-1). The philosophy acknowledges diversity among family structures and backgrounds; family goals, dreams, strategies, and actions; and family support, service, and information needs (Ahmann, 1994).*

BOX 27-1
The Key Elements of Family-Centered Care

Incorporating into policy and practice the recognition that the *family is the constant* in a child's life while the service systems and support personnel within those systems fluctuate

Facilitating *family/professional collaboration* at all levels of hospital, home, and community care:
- Care of an individual child
- Program development, implementation, and evaluation
- Policy formation

Exchanging complete and unbiased information between family members and professionals in a supportive manner at all times

Incorporating into policy and practice the recognition and *honoring of cultural diversity*, strengths, and individuality within and across all families, including *ethnic, racial, spiritual, social, economic, educational,* and *geographic diversity*

Recognizing and respecting *different methods of coping* and implementing comprehensive policies and programs that provide *developmental, educational, emotional, environmental, and financial support* to meet the diverse needs of families

Encouraging and facilitating *family-to-family support* and networking

Ensuring that *home, hospital,* and *community service* and *support systems* for children needing specialized health and developmental care and their families are *flexible, accessible, and comprehensive* in responding to diverse family-identified needs

Appreciating families as families and children as children, recognizing that they possess a wide range of strengths, concerns, emotions, and aspirations beyond their need for specialized health and developmental services and support

From Shelton TL, Stepanek JS: *Family-centered care for children needing specialized health and developmental services*, Bethesda, Md, 1994, Association for the Care of Children's Health.

Two basic concepts in this process are enabling and empowerment. Professionals *enable* families by creating opportunities and means for all family members to display their present abilities and competencies and to acquire new ones that are necessary to meet the needs of the child and family. **Empowerment** describes the interaction of professionals with families in such a way that families maintain or acquire a sense of control over their family lives and attribute positive changes that result from helping behaviors that foster their own strengths, abilities, and actions (Dunst, Trivette, and Deal, 1988).

The *parent-professional partnership*† is a powerful mechanism for enabling and empowering families. Parents serve as

*Resources on family-centered care are available from the **Association for Care of Children's Health,** 7910 Woodmont Ave., Suite 300, Bethesda, MD 20814; (301) 654-6549. A facilitator's guide, *Recognizing Family-Centered Care*, and other publications are available from **Project Copernicus,** 2911 E. Biddle St., Baltimore, MD 21213; (410) 550-9700.

†For information about parent-professional partnerships, a free pamphlet, *Equals in This Partnership*, is available from **The National Center for Infants, Toddlers, and Families,** 34 15th Street NW, Washington, DC, 20005-1013, (202) 638-1144.

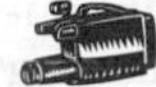
For additional information, please view "Family-Centered Care" in *Whaley and Wong's Pediatric Nursing Video Series*, St. Louis, 1996, Mosby; (800) 426-4545.

respected equals with professionals† and have the rightful role in deciding what is important for themselves and their family; the professional's role is to support and strengthen the family's ability to nurture and promote its members' development in a way that is both enabling and empowering.

Partnerships imply the belief that partners are capable individuals who become more capable by sharing knowledge, skills, and resources in a manner that benefits all participants. Collaboration is viewed as a continuum. Families have the option of being anywhere along that continuum, depending on the strengths and needs of the child, the family, and the professionals who are involved (Shelton, Jeppson, and Johnson, 1987). The nurse can help *every* family, including those with a previous history of serious personal and/or family problems, to identify their strengths, build on them, and assume a comfortable level of participation. Although caring for the family is strongly emphasized throughout the text, it is also highlighted in features such as Cultural Considerations and Family Home Care boxes.

Atraumatic Care

Although tremendous advances have been made in pediatric care, much of what is done to children to cure illness and prolong life is traumatic, painful, upsetting, and frightening. Unfortunately, minimizing the trauma of medical interventions has not kept pace with the technologic advances. With knowledge of the stressors imposed on ill children and their families and armed with interventions shown to be safe and effective in eliminating or reducing the stressors, health professionals must direct their attention to providing care that is as atraumatic as possible.

Atraumatic care is the provision of therapeutic care in settings, by personnel, and through the use of interventions that eliminates or minimizes the psychologic and physical distress experienced by children and their families in the health care system. **Therapeutic care** encompasses the prevention, diagnosis, treatment, or palliation of chronic or acute conditions. *Setting* refers to whatever place that care is given—the home, the hospital, or any other health care setting. *Personnel* include anyone directly involved with providing therapeutic care. *Interventions* range from psychologic approaches such as preparing children for procedures to physical interventions such as providing space for a parent to room in. *Psychologic distress* may include anxiety, fear, anger, disappointment, sadness, shame, or guilt. *Physical distress* may range from sleeplessness and immobilization to the experience of disturbing sensory stimuli, such as pain, temperature extremes, loud noises, bright lights, or darkness. Simply, atraumatic care is concerned with the who, what, when, where, why, and how of any procedure performed on a child for the purpose of preventing or minimizing psychologic and physical stress (Wong, 1989).

The overriding goal in providing atraumatic care is *first, do no harm.* Three principles provide the framework for achieving this goal: (1) prevent or minimize the child's separation from the family; (2) promote a sense of control; and (3) prevent or minimize bodily injury and pain. Examples of providing atraumatic care include fostering the parent-child relationship during hospitalization, preparing the child before any unfamiliar treatment or procedure, controlling pain, allowing the child privacy, providing play activities for expression of fear and aggression, minimizing loss of control, and respecting cultural differences.

Throughout this text the concept of atraumatic care is an integral part of all discussions of nursing care. Selected examples are highlighted in Atraumatic Care boxes. Many other boxes and tables focusing on culture, family teaching, research, and critical thinking incorporate aspects of providing care as atraumatically as possible. Chapter 40, Reaction to Illness and Hospitalization, is organized according to the principles of providing atraumatic care.

Primary Nursing

Part of the trend in nursing practice, particularly in pediatrics, is a deeper commitment to patient accountability. One of the outgrowths of this has been the movement toward **primary nursing,** which involves 24-hour responsibility and accountability by one nurse for the care of a small group of patients. The primary nurse becomes the bedside nurse, with few if any duties delegated to other staff. If responsibilities are shared, it is usually with an associate primary nurse who maintains continuity of care when the primary nurse is not working.

One of the traditional problems with primary nursing is providing consistency in scheduling the same nurse and associate. An approach that minimizes this difficulty is to designate one primary nurse and as many associates as are needed to ensure that the same group of nurses care for the child. This group of nurses forms the *primary core.* One nurse is assigned to the patient for each shift, and additional nurses are assigned for these individuals' days off. By identifying the primary core for a specific period in advance, all the nurses working with the child can plan care jointly, with the primary nurse maintaining overall responsibility.

The philosophy of primary care is supported throughout the discussion of nursing of children. In some instances the one-to-one relationship between child and nurse is emphasized because of its therapeutic benefit, such as in nonorganic failure to thrive. However, primary nursing is universally a supportive intervention in pediatric nursing because it provides a consistent caregiver for the child and focuses on the family unit as an integral component in the planning and implementation of care.

Case Management*

Nursing case management is an extension of primary nursing (Weinstein, 1991). As a general concept, **case management** is a care delivery system that balances cost and quality and was created in response to pressure from payers to provide care in a more cost-effective manner. Although the movement to case management began in adult care, it was quickly adapted to pediatric care. Simultaneously, benefits to case management, such as improved patient/family satisfaction, decreased fragmentation of care, and the ability to describe and measure outcomes for a homogenous group of patients, became apparent.

Case management is not a new concept. It has been used in outpatient settings, primarily by assigning a case manager to a particular patient or group of patients. The new model includes a timeline for care as a component of the

*Annette C. Bollig, MSN, RN, wrote this section.

process. These timelines for care have a variety of names: critical paths, guidelines for care, case management plans, Caremaps,* coordinated care plans, or other titles that are agreed on within a specific agency. Regardless of the name given to the timeline, these are multidisciplinary plans that include all of the components of care for an episode or multiple episodes of illness, as well as the outcomes that are expected as a result of delivering that care. They can be confined to inpatient care or can include the entire continuum of care, including home care (see also Chapter 40).

Concurrent with the movement to provide care in a systematic manner have been efforts by professional and government organizations to develop *clinical practice guidelines* for the care of an illness, disease, or related problem. Although timelines for care are usually developed within an institution and reflect local practice patterns, clinical guidelines are being developed on a national level that reflect the research that has been conducted relative to a specific disease or illness. A federal agency that is developing clinical guidelines is the *Agency for Health Care Policy and Research (AHCPR).*†

As the movement for providing care based on guidelines continues, institutions will be challenged to incorporate clinical guidelines into the timelines for care that are developed locally. The result of this effort will mean that professionally developed clinical guidelines will be integrated into practice at the local level.

Because of the movement to provide care based on clinical guidelines, it is expected that in the future, payment for health care will also be tied to clinical guidelines. This effort will provide encouragement for care to be provided in the most cost-effective manner while ensuring that care is based on guidelines that reflect current research rather than traditional practice.

With the present efforts to improve the health care system in the United States and to provide universal health coverage while controlling costs, managed care has become a key model in health care reform. Nurses should take an active role in being part of the final plan and in creating opportunities for the profession to be a leader, not a follower, in delivery of care (Hemphill and Biester, 1994).

ROLE OF THE PEDIATRIC NURSE

Therapeutic Relationship

The establishment of a therapeutic relationship is the essential foundation for providing quality nursing care (Price, 1993). Pediatric nurses need to be meaningfully related to children and their families and yet separate enough to distinguish their own feelings and needs. In a **therapeutic relationship,** caring, well-defined boundaries separate the nurse from the child and family. These boundaries are positive and professional, and promote the family's control over the child's health care (Barnsteiner and Gillis-Donovan, 1990). Both the nurse and the family are empowered, and open communication is maintained. In a **nontherapeutic relationship,** these boundaries are blurred, and many of the nurse's actions may serve personal needs, such as a need to feel wanted and involved, rather than the family's needs.

Relevant in all settings, a family-centered approach to nursing practice is most obvious in the home care arena. However, it is in the home care setting where nurses face the greatest challenge in determining the boundary between a collaborative relationship with the family and becoming part of the family system. Several factors challenge the maintenance of such clear boundaries: the informal home environment, the casual social conversations that occur with family members throughout the day, the participation by family members in care of the child, and the attempt by some families to reduce the stress of having a stranger in the home by incorporating the nurse as a member of the family.

Exploring whether relationships with patients are therapeutic or nontherapeutic can help nurses identify problem areas early in their interactions with children and families. Although questions for exploring types of involvement can be labeled negative or positive, no one action makes a relationship therapeutic or nontherapeutic. For example, a nurse may spend additional time with the family but still recognize his or her own needs and maintain professional separateness. An important clue to nontherapeutic relationships is the staff's concerns about their peer's actions with the family.

Family Advocacy/Caring

Although the nurse is responsible to self, the profession, and the institution of employment, the primary responsibility is to the consumer of nursing services, the child and family. The nurse must work with members of the family, identifying *their* goals and needs, and plan interventions that best meet the defined problems. As an advocate, the nurse assists children and their families in making informed choices and acting in the child's best interest (Rushton, 1993). Advocacy involves ensuring that families are aware of all available health services, informed adequately of treatments and procedures, involved in the child's care, and encouraged to change or support existing health care practices. The United Nations Declaration of the Rights of the Child (Box 27-2) provides guidelines for nursing practice to ensure that every child receives optimum care. The nurse uses this knowledge to adapt care for the child's optimum physical and emotional well-being.

BOX 27-2
United Nations' Declaration of the Rights of the Child

All children need:
- To be free from discrimination
- To develop physically and mentally in freedom and dignity
- To have a name and nationality
- To have adequate nutrition, housing, recreation, and medical services
- To receive special treatment if handicapped
- To receive love, understanding, and material security
- To receive an education and develop his or her abilities
- To be the first to receive protection in disaster
- To be protected from neglect, cruelty, and exploitation
- To be brought up in a spirit of friendship among people

*Caremap is a registered trademark of the **Center for Case Management, Inc.,** South Natick, MA.

†To order guidelines, contact **AHCPR Publications Clearinghouse,** PO Box 8547, Silver Spring, MD 20907; (800) 358-9295.

As nurses care for children and families, they must demonstrate *caring*, expressing compassion and empathy for others. Aspects of caring embody the concept of atraumatic care and the development of a therapeutic relationship with clients. Parents perceive caring as a sign of quality nursing care, which is often focused on the nontechnical needs of the child and family. Parents describe "personable" care as actions by the nurse, including acknowledging the parent's presence, listening, making the parent feel comfortable in the hospital environment, involving the parent and child in the nursing care, showing interest and concern for their welfare, showing affection and sensitivity to the parent and child, communicating with them, and individualizing the nursing care. Parents perceive "personable" nursing care as being integral to establishing a positive relationship (Price, 1993).

The nurse is aware of the needs of children and works with all caregivers to ensure that these fundamental requirements are met. This often necessitates that the nurse expand the boundaries of practice to less traditional settings. The nurse may be involved in education, political/legislative change, rehabilitation, screening, administration, and even engineering and architecture. Regardless of how removed from direct patient care individual nurses become, they continue to foster health care practices that promote the well-being of children by incorporating knowledge of child growth and development into particular roles of practice. For example, as educator the nurse has the primary responsibility of helping others learn about and care for children. Their audience may be other nurses, parents, schoolteachers, other members of the health team, or the general public. In some states nurses are involved in mass media programs for immunization of all children.

Disease Prevention/Health Promotion

The trends toward health care have been prevention of illness and maintenance of health, rather than treatment of disease or disability. Nursing has kept pace with this change, especially in the area of child care. In 1965, specialized **pediatric nurse practitioner (PNP)** programs began to develop that have led to several specialized ambulatory or primary care roles for nurses. The thrust of these programs has been to educate nurses beyond the basic preparational stage in areas of child health maintenance so that all children can receive high-quality care (Lancaster and Lancaster, 1993). The practitioner programs have expanded to prepare school nurse, developmental, and oncology pediatric nurse practitioners. Although the curriculum varies, the course content generally includes history taking, physical diagnosis, growth and development, health education, pharmacology, counseling, common childhood problems, and planning care for individuals and groups. Most of these programs are now part of graduate nursing education.

The **clinical nurse specialist (CNS)** role has been developed in an attempt to provide expert nursing care. In addition, the CNS serves as a role model for the staff's clinical practice, as a researcher to validate nursing observations and interventions, as a change agent within the health care system, and as a consultant/teacher to the health care team (Naylor and Brooten, 1993). The clinical specialist is competent in providing nursing care during all stages of illness or wellness and functions in any of the settings where patients may be found—the hospital, home, community, clinic, or long-term facility. The CNS role has developed within each of the traditional specialty areas and includes subspecialties, such as cardiovascular, oncologic, and neurologic pediatric CNS. The educational preparation includes a graduate degree in nursing. Several graduate programs now combine the PNP and CNS roles. Although the title for the merged roles varies, these nurses are commonly called **advanced nurse practitioners (ANP** or **ARNP)** (Jackson, 1995).

Every nurse involved with child care must practice preventive health. Regardless of the identified problem, the role of the nurse is to plan care that fosters every aspect of growth and development. Based on a thorough assessment process, problems related to nutrition, immunizations, safety, dental care, development, socialization, discipline, or schooling often become obvious. Once the problem is identified, the nurse acts to intervene directly or to refer the family to other health persons or agencies.

The best approach to prevention is education and anticipatory guidance. An appreciation of the hazards or conflicts of each developmental period enables the nurse to guide parents regarding childrearing practices aimed at preventing potential problems. One of the most significant examples is safety. Since each age-group is at risk for special types of injuries, preventive teaching can help prevent most injuries, thus significantly lowering permanent disability and mortality from injuries in children.

Prevention also involves less obvious aspects of child care. Besides preventing physical disease or injury, the nurse's role is also to promote mental health. For example, it is not sufficient to administer immunizations without regard for the psychologic trauma associated with the procedure. Optimum health involves the practice of good medicine with a humane approach to health care; the nurse is often the one professional capable of ensuring "humanity."

Health Teaching

Health teaching is inseparable from family advocacy and prevention. Health teaching may be a direct goal of the nurse, such as during parenting classes, or may be indirect, such as helping parents and children understand a diagnosis or medical treatment, encouraging children to ask questions about their bodies, referring families to health-related professional or lay groups, supplying patients with appropriate literature, and providing anticipatory guidance.

Health teaching is often one area in which nurses need preparation and practice with competent role models, because it involves transmitting information at the child and family's level of understanding and desire for information. As an effective educator, the nurse focuses on giving appropriate health teaching with generous feedback and evaluation to promote learning.

Support/Counseling

Attention to emotional needs requires support and sometimes counseling. Often the role of child advocate or health teacher is supportive by the very nature of the individualized approach. Support can be offered in many ways, the most common of which include listening, touching, and physical presence. The last two are most helpful with children because they facilitate nonverbal communication.

Counseling involves a mutual exchange of ideas and opinions that provides the basis for mutual problem solving. It involves support, as well as teaching, techniques to foster expression of feelings or thoughts, and approaches to help the family cope with stress. Optimally, counseling not only helps resolve a crisis or problem, but also enables the family to attain a higher level of functioning, greater self-esteem, and closer relationships. Although counseling is often the role of nurses in more specialized areas, counseling techniques are discussed in various sections of the text to help students and nurses cope with immediate crises and refer families for additional professional assistance.

Restorative Role

The most basic of all nursing roles is the restoration of health through caregiving activities. Nurses are intimately involved with meeting the physical and emotional needs of children, including feeding, bathing, toileting, dressing, security, and socialization. Although they are responsible for instituting physicians' orders, they are also held singularly accountable for their own actions and judgments regardless of written orders.

A significant aspect of restoration of health is continual assessment and evaluation of physical status. Indeed, the concentrated focus throughout the text on physical assessment, pathophysiology, and scientific rationale for therapy is to assist the nurse in decision making regarding health status. The nurse must be aware of normal findings in order to intelligently identify and document deviations. In addition, the pediatric nurse never loses sight of the emotional and developmental needs of the individual child, which can significantly influence the course of the disease process.

Coordination/Collaboration

The nurse, as a member of the health team, collaborates and coordinates nursing services with the activities of other professionals. Working in isolation does not serve the child's best interest. First, the concept of "holistic care" can only be realized through a unified interdisciplinary approach. Second, being aware of individual contributions and limitations to the child's care, the nurse must collaborate with other specialists to provide for high-quality health services. Failure to recognize limitations can be nontherapeutic at best and destructive at worst. For example, the nurse who feels competent in counseling but who is really inadequate in this area may not only prevent the child from dealing with a crisis but may also impede future success with a qualified professional.

Even nurses who practice in isolated geographic areas widely separated from other health professionals cannot be considered independent. Every nurse works interdependently with the child and family, collaborating on needs and interventions so that the final care plan is one that truly meets the child's needs. Unfortunately, this is one aspect of collaboration and coordination that is lacking in health care planning. Often numerous disciplines work together to formulate a comprehensive approach without consulting with clients regarding their ideas or preferences. The nurse is in a vital position to include consumers in their care, either directly or indirectly, by communicating their thoughts to the health team.

Ethical Decision Making*

Ethical dilemmas arise when competing moral considerations underlie various alternatives. Parents, nurses, physicians, and other health care team members may reach different but morally defensible decisions by assigning different weight to the competing moral values. These competing moral values may include *autonomy*, the patient's right to be self-governing; *nonmaleficence*, the obligation to minimize or prevent harm; *beneficence*, the obligation to promote the patient's well-being; and *justice*, the concept of fairness (Erlen and Burns, 1992). Thus nurses must determine the most beneficial or least harmful action within the framework of societal mores, professional practice standards, the law, institutional rules, religious traditions, the family's value system, and the nurse's personal values.

When ethical conflicts occur, nurses may experience conflicting loyalties to their profession, colleagues, patients and families, institutions, and society. Moreover, the nurse's role in ethical decision making can be ambiguous. A nurse may be obliged to carry out procedures based on physician orders or hospital policy that are inconsistent with the patient's best interest. At times, members of the health care team do not seek the nurse's input or involvement, leaving the nurse with incomplete information about the clinical situation or without a voice in decision making.

The role of nurses as members of the health care team justifies their participation in collaborative ethical decision making. Nurses routinely use systematic problem-solving skills, known as the nursing process, to resolve clinical problems. Each decision requires the nurse to collect pertinent physiologic and psychosocial data, assess relevant values held by the patient and family, and incorporate those data into a plan of care. Each of these activities is a crucial component of ethical decision making.

Furthermore, since nurses spend the most time directly caring for the child, they are in a unique position to provide insight about the patient's condition and response to therapy. In addition, they assist families in dealing with their grief and stress and often interpret information regarding the child's condition, prognosis, and treatment options to help families make informed decisions. Because of their relationship to families, nurses are often able to represent the child's and parent's values, beliefs, and preferences, thus serving as an important liaison for communication between the family and other health team members.

The nurse can also use the professional code of ethics for guidance. A code of ethics provides one means for professional self-regulation. The Code for Nurses by the American Nurses' Association focuses on the nurse's accountability and responsibility to the client and emphasizes the nursing role as an independent professional role that upholds its own legal liability (Box 27-3).

Nurses must prepare themselves systematically for collaborative ethical decision making. This can be accomplished through formal coursework, continuing education, contemporary literature, and working to establish an environment conducive to ethical discourse. Moreover, nurses must be knowledgeable about mechanisms for dispute resolution, case review by ethics committees, procedural safeguards, state statutes, and case law.

Research

Practicing nurses should contribute to research, since they are the individuals observing human responses to health and illness. Unfortunately, few nurses systematically record or an-

*Cindy Hylton Rushton, PhD, RN, C, FAAN, wrote this section.

alyze such observations. For example, pediatric nurses devise innovative methods to encourage children to comply with treatments. Only if these interventions are clinically evaluated and shared with other nurses, especially through publications, can a body of knowledge on nursing practice develop.

Research also implies a questioning of *why* something is effective and *if* there is a better approach. Evaluation is essential to the nursing process, and research is one of the best ways to accomplish this. Therefore nurses need to be more involved in research and in applying research findings to their practice. Throughout the text, research relevant to nursing of children and families is incorporated as appropriate. Research findings are presented to encourage nurses to base their practice on theoretic foundations, not tradition.

Health Care Planning

Up to this point, the nurse's role has been viewed through the nucleus of a family. However, the nursing role is far more extensive and includes the community or society as a whole. Traditionally, nurses have been involved in public health care, on either a continuous or an episodic basis. Rarely, however, have nurses been involved in health care planning, especially on a political or legislative level. Their role must also involve the decision-making body of government. Nursing, as the largest health care profession, needs to have a voice, especially as family/consumer advocate. This does not mean that the nurse must hold public office. Rather, it suggests knowledge and awareness of community needs, interest in government formulation of bills, support of politicians to ensure passage (or rejection) of significant legislation, and active involvement in groups dedicated to the welfare of children, such as professional nursing societies, parent-teacher organizations, parent support groups, religious organizations, and voluntary organizations.

BOX 27-3

Code for Nurses

1. The nurse provides services with respect for human dignity and the uniqueness of the client unrestricted by considerations of social or economic status, personal attributes, or the nature of health problems.
2. The nurse safeguards the client's right to privacy by judiciously protecting information of a confidential nature.
3. The nurse acts to safeguard the client and the public when health care and safety are affected by the incompetent, unethical, or illegal practice of any person.
4. The nurse assumes responsibility and accountability for individual nursing judgments and actions.
5. The nurse maintains competence in nursing.
6. The nurse exercises informed judgment and uses individual competence and qualifications as criteria in seeking consultation, accepting responsibilities, and delegating nursing activities to others.
7. The nurse participates in activities that contribute to the ongoing development of the profession's body of knowledge.
8. The nurse participates in the profession's efforts to implement and improve standards of nursing.
9. The nurse participates in the profession's efforts to establish and maintain conditions of employment conducive to high-quality nursing care.
10. The nurse participates in the profession's effort to protect the public from misinformation and misrepresentation and to maintain the integrity of nursing.
11. The nurse collaborates with members of the health professions and other citizens in promoting community and national efforts to meet the health needs of the public.

American Nurses' Association, 1976, 1985. Reproduced with permission of the American Nurses' Association.

Health care planning involves not only providing new services, but also promoting the highest quality of existing ones. Nursing needs to ensure the excellence of its own profession through each individual member, who practices according to the Code of Nurses and standards of practice. A **standard of practice** is the level of performance that is expected of a professional. Pediatric nurses are obligated to follow the *Standards of Maternal-Child Health Nursing* and specific standards for their specialty, such as pediatric oncology nursing or school nursing.* They should also be involved in making certain their colleagues implement the standards, through education, role modeling, and supervision.

Throughout the text the highest standards of nursing practice are continually reflected in the emphasis on thorough assessment, focus on scientific rationale as the basis for care, summary of nursing care goals and responsibilities, and comprehensive discussion of growth and development. Family-centered principles are continually evident in the consideration of dynamics affecting the child, parents, siblings, and extended members. The nurse is viewed as a vital component of the health care delivery system. Although nursing functions are clearly outlined, nursing responsibilities must be equally emphasized.

FUTURE TRENDS

The present shift in focus from treatment of disease to promotion of health is likely to further expand nurses' roles in ambulatory care, with prevention and health teaching receiving a major emphasis. As prospective payment becomes a certainty in pediatric care, the need for home care and community health services will necessitate that nurses become more independent and highly skilled beyond the traditional care settings. Both of these trends are illustrated throughout the book, with increased emphasis on prevention through anticipatory guidance, child health and family assessment, and discharge planning and home care. As changing social policy shapes the expanding health care arena, the focus of nursing care is no longer what nurses *do for* families, but rather what they *do with* them (Plotnick and Presler, 1996). Therefore the philosophy of family-centered care is no longer an option but a mandate.

Technologic advances will also influence pediatric nurses' roles. Increasing technical skills related to patient care, as well as the demand for computer knowledge in the work setting, are inevitable future trends. As more positions are created in the health care system that do not require a nursing background, such as "patient care educator," or unlicensed assistive personnel, nurses will be required to continually update their knowledge and prove their unique contribution. **Unli-**

*Available from the **Association of Pediatric Oncology Nurses,** 4700 W. Lake Ave., Glenview, IL 60025-1485, (708) 375-4700, fax (708) 375-4777; and the **National Association of School Nurses,** Lamplighter Lane, P.O. Box 1300, Scarborough, ME 04074, (207) 883-2117.

censed assistive personnel (UAP) "are individuals who are trained to function in an assistive role to the registered professional nurse in the provision of [student] care activities as delegated by and under the supervision of the registered professional nurse" (American Nurses Association, 1994).

> **Nursing ALERT**
>
> When the registered nurse determines that someone who is not licensed to practice nursing can safely provide a selected nursing activity or task for a patient and delegates that activity to the individual, the nurse remains responsible and accountable for the care provided.

Changing demographics will also affect pediatric nursing. The actual number of children in the United States under the age of 18 years will increase from 64.3 million in 1990 to an estimated 78 million in 2020, but their relative importance in terms of proportion of the total population will decrease from 26% to 24%. In other words, the adult population is growing faster than the pediatric population. Accompanying this trend is a decrease in younger children and an increase in older children, as well as a decrease in the Caucasian population with an increase in minority groups. For example, Caucasian births are expected to decline in the 1990s, African-American births are projected to rise, and the largest increases will occur in Hispanic (70%) and Asian (50%) births (Guyer et al, 1995). Such changes will impact the delivery of health care, with problems of adolescents and minority groups taking on more significance. As the elderly make up a larger percentage of the population, health care dollars will be split between the youngest and the oldest groups, with shrinking resources having to meet the needs of both. Nurses will need to keep abreast of developments in adolescent medicine and continually adapt their care to the cultural milieu in which they practice. An ever-present challenge will be cost containment without sacrificing quality care.

Key Points

- *Healthy People 2000* sets the health care objectives for the 1990s and focuses on prevention as the method of achieving its goals.
- Although the infant mortality rate in the United States is at an all-time low, the United States lags significantly behind most other well-developed countries.
- Birth weight is the leading determinant of neonatal death in developed countries.
- Injuries are the leading cause of death in children over age 1 year, with the majority resulting from motor vehicle injuries.
- Childhood morbidity encompasses acute illness, chronic disease, and disability.
- Of childhood illness, 80% are attributable to infections, with respiratory tract infections occurring two to three times as often as all other illnesses combined.
- The "new morbidity," or "pediatric social illness," refers to behavioral, social, and educational problems that can significantly alter a child's health.
- The study of pediatrics began in the last half of the 1800s under the influence of Abraham Jacobi, who is referred to as the Father of Pediatrics.
- The work of Lillian Wald, a social reformer, has had far-reaching effects on child health and nursing. She started visiting nurse services in New York City and was instrumental in establishing the role of the first full-time school nurse.
- Primary nursing involves care and accountability by one nurse for a small patient population.
- The philosophy of **family-centered care** recognizes the family as the constant in a child's life and that service systems and personnel must support, respect, encourage, and enhance the strength and competence of the family.
- The pediatric nurse's roles include a therapeutic relationship, family advocacy, disease prevention/health promotion, health teaching, support-counseling, coordination/collaboration, ethical decision making, research, and health care planning.
- With the shift in focus from treatment of disease to promotion of health, nurses' roles may expand in ambulatory care, with emphasis on prevention and health teaching.
- Changing demographics will result in greater significance of adolescents' and minority groups' problems and decreasing resources for health care.

References

Ahmann E: Family-centered care: the time has come, *Pediatr Nurs* 20(1):52-53, 1994.

American Academy of Pediatrics, Committee on Early Childhood, Adoption, and Dependent Care: Initial medical evaluation of an adopted child, *Pediatrics* 88(3):642-644, 1991.

American Academy of Pediatrics, Committee on Injury and Poison Prevention: Bicycle helmets, *Pediatrics* 95(4):609-610, 1995.

American Academy of Pediatrics, Committee on Psychosocial Aspects of Child and Family Health: The pediatrician and the "new morbidity," *Pediatrics* 92(5):731-733, 1993.

American Nurses Association: *Nursing's social policy statement*, Washington, DC, 1995, American Nurses Publishing.

American Nurses' Association: *Registered professional nurses & unlicensed assistive personnel*, Washington, DC, 1994, American Nurses Publishing.

Barnsteiner J, Gillis-Donovan J: Being related and separate: a standard for therapeutic relationships *MCN* 15(4):223-228, 1990.

Child health USA '94, US Department of Health and Human Services, Public Health Service, Health Resources and Services Administration, Maternal and Child Health Bureau, DHHS Pub. No. HRSA-MCH-95-1, Washington, DC, July 1995.

Christoffel K et al: Psychosocial factors in childhood pedestrian injury: a matched case-control study, *Pediatrics* 97(1):33-42, 1996.

Cone TE Jr: Highlights of two centuries of American pediatrics, 1776-1976, *Am J Dis Child* 130:762-775, 1976.

Division of Injury Control, Center for Environmental Health and Injury Control, Centers for Disease Control: Childhood injuries in the United States, *Am J Dis Child* 144(6):627-646, 1990.

Dunst C, Trivette C, Deal A: *Enabling and empowering families*, Cambridge, Mass, 1988, Brookline Books.

Erlen JA, Burns JA: Demystifying ethical decision making, *Orthop Nurs* 11(1):49-53, 1992.

Gortmaker S et al: Chronic conditions, socioeconomic risks, and behavioral problems in children and adolescents, *Pediatrics* 85(3):267-276, 1990.

Guyer B et al: Annual summary of vital statistics—1994, *Pediatrics* 96(6):1029-1039, 1995.

Healthy people, 2000—national health promotion and disease prevention objectives, GPO 017-001-00474-0, Washington, DC, 1991, US Public Health Service.

Hemphill NP, Biester DJ: Case management in a reformed health care system, *J Pediatr Nurs* 9(2):124-125, 1994.

Jackson PL: Opportunities and challenges for pediatric nurse practitioners, *Pediatr Nurs* 21(1):43-46, 1995.

Johnson BH, McGonigel M, Kaufmann R, editors: *Guidelines and recommended practices for the Individualized Family Service Plan*, Washington, DC, 1989, Association for the Care of Children's Health.

Khoury MJ, Erickson JD: Improved ascertainment of cardiovascular malformations in infants with Down's syndrome, Atlanta, 1968 through 1989: implications for the interpretation of increasing rates of cardiovascular malformations in surveillance systems, *Am J Epidemiol* 136(12):1457–1464, 1992.

Kochanek KD, Hudson BL: Advance report of final mortality statistics, 1992, *Mon Vit Stat Rep* 43(6):65, Hyattsville, Md, 1995, National Center for Health Statistics.

Lancaster J, Lancaster W: Nurse practitioners: health care providers whose time has come, *Fam Community Health* 16(2):1-8, 1993.

Mason JO, McGinnis JM: Healthy people 2000: an overview of the national health promotion and disease prevention objectives, *Public Health Rep* 105(5):441-446, 1990.

Mili F et al: Prevalence of birth defects among low–birth weight infants, *Am J Dis Child* 145(11):1313-1318, 1991.

Naeye RL: Race and infant mortality, *Am J Dis Child* 147(10):1030-1031, 1993.

Nakamura RM and others: Excess infant mortality in an American Indian population, 1940-1990, *JAMA* 266(16):2244-2248, 1991.

Naylor MD, Brooten D: The roles and functions of clinical nurse specialists, *Image J Nurs Sch* 25(1):73-78, 1993.

Pless I: *Morbidity and mortality among the young*. In Hoekelman RA et al, editors: *Primary pediatric care*, ed 2, St Louis, 1992, Mosby.

Plotnick J, Presler B: Rugged individualism and compassion: the foundation of public policy, *MCN* 21(1):20-33, 1996.

Price PJ: Parents' perceptions of the meaning of quality nursing care, *Adv Nurs Sci* 16(1):33-41, 1993.

Rachuba L, Stanton B, Howard D: Violent crime in the United States, *Arch Pediatr Adolesc Med* 149(9):953-960, 1995.

Rushton CH: Child/family advocacy: ethical issues, practical strategies, *Crit Care Med* 21(9):S387, 1993.

Schmidt WM: Health and welfare of colonial American children, *Am J Dis Child* 130:694-701, 1976.

Schoendorf KC et al: Mortality among infants of black as compared with white college-educated parents, *N Engl J Med* 326(23):1522-1526, 1992.

Shelton T, Jeppson E, Johnson B: *Family-centered care for children with special health care needs*, Washington, DC, 1987, Association for the Care of Children's Health.

Wegman ME: Annual summary of vital statistics—1993, *Pediatrics* 94(6):792-803, 1994.

Weinstein R: Hospital case management: the path to empowering nurses, *Pediatr Nurs* 17(3):289-293, 1991.

Wilcox AJ, Skjaerven R: Birth weight and perinatal mortality: the effect of gestational age, *Am J Public Health* 82(3):378-382, 1992.

Wong D: *Principles of atraumatic care*. In Feeg V, editor: *Pediatric nursing: forum on the future: looking toward the 21st century*, Pitman, NJ, 1989, Anthony J Jannetti.

Bibliography

Mortality and Morbidity

Bass JL et al: Childhood injury prevention counseling in primary care settings: a critical review of the literature, *Pediatrics* 92(4):544-550, 1993.

Blum RW et al: American Indian—Alaska native youth health, *JAMA* 267(12):1637-1644, 1992.

Dannenberg AL, Vernick JS: A proposal for the mandatory inclusion of helmets with new children's bicycles, *Am J Public Health* 83(5):644-646, 1993.

Fingerhut LA, Jones C, Makuc D: *Firearm and motor vehicle injury mortality—variations by state, race, and ethnicity: United States, 1990-91*, Advance data from vital and health statistics, No 242, Hyattsville, Md, 1994, National Center for Health Statistics.

Hall JR et al: Traumatic death in urban children, revisited, *Am J Dis Child* 147(1):102-107, 1993.

Igoe JB: Healthy people 2000, *Pediatr Nurs* 16(6):584-586, 1990.

Jones NE: Childhood injuries: an epidemiologic approach, *Pediatr Nurs* 18(3):235-239, 1992.

Jones NE: Childhood residential injuries, *MCN* 18(3):168-172, 1993.

Kliegman RM: Perpetual poverty: child health and the underclass, *Pediatrics* 89(4):710-713, 1992.

Lenaghan P: Healthy people 2000, *J Emerg Nurs* 18(5):480-481, 1992.

Mandelbaum JL: Child survival: what are the issues? *J Pediatr Health Care* 6(3):132-137, 1992.

Sewell KH, Gaines SK: A developmental approach to childhood safety education, *Pediatr Nurs* 19(5):464-466, 1993.

Society of Pediatric Nurses (SPN): Policy statement on pediatric firearm injuries, *SPN News* 4(1):7, 1995.

Society of Pediatric Nurses (SPN): Policy statement on pediatric injury prevention, *SPN News* 4(1):6, 1995.

Swartz MK: The handgun as a consumer product, *J Pediatr Health Care* 8(6):288-290, 1994.

Yanhauer A: A classic study of infant mortality—1911-1915, *Pediatr* 94(6):874-877, 1994.

Zadinsky JK, Boettcher JH: Preventability of infant mortality in a rural community, *Nurs Res* 41(4):223-227, 1992.

Evolution of Child Health Care

Arnold L et al: Lessons from the past, *MCN* 14(2):75-82, 1989.

Burns M, Thornam CB: Broadening the scope of nursing practice: federal programs for children, *Pediatr Nurs* 19(6):546-552, 1993.

Cone TE, Jr: *History of American pediatrics*, Boston, 1980, Little, Brown.

DeGraw C et al: Public law 99-457: new opportunities to serve young children with special needs, *J Pediatr* 113(6):971-974, 1988.

Farel A: Public health in early intervention: historic foundations for contemporary training, *Inf Young Child* 1(1):63-70, 1988.

Gale C: Inadequacy of health care for the nation's chronically ill children, *J Pediatr Health Care* 3(1):20-27, 1989.

Harvey B: New series of essays on pediatric history, *Pediatrics* 92(3):467-468, 1993.

Inglis AD: United States maternal and child health services, *Neonatal Network* 9(8):35-43, 1991.

McMillan JA: What we must do for children in the 1990s, *Contemp Pediatr* 7(7):28-50, 1990.

Oberg C: Medically uninsured children in the United States: a challenge to public policy, *Pediatrics* 85(5):824-833, 1990.

Velsor-Friedrich B: The federal government and child health, *J Pediatr Nurs* 5(1):56-58, 1990.

Williams BC, Miller CA: Preventive health care for young children: findings from a 10-country study and directions for United States policy, *Pediatrics* 89(5, suppl):983-998, 1992.

Pediatric Nursing

Barnsteiner JH et al: Defining and implementing a standard for therapeutic relationships, *J Holistic Nurs* 12(1):35-48, 1994.

Bell PL: Neonatal case management: a challenge for advanced practice nurses, *J Perinat Neonatal Nurs* 8(2):48-56, 1994.

Betz CL: Will nursing education respond to the changes in health care?, *J Pediatr Nurs* 10(2):81, 1995.

Bottorff JL: Nursing: a practice science of caring, *Adv Nurs Sci* 14(1):26-39, 1991.

Broome ME: A commentary on confronting the challenges, *Pediatr Nurs* 21(1):49-50, 1995.

Clochesy JM et al: Preparing advanced practice nurses for acute care, *Am J Crit Care* 3(4):255-259, 1994.

Delegation of School Health Services to Unlicensed Assistive Personnel: A position paper of the National Association of State School Nurse Consultants, *J School Nurs* 11(4):13-16, 1995.

El-Sherif C: Nurse practitioners—where do they belong within the organizational structure of the acute care setting? *Nurs Practitioner* 20(1):62-65, 1995.

Engleman SG: From myths to a critical path: what happens when someone asks why? *J Pediatr Nurs* 10(1):69-71, 1995.

Feeg VD: The future of pediatric nursing: anticipating the health care needs of children, *Imprint* 37(4):70-77, 1990.

Fein EZ: Keeping expert nurses expert, *MCN* 19(6):305-308, 1994.

Fenton M, Brykezynski K: Qualitative distinctions and similarities in the practice of clinical nurse specialists and nurse practitioners, *J Profess Nurs* 9:313-326, 1993.

Fry-Revere S: Ethics consultation: an update on accountability issues, *Neonatal Intens Care* 7(4):58-64, 1994.

Harper DC: Advanced practice nursing: changes on the horizon, *Pediatr Nurs* 21(1):41-42, 1995.

Hinds PS: Crossing the lines of professionalism, *J Pediatr Oncol Nurs* 11(4):137, 1994.

Hylton Rushton C, Armstrong L, McEnhill M: Establishing therapeutic boundaries as patient advocates, *Pediatr Nurs* 22(3):185–189, 1996.

Jerome JM, Ferraro-McDuffie AR: Nurse self-awareness in therapeutic relationships, *Pediatr Nurs* 18(2):153-156, 1992.

Keefe MR: An integrated approach to incorporating research findings into practice, *MCN* 18(2):65-70, 1993.

Kolcaba KY: The art of comfort care, *Image J Nurs Sch* 27(4):287-289, 1995.

Kowalski K et al: The high-touch paradigm: a 21st century model for maternal-child nursing, *MCN* 21(1):43-50, 1996.

Miltenberger-Olsen G: I am a nurse: a historical perspective, Bixby, Okla, 1995, Angel Wings Publishing.

Naylor M, Brooten D: The roles and functions of clinical nurse specialists, *Image J Nurs Scholarship* 25:73-78, 1993.

Pearson L: Annual update of how each state stands on legislative issues affecting advanced nursing practice, *Nurs Practition* 20(1):13-18, 1995.

Rushton CH, Infante MD: Keeping secrets: the ethical and legal challenges, *Pediatr Nurs* 21(5):479-482, 1995.

Totka JP: Exploring the boundaries of pediatric practice: nurse stories related to relationships, *Pediatr Nurs* 22(3):191–196, 1996.

Winslow EH: How patients define caring may surprise you. *AJN* 94(6):57-58, 1994.

Case Management

Crummette BD, Boatwright DN: Case management in inpatient pediatric nursing, *Pediatr Nurs* 17(5):469-73, 1991.

Davis B, Steele S: Case management for young children with special health care needs, *Pediatr Nurs* 17(1):15-20, 1991.

Elizondo AP: Nursing case management in the neonatal intensive care unit, part 2: developing critical pathways, *Neonat Net* 14(1):11-19, 1995.

Kaufman J: Case management services for children with special health care needs: a family-centered approach, *J Case Manag* 1(2):53-56, 1992.

Lewis CC et al: Care management for children who are medically fragile/technology-dependent, Issues *Comprehens Pediatric Nurs* 15(2):73-91, 1992.

Lynam L: Case management and critical pathways: friend or foe? *Neonat Net* 13(8):48-49, 51, 1994.

Patterson J: The role of nurse manager in a case management delivery system, *Pediatr Nurs* 17(3):282, 1991.

Smith LD: Continuity of care through nursing case management of the chronically ill child, *Clin Nurs Specialist* 8(2):65-68, 1994.

Steele S: Nurse and parent collaborative case management in a rural setting, *Pediatr Nurs* 19(6):612-615, 1993.

CHAPTER 28

Social, Cultural, and Religious Influences on Child Health Promotion

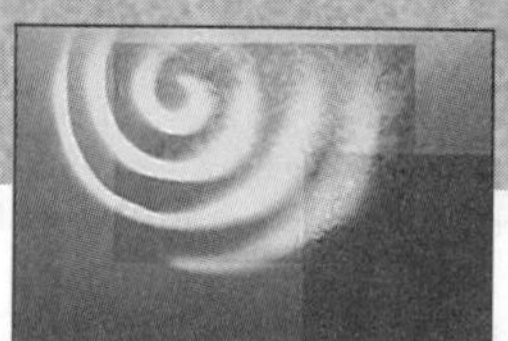

CULTURE, P. 800
Social roles, p. 801
Subcultural influences, p. 801
The child and family in North America, p. 805
Cultural shock, p. 806
CULTURAL/RELIGIOUS INFLUENCES ON HEALTH CARE, P. 806
Susceptibility to health problems, p. 806
Customs and folkways, p. 808
Health beliefs and practices, p. 811
Religious beliefs, p. 813
Importance of culture and religion to nurses, p. 813

Culture

A **culture** is a pattern of assumptions, beliefs, and practices that unconsciously frames or guides the outlook and decisions of a group of people (Buchwald et al, 1994). Culture differs from both race and ethnicity. Race is defined as a division of mankind possessing traits that are transmissible by descent and sufficient to characterize it as a distinct human type. One method of classifying race, based on skin color, is caucasoid (white), negroid (black), and mongoloid (yellow). **Ethnicity** is the affiliation of a set of persons who share a unique cultural, social, and linguistic heritage. **Socialization** is the process by which children acquire the beliefs, values, and behaviors of a given society in order to function within that group.

A culture is composed of individuals who share a set of values, beliefs, practices (language, dress, diet, health care), social relationships, law, politics, economics, and norms of behavior that is learned, integrative, social, and satisfying (Habayeb, 1995). Culture is not a surface veneer that covers a basic outlook shared by all human beings but an ingrained orientation to life that serves as a frame of reference for individual perception and judgment. People from one culture differ from those in other cultures in the ways they think, solve problems, perceive, and structure the world. Essentially, culture incorporates experiences of the past, influences thought and action in the present, and transmits these traditions to future group members. Adaptation is necessary, however, for the culture to survive in an ever-changing world. Consciously and unconsciously, the members abandon, modify, or assume new patterns to meet the needs of the group.

The culture in which children are reared determines the type of food they will eat, the language they will speak, the ideals of behavior they will follow, and the way they will conduct themselves in social roles. Even children's play and their types of games are culturally determined. To be acceptable members of the culture, children must learn how the culture expects them to behave toward others in the group. In turn, they learn how they can expect others to behave toward them. This cultural understanding is typically established in children by age 5 years (Lynch, 1992).

Related to the large culture are many **subcultures**, those smaller groups within a culture that possess many characteristics of the larger culture while contributing their own particular values. Subcultural influences are discussed in more detail later in the chapter.

The culture fosters and reinforces those behaviors deemed desirable and appropriate; it attempts to depress or extinguish those at conflict with cultural norms. Cultures and subcultures contribute to the uniqueness of child members in such a subtle way and at such an early age that children grow up to think that their beliefs, attitudes, values, and practices are the "correct" or "normal" ones; those of other cultures may be viewed as "deviant" or "wrong." A set of values learned in childhood is apt to characterize children's attitudes and behavior for life.

The manner and sequence of the growth and development phenomenon are universal and fundamental features of all children; however, the variations in behavioral responses that children display to similar events are believed to be determined by cultures. Inborn temperament and modes of behavior that prompt children to behave in their own preferred and highly individual manner may be in harmony or in conflict with the culture. Such forces as heredity and maturation impose limits on the influence that parents and other social groups may bring to bear.

SOCIAL ROLES

Much of children's self-concept is derived from their ideas about their social roles. Roles are cultural creations; therefore the culture prescribes patterns of behavior for persons in a variety of social positions. All persons who hold similar social positions have the obligation to behave in a particular manner. A role prohibits some behaviors and allows others. Because it delineates and clarifies roles, the culture is a significant influence on the development of children's self-concept.

A social group consists of a system of roles carried out in both primary and secondary groups. A *primary group* is characterized by intimate, continued face-to-face contact, mutual support of the members, and the ability to order or constrain a considerable proportion of individual members' behavior. Two such groups are the family and the peer group, both of which exert a great deal of influence on the child. Some communities (e.g., contemporary rural, religious, or ethnic communities) also exert a strong primary-group influence.

Secondary groups are groups that have limited, intermittent contact and in which there is generally less concern for members' behavior. These groups offer little in terms of support or pressure toward conformity except in rigidly limited areas. Examples of secondary groups are professional associations and church organizations (also considered in relation to subgroups). The childrearing orientation in a secondary-group environment, such as urban communities, differs considerably from that of a primary-group community. An urban community is dynamic and rapidly changing; therefore many of the traditional behaviors and values do not meet its needs. Consequently, parents are often uncertain about what to teach their children. They may wish to rear their children with values consistent with their own, but the differences in experience between the generations are too great. As a result, they often grant their children autonomy in some areas of decision making early in the developmental process, and other secondary groups assume a greater influence. The children are exposed to an assortment of social groups with diverse sets of values and expectations.

Guilt and Shame Orientation

Conditioning children to feel either guilt or shame for misdeeds is a technique used by a culture to control social behavior—to internalize the norms and expectations of others. Some cultural groups value a well-developed conscience (superego) and condition their children to feel guilt following wrongdoing. Offenders get an uncomfortable physical feeling and want to purge themselves. Since guilt is based within the individual, successful conditioning produces self-regulated persons who punish themselves without their being caught in the act of wrongdoing.

In many cultural groups guilt is lacking, and social controls are based on the use of shame. Offenders do not want anyone to see them when they have been found guilty of a wrongful deed. Sometimes children in these groups learn that anything is acceptable as long as one is not caught; the shame results when the forbidden act is found out by others.

Although both techniques are used by members of both primary- and secondary-group communities, shame is apt to be more successful in a primary-group community because most behaviors are quite public. In secondary-group communities it is less effective; persons are not as apt to be caught and, if caught, can withdraw and join a group that is unaware of the misdeed. Guilt probably has a greater influence on behavior in urban communities, although many authorities believe that the trend in urban North America is shifting away from a guilt orientation. Rapid changes in North American culture leave parents unsure of their own values; therefore much of their function is abandoned to the school and peers. Peers are notorious for using shame as a disciplinary technique.

SUBCULTURAL INFLUENCES

Except in rare situations, children grow and develop in a blend of cultures and subcultures. In a large, complex society such as the United States, different groups have their own set of standards, values, and expectations within the collective ways of the large culture. Although many cultural differences are related to geographic boundaries, subcultures are not always restricted by location.

Children's membership in a cultural subgroup is, for the most part, involuntary. They are born into a family with a specific ethnic and/or racial heritage, socioeconomic level, and religious beliefs. Although in the complex North American society there are countless subcultures and considerable variation in the way of life, those subcultures that seem to exert the greatest influence on childrearing are ethnicity, social class, and occupational role. In addition, schools and peer-group subcultures are strong influences in the socialization of the child.

Ethnicity

Ethnicity is the classification of or affiliation with any of the basic groups or divisions of mankind or any heterogeneous population differentiated by customs, characteristics, language, or similar distinguishing factors. Ethnic differences extend to many areas and include such manifestations as family structure, language, food preferences, moral codes, and expression of emotion.

To establish their place in the group, children learn how to adhere to a mode of behavior that is in accordance with standards distinctive to the group and how they can expect others to behave toward them. They take their cues from observing and imitating those to whom they are exposed. For example, children of a racial minority form a perception of their role as a group member by observing the manner in which role models within the subgroup respond to treatment by people outside the subgroup. When they see group members display an attitude of inferiority, they assume this to be the appropriate behavior. These perceptions are then incorporated into their own self-concept.

In the United States the cross-cultural lines are becoming blurred as subcultures are assimilated and blended into the larger culture (Fig. 28-1). Although ethnic differences in childrearing are probably diminishing, they remain important. It is particularly difficult for persons to attempt to maintain an identity with a subculture while living and conforming to the requirements of the dominant culture. Universal

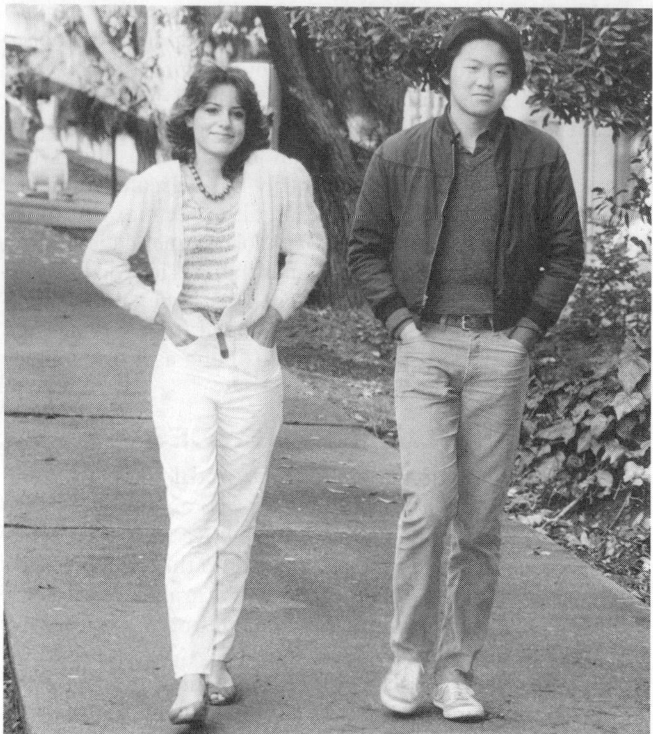

Fig. 28-1 Youngsters from different cultural backgrounds interact within the larger culture.

customs and language used in commercial and educational systems are different from those of the minority culture. Often the values are in conflict. Consequently, children reared in this environment are confused about roles and values, and they usually adopt those of the more influential or higher-status culture. Youth, in particular, are influenced by the locally dominant group.

The term **ethnocentrism** refers to the emotional attitude that one's own ethnic group is superior to others; that one's values, beliefs, and perceptions are the correct ones; and that the group's ways of living and behaving are the best way. Ethnic stereotyping or labeling stems from ethnocentric views of people (Friedman, 1990). Ethnocentrism implies that all other groups are inferior and that their ways are not in the best interests of the group. This attitude strongly influences the ability of one person to evaluate the beliefs and behaviors of others objectively. This inherent viewpoint of individuals tends to bias their interpretation and understanding of the behavior of others.

Social Class/Occupation

Although there are expectations, probably the greatest influence on childrearing practices and their consequences is the social class of the family into which a child is born. Differences in childrearing goals and practices, as well as attitudes toward health, have been found to be greater between social classes than between races or ethnic groups. In North America social class and socioeconomic level are essentially synonymous and are most easily determined by occupation; for example, the upper middle class consists primarily of professional and business people, almost all with a college education. The working class includes employees in manufacturing, trades, and service occupations who have a high school education. In the lower class the breadwinners are typically unskilled laborers or unemployed families who may or may not be on public assistance (Elkin and Handel, 1989). Since children are reared differently by parents who vary in respect to these factors, social class can be expected to produce substantial variation in their upbringing.

Middle and upper class. Children from these classes live in an enriched environment that provides material comforts and broader opportunities. The parents are usually educated beyond high school and have occupations that require judgment, creativity, and resourcefulness. These attributes are fostered in their children. Other authority figures such as teachers are usually from a middle-class background and have activities and expectations for the children that are similar to those of the parents.

Most middle-class parents are future oriented, have higher educational and occupational aspirations for their children, and use long-range planning to meet these goals (Shaffer, 1985). Middle-class parents typically encourage their children in activities that foster achievement, such as music lessons, athletics, and scouting, in the belief that this will make them well-rounded, self-directed adults.

In the area of discipline, middle-class parents are more apt to use manipulative techniques such as reasoning and drawing on the child's sense of guilt. They tend to scold and use isolation rather than physical punishment. There is more concern regarding the *intent* of the act than the *consequence of* the act.

It is believed that upper-class parents are more permissive and foster desirable behavior through positive reinforcement. However, much of the actual child care in upper-class families is delegated to surrogates, such as housekeepers, nannies, or private schools. The parent serves as an arbitrator between the children and the caregivers.

Lower and working class. The uncertainty of their life leads members of the lower classes to be present oriented; that is, to take advantage of gratification when possible. This orientation is distinctly different from that of most members of the middle class, who may be more willing to delay gratification to achieve a long-term goal.

Children in lower-class families encounter major educational disadvantages, reflected in the high incidence of academic failure and attendant dropout rate. Some of the major educational disadvantages many children from the lower social class encounter include the following:

- Parents are more likely to value the concrete and tangible rather than the abstract and are therefore less inclined to encourage these qualities in their children.
- Parents are less likely to read to the child or encourage educational play because of their own educational level.
- No role models may be available to support the value of education.
- Inadequate funding and/or poor quality of education may exist in neighborhood schools.
- Poor health and inadequate nutrition of the children is common.

- Parents are more likely to have limited communication skills such as simple grammar, inability to express abstractions, and ethnic dialects, which hamper interactions with teachers from middle-class backgrounds.

Parents from lower and working classes are generally tradition oriented, stressing obedience and conformity to parental values and external regulations. The most frequently used form of discipline for undesirable behavior is physical punishment. Parents are usually less interested in the direction of children's activities than in conduct; they are more concerned that children stay out of trouble.

With better job security through unionization, unemployment compensation, and other welfare features, some segments of the lower classes are finding life more predictable. They are less apt to seize gratifications lest the opportunity vanish and are beginning to develop long-range goals, including an increased interest in education for their children.

Poverty

A subcultural influence closely related to but different from social class is the condition known as poverty. It is a relative concept and is usually associated with the general standards of a population. The term **poverty** implies both visible and invisible impoverishment. *Visible poverty* refers to lack of money or material resources, which includes insufficient clothing, poor sanitation, and deteriorating housing. *Invisible poverty* refers to social and cultural deprivation such as limited employment opportunities, inferior educational opportunities, lack of or inferior medical services and health care facilities, and an absence of public services.

The very poor in the society who consistently exist on or below the poverty level live in a perpetual state of despair. Their limited skills give them no bargaining power in the job market, and the education needed to improve their status is beyond them. The poor desire better things for their children but are trapped in a circular pattern that perpetuates their life condition. Their powerlessness to control their fate or condition is a source of fatalism and resignation that is characteristic of the group in general. Optimism, when it is manifested, is more likely to be expressed in terms of luck or chance. This fatalistic attitude, which significantly impedes occupational and educational aspirations, also inhibits the poor from seeking health care or practicing preventive health care measures.

Factors related to poverty. Throughout the United States there are groups of people, geographically segregated, who constitute what are known as "pockets of poverty." These are seen in the dense urban areas, such as the ghettos, and many rural areas, especially those that are geographically isolated from the needed facilities and services. The nonurbanized regions identified as poverty areas in the United States are Appalachia, the deep South, the lower Southwest, and northern New England.

Certain ethnic or racial groups are overrepresented in the impoverished population. The most obvious of these are African-Americans, Hispanics, and Native Americans.

Homelessness. One of the most pressing problems in the United States is the growing number of homeless families. Homeless individuals are those persons who lack resources and community ties necessary to provide for their own adequate shelter. In the past the homeless population traditionally included single adults, mostly men. Currently, the fastest growing segment of the homeless population consists of families, constituting at least one third of the people without homes throughout the United States. The largest group includes single mothers from minority groups with two or three young children. Homeless two-parent families are mostly Caucasian with fewer children.

Many families are becoming homeless because of physical abuse, substance abuse, disagreements with the landlord, poor living conditions, job layoffs, low income, parental mental illness, domestic conflict, and unexpected family or economic crises. Most families move into homelessness gradually after family members and friends are no longer willing to provide housing (Davidhizar and Frank, 1992).

Another group of homeless children are the "runaway" and "throwaway" adolescents. In the United States this group numbers between 250,000 and 500,000. Many runaways are victims of physical and sexual abuse and leave home because of long-term family or school problems.

Migrant families. One of the most disadvantaged groups is migrant farm workers and their children. The low position of these families on the economic scale and their mobile existence subject them to inadequate sanitation, substandard housing, social isolation, and lack of educational and medical facilities. This life style is especially deleterious to the children. For example, children are apt to live in a number of localities and attend a variety of schools in the course of a year with no continuity in either education or health care. In addition, most migrant families have no health care insurance. Because both parents work in the fields, children receive little adult supervision; therefore accident rates are high, and meals are erratic. Except where prohibited by law, children are even recruited to work in the fields along with the adults. Some migrants have a home base to which they return at the end of a growing season; others travel continuously, migrating north in summer and south in winter.

Affluence

On the opposite end of the socioeconomic spectrum are the children of affluent members of society. Although they can live within the warmth of a positive family relationship, many of them appear to be just as deprived as poverty-stricken children. Wealth does not provide protection against many of life's problems and disappointments, especially in the area of parent-child relationships. Like their counterparts in the poverty groups, children of the affluent may suffer from discrimination, inadequate parenting, or unsatisfactory role models.

Children of the wealthy suffer most from lack of parental contact. There may be long separations from loving, caring parents because of social or business interests. Even their places of residence contribute to their isolation and loneliness. Paid parent surrogates, including servants, sports professionals (such as tennis or swimming instructors), and private school personnel, provide them with adult companionship and authority. During the early years many wealthy children form stronger attachments to these people than to their parents. However, as the children grow older, they become aware of class distinctions. They realize that they must separate from these early relationships to form bonds with individuals in their class. Parents may begin involving the older adolescent in the family business and in adult social activities. But for many young people a meaningful life with their family has come too late. They feel lonely, isolated, and unloved (Adams, 1991).

Many children from wealthy families, like those from poor families, seem to thrive and flourish, making positive contributions to their families and society. However, some grow up to display boredom and a lack of motivation or self-discipline. They are suspicious of others, finding it difficult to believe they are liked for themselves and not for their money or position, and they do not trust others enough to enter into true friendships. Affluent children may also fail to acquire skills to handle responsibility and money.

Religion

Probably the most influential factor in shaping the culture of the United States is the Judeo-Christian faith. Many immigrants came to the country for religious freedom and established a religious and moral atmosphere that persists today. However, there are individual differences that are part of the general culture.

The religious orientation of the family dictates a code of morality and influences the family's attitudes toward education, male and female role identity, and beliefs regarding their ultimate destiny (Fig. 28-2). It may also determine the school that the children attend, the companions with whom they associate, and often their mate selection.

In a few instances, such as in the Mennonite and Amish communities, religion is the basis of a common way of life that determines where and how the children are reared.

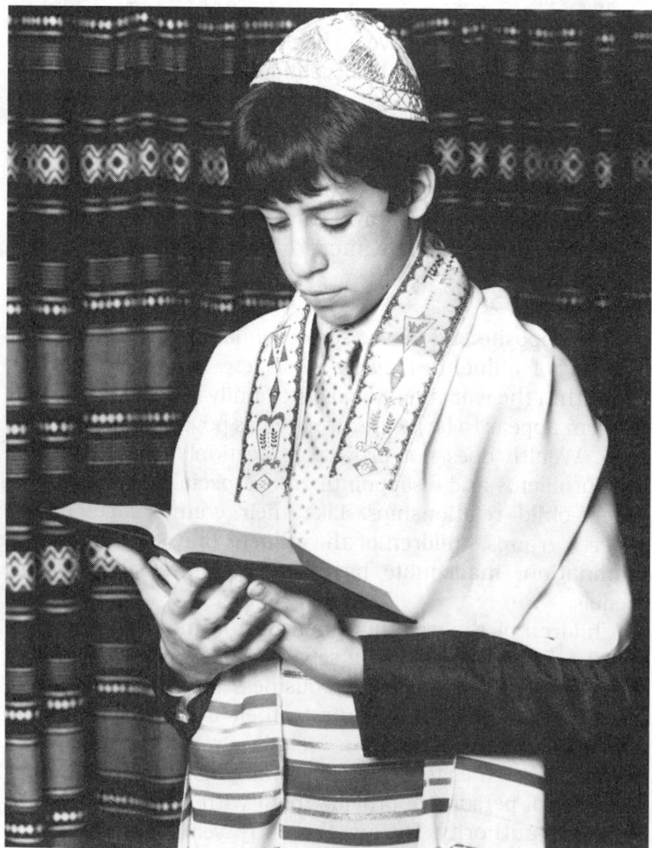

Fig. 28-2 A boy during his bar mitzvah ceremony.

Schools

Next to the family, the schools exert the major force in providing continuity between generations by conveying a vast amount of culture from the older members to the young. In this way children are prepared to carry out the traditional social roles they are expected to assume as adults in society. School rules and regulations regarding attendance, authority relationships, and the system of sanctions and rewards based on achievement transmit to the child the behavioral expectations of the adult world of employment and relationships. School is often the only institution in which children systematically learn about the negative consequences of behaviors that deviate from social expectations. Through education individuals in the lower classes are offered the opportunity for further education and the capacity to move up in the social strata.

Traditionally the socialization process of school has begun when the child enters kindergarten or first grade. Today, with almost 60% of mothers of preschool children working outside the home, this socialization process begins much earlier for a significant number of children in a variety of child care settings.

Peer Cultures

Peer groups also have an impact on the socialization of children (Fig. 28-3). Peer relationships become increasingly important and influential as children proceed through school. In school, children have what can be regarded as a culture of

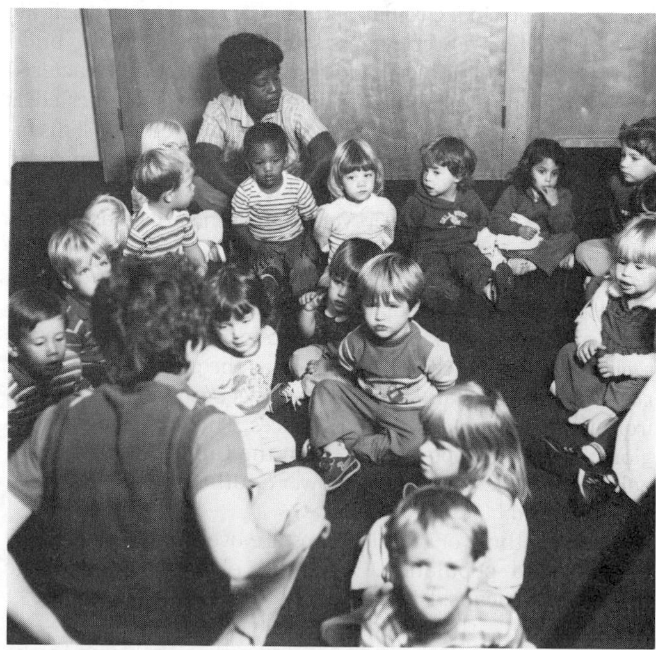

Fig. 28-3 Children from a variety of cultural and ethnic backgrounds begin to socialize in the child care setting.

their own. It is most apparent in the school and in the unsupervised play group. The play group presents this culture in a much purer form than does the school, which is partly produced by adults.

During their lives children are exposed to value systems such as those of the family, ethnic group, and social class. In peer-group interaction they are confronted with a variety of these sets of values. The values imposed by the peer group are especially compelling because children must accept and conform to them in order to be accepted as members of the group. When the peer values are not too different from those of family and teachers, the mild conflict created by these small differences serves to separate children from the adults in their lives and to strengthen the feeling of belonging to the peer group.

The kind of socialization provided by the peer group depends on the special subculture that develops from the background, interests, and capabilities of its members. Some groups support school achievement, others focus on athletic prowess, and still others are decidedly antithetic to educative goals. Scholastic achievement is strongly related to the value system of the peer groups. Many conflicts between teachers and students and between parents and students can be attributed to fear of rejection by peers. A conflict between what is expected from parents regarding academic achievement and what is expected from the peer culture may be especially pronounced in high school.

Although it has neither the traditional authority of the parents nor the legal authority of the schools for teaching information, the peer group manages to convey a substantial amount of information to its members, especially about taboo subjects, such as sex and drugs. Through peer relationships, children learn ways to deal with dominance and hostility and to relate with persons in positions of leadership and authority. The peer subculture relieves boredom and provides recognition that individual members do not receive from teachers and other authority figures.

The peer-group culture has secrets, mores, and codes of ethics with which they promote feelings of group solidarity and detachment from adults. Traditions and folkways are transferred from "generation to generation" of schoolchildren and have a great influence over the behavior of all group members.

Biculture

Some children are exposed to the values, role relationships, and life-styles of two cultures—a virtual "straddling" of two cultures. Although sometimes observed in play groups, this background is usually not a significant factor until children enter school. Children of one culture must unlearn some of the established practices of the culture in order to become socialized in the other, especially in role relationships. For example, children from Hispanic and Asian cultures are taught to look away when scolded; in U.S. schools the teacher expects direct eye contact—"Look at me when I speak to you" (Sloat and Matsuura, 1990). Children learn new roles and social behavior more rapidly than their adult counterparts.

This biculture is particularly marked in language differences. The bilingual child is said to be at a disadvantage in school situations of the dominant culture, especially a culture in which there is controversy over bilingual education. Those supporting bilingual education adhere to the principle that children will understand more readily and perform more realistically (especially in testing situations) if learning is directed in their own language; others contend that children living in a dominant culture should adopt the ways of that culture, including language.

THE CHILD AND FAMILY IN NORTH AMERICA

North America is an aggregate of numerous cultures that are blended with the unique heritage of pioneering frontiersmen. There has always been a basic optimistic view of the world, a belief that things can be better and that the children can and will be better off than the parents. This hopeful outlook and a general future orientation, together with the possibility of upward social mobility, have created a pervasive overall attitude of optimism. Increasing development of self-confidence and autonomy in children is fostered and encouraged. Children are generally permitted a greater degree of freedom than in more tradition-oriented cultures, where individuals remain in one class for life.

Family life in North America is characterized by increasing geographic and economic mobility. There is less reliance on tradition, families are fragmented, and there is limited opportunity to transmit and acquire the traditional and accepted customs of a culture. Consequently, young adults rely to a greater extent on the professed experts, peers, and mass media for acquisition of acceptable patterns of behavior, including childrearing practices. Conflicting information can be a source of confusion and frustration as parents attempt to determine the comparatively stable, essential components of the culture and transmit these to their children.

Children in North America grow up with a number of adults who differ from one another but who all provide input as role models, teachers, and standards for behavior. Most children live in some form of nuclear family located in sharply differentiated neighborhoods determined by income and ethnic status within a highly technical, largely urban society. Class differences in childrearing persist, but they are becoming less divergent as a result of the increased homogeneity of the culture.

Cultural Considerations 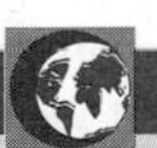

CLASSIFICATION OF MINORITY GROUPS

The definition of various minority groups is not universal. In the 1990 U.S. census form, blacks included persons identified, for example, as African- or Afro-American, Haitian, Jamaican, West Indian, or Nigerian. Persons of Spanish/Hispanic origin included Mexican, Mexican-American, Chicano, Puerto Rican, Cuban, Argentinean, Columbian, Costa Rican, Dominican, Ecuadoran, Guatemalan, Honduran, Nicaraguan, Peruvian, and Salvadoran persons, as well as persons from other Spanish-speaking countries, the Caribbean, or Central or South America. Mexican-American referred only to persons of Mexican origin or ancestry. In some writings the term Latino refers to individuals from Mexico and Central America (Friedman, 1990). *Asian* or *Pacific Islander* groups include Chinese, Japanese, Hawaiian, Filipino, Vietnamese, Korean, Asian Indian, Guamanian, and Samoan (Martin, 1995).

Minority-Group Membership

The United States has more racial, ethnic, and religious minority groups than any other country. Ethnic minority groups are becoming increasingly important because it is anticipated that these groups will produce children at a faster rate than will the majority Caucasian population. Consequently, the minority population is increasing while the majority Caucasian population is decreasing. African-Americans are the largest minority group, followed closely by Hispanics. By the year 2000 one in every four Americans will be black, Hispanic, or Asian (Fleming, 1989). (See the Cultural Considerations box on p. 805.)

One of the difficulties with including diverse groups of people under ethnic labels such as African-American, Asian, or Hispanic is that the groups can differ tremendously in their own cultural heritage. Just as the majority Caucasian population differs according to various subcultures such as socioeconomic status and occupation, so do the minority groups.

Nursing ALERT

Generalizations made about an ethnic group may not apply to certain groups and individuals.

When minority groups immigrate to another country, a certain degree of cultural/ethnic blending occurs through the process of **acculturation**—those gradual changes produced in a culture by the influence of another culture that cause one or both cultures to be more similar to the other. However, the changes occur to various degrees in different families and groups. At one time it was believed that the great diversity among the ethnic groups in the United States would result in a great "melting pot" where the differences among different cultures would eventually diminish to produce a homogeneous society. However, this does not appear to be the case. Many groups continue to identify with their traditional heritage while adapting to the ill-defined concept of the "American way."

Early in life children become aware of their racial or ethnic status and of the discriminatory attitudes of the majority culture toward their group. The direct effects of discrimination are anger and low self-esteem, which become manifest in a variety of behaviors. Inner conflicts and suppressed hostility that focus children's attention inward may be factors in the failure of many children to achieve in other areas.

Evidence indicates that changes in attitudes are slowly taking place in some groups and in some places. With growing awareness, interest, and understanding by increasing numbers of the majority group, which has accompanied the emergence of racial and ethnic pride, minority-group children are becoming more secure and confident in their racial or ethnic identity.

CULTURAL SHOCK

The term *cultural shock* describes the "feelings of helplessness and discomfort and a state of disorientation experienced by an outsider attempting to comprehend or effectively adapt to a different cultural group because of differences in cultural practices, values, and beliefs" (Leininger, 1978). This state occurs with both clients and health care providers who move from one cultural setting to another. It can happen to persons who immigrate to a new country or persons from a subcultural group who must adjust to the ways of an unfamiliar subgroup (such as children entering the school subculture or consumers who enter the hospital subculture). Cultural shock is characterized by the inability to respond to or function in a new or strange situation.

Numerous factors influence reactions to a new environment. Language barriers, including dialects and jargon (such as medical language) specific to a subcultural group, inhibit effective communication. Habits and customs (such as different role behaviors or etiquette) and differences in attitudes and beliefs are puzzling to the stranger in the new environment. The outsider experiences an intense sense of isolation and feelings of loneliness and nonrelatedness. Nurses entering an unfamiliar cultural situation can reduce the cultural shock by becoming familiar with the cultural groups with which they work and by learning tolerance of the values, beliefs, and customs of these groups. See the Critical Thinking Q & A on p. 809.

Nursing ALERT

Because American cultures and subcultures can be so diverse, it is essential that nurses be aware of and knowledgeable about the predominant groups in his or her locality and apply the knowledge in their practice.

Cultural/Religious Influences on Health Care

SUSCEPTIBILITY TO HEALTH PROBLEMS

Some groups of people are more susceptible than others to certain illnesses. An innate susceptibility is acquired through generations of evolutionary changes that take place within constrained or segregated populations. The proximity to disease, environmental factors, and the general physical status are significant factors associated with health problems.

Hereditary Factors

The genetic constitution of individuals as groups influences the degree to which they are susceptible to a specific disorder. It may be the result of an inherent lack of resistance to a disease organism, a trait that is an advantage in one environment but places the possessor at a disadvantage in another, or the consequence of intermarriage within a relatively narrow range of geographic, ethnic, or religious restrictions.

A number of conditions show ethnic or racial differences. For example, Tay-Sachs disease affects primarily Ashkenasi Jewish families, particularly those of Northeastern European origin, whereas Sephardic Jewish families appear to be no more at risk for the disease than are other populations. The incidence of cystic fibrosis is highest in whites and almost nonexistent in Asians, and the rare affected blacks are usually in areas where there is apt to be mixed ancestry. A classic disorder of blacks, especially Africans, is sickle cell disease (see

Chapter 46); however, the incidence of cardiovascular disease, pneumonia, and diabetes is also high among blacks. Native Americans have particularly high rates of tuberculosis, diarrhea, alcoholism, and suicide. Racial and ethnic differences are further considered in relation to diseases and defects as they are discussed throughout the book.

Common food items and drugs may cause health problems in certain ethnic groups. For example, persons of Mediterranean, African, Near Eastern, and Asian origin frequently have glucose-6-phosphate dehydrogenase (G-6-PD) deficiency. They may develop acute hemolytic anemia after they ingest fava (horse or broad) beans or certain drugs such as aspirin preparations, sulfonamides, or primaquine. Other groups, especially southern Europeans, Jews, Arabs, blacks, Asians, and Native Americans, have a deficiency of lactase, the enzyme needed to metabolize lactose.

Physical characteristics. Among racial groups there are observable differences in physical appearance. The most obvious are skin and hair coloring and texture. Skin color is determined by the amount of melanin pigment present in the skin. Persons from countries located near the equator have darkly pigmented skin, which serves to protect the skin from the year-round exposure to the sun's rays; persons from the northern countries have very light skin, which provides for maximum exposure to the sun's rays (necessary for vitamin D metabolism) during the short daylight hours. There can be wide variations in skin color between these two extremes in terms of geographic origin or from intermixing of dark and light skin color. As a consequence of the dark pigmentation, the detection of skin color changes (e.g., vasomotor alterations, cyanosis, jaundice) can be difficult and requires modification of assessment techniques (see Table 32-9).

Variations in the newborn are often related to racial or ethnic origin. For example, newborn infants of Asian and African-American parents are smaller than infants of Caucasian parentage, and bluish pigmented areas (mongolian spots) on the sacral region are a common observation on Asian, Native American, and Mexican-American infants.

Evaluation of stature and body build reveals some racial tendencies. Children from Asian countries are commonly smaller, falling below the 10th percentile on weight and height charts used for children in the United States (Baze, 1991). This difference in stature can lead to misinterpretation of health status and capabilities. A small child may appear very intelligent for body size but be of average mental ability for age.

Socioeconomic Factors

The most overwhelming adverse influence on health is socioeconomic status. A higher percentage of lower-class individuals are suffering from some health problem at any one time than are those in any other group.

In the lower classes children are less likely to be immunized against preventable diseases than are children in the upper and middle classes. Lack of funds or inaccessibility to health services inhibits treatment for any but severe illness or injury. Sometimes health care is inadequate because of ignorance. In some areas a disorder is so commonplace that it is looked on as unavoidable; it is not recognized as something that requires (or is amenable to) treatment. The parents may not have information regarding causes, treatment, outcome of the illness, or preventive measures.

Poverty. A high correlation between poverty and the prevalence of illness has long been observed. Impoverished families suffer from poor nutrition; without medical insurance they have little if any preventive health care, inadequate health maintenance, and very limited access to medical treatment. One of the most significant health problems related to poverty is a high infant mortality rate. Day-to-day needs of food, clothing, and lodging take precedence over health care as long as the ailing person feels able to perform activities of daily living.

Poor families are denied access to many health institutions for emergency or other hospital care. Frequently they must travel long distances to service centers that are willing to assume their care. In an emergency they must find money for taxi fare, borrow an automobile, or seek other means of transportation. They must find care for dependents, such as other infants and small children, or have them accompany them when taking the ill child for care. Families tend to delay preventive care indefinitely unless health services are relatively accessible. They are more likely to consult folk practitioners or other persons within their community.

Poor nutrition accounts for many health problems in the lower classes. Lack of funds and knowledge results in a diet that may be seriously lacking in essential food substances, especially protein, vitamins, and iron. This inadequate diet often leads to nutritional deficiency disorders and growth retardation in children. In many the total intake is insufficient to support normal growth. Unstructured eating patterns and irregularly scheduled mealtimes may also contribute to erratic food intake and a proportionately larger consumption of nonnourishing snacks, which can result in excessive weight gain.

Because of deficient preventive care, dental problems are more prevalent. Lack of standard immunizations, together with reduced resistance from poor nutrition, renders the exposed children in poor segments of the population vulnerable to communicable diseases. Poor sanitation and crowded living conditions also contribute to the higher incidence and perpetuation of illness. In general, poor people become ill more frequently and remain ill for longer periods of time than do persons in the general population.

Homelessness. Homeless children experience all of the health problems associated with poverty, as well as other types of disorders. Lack of a permanent dwelling deprives children of the most basic necessities for proper growth and development. Homelessness disrupts a child's friendships and schooling. Homeless children suffer from physical and mental disorders that exceed those found in poor children who have a permanent residence (Bassuk and Rosenberg, 1990), and they are particularly vulnerable for early initiation of and sustained participation in substance-abuse behaviors (Wagner, Melragon, and Menke, 1993).

Migrant families. Migrants generally suffer more illness, both acute and chronic, than does the general population. They are subject to unhealthy environments, poverty, and insufficient medical care; their health-seeking behavior in general is an illness- or injury-oriented recourse to medical care. The health problems of migrant children appear to be dental caries, upper respiratory tract infections, otitis media, scabies and lice, intestinal parasites, pesticide exposure, injuries, teenage pregnancy, and growth and development delay (American Academy of Pediatrics, 1989). Affected persons will postpone seeking care for themselves or their children until physical pain or suffering is almost unbearable.

When medical care is provided to a migrant family, follow-up care is usually impossible because of their transient lifestyle. Compliance to medical therapies is primarily related to accessibility and availability. For example, medications provided by health workers are more likely to be taken than those that must be obtained at a pharmacy. In addition, medications are often discontinued following self-perceived recovery. Compliance is more likely if treatment regimens do not interfere with work or family responsibilities.

CUSTOMS AND FOLKWAYS

Nurses must be aware of the need to consider cultural differences in clients when providing health care. An understanding of the various beliefs regarding the causation of illness and disease, as well as traditional health practices, is essential to successful intervention. The more nurses know about the values, beliefs, and customs of other ethnic groups, the better able they are to meet the needs of these families and to gain their cooperation and compliance.

Cultural Relativity

Although clinical characteristics of a disease or condition are essentially the same across cultures, how a child or family interprets or experiences the disease varies. Culture as an influence is one obvious explanation for variance. **Cultural relativity** is the concept that any behavior must be judged first in relation to the context of the culture in which it occurs. Nurses must first relate to the family's perceptions and interpretations of experiences from the family's background and cultural belief system before they can effectively intervene.

Some cultures, for example, may view a chronic illness or disability as affecting only particular aspects of a child's life, and the child as a whole is viewed as normal. In contrast, Chinese families more frequently describe the illness as having global effects on many aspects of the child's present and future life (Elfert, Anderson, and Lai, 1991). These contrasting views may result in a difference in goals and expectations parents have for their children.

In some cultures the child's gender may influence a family's perception of the implications of an illness or disability. For example, in the Arabic and Asian cultures the male child is held in higher esteem than the female child. This also holds true for some families of Jewish, Italian, Greek, and Indian origin. The male child may receive better health care and more food, because this is the child who will take care of his parents in their old age (Issacs, 1989).

Defining disease or signs and symptoms of illness is also influenced by culture. Some cultures, for example, perceive diarrhea as a cleansing of the body that is essential for health maintenance and illness prevention and/or cure. Furthermore, signs or symptoms resulting from diarrhea and ensuing dehydration, such as malaise, fever, anorexia, and irritability, may be viewed as separate illness entities.

Nurses can often recognize a family's health-related cultural perceptions and interpretations through discussion and observation. Implications of these perceptions should be explored and considered when effective culturally appropriate interventions are being planned.

Relationships with Health Care Providers

The manner of relating with health care providers differs considerably among cultural groups. One area of conflict to some nurses is the attitude toward time and waiting that is part of some cultures. For example, African-Americans are very flexible in their time orientation; an African-American family may be late for or miss appointments because other issues take precedence over the appointment, and they may not communicate this to the health agency. Hispanics, too, have a very relaxed view of time. Whereas the dominant culture in the United States says that "time flies," the Hispanic says, "time walks." The Japanese, on the other hand, consider time to be valuable and to be used wisely. They tend to be punctual for medical appointments and persistent in following prescribed regimens. A Vietnamese family will subordinate time to values considered to be more significant, such as propriety. They may be late for an appointment because of an overextended visit by a friend in their home. In general, Asian-Americans view the American focus on time as offensive.

In many cultural groups the mother assumes the responsibility for health care; in others both parents are involved equally in relationships with health workers. A somewhat different approach is apparent in some of the Asian cultures. For example, the father in Vietnamese families, as unquestioned head of the family, is traditionally the family member who interacts with persons, including health care providers, outside the family unit (Fig. 28-4).

In the Hispanic family the father, as head of the house, makes decisions regarding illness and treatment of family members, but the grandmother in the extended family is consulted regarding child care. Usually the family confers with other members before reaching a decision regarding treatment or hospitalization of a child. The Arab family also relies on others to give advice and guidance in a time of crisis (see the Critical Thinking Q & A on p. 809). A Japanese father may appear to be passive and uninvolved but actually is involved according to his own cultural standards.

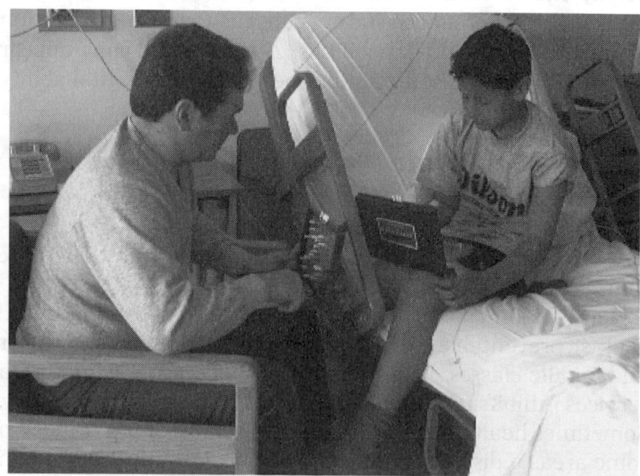

Fig. 28-4 A father with his hospitalized child.

Critical Thinking Q & A

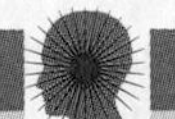

REDUCING CULTURAL SHOCK

A woman from the Middle East is visiting her child who is hospitalized for a serious illness. Her husband left for home a short time ago to wash and change clothes. She speaks little English. You need to obtain consent from her for an emergency procedure. She is hesitant and refuses to sign the consent form. You:

1. Document that the mother refuses to sign the consent form and inform the physician that the procedure cannot be done
2. Realize that she may be hesitant to sign for consent without her husband's presence, since her culture requires the male to make the decisions for the welfare of the family members
3. Explain to her that you cannot help her child unless she signs for permission to do so
4. Realize that she may not understand what you're saying and try to find an interpreter

The correct answer is two. In the Arab culture men typically make the decisions, and wives are expected to support that decision. Trying to find an interpreter or intimidating her to sign does not address the main issue of the Arab cultural tradition. Although in emergency cases, treatment is often approved by the institution or state if a physician documents treatment is necessary and that any delay in treatment may jeopardize the health of the child; in this situation contacting the father first is appropriate.

Nursing ALERT

In working with families, it is essential for nurses to identify key members—failure to include these significant individuals in teaching can seriously hinder adherence to the plan of care.

Nurses should make themselves aware of any specific attitudes regarding the manner of approach to a child in a given culture. Navajo Indians do not like a stranger near their infants. It is feared that the stranger may "witch" the child and cause him or her harm. On the other hand, if a stranger, particularly a woman, lavishes attention on a Latino infant but fails to touch the child, he or she will develop symptoms of the "evil eye" (see p. 811). Vietnamese and Korean families may become upset if a newborn is admired at length for fear the evil spirits will overhear and desire the infant.

Some ethnic groups such as the Amish consider a child's admission to the hospital a family affair, with all members gathering to support and console the child and parents. In others such as the Samoan family, the family is willing to relinquish the care of the child to the hospital authority without interference. Their visits with the child are short, although intense, but this behavior may be misinterpreted by the hospital staff as disinterest or abandonment.

Nurses who are members of a majority culture may encounter tension and distrust in a child from a minority culture as a result of the child's learned conception or relationships with other persons in the majority group. Based on these perceptions, minority children often suspect that nurses may have hostile feelings toward them and fear ill treatment. When such children are hospitalized, this feeling compounds the feelings of loneliness, helplessness, and retribution that accompany fearful happenings and separation from families. The reverse situation may be encountered by a nurse from a minority culture attempting to meet the needs of a child who has been conditioned to view the nurse's cultural or ethnic group.

BOX 28-1
Helpful Communication Tools

1. Have a series of audio and audiovisual recordings in several languages designed to greet and familiarize the family with the hospital.
2. In the event an interpreter is not available, develop a multilingual booklet containing illustrations of commonly used phrases and hospital routines.
3. Have legal consent forms and explanations of common diagnostic tests available in several languages.
4. Keep cards with common greetings, phrases, and names of body parts in the family's language with the patient's chart, for example, *miseries* (pain) and *locked bowels* (constipation) in black people and *caida de la mollera* (fallen fontanel from dehydration), *susto* (fright), *dolor, duele,* or *lele* (pain), and *la diarrhea* (diarrhea) in Hispanics.
5. Develop a cultural reference manual that includes a brief description of the culture; their views on matters such as health, illness, and diet; and a list of interpreters and ethnic community services or other sources for quick reference (Kuensting and Sanders, 1995).

Communication. Communication may be a source of distress and misunderstanding between persons from different ethnic groups, especially if the languages are different (Box 28-1). Ideally, conversations with families who are unable to speak the dominant language are best conducted by a health care worker who speaks the language of the family. If this is not possible, it may be necessary to use an interpreter (see Communicating with Families Through an Interpreter, Chapter 31).

Some persons with poor or limited language comprehension may simply smile and nod in agreement if they do not understand the questions or directives. It is vital that the family fully understand all implications of a child's care and management before they sign permits for special procedures or assume responsibility for the child's care. It is not uncommon for a Vietnamese or a Japanese family to indicate "yes" when in fact they mean "no" in order to avoid social disharmony. They tend to use indirectness rather than confrontation and may become evasive when direct questioning makes them feel uncomfortable.

Nonverbal communication is a practiced art in many Native American tribes, and the members are highly sensitive to body language. They emphasize periods of silence to formulate thoughts in preparation for speech and often remain silent after listening to statements by others in order to properly assimilate what has been said. Interruption, interjection, or haste to arrive at abrupt conclusions is perceived as immature behavior.

The level of comfort with body space or distance from others varies among cultures. Anglos are generally comfortable at an arm's length, Hispanics tend to get closer, and Asians prefer a greater distance.

Eye contact is viewed differently in cultures. Although Anglos are advised to look people straight in the eye, it is not uncommon for persons in some ethnic groups to avoid eye contact and become uncomfortable when conversing with health workers. A Vietnamese patient may not look directly into the nurse's eyes, as a sign of respect. Some Native Americans will make eye contact during the initial greeting, but continued, unwavering eye contact is considered insulting and disrespectful. Asians may consider eye contact a sign of hostility or impoliteness.

Gestures also may have different meanings. For example, some Asians consider finger or foot pointing disrespectful. Native Americans consider vigorous handshaking a sign of aggression, whereas to Anglos the gesture is a sign of good will.

Families may be reluctant to question or otherwise initiate contact with health professionals. In the Asian cultures, for example, it is considered a sign of disrespect to question those who are viewed as persons of authority. A Japanese family may wait silently rather than ask or question. They believe that the health professionals know best and will meet their needs without being asked. It is also important to avoid criticism. Criticism can cause Asians to "lose face," or to feel ashamed, which is highly undesirable.

Families may have poor language comprehension. Many persons are able to read and write English better than they can speak or understand it. Also, the dominant language usually takes over in anxiety-provoking situations, even in persons who are able to communicate satisfactorily under ordinary circumstances.

The expression of emotion also varies ethnically. In some cultures (e.g., Latin or Jewish) emotions are expressed openly, and members are accustomed to sharing their sorrows and joys with family and friends. Conversely, Nordic and Asian groups are more restrained.

Health care providers generally ask questions and use handouts, booklets, and—particularly with children—dolls and pictures as communication aids. This is uncommon in some cultures. For example, Native American healers ask few questions and do not use forms. In some cultures it is inappropriate or considered taboo to look at the inside of the body, even in pictures, or to use dolls or puppets (Malach and Segel, 1990). Nurses need to consider both verbal and nonverbal communication techniques to interact effectively with children and their families from different cultures (see Guidelines for Culturally Sensitive Interactions, p. 869).

Food Customs

Food customs and symbolism are an integral part of various cultural, ethnic, and religious groups. Although in a large country such as the United States most persons have adopted the eclectic food habits that have evolved over countless generations, many ethnic and geographic food traditions and preferences are retained. Special holidays, ceremonies, and life experiences such as births, birthdays, weddings, and death are often marked by special food items or feasts. In many cultures specific food practices are followed during pregnancy in the belief that certain foods damage the developing fetus.

The distinctive food customs of ethnic groups are a product of their native environment, determined by availability. Fish is a staple food of persons living near the ocean. Fruit and vegetable preferences are directly related to the climate in which they grow naturally or can be cultivated. The types of grain that are ethnically associated are also those that grow best in the native lands. For example, rice is the staple grain of Asians. The diet of the Eskimo is predominantly fish and meat, depending on which is the most easily procured in the area. Even in the continental United States there are regional favorites such as rice, hominy grits, and okra in the southern states. In some cultures food is highly spiced; in others foods tend to be bland. Table 28-1 lists the food items common to most cultures and can be used to select foods that most children know and like.

There are a number of restrictions related to food items. Some have a physiologic origin, such as lack of dairy foods in the diets of some persons of African or Asian ancestry in whom a hereditary lactase deficiency prevents digestion of foods containing lactose. Others have religious restrictions, such as kosher foods and food preparation of the Orthodox Jewish faith and the vegetarian diet of Seventh-Day Adventists (see Vegetarian Diets, Chapter 44).

Children in a strange environment such as the hospital feel much more comfortable when they are served familiar foods. Hospital food often tastes strange and bland. The family may be concerned that their child is not receiving foods appropriate to their culture and beliefs. Where possible, it is advisable to provide children's ethnic foods or allow families to bring favorite foods. Concern for differences in food habits and patterns projects an attitude of respect for the family's ethnic or religious heritage.

TABLE 28-1 Foods common to most ethnic food patterns

MEAT AND ALTERNATIVES	MILK AND MILK PRODUCTS	GRAIN PRODUCTS	VEGETABLES	FRUITS	OTHERS
Pork*	Milk	Rice	Carrots	Apples	Fruit juices
Beef	Ice cream	White bread	Cabbage	Bananas	
Chicken	Yogurt	Noodles, macaroni, spaghetti	Green beans	Oranges	
Eggs		Dry cereal	Greens (especially spinach)	Peaches	
Beans			Sweet potatoes or yams	Pears	
			Tomatoes		

From Endres JB, Rockwell RE: *Food, nutrition, and the young child*, St. Louis, 1980, Mosby, p. 180.
*May be restricted because of religious custom.

HEALTH BELIEFS AND PRACTICES

Health Beliefs

Beliefs related to the cause of illness and the maintenance of health are an integral part of the cultural heritage of families. Often inseparable from religious beliefs, they influence the way that families cope with health problems and the way that they respond to health care providers. Predominant among most cultures are beliefs related to natural forces, supernatural forces, and imbalance between forces.

Natural forces. The most common natural forces held responsible for ill health if the body is not adequately protected include cold air entering the body, impurities in the air, or other natural sources. For example, a Chinese mother may overdress her infant in an effort to keep cold wind from entering the child's body. The Chinese believe that cold weather, rain, and wind are responsible for "cold" conditions.

In the African-American culture natural phenomena such as phases of the moon, seasons of the year, and planet positions are believed to affect the body and its processes. Therefore health maintenance is strongly associated with the ability to read "the signs." Most Native Americans consider health to be a state of harmony with nature and the universe.

Supernatural forces. High on the list of causes of illness are forces beyond comprehension and logical explanation. Evil influences such as voodoo, witchcraft, or evil spirits are viewed in some cultures as causes of adverse health, especially those illnesses that cannot be explained by other means.

A health belief that is common among people from Latin American, Mediterranean, Near Eastern, some Asian, and some African societies is the concept of the *evil eye* (*mal ojo* is the Hispanic term). It is part of the concept of health as a state of balance; illness is a state of imbalance (see p. 809). Strength and power are associated with the evil eye. Therefore, as long as an individual's strength and weakness remain in balance, he or she is unlikely to become a victim of the evil eye. Weaknesses are not necessarily physical. For example, an excess of some emotion, such as envy, can create a weakness. Infants and small children, because of immature development of their internal strength-weakness states, are especially vulnerable to the gaze of the evil eye. Consequently, the evil eye concept serves to rationalize an inexplicable onset of illness in children who display such symptoms as restlessness, crying, diarrhea, vomiting, and fever.

Although seldom expressed to health care providers, the belief that a witch can cast a spell over others at the request of someone who wishes them ill is found in Hispanic, African, and Australian aboriginal cultures. The victim is often tortured in effigy by pins driven into a doll at the location where the intended victim is to be hurt. "Voodoo deaths" have occurred from the victim's belief in the curse and may result from dehydration as the victim gives up the will to live and refuses to drink (Chidester, 1990).

Imbalance of forces. The concept of balance or equilibrium is widespread throughout the world. One of the most common imbalances supported by the Hispanic, Filipino, Chinese, and Arab cultures is that which exists between "hot" and "cold." Hot and cold describe certain properties and conditions completely unrelated to temperature. Diseases, areas of the body, foods, and illnesses are classified as either "hot" or "cold." In Chinese health belief the forces are termed *yin (cold)* and *yang (hot)*. To maintain health, these hot and cold forces must be kept in balance.

Illness is treated by restoring normal balance through the application of appropriate "hot" or "cold" remedies. A "cold" condition such as a respiratory disease is believed to be caused by exposure to cold weather, rain, or cold wind entering the body; it is treated by administration of "hot" foods, herbs, or drugs. Menstruation is considered to be a "hot" condition; therefore women are cautioned against ingesting "hot" foods, which might increase menstrual flow or produce cramping. Ingesting too much of either "hot" or "cold" foods can also be interpreted as a cause of illness.

Health care workers who are aware of this belief are better able to understand why some persons refuse to eat certain foods. It is possible to help families devise a diet that contains the necessary balance of basic food groups prescribed by the medical subculture while conforming to the beliefs of the ethnic subculture.

Health Practices

There are numerous similarities among cultures regarding prevention and treatment of illness. All cultures have some types of home remedies that they apply before seeking help from other persons. Within the ethnic community folk healers who are endowed with the ability to "cure" maladies are sought for special situations and when home remedies are unsuccessful. There is the *curandero* (male) or *curandera* (female) of the Mexican-American community whose healing powers are believed to be a gift from God. The Asian consults an herbalist, knowledgeable in medicines, and/or an ethnic physician practiced in Asian therapies, including acupuncture, acupressure, and moxibustion (application of heat). Native Americans consult a variety of healers with specific skills and knowledge. Specialized medicine persons diagnose illness, provide nonsacred treatments (usually by way of massage and herbs), and care for souls. Other specialists perform sacred services or affect cues through spiritual means.

The folk healers are very powerful persons in their community. They "speak the language" of the family who seeks help and often combine their rituals and potions with prayer and entreaties to God. They also are able to create an atmosphere conducive to successful management. Furthermore, they exhibit a sincere interest in the family and their problem.

Some folk remedies are compatible with the medical regimen and can be used to reinforce the treatment plan. For example, most of the foods contraindicated for persons with peptic ulcers are "hot" foods and would be avoided because of their belief systems. Also, aspirin (a "hot" medication) is an appropriate therapy for "cold" diseases such as the common cold and arthritis. It is not uncommon to discover that a folk prescription has a scientific basis. However, numerous health remedies or preventive practices have no specific basis, such as the use of garlic or *asafetida* (a fetid gum resin of various oriental plants) that is worn around the neck to prevent contagious diseases. Also, the wearing of copper or silver bracelets to protect the wearer as he or she grows has no scientific basis. Practices that do no harm should be respected.

To overcome the effect of the evil eye usually requires spe-

BOX 28-2
Cultural Practices Possibly Considered Abusive by the Dominant Culture

Coining—A Vietnamese practice that may produce weltlike lesions on the child's back when a coin, held on edge, is repeatedly rubbed lengthwise on the oiled skin to rid the body of the disease.

Cupping—An Old World practice (also practiced by the Vietnamese) of placing a container (e.g., tumbler, bottle, jar) containing steam against the skin surface to "draw out the poison" or other evil element. When the heated air within the container cools, a vacuum is created that produces a bruiselike blemish on the skin directly beneath the mouth of the container.

Burning or **moxibustion**—A practice of some Southeast Asian groups where small areas of skin are burned to treat enuresis and temper tantrums.

Forced kneeling—A child discipline measure of some Caribbean groups where a child is forced to kneel for a long period of time.

Genital gestures and practices—Teluga-speaking people of central southern India touch and kiss the penis as a sign of greeting that honors the son over the daughter; the gestures are not erotic or sexual communications (Money, Prakasam, and Joshi, 1991).

Topical garlic application—A practice of Yemenite Jews in which crushed garlic cloves or garlic-petroleum jelly plaster is applied to the wrists to treat infectious disease; the practice can result in blisters or garlic burns.

Traditional remedies that contain lead—*Greta* and *azarcon* (Mexico; used for digestive problems), *paylooah* (Southeast Asia; used for rash or fever), and *surma* (India; used as a cosmetic to improve eyesight).

Traditional remedy that contains mercury—*Azoque* (Spanish word for quicksilver; used for diarrhea).

cialized rituals conducted by the appropriate practitioner. For example, the Chicano curandera ascertains that the condition is truly the result of the evil eye by performing an assessment ritual and then, with a confirmed diagnosis, performs a curative ritual. Sometimes the faith in the folk practitioner results in a delay in obtaining needed medical treatment, although the practitioner will usually suggest medical care if his or her ministrations are unsuccessful.

Health practices of different cultures may also present problems in assessment and interpretation. For example, certain cultural practices or remedies can be misdiagnosed as evidence of "child abuse" by uninformed professionals (Box 28-2). It is important to explain why these and other familiar remedies may now be considered harmful. Families need to understand how such practices can place them in jeopardy with child protective services and to explore alternative measures that are more acceptable to the dominant culture (Hayes and Dreher, 1991).

Cultural health remedies that are detrimental to health include eating clay, excessive amounts of salt, or compounds that contain lead or mercury. A careful history can reveal these remedies, but it may require the collaboration of a folk healer to convince a user to stop the practice.

Faith healing and religious rituals are closely allied with many folk-healing practices. Wearing of amulets, medals, and other religious relics believed by the culture to protect the individual and facilitate healing is a common practice. It is important for health workers to recognize the value of this practice and keep the items where the family has placed them or nearby. It offers comfort and support and rarely impedes medical and nursing care. If an item must be removed during a procedure, it should be replaced, if possible, when the procedure is completed. The reason for its temporary removal is explained to the family, and they are reassured that their wishes will be respected (see the Family Focus box above).

Nurses can be most effective by operating from a multicultural perspective. Adopting a multicultural perspective means using appropriate aspects of each health cultural orientation under consideration to develop culturally acceptable health care interventions.

Family Focus

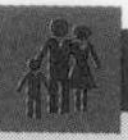

CULTURAL AWARENESS

I am a pediatric emergency nurse with a high regard for cultural diversities and a respect for healing practices and beliefs. I even made a manual for my emergency department that contains some of the information needed to help us to understand and communicate with subcultures in the urban community that we serve. Although I learned a great deal putting this manual together, it doesn't come close to the lesson I learned with the following experience:

A 15-month-old Bosnian female in status epilepticus was carried in by her parents. They were very frightened and spoke very little English. I learned that the child had received a measles, mumps and rubella (MMR) immunization the day before. As I proceeded to unwrap her from the blanket she was in, I quickly assessed the airway, breathing, and circulation (ABCs). I noticed that she was very warm (probably a febrile seizure), and a rag soaked in alcohol was tied around each thigh (this was odd). Focusing on her potential airway compromise and trying to calm the parents, I proceeded to put an oxygen mask on her, undress her for a full assessment, and remove the alcohol rags. I spoke to the parents all the while in a calm, soothing voice. Once an IV was established and I gave her Ativan, the seizures stopped. So did the communication between her parents and me. I noticed that they would no longer give me eye contact and that the mother would not even speak to me after the seizures stopped. It wasn't until I was returning to the department from admitting her that I realized why they might have stopped communicating with me . . . I removed the rags! Had I only thought to replace the rags or asked their permission to remove the rags, things may have been different.

Laura L. Kuensting, RN
Cardinal Glennon Children's Hospital
St. Louis, Mo.

Nursing ALERT

Avoid directly criticizing traditional health cultural beliefs and practices as wrong or harmful or implying that biomedical measures are uniformly correct and effective and the only way to prevent illness or treat sickness. Such criticisms usually result in rejection of both biomedical health care practitioners and their health teaching. When folk practices do not interfere with the welfare of the patient, they need not be discouraged. Often a compromise can be reached that accomplishes the goal of the nurse while maintaining the dignity and self-esteem of the child and family.

RELIGIOUS BELIEFS

Religion influences the life-style of most cultures. Among many groups illness, injury, or death is believed to be sent by God as a punishment for sin. Some may believe that health workers will be unable to help a person whom God is punishing and may express a fatalistic attitude toward treatment, stating that it is "will of God." Others view it as a test of strength, like the testing of Job in the Bible, and strive to remain faithful and overcome the conflicts.

Religious affiliation has implications for many health-related functions and procedures. It is comforting for the family of an ill child to have this need recognized and respected. Nurses need to determine if there are any special considerations, including dietary restrictions, related to spiritual practices that are important to the family. Family members are asked whether they want a clergy member present and whether they prefer hospital staff to call or prefer to do this on their own. Children will rarely voice a need for spiritual support. Nurses need to listen closely for indirect references such as "God doesn't care what happens to people" (Clutter, 1991).

It is also important to determine the wishes of the family regarding baptism, rites or practices related to death, and other religious rituals (such as circumcision, prayer, communion, or use of amulets or icons). Religion, which offers families understanding and spiritual support, is a valuable asset to health care. Characteristics of selected religions with beliefs that affect health care are outlined in Table 28-2.

IMPORTANCE OF CULTURE AND RELIGION TO NURSES

To begin to understand and to deal effectively with families in a multicultural community or in a unicultural community that is different from one's own, nurses need to be aware of their own attitudes and values regarding a way of life, including health practices. Nurses, too, are a product of their own cultural background. They also need to recognize that they are part of the "nursing culture." Nurses function within the framework of a professional culture with its own values and traditions and, as such, become socialized into their professional culture in their educational program and later in their work environments and professional associations (Friedman, 1990).

Frequently nurses and other health care workers are not aware of their own cultural values and how those values influence their thoughts and actions. Those who are aware of their own culturally founded behavior are more sensitive to cultural behavior in others. To recognize that a behavior may be characteristic of a culture rather than an "abnormal" behavior places nurses at an advantage in their relationships with families. When nurses respect the cultural differences of a family, they are better able to determine whether the behavior is distinctive to the individual or a characteristic of the culture.

Cultural standards and values, the family structure and function, and past experiences with health care influence a family's feelings and attitudes toward health, their children, and health care delivery systems. It is often difficult for nurses to be nonjudgmental and objective in working with families whose behaviors and attitudes differ from or conflict with their own. Being aware of one's own feelings and attitudes and respecting those of the family are essential to a helping relationship and achievement of nursing goals. Relying on one's own values and experiences for guidance can result only in frustration and disappointment. It is one thing to know what is needed to deal with a health problem; it is often quite another to implement a fruitful course of action unless nurses work within the cultural and socioeconomic framework of the family. See the Critical Thinking Q & A above.

It is beneficial to adapt ethnic practices to the health needs of the family rather than attempt to change long-standing beliefs. To aid their efforts to understand and respect the cultural beliefs of families, nurses should have a readily available resource file containing pertinent information about the cultural and subcultural characteristics of the community in which they practice (e.g., traditional practices related to infant feeding practices and the time and manner of weaning and toilet training). Bridging cultural gaps in delivery of health care to children requires the establishment of a close relationship with families and other influential persons in the community (such as the local folk healer) and periodic assessment of one's own attitudes and behaviors and those of other health workers toward people of other racial or ethnic origins.

Some characteristics of selected cultures are outlined in Table 28-3.

Tables 28-2 and 28-3 are presented as beginning frameworks for practicing transcultural nursing. Nurses must assess the cultural and religious practices of families to identify how these practices are similar to and different from those of their own cultural and religious backgrounds. Guidelines for assessing cultural and religious practices of families are described in Box 31-5 on p. 883.

Critical Thinking 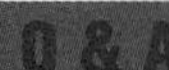 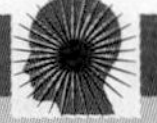

CULTURAL PRACTICES

Knowledge of cultural practices in a locality can be as important as knowledge of communicable diseases. This knowledge:

1. Is not valuable unless the nurse uses it to assess contributing cultural factors that may aid or hinder the care of the child and family
2. It is not helpful unless the nurse is part of the culture
3. Is only valuable in making nurses aware of diversities in care
4. Is learned only from reading about the traditional beliefs and practices of cultural groups

The correct answer is one. Information about a culture is not valuable unless you apply the knowledge to the situation. A nurse does not need to be a part of a culture to be aware of differences and to respect its practices. Although cultural knowledge may be helpful in awareness of diversities in practices and care, putting the knowledge to *use* is the challenge and the goal. Information about cultures is learned from a variety of methods (e.g., observation, previous experience/interactions, television, journals, textbooks, and travel).

Nursing ALERT

These generalizations are presented to help nurses learn the unique beliefs and practices of various groups and are not meant to be stereotypes of any group. It is critical to remember that no cultural group is homogeneous, every racial and ethnic group contains great diversity, and knowledge of a culture may not reflect an individual member's beliefs (Nance, 1995).

TABLE 28-2 Religious beliefs that affect nursing care

BELIEFS ABOUT BIRTH AND DEATH	BELIEFS ABOUT DIET AND FOOD PRACTICES	BELIEFS REGARDING MEDICAL CARE	COMMENTS
Adventist (Seventh-Day Adventist; Church of God)			
Birth: Opposed to infant baptism Baptism by immersion in adulthood *Death:* Desires baptism before death	Meat prohibited in some groups No alcohol, coffee, or tea	Some believe in divine healing and practice anointing with oil and use of prayer May desire communion or baptism when ill Believe in man's choice and God's sovereignty Some oppose hypnosis as therapy	Sabbath: Saturday for many Accept Bible literally
Baptist (27 groups)			
Birth: Opposed to infant baptism Believers baptized by immersion as adults *Death:* Counsel and prayer with clergy, family, patient	Some groups discourage coffee, tea, and alcohol	"Laying on of hands" (some) May encounter some resistance to some therapies, such as abortion Believe God functions through physician Some believe in predestination; may respond passively to care	Fundamentalist and conservative groups accept Bible as inspired word of God
Black Muslim			
Birth: No baptism *Death:* Carefully prescribed procedure for washing and shrouding dead	Prohibit alcohol, pork, and foods traditional among African-Americans (e.g., corn bread, collard greens)	Faith healing unacceptable Always maintain personal habits of cleanliness	General adherence to Muslim tenets overlaid, in many instances, by antagonism to Caucasians, especially Christians and Jews Do not indulge in activities (such as sleeping) more than is necessary to health
Buddhist Churches of America			
Birth: No infant baptism Infant presentation *Death:* Last rite chanting often practiced at bedside soon after death Priest should be contacted	No requirements or restrictions Some sects are strictly vegetarian Discourage use of alcohol and drugs	Illness believed to be a trial to aid development of soul; illness due to Karmic causes May be reluctant to have surgery or certain treatments on holy days Cleanliness believed to be of great importance Family may request Buddhist priest for counseling	Optimistic outlook; teach ways to overcome fears, anxieties, apprehension
Church of Christ Scientist (Christian Science)			
Birth: No baptism *Death:* No last rites	No requirements or restrictions	Deny the existence of health crisis; see sickness and sin as errors of mind that can be altered by prayer Oppose human intervention with drugs or other therapies; however, accept legally required immunizations Many adhere to belief that disease is a human mental concept that can be dispelled by "spiritual truth" to extent that they refuse all medical treatment	Many desire services of practitioner or reader; will sometimes refuse even emergency treatment until they have consulted a reader Unlikely to donate organs for transplant

Data from Carpenito, 1992; Conley, 1990; Kozier and Erb, 1995; Spector, 1985; personal communications.

TABLE 28-2 Religious beliefs that affect nursing care—cont'd

BELIEFS ABOUT BIRTH AND DEATH	BELIEFS ABOUT DIET AND FOOD PRACTICES	BELIEFS REGARDING MEDICAL CARE	COMMENTS
Church of Jesus Christ of Latter Day Saints (Mormon)			
Birth: No baptism at birth Infant is "blessed" by church official at first opportunity after birth (in church) Baptism by immersion at 8 years *Death:* No special rites but may desire presence of church elders during any acute illness, when condition worsens, when undergoing risky or frightening tests or procedures, when feeling sick enough to die, or when dying	Prohibit tea, coffee, alcohol Encourage sparing use of meats Fasting for 24 hours on first Sunday each month (from after evening meal Saturday until evening meal on Sunday)	Devout adherents believe in divine healing through anointment with oil and "laying on of hands" by church officials (elders) Medical therapy not prohibited	Married adults wear special undergarments May request Sacrament on Sunday while in hospital Financial support for sick available through well-funded welfare system Discourage cremation Discourage use of tobacco
Eastern Orthodox (e.g., Turkey, Egypt, Syria, Rumania, Bulgaria, Cyprus, Albania)			
Birth: Most believe in infant baptism by immersion 8 to 40 days after birth *Death:* Last rites obligatory for impending death	Restrictions depend on specific sect	Annointment of the sick No conflict with medical science	Discourage cremation
Episcopal (Anglican)			
Birth: Infant baptism mandatory; urgent if poor prognosis *Death:* Last rites available but not mandatory	Abstain from meat on fast days May fast on Wednesday, Friday, during Lent, and before Christmas Some feast for 6 hours before receiving Holy Communion	Some believe in spiritual healing Rite for anointing sick available but not mandatory	Religions icons very important Communion four times yearly: Christmas, Easter, June 30, and August 15; may be mandatory for some
Friends (Quakers)			
Birth: No baptism Infant's name recorded in official book	No requirements or restrictions Most practice moderation Avoid alcohol and illicit drugs	No special rites or restrictions	Believe in plain speech and dress Pacifists
Greek Orthodox			
Birth: Baptism considered important Performed 40 days after birth If not possible to baptize by sprinkling or immersion, church allows child baptism "in the air" by moving the child in the form of a cross as appropriate words are said *Death:* Last rites, administration of Sacrament of Holy Communion Should be performed while dying person is still conscious	Church-prescribed fast periods—usually occur on Wednesday, Friday, and during Lent; consist of avoiding meat and (in some cases) dairy products If health is compromised, priest may be contacted to convince family to forego fasting	Each health crisis handled by ordained priest; deacon may also serve in some cases Holy Communion administered in hospital Some may desire Sacrament of the Holy Unction performed by priest	Oppose euthanasia Believe every reasonable effort should be made to preserve life until termination by God Discourage autopsies that may cause dismemberment Prefer burial to cremation

Continued.

TABLE 28-2 Religious beliefs that affect nursing care—cont'd

BELIEFS ABOUT BIRTH AND DEATH	BELIEFS ABOUT DIET AND FOOD PRACTICES	BELIEFS REGARDING MEDICAL CARE	COMMENTS
Hindu			
Birth: No ritual *Death:* Special prescribed rites Priest pours water into the mouth of dead child, ties a thread around neck or wrist to signify blessing (should not be removed) Family washes body and is particular about who touches body	Many dietary restrictions Beef and veal not eaten Some strict vegetarians	Illness or injury believed to represent sins committed in previous life Accept most modern medical practices	Cremation preferred
Islam (Muslim/Moslem)			
Birth: No baptism *Death:* Patient must confess sins and beg forgiveness before death; family should be present Family washes and prepares body, then turns it to face Mecca Only relatives and friends may touch body	Prohibit all pork products and any meat that is not ritually slaughtered Daylight fasting practiced during ninth month of Muhammadan year (Ramadan) Strict Muslims do not use alcohol or mind-altering drugs	Faith healing not acceptable unless psychologic condition of patient is deteriorating; performed for morale Ritual washing after prayer; prayer takes place five times daily (on rising, midday, afternoon, early evening, and before bed); during prayer, face Mecca and kneel on prayer rug	Older Muslims often have a fatalistic view that may interfere with compliance to therapy May oppose autopsy
Jehovah's Witness			
Birth: No baptism *Death:* No last rites	Eat nothing to which blood has been added; can eat animal flesh that has been drained	Adherents are generally absolutely opposed to blood transfusions, including banking of own blood; individuals can sometimes be persuaded in emergencies May be opposed to use of albumin, globulin, factor replacement (hemophilia), vaccines	Often possible to obtain a court order appointing a hospital official as temporary guardian to consent to a child's transfusion when parents refuse consent Autopsy approved only as required by law
Judaism (Orthodox and Conservative)			
Birth: No baptism Ritual circumcision of male infants on eighth day; performed by Mohel (ritual circumciser familiar with Jewish law and aseptic technique) Reform Jews favor ritual circumcision, but not as a religious imperative *Death:* Remains are ritually washed by members of the Ritual Burial Society Burial should take place as soon as possible	Numerous dietary kosher laws exist that may be influenced by local practices and family and cultural tradition Allowed only meat from animals that are vegetable eaters, are cloven hoofed, chew their cud, and are ritually slaughtered; fish that have scales and fins Prohibit any combination of meat and milk; milk products served first can be followed by meat in a few minutes, but milk may not be consumed for several hours after eating meat Fasting for 24 hours is part of Yom Kippur observance Matzo replaces leavened bread during Passover week	May resist surgical procedures during Sabbath, which extends from sundown Friday until sundown Saturday Seriously ill and pregnant women are exempt from fasting Illness is grounds for violating dietary laws (e.g., patient with congestive heart failure does not have to use kosher meats, which are high in sodium)	Oppose all forms of mutilation, including autopsy; body parts not donated or removed; amputated limbs, organs, or surgically removed tissues should be made available to family for burial Donation or transplantation of organs requires rabbinical consent May oppose prolongation of life after irreversible brain damage
Lutheran			
Birth: Baptize only living infants shortly after birth *Death:* Last rites optional	No requirements or restrictions	If grave prognosis, family may request anointing and blessing of sick or visit by church official	Accept scientific developments
Mennonite (Similar to Amish)			
Birth: No baptism in infancy Baptism during early or middle teens	No requirements or restrictions	No illness rituals Deep concern for dignity and self-determination of individual that would conflict with shock treatment or medical treatment affecting personality or will	

TABLE 28-2 Religious beliefs that affect nursing care—cont'd

BELIEFS ABOUT BIRTH AND DEATH	BELIEFS ABOUT DIET AND FOOD PRACTICES	BELIEFS REGARDING MEDICAL CARE	COMMENTS
Methodist			
Birth: Baptism may be at birth or performed on children or adults *Death:* No ritual	No requirements or restrictions	Communion may be requested before surgery or similar crisis	Encourage donation of body or body parts to medical science
Nazarene			
Birth: Baptism optional *Death:* No last rites	No requirements or restrictions Alcohol prohibited	Church official administers communion and laying on of hands Adherents believe in divine healing but not exclusive of medical treatment	Cremation permitted
Pentecostal (Assembly of God, Four-Square)			
Birth: No baptism at birth Baptism by complete immersion after age of accountability *Death:* No last rites	Abstain from alcohol, eating blood, strangled animals, or anything to which blood has been added Some individuals may resist pork	No restrictions regarding medical care Deliverance from sickness is provided for in atonement; may pray for divine intervention in health matters and seek God in prayer for themselves and others when ill	Some insist illness is divine punishment; most consider it an intrusion of Satan Practice glossolalia (speaking in tongues)
Orthodox Presbyterian			
Birth: Infant baptism by sprinkling *Death:* Last rites not a sacramental procedure; scripture reading and prayer	No requirements or restrictions	Communion administered when appropriate and convenient Blood transfusion accepted when advisable Pastor or elder should be called for ill person Believe science should be used for relief of suffering	Full forgiveness granted for any illness connected with a sin
Roman Catholic			
Birth: Infant baptism by sprinkling mandatory; especially urgent in poor prognosis, when it may be performed by anyone *Death:* Rite for anointing of the sick is mandatory Family or patient may request anointing if prognosis is grave	Fasting and abstaining from meat mandatory on Ash Wednesday and Good Friday; fasting optional during Lent; no meat on Fridays during Lent as general rule Children and most hospital patients exempt from fasting (eating only one full meal and no eating between meals) Some older Catholics may adhere to older rule of no meat on Friday	Encourage anointing of sick, although this may be interpreted by older members of church as equivalent to the old terminology "extreme unction" or "last rites"; they may require careful explanation if reluctance is associated with fear of imminent death Traditional church teaching does not approve of contraceptives or abortion	Family may request that major amputated limb be buried in consecrated ground Transplant accepted as long as loss of organ does not deprive donor of life or functional integrity of body Autopsy acceptable Religious articles, especially medals worn on the body, important and should be removed only when necessary and replaced as soon as possible
Russian Orthodox			
Birth: Baptism by priest only *Death:* Traditionally after death arms are crossed, fingers set in a cross	No meat or dairy products on Wednesday and Friday and during Lent	Cross necklace is important and should be removed only when necessary and replaced as soon as possible Adherents believe in divine healing, but not exclusive of medical treatment	Opposed to autopsy, embalming, or cremation
Unitarian Universalist			
Birth: Some practice infant baptism; most consider it unnecessary *Death:* No ritual	No requirements or restrictions	Believe God helps those who help themselves Some may prefer not to have clergy visit them in hospital	Cremation preferred to burial

TABLE 28-3 Cultural characteristics related to health care of children

CULTURAL GROUP	HEALTH BELIEFS	HEALTH PRACTICES
Asian-Americans		
Chinese	A healthy body is viewed as gift from parents and ancestors and must be cared for Health is one of the results of balance between the forces of *yin* (cold) and *yang* (hot), energy forces that rule the world Illness is caused by imbalance Blood is source of life and is not regenerated *Chi* is innate energy Lack of *chi* and blood results in deficiency that produces fatigue, poor constitution, and long illness	Goal of therapy is to restore balance of *yin* and *yang* Acupuncturist applies needles to appropriate meridians identified in terms of *yin* and *yang* Acupressure and *tai chi* are replacing acupuncture in some areas Moxibustion is application of heat to skin over specific meridians Wide use of medicinal herbs procured and applied in prescribed ways Folk healers are herbalist, spiritual healer, temple healer, fortune healer Meals may or may not be planned to balance hot and cold Milk intolerance is relatively common Use of condiments (e.g., monosodium glutamate and soy sauce) may create difficulty with some diet regimens (e.g., low-salt diets)
Japanese	Three major belief systems: *Shinto* religious influence Humans are inherently good Evil is caused by outside spirits Illness is caused by contact with polluting agents (e.g., blood, corpses, skin diseases) Chinese and Korean influence Health is achieved through harmony and balance between self and society Disease is caused by disharmony with society and not caring for body Portuguese influence Germ theory of disease is upheld	Believe evil is removed by purification Energy is restored by means of acupuncture, acupressure, massage, and moxibustion along affected meridians *Kampō* medicine is practiced—use of natural herbs Diseased parts are removed Trend is to use both Western and Oriental healing methods Care for disabled is viewed as family's responsibility Pride is taken in child's good health Preventive care, medical care for illness—are sought Some food combinations may be avoided (e.g., milk and cherries, watermelon and crab) and pickled plums are believed to have special properties
Vietnamese	Good health is considered to be balance between *yin* (cold) and *yang* (hot) Person's life has been predisposed toward certain phenomena by cosmic forces Health is the result of harmony with existing universal order; harmony attained by pleasing good spirits and avoiding evil ones Belief in *am duc*, the amount of good deeds accumulated by ancestors Many use rituals to prevent illness Some restrictions are practiced to prevent incurring wrath of evil spirits	Family uses all means possible before using outside agencies for health care Fortune-tellers determine event that caused disturbance Temple is visited to procure divine instruction Use astrologer to calculate cyclic changes and forces Health is regarded as family responsibility; outside aid is sought when resources run out Certain illnesses are considered only temporary (such as pustules, open wounds) and ignored Generalist health healers are sought Special diets used to prevent illness and promote health Lactose intolerance is prevalent
Filipinos	God's will and supernatural forces govern universe Illness, accidents, and other misfortunes are God's punishment for violations of His will "Hot" and "cold" balance and imbalance are widely accepted as cause of health and illness	Some use amulets as a shield from witchcraft or as good luck pieces Catholics subsitute religious medals and other items

Data from Anderson and Fenichel, 1989; Bloch, 1983; Char, 1981; Chen-Louie, 1983; DeSantis, 1988; Ehling, 1981; Greathouse and Miller, 1981; Hashizume and Takano, 1983; Holland and Sweeney, 1985; Hollingsworth, Brown, and Brooten, 1980; Lacay, 1981; Monrroy, 1983; Orque, 1983a, 1983b; Randall-David, 1989; Sodetaini-Shebata, 1981.

TABLE 28-3 Cultural characteristics related to health care of children—cont'd

FAMILY RELATIONSHIPS	COMMUNICATION	COMMENTS
Extended family pattern common Strong concept of loyalty of young to old Respect for elders taught at early age—acceptance without questioning or talking back Children's behavior a reflection on family Family and individual honor and "face" important Self-reliance and self-restraint highly valued; self-expression repressed Males valued more highly than females; women submissive to men in family	Open expression of emotions unacceptable Often smile when they do not comprehend	Do not react well to painful diagnostic workup; are especially upset by drawing of blood Deep respect for their bodies and believe it best to die with bodies intact; therefore may refuse surgery Believe in reincarnation Older members fear hospitals; often believe hospital is a place to go to die Children sometimes breastfed for up to 4 or 5 years*
Close intergenerational relationships Family provides anchor Family tends to keep problems to self Value self-control and self-sufficiency Concept of *haji* (shame) imposes strong control; unacceptable behavior of children reflects on family Many adopt practices of contemporary middle class Concern for child's missing school may result in sending to school before fully recovered from illness	*Issei*—born in Japan; usually speak Japanese only *Nisei, Sansei,* and *Yonsei* have few language difficulties New immigrants able to read and write English better than able to speak or understand it Make significant use of nonverbal communication with subtle gestures and facial expression Tend to suppress emotions Will often wait silently	Generational categories: *Issei*—1st generation to live in United States *Nisei*—2nd generation *Sansei*—3rd generation *Yonsei*—4th generation *Issei* and *Nissei*—tolerant and permissive childrearing until 5 or 6, then emphasis on emotional reserve and control Cleanliness highly valued Time considered valuable and used wisely Tendency to practice emotional control may make assessment of pain more difficult
Family revered institution Multigenerational families Family chief social network Children highly valued Individual needs and interests subordinate to those of family group Father main decision maker Women taught submission to men Parents expect respect and obedience from children	Many immigrants are not proficient in speaking and understanding English May hesitate to ask questions Questioning authority sign of disrespect; asking questions considered impolite Use indirectness rather than forthrightness in expressing disagreement May avoid eye contact with health professionals as a sign of respect	Consider status more important than money Children taught emotional control Time concept more relaxed—consider punctuality less significant than other values (i.e., property) Place high value on social harmony
Family highly valued, with strong family ties Multigenerational family structure common, often with collateral members as well Personal interests are subordinated to family interests and needs Members avoid any behavior that would bring shame on the family	Immigrants and older persons may not be able to speak or understand English	Tend to have a fatalistic outlook on life Believe time and providence will solve all

*Most Asian cultures consider the child 1 year old at the time of birth. Traditional Chinese custom adds 1 year on January 1, regardless of the birthday—a child born in December is 2 years old the next January.

Continued.

TABLE 28-3 Cultural characteristics related to health care of children—cont'd

CULTURAL GROUP	HEALTH BELIEFS	HEALTH PRACTICES
African-Americans	Illness classified as: Natural—affected by forces of nature without adequate protection (e.g., cold air, pollution, food and water) Unnatural—evil influences (e.g., witchcraft, voodoo, hoodoo, hex, fix, rootwork); symptoms often associated with eating Serious illness sent by God as punishment (e.g., parents punished by illness or death of child) Believe serious illness can be avoided May resist health care because illness is "will of God"	Self-care and folk medicine very prevalent Folk therapies usually religious in origin Attempt home remedies first; poorer people do not seek help until illness is serious Usually seek help from: "Old lady"—woman in community with a common knowledge of herbs; consulted regarding pediatric care Spiritualist—has received gift from God for healing incurable diseases or solving personal problems; strongly based on Christianity Priest (voodoo priest/priestess)—most powerful healer Root doctor—meets need for herbs, oils, candles, and ointments Prayer is common means for prevention and treatment
Haitians*	Illnesses have a supernatural or natural origin Supernatural illness are caused by angry voodoo spirits, enemies, or the dead, especially deceased ancestors Natural illnesses are based on conceptions of natural causation: Irregularities of blood volume, flow, purity, viscosity, color and/or temperature (hot/cold) Gas *(gaz)* Movement and consistency of mother's milk Hot/cold imbalance in the body Bone displacement Movement of diseases Health is maintained by good dietary and hygienic habits	Health is a personal responsibility Foods have properties of "hot"/"cold" and "light"/"heavy" and must be in harmony with one's life cycle and bodily states Natural illnesses are treated by home remedies first Supernatural illness are treated by healers: voodoo priest *(houngan)* or priestess *(mambo)*, midwife *(fam saj)*, and herbalist or leaf doctor *(dokte fey)* Amulets and prayer are used to protect against illness due to curses or willed by evil people
Hispanic Americans Mexican-Americans (Latinos, Chicanos, Raza-Latinos)	Health beliefs have strong religious association Believe in body imbalance as a cause of illness, especially imbalance between *caliente* (hot) and *frio* (cold) or "wet" and "dry" Some maintain good health is a result of "good luck"—a reward for good behavior Illness is prevented by performing properly, eating proper foods, and working proper amount of time; accomplished through prayer, wearing religious medals or amulets, and sleeping with relics at home Illness is a punishment from God for wrongdoing, forces of nature, and the supernatural	Seek help from *curandero* or *curandera*, especially in rural areas Curandero(a) receives his/her position by birth, apprenticeship, or a "calling" via dream or vision Treatments involve use of herbs, rituals, and religious artifacts Practice for severe illness—make promises, visit shrines, offer medals and candles, offer prayers Adhere to "hot" and "cold" food prescriptions and prohibitions for prevention and treatment of illness
Puerto Ricans	Subscribe to the "hot-cold" theory of causation of illness Believe some illness caused by evil spirits and forces	Infrequent use of health care systems Seek folk healers—use of herbs, rituals Consult spiritualist medium for mental disorders *Santeria* is system and practitioners are called *santeros* Treatments classified as "hot" or "cold"

*This section was written by Lydia DeSantis, Ph.D., R.N.

TABLE 28-3 Cultural characteristics related to health care of children—cont'd

FAMILY RELATIONSHIPS	COMMUNICATION	COMMENTS
Strong kinship bonds in extended family; members come to aid of others in crisis Less likely to view illness as a burden Augmented families common (unrelated persons living in same household) Place strong emphasis on work and ambition Sex-role sharing among parents Elderly members respected	Alert to any evidence of discrimination Place importance on nonverbal behavior May use nonstandard English or "black English" Use "testing" behaviors to assess personnel in health care situations before seeking active care Best to use simple, direct, but caring approach	High level of caution and distrust of majority group Social anxiety related to tradition of humiliation, oppression, and loss of dignity Will elect to retain dignity rather than seek care if values are compromised Strong sense of peoplehood High incidence of poverty Black minister a strong influence in black community Visits by family minister are sought, expected, and valued in helping to cope with illness and suffering
Maintenance of family reputation is paramount Lineal authority supreme; children in a subordinate position in family hierarchy Children valued for parental social security in old age and expected to contribute to family welfare at an early age Children viewed as "gifts from god" and treated with indulgence and affection	Recent immigrants and older persons may speak only Haitian creole May prefer family/friends to act as translators and confidants Often smile and nod in agreement when they do not understand Quiet and gentle communication style and lack of assertiveness lead health care providers to falsely believe they comprehend health teaching and are compliant Will not ask questions if health care provider is busy or rushed	Will use biomedical and ethnomedical (folk) systems simultaneously Resistant to dietary and work restrictions Adherence to prescribed treatments directly related to perceived severity of illness
Traditionally men considered breadwinners and key decision makers in matters outside the home; women considered homemakers Males considered big and strong *(macho)* Strong kinship; extended families include *compadres* (godparents) established by ritual kinship Children valued highly and desired, taken everywhere with family Many homes contain shrines with statues and pictures of saints Elderly treated with respect	May use nonstandard English Most bilingual; many only speak Spanish May have a strong preference for native language and revert to it in times of stress May shake hands or engage in introductory embrace Interpret prolonged eye contact as disrespectful	High degree of modesty—often a deterrent to seeking medical care and open discussions of sex Youngsters often reluctant to share communal showers in schools Relaxed concept of time—may be late for appointments More concerned with present than with future and therefore may focus on immediate solutions rather than long-term goals Magicoreligious practices common May view hospital as place to go to die
Family usually large and home centered—the core of existence Father has complete authority in family—family provider and decision maker Wife and children subordinate to father Children valued—seen as a gift from God Children taught to obey and respect parents; corporal punishment to ensure obedience	May use nonstandard English Spanish speaking or bilingual Strong sense of family privacy—may view questions regarding family as impudent	Relaxed sense of time Pay little attention to *exact* time of day Suspicious and fearful of hospitals

Continued.

TABLE 28-3 Cultural characteristics related to health care of children—cont'd

CULTURAL GROUP	HEALTH BELIEFS	HEALTH PRACTICES
Cuban-Americans*	Prevention and good nutrition are related to good health	Diligent users of the medical model, in part because of aggressive public health practices on the island before and after the revolution Eclectic health-seeking practices, including preventive measures, extensive use of the medical model, and, in some instances, folk medicine of both religious and nonreligious origins; home remedies; in many instances seek assistance of *santeros* (Afro-Cuban healers) and spiritualists to complement medical treatment Nutrition is important; parents show overconcern with eating habits of their children and spend a considerable part of the budget on food; traditional Cuban diet is rich in meat and starch; consumption of fresh vegetables added in United States
Native American (numerous tribes)	Believe health is state of harmony with nature and universe Respect of bodies through proper management All disorders believed to have aspects of supernatural Violation of a restriction or prohibition thought to cause illness Fear of witchcraft May carry objects believed to guard against witchcraft Theology and medicine strongly interwoven	Medicine persons: Altruistic persons who must use powers in purely positive ways Persons capable of both good and evil—perform negative acts against enemies Diviner-diagnosticians—diagnose but do not have powers or skill to implement medical treatment Specialists—use herbs and curative but nonsacred medical procedures Medicine persons—use herbs and ritual Singers—cure by the power of their song obtained from supernatural beings; effect cures by laying on of hands

*This section was written by Mercedes Sandaval, Ph.D.

Key Points

- A culture is composed of individuals with a set of values, beliefs, practices, and information that is learned, integrative, social, and satisfying.
- Nurses have a responsibility to understand the influence of culture, race, and ethnicity on the development of social and emotional relationships, childrearing practices, and attitudes toward health.
- Socialization is the process by which children acquire the beliefs, values, and behaviors considered desirable or appropriate by the culture.
- A child's self-concept evolves from ideas about his or her social roles.
- Guilt and shame are two behaviors commonly conditioned in children to control social behavior.
- Important subcultural influences on children include ethnicity, social class, poverty, affluence, occupation, religion, schools, peers, and biculture.
- Membership in a minority group presents special challenges for children, although changes in societal attitudes are slowly taking place.
- Cultural shock refers to a person's feeling of helplessness and disorientation while trying to adapt to a different cultural group and its practices, values, and beliefs.
- A child's physical characteristics and susceptibility to health problems are strongly related to ethnic and cultural variations of hereditary and socioeconomic forces.
- Cultural beliefs related to the course of illness and maintenance of health may focus on natural forces, supernatural forces, or imbalance of forces.
- In planning and implementing patient care, nurses need to strive to adapt ethnic practices to the family's health needs rather than attempt to change long-standing beliefs.
- No cultural group is homogeneous, and every racial and ethnic group contains great diversity.

TABLE 28-3 Cultural characteristics related to health care of children—cont'd

FAMILY RELATIONSHIPS	COMMUNICATION	COMMENTS
Strong family ties with mother and father kinships Children supported and assisted by parents long after becoming adults Elderly cared for at home	Most are bilingual (English/Spanish), except for segments of the senior population	In less than 30 years Cubans have been able to obtain a higher standard of living than other Hispanic groups in United States Have been able to retain many of their former social institutions: e.g., bilingual and private schools, clinics, social clubs, the family as an extended network of support Many do not feel discriminated against nor harbor feelings of inferiority with respect to Anglo-Americans or "mainstream" population
Extended family structure—usually includes relatives from both sides of family Elder members assume leadership roles	Most continue to speak their Indian language, as well as English Nonverbal communication	Time orientation—present Respect for age Going to hospital associated with illness or disease; therefore may not seek prenatal care, since pregnancy viewed as natural process Tend to take time to form an opinion of professionals

References

Adams PJ: *Effects of poverty and affluence.* In Hendee WR: *The health of adolescents,* San Francisco, 1991, Jossey-Bass.

American Academy of Pediatrics: Health care for children of migrant families, *Pediatrics* 84(4):739-740, 1989.

Anderson P, Fenichel D: *Serving culturally diverse families of infants and toddlers with disabilities,* Washington, DC, 1989, National Center for Clinical Infant Programs.

Bassuk EL, Rosenberg L: Psychosocial characteristics of homeless children and children with homes, *Pediatrics* 85(3):257-261, 1990.

Baze S: *Measuring physical growth.* In Smith D, editor: *Comprehensive child and family nursing skills,* St Louis, 1991, Mosby.

Bloch B: *Nursing care of black patients.* In Orque MS, Bloch B, Monrroy LSA, editors: *Ethnic nursing care,* St Louis, 1983, Mosby.

Buchwald D et al: Caring for patients in a multicultural society, *Patient Care* 28(11):105-120, 1994.

Carpenito LJ: *Nursing diagnosis: application to clinical practice,* ed 4, Philadelphia, 1992, JB Lippincott.

Char EL: *The Chinese American.* In Clark AL, editor: *Culture and childrearing,* Philadelphia, 1981, FA Davis.

Chen-Louie T: *Nursing care of Chinese American patients.* In Orque MS, Bloch B, Monrroy LSA, editors: *Ethnic nursing care,* St Louis, 1983, Mosby.

Chidester D: *Patterns of transcendence: religion, death, and dying,* Belmont, Calif, 1990, Wadsworth.

Clutter L: *Fostering spiritual care for the child and family.* In Smith D, editor: *Comprehensive child and family nursing skills,* St Louis, 1991, Mosby.

Conley L: Childbearing and childrearing practices in Mormonism, *Neonatal Network* 9(3):41-48, 1990.

Davidhizar R, Frank B: Understanding the physical and psychosocial stressors of the child who is homeless, *Pediatr Nurs* 18(6):559-562, 1992.

DeSantis L: Cultural factors affecting newborn and infant diarrhea, *J Pediatr Nurs* 3(6):391-398, 1988.

Ehling MB: *The Mexican American (El Chicano).* In Clark AL, editor: *Culture and childrearing,* Philadelphia, 1981, FA Davis.

Elfert H, Anderson J, Lai M: Parents' perceptions of children with chronic illness: a study of immigrant Chinese families, *J Pediatr Nurs* 6(2):114-120, 1991.

Elkin F, Handel G: *The child and society: the process of socialization,* New York, 1989, Random House.

Fleming J: Meeting the challenge of culturally diverse populations, *Pediatr Nurs* 15(6):566, 634, 1989 (guest editorial).

Freidman M: Transcultural family nursing: application to Latino and black families, *Pediatr Nurs* 5(3):214-222, 1990.

Greathouse B, Miller VG: *The black American.* In Clark AL, editor: *Culture and childrearing,* Philadelphia, 1981, FA Davis.

Habayeb GL: Cultural diversity: a nursing concept not yet reliably defined, *Nurs Outlook* 43(5):224-227, 1995.

Hayes J, Dreher C: *Providing culturally sensitive care.* In Smith D, editor: *Comprehensive child and family nursing skills,* St Louis, 1991, Mosby.

Holland S, Sweeney E: *Vietnamese children and families: the impact of culture,* Washington, DC, 1985, Association for Care of Children's Health.

Hollingsworth AO, Brown LP, Brooten DA: The refugees and childbearing: what to expect, *RN* 43(11):45-48, 1980.
Issacs P: Growth parameters and blood values in Arabic children, *Pediatr Nurs* 15(6):579-583, 1989.
Kozier B, Erb G: *Fundamentals of nursing*, ed 5, Menlo Park, Calif, 1995, Addison-Wesley.
Kuensting L, Sanders G, editors: *Cultural considerations*, Park Ridge, Ill, 1995, Emergency Nurses Association.
Lacay G: *The Puerto Rican in mainland America*. In Clark AL, editor: *Culture and childrearing*, Philadelphia, 1981, FA Davis.
Leininger M: *Transcultural nursing*, New York, 1978, John Wiley & Sons.
Lynch E: *From cultural shock to cultural learning*. In Lynch E, Hanson M, editors: *Developing cross-cultural competence*, Baltimore, 1992, Paul H Brookes.
Malach F, Segel N: Perspectives on health care delivery systems for American Indian families, *Child Health Care* 19(4):219-228, 1990.
Martin JA: Birth characteristics for Asian or Pacific Islander subgroups, 1992, *Monthly vital statistics report*, 43(10, suppl):28-53, 1995, National Center for Health Statistics.
Money K, Prakasam K, Joshi V: Transcultural developmental sexology: genital greeting versus child molestation, *Issues Child Abuse Accusations* 9(4):215-216, 1991.
Monrroy LSA: *Nursing care of Raza/Latina patients*. In Orque MS, Bloch B, Monrroy LSA, editors: *Ethnic nursing care*, St Louis, 1983, Mosby.
Nance TA: Intercultural communication: finding common ground, *J Obstet Gynecol Neonatal Nurs* 24(3):249-255, 1995.
Orque MS: *Nursing care of Filipino American patients*. In Orque MS, Bloch B, Monrroy LSA, editors: *Ethnic nursing care*, St Louis, 1983a, Mosby.
Orque MS: *Nursing care of South Vietnamese patients*. In Orque MS, Bloch B, Monrroy LSA, editors: *Ethnic nursing care*, St Louis, 1983b, Mosby.
Randall-David E: *Strategies for working with culturally diverse communities and clients*, Washington, DC, 1989, Association for the Care of Children's Health.
Shaffer DC: *Developmental psychology: theory, research, and application*, Monterey, Calif, 1985, Brooks/Cole Publishing Co.
Sloat A, Matsuura W: *Intercultural communication*. In Craft M, Denehy J, editors: *Nursing interventions for infants and children*, Philadelphia, 1990, WB Saunders.
Sodetani-Shibata AE: *The Japanese American*. In Clark AL, editor: *Culture and childrearing*, Philadelphia, 1981, FA Davis.
Spector RE: *Cultural diversity in health and illness*, ed 2, New York, 1985, Appleton-Century Crofts.
Wagner J, Melragon B, Menke E: Homeless children: interdisciplinary drug prevention intervention, *J Child Adolesc Psychiatr Ment Health Nurs* 6(1):22-30, 1993.

Bibliography

General

Ahmann E: "Chunky stew": appreciating cultural diversity while providing health care for children, *Pediatr Nurs* 20(3):320-322, 1994.
Anderson JM: Health care across cultures, *Nurs Outlook* 38(3):136-139, May/June, 1990.
Bauwens EE, Anderson S: *Social and cultural influences on health care*. In Stanhope M, Lancaster J, editors: *Community health nursing*, ed 3, St Louis, 1992, Mosby.
Buchwald D et al: Five vignettes of cross-cultural care, *Patient Care* 29(11):120-123, 1994.
Chan S: Early intervention with culturally diverse families of infants and toddlers with disabilities, *Inf Young Child* 3(2):78-87, 1990.
Choi ES, Hamilton RK: The effects of culture on mother-infant interaction, *J Obstet Gynecol Neonatal Nurs* 15:256-261, 1986.
Conatser C: Effect of wealth on approach to patient care, *J Assoc Pediatr Oncol Nurses* 3(2):14-19, 1986.
Culture and nursing practice: an applied view, *Holistic Nurs Pract* 6(3):entire issue, 1992.
Evans V: *Sociodemographic trends toward the 21st century*. In Feeg V, editor: *Pediatric nursing: forum on the future: looking toward the 21st century*, Pitman, NJ, 1989, Anthony J Jannetti.
Giger J, Davidhizar R: *Transcultural nursing: assessment and intervention*, St Louis, 1991, Mosby.
Juarez G: Controlling pain: when culture clashes with pain control, *Nursing '95* 25(5):90, 1995.
Kohn S: Dismantling sociocultural barriers to care, *Healthcare Forum J* 38(3):30-33, 1995.
Olness K: *Cultural issues in primary pediatric care*. In Hoekelman RA: *Primary pediatric care*, ed 2, St Louis, 1992, Mosby.
Shulsinger E: Needs of sheltered homeless children, *J Pediatr Health Care* 4(3):136-140, 1991.
Tripp-Reimer T, Afifi LA: Cross-cultural perspectives on patient teaching, *Nurs Clin North Am* 24(3):613-619, 1989.
Tripp-Reimer T, Brink PJ, Saunders JM: Cultural assessment: content and process, *Nurs Outlook* 32:78-82, 1984.
Tseng W, Hsu J: *Culture and family*, Binghamton, NY, 1990, Haworth Press.

Religion

Abbott DA, Berry M, Meredith WH: Religious beliefs and practice: a potential asset in helping families, *Fam Relations* 39(4):443-448, 1990.
Adams CE and others: The effects of religious beliefs on the health care practices of the Amish, *Nurs Pract* 11(3):58-67, 1986.
Carson V: *Spiritual dimensions of nursing practice*, Philadelphia, 1989, WB Saunders.
Conley L: Childbearing and childrearing practices in Mormonism, *Neonatal Network* 9(3):41-48, 1990.
Gershan JA: Judiac ethical beliefs and customs regarding death and dying, *Crit Care Nurse* 5(1):32-34, 1985.
Masulis K: When parents refuse treatment for their children . . . Jehovah's Witnesses, *J Christ Nurs* 4(2):10-12, 1987.
O'Rourke K: Pain relief: the perspective of Catholic tradition, *J Pain Symptom Manage* 7(8):485-491, 1992.
Randall-David E: *Strategies for working with culturally diverse communities and clients*, Washington, DC, 1989, Association for the Care of Children's Health.
Roberson MHB: The influence of religious beliefs on health choices of Afro-Americans, *Top Clin Nurs* 7(3):57-63, 1985.
Shelly JA: Spiritual care: planting seeds of hope, *Crit Care Update* 9(2):7-15, 1982.
Sodestrom KE, Martinson IM: Patients' spiritual coping strategies: a study of nurse and patient perspectives, *Oncol Nurs Forum* 14(2):41-46, 1987.
Swan R: The law should protect all children . . . children in faith-healing sects, *J Christ Nurs* 4(2):40, 1987.
Thurkauf GE: Understanding the beliefs of Jehovah's Witnesses, *Focus Crit Care* 16(3):199-204, 1989.

Specific Ethnic Groups

Berne AS and others: A nursing model for addressing the health needs of homeless families, *Image J Nurs Sch* 22(1):8-13, 1990.
Bishop S: The mental health of children and families in rural America, *J Child Adolesc Psychiatr Ment Health Nurs* 3(3):77-78, 1990.

Cheadle A et al: Relationship between socioeconomic status, health status, and lifestyle practices of American Indians: evidence from a plains reservation population, *Public Health Rep* 109(3):405-413, 1994.

Davis RE: The heart and soul of Puerto Rican community: caring and caregivers, *J Multicult Nurs* 1(2):21-27, 1994.

de Leon Siantz M: Correlates of maternal depression among Mexican-American migrant farmworker mothers, *Child Adolesc Psychiatr Ment Health Nurs* 3(1):9-13, 1990.

DeSantis L: Cultural factors affecting newborn and infant diarrhea, *J Pediatr Nurs* 3(6):391-398, 1988.

Desantis L: Infant feeding practices of Haitian mothers in South Florida: cultural beliefs and acculturation, *Matern Child Nurs J* 15:77-89, 1986.

Duque MC: Caring for Colombian children with the realm of health and disease, *J Pediatr Nurs* 9(3):213-216, 1994.

Egan MG: A family assessment challenge: refugee youth and foster family adaptation, *Top Clin Nurs* 7(3):64-69, 1985.

Foreman JT: *Susto* and the health needs of the Cuban refugee population, *Top Clin Nurs* 7(3):40-47, 1985.

Hansen M, Resnick L: Health beliefs, health care, and rural Appalachian subcultures from an ethnographic perspective, *Fam Community Health* 13(1):1-10, 1990.

Hashizume S, Takano J: *Nursing care of Japanese patients.* In Orque MS, Bloch B, Monrroy LSA, editors: *Ethnic nursing care,* St Louis, 1983, Mosby.

Marrio EB, Hall RR: Asian family traditions and their influence in transcultural health care delivery, *Child Health Care* 15(3):172-177, 1987.

Martinson IM: *The challenge of culturally diverse pediatric clients.* In Feeg V, editor: *Pediatric nursing: forum on the future: looking toward the 21st century,* Pitman, NJ, 1989, Anthony J Jannetti.

Mattson S, Lew L: Culturally sensitive prenatal care for Southeast Asians, *JOGNN* 21(1):48-54, 1992.

Pass CM: Psychological factors, childbearing, and black female adolescents, *J Pediatr Nurs* 1:247-259, 1986.

Powell D, Zambrana R, Silva-Palacios V: Designing culturally responsive parent programs: a comparison of low-income Mexican and Mexican-American mothers' preferences, *Fam Relations* 39(3):298-304, 1990.

Ramirez AG: A media-based acculturation scale for Mexican-Americans: application to public health education programs, *Fam Community Health* 9(3):63-71, 1986.

Rescoria L, Parker R, Stolley P: Ability, achievement, and adjustment in homeless children, *Am J Orthopsychiatry* 61(2):210-220, 1991.

Rosenburg JA: Health care for Cambodian children: integrating treatment plans, *Pediatr Nurs* 12:118-125, 1986.

Rozendal N: Understanding Italian American cultural norms, *J Psychosoc Nurs Ment Health Serv* 25(2):29-35, 1987.

van Breda A: Health issues facing Native American children, *Pediatr Nurs* 15(6):575-577, 1989.

Wood D: Homeless children: their evaluation and treatment, *J Pediatr Health Care* 3(4):194-199, 1989.

CHAPTER 29

Family Influences on Child Health Promotion

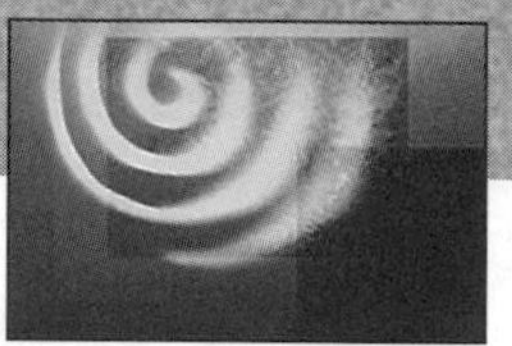

GENERAL CONCEPTS, P. 826
Definition of family, p. 826
Family nursing interventions, p. 826

FAMILY ROLES, RELATIONSHIPS, AND STRENGTHS, P. 827
Parental roles, p. 827
Role learning, p. 828
Family size and configuration, p. 828
Family strengths, p. 830

PARENTING, P. 831

SPECIAL PARENTING SITUATIONS, P. 835
Parenting the adopted child, p. 835
Parenting and divorce, p. 837
Single parenting, p. 839
Parenting in reconstituted families, p. 840
Parenting in dual-earner families, p. 840
Accommodationg contemporary parenting situations, p. 840

General Concepts

DEFINITION OF FAMILY

The term **family** has been defined in a number of ways and for a number of purposes according to an individual's own frame of reference or value judgment, or the discipline. For example, biology describes the family as fulfilling the biologic function of perpetuation of the species. Psychology emphasizes the interpersonal aspects of the family and its responsibility for personality development. Economics views the family as a productive unit that provides for material needs, and sociology depicts it as the social unit that reacts with the larger society. Others define family in relation to the persons who make up the family unit; the most common types of relationships are *consanguineous* (blood relationships), *affinal* (marital relationships), and *family of origin* (the family unit a person is born into).

Traditionally a family has been conceptualized as a group, with the belief that both a mother and a father are needed to rear a child. Nearly all societies grant a very high rank to the married status, but in today's society a broad definition of the family is needed, such as "a group of people, living together or in close contact, who take care of one another and provide guidance for their dependent members." Most important, for any given patient, "family" is whatever the patient considers it to be (Patterson, 1995) (see the Critical Thinking Q & A box on p. 827, left).

Nursing of infants and children is intimately involved with care of the child *and* the family. Consequently, nurses must be aware of the functions of the family, various types of family structures, and theories that provide a foundation for understanding the changes within a family and for directing family-oriented interventions.

FAMILY NURSING INTERVENTIONS

In working with children, nurses must include family members in their plan of care. In essence, the *patient is the family.* To discover family dynamics and the unit's strengths and weaknesses, a thorough family assessment is needed (see Chapter 31). The interventions nurses use with families depend on their theoretic model of the family. For example, in family systems theory the focus is on the interactions of the members rather than on an individual member. In this case it is essential to use group dynamics to involve all members in the intervention process and to be a skillful communicator (see the Critical Thinking Q & A box on p. 827, right). Systems theory also presents an excellent opportunity for anticipatory guidance. Because each member of the family reacts to every stress experienced by that system, such as the birth of a child, nurses can intervene to help the family prepare for and cope with the change. At each stress point there is the opportunity for change and learning because families are more open to interventions at this time (Brazelton, 1995).

In the family stress theory, crisis intervention strategies are used, and the chief focus is on helping members cope with the challenging event. In the developmental theory a primary nursing function is to provide anticipatory guidance that prepares members for transition to the next family stage.

Critical Thinking Q & A

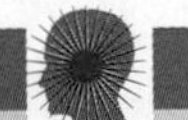

FAMILY STRUCTURE

As the nurse, you are interviewing the mother of John, a school-age boy. The mother says their family consists of herself, her son, her lesbian partner, and two foster children. John's father lives in another state and has no contact with him. John has one grandparent, who lives in another city in a nursing home. When planning care for John and his family, John's family should be considered to be which of the following?

1. Nuclear family of mother, father, and son
2. Single-parent family of mother and son
3. Extended family of mother, father, grandparent, and son
4. Family members identified by the mother

The best answer is four. The family defines its own members. In this situation, John's family consists of those people who live in his home. Traditionally, family composition has referred to either nuclear or extended families. However, many alternative family structures such as John's occur. The nurse needs to recognize that not all families are traditional in their membership.

Nurses use a variety of strategies when working with families (Box 29-1). It is important for nurses to be aware of their degree of professional competence in using family nursing interventions. An important nursing role is to recognize situations in which a referral to more specialized services is required.

Family Roles, Relationships, and Strengths

Each individual has a position, or status, in the family structure and plays culturally and socially defined roles in interactions within the family group. Each family has its own traditions and values and sets its own standards for interaction within and outside the group. Each determines the experiences the children should have, those from which they are to be shielded, and how each of these experiences meets the needs of family members. Where family ties are strong, social control is highly effective, and most members conform to their roles willingly and with commitment. Conflicts arise when people do not fulfill their roles in ways that meet the expectations of other family members either because they are unaware of the expectations or because they choose not to meet them.

PARENTAL ROLES

In all family groups the socially recognized status of father and mother exists with socially sanctioned roles that prescribe appropriate sexual behavior and childrearing responsibilities. The guides for behavior in these roles serve to control sexual conflict in society and provide for prolonged care of children. The degree to which parents are committed and the way they play their roles are influenced by their unique socialization experience.

Critical Thinking Q & A

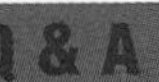

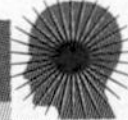

FAMILY THEORIES

As the school nurse, you are working with a family that consists of a mother, a father, and their 10-year-old son and 16-year-old daughter. The daughter, Jenny, has stopped going to school this week. She has had many conflicts with her parents, and her relationship with her father is very strained. He recently took away her driving privileges because of curfew violations. Jenny says she is quitting school if she cannot drive. Which of the following three family theories would you apply when working with this family?

1. Developmental theory
2. Family stress theory
3. Family system theory

The best answer is three. In family system theory the family is viewed as a system that continually interacts with its members. Family interactions rather than individual members are viewed as the source of the problems. Although developmental and family stress theories could be applied, the family is experiencing an interaction problem more than a developmental or stress-related problem.

BOX 29-1
Family Nursing Interventions

- Behavior modification
- Contracting
- Case management/coordination
- Collaborative strategies
- Counseling, including support, cognitive reappraisal, and reframing
- Empowering families through active participation
- Environmental modification
- Family advocacy
- Family crisis intervention
- Networking, including use of self-help groups and social support
- Providing information and technical expertise
- Role modeling
- Role supplementation
- Teaching strategies, including stress management, life-style modifications, and anticipatory guidance

From Friedman MM: *Family nursing: theory and practice,* ed 3, Norwalk, Conn, 1992, Appleton & Lange.

Role definitions are changing as a result of changing economy and the women's liberation movement. Women are achieving equality with men in education, more women are entering the labor force, and the number of women who choose to have fewer children or none at all is increasing. During childhood, particularly in the upper and middle classes, the trend is toward deemphasizing the basic male-female characteristics of aggression, dependence, and achievement. As the role of the woman changes, there must necessarily be a change in the complementary role of the man. Fathers are taking a more active role in childrearing and household activities, particularly in middle-class families. Marital roles remain most segregated in the lower classes. A redefinition of gender roles in the American family is taking place, but a cultural lag of the persisting traditional role definitions creates conflicts in many of these families.

ROLE LEARNING

Roles are learned through the socialization process. During all stages of development, children learn and practice (through interaction with others and in their play) a set of social roles and something of the characteristics of other roles. They behave in patterned and more or less predictable ways because they learn roles that define mutual expectations in typical and recurring social relationships. Role conceptions are transmitted by socializing agents (parents, peers, authority figures) who use positive and negative sanctions to ensure conformity to their norms.

In some cultures the role behavior expected of children conflicts with desirable adult behavior. For example, in the United States children are expected to be submissive in childhood but dominant as adults. This conflict of expectations is known as *role discontinuity.* Other cultures value the same behaviors, such as courage and aggression, both in children and adults; this provides *role continuity.*

Role structuring initially takes place within the family unit, where the children fulfill a set of roles and respond to the complementary roles of their parents and other family members. The roles of the children are shaped primarily by the parents, who apply direct or indirect pressures in an attempt to induce or force children into the desired patterns of behavior. Each set of parents has its own techniques, and each determines the course that the process of socialization is to follow (see Limit-Setting and Discipline, p. 833).

Research indicates that birth order influences the role each sibling is assigned within the family (Hoopes and Harper, 1987). When children enter a particular family, they sense the physical, social, and emotional values associated with their own specific roles. They then develop characteristic response patterns to fulfill their roles. Each sibling position role is created to meet both the family's and the individual's needs (Box 29-2).

Children respond to life situations according to behaviors learned in reciprocal transactions. As they acquire important role-taking skills, their relationships with others change. They become proficient at understanding others as they acquire the ability to discriminate their own perspectives from those of others. Children who get along well with others and attain status in the peer group have well-developed role-taking skills.

FAMILY SIZE AND CONFIGURATION

The size and composition of the family directly influence child development. No two children grow in exactly the same environment, although identical twins most nearly approximate this. For example, in a nuclear family with two children—even of the same gender—one child lives in a family with an older sibling, whereas the other child is reared in a family with a younger sibling. In a family in which there is a 10-year age span among the children, one child may be born to a 20-year-old mother and the other to a 30-year-old mother. For each child the environment is different.

Family Size

Parenting practices differ between small and large families. In small families more emphasis is placed on the individual development of the children. Parenting is intensive rather than extensive, and there is constant pressure to measure up to family expectations. Children's development and achievement are measured against that of other children in the neighborhood and social class. In small families there is more democratic participation by the children than in larger families.

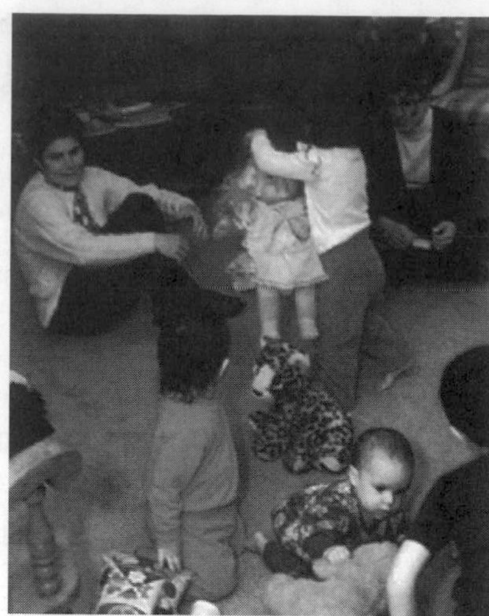

Fig. 29-1 Innumerable relationships and activities are possible in a large family.

Children in large families are able to adjust to a variety of changes and crises. There is more emphasis on the group and less on the individual (Fig. 29-1). Cooperation is essential, often because of economic necessity. The large number of persons sharing a limited amount of space requires a greater degree of organization, administration, and authoritarian control. The control is wielded by a dominant family member—a parent or an older child. Because the number of children reduces the intimate, one-to-one contact between the parent and any individual child, siblings may turn to each other to have their needs met. Individual children may adopt specialized roles in an attempt to gain recognition in the family.

Discipline is often administered by older siblings in large families. Siblings are usually better attuned to what constitutes misbehavior, and sibling disapproval or ostracism is often more meaningful than parental measures. Large families seem to generate a sense of security in the children fostered by sibling support and cooperation. However, adolescents from a large family are more peer oriented than family oriented.

Spacing of Children and Ordinal Position

Age differences between siblings affect the childhood environment but to a lesser extent than does the gender of the siblings. The arrival of a sibling has the greatest impact on the older child, and a 2- to 4-year difference in age appears to be most threatening. When the older child is very young, the self-image is too immature to be threatened. At an older age the child is better able to understand the situation and therefore is less likely to see the newcomer as a threat, although the child does feel the loss of the only-child status. Studies reveal that there is more affection and less rivalry or hostility when children are spaced 4 or more years apart (Lobato, 1990).

BOX 29-2
Influence of Ordinal Position on Children

Firstborn children
Are more achievement oriented
Are more dominant
Receive more physical punishment
Are allowed to show more aggression to siblings
Have stronger consciences, are more self-disciplined and inner directed
Are more socially anxious
Are prone to feelings of guilt
Identify more with parents than with peers
Are more conservative
Are subject to greater parental expectations
Begin to speak earlier in life
Demonstrate higher intellectual achievement
Plan better and experience fewer frustrations
Are likely to be most wanted

Middle children
Have more demands made on them for household help
Are praised less often
Receive less of parents' time
Learn to compromise and be adaptable
Are less stimulated toward achievement
Are more difficult to characterize because of a variety of positions in family

Youngest children
Are less dependent than firstborn children
Are less tense, more affectionate, and more good-natured
Tend to identify more with peer group than with parents
Are more flexible in their thinking
Are popular with classmates
Have fewer demands placed on them for household help

Only children
Resemble firstborn children
Are more mature and cultivated
Experience greater parental pressure for mature behavior and achievement
Demonstrate superiority in language facility
Rarely develop into stereotype of spoiled, selfish child
Often enjoy a rich fantasy life as a result of isolation

In general, the narrower the spacing between siblings, the more the children influence one another, especially in emotional characteristics; the wider the spacing, the greater the influence of the parents. This is not to say that bonds are nonexistent between siblings with large age spans or that siblings with only a year or two difference in age will always feel a strong bond. However, high accessibility during these developmentally formative years is the almost routine accompaniment of an influential sibling relationship. High-access siblings are generally close in age and the same gender, which promotes access to common life events. They often attend the same school, play with the same friends, date in the same circle, and share a common bedroom and clothing.

It has also been observed for some time that the birth position of children affects their personalities. Parents treat children differently, and sibling interactions are different depending on the children's position within the family. The major influences of ordinal position on children are presented in Box 29-2. However, children vary tremendously; these generalizations represent averages and do not apply in all situations.

Sibling Interaction

Most children have at least one brother or sister. Asked why they chose to have a second child, most parents give as their primary reason the fact that they did not want their firstborn to be an only child (Lobato, 1990). Right or wrong, many people believe that children develop best within the company of other children.

Perhaps the most unique feature of the sibling relationship is its duration. Likely the longest relationship shared with another human being, the sibling relationship lasts through a lifetime, often 50 to 80 years, as compared with the child-parent relationship of approximately 30 to 50 years. Siblings spend long periods of time together and come to know each other—at their best and worst—extremely well.

Sibling functions. Siblings exert power, exchange services, and express feelings in reciprocal ways that are often not revealed explicitly in the presence of parents. They see themselves in their brother or sister, experience life vicariously through their sibling's behavior, and begin to expand on their own possibilities. Siblings can also be touchstones for what the other would *not* like to be, and they tend to use each other as yardsticks for comparison. They are sounding boards for one another; they offer a safe forum for experimenting with new behaviors and roles before using either with parents or nonfamily peers.

Brothers and sisters provide each other with tangible services (e.g., lending money, clothing, toys, sports equipment, teaching a skill), help with childhood problems, provide support in dealing with parents or others outside the family, and may provide an introduction to a new friendship group. Children learn to negotiate and bargain, and sometimes to manipulate. They learn about sharing, competition, rivalry, and compromise. Siblings can also protect one another from parental-executive abuse of power and can form a coalition to deal with the issues of authority, power, and emotional support. Negotiating with parents is stronger when siblings act together rather than singly.

Siblings interpret the outside world for each other and perform genuine educative functions for the parents. A related function is pioneering, wherein one sibling initiates a process, thereby giving permission to the others to follow accordingly. Patterns may include breaking explicit family rules, taking new developmental pathways (such as leaving the family), or adopting different moral/political codes and life-styles.

Tattling can be an important lever in sibling interactions. On the other hand, there is often a conspiracy of silence among siblings, leaving the parents feeling isolated and excluded. A willingness to make and maintain each other's privacy often serves as a powerful bond of loyalty among the children. It is this loyalty that often distinguishes the relationship between siblings from that between friends.

More active sibling relationships. Sibling relationships vary among cultures. Certain factors, however, may be giving the sibling relationship greater significance in North America than in the past. Shrinking family size, longer life spans, divorce and remarriage, geographic mobility, maternal employment, alternative sources of child care, competitive pressures, stress, and various forms of parental insufficiency may be propelling siblings into greater contact and emotional interdependence than ever before.

For example, siblings often join forces to confront the trauma of divorce. They often rely on each other for support when parents remarry. The large number of working mothers means that many young siblings today have large amounts of time when their relationship is not monitored by a personally committed adult. Often an older sibling is required to baby-sit, which results in children spending more and more time together unsupervised. In a worried, mobile, high-stress, fast-paced, parent-absent society, children often turn to a sibling to meet their need for contact, constancy, and permanency.

Multiple Births

A deviation in early development that occurs with variable frequency is multiple births. Twins are not uncommon in the population, but triplets are rare, and quadruplets or quintuplets are extremely unusual. In any of these situations the offspring can be of like or unlike gender (i.e., derived from a single ovum, from multiple ova, or a combination of the two, which can involve one or more cell divisions). The cause of twinning is unknown, but the increase in the number of larger multiples (quintuplets, sextuplets) during recent years has been associated with fertility-enhancing techniques (ovulation-inducing drugs and assisted reproductive techniques such as in-vitro fertilization) (Ventura et al, 1995).

BOX 29-3
Characteristics of Twins

Monozygotic (MZ, identical twins)	Dizygotic (DZ, fraternal twins)
Result of one fertilized ovum that became separated early in development	Result of fertilization of two ova
Alike physically and genetically	Differ physically and genetically
Same gender	May be like or opposite gender
Frequency	Frequency:
Occurs uniformly in all populations	Varies among races (highest—blacks, lowest—Asians, intermediate—whites)
Unaffected by maternal age	More common with advancing maternal age (maximum at age 35-39, then decreases rapidly)
Tendency unaffected by heredity	Marked familial tendency Expressed only in the female Fathers appear to transmit disposition toward double ovulation to daughters
Similar behavior	Dissimilar behavior; more sibling rivalry

Twins are of two distinct types: identical, or monozygotic (MZ); and fraternal, or dizygotic (DZ) (Box 29-3). In the United States the overall twinning rate is approximately 1 in 80 pregnancies and consists of one-third MZ and two-thirds DZ twins.

A special type of sibling relationship is observed in twins, although their tendencies to get along with each other and to quarrel are not too different from those of any other two siblings, especially if they are different-gender fraternal twins. Twins generally tend to work out a relationship that is reasonably satisfactory to both and demonstrate early independence from parental attention. They develop a remarkable capacity for cooperative play and considerable loyalty and generosity toward each other. It is not uncommon for them to evolve a private language between themselves that may interfere with development of the family language.

In a twinship, one member of the pair, to a greater or lesser extent, is more dominant, outgoing, and assertive than the other, often to the consternation of their parents. However, the seemingly more passive twin is able to accomplish as much and get his or her way as often as the more assertive twin.

Identical twins differ in their response to the tendency of some parents to treat twins exactly alike. The present philosophy is to determine the degree to which the children demonstrate an inclination toward togetherness. Some twins thrive best when they are constantly in each other's company; others prefer more individuality and separateness. The conservative approach is to allow the children to follow their natural inclinations. Early years of togetherness are often the basis of the children's security. To separate them too early may produce unnecessary stresses. The tendency is to foster individual differences as they are evidenced to ease the process of separation when it becomes advisable.

Parents of twins have numerous adjustments to make, from difficulty in attachment and bonding (see Chapter 19) to the stresses of the heavy work load and monetary expenses. The National Organization of Mothers of Twins Clubs, Inc.,* has local chapters throughout the United States and Canada and offer information and support to parents of twins and is highly recommended as a resource for all new parents of twins. The Twins Foundation†—an organization founded by a group of twins and designed to aid twins and other multiples —is recommended for older children.

FAMILY STRENGTHS

Increasing interest has been shown in the family characteristics that seem to help families function effectively. Experts suggest that there are approximately 12 major, nonmutually exclusive qualities of strong families (Box 29-4). They caution that not all strong families are characterized by the presence of all 12 qualities but that a combination of qualities appears to define strong families (Dunst, Trivette, and Deal, 1988). Knowledge of these factors guides the nurse at each step of the nursing process. The nurse is better able to predict the ways in which families may cope and respond to a stressful event, provide individualized support that builds on family strengths and unique functioning style, and assist family members in obtaining appropriate resources.

*P.O. Box 23188, Albuquerque, NM 87192-1188; (505) 275-0955.
†P.O. Box 6043, Providence, RI 02904-6043; (401) 729-1000.

BOX 29-4
Qualities of Strong Families

1. A belief and sense of *commitment* toward promoting the well-being and growth of individual family members, as well as that of the family unit
2. *Appreciation* for the small and large things that individual family members do well and *encouragment* to do better
3. Concentrated effort to spend *time* and do things together, no matter how formal or informal the activity or event
4. A sense of *purpose* that permeates the reasons and basis for "going on" in both bad and good times
5. A sense of *congruence* among family members regarding the value and importance of assigning time and energy to meet needs
6. The ability to *communicate* with one another in a way that emphasizes positive interactions
7. A clear set of *family rules, values,* and *beliefs* that establishes expectations about acceptable and desired behavior
8. A varied repertoire of *coping strategies* that promotes positive functioning in dealing with both normative and nonnormative life events
9. The ability to engage in *problem-solving* activities designed to evaluate options for meeting needs and procuring resources
10. The ability to be *positive* and see the positive in almost all aspects of their lives, including the ability to see crises and problems as an opportunity to learn and grow
11. *Flexibility* and *adaptability* in the roles necessary to procure resources to meet needs
12. A *balance* between the use of internal and external family resources for coping and adapting to life events and planning for the future

From Dunst C, Trivette C, Deal A: *Enabling and empowering families: principles and guidelines for practice,* Cambridge, Mass, 1988, Brookline Books.

Parenting

MOTIVATION FOR PARENTHOOD

A dominant characteristic in all societies is that adults are expected to become parents and to be gratified by the experience. Pressures of tradition, sentiment regarding the state of motherhood, and religious exhortations to fulfill divine commands of fertility profoundly influence decision making because conformity to social-role expectations is a strong influence in family planning.

Although many pregnancies are unplanned, there are numerous reasons why couples decide to initiate a pregnancy. Many consider children a normal part of marriage, others see them as proof of their adulthood, some desire heirs for the family name and fortune, and a few want to fulfill a parent's wish for grandchildren. Having a child in an attempt to save an unstable marriage is a poor reason that usually fails in its goal. However, in most instances the couple sincerely wishes to become parents.

Factors that are likely to influence family size are social class, religion, race, type of conjugal-role relationships, and the social-psychologic aspects of sexual relations. Of course, how effectively the couple practices contraception may determine whether the family size remains as planned. Also, in the case of divorce and remarriage an individual may decide to have more children with the new spouse.

PREPARATION FOR PARENTHOOD

The basic goals of parenting are to promote the physical survival and health of the children, to foster the skills and abilities necessary to be a self-sustaining adult, and to foster behavioral capabilities for maximizing cultural values and beliefs. However, new parents approach parenthood with meager experience and scant knowledge, although no other task can compare, in overall consequences, with that of rearing a human being. Parents learn by trial and error, committing the same mistakes that have been committed by countless other parents, but they somehow manage to accomplish the task and become more skilled with each additional child. Tradition rather than rational planning furnishes the chief norms for childrearing. Experience in having been nurtured as a child is an essential component of successful parenting.

Their own parents are probably the only persons that parents observe intimately in the parental role; this results in a *generational continuity*—parents rear their own children in much the same way as they themselves were reared. Other essential skills and knowledge parents need to feel more comfortable in the parenting role include a basic understanding of childhood growth and development, bathing, feeding, use of play, and interpersonal communication skills. All of this information is integrated throughout this text.

TRANSITION TO PARENTHOOD

Although there is disagreement regarding whether the birth of a couple's first child should be labeled a crisis, the early weeks of an infant's life call for a couple to make drastic adjustments. Although the parents have anticipated and perhaps prepared for the child's arrival, birth means the sudden imposition of totally dependent care 24 hours a day for the new member of the family. It may very well be a crisis if the event is perceived as disturbing old habits and relationships and eliciting new responses. It requires role changes, destroys or significantly modifies former relationships, and means adjusting to new role realignments. Whereas previously the roles of a couple were husband and wife, they now become, in addition, father and mother. It is difficult to adjust to being parents, but it is a normal human experience and a tool for personal growth.

The birth of an infant is a highly significant event that alters the behavior of both mothers and fathers. No amount of preparation can truly and fully prepare prospective parents for the constant and immediate needs of an infant. However, certain factors influence the transition to the parental role. One factor in which the cultural trend has changed in recent years is parental age. The most satisfactory age for childrearing has been established as the years between 18 and 35. During this time parents are considered to be in optimum health, with a predicted life span that allows sufficient time and vigor to raise a family. However, the age at which parents begin their families has changed over the last few decades in the United States, with a substantial increase in the birth rate for women 30 to 44 years of age and a slight decline for women ages 18 to 29 years of age (Ventura et al, 1995).

Other factors influencing the transition to the parental role include the following:

- First-time parents who have had parenting education experience less stress in the transition than do those who have not (Gage and Christensen, 1991).
- Parents with previous experience, such as another child, appear to be more relaxed and have less conflict in disciplinary relationships, and they are more aware of normal growth and development expectations.
- Fathers who are highly involved with their child often feel more comfortable and successful in the parenting role (Fig. 29-2).
- The amount of stress experienced by one or both parents may interfere with the ability to exhibit patience and understanding or to otherwise cope with their children's behavior.
- Special characteristics of the infant, such as a temperamentally difficult infant, can cause the parents to lose confidence and doubt their abilities. Also, an infant with special care needs, such as those associated with a disability, can be a significant source of added stress.
- Marital relationships can have a negative effect on parental transition, because marital tension or strife can alter caregiving routines and interfere with enjoyment of the infant. Conversely, parents who support and encourage one another serve as a positive influence on establishing a satisfying parental role. The best single predictor of postpartum marital adjustment is the couple's level of marital adjustment during pregnancy (Wallace and Gotlib, 1990).

Support Systems

Successful adaptation to the stress of transition to parenthood involves at least two types of family resources (McCubbin and Patterson, 1982). First are the *internal resources* of the family, such as adaptability and integration. Changing from an orderly, predictable life to a relatively disordered, unpredictable one is a universal adaptation families must make. Rigid schedules are impossible to maintain, and former activities must be curtailed or abandoned. *Adaptation* is reflected in learning to be patient, becoming better organized, and becoming more flexible. *Integration* involves an attempt of the couple to continue some activities they engaged in before they became parents. In this way couples are able to maintain a sense of continuity and appreciate the importance of the husband-wife relationship.

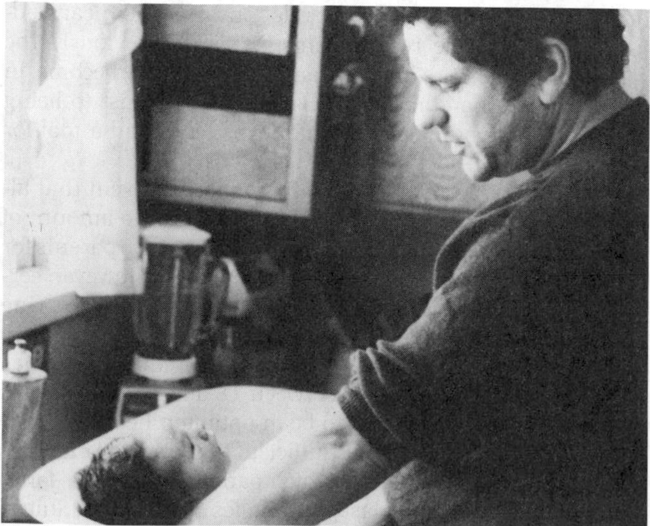

Fig. 29-2 Fathers who assume care of their children may feel more comfortable and successful in their parenting role.

The second type of resource for coping with stress is the use of **coping strategies** that strengthen the organization and functioning of the family. These strategies include the use of community resources, the use of social support, and the adoption of a future orientation. Interpersonal supports that provide information, advice, and caretaking are derived from friends, relatives, and neighbors. Relationships with family, friends, and community are essential. For fathers, positive work relationships seem to be especially important; for mothers, activities with friends are important (Daniels and Moos, 1988). Arranging for time away from the child or children is also beneficial. Fathers can assume care of the family to allow the mother some time to herself at home or away from the home, even if just for an afternoon or evening. Adoption of a future orientation provides reassurance to parents that things will get better, that they will cope, and that it is realistic to plan for the time when they will be able to engage in self-fulfilling activities.

It is also reassuring to know that others experience ambivalent feelings toward parenthood and share the same difficulties and frustrations. Exchanging ideas and experiences with other parents provides an opportunity to voice concerns and to learn new ways of coping with the multiple problems of childrearing. Whether it is family, friends, or community resources, parents need persons to whom they can turn for advice, comfort, and assistance—parents with whom they can share the joys and difficulties of childrearing.

PARENTING BEHAVIORS

Parental Styles of Control

Although there are variations and degrees in parenting styles, they can generally be described as either authoritarian, permissive, or authoritative. **Authoritarian,** or *dictatorial,* parents try to control their children's behavior and attitudes through unquestioned mandates. They establish rules and regulations or a standard of conduct that they expect to be followed rigidly and unquestioningly. They value and reward absolute obedience, mute acceptance of their word, and unfailing respect for the family's principles and beliefs. They forcefully punish any behavior that is contrary to parental standards. Parental authority is exercised with little explanation and little involvement of the child in decision making. The message is: "Do it because I say so."

Punishment need not be corporal but may be stern withdrawal of love and approval. Careful training often results in rigidly conforming behavior in the children, who tend to be sensitive, shy, self-conscious, retiring, and submissive. They are more apt to be courteous, loyal, honest, and dependable but docile. These behaviors are more typically observed when parental arbitrary power assertion is accompanied by close supervision and a reasonable level of affection. If not, arbitrary power assertion is more likely to be associated with both defiant and antisocial behavior.

Permissive, or *laissez-faire,* parents exert little or no control over their children's action. These well-meaning parents sometimes confuse permissiveness with license. They avoid imposing their own standards of conduct and allow their children to regulate their own activity as much as possible. These parents consider themselves to be resources for the children, not role models. If rules do exist, the parents explain the underlying reason, encourage the children's opinions, and consult them in decision-making processes. They employ lax, inconsistent discipline, do not set sensible limits, and do not prevent the children from upsetting the home routine. The parents rarely punish the children because most behavior is considered acceptable. Consequently, the children, in effect, control the parents. Children of submissive parents are often disobedient, disrespectful, irresponsible, aggressive, and generally defiant of authority.

Authoritative, or *democratic,* parents combine childrearing practices from both of the foregoing extremes. They direct their children's behavior and attitudes by emphasizing the reason for rules and negatively reinforcing deviations. They respect the individuality of each of their children and allow them to voice their objections to family standards or regulations. Parental control is firm and consistent but tempered with encouragement, understanding, and security. Control is focused on the issue, not on withdrawal of love or fear of punishment. These parents foster "inner-directedness," a conscience that regulates behavior on the basis of feelings of guilt or shame for wrongdoing, not on fear of being caught or punished. Parents' realistic standards and reasonable expectations produce children with high self-esteem who are self-reliant, assertive, inquisitive, content, and highly interactive with other children.

The most successful type of childrearing seems to be the authoritative method. Parents do not set rigid, arbitrary limits but maintain firm control, particularly in areas of parent-child disagreement. Permissiveness is tempered with reasonable and consistent limit-setting. Parental power is shared, and both parents provide leadership but listen to what the children think.

LIMIT-SETTING AND DISCIPLINE

In its broadest sense, **discipline** means to teach or refers to a set of rules governing conduct. In a narrower sense, it refers to the action taken to enforce the rules following noncompliance. **Limit-setting** refers to establishing the rules or guidelines for behavior. Generally, the clearer the limits that are set and the more consistently they are enforced, the less need there is for disciplinary action.

Therefore the initial goal for the family is for the nurse to help parents establish realistic and concrete "rules." Limit-setting and discipline are positive, necessary components of childrearing and serve several useful functions as they help children do the following:

- Test their limits of control
- Achieve in areas appropriate for mastery at their level
- Channel undesirable feelings into constructive activity
- Protect themselves from danger
- Learn socially acceptable behavior

Children want and need limits. Unrestricted freedom is a tremendous threat to their security and safety. Through testing the limits imposed on them, children learn the extent to which they can manipulate their environment, and they gain reassurance from knowing that others will be there to protect them from potential harm.

Minimizing Misbehavior

The goals of or reasons for misbehavior may include attention, power, defiance, and a display of inadequacy (the child misses classes because of a fear that he or she is unable to do the work). Children may also misbehave because the rules are not clear or consistently applied. Acting-out behavior, such as a temper tantrum, may represent uncontrolled frustration, anger, depression, or pain.

The best approach is to structure interactions with children so that unacceptable behavior is prevented or minimized. Although many parents devise strategies that are most effective for their child, general guidelines include those listed in the Home Care box below.

Types of Discipline

Regardless of the type of discipline used, certain principles are essential in ensuring the efficacy of the approach (see the

Home Care

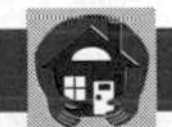

MINIMIZING MISBEHAVIOR

Set realistic goals for acceptable behavior and expected achievements.
Structure opportunities for small successes to lessen feelings of inadequacy.
Praise children for desirable behavior with attention and verbal approval.
Structure the environment to prevent unnecessary difficulties (e.g., place fragile objects in an inaccessible area)
Set clear and reasonable rules; expect the same behavior regardless of the circumstances. If exceptions are made, clarify that the change is for one time only.
Teach desirable behavior through example, such as using a quiet, calm voice rather than screaming.
Review expected behavior before special or unusual events, such as visiting a relative or eating dinner in a restaurant.
Phrase requests for appropriate behavior positively, such as "Put down the book," rather than "Don't touch the book."
Call attention to unacceptable behavior as soon as it begins; use distraction to change the behavior or offer alternatives to annoying actions, such as a quiet toy for one that is excessively noisy.
Give advance notice or "friendly reminders" such as "When the TV program is over, it is time for dinner" or "I'll give you to the count of three and then we need to go."
Be attentive to situations that increase the likelihood of misbehaving, such as overexcitement or fatigue or decreased personal tolerance to minor infractions.
Offer sympathetic explanations for not granting a request, such as "I am sorry I can't read you a story now, but I need to finish dinner. Then we can spend time together."
Keep any promises made to children.
Avoid outright conflicts; temper discussions with statements such as "Let's talk about it and see what we can decide together" or "I need to think about it first."
Provide children with opportunities for power and control.

Guidelines

IMPLEMENTING DISCIPLINE

Consistency—Implement disciplinary action exactly as agreed on and for each infraction.

Timing—Initiate discipline as soon as child misbehaves; if delays are necessary, such as to avoid embarrassment, verbally disapprove of the behavior and state that disciplinary action will be implemented.

Commitment—Follow through with the details of the discipline, such as timing of minutes; avoid distractions that may interfere with the plan, such as telephone calls.

Unity—Make certain that all caregivers agree on the plan and are familiar with the details to prevent confusion and alliances between the child and one parent.

Flexibility—Choose disciplinary strategies that are appropriate to child's age, temperament, and the severity of the misbehavior.

Planning—Plan discipline strategies in advance and prepare child if feasible (e.g., explain use of time-out); for unexpected misbehavior, try to discipline when you are calm.

Behavior-orientation—Always disapprove of the behavior, not the child, with such statements as "That was a wrong thing to do. I am unhappy when I see behavior like that."

Privacy—Administer discipline in private, especially with older children who may feel ashamed in front of others.

Termination—Once the discipline is administered, consider child as having a "clean slate" and avoid bringing up the incident or lecturing.

Guidelines box above). To deal with misbehavior, parents need to implement appropriate disciplinary action. Numerous approaches are available, and some have definite advantages over others.

Reasoning involves explaining why an act is wrong and is usually appropriate for older children, especially when moral issues are involved. However, young children cannot be expected to "see the other side" because of their egocentrism.

Children in the preoperative stage of cognitive development (toddlers and preschoolers) have a limited ability to distinguish between their point of view and those of others (Blum et al, 1995). Sometimes children use the "reasoning" as a way of gaining attention. For example, they may misbehave in order for the parents to give them a lengthy explanation of the wrongdoing because negative attention is better than none. When children use this technique, parents may need to end the explanation by stating, "This is the rule, and this is how I expect you to behave. I won't explain it any further."

Unfortunately, reasoning is often combined with *scolding,* which sometimes takes the form of shame or criticism. For example, the parent may state, "You are a bad boy for hitting your brother." Children take such remarks seriously and personally, believing that *they* are bad.

Nursing ALERT

When reprimanding children, focus only on the misbehavior, not on the child. Use of "I" messages rather than "you" messages expresses personal feelings without accusation or ridicule. For example, an "I" message attacks the behavior—"I am upset when Johnny is punched; I don't like to see him hurt"—not the child.

Positive and negative reinforcement is the basis of *behavior modification* theory—behavior that is rewarded will be repeated; behavior that is not, will be extinguished. Using *rewards* is a positive approach; by encouraging children to behave in specified ways, the tendency to misbehave is lessened. With young children, using paper stars is very effective. For older children the "token system" is appropriate, especially if a certain number yields a special reward such as a trip to the movies or a new book. In planning a reward system, the expected behaviors must be clearly explained to the child, and the rewards must be reinforcing. A chart should be used to record the stars or tokens, and every earned reward should be promptly given. Verbal approval should always accompany material rewards.

Consistently *ignoring* behavior will eventually extinguish or minimize the act. Although this approach sounds very simple, it is often difficult to implement consistently. Parents often "give in" and resort to previous patterns of discipline. Consequently, the behavior is actually reinforced because the child learns that persistence gains parental approval.

The strategy of *consequences* involves allowing children to experience the results of their misbehavior and includes the following three types:

1. **Natural**—Those that occur without any intervention, such as being late and missing dinner
2. **Logical**—Those that are directly related to the rule, such as not being allowed to play with another toy until the used ones are put away
3. **Unrelated**—Those that are imposed deliberately, such as no playing until homework is completed or the use of time-out

Natural or logical consequences are preferred but are effective only when they are meaningful to children. For example, the natural consequence of living in a messy room may do little to encourage cleaning up, but allowing no friends over until the room is neat can be very motivating! Withdrawing privileges is often an unrelated consequence. After the child experiences the consequence, the parent should refrain from any comment, because the usual tendency is for the child to try to place blame for imposing the rule.

Time-out is actually a refinement of the common practice of "sending the child to his or her room" and is a type of unrelated consequence. It is also based on the premise of removing the reinforcer (i.e., the satisfaction or attention the child is receiving from the activity). When placed in an unstimulating and isolated place, children become bored and consequently agree to behave in order to reenter the family group (Fig. 29-3). Time-out avoids many of the problems of other disciplinary approaches because no physical punishment is involved, no reasoning or scolding is given, and the parent is usually not present for all of the time-out, facilitating his or her ability to consistently apply the punishment. It also offers both the child and the parent a "cooling off" time. To be effective, time-out must be planned in advance (see the Home Care box on p. 835).

Corporal punishment most often takes the form of spanking. Based on the principles of aversive therapy, inflicting pain through spanking causes a dramatic short-term decrease in the behavior. However, there are some serious flaws in this approach: (1) it teaches children that violence is acceptable, (2) many times the spanking is the result of parental rage and

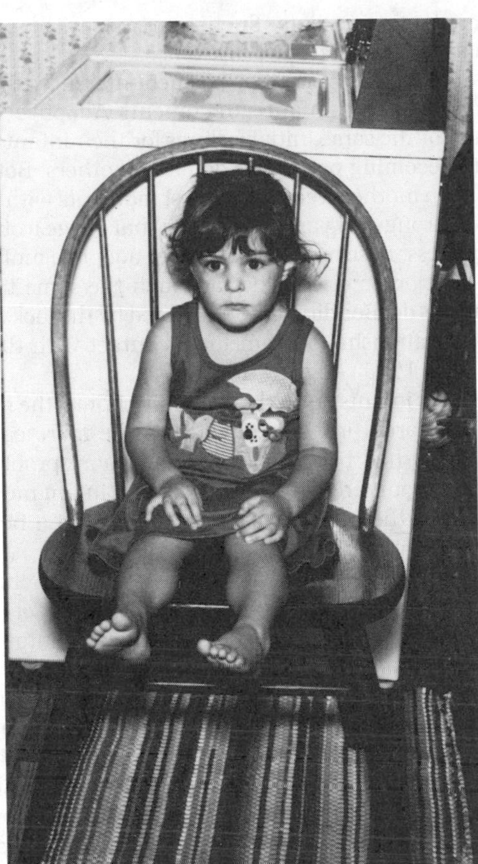

Fig. 29-3 Time-out is an excellent disciplinary strategy for young children.

may physically harm the child, and (3) children become "accustomed" to spanking, requiring more severe corporal punishment each time. Consequently, parents may use paddles, whips, belts, or other objects, or they may eliminate a spanking because of their unwillingness to "hit the child harder," a practice that may prolong the behavior.

Spanking can result in severe physical injury and even death (Eichelberger, Beal, and May, 1991). Nevertheless, corporal punishment is often exempted from the category of assault, even when it produces specific injuries, which may be treated as "accidental" or "incidental" to discipline (Garbarino et al, 1992).

Even when corporal punishment does not involve serious physical damage to children, the psychologic impact may be great (Hyman et al, 1985). It can also interfere with effective parent-child interactions; children who receive corporal punishment are less likely to learn what they *should* do, because the focus is on what they *should not* do (Nelms, 1993). In addition, the misbehavior is likely to occur when the parent is not around because children have not learned to behave well for their own sake. Parental use of corporal punishment has also been found to interfere with the child's development of moral reasoning (Finkelhor et al, 1983).

The use of corporal punishment, a model of violent behavior, has been questioned more of late in conjunction with concern regarding increasing violence in contemporary society. Unfortunately, in many parts of the United States the practice of corporal punishment continues to play a role in the public education of schoolchildren.

Home Care 

USING TIME-OUT

Select an area for time-out that is safe, convenient, and unstimulating but where the child can be monitored, such as the bathroom, hallway, or laundry room; avoid frightening areas such as a cellar or dark closet.
Determine what behaviors warrant a time-out.
Make sure children understand the "rules" and how they are expected to behave.
Explain to children the process of time-out:
- When they misbehave, they will be given *one* warning.
- If they do not obey, they will be sent to the place designated for time-out.
- They are to sit there for a specified period of time.
- If they cry, refuse, or display any disruptive behavior, the time-out period will begin *after* they quiet down.
- When they are quiet for the duration of the time, they can then leave the room.

A rule for the length of time-out is, *1 minute per year of age;* to record the time, use a kitchen timer with an audible bell rather than a watch.
Implement time-out in a public place by selecting a suitable area or explain to children that time-out will be spent immediately on returning home and mark their hand with a felt-tip pen as a reminder.

Special Parenting Situations

Parenting is a demanding task under the most ideal circumstances, but when parents and children are faced with situations that deviate from what is considered to be the norm, the potential for family disruption is increased. Some of the issues commonly encountered are divorce, single parenthood, reconstituted families, adoption, and dual-career families. The problems associated with children of alcoholic parents, parents with physical disabilities, homeless parents, or incarcerated parents are ones that are not addressed in the following discussions but are topics that the reader may wish to investigate.

PARENTING THE ADOPTED CHILD

Adoption establishes the legal relationship of parent and child between persons who are not so related by birth, with the same rights and obligations that exist between children and their biologic parents. In healthy families, the ties of affection between the adoptive parents and their children are just as strong as biologic ties.

Although most adoptions are by couples who have been unable to have children of their own, many people—including single, divorced, and widowed persons—consider adoption for other reasons. There are some who feel a responsibility to provide a home for a child who needs one; others are able to have more children of their own but are seriously concerned about overpopulation and elect to increase their family through adoption; many are families who are finding "room for one more" with whom to share their love. Almost half of the adoptable children in the United States are adopted by relatives, either extended family members or stepparents.

The Adoptive Family

Most problems faced by adoptive parents are no different from those encountered by biologic parents. All parents want to be good parents, but this desire is often intensified in adoptive parents. Adoptive parents have been portrayed as more apprehensive and insecure than biologic parents and in need of more assistance. However, adoptive parents may feel the need for less assistance than biologic parents. This feeling is probably a result of the adoptive parents' completely voluntary decision to become parents, the relatively long time they have had to prepare for parenting, and the maturity associated with adopting (Edwards, 1987).

Unlike biologic parents, who prepare for their child's birth with prenatal classes and the support of friends and relatives, adoptive parents may have few sources of support and preparation for the new addition to their family (Koepke et al, 1991). Nurses who offer services to adoptive parents can provide the information, support, and reassurance needed to reduce parental anxiety regarding the adoptive process and can refer them to state parental support groups that provide guidance for adoptive parents. Such sources can be contacted through a state or county welfare office.

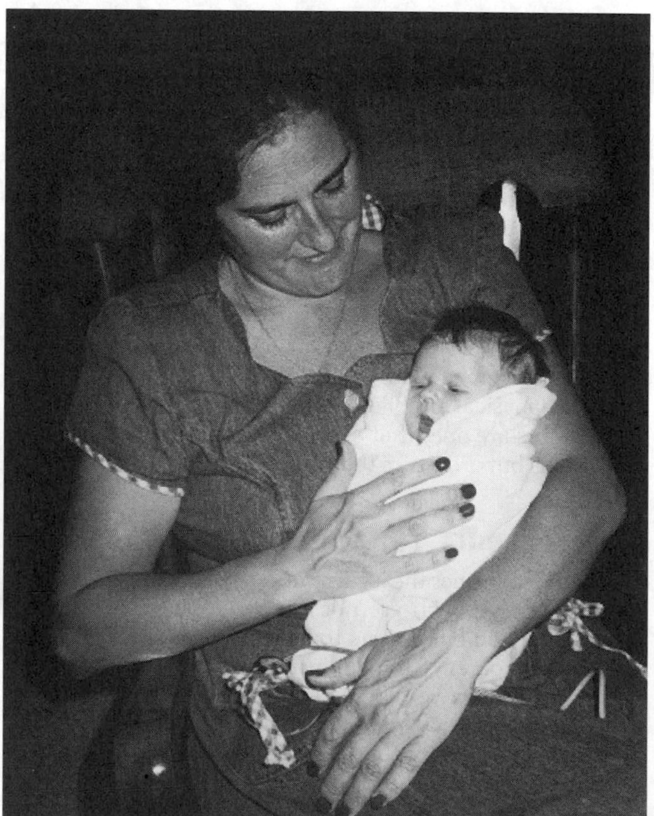

Fig. 29-4 Adoptive parents are often "instant parents." Both they and the child need time to learn about each other.

An initial concern that may be encountered by the adopting family is parent-infant attachment. Adoptive mothers have many of the same initial feelings for their infants and reactions to becoming parents as do birth mothers. Both adoptive and birth mothers react to the first moments with their infants with strong and varied emotions that range from happiness to distress. Research indicates that adoptive mothers are likely to develop emotional ties at much the same time that birth mothers do. Bonding is not hindered by the lack of either a biologic relationship or immediate contact with the infant (Koepke et al, 1991) (Fig. 29-4).

The sooner infants enter their adoptive home, the better for purposes of parent-infant attachment. The more caregivers the infant has had before adoption, the more problems are likely to be encountered in attachment. The infant must break the bond with the previous caregiver and form a new bond with the adoptive parents.

One of the difficulties of rearing adopted older children is helping them to deal with having had another set of parents. Children who are adopted after 2 years of age maintain an image of previous parenting persons. In addition to their biologic parents, the children may have lost siblings, grandparents, friends, and personal possessions. Often they have lived in several foster homes in which they formed attachments. They need time and assistance in working through the grief process that is an integral part of any loss. At the same time, they must adjust to a new household and relationships. Children who have experienced many losses and disappointments find adjustment more difficult and take longer to overcome the fear of rejection and to develop affectionate ties to the new family. They grieve for those they left behind and may be afraid to love in case they must again move on.

Another area of special concern to adoptive parents is the task of telling children that they are adopted. Unfortunately, there are no clear-cut guidelines for parents to follow in determining precisely when children are ready for the information, and parents are naturally reluctant to present the child with such unsettling news. However, it is an important aspect of their parental responsibilities; although parents may be tempted to withhold the fact from the child, it is an essential component of the child's identity. Most authorities believe that children should be informed at a young enough age so that as they grow older, they do not remember a time when they did not know they were adopted (see the Critical Thinking Q & A on p. 837).

Parents can anticipate some behavior changes following the disclosure—especially in older children. Children may use the fact of their adoption as a weapon to manipulate and threaten parents. There is the inevitable "My real mother would not treat me like this," or "You don't love me as much because I'm adopted." Statements such as these hurt parents and increase their feelings of insecurity so that as parents they may become overly permissive. Adopted children need the same undemanding love as any other child, combined with firm discipline and limit-setting.

The adolescent years may also present special challenges. The normal confrontations of adolescents and parents may assume more painful aspects in adoptive families. Adolescents may use their adoption as a tool in defying parental authority

Critical Thinking Q & A 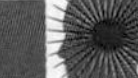

PARENTING THE ADOPTED CHILD

Twelve-month-old Justin was adopted at birth. His parents tell you that they wonder when to tell Justin that he is adopted. As the nurse, what advice would you give Justin's parents?

1. Reassure them that since Justin was adopted at birth they do not need to tell him he was adopted.
2. Give Justin's parents some books and pamphlets about adoption so that they can decide on their own what to do.
3. Recommend that they tell Justin in a matter-of-fact manner and at an early age so that he always knows he was adopted.
4. Suggest that they not tell Justin until he reaches early adolescence and can better understand this information.

The best answer is three. Being adopted can be viewed by the adoptee as part of his unique heritage. Justin's parents chose to have him join the family as a welcomed member. Babies and children join families in many ways, such as biologic heritage or blending of families. Sharing the story of adoption is an important parental responsibility and can be handled much like sharing birth experiences with a biologic child. Most authorities believe that children should be informed at a young enough age so that as they grow older, they do not remember a time when they did not know they were adopted. Waiting until adolescence is too late. Children have a more difficult adjustment if disclosure occurs when they are older. Giving Justin's parents resources about adoption is appropriate; however, because they have asked you as the nurse for guidance, a more direct approach is best.

or as a justification for aberrant behavior. As they attempt to master the task of identity formation, the feeling of abandonment by their natural parents may come to awareness or may be intensified. During this time adopted children may feel the need to discover the identity of their biologic parents to define themselves and their identity—one of the major tasks of adolescent development. Gender differences in reaction to adoption may surface. It has been shown that girls may have more difficulty accepting their sexuality because they may not be able to identify with a nonfertile female parent. It is important for parents to reassure their children that they understand the feelings of needing to search for one's identity.

Cross-Racial and International Adoption

The adoption of children of racial backgrounds different from that of the family is relatively commonplace. In addition to the problems faced by adopted children of any age, children of a cross-racial adoption must deal with their differentness. It is advised that parents who adopt such children do everything to preserve the adopted children's racial heritage.

Although the children are full-fledged members of an adopting family and citizens of the adopted country, those with a foreign appearance or other decided racial characteristics may create dilemmas outside the family. Strangers, or even relatives and friends, may make thoughtless comments and talk about the children as though they were not members of the family. It is vital that the family make it clear to others that this is their child and a cherished member of the family.

In international adoptions the medical information the parents receive may be quite complete or very sketchy (Hostetter and Johnson, 1989). Many internationally adopted children were born prematurely, and common health problems such as infant diarrhea and malnutrition may delay growth and development. Such children may have serious or multiple health problems. Many foreign-born children have not been immunized adequately (American Academy of Pediatrics, 1991). Cultural practices such as constant holding rather than letting the child explore may further affect the child's progress. Regardless of age, some internationally adopted children may experience temporary adjustment problems. In addition to giving advice on medical management, nurses should provide these parents with opportunities to discuss their feelings and situations.

PARENTING AND DIVORCE

Since the mid-1960s there has been a marked change in the stability of families, which is reflected in increased rates of divorce, single parenthood, and remarriage. In 1994 the divorce rate for the United States was 4.6 per 1000 total population (Singh et al, 1995). The divorce rate has changed very little since 1987. In the previous decade the rate increased almost yearly, with a peak in 1979. Although almost one half of all divorcing couples are childless, more than 1 million children experience divorce each year, and most of the children are very young.

During a divorce, the coping abilities of the parents may be compromised. The parents may be much too preoccupied with their own feelings, needs, and life changes to be available to and supportive of their children. Newly employed parents, usually mothers, are likely to leave children with new caregivers, in strange settings, or alone after school. The parent may also spend more time away from home searching for or establishing new relationships. Sometimes, however, the adult feels frightened and alone and begins to depend on the child as a substitute for the absent parent. This dependence places an enormous burden on the child.

Common characteristics in the custodial household following separation and divorce include disorder, coercive types of control, inflammable tempers in both parents and children, reduced parental competence, a greater sense of parental helplessness, poorly enforced discipline, and diminished regularity in enforcing household routines. Noncustodial parents also are seldom prepared for the role of visitor and may not have a residence suitable for children's visits. They may be concerned about maintaining the arrangement over the years to follow.

Impact of Divorce on Children

The results of numerous studies show that divorce has a profound effect on children. Long-term studies indicate that many youngsters suffer for years from psychologic and social difficulties associated with continuing and/or new stresses in the postdivorce family. A main outcome is heightened anxiety about forming enduring relationships as young adults (Wallerstein, 1991). Even when a divorce is amiable and open, children may recall parental separation with the same emotions felt by victims of a natural disaster: loss, grief, and vulnerability to forces beyond their control (Tuttle, 1992).

The impact of divorce on children depends on a variety of factors, including the age and gender of the children, the outcome of the divorce, and the quality of the parent-child relationship and parental care during the years following the divorce. Family characteristics appear to be more critical to children's well-being than specific child characteristics such as age or gender. The most important factor is continuing conflict between the divorced parents (Amato and Keith, 1991; Wallerstein and Johnston, 1990). Children cope better when parents adopt an attitude of "together for the child while separate for us" (Leung and Robson, 1990). High levels of ongoing family conflict are related to problems of social development, emotional stability, and cognitive skills for the child.

Complications sometimes associated with divorce include efforts on the part of one parent to subvert the child's loyalties to the other, abandonment to other caregivers, and adjustment to a stepparent. In the majority of divorce cases the mother receives custody of the child; this has an effect on the male child's identification with a father figure, in addition to all of the other ramifications of living in a family without a father or in a single-parent family. Many divorced mothers with young children move in with parents, other relatives, or friends in some type of dependent or sharing arrangement.

Children may feel a sense of shame and embarrassment concerning the family situation. Such feelings cause children to see themselves as different, inferior, or unworthy of love, especially if they feel any responsibility for the family dissolution. Although the social stigma attached to divorce no longer produces the emotions it has in the past, it may still exist in some small towns and can reinforce children's negative self-image. The lasting effects of divorce depend on the children's and the parents' adjustment to the transition from an intact family to a single-parent family and, often, to a reconstituted family.

Although most studies have concentrated on the negative effects of divorce on youngsters, positive outcomes of divorce have been reported. A successful postdivorce family, either as a single-parent or reconstituted family, can improve the quality of life for adults and children. Living with conflict is resolved, and a better relationship with one or both parents may result. Children may also have less contact with a disturbed parent. Greater maturity, independence, and a commitment to sustaining relationships are also positive outcomes (Wallerstein and Johnston, 1990). However, emotional adjustment is closely associated with the child's personal adjustment before the divorce (Demo and Acock, 1988).

BOX 29-5

Feelings and Behaviors of Children Related to Divorce

Infancy

Effects of reduced mothering or lack of mothering
Increased irritability
Disturbance in eating, sleeping, and elimination
Interference with attachment process

Early preschool children (ages 2-3 years)

Frightened and confused
Blame themselves for the divorce
Fear of abandonment
Increased irritability, whining, tantrums
Regressive behaviors (e.g., thumb-sucking, loss of elimination control)
Separation anxiety

Later preschool children (ages 3-5 years)

Fear of abandonment
Blame themselves for the divorce; decreased self-esteem
Bewilderment regarding all human relationships
Become more aggressive in relationships with others (e.g., siblings, peers)
Engage in fantasy to seek understanding of the divorce

Early school-age children (ages 5-6 years)

Depression and immature behavior
Loss of appetite and sleep disorders
May be able to verbalize some feelings and understand some divorce-related changes
Increased anxiety and aggression
Feel abandoned by departing parent

Middle school-age children (ages 6-8 years)

Panic reactions
Feelings of deprivation—loss of parent, attention, money, and secure future
Profound sadness, depression, fear, and insecurity
Feelings of abandonment and rejection
Fear regarding the future
Difficulty expressing anger at parents
Intense desire for reconciliation of parents
Impaired capacity to play and enjoy outside activities
Decline in school performance
Altered peer relationships—become bossy, irritable, demanding, and manipulative
Frequent crying, loss of appetite, sleep disorders
Disturbed routine, forgetfulness

Later school-age children (ages 9-12 years)

More realistic understanding of divorce
Intense anger directed at one or both parents
Divided loyalties
Able to express feelings of anger
Ashamed of parental behavior
Feel the need for revenge; may wish to punish the parent they hold responsible
Feel lonely, ejected, and abandoned
Altered peer relationships
Decline in school performance
May develop somatic complaints
May engage in aberrant behavior such as lying, stealing
Temper tantrums
Dictatorial attitude

Adolescents (ages 12-18 years)

Able to disengage themselves from parental conflict
Feel a profound sense of loss—of family, childhood
Feelings of anxiety
Worry about themselves, parents, siblings
Express anger, sadness, shame, embarrassment
May withdraw from family and friends
Disturbed concept of sexuality
May engage in acting-out behaviors

Age- and gender-related responses to divorce. Previously it was believed that divorce had a greater impact on younger children, but more recent observations indicate that divorce constitutes a major disruption for children in all age groups. The feelings and behaviors of children may differ according to age (Box 29-5) and gender, but also suffer stresses second only to the stress produced by the death of a parent.

Although considerable research has looked at gender differences in children's adjustments to divorce, the findings are not conclusive. In general, it appears that boys have more problematic behavior than girls after divorce. Postdivorce parenting difficulties also tend to be greater with sons than with daughters and typically begin before the divorce (Shaw, Emery, and Tuer, 1993).

Telling the children. Parents are understandably hesitant to tell children about their decision to divorce. A vast majority of parents neglect to discuss with their preschool children either the divorce or the inevitable changes it brings. Without preparation, even children who remain in the family home are confused by the parental separation, and this confusion seems to overpower any soothing effects that remaining in the home may have (Stirtzinger and Cholvat, 1990).

Most likely, the children are already experiencing vague, uneasy feelings that are more difficult to cope with than being told truthfully about the situation. If possible, the initial disclosure should include both parents and all siblings, followed by later discussions with each child individually. Ample time should be set aside for the discussions, and they should take place during a period of calm, not after an argument. Parents who physically hold or touch their children provide them with a reassuring feeling of warmth. The discussions should include the reason for the divorce—minimizing blame—and reassurance that the divorce is not the fault of the children. Children may feel guilty, as though they have somehow failed or are being punished for misbehavior. They wonder what role they played in the divorce or failure to keep the family together.

Parents need not fear crying in front of the children; it gives the children permission to cry also. Children need to ventilate their feelings. They normally feel anger and resentment and should be allowed to communicate these feelings without punishment. They also have feelings of terror and abandonment and long for consistency and order in their lives. They need to know where they will live, who will take care of them, if they will be with their siblings, and if there will be enough money to live on. The children may also fear that if the parents have stopped loving each other, they could also stop loving them. Their need for assurance of love is tremendous at this time.

Custody and Parenting Partnerships

Traditionally the mother has been given custody of the children when parents separate. Now both parents and the courts are seeking alternatives. The present belief is that neither fathers nor mothers should be awarded custody automatically but that custody should be awarded to the parent who is best able to provide for the children's welfare. In certain situations children experience severe stress when living or spending time with a certain parent.

Although in most divorce cases the mother still receives custody of the child with visitation agreements for the father, more courts are now awarding custody to fathers. Men usually make more money and can offer more material benefits than many women are able to provide. The incidence of delinquent support payments to custodial mothers is a matter of universal knowledge and concern.

Often overlooked are the changes that may occur in the children's relationships with other relatives, especially grandparents. Grandparents on the noncustodial side are often kept from their grandchildren; those on the custodial side may be overwhelmed by their adult child's return to the household with grandchildren.*

Two less common custody arrangements are divided custody and joint custody. **Divided,** or **split custody** means that each parent is awarded custody of one or more of the children, thereby separating siblings. For example, sons might live with the father and daughters with the mother. **Joint custody** takes one of two forms. In *joint physical custody* the parents alternate the physical care and control of the children on a reasonably equitable basis while maintaining shared parenting responsibilities legally. This type of custody arrangement works well for families who live close to each other and whose occupations allow an active role in the care and rearing of the children. In *joint legal custody*, the children reside with one parent, but both parents are the children's legal guardians and both participate in childrearing (Arditti, 1992).

Co-parenting offers substantial benefits for the family: children can be close to both parents, and life wih each parent can be more normal as opposed to a disciplinarian mother and a recreational father. However, to be successful, the parents must place a high value on the commitment to provide as normal parenting as possible and be able to separate their marital conflicts from the parenting roles. No matter what type of custody arrangement is awarded, the primary consideration is the welfare of the children.

SINGLE PARENTING

Single-parent status is acquired by means of divorce, separation, or death or through the birth or adoption of a child by a single person. Although divorce rates have stabilized, the number of single-parent households continues to rise. Today, one child in four lives in a single-parent family, with the majority of single parents being women (Center for the Study of Social Policy, 1993).

Managing shortages of money, time, and energy are major concerns of single parents. Studies repeatedly confirm the financial difficulties of single-parent families, particularly in the case of single mothers. (The average income of single-mother families is 60% that of single-father families; in addition, only 31% of mother-headed households receive any child support or alimony [Center for the Study of Social Policy, 1993].) In fact, the stigma of poverty may be more keenly felt than the discrimination associated with being a single parent (Richards, 1989). In addition, these families are often forced by their financial status to live in communities in which inadequate housing and personal safety are concerns. When relo-

Grandparents*, a newsletter for grandparents in divided families, is published by **Scarsdale Family Counseling Service, 405 Harwood Building, Scarsdale, NY 10583; (914) 723-3281.

cation is necessary, families may need to move away from friends and neighbors who have been sources of emotional support. Many single parents have trouble arranging for adequate child care, and care for sick children is especially difficult to obtain. Single mothers trying to balance work, chores, and child care may often give up personal activities, recreation, and even rest.

Fathers who have custody of their children have many of the same problems as divorced mothers. They often feel overburdened by the responsibility, are depressed, and are concerned about their ability to cope with the emotional needs of their children, especially the needs of girls. They find it difficult at first to coordinate household tasks, school visits, and other activities associated with managing a household alone. Fathers often demand more assistance with household tasks and more independence from their children than custodial mothers do, and they are likely to make use of alternative caregiving and support systems.

Supports and resources for single-parent families include health care services that are open evenings and weekends, high-quality child care, respite child care to relieve parental exhaustion and burnout, and parent enhancement centers for advancing education and job skills, providing recreational activities, and offering parenting education. Groups for single-parent fathers and grandparents who are primary caregivers are also important (Strett, 1989). There is a need on the part of the parent for social contacts and a life separate from the children for the emotional growth of both the parent and the children. The single parent can find support and encouragement from Parents Without Partners, Inc.,* an organization designed to meet the needs of this increasingly important group.

PARENTING IN RECONSTITUTED FAMILIES

In the United States approximately half of all children in homes in which parents have divorced will experience yet another major change in their lives within 3 years of a divorce—a return to a nuclear family and the sudden acquisition of a stepparent when the custodial parent remarries (Hetherington, Stanley-Hagen, and Anderson, 1989). The entry of a stepparent into a ready-made family requires adjustments for all family members. Some obstacles to the role adjustments and family problem solving include the disruption of previous life-styles and interaction patterns, complexity in the formation of new ones, and lack of social supports. Despite these problems, most children from divorced families want to live in a two-parent home.

The term *parenting coalition* has been suggested to describe the situation in which there are more than two parents for a child, such as in stepfamilies (Visher and Visher, 1989). This term implies the need for cooperation rather than competition between the biologic parents and the stepparents. Cooperative parenting relationships can allow more time for each set of parents to be alone to establish their own relationship. Under ideal circumstances, power conflicts between the two households can be reduced, and tension and anxiety can be lessened for all family members. In addition, the children's self-esteem can be increased, and there is a greater likelihood of continued contact with grandparents. The development of a parenting coalition requires time. Flexibility, mutual support, and open communication are critical in successful relationships in stepfamilies and stepparenting situations (Rosen, 1987).

Unfortunately, stepfamilies usually do not seek help to prevent problems from arising. Typically, information and counseling are sought only when problems have surfaced and can no longer be ignored. A preventive rather than remedial approach to stepfamilies and stepparenting is needed (Ganong and Coleman, 1989) (see the Family Focus box above).

Family Focus

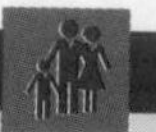

BLENDED FAMILIES AND LIVING "IN STEP"

Let relationships develop slowly and naturally. Do not expect too much too soon from the children, your spouse, or yourself.
Do not criticize or belittle lost (or new) parents or try to erase or replace them. Stepparents are additional parents.
Expect confused feelings, anxieties, competition for attention, bids for loyalty. Decide on standards of discipline and behavior and stick to them.
Communicate. Do not pretend everything is fine if it is not. Look at problems squarely and deal with them openly.
If you need help, admit it and get it. Read a book, get counseling, join a support group, call a family meeting.

From Stein B: Yours, mine, and ours: a look at stepfamilies, *Growing Parent* 12(9):1-5, 1984.

PARENTING IN DUAL-EARNER FAMILIES

No change in family life-style has had more impact than the large numbers of women entering the workplace. As women have moved away from the traditional homemaker pattern, the number of dual-earner families has increased dramatically. In 1993 54% of mothers with children under 3 years of age were in the civilian labor force; 64% of women with children 3 to 5 years of age were employed (Children's Defense Fund, 1994). This trend is unlikely to diminish. As a result, the family is subjected to considerable stress as members attempt to meet the challenge of the often competing demands of occupational needs and those regarded as necessary for a rich family life.

Nurses play an important role in helping families find suitable sources of child care and prepare children for this experience (see Alternate Child Care Arrangements, Chapter 33).

ACCOMMODATING CONTEMPORARY PARENTING SITUATIONS

During recent years both the private and government sectors have noted some of the problems faced by contemporary families. Many of these issues involve working parents. For example, perhaps one of the greatest stressors for working single-parent or dual-earner families is when a child becomes ill. Frequency of childhood illness, exclusion practices of most licensed child-care programs, and employers' limited sick leave policies are contributing factors (Jordan, 1986). Al-

*International Headquarters, 401 N. Michigan Avenue, Chicago, IL 60611-4267; (312) 644-6610.

though the preferred type of care for the sick child is that provided by the parents at home, families have a variety of options, including in-home care by a trained provider other than the child's parent, care by a relative, on-site care in the child's usual program, and care in a separate, specialized group day care setting for mildly ill children (Giebink, 1993).

Sick child care in a group setting is becoming popular in many communities. Although standards and criteria for such settings have been established (Smith, Shillam, and Zimmerman, 1989), research is needed to determine outcomes for children.

Some employers have become more family focused and give parents time off to be with their sick children. Increasing numbers are also more generous in the amount of time they offer parents—fathers as well as mothers—to remain at home after the birth or adoption of a child. More flexible work schedules and family-oriented legislation can also ease the burden of managing family and work responsibilities (Arnold and Brecht, 1990). The passage of the Family and Medical Leave Act (FMLA) in 1993 set the stage for a greater focus on the issues that contemporary American families face. Under this law, parents are guaranteed time away from work without pay and without jeopardizing their employment to care for their children in certain situations.

Role definitions are often altered to arrange an equitable division of time and labor and to resolve conflicts between earlier and later norms, especially those related to the traditional norms of the culture. Overload is a common source of stress in a dual-earner family, and social activities are significantly curtailed. Time demands and scheduling are major problems, and when there are children, the demands can be even more intense. Dual-earner couples may increase the strain on themselves to avoid creating stress for their children, but there is no evidence to indicate that the dual-earner life-style as such is stressful to children. However, the stress experienced by the parents may affect the children indirectly.

Working Mothers

Even though working mothers have become the norm in the United States, disapproving attitudes from some health care workers and some child-care books, lack of a national policy on child care, and "scripts" from their own childhood of being cared for by an at-home mother contribute to the torn and guilty feelings many working mothers experience (Balk and Christoffel, 1988).

Fathers are taking a more active role in child care. By 1991 one of every five preschool children (under age 5) was cared for by the father while the mother worked outside the home (O'Connell, 1993).

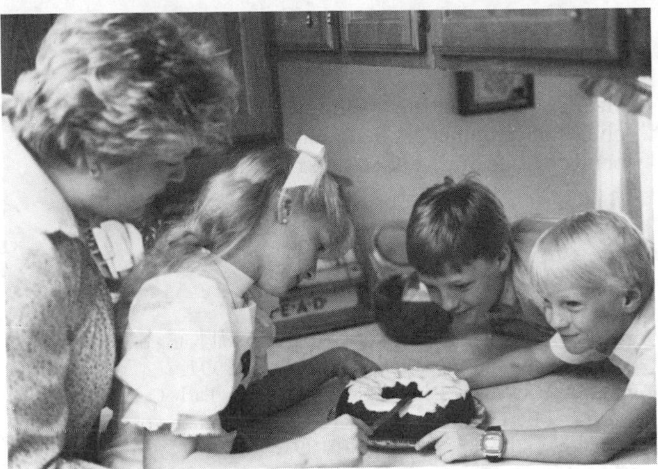

Fig. 29-5 Many working mothers take every opportunity to engage in activities with their children.

The quality of child care is a persistent concern for all working parents. However, mothers are more likely than fathers to adjust their work schedule to accommodate child-care needs. Even in familes in which the father is the primary caregiver while the mother is at work, 40% of mothers adjusted their work hours to meet child care needs, compared with 6% of fathers (O'Connell, 1993).

The mother's status as a working woman has not been found consistently to have either positive or negative effects on children's development and educational outcomes (Balk and Christoffel, 1988) (Fig. 29-5). Working women who scored high on measures of emotional well-being, sensitivity to and acceptance of their children, satisfaction with nonwork time, and positive feelings about their marriage were more likely to have securely attached infants, regardless of child-care arrangements (Belsky, 1988). One consistent finding is that the "consequences of maternal employment" (mental health, marital satisfaction, children's well-being) are favorable when the woman's employment status is consistent with her and her partner's preferences about it (Spitzke, 1988). The economic background of the family also interacts with the effects of the type of child care and its psychologic outcomes (Friedman et al, 1994).

Key Points

- Because there is no agreement about the definition of *family*, a family is what the patient considers it to be.
- Although the traditional family structure has been nuclear or extended, in recent years other forms such as the single-parent family have emerged.
- Family size and positioning within the family structure have a strong impact on a child's development.
- Interpersonal skills and a basic understanding of childhood growth and development are two essential areas of focus for parents.
- Parents tend to predominate in one of three types of parental control: authoritarian, permissive, and authoritative.
- Three areas of special concern to adoptive families include

the initial attachment process, the risk of telling the children they are adopted, and identity formation during adolescence.

- Marital factors within the home significantly influence a child's development. The impact of divorce on a child depends on age and gender, outcome, and quality of the parent-child relationship and parental care following the divorce.
- Single-parenting and stepparenting create adjustment difficulties and add stress to the already demanding parental role. Significant numbers of children will live in a single-parent reconstituted family at some point.

References

Amato PR, Keith B: Parental divorce and the well-being of children: a meta-analysis, *Psychol Bull* 110(1):26-46, 1991.

American Academy of Pediatrics, Committee on Early Childhood, Adoption and Dependent Care: Initial medical evaluation of an adopted child, *Pediatrics* 88(3):642-644, 1991.

Arditti J: Differences between fathers with joint custody and noncustodial fathers, *Am J Orthopsychiatry* 62(2):186-195, 1992.

Arnold L, Brecht M: Legislative issues affecting parenting: an overview of current policies, *J Perinat Neonat Nurs* 4(2):24-32, 1990.

Balk S, Christoffel K: Advising the working mother, *Contemp Pediatr* 5(9):56-85, 1988.

Belsky J: The "effects" of infant day care reconsidered, *Early Childhood Res Q* 3(3):235-272, 1988.

Blum NJ et al: Disciplining young children: the role of verbal instructions and reasoning, *Pediatrics* 96(2):336-341, 1995.

Brazelton TB: Working with families: opportunities for early intervention, *Pediatr Clin North Am* 42(1):1-10, 1995.

Center for the Study of Social Policy: *Kids count*, Washington, DC, 1993, Annie E Casey Foundation.

Children's Defense Fund: *The state of America's children 1994*, Washington, DC, 1994, CDF.

Daniels D, Moos R: Exosystem influences on family and child functioning, *J Soc Behav Pers* 3(4):113-133, 1988.

Demo D, Acock A: The impact of divorce on children, *J Marriage Fam* 50:619-648, 1988.

Dunst C, Trivette C, Deal A: *Enabling and empowering families: principles and guidelines for practice*, Cambridge, Mass, 1988, Brookline Books.

Edwards J: Perceived needs of adoptive and biologic parents, *Issues Compr Pediatr Nus* 10:223-234, 1987.

Eichelberger S, Beal D, May R: Hypovolemic shock in a child as a consequence of corporal punishment, *Pediatrics* 87(4):570-571, 1991.

Finkelhor D et al: *The dark side of families: current family violence research*, Newport, Calif, 1983, Sage Publications.

Friedman SL et al: Effects of child care on psychological development: issues and future directions for research, *Pediatrics* 94(suppl 6, part 2 of 2):1069-1070, 1994.

Gage M, Christensen D: Parental role socialization and the transition to parenthood, *Fam Relations* 40(3):332-337, 1991.

Ganong L, Coleman M: Preparing for remarriage: anticipating the issues, seeking solutions, *Fam Relations* 38:28-33, 1989.

Garbarino J ct al: *Children in danger: coping with the consequences of community violence*, San Francisco, 1992, Jossey-Bass.

Giebink G: Care of the ill child in day-care settings, *Pediatrics* 91(1, pt 2):229-233, 1993.

Hetherington EM, Stanley-Hagan M, Anderson ER: Marital transitions: a child's perspective, *Am Psychologist* 44(2):303-312, 1989.

Hoopes M, Harper J: *Birth order roles and sibling patterns in individual and family therapy*, Rockville, Md, 1987, Aspen.

Hostetter M, Johnson D: International adoption: an introduction for physicians, *Am J Dis Child* 143:325-332, 1989.

Hyman I et al: *Child abuse in the schools: community and judicial attitudes.* Paper presented at the 62nd annual meeting of the American Orthopsychiatric Association, New York, April 24, 1985.

Jordan A: The unresolved child care dilemma: care of the acutely ill child, *Rev Infect Dis* 8(4):626-630, 1986.

Koepke J et al: Becoming parents: feelings of adoptive mothers, *Pediatr Nurs* 17(4):333-336, 1991.

Leung AK, Robson WL: Children of divorce, *J R Soc Health* 110(5):161-163, 1990.

Lobato D: *Brothers, sisters, and special needs*, Baltimore, Md, 1990, Paul H Brookes.

McCubbin HI, Patterson JM: *Family adaptation to crisis.* In McCubbin HI, Cauble E, Patterson JM, editors: *Family stress, coping, and social support*, Springfield, Ill, 1982, Charles C Thomas.

Nelms B: Discipline: what do you recommend? *J Pediatric Health Care* 7(1):1-2, 1993.

O'Connell M: *Where's papa? Fathers' role in child care*, Washington, DC, 1993, Population Reference Bureau.

Patterson J: Promoting resilience in families experiencing stress, *Pediatr Clin North Am* 42(1):47-63, 1995.

Richards L: The precarious survival and hard-won satisfaction of white single-parent families, *Fam Relations* 38:396-403, 1989.

Rosen M: *Stepfathering*, New York, 1987, Ballatine Books.

Shaw DS, Emery RE, Tuer MD: Parental functioning and children's adjustment in families of divorce: a prospective study, *J Abnorm Child Psychol* 21(1):119-134, 1993.

Singh GK et al: Annual summary of births, marriages, divorces, and deaths: United States, 1994. *Monthly vital statistics report*, vol 43, no 13, Hyattsville, Md, National Center for Health Statistics, 1995.

Smith K, Shillam P, Zimmerman F: Standards and criteria: group child care for sick children, *Pediatr Nurs* 15(6):600-602, 1989.

Spitzke G: Women's employment and family relations: a review, *J Marriage Fam* 50(3):595-618, 1988.

Stirtzinger R, Cholvat L: Preschool age children of divorce: transitional phenomena and the mourning process, *Can J Psychiatry* 35:506-514, 1990.

Strett R: Support services for single parents, *Early Childhood Update* 5:6, Winter 1989.

Tuttle G: Divorce: how are the children coping? *Can Nurse* 88(11):13-16, 1992.

Ventura SJ et al: Advance report of final natality statistics, 1993. *Monthly vital statistics report*, vol 44, no 3, supp, Hyattsville, Md, National Center for Health Statistics, 1995.

Visher E, Visher J: Parenting coalitions after remarriage: dynamics and therapeutic guidelines, *Fam Relations* 38:65-70, 1989.

Wallace P, Gotlib I: Marital adjustment during the transition to parenthood: stability and predictors of change, *J Marriage Fam* 52(1):21-29, 1990.

Wallerstein JS: The long-term effects of divorce on children: a review, *J Am Acad Child Adolesc Psychiatry* 30(3):349-360, 1991.

Wallerstein JS, Johnston JR: Children of divorce: recent findings regarding long-term effects and recent studies of joint and sole custody, *Pediatr Rev* 11(7):197-204, 1990.

Bibliography

General

Aldous J: Family development and the life course: two perspectives on family change, *J Marriage Fam* 52(3):571-583, 1990.

Beutler IF et al: The family realm: theoretical contributions for understanding its uniqueness, *J Marriage Fam* 51(3):805-815, 1989.

Bornstein MH, editor: *Handbook of parenting*, vol 1-4, Hillshale, NJ, 1995, Lawrence Erlbaum Associates.

Cohen WI: Family-oriented pediatric care: taking the next step, *Pediatr Clin North Am* 42(1):11-20, 1995.

Friedman M: *Family nursing: theory and practice*, ed 3, Norwalk, Conn, 1992, Appleton-Century-Crofts.

Gillis CL et al, editors: *Toward a science of family nursing*, Menlo Park, Calif, 1989, Addison-Wesley.

Glick PC: Fifty years of family demography: a record of social change, *J Marriage Fam* 50(4):861-873, 1988.

Green M: No child is an island: contextual pediatrics and the "new" health supervision, *Pediatric Clin North Am* 42(1):79-88, 1995.

Kune-Karrer BM, Taylor EH: Toward multiculturality: implications for the pediatrician, *Pediatr Clin North Am* 42(1):21-30, 1995.

Lavee Y, Olson D: Family types and response to stress, *J Marriage Fam* 53(3):786-788, 1991.

MacPhee M: The family systems approach and pediatric nursing care, *Pediatr Nurs* 21(5):417-423, 437, 1995.

Schor EL: The influence of families on child health: family behaviors and child outcomes, *Pediatr Clin North Am* 42(1):89-102, 1995.

Smoyak SA: *Changing American families*. In Hoekelman RA et al, editors: *Primary pediatric care*, ed 2, St Louis, 1992, Mosby.

Family Constellations/Parenting

Carter-Jessop L, Yoos L: Parental thinking: assessment and applications in nursing, *Maternal Child Nurs J* 22(2): 49-55, 1994.

Christopherson ER: Discipline, *Pediatr Clin North Am* 39:395-412, 1992.

Gellerstedt ME, leRoux P: Beyond anticipatory guidance: parenting and the family life cycle, *Pediatr Clin North Am* 42(1):65-78, 1995.

Howard BJ: Discipline in early childhood, *Pediatr Clin North Am* 38:1351-1396, 1991.

Patterson JM, Garwick AW: Levels of meaning in family stress theory, *Fam Pract* 33:287-304, 1994.

Simons R et al: Husband and wife differences in determinants of parenting: a social learning/exchange model of parental behavior, *J Marriage Fam* 52(2):375-392, 1990.

Visher JS, Visher EB: Beyond the nuclear family: resources and implications for pediatricians, *Pediatr Clin North Am* 42(1):31-46, 1995.

Special Parenting Situations

Amato P: The "child of divorce" as a person prototype: bias in the recall of information about children in divorced families, *J Marriage Fam* 53(1):59-69, 1991.

Anable KE: Children of divorce: ways to heal the wounds, *Clin Nurs Spec* 5(3):133-137, 1991.

Arditti JA: Noncustodial fathers: an overview of policy and resources, *Fam Relations* 39(4):460-465, 1990.

Benin M, Edwards D: Adolescents' chores: the differences between dual- and single-career families, *J Marriage Fam* 52(2):361-373, 1990.

Bray JH, Berger SH: Noncustodial father and paternal grandparent relationship in stepfamilies, *Fam Relations* 39(4):414-419, 1990.

Brazelton TB: Putting a child in day care: issues for working parents, *Pediatrics* 91(1, pt 2):271-272, 1993.

Bredekamp S: Day-care standards: need and impact, *Pediatrics* 91 (1, pt 2):234-236, 1993.

Brubeck D, Beer J: Depression, self-esteem, suicide ideation, death anxiety, and GPA in high school students of divorced and non-divorced parents, *Psychol Rep* 71(3, pt I): 755-763, 1992.

Caldwell BM: Impact of day care on the child, *Pediatrics* 91(1, pt 2):225-228, 1993.

Christensen DH, Dahl CM, Rettig KD: Noncustodial mothers and child support: examining the larger context, *Fam Relations* 39(4):388-394, 1990.

Day care for early preschool children: implications for the child and family, *Am J Psychiatry* 150(8):1281-1287, 1993.

Depner CE, Bray JH: Modes of participation for noncustodial parents: the challenge for research, policy, practice and education, *Fam Relations* 39(4):378-381, 1990.

Dvoskin AG: *Child custody*. In Hoekelman RA et al, editors: *Primary pediatric care*, ed 2, St Louis, 1992, Mosby.

Fairchild MW, Zebal BH: *Children of divorce*. In Hoekelman RA et al, editors: *Primary pediatric care*, ed 2, St Louis, 1992, Mosby.

Ferreiro BW: Presumption of joint custody: a family policy dilemma, *Fam Relations* 39(4):420-426, 1990.

Garvin V, Leber D, Kalter N: Children of divorce: predictors of change following preventive intervention, *Am J Orthopsychiatry* 61(3):438-447, 1991.

Hajal F, Rosenberg D: The family life cycle in adoptive families, *Am J Orthopsychiatry* 61(1):78-85, 1991.

Healy JM Jr, Malley JE, Stewart AJ: Children and their fathers after parental separation, *Am J Orthopsychiatry* 60(4):531-543, 1990.

Johnston JR: Role diffusion and role reversal: structural variation in divorced families and children's functioning, *Fam Relations* 39(4):405-413, 1990.

Melnyk BM: Changes in parent-child relationships following divorce, *Pediatr Nurs* 17(4):337-341, 1991.

Menaghan D, Parcel T: Parental employment and family life: research in the 1980s, *J Marriage Fam* 52(4):1079-1098, 1990.

Nickman SL: *Adoption and foster care*. In Hoekelman RA et al, editors: *Primary pediatric care*, ed 2, St Louis, 1992, Mosby.

Richman JM, Chapman MV, Bowen GL: Recognizing the impact of marital discord and parental depression on children: a family-centered approach, *Pediatr Clin North Am* 42(1):167-180, 1995.

Schwartzberg AZ: The impact of divorce on adolescents, *Hosp Community Psychiatry* 43(6):634-637, 1992.

Shaw DS: The effects of divorce on children's adjustment: review and implications, *Behav Modif* 15(4):456-485, 1991.

Tiedje LB, Collins C: Combining employment and motherhood, *MCN* 14:9-14, 1989.

Tschann J et al: Family process and children's functioning during divorce, *J Marriage Fam* 51:431-444, 1990.

Volling B, Belsky J: Multiple determinants of father involvement during infancy in dual-earner and single-career families, *J Marriage Fam* 53(2):461-474, 1991.

Wallerstein JS, Blakeslee S: *Second chances: men, women, and children a decade after divorce*, New York, 1989, Ticknor & Fields.

CHAPTER 30

Developmental Influences on Child Health Promotion

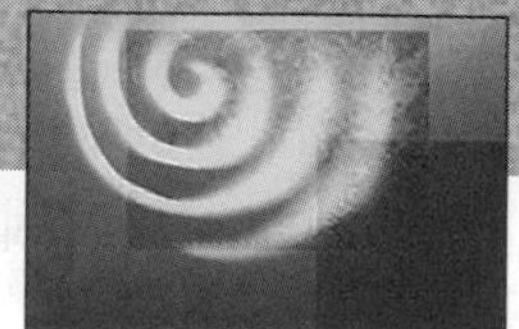

GROWTH AND DEVELOPMENT, P. 844
Foundations of growth and development, p. 844
Biologic growth and physical development, p. 846
Physiologic changes, p. 848
Temperament, p. 849

DEVELOPMENT OF PERSONALITY AND MENTAL FUNCTION, P. 850
Theoretic foundations of personality development, p. 850
Theoretic foundations of mental development, p. 852
Development of self-concept, p. 854

ROLE OF PLAY IN DEVELOPMENT, P. 855
Classification of play, p. 855
Functions of play, p. 857
Toys, 858

SELECTED FACTORS THAT INFLUENCE DEVELOPMENT, P. 858

Growth and Development

FOUNDATIONS OF GROWTH AND DEVELOPMENT

Growth and development, usually referred to as a unit, expresses the sum of the numerous changes that take place during the lifetime of an individual. The entire course is a dynamic process that encompasses several interrelated dimensions:

Growth—an increase in number and size of cells as they divide and synthesize new proteins; results in increased size and weight of the whole or any of its parts

Development—a gradual change and expansion; advancement from lower to more advanced stages of complexity; the emerging and expanding of the individual's capacities through growth, maturation, and learning

Maturation—an increase in competence and adaptability; aging; usually used to describe a qualitative change; a change in the complexity of a structure that makes it possible for that structure to begin functioning; to function at a higher level

Differentiation—processes by which early cells and structures are systematically modified and altered to achieve specific and characteristic physical and chemical properties; sometimes used to describe the trend of mass to specific; development from simple to more complex activities and functions

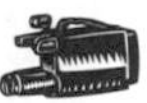

For additional information, please view "Growth and Development" in *Whaley and Wong's Pediatric Nursing Video Series,* St Louis, 1996, Mosby; (800)426-4545.

Stages of Development

Most authorities in the field of child development conveniently categorize child growth and behavior into approximate age stages or in terms that describe the features of an age group. The age ranges of these stages are admittedly arbitrary, and, since they do not take into account individual differences, cannot be applied to all children with any degree of precision. However, this categorization affords a convenient means to describe the characteristics associated with the majority of children at periods when distinctive developmental changes appear and specific developmental tasks must be accomplished. (A **developmental task** is a set of skills and competencies peculiar to each developmental stage that children must accomplish or master in order to deal effectively with the environment.) It is also significant for nurses to know that there are characteristic health problems peculiar to each major phase of development. The sequence of descriptive age periods and subperiods that are used here and elaborated in subsequent chapters is listed in Box 30-1.

Patterns of Growth and Development

There are definite and predictable patterns in growth and development that are continuous, orderly, and progressive. These patterns, which are sometimes referred to as trends or

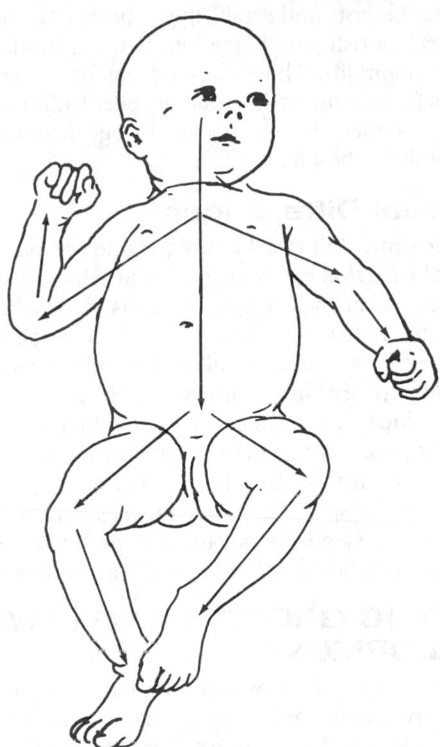

Fig. 30-1 Directional trends in growth.

principles, are universal and basic to all human beings. Although they are more apparent with respect to physical growth, most of these patterns apply to psychologic and social growth as well. Growth and development follow predetermined trends in direction, sequence, and pace, but each human being accomplishes these in a manner and time unique to that individual.

Directional trends. Growth and development proceed in regular, related directions or gradients and reflect the physical development and maturation of neuromuscular functions (Fig. 30-1). The first pattern is the **cephalocaudal,** or *head-to-tail,* direction; that is, the head end of the organism develops first and is very large and complex, whereas the lower end is small and simple and takes shape at a later period. Infants achieve structural control of the head before they have control of the trunk and extremities, hold their back erect before they stand, use their eyes before their hands, and gain control of their hands before they have control of their feet.

Second, the **proximodistal,** or *near-to-far,* trend applies to the midline-to-peripheral concept. In the infant, shoulder control precedes mastery of the hands, the whole hand is used as a unit before the fingers can be manipulated, and the central nervous system develops more rapidly than the peripheral nervous system.

These trends or patterns are bilateral and appear symmetric—each side develops in the same direction and at the same rate as the other. For some of the neurologic functions, this symmetry is only external because of unilateral differentiation of function at an early stage of postnatal development. For example, by the age of approximately 5 years the child has demonstrated a decided preference for the use of one hand over the other, although previously either one had been used.

The third trend, **differentiation,** describes development from simple operations to more complex activities and functions. From very broad, global patterns of behavior, more spe-

BOX 30-1

Developmental Age Periods

Prenatal period: Conception to birth

Germinal: Conception to approximately 2 weeks

Embryonic: 2 to 8 weeks

Fetal: 8 to 40 weeks (birth)

A rapid growth rate and total dependency make this one of the most crucial periods in the developmental process. The relationship between maternal health and certain manifestations in the newborn emphasizes the importance of adequate prenatal care to the health and well-being of the infant.

Infancy period: Birth to 12 or 18 months

Neonatal: Birth to 27 or 28 days

Infancy: 1 to approximately 12 months

The infancy period is one of rapid motor, cognitive, and social development. Through mutuality with the caregiver (parent), the infant establishes a basic trust in the world and the foundation for future interpersonal relationships. The critical first month of life, although part of the infancy period, is often differentiated from the remainder because of the major physical adjustments to extrauterine existence and the psychologic adjustment of the parent.

Early childhood: 1 to 6 years

Toddler: 1 to 3 years

Preschool: 3 to 6 years

This period, which extends from the time the children attain upright locomotion until they enter school, is characterized by intense activity and discovery. It is a time of marked physical and personality development. Motor development advances steadily. Children at this age acquire language and wider social relationships, learn role standards, gain self-control and mastery, develop increasing awareness of dependence and independence, and begin to develop a self-concept.

Middle childhood: 6 to 11 or 12 years

Frequently referred to as the "school age," this period of development is one in which the child is directed away from the family group and is centered around the wider world of peer relationships. There is steady advancement in physical, mental, and social development, with emphasis on developing skill competencies. Social cooperation and early moral development take on more importance with relevance for later life stages. This is a critical period in the development of a self-concept.

Later childhood: 11 to 19 years

Prepubertal: 10 to 13 years

Adolescence: 13 to approximately 18 years

The tumultuous period of rapid maturation and change known as adolescence is considered to be a traditional period that begins at the onset of puberty and extends to the point of entry into the adult world—usually high school graduation. Biologic and personality maturation are accompanied by physical and emotional turmoil, and there is redefining of the self-concept. In the late adolescent period the child begins to internalize all previously learned values and to focus on an individual, rather than a group, identity.

cific, refined patterns emerge. All areas of development (physical, mental, social, and emotional) proceed in this direction. Generalized development precedes specific or specialized development; gross, random muscle movements take place before fine muscle control.

Sequential trends. In all dimensions of growth and development there is a definite, predictable sequence, with each child normally passing through every stage. Children crawl before they creep, creep before they stand, and stand before they walk. Later facets of the personality are built on the early foundation of trust. The child babbles, then forms words and, finally, sentences; writing emerges from scribbling.

Developmental pace. Although there is a fixed, precise order to development, it does not progress at the same rate or pace. There are periods of accelerated growth and periods of decelerated growth in both total body growth and the growth of subsystems. The rapid growth before and after birth gradually levels off throughout early childhood. Growth is relatively slow during middle childhood, markedly increases at the beginning of adolescence, and levels off in early adulthood. Each child grows at his or her own pace. Marked differences are observed between children as they reach and surmount developmental milestones.

Sensitive periods. There are limited times during the process of growth when the organism will interact with a particular environment in a specific manner. Periods termed *critical, sensitive, vulnerable,* and *optimal* are those times in the lifetime of an organism when it is more susceptible to positive or negative influences.

The quality of interactions during these sensitive periods determines whether the effects on the organism will be beneficial or harmful. For example, physiologic maturation of the central nervous system is influenced by adequacy and timing of contributions from the environment, such as stimulation and nutrition.

Psychologic development also appears to have sensitive periods when an environmental event has maximal influence on the developing personality. For example, primary socialization occurs during the first year when the infant makes the initial social attachments and establishes a basic trust in the world. A warm relationship with a parent figure is fundamental to a healthy personality. The same concept might be applied to readiness for learning skills such as toilet training or reading. In these instances there appears to be an opportune time when the skill is best learned.

Individual Differences

Each child grows in his or her unique and personal way. Great individual variation exists at the age at which developmental milestones are reached. The sequence is predictable; the exact timing is not. Rates of growth vary, and measurements are defined in terms of ranges to allow for individual differences. Some children are fast growers, others are moderate, and some are slower to reach maturity. Periods of fast growth, such as the pubescent growth spurt, may begin earlier or later in some children than in others. Children may grow fast or slow during the spurt and may finish sooner or later than other children. Gender is an influential factor because girls seem to be more advanced in physiologic growth at all ages.

BIOLOGIC GROWTH AND PHYSICAL DEVELOPMENT

As children grow, their external dimensions change. These changes are accompanied by corresponding alterations in structure and function of internal organs and tissues that reflect the gradual acquisition of physiologic competence. Each part has its own rate of growth, which may be directly related to alterations in the size of the child (e.g., the heart rate). Skeletal muscle growth approximates whole body growth; brain, lymphoid, adrenal, and reproductive tissues follow distinct and individual patterns. When there has been a secondary cause of growth deficiency, such as severe illness or acute malnutrition, recovery from the illness or the establishment of an adequate diet will produce a dramatic acceleration of the growth rate that usually continues until the child's individual growth pattern is resumed.

External Proportions

Variations in the growth rate of different tissues and organ systems produce significant changes in body proportions during childhood. The cephalocaudal trend of development is

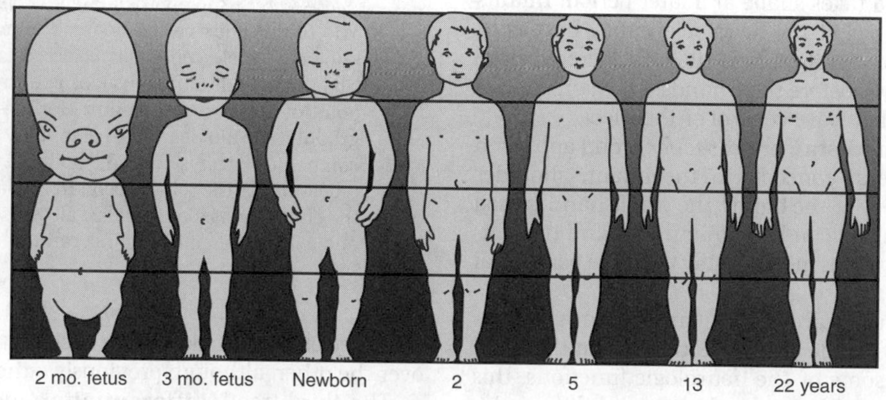

Fig. 30-2 Changes in body proportions from before birth to adulthood. (From Crouch JE, McClintic JR: *Human anatomy and physiology,* ed 2, New York, 1976, John Wiley & Sons.)

most evident in total body growth, as indicated by these changes (Fig. 30-2). During fetal development the head is the fastest growing body part. During infancy growth of the trunk predominates; the legs are the most rapidly growing part during childhood; in adolescence the trunk once again elongates. In the newborn infant the lower limbs are one third the total body length but only 15% of the total body weight; in the adult the lower limbs constitute one half of the total body weight and 30% or more of the total body weight. As growth proceeds, the midpoint in head-to-toe measurements gradually descends from a level even with the umbilicus at birth to the level of the symphysis pubis at maturity.

Biologic Determinants of Growth and Development

The most prominent feature of childhood and adolescence is physical growth. Throughout development various tissues in the body undergo changes in growth, composition, and structure. In some tissues the changes are continuous (e.g., bone growth and dentition); in others significant alterations occur at specific stages (e.g., appearance of secondary sex characteristics). When these measurements are compared with standardized norms, a child's developmental progress can be determined with a high degree of confidence (Table 30-1).

Linear growth, or *height*, occurs almost entirely as a result of skeletal growth and is considered a stable measurement of general growth. Growth in height is not uniform throughout life but ceases when maturation of the skeleton is complete. The maximum growth in length occurs before birth, but the newborn continues to grow at a rapid, though slower, rate. Adult height can be estimated by doubling the child's height at the age of 2 years.

At birth, *weight* is more variable than height and is, to a greater extent, a reflection of the intrauterine environment. The average newborn weighs from 3175 to 3400 g (7 to 7$^1/_2$ pounds). In general, the birth weight doubles by 4 to 7 months of age and triples by the end of the first year. By the end of the second year it usually quadruples. After this point the "normal" rate of weight gain, just as the growth in height, assumes a steady annual increase of approximately 2 to 2.75 kg (4.4 to 6 pounds) per year until the adolescent growth spurt.

Both *bone age* determinants and state of *dentition* are used as indicators of development. Since both are discussed elsewhere, neither is elaborated here (see next section for bone age; see also Chapters 33 and 34 for dentition).

Skeletal Growth and Maturation

The most accurate measure of general development is **skeletal age** or **bone,** the radiologic determination of osseous maturation. Skeletal age appears to correlate more closely with other measures of physiologic maturity (such as onset of menarche) than with chronologic age or height. This "bone age" is determined by comparing the mineralization of ossification centers and advancing bony form to age-related standards.

Bone formation begins during the second month of fetal life when calcium salts are deposited in the intercellular substance (matrix) to form calcified cartilage first and then true bone. There are some differences in this bone formation. In small bones the bone continues to form in the center, and cartilage continues to be laid down on the surfaces. In long bones the ossification begins in the *diaphysis* (the long central portion of the bone) and continues in the *epiphysis* (the end por-

TABLE 30-1 General trends in height and weight gain during childhood

AGE GROUP	WEIGHT*	HEIGHT*
Infants		
Birth–6 months	Weekly gain: 140-200 g (5-7 oz) Birth weight doubles by end of first 4-7 months†	Monthly gain: 2.5 cm (1 inch)
6-12 months	Weight gain: 85-140 g (3-5 oz) Birth weight triples by end of first year	Monthly gain: 1.25 cm ($^1/_2$ inch) Birth length increases by approximately 50% by end of first year
Toddlers	Birth weight quadruples by age 2$^1/_2$ Yearly gain: 2-3 kg (4$^1/_2$ - 6$^1/_2$ lb)	Height at age 2 is approximately 50% of eventual adult height Gain during second year: about 12 cm (4$^3/_4$ inches) Gain during third year: about 6-8 cm (2$^3/_8$ - 3$^1/_4$ inches)
Preschoolers	Yearly gain: 2-3 kg (4$^1/_2$ - 6$^1/_2$ lb)	Birth length doubles by age 4 Yearly gain: 5-7.5 cm (2-3 inches)
School-age children	Yearly gain: 2-3 kg (4$^1/_2$ - 6$^1/_2$ lb)	Yearly gain after age 7: 5 cm (2 inches) Birth length triples by about age 13
Pubertal growth spurt		
Females—10-14 years	Weight gain: 7-25 kg (15-55 lb) Mean: 17.5 kg (38$^1/_8$ lb)	Height gain: 5-25 cm (2-10 inches); approximately 95% of mature height achieved by onset of menarche or skeletal age of 13 Mean: 20.5 cm (8$^1/_4$ inches)
Males—11-16 years	Weight gain: 7-30 kg (15-65 lb) Mean: 23.7 kg (52$^1/_8$ lb)	Height gain: 10-30 cm (4-12 inches); approximately 95% of mature height achieved by skeletal age of 15 years Mean: 27.5 cm (11 inches)

*Yearly height and weight gains for each age-group represent averaged estimates from a variety of sources.
†Data from Jung G, Czajka-Narins DM: *Am J Clin Nutr* 42:182-189, 1985.

tions of the bone). Between the diaphysis and the epiphysis an *epiphyseal cartilage plate* unites with the diaphysis by columns of spongy tissue, the *metaphysis*. Active growth in length takes place in the epiphyseal growth plate. Interference with this growth site by trauma or infection can result in deformity.

The first centers of ossification appear in the 2-month-old embryo, and at birth the number is approximately 400, about half the number at maturity. New centers appear at regular intervals during the growth period and provide the basis for assessment of bone age. Postnatally the earliest centers to appear (at 5 to 6 months of age) are those of the capitate and hamate bones in the wrist. Therefore radiographs of the hand and wrist provide the most useful areas for screening to determine skeletal age, especially before age 6 years. These centers appear earlier in girls than in boys.

Neurologic Maturation

In contrast to other body tissues, which grow rapidly after birth, the nervous system grows proportionately more rapidly before birth. Two periods of rapid brain cell growth occur during fetal life: a dramatic increase in the number of neurons between 15 and 20 weeks of gestation and another increase at 30 weeks, which extends to 1 year of age. The rapid growth of infancy continues during early childhood and then slows to a more gradual rate during later childhood and adolescence.

It is believed that no new nerve cells appear after the sixth month of fetal life. Postnatal growth consists of increasing the amount of cytoplasm around the nuclei of existing cells, increasing the number and intricacy of communications with other cells, and advancing their peripheral axions to keep pace with expanding body dimensions. This allows for increasingly complex movement and behavior. Neurophysiologic changes also provide the foundation for language, learning, and behavior development. Neurologic or electroencephalographic development is sometimes used as an indicator of maturational age in the early weeks of life.

Lymphoid Tissues

Lymphoid tissues contained in the lymph nodes, thymus, spleen, tonsils, adenoids, and blood lymphocytes follow a growth pattern unlike that of other body tissues. These tissues are small in relation to total body size, but they are well developed at birth. They increase rapidly to reach adult dimensions by 6 years of age and continue to grow. At about age 10 to 12 years they reach a maximum development that is approximately twice their adult size. This is followed by a rapid decline until adult dimensions are achieved by the end of adolescence.

Development of Organ Systems

All tissues and organ systems undergo changes during development. Some are striking; others are more subtle. Many have implications for assessment and care. Since the major importance of these changes relates to their dysfunction, the developmental characteristics of various systems and organs are discussed throughout the book as they relate to these areas. Physical characteristics and physiologic changes that vary with age are included in age-group descriptions.

PHYSIOLOGIC CHANGES

Physiologic changes that take place in all organs and systems are discussed as they relate to dysfunction. Others such as pulse and respiratory rates and blood pressure, are an integral part of physical assessment (see Chapter 32). In addition, there are changes in basic functions, including metabolism, temperature, and patterns of sleep and rest.

Metabolism

The rate of metabolism when the body is at rest (**basal metabolic rate**, or **BMR**) demonstrates a distinctive change throughout childhood. Highest in the newborn infant, the BMR closely relates to the proportion of surface area to body mass, which changes as the body increases in size. In both sexes the proportion decreases progressively to maturity. The BMR is slightly higher in boys at all ages and further increases during pubescence over that in girls.

The rate of metabolism determines the caloric requirements of the child. The basal energy requirement of infants is about 108 kcal/kg of body weight and decreases to 40 to 45 kcal/kg at maturity (Table 30-2). Water requirements remain at approximately 1.5 ml per calorie of energy expended throughout life. Children's energy needs vary considerably at different ages and with changing circumstances. The energy requirement to build tissue steadily decreases with age, following the general growth curve; however, energy needs vary with the individual child and may be considerably more. For short periods (e.g., during strenuous exercise) and more prolonged periods (e.g., illness), the needs can be very high. During illness each degree of fever increases the basal metabolism 10%, with a corresponding fluid requirement.

Temperature

Body temperature, reflecting metabolism, displays the same decrement from infancy to maturity (see the Appendix). Following the unstable regulatory ability in the neonatal period, heat production steadily declines as the infant grows into childhood. Individual differences of 0.5° to 1° F are normal, and occasionally a child normally displays an unusually high

TABLE 30-2 Recommended daily requirements for calories and protein through adolescence*

AGE (YEARS)	ENERGY ALLOWANCE (kcal/kg)	PROTEIN (g)
Infants		
0-$^1/_2$	108	13
$^1/_2$-1	98	14
Children		
1-3	102	16
4-6	90	24
7-10	70	28
Males		
11-14	55	45
15-18	45	49
Females		
11-14	47	46
15-18	40	44

*Data from Food and Nutrition Board: *Recommended daily allowances*, ed 10, Washington, DC, 1989, National Academy Press.

or low temperature. Beginning at approximately 12 years of age, the temperature in girls remains relatively stable, whereas in boys it continues to fall for a few years longer. Females maintain a temperature slightly above that of males throughout life.

Even with improved temperature regulation, infants and young children are highly susceptible to temperature fluctuations. Body temperature responds to changes in environmental temperature and is increased with active exercise, crying, and emotional upset. Infections can cause a higher and more rapid temperature increase in infants and young children than in older children. In relation to body weight, an infant produces more heat per unit than do children near maturity. Consequently, during active play or when heavily clothed, an infant or small child is likely to become overheated.

Sleep and Rest

Sleep, a protective function in all organisms, allows for repair and recovery of tissues following activity. As in most aspects of development, there is wide variation among individual children in the amount and distribution of sleep at various ages. As children mature, there is a change in the total time they spend in sleep and in the amount of time they spend in deep sleep.

Newborn infants sleep much of the time that is not occupied with feeding and other aspects of their care. As infants grow older, the total time spent in sleep gradually decreases, they remain awake for longer periods, and they sleep longer at night. During the latter part of the first year, most children sleep through the night and take one or two naps during the day. By the time they are 12 to 18 months old, most children have eliminated the second nap. After age 3 years the child has usually given up daytime naps except in cultures in which an afternoon nap or siesta is customary. During ages 4 to 10 sleep time declines slightly and then increases somewhat during the pubertal growth spurt. The changes in length of sleep at different ages is shown in Fig. 30-3.

There is a change in the quality of sleep as children mature. The time spent in deep, restful sleep increases from 50% in infancy to 80% in the older child.

TEMPERAMENT

Defined as "the manner of thinking, behaving, or reacting characteristic of an individual" (Chess and Thomas, 1985), **temperament** refers to the way in which a person deals with life. From the time of birth, children exhibit marked individual differences in the way they respond to their environment and the way others, particularly the parents, respond to them and their needs. A generic basis has been suggested for some differences in temperament. Nine characteristics of temperament have been identified through interviews with parents (Box 30-2). Temperament refers to behavioral tendencies, not to discrete behavioral acts. There are no implications of good or bad. Most children can be placed into one of three common categories based on their overall pattern of temperamental attributes:

The easy child. Easy-going children are even tempered, are regular and predictable in their habits, and have a positive approach to new stimuli. They are open and adaptable to change and display a mild to moderately intense mood that is typically positive. Approximately 40% of children fall into this category.

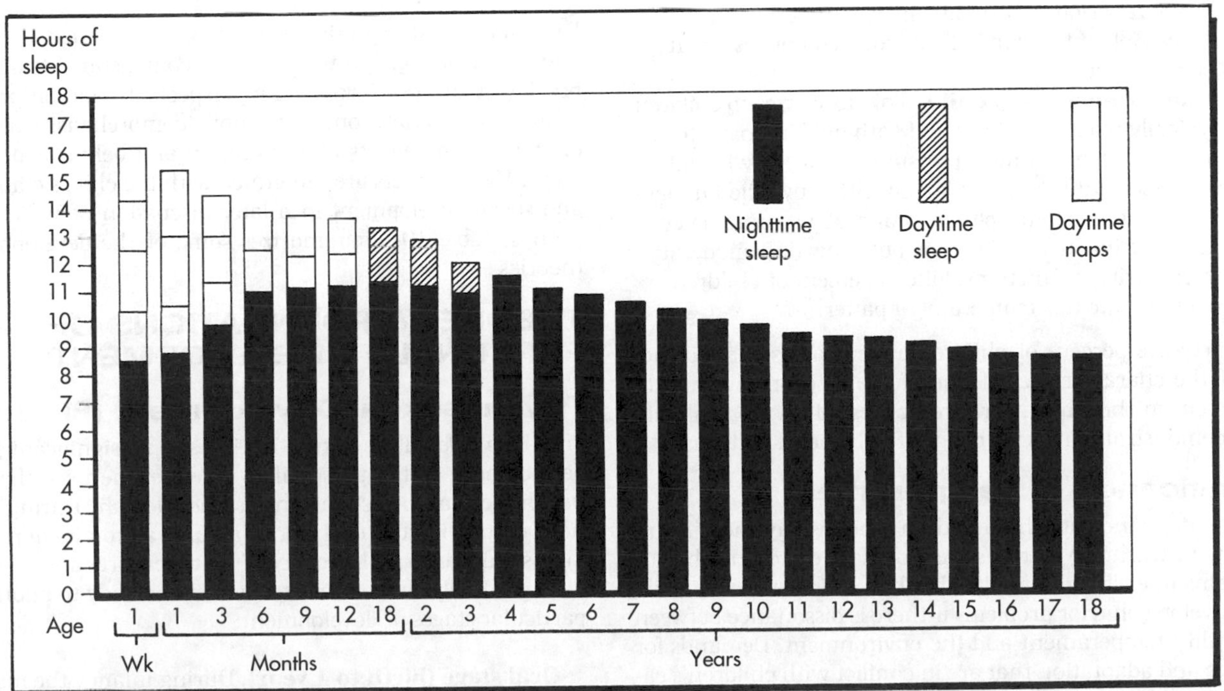

Fig. 30-3 Changes in number of hours of sleep with increasing age. (Modified from Ferber R: *Solve your child's sleep problems*, New York, 1985, Simon & Schuster.)

BOX 30-2
Attributes of Temperament

Activity—level of physical motion during activity, such as sleep, eating, play, dressing, and bathing
Rhythmicity—regularity in the timing of physiologic functions such as hunger, sleep, and elimination
Approach-withdrawal—nature of initial responses to a new stimulus such as people, situations, places, foods, toys, and procedures (*Approach* responses are positive and are displayed by activity or expression; *withdrawal* responses are negative expressions or behaviors.)
Adaptability—ease or difficulty with which the child adapts or adjusts to new or altered situations
Threshold of responsiveness (sensory threshold)—amount of stimulation, such as sounds or light, required to evoke a response in the child
Intensity of reaction—energy level of the child's reactions, regardless of quality or direction
Mood—amount of pleasant, happy, friendly behavior compared with unpleasant, unhappy, crying, unfriendly behavior exhibited by the child in various situations
Distractibility—ease with which a child's attention or direction of behavior can be diverted by external stimuli
Attention span and persistence—length of time a child pursues a given activity *(attention)* and the continuation of an activity in spite of obstacles *(persistence)*

The difficult child. Difficult children are highly active, irritable, and irregular in their habits. Negative withdrawal responses are typical, and they require a more structured environment. These children adapt slowly to new routines, people, or situations. Mood expressions are usually intense and primarily negative. They exhibit frequent periods of crying, and frustration often produces violent tantrums. This group comprises about 10% of children.

The slow-to-warm-up child. Slow-to-warm-up children typically react negatively and with mild intensity to new stimuli and, unless pressured, adapt slowly with repeated contact. They respond with only mild but passive resistance to novelty or changes in routine. They are quite inactive and moody but show only moderate irregularity in functions. Fifteen percent of children demonstrate this temperament pattern.

Thirty-five percent of children either have some, but not all, of the characteristics of one of the categories or are inconsistent in their behavioral responses. Many normal children demonstrate this wide range of behavioral patterns.

Significance of Temperament

Observations indicate that children who display the difficult or slow-to-warm-up patterns are more vulnerable to behavior problems in early and middle childhood. However, any child can develop behavior problems if there is dissonance between the child's temperament and the environment. Demands for change and adaptation that are in conflict with children's capacities can become excessively stressful. However, authorities emphasize that it is not children's temperament patterns that place them at risk but the *degree of fit* between children and their environments, specifically their parents, that determines the degree of vulnerability. The greater the difference between the child's temperament and the ability of the parents to accept and deal with the behavior, the greater the likelihood of subsequent behavior problems. Since temperament is identified primarily by parental perceptions, a child described as difficult at one time may be perceived as easy at a later date (Wolk et al, 1992). (For example, see Failure to Thrive, Chapter 33.)

Child temperament appears to be a relevant factor in parental adjustment. Difficult child temperament has been directly related to maternal distress, discomfort in the role of parent, poor spousal relationships, and negative changes in way of life (Sheeber and Johnson, 1992).

Early identification of temperament provides a useful tool for caregivers in anticipating probable areas of difficulty or risk associated with development. For example, "difficult" children may be prone to colic in infancy, and active children require more vigilance to prevent injury. Also, school entry will require different approaches for children with different temperaments.

Several parental questionnaires have been devised to facilitate assessment of temperament. Nurses who use these assessment tools are better able to help parents interpret their child's behavior and to provide anticipatory guidance regarding numerous aspects of childrearing.

Development of Personality and Mental Function

Personality and cognitive skills develop in much the same manner as biologic growth—new accomplishments build on previously mastered skills. Many aspects depend on physical growth and maturation. This is not a comprehensive account of the multiple facets of personality and behavior development. Many aspects are integrated with the child's emotional and social development in a later discussion of various age groups. Table 30-3 summarizes some of the developmental theories.

THEORETIC FOUNDATIONS OF PERSONALITY DEVELOPMENT

Psychosexual Development (Freud)

Freud considered the sexual instincts to be significant in the development of the personality. However, he used the term **psychosexual** to describe any *sensual pleasure.* During childhood certain regions of the body assume a prominent psychologic significance as the source of new pleasures and new conflicts gradually shifts from one part of the body to another at particular stages of development:

Oral stage (birth to 1 year). During infancy the major source of pleasure seeking is centered on oral activities such as sucking, biting, chewing, and vocalizing. Children may prefer one of these over the others, and the

TABLE 30-3 Summary of personality, cognitive, and moral development theories

STAGE/AGE	PSYCHOSEXUAL STAGES (FREUD)	PSYCHOSOCIAL STAGES (ERIKSON)	COGNITIVE STAGES (PIAGET)	MORAL JUDGMENT STAGES (KOHLBERG)
Infancy Birth to 1 year	Oral-sensory	Trust vs. mistrust	Sensorimotor (birth to 2 years)	
Toddlerhood 1-3 years	Anal-urethral	Autonomy vs. shame and doubt	Preoperational thought, preconceptual phase (transductive reasoning, e.g., specific to specific) (2-4 years)	Preconventional (premoral) level Punishment and obedience orientation
Early childhood 3-6 years	Phallic-locomotion	Initiative vs. guilt	Preoperational thought, intuitive phase (transductive reasoning) (4-7 years)	Preconventional (premoral) level Naive instrumental orientation
Middle childhood 6-12 years	Latency	Industry vs. inferiority	Concrete operations (inductive reasoning and beginning logic) (7-11 years)	Conventional level Good-boy, nice-girl orientation Law-and-order orientation
Adolescence 12-18 years	Genitality	Identity and repudiation vs. identity confusion	Formal operations (deductive and abstract reasoning) (11-15 years)	Postconventional or principled level Social-contract orientation Universal ethical principle orientation (no longer included in revised theory)

preferred method of oral gratification can provide some indication of the personality they develop.

Anal stage (1 to 3 years). Interest during the second year of life centers in the anal region as sphincter muscles develop and children are able to withhold or expel fecal material at will. At this stage the climate surrounding toilet training can have lasting effects on children's personalities.

Phallic stage (3 to 6 years). During the phallic stage the genitals become an interesting and sensitive area of the body. Children recognize differences between the sexes and become curious about the dissimilarities. This is the period around which the controversial issues of the Oedipus and Electra complexes, penis envy, and castration anxiety are centered.

Latency period (6 to 12 years). During the latency period children elaborate on previously acquired traits and skills. Physical and psychic energy are channeled into acquisition of knowledge and vigorous play.

Genital stage (age 12 and over). The last significant stage begins at puberty with maturation of the reproductive system and production of sex hormones. The genital organs become the major source of sexual tensions and pleasures, but energies are also invested in forming friendships and preparation for marriage.

Psychosocial Development (Erikson)

The most widely accepted theory of personality development is that advanced by Erikson (1963). Although built on Freudian theory, it is known as **psychosocial development** and emphasizes a healthy personality as opposed to a pathologic approach. Erikson also uses the biologic concepts of critical periods and epigenesis, describing key conflicts or core problems that the individual strives to master during critical periods in personality development. Successful completion or mastery of each of these core conflicts is built on the satisfactory completion or mastery of the previous core.

Each psychosocial stage has two components—the favorable and the unfavorable aspects of the core conflict—and progress to the next stage depends on resolution of this conflict. No core conflict is ever mastered completely but remains a recurrent problem throughout life. No life situation is ever secure. Each new situation presents the conflict in a new form. For example, when children who have satisfactorily achieved a sense of trust encounter a new experience (e.g., hospitalization), they must again develop a sense of trust in those responsible for their care to master the situation. Erikson's life span approach to personality development consists of eight stages; however, only the first five relating to childhood are included here:

Trust vs. mistrust (birth to 1 year). The first and most important attribute to develop for a healthy personality is a basic *trust*. Establishment of basic trust dominates the first year of life and describes all the child's satisfying experiences at this age. Corresponding to Freud's oral stage, it is a time of "getting" and "taking in" through all the senses. It exists only in relation to something or someone; therefore consistent, loving care by a mothering person is essential to development of trust. *Mistrust* develops when trust-promoting experiences are deficient or lacking or when basic needs are inconsistently or inadequately met. Although shreds of mistrust are sprinkled throughout the personality, from a basic trust in parents stems trust in the world, other people, and oneself. The result is *faith* and *optimism*.

Autonomy vs. shame and doubt (1 to 3 years). Corresponding to Freud's anal stage, the problem of *autonomy* can be symbolized by the holding on and letting go of the sphincter muscles. The development of autonomy during the toddler period is centered around children's increasing ability to control their bodies, themselves, and their environment. They want to do things for themselves, using their newly acquired motor skills of walking, climbing, and manipulating and their mental powers of selection and decision making. Much of their learning is acquired through imitating the activities and behavior of others. Negative feelings of *doubt* and *shame* arise when children are made to feel small and self-conscious, when their choices are disastrous, when others shame them, or when they are forced to be dependent in areas in which they are capable of assuming control. The favorable outcomes are *self-control* and *willpower.*

Initiative vs. guilt (3 to 6 years). The stage of *initiative* corresponds to Freud's phallic stage and is characterized by vigorous, intrusive behavior, enterprise, and a strong imagination. Children explore the physical world with all their senses and powers. They develop a conscience. No longer guided only by outsiders, there is an inner voice that warns and threatens. Children sometimes undertake goals or activities that are in conflict with those of parents or others, and being made to feel that their activities or imaginings are bad produces a sense of *guilt.* Children must learn to retain a sense of initiative without impinging on the rights and privileges of others. The lasting outcomes are *direction* and *purpose.*

Industry vs. inferiority (6 to 12 years). The stage of *industry* is the latency period of Freud. Having achieved the more crucial stages in personality development, children are ready to be workers and producers. They want to engage in tasks and activities that they can carry through to completion; they need and want real achievement. Children learn to compete and cooperate with others, and they learn the rules. It is a decisive period in their social relationships with others. Feelings of *inadequacy* and *inferiority* may develop if too much is expected of them or if they believe they cannot measure up to the standards set for them by others. The ego quality developed from a sense of industry is *competence.*

Identity vs. role confusion (12 to 18 years). Corresponding to Freud's genital period, the development of *identity* is characterized by rapid and marked physical changes. Previous trust in their bodies is shaken, and children become overly preoccupied with the way they appear in the eyes of others as compared with their own self-concept. Adolescents struggle to fit the roles they have played and those they hope to play with the current roles and fashions adopted by their peers, to integrate their concepts and values with those of society, and to come to a decision regarding an occupation. Inability to solve the core conflict results in *role confusion.* The outcome of successful mastery is *devotion* and *fidelity* to others and to values and ideologies.

THEORETIC FOUNDATIONS OF MENTAL DEVELOPMENT

Cognitive Development (Piaget)

The term **cognition** refers to the process by which developing individuals become acquainted with the world and the objects it contains. Children are born with inherited potentials for intellectual growth, but they must develop into that potential through interaction with the environment.

Cognitive development consists of age-related changes that occur in mental activities. The best-known theory regarding children's thinking, and a more comprehensive developmental theory than those already described, was developed by the Swiss psychologist Jean Piaget (1969). According to Piaget, intelligence enables individuals to make adaptations to the environment that increase the probability of survival and to establish and maintain equilibrium with the environment through their behavior.

Piaget proposed three stages of reasoning: (1) intuitive, (2) concrete operational, and (3) formal operational. When they enter the stage of concrete logical thought at about age 7 years, children are able to make logical inferences, classify, and deal with quantitative relationships about concrete things. Not until adolescence are they able to reason abstractly with any degree of competence. Each stage is derived from and builds on the accomplishments of the previous stage in a continuous, orderly process. The course of intellectual development is both maturational and invariant and is divided into the following stages (ages are approximate):

Sensorimotor (birth to 2 years). The sensorimotor stage of intellectual development consists of six substages (see Cognitive Development [Piaget], Chapters 33 and 34) that are governed by sensations by which simple learning takes place. Children progress from reflex activity through simple repetitive behaviors to imitative behavior. They develop a sense of "cause and effect" as they direct behavior toward objects. Problem solving is primarily trial and error. They display a high level of curiosity, experimentation, and enjoyment of novelty and begin to develop a sense of self as they are able to differentiate themselves from their environment. They become aware that objects have *permanence*—that an object exists even though it is no longer visible. Toward the end of the sensorimotor period children begin to use language and representational thought.

Preoperational (2 to 7 years). The predominant characteristic of the preoperational stage of intellectual development is *egocentrism,* which in this sense does not mean selfishness or self-centeredness, but the inability to put oneself in the place of another. Children interpret objects and events, not in terms of general properties, but in terms of their relationships or their use to them. They are unable to see things from any perspective other than their own; they cannot see another's point of view, nor can they see any reason to do so (see Cognitive Development [Piaget], Chapter 35).

Preoperational thinking is concrete and tangible. Children cannot reason beyond the observable, and they lack the ability to make deductions or generalizations. Thought is dominated by what they see, hear, or otherwise experience. However, they are increasingly able to use language and symbols to represent objects in their environment. Through imaginative play, questioning, and other interacting, they begin to elaborate concepts and to make simple associations between ideas. In the latter stage of this period their reasoning is *intuitive* (e.g., the stars have to go to bed as they do), and they are only beginning to deal with problems of weight, length, size, and time. Reasoning is also *transductive*—because two events occur together, they cause each other, or knowledge of one characteristic is transferred to another (e.g., all women with big bellies have babies).

Concrete operations (7 to 11 years). At this age thought becomes increasingly logical and coherent. Children are able to classify, sort, order, and otherwise organize facts about the world to use in problem solving. They develop a new concept of permanence—*conservation* (see Cognitive Development [Piaget], Chapter 36). That is, they realize that physical factors such as volume, weight, and number remain the same, even though outward appearances are changed. They are able to deal with a number of different aspects of a situation simultaneously. They do not have the capacity to deal in abstraction; they solve problems in a concrete, systematic fashion based on what they can perceive. Reasoning is *inductive.* Through progressive changes in thought processes and relationships with others, thought becomes less self-centered. They can consider points of view other than their own. Thinking has become socialized.

Formal operations (11 to 15 years). Formal operational thought is characterized by adaptability and flexibility. Adolescents can think in abstract terms, use abstract symbols, and draw logical conclusions from a set of observations. For example, they can solve the question: if A > B and B > C, which symbol is the largest?; the answer is A. They can make hypotheses and test them; they can consider abstract, theoretic, and philosophic matters. Although they may confuse the ideal with the practical, most contradictions in the world can be dealt with and resolved.

Language Development

Children are born with the mechanism and capacity to develop speech and language skills. However, they will not speak spontaneously. The environment must provide a means for them to acquire these skills. Speech requires intact physiologic structure and function (including respiratory, auditory, and cerebral) plus intelligence, a need to communicate, and stimulation.

The rate of speech development varies from child to child and is directly related to neurologic competence and cognitive development. Gesture precedes speech, and in this way a small child communicates satisfactorily. As speech develops, gesture recedes but never disappears entirely. At all stages of language development, children's comprehension vocabulary (what they understand) is greater than their expressed vocabulary (what they can say), and this development reflects a continuing process of modification that involves both the acquisition of new words and the expanding and refining of word meanings previously learned. By the time they begin to walk, children are able to attach a name to objects and persons.

The first parts of speech used are nouns, sometimes verbs (e.g., "go"), and combination words (such as "bye-bye"). Responses are usually structurally incomplete during the toddler period, although the meaning is clear. Next adjectives and adverbs are used to qualify nouns, followed by adverbs to qualify nouns and verbs. Later, pronouns and gender words are added (such as "he" and "she"). By the time children enter school, they are able to use simple, structurally complete sentences that average five to seven words.

Moral Development (Kohlberg)

Children also acquire moral reasoning in a developmental sequence. Moral development, as described by Kohlberg (1968), is based on cognitive developmental theory and consists of the following three major levels, each of which has two stages:

Preconventional level. The preconventional level of moral development parallels the preoperational level of cognitive development and intuitive thought. Culturally oriented to the labels of good/bad and right/wrong, children integrate these in terms of the physical or pleasurable consequences of their actions. At first children determine the goodness or badness of an action in terms of its consequences. They avoid punishment and obey without question those who have the power to determine and enforce the rules and labels. They have no concept of the basic moral order that supports these consequences. Later children determine that the right behavior consists of that which satisfies their own needs (and sometimes the needs of others). Although elements of fairness, give and take, and equal sharing are evident, they are interpreted in a very practical, concrete manner with loyalty, gratitude, or justice.

Conventional level. At the conventional stage children are concerned with conformity and loyalty. They value the maintenance of family, group, or national expectations, regardless of consequences. Behavior that meets with approval and pleases or helps others is considered to be good. One earns approval by being "nice." Obeying the rules, doing one's duty, showing respect for authority, and maintaining the social order are the correct behaviors. This level is correlated with the stage of concrete operations in cognitive development.

Postconventional, autonomous, or principled level. At the postconventional level the individual has reached the cognitive stage of formal operations. Correct behavior tends to be defined in terms of general individual rights and standards that have been examined and agreed on by the entire society. Although procedural rules for reaching consensus become important with emphasis on the legal point of view, there is also emphasis on the possibility for changing law in terms of societal needs and rational considerations.

The most advanced level of moral development is one in which self-chosen ethical principles guide decisions of conscience. These are abstract and ethical but universal principles of justice and human rights with respect for the dignity of persons as individuals. It is believed that few persons reach this stage of moral reasoning.

Spiritual Development

Spiritual beliefs are closely related to the moral and ethical portion of the child's self-concept and, as such, must be considered as part of the child's basic needs assessment. Children need to have meaning, purpose, and hope in their lives. Also, the need for confession and forgiveness is present, even in very young children. Extending beyond religion (an organized set of beliefs and practices), spirituality affects the whole person: mind, body, and spirit (Clutter, 1991). Fowler (1974) has identified seven stages in the development of faith, four of which are closely associated with and parallel cognitive and psychosocial development in childhood:

Stage 0: Undifferentiated. This stage of development encompasses the period of infancy during which children have no concept of right or wrong, no beliefs, and no convictions to guide their behavior. However, the beginnings of a faith are established with the development of basic trust through their relationships with the primary caregiver.

Stage 1: Intuitive-projective. Toddlerhood is primarily a time of imitating the behavior of others. Children imitate the religious gestures and behaviors of others without comprehending any meaning or significance to the activities. During the preschool years children assimilate some of the values and beliefs of their parents. Parental attitudes toward moral codes and religious beliefs convey to children what they consider to be good and bad. Children still imitate behavior at this age and follow parental beliefs as part of their daily lives rather than through an understanding of their basic concepts.

Stage 2: Mythical-literal. Through the school-age years, spiritual development parallels cognitive development and is closely related to children's experiences and social interaction. Most have a strong interest in religion during the school-age years. The existence of a deity is accepted, and petitions to an omnipotent being are important and expected to be answered; good behavior is rewarded, and bad behavior is punished. Their developing conscience bothers them when they disobey. They have a reverence for thoughts and matters and are able to articulate their faith. They may even question its validity.

Stage 3: Synthetic-convention. As children approach adolescence, however, they become increasingly aware of spiritual disappointments. They recognize that prayers are not always answered (at least on their own terms) and may begin to abandon or modify some religious practices. They begin to reason, to question some of the established parental religious standards, and to drop or modify some religious practices.

Stage 4: Individuating-reflexive. Adolescents become more skeptical and begin to compare the religious standards of their parents with those of others. They attempt to determine which to adopt and incorporate into their own set of values. They also begin to compare religious standards with the scientific viewpoint. It is a time of searching rather than reaching. Adolescents are uncertain about many religious ideas but will not achieve profound insights until late adolescence or early adulthood.

DEVELOPMENT OF SELF-CONCEPT

The term **self-concept** includes all the notions, beliefs, and convictions that constitute an individual's self-knowledge and that influence that individual's relationships with others. It is not present at birth but develops gradually as a result of unique experiences within the self, with significant others, and with the realities of the world. However, an individual's self-concept may or may not reflect reality.

In infancy the self-concept is primarily an awareness of one's independent existence learned in part as a result of social contacts and experiences with others. The process becomes more active during toddlerhood as children explore the limits of their capacities and the nature of their impact on others. School-age children are more aware of differences among people, are more sensitive to social pressures, and become more preoccupied with issues of self-criticism and self-evaluation. During early adolescence children focus more on physical and emotional changes taking place and on peer acceptance. The self-concept is crystallized during later adolescence as young people organize their self-concept around a set of values, goals, and competencies acquired throughout childhood.

Body Image

A vital component of self-concept, **body image** refers to the subjective concepts and attitudes that individuals have toward their own bodies. It consists of the physiologic (the perception of one's physical characteristics), psychologic (values and attitudes toward the body, abilities, and ideals), and social nature of one's image of self (the self in relation to others). All three of the components interrelate with each other. Body image is a complex phenomenon that evolves and changes during the process of growth and development. Any actual or perceived deviation from the "norm" (no matter how this is interpreted) is cause for concern. The extent to which a characteristic, defect, or disease affects children's body image is influenced by the attitudes and behavior of those around them.

The significant others in their lives exert the most important and meaningful impact on children's body image. Labels that are attached to them (such as "skinny," "pretty," or "fat") or body parts (such as "ugly mole," "bug eyes," or "yucky skin") are incorporated into the body image. Because they lack the understanding of deviations from the physical standard or norm, children notice prominent differences in others and unwittingly make "rude" and often cruel remarks about such minor deviations as large or widely spaced front teeth, large or small eyes, moles, or extreme variations in height.

Infants receive input about their bodies through self-exploration and sensory stimulation from others. As they begin to manipulate their environment, they become aware of their bodies as separate from others. Toddlers learn to identify the various parts of their bodies and are able to use symbols to represent objects. Preschoolers become aware of the wholeness of their bodies and discover the genitals. Exploration of the genitals and the discovery of differences between the sexes become important. There is only a vague concept of internal organs and function (Selekman, 1983).

School-age children begin to learn about internal body structure and function and become aware of differences in body size and configuration. They are highly influenced by the cultural norms of society and current fads. Children whose bodies deviate from the norm are often criticized or ridiculed.

Adolescence is the age when children become most concerned about the physical self. The familiar body changes and the new physical self must be integrated into the self-concept. Adolescents face conflicts over what they see and what they visualize as the ideal body structure. Body image formation during adolescence is a crucial element in the shaping of identity, the psychosocial crisis of adolescence.

Self-Esteem

The term **self-esteem** refers to a personal, subjective judgment of one's worthiness derived from and influenced by the social groups in the immediate environment and individuals' perceptions of how they are valued by others. Self-esteem changes with development. Highly egocentric toddlers are unaware of any difference between competence and social approval. Preschool and early school-age children, on the other hand, are increasingly aware of the discrepancy between their competencies and the abilities of more advanced children. The acceptance of adults and peers outside the family group becomes more important to them. Positive feedback enhances their self-esteem; they are vulnerable to feelings of worthlessness and are anxious about failure.

As children's competencies increase and they develop meaningful relationships, their self-esteem rises. Their self-esteem is again at risk during early adolescence when they are defining an identity and sense of self in the context of their peer group. Unless children are continually made to feel incompetent and of little worth, a decrease in self-esteem during vulnerable times is only temporary. Children assess the following aspects of themselves in forming an overall evaluation of their self-esteem (Sieving and Zirbel-Donisch, 1990):

Competence: How adequate are my cognitive, physical, and social skills?
Sense of control: How well can I complete tasks needed to produce desired actions? Is someone or something specific vs. luck or chance responsible for my successes and failures?
Moral worth: How closely do my actions and behaviors meet moral standards that have been set?
Worthiness of love and acceptance: How worthy am I of love and acceptance from parents, other significant adults, siblings, and peers?

Factors that influence the formation of a child's self-esteem include (1) the child's temperament and personality, (2) abilities and opportunities available to accomplish age-appropriate developmental tasks, (3) significant others, and (4) social roles assumed and the expectations of these roles (see also Psychosocial History, Chapter 31).

Role of Play in Development

Through the universal medium of **play** children learn what no one can teach them. They learn about their world and how to deal with this environment of objects, time, space, structure, and people. They learn about themselves operating within that environment—what they can do, how to relate to things and situations, and how to adapt themselves to the demands society makes on them. Play is the *work* of the child. In play children continually practice the complicated, stressful processes of living, communicating, and achieving satisfactory relationships with other people.

CLASSIFICATION OF PLAY

From a developmental point of view, patterns of children's play can be categorized according to content and social character. In both there is an additive effect; each builds on past accomplishments, and some element of each is maintained throughout life. At each stage in development the new predominates.

Content of Play

The content of play involves primarily the physical aspects of play, although social relationships cannot be ignored. The content of play follows the directional trend of the simple to the complex:

Social-affective play. Play begins with social-affective play, wherein infants take pleasure in relationships with people. As adults talk, touch, nuzzle, and in various ways elicit a response from an infant, the infant soon learns to provoke parental emotions and responses with such behaviors as smiling, cooing, or initiating games and activities. The type and intensity of the adult behavior with children vary among cultures.
Sense-pleasure play. Sense-pleasure play is a nonsocial stimulating experience that originates from without. Objects in the environment—light and color, tastes and odors, textures and consistencies—attract children's attention, stimulate their senses, and give pleasure. Pleasurable experiences are derived from handling raw materials (water, sand, food), from body motion (swinging, bouncing, rocking), and from other uses of senses and abilities (smelling, humming) (Fig. 30-4).
Skill play. Once infants have developed the ability to grasp and manipulate, they persistently demonstrate and exercise their newly acquired abilities through skill play, repeating an action over and over again. The element of sense-pleasure play is often evident in the practicing of a new ability, but all too frequently the determination to conquer the elusive skill produces pain and frustration (e.g., learning to ride a bicycle).
Unoccupied behavior. In unoccupied behavior children are not playful but focus their attention momentarily on anything that strikes their interest. Children day-

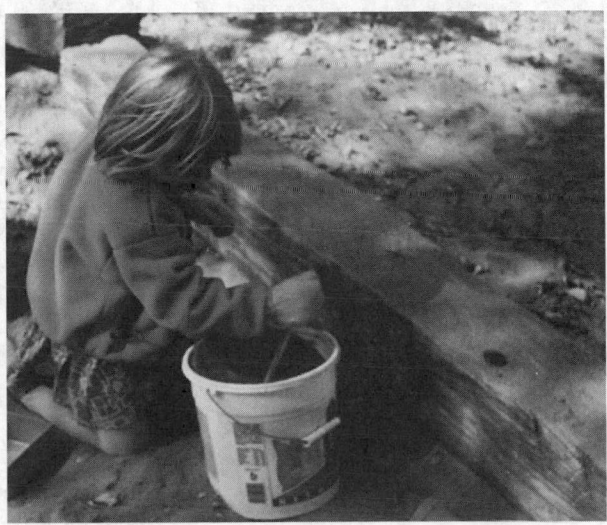

Fig. 30-4 Children derive pleasure from handling raw materials.

dream, fiddle with clothes or other objects, or walk aimlessly. This role differs from that of onlookers, who actively observe the activity of others.

Dramatic, or pretend, play. One of the vital elements in children's process of identification is dramatic play, also known as symbolic or pretend play. It begins in late infancy (11 to 13 months) and is the predominant form of play in the preschool child. Once children begin to invest situations and people with meanings and to attribute affective significance to the world, they can pretend and fantasize almost anything. By acting out events of daily life, children learn and practice the roles and identities modeled by the members of their family and society. Children's toys, replicas of the tools of society, provide a medium for learning about adult roles and activities that may be puzzling and frustrating to them. Interacting with the world is one way children get to know it. The simple, imitative, dramatic play of the toddler such as using the telephone, driving a car, or rocking a doll evolves into more complex, sustained dramas of the preschooler, which extend beyond common domestic matters to the wider aspects of the world and the society such as playing police officer, storekeeper, teacher, or nurse. Older children work out elaborate themes, act out stories, and compose plays (Fig. 30-5).

Games. Children in all cultures engage in games alone and with others. Solitary activity involving games begins as very small children participate in repetitive activities and progress to more complicated games that challenge their independent skills, such as solving puzzles, solitaire, and computer or video games. Very young children participate in simple *imitative games,* such as pat-a-cake and peekaboo. Preschool children learn and enjoy *formal games* that begin with ritualistic, self-sustaining games such as ring-around-a-rosy and London Bridge. With the exception of some simple board games, preschool children do not engage in *competitive games.* Preschoolers hate to lose and will try to cheat, want to change rules, or demand exceptions and opportunities to change their moves. School-age children and adolescents enjoy competitive games, including cards, checkers, chess, and physically active games such as baseball.

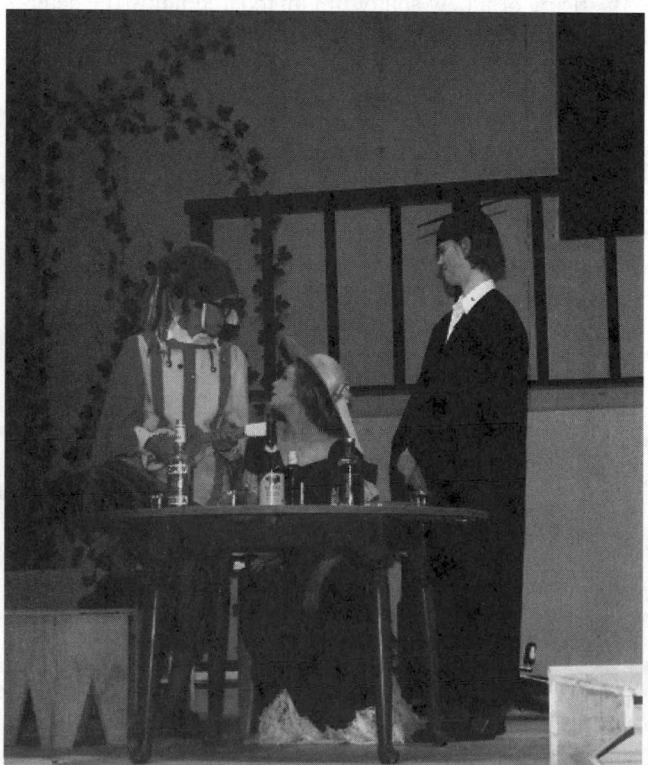

Fig. 30-5 Older children enjoy being in plays.

Social Character of Play

The play interactions of infancy are between the child and an adult. Children continue to enjoy the company of an adult but are increasingly able to play alone. As age advances, interaction with age-mates increases in importance and becomes an essential part of the socialization process. Through interaction, highly egocentric infants, unable to tolerate delay or interference, ultimately acquire concern for others and the ability to delay gratification or even to reject gratification at the expense of another. A pair of toddlers engage in considerable combat because their personal needs cannot tolerate delay or compromise. By the time they reach age 5 or 6 years, children are able to arrive at a compromise or make use of arbitration, usually after they have attempted but failed to gain their own way. Through continued interaction with peers and the growth of conceptual abilities and social skills, children are able to increase participation with others in the following types of play:

Onlooker play. During onlooker play children watch what other children are doing but make no attempt to enter into the play activity. There is an active interest in observing the interaction of others but no movement toward participating. Watching an older sibling bounce a ball is a common example of the onlooker role.

Solitary play. During solitary play children play alone with toys different from those used by other children in the same area. They enjoy the presence of other children but make no effort to get close to or speak to them. Their interest is centered on their own activity, which they pursue with no reference to the activities of the others.

Parallel play. During parallel activities children play independently but among other children. They play with toys like those the children around them are using, but as each child sees fit, neither influencing nor being influenced by the other children. Each plays beside, but not with, other children (Fig. 30-6). There is no group association. Parallel play is the characteristic play of toddlers, but it may also occur in other groups of any age. Individuals who are involved in a creative craft with each person separately working on an individual project are engaged in parallel play.

Associative play. In associative play children play together and are engaged in a similar or even identical activity, but there is no organization, division of labor,

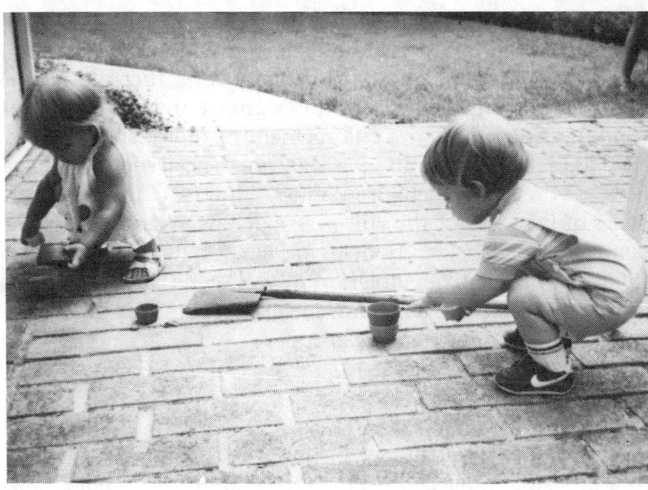

Fig. 30-6 Parallel play.

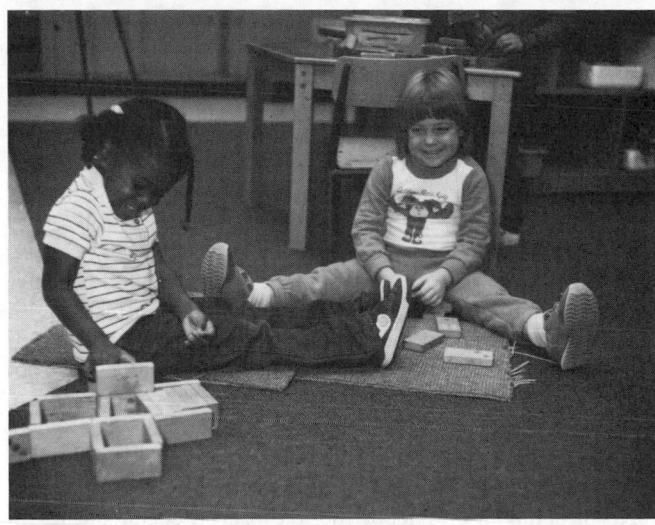

Fig. 30-7 Associative play.

leadership assignment, or mutual goal. Children borrow and lend play materials, follow each other with wagons and tricycles, and sometimes attempt to control who may or may not play in the group. Each child acts according to his or her own wishes; there is no group goal (Fig. 30-7). For example, two children play with dolls, borrowing articles of clothing from each other and engaging in similar conversation, but neither directs the other's actions or establishes rules regarding the limits of the play session. There is a great deal of behavioral contagion: when one child initiates an activity, the entire group follows the example.

Cooperative play. Cooperative play is organized, and children play in a group *with* other children (Fig. 30-8). They discuss and plan activities for the purposes of accomplishing an end—to make something, to attain a competitive goal, to dramatize situations of adult or group life, or to play formal games. The group is loosely formed, but there is a marked sense of belonging or not belonging. The goal and its attainment require organization of activities, division of labor, and playing roles. The leader-follower relationship is definitely established, and the activity is controlled by one or two members who assign roles and direct the activity of the others. The activity is organized to allow one child to supplement another's function in order to complete the goal.

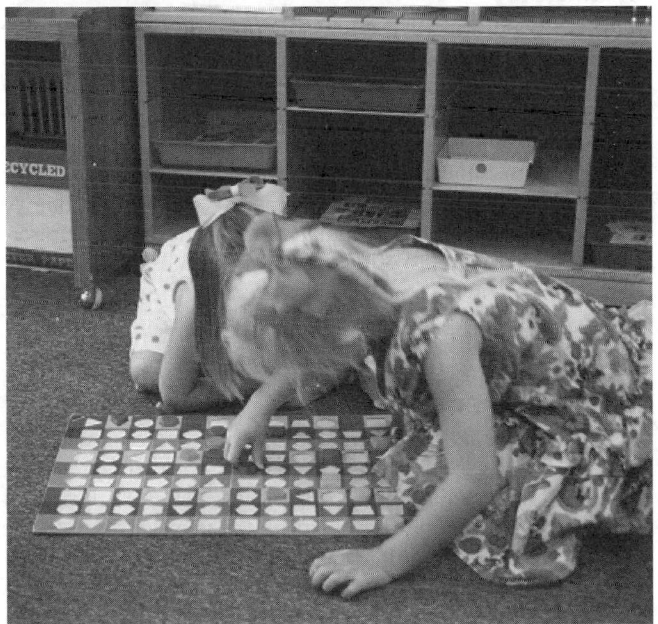

Fig. 30-8 Cooperative play.

FUNCTIONS OF PLAY

Sensorimotor Development

Sensorimotor activity is a major component of play at all ages and is the predominant form of play in infancy. Active play is essential for muscle development and serves a useful purpose as a release for surplus energy. Through sensorimotor play children explore the nature of the physical world. Infants gain impressions of themselves and their world through tactile, auditory, visual, and kinesthetic stimulation. Toddlers and preschoolers revel in body movement and exploration of things in space. With increasing maturity sensorimotor play becomes more differentiated and involved. Whereas very young children run for the sheer joy of body movement, older children incorporate or modify the motions into increasingly complex and coordinated activities such as races, games, skating, and bicycle riding.

Intellectual Development

Through exploration and manipulation children learn colors, shapes, sizes, textures, and the significance of objects. They learn the significance of numbers and how to use them; they learn to associate words with objects; and they develop an understanding of abstract concepts and spatial relationships such as *up, down, under,* and *over.* Activities such as puzzles and games help them develop problem-solving skills. Books, stories, films, and collections expand knowledge and provide enjoyment as well. Play provides a means to practice and expand language skills. Through play children continually rehearse past experiences to assimilate them into new perceptions and relationships. Play helps children comprehend the world in which they live and distinguish between fantasy and reality.

Socalization

From very early infancy children show interest and pleasure in the company of others. Their initial social contact is with the mothering person, but through play with other children they learn to establish social relationships and solve the problems associated with these relationships. They learn to give and take, which is more readily learned from critical peers than from the more tolerant adults. They learn the sex role that society expects them to fulfill, as well as approved patterns of behavior and deportment. Closely associated with socialization is development of moral values and ethics. Children learn right from wrong, the standards of the society, and to assume responsibility for their actions.

Creativity

In no other situation is there more opportunity to be creative than in play. Children can experiment and try out their ideas in play through every medium at their disposal, including raw materials, fantasy, and exploration. Creativity is stifled by pressure toward conformity; therefore striving for peer approval may inhibit creative endeavors in the school-age or adolescent child. Creativity is primarily a product of solitary activity; yet creative thinking is often enhanced in group settings where listening to others' ideas stimulates further exploration of one's own ideas. Once children feel the satisfaction of creating something new and different, they transfer this creative interest to situations outside the world of play.

Self-Awareness

Beginning with active explorations of their bodies and awareness of themselves as separate from the mother, the process of self-identity is facilitated through play activities. Children learn who they are and their place in the world. They become increasingly able to regulate their own behavior, to learn what their abilities are, and to compare their abilities with those of others. Through play children are able to test their abilities, to assume and try out various roles, and to learn the effect their behavior has on others.

Therapeutic Value

Play is therapeutic at any age. It provides a means for release from the tension and stress encountered in the environment. In play children can express emotions and release unacceptable impulses in a socially acceptable fashion. Children are able to experiment and test fearful situations and can assume and vicariously master the roles and positions that they are unable to perform in the world of reality. Children reveal much about themselves in play. Through play children are able to communicate to the alert observer the needs, fears, and desires that they are unable to express with their limited language skills. Throughout their play children need the acceptance of adults and their presence to help them control aggression and to channel their destructive tendencies.

Moral Value

Although children learn at home and at school the behaviors considered right and wrong in the culture, the interaction with peers during play contributes significantly to their moral training. Nowhere is the enforcement of moral standards so rigid as in the play situation. If they are to be acceptable members of the group, children must adhere to the accepted codes of behavior of the culture—e.g., fairness, honesty, self-control, and consideration for others. Children soon learn that their peers are less tolerant of violations than are adults and that to maintain a place in the play group, they must conform to the standards of the group.

TOYS

The type of toys chosen by and/or provided for children can facilitate their development in the areas just described. Toys that are small replicas of the culture and its tools help them assimilate their culture. Toys that require pushing, pulling, rolling, and manipulating teach them about physical properties of the items and help to develop muscles and coordination. Rules and the basic elements of cooperation and organization are learned through board games.

Because they can be used in a variety of ways, raw materials with which children can use their own creativity and imaginations are sometimes superior to ready-made items. For example, building blocks can be used to construct a variety of things, to count, and to learn shapes and sizes.

Toy Safety

Selection of toys and play equipment is a joint effort between parents and children, but evaluation of their safety is the responsibility of the adult. Government agencies do not inspect and police all toys on the market. Therefore adults who purchase, supervise purchases, or allow children to use play equipment need to evaluate such equipment for its safety, including toys that are gifts or those that are purchased by the children themselves (see the Home Care box on p. 859). They should also be alert to notices of toys determined to be defective and recalled by the manufacturers. Parents and health workers can obtain information on a variety of recalled products and can report potentially dangerous toys and child products to the U.S. Consumer Product Safety Commission (CPSC)* or, in Canada, the Canadian Toy Testing Council.†

Selected Factors that Influence Development

HEREDITY

Inherited characteristics have a profound influence on development. The sex of the child, determined by random selection at the time of conception, directs both the pattern of growth and the behavior of others toward the child. In all cultures, attitudes and expectations are different with respect to the sex of

*CPSC hotline: (800) 638-CPSC.

†22 Hamilton Ave. North, Ottawa, Ontario, Canada K1Y 1V6; (613) 729-7101.

Home Care

TOY SAFETY*

Selection

Select toys that suit the skills, abilities, and interests of children.

Select toys that are safe for the specific child; look for a label that indicates the intended age group. Toys that are safe for one age may not be safe for another.

- For infants, toddlers, and all children who still mouth objects, avoid toys with small parts that may pose a fatal choking or aspiration hazard. Toys in this category are usually labeled: "Not recommended for children under 3 years."
- For infants avoid toys with strings or cords that are 7 inches or longer, since they may cause strangulation.
- For all children under 8 years, avoid electric toys with heating elements.
- For children under 5 years, avoid arrows or darts.

Check for safety labels such as "flame retardant" or "flame resistant."

Select toys durable enough to survive rough play; look for sturdy construction such as tightly secured eyes, nose, or small parts.

Select toys light enough that they will not cause harm if one falls on a child.

Look for toys with smooth, rounded edges. Avoid toys with sharp edges that can cut or that have sharp points. Points on the inside of the toy can puncture if the toy is broken.

Avoid toys with any shooting or throwing objects that can injure eyes.

- This includes toys in which other missiles, such as sticks or pebbles, might be used as substitutes for the intended projectiles.
- Arrows and darts used by children should have blunt tips and be manufactured from resilient materials; make certain tips are securely attached.

Make certain that materials in toys are nontoxic.

Avoid toys that make loud noises that might be damaging to a child's hearing.

- Even some squeaking toys are too loud when held close to the ear.
- If selecting caps for cap guns, look for the label required by Federal law to be on boxes or packages of caps that states: "Warning—Do not fire closer than 1 foot to the ear. Do not use indoors."

Make certain that arrows or darts have soft tips, rubber suction cups, or other protective tips. Check to be certain that tips are secure.

If selecting a toy gun, be certain that the barrel or the entire gun is brightly colored to avoid being mistaken as a real gun.

Check toy instructions for clarity. They should be clear to an adult and, when appropriate, to the child.

Supervision

Maintain a safe play environment.

- Remove and discard plastic wrappings on toys immediately; they could suffocate a child.
- Remove large toys, bumper pads, and boxes from playpens; an adventuresome child can use such items as a means of climbing or falling out.

Set "ground rules" for play.

Supervise young children closely during play.

Teach children how to use toys properly and safely.

Instruct older children to keep their toys away from younger brothers, sisters, and friends.

Keep children who are playing with riding toys away from stairs, hills, traffic, and swimming pools.

Establish and enforce rules regarding protective gear.

- Insist that children wear helmets when using bicycles, skateboards, or in-line skates.
- Insist that children wear gloves and wrist, elbow, and knee pads when using skateboards or in-line skates.

Instruct children on electrical safety.

- Teach children the proper way to unplug an electric toy—pull on the plug, not the cord.
- Teach children to beware of electrical appliances and even electrically operated playthings; frequently children are unfamiliar with the hazards of electricity in association with water.

Teach children the safe use of utensils that under certain circumstances can cause injury—scissors, knives, needles, heating elements, or loops, long string, or cord.

Maintenance

Inspect old and new toys regularly for breakage, loose parts, and other potential hazards.

- Look for jagged or sharp edges or broken parts that might constitute a choking hazard.
- Check movable parts to make certain they are attached securely to the toys; sometimes pieces that are safe when attached to the toy become a danger when detached.
- Examine all outdoor toys regularly for rust and weak or sharp parts that could become a danger to a child.
- Check electrical cords and plugs for cracked or fraying parts.

Maintain toys in good repair, without signs of possible hazards such as sharp edges, splinters, weak seams, or rust.

- Make repairs immediately, or discard out of reach of children.
- Sand sharp wooden toys or splintered surfaces smooth.
- Use only paint labeled "nontoxic" to repaint toys, toy boxes, or children's furniture.

Storage

Provide a safe place for children to store toys.

Select a toy chest or toy box that is ventilated, is free of self-locking devices that could trap a child inside, and has a lid designed not to pinch a child's fingers or fall on a child's head.

If containers other than toy chests are used for storage purposes, they should be fitted with spring-loaded support devices if they have a hinged lid to avoid entrapment and suffocation.

Teach children to store toys safely in order to prevent accidental injury from stepping, tripping, or falling on a toy.

Playthings meant for older children and adults should be safely stowed away on high shelves, in locked closets, or in other areas unavailable to younger children.

*Another helpful resource is *Toy Safety: Guidelines for Parents* from American Academy of Pediatrics, Division of Publications, 141 Northwest Point Blvd, P.O. Box 927, Elk Grove Village, IL 60009-0927; (800) 433-9016.

the child. Sex plus other hereditary determinants strongly affects the end result of growth and the rate of progress toward it. There is a high correlation between parent and child with regard to traits such as height, weight, and rate of growth. Most physical characteristics, including shape and form of features, body build, and physical peculiarities, are inherited and can influence the way in which children grow and interact with their environment. Many dimensions of personality, such as temperament, activity level, responsiveness, and a tendency toward shyness, are believed to be inherited.

Differences in health and vigor of children may be attributed to hereditary traits. An inherited physical or mental disorder will alter or modify a child's physical and/or emotional growth and interactions. The extent to which disabling conditions interfere with the child's growth and well-being is considered in relation to numerous disabilities throughout the remainder of the book.

NEUROENDOCRINE FACTORS

It has been suggested there may be a growth center in the hypothalamic region responsible for maintaining genetically determined growth patterns. Some functional relationship is believed to exist between the hypothalamus and the endocrine system that influences growth. There is also evidence, based on observations of denervated skeletal muscles, that the peripheral nervous system may influence growth, because muscles deprived of nerve supply degenerate. Many of these effects are not sufficiently explained by disuse or diminished blood supply.

Probably all hormones affect growth in some fashion. Three hormones—growth hormone, thyroid hormone, and androgens—when given to persons deficient in these hormones, stimulate protein anabolism and thereby produce retention of elements essential for building protoplasm and bony tissue. It appears that each of the hormones that has a significant influence on growth manifests its major effect at a different period of growth (see Chapter 49).

NUTRITION

Nutrition is probably the single most important influence on growth. Dietary factors regulate growth at all stages of development, and their effects are exerted in numerous and complex ways. During the rapid prenatal growth period, faulty nutrition may influence development from the time of implantation of the ovum until birth. During infancy and childhood the demand for calories is relatively great, as evidenced by the rapid increase in both height and weight. At this time protein and caloric requirements are higher than at almost any period of postnatal development. As the growth rate slows with its concomitant decrease in metabolism, there is a corresponding reduction in caloric and protein requirements (Table 30-2).

Growth is uneven during the periods of childhood between infancy and adolescence when there are plateaus and small growth spurts. The child's appetite will fluctuate in response to these variations until the turbulent growth spurt of adolescence, when adequate nutrition is extremely important but may be subjected to numerous emotional influences. Adequate nutrition is closely related to good health throughout life, and an overall improvement in nourishment is evidenced by the gradual increase in size and early maturation of children in this century.

INTERPERSONAL RELATIONSHIPS

Relationships with significant others play a critical role in development, particularly in emotional, intellectual, and personality development. Not only do the quality and quantity of contacts with other persons exert an influence on the growing child, but the widening range of contacts is essential to learning and the development of a healthy personality.

The mothering person is unquestionably the single most influential person during early infancy. This person is the one who meets the infant's basic needs of food, warmth, comfort, and love. He or she provides stimulation for the child's senses and facilitates his or her expanding capacities. Through this person, the child learns to trust the world and feel secure to venture in increasingly wider relationships.

It is generally the parents who are most influential in helping the child to assume sex-role identification. Parents define and reinforce acceptable sex-role behavior and provide sex-appropriate role models for the child. In the absence of a sex-role model in the family setting, the child may adopt some characteristics of the opposite-sex parent or sibling. Frequently the child identifies with a teacher or other significant person of the same sex.

Siblings are children's first peers, and the way in which they learn to relate to each other affects later interactions with peers outside the family group. The sphere of persons from whom children seek approval widens to include other members of their family, their peers, and, to a lesser extent, other authority figures (e.g., teachers). The increasing importance of the peer group in determining the behavior of school-age children and adolescents is well documented (Fig. 30-9).

When children fail to have quality interpersonal relationships with "mothering" persons, they experience **emotional**

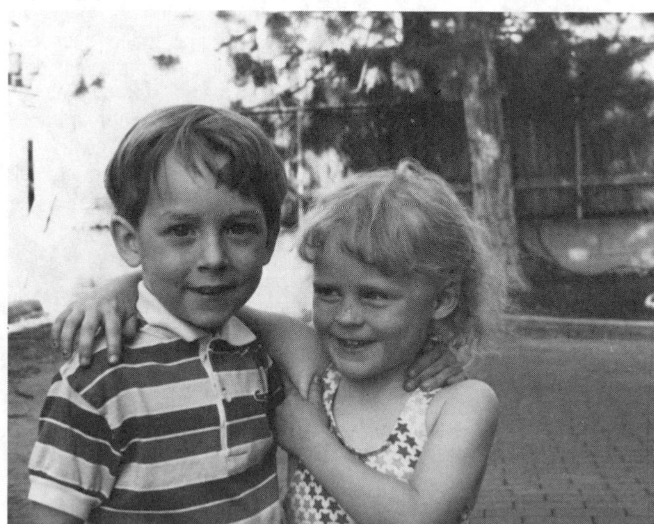

Fig. 30-9 Peers become increasingly important as children develop friendships outside the family group.

deprivation. The most prominent feature of emotional deprivation, particularly during the first year, is developmental retardation. Much of the information regarding the adverse effects of interpersonal influences on development has been acquired through retrospective studies of gross deprivation and trauma. The most notable instances involved homeless infants who were placed in institutions for care. Those infants, who did not receive consistent mothering care, failed to gain weight even with an adequate diet; were pale, listless, and immobile; and were unresponsive to stimuli that usually elicit a response such as smiling or cooing in the normal infant. If emotional deprivation continues for a sufficient length of time, the child may not survive infancy.

Although the most remarkable examples of emotional deprivation were first recognized among infants in institutions, the term *masked deprivation* has been used to describe children reared in homes where there is a distorted parent-child relationship or otherwise disordered home environment. Infants do not thrive if the caregiving person is hostile, fearful of handling them, or indifferent to them and their needs. Such children exhibit poor growth, even though they are apparently free of physical disease. Growth retardation in these children is believed to be caused by a psychologically induced endocrine imbalance that interferes with growth. These same infants and children display "catch-up" growth in a changed environment. (See Failure to Thrive, Chapter 33.)

SOCIOECONOMIC LEVEL

Evidence indicates that the socioeconomic level of children's families has a significant impact on growth and development. At all ages children from upper- and middle-class families are taller than comparative children of families in the lower socioeconomic strata.

The cause of these differences is less definite, although the poorer health and nutrition of lower socioeconomic levels are probably significant factors. Nutritious food sources (especially proteins) are scarce, and other factors (e.g., larger family size and regularity in eating, sleeping, and exercise) may play a role.

Families from lower socioeconomic groups may lack the knowledge or resources needed to provide the safe, stimulating, and enriched environment that fosters optimum development for children. They may be unable to move from unsafe neighborhoods where drug traffic and drive-by shootings are the norm. The effects on the emotional development of children living under these conditions have been compared with those experienced by children living in war zones.

DISEASE

Altered growth and development is one of the clinical manifestations in a number of hereditary disorders. Growth impairment is particularly marked in skeletal disorders, such as the various forms of dwarfism and at least one of the chromosomal anomalies (Turner syndrome). Many of the disorders of metabolism, such as vitamin D–resistant rickets, the mucopolysaccharidoses, and the numerous endocrine disorders, interfere with the normal growth pattern. In other disorders the tendency is toward the upper percentile of height (e.g., Klinefelter syndrome and Marfan syndrome).

Many chronic illnesses that are associated with varying degrees of growth failure are congenital cardiac anomalies and respiratory disorders such as cystic fibrosis. Any disorder characterized by the inability to digest and absorb body nutrients will have an adverse effect on growth and development.

ENVIRONMENTAL HAZARDS

Hazards in the environment are a source of concern to health care providers and others interested in health and safety. Physical injuries are the most prevalent consequences of environmental dangers, and these are discussed extensively throughout the book as they apply in relation to age, specific hazards, and selected physical disabilities.

The harmful agents most often associated with health risks are chemicals and radiation. Water, air, and food contamination from a variety of origins is well documented. Significant sources of exposure are substances in the immediate environment such as lead and asbestos, chemicals secreted in breast milk (especially prescribed drugs and nicotine), and contamination within well-insulated homes (especially from disinfectants or burning of substances that produce toxic fumes). Passive inhalation of tobacco smoke by infants and children is a hazard at all stages of development. The harmful effects of large doses of radiation are unquestioned, although the effects of low-dose or short-term radiation are debatable, as are the safe vs. harmful dosage levels.

STRESS IN CHILDHOOD

Defined from both a physiologic and an emotional point of view, essentially **stress** is "an imbalance between environmental demands and a person's coping resources that . . . disrupts the equilibrium of the person" (Masten et al, 1988).

Although all children experience stress, some youngsters appear to be more vulnerable than others. Children's age, temperament, life situation, and state of health affect their vulnerability, reactions, and ability to handle stress. Also, the responses to a stressor can be behavioral, psychologic, or physiologic. It is impossible, unrealistic, and undesirable to protect children from stress, but providing them with interpersonal security helps them develop coping strategies for dealing with stress. The concept of an *emotional bank,* in which deposits, as well as withdrawals, can be made can help parents and caregivers maintain a proper perspective regarding the effects of stress and coping (Usdin, 1988). Children with a positive balance in the account can tolerate significant withdrawal experiences. For children with a low balance, even a minor withdrawal may bankrupt the account, causing it to be overdrawn.

Parents and other caregivers can try to recognize signs of stress in order to help children deal with stresses before they become overwhelming. Signs of stress take many forms but are typically the same ones seen in children who are abused (see Chapter 35) or depressed (see Chapter 36). If a number of stresses are imposed on children at the same time, the children are more vulnerable. When a succession of stresses produces an excessive stress load, children may experience a serious change in health and/or behavior.

It is most important that parents and persons working with children understand the nature of childhood stress and ways it can be recognized or anticipated. Caregivers must *listen* to children so they are aware of children's fears and concerns and let them know that they are important and that what they say matters. Physical contact is comforting and reassuring to children. Simply holding, touching, or hugging children is both relaxing and comforting and facilitates communication. Spending unhurried time with children, sharing family outings and vacations, and exposing children to positive influences help build children's strengths and security. Solid supportive interpersonal relationships are essential to the psychologic well-being of children.

Coping

Coping refers to a special class of individual reactions to stressors—specifically, a reaction to a stressor that resolves, reduces, or replaces the affect state classified as stressful. Children, like adults, respond to everyday stress by trying to change the circumstances or to adjust to circumstances the way they are. **Coping strategies** are the specific ways in which children cope with stressors, as distinguished from **coping styles,** which are relatively unchanging personality characteristics or outcomes of coping (Ryan-Wenger, 1992). Any strategy that provides relaxation is effective in reducing stress, and most children have their own natural methods, such as withdrawal, physical activity, reading, listening to music, working on a project, or taking a nap. Some turn to parents to resolve their problems, or they may develop socially unacceptable strategies such as cheating, stealing, or lying.

Children can be taught stress-reduction techniques to use in coping. First, they must be helped to recognize signs of tension in themselves and then taught any of a variety of appropriate strategies—special exercises, relaxation and breathing, mental imagery, and numerous other simple activities. Also, parents and other caregivers can anticipate possible stress-provoking events and prepare children for coping by role playing a scenario or "talking it through" beforehand. Most of the stress-reducing strategies discussed in Chapter 41 in relation to managing pain are effective for any stress situation.

Probably the most useful tool that children can learn is how to solve problems. When children can view any new situation as a problem to be solved and an opportunity to learn, they are not vulnerable to the control of others. It provides them with a sense of mastery over their own lives and reinforces the fact that they have within themselves the ability and information to handle whatever comes their way. Problem-solving skill gives them the confidence to know where and how to seek help when they need it.

INFLUENCE OF THE MASS MEDIA

Media can have an enormous influence on the developing child. Children may identify closely with people or characters portrayed in reading materials, movies, videos, and television programs and commercials. Today children tend to select media figures as their ideal role models, whereas in the past the majority of children chose their parents or parent surrogates as the people they most wanted to be like (Duck, 1990). This trend can be viewed as a grave concern or a magnificent opportunity to promote positive role models. There is no doubt that the communications media provide children with a means for extending their knowledge about the world in which they live and have contributed to narrowing the differences between classes.

Reading Materials

The oldest form of mass media (i.e., books, newspapers, and magazines) contribute to children's competence in almost every direction, as well as providing enjoyment. Recognition of the impact that reading matter used in the schools has on the value system and socialization processes has prompted reevaluation of the content of textbooks in terms of the biased presentation of male and female role models, the sugar-coated view of life situations, and the biased history of minority groups.

Fairy tales, for generations the mainstay of young children's literature, for a time suffered condemnation as being sexist, overly violent in content, and riddled with unfavorable stereotypes such as the wicked stepmother, dwarfs, and physical unattractiveness associated with evil. They are now believed to provide an excellent medium for explaining puzzling and important topics such as death, stepparents, and inner feelings and turmoils. Although they do not provide solutions, fairy tales confront children with emotional predicaments and offer suggestions for dealing with them.

Comic books and other pulp reading material have been popular in every generation, usually at the expense of literature provided by schools, libraries, and parents. Many children have nothing else to read. The easy reading, quick action, and adventure in brief episodes seem to fulfill a need for children who are striving to understand both aggression in others and their own impulses. Reading ability, intelligence, and school adjustment apparently have no relationship to the number and type of comic books read. Most comic books appear to be relatively harmless to the majority of children and may be beneficial. Comic books seem to have only a minor influence on acquisition of beliefs, values, and behaviors. The popularity of this medium has prompted some educators to encourage translations of literature into comic book form to stimulate students' interest in the classics.

Movies

Movies, although usually not closely bound to reality, often portray an assortment of socially approved behaviors. Such movies perhaps make a contribution to children's value systems and provide opportunities for desirable social learning. On the other hand, children, especially adolescents, flock to the "macho" movies and those in which the heroes resort to violent resolution of problems, such as the use of karate techniques and wild car chases. The carry-over of these influences into daily life and relationships may account, in part, for the increase in violent behavior of young persons.

Another concern is the number of "slasher" and R-rated movies available to children and teenagers in theaters, on cable television, and on videocassettes. The content of movies has changed markedly during the past few years, with mutilation as a major theme. For children who are unable to distinguish between reality and fantasy, these films play on their deepest fears, resulting in bedtime fears, nightmares, and a fearful view of the world (Schmitt, 1989).

Young children can be frightened by some of the movies considered to be safe for family viewing. For example, the villainous witches in *Snow White* and the *Wizard of Oz* can be terrifying figures. Also, some of the classic Disney movies such as *Snow White* and *Cinderella,* which depict stepmothers as evil, destructive persons, can have a negative effect on children-stepmother relationships or can be confusing to children who have developed a positive relationship with a stepmother. Children as young as 4 years can recognize that cartoons are "make believe," but children as old as age 6 continue to assume that noncartoon features are at least roughly analogous to social reality (Downs, 1990). Parents can use viewing films as opportunities to open discussion, provide explanations, and explore difficult or troubling concepts or events.

Television

The medium with the most impact on children in North America today is television, which has become one of the most significant socializing agents in the lives of young children. The average child in the United States spends more time watching television than in any other activity except sleeping: 25 hours per week for children 2 to 5 years old, 22 hours for children 6 to 12 years old, and 23 hours for 12 to 17-year-olds. These figures do not include videocassette recorder (VCR) use (American Academy of Pediatrics, 1990).

The content of programs and commercials provides multiple sources for acquiring information, modeling behaviors, and observing value orientations. Besides producing a leveling effect on class differences in general information and vocabulary, TV exposes children to a wider variety of topics and events than they encounter in day-to-day life. Television always has time to talk to children and is a form of access to the adult world.

Most researchers have concluded that protracted television viewing can have detrimental effects on children. Increased verbal and physical aggressive behavior, reduced persistence at problem solving, greater sex-role stereotyping, and reduced creativity have been reported repeatedly.

Excessive television viewing has also been linked to obesity and high blood cholesterol levels in children (Gortmaker, Dietz, and Cheng, 1990). The passive activity is frequently accompanied by eating—in many cases high-calorie snacks. Furthermore, children may expend tremendous mental energy processing the audiovisual messages from TV, which may be very exhausting and make them less likely to engage in physical activity later. Television viewing has a fairly profound effect of lowering the metabolic rate and may be a mechanism for the relationship between obesity and the amount of television viewing (Klesges, Shelton, and Klesges, 1993).

TV programs and commercials, like movies, contain many implicit and explicit messages that promote alcohol consumption, smoking, violence, and promiscuous or unsafe sexual activity. An area of increasing concern is Music Television (MTV), especially when heavy metal rock groups, whose lyrics and videos sensationalize violent sex, suicide, and satanism, are featured. Although no clear evidence documents a relationship between television viewing and sexual activity or the use of alcohol or tobacco, the frequency of adolescent pregnancy and sexually transmitted diseases, the prevalence of alcohol-related deaths among adolescents, and the popularity of smoking among youth represent major sources of concern and speculation.

On the positive side, television has been shown to be a positive influence on children's abilities to deal with a variety of social issues such as divorce, the arrival of a new baby, discrimination, honesty, and helpfulness. Children who view educational programming (such as "Mister Rogers' Neighborhood" and "Sesame Street") for a long period of time become more affectionate, considerate, cooperative, and helpful toward their playmates. The ways that minority and ethnic characters are portrayed on television can have an impact on the way the majority culture views minority persons and on the self-image of minority children.

Many parents are concerned about the effects of television viewing on their children, and most would like information regarding its use (Bernard-Bonnin, 1991). Parents need to supervise the amount and type of TV programs their children watch and to teach their children how to watch TV (see the Home Care box above).

Home Care

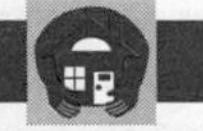

TELEVISION VIEWING

- Provide a positive role model by developing television substitutes such as reading, athletics, physical conditioning, and hobbies.
- Construct a time chart of child's activities (homework, TV viewing, scheduled outside activities, playing with a friend).
- Discuss with child what both believe to be a balanced set of activities.
- At the beginning of each week select appropriate programs from television schedules.
- Allow child to select programs from this approved list.
- Limit child's viewing to 2 hours or less per day.
- Rule out TV at specific times (e.g., before breakfast or on school nights).
- Make a list of alternative activities (e.g., riding a bicycle, reading a book, or working on a hobby).
- Require that child choose to do something from this list before watching TV.
- Watch programs with child.
- Discuss program and commercial content with child:
  - Distinguish between the real and the unreal.
  - Correlate consequences with actions.
  - Point out subtle messages.
  - Explore alternatives to aggressive conflict resolution.
  - Stress purpose of program (e.g., entertainment, education).
  - Explain likes and dislikes.
- Turn the TV off after the selected program is over.
- Monitor cable and pay TV selections; use a lockbox if necessary.
- Limit use of TV as a safe distraction to potentially stressful times (e.g., keeping the children occupied while the parent gets organized after a difficult day).

Key Points

- Growth describes a change in quantity and occurs when cells divide and synthesize new proteins.
- Maturation, a qualitative change, describes the aging process or an increase in competence and adaptability.
- Differentiation refers to a biologic description of the processes by which early cells and structures are modified and altered to achieve specific and characteristic physical and chemical properties.
- Development involves change from a lower to a more advanced stage of complexity.
- The five major developmental periods are prenatal, infancy, early childhood, middle childhood, and later childhood (pubescence and adolescence).
- Growth and development proceed in predictable patterns of direction, sequence, and pace.
- The directional trends in growth and development are cephalocaudal, proximodistal, and mass to specific.
- Physical development includes increase in height and weight and changes in body proportion, dentition, and some body tissues.
- The three broad classifications of child temperament are the easy child, the difficult child, and the slow-to-warm-up child.
- The developmental theories most widely used in explaining child growth and development are Freud's psychosexual stages, Erikson's stages of psychosocial development, Piaget's stages of cognitive development, and Kohlberg's stages of moral development.
- Development of self-concept occurs through children's interactions and observations of their own experiences with others and with the environment.
- Play is one of the most important media through which children learn about themselves, others, and their environment.
- Factors influencing development include heredity, neuroendocrine factors, nutrition, interpersonal relationships, socioconomic status, disease, stress, and mass media.

References

American Academy of Pediatrics, Committee on Communications: Children, adolescents and television, *Pediatrics* 85(6):1119-1120, 1990.

Bernard-Bonnin A et al: Television and the 3- to 10-year-old child, *Pediatrics* 88(1):48-54, 1991.

Chess S, Thomas A: Temperamental differences: a critical concept in child health care, *Pediatr Nurs* 11:167-171, 1985.

Clutter L: *Fostering spiritual care for the child and family.* In Smith DP et al, editors: *Comprehensive child and family nursing skills,* St Louis, 1991, Mosby.

Downs A: Children's judgments of televised events: the real versus pretend distinction, *Percept Mot Skills* 70:779-782, 1990.

Duck J: Children's ideals: the role of real-life versus media figures, *Aust J Psychol* 42:19-29, 1990.

Erikson EH: *Childhood and society,* ed 2, New York, 1963, WW Norton.

Fowler JW: Toward a developmental perspective on faith, *Religious Educ* 69:207-219, 1974.

Gortmaker S, Dietz W, Cheng L: Inactivity, diet, and the fattening of America, *J Am Diet Assoc* 90(9):1247-1252, 1990.

Jung FE, Czajka-Narins DM: Birth weight doubling and tripling times: an updated look at the effects of birth weight, sex, race and type of feeding, *Am J Clin Nutr* 42:182-189, 1985.

Klesges R, Shelton M, Klesges I: Effects of television on metabolic rate: potential implications for childhood obesity, *Pediatrics* 91(2):281-286, 1993.

Kohlberg L: *Moral development.* In Sills DL, editor: *International encyclopedia of the social sciences,* New York, 1968, Macmillan.

Masten A et al: Competence and stress in school children: moderating effects of individual and family qualities, *J Child Psychol Psychiatry* 29:747-764, 1988.

Piaget J: *The theory of stages in cognitive development,* New York, 1969, McGraw-Hill.

Ryan-Wenger N: A taxonomy of children's coping strategies: a step toward theory development, *Am J Orthopsychiatry* 62(2):256-263, 1992.

Schmitt BD: Nightmares on main street, *Am J Dis Child* 143:649, 1989 (editorial).

Selekman J: The development of body image in the child: a learned response, *Top Clin Nurs* 5(1):13-21, 1983.

Sheeber L, Johnson J: Child temperament, maternal adjustment, and changes in family life style, *Am J Orthopsychiatry* 62(2):178-185, 1992.

Sieving R, Zirbel-Donisch S: Development and enhancement of self-esteem in children, *J Pediatr Health Care* 4(6):290-296, 1990.

Usdin G: Investing in the "emotional bank" concept, *Child Teens Today* 8(6):7, 1988.

Wolk S et al: Factors affecting parents perceptions of temperament in early infancy, *Am J Orthopsychiatry* 62(1):71-82, 1992.

Bibliography

Allen LH et al: The interactive effects of dietary quality on the growth and attained size of young Mexican children, *Am J Clin Nutr* 56(2):353-364, 1992.

Baillargeon R, DeVos J: Object permanence in young infants: further evidence, *Child Dev* 62(6):1227-1246, 1991.

Bantz DL, Siktberg L: Teaching families to evaluate age-appropriate toys, *J Pediatr Health Care* 7:111-114, 1993.

Brown MS et al: Type A behavior in children: what a pediatric nurse practitioner needs to know, *J Pediatr Health Care* 3:131-136, 1989.

Busen NH: Societal values: a cause of stress in children, *J Pediatr Health Care* 2:300-306, 1988.

Carey WB: Temperament: a tool for coping with problem behavior, *Contemp Pediatr* 6(1):139-153, 1989.

Chess S, Thomas A: Temperamental differences: a critical concept in child health care, *Pediatr Nurs* 11:167-171, 1985.

Chess S, Thomas A: *Temperament in clinical practice,* New York, 1986, Guilford Press.

Derksen OJ et al: Children and the influence of the media, *Prim Care* 21(4):747-758, 1994.

Dixon SD, Stein MT: *Encounters with children: pediatric behavior and development,* ed 2, St Louis, 1992, Mosby.

Fabes RA, Eisenberg N: Young children's coping with interpersonal anger, *Child Dev* 63(1):116-128, 1992.

Flavell JH et al: Young children's understanding of different types of beliefs, *Child Dev* 63(4):960-977, 1992.

Health L, Bresolin L, Rinaldi R: Effects of media violence on children: a review of the literature, *Arch Gen Psychiatry* 46(4):376-379, 1989.

Henry J, Giordano B: Introduction—assessment of growth in infants and children: normal and abnormal pattern, *J Pediatr Health Care* 5:289-290, 1992.

Hobbie C: Relaxation-techniques for children and young people, *J Pediatr Health Care* 3:83-87, 1989.

Holaday B et al: Vygotsky's zone of proximal development: implications for nurse assistance of children's learning, *Issues Compr Pediatr Nurs* 17(1):15-27, 1994.

Houldin A, Fullard W, Heverly M: Toddler temperament and the quality of the child-rearing environment, *Pediatr Nurs* 15(5):491-496, 544, 1989.

Jessee PO: Nurses, children, and play, *Issues Compr Pediatr Nurs* 15(4):261-269, 1992.

Klein J et al: Adolescents' risky behavior and mass media use, *Pediatrics* 92(1):24-31, 1993.

Levine MD, Carey WB, Crocker AC: *Developmental-behavioral pediatrics,* ed 2, Philadelphia, 1992, WB Saunders.

Lewis M, Alessandri SM, Sullivan MW: Differences in shame and pride as a function of children's gender and task difficulty, *Child Dev* 63(3):630-638, 1992.

Lillard AS: Pretend play skills and the child's theory of mind, *Child Dev* 64(2):348-371, 1993.

Marino BL: Studying infant and toddler play, *J Pediatr Nurs* 6(1):16-20, 1991.

Mebert CJ: Dimensions of subjectivity in parents' ratings of infant temperament, *Child Dev* 62(2):352-361, 1991.

Morrow JD: The eyes have it: visual attention as an index of infant cognition, *J Pediatr Health Care* 7:150-155, 1993.

Robinson TN et al: Does television viewing increase obesity and reduce physical activity? Cross-sectional and longitudinal analyses among adolescent girls, *Pediatrics* 91:273-280, 1993.

Rollins J: *Meeting the child's developmental needs through play.* In Smith DP et al, editors: *Comprehensive child and family nursing skills,* St Louis, 1991, Mosby.

Rollins J: Nurses as gangbusters: a response to gang violence in America, *Pediatr Nurs* 19(6):559-567, 1993.

Sahler OJZ: *Theories and concepts of development as they relate to pediatric practice.* In Hoekelman RA et al, editors: *Primary pediatric care,* ed 3, St Louis, 1997, Mosby.

Sameroff AJ et al: Stability of intelligence from preschool to adolescence: the influence of social and family risk factors, *Child Dev* 64(1):80-97, 1993.

Shapiro CM, Flanigan MJ: Function of sleep, *Br Med J* 306:383-385, 1993.

Sieving R, Zirbel-Donisch S: Development and enhancement of self-esteem in children, *J Pediatr Health Care* 4(6):290-296, 1990.

Smitherman C: The lasting impact of fetal alcohol syndrome and fetal alcohol effect on children and adolescents, *J Pediatr Health Care* 8:121-126, 1994.

Stein KF: Schema model of self-concept, *Image J Nurs Scholarship* 27(3):187-193, 1995.

St Peters M et al: Television and families: what do young children watch with their parents? *Child Dev* 62(6):1409-1423, 1991.

Strayer J: Children's concordant emotions and cognitions in response to observed emotions, *Child Dev* 64(1):188-201, 1993.

Thomas RM: *Comparing theories of child development,* ed 3, Belmont, Calif, 1992, Wadsworth.

CHAPTER 31

Communication and Health Assessment of the Child and Family

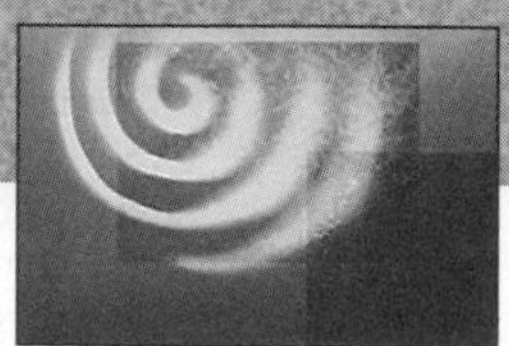

COMMUNICATION, P. 866

Verbal communication, p. 866

Nonverbal communication—paralanguage, p. 867

GUIDELINES FOR COMMUNICATION AND INTERVIEWING, P. 867

Establishing a setting for communication, p. 867

COMMUNICATING WITH FAMILIES, P. 868

Communicating with parents, p. 868

Communicating with children, p. 872

Communication techniques, p. 875

HISTORY TAKING, P. 875

Performing a health history, p. 875

FAMILY ASSESSMENT, P. 882

NUTRITIONAL ASSESSMENT, P. 885

Communication

The forms of communication may be verbal, nonverbal, or abstract. **Verbal communication** may involve language and its expression; vocalizations in the form of laughs, moans, or squalls; or the implications of what is not said in light of what has been said. **Nonverbal communication** is often called body language and includes gestures, movements, facial expressions, postures, and reactions. **Abstract communication** takes the form of play, artistic expression, symbols, photographs, and choice of clothing. Because it is possible to exert greater conscious control over verbal communication, it is a less reliable indicator of true feelings, especially with children.

Many factors influence the communication process. To be successful (gratifying), communication must be appropriate to the situation, properly timed, and clearly delivered. This implies that nurses understand and use techniques of effective communication, including listening. Verbal and nonverbal messages must be congruent; that is, two or more messages sent via different levels must not be contradictory.

VERBAL COMMUNICATION

Words shape reality and thus hold tremendous power. A person can change another person's perception of reality by the choice of words that are used. For example, if the diagnosis of cancer is always referred to as a tumor, cyst, malignancy, or carcinoma, patients may never really know that they have cancer. Consequently, they may assume less responsibility for their care than if they were aware of the seriousness of the condition. By learning to recognize how patients and health professionals use language to manipulate reality, a person can also learn how to change perceptions and communicate more effectively.

Avoidance Language

The most common way that people try to alter reality is by avoiding words that truly describe it. For example, euphemisms such as "passed on" are used instead of "death." Avoidance language indicates that a person wants to hide something, particularly feelings. As a rule, accepting a person's use of euphemisms only serves to perpetuate the fears and never helps the person deal with them. In contrast, the use of straightforward, precise, descriptive language lends perspective to the situation and allows the person to discuss the fears. Imagined fears are usually worse than reality.

Distancing Language

People may use impersonal words such as "it" or "others" to shield themselves from the painful reality of a situation. For example, parents may state that they know *someone* with a child who is slow, when they may actually be talking about personal fears regarding *their* child. By realizing that the parents may need to talk about this difficult subject, the nurse can provide sensitive statements that ease them into discussing their situation.

One of the dangers in supporting distancing language is that the person may effectively deny that a problem exists. To

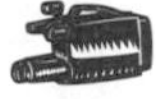

For additional information, please view "Communicating with Children and Families" in *Whaley and Wong's Pediatric Nursing Video Series*, St Louis, 1996, Mosby; (800) 426-4545.

return to the previous example, if the issue of retardation is never approached directly but is allowed to be "someone else's problem," the parents may not be able to make decisions for special schools or individualized training.

Sometimes distancing is desirable because the topic may be too painful to discuss directly. The use of the third-person technique may be very therapeutic in allowing an individual the opportunity to indirectly approach a subject and receive feedback but still remain in control.

NONVERBAL COMMUNICATION—PARALANGUAGE

In addition to the spoken word, messages are also relayed through nonverbal means, or **paralanguage**—the pitch, pause, intonation, rate, volume, and stress apparent in speech. Young children become very adept at understanding paralanguage; long before they know the meaning of words, they sense anxiety or fear by the rise in pitch or the accelerated rate of the parent's voice. By careful observation of the spoken word, nurses can better understand the meaning of another's verbal message and more accurately control their own paralanguage.

Because most people do not exert conscious control over their paralanguage, it is a valuable clue to feelings and concerns. For example, *pausing* may signify a need to formulate thoughts, recall information, or fabricate a story. Frequent pauses often make the speaker sound unsure. Long pauses may mean that the individual needs more information.

Rate is another characteristic that gives unspoken messages. Talking too fast usually makes the speaker sound glib and insensitive. Talking slowly with a firm tone and appropriate pauses conveys authority. Therefore a person is much more likely to "hear" instructions if the latter approach is used. Children in particular respond attentively to a slow, even, steady voice.

Confirming and Disconfirming Behaviors

People respond to each other through *confirming behaviors,* such as nodding the head, using direct eye contact, repeating or requesting clarification, and making appropriate comments, or *disconfirming behaviors,* such as tapping fingers or a foot, turning away from the speaker, avoiding eye contact, and interrupting (Heineken and Roberts, 1983). Because there is a reciprocal relationship between such behaviors, nurses need to use confirming behaviors to receive confirmation in return. This "mirroring" effect is particularly evident in children because of their sensitivity to nonverbal cues.

Guidelines for Communication and Interviewing

The most widely used method of communicating with parents on a professional basis is the interview process. Interviewing, unlike social conversation, is a specific form of goal-directed communication. As nurses converse with children and adults, they focus on the individuals to determine the type of persons they are, their usual mode of handling problems, whether help is needed, and the way in which they react to counseling. Developing interviewing skills requires time and practice, but following some guiding principles can facilitate this process.

ESTABLISHING A SETTING FOR COMMUNICATION

Appropriate Introduction

Nurses should introduce themselves to and ask the name of each family member who is present. Address parents or other adults using their appropriate titles, such as "Mr." and "Mrs.," unless they specify a preferred name. Record the preferred name on the health record. Using formal address or preferred names rather than first names or "mom" or "dad," conveys respect and regard for the parents or other caregivers and the critical role they play in the lives of their children (Leff and Walizer, 1992).

At the beginning of the visit, include children in the interaction by asking them their name, age, and other information. Nurses often direct all questions to adults, even when children are old enough to speak for themselves. This serves to terminate one extremely valuable source of information, the patient. When the child is included, follow the general rules for communicating with children (p. 876).

Role Clarification and Explanation of the Interview

During the introduction it is also necessary to clarify the nurse's particular role in the health setting. For example, nurses performing interviews may be pediatric nurse practitioners (PNPs), inpatient staff nurses, clinic nurses, office nurses, visiting nurses, or school nurses. A parent is much more likely to reveal personal information about the child and family if the relevance and importance of the interview are stressed. Otherwise, parents may refuse to elaborate on certain areas because they believe it has no bearing on the "problem." In addition, because more than one member of the health team may take a history during the course of a hospital admission, it is important to clarify the reason for each interview.

Another reason for role clarification is education of the health consumer. With expanded roles in nursing, it is not unusual for families to think that the examiner is a physician rather than a nurse. Role clarification is especially important because some parents may feel deceived if they later are made aware of the nurse's identity. Because the general consumer acceptance of PNPs has been very favorable, it is also important that PNPs acknowledge their expertise by emphasizing their role.

Preliminary Acquaintance

To make the family feel at ease and to develop rapport, begin the interview with some general conversation. The opening statements should be general but still informative. Comments such as "How have things been since your last visit?" "Tell me about Johnny," or (to the child) "What do you think is going to happen today?" allow the parent or child to express the main concern in a casual, relaxed atmosphere.

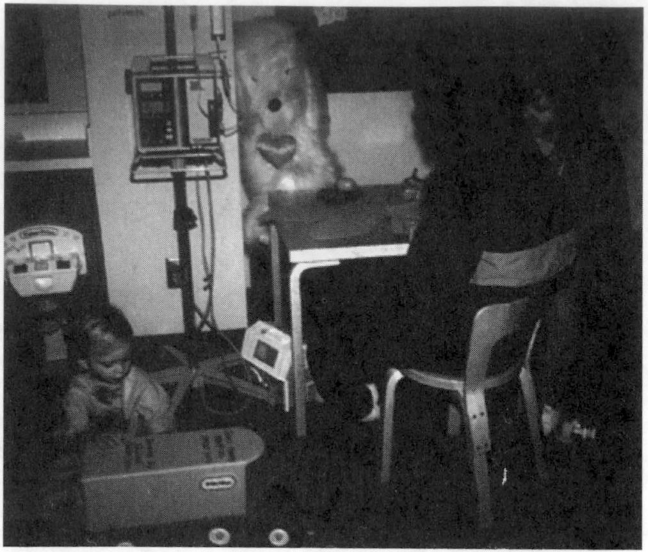

Fig. 31-1 Child plays while nurse interviews parent.

Critical Thinking Q & A

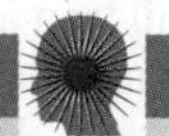

THE INTERVIEW

During your interview with Ms. Gaines, $2^1/_2$-year-old Jesse continually interrupts the conversation. Although Ms. Gaines has told her several times to be quiet, the interruptions continue. Frustrated, the mother states firmly, "If you don't be good, the nurse will give you a shot." Jesse begins to cry softly and hugs her mother's legs. Your most appropriate response is which of the following:

1. State, "Ms. Gaines, don't threaten Jesse that way. Her behavior isn't bothering me."
2. Do nothing, because Jesse has become quiet.
3. State, "Jesse, nurses don't give needles because children are not being quiet. Here are paper and crayons to draw some pictures while your mom and I talk."
4. Hug Jesse and give her crayons and paper to draw.

The correct answer is three. The threat of injections or other painful or frightening procedures should never be used to gain a child's cooperation. You want to reassure Jesse about this but at the same time reinforce the need for her to be quiet. Providing play materials helps keep her occupied.

Although the other responses may seem appropriate, they fail to remove the threat of a "shot" to Jesse. In particular, the first response can alienate your relationship with the parent. It also dismisses the issue that the interruptions *do* bother Ms. Gaines and most likely affect the quality of the interview.

The preliminary acquaintance conversation also reveals how responsive the informant may be to questions. For example, using open-ended statements, such as "Tell me about the baby," may lead the parent into a lengthy detailed discussion. In this case direct questions toward specific answers to avoid irrelevant remarks. At other times a parent may respond to open-ended questions with only minimal information, in which case continue to use open-ended questions rather than "yes" or "no" type questions.

Assurance of Privacy and Confidentiality

The place where the interview is conducted is almost as important as the interview itself. The physical environment should allow for as much privacy as possible, with distractions such as interruptions, noise, or other visible activity kept to a minimum. At times it may be necessary to turn off a television or radio. The environment should also have some play provision for young children to keep them occupied during the parent-nurse interview (Fig. 31-1). Parents who are constantly interrupted by their children are unable to concentrate fully on the questions asked of them and tend to give short answers to terminate the interview as quickly as possible (see the Critical Thinking Q & A box to the left).

Confidentiality is another essential component of the initial phase of the interview. Because the interview is usually shared with other members of the health team or the teacher (as in the case of students), be certain to inform the parents of the confidential limits of the conversation. If there is concern regarding confidentiality in a situation, such as talking to a parent suspected of child abuse or a teenager contemplating suicide, deal with this directly and inform the person that in such instances confidentiality cannot be ensured.

Communicating with Families

COMMUNICATING WITH PARENTS

Although the parent and child are separate and distinct individuals, relationships with the child are often mediated via the parent, particularly in the case of younger children. For the most part, information about the child is acquired by direct observation or is communicated to the nurse by the parent. Usually it can be assumed that because of the close contact with the child, the parent gives reliable information. Making an assessment of the child requires input from the child (verbal and nonverbal), information from the parent, and the nurse's own observations of the child and interpretation of the relationship between the child and the parent. Counseling and guidance must be directed to the caregiver of infants and small children; when children are old enough to be active participants in their own health maintenance, the parent becomes a collaborator in health care.

Encouraging the Parent to Talk

Interviewing the parent not only offers the opportunity to determine the health and developmental status of the child but also offers information about factors that influence the child's life. Whatever the parent sees as a problem should be a concern of the nurse. These problems are not always easy to identify. Nurses need to be alert for clues and signals by which a parent communicates worries and anxieties. Careful phrasing with broad open-ended questions such as "What is Jimmy eating now?" provides more information than several single-answer questions such as "Is Jimmy eating what the rest of the family eats?"

Sometimes the parent will take the lead without prompting. At other times it may be necessary to direct another question on the basis of an observation such as "Connie seems unhappy today" or "How do you feel when David cries?" If the parent appears to be tired or distraught, consider asking, "What do you do to relax?" or "What help do you have with the children?" A comment such as "You handle the baby very well. What types of experience have you had with babies?" to new parents who appear comfortable with their first child gives positive reinforcement and provides an opening for any questions they might have regarding the care of the infant. Often all that is required to keep parents talking is a nod or saying "yes" or "uh-huh."

When attempting to elicit feelings and covert problem areas, avoid closed-ended questions that begin with "Does . . . ," "Did . . . ," or "Is . . . ," which usually require only a single response. In addition, asking questions such as "Does your son have any problems at school?" subtly implies a lack of parental skills and evokes defensiveness. Instead say, "What . . . ," "How . . . ," "Tell me about . . . ," and encourage elaboration with "You were saying . . . ," "You say that . . . ," or by reflecting a key word. Open-ended questions are nonthreatening and encourage description.

Directing the Focus

The ability to direct the focus of the interview while allowing for maximum freedom of expression is one of the most difficult goals in effective communication. One approach is the use of open-ended or broad questions followed by guiding statements. For example, if the parent proceeds to list the other children by name, say, "Tell me their ages, too." If the parent continues to describe each child in-depth (which is not the purpose of the interview), redirect the focus by stating, "Let's talk about the other children later. You were beginning to tell me about Paul's activities at school." This approach conveys interest in the other children but focuses the assessment on the patient.

In the event that the parent has suggested that a problem exists with one of the other children, reintroduce this subject at the end of the interview to assess the need for further family follow-up. Saying to the parent, "Before, you were mentioning that your older son is having trouble in school. Tell me what you see as the problem," reintroduces this subject but only in terms of the possible problem.

Listening and Cultural Awareness

Listening is the most important component of effective communication. When listening is truly aimed at understanding the patient, it is an active process that requires concentration and attention to all aspects of the conversation—verbal, nonverbal, and abstract. Major blocks to listening are environmental distraction and premature judgment.

The attitudes and feelings of the nurse are easily injected into an interview. Nurses' perceptions of a parent's behavior are often influenced by their own perceptions, prejudices, and assumptions, which may include racial, religious, and cultural stereotypes. What may be interpreted as passive hostility or disinterest in a parent may be shyness or an expression of anxiety. For example, in Western cultures eye contact and directness are signs of paying attention. However, in many non-Western cultures, including that of Native Americans, directness such as looking someone in the eye is considered rude.

Guidelines

CULTURALLY SENSITIVE INTERACTIONS

Nonverbal strategies

Invite family members to choose where they would like to sit or stand, allowing them to select a comfortable distance.
Observe interactions with others to determine which body gestures (e.g., shaking hands) are acceptable and appropriate. Ask when in doubt.
Avoid appearing rushed.
Be an active listener.
Observe for cues regarding appropriate eye contact.
Learn the appropriate use of pauses or interruptions for different cultures.
Ask for clarification if nonverbal meaning is unclear.

Verbal strategies

Learn proper terms of address.
Use a positive tone of voice to convey interest.
Speak slowly and carefully, not loudly, when families have poor language comprehension.
Encourage questions.
Learn basic words and sentences of family's language, if possible.
Avoid professional terms.
When asking questions, tell the family why the questions are being asked, the way in which the information they provide will be used, and how it might benefit their child.
Repeat important information more than once.
Always give the reason or purpose for a treatment or prescription.
Use information written in the family's language.
Offer the services of an interpreter when necessary (see p. 871.)
Learn from families and representatives of their culture methods of communicating information without creating discomfort.
Address intergenerational needs (e.g., family's need to consult with others).
Be sincere, open, and honest and, when appropriate, share personal experiences, beliefs, and practices to establish rapport and trust.

Children are taught to avert their gaze and to look down when being addressed by an adult, especially one with authority (Sloat and Matsuura, 1990). Therefore judgments about "listening," as well as verbal interactions, need to be made with an appreciation of cultural differences (see the Guidelines box above; see Chapter 28).

Although it is necessary to make some preliminary judgments, listen with as much objectivity as possible by clarifying meanings and attempting to see the situation from the parent's point of view. Effective interviewers use conscious control over their reactions and responses and the techniques they use.

Use of minimum verbal activity with active listening facilitates parent involvement. It is tempting to spend time explaining, describing, and interpreting health information when the opportunity presents itself. However, it is possible to provide effective health education by properly timing the information and presenting only as much as is necessary at the moment.

Careful listening facilitates the use of clues, verbal leads, or signals from the interviewee to move the interview along. Frequent references to an area of concern, repetition of certain key words, or a special emphasis on something or someone serves as cues to the interviewer for the direction of inquiry. Concerns and anxieties are usually mentioned in a casual, offhand manner. Even though they are casual, they are important and deserve careful scrutiny to identify problem areas. For example, a parent who is concerned about a child's habit of bed-wetting may casually mention that the child's bed was "wet this morning."

Because the interview is almost always triangular—between the nurse, parent, and child—the parent may wish to convey information in such a way as to prevent the child from hearing it. Active listening is required of the nurse to hear the unspoken message. The following example illustrates this point:

> During a routine health visit, the nurse performed a complete history and physical examination on a 4-year-old girl. The child was accompanied by her mother, who appeared to be a reliable, well-informed, and talkative informant. During the child's birth history, the mother gave all the information asked. However, during the family history, the mother stated to the nurse, "I had a hysterectomy 6 years ago." Because the nurse gave no indication of acknowledging the significance of this statement, the mother repeated it, only this time she stressed the "6 years." The nurse, who had not been listening as attentively as she should have, realized that the mother was telling her something very important. The mother raised her eyebrows and gently shook her head "no," warning the nurse not to explore this area too openly. The nurse correctly read the cues and stated, "Let's return to your health history later."
>
> At the completion of the physical examination, the nurse brought the child to the health center's playroom and took the opportunity to investigate this contradictory information of a "4-year-old child born to a woman with a hysterectomy 6 years ago." The mother revealed that the child was adopted. The mother was greatly concerned about the fact that the child was unaware of this and requested the nurse's advice.
>
> Fortunately, the nurse had "listened" carefully enough to realize the significance of this woman's concern and allowed her the opportunity to discuss it in private.

Listening is also helpful in assessing reliability. For example, the answers elicited at the beginning of the interview may differ from those at the end, when the parent feels more confident in revealing problems. It is important to identify any discrepancies and reintroduce those topics for further investigation.

Using Silence

Silence as a response is often one of the most difficult interviewing techniques to learn. It requires a sense of confidence and comfort on the part of the interviewer to allow the interviewee space in which to think without interruptions. Silence permits the interviewee to sort out thoughts and feelings and search for responses to questions. It also allows for the sharing of feelings in which two or more people absorb the emotion to its depth.

Sometimes it is necessary to break the silence and reopen communication. Do this in a way that encourages the person to continue talking about what is considered important. Breaking a silence by introducing a new topic or by prolonged talking essentially terminates the interviewee's opportunity to use the silence. Suggestions for breaking the silence include statements such as "Is there anything else you wish to say?" "I see you find it difficult to continue; how may I help?" or "I don't know what this silence means. Perhaps there is something you would like to put into words but find difficult to say."

Being Empathic

Empathy is the capacity to understand what another person is experiencing from within that person's frame of reference; it is often described as the ability to put oneself in another's shoes. The essence of empathic interaction is accurately understanding another's feelings (Bellet and Maloney, 1991). Empathy differs from **sympathy,** which involves *having* feelings or emotions in common with another person rather than *understanding* those feelings. Sympathy is not therapeutic in the helping relationship because it leads to feeling emotionally overinvolved and potentially to professional burnout (Holden, 1990).

Of the different types of support such as empathy, encouragement, or reassurance, empathy is the most beneficial but least used form (Wissow, Roter, and Wilson, 1994). Some individuals are naturally empathic; however, empathy can be learned by attending to the verbal and nonverbal language of the interviewee. *Neurolinguistic programming (NLP)* is concerned with the *manner* of accessing and understanding information and is an excellent method of increasing empathic communication. Although people may use all of the following sensory modalities to communicate, usually one modality predominates: visual, auditory, or kinesthetic. The specific sensory mode is identified by observing the type of verbs, adjectives, and adverbs the person uses and then using this mode in responding to the individual. For example, if a person using the visual mode states, "I can't *see* why you have to perform these procedures on my child," a response using the same mode is, "What do you *see* as the reason for them?"

Defining the Problem

To arrive at a solution to a problem, the nurse and the parent must agree that a problem exists. Sometimes the parent may believe that there is a problem that the nurse is unable to see. For example, a mother was overly concerned about every small sniffle, sneeze, or cough in her infant, who had been carefully examined and found to be healthy with no evidence of a respiratory problem. On careful questioning, the nurse discovered that a previous child had died of pneumonia in infancy. Consequently, the nurse was better able to understand the mother's concern and could help the mother deal with her special anxieties about her infant; the nurse could also teach her how to recognize any need for concern.

Occasionally a problem is identified that the parent denies exists. In this case pursue the situation and either find a way to deal with it or enlist the aid of other health team members. For example, the parents of a child with Down syndrome may refuse to believe that their child is different from any other child of the same age. They may say, "He is just a little slow," or "All the child needs to do is to try harder." A child with an obvious behavior problem may be described by the parents as "stubborn." Such statements may be clues that the parents have not progressed past the stage of denial in adjusting to the condition.

Solving the Problem

Once the problem is identified and agreed on by the parent and the nurse, they can begin to arrive at a solution. A parent who is included in the problem-solving process is more apt to follow through with a course of action. Questions such as "What have you tried so far?" or "What have you thought about doing?" provide leads for exploration and give the parents the feeling that their ideas and solutions are worthwhile. These ideas can be followed by "What prevents you from trying that?" "That sounds like a good plan," and "You seem to be stumped. Have you considered trying this?" Such approaches encourage active participation and reinforce rather than belittle parents' efforts to solve their problems.

Sometimes parents arrive at a solution that the nurse does not consider the best alternative. If it can be ascertained that it will do no harm and if the parents are convinced of its merits, it is usually best to allow them to continue with the plan. A course of action is more likely to be carried out when parents can reach their own conclusions. However, when parental decisions may be hazardous, nurses are obligated to discuss the risks with the family and try to reach a more beneficial solution. Whenever possible, decisions should be those of the parents, with the nurse serving as a *facilitator* in problem solving.

Providing Anticipatory Guidance

The ideal way to handle a situation is to deal with it *before* it becomes a problem. The best preventive measure is anticipatory guidance. Traditionally, anticipatory guidance has focused on providing families with information on normal growth and development, as well as nurturing childrearing practices. For example, one of the most significant areas in pediatrics is injury prevention. Beginning prenatally, parents need specific instructions on home safety. Because of the child's maturing developmental skills, home safety changes must be implemented early to minimize risks to the child.

Many normal developmental changes can disturb unprepared parents, such as a toddler's diminished appetite, negativism, altered sleeping patterns, and anxiety toward strangers. Such topics are discussed in the chapters on health promotion to provide the nurse with knowledge to counsel parents.

However, anticipatory guidance should extend beyond giving information and toward empowering families to use the information as a means of building competence in their parenting abilities. To achieve this level of anticipatory guidance the following must be done (Gorzka et al, 1991):

- Base interventions on needs identified by the family, not by the professional
- View the family as competent or as having the ability to be competent
- Provide opportunities for the family to achieve competence

BOX 31-1

Blocks to Communication

Socializing
Giving unrestricted and sometimes unasked-for advice
Offering premature or inappropriate reassurance
Giving overready encouragement
Defending a situation or opinion
Using stereotyped comments or cliches
Limiting expression of emotion by asking directed, closed-ended questions
Interrupting and finishing the person's sentence
Talking more than the interviewee
Forming prejudged conclusions
Deliberately changing the focus

Signs of information overload

Long periods of silence
Wide eyes and fixed facial expression
Constant fidgeting or attempting to move away
Nervous habits (e.g., tapping, playing with hair)
Sudden disruptions (e.g., asking to go to the bathroom)
Looking around
Yawning, eyes drooping
Frequently looking at a watch or clock
Attempting to change topic of discussion

Avoiding Blocks to Communication

A number of blocks to communication can adversely affect the quality of the helping relationship. Many of these blocks are initiated by the interviewer, such as giving unrestricted advice or forming prejudged conclusions. Another type of block occurs primarily with the interviewees and deals with information overload. When individuals are presented with too much information or information that is overwhelming, they often demonstrate signals of increasing anxiety or decreasing attention. Such signals should alert the interviewer to give less information or to clarify what has been said. Some of the more common blocks to communication, including signs of information overload, are listed in Box 31-1.

Communication blocks can be corrected by careful analysis of the interview process. One of the best methods for improving interviewing skills is audiotape or videotape feedback. With supervision and guidance, the interviewer can recognize the blocks and consciously avoid them.

Communicating With Families Through an Interpreter

Sometimes communication is impossible because two people speak different languages. In this case it is necessary to obtain information through a third party, the interpreter. When an interpreter is used, the same guidelines for interviewing are used. Specific guidelines for using an adult interpreter are presented in the Guidelines box on p. 872.

Communicating with families through an interpreter requires sensitivity to cultural, legal, and ethical considerations. For example, in some cultures using a child as an interpreter is considered an insult to an adult, because children are expected to show respect by not questioning their elders. In some cultures class differences between the interpreter and the family may cause the family to feel intimidated and less inclined to offer information. Therefore choose the translator

Guidelines

USING AN INTERPRETER

Explain to the interpreter the reason for the interview and the type of questions that will be asked.
Clarify whether a detailed or brief answer is required and whether the translated response can be general or literal.
Introduce the interpreter to the family and allow some time before the actual interview so that they can become acquainted.
Communicate directly with family members when asking questions to reinforce interest in them and to observe nonverbal expressions, but do not ignore the interpreter.
Pose questions to elicit only one answer at a time, such as "Do you have pain?" rather than "Do you have any pain, tiredness, or loss of appetite?"
Refrain from interrupting the family member and interpreter while they are conversing.
Avoid commenting to the interpreter about family members, because they may understand some English.
Be aware that some medical words, such as "allergy," may have no similar word in another language; avoid medical jargon whenever possible.
Respect cultural differences; it is often best to pose questions about sex, marriage, or pregnancy indirectly—ask about "child's father" rather than "mother's husband."
Allow time following the interview for the interpreter to share something that he or she believed could not be said earlier; ask about the interpreter's impression of nonverbal clues to communication and the family members' reliability or ease in revealing information.
Arrange for the family to speak with the same interpreter on subsequent visits whenever possible.

carefully, and provide time for the interpreter and family to establish rapport.

Issues of legal and ethical concerns may also arise. For example, in obtaining informed consent through an interpreter, it is important that the family be fully informed of all aspects of the particular procedure to which they are consenting. Issues of confidentiality may arise when family members related to another patient are asked to interpret for the family, thus revealing sensitive information that may be shared with other families on the unit.

When no one else is available to translate, children within the family are often asked to assume this role. In this situation it is important to stress *literal* translation of parent responses. To maximize correct translations, it may be necessary to interrupt the parent and ask the child to translate every few sentences. When using children as interpreters, ask questions directed at specific answers and assess the interpreted translation in terms of nonverbal expressions of communication.*

Nursing ALERT

When using translated materials such as a health history form, be sure the informant is literate in the foreign language.

*Interpreting services are also available through **American Telephone and Telegraph (AT&T)** by calling (800) 628-8486 or (800) 752-6096.

COMMUNICATING WITH CHILDREN

Although the greatest amount of verbal communication may usually be carried out with the parent, do not exclude the child during the interview. Pay attention to infants and younger children through play or by occasionally directing questions or remarks to them. Include older children as active participants.

In communication with children of all ages, the nonverbal components of the communication process convey the most significant messages. It is difficult to disguise feelings, attitudes, and anxiety when relating to children. They are very alert to surroundings and attach meaning to every gesture and move that is made. This is particularly true with very young children.

Active attempts to make friends with children before they have had an opportunity to evaluate an unfamiliar person tend to increase their anxiety. A helpful tactic is to continue to talk to the child and parent but go about activities that do not involve the child directly, thus allowing the child to observe from a safe position. If the child has a special toy or doll, "talk" to the doll first. Ask simple questions such as "Does your teddy bear have a special name?" to ease the child into conversation. Other guidelines for communicating with children are presented in the Guidelines box on p. 873. Specific guidelines for preparing children for procedures, a common nursing function, are discussed in Chapter 42.

Communication Related to Development of Thought Processes

The normal development of language and thought offers a frame of reference in knowing how to communicate with children. Thought processes progress from concrete to functional and finally to abstract, formal operations.

Infancy. Because they are unable to use words, infants primarily use and understand nonverbal communication. Infants communicate their needs and feelings through nonverbal behaviors and vocalizations that can be interpreted by someone who is around them for a sufficient amount of time. Infants smile and coo when content and cry when distressed. Crying is provoked by unpleasant stimuli from inside or outside, such as hunger, pain, body restraint, or loneliness. Adults interpret this response to mean that an infant needs something and consequently try to alleviate the discomfort and reduce tension. Crying (or the desire to cry) persists as a part of everyone's communication repertoire.

Infants respond to adults' nonverbal behaviors. They become quiet when they are cuddled, patted, or receive other forms of gentle, physical contact. They derive comfort from the sound of a voice, even though they do not understand the words that are spoken. Until infants reach the age at which they experience stranger anxiety, they readily respond to any firm, gentle handling and quiet, calm speech. Loud, harsh sounds and sudden movements are frightening.

Older infants' attentions are centered on themselves and their parents; therefore any stranger is a potential threat until proved otherwise. Holding out the hands and asking the child to "come" is seldom successful, especially if the infant is with the parent. If infants must be handled, simply pick them up firmly without gestures. Observe the position in which the parent holds the infant. Most infants have learned to prefer a

Guidelines

COMMUNICATING WITH CHILDREN

- Allow children time to feel comfortable.
- Avoid sudden or rapid advances, broad smiles, extended eye contact, or other gestures that may be seen as threatening.
- Talk to the parent if the child is initially shy.
- Communicate through transition objects such as dolls, puppets, or stuffed animals before questioning a young child directly.
- Give older children the opportunity to talk without the parents present.
- Assume a position that is at eye level with the child (Fig. 31-2).
- Speak in a quiet, unhurried, and confident voice.
- Speak clearly, be specific, and use simple words and short sentences.
- State directions and suggestions *positively*.
- Offer a choice only when one exists.
- Be honest with children.
- Allow them to express their concerns and fears.
- Use a variety of communication techniques.

particular position and manner of handling. In general, infants are more at ease upright than horizontal. Hold infants so that they can see their parents. Until they have developed the understanding that an object (in this case the parent) removed from sight can still be present, they have no way of knowing that the object is still there.

Early childhood. Children under 5 years of age are egocentric. They see things only in relation to themselves and from their point of view. Therefore focus communication on *them.* Tell them what they can do or how they will feel. Experiences of others are of no interest to them. It is futile to use another child's experience as an attempt to gain the cooperation of very small children. Allow them to touch and examine articles that will come in contact with them. A stethoscope bell will feel cold; palpating a neck might tickle. Although they have not yet acquired sufficient language skills to express their feelings and wants, toddlers are able to communicate effectively with their hands to transmit ideas without words. They push away an unwanted object, pull another person to show them something, point, and cover the mouth that is saying something they do not wish to hear.

Everything is direct and concrete to small children. They are unable to work with abstractions, and they interpret words literally. Analogies escape them because they are unable to separate fact from fantasy. For example, they attach literal meaning to such common phrases as "two-faced," "sticky fingers," or "coughing your head off." Children who are told they will get "a little stick in the arm" may not be able to envision an injection (Fig. 31-3). Therefore avoid using a phrase that might be misinterpreted by a small child (see the Guidelines box under Preparation for Procedures, Chapter 42).

Use language that is consistent with the child's developmental level. For example, in talking with a toddler, use simple, *short* sentences, repeat words that are *familiar* to the child, and limit descriptions to *concrete* explanations. Be certain that nonverbal messages are consistent with words and actions.

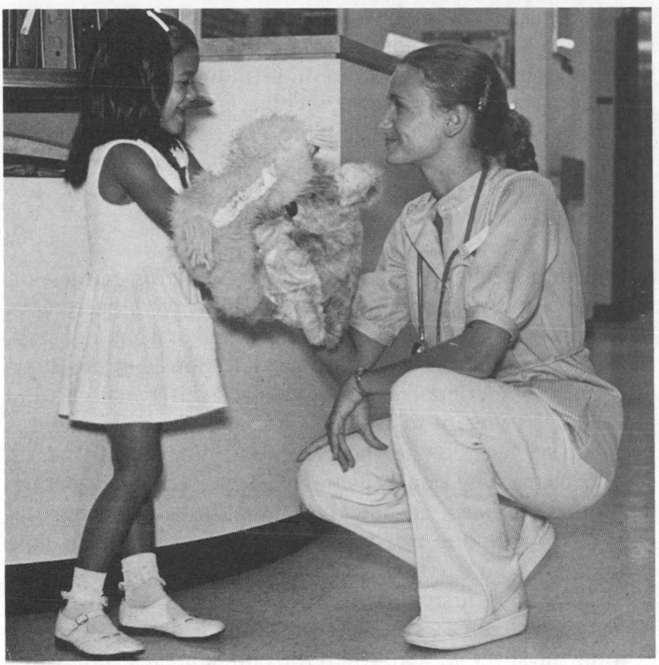

Fig. 31-2 Nurse assumes position at child's level.

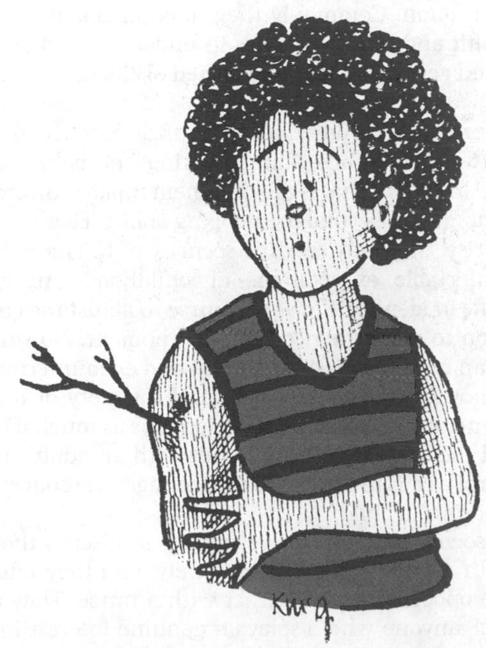

Fig. 31-3 To a young child the expression " a little stick in the arm" is taken literally.

For example, do not smile while doing something painful; children may think you enjoy hurting them.

Young children assign human attributes to inanimate objects. Consequently, they fear that objects may jump, bite, cut, or pinch all by themselves. Children do not know that these devices are unable to perform without human direction. To minimize their fear, keep unfamiliar equipment out of view until it is needed.

School-age years. Younger school-age children rely less on what they see and more on what they know when faced with new problems. They want explanations and reasons for everything but require no verification beyond that. They are interested in the functional aspect of all procedures, objects, and activities. They want to know why an object exists, why it is used, how it works, and the intent and purpose of its user. They need to know what is going to take place and why it is being done to *them* specifically. For example, to explain a procedure such as taking a blood pressure, show the child how squeezing the bulb pushes air into the cuff and makes the "silver" in the tube go up. Let the child operate the bulb. An explanation for the reason might be as simple as "I want to see how far the silver goes up when the cuff squeezes your arm." Consequently, the child becomes an enthusiastic participant.

School-age children have a heightened concern about body integrity. Because of the special importance and value they place on their body, they are overly sensitive to anything that constitutes a threat or suggestion of injury to it. This concern extends to their possessions also, and therefore they may appear to overreact to loss or threatened loss of treasured objects. Helping children to voice their concerns enables the nurse to provide reassurance and to implement activities that reduce their anxiety.

Older children have an adequate and satisfactory use of language. They still require relatively simple explanations, but their ability to think concretely can facilitate communication and explanation. Commonly they have sufficient experience with health and health workers to understand what is transpiring and generally what is expected of them.

Adolescence. As children move into adolescence, they fluctuate between child and adult thinking and behavior. They are riding a current that is moving them rapidly toward a maturity that may be beyond their coping ability. Therefore when tensions rise, they may seek the security of the more familiar and comfortable expectations of childhood. Anticipating these shifts in identity allows the nurse to adjust the course of interaction to meet the needs of the moment. No single approach can be relied on consistently, and encountering cooperation, hostility, anger, bravado, and a variety of other behaviors and attitudes can be expected. It is as much a mistake to regard the adolescent as an adult with an adult's wisdom and control as it is to confine to the teenager the concerns and expectations of a child.

Adolescents often are more willing to discuss their concerns with an adult outside the family, and they often welcome the opportunity to interact with a nurse. They are accepting of anyone who displays a genuine interest in them. However, adolescents are quick to reject persons who attempt to impose their values on them, whose interest is feigned, or who appear to have little respect for who they are and what they think or say.

As with all children, adolescents need to express their feelings. Generally, they talk quite freely when given an opportunity. However, what adolescents say cannot always be taken at face value. When emotional factors are involved, the feelings that are interjected into words are as significant as the words that are used. To give support, be attentive, try not to interrupt, and avoid comments or expressions that convey disapproval or surprise. Avoid prying and asking embarrassing questions, and resist any impulse to give advice. Adolescents often reveal their feelings or a source of concern or ask a question when they are involved in routine matters such as a physical assessment.

Teenagers characteristically have a language and culture all their own that further sets them apart. To avoid misinterpretation, clarify terms frequently. Occasionally adolescents refuse to answer or answer only in monosyllables. Usually this happens when they are opposed to the contact or do not yet feel safe enough to reveal themselves. In this instance confine discussions to irrelevant topics to reduce the element of threat until such time as they feel more secure. Be alert for signals that indicate they are ready to talk. The major sources of concern for adolescents are attitudes and feelings toward sex, substance abuse, relationships with parents, peer-group acceptance, and developing a sense of identity.

Interviewing the adolescent presents some special situations. The first may be whether to talk with the adolescent alone, with the adolescent and parents together, or with each individually. Of course, if the adolescent is alone there is no question except whether to suggest to the teenager that the parents may be interviewed at another time. If the parents and teenager are together, talking with the adolescent first has the advantage of immediately identifying with the young person, thus fostering the interpersonal relationship. However, talking with the parents initially may provide insight into the family relationship. In either case, give both parties an opportunity to be included in the interview. If time constraints are important, such as during history taking, clarify

Guidelines

COMMUNICATING WITH ADOLESCENTS

Build a foundation

Spend time together.
Encourage expression of ideas and feelings.
Respect their views.
Tolerate differences.
Praise good points.
Respect their privacy.
Set a good example.

Communicate effectively

Give undivided attention.
Listen, listen, listen.
Be courteous, calm, and open-minded.
Try not to overreact. If you do, take a break.
Avoiding judging or criticizing.
Avoid the "third degree" of continuous questioning.
Choose important issues when taking a stand.
After taking a stand:
- Think through all options.
- Make expectations clear.

these matters at the onset to avoid appearing to "take sides" by talking more with one person than with the other.

Confidentiality is of great importance when interviewing adolescents. Explain to parents and teenagers the limits of confidentiality, specifically that young persons' disclosures will not be shared unless they indicate a need for intervention, as in the case of suicidal behavior.

Another dilemma in interviewing adolescents is that two views of a problem commonly exist—the teenager's and the parent's. Clarification of the problem is a major task. However, providing both parties with an opportunity to discuss their perceptions in an open and unbiased atmosphere can, by itself, be therapeutic. Demonstrating positive communication skills can help families communicate more effectively (see the Guidelines box on p. 874).

COMMUNICATION TECHNIQUES

In addition to conventional interviewing methods such as reflection and open-ended questions, a number of techniques encourage family members to express their thoughts and feelings in a less directive and confrontational manner. Several approaches are projective—they present nonspecific material that enables individuals to externalize or project inner aspects of themselves to others.

A variety of verbal techniques can be used to encourage communication. Some of these techniques can be used to pose questions or explore concerns in a less threatening manner. Others can be presented as "word games," which are often well received by children. However, for many children and adults, talking about feelings is difficult, and verbal communication may be more stressful than supportive. In such instances several nonverbal techniques can be used to encourage communication.

Both verbal and nonverbal techniques are described in Box 31-2. Because of the importance of play in communicating with children, play is discussed more extensively in the following section. Any of the verbal or nonverbal techniques can give rise to strong feelings that surface unexpectedly. Be prepared to handle them or to recognize when issues go beyond your ability to deal with them. At that point, consider an appropriate referral.

Play

Play is a universal language of children. It is one of the most important forms of communication and can be an effective technique in relating to children. Clues about physical, intellectual, and social developmental progress can often be gleaned from the form and complexity of a child's play behaviors. Play requires a minimum of equipment or none at all. Therapeutic play is often used to reduce the trauma of illness and hospitalization (Chapter 41) and to prepare children for therapeutic procedures (Chapter 42).

Because their ability to perceive precedes their ability to transmit, small infants respond to activities that register on their senses. Patting, stroking, and other skin play convey messages. Repetitive actions such as stretching infants' arms out to the side while they are lying on their back and then folding them across the chest or raising and revolving the legs in a bicycling motion will elicit pleasurable sounds. Colorful items to catch the eye or interesting sounds such as a ticking clock, chimes, bells, or singing can be used to attract children's attention.

Older infants respond to simple games. The old game of peekaboo is an excellent means of initiating communication with infants while maintaining a "safe," nonthreatening distance. After this intermittent eye-to-eye contact, the nurse is no longer viewed as a stranger but as someone who is a friend. This communication can be followed by touch games. Clapping an infant's hands together for pat-a-cake or wiggling the toes for "this little piggy" delights an infant or small child. Much of the nursing assessment can be carried out with the use of games and simple play equipment while the infant remains in the safety of the parent's arms or lap. Talking to a foot or other part of the child's body is an effective tactic.

The nurse can capitalize on the natural curiosity of small children by playing games such as "Which hand do you take?" and "Guess what I have in my hand" or by manipulating items such as a flashlight or stethoscope. Finger games are very useful. More elaborate materials such as puppets and replicas of familiar or unfamiliar items serve as excellent means to communicate with small children. The variety and extent are limited only by the nurse's imagination.

Through play children reveal their perceptions of interpersonal relationships with their family, friends, or hospital personnel. Children may also reveal the wide scope of knowledge they have acquired from listening to others around them. For example, through needle play, children may disclose how carefully they have watched each procedure by precisely duplicating the technical skills. They may also reveal how well they remember those who performed procedures. One child who painstakingly reenacted every detail of a tedious medical procedure also played the role of the physician who had repeatedly shouted at her to be still for the long ordeal. Her anger at him was most evident during the play session and revealed the cause for her abrupt withdrawal and passive hostility toward the medical and nursing staff following the test.

Play sessions serve not only as assessment tools for determining children's awareness and perception of their illness but also as methods of intervention and evaluation. In the previous example, when the child revealed anger toward the physician, the nurse acted the part of the patient but this time did not accept the physician's harsh commands to stay still. Instead the nurse said to the physician all the things the child had wished she could say.

Subsequent play sessions can also be used for evaluation of the child's progress. A change in the type of drawing or the theme of the play may indicate progression toward or away from the ability to deal with anxiety.

History Taking

PERFORMING A HEALTH HISTORY

The format used for history taking may be (1) *direct*—the nurse asks for information via direct interview with the informant, or (2) *indirect*—the informant supplies the information by completing some type of questionnaire. The direct method is superior to the indirect approach or a combination of both. However, in view of time constraints, the direct approach is not always practical. If the direct approach cannot be used, review parents' written responses and question them regarding any unusual answers. The categories listed in Box 31-3 encompass children's current and past health status and information about their psychosocial environment.

BOX 31-2
Creative Communication Techniques with Children

VERBAL TECHNIQUES

"I" messages

Relate a feeling about a behavior in terms of "I."
Describe the effect the behavior had on the person.
Avoid the use of "you."
"You" messages are judgmental and provoke defensiveness.
Example: "You" message—"You are being very uncooperative about doing your treatments."
Example: "I" message—"I am concerned about how the treatments are going because I want to see you get better."

Third-person technique

Involves expressing a feeling in terms of a third person ("he," "she," "they").
Is less threatening than directly asking children how they feel because it gives them an opportunity to agree or disagree without being defensive.
Example: "Sometimes when a person is sick a lot, he feels angry and sad because he cannot do what others can." Either wait silently for a response or encourage a reply with a statement such as "Did you ever feel that way?"
This approach allows children three choices: (1) to agree and, hopefully, express how they feel; (2) to disagree; or (3) to remain silent, in which case they probably have such feelings but are unable to express them at this time.

Facilitative responding

Involves careful listening and reflecting back to patients the feelings and content of their statements.
Responses are empathic and nonjudgmental and legitimize the person's feelings.
Formula for facilitative responses: "You feel ______________ because ______________."
Example: If child states, "I hate coming to the hospital and getting needles," a facilitative response is, "You feel unhappy because of all the things that are done to you."

Storytelling

Uses the language of children to probe into areas of their thinking while bypassing conscious inhibitions or fears.
Simplest technique is asking children to relate a story about an event, such as "being in the hospital."
Other approaches:
Show children a picture of a particular event, such as a child in a hospital with other people in the room, and ask them to describe the scene.
Cut out comic strips, remove words, and have the child add statements for scenes.

Mutual storytelling

Reveals the child's thinking and attempts to change the child's perceptions or fears by retelling a somewhat different story (more therapeutic approach than storytelling).
Begins by asking the child to tell a story about something, followed by another story told by the nurse that is similar to the child's tale but with differences that help the child in problem areas.
Example: The child's story is about going to the hospital and never seeing his or her parents again. The nurse's story is also about a child (using different names but similar circumstances) in a hospital whose parents visit everyday in the evening after work until the child is better and goes home with them.

Bibliotherapy

Uses books in a therapeutic and supportive process.*
Provides children with an opportunity to explore an event that is similar to their own but sufficiently different to allow them to distance themselves from it and remain in control.
General guidelines for using bibliotherapy are the following:
Assess the child's emotional and cognitive development in terms of readiness to understand the book's message.
Be familiar with the book's content (intended message or purpose) and the age for which it is written.
Read the book to the child if the child is unable to read.
Explore the meaning of the book with the child by having the child do the following:
Retell the story
Read a special section with the nurse or parent
Draw a picture related to the story and discuss the drawing
Talk about the characters
Summarize the moral or meaning of the story

Dreams

Often reveal unconscious and repressed thoughts and feelings.
Ask the child to talk about a dream or nightmare.
Explore with the child what meaning the dream could have.

"What if" questions

Encourage the child to explore potential situations and to consider different problem-solving options.
Example: "What if you got sick and had to go the hospital?" Children's responses reveal what they know already and what they are curious about and provide an opportunity for helping children learn coping skills, especially in potentially dangerous situations.

Three wishes

Involves asking, "If you could have any three things in the world, what would they be?"
If the child answers, "That all my wishes come true," ask the child for specific wishes.

Rating game

Uses some type of rating scale (numbers, sad to happy faces) to rate an event or feeling.
Example: Instead of asking youngsters how they feel, ask how their day has been "on a scale of 1 to 10, with 10 being the best."

Word association game

Involves stating key words and asking children to say the first word they think of when they hear the word.
Start with neutral words and then introduce more anxiety-producing words, such as "illness," "needles," "hospitals," and "operation."
Select key words that relate to some relevant event in the child's life.

Sentence completion

Involves presenting a partial statement and having the child complete it.
Some sample statements are the following
The thing I like best (least) about school is ______________.
The best (worst) age to be is ______________.
The most (least) fun thing I ever did was ______________.

* See resources for children's books in the Bibliography at the end of this chapter.

BOX 31-2
Creative Communication Techniques with Children—cont'd

The thing I like most (least) about my parents is ________.
The one thing I would change about my family is ________.
If I could be anything I wanted, I would be ________.
The thing I like most (least) about myself is ________.

Pros and cons

Involves selecting a topic, such as "being in the hospital," and having child list "five good things and five bad things" about it.
Is an exceptionally valuable technique when applied to relationships, such as things family members like and dislike about each other.

NONVERBAL TECHNIQUES

Writing

Is an alternative communication approach for older children and adults.
Specific suggestions include the following:
Keep a journal or diary.
Write down feelings or thoughts that are difficult to express.
Write "letters" that are never mailed (a variation is making up a "pen pal" to write to).
Keep an account of the child's progress from both a physical and an emotional viewpoint.

Drawing

Is one of the most valuable forms of communication—both nonverbal (from looking at the drawing) and verbal (from the child's story of the picture).
Children's drawings tell a great deal about them because they are projections of their inner selves.
Spontaneous drawing involves giving child a variety of art supplies and providing the opportunity to draw.
Directed drawing involves a more specific direction, such as "draw a person" or the "three themes" approach (state three things about the child and ask the child to choose one and draw a picture).

Guidelines for evaluating drawings

Use spontaneous drawings and evaluate more than one drawing whenever possible.
Interpret drawings in light of other available information about the child and family.
Interpret drawings as a whole rather than focusing on specific details of the drawing.
Consider individual elements of the drawing that may be significant:
Gender of figure drawn first—Usually relates to child's perception of own gender role
Size of individual figures—Expresses importance, power, or authority
Order in which figures are drawn—Expresses priority in terms of importance
Child's position in relation to other family members—Expresses feelings of status or alliance
Exclusion of a member—May denote feeling of not belonging or a desire to eliminate
Accentuated parts—Usually express concern for areas of special importance (e.g., large hands may be a sign of aggression)
Absence of or rudimentary arms and hands—Suggest timidity, passivity, or intellectual immaturity; tiny, unstable feet may be an expression of insecurity, and hidden hands may mean guilt feelings
Placement of drawing on the page and type of stroke—Free use of paper and firm, continuous strokes express security, whereas drawings restricted to a small area and lightly drawn in broken or wavering lines may be a sign of insecurity
Erasures, shading, or cross-hatching—Expresses ambivalence, concern, or anxiety about a particular area

Magic

Uses simple magic tricks to help establish rapport with a child, encourage compliance with health interventions, and provide effective distraction during painful procedures.
Although the "magician" talks, no verbal response from the child is required.

Play

Is the universal language and "work" of children.
Tells a great deal about children because they project their inner selves through the activity.
Spontaneous play involves giving the child a variety of play materials and providing the opportunity to play.
Directed play involves a more specific direction such as providing medical equipment or a dollhouse for focused reasons (e.g., exploring child's fear of injections or exploring family relationships).

Identifying Information

Much of the identifying information may already be available from other recorded sources. However, if the parent and youngster seem anxious, use this opportunity to ask about such information to help them feel more comfortable.

Informant. One of the important elements of identifying information is the informant, the person(s) who furnished the information. Record (1) who the person is (child, parent, or other), (2) an impression of reliability and willingness to communicate, and (3) any special circumstances, such as the use of an interpreter or conflicting answers by more than one person.

Chief Complaint

The chief complaint is the specific reason for the child's visit to the clinic, office, or hospital. It may be viewed as the theme, with the present illness as the description of the problem. The chief complaint is elicited by asking open-ended neutral questions such as "What seems to be the matter?" "How may I help you?" or "Why did you come here today?" Avoid labeling-type questions such as "How are you sick?" or "What is the problem?" because it is possible that the reason for the visit is not an illness or problem.

Occasionally it is difficult to isolate one symptom or problem as the chief complaint because the parent may identify many. In this situation be as specific as possible when asking

BOX 31-3
Outline of a Pediatric Health History

Identifying information

1. Name
2. Address
3. Telephone
4. Birthdate and place
5. Race/ethnic group
6. Gender
7. Religion
8. Date of interview
9. Informant

Chief complaint (CC)—To establish the major *specific* reason for the child's and parents' seeking professional health attention

Present illness (PA)—To obtain *all* details related to the chief complaint

Past history (PH)—To elicit a profile of the child's previous illnesses, injuries, or operations

1. Birth history (pregnancy, labor, and delivery, perinatal history)
2. Previous illnesses, injuries, or operations
3. Allergies
4. Current medications
5. Immunizations
6. Growth and development
7. Habits

Review of systems (ROS)—To elicit information concerning any potential health problem

1. General
2. Integument
3. Head
4. Eyes
5. Ears
6. Nose
7. Mouth
8. Throat
9. Neck
10. Chest
11. Respiratory
12. Cardiovascular
13. Gastrointestinal
14. Genitourinary
15. Gynecologic
16. Musculoskeletal
17. Neurologic
18. Endocrine

Family medical history—To identify the presence of genetic traits or diseases that have familial tendencies and to assess exposure to a communicable disease in a family member and family habits that may affect the child's health, such as smoking and other chemical use

Psychosocial history—To elicit information about the child's self-concept

Sexual history—To elicit information concerning the child's sexual concerns and/or activities and any pertinent data regarding adults' sexual activity that influence the child

Family history—To develop an understanding of the child as an individual and as a member of a family and a community

1. Family composition
2. Home and community environment
3. Occupation and education of family members
4. Cultural and religious traditions
5. Family function and relationships

Nutritional assessment—To elicit information on the adequacy of the child's nutritional intake and need

1. Dietary intake
2. Clinical examination

questions. For example, asking informants to state which *one* problem or symptom prompted them to seek help now may help them focus on the most immediate concern.

Present Illness

The history of the present illness* is a narrative of the chief complaint from its earliest onset through its progression to the present. Its four major components are (1) the details of *onset,* (2) a complete *interval* history, (3) the *present* status, and (4) the reason for seeking help *now.* The focus of the present illness is on all factors relevant to the main problem, even if they have disappeared or changed during the onset, interval, and present.

Analyzing a symptom. Because pain is often the most characteristic symptom denoting the onset of a physical problem, it is used as an example for analysis of a symptom. Assessment includes (1) type, (2) location, (3) severity, (4) duration, and (5) influencing factors (see the Guidelines box on p. 879, left; see also Pain Assessment, Chapter 41).

Past History

The past history contains information relating to all previous aspects of the child's health status and concentrates on several areas that are ordinarily deleted in the history of an adult, such as birth history, detailed feeding history, immunizations, and growth and development. Because a great deal of data are included in this section, use a combination of open-ended and fact-finding questions. For example, begin interviewing for each section with an open-ended statement, such as "Tell me about your child's birth," to provide the informants with the opportunity to relate what they think is most important. Ask fact-finding questions related to specific details whenever necessary to focus the interview on certain topics.

Birth history. The birth history includes all data concerning (1) the mother's health during pregnancy, (2) the labor and delivery, and (3) the infant's condition immediately after birth. Because prenatal influences have significant effects on a child's physical and emotional development, a thorough investigation of the birth history is essential. Because parents may question what relevance pregnancy and birth have on the child's present condition, particularly if the child is past infancy, explain why such questions are included. An appropriate statement may be, "I will be asking you some questions about your pregnancy and . . . (refer to child by name) birth. Your answers will give me a more complete picture of his (or her) overall health."

Because emotional factors also affect the outcome of pregnancy and the subsequent parent-child relationship, investigate (1) concurrent crises during pregnancy, and (2) prenatal attitudes toward the fetus. It is best to approach the topic of parental acceptance of pregnancy through indirect questioning. Asking parents if the pregnancy was planned is a leading statement because they may respond affirmatively for fear of criticism if the pregnancy was unexpected. Rather, encourage parents to disclose their true reactions by referring to specific

*The term *illness* is used in its broadest sense to denote any problem of a physical, emotional, or psychosocial nature. It is actually a history of the chief complaint.

Guidelines

ANALYZING THE SYMPTOM: PAIN

Type—Be as specific as possible. With young children, asking the parents how they know the child is in pain may help describe its type, location, and severity. For example, a parent may state, "My child must have a severe earache because she pulls at her ears, rolls her head on the floor, and screams. Nothing seems to help." Help older children describe the "hurt" by asking them if it is sharp, throbbing, dull, aching, or stabbing. Record whatever words they use in quotes.

Location—Be specific. "Stomach pains" is too general a description. Children can better localize the pain if they are asked to "point with one finger to where it hurts" or to "point to where Mommy or Daddy would put a Band-Aid." Determine if the pain radiates by asking, "Does the pain stay there or move? Show me with your finger where the pain goes."

Severity—Best determined by finding out how it affects the child's usual behavior. Pain that prevents a child from playing, interacting with others, sleeping, and eating is most often severe. Assess pain intensity using a rating scale, such as a numeric scale or faces scale (see Table 41-2).

Duration—Include the duration, onset, and frequency. Describe in terms of activity and behavior, such as "pain lasted all night because child refused to sleep and cried intermittently."

Influencing factors—Include anything that causes a change in the type, location, severity, or duration of the pain: (1) precipitating events (those that cause or increase the pain), (2) relieving events (those that lessen the pain, such as medications), (3) temporal events (times when the pain is relieved or increased), (4) positional events (standing, sitting, lying down), and (5) associated events (meals, stress, coughing).

facts relating to the pregnancy, such as the spacing between offspring, an extended or short interval between marriage and conception, or the concurrent experience of pregnancy and adolescence. The parent can choose to explore such statements with further explanations or, for the moment, may not be able to reveal such feelings. If the parent remains silent, refocus on this topic later in the interview.

Dietary history. Because parental concerns are common and nursing interventions are important in ensuring optimum nutrition, the dietary history is discussed in detail at the end of this chapter.

Previous illnesses, injuries, and operations. When inquiring about past illnesses, begin with a general statement such as "What other illnesses has your child had?" Because parents are most likely to recall serious health problems, ask specifically about colds, earaches, and childhood diseases such as measles, rubella (German measles), chickenpox, mumps, pertussis (whooping cough), diphtheria, tuberculosis, scarlet fever, strep throat, tonsillitis, or allergic manifestations.

In addition to illnesses, ask about injuries that required medical intervention, operations, and any other reason for

Guidelines

TAKING AN ALLERGY HISTORY

Ask the following questions:

- Are you allergic to any medication or other product, such as latex (e.g., rubber gloves, balloons, catheters)? If yes, what is (are) you allergic to and in what form?
- What type of reaction did you have?
- How soon after the therapy was started or you came in contact with the product did this occur?
- How long ago did the reaction occur?
- Who told you that it was an allergic reaction?
- Have you taken this product or other drugs of similar class after this reaction occurred? If yes, did you experience similar problems?

Modified from Pau A, Morgan J, Terlingo A: Drug allergy documentation by physicians, nurses and medical students, *Am J Hosp Pharm* 46(3):570-573, 1989.

hospitalization, including the dates of each incident. It is important to focus on injuries such as accidental falls, poisonings, chokings, or burns, because these injuries may be a potential area for parental guidance.

Allergies. Ask about commonly known allergic disorders, such as hay fever and asthma, and about unusual reactions to drugs, food, latex products (see Spina Bifida, Chapter 52), or other contact agents such as poisonous plants, animals, household products, or fabrics. If asked appropriate questions, most people can give reliable information about drug reactions (see the Guidelines box above).

Nursing ALERT

Information about allergic reactions to drugs or other products is essential. Failure to document a serious reaction places the child at risk if the agent is given.

Current medications. Inquire about current drug regimens, including vitamins, antipyretics (especially aspirin), antibiotics, antihistamines, decongestants, or antitussives. List all medications, including name, dose, schedule, duration, and reason for administration. Parents are often unaware of the actual name of the drug. Whenever possible, ask parents to bring the containers with them to the next visit, or ask them for the name of the pharmacy and call for a list of all the child's recent prescription medications. However, this list will not include over-the-counter medications.

Immunizations. A record of all immunizations is essential. Because many parents are unaware of the exact name and date of each immunization, the most reliable source of information is a hospital, clinic, or private practitioner's record. All immunizations and "boosters" are listed, stating (1) the name of the specific disease, (2) the number of injections, (3) the dosage (sometimes lesser amounts are given if a reaction is anticipated), (4) the ages when administered, and (5) the occurrence of any reaction following the immunization.

Nursing ALERT

Inquire about previous administration of any horse or other foreign serum, recent administration of gamma globulin or blood transfusion, and anaphylactic reactions to neomycin or chicken eggs.

Growth and development. The most important previous growth patterns to record are (1) approximate weight at 6 months, 1 year, 2 years, and 5 years of age; (2) approximate length at ages 1 and 4 years; and (3) dentition, including age of onset, number of teeth, and symptoms during teething. Developmental milestones include (1) age of holding up head steadily, (2) age of sitting alone without support, (3) age of walking without assistance, (4) age of saying first words with meaning, (5) present grade in school, (6) scholastic grades, and (7) interaction with other children, peers, and adults.

Use specific and detailed questions when inquiring about each developmental milestone. For example "sitting up" can mean many different activities, such as sitting propped up, sitting in someone's lap, sitting with support, sitting up alone but in a hyperflexed position for assisted balance, or sitting up unsupported with the back slightly rounded. A clue to a misunderstanding of the requested activity may be an unusually early age of achievement (see Developmental Assessment, Chapter 32).

Habits. Habits are an important area to explore (Box 31-4). Parents often express concerns during this part of the history. Encourage their input by saying, "Please tell me any concerns you have about your child's habits, activities, or development." Investigate further any concerns that are expressed.

One of the most common concerns relates to sleep. Many children develop a normal sleep pattern, and all that is required during the assessment is a general overview of nighttime sleep and nap schedules. However, a number of children also develop sleep problems (see Chapters 33 and 35). When sleep problems occur, a more detailed sleep history is required to guide appropriate interventions.*

Habits related to the use of chemicals apply primarily to older children and adolescents. If a youngster admits to smoking, drinking, or drug use, ask about the quantity and frequency. Questions such as "Have you ever had a drinking or drug problem?" or "When was the last time you had a drink or took drugs?" may yield more reliable data than questions such as "How much do you drink?" or "How often do you drink or take drugs?"

Clarify that "drinking" includes all types of alcohol, such as beer and wine. When quantities such as a "glass" of wine or a "can" of beer are given, ask about the size of the container.

If older children deny the use of chemical substances, inquire about past experimentation. Asking, "You mean you never tried to smoke or drink?" implies that the nurse expects some such activity, and the youngster may be more inclined to answer truthfully. Be aware of the confidential nature of such questioning, the adverse effect that the parents' presence may have on the adolescent's willingness to answer, and that self-report may not be an accurate account of chemical abuse.

*A sleep history and a sleep chart for the family to record the child's daily sleep and wake activities is available in Wong DL: *Wong and Whaley's clinical manual of pediatric nursing*, ed 4, St Louis, 1996, Mosby.

BOX 31-4
Habits to Explore During Health Interview

Behavior patterns, such as nail-biting, thumb-sucking, pica (habitual ingestion of nonfood substances), rituals ("security" blanket or toy), and unusual movements (head-banging, rocking, overt masturbation, and walking on toes)
Activities of daily living, such as hour of sleep and arising, duration of nighttime sleep and naps, type and duration of exercise, regularity of stools and urination, age of toilet training, and occurrences of daytime or nighttime bed-wetting
Unusual disposition, as well as response to frustration
Use or abuse of alcohol, drugs, coffee, or tobacco products

Review of Systems

The review of systems is a specific review of each body system, similar to the order of the physical examination (see the Guidelines box on p. 881). Often the history of the present illness provides a complete review of the system involved in the chief complaint. Because asking questions about other body systems may appear unrelated and irrelevant to the parents or child, precede the questioning with an explanation of why the data are needed (similar to the explanation concerning the relevance of the birth history), and reassure that the child's main problem has not been forgotten.

Begin the review of a specific system with a broad statement such as "How has your child's general health been?" or "Has your child had any problems with his eyes?" If the parent states that there have been past problems with some body function, pursue this with an encouraging statement such as "Tell me more about that." If the parent denies any problems, query for specific symptoms such as "No headaches, bumping into objects, or squinting?" If the parent reconfirms the absence of such symptoms, record positive statements in the history, such as "Mother denies headaches, bumping into objects, or squinting." In this way, anyone who reviews the health history is aware of exactly what symptoms were investigated.

Family Medical History

The family medical history is used primarily for the purpose of discovering the potential existence of hereditary or familial diseases in the parents and child. In general, it is confined to first-degree relatives (parents, siblings, grandparents, and immediate aunts and uncles). Information for each family member includes age, marital status, state of health if living, cause of death if deceased, and any evidence of the following conditions: heart disease, hypertension, cancer, diabetes mellitus, obesity, congenital anomalies, allergy, asthma, seizures, tuberculosis, sickle cell disease, mental retardation, mental disorders such as depression or psychosis, emotional problems, syphilis, or rheumatic fever. Confirm the accuracy of the reported disorders by inquiring about the symptoms, course, treatment, and sequelae of each diagnosis.

Guidelines

REVIEW OF SYSTEMS

General—overall state of health, fatigue, recent and/or unexplained weight gain or loss (period of time for either), contributing factors (change of diet, illness, altered appetite), exercise tolerance, fevers (time of day), chills, night sweats (unrelated to climatic conditions), frequent infections, general ability to carry out activities of daily living

Integument—pruritus, pigment or other color changes, acne, eruptions, rashes (location), tendency for bruising, petechiae, excessive dryness, general texture, disorders or deformities of nails, hair growth or loss, hair color change (for adolescent, use of hair dyes or other potentially toxic substances such as hair straighteners)

Head—headaches, dizziness, injury (specific details)

Eyes—visual problems (ask about behaviors indicative of blurred vision such as bumping into objects, clumsiness, sitting very close to television, holding a book close to face, writing with head near desk, squinting, rubbing the eyes, bending head in an awkward position), cross-eye (strabismus), eye infections, edema of lids, excessive tearing, use of glasses or contact lenses, date of last optic examination

Nose—nosebleeds (epistaxis), constant or frequent running or stuffy nose, nasal obstruction (difficulty in breathing), alteration or loss of sense of smell

Ears—earaches, discharge, evidence of hearing loss (ask about behaviors such as need to repeat requests, loud speech, inattentive behavior), results of any previous auditory testing

Mouth—mouth breathing, gum bleeding, toothaches, tooth-brushing, use of fluoride, difficulty with teething (symptoms), last visit to dentist (especially if temporary dentition is complete), response to dentist

Throat—sore throats, difficulty in swallowing, choking (especially when chewing food—may be from poor chewing habits), hoarseness, or other voice irregularities

Neck—pain, limitation of movement, stiffness, difficulty in holding head straight (torticollis), thyroid enlargement, enlarged nodes or other masses

Chest—breast enlargement, discharge, masses, enlarged axillary nodes (for adolescent female, ask about breast self-examination)

Respiratory—chronic cough, frequent colds (number per year), wheezing, shortness of breath at rest or on exertion, difficulty in breathing, sputum production, infections (pneumonia, tuberculosis), date of last chest x-ray examination, and skin reaction from tuberculin testing

Cardiovascular—cyanosis or fatigue on exertion, history of heart murmur or rheumatic fever, anemia, date of last blood count, blood type, recent transfusion

Gastrointestinal (much of this in regard to appetite, food tolerance, and elimination habits has been asked elsewhere)—nausea, vomiting (not associated with eating, may be indicative of brain tumor or increased intracranial pressure), jaundice or yellowing skin or sclera, belching, flatulence, recent change in bowel habits (blood in stools, change of color, diarrhea, or constipation)

Genitourinary—pain on urination, frequency, hesitancy, urgency, hematuria, nocturia, polyuria, unpleasant odor to urine, force of stream, discharge, change in size of scrotum, date of last urinalysis (for adolescent, sexually transmitted disease, type of treatment; for male adolescent, ask about testicular self-examination)

Gynecologic—menarche, date of last menstrual period, regularity or problems with menstruation, vaginal discharge, pruritus, date and result of last Pap smear (include obstetric history as discussed under birth history when applicable); if sexually active, type of contraception, sexually transmitted disease, type of treatment

Musculoskeletal—weakness, clumsiness, lack of coordination, unusual movements, back or joint stiffness, muscle pains or cramps, abnormal gait, deformity, fractures, serious sprains, activity level

Neurologic—seizures, tremors, dizziness, loss of memory, general affect, fears, nightmares, speech problems, any unusual habits

Endocrine—intolerance to weather changes, excessive thirst and/or urination, excessive sweating, salty taste to skin, signs of early puberty

Geographic location. One of the important areas to explore when assessing the family health history is geographic location, including the birthplace and travel to different areas in or outside of the country for identification of possible exposure to endemic diseases. Although the primary interest focuses on the child's temporary residence in various localities, also inquire about close family members' travel, especially during tours of military service or business trips. Children are especially susceptible to parasitic infestation in areas of poor sanitary conditions and to vectorborne diseases, such as those from mosquitoes or ticks in warm and humid or heavily wooded regions.

Psychosocial History

In the traditional medical history a personal and social section is included that concentrates on children's personal status, such as school adjustment and any unusual habits, and on the family and home environment. Because several personal aspects are covered under development and habits and the social aspects are discussed in detail under Family Assessment, only those issues related to children's ability to cope and their general view of themselves in terms of self-concept are presented here (see Development of Self-Concept, Chapter 30).

Through observation obtain a general idea of how children handle themselves in terms of confidence in dealing with others, ability to answer questions, and coping with new situations. Observe the parent-child relationship for the types of messages sent to children about their coping skills and self-worth. Do the parents treat the child with respect, focusing on strengths, or is the interaction one of constant reprimands, with emphasis on weaknesses and faults? Do the parents help the child learn new coping strategies or support the ones the child uses?

Messages about body image are also conveyed through the parent-child interaction. Do the parents label the child and body parts, such as "bad boy," "skinny legs," or "ugly scar"? Do the parents handle the child gently, using soothing touch to calm an anxious child, or do they treat the child roughly, using slaps or restraint to force compliance? If the child touches certain parts of the body, such as the genitals, do the parents make comments that suggest a negative connotation?

With older children, many of the communication strategies discussed earlier in the chapter are useful in eliciting more definitive information about their coping and self-concept. Children can write down five things they like and dislike about themselves. Sentence completion statements such as "The thing I like best (or worst) about myself is ______," "If I could change one thing about myself, it would be ______," or "When I am scared, I ______," can be used.

Sexual History

The sexual history is an essential component of an adolescent's health assessment. The history uncovers areas of concern related to sexual activity, alerts the nurse to circumstances that may indicate screening for sexually transmitted diseases or testing for pregnancy, and provides information related to the need for sexual counseling, such as safe sex practices.

One approach toward initiating a conversation about sexual concerns is to begin with a history of peer interactions. Open-ended statements such as "Tell me about your social life," or "Who are your closest friends?" generally lead into a discussion of dating and sexual issues. To probe further, include questions about the adolescent's attitudes on such topics as sex education, "going steady," "living together," and premarital sex. Phrase questions to reflect concern rather than judgment or criticism of sexual practices.

In any conversation regarding sexual history, be aware of the language that is used in either eliciting or conveying sexual information. For example, avoid asking if the adolescent is "sexually active," because this term is broadly defined. "Are you having sex with anyone?" is probably the most direct and best understood question. Because homosexual experimentation may occur, refer to all sexual contacts in nongender terms such as "anyone" or "partners" rather than "girlfriends" or "boyfriends."

A detailed account of sexual partners is needed if the patient has a history, displays any of the symptoms, or asks for treatment of a sexually transmitted disease. A difficult but necessary part of the interview is to determine the sites of possible infection. Because sexual diseases can be contracted at any of the body orifices, inform the adolescent that a sexually transmitted disease can be acquired without visible signs of disease at nongenital sites.

Family Assessment

Assessment of the family structure and function is an important component of the history-taking process. Because the quality of the functional relationship between the child and family members is a major factor in emotional and physical health, family assessment is discussed separately and in greater detail apart from the more traditional health history.

Family assessment is the collection of data about the composition of the family and the relationships among its members. In its broadest sense **family** refers to all those individuals who are considered by the family member to be significant to the nuclear unit, including relatives, friends, and other social groups such as the school and church. Although family assessment is not family therapy, it can be and often is therapeutic. Involving family members in discussing family characteristics and activities often stimulates productive discussion and insight into family dynamics and relationships.

Because of the time involved in performing an in-depth family assessment as presented here, be selective in deciding when knowledge of family function may facilitate nursing care. During brief contacts with families a full assessment is not appropriate, and screening with one or two questions from each category may reflect the health of the family system or the potential need for additional assessment. Indications for performing a comprehensive family assessment are children receiving comprehensive well-child care, experiencing major stressful life events (e.g., chronic illness, disability, parental divorce, or death of a family member), requiring extensive home care, with developmental delays, with repeated accidental injuries and those with suspected child abuse, and with behavioral or physical problems that suggest family dysfunction as the etiology.

ASSESSMENT OF FAMILY STRUCTURE

Family structure refers to the composition of the family—who lives in the home—and those social, cultural, religious, and economic characteristics that influence the child's and family's overall psychobiologic health (see Chapters 28 and 29). Because the information elicited in this part of the history is often the most personal and confidential, include it toward the end of the interview, when rapport is well established.

The most common method of eliciting information on the family structure is interviewing family members. The principal areas of concern (Box 31-5) are (1) family composition, (2) home and community environment, (3) occupation and education of family members, and (4) cultural and religious traditions.

Nursing ALERT

In assessing family composition it is sometimes difficult to ascertain the status of the adult relationships. If the parent fails to mention the other parent, ask, "Where is the child's father (or mother)?" Avoid saying "husband" or "wife" because this assumes that only marital relationships exist.

Several structural assessment tools can be used to collect and record data about the family composition and environment. As with the interview method, such tools also provide information about relationships, although several additional methods should be used to assess family function.

A **sociogram** is a drawing of circles that indicates the significant persons in an individual's life; its use is appropriate for adults and children as young as 5 years of age. The person is given blank paper and a pencil with the following instructions: "Draw a circle to represent you. Around the circle draw circles to represent the most significant persons in your life and label each. Draw the circles in proximity to your circle to represent closeness. For example, the person who is most sig-

BOX 31-5
Family Assessment Interview

GENERAL GUIDELINES FOR FAMILY INTERVIEW

Schedule the interview with the family at a time that is most convenient for all parties; include as many family members as possible; clearly state the purpose of the interview.
Begin the interview by asking each person's name and their relationship to each other.
Restate the purpose of the interview and the objective.
Keep the initial conversation general to put members at ease and to learn the "big picture" of the family.
Identify major concerns and reflect these back to the family to be certain that all parties perceive the same message.
Terminate the interview with a summary of what was discussed and a plan for additional sessions if needed.

STRUCTURAL ASSESSMENT AREAS

Family Composition

Immediate members of the household (names, ages, and relationships)
Significant extended family members
Previous marriages, separations, deaths of spouses, or divorces

Home and Community Environment

Type of dwelling/number of rooms/occupants
Sleeping arrangements
Number of floors, accessibility of stairs, elevators
Adequacy of utilities
Safety features (fire escape, smoke detector, guardrails on windows, use of car restraint)
Environmental hazards (e.g., chipped paint, poor sanitation, pollution, heavy street traffic)
Availability and location of health facilities, schools, play areas
Relationship with neighbors
Recent crises or changes in home
Child's reaction/adjustment to recent stresses

Occupation and Education of Family Members

Types of employment
Work schedules
Work satisfaction
Exposure to environmental/industrial hazards
Sources of income and adequacy
Effect of illness on financial status
Highest degree or grade level attained

Cultural and Religious Traditions

Religious beliefs and practices
Cultural/ethnic beliefs and practices
Language spoken in home

Assessment questions include the following:

Does the family identify with a particular religious/ethnic group? Are both parents from that group?
How is religious/ethnic background part of family life?
What special religious/cultural traditions are practiced in the home (e.g., food choices and preparation)?
Where were family members born, and how long have they lived in this country?
What language does the family speak most often?
Do they speak/understand English?
What do they believe causes health or illness?
What religious/ethnic beliefs influence the family's perception of illness and its treatment?
What methods are used to prevent/treat illness?
How does the family know when a health problem needs medical attention?
Who is the person the family contacts when a member is ill?
Does the family rely on cultural/religious healers or remedies? If so, ask them to describe the type of healer or remedy.
Who does the family go to for support (clergy, medical healer, relatives)?
Does the family experience discrimination because of their race, beliefs, or practices? Ask them to describe.

FUNCTIONAL ASSESSMENT AREAS

Family Interactions and Roles

Interactions refer to ways family members relate to each other
Chief concern is amount of intimacy and closeness among the members, especially spouses
Roles refer to behaviors of people as they assume a different status or position

Observations include the following:

Family members' responses to each other (cordial, hostile, cool, loving, patient, short-tempered)
Obvious roles of leadership vs. submission
Support and attention shown to various members

Assessment questions include the following:

What activities does the family perform together?
Whom do family members talk to when something is bothering them?
What are members' household chores?
Who usually oversees what is happening with the children, such as at school or concerning their health?
How easy or difficult is it for the family to change or accept new responsibilities for household tasks?

Power, Decision Making, and Problem Solving

Power refers to individual member's control over others in family; manifested through family decision making and problem solving
Chief concern is clarity of boundaries of power between parents and children
One method of assessment involves offering a hypothetical conflict or problem, such as a child failing school, and asking family how they would handle this situation

Assessment questions include the following:

Who usually makes the decisions in the family?
If one parent makes a decision, can the child appeal to the other parent to change it?
What input do children have in making decisions or discussing rules?
Who makes and enforces the rules?
What happens when a rule is broken?

Communication

Concerned with clarity and directness of communication patterns

Observations include the following:

Who speaks to whom
If one person speaks for another or interrupts
If members appear disinterested when certain individuals speak
If there is agreement between verbal and nonverbal messages
Further assessment includes periodically asking family members if they understood what was just said and to repeat the message

Continued.

BOX 31-5
Family Assessment Interview—cont'd

Assessment questions include the following:

How often do family members wait until others are through talking before "having their say?"
Do parents or older siblings tend to lecture and preach?
Do parents tend to talk "down" to the children?

Expression of Feelings and Individuality

Concerned with personal space and freedom to grow with limits and structure needed for guidance
Observing patterns of communication offers clues to how freely feelings are expressed

Assessment questions include the following:

Is it OK for family members to get angry or sad?
Who gets angry most of the time? What do they do?
If someone is upset, how do other family members try to comfort this person?
Who comforts specific family members?
When someone wants to do something, such as try out for a new sport or get a job, what is the family's response (offer assistance, discouragement, or no advice)?

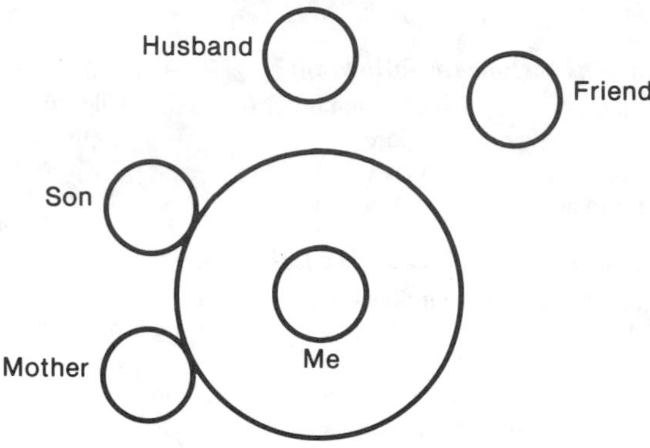

Fig. 31-4 Sociogram of mother with strong, unresolved grief feelings regarding loss of child.

nificant is the circle closest to you." Family members can label the relationships as supportive with a plus sign or negative with a minus sign.

Not only is the sociogram a portrait of the person's significant relationships, it may also uncover unresolved relationships (Fig. 31-4). After completing the sociogram, encourage the family to explore their feelings further with questions such as the following:

- How would you change the circles to improve relationships?
- How do you think you could accomplish these changes?
- If one person in the circle were to change, what effect do you think that would have on others in the circle?

ASSESSMENT OF FAMILY FUNCTION

Family function is concerned with how family members behaves toward one another and with the quality of the relationships. It is considered the most important component in determining "family health." Assessment of function requires more skill on the part of the interviewer than does assessment of structure and is best approached after structure has been assessed. As in assessment of family structure, the more traditional method of eliciting information on family function is to interview family members. The principal areas of concern are discussed in Box 31-5.

In addition to observing and interviewing the family to assess family function, several other methods are available and should be used as needed to obtain a comprehensive assessment. The following section discusses selected instruments that are reliable and valid but require little or no formal training and minimal time to administer.

The *Family APGAR (FAPGAR)* is a brief screening questionnaire designed to reflect a family member's satisfaction with the functional state of the family (Smilkstein, Ashworth, and Montano, 1982) (see the Appendix). The acronym APGAR is for Adaptation, Partnership, Growth, Affection, and Resolve (commitment). The acronym was chosen because it is familiar to health professionals, but it bears no relationship to the Apgar scoring system for newborns.

The questions in Box 31-6 can be used in the interview without the APGAR ratings to elicit similar types of information. It can be completed in approximately 5 minutes, can be used by families with traditional and alternative life-styles and from different cultures, and is appropriate for children age 10 years or older. Separate forms have been designed to assess relationships with friends and fellow workers, because these groups represent other significant sources of support.

The responses to the five questions are scored as follows: "Almost always"—2; "Some of the time"—1; and "Hardly ever"—0. Each score is totaled. Scores of 7 to 10 suggest a highly functional family; 4 to 6, a moderately dysfunctional family; and 0 to 3, a severely dysfunctional family. Also, a low score in any single item could signal family dysfunction. The family APGAR is not recommended for use with individuals from enmeshed (overly close) or "psychosomatic" families. Persons with health problems such as asthma, atopic dermatitis, or irritable bowel syndrome may report falsely high scores (Smilkstein, 1993).

Undoubtedly the richest environment for observing a child's development and interactions with family members is the home. Two tools that can be used to assess the child's home environment are the *Home Observation for Management of the Environment (HOME) Inventory** (Caldwell and Bradley, 1984) and the *Home Screening Questionnaire (HSQ)*†

*The forms and an administration manual are available for a fee from the **Center for Research on Teaching and Learning,** College of Education, University of Arkansas at Little Rock, 2801 S. University Ave., Little Rock, AK 72204; (501) 569-3422.

†The forms and manual are available for a fee from **Denver Developmental Materials, Inc.,** P.O. Box 6919, Denver, CO 80206-0919; (303) 355-4729 or (800) 419-4729.

BOX 31-6
Family APGAR

Definition	Functions Measured by the Family APGAR	Relevant Open-Ended Questions
Adaptation is the use of intrafamilial and extrafamilial resources for problem solving when family equilibrium is stressed during a crisis.	How resources are shared, or the degree to which a member is satisfied with the assistance received when family resources are needed	How have family members aided each other in time of need? In what way have family members received help or assistance from friends and community agencies?
Partnership is the sharing of decision making and nurturing responsibilities by family members.	How decisions are shared, or the member's satisfaction with mutuality in family communication and problem solving	How do family members communicate with each other about such matters as vacations, finances, medical care, large purchases, and personal problems?
Growth is the physical and emotional maturation and self-fulfillment that is achieved by family members through mutual support and guidance.	How nurturing is shared, or the member's satisfaction with the freedom available within the family to change roles and attain physical and emotional growth or maturation	How have family members changed during the past years? How has this change been accepted by family members? In what ways have family members aided each other in growing or developing independent life-styles? How have family members reacted to your desire for change?
Affection is the caring or loving relationship that exists among family members.	How emotional experiences are shared, or the member's satisfaction with the intimacy and emotional interaction that exists in the family	How have members of your family responded to emotional expressions, such as affection, love, sorrow, or anger?
Resolve is the commitment to devote time to other members of the family for physical and emotional nurturing. It also usually involves a decision to share wealth and space.	How time (and space and money) is shared, or the member's satisfaction with the time commitment that has been made to the family by its members	How do members of your family share time, space, and money?

Modified from Smilkstein G: The Family APGAR: a proposal for a family function test and its use by physicians, *J Fam Pract* 6(6):1231-1239, 1978.

(Frankenburg and Coons, 1986). Both are divided into two age groups—birth to 3 years of age and 3 to 6 years of age. HOME has an additional inventory for children ages 6 to 10 years. Forms are also available for children with moderate-to-severe disabilities in each of the three age groups for visual, auditory, orthopedic, and cognitive impairments. The HOME Inventory assesses the quality and quantity of the social, emotional, and cognitive support that is available to children in their home environment, including low income families and low-birth-weight children (Bradley et al, 1994).

Some of the HOME items require direct observation, whereas others necessitate questioning of the parents. Each item receives a "yes" or "no" response. The number of "yes" responses correlates with the amount of appropriate environmental stimulation. Any "no" responses indicate possible areas for intervention and counseling. Use of HOME requires approximately a 1-hour home visit with both the child and the major caregiver.

The HSQ was developed using HOME as a guide. The 0- to 3-year form consists of 30 items plus a checklist of toys available to the child in the home. The 3- to 6-year form has 34 items and a similar toy checklist. The questions are written at approximately a third- to sixth-grade reading level and, unlike the HOME, can be completed by the parents in any setting in approximately 15 to 20 minutes. Scoring directions are detailed in the manual and are based on credits for different answers. For each age group there is a minimum score for determining suspect or nonsuspect results.

Nutritional Assessment

DIETARY INTAKE

Knowledge of the child's dietary intake is a useful and practical component of a nutritional assessment. However, it is also one of the most difficult factors to assess. Individuals' recall of food consumption, especially amounts eaten, is often unreliable. In addition, people may be hesitant to reveal their eating patterns if they sense criticism from the nurse. People from different cultures may have difficulty adequately describing the types of food they eat. Despite these obstacles, a food intake record is essential. Several methods are available.

Regardless of the format used in recording food intake, every nutritional assessment should begin with a *dietary history*. The exact questions used to elicit a dietary history vary with the child's age. In general, the younger the child, the more specific and detailed the history should be. Box 31-7 provides a sample dietary history for children with additional questions regarding infant feeding.

BOX 31-7
Dietary History

What are the family's usual mealtimes?
Do family members eat together or at separate times?
Who does the family grocery shopping and meal preparation?
How much money is spent to buy food each week?
How are most foods prepared—baked, broiled, fried, other?
How often does the family or your child eat out?
What types of restaurants do you go to?
What types of food does your child typically eat at restaurants?
Does your child eat breakfast regularly?
Where does your child eat lunch?
What are your child's favorite foods, beverages, and snacks?
What are the average amounts eaten per day?
What foods are artificially sweetened?
What are your child's snacking habits?
When are sweet foods usually eaten?
What are your child's toothbrushing habits?
What special cultural practices are followed? What ethnic foods are eaten?
What foods and beverages does your child dislike?
How would you describe your child's usual appetite (hearty eater, picky eater)?
What are your child's feeding habits (breast, bottle, cup, spoon, eats by self, needs assistance, any special devices)?
Does your child take vitamins or other supplements? Do they contain iron or fluoride?
Are there any known or suspected food allergies? Is your child on a special diet?
Has your child lost or gained weight recently?
Are there any feeding problems (excessive fussiness, spitting up, colic, difficulty sucking or swallowing)? Are there any dental problems or appliances, such as braces, that affect eating?
What types of exercise does your child do regularly?
Is there a family history of cancer, diabetes, heart disease, high blood pressure, or obesity?

Additional Questions About Infants

What was the infant's birth weight? When did it double? Triple?
Was the infant premature?
Are you breastfeeding or have you breastfed your infant? For how long?
If you use a formula, what is the brand?
How long has the infant been taking it?
How many ounces does the infant drink each day?
Are you giving the infant cow's milk (whole, low-fat, skimmed)?
When did you start?
How many ounces does the infant drink each day?
Do you give your infant extra fluids (water, juice)?
If the infant takes a bottle to bed at nap or nighttime, what is in the bottle?
At what age did you start cereal, vegetables, meat or other protein sources, fruit/juice, finger food, table food?
Do you make your own baby food or use commercial foods, such as infant cereal?
Does the infant take a vitamin/mineral supplement? If so, what type?
Has the infant shown an allergic reaction to any food(s)? If so, list the foods and describe the reaction.
Does the infant spit up frequently, have unusually loose stools, or have hard, dry stools? If so, how often?
How often do you feed your infant?
How would you describe your infant's appetite?

The broad overview elicited from the dietary history can be helpful in evaluating food frequency records (Box 31-8). It also is concerned with financial and cultural factors that influence food selection and preparation (See the Cultural Considerations box below).

The most common and probably the easiest method of assessing daily intake is the *24-hour recall.* The child or parent recalls every item eaten in the past 24 hours and the approximate amounts. The 24-hour recall is most beneficial when it represents a typical day's intake. Some of the difficulties with a daily recall are the family's inability to remember exactly what was eaten and inaccurate estimation of portion size. To increase accuracy of reporting portion sizes, the use of food models and additional questioning are recommended. In general, this method is most useful in providing *qualitative* information about the child's diet.

Cultural Considerations

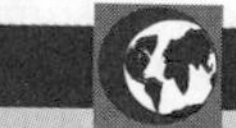

FOOD PRACTICES

Because cultural practices are very prevalent in food preparation, consider carefully the types of questions that are asked and the judgments made in regard to counseling. For example, some cultures such as Hispanic, black, and Native American include many vegetables, legumes, and starches in their diet that together provide sufficient essential amino acids, even though the actual amount of meat or dairy protein is low. (See Chapter 28).

To improve the reliability of the daily recall, the family can complete a *food diary* by recording every food and liquid consumed for a certain number of days. A 3-day record consisting of 2 weekdays and 1 weekend day is representative for most people. Providing specific charts to record intake can improve compliance. The family should record items immediately after eating.

A *food frequency questionnaire or record* (Box 31-8) provides information about the number of times in a day, week, or month a child consumes items from the different food groups. In general, it provides more of a qualitative overview but has the advantage of avoiding recall based on a "typical" day. It can be especially useful when verifying a food history or diary.

CLINICAL EXAMINATION

A significant amount of information regarding nutritional deficiencies is elicited from a clinical examination, especially from assessing the skin, hair, teeth, gums, lips, tongue, and eyes. Hair, skin, and mouth are vulnerable because of the rapid turnover of epithelial and mucosal tissue. Table 31-1 summarizes clinical signs of possible nutritional deficiency or excess. Few are diagnostic for a specific nutrient, and if suspi-

BOX 31-8
Food Frequency Record*

Food Group	Number of Servings (Day, Week)	Serving Size (in Cup, Tablespoon, or Ounce Portions)	Food Group	Number of Servings (Day, Week)	Serving Size (in Cup, Tablespoon, or Ounce Portions)
Breads/cereals/rice/pasta			***Milk/cheese/yogurt***		
Bread, tortilla			Milk		
Cooked pasta, rice, hot cereal			Cheese		
Dry cereal (not presweetened)			Yogurt		
Crackers			Pudding		
Muffins			Ice cream		
Other			Other		
Vegetables			***Other protein foods***		
Yellow or orange			Meat		
Green/leafy			Fish		
Other			Poultry		
			Egg		
			Peanut butter		
			Legumes (dried beans, peas)		
			Nuts		
			Other		
Fruits/juice			***Fats/oils/sweets***		
Citrus (orange, grapefruit, strawberries, lemon, lime, tangerine)			Butter, oil, margarine, mayonnaise, salad dressing		
Noncitrus			Soda, punch		
Other			Cake/cookie, etc.		
			Candy		
			Presweetened cereal		

*For comparison of actual intake with recommended intake, see Food Guide Pyramid, Fig. 44-1.

cious signs are found, they must be confirmed with dietary and biochemical data. Generally, the clinical examination does not reveal children *at risk* for a deficiency or excess.

Anthropometry, an essential parameter of nutritional status, is the measurement of height, weight, head circumference (in young children), proportions, skinfold thickness, and arm circumference. Height and head circumference reflect past nutrition, whereas weight, skinfold thickness, and arm circumference reflect present nutritional status, especially of protein and fat reserves. Skinfold thickness is a measurement of the body's fat content, because approximately one half of the body's total fat stores are directly beneath the skin. The upper arm muscle circumference is correlated with measurements of total muscle mass. Because muscle serves as the body's major protein reserve, this measurement is considered an index of the body's protein stores. Ideally growth measurements are recorded over time, and comparisons are made regarding the *velocity* of growth based on previous and present values. Techniques for anthropomorphic measurement are discussed in Chapter 32.

Numerous *biochemical tests* are available for assessing nutritional status and include analysis of plasma, blood cells, urine, or tissues from liver, bone, hair, and fingernails. Many of these tests are complicated and are not performed routinely. Common laboratory procedures for nutritional status include measurement of hemoglobin, hematocrit, transferrin, albumin, creatinine, and nitrogen. Laboratory values for these tests and more specific nutrient measurements are given in the Appendix.

EVALUATION OF NUTRITIONAL ASSESSMENT

After collecting the data needed for a thorough nutritional assessment, evaluate the findings to plan appropriate counseling. From the data, assess whether the child is (1) malnourished, (2) at risk for becoming malnourished, or (3) well nourished with adequate reserves.

Analyze the daily food diary for the variety and amounts of foods suggested in the Food Guide Pyramid (see Fig. 44-1). For example, if the list includes no vegetables, inquire about this

TABLE 31-1 Clinical assessment of nutritional status

EVIDENCE OF ADEQUATE NUTRITION	EVIDENCE OF DEFICIENT OR EXCESS NUTRITION	DEFICIENCY/EXCESS*
General growth		
Within 5th and 95th percentiles for height, weight, and head circumference	Below 5th or above 95th percentiles for growth	Protein, calories, fats, and other essential nutrients, especially A, pyridoxine, niacin, calcium, iodine, manganese, zinc
Steady gain with expected growth spurts during infancy and adolescence	Absence of or delayed growth spurts; poor weight gain	
Sexual development appropriate for age	Delayed sexual development	Excess vitamin A, D
Skin		
Smooth, slightly dry to touch	Hardening and scaling	Vitamin A
Elastic and firm	Seborrheic dermatitis	Excess niacin
Absence of lesions	Dry, rough, petechiae	Riboflavin
Color appropriate to genetic background	Delayed wound healing	Vitamin C
	Scaly dermatitis on exposed surfaces	Riboflavin, vitamin C, zinc
	Wrinkled, flabby	Niacin
	Crusted lesions around orifices, especially nares	Protein and calories
		Zinc
	Pruritus	Excess vitamin A, riboflavin, niacin
	Poor turgor	Water, sodium
	Edema	Protein, thiamin
		Excess sodium
	Yellow tinge (jaundice)	Vitamin B_{12}
		Excess vitamin A, niacin
	Depigmentation	Protein, calories
	Pallor (anemia)	Pyridoxine, folic acid, vitamin B_{12}, C, E (in premature infants), iron
		Excess vitamin C, zinc
	Paresthesia	Excess riboflavin
Hair		
Lustrous, silky, strong, elastic	Stringy, friable, dull, dry, thin	Protein, calories
	Alopecia	Protein, calories, zinc
	Depigmentation	Protein, calories, copper
	Raised areas around hair follicles	Vitamin C
Head		
Even molding, occipital prominence, symmetric facial features	Softening of cranial bones, prominence of frontal bones, skull flat and depressed toward middle	Vitamin D
Fused sutures after 18 months	Delayed fusion of sutures	Vitamin D
	Hard tender lumps in occiput	Excess vitamin A
	Headache	Excess thiamin
Neck		
Thyroid not visible, palpable in midline	Thyroid enlarged; may be grossly visible	Iodine
Eyes		
Clear, bright	Hardening and scaling of cornea and conjunctiva	Vitamin A
Good night vision	Night blindness	
Conjunctiva—pink, glossy	Burning, itching, photophobia, cataracts, corneal vascularization	Riboflavin
Ears		
Tympanic membrane—pliable	Calcified (hearing loss)	Excess vitamin D

*Nutrients listed are deficient unless specified as excess.

TABLE 31-1 Clinical assessment of nutritional status—cont'd

EVIDENCE OF ADEQUATE NUTRITION	EVIDENCE OF DEFICIENT OR EXCESS NUTRITION	DEFICIENCY/EXCESS*
Nose		
Smooth, intact nasal angle	Irritation and cracks at nasal angle	Riboflavin Excess vitamin A
Mouth		
Lips—smooth, moist, darker color than skin	Fissures and inflammation at corners	Riboflavin Excess vitamin A
Gums—firm, coral pink color, stippled	Spongy, friable, swollen, bluish red or black color, bleed easily	Vitamin C Niacin
Mucous membranes—bright pink, smooth, moist	Stomatitis	Niacin, riboflavin, folic acid
Tongue—rough texture, no lesions, taste sensation	Glossitis Diminished taste sensation	Zinc Excess fluoride Vitamin A, C, D, calcium, phosphorus Excess carbohydrates
Teeth—uniform white color, smooth, intact	Brown mottling, pits, fissures Defective enamel Caries	
Chest		
In infants, shape is almost circular	Depressed lower portion of rib cage	Vitamin D
In children, lateral diameter increases in proportion to anteroposterior diameter	Sharp protrusion of sternum	
Smooth costochondral junctions	Enlarged costochondral junctions	Vitamin C, D
Breast development—normal for age	Delayed development	See General Growth, especially zinc
Cardiovascular system		
Pulse and blood pressure within normal limits	Palpitations Rapid pulse	Thiamin Potassium Excess thiamin
	Arrhythmias	Magnesium, potassium Excess niacin, potassium
	Increased blood pressure Decreased blood pressure	Excess sodium Thiamin; excess niacin
Abdomen		
In young children, cylindric and prominent	Distended, flabby, poor musculature Prominent, large	Protein, calories Excess calories
Older children, flat	Potbelly, constipation	Vitamin D
Normal bowel habits	Diarrhea	Niacin Excess vitamin C
	Constipation	Excess calcium, potassium
Musculoskeletal system		
Muscles—firm, well-developed, equal strength bilaterally	Flabby, weak, generalized wasting Weakness, pain, cramps	Protein, calories Thiamin, sodium, chloride, potassium, phosphorus, magnesium Excess thiamin
	Muscle twitching, tremors Muscular paralysis	Magnesium Excess potassium
Spine—cervical and lumbar curves (double S curve)	Kyphosis, lordosis, scoliosis Bowing of extremities, knock-knees	Vitamin D Vitamin D, calcium, phosphorus
Extremities—symmetric; legs straight with minimum bowing	Epiphyseal enlargement Bleeding into joints and muscles, joint swelling, pain	Vitamin A, D Vitamin C
Joints—flexible, full range of motion, no pain or stiffness	Thickening of cortex of long bones with pain and fragility, hard tender lumps in extremities	Excess vitamin A
	Osteoporosis of long bones	Calcium; excess vitamin D

*Nutrients listed are deficient unless specified as excess.

Continued.

TABLE 31-1 Clinical assessment of nutritional status—cont'd

EVIDENCE OF ADEQUATE NUTRITION	EVIDENCE OF DEFICIENT OR EXCESS NUTRITION	DEFICIENCY/EXCESS*
Neurologic system		
Behavior—alert, responsive, emotionally stable	Listless, irritable, lethargic, apathetic (sometimes apprehensive, anxious, drowsy, mentally slow, confused)	Thiamin, niacin, pyridoxine, vitamin C, potassium, magnesium, iron, protein, calories Excess vitamin A, D, thiamin, folic acid, calcium
	Masklike facial expression, blurred speech, involuntary laughing	Excess manganese
Absence of tetany, convulsions	Convulsions	Thiamin, pyridoxine, vitamin D, calcium, magnesium Excess phosphorus (in relation to calcium)
Intact peripheral nervous system	Peripheral nervous system toxicity (unsteady gait, numb feet and hands, fine motor clumsiness)	Excess pyridoxine
Intact reflexes	Diminished or absent tendon reflexes	Thiamin, vitamin E

*Nutrients listed are deficient unless specified as excess.

rather than assume that the child dislikes vegetables, because it could be that none were served on that day. Also, evaluate the information in terms of the family's ethnic practices and financial resources. Encouraging increased protein intake with additional meat may be unfeasible for families on a limited budget or in conflict with food practices that use meat sparingly, such as in Asian meal preparation.

Compare findings from clinical examination and anthropometry with the data obtained from the dietary intake. For example, signs of anemia and a dietary record of iron-poor foods suggest laboratory analysis of hemoglobin, hematocrit, and transferrin. Refer any suspicious findings for further evaluation.

Key Points

- Communication, the most important skill nurses must possess in the care of children, has verbal, nonverbal, and abstract components.
- To effectively establish a setting for communication, nurses must make an appropriate introduction, clarify their role and the purpose of the interview, and ensure privacy and confidentiality.
- When communicating with parents, nurses need to encourage parental involvement, listen carefully, use silence, and be empathic.
- Communication with children must reflect their developmental stage.
- Verbal communication techniques that have proved to be effective include the third-person technique, facilitative responding, storytelling, bibliotherapy, the use of "what if" questions, and other word games.
- Nonverbal communication with children may take the form of writing, drawing, magic, and play.
- The objectives of performing a health history are to identify pertinent information, determine the chief complaint, analyze the present illness, secure the past history, review biologic systems, and record a family medical history and child psychosocial and sexual history.
- Family assessment is the collection of data about family composition and relationships among its members; it also focuses on home and community environment, occupation and education, and cultural and religious traditions.
- The family function interview examines interaction and roles, power, decision making, problem solving, communication, and expression of feelings and individuality.
- Nutritional assessment is performed by determination of dietary intake, clinical examination, and biochemical analysis.

References

Bellet PS, Maloney MJ: The importance of empathy as an interviewing skill in medicine, *JAMA* 266(13):1831-1832, 1991.

Bradley RH et al: A reexamination of the association between HOME scores and income, *Nurs Res* 43(5):260-266, 1994.

Caldwell B, Bradley R: *Home observation for measurement of the environment,* rev ed, Little Rock, Ark, 1984, University of Arkansas.

Frankenburg W, Coons C: Home Screening Questionnaire: its validity in assessing home environment, *J Pediatr* 108(4):624-626, 1986.

Gorzka PA et al: Parenting: categories for anticipatory guidance, *J Child Adolesc Psychiatr Ment Health Nurs* 4(1):16-19, 1991.

Heineken J, Roberts FB: Confirming, not disconfirming: communicating in a more positive manner, *MCN* 8(1):78-80, 1983.

Holden RJ: Empathy: the art of emotional knowing in holistic nursing care, *Holistic Nurs Pract* 5(1):70-79, 1990.

Leff P, Walizer E: *Building the healing partnership,* Cambridge, Mass, 1992, Brookline Books.

Sloat A, Matsuura W: *Intercultural communication.* In Craft M, Denehy J, editors: *Nursing interventions for infants and children,* Philadelphia, 1990, WB Saunders.

Smilkstein G: Family APGAR analyzed, *Fam Med* 25(5):293-294, 1993 (letter to the editor).

Smilkstein G, Ashworth C, Montano D: Validity and reliability of the family APGAR as a test of family function, *J Fam Pract* 15(2):303-311, 1982.

Wissow LS, Roter DL, Wilson MEH: Pediatrician interview style and mother's disclosure of psychosocial issues, *Pediatrics* 93(2):289-295, 1994.

Bibliography

Communication Strategies/Health Interview

Able-Boone H, Dokecki P, Smith M: Parent and health care provider communication and decision making in the intensive care nursery, *Child Health Care* 18(3):113-141, 1989.

Andrist L: Taking a sexual history and educating clients about safe sex, *Nurs Clin North Am* 23(4):959-973, 1988.

Baretich D, Stephenson P, Igoe J: Using art to understand children's perceptions of roles in physician's office visits, *Pediatr Nurs* 15(4):356-360, 1989.

Barnes LP: Strategies for using interviewing skills in patient teaching, *MCN* 19(6):311, 1994.

Barnsteiner JH, Gillis-Donovan J: Being related and separate: a standard for therapeutic relationships, *MCN* 15.223-228, 1990.

Boyle WE Jr, Hoekelman RA: *The pediatric history.* In Hoekelman RA et al, editors: *Primary pediatric care,* ed 3, St Louis, 1997, Mosby.

Brantly DK: Communicating with children: age-related techniques. In Smith D et al, editors: *Comprehensive child and family nursing skills,* St Louis, 1991, Mosby.

Brantly DK: *Conducting an interview.* In Smith D et al, editors: *Comprehensive child and family nursing skills,* St Louis, 1991, Mosby.

Brantly DK: Conducting the psychosocial assessment of the child. In Smith D et al, editors: *Comprehensive child and family nursing skills,* St Louis, 1991, Mosby.

Buchwald D et al: The medical interview across cultures, *Patient Care* 27(7):141-166, 1993.

Butz A, Alexander C: Use of health diaries with children, *Nurs Res* 40(1):59-61, 1991.

Byrnes K: Conducting the pediatric health history: a guide, *Pediatr Nurs* 22(2):135-137, 1996.

Cassell E, Coulehan J, Putnam S: Making good interview skills better, *Patient Care* 23(6):145-148, 1989.

Crowther, D: Metacommunications: a missed opportunity, *J Psychosoc Nurs* 29(4):13-16, 1991.

Denehy J: *Communicating with children through drawings.* In Craft M, Denehy J, editors: *Nursing interventions for infants and children,* Philadelphia, 1990, WB Saunders.

DiLeo JH: *Children's drawings as diagnostic aids,* New York, 1980, Brunner/Mazel.

DiLeo JH: *Interpreting children's drawings,* New York, 1983, Brunner/Mazel.

Dunst C, Trivette C, Deal A: *Enabling and empowering families: principles and guidelines for practice,* Cambridge, Mass, 1988, Brookline Books.

Elizabath J: Form of address: an addition to history taking? *Br Med J* 298(6668):257, 1989.

Faber A, Mazlish E: *How to talk so kids will listen and listen so kids will talk,* New York, 1980, Avon Books.

Fochtman D: Therapeutic relationships, *J Pediatr Oncol Nurs* 8(1):1-2, 1991.

Freeman M: Therapeutic use of storytelling for older children who are critically ill, *Child Health Care* 20(4):208-215, 1991.

Garbarino J et al: *What children can tell us: eliciting, interpreting, and evaluating information from children,* San Francisco, 1989, Jossey-Bass.

Gaynard L, Goldberger J, Laidley L: The use of stuffed, body-outline dolls with hospitalized children and adolescents, *Child Health Care* 20(4):216-224, 1991.

Green M: 20 interview questions that work, *Contemp Pediatr* 9(11):47-71, 1992.

Hahn K: Therapeutic storytelling: helping children learn and cope, *Pediatr Nurs* 13(3):175-178, 1987.

Hart R et al: *Therapeutic play activities for hospitalized children,* St Louis, 1992, Mosby.

Hauck MR: Cognitive abilities of preschool children: implications for nurses working with young children, *J Pediatr Nurs* 6(4):230-245, 1991.

Hudson C et al: Storytelling: a measure of anxiety in hospitalized children, *Child Health Care* 16(2):118-122, 1987.

Johnson B: Children's drawings as a projective technique, *Pediatr Nurs* 16(1):11-16, 1990.

Kramer N: Comparison of therapeutic touch and casual touch in stress reduction of hospitalized children, *Pediatr Nurs* 16(5):483-485, 1990.

Lynn M: Projective technique: a way of getting "hidden" information, Part 1, *J Pediatr Nurs* 1(6):58-60, 1986.

Messinger R, Davidson PN, Hoekelman RA: *Communication with parents and patients.* In Hoekelman RA et al, editors: *Primary pediatric care,* ed 3, St Louis, 1997, Mosby.

Nance TA: Intercultural communication: finding common ground, *J Obstet Gynecol Neonatal Nurs* 24(3):249-255, 1995.

O'Malley ME, McNamara ST: Children's drawings: a preoperative assessment tool, *AORN J* 57(5):1074-1089, 1993.

Rollins J: Childhood cancer: siblings draw and tell, *Pediatr Nurs* 16(1):21-27, 1990.

Stevens NV: *Obtaining a health history.* In Smith D et al, editors: *Comprehensive child and family nursing skills,* St Louis, 1991, Mosby.

Sunde ER, Mabe PA, Josephson A: Difficult parents: from adversaries to partners, *Clin Pediatr* 32(4):213-219, 1993.

Thompson SW: Communication techniques for allaying anxiety and providing support for hospitalized children, *J Child Adolesc Psychiatry Ment Health Nurs* 4(3):119-122, 1992.

Tiedman M, Simon K, Clatworthy S: *Communicating through therapeutic play.* In Craft M, Denehy J, editors: *Nursing interventions for infants and children,* Philadelphia, 1990, WB Saunders.

Tuffnell DJ et al: Use of translated written material to communicate with non–English-speaking patients, *Br Med J* 309(6960):992, 1994.

Vezeau T: Storytelling: a practitioner's tool, *MCN* 18:193-196, 1993.

Walker C: Use of art and play therapy in pediatric oncology, *J Pediatr Oncol Nurs* 6(4):121-126, 1989.

Winkelstein M: Fostering positive self-concept in the school-age child, *Pediatr Nurs* 15(3):229-233, 1989.

Family Assessment

Birenbaum LK: Measurement of family coping, *J Pediatr Oncol Nurs* 8(1):39-42, 1991.

Bradley R, Caldwell B: Using the home inventory to assess the family environment, *Pediatr Nurs* 14(2):97-103, 1988.

Brantly DK: Conducting a psychosocial assessment of the family. In Smith D et al, editors: *Comprehensive child and family nursing skills,* St Louis, 1991, Mosby.

Coleman WL: The first interview with a family, *Pediatr Clin North Am* 42(1):119-130, 1995.

Danielson CB, Hamel-Bissell B, Winstead-Fry P: *Families, health, and illness,* St Louis, 1993, Mosby.
Donelly E: Family health assessment, *Home Health Nurse* 11(2):30-37, 1993.
Gilliss C et al: *Toward a science of family nursing,* Menlo Park, Calif, 1989, Addison-Wesley.
Lapp C, Diemert C, Enestvedt R: Family-based practice: discussion of a tool merging assessment with intervention, *Fam Community Health* 12(4):21-28, 1990.
Lotas M et al: The HOME Scale: The influence of socioeconomic status on the evaluation of the home environment, *Nurs Res* 41(6):338-341, 1992.
Martinson I: *The challenge of culturally diverse pediatric clients.* In *Pediatric nursing: forum on the future: looking toward the 21st century,* Pitman, NJ, 1989, Anthony J Jannetti.
McCubbin H, McCubbin M: *Family system assessment in health care.* In McCubbin H, Thompson A, editors: *Family assessment inventories for research and practice,* ed 2, Madison, Wis, 1991, The University of Wisconsin—Madison.
Rosenbaum J: A cultural assessment guide: learning cultural sensitivity, *J Can Nurs Assoc* 87(4):32-33, 1991.
Speer J, Sachs B: Selecting the appropriate family assessment tool, *Pediatr Nurs* 11(5):349-355, 1985.
Touliatos J, Perlmutter B, Straus M, editors: *Handbook of family measurement techniques,* London, 1990, Sage Publications.
Wright L, Leahey M: *Nurses and families: a guide to family assessment and intervention,* Philadelphia, 1984, FA Davis.

Nutritional Assessment

American Academy of Pediatrics, Committee on Nutrition: *Pediatric nutrition handbook,* Elk Grove Village, Ill, 1993, The Academy.
Basch C et al: Validation of mothers' reports of dietary intake by four- to seven-year-old children, *Am J Public Health* 80(11):1314-1317, 1990.
Benjamin D: Laboratory tests and nutritional assessment: protein-energy status, *Pediatr Clin North Am* 36(1):139-161, 1989.
Buzzard IM, Willet WC, editors: First international conference on dietary assessment methods: assessing diets to improve world health, *Am J Clin Nutr* 59 (suppl 1): entire issue, 1994.
Kristal A et al: Development and validation of a food use checklist for evaluation of community nutrition interventions, *Am J Public Health* 80(11):1318-1322, 1990.
Liguori R: *Assessing nutritional status.* In Smith D et al, editors: *Comprehensive child and family nursing skills,* St Louis, 1991, Mosby.
Pipes PL, Trahms CM: *Nutrition in infancy and childhood,* ed 5, St Louis, 1995, Mosby.
Simko M, Cowell C, Hreha M: *Practical nutrition: a quick reference for the health care practitioner,* Rockville, Md, 1989, Aspen.

Bibliotherapy

Association for the Care of Children's Health: *Books for children and teenagers about hospitalization, illness, and disabling conditions,* Washington, DC, 1987, The Association.
Berg PJ, Devlin MK, Gedaly-Duff V: Bibliotherapy with children experiencing loss, *Issues Compr Pediatr Nurs* 4:37-50, 1980.
Cohen L: "Here's something I want you to read," *RN* 55(10):56-59, 1992.
Cuddigan M, Hanson MB: *Growing pains: helping children deal with everyday problems through reading,* Chicago, 1988, American Library Association.
Dreyer S: *The Bookfinder 4: when kids need books,* Circle Pines, Minn, 1989, American Guidance Service.
Fassler J: *Helping children cope: mastering stress through books and stories,* London, 1978, The Free Press.
Fosson A, Husband E: Bibliotherapy for hospitalized children, *South Med J* 77(3):342-346, 1984.
Oppenheim J, Brenner B, Boegehold B: *Choosing books for kids,* New York, 1986, Ballantine Books.
Wallace NE: Special books for special children, *Child Health Care* 12(1):34-36, 1983.

CHAPTER 32

Physical and Developmental Assessment of the Child

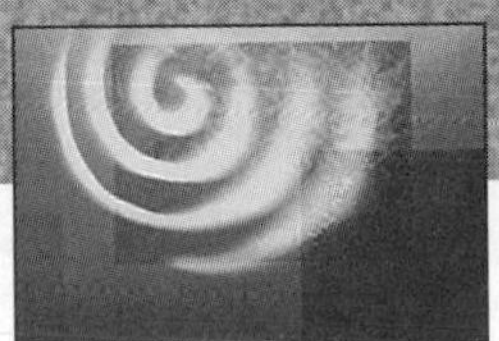

GENERAL APPROACHES TOWARD EXAMINING THE CHILD, P. 893

PHYSICAL EXAMINATION, P. 896

Growth measurements, p. 896
Physiologic measurements, p. 900
General appearance, p. 905
Skin, p. 906
Lymph nodes, p. 907
Head and neck, p. 907
Eyes, p. 908
Ears, p. 914
Nose, p. 918
Mouth and throat, p. 918
Chest, p. 920
Lungs, p. 921
Heart, p. 922
Abdomen, p. 924
Genitalia, p. 926
Anus, p. 928
Back and extremities, p. 928
Neurologic assessment, p. 930

DEVELOPMENTAL ASSESSMENT, P. 931

Denver II, p. 931
Revised Prescreening Developmental Questionnaire (R-PDQ), p. 934
Developmental screening and interpretation, p. 934

General Approaches Toward Examining the Child

SEQUENCE OF THE EXAMINATION

Ordinarily the sequence for examining patients follows a head-to-toe direction. The main function of such a systematic approach is to provide a general guideline for assessment of each body area to minimize omitting segments of the examination. The standard recording of data also facilitates exchange of information among different professionals. The typical organization of a physical examination is indicated in the chapter outline. In examining children, this orderly sequence is often altered to accommodate the child's developmental needs, although the examination is recorded following the head-to-toe model. Using developmental and chronologic age as the main criteria for assessing each body system accomplishes several goals:

1. Minimizes stress and anxiety associated with assessment of various body parts
2. Fosters a trusting nurse-child-parent relationship
3. Allows for maximum preparation of the child
4. Preserves the essential security of the parent-child relationship, especially with young children
5. Maximizes the accuracy and reliability of assessment findings

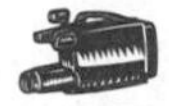

For additional information, please view "Pediatric Assessment" in *Whaley and Wong's Pediatric Nursing Video Series*, St Louis, 1996, Mosby; (800) 426-4545.

PREPARATION OF THE CHILD

Although the physical examination consists of painless procedures, to a child the use of a tight arm cuff, probes in the ears and mouth, pressing on the abdomen, and listening to the chest with a cold piece of metal can be considerably stressful. Therefore the same considerations discussed in Chapter 42 for preparing children for procedures are followed here. In addition to that discussion, general guidelines related to the examining process are presented in Box 32-1. The physical examination should be as pleasant as possible, as well as educational. For example, with preschool and older children, the nurse can use a detailed drawing or anatomically correct doll to help them learn about their bodies (Vessey, Braithwaite, and Weidmann, 1990). The "paper-doll" technique is a useful approach to teaching children about the part of the body that is being examined (Fig. 32-1). At the conclusion of the visit, the child can bring home the paper doll as a memento of the experience.

In most instances, children cooperate best when their parents remain with them. There are occasions, however, when older children, particularly adolescents, prefer to be examined alone, such as during the genital examination. Often the child being examined is also accompanied by a sibling, who may be disruptive because of boredom. A helpful tactic is to involve

BOX 32-1

General Guidelines For Performing Pediatric Physical Examination

- Perform examination in appropriate, nonthreatening area.
  - Have room well lit and decorated with neutral colors.
  - Have room temperature comfortably warm.
  - Place all strange and potentially frightening equipment out of sight.
  - Have some toys, dolls, stuffed animals, and games available for child.
  - If possible, have rooms decorated and equipped for different-age children.
  - Provide privacy, especially for school-age children and adolescents.
- Provide time for play and becoming acquainted.
- Observe behaviors that signal child's readiness to cooperate:
  - Talking to nurse
  - Making eye contact
  - Accepting offered equipment
  - Allowing physical touching
  - Choosing to sit on examining table rather than parent's lap
- If signs of readiness are not observed, use the following techniques:
  - Talk to parent while essentially "ignoring" child; gradually focus on child or a favorite object, such as a doll.
  - Make complimentary remarks about child, such as appearance, dress, or a favorite object.
  - Tell a funny story or play a simple magic trick.
  - Have a nonthreatening "friend" available, such as a hand puppet to "talk" to child for the nurse (see Fig. 32-22, *A*).
- If child refuses to cooperate, use the following techniques:
  - Assess reason for uncooperative behavior; consider that a child who is unduly afraid may have had a previous traumatic experience.
  - Try to involve child and parent in process.
  - Avoid prolonged explanations about examining procedure.
  - Use a firm, direct approach regarding expected behavior.
  - Perform examination as quickly as possible.
  - Have attendant gently restrain child.
  - Minimize any disruptions or stimulation.
    - Limit number of people in room.
    - Use isolated room.
    - Use quiet, calm, confident voice.
- Begin examination in a nonthreatening manner for young children or children who are fearful:
  - Use those activities that can be presented as games, such as test for cranial nerves (see Table 32-12) or parts of developmental screening tests (p. 931).
  - Use approaches such as "Simon says" to encourage child to make a face, squeeze a hand, stand on one foot, and so on.
  - Use "paper-doll" technique.
    - Lay child supine on an examining table or floor that is covered with a large sheet of paper.
    - Trace around child's body outline.
    - Use body outline to demonstrate what will be examined, such as drawing a heart and listening with the stethoscope before performing the activity on child.
- If several children in the family will be examined, begin with the most cooperative child to provide modeling of desired behavior.
- Involve child in examination process:
  - Provide choices, such as sitting on table or in patient's lap.
  - Allow child to handle or hold equipment.
  - Encourage child to use equipment on a doll, family member, or examiner.
  - Explain each step of the procedure in simple language.
- Examine child in a comfortable and secure position:
  - Sitting in parent's lap
  - Sitting upright if in respiratory distress
- Proceed to examine the body in an organized sequence (usually head to toe) with the following exceptions:
  - Alter sequence to accommodate needs of different-age children (see Table 32-1).
  - Examine painful areas last.
  - In emergency situation, examine vital functions (airway, breathing, and circulation) and injured area first.
- Reassure child throughout examination, especially about bodily concerns that arise during puberty.
- Discuss findings with family at end of examination.
- Praise child for cooperation during examination; give reward such as a small toy or sticker.

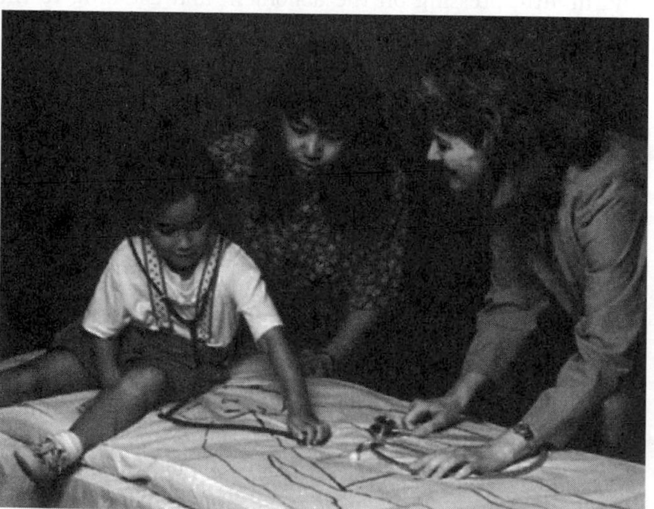

Fig. 32-1 Using paper-doll technique to prepare child.

the sibling in the examination by allowing the child to hold the stethoscope or a tongue blade and praising the child for the "help" during the assessment.

Table 32-1 summarizes guidelines for positioning, preparing, and examining children at various ages. Since no child fits precisely into one age category, it may be necessary to vary the approach after a preliminary assessment of the child's developmental achievements and needs. Even when the best approach is used, many toddlers are uncooperative and unable to be consoled for much of the physical examination. However, some seem intrigued by the new surroundings and unusual equipment and respond more like preschoolers than toddlers. Likewise, some early preschoolers may require more of the "security measures" employed with younger children, such as continued parent-child contact, and less of the preparatory measures used with preschoolers, such as playing with the equipment before and during the actual examination (Fig. 32-2).

Although the variations in the general approaches are numerous, some of them are elaborated here because they are

TABLE 32-1 Age-specific approaches to physical examination during childhood

POSITION	SEQUENCE	PREPARATION
Infant		
Before sits alone: supine or prone, preferably in parent's lap; before 4 to 6 months: can place on examining table After sits alone: use sitting in parent's lap whenever possible If on table, place with parent in full view	If quiet, auscultate heart, lungs, abdomen Record heart and respiratory rates Palpate and percuss same areas Proceed in usual head-toe direction Perform traumatic procedures last (eyes, ears, mouth [while crying]) Elicit reflexes as body part examined Elicit Moro reflex last	Completely undress if room temperature permits Leave diaper on male Gain cooperation with distraction, bright objects, rattles, talking Smile at infant; use soft, gentle voice Pacify with bottle of sugar water or feeding Enlist parent's aid for restraining to examine ears, mouth Avoid abrupt, jerky movements
Toddler		
Sitting or standing on/by parent Prone or supine in parent's lap	Inspect body area through play: "count fingers," "tickle toes" Use minimal physical contact initially Introduce equipment slowly Auscultate, percuss, palpate whenever quiet Perform traumatic procedures last (same as for infant)	Have parent remove outer clothing Remove underwear as body part examined Allow to inspect equipment; demonstrating use of equipment usually ineffective If uncooperative, perform procedures quickly Use restraint when appropriate; request parent's assistance Talk about examination if cooperative; use short phrases Praise for cooperative behavior
Preschool child		
Prefer standing or sitting Usually cooperative prone/supine Prefer parent's closeness	If cooperative, proceed in head-toe direction If uncooperative, proceed as with toddler	Request self-undressing Allow to wear underpants if shy Offer equipment for inspection; briefly demonstrate use Make up "story" about procedure: "I'm seeing how strong your muscles are" (blood pressure). Use paper-doll technique Give choices when possible Expect cooperation; use positive statements: "Open your mouth"
School-age child		
Prefer sitting Cooperative in most positions Younger child prefers parent's presence Older child may prefer privacy	Proceed in head-toe direction May examine genitalia last in older child Respect need for privacy	Request self-undressing Allow to wear underpants Give gown to wear Explain purpose of equipment and significance of procedure, such as otoscope to see eardrum, which is necessary for hearing Teach about body functioning and care
Adolescent		
Same as for school-age child Offer option of parent's presence	Same as older school-age child	Allow to undress in private Give gown Expose only area to be examined Respect need for privacy Explain findings during examination: "Your muscles are firm and strong." Matter-of-factly comment about sexual development: "Your breasts are developing as they should be." Emphasize normalcy of development Examine genitalia as any other body part; may leave to end

more common. For example, the suggested sequence may change considerably when the child is in pain or when obvious physical defects are present. In either situation, examine the affected area last to minimize distress early in the examination and to focus on normal, healthy, or functioning body parts.

Positioning may also be altered because of physical distress. For example, the child who is having difficulty breathing may not be able to lie down; thus perform as much of the physical examination as possible with the child in a sitting or slightly reclining position, or complete the examination at another time.

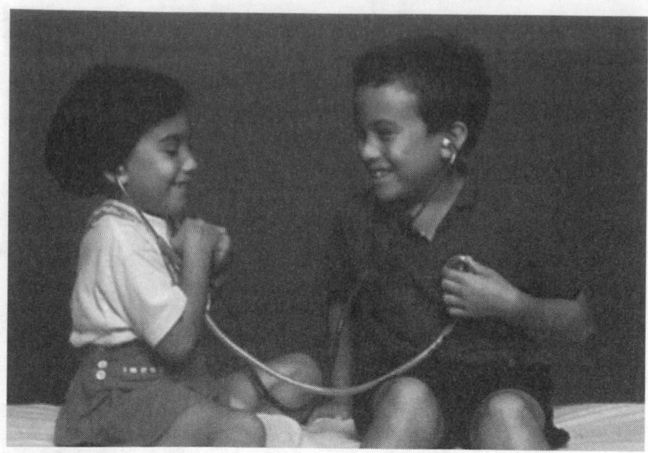

Fig. 32-2 Preparing children for physical examination.

Physical Examination

Although the approach to and sequence of the physical examination differ according to the child's age, the following discussion outlines the traditional model for physical assessment. Although the focus includes all pediatric age-groups, the reader is referred to Chapter 22 for a detailed discussion of a newborn assessment. Since the physical examination is a vital part of preventive pediatric care, the schedule for periodic health assessments is given in Box 32-2.

GROWTH MEASUREMENTS

Measurement of physical growth in children is a key element in evaluation of their health status. Physical growth parameters include weight, height (length), skinfold thickness, arm circumference, and head circumference. Values for these growth parameters are plotted on percentile charts, and the child's measurements in percentiles are compared with those of the general population.

BOX 32-2

Child Preventive Care Timeline

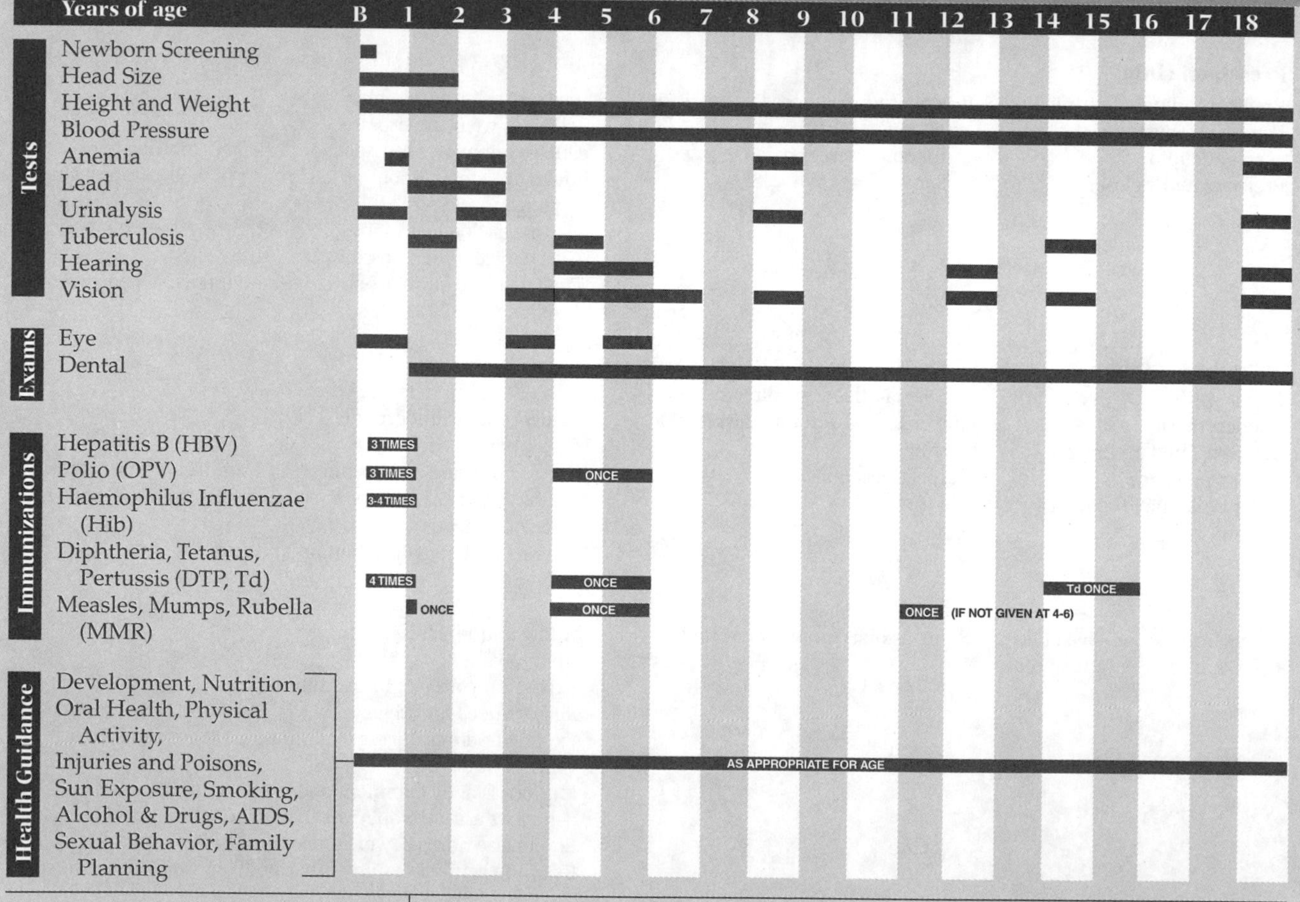

	Years of age	B	1	2	3	4	5	6	7	8	9	10	11	12	13	14	15	16	17	18
Tests	Newborn Screening	■																		
	Head Size	■	■																	
	Height and Weight	■	■	■	■	■	■	■	■	■	■	■	■	■	■	■	■	■	■	■
	Blood Pressure				■	■	■	■	■	■	■	■	■	■	■	■	■	■	■	■
	Anemia	■		■						■										■
	Lead		■	■																
	Urinalysis	■		■						■										■
	Tuberculosis		■			■										■				
	Hearing					■	■							■						■
	Vision				■	■	■	■		■				■		■				■
Exams	Eye	■			■		■													
	Dental		■	■	■	■	■	■	■	■	■	■	■	■	■	■	■	■	■	■
Immunizations	Hepatitis B (HBV)	3 TIMES																		
	Polio (OPV)	3 TIMES				ONCE	ONCE													
	Haemophilus Influenzae (Hib)	3-4 TIMES																		
	Diphtheria, Tetanus, Pertussis (DTP, Td)	4 TIMES				ONCE	ONCE									Td ONCE	Td ONCE			
	Measles, Mumps, Rubella (MMR)		ONCE			ONCE	ONCE						ONCE (IF NOT GIVEN AT 4-6)							
Health Guidance	Development, Nutrition, Oral Health, Physical Activity, Injuries and Poisons, Sun Exposure, Smoking, Alcohol & Drugs, AIDS, Sexual Behavior, Family Planning	AS APPROPRIATE FOR AGE	■	■	■	■	■	■	■	■	■	■	■	■	■	■	■	■	■	■

KEY: ■ Recommended by all major authorities. ■ Recommended by some major authorities.

Please note: Children with special risk factors may need more frequent and additional types of preventive care. Some examples:

RISK FACTOR	PREVENTIVE SERVICES NEEDED
Exposure to TB	TB test
Sexually active	Pap test (females); syphilis, gonorrhea, chlamydia tests
High-risk sexual behavior	AIDS test, hepatitis immunization
Drug abuse	AIDS, TB tests, hepatitis immunization

From *Child health guide: put prevention into practice,* US Department of Health and Human Services, undated, pp. 20-21.

The most commonly used growth charts in the United States are from the National Center for Health Statistics (NCHS) and are available for boys and girls ages (see the Appendix):

1. **Birth to 36 months**—records weight by age, recumbent length by age, weight for length, and head circumference by age
2. **Two to 18 years**—records weight by age, stature by age
3. **Prepubescence**—records weight for stature

Nursing ALERT

The prepubescent charts are only appropriate for plotting values for prepubescent boys and girls, regardless of chronologic age, and not for any child showing signs of pubescence, such as breast budding, testicular enlargement, or growth of axillary or pubic hair.

Two sets of charts include data for children ages 2 to 3 years; the major difference between the two charts is that one set (birth to 36 months) is based on **recumbent length** (length while lying supine), and the other set (2 to 18 years) uses **stature** (standing height). These two methods of measuring length are not equivalent. Measurements using recumbent length are greater by as much as 2 cm, or nearly 1 inch, in this age-group than measurements obtained using stature. This amount of difference between measurements can lead to an erroneous conclusion of delayed growth if length is plotted during one visit and stature during the next visit on the birth to 36-month chart.

Nursing ALERT

Plot only recumbent length on the birth to 36-month NCHS growth charts and stature on the 2- to 18-year growth charts.

The NCHS growth charts use the 5th and 95th percentiles as criteria for determining which children are outside the normal limits for growth. In general, those whose height or weight falls below the 5th percentile are considered underweight or small in stature; those whose measurements are above the 95th percentile are considered overweight or large in stature.

Overall evaluation of growth requires judgment in interpretation of growth percentiles. Generally, children whose height or weight falls below the 5th percentile or above the 95th percentile should be followed closely. However, small or large size may be genetic (Fig. 32-3) (see the Cultural Considerations box to the right). Comparing children's growth trends with those of their parents is essential in evaluating adequate growth.

Breastfed infants grow slower than bottle-fed infants, especially during the second half of the first year. This slower growth is normal, although it may be at or below the 5th percentile (Dewey et al, 1993). Since the NCHS charts used a sample of children who were mainly bottle-fed, the growth percentiles for breastfed infants must be carefully interpreted.

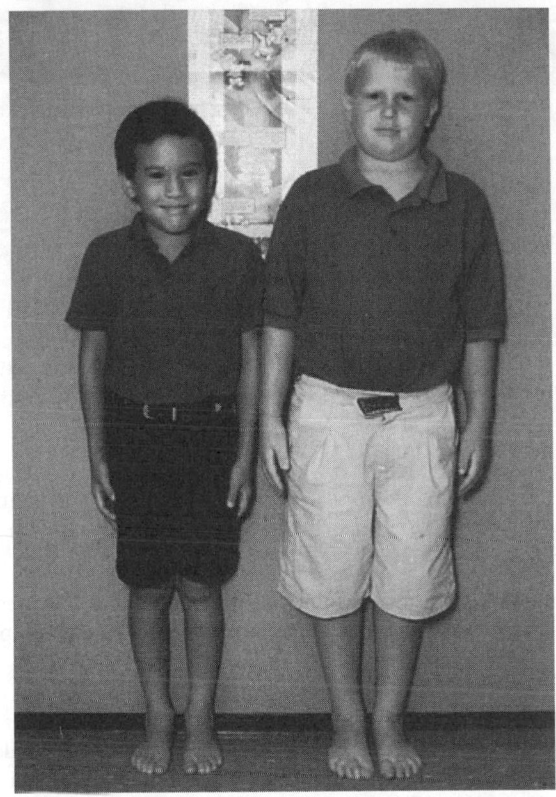

Fig. 32-3 These children of identical age (8 years) are markedly different in size. The child on the left, of Asian descent, is at the 5th percentile for height and weight. The child on the right is above the 95th percentile for height and weight. However, both children demonstrate normal growth patterns.

Cultural Considerations

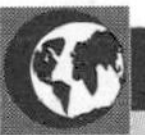

ETHNIC DIFFERENCES IN GROWTH

A potential concern with the U.S. growth charts is their accuracy in evaluating the growth of children from different ethnic and socioeconomic backgrounds. Research findings indicate that these growth charts can serve as a reference guide for all racial or ethnic groups if used from the perspective that different groups of children have varying normal distributions on the growth curves. The NCHS charts are accurate for African-American children because this group was included in the sample population. There are special growth charts for Chinese children.

Children whose growth may be questionable include the following:

- Children whose height and weight percentiles are widely disparate (e.g., height in the 10th percentile and weight in the 90th percentile, especially with above-average skinfold thickness)
- Children who fail to show the expected growth rates in height and weight, especially during the rapid growth periods of infancy and adolescence (Table 32-2)

TABLE 32-2 Expected growth rates at various ages

AGE	EXPECTED GROWTH RATE (IN CM/YEAR)
1 to 6 months	18-22
6 to 12 months	14-18
2nd year	11
3rd year	8
4th year	7
5th to 10th years	5-6

From *Human growth and growth disorders: an update*, San Francisco, 1989, Genentech.

- Children who show a sudden increase, except during puberty, or decrease in a previously steady growth pattern

Since growth is a continuous but uneven process, the most reliable evaluation lies in comparison of growth measurements over a prolonged time.

Length

The term *length* refers to measurements taken when children are supine (also referred to as *recumbent length*). Until children are 24 months old (36 months if the birth to 36-month chart is used), measure recumbent length. Because of the normally flexed position during infancy, fully extend the body by (1) holding the head in midline, (2) grasping the knees together gently, and (3) pushing down on the knees until the legs are fully extended and flat against the table. If using a measuring board, place the head firmly at the top of the board and the heels of the feet firmly against the footboard.

If such a measuring device is not available, measure length by placing the child on a paper-covered surface, marking the end points of the top of the head and the heels of the feet, and measuring between these two points (Fig. 32-4). For accurate measurement hold the writing utensil at a right angle to the table when marking the cephalic point; position the feet with the toes pointing directly to the ceiling when marking the heel point. Regardless of the method used, have someone assist in holding the child's head in midline while you extend the legs and take the measurements.

Height

The term *height* (or stature) refers to the measurement taken when children are standing upright. Measure height by having the child, with shoes removed, stand as tall and straight as possible, with the head in midline and the line of vision parallel to the ceiling or floor. Be sure the child's back is to the wall or other vertical flat surface, with the heels, buttocks, and back of the shoulders touching the wall and the medial malleoli touching if possible (Fig. 32-5). Check for and correct bending of the knees, slumping of the shoulders, or raising of the heels of the feet. Normally height is less if measured in the afternoon than in the morning. To minimize this variation, apply modest upward pressure under the jaw or the mastoid processes behind the ear.

For the most accurate measurement, use a wall-mounted

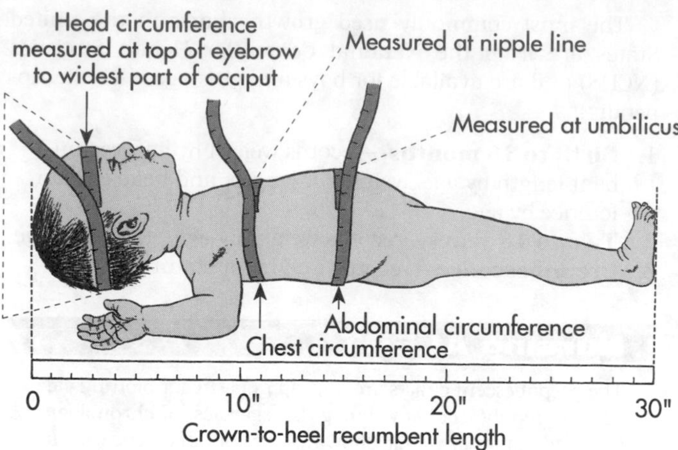

Fig. 32-4 Measurement of head, chest, and abdominal circumference and crown-to-heel (recumbent) length.

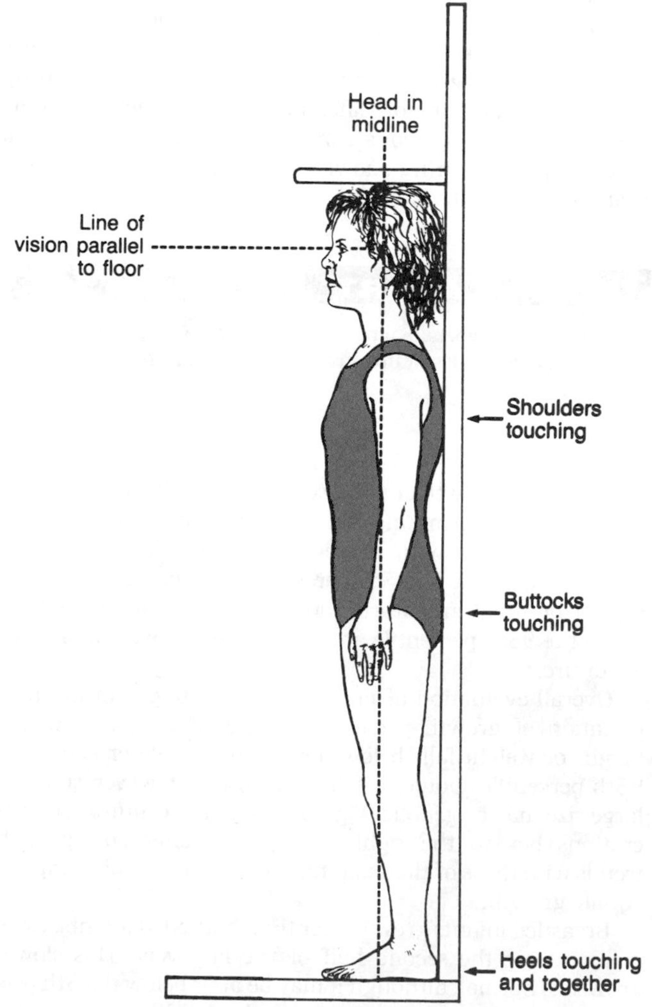

Fig. 32-5 Measurement of height. (Redrawn from *Human growth and growth disorders: an update*, San Francisco, 1989, Genentech.)

unit (*stadiometer*). The movable measuring rod of platform scales is accurate only if it maintains a parallel position to the floor and rests securely on the topmost part of the head. To improvise a flat surface for measuring length, attach a paper or metal tape or yardstick to the wall, position the child adjacent to the tape, and place a three-dimensional object such as a thick book or box, on top of the head. Rest the side of the object firmly against the wall to form a right angle. Measure length or stature to the nearest 1 mm or $\frac{1}{8}$ inch.

Weight

Weight is measured with an appropriately sized beam balance scale, which measures weights to the nearest 10 g or $\frac{1}{2}$ ounce for infants and 100 g or $\frac{1}{4}$ pound for children. Before the child is weighed, the scale is balanced by setting it at zero and noting if the balance registers exactly in the middle of the mark. If the end of the balance beam rises to the top or bottom of the mark, more or less weight, respectively, is added. Some scales are designed to allow for self-correction, but others need to be recalibrated by the manufacturer. Scales vary in their accuracy; infant scales tend to be more accurate than adult platform scales, and newer scales tend to be more accurate than older ones, especially at the upper levels of weight measurement. When precise measurements are needed, two nurses should take the weight independently, and if there is a discrepancy, a third reading should be taken (Burke, Roberts, and Maloney, 1988).

Take measurements in a comfortably warm room. When the birth to 36-month growth charts are used, children should be weighed nude. Older children are usually weighed while wearing their underpants or a light gown. However, with all children, always respect their privacy. If the child must be weighed wearing some article of clothing or some type of special device, such as a prosthesis or an armboard for an intravenous device, note this when recording the weight. Children who are measured for recumbent length are usually weighed on an infant platform scale and placed in a lying-down or sitting position. When weighing children, place your hand lightly above the body of the infant to prevent the child from accidentally falling off the scale (Fig. 32-6, *A*) or stand close to the toddler, ready to prevent a fall (Fig. 32-6, *B*). For maximum asepsis, cover the scale with a clean sheet of paper between each child's measurement.

Guidelines 

MEASURING TRICEPS SKINFOLD THICKNESS

- With child's right arm flexed 90 degrees at elbow, mark midpoint between acromion and olecranon on posterior aspect of arm.
- With arm hanging freely, grasp a fold of skin between thumb and forefinger 1 cm above midpoint.
- Gently pull fold away from underlying muscle and continue to hold until measurement is completed.
- Place caliper jaws over skinfold at midpoint mark and follow directions for using the device.
- Estimate reading to nearest 1 mm, 2 to 3 seconds after applying pressure.
- Take measurements until duplicates agree within 1 mm.

Skinfold Thickness and Arm Circumference

Measures of relative weight and stature cannot distinguish between adipose (fat) tissue or muscle. One convenient measure of body fat is *skinfold thickness*, which is increasingly recommended as a routine measurement (see also Anthropometry, Chapter 31). Skinfold thickness is measured with special calipers such as the Lange calibers. The most common sites for measuring skinfold thickness are the triceps (most practical for routine clinical use), subscapula, suprailiac, abdomen, and upper thigh. For greatest reliability the exact procedure for measurement must be followed and the average of at least two measurements of one site recorded (see the Guidelines box above).

Arm circumference is an indirect measure of muscle mass. Measurement of arm circumference follows the same procedure for skinfold thickness except measure the midpoint with a paper or steel tape. Place the tape vertically along the posterior aspect of the upper arm to the acromial process and to the olecranon process; half the measured length is the midpoint.

A 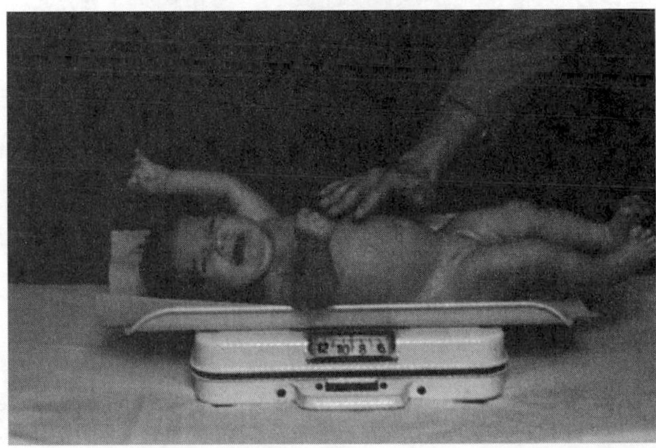

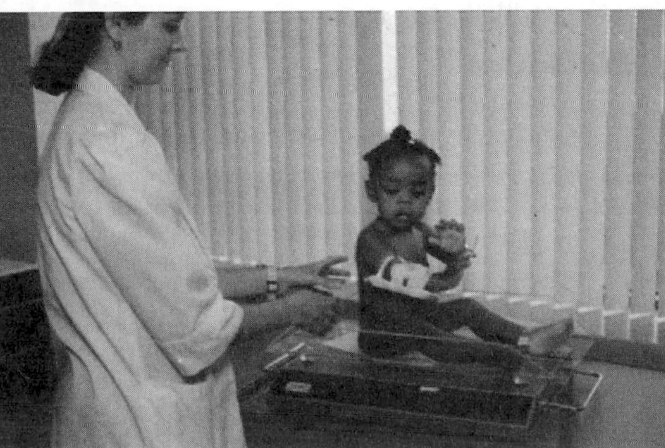 B

Fig. 32-6 **A,** Infant on scale. **B,** Toddler on scale. Note presence of nurse to prevent falls.

Percentiles for triceps skinfold and arm circumference in children are listed in the Appendix and may be used as reference data. However, the percentiles are not standards or norms, because values between the 5th and 95th percentiles are not ranges of normal.

Head Circumference

Measure head circumference in children up to 36 months of age and in any child whose head size is questionable. Measure the head at its greatest circumference, usually slightly above the eyebrows and pinna of the ears and around the occipital prominence at the back of the skull (see Fig. 32-4). Since head shape can affect the location of the maximum circumference, more than one measurement at points above the eyebrows may need to be taken to obtain the most accurate measure. Use a paper or metal tape because a cloth tape can stretch and give a falsely small measurement. For greatest accuracy, use devices with tenths of a centimeter, since the percentile charts have only 0.5 cm increments.

Plot the head size on the appropriate growth chart under head circumference. Generally, head and chest circumferences are equal at about 1 to 2 years of age. During childhood chest circumference exceeds head size by about 5 to 7 cm (2 to 3 in) (for newborns see Physical Assessment, Chapter 22).

PHYSIOLOGIC MEASUREMENTS

Physiologic measurements, key elements in evaluating physical status of vital functions, include temperature, pulse, respiration, and blood pressure. Compare each physiologic recording with normal values for that age-group (see the Appendix). In addition, compare the values taken on preceding health visits with present recordings. For example, a falsely elevated blood pressure reading may not indicate hypertension if previous recent readings have been within normal limits. The isolated recording may indicate some stressful event in the child's life.

As in most procedures carried out with children, older children and adolescents are treated much the same as are adults. However, special consideration must be given to preschool children (see the Atraumatic Care box below).

For best results in taking vital signs of infants, count respirations first, before the infant is disturbed, take the pulse next, and measure temperature last. If vital signs cannot be taken without disturbing the child, record the child's behavior (e.g., crying) along with the measurement.

Temperature

Temperature can be measured at several sites in the body via the oral, rectal, axillary, skin, or tympanic membrane route (Fig. 32-7). Recent substitutes for the traditional mercury thermometer are the electronic thermometer, the tympanic membrane sensor, the Tempa-Dot, the plastic strip, and the digital thermometer. These devices offer the advantages of measuring temperature rapidly and/or avoiding oral or rectal intrusion (Table 32-3). Although the accuracy of these instruments differs, accuracy is decreased to a greater extent if correct technique is not used (Pontious et al, 1994b).

No universal agreement exists regarding the length of time mercury thermometers should be kept in place. Recommendations based on research are 7 minutes for an oral reading, 4 minutes for a rectal reading, and 5 minutes for an axillary reading. However, these times may vary widely within practice settings and may not represent clinically significant differences from temperature readings taken for shorter intervals.

Atraumatic Care

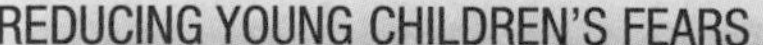

REDUCING YOUNG CHILDREN'S FEARS

Young children, especially preschoolers, fear intrusive procedures because of their poorly defined body boundaries. Therefore avoid invasive procedures, such as measuring rectal temperature, whenever possible. Also, avoid using the word "take" when measuring vital signs, since young children interpret words literally and may think that their temperature or other function will be taken away. Instead, say, "I want to know how warm you are."

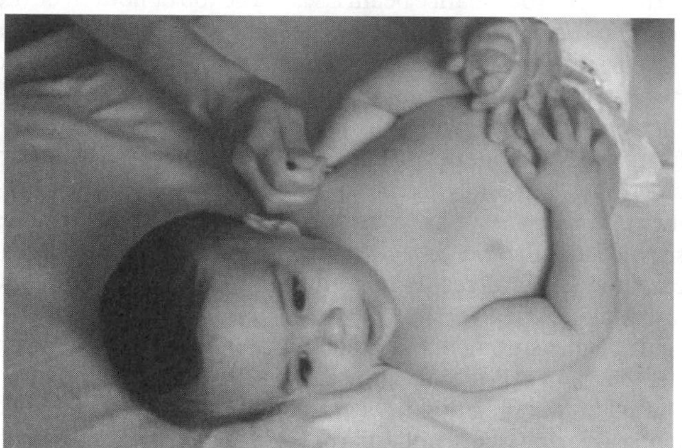

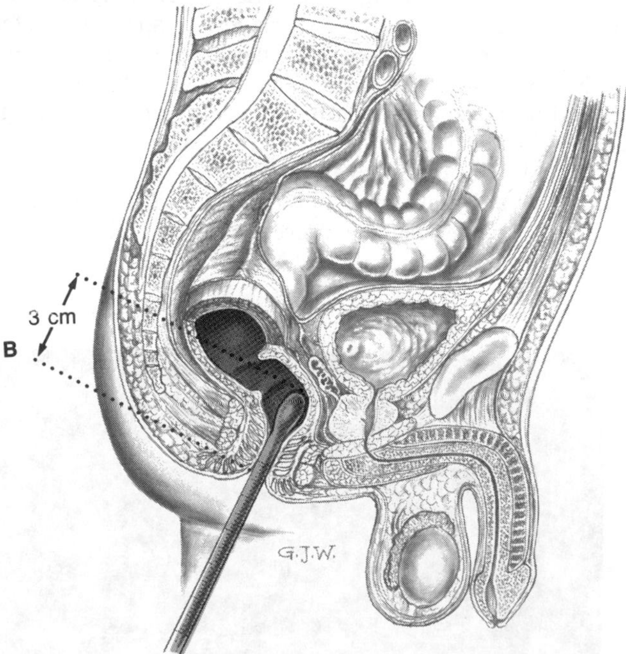

Fig. 32-7 **A,** Position for taking axillary temperature. **B,** Cross section of rectum illustrates curve at approximately 3 cm from anus, where risk of perforation from thermometer is greatest in infants up to 3 months of age.

TABLE 32-3 Comparison of body temperature techniques

DESCRIPTION/PROCEDURE	COMMENTS
Mercury glass thermometer	
Heat causes mercury to expand and rise in glass tube	Only difference in selection of mercury thermometers is that rectal type has more rounded tip as compared with oral type, which has more slender, elongated tip Appropriate length of time mercury thermometer should remain in place for accurate measurement of temperature is controversial; a general rule is to leave thermometer in place about 3 minutes, or follow agency policy If in doubt about the optimum length of insertion time, reinsert the mercury thermometer after the first reading, for a short time and recheck the scale for a rise. If the value is increased, reinsert the thermometer until the next reading is the same as the previous reading.
Oral temperature	
Place under tongue in right or left posterior sublingual pocket, not in front of tongue; have child keep mouth closed without biting on thermometer	Sublingual site indicates rapid changes in core body temperature *better* than rectal site Several factors affect temperature of mouth, such as hot or cold beverages, smoking, open-mouth breathing, and ambient temperature Oxygen by mask lowers oral temperature, but clinical significance of difference is questionable
Axillary temperature	
Place under arm with tip in center of axilla and kept close to skin, not clothing; hold child's arm firmly against side (Fig. 32-7, *A*)	Recommended for children who object strongly to rectal temperature but for whom an oral temperature is not feasible Has advantage of avoiding intrusive procedure and eliminating risk of rectal perforation and possible peritonitis May be affected by poor peripheral perfusion (lower value) or use of radiant warmers or brown fat in cold-stressed neonates (higher value)
Rectal temperature	
Place well-lubricated tip not more than 2.5 cm (1 inch) into rectum; securely hold thermometer close to anus May place child in side-lying, supine, or prone position (i.e., supine with knees flexed toward abdomen); cover penis, because procedure often stimulates urination A small child may be placed prone across parent's lap	Taken only when no other route or device can be used (e.g., in children whose mental age or temperament prevents cooperation and understanding instructions, agitated children, and those who have had oral or axillary injuries or surgery) Not recommended, because core temperature is not obtained unless thermometer is inserted to depth of at least 5 cm, which incurs risk of rectal perforation, especially in infants less than 3 months of age, since colon curves at depth of 3 cm (Fig. 32-7, *B*); also not recommended in anyone who has had rectal surgery, or in children with diarrhea or those receiving chemotherapy that affects mucosa Stool in rectum and less blood flow to area affects accuracy, especially in measuring changes in body temperature
Electronic thermometer	
Senses temperature with electronic component called thermistor mounted at tip of plastic and stainless steel probe, which is connected to electronic recorder; temperature measurement appears on digital display within 60 seconds Place probe in mouth, axilla, or rectum as with mercury thermometer	Ideally suited to pediatric use because plastic sheath is unbreakable, and child's mouth can remain open when oral temperature is taken
Infrared thermometry	
Infrared thermometer measures thermal radiation from axilla, ear canal opening, or tympanic membrane; temperature measurement appears on digital display in about 1 second	

Continued.

TABLE 32-3 Comparison of body temperature techniques—cont'd

DESCRIPTION/PROCEDURE	COMMENTS
Tympanic membrane sensor	
Insert covered probe tip gently in ear canal pointing toward midpoint between opposite eyebrow and sideburns (Terndrup and Rajk, 1992) For most accurate results, straighten ear canal for sensor to measure heat from drum, not sides of canal (see Fig. 32-20), take three measurements, and record highest reading Most models use "offsets" or internal calculations that transform ear temperature into supposedly equivalent oral or rectal temperatures	Tympanic membrane is excellent site because both eardrum and hypothalamus (temperature-regulating center) are perfused by same circulation Sensor is unaffected by cerumen; presence of suppurative or nonsuppurative otitis media does not significantly affect measurement; ear against surface, i.e., mattress, may be higher in temperature than exposed ear; warm ambient temperature may increase aural temperature Procedure is well-accepted by infants and children Because of difficulty with correct placement in young infants' ears, accuracy may be affected (Weiss, Poeltler, and Gocka, 1993)
Ear sensor (OTOTEMP)*	
Measures infrared heat energy radiating from canal opening, scans canal for highest temperature reading, and then calculates arterial temperature (correlates highly with core or internal body temperature) Insert hemispherical probe in ear opening; ear tug is not necessary	Available in two sizes; smaller size of LighTouch Pedi-Q is for smaller children Does not calculate offsets; therefore reading is only for arterial temperature (not equivalent to other sites)
Axillary sensor (Ototemp LighTouch Neonate)*	
Measures infrared heat energy radiating from axilla Touch covered probe to axilla, depress and release button, remove and read	Can be used on wet skin, in incubators, or under radiant heaters, warming pads, or other heat sources
Digital thermometer	
Consists of probe that connects to microprocessor chip, which translates signals into degrees and sends temperature measurement to digital display Used like oral mercury thermometer	More accurate and easier to read, but somewhat more expensive than mercury or plastic strip thermometer
Tempa-dot	
Single-use disposable thermometer with specific chemical mixture in each circle that changes color to measure temperature in increments of two tenths of a degree Used like mercury thermometer; kept in mouth (1 minute), axilla (3 minutes), and rectum (3 minutes); color change is read 10-15 seconds after removing thermometer	Found to be accurate and reliable for children with and without fever, especially for temperature below 38° C (100.4° F) (Pontious et al, 1994a, 1994b) Easier to read than mercury or plastic strip thermometer Safer than glass thermometers (disposable and flexible) Read thermometer away from heat source (e.g., radiant warmer) If unused thermometer changes color from storage in warm area (above 35° C [95° F]), place in freezer for 1 hour, then at room temperature for 24 hours before using
Plastic strip thermometer (Thermograph)	
Changes color in response to sensed temperature changes Place strip on forehead until color change occurs; usually takes less than 15 seconds Some strips are used like oral mercury thermometer	Accuracy is variable; best used for screening Advantages for home use include simple instructions and minimal cost Can provide continuous measurement without disturbing child

*Manufactured by Exergen Corporation, One Bridge Street, Newton, MA 02158; (800) 422-3006, (617) 527-6660, FAX (617) 527-6590.

Normal body temperature registers 37.0° C (98.6° F) through the oral route. Traditionally it has been assumed that rectal temperatures are 1° F higher and axillary temperatures are 1° F lower than oral temperatures. However, it has been demonstrated that this difference is considerably less (Pontious et al, 1994a). Because of these variations, chart the route along with the recorded temperature reading.

Whenever a child feels extra warm to the touch, measure the temperature even if it was normal only a short time before. Other signs of increased body temperature are flushed skin, increased respiratory and heart rate, malaise, and a "glassy look" to the eyes.

Pulse

A satisfactory pulse can be taken radially in children over 2 years of age. However, in infants and young children the api-

TABLE 32-4 Grading of pulses

GRADE	DESCRIPTION
0	Not palpable
+1	Difficult to palpate, thready, weak, easily obliterated with pressure
+2	Difficult to palpate, may be obliterated with pressure
+3	Easy to palpate, not easily obliterated with pressure (normal)
+4	Strong, bounding, not obliterated with pressure

TABLE 32-5 Commonly available blood pressure cuffs

CUFF NAME*	BLADDER WIDTH (CM)	BLADDER LENGTH (CM)
Newborn	2.5-4.0	5.0-9.0
Infant	4.0-6.0	11.5-18.0
Child	7.5-9.0	17.0-19.0
Adult	11.5-13.0	22.0-26.0
Large arm	14.0-15.0	30.5-33.0
Thigh	18.0-19.0	36.0-38.0

From Report of the Second Task Force on Blood Pressure Control in Children—1987, *Pediatrics* 79(1):1-25, 1987.
*Cuff name does not guarantee that the cuff will be appropriate size for a child within that age range.

cal impulse (heard through a stethoscope held to the chest at the apex of the heart) is more reliable. (See Fig. 32-29 for location of pulses.) Count the pulse for 1 full minute in infants and young children because of possible irregularities in rhythm. However, when frequent apical rates are needed, use shorter counting times (e.g., 15- or 30-second intervals). For greater accuracy, measure the apical rate while the child is asleep; record the child's behavior along with the rate. Pulses may be graded according to the criteria in Table 32-4. Compare radial and femoral pulses at least once during early infancy to detect the presence of circulatory impairment such as coarctation of the aorta. (See the Appendix for normal rates for pediatric age groups.)

Respiration

Count the respiratory rate in the same manner as for the adult patient. However, in infants, observe abdominal movements, since respirations are primarily diaphragmatic. Since the movements are irregular, count them for 1 full minute for accuracy (see also p. 921). (See the Appendix for normal respiratory rates in children.)

Blood Pressure

Blood pressure (BP) measurement by noninvasive methods is part of a routine vital sign determination. BP should be measured annually in children 3 years of age through adolescence, and in children with symptoms of hypertension, children in emergency rooms and intensive care units, and high-risk infants (Report of the Second Task Force, 1987). Several authorities also recommend routine measurements in low-risk neonates (Seidel, Rosenstein, and Pathak, 1993).

Measurement devices. The most common method of measuring BP uses *auscultation* and either a *mercury-gravity* or *aneroid sphygmomanometer.* Both types are reliable and accurate, but the mercury-gravity manometer does not require recalibration as does the aneroid type.

BP can also be measured using electronic devices that employ oscillometric or Doppler techniques. In *oscillometry*, pressure changes are transmitted through the arterial wall to the pressure cuff, and the oscillations are detected by a pressure-sensitive indicator. Oscillometers have digital readouts for systolic, diastolic, and *mean arterial pressures (MAP)*, and pulse. The MAP is not the same as the mean BP (arithmetic average of systolic and diastolic pressures). Rather, it is a value somewhat lower than the arithmetic mean. BP readings using oscillometry such as Dinamap are generally higher and correlate better with direct radial artery values than measurements using auscultation (see Table 32-8, p. 905). Oscillometry also eliminates common problems found with the auscultation method, such as deflating the cuff too rapidly, not hearing the softest sounds, and rounding numbers for the Korotkoff sounds.

The *Doppler ultrasound* translates changes in ultrasound frequency caused by blood movement within the artery to audible sound by means of a transducer in the cuff. The Doppler is useful for systolic pressure measurement but is unreliable for diastolic pressure measurement. Oscillometric and Doppler instruments are useful in measuring BP in infants and have largely replaced the flush method, which reflects only the mean BP, and the auscultatory method.

Selection of cuff. No matter what type of noninvasive technique is used, the most important factor in accurately measuring BP is the use of an appropriately sized cuff (*cuff size* refers only to the inner inflatable bladder, not the cloth covering). Unfortunately, authorities disagree on the correct method for determining cuff size. The Report of the Second Task Force (1987) recommends cuff size based on *limb length* (Table 32-5):

- Width sufficient to cover approximately 75% of upper arm between top of shoulder and olecranon
- Length sufficient to completely encircle circumference of limb with or without overlapping
- Enough room at antecubital fossa to place bell of stethoscope
- Enough room at upper edge of cuff to prevent obstruction of axilla

The American Heart Association (Frohlich et al, 1988) recommends a method based on *limb circumference* (Table 32-6):

- Width 40% to 50% of limb circumference; measured at upper arm midway between top of shoulder and olecranon
- Length sufficient to completely or nearly completely encircle circumference of limb without overlapping

Using limb length for selecting cuff width may produce satisfactory BP readings in children with average weight for height, but inaccurate readings in children with thick arms.

TABLE 32-6 Recommended bladder dimensions for blood pressure cuffs

ARM CIRCUMFERENCE AT MIDPOINT (CM)	CUFF NAME*	BLADDER WIDTH (CM)	BLADDER LENGTH (CM)
5-7.5	Newborn	3	5
7.5-13	Infant	5	8
13-20	Child	8	13
24-32	Adult	13	24
32-42	Wide adult	17	32
42-50	Thigh	20	42

From Frohlich ED et al: Recommendations for human blood pressure determination by sphygmomanometers: report of a special task force appointed by the Steering Committee, American Heart Association, *Circulation* 77:501A, 1988.

*Cuff name does not guarantee that the cuff will be appropriate size for a child within that age range.

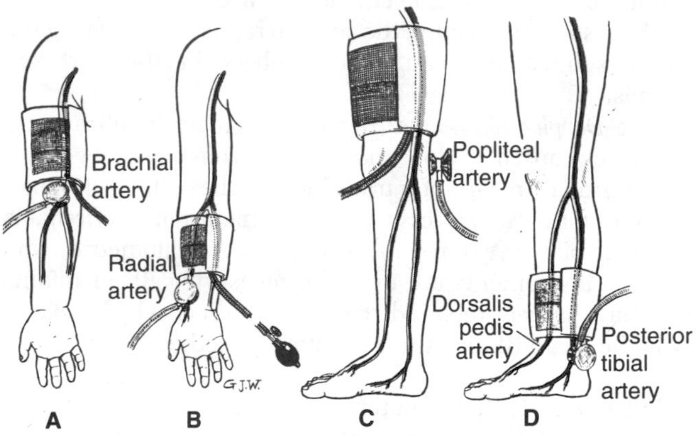

Fig. 32-8 Sites for measuring blood pressure. **A**, Upper arm. **B**, Lower arm or forearm. **C**, Thigh. **D**, Calf or ankle.

Using limb circumference for selecting cuff width more accurately reflects direct arterial BP than using limb length, because this method takes into account the varying thickness of the arm and the amount of pressure required to compress the artery (Park and Guntheroth, 1989). For measurement sites other than the upper arms, the limb circumference guidelines can be used, although the shape of the limb (i.e., conical shape of the thigh) may prevent appropriate placement of the cuff and inaccurately reflect intraarterial BP (Fig 32-8).

Cuffs that are either too narrow or too wide affect the accuracy of BP measurements, although wide cuffs tend to affect BP readings less. If the cuff is too small, the reading on the device is falsely high. If the cuff is too large, the reading is falsely low.

Nursing ALERT

In choosing cuff sizes, use an appropriately sized cuff. When the correct size is not available, use an oversized cuff rather than an undersized one or use another site that more appropriately fits the cuff size. Do not choose a cuff based on the name of the cuff (i.e., an "infant" cuff may be too small for some infants).

TABLE 32-7 Differences in oscillometric systolic BP between arm and lower extremity sites in normal children

	SYSTOLIC BP × (MEAN ± SD)	
AGE-GROUP (YEARS)	ARM-THIGH	ARM-CALF
4-8	−7.1±6.8	−9.3± 7.4
9-16	−2.4±7.7	−5.0±26.9

From Park M, Lee D, Johnson GA: Oscillometric blood pressures in the arm, thigh, and calf in healthy children and those with aortic coarctation, *Pediatrics* 91(4):761-765, 1993.

When another site is used, BP measurements using noninvasive techniques may differ. Generally, systolic pressure in the lower extremities (thigh or calf) is greater than pressure in the upper extremities, and systolic BP in the calf is higher than that in the thigh. These differences are listed in Table 32-7 and apply to oscillometric measurements taken on the right extremities with the child supine and the cuff size based on the circumference method (Park, Lee, and Johnson, 1993).

Nursing ALERT

Compare blood pressure in the upper and lower extremities at least once to detect abnormalities such as coarctation of the aorta, in which the lower extremity pressure is less than the upper extremity pressure.

Measurement and interpretation. Measuring and interpreting BP in infants and children requires additional attention to correct procedure because (1) limb sizes vary and cuff selection must accommodate the circumference; (2) excessive pressure on the antecubital fossa affects the Korotkoff sounds; (3) children easily become anxious, which can elevate BP; and (4) BP values change with age and growth. Larger children, especially in terms of height, have higher normal BPs than smaller children of the same age.

Although the technique of BP measurement in children is generally the same as that used for adults (see the Guidelines box on p. 905), some aspects of the procedure are especially important. Because children are easily upset by unfamiliar procedures, prepare them for BP measurement. For children of preschool age and above, explain each step of the procedure and tell them how the cuff will feel, such as a tight feeling or an arm hug. Use explanations such as "I want to see how strong your muscle is" or "Let's watch the silver rise in the tube."

Since the child should be quiet and relaxed during the procedure, measure BP before performing any anxiety-producing procedures. Infants and small children may be more quiet if the reading is taken while they are sitting in the parent's lap.

Use a pediatric stethoscope and bell for hearing BP sounds in small children and infants. If ausculation is not possible, obtain a systolic reading by palpation; measure the point at which the pulse at the radial or brachial artery reappears as the cuff is deflated.

Guidelines

MEASURING BLOOD PRESSURE

Use an appropriately sized cuff.
Use same position, preferably sitting, and right arm for brachial artery site (Fig. 32-8, *A*).
Use alternate site as needed to accommodate available cuff sizes:
- Use smaller size on forearm: place cuff above wrist and auscultate radial artery (Fig. 32-8, *B*).
- Use larger size on thigh: place cuff above knee and auscultate popliteal artery (Fig. 32-8, *C*).
- Use larger size on calf: place cuff above malleoli or at mid-calf and auscultate posterior tibial or dorsal pedal artery (Fig. 32-8, *D*).

Position limb at level of heart.
Rapidly inflate cuff to about 20 mm Hg above point at which radial pulse disappears.
Release cuff pressure at a rate of about 2 to 3 mm Hg/sec during auscultation of artery.
Read mercury-gravity manometer at eye level.
Record systolic value as onset of a clear tapping sound (first Korotkoff sound).
Record diastolic pressure as:
- Fourth Korotkoff sound (K4) (low-pitched, muffled sound) for children up to age 12 years
- Fifth Korotkoff sound (K5) (disappearance of all sound) for children ages 13 to 18 years

Record also limb, position, cuff size, and method of measurement.
If using electronic monitor, follow manufacturer's instructions and guidelines for correct cuff size.
- With oscillometric device (i.e., Dinamap), can use all four limb sites, but reserve the thigh for last, since it is the most uncomfortable.
- Stabilize limb during cuff deflation, since movement interferes with the device's ability to measure BP accurately.

The average BP readings at various ages throughout childhood using sphygmomanometry are listed in the Appendix, and readings using oscillometry are listed in Table 32-8. A ***normal BP*** is defined as a systolic and diastolic BP less than the 90th percentile for age and gender (Box 32-3). (See also Hypertension in Chapter 45.)

TABLE 32-8 Normative dinamap BP values (systolic/diastolic, mean arterial pressure in parentheses)

AGE-GROUP	MEAN	90TH PERCENTILE	95TH PERCENTILE
Newborn (1-3 days)	65/41(50)	75/49(59)	78/52(62)
1 month to 2 years	95/58(72)	106/68(83)	110/71(86)
2-5 years	101/57(74)	112/66(82)	115/68(85)

From Park M, Menard S: Normative oscillometric blood pressure values in the first 5 years in an office setting, *Am J Dis Child* 143(7):860-864, 1989.

BOX 32-3
Estimating Average Blood Pressure Measurements

Use the following quick formula for average **systolic BP** using auscultation:

1 to 7 years: age in years + 90

8 to 18 years: (2 × age in years) + 83

Use the following formula for average **diastolic BP** using auscultation:

1 to 5 years: 56

6 to 18 years: age in years +52

Nursing ALERT

Published norms for BP are valid only if the same method of measurement (auscultation and limb length for cuff size) is used in clinical practice.

GENERAL APPEARANCE

The general appearance of the child is a cumulative, subjective impression of the child's physical appearance, state of nutrition, behavior, personality, interactions with parents and nurse (also siblings if present), posture, development, and speech. Although general appearance is recorded in the beginning of the physical examination, it encompasses all the observations of the child during the interview and physical assessment.

Note the *facies*, the facial expression and appearance of the child. For example, the facies may give clues to children who are in pain; have difficulty breathing; feel frightened, discontent, or happy; are mentally deficient; or are acutely ill.

Observe the *posture, position,* and types of *body movement.* The child with hearing or vision loss may characteristically tilt the head in an awkward position to hear or see better. The child in pain may favor a body part. The child with low self-esteem or a feeling of rejection may assume a slumped, careless, and apathetic pose or posture. Likewise, a child with confidence, a feeling of self-worth, and a sense of security usually demonstrates a tall, straight, well-balanced posture. While observing such "body language," do not interpret too freely but rather record objectively.

Note the child's *hygiene* in terms of cleanliness; unusual body odor; the condition of the hair, neck, nails, teeth, and feet; and the condition of the clothing. Such observations are excellent clues to possible instances of neglect, inadequate financial resources, housing difficulties (e.g., no running water), or lack of knowledge concerning children's needs.

General appearance includes an overall impression of the child's state of *nutrition.* This impression is more than a statement describing body weight or stature, such as "slender and tall." It is an estimation of the quality, as well as the quantity, of nutritional intake. For example, two children can be of the same height and weight, yet one can appear overweight because of flabby, loose skin, whereas the other child appears strong, robust, and well-built because of firm, well-defined musculature. Likewise, a small, slender child may be well-nourished with no signs of chronic undernutrition, such as bony prominences, protuberant abdomen, flat buttocks, gaunt facies, and poor muscle tone with evidence of wasting.

Compare your impression of the nutritional state with the parents' history of feeding practices. Discrepancies between the two "impressions" may be a valuable area for nutritional counseling. For example, parents who believe that their child is too thin and eats too little, despite evidence of adequate growth and physical signs of proper nutrition, may find it helpful to keep a daily diary to calculate the child's cumulative food intake. Many parents are surprised at the quantity of food ingested, even though the amounts at each meal or snack are small.

Behavior includes the child's personality, level of activity, reaction to stress, requests, frustration, interactions with others (primarily the parent and nurse), degree of alertness, and response to stimuli. Some mental questions that serve as reminders for observing behavior include: What is the child's overall personality? Does the child have a long attention span or is he or she easily distracted? Can the child follow two or three commands in succession without the need for repetition? What is the youngster's response to delayed gratification or frustration? Is eye-to-eye contact used during conversation? What is the child's reaction to the nurse and family members? Is the child quick or slow to grasp explanations?

Development can be assessed by carefully observing the child, but verify your impressions with screening tests. Various tests for assessing development, speech, vision, and hearing are discussed later in this chapter and in Chapter 39.

Record an overall estimate of the child's speech development, motor skills, degree of coordination, and recent area of achievement under general appearance. For example, the following statement may apply to an 18-month-old child: "Motor development advanced for age; climbs, runs, jumps (most recent motor skill), manipulates small objects with ease; excellent coordination and balance; beginning to name many objects; uses two-word phrases; and enjoys 'talking' to self and others."

SKIN

Skin is assessed for color, texture, temperature, moisture, and turgor. Examination of the skin and its accessory organs primarily involves inspection and palpation. The normal color in light-skinned children varies from a milky-white and rose color to a deeply hued pink color. Dark-skinned children such as those of Native American, Hispanic, or African-American descent have inherited various brown, red, yellow, olive-green, and bluish tones in their skin. Oriental people have skin that normally has a yellow tone.

Several variations in skin color can occur, some of which warrant further investigation. The types of color change and their appearance in children with light or dark skin are summarized in Table 32-9.

Normally the skin *texture* of young children is smooth and slightly dry, not oily or clammy. Evaluate skin *temperature* by symmetrically feeling each part of the body and comparing upper areas with lower ones. Note any difference in temperature.

Determine **tissue turgor,** or the amount of elasticity in the skin, by grasping the skin on the abdomen between the thumb and index finger, pulling it taut, and quickly releasing it. Elastic tissue immediately assumes its normal position without residual marks or creases. In children with poor skin turgor the skin remains suspended or tented for a few seconds before slowly falling back on the abdomen. Skin turgor is one of the best estimates of adequate hydration and nutrition.

Accessory Structures

Inspection of the accessory structures of the skin may be performed while the skin is being examined or when the scalp and extremities are being assessed.

Inspect the *hair* for color, texture, quality, distribution, and elasticity. Children's scalp hair is usually lustrous, silky, strong, and elastic. Genetic factors affect the appearance of hair. For example, the hair of black children is usually curlier and coarser than that of white children. Hair that is stringy, dull, brittle, dry, friable, and depigmented may suggest poor nutrition. Record any bald or thinning spots. Loss of hair in infants may indicate lying in the same position and may be a clue for counseling parents concerning the child's stimulation needs.

Inspect the hair and scalp for general cleanliness. Various ethnic groups condition their hair with oils or lubricants, which, if not thoroughly washed from the scalp, clog the sebaceous glands, causing scalp infections. Also examine the area for lesions, scaliness, evidence of infestation, such as lice or ticks, and signs of trauma, such as ecchymosis, masses, or scars.

In children who are approaching puberty, look for growth of secondary hair as a sign of normally progressing pubertal changes. Note precocious or delayed appearance of hair growth because although not always suggestive of hormonal dysfunction, it may be of great concern to the early- or late-maturing adolescent.

Inspect the *nails* for color, shape, texture, and quality. Normally the nails are pink, convex, smooth, and hard but flexible (not brittle). The edges, which are usually white, should extend over the fingers. Dark-skinned individuals may have more deeply pigmented nail beds. Short, ragged nails are typical of habitual biting. Uncut, dirty nails are a sign of poor hygiene.

Each individual has a distinct set of handprints and footprints. The patterns, or **dermatoglyphics,** are unique to the

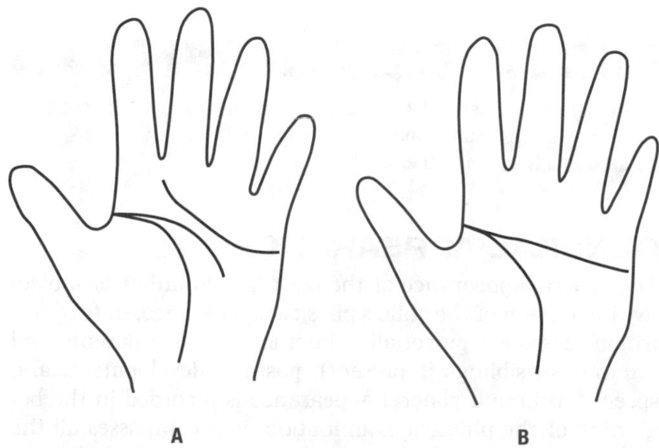

Fig. 32-9 Examples of flexion creases on palm. **A,** Normal. **B,** Transpalmar crease.

TABLE 32-9 Differences in color changes of racial groups

DESCRIPTION	APPEARANCE IN LIGHT SKIN	APPEARANCE IN DARK SKIN
Cyanosis		
A bluish tone through skin reflects reduced (deoxygenated) hemoglobin	Bluish tinge, especially in palpebral conjunctiva (lower eyelid), nail beds, earlobes, lips, oral membranes, soles, and palms	Ashen gray lips and tongue
Pallor		
Paleness may be a sign of anemia, chronic disease, edema, or shock	Loss of rosy glow in skin, especially face	Ashen-gray appearance in black skin More yellowish-brown color in brown skin
Erythema		
Redness may be result of increased blood flow from climatic conditions, local inflammation, infection, skin irritation, allergy, or other dermatoses or may be caused by increased numbers of red blood cells as a compensatory response to chronic hypoxia	Redness easily seen anywhere on body	Much more difficult to assess; rely on palpation for warmth or edema
Ecchymosis		
Large, diffuse areas, usually black and blue in color, are caused by hemorrhage of blood into skin; are typically result of injuries	Purplish to yellow-green areas; may be seen anywhere on skin	Very difficult to see unless in mouth or conjunctiva
Petechiae		
Same as ecchymosis except for size: small, distinct pinpoint hemorrhages 2 mm or less in size; can denote some type of blood disorder, such as leukemia	Purplish pinpoints most easily seen on buttocks, abdomen, and inner surfaces of the arms or legs	Usually invisible except in oral mucosa, conjunctiva of eyelids, and conjunctiva covering eyeball
Jaundice		
Yellow staining of the skin usually caused by bile pigments	Yellow staining seen in sclera of eyes, skin, fingernails, soles, palms, and oral mucosa	Most reliably assessed in sclera, hard palate, palms, and soles

individual and vary a great deal in detail and complexity. The palm normally shows three flexion creases (Fig. 32-9, *A*). In some situations such as Down syndrome the two distal horizontal creases are fused to form a single horizontal crease, the *single palmar crease* or *transpalmar crease* (Fig. 32-9, *B*). If grossly abnormal lines or folds are observed, sketch a picture to describe them and refer the finding to a specialist for further investigation.

LYMPH NODES

Lymph nodes are usually assessed when the part of the body in which they are located is examined. Although the body's lymphatic drainage system is extensive, the usual sites for palpating accessible lymph nodes are shown in Fig. 32-10.

Palpate nodes by using the distal portion of the fingers and gently but firmly pressing in a circular motion along the regions where nodes are normally present. During assessment of the nodes in the head and neck, tilt the child's head upward slightly but without tensing the sternocleidomastoid or trapezius muscles. This position facilitates palpation of the *submental, submaxillary, tonsillar,* and *cervical nodes.* Palpate the *axillary nodes* with the arms relaxed at the side but slightly abducted. Assess the *inguinal nodes* with the child in the supine position. Note size, mobility, temperature, and tenderness, as well as reports by the parents regarding any visible change of enlarged nodes. In children, small, nontender, movable nodes are usually normal. Tender, enlarged, warm lymph nodes generally indicate infection or inflammation proximal to their location. Report such findings for further investigation.

HEAD AND NECK

Observe the head for general *shape* and *symmetry.* A flattening of one part of the head, such as the occiput, may indicate that the child continually lies in this position. Marked asymmetry is usually abnormal and may indicate premature closure of the sutures (craniosynostosis).

Note *head control* in infants and *head posture* in older children. Most infants by 4 months of age should be able to hold the head erect and in midline when in a vertical position.

Nursing ALERT

Significant head lag after 6 months of age strongly indicates cerebral injury and is referred for further evaluation.

Evaluate range of motion by asking the older child to look in each direction (to either side, up, and down) or manually putting the younger child through each position. Limited

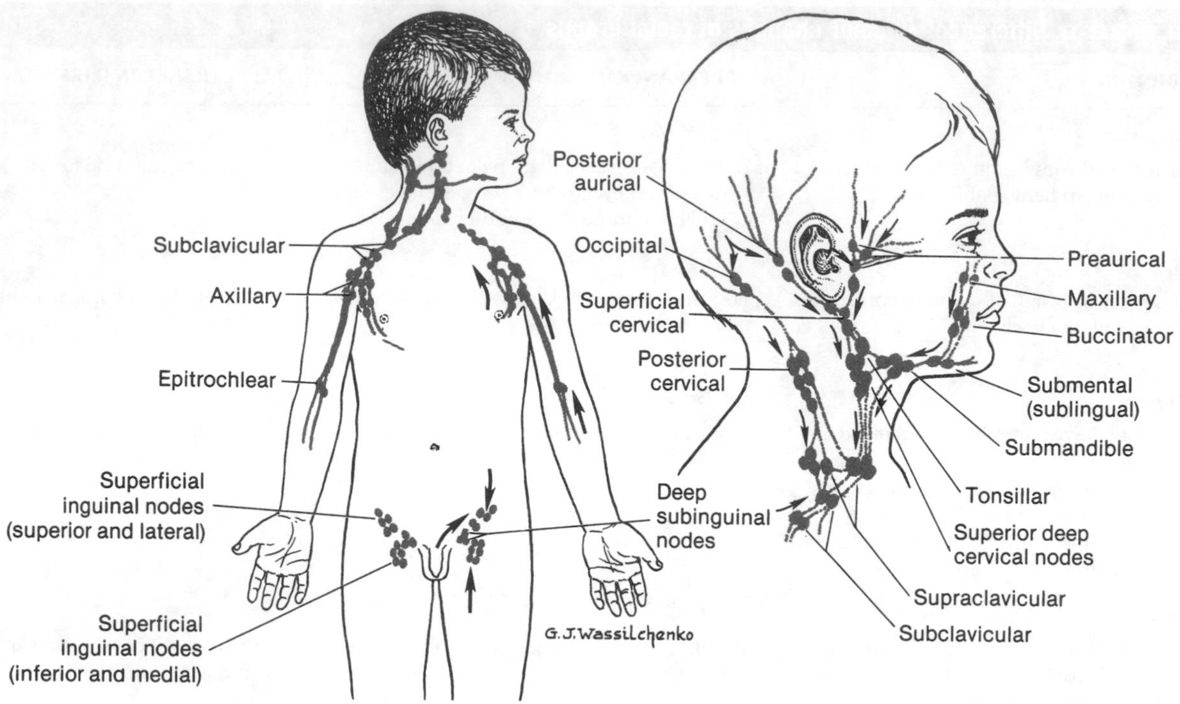

Fig. 32-10 Location of superficial lymph nodes. Arrows indicate directional flow of lymph.

range of motion may indicate *wryneck*, or *torticollis*, a result of injury to the sternocleidomastoid muscle, in which the child holds the head to one side with the chin pointing toward the opposite side.

Nursing ALERT

Hyperextension of the head (opisthotonos) with pain on flexion is a serious indication of meningeal irritation and is referred for immediate medical evaluation.

Palpate the *skull* for patent sutures, fontanels, fractures, and swellings. Normally the posterior fontanel closes by the second month of life and the anterior fontanel fuses between 12 and 18 months of age. Early or late closure is noted, since either may be a sign of a pathologic condition. For a more detailed discussion of the cranial bones, see Chapter 22.

While examining the head, observe the *face* for symmetry, movement, and general appearance. Ask the child to "make a face" to assess symmetric movement and disclose any degree of paralysis. Note any unusual facial proportion such as an unusually high or low forehead, wide- or close-set eyes, or a small, receding chin.

In addition to assessment of the head and neck for movement, inspect the neck for size and palpate for associated structures. The neck is normally short with skinfolds between the head and shoulders during infancy; however, it lengthens during the next 3 to 4 years.

Nursing ALERT

If any masses are detected in the neck, report them for further investigation. Large masses can block the airway.

EYES

Inspection of External Structures

Inspect the *lids* for proper placement on the eye. When the eye is open, the upper lid should fall between the upper iris and the top portion of the pupil. When the eyes are closed, the lids should completely cover the cornea and sclera (Fig. 32-11).

Determine the general slant of the *palpebral fissures* or lids by drawing an imaginary line through the two points of the medial canthus and across the outer orbit of the eyes and aligning each eye on the line. Usually the palpebral fissures lie horizontally. However, in Asian persons the slant is normally upward.

Also inspect the lining of the lids, the *palpebral conjunctiva*. To examine the lower conjunctival sac, pull the lid down while the patient looks up. To evert the upper lid, hold the upper lashes and gently pull *down* and *forward* as the child looks down. Normally the conjunctiva appears pink and glossy. Vertical yellow striations along the edge are the *meibomian* or *sebaceous glands* near the hair follicle. Located in the inner or medial canthus and situated on the inner edge of the upper and lower lids is a tiny opening, the *lacrimal punctum*. Note any excessive tearing or inflammation of the lacrimal apparatus.

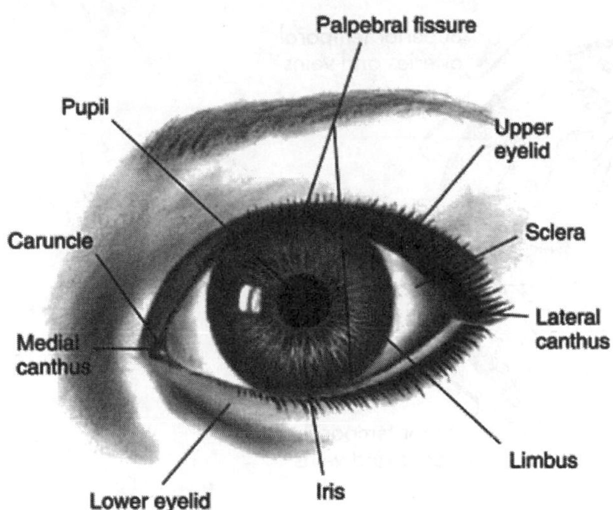

Fig. 32-11 External structure of eye.

The *bulbar conjunctiva,* which covers the eye up to the limbus or junction of the cornea and sclera, should be transparent. The *sclera* or white covering of the eyeball, should be clear. Tiny black marks in the sclera of heavily pigmented individuals are normal.

The *cornea,* or covering of the iris and pupil, should be clear and transparent. Any opacities are recorded, since they can be signs of scarring or ulceration, which can interfere with vision. The best way to test for opacities is to illuminate the eyeball by shining a light at an angle (obliquely) toward the cornea.

Compare the *pupils* for size, shape, and movement. They should be round, clear, and equal. Test their *reaction to light* by quickly shining a source of light toward the eye and removing it. As the light approaches, the pupils should constrict; as the light fades, the pupils should dilate. Test *accommodation,* or the focusing ability of the eyes to produce clear vision at different distances, by having the child look at a bright, shiny object at a distance and quickly moving the object toward the face. The pupils should constrict as the object is brought near the eye. Normal findings on examination of the pupils may be recorded as *PERRLA,* which means *pupils equal, round, react to light and accommodation.*

Inspect the *iris* for color, size, and clarity. Permanent eye color is usually established by 6 to 12 months of age. As the iris and pupil are inspected, look for the *lens.* Normally the lens is not visible through the pupil.

Inspection of Internal Structures

The ophthalmoscope permits visualization of the interior of the eyeball with a system of lenses and a high-intensity light. The lenses permit clear visualization of eye structures at different distances from the nurse's eye and correct visual acuity differences in the examiner and child. Use of the ophthalmoscope requires practice to know which lens setting produces the clearest image.

The ophthalmic and otic head are usually interchangeable on one "body" or handle, which encloses the power source, either disposable or rechargeable batteries. Practice changing the heads, which snap on and are secured with a quarter turn, and replacing the batteries and light bulbs. Nurses who are not directly involved in physical assessment are often responsible for ensuring that the equipment functions properly.

Preparing the child. Prepare the child for the ophthalmic examination by showing the child the instrument, demonstrating the light source and how it shines in the eye, and explaining the reason for darkening the room. For infants and young children who do not respond to such explanations, use distraction to encourage them to keep their eyes open. Forcibly parting the lids results in an uncooperative, watery-eyed child and a frustrated nurse. Usually, with some practice, the nurse can elicit a red reflex almost instantly while approaching the child and may also gain a momentary inspection of the blood vessels, macula, or optic disc.

Funduscopic examination. Fig. 32-12 shows the structures of the back of the eyeball, or the *fundus.* The fundus is immediately apparent as the *red reflex.* The intensity of the color increases in darkly pigmented individuals.

Nursing ALERT

A brilliant, uniform red reflex is an important sign because it virtually rules out almost all serious defects of the cornea, aqueous chamber, lens, and vitreous chamber. Any dark shadows or opacities are recorded because they indicate some abnormality in any of these structures.

As the ophthalmoscope is brought closer to the eye, the most conspicuous feature of the fundus is the *optic disc,* the area where the blood vessels and optic nerve fibers enter and exit from the eye. The color of the disc is creamy pink; it is lighter in color than the surrounding fundus. Normally it is round or vertically oval.

After the optic disc is located, the area is inspected for *blood vessels.* The central retinal artery and vein appear in the depths of the disc and emanate outward with visible branching. The *veins* are darker in color and about one fourth larger in size than the *arteries.* Normally the branches of the arteries and veins cross each other.

Other structures that may be seen are the *macula,* the area of the fundus with the greatest concentration of visual receptors, and, in the center of the macula, a minute glistening spot of reflected light called the *fovea centralis;* this is the area of most perfect vision.

Vision Testing

Several tests are available for assessing vision. This discussion focuses on four areas: (1) binocularity, (2) visual acuity, (3) peripheral vision, and (4) color vision. The reader is referred to Chapter 39 for behavioral and physical signs that indicate visual impairment.

Binocularity. Normally, by the age of 3 to 4 months, children achieve the ability to fixate on one visual field with both eyes simultaneously **(binocularity)**. One of the most important tests for binocularity is alignment of the eyes to detect

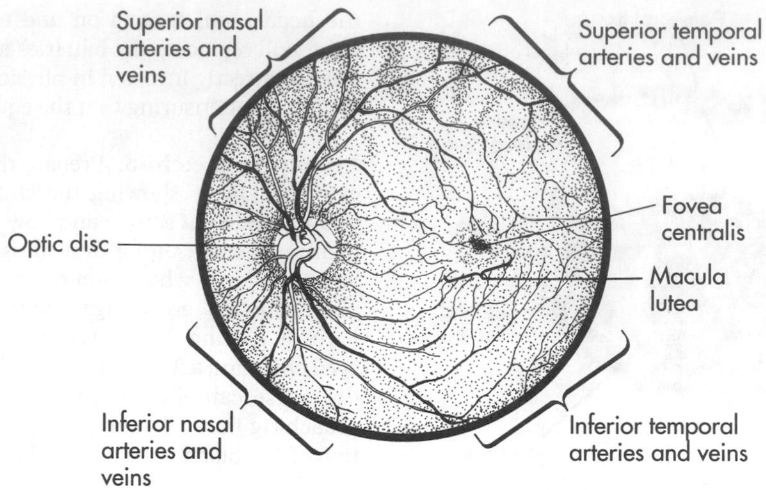

Fig. 32-12 Structures of fundus.

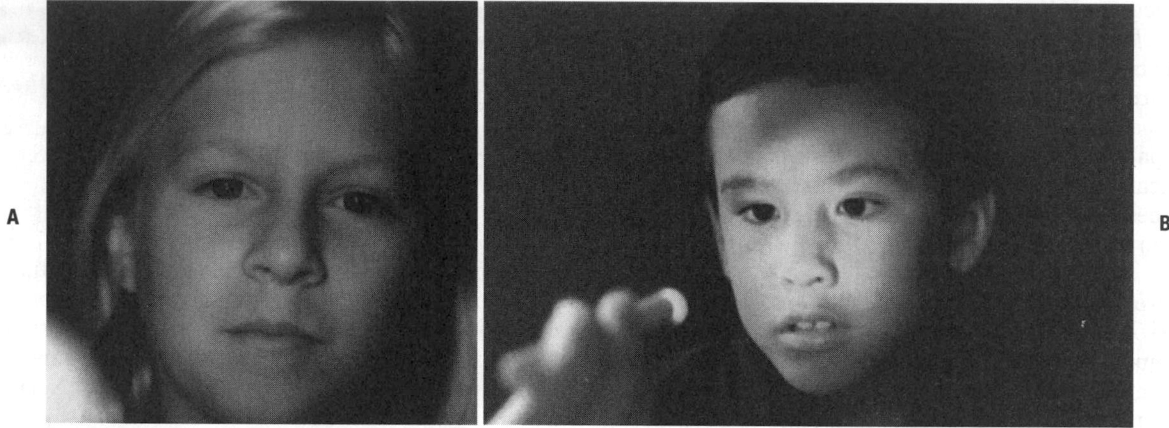

Fig. 32-13 **A,** Corneal light reflex test demonstrating orthophoric eyes. **B,** Pseudostrabismus. Inner epicanthal folds cause eyes to appear malaligned; however, corneal light reflexes fall perfectly symmetrically.

nonbinocular vision, or **strabismus.** In strabismus, or "cross-eye," one eye deviates from the point of fixation. If the malalignment is constant, the weak eye becomes "lazy," and the brain eventually suppresses the image produced by that eye. If strabismus is not detected and corrected by age 4 to 6 years, blindness from disuse, known as *amblyopia,* may result.

Two tests commonly used to detect malalignment are the corneal light reflex and the cover tests. In the *corneal light reflex test* (also called *red reflex gemini test* or *Hirschberg test*), shine a flashlight or the light of the ophthalmoscope directly into the patient's eyes from a distance of about 40.5 cm (16 inches). If the eyes are *orthophoric,* or normal, the light falls symmetrically within each pupil (Fig. 32-13, *A*). If the light falls off center in one eye, the eyes are malaligned. *Epicanthal folds,* excess folds of skin that extend from the roof of the nose to the inner termination of the eyebrow and that partially or completely overlap the inner canthus of the eye, may give a false impression of malalignment (*pseudostrabismus*) (Fig. 32-13, *B*). Epicanthal folds are often found in Asian children.

In the *cover test,* one eye is covered, and the movement of the *uncovered eye* is observed while the child looks at a near (33 cm, or 13 inches) or distant (50 cm, or 20 inches) object. If the uncovered eye does not move, it is aligned. If the uncovered eye moves, a malalignment is present because when the stronger eye is temporarily covered, the weaker eye attempts to fixate on the object.

In the *uncover test,* occlusion is shifted back and forth from one eye to the other, and movement of the *covered* eye is observed as soon as the occluder is removed while the child focuses on a point in front of him or her. If normal alignment is present, shifting the cover from one eye to the other will not cause movement of the covered eye. If malalignment is present, the covered eye will move from its position when covered to a straight position when uncovered. This test takes more practice than the other cover test because the occluder must be moved back and forth quickly and accurately to see the eye

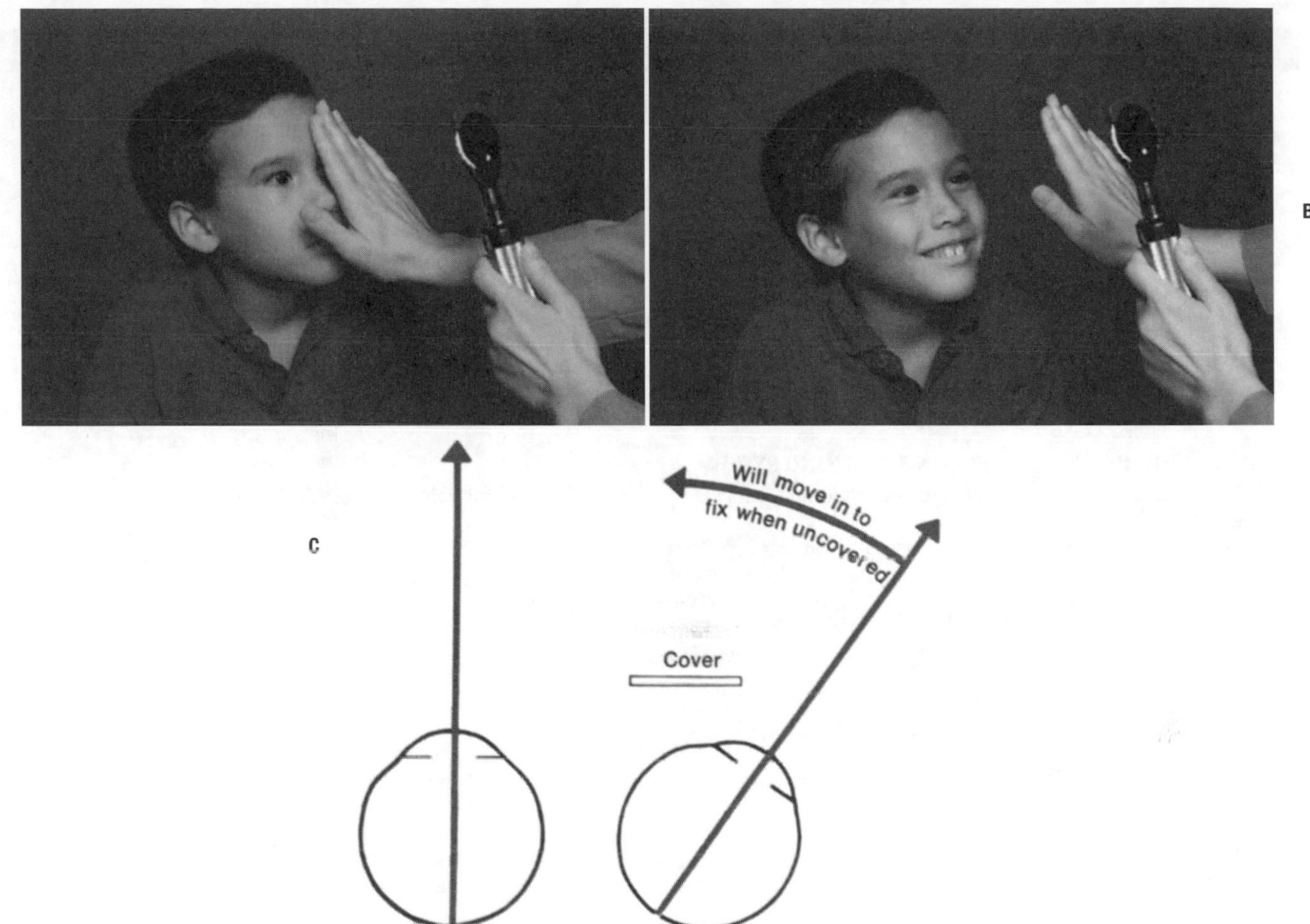

Fig. 32-14 Uncover test for strabismus. **A,** Eye is occluded, child is fixating on light source. **B,** If eye does not move when uncovered, eyes are aligned. **C,** Exophoria. As eye is uncovered, it shifts to fixate on object. (**C** from Prior JA, Silberstein JS, Stang JM: *Physical diagnosis: the history and examination of the patient,* ed 6, St Louis, 1981, Mosby.)

move. Since deviations can occur at different ranges, it is important to perform the cover tests at both close and far distances.

The cover test is usually easier to perform if the examiner uses his or her own hand rather than a card-type occluder (Fig. 32-14). Attractive occluders fashioned like an ice cream cone or happy face lollipop cut from cardboard are also well-received by young children.

Visual acuity testing in children beyond infancy. The most common test for measuring visual acuity (the ability to see near and far objects clearly) is the *Snellen Letter chart,* which consists of lines of letters of decreasing size (see the Appendix). Each line is given a value; for example, line 7 is "20."

During testing, children stand 20 feet from the chart (with heels at the 20-foot line) and read each line. If they can read line 7, they have 20/20 vision, the accepted standard for normal acuity. If they can read only line 2, they have 20/100 vision—they are able to see at a distance of 20 feet what people with 20/20 or normal eyesight can see at 100 feet.

Other letter or symbol screening tests are described in Table 32-10. Many of the tests that are suitable for preschoolers can also be used for difficult-to-test children, such as those with developmental delays. The *Snellen symbol chart* is frequently used to screen preschool children (see the Appendix). However, many young children have difficulty because of confusion in identifying the direction of the E, rather than inability to see the symbol clearly. To avoid this problem, the *Blackbird Preschool Vision Screening System* was developed by a nurse (Fig. 32-15). The screening system uses a modified E that resembles a bird and a story about the Blackbird to help engage children's attention. Testing is done with flash cards or a wall-mounted chart, and the children are instructed to indicate the direction of the bird's flight. Some have reported a higher percentage of children successfully tested with the Blackbird System than with the Snellen E (Sato-Viacrucis, 1985). The Blackbird System also contains guidelines for vision screening the noncommunicative, nonreaders, or non-English-speaking children to assist screeners with more difficult-to-test populations, and the *Blackbird Storybook Home Eye Test* is designed for parents to prescreen young children at home.

TABLE 32-10 Letter or symbol vision acuity tests

DESCRIPTION	COMMENTS*
SNELLEN LETTER†	
Uses letters of the English alphabet for testing at 20 feet	Suitable for most children above the second grade who are familiar with reading the alphabet
SNELLEN E†	
Uses the capital letter E pointing in four directions; children "read" the chart by showing the direction of the letter E or using a large duplicate E to match the chart E at 20 feet	For illiterate or non-English-speaking people, preschool children, and grade 1 Preschool children often have difficulty with direction despite adequate vision
HOME EYE TEST FOR PRESCHOOLERS‡	
Uses a large letter E for demonstration and an E chart for testing at 10 feet	Designed for use by parents for children ages 3 to 6 years
BLACKBIRD PRESCHOOL VISION SCREENING SYSTEMS§	
Uses a modified E to resemble a flying bird; children identify which way the bird is flying Uses flash cards, story-telling, and disposable cardboard eyeglass occluders	Designed for children as young as 3 years
BLACKBIRD STORYBOOK HOME EYE TEST§	
Similar to above	Designed for use by parents for children as young as $2^1/_2$ years
HOTV OR MATCHING SYMBOL†	
Uses the four letters H, O, T, and V on a chart for testing at 10 or 20 feet Child names the letters on the chart or matches them to a demonstration card	Suitable for children as young as 3 years Avoids the problem with image reversal and eye-hand coordination that can occur with the letter E
FAYE SYMBOL CHART†	
Uses pictures of a house, apple, and umbrella on a chart for testing at 10 feet	Suitable for children as young as 27 to 30 months
DENVER EYE SCREENING TEST (DEST)||	
Uses single cards for the letter E, one for demonstration and one for testing at 15 feet Also uses Allen Picture Cards (a tree, birthday cake, horse and rider, telephone, car, house, and teddy bear) for testing at 15 feet	Suitable for children $2^1/_2$ years and older May be reliably used with cooperative children from the age of 24 months
DOT TEST†	
Uses a series of different-sized dots; child points to one of the nine dots randomly positioned on a disk	Suitable for children as young as 24 months

*Ages for testing are based on published reports. Proper instruction of young children is essential for successful screening.
†Available from Good-Lite Co., 1540 Hannah Ave., Forest Park, IL 60130; (708) 366-3860.
‡Available from the National Society to Prevent Blindness, 500 E. Remington Rd., Schaumburg, IL 60173; (800) 331-2020.
§Available from Blackbird Vision Screening System, P.O. Box 277424, Sacramento, CA 95827; (800) 363-6884.
||Available from Denver Developmental Materials, Inc., P.O. Box 6919, Denver, CO 80206-0919; (303) 355-4729.

Although most chart tests are designed for testing at 20 feet, modifications can be made for testing at closer ranges because it is easier to engage children's attention at a closer range, and the charts require less space for the screening lane. Measurements at closer range are converted to the standard 20-foot scale by multiplying the two numbers by the number that converts the first one to 20. For example, 10/25 is equivalent to 20/50. When closer ranges are used, proper positioning of the child (e.g., with heels on the 10-foot mark) is essential. Because young children are active, their tendency to move or lean forward can affect the testing more at close distances than at farther ones. (See Critical Thinking Q & A box on p. 913).

There are no universal criteria for referring children when using Snellen charts. The *National Society to Prevent Blindness* (1988) recommends the following criteria for referral of children for a complete eye examination:

1. Three-year-old children with vision in either eye of 20/50 or less (inability to correctly identify one more than half the symbols on the 40-foot line) or a two-line difference in visual acuity between the eyes in the passing range (e.g., 20/20 in one eye and 20/40 in the other eye)
2. All other ages and grades with vision in either eye of 20/40 or less (inability to correctly identify one more than half the symbols on the 30-foot line)

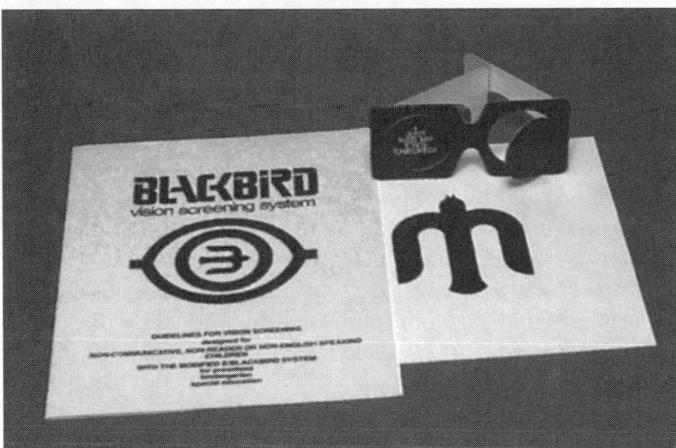

Fig. 32-15 Blackbird Vision Screening System. Note Blackbird symbol and special "eyeglass" occluder.

3. All children who consistently show any signs of possible visual disturbances, regardless of visual acuity (see Chapter 39)

Visual acuity testing in infants and difficult-to-test children. In newborns vision is tested mainly by checking for *light perception* by shining a light into the eyes and noting responses such as pupillary constriction, blinking, following the light to midline, increased alertness, or refusal to open the eyes after exposure to the light. Although the simple maneuver of checking light perception and eliciting the pupillary light reflex indicates that the anterior half of the visual apparatus is intact, it does not confirm that the infant can see. In other words, this test does not assess whether the brain receives the visual message and interprets the signals.

Another test of visual acuity is the infant's ability to fix on and follow a target. Although any brightly colored or patterned object can be used, the human face is excellent. Hold the infant upright while moving your face slowly from side to side.

Nursing ALERT

If visual fixation and following are not present by 3 to 4 months of age, further ophthalmologic evaluation is needed.

Other signs that may indicate visual loss include fixed pupils, marked strabismus, constant nystagmus, setting-sun sign, and slow lateral movements. Unfortunately, it is very difficult to test each eye separately; the presence of such signs in one eye could indicate unilateral blindness.

Special tests are available for testing infants and other difficult-to-test children to assess acuity and/or confirm blindness. For example, in *visually evoked potentials*, the eyes are stimulated with a bright light or pattern, and electrical activity to the visual cortex is recorded through scalp electrodes. Acuity is assessed by using progressively smaller patterns.

Peripheral vision. In children who are old enough to cooperate, estimate *peripheral vision*, or the visual field of each eye,

Critical Thinking Q & A

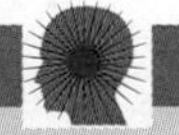

VISION SCREENING

Your nursing class will be assisting with EPSDT (Early Periodic Screening, Diagnosis, and Treatment) screens for preschoolers. You are responsible for setting up the area for visual screening. You will need all of the following equipment *except:*

1. Snellen acuity charts
2. Pirate patches
3. Penlights
4. A paper or metal tape measure

The correct answer is one. The Snellen chart is inappropriate because it uses letters, and it cannot be assumed that preschoolers know their alphabet. The "Lazy E" acuity chart is not ideal, because preschoolers may not have the perceptual abilities needed to determine which direction the "legs" of the E are pointing. A picture acuity chart or the Blackbird system should be used with this population. Pirate patches serve as eye occluders and are needed for assessing acuity and alignment. Penlights are needed for assessing corneal light reflex and pupil reactivity. A non-stretchable tape measure is used to determine the correct distance for assessing acuity when using an eye chart.

Contributed by Judith A. Vessey, RN, C, PhD.

by having children fixate on a specific point directly in front of them as an object, such as a finger or a pencil, is moved from beyond the field of vision into the range of peripheral vision. Check each eye separately and for each quadrant of vision. As soon as children see the object, have them say "stop." At that point measure the angle from the anteroposterior axis of the eye (straight line of vision) to the peripheral axis (point at which the object is first seen). Normally, children see about 50 degrees upward, 70 degrees downward, 60 degrees nasalward, and 90 degrees temporally. Limitations in peripheral vision may indicate blindness from damage to structures within the eye or to any of the visual pathways.

Color vision. Another important test is for color vision. It is estimated that 8% to 10% of white males and less than half that percentage of black males inherit the X-linked disorder known as *color vision deficit* (less acceptable term, *color blindness*). From 0.5% to 1% of white females are affected. Although the severity of impaired perception of color varies considerably, the two most common types are *protanomaly*, in which the child confuses gray with pink or pale blue with green, and *deuteranomaly*, in which the child confuses gray with pale purple or green. In most of these individuals the color vision deficit causes no major problems. However, some of the difficulties encountered by individuals with more severe deficits may be inability to distinguish amber or red traffic lights, failure to see a red brake light on the rear of a car, difficulty in distinguishing green traffic lights from certain types of incandescent street lamps, and a poor sense of color coordination of clothing. For school-age children the greatest difficulty lies in performance of academic skills that use color as a visual aid. Adolescents may be ineligible for certain vocational opportunities, such as electronics, photography, printing, interior decorating, pharmaceuticals, textiles, police work, and several types of military service.

The tests available for color vision include the *Ishihara test* and the *Hardy-Rand-Rittler (HRR) test.* Each consists of a series of cards (pseudoisochromatic) on which is printed a color field composed of spots of a certain "confusion" color. Against the field is a number or symbol similarly printed in dots but of a color likely to be confused with the field color by the person with a color vision deficit. As a result, the figure or letter is invisible to an affected individual but is clearly seen by a person with normal vision. By using the HRR test, which uses symbols rather than numbers, reliable testing can be done on children as young as 3 years of age (Kovalesky, 1985). Nurses administering the test must be familiar with the testing materials and should be able to inform the parents of the disorder's effects on practical areas of living, its genetic transmission, and its irreversibility.

EARS

Inspection of External Structures

The entire external earlobe is called the *pinna,* or *auricle,* and is located on each side of the head. Measure the *height* alignment of the pinna by drawing an imaginary line from the outer orbit of the eye to the occiput or most prominent protuberance of the skull. The top of the pinna should meet or cross this line. Low-set ears are commonly associated with renal anomalies or mental retardation. Measure the *angle* of the pinna by drawing a perpendicular line from the imaginary horizontal line and aligning the pinna next to this mark. Normally the pinna lies within a 10-degree angle of the vertical line (Fig. 32-16). If it falls outside this area, record the deviation and look for other anomalies.

Normally the pinna extends slightly outward from the skull. Except in newborn infants, ears that are flat against the head or protruding away from the scalp may indicate problems. Flattened ears in infants may suggest a frequent side-lying position and, just as with isolated areas of hair loss, may be a clue to investigating parents' understanding of the child's stimulation needs.

Inspect the *skin* surface around the ear for small openings, extra tags of skin, or sinuses. If a sinus is found, note this, since it may represent a fistula that drains into some area of the neck or ear. Cutaneous tags represent no pathologic process but may cause parents concern in terms of the child's appearance.

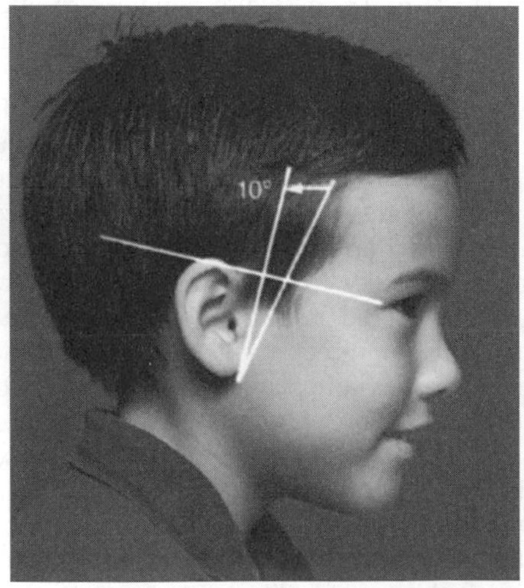

Fig. 32-16 Ear alignment.

Also assess the ear for general *hygiene.* An otoscope is not necessary for looking into the external canal to note the presence of *cerumen,* a waxy substance produced by the ceruminous glands in the outer portion of the canal. Cerumen is usually yellow-brown and soft. If an otoscope is used and any discharge is seen, its color and odor are noted. Prevent transmitting potentially infectious material to the other ear or to another child through handwashing and using disposable specula or sterilizing reusable specula between each examination.

Inspection of Internal Structures

The head of the otoscope permits visualization of the tympanic membrane by use of a bright light, a magnifying glass, and a speculum. Some otoscopes have an attachment for a pneumonic device to insert air into the canal to determine membrane compliance (movement). The speculum, which is inserted into the external canal, comes in a variety of sizes to accommodate different canal widths. The largest speculum that fits comfortably into the ear is used to achieve the greatest area of visualization. The lens, or magnifying glass, is movable, allowing the examiner to insert an object such as a curette into the ear canal through the speculum while still viewing the structures through the lens.

Positioning the child. Before beginning the otoscopic examination, position the child properly and restrain if necessary. Older children usually cooperate and do not need restraint. However, prepare them for the procedure by allowing them to play with the instrument, demonstrating how it works, and stressing the importance of remaining still. A helpful suggestion is to let them observe you examining the parent's ear. Restraint is needed for younger children because the ear examination upsets them (see the Atraumatic Care box below).

As you insert the speculum into the meatus, move it around the outer rim to accustom the child to the feel of something entering the ear. If examining a painful ear, touch a nonpainful part of the affected ear, then examine the unaffected ear, and finally return to the painful ear. By this time the child is usually less fearful of anything causing discomfort to the ear and will cooperate more.

For their protection and safety, infants and toddlers must be restrained for the otoscopic examination. There are two general positions of restraint. In one the child is seated sideways in the parent's lap with one arm "hugging" the parent

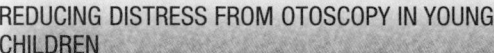

Atraumatic Care

REDUCING DISTRESS FROM OTOSCOPY IN YOUNG CHILDREN

Make examining the ear a game by explaining that you are looking for a "big elephant" in the ear. This kind of "fairy tale" is an absorbing distraction and usually elicits cooperation. After the ear has been examined, clarify that "looking for elephants" was only pretending and thank the child for letting you look in his or her ear.

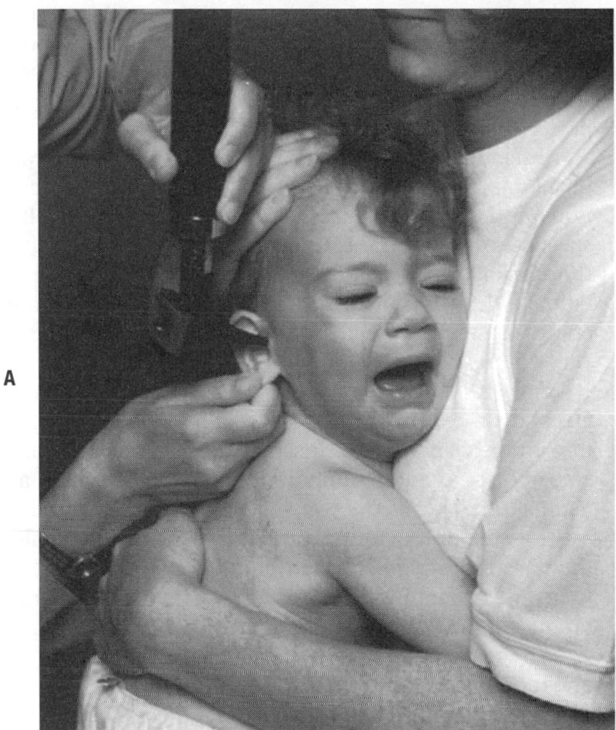

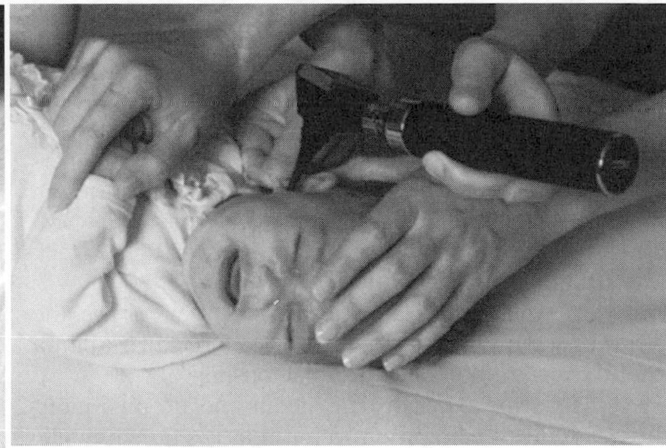

Fig. 32-17 Position for restraining child, **A,** and infant, **B,** during otoscopic examination.

and the other arm at the side. The ear to be examined is toward the nurse. With one arm the parent holds the child's head firmly against his or her chest, and with the other arm "hugs" the child, thereby securing the child's free arm. The ear is examined using the same procedure for holding the otoscope as described later (Fig. 32-17, *A*).

The other position involves placing the child on the side, back, or abdomen with the arms at the side and the head turned so that the ear to be examined points toward the ceiling. Lean over the child and use the upper part of the body to restrain the arms and upper trunk movements, and the examining hand to stabilize the head. This position is practical for young infants or for older children who need minimal restraining, but it may not be feasible for other children who protest vigorously. For safety enlist the parent's or an assistant's help in immobilizing the head by firmly placing one hand above the ear and the other on the child's side, back, or abdomen (Fig. 32-17, *B*).

With cooperative children examine the ear with the child in a side-lying, sitting, or standing position. One disadvantage to standing is that the child may "walk away" as the otoscope enters the canal. If the child is standing or sitting, tilt the head slightly toward the child's opposite shoulder to achieve a better view of the drum (Fig. 32-18).

With the thumb and forefinger of the free (usually nondominant) hand, grasp the auricle. For the two positions of restraint, hold the otoscope upside down at the junction of its head and handle with the thumb and index finger. Place the other fingers against the skull to allow the otoscope to move with the child in case of sudden movement. In examining a cooperative child, hold the handle with the otic head upright or upside down. Use the dominant hand to examine both ears or reverse hands for each ear, whichever is more comfortable.

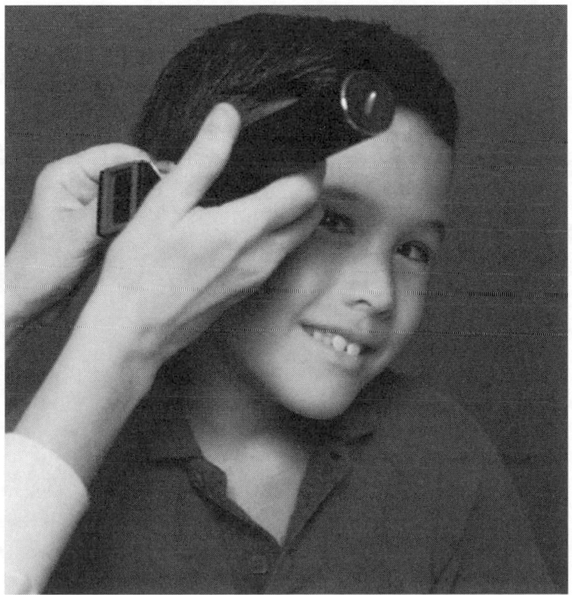

Fig. 32-18 Positioning head by tilting it toward opposite shoulder for full view of tympanic membrane.

Before using the otoscope, visualize the external ear and the tympanic membrane as being superimposed on a clock (see Fig. 32-19). The numbers become important geographic landmarks. Introduce the speculum into the meatus between the 3 and 9 o'clock positions in a *downward* and *forward* position. Because the canal is curved, the speculum does not permit a panoramic view of the tympanic membrane unless the canal is straightened. In infants the canal curves upward. Therefore pull the pinna *down* and *back* to the 6 to 9 o'clock range to straighten the canal (Fig. 32-20, *A*).

With older children, usually those over 3 years of age, the canal curves downward and forward. Therefore pull the pinna *up* and *back* toward a 10 o'clock position (Fig. 32-20, *B*). If there is difficulty in visualizing the membrane, try repositioning the head, introducing the speculum at a different angle, and pulling the pinna in a slightly different direction. Do not insert the speculum past the cartilaginous (outermost) portion of the canal, usually a distance of 0.60 to 1.25 cm (1/4 to 1/2 inch) in older children. Insertion of the speculum into the posterior or bony portion of the canal causes pain.

In neonates and young infants the walls of the canal are pliable and floppy because of the underdeveloped cartilaginous and bony structures. Therefore the very small 2 mm speculum usually needs to be inserted deeper into the canal than in older children. Great care must be exercised not to damage the walls or drum. For this reason, only an experienced examiner should insert an otoscope into the ears of very young infants.

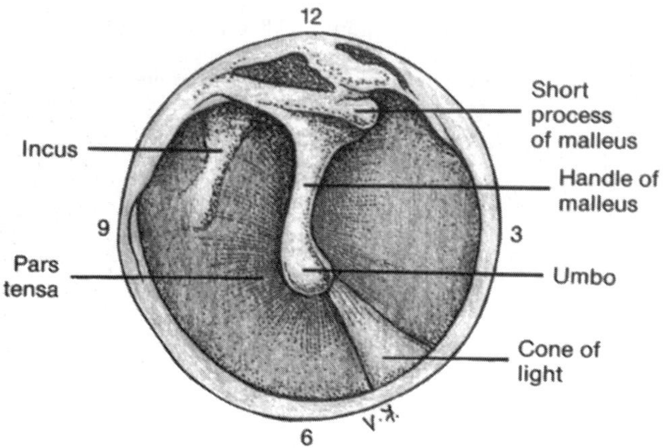

Fig. 32-19 Landmarks of tympanic membrane with "clock" superimposed. (Modified from Potter PA, Perry AG: *Basic nursing: theory and practice,* ed 2, St Louis, 1991, Mosby.)

Otoscopic examination. As you introduce the speculum into the external canal, inspect the walls of the canal, the color of the tympanic membrane, the light reflex, and the usual landmarks of the bony prominences of the middle ear.

The *walls* of the external auditory canal are pink, although they are more pigmented in dark-skinned children. Minute hairs are evident in the outermost portion, where cerumen is produced. Note signs of irritation, foreign bodies, or infection.

Foreign bodies in the ear are not uncommon in children and range from erasers to beans. Symptoms may include pain, discharge, and affected hearing. Soft objects such as paper or insects can be removed with forceps. Small, hard objects such as pebbles can be removed with a suction tip, a hook, or irrigation. However, irrigation is contraindicated if the object is vegetative matter, such as beans or pasta, which swells when in contact with fluid.

Nursing ALERT

If there is any doubt about the type of object in the ear and the appropriate method to remove it, refer the child to the appropriate practitioner.

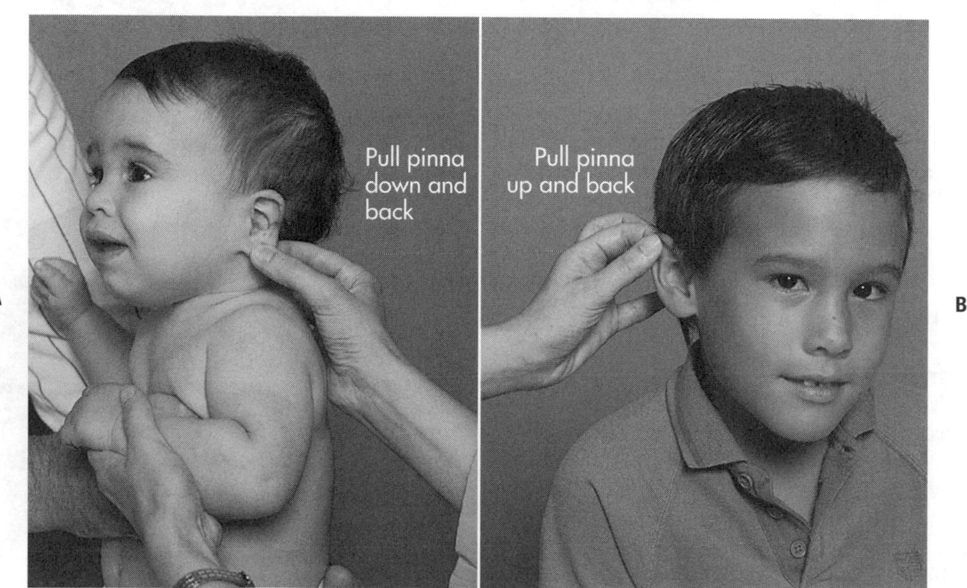

Fig. 32-20 Positioning of eardrum in infant, **A**, and in child over 3 years of age, **B**.

TABLE 32-11 Selected hearing and tympanic membrane compliance tests*

DESCRIPTION	COMMENTS
Clinical hearing tests	
In newborns elicit the startle reflex and observe other neonatal responses to loud noises, such as facial grimaces, blinking, gross motor movement, quiet if crying or crying if quiet, opening the eyes, or ceasing sucking activity. During infancy note child's reaction to a noise. Stand about 18 inches away from infant, to the side, and out of child's peripheral field of vision. With the room silent and infant sitting in parent's lap, distracted by some object, make a voice sound such as "ps" or "phth" (high-pitched) or "oo" (low-pitched), ring a bell or a rattle, or rustle tissue paper.	An objective sign of alerting to sound may be an increase in heart rate or respiratory rate. Absence of alerting behaviors suggests hearing loss. Eliciting the startle reflex is used only in infants from birth to 4 months. Test is usually inadequate for children beyond infancy because of their tendency to ignore sounds or be distracted.
Crib-o-gram	
Neonatal screening tool that analyzes hearing responses by comparing the infant's motor activity before, during, and after a sound is introduced. A motion-sensitive transducer is placed beneath the mattress, and a microprocessor "reads" the infant's movements.	Both administration of the test and its scoring are totally automated. The test is repeated several times to increase reliability. A consistent change in activity that coincides with the test sound is scored as a pass. Neonates who are premature or ill may not respond to sound despite adequate hearing.
Tympanometry	
Measures tympanic membrane compliance (or mobility) and estimates middle ear air pressure. A soft rubber cuff is pressed over the external canal to produce an airtight seal; an automatic reading of air pressure registers on the machine.	Detects middle ear disease and abnormalities but does not indicate the degree of hearing loss or the interpretation of sound. Difficult to perform in young children because of inability to maintain an adequate seal or excessive movement by the child.
Conduction tests	
Rinne test—Stem of tuning fork is placed against the mastoid bone until the sound ceases to be audible. Tuning fork is then moved so that the prongs are held near, but not touching, the auditory meatus. Child should again hear the sound *(Rinne positive)*. If sound is not again audible *(Rinne negative)*, some abnormality is interfering with the conduction of air through the external and middle chambers.	Requires the cooperation and ability of the child to signal when the sound is no longer audible and when it is again heard. Not useful for most children before preschool age.
Weber test—Stem of tuning fork is held in the midline of the head. Child should hear the sound equally in both ears *(Weber positive)*. With air conductive loss, child will hear the sound better in the affected ear *(Weber negative)*.	Often not suitable for young children because of their difficulty in discriminating between "better, more, or less."
Audiometry	
Electrical audiometer measures the threshold of hearing for puretone frequencies and loudness. A sound is transmitted to the child's ear and reduced until child indicates the sound is no longer heard; this procedure is repeated for several sounds covering the range found in conversation. In an air conduction audiogram the sounds are transmitted through earphones. In a bone conduction audiogram the sounds are passed through a plaque placed over the mastoid bone.	Provides valuable information regarding the severity of the hearing loss, the sound cycles involved, and the possible location of the defect. Requires specialized training of personnel, expensive equipment, and cooperation from the child in terms of confirming the perception of sound. For children ages 24 months to about 5 years, play audiometry can be used; it is based on behavior modification and involves reinforcement for correct response.
Evoked otoacoustic emissions (EOAES)	
Special OAE analyzer delivers a rapid series of clicks to the ear through a probe fitted with a tympanometry tip that is inserted closely in the external auditory canal. The presence of OAEs, defined as sound energy emitted by the cochlea that is believed to be generated by the movement of the outer hairs of the organ of Corti, is usually associated with normal or near-normal cochlear sensitivity; their absence indicates a hearing loss of at least 20-25 dB, provided there is no conductive dysfunction (Abdo, Feghali, and Stapells, 1993)	Preferred method of screening neonates for sensorineural hearing loss (ototoxicity and noise-induced hearing loss). Requires specialized equipment. Minimal training is required. Infants must be in a quiet sleep for testing. Results do not indicate severity of cochlear damage; should be followed by BAER (see below).
Brainstem-auditory evoked response (BAER)	
Through electrode wires attached to the infant's or child's scalp, electrical or brain wave potentials generated within the auditory system are transmitted to a computer for analysis. Following repetitive acoustic stimulation, the waveforms from a normal sleeping or quiet infant consist of several peaks and valleys that reflect activations of neural structures of the brain.	Requires specialized training of personnel and expensive equipment.

*Any child who is suspected of a hearing loss because of poor performance using screening tests is referred for special audiometric or BAER testing.

The *color* of the *tympanic membrane* is a translucent, light pearly pink or gray. Note marked erythema (which may indicate suppurative otitis media), a dull nontransparent grayish color (sometimes suggestive of serious otitis media), or ashen-gray areas (signs of scarring from a previous perforation). A black area usually suggests a perforation of the membrane that has not healed.

The characteristic tenseness and slope of the tympanic membrane cause the light of the otoscope to reflect at about the 5 or 7 o'clock position. The *light reflex* is a fairly well-defined cone-shaped reflection, which normally points away from the face.

The *bony landmarks* of the drum are formed by the *umbo*, or tip of the malleus bone. It appears as a small, round, opaque concave spot near the center of the drum. The *manubrium* (long process or handle) of the malleus appears to be a whitish line extending from the umbo upward to the margin of the membrane. At the upper end of the long process near the 1 o'clock position (in the right ear) is a sharp, knoblike protuberance, representing the *short process* of the malleus. Note the absence of the light reflex or loss or abnormal prominence of any of these landmarks.

Auditory Testing

Several types of hearing tests are available (Table 32-11). Some of them, such as audiometric testing, involve specialized equipment that measures the degree of hearing loss. Others such as tests for the startle reflex in neonates are rough estimations of perception of sound. The nurse must operate under a high index of suspicion for those children who may have conditions associated with hearing loss and who may have developed behaviors that indicate auditory impairment. Types of hearing loss, causes, clinical manifestations, and appropriate treatment are discussed in Chapter 39.

NOSE

Inspection of External Structures

The nose is located in the middle of the face just below the eyes and above the lips. Compare its placement and alignment by drawing an imaginary vertical line from the center point between the eyes down to the notch of the upper lip. The nose should lie exactly vertical to this line, with each side exactly symmetric. Note its location, any deviation to one side, and asymmetry in overall size and in diameter of the nares (nostrils). The *bridge* of the nose is sometimes flat in Asian and black children. Observe the *alae nasi* for any sign of flaring, which indicates respiratory difficulty. Always report any flaring of the alae nasi. Fig. 32-21 illustrates the usual landmarks used in describing the external structures of the nose.

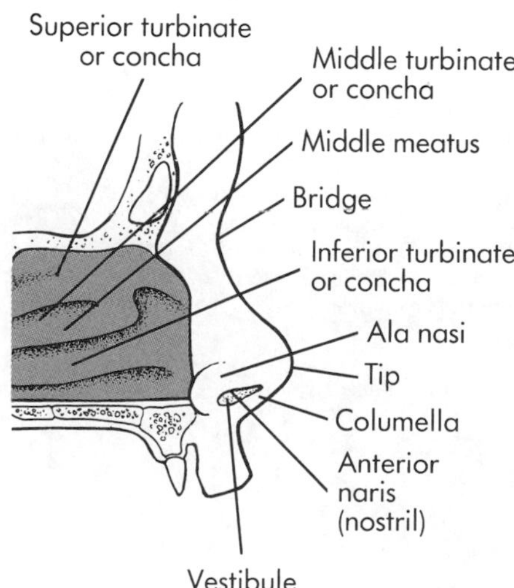

Fig. 32-21 External landmarks and internal structures of nose.

Inspection of Internal Structures

Inspect the *anterior vestibule* of the nose is by pushing the tip upward, tilting the head backward, and illuminating the cavity with a flashlight or otoscope without the attached ear speculum.

Note the *color* of the *mucosal lining*, which is normally redder than the oral membranes, as well as any swelling, discharge, dryness, or bleeding. There should be no discharge from the nose.

On looking deeper into the nose, inspect the *turbinates* or *concha*, plates of bone that jut into the nasal cavity and are enveloped by mucous membrane. The turbinates greatly increase the surface area of the nasal cavity as air is inhaled. The spaces or channels between the turbinates are called *meatus* and correspond to each of the three turbinates. Normally the front end of the inferior and middle turbinate and the middle meatus are seen. They should be the same color as the lining of the vestibule.

Inspect the *septum*, which should divide the vestibules equally. Note any deviation, especially if it causes an occlusion of one side of the nose. A perforation may be evident within the septum. If this is suspected, shine the light of the otoscope into one naris and look for admittance of light through the perforation to the other nostril.

Since olfaction is an important function of the nose, testing for smell may be done at this point or as part of cranial nerve assessment (see Table 32-12, p. 932).

MOUTH AND THROAT

With a cooperative child, almost the entire examination of the mouth and throat can be accomplished without the use of a tongue blade. Ask the child to open the mouth wide, to move the tongue in different directions for full visualization, and to say "ahh," which depresses the tongue for full view of the back of the mouth (tonsils, uvula, and oropharynx). For a closer look at the buccal mucosa or lining of the cheeks, ask

Atraumatic Care

ENCOURAGING OPENING THE MOUTH FOR EXAMINATION

- Perform the examination in front of a mirror.
- Let child first examine someone else's mouth, such as the parent, the nurse, or a puppet (Fig. 32-22, *A*) and then examine the child's mouth.
- Instruct child to tilt the head back slightly, breathe deeply through the mouth, and hold the breath; this action lowers the the tongue to the floor of the mouth without using a tongue blade.

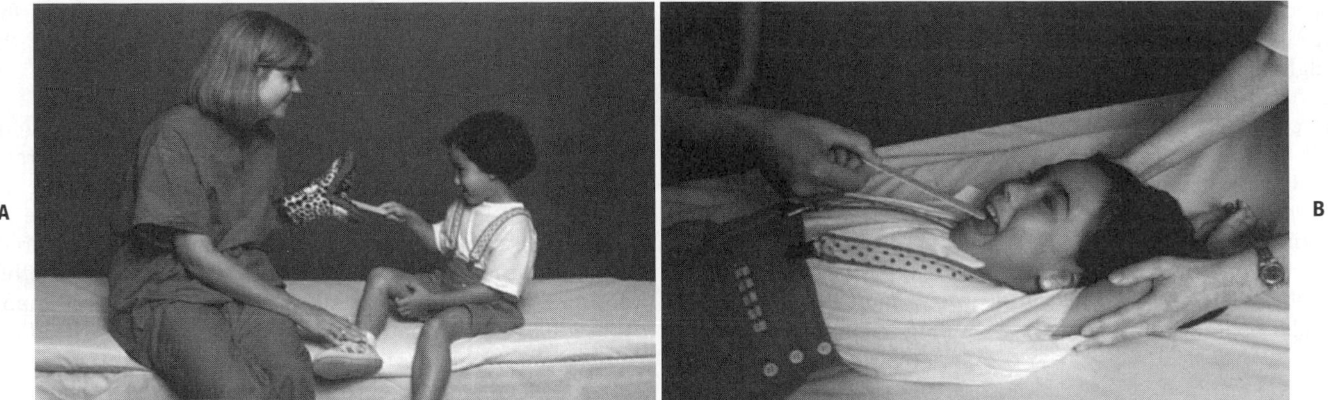

Fig. 32-22 **A,** Encouraging child to cooperate. **B,** Positioning child for examination of mouth.

children to use their fingers to move the outer lip and cheek to one side (see the Atraumatic Care box on p. 918).

Infants and toddlers, however, usually resist attempts to keep the mouth open. Because inspecting the mouth is an upsetting part of the examination, leave it to the end of the physical examination (along with examination of the ears) or do it during episodes of crying. However, the use of a tongue blade (preferably flavored) to depress the tongue is necessary. Place the tongue blade along the *side* of the tongue, not in the center back area where the gag reflex is elicited. Fig. 32-22, *B,* illustrates proper positioning of the child for the oral examination.

The major structure of the exterior of the mouth is the *lips.* The lips should be moist, soft, smooth, and pink, the color of a deeper hue than the surrounding skin. The lips should be symmetric when relaxed or tensed. Assess symmetry when the child talks or cries.

Inspection of Internal Structures

The major structures that are visible within the oral cavity and oropharynx are the mucosal lining of the lips and cheeks, gums or gingiva, teeth, tongue, palate, uvula, tonsils, and posterior oropharynx (Fig. 32-23). Inspect all areas lined with *mucous membranes* (inside the lips and cheeks, gingiva, underside of tongue, palate, and back of pharynx) for color, any areas of white patches or ulceration, bleeding, sensitivity, and moisture. The membranes should be bright pink, smooth, glistening, uniform, and moist.

Inspect the *teeth* for number in each dental arch, for hygiene, and for occlusion or bite (see also Teething, Chapter 33). Discoloration of tooth enamel with obvious plaque (whitish coating on the surface of the teeth) is a sign of poor dental hygiene and indicates a need for counseling. Brown spots in the crevices of the crown of the tooth or between the teeth may be caries (cavities). Chalky white to yellow or brown areas on the enamel may indicate fluorosis (excessive fluoride ingestion). Teeth that appear greenish black may be stained temporarily from ingestion of supplemental iron.

Examine the *gums (gingiva)* surrounding the teeth. The color is normally coral pink, and the surface texture is stippled, similar to the appearance of orange peel. In dark-

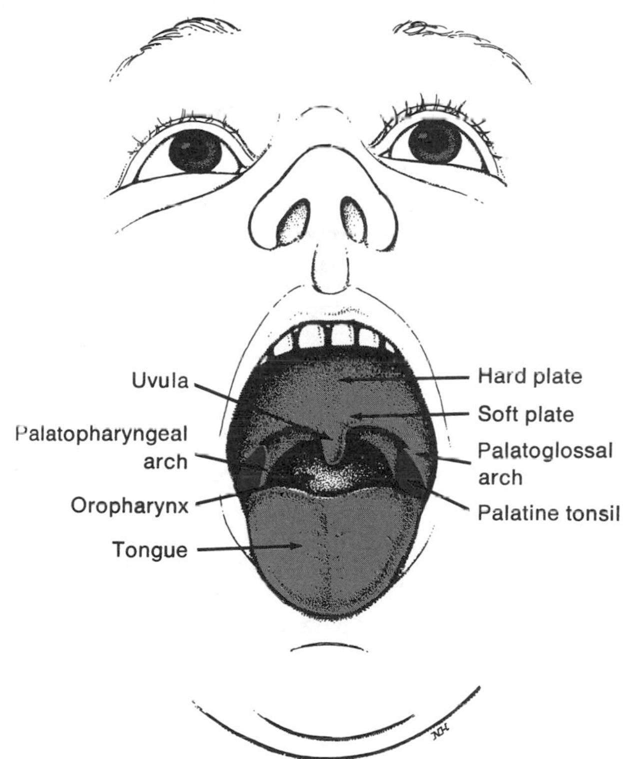

Fig. 32-23 Interior structures of mouth.

skinned children, the gums are more deeply colored, and a brownish area is often observed along the gum line.

Inspect the *tongue* for the presence of papillae, small projections that contain several taste buds and give the tongue its characteristic rough appearance. Note the size and mobility of the tongue. Normally the tip of the tongue should extend to the lips or beyond.

The roof of the mouth consists of the *hard palate,* which is located near the front of the oral cavity, and the *soft palate,* which is located toward the back of the pharynx and which has a small midline protrusion called the *uvula.* Carefully inspect the palates to be sure that they are intact. The arch of the palate should be dome-shaped. A narrow, flat roof or a high, arched palate affects the placement of the tongue and can cause feeding and speech problems. Test movement of the uvula by eliciting a gag reflex. It should move upward to close off the nasopharynx from the oropharynx.

Examine the oropharynx and note the size and color of the *palatine tonsils.* They are normally the same color as the surrounding mucosa, glandular, rather than smooth in appearance, and barely visible over the edge of the palatoglossal arches. The size of the tonsils varies considerably during childhood. However, report any swelling, redness, or white areas on the tonsils.

CHEST

Inspect the chest for size, shape, symmetry, movement, breast development, and the presence of the bony landmarks formed by the ribs and sternum. The *rib cage* consists of twelve ribs and the sternum, or breast bone, located in the midline of the trunk (Fig. 32-24). The *sternum* is composed of three main parts. The *manubrium,* the uppermost portion, can be felt at the base of the neck at the *suprasternal notch.* The largest segment of the sternum is the *body,* which forms the *sternal angle (angle of Louis)* as it articulates with the manubrium. At the end of the body is a small, movable process called the *xiphoid.* The angle of the costal margin as it attaches to the sternum is called the *costal angle* and is normally about 45 to 50 degrees. These bony structures are important landmarks in the location of ribs and intercostal spaces.

Intercostal spaces (ICS) are the spaces between the ribs. They are numbered according to the rib directly *above* the space. For example, the space immediately below the second rib is the second intercostal space.

The *thoracic cavity* is also divided into segments by drawing imaginary lines on the chest and back. Fig. 32-25 illustrates the anterior, lateral, and posterior divisions. Measure the *size* of the chest by placing the measuring tape around the rib cage at the nipple line (see Fig. 32-4). For greatest accuracy take two measurements, one during inspiration and the other during expiration, and record the average. Chest size is important mainly in comparison with its relationship to head circumference, which is discussed on p. 900. Always report marked disproportions because most are caused by abnormal head growth, although some may be the result of altered chest shape, such as *barrel chest* (chest is round) or *pigeon chest* (sternum protrudes outward).

During infancy the *shape* of the chest is almost circular, with the anteroposterior (front-to-back) diameter equaling the transverse or lateral (side-to-side) diameter. As the child grows, the chest normally increases in the transverse direction, causing the anteroposterior diameter to be less than the lateral diameter. Note the *angle* made by the lower costal margin and the sternum, and palpate the junction of the ribs to the costal cartilage (costochondral junction) and sternum, which should be fairly smooth.

Movement of the chest wall should be symmetric bilaterally and coordinated with breathing. During inspiration, the chest rises and expands, the diaphragm descends, and the costal an-

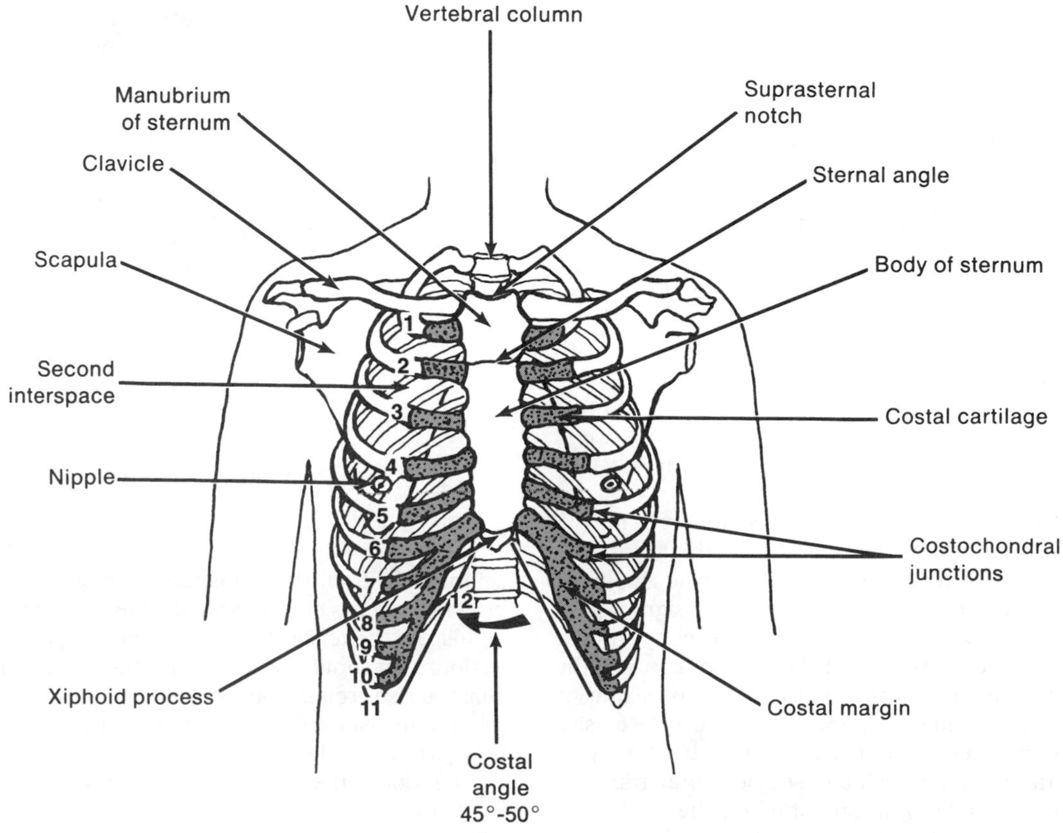

Fig. 32-24 Rib cage.

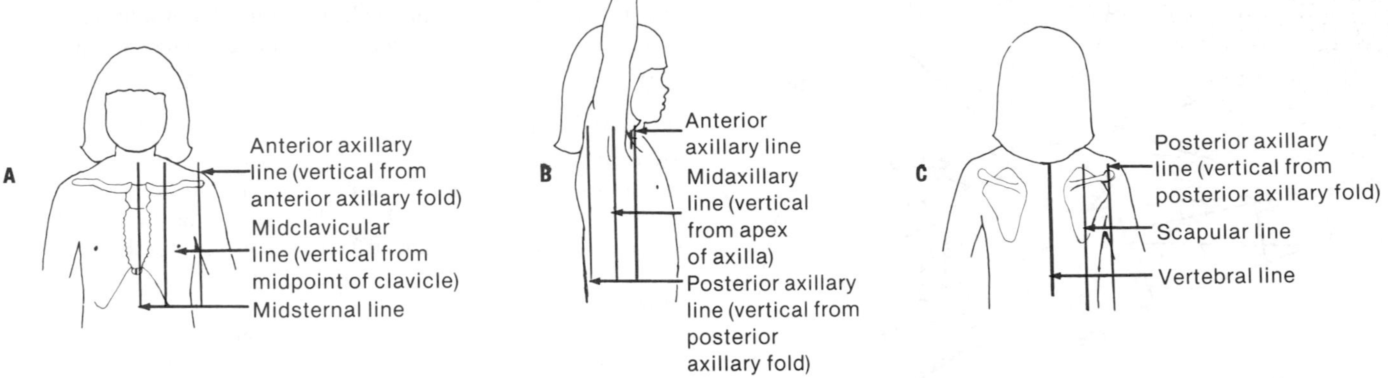

Fig. 32-25 Imaginary landmarks of chest. **A,** Anterior. **B,** Right lateral. **C,** Posterior.

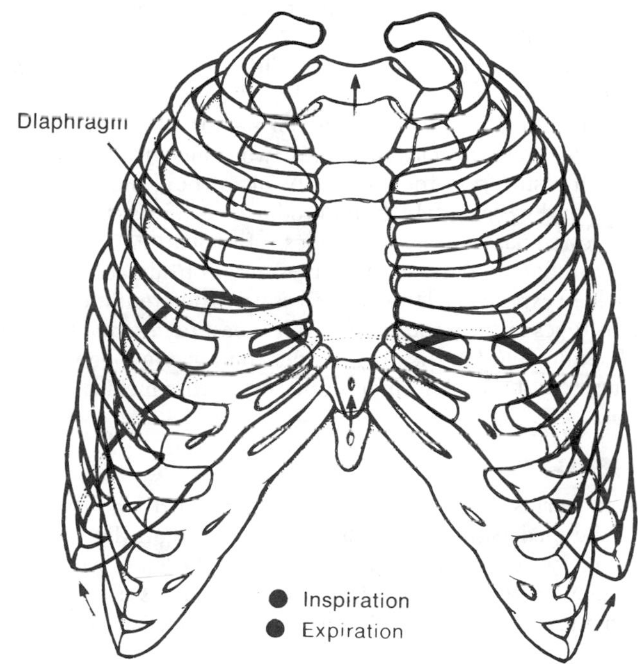

Fig. 32-26 Movement of chest during respiration.

gle increases. During expiration, the chest falls and decreases in size, the diaphragm rises, and the costal angle narrows (Fig. 32-26). In children under 6 or 7 years of age, respiratory movement is principally abdominal or diaphragmatic. In older children, particularly females, respirations are chiefly thoracic. In either type, the chest and abdomen should rise and fall together. Always report any asymmetry of movement.

While inspecting the skin surface of the chest, observe the position of the *nipples,* as well as any evidence of *breast development.* Normally the nipples are located slightly lateral to the midclavicular line between the fourth and fifth ribs. Note symmetry of nipple placement and normal configuration of a darker pigmented areola surrounding a flat nipple in the prepubertal child.

Pubertal breast development usually begins in girls between 10 and 14 years of age (see Chapter 37). Record early (precocious) or delayed breast development, as well as evidence of any other secondary sexual characteristics. In males *breast enlargement (gynecomastia)* may be caused by hormonal or systemic disorders, but more commonly it is a result of adipose tissue from obesity or a transitory body change during early puberty. In either situation investigate the child's feelings regarding breast enlargement.

In adolescent females who have achieved sexual maturity, palpate the breasts for evidence of any masses or hard nodules. Use this opportunity to discuss the importance of routine self-breast examination so that it becomes a practiced habit during later years. Emphasize that most palpable masses are benign to decrease any fear or concern that results when a mass is felt.

LUNGS

The *lungs* are situated inside the thoracic cavity, with one lung on each side of the sternum. Each lung is divided into an *apex,* which is slightly pointed and rises above the first rib; a *base,* which is wide and concave and rides on the dome-shaped diaphragm; and a body, which is divided into *lobes.* The right lung has three lobes: the upper, middle, and lower. The left lung has only two lobes, the upper and lower, because of the space occupied by the heart (Fig. 32-27).

Inspection of the lungs primarily involves observation of respiratory movements, which are discussed on p. 903. Evaluate respirations for rate (number per minute), rhythm (regular, irregular, or periodic), depth (deep or shallow), and quality (effortless, automatic, difficult, or labored). Note the character of breath sounds such as noisy, grunting, snoring, or heavy.

Evaluate respiratory movements by placing each hand flat against the back or chest with the thumbs in midline along the lower costal margin of the lungs. The child should be sitting during this procedure and, if cooperative, should take several deep breaths. During respiration your hands will move with the chest wall. Assess the amount and speed of respiratory excursion and note any asymmetry of movement.

Experienced examiners may percuss the lungs. The anterior lung is percussed from apex to base, usually with the child in the supine or sitting position. Each side of the chest is percussed in sequence to compare the sounds. When the posterior lung is percussed, the procedure and sequence are the

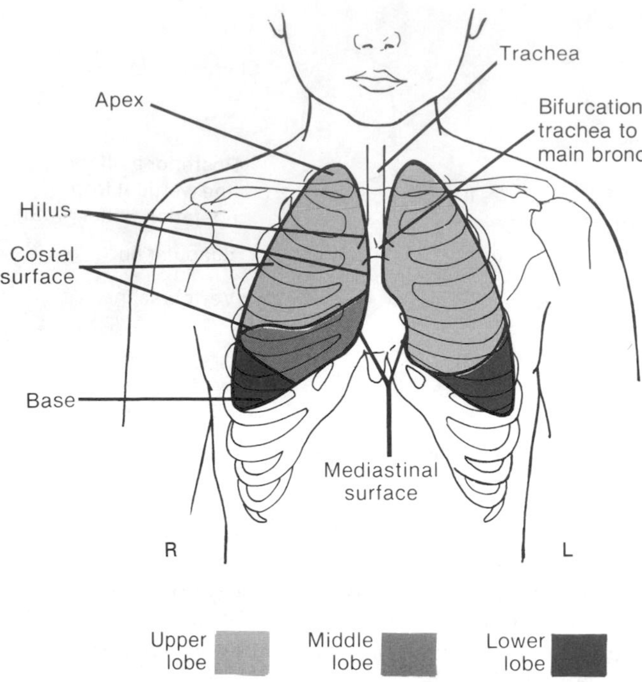

Fig. 32-27 Location of lobes of lungs within thoracic cavity.

Guidelines

EFFECTIVE AUSCULTATION

Make sure child is relaxed and not crying, talking, or laughing. Record if child is crying.
Check that room is comfortable and quiet.
Warm stethoscope before placing it against skin.
Apply firm pressure on chestpiece but not enough to prevent vibrations and transmission of sound.
Avoid placing stethoscope over hair or clothing, moving it against skin, breathing on tubing, or sliding fingers over chestpiece, which may cause sounds that falsely resemble pathologic findings.
Use a symmetric and orderly approach to compare sounds.

Atraumatic Care

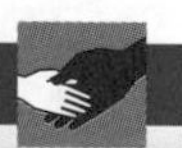

ENCOURAGING DEEP BREATHS

Ask child to "blow out" the light on an otoscope or pocket flashlight; discreetly turn off the light on the last try so that the child feels successful.
Place a cotton ball in child's palm; ask child to blow the ball into the air and have parent catch it.
Place a small tissue on the top of a pencil and ask child to blow the tissue off.
Have child blow a pinwheel, a party horn, or bubbles.

same, although the child should be sitting. Resonance is heard over all the lobes of the lungs that are not adjacent to other organs. Any deviation from the expected sound is recorded and reported.

Auscultation

Auscultation involves using the stethoscope to evaluate breath sounds (see the Guidelines box to the left). Breath sounds are best heard if the child inspires deeply (see the Atraumatic Care box below, left). In the lungs breath sounds are classified as vesicular, bronchovesicular, or bronchial (Box 32-4).

Absent or *diminished breath sounds* are always an abnormal finding warranting investigation. Fluid, air, or solid masses in the pleural space all interfere with the conduction of breath sounds. Diminished breath sounds in certain segments of the lung can alert the nurse to pulmonary areas that may benefit from chest physiotherapy. Increased breath sounds following pulmonary therapy indicate improved passage of air through the respiratory tract.

Various pulmonary abnormalities produce *adventitious sounds* that are not normally heard over the chest. These sounds occur in addition to normal or abnormal breath sounds. They are classified into two main groups: *crackles*, which result from the passage of air through fluid or moisture, and *wheezes*, which are produced as air passes through narrowed passageways, regardless of the cause, such as exudate, inflammation, spasm, or tumor. Considerable practice with an experienced tutor is necessary to differentiate the various types of lung sounds. Often it is best to describe the type of sound heard in the lungs rather than trying to label it. Always report any abnormal sounds for further medical evaluation.

HEART

The heart is situated in the thoracic cavity between the lungs in the mediastinum and above the diaphragm (Fig. 32-28). About two thirds of the heart lies within the left side of the rib cage, with the other third on the right side as it crosses the sternum. The heart is positioned in the thorax like a trapezoid:

BOX 32-4
Classification of Normal Breath Sounds

Vesicular breath sounds

Heard over entire surface of lungs, with exception of upper intrascapular area and area beneath manubrium.
Inspiration is louder, longer, and higher pitched than expiration.
Sound is soft, swishing noise.

Bronchovesicular breath sounds

Heard over manubrium and in upper intrascapular regions where trachea and bronchi bifurcate.
Inspiration is louder and higher in pitch than in vesicular breathing.

Bronchial breath sounds

Heard only over trachea near suprasternal notch.
Inspiratory phase is short, and expiratory phase is long.

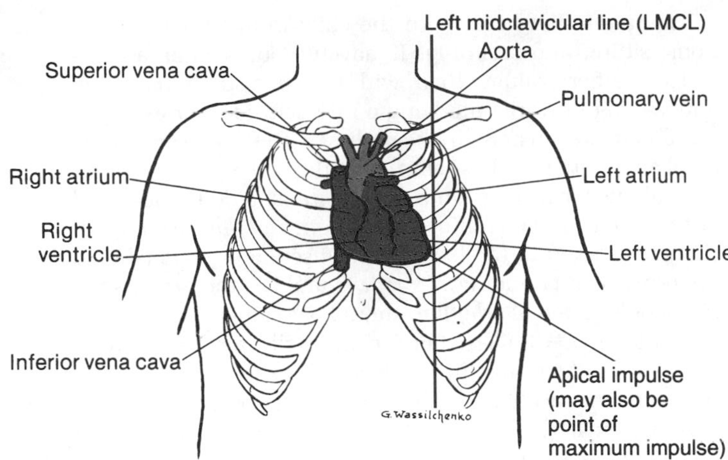

Fig. 32-28 Position of heart within thorax.

Vertically along the right sternal border (RSB) from the second to the fifth rib

Horizontally (long side) from the lower right sternum to the fifth rib at the left midclavicular line (LMCL)

Diagonally from the left sternal border (LSB) at the second rib to the LMCL at the fifth rib

Horizontally (short side) from the RSB and LSB at the second intercostal space (ICS)—base of the heart

Inspection is best done with the child sitting in a semi-Fowler position. Look at the anterior chest wall from an angle, comparing both sides of the rib cage with each other. Normally, they should be symmetric. In children with thin chest walls, a pulsation may be visible. Since comprehensive evaluation of cardiac function is not limited to the heart, also consider other findings such as the presence of all pulses (especially the femoral pulses) (Fig. 32-29), distended neck veins, clubbing of the fingers, peripheral cyanosis, edema, blood pressure, and respiratory status.

Use palpation to determine the location of the *apical impulse (AI)*, the most lateral cardiac impulse that may correspond to the apex. The AI is found:

- Just lateral to the left MCL and fourth ICS in children <7 years of age
- At the left MCL and fifth ICS in children >7 years of age

Although the AI gives a general idea of the size of the heart (with enlargement, the apex is lower and more lateral), its normal location is quite variable, making it a rather unreliable indicator of heart size.

The *point of maximum intensity (PMI)*, as the name implies, is the area of most intense pulsation. Usually, the PMI is located at the same site as the AI, but it can occur elsewhere. For this reason, the two terms should not be used synonymously.

Assess *capillary filling time*—an important test for peripheral circulation by pressing the skin lightly on a central site such as the forehead or a peripheral site such as the top of the hand to produce a slight blanching. The time it takes for the blanched area to return to its original color is the *capillary refill time*.

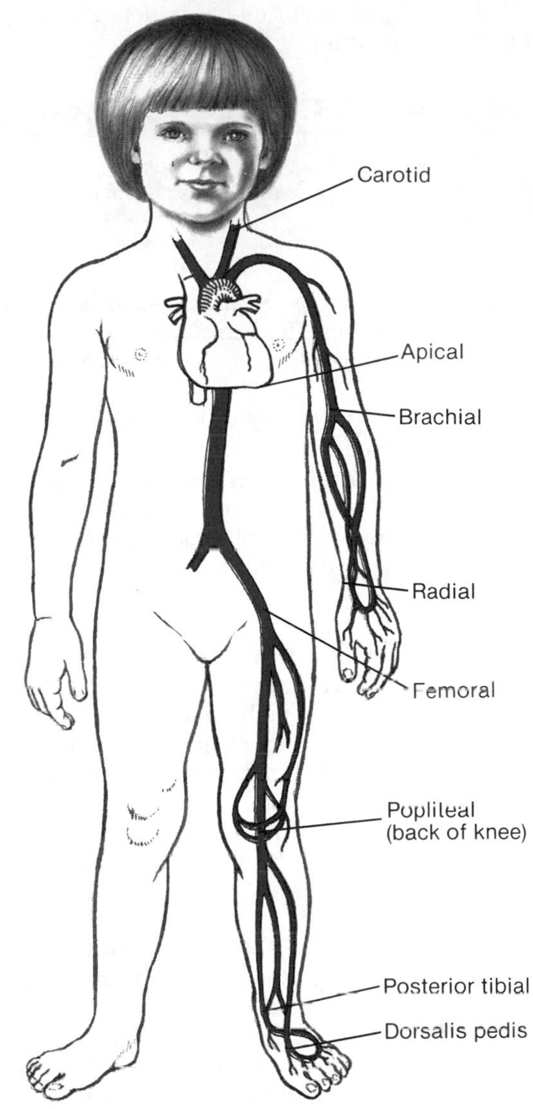

Fig. 32-29 Location of pulses.

Nursing ALERT

Capillary refill should be brisk—in less than 2 seconds; prolonged refill may be associated with poor systemic perfusion, as well as a cool temperature.

Auscultation

Origin of heart sounds. The heart sounds are produced by the opening and closing of the valves and the vibration of blood against the walls of the heart and vessels. Normally, two sounds—S_1 and S_2—are heard, which correspond respectively to the familiar "lub dub" often used to describe the sounds. S_1 is caused by closure of the *tricuspid* and *mitral valves* (sometimes called the *atrioventricular valves*). S_2 is the result of closure of the *pulmonic* and *aortic valves* (sometimes called *semilunar valves*). Normally the split of the two sounds in S_2 is distinguishable and widens during inspiration. *Physiologic splitting* is a significant normal finding.

Nursing ALERT

"Fixed splitting," in which the split in S_2 does not change during inspiration, is an important diagnostic sign of atrial septal defect.

Two other heart sounds—S_3 and S_4—may be produced. S_3 is normally heard in some children; S_4 is rarely heard as a normal heart sound; usually it indicates the need for further cardiac evaluation.

Another important category of heart sounds is *murmurs,* sounds that are produced by vibrations within the heart chambers or in the major arteries from the back-and-forth flow of blood. The description and classification of murmurs are skills that require considerable practice and training. Consult with an experienced practitioner whenever a murmur is identified or suspected.

Differentiating normal heart sounds. Fig. 32-30 illustrates the approximate anatomic position of the valves within the heart chambers. Note that the anatomic location of valves does not correspond to the area where the sounds are heard best. The auscultatory sites are located in the direction of the blood flow through the valves.

Normally S_1 is louder at the apex of the heart in the mitral and tricuspid area, and S_2 is louder near the base of the heart in the pulmonic and aortic area. Listen to each sound by inching down the chest. To distinguish between S_1 or S_2 heart sounds, simultaneously palpate the carotid pulse with the index and middle finger and listen to the heart sounds; S_1 is synchronous with the carotid pulse. The following areas should also be auscultated for sounds such as murmurs, which may radiate to these sites: the sternoclavicular area above the clavicles and manubrium, the area along the sternal border, the area along the left midaxillary line, and the area below the scapulae.

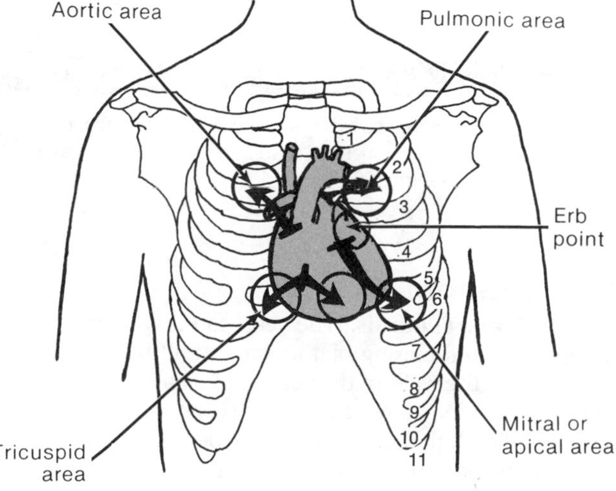

Fig. 32-30 Direction of heart sounds for anatomic valve sites and areas (circled) for auscultation.

Auscultate the heart with the child in at least two positions: sitting and reclining. If adventitious sounds are detected, further evaluate them with the child standing, sitting and leaning forward, and lying on the left side. For example, atrial sounds such as S_4 are heard best with the person in a recumbent position and usually fade if the person sits or stands.

Evaluate for heart sounds (1) *quality* (should be clear and distinct, not muffled, diffuse, or distant); (2) *intensity,* especially in relation to the location or auscultatory site (should not be weak or pounding); (3) *rate* (should be the same as the radial pulse); and (4) *rhythm* (should be regular and even). A particular arrhythmia that occurs normally in many children is *sinus arrhythmia,* in which the heart rate increases with inspiration and decreases with expiration. Differentiate this rhythm from a truly abnormal arrhythmia by having children hold their breath. In sinus arrhythmia, cessation of breathing causes the heart rate to remain steady.

ABDOMEN

Examination of the abdomen involves inspection, followed by auscultation and then palpation. Palpation is performed last because it may distort the normal abdominal sounds. Knowledge of the anatomic placement of the abdominal organs is essential to differentiate normal, expected findings from abnormal ones (Fig. 32-31).

For descriptive purposes divide the abdominal cavity into four quadrants by drawing a vertical line midway from the sternum to the pubic symphysis and a horizontal line across the abdomen through the umbilicus. Each section is named as follows:

- Left upper quadrant (LUQ)
- Left lower quadrant (LLQ)
- Right upper quadrant (RUQ)
- Right lower quadrant (RLQ)

Inspection

Note the *contour* of the abdomen with the child erect and supine. Normally the abdomen of infants and young children is quite cylindric and, in the erect position, fairly prominent because of the physiologic lordosis of the spine. In the supine position the abdomen appears flat. In a healthy child a midline protrusion is usually a variation of normal muscular development.

Nursing ALERT

A tense, boardlike abdomen is a serious sign of paralytic ileus and intestinal obstruction.

The *skin* covering the abdomen should be uniformly taut, without wrinkles or creases. Sometimes silvery, whitish striae ("stretch marks") are seen, especially if the skin has been stretched as in obesity. Superficial veins are usually visible in light-skinned, thin infants, but distended veins are an abnormal finding.

Observe movement of the abdomen. Normally, chest and abdominal movements are synchronous. In infants and thin children *peristaltic waves* may be visible through the abdominal wall; they are best observed by standing at eye level to and across from the abdomen. Always report this finding.

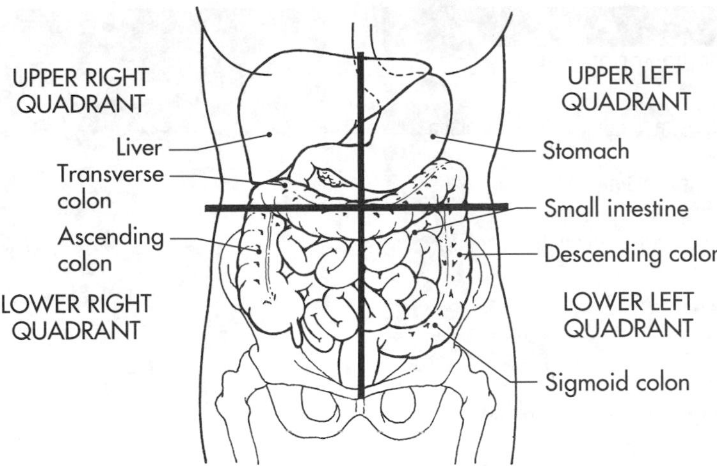

Fig. 32-31 Location of structures in abdomen. Cross rules divide cavity into quadrants.

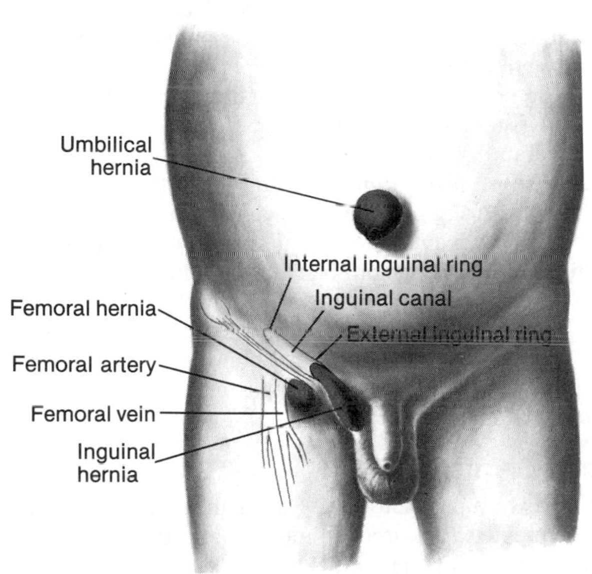

Fig. 32-32 Location of hernias.

Examine the *umbilicus* for size, hygiene, and evidence of any abnormalities such as hernias. The umbilicus should be flat or only slightly protruding. If a herniation is present, palpate the sac for abdominal contents and estimate the approximate size of the opening. *Umbilical hernias* are common in infants, especially in black children.

Hernias may exist elsewhere on the abdominal wall (Fig. 32-32). An *inguinal hernia* is a protrusion of peritoneum through the abdominal wall in the inguinal canal. It occurs mostly in males, is often bilateral, and may be visible as a mass in the scrotum. To locate a hernia, slide the little finger into the external inguinal ring at the base of the scrotum and ask the child to cough. If a hernia is present, it will hit the tip of the finger. If the child is too young to cough, have the child blow up a balloon or laugh to raise the intraabdominal pressure sufficiently to demonstrate the presence of an inguinal hernia.

A *femoral hernia,* which occurs more often in girls, is felt or seen as a small mass on the anterior surface of the thigh just below the inguinal ligament in the femoral canal (a potential space medial to the femoral artery). Feel for a hernia by placing the index finger of your right hand on the child's right femoral pulse (left hand for left pulse) and the middle ring finger flat against the skin toward the midline. The ring finger lies over the femoral canal, where the herniation occurs. Palpation of hernias in the pelvic region is often part of the examination of genitalia.

Auscultation

The most important finding to listen for is **peristalsis,** or *bowel sounds,* which sound like short metallic clicks and gurgles. Their frequency per minute should be recorded (e.g., five bowel sounds per minute). Bowel sounds may be stimulated by stroking the abdominal surface with a fingernail. Report absence of bowel sounds or hyperperistalsis, since either usually denotes an abdominal disorder.

Palpation

Two types of palpation are performed: superficial and deep. In *superficial palpation* lightly place the hand against the skin and feel each quadrant, noting any areas of tenderness, muscle tone, and superficial lesions, such as cysts. Since superficial palpation is often perceived as tickling, several techniques can be used to minimize this sensation and provide relaxation (see the Atraumatic Care box on p. 926). Admonishing the child to stop laughing only draws attention to the sensation and decreases cooperation.

Deep palpation is used for palpating organs and large blood vessels and for detecting masses and tenderness that were not discovered during superficial palpation. Palpation usually begins in the lower quadrants and proceeds upward to avoid missing the edge of an enlarged liver or spleen. Except for palpating the liver, successful identification of other organs such as the spleen, kidney, and part of the colon, requires considerable practice with tutored supervision. Report any questionable mass.

The lower edge of the *liver* is sometimes felt in infants and young children as a superficial mass 1 to 2 cm (0.4 to 0.8

Atraumatic Care

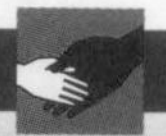

PROMOTING RELAXATION DURING ABDOMINAL PALPATION

- Position child comfortably, such as in a semireclining position in the parent's lap, with knees flexed.
- Warm the hands before touching the skin.
- Use distraction such as telling stories or talking to child.
- Teach child to use deep breathing and to concentrate on an object.
- Give infant a bottle or pacifier.
- Begin with light, superficial palpation and gradually progress to deeper palpation.
- Palpate any tender or painful areas last.
- Have child hold the parent's hand and squeeze it if palpation is uncomfortable.
- Use the nonpalpating hand to comfort child such as placing the free hand on the child's shoulder while palpating the abdomen.
- To minimize sensation of tickling during palpation:
  - Have children "help" with palpation by placing their hand over the palpating hand.
  - Have them place their hand on the abdomen with the fingers spread wide apart, and palpate between their fingers.

inch) below the right costal margin (the distance is sometimes measured in fingerbreadths). Normally the liver descends during inspiration as the diaphragm moves downward. Do not mistake this downward displacement as a sign of liver enlargement.

Nursing ALERT

If the liver is palpable 3 cm below the right costal margin or the spleen is palpable more than 2 cm below the left costal margin, these organs are enlarged—a finding that is always reported for further medical investigation.

Palpate the *femoral pulses* by placing the tips of two or three fingers (index, middle, and/or ring) along the inguinal ligament about midway between the iliac crest and pubic symphysis. Feel both pulses simultaneously to make certain that they are equal and strong (Fig. 32-33).

Nursing ALERT

Absence of femoral pulses is a significant sign of coarctation of the aorta and is referred for medical evaluation.

GENITALIA

Examination of genitalia conveniently follows assessment of the abdomen while the child is still supine. In adolescents inspection of the genitalia may be left to the end of the examination. The best approach is to examine the genitalia matter-of-factly, placing no more emphasis on this part of the assessment than on any other segment. It helps to relieve children's and parents' anxiety by telling them the results of the findings, for example, "Everything looks fine here."

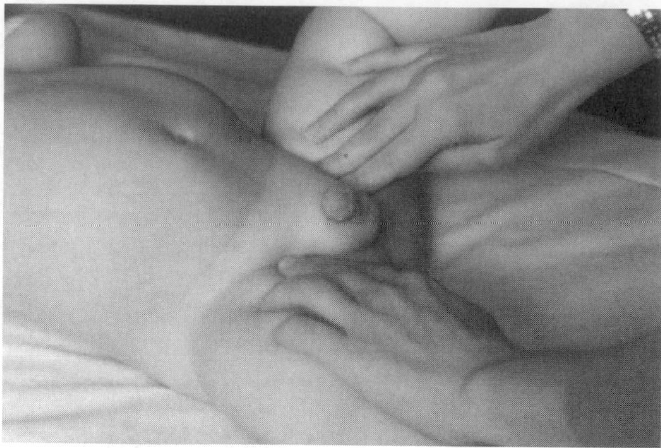

Fig. 32-33 Palpating for femoral pulses.

If it is necessary to ask questions about discharge or difficulty in urinating, respect the child's privacy by covering the lower abdomen with the gown or underpants. To prevent embarrassing interruptions, keep the door or curtain closed and post a "do not disturb" sign. Have a drape ready to cover the genitalia if someone enters the room.

In examining the genitalia, wear gloves whenever touching body substances. It might be helpful for the adolescent to know that wearing gloves also prevents skin-to-skin contact.

The genital examination is an excellent time for eliciting questions of concern about body functioning or sexual activity. Also use this opportunity to increase or reinforce the child's knowledge of reproductive anatomy by naming each body part and explaining its function. For males, this part of the health assessment is an opportune time to teach self-testicular examination.

Male Genitalia

Note the external appearance of the glans and shaft of the penis, the prepuce, the urethral meatus, and the scrotum (Fig. 32-34). The size of the *penis* is generally small in infants and young boys until puberty, when it begins to increase in both length and width. Be familiar with normal pubertal growth of the external male genitalia to compare the findings with the expected sequence of maturation (see Chapter 37).

Examine the *glans* (head of the penis) and *shaft* (portion between the perineum and prepuce) for signs of swelling, skin lesions, inflammation, or other irregularities. Any of these signs may indicate underlying disorders, especially sexually transmitted diseases.

The *urethral meatus* is carefully inspected for location and evidence of discharge. Normally it is centered at the tip of the glans.

Hair distribution is also noted. Normally before puberty, no pubic hair is present. Soft downy hair at the base of the penis is an early sign of pubertal maturation. In older adolescents hair distribution is diamond-shaped from the umbilicus to the anus.

The location and size of the *scrotum* are noted. The scrota hang freely from the perineum behind the penis, and the left scrotum normally hangs lower than the right. In infants the scrota appear large in relation to the rest of the genitalia. The

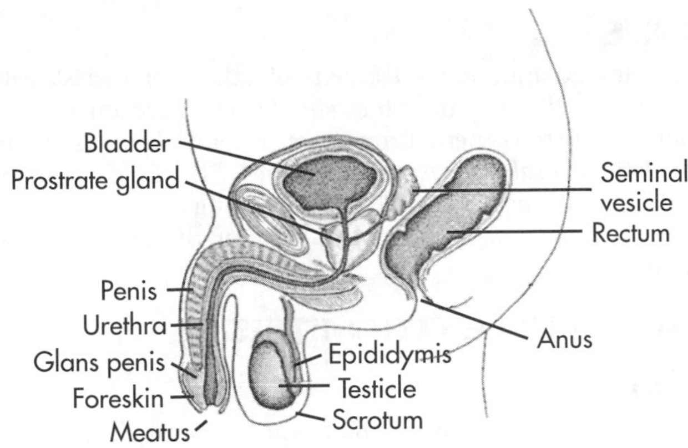

Fig. 32-34 Major structures of genitalia in uncircumcised postpubertal male.

skin of the scrotum is loose and highly rugated (wrinkled). During early adolescence the skin normally becomes redder and coarser. In dark-skinned children the scrota are usually more deeply pigmented.

Palpation of the scrotum includes identification of the testes, epididymis, and, if present, inguinal hernias. The two *testes* are felt as small ovoid bodies about 1.5 to 2 cm (0.6 to 0.8 inch) long—one in each scrotal sac. They do not enlarge until puberty, when they approximately double in size.

Palpating for the presence of the testes requires avoiding to stimulation of the **cremasteric reflex.** When stimulated by cold, touch, emotional excitement, or exercise, the reflex pulls the testes higher into the pelvic cavity. Several measures are useful in preventing the cremasteric reflex during palpation of the scrotum. First, warm the hands. Second, if the child is old enough, examine him in a tailor or "Indian" position, which stretches the muscle, preventing its contraction (Fig. 32-35, *A*). Third, block the normal pathway of ascent of the testes by placing the thumb and index finger over the upper part of the scrotal sac along the inguinal canal (Fig. 32-35, *B*). If there is any question concerning the existence of two testes, place the index and middle fingers in a scissors fashion to separate the right and left scrotum. If after using these techniques the testes have not been palpated, feel along the inguinal canal and perineum to locate masses that may be undescended testes. Although undescended testes may descend at any time during childhood and are checked at each visit, failure to palpate testes is reported.

Female Genitalia

The examination of female genitalia is limited to inspection and palpation of external structures. If a vaginal examination is required, an appropriate referral is made unless the nurse is qualified to perform the procedure. A convenient position for examination of the genitalia involves placing the young child supine on the examining table or in a semi-reclining position on the parent's lap with the feet supported on your knees as you sit facing the child. Divert the child's attention from the examination by instructing her to try to keep the soles of her feet pressed against each other. Separate the labia majora with the thumb and index finger and retract outward to expose the labia minora, urethral meatus, and vaginal orifice.

Examine the female genitalia for size and location of the structures of the *vulva* or *pudendum* (Fig. 32-36). The *mons pubis* is a pad of adipose tissue over the symphysis pubis. At puberty the mons is covered with hair, which extends along the labia. The usual pattern of female *hair distribution* is an inverted triangle. The appearance of soft downy hair along the labia majora is an early sign of sexual maturation.

Note the size and location of the *clitoris.* It is a small erectile organ located at the anterior end of the labia minora. It is covered by a small flap of skin, the *prepuce.*

The *labia majora* are two thick folds of skin running posteriorly from the mons to the posterior commissure of the vagina. Internal to the labia majora are two folds of skin called the *labia minora.* Although the labia minora are usually prominent in the newborn, they gradually atrophy, which makes them almost invisible until their enlargement during puberty.

The inner surface of the labia should be pink and moist. Note the size of the labia and any evidence of fusion, which may suggest male scrota. Normally no masses are palpable within the labia.

The *urethral meatus* is located posterior to the clitoris and is surrounded by Skene glands and ducts. Although not a

A

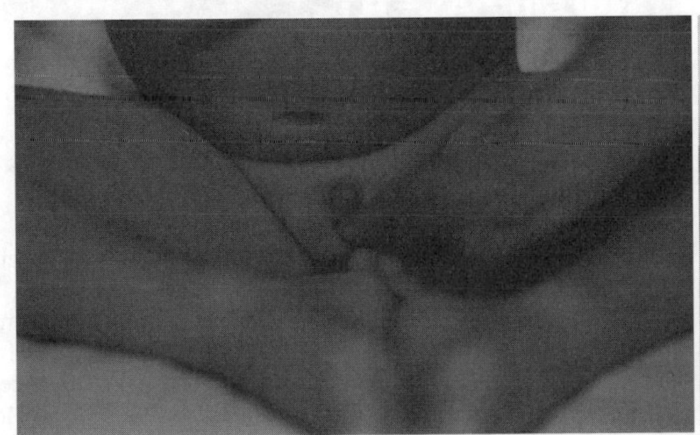

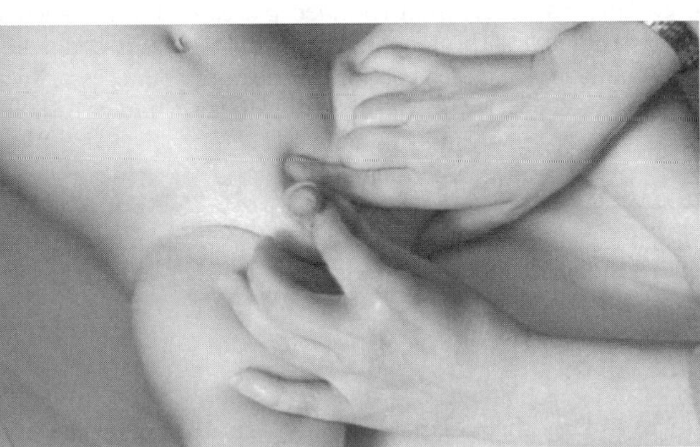

B

Fig. 32-35 **A,** Preventing cremasteric reflex by having child sit in "tailor" position. **B,** Blocking inguinal canal during palpation of scrotum for descended testes.

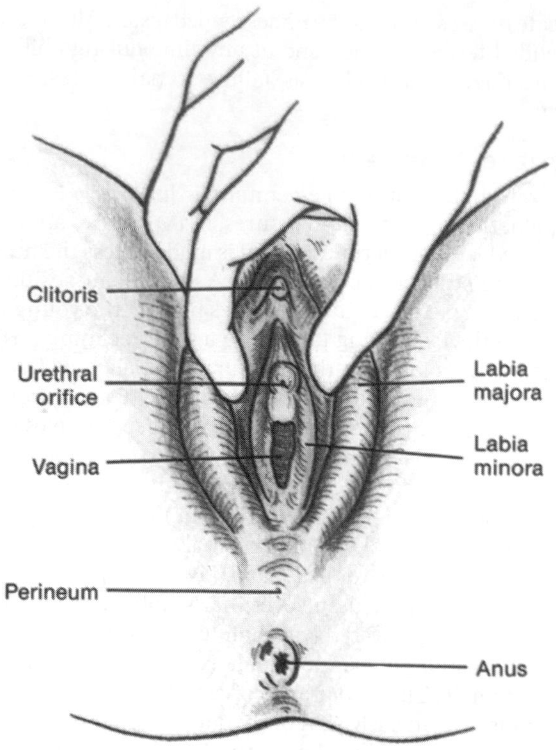

Fig. 32-36 External structures of genitalia in postpubertal female. Labia are spread to reveal deeper structures. (From Potter PA, Perry AG: *Basic nursing: theory and practice,* ed 3, St Louis, 1995, Mosby.)

prominent structure, the meatus appears as a small V-shaped slit. Note its location, especially if it opens from the clitoris or inside the vagina. Gently palpate the glands, which are common sites of cysts and sexually transmitted lesions.

The *vaginal orifice* is located posterior to the urethral meatus. Its appearance varies depending on individual anatomy and sexual activity. Ordinarily, examination of the vagina is limited to inspection. In virgins a thin crescent-shaped or circular membrane, called the *hymen,* may cover part of the vaginal opening. In some instances it completely occludes the orifice. After rupture, small rounded pieces of tissue called *caruncles* remain. Although an imperforate hymen denotes lack of penile intercourse, a perforate one does not necessarily indicate sexual activity (see also Sexual Abuse, Chapter 35).

Nursing ALERT

In females who have been circumcized, the genitalia will appear different. Do not show surprise or disgust, but note the appearance and discuss the procedure with the young woman.

Surrounding the vaginal opening are *Bartholin glands,* which secrete a clear, mucoid fluid into the vagina for lubrication during intercourse. Palpate the ducts for cysts. Also note the discharge from the vagina, which is usually clear or white.

ANUS

Following examination of the genitalia, the anal area is easily examined, although the child should be placed on the abdomen. Note the general firmness of the *buttocks* and symmetry of the *gluteal folds.* Assess the tone of the anal sphincter by eliciting the *anal reflex.* Gently scratching the anal area results in an obvious quick contraction of the external anal sphincter.

BACK AND EXTREMITIES

Spine

The general *curvature* of the spine is noted. Normally the back of a newborn is rounded or C-shaped from the thoracic and pelvic curves. The development of the cervical and lumbar curves approximates development of various motor skills, such as cervical curvature with head control, and gives the older child the typical double-S curve.

Marked curvatures in posture are abnormal (see Fig. 51-18). **Scoliosis,** lateral curvature of the spine, is an important childhood problem, especially in females. Although scoliosis may be identified by observing and palpating the spine and noting a sideways displacement, more objective tests include the following:

1. With the child standing erect, clothed only in underpants (and bra if older girl), observe from behind, noting asymmetry of the shoulders and hips.
2. With the child bending forward so that the back is parallel to the floor, observe from the side, noting asymmetry or prominence of the rib cage.

A slight limp, a crooked hemline, or complaints of a sore back are other signs and symptoms of scoliosis.

Inspect the *back,* especially along the spine, for any tufts of hair, dimples, or discoloration. *Mobility* of the vertebral column is easily assessed in most children because of their propensity for constant motion during the examination. However, mobility can be tested by asking the child to sit up from a prone position or to do a modified sit-up exercise.

Movement of the cervical spine is an important diagnostic sign of neurologic problems such as meningitis. Normally movement of the head in all directions is effortless.

Nursing ALERT

Hyperextension of the neck and spine, or *opisthotonos,* which is accompanied by pain when the head is flexed, is always referred for immediate medical evaluation.

Extremities

Inspect each extremity for symmetry of length and size; refer any deviation for orthopedic evaluation.

Count the fingers and toes to be certain of the normal number. This is so often taken for granted that an extra digit (*polydactyly*) or fusion of digits (*syndactyly*) may go unnoticed.

Inspect the arms and legs for *temperature* and *color,* which should be equal in each extremity, although the feet may normally be colder than the hands.

Assess the *shape* of bones. Several variations of bone shape

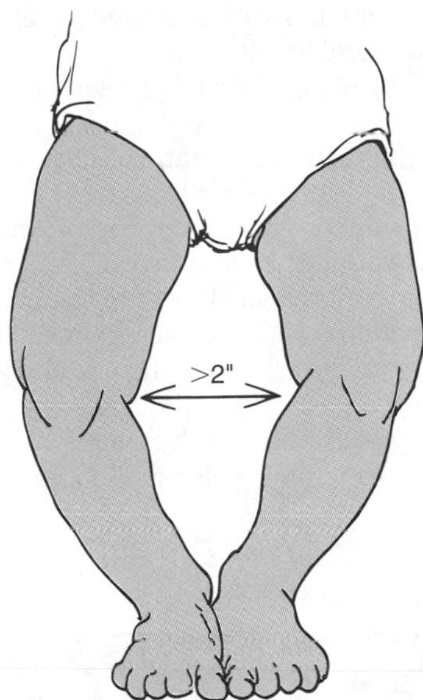

Fig. 32-37 Bowleg.

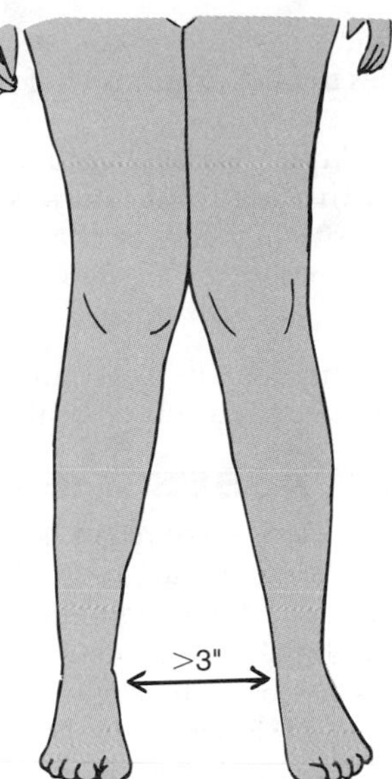

Fig. 32-38 Knock-knee.

may be observed in children. Although many of them cause parents concern, most are benign and require no treatment. *Bowleg*, or *genu varum*, is lateral bowing of the tibia. It is clinically present when the child stands with the medial malleoli (rounded prominence on either side of the ankle) opposite each other and the space between the knees is greater than approximately 5 cm (2 inches) (Fig. 32-37). Toddlers are usually bowlegged after beginning to walk until all their lower back and leg muscles are well-developed. Unilateral or asymmetric bowlegs that are present beyond the age of 2 to 3 years, particularly in black children, may represent pathologic conditions requiring further investigation.

Knock-knee, or *genu valgum*, appears as the opposite of bowleg, in that the knees are close together but the feet are spread apart. It is determined clinically by using the same method as for genu varum but by measuring the distance between the malleoli, which normally should be less than 7.5 cm (3 inches) (Fig. 32-38). Knock-knee is normally present in children from about 2 to 7 years of age. Knock-knee that is excessive, asymmetric, accompanied by shortened stature, or evident in a child nearing puberty requires further evaluation.

Next, inspect the *feet*. Infants' and toddlers' feet appear flat because the foot is normally wide and the arch is covered by a fat pad. Development of the arch occurs naturally from the action of walking. Normally at birth the feet are held in a valgus (outward) or varus (inward) position. To determine whether a foot deformity at birth is the result of intrauterine position or development, scratch the outer, then inner, side of the sole. If the foot position is self-correctable, it will assume a right angle to the leg. As the child begins to walk, the feet turn outward less than 30 degrees and inward less than 10 degrees.

Toddlers have a "toddling" or broad-based gait, which facilitates walking by lowering the center of gravity. As the child reaches preschool age, the legs are brought closer together. By school age the walking posture is much more graceful and balanced.

The most common gait problem in young children is *pigeon toe*, or *toeing in*, which usually results from torsional deformities, such as internal tibial torsion (abnormal rotation or bowing of the tibia). Tests for tibial torsion include measuring the thigh-foot angle, which requires considerable practice for accuracy.

Elicit the *plantar* or *grasp reflex* by exerting firm but gentle pressure with the tip of the thumb against the lateral sole of the foot from the heel upward to the little toe and then across to the big toe. The normal response in children who are walking is flexion of the toes. *Babinski sign*, dorsiflexion of the big toe and fanning of the other toes, is normal during infancy but abnormal after about 1 year of age or when locomotion begins.

Joints

Evaluate the joints for *range of motion*. Normally this requires no specific testing if the nurse has been observant of the child's movements during the examination. However, the hips should be routinely investigated in infants for congenital dislocation. Signs of congenital hip dislocation are discussed in Chapter 51. Report any evidence of joint immobility or hyperflexibility.

Palpate the joints for *heat*, *tenderness*, and *swelling*. These signs, as well as redness over the joint, warrant further investigation.

Muscles

Note symmetry and quality of muscle development, tone, and strength. Observe *development* by looking at the shape and contour of the body in both a relaxed and a tensed state. Estimate *tone* by grasping the muscle and feeling its firmness when it is relaxed and contracted. A common site for testing tone is the biceps muscle of the arm. Children are usually willing to "make a muscle" by clenching their fist.

Estimate *strength* by having the child use an extremity to push or pull against resistance, as in the following examples:

Arm strength. Child holds the arms outstretched in front of the body and tries to raise the arms while downward pressure is applied.

Hand strength. Child shakes hands with nurse and squeezes one or two fingers of the nurse's hand.

Leg strength. Child sits on a table or chair with the legs dangling and tries to raise the legs while downward pressure is applied.

Note symmetry of strength in the extremities, hands, and fingers, and report evidence of paresis or weakness.

NEUROLOGIC ASSESSMENT

The assessment of the nervous system is the broadest and most diverse part of the examining process, since every human function, both physical and emotional, is controlled by neurologic impulses. Much of the neurologic examination has already been discussed, such as assessment of behavior, sensory testing, and motor functioning. The following focuses on a general appraisal of cerebellar functioning, deep tendon reflexes, and the cranial nerves.

Cerebellar Functioning

The cerebellum controls balance and coordination. Much of the assessment of cerebellar functioning is included in observing the child's posture, body movements, gait, and development of fine and gross motor skills. Tests such as balancing on one foot and the heel-to-toe walk assess balance. Test *coordination* by asking the child to reach for a toy, button clothes, tie shoes, or draw a straight line on a piece of paper, provided the child is old enough to do these activities. Coordination can also be tested by any sequence of rapid successive movements, such as quickly touching each finger with the thumb of the same hand.

Several tests for cerebellar function are described in Box 32-5 and can be performed as games. When the Romberg test is done, stay beside the child if there is a possibility that the child may fall. School-age children should be able to perform these tests, although, in the finger-to-nose test, preschoolers normally can only bring the finger within 5 to 7.5 cm (2 to 3) inches of the nose. Difficulty in performing these exercises indicates poor sense of position (especially with the eyes closed) and incoordination (especially with the eyes opened).

Reflexes

Testing reflexes is an important part of the neurologic examination. Persistence of primitive reflexes (see Chapter 22), loss of reflexes, or hyperactivity of deep tendon reflexes is usually the result of a cerebral insult.

Elicit reflexes by using the rubber head of the reflex hammer, flat of the finger, or side of the hand. If the child is easily frightened by equipment, use a hand or finger. Although testing reflexes is a simple procedure to perform, the child may inhibit the reflex by unconsciously tensing the muscle. To avoid tensing, distract younger children with toys or talk to them. To divert their attention away from the testing and cause involuntary relaxation of the muscles, have older children grasp their two hands in front of them and try to pull them apart.

Deep tendon reflexes are stretch reflexes of a muscle. The most common deep tendon reflex is the *knee jerk,* or *patellar*

BOX 32-5
Tests for Cerebellar Function

Finger-to-nose test. With child's arm extended, ask child to touch the nose with the index finger with eyes open and then closed.

Heel-to-shin test. While standing, have child run the heel of one foot down the shin or anterior aspect of the tibia of the other leg, both with eyes opened and then closed.

Romberg test. With eyes closed, have child stand with heels together; falling or leaning to one side is abnormal and is called *Romberg sign.*

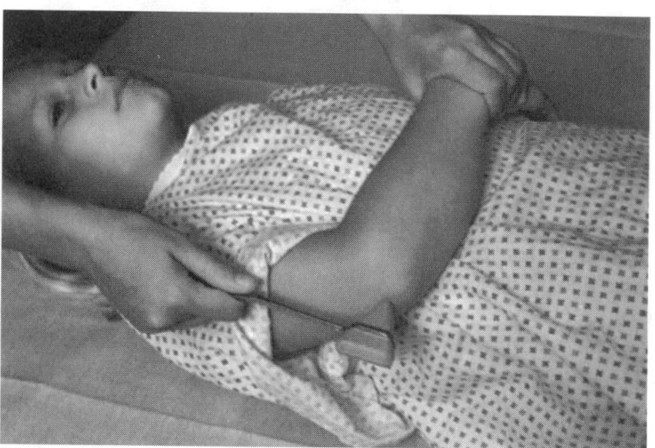

Fig. 32-39 Testing for triceps reflex. Child is placed supine, with forearm resting over chest, and triceps tendon is struck. Alternate procedure: child's arm is abducted, with upper arm supported and forearm allowed to hang freely. Triceps tendon is struck. Normal response is partial extension of forearm.

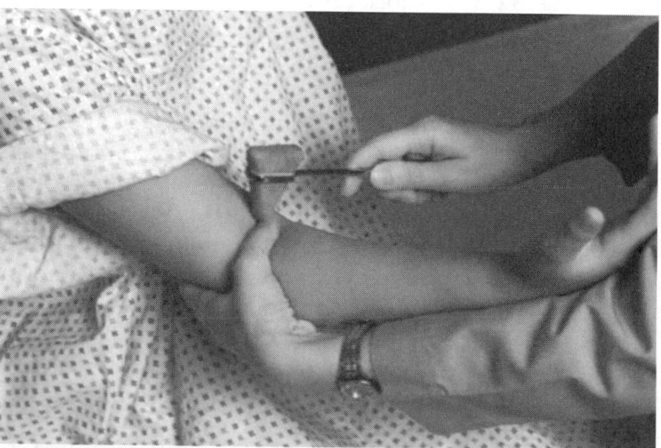

Fig. 32-40 Testing for biceps reflex. Child's arm is held by placing partially flexed elbow in examiner's hand with thumb over antecubital space. Examiner's thumbnail is struck with hammer. Normal response is partial flexion of forearm.

reflex (this is sometimes called the *quadriceps reflex*). The reflexes normally elicited are described in Figs. 32-39 to 32-42. Report any diminished or hyperreflexic response for further evaluation.

Cranial Nerves

Assessment of the cranial nerves is an important area of neurologic assessment (Table 32-12). With young children present the tests as games to encourage trust and security at the beginning of the examination. Or include the cranial nerve test when each "system" is examined, such as tongue movement and strength, gag reflex, swallowing, and position of the uvula during examination of the mouth.

Developmental Assessment

One of the most essential components of a complete health appraisal is assessment of developmental functioning. *Screening procedures* are designed to identify quickly and reliably those children whose developmental level is below normal for their age and who therefore require further investigation. They also provide a means of recording objective measurements of present developmental functioning for future reference. Since the passage of P.L. 99-457, the Education of the Handicapped Act Amendments of 1986, much greater emphasis is placed on developmental assessment of children with disabilities, and nurses can play a vital role in providing this service. All of the procedures discussed in this section can be administered in a variety of settings—home, school, day-care center, hospital, practitioner's office, or clinic.

DENVER II

The most widely used developmental screening tests for young children have been the series of tests developed by Dr. William Frankenburg and his colleagues in Denver, Colorado. The oldest and best known, the *Denver Developmental Screening Test (DDST)* and its revision, the *DDST-R* have been revised, restandardized, and renamed the *Denver II.* Before administering the Denver II, the examiner should be trained by, and receive a certificate from, a master instructor who has been trained by the Denver faculty.* The Denver II differs from the

*Forms and complete instructions are available from **Denver Developmental Materials, Inc.**, P.O. Box 6919, Denver, CO 80206-0919; (303) 355-4729. The DDST and DDST-R are no longer available, since they have been replaced by the DENVER II.

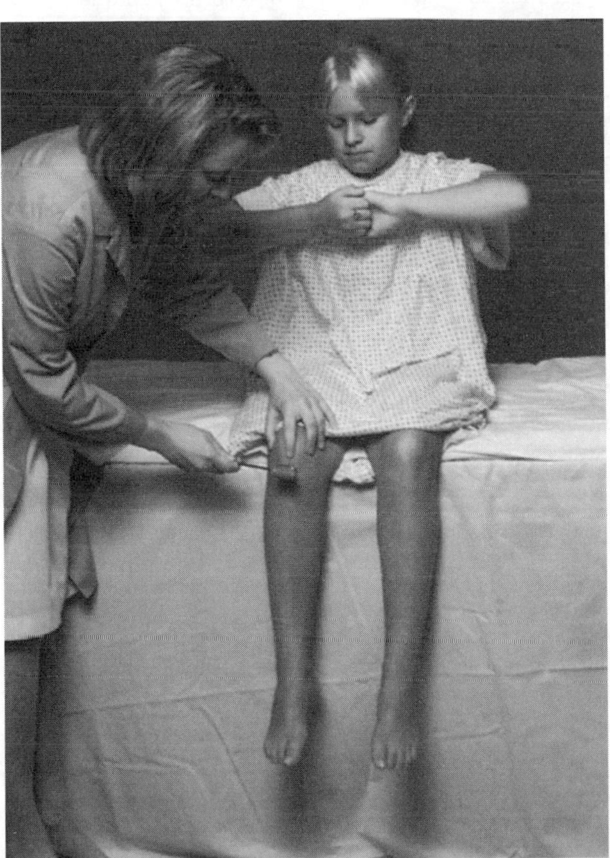

Fig. 32-41 Testing for patellar, or knee jerk, reflex, using distraction. Child sits on edge of examining table (or on parent's lap) with lower legs flexed at knee and dangling freely. Patellar tendon is tapped just below kneecap. Normal response is partial extension of lower leg.

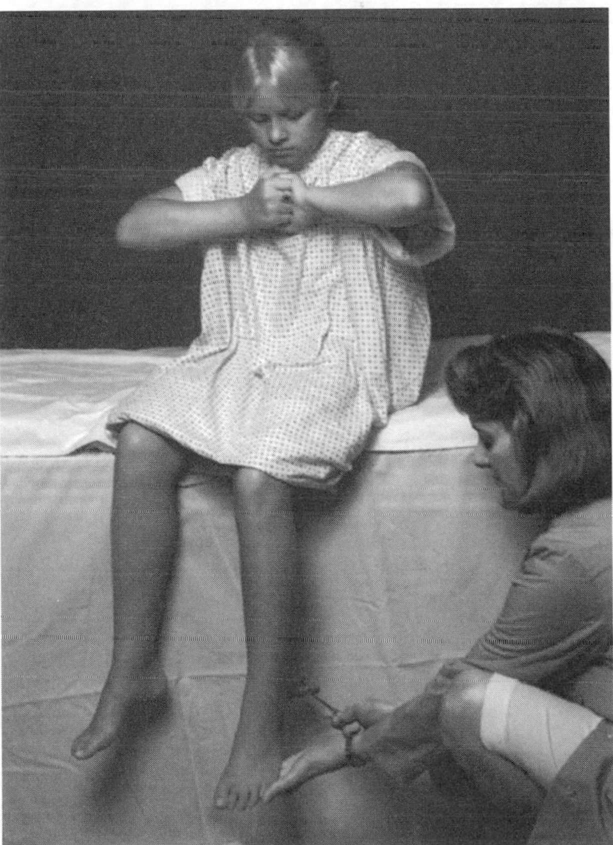

Fig. 32-42 Testing for Achilles reflex. Same position employed in eliciting knee jerk reflex is used. Foot is supported lightly in examiner's hand, and Achilles tendon is struck. Normal response is plantar flexion of foot (foot pointing downward).

TABLE 32-12 Assessment of cranial nerves

DISTRIBUTION/FUNCTION	TEST
I—Olfactory nerve	
Olfactory mucosa of nasal cavity Smell	With eyes closed, have child identify odors such as coffee, alcohol from a swab, or other smells; test each nostril separately
II—Optic nerve	
Rods and cones of retina, optic nerve Vision	Check for perception of light, visual acuity, peripheral vision, color vision, and normal optic disc
III—Oculomotor nerve	
Extraocular muscles (EOM) of eye: Superior rectus (SR)—moves eyeball up and in Inferior rectus (IR)—moves eyeball down and in Medial rectus (MR)—moves eyeball nasally Inferior oblique (IO)—moves eyeball up and out	Have child follow an object (toy) or light in the six cardinal positions of gaze (see Fig. 32-43)
Pupil constriction and accommodation	Perform PERRLA
Eyelid closing	Check for proper placement of lid
IV—Trochlear nerve	
Superior oblique muscle (SO)—moves eye down and out	Have child look down and in (Fig. 32-43)
V—Trigeminal nerve	
Muscles of mastication	Have child bite down hard and open jaw; test symmetry and strength
Sensory: face, scalp, nasal and buccal mucosa	With child's eyes closed, see if child can detect light touch in the mandibular and maxillary regions Test corneal and blink reflex by touching cornea lightly (approach from the side so that child does not blink before cornea is touched)
VI—Abducens nerve	
Lateral rectus (LR) muscle—moves eye temporally	Have child look toward temporal side (Fig. 32-43)
VII—Facial nerve	
Muscles for facial expression	Have child smile, make funny face, or show teeth to see symmetry of expression
Anterior two thirds of tongue (sensory)	Have child identify a sweet or salty solution; place each taste on anterior section and sides of protruding tongue; if child retracts tongue, solution will dissolve toward posterior part of tongue
VIII—Auditory, acoustic, or vestibulocochlear nerve	
Internal ear Hearing/balance	Test hearing; note any loss of equilibrium or presence of vertigo
IX—Glossopharyngeal nerve	
Pharynx, tongue	Stimulate posterior pharynx with a tongue blade; child should gag
Posterior one third of tongue (sensory)	Test sense of sour or bitter taste on posterior segment of tongue
X—Vagus nerve	
Muscles of larynx, pharynx, some organs of gastrointestinal system, sensory fibers of root of tongue, heart, lung, and some organs of gastrointestinal system	Note hoarseness of voice, gag reflex, and ability to swallow Check that uvula is in midline; when stimulated with a tongue blade, should deviate upward and to stimulated side
XI—Accessory nerve	
Sternocleidomastoid and trapezius muscles of shoulder	Have child shrug shoulders while applying mild pressure; with examiner's hands placed on shoulders, have child turn head against opposing pressure on either side; note symmetry and strength
XII—Hypoglossal nerve	
Muscles of tongue	Have child move tongue in all directions; have child protrude tongue as far as possible; note any midline deviation Test strength by placing tongue blade on one side of tongue and having child move it away

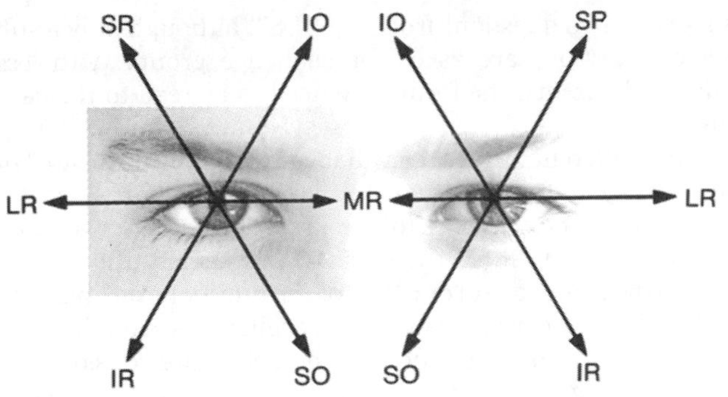

SR IO IO SP
LR MR LR
IR SO SO IR

Fig. 32-43 Testing cardinal positions of gaze.

DDST in items, test form, interpretation, and referral (see the Appendix). The previous total of 105 items has been increased to 125, including an increase from 21 DDST to 39 Denver II language items. Previous items that were difficult to administer and/or interpret have been either modified or eliminated. Many items that were previously tested by parental report now require observation by the examiner.

Each item was evaluated to determine if significant differences exist on the basis of gender, ethnic group, maternal education, and place of residence. Items for which clinically significant differences exist were replaced, or if retained, are discussed in the Technical Manual. When evaluating children delayed on one of these items, the examiner can look up norms for the subpopulations to consider if the delay may be a result of sociocultural or environmental differences.

The items on the test form are arranged in the same format as the DDST-R. The norms for the distribution bars were updated with the new standardization data but retain the 25th, 50th, 75th, and 90th percentile divisions. The test form contains a place to rate the child's behavioral characteristics (compliance, interest in surroundings, fearfulness, and attention span).

To determine relative areas of advancement and areas of delay, sufficient items should be administered to establish the basal and ceiling levels in each sector. By scoring appropriate items as "pass," "fail," "refusal," or "no opportunity," and relating such scores to the age of the child, each item can be interpreted as described in Box 32-6. To identify cautions, all items intersected by the age line are administered. To screen solely for developmental delays, only the items located totally to the *left* of the child's age line are administered. Criteria for referral are based on the availability of resources in the community (Box 32-6).

Research on the Denver II's validity and accuracy is in its beginning stages. One study found that most children with even subtle developmental problems were identified. However, almost half of the children without developmental problems received suspect scores, resulting in a high rate of overreferrals (Glascoe et al, 1992). To minimize overreferrals, a decision for referral depends not only on the results of the Denver II, but also on the practitioner's clinical judgment after considering the child's developmental history; general health status; social, cultural, and emotional environment; and the availability of local resources for diagnosis and treatment (Frankenburg, 1994a).

BOX 32-6
Denver II Scoring

Interpretation of Denver II Scores

Advanced: Passed an item completely to the *right* of the age line (passed by less than 25% of children at an age older than the child)
OK: Passed, failed, or refused an item intersected by the age line between the 25th and 75th percentiles
Caution: Failed or refused items intersected by the age line on or between the 75th and 90th percentiles
Delay: Failed an item completely to the *left* of the age line; refusals to the left of the age line may also be considered delays, since the reason for the refusal may be inability to perform the task

Interpretation of Test

Normal: No delays and a maximum of one caution
Suspect: One or more delays and/or two or more cautions
Untestable: Refusals on one or more items completely to the left of the age line or on more than one item intersected by the age line in the 75% to 90% area

Recommendations for Referral for Suspect and Untestable Tests

Rescreen in 1 to 2 weeks to rule out temporary factors.
If rescreen is suspect or untestable, use clinical judgment based on the following: number of cautions and delays; which items are cautions and delays; rate of past development; clinical examination and history; availability of referral resources.

Although it is not the purpose of this discussion to detail the instruction manual, some points concerning preparation, administration, and interpretation of the Denver II are important to stress. Before beginning the screen, ask if the child was born prematurely and correctly calculate the adjusted age. Up to 24 months of age, allowances are made for infants born prematurely by subtracting the number of weeks of missed gestation from their present age and testing them at the adjusted age. For example, a 16-week-old infant who was born 4 weeks early is tested at a 12-week adjusted age level. Explain to the parents and child, if appropriate, that the screenings are *not* intelligence tests but a method of showing what the child can do at a particular age. Emphasize that the child is *not* expected to perform each item on the test.

Tell the parent before the screening begins that the results of the child's performance will be explained after all the items have been concluded. It is the nurse's responsibility to properly inform parents of any testing or screening procedure before its administration so that they are fully aware of its purpose and intent.

Prepare toddlers and preschoolers for the procedure by presenting it as a game. Often, the Denver II is an excellent way to begin a health appraisal because it is nonthreatening, requires no painful or unfamiliar procedures, and capitalizes on the child's natural activity of play. Since children are easily distracted, perform each item quickly and present only one toy from the kit at a time. After that toy's purpose is concluded, such as building a tower of blocks or identifying its color, replace the toy in the bag and take out another one.

Other temporary factors that may interfere with the child's performance include fatigue, illness, fear, hospitalization, separation from the parent, or general unwillingness to perform the activities. In addition, undiagnosed mental retardation, hearing loss, vision loss, neurologic impairment, or a familial pattern of slow development greatly influences the child's performance.

Following completion of the Denver II, ask the parent if the child's performance was typical of behavior at other times. If the parent replies affirmatively and the child's cooperation was satisfactory, explain the results, emphasizing all successful items first, then those items failed but which the child was not expected to pass, and finally those items that indicate delays. If the parent replies that the child's performance was not typical of usual behavior, it is best to defer any scoring or discussion of results, especially if the refusals yield a suspect score. In this situation reschedule testing for a time when the child is more likely to cooperate.

In explaining a normal score, focus on how well the child performed and reinforce the parents' efforts in satisfactorily stimulating their child. In addition to assessing the child's present developmental level, the Denver II can be used to guide parents toward those activities that are appropriate, although not necessarily expected, for the child's age. By testing for items to the right of the age line (ones child is not expected to perform), children with advanced development, who may be gifted, can be identified.

In explaining delays, carefully note the parent's response, especially casual acceptance, such as "He'll catch up," or questions such as "Does this mean my child is retarded?" Be aware of personal anxieties during these situations and refrain from giving glib reassurances, such as "I'm sure he will do better the next time." Rather, respond honestly to parents' questions, yet with appropriate flexibility and concern, stressing the need for further developmental testing.

REVISED PRESCREENING DEVELOPMENTAL QUESTIONNAIRE (R-PDQ)

The R-PDQ is a revision of the original PDQ (Frankenburg, Fandal, and Thornton, 1987). Advantages of the R-PDQ include the addition and arrangement of items to be more age-appropriate, simplified parent scoring, and easier comparison with Denver Developmental Screening Test (DDST) norms for professionals. The R-PDQ is a parent-answered prescreen consisting of 150 questions from the DDST, although only a subset of questions are asked for each age group. With less-educated parents, the form may need to be read to the caregiver.

Four different forms are available and are selected based on age: orange (0 to 9 months), purple (9 to 24 months), gold (2 to 4 years), and white (4 to 6 years). The caregiver answers the questions until (1) three "NOs" are circled (they do not have to be consecutive) or (2) all of the questions on both sides of the form have been answered. Scoring is based on the number of delays. Children who have no delays are considered to be developing normally. If a child has one delay, the caregiver is provided with age-appropriate developmental activities to pursue with the child and a rescreen with the R-PDQ is done 1 month later. If on rescreening, a child has one or more delays, the Denver II is administered as soon as possible. If a child has two or more delays on the first screening with the R-PDQ, the Denver II is administered as soon as possible.

DEVELOPMENTAL SCREENING AND INTERPRETATION

Although screening tests are an effective method of applying the knowledge of children's expected rate of development to a large segment of the population, they are only as successful as the individual's expertise in administering them. Since many of the screening tests are devised to be used by paraprofessionals, there are inherent risks in screening if such individuals are not properly trained or supervised. For example, false-positives can label the child as developmentally delayed and cause problems that otherwise might not have existed. False-negatives can prevent children with problems from receiving the help they need.

Nurses administering developmental screening or supervising paraprofessionals' testing need to assess the child's "whole picture" and not rely solely on any screening procedure. Development, like growth and health, is a dynamic process. Tests such as the Denver II should be used as part of *developmental surveillance,* a continuous comprehensive primary health care approach that includes the parents as partners with professionals (Frankenburg, 1994b). Evaluation of the child's total well-being is the result of evaluating data from a comprehensive health and family history, physical examination, and developmental screening.

Key Points

- The most common approach to examining children follows a head-to-toe sequence.
- Growth measurements during the physical examination focus on length, height, weight, skinfold thickness, and arm and head circumference. Assessment of growth is measured against standard growth charts to determine a child's status in comparison with other children of the same age.
- Measurements of temperature, pulse, respiration, and blood pressure constitute the physiologic approach to assessment.
- The general appearance of a child is a cumulative, subjective impression of physical appearance, state of nutrition, behavior, personality, interactions with parents and nurse, posture, development, and speech.
- Assessment of the skin, which primarily involves inspection and palpation, focuses on color, texture, temperature, moisture, and turgor. The nurse needs to be aware of both physiologic and ethnic factors that may affect these areas.
- In assessment of the lymph nodes, the nurse examines, by palpation, the part of the body in which the glands are located.
- The head is inspected for shape, symmetry, mobility, and head control.

- Examination of the eyes includes placement and alignment, inspection of external and internal structures, and vision testing.
- Ears are examined for placement and alignment, inspection of external and internal structures, and auditory testing.
- The lungs are examined by methods of inspection, palpation, percussion, and auscultation.
- Auscultation is the most important procedure for examining the heart.
- Abdominal assessment follows an orderly sequence of inspection, auscultation, and palpation, since palpation may distort normal abdominal sounds.
- Examination of the genitalia may provoke anxiety in the child, and the nurse must avoid any transference of anxiety.
- Neurologic assessment addresses behavior; motor, sensory, and cerebellar functioning; reflexes; and cranial nerves.
- The Denver II, a major revision and a restandardization of the DDST, differs from the DDST in items included in the test, the test form, and the interpretation of scoring.

References

Abdo MH, Feghali JG, Stapells DR: Transient evoked otoacoustic emissions: clinical applications and technical considerations, *Int J Pediatr Otorhinolaryngol* 25:61-71, 1993.

Burke S, Roberts C, Maloney R: Infant and child weights: reliability and validity of scales, *Issues Compr Pediatr Nurs* 11(4):241-249, 1988.

Dewey KG et al: Growth of breast-fed infants deviates from current reference data: a pooled analysis of U.S., Canadian, and European data sets, *Pediatrics* 96(3): 495-503, 1995.

Frankenburg WK: Preventing developmental delays: is developmental screening sufficient? I. Developmental screening and the Denver II, *Pediatrics*, 93(4):586-589, 1994a.

Frankenburg WK: Preventing developmental delays: is developmental screening sufficient? II. Partners in health care, *Pediatrics* 93(4)589 593, 1994b.

Frankenburg WK, Fandal A, Thornton S: Revision of Denver Prescreening Developmental Questionnaire, *J Pediatr* 110(4):653-657, 1987.

Frohlich E et al: Recommendations for human blood pressure determination by sphygmomanometers: report of a special task force appointed by the Steering Committee, American Heart Association, *Circulation* 77:501A, 1988.

Glascoe FP et al: Accuracy of the Denver-II in developmental screening, *Pediatrics* 89:1221-1225, 1992.

Kovalesky A: *Nurses' guide to children's eyes,* New York, 1985, Grune & Stratton.

National Society to Prevent Blindness: *Guide to testing distance visual acuity,* Schaumburg, Ill., 1988, The Society.

Park JK, Guntheroth WG: Accurate blood pressure measurement in children, *Am J Noninvas Cardiol* 3:297-309, 1989.

Park M: *Pediatric cardiology for the practitioner,* ed 2, St Louis, 1988, Mosby.

Park M, Lee D, Johnson GA: Oscillometric blood pressures in the arm, thigh, and calf in healthy children and those with aortic coarctation, *Pediatrics* 91(4):761-765, 1993.

Pontious S et al: Accuracy and reliability of temperature measurement in the emergency department by instrument and site in children, *Pediatr Nurs* 20(1):58-63, 1994b.

Pontious S et al: Accuracy and reliability of temperature measurement by instrument and site, *J Pediatr Nurs* 9(2):114-123, 1994a.

Report of the Second Task Force on blood pressure control in children—1987, *Pediatrics* 79(1):1-25, 1987.

Sato-Viacrucis K: The evolution of the Snellen E to the Blackbird, *School Nurse,* pp 18-19, Spring 1985.

Seidel HM, Rosenstein BJ, Pathak A: *Care of the full term newborn,* St Louis, 1993, Mosby.

Terndrup TE, Rajk J: Impact of operator technique and device on infrared emission detection tympanic thermometry, *J Emerg Med* 10:683-687, 1992.

Vessey J, Braithwaite K, Widemann M: Teaching children about their internal bodies, *Pediatr Nurs* 16(1):29-33, 1990.

Weiss ME, Poeltler D, Gocka I: Infrared tympanic thermometry for neonatal temperature assessment, *JOGNN* 23(9):798-804, 1993.

Bibliography

Physical Assessment

Barness LA: *Manual of pediatric physical diagnosis,* ed 6, St Louis, 1991, Mosby.

Beach PS, McCormick DP: Editorial comment: clinical applications of ear thermometry, *Clin Pediatr* 30(4, suppl):3-4, 1991.

Betts PR, Voss LD, Bailey BJR: Measuring the heights of very young children, *Br Med J* 304:1351-1352, 1992.

Bowers A, Thompson J: *Clinical manual of health assessment,* ed 4, St Louis, 1992, Mosby.

Combs JT: Two useful tools for exploring the middle ear, *Contemp Pediatr* 10(11):60-75, 1993.

Crouch ER Jr, Crouch ER: Pediatric vision screening: Why? When? What? How? *Contemp Pediatr* 8:9-30, 1991.

Cunningham DR: *Auditory screening.* In Hoekelman RA et al, editors: *Primary pediatric care,* ed 2, St Louis, 1992, Mosby.

Elvik SL: Vaginal discharge in the prepubertal girl, *J Pediatr Health Care* 4:181-185, 1990.

Engel J: *Pocket guide to pediatric assessment,* ed 3, St Louis, 1997, Mosby.

Erickson RS et al: Accuracy of infrared ear thermometry and traditional temperature methods in young children, *Heart Lung* 23(3):181-195, 1994.

Gemberling C: The adolescent gynecologic examination: an overview, *J Pediatr Health Care* 1(3):141-151, 1987.

Greene J: Making adolescent space in a pediatric office, *Pediatr Nurs* 15(4):402-404, 1989.

Gundy JH: *The pediatric physical examination.* In Hoekelman RA et al, editors: *Primary pediatric care,* ed 2, St Louis, 1992, Mosby.

Haddock BJ, Merrow DL, Swanson MS: The falling grace of axiliary temperatures, *Pediatr Nurs* 22(2): 121-125, 1996.

Henry JJ: Routine growth monitoring and assessment of growth disorders, *J Pediatr Health Care* 6(5):291-301, 1992.

Hinton A, Moore-Gillon V: Recent advances: otorhinolaryngology, *Brit Med J* 309:651-654, 1994.

Johnson A, Stayte M, Wortham C: Vision screening at 8 and 18 months, *Br Med J* 299:545-549, 1989.

Killam P: Orthopedic assessment of young children: developmental variations, *Nurse Pract* 14(7):27-28, 1989.
Kronmiller J: Oral soft tissue abnormalities in children, *Pediatr Nurs,* 13(3):161-165, 1987.
Lieber MT, Taub AS: Common foot deformities and what they mean for parents, *MCN* 13(1):47-50, 1988.
Linley JF: Screening children for common orthopedic problems, *Am J Nurs* 87(10):1312-1316, 1987.
MacPhee M, Mori C: Teaching nurses about neuromotor development: an evaluative study, *Pediatr Nurs* 17(5):438-442, 444, 1991.
Mason KJ: Pediatric orthopaedics: development norms, *Orthop Nurs* 8(4):45-50, 1989.
Norton SJ: Application of transient evoked otoacoustic emissions to pediatric populations, *Ear Hear* 14(1):64-73, 1993.
Olk D: Quieting the disruptive sibling, *Contemp Pediatr* 6(10):116, 1989.
Pandit JC: Testing acuity of vision in general practice: reaching recommended standard, *Brit Med J* 309(6966):1408, 1994.
Petersen-Smith A et al: Comparison of aural infrared with traditional rectal temperatures in children from birth to age three years, *J Pediatr* 125(1):83-85, 1994.
Pickering TG: Blood pressure measurement and detection of hypertension, *Lancet* 344(8914):31-35, 1994.
Pineyard BJ: Assessment of infant growth, *J Pediatr Health Care* 6(5):302-308, 1994.
Roche A, Guo S, Moore W: Weight and recumbent length from 1 to 12 mo of age: reference data for 1-mo increments, *Am J Clin Nur* 49:599-607, 1989.
Roche A and others: Head circumference reference data: birth to 18 years, *Pediatrics* 79(5):706-712, 1987.
Sackett DL, Rennie D: The science of the art of the clinical examination, *JAMA* 267(19):2650-2652, 1992.
Sanet R, Ellis G: What is the most effective vision screening tool to use with preschool-age children in early childhood programs? *School Nurse* 6:27-31, 1990.
Schubiner H: Preventive health screening in adolescent patients, *Prim Care* 16(1):211-230, 1989.
Schuman AJ: Taking the pain—and fear—out of office visits, *Contemp Pediatr* 8(4):81-87, 1991.
Seidel H et al: *Mosby's guide to physical examination,* ed 3, St Louis, 1995, Mosby.
Stata K: Improving hearing screening programs in the elementary school, *School Nurse* 4(3):16-19, 1988.
Strahlman ER: *Vision screening.* In Hoekelman RA et al, editors: *Primary pediatric care,* ed 3, St Louis, 1997, Mosby.
Sullivan L: How effective is preschool vision, hearing, and developmental screening? *Pediatr Nurs* 14(3):181-183, 1988.
Tolmas HC: Adolescent pelvic examination: an effective practical approach, *Am J Dis Child* 145:1269-1271, 1991.
Tsesis VA: Creating the virtual office, *Contemp Pediatr* 12(2):103-109, 1995.
Wasserman RC: Screening for vision problems in pediatric practice, *Pediatr Rev* 13(1):4-5, 1992.
Wells N et al: Does tympanic temperature measure up? *MCN* 20(2):95-100, 1995.
Wong DL: The paper-doll technique, *Pediatr Nurs* 7(6):39-40, 1981.
Yacone-Morton L: Cardiac assessment, *RN* 54(12):28-34, 1991.

Developmental Assessment

Adesman AR: Is the Denver II Developmental Test worthwhile? *Pediatrics* 90(6):1009-1010, 1992 (letter to the editor).
Allen MC, Alexander GR: Gross motor milestones in preterm infants: correction for degree of prematurity, *J Pediatr* 116(6):955-959, 1990.
Casey PH, Swanson M: A pediatric perspective of developmental screening in 1993, *Clin Pediatr* 32(4):209-212, 1993.
Casey PH et al: Developmental intervention: a pediatric clinical review, *Pediatr Clin North Am* 33(4):899-923, 1986.
Dworkin P: British and American recommendations for developmental monitoring: the role of surveillance, *Pediatrics* 84(6):1000-1010, 1989.
Dworkin P: Developmental screening—expecting the impossible? *Pediatrics* 83(4):619-621, 1989.
Finney JW, Weist MD: Behavioral assessment of children and adolescents, *Pediatr Clin North Am* 39(3):369-378, 1992.
First LR, Palfrey JS: The infant or young child with developmental delay, *New Eng J Med* 330(7):478-483, 1994.
Frankenburg WK, Chen J, Thornton S: Common pitfalls in the evaluation of developmental screening tests, *J Pediatr* 113(5):1110-1113, 1988.
Frankenburg WK, Thornton S: A child development program for a busy office practice, *Contemp Pediatr* 6(2):90-106, 1989.
Glascoe F, Byrne K: Is the Denver II Developmental Test worthwhile? *Pediatrics* 90(6):1010-1011, 1992 (reply to the editor).
Meisels SJ: Can developmental screening tests identify children who are developmentally at risk? *Pediatrics* 83(4):578-585, 1989.
Ouden LD: Is it correct to correct? Developmental milestones in 555 "normal" preterm infants compared with term infants, *J Pediatr* 118(3):399-404, 1991.
Squires JK, Nickel R, Bricker D: Use of parent-completed developmental questionnaires for child-find and screening, *Infants Young Child* 3(2):46-57, 1990.
Steele SM: Assessing developmental delays in preschool children, *J Pediatr Health Care* 2(3):141-145, 1988.
Wade GH: Update on the Denver II, *Pediatr Nurs* 18(2):140-141, 1992.

CHAPTER 33

The Infant and Family

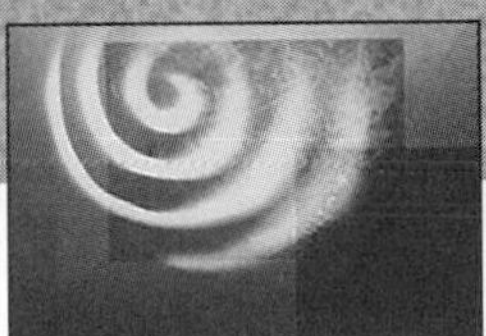

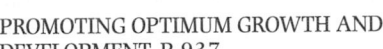

PROMOTING OPTIMUM GROWTH AND DEVELOPMENT, P. 937

Biologic development, p. 937
Psychosocial development, p. 943
Cognitive development, p. 943
Development of body image, p. 944
Social development, p. 944
Temperament, p. 948
Coping with concerns related to normal growth and development, p. 948

PROMOTING OPTIMUM HEALTH DURING INFANCY, P. 956

Nutrition, p. 956
Sleep and activity, p. 959
Dental health, p. 961
Immunizations, p. 961
Injury prevention, p. 970
Anticipatory guidance—care of families, p.977

SPECIAL HEALTH PROBLEMS, P. 979

Feeding difficulties, p. 979
Failure to thrive (FTT), p. 980
Disorders of unknown etiology, p. 984
Sudden infant death syndrome (SIDS), p. 984
Apnea of infancy (AOI), p. 986
Autism, p. 988

Promoting Optimum Growth and Development

BIOLOGIC DEVELOPMENT

At no other time in life are physical changes and developmental achievements so dramatic as during infancy. All major body systems undergo progressive maturation, and there is concurrent development of skills that increasingly allows infants to respond to and cope with the environment. Acquisition of these fine and gross motor skills occurs in an orderly head-to-toe and center-to-periphery (cephalocaudal-proximodistal) sequence.

Proportional Changes

During the first year *growth* is very rapid, especially during the initial 6 months. Infants gain 680 g (1.5 pounds) a month until age 5 months, when the birth weight has at least doubled. An average weight for a 6-month-old child is 7.26 kg (16 pounds). Weight gain slows during the second 6 months. By 1 year of age the infant's birth weight has tripled, for an average weight of 9.75 kg (21.5 pounds). Infants who are breastfed beyond 4 to 6 months of age typically gain less weight than those who are bottle-fed (Dewey et al, 1993).

Height increases by 2.5 cm (1 inch) a month during the first 6 months and also slows during the second 6 months. Increases in length occur in sudden spurts, rather than in a slow gradual pattern (Lampl, Veldhuis, and Johnson, 1992). Average height is 65 cm (25½ inches) at 6 months and 74 cm (29 inches) at 12 months. By 1 year the birth length has increased by almost 50%. The increase in length occurs mainly in the trunk, rather than in the legs, and contributes to the characteristic physique of the infant.

Head growth is also rapid. During the first 6 months head circumference increases approximately 1.5 cm (0.6 inch) a month but decreases to only 0.5 cm (0.2 inch) monthly during the second 6 months. The average size is 43 cm (17 inches) at 6 months and 46 cm (18 inches) at 12 months. By 1 year head size has increased by almost 33%. Closure of the cranial sutures occurs, with the posterior fontanel fusing by 6 to 8 weeks of age and the anterior fontanel closing by 12 to 18 months of age.

The expanding head size reflects the growth and differentiation of the *nervous system*. By the end of the first year the brain has increased in weight about two and one half times. The maturation of the brain is exhibited in the dramatic developmental achievements of infancy (Table 33-2). The primitive reflexes are replaced by voluntary, purposeful movement. As myelinization occurs, the righting reflexes appear, as does the protective parachute reflex (Fig. 33-1), in which the hands and fingers extend forward, as in a protective response during a fall, when the infant is suddenly thrust downward while being held horizontally.

The *chest* assumes a more adult contour, with the lateral diameter becoming larger than the anteroposterior diameter. The chest circumference approximately equals the head cir-

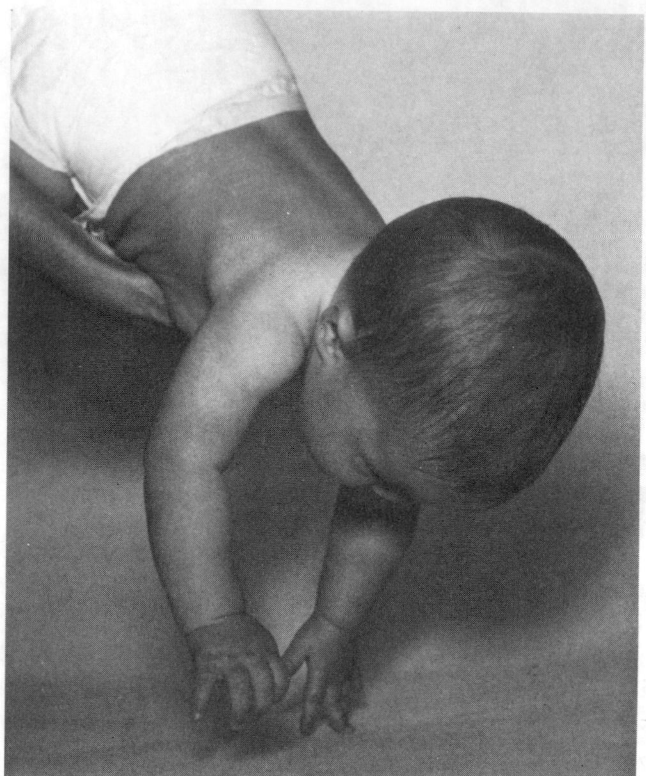

Fig. 33-1 Parachute reflex.

cumference by the end of the first year. The *heart* grows less rapidly than does the rest of the body. Its weight is usually doubled by 1 year of age, in comparison with body weight, which triples during the same period. The size of the heart is still large in relation to the chest cavity; its width is about 55% of the width of the chest.

Maturation of Systems

Most organ systems change and grow during infancy. The *respiratory* rate slows somewhat (see the Appendix) and is relatively stable. Respiratory movements continue to be abdominal. Several factors predispose the infant to more severe and acute respiratory problems. The close proximity of the trachea to the bronchi and its branching structures rapidly transmits an infectious agent from one anatomic location to another.

Although the lumen of the trachea and bronchi enlarges during infancy, it remains small in comparison with the total size of the lung, maintaining high resistance to the volume of air inspired. The small airways are readily blocked by edema, mucus, or a foreign body. The flexible rib cage has less elastic recoil, and during respiratory distress the work of breathing is increased. The short, straight eustachian tube closely communicates with the ear, allowing infection to ascend from the pharynx to the middle ear. In addition, the inability of the immune system to produce *immunoglobulin A* (IgA) in the mucosal lining provides less protection against infection in infancy than during later childhood.

The *heart* rate slows (see the Appendix) and frequently displays *sinus arrhythmia* (rate increases with inspiration and decreases with expiration). Blood pressure also changes during infancy (see the Appendix). Systolic pressure rises during the first 2 months as a result of the increasing ability of the left ventricle to pump blood into the systemic circulation. Diastolic pressure decreases during the first 3 months and then gradually rises to values close to those at birth. Fluctuations in blood pressure occur during varying states of activity and emotion.

Significant *hemopoietic changes* occur during the first year (see the Appendix). *Fetal hemoglobin* (HgF) is the primary hemoglobin for the first 2 to 3 months, with adult hemoglobin steadily increasing through the first half of infancy. Fetal hemoglobin results in shortened survival of red blood cells (RBCs) and thus a decreased number of RBCs. A common result at 2 to 3 months of age is *physiologic anemia.* High levels of HgF are thought to depress the production of *erythropoietin,* a hormone released by the kidney that stimulates RBC production.

Maternal iron stores are present for the first 5 to 6 months and then gradually diminish; that diminution also accounts for lowered hemoglobin levels toward the end of the first 6 months. The occurrence of physiologic anemia is not affected by an adequate supply of iron. However, when erythropoiesis is stimulated, iron supplies are necessary for formation of hemoglobin.

The *digestive processes* are immature at birth. Saliva is secreted in small amounts, but the majority of all digestive processes do not begin functioning until age 3 months, when drooling is common because of the poorly coordinated swallowing reflex. The enzyme *ptyalin* (also called *amylase*) is present in small amounts but usually has little effect on the foodstuff because of the small amount of time the food stays in the mouth. Digestion in the stomach consists primarily of the action of hydrochloric acid and rennin, an enzyme that acts specifically on the casein in milk to form curds, which are coagulated semisolid particles of milk. The curds cause the milk to be retained in the stomach long enough for digestion to occur.

Digestion also takes place in the duodenum, where pancreatic enzymes and bile begin to break down protein and fat. Secretion of the pancreatic enzyme *amylase,* which is needed for digestion of complex carbohydrates, is deficient until about the fourth to sixth month of life. *Lipase* is also limited, and infants do not achieve adult levels of fat absorption until 4 to 5 months of age. *Trypsin* is secreted in sufficient quantities to catabolize protein into polypeptides and some amino acids.

The immaturity of the digestive processes is evident in the appearance of stools. During infancy solid foods, such as peas, carrots, corn, and raisins, are passed incompletely broken down in the feces. An excess quantity of fiber disposes the child to loose, bulky stools. Breastfed infants have twice as many stools as formula-fed infants.

Throughout infancy the stomach enlarges to accommodate a greater volume of food. By the end of the first year the infant is able to tolerate three meals a day and a before-bedtime feeding (breast or bottle), and may have one or two bowel movements daily. However, with any type of gastric irritation the infant is vulnerable to diarrhea, vomiting, and dehydration (see Chapter 43).

Paralleling the ability of the gastrointestinal system to digest and absorb more complex foodstuff is the process of tooth eruption. *Tooth eruption* occurs in a fairly orderly sequence beginning at about 6 to 7 months of age (see discussion of teething on p. 954).

The *liver* is the most immature of all the gastrointestinal organs throughout infancy. The ability to conjugate bilirubin and to secrete bile is achieved after the first couple of weeks of life. However, the capacities for *gluconeogenesis*, formation of plasma protein and ketones; storage of vitamins; and deamінization of amino acids remain relatively immature for the first year of life.

The *immunologic system* undergoes numerous changes during the first year. The newborn receives significant amounts of maternal IgG, which confers immunity for about 3 months against antigens to which the mother was exposed. During this time the infant begins to synthesize IgG, and about 40% of adult levels are reached by 1 year of age. Significant amounts of IgM are produced at birth, and adult levels are reached by 9 months of age. The production of IgA is much more gradual, and maximum levels are not attained until puberty.

During infancy *thermoregulation* becomes more efficient as the ability of the skin to contract and muscles to shiver in response to cold increases. The peripheral capillaries respond to change in ambient temperature to regulate heat loss. In response to cold the capillaries constrict, conserving core body temperature and decreasing potential evaporative heat loss from the skin surface. In response to heat the capillaries dilate, decreasing internal body temperature through evaporation, conduction, and convection. Shivering causes the muscles and muscle fibers to contract, generating metabolic heat, which is distributed throughout the body. Accumulation of adipose tissue during the first 6 months serves to insulate the body against heat loss.

At birth 75% of the infant's *body weight* is water and there is an excess of extracellular fluid (ECF). As the percentage of body water decreases, so does the amount of ECF—from 40% at term to 20% in adulthood. The high proportion of ECF, which is composed of blood plasma, interstitial fluid, and lymph, predisposes the infant to a more rapid loss of total body fluid and consequently dehydration.

The immaturity of the *renal structures* also predisposes the infant to dehydration. Complete maturity of the kidney occurs during the latter half of the second year. Before this time the filtration capacity of the glomeruli is reduced. Urine is voided frequently and has a low specific gravity (1.000 to 1.010).

Auditory acuity is at adult levels during infancy. Visual acuity begins to improve, and binocular fixation is established. **Binocularity,** or the fixation of two ocular images into one cerebral picture *(fusion)*, begins to develop by 6 weeks of age and should be well established by age 4 months. *Depth perception (stereopsis)* begins to develop by age 7 to 9 months but may exist earlier as an innate safety mechanism against accidental falling.

Fine Motor Behavior

Fine motor behavior includes the use of the hands and fingers in the prehension (grasp) of an object. Grasping occurs during the first 2 to 3 months as a reflex and gradually becomes voluntary. At 1 month the hands are predominantly closed and by 3 months are mostly open. By this time infants demonstrate a desire to grasp an object, but they "grasp" it more with the eyes than with the hands. If a rattle is placed in the hand, the infant will actively hold onto it. By 4 months the infant regards both a small pellet and the hands and looks from the object to the hands and back again. By 5 months the infant is able to grasp an object voluntarily.

Gradually the palmar grasp (using the whole hand) is replaced with a pincer grasp (using the thumb and index finger). By 8 to 9 months the infant uses a crude pincer grasp but by 11 months has progressed to a neat pincer grasp (Fig. 33-2).

By 6 months infants have increased manipulative skill.

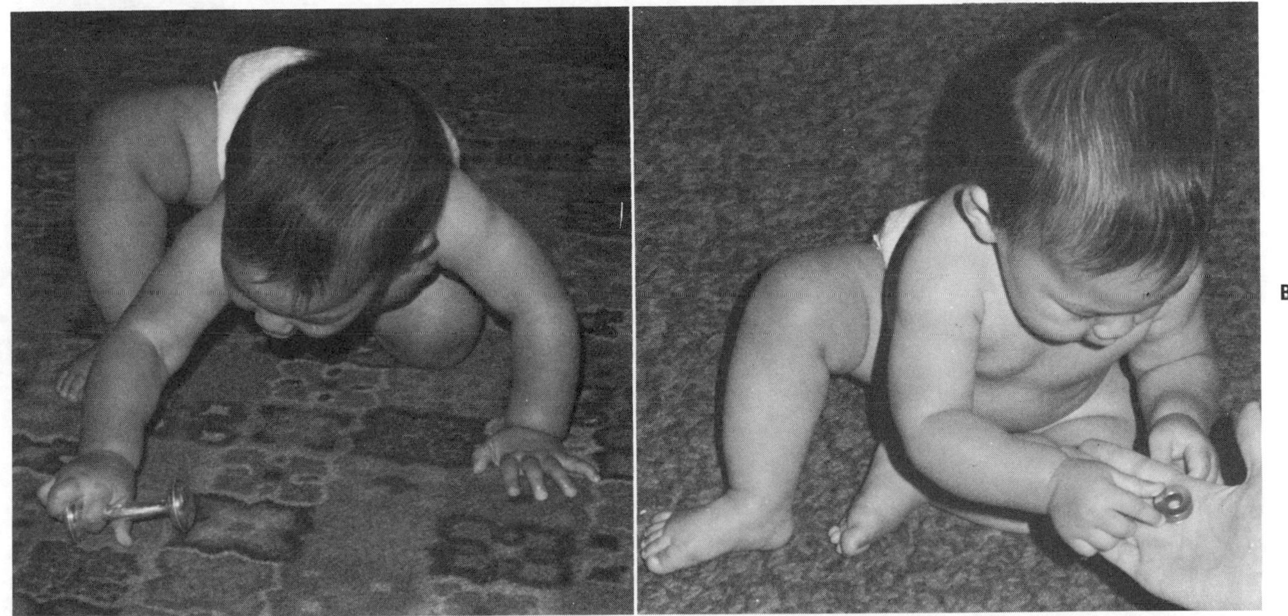

Fig. 33-2 **A,** Crude pincer grasp at 8 to 10 months. **B,** Neat pincer grasp at 10 to 11 months.

They hold their bottle, grasp feet and pull them to the mouth, and feed themselves a cracker. By 7 months they transfer objects from one hand to the other, use one hand for grasping, and hold a cube in each hand simultaneously. They enjoy banging objects and will explore the movable parts of a toy.

By 10 months the pincer grasp is sufficiently established to enable infants to pick up a raisin and other finger foods. They can deliberately let go of an object and offer it to someone. By 11 months they put objects into a container and like to remove them. By 1 year infants try to build a tower of two blocks but fail.

Gross Motor Development

Head control. The full-term newborn can momentarily hold the head in midline and parallel when the body is suspended ventrally and can lift and turn the head from side to side when prone. This is not the case when the infant is lying prone on a pillow or soft surface; infants do not have the head control to lift their head out of the depression of the object and therefore risk suffocation (see Sudden Infant Death Syndrome, p. 984). However, marked head lag is evident when the infant is pulled from a lying to a sitting position. By 3 months of age infants can hold their head well beyond the plane of the body, and by 4 months of age they can lift the head and front portion of the chest about 90 degrees above the table, bearing their weight on the forearms. Only slight head lag is evident when the infant is pulled from a lying to a sitting position, and by 4 to 6 months head control is well established (Figs. 33-3 and 33-4).

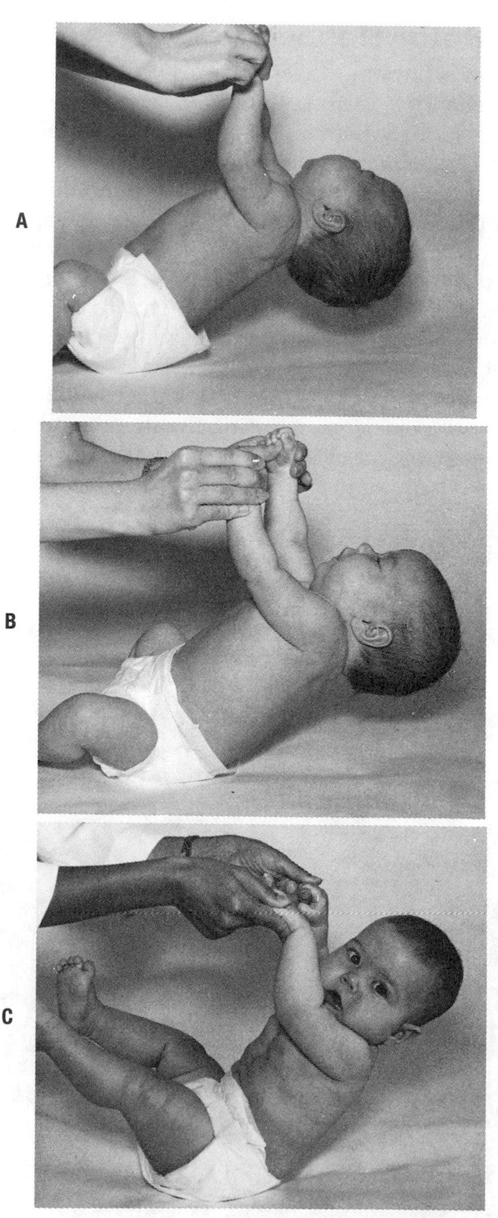

Fig. 33-3 Head control while pulled to sitting position. **A,** Complete head lag at 1 month. **B,** Partial head lag at 2 months. **C,** Almost no head lag at 4 months.

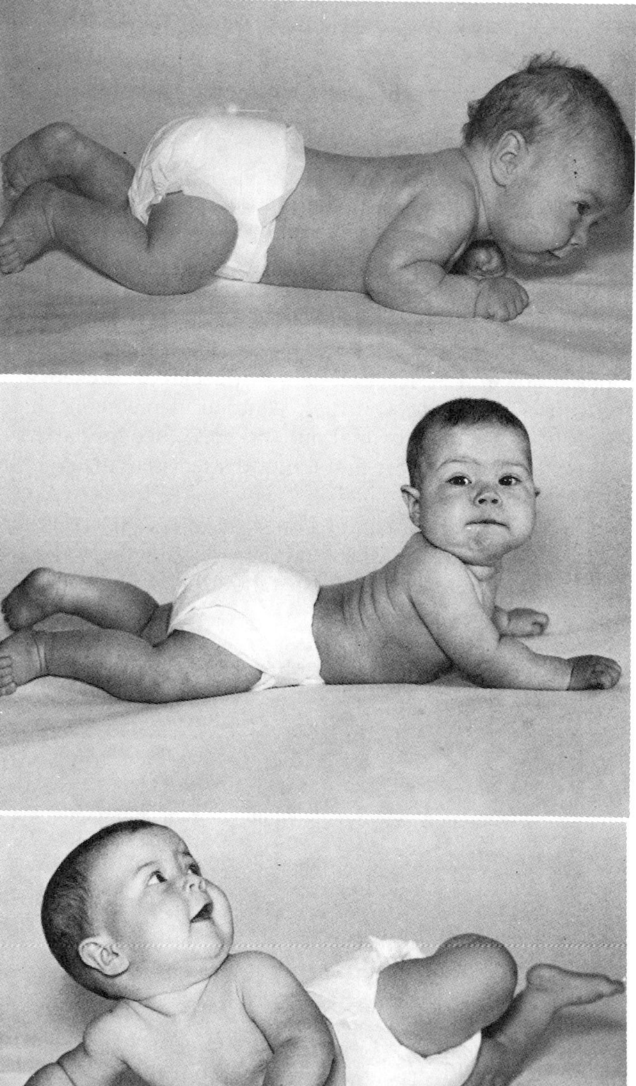

Fig. 33-4 Head control while prone. **A,** Infant momentarily lifts head at 1 month. **B,** Infant lifts head and chest 90 degrees and bears weight on forearms at 4 months. **C,** Infant lifts head, chest, and upper abdomen and can bear weight on hands at 6 months. Note how this position facilitates turning from abdomen to back.

Nursing ALERT

Any child who displays head lag at 6 months of age should have a developmental/neurologic evaluation.

Rolling over. Newborns may roll over accidentally because of their rounded back. The ability to turn willfully from the abdomen to the back occurs at 5 months and from the back to the abdomen at 6 months. It is noteworthy that the parachute reflex (see Fig. 33-1), which elicits a protective response to falling, appears at 7 months.

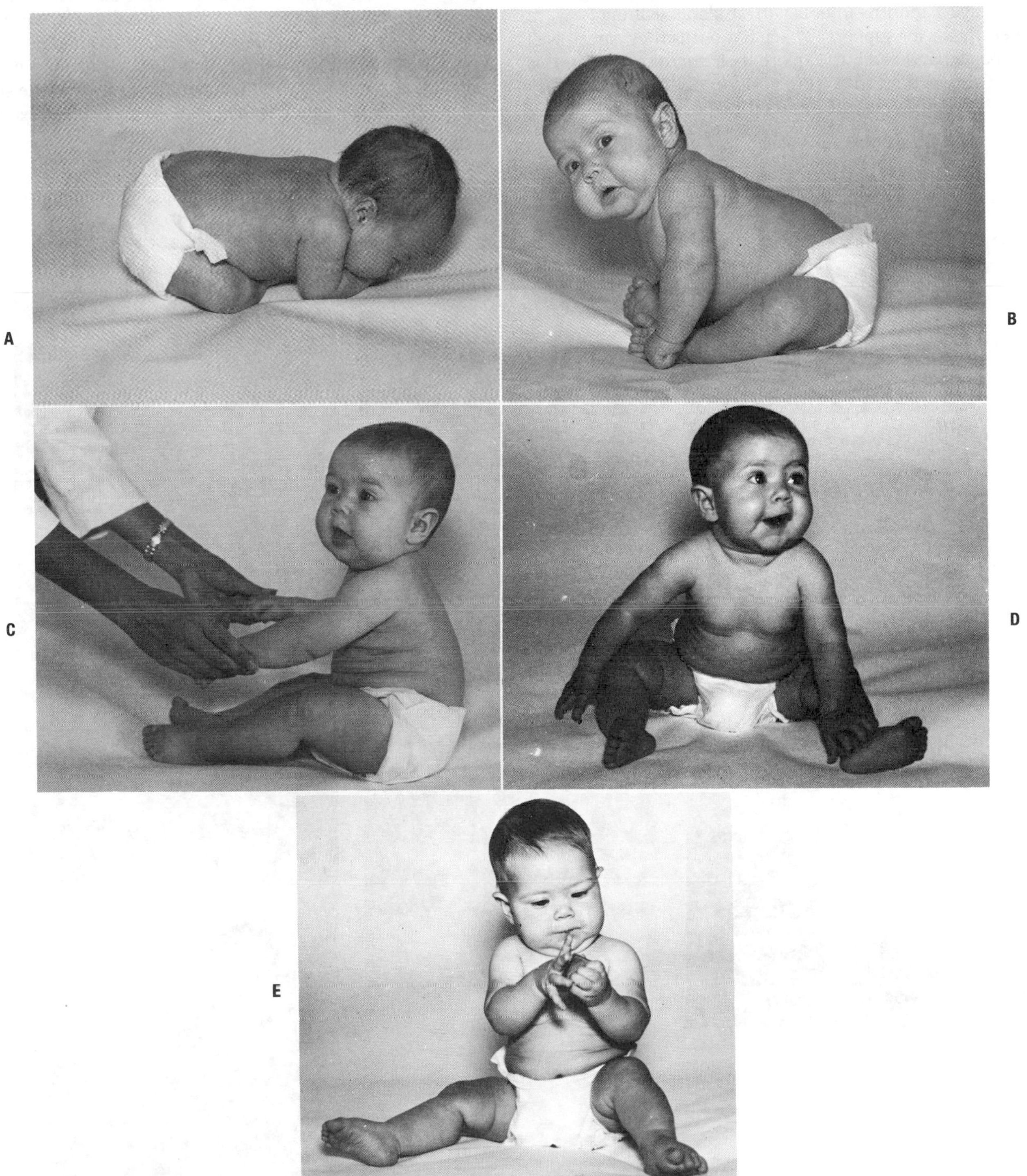

Fig. 33-5 Development of sitting. **A,** Back is completely rounded, and infant has no ability to sit upright at 1 month. **B,** Back is still rounded, but infant can sit up momentarily with some head control at 2 months. **C,** Back is rounded only in lumbar area, and infant is able to sit erect with good head control at 4 months. **D,** Infant can sit alone, leaning on hands for support, at 7 months. **E,** Infant sits without support at 8 months. Note the transferring of objects that occurs at 7 months.

Sitting. The ability to sit follows progressive head control and straightening of the back, as shown in Fig. 33-5. For the first 2 to 3 months the back is uniformly rounded. The convex cervical curve forms at about 3 to 4 months when head control is established. The convex lumbar curve appears when the child begins to sit, at about age 4 months. As the spinal column straightens, the infant can be propped in a sitting position. By age 7 months infants can sit alone, leaning forward on their hands for support. By age 8 months they can sit well unsupported and begin to explore their surroundings in this position rather than in a lying position. By 10 months they can maneuver from a prone to a sitting position.

Locomotion. Locomotion involves acquiring the ability to bear weight, propel forward on all four extremities, stand upright with support, and finally walk alone (Fig. 33-6). Following a *cephalocaudal* pattern, infants 4 to 6 months old have increasing coordination in their arms. In initial locomotion infants propel themselves backward by pushing with the arms. By 6 to 7 months infants are able to bear all their weight on their legs, with assistance. *Crawling* (propelling forward with belly on floor) progresses to *creeping* on hands and knees (with belly off floor) by 9 months. At this time they stand while holding onto furniture and can pull themselves to the standing position but are unable to maneuver back down, except by

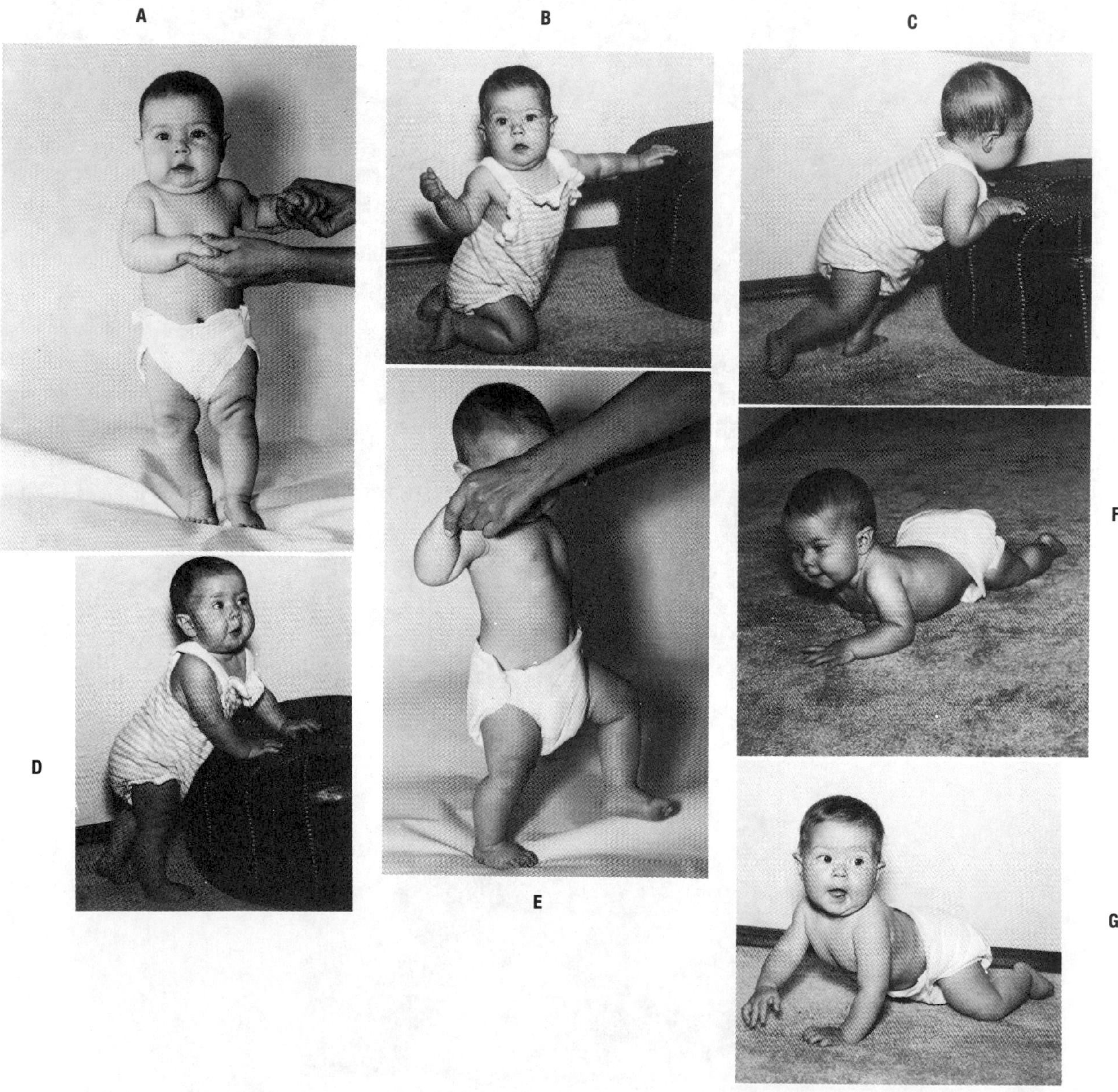

Fig. 33-6 Development of locomotion. **A,** Infant bears full weight on feet by 7 months. **B,** Infant can maneuver from sitting to kneeling position. **C,** Infant can pull self to standing position, and **D,** can stand holding onto furniture at 9 months. **E,** While standing, infant takes deliberate step at 10 months. **F,** Infant crawls with abdomen on floor and pulls self forward, and then, **G,** creeps on hands and knees at 9 months.

falling. By 11 months they walk while holding onto furniture or with both hands held, and by 1 year they may be able to walk with one hand held. A number of infants attempt their first independent steps by their first birthday.

PSYCHOSOCIAL DEVELOPMENT

Developing a Sense of Trust (Erikson)

Erikson's phase 1 (birth to 1 year) is concerned with *acquiring a sense of trust* while overcoming a sense of *mistrust.* The trust that develops is a trust of self, of others, and of the world. Infants "trust" that their feeding, comfort, stimulation, and caring needs will be met. The crucial element for the achievement of this task is the *quality* of both the parent (caregiver)–child relationship and the care the infant receives. The provision of food, warmth, and shelter by itself is inadequate for the development of a strong sense of self. The infant and parent must jointly learn to meet their needs satisfactorily in order for mutual regulation of frustration to occur. When this synchrony fails to develop, mistrust is the eventual outcome.

Failure to learn "delayed gratification" leads to mistrust. It can result from too much or too little frustration. If parents always meet their children's needs before the children signal their readiness, infants will never learn to test their ability to control the environment. If the delay is prolonged, infants will experience constant frustration and eventually mistrust others' efforts to satisfy them. Therefore, consistency of care is essential.

The trust acquired in infancy is foundational for all the succeeding phases. It allows infants feelings of physical comfort and security, which assist them in experiencing unfamiliar, unknown situations with a minimum of fear. Erikson has divided the first year of life into two oral/social stages. During the first 3 to 4 months, food intake is the most important social activity in which the infant engages. The newborn can tolerate little frustration or delay of gratification. Primary *narcissism* (total concern for oneself) is at its height.

However, as bodily processes such as vision, motor movements, and vocalization are better controlled, infants use more advanced behaviors to interact with others. For example, rather than crying, infants may put their arms up to signify a desire to be held.

The next social modality involves a mode of reaching out to others through *grasping.* Initially grasping is reflexive, but even as a reflex it has a powerful social meaning for the parents. The reciprocal response to the infant's grasping is the parents' holding on and touching. There is pleasurable tactile stimulation for both the child and the parents.

Tactile stimulation is extremely important in the total process of acquiring trust. The degree of mothering skill, the quantity of food, or the length of sucking does not determine the quality of the experience. Rather, it is the total nature of the quality of the interpersonal relationship that influences the infant's formulation of trust.

During the second stage, the more active and aggressive modality of *biting* occurs. Infants learn that they can hold onto what is their own and can more fully control their environment. During this stage infants may be confronted with one of their first conflicts. If they are breastfeeding, they quickly learn that biting causes withdrawal of the nipple and anxiety in the mother. Yet biting also brings internal relief from teething discomfort and a sense of power or control.

This conflict may be solved in a variety of ways. The mother may wean the infant from the breast and begin bottle-feeding, or the infant may learn to bite substitute "nipples," such as a pacifier, and retain pleasurable breastfeeding. The successful resolution of this conflict strengthens the mother-child relationship because it occurs at a time when infants are recognizing the mother as the most significant person in their life.

COGNITIVE DEVELOPMENT

The Sensorimotor Phase (Piaget)

The theory most frequently used to explain *cognition,* or the ability to know, is that of Piaget. The period of birth to 24 months is termed the *sensorimotor phase* and is composed of six stages; however, inasmuch as this discussion is concerned with the period from birth to 12 months, only the first four stages are discussed. The last two stages occur during the toddler period of 12 to 24 months and are discussed in Chapter 34.

During the sensorimotor phase the infant progresses from reflex behavior to simple repetitive acts to imitative activity. Three crucial events take place during this phase.

First infants learn to separate themselves from other objects in the environment. They realize that others besides them control the environment and that certain readjustments must take place for mutual satisfaction to occur. This coincides with Erikson's concept of the formation of trust and mutual regulation of frustration.

The second major accomplishment is achievement of the concept of **object permanence,** or the realization that objects that leave one's visual field still exist. A typical example of the development of object permanence is when infants are able to pursue objects they observe being hidden under a pillow or behind a chair (Fig. 33-7). This skill develops at ap-

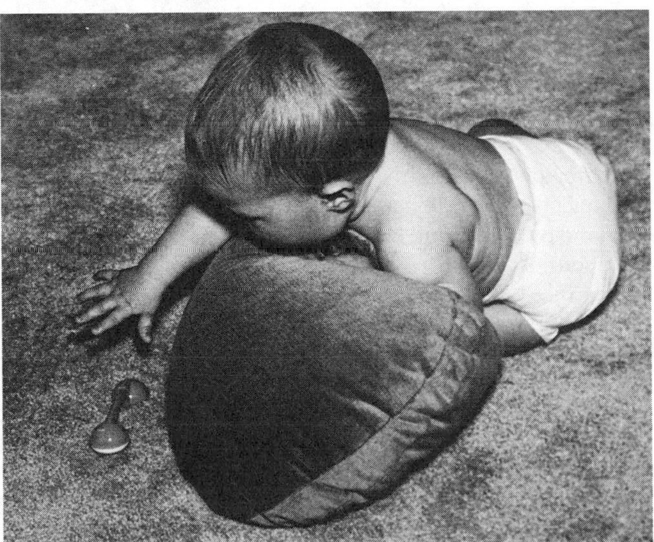

Fig. 33-7 Nine-month-old infant actively searches for object hidden behind pillow.

proximately 9 to 10 months of age, a period that also corresponds to the time of increased locomotion skills.

The last major intellectual development of this period is the ability to use *symbols* or *mental representation.* The use of symbols allows the infant to think of an object or situation without actually experiencing it. The recognition of symbols is the beginning of understanding time and space.

The four stages of Piaget's theory of cognitive development that affect infants are as follows:

Stage I: Use of reflexes. The first stage, from birth to 1 month, is identified by the *use of reflexes.* At birth the infant's individuality and temperament are expressed through the physiologic reflexes of sucking, rooting, grasping, and crying. The repetitious nature of the reflexes, along with the continuing myelinization of the brain, are the beginning of associations between an act and a sequential response. When infants cry because of hunger, a nipple is put into the mouth, and they suck, feel satisfaction, and sleep.

Stage II: Primary circular reactions. This stage marks the beginning of the replacement of reflexive behavior with voluntary acts. During this period from 1 to 4 months, activities such as sucking or grasping become deliberate acts that elicit certain responses. Infants incorporate and adapt their reactions to the environment and recognize the stimulus that produces a response. Previously they would cry until the nipple was presented to the mouth. Now they associate the nipple with the sound of the parent's voice. They accommodate this new piece of information and adapt by ceasing to cry when they hear the voice, before they receive the nipple.

Stage III: Secondary circular reactions. The third stage is a continuation of the previous one and lasts until 8 months of age. In this stage the circular primary reactions are intentionally repeated and prolonged for the response that results. Grasping and holding now become shaking, banging, and pulling. Shaking is performed to hear a noise, not solely for the pleasure of shaking. Quality and quantity of an act become evident. "More" or "less" shaking produces different responses. Causality, time, deliberate intention, and one's separateness from the environment begin to develop.

Three new processes of human behavior—imitation, play, and affect—occur. *Imitation* requires the differentiation of behaviors. By the second half of the first year, the infant can imitate sounds and simple gestures. *Play* becomes evident as the infant takes pleasure in performing a mastered act. Many of the infant's waking hours are absorbed in sensorimotor play. *Affect,* an outward manifestation of emotion and feeling, is seen as the infant develops.

Object permanence begins to develop at this time. During the first 6 months infants believe that an object exists only for as long as they can visually perceive it: in other words, out of sight, out of mind. When the object continues to be present or remembered even though it is beyond the range of perception, affect to external objects is evident. Object permanence is a critical component of parent-child attachment and is seen in the development of stranger anxiety at 6 to 8 months of age (p. 948).

Stage IV: Coordination of secondary schemata and its application to new situations. During the fourth sensorimotor stage, infants use previous behavioral achievements primarily as the foundation for adding new intellectual skills to their expanding repertoire. This stage from 9 to 12 months is largely transitional. Increasing motor skills allow for greater exploration of the environment. The child begins to discover that hiding an object does not mean that it is gone and that removing an obstacle will reveal the object (Fig. 33-7). This marks the beginning of intellectual reasoning. Furthermore, children can experience an event by *observing* it, and they begin to associate symbols with events, such as "bye-bye" with "going in the car," but the classification is purely their own. Unlike in the second stage, where the infant learned from the type of interaction between objects or individuals, in this stage the child learns from the object itself. Intentionality is further developed in that now infants will actively attempt to remove a barrier to their desired (or undesired) action. If something is in their way, they will attempt to climb over it or push it away. Previously an obstacle would cause them to give up any further attempt to achieve their desired goal.

DEVELOPMENT OF BODY IMAGE

The development of body image parallels sensorimotor development. Infants' kinesthetic and tactile experiences are the first perceptions of their body, and the mouth is the principal area of pleasurable sensations. Other parts of the body are primarily objects of pleasure—the hands and fingers to suck and the feet to play with. As physical needs are met, they feel comfort and satisfaction with their body. Verbal and nonverbal (touch) messages conveyed by the caregivers reinforce these feelings. For example, when infants smile, they receive emotional satisfaction from others who smile back.

The development of object permanence is basic to the development of self-image. By the end of the first year infants recognize that they are distinct from their parents. At the same time, there is increasing interest in their image, especially in the mirror (Fig. 33-8). As motor skills develop, they learn that parts of the body are useful; for example, the hands carry objects to the mouth and the legs help them move to different locations. All of these achievements transmit messages to them about themselves. It is therefore important to transmit positive messages to infants about their bodies.

SOCIAL DEVELOPMENT

Infants' social development is initially influenced by their reflexive behavior, such as the grasp, and eventually depends primarily on the interaction between them and the principal caregivers. *Attachment* to the parent is increasingly evident during the second half of the first year. In addition, tremendous strides are made in communication and personal-social behavior. Whereas crying and reflexive behavior are methods to meet one's needs in the neonatal period, the social smile is an early step in social communication. This has a profound effect on family members and is a tremendous stimulus for evoking continued responses from others. By 4 months infants laugh aloud.

Play is a major socializing agent and provides stimulation needed to learn from and interact with the environment. By

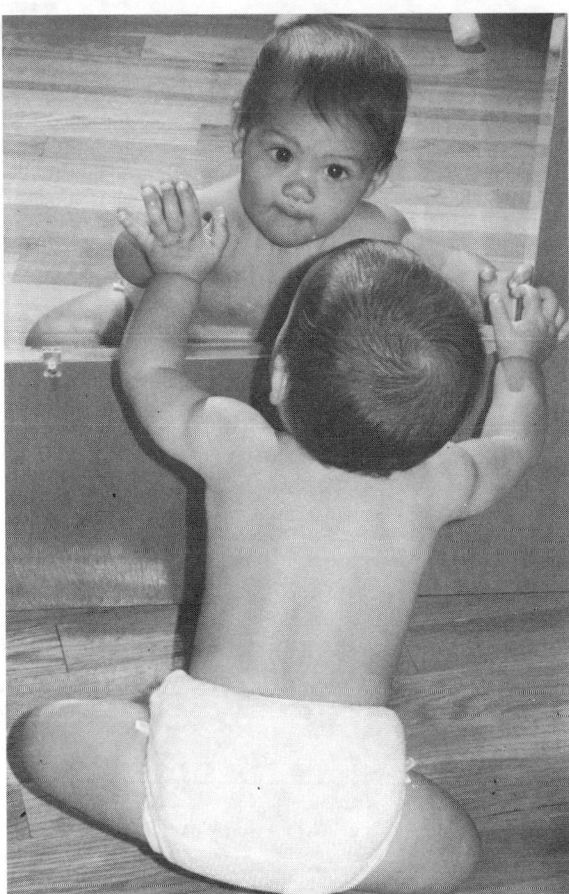

Fig. 33-8 Nine-month-old infant enjoying own image in mirror.

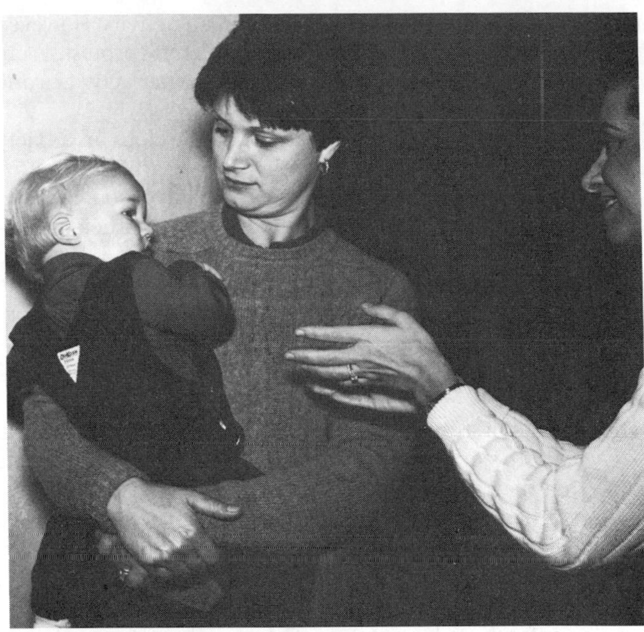

Fig. 33-9 Behaviors related to fear of strangers include clinging to the parent and turning away from the stranger.

age 6 months infants are very personable. They play games such as peekaboo when their head is hidden in a towel; they signal their desire to be picked up by extending their arms; and they show displeasure when a toy is removed or their face is washed.

Attachment

Several components are crucial in the process of attachment. Some of them, such as the maternal sensitive period and paternal engrossment, are discussed in Chapter 22 and emphasize the importance of the first hour and days of life. The following is a discussion of attachment after the neonatal period. Although the word *mother* is frequently used, it does not refer exclusively to the biologic mother but to the consistent caregiver with whom the child relates more than anyone else. In light of the changing social climate, this may very well be the father. Studies on father–child attachment demonstrate that similar stages occur as in mother attachment, and that fathers are more involved in child care when mothers are employed outside the home (although mothers continue to do the majority of infant care) (Jones and Heermann, 1992).

During infancy attachment progresses with the child assuming an increasingly significant role. Two components of cognitive development are required for attachment: (1) the ability to discriminate the mother from other individuals and (2) the achievement of object permanence. Both of these processes prepare the infant for an equally important aspect of attachment—separation from the parent.

During the formation of attachment to the parent, the infant progresses through four distinct but overlapping stages. For the first few weeks infants respond indiscriminately to anyone. Attachment is facilitated by eye contact during feedings and being held close to the caregiver's body. Beginning at about 8 to 12 weeks of age, infants cry, smile, and vocalize more to the mother than to anyone else but continue to respond to others, whether familiar or not. At about age 6 months infants show a distinct preference for the mother. They follow her more, cry when she leaves, enjoy playing with her more, and feel most secure in her arms. About 1 month after showing attachment to the mother, many infants begin attaching to other members of the family, most often the father.

Infants acquire other developmental behaviors that influence the attachment process. These include (1) differential crying, smiling, and vocalization (more to the mother than to anyone else); (2) visual-motor orientation (looking more at the mother even if she is not close); (3) crying when the mother leaves the room; (4) approach through locomotion (crawling, creeping, or walking); (5) clinging (especially in the presence of a stranger); and (6) exploring away from the mother while using her as a secure base.

Stranger fear. As infants develop the ability to differentiate among individuals, they learn to distinguish their mother or other primary caregiver from other individuals by 5 to 6 months of age. This cognitive awareness results in a preference for "mother" and is demonstrated by behaviors typical of stranger anxiety, such as clinging to the parent, crying, and turning away from the stranger (Fig. 33-9).

Family members, such as grandparents, often describe this behavior as an indication that the child is "spoiled." This is not the case. This process results from improving cognitive development and peaks at 8 months of age. Because object permanence is just beginning to develop, infants may not notice the mother's absence if they are absorbed in an activity. However, when they become aware of her absence, they protest. From this point onward they become very alert to her activities and whereabouts.

Along with stranger anxiety, the child develops an anxiety related to separation from the mother. This manifests itself by later infancy and lasts throughout early toddlerhood. By 11 to 12 months infants are able to anticipate the mother's imminent departure by watching her behaviors and begin to protest *before* she leaves. At this point many parents learn to postpone alerting the child to their departure until just before leaving.

Language Development

The infant's first means of verbal communication is crying. They learn to signal displeasure before pleasure. Many parents state that they can distinguish between different types of crying and from these messages are able to interpret the infant's needs. However, crying can be a source of acute distress for parents, especially the unconsolable crying of colic (see p. 979). Parents benefit from an explanation of the variability of crying among infants and assurance that periods of "unexplained fussiness" are normal. Some parents may need guidance in consoling techniques, such as holding, swaddling, massaging, caressing, rocking, walking, or stimulating sucking. During the end of the first year infants cry for attention, from fear, especially stranger fear, and from frustration, usually in response to their developing but inadequate motor skills.

Nursing ALERT

Be alert to parent reports about maternal postpartum depression and infant crying because these concerns may indicate a stressed mother–infant relationship (Miller, Barr, and Eaton, 1993).

Family Focus

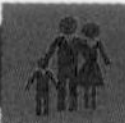

CHILD'S DEVELOPING LANGUAGE SKILLS

During the acquisition of new language skills the child temporarily may give up other recently learned sounds or words. This is often distressing for parents, who have waited in anticipation for the words "dada" or "mama," since these sounds are commonly replaced by other vocalizations and may not be repeated for several weeks. Nurses should reassure parents that the child will again say these special words, and with increased meaning.

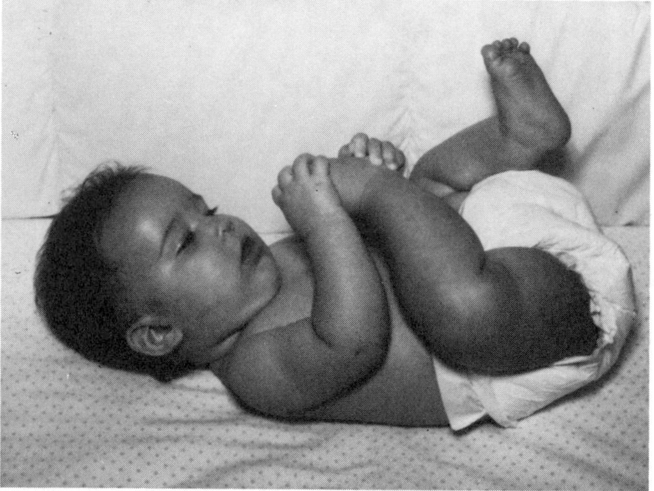

Fig. 33-10 During early infancy body parts are primarily objects of pleasure for the child.

Vocalizations heard during crying eventually become some syllables and words (e.g., the "mama" heard during vigorous crying). Infants vocalize as early as 5 to 6 weeks of age by making small throaty sounds. By 2 months they make single vowel sounds, such as *ah, eh,* and *uh.* By 3 to 4 months the consonants *n, k, g, p,* and *b* are added, and infants coo, gurgle, and laugh aloud. By 8 months they imitate sound, add the consonants *t, d,* and *w,* and combine syllables such as "dada"; but they do not ascribe meaning to the word until 10 to 11 months of age (see the Family Focus box above). By 9 to 10 months they comprehend the meaning of the word "no" and obey simple commands. By age 1 year they can say three to five words with meaning.

Play

Play mirrors all of the developmental tasks and allows children to experiment safely with their newly learned skills. Play during infancy represents the various social and cognitive modalities proposed by Erikson and Piaget. From shortly after birth, the senses of hearing and touch are the only ones fully developed. Therefore stimulation is geared to them. Being held or rocked and listening to a musical mobile are ideal at this time.

Infants' activity is primarily narcissistic, revolving around their own body. At 2 months of age infants will look at their extended hand as if it were an unfamiliar object. At about age 6 months infants play with their feet and find fingers excellent nipple substitutes (Fig. 33-10). During this time the ability to grasp is well under voluntary control, and everything is reached for and brought to the mouth for inquisitive exploration. When the pincer grasp is mastered, infants are absorbed with growing independence, refusing to allow others to feed them.

Play reflects infants' social development and their increasing awareness of the environment. From birth to age 3 months the infant's response to the environment is global and largely undifferentiated. Play is dependent; pleasure is demonstrated by a quieting attitude (age 1 month), later by a smile (age 2 to 3 months), and then by a squeal (age 3 to 4 months). By age 3 to 6 months infants show more discriminate interest in the stimuli presented to them and begin to play alone with a rattle or soft stuffed toy or to play with someone else. There is much more interaction during play. By 4 months of age they laugh aloud, show preference for certain toys, and are excited when food or a favorite object is given to them.

By 6 months to 1 year of age, play is more sophisticated

TABLE 33-1 Play during infancy

AGE (MONTHS)	VISUAL STIMULATION	AUDITORY STIMULATION	TACTILE STIMULATION	KINETIC STIMULATION
Suggested Activities				
Birth-1	Look at infant at close range Hang bright, shiny object within 20-25 cm (8-10 inches) of infant's face and in midline Hang mobiles with black-and-white contrast designs	Talk to infant, sing in soft voice Play music box, radio, television Have ticking clock or metronome nearby	Hold, caress, cuddle Keep infant warm May like to be swaddled	Rock infant, place in cradle Use carriage for walks
2-3	Provide bright objects Make room bright with pictures or mirrors on walls Take infant to various rooms while doing chores Place infant in infant seat for vertical view of environment	Talk to infant Include in family gatherings Expose to various environmental noises other than those of home Use rattles, wind chimes	Caress infant while bathing, at diaper change Comb hair with a soft brush	Use infant swing Take in car for rides Exercise body by moving extremities in swimming motion Use cradle gym
4-6	Place infant in front of unbreakable mirror Give brightly colored toys to hold (small enough to grasp)	Talk to infant, repeat sounds infant makes Laugh when infant laughs Call infant by name Crinkle different papers by infant's ear Place rattle or bell in hand	Give infant soft squeeze toys of various textures Allow to splash in bath Place nude on soft furry rug and move extemities	Use swing or stroller Bounce infant in lap while holding in standing position Support infant in sitting position, let infant lean forward to balance self Place infant on floor to crawl, roll over, sit
6-9	Give infant large toys with bright colors, movable parts, and noisemakers Place unbreakable mirror where infant can see self Play peekaboo, especially hiding face in a towel Make funny faces to encourage imitation Give ball of yarn or string to pull apart	Call infant by name Repeat simple words such as "dada," "mama," "bye-bye" Speak clearly Name parts of body, people, and foods Tell infant what you are doing Use "no" only when necessary Give simple commands Show how to clap hands, bang a drum	Let infant play with fabrics of various textures Have bowl with foods of different size and textures to feel Let infant "catch" running water Encourage "swimming" in large bathtub or shallow pool Give wad of sticky tape to manipulate	Hold upright to bear weight and bounce Pick up, say "up" Put down, say "down" Place toys out of reach; encourage infant to get them Play pat-a-cake
6-12	Show infant large pictures in books Take infant to places where there are animals, many people, different objects (shopping center) Play ball by rolling it to child, demonstrate "throwing" it back Demonstrate building a two-block tower	Read infant simple nursery rhymes Point to body parts and name each one Imitate sounds of animals	Give infant finger foods of different textures Let infant mess and squash food Let infant feel cold (ice cube) or warm objects; say what temperature each is Let infant feel a breeze (fan blowing)	Give large push-pull toys Place furniture in a circle to encourage cruising Turn in different positions
Suggested Toys				
Birth-6	Nursery mobiles Unbreakable mirrors See-through crib bumpers Contrasting colored sheets	Music boxes Musical mobiles Crib dangle bells Small-handled clear rattle	Stuffed animals Soft clothes Soft or furry quilt Soft mobiles	Rocking crib/cradle Weighted or suction toy Infant swing (wind-up)
6-12	Various colored blocks Nested boxes or cups Books with rhymes and bright pictures Strings of big beads Simple take-apart toys Large ball Cup and spoon Large puzzles Jack-in-the box	Rattles of different sizes, shapes, tones, and bright colors Squeaky animals and dolls Records with light, rhythmic music	Soft, different-textured animals and dolls Sponge toys, floating toys Squeeze toys Teething toys Books with textures and objects, such as fur and zipper	Push-pull toys Baby swing Activity box for crib

and involves sensorimotor skills. Actual games are played, such as peekaboo, pat-a-cake, verbal repetition, and imitation of simple gestures in response to demonstration. Play is much more selective, not only in terms of specific toys but also in terms of "playmates." Although play is solitary or one-sided, infants choose with whom they will interact. At 6 to 8 months of age they usually refuse to play with strangers until they begin to know them. Parents are definite favorites.

Stimulation is as important for developmental growth as food is for biologic growth. Knowledge of developmental milestones allows nurses to guide parents regarding proper play for infants. It is not sufficient to place a mobile over a crib and toys in a playpen for a child's optimal social, emotional, and intellectual development. Play must provide interpersonal contact, as well as recreational and educational stimulation. Infants need to be *played with,* not merely allowed to *play.* Although the type of play infants engage in is called *solitary,* this is a figurative, not literal, term to denote one-sided play. The kind of toy given to the child is much less important than the quality of personal interaction that occurs.

Table 33-1 lists play activities that are appropriate for the developmental level of the infant in view of motor, language, and personal-social achievements. Although the activities are grouped according to the major mode of stimulation provided, there is overlap in many instances. In addition, play activities suggested for one age group may be appropriate for an older age group but are generally inappropriate for a younger age group. The most important component of play is safety.

TEMPERAMENT

The infant's temperament or behavioral style influences the kind of interaction that occurs between the child and parents and other family members (see general discussion of temperament in Chapter 30). In assessing a child's temperament, the parents' perception of the child and the degree of *fit* between their expectations and the child's actual temperament are important. The more dissonance or lack of harmony between the child's temperament and the parent's ability to accept and deal with the behavior, the more risk for subsequent parent–child conflicts.

The *Infant Temperament Questionnaire (ITQ)* (Carey and McDevitt, 1978) can be used as a screening tool with parents. The questionnaire focuses on nine temperament variables, but the 95 questions relate specifically to activities such as sleep, feeding, play, diapering, and dressing. The scores from the ITQ help identify the child's temperament style.

With knowledge of the infant's temperament, nurses are better able to (1) provide parents with background information that will help them see their child in a better perspective, (2) offer a more organized picture of their child's behavior and possibly reveal distortions in their perceptions of the behavior, and (3) guide parents regarding appropriate childrearing techniques (Chess and Thomas, 1985).

Childrearing Practices Related to Temperament

Most parents realize that their infant is born with unique characteristics, and few parents of difficult infants need to be told of the challenge of caring for them. However, very few parents are aware of the significance of the temperamental characteristics and of constructive approaches to dealing with them. The following are examples of interventions that promote more positive parenting of infants with different temperament styles.

> **Family Focus** 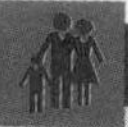
>
> DIFFICULT TEMPERAMENT AND PRETERM INFANTS
>
> **Parents typically rate preterm, low-birth-weight infants as being more difficult than full-term infants. Parents are often concerned that the difficult temperament is permanent and results from the many negative and painful hospital experiences. The family can be reassured that although these infants may be difficult to parent for the first 6 months of corrected age (chronologic age minus amount of prematurity), no particular perinatal event is responsible. Also, over time the infants tend to become less difficult (Gennaro, Medoff-Cooper, and Lotas, 1992).**

Difficult children may respond better to scheduled feedings and structured caregiving routines than demand feedings and frequent changes in daily routines. These children sleep less and may need more structured approaches to bedtime to prevent bedtime problems. *Highly distractible children* may require additional soothing measures such as swinging, rocking, or being carried in a pack that the parent wears across the chest or back. Children with *high activity* levels require vigilant watching, and parents need to take extra precautions in safeguarding the home. These children benefit from increased opportunities for gross motor activity to channel their energy constructively.

The *slow-to-warm-up child* may demonstrate more stranger fear than other children and may require more gradual and frequent preparation for new situations, such as substitute child care. Even the *easy child* can present problems in that the parents may need reminders to feed the child who sleeps for prolonged intervals and rarely cries. They may have to "retrain" the child because of the ease of developing troublesome habits, such as keeping the child up late or sleeping with the youngster.

Appropriate counseling based on awareness of the child's temperament can greatly enhance the quality of interaction between parents and infant. Even just letting parents know that "difficult" traits are innate can relieve feelings of guilt and incompetence (see the Family Focus box above).

■ ■ ■

A summary of growth and development during infancy is presented in Table 33-2. Although all milestones are important, some represent essential integrative aspects of development that lay the foundation for the achievement of more advanced skills. These essential milestones are designated by a bullet (■) in the chart. The table represents the *average* monthly age at which various skills are attained. It must be remembered that although the sequence is the same, the rate will vary among children.

COPING WITH CONCERNS RELATED TO NORMAL GROWTH AND DEVELOPMENT

Separation and Stranger Fear

During infancy a number of fears can appear. However, the fear that causes parents most concern is related to the child's fear of strangers and separation. Although erroneously interpreted by some as signs of undesirable, antisocial behavior, **stranger fear** and **separation anxiety** are important components of a strong, healthy parent-child attachment. However, this period can present difficulties for parent and child. Parents may be more hesitant to leave the child with others because the older infant protests violently against having a baby-sitter. To accustom the infant to new people, parents are encouraged to have close friends or relatives visit often. This provides other persons with whom the child is comfortable and who can give parents time for themselves.

Infants also need opportunities to experience strangers safely. Usually toward the end of the first year, infants begin to venture away from the parent and demonstrate curiosity about strangers. If allowed to explore at their own rate, many infants will eventually "warm up." If parents hold the child away from their face, the infant can observe while maintaining close physical contact. The best approach for the stranger (who may be the nurse) is to talk to the parent, talk softly, meet the child at eye level (to appear smaller), maintain a safe distance from the infant, and avoid sudden, intrusive gestures, such as holding the arms out and smiling broadly.

Parents also may wonder whether they should encourage the child's clinging, dependent behavior, especially if there is pressure from others who view this as "spoiling." Parents need to be reassured that such behavior is healthy, desirable, and necessary for the child's optimal emotional development. If parents can reassure the infant of their presence, the infant will learn to realize that they are still there even if not physically present. Talking to infants when leaving the room, allowing them to hear one's voice on the telephone, and using transitional objects, such as a favorite blanket or toy, reassures them of the parent's continued presence.

Alternate Child Care Arrangements

For many parents, especially working mothers, the need for locating safe and competent child care facilities for the infant is an increasingly difficult problem—one that is compounded by the number of mothers working outside the home. Over the past 30 years there has been a marked shift in child care arrangements, with fewer children being cared for at home and more children being cared for in group centers or other settings.

The basic types of care are in-home care, in either the parent's or another caregiver's home, and center-based care, usually in a daycare center. *In-home* care may consist of a full-time baby-sitter who lives in the home, a full-time baby-sitter who goes to the home, cooperative arrangements such as exchange baby-sitting, and family day care. A licensed *family day care home* typically provides care and protection for up to five children for part of a 24-hour day. *Center-based group care* usually refers to a day care facility that provides care for six or more children, for 6 or more hours in a 24-hour day. *Work-based group care* is another option that is becoming increasingly popular as employers recognize the benefit of high-quality and convenient child care to their employees. *Sick-child care* may also be available for times the youngster is ill. Such programs are often located in community hospitals (Landis and Chang, 1991).

Nurses may provide guidance to parents in selecting suitable, well-qualified facilities or individuals to care for their child. The decision to leave an infant in another's care often engenders doubt and guilt in the parent, despite reassurance that the provision of competent, loving care by someone other than the parent is not detrimental to the child's future development. Therefore, any assistance is often appreciated.

Guidelines for selecting child care facilities are discussed in Chapter 35 under Preschool or Kindergarten Experience. The same conscientious attention should be applied to locating competent baby-sitters. References are essential, and there is no substitute for observing the interaction between the individual and the child. Although very young infants need little if any preparation for the introduction of a new caregiver, older infants may benefit from gradual placement to reduce stranger fear. At all times the parent should have the right to visit the child, and regular conferences should be established to review the child's progress.

Limit Setting and Discipline

As infants' motor skills advance and mobility increases, parents are faced with the need to set safe limits (see discussion of nurse's role in injury prevention on p. 977). Although there are numerous disciplinary techniques, some are more appropriate for this age than others. Parents can begin discipline by using a negative voice and stern eye contact. When the child engages in unacceptable activity, play should be stopped and a firm voice should be used. Corporal punishment is not recommended. Although parents may be concerned with starting discipline during infancy, it is important to stress that the earlier effective disciplinary methods are employed, the easier it is to continue these approaches. The most important components of discipline are consistency and appropriateness. The same behaviors must consistently be acknowledged in the same way, and the degree of limit setting must be appropriate to the child's developmental level (See also Limit Setting and Discipline, Chapter 29.)

Thumb-Sucking and Use of Pacifier

Sucking is the infant's chief pleasure, and it may not be satisfied by breastfeeding or bottle-feeding. It is such a strong need that infants who are deprived of sucking, such as those with a cleft lip repair, will suck on their tongue. Some newborns are born with sucking pads on their fingers from in utero sucking activity. Several benefits of nonnutritive sucking have been documented, such as increased weight gain in preterm infants, decreased crying, and increased behavioral organization (Pickler and Frankel, 1995).

Problems arise when parents are concerned about sucking of fingers, thumb, or pacifier and attempt to restrain this natural tendency. Before offering advice, nurses should investigate the parents' feelings and base guidance on this information (see the Critical Thinking Q & A box on p. 956).

During infancy and early childhood, there is no need to restrain nonnutritive sucking. Malocclusion may occur if thumb-sucking persists past 4 years of age or when the permanent teeth erupt. There is probably less dental displacement with the use of a pacifier than with the use of a hard, rigid finger. Pacifiers may be relinquished earlier than thumbs because they are less readily available. If the child uses a pacifier, safety considerations in purchasing one must be stressed (see p. 970).

Some evidence suggests that the early introduction of a pacifier (during the first month) may shorten the duration of

Text continued on p. 954.

TABLE 33-2 Growth and development during infancy*

AGE (MONTHS)	PHYSICAL	GROSS MOTOR	FINE MOTOR
1	Weight gain of 150 to 210 g weekly for first 6 months Height gain of 2.5 cm (1 inch) monthly for first 6 months Head circumference increases by 1.5 cm (1/2 inch) monthly for first 6 months Primitive reflexes present and strong Doll's eye reflex and dance reflex fading Obligatory nose breathing (most infants)	■ Assumes flexed position with pelvis high but knees not under abdomen when prone (at birth, knees flexed under abdomen) ■ Can turn head from side to side when prone, lifts head momentarily from bed (see Fig. 33-4, *A*) Has marked head lag, especially when pulled from lying to sitting position (see Fig. 33-3, *A*) Holds head momentarily parallel and in midline when suspended in prone position Assumes asymmetric tonic neck reflex position when supine When held in standing position, body limp at knees and hips In sitting position, back is uniformly rounded, head control absent (see Fig. 33-5, *A*)	Hands predominantly closed Grasp reflex strong Hand clenches on contact with rattle
2	Posterior fontanel closed Crawling reflex disappears	■ Assumes less flexed position when prone—hips flat, legs extended, arms flexed, head to side Less head lag when pulled to sitting position (see Fig. 33-3, *B*) Can maintain head in same plane as rest of body when held in ventral suspension When prone, can lift head almost 45 degrees off table When held in sitting position, head is held up but bobs forward (see Fig. 33-5, *B*) Assumes asymmetric tonic neck reflex position intermittently	Hands frequently open Grasp reflex fading
3	■ Primitive reflexes fading	Able to hold head more erect when sitting, but still bobs forward Has only slight head lag when pulled to sitting position Assumes symmetric body positioning Able to raise head and shoulders from prone position to a 45- to 90-degree angle from table; bears weight on forearms When held in standing position, able to bear slight fraction of weight on legs Regards own hand	■ Actively holds rattle but will not reach for it Grasp reflex absent Hands kept loosely open Clutches own hand; pulls at blankets and clothes
4	Drooling begins ■ Moro, tonic neck, and rooting reflexes have disappeared	■ Has almost no head lag when pulled to sitting position (see Fig. 33-3, *C*) ■ Balances head well in sitting position (see Fig. 33-5, *C*) Back less rounded, curved only in lumbar area Able to sit erect if propped up Able to raise head and chest off surface to angle of 90 degrees (see Fig. 33-4, *B*) Assumes predominant symmetric position ■ Rolls from back to side	■ Inspects and plays with hands; pulls clothing or blanket over face in play Tries to reach objects with hand but overshoots Grasps object with both hands Plays with rattle placed in hand, shakes it, but cannot pick it up if dropped Can carry objects to mouth

*Bullets indicate milestones that represent essential integrative aspects of development that lay the foundation for the achievement of more advanced skills.
†Degree of visual acuity varies according to vision measurement procedure used.

TABLE 33-2 Growth and development during infancy*—cont'd

SENSORY	VOCALIZATION	SOCIALIZATION/COGNITION
▪ Able to fixate on moving object in range of 45 degrees when held at a distance of 20-25 cm (8-10 in) Visual acuity approaches 20/100† Follows light to midline Quiets when hears a voice	Cries to express displeasure Makes small throaty sounds Makes comfort sounds during feeding	Is in sensorimotor phase—stage I, use of reflexes (birth-1 month), and stage II, primary circular reactions (1-4 months) Watches parent's face intently as she or he talks to infant
Binocular fixation and convergence to near objects beginning When supine, follows dangling toy from side to point beyond midline Visually searches to locate sounds Turns head to side when sound is made at level of ear	▪ Vocalizes, distinct from crying Crying becomes differentiated Coos Vocalizes to familiar voice	▪ Demonstrates social smile in response to various stimuli
▪ Follows object to periphery (180 degrees) ▪ Locates sound by turning head to side and looking in same direction Begins to have ability to coordinate stimuli from various sense organs	▪ Squeals aloud to show pleasure Coos, babbles, chuckles Vocalizes when smiling "Talks" a great deal when spoken to Less crying during periods of wakefulness	Displays considerable interest in surroundings Ceases crying when parent enters room Can recognize familiar faces and objects, such as feeding bottle Shows awareness of strange situations
Able to accommodate to near objects Binocular vision fairly well established Can focus on a 1.25 cm (½ in) block Beginning eye-hand coordination	Makes consonant sounds *n, k, g, p, b* ▪ Laughs aloud Vocalization changes according to mood	Is in stage III, secondary circular reactions Demands attention by fussing; becomes bored if left alone Enjoys social interaction with people Anticipates feeding when sees bottle or mother, if breastfeeding Shows excitement with whole body, squeals, breathes heavily Shows interest in strange stimuli Begins to demonstrate memory

Continued.

TABLE 33-2 Growth and development during infancy*—cont'd

AGE (MONTHS)	PHYSICAL	GROSS MOTOR	FINE MOTOR
5	Beginning signs of tooth eruption Birth weight doubles	No head lag when pulled to sitting position When sitting, able to hold head erect and steady Able to sit for longer periods when back is well supported Back straight When prone, assumes symmetric positioning with arms extended ■ Can turn over from abdomen to back When supine, puts feet to mouth	■ Able to grasp objects voluntarily Uses palmar grasp, bidextrous approach Plays with toes Takes objects directly to mouth Holds one cube while regarding a second
6	Growth rate may begin to decline Weight gain of 90 to 150 g (3 to 5 ounces) weekly for next 6 months Height gain of 1.25 cm (1/2 inch) monthly for next 6 months ■ Teething may begin with eruption of two lower central incisors ■ Chewing and biting occur	When prone, can lift chest and upper abdomen off table, bearing weight on hands (see Fig. 33-4, *C*) When about to be pulled to a sitting position, lifts head Sits in high chair with back straight Rolls from back to abdomen When held in standing position, bears almost all of weight Hand regard absent	Resecures a dropped object Drops one cube when another is given Grasps and manipulates small objects Holds bottle Grasps feet and pulls to mouth
7	Eruption of upper central incisors	When supine, spontaneously lifts head off table ■ Sits, leaning forward on both hands (see Fig. 33-5, *D*) When prone, bears weight on one hand Sits erect momentarily Bears full weight on feet (see Fig. 33-6, *A*) When held in standing position, bounces actively	■ Transfers object from one hand to the other (see Fig. 33-5, *E*) Has unidextrous approach and grasp Holds two cubes more than momentarily Bangs cube on table Rakes at a small object
8	Begins to show regular patterns in bladder and bowel elimination Parachute reflex appears (see Fig. 33-1)	■ Sits steadily unsupported (see Fig. 33-5, *E*) Readily bears weight on legs when supported; may stand holding onto furniture Adjusts posture to reach an object	Has beginning pincer grasp using index, fourth, and fifth fingers against lower part of thumb Releases objects at will Rings bell purposely Retains two cubes while regarding third cube Secures an object by pulling on a string Reaches persistently for toys out of reach
9	Eruption of upper lateral incisor may begin	Creeps on hands and knees Sits steadily on floor for prolonged time (10 minutes) Recovers balance when leans forward but cannot do so when leaning sideways ■ Pulls self to standing position and stands holding onto furniture (see Fig. 33-6, *B-D*)	■ Uses thumb and index finger in crude pincer grasp (see Fig. 33-2) Preference for use of dominant hand now evident Grasps third cube Compares two cubes by holding them together

TABLE 33-2 Growth and development during infancy*—cont'd

SENSORY	VOCALIZATION	SOCIALIZATION/COGNITION
Visually pursues a dropped object Is able to sustain visual inspection of an object Can localize sounds made below the ear	Squeals Makes vowel cooing sounds interspersed with consonant sounds (e.g., *ah-goo*)	Smiles at mirror image Pats bottle or breast with both hands More enthusiastically playful, but may have rapid mood swings Is able to discriminate strangers from family Vocalizes displeasure when object taken away Discovers parts of body
Adjusts posture to see an object Prefers more complex visual stimuli Can localize sounds made above the ear Will turn head to the side, then look up or down	■ Begins to imitate sounds ■ Babbling resembles one-syllable utterances,—*ma, mu, da, di, hi* Vocalizes to toys, mirror image Takes pleasure in hearing own sound (self-reinforcement)	Recognizes parents; begins to fear strangers Holds arms out to be picked up Has definite likes and dislikes Begins to imitate (cough, protrusion of tongue) Excites on hearing footsteps Laughs when head is hidden in a towel ■ Briefly searches for a dropped object (object permanence beginning) Frequent mood swings—from crying to laughing with little or no provocation
■ Can fixate on very small objects Responds to own name Localizes sound by turning head in a curving arch Beginning awareness of depth and space Has taste preferences	■ Produces vowel sounds and chained syllables *baba, dada, kaka* Vocalizes four distinct vowel sounds "Talks" when others are talking	■ Increasing fear of strangers; shows signs of fretfulness when mother disappears Imitates simple acts and noises Tries to attract attention by coughing or snorting Plays peekaboo Demonstrates dislike of food by keeping lips closed Exhibits oral aggressiveness in biting and mouthing Demonstrates expectation in response to repetition of stimuli
	Makes consonant sounds *t, d,* and *w* Listens selectively to familiar words Utterances signal emphasis and emotion Combines syllables, such as *dada*, but does not ascribe meaning to them	Increasing anxiety over loss of parent, particularly mother, and fear of strangers Responds to "no" Dislikes dressing, diaper change
Localizes sounds by turning head diagonally and directly toward sound Depth perception increasing	Responds to simple verbal commands Comprehends "no-no"	Parent (mother) is increasingly important for own sake Shows increasing interest in pleasing parent Begins to show fears of going to bed and being left alone Puts arms in front of face to avoid having it washed

Continued.

TABLE 33-2 Growth and development during infancy*—cont'd

AGE (MONTHS)	PHYSICAL	GROSS MOTOR	FINE MOTOR
10	Labyrinth-righting reflex is strongest—when infant is in prone or supine position, is able to raise head	Can change from prone to sitting position Stands while holding onto furniture, sits by falling down Recovers balance easily while sitting While standing, lifts one foot to take a step (see Fig. 33-6, *E*)	Crude release of an object beginning Grasps bell by handle
11	Eruption of lower incisors may begin	When sitting, pivots to reach toward back to pick up an object ▪ Cruises or walks holding onto furniture or with both hands held	Explores objects more thoroughly (e.g., clapper inside bell) Has neat pincer grasp (see Fig. 33-2, *B*) Drops object deliberately so it will be picked up Puts one object after another into a container (sequential play) Able to manipulate an object to remove it from tight-fitting enclosure
12	▪ Birth weight tripled ▪ Birth length increased by 50% Head and chest circumference equal (head circumference 46.5 cm [18 ½ inches]) Has total of six to eight deciduous teeth Anterior fontanel almost closed Landau reflex fading Babinski reflex disappears Lumbar curve develops; lordosis evident during walking	▪ Walks with one hand held Cruises well ▪ May attempt to stand alone momentarily; may attempt first step alone Can sit down from standing position without help	Releases cube in cup Attempts to build two-block tower but fails Tries to insert a pellet into a narrow-necked bottle but fails Can turn pages in a book, many at a time

breastfeeding. Possible explanations include less stimulation of the breasts and less milk production or a sign that breastfeeding difficulties already exist (Victora et al, 1993).

To decrease dependence on nonnutritive sucking in young infants, sucking pleasure can be increased by prolonging feeding time. A small-holed, firm nipple causes stronger sucking and slower feeding. Also, the parent's excessive use of the pacifier to calm the child should be explored. It is not unusual for parents to place a pacifier in the infant's mouth as soon as crying begins, thus reinforcing a pattern of distress relief.

Thumb-sucking reaches its peak at 18 to 20 months of age and is most prevalent when the child is hungry or tired. Persistent thumb-sucking in a listless, apathetic child always warrants investigation. It may be a sign of an emotional problem between parent and child or of boredom, isolation, and lack of stimulation.

Teething

One of the more difficult periods in the infant's (and parents') life is the eruption of the deciduous (primary) teeth, often referred to as teething. The age of tooth eruption shows considerable variation among children, but the order of their appearance is fairly regular and predictable (Fig. 33-11). The first primary teeth to erupt are the lower central incisors,

TABLE 33-2 Growth and development during infancy*—cont'd

SENSORY	VOCALIZATION	SOCIALIZATION/COGNITION
	■ Says "dada," "mama" with meaning Comprehends "bye-bye" May say one word (e.g., "hi," "bye," "no")	Inhibits behavior to verbal command of "no-no" or own name Imitates facial expressions, waves bye-bye Extends toy to another person but will not release it ■ Develops object permanence Repeats actions that attract attention and cause laughter Pulls clothes of another to attract attention Plays interactive games such as pat-a-cake Reacts to adult anger, cries when scolded Demonstrates independence in dressing, feeding, locomotive skills, and testing of parents Looks at and follows pictures in a book
	Imitates definite speech sounds	Experiences joy and satisfaction when a task is mastered Reacts to restrictions with frustration Rolls ball to another on request Anticipates body gestures when a familiar nursery rhyme or story is being told (e. g., holds toes and feet in response to "This little piggy went to market") Plays game up-down, "so big," or peek-aboo Shakes head for "no"
Discriminates simple geometric forms (e.g., circle) Amblyopia may develop with lack of binocularity Can follow rapidly moving object Controls and adjusts response to sound; listens for sound to recur	■ Says three to five words besides "dada," "mama" Comprehends meaning of several words (comprehension always precedes verbalization) Recognizes objects by name Imitates animal sounds Understands simple verbal commands (e.g., "Give it to me," "Show me your eyes")	Shows emotions such as jealousy, affection (may give hug or kiss on request), anger, fear Enjoys familiar surroundings and explores away from parent Is fearful in strange situation; clings to parent May develop habit of "security blanket" or favorite toy Has increasing determination to practice locomotor skills ■ Searches for an object even if it has not been hidden, but searches only where object was last seen

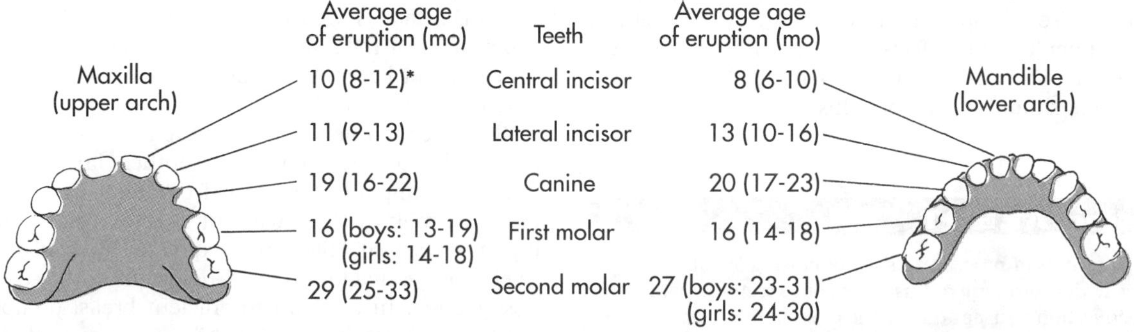

Fig. 33-11 Sequence of eruption of primary teeth. *Range represents ±1 standard deviation or 67% of subjects studied. (Data from McDonald RE, Avery DR: *Dentistry for the child and adolescent,* ed 6, St. Louis, 1994, Mosby.)

Critical Thinking Q & A 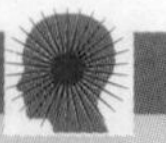

THUMB-SUCKING

During a well-child visit you observe that Mrs. Lopez persistently takes the thumb out of the mouth of her 10-month-old daughter, Maria. You ask whether she has concerns about the thumb-sucking. She replies, "Of course. Her teeth are coming in so nice and straight and I don't want the thumb to make them crooked." An appropriate response is:

1. Sucking on a thumb or pacifier is common in young children, especially in infants. It satisfies their need to suck and helps them comfort themselves. Sometimes, making an issue of the sucking can cause it to last longer.
2. Thumb-sucking is perfectly normal and children stop when they are ready, so don't worry about it.
3. If thumb-sucking continues when most of her teeth are in, it will make them crooked. But we don't need to worry about it now.
4. You are right to be concerned. Let her suck longer on the bottle to satisfy her sucking needs.

The correct answer is one. The response provides factual information in a nonjudgmental manner that invites further discussion. Options two and three are partly correct in regard to thumb-sucking but offer premature reassurance. Option four is incorrect and at 10 months of age, infants should be relying less, not more, on bottle-feeding, which can lead to ingestion of excessive amounts of milk, juice, or other sweetened beverages in place of solid foods; as well as to dental caries (see *Weaning,* p. 959, and *Dental Health,* p. 961).

which appear at approximately 6 to 8 months of age. These are followed closely by the upper central incisors. A quick guide to assessment of deciduous teeth during the first 2 years is: *age of the child in months − 6 = number of teeth.* For example: 8 months of age − 6 = 2 teeth at this age.

Teething is a physiologic process, and as the crown of the tooth breaks through the periodontal membrane, some discomfort may be experienced. Some children show minimal evidence of teething, such as drooling, increased finger-sucking, or biting on hard objects. Others are very irritable, have difficulty sleeping, and refuse to eat. Generally, signs of illness such as high fever, vomiting, or diarrhea are not symptoms of teething but of illness. However, as many parents report, a low-grade fever is common in the 4- to 19-day period before the day of tooth eruption (Jaber et al, 1992).

Cold is soothing. Giving the child a frozen teething ring or an ice cube securely wrapped in a washcloth helps relieve the inflammation. Several nonprescription topical anesthetic ointments are available, (e.g., Baby Orajel). If these are used, parents are advised to apply them correctly. In the event of persistent irritability that affects sleeping and feeding, systemic analgesics, such as acetaminophen, can be given judiciously. Parents should know that this is a temporary measure.

Nursing ALERT

Teething powders or procedures such as cutting or rubbing the gums with aspirin are not used to reduce teething pain, because ingestion or aspiration of the powder, infection or irritation of the tissue, or aspiration of the aspirin can occur.

Infant Shoes

Many parents are unaware of the types of shoes that are appropriate for the older infant and buy expensive infant shoes because of misleading advertising claims. Inflexible shoes that have hard soles can be detrimental by delaying walking, aggravating intoeing and outtoeing, and impeding the development of supportive foot muscles. Counseling parents regarding footwear should begin when infants are 6 months old, well before they are standing or walking.

When children begin walking, the main reason for wearing shoes is *protection.* To provide protection, the shoe should retain its fit, be made of durable material with a smooth interior and few construction seams to irritate the skin, and be soft and flexible, especially in the toe area. A high-top shoe is not necessary for support but may be helpful in keeping the foot in the shoe. A good shoe conforms to the shape of the foot, with a rounded toe area and sufficient toe room. Inexpensive but well-constructed sneakers or soft-leather moccasin-type shoes are adequate for walking infants.

Even if the shoes are fitted properly, frequent changes are needed to accommodate the infant's rapidly growing feet. Shoe size changes at approximately 3-month intervals from 12 to 36 months of age; during this time the child's foot should be measured every 3 months. Curled toes when shoes are removed and redness and irritation of the skin on the bottom of the toes indicate the need for a larger size.

Promoting Optimum Health During Infancy

NUTRITION

The First 6 Months

The decision to breast- or bottle-feed the infant is highly individual and is discussed in Chapter 24. This section is primarily concerned with nutrition during infancy.

Human milk is the most desirable and complete diet for the infant for the first 6 months. The normal infant receiving breast milk from a well-nourished mother needs no specific vitamin and mineral supplements, with the exception of fluoride in a dose of 0.25 mg daily (regardless of the fluoride content of the local water supply) and iron by 4 to 6 months of age (when fetal iron stores are depleted) (Calvo, Galinda, and Aspres, 1992; Position statement, 1992). Supplements of 400 IU of vitamin D daily may be indicated if the mother's vitamin D intake is inadequate. Some authorities also suggest supplements if the infant does not receive adequate exposure to ultraviolet light (American Academy of Pediatrics, Committee on Nutrition, 1995).

Employed mothers can continue breastfeeding with guidance and encouragement. Most mothers find that a program of breast-pumping when away from home and bottle-feeding of breast milk, with or without supplemental formula feedings, is successful. Milk can be expressed by hand or pump and safely refrigerated for up to 24 hours. After that time freezing is suggested. In addition to efficient breast-pumping, these mothers also cite the need for child care by a trusted agency or individual and support and assistance from significant others.

Like all breastfeeding mothers, these women must have proper nutrition and rest for lactation. With a schedule of work and child care, careful planning is required to manage the demands of both responsibilities successfully.

An acceptable alternative to breastfeeding is commercial iron-fortified formula. Like human milk, it supplies all the nutrients needed by the infant for the first 6 months.

Commercially prepared vitamin/iron preparations with or without fluoride are available to meet the specific needs of the infant. Unmodified whole cow's milk, low-fat cow's milk, and imitation milks are not acceptable as a major source of nutrition for infants because of their altered ability to be digested, increased risk of contamination, and lack of components needed for appropriate growth. Whole milk may cause occult gastrointestinal bleeding and iron deficiency anemia in infants.

Nursing ALERT

Whole milk should not be introduced to infants until after 1 year of age (American Academy of Pediatrics, Committee on Nutrition, 1995).

The amount of formula per feeding and the number of feedings per day vary among infants. In general, the number of feedings decreases from six at 1 month of age to four to five at 6 months. Regardless of the number of feedings, the total amount of formula ingested should not exceed 960 ml per day. Parents should be cautioned concerning excessive use of juices and nonnutritive drinks (e.g., Kool-Aid) during this period.

The addition of solid foods before 4 to 6 months of age is not recommended, although mothers may receive conflicting advice from other women (e.g., their mothers), who cared for children during the era of early introduction of solids. During the early months solid foods are not compatible with the ability of the gastrointestinal tract and nutritional needs of the infant. Feeding solids to young infants exposes them to food antigens that may produce food-protein allergy. In addition, the infant is not ready developmentally. The extrusion (protrusion) reflex is strong and pushes food out of the mouth, and infants instinctively suck when given food. Because of their limited range-of-motor abilities, infants are unable to push food away or avoid feeding deliberately. Therefore, early introduction of solids is a type of forced feeding.

The Second 6 Months

During the second half of the first year human milk or formula continues to be the primary source of nutrition. If breastfeeding is discontinued, commercial iron-fortified formula should be substituted. Formulas specially marketed for older infants offer no advantages for infants.

The major change in feeding habits is the addition of solid foods to the infant's diet. Physiologically and developmentally, the infant is in a transition period at 4 to 6 months of age. By this time the gastrointestinal tract has matured sufficiently to handle more complex nutrients and is less sensitive to potentially allergenic foods. Tooth eruption is beginning and facilitates biting and chewing. The extrusion reflex has disappeared, and swallowing is more coordinated to allow the infant easily to accept solids. Head control is well developed, permitting infants to sit with support and purposely turn the head away to communicate lack of interest in food. Voluntary grasping and improved eye-hand coordination gradually allow infants to pick up "finger" foods and feed themselves. Their increasing sense of independence is evident in their desire to hold their own bottle and try to "help" during feeding.

Selection and Preparation of Solid Foods

The choice of foods to introduce first is variable but should be based on the reasons for feeding, such as supplying nutrients not found in formula or breast milk. Infant cereal is generally introduced first because of its high iron content (7 mg of iron per 3 tablespoons of dry cereal). There are several types of commercially prepared infant cereals, such as rice, barley, oatmeal, and high-protein cereals, but rice is usually suggested as an initial food because of its digestibility and low allergenic potential.

Infant cereal is mixed with formula until whole milk is given. If the infant is breastfed, the cereal is mixed with expressed breast milk or water. After 6 months of age, fruit juices can be mixed with the dry cereal; the vitamin C content of the juice enhances the absorption of iron in the cereal. Because of their benefit as a source of iron, infant cereals should be continued until the child is 18 months of age.

Fruit juice can be offered for its rich source of vitamin C and as a substitute for milk for one feeding a day. Large quantities of certain juices, such as apple, pear, prune, sweet cherry, peach, and grape, are avoided because they may cause abdominal pain, diarrhea, or bloating in some children (American Academy of Pediatrics, Committee on Nutrition, 1991). Because vitamin C is naturally destroyed by heat, juice is not warmed. Containers of juice are always kept covered and refrigerated to prevent further vitamin loss.

Nursing ALERT

Offer fruit juice from a cup, rather than a bottle, to prevent the development of "nursing" caries (see Low-Cariogenic Diet, Chapter 34).

The addition of other foods is arbitrary. A common sequence is strained fruits followed by vegetables and finally meats. If foods are introduced early, citrus fruits, meats, and eggs are still delayed until after 6 months of age because of their potential to result in allergy. At 6 months foods such as a cracker or zwieback can be offered as a type of finger and teething food. By 8 to 9 months junior foods and nutritious finger foods, such as a firmly cooked vegetable, raw pieces of fruit (except grapes), or cheese, can be given. By 1 year well-cooked table foods are served.

Commercially prepared baby foods are the most commonly used types of food served to infants in the United States. They are convenient and contain no added salt or sugar, but are relatively expensive. An alternative is preparing baby foods at home, which is a simple and inexpensive process. Fruits and vegetables can be steamed in a small amount of water and pureed in a blender or food processor. Many of them, such as ripe banana, can be mashed fine with a fork. Fruits such as apples or pears require little or no water in the cooking process. Vegetables such as carrots, potatoes, and string beans require additional water in the cooking and blending process. Preferably, home-prepared infant foods should be fresh or frozen, because canned foods, other than those prepared for infants, may have excessive sodium or sugar or be a source of lead from the container. There is no evidence that the addition of salt to foods such as peas increases the infant's acceptance of the new food (Sullivan and Birch, 1994).

Introduction of Solid Foods

When the spoon is first introduced to infants, they are likely to push it away and appear dissatisfied. Some patience and skill are required to overcome this initial response, especially if the extrusion reflex is still present. A small-bowled, straight, and long-handled spoon, similar to a demitasse spoon, allows a small portion of food to be placed toward the back of the tongue. If food is placed on the front of the tongue and pushed out, it is simply scooped up and refed to the infant. As children become accustomed to the spoon, they will more eagerly accept the food and will eventually open their mouth in anticipation (or keep it closed in dislike). Since the first introduction of food is a new experience, the spoon feeding should be attempted before or after ingestion of a small amount of breast milk or formula to associate this new experience with a pleasurable and satisfying experience. Trying to introduce a new food *after* the entire milk feeding is usually useless, since the infant is satiated and has no inclination to try something new.

After several spoon feedings, new food can be introduced at the beginning of a meal. It is best to introduce many new foods during the first year, when the infant is more likely to eat them because of a hearty appetite resulting from a rapid growth rate.

Each new food is introduced at intervals of 4 to 7 days to allow for identification of food allergies. New foods are offered in small amounts, from 1 teaspoon to 1 to 2 tablespoons. As the amount of solid food increases, the quantity of milk is decreased to less than a liter a day to prevent overfeeding.

Home Care

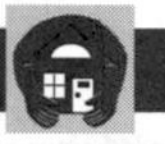

INTRODUCING SOLID FOODS TO INFANTS*

Introduce solids when infant is hungry.

Begin spoon feeding by pushing food to back of tongue because of infant's natural tendency to thrust the tongue forward.

Use a small spoon with a straight handle; begin with 1 or 2 teaspoons of food; gradually increase to a couple of tablespoons per feeding.

Introduce one food at a time, usually at intervals of 4 to 7 days to allow for identification of food allergies.

As the amount of solid food increases, decrease the quantity of milk to prevent overfeeding.

Do not introduce foods by mixing them with formula in the bottle.

*A recommended resource is *Starting Solids: a Guide for Parents and Child Care Providers,* available from the National Association of Pediatric Nurse Associates and Practitioners (NAPNAP), 1101 Kings Highway North, Suite 206, Cherry Hill, NJ 08034-1931.

Food should not be mixed in the bottle and fed through a nipple with a large hole. This deprives the child of the pleasure of learning new tastes and developing a discriminating palate. It can also cause problems with poor chewing of food later in life, since this experience would be lacking. A summary of the principles that govern the introduction of new foods is given in the Home Care box below, left.

Nursing ALERT

Although microwaving of bottles and baby food is not recommended, it remains a common practice. Guidelines have been developed for microwave heating of refrigerated formula and these should be given to the family (see the Home Care box below, right).

The infant's first tries at self-feeding or cup feeding are sloppy experiences. Finger foods such as soft fruits or vegetables are just as good playthings as food; they can be squeezed, smeared, squashed, and thoroughly painted on oneself, others, and the surrounding environment. However, all of this is part of learning, and mastery follows many accidents.

If parents find this experience distressing, a few suggestions may prove helpful. The feeding area should have a floor that can be easily wiped and is relatively far from walls, upholstered furniture, or drapes. A hand-held portable vacuum is helpful in cleaning up crumbs. Messes are confined to one area if the child is seated in a high chair rather than allowed to crawl or walk around while drinking or eating. Infants should be expected to get themselves covered with food; therefore a large bib (plastic can be wiped easily but needs to be removed after feeding) should be used, as well as washable clothes that are easily removed. High chairs can be thoroughly cleaned in a shower. Outdoor dining provides an excellent opportunity for practicing with a cup, spoon, or fingers

Home Care

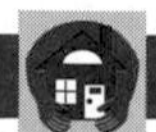

GUIDELINES FOR MICROWAVE HEATING OF REFRIGERATED INFANT FORMULA

Prior to heating

- Heat only 4 oz or more
- Heat only *refrigerated* formula
- Always *stand* the bottle up
- Always leave bottle top *uncovered* to allow heat to escape

Heating instructions (full power)

- 4-oz Bottles
  Heat for no more than 30 seconds
- 8-oz Bottles
  Heat for no more than 45 seconds

Serving instructions

- Always replace nipple assembly; *invert* 10 times (vigorous shaking is unnecessary)
- Formula should be cool to the touch; formula warm to the touch may be too hot to serve
- Always *test* formula; place several drops on tongue or on top of the hand (not the inside wrist)

From Sigman-Grant M, Bush G, and Anantheswaran, R: Microwave heating of infant formula: a dilemma resolved, *Pediatrics* 90(3):414, 1992.

because accidents are simple to hose or sweep away. Children cannot be pressured into eating neatly or developing table manners before manipulative skill is acquired.

Preventing Obesity

The most prevalent nutritional disorder in the United States is overeating, and prevention begins early. From infants' first feeding parents should allow their children to regulate the amount of formula they desire. No attempt should be made to encourage infants to finish the last drop or, later, to clean the plate.

Often, eating habits are controlled by the sociocultural background of the family, rather than by their knowledge of well-balanced nutrition. Common myths such as "a fat baby is a healthy baby" are difficult to dispel. In some cultures overweight infants are regarded as a sign of good mothering, and any suggestion regarding altering the child's weight is threatening to the parent. Understanding cultural values is important in effecting change through counseling.

If too much formula or milk is the problem, several strategies can be used to reduce the intake, although the nurse must caution parents not to restrict food/formula intake excessively. A commercial formula (Advance)* is available that provides 20% fewer calories than regular formula or whole cow's milk. Other strategies are to substitute water for a bottle of formula or use a smaller-hole nipple to prolong sucking with less intake. The objective is not for the infant to lose weight but to slow weight gain until the weight is appropriate for age and height.

Nursing ALERT

Dietary fat should not be restricted. Substituting skim or low-fat milk is unacceptable, because the essential fatty acids are inadequate and the solute concentration of protein and electrolytes, such as sodium, is too high.

The selection of solid foods is also an important aspect of controlling obesity. Approximately 20% of commercial baby foods contain less than 50 kcal/100 g, whereas another 20% contain more than 100 kcal/100 g. Choosing low-calorie foods can significantly lower the daily caloric intake without actually decreasing the total quantity of food. The use of sweet foods is kept to a minimum by not adding sugar to the formula or cereal and avoiding finger foods such as cookies. Other foods rich in calories that should be restricted in serving size rather than eliminated include butter, cream, ice cream, pudding, and chocolate.

Parents are encouraged to interpret the infant's signals of discomfort and intervene in ways other than through feeding. Crying, fussiness, and sucking do not necessarily indicate hunger. Rocking, stroking, holding, and offering a toy or a pacifier may be more appropriate than automatically responding with food.

Weaning

Defined as the process of giving up one method of feeding for another, **weaning** usually refers to relinquishing the breast or bottle for a cup. In Western societies this is generally regarded as a major task for infants and is frequently seen as a potentially traumatic experience. It is psychologically significant because the infant is required to give up a major source of oral pleasure and gratification.

There is no one time for weaning that is best for every child, but most infants show signs of readiness during the second half of the first year. They have learned that good things come from a spoon. Their increasing desire for freedom of movement may lessen their desire to be held close for feedings. They are acquiring more control over their actions and can easily manipulate a cup to their lips (even if it is held upside down!). Imitation becomes a powerful motivator by age 8 or 9 months, and they enjoy using a cup or glass as others do.

Weaning should be gradual, with one bottle-feeding or breastfeeding being replaced at a time. The last feeding to be discontinued is usually the nighttime one. If breastfeeding is terminated before 5 or 6 months of age, weaning should be to a bottle to provide for the infant's continued sucking needs. If breastfeeding is discontinued later, weaning can be directly to a cup, especially by 12 to 14 months of age.

SLEEP AND ACTIVITY

Sleep patterns vary among infants, and active infants typically sleep less than placid children. Generally, by 3 to 4 months of age most infants have developed a nocturnal pattern of sleep that lasts from 9 to 11 hours. The total daily sleep is about 15 hours. The number of naps per day varies, but by the end of the year infants may take one or two naps. Breastfed infants usually sleep for less prolonged periods, especially during the night, than do bottle-fed infants. Because of the trend toward breastfeeding, sleep norms such as those described previously, which were based primarily on bottle-fed infants, may no longer be relevant. Because of the possible association between the prone position and risk of sudden infant death syndrome (SIDS) (see Chapter 33), infants should be placed supine or side lying until they roll over on their own.

Most infants are naturally active and need no encouragement to be mobile. However, problems can arise when devices such as playpens, strollers, commercial swings, and walkers are used excessively. These restrict movement and prevent infants from exploring and developing gross motor skills. Contrary to popular belief, walkers do not enhance coordination and are dangerous if tipped over or placed near stairs. The American Academy of Pediatrics, Committee on Injury and Poison Prevention (1995), recommends a ban on the sale of infant walkers.

Nursing ALERT

Formal infant exercise programs do not provide any long-term benefit to normal infants, and the possibility for damage to the infant's skeletal system exists. For these reasons, such programs are not recommended (American Academy of Pediatrics, 1988).

Sleep Problems

Concerns regarding sleep are common during infancy. Sometimes they are as basic as parents' questioning whether the in-

*Manufactured by Ross Laboratories, Columbus, OH.

TABLE 33-3 Selected sleep disturbances during infancy and early childhood

DISORDER/DESCRIPTION	MANAGEMENT
Nighttime feeding*	
Child has a prolonged need for middle-of-night bottle-feeding or breastfeeding Child goes to sleep at the breast or with a bottle Awakenings are frequent (may be hourly) Child returns to sleep after feeding; other comfort measures (e.g., rocking or holding) are usually ineffective	Increase daytime feeding intervals to 4 hours or more (may need to be done gradually) Offer last feeding as late as possible at night; may need to reduce amount of formula or length of breastfeeding gradually Offer no bottles in bed Put to bed *awake* When child is crying, check at progressively longer intervals each night; reassure child but do not hold, rock, take to parent's bed, or give bottle or pacifier
Developmental night crying	
Child aged 6-12 months with undisturbed nighttime sleep now awakes abruptly; may be accompanied by nightmares	Reassure parents that this is temporary phase Enter room immediately to check on child but keep reassurances *brief* Avoid feeding, rocking, taking to parent's bed, or any other routine that may initiate trained night crying
Trained night crying* (inappropriate sleep associations)	
Child typically falls asleep in place other than own bed, e.g., rocking chair or parent's bed, and is taken to own bed while asleep; upon awakening, cries until usual routine is instituted, e.g., rocking	Put child in own bed when *awake* If possible, arrange separate sleeping area from other family members When child is crying, check at progressively longer intervals each night; reassure child but do not resume usual routine
Refusal to go to sleep*	
Child resists bedtime and leaves room repeatedly Nighttime sleep may be continuous, but frequent awakenings and refusal to return to sleep may occur and become a problem if parent allows child to deviate from usual sleep pattern	Evaluate if hour of sleep is too early (child may resist sleep if not tired) Assist parents in establishing consistent before-bedtime routine and enforcing consistent limits regarding child's bedtime behavior If child persists in leaving bedroom, close door for progressively longer periods Use reward system with child to provide motivation
Nighttime fears	
Child resists going to bed or wakes during the night because of fears Child seeks parent's physical presence and with parent nearby, falls asleep easily, unless fear is overwhelming	Evaluate if hour of sleep is too early (child may fantasize when nothing to do but think in dark room) Calmly reassure the frightened child; keeping a nightlight on may be helpful Use reward system with child to provide motivation to deal with fears Avoid patterns that can lead to additional problems, e.g., sleeping with child or taking child to parent's room If child's fear is overwhelming, consider desensitization, e.g., progressively spending longer periods alone; consult professional help for protracted fears Distinguish between nightmares and sleep terrors (confused partial arousals) (see Sleep Problems, Chapter 35)

Modified from Ferber R: Behavioral "insomnia" in the child, *Psychiatr Clin North Am* 10(4):641-653, 1987.
*Guidelines for parents in dealing with these sleep problems are in Wong DL: *Wong and Whaley's clinical manual of pediatric nursing,* ed 4, St Louis, 1996, Mosby.

fant needs additional sleep. In this case it is best to investigate the reason for their concern, stressing the individual needs of each child. Infants who are active during wakeful periods and who are growing normally are sleeping a sufficient amount of time.

However, there are a number of more serious concerns that require intervention. Sleep disturbances of physiologic origin are rare, with the exception of colic. The more common sleep disturbances are a learned pattern or developmental characteristic of some infants (Table 33-3). Although many families may report sleep problems that are typical of these patterns, interventions are offered *only* when the pattern is disruptive to the family (see the Cultural Considerations box on p. 961).

However, when a sleeping problem is presented, a careful assessment is essential. Charting sleep habits both before and after interventions is also an important strategy.* Questions regarding the frequency and duration of waking, the usual bedtime routine, the number of nighttime feedings, the perceived problem (e.g., how much disruption the behavior gen-

*A sleep history and a 2-week sleep record for families are available in Wong DL: *Wong and Whaley's clinical manual of pediatric nursing,* ed 4, St Louis, 1996, Mosby.

Cultural Considerations

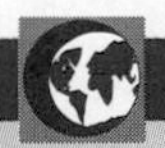

THE FAMILY BED

Cosleeping, or the "family bed," in which parents allow the children to sleep with them, is a relatively common and accepted practice, especially among African-American, Hispanic, and Asian families, such as the Japanese (Schachter et al, 1989). Other groups that are adopting cosleeping include (1) single parents, whose need for company may encourage this practice; (2) working parents, who desire the closeness at night that was lost during the day; and (3) parents who have had an issue about sleep or separation in their own past (Brazelton, 1990).

erates), and the attempted interventions are important in planning effective approaches designed for the specific sleep problem. A common suggestion given for any type of sleep problem—"let the child cry until falling asleep"—is very difficult to implement and is inappropriate for certain conditions. Once the parents relent and console the child, they have only reinforced the crying.

An equally effective and more atraumatic approach to night crying, known as *graduated extinction,* is to let the child cry for progressively longer times between *brief* parental interventions that consist only of reassurance, not rocking, holding, or using the bottle or pacifier. For example, the parents may check on the child every 5 minutes during the first night and progressively extend this interval by 5 minutes on successive nights (Ferber, 1985).

Families who cannot tolerate the unexpected crying spells while everyone else is asleep can try the two-step approach. Graduated extinction is used during naps and at bedtime until the parents retire. If the child cries during the night, the parents use comforting measures. However, once the child is partially trained, step 2—the use of graduated extinction at all times (Schmitt, 1992)—is initiated.

The best way to prevent sleep problems is to encourage parents to establish bedtime rituals that do not foster problematic patterns. One of the most constructive is placing infants *awake* in their own crib. When infants are accustomed to falling asleep somewhere else, such as in their parent's arms, and then being transferred to their crib, they awaken in unfamiliar surroundings and are unable to fall asleep until the routine is repeated (Anders, Halpern, and Hua, 1992). Also, the bed should be used for sleeping only—not as a playpen. It is advisable not to hang playthings over or on the bed; in this way the child associates the bed with sleep, not with activity. Although the interventions described previously and in Table 33-3 are usually successful, it is much easier to prevent the problem with appropriate counseling during the early months of the infant's life.

DENTAL HEALTH

Good dental hygiene begins as soon as the primary teeth erupt. The teeth and gums are initially cleaned by wiping them with a damp cloth; toothbrushing is too harsh for the tender gingiva. The infant can be stabilized by cradling with one arm and using the free hand to cleanse the teeth. Oral hygiene can be made pleasant by singing or talking to the infant. There are no clear guidelines as to when toothbrushing should begin. However, it is generally recommended that, as more teeth erupt and the infant adjusts to the routine of cleaning, a small, soft-bristled toothbrush be used. Water is preferred to toothpaste, which the infant will swallow; if the toothpaste is fluoridated, the infant will ingest excessive amounts (Nowak, 1993).

Fluoride, an essential mineral for building caries-resistant teeth, is needed from 6 months of age if the infant does not receive water with an adequate fluoride content. The American Academy of Pediatrics, Committee on Nutrition (1995) no longer recommends fluoride supplementation from birth to 6 months. Also, the fluoride dosage has been decreased from earlier recommendations because of an increased occurrence of dental fluorosis resulting from excessive fluoride ingestion (see Table 34-2).

Dietary considerations are also important because habits begun during infancy tend to continue into later years. Foods with concentrated sugar are used sparingly (if at all) in the infant's diet. The practice of coating pacifiers with honey or using commercially available hard-candy pacifiers is discouraged. Besides being cariogenic, honey also may cause infant botulism, and parts of the candy pacifier can be aspirated (see p. 970). Parents need to be counseled regarding the detrimental effects of frequent and prolonged bottle-feeding or breast-feeding during sleep, when the sweet milk or other fluid, such as juice, bathes the teeth, producing *nursing caries.* (See also Chapter 34 for a more extensive discussion of dental care, including nursing caries.)

IMMUNIZATIONS

One of the most dramatic advances in pediatrics has been the decline of infectious diseases over the past 60 years because of the widespread use of **immunization** for preventable diseases. Although many of the presently available immunizations can be given to individuals of any age, the recommended primary schedule begins during infancy and, with the exception of boosters, is completed during early childhood. Therefore, the discussion of childhood immunizations for diphtheria, tetanus, pertussis (DTP) or acellular pertussis (DTaP); polio (IPV or OPV); measles, mumps, rubella (MMR); *Haemophilus influenzae* type b (Hib); hepatitis B virus (HBV); and chickenpox (varicella zoster virus [VZV]) is included under health promotion during infancy. Selected vaccines that are generally reserved for children considered at high risk for the disease are discussed here and as appropriate throughout the text. (See also Communicable Diseases, Chapter 35, for a discussion of several of the diseases for which vaccines are available.)

Unfounded fears regarding side effects of vaccines, especially DTP, have also had an impact on immunization rates and vaccine production. Concerns that DTP vaccine causes SIDS and pertussis vaccine results in permanent neurologic damage have caused many families to bring lawsuits against vaccine producers, causing a drastic increase in vaccine costs and at one time prompting some manufacturers to stop vaccine production. The Institute of Medicine (IOM) (1993) found no evidence that diphtheria and tetanus toxoids cause encephalopathy, infantile spasms, or SIDS. They did find a relationship between DTP vaccination and acute encephalopathy occurring within 7 days of the vaccination. This association occurs rarely—at a rate of 0 to 10.5/million immunizations—and probably occurs in children with an underlying neurologic disorder.

Practitioners are required to inform families fully of the risks and benefits of the vaccines. The U.S. Public Health Service has developed a series of vaccine information pamphlets (VIPs). Health professionals need to be aware of the importance of providing parents with sufficient time to read the information, discussing the vaccines to determine caregivers' understanding of the material, addressing parents' concerns, and dispelling unfounded fears. Since nurses frequently administer vaccines during health supervision visits, they may have the responsibility for adequately informing parents of the nature, prevalence, and risks of the disease; the type of immunization product to be used; the expected benefits; the risk of side effects; and the need for accurate immunization records. Referring to immunizations as "baby shots" and limiting the discussion to vague statements about the vaccines are unacceptable practices.

Schedule for Immunizations

In the United States two organizations—the Advisory Committee on Immunization Practices (ACIP) of the U.S. Public Health Service Centers for Disease Control and Prevention (CDC) and the Committee on Infectious Diseases of the American Academy of Pediatrics (AAP)—govern the recommenda-

TABLE 33-4 Recommended childhood immunization schedule United States, January - December 1997

Vaccines[1] are listed under the routinely recommended ages. Bars indicate range of acceptable ages for vaccination. Shaded bars indicate *catch-up vaccination:* at 11-12 years of age, hepatitis B vaccine should be administered to children not previously vaccinated, and Varicella vaccine should be administered to children not previously vaccinated who lack a reliable history of chickenpox.

AGE → / VACCINE ↓	BIRTH	1 MO	2 MOS	4 MOS	6 MOS	12 MOS	15 MOS	18 MOS	4-6 YRS	11-12 YRS	14-16 YRS
Hepatitis B[2,3]	Hep B-1	Hep B-1	Hep B-1								
		Hep B-2	Hep B-2	Hep B-2							
					Hep B-3	Hep B-3	Hep B-3	Hep B-3		Hep B[3]	
Diphtheria, Tetanus, Pertussis[4]			DTaP or DTP	DTaP or DTP	DTaP or DTP		DTaP or DTP[4]	DTaP or DTP[4]	DTaP or DTP	Td	Td
H. influenzae type b[5]			Hib	Hib	Hib 5	Hib[5]	Hib[5]				
Polio[6]			Polio[6]	Polio		Polio[6]	Polio[6]	Polio[6]	Polio		
Measles, Mumps, Rubella[7]						MMR	MMR		MMR[7] or	MMR[7]	
Varicella[8]						Var	Var	Var		Var[8]	

From *Pediatrics* 99(1):137-138, 1997. Approved by the Advisory Committee on Immunization Practices (ACIP), the American Academy of Pediatrics (AAP), and the American Academy of Family Physicians (AAFP).

[1]This schedule indicates the recommended age for routine administration of currently licensed childhood vaccines. Some combination vaccines are available and may be used whenever administration of all components of the vaccine is indicated. Providers should consult the manufacturers' package inserts for detailed recommendations.

[2]*Infants born to HBsAg-negative mothers* should receive 2.5 μg of Merck vaccine (Recombivax HB) or 10 μg of SmithKline Beecham (SB) vaccine (Engerix-B). The 2nd dose should be administered ≥1 mo after the 1st dose.
Infants born to HBsAg-positive mothers should receive 0.5 ml hepatitis B immune globulin (HBIG) within 12 hr of birth, and either 5 μg of Merck vaccine (Recombivax HB) or 10 μg of SB vaccine (Engerix-B) at a separate site. The 2nd dose is recommended at 1-2 mos of age and the 3rd dose at 6 mos of age.
Infants born to mothers whose HBsAg status is unknown should receive either 5 μg of Merck vaccine (Recombivax HB) or 10 μg of SB vaccine (Engerix-B) within 12 hrs of birth. The 2nd dose of vaccine is recommended at 1 mo of age and the 3rd dose at 6 mos of age. Blood should be drawn at the time of delivery to determine the mother's HBsAg status; if it is positive, the infant should recieve HBIG as soon as possible (no later than 1 wk of age). The dosage and timing of subsequent vaccine doses should be based upon the mother's HBsAg status.

[3]Children and adolescents who have not been vaccinated against hepatitis B in infancy may begin the series during any childhood visit. Those who have not previously received 3 doses of hepatitis B vaccine should initiate or complete the series during the 11-12-year-old visit. The 2nd dose should be administered at least 1 mo after the 1st dose, and the 3rd dose should be administered at least 4 mos after the 1st dose and at least 2 mos after the 2nd dose.

[4]DTaP (diphtheria and tetanus toxoids and acellular pertussis vaccine) is the preferred vaccine for all doses in the vaccination series, including completion of the series in children who have received ≥1 dose of whole-cell DPT vaccine. Whole-cell DTP is an acceptable alternative to DTaP. The 4th dose of DTaP may be administered as early as 12 months of age, provided 6 months have elapsed since the 3rd dose, and if the child is considered unlikely to return at 15-18 mos of age. Td (tetanus and diptheria toxoids, absorbed, for adult use) is recommended at 11-12 years of age if at least 5 years have elapsed since the last dose of DTP, DTaP, or DT. Subsequent routine Td boosters are recommended every 10 years.

[5]Three *H. influenzae* type b (Hib) conjugate vaccines are licensed for infant use. If PRP-OMP (PedvaxHIB [Merck]) is administered at 2 and 4 mos of age, a dose at 6 mos is not required. After completing the primary series, any Hib conjugate vaccine may be used as a booster.

[6]Two poliovirus vaccines are currently licensed in the US: Inactivated poliovirus vaccine (IPV) and oral poliovirus vaccine (OPV). The following schedules are all acceptable by the ACIP, The AAP, and the AAFP, and parents and providers may choose among them:

1. IPV at 2 and 4 mos; OPV at 12-18 mos and 4-6 yr
2. IPV at 2, 4, 12-18 mos, and 4-6 yr
3. OPV at 2, 4, 6-18 mos, and 4-6 yr

The ACIP routinely recommends schedule 1. IPV is the only poliovirus vaccine recommended for immunocompromised persons and their household contacts.

[7]The 2nd dose of MMR is routinely recommended at 4-6 yrs of age or at 11-12 yrs of age, but may be administered during any visit, provided at least 1 mo has elapsed since receipt of the 1st dose and that both doses are administered at or after 12 months of age.

[8]Susceptible children may receive Varicella vaccine (Var) at any visit after the first birthday, and those who lack a reliable history of chickenpox should be immunized during the 11-12 year-old visit. Children ≥ 13 years of age should receive 2 doses, at least 1 mos apart.

tions for immunization policies and procedures. In Canada, recommendations are from the National Advisory Committee on Immunization under the authority of the Minister of National Health and Welfare. Because ACIP is concerned primarily with national health issues and the Committee on Infectious Diseases formulates its recommendations for infants and children who receive regular health care, there are occasionally different perspectives in each group's recommendations. The policies of each committee are recommendations, not rules, and they change as a result of advances in the field of immunology. Nurses need to realize the purpose of each organization; to view immunization practices in light of the needs of an individual child, as well as the community; and to keep informed of the latest advances and changes in policy.

The recommended age for beginning primary immunizations of infants is at birth (Table 33-4). Children born prematurely should receive the *full dose* of each vaccine at the appropriate chronologic age. If the infant is hospitalized, oral poliovirus vaccine (OPV) is initiated after discharge to prevent transmission of OPV in the nursery. Recommended schedules for children not immunized during infancy are included in Table 33-5. Tables 33-6 and 33-7 describe immunization schedules for Canadian children. Children who began primary immunization at the recommended age but who fail to receive all the doses do not have to begin the series again, but receive only the missed doses. In situations when there is doubt that the child will return for immunization according to the optimum schedule, HBV, DTaP or DTP, OPV, or inactivated poliovirus vaccine (IPV), MMR, and Hib vaccines can be administered simultaneously. However, parenteral vaccines are given in separate syringes in different injection sites (American Academy of Pediatrics, 1994).

Recommendations for Routine Immunizations

Hepatitis B virus (HBV). HBV, a potentially fatal viral infection that eventually causes cirrhosis or liver cancer during adulthood, is an important pediatric disease, because HBV infections occurring during childhood and adolescence can lead

TABLE 33-5 Recommended immunization schedules for children not immunized in the first year of life in the United States

RECOMMENDED TIME/AGE	IMMUNIZATION(S)*,†	COMMENTS
Younger than 7 years		
First visit	DTP, Hib, HBV‡, MMR, OPV, VZV	If indicated, tuberculin testing may be done at same visit If child is 5 years of age or older, Hib is not indicated
Interval after first visit:		
1 month	DTP, HBV	OPV may be given if accelerated poliomyelitis vaccination is necessary, such as for travelers to areas where polio is endemic
2 months	DTP, Hib‡, OPV	Second dose of Hib is indicated only in children whose first dose was received when younger than 15 months
≥8 months	DTP or DTAP§, HBV, OPV	OPV is not given if the third dose was given earlier
4-6 years (at or before school entry)	DTP or DTAP§, OPV	DTP or DTaP is not necessary if the fourth dose was given after the fourth birthday; OPV is not necessary if the third dose was given after the fourth birthday
11-12 years	MMR	At entry to middle school or junior high school
10 years later	Td	Repeat every 10 years throughout life
7 Years and older||, ¶		
First visit	HBV#, OPV, MMR, Td, VZV	After the 13th birthday, 2 doses of VZV are required 4 to 8 weeks apart.
Interval after first visit:		
2 months	HBV#, OPV, Td	OPV may also be given 1 month after the first visit if accelerated poliomyelitis vaccination is necessary
8-14 months	HBV#, OPV, Td	OPV is not given if the third dose was given earlier
11-12 years	MMR	At entry to middle school or junior high
10 years later	Td	Repeat every 10 years throughout life

From American Academy of Pediatrics: *Report of the Committee on Infectious Diseases*, ed 23, Elk Grove Village, Ill, 1994, The Academy. American Academy of Pediatrics, Committee on Infectious Diseases: Recommendations for the use of live attenuated varicella vaccine, *Pediatrics* 95(5):791-796, 1995.

*Abbreviations for vaccines are on p. 961. If all needed vaccines cannot be administered simultaneously, priority should be given to protecting the child against those diseases that pose the greatest immediate risk. In the United States these diseases for children younger than 2 years usually are measles and *Haemophilus influenzae* type b infection; for children older than 7 years, they are measles, mumps, and rubella (MMR).

†DTP or DTaP, HBV, Hib, MMR, VZV, and OPV can be given simultaneously at separate sites if failure of the patient to return for future immunizations is a concern.

‡Any licensed Hib conjugate vaccine may be used.

§DTaP is not currently licensed for use in children younger than 15 months of age and is not recommended for primary immunization (i.e., first 3 doses) at any age.

||If person is 18 years or older, routine poliovirus vaccination is not indicated in the United States.

¶Minimal interval between doses of MMR is 1 month.

#Priority should be given to hepatitis B immunization of adolescents.

TABLE 33-6 Routine primary immunization schedule for infants and children in Canada

AGE	IMMUNIZATION AGAINST				
2 months	Diphtheria	Pertussis	Tetanus	Poliomyelitis	*Haemophilus influenzae* b*
4 months	Diphtheria	Pertussis	Tetanus	Poliomyelitis	*Haemophilus influenzae* b
6 months	Diphtheria	Pertussis	Tetanus	Poliomyelitis†	*Haemophilus influenzae* b
12 months	Measles	Mumps	Rubella		
18 months	Diphtheria	Pertussis	Tetanus	Poliomyelitis	*Haemophilus influenzae* b
4-6 years	Diphtheria	Pertussis	Tetanus	Poliomyelitis	
14-16 years	Diphtheria‡		Tetanus‡	Poliomyelitis†	

From National Advisory Committee on Immunization: *Canadian Immunization guide,* ed 4, Canada, 1993, Authority of the Minister of National Health and Welfare, Health Protection Branch, Laboratory Centre for Disease Control.
*Hib schedule shown is for HbOC or PRP-T vaccine. If PRP-OMP is used, give at 2, 4, and 12 months of age.
†Omit this dose of OPV if used exclusively.
‡Td (tetanus and diphtheria toxoid), a combined adsorbed "adult-type" preparation for use in persons ≥ 7 years of age, contains less diphtheria toxoid than preparations given to younger children and is less likely to cause reactions in older persons. Repeat every 10 years throughout life.

TABLE 33-7 Routine immunization schedules for children not immunized in early infancy in Canada

TIMING	IMMUNIZATION AGAINST				
For children 7 years of age and younger					
First visit	Diphtheria	Pertussis	Tetanus	Poliomyelitis	*Haemophilus influenzae* b
	Measles§	Mumps§	Rubella§		
2 months later	Diphtheria	Pertussis	Tetanus	Poliomyelitis	*Haemophilus influenzae* b||
2 months later	Diphtheria	Pertussis	Tetanus	Poliomyelitis†	
6-12 months later	Diphtheria	Pertussis	Tetanus	Poliomyelitis	*Haemophilus influenzae* b||
4-6 years¶	Diphtheria	Pertussis	Tetanus	Poliomyelitis	
14-16 years	Diphtheria‡	Tetanus‡	Poliomyelitis†		
For children 7 years of age and older					
First visit	Diphtheria‡		Tetanus‡	Poliomyelitis	
	Measles	Mumps	Rubella		
2 months later	Diphtheria‡		Tetanus‡	Poliomyelitis	
6-12 months later	Diphtheria‡		Tetanus‡	Poliomyelitis	
10 years later	Diphtheria‡		Tetanus‡		

From National Advisory Committee on Immunization: *Canadian immunization guide,* ed 4, Canada, 1993, Authority of the Minister of National Health and Welfare, Health Protection Branch, Laboratory Centre for Disease Control.
*,†,‡See Table 33-6.
§Delay until subsequent visit if child is <12 months of age.
||Recommended schedule and number of doses depend on the product used and the age of the child when vaccination is begun. Not required past age 5.
¶Omit these doses if the previous doses of DTP and polio were given after the fourth birthday.

to these consequences. Up to 90% of infants infected perinatally and 25% to 50% of children infected before age 5 years will become HBV carriers. In addition, the incidence of HBV infection increases rapidly during adolescence (American Academy of Pediatrics, 1992). Despite the availability of a safe, effective vaccine, new cases have increased about 50% during the last decade. Past immunization strategies targeted several high-risk groups, including health care workers and others in contact with blood and body fluids, recipients of certain blood products (such as those with hemophilia), heterosexuals with multiple partners, sexually active homosexual and bisexual males, intravenous drug abusers, immigrants from countries where HBV is widespread, and children born to mothers who are HBV surface antigen (HBsAg) positive. To improve immunization rates, current recommendations include immunizations for all newborns, as well as several high-risk groups (Centers for Disease Control and Prevention, 1994). The American Academy of Pediatrics (1994) also encourages the routine immunization of all adolescents against HBV when feasible.

The vaccine is given intramuscularly in the vastus lateralis in neonates but may be given in the deltoid muscle during later infancy. Regardless of age, the dorsogluteal site is avoided because it has been associated with low antibody seroconversion rates, indicating a reduced immune response (Zuckerman, Cockcroft, and Zuckerman, 1992). It can be safely administered simultaneously at a separate site with DTP, MMR, and Hib vaccines. Dosage depends on the child's age and type of vaccine used (Table 33-5).

Diphtheria. Diphtheria vaccine is commonly administered intramuscularly (1) in combination with tetanus and pertus-

TABLE 33-8 Guide to tetanus prophylaxis in routine wound management, 1991

HISTORY OF ADSORBED TETANUS TOXOID (DOSES)	CLEAN, MINOR WOUNDS		ALL OTHER WOUNDS*	
	TD†	TIG	TD†	TIG
Unknown or < three	Yes	No	Yes	Yes
≥ Three‡	No§	No	No||	No

From Recommendations of the Immunization Practices Advisory Committee (ACIP): Diphtheria, tetanus, and pertussis: recommendations for vaccine use and other preventive measures, *MMWR* 40(RR-10):1-28, 1991.
*Such as, but not limited to, wounds contaminated with dirt, feces, soil, and saliva; puncture wounds; avulsions; and wounds resulting from missiles, crushing, burns, and frostbite.
†For children <7 years old; DTP (DT, if pertussis vaccine is contraindicated) is preferred to tetanus toxoid alone. For persons ≥7 years of age, Td is preferred to tetanus toxoid alone.
‡If only three doses of *fluid* toxoid have been received, then a fourth dose of toxoid, preferably an adsorbed toxoid, should be given.
§Yes, if >10 years since last dose.
||Yes, if >5 years since last dose. (More frequent boosters are not needed and can accentuate side effects.)

sis vaccines (DTP or DTaP) or DTP and Hib vaccines for children younger than 7 years of age, (2) in a combined vaccine with tetanus (DT) for children younger than 7 years of age who have some contraindication for receiving pertussis vaccine, (3) in smaller doses (15% to 20% of that in DTP or DT) with tetanus vaccine (Td) for use in children age 7 years and older, or (4) as a single antigen when combined antigen preparations are not indicated. Although the diphtheria vaccine does not produce absolute immunity, when it is given according to the recommended schedule, protective antitoxin persists for 10 years or more.

Tetanus. Three forms of tetanus vaccine—tetanus toxoid, tetanus immune globulin (TIg) (human), and tetanus antitoxin (usually horse serum)—are available. Tetanus toxoid is used for routine primary immunization, usually in one of the combinations listed and provides protective antitoxin levels for 10 years or more.

For wound management, passive immunity is available with TIG or animal-source antitoxin. However, because the risk of severe reaction, such as anaphylactic shock or serum sickness, to the foreign substances of animal serum is always greater, the choice is TIG. In persons with a history of two previous doses of tetanus toxoid, a booster dose of the toxoid can be given. When tetanus toxoid and TIG are given concurrently, separate syringes and different intramuscular sites are used. Table 33-8 presents a summary of the recommended procedure for tetanus prophylaxis in wound management.

Pertussis. Pertussis vaccine is recommended for all children 6 weeks through 6 years of age (up to the seventh birthday) who have no neurologic contraindications to its use. It is not given to children 7 years or older because the risk of receiving the vaccine increases as the incidence, severity, and fatality of the disease decrease.

Currently, two forms of pertussis vaccine are available for intramuscular administration in the United States. The *whole-cell pertussis vaccine* is prepared from inactivated cells of *Bordetella pertussis* and contains multiple antigens. In contrast, the *acellular pertussis vaccine* contains one or more immunogens derived from the *B. pertussis* organism. The highly purified acellular vaccine is associated with fewer local and systemic reactions than those occurring with the whole-cell vaccine in children of similar age. The acellular vaccine (DTaP [ACEL-IMUNE or Tripedia]) is preferred for use at all ages, but the DTP is an acceptable alternative (American Academy of Pediatrics, 1997a; 1997b).

Polio. There are two polio vaccines, the trivalent form of *OPV* (developed by Sabin) and the *IPV* (developed by Salk) OPV has been used in the United States because the live virus can be shed to contacts, who become immunized through this exposure. However, OPV has caused vaccine-associated paralysis in both recipients and contacts. IPV is now being recommended for this reason (American Academy of Pediatrics, 1997c).

IPV has the disadvantage of being given by subcutaneous injection and producing less immunity. In the United States an enhanced-potency form of IVP is used.

Each of the following immunization schedules is acceptable: (1) *sequential*—IPV at 2 and 4 months, OPV at 12 to 18 months and 4 to 6 years; (2) *IPV only*—IPV at 2, 4, and 12 to 18 months and at 4 to 6 years; (3) *OPV only*—OPV at 2, 4, and 6 to 18 months and at 4 to 6 years. Parents and practitioners may choose among these schedules. The sequential schedule is now recommended for most children. IPV is the only poliovirus vaccine recommended for immunocompromised persons and their household contacts (American Academy of Pediatrics, 1997a).

Measles. Because of the presence of maternal antibodies, measles (rubeola) virus vaccine was usually delayed until 15 months of age for infants who live in communities where the disease is not prevalent. However, it can now be given at 12 to 15 months of age. During the course of measles outbreaks, the vaccine can be given any time after 6 months of age, followed by a second inoculation after age 12 months.

Because of continued outbreaks of measles among unvaccinated preschool-age children and among vaccinated school-age children and college students, a second measles immunization is recommended before school entry at 4 to 6 years of age or at 11 to 12 years of age. It is given subcutaneously with vaccines for mumps and rubella (MMR).

Mumps. Mumps virus vaccine is recommended for children at 12 to 15 months of age and is typically given in combination with measles and rubella. It should not be administered to infants younger than 12 months because persisting maternal antibodies can interfere with the immune response. It is administered subcutaneously in the combined MMR vaccine.

Rubella. Rubella is a relatively mild infection in children, but in a pregnant woman it presents serious risks to the developing fetus. Therefore the aim of rubella immunization is actually protection of the unborn child rather than the recipient of the immunization.

Rubella immunization is recommended for all children at 12 to 15 months of age and is administered in a combined form with measles and mumps vaccine. Increased emphasis should also be placed on vaccinating all unimmunized prepubertal children and susceptible adolescents and adult women in the childbearing age group.

Because the live attenuated virus may cross the placenta and present a risk to the developing fetus, rubella vaccine is not given to any pregnant woman. Although this is standard practice, current evidence from women who received the vaccine while pregnant and delivered unaffected offspring indicates that the risk to the fetus is negligible (Centers for Disease Control and Prevention, 1994). In addition, there is no reported danger of administering rubella vaccine to a child if the mother is pregnant. It is administered subcutaneously in the combined MMR vaccine.

Haemophilus influenzae type b (Hib). Hib conjugate vaccines provide protection against a number of serious infections caused by Hib, especially bacterial meningitis, epiglottitis, bacterial pneumonia, septic arthritis, and sepsis. (Hib is not associated with the viruses that cause influenza, or "flu.")

The following Hib conjugate vaccines are available:

- Diphtheria toxoid conjugate (PRP-D) (ProHIBit)
- Diphtheria CRM_{197} protein conjugate (PRP-HbOC) (Hib-TITER)
- Meningococcal protein conjugate (PRP-OMP) (Pedvax HIB)
- PRP conjugate with tetanus toxoid (PRP-T) (ActHIB and OmniHIB)
- HibTITER is also combined in a vaccine with DTP (Tetramune)

These conjugate vaccines connect Hib to a nontoxic form of another organism, such as meningococcal protein or diphtheria protein. There is *no* antibody response to these nontoxic proteins, but they significantly improve the antibody response to Hib, especially in infants.

HbOC or PRP-T is recommended at 2, 4, and 6 months of age, with a booster at 12 to 15 months. Only two doses of PRP-OMP are required—at ages 2 to 6 months, administered at least 2 months apart, with a booster at 12 to 15 months. PRP-D is not licensed for use in infants under 12 months. When possible, the Hib conjugate vaccine used at the first vaccination should be used for all subsequent vaccinations in the primary series. When either a Hib vaccine or Tetramune is used, the vaccine is administered by intramuscular (IM) injection using a separate syringe and at a separate site from any concurrent vaccinations.

Children less than age 2 years who experience an Hib-related illness still need to be immunized; the vaccine is not recommended for children over age 5 years except for those with chronic conditions that affect their immune function.

Varicella. The live virus varicella zoster (VZ) or chickenpox vaccine is recommended for all children between 12 and 18 months of age and all older susceptible children, up to age 12 years. The dose is 0.5 ml, given subcutaneously, with one dose for children 12 months to 12 years and two doses for youngsters after the thirteenth birthday. The vaccine must be kept frozen in the lyophilized form (stable particles that readily go into solution) and used immediately after being reconstituted to ensure maximum response.

In a small number of immunized children chickenpox may develop. However, the disease is mild; children have fewer lesions and less itching, fever, or headache, and more than half have no symptoms other than the rash. The contagiousness of the infection is also significantly reduced (American Academy of Pediatrics, Committee on Infectious Diseases, 1995).

Recommendations for Selected Immunizations

Several additional vaccines are recommended for children at high risk for particular diseases. Most of these children have chronic disorders or impaired immune systems that make them more susceptible to certain infections than the general population. Selected immunizations are presented in Table 33-9. Others, such as the rabies vaccine, are discussed elsewhere in this text.

Reactions

Vaccines for routine immunizations are among the safest and most reliable drugs available. However, minor side effects do follow many of the immunizations, and a serious reaction may rarely result from the vaccine.

With inactivated antigens, such as DTP, side effects are most likely to occur within a few hours or days of administration and are usually limited to local tenderness, erythema, and swelling at the injection site; low-grade fever; and behavioral changes (drowsiness, fretfulness, decrease in eating, prolonged or unusual cry). Local reactions tend to be less severe when the deltoid site is used rather than the vastus lateralis and when a needle of sufficient length to deposit the vaccine in the muscle is used (see the Atraumatic Care box on p. 970). Rarely, more severe reactions may occur. Especially with pertussis these may include loss of consciousness, convulsions, persistent inconsolable crying episodes, generalized or focal neurologic signs, fever (temperature at or above 40.5° C [105° F]), and systemic allergic reaction. Reactions to DTP tend to be more severe if they occurred with a previous immunization.

Nursing ALERT

Recommend prophylactic use of acetaminophen at time of DTP immunization and every 4 to 6 hours for a total of 3 doses

Advise parents to notify practitioner *immediately* of any unusual side effects.

Reactions to DTP tend to be more severe if they occurred with a previous immunization.

TABLE 33-9 Recommendations for selected nonmandated vaccines

DESCRIPTION	ADMINISTRATION/PRECAUTIONS
Influenza virus vaccine	
Affords protection against strains of influenza Recommended for children age 6 months and older with chronic disorders of cardiovascular or pulmonary system, including asthma, whose severity warranted regular medical care or hospitalization during preceding year; other eligible children include those with diabetes mellitus, renal dysfunction, anemia, immunosuppression, human immunodeficiency virus (HIV) infection, or long-term aspirin therapy (because of risk of development of Reye syndrome after influenza infection)	Administered in fall, preferably November; repeated yearly Intramuscular injection; 2 doses of split vaccine at least 4 weeks apart for children age 12 years or younger; 1 dose of split or whole vaccine for children over 12 years of age Contraindicated in persons with anaphylactic hypersensitivity to eggs May be given simultaneously with other childhood immunizations but at separate site
Pneumococcal polysaccharide vaccine (Pneumovax; PNU-IMUNE)	
Affords protection against 23 types of *Streptococcus pneumoniae* Recommended for children age 2 years and older with sickle cell disease, functional or anatomic asplenia, nephrotic syndrome, human immunodeficiency virus (HIV) infection, and Hodgkin disease before beginning cytoreduction therapy	Subcutaneous or intramuscular injection Revaccination is not recommended Should be deferred during pregnancy
Meningococcal polysaccharide vaccine (Menomune)	
Affords protection against *Neisseria meningitidis;* serogroups A, C, Y, and W-135. Recommended for children 2 years and older with terminal complement deficiencies and anatomic or functional asplenia	Subcutaneous injection Duration of protection unknown Safety during pregnancy not established
Hepatitis A virus vaccine (HAVRIX, Vaqta)	
Affords protection against hepatitis A virus Recommended for children ages 2 years and older who are at high risk for contracting hepatitis A: travelers to hepatitis A endemic areas; military personnel; ethnic and geographic populations with cyclic hepatitis A epidemics, such as Native American and Alaskan communities; homosexuals; IV-drug users and noninjection street-drug users; chronic liver disease patients; individuals with occupational risk of exposure, such as child-care and institutional workers, as well as primate-animal handlers; and laboratory workers who handle live hepatitis A virus.	HAVRIX: intramuscular injection, 2 doses, 1 month apart, any time between 2 to 18 years; booster dose should be given 6 to 12 months after the second dose Vaqta: requires only one injection between ages 2 and 17 years, followed by a booster dose 6-12 months later.

Hib vaccine is one of the safest vaccines available but may be associated with low-grade fever and mild local reactions at the site of subcutaneous injection, which resolve rapidly. Fever (temperature more than 38.5° C [101.3° F]) may rarely occur. HBV is equally well tolerated.

Unlike the inactivated antigens, live attenuated virus vaccines such as MMR and OPV multiply for days or weeks, and unfavorable reactions and "vaccine-associated" disorders can occur for a period of 30 to 60 days. However, they are usually mild, although reactions to rubella tend to be more troublesome in older children and adults. The varicella vaccine produces minimal reactions, especially during adolescence. Adolescents may experience pain, tenderness, or redness at the injection site and a mild vaccine-associated maculopapular or varicellaform rash at the injection site or elsewhere.

Contraindications/Precautions

Nurses need to be aware of the reasons for withholding immunizations—both for the child's safety in terms of preventing reactions and for the child's maximum benefit from receiving the vaccine. Unfounded fears and lack of knowledge regarding contraindications can needlessly prevent a child from having protection from life-threatening diseases. The contraindications to and precautions for the usual childhood vaccines are presented in Table 33-10.

Administration

The principal precautions in administering immunizations include proper storage of the vaccine to protect its potency and institution of recommended procedures for injection. The nurse must be familiar with the manufacturer's directions for storage and reconstitution of the vaccine. For example, if the vaccine is to be refrigerated, it should be stored on a center shelf, not on the door, where frequent temperature decreases from opening the refrigerator can alter the vaccine's potency. For protection against light the vial can be wrapped in aluminum foil. Periodic checks are established to ensure that no vaccine is used after its expiration date.

The DTP vaccines contain the adjuvant alum to retain the antigen at the depot site and prolong the stimulatory effect.

TABLE 33-10 Contraindications and precautions to vaccination*

TRUE CONTRAINDICATIONS AND PRECAUTIONS	NOT CONTRAINDICATIONS (VACCINES MAY BE ADMINISTERED)
General for all vaccines (DTP/DTaP, OPV, IPV, MMR, Hib, Hepatitis B, VZV)	
Contraindications	***Not contraindications***
Anaphylactic reaction to a vaccine contraindicates further doses of that vaccine Anaphylactic reaction to a vaccine constituent contraindicates the use of vaccines containing that substance Moderate or severe illnesses with or without a fever	Mild to moderate local reaction (soreness, redness, swelling) following a dose of an injectable antigen Mild acute illness with or without low-grade fever Current antimicrobial therapy Convalescent phase of illnesses Prematurity (same dosage and indications as for full-term infants) Recent exposure to an infectious disease History of penicillin or other nonspecific allergies or family history of such allergies
Diphtheria, tetanus, pertussis, or acellular pertussis (DTP/DTaP)	
Contraindications	***Not contraindications***
Encephalopathy within 7 days of administration of previous dose of DTP	Temperature of <40.5° C (105° F) following a previous dose of DTP Family history of seizures‡ Family history of sudden infant death syndrome Family history of an adverse event following DTP administration
Precautions†	
Fever of ≥40.5° C (105° F) within 48 hours after vaccination with a prior dose of DTP Collapse or shocklike state (hypotonic-hyporesponsive episode) within 48 hours of receiving a prior dose of DTP Seizures within 3 days of receiving a prior dose of DTP Persistent, inconsolable crying lasting ≥3 hours within 48 hours of receiving a prior dose of DTP	
Oral polio (OPV)§	
Contraindications	***Not contraindications***
Infection with HIV or a household contact with HIV Known altered immunodeficiency (hematologic and solid tumors; congenital immunodeficiency; and long-term immunosuppressive therapy) Immunodeficient household contact	Breastfeeding Current antimicrobial therapy Diarrhea
Precaution†	
Pregnancy	
Inactivated polio (IPV)	
Contraindication	
Anaphylactic reaction to neomycin or streptomycin	
Precaution†	
Pregnancy	

From Centers for Disease Control and Prevention: General recommendations on immunization: recommendations of the Advisory Committee on Immunization Practices (ACIP), *MMWR* 43(RR-1):24-25, 1994 and American Academy of Pediatrics: Committee on Infectious Diseases: Recommendations for the use of live attenuated varicella vaccine, *Pediatrics* 95(5):791-796, 1995.

*This information is based on the recommendations of the Advisory Committee on Immunization Practices (ACIP) and those of the Committee on Infectious Diseases (Red Book Committee) of the American Academy of Pediatrics (AAP). Sometimes these recommendations vary from those contained in the manufacturer's package inserts. For more detailed information, providers should consult the published recommendations of the ACIP, the AAP, and the manufacturer's package inserts.

†The events or conditions listed as precautions, although not contraindications, should be carefully reviewed. The benefits and risks of administering a specific vaccine to an individual under the circumstances should be considered. If the risks are believed to outweigh the benefits, the vaccination should be withheld; if the benefits are believed to outweigh the risks (e.g., during an outbreak or foreign travel), the vaccination should be administered. Whether and when to administer DTP to children with proven or suspected underlying neurologic disorders should be decided on an individual basis. It is prudent on theoretic grounds to avoid vaccinating pregnant women. However, if immediate protection against poliomyelitis is needed, OPV is preferred, although IPV may be considered if full vaccination can be completed before the anticipated imminent exposure.

‡Acetaminophen given before administering DTP and thereafter every 4 hours for 24 hours should be considered for children with a personal or family history of seizures in siblings or parents.

§No data exist to substantiate the theoretic risk of a suboptimal immune response from the administration of OPV and MMR within 30 days of each other.

TABLE 33-10 Contraindications and precautions to vaccination*—cont'd

TRUE CONTRAINDICATIONS AND PRECAUTIONS	NOT CONTRAINDICATIONS (VACCINES MAY BE ADMINISTERED)
Measles, mumps, rubella (MMR)§	
Contraindications	***Not contraindications§***
Anaphylactic reactions to egg ingestion and to neomycin|| Pregnancy Known altered immunodeficiency (hematologic and solid tumors, congenital immunodeficiency, and long-term immunosuppressive therapy)	Tuberculosis or positive PPD skin test result Simultaneous TB skin testing¶ Breastfeeding Pregnancy of mother of recipient Immunodeficient family member or household contact Infection with HIV Nonanaphylactic reactions to eggs or neomycin
Precautions†	
Recent immune globulin (Ig) administration Immune globulin products and MMR should not be given simultaneously; if unavoidable, give at different sites and revaccinate or test for seroconversion in 3 months; if Ig is given first, MMR should not be given for at least 3 to 6 months, depending on the dose; if MMR is given first, Ig should not be given for 2 weeks	
Haemophilus influenzae Type B (Hib)	
Contraindication	***Not a contraindication***
Nonidentified	History of Hib disease
Hepatitis B virus (HBV)	
Contraindication	***Not a contraindication***
Anaphylactic reaction to common baker's yeast	Pregnancy
Varicella zoster virus (VZV)	
Contraindications	***Not contraindications***
Immunocompromised individuals, such as those with congenital immunodeficiency, blood dyscrasias, leukemia, lymphoma, symptomatic HIV infection, and malignancy for which they are receiving immunosuppressive therapy Asymptomatic HIV infection Individuals who are receiving high doses of systemic corticosteroids (2 mg/kg/day or more of prednisone, or its equivalent or 20 mg/day of prednisone if their weight is >10 kg) for >1 month (interval of 1 month or more after discontinuation of steroid use is probably sufficient to administer vaccine safely) Pregnancy Anaphylactoid reaction to neomycin	Presence of immunodeficient or HIV-seropositive family member Children receiving only inhaled steroids Pregnancy of family member Nonanaphylactoid reactions to neomycin, such as contact dermatitis
Precautions	
Immunization should be considered when child with acute lymphocytic leukemia has been in continuous remission for at least 1 year and has lymphocyte count over 700/μl and platelet count over 100,000/μl 24 hours before vaccination Children with no history of varicella who are receiving systemic steroids for conditions such as nephrosis and asthma may be immunized if not otherwise immunosuppressed, assuming that they are receiving <2 mg/kg/day of prednisone or its equivalent (or <20 mg/day if their weight is >10 kg) When postpubertal females are immunized, pregnancy should be avoided for 1 month after immunization. May be considered for VZV-susceptible nursing mother, if risk for exposure to natural VZV is high Should not be administered within at least 5 months after receipt of any form of immune globulin or other blood product Salicylates should not be administered for 6 weeks after varicella vaccine because of the associations among Reye syndrome, natural varicella, and salicylates	

||Persons with a history of anaphylactic reactions following egg ingestion should be vaccinated only with caution. Protocols have been developed for vaccinating such persons and should be consulted.

¶Measles vaccination may temporarily suppress tuberculin reactivity. If testing cannot be done the day of MMR vaccination, the test should be postponed for 4 to 6 weeks.

Atraumatic Care

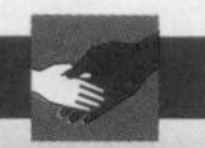

IMMUNIZATIONS

To minimize local reactions from DTP vaccines:
- Select a needle of adequate length (1 inch in infants) to deposit the antigen deep in the muscle mass
- Inject into the vastus lateralis or ventrogluteal muscle; the deltoid may be used in children 18 months or older (except for HBV, deltoid may be used during later infancy)
- Use an air bubble to clear the needle after injecting the vaccine (theoretically beneficial but unproved)

To minimize pain*
- Apply the topical anesthetic EMLA to the injection site for a minimum of 1 hour, preferably for up to 2 hours for greater penetration
- In preschool children use distraction, such as telling the child to "take a deep breath and blow and blow and blow until I tell you to stop"

Note: Changing the needle on the syringe after drawing up the vaccine and before injecting it has not been shown to be effective in decreasing local reactions.

*See also Pain Management, Chapter 25.

Because subcutaneous or intracutaneous injection of the adjuvant can cause local irritation, inflammation, or abscess formation, excellent intramuscular injection technique must be used (see the Atraumatic Care box above).

The total series requires a number of injections, and every attempt is made to rotate the sites and administer the injections as painlessly as possible (see discussion on intramuscular injections in Chapter 41). When two or more injections are given at separate sites, the order of injections is arbitrary. Some practitioners suggest injecting the less painful one first. Some believe this is DTP, whereas others suggest the MMR or Hib vaccine. Still others advocate injecting at two sites simultaneously (requires two operators). Research is needed to determine which sequence is least painful. Since allergic reactions can occur after injection of vaccines, appropriate precautions are taken (see Anaphylaxis, Chapter 45).

Another important nursing responsibility is accurate documentation. Each child should have an immunization record for parents to keep, especially for families who move frequently. The following information is documented on the medical record: day, month, and year of administration; manufacturer and lot number of vaccine; and name, address, and title of the person administering the vaccine. Additional data to record are the site and route of administration and evidence that the parent or legal guardian gave informed consent before the immunization was administered. Any adverse reaction after the administration of any vaccine is reported to the Vaccine Adverse Event Reporting System (VAERS).*

INJURY PREVENTION

Injuries are a major cause of death during infancy, especially for children 6 to 12 months old. Constant vigilance, awareness, and supervision are essential as the child gains increased locomotor and manipulative skills that are coupled with an insatiable curiosity about the environment. Table 33-11 lists the major developmental achievements of each period during infancy and the appropriate injury prevention plan.

Aspiration of Foreign Objects

Asphyxiation by foreign material in the respiratory tract, combined with mechanical suffocation, is the leading cause of fatal injury in children younger than 1 year of age. The size, shape, and consistency of foods or objects are important determinants of fatal obstruction. For example, small spheric or cylindric and pliable objects (less than 3.2 cm) are more likely to obstruct the airway completely. Unfortunately, common household items can be deadly to infants.

As soon as infants have the ability to find the mouth, they are vulnerable to aspiration of small objects, such as those left within reach or removable parts of objects that may on initial inspection appear safe. All toys must be carefully inspected for potential danger. Rattles, for example, have small beads in them to produce noise. A broken or cracked rattle can be dangerous because the beads can be aspirated while the infant has the toy in the mouth. Stuffed animals are another potentially dangerous toy if any of the parts, such as the eyes or nose, is a removable button or plastic piece. An active infant can grab a low-hanging mobile and quickly chew off a small piece. As soon as the infant crawls or plays on the floor, the floor must be kept free of any small articles that can be picked up and swallowed, such as coins.

When infant *clothes* are purchased, the type of closure is important. A front button can be pulled off easily and swallowed. Safety pins for diapers are kept closed and away from the dressing table. Even though a young infant may not search for them, practicing this good habit from the beginning prevents future injuries.

Food items are the second most common cause of aspiration, and the most frequent offenders are hot dogs, candy, nuts, and grapes. When new foods are given to the child, nuts, hard candies, marshmallows, large amounts of peanut butter, or fruits with pits or seeds are avoided. When traveling, especially in airplanes, or entertaining, snack foods such as peanuts and popcorn are kept away from young children. If given to young children, hot dogs must be cut into small, irregular pieces rather than served whole or sliced into sections, because their size (diameter), round shape, and consistency allow for complete occlusion of the airway. Perhaps the most dangerous food is dried beans, which, if aspirated, enlarge when they come in contact with the wet mucosa and block the airway.

Pacifiers can also be dangerous because the entire object may be aspirated if it is small or the nipple and shield may become detached from the handle and become lodged in the pharynx. Improvised pacifiers, such as those commonly made in hospitals from a padded nipple, also present dangers. The nipple may separate from the plastic collar and be aspirated. In addition, parents may continue to offer this pacifier to the infant at home. To prevent the hazards of improvised pacifiers, hospitals should use only safe commercial types. Candy pacifiers pose dangers because the candy portion can dislodge from the circular base and be aspirated. To be safe, pacifiers should have (Nowak, 1993) (Fig. 33-12) the following:

- Sturdy one-piece construction with material that is nontoxic, flexible, and firm but not brittle
- An easily grasped handle

* For information call (800) 822-7967.

TABLE 33-11 Injury prevention during infancy

Age: Birth-4 Months

Major developmental accomplishments

Involuntary reflexes, such as the crawling reflex, may propel infant forward or backward and the startle reflex may cause the body to jerk

May roll over

Increasing eye-hand coordination and voluntary grasp reflex

Injury Prevention

Aspiration

Not as great a danger to this age group, but should begin practicing safeguarding early (see under 4-7 Months)

Never shake baby powder directly on infant; place powder in hand and then on infant's skin; store container closed and out of infant's reach

Hold infant for feeding; do not prop bottle

Know emergency procedures for choking*

Use pacifier with one-piece construction and loop handle

Suffocation/Drowning

Keep all plastic bags stored out of infant's reach; discard large plastic garment bags after tying in a knot

Do not cover mattress with plastic

Use a firm mattress and loose blankets; no pillows

Make sure crib design follows federal regulations and mattress fits snugly†

Position crib away from other furniture and away from radiators

Avoid sleeping in bed with infant

Do not tie pacifier on a string around infant's neck

Remove bibs at bedtime

Never leave infant alone in bath

Do not leave infant under 12 months alone on adult or youth mattress

Falls

Always raise crib rails

Never leave infant on a raised, unguarded surface

When in doubt as to where to place child, use the floor

Restrain child in infant seat and never leave child unattended while the seat is resting on a raised surface

Avoid using a high chair until child can sit well with support

Poisoning

Not as great a danger to this age group, but should begin practicing safeguards early (see under 4-7 Months)

Burns

Install smoke detectors in home

Use caution when warming formula in microwave oven; always check temperature of liquid before feeding

Check bathwater

Do not pour hot liquids when infant is close by, such as sitting on lap

Beware of cigarette ashes that may fall on infant

Do not leave infant in the sun for more than a few minutes; keep exposed areas covered

Wash flame-retardant clothes according to label directions

Use cool-mist vaporizers

Do not leave child in parked car

Check surface heat of car restraint before placing child in seat

Motor vehicles

Transport infant in federally approved, rear-facing car seat that is not placed by an air bag safety device*

Do not place infant on the seat or in lap

Do not place child in a carriage or stroller behind a parked car

Bodily damage

Avoid sharp, jagged objects

Keep diaper pins closed and away from infant

Age: 4-7 months

Major developmental accomplishments

Rolls over

Sits momentarily

Grasps and manipulates small objects

Resecures a dropped object

Has well-developed eye-hand coordination

Can focus on and locate very small objects

Mouthing is very prominent

Can push up on hands and knees

Crawls backward

Injury prevention

Aspiration

Keep buttons, beads, syringe caps, and other small objects out of infant's reach

Keep floor free of any small objects

Do not feed infant hard candy, nuts, food with pits or seeds, or whole or circular pieces of hot dog

Exercise caution when giving teething biscuits, because large chunks may be broken off and aspirated

Do not feed infant while child is lying down

Inspect toys for removable parts

Keep baby powder, if used, out of reach

Avoid storing large quantities of cleaning fluid, paints, pesticides, and other toxic substances

Discard used containers of poisonous substances

Do not store toxic substances in food containers

Discard used button-sized batteries; store new batteries in safe area

Know telephone number of local poison control center (usually listed in front of telephone directory)

Suffocation

Keep uninflated balloons out of reach

Remove all crib toys that are strung across crib or playpen when child begins to push up on hands or knees or is 5 months old

Falls

Restrain in a high chair

Keep crib rails raised to full height

Poisoning

Make sure that paint for furniture or toys does not contain lead

Place toxic substances on a high shelf or in locked cabinet

Hang plants or place on high surface rather than on floor

*Home care instructions for care of the choking infant and for use of child safety seats are available in Wong DL: *Wong and Whaley's clinical manual of pediatric nursing*, ed 4, St Louis, 1996, Mosby.

†Information available from U.S. Consumer Product Safety Commission; (800) 638-CPSC.

Continued.

TABLE 33-11 Injury prevention during infancy—cont'd

Injury prevention—cont'd	
Burns Keep faucets out of reach Place hot objects (cigarettes, candles, incense) on high surface Limit exposure to sun; apply sunscreen Motor vehicles See under Birth-4 Months	*Bodily damage* Give toys that are smooth and rounded, preferably made of wood or plastic Avoid long, pointed objects as toys Avoid toys that are excessively loud Keep sharp objects out of infant's reach
Age: 8-12 Months	
Major Developmental Accomplishments	
Crawls/creeps Stands, holding onto furniture Stands alone Cruises around furniture Walks Climbs Pulls on objects	Throws objects Is able to pick up small objects; has pincer grasp Explores by putting objects in mouth Dislikes being restrained Explores away from parent Increasing understanding of simple commands and phrases
Injury prevention	
Aspiration Keep lint and small objects off floor, furniture, and out of reach of children Take care in feeding solid table food to ensure that very small pieces are given Do not use beanbag toys or allow child to play with dried beans See also under 4-7 Months *Suffocation/Drowning* Keep doors of ovens, dishwashers, refrigerators, coolers, and front-loading clothes washers and dryers closed at all times If storing an unused appliance, such as a refrigerator, remove the door Supervise contact with inflated balloons; immediately discard popped balloons and keep uninflated balloons out of reach Fence swimming pools Always supervise when near any source of water, such as cleaning buckets, drainage areas, toilets Keep bathroom doors closed Eliminate unnecessary pools of water Keep one hand on child at all times when in tub	*Falls* Fence stairways at top and bottom if child has access to either end† Dress infant in safe shoes and clothing (soles that do not "catch" on floor, tied shoelaces, pant legs that do not touch floor) Avoid using infant walkers Ensure that furniture is sturdy enough for child to pull self to standing position and cruise *Poisoning* Administer medications as a drug, not as a candy Do not administer medications unless so prescribed by a practitioner Replace medications and poisons immediately after use; replace caps properly if a child-protector cap is used Have syrup of ipecac in home; use only if advised *Burns* Place guards in front of or around any heating appliance, fireplace, or furnace Keep electrical wires hidden or out of reach Place plastic guards over electrical outlets; place furniture in front of outlets Keep hanging tablecloths out of reach (child may pull down hot liquids or heavy or sharp objects)

- A mouthguard that cannot be separated from the nipple, has two ventilating holes, and is too large to be aspirated
- No detachable ribbon or string
- A label warning against tying the pacifier around the infant's neck

Using a syringe to measure and dispense oral liquid medications to young children accurately has become common practice. However, the *syringe cap* is a potential aspiration hazard. As a precaution, keep parts of medication devices out of the reach of children and be certain the cap is removed before dispensing medication.

Even safety devices can be dangerous. To prevent tampering, items (such as baby food jars) may be covered with a plastic oversleeve. The *tear-down strip* can be aspirated and is very difficult to locate because it is clear.

Another hazardous substance if aspirated is *baby powder*, which is usually a mixture of talc (hydrous magnesium silicate) and other silicates. Although the use of talc has been discouraged, it is a common baby care product and can cause severe and often fatal aspiration pneumonia. One of the factors involved in talc aspiration is the similar appearance of baby powder containers and nursing bottles. Talc containers often become favorite playthings and are placed in the mouth. Improper use of powder by sprinkling it directly on the skin creates a cloud of talc dust that is easily inhaled. Parents are advised of the danger of baby powder and are discouraged from using it. If they prefer to use a powder, a cornstarch preparation can be substituted (see Diaper Dermatitis, Chapter 49). Whenever a powder is used, it is placed in the hand and then applied to the skin, never shaken directly from the container to the skin. The container is kept closed and immediately stored in a safe place, especially away from curious tod-

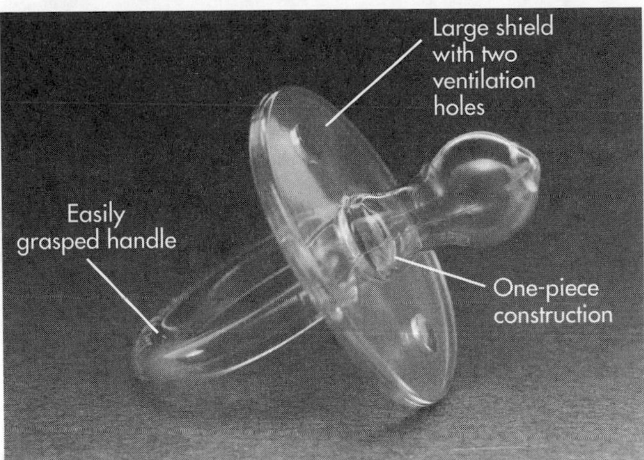

Fig. 33-12 Design of safe pacifier.

dlers, who often imitate caregiving activities and may accidentally shake it on the infant.

Suffocation

Mechanical suffocation includes suffocation by covering of the airway (i.e., mouth and nose), by pressure on the throat and chest, and by exclusion of air, such as by refrigerator entrapment. Nonfood items cause the majority of deaths in young children. *Latex balloons,* whether partially inflated, uninflated, or popped, are the leading cause of pediatric choking deaths from children's products (Holida, 1993). They should be kept away from infants and young children. Even the practice of inflating latex gloves to amuse children in health care settings may pose a danger.

Nursing ALERT

Encourage adults to:
Blow up balloons for children
Supervise balloon play
Pick up and dispose of broken balloon pieces
Warn older children of dangers of chewing or sucking on balloons
Substitute Mylar balloons for latex balloons

In addition, the accessibility of plastic linings of diapers used on the infant and/or on dolls is especially dangerous to young children.

The *bed* or *crib* poses a number of hazards. An infant who is placed in a bed under blankets and sheets that are tucked in can be caught under them and be unable to wriggle free. Baby pillows filled with plastic foam beads that make them resemble small bean bags are dangerous; very young infants are suffocated when the pillow contours to the face and blocks the airway. There are potential dangers in adults' sleeping with a small infant because of the possibility of their rolling over and smothering the child.

Infant strangulation may occur if the infant's head becomes caught between the crib slats and mattress or objects close to the crib. Suffocation deaths are not confined to cribs; ill-fitting mattresses in adult or youth beds, bunk beds, and waterbeds have also been reported. According to federal regulation the distance between crib slats should not be more than $2^3/_8$ inches (about 6 cm), roughly the width of three adult fingers. Mattresses and bumper pads should fit snugly against the slats. A general rule is that if two adult fingers can be placed between the mattress and crib or bed side, the mattress is too small. A temporary solution is to place large, rolled towels in the space to create a snug fit.

Corner post extensions on cribs are another source of strangulation. Children have died when their clothing caught on raised corner posts as they climbed out of the crib. Voluntary manufacturing standards state the corner post extensions should not exceed $^1/_{16}$ inch. However, the safety of *any* extension is questionable. Decorative extensions need to be removed from cribs. Ideally, information regarding correct crib design should be given prenatally before parents have purchased or borrowed a crib.*

Mesh-sided playpens and cribs can be hazards if the sides are left in the lowered position. Infants have suffocated when they fell off the edge of the mattress and the head or chest was compressed between the floorboard and mesh side. Parents should be advised of this danger and encouraged *always* to keep the sides locked securely in the up position whenever the child is in the playpen or crib.

The crib should be positioned away from large furniture, because children who crawl out of the crib may become caught between the two objects. Cribs should also be located away from windows, where drape or blind cords can become wrapped around the infant's neck.

Another cause of suffocation is *plastic bags.* Large plastic bags used over garments are very lightweight and can easily and quickly be wrapped around the head of an active infant or pressed against the face. Pillows and mattresses should not be covered with plastic for this reason. Older infants may play with a plastic bag and accidentally pull it over their heads. Because plastic is nonporous, suffocation takes place in a matter of minutes.

Cords either near the infant or tied around the infant's neck can potentially cause strangulation. Bibs are removed at bedtime, and objects such as pacifiers are never hung on a string around the infant's neck. This is a common practice in some cultures that can be remedied by attaching a *short* string tied to a pacifier and pinning the string on the child's shirt.

Toys that have strings attached, such as a telephone, or toys that are tied to cribs or playpens can be hazards because the string can become wrapped around the child's neck or the child can become entrapped in the toy. As a precaution, all cords should be less than 30 cm (12 inches) long. Crib toys should be hung high enough that the infant cannot become entangled in them or should no longer be used once the child is able to reach them.

Restraining straps, if applied too loosely or left unfastened, can be a hazard. For example, a child may slide off a high

*The booklet *It Hurts When They Cry* gives basic information on hazards, safety features, and proper use of nursery furniture and equipment. It is available at no charge from **U.S. Consumer Product Safety Commission,** Publication Request, Washington, DC 20207; (800) 638-2772. Additional free information is available from the **Danny Foundation,** 3158 Danville Blvd; P.O. Box 680, Alamo, CA 94507; (800) 83-DANNY.

chair beneath the tray and become strangled on the loose strap. All straps should be fastened securely.

Motor Vehicle Injuries

Automobile injuries are the leading cause of accidental death in children older than 1 year of age. However, a significant number of infants are injured or die from improper restraint within the vehicle, most often from riding on the lap of another occupant. All infants must be secured in a federally approved restraint rather than held or placed on the seat of the car. There is no safe alternative.

Infant restraints are designed either as an infant-only model (Fig. 33-13) or as a convertible infant-toddler model. Either restraint is a semireclined seat that faces the *rear* of the car. A rear-facing car seat provides the very best protection for the disproportionately heavy head and the weak neck of a young child. This position minimizes the stress on the neck by spreading the forces of a frontal crash over the entire back, neck, and head; the spine is supported by the back of the car seat. If the seat were faced forward, the head would whip forward as a result of the force of the crash, creating enormous stress on the neck.

Nursing ALERT

Infants should face the rear from birth to 20 pounds and as close to 1 year of age as possible.

The restraint is anchored to the vehicle with the car seat belt and has a harness system for restraining the infant. Some harness systems require a clip to keep the shoulder straps correctly positioned. Although many infant restraints can be recliners, they are only used in the car in the position specified by the manufacturer.

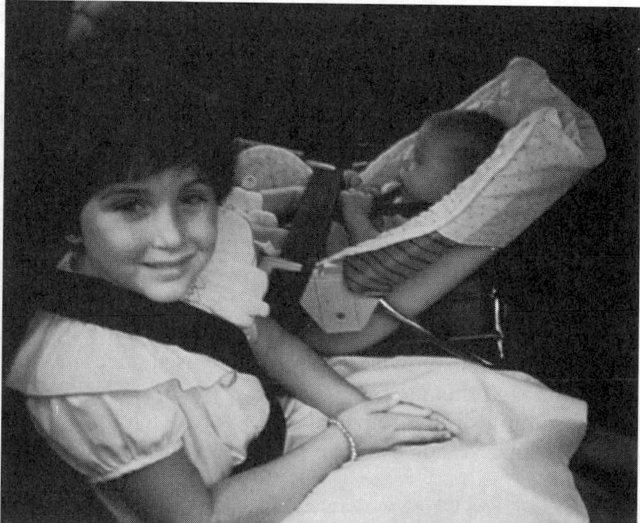

Fig. 33-13 Federally approved infant car restraint. Note placement in middle of back seat and use of car lap/shoulder belt for older child.

Nursing ALERT

Infant safety seats must not be placed in the front seat of a car equipped with an air bag on the passenger side. The safest place to ride for infants and children (even through school age) is in the back seat, properly restrained. If, in an emergency, a child must ride in the front seat, the vehicle seat should be moved back as far as it can go, away from the air bag (American Academy of Pediatrics, 1997).

For restraints to be effective, they must be used properly. Dressing the infant in an outfit with sleeves and legs allows the harness to hold the child securely in the seat. A small blanket or towel rolled tightly can be placed on either side of the head to minimize movement and keep the infant's hips against the back of the seat. Padding between the infant's legs and crotch is added to prevent slouching. Thick, soft padding is not placed under the infant or behind the back because during the impact the padding will compress, leaving the harness straps loose. (For further discussion of restraints see Chapter 34.)

Falls

Falls are most common after 4 months of age when the infant has learned to roll over, but they can occur at any age. Newborns are normally active, assume a flexed position, and have crawling reflexes that can propel them forward. The best advice is never to place a child unattended on a raised surface that has no type of guardrail. When in doubt, the safest place is the floor. Even though young infants cannot climb over a partially raised crib rail, it is best to form a habit of raising the rail all the way, because someday that infant will be able to climb out. Crib sides should have a latching device that cannot be easily released. The welds attaching the crib corner locks to the corner posts should not be cracked or broken. If the welds are damaged, the bedspring could fall to the floor. Ideally, cribs should be placed on carpeted, not hard, floors.

Another danger area for falling is a *changing table*, which is usually high and narrow. Although these tables have a restraining belt, children are never left unattended, even when restrained. The best way to prevent having to leave is to arrange the area with all necessary articles within easy reach so that the child is always in full sight of the caregiver. It takes only a fraction of a second for an infant to fall off. During the latter half of the first year, infants usually resist dressing and diapering and may be difficult to manage. If there is danger that the child is strong enough to resist restraining, the infant should be changed on a safer surface, such as a clean floor.

Infant seats, high chairs, walkers, and *swings* present additional opportunities for falls. If the infant seat is placed on a table, the child should never be left unrestrained or unattended. The same rule is essential for other baby equipment, particularly when the child has learned to crawl and to stand up. Small infants can slip through a high chair if a protective harness is not used. The danger of falls from being unrestrained applies to shopping carts as well (Tully, 1993). High chairs are designed for older infants who can sit well and who are tall enough to have the tray at the level of the chest or abdomen. Infant walkers are responsible for a number of different types of injuries that occur because the walker tipped over or fell down stairs. Parents need to be warned of these dangers and encouraged to keep a constant vigil on their child's activities. The American Academy of Pediatrics Committee on Injury and Poison Prevention (1995) does not recommend the use of walkers.

Once infants are mobile, they should not be allowed to crawl unsupervised on any raised surface, near stairs, or near any water reservoir. Gates should be used at the *bottom* and *top* of *stairs*, because both present dangers to the crawling and climbing infant. However, certain types of gates can present hazards. Freestanding enclosures constructed of criss-crossed wood slats that expand and contract can trap the head or neck when children attempt to climb over them. If these types of gates are used, they must be securely fastened to prevent mobility of the slats.

As children begin to pull themselves to a standing position, *heavy objects*, such as unsturdy furniture or any free-standing item (e.g., wrought iron fish tank stands or concrete birdbath), can be extremely dangerous if pulled down on top of the child. To prevent injury from furniture tipping over, TVs should be placed on lower furniture, as far back as possible. Angle braces or anchors can secure furniture to walls.

Sometimes even when the environment is made safe, infants may literally trip over their own feet from *clothing*. Slippery socks; hard, slick soles on shoes or rubber soles that can catch, especially on a carpet; and long pants or pajama bottoms can easily upset a child's balance. Such dangers need to be pointed out to parents, especially when infants are taking their first steps.

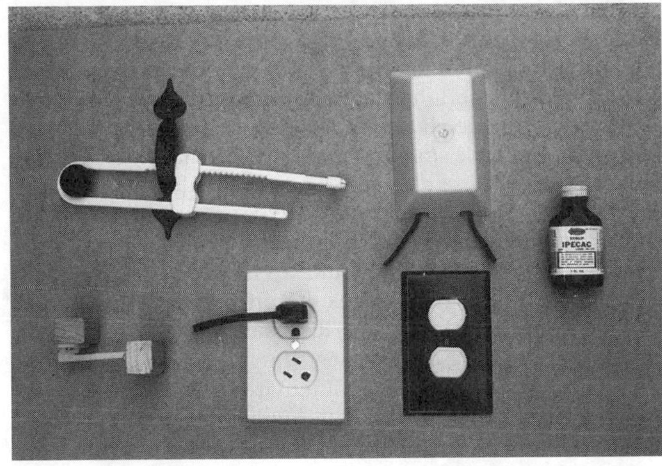

Fig. 33-14 Safety demonstration board. *Clockwise from lower left:* Cabinet latches, shock guard for electrical outlet, syrup of ipecac, and two types of outlet covers (white cover is passive device that automatically covers outlet when plug is removed).

Poisoning

Poisoning is one of the major causes of death in children younger than 5 years of age. The highest incidence occurs in those in the 2-year-old group; the second highest incidence, in 1-year-old children. Infants who do not crawl are relatively free from danger of poisonous agents by virtue of immobility. However, once locomotion begins, danger from poisoning is present almost everywhere. There are more than 500 toxic substances in the average home, and about a third of all poisonings occur in the kitchen.

The major reason for ingestion of poisons is *improper storage*. To protect the infant, toxic agents should not be placed on a low shelf, table, or floor. Drugs that are kept in a purse pose additional dangers; if the purse is given to infants to play with, they may open it and ingest the drug. Another unrecognized hazard is that during diaper changes infants are near many toxic substances such as ointments, creams, oils, and talc. Parents may even hand infants a potentially poisonous object to quiet them. Such dangers need to be stressed to parents, and toys need to be kept at diapering areas to minimize risks.

Plants are another source of poisoning for infants. Plants are frequently placed on the floor, and the leaves or flowers are attractive and easy to pull off. More than 700 species of plants are known to have caused illness or death.

Another danger is ingestion of *button-sized batteries* that are used in devices such as hearing aids, calculators, watches, and cameras. Because they are bright and shiny, they are attractive to children. However, they can cause severe morbidity, even death, if lodged in the esophagus. The strong alkali in a battery can leak and cause a severe caustic burn. As a precaution small batteries must be safely stored and discarded where young children cannot easily retrieve them.

Not all poisonings result from ingestion—*inhalation* is another possible route, such as inhaling chlorine vapors from household cleaning or pool supplies. Recent concern has addressed passive cocaine toxicity in young children exposed to freebase cocaine ("crack") smoking by adults. Children should be protected from environments where these toxins exist (for a discussion of passive cigarette smoking, see Chapter 42).

The only sure way to prevent poisoning is to remove toxic agents; that means placing them high out of the infant's reach. However, because crawling infants soon become climbing toddlers, it is best to keep all toxic agents, especially drugs, in a locked cabinet. Special plastic hooks can be attached to the inside of cabinet doors to keep them securely closed (see Fig. 33-14). Firm thumb pressure is required to unlatch the hook, and small children are usually unable to manipulate them. Locks are best, but for frequently used cleaning agents, such as those often kept under a kitchen sink, hooks are a practical alternative.

With several hundred toxic substances in each house, locking up all potentially toxic substances could present a problem; however, careful planning can help. Having a large surplus of cleaning agents, furniture polishes, laundry additives, paints, insecticides, and solvents should be avoided. Used poison containers should be promptly discarded and not used to store another poison without adequately marking the package. Any potentially hazardous substance should not be stored in any type of food container. A popular container used to store toxic liquids is a soda bottle. A child who is unaware of the dangerous contents is vulnerable for poisoning. Parents should know the location of local poison control centers and call them in the event of a suspected poisoning. Emergency measures for poisoning are discussed in Chapter 43.

Burns

Burns such as scalding from water that is too hot, excessive sunburn, and burns from house fires, electrical wires, sockets, and heating elements such as radiators, registers, and floor furnaces cause a significant number of deaths and many more injuries in infants. The infant's skin is particularly sensitive to irritation, and the mechanisms for temperature preception are not completely developed. As a general precaution, all homes should have smoke alarms installed near the bedroom areas.

Scald burns from *hot tap water* can be prevented by lowering the hot water heater to a safe temperature of 49° C (120° F). In addition, the bathwater should be checked before the infant is immersed. Scalds can also result from bathing infants in the kitchen sink when the garbage disposal, occluded with debris, causes the draining dishwasher effluent to back up into the sink. The temperature of the effluent from a dishwasher is typically that of the maximum water temperature of the household water heater, but many dishwashers are equipped with heating elements that heat water to a temperature that is even higher. As a precaution, instruct caregivers to avoid bathing small children in the kitchen sink while the dishwasher is running.

If formula or food is warmed in a *microwave oven*, it must be checked before feeding because the container may remain cool while the contents are hot. Another danger is explosion of the bottle from the buildup of steam. Because of these dangers, microwaving infant formula or food should be avoided or done according to the guidelines on p. 958. The handles of cooking utensils should be turned toward the back of the stove. When the infant is underfoot, pouring hot liquids and cooking with hot oil are avoided. Hanging tablecloths are also placed out of the infant's reach to prevent pulling hot items off the table.

Sunburn can be a source of a first- or second-degree burn. Exposure to direct sunlight should be avoided. When infants are in the sun, the body, especially the face and head, should be covered. Sunscreen can be used on older infants (see Sunburn, Chapter 49). Although black-skinned infants burn less readily, their thin skin can become sunburned and needs protection.

Electrical outlets should be covered with protective plastic caps that prevent the child from sucking on the outlet or putting objects such as hairpins into it (Fig. 33-14). Live wires are placed out of reach so that curious infants cannot chew on them and break the rubber coating (Fig. 33-15). Infants should not be allowed to play near television sets, stereo units, or other appliances, whether these units are on or off; infants cannot determine when the appliance is safe.

Any *heat-producing element* should have a guard placed in front of it. Fireplaces should be well screened because they are very appealing and within easy access. Small portable heaters should be placed on a high surface. Floor furnaces should have barrier gates to prevent children from crawling or walking over them. Burning cigarettes, candles, and incense are kept out of reach, and infants should not be held by a smoking adult, because falling ashes are a hazard, especially to the eyes. Heated-mist vaporizers are a source of burns and should not be used. If humidity is needed, only cool mist vaporizers are safe.

By law, all infant sleepwear must be flame retardant. Unfortunately, this does not apply to all *infant clothing*. Flame-retardant fabric must never be viewed as the ultimate protection against burns. Repeated washing reduces the flame-retardant properties, and the use of soap or bleach destroys the protection. Detergent should be used for washing flame-retardant clothing, but infants who are sensitive to such agents are unprotected when their clothing is washed even with a mild soap. If sleepwear is home sewn, parents are advised to look for specially treated flame-retardant fabric.

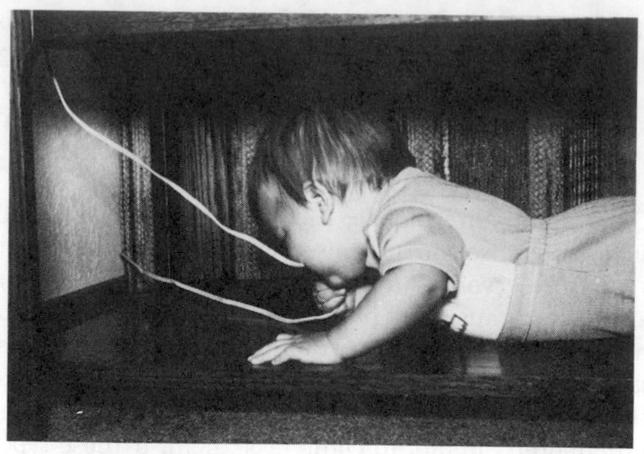

Fig. 33-15 Crawling infants can find hazardous electrical wires even in "hidden" areas.

Another type of thermal injury occurs when children are exposed to excessive heat during confinement in poorly ventilated *vehicles*. The practice of leaving the windows open a couple of inches is not protective. The nurse should caution parents never to leave children in parked cars, especially when the automobile is in direct sunlight.

Children can also be burned by overheated metal hardware and vinyl seats in cars parked in the sun. As a precaution the surface heat of car restraints should be determined before placing children in them. Covering the restraints and hardware (such as metal latches on seat belts) may be necessary to prevent skin burns. An additional safeguard is buying a light-colored restraint, which absorbs less heat.

Drowning

Drowning in this age group can occur in only inches of water. Consequently, infants should never be left unsupervised in a bathtub or hot tub or near a source of water such as a swimming pool, lake, toilet, or bucket. Organized swimming instruction is not recommended for children under 4 years of age, because it may lead to a false sense of security. No infant can be expected to learn the elements of water safety or to react appropriately in an emergency. Therefore all young children need to be considered at risk when near water (American Academy of Pediatrics, Committee on Injury and Poison Prevention, 1993). Infants and toddlers are also at increased risk of infection and convulsions from swallowing large amounts of water.

Bodily Damage

Injuries can occur in numerous ways. Sharp, jagged-edged objects can cause wounds in the skin. Long-pointed articles, such as the common toothpick or fork, can be poked into the eye or ear, causing serious damage. Such articles should be safely stored away from the infant's reach; forks are best avoided for self-feeding until the child has mastered the spoon, usually by age 18 months.

In addition to hazards such as aspiration from toys, small articles can be placed in the ear or nose, and excessive noise from toys can result in sensorineural hearing loss. Although toys with the highest noise levels are model airplanes, air guns, toy cap guns, and firecrackers, even common squeaking toys used by young children may be harmful if placed close to the ear.

Even clothes and hair can present dangers to infants who cannot call attention to the problem. For example, constriction injuries can result from excessively tight bands on socks, as well as fibers of hair or thread wrapped tightly around appendages, usually toes or fingers.

Another frequently unrecognized danger to infants is animal attacks. Helpless infants, as newcomers to the home, can provoke jealousy in animals, especially dogs and cats. However, unprovoked attacks by ferrets and roosters have also been reported. Parents must be constantly vigilant to protect the child from household pets and farm animals (see Animal Bites, Chapter 49).

Nurse's Role in Injury Prevention

When the potential environmental dangers to which infants are vulnerable are considered, the task of preventing these injuries only begins to be appreciated. Nurses must be aware of the possible causes of injury in each age group in order for *anticipatory* preventive teaching to occur. For example, the guidelines for injury prevention during infancy presented in Table 33-10 should be discussed *before* the child reaches the susceptible age group. Preventive teaching ideally occurs during pregnancy. Inasmuch as two-thirds of all injuries to children occur in the home, the importance of safety cannot be overemphasized. The Home Care box on p. 978 summarizes a home safety checklist that can be presented to parents to increase their awareness of danger areas in the home and assist them in implementing safety devices and practices *before* their absence can inflict injury on infants. In addition, displays such as a safety demonstration board (Fig. 33-14) can be helpful in familiarizing parents with inexpensive, commercial devices that can be used in the home to prevent injuries.

To help parents appreciate the dangers present in their home to young children, suggest that they get eye level with the floor to survey the environment from a child's view.

Injury prevention requires protection of the child and education of the caregiver. Nurses in ambulatory care settings, health maintenance centers, or visiting nurse agencies are in a most favorable position for injury education. This does not exclude nurses in inpatient facilities, who can use visiting times as an excellent opportunity for discussing this topic.

One approach to teaching injury prevention is to relate why children in various age groups are prone to specific types of injuries. Stressing prevention is just as important as emphasizing the *why* of the injury. However, injury prevention must also be practical. Asking parents for their ideas leads to realistic suggestions that can be followed. For instance, bathroom cleaning agents, cosmetics, and personal care items can be placed on a top shelf in the linen closet, and towels or sheets can be stored on the lower shelves and floor.

If an injury has occurred, the nurse should not be quick to admonish the parent. Injuries do not always indicate neglect. It is a difficult task to watch children carefully without overprotecting or unnecessarily confining them. Small falls help children learn the dangers of heights. Touching a hot object once can emphasize to the child the pain of a burn. Allowing children to explore while maintaining consistent, age-appropriate limits is sound advice.

Parents need to remember that infants and young children cannot anticipate danger or understand when it is or is not present. A dead electrical wire may present no actual harm, but if the child is allowed to play with it, a poor behavior is enforced and will be practiced when the child encounters a live wire. Although it is always wise to explain why something is dangerous, it must be remembered that small children need to be physically removed from the situation.

It is not easy to teach safety, supervise closely, and refrain from saying "no" a hundred times a day. Parents become acutely aware of this dilemma as soon as the infant learns to crawl. Preventing injuries to children is usually the first reason for limit setting and discipline, but limits are also set to prevent damage to valuable household objects. When small children are in the home, dangerous objects must be removed or guarded and valuable articles placed out of reach.

When children are taught the meaning of "no," they should also be taught what "yes" means. Children should be praised for playing with suitable toys, their efforts at behaving or listening should be reinforced, and recreational toys that are innovative and creative should be provided for them. Infants love to tear paper and avidly pursue books, magazines, or newspapers left on the floor. Instead of always scolding them for destroying a valued book, child-safe books (such as those constructed of fabric) can be kept available for them to play with. If they enjoy pots and pans, a cabinet can be arranged with safe utensils for them to explore.

One additional factor must be stressed concerning injury prevention and education. Children are imitators; they copy what they see and hear. *Practicing safety teaches safety,* which applies to parents and their children and to nurses and their clients. Saying one thing but doing another confuses children and can lead to difficulties as the child grows older.

ANTICIPATORY GUIDANCE—CARE OF FAMILIES

Childrearing is no easy task; it presents challenges to new parents as well as to "seasoned" parents. With society's changing roles and mores, combined with a highly mobile population, there is little stability for traditional role models and time-honored methods of raising children. As a result, parents look more to professionals for guidance. Nurses are in an advantageous position to render assistance and suggestions. Every phase of a child's life has its particular traumas—toilet training for toddlers, unexplained fears for preschoolers, or identity crises for adolescents. For parents of an infant some challenges center around dependency, discipline, increased mob ity, and safety. Major areas for parental guidance d first year are listed in the Home Care box on p.

Home Care

CHILD SAFETY HOME CHECKLIST

Safety: fire, electrical, burns

- ☐ Guards in front of or around any heating appliance, fireplace, or furnace (including floor furnace)*
- ☐ Electrical wires hidden or out of reach*
- ☐ No frayed or broken wires; no overloaded sockets
- ☐ Plastic guards or caps over electical outlets, furniture in front of outlets*
- ☐ Hanging tablecloths out of reach, away from open fires*
- ☐ Smoke detectors tested and operating properly
- ☐ Kitchen matches stored out of child's reach*
- ☐ Large, deep ashtrays throughout house (if used)
- ☐ Small stoves, heaters, and other hot objects (cigarettes, candles, coffee pots, slow cookers) placed where they cannot be tipped over or reached by children
- ☐ Hot water heater set at 49° C (120° F) or lower
- ☐ Pot handles turned toward back of stove, center of table
- ☐ No loose clothing worn near stove
- ☐ No cooking or eating hot foods or liquids with child standing nearby or sitting in lap
- ☐ All small appliances, such as iron, turned off, disconnected, and placed out of reach when not in use
- ☐ Cool, not hot, mist vaporizer used
- ☐ Fire extinguisher available on each floor and checked periodically
- ☐ Electric fuse box and gas outlet accessible
- ☐ Family escape plan in case of a fire practiced periodically; fire escape ladder available on upper-level floors
- ☐ Telephone number of fire or rescue squad and address of home with nearest cross street posted near phone

Safety: suffocation and aspiration

- ☐ Small objects stored out of reach*
- ☐ Toys inspected for small removable parts or long strings*
- ☐ Hanging crib toys and mobiles placed out of reach
- ☐ Plastic bags stored away from young child's reach, large plastic garment bags discarded after tying in knots*
- ☐ Mattress or pillow not covered with plastic or in manner accessible to child*
- ☐ Crib design according to federal regulations (crib slats less than 2$^{3}/_{8}$ inches [6 cm] apart) with snug-fitting mattress*†
- ☐ Crib positioned away from other furniture or windows*
- ☐ Portable playpen gates up at all times while in use*
- ☐ Accordion-style gates not used*
- ☐ Bathroom doors kept closed and toilet seats down*
- ☐ Faucets turned off firmly*
- ☐ Pool fenced with locked gate
- ☐ Proper safety equipment at poolside
- ☐ Electric garage door openers stored safely and garage door adjusted to rise when door strikes object
- ☐ Doors of ovens, trunks, dishwashers, refrigerators, and front-loading clothes washers and dryers kept closed*
- ☐ Unused appliance, such as a refrigerator, securely closed with lock or doors removed*
- ☐ Food served in small noncylindric pieces*
- ☐ Toy chests without lids or with lids that securely lock in open position*
- ☐ Buckets and wading pools kept empty when not in use*
- ☐ Clothesline above head level
- ☐ At least one member of household trained in basic life support (CPR), including first aid for choking‡

Safety: poisoning

- ☐ Toxic substances, including batteries, placed on a high shelf, preferably in locked cabinet
- ☐ Toxic plants hung or placed out of reach*
- ☐ Excess quantities of cleaning fluid, paints, pesticides, drugs, and other toxic substances not stored in home
- ☐ Used containers of poisonous substances discarded where child cannot obtain access
- ☐ Telephone number of local poison control center and address of home with nearest cross street posted near phone
- ☐ Syrup of ipecac in home containing two doses per child
- ☐ Medicines clearly labeled in childproof containers and stored out of reach
- ☐ Household cleaners, disinfectants, and insecticides kept in their original containers, separate from food and out of reach
- ☐ Smoking in areas away from children

Safety: falls

- ☐ Nonskid mats, strips, or surfaces in tubs and showers
- ☐ Exits, halls, and passageways in rooms kept clear of toys, furniture, boxes, or other items that could be obstructive
- ☐ Stairs and halls well lighted, with switches at both top and bottom
- ☐ Sturdy handrails for all steps and stairways
- ☐ Nothing stored on stairways
- ☐ Treads, risers, and carpeting in good repair
- ☐ Glass doors and walls marked with decals
- ☐ Safety glass used in doors, windows, and walls
- ☐ Gates on top and bottom of staircases and elevated areas, such as porch, fire escape*
- ☐ Guardrails on upstairs windows with locks that limit height of window opening and access to areas such as fire escape*
- ☐ Crib side rails raised to full height; mattress lowered as child grows*
- ☐ Restraints used in high chairs, walkers, or other baby furniture; preferably walkers not used*
- ☐ Scatter rugs secured in place or used with nonskid back
- ☐ Walks, patios, and driveways in good repair

Safety: bodily injury

- ☐ Knives, power tools, and unloaded firearms stored safely or placed in locked cabinet
- ☐ Garden tools returned to storage racks after use
- ☐ Pets properly restrained and immunized for rabies
- ☐ Swings, slides, and other outdoor play equipment kept in safe condition
- ☐ Yard free of broken glass, nail-studded boards, other litter
- ☐ Cement birdbaths placed where young child cannot tip them over*

*Safety measures are specific for homes with young children. All safety measures should be implemented in homes where children reside and visit frequently, such as those of grandparents or baby-sitters.

†Federal regulations are available from U.S. Consumer Product Safety Commission; (800) 638-CPSC.

‡Home care instructions for infant cardiopulmonary resuscitation and infant/child choking are available in Wong DL: *Wong and Whaley's clinical manual of pediatric nursing,* ed 4, St. Louis, 1996, Mosby.

Home Care

GUIDANCE DURING INFANT'S FIRST YEAR

First 6 months

Understand each parent's adjustment to newborn, especially mother's postpartal emotional needs.
Teach care of infant and assist parents to understand his or her individual needs and temperament and that the infant expresses wants through crying.
Reassure parents that infant cannot be spoiled by too much attention during the first 4 to 6 months.
Encourage parents to establish a schedule that meets their needs and the child's.
Help parents understand infant's need for stimulation in environment.
Support parents' pleasure in seeing child's growing friendliness and social response, especially smiling.
Plan anticipatory guidance for safety.
Stress need for immunization.
Prepare for introduction of solid foods.

Second 6 months

Prepare parents for child's "stranger fear."
Encourage parents to allow child to cling to them and avoid long separation from either.
Guide parents concerning discipline because of infant's increasing mobility.
Encourage use of negative voice and eye contact rather than physical punishment as a means of discipline.
Encourage showing most attention when infant is behaving well, rather than when infant is crying.
Teach injury prevention because of child's advancing motor skills and curiosity.
Encourage parents to leave child with suitable caregiver to allow some free time.
Discuss readiness for weaning.
Explore parents' feelings regarding infant's sleep patterns.

Special Health Problems

FEEDING DIFFICULTIES

Regurgitation and "Spitting Up"

The return of small amounts of food after a feeding is a common occurrence during infancy. It should not be confused with actual vomiting, which can be associated with a number of disturbances, both insignificant and serious (see Chapter 44). For clarification the following terms are defined:

Spitting up—Dribbling of unswallowed formula from the infant's mouth immediately after a feeding
Regurgitation—Return of undigested food from the stomach, usually accompanied by burping

The insignificance of regurgitation or spitting up should be explained to parents, especially to those who are concerned. It can be reduced by some simple measures, such as frequent burping during and after feeding, minimal handling at feeding and after, and positioning of the child on the right side with the head slightly elevated after feeding. The inconvenience of spitting up is managed with the use of absorbent bibs on the infant and protective cloths on the parent.

Sometimes, frequent dribbling of formula causes excoriation of the corners of the mouth, chin, and neck. Keeping the area dry prevents skin breakdown but can be difficult. Helpful suggestions include applying a thin film of petrolatum or A & D ointment to the affected areas after cleansing and using absorbent nonplastic-lined terrycloth bibs that are changed frequently.

Paroxysmal Abdominal Pain (Colic)

Colic is generally described as paroxysmal abdominal pain or cramping that is manifested by loud crying and drawing the legs up to the abdomen. Other definitions include variables such as duration of cry greater than 3 hours a day and parental dissatisfaction with the child's behavior. Colic is more common in infants under the age of 3 months than in older infants, and infants with "difficult" temperaments are more likely to be colicky. Despite the obvious behavioral indications of pain, the child tolerates the formula well, gains weight, and thrives.

Among the theories that have been investigated as potential causes are too rapid feeding, overeating, swallowing of excessive air, improper feeding technique (especially in positioning and burping), and emotional stress or tension between parent and child. Although all of these may occur, there is no evidence that one factor is consistently present. In some infants colic may be a sign of cow's milk allergy or intolerance, and eliminating cow's milk products from the infant's diet and the diet of lactating mothers can reduce the symptoms. (See cow's milk allergy, Chapter 44.) Parental smoking has also been associated with colic.

Therapeutic management. Management of colic should begin with an investigation of diagnosable causes, such as cow's milk allergy. If a sensitivity to cow's milk is strongly suspected, a trial substitution of another formula, such as a casein hydrolysate (Nutramigen), is warranted. Soy formulas are avoided because of the possibility of sensitivity to soy protein as well. When no specific cause can be found, the supportive measures discussed under Nursing Considerations are employed.

The use of drugs, including sedatives, antispasmodics antihistamines, and antiflatulents, is sometimes recommended. The most commonly used sedatives are phenobarbitol and hydroxyzine hydrochloride (Atarax).

Nursing ALERT

The antispasmodic dicyclomine hydrochloride (Bentyl) is not recommended for infants under 6 months of age because of rare instances of death.

Nursing care management. The initial step in managing colic is to take a thorough, detailed history of the usual daily events. Areas that should be stressed include the following: (1) diet of the breastfeeding mother; (2) time of day when attacks occur; (3) relationship of the attacks to feeding time;

Home Care

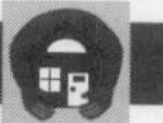

RELIEVING COLIC

Place infant prone over a covered hot-water bottle, heated towel, or covered heating pad.
Massage abdomen.
Change infant's position frequently; walk with child's face down and body across the parent's arm, with the hand under the abdomen applying gentle pressure (Fig. 33-16).
Use a front carrier for transporting infant.
Swaddle tightly with a soft, stretchy blanket.
Place in a wind-up swing.
Take for car rides or outside for a change in environment.
Use a commercial device* in the crib that simulates the vibration and sound of a car ride.
Provide smaller, frequent feedings; burp during and after feedings using the shoulder position, and place in an upright seat after feedings.
Introduce a pacifier for added sucking.
In breastfed infants, mother should avoid all milk products for a trial period.
If household members smoke, avoid smoking near infant; preferably confine smoking activity to outside home.
If nothing reduces the crying, place infant in crib and allow to cry; periodically hold and comfort child and put down again.

*Sweet Dreams, Inc., SleepTight Order Department, 4710 E. Walnut St., Westerville, Ohio 43081; (800) NO COLIC ([800] 662-6542).

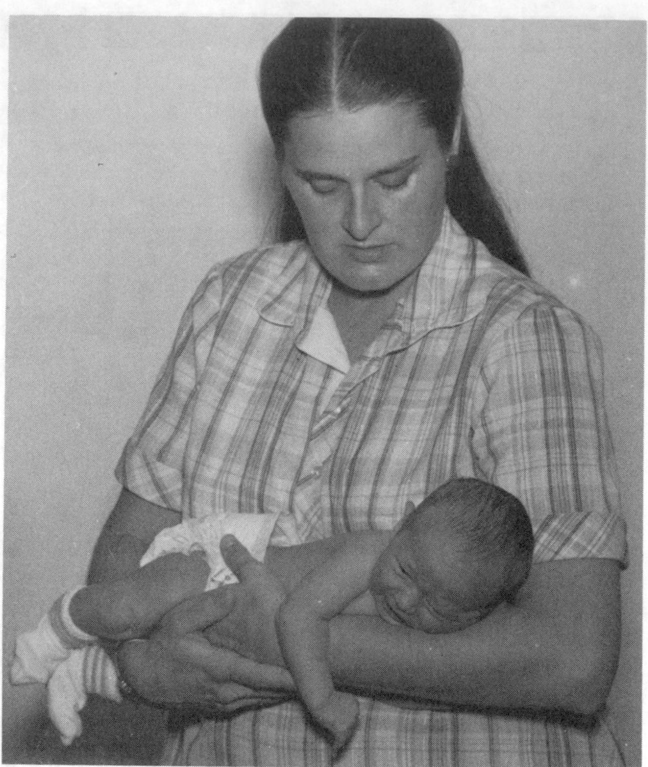

Fig. 33-16 The "colic carry" may be comforting to an infant with colic.

(4) presence of specific family members during attacks, and habits, such as smoking by family members; (5) activity of the mother or usual caregiver before, during, and after the crying; (6) characteristics of the cry (duration, intensity); and (7) measures used to relieve the crying and their effectiveness. Of special emphasis is a careful assessment of the feeding process via *demonstration* by the parent.

If milk sensitivity is suspected, bottle-fed infants and breastfeeding mothers should follow a milk-free diet for a minimum of 5 days in an attempt to reduce symptoms in the infant. Mothers should be cautioned that some nondairy creamers may contain calcium caseinate, a cow's milk protein. If this approach is helpful, lactating mothers may need calcium supplements to meet the body's requirement. Bottle-fed infants may improve with the same dietary modifications as for the child with cow's milk allergy.

More often than not, no change is required in feeding practices. When no cause can be identified, it is preferable to determine the time of the onset of crying and attempt to manipulate the circumstances associated with it. For example, some infants have episodes of colic around the family's dinner time, when all household members are home and the mother is preoccupied with cooking. The overstimulating, more tense atmosphere may upset the infant. Encouraging someone else to prepare dinner or the mother to prepare dinner earlier in the day and feed the infant in a more quiet area of the house may help reverse the environmental conditions that may have provoked the attack of colic. Other approaches for relieving colic are listed in the Home Care box above. Parents are encouraged to try as many of these approaches as possible, because not all are effective for every infant (see also the Family Focus and Critical Thinking Q & A boxes on p. 981).

Failure to Thrive (FTT)

FTT is a sign of inadequate growth resulting from inability to obtain and/or use calories required for growth. FTT has no universal definition, although one of the more common parameters is a weight (and sometimes height) that falls below the 5th percentile for the child's age. Some authorities prefer the 3rd percentile as a criterion, but the widely used National Center for Health Statistics growth charts include only the 5th, not the 3rd, percentile in their measurements. Growth measurements alone are not used to diagnose children with FTT. Rather, the finding of a persistent deviation from an established growth curve is cause for concern.

Three general categories of failure to thrive are:

Organic failure to thrive (OFTT)—result of a physical cause, such as congenital heart defects, neurologic lesions, microcephaly, chronic renal failure, gastroesophageal reflux, malabsorption syndrome, endocrine dysfunction, cystic fibrosis, or acquired immunodeficiency syndrome (AIDS).

Nonorganic failure to thrive (NFTT)—has a definable cause that is unrelated to disease. NFTT is most often the result of psychosocial factors, such as inadequate nutritional knowledge of the parent; deficiency in maternal care or a disturbance in maternal-child attachment; or a disturbance in the child's ability to separate from the parent, leading to food refusal to maintain attention.

Idiopathic failure to thrive—unexplained by the usual organic and environmental causes but may also be

Family Focus 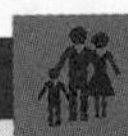

COLIC

Although colic is considered a minor ailment, the presence of a colicky, crying, irritable infant can have an intense emotional impact on parent-child attachment and family relationships. Parents, especially mothers, often relate histories of a daily routine that is laden with feelings of frustration, anger, despair, and helplessness. A vicious circle ensues in which the parent's own anxiety may be transferred to the infant, further increasing the tension, irritability, and crying.

One of the most important areas of nursing concern is the support of parents during the colic period. It should be stressed that despite the crying and obvious pain, the infant is doing well. Colic disappears spontaneously, usually by 3 months of age, although guarantees should never be given, because it may continue much longer. The parent, especially the mother, should be encouraged to leave the house and arrange for some free time. Most important, it should be emphasized that colic does not indicate poor or inadequate parenting. Parents' negative feelings toward the infant and insecurities regarding their parenting abilities are normal. Parents are encouraged to talk about such feelings, since active listening may do more to relieve the colic syndrome than offering stereotyped advice, remedies, and glib statements such as "Don't worry about it; your child will eventually outgrow the colicky spells."

Critical Thinking  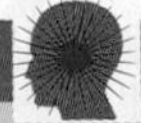

COLIC

During a routine clinic visit you notice that the mother of a 2-month-old infant appears very tired, readily becomes confused answering simple questions, and casually mentions that the infant cries much more than her first child did and for no apparent reason. You direct the focus of the interview on the infant's behavior preceding the crying spells; feeding habits, including dietary history; and patterns of sleep. The mother suspects that the infant has colic. The best response to this mother is:

1. "Well, Dr. Smith will be in shortly, and you can discuss this with her."
2. "You must feel frustrated about this situation; can you tell me more about your concerns?"
3. "Colic is a complex problem for which there are few solutions other than giving the child medications and tolerating the crying the best way possible."
4. "We have some pamphlets on colic in the lobby; after you see the doctor, be sure to pick one up and read it at home."

The correct answer is two. This allows the mother time to express her feelings about the colicky infant, as well as her own fears about childrearing and possible inadequacies, and opens the door for a discussion of some solutions to the problem. The other options end the discussion and suggest that the mother or another health professional is responsible for a solution.

classified as NFTT. Both categories of NFTT account for the majority of cases of FTT.

Traditionally the category of NFTT has implied a disturbance in the parent-child interaction. However, this is not always the case. Many other factors can lead to inadequate feeding of the infant, such as the following:

Poverty—lack of funds to buy sufficient food; may dilute formula to extend available supply

Health beliefs—use of fad diets; excessive concern with preventing conditions such as obesity, hypercholesterolemia, or nursing caries

Inadequate nutritional knowledge—cultural confusion of newly arrived immigrants who are unaware of appropriate food selections in American markets; parents with cognitive impairment

Family stress—overwhelming involvement with another chronically ill child; any number of other stresses (financial, marital, excessive parenting and employment responsibilities, depression, chemical abuse, acute grief)

Feeding resistance—result of nonoral nutritional therapy early in life

Insufficient breast milk—result of a number of different causes (fatigue, illness, poor release of milk, insufficient glandular tissue, lack of maternal confidence)

In these instances parent education and provision of necessary supports (financial or psychosocial) are successful in correcting the reason for the malnutrition. Dealing with families in which a child has NFTT because of a parent-child disturbance is much more difficult and is the focus of the nursing care discussion on p. 982.

Diagnostic evaluation. Diagnosis is initially made from evidence of growth retardation. If FTT is recent, the weight, but not the height, is below accepted standards (usually the 5th percentile); if FTT is long-standing, both weight and height are depressed, indicating chronic malnutrition. Additional diagnostic procedures include a complete health and dietary history, physical examination for evidence of organic causes, developmental assessment, and a family assessment. Other tests are selected *only* as indicated to rule out organic problems. To prevent the overuse of diagnostic procedures, NFTT should be considered *early* in the differential diagnosis.

Therapeutic management. Regardless of the cause of FTT, the treatment is directed at reversing the malnutrition. The goal is to provide sufficient calories to support "catch-up" growth—a rate of growth greater than the expected rate for age. Any coexisting medical problems are treated.

In most cases of NFTT, a multidisciplinary team of physician, nurse, dietitian, child-life specialist, and social worker or mental health professional is needed to deal with the multiple psychologic problems. Efforts are made to relieve any additional stresses on the family, such as referrals to welfare agencies or supplemental food programs.

Prognosis. The prognosis for NFTT is related to the cause. If the parents have simply been ignorant of the infant's needs, teaching may remedy the child's limited caloric intake and permanently reverse the growth failure. Inadequate or decreased feeding periods by the infant's primary caregiver are often observed as the cause of NFTT in conjunction with family disorganization. When family dysfunction is extensive, the prognosis is uncertain. Factors related to poor prognosis are severe feeding resistance, lack of awareness in and cooperation from the parent(s), low family income, low maternal educational level, and early age of onset of NFTT. Many of these children are below normal in intellectual development, have poorer language development and less well developed reading skills, attain lower social maturity, and have a higher incidence of behavioral disturbances. Such findings indicate that a long-term plan is needed for the optimal development of these children.

Nursing Care Management

Assessment

Nurses play a critical role in the diagnosis of NFTT through their assessment of the child, parents, and family interaction. Knowledge of the characteristics of children with NFTT and their families is essential in helping identify these children and hastening the confirmation of a correct diagnosis (Box 33-1). Accurate assessment of initial weight and height and daily weight, as well as recording of all food intake, is vital. The feeding behavior of the child is documented, as well as the parent-child interaction during feeding, other caregiving activities, and play. (See also Nutritional Assessment, Chapter 31.) The approximate developmental age should be assessed on admission by administering an appropriate developmental test. Only after objective measurements are available is a plan of care for stimulation outlined.

The nursing admission history and ongoing assessment should also focus on the following characteristics that have been identified in many of these children and their parents.

The child. Besides the obvious signs of malnutrition and delayed development, children with NFTT (Box 33-1) may interact differently from children with OFTT. They display intense interest in inanimate objects, such as toys, and much less interest in social interactions. They are vigilant of people at a distance but become increasingly distressed as they approach them. They dislike being touched or held and avoid face-to-face contact. However, when they are held, they protest briefly on being put down and are apathetic when left alone.

Frequently there is a history of difficult feeding, vomiting, sleep disturbance, and excessive irritability. Habit patterns such as crying during feedings, vomiting, hoarding food in the mouth, ruminating after feeding, refusing to switch from liquids to solids, and demonstrating aversion behavior, such as turning from food or spitting food, become attention-seeking mechanisms to prolong the attention received at mealtime. In addition, chronic reduction in calories can lead to appetite depression, which compounds the problem.

A feature of many children with NFTT is their irregularity (low rhythmicity) in activities of daily living. Some of these children typify the "difficult" temperament pattern. However, another type is the passive, sleepy, lethargic infant who does not wake up for feedings. Parents who have been advised of "demand feeding schedules" may be unsure of whether to wake the child or let the child sleep. Because of their inexperience and lack of guidance, parents may develop a pattern of infrequent feeding that is inadequate to meet the infant's nutritional needs. Such a pattern is particularly detrimental to the breastfeeding infant, in whom frequent nursing is essential to an adequate milk supply. Such characteristics in a child do not necessarily result in NFTT. Rather, a complex set of variables is significant, such as the degree of *fit* between the child's temperament and that of the parents. Since the personalities of infants can have definite effects on the parent-child attachment process, identifying such situations of disharmony may be one approach to prevention and anticipatory guidance.

BOX 33-1
Clinical Manifestations of Nonorganic Failure to Thrive

Growth failure—below 5th percentile in weight only or weight and height
Developmental retardation—social, motor, adaptive, language
Apathy
Poor hygiene
Withdrawn behavior
Feeding or eating disorders, such as vomiting, anorexia, pica, rumination
No fear of strangers (at age when stranger fear is normal)
Avoidance of eye contact
Wide-eyed gaze and continual scan of the environment ("radar gaze")
Stiff and unyielding or flaccid and unresponsive
Minimal smiling

The parents. Some parents are at increased risk for attachment problems because of (1) isolation and social crisis, (2) inadequate support systems, and (3) poor parenting as a child. Other factors that should be considered are lack of education; physical and mental health problems, such as retardation, depression, or drug dependence; immaturity, especially in adolescent parents; and lack of commitment to parenting, such as giving higher priority to career goals. Frequently these parents and their families are under stress and in multiple chronic emotional, social, and financial crises.

Nursing Diagnoses

A number of nursing diagnoses are prominent in the nursing care of the child with NFTT. The most common nursing diagnoses are as follows:

- Altered nutrition: less than body requirements related to
  Deprivation of necessities
  Emotional deprivation
- Altered growth and development related to
  Socially restricted environment (infant deprivation)
  Physical neglect
- Altered parenting related to (specify, e.g., knowledge deficit, poverty)

If an organic cause is found, additional nursing diagnoses may be related to care specific for that disorder, such as heart disease.

Planning

Planning needs to begin as soon as possible on admission. The highest-priority nursing goal is providing the infant with sufficient nutrients for growth. More specific nursing care depends on the identified cause of FTT. If an organic cause is confirmed, care is related primarily to management of the dis-

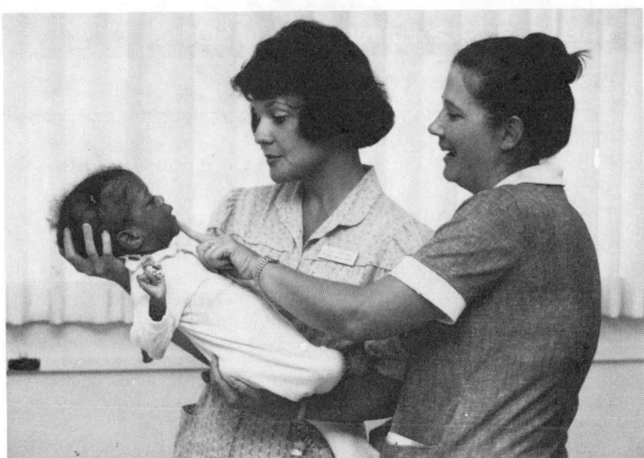

Fig. 33-17 A consistent nurse is important in developing trust in infants with nonorganic failure to thrive.

order. If the problem is one of inadequate knowledge regarding child feeding, parental education is required. When serious psychosocial factors are involved, hospitalization is needed and additional interventions are required to meet the needs of both the child and the family. The following are goals for the hospitalized child with NFTT and the family:

1. The child will experience weight gain.
2. The child will demonstrate positive response to developmental stimulation.
3. The family will demonstrate ability to provide appropriate care to child.
4. The family will receive adequate support and home services.

Implementation

Since part of the difficulty between parent and child are dissatisfaction and frustration, the child should have a consistent primary nurse for all three shifts (Fig. 33-17). Only the same nurse caring for the child over a period of time can learn to perceive the child's cues and reverse the cycle of dissatisfaction, especially in the area of feeding. Since these children are not ill with any physical disorder but debilitated from general malnutrition, they should be placed in a room with noninfectious children of a similar age.

Because many of these children are responding to stimuli that have led to the negative feeding patterns, the first goal is to structure the feeding environment to encourage eating. Initially staff members may need to feed these children to assess thoroughly the difficulties encountered during the feeding process and to devise strategies that eliminate or minimize such problems. General guidelines for the feeding process are outlined in the Guidelines box above.

Foods appropriate to the child's age are selected. To increase caloric intake, supplements, such as Polycose or powdered milk, can be added to foods, and powdered commercial formula can be prepared to yield 24 cal/oz rather than 20 cal/oz.

Besides attending to the physical needs of the child, the nurse must plan care for appropriate developmental stimulation. Once an approximate developmental age is established, a planned program of play is begun. Ideally a child-life specialist is involved to implement and supervise the stimulation program. Every effort is made to teach the parent how to play and interact with the child.

Nursing care of these children involves a "systems" approach. In other words, for the entire family to become healthy, each member must be helped to change. Care of the parents is aimed at helping them increase their feelings of self-esteem through positive, successful parenting skills. Initially this necessitates providing an environment in which they feel welcomed and accepted. Because these parents are often distrustful of authority figures, it may take some time before they develop any trust toward the nurse. One approach is to empathize with the parent about the difficulties of childrearing. For example, the nurse may state that many parents find adjusting to parenthood a trying time or that the demands of caring for an infant can become overwhelming.

Guidelines

FEEDING CHILDREN WITH NONORGANIC FAILURE TO THRIVE

Provide a primary core of staff to feed the child. The same nurses are able to learn the child's cues and respond consistently.

Provide a quiet, unstimulating atmosphere. A number of these children are very distractible, and their attention is diverted with minimal stimuli. Older children do well at a feeding table; younger children should always be held.

Maintain a calm, even temperament throughout the meal. Negative outbursts may be commonplace in this child's habit formation. Limits on eating behavior definitely need to be provided, but they should be stated in a firm, calm tone. If the nurse is hurried or anxious, the feeding process will not be optimized.

Talk to the child by giving directions about eating. "Take a bite, Lisa" is appropriate and directive. The more distractible the child, the more directive the nurse should be to refocus attention on feeding. Positive comments about feeding are given.

Be persistent. This is perhaps one of the most important guidelines. Parents often give up when the child begins negative feeding behavior. Calm perseverance through 10 to 15 minutes of food refusal will eventually diminish negative behavior. Although forced feeding is avoided, "strictly encouraged" feeding is essential.

Maintain a face-to-face posture with the child when possible. Encourage eye contact and remain with the child throughout the meal.

Introduce new foods slowly. Often these children have been exclusively bottle-fed. If acceptance of solids is a problem, begin with pureed food and, once it is accepted, advance to junior and regular solid foods.

Follow the child's rhythm of feeding. The child will set a rhythm when the previous conditions are met.

Develop a structured routine. Disruption in their other activities of daily living has great impact on feeding responses, so bathing, sleeping, dressing, and playing, as well as feeding, are structured. The nurse should feed the child in the same way and place as often as possible. The length of the feeding should also be established (usually 30 minutes).

Teaching infant care techniques to the parents is begun through *example* and *demonstration*, not through lecturing. As the nurse perceives the infant's cues, these are emphasized to the parents. For example, during a feeding the nurse may comment that the infant is still hungry because the child sucks vigorously and looks at the nurse. When the infant is satisfied, the nurse points out that the infant is signaling this by releasing the strong suck, closing the eyes, and breathing deeply and more slowly. By example, the child is gently placed into the crib for a nap.

At the same time, the parents are offered an opportunity to care for the infant without having demands made on them. For example, the nurse suggests that at the next feeding one of the parents offer the child the bottle. Whenever the parents participate, they are praised and encouraged to continue caring for the child.

Plans are made to continue these interventions at home. A public health or home health referral is made, and if a foster grandparent is included, this person should also visit the family. Social agencies that can provide financial or housing assistance to lessen the stress of everyday life are also contacted.

Evaluation

The effectiveness of nursing interventions is determined by continual reassessment and evaluation of care, based on the following observational guidelines and expected outcomes:

1. Record weight and caloric intake daily; document child's reaction to feeding environment; review notes to see whether changes were made as necessary to improve eating and whether consistent group of nurses fed child.
2. Perform developmental screening tests as needed.
3. Document parents' relationship with child, staff and other supportive individuals. Note length of time parents visit, appointments kept with referral services, and any requests for help.
4. Keep a record of all client teaching and note whether outcome behaviors were met.

Expected outcomes:

1. Child gains weight (specify) (usually a minimum of 1 to 2 oz/day).
2. Child displays a positive response to interventions (e.g., social smile).
3. Family demonstrates ability to provide appropriate care to child.
4. Family experiences reduction of anxiety and follows through on programs and activities.

See also Nursing Care Plan: The Child with Nonorganic Failure to Thrive.*

DISORDERS OF UNKNOWN ETIOLOGY

Sudden Infant Death Syndrome (SIDS)

SIDS is defined as the sudden death of an infant under 1 year of age that remains unexplained after a complete postmortem examination, including an investigation of the death scene and a review of the case history. It is the leading cause of death in children between the ages of 1 month and 1 year and claims the lives of 7000 infants annually. Table 33-12 summarizes the major epidemiologic characteristics of SIDS.

TABLE 33-12 Epidemiology of SIDS

FACTORS	OCCURRENCE
Incidence	1.4:1000 live births
Peak age	2 to 4 months; 95% occur by 6 months
Sex	Higher percentage of males affected
Time of death	During sleep
Time of year	Increased incidence in winter; peak in January
Racial	Greater incidence in Native Americans and blacks, followed by whites, Asians, and Hispanics
Socioeconomic	Increased occurrence in lower socioeconomic class
Birth	Higher incidence in: Premature infants, especially infants of low birth weight Multiple births* Neonates with low Apgar scores Infants with central nervous system disturbances and respiratory disorders such as bronchopulmonary dysplasia Increasing birth order (subsequent siblings as opposed to firstborn child) Infants with a recent history of illness
Sleep habits	Prone position; use of soft bedding; overheating (thermal stress)
Feeding habits	Lower incidence in breastfed infants
Siblings	May have greater incidence
Maternal	Young age; cigarette smoking, especially during pregnancy; substance abuse (heroin, methadone, cocaine)

*Although a rare event, simultaneous death of twins from SIDS can occur.

Cause. Numerous theories have been proposed regarding the cause of SIDS; however, the cause is unknown. The most compelling hypothesis is that SIDS is related to a brainstem abnormality in the neurologic regulation of cardiorespiratory control. Abnormalities include prolonged sleep apnea, increased frequency of brief inspiratory pauses, excessive periodic breathing, and impaired arousal responsiveness to increased carbon dioxide or decreased oxygen. However, sleep apnea is not the cause of SIDS. The vast majority of infants with apnea do not die, and only a minority of SIDS victims have documented *apparent life-threatening events (ALTEs)* (see Apnea of Infancy, p. 986). A theory that has been disproved associated SIDS with diphtheria, tetanus, and pertussis vaccines. The role of maternal smoking, or exposure to secondhand smoke in the house, has been postulated, yet no conclusive evidence has pointed to that as the single cause of SIDS.

Studies from countries other than the United States link sleep habits with an increased risk of SIDS. Sleeping in the

*In Wong DL: *Wong and Whaley's clinical manual of pediatric nursing*, ed 4, St Louis, 1996, Mosby.

prone position may cause oropharyngeal obstruction or affect the thermal balance or arousal state. Whether sleeping in the prone position is in itself a risk factor or whether it depends on some other condition, such as sleeping on soft bedding, is unknown. Another postulated theory is that SIDS may be caused by rebreathing of CO_2. Infants sleeping prone may be unable to move their heads to the side, thus increasing the risk of suffocation and lethal rebreathing (Kemp and others, 1993).

Nursing ALERT

Such findings have important implications for practices that may reduce the risk of SIDS, such as encouraging supine or side-lying sleeping positions; avoiding soft, moldable mattresses and pillows; and avoiding overheating during sleep. The American Academy of Pediatrics recommends the supine or side-lying sleep position for healthy infants (Infant sleep position, 1994). Infants with breathing problems or excessive vomiting should continue to sleep prone on a firm surface mattress or bedding.

Although the cause is unknown, autopsies reveal consistent pathologic findings, such as pulmonary edema and intrathoracic hemorrhages, that confirm the diagnosis of SIDS. Consequently, all infants suspected of dying of SIDS should have an autopsy, and these findings shared with the parents as soon as possible after the death.

Children at risk for SIDS. Certain groups of children are at increased risk for SIDS. These groups include the following:

1. Infants with one or more severe ALTEs requiring cardiopulmonary resuscitation (CPR) or vigorous stimulation
2. Preterm infants who continue to have pathologic apnea at the time of hospital discharge
3. Siblings of two or more SIDS victims
4. Infants with certain types of diseases or conditions, such as central hypoventilation

Home monitoring and/or the use of respiratory stimulant drugs is recommended for these groups of children. No diagnostic tests exist to predict which infants, including those in the groups discussed, will survive or die, and home monitoring is no guarantee of survival. At the present time, strategies to prevent SIDS are best directed at decreasing known or suspected risk factors, such as mothers seeking adequate prenatal care and avoiding cigarette smoking and drug abuse both before and after the child's birth. In addition, adherence to the guidelines for nonprone sleeping in healthy term infants is a positive step for the prevention of SIDS.

Whether subsequent siblings of the SIDS infant are at increased risk for SIDS is unclear. Even if the increased risk is correct, families have a 99% chance that their subsequent child will *not* die of SIDS. Home monitoring is not recommended for this group of children but is often used by practitioners.

Nursing care management. Loss of a child from SIDS presents several crises with which the parents must cope. In addition to grief and mourning for the death of their child, the parents must face a tragedy that was extremely sudden, unexpected, and unexplained. The psychologic intervention for the family must deal with these additional variables. This discussion focuses primarily on the objectives of care for families experiencing SIDS, rather than on the process of grief and mourning, which is explored in Chapter 39.

One approach to delineating the nursing care plan for these families is to base it on the usual sequence of events that occurs after the infant is found. This approach encompasses the different areas in which nurses may be involved with the family.

Finding the infant. Usually it is the mother who finds the child dead in the crib. Typically the child is in a disheveled bed, with blankets over the head, and huddled into a corner. Frothy, blood-tinged fluid fills the mouth and nostrils, and the infant may be lying face down in the secretions, suggesting that he or she bled to death. The diaper is wet and full of stool, as is consistent with a cataclysmic type of death. The hands may be clutching the sheets, as if the child were in distress before death. The initial appearance of the child combined with the shock of such an unexpected event adds to the horror that the parents must face.

Frequently the mother is alone and must deal with her initial shock, panic, grief, questions of the other siblings, and the decision of where to find help. The first persons to arrive may be the police and ambulance attendants. Ideally they will handle the situation by asking few questions; giving *no* indication of wrongdoing, abuse, or neglect; making sensitive judgments concerning the resuscitation efforts for the child; and comforting the members of the family as much as possible. These individuals should be properly informed about SIDS in order to recognize its characteristic signs and tell parents that their child probably died of a disease called sudden infant death syndrome, which cannot be predicted or prevented. A compassionate, sensitive approach to the family during the very first few minutes can help spare them some of the overwhelming guilt and anguish that frequently follow this type of death.

Arriving at the emergency room. The first contact that nurses typically have with these families is in the emergency room, when the infant is seen by a physician in order to be pronounced dead. Usually there is no attempt at resuscitation. During the time in the emergency room several aspects warrant special consideration. Parents are asked only factual questions, such as when they found the infant, how he or she looked, and whom they called for help. Any remarks that may suggest responsibility, such as why they didn't go in earlier, didn't they hear the infant cry out, was the head buried in a blanket, or were the other siblings jealous of this child, are avoided.

The events that took place when help arrived are discussed. If resuscitation was attempted, the infant may have fractured ribs, internal bleeding, and traumatic bruising, which can simulate physical abuse. Also, if statements were made that were misguided, such as "This looks like suffocation," they can be corrected before parents harbor them in their minds as indications of their guilt. The discussion of an autopsy should be presented at this time, emphasizing that a diagnosis cannot be confirmed until the postmortem examination is completed. Instructions about the autopsy and funeral arrangements may need to be repeated or put in writing. If the mother was breastfeeding, she needs information about abrupt discontinuation of lactation.

Another important aspect of compassionate care for these parents is allowing them to say good-bye to their child. Before they go into the examining room, any blood or emesis is removed from the child, the body is covered partially with a sheet or blanket, and the room is put in order, especially if instruments and equipment were used. These are the parents' last moments with their child, and they should be as quiet, meaningful, peaceful, and undisturbed as possible. The child's belongings are packaged for the parents to take home if they wish. Because the parents leave the hospital without their infant, it is helpful to accompany them to the car or arrange for someone else to take them home.

Returning home. When the parents return home, they should be visited by a competent, qualified professional as soon after the death as possible. Printed material that contains excellent information about SIDS (available from the national organizations*) should be provided.

During the initial visit the parents are helped to gain an intellectual understanding of the disease. The nursing objectives are to assess what the parents have been told, what they think happened, and how they have explained this to the other siblings, other family members, and friends.

Some parents are able to discuss their feelings openly, and the nurse supports this coping skill. However, others may be reluctant to express their grief, and the nurse may help these parents bring their feelings out into the open.

The nurse can encourage the expression of emotions by asking about crying and feeling sad, angry, or guilty. It is an attempt to provoke a display of emotion, not just an admission of a feeling. During this session the parents should be helped to explore their usual coping mechanisms and, if these are ineffectual, to investigate new approaches. For example, one parent may refrain from discussing the death for fear of upsetting the other parent, but each may need to hear how the other feels.

The number of visits and plans for subsequent intervention need to be flexible. For example, the siblings may initially appear accepting of the explanation and well adjusted but may later refuse to go to sleep or ask questions about graves or funerals, indicating their need for further help in dealing with the death. Parents facing the question of a subsequent child will need support. Both the birth of a subsequent child and the survival of that child, especially past the age of death of the previous child, are important transitional stages for parents.

Since the mourning process may take *at least* a year for completion of acceptance and social reorganization, nurses should call on the family periodically to evaluate their progress. Many families receive much solace and support from talking to other parents who have lost a child to SIDS.

***Sudden Infant Death Syndrome Clearinghouse,** 8201 Greensboro Dr., Suite 600, McLean, VA 22102, (703) 821-8955; **American Sudden Infant Death Syndrome (SIDS) Institute,** 275 Carpenter Dr., Suite 100, Atlanta, GA 30328, (800) 232-SIDS (in Georgia, [800] 847-SIDS); **The Sudden Infant Death Syndrome Alliance,** 10500 Little Patuxent Parkway, Suite 420, Columbia, MD 21044, (800) 221-SIDS.

Apnea of Infancy (AOI)

Apnea of infancy (AOI) generally refers to pathologic apnea in infants of more than 37 weeks' gestation. The clinical presentation of AOI is an *ALTE* (previously referred to by the inaccurate and misleading expression, "near-miss SIDS") that is described as:

- Frightening to the observer, who fears the child died or would have died without vigorous intervention
- Some combination of:
  - Apnea—cessation of breathing for 20 seconds or more; usually central but occasionally obstructive
  - Color change—cyanosis or pallor, but sometimes plethora
  - Marked change in muscle tone—usually extreme limpness
  - Choking or gagging

AOI can be a symptom of many disorders, including sepsis, seizures, upper airway abnormalities, gastroesophageal reflux, hypoglycemia or other metabolic problems, impaired regulation of breathing during sleep or feeding, or a result of intentional poisoning by a caregiver. However, in about half the cases no cause is identified. Infants with a history of ALTEs are at increased risk for SIDS, but these children constitute less than 7% of all SIDS victims. A diagnosis of AOI is made when no identifiable cause for the ALTE is found (Keens and Ward, 1993).

Diagnostic evaluation. The most widely used test is continuous recording of cardiorespiratory patterns (cardiopneumogram or pneumocardiogram). Four-channel or multichannel pneumocardiograms monitor heart rate, respirations (chest impedance), nasal airflow, and oxygen saturation. A more sophisticated test, polysomnography ("sleep test"), also records brain waves, eye and body movements, esophageal manometry, and end-tidal carbon dioxide measurements. However, none of these tests can predict risk. Some children with normal results may still have subsequent apneic episodes.

Therapeutic management. Treatment usually involves continuous home monitoring of cardiorespiratory rhythms and/or the use of methylxanthines (respiratory stimulant drugs, such as theophylline or caffeine). Therapeutic levels are typically 6 to 10 or 13 μg/ml of theophylline and 10 to 20 μg/ml of caffeine. The criteria for discontinuing the monitoring is based on the infant's clinical condition. A general guideline for discontinuation is when infants with ALTEs have gone 2 or 3 months without significant numbers of episodes requiring intervention.

Nursing ALERT

The concentration of theophylline required for apnea is less than that required for bronchodilation.

Nursing care management. The diagnosis of AOI engenders great anxiety and concern in parents, and the institution of home monitoring presents additional physical and emotional burdens. If monitoring is required, the nurse can be a

Critical Thinking Q & A

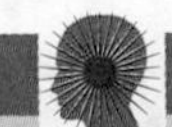

HOME APNEA MONITORING

A family has just taken their newborn home with an apnea monitor. The diagnosis is apnea of prematurity. You are the nurse making the first home visit. You should expect to find all of the following except:

1. The parent appears knowledgeable of monitor use, responses to alarms, and CPR.
2. The infant's respiratory status is stable and color is good.
3. The monitor is plugged into an extension cord.
4. The family appears anxious.

The correct answer is three. No medical equipment should be plugged into extension cords. If necessary, furniture and equipment should be rearranged so that an appropriate outlet can be used. Regarding the other answers, parents should be well trained in caring for the child on an apnea monitor before being sent home. The nurse should usually only need to review procedures. However, if parents do not have the necessary information and skills, training should be a priority on the first home visit. Anxiety is common for the first 4 to 8 weeks of home apnea monitoring. With a diagnosis of apnea of prematurity, the infant should appear healthy and should not exhibit respiratory distress. Signs to the contrary necessitate immediate contact with the family's practitioner.

major source of support to the family in terms of education about the equipment, observation of the infant's status, and immediate intervention during apneic episodes, including CPR (see the Critical Thinking Q & A above). To help the family cope with the numerous procedures they must learn, adequate preparation before discharge and written instructions are essential.*

Several types of home monitors are available, and most hospitals select the model that the infant will use at home. Nurses, especially those involved in the care at home, must become familiar with the equipment, including its advantages and disadvantages. Safety is a major concern, since monitors can cause electrical burns and electrocution. The following precautions are recommended:

1. Remove leads from infant when not attached to monitor.
2. Unplug power cord from electrical outlet when cord is not plugged into monitor.
3. Use safety covers on electrical outlets to discourage children from inserting objects into a socket.

Siblings should also be supervised when near the infant and taught that the monitor is not a play object. Other safety practices include informing local utility and rescue squads of the home monitoring in case of an emergency. Telephone numbers for these services should be posted near all telephones in the home.

Caregivers need detailed information regarding proper attachment of the electrodes to the infant's chest with impedance monitors that detect chest movement. The electrodes are placed in the midaxillary line, at a space one or two fingerbreadths below the nipple (Fig. 33-18). Adhesive electrodes are attached directly to the skin. For home use, electrodes attached to a belt that is placed around the child's trunk are preferred. The belt is positioned so that the electrodes contact the skin in the same area as shown in Fig. 33-18. Newer technology monitors have memory chips that allow for event recording; this may prove to be an effective tool in evaluating the use of the monitor and reported frequency of alarms (Ahmann, Meny, and Fink, 1992).

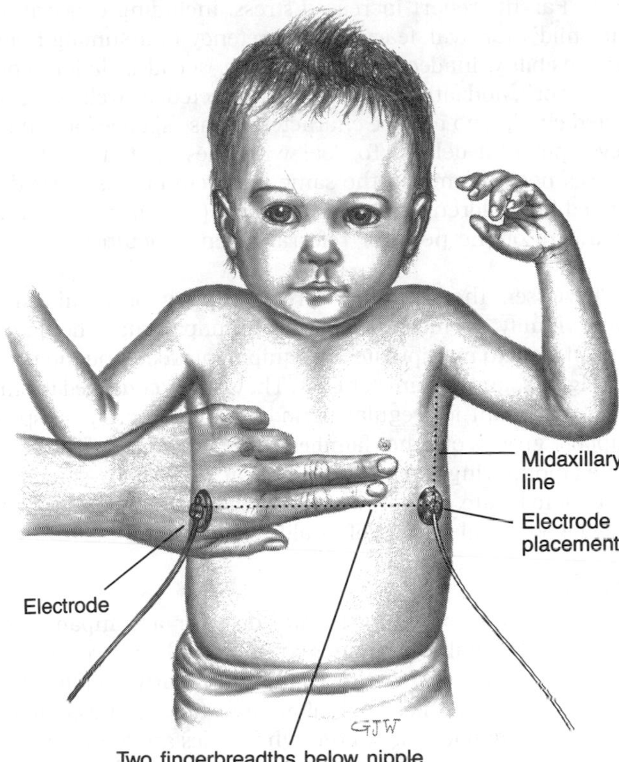

Fig. 33-18 Electrode placement for apnea monitoring. In small infants one fingerbreadth may be used.

Monitors are effective only if they are used. They do not prevent death but alert the caregiver to the ALTE in time to intervene. The need to use the monitor and to respond appropriately to alarms must be stressed. Noncompliance can result in the infant's death.

Nursing ALERT

If the infant is apneic, gently stimulate trunk by patting or rubbing it. If the infant is prone, turn to the back and flick the feet. If there is still no response, begin CPR. Never vigorously shake the child. No more than 15 to 30 seconds is spent on stimulation before implementing CPR.

Family support. Although AOI is not a chronic illness, many of the stresses observed during the monitoring period are characteristic of those of families with chronically ill chil-

*Home care instructions for apnea monitoring and CPR are available in Wong DL: *Wong and Whaley's clinical manual of pediatric nursing,* ed 4, St Louis, 1996, Mosby. Educational materials may also be obtained from the **American SIDS Institute.**

dren. Parents report increased stress, including concern for the child's survival, fear of incompetency in assuming home responsibility, inadequate respite care, social isolation, constant work, and fatigue. Siblings are affected, as well as the affected child, who may be characterized as "spoiled" and have developmental delays. To deal with these potential effects, nurses need to employ the same interventions as those discussed for children with chronic illness (see Chapter 38) and be aware of the need for referral when difficulties are suspected.

To lessen the continuous responsibility of monitoring, other family members, such as grandparents, should be taught how to manipulate the equipment, read and interpret the signals, and administer CPR. They are encouraged to stay with the infant for regular periods to allow parents respite. Support groups of other families who have successfully completed monitoring can also be of benefit. Since baby-sitters are difficult to locate, support group members or nursing students may be potential sources of qualified caregivers.

Autism

Autism, a complex developmental disorder accompanied by severe and usually permanent intellectual and behavioral deficits, is manifested during infancy and early childhood. It occurs in 1:2500 children, is about four times more common in males than in females (although females are more severely affected), and is not related to socioeconomic level, race, or religion.

Etiology. The cause of autism is an unsolved and controversial question. However, considerable evidence supports a biologic cause. Individuals with autism may have abnormal electroencephalograms, seizures, delayed development of hand dominance, persistence of primitive reflexes, metabolic abnormalities (elevated blood serotonin), and cerebellar vermal hypoplasia (part of the brain involved in regulating motion and some aspects of memory).

There is also strong evidence for a genetic basis that in twins is consistent with an autosomal recessive pattern of inheritance. Twin studies demonstrate a very high concordance (96%) for monozygotic (identical) twins and a 24% concordance for dizygotic (nonidentical) twins. In addition, between 5% and 16% of males with autism are positive for the fragile X chromosome (see Fragile X Syndrome, Chapter 39).

Clinical manifestations diagnostic evaluation. Children with autism demonstrate several peculiar and bizarre characteristics, primarily in social interactions, communication, and behavior. The clinical manifestations typically seen in children with autism are described in the Box 33-2. The majority of children with autism are mentally retarded, with scores typically in the moderate to severe range. More females than males tend to have very low intelligence scores. Despite relatively severe mental retardation, some children with autism (known as *savants*) excel in particular areas, such as art, music, memory, mathematic calculation, or perceptual skills, such as puzzle building.

Prognosis. Autism is a severely disabling condition. Only about 1% to 2% of the autistic population ultimately achieve independence, with the majority requiring lifelong supervision. Aggravation of psychiatric symptoms occurs in about half the children during adolescence, with girls having a tendency for continued deterioration. The prognosis is most favorable for children with communicative speech development by age 6 years and an intelligence quotient above 50 at the time of diagnosis. Early recognition of behaviors associated with autism is critical in order to implement appropriate interventions and family involvement.

BOX 33-2
Clinical Manifestations of Autism

Social Relations and Behavior

Extreme interpersonal isolation
Intense, abnormal concern for preservation of sameness
Unyielding to cuddling and holding
Do not respond to verbal stimulation
Bizarre attachment to mechanical objects
Odd repetitive behaviors, such as flicking a light switch on and off
Difficult to manage; passive or irritable
Frequent temper tantrums and/or self-destructive behavior

Development

Mental retardation, usually severe
May have advanced gross motor skills
Normal to hyperactive
May have exceptional ability (e.g., memory)
Poor suck and feeding responses

Language

Echolalia or parrot speech (automatic repetition of words spoken to them)
Pronominal reversal (tendency to use "you" for "I")
Literal, concrete use of words (e.g., "in" to mean "door")

Sensory/Perceptual Processes

Sensory deficits even though vision and hearing intact
Act as if deaf, yet may be overly sensitive to sound
Hyposensitive or hypersensitive to pain
Have aversion to touch

Nursing care management. Therapeutic intervention for the child with autism is a specialized area involving professionals with advanced training. Numerous therapies have been employed; the most promising results have been through highly structured and intensive behavioral modification programs. In general, the objective is to increase social awareness of others, teach verbal communication, and decrease unacceptable behavior. However, the vast majority of these children need assistance and supervision throughout adulthood, although early diagnosis and early educational treatment positively influence the child's future development.

When these children are hospitalized, the parents are essential to planning care and ideally should stay with the child as much as possible. Decreasing stimulation by using a private or semiprivate room, avoiding extraneous auditory and visual distraction, and encouraging the parents to bring in possessions the child is attached to may lessen the disruptiveness of hospitalization. Since physical contact often upsets these children, minimum holding may be necessary to prevent behavioral outbursts.

Care must be taken when performing procedures on, administering medicine to, or feeding these children, since they are often either fussy eaters who may willfully starve themselves or gag to prevent eating or indiscriminate hoarders, swallowing any available edible or inedible items, such as a thermometer. Their disturbing sleep patterns may also pose problems in a hospital setting. A thorough assessment of the child's usual routine and activities can help maintain an environment that is more manageable and conducive to physical recovery.

A key principle in working with these children is establishing trust. They need to be introduced slowly to new situations, with visits with staff caregivers kept short whenever possible. Because these children have difficulty organizing their behavior and redirecting their energy, they need to be told directly what to do. Communication should be at the child's developmental level, brief, and concrete. Only one request is given at a time, such as "sit on bed."

Family support. Autism, like so many other chronic conditions, involves the entire family and often becomes "a family disease." Unfortunately, the psychogenetic theory, popular in the 1960s especially among psychoanalysts, had portrayed the parents as detached, cold individuals. Although the psychogenetic theory is unsupported by current findings, it has caused many public misconceptions about these families and greatly intensified many parents' guilt. Nurses can help alleviate the guilt and shame often associated with this disorder by stressing what is known from a biologic standpoint, as well as how little is known about the cause of autism.

Parents need expert counseling early in the course of the disorder and should be referred to the Autism Society of America (ASA).* ASA is the most efficient clearinghouse for information about education, treatment programs and techniques, and facilities such as camps and group homes. There is also a siblings group called SHARE (Siblings Helping Persons with Autism Through Resources and Energy).

As much as possible, the family is encouraged to care for the child in the home. With the help of family support programs in many states, families are often able to provide home care and assist with the educational services the child needs. As the young person approaches adulthood, the family may require assistance in locating a long-term care facility for the affected adult (see also Chapter 39).

*7910 Woodmont Ave., Suite 650, Bethesda, Md 20814.

Key Points

- Biologic development of the child encompasses sensory changes, including binocularity and depth perception; maturation of biologic systems; fine motor development; and gross motor development.
- Erikson's theory of psychosocial development (birth to 1 year) is concerned with acquiring a sense of trust while overcoming a sense of mistrust.
- Piaget's theory of cognitive development, as it applies to the infant, focuses on the sensorimotor phase, which includes the use of reflexes, primary circular reactions, secondary circular reactions, and coordination of secondary schemata and their application to new situations.
- Development of body image begins in infancy; by 1 year of age infants recognize that they are distinct from their parents.
- Social development of the infant is guided by attachment, language development, personal-social behavior, and participation in play.
- Temperament is an important indicator of the kind of interaction that occurs between the child and parents and siblings.
- Parents are faced with many concerns, including infant fears, child care, limit setting and discipline, thumb-sucking and pacifier use, teething, and choice of infant shoes.
- Breast milk or formula is the most desirable food for the infant during the first 6 months, followed by gradual introduction of solid food during the second 6 months. Whole milk is not recommended until after 12 months.
- Fluoride supplements and appropriate dietary intake promote good dental hygiene.
- Infants may be prone to sleep disturbances, and the nurse should instruct the parents, after careful assessment, in adjusting the infant's schedule.
- Recommended routine immunizations include those for diphtheria, tetanus, pertussis, polio, measles, mumps, rubella, *Haemophilus influenzae* type b, hepatitis B virus, and varicella.
- Recommended immunizations for selected groups of children are influenza virus, pneumococcal, and meningococcal vaccines, and the hepatitis A virus.
- Because injuries are a major cause of death during infancy, parents should be alerted to motor vehicle, aspiration, suffocation, burn, drowning, falling, poisoning, and bodily injuries.
- Treatment of colic may involve change in feeding practices, correction of a stressful environment, and support of the parent.
- Failure to thrive may be classified as organic, resulting from some physical cause, or nonorganic, resulting from psychosocial factors involving the child and caregiver (e.g., maternal deprivation), environmental causes (e.g., inadequate parental knowledge of child feeding), or unexplained causes.
- Sudden infant death syndrome is the leading cause of death in children between the ages of 1 week and 1 year.
- The primary nursing responsibility in care associated with sudden infant death and other conditions of unknown cause is emotional support of the family.
- Children with apnea of infancy receive home monitoring to alert the family to an apparent life-threatening event.
- Autism is a lifelong developmental disorder that is characterized by severe cognitive and social retardation, bizarre behavior, and gross language deficits.

References

Ahmann E, Meny RG, Fink RJ: Use of home apnea monitors, *JOGNN* 21(5):394-399, 1992.

American Academy of Pediatrics, Air bag safety issues examined, *AAP News* 13(1):1, 13, 1997.

American Academy of Pediatrics, Committee on Infectious Diseases: Universal hepatitis B immunization, *Pediatrics* 89(4):795-800, 1992.

American Academy of Pediatrics, Committee on Infectious Diseases: *Haemophilius influeanzae* type b conjugate vaccines: *Pediatrics* 92(3):480-488, 1993.

American Academy of Pediatrics, Committee on Infectious Diseases: 1994 red book: report of the Committee on Infectious Diseases, ed 23, Elk Grove Village, Ill, 1994, The Academy.

American Academy of Pediatrics, Committee on Infectious Diseases: Recommendations for the use of live attenuated varicella vaccine, *Pediatrics* 95(5):791-795, 1995.

American Academy of Pediatrics, Committee on Infectious Diseases: Recommended childhood immunization schedule—United States, January-December 1997, *Pediatrics* 99(1):136,1997a.

American Academy of Pediatrics, Committee on Infectious Diseases: Acellular pertussis vaccine: recommendations for use as the initial series in infants and children, *Pediatrics* 99(2):282-287, 1997b.

American Academy of Pediatrics, Committee on Infectious Diseases: Poliomyelitis prevention: recommendations for use of inactivated poliovirus vaccine, *Pediatrics* 99(2):300-305, 1997c.

American Academy of Pediatrics, Committee on Injury and Poison Prevention: Drowning in infants, children and adolescents, *Pediatrics* 92(2):292-294, 1993.

American Academy of Pediatrics, Committee on Injury and Poison Prevention: Injuries associated with infant walkers, *Pediatrics* 95(5):778-780, 1995.

American Academy of Pediatrics, Committee on Nutrition: Policy statement: the use of fruit juice in the diets of young children, *AAP News* 7(2):11, 1991.

American Academy of Pediatrics, Committee on Nutrition: Fluoride supplementation for children, *Pediatrics* 95(5):777, 1995.

American Academy of Pediatrics, Committee on Sports Medicine: Infant exercise programs, *Pediatrics* 82(5):800, 1988.

American Public Health Association and American Academy of Pediatrics: *Caring for our children: national health and safety performance standards: guidelines for out-of-home child care programs,* Washington, DC, 1992, The Association.

Anders TF, Halpern LF, Hua J: Sleeping through the night: a developmental perspective, *Pediatrics* 90(4):554-560, 1992.

Brazelton T: Parent-infant cosleeping revisited, *Ab Initio* 2(1):1-7, 1990.

Calvo EB, Galindo AC, Aspres NB: Iron status in exclusively breastfed infants, *Pediatrics* 90(3):375-379, 1992.

Carey WB, McDevitt SC: Revision of the infant temperament questionnaire, *Pediatrics* 61(5):735-739, 1978.

Centers for Disease Control and Prevention: General recommendations on immunization: recommendations of the Advisory Committee on Immunization Practices (ACIP), *MMWR* 43(RR-1):1-38, 1994.

Chess S, Thomas A: Temperamental differences: a critical concept in child health care, *Pediatr Nurs* 11(3):167-171, 1985.

Dewey KG et al: Breast-fed infants are leaner than formula-fed infants at 1 year of age: the DARLING study, *Am J Clin Nutr* 57(2):140-145, 1993.

Ferber R: *Solve your child's sleep problems,* New York, 1985, Simon & Schuster.

Genarro S, Medoff-Cooper B, Lotas M: Perinatal factors and infant temperament: a collaborative approach . . . common variables of three studies examined, *Nurs Res* 41(6):375-377, 1992.

Holida DL: Latex balloons: they can take your breath away, *Pediatr Nurs* 19(1):39-43, 68, 1993.

Infant sleep position and sudden infant death syndrome (SIDS) in the United States: joint commentary from the American Academy of Pediatrics and selected agencies of the federal government, *Pediatrics* 93(5):820, 1994.

Institute of Medicine: *Adverse events associated with childhood vaccines,* Washington, DC, 1993, National Academy Press.

Jaber L, Cohen IJ, Mor A: Fever associated with teething, *Arch Dis Child* 67(2):233-234, 1992.

Jones L, Heermann J: Parental division of infant care: contextual influences and infant characteristics, *Nurs Res* 41(4):228-234, 1992.

Keens TG, Ward SLD: Apnea spells, sudden death, and the role of the apnea monitor, *Pediatr Clin North Am* 40(5):897-911, 1993.

Kemp JS et al: Unintentional suffocation by rebreathing: a death scene and physiologic investigation of a possible cause of sudden infant death, *J Pediatr* 122(6):874-880, 1993.

Lampl M, Veldhuis JD, Johnson ML: Saltation and stasis: a model of human growth, *Science* 258(5083):801-803, 1992.

Landis SE, Chang A: Child care options for ill children, *Pediatrics* 88(4):705-718, 1991.

Miller A, Barr R, Eaton W: Crying and motor behavior of six-week-old infants and postpartum maternal mood, *Pediatrics* 92(4):551-558, 1993.

Nowak AJ: What pediatricians can do to promote oral health, *Contemp Pediatr* 10(4):90-106, 1993.

Pickler R, Frankel H: The effect of non-nutritive sucking on preterm infants' behavioral organization and feeding performance, *Neonatal Network* 14(2):83, 1995.

Position statement: infant feeding, *Clin Pediatr* 31(8):510, 1992.

Schachter F et al: Cosleeping and sleep problems in Hispanic-American urban young children, *Pediatrics* 84(3):522-530, 1989.

Schmitt BD: The "two-step" approach to infant sleep problems, *Contemp Pediatr* 9(11):37-38, 1992.

Sullivan SA, Birch LL: Infant dietary experience and acceptance of solid foods, *Pediatrics* 93(2):271-277, 1994.

Tully S: Injuries to children in shopping carts, *AAP News* 9(6):11, 1993.

Victora CG et al: Use of pacifiers and breastfeeding duration, *Lancet* 341(8842):404-406, 1993.

Zuckerman JN, Cockcroft A, Zuckerman AJ: Site of injection for vaccination, *Br Med J* 305(6862):1158, 1992.

Bibliography

Growth and Development

Belfer M: Body image: impacts and distortions. In Levine M et al, editors: *Developmental-behavioral pediatrics,* ed 2, Philadelphia, 1992, WB Saunders.

Erikson E: *Childhood and society,* ed 2, New York, 1963, WW Norton.

Friendly DS: Developmental of vision in infants and young children, *Pediatr Clin North Am* 40(4):693-703, 1993.

Garmezy N, Rutter M, editors: *Stress, coping, and development in children,* New York, 1989, McGraw-Hill.

Knobloch H, Stevens F, Malone AF: *Manual of developmental diagnosis,* Hagerstown, Penn, 1980, Harper & Row.

Maier H: *Three theories of child development,* ed 3, New York, 1988, Harper & Row.

Marino B: Assessments of infant play: applications to research and practice, *Issues Compr Pediatr Nurs* 11(4):227-240, 1988.
Piaget J: *The construction of reality in the child,* New York, 1975, Ballantine Books.
Seligman S: Emotional and social development in infancy and early childhood, *Early Child Update* 5(4):1-2, 1989.
Singhi P, Radhika S: Kiss: a developmental milestone or a culture-determined skill? *Am J Dis Child* 146(6):663-664, 1992.
Vaughan III VC: Assessment of growth and development during infancy and early childhood, *Pediatr Rev* 13(3):88-97, 1992.

Attachment/Temperament/Parenting

Calkins SD, Fox NA: The relations among infant temperament, security of attachment, and behavioral inhibition at twenty-four months, *Child Dev* 63(6):1456-1472, 1992.
Coffman S et al: Temperament and interactive effects: mothers and infants in a teaching situation, *Issues Compr Pediatr Nurs* 15:169-182, 1992.
Coffman S et al: Infant mother attachment: relationships to maternal responsiveness and infant temperament, *J Pediatr Nurs* 10(1):9-18, 1995.
Graham MV: Parental sensitivity to infant cues: similarities and differences between mothers and fathers, *J Pediatr Nurs* 8(6):376-384, 1993.
Harris E, Weston D, Lieberman A: Quality of mother-infant attachment and pediatric health care use, *Pediatrics* 84(2):248-254, 1989.
Isabella RA: Origins of attachment: maternal interactive behavior across the first year, *Child Dev* 64(2):605-621, 1993.
Koniak-Griffin D, Rummell M: Temperament in infancy: stability, change, and correlates, *Matern Child Nurs J* 17(1):25-40, 1988.
Wasserman R et al: Infant temperament and school age behavior: 6-year longitudinal study in the pediatric practice, *Pediatrics* 85(5):801-807, 1990.

Concerns Related to Growth and Development

For bibliography on day care, see Chapter 35.
Castiglia P: Thumb sucking, *J Pediatr Health Care* 2(6):322-323, 1988.
Clutter L: Helping parents prepare for travel and vacations with children, *Pediatr Nurs* 14(3):211-215, 1988.
Friman PC: Concurrent habits: what would Linus do with his blanket if his thumb-sucking were treated? *Am J Dis Child* 144(12):1316-1318, 1990.
Glendon M: If the shoe fits . . . wear it, *Pediatr Nurs* 13(4):230-271, 1987.
Solomon R, Martin K: Can you spoil an infant? A primary care survey, *Am J Dis Child* 144(4):426-427, 1990.

Nutrition

Finberg L: How good a food for humans is cow's milk? *Am J Dis Child* 146(12):1432, 1992.
Fomon SJ: *Nutrition of normal infants,* St Louis, 1993, Mosby.
Fuchs GL et al: Iron status and intake of older infants fed formula vs cow milk with cereal, *Am J Clin Nutr* 58:343-348, 1993.
Lawrence RA: *Breast feeding: a guide for the medical profession,* ed 4, St Louis, 1994, Mosby.
Lawrence R: The clinician's role in teaching proper infant feeding techniques, *J Pediatr* 126:5112-5117, 1995.
McCain GC: Promotion of preterm infant nipple feeding with non-nutritive sucking, *J Pediatr Nurs* 10(1):3-8, 1995.
Nemethy M, Clore E: Microwave heating of infant formula and breast milk, *J Pediatr Health Care* 4(3):131-135, 1990.
Pipes PL, Trahms CM: *Nutrition in infancy and childhood,* ed 5, St Louis, 1993, Mosby.
Schmitt BD: When weaning is delayed, *Contemp Pediatr* 7(6):67-68, 1990.
Sigman-Grant M, Bush G, Anantheswaran R: Microwave heating of infant formula: a dilemma resolved, *Pediatrics* 90(3):412-415, 1992.
Snow LS, Fry ME: Formula feeding in the first year of life, *Pediatr Nurs* 16(5):442-446, 1990.
Sullivan PB: Cows' milk induced intestinal bleeding in infancy, *Arch Dis Child* 68(2):240-245, 1993.
Weigley ES: Changing patterns in offering solids to infants, *Pediatr Nurs* 16(5):439-441, 1990.
Worobey J, Lewis M: Behavioral differences in response to stress between breast- and bottle-fed infants, *Top Clin Nutr* 7(3):48-55, 1992.

Sleep and Activity

Adair R et al: Reduced night waking in infancy: a primary care intervention, *Pediatrics* 89(4):585-588, 1992.
Adams L, Rickert V: Reducing bedtime tantrums: comparison between positive routines and graduated extinction, *Pediatrics* 84(5):756-761, 1989.
Balsmeyer B: Sleep disturbances of the infant and toddler, *Pediatr Nurs* 16(5):447-452, 1990.
Bardossi K: Getting kids to bed: how tough is too tough? *Contemp Pediatr* 8(1):97-105, 1991.
Horne J: Sleep and its disorders in children, *J Child Psychol Psychiatry* 33(3):473-487, 1992.
Jaffa T et al: Sleep disorders in children, *Br Med J* 306(6878):640-643, 1993.
Schmitt BD: When your child refuses to go to bed, *Contemp Pediatr* 6(7):70-71, 1989.
Schmitt BD: How to help the trained night feeder, *Contemp Pediatr* 9(11):41-49, 1992.

Dental Health

For bibliography, see Chapter 34.

Immunizations

Abbotts B, Osborn LM: Immunization status and reasons for immunization delay among children using public health immunization clinics, *Am J Dis Child* 147:965-968, 1993.
Ad Hoc Working Group for the Development of Standards for Pediatric Immunization Practices: Standards for pediatric immunization practices, *JAMA* 269(14):1817-1822, 1993.
Adams WG et al: Decline of childhood *Haemophilus influenzae* type b (Hib) disease in the Hib vaccine era, *JAMA* 269(2):221-226, 1993.
American Academy of Pediatrics, Committee on Practice and Ambulatory Medicine: Implementation of the immunization policy (S94-26), *Pediatrics* 96(2):360-361, 1995.
Brown J et al: Missed opportunities in preventive pediatric health care: immunizations or well-child care visits? *Am J Dis Child* 147(10):1081-1084, 1993.
Caulfield M: Hepatitis B: a disease needing a vaccine or a vaccine needing a disease? *Clin Pediatr* 32(7):443-444, 1993.
Peter G: Childhood immunizations, *New Engl J Med* 327(25):1794-1800, 1992.
Zanga JR: Should there be a universal childhood vaccination against hepatitis B? II. A rebuttal, *Pediatr Nurs* 19(5):451-452, 1993.
Zell ER et al: Low vaccination levels of U.S. preschool and school-age children, *JAMA* 271(11):833-839, 1994.

Injury Prevention

For additional citations, see Chapters 1 and 34.
Agran PF, Winn DG, Castillo DN: On-lap travel: still a problem in motor vehicles, *Pediatrics* 90(1):27-29, 1992.
Air-bag–associated fatal injuries to infants and children riding in front passenger seats—United States, *MMWR* 44(45):845-846, 1995.
Botash A: Syringe caps: an aspiration hazard, *Pediatrics* 90(1):92-93, 1992.
Children and waterbeds, *Pediatr Nurs* 17(6):577, 1991 (letter and reply).
Coppens N: Parental responses to children in unsafe situations, *Pediatr Nurs* 16(6):571-574, 1990.

Gielen AC, Collins B: Community-based interventions for injury prevention, *Fam Community Health* 15(4):1-11, 1993.

Jones NE: Prevention of childhood injuries. II. Recreational injuries, *Pediatr Nurs* 18(6):619-621, 1992.

Gunn WJ et al: Injuries and poisonings in out-of-home child care and home care, *Am J Dis Child* 145(7):779-781, 1991.

Ramsey K, Goldbach R, Stephenson S: Near fatal aspiration of a candy pacifier, *Pediatrics* 84(1):126-127, 1989.

Sheridan R, Sheridan M, Tompkins R: Dishwasher effluent burns in infants, *Pediatrics* 91(1):142-143, 1993.

Stewart DD: Child passenger safety: current technical issues for advocates and professionals, *Fam Community Health* 15(4):12-27, 1993.

Colic

Barr RG et al: The crying of infants with colic: a controlled empirical description, *Pediatrics* 90(1):14-21, 1992.

Hill DJ et al: Charting infant distress: an aid to defining colic, *J Pediatr* 121(5):755-758, 1992.

Jacobson D and Melvin N: A comparison of temperament and maternal bother in infants with and without colic, *J Pediatr Nurs* 10(3):181-187, 1995.

MacPhee M, Mori C, Goldson E: Change in the hospital setting: adopting a team approach for nonorganic failure-to-thrive, *J Pediatr Nurs* 9(4):218-225, 1994.

Treem WR: Infant colic: a pediatric gastroenterologist's perspective, *Pediatr Clin North Am* 41(5):1121-1138, 1994.

Weizman Z et al: Efficacy of herbal tea preparation in infantile colic, *J Pediatr* 122(4):650-652, 1993.

Failure to Thrive

Bithoney WG, Dubowitz H, Egan H: Failure to thrive/growth deficiency, *Pediatr Rev* 13(12):453-459, 1992.

Bithoney WG, Rathbun J: Failure to thrive. In Levine MD et al, editors: *Developmental-behavioral pediatrics*, ed 2, Philadelphia, 1992, WB Saunders.

Kelleher KJ et al: Risk factors and outcomes for failure to thrive in low birth weight preterm infants, *Pediatrics* 91(5):941-948, 1993.

Klein M: The home health nurse clinician's role in the prevention of nonorganic failure to thrive, *J Pediatr Nurs* 5(2):129-135, 1990.

Maggioni A, Lifshitz F: Nutritional management of failure to thrive, *Pediatr Clin North Am* 42(4):791-809, 1995.

Sudden Infant Death Syndrome/Apnea of Infancy

Bignall J: Decline in sudden infant deaths, *Lancet* 341:887, 1993.

Freed GE et al: Sudden infant death syndrome prevention and an understanding of selected clinical issues, *Pediatr Clin North Am* 41(5):967-990, 1994.

Hunziker U, Barr R: Increased carrying reduces infant crying: a randomized controlled trial, *Pediatrics* 77(5):641-648, 1986.

Hunt CE: Infant sleeping position: back to the bench, *Arch Pediatr Adolesc Med* 148(2):131-133, 1994.

Infant sleep position and sudden infant death syndrome (SIDS) in the United States: joint commentary from the American Academy of Pediatrics and selected agencies of the federal government, *Pediatrics* 93(5):820, 1994.

Schoendorf KC, Kiely JL: Relationship of sudden infant death syndrome to maternal smoking during and after pregnancy, *Pediatrics* 90(6):905-908, 1992.

Spinner S et al: Recent advances in home apnea monitoring, *Neonatal Netw* 14(8):39-46, 1995.

Stevens MS: Parents coping with infants requiring home cardiorespiratory monitoring, *J Pediatr Nurs* 9(1):2-12, 1994.

Autism

Baerg KL: Effective communication with autistic children, *Rehabil Nurs* 16(2):88-90, 1991.

Christian WP: Childhood autism. In Levine M et al, editors: *Developmental-behavioral pediatrics*, ed 2, Philadelphia, 1992, WB Saunders.

Denekla MB, James LS: An update on autism: a developmental disorder, *Pediatrics* 87(5, suppl):751-796, 1991.

Mulick JA, Jacobson JW, Kobe FH: Anguished silence and helping hands: autism and facilitated communication, *Skeptical Inquirer* 17(3):270-280, 1993.

Stone WL and others: Early recognition of autism: parental reports vs clinical observation, *Arch Pediatr Adolesc Med* 148:174-179, 1994.

Tuchman R, Gilman J: Pharmacotherapy of pervasive developmental disorders, *Int Pediatr* 8(2):211-218, 1993.

Zimmerman AW, Frye VH, Potter NT: Immunological aspects of autism, *Int Pediatr* 8(2):199-204, 1993.

CHAPTER 34

The Toddler and Family

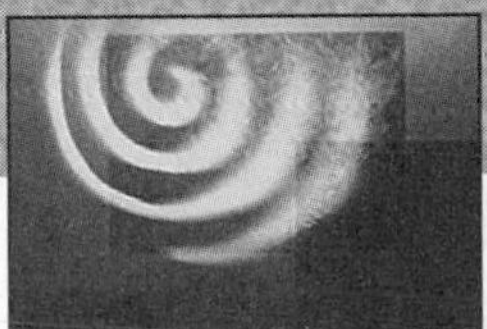

PROMOTING OPTIMUM GROWTH AND DEVELOPMENT, P. 993

Biologic development, p. 993
Psychosocial development, p. 994
Cognitive development, p. 995
Spiritual development, p. 996
Development of body image, p. 997
Development of sexuality, p. 997
Social development, p. 998
Coping with concerns related to normal growth and development, p. 999

PROMOTING OPTIMUM HEALTH DURING TODDLERHOOD, P. 1003

Nutrition, p. 1003
Sleep and activity, p. 1004
Dental health, p. 1004
Injury prevention, p. 1006

Promoting Optimum Growth and Development

The term *terrible twos* has often been used to describe the toddler years, the period from 12 to 36 months of age. It is a time of intense exploration of the environment as children attempt to find out how things work and how to control others through temper tantrums, negativism, and obstinacy. Although this can be a challenging time for parents and child as each learns to know the other better, it is an extremely important period for developmental achievement and intellectual growth.

BIOLOGIC DEVELOPMENT

Proportional Changes

Growth slows considerably during toddlerhood. The average *weight* gain is 1.8 to 2.7 kg (4 to 6 pounds) per year. The average weight at 2 years is 12 kg (27 pounds). The birth weight is quadrupled by $2^1/_2$ years of age. The rate of increase in height also slows. The usual increment is an addition of 7.5 cm (3 inches) per year and occurs mainly in elongation of the legs rather than the trunk. The average *height* of a 2-year-old is 86.6 cm (34 inches). In general, adult height is about twice the 2-year-old child's height. Accurate measurement of height and weight during the toddler years should reveal a steady growth curve that is *steplike* in nature rather than linear (straight), which is characteristic of the growth spurts during the early childhood years.

The rate of increase in *head circumference* slows somewhat by the end of infancy, and head circumference is usually equal to chest circumference by 1 to 2 years of age. The usual total increase in head circumference during the second year is 2.5 cm (1 inch). Then the rate of increase slows until at age 5 years the increase is less than 1.25 cm ($^1/_2$ inch) per year. The anterior fontanel closes between 12 and 18 months of age.

Chest circumference continues to increase in size and exceeds head circumference during the toddler years. Its shape also changes as the transverse, or lateral, diameter exceeds the anteroposterior diameter. After the second year the chest circumference exceeds the abdominal measurement, which, in addition to the growth of the lower extremities, gives the child a taller, leaner appearance. However, the toddler retains a squat, "pot-bellied" appearance because of the less well developed abdominal musculature and short legs (Fig. 34-1). The legs retain a slightly bowed or curved appearance during the second year from the weight of the relatively large trunk.

Sensory Changes

Visual acuity of 20/20 is achieved during the toddler years, although 20/40 is considered acceptable. Full binocular vision is well developed, and any evidence of persistent strabismus requires professional attention as early as possible to prevent amblyopia. Depth perception continues to develop but, because of the child's lack of motor coordination, falls from heights continue to be a persistent danger.

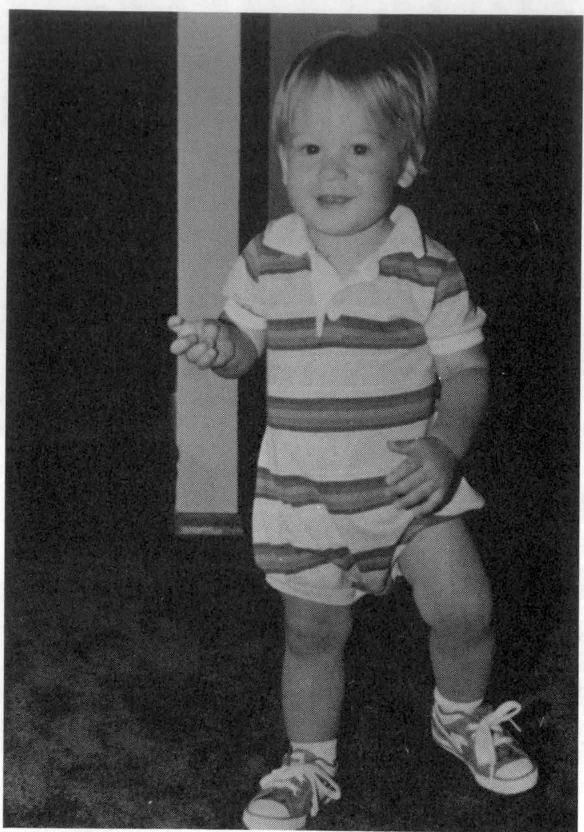

Fig. 34-1 Typical toddling gait.

The senses of *hearing, smell, taste,* and *touch* become increasingly well developed, coordinated with each other, and associated with other experiences. All of the senses are used to explore the environment. Toddlers will visually inspect an object by turning it over; they may taste it, smell it, and touch it several times before they are satisfied with their investigation. They will shake it to see if it makes noise and vigorously test its durability.

Another example of the integrated function of the senses is the toddler's development of specific *taste preferences.* The child is much less likely than infants to try a new food because of its appearance, smell, or taste.

Maturation of Systems

Most of the physiologic systems are relatively mature by the end of toddlerhood. Volume of the *respiratory tract* and growth of associated structures continue to increase during early childhood, lessening some of the factors that predisposed the child to frequent and serious infections during infancy. The internal structures of the ear and throat continue to be short and straight, and the lymphoid tissue of the tonsils and adenoids continues to be large. As a result, otitis media, tonsillitis, and upper respiratory tract infections are common.

The respiratory and heart rates slow, and the blood pressure increases (see the Appendix). Respirations continue to be abdominal. Under conditions of moderate variation in temperature, the toddler rarely has the difficulties of the young infant in maintaining *body temperature.* The mature functioning of the renal system serves to conserve fluid under times of stress, decreasing the risk of dehydration.

The *digestive processes* are fairly complete by the beginning of toddlerhood. The acidity of the gastric contents continues to increase and has a protective function, since it is capable of destroying many types of bacteria. Stomach capacity increases to allow for the usual schedule of three meals a day.

One of the more prominent changes of the gastrointestinal system is the voluntary control of elimination. With complete myelination of the spinal cord, control of the anal and urethral sphincters is gradually achieved. The physiologic ability to control the sphincters probably occurs somewhere between ages 18 and 24 months. Bladder capacity also increases considerably. By 14 to 18 months of age the child is able to retain urine for up to 2 hours or longer.

The *defense mechanisms* of the skin and blood, particularly phagocytosis, are much more efficient in toddlers than in infants. The production of antibodies is well established. However, many young children demonstrate a sudden increase in colds and minor infections when entering group situations such as daycare because of their exposure to pathogens.

Gross and Fine Motor Development

The major *gross motor skill* during the toddler years is the development of locomotion. By 12 to 13 months of age toddlers walk alone using a wide stance for extra balance; and by 18 months they try to run but fall easily. Between 2 and 3 years of age refinement of the upright, biped position is evident in improved coordination and equilibrium. Toddlers at age 2 can walk up and down stairs, and by age $2^1/_2$ years they can jump, using both feet, stand on one foot for a second or two, and manage a few steps on tiptoe. By the end of the second year they can stand on one foot, walk on tiptoe, and climb stairs with alternate footing.

Fine motor development is demonstrated in increasingly skillful manual dexterity. For example, by age 12 months they are able to grasp a very small object but are unable to release it at will. At 15 months they can drop a pellet into a narrow-necked bottle. Casting or throwing objects and retrieving them become almost obsessive activities at about 15 months. By 18 months of age toddlers can throw a ball overhand without losing their balance.

Mastery of gross and fine motor skills is evident in all phases of the child's activity such as play, dressing, language comprehension, response to discipline, social interaction, and proneness to injuries. Activities occur less in isolation and more in conjunction with other physical and mental abilities to produce a purposeful result. For example, the toddler walks to reach a new location, releases a toy to choose a new one, and scribbles to look at the image produced. The possibilities of the exploration, investigation, and manipulation of the environment—and its hazards—are endless.

PSYCHOSOCIAL DEVELOPMENT

Toddlers are faced with the mastery of several important tasks. If the need for basic trust has been satisfied, they are ready to give up dependence for control, independence, and autonomy. Some of the specific tasks to be dealt with include the following:

- Differentiation of self from others, particularly the mother
- Toleration of separation from parent
- Ability to withstand delayed gratification

- Control over bodily functions
- Acquisition of socially acceptable behavior
- Verbal means of communication
- Ability to interact with others in a less egocentric manner

Mastery of these goals is only begun during late infancy and the toddler years, and such tasks as developing interpersonal relationships with others may not be completed until adolescence. However, crucial foundations for successful completion of such developmental tasks are laid during these early formative years.

Developing a Sense of Autonomy (Erikson)

According to Erikson, the developmental task of toddlerhood is acquiring a sense of **autonomy** while overcoming a sense of *doubt* and *shame*. As infants gain trust in the predictability and reliability of their parents, environment, and interaction with others, they begin to discover that their behavior is their own and that it has a predictable, reliable effect on others. However, although they realize their will and control over others, they are confronted with the conflict of exerting autonomy and relinquishing the much enjoyed dependence on others. Exerting their will has definite negative consequences, whereas retaining dependent, submissive behavior is generally rewarded with affection and approval. However, continued dependency creates a sense of doubt regarding their potential capacity to control their actions. This doubt is compounded by a sense of shame for feeling this urge to revolt against others' will and a fear that they will exceed their own capacity for manipulating the environment.

Just as the infant has the social modalities of grasping and biting, the toddler has the newly gained modality of holding on and letting go. To hold on and let go is evident with the use of the hands, mouth, eyes, and, eventually, the sphincters, when toilet training is begun. These social modalities are expressed constantly in the child's play activities such as casting or throwing objects; taking objects out of boxes, drawers, or cabinets; holding on tighter when someone says, "No, don't touch"; and spitting out food as taste preferences become very strong.

Several characteristics, especially negativism and ritualism, are typical of toddlers in their quest for autonomy. As toddlers attempt to express their will, they often act with **negativism,** the persistent negative response to requests. The words "no" or "me do" can be the sole vocabulary. Emotions become very strongly expressed, usually in rapid mood swings. One minute toddlers can be engrossed in an activity, and the next minute they might be violently angry because they are unable to manipulate a toy or open a door. If scolded for doing something wrong, they can have a temper tantrum and almost instantaneously pull at the parent's legs to be picked up and comforted. Often these swift changes are difficult for parents to understand and cope with. Many parents find the negativism exasperating and, instead of dealing constructively with it, give into it, which further threatens children in their search for learning acceptable methods of interacting with others (see Negativism, p. 1002).

In contrast to negativism, which frequently disrupts the environment, **ritualism,** the need to maintain sameness and reliability, provides a sense of comfort. Toddlers can venture out with security when they know that familiar people, places, and routines still exist. One can easily understand why change such as hospitalization represents such a threat to these children. Without the comfortable rituals, there is little opportunity to exert autonomy. Consequently, dependency and regression occur (see Regression, p. 1003).

Erikson focuses on the development of the *ego,* which may be thought of as reason or common sense, during this phase of psychosocial development. There is a struggle as the child deals with the impulses of the *id* and attempts to tolerate frustration and learn socially acceptable ways of interacting with the environment. The ego is evident as the child is able to tolerate delayed gratification.

There is also a rudimentary beginning of the *superego,* or conscience, which is the incorporation of the morals of society and the process of acculturation. With the development of the ego, children further differentiate themselves from others and expand their sense of trust within themselves. But as they begin to develop awareness of their own will and capacity to achieve, they also become aware of their ability to fail. This ever-present awareness of potential failure creates doubt and shame. Successful mastery of the task of autonomy necessitates opportunities for self-mastery while withstanding the frustration of necessary limit-setting and delayed gratification. Opportunities for self-mastery are present in appropriate play activities, toilet training, the crisis of sibling rivalry, and successful interactions with significant others.

COGNITIVE DEVELOPMENT

Sensorimotor and Preconceptual Phase (Piaget)

The period from 12 to 24 months of age is a continuation of the final two stages of the sensorimotor phase. During this time the cognitive processes develop rapidly and at times seem similar to those of mature thinking. However, reasoning skills are still quite primitive and need to be understood to effectively deal with the typical behaviors of this age group.

Tertiary circular reactions. In the fifth stage (13 to 18 months of age), the child uses active experimentation to achieve previously unattainable goals. Newly acquired physical skills are increasingly important for the function they serve rather than for the acts themselves. The child incorporates the old learning of secondary circular reactions with new skills and applies the combined knowledge to new situations, with emphasis on the results of the experimentation. In this way there is the beginning of rational judgment and intellectual reasoning. During this stage there is further differentiation of oneself from objects. This is evident in the child's increasing ability to venture away from the parent and to tolerate longer periods of separation.

Awareness of a causal relationship between two events is apparent. After flipping a light switch, toddlers are aware that a reciprocal response occurs. However, they are not able to transfer that knowledge to new situations. Therefore, every time they see what appears to be a light switch, they must reinvestigate its function. Such behavior demonstrates the beginning of categorizing data into distinct classes, subclasses, and so on. There are innumerable examples of this type of behavior as toddlers continuously explore the same object each time it appears in a new place.

Because classification of objects is still rudimentary, the appearance of an object denotes its function. For example, if the child's toys are stored in a paper bag or large container, that toy receptacle is no different from the garbage pail or laundry basket. If allowed to turn over the toy receptacle, the child will just as quickly do the same to other similar containers because, in the child's mind, there is no difference. Expecting the child to judge which receptacles are permissible to explore and which are not is inappropriate for this age group. Instead, the forbidden object such as the garbage pail should be placed out of reach.

The discovery of objects as objects leads to the awareness of their spatial relationships. Children are able to recognize different shapes and their relationship to each other. For example, they can fit slightly smaller boxes into each other (nesting) and can place a round object into a hole, even if the board is turned around, upside down, or reversed. Children are also aware of space and the relationship of their body to dimensions such as height. They will stretch and stand on a low stair or stool to reach an object.

Object permanence has also advanced. Although they still cannot find an object that has been invisibly displaced or moved from under one pillow to another without their seeing the change, toddlers are increasingly aware of the existence of objects behind closed doors, in drawers, and under tables. Parents are usually acutely aware of this developmental achievement and find high places and locked cabinets the only places inaccessible to toddlers.

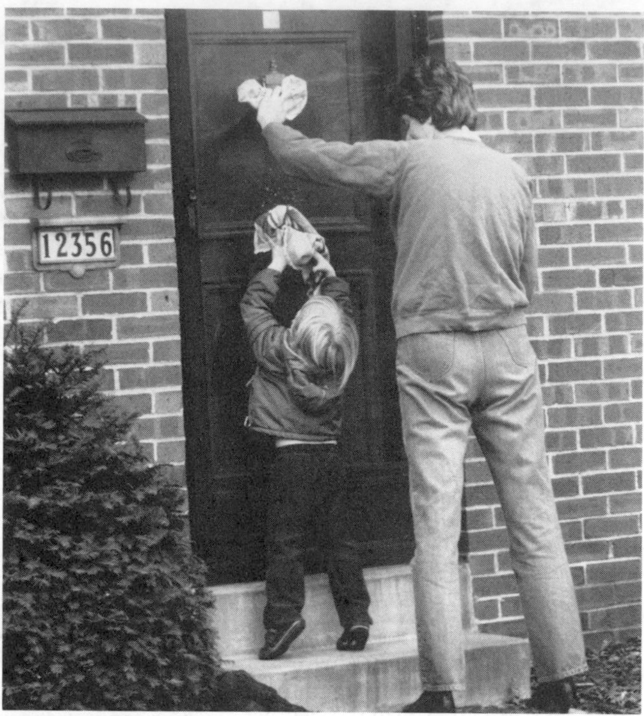

Fig. 34-2 Domestic mimicry and sex-role behavior are common during toddlerhood.

Invention of new means through mental combinations. From ages 19 to 24 months the child is in the final sensorimotor stage. During this stage the child completes the more primitive, autistic thought processes of infancy and is prepared for the more complex mental operations that occur during the phase of preoperational thought. One of the most dramatic achievements of this stage is in the area of object permanence. Children will now actively search for an object in several potential hiding places. In addition, they can infer a cause when only experiencing the effect. They can infer that an object was hidden in any number of places even if they only saw the original hiding place.

Imitation displays deeper meaning and understanding. There is greater symbolization to imitation. The child is acutely aware of others' actions and attempts to copy them in gestures and in words. *Domestic mimicry* (imitating household activities) and sex-role behavior become increasingly common during this period and during the second year. Identification with the parent of the same sex becomes apparent by the second year and represents the child's intellectual ability to differentiate different models of behavior and to imitate them appropriately (Fig. 34-2).

The concept of time is still embryonic, but children have some sense of timing in terms of anticipation, memory, and the limited ability to wait. They may listen to the command, "Just a minute," and behave appropriately. However, their sense of timing is exaggerated—1 minute can seem like an hour. Toddlers' limited attention spans also indicate their sense of immediacy and concern for the present.

Preconceptual phase. At approximately 2 years of age the child enters the preconceptual phase of cognitive development, which lasts until about age 4. The preconceptual phase is a subdivision of the preoperational phase, which spans ages 2 to 7 years. The preconceptual phase is primarily one of transition that bridges the purely self-satisfying behavior of infancy and the rudimentary socialized behavior of latency. *Preoperational thought* implies that children cannot think in terms of *operations*—the ability to manipulate objects in relation to each other in a logical fashion. Rather, toddlers think primarily on the basis of their perception of an event. Problem solving is based on what they see or hear directly rather than on what they recall about objects and events. Several characteristics are unique to preoperational thought (Box 34-1).

Within the second year the child increasingly uses language symbolically and is concerned with the "why" and "how" of things. For example, a pencil is "something to write with" and food is "something to eat." However, such mental symbolization is closely associated with prelogical reasoning. For instance, a needle is "something that hurts." Such painful experiences take on new significance, since memory is associated with the specific event and fears are likely to develop, such as resistance to people who wear white uniforms or rooms that look like the practitioner's office. Because of the vulnerability of these early years, it is essential to prepare children for new experiences, whether it is a new baby-sitter or a visit to the dentist.

SPIRITUAL DEVELOPMENT

Toddlers have only a vague idea of God and religious teachings because of their immature cognitive processes. However, routines such as saying prayers before meals or at bedtime can be very important and comforting. Near the end of toddler-

BOX 34-1
Characteristics of Preoperational Thought

Egocentrism—Inability to envision situations from perspectives other than one's own

Example: If a person is positioned between the toddler and another child, the toddler, who is facing the person, will explain that both children can see the middle person's face. The young child is unable to realize that the other person views the middle person from a different perspective, the back.

Implication: Avoid moralizing about "why" something is wrong if it requires an understanding of someone else's feelings or opinion. Telling a child to stop hitting because hitting hurts the other person is often ineffective because, to the aggressor, it feels good to hit someone else. Instead, emphasize that hitting is not allowed.

Transductive—Reasoning from the particular to the particular

Example: Child refuses to eat a food because something previously eaten did not taste good.

Implication: Accept child's reasoning; offer refused food at different time.

Global organization—Changing any one part of the whole changes the entire whole

Example: Child refuses to sleep in room because location of bed is changed.

Implication: Accept child's reasoning; use same bed position or introduce change slowly.

Centration—Focusing on one aspect rather than considering all possible alternatives

Example: Child refuses to eat a food because of its color, even though its taste and smell are acceptable.

Implication: Accept child's reasoning.

Animism—Attributing lifelike qualities to inanimate objects

Example: Child scolds stairs for making child fall down.

Implication: Join child in the "scolding." Keep frightening objects out of view.

Irreversibility—Inability to undo or reverse the actions initiated physically

Example: When told to stop doing something, such as talking, child is unable to think of positive activity.

Implication: State requests or instructions *positively* (e.g., "Be quiet.")

Magical—Believing that thoughts are all-powerful and can cause events

Example: Child wishes someone died; then if the person dies, child feels at fault because of the "bad" thought that made the death happen.

Calling children "bad" because they did something wrong makes children feel as if they are bad.

Implication: Clarify that thoughts do not make things happen and that child is not responsible.

Use "I" messages rather than "you" messages to communicate thoughts, feelings, expectations, or beliefs without imposing blame or criticism. Emphasize that the act is bad, not the child.

Inability to conserve—Inability to understand the idea that a mass can be changed in size, shape, volume, or length without losing or adding to the original mass (instead, children judge what they see by the immediate perceptual clues given to them)

Example: If two lines of equal length are presented in such a way that one appears longer than the other, child will state that one line is longer even if child measures both lines with a ruler or yardstick and finds that each has the same length.

Implication: Change the most obvious perceptual clue to reorient child's view of what is seen. For example, give medicine in a small medicine cup, rather than a large cup, since child will imagine that the large vessel contains more liquid. If child refuses the medicine in the small cup, pour it into a large cup, because the liquid will appear to be less in a tall, wide container.

Give a large flat cookie rather than a thick small one, or do the reverse with meat or cheese; child will usually eat larger size of favorite food and smaller size of less favorite food.

hood, when children use preoperational thought, there is some advancement of their understanding of God. Religious teachings, such as reward or fear of punishment (heaven or hell) and moral development (see discussion in Chapter 30), may influence their behavior.

DEVELOPMENT OF BODY IMAGE

As in infancy, the development of body image closely parallels cognitive development. With increasing motor ability toddlers recognize the usefulness of body parts and gradually learn their respective names. They also learn that certain parts of the body have various meanings; for example, during toilet training the genitals become significant, and cleanliness is emphasized. By 2 years of age there is recognition of sexual differences and reference to self by name and then by pronoun.

Once they begin preoperational thought, toddlers can use symbols to represent objects, but their thinking may lead to inaccuracies. For example, if someone who is pregnant is called "fat," they will describe all "fat" women as having babies. There is a beginning recognition of words used to describe physical appearance, such as "pretty," "handsome," or "big boy." Such expressions eventually influence how children view their own bodies.

Although there has been little research done on body-image development in young children, it is evident that body integrity is poorly understood and that intrusive experiences are threatening. For example, toddlers forcefully resist procedures such as examining the ear or mouth and taking a rectal temperature. Toddlers also have unclear body boundaries and may associate nonviable parts such as feces with essential body parts. This can be seen in a toddler who is upset by flushing the toilet and watching the stool disappear.

Nurses can assist parents in fostering a positive body image in their child by encouraging them to avoid negative labels such as "skinny arms" or "chubby legs"—self-perceptions that can last a lifetime. Body parts, especially those related to elimination and reproduction, should be called by their correct names. Respect for the body should be practiced.

DEVELOPMENT OF SEXUALITY

Just as toddlers explore their environment, they also explore their bodies and find that touching certain body parts is pleasurable. Genital fondling (masturbation) can occur and involves manual stimulation, as well as posturing movements (especially in young girls) such as tightening of the thighs or mechanical pressure applied to the pubic or suprapubic area (Lidster and Horsburgh, 1994). Other demonstrations of sensual activities include rocking, swinging, and hugging people and toys. Parental reactions to toddlers' sexual behavior will influence the children's own attitudes and should be accepting rather than critical.

Children in this age group are learning vocabulary associated with anatomy, elimination, and reproduction. Certain associations between words and functions become significant and can influence future sexual attitudes. For example, if parents refer to the genitals as dirty, especially in the context of elimination, this association between "genitals" and "dirty" may be transferred to sexual functions.

Sex-role differences become obvious to children and are evident in much of their imitative play. Early attitudes are formed about affectional behaviors between adults from observing parental and other adult sexual/sensual activities. (See also Sex Education, Chapter 35.)

SOCIAL DEVELOPMENT

A major task of the toddler period is differentiation of self from significant others, usually the mother. The differentiation process consists of two phases: **separation,** the children's emergence from a symbiotic fusion with the mother, and **individuation,** those achievements that mark children's assumption of their individual characteristics in the environment. Although the process begins during the latter half of infancy, the major achievements occur during the toddler years.

Toddlers have an increased understanding and awareness of object permanence and some ability to withstand delayed gratification and tolerate moderate frustration. As a result, toddlers react differently to strangers than do infants. The appearance of unfamiliar persons does not represent such a significant threat to their attachment to mother. They have learned from experience that parents exist when physically absent. Repetition of events such as going to bed without the parents but waking to find them there again reinforces the reliability of such brief separations. Consequently, toddlers are able to venture away from their parents for brief periods of time because of the security of knowing that the parents will be there when they return.

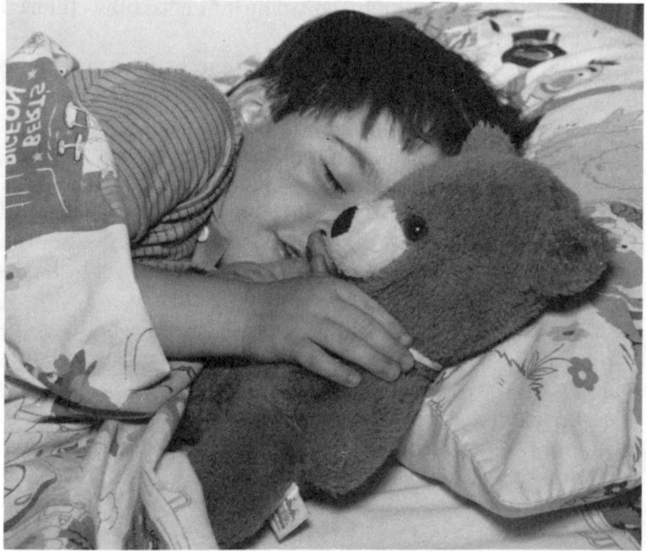

Fig. 34-3 Transitional objects such as a warm and fuzzy stuffed animal are sources of security to a toddler.

Transitional objects such as a favorite blanket or toy provide security for children, especially when they are separated from parents, dealing with a new stress, or just fatigued (Fig. 34-3). Security objects often become so important to toddlers that they refuse to have them taken away. Such behavior is normal; there is no need to discourage this tendency. During separations such as daycare, hospitalization, or even staying overnight with a relative, transitional objects should be provided to minimize any feelings of fear or loneliness.

Learning to tolerate and master brief periods of separation is an important developmental task of children in this age group. In addition, it is a necessary component of parenting, since brief periods of separation allow parents to recoup their energy and patience and to minimize directing their irritations and frustrations at the children.

Language Development

The most striking characteristic of language development during early childhood is the increasing level of comprehension. Although the number of words acquired—from about 4 at 1 year of age to approximately 300 at age 2 years—is notable, *the ability to comprehend and understand speech is much greater than the number of words the child can say.* This is particularly evident in bilingual families, where the vocabulary may be delayed, but comprehension in either language is appropriate.

At age 1 year the child uses one-word sentences or holophrases. The word "up" can mean "pick me up" or "look up there." For the child the one word conveys the meaning of a sentence, but to others it may mean many things or nothing. At this age about 25% of the vocalizations are intelligible. By the age of 2 years the child uses multiword sentences by stringing together two or three words, such as the phrases, "mama go bye-bye" or "all gone," and approximately 65% of the speech is understandable.

Personal-Social Behavior

One of the most dramatic aspects of development in the toddler is personal-social interaction. Parents frequently wonder why their manageable, docile, lovable infant has turned into a determined, strong-willed, volatile-tempered little tyrant. In addition, the tyrant of the "terrible twos" can swiftly and unpredictably revert back to the adorable infant. All of this is part of "growing up" and is evident in such areas as dressing, feeding, playing, and establishing self-control.

Toddlers are developing skills of independence, which are evident in all areas of behavior. By 15 months children feed themselves, drink well from a covered cup, and manage a spoon, with considerable spilling. By 24 months they use a spoon well and by 36 months may be using a fork. Between ages 2 and 3 years they eat with the family and like to help with chores such as setting the table or removing dishes from the dishwasher, but they lack table manners and may find it difficult to sit through the family's entire meal.

In dressing, toddlers also demonstrate strides in independence. The 15-month-old child helps by putting the arm or foot out for dressing and pulls shoes and socks off. The 18-month-old child removes gloves, helps with pullover shirts, and may be able to unzip. By age 2 years the toddler removes most articles of clothing and puts on socks, shoes, and pants without regard for right or left and back or front. Help is still needed to fasten clothes.

Play

Play magnifies the toddler's physical and psychosocial development. Interaction with people becomes increasingly important. The solitary play of infancy progresses to **parallel play**—the toddler plays alongside, not with, other children. Although sensorimotor play is still prominent, there is much less emphasis on the exclusive use of one sensory modality. The toddler inspects the toy, talks to the toy, tests its strength and durability, and invents several uses for it. Imitation is one of the most distinguishing characteristics of play and enriches children's opportunity to engage in fantasy. With less emphasis on sex-stereotyped toys, play objects such as dolls, carriages, dollhouses, dishes, cooking utensils, child-sized furniture, trucks, and dress-up clothes are suitable for both sexes (Fig. 34-4).

Increased locomotive skills make push-pull toys, stick horses, straddle trucks or cycles, a small, low gym and slide, varied-size balls, and rocking horses appropriate for the energetic toddler. Finger paints, thick crayons, chalk, blackboard, paper, and puzzles with large, simple pieces use the child's developing fine motor skills. Interlocking blocks in varied sizes and shapes provide hours of fun and during later years are useful objects for creative and imaginative play.

Talking is a form of play for the toddler, who enjoys musical toys such as play phonographs, "talking" dolls and animals, and play telephones. Appropriate children's television programs are excellent for children in this age group, who learn to associate words with visual images. Toddlers also enjoy "reading" stories from a picture book and imitating the sounds of animals.

Tactile play is also important for the exploring toddler. Water toys, a sandbox with pail and shovel, finger paints, soap bubbles, and clay provide excellent opportunities for free creative and manipulative recreation. Adults sometimes forget the fascination of feeling slippery cream such as whipped cream or pudding, catching airy bubbles, squeezing and reshaping clay, or smearing paints. These types of unstructured activities are as important as educational play to allow children freedom of expression.

Selection of appropriate toys must involve safety factors, especially in relation to size and sturdiness. The oral activity of toddlers makes them at risk for aspirating small objects or ingesting toxic substances. Parents need to be especially vigilant of toys played with in other children's homes or those of older siblings. Toys are a potential source of serious bodily damage to toddlers, who may have the physical strength to manipulate them but not the knowledge to appreciate their danger (see Home Care: Toy Safety, Chapter 30).

Table 34-1 summarizes the major features of growth and development for the age groups of 15, 18, 24, and 30 months.

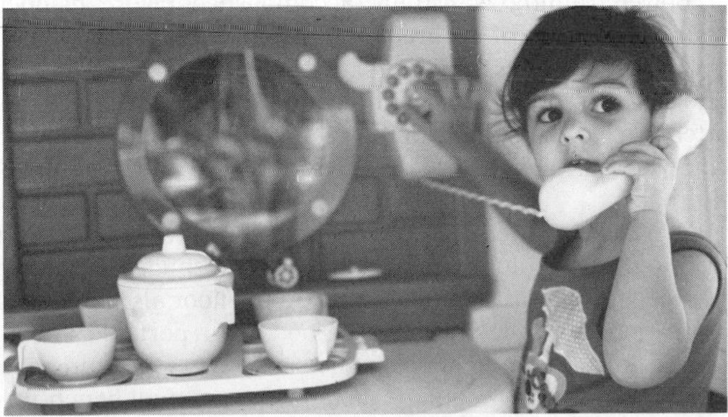

Fig. 34-4 Imitative play is common during the toddler years.

COPING WITH CONCERNS RELATED TO NORMAL GROWTH AND DEVELOPMENT

Toilet Training

One of the major tasks of toddlerhood is toilet training. Voluntary control of the anal and urethral sphincters is achieved sometime after the child is walking, probably between ages 18 and 24 months. However, complex psychophysiologic factors are required for readiness. The child must be able to recognize

Guidelines 

ASSESSING TOILET TRAINING READINESS

Physical readiness

- Voluntary control of anal and urethral sphincters, usually by 18 to 24 months of age
- Ability to stay dry for 2 hours; decreased number of wet diapers; waking dry from nap
- Regular bowel movements
- Gross motor skills of sitting, walking, and squatting
- Fine motor skills to remove clothing

Mental readiness

- Recognizes urge to defecate or urinate
- Verbal or nonverbal communicative skills to indicate when wet or has urge to defecate or urinate
- Cognitive skills to imitate appropriate behavior and follow directions

Psychologic readiness

- Expresses willingness to please parent
- Able to sit on toilet for 5 to 10 minutes without fussing or getting off
- Curiosity about adults' or older sibling's toilet habits
- Impatience with soiled or wet diapers; desire to be changed immediately

Parental readiness

- Recognizes child's level of readiness
- Willing to invest the time required for toilet training
- Absence of family stress or change such as a divorce, moving, new sibling, or imminent vacation

TABLE 34-1 Growth and development during toddler years

AGE (MONTHS)	PHYSICAL	GROSS MOTOR	FINE MOTOR
15	Steady growth in height and weight Head circumference 48 cm (19 inches) Weight 11 kg (24 pounds) Height 78.7 cm (31 inches)	Walks without help (usually since age 13 months) Creeps up stairs Kneels without support Cannot walk around corners or stop suddenly without losing balance Assumes standing position without support Cannot throw ball without falling	Constantly casts objects to floor Builds tower of two cubes Holds two cubes in one hand Releases a pellet into a narrow-necked bottle Scribbles spontaneously Uses cup well but rotates spoon
18	Physiologic anorexia from decreased growth needs Anterior fontanel closed Physiologically able to control sphincters	Runs clumsily, falls often Walks up stairs with one hand held Pulls and pushes toys Jumps in place with both feet Seats self on chair Throws ball overhand without falling	Builds tower of three to four cubes Release, prehension, and reach well developed Turns pages in a book two or three at a time In drawing, makes stroke imitatively Manages spoon without rotation
24	Head circumference 49 to 50 cm (19.5 to 20 inches) Chest circumference exceeds head circumference Lateral diameter of chest exceeds anteroposterior diameter Usual weight gain of 1.8 to 2.7 kg (4 to 6 pounds) Usual gain in height of 10 to 12.5 cm (4 to 5 inches) Adult height approximately double height at 2 years of age May have achieved readiness for beginning daytime control of bowel and bladder Primary dentition of 16 teeth	Goes up and down stairs alone with two feet on each step Runs fairly well, with wide stance Picks up object without falling Kicks ball forward without overbalancing	Builds tower of six to seven cubes Aligns two or more cubes like a train Turns pages of book one at a time In drawing, imitates vertical and circular strokes Turns doorknob, unscrews lid
30	Birth weight quadrupled Primary dentition (20 teeth) completed May have daytime bowel and bladder control	Jumps with both feet Jumps from chair or step Stands on one foot momentarily Takes a few steps on tiptoe	Builds tower of eight cubes Adds chimney to train of cubes Good hand-finger coordination; holds crayon with fingers rather than fist Moves fingers independently In drawing, imitates vertical and horizontal strokes, makes two or more strokes for cross

the urge to let go and hold on and be able to communicate this sensation to the parent. In addition, there is probably some necessary motivation in the desire to please the parent by holding on, rather than pleasing oneself by letting go.

Usually physiologic and psychologic readiness is not complete until 18 to 24 months of age. By this time the child has mastered the majority of essential gross motor skills, can communicate intelligibly, is less in conflict with self-assertion and negativism, and is aware of the ability to control the body and please the parent. One of the most important responsibilities of nurses is to help parents identify the readiness signs in their child (see the Guidelines box on p. 999).*

*A helpful brochure is *Toilet Training: A Parent's Guide,* available from the **American Academy of Pediatrics,** 141 Northwest Point Blvd., P.O. Box 927, Elk Grove Village, IL 60009-0927; (800) 433-9016.

Bowel training is usually accomplished before bladder training because of its greater regularity and predictability. There is a stronger sensation for defecation than for urination, and the sensation of defecation can be brought to the child's attention. In fact, nighttime bladder training may not be completed until 4 or 5 years of age, and even later training is normal.

A number of techniques can be helpful when initiating training. A freestanding potty-chair allows children a feeling of security. Planting the feet firmly on the floor also facilitates defecation (Stark, 1994). Another option is a portable seat attached to the regular toilet, which may ease the transition from potty-chair to regular toilet. Placing a small bench under the feet helps to stabilize the child's position. It is probably best to keep the potty in the bathroom and to let the child observe the excreta being flushed down the toilet to associate

TABLE 34-1 Growth and development during toddler years—cont'd

SENSORY	LANGUAGE	SOCIALIZATION
Able to identify geometric forms; places round object into appropriate hole Binocular vision well developed Displays an intense and prolonged interest in pictures	Uses expressive jargon Says four to six words, including names "Asks" for objects by pointing Understands simple commands May use head-shaking gesture to denote "no" Uses "no" even while agreeing to the request	Tolerates some separation from parent Less likely to fear strangers Beginning to imitate parents, such as cleaning house (sweeping, dusting), folding clothes May discard bottle Manages spoon but rotates it near mouth Kisses and hugs parents, may kiss pictures in a book Expresses emotions, has temper tantrums
	Says 10 or more words Points to a common object, such as a shoe or ball, and to two or three body parts	Great imitator (domestic mimicry) Takes off gloves, socks, and shoes and unzips Temper tantrums may be more evident Beginning awareness of ownership ("my toy") May develop dependency on transitional objects such as "security blanket"
Accommodation well developed In geometric discrimination, able to insert square block into oblong space	Has vocabulary of approximately 300 words Uses two- to three-word phrases Uses pronouns "I," "me," "you" Understands directional commands Gives first name; refers to self by name Verbalizes need for toileting, food, or drink Talks incessantly	Stage of parallel play Has sustained attention span Temper tantrums decreasing Pulls people to show them something Increased independence from parent Dresses self in simple clothing
	Gives first and last name Refers to self by appropriate pronoun Uses plurals Names one color	Separates more easily from parent In play, helps put things away, can carry breakable objects, pushes with good steering Begins to notice sex differences; knows own sex May attend to toilet needs without help, except for wiping

these activities with usual practices. If a potty-seat is not available, having the child sit *facing* the toilet tank provides added support. Boys may begin toilet training in the stand-up position or by sitting on a potty-chair or toilet. Imitating father is a powerful motivating force (Fig. 34-5).

Practice sessions should be limited to 5 or 10 minutes, a parent should stay with the child, and sanitary habits should be used after every session. Children should be praised for cooperative behavior and/or successful evacuation. It is helpful to dress children in easily removed clothing; to use training pants, "pull-on" diapers, or panties; and to encourage imitation by watching others. Forcing children to sit on the potty-chair or toilet for long periods, spanking them for having accidents, and other methods of negative control should be avoided. Daytime accidents are common, particularly during periods of intense activity. Young children become so engrossed in play activity that if they are not reminded, they will wait until it is too late to reach the bathroom. Therefore frequent reminders and trips to the toilet are necessary.

Sibling Rivalry

The natural jealousy and resentment of children to a new child in the family is referred to as *sibling rivalry*. The arrival of a new infant represents a crisis for even the best-prepared toddlers. It is not the infant that toddlers hate or resent but the changes that this additional sibling produces, especially the separation from mother during the birth. The parents now share their love and attention with someone else, the usual routine is disrupted, and toddlers may lose their crib and/or room—all at a time when they thought they were in control of their world. Sibling rivalry tends to be most pronounced in the firstborn, who experiences *dethronement* (loss of sole

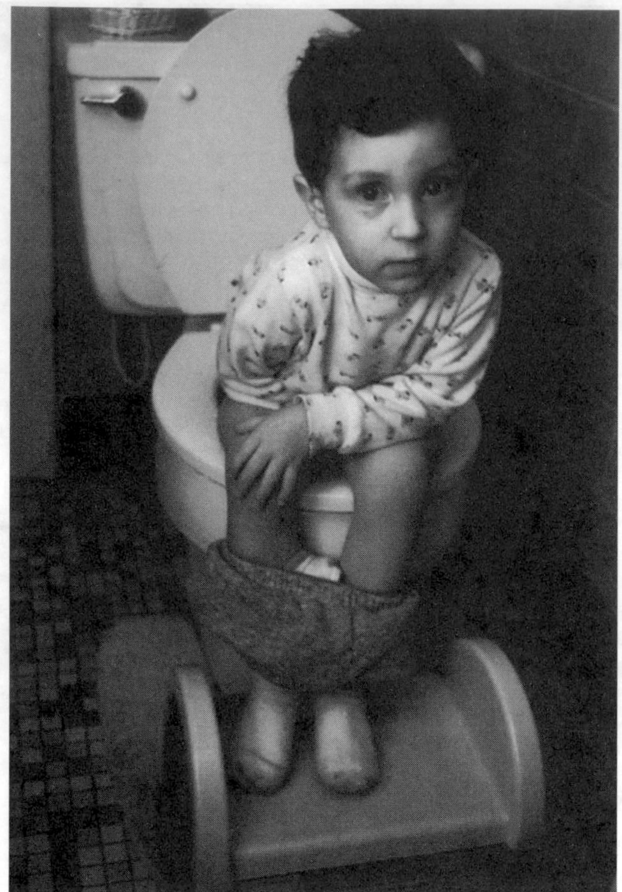

Fig. 34-5 Boys may begin toilet training sitting on a toilet. Note feet on small bench.

parental attention). It also seems to be most difficult for young children, particularly in terms of mother-child interaction.

Preparation of children for the birth of a sibling is quite individual, but age dictates some important considerations. Time for toddlers is a vague concept. Tomorrow could be yesterday or next week, and a month from now could be never. Preparing children too soon for the birth may lessen their interest by the time the event occurs. A good time to start talking about the new baby is when toddlers become aware of the pregnancy and the changes taking place in the home in anticipation of the new member.

Toddlers need to have a realistic idea of what the newborn will be like. Telling them that a new playmate will come home soon sets up unrealistic expectations. Rather, parents should stress the activities that will take place when the baby arrives home, such as diapering, bottle- or breast-feeding, bathing, and dressing. At the same time, parents should emphasize which routines will stay the same, such as reading stories or going to the park. If toddlers have had no contact with an infant, it is a good idea to introduce them to one, if feasible. Providing a doll on which toddlers can imitate parental behaviors is another excellent strategy. They can tend to the doll's needs (diapering, feeding) at the same time the parent is performing similar activities for the infant.

A new sibling in the home is stressful; any additional stresses for the toddler should be avoided or minimized. For example, moving the toddler to a regular bed or to a different room should be done well in advance of the infant's arrival.

Pregnancy is an abstraction for toddlers. They need concrete illustrations of how the baby is growing inside the mother. It is an excellent opportunity for introducing aspects of reproduction and sexuality. Seeing simple pictures of the uterus and fetus and feeling the fetus move help the child feel involved in the experience. Children also benefit from "siblings" classes that may be part of prenatal sessions.

When the new baby arrives, toddlers keenly feel the changed focus of attention. Visitors may initiate problems when they inadvertently shower the infant with attention and presents while neglecting the older child. Parents can minimize this by alerting visitors to the toddler's needs, having small presents on hand for the toddler, and including the child in the visit as much as possible.

How children exhibit jealousy is complex. Some will overtly hit the infant, push the child off mother's lap, or pull the bottle or breast from the infant's mouth. More often the expressions of hostility and resentment are more subtle and covert. Toddlers may verbally express a wish that the infant "go back inside mommy," or they will revert to more infantile forms of behavior such as demanding a bottle, soiling their underpants, clinging for attention, using baby talk, or aggressively acting out toward others. For this reason, parents must protect infants by supervising the interaction between the siblings.

Temper Tantrums

Toddlers may assert their independence by violently objecting to discipline. They may lie down on the floor, kick their feet, and scream at the top of their lungs. Some have learned the effectiveness of holding their breath until the parent relents. Although holding one's breath may cause fainting from the lack of oxygen, the accumulation of carbon dioxide will stimulate the respiratory control center, resulting in no physical harm.

The best approach toward extinguishing such attention-seeking behavior is to ignore it, provided the behavior is not injuring the child, such as violently banging the head on the floor. However, the parent should remain close by. When the tantrum has subsided, the child needs to feel some control and security. At this time a toy or a favorite activity can be substituted for the ungranted request. (See also Limit Setting and Discipline in Chapter 29.)

Frequently temper tantrums can be avoided by giving the child advance warning of a request. For example, a popular time for tantrums is before bed. Active toddlers often have trouble slowing down and when placed in bed, resist staying there. One approach is to establish limited rituals that signal readiness for bed such as a bath or story. Parents can reinforce the pattern by stating, "After this story it is bedtime," and consistently carrying out the routine.

Negativism

One of the more difficult aspects of rearing children in this age group is their persistent "no" response to every request. The negativism is not an expression of being fresh or insolent, but a necessary assertion of self-control. One method of dealing with the negativism is reducing the opportunities for a "no" answer. Asking the child, "Do you want to go to sleep now?" is an almost certain example of a question that will be answered with an emphatic "no." Instead, tell the child that it is time to go to sleep and proceed accordingly.

In their attempt to exert control, children like to make choices. When confronted with appropriate choices, such as, "You may have a peanut butter and jelly sandwich or chicken noodle soup for lunch," they are more likely to choose one rather than automatically say no. However, if their response is negative, parents should make the choice for the child.

Regression

The retreat from one's present pattern of functioning to past levels of behavior is referred to as **regression.** It usually occurs in instances of discomfort or stress when one attempts to conserve psychic energy by reverting to patterns of behavior that were successful in earlier stages of development. Regression is common in toddlers, because almost any additional stress hinders their ability to master present developmental tasks. Any threat to their autonomy such as illness, hospitalization, separation, or adjustment to a sibling, represents a need to revert to earlier forms of behavior, such as increased dependency; refusal to use the potty-chair; temper tantrums; demand for the bottle, stroller, or crib; and loss of newly learned motor, language, social, and cognitive skills.

At first such regression appears acceptable and comfortable for children, but the loss of newly acquired achievements is frightening and threatening because children are aware of their total helplessness in the recent past. Parents, too, become frightened of regressive behavior and frequently in their efforts to deal with it force the child to cope with an additional source of stress—the pressure to live up to expected standards.

When regression does occur, the best approach is to ignore it while praising existing patterns of appropriate behavior. Regression is a child's way of saying, "I can't cope with this present stress and perfect this skill as well, but I will if given patience and understanding." For this reason it is advisable not to attempt new areas of learning when an additional crisis is present or expected, such as beginning toilet training shortly before a sibling is born or attempting new areas of learning during a brief period of hospitalization.

Promoting Optimum Health During Toddlerhood

NUTRITION

During the period from 12 to 18 months of age, the growth rate slows, decreasing the child's need for calories, protein, and fluid. However, the protein (1.2 g/kg) and caloric (102 kcal/kg) requirements are still relatively high to meet the demands for muscle tissue growth and high activity level (Forgac, 1995). The need for minerals such as iron, calcium, and phosphorus is still high, particularly when one considers the poor food habits of children in this age group and the increased mineralization within bones.

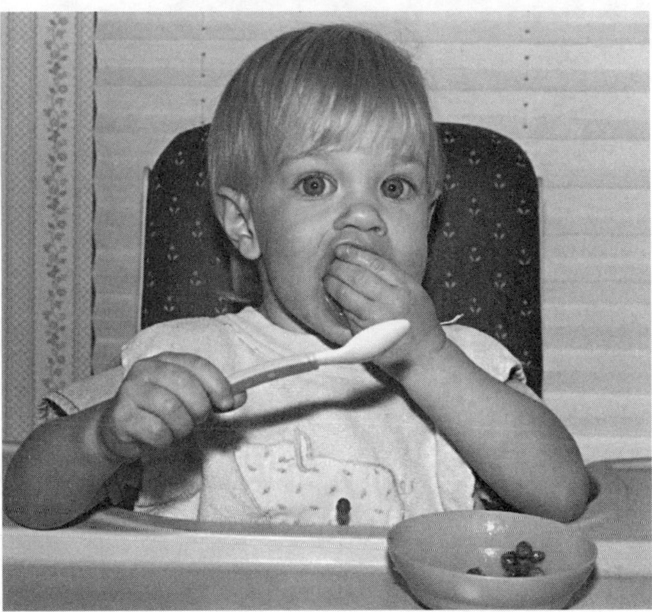

Fig. 34-6 Toddlers will often hold a spoon but continue to eat with their fingers.

At approximately 18 months of age, most toddlers manifest this decreased nutritional need with a decreased appetite, a phenomenon known as *physiologic anorexia.* They become picky, fussy eaters with strong taste preferences. They may eat large amounts one day and almost nothing the next. They are increasingly aware of the nonnutritive function of food: the pleasure of eating, the social aspect of mealtime, and the control of refusing food. They are influenced by factors other than taste when choosing food. If a family member refuses to eat something, toddlers are likely to imitate that response. If the plate is overfilled, they are likely to push it away, overwhelmed by its size. If food does not appear or smell appetizing, they will probably not agree to try it. In essence, mealtime is more closely associated with psychologic components than with nutritional ones.

Developmentally, by 12 months of age most children are eating the same food prepared for the rest of the family. Some may have mastered using a cup with occasional spilling, although most cannot adeptly use a spoon until 18 months of age or later and generally prefer using their fingers (Fig. 34-6).

Nutritional Counseling

Eating habits established in the first 2 or 3 years of life tend to have lasting effects on subsequent years. If food is used as a reward or sign of approval, a child may overeat for nonnutritive reasons. If food is forced and mealtime is consistently unpleasant, the usual pleasure associated with eating may not develop. Mealtimes should be enjoyable rather than times for discipline or family arguments. The social aspect of mealtime may be distracting for young children; therefore an earlier feeding hour may be appropriate. Young children are unable to sit through a long meal and become fidgety and disruptive.

BOX 34-2
Sample Menu for Toddlers Based on Food Guide Pyramid*

Breakfast	$^{1}/_{2}$ cup dry, unsweetened cereal $^{1}/_{2}$ cup orange juice 4 oz low-fat milk
Snack	$^{1}/_{2}$-1 whole banana
Lunch	1 tbsp peanut butter 2 tsp all-fruit preserves 1 slice whole-wheat bread 2 tbsp peas 4 oz low-fat milk
Snack	2 graham crackers 4 oz low-fat milk
Dinner	1 chicken leg, roasted without skin $^{1}/_{4}$-$^{1}/_{2}$ cup macaroni and cheese 2 tbsp green beans, cooked 2 tbsp carrots, cooked 4-6 oz low-fat milk
Snack	$^{1}/_{2}$ cup frozen yogurt
Total Servings	
Bread, cereal, rice, pasta	6-7
Vegetable	3
Fruit	3-4
Milk, yogurt, cheese	2-3
Meat, poultry, fish, dried beans, eggs, nuts	2

*Use fats, oils, and sweets sparingly. Increase fluids with servings of water. Serving sizes are minimums for nutritional adequacy. Many children eat more.

This is particularly common when children are brought to the table just after active play. Calling them in from play 15 minutes before mealtime allows them ample opportunity to get ready for eating while settling down their active minds and bodies.

The method of serving food also takes on more importance during this period. Toddlers need to feel control and achievement in their abilities. Giving them large, adult-size portions can overwhelm them. In general, what is eaten is much more significant than how much is consumed. Small amounts of meat and vegetables supply greater food value than a large consumption of bread or potato. Serving sizes need to be appropriate for age (Box 34-2). A general guide to the serving size of food is 1 tablespoon of solid food per year of age or one fourth to one third the adult portion size. Young children tend to like less spicy, bland food, although this is a culturally determined preference. Substitutions can be provided for foods that they do not enjoy, although this practice should not cater to all their desires. Frequent nutritious snacks can replace a meal. "Grazing"—nibbling and snacking—is a good way to ensure proper nutrition, provided appropriate foods are offered.

The ritualism of this age also dictates certain principles in feeding practices. Toddlers like the same dish, cup, or spoon every time they eat. They may reject a favorite food simply because it is served in a different dish. If one food touches another, they often refuse to eat it. Mixed foods such as stews or casseroles are rarely favorites. Since toddlers are unpredictable in their table manners, it is best to use plastic dishes and cups for both economy and safety. For some children a regular meal-time schedule also helps satisfy their desire and need for predictability and ritualism.

Most children by 12 months of age are eating the same food prepared for the rest of the family. However, appetite and food preferences are sporadic. Often the interest in food parallels a growth spurt, so that periods of good eating are interspersed with phases of poor eating. "Food jags" are common.

Such food fads do not ensure a well-balanced diet, but attempts to alter them are usually unsuccessful. It is preferable to accept such extremes and offer other foods in small portions. Introducing at least three items from the different food groups at each meal helps develop a variety of taste preferences and well-balanced eating habits.

SLEEP AND ACTIVITY

Total sleep decreases only slightly during the second year and averages about 12 hours a day. Most children take one nap a day, and by the end of the second or third year many relinquish this habit. The activity level is high, and there is rarely a problem with too little physical exercise, provided inappropriate restrictions are not instituted. With increasing numbers of young children being cared for outside the home, attention to the kinds of activity provided is important. For example, children with high activity levels may benefit from an environment in which outdoor play is encouraged.

Sleep problems are common, especially going to bed and falling asleep, and are probably related to fears of separation. Bedtime rituals (same hour of sleep, snack, quiet activity) are helpful, and transitional objects such as a favorite stuffed animal or blanket can help ease the child's insecurity at bedtime (Fig. 34-3).

DENTAL HEALTH

Regular Dental Examinations

Ideally the child should see a dentist (or pedodontist, a pediatric dentist) soon after the first teeth erupt and no later than age $2^{1}/_{2}$ years, when primary dentition is completed. Initial visits to the dentist should be nontraumatizing. Since toddlers react negatively to new and potentially frightening experiences, the initial visit can center around meeting the dentist, seeing the equipment, and sitting in the chair. If the child is cooperative, the dentist may just look at the teeth but reserve a more thorough examination for another visit. Modeling, in which the child observes procedures performed on the parent or a cooperative sibling, can also be effective.

Removal of Plaque

The objective of oral hygiene is removal of **plaque,** soft bacterial deposits that adhere to the teeth and cause *dental caries (decay* or *cavities)* and *periodontal (gum) disease.* The most effective methods for plaque removal are brushing and flossing.

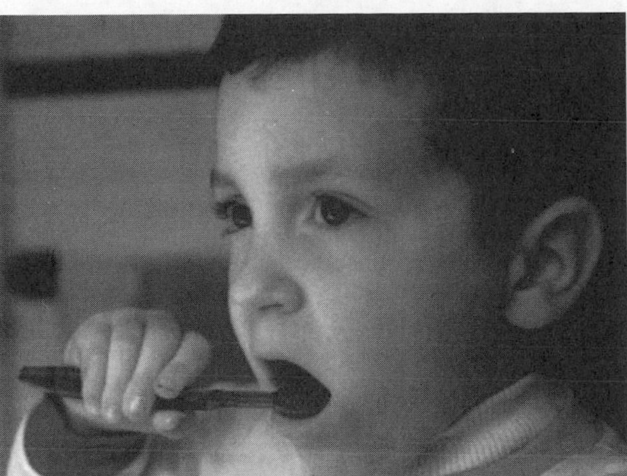

Fig. 34-7 Young children can participate in toothbrushing, but parents need to thoroughly brush all teeth.

Several brushing techniques exist, although there is no universal agreement regarding the best method. One that is suitable for cleaning the primary teeth is the scrub method. The tips of the bristles are placed firmly at a 45-degree angle against the teeth and gums and moved back and forth in a vibratory motion. The ends of the bristles should be wiggling but not moving forcefully back and forth, which can damage the gums and enamel. All the surfaces of the teeth are cleaned in this manner except the lingual (inner) surfaces of the anterior teeth. To clean these surfaces, the toothbrush is placed vertical to the teeth and moved up and down. Only a few teeth are brushed at one time, using six to eight strokes for each section. A systematic approach is used so that all surfaces are thoroughly cleaned (Fig. 34-7).

For young children the most effective cleaning is done by parents. Several positions can be used that facilitate access to the mouth and help stabilize the head for comfort:

- Stand with child's back toward adult. (When done in front of a bathroom mirror, both child and adult can see what is being done in the mirror.)
- Sit on a couch or bed with child's head resting in adult's lap.
- Sit on the floor or a stool with child's head resting between adult's thighs.

With all positions, use one hand to cup the chin and one to brush the teeth. For easier access to back teeth, the mouth is held partially open.

For effective cleaning, a small toothbrush with soft, rounded, multitufted nylon bristles that are short and uniform in length is recommended. Nylon bristles dry more rapidly after use and retain their shape better than natural bristles. Toothbrushes are replaced as soon as the bristles are frayed or bent. With young children, brushing may be more easily accomplished using only water, since many children dislike the foam from toothpaste and the foam interferes with visibility. There is also the danger of swallowing fluoridated

TABLE 34-2 Fluoride supplementation*

AGE	WATER FLUORIDE CONTENT (IN PPM)†		
	<0.3	0.3-0.6	>0.6
Birth–6 months	0	0	0
6 months–3 years	0.25	0	0
3–6 years	0.50	0.25	0
6–16 years	1.00	0.50	0

From American Academy of Pediatrics, Committee on Nutrition: Fluoride supplementation for children, *Pediatrics* 95(5): 777, 1995.
*Fluoride daily doses are given in milligrams.
†*PPM*, Parts per million.

toothpaste (see following discussion under Fluoride). When using toothpaste, children should select the flavor they like to encourage the brushing habit.

After the teeth have been cleaned, they should be flossed with dental floss to remove plaque and debris from between the teeth and below the gum margin, where brushing is ineffective. Since young children do not have the dexterity to manipulate the floss, parents are taught the procedure.

A disclosing agent is helpful in identifying areas of the teeth where plaque accumulates. It also helps motivate children to clean their teeth because plaque is difficult to see. After cleaning, the mouth is inspected to ensure that all traces of plaque have been removed. Where plaque remains, the teeth are rebrushed.

Ideally the teeth should be cleaned after each meal and especially before bedtime, and the child should be given nothing to eat or drink after the night brushing except water. When brushing is impractical, the "swish-and-swallow" method of cleaning the mouth is taught: with a mouthful of water the child rinses the mouth and swallows, repeating the procedure three or four times.

Fluoride

Fluoride, a mineral, reduces the incidence of tooth decay and is found in water, foods, or drinks in which fluoridated water was used as part of the processing system. Because the water fluoridation process and fluoride toothpaste manufacturing are almost impossible to unify in the United States, the dosage of fluoride supplements has been lowered to reduce the incidence of fluorosis. Increased fluoride ingestion leads to enamel protein retention, hypomineralization of the enamel and dentin, and disturbance of crystal formation. The effects caused by this change range from merely discernible white fiberlike lines or spots to gray-brown stains or pitted areas.

It is now recommended that fluoride supplementation be withheld from birth to 6 months and decreased in dosage from 6 months to 6 years of age. Supplements are not needed if the water supply has adequate fluoride. The level of fluoride in water has been decreased from the earlier recommendation of 0.7 to 0.6 parts per million (Table 34-2) (American Academy of Pediatrics, 1995).

Nurses have a responsibility to ensure an optimal fluoride regimen for children and to counsel families regarding correct use of supplements. The nurse should have a knowledge of the fluoride content of the community water supply and provide instruction to parents regarding correct administration of fluoride drops or tablets. Supplements should remain in the mouth for 30 seconds before swallowing and be taken on an empty stomach. Afterward the child should not drink or eat for 30 minutes. All fluoride products (toothpaste, supplements, and rinse) need to be stored away from young children to prevent poisoning. If the water supply is fluoridated, parents are encouraged to use water to prepare drinks and foods (Serwint et al, 1993).

Low-Cariogenic Diet

Diet is critical to developing good teeth because the carious process depends primarily on fermentable sugars, especially sucrose. Refined table sugar, honey, molasses, corn syrup, and dried fruits such as raisins are highly cariogenic.

Ideally such foods should be eliminated. However, since this is impractical, some suggestions can be helpful. First, *the frequency with which sugar is consumed is more important than the total amount eaten.* Therefore, when sweets are eaten, they are less damaging if consumed immediately after a meal rather than as a snack between meals. When sweets are served as the dessert, the teeth can be cleaned afterward, decreasing the amount of time the sugar is in the mouth.

Second, the form of sugar is important. The more cariogenic foods are those that are sticky or hard, since they remain in the mouth longer. Consequently, sucking on lollipops is more cariogenic than eating a chocolate bar. Sometimes the source of the sugar is "hidden," such as in numerous prescription and nonprescription drugs and in many popular cereals, including the "all-natural" variety. Reading food labels is essential in eliminating sources of sucrose. Some snacks do not contribute to tooth decay. Aged cheeses, such as cheddar, may alter the pH and retard bacterial growth. Sugarless gum chewed after eating may actually protect against cavities by stimulating saliva that neutralizes acid. The artificial sweeteners saccharin and aspartame are noncariogenic; sorbitol has low cariogenic potential.

A special form of tooth decay in children between 18 months and 3 years of age is **nursing caries** (also called **nursing bottle caries or bottle-mouth caries**), which occurs when the child is routinely given a bottle of milk or juice at nap or bedtime or uses the bottle as a pacifier while awake. Frequent nocturnal breast-feeding for prolonged periods also leads to extensive destruction of the teeth. The practice of coating pacifiers in honey can also contribute to caries and may be a potential source of botulism poisoning. As the sweet liquid pools in the mouth, the teeth are bathed for several hours in this cariogenic environment. The maxillary (upper) incisors and molars are affected most, since the mandibular (lower) incisors are protected by the lower lip, tongue, and saliva. Severely decayed teeth may require the application of stainless steel bands to preserve the spacing until the permanent teeth erupt.

Prevention involves eliminating the bedtime bottle completely, feeding the last bottle before bedtime, substituting a bottle of water for milk or juice, not using the bottle as a pacifier, and never coating pacifiers in sweet substances. Juice in bottles, especially commercially available ready-to-use bottles, is discouraged, since the beverage is especially damaging because the sugar is more readily converted to acid. Juice should always be offered in a cup to avoid prolonging the bottle-feeding habit. Nurses are in an excellent position to counsel parents regarding the dangers of this habit and other aspects of dental care.*

INJURY PREVENTION

Injuries cause more deaths in the age group 4 years and younger than in any other childhood period except adolescence. The injury death rate has remained relatively unchanged during the past decade; however, the corresponding rates from all other causes of death combined have declined significantly. Injury's prominence as the leading cause of death among toddlers and preschoolers underscores the need to emphasize safety awareness among parents. Child protection and parent education are key determinants in injury prevention.

A major factor in the critical increase of injuries during early childhood is the unrestricted freedom achieved through locomotion combined with an unawareness of danger within the environment. Specific categories of injuries and appropriate prevention are best understood by associating them with the major developmental achievements of young children (Table 34-3). The discussions of injuries in Chapters 27 and 33 are also relevant to safety concerns at this age.

Motor Vehicle Injuries

Motor vehicle injuries cause more accidental deaths in all pediatric age groups after age 1 year than any other type of injury or disease and are responsible for almost one half of all accidental deaths among children ages 1 to 4 years. Many of the deaths are caused by injuries within the car when restraints have not been used or have been used improperly. Approved restraints properly installed and applied can reduce the majority of fatalities and injuries (Osberg and DiScala, 1992).

Nurses have a responsibility for educating parents regarding the importance of car restraints and their proper use. Five types of restraints are available: (1) infant-only devices, (2) convertible models for both infants and toddlers, (3) boosters, (4) safety belts, and (5) devices for children with special needs (see Chapter 38). The infant restraints are discussed in Chapter 33; the convertible restraints and boosters are included here.

The *convertible restraint* is suitable for infants in the rear-ward-facing position and for toddlers in the forward-facing position (Fig. 34-8). The transition point for switching to the forward-facing position is defined by the manufacturer but is generally at a body weight of at least 9 kg (20 pounds) and 1 year of age. Convertible safety seats should be used until the child weighs at least 18 kg (40 pounds). The restraint consists of a molded hard plastic or metal frame with energy-absorbing padding and a special harness system designed to

---

*Sources of information about nursing bottle caries and other aspects of child dental health include **National Institute of Dental Research,** NIH, Building 31, Room 2 C35, 31 Center Drive MSC 2290, Bethesda, MD 20892-2290, (301) 496-4261; **American Society of Dentistry for Children,** 211 E. Chicago Ave., Suite 1036, Chicago, IL 60611, (312) 337-2169 or 800-544-2174 (outside Illinois); **American Dental Association,** 211 E. Chicago Ave., Chicago, IL 60611, (312) 440-2500 or 800-621-8099 (outside Illinois); and **Canadian Dental Association,** 1815 Alta Vista Dr., Ottawa, Ontario K1G, (613) 523-1770. Guidelines for children's dental care are available in Wong DL: *Wong and Whaley's clinical manual of pediatric nursing,* ed 4, St Louis, 1996, Mosby.

TABLE 34-3 Injury prevention during early childhood

DEVELOPMENTAL ABILITIES RELATED TO RISK OF INJURY	INJURY PREVENTION
	Motor vehicles
Walks, runs, and climbs Can open doors and gates Can ride tricycle Can throw ball and other objects	Use federally approved car restraint; if restraint is not available, use lap belt Supervise child while playing outside Do not allow child to play on curb or behind a parked car Do not permit child to play in pile of leaves, snow, or large cardboard container in trafficked area Supervise tricycle riding Lock fences and doors if not directly supervising children Teach child to obey pedestrian safety rules Obey traffic regulations; cross only at crosswalks and only when traffic signal indicates it is safe Stand back a step from the curb until it's time to cross Look left, right, and left again and check for turning cars before crossing street Use sidewalks; when there is no sidewalk, walk on the left, facing traffic Wear light colors at night, and attach fluorescent material to clothing
	Drowning
Can explore if left unsupervised Has great curiosity Helpless in water; unaware of its danger; depth of water has no significance	Supervise closely when near any source of water Keep bathroom doors closed Have fence around swimming pool and lock gate Teach swimming and water safety
	Burns
Can reach heights by climbing, stretching, and standing on toes Pulls objects Explores any holes or opening Can open drawers and closets Unaware of potential sources of heat or fire Plays with mechanical objects	Turn pot handles toward back of stove Place electric appliances, such as coffee maker and popcorn machine, toward back of counter Place guardrails in front of radiators, fireplaces, or other heating elements Store matches and cigarette lighters in locked or inaccessible area; discard carefully Place burning candles, incense, hot foods, and cigarettes out of reach Do not let tablecloth hang within child's reach Do not let electric cord from iron or other appliance hang within child's reach Cover electrical outlets with protective plastic caps Keep electrical wires hidden or out of reach Do not allow child to play with electrical appliance, wires, or lighters Stress danger of open flames; teach what "hot" means Always check bathwater temperature; adjust water heater temperature to 49° C (120° F) or lower; do not allow children to play with faucets Apply a sunscreen when child is exposed to sunlight
	Poisoning
Explores by putting objects in mouth Can open drawers, closets, and most containers Climbs Cannot read labels Does not know safe dose or amount	Place all potentially toxic agents out of reach or in a locked cabinet Caution against eating nonedible items such as plants Replace medications or poisons immediately; replace child-resistant closures properly Administer medications as a drug, not as a candy Do not store large surplus of toxic agents Promptly discard empty poison containers; never reuse to store a food item or other poison Teach child not to play in trash containers Never remove labels from containers of toxic substances Have syrup of ipecac in home; use only if advised Know number and location of nearest poison control center (usually listed in front of telephone directory)
	Falls
Can open doors and some windows Goes up and down stairs Depth perception unrefined	Keep screen in window, nail securely, and use guardrail Place gates at top and bottom of stairs Keep doors locked or use child-proof doorknob covers at entry to stairs, high porch, or other elevated area, including laundry chute Remove unsecured or scatter rugs

Continued.

TABLE 34-3 Injury prevention during early childhood—cont'd

DEVELOPMENTAL ABILITIES RELATED TO RISK OF INJURY	INJURY PREVENTION
	Falls
	Apply nonskid bath mat or decals in bathtub or shower
	Keep crib rails fully raised and mattress at lowest level
	Place carpeting under crib and in bathroom
	Keep large toys and bumper pads out of crib or playpen (child can use these as "stairs" to climb out), then move to youth bed when child is able to climb out of crib
	Avoid using walkers, especially near stairs
	Dress in safe clothing (soles that do not "catch" on floor, tied shoelaces, pant legs that do not touch floor)
	Keep child restrained in vehicles; never leave unattended in shopping cart
	Supervise at playgrounds; select play areas with soft ground cover and safe equipment
	Choking and suffocation
Puts things in mouth May swallow hard or nonedible pieces of food	Avoid large, round chunks of meat, such as whole hot dogs (slice lengthwise into short pieces)
	Avoid fruit with pits, fish with bones, dried beans, hard candy, chewing gum, nuts, popcorn, grapes, marshmallows
	Choose large sturdy toys without sharp edges or small removable parts
	Discard old appliances (e.g., refrigerators, ovens); if storing an old appliance, remove the door
	Keep automatic garage door transmitter in inaccessible place
	Select safe toy boxes or chests without heavy, hinged lids
	Bodily damage
Still clumsy in many skills Easily distracted from tasks Unaware of potential danger from strangers or other people	Avoid giving sharp or pointed objects—such as knives, scissors, or toothpicks—especially when walking or running
	Do not allow lollipops or similar objects in mouth when walking or running
	Teach safety precautions (e.g., to carry knife or scissors with pointed end away from face)
	Store all dangerous tools, garden equipment, and firearms in locked cabinet
	Be alert to danger of supervised animals and household pets
	Use safety glass and decals on large glassed areas, such as sliding glass doors
	Teach child name, address, and phone number and to ask for help from appropriate people (cashier, security guard, policeman) if lost; have identification on child (shown in clothes, inside shoe)
	Teach stranger safety
	Avoid personalized clothing in public places
	Never go with a stranger
	Tell parents if anyone makes child feel uncomfortable in any way
	Always listen to child's concerns regarding others' behavior
	Teach child to say "no" when confronted with uncomfortable situations

hold the child firmly in the seat and distribute the forces to body areas that can withstand the impact.

Boosters are not restraint systems like the convertible devices because they depend on the vehicle belts to hold the child and booster in place. Boosters are of two types: *a low-shield model* that primarily uses a lap belt (Fig. 34-9) and a *belt-positioning model* that uses a lap/shoulder belt. The combination lap/shoulder belt is preferred to the shield (lap belt) model (American Academy of Pediatrics, 1996).

Some older-model restraints require the use of a top anchor (tether) strap to prevent the child from pitching forward in a crash. If the tether strap is not used, up to 90% of the restraint's protection is lost. Instructions for proper installation of the tether strap and permanent bracket are included with the car restraint. Cars with free-sliding latchplates on the lap/shoulder belt require the use of a metal locking clip to keep the belt in a tight-holding position. The locking clip is threaded onto the belt above the latchplate (inset, Fig. 34-8). If parents have newer cars with automatic lap/shoulder belts, they need to have additional lap belts installed to properly secure the restraint.

Children should use specially designed car restraints until they weigh at least 27 kg (60 pounds) or are 8 years old (American Academy of Pediatrics, 1996). Children who outgrow the convertible restraint may still be able to ride safely in a booster seat until the midpoint of the head is higher than

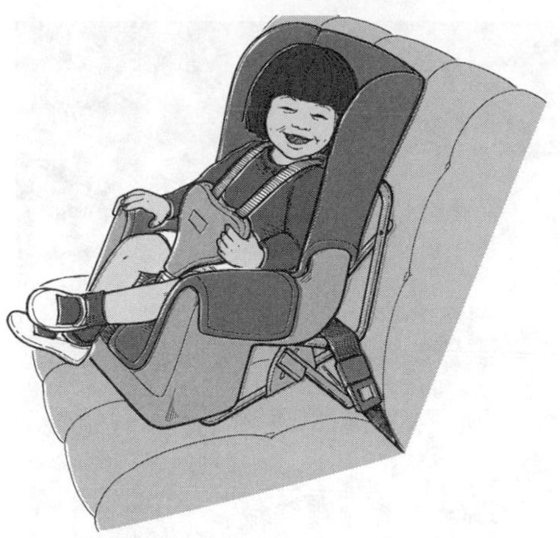

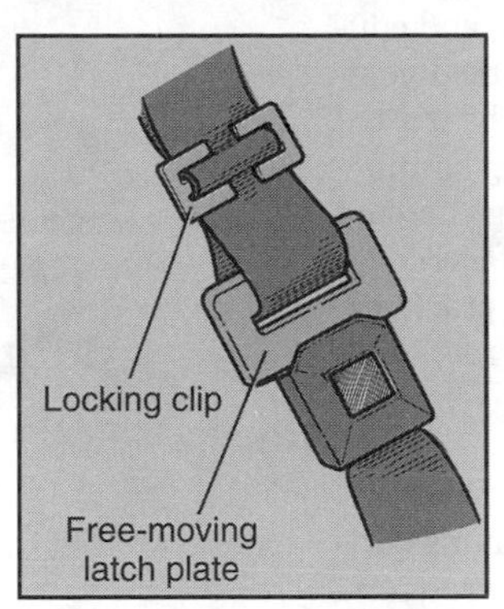

Fig. 34-8 Convertible seat in forward-facing position for older infants and children. **Inset,** Use of locking clip.

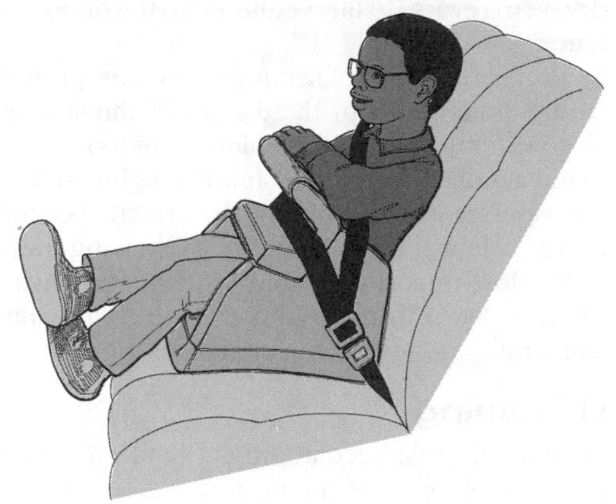

Fig. 34-9 Automobile booster seat. Note placement of shoulder strap (away from neck or face).

the vehicle seat back. If a car safety seat is not available, the lap belt provides more protection than no restraint (except for infants, where there is no safe alternative to approved restraint devices). Shoulder-only automatic belts are designed to protect adults. Children should use the manual shoulder belts in the rear seat. Air bags do not take the place of child safety seats or seat belts. The safest area of the car for children is the back seat. Children should not ride in the front seat of a car with a passenger-side airbag (American Academy of Pediatrics, 1997).

Nursing ALERT

Safety belts should be worn low on the hips, snug, and not on the abdominal area. Children should be taught to sit up straight to allow for proper fit. The shoulder belt is used *only* if it does not cross the child's neck or face.

For any restraint to be effective, it must be used consistently and properly. Examples of misuse include misrouting the vehicle seat belt through the restraint, failing to use the vehicle seat belt to secure the restraint, failing to use a tether strap, failing to use the restraint's harness system, and incorrectly positioning the child, especially facing infants forward instead of rearward (Graham, Kittredge, and Stuemky, 1992). To address these issues, nurses must stress correct use of car restraints and rules that ensure compliance (see the Home Care box to the right). Children riding in car safety seats are generally much better behaved than children left unrestrained, which can be a major benefit to parents and should be emphasized as an additional advantage of restraints.*

Injuries may also occur during sudden stops when objects are left unrestrained. On sudden impact a loose ball becomes

Home Care 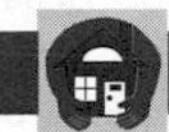

USING CAR SAFETY SEATS

Read manufacturer's directions and follow them exactly.
Anchor safety seat securely to car's seat and apply harness snugly to child.
Do not place safety seat in the front seat of a car equipped with a passenger-side air bag.
Do not start the car until *everyone* is properly restrained.
Always use the restraint, even for short trips.
If child begins to climb out or undo the harness, firmly say, "No." It may be necessary to stop the car to reinforce the expected behavior. Use rewards such as stars or stickers to encourage cooperative behavior.
Encourage child to help attach buckles, straps, and shields; but always double-check fastenings.
Decrease boredom on long trips. Keep soft toys in the car for quiet play, talk to child, and point out objects and teach child about them. Stop periodically. If child wishes to sleep, make sure child stays in the restraint.
Insist that others who transport children also follow these safety rules.

a projectile missile. Therefore all items should be secured or stored in the trunk.

Children over 3 years of age are often involved in pedestrian traffic injuries. Because of their gross motor skills of walking, running, and climbing and their fine motor skills of opening doors and fence gates, they are likely to be in hazardous areas when unsupervised. Because they are unaware of danger and unable to approximate the speed of a car, they are hit by moving vehicles. Running after a ball, playing in a pile of leaves or snow or inside a cardboard box, riding a tricycle, and playing behind a parked car or near the curb are common activities that may result in a vehicular tragedy. A precaution when children are playing in driveways is attaching a pole with a bright flag to the tricycle so the flag is high enough to be visible through an automobile's back window. Another safeguard is the use of a device that beeps when the vehicle is

*__American Academy of Pediatrics.__ 141 Northwest Point Blvd., P.O. Box 927, Elk Grove Village, IL 60007, (800) 433-9016; and local division of traffic safety or **Department of Transportation, National Highway Traffic Safety Administration,** (800) 424-9393. Guidelines for car seat safety are available in Wong DL: *Wong and Whaley's clinical manual of pediatric nursing,* ed 4, St Louis, 1996, Mosby.

driven in reverse to alert children to the oncoming car, van, or truck.

Preventing vehicular injuries involves protecting and educating children about the danger of moving or parked vehicles. Although preschool children are too young to be trusted to always obey, the parent should emphasize looking for moving vehicles before crossing the street, recognizing the stop and go colors of traffic lights, and following traffic officers' signals. Most important, what is preached must be practiced. Children learn through imitation, and consistency reinforces learning.

Drowning

Drowning, ranks second among boys and third among girls ages 1 to 4 years as a cause of accidental death; drowning from water transportation is excluded from these statistics. With well-developed skills of locomotion, toddlers are able to reach potentially dangerous areas such as bathtubs, toilets, buckets, swimming pools, hot tubs, and lakes. Their intense drive for exploration and investigation, combined with an unawareness of the danger of water and their helplessness in water, makes drowning always a viable threat. It is also one category of injuries that results in death within minutes, diminishing the chance for rescue and survival. Supervising children when near any source of water is essential; teaching swimming and water safety can be helpful but cannot be regarded as sufficient protection.

Burns

Burns rank second to motor vehicle injuries among girls and third among boys in this age group as a cause of accidental death. Their ability to climb, stretch, and reach objects above their head makes any hot surface a potential source of danger. Scalds from children pulling pots on top of themselves are a major source of burns. As a precaution, pot handles should be turned toward the back of the stove. Ideally, the knobs for controlling the range burners should be out of reach, not on the front panel where nimble fingers can turn them on and accidentally touch the hot burner. Oven doors should be closed whenever the oven is turned on or when it is cooling. The outside of doors of automatic self-cleaning ovens may become hot and, if touched, could cause a burn. Other sources of heat, such as radiators, fireplaces, accessible furnaces, kerosene heaters, or wood-burning stoves, should have guards placed in front of them. The tops of some of these heaters are designed to become hot enough to boil water to provide humidity. They are hazardous if touched or if the pan of water is spilled. Portable electric heaters must be placed in a high area, well out of reach of climbing young children.

Hot objects such as candles, incense, cigarettes, pots of tea or coffee, or irons must be placed away from children. The flame of a candle and the smoke of a cigarette invite investigation. Ashtrays with a center well are preferred to prevent the cigarette from falling off the rim, and adults should try not to smoke, cook, or drink hot liquids when children are physically close. If tablecloths are used, the edges should be placed out of reach to prevent injuries from both burns and falling objects.

Flame burns represent one of the most fatal types of burns and commonly occur when children play with matches and accidentally set themselves (and the home) on fire. To prevent flame burns, matches and lighters must be stored safely away from children, and parents need to teach children the dangers of playing with such objects. In addition, smoke detectors should be installed in all homes to alert the occupants of a fire. A safety plan for immediate escape is also essential.

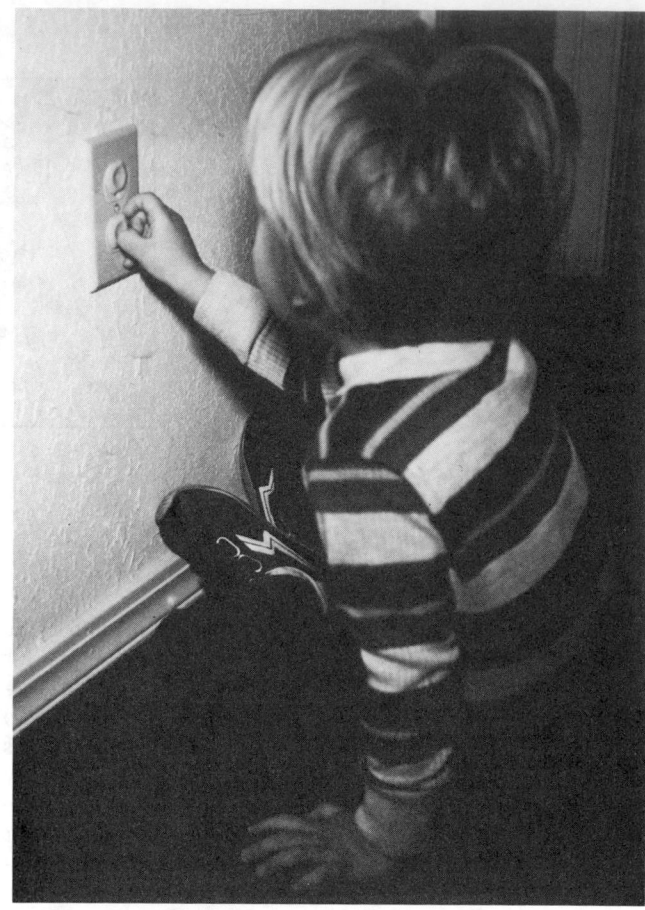

Fig. 34-10 Special plastic caps in electrical sockets prevent young fingers from exploring dangerous areas.

Electrical burns also represent an immediate danger to children. Because preschoolers' can manipulate small, thin objects, they are able to insert paper clips or other conductive articles into electrical sockets. Young toddlers may explore outlets and wires by mouthing them. Since water is an excellent conductor, the chance for a severe circumoral electrical burn is great. Protective guards should be plugged into electrical outlets when not in use (Fig. 34-10), or furniture should be placed in front of them to make them inaccessible when feasible. Children should not be allowed to play with electrical cords or appliances, which should be kept out of reach as much as possible.

An example of an appliance that interests children and can present a hazard is an electric popcorn popper. Children can become so excited by the popping that they may inadvertently pull the electric cord and popper off the table, resulting in a burn from contact with the hot oil, corn, or appliance.

Scald burns are the most common type of thermal injury in children. A scalding burn is often caused by high-temperature tap water, which children come in contact with either as a result of turning on the hot-water faucet, falling into a bathtub of hot water, or deliberate abuse. Always supervising youngsters when they are near tap water and checking bathwater temperatures are methods of prevention. Limiting household water temperatures to lower than 49° C (120° F) is also recommended. At this temperature it takes 10 minutes of exposure to the water to cause a full-thickness burn. Conversely, water temperatures of 54° C (130° F), the usual setting of most water heaters, expose household members to the risk of full-thickness burns within 30 seconds. Nurses can help prevent such burns by advising parents of this common household danger and recommending that they readjust the water heater to a safe temperature. A meat or candy thermometer is a convenient way to measure water temperature. An easy-to-read hot-water gauge that changes color to show water temperatures between 120° F and 150° F is also available; it shows a "hot," "cool," or "OK" water temperature. A special device can also be added to the faucet that reduces the water flow once the set temperature is reached.

Poisoning

Ingestion of toxic agents is common during early childhood. The highest incidence occurs in children in the 2-year-old age group. Although in many instances poisoning does not result in mortality, it may cause significant morbidity, such as esophageal stricture from lye ingestion. Mouthing activity continues to be prevalent after 1 year of age, and exploring objects by tasting them is part of children's curious investigation. Almost every nonfood substance is potentially harmful, including many house plants, and by 2 years of age toddlers are able to climb most heights, open most drawers or closets, and unscrew most lids. By trial and error younger children also manage to undo tops of bottles, plastic containers, aerosol cans, and jars, including those with child-resistant closures. In addition, pharmacists often transfer drugs to regular containers for the elderly, who may have difficulty with child-resistant closures. Newer forms of drugs such as transdermal patches and cough-suppressant lozenges have created additional dangers, since they are not packaged with safety caps and the lozenges look like candy.

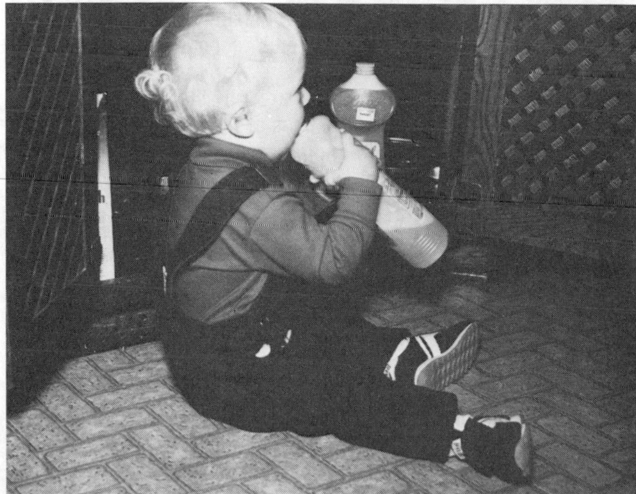

Fig. 34-11 Children are most likely to ingest substances that are on their level such as cleaning agents stored under sinks, rat poison, plants, or diaper pail deodorants.

The major reason for poisoning is improper storage (Fig. 34-11). The guidelines suggested in Chapter 33 apply to children in this age group as well. However, unlike the infant who was confined to certain heights and unable to unlatch inventive locks, young children manage to find access to many high-level, tight-security places. For this age group only a locked cabinet is safe.

Parents should have two doses of ipecac syrup for each child in the home, know its proper use and administration in case of a poisoning, and have the phone number and location of the nearest poison control center. Emergency and preventive measures for accidental poisoning are discussed in Chapter 44.

Falls

Falls are still a hazard to children in this age group, although by the later part of early childhood gross and fine motor skills are well developed, decreasing the incidence of falls down stairs or from chairs. However, playground injuries are common. Children need to be taught safety at play areas, such as no horseplay on high slides or jungle gyms, *sitting* on swings, and staying away from moving swings. Passive prevention includes placement of grass, sand, or wood chips under play equipment. Swing seats should be made of plastic, canvas, or rubber and have smooth or rounded edges. Slides should not exceed an incline of 30 degrees, have evenly spaced rungs for climbing, and have protective "tunnels."

The climbing and running of the typical toddler are complicated by the child's total neglect for and lack of appreciation of danger. Gates must be placed at both ends of stairs. Accessible windows that are left open during warm weather must be screened or guarded with a rail. Falling from open windows is a major cause of accidental death in urban, lower socioeconomic groups. Doors leading to stairwells or porches must be locked, since preschool children can easily open them. Laundry chutes are another potential danger and typically are not locked because of their frequent use. A convenient type of lock is a sliding bar or hook that can be attached to the door and frame at a level higher than the child can reach.

Cribs and vehicles are other sources of falls. To avoid injury, crib rails should be fully raised, the mattress should be kept at the lowest position, and toys or bumper pads that may be used as steps to climb out should be removed. Ideally the floor should be carpeted. Once children reach a height of 89 cm (35 inches), they should sleep in a bed rather than a crib. If a bunk bed is selected, parents should be aware of possible dangers: falls and head entrapment between the mattress and guardrail or between the supporting mattress slats. If the beds are constructed of tubular metal, parents should check for breaks or cracks in the metal and welds, which may lead to collapse and injury. Children who sleep on the top bunk should be 6 years or older.

Children who are unrestrained can fall from high chairs, shopping carts, carriages, and car seats. Therefore proper restraint and adequate supervision are essential.

Clothing can also increase the chance of falling. Slippery shoes or socks, rubber-soled shoes that "catch" on the floor and rug, and loose or cuffed pants can easily make a child fall.

Simple safety measures such as checking clothing and shoes, keeping shoelaces tied with double knots, or using self-adhering closures, can prevent accidents.

Aspiration and Suffocation

Usually by 1 year of age children chew well, but they may have difficulty with large pieces of food such as meat and whole hot dogs and with hard foods such as nuts or dried beans. Young children cannot discard pits from fruit or bones from fish. It takes practice to learn how to chew gum without swallowing it. Therefore the same precautions as discussed for infants regarding food selection must be implemented (see Chapter 33).

Play objects for toddlers must still be chosen with an awareness of danger from small parts. Large, sturdy toys without sharp edges or removable parts are safest. Coins, paper clips, pins, bells, button batteries, pull-tabs on cans, thumbtacks, nails, screws, jewelry (especially pierced earrings), and all types of pins are common household objects that can cause significant harm if swallowed or aspirated. Because of the danger of aspiration, parents should be taught emergency procedures for choking (see Airway Obstruction, Chapter 43).*

*Home care instructions on caring for the choking child are available in Wong DL: *Wong and Whaley's clinical manual of pediatric nursing*, ed 4, St Louis, 1996, Mosby.

Another cause of death by traumatic asphyxiation is from electrically operated garage doors. Young children playing in the garage may become trapped under the door. Although the automatic doors should reverse when striking an object, they may not do so when hitting a flexible object or one that is very close to the ground. Precautions include placing controls where they are inaccessible to children, such as high on a wall and in a locked car, and instructing children that the transmitter is not a toy. Periodically the door should be checked to determine if it returns when striking an object.

Suffocation from causes seen during infancy is less frequent, but old refrigerators, ovens, and other large appliances are an ever-present threat. Toddlers can climb inside these appliances and, if they close the door behind them, can be trapped inside. Discarding old appliances or removing all doors during storage prevents such tragic deaths. Toddlers may also suffocate when unsafe toy box lids accidentally close on their head or neck. Parents should be advised of this danger and encouraged to buy storage chests with lightweight, removable covers.

Bodily Damage

Toddlers are still clumsy in many of their skills and can seriously harm themselves when walking while holding a sharp or pointed object or having food or objects such as spoons in their mouths. Preventing such occurrences is the best approach with toddlers. With preschoolers teaching safety is

Home Care

GUIDANCE DURING TODDLER YEARS

Ages 12 to 18 months

Prepare parents for expected behavioral changes of toddler, especially negativism and ritualism.

Assess present feeding habits and encourage gradual weaning from bottle and increased intake of solid foods.

Stress expected feeding changes of physiologic anorexia, presence of food fads and strong taste preferences, need for scheduled routine at mealtimes, inability to sit through an entire meal, and lack of table manners.

Assess sleep patterns at night, particularly habit of a bedtime bottle, which is a major cause of dental caries, and procrastination behaviors that delay hour of sleep.

Prepare parents for potential dangers of the home, particularly motor vehicle, poisoning, and falling injuries; give appropriate suggestions for safeproofing the home.

Discuss need for firm but gentle discipline and ways in which to deal with negativism and temper tantrums; stress positive benefits of appropriate discipline.

Emphasize importance for both child and parents of brief, periodic separations.

Discuss new toys that use developing gross and fine motor, language, cognitive, and social skills.

Emphasize need for dental supervision, types of basic dental hygiene at home, and food habits that predispose to caries; stress importance of supplemental fluoride.

Ages 18 to 24 months

Stress importance of peer companionship in play.

Explore need for preparation for additional sibling; stress importance of preparing child for new experiences.

Discuss present discipline methods, their effectiveness, and parents' feelings about child's negativism; stress that negativism is important aspect of developing self-assertion and independence and is not a sign of spoiling.

Discuss signs of readiness for toilet training; emphasize importance of waiting for physical and psychologic readiness.

Discuss development of fears, such as darkness or loud noises, and of habits, such as security blanket or thumbsucking; stress normalcy of these transient behaviors.

Prepare parents for signs of regression in time of stress.

Assess child's ability to separate easily from parents for brief periods of separation under familiar circumstances.

Allow parents opportunity to express their feelings of weariness, frustration, and exasperation; be aware that it is often difficult to love toddlers at times when they are not asleep!

Point out some of the expected changes of the next year, such as longer attention span, somewhat less negativism, and increased concern for pleasing others.

Ages 24 to 36 months

Discuss importance of imitation and domestic mimicry and need to include child in activities.

Discuss approaches toward toilet training, particularly realistic expectations and attitude toward accidents.

Stress uniqueness of toddlers' thought processes, especially through their use of language, poor understanding of time, causal relationships in terms of proximity of events, and inability to see events from another's perspective.

Stress that discipline still must be quite structured and concrete and that relying solely on verbal reasoning and explanation leads to injuries, confusion, and misunderstanding.

Discuss investigation of preschool or daycare center toward completion of second year.

most important. The child should be taught that when walking with a pointed object such as a knife or scissors, the pointed end is held away from the face. Dangerous garden or workshop equipment and all firearms should be stored in a locked cabinet. Power lawn mowers are especially dangerous, and young children should not be allowed in an area where a mower is being used; nor should they be taken for a ride on a mower or allowed to operate the device. Safety education should include respect for firearms and their proper and appropriate use, including nonpowder guns such as air guns and rifles, which cause serious penetrating injuries (Lie et al, 1994). In addition, the child should be warned of and protected against potential danger from animals (see Bodily Damage, Chapter 33, and Animal Bites, Chapter 50).

Toys can be a source of danger, and safety must be a prime consideration when selecting toys (see Home Care: Toy Safety, Chapter 30). Most toys have age ranges written on them to designate their safety, but this information must be used with knowledge of the specific child's readiness.

Household safety should be practiced and includes the usual precautions recommended for any age group (see Home Care: Child Safety Home Checklist, Chapter 33).

Additional safeguards for young children are the use of safety glass in doors, windows, and tabletops and the application of decals on glassed areas to lessen the likelihood of running through glass. Also, children should not be allowed to run, jump, wrestle, or play ball near glass structures (Armstrong and Molyneux, 1992).

ANTICIPATORY GUIDANCE—CARE OF FAMILIES

Understanding toddlers is fundamental to successful childrearing. Nurses, particularly those in ambulatory or child health centers, are in a favorable position to assist parents in meeting the tasks and needs of children in this age group. Prevention yields better results than treatment. Anticipatory guidance is paramount if one wishes to prevent future problems (see the Home Care box on p. 1012). Advice is sometimes not the sole answer. Actual assistance, such as being available for home visiting or telephone consulting, should be part of the nurse's flexible repertoire of interventions. Whether parents are experiencing the rearing dilemmas of a first or a subsequent child, they benefit from sharing their feelings, frustrations, and satisfactions. They need adult companionship, freedom from childrearing responsibilities, and periodic separations from their children. Part of a nurse's responsibility is to provide opportunities for parents to express their feelings and meet their physical, mental, and spiritual needs.

Key Points

- The toddler stage, extending from 12 to 36 months, is a period of intense exploration of the environment.
- Biologic development during the toddler years is characterized by the acquisition of fine and gross motor skills that allow children to master a wide variety of activities.
- Although most of the physiologic systems are mature by the end of toddlerhood, development of certain areas of the brain is still occurring, allowing for greater intellectual capacity.
- Locomotion is the major gross motor skill acquired during toddlerhood, followed by increased eye-hand coordination.
- Specific tasks in the psychosocial development of a toddler include differentiating self from others, tolerating separation from parent, coping with delayed gratification, controlling bodily functions, acquiring socially acceptable behavior, verbally communicating, and interacting with others in a less egocentric manner.
- According to Erikson, the major developmental task of toddlerhood is acquiring a sense of autonomy while overcoming a sense of doubt and shame.
- Language is the major cognitive achievement in toddlerhood.
- In Piaget's sensorimotor and preconceptual phases of development, the toddler experiments by incorporating the old learning of secondary circular reactions with new skills and applies this knowledge to new situations. There is the beginning of rational judgment, an understanding of causal relationships, and discovery of objects as objects.
- Preconceptual thought is characterized by egocentricism, centration, global organization of thought processes, animism, and irreversibility.
- Development of body image occurs with increasing motor ability, at which point toddlers recognize the importance and capacity of body parts.
- The two phases of differentiation of self from significant others are separation and individuation.
- The most striking characteristic of language development during early childhood is the increasing level of comprehension.
- Parental concerns during the toddler years include toilet training; coping with sibling rivalry; and dealing with temper tantrums, negativism, and regression.
- Nutrition is important at this stage because eating habits established in toddlerhood tend to have lasting effects in subsequent years.
- Regular dental examinations, fluoride supplementation, removal of plaque, and provision of a low-cariogenic diet promote optimum dental health.
- Because of increased locomotion, toddlers are at high risk for sustaining injuries. Fatal injuries are primarily the result of motor vehicle accidents, drownings, and burns.

References

American Academy of Pediatrics: Air bag safety issues examined, AAP News 13(1):1,13, 1997

American Academy of Pediatrics, Committee on Injury and Poison Prevention: Selecting and using the most appropriate car seat safety seats for growing children: guidelines for counseling parents, *Pediatrics* 97(5):761-763, 1996.

American Academy of Pediatrics, Committee on Nutrition: Fluoride supplementation for children, *Pediatrics* 95(5):777, 1995.

Armstrong AM, Molyneux E: Glass injuries to children, *Br Med J* 304(6823):360, 1992.

Forgac MT: Timely statement of the American Dietetic Association: dietary guidance for healthy children, *J Am Dietetic Assoc* 95(3):370, 1995.

Graham CJ, Kittredge O, Stuemky JH: Injuries associated with child safety seat misuse, *Pediatr Emerg Care* 8:351-353, 1992.

Lidster CA, Horsburgh ME: Masturbation—beyond myth and taboo, *Nurs Forum* 29(3):18-27, 1994.

Lie L et al: American Public Health Association/American Academy of Pediatrics Injury Prevention Standards, *Pediatrics* 94(6 Pt 2):1046-1048, 1994.

Osberg JS, Di Scala C: Morbidity among pediatric motor vehicle crash victims: the effectiveness of seat belts, *Am J Public Health* 82(3):422-425, 1992.

Serwint JR and others: Child-rearing practices and nursing caries, *Pediatrics* 92(2):233-237, 1993.

Stark M: Assessment and management of the care of children with nocturnal enuresis: guidelines for primary care, *Nurs Pract Forum* 5(3):170-176, 1994.

Bibliography

Growth and Development

Dixon SD, Stein MT: *Encounters with children: a practical guide to pediatric behavior and development,* ed 2, St Louis, 1992, Mosby.

Fina DK: The spiritual needs of pediatric patients and their families, *AORN J* 62 (4):556-564, 1995.

Gross D, Tucker S: Parenting confidence during toddlerhood: a comparison of mothers and fathers, *Nurs Pract: Am J Primary Health Care* 19(10):25, 29-30, 33-34, 1994.

Howard BT: Growing together: the toddler years need not be turbulent, *Contemp Pediatr* 7(6):21-40, 1990.

King EH, Logsdon DA, Schroeder SR: Risk factors for developmental delay among infants and toddlers, *Child Health Care* 21(1):39-52, 1992.

Zuckerman BS, Frank DA: Infancy and toddler years. In Levine MD et al, editors: *Developmental-behavioral pediatrics,* ed 2, Philadelphia, 1992, WB Saunders.

Toilet Training

Berk L, Friman P: Epidemiologic aspects of toilet training, *Clin Pediatr* 29(5):278-282, 1990.

Brooks JG: I'm a big kid now: a book about toilet training, Neenah, Wis, 1992, Kimberly Clark.

Loening-Baucke V: Management of chronic constipation in infants and toddlers, *Am Fam Physician* 49(2):397-400, 411-413, 1994.

Maleham T: A dry run . . . night-time continence—with help from some cartoon characters, *Nurs Times* 89(30):66, 68, 1993.

Stadtler AC: Preventing encopresis, *Pediatr Nurs* 15(3):282-284, 1989.

Sibling Rivalry

Castiglia PT: Sibling rivalry, *J Pediatr Health Care* 3(1):52-54, 1989.

Lansky V: *A new baby at Koko bear's house,* Deephaven, Minn, 1990, The Book Peddlers.

Leung, AK, Robson LM: Sibling rivalry, *Clin Pediatr* 30(5):314-317, 1991.

Pakula, LC: Sibling rivalry, *Pediatr Rev* 13(2):72-73, 1992.

Schmitt BD: Sibling rivalry toward a new baby, *Contemp Pediatr* 7(3):111-112, 1990.

Negativism/Temper Tantrums

Blum NJ et al: Disciplining young children: the role of verbal instructions and reasoning, *Pediatrics* 96(2 Pt 1):336-341, 1995.

Brayden RM, Poole SR: Common behavioral problems in infants and children, *Prim Care* 22(1):81-97, 1995.

Gross D, Conrad B: Temperament in toddlerhood, *J Pediatr Nurs* 10(3):146-151, 1995.

Needlman R, Howard B, Zuckerman B: Temper tantrums: when to worry, *Contemp Pediatr* 6(8):12-34, 1989.

Schmitt BD: The stubborn toddler who just says "No," *Contemp Pediatr* 7(4):71-72, 1990.

Socolar RR, Stein RE: Spanking infants and toddlers: maternal belief and practice, *Pediatrics* 95(1):105-111, 1995.

Nutrition

American Academy of Pediatrics, Committee on Nutrition: *Pediatric nutrition handbook,* Elk Grove Village, Ill, 1993, The Academy.

Feeney B: Teaching aid . . . child health, nutrition, *Nurs Times* 91(10)42-44, 1995.

Lucas B: Nutrition in childhood. In Mahan LK, Arlin MT: *Krause's food, nutrition, and diet therapy,* ed 8, Philadelphia, 1992, WB Saunders.

McGarr B, Dwyer J, Holland HM: Delivering nutrition services in early intervention in rural areas, *Infants & Young Child* 7(3):52-62, 1995.

Pipes P, Trahms CM: *Nutrition in infancy and childhood,* ed 5, St Louis, 1993, Mosby.

Satter E: Feeding dynamics: helping children to eat well, *J Pediatr Health Care* 9(4):178-184, 1995.

Schmitt BD: A commonsense approach to sweets, *Contemp Pediatr* 8(9):63-65, 1991.

Dental Health

American Academy of Pediatric Dentistry: *Recommendations for preventive pediatric dental care,* Chicago, May 1992, The Academy.

Johnsen DC: The role of the pediatrician in identifying and treating dental caries, *Pediatr Clin North Am* 38(5):1173-1181, 1991.

Jones KF, Berg JH, Coody D: Update in pediatric dentistry, *J Pediatr Health Care* 8(4):160-167. 1994.

Lloyd S: Developments in oral health: teaching parents to look after children's teeth, *Prof Care Mother Child* 4(2):34-36, 1994.

McDonald RE, Avery DR: *Dentistry for the child and adolescent,* ed 6, St Louis, 1994, Mosby.

Nowak AJ: What pediatricians can do to promote oral health, *Contemp Pediatr* 10(4):90-106, 1993.

Ogasawara T, Watanabe T, Kasahara H: Readiness for toothbrushing of young children, *J Dent Child* 59(5):353-359, 1992.

Schulte JR, Druyan ME, Hagen JC: Early childhood tooth decay, *Clin Pediatr* 31(12):727-730, 1992.

Von Burg MM, Sanders BJ, Weddell JA: Baby bottle tooth decay: a concern for all mothers, *Pediatr Nurs* 21(6):515-519, 1995.

Injury Prevention

Accident Facts, Chicago, 1995, National Safety Council.

Agran P, Winn D, Castillo D: Unsupervised children in vehicles: a risk for pediatric trauma, *Pediatrics* 87(1):70-73, 1991.

American Academy of Pediatrics, Committee on Injury and Poison Prevention: Children in pickup trucks, *Pediatrics* 88(2):393-394, 1991.

American Academy of Pediatrics Committee on Injury and Poison Prevention: Injuries associated with infant walkers, *Pediatrics* 95(5):778-780, 1995.

Bull MJ, Stroup KB, Doll JP: A parent guide: selecting and using car safety seats, *Contemp Pediatr* 7(7):113-118, 1990.

Bull MJ et al: Establishing special needs car seat loan program, *Pediatrics* 85(4):540-547, 1990.

Christoffel KK, Naureckas SM: Firearm injuries in children and adolescents: epidemiology and preventive approaches, *Curr Opin Pediatr* 6(5):519-524, 1994.

Gielen AC et al: In-home injury prevention practices for infants and toddlers: the role of parental beliefs, barriers, and housing quality, *Health Educ Q* 22(1):85-95, 1995.

Johnston C, Rivara FP, Soderberg R: Children in car crashes: analysis of data for injury and use of restraints, *Pediatrics* 93(6 Pt 1):960-965, 1994.

McFadden EA: Equipment safety for infants and children: beyond clinical practice, *J Pediatr Nurs* 9(5):335-336, 1994.

Schubert W, Ahrenholz DH, Solem LD: Burns from hot oil and grease: a public health hazard, *J Burn Care Rehabil* 11(6):558-562, 1990.

Sewell KH, Gaines SK: A developmental approach to childhood safety education, *Pediatr Nurs* 19(5):464-466, 1993.

Stuy M, Green M, Doll J: Child care centers: a community resource for injury prevention, *J Dev Behav Pediatr* 14(4):224-229, 1993.

Stylianos S, Eichelberger MR, Pediatric trauma: prevention strategies, *Pediatr Clin North Am* 40(6):1359-1368, 1993.

Swartz MK: Playground safety, *J Pediatr Health Care* 6(3):161-162, 1992.

CHAPTER 35

The Preschooler and Family

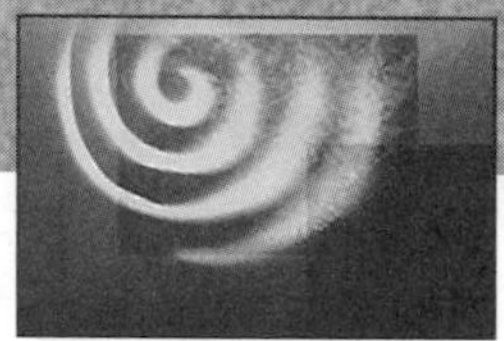

PROMOTING OPTIMUM GROWTH AND DEVELOPMENT, P. 1016

Biologic development, p. 1016
Psychosocial development, p. 1017
Cognitive development, p. 1017
Moral development, p. 1018
Spiritual development, p. 1018
Development of body image, p. 1018
Development of sexuality, p. 1018
Social development, p. 1018
Coping with concerns related to normal growth and development, p. 1021

PROMOTING OPTIMUM HEALTH DURING THE PRESCHOOL YEARS, P. 1025

Nutrition, p. 1025
Sleep and activity, p. 1026
Dental health, p. 1027
Injury prevention, p. 1027

SPECIAL HEALTH PROBLEMS, P. 1028

Communicable diseases, p. 1028
Child maltreatment, p. 1039

Promoting Optimum Growth and Development

The combined biologic, psychosocial, cognitive, spiritual, and social achievements during the *preschool period* (3 to 5 years of age) prepare preschoolers for their most significant change in life-style—entrance into school. Their control of bodily systems, experience of brief and prolonged periods of separation, ability to interact cooperatively with other children and adults, use of language for mental symbolization, and increased attention span and memory ready them for the next major period—the school years. Successful achievement of previous levels of growth and development is essential for preschoolers to refine many of the tasks that were mastered during the toddler years.

BIOLOGIC DEVELOPMENT

The rate of physical growth slows and stabilizes during the preschool years. The average *weight* at 3 years is 14.6 kg (32 pounds), at 4 years 16.7 kg (36.75 pounds), and at 5 years 18.7 kg (41.25 pounds). The average weight gain remains about 2.3 kg (5 pounds) per year.

Growth in *height* also remains steady at a yearly increase of 6.75 to 7.5 cm (2.5 to 3 inches) and generally occurs in elongation of the legs rather than of the trunk. The average height at 3 years is 95 cm (37.25 inches), at 4 years 103 cm (40.5 inches), and at 5 years 110 cm (43.25 inches).

Physical proportions no longer resemble those of the squat, potbellied toddler. The preschooler is slender but sturdy, graceful, agile, and posturally erect. There is little difference in physical characteristics according to sex, except as dictated by such factors as dress and hairstyle.

Most *body systems* are mature and stable and can adjust to moderate stress and change. During this period most children are toilet trained. Motor development consists for the most part of increases in strength and refinement of previously learned skills such as walking, running, and jumping. However, muscle development and bone growth are still far from mature. Excessive activity and overexertion can injure delicate tissues. Good posture, appropriate exercise, and adequate nutrition and rest are essential for optimum development of the musculoskeletal system.

Gross and Fine Motor Behavior

Walking, running, climbing, and jumping are well established by age 36 months. Refinement in eye-hand and muscle coordination is evident in several areas. At age 3 the preschooler rides a tricycle, walks on tiptoe, balances on one foot for a few seconds, and broad jumps. By age 4 the child skips and hops proficiently on one foot (Fig. 35-1) and catches a ball reliably. By age 5, the child skips on alternate feet, jumps rope, and begins to skate and swim.

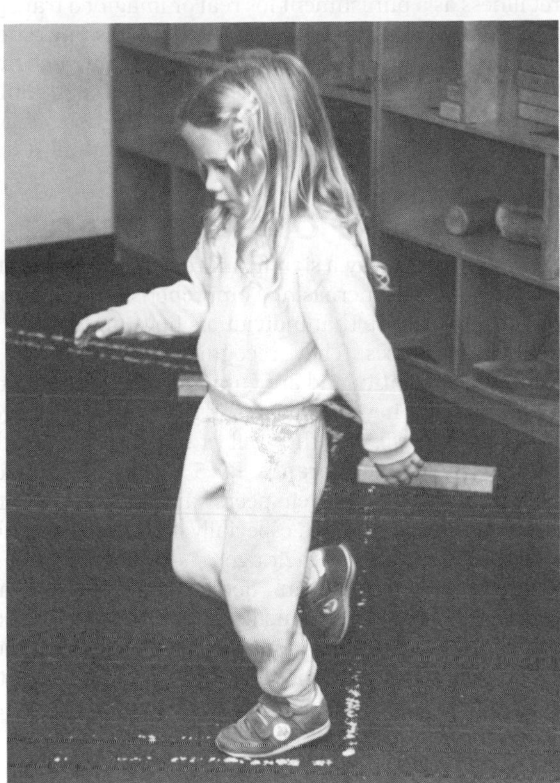

Fig. 35-1 A 4-year-old child has sufficient balance to walk or hop on one foot.

Fine motor development is evident in the child's increasingly skillful manipulation, such as in drawing and dressing. These skills provide readiness for learning and independence for entry into school.

PSYCHOSOCIAL DEVELOPMENT

Developing a Sense of Initiative (Erikson)

If preschoolers have mastered the tasks of the toddler period, they are ready to face the developmental endeavors of this stage. The chief psychosocial task of the preschool period is acquiring a **sense of initiative.** Children are in a stage of energetic learning. They play, work, and live to the fullest and feel a real sense of accomplishment and satisfaction in their activities. Conflict arises when children overstep the limits of their ability and inquiry and experience a sense of *guilt* for not having behaved or acted appropriately. Feelings of guilt, anxiety, and fear may also result from thoughts that differ from expected behavior.

A particularly stressful thought is wishing one's parent dead. As a sense of rivalry or competition develops between the child and same-sex parent, the child may think of ways to get rid of the interfering parent. In most situations this rivalry is resolved by strongly identifying with the same-sex parent and peers during the school years. However, if that parent dies before the identification process is completed, the preschooler can be overwhelmed with feelings of guilt for having wished and therefore "caused" the death. Clarifying for children that wishes cannot and do not make events occur is essential in helping them overcome their guilt and anxiety.

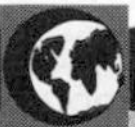

Cultural Considerations

LEARNING SOCIOCULTURAL MORES

Developing a conscience implies *learning the sociocultural mores* of the family's heritage. Depending on the type of attitudes conveyed, children will learn not only appropriate behaviors but also tolerant, biased, or prejudiced values concerning their ethnic, religious, and social background and those of other groups. Much of this influence may remain dormant until they associate with children or adults of a different heritage. Then, depending on the particular group, children may be accepted or isolated for their attitudes.

Development of the *super-ego* or **conscience** begins toward the end of the toddler years and is a major task for preschoolers (see the Cultural Considerations box above). Learning right from wrong and good from bad is the beginning of morality (see Moral Development).

COGNITIVE DEVELOPMENT

One of the tasks related to the preschool period is readiness for school and scholastic learning. Many of the thought processes of this period are crucial for achieving such readiness, and it is intentional that the child begins school between ages 5 and 6 rather than at an earlier age.

Preoperational Phase (Piaget)

Piaget's cognitive theory actually does not include a period specifically for children 3 to 5 years old. The *preoperational phase* comprises the age span from 2 to 7 years and is divided into two stages: the *preconceptual phase,* ages 2 to 4, and the phase of **intuitive thought,** ages 4 to 7. One of the main transitions during these two phases is the shift from totally egocentric thought to social awareness and the ability to consider other viewpoints. However, egocentricity is still evident. (For a review of the characteristics of preoperational thought, see Chapter 34.)

Language continues to develop during the preschool period. Speech remains primarily a vehicle of egocentric communication. Preschoolers assume that everyone thinks as they do and that a brief explanation of their thinking makes the entire thought understood by others. Because of this self-referenced, egocentric verbal communication, it is frequently necessary to explore and understand the young child's thinking through other non-verbal approaches. For children in this age group, the most enlightening and effective method is **play,** which becomes the child's way of understanding, adjusting to, and working out life's experiences.

Preschoolers increasingly use language without comprehending the meaning of words, particularly concepts of right and left, causality, and time. Children may use the concepts correctly but only in the circumstances in which they have learned them. For example, they may know how to put on shoes by remembering that the buckle is always on the outside of the foot. However, if different shoes have no buckles, they cannot reason which shoe fits which foot. In other words, they do not understand the concept of *right and left.*

Superficially, *causality* resembles logical thought. Preschoolers explain a concept as they heard it described by others, but their understanding is limited. An example is the concept of time. Since *time* is still incompletely understood, the child interprets it according to his or her own frame of reference, such as "A long time means until Christmas." Consequently, time is best explained in relationship to an event, such as "Your mother will visit you after you finish your lunch." Avoiding words such as "tomorrow," "next week," or "Tuesday" to express when an event is expected to occur and associating time with usual expected daily occurrences help children learn about temporal relationships while increasing their trust in others' predictions.

Preschoolers' thinking is often described as ***magical thinking.*** Because of their egocentrism and transductive reasoning, they believe that thoughts are all-powerful. Such thinking places them in the vulnerable position of feeling guilty and responsible for bad thoughts, which may coincide with the occurrence of a wished event. Their inability to logically reason the cause and effect of illness or an injury makes it especially difficult for them to understand such events.

MORAL DEVELOPMENT

Preconventional or Premoral Level (Kohlberg)

Young children's development of moral judgment is at the most basic level. There is little, if any, concern for why something is wrong. They behave because of the freedom or restriction that is placed on actions. In the *punishment and obedience orientation* children (ages about 2 to 4 years) judge whether an action is good or bad depending on whether it results in reward or punishment. If children are punished for it, the action is bad. If they are not punished, the action is good, regardless of the meaning of the act. For example, if parents allow hitting, the child will perceive that hitting is good because it is not associated with punishment.

From approximately 4 to 7 years of age children are in the stage of *naive instrumental orientation,* in which actions are directed toward satisfying their needs and less frequently the needs of others. There is a very concrete sense of justice. Reciprocity or fairness involves the philosophy of "You scratch my back and I'll scratch yours," with no thought of loyalty or gratitude (Thomas, 1996).

SPIRITUAL DEVELOPMENT

Children's knowledge of faith and religion is learned from significant others in their environment, usually from the parents and their religious practices. However, young children's understanding of spirituality is influenced by their cognitive level. Preschoolers have a concrete conception of a God with physical characteristics who is often like an imaginary friend. They understand simple Bible stories and memorize short prayers, but their understanding of the meaning of these rituals is limited. They benefit from concrete representations of religious practices such as picture Bible books and small statues such as those of the Nativity scene.

Development of the conscience is strongly linked to spiritual development. At this age children are learning right from wrong and behave correctly to avoid punishment. Wrongdoing provokes feelings of guilt, and preschoolers often misinterpret illness as a punishment for real or imagined transgressions. It is important that children view God as one who bestows unconditional love rather than as a judge of good or bad behavior. Praying to God and observing religious traditions, (e.g., prayers before meals or bedtime) can help children through stressful periods such as hospitalization (Clutter, 1991).

DEVELOPMENT OF BODY IMAGE

The preschool years play a significant role in the development of body image. With increasing comprehension of language, preschoolers recognize that individuals have undesirable and desirable appearances. They recognize differences in skin color and racial identity and are vulnerable to learning prejudices and biases. They are aware of the meaning of words such as *pretty* or *ugly,* and they reflect the opinions of others regarding their own appearance. By 5 years of age children compare their size with their peers' and can become conscious of being large or short, especially if others refer to them as "so big" or "so little" for their age.

Despite the advances in body image development, preschoolers have poorly defined body boundaries and little knowledge of their internal anatomy. Intrusive experiences are frightening, especially those that disrupt the integrity of the skin such as injections and surgery. There is a fear that if the skin is "broken," all their blood and "insides" can leak out. Therefore bandages are critical to "keeping everything from coming out."

DEVELOPMENT OF SEXUALITY

Sexual development during these years is a very important phase in a person's overall sexual identity and beliefs. Preschoolers are forming strong attachments to the opposite-sex parent while identifying with the same-sex parent.

As sexual identity is developing beyond gender recognition, modesty as well as fears of mutilation, may become a concern. There is sex-role imitation, and "dressing up" like Mommy or Daddy is an important activity. Attitudes and responses of others to role playing can condition the child to views of self or others. For example, comments such as "Boys shouldn't play with dolls" can influence a boy's self-concept of masculinity.

Sexual exploration may be more pronounced now than ever before, particularly in terms of exploring and manipulating the genitals. Questions about sexual reproduction may come to the forefront in the preschooler's search for understanding (see Sex Education, Chapters 35 to 37).

SOCIAL DEVELOPMENT

During the preschool period the **individuation-separation** process is completed. Preschoolers have overcome much of the anxiety associated with strangers and the fear of separation of earlier years. They relate to unfamiliar people easily and tolerate brief separations from parents with little or no protest. However, they still need parental security, reassurance, guidance, and approval, especially when entering preschool or elementary school. Prolonged separation such as that imposed by illness and hospitalization is difficult, but preschoolers respond very well to anticipatory preparation and concrete explanation. They can cope with changes in daily routine much better than toddlers; however, they may develop more imaginary fears. They gain security and comfort from familiar objects such as toys, dolls, or photographs of family members. They are able to work through many of their unresolved fears, fantasies, and anxieties through play, especially if guided with appropriate play objects (e.g., dolls or puppets) that represent family members, medical and nursing staff, and other children.

Language

Compared to toddlerhood, language during the preschool years is more sophisticated and complex. Both cognitive ability and environment, particularly consistent role models, influence vocabulary, speech, and comprehension. Language becomes a major mode of communication and social interaction. Vocabulary increases dramatically, from 300 words at age 2 to over 2100 words at the end of 5 years. Sentence structure, grammatical usage, and intelligibility also advance to a more adult level.

Children between the ages of 3 and 4 form sentences of about three to four words and include only the most essential words to convey a meaning. Such speech is often termed **telegraphic** for its brevity in length. Three-year-old children ask many questions and use plurals, correct pronouns, and the past tense of verbs. They name familiar objects such as animals, parts of the body, relatives, and friends. They can give and follow simple commands. They talk incessantly, regardless of whether anyone is listening or answering them. They enjoy musical or talking toys or dolls and imitate new words proficiently.

From ages 4 to 5 preschoolers use longer sentences of four to five words and use more words to convey a message, such as prepositions, adjectives, and a variety of verbs. They follow simple directional commands such as "Put the ball on the chair," but can carry out only one request at a time. They answer questions such as "What do you do when you are hungry?" by describing the appropriate action. The pattern of asking questions is at its peak, and children usually repeat the question until they receive an answer.

By the end of age 5 children can use all parts of speech correctly, except for deviations from the rule. They can define simple things by describing their use, shape, or general category of classification, rather than simply describing their outward appearance. For example, they define a ball as "round, something you bounce, or a toy," rather than by its color. They can give some opposites, such as "If Mommy is a woman, Daddy is a man." By the time they are 6 years old, they can describe an object according to its composition, such as "A spoon is made of metal."

Personal-Social Behavior

The pervasive ritualism and negativism of toddlerhood gradually diminish during the preschool years. Although self-assertion is still a major theme, preschoolers demonstrate their sense of autonomy differently. They are able to verbalize their request for independence and perform independently because of their much-refined physical and cognitive development. By 4 or 5 years of age they need little if any assistance with dressing, eating, or toileting (Fig. 35-2). They can also be trusted to obey warnings of danger, although 3- or 4-year-old children may exceed their boundaries at times.

They are also much more sociable and willing to please. They have internalized many of the standards and values of the family and culture. However, by the end of early childhood they begin to question parental values and compare them with those of their peer group and other authority figures; as a result, they may be less willing to abide by the family's code of conduct. Preschoolers become increasingly aware of their position and role within the family. Although this is a more secure age for experiencing the addition of another sibling, relinquishing the position of first or youngest is still difficult and requires appropriate preparation (see Sibling Rivalry, Chapter 34).

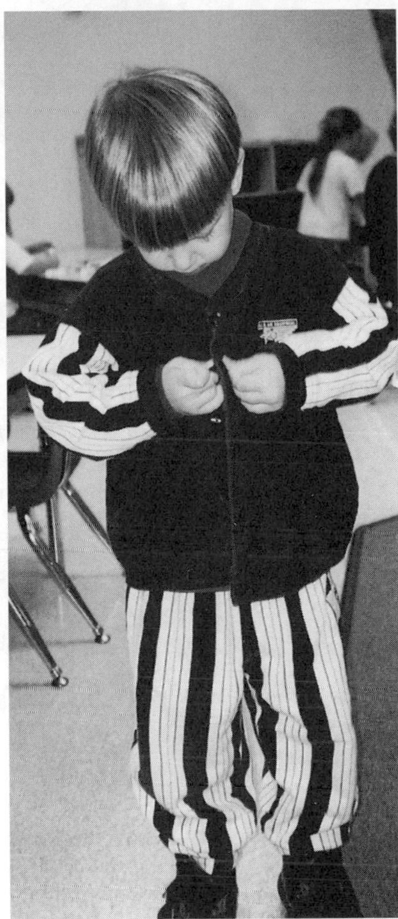

Fig. 35-2 Most preschoolers are able to dress themselves but need help with more difficult items of clothing.

Play

Various types of play are typical of this period, but preschoolers especially enjoy **associative play**—group play in similar or identical activities but without rigid organization or rules. Play should provide for physical, social, and mental development.

Play activities for physical growth and refinement of motor skills include jumping, running, and climbing. Tricycles, scooter trucks, wagons, gym and sports equipment, sandboxes, wading pools, and winter sleds can help develop muscles and coordination. Activities such as swimming, skating,

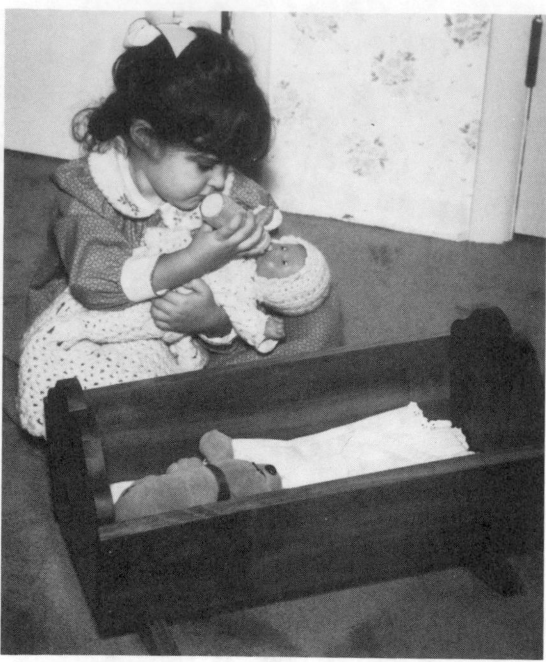

Fig. 35-3 Imaginative and dramatic play is typical of preschoolers, who enjoy using fantasy.

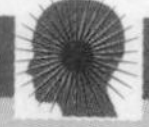

Critical Thinking Q & A

IMITATIVE PLAY

In her bedroom 4-year-old Juanita is playing with her dolls. She pretends one doll is "Mommy" and is talking on the telephone: "Be quiet! Can't you see that I am busy? This is an important call. Go away." She hangs up the phone and chooses another doll, pokes it, and cries, "You're bad. Mommy doesn't like you."

Juanita's mother, Mrs. Ortiz, hears this play conversation and realizes she says similar things to Juanita when she is on the telephone. What advice would you give Mrs. Ortiz:

1. Reassure her that imitation is a normal and healthy activity in 4-year-olds.
2. Suggest that she use a telephone recorder to return calls at more convenient times.
3. Inquire about her reactions to the play conversation and discuss possible ways to avoid the situation.
4. Refer the child to a psychologist for further assessment of the apparent child-mother conflict.

The best answer is three. You want to capitalize on the mother's awareness of the possible messages the child's play has revealed. Your goal is also to empower the parent to find reasonable options that accommodate her life-style.

Although a telephone recorder is one option, it may not be the best one. Although this play behavior is typical of preschoolers, premature reassurance will not address the issue or solutions. More assessment is needed before suggesting a referral.

and skiing teach safety, as well as muscle development and coordination.

Manipulative, constructive, creative, and educational toys provide for quiet activities, fine motor development, and self-expression. Easy construction sets, large blocks of various sizes and shapes, a counting frame, alphabet or number flash cards, paints, crayons, simple carpentry tools, musical toys, illustrated books, simple sewing or handicraft sets, large puzzles, and clay are suitable toys. Electronic games and educational computer programs are especially valuable in helping children learn basic skills such as letters and simple words.

Probably the most characteristic and pervasive preschool activity is **imitative,** imaginative, and dramatic **play.** Dress-up clothes, dolls, housekeeping toys, dollhouses, play-store toys, telephones, farm animals and equipment, village sets, trains, trucks, cars, planes, hand puppets, and doctor and nurse kits provide hours of self-expression (Fig. 35-3). Probably at no other time is the reproduction of adult behavior so faithful and absorbing as in 4- and 5-year-old children (see the Critical Thinking Q & A box above). Toward the end of the preschool period, children are less satisfied with make-believe or pretend objects and enjoy actually doing the activity such as cooking and carpentry.

Television and videotapes also have their places in children's play, although each should only be one part of children's total repertoire of social and recreational activities. Parents and other caregivers should supervise selection of programs, preview programs for appropriateness, and schedule hours for television viewing. (See the discussion on television, including the Home Care box, in Chapter 30.)

Play is so much a part of the young child's life that reality and fantasy become blurred. The make-believe is reality during play and only becomes fantasy when the toys are put away or the dress-up clothes are removed. It is no wonder that **imaginary playmates** are so much a part of this age period.

The appearance of imaginary companions usually occurs between the ages of 2½ to 3 years, and for the most part such playmates are relinquished when the child enters school. There seems to be a relationship between the level of intelligence and the presence of the imaginary companion. The more intelligent children tend to have the more vivid and complex pretend playmates.

Imaginary companions serve many purposes—they become friends in times of loneliness, they accomplish what the child is still attempting, and they experience what the child wants to forget or remember. It is not unusual for the "friend" to have a myriad of vices and to be blamed for wrongdoing. Sometimes the child hopes to escape punishment by saying, "My friend Brian broke the glass." At other times the child may fantasize that the companion misbehaved and play the role of parent. This becomes a way of assuming control and authority in a safe situation.

Parents often worry about the imaginary playmates, not realizing how normal and useful they are. They need to be reassured that children's fantasy is a sign of health that helps them differentiate between pretend and reality. Parents can acknowledge the presence of the imaginary companion by calling him or her by name and even agreeing to simple requests such as setting an extra place at the table, but they should not allow the child to use the playmate to avoid punishment or responsibility. For example, if the child blames the companion for messing a room, parents need to state clearly that the child is the only one they see and therefore the child is responsible for cleaning up (see the Critical Thinking Q & A box on p. 1021). The major developmental achievements for children ages 3 to 5 are summarized in Table 35-1.

Critical Thinking Q & A

IMAGINARY PLAYMATES

Mrs. Petner tells you, the nurse, that her 2½ year-old daughter, Kimberly, has an imaginary playmate named Alison. She was not very concerned about this until Kimberly started putting a plate on the table for Alison at mealtimes. Your best reply is which of the following?

1. "This is highly unusual behavior for children this age and indicates giftedness."
2. "This is normal for children this age, and it is fine to allow her to set a place for her imaginary playmate."
3. "It is best not to allow Kimberly to include her imaginary playmate in activities such as mealtimes."
4. "It is important that Kimberly separate reality from fantasy, and a referral to a mental health professional is indicated."

The best answer is two. Imaginary playmates are normal at this age and serve many purposes. Parents can acknowledge the presence of an imaginary companion as long as the child does not use the playmate to avoid punishment or responsibility. A referral is not necessary. Although the child may be gifted, this one behavior does not indicate that this is true.

COPING WITH CONCERNS RELATED TO NORMAL GROWTH AND DEVELOPMENT

Preschool and Kindergarten Experience

During the preschool years many children attend some type of early childhood program, usually preschool or a daycare center. Group care has become commonplace with the large number of mothers presently employed outside the home (see Alternate Child Care Arrangements, Chapter 33). The effects of early education and stimulation on children have increasingly gained recognition and importance (for a discussion of the effects of daycare on young children, see Working Mothers, Chapter 29). Since social development widens to include age-mates and other significant adults, preschool provides an excellent vehicle for expanding children's experiences with others. It also is an excellent preparation for entrance into elementary school.

In preschool or daycare centers children are exposed to opportunities for learning group cooperation, adjusting to various sociocultural differences, and coping with frustration, dissatisfaction, and anger. If activities are tailored to provide mastery and achievement, children increasingly have feelings of success, self-confidence, and personal competence. Whether or not structured learning is imposed is less important than the social climate, type of guidance, and attitude toward the children that is fostered by the teacher or leader. With a teacher who is aware of preschoolers' developmental abilities and needs, children will learn from the activity that is provided. Most programs incorporate a daily schedule of quiet play, active outdoor activity, group activities such as games and projects, creative or free play, and snack and rest periods.

Preschool is particularly beneficial for children who lack a peer-group experience such as an only child and for children from impoverished homes. It also is an excellent preparation for kindergarten.

One of the issues that parents face is the child's readiness for preschool or kindergarten. There are no absolute indicators for school readiness, but children's social maturation, especially attention span, is as important as their academic readiness. Using a developmental screening tool that addresses cognitive (especially language), social, and physical milestones can identify children who may benefit from diagnostic testing.

Nurses can be helpful in guiding parents in locating suitable facilities with a well-qualified staff. State licensing agencies can help parents identify daycare centers that accept children of specific age groups and are conveniently located. State-licensed programs are supposed to abide by established standards, which represent the *minimum* requirements and safeguards. However, enforcement of the standards is sometimes inadequate. Early childhood programs may also belong to a voluntary accreditation system, the National Academy of Early Childhood Programs, which serves as a model for *optimum* care.* References from other parents are also helpful, provided they have investigated the center carefully.

Other areas for parents to evaluate are the center's daily program, teacher qualifications, student/staff ratio, discipline policy, environmental safety precautions, provision of meals, sanitary conditions, adequate indoor/outdoor space per child, and fee schedule. In terms of an overall evaluation there *is no substitute for a personal observation of the facility.* Parents should arrange to meet the director and some of the employees, especially those who would be caring for the child. Developing a checklist may be helpful to systematically evaluate the center and make comparisons with other facilities.

One of the areas that is increasingly important in selecting child care centers is the agency's health practices. Substantial evidence shows that children in daycare centers, especially those under 3 years of age, have more illnesses, especially diarrhea, hepatitis A, meningitis, otitis media, respiratory tract infections, and cytomegalovirus, than children not in daycare centers.

Nurses play an important role in infection control. Not only can they advise parents regarding the evaluation of a center's sanitary practices, but they can also take an active part in educating staff in measures to minimize transmission of infection. For example, in centers caring for children who are not toilet trained, reducing environmental contamination with urine and feces is an important infection control issue (Fig. 35-4).

Children need preparation for the preschool or kindergarten experience.† For young children it represents a change from their usual home environment and prolonged separation from parents.

Before the child begins the school experience, the parents should present the idea as exciting and pleasurable. Talking to the child about activities such as painting, building with blocks, or enjoying swings and other outdoor equipment al-

*Information about the accreditation criteria and procedures of the National Academy of Early Childhood Programs is available from the **National Association for the Education of Young Children,** 1834 Connecticut Ave., N.W., Washington, DC 20009; (202) 232-8777 or (800) 424-2460. These criteria are excellent guidelines for evaluating preschools or daycare centers.

†Recommended books for preparing young children for daycare or school include Rogers F: *Going to Day Care* and *When Your Child Goes to School,* GP Putnam's Sons.

TABLE 35-1 Growth and development during preschool years

AGE (YEARS)	PHYSICAL	GROSS MOTOR	FINE MOTOR	LANGUAGE
3	Usual weight gain of 1.8 to 2.7 kg (4 to 6 pounds) Average weight of 14.6 kg (32 pounds) Usual gain in height of 7.5 cm (3 inches) Average height of 95 cm (37.25 inches) May have achieved nighttime control of bowel and bladder	Rides tricycle Jumps off bottom step Stands on one foot for a few seconds Goes up stairs using alternate feet, may still come down using both feet on step Broad jumps May try to dance, but balance may not be adequate	Builds tower of nine or ten cubes Builds bridge with three cubes Adeptly places small pellets in narrow-necked bottle In drawing, copies a circle, imitates a cross, names what has been drawn, cannot draw stick figure but may make circle with facial features	Has vocabulary of about 900 words Uses primarily "telegraphic" speech Uses complete sentences of three or four words Talks incessantly, regardless of whether anyone is paying attention Repeats sentence of six syllables Asks many questions
4	Pulse and respiration rates decrease slightly Growth rate is similar to that of previous year Average weight of 16.7 kg (36.75 pounds) Average height of 103 cm (40.5 inches) Length at birth is doubled Maximum potential for development of amblyopia	Skips and hops on one foot Catches ball reliably Throws ball overhand Walks downstairs using alternate footing	Uses scissors successfully to cut out picture following outline Can lace shoes, but may not be able to tie bow In drawing, copies a square, traces a cross and diamond, adds three parts to stick figure	Has vocabulary of 1500 words or more Uses sentences of four to five words Questioning is at peak Tells exaggerated stories Knows simple songs May be mildly profane if associates with older children Obeys four prepositional phrases, such as "under," "on top of," "beside," "in back of," or "in front of" Names one or more colors Comprehends analogies, such as, "If ice is cold, fire is ______"
5	Pulse and respiration rates decrease slightly Average weight of 18.7 kg (41.25 pounds) Average height of 110 cm (43.25 inches) Eruption of permanent dentition may begin Handedness is established (about 90% are righthanded)	Skips and hops on alternate feet Throws and catches ball well Jumps rope Skates with good balance Walks backward with heel to toe Jumps from height of 12 inches and lands on toes Balances on alternate feet with eyes closed	Ties shoelaces Uses scissors, simple tools, or pencil very well In drawing, copies a diamond and triangle; adds seven to nine parts to stick figure; prints a few letters, numbers, or words such as first name	Has vocabulary of about 2100 words Uses sentences of six to eight words, with all parts of speech Names coins (e.g., nickel, dime) Names four or more colors Describes drawing or pictures with much comment and enumeration Knows names of days of week, months, and other time-associated words Knows composition of articles, such as, "A shoe is made of ______" Can follow three commands in succession

TABLE 35-1 Growth and development during preschool years—cont'd

SOCIALIZATION	COGNITION	FAMILY RELATIONSHIPS
Dresses self almost completely if helped with back buttons and told which shoe is right or left Pulls on shoes Has increased attention span Feeds self completely Can prepare simple meals such as cold cereal and milk Can help to set table; can dry dishes without breaking any May have fears, especially of dark and going to bed Knows own sex and sex of others Play is parallel and associative; begins to learn simple games but often follows own rules; begins to share	Is in preconceptual phase Is egocentric in thought and behavior Has beginning understanding of time; uses many time-oriented expressions, talks about past and future as much as about present, pretends to tell time Has improved concept of space as demonstrated in understanding of prepositions and ability to follow directional command Has beginning ability to view concepts from another perspective	Attempts to please parents and conform to their expectations Is less jealous of younger sibling; may be opportune time for birth of additional sibling Is aware of family relationships and sex-role functions Boys tend to identify more with father or other male figure Has increased ability to separate easily and comfortably from parents for short periods
Very independent Tends to be selfish and impatient Aggressive physically as well as verbally Takes pride in accomplishments Has mood swings Shows off dramatically, enjoys entertaining others Tells family tales to others with no restraint Still has many fears Play is associative Imaginary playmates are common Uses dramatic, imaginative, and imitative devices Sexual exploration and curiosity demonstrated through play, such as being "doctor" or "nurse"	Is in phase of intuitive thought Causality is still related to proximity of events Understands time better, especially in terms of sequence of daily events Unable to conserve matter Judges everything according to one dimension such as height, width, or order Immediate perceptual clues dominate judgment Is beginning to develop less egocentrism and more social awareness May count correctly but has poor mathematic concept of numbers Obeys because parents have set limits, not because of understanding of right or wrong	Rebels if parents expect too much, such as impeccable table manners Takes aggression and frustration out on parents or siblings Do's and don'ts become important May have rivalry with older or younger siblings; may resent older sibling's privileges and younger sibling's invasion of privacy and possessions May "run away" from home Identifies strongly with parent of opposite sex Is able to run simple errands outside the home
Less rebellious and quarrelsome than at age 4 years More settled and eager to get down to business Not as open and accessible in thoughts and behavior as in earlier years Independent but trustworthy; not foolhardy; more responsible Has fewer fears; relies on outer authority to control world Eager to do things right and to please; tries to "live by the rules" Has better manners Cares for self totally, occasionally needing supervision in dress or hygiene Not ready for concentrated close work or small print because of slight farsightedness and still unrefined eye-hand coordination Play is associative; tries to follow rules but may cheat to avoid losing	Begins to question what parents think by comparing them with age-mates and other adults May notice prejudice and bias in outside world Is more able to view other's perspective, but tolerates differences rather than understanding them May begin to show understanding of conservation of numbers through counting objects regardless of arrangement Uses time-oriented words with increased understanding Very curious about factual information regarding world	Gets along well with parents May seek out parent more often than at age 4 years for reassurance and security, especially when entering school Begins to question parents' thinking and principles Strongly identifies with parent of same sex, especially boys with their fathers Enjoys activities such as sports, cooking, shopping with parent of same sex

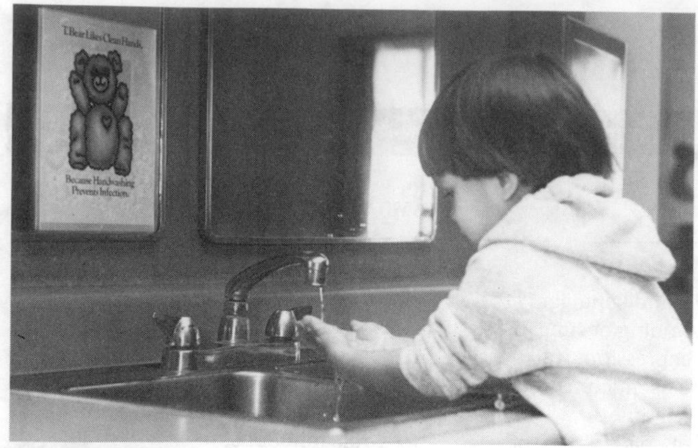

Fig. 35-4 Thorough handwashing is the single most effective method of preventing infection.

lows the child to fantasize about the forthcoming event in a positive manner. When the first day of school arrives, the parents should behave confidently. Such behavior requires parents to have resolved their own feelings regarding the experience.

Parents should introduce their child to the teacher and the facility. In some instances it is helpful to remain for at least some part of the first day until the child is comfortable and at ease. Other specific actions that can help lessen separation anxiety include providing the school with detailed information about the child's home environment such as familiar routines, favorite activities, food preferences, names of siblings or pets, and personal habits. Such information helps the child feel familiar in the strange surroundings. When schools automatically request this information, the parent has a valuable clue to evaluating the quality of the program, since the request represents the staff's awareness of each child's needs. Transitional objects such as a favorite toy, may also help the child bridge the gap from home to school.

Sex Education

Preschoolers have experienced a tremendous amount of information during their short lifetimes. Although their thinking may not be mature, they search constantly for explanations and reasons that are logical and reasonable to them. The word "why" seems to supplant the word "no," which was common in toddlerhood. It is only natural that as they learn about "me," they will also want to know "why me," and "how me." Questions such as "Where do babies come from?" are as casual as "What makes it rain?" or "Who is that?" It is the *way* in which questions about procreation are answered that conditions children, even the youngest, to separate these questions from others about their world.

Two rules govern answering sensitive questions about topics such as sex. The first is to *find out what children know and think.* By investigating the theories children have produced as a reasonable explanation, parents can not only give correct information but also help children understand why their explanation is inaccurate. Another reason for ascertaining what the child thinks before offering any information is that the "unasked for" answer may be given. For example, 4-year-old Sally asked her father, "Where did I come from?" Both parents quickly took this inquiry as a clue for offering sex education. After the explanation, Sally exclaimed, "I don't know about all that! All I know is Mary came from New York and I want to know where I was born."

The second rule for giving information is to be *honest.* It is true that much of the correct information will be forgotten or misunderstood by the preschooler, but what is more important is that the correct information can be restated until the child absorbs and comprehends the facts. Even though the correct anatomic words may be hard to pronounce or even more difficult to remember, they become foundational content for explaining other concepts later on.

Honesty does not imply imparting to children every fact of life or allowing excessive permissiveness in sexual curiosity. When children ask one question, they are looking for one answer. When they are ready, they will ask about the other "unfinished" parts of the story. Sooner or later they will wonder how the "sperm meets the egg" and "how the baby gets out," but it is best to wait until they ask.

Regardless of whether children are given sex education, they will engage in games of sexual curiosity and exploration. At about 3 years of age children are aware of the anatomic differences between the sexes and are very concerned with how the other "works." This is not really "sexual" curiosity, because many children are still unaware of the reproductive function of the genitals. Their curiosity is for the eliminative function of the anatomy. Little boys wonder how girls can urinate without a penis, so they watch girls go to the bathroom. Since they cannot see anything but the stream of water coming out, they want to observe further for what makes it come out. "Doctor play" is often a game invented for just such investigation. Little girls are no less curious about boys' anatomy. It is very intriguing to have a closer inspection of this "thing" that girls do not have.

One question that parents often have is how to handle such sexual curiosity. A positive approach is to neither condone nor condemn the sexual curiosity but to express that if children have questions, they should ask the parents, and then encourage them to engage in some other activity. In this way children can be helped to understand that there are ways that their sexual curiosity can be satisfied other than through playing investigative games. This in no way condemns the act but stresses alternate methods to seek solutions and answers. Allowing children unrestricted permissiveness only intensifies their anxiety and concern, since exploring and searching usually yield little evidence to satisfy their curiosity.

Another concern for some parents is *masturbation,* or self-stimulation of the genitals. This occurs at any age for a variety of reasons and, if not excessive, is normal and healthy. It is most common at 4 years of age and during adolescence (Leung and Robson, 1993). For preschoolers it is a part of sexual curiosity and exploration. If parents are concerned about masturbation in their children, it is essential for nurses to investigate the circumstances associated with the activity, because it may be an expression of anxiety, boredom, or unresolved conflicts. For example, a boy who repeatedly touches his penis is not masturbating for pleasure but may be reassuring himself that it is intact. Also, children who openly and publicly masturbate are inviting a reaction, such as discipline, punishment, or criticism. They may be overwhelmed by their sexual feelings and asking others to help them channel them into more constructive outlets. Since masturbation, like other forms of sex play, is a private act, parents should emphasize this to children as part of teaching them socially acceptable behavior.

Fears

The greatest number and variety of real and imagined fears are present during the preschool years and include fear of the dark, being left alone (especially at bedtime), animals (particularly large dogs and snakes), ghosts, sexual matters (castration), and objects or persons associated with pain. Parents often become perplexed about handling the fears because no amount of logical persuasion, coercion, or ridicule will send away the ghosts, boogeymen, monsters, and devils.

The best way to help children overcome their fears is by actively involving them in finding practical methods to deal with the frightening experience. This may be as simple as keeping a night light on in the child's bedroom for assurance that no monsters lurk in the dark. Exposing children to the feared object in a safe situation also provides a type of conditioning or **desensitization.** For instance, children who are afraid of dogs should never be forced to approach or touch one, but they may be gradually introduced to the experience by watching other children play with the animal. This type of modeling (i.e., demonstrating fearlessness in others) can be very effective if the child is allowed to progress at his or her own rate.

Usually by 5 or 6 years of age children relinquish these old fears. Explaining the developmental sequence of fears and their gradual disappearance may help parents feel more secure in handling preschoolers' fears. Sometimes fears do not subside with simple measures or developmental maturation. When children experience severe fears that disrupt family life, professional help is required.

Speech Problems

The most critical period for speech development occurs between 2 and 4 years of age. During this period children are using their rapidly growing vocabulary faster than they can produce the words. This failure to master sensorimotor integrations results in ***stuttering*** or ***stammering*** as children try to say the word they are already thinking about. This dysfluency in speech pattern is a *normal* characteristic of language development.

However, when parents or other significant persons place undue emphasis or stress on this pattern of **dysfluency,** an abnormal speech pattern may result. Chances for reversal of stuttering are good until about 5 years of age. Therefore prevention must begin early.

Nursing ALERT

Dysfluency must be arrested before children develop an awareness or anticipation of the difficulty and begin to mistrust their speech skills.

The nurse should discuss with parents the normal dysfluencies in children's speech. When stuttering does occur, families are advised to use the suggestions listed in the Home Care box above to avoid inadvertently reinforcing this pattern. If excessive concern on the part of the parent or frustration and struggling by the child are noted, the child is referred for language and speech evaluation.

Home Care 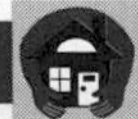

DEALING WITH STUTTERING IN CHILDREN

To be encouraged

Viewing hesitancy and dysfluency as a normal part of speech development
Giving child plenty of time and the impression of not being rushed or in a hurry
Looking directly at child while he or she is talking; being patient and never ridiculing or criticizing
Setting a good example by speaking clearly and articulating well
Identifying situations when stuttering increases and avoiding them or ignoring the hesitancy
Capitalizing on periods of fluent speech with positive reinforcement such as singing songs or repeating nursery rhymes

To be avoided

The natural tendency to "help" by supplying word when child is having a block
Telling child to stop or start over, to think before speaking, or to take it easy and go slowly
Showing great concern, embarrassment, or disapproval for hesitancy
Doing *anything* that emphasizes stuttering and calls child's attention to speech skills
Promising reward for proper speech

Children who are pressured into producing sounds ahead of their developmental level may develop **dyslalia** (articulation problems) or revert to using infantile speech. Prevention involves discussing with parents the usual achievement of speech production during childhood. The *Denver Articulation Screening Examination (DASE)* is an excellent tool to assess articulation skills in the child and to explain to parents the expected progression of sounds (see Appendix). The DASE is a reliable, effective screening tool because it requires only 10 minutes to perform and it is designed to discriminate between significant delay and normal variations in the acquisition of speech sounds.

Promoting Optimum Health During the Preschool Years*

NUTRITION

Nutritional requirements for preschoolers are fairly similar to those for toddlers. The requirement for calories per unit of

*For a more comprehensive understanding, the reader is urged to also review the material presented in Chapter 34 under Promoting Optimum Health During Toddlerhood.

body weight continues to decrease slightly to 90 kcal/kg for an average daily intake of 1800 calories. Fluid requirements may also decrease slightly to about 100 ml/kg daily but depend on the activity level, climatic conditions, and state of health. The protein requirements are 1.2 g/kg for an average daily consumption of 24 g (Food and Nutrition Board, 1989). A moderately reduced fat diet may be recommended for healthy preschool children. However, it is important that the diet not be deficient in nutrients such as calcium (Shea et al, 1993).

Some preschoolers still have food habits that are typical of toddlers, such as food fads and strong taste preferences. When children reach 4 years of age, they seem to enter another period of finicky eating, which is generally characteristic of the more rebellious and rowdy behavior of children in this age group. By age 5 children are more agreeable to trying new foods, especially if encouraged by an adult who allows the child to help with food preparation or experiments with a new taste or different dish (Fig. 35-5). Mealtimes can become battlegrounds if parents expect perfect table manners. Usually the 5-year-old child is ready for the "social" side of eating, but the 3- or 4-year-old child still has difficulty sitting quietly through a long family meal.

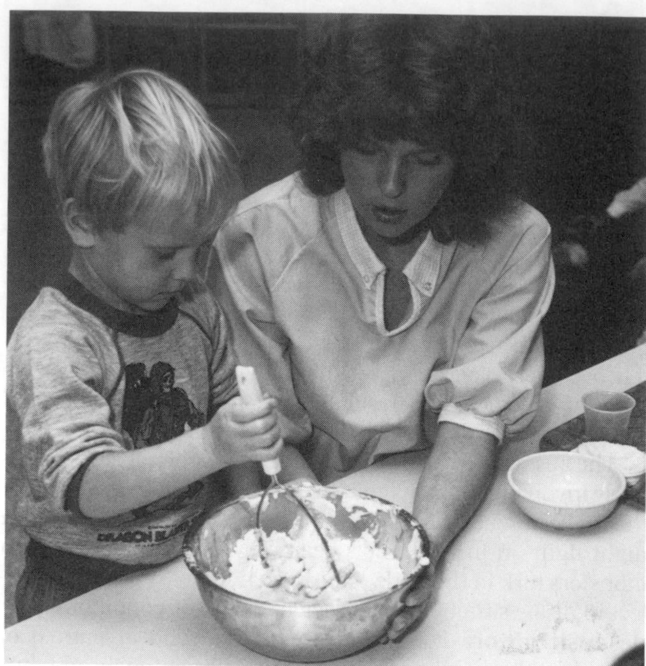

Fig. 35-5 Preschool-age children enjoy helping adults and are more likely to try new foods if they can assist in the preparation.

The amount and variety of foods consumed by young children vary greatly from day to day. Consequently, parents sometimes worry about the quantity of food preschoolers consume. In general, the quality is much more important than the quantity, a fact that should be stressed during nutritional counseling. There is some evidence that children self-regulate their caloric intake. If they eat less at one meal, they will compensate at another meal or snack (Birch et al, 1991; Shea et al, 1992). Also, children's likes and dislikes may be related to genetic sensitivity to tastes (Anliker et al, 1991).

One approach toward lessening this parental concern is advising parents to keep a weekly record of everything the child eats. In particular, the need for measuring the amount of food, such as setting aside ½ cup of vegetables, and serving the child from this premeasured amount is stressed. This provides a more accurate estimate of food intake at each meal. Usually by the end of the week, when they look at the food chart, parents are amazed at how much the child has consumed. In general, preschoolers consume only slightly more than toddlers, or about half of an adult's portion.

SLEEP AND ACTIVITY

Sleep patterns vary widely, but the average preschooler sleeps about 12 hours a night and infrequently takes daytime naps. Activity levels continue to be high, although quiet activities such as television are increasingly appealing and can become an unhealthy substitute for active play. Preschoolers' increased gross motor abilities and coordination provide them with the opportunity to engage in many sports, if only at a novice level. Whether young children should begin formalized training in an activity at this early age is controversial. The American Academy of Pediatrics (1992) recommends that children's readiness to participate in organized sports should be determined individually. The decision should be based on the child's (not the parent's) motivation and enjoyment. The American Academy of Pediatrics encourages free play, a variety of physical activities, a noncompetitive atmosphere, and emphasis on fun and safety.

Sleep Problems*

The preschool years are a prime time for sleep problems. Young children sometimes have trouble going to sleep, especially after so much activity and stimulation during the day. Others may develop bedtime fears, wake during the night, or have nightmares or sleep terrors. Still others may prolong the inevitable through elaborate rituals. Children with reported sleep problems may be more likely to have a difficult temperament than those without sleep disturbances (Atkinson et al, 1995).

Recommendations for sleep disturbance are offered only *after* a thorough assessment of the problem has been completed. Cultural traditions may dictate sleep practices that are contrary to certain well-accepted professional recommendations. Therefore parents' perceptions of a sleep habit may not be considered a problem (see the Cultural Considerations box on p. 1027).

Interventions can differ greatly; for example, **nightmares** (scary dreams that are followed by full waking) and **sleep terrors** (partial arousal from deep, nondreaming sleep) require very different approaches. Although sleep terrors require no intervention (the best approach is to remain uninvolved so that the child remains asleep), nightmares respond best to the following interventions:

- Accept dream as real fear.
- Sit with child; offer comfort, assurance, and sense of protection.

*Guidelines for helping parents deal with sleep problems are available in Wong DL: *Wong and Whaley's clinical manual of pediatric nursing*, ed 4, St Louis, 1996, Mosby.

Cultural Considerations 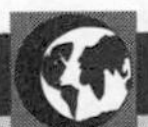

CO-SLEEPING

Although many experts recommend that infants and children be trained to always sleep in their own crib or bed, co-sleeping, or the "family bed" (in which parents allow the children to sleep with them or the siblings to sleep together in one bed), is a relatively common and accepted cultural practice, especially among black, Hispanic, and Asian families such as the Japanese. Other groups that are adopting co-sleeping include (1) single parents, whose need for company may encourage this practice; (2) working parents, who desire the closeness at night that was lost during the day; and (3) parents who have had an issue about sleep or separation in their own past (Brazelton, 1992).

- Lie down with child or take to own bed *only* if child is not calmed by other measures and understands this is a special occasion.
- Consider professional counseling for recurrent nightmares unresponsive to above approaches.

For children who delay going to bed, a recommended approach involves counseling parents about the importance of a consistent bedtime ritual. Attention-seeking behavior is ignored, and the child is not taken into the parents' bed or allowed to stay up past a reasonable hour. Other measures that may be helpful include keeping a light on in the room, providing transitional objects, such as a favorite toy, or leaving a drink of water by the bed.

Helping children slow down *before* bedtime also contributes to less resistance to going to bed. One approach is to establish limited rituals that signal readiness for bed such as a bath or story. Parents can reinforce the pattern by stating, "After this story it is bedtime," and consistently carrying out the routine. If extra stimulation such as having visitors arrive at bedtime is disruptive to children's routine, it is advisable to settle children in bed beforehand.

DENTAL HEALTH

By the beginning of the preschool period, the eruption of the deciduous teeth is complete. Dental care is essential to preserve these temporary teeth and to teach good dental habits (see Chapter 34). Although preschoolers' fine motor control is improved, they still require assistance and supervision with brushing, and flossing should be done by parents. Professional care and prophylaxis, especially fluoride supplements, should be continued. If children are cared for away from home, parents are encouraged to monitor the dental care provided by others, including the diet to keep cariogenic foods to a minimum.

INJURY PREVENTION

Because of improved gross and fine motor skills, coordination, and balance, preschoolers are less prone to falls than are toddlers. They tend to be less reckless, to listen more to parental rules, and to be aware of potential dangers, such as hot objects, sharp instruments, and dangerous heights. Putting objects in the mouth as part of exploration has all but ceased, although poisoning is still a danger. Pedestrian motor vehicle injuries increase because of activities such as playing in the street, riding tricycles, running after balls, or forgetting safety regulations when crossing streets.

In general, the guidelines suggested for injury prevention in Table 34-3 apply to children in this age group as well. However, emphasis is now on *education* for safety and potential hazards, in addition to appropriate protection. Since preschoolers are great imitators, it is especially essential that parents set a good example by "practicing what they preach." Children quickly observe discrepancies in what they are told to do and what they see others do. Establishing habits at this time, such as wearing bicycle helmets, can create long-term safety behaviors.

Home Care 

GUIDANCE DURING PRESCHOOL YEARS

Age 3 years

Prepare parents for child's increasing interest in widening relationships.
Encourage enrollment in preschool.
Emphasize importance of setting limits.
Prepare parents to expect exaggerated tension-reduction behaviors such as need for "security blanket."
Encourage parents to offer child choices when child vacillates.
Expect marked changes at $3\frac{1}{2}$ years, when child becomes less coordinated (motor and emotional), becomes insecure, and exhibits emotional extremes.
Prepare parents for normal dysfluency in speech and advise them to avoid focusing on the pattern.
Prepare parents to expect extra demands on their attention as a reflection of child's emotional insecurity and fear of loss of love.
Warn parents that equilibrium of 3-year-old will change to aggressive, out-of-bounds behavior of 4-year-old.
Anticipate more stable appetite with more food selections.
Stress need for protection and education of child to prevent injury (see Injury Prevention, Chapter 34)

Age 4 years

Prepare for more aggressive behavior, including motor activity and offensive language.
Prepare parents to expect resistance to parental authority.
Explore parental feelings regarding child's behavior.
Suggest some kind of respite for primary caregivers, such as placing child in preschool for part of the day.
Prepare for increasing sexual curiosity.
Emphasize importance of realistic limit-setting on behavior and appropriate discipline techniques.
Prepare parents for highly imaginary 4-year-old who indulges in "tall tales" (to be differentiated from lies) and for child's imaginary playmates.
Expect nightmares or an increase in them and suggest they make sure child is fully awakened from a frightening dream.
Provide reassurance that a period of calm begins at 5 years of age.

Age 5 years

Expect tranquil period at 5 years.
Prepare child for entrance into school environment.
Make sure immunizations are up to date before entering school.
Suggest that nonemployed mothers (or fathers if appropriate) consider own activities when child begins school.
Suggest swimming lessons.

ANTICIPATORY GUIDANCE—CARE OF FAMILIES

The preschool years present fewer childrearing difficulties than earlier years, and this stage of development is facilitated by appropriate anticipatory guidance in the areas already discussed (see the Home Care box on p. 1027). There is a shift in childrearing practices from protection to education. Whereas injury prevention previously focused on safeguarding the immediate environment with less emphasis on reasoning, now the protective guardrails or electrical outlet caps may be substituted with verbal explanations of why danger exists and how to avoid it with appropriate judgment and understanding.

During this period an emotional transition between parent and child is also occurring. Although children are still attached to their parents and accepting of all parental values and beliefs, they are nearing the period of life when they will question previous teachings and prefer the companionship of peers. Entry into school marks a separation from home for parents, as well as for children. Parents need help in adjusting to this change, particularly if the mother has focused her daily activity primarily on home responsibilities. As preschoolers begin preschool or elementary school, mothers may need to seek activities beyond the family such as community involvement or pursuing a career. In this way all family members are adjusting to change, which is part of the process of growth and development.

Special Health Problems

COMMUNICABLE DISEASES

Young children are especially susceptible to infectious disease, and a number of disorders occur predominantly during these early years. The incidence of childhood communicable diseases has declined greatly since the advent of immunizations. Serious complications resulting from such infections have been further reduced with the use of antibiotics and antitoxins. However, infectious diseases do occur, and nurses must be familiar with the infectious agent in order to recognize the disease and institute appropriate preventive and supportive interventions. See also Chapter 50 for a discussion of nursing care for dermatologic conditions.

Nursing Care Management

Assessment

Identification of the infectious agent is of primary importance to prevent exposure to susceptible individuals. Nurses in ambulatory care settings, child care centers, and schools are often the first persons to see signs of a communicable disease such as a rash or sore throat. The nurse must operate under a high index of suspicion for common childhood diseases in order to identify potentially infectious cases and to recognize diseases that require medical intervention. An example is the common complaint of sore throat. Although most often a symptom of a minor viral infection, it can signal diphtheria or a streptococcal infection, such as scarlet fever. Each of these bacterial conditions requires appropriate medical treatment to prevent serious sequelae.

Assessment of the following is helpful in identifying potentially **communicable diseases:** (1) recent exposure to a known case; (2) **prodromal symptoms** (symptoms that occur between early manifestations of the disease and its overt clinical syndrome) or evidence of constitutional symptoms such as a fever or rash (Table 35-2); (3) immunization history; and (4) history of having the disease. Since immunizations are available for several of the diseases and in almost each case an attack confers lifelong immunity, the possibility of many infectious agents can be eliminated based on these two criteria.

Nursing Diagnoses

A number of nursing diagnoses are prominent in the nursing care of the child with a communicable disease, and others specific to individual cases become evident. The most common nursing diagnoses are presented in the Nursing Care Plan on p. 1038.

Planning

In addition to identification of the communicable disease (see Assessment), the principal goals are as follows:

1. The child will not spread the infection to others.
2. The child will not experience complications.
3. The child will have minimal discomfort.
4. The child and family will receive adequate emotional support.

Implementation

Prevent spread. Prevention consists of two components: prevention of the disease and control of its spread to others. Primary prevention rests almost exclusively on immunization. (The nurse's role in immunization of children is discussed in Chapter 33.)

Control measures to prevent spread of the disease include appropriate techniques to reduce risk of cross-transmission of infectious organisms between patients and to protect health care workers from organisms harbored by patients. If the child is hospitalized, the facility's policies for infection control are followed (see Chapter 42). The most important procedure to stress is handwashing. Persons directly caring for the child or handling contaminated articles must wash their hands before beginning care of another patient. The child is instructed to practice good handwashing technique after toileting and before eating. For those diseases spread by droplets, the nurse instructs parents in measures aimed at reducing airborne transmission. The child who is old enough should use a tissue to cover the face during coughing or sneezing; otherwise the parent should cover the child's mouth with a tissue and then discard it. The usual hygiene measures of not sharing eating and drinking utensils are stressed to the family.

Nursing ALERT

If a child is admitted to the hospital with an undiagnosed exanthema, strict isolation is instituted until a diagnosis is confirmed. Childhood communicable diseases requiring strict isolation are diphtheria and chickenpox.

Prevent complications. Although most youngsters recover without any difficulty, certain groups of children are at risk for serious, even fatal, complications from communicable diseases, especially the viral diseases of chicken pox and erythema infectiosum (EI). Children with an immunodeficiency—those receiving steroid or other immunosuppressive therapy, those with a generalized malignancy such as leukemia or lymphoma, or those with an immunologic disorder—are at risk for viremia from replication of the *varicella-zoster virus (VZV)** in the blood. VZV is so named because it causes two distinct diseases: *varicella (chickenpox)* and *zoster (herpes zoster* or *shingles)*. Varicella occurs primarily in children under 15 years of age. However, it leaves the threat of herpes zoster, an intensely painful varicella that is localized to a single dermatome (body area innervated by a particular segment of the spinal cord) (Straus, 1993). Patients who are immunocompromised and healthy infants under 1 year of age (who also have reduced immunity) are at a higher risk for reactivation of VZV, causing herpes zoster, probably as a result of a deficiency in cellular immunity (Terada et al, 1994).

Children with hemolytic disease such as sickle cell disease are at risk for aplastic anemia from EI. The *human parvovirus (HPV)* infects and lyses red blood cell precursors, thus interrupting the production of red blood cells. Therefore, in patients who need increased red blood cell production to maintain normal cell volumes, the virus may precipitate a severe aplastic crisis. Because the fetus depends on a high rate of red blood cell production and has an immature immune system, it may develop severe anemia as a result of HPV infection in the mother.

Nursing ALERT

High-risk children who have signs of these communicable diseases are referred to the practitioner immediately. School nurses are responsible for warning parents about recent outbreaks of these communicable diseases to prevent susceptible children's exposure to known cases. In most instances high-risk children are kept out of school until the outbreak is over.

Prevention of complications from diseases such as diphtheria and scarlet fever necessitates compliance with antibiotic therapy. With oral preparations the need to complete the entire course of therapy is stressed (see Compliance, Chapter 42). Varicella-zoster immune globulin (VZIG) may be given to high-risk children after exposure to chickenpox to prevent the development of varicella. The antiviral agent acyclovir (Zovirax) may be used to treat varicella infections. It is effective in decreasing the number of lesions; shortening the duration of fever; and decreasing itching, lethargy, and anorexia (Dunkle et al, 1991). Recent evidence suggests that vitamin A supplementation reduces both morbidity and mortality in measles and that all children with severe measles should be given vitamin A supplements (Glasziou and MacKerras, 1993).

*Educational materials for health care providers and families may be obtained from the **Varicella Zoster Virus Research Foundation,** 40 East 72nd St., New York, NY 10021; or by calling Burroughs Wellcome Co at 1-800-843-8889.

A single oral dose of 200,000 IU for children at least 1 year old (half that dose for children 6 to 12 months of age) is recommended. The higher dose may be associated with vomiting and headache for a few hours. The dose should be repeated the next day and at 4 weeks for children with ophthalmologic evidence of vitamin A deficiency (American Academy of Pediatrics, 1993b).

Nursing ALERT

Although the risk of vitamin A toxicity from these doses (they are 100 to 200 times the recommended dietary allowance) is very low, nurses should instruct parents on safe storage of the drug. Ideally vitamin A should be dispensed in the age-appropriate unit dose to prevent excessive administration and possible toxicity.

Provide comfort. Many of the communicable diseases cause skin manifestations that are bothersome to the child. The chief discomfort from most of the rashes is itching, and measures such as cool baths (usually without soap) and lotions such as calamine are helpful.

Nursing ALERT

When lotions with active ingredients such as diphenhydramine in Caladryl are used, they are applied sparingly, especially over open lesions where excessive absorption can lead to drug toxicity, and in children simultaneously receiving oral diphenhydramine.

To avoid overheating, which increases itching, children should wear lightweight, loose, nonirritating clothing and keep out of the sun. If the child persists in scratching, the nails are kept short and smooth; mittens and clothes with long sleeves or legs may be needed. For severe itching, antipruritic medication such as diphenhydramine (Benadryl) or hydroxyzine (Atarax) may be required, especially when the child desires to sleep.

An elevated temperature is common, and both antipyretic medicine (acetaminophen or Children's Motrin) and environmental manipulation are implemented (see Controlling Elevated Temperature, Chapter 42). Acetaminophen is effective in lowering the fever, but evidence suggests that in chickenpox the medication does not significantly reduce the symptoms of itching, anorexia, abdominal pain, fussiness, or vomiting and that it may delay scabbing of the lesions (Doran et al, 1989).

A sore throat, another frequent symptom, is managed with lozenges, saline rinses (if the child is old enough to cooperate), and analgesics. Since most children are anorectic during an illness, bland foods and increased liquids are usually preferred. During the early stages of the disease children voluntarily curtail their activity, and although bed rest is beneficial, it should not be imposed unless specifically indicated (e.g., in pertussis). During periods of irritability, quiet activity (e.g., reading, music, television, puzzles, coloring) helps distract children from the discomfort.

Text continued on p. 1036.

TABLE 35-2 Communicable diseases of childhood

DISEASE
Chickenpox (Varicella) (Fig. 35-6) **Agent:** Varicella zoster virus (VZV) **Source:** Primary secretions of respiratory tract of infected persons; to a lesser degree skin lesions (scabs not infectious) **Transmission:** Direct contact, droplet (airborne) spread, and contaminated objects **Incubation period:** 2 to 3 weeks, usually 13 to 17 days **Period of communicability:** Probably 1 day before eruption of lesions (prodromal period) to 6 days after first crop of vesicles when crusts have formed
Diphtheria **Agent:** *Corynebacterium diphtheriae* **Source:** Discharges from mucous membranes of nose and nasopharynx, skin, and other lesions of infected person **Transmission:** Direct contact with infected person, a carrier, or contaminated articles **Incubation period:** Usually 2 to 5 days, possibly longer **Period of communicability:** Variable; until virulent bacilli are no longer present (identified by three negative cultures); usually 2 weeks but as long as 4 weeks

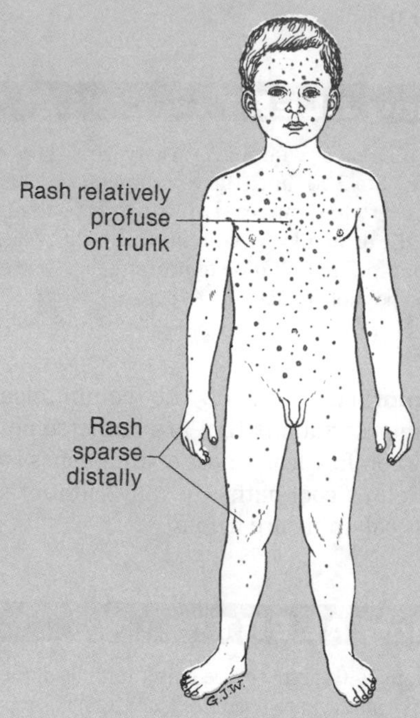

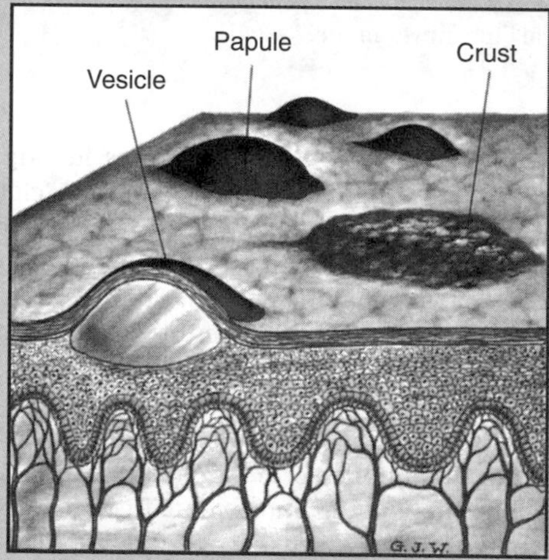

Simultaneous stages of lesions in chickenpox

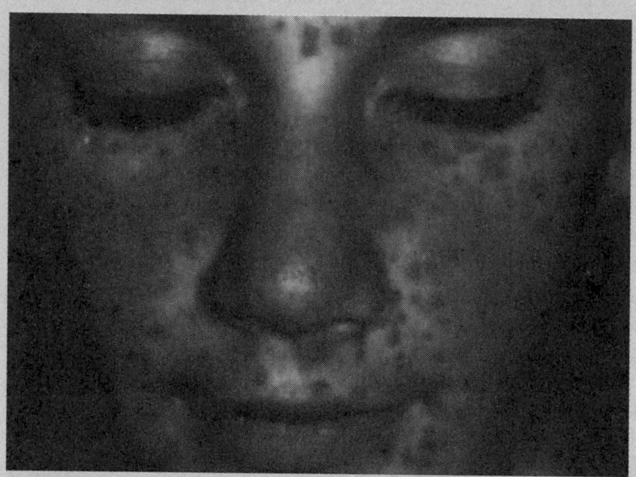

Fig. 35-6 Chickenpox (varicella). (Clinical view from Habif TP: *Clinical dermatology: a color guide to diagnosis and therapy*, ed 2, St Louis, 1990, Mosby.)

CLINICAL MANIFESTATIONS	THERAPEUTIC MANAGEMENT/COMPLICATIONS	NURSING CONSIDERATIONS
Prodromal stage: Slight fever, malaise, and anorexia for first 24 hours; rash highly pruritic; begins as macule, rapidly progresses to papule and then vesicle (surrounded by erythematous base, becomes umbilicated and cloudy, breaks easily and forms crusts); all three stages (papule, vesicle, crust) present in varying degrees at one time **Distribution:** Centripetal, spreading to face and proximal extremities but sparse on distal limbs and less on areas not exposed to heat (i.e., from clothing or sun) **Constitutional signs and symptoms:** Elevated temperature from lymphadenopathy, irritability from pruritus	**Specific:** Antiviral agent acyclovir (Zovirax) varicella-zoster immune globulin (VZIG) after exposure in high-risk children **Supportive:** Diphenhydramine hydrochloride or antihistamines to relieve itching; skin care to prevent secondary bacterial infection **Complications:** Secondary bacterial infections (abscesses, cellulitis, pneumonia, sepsis) Encephalitis Varicella pneumonia Hemorrhagic varicella (tiny hemorrhages in vesicles and numerous petechiae in skin) Chronic or transient thrombocytopenia	Maintain strict isolation in hospital Isolate child in home until vesicles have dried (usually 1 week after onset of disease), and isolate high-risk children from infected children Administer skin care: give bath and change clothes and linens daily; administer topical application of calamine lotion; keep child's fingernails short and clean; apply mittens if child scratches Keep child cool (may decrease number of lesions) Lessen pruritus; keep child occupied Remove loose crusts that rub and irritate skin Teach child to apply pressure to pruritic area rather than scratching it If older child, reason with child regarding danger of scar formation from scratching Avoid use of aspirin; use of acetaminophen controversial (see p. 1029)
Vary according to anatomic location of pseudomembrane **Nasal:** Resembles common cold, serosanguineous mucopurulent nasal discharge without constitutional symptoms; may be frank epistaxis **Tonsillar/pharyngeal:** Malaise; anorexia; sore throat; low-grade fever; pulse increased above expected for temperature within 24 hours; smooth, adherent, white or gray membrane; lymphadenitis possibly pronounced (bull's neck); in severe cases, toxemia, septic shock, and death within 6 to 10 days **Laryngeal:** Fever, hoarseness, cough, with or without previous signs listed; potential airway obstruction, apprehensive, dyspneic retractions, cyanosis	Antitoxin (usually intravenously); preceded by skin or conjunctival test to rule out sensitivity to horse serum Antibiotics (penicillin or erythromycin) Complete bed rest (prevention of myocarditis) Tracheostomy for airway obstruction Treatment of infected contacts and carriers **Complications:** Myocarditis (second week) Neuritis	Maintain strict isolation in hospital Participate in sensitivity testing; have epinephrine available Administer antibiotics; observe for signs of sensitivity to penicillin Administer complete care to maintain bed rest Use suctioning as needed Observe respirations for signs of obstruction Administer humidified oxygen if prescribed

Continued.

TABLE 35-2 Communicable diseases of childhood—cont'd

DISEASE

Erythema infectiosum (Fifth disease)
Agent: Human parvovirus B19 (HPV)
Source: Infected persons
Transmission: Unknown; possibly respiratory secretions and blood
Incubation period: 4 to 14 days, may be as long as 20 days
Period of communicability: Uncertain but before onset of symptoms in most children; also for about 1 week after onset of symptoms in children with aplastic crisis

Exanthema subitum (Roseola)
Agent: Human herpes virus type 6 (HHV-6)
Source: Unknown
Transmission: Unknown (virtually limited to children between 6 months and 2 years of age)
Incubation period: Unknown
Period of communicability: Unknown

Measles (Rubeola)
Agent: Virus
Source: Respiratory tract secretions, blood, and urine of infected person
Transmission: Usually by direct contact with droplets of infected person
Incubation period: 10 to 20 days
Period of communicability: From 4 days before to 5 days after rash appears but mainly during prodromal (catarrhal) stage

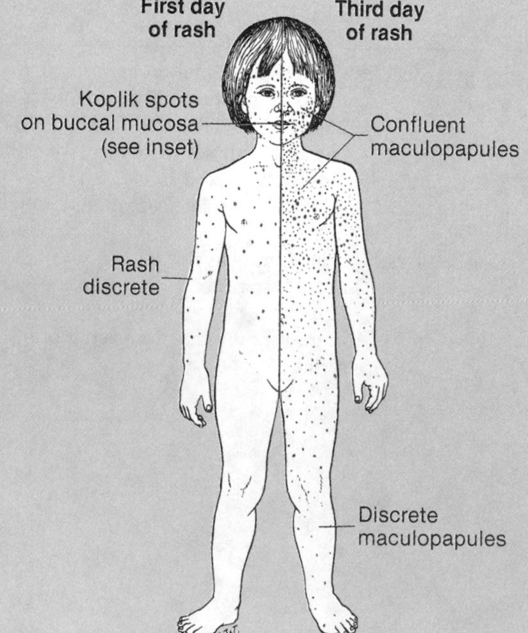

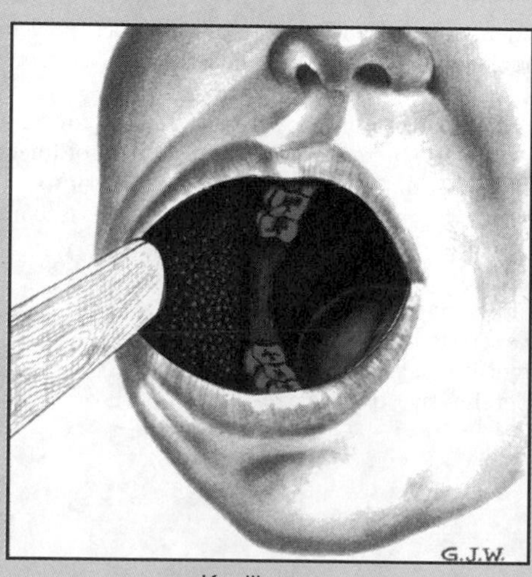

Koplik spots

CLINICAL MANIFESTATIONS	THERAPEUTIC MANAGEMENT/COMPLICATIONS	NURSING CONSIDERATIONS
Rash appears in three stages: I—Erythema on face, chiefly on cheeks, "slapped face" appearance; disappears by 1 to 4 days II—About 1 day after rash appears on face, maculopapular red spots appear, symmetrically distributed on upper and lower extremities; rash progresses from proximal to distal surfaces and may last a week or more III—Rash subsides but reappears if skin is irritated or traumatized (sun, heat, cold, friction) In children with aplastic crisis, rash is usually absent; and prodromal illness includes fever, myalgia, lethargy, nausea, vomiting, and abdominal pain	**Symptomatic and supportive:** Antipyretics, analgesics, antiinflammatory drugs Possible blood transfusion for transient aplastic anemia **Complications:** Self-limited arthritis and arthralgia (arthritis may become chronic) (Nocton et al, 1993) May result in fetal death if mother infected during pregnancy, but no evidence of congenital anomalies Aplastic crisis in children with hemolytic disease or immune deficiency Myocarditis (rare)	Isolation of child not necessary, except hospitalized child (immunosuppressed or with aplastic crises) suspected of HPV infection is placed on respiratory isolation and universal precautions Pregnant women: need not be excluded from workplace where HPV infection is present; should not care for patients with aplastic crises; explain low risk of fetal death to those in contact with affected children
Persistent high fever for 3 to 4 days in child who appears well Precipitous drop in fever to normal with appearance of rash **Rash:** Discrete rose-pink macules or maculopapules appearing first on trunk, then spreading to neck, face, and extremities; nonpruritic, fades on pressure, lasts 1 to 2 days **Associated signs and symptoms:** Cervical/postauricular lymphadenopathy, injected pharynx, cough, coryza	Nonspecific Antipyretics to control fever **Complications:** Recurrent febrile seizures (possibly from latent infection of central nervous system that is reactivated by fever) Encephalitis (rare)	Teach parents measures for lowering temperature (antipyretic drugs) If child is prone to seizures, discuss appropriate precautions, possibility of recurrent febrile seizures (Kondo et al, 1993)
Prodromal (catarrhal) stage: Fever and malaise, followed in 24 hours by coryza, cough, conjunctivitis, Koplik spots (small, irregular red spots with a minute, bluish white center first seen on buccal mucosa opposite molars 2 days before rash); symptoms gradually increase in severity until second day after rash appears, when they begin to subside **Rash:** Appears 3 to 4 days after onset of prodromal stage; begins as erythematous maculopapular eruption on face and gradually spreads downward; more severe in earlier sites (appears confluent) and less intense in later sites (appears discrete); after 3 to 4 days assumes brownish appearance, and fine desquamation occurs over areas of extensive involvement **Constitutional signs and symptoms:** Anorexia, malaise, generalized lymphadenopathy	Vitamin A supplementation (see p. 1029) **Supportive:** Bed rest during febrile period; antipyretics Antibiotics to prevent secondary bacterial infection in high-risk children **Complications:** Otitis media Pneumonia Bronchiolitis Obstructive laryngitis and laryngotracheitis Encephalitis	Isolation until fifth day of rash; if hospitalized, institute respiratory precautions Maintain bed rest during prodromal stage; provide quiet activity **Fever:** Instruct parents to administer antipyretics; avoid chilling; if child is prone to seizures, institute appropriate precautions (fever spikes to 40° C [104° F] between fourth and fifth days) **Eye care:** Dim lights if photophobia present; clean eyelids with warm saline solution to remove secretions or crusts; keep child from rubbing eyes; examine cornea for signs of ulceration **Coryza/cough:** Use cool mist vaporizer; protect skin around nares with layer of petrolatum; encourage fluids and soft, bland foods **Skin care:** Keep skin clean; use tepid baths as necessary

Continued.

TABLE 35-2 Communicable diseases of childhood—cont'd

DISEASE
Mumps **Agent:** Paramyxovirus **Source:** Saliva of infected persons **Transmission:** Direct contact with or droplet spread from an infected person **Incubation period:** 14 to 21 days **Period of communicability:** Most communicable immediately before and after swelling begins
Pertussis (Whooping cough) **Agent:** *Bordetella pertussis* **Source:** Discharge from respiratory tract of infected persons **Transmission:** Direct contact or droplet spread from infected person; indirect contact with freshly contaminated articles **Incubation period:** 5 to 21 days, usually 10 **Period of communicability:** Greatest during catarrhal stage before onset of paroxysms and may extend to fourth week after onset of paroxysms
Poliomyelitis **Agent:** Enteroviruses, three types: type 1—most frequent cause of paralysis, both epidemic and endemic; type 2—least frequently associated with paralysis; type 3—second most frequently associated with paralysis **Source:** Feces and oropharyngeal secretions of infected persons, especially young children **Transmission:** Direct contact with persons with apparent or inapparent active infection; spread is via fecal-oral and pharyngeal-oropharyngeal routes **Incubation period:** Usually 7 to 14 days, with range of 5 to 35 days **Period of communicability:** Not exactly known; virus is present in throat and feces shortly after infection and persists for about 1 week in throat and 4 to 6 weeks in feces

CLINICAL MANIFESTATIONS	THERAPEUTIC MANAGEMENT/COMPLICATIONS	NURSING CONSIDERATIONS
Prodromal stage: Fever, headache, malaise, and anorexia for 24 hours, followed by earache that is aggravated by chewing **Parotitis:** By third day, parotid gland(s) (either unilateral or bilateral) enlarges and reaches maximum size in 1 to 3 days; accompanied by pain and tenderness **Other manifestations:** Submaxillary and sublingual infection, orchitis, and meningoencephalitis	**Symptomatic and supportive:** Analgesics for pain and antipyretics for fever Intravenous fluid may be necessary for child who refuses to drink or vomits because of meningoencephalitis **Complications:** Sensorineural deafness Postinfectious encephalitis Myocarditis Arthritis Hepatitis Epididymoorchitis Sterility (extremely rare in adult males)	Isolation during period of communicability; institute respiratory precautions during hospitalization Maintain bed rest during prodromal phase until swelling subsides Give analgesics for pain; if child is unwilling to chew medication, use elixir form Encourage fluids and soft, bland foods; avoid foods requiring chewing Apply hot or cold compresses to neck, whichever is more comforting To relieve orchitis, provide warmth and local support with tight-fitting underpants (stretch bathing suit works well)
Catarrhal stage: Begins with symptoms of upper respiratory tract infection such as coryza, sneezing, lacrimation, cough, and low-grade fever; symptoms continue for 1 to 2 weeks, when dry, hacking cough becomes more severe **Paroxysmal stage:** Cough most often occurs at night and consists of short, rapid coughs followed by sudden inspiration associated with a high-pitched crowing sound or "whoop"; during paroxysms cheeks become flushed or cyanotic, eyes bulge, and tongue protrudes; paroxysm may continue until thick mucous plug is dislodged; vomiting frequently follows attack; stage generally lasts 4 to 6 weeks, followed by convalescent stage	Antimicrobial therapy (e.g., erythromycin) Administration of pertussis-immune globulin **Supportive treatment:** Hospitalization required for infants, children who are dehydrated, or those who have complications Bed rest Increased oxygen intake and humidity Adequate fluids Intubation possibly necessary **Complications:** Pneumonia (usual cause of death) Atelectasis Otitis media Convulsions Hemorrhage (subarachnoid, subconjunctival, epistaxis) Weight loss and dehydration Hernia Prolapsed rectum	Isolation during catarrhal stage; if hospitalized, institute respiratory precautions Maintain bed rest as long as fever present Keep child occupied during day (interest in play associated with fewer paroxysms) Reassure parents during frightening episodes of whooping cough Provide restful environment and reduce factors that promote paroxysms (dust, smoke, sudden change in temperature, chilling, activity, excitement); keep room well ventilated Encourage fluids; offer small amount of fluids frequently; refeed child after vomiting Provide high humidity (humidifier or tent); suction gently but often to prevent choking on secretions Observe for signs of airway obstruction (increased restlessness, apprehension, retractions, cyanosis) Involve public health nurse if child cared for at home
May be manifested in three different forms: **Abortive or inapparent**—Fever, uneasiness, sore throat, headache, anorexia, vomiting, abdominal pain; lasts a few hours to a few days **Nonparalytic**—Same manifestations as abortive but more severe, with pain and stiffness in neck, back, and legs **Paralytic**—Initial course similar to nonparalytic type, followed by recovery and then signs of central nervous system paralysis	No specific treatment, including antimicrobials or gamma globulin Complete bed rest during acute phase Assisted respiratory ventilation in case of respiratory paralysis Physical therapy for muscles following acute stage **Complications:** Permanent paralysis Respiratory arrest Hypertension Kidney stones from demineralization of bone during prolonged immobility	Maintain complete bed rest Administer mild sedatives as necessary to relieve anxiety and promote rest Participate in physiotherapy procedures (use of moist hot packs and range-of-motion exercises) Position child to maintain body alignment and prevent contractures or decubiti; use footboard Encourage child to move; administer analgesics for maximum comfort during physical activity Observe for respiratory paralysis (difficulty in talking, ineffective cough, inability to hold breath, shallow and rapid respirations); report such signs and symptoms to practitioner; have tracheostomy tray at bedside

Continued.

TABLE 35-2 Communicable diseases of childhood—cont'd

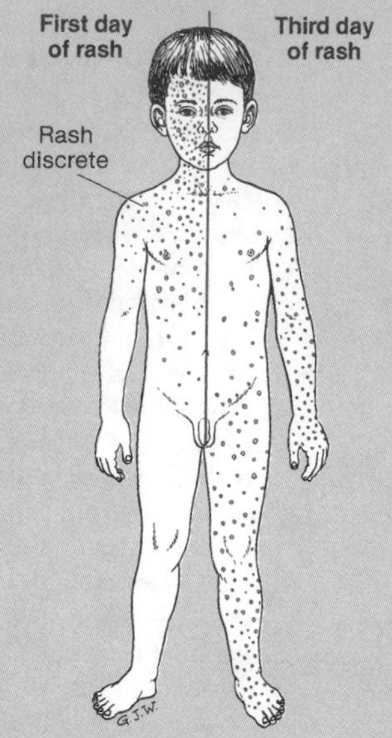

DISEASE

Rubella (German measles)

Agent: Rubella virus

Source: Primarily nasopharyngeal secretions of person with apparent or inapparent infection; virus also present in blood, stool, and urine

Transmission: Direct contact and spread via infected person; indirectly via articles freshly contaminated with nasopharyngeal secretions, feces, or urine

Incubation period: 14 to 21 days

Period of communicability: 7 days before to about 5 days after appearance of rash

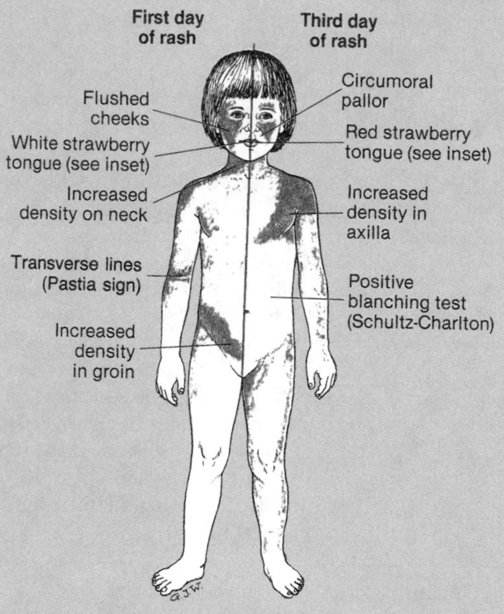

Scarlet fever (Fig. 35-7)

Agent: Group A β-hemolytic streptococci

Source: Usually from nasopharyngeal secretions of infected persons and carriers

Transmission: Direct contact with infected person or droplet spread; indirectly by contact with contaminated articles, ingestion of contaminated milk or other food

Incubation period: 2 to 4 days, with range of 1 to 7 days

Period of communicability: During incubation period and clinical illness approximately 10 days; during first 2 weeks of carrier phase, although may persist for months

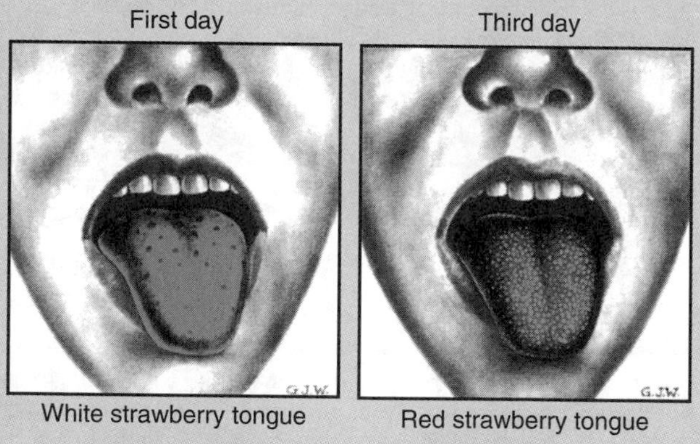

Fig. 35-7 Scarlet fever.

Support child and family. Most communicable diseases are benign, but they produce considerable concern and anxiety for some parents. Often the occurrence of a disease such as chickenpox is the first time the child is acutely uncomfortable. Parents need assistance to cope effectively with manifestations of the illness such as intense itching. Sometimes a visiting nurse may help the family develop a plan of care and encourage compliance with any treatments.

The family and child need reassurance that recovery from the disease is generally rapid. However, visible signs of the dermatosis may be present for some time after the child is well enough to resume usual activities. When the disease involves noticeable signs, such as the crusts of chickenpox, the child may benefit from preparation before returning to school. For example, the parent can discuss the child's physical appearance with the teacher and/or school nurse and request that they explain the child's condition to classmates.

CLINICAL MANIFESTATIONS	THERAPEUTIC MANAGEMENT/COMPLICATIONS	NURSING CONSIDERATIONS
Prodromal stage: Absent in children, present in adults and adolescents; consists of low-grade fever, headache, malaise, anorexia, mild conjunctivitis, coryza, sore throat, cough, and lymphadenopathy; lasts for 1 to 5 days, subsides 1 day after appearance of rash **Rash:** First appears on face and rapidly spreads downward to neck, arms, trunk, and legs; by end of first day body is covered with a discrete, pinkish red maculopapular exanthema; disappears in same order as it began and is usually gone by third day **Constitutional signs and symptoms:** Occasionally low-grade fever, headache, malaise, and lymphadenopathy	No treatment necessary other than antipyretics for low-grade fever and analgesics for discomfort **Complications:** Rare (arthritis, encephalitis, or purpura); most benign of all childhood communicable diseases; greatest danger is teratogenic effect on fetus	Reassure parents of benign nature of illness in affected child Use comfort measures as necessary Isolate child from pregnant women
Prodromal stage: Abrupt high fever, pulse increased out of proportion to fever, vomiting, headache, chills, malaise, abdominal pain **Enanthema:** Tonsils enlarged, edematous, reddened, and covered with patches of exudate; in severe cases appearance resembles membrane seen in diphtheria; pharynx is edematous and beefy red; during first 1 to 2 days tongue is coated and papillae become red and swollen (white strawberry tongue); by fourth or fifth day white coat sloughs off, leaving prominent papillae (red strawberry tongue); palate is covered with erythematous punctate lesions **Exanthema:** Rash appears within 12 hours after prodromal signs; red pinhead-sized punctate lesions rapidly become generalized but are absent on face, which becomes flushed with striking circumoral pallor; rash is more intense in folds of joints; by end of first week desquamation begins (fine, sandpaper-like on torso; sheetlike sloughing on palms and soles), which may be complete by 3 weeks or longer	Treatment of choice is a full course of penicillin (or erythromycin in penicillin-sensitive children); fever should subside 24 hours after beginning therapy Antibiotic therapy for newly diagnosed carriers (nose or throat cultures positive for streptococci) **Supportive measures:** Bed rest during febrile phase, analgesics for sore throat **Complications:** Otitis media Peritonsillar abscess Sinusitis Glomerulonephritis Carditis, polyarthritis (uncommon)	Institute respiratory precautions until 24 hours after initiation of treatment Ensure compliance with oral antibiotic therapy (intramuscular benzathine penicillin G [Bicillin] may be given if parents' reliability in giving oral drugs is questionable) Maintain bed rest during febrile phase; provide quiet activity during convalescent period Relieve discomfort of sore throat with analgesics, gargles, lozenges, antiseptic throat sprays (Chloraseptic), and inhalation of cool mist Encourage fluids during febrile phase; avoid irritating liquids (citrus juices) or rough foods; when child is able to eat, begin with soft diet Advise parents to consult practitioner if fever persists after beginning therapy Discuss procedures for preventing spread of infection

Nursing ALERT

The occurrence of a communicable disease provides the opportunity to ask parents about the child's immunization status and to reinforce the benefits of vaccines for children.

Evaluation

The effectiveness of nursing interventions is determined by continual reassessment and evaluation of care based on the following observational guidelines and expected outcomes:

1. Observe or inquire about family members' use of control measures; observe for signs of disease in household contacts.
2. Monitor vital signs, especially temperature; inquire about the identification of high-risk contacts and appropriate isolation of the contact; observe or inquire about compliance with antibiotic or antiviral therapy.
3. Inquire about effectiveness of comfort measures.
4. Interview family and child regarding their feelings and concerns, especially when child returns to school.

Nursing Care Plan

CHILD WITH A COMMUNICABLE DISEASE

Nursing Diagnosis: Risk for infection related to susceptible host and infectious agents

Expected outcome: Infection remains confined to original source.

• **NURSING INTERVENTIONS/*RATIONALES***

Institute appropriate infection control practices as recommended by the Centers for Disease Control and Prevention (see Chapter 42) *to prevent spread of microorganisms.* **(Scrupulous handwashing by all who have contact with the infected child is critical in control of the disease).**

Work with family and public health nurse *to ensure adherence to infection control practices and therapeutic regimens if individual is treated in the home.*

Report disease to health department to monitor outbreak.

Identify susceptible individuals in community (i.e., high-risk children, close contacts of infected child) who may require prophylactic treatment or need to practice careful avoidance and close monitoring practices *to prevent contracting the disease.*

Promote public education and service programs (i.e., immunization, food handling, animal control, screening) *that aim at prevention/spread of communicable disease on community level.*

Nursing Diagnosis: Risk for injury related to disease complications, trauma to skin from scratching

Expected outcomes: Patient will show no evidence of complications; skin remains intact.

• **NURSING INTERVENTIONS/*RATIONALES***

Involve child and parents in planning and carrying out therapeutic regimen (e.g., bed rest, hydration, feeding, prescribed medications) *to increase compliance.*

Monitor vital signs and appropriate laboratory values, make ongoing assessments of appropriate systems *to detect early signs of potential complications (ear, eye, respiratory infections; seizures, central nervous system involvement; myocarditis, arthritis, hepatitis).* Observe skin *to detect signs of scratching, trauma, infection.*

Institute seizure precautions *if febrile convulsions are a possible complication.*

Maintain good body hygiene; use antipruritics, lotions as needed; keep child's fingernails trimmed, use mittens or restraints, cover affected areas; keep skin cool *to prevent scratching, relieve itching,* and *reduce risk of trauma and secondary infection of lesions.*

Offer small frequent sips of child's favorite liquids and water *to ensure hydration* and frequent small feedings of favorite soft, bland foods (soups, ice cream, pudding, gelatin) *to reduce anorexia, nausea and vomiting.*

Nursing Diagnosis: Pain related to skin lesions, malaise

Expected outcome: Patient will exhibit minimum signs of discomfort.

• **NURSING INTERVENTIONS/*RATIONALES***

Use comfort measures such as vaporizer, gargles, and lozenges *to keep membranes moist;* petrolatum *for chapped lips;* saline *to cleanse crusted eyes;* cool moist cloths, tepid baths, and lotion *to relieve itching skin.*

Use nonpharmacologic techniques (i.e., distraction, relaxation, guided imagery, positive self-talk, thought stopping) *for pain reduction.*

Administer analgesics, antipyretics, and antipruritics per physician order *to relieve pain, fever, itching.* **(Do not use salicylates because of possible risk of Reye syndrome)**

Nursing Diagnosis: Social isolation related to environmentally imposed constraints secondary to communicable disease

Expected outcomes: Patient will interact in socially acceptable and developmentally appropriate manner and participate in meaningful diversional activity.

• **NURSING INTERVENTIONS/*RATIONALES***

Explain reasons for confinement *to enhance child's understanding.*

Enlist child's assistance with enforcing restrictions *to provide increased sense of control.*

Allow child to examine and play with any needed isolation supplies (i.e., gown, gloves, mask) *to relieve fears, increase sense of control.*

Have staff identify themselves to child before donning any required protective clothing *to increase child's trust in caregivers.*

Encourage parents to remain with child during hospitalization *to decrease separation and feelings of isolation.*

Encourage contact with peers and siblings by telephone *to maintain social interaction and reduce sense of isolation.*

Plan specific periods of developmentally appropriate diversional activity suited to child's physical condition and energy level *to decrease feelings of boredom and negative self-absorption.*

Expected outcomes:
See the Nursing Care Plan on p. 1038.

Child Maltreatment

The broad term **child maltreatment** includes intentional physical abuse or neglect, emotional abuse or neglect, and sexual abuse of children, usually by adults. It is one of the most significant social problems affecting children. In 1993 about 2.9 million children were reported as victims of child abuse and neglect to child protective services in the United States. However, this does not represent the number of children actually maltreated. Of these reported cases, about 35% were found to be substantiated or indicated (*In Fact…*, undated). It is also likely that many other abuse cases are never brought to the attention of the authorities. Consequently, the best available statistics only partially reflect the true incidence of child maltreatment. According to the National Center on Child Abuse and Neglect (NCCAAN) (1993), the following statistics represent the incidence of child maltreatment in the United States*: emotional neglect, 3.2 per 1000; emotional abuse, 3 per 1000; educational abuse, 4.5 per 1000; physical neglect, 8.1 per 1000; physical abuse, 4.9 per 1000; and sexual abuse, 2.1 per 1000. About 2000 children die from abuse or neglect each year; most of these children are under 4 years of age (A Nation's Shame, 1995).

CHILD NEGLECT

Child neglect is the most common form of maltreatment. About one half of all reported cases are associated with deprivation of necessities, and over one third of deaths from maltreatment are in this group. Neglect is generally defined as the failure of a parent or other person legally responsible for the child's welfare to provide for the child's basic needs and an adequate level of care (Council on Scientific Affairs, 1985).

Little is known about the etiology of neglect, although it appears that many of the risk factors identified in physical abuse apply to neglect as well (see the following discussion). Ignorance of the child's needs and a lack of resources are important contributing factors. For example, neglectful parents often demonstrate poor parenting skills. They may be unaware that an infant needs to be fed every 3 to 4 hours, may not know what to feed the child, and may have insufficient funds to buy food. The most serious lack of knowledge is failure to recognize emotional nurturing as an essential need of children. (See also Failure to Thrive, Chapter 33.)

Types of Neglect

Neglect takes many forms and can be classified broadly as physical or emotional maltreatment. **Physical neglect** involves the deprivation of necessities such as food, clothing, shelter, supervision, medical care, and education. **Emotional neglect** generally refers to failure to meet the child's needs for affection, attention, and emotional nurturance. It may also include lack of intervention for or fostering of maladaptive behavior such as delinquency or substance abuse. **Emotional abuse,** an even more difficult aspect of maltreatment to define, refers to the deliberate attempt to destroy or significantly impair a child's self-esteem or competence. Emotional abuse may take the following forms: rejecting, isolating, terrorizing, ignoring, or corrupting the child.

PHYSICAL ABUSE

The deliberate infliction of physical injury on a child, usually by the child's caregiver, is termed **physical abuse.** Minor physical injury is responsible for more reported cases of maltreatment than major physical injury, but major physical abuse causes more deaths. Despite the importance of the problem, a universally accepted definition of what constitutes minor and major physical abuse does not exist. Rather, each state in the United States defines abuse according to its individual reporting laws.

Munchausen Syndrome by Proxy

One of the more unusual and perplexing types of abuse, usually physical, is Munchausen syndrome by proxy (MSP), which refers to illness that one person fabricates or induces in another person. In children, it is usually the mother who fabricates signs and symptoms of illness in her child, the proxy, to gain attention from the medical staff. Rarely the father may be the perpetrator (Jones et al, 1993). MSP can take many forms, such as adding maternal blood to the child's urine to simulate hematuria, presenting a fictitious medical history, chronic poisoning of the child, or suffocating the child to cause apnea and seizures. Another form of MSP is alleging that the child has been sexually abused by someone else to gain recognition as the child's protector.

Such cases are often very difficult to confirm and require a high index of suspicion to protect the children. Warning signs of MSP include:

- Unexplained, prolonged, recurrent, or extremely rare illness
- Discrepancies between clinical findings and history
- Illness unresponsive to treatment
- Signs and symptoms occurring only in parent's presence
- Parent knowledgeable about illness, procedures, and treatments
- Parent very interested in interacting with health team members
- Parent very attentive toward child (refuses to leave hospital)
- Family members with similar symptoms

Consequences for children with MSP can be serious. They often undergo needless and painful medical procedures and treatments. The parent's actions may induce a serious illness in children; one that is fatal in almost 10% of the cases (Wilde and Pedroni, 1993). Children may develop chronic invalidism, accepting the illness story and believing themselves to be ill. Finally, they may develop MSP as an adult. Even when some of these children are removed from the home, they continue to suffer severe psychologic trauma. Other siblings remaining in the home may become substitute victims.

---

*Additional information is available from the **Clearinghouse on Child Abuse and Neglect Information,** P.O. Box 1182, Washington, DC 20013-1182; (703) 385-7565 or (800) FYI-3366.

Factors Predisposing to Physical Abuse

The exact cause of child abuse is not known, although three factors—parental characteristics, characteristics of the child, and environmental characteristics—influence the potential for abuse. However, no one factor or group of factors is predictive of abuse. Rather, the interaction of these factors is thought to increase the risk of abuse occurring in a particular family.

Parental characteristics. Extensive research has focused on parental characteristics that distinguish abusive parents from nonabusive parents. Unfortunately the findings from most of these studies provide conflicting evidence. For example, it is commonly believed that abusive parents were abused as children. However, few studies support this relationship. Although physical punishment tends to occur in abusive parents' childhood, most of the parents were not physically abused as children. However, abusive parents who report that they were severely punished as children are much more likely to injure their own children (Kotelchuck, 1982). If the abuse was not overt physical violence, abusive parents typically recall their punishment as unfair and severe, and they characterize their relationship with their parents as negative. Abusive parents tend to have difficulty controlling aggressive impulses, and the free expression of violence is one of the most consistent qualities of these families (Altemeier et al, 1982).

Another finding is that abusive families are often more socially isolated and have fewer supportive relationships than nonabusive parents. Children of teenage mothers are more at risk of abuse than those from older mothers (Stier et al, 1993). With little or no available support system and the presence of concurrent stresses imposed by the child or environment, these parents are extremely vulnerable to additional crises of any nature and literally strike out at the child as a method of releasing their increasing frustration and anxiety.

Other factors identified in abusive parents include low self-esteem and less than adequate maternal functioning. Although inadequate knowledge of childrearing is often cited as a characteristic of abusive parents, research findings do not consistently support this belief. However, this does not mean that these parents cannot benefit from learning more constructive ways of rearing their children, especially nonviolent discipline methods.

Characteristics of the child. The child also unintentionally contributes to the abusive situation. In families of two or more children usually only one child is the victim of abuse. This child's temperament, position in the family, additional physical needs if ill or disabled, activity level, or degree of sensitivity to parental needs all contribute to the potential for physical abuse. For example, one child may not be abused if he or she fits into the "easy-child pattern," whereas another sibling with a difficult temperament may add to the parent's stress sufficiently to precipitate an abusive act. However, temperament alone is not the critical factor; rather, it is the "fit" or compatibility between the child's temperament and the parent's ability to deal with that behavioral style.

Occasionally the abused child is illegitimate, unwanted, brain damaged (especially in situations in which the parents cannot accept the retardation), hyperactive, or physically disabled. Sometimes children are abused because they remind the parent of someone the parent dislikes, such as a younger brother or sister who received all the attention from their own parents. Premature infants may be at risk for maltreatment because of the failure of parent-child bonding during early infancy. Often a difficult pregnancy, labor, or delivery is a predisposing factor in abuse, especially when the infant is born prematurely or with congenital anomalies.

Although one child is usually the victim in an abusive family, removing that child from the home often places the other siblings at risk for abuse. Child maltreatment usually is not confined to one child because of a disturbed parent-child relationship but is a result of a family in distress. Therefore no child is safe if left in the abusive environment unless the parents can be helped to learn new parenting skills and to meet their needs and release their frustration through alternatives other than attacking their children.

Environmental characteristics. The environment is a significant part of the potential abusive situation. Typically the environment is one of chronic stress, including problems of divorce, poverty, unemployment, poor housing, frequent relocation, alcoholism, and drug addiction. Increased exposure between children and parents, such as that which occurs in crowded living conditions, also increases the likelihood of abuse.

Although abuse has been reported mostly from lower socioeconomic populations, child abuse is by no means a problem of any one societal group. It spans all educational, social, and economic levels. Certainly stresses imposed by poverty predispose lower socioeconomic families to abusive situations, and abuse in these groups is more apt to be reported. However, concealed crises can also be present in upper-class families. For example, a wealthy family experiencing major life changes such as rehousing, the birth of an additional child, or marital discord may have sufficient environmental stressors imposed on them to produce a potentially abusive situation. Wealthy families may be so overinvolved with commitments outside the home that abuse may be inflicted by substitute caregivers. Nurses need to be aware of such factors in order to identify the less obvious examples of child abuse and neglect.

SEXUAL ABUSE

Sexual abuse is one of the most devastating types of child maltreatment, and current estimates indicate that it has increased significantly during the past decade. However, the increased rate of reporting may not reflect a true increase in prevalence of sexual abuse, but may be due to changes in legislation and in society's attitudes toward women and children (Feldman et al, 1991). The number of reported occurrences was approximately 14% of all child maltreatment cases in 1993 (*In Fact...*, undated), but many authorities believe that this figure represents only a small percentage of the actual incidence.

As with all forms of child maltreatment, no universal definition for sexual abuse exists. The Child Abuse and Prevention Act (Public Law 100-294) defines **sexual abuse** as "the use, persuasion, or coercion of any child to engage in sexually explicit conduct (or any simulation of such conduct) for producing any visual depiction of such conduct, or rape, molestation, prostitution, or incest with children."

Sexual abuse includes several types of sexual maltreatment, including the following (see also Rape, Chapter 11; Sexual abuse, Chapter 11).

Incest—any physical sexual activity between family members; blood relationship is not required (abusers can include stepparents, nonrelated siblings, grandparents, uncles, and aunts); does not include sexual relations between legally sanctional partners such as spouses

Molestation—a vague term that includes "indecent liberties" such as touching, fondling, kissing, single or mutual masturbation, or oral-genital contact

Exhibitionism—indecent exposure, usually exposure of the genitals by an adult male to children or female adults

Child pornography—arranging and photographing in any media sexual acts involving children, alone or with adults or animals, regardless of consent by the child's legal guardian; also may denote distribution of such material in any form with or without profit

Child prostitution—involving children in sex acts for profit and usually with changing partners

Pedophilia—literally means "love of child" and does not denote a type of sexual activity but the preference of an adult for prepubertal children as the means of achieving sexual excitement

Characteristics of Abusers and Victims

Anyone, including siblings and mothers, can be sexual abusers, but a typical abuser is a male that the victim knows. Offenders come from all levels of society. Some are prominent persons in the community, and some, especially in the case of pedophiliacs (also called "child molesters"), are in positions such as teaching and coaching where they work closely with children.

Pornography and prostitution may involve strangers, as well as the children's own parents. There are no typical characteristics of these offenders, although the abused children tend to be runaways—young adolescents who engage in these activities to obtain money for food, shelter, drugs, and alcohol. Incestuous relationships between father or stepfather and daughter are generally prolonged, and the victims are usually reluctant to report the situation because of fear of retaliation and fear that they will not be believed. Typically incestuous relationships begin later than other forms of child abuse, and the average age of the victim is 9 years (Highlights, 1988). The eldest daughter is usually abused, but in her absence another sister is substituted. Sibling incest may also occur (Gilbert, 1992). Sexual abuse by relatives with a strong emotional bond with the victim is the most devastating to the child.

Boys are also victims of both intrafamilial and extrafamilial abuse. Males are much less likely to report abuse, and they may suffer much greater emotional harm from incestuous relationships, especially between mother and son, than female victims. Boys are likely to be subjected to anal penetration and oral-genital contact, to have subtle physical findings, and to be abused by a father, stepfather, or mother's boyfriend.

Initiation and Perpetuation of Sexual Abuse

The cycle of sexual abuse often starts innocently, unless it involves an isolated attack, such as rape. Often offenders spend time with the victims to gain their trust before initiating any sexual contact. Most victims are then pressured into being an accessory to the sexual activity through various means (Box 35-1) and may be unaware that sexual activity is part of the offer. Children may not reveal the truth for fear that their parents would not believe them if they told—especially if the offender is a trusted member of the family. Some fear they will be blamed for the situation, and many young children with limited vocabulary have difficulty describing the activity when they do have the courage or opportunity to reveal the abuse.

Seductiveness by the child does not initiate incest. Most young girls experiment in seduction, especially during the preschool years, but the father's response normally differentiates this playfulness from overt sexual invitation. Although the reasons for incest are complicated and can occur in various family types, it does not occur in healthy families. Most incestuous relationships are directly tied to sexual maladjustment and estrangement between husband and wife. Most begin following the cessation of sexual relationships with the usual partner. Most fathers experience little guilt, and many wives at some level are aware of the incestuous affair. The wife may react by tolerating the situation or may resort to use of denial; some remain unaware of the activity. Consequently, the home offers little protection to young victims, since abusers have easy access to their victims and the children feel they cannot reveal their secret to other family members. However, not all incestuous relationships follow this pattern of silence. Currently, reports of father-daughter incest during child custody conflicts have become more common and have raised serious concerns regarding the possibility of false accusation. Rather than tolerating or denying the child's sexual abuse, the other parent (usually the mother) is typically the chief accuser. (See the Family Focus box on p. 1042.)

BOX 35-1
Methods Used to Pressure Children Into Sexual Activity

The child is offered gifts or privileges.

The adult misrepresents moral standards by telling the child that it is "okay to do."

Isolated and emotionally and socially impoverished children are enticed by adults who meet their needs for warmth and human contact.

The successful sex offender pressures the victim into secrecy regarding the activity by describing it as a "secret between us" that other people may take away if they find out.

The offender plays on the child's fears, including fear of punishment by the offender, fear of repercussions if the child tells, and fear of abandonment or rejection by the family.

Family Focus

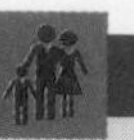

FALSE ALLEGATIONS OF ABUSE

Although most concern among health professionals is to detect child abuse early and to protect the child from further abuse, prevention of abuse must also include prevention of false allegations of abuse. Although some degree of overreporting is expected because the law requires the reporting of suspected maltreatment, the degree of overreporting is considered unreasonably high. Under the present child abuse laws, child protective services have the authority to remove a child from the home solely on the basis of allegations made to an abuse hotline (Radko, 1993).

Despite the fact that more than half of all reports are unfounded, little attention has been directed to the problem of false accusations and its devastating consequences such as removal of the child from the home, termination of parental rights, public ridicule of the family, loss of employment, and excessive legal fees to regain custody of the child. Nurses play a critical role in carefully documenting all evidence of abuse, giving alleged offenders the opportunity to present their account of the incident, and recognizing diseases or cultural practices that may be confused with abuse (Wong, 1987). In the unfortunate event that a family is wrongly accused of abuse, they may benefit from the services of the **National Association of State Victims of Child Abuse Legislation (VOCAL) Organizations,*** a support group for persons who have experienced false accusations. Another organization that may be helpful to family members who have been accused of sexual abuse by their adult children is the **False Memory Syndrome (FMS) Foundation.†** The research and educational institution is dedicated to understanding and preventing allegations of abuse based on "false" memories. In recent years adult children, primarily women, claim to suddenly remember childhood sexual abuse, usually by fathers. The abuse is said to have been repressed for many years, but the memory is recovered with the help of a therapist (Loftus, 1995).

*1030 G. St., Suite 200, Sacramento, CA 95814.
†3508 Market St., Suite 128, Philadelphia, PA 19104, (215) 387-1865.

Nursing Care Management

Assessment

One of the most critical responsibilities of all health professionals is identifying abusive situations as early as possible. The characteristics that may predispose members of some families to commit abuse can serve as a framework for assessing vulnerability but are never predictive of actual abuse.

Nursing ALERT

Nurses must be aware of their biases regarding child abuse. Studies show that nurses are less likely to report abuse when the child is female and from a middle-income, as opposed to lower-income, family (Pillitteri et al, 1992); are significantly less comfortable dealing with sexual abuse, abuse of infants, and fathers as the abusers (Seidl et al, 1993); and have greater discomfort in dealing with abusers of children with disabilities than abusers of children without disabilities (Stanton et al, 1994).

Guidelines

TALKING WITH CHILDREN WHO REVEAL ABUSE

Provide a private time and place to talk.
Do not promise not to tell; tell them that you are required by law to report the abuse.
Do not express shock or criticize their family.
Use their vocabulary to discuss body parts.
Avoid using any leading statements that can distort their report.
Reassure them that they have done the right thing by telling.
Tell them that the abuse is not their fault, that they are not bad or to blame.
Determine their immediate need for safety.
Let the child know what will happen when you report.

Rather, a thorough physical examination and a careful, detailed history are the diagnostic tools needed to identify abuse. Nurses have a very special role because they may be the first person to see the child and parent and are the consistent caregivers if the child is hospitalized (see the Guidelines box above).

Evidence of maltreatment. Recognition of abuse or neglect necessitates a familiarity with both physical and behavioral signs that suggest maltreatment (Box 35-2). No one indicator can diagnose maltreatment; rather it is a pattern or combination of indicators that should arouse suspicion and further investigation. In addition, signs of possible abuse must be coupled with an understanding of diseases such as bleeding disorders, osteogenesis imperfecta, or sudden infant death syndrome and cultural practices such as cupping or coin rubbing (see Health Practices, Chapter 28) that may mimic physical abuse. Unintentional injuries may also be wrongly diagnosed as abuse, such as burns from metal buckles on car seats, lacerations from seat belts, or retinal hemorrhage after cardiopulmonary resuscitation. Normal variants such as mongolian spots and congenital anomalies of genitalia can be mistaken for abuse.

Not all forms of physical abuse demonstrate obvious signs. Violent shaking of children (*shaken baby syndrome [SBS]*) can cause fatal intracranial trauma without signs of external head injury (American Academy of Pediatrics, 1993a). Nurses should suspect SBS in infants less than 1 year of age who present with subdural and/or retinal hemorrhages in the absence of external signs of trauma (Chiocca, 1995).

Nursing ALERT

Stress to parents and other caregivers the dangers of shaking infants (can cause shaken baby syndrome [SBS]). Advise against shaking as a method of burping or waking infant, tossing infant in air, and shaking infant when feeling angry or tense.

If MSP is suspected, nurses play an important role in monitoring the parent's activities to identify instances of causing the children's symptoms. Using a hidden video camera to document the parent's behavior is becoming a more common diagnostic procedure, but the parent's right of privacy must be considered (Wilde and Pedroni, 1993).

BOX 35-2
Clinical Manifestations of Potential Child Maltreatment

Physical neglect

Suggestive physical findings

Failure to thrive
Signs of malnutrition, such as thin extremities, abdominal distention, lack of subcutaneous fat
Poor personal hygiene, especially of teeth
Unclean and/or inappropriate dress
Evidence of poor health care, such as nonimmunized status, untreated infections, frequent colds
Frequent injuries from lack of supervision

Suggestive behaviors

Dull and inactive; excessively passive or sleepy
Self-stimulatory behaviors, such as finger-sucking or rocking
Begging or stealing food (in older child)
Absenteeism from school (in older child)
Drug or alcohol addiction (in older child)
Vandalism or shoplifting (in older child)

Emotional Abuse and Neglect

Suggestive physical findings

Failure to thrive
Feeding disorders, such as rumination
Enuresis
Sleep disorders

Suggestive behaviors

Self-stimulatory behaviors, such as biting, rocking, sucking
During infancy, lack of social smile and stranger anxiety
Withdrawal
Unusual fearfulness
Antisocial behavior such as destructiveness, stealing, cruelty
Extremes of behavior such as overcompliant and passive or aggressive and demanding
Lags in emotional and intellectual development, especially language
Suicide attempts

Physical abuse

Suggestive physical findings

Bruises and welts
- On face, lips, mouth, back, buttocks, thighs, or areas of torso
- Regular patterns descriptive of object used such as belt buckle, hand, wire hanger, chain, wooden spoon, squeeze or pinch marks
- May be present in various stages of healing

Burns
- On soles of feet, palms of hands, back, or buttocks
- Patterns descriptive of object used such as round cigar or cigarette burns; "glovelike," sharply demarcated areas from immersion in scalding water; rope burns on wrists or ankles from being bound; burns in the shape of an iron, radiator, or electric stove burner
- Absence of "splash" marks and presence of symmetric burns
- Stun gun injury—lesions circular, fairly uniform (up to 0.5 cm), and paired about 5 cm apart (Frechette and Rimsza, 1992).

Fractures and dislocations
Skull, nose, or facial structures
- Injury may denote type of abuse, such as spiral fracture or dislocation from twisting of an extremity or whiplash from shaking the child
- Multiple new or old fractures in various stages of healing

Lacerations and abrasions
- On backs of arms, legs, torso, face, or external genitalia
- Unusual symptoms such as abdominal swelling, pain, and vomiting from punching
- Descriptive marks such as from human bites or pulling the hair out

Chemical
- Unexplained repeated poisoning, especially drug overdose
- Unexplained sudden illness, such as hypoglycemia from insulin administration

Suggestive behaviors

Wariness of physical contact with adults
Apparent fear of parents or going home
Lying very still while surveying environment
Inappropriate reaction to injury, such as failure to cry from pain
Lack of reaction to frightening events
Apprehension when hearing other children cry
Indiscriminate friendliness and displays of affection
Superficial relationships
Acting-out behavior such as aggression to seek attention
Withdrawal behavior

Sexual abuse

Suggestive physical findings

Bruises, bleeding, lacerations or irritation of external genitalia, anus, mouth, or throat
Torn, stained, or bloody underclothing
Pain on urination or pain, swelling, and itching of genital area
Penile discharge
Sexually transmitted disease, nonspecific vaginitis, or venereal warts
Difficulty in walking or sitting
Unusual odor in the genital area
Recurrent urinary tract infections
Presence of sperm
Pregnancy in young adolescent

Suggestive behaviors

Sudden emergence of sexually related problems, including excessive or public masturbation, age-inappropriate sexual play, promiscuity, or overtly seductive behavior
Withdrawn, excessive daydreaming
Preoccupied with fantasies, especially in play
Poor relationships with peers
Sudden changes such as anxiety, loss or gain of weight, clinging behavior
In incestuous relationships, excessive anger at mother for not protecting daughter
Regressive behavior such as bed-wetting or thumb-sucking
Sudden onset of phobias or fears, particularly fears of the dark, men, strangers, or particular settings or situations (e.g., undue fear of leaving the house or staying at the day care center or the baby-sitter's house)
Running away from home
Substance abuse, particularly of alcohol or mood-elevating drugs
Profound and rapid personality changes, especially extreme depression, hostility, and aggression (often accompanied by social withdrawal)
Rapidly declining school performance
Suicidal attempts or ideation

Neglect and emotional abuse. Neglect from deprivation of necessities is easier to identify than emotional neglect or abuse because physical signs are usually evident. Although emotional maltreatment may be readily suspected, it is very difficult to substantiate. Physical signs are often nonspecific, and nurses must rely on behavioral indicators, which range from depression to acting-out behavior, to help identify a possibly abusive situation. Any persistent and unexplained change in the child's behavior is an important clue to possible emotional abuse.

Sexual abuse. Identifying instances of sexual abuse is particularly difficult because frequently few if any obvious physical indications of the activity may exist. Also, many individuals are hesitant to believe children and unwilling to report incidents. Even health professionals are sometimes at fault when they perform cursory physical examinations of the genitalia and ignore behavior or verbal comments that suggest abuse. When sexual abuse is suspected, other children in the family should also be evaluated, since multiple victims are not uncommon.

Unfortunately there is no typical profile of the victim, and there must be a high index of suspicion to identify these children. Physical signs vary and may include any of those listed for sexual abuse in Box 35-2. The victim may exhibit various behavioral manifestations. Unfortunately none of these behaviors is diagnostic of sexual abuse. When abused children exhibit these behaviors, the signs may be incorrectly attributed to the normal stresses of childhood, especially in older school-age children or adolescents. Even signs considered most predictive of sexual abuse such as certain genital findings, sexually inappropriate behavior for age, enactment of adult sexual activity, and intense focus on sexual activity (e.g., masturbation) do not always indicate that sexual abuse has occurred. For example, many genital findings that have been reported as conclusive or highly suspect for sexual abuse, such as vaginal opening >4 mm, hymenal tears, reflex anal dilation, and condylomata acuminata (anogenital or venereal warts) may be found in unabused prepubertal children (Wong, 1991). Also, abused children may not demonstrate more knowledge of sexual activity than nonabused children. However, one difference in the abused children's explanation of sexual activity may be unusual affective responses. For example, abused children may relate stories that include fear of going to sleep or of being with a parent (Gordon, Schroeder, and Abrams, 1990).

History pertaining to the incident. In addition to observable evidence of abuse, the type of history revealed by the parents or other caregiver such as the baby-sitter or mother's boyfriend, is a significant factor. Areas of the history that should arouse suspicion of abuse are summarized in Box 35-3.

Nursing ALERT

Incompatibility between the history and the injury is probably the most important criterion on which to base the decision to report suspected abuse.

BOX 35-3

Warning Signs of Abuse

Physical evidence of abuse and/or neglect, including previous injuries
Conflicting stories about the "accident" or injury from the parents or others
Cause of injury blamed on sibling or other party
An injury inconsistent with the history, such as a concussion and broken arm from falling off a bed
History inconsistent with child's developmental level, such as a 6-month-old turning on the hot water
A complaint other than the one associated with signs of abuse (e.g., a chief complaint of a cold when there is evidence of first- and second-degree burns)
Inappropriate response of caregiver, such as an exaggerated or absent emotional response; refusal to sign for additional tests or agree to necessary treatment; excessive delay in seeking treatment; absence of the parents for questioning
Inappropriate response of child, such as little or no response to pain; fear of being touched; excessive or lack of separation anxiety; indiscriminate friendliness to strangers
Child's report of physical or sexual abuse
Previous reports of abuse in the family
Repeated visits to emergency facilities with injuries

An important point to remember when taking a history is that maltreated children rarely betray their parents by admitting to the abuse they received. If questioned, they will repeat the same story as the parents and try to defend their parents' actions. If the interviewer directly accuses the parents of abuse, the child may accept responsibility for the act in an attempt to vindicate the parents from the accusation. Whether children respond in this way out of fear is uncertain. However, children do fear losing whatever security and love they have. Between abusive acts children may receive some measure of attention and love from the parents. If they betray the parents, they may lose this and be uncertain or fearful of the consequences such as foster care. Preserving the present situation may be less frightening than the unknown future.

The *disclosure of sexual abuse* can occur in a variety of ways—the act is observed by others, resulting in a direct confrontation; the child tells someone such as a parent of a friend; visible clues of the relationship are observed, such as an accumulation of coins, gifts, or candy; or more obvious clues are seen, such as a child coming home disheveled or becoming pregnant; and physical or behavioral signs and symptoms are observed. Children usually describe the experience in terms of whether it was unpleasant, painful, or pleasurable (usually a response to hand-genital contact); some indicate no reaction. Young children often feel no guilt or shame because the act is pleasurable and they are unaware of its inappropriateness.

Nursing ALERT

When children report potentially sexually abusive experiences, their reports need to be taken seriously, but also cautiously to avoid alarming the child or falsely accusing a person.

Children's reports of sexual abuse may vary from contradictory stories to unwavering versions of the experience. Although their stories may sound contradictory, this may reflect the child's experiences in several instances of abuse. Also, children who repeatedly tell identical facts may have been prompted to do so. Increasing evidence suggests that the types of interrogation children are exposed to after they report sexual abuse shape their thinking. Through the use of leading questions, closed questions (those requiring yes or no answers), intimidation, prodding, and selective reinforcement for certain answers, children begin to tell stories that never occurred. Eventually they may come to experience the tale as reality (Wakefield and Underwager, 1989).

Parental behaviors. Certain behavioral responses of the parents to their child and to the interviewer should alert the nurse to the possibility of maltreatment. Although no one pattern of behaviors is characteristic of these parents, some responses follow. Abusive parents have difficulty in showing concern toward their child. They are unable to comfort the child and give no indication of realizing how the child may feel, physically or emotionally. Instead they are critical of and angry with the child for being injured. They maintain that the child is responsible for the injury, and, if asked any question regarding their responsibility to protect or supervise the child, they become hostile and aggressive. They act as if the child's injury is an assault on them. Their entire perception of the incident is in terms of how it affects them, not the child, which is an indication of their preoccupation with their own needs and of their inability to give support to others.

During the child's hospitalization they may not become involved in the child's care and may show little concern for his or her progress, eventual discharge, or need for follow-up care. However, if they are pressured during interrogation, they immediately demand to take the child home, regardless of the child's readiness for discharge.

Families respond to sexual abuse with a wide variety of emotional reactions, which range from not believing the child to being very supportive. Parents and other family members may display the same type of emotional responses as the victim such as inability to eat or sleep and somatic complaints such as headache. In the acute emotional phase parents need to blame someone. The three common targets are the offender, the child, and themselves. The parents commonly express anger at the child for "stupid" behavior and may even restrict the child's privileges as punishment. When the victim is a girl, the parents may question her sexual provocation of the event. Self-blaming parents assume full responsibility, believing that they have been inadequate parents or should not have allowed the child to go out. When a baby-sitter or trusted relative is involved in the assault and the child's complaint has not been believed until gross evidence is presented, the parents are often devastated by guilt.

Child behaviors. Abused children's responses to their parents or the injury may also support the suspicion of abuse. Although no one pattern is typical, extremes of behavior may be observed. Children may be very unresponsive to the parent or excessively clinging and intolerant of separation. There may be overattachment to the abusive parent, possibly in the hope of preventing any upset that may precipitate anger and another attack. During care of the injury children may be passive and accepting of the discomfort or uncooperative and fearful of any physical contact. Some children maintain a wary watchfulness of all strangers; some shy away from strangers as if frightened; others are unusually affectionate and outgoing.

Nursing Diagnoses

A number of nursing diagnoses are prominent in the nursing care of the maltreated child and family, and others specific to individual cases become evident. The most common nursing diagnoses are outlined in the Nursing Care Plan on p. 1048.

Planning

The main nursing goals related to child maltreatment are as follows:

1. The child will be protected from further abuse.
2. The child and family will receive adequate support.
3. The hospitalized child and family, including foster parents if appropriate, will be prepared for discharge.
4. The child will not experience any maltreatment.

Implementation

Protect child from further abuse. Initially identification of instances of suspected abuse or neglect is essential. The nurse may come in contact with abused children in an emergency room, practitioner's office, home, day care center, or school.

Nursing ALERT

The priority is to remove the child from the abusive situation to prevent further injury.

All states and provinces in North America have laws for mandatory reporting of child maltreatment. Suspected child abuse is reported to the local authorities.* Referrals usually come to the Bureau of Child Welfare and are assigned to a caseworker in an agency such as the Child Protective Services (CPS). Once a referral has been made, a caseworker is assigned to investigate the report. Based on the findings, the child is left in the home or temporarily removed.

A court proceeding may be necessary before the child can be placed outside the home or when parental rights are to be terminated. When the courts are involved, they usually require firsthand testimony by the referring parties. Nurses may be subpoenaed to appear in court, or their notes may be introduced as evidence in court hearings. Accurate and factual documentation is essential. A suggested outline for recording pertinent assessment data is presented in the Guidelines box on p. 1046. Behaviors are described, not interpreted, and are recorded daily to establish a progress record. Conversations

*Telephone numbers are usually listed under "Child Abuse" in the business white pages of the local directory, or call the emergency child abuse hotline: (800) 422-4453 ([800] 4-A-CHILD).

Guidelines

RECORDING ASSESSMENT DATA IN SUSPECTED ABUSE

History of Injury

1. Date, time, and place of occurrence
2. Sequence of events with recorded times
3. Presence of witnesses, especially person caring for child at time of incident
4. Time lapse between occurrence of injury and initiation of treatment
5. Interview with child when appropriate, including verbal quotations and information from drawing or other play activities
6. Interview with parent, witnesses, or other significant persons, including verbal quotations
7. Description of parent-child interactions (verbal interactions, eye contact, touching, parental concern)
8. Name, age, and condition of other children in home (if possible)

Physical Examination

1. Location, size, shape, and color of bruises; approximate location, size, and shape on drawing of body outline
2. Distinguishing characteristics such as a bruise in the shape of a hand; round burn (possibly caused by cigarette)
3. Symmetry or asymmetry of injury; presence of other injuries.
4. Degree of pain; any bone tenderness
5. Evidence of past injuries; general state of health and hygiene
6. Developmental level of child; perform screening test (see Developmental Assessment, Chapter 32)

between the nurse, child, and parent are recorded verbatim as much as possible.

Support child. Frequently children suspected of abuse are hospitalized for medical management of their injuries. When the sexually abused child has been physically harmed, the care is consistent with that provided a rape victim (see Chapter 11). Regardless of the type of abuse, their needs are the same as those of any hospitalized child. The child should be treated as a child with the usual physical needs, developmental tasks, and play interests—not as a dramatic victim of abuse. The nurse is the child's advocate in this goal. The nurse also encourages the child's relationship with the parents. *The nurse does not become a substitute parent to the exclusion of the child's natural parents.* Such an intent only intensifies the parents' feelings of inadequacy, worthlessness, and isolation. It in no way helps them understand their child or promotes their trust in health professionals. The goal of the *consistent* nurse-child relationship is to provide a role model for the parents in helping them to relate positively and constructively to their child and to foster a therapeutic environment for the child in his or her reprieve from the abusing situation.

Sexual abuse. The type of care needed by the child depends on the circumstances of the sexual abuse. It varies from reassurance and support when the act involves exhibitionism to long-term counseling in incestuous situations. In *interviewing* these children, nurses must be very careful to avoid biasing the child's retelling of the events. Some experts suggest that health professionals limit the interview to the child's physical and mental health concerns and leave the topics of the family's social, legal, or other problems to the police or CPS personnel (Koop, 1988).

In preparation for an interview, every effort is made to make the child feel comfortable with appropriate introductions and to avoid duplicating the behaviors typically used by offenders, such as touching the child without permission. The interview is conducted in a quiet and private location, preferably a neutral place such as a school playroom or office, and not where the abuse occurred. Neutral questions are asked first, such as the child's reaction to the hospital (if appropriate). Then the incident is discussed in general terms. The interview should include such nonleading questions as, "Do you know why you were brought to the hospital?" "Do you know what will happen here?" or "How do you feel about being here?" Later the question, "Can you tell me what happened?" and other questions may elicit an account of the incident. Sometimes the parents are able to help the child describe the incident, and questions can then be directed to the circumstances of the assault. Questions should progress chronologically and proceed from the nonsexual to the more sexual content. If the child shows evidence of becoming too upset, the focus is redirected toward more neutral and less emotionally laden areas.

Children are given the opportunity to ask questions, but if they are hesitant, they are never pressured into talking. Young children in particular lack the verbal skills to describe body parts adequately. These children may benefit from play situations that provide opportunities for disclosure such as drawing or playing with puppets or anatomically correct dolls or with dollhouses.

Considerable controversy exists regarding the use of children's *drawings* and *anatomically correct dolls* as *diagnostic* tests for sexual abuse. The presence of genitalia on a human figure drawing or sexual play with the dolls does not prove sexual abuse; the children's description and explanation of the drawing or play are more relevant than the content. Genitalia on drawings and sexual doll play may raise suspicion of abuse but are not diagnostic (Wakefield and Underwager, 1989).

Support family. One of the most difficult, yet essential, components of success with abusive parents is the quality of the *therapeutic relationship.* It must be one of genuine concern and treatment, not one of accusation and punishment. Nurses must examine their personal feelings toward these parents, particularly when sexual abuse is present. A therapeutic approach is to view the parent as the patient and the child as the victim of abuse. Unless the nurse's attitude is positive, abusive parents will not be motivated to change, since they will not be working with a trusting person who demonstrates the kind of behavior that is being asked of them.

When parental ignorance of childrearing practices has played a part in the abuse, the nurse can educate the parent regarding *children's physical and emotional needs.* Because of the parents' own childrearing, they may not be aware of nonviolent methods of discipline such as time-out or consequences. They may also need help in dealing with their frustration so that they do not vent anger on the child. Since these parents may be sensitive to criticism or domination and already possess a very low self-esteem, teaching is implemented through demonstration and example rather than through lecturing. Any *competent parenting abilities* they demonstrate are praised to promote their sense of parental adequacy.

Sexual abuse. Care of the family also depends on the circumstances of the sexual abuse. With a nonparent offender the family may be more able to support the child than if incest were involved. Family members are encouraged to express their feelings of anger, guilt, shame, and/or embarrassment but are also cautioned to avoid displacing such feelings on the child. For example, it is easy for parents to admonish the child with a statement such as, "We told you never to go with strangers," which makes the child feel responsible.

Family members are advised to encourage the child to resume normal activities and to observe the child for signs of distress (see Posttraumatic Stress Disorder, Chapter 36). Children express their feelings primarily through behavior. Parents should be alert for changes in behavior that indicate distress resulting from the incident, such as remaining in the house, refusing to go to school, changes in sleeping patterns, and frequency of dreams and nightmares. Children are encouraged to talk about these feelings and nightmares, since the more they can talk about the experience, the more they are able to gain control over it.

Referral. Referral to appropriate agencies is also essential. Most abusive parents tend to live in poverty, and the daily stresses imposed by their life-style are overwhelming. Resources for financial aid, improved housing, and child care should be sought. Self-help groups also provide important services. Such groups as Parents Anonymous* (a group for parents who have abused or fear that they may abuse their child, but only in terms of physical abuse, not sexual abuse) and Parents United International, Inc.† (a group devoted to helping sexually abused families) are very accepting and nonjudgmental, because everyone has been in the same position.

There is no way to predict which families will be successfully rehabilitated. With father-daughter incest, however, the best results occur when the father accepts full responsibility for the act, the mother acknowledges her role in failing to protect the child, and the child is able to understand and forgive the parents and develop a positive self-image despite the traumatic experience.

Plan for discharge. Discharge planning should begin as soon as the legal disposition for placement has been decided, which may be temporary foster home placement, return to the parents, or permanent termination of parental rights. The latter is the most drastic solution, but it is necessary in situations of repeated, life-threatening abuse. Whenever children are sent to a foster home or juvenile institution, they must be allowed an opportunity to express their feelings. No matter how severe the abuse, they usually mourn the loss of their parents. They need help to understand why they must not return home and that this new home is in no way a punishment. Whenever possible, foster parents are encouraged to visit in the hospital, and the nurse should take an active role in helping them understand the child. It is unfortunate that some abused children live in torment as they are sent from one foster home to another, sometimes enduring worse circumstances than those that existed in their original home. Only through constant evaluation of the placement residence and the child's adjustment to a new environment can the vicious circle of abuse, abandonment, and neglect be stopped.

Prevent abuse. Prevention of child maltreatment has been an extremely difficult goal. Programs aimed at identifying potential abusers and instituting supportive intervention before the occurrence of an abusive act have met with variable success. However, nurses have played an important role in such

*520 S. Lafayette, Park Plaza, Suite 316, Los Angeles, CA 90057.
†P.O. Box 952, San Jose, CA 95108; (408) 453-7616.

Home Care

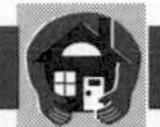

PREVENTING OR DEALING WITH SEXUAL ABUSE OF CHILDREN

Sexual assault of children is much more common than most people realize. It may be preventable if children are prepared properly. *To provide protection and preparation:*
- Pay careful attention to who is around children. (Unwanted touch *may* come from someone liked and trusted.)
- Back up a child's right to say "no."
- Encourage communication by taking seriously what children *say.*
- Take a second look at signals of potential danger.
- Refuse to leave children in the company of those not trusted.
- Include information about sexual assault when teaching about safety.
- Provide specific definitions and examples of sexual assault.
- Remind children that even "nice" people sometimes do mean things.
- Urge children to tell about *anybody* who causes them to be uncomfortable.
- Prepare children to deal with bribes and threats, as well as possible physical force.
- Virtually eliminate secrets between children and parents.
- Teach children how to say "no," ask for help, and control who touches them and how.
- Model self-protective and limit-setting behavior for children.

Should it ever become necessary to *help a child recover from a sexual assault:*
- Listen carefully to understand children.
- Support the child for telling by praise, belief, sympathy, and lack of blame.
- Know local resources and choose help carefully.
- Provide opportunities to talk about the assault.
- Provide opportunities for the entire family to go through a recovery process.

Sexual assault affects everyone. *To help deal with this social problem:*
- Provide sympathetic care and support to those who have been victimized.
- Recognize that offenders do not change without intervention.
- Organize neighborhood programs to support each other's efforts to protect children.
- Encourage schools to provide information about sexual assault as a problem of health and safety.
- Organize community groups to support educational treatment and law enforcement programs.

Modified from Adams C, Fay J: *No more secrets: protecting your child from sexual assault,* San Luis Obispo, Calif, 1981, Impact.

programs. For example, prenatal and infancy home visiting by nurses to primiparas who were either teenagers, unmarried, or of low socioeconomic status resulted in significantly fewer reports of child abuse during the first 2 years (Olds et al, 1986). The nurses provided information on normal child growth and development and routine health care needs, served as informal support persons, and referred families to appropriate services when a need for assistance was identified.

Such programs provide models that can be used to reduce factors known to increase the risk of abuse. However, nurses in a variety of settings can implement similar activities. Nurses in prenatal clinics can prepare expectant families for the adjustment of parenthood. Nursery and postpartum nurses can foster the attachment process by encouraging parents to hold and look at their infant. In neonatal intensive care units nurses can minimize the effects of separation by encouraging parents to visit, and they can help them become comfortable in the child's care. Those in ambulatory settings can teach parents appropriate methods of bathing, feeding, toileting, disciplining, and preventing injuries, while stressing the normal needs and developmental characteristics of children. Nurses need to be sensitive to the parents' needs for attention, reassurance, and reinforcement. Nurses need to know what kinds of community services are available, including self-help groups, and make timely referrals.

Sexual abuse. Unlike preventive efforts for neglect and physical abuse, which have been aimed at the potential offender, *prevention of child sexual abuse* has centered on education of children to protect themselves. Currently there is much controversy regarding the effectiveness of these pro-

Nursing Care Plan

CHILD WHO IS MALTREATED

Nursing Diagnosis: Risk for trauma related to characteristics of environment, child, caregiver(s)

Expected Outcome: **Patient will exhibit no evidence of further injury or neglect.**

• **NURSING INTERVENTIONS/*RATIONALES***

Identify children at risk for potential abuse *to initiate preventive measures.*

Identify signs of maltreatment and implement measures *to prevent further maltreatment* (i.e., report suspicions to appropriate authorities; assist in removing child from unsafe environment and establishing in a safe environment; institute strict supervision if child is hospitalized).

Keep factual records (i.e., child's physical condition, behavioral responses; family responses; description of environment) *for documentation of maltreatment.*

Help child to recognize situations that place them at risk for sexual abuse and teach assertive responses *to discourage abuse.*

Refer family to appropriate social agencies for assistance with finances, food, shelter, clothing, health care *to help prevent neglect.*

Participate in multidisciplinary team efforts *to assess for continued abuse or neglect and make decisions about removal from and return to the environment.*

Nursing Diagnosis: Fear/anxiety related to repeated maltreatment, powerlessness, potential loss of parents

Expected Outcome: **Patient will exhibit decreasing evidence of distress.**

• **NURSING INTERVENTIONS/*RATIONALES***

Provide consistent caregivers and therapeutic environment during hospitalization *to build trust and relieve stress.*

Provide support to child (i.e., treat child as someone with the usual age-appropriate physical, developmental, and social needs; avoid interrogation; ask permission to touch child; show attention to praise child's abilities and appropriate behaviors; give child opportunity to talk and ask questions without pressure to do so; use play to promote self expression) *to decrease anxieties and increase confidence.*

Nursing Diagnosis: Altered parenting related to child, caregiver, or situational characteristics that precipitate abusive behavior

Expected Outcome: **Patient will exhibit evidence of changing parenting behaviors.**

• **NURSING INTERVENTIONS/*RATIONALES***

Provide support to family (i.e., interactions with parents that reflect care and concern rather than accusation and punishment; encourage parent-child relationship; do not usurp parental role; rather provide a role model for constructive interaction with the child) *to establish trust and provide motivation for change.*

Assess parent-childrearing beliefs and practices *to establish baseline for teaching.*

Teach realistic expectations of child behavior and capabilities, emphasizing alternative methods of discipline such as reward, time out *to give parents alternatives to verbal or physical abusive behavior.*

Identify appropriate developmental issues (i.e., toilet training, toddler negativism, independence seeking) that may trigger abuse and help parents work out specific methods for management of the issue *to provide concrete approaches to timely issues.*

Use demonstration, role-modeling approaches rather than lecture or authoritarian approach *to overcome lack of self-esteem and sensitivity to criticism and establish trust.*

Praise competent parenting behaviors *to increase confidence in parenting abilities.*

Refer parent(s) to appropriate sources for classes on how to parent; counseling to explore abuse patterns; support groups *to decrease chances of repeat abuse.*

grams. The main issue is whether young children should be expected to participate in their own protection. Some experts suggest that in the struggle between sexual offender and potential child victim, most factors favor the adult, who has superior knowledge, strength, and skill to overcome most children's efforts at self-protection (Conte, Wolf, and Smith, 1989). Clearly sexual abuse prevention is more than teaching children to say "no" or to recognize their right not to be touched in "private places." It is equally important to teach children safety in terms of potential risk situations. Several suggestions for parents regarding protecting and educating children against possible molestation are presented in the Home Care box on p. 1047.

The nurse is frequently in a position to discuss this topic with parents as part of health maintenance and to provide guidelines. Books are available for parents that describe sexual abuse and its prevention.* Helpful games such as "What if the baby-sitter wants to wrestle and hug but tells you to keep it a secret?" can be used to explore dangerous situations in advance and help children learn the importance of saying "no." They need reassurance that no matter what the other person says or does, the parents want to know about it and will not punish them. Even if children do participate in the activity before telling the parents, they must be reassured that it was not their fault.

*Sources of information are the **National Committee for Prevention of Child Abuse,** Publishing Department, 332 S. Michigan Ave., Suite 1600, Chicago, IL 60604-4357, (312) 663-3520; **C. Henry Kempe National Center for the Prevention and Treatment of Child Abuse and Neglect,** 1205 Oneida St., Denver, CO 80220, (303) 321-3963; **American Association for Protecting Children, American Humane Association,** 63 Inverness Dr. E., Englewood, CO 80112, (800) 227-4645 (outside Colorado) or (303) 792-9900; and **National Resource Center on Child Sexual Abuse,** 107 Lincoln St., Huntsville, AL 35801, (800) 543-7006.

In addition, parents need to be made aware that "nice" people, including friends and relatives, can be offenders; parents should carefully observe how others act toward the child. A sudden change in the child's behavior and a response such as "I don't like Uncle anymore" are clues to investigate the relationship. In the event of any doubt, further solitary encounters with this person and the child should be prevented. It is sometimes to the child's great misfortune that parents do not take certain comments seriously, such as "He hugs me too tight" or "I don't want to go with him." Casual parental statements such as "He just loves you" or "You do whatever adults tell you to do" can place children in jeopardy. Health professionals can alert parents to such dangers and guide them toward an appreciation of the problem, providing concrete guidelines toward child education and protection.

Evaluation

The effectiveness of nursing interventions is determined by continual reassessment and evaluation of care based on the following observational guidelines and expected outcomes:

1. Observe child for additional physical and behavioral evidence of abuse; observe child's reactions to health professionals; if child is hospitalized, check staffing patterns for schedule of consistent group of nurses caring for child.
2. Interview parents regarding their knowledge of children's physical and development needs.
3. Interview child regarding feelings about returning home or placement outside the home.
4. Investigate community programs aimed at preventing child maltreatment.

Expected outcomes:
See the Nursing Care Plan on p. 1048.

Key Points

- The preschool years comprise the period from 3 to 5 years of age, a time that is considered critical for emotional and psychologic development.
- Biologic development in the preschool period is characterized by mature body systems and refinement in gross and fine motor behavior, as evidenced by participation in activities such as running, riding a bicycle, and drawing.
- According to Erikson, acquiring a sense of initiative is the chief psychosocial task of the preschooler. Development of the superego occurs during this period, and conscience begins to emerge.
- According to Piaget, the preschool age is characterized by intuitive or prelogical thinking and a move toward logical thought processes through advanced, complex learning; language; and understanding of causality.
- The seeds of moral development are planted during the preschool period. According to Kohlberg, children are in the stage of naive instrumental orientation, in which they are concerned with satisfying their own needs and, less frequently, the needs of others.
- Social development includes further individuation-separation; more sophisticated language; greater independence; and more complex, imaginative forms of play.
- Areas of special concern to parents during the preschool period are preschool and kindergarten experience, sex education, fears, and speech problems.
- In selecting a school, parents should inquire about daily programs, teacher qualifications, accreditation, student/staff ratio, safety, meals, fees, and health practices.
- Two rules that govern answering questions about sex and other sensitive issues are to find out what the child thinks and to be honest.
- Fears constitute a great part of the preschool period; objects, potential annihilation, and parent-induced fears are common sources.
- Hesitancy or nonfluency in speech patterns is a normal characteristic of language development. Speech problems can occur when parents express excessive concern over this pattern.

- Health promotion continues to be directed toward proper nutrition, adequate sleep, proper dental care, and injury prevention.
- Although the incidence of childhood communicable diseases has declined because of immunizations, these diseases do occur and can cause serious complications.
- Nursing goals in the treatment of a communicable disease are identification, prevention of transmission, provision of comfort, and prevention of complications.
- Child maltreatment may take the form of physical abuse or neglect, emotional abuse or neglect, or sexual abuse.
- Parental, child, and environmental characteristics are criteria that may predispose children to maltreatment.
- Identification of abuse entails securing evidence of maltreatment, taking a history pertaining to the incident, and assessing parental and child behaviors.
- The reported incidence of sexual abuse has increased in the last decade; common forms are incest, molestation, rape, exhibitionism, child pornography, child prostitution, and pedophilia.

References

Altemeier WA III et al: Antecedents of child abuse, *J Pediatr* 100(5):823-829, 1982.

American Academy of Pediatrics, Committee on Sports Medicine and Fitness: Fitness, activity, and sports participation in the preschool child, *Pediatrics* 90(6):1002-1004, 1992.

American Academy of Pediatrics, Committee on Child Abuse and Neglect: Shaken baby syndrome—inflicted cerebral trauma, *Pediatrics* 92(2):872-873, 1993a.

American Academy of Pediatrics, Committee on Infectious Diseases: Vitamin A treatment of measles, *Pediatrics* 91(5):1014-1015, 1993b.

Anliker JA et al: Children's food preferences and genetic sensitivity to the bitter taste of 6-*n*-propylthiouracil (PROP), *Am J Clin Nutr* 54(2):316-320, 1991.

Atkinson E et al: Sleep disruption in young children, *Child Care, Health Dev* 21(4):233-246, 1995.

Birch LL et al: The variability of young children's energy intake, *N Engl J Med* 324(4):232-235, 1991.

Brazelton TB: *Touchpoints,* Reading, Mass, 1992, Addison-Wesley.

Chiocca EM: Shaken baby syndrome; a nursing perspective, *Pediatr Nurs* 21(1):33-38, 1995.

Clutter L: Fostering spiritual care for the child and family. In Smith D et al, editors: *Comprehensive child and family nursing skills,* St Louis, 1991, Mosby.

Conte J, Wolf S, Smith T: What sexual offenders tell us about prevention strategies, *Child Abuse Negl* 13:293-301, 1989.

Council on Scientific Affairs: AMA diagnostic and treatment guidelines concerning child abuse and neglect, *JAMA* 254(6):796-800, 1985.

Doran T et al: Acetaminophen: more harm than good for chickenpox? *J Pediatr* 114(6):1045-1048, 1989.

Dunkle LM et al: A controlled trial of acyclovir for chickenpox in normal children, *N Engl J Med* (325):1539-1544, 1991.

Feldman W et al: Is childhood sexual abuse really increasing in prevalence? An analysis of the evidence, *Pediatrics* 88(1):29-33, 1991.

Food and Nutrition Board, National Research Council: *Recommended dietary allowances,* ed 10, Washington, DC, 1989, National Academy Press.

Frechette A, Rimsza ME: Stun gun injury: a new presentation of the battered child syndrome, *Pediatrics* 89(5):898-901, 1992.

Gilbert CM: Sibling incest: a descriptive study of family dynamics, *J Child Adolesc Psychiatr Ment Health Nurs* 5(1):5-9, 1992.

Glasziou PP, Mackerras DEM: Vitamin A supplementation in infectious diseases: a meta-analysis, *Br Med J* 306(6874):366-370, 1993.

Gordon B, Schroeder C, Abrams M: Children's knowledge of sexuality: a comparison of sexually abused and nonabused children, *Am J Orthopsychiatry* 60(2):250-257, 1990.

Highlights of official child neglect and abuse reporting 1986, Denver, 1988, The American Humane Association.

In Fact...answers to frequently asked questions on child abuse and neglect, Washington, DC, undated, National Clearinghouse on Child Abuse and Neglect Information.

Jones VF et al: The role of the male caretaker in Munchausen syndrome by proxy, *Clin Pediatr* 32:245-247, 1993.

Kondo K et al: Association of human herpesvirus-b infection of the central nervous system with recurrence of febrile convulsions, *J Infect Dis* 167(5):1197-1200, 1993.

Koop CE: *The surgeon general's letter on child sexual abuse,* Rockville, Md, 1988, US Department of Health and Human Services, Public Health Service, Health Resources and Services Administration, Bureau of Maternal and Child Health and Resources Development, Office of Maternal and Child Health.

Kotelchuck M: Child abuse and neglect: prediction and misclassification. In Starr RH, editor: *Child abuse prediction policy implications,* Cambridge, Mass, 1982, Ballinger.

Leung A, Robson W: Childhood masturbation, *Clin Pediatr* 32(4):238-241, 1993.

Loftus E: Remembering dangerously, *Sketical Inquirer* 19(2):20-29, 1995.

National Center on Child Abuse and Neglect: *A coordinated response to child abuse and neglect: a basic manual,* Washington, DC, 1993, National Center.

A nation's shame: fatal child abuse and neglect in the United States, Washington, DC, 1995, US Advisory Board on Child Abuse and Neglect.

Nocton JJ et al: Human parvovirus-associated arthritis in children, *J Pediatr* 122(2):186-190, 1993.

Olds DL et al: Preventing child abuse and neglect: a randomized trial of nurse home visitation, *Pediatrics* 78(1):65-78, 1986.

Pillitteri A et al: Parent gender, victim gender, and family socioeconomic level influences on the potential reporting by nurses of physical child abuse, *Issues Compr Pediatr Nurs* 15:239-247, 1992.

Radko K: Child abuse: guilty until proven innocent or legalized governmental child abuse, *Issues Child Abuse Accus* 5(2):96-101, 1993.

Seidl AH et al: Nurses' attitudes toward the child victims and the perpetrators of emotional, physical, and sexual abuse, *Issues Child Abuse Accus* 5(1):28-38, 1993.

Shea S et al: Variability and self-regulation of energy intake in young children in their everyday environment, *Pediatrics* 90:542-546, 1992.

Shea S et al: Is there a relationship between dietary fat and stature or growth in children three to five years of age? *Pediatrics* 92:579-586, 1993.

Stanton M et al: Nurses' attitudes toward emotional, sexual, and physical abusers of children with disabilities, *Rehabil Nurs* 19(4):214-218, 1994.

Stier DM et al: Are children born to young mothers at increased risk of maltreatment? *Pediatrics* 91(3):642-648, 1993.

Straus SE: Shingles: sorrows, salves, and solutions, *JAMA* 269(14): 1836-1839, 1993.

Terada K et al: Varicella-zoster virus (VZV) reactivation is related to the low response of VZV-specific immunity after chickenpox in infancy, *J Infect Dis* 169:650-652, 1994.

Thomas RM: *Comparing theories of child development,* ed 4, Pacific Grove, Calif, 1996, Brooks-Cole.

Wakefield H, Underwager R: Interrogation of children, *Issues Child Abuse Accus* 1(1):14-28, 1989.

Wilde JA, Pedroni AT Jr: Privacy rights in Munchausen syndrome, *Contemp Pediatr* 10(1):83-91, 1993.

Wong DL: False allegations of child abuse: the other side of the tragedy, *Pediatr Nurs* 13(5):329-333, 1987.

Wong DL: The "evidence" is shaky at best, *Am J Nurs* 9(2):18, 1991.

Bibliography

Growth and Development

Ames LB, Ilg FI: *Your three-year-old: friend or enemy*, New York, 1980, Delacorte Press.

Ames LB, Ilg FI: *Your four-year-old: wild and wonderful*, New York, 1981, Delacorte Press.

Ames LB, Ilg FI: *Your five-year-old: sunny and serene*, New York, 1981, Delacorte Press.

Blum NJ et al: Disciplining your children: the role of verbal instructions and reasoning, *Pediatrics* 96(2):336-341, 1995.

Dixon SD, Stein MT: *Encounters with children: a practical guide to pediatric behavior and development*, ed 2, St Louis, 1992, Mosby.

Hauck MR: Cognitive abilities of preschool children: implications for nurses working with young children, *J Pediatr Nurs* 6(4):230-235, 1991.

Howard BJ: Growing together; learning independence in the preschool years, *Contemp Pediatr* 7(7):11-26, 1990.

Lavigne JB et al: Behavioral and emotional problems among preschool children in pediatric primary care: prevalence and pediatricians' recognition, *Pediatrics* 91(3):649-655, 1993.

Lowrey G: *Growth and development of children*, ed 8, St Louis, 1986, Mosby.

Lyytinen P: Developmental trends in children's pretend play, *Child Care Health Dev* 17(1):25, 1991.

Morrison CD, Bundy AC, Fisher AG: The contribution of motor skills and playfulness to the play performance of preschoolers, *Am J Occup Ther* 45(8):687-694, 1991.

Prior M et al: Sex differences in psychological adjustment from infancy to 8 years, *J Am Acad Child Adolesc Psychiatry* 32(2):291-304, 1993.

Rugg HA, Saltarelli LM: Exploratory play with objects: basic cognitive processes and individual differences, *New Dir Child Dev* (59):5-16, 1993.

Shonkoff JP: Preschool. In Levine MD et al, editors: *Developmental-behavioral pediatrics*, Philadelphia, 1992, WB Saunders.

Preschool and Kindergarten Experience

Byrd RS, Weitzman ML: Predictors of early grade retention among children in the United States, *Pediatrics* 93(3):481-487, 1994.

Casey PH, Evans LD: School readiness: an overview for pediatricians, *Pediatr Rev* 14(1):4-10, 1993.

Karp R et al: Growth and academic achievement in inner-city kindergarten children, *Clin Pediatr* 31(6):336-340, 1992.

Martin S, Ramey C, Ramey S: The prevention of intellectual impairment in children of impoverished families: findings of a randomized trial of educational day care, *Am J Public Health* 80:844-847, 1990.

Oberklaid F et al: Predicting preschool behavior problems from temperament and other variables in infancy, *Pediatrics* 91(1):113-120, 1993.

Palmer DJ et al: An exploratory study of the structure and validity of pediatric examination of educational readiness, *Dev Behav Pediatr* 11(6):317-321, 1990.

Robinson J: *Is your child ready for school?* New York, 1990, Simon & Schuster.

Wilson DA, Knudtson MD: Assessing school readiness through the school-entry screening exam, *Nurs Pract* 17(9):24-26, 29-30, 33, 1992.

Sex Education

Aquilino ML, Ely J: Parents and the sexuality of preschool children, *Pediatr Nurs* 11(1):41-46, 1985.

Calderone MS: Sexual health and the child, *Compr Ther* 6(12):3-7, 1980.

Castiglia PT: Masturbation, *J Pediatr Health Care* 2(2):111-112, 1988.

Masters WH, Johnson VE, Kolodny RC: *Human sexuality*, ed 3, Glenview, Ill, 1988, Scott, Foresman.

Speech Problems

Biro P, Thompson M: Screening young children for communication disorders, *MCN* 9(6):410-413, 1984.

Goldberg R: Identifying speech and language delays in children, *Pediatr Nurs* 15(4):252-259, 1984.

Pastore DR: Stuttering. In Hoekelman R et al, editors: *Primary pediatric care*, ed 2, St Louis, 1992, Mosby.

Schmitt BD: Does your child have a stuttering problem? *Contemp Pediatr* 8(3):83-84, 1991.

Sleep Problems

Beltramini A, Hertzig M: Sleep and bedtime behavior in preschool-aged children, *Pediatrics* 71(2):153-158, 1983.

Clore ER, Hibel J: The parasomnias of childhood, *J Pediatr Health Care* 7(1):12-16, 1993.

Crawford W, Bennet R, Hewitt K: Sleep problems in pre-school children, *Health Visit* 62(3):79-81, 1989.

DiMario F, Enery ES, III: The natural history of night terrors, *Clin Pediatr* 26(10):505-511, 1987.

Edgil A et al: Sleep problems of older infants and preschool children, *Pediatr Nurs* 11(2):87-89, 1985.

Gates D, Morwessel N. Night terrors: strategies for family coping, *J Pediatr Nurs* 4(1):48-53, 1989.

Jimmerson KR: Maternal, environmental, and temperamental characteristics of toddlers with and toddlers without sleep problems, *J Pediatr Health Care* 5(2):71-77, 1991.

Leung AK, Robson WL: Nightmares, *J Natl Med Assoc* 85(3):233-235, 1993.

McMenamy C, Katz RC: Brief parent-assisted treatment for children's nighttime fears, *J Dev Behav Pediatr* 10(3):145-148, 1989.

Pagel J: Nightmares, *Am Fam Physician* 39(3):145-148, 1989.

Stores G: Sleep problems, *Arch Dis Child* 67(12):1420-1421, 1992.

Communicable Diseases

American Academy of Pediatrics Committee on Infectious Diseases: *1994 Red book: report of the committee on infectious diseases*, ed 23, Elk Grove Village, Ill, 1994, The Academy.

Cromer BA et al: Unrecognized pertussis infection in adolescents, *Am J Dis Child* 147:575-577, 1993.

Feder HM: Fifth disease, *N Engl J Med* 331(16):1062, 1994.

Gurevich I: Fifth disease and other parvovirus B 19 infections, *Heart Lung* 20(4):342-344, 1991.

Kerfoot F: The perils of pertussis, *J Pediatr Nurs* 4(4):277, 1989.

Stevenson L, Brooke DS: Roseola (human herpesvirus 6), *J Pediatr Health Care* 8(6):283, 1994.

Child Maltreatment

Alexander R et al: Incidence of impact trauma with cranial injuries ascribed to shaking, *Am J Dis Child* 144:724-726, 1990.

Alexander R and others: Serial abuse in children who are shaken, *Am J Dis Child* 144(1):58-60, 1990.

American Academy of Pediatrics, Committee on Bioethics: Religious exemptions from child abuse statutes, *Pediatrics* 81(1):169-171, 1988.

American Academy of Pediatrics, Committee on Child Abuse and Neglect and Committee on Community Health Services: Investigation and review of unexpected infant and child deaths, *Pediatrics* 92(5):734-735, 1993.

American Academy of Pediatrics, Committee on Early Childhood, Adoption, and Dependent Care: Developmental issues in foster care for children, *Pediatrics* 91(5):1007-1009, 1993.

American Academy of Pediatrics, Task Force on Child Abuse and Neglect: Public disclosure of private information about victims of abuse, *Pediatrics* 82(3):387, 1988.

Anderson CL: The parenting profile assessment: screening for child abuse, *Appl Nurs Res* 6(1):31-3, 1993.

Andrews AB: Developing community systems for the primary prevention of family violence, *Fam Community Health* 16(4):1-9, 1994.

Baldwin MA: Munchausen syndrome by proxy: neurological manifestations, *J Neurosci Nurs* 26(1):18-23, 1994.

Berenson AB: Appearance of the hymen at birth and one year of age: a longitudinal study, *Pediatrics* 91(4):820-825, 1993.

Berkowitz CD: Child sexual abuse, *Pediatr Rev* 13(12):443-452, 1992.

Besharov DJ: *Recognizing child abuse: a guide for the concerned,* New York, 1990, MacMillan.

Brucker JM: Battered child syndrome: educating the pediatric nurse, *J Pediatr Nurs* 6(6):428-429, 1991.

Burgess A, Hartman C, Kelley S: Assessing child abuse: the triads checklist, *J Psychosoc Nurs* 28(4):6-14, 1990.

Coleman L: Medical examination for sexual abuse: have we been misled? *Issues Child Abuse Accus* 1(3):1-9, 1989.

Dubowitz H, Black M, Harrington D: The diagnosis of child sexual abuse, *Am J Dis Child* 146(6):688-693, 1992.

Goldson E: The affective and cognitive sequelae of child maltreatment, *Pediatr Clin North Am* 38(6):1481-1496, 1991.

Hochhauser KG, Richardson RA: Munchausen syndrome by proxy: an exploratory study of pediatric nurses' knowledge and involvement. *J Pediatr Nurs* 9(5):313-320, 1994.

Horsham P: Child sexual abuse: what parents need to know, *Can Nurse* 88(8):32-35, 1992.

Hyden PW, Gallagher TA: Child abuse intervention in the emergency room, *Pediatr Emerg Med* 39(5):1053-1081, 1992.

Kelley SJ: Parental stress response to sexual abuse and ritualistic abuse of children in day-care centers, *Nurs Res* 39(1):25-29, 1990.

Kelley SJ: Methodological issues in child sexual abuse research, *J Pediatr Nurs* 6(1):21-29, 1991.

Kemper KJ et al: Screening for maternal experiences of physical abuse during childhood, *Clin Pediatr* 33(6):333-339, 1994.

Lesniak LP: Penetrating the conspiracy of silence: identifying the family at risk for incest, *Fam Community Health* 16(2):66-76, 1993.

Lewin L: Establishing a therapeutic relationship with an abused child, *Pediatr Nurs* 16(3):263-264, 1990.

McCann J et al: Comparison of genital examination techniques in prepubertal girls, *Pediatrics* 85(2):182-187, 1990.

McCann J et al: Genital findings in prepubertal girls selected for nonabuse: a descriptive study, *Pediatrics* 86(3):428-439, 1990.

Middleton C: Controversy . . . in best interests of the child!!! . . ., *Child Care, Health Dev* 21(4):271-285, 1995.

Old D et al: Effects of prenatal and infancy nurse home visitation on surveillance of child maltreatment, *Pediatrics* 95(3):365-372, 1995.

Osborn M, Bryan S: Patient care guidelines: evidentiary examination in sexual assault, *J Emerg Nurs* 15(3):284-290, 1989.

Paradise JE: Predictive accuracy and the diagnosis of sexual abuse: a big issue about a little tissue, *Child Abuse Negl* 13:169-176, 1989.

Post CA: Play therapy with an abused child: a case study, *J Child Adolesc Psychiatr Ment Health Nurs* 3(1):34-36, 1990.

Saucier BL: The effects of play therapy on developmental achievement levels of abused children, *Pediatr Nurs* 15(1):27-30, 1989.

Schwab NC: Child abuse and neglect: legal and clinical implications for school nursing practice, *School Nurse* 5(4):17-28, 1989.

Senner A, Ott M: Munchausen syndrome by proxy, *Issues Compr Pediatr Nurs* 12(5):345-357, 1989.

CHAPTER 36

The School-Age Child and Family

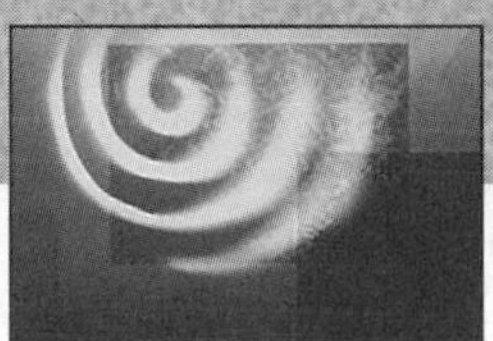

PROMOTING OPTIMUM GROWTH AND DEVELOPMENT, P. 1053

Biologic development, p. 1053
Psychosocial development, p. 1055
Cognitive development (Piaget), p. 1056
Moral development (Kohlberg), p. 1057
Spiritual development, p. 1057
Social development, p. 1057
Developing a self-concept, p. 1060
Coping with concerns related to normal growth and development, p. 1060
Summary of growth and development, p. 1063

PROMOTING OPTIMUM HEALTH DURING THE SCHOOL YEARS, P. 1063

Nutrition, p. 1063
Sleep and rest, p. 1063
Exercise and activity, p. 1065
Dental health, p. 1066
Sex education, p. 1068
School health, p. 1068
Injury prevention, p. 1069
Anticipatory guidance—care of families, p. 1069

SPECIAL HEALTH PROBLEMS, P. 1072

Health problems related to sports participation, p. 1072
Altered growth and maturation, p. 1073

Tall or short stature, p. 1073
Sex chromosome abnormalities, p. 1074

Disorders with behavioral components, p. 1075

Attention deficit hyperactivity disorder and learning disability, p. 1075
Enuresis, p. 1077
Encopresis, p. 1077
Posttraumatic stress disorder, p. 1078
School phobia, p. 1078
Recurrent abdominal pain, p. 1079
Conversion reaction, p. 1079
Childhood depression, p. 1079
Childhood schizophrenia, p. 1080

Promoting Optimum Growth and Development

The segment of the life span that extends from age 6 years to approximately age 12 years has various labels, each of which describes an important characteristic of the period. These middle years are most often referred to as *school-age* or the *school years.* This period begins with entrance into the wider sphere of influence represented by the school environment, which has a significant impact on development and relationships. This is when the child affiliates with age-mates and learns the culture of childhood. With peer groups, children establish the first close relationships outside the family group.

Physiologically the middle years begin with the shedding of the first deciduous tooth and end at puberty with the acquisition of the final permanent teeth (with the exception of the wisdom teeth). During the preceding 5 to 6 years the child has progressed from a helpless infant to a sturdy, complicated individual with the capacity to communicate, conceptualize in a limited way, and become involved in complex social and motor behavior. Physical growth has been equally rapid. In contrast, the period of middle childhood, between the rapid growth of early childhood and the prepubescent growth spurt, is a time of gradual growth and development with steadier and more even progress in both physical and emotional aspects.

BIOLOGIC DEVELOPMENT

During middle childhood, growth in height and weight assumes a slower but steady pace as compared with the earlier years. Between ages 6 and 12 years, children grow an average of 5 cm (2 inches) per year to gain 30 to 60 cm (1 to 2 feet) in height and almost double their weight, increasing 2 to 3 kg ($4^1/_2$ to $6^1/_2$ pounds) per year. The average 6-year-old child is about 116 cm (45 inches) tall and weighs about 21 kg (46 pounds); the average 12-year-old child stands about 150 cm (59 inches) tall and weighs approximately 40 kg (88 pounds). During this period, girls and boys differ very little in size, although boys tend to be slightly taller and somewhat heavier

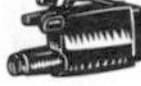

*For addditional information, please view "Growth and Development" in *Whaley and Wong's Pediatric Nursing Video Series*, St Louis, 1996, Mosby; (800)426-4545.

than girls. Toward the end of the school-age years, both boys and girls begin to increase in size. Because many girls begin puberty midway through this school-age period, most girls surpass boys in both height and weight by the end of the school-age years (to the acute discomfort of both girls and boys).

Proportional Changes

School-age children are more graceful and steadier on their feet than they were as preschoolers. Their body proportions take on a slimmer look, with longer legs, varying body proportion, and a lower center of gravity. Posture improves over that of the preschool period to facilitate locomotion and efficiency in using the arms and trunk. These proportions make climbing, bicycle riding, and other activities much easier. Fat gradually diminishes, and its distribution patterns change, contributing to the thinner appearance of the child during the middle years.

Accompanying the skeletal lengthening and fat diminution is an increase in the percentage of body weight represented by muscle tissue. By the end of this period, both boys and girls double their strength and physical capabilities, and their steady and relatively consistent acquisition of refined coordination increases their poise and skill. However, this increased strength can be misleading. Although strength increases, muscles are still functionally immature when compared with those of the adolescent, and they are more readily damaged by muscular injury caused by overuse.

The most pronounced changes, and those that are the best indicators of increasing maturity in children, are a decrease in head circumference in relation to standing height, a decrease in waist circumference in relation to height, and an increase in leg length related to height. These observations often provide a clue to a child's degree of physical maturity that has proved useful in predicting readiness for meeting the demands of school. There appears to be a correlation between physical indications of maturity and success in school.

Facial changes. Certain physiologic and anatomic characteristics are typical of children in the years of middle childhood. Facial proportions change as the face grows faster in relation to the remainder of the cranium. The skull and brain grow very slowly during this period and increase little in size thereafter. Because all of the primary (deciduous) teeth are lost during this age span, middle childhood is sometimes known as the *age of the loose tooth* (Fig. 36-1) and the early years of middle childhood as the *ugly duckling stage,* when the new secondary (permanent) teeth appear to be much too large for the face.

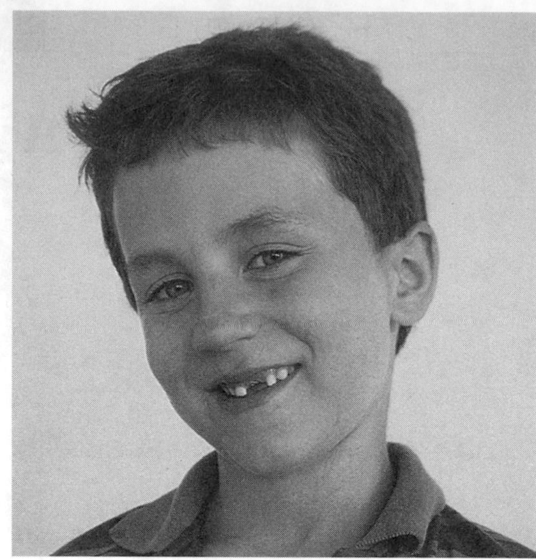

Fig. 36-1 Middle childhood is the stage of development when deciduous teeth are shed.

Maturation of Systems

Maturity of the gastrointestinal system is reflected in fewer stomach upsets, better maintenance of blood glucose levels, and an increased stomach capacity, which permits retention of food for longer periods of time. The school-age child does not need to be fed as carefully, as promptly, or as frequently as before. Caloric needs are less than they were in the preschool years.

Physical maturation is evidenced in other body tissues and organs. *Bladder capacity,* although differing widely among individual children, is generally greater in girls than in boys. The *heart* grows more slowly during the middle years and is smaller in relation to the rest of the body than at any other period of life. Heart and respiratory rates steadily decrease, and blood pressure increases from ages 6 to 12 years (see the Appendix).

The *immune system* becomes more competent in its ability to localize infections and to produce an antibody-antigen response (Miller, 1989).

Bones continue to ossify throughout childhood but yield to pressure and muscle pull more than mature bones. Children should have ample opportunity to move around, and they should observe appropriate caution in carrying heavy loads. For example, they should shift books from one arm to the other, and those who carry tote bags slung from the shoulders should alternate the load from one shoulder to the other to avoid developing a low shoulder or spinal curvature.

There are wider differences between children at the end of middle childhood than at the beginning; such differences are sometimes striking. These differences become increasingly apparent and, if extreme or unique, may create emotional problems unless the associated characteristics of height and weight relationships, rapid or slow growth, and other important features of development are recognized and explained to children and their families. Physical maturity is not necessarily correlated with emotional and social maturity. Seven-year-old children who look like 10-year-old children will, in fact, think and act like 7-year-old children. To expect behavior appropriate for 10-year-old children from them is unrealistic and can be detrimental to their development of competence and self-esteem. Conversely, to treat 10-year-old children as though they were 7 years old is an equal disservice to them.

Prepubescence

Preadolescence is the period that begins toward the end of middle childhood and ends with the thirteenth birthday. Since puberty signals the beginning of the development of secondary sex characteristics, **prepubescence,** the 2-year period that precedes puberty, typically occurs during preadolescence.

Toward the end of middle childhood the discrepancies in growth and maturation between boys and girls begin to be apparent. On the average there is a difference of approximately 2 years between girls and boys in the age of onset of pubescence. This is a period of rapid growth in height and weight, especially for girls.

There is no universal age at which children assume the characteristics of prepubescence. The first physiologic signs begin to appear at about 9 years of age (particularly in girls) and are usually clearly evident in 11- to 12-year-old children. Although the preadolescent child does not want to be different, at this age the variability in physical growth and physiologic changes between children of the same sex and between the two sexes is often striking. This variability, especially in relation to the onset of secondary sexual characteristics, is of utmost concern to the preadolescent. Either early or late appearance of these characteristics can be a source of embarrassment and uneasiness to both sexes.

Preadolescence is a time when considerable overlapping of developmental characteristics occurs, with elements of both middle childhood and early adolescence. However, there are sufficient unique characteristics to set this period apart as an age category. Generally, the earliest age at which **puberty** begins is 10 years in girls and 12 years in boys, although there has been an increase in the number of girls reaching puberty at age 9 years. The average age of puberty in girls is 12 years; for boys it is 14 years. Boys experience little visible sexual maturation during preadolescence.

PSYCHOSOCIAL DEVELOPMENT

Middle childhood is the period of psychosexual development that Freud described as the latency period, a time of tranquility between the oedipal phase of early childhood and the eroticism of adolescence. During this time, children experience relationships with same gender peers following the indifference of earlier years and preceding the heterosexual fascination that accompanies puberty.

Developing a Sense of Industry (Erikson)

Successful mastery of Erikson's first three stages of psychosocial development is probably the most important accomplishment in terms of development of a healthy personality (Erikson, 1963). Successful completion of these stages requires a loving environment within a stable family unit. The child is now prepared to engage in experiences and relationships beyond this intimate group.

It has been suggested that the individual's fundamental attitude toward work is established during middle childhood. A *sense of industry,* for which a more descriptive term is *stage of accomplishment,* is achieved somewhere between age 6 years and adolescence. School-age children are eager to develop skills and participate in meaningful and socially useful work. Children acquire a sense of industry through both formal and self-directed education.

Interests expand in the middle years, and with a growing sense of independence, the child wants to engage in tasks that can be carried through to completion (Fig. 36-2). During this time, children receive the systematic instruction prescribed by their individual cultures and develop the skills needed to become useful, contributing members of their social communities. They gain a great deal of satisfaction from independent behavior in exploring and manipulating their environment and from interaction with peers. Often the acquisition of skills is a means for achieving success in social activities. Reinforcement in the form of grades, material rewards, additional privileges, and recognition provide encouragement and stimulation.

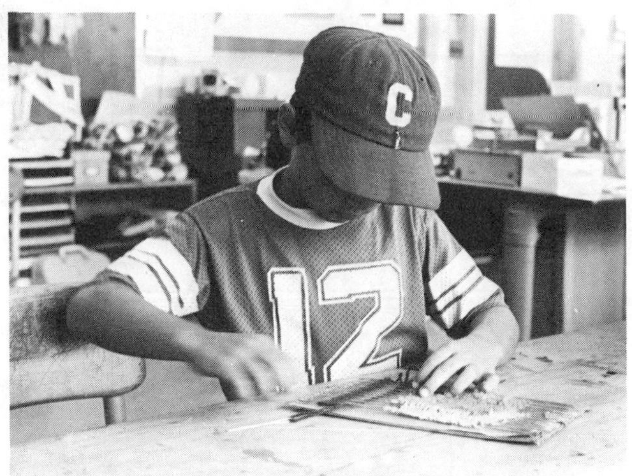

Fig. 36-2 School-age children are motivated to complete tasks working alone.

A sense of accomplishment also involves the ability to cooperate and to compete with others—to cope more effectively with people. Middle childhood is when children learn the value of doing things with others and the benefits derived from division of labor in the accomplishment of goals. Peer approval is a strong motivating power.

The danger inherent in this period of personality development is the occurrence of situations that might result in a sense of *inferiority.* This may happen if the previous stages have not been successfully achieved or if the child is incapable of or unprepared for assuming the responsibilities associated with developing a sense of accomplishment. Feelings of inferiority or lack of worth can be derived from children themselves or from the social environment. Children with chronic disabilities may be at a disadvantage for the acquisition of certain skills and at risk for feeling inferior. However, no child can do well in everything, and children must learn that they will not be able to master each skill they attempt. All children, even children who in most instances have positive attitudes toward work and their own capabilities, feel some degree of inferiority with regard to a specific skill that they cannot master.

Children need and want real achievement. When they have access to tasks that must be done, that they are able to do well despite individual differences in their innate capacities and emotional development, and for which they are suitably rewarded, children can achieve a sense of industry and accomplishment.

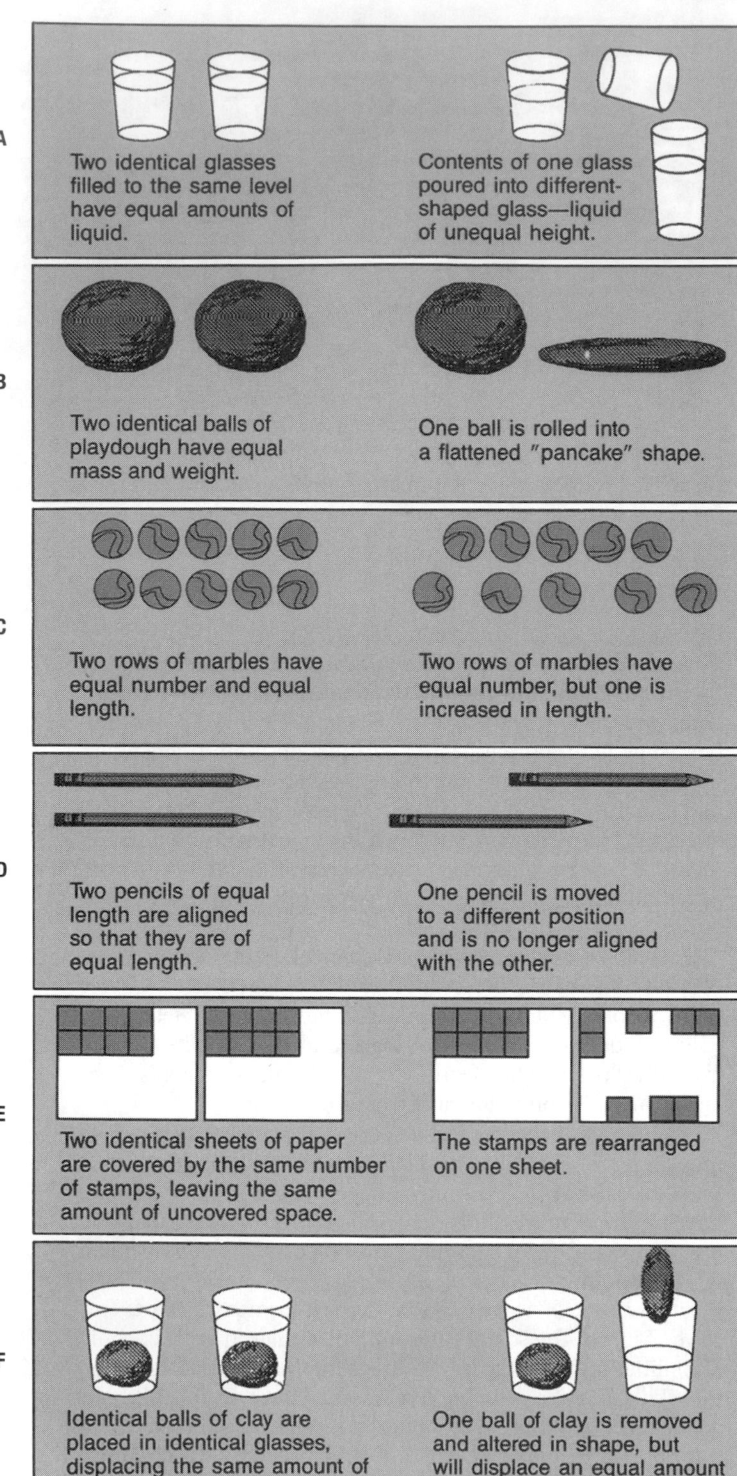

Fig. 36-3 Common examples that demonstrate the child's ability to conserve. The child who has mastered conservation recognizes that the properties of objects are constant despite changes in shape or arrangement. Different aspects of this concept are mastered at different ages. (The ages listed are only approximate.) **A,** Liquids (5 to 7 years). **B,** Mass (5 to 7 years) and weight (9 to 10 years). **C,** Number (5 years). **D,** Length (6 to 7 years). **E,** Area (9 to 10 years). **F,** Volume (9 to 12 years).

COGNITIVE DEVELOPMENT (PIAGET)

When children enter the school-age years, they begin to acquire the ability to relate a series of happenings to mental representations that can be expressed both verbally and symbolically. Piaget describes this stage of development as *concrete operations,* when children are able to use thought processes to experience events and actions. The rigid, egocentric outlook of the preschool years is replaced by thought processes that allow children to see things from the point of view of another.

During this stage, children develop an understanding of relationships between things and ideas. They progress from making judgments based on what they see *(perceptual thinking)* to making judgments based on what they reason *(conceptual thinking)*. They are increasingly able to master symbols and to use their memory store of past experiences in evaluating and interpreting the present.

One of the major cognitive tasks of school-age children is mastering the concept of *conservation* (Fig. 36-3). At an early age (about 5 to 7 years), they grasp the concept of reversibility of numbers as a basis for simple mathematic problems (e.g., $2 + 4 = 6$ and $6 - 4 = 2$). They learn that certain properties of the environment are not changed simply by altering their arrangement in space, and they become able to resist perceptual cues that suggest such alterations in the physical state of an object. For example, they recognize that changing the shape of a substance such as a lump of clay does not alter its total mass. They no longer perceive a tall, thin glass of water as containing a greater volume than a short, wide glass; they can distinguish between the weight of items regardless of their size. They recognize that size is not necessarily related to weight or volume. There appears to be a developmental sequence in children's capacity to conserve matter. Conservation of mass usually is accomplished earliest, weight some time later, and volume last.

School-age children also develop classification skills and can group and sort objects according to the attributes that they share, place things in a sensible and logical order, and, in doing so, hold a concept in mind while making decisions based on that concept. It is characteristic of middle childhood that children derive a great deal of enjoyment from classifying and ordering their environment. They become occupied with numerous and varied collections of objects, such as stickers, stamps, shells, dolls, cars, stones, and anything that is classifiable. They even begin to order friends and relationships (e.g., first best friend, second best friend).

They develop the ability to understand relational terms and concepts, such as bigger and smaller; darker and paler; heavier and lighter; to the right of and to the left of; first, last, and intermediate relationships (fourth, second, and so on); and more than and less than. They can see family relationships in terms of reciprocal roles (e.g., to be a brother, one must have a sibling).

They learn the alphabet and the ever-widening world of symbols called words that can be arranged in terms of structure and their relationship to the alphabet. They learn to tell time, to see the relationship of events in time (history) and places in space (geography), and to combine time and space relationships (geology and astronomy).

The most significant skill, the ability to read, is acquired during the school-age years and becomes the most valuable tool for independent inquiry. Children's capacity for exploration, imagination, and expansion of knowledge is enhanced by the ability to read as they progress from the repetition and confusion of early efforts to increasing facility and comprehension.

MORAL DEVELOPMENT (KOHLBERG)

As children move from egocentrism to the more logical patterns of thought, they also move through stages in the development of conscience and moral standards. Young children do not believe that standards of behavior come from within themselves but that rules are established and set down by others. During the preschool years, children, to some extent, adopt and internalize the moral values of their parents. They learn the standards for acceptable behavior, act according to these standards, and feel guilty when they violate the standards. Although children who are 6 or 7 years of age know the rules and behaviors expected of them, they do not understand the reasons behind them. Rewards and punishments guide their judgment; a "bad act" is one that breaks a rule or does harm. Young children may believe that what other people tell them to do is right and that what they think of themselves is wrong. Consequently, children 6 or 7 years old are more likely to interpret accidents and misfortunes as punishment for misdeeds or "bad" acts.

Older school-age children are able to judge an act by the intentions that prompted it rather than just by the consequences. Rules and judgments become less absolute and authoritarian and begin to be founded more on the needs and desires of others. For older children a rule violation is apt to be viewed in relation to the total context in which it appears; reactions are influenced by the situation as well as by the morality of the rule itself. Whereas a younger child can judge an act only according to whether it is right or wrong, older children will take into account a different point of view to make a judgment. They are able to understand and accept the concept of treating others as they would like to be treated.

SPIRITUAL DEVELOPMENT

Children at this age think in very concrete terms but are avid learners and have a great desire to learn about their God. They picture God as human and tend to describe him in terms of character traits such as loving and helping. He is a very important person in the lives of many children. They are fascinated by the concepts of hell and heaven, and, with a developing conscience and concern about rules, they fear going to hell for misbehavior. School-age children want and expect to be punished for misbehavior and, if given the option, tend to choose a punishment that "fits the crime." Often they view illness or injury as a punishment for a real or imagined misdeed. The beliefs and ideals of family and religious personages are more influential than those of their peers in matters of faith.

School-age children begin to learn the difference between the natural and the supernatural but have difficulty understanding abstractions. Consequently, religious concepts must be presented to them in concrete terms. They are comforted by prayer or other religious rituals, and if they are a part of their daily lives, these activities can help them cope with threatening situations. Their petitions to their God in prayers tend to be for very tangible rewards. Although younger children expect their prayers to be answered, as they get older, they begin to recognize that this does not always occur and become less concerned when prayers are not answered. They are able to discuss their feelings about their faith and how it relates to their lives (see the Cultural Considerations box above).

Cultural Considerations 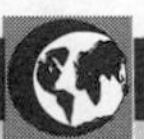

RELIGIOUS ORIENTATION

Many schools and communities have a Judeo-Christian orientation toward prayer, holidays, and values. This may result in conflict and discomfort for children of other religious/ethnic groups. Sensitivity must be exercised so as not to offend and confuse children from other religious backgrounds, such as those of the Buddhist, Hindu, and Muslim faiths.

SOCIAL DEVELOPMENT

One of the most important socializing agents in the life of the school-age child is the peer group. Together, members explore ideas and the physical environment around them. In addition to parents and the schools, the peer group manages to convey a substantial amount of material to its members. Children have a culture all their own, with secrets, mores, and codes of ethics with which they promote feelings of group solidarity and detachment from adults. Through peer relationships, children learn ways in which to deal with dominance and hostility and to relate to persons in positions of leadership and authority.

Identification with peers appears to be a strong influence in the child's gaining independence from parents. The aid and support of the group provide the child with enough security to risk the moderate parental rejection brought about by each small victory in the development of independence.

Much of the child's concept of the appropriate gender role is acquired through relationships with peers. During the early school years there is little difference relative to gender in the play experiences of children. Games and many other activities are shared by both girls and boys. However, in the later school years the differences become marked.

Social Relationships and Cooperation

Daily relationships with age-mates provide the most important social interactions in the life of school-age children. For the first time, children are able to join in group activities with unrestrained enthusiasm and steady participation. Previous interactions had been limited to short periods under considerable adult supervision. With increased skills and wider opportunities, children are able to become involved with one or several peer groups in which they can gain status as respected members.

Valuable lessons are learned from daily interactions with age-mates. First, children learn to appreciate the numerous and varied points of view that are represented in the peer group. As children interact with peers who see the world in ways that are somewhat different from the way they see it, they become aware of the limits of their own point of view. Because age-mates are peers and are not forced to accept each other's ideas as they are expected to accept those of adults,

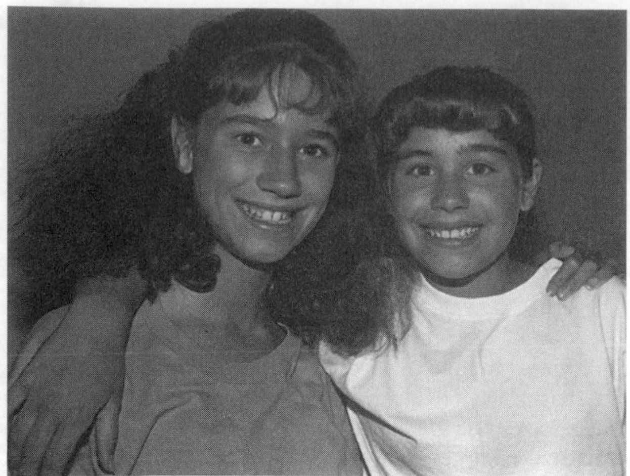

Fig. 36-4 School age is the time when children have "best friends."

other children have a significant influence on decreasing the egocentric outlook of the child. Consequently, children learn to argue, persuade, bargain, cooperate, and compromise in order to maintain friendships.

Second, children become increasingly sensitive to the social norms and pressures of the peer group. The peer group establishes standards for acceptance and rejection, and children may be willing to modify their behavior to be accepted by the group. The need for peer approval becomes a powerful influence toward conformity. Children learn to dress, talk, and behave in a manner acceptable to the group. A variety of roles, such as class joker or class hero, may be assumed by individual children to gain approval from the group.

Third, the interaction among peers leads to the formation of intimate friendship between same-gender peers. The school-age period is when children have "best friends" with whom they share secrets, private jokes, and adventures; they come to one another's aid in times of trouble. In the course of these friendships, children also fight, threaten, break up, and reunite. These dyadic relationships, in which the child experiences love and closeness for a peer, seem to be important as a foundation for heterosexual relationships in adulthood (Fig. 36-4).

Clubs and peer groups. One of the outstanding characteristics of middle childhood is the formation of formalized groups, or clubs. A prominent feature of many of these groups is the rigid rules imposed on the members. There is an exclusiveness in the selection of persons who have the privilege of joining. Acceptance in the group is often determined on a pass-fail basis according to social or behavioral criteria. Conformity is the core of the group structure. There are often secret codes, shared interests, and special modes of dress, and each child must abide by a standard of behavior established by the members. Understanding of and conformity to the rules provide children with feelings of security and relieve them of the responsibility of making decisions. By merging their identities with those of their peers, children are able to move from the family group to an outside group as a step toward seeking further independence. They substitute conformity to a peer-group pattern for conformity to a family pattern while they are still too shaky and insecure to function independently.

During the early school-age years, groups are rather small and loosely organized with changing membership and little formal structure. The more prolonged cohesiveness characteristic of groups or cliques in later school years is not obvious. As a rule, girls' groups are less formalized than boys', and, although there may be a mixture of both genders in the earlier school years, the groups of later school years are composed predominantly of children of the same gender. Common interests are a frequent basis around which a group is structured.

This is also a time for overnight or day camp, during which time children learn that there may be different rules in different settings. Camp counselors may be the only other adults besides parents (and occasionally teachers) who require children to take responsibility for their physical cleanliness and personal belongings, but they also expect the children to cooperate with fellow campers and function as a unit.

Although peer-group identification and association are essential to a child's socialization, there can be dangers inherent in strong peer-group attachment. Peer pressures may force children into taking risks, even against their better judgment. Peer-group activities that result in unacceptable, unlawful, or criminal *gang violence* are increasing in the United States and represent a significant challenge for health professionals and teachers who work with children (Rollins, 1993).

Relationships with Families

Although the peer group is highly influential and necessary to normal child development, parents are still the primary influence in shaping the child's personality, setting standards for behavior, and establishing value systems. It is the family values that usually predominate when parental and peer value systems come into conflict. Although children may appear to reject parental values while testing the new values of the peer group, ultimately they will retain and incorporate into their own value systems the parental values they have found to be of worth.

Peer associations seem to remain within the social class systems. Not infrequently, there may be discrimination in membership based on ethnic or racial origin.

Children want to spend more time in the company of peers and may seem eager to leave the house; they often prefer activities of the peer group to family activities. This can be very disturbing to parents. Children become intolerant and critical of parents and their ways when they deviate from those of the group. Children discover that parents can be wrong, and they begin to question the knowledge and authority of parents, who previously were considered to be all-knowing and all-powerful.

Although increased independence is the goal of middle childhood, children are not ready to abandon parental control. They need and want restrictions placed on their behavior; they are not yet prepared to cope with all the problems of their expanding environment. They feel more secure knowing that there is an authority greater than themselves to implement controls and restrictions. Children may complain loudly about the restrictions and try their best to break down parental barriers, but they are uneasy if they succeed in doing so. They respect the adults on whom they can rely to prevent them from acting on each and every urge. Children sense in this behavior an expression of love and concern for their welfare.

Children also need their parents as adults, not as pals. Sometimes parents, hurt at their children's rejection, attempt to maintain their love and gratitude by assuming the role of "pals." Children need the stable, secure strength provided by mature adults to whom they can turn during troubled relationships with peers or stressful changes in their world. During a disruption in their lives, such as times of failure, periods of illness, or a move that separates them from the security of friends, children need the firm, secure anchor of parental interest and concern. With a secure base in a loving family, children are able to develop the self-confidence and maturity needed to break loose from the group and stand independently.

Play

As children enter the school years, their play takes on new dimensions that reflect a new stage of development. Not only does play involve increased physical skill, intellectual skill, and fantasy, but as children form groups and cliques, they begin to develop a sense of belonging to a team or club. To belong to a group is of vital importance; clubs, secret societies, and organizations, such as Scouts, are part of the culture of childhood.

Rules and ritual. The need for conformity in middle childhood is strongly manifested in the activities and games so important in the life of school-age children. Up to this point, they have played games they have invented themselves, or they have played in the company of a friend or an adult, when rules more or less evolved with the game. Now they begin to see the need for rules, and the games they begin to play have fixed and unvarying rules that may be bizarre and extraordinarily rigid (especially those made up by the group).

Conformity and ritual permeate the play of school-age children. Not only are they present in games, but they are also evident in much of the children's behavior and language. Childhood is full of chants and taunts, such as "Eeeny, meeny, miney, mo," "Last one is a rotten egg," and "Step on a crack, break your mother's back." Children derive a great deal of pleasure and power from such sayings, which have been handed down with few changes through generations.

Team play. A more complex form of play that evolves from the need for peer interaction is the team game and sports that are part of the early school years. The rules of a team game may require the presence of a referee, umpire, or person of authority so that the rules can be followed more accurately. Through team play, children learn to modify or exchange personal goals for goals of the group and come to see the concept of division of labor as an effective strategy for attaining a goal. They learn about the nature of competition and the importance of winning—an attribute highly valued in the United States.

Team play can also contribute to children's social, intellectual, and skill growth. Children will work hard to develop the skills needed to become team members, to improve their contribution to the group effort, and to anticipate the consequences of their behavior for the group. Team play helps stimulate cognitive growth as children are called on to learn many complex rules, make judgments about those rules, plan strategies, and assess the strengths and weaknesses of members of their own team and members of the opposing team.

Quiet games and activities. Although the play of school-age children is highly active, they also enjoy many quiet and solitary activities. The middle years are the time for collections, which constitute another ritual. The early school-age child's collections are an odd assortment of unrelated objects in messy, disorganized piles. Collections of later years are more orderly and selective, and they are organized neatly in scrapbooks, on shelves, or in boxes.

School-age children become fascinated with increasingly complex board or card games, such as Monopoly and rummy, that they can play with a best friend, family members, or a group. As in all games, their adherence to rules is fanatic. There is usually much discussion and argument, but the disagreement is easily resolved through reading the appropriate rule of the game.

The newly acquired skill of reading becomes increasingly satisfying as school-age children are able to expand their knowledge of the world through books (Fig. 36-5). School-age children never tire of stories, and just like preschool children, they love to have stories read aloud. Sewing, cooking, carpentry, gardening, and creative activities such as painting are other activities often enjoyed. Many creative skills, such as music and art, as well as athletic skills, such as swimming, horseback riding, dancing, and skating, are learned and delighted in during childhood and continue to be enjoyed into adolescence and adulthood.

Ego mastery. Play also affords children the means to acquire representational mastery over themselves, their environment, and others. Through play, they can feel as big, as powerful,

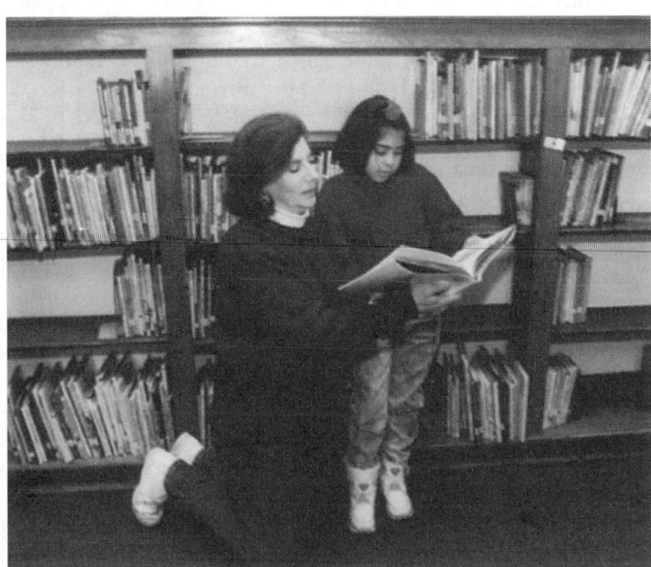

Fig. 36-5 Selecting a book with the assistance of an adult.

and as skillful as their imaginations will allow, and they can attain vicarious mastery and power over whomever and whatever they choose. They need to feel in control in their play. Schoolchildren still need the opportunity to use large muscles in exuberant outdoor play and the freedom to exert their newfound autonomy and initiative. They need space in which to exercise large muscles and to work off tensions, frustrations, and hostility. Physical skills practiced and mastered in play help them develop a feeling of personal competence, which contributes to a sense of accomplishment and helps provide a place of status in the peer group.

DEVELOPING A SELF-CONCEPT

The term *self-concept* refers to a conscious awareness of various self-perceptions, such as one's physical characteristics, abilities (as determined by the sense of industry), values, self-ideals and expectancy, and idea of self in relation to others. It also includes one's body image, sexuality, and self-esteem. Although primary caregivers continue to impart the greatest influence on children's self-evaluation, during middle childhood the opinions of peers and teachers provide further input. With the emphasis on skill building and broadened social relationships, children are continually occupied in the process of self-evaluation.

The significant adults in children's lives can often manage, unobtrusively, to manipulate children's environments so that they meet with success. Each small success increases children's self-image. The more positive they feel about themselves, the more confident they feel in trying again for success. All children profit from feeling that they are in some way special to a significant adult. A positive self-concept makes children feel likable, worthwhile, and able to make a valuable contribution to their world. Such feelings lead to self-respect, self-confidence, and a general sense of happiness. Negative feelings about one's self-concept lead to self-doubt.

Developing a Body Image

School-age children have a relatively accurate and positive perception of their physical selves, but in general, they like their physical selves less as they grow older. The head appears to be the most important part of the school-age child's perceived image of self, with hair and eye color the characteristics used most commonly to describe the physical self.

Body image is influenced, but not solely determined, by significant others. The number of significant others influencing perception of physical self increases with age. Children are acutely aware of bodies—their own, those of their peers, and those of adults—and are acutely aware of deviations from the norm. It is important that children know body functions and that adults correct misinformation children may have about the body (e.g., what is fat).

At this time, physical impairments, such as hearing or visual defects, ears that "stick out," or birthmarks, assume greater importance. Increasing awareness of these differences, especially when accompanied by unkind comments and taunts from other children, may cause a child to feel inferior and less desirable. This is especially true if the defect interferes with the child's ability to participate in childhood games and activities. When children are teased or criticized about being different, the effect can be lasting.

COPING WITH CONCERNS RELATED TO NORMAL GROWTH AND DEVELOPMENT

School Experience

The school serves as the agent for transmitting the values of the society to each succeeding generation of children and as the setting for most of their relationships with peers. As a socializing agent second only to the family, schools exert a profound influence on the social development of children.

School entrance causes a sharp break in the structure of the child's world. For many children it is their first experience in conforming to a group pattern imposed by an adult who is not a parent and who has responsibility for too many children to be constantly aware of each child as an individual. Children want to go to school and usually adapt to the new conditions with little difficulty. Successful adjustment is directly related to the physical and emotional maturity of the child and to the parent's readiness to accept the separation associated with school entrance. Unfortunately, some parents express their subconscious attempts to delay the child's maturity by clinging behavior, particularly with their youngest child.

By the time they enter school the majority of children have a fairly realistic concept of what school involves. Most children have had experience with kindergarten, and some with preschool as well. However, the extent to which they are prepared differs. Middle-class children have fewer adjustments to make and less to learn about expected behavior, since the school tends to reflect dominant middle-class customs and values.

Classmates have a significant impact on the socialization of individual children. School is usually the first time that most children become members of a large group of individuals their own age. Peer relationships become increasingly important and influential as children proceed through school. The kind of influence exerted by the peer group depends on the background, interests, and abilities of the individual child.

Teachers. To facilitate the transition from home to school, teachers should have personality characteristics that allow them to deal with the problems of young children. Children respond best to teachers with attributes that they would desire in a warm, loving parent. As a parent surrogate, the teacher in the early grades performs many of the activities formerly assumed by the parent, such as recognizing children's personal needs (such as a need to go to the bathroom or for help with clothing) and helping to develop their social behavior (e.g., manners).

Teachers, like parents, are concerned about the psychologic and emotional welfare of the child. Although the functions of teachers and parents differ, both place constraints on behavior and both are in a position to enforce standards of conduct. However, the teacher's primary responsibility is to stimulate and guide children's intellectual development, as opposed to providing for their physical welfare beyond the school setting. The teacher shares the parental influence in determining the child's attitudes and values.

Teachers serve as models with whom children identify and whom they try to emulate. Teacher approval is sought; teacher disapproval is avoided. The teacher is a very signifi-

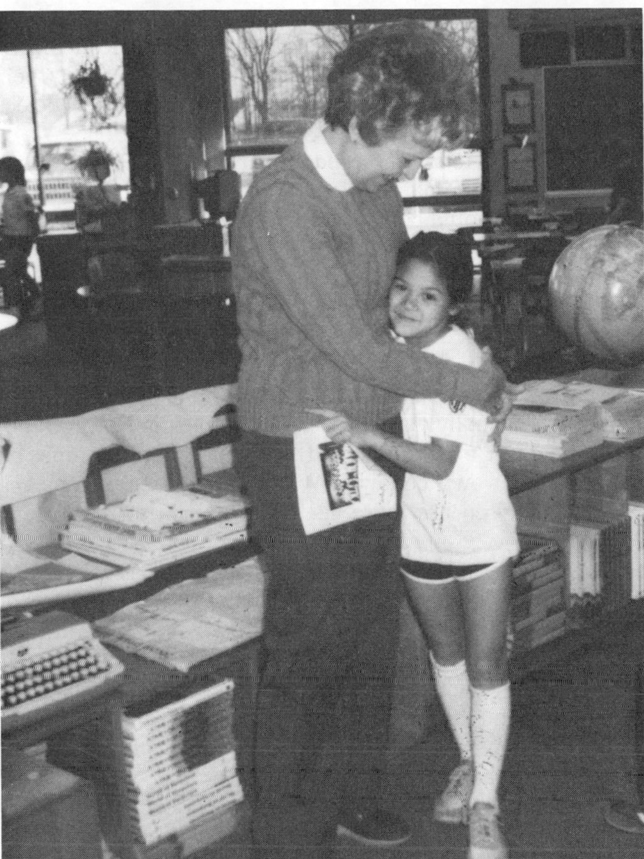

Fig. 36-6 Children can develop close relationships with their teachers.

cant person in the life of the child during the early school years and hero worship of a teacher may extend into late childhood and preadolescence (Fig. 36-6). Learner-centered behaviors on the part of teachers, such as making supportive statements that reassure or commend children, making accepting and clarifying statements that help children refine ideas and feelings to provide a sense of being understood, and providing constructive assistance that aids children with their own problem solving, all contribute to the expansion and development of a positive self-concept.

Parents. Parents share responsibility with the schools for helping children achieve their maximum potential. There are numerous ways in which parents can supplement the school (see the Home Care box to the right).

Cultivating responsibility is the goal of parental assistance. Being responsible for schoolwork helps children learn to keep promises, meet deadlines, and succeed at their jobs as adults. Responsible children may occasionally ask for help (e.g., with a spelling list), but usually they like to think through their work by themselves. Excessive pressure or lack of encouragement from parents may inhibit the development of these desirable traits (Schmitt, 1990b).

Home Care

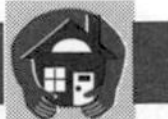

HELPING CHILDREN IN SCHOOL

General guidelines

Be supportive—through companionship share ideas and thoughts.
Be positive—every child should experience some success each day.
Share an interest in reading—use the library, discuss books they are reading.
Support and encourage activity rather than passivity.
Encourage originality—help children make their own projects from discarded articles or other available materials.
Foster the development of hobbies and collections.
Encourage children to wonder and reflect during free time.
Encourage family experiences and trips to places of interest.
Encourage questions—help children discover sources for information or places in which to explore and investigate.
Stimulate creative thinking and problem solving—help children try out new solutions to problems without fear of making mistakes.
Use rewards rather than punishment.

Specific guidelines

Meet the teacher at the beginning of the school year and plan to visit the school to see what is taught and expected.
Send the child to school every day—teachers are concerned when parents make other plans for their children; it conveys the impression that school is unimportant.
Demonstrate an interest in what the child is learning.
Demonstrate an interest in content and growth more than in grades.
Make it clear to the child that schoolwork is between the child and the teacher; teacher and child should set goals for better school performance to allow the child to feel responsible for school successes and failures.
Take advantage of situations that support and reinforce school learning.
Share information with teachers that will help them understand the child better.
Communicate with the teacher if there appears to be a problem—avoid waiting for a scheduled conference.
Provide a quiet, well-lighted area for study that is safe from interruption; do not allow television.
Avoid dictating a study time, but do enforce rules, such as no television until homework is done; accept the child's word that the work is complete.
Focus any help with homework on explaining the question, not giving the answer.
Teach the child to break large tasks (such as a report) into smaller manageable tasks spread over the allotted time rather than attempt the entire project the night before it is to be completed.
Limit home tutoring to special circumstances, such as when the teacher requests parental assistance after a child's prolonged absence.
Request special help for children with learning problems.
Support the school staff by showing respect for both the school system and the teacher, especially in the child's presence.

Latchkey Children

The term **latchkey children** is used to describe children in elementary school who spend some amount of time, before or after school, without supervision of an adult or an older adolescent. The increasing numbers of single-parent families and working mothers, together with the lack of available child care, has created a stress-provoking situation for a large number of schoolchildren. Some of these children may also have a chronic illness (Holaday, Turner, Henson, and Swan, 1994).

The effect on these children varies. Inadequate adult supervision after school leaves children at greater risk for injury and delinquent behavior. In some instances, outside activities are curtailed and relationships with peers may be significantly diminished. Many latchkey children feel lonelier, more isolated, and more fearful than children who have someone to care for them. To cope with their fears and anxieties while alone, these children may devise strategies such as hiding, playing the television at loud volume, or using pets as a source of comfort.

Many communities and persons concerned about their welfare are trying to help children and their parents deal with this potentially serious problem. School-age care programs have been implemented by some communities and employers. It is important to teach self-help skills to these children and provide telephone check-in and reassurance programs.

Limit Setting and Discipline

Numerous factors influence the amount and manner of discipline and limit setting imposed on school-age children: the psychosocial maturity of the parents, the childhood and childrearing experiences of the parents, the temperament of the children, the context of the children's misconduct, and the response of the children to rewards and punishments. As children are increasingly able to see a situation from the point of view of another, they are able to understand the effects of their reactions on others and themselves.

Disciplinary techniques should help children control their own behavior. Reasoning is an effective technique for this age group. With advancing cognitive skills, they can benefit from more complex types of disciplinary strategies. For example, withholding privileges, requiring compensation, imposing penalties, and contracting can be used with great success. Problem solving is the best approach to limit setting, and children themselves can be included in the process of determining appropriate disciplinary measures.

Dishonest Behavior

During middle childhood it is not uncommon for children to engage in what is considered to be antisocial behavior. Lying, stealing, and cheating may become manifest in previously well-behaved children. It is especially disturbing to parents, who may have difficulty coping with this behavior.

Lying can occur for a number of reasons. Preschool children often have difficulty distinguishing between fact and fantasy. By the time they reach school age, they still "tell stories" but can distinguish between what is real and what is make-believe. If not, they need to be taught to distinguish between fantasy and reality. Often children exaggerate a story or situation as a means to impress their family or friends.

Young children will lie to escape punishment or get out of some difficulty even when the evidence of their misbehavior is before their eyes. Older children may lie in order to meet expectations set by others to which they have been unable to measure up. However, most children are very concerned with the wrongness of lying and cheating—especially in their friends. They are quick to tell on others when they detect cheating.

Parents need to be reassured that all children lie sometimes and that they often have difficulty separating fantasy from reality. Parents should be helped to understand the importance of their own behavior as role models and of being truthful in their relationships with children.

Cheating is most common in young children ages 5 to 6 years. They find it difficult to lose at a game or contest, and so they cheat to win. They have not yet acquired the full realization of the wrongness of this behavior and do it almost automatically. It usually disappears as they mature. However, because children model observed behaviors, parents must be aware of their own behavior. When parents set examples of honesty, children are more likely to conform to these standards.

Like other ethically related behavior, *stealing* is not an unexpected event in the younger child. Between 5 and 8 years of age, children's sense of property rights is limited, and they tend to take something simply because they are attracted to it or to take money for what it will buy. They are equally likely to give away something valuable that belongs to them. When young children are caught and punished, they are penitent—they "didn't mean to" and "promise never to do it again," but it is quite likely that they will repeat the performance the following day. Often they not only steal but lie about it as well or attempt to justify the act with excuses. It is seldom helpful to trap children into admission by asking directly if they committed the offense. Children do not take on such responsibility until nearer the end of middle childhood.

There are several reasons why children steal: a lack of a sense of property rights, an attempt to acquire the means with which to bribe favors from other children, a strong desire to own the coveted item, or a means for revenge in order to "get back at someone" (usually a parent) for what they consider to be unfair treatment. Older children may steal to supplement an inadequate income from other sources. Sometimes stealing is an indication that something is seriously wrong or lacking in the child's life. For example, children may steal to make up for love or another satisfaction that they feel is lacking.

In most situations it is best not to attempt to find a hidden or deep meaning to the stealing. An admonition, together with an appropriate and reasonable punishment, such as having the older child pay back the money or return the stolen items, ordinarily takes care of most cases. Many children can be taught to respect the property rights of others with little difficulty despite the temptations and opportunities presented to them. If children's personal rights are respected, they are more likely to respect the rights of others. Some children simply need more time to learn the importance of the culture's rules regarding private property.

Stress and Fear

Children today face more stresses than have children in previous generations. Many children are stressed by conflict within the home and have constant anxiety regarding the separation that these disruptions can cause. The school environment is another stressful experience for some children. Competition with classmates for grades and teacher recognition and being labeled as "stupid" or "learning disabled" can result in emotional discomfort. Increasing violence within the family and school also serves as a stressor for children.

To help children cope with the stresses in their lives, the parent, teacher, or health worker must be able to recognize signs that indicate a child is undergoing stress and identify the source promptly.

Nursing ALERT

The nurse who observes the following signs of stress in a child should explore the situation further:

- Stomach pains or headache
- Sleep problems
- Bed-wetting
- Changes in eating habits
- Aggressive or stubborn behavior
- Reluctance to participate
- Regression to earlier behaviors (e.g., thumb-sucking)

Children must be taught how to recognize signs of stress in themselves, such as a pounding heart, rapid breathing, or butterflies in the stomach. Once they are able to recognize that they are stressed, they can employ techniques for managing their stress. Probably the most useful technique is to help them plan a means for dealing with any stress through problem solving.

A wide variety and degree of anxiety symptoms, including fear of the dark, excessive worry about past behavior, self-consciousness, social withdrawal, and an excessive need for reassurance, are considered normal developmental events for children (Bell-Dolan, Last, and Strauss, 1990). School-age children are less fearful of body safety than they were as preschoolers, although they still fear being hurt, kidnapped, or having to undergo surgery. They also fear death and are fascinated by all the aspects of death and dying. There is a lessening of the fear of noises, darkness, storms, and dogs. Most of the new fears that trouble school-age children are related to school and family.

SUMMARY OF GROWTH AND DEVELOPMENT

The preceding stages of child development demonstrate individuality in the patterns of development. Each child has a unique developmental pattern; therefore any attempt to describe the typical child can only represent an average and should not be considered absolute criteria for any given child. A summary of growth and development in middle childhood is presented in Table 36-1.

Promoting Optimum Health During the School Years

When school-age children enter school, they leave the relatively protected environment of home and neighborhood and experience interpersonal contacts with a larger number of children. Many childhood illnesses can be prevented or lessened by careful health supervision. The body's natural defenses against illness can be supported through careful attention to diet, rest, and exercise and protection from extreme mental and physical stress.

NUTRITION

Although caloric needs are diminished in relation to body size during middle childhood, resources are being laid down for the increased growth needs of the adolescent period. It is important to impress on children and their parents the value of a diet that is balanced to promote growth. Since children usually eat as the family does, the quality of their diet depends to a large extent on the family's pattern of eating.

Likes and dislikes established at an early age continue in middle childhood, although the propensity for single food preferences begins to end and children acquire a taste for an increasing variety of foods. However, with the easy availability of fast-food restaurants, the influence of the mass media, and the temptation of an immense variety of "junk food," it is all too easy for children to fill up on empty calories—foods that do not promote growth, such as sugars, starches, and excess fats. The easy availability of high-calorie foods, combined with the tendency toward more sedentary activities, is contributing to an increasing prevalence of childhood obesity. This problem is discussed further in Chapter 37.

Parents do not know what their children eat when they are away from home. A parent may pack a lunch to be eaten at school but be unaware of how much is eaten, traded, sold, or thrown away. Nutrition education can and should be integrated with other classroom learning throughout the child's school years. In school the Food Guide Pyramid and the elements of a wholesome diet are learned, as well as how food products are grown, processed, and prepared. The school nurse can take an active role in nutrition education by working with teachers to plan and implement units on nutrition instruction and with parents and children to give nutritional guidance.

SLEEP AND REST

The amount of sleep and rest that is required during middle childhood is a highly individual matter. There is no specific amount needed by a child at any given age. The amount depends, rather, on the child's age, the activity level, and other factors, such as state of health. The growth rate has slowed; therefore less energy is expended in growth than was expended during the preceding periods.

During the school years, children usually do not require a nap, but they spend 8 to $9\frac{1}{2}$ hours in bed and sleep approximately 95% of that time (Coble et al, 1987). Although there are fewer bedtime problems with advancing years, there are still occasional difficulties associated with the necessary bedtime ritual. Usually there is little problem for children 6 and 7 years old, and the task of going to bed can be facilitated by encouraging quiet activity before bedtime, such as coloring and reading. However, most children in middle childhood must be reminded often to go to bed; 8- to 9-year-old and 11-year-old children are particularly resistant. Often children are unaware that they are tired; if they are allowed to remain up later than usual, they are fatigued the following day. Sometimes the bedtime resistance can be resolved by allowing a later bedtime in deference to the child's advancing age.

TABLE 36-1 Growth and development during school-age years

AGE (YEARS)	PHYSICAL AND MOTOR	MENTAL	ADAPTIVE	PERSONAL-SOCIAL
6	Growth and weight gain continues slowly Weight: 16-23.6 kg (35½-58 lb); height: 106.6-123.5 cm (42-48 inches) Central mandibular incisors erupt Loses first tooth Gradual increase in dexterity Active age; constant activity Often returns to finger feeding More aware of hand as a tool Likes to draw, print, and color Vision reaches maturity	Develops concept of numbers Counts 13 pennies Knows whether it is morning or afternoon Defines common objects such as fork and chair in terms of their use Obeys triple commands in succession Knows right and left hands Says which is pretty and which is ugly in a series of drawings of faces Describes the objects in a picture rather than simply enumerating them Attends first grade	At table, uses knife to spread butter or jam on bread At play, cuts, folds, pastes paper toys, sews crudely if needle is threaded Takes bath without supervision; performs bedtime activities alone Reads from memory; enjoys oral spelling game Likes table games, checkers, simple card games Giggles a lot Sometimes steals money or attractive items Has difficulty owning up to misdeeds Tries out own abilities	Can share and cooperate better Has great need for children of own age Will cheat to win Often engages in rough play Often jealous of younger brother or sister Does what adults are seen doing May have occasional temper tantrums Is a boaster Is more independent, probably influence of school Has own way of doing things Increases socialization
7	Begins to grow at least 5 cm (2 inches) a year Weight: 17.7-30 kg (39-66½ lb); height: 111.8-129.7 cm (44-51 inches) Maxillary central incisors and lateral mandibular incisors erupt More cautious in approaches to new performances Repeats performances to master them Jaw begins to expand to accommodate permanent teeth	Notices that certain parts are missing from pictures Can copy a diamond Repeats three numbers backward Develops concept of time; reads ordinary clock or watch correctly to nearest quarter hour; uses clock for practical purposes Attends the second grade More mechanical in reading; often does not stop at the end of a sentence, skips words such as *it, the,* and *he*	Uses table knife for cutting meat; may need help with tough or difficult pieces Brushes and combs hair acceptably without help May steal Likes to help and have a choice Is less resistant and stubborn	Is becoming a real member of the family group Takes part in group play Boys prefer playing with boys; girls prefer playing with girls Spends a lot of time alone; does not require a lot of companionship
8-9	Continues to grow at 5 cm (2 inches) a year Weight: 19.6-39.6 kg (43-87 lb); height: 117-141.8 cm (46-56 inches) Lateral incisors (maxillary) and mandibular cuspids erupt Movement fluid; often graceful and poised Always on the go; jumps, chases, skips Increased smoothness and speed in fine motor control; uses cursive writing Dresses self completely Likely to overdo; hard to quiet down after recess More limber; bones grow faster than ligaments	Gives similarities and differences between two things from memory Counts backward from 20 to 1; understands concept of reversibility Repeats days of the week and months in order; knows the date Describes common objects in detail, not merely their use Makes change out of a quarter Attends third and fourth grades Reads more; may plan to wake up early just to read Reads classic books, but also enjoys comics More aware of time; can be relied on to get to school on time Can grasp concepts of parts and whole (fractions)	Makes use of common tools such as hammer, saw, or screwdriver Uses household and sewing utensils Helps with routine household tasks such as dusting, sweeping Assumes responsibility for share of household chores Looks after all of own needs at table Buys useful articles; exercises some choice in making purchases Runs useful errands Likes pictorial magazines Likes school; wants to answer all the questions Is afraid of failing a grade; is ashamed of bad grades Is more critical of self Takes music and sports lessons	Is easy to get along with at home Likes the reward system Dramatizes Is more sociable Is better behaved Is interested in boy-girl relationships but will not admit it Goes about home and community freely, alone or with friends Likes to compete and play games Shows preference in friends and groups Plays mostly with groups of own sex but is beginning to mix Develops modesty Compares self with others Enjoys Scouts, group sports

TABLE 36-1 Growth and development during school-age years—cont'd

AGE (YEARS)	PHYSICAL AND MOTOR	MENTAL	ADAPTIVE	PERSONAL-SOCIAL
		Understands concepts of space, cause and effect, nesting (puzzles), conservation (permanence of mass and volume) Classifies objects by more than one quality; has collections Produces simple paintings or drawings		
10-12	*Boys:* Slow growth in height and rapid weight gain; may become obese in this period Weight: 24.3-58 kg (54-128 lb); height: 127.5-162.3 cm (50-64 inches) Posture is more similar to an adult's; will overcome lordosis *Girls:* pubescent changes may begin to appear; body lines soften and round out Remainder of teeth will erupt and tend toward full development (except wisdom teeth)	Writes brief stories Attends fifth to seventh grades Writes occasional short letters to friends or relatives on own initiative Uses telephone for practical purposes Responds to magazine, radio, or other advertising Reads for practical information or own enjoyment—stories or library books of adventure or romance, or animal stories	Makes useful articles or does easy repair work Cooks or sews in small way Raises pets Washes and fixes own hair Is responsible for a thorough job of cleaning hair, but may need reminding to do so Is sometimes left alone at home for an hour or so Is successful in looking after own needs or those of other children left in his or her care	Loves friends; talks about them constantly Chooses friends more selectively; may have a "best friend" Loves conversation Develops beginning interest in opposite sex Is more diplomatic Likes family; family really has meaning Likes mother and wants to please her in many ways Demonstrates affection Likes dad, too; he is adored and idolized Respects parents

Twelve-year-old children usually offer no difficulty in relation to bedtime. Some even retire early to enjoy slow preparations for bed, to read, or to listen to music.

EXERCISE AND ACTIVITY

The improved capabilities and adaptability of the school-age child permit greater speed and effort in motor activities; larger, stronger muscles permit longer and increasingly strenuous play without exhaustion. During middle childhood, youngsters acquire the coordination, timing, and concentration that are required to participate in adult-type activities, even though they may be deficient in the strength, stamina, and control of the adolescent and adult. Consequently, a larger amount of physical activity should be expected and encouraged during the school years. However, it must be kept in mind that although school-age children are large and appear to be strong, they may not be ready for strenuous competitive athletics.

All growing children need some regular exercise and should be afforded opportunities for various kinds that provide satisfying experiences to meet individual likes and dislikes. Appropriate activities that promote coordination and development during the school-age years include running, jumping rope, swimming, skating, and bicycle riding. Positive reinforcement achieved by experiencing increasingly smooth, rhythmic, and efficient use of the body conditions the child toward regular physical activity.

Exercise is essential for developmental progress in a number of areas, including muscle development and tone, refinement of balance and coordination, increased strength and endurance, and stimulation of body functions and metabolic processes. Children need ample space in which to run, jump, skip, and climb, and safe facilities and equipment to use both indoors and outdoors.

Children with disabling conditions or those who hesitate to become involved in active play, such as obese children, require special assessment and help so that activities that will appeal to them, that are compatible with their limitations, and that, at the same time, meet their developmental needs can be determined.

Sports

A great deal of controversy has surrounded the trend toward earlier participation in competitive athletics and the amount and type of competitive sports that are appropriate for children in the elementary grades. The current view is that virtually every child is suited for some type of sport, and authorities do not discourage participation if children are matched to the type of sport appropriate to their abilities and to their physical and emotional constitution. School-age children enjoy competition, and when those involved with children in this age-group understand children's physical limitations and teach them the proper techniques and safety measures necessary to avoid injury to developing bones and muscles, a safe and appropriate sport can be found for even the most unskilled and noncompetitive child (Fig. 36-7).

Various acceptable sports activities are available to school-age children (e.g., baseball, soccer, gymnastics, swimming). Equipment should be maintained in safe condition, and protective apparatus should be worn to prevent serious injury (see Traumatic Injury, Chapter 51).

During the school-age years, girls have the same basic body structure as boys and thus have a similar response to systematic exercise training. At puberty, when boys become larger and have more muscle mass, it is usually recommended that girls compete only against other girls. Before puberty there is no essential difference in strength and size between girls and boys, making these precautions unnecessary (Metcalf and Roberts, 1993).

The American Academy of Pediatrics, Committee on Sports Medicine and Committee on School Health (1989) recommends that preadolescence is a time to teach fundamental motor skills; develop fitness in a practical, safe, and gradual manner; and promote desired attitudes and values. Activities should include both practice sessions and unstructured play; the actual game or event should be managed in a manner that stresses mastery of the sport and enhancement of self-image rather than winning or pleasing others. All children should have an opportunity to participate, and special ceremonies should recognize all participants rather than individuals.

A

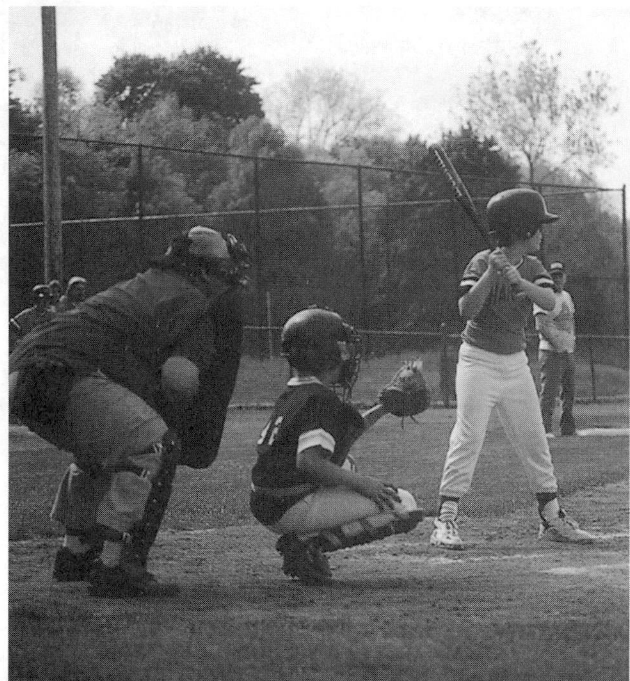

B

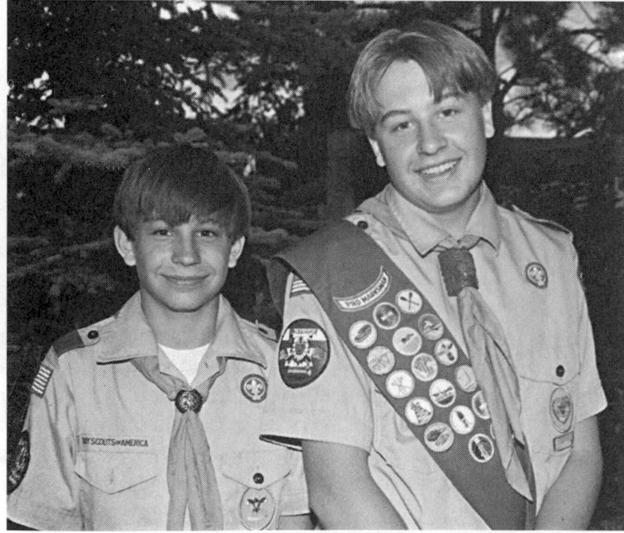

Fig. 36-7 The activities engaged in by school-age children vary according to interest and opportunity. **A,** Baseball. **B,** Scouting.

Acquisition of Skills

School-age children also demonstrate increasing capacities in fine muscle facility and complex artistic skills. Handedness is well established by the beginning of the school years, and children make great strides in writing and drawing during this age period. It is a time of energetic and vibrant creative productivity. With the tools of language and reading, children can create poems, stories, and plays. With more advanced fine motor skills, they are able to master an unlimited variety of handicrafts, such as ceramics, needlework, wood carving, and beadwork. They avidly pursue these skills in solitude, with a friend, or in programs offered through organized groups such as boys' or girls' clubs, Scouting, or special interest groups, which use crafts or other activities as a means to occupy, entertain, and educate children (Fig. 36-7).

School-age children can assume responsibility for their own needs, although their distaste for soap and water and "dress" clothes is legendary. School-age children can and want to assume their share of household tasks, which usually are related to the male and female roles defined by their culture, and many assume responsibility for tasks outside the home, such as baby-sitting, mowing lawns, or paper routes.

DENTAL HEALTH

The first permanent (secondary) teeth erupt at about 6 years of age, beginning with the 6-year molar, which erupts posterior to the deciduous molars. The others appear in approximately the same order as eruption of the primary teeth (see Teething, Chapter 33) and follow shedding of the deciduous teeth (Fig. 36-8). With the appearance of the second permanent (12-year) molar, most of the permanent teeth are present. Permanent dentition is somewhat more advanced in girls than it is in boys.

Since it is during the school-age years that the permanent teeth erupt, good dental hygiene and regular attention to dental caries are vital parts of health supervision during this period (see Dental Health, Chapter 34). Correct brushing techniques should be taught or reinforced, and the role that fermentable carbohydrates play in producing dental caries should be emphasized. It is also important to be alert to possible malocclusion problems that may result from irregular eruption of permanent teeth and that may impair function. Regular dental supervision and continued fluoride supplementation are as essential as regular medical supervision and should be an integral part of the health maintenance program.

The most effective means of preventing dental caries is

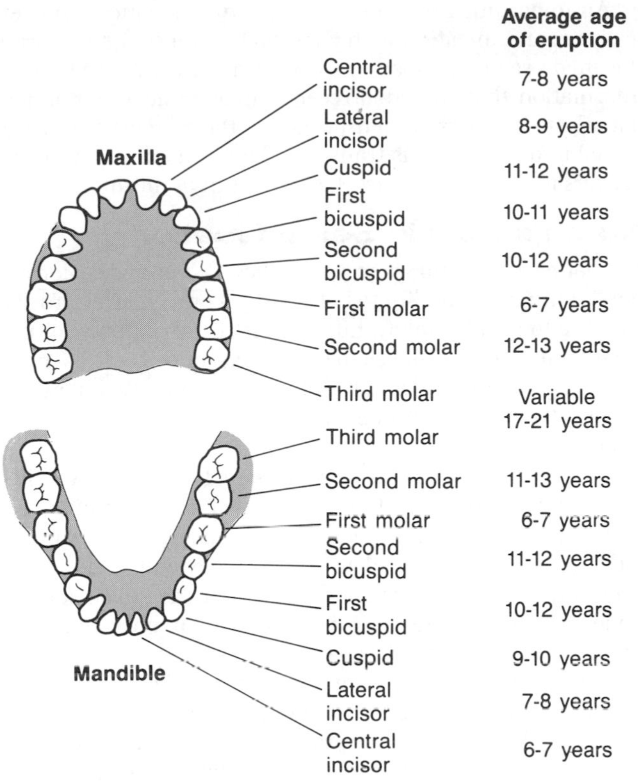

Maxilla

	Average age of eruption
Central incisor	7-8 years
Lateral incisor	8-9 years
Cuspid	11-12 years
First bicuspid	10-11 years
Second bicuspid	10-12 years
First molar	6-7 years
Second molar	12-13 years
Third molar	Variable 17-21 years
Third molar	
Second molar	11-13 years
First molar	6-7 years
Second bicuspid	11-12 years
First bicuspid	10-12 years
Cuspid	9-10 years
Lateral incisor	7-8 years
Central incisor	6-7 years

Mandible

Fig. 36-8 Sequence of eruption of secondary teeth. (Data from McDonald RE, Avery DR: *Dentistry for the child and adolescent*, ed 6, St Louis, 1994, Mosby).

proper oral hygiene. Children should be taught to carry out their own dental care with the supervision and guidance of the parents. Parents should learn the brushing technique along with their children, and they should inspect their children's efforts until the children can assume full responsibility.

Teeth should be brushed after meals, after snacks, and at bedtime. Children who brush their teeth frequently and become accustomed to the feel of a clean mouth at an early age usually maintain the habit throughout life. For the school-age child with mixed and permanent dentition the best toothbrush is one of soft nylon bristles with an overall length of about 21 cm. Numerous methods of brushing the teeth have been described and recommended for children, but there is no conclusive evidence that one method is superior to another. The thoroughness of the cleaning is more important than the specific technique used. The dentist will assess all factors, such as manipulative skills and any special needs of the child, and suggest the most appropriate brushing technique and regimen. Brushing is followed by flossing. Flossing is done by the parents until children acquire the manual dexterity needed. Most children are not able to floss properly until about 8 or 9 years of age.

Dental Problems

Limited or inadequate dental care results in the most prevalent of all childhood health problems: dental caries, malocclusion, and periodontal disease. Trauma, especially **tooth evulsion** is also an important problem. All of these conditions benefit from early intervention to prevent tooth loss.

Dental caries (cavities) is one of the most common chronic diseases that afflict humans at all ages; it is the principal oral problem in children and adolescents. Reducing the incidence and consequences of the disorder is of great importance in childhood because dental caries, if untreated, results in total destruction of the involved teeth. The ages of greatest vulnerability are 4 to 8 years for the primary dentition and 12 to 18 years for the secondary or permanent dentition.

Dental caries is a multifactorial disease; it involves susceptible teeth, cariogenic microflora, and an appropriate oral environment. The incidence of lesions and the likelihood of progressive invasion vary considerably and depend on a number of factors being present in the right combination. Oral inspection is an integral part of the nursing assessment of the child. If there is any evidence of dental caries or other unhealthy state, the child is referred for dental services. An alarming number of children do not receive regular dental supervision, and a significant number reach adulthood without having been examined or treated by a dentist.

Periodontal disease, inflammatory and degenerative conditions involving the gums and tissues supporting the teeth, often begins in childhood and accounts for a significant amount of tooth loss in adulthood. The more common periodontal problems are *gingivitis* (simple inflammation of the gums) and *periodontitis* (inflammation of the gums and loss of connective tissue and bone in the supporting structures of the teeth).

The most prevalent periodontal disease, gingivitis, is a reversible inflammatory disease that begins very early in many children and is most often associated with the buildup of plaque on the teeth. Changes take place in the plaque bacteria, in both type and number of organisms, causing them to release various destructive exotoxins, enzymes, and other noxious agents. They act to produce an inflammatory reaction in the gingival tissues, causing the gums to become red, edematous, tender, and subject to bleeding at the slightest irritation. Management is directed toward prevention by conscientious brushing and flossing, including the use of fluoride. The child should see the dentist at any signs of inflammation or irritation.

Malocclusion occurs when teeth of the upper and lower dental arches do not approximate in the proper relationships; the physiologic function of chewing is less effective and the cosmetic effect is less pleasing. Teeth that are uneven, crowded, or overlapping or are otherwise unable to meet their counterparts in the opposite jaw in the appropriate relationships may be predisposed to disease in later years.

Orthodontic treatment is usually most successful when it is started in the later school-age years or the early teenage years, after the last primary teeth have been shed and before growth ceases. However, referral should be made as soon as malocclusion is evident, since some deformities can be corrected at an earlier age.

Dental injury may occur in childhood and includes fractures of varying degrees of severity, chipping, dislocation, or evulsion. All tooth injuries require prompt treatment by a competent dentist to prevent permanent displacement or loss. Delayed examination and diagnosis of tooth damage can result in infection or pulp involvement. Also, because it can affect the remaining teeth, replacement of the lost tooth is

EMERGENCY

EVULSED TOOTH

Recover tooth.
Hold tooth by crown; avoid touching root area.
If tooth is dirty, rinse it gently under running water or saline solution; be sure to insert stopper in sink or basin (to avoid tooth loss).
Insert tooth into socket.
Have child maintain tooth in place.
Transport child to dentist immediately.
Avoid sudden stops or sharp turns to prevent dislodging tooth.

If reluctant to reimplant tooth:

Place evulsed tooth in suitable medium for transport:
1. Cold milk
2. Saliva—under child's or parent's tongue

If child is holding tooth in the mouth, avoid sudden stops to prevent swallowing tooth.
DON'T FORGET TO TAKE TOOTH.

needed to maintain normal alignment and position of the other teeth.

A tooth that is *evulsed* (avulsed, exarticulated, or "knocked out") should be replanted by the child, parent, or nurse and stabilized as soon as possible so that the blood supply to the tooth can be reestablished and the tooth kept alive (see the Emergency box above). If the tooth is replaced within 30 minutes, there is a 70% chance that it will become reattached and roots will not resorb or the crown exfoliate. Evulsed primary teeth are usually not reimplanted.

As with all mouth trauma, an evulsed tooth causes a large amount of bleeding, which is most distressing to the child. Bleeding is frightening to children and their families; therefore the nurse or anyone who is faced with dental trauma should be prepared to cope with the emotionality that accompanies tooth evulsion. Using a calm approach and providing gentle reassurance to the child requires only a moment and goes a long way toward reducing anxiety.

SEX EDUCATION

Evidence indicates that many children experience some form of sex play during or before preadolescence as a response to normal curiosity, not as a result of love or sexual urge. Children are experimentalists by nature, and this play is incidental and transitory. Any adverse emotional consequences or guilt feelings depend on how the behavior is managed by the parents, if it is discovered, or whether children view their actions as wrong in the eyes of significant persons, particularly the parents (Levine, 1992).

The child's attitude toward sex is acquired indirectly at a very early age. Initial curiosity about differences in body structure between boys and girls and between children and adults arises in the preschool years. Middle childhood is an ideal time for formal sex education, and many authorities believe that the topic is best presented from a life-span approach. Information about sexual maturation and the process of reproduction helps to minimize the child's uncertainty, embarrassment, and feelings of isolation that often accompany puberty.

An important component of ongoing sex education is effective communication with parents. If parents either repress the child's sexual curiosity or avoid dealing with it, the sexual information that the child receives may be acquired almost entirely from peers. When peers are the primary source of sexual information, it is transmitted and exchanged in secret conversation and contains a large amount of misinformation.

Nurse's Role in Sex Education

No matter where nurses practice, they can provide information on human sexuality to both parents and children. To discuss the topic adequately, nurses must have not only an understanding of the physiologic aspects of sexuality and a knowledge of cultural and societal values, but also an awareness of their own attitudes, feelings, and biases about sexuality.

When sexual information is presented to school-age children, sex and sexuality should be treated as a normal part of growth and development. Questions should be answered honestly, matter-of-factly, and to the same extent as questions about other topics. Answers should be at the child's level of understanding. There may be times when boys and girls should be taught content separately.

Children need help to differentiate sex and sexuality. Exercises on clarifying values, identifying role models, engaging in problem-solving skills, and practicing responsibility are important prerequisites to the sexual information needed in early adolescence. In addition, children need to have much of the sexual information that is provided to them via the media or jokes explained and defused. Information concerning the acquired immunodeficiency syndrome (AIDS) should be presented in simple, accurate terms and should focus on how the AIDS virus is transmitted (Schonfeld et al, 1993).

Preadolescents need more precise information. They are interested in concrete information, such as "What if I start my period in the middle of class?" or "How can I keep people from telling I have an erection?" It is important to tell them what they want to know and what they can expect to happen as they mature sexually.

During encounters with parents, nurses can be open and available for questions and discussion. They can set an example by the language they use in discussing body parts and their function and by the way in which they deal with problems that have emotional overtones, such as exploratory sex play and masturbation. Parents need help to understand normal behaviors and to view sexual curiosity in their children as a part of the developmental process. Assessing the parents' level of knowledge and understanding of sexuality provides cues to their need for supplemental information that will better prepare them for the increasingly complex explanations that will be needed as their children grow older.

SCHOOL HEALTH

Child health maintenance is ultimately the responsibility of the parents; however, the public schools and health departments in the United States have contributed to the improvement of child health by providing a healthful school environment, health services, and health education that emphasizes sound health practices. Most of these functions constitute major components of community health services and involve large amounts of public funds and large numbers of health professionals, including nurses.

A school health program is involved in ongoing health maintenance through assessment, screening, and referral activities. Routine health services provided by most schools include health appraisal, emergency care, safety education, communicable disease control, counseling, and follow-up care. The health education of schoolchildren is primarily directed toward providing knowledge of health and influencing habits, attitudes, and conduct in relation to health and injury prevention.

Traditionally, school nurses have been viewed from a limited perspective that placed them in the role of disease detector, applier of bandages, and official caregiver in cases of illness and injury. Although these are still important functions, this traditional role is acquiring much broader dimensions. School nurses are being prepared to provide primary health care on a broader scale, including the assessment of physical, psychomedical, psychoeducational, behavioral, and learning disorder problems, and to offer comprehensive well-child care. Many health care reformers are also proposing that school health services be enlarged beyond meeting the needs of schoolchildren to meet those of their families and the community (Igoe, 1993). School nurse practitioners will play an essential role in these school-based centers.

Since the passage of Public Laws 94-142 and 99-457, which require the integration of children with chronic illness or disability into the regular classrooms, school health services are also responsible for the medical and nursing needs of these children. School nurse practitioners are vital to the development, implementation, and evaluation of health care plans and programs for these children. Unfortunately, not all schools have a school nurse, and the use of unlicensed assistive personnel (UAP) is increasing. School nurses are faced with the delegation to and supervision of UAP (Delegation, 1995).

INJURY PREVENTION

Because school-age children have developed more refined muscular coordination and control and can apply their cognitive capacities to a more judicious course of action, the incidence of injury is diminished in children in this age group when compared with the incidence in early childhood.

The most common cause of severe injury and death in school-age children is motor vehicle accidents—either as pedestrian or passenger. Nurses must continue to emphasize the importance of the three automobile safety measures that have been found to reduce the severity of injuries: effective restraint systems, door-lock mechanisms, and appropriate passenger seating locations in the motor vehicle.

The school-age child's desire for riding bicycles increases the risk of injury on streets and byways. Other serious injuries include accidents on skateboards, trampolines, sleds, skates, skis, and other sports equipment. All-terrain vehicles (ATVs), popular with children under 16 years of age, are unstable, difficult to handle, and responsible for an increasing number of childhood injuries (Dolan, Knapp, and Andres, 1989).

Most injuries occur in or near the home or school. The most effective means of prevention is education of the child and family regarding the hazards of risk taking and improper use of the equipment. Safety helmets, protective eye and mouth shields, and protective padding are strongly recommended for children engaged in active sports, even though they may not be required equipment. For example, falls from bicycles, ATVs, and skating devices cause a significant number of head injuries in school-age children. Since head injury is the major cause of bicycle-related fatalities, probably the single most important aspect of bicycle safety is to encourage the rider to wear a protective helmet (Fig. 36-9; American Academy of Pediatrics, 1995). Physically active school-age children are highly susceptible to cuts and abrasions, and the incidence of childhood fractures, strains, and sprains is noteworthy. The incidence is significantly higher in school-age boys than in school-age girls. Injuries of a serious nature are discussed as appropriate elsewhere in the book—burns (Chapter 50), eye trauma (Chapter 39), near-drowning (Chapter 48), and head injuries (Chapter 48). The prevalence of injuries depends on the dangers present in the environment, the protection offered by adults, and the behavior patterns of the children. See Table 36-2 for the major developmental accomplishments and suggestions for prevention, and see the Home Care boxes on p. 1071 for bicycle safety and skateboard and in-line skating safety.

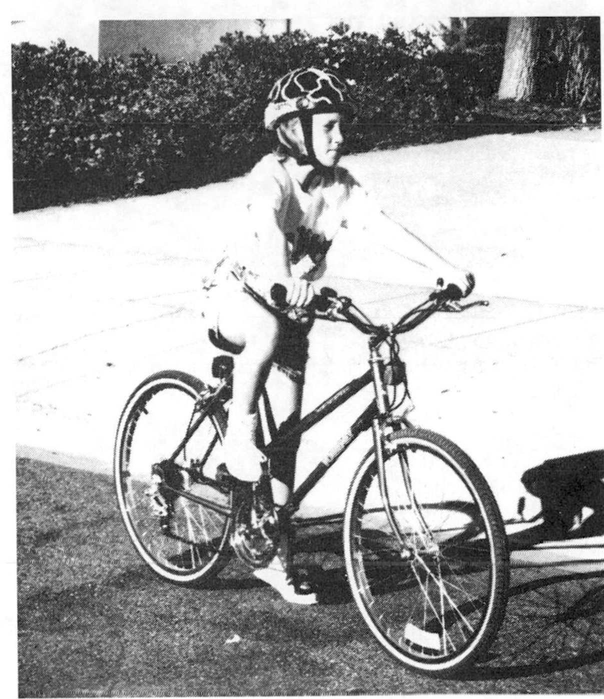

Fig. 36-9 The right-size bike is important; the child should be able to sit on the bike and place balls of both feet on the ground. Foot should comfortably reach and manipulate the pedal in the down position. Wearing a protective helmet is mandatory. Helmet should sit on top of the head in a level position and should not rock back and forth or side to side. The strap should always be fastened securely under the chin.

ANTICIPATORY GUIDANCE—CARE OF FAMILIES

Parents of the school-age child find themselves in the position of sharing their child's time with the increasingly important peer group. It is through early peer relationships that children begin to prepare for moving from narrow, sheltered family relationships to a broader world of relationships and increased independence. Parents must learn to provide support as un-

TABLE 36-2 Injury prevention during school-age years

DEVELOPMENTAL ABILITIES RELATED TO RISK OF INJURY	INJURY PREVENTION
Is increasingly involved in activities away from home Is excited by speed and motion Is easily distracted by environment Can be reasoned with	**Motor vehicles** Educate child regarding proper use of seat belts while a passenger in a vehicle Maintain discipline while a passenger in a vehicle (e.g., keep arms inside, do not lean against doors or interfere with driver) Emphasize safe pedestrian behavior Insist on wearing safety apparel (e.g., helmet) where applicable, such as riding bicycle, motorcycle, moped, and ATVs (see the Home Care boxes on p. 1071)
Is apt to overdo May work hard to perfect a skill Has cautious, but not fearful, gross motor actions Likes swimming	**Drowning** Teach child to swim Teach basic rules of water safety Select safe and supervised places to swim Check sufficient water depth for diving Swim with a companion Use an approved flotation device in water or boat Advocate for legislation requiring fencing around pools Learn cardiopulmonary resuscitation (CPR)
Has increasing independence Is adventuresome Enjoys trying new things	**Burns** Instruct child in behavior in areas involving contact with potential burn hazards (e.g., gasoline, matches, bonfires or barbecues, lighter fluid, firecrackers, cigarette lighters, cooking utensils, chemistry sets); avoid climbing or flying kite around high-tension wires Instruct child in proper behavior in the event of fire (e.g., fire drills at home, school, and so on) Teach child safe cooking (use low heat, avoid any frying, be careful of steam burns, scalds, or exploding foods, especially from microwaving)
Adheres to group rules May be easily influenced by peers Strong allegiance to friends	**Poisoning** Educate child regarding hazards of taking nonprescription drugs and chemicals, including aspirin and alcohol Teach child to say "no" if offered illegal or dangerous drugs or alcohol Keep potentially dangerous products in properly labeled receptacles—preferably out of reach

Has increased physical skills
Needs strenuous physical activity
Is interested in acquiring new skills and perfecting attained skills
Is daring and adventurous, especially with peers
Frequently plays in hazardous places
Confidence often exceeds physical capacity
Desires group loyalty and has strong need for friends' approval
Attempts hazardous feats
Accompanies friends to potentially hazardous facilities
Delights in physical activity
Is likely to overdo
Growth in height exceeds muscular growth and coordination
	Bodily damage
	Help provide facilities for supervised activities
	Encourage playing in safe places
	Keep firearms safely locked up except during adult supervision
	Teach proper care of, use of, and respect for devices with potential danger (power tools, firecrackers, and so on)
	Teach children not to tease or surprise dogs, invade their territory, take dogs' toys, or interfere with dogs' feeding
	Stress eye, ear, or mouth protection when using potentially hazardous objects or devices or when engaged in potentially hazardous sports
	Teach safety regarding use of corrective devices (glasses); if child wears contact lenses, monitor duration of wear to prevent corneal damage
	Stress careful selection, use, and maintenance of sports and recreation equipment, such as skateboards and in-line skates (see the Home Care box on p. 1071)
	Emphasize proper conditioning, safe practices, and use of safety equipment for sports or recreational activities
	Caution against engaging in hazardous sports, such as those involving trampolines
	Use safety glass and decals on large glassed areas, such as sliding glass doors
	Teach name, address, and phone number and to ask for help from appropriate people (cashier, security guard, police) if lost; have identification on child (sewn in clothes, inside shoe)
	Teach personal safety:
	  Avoid personalized clothing in public places
	  Never go with a stranger
	  Tell parents if anyone makes child feel uncomfortable in any way
	  Always listen to child's concerns regarding others' behavior
	  Say "no" when confronted with uncomfortable situations

Home Care

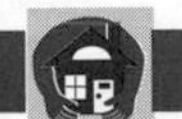

BICYCLE SAFETY

Always wear properly fitted bicycle helmet that is approved by Snell or the American National Standards Institute (ANSI) (Fig. 36-9); replace damaged helmet.
Ride bicycles with traffic and away from parked cars.
Ride single file.
Walk bicycles through busy intersections only at crosswalks.
Give hand signals well in advance of turning or stopping.
Keep as close to the curb as practical.
Watch for drain grates, potholes, soft shoulders, and loose dirt or gravel.
Keep both hands on handlebars, except with signaling.
Never ride double on a bicycle.
Do not carry packages that interfere with vision or control; do not drag objects behind bike.
Watch for and yield to pedestrians.
Watch for cars backing up or pulling out of driveways; be especially careful at intersections.
Look left, right, then left before turning into traffic or roadway.
Never hitch a ride on a truck or other vehicle.
Learn rules of the road and respect for traffic officers.
Obey all local ordinances.
Wear shoes that fit securely while riding.
Wear light colors at night and attach fluorescent material to clothing and bicycle.
Be certain the bicycle is the correct size for rider.
Equip bicycle with proper lights and reflectors.
Have the bicycle inspected to ensure good mechanical condition.
Children riding as passengers must wear appropriate-size helmets in specially designed protective seats.

From American Academy of Pediatrics, Comittee on Injury and Poison Prevention: Bicycle helmets, *Pediatrics* 95(4):609-610, 1995.

Home Care

SKATEBOARD AND IN-LINE SKATE SAFETY

Children younger than 5 years of age should not use skateboards or in-line skates. They are not developmentally prepared to protect themselves from injury.
Children who ride skateboards or in-line skates should wear helmets and protective equipment, especially on knees, wrists, and elbows, to prevent injury.
Skateboards and in-line skates should never be ridden near traffic. Their use should be prohibited on streets and highways. Activities that bring skateboards together (e.g., "catching a ride") are especially dangerous.
Some types of use, such as riding homemade ramps on hard surfaces, may be particularly hazardous.

Modified from American Academy of Pediatrics, Committee on Injury and Poison Prevention: Skateboard injuries, *Pediatrics* 95(4):611-612, 1995.

Home Care

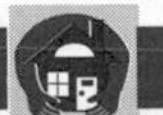

GUIDANCE DURING SCHOOL YEARS

Age 6 years

Prepare parents to expect strong food preferences and frequent refusal of specific food items.
Prepare parents to expect increasingly ravenous appetite.
Prepare parents for emotionality as child experiences erratic mood changes.
Help parents anticipate continued susceptibility to illness.
Teach injury prevention and safety, especially bicycle safety.
Encourage parents to respect child's need for privacy and to provide a separate bedroom for child, if possible.
Prepare parents for child's increasing interests outside the home.
Help parents understand the need to encourage child's interactions with peers.

Ages 7 to 10 years

Prepare parents to expect improvement in health with fewer illnesses, but warn them that allergies may increase or become apparent.
Prepare parents to expect an increase in minor injuries.
Emphasize caution in selecting and maintaining sports equipment and reemphasize safety.
Prepare parents to expect increased involvement with peers and interest in activities outside the home.
Emphasize the need to encourage independence while maintaining limit setting and discipline.
Prepare mothers to expect more demands at 8 years.
Prepare fathers to expect increasing admiration at 10 years; encourage father-child activities.
Prepare parents for prepubescent changes in girls.

Ages 11 to 12 years

Help parents prepare child for body changes of pubescence.
Prepare parents to expect a growth spurt in girls.
Make certain child's sex education is adequate with accurate information.
Prepare parents to expect energetic but stormy behavior at 11 years to become more even tempered at 12 years.
Encourage parents to support child's desire to "grow up" but to allow regressive behavior when needed.
Prepare parents to expect an increase in masturbation.
Instruct parents that the amount of rest the child needs may increase.
Help parents educate child regarding experimentation with potentially harmful activities.

Health guidance

Help parents understand the importance of regular health and dental care for the child.
Encourage parents to teach and model sound health practices—including diet, rest, activity, and exercise.
Stress the need to encourage children to engage in appropriate physical activities.
Emphasize providing a safe physical and emotional environment.
Encourage parents to teach and model safety practices.

obtrusively as possible without feeling rejected, hurt, or angry. The nurse can help parents of the school-age child by providing anticipatory guidance and reassurance throughout this period of child development and maturation (see the Home Care box on p. 1071, right).

Special Health Problems

HEALTH PROBLEMS RELATED TO SPORTS PARTICIPATION

Every sport has some potential for injury to the participant—whether the youngster engages in serious competition or participates for enjoyment. Serious injury can occur during rough contact sports or to persons who are not physically prepared for the activity. The risk of injury is greater if the youngster's body build is not suited to the sport, if the muscles and support systems (respiratory and cardiovascular) are insufficiently conditioned to withstand the rigors of the physical stress, or if the youngster lacks the insight and judgment to recognize when an activity is beyond his or her capabilities. More injuries occur during recreational sports participation than in organized athletic competition.

Not only does the activity itself pose a hazard of greater or lesser degree (Fig. 36-10), but the environment and the sports or recreational equipment present additional risks. Children participate in physical activity in various environments, both indoors and outdoors, on floors, on the ground, on snow, on or beneath water surfaces, and sometimes in free air space. These activities frequently involve equipment that intensifies the risk factor.

Acute overload injuries occur suddenly during an activity and produce immediate symptoms. They can be caused by a blow or overstretching, twisting, or sudden stress to tissues.

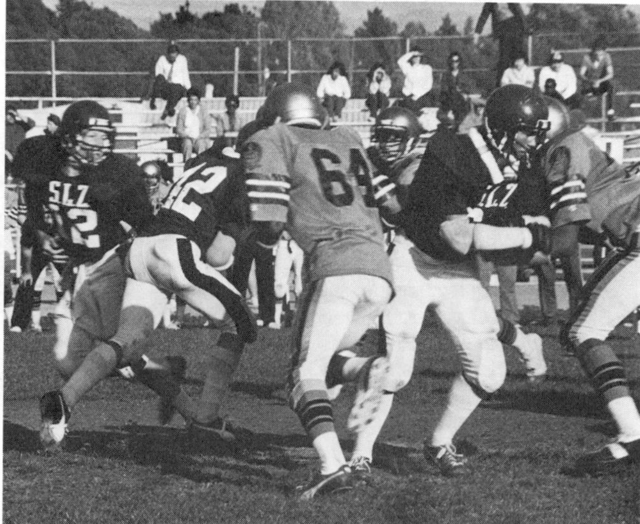

Fig. 36-10 Football is an example of a strenuous collision sport.

For descriptions and management of traumatic injuries, see Chapter 51.

Overuse Syndromes

To excel in sports the young athlete is forced to train longer, harder, and earlier in life than previously. The rewards are an increased level of fitness, better performances, faster times, and the satisfaction of attaining a personal goal. However, the risk of overuse injury is always present and can be related to several factors: training errors, muscle-tendon imbalance, anatomic malalignment, incorrect footwear or playing surface, an associated disease state, and growth.

The common feature in overuse injuries is the repetitive microtrauma that occurs to a particular anatomic structure when the same movements are performed over a long period of time. The end result is inflammation of the involved structure with complaints of pain, tenderness, swelling, and disability. Examples of overuse syndromes include "Little League elbow" (tendinitis and osteochondritis from repetitive throwing), "tennis elbow" (lateral epicondylitis from repetitive elbow strain), and Osgood-Schlatter disease (traction apophysitis of tibial tubercle).

Stress fractures. Stress fractures occur as a result of repeated muscle contraction and are seen most often in repetitive weightbearing sports such as running, gymnastics, and basketball. They occur less often in swimmers. The most common symptoms are a sharp, persistent, progressive pain or a deep, persistent, dull ache located over the bone. Sometimes there is pain on impact (heel strike), but the most important clinical sign is pain over the involved bony surface. Diagnosis is established on the basis of clinical observation. Occasionally a bone scan may be needed.

Therapeutic management. Development of inflammation is common to all overuse syndromes; therefore the management is directed toward rest or alteration of activities, physical therapy, and medication. Rest is the primary therapy and is usually interpreted as reduced activity and the use of alternative exercise—*not* bed rest or immobilization with casting. The primary purpose is to alleviate the repetitive stress that initiated the symptoms. It is important to keep the youngster mobile. Training can be continued with alternative exercise that maintains conditioning without aggravating the injury. For example, pool running (treading water in the deep end of a pool) can use the same movements as running but without the weight bearing.

Other modalities include cryotherapy and cold whirlpools. Sometimes taping, bracing, splinting, and other orthotics are employed (treatment is very specific to the injury). Medications such as nonsteroidal antiinflammatory drugs are prescribed for discomfort. Topical medications are of questionable value.

Nurse's Role in Sports for Children and Adolescents

Nurses may become involved in sports activities in the areas of preparation and evaluation for activities, prevention of injury, treatment of injuries, and rehabilitation after injury. Selecting an appropriate sport for both recreation and competition is a joint effort of youngster, parents, and health professionals.

The best approach to counseling children and parents regarding sports participation is to encourage activities that are most likely to provide pleasure and physical benefits throughout childhood and into adulthood. Exposure to various sports activities is probably better for young children than limiting them to one sport. Parents should be cautioned against overprogramming children so that the children have ample time for other activities and associations.

When children sustain athletic injuries, nurses are often responsible for instructing the children and their parents regarding care. Instructions (e.g., schedule for appointments, application of ice, and any restrictions in activity) should be made clear and preferably be accompanied by written directions. The importance of taking medications as prescribed is emphasized, since they may be needed for an extended period of time and compliance may be difficult.

Prevention of sports injuries is probably the most important aspect of any athletic program. Children should be suited to the activity, and the environment and equipment should be safe for physical activity. Children should be adequately prepared for the sport, especially if it requires strenuous and/or continuous physical exertion. Nurses collaborate with coaches and athletic trainers to ensure that safety measures are carried out. Stretching exercises, warming up and cooling down activities, and an appropriate training program are only some of the requisites for safe participation. Protective measures, such as pads, taping, wrapping, or other devices, are employed for areas at risk. Nurses are also on the alert for environmental safety risks.

ALTERED GROWTH AND MATURATION

The absence of physical and/or sexual maturation at a time when other children are experiencing positive evidence of sexual development and its associated spurt in growth and physical strength is a matter of concern to both the parents and their affected child. Fortunately, in most instances the delay in development is a simple physiologic or **constitutional delay** that merely represents one end of the normal genetically influenced variation of pubertal growth. These children will go through a delayed but normal puberty to finally catch up, in their late teens, with their more rapidly developing age-mates. Less benign causes of delayed development may be of endocrine origin or chromosomal aberrations. In other situations, delayed development may result from chronic diseases (such as malabsorption or chronic asthma) that are serious enough to retard the developmental process or environmental factors (such as stress or poor nutrition).

Serial measurements of growth are plotted periodically on standard growth charts to determine the pattern of growth and to compare the individual child with the norm for that particular age group. When assessing children in the extremes of height ranges, it is important to compare their height with the height of their parents and siblings.

Tall or Short Stature

Tall stature. Despite the fact that the average height of both boys and girls is steadily increasing, there is still a small group of children who, because of some organic disorder or a familial tendency, are excessively tall when compared with their contemporaries. To some, especially boys, it may be a source of pride; to others, especially girls, it may be a source of intense anxiety and a severe social handicap.

When the rate of height change before puberty suggests the probability of excessive adult height, treatment with hormones may be considered, although there is a great deal of controversy regarding their use for this purpose. The use of estrogens has proved effective in controlling height when therapy is initiated before menarche and before the end of the adolescent growth spurt that normally precedes menarche. The selection of children for hormonal therapy is based on careful evaluation of physical, psychologic, and social factors.

Short stature. Short stature is a nonspecific finding that may be the first manifestation of a serious disorder, or it may be of no consequence medically. From a worldwide point of view the most common cause of short stature and/or delayed development is probably inadequate nutrition; however, the major disorders that produce delayed development are chronic diseases, endocrine dysfunction, and syndromes of primary gonadal failure.

Chronic diseases can interfere with growth, but unless the illness is unduly prolonged, catch-up growth will occur. Diseases and disorders that usually cause some degree of growth delay include asthma, cystic fibrosis, gastrointestinal diseases (such as parasitic infections), malabsorption syndromes, cardiac anomalies, and chronic renal disturbances. The duration of the illness is more significant than the intensity in terms of the effect on growth, although the precise length of time necessary to affect growth permanently has not been determined.

Skeletal disorders that affect growth in stature are principally those described as dwarfism. Most are caused by various congenital defects and disorders, such as achondroplasia, and by some of the inborn errors of metabolism, such as Hurler or Hunter syndrome.

Psychosocial or *deprivation dwarfism* is a stress-induced growth failure that appears to be more common than previously thought. It is defined as growth retardation in children over 2 years of age caused by environmental (emotional) stress and is associated with a marked delay in physical growth, delayed developmental skills, and immature behavior. When these children are removed from the deprived environment, their growth proceeds at a normal or increased rate. (See Failure to Thrive, Chapter 33, and Child Maltreatment, Chapter 35.)

Management consists of continued medical observation, attention to general health and nutrition, and psychologic support. Where growth delay is accompanied by poor self-esteem, many authorities recommend hormonal therapy. Testosterone in carefully regulated doses has proved effective in some cases. Growth hormone is capable of increasing height and is used to treat growth hormone deficiency. Its use with children who have constitutional delay is highly controversial (see Hypopituitarism, Chapter 49).

Nursing care management. Deviation from the normal course of puberty is always of concern to the affected youngster, and to some it assumes monumental proportions. Most of the problems of delayed development are caused by simple constitutional delay of puberty, and in this situation the child can be assured that the normal course of events will eventually take place.

One of the difficulties related to a size that is incongruent with chronologic and mental age is the manner in which others, especially adults, relate to the child. People quite naturally respond to children with short stature as though they are younger than their age. Consequently, these children often react with babyish or juvenile behavior, thus setting in motion a circular pattern of behavior and response. Conversely, children who are tall or physically advanced for their age are frequently treated as though they are more advanced than their years. They are often considered to be retarded or behaviorally immature when they actually perform according to the normal behavioral expectations for their age.

Listening to distressed youngsters and conveying to them interest and concern are prerequisite to any successful intervention. Counseling and therapy are individualized to meet the needs of each child. Encouraging these children to accentuate the positive aspects of their bodies and personalities with sound health practices and good grooming helps foster a more positive self-image.

Sex Chromosome Abnormalities

Compared with most hereditary disorders, sex chromosome abnormalities are encountered with relatively high frequency. Most are caused by an alteration in sex chromosome number, some of which are listed in Table 36-3. The more common of these are Turner and Klinefelter syndromes. Some general characteristics of sex chromosome abnormalities are as follows:

1. There is a direct relationship between the male or female body type and the presence or absence of a Y chromosome. It appears that the Y chromosome is essential for the development of male characteristics.
2. The severity of defects is not related to the number of extra X chromosomes, except for mental retardation, which increases proportionately with each X chromosome.
3. The presence of more than one Y chromosome appears to have variable but as yet not well-defined effects on an individual.
4. The majority of these conditions are caused by nondisjunction.

Turner syndrome. Turner syndrome is caused by absence of one of the X chromosomes; as a result, the number of chromosomes in these girls is 45—44 pairs of autosomes and 1 X chromosome (45,X). The incidence of the condition in the population has been estimated at 1 in 2500 female births. Although this disorder is often recognized at birth with the signs of a webbed neck, low posterior hairline, widely spaced nipples, and edema of the hands and feet, it is diagnosed most frequently at puberty because of three outstanding features: short stature, sexual infantilism, and amenorrhea.

Girls with Turner syndrome will always be sterile. They have been found to have difficulty with peer relationships and understanding social cues. They exhibit more behavioral problems, especially in relation to immature, socially isolated behavior. Definitive diagnosis is confirmed on the basis of a negative sex chromatin test; chromosomal analysis is rarely necessary.

Therapy is always individualized for these girls and consists primarily of hormone treatment and psychologic counseling for both child and parents. Linear growth often can be increased by the administration of growth hormone, provided therapy is begun early. Estrogen therapy is initiated during the usual time for puberty to promote the development of secondary sex characteristics. Responses to estrogen therapy vary from girl to girl, but gradual feminization is accomplished to some degree in most individuals.

TABLE 36-3 Common sex chromosome abnormalities

SYNDROME	CHROMOSOMAL NOMENCLATURE	PHENOTYPE	INCIDENCE (LIVE BIRTHS)	CLINICAL MANIFESTATIONS
Turner	45,X or 45,XO	Female	1:2500 female births*	Short stature; webbed neck; low posterior hairline; shield-shaped chest with widely spaced nipples; sterile; no development of secondary sex characteristics; learning disabled
Triple X or superfemale	47,XXX (can also be 48,XXXX or 49,XXXXX)	Female	1:850-1250 female births	Normal female characteristics; usually tall; variable mental capacity and behavior, at risk for impaired learning; fertile
XYY male	47,XYY (can also be 48,XYYY or mosaic)	Male	1:900 male births*	Usually normal sexual development; tendency to be tall with long head; poor coordination; may demonstrate aberrant behavior
Klinefelter	47,XXY (48,XXYY, 48,XXXY, 49,XXXXY, and so on, mosaics)	Male	1:850 male births*	Tall with long legs; hypogenitalism; sterile; male secondary sex characteristics may be deficient; may demonstrate aberrant behavior; learning disabled; possible gynecomastia
Fragile X (see also Chapter 39)	46,XY or 46,XX	Predominantly male	Not established	Normocephaly or macrocephaly; prominent mandible; large ears; macroorchidism; mental retardation

*Data from Nora JJ, Fraser FC: *Medical genetics: principles and practice*, ed 3, Philadelphia, 1989, Lea & Febiger.

Klinefelter syndrome. The most common of all chromosomal abnormalities, Klinefelter syndrome, is caused by the presence of one or more additional X chromosomes. The majority of males with this syndrome have a chromosomal complement of 47,XXY. In young boys this disorder is seldom seen before puberty, at which time varying degrees of failure of adolescent virilization occur. Some males are not detected until they appear for evaluation for infertility. All have absence of sperm in the semen (azoospermia), small testes, and defective development of secondary sex characteristics. The incidence of Klinefelter syndrome is estimated to be approximately 1 in 850 live male births. In 80% of these boys there is a chromatin-positive buccal smear, and the extra chromosome is apparent on chromosomal analysis.

Cognitive impairment of varying degrees is a frequent finding and appears to have a direct relationship to the number of X chromosomes in the cells. Boys with Klinefelter syndrome may also have gross motor skill difficulties, developmental language delay, poor verbal skills, and reduced auditory memory. Shyness, passivity, behavioral problems, and school difficulties are often associated with the disorder, but this may be related to the difference in body build and delayed development.

The major effort in medical treatment is directed toward enhancing the masculine characteristics through the administration of male hormones, principally testosterone. Cosmetic surgery will eliminate embarrassment for the boy with gynecomastia.

Nursing care management. The nursing care of children with Turner or Klinefelter syndrome is primarily supportive. Nurses assist in diagnosis, explain tests and therapies to children and families, and provide support and encouragement. Since both disorders render the individual unable to reproduce, psychologic counseling, as well as modification of sex education, will be an important aspect of care. Marriage and sexual relationships are still possible, and alternative reproductive options, such as artificial insemination and adoption, should be discussed.

DISORDERS WITH BEHAVIORAL COMPONENTS

Attention Deficit Hyperactivity Disorder and Learning Disability

Attention deficit hyperactivity disorder (ADHD) refers to developmentally inappropriate degrees of inattention, impulsiveness, and hyperactivity. The symptoms of ADHD must have been present before the age of 7 years and must be present in at least two settings. In addition, "the persistence of developmentally inappropriate and marked inattention must not be a symptom of another disorder" (American Psychiatric Association, 1994). **Learning disability (LD)** refers to a heterogeneous group of disorders manifested by significant difficulties in the acquisition and use of listening, speaking, reading, writing, reasoning, mathematic abilities, or social skills.

ADHD and LD conditions affect every aspect of the child's life but are most obvious in the classroom. Early identification of affected children is needed, since the characteristics of the disorder significantly interfere with the normal course of

BOX 36-1
Diagnostic Criteria for ADHD

A. Either 1 or 2:
  1. Six (or more) of the following symptoms of *inattention* have persisted for at least 6 months to a degree that is maladaptive and inconsistent with developmental level:

     Inattention
     a. Often fails to give close attention to details or makes mistakes in schoolwork, work, or other activities
     b. Often has difficulty sustaining attention in tasks or play activities
     c. Often does not seem to listen when spoken to directly
     d. Often does not follow through on instructions and fails to finish schoolwork, chores, or duties in the workplace (not due to oppositional behavior or failure to understand instructions)
     e. Often has difficulty organizing tasks and activities
     f. Often avoids, dislikes, or is reluctant to engage in tasks that require sustained mental effort (such as schoolwork or homework)
     g. Often loses things necessary for tasks or activities (e.g., toys, school assignments, pencils, books, or tools)
     h. Is often easily distracted by extraneous stimuli
     i. Is often forgetful in daily activities
  2. Six (or more) of the following symptoms of *hyperactivity-impulsivity* have persisted for at least 6 months to a degree that is maladaptive and inconsistent with developmental level:

     Hyperactivity
     a. Often fidgets with hands or feet or squirms in seat
     b. Often leaves seat in classroom or in other situations in which remaining seated is expected
     c. Often runs about or climbs excessively in situations in which it is inappropriate (in adolescents or adults, may be limited to subjective feelings of restlessness)
     d. Often has difficulty playing or engaging in leisure activities quietly
     e. Is often "on the go" or often acts as if "driven by a motor"
     f. Often talks excessively

     Impulsivity
     g. Often blurts out answers before questions have been completed
     h. Often has difficulty awaiting turn
     i. Often interrupts or intrudes on others (e.g., butts into conversations or games)

B. Some hyperactive-impulsive or inattentive symptoms that caused impairment were present before age 7 years.
C. Some impairment from the symptoms is present in two or more settings (e.g., at school, work, and home).
D. There must be clear evidence of clinically significant impairment in social, academic, or occupational functioning.
E. The symptoms do not occur exclusively during the course of or are not accounted for by another mental disorder.

From American Psychiatric Association: *Diagnostic and statistical manual of mental disorders*, ed 4 (DSM IV), Washington, DC, 1994, American Psychiatric Association.

emotional and psychologic development. Many children develop maladaptive behavior patterns that impede psychosocial adjustment while they try to cope with cognitive dysfunction. Their behavior evokes negative responses from others, and repeated exposure to negative feedback adversely affects their self-concept. Constant failure despite honest effort can also affect their self-esteem.

Diagnostic evaluation. The behaviors exhibited by the child with ADHD are not unusual aspects of child behavior. The difference lies in the quality of motor activity and developmentally inappropriate inattention, impulsivity, and hyperactivity the child displays. The manifestations may be numerous or few, mild or severe, and will vary with the developmental level of the child. Any given child will not have every manifestation that is characteristic of the syndrome. The diagnostic criteria established by the American Psychiatric Association (1994) for identifying the child with ADHD are outlined in Box 36-1.

A comprehensive battery of tests is needed to confirm a learning disability. These include intelligence tests (these children tend to have normal or above-average intelligence quotients [IQs]), hand-eye coordination tests, and measurements of auditory and visual perception, comprehension, and memory. Often there is a wide gap between verbal and performance scores on IQ tests.

Therapeutic management. Management of the child with ADHD or LD usually involves multiple approaches that include family education and counseling, medication, proper classroom placement, environmental manipulation, and sometimes psychotherapy for the child.

Medication. Many drugs have been advocated for the management of symptoms of ADHD. The most commonly prescribed medications are dextroamphetamine (Dexedrine) or methylphenidate (Ritalin). However, not all children benefit from medications. Children taking stimulant medication may have symptoms that include nervousness, insomnia, and decreased appetite with subsequent weight loss. Long-term use of dextroamphetamine may result in suppression of growth (see the Critical Thinking Q & A box to the right).

Environmental manipulation. The child's environment is simplified by decreasing external stimuli and distractions, reducing alternatives, and encouraging desired patterns of behavior. Parents need to develop firm but reasonable limits and provide a stable and predictable environment with regular routines of sleeping, eating, working, and playing.

Classroom education. Special activities in the schools are designed to offer a direct attack on such areas of deficit as visual perception, auditory perception, and other areas involving integration and coordination. The purpose of programs for children with special learning disabilities is to assist them toward more successful achievement, personal adjustment, and eventual retention in the regular classroom. However, according to Public Law 94-142, The Education for All Handicapped Children's Act, children with ADHD or LD must receive free public education in the least restrictive environment (see Chapters 27 and 38).

Course of ADHD. In the majority of affected children the disorder is relatively stable through early adolescence. In most individuals, symptoms diminish during late adolescence and adulthood, although a minority experience the full complement of symptoms of ADHD into middle adulthood. Other adults may no longer have the full disorder but still retain some symptoms that cause functional impairment (American Psychiatric Association, 1994).

Children with LD grow up to be adults with LD. The goal is to help them identify their area of weakness and to compensate for it.

Nursing care management. Nurses are active participants in all aspects of management of the child with ADHD or LD. Nurses in the community setting work with families in the home and with school personnel on a long-term basis to help plan and implement therapeutic regimens and to evaluate the effectiveness of therapy. They should explain that children taking stimulant medication need to have it administered in the morning to maximize its effectiveness in the classroom and to decrease its insomnia-producing potential. Parents benefit from practical, specific strategies for helping children with ADHD, such as the need for structure and consistency in dressing, meals, sleep, and discipline (Comfort, 1992).

Nurses must understand which type of LD a child has in order to best provide direction for the child, parents, and teachers. Children with an auditory perceptual deficit appear

Critical Thinking Q & A

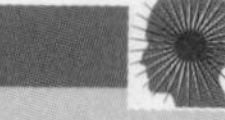

ADHD

Johnnie, age 8 years, is a third grader who was diagnosed with ADHD 1 year ago. Johnnie has been taking the drug methylphenidate (Ritalin) for the past year. Which of the following behaviors indicates that Johnnie may need to have the administration times of his medications changed?

1. For the past week, Johnnie has not eaten his lunch. He states that he is not hungry.
2. During this school year, Johnnie's math grade has increased from a letter grade of D to a grade of B.
3. Johnnie's mother told the school nurse that Johnnie has been sleeping very well at night.
4. During the past year, Johnnie's teacher has noted that Johnnie has been socializing more with his classmates and that he now has a "best friend."

The correct answer is one. Children taking stimulant medications often experience positive effects such as improvement in school work and increasing self-confidence in social skills. However, there are also negative side effects for some of the drugs used to treat ADHD. For example, side effects for methylphenidate include nervousness, decreased appetite, and insomnia. The absorption rate of methylphenidate is increased when this drug is taken with meals; therefore side effects such as decreased appetite may become more pronounced when the medication is taken with meals. Side effects can be alleviated by changing the times when the drug is administered or by switching to a sustained time-release form of the drug that can be given once a day in the morning. When evaluating a child's response to the medication, it is important to obtain reports from the child's teacher, the school nurse, and the parents. Information concerning the child's behavior in at least two settings should be obtained before adjustments are made in the medication dosage or scheduling.

unable to follow directions or to comprehend large amounts of verbal teaching. These children need to be taught with diagrams, pictures, demonstration, and written lists. Children with a visual perceptual deficit may have difficulty reading, lining up numbers for mathematic operations, or judging distance. These children may have dyslexia (letter reversals) and do better with demonstration and a verbal approach. Children with an integrative deficit may have difficulty sequencing data or storing and retrieving sensory data. Multisensory techniques should be used, and comprehension should be checked frequently throughout instruction. Children with motor deficits may need to use computers in the classroom, since their handwriting will *not* improve. They may need to find alternatives to physical competition that requires coordination of movement (Selekman, 1991).

Enuresis

Enuresis (bed-wetting) is a common and troublesome disorder that is difficult to define because of the variable ages at which children achieve bladder control. In a broad sense the disorder can be defined as repeated involuntary urination (usually nocturnal) in children who are beyond the age when voluntary bladder control should normally have been acquired. The chronologic or developmental age of the child must be at least 5 years. The voiding of urine must occur at least twice a week for at least 3 months. Enuresis affects 5 million children in the United States and is more common in boys than in girls (Houts, 1991). Enuresis is primarily an alteration of neuromuscular bladder functioning and is often benign and self-limiting. Nocturnal bed-wetting usually ceases when the child is 6 to 8 years of age, although it sometimes continues into adolescence (see the Cultural Considerations box to the right).

Organic causes that may be related to enuresis should be ruled out before psychogenic factors are considered. These include structural disorders of the urinary tract, urinary tract infection, neurologic deficits, disorders that increase the normal output of urine, such as diabetes, and disorders such as chronic renal failure or sickle cell disease that impair the concentrating ability of the kidneys.

A bladder volume of 300 to 350 ml is sufficient to hold a night's urine. The bladder capacity of a child can be determined by having the child void in a measuring cup after holding urine for as long as possible. Normal bladder capacity (in ounces) is the child's age plus 2 ounces (e.g., a 6-year-old's normal capacity is 8 ounces) (Schmitt, 1990a).

In some cases the enuresis is influenced by emotional factors, although it is doubtful that they are causative factors. Parents report that these children sleep more soundly than other children; however, the depth of sleep has not been identified as the cause of nocturnal enuresis (Rappaport, 1993).

Enuresis has a strong familial tendency. The predominant symptom is urgency that is immediate and accompanied by acute discomfort, restlessness, and sometimes urinary frequency.

Various therapeutic techniques are employed in the management of enuresis. These include drugs, bladder training, restriction or elimination of fluids after the evening meal, interruption of sleep to void, and some type of electrical device designed to establish a conditioned reflex response to waken the child at the initiation of voiding.

Cultural Considerations 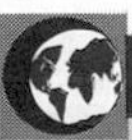

ENURESIS

The age at which children attain urinary continence varies widely. For example, Caucasian children in the United States tend to achieve continence earlier than African-American children. In addition, children in Great Britain and Sweden appear to attain continence slightly earlier than children in the United States, and in the extreme, the East African Digos often achieve bladder control by the age of 12 months. Therefore practitioners must be sensitive to the differences among groups before labeling a child enuretic (Rappaport, 1992).

Anticholinergic drugs, especially oxybutynin, reduce uninhibited bladder contractions and may be helpful for children with daytime urinary frequency. Desmopressin (DDAVP) nasal spray, an analog of vasopressin, reduces nighttime urine output to a volume less than functional bladder capacity.

Nursing care management. No matter what techniques are employed, the nurse can help both children and parents understand the problem of enuresis, the treatment plan, and the probable difficulties they may encounter in the process. More importantly, the nurse can provide consistent support and encouragement to help sustain them through the inconsistent and unpredictable treatment process. Children need to believe that they are helping themselves and to sustain feelings of confidence and hope.

Encopresis

Encopresis is the repeated voluntary or involuntary passage of feces of normal or near-normal consistency into places not appropriate for that purpose according to the individual's own sociocultural setting. The fecal incontinence must not result from any physiologic effect, such as a laxative, or a general medical condition. The fecal incontinence may be related to emotional problems. The disorder is less common than enuresis, but the two may co-exist.

Primary encopresis is identified by age 4 years when the child has not achieved fecal continence. Secondary encopresis is fecal incontinence occurring in a child over 4 years of age after a period of established fecal continence. Predisposing factors seem to be inconsistent toilet training and psychosocial stress, such as entering school or the birth of a sibling. The disorder is more common in boys than in girls. Incontinence commonly occurs secondary to constipation, painful impaction, or retention of feces with subsequent overflow. It is not unusual for soiling to take place after bathing because of reflex stimulation.

School performance and attendance are affected as the child's offensive odor becomes a target for scorn and derision from classmates. This causes further withdrawal and other behavioral manifestations. Therapeutic management consists of determining the cause of the soiling and applying appropriate interventions to correct the problem. It may involve dietary changes, relief of a fecal impaction, and/or behavioral therapy. Often, psychotherapeutic intervention with the child and family becomes necessary.

Family Focus 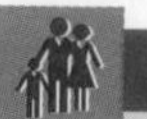

HELPING FAMILIES UNDERSTAND ENCOPRESIS

The prevailing attitude of nurses toward the family of a child with encopresis should be one of no-fault, thus relieving the guilt of both parents and child. Since parents and children are often reluctant to volunteer information, direct questioning about the soiling is more successful. Parents are usually relieved to know that other parents share this problem and are surprised to know that functional changes that take place as the condition develops make control of seepage impossible. Many parents complain that their children soil because they do not take time from play for a bowel movement. Actually the children may be unaware of a prior sensation and unable to control the urge once it begins. They may be so accustomed to bowel accidents that they are unable to smell or feel it and even deny soiling when it occurs.

Nursing care management. The nursing care of the child with encopresis involves primarily education and support of the family, as well as treatment of existing constipation. Families are taught the physiology of normal defecation, toilet training as a developmental process, and the treatment outlined for the particular family. Family counseling is directed toward reassurance that most problems resolve successfully, although relapses during periods of stress are possible (see the Family Focus box above).

Posttraumatic Stress Disorder

Posttraumatic stress disorder (PTSD) is commonly observed after an overwhelming stimulus (e.g., physical abuse or experiencing a sibling dying while in the child's care). Disasters initiate similar psychologic effects, and PTSD has been diagnosed in many children who have experienced such events. Children with PTSD tend to relive or visualize traumatic experiences for years and retain some fear specific to the event. They continue to function as always but have a feeling of foreboding regarding the future. The way in which children react depends on what resources the individual child brings to the situation—coping strategies used, defense mechanisms summoned, and the child's social environment. Although studies indicate that children do not outgrow the trauma, they can be helped to overcome their sense of hopelessness.

The response to the event takes place in three stages. The *initial response* to the stressor is intense arousal, which usually lasts for a few minutes to 1 or 2 hours. The stress hormones are at the maximum as the individual prepares for "fight or flight." A prolonged arousal phase may indicate psychosis.

The *second phase*, which lasts approximately 2 weeks, is one in which defense mechanisms are mobilized. It is a period of quiescence in which the event appears to have produced no impression. The victims feel numb, and stress hormone secretion is absent. The reaction is outside their awareness, not well controlled, and involves some type of behavioral pattern. Defense mechanisms are less adaptive to specific situations and may not be what the situation demands. Denial that anything is wrong is a frequently observed defense mechanism.

The *third phase* is one of coping, which normally extends over 2 to 3 months. It is one of consciously directed inquiry. The victims want to know what happened and appear to be getting worse, when actually they are getting better. Numerous psychologic symptoms may be apparent, such as depression, repetitive phenomenon, phobic symptoms, anxiety symptoms, and conversion reactions. Children frequently display repetitive actions. They play out the situation over and over again in an attempt to come to terms with their fear. Flashbacks are common. This phase can be self-perpetuating, and a prolonged reaction can develop into an obsession with the traumatic event. Some traumatic effects remain indefinitely (Terr, 1989).

Nursing care management. Children need to deal with any traumatic event; much depends on the intensity of the event and their reaction to it. They usually react in much the same manner as their caregivers (contagious pathology); therefore it is important to be aware of these reactions also. In the second, or defense, phase of the PTSD the appropriateness of the defense mechanism must be assessed, and children must be assisted in applying their defense. If children do not engage in some catharsis, or if their defense phase is prolonged, they may need referral for special psychologic help.

Coping is a learned response, and children in the third phase can be helped to use their coping strategies to deal with their fear. Children usually are willing to accept reasoning. Those who are assisted in their catharsis and allowed expression will survive without serious lasting effects. It is important for children to be reassured regarding the randomness of an event such as a playground shooting, rape, attack, or natural disaster (e.g., hurricane, earthquake). They should be encouraged to play out the stress and/or discuss their feelings about the event. If they cannot do this, they may become obsessed with the traumatic event and need professional help. Conversion reactions are common obsessive behaviors in children.

Children need professional help if any of the phases of PTSD are prolonged. Boys tend to have a prolonged defense phase more often than girls. Occasionally the event will be unrecognized, and the affected child will engage in what is considered unusual behavior. Children exhibiting any sudden change in behavior must be assessed for a traumatic event—"Did something happen?" When the change in behavior is traced to a traumatic event, treatment can be implemented.

School Phobia

Children, other than beginning students, who resist going to school because of dread of the school situation, concerns with leaving home, or both, are said to have school phobia. Anxiety—especially anxiety over separation from the parent, usually the mother—that frequently verges on panic is a constant manifestation. Some children are afraid the parent will not be home when they get there. Simple reassurance is often sufficient for these children.

Physical symptoms are prominent and may affect any part of the body (e.g., anorexia, nausea, vomiting, diarrhea, dizziness, headache, leg pains, abdominal pains, or even a low-grade fever). A striking feature of school phobia is the prompt subsiding of symptoms when it is evident that the child can remain at home. Another significant observation is absence of symptoms on weekends and holidays unless they are related to other places such as Sunday school or parties. Occasional mild reluctance is not uncommon among schoolchildren, but if the fear continues for longer than a few days, it must be considered as a serious problem—a warning of an important personality problem.

Nursing care management. The interventions for school phobia depend on the cause. The primary goal is to return the child to school. The longer a child is permitted to stay out of school, the more difficult it is to reenter. Parents must be convinced gently but firmly that *immediate* return is essential and that it is their responsibility to insist on school attendance.

The child with severe symptoms may require modified school attendance, such as part-time class attendance and spending time in the counselor's or nurse's office, then getting homework from the teacher after class. It may be necessary for a parent to attend class with the child. If the problem persists, professional help is recommended.

Recurrent Abdominal Pain

Recurrent abdominal pain (RAP) is one of the somatic complaints of childhood that is almost always attributed to a psychogenic etiology, although it can be a symptom of either psychosomatic or organic disease. Children with RAP have real pain that the child usually locates in the periumbilical area. However, on palpation the pain is more likely to be experienced in the epigastric area or in the lower right or left quadrant and is accompanied by vague tenderness without muscle guarding. The pain is irregular in time, duration, and intensity and is associated with either loose or pellet-formed stools. Other symptoms that may accompany the abdominal pain are headache, pallor, dizziness, and dysuria.

Support for the psychologic aspects of this disorder is based on observations of aggravation of symptoms during times of tension or stress. Children with RAP tend to be highly sensitive, to have a poor self-image, and to be uncomfortable with expressions of anger or argument, especially from those persons who are significant in their life. School attendance is adversely affected, and these children generally exhibit poor learning performance. It is not uncommon for symptoms to be aggravated during school days.

Treatment is difficult. Hospitalization may be necessary, and the child commonly shows improvement in the hospital environment. Initial efforts are directed toward ruling out organic causes of the pain, relieving discomfort, and attempting to determine the situations that precipitate attacks. A high-fiber diet and bowel training are emphasized. When simple measures are ineffective, an antispasmodic drug such as propantheline bromide may be prescribed to relieve the muscle spasm.

Nursing care management. Once the diagnosis has been established, the parents and child need an explanation of the pain, which can be compared to a skeletal muscle cramp or "charley horse" for easier comprehension. Reassurance that the symptoms are not unique to their child and that the pain can be expected to subside is helpful in relieving parental fears and anxieties. When parents are reassured that there is no organic cause of the pain, they will need some guidance regarding what they can do during a painful episode. All too often they feel helpless and anxious, which tends to compound the child's distress.

The simple expedient of having the child rest in a peaceful, quiet environment and providing comfort will often relieve the symptoms in a short time. A heating pad may also help ease the discomfort. Teaching children relaxation exercises and guided imagery may also be helpful (see Pain Management, Chapter 41). If pain is not relieved by these simple measures, the parents are taught how to administer antispasmodics, if prescribed. For example, if pain is precipitated by meals, having the child take the medication 20 to 30 minutes before mealtime may prevent an episode.

The most valuable measures that the nurse can provide are support and reassurance to the family. When open communication is established and families are able to see a relationship between stress-provoking situations and the child's symptoms, the chance for remedial action is enhanced. Follow-up care and continued support are essential because the symptoms tend to remit and exacerbate; therefore the availability of a supportive health professional can be a source of comfort to the child and family.

Conversion Reaction

Conversion reaction, also known as hysteria, hysterical conversion reaction, and childhood hysteria, is a psychophysiologic disorder with a sudden onset that can usually be traced to a precipitating environmental event. Once considered rare in childhood, the diagnosis of conversion reaction occurs more often than has generally been acknowledged. In childhood the disorder is observed with equal frequency in both genders, but girls with the disorder outnumber affected boys during adolescence.

The manifestations involve primarily the voluntary musculature and special senses and include abdominal pain, fainting, pseudoseizures, paralysis, headaches, and visual field restriction. The most commonly observed symptom is seizure activity, which can be differentiated from symptoms of neurogenic origin by formal tests, the most useful of which is the finding of a normal electroencephalogram.

Before the onset of symptoms, nearly all children with conversion reaction have experienced a major family crisis, such as loss of a parent or other significant person through death, divorce, or moving.

Nursing care management. Nursing care is similar to that for the child with RAP.

Childhood Depression

Depression in childhood is often difficult to detect. Children may be unable to express their feelings and tend to act out their problems and concerns. Some states of depression are temporary (e.g., acute depression precipitated by a traumatic event). This might include a period of hospitalization, loss of a parent through death or separation, or loss of a significant relationship with something (a pet), someone (a friend or family member), or a place (move from a familiar home, neighborhood, or city). The characteristics of children with depression are outlined in Box 36-2. The child tends to spend more time in solitary activities, especially television viewing, and schoolwork is impaired. Some children become more dependent and clinging; others become more aggressive and disruptive. The manifestations may last a few days or weeks, usually resolving spontaneously.

BOX 36-2
Characteristics of Children with Depression

Behavior
Predominantly sad facial expression with absence or diminished range of affective response
Solitary play, work, or tendency to be alone; disinterest in play
Lowered grades in school; lack of interest in doing homework or achieving in school
Diminished motor activity; tiredness
Change in appetite resulting in weight loss or gain
Alterations in sleeping pattern
Tearfulness or crying

Internal states
Utterance of statements reflecting lowered self-esteem, sense of hopelessness, or guilt
Suicidal ideations

Physiology
Constipation
Nonspecific complaints of not feeling well
Lowered urinary excretion of 30, methoxy-4-hydroxyphenylglycol (MHPG)
Abnormal dexylmethazone suppression test (DST)
Hypersecretion of growth hormone during sleep
Blunting of growth hormone to insulin-induced hypoglycemia, suggestive of endogenous depression

Modified from Brantly DK, Takacs DJ: Anxiety and depression in preschool and school-aged children. In Clunn PA, editor: *Child psychiatric nursing*, St Louis, 1991, Mosby.

More serious and less common are depressive responses to more chronic stress and loss; these are frequently observed in children with chronic illness or disability. There is usually no apparent precipitating event, but there is often a history of frequent disruptions in important relationships. Manifestations are as varied as those observed in acute depression but occur more frequently and extend over a longer period of time.

Nursing care management. The management of childhood depression is usually psychotherapeutic and highly individualized. Nurses should be aware that depression is a problem that can easily be overlooked in the child and one that can interrupt normal growth and development. Recognizing depression and making appropriate referrals are important nursing functions. Identification of the depressed child requires a careful history (health, growth and development, social, and family health), interviews with the child, and observations by the nurse, parents, and teachers (see also Suicide, Chapter 37.)

Childhood Schizophrenia

Childhood schizophrenia refers to severe deviations in ego functioning and is a term generally reserved for psychotic disorders that appear after the first 4 or 5 years of life. Schizophrenia in adults occurs with relative frequency, and although childhood psychosis is not as common, it is by no means rare.

Childhood schizophrenia is characterized by a gradual onset of neurotic symptoms that show wide variation according to each affected child's developmental level, the age of onset, the nature of early childhood experiences, and the type of defense mechanisms used. However, the basic core disturbance is the child's lack of contact with reality and the subsequent development of a personal world. Secondary characteristics represent impairment in a wide number of areas of development, including cognition, perception, emotion, language, and physical motor control. The most common manifestations involve language disturbances, impaired interpersonal relationships, and inappropriate affect (outward expression of emotion).

Nursing care management. Nursing of psychotic children is a highly specialized area, but since these problems are being recognized with increasing frequency, nurses should be alert to the possibility. A child who consistently demonstrates abnormal behavior should be referred for evaluation.

Key Points

- Middle childhood, also known as the school years, is a comfortable period of life that extends from 6 to 12 years of age.
- Although slower than previous years, there is a steady gain in height and weight with maturation of body systems; primary teeth are lost and replaced by permanent teeth.
- School-age children develop what Erikson terms a sense of industry or accomplishment.
- School-age children, although having a limited capacity for abstract thought, can use their thought processes in solving more complex problems, make judgments based on reasoning, and see a situation from the point of view of another.
- The child develops a conscience and is able to understand and adhere to rules and standards set by others.
- Entertaining different points of view, becoming sensitive to social norms, and forming peer friendships are the most important features of social development during the school years.
- Cooperative play, team activities, and acquisition of skills are prime elements of play during the school years; rules and rituals assume greater importance.
- School-age children become proficient at many types of activities.
- Typical parental concerns during middle childhood are beginning separation from the family unit, dishonest behavior, and scholastic achievement.

- Optimum nutrition is often hampered by an affinity for and availability of junk foods, irregular family meals, and schedules of working parents.
- Dental care continues to be important; dental problems include caries, periodontal disease, malocclusion, and tooth evulsion.
- Increased socialization, earlier pubertal development, and constant media exposure make the school years an ideal time for sex education.
- School health ideally offers programs that include health appraisal, emergency care, safety education, communicable disease control, counseling, guidance, and health education with adjustment to individual student needs.
- Injury prevention is directed toward safety education, provision of safe play areas and equipment, and well-supervised sports activities.
- Participation in sports predisposes children and adolescents to both acute injuries and overuse syndromes.
- Alterations in growth and maturation may be manifest in short or tall stature, precocious puberty, and delayed sexual development.
- Tools for assessment of growth include a family history, previous growth patterns, physical examination, bone age determination, and endocrine studies.
- Effective therapies for attention deficit hyperactivity disorder and learning disabilities usually involve a multiple approach: family education and counseling, medication, remedial education, environmental manipulation, and psychotherapy.
- Behavior problems in middle childhood can result from attention deficit hyperactivity disorder, enuresis, encopresis, posttraumatic stress disorder, school phobia, recurrent abdominal pain, childhood depression, conversion reaction, and childhood schizophrenia.

References

American Academy of Pediatrics, Committee on Injury and Poison Prevention: Bicycle helmets, *Pediatrics* 95(4):609-610, 1995.

American Academy of Pediatrics, Committee on Sports Medicine and Committee on School Health: Organized athletics for preadolescent children, *Pediatrics* 84:583-584, 1989.

American Psychiatric Association: *Diagnostic and statistical manual of mental disorders,* ed 4 (DSM-IV), Washington, DC, 1994, American Psychiatric Association.

Bell-Dolan D, Last C, Strauss C: Symptoms of anxiety disorders in normal children, *J Am Acad Child Adolesc Psychiatry* 29:759-765, 1990.

Coble PA et al: *EEG sleep of healthy children 6 to 12 years of age.* In Guilleminault C, editor: *Sleep and its disorders in children,* New York, 1987, Raven Press.

Comfort RL: Living with an unconventional child, *J Pediatr Health Care* 6(3):114-120, 1992.

Delegation of School Health Services to Unlicensed Assistive Personnel: A position paper of National Association of State School Nurse Consultants, *J School Nurse* 11(4):13-16, 1995.

Dolan MA, Knapp JF, Andres J: Three-wheel and four-wheel all-terrain vehicle injuries in children, *Pediatrics* 84:694-698, 1989.

Erikson EH: *Childhood and society,* ed 2, New York, 1963, WW Norton.

Holaday B, Turner-Henson A, Swan, JH: Chronically-ill latchkey children, *Clin Pediatr* 33(5):303-306, 1994.

Houts AC: Nocturnal enuresis as a biobehavioral problem, *Behav Ther* 22:133-151, 1991.

Igoe JB: School-linked family health centers in health care reform, *Pediatr Nurs* 19:67-68, 1993.

Levine MD: *Middle childhood.* In Levine MD et al: *Developmental-behavioral pediatrics,* ed 2, Philadelphia, 1992, WB Saunders.

Metcalf JH, Roberts SO: Strength training and the immature athlete: an overview, *Pediatr Nurs* 19:325-332, 1993.

Miller ME: *Immunodeficiency of immaturity.* In Stiehm R: *Immunologic disorders in infants and children,* Philadelphia, 1989, WB Saunders.

Rappaport LA: *Enuresis.* In Levine M et al: *Developmental-behavioral pediatrics,* ed 2, 1992, WB Saunders.

Rappaport LA: The treatment of nocturnal enuresis—where are we now? *Pediatrics* 92:465-466, 1993.

Rollins JA: Nurses as gangbusters: a response to gang violence in America, *Pediatr Nurs* 19:559-567, 1993.

Schmitt B: Nocturnal enuresis: finding the treatment that fits the child, *Contemp Pediatr* 7(9):70-97, 1990a.

Schmitt B: Preventing problems with schoolwork, *Contemp Pediatr* 7(9):31-32, 1990b.

Schonfeld DJ et al: Understanding of acquired immunodeficiency syndrome by elementary school children—a developmental survey, *Pediatrics* 92:389-395, 1993.

Selekman J: *Primary care of the child with a learning disability.* In Jackson P, Vessey J: *Primary care of children with chronic conditions,* St Louis, 1991, Mosby.

Terr L: Traumatic events in childhood have lasting effects, *AAP News* 5(5):1, 1989.

Bibliography

General

Adger H, DeAngelis C: Sexuality education: our schools can do better, *Contemp Pediatr* 6(10):56-67, 1989.

Carey WB: Temperament issues in the school-aged child, *Pediatr Clin North Am* 39:537-549.1992.

Dixon SD, Stein MT: *Encounters with children: pediatric behavior and development,* ed 2, St Louis, 1992, Mosby.

Dworkin PH: Behavior during middle childhood: developmental themes and clinical issues, *Pediatr Ann* 18:347-355, 1989.

Eiden H, Thomas M, Fosarelli P: A teaching tool for children in self-care, *J Pediatr Health Care* 1:292-297, 1987.

Feldman H: The development of thinking skills in school-age children, *Pediatr Ann* 18:356-362, 1989.

Guilleminault C: *Disorders of arousal in children: somnambulism and night terrors.* In Guilleminault C, editor: *Sleep and its disorders in children,* New York, 1987, Raven Press.

Landman GB: Language development from six to twelve, *Pediatr Ann* 18:373-379, 1989.

Sandler A: Social development in middle childhood, *Pediatr Ann* 18:380-387, 1989.

Vessey JA, Braithwaite KB, Wiedmann M: Teaching children about their internal bodies, *Pediatr Nurs* 16:29-33, 1990.

Winkelstein ML: Fostering positive self-concept in the school-age child, *Pediatr Nurs* 15:229-233, 1989.

Wynn D, Schmidt CK, Alvin RM: Test-retest reliability of a body knowledge instrument in school-age children, *Matern Child Nurs J* 22:56-64, 1994.

Health Promotion

American Academy of Pediatrics, Committee on School Health: *School health: a guide for health professionals,* Elk Grove Village, Ill, 1987, American Academy of Pediatrics.
American Academy of Pediatrics, Committee on Sports Medicine and Committee on School Health: Physical fitness and the schools, *Pediatrics* 80:449-450, 1987.
Bailey-Britton AM: The relationship between health and academic performance in school-age children, *Issues Compr Pediatr Nurs* 10:273-289, 1987.
Bausell RB: A national survey assessing pediatric preventive behaviors, *Pediatr Nurs* 11:438-444, 1985.
Cowell JM et al: School health services: a hub of services to children and their families, *Pediatr Nurs* 17:86-88, 1991.
Ferber R: Sleep schedule–dependent causes of insomnia and sleepiness in middle childhood and adolescence, *Pediatrician* 17:13-20, 1990.
Giordana BP, Igoe JB: Health promotion: the new frontier, *Pediatr Nurs* 17:490-492, 1991.
Hester ND: Health concerns of school-age children. *Issues Compr Pediatr Nurs* 10:251-262, 1987.
Pidgeon V, Olson S: A comparison of illness concepts of school-age children and adolescents, *Issues Compr Pediatr Nurs* 9:209-221, 1986.
Pipes PL: *Nutrition in infancy and childhood,* ed 5, St Louis, 1993, Mosby.
Scanlon BJ: An holistic approach to school dental health, *J Sch Nurs* 7:12-15, 1991.

School Health

American Academy of Pediatrics, Committee on School Health: Guidelines for the administration of medication in school, *Pediatrics* 92:499-500, 1993.
Fryer GE, Igoe JB: A relationship between availability of school nurses and child well-being, *J School Nurs* 11(3):12-16, 18, 1995.
Farren M, McKevitt RK: *Nursing roles in school health.* In Hoekelman RA et al: editors: *Primary pediatric care,* ed 2, St Louis, 1992, Mosby.
Garbarino J et al: *Children in danger: coping with the consequences of community violence,* San Francisco, 1992, Jossey-Bass.
Groves BM et al: Silent victims: children who witness violence, *JAMA* 269:261-264, 1993.
Igoe JB: Healthy long-term attitudes on personal health can be developed in school-age children, *Pediatrician* 15:127-136, 1988.
Kornguth ML: School illnesses: who's absent and why? *Pediatr Nurs* 16:95-99, 1990.
Lear JG: Building a health/education partnership: the role of school-based health centers, *Pediatr Nurs* 18(2):172-173, 1992.
MacBriar BR et al: Development of a health concerns inventory for school-age children, *J School Nurs* 11(3):25-29, 1995.
Meeker R et al: A comprehensive school health initiative, *Image J Nurs Sch* 18:86-91, 1986.
Mudd KE, Noone SA: Management of severe food allergy in the school setting, *J School Nurs* 11(3):30-32, 1995.
Velsor-Friedrich B: Schools and health. II. School-based clinics, *J Pediatr Nurs* 10(1):62-63, 1995.

Injury Prevention

American Academy of Pediatrics, Committee on Accident and Poison Prevention: All-terrain vehicles: two-, three-, and four-wheeled unlicensed motorized vehicles, *Pediatrics* 79:306-308, 1987.
American Academy of Pediatrics, Committee on Accident and Poison Prevention: Injuries related to "toy" firearms, *Pediatrics* 79:473-474, 1987.
American Academy of Pediatrics, Committee on Accident and Poison Prevention: Bicycle helmets, *Pediatrics* 85:229-230, 1990.
American Academy of Pediatrics, Committee on Injury and Poison Prevention: Skateboard injuries, *Pediatrics* 95(4):611-612, 1995.
Boyce WT, Sobolewski S: Recurrent injuries in school children, *Am J Dis Child* 143:338-342, 1989.
Christoffel KK: Child passenger safety, *Am J Dis Child* 143:1271-1272, 1989.
Council on Scientific Affairs, American Medical Association: Council report: helmets and preventing motorcycle- and bicycle-related injuries, *JAMA* 272(19):1535-1538, 1994.
Jones NE: Childhood injuries: an epidemiologic approach, *Pediatr Nurs* 18:235-239, 1992.
Cushman R et al: Helmet promotion in the emergency room following a bicycle injury: a randomized trial, *Pediatrics* 88:43-47, 1991.
Jones NE: Prevention of childhood injuries. I. Motor vehicle injuries, *Pediatr Nurs* 18:380-382, 1992.
Jones NE: Prevention of childhood injuries. II. Recreational injuries, *Pediatr Nurs* 18:619-621, 1992.
Lee EJ: Accident reports: survey of high school injuries, *Pediatr Nurs* 13:151-154, 1987.
Rivara FP et al: Attitudes and practices toward children as pedestrians, *Pediatrics* 84:1017-1021, 1989.
Schor EL: Unintentional injuries: patterns within families, *Am J Dis Child* 141:1280-1284, 1987.
Selbst SM, Alexander D, Ruddy R: Bicycle-related injuries, *Am J Dis Child* 141:140-144, 1987.
Senturia YD, Christoffel KK, Donovan AA: Children's household exposure to guns: a pediatric practice-based survey, *Pediatrics* 93(3):469-475, 1994.
Wilson MH: Preventing injury in the "middle years," *Contemp Pediatr* 6(6):20-54, 1989.

Disorders Related to Sports

American Academy of Pediatrics, Committee on Sports Medicine: Amenorrhea in adolescent athletes, *Pediatrics* 84:394-395, 1989.
American Academy of Pediatrics, Committee on Sports Medicine: Knee brace use by athletes, *Pediatrics* 85:228, 1990.
Backous DD et al: Soccer injuries and their relation to physical maturity, *Am J Dis Child* 142:839-842, 1988.
Council on Scientific Affairs: Drug abuse in athletes, *JAMA* 259:1703-1705, 1988.
Goldberg B et al: Injuries in youth football, *Pediatrics* 81:255-261, 1988.
Hergenroeder AC: Diagnosis and treatment of ankle sprains, *Am J Dis Child* 144:809-814, 1990.
Kris-Etherton PM: Nutrition and athletic performance, *Contemp Nutr* 14(8), 1989.
Mansfield MJ, Emans SJ: Growth in female gymnasts: should training decrease during puberty? *J Pediatr* 122:237-240, 1993.
McLain LG, Reynolds S: Sports injuries in a high school, *Pediatrics* 84:446-450, 1989.
Ostrum G: Sports-related injuries in youth: prevention is the key and nurses can help, *Pediatr Nurs* 19:333-342, 1993.
Pratt M: Strength, flexibility, and maturity in adolescent athletes, *Am J Dis Child* 143:560-563, 1989.
Rowland TW, Kelleher JF: Iron deficiency in athletes, *Am J Dis Child* 143:197-200, 1989.
Runyan CW, Gerkin EA: Epidemiology and prevention of adolescent injury: a review and research agenda, *JAMA* 262:2273-2279, 1989.
Terney R, McLain LG: The use of anabolic steroids in high school students, *Am J Dis Child* 144:99-103, 1990.
Yelverton GA: Anabolic steroids, *Pediatr Nurs* 15:63, 1989.

Altered Growth and/or Maturation

Bercu B: Growth hormone treatment and the short child: to treat or not to treat, *J Pediatr Health Care* 110:991-995, 1987.
Henry JJ: Routine growth monitoring and assessment of growth disorders, *J Pediatr Health Care* 6:291-301, 1992.
Mandoki M, Sumner G: Klinefelter syndrome: the need for early identification and treatment, *Clin Pediatr* 30(3):161-164, 1991.
Moore KC et al: Clinical diagnoses of children with extremely short

stature and their response to growth hormone, *J Pediatr* 122:687-692, 1992.

Rapaport R et al: Immune functions during treatment of growth hormone-deficient children with biosynthetic human growth hormone, *Clin Pediatr* 30(1):22-27, 1991.

Rohn R: Comparative heights of mothers and fathers whose children are short, *Am J Dis Child* 144(9):995-997, 1990.

Schwartz ID, Root AW: Puberty in girls: early, incomplete, or precocious? *Contemp Pediatr* 7(1):147-156, 1990.

Stabler B: Psychosocial outcomes of short stature, *Pediatr Rounds* 2:5-7, 1993.

Walker J and others: Treatment of short normal children with growth hormone—a cautionary tale? *Lancet* 336:1331-1334, 1990.

Enuresis/Encopresis

Castiglia PT: Encopresis, *J Pediatr Health Care* 1:335-337, 1987.

Castiglia PT: Nocturnal enuresis, *J Pediatr Health Care* 1:280-282, 1987.

Corkery J: Nintendo power, *Am J Dis Child* 144(9):959, 1990.

Friman PC, Warzak WJ: Nocturnal enuresis: a prevalent, persistent, yet curable parasomnia, *Pediatrician* 17:38-45, 1990.

Gibson LY: Bedwetting: a family's recurrent nightmare, *Am J Matern Child Nurs* 14:270-272, 1989.

Miller K: Concomitant nonpharmacologic therapy in the treatment of primary nocturnal enuresis, *Clin Pediatr* 32:32-37, 1993.

Piazza C et al: Reinforcement of incontinent stools in the treatment of encopresis, *Clin Pediatr* 30(1):28-32, 1991.

Rushton H: Nocturnal enuresis: epidemiology, evaluation, and current available treatment options, *J Pediatr* 114:691-696, 1989.

Stroh SE, Stern HP, McCarthy SG: Fecal incontinence in children: a clinical update, *Am J Matern Child Nurs* 14:252-254, 1989.

Terho P: Desmopressin in nocturnal enuresis, *J Urol* 145:818-820, 1991.

Behavior Disorders

Carpenter WT, Buchanan RW: Medical progress: schizophrenia, *N Engl J Med* 330:681-690, 1994.

Castiglia P: School phobias/school avoidance, *J Pediatr Health Care* 7:229-232, 1993.

Conway A, Bernardo L, Tontala K: The effects of disasters on children: implications for emergency nurses, *J Emerg Nurs* 16(6):393-397, 1990.

Davis B: Loneliness in children and adolescents, *Issues Compr Pediatr Nurs* 13(1):59-69, 1990.

Hodgman C et al: Managing depression in children, *Patient Care* 27:51-60, 1993.

Jacobson J: The relationship between social support and depression in adolescents, *J Child Adolesc Psychiatr Ment Health Nurs* 4(1):20-24, 1991.

Lipovsky JA: Posttraumatic stress disorder in children, *Fam Community Health* 14(3):42-51, 1991.

Puskar K, Dvorsak K: Relocation stress in adolescents: helping teenagers cope with a moving dilemma, *Pediatr Nurs* 17(3):295-297, 1991.

Weller EB, Weller RA: Pediatric management of depression, *Pediatr Ann* 18:104-113, 1989.

Wyllie R, Kay M: Causes of recurrent abdominal pain, *Clin Pediatr* 32:369-371, 1993.

Attention Deficit Hyperactivity Disorder/ Learning Disabilities

Adesman AR, Wender EH: Improving the outcome for children with ADHD, *Contemp Pediatr* 8(3):122-139, 1991.

Amaya-Jackson L, Cantwell D: Controversies in psychopharmacological management of attention deficit and related disorders, *Int Pediatr* 6(2):176-183, 1991.

American Academy of Pediatrics: Learning disabilities, dyslexia, and vision, *Pediatrics* 90:124-126, 1992.

Castiglia P: Dyslexia, *J Pediatr Health Care* 4(4):206-208, 1990.

Murphy MA, Hagerman RJ: Attention deficit hyperactivity disorder in children: diagnosis, treatment, and follow-up, *J Pediatr Health Care* 6(1):2-11, 1992.

Smitherman CH: A drug to ease attention deficit-hyperactivity disorder, *Am J Matern Child Nurs* 15(6):362-365, 1990.

Vatz RE, Weinberg LS: Treatment of attention-deficit hyperactivity disorder, *JAMA* 269:2368, 1993.

Voeller K: The neurological basis of attention deficit hyperactivity disorder, *Int Pediatr* 5(2):171-176, 1990.

CHAPTER 37

The Adolescent and Family

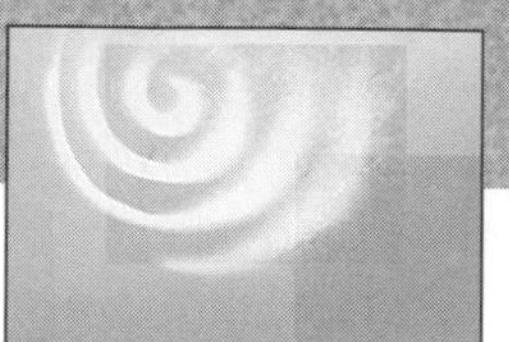

PROMOTING OPTIMUM GROWTH AND DEVELOPMENT, P. 1084

Biologic development, p. 1084
Psychosocial development, p. 1089
Cognitive development (Piaget), p. 1090
Moral development (Kohlberg), p. 1090
Spiritual development, p. 1090
Social development, p. 1091
Development of self-concept and body image, p. 1094

PROMOTING OPTIMUM HEALTH DURING ADOLESCENCE, P. 1097

Immunizations, p. 1098
Nutrition, p. 1098
Sleep and rest, p. 1099
Exercise and activity, p. 1099
Dental health, p. 1099
Personal care, p. 1099
Stress reduction, p. 1100
Sexuality education and guidance, p. 1101
Injury prevention, p. 1102
Anticipatory guidance—care of families, p. 1104

SPECIAL HEALTH PROBLEMS, P. 1104

Disorders related to the reproductive system, p. 1104
Amenorrhea, p. 1104
Dysmenorrhea, p. 1105
Vaginitis, p. 1105
Disorders of the male reproductive system, p. 1105
Gynecomastia, p. 1106
Eating disorders, p. 1106
Obesity, p. 1106
Anorexia nervosa, p. 1109
Bulimia, p. 1110
Disorders with behavioral components, p. 1111
Smoking, p. 1111
Substance abuse, p. 1112
Suicide, p. 1115

Promoting Optimum Growth and Development

Adolescence is a period of transition between childhood and adulthood—a time of rapid physical, cognitive, social, and emotional maturing as the youngster prepares for adulthood. The precise boundaries of adolescence are difficult to define, but this period is customarily viewed as beginning with the gradual appearance of secondary sex characteristics at about 11 or 12 years of age and ending with cessation of body growth at 18 to 20 years.

Several terms are commonly used in reference to this particular stage of growth and development. **Puberty** primarily refers to the maturational, hormonal, and growth process that occurs when the reproductive organs begin to function and the secondary sex characteristics develop. This process is sometimes divided into three stages: **prepubescence,** the period of about 2 years immediately before puberty when the child is developing preliminary physical changes that herald sexual maturity; **puberty,** the point at which sexual maturity is achieved, marked by the first menstrual flow in girls but by less obvious indications in boys; and **postpubescence,** a 1- to 2-year period following puberty during which skeletal growth is completed and reproductive functions become fairly well established. **Adolescence,** which literally means "to grow into maturity," is generally regarded as the psychologic, social, and maturational process initiated by the pubertal changes. It involves three distinct subphases: *early adolescence* (ages 11 to 14 years), *middle adolescence* (ages 15 to 17 years), and *late adolescence* (ages 18 to 20 years). Adolescence tends to begin and end earlier in girls than in boys. The term *teenage years* is used synonymously with *adolescence* to describe ages 13 through 19 years.

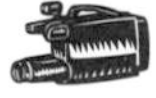

For additional information, please view "Growth and Development"in *Whaley and Wong's Pediatric Nursing Video Series,* St Louis, 1996, Mosby; (800) 426-4545.

BIOLOGIC DEVELOPMENT

The physical changes of puberty are primarily the result of hormonal activity under the influence of the central nervous system, although all aspects of physiologic functioning are mutually interacting. The very obvious physical changes are noted in increased physical growth and in the appearance and development of secondary sex characteristics; less obvious are physiologic alterations and neurogonadal maturity, accompanied by the ability to procreate. Physical distinction between the genders is determined on the basis of distinguishing characteristics: *primary sex characteristics* are the external and internal organs that carry out the reproductive functions (e.g., ovaries, uterus, breasts, and penis); *secondary sex characteristics* are the changes that occur throughout the body as a result of the hormonal change (e.g., voice alterations, development of facial and pubertal hair, and fat deposits) but play no direct part in reproduction.

Hormonal Changes of Puberty

It is generally accepted that the events of puberty are caused by hormonal influences and controlled by the anterior pituitary (adenohypophysis) in response to a stimulus from the hypothalamus. Stimulation of the gonads has a dual function: (1) production and release of gametes—production of sperm in the male and maturation and release of ova in the female—and (2) secretion of gender-appropriate hormones—estrogen and progesterone from the ovaries (female) and testosterone from the testes (male).

Sex hormones. Sex hormones are secreted by the ovaries, testes, and adrenals; they are produced in varying amounts by both genders throughout the life span. The adrenal cortex is responsible for the small amounts secreted before the pubescent years, but the sex hormone production that accompanies maturation of the gonads is responsible for the variety of biologic changes observed during puberty.

Estrogen, the feminizing hormone, is found in low quantities during childhood; it is secreted in slowly increasing amounts until about age 11 years. In males this gradual increase continues through maturation. In females the onset of estrogen production in the ovary causes a pronounced increase that continues until about 3 years after the onset of menstruation, at which time it reaches a maximum level that continues throughout the reproductive life of the female.

Androgens, the masculinizing hormones, are also secreted in small and gradually increasing amounts up to about 7 or 9 years of age, at which time there is a more rapid increase in both genders, especially boys, until about age 15 years. These hormones appear to be responsible for most of the rapid growth changes of early adolescence. With the onset of testicular function the level of androgens (principally **testosterone**) in males increases over that in females and continues to increase until a maximum is attained at maturity.

Sexual Maturation

The visible evidence of sexual maturation is achieved in orderly sequence, and the state of maturity can be estimated on the basis of the appearance of these external manifestations. The age at which these changes are observed and the time required to progress from one stage to another may vary considerably among children. The time from the appearance of breast buds to full maturity may be $1^1/_2$ to 6 years for adolescent girls; it may take 2 to 5 years for male genitalia to reach adult size. The stages of the development of secondary sex characteristics and genital development have been defined as a guide for estimating sexual maturity and are commonly referred to as the *Tanner stages.* The usual sequence of appearance of maturational changes is presented in Box 37-1.

BOX 37-1
Usual Sequence of Maturational Changes

Girls	Boys
Breast changes Rapid increase in height and weight Growth of pubic hair Appearance of axillary hair Menstruation (usually begins 2 years after first signs) Abrupt deceleration of linear growth	Enlargement of testicles Growth of pubic hair, axillary hair, hair on upper lip, hair on face and elsewhere on body (facial hair usually appears about 2 years after appearance of pubic hair) Rapid increase in height Changes in the larynx and, consequently, the voice (usually take place along with growth of penis) Nocturnal emissions Abrupt deceleration of linear growth

Sexual maturation in girls. In most girls the initial indication of puberty is the appearance of breast buds, an event known as *thelarche,* which occurs between ages 9 and 13.5 years. (Fig. 37-1). This is followed in approximately 2 to 6 months by growth of pubic hair on the mons pubis, known as *adrenarche* (Fig. 37-2).

The initial appearance of menstruation, or **menarche,** occurs about 2 years after the appearance of the first pubescent changes, approximately 9 months after attainment of peak height velocity and 3 months after attainment of peak weight velocity. Menarche has been related to a critical gain in body fat content (more fat content, earlier menarche), although this is controversial. The normal age range of menarche is usually 10.5 to 15 years, with the average age being 12.8 years for North American girls. Initial menstrual periods are usually scanty, irregular, and anovulatory. Ovulation and regular menstrual periods usually occur 6 to 14 months after menarche. Girls may be considered to have *pubertal delay* if breast development has not occurred by age 13 years or if menarche has not occurred within 4 years of the onset of breast development.

Sexual maturation in boys. The first pubescent changes in boys are testicular enlargement accompanied by thinning, reddening, and increased looseness of the scrotum (Fig. 37-3). These events usually occur between 9.5 and 14 years of age. Early puberty is also characterized by the initial appearance of pubic hair. Penile enlargement begins, and testicular enlargement and pubic hair growth continue throughout midpuberty. During this period there is also increasing muscularity, early voice changes, and development of early facial hair. Temporary breast enlargement and tenderness **(gynecomastia),** are common during midpuberty, occurring in up to one half of boys (see the Critical Thinking Q&A box

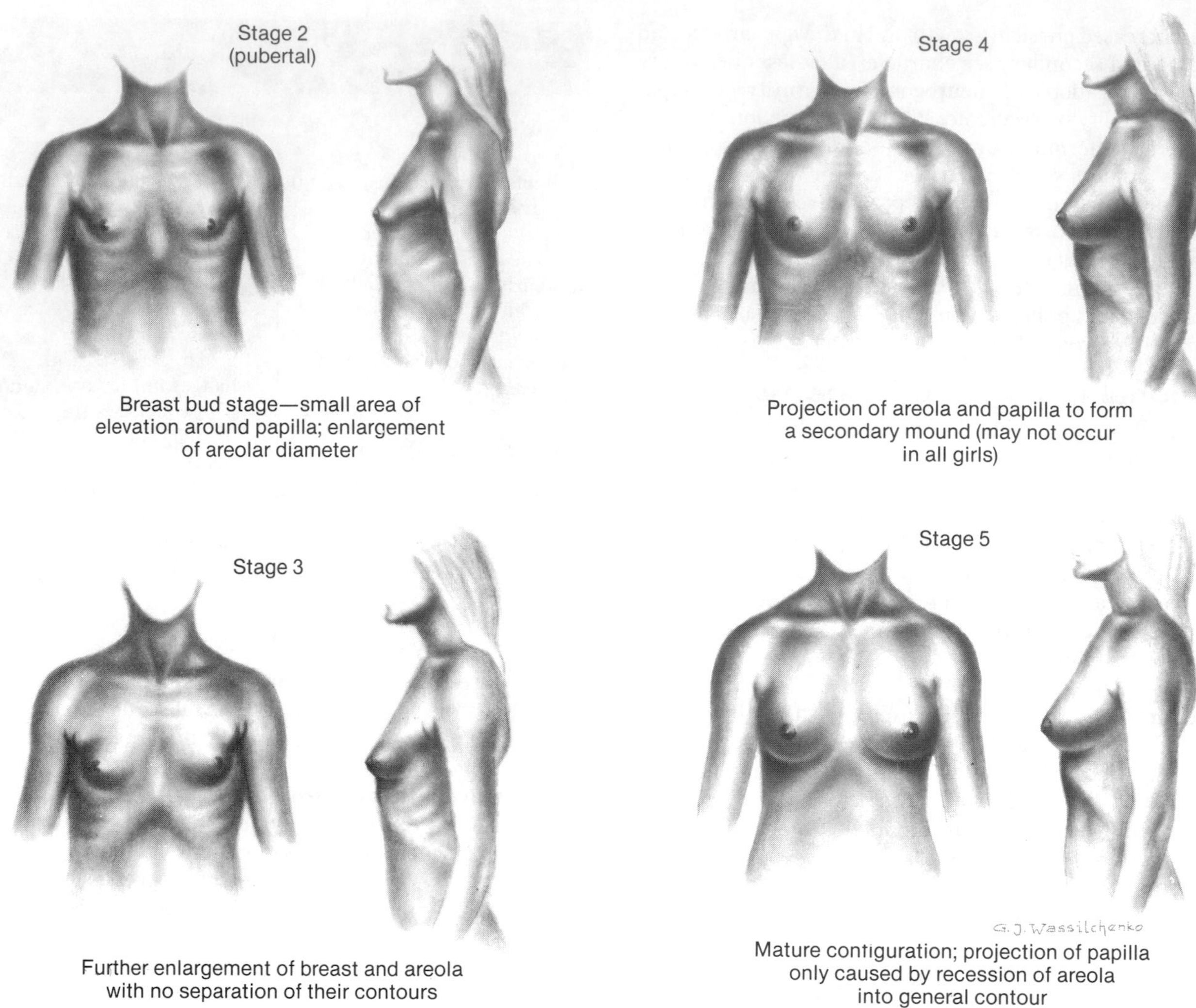

Stage 2
(pubertal)
Breast bud stage—small area of elevation around papilla; enlargement of areolar diameter
Stage 4
Projection of areola and papilla to form a secondary mound (may not occur in all girls)
Stage 3
Further enlargement of breast and areola with no separation of their contours
Stage 5
G. J. Wassilchenko
Mature configuration; projection of papilla only caused by recession of areola into general contour

Fig. 37-1 Development of the breast in girls—average age span, 11 to 13 years. Stage 1 (prepubertal—elevation of papilla only) is not shown. (Modified from Marshall WA, Tanner JM: *Arch Dis Child* 44:291, 1969; and Daniel WA, Paulshock BZ: *Patient Care*, pp. 122-124, May 13, 1979.)

on p. 1088). The spurts in height and weight occur concurrently toward the end of midpuberty. For most boys, breast enlargement disappears within 2 years. By late puberty there is a definite increase in the length and width of the penis, testicular enlargement continues, and first ejaculation occurs. Axillary hair develops and facial hair extends to cover the anterior neck. Final voice changes occur secondary to the growth of the larynx. Concerns about *pubertal delay* should be considered for boys who exhibit no enlargement of the testes or scrotal changes by ages 13.5 to 14 years or if genital growth is not complete 4 years after the testicles begin to enlarge.

Physical Growth

A constant phenomenon associated with sexual maturation is a dramatic increase in growth. The final 20% to 25% of height is achieved during puberty, and most of this growth occurs during a 24- to 36-month period—the adolescent *growth spurt*. This accelerated growth occurs in all children but, as in other areas of development, is highly variable in age of onset, duration, and extent. The growth spurt begins earlier in girls, usually between ages 9.5 and 14.5 years; on the average it begins between ages 10.5 and 16 years in boys. During this period the average boy will gain 10 to 30 cm (4 to 12 inches) in height and 7 to 30 kg (15 to 65 pounds) in weight; the average girl, in whom the growth spurt is slower and less extensive, will gain 5 to 20 cm (2 to 8 inches) in height and 7 to 25 kg (15 to 55 pounds) in weight. Growth in height typically ceases 2 to 2.5 years after menarche in girls and at age 18 to 20 years in boys.

This increase in size is acquired in a characteristic sequence of changes. Growth in length of the extremities and neck precedes growth in other areas, and, since these parts are first to reach adult length, the hands and feet appear larger than normal during adolescence. Increases in hip and chest breadth take place in a few months, followed several months later by an increase in shoulder width. These changes are followed by increases in length of the trunk and depth of the chest. It is this sequence of changes that is responsible for

Stage 1
(prepubertal)

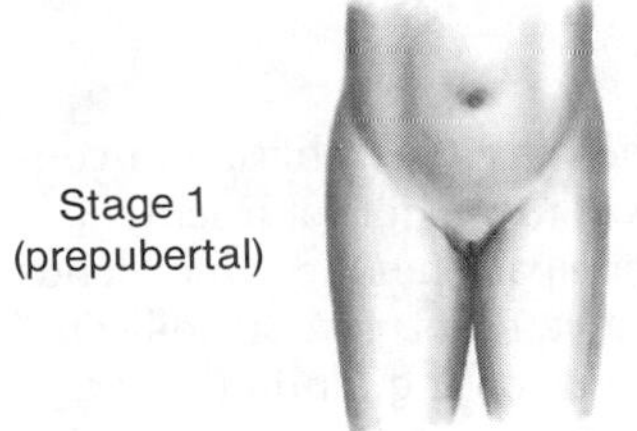

No pubic hair; essentially the same as during childhood; no distinction between hair on pubis and over the abdomen

Stage 2

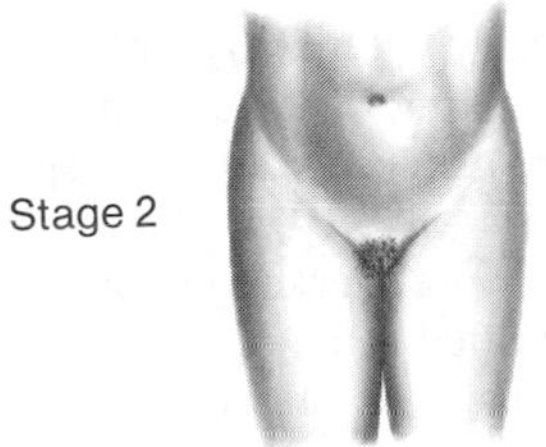

Sparse growth of long, straight, downy, and slightly pigmented hair extending along labia; between stages 2 and 3 begins to appear on pubis

Stage 3

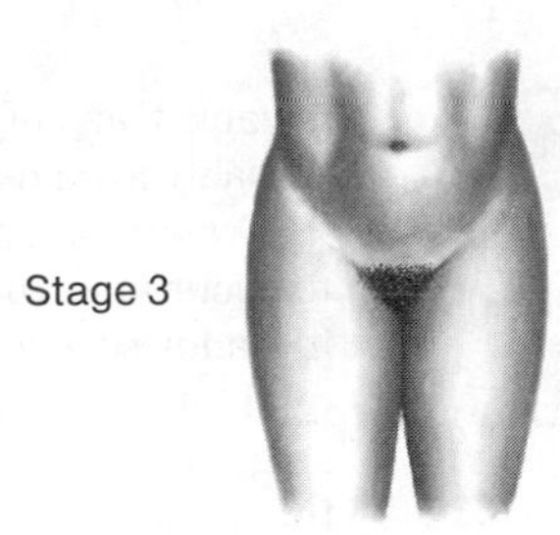

Hair darker, coarser, and curly and spread sparsely over entire pubis in the typical female triangle

Stage 4

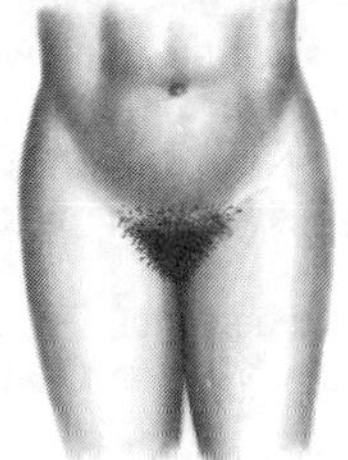

Pubic hair denser, curled, and adult in distribution but less abundant and restricted to the pubic area

Stage 5

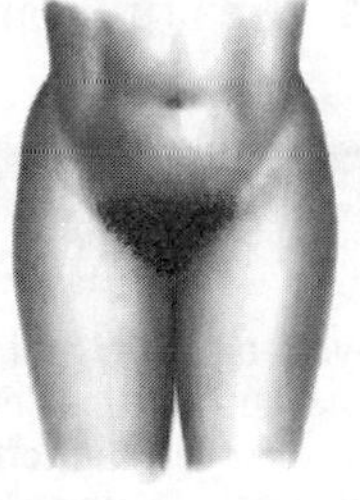

Hair adult in quantity, type, and pattern with spread to inner aspect of thighs

Fig. 37-2 Growth of pubic hair in girls—average age span for stages 2 through 5, 11 to 14 years. (Modified from Marshall WA, Tanner JM: *Arch Dis Child* 44:291, 1969; and Daniel WA, Paulshock BZ: *Patient Care*, pp. 122-124, May 13, 1979.)

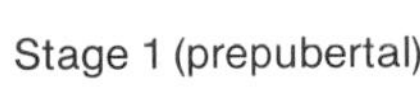

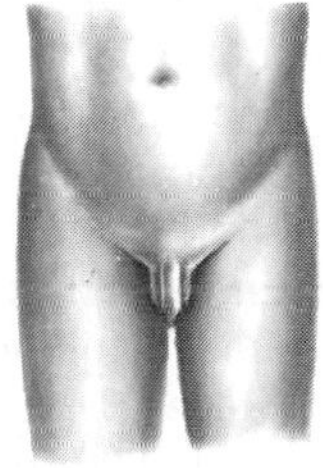

No pubic hair; essentially the same as during childhood; no distinction between hair on pubis and over the abdomen

Stage 2 (pubertal)

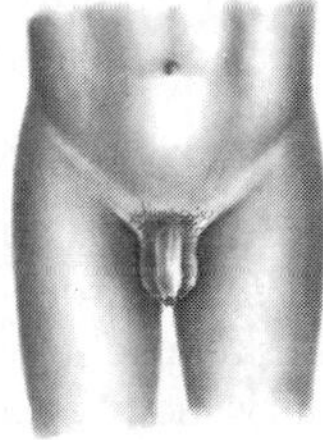

Initial enlargement of scrotum and testes; reddening and textural changes of scrotal skin; sparse growth of long, straight, downy, and slightly pigmented hair at base of penis

Stage 3

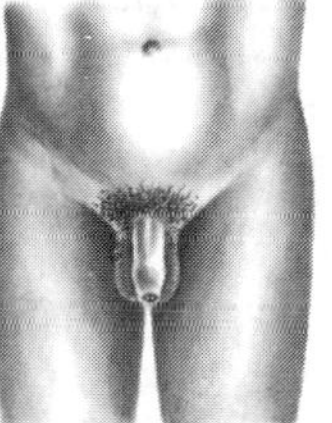

Initial enlargement of penis, mainly in length; testes and scrotum further enlarged; hair darker, coarser, and curly and spread sparsely over entire pubis

Stage 4

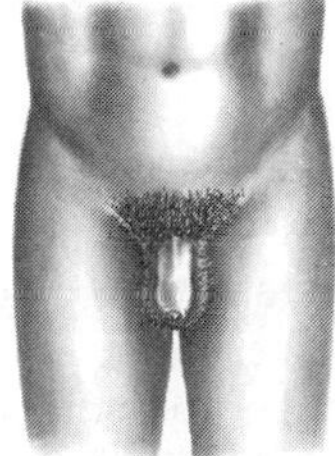

Increased size of penis with growth in diameter and development of glans; glans larger and broader; scrotum darker; pubic hair more abundant with curling but restricted to pubic area

Stage 5

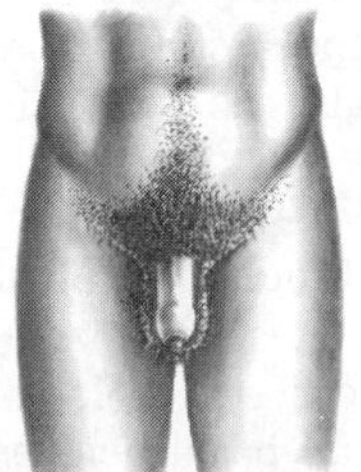

Testes, scrotum, and penis adult in size and shape; hair adult in quantity and type with spread to inner surface of thighs

Fig. 37-3 Developmental stages of secondary sex characteristics and genital development in boys—average age span, 12 to 16 years. (Modified from Marshall WA, Tanner JM: *Arch Dis Child* 44:291, 1969; and Daniel WA, Paulshock BZ: *Patient Care*, pp. 122-124, May 13, 1979.)

Critical Thinking Q & A 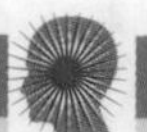

EMBARRASSING BODY CHANGES

Twelve-year-old Sam and his mother arrive at the clinic for Sam's checkup for a health clearance to attend summer camp. "What are you looking forward to most about going to camp, Sam?" you ask. "Nothing," Sam replies. "I don't even want to go."

"Sam's just getting lazy," said his mother. "His physical education (PE) teacher called the other night and said that Sam has used every excuse in the world to get out of participating in class." She continued, "He even wants to quit the swim team. All he wants to do is sit around and watch television and eat. Look at him. His laziness and all the food is beginning to show." You glance over at Sam and see a slight pouch and enlarged breasts through his T-shirt. Your most appropriate response would be:

1. "Sam, you are at a time in your life when you want and really need to eat, but if you don't stay active, you will become overweight.
2. "Sam, I see that you have something in common with many boys your age. On the way to becoming a man, some boys get enlarged and tender breasts for a short time."
3. "Sam, I see why you don't want to go to camp; you're afraid the other kids will make fun of you."
4. "Sam, you should go to camp. It will be lots of fun and you will be able to work off some of the extra pounds you've gained."

Answer two is the most appropriate response. Sam has gynecomastia. You surmise that he is embarrassed or perhaps even being teased about the condition. He needs to remove his shirt—further exposing his "problem"—during swim team practice or meets, and during showers after PE classes. This is probably why he has avoided both activities and is not looking forward to attending summer camp. The other three answers deny Sam the information he needs to adapt to this troublesome but temporary change in his body.

the characteristic long-legged, gawky appearance of the early adolescent child.

Gender Differences in General Growth Patterns

Gender differences in general growth and distribution patterns are apparent in skeletal growth, muscle mass, adipose tissue, and skin. Skeletal growth differences between boys and girls are apparently a function of hormonal effects at puberty and are evident primarily in limb length. The earlier cessation of growth in girls is caused by epiphyseal unity under the potent effect of estrogen secretion, and the hormonal effect on female bone growth is much stronger than the similar effect of testosterone in males. In boys the prolonged growth period before puberty and the less rapid epiphyseal closure are reflected in their greater overall height and longer arms and legs. Other skeletal differences are increased shoulder width in boys and broader hip development in girls.

Hypertrophy of the laryngeal mucosa and enlargement of the larynx and vocal cords occur in both boys and girls to produce voice changes. Girls' voices become slightly deeper and considerably fuller, but the effect in boys is striking. The "change of voice" in adolescent boys is one of the most noticeable traits of puberty, with the voice often shifting uncontrollably from deep to high tones in the middle of a sentence.

Growth of lean body mass, principally muscle, which tends to occur after the bone growth spurt, takes place steadily during adolescence. Lean body mass is both quantitatively and qualitatively greater in males than in females at comparable stages of pubertal development. Muscle development, under the influence of androgenic hormones, increases steadily. Muscles become remarkably well developed in boys, whereas in girls muscle mass increase is proportionate to general tissue growth.

Nonlean mass, primarily fat, is also increased but follows a less orderly pattern. There may be a transient increase in subcutaneous fat just before the skeletal growth spurt, especially in boys. This is followed 1 to 2 years later by a modest to marked decrease, again more marked in boys. Later, variable amounts of fat are deposited to fill out and contour the mature physique in patterns characteristic of the adolescent's gender, particularly in the regions over the thighs, hips, and buttocks and around the breast tissue.

Hormonal influences during puberty cause an acceleration in growth and maturation of the skin and its structural appendages. Sebaceous glands become extremely active at this time, especially those on the genitals and in the "flush areas" of the body (i.e., the face, neck, shoulders, and upper back and chest). This increased activity and the structural nature of the glands are extremely important in the pathogenesis of a common problem of puberty: acne (see Chapter 50). The eccrine sweat glands, present almost everywhere on the human skin, become fully functional and respond to emotional as well as thermal stimulation. Heavy sweating appears to be more pronounced in boys than in girls. The apocrine sweat glands, nonfunctional in childhood, reach secretory capacity during puberty. Unlike the eccrine sweat glands, the apocrine glands are limited in distribution and grow in conjunction with hair follicles in the axillae, around the areola of the breast, around the umbilicus, on the external auditory canal, and in the genital and anal regions. Apocrine glands secrete a thick substance as a result of emotional stimulation that, when acted on by surface bacteria, becomes highly odoriferous.

Body hair assumes very characteristic distribution patterns and changes texture during puberty. Under the influence of gonadal and adrenal androgens, hair coarsens, darkens, and lengthens at sites related to secondary sex characteristics. Pubic and axillary hair appears in both genders, although pubic hair is more extensive in males than in females. Beard, mustache, and body hair on the chest, upward along the linea alba, and sometimes on other areas (such as the back and shoulder) appears in males and is androgen dependent. Extremity hair appears in varying amounts in both males and females but is also more prolific in the male.

Physiologic Changes

A number of physiologic functions are altered in response to some of the pubertal changes. The size and strength of the heart, blood volume, and systolic blood pressure increase, whereas the pulse rate and basal heat production decrease (see the Appendix). Blood volume, which has increased steadily during childhood, reaches a higher value in boys than in girls, a fact that may be related to the increased muscle mass in pubertal boys. Adult values are reached for all formed elements of the blood. Respiratory rate and basal metabolic rate, decreasing steadily throughout childhood, reach the adult rate in adolescence. Respiratory volume and vital capacity are increased, and to a far greater extent in males than in females. During this period, physiologic responses to exercise change drastically—performance improves, especially in boys, and the body is able to make the physiologic adjustments needed for normal functioning after exercise is completed. These capabilities result from the increased size and strength of muscles and the increased level of cardiac, respiratory, and metabolic functioning.

PSYCHOSOCIAL DEVELOPMENT

Developing a Sense of Identity (Erikson)

Traditional psychosocial theory holds that the developmental crisis of adolescence leads to the formation of a sense of identity (Erikson, 1963). Throughout childhood, individuals have been going through the process of identification as they concentrate on various parts of the body at specific times. During infancy, children identify themselves as being separate from the mother; during early childhood, they establish a gender role identification with the appropriate-gender parent; and in later childhood, they establish who they are in relation to others. In adolescence, they come to see themselves as distinct individuals, somehow unique and separate from every other individual.

The early period of adolescence begins with the onset of puberty and extends to relative physical and emotional stability at or near graduation from high school. During this time the adolescent is faced with the crisis of *group identity* vs. alienation. In the period that follows the individual hopes to attain autonomy from the family and develop a sense of *personal identity* as opposed to role diffusion. A sense of group identity appears to be essential as a prelude to a sense of personal identity. Young adolescents must resolve questions concerning relationships with a peer group before they are able to resolve questions about who they are in relation to family and society.

Group identity. During the early stage of adolescence the pressure to belong to a group is intensified. Teenagers find it essential to have a group to which they feel they can belong and which provides them with status. Belonging to a crowd helps adolescents define the differences between themselves and their parents. They dress as the group dresses and wear makeup and hairstyles according to group criteria—all of which are different from those of the parental generation. Language, music, and dancing reflect a culture that is exclusive to the adolescent. When adults begin to emulate these fashions and interests, the style changes immediately. The evidence of adolescent conformity to the peer group and nonconformity to the adult group provides teenagers with a frame of reference in which they can display their own self-assertion while they reject the identity of their parents' generation. To be different is to be unaccepted and alienated from the group.

Individual identity. The quest for personal identity is part of the ongoing identification process. As youngsters establish identity within a group, they are also attempting to incorporate multiple body changes into a concept of the self. Body awareness is part of self-awareness, and for some time the adolescent will engage in assimilating the self represented by this dimension. In this search for identity, adolescents consider the relationships that have developed between themselves and others in the past, as well as the directions they hope to be able to take in the future.

Significant others hold certain expectations for the behavior of the adolescent. Often these expectations or demands are persistent enough to result in certain decisions that might be made differently or not at all if the individual could be solely responsible for identity formation. It is all too easy to slip into the roles that are expected by these external influences without incorporating personal goals or questioning these decisions in relation to the developing personality. Thus individuals may become what parents or others wish them to be based on these premature decisions. Also, young persons might form a negative identity when society or their culture provides them with a self-image that is contrary to the values of the community. Labels such as "juvenile delinquent" or "failure" are applied to certain adolescents, who then accept and live up to these labels with behaviors that validate and strengthen them.

The process of evolving a personal identity is time-consuming and fraught with periods of confusion, depression, and discouragement. Determining an identity and a place in the world is a critical and perilous feature of adolescence (see the Critical Thinking Q & A box below). However, as

Critical Thinking Q & A 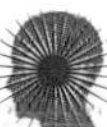

DISCUSSING THE FUTURE

Jeremy, age 17 years, will be graduating from high school in the spring. His mother, a single parent, tells you that she is concerned because the time is quickly approaching and Jeremy has made no plans for what he will do with his life after graduation. Whenever Jeremy mentions the topic, his mother tells him, "This is what you must do" and begins to outline the steps he must take. Jeremy just walks away. She asks, "What should I do?" Your most appropriate advice to Jeremy's mother is:

1. "Think about Jeremy's interests and what he has been successful doing in the past. Arrange for him to speak to someone whose career builds on those interests."
2. "Continue to tell him what he must do. Eventually you will get through to him and he will listen."
3. "Be open and available to him. Tell him what you think, but not what to do."
4. "You are wise to be concerned. We need to arrange some counseling for Jeremy."

The correct answer at this stage is number three. Most adolescents want adult guidance and help, and messages are more likely to be heard if presented in an open-ended, nonjudgmental, nondictatorial fashion. Teenagers are unlikely to discuss their concerns on a timetable. Parents create the time and space and then wait. Parents who are available and willing to listen generally find that their adolescents are eager to talk. Answer number one could be a good second step if Jeremy and his mother explore his interests together. Answer number two is disrespectful to Jeremy, has not worked in the past, and likely will not work in the future. Answer number four may be necessary at a later time if other strategies fail.

the pieces are gradually shifted and settled into place, a positive identity eventually emerges from the confusion. Role diffusion results when the individual is unable to formulate a satisfactory identity from the multiplicity of aspirations, roles, and identifications.

Sex-role identity. Adolescence is the time for consolidation of a sex-role identity. During early adolescence the peer group begins to communicate some expectations regarding heterosexual relationships, and as development progresses, adolescents encounter expectations for mature sex-role behavior from both peers and adults. Expectations such as these vary from culture to culture, among geographic areas, and among socioeconomic groups.

Emotionality. Adolescents vacillate in their emotional states and between considerable maturity and childlike behavior. One minute they are exuberant and enthusiastic; the next minute they are depressed and withdrawn. Unpredictable, but essentially normal, outbursts of primitive behavior appear as the teenager loses control over instinctual drives. As the tension is relieved, emotion is brought under control and individuals retreat to review what has happened, to attempt to master their anger, and in the overall process to grow in their ability to control their emotions and gain from the new experience. Because of these "tantrums" and mood swings, adolescents are often labeled as unstable, inconsistent, and unpredictable. Little things can cause an emotional upheaval and, depending on the teenager's interpretation, can mean a great deal.

Teenagers are better able to control their emotions in later adolescence. They can approach problems more calmly and rationally, and although they are still subject to periods of depression, their feelings are less vulnerable and they begin to demonstrate the more mature emotions of later adolescence. Whereas early adolescents react immediately and emotionally, older adolescents can control their emotions until socially acceptable times and places for expression present themselves. They are still subject to heightened emotion, and when it is expressed, their behavior reflects feelings of insecurity, tension, and indecision.

COGNITIVE DEVELOPMENT (PIAGET)

Cognitive thinking culminates with the capacity for *abstract thinking.* This stage, the period of *formal operations,* is Piaget's fourth and last stage. Adolescents are no longer restricted to the real and actual, which was typical of the period of concrete thought; they are also concerned with the possible. They now think beyond the present. Without having to center attention on the immediate situation, they can imagine a sequence of events that might occur, such as college and occupational possibilities; how things might change in the future, such as relationships with parents; and the consequences of their actions, such as dropping out of school. At this time, their thoughts can be influenced by logical principles rather than just their own perceptions and experiences. They now become increasingly capable of scientific reasoning and formal logic.

They are capable of mentally manipulating more than two categories of variables at the same time. For example, they can consider the relationship between speed, distance, and time in planning a trip. They can detect logical consistency or inconsistency in a set of statements and evaluate a system or set of values in a more analytic manner. For instance, they question the parent who insists on honesty in the youngster but at the same time cheats on an income tax report or expense account.

Young people are now able to think about both their own thinking and the thinking of others. They wonder what opinion others have of them, and they are increasingly able to imagine the thoughts of others. With this capacity comes the ability to differentiate between others' thoughts and their own and to interpret thoughts of others more accurately. Thus they are able to understand that few concepts are absolute or independent of other influencing factors. As they come to know that other cultures and communities have different norms and standards from their own, it becomes easier to accept members of these other cultures, and the decision to behave in their own culture in an accepted manner becomes a more conscious commitment to that culture.

MORAL DEVELOPMENT (KOHLBERG)

Whereas younger children merely accept the decisions or point of view of adults, adolescents, to gain autonomy from adults, must substitute their own set of morals and values. When old principles are challenged but new and independent values have not yet emerged to take their place, young people search for a moral code that preserves their personal integrity and guides their behavior, especially in the face of strong pressure to violate the old beliefs. Their decisions involving moral dilemmas must be based on an internalized set of moral principles that provides them with the resources to evaluate the demands of the situation and to plan a course of action that is consistent with their ideals.

Late adolescence is characterized by a serious questioning of existing moral values and their relevance to society and the individual. Adolescents can easily take the role of another. They understand duty and obligation based on reciprocal rights of others, as well as the concept of justice that is founded on making amends for misdeeds and repairing or replacing what has been spoiled by wrongdoing. However, they seriously question established moral codes, often as a result of observing that adults verbally ascribe to a code but do not adhere to it.

SPIRITUAL DEVELOPMENT

As youngsters move toward independence from parents and other authorities, some begin to question the values and ideals of their families. Others cling to these values as a stable element in their lives as they struggle with the conflicts of this turbulent period. Adolescents need to work out these conflicts for themselves, but they also need support from authority figures and/or peers for their resolution. Often the peer group is more influential than parents, although values acquired during the formative years are usually maintained.

Adolescents are capable of understanding abstract concepts and of interpreting analogies and symbols. They are able to empathize, philosophize, and think logically. Most are searching for ideals and speculate about illogical statements and conflicting ideologies. Their tendency toward introspection and emotional intensity at this age often makes it difficult for others to know what they are thinking. They tend to keep their thoughts private, fearing that no one will understand these feelings that they perceive to be unique and special. Yet it is not uncommon for them to reveal deep spiritual concerns. They need support and encouragement in their struggle for understanding and the freedom to question without censure.

Young people may reject formal worship services but engage in individual worship in the privacy of their room. They may need to explore the concept of the existence of God. Comparing their religion with that of others may result in their questioning their own beliefs but ultimately results in formulating and solidifying their spirituality.

SOCIAL DEVELOPMENT

To achieve full maturity, adolescents must free themselves from family domination and define an identity independent of parental authority. However, this process is fraught with ambivalence on the part of both teenagers and their parents. Adolescents want to grow up and to be free of parental restraints; yet they are fearful as they try to comprehend the responsibilities that are linked with independence. Feelings of immortality and exemption from the consequences of risk-taking behavior, although viewed as negative, can serve an important developmental function at this time. These feelings can give adolescents the courage to separate from their parents and become independent (Prothrow-Stith, 1993). Part of this emancipation involves developing social relationships outside the family that help teenagers identify their role in society. Adolescence is a time of intense sociability and often a time of equally intense loneliness. Acceptance by peers, a few close friends, and the secure love of a supportive family are requisites for the interpersonal maturation process.

Relationships with Parents

During adolescence the parent-child relationship changes from one of protection-dependency to one of mutual affection and equality. The process of achieving independence often involves turmoil and ambiguity as both parent and adolescent learn to play new roles and work toward this end while, at the same time, resolving the often painful series of rifts essential to establishing the ultimate relationships.

Most of the behavior observed in the adolescent is related to the struggle for independence and the external restrictions and checks that are placed on this spontaneous maturation process. On the one hand, adolescents are accepted as maturing preadults. They are allowed privileges heretofore denied, and they are provided with increasing responsibilities. On the other hand, because of their unpredictability and insecurity in evaluating situations and making sound judgments, they must conform to regulations and restrictions set by adults. This state of affairs is particularly exemplified by the struggle between parents and adolescents concerning the nightly curfew.

As teenagers assert their rights for grown-up privileges, they frequently create tensions within the home. They resist parental control, and conflicts can arise from almost any situation or any subject. Some of the favorite topics of dispute include use of the telephone, manners, dress, chores and duties, homework, disrespectful behavior, friendships, dating, money, automobiles, drinking and/or drugs, smoking, and time schedules. Present in these areas of conflict are the overriding argument that "Everyone else has one" or is allowed the desired item or privilege and the ever-present assertions that "You don't understand me or trust me" and "You always treat me like a baby." Spoken or unspoken, parents' reactions consist of "Is this all the thanks I get for what I have done, or am doing, for you?"

The teenager's earliest attempts to achieve emancipation from parental controls are manifested in a period of rejection of the parents. Adolescents are critical, argumentative, and generally remote with both parents. They absent themselves from home and family activities and spend an increasing amount of time with the peer group. They confide less in their parents. This rejection is not consistent, however, and varies with mood changes.

With advancing adolescence, teenagers become more competent, and with this competence comes a need for more autonomy. However, although they are psychologically better prepared for independence, they are often thwarted in their efforts by lack of money or by other parental barriers. Much conflict arises in relation to the teenager's outside activities and the elements of privacy and trust. Too many parents believe that they must know all of their adolescent's activities and feelings; they may go through the teenager's belongings in an attempt to find out what the youngster is doing. However, to gain the respect and trust of adolescents, parents must respect their youngster's privacy, as well as show an honest and sincere interest in what the adolescent believes and feels (see the Family Focus box below).

The recent trends in society in terms of equality and relaxation of previous moral standards have made the adjustments of teenagers and parents increasingly difficult. The so-called

Family Focus 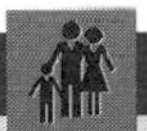

COMMUNICATION WITH TEENAGERS—THE ART OF LISTENING

Conflicts between parents and their adolescents often result from a very natural characteristic of parenthood: the desire to protect one's offspring from harm or from simply doing something "stupid," embarrassing, or that they may later regret. Teenagers sometimes bounce their thoughts and ideas off adults. Sometimes they really want some feedback; other times, they simply want to elicit a reaction.

I found it easy to listen openly, thoughtfully, and without interrupting when my teenagers' friends discussed troublesome topics. However, one day, when one of my own teenagers had a similar conversation with me, the parent part kicked in. I felt responsible and spoke my piece on the spot. This brought communication to a halt and resulted in defensiveness. It was a long time before my child tried to talk to me about anything controversial again.

The next time one of my teenagers started a similar conversation, I decided to try to trick myself. Throughout the entire conversation, I told myself over and over again to act as if this were not my teenager, but someone else's child. I found this actually worked quite well and I was able to listen without interrupting. I continued to use the system, at times with more success than others.

Mother of four

generation gap is widening in relation to a number of attitudes, values, and beliefs. Parents can no longer find guidance from their own experiences in understanding the needs of today's teenagers.

Relationships with Peers

Although parents remain the primary influence in their lives, for the majority of adolescents peers assume a more significant role in adolescence than they did during childhood. The peer group serves as a strong support to teenagers, individually and collectively, providing them with a sense of belonging and a feeling of strength and power. It forms that transitional world between dependence and autonomy.

Peer group. Adolescents are usually social, gregarious, and group minded. Thus the peer group has an intense influence on adolescents' self-evaluation and behavior. To gain acceptance by a group, younger teenagers tend to conform completely in such things as mode of dress, hairstyle, taste in music, and vocabulary, often at the expense of individuality and self-assertion. The teenagers' entire being is measured by the reactions of their peers.

The school is psychologically important to adolescents as a focus of social life. Teenagers usually distribute themselves into a relatively predictable social hierarchy. They know to which group they and others belong.

Within the larger groups are smaller, distinct, and rather exclusive crowds or cliques of selected close friends, based on common tastes, interests, and background, who are emotionally attached to each other. Although cliques may become formalized, most remain informal and small. But each has an identifying feature that proclaims its difference from others and its solidarity within itself, in much the same manner as the adolescent generation as a whole sets itself apart from the adult generation. Cliques are usually made up of one gender, and girls tend to be more cliquish than boys and to have a greater need for close friendships (Fig. 37-4). Within the intimacy of the group, adolescents gain support in learning about themselves, consideration for the feelings of others, and increased ego development and self-reliance.

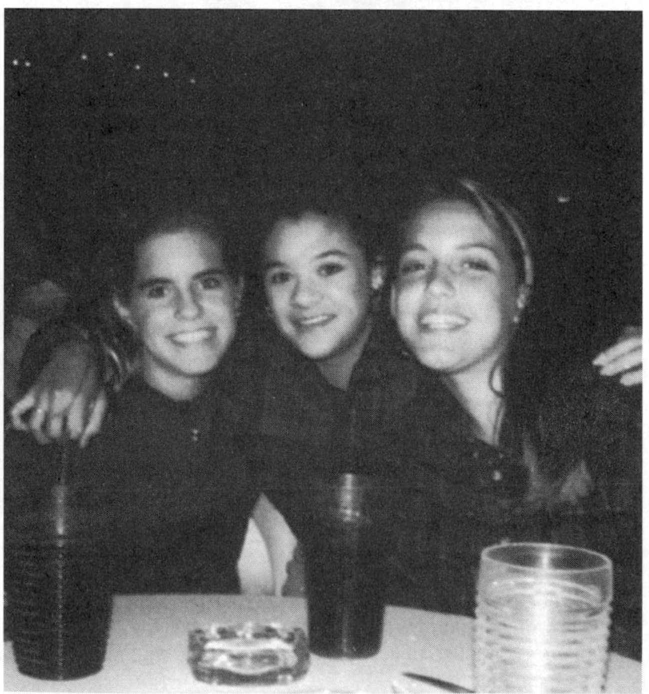

Fig. 37-4 Teenagers like to gather in small groups.

To belong is of utmost importance; thus adolescents behave in a way that will ensure their establishment in a group. Adolescents are highly susceptible to social approval, acceptance, and demands. To be ignored or criticized by peers creates feelings of inferiority, inadequacy, and incompetence.

Best friends. Personal friendships of the one-on-one variety usually develop between like-gender adolescents. This relationship is closer and more stable than it is in middle childhood, and it is important in the quest for identity. A best friend is the best audience on whom to try out possible roles and identities that an adolescent wants to test. Best friends may try a role together, each providing support for the other. Each cares about what the other thinks and feels. Since a sense of intimacy grows within a permanent relationship, the stability of this like-gender friendship is an important link in the progress toward an intimate heterosexual relationship in young adulthood.

Heterosexual Relationships

During adolescence, relationships with members of the opposite gender take on new importance. Although there seems to be a trend toward earlier dating, on the *average*, dating activities begin in the seventh and eighth grades and are usually "crowd" dates at organized school functions. For example, a group of girls just happens to be around a certain group of boys at most activities. During high school, crowd dates are still popular, but now there is more pairing off of couples. Double-dating and then single-pair dating follow group dating. Most adolescents are dating to some degree by the time they leave high school.

The type and degree of seriousness of heterosexual relationships vary. The initial stage is usually noncommittal, extremely mobile, and seldom characterized by any deep romantic attachments. Crushes, those strong feelings of attachment to an important or well-liked adult in the youngster's life who embodies the qualities considered most valuable by the adolescent, are common in early adolescence; they constitute one of the earliest "love" attachments.

During early midadolescence, as their sexual capacity is evolving, young boys may feel the need to test the power of their sexuality by numerous exploits and conquests. It may be a response to inner sexual pressures or a need to conform to group expectations. With advancing adolescence and a firmer sexual identity, steady dating and boy-girl love relationships with deeper commitment become more numerous. The relationship continues until misunderstanding or boredom ends the association, and the process is often repeated with another partner.

Authorities disagree regarding the value of early opposite-gender relationships in the development of a sexual identity. Some believe that longer like-gender relationships are necessary to fully develop the characteristics of one's own gender, whereas others believe that dating provides adolescents with

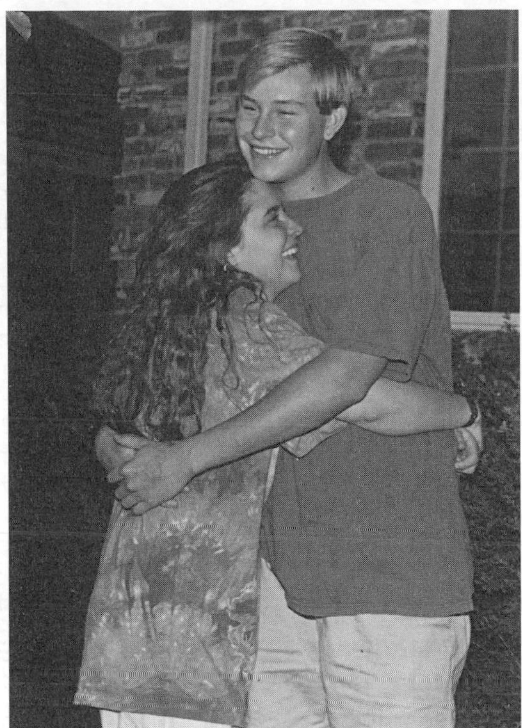

Fig. 37-5 Heterosexual friendships are characteristic of adolescence.

experience in human relationships, promotes social skills, and enhances their ability to choose a mate wisely (Fig. 37-5).

Sexual activity. Since puberty occurs at earlier ages than it did a half-century ago, and since the line between sexuality and sex is blurred, sexual activity among adolescents is an area that must be addressed. Masturbatory activity usually begins at puberty. Although both genders engage in this behavior, it is more commonly reported by boys. Masturbation provides an opportunity for sexual self-exploration before the development of regular social-sexual interaction with another individual. Participation in this behavior is greatly influenced by learned cultural attitudes, religion, and sex-role expectations.

During adolescence, most youngsters indulge in kissing and petting, the traditional first steps in the sequence of heterosexual activity. In addition, a greater proportion of teenagers are sexually experienced with each successive year of adolescence. About one third of males and one fourth of females have had sexual intercourse by age 15 years; by the age of 18 or 19 years, three quarters of American youth have had sexual relations with another person (Seidman and Rieder, 1994).

Adolescents engage in sexual relationships for pleasurable sensations, to satisfy sexual drives, to satisfy curiosity, as a conquest, as an expression of some degree of affection, or from the inability to withstand pressures to conform. Often the urge to belong to and gain reassurance from a group and the wish to really belong to someone provoke a series of increasingly intimate physical contacts with a favored boyfriend or girlfriend, with each contact being more sexually provocative than the last. Eventually sexual intercourse becomes established as a behavior pattern and a method for ensuring social participation—or even as an end in itself. Early dating can involve an adolescent pair in a close sexual relationship before they are ready for intimacy.

The current trend toward greater permissiveness regarding adolescent sexual behavior will undoubtedly have an effect on the adolescent developmental experience. However, the recent concern with transmission of acquired immunodeficiency syndrome (AIDS) may influence these sexually permissive attitudes. It has been predicted that attitudes toward sex will shift from a moral context to a predominantly health context within a few years. Unfortunately, many adolescents cling to the fallacy that heterosexual behaviors are AIDS free.

Homosexuality in Adolescents

The development of homosexuality during childhood or adolescence has been greatly ignored and thought to be either a transient experience or a pathologic event. The pediatric community has recognized the special needs of these adolescents in order to foster a healthy transition during this period.

Confusion about sexual orientation is common in adolescence. However, most adolescents who participate in homosexual activity or have homosexual feelings do not become gay or lesbian adults (Friedman and Downey, 1994). Nurses need to recognize the potential for same-gender attraction and to be sensitive to the fact that not all youths will be involved in heterosexual relationships. Nurses must also evaluate their own attitudes and beliefs about homosexuality to determine their own comfort level in providing health care to gay or lesbian youths.

In addition to all the normal tasks of adolescence, gay males and females have their own unique issues of identity formation. This process, which can begin as early as preadolescence, has been called "coming out" and does not refer to any particular event or time, but to a series of events that lead adolescents to establish an integrated sense of who they are.

Interests and Activities

During early adolescence the interests and activities of girls and boys are in rather sharp contrast. Boys spend a great deal of time in active sports or "just going out with the guys." They enjoy hobbies and clubs, and television and video or computer games take up a good part of their time. Girls and mixed-gender activities are of interest to boys but do not become prominent concerns until their development more nearly approaches that of the more rapidly maturing girls. As their bodies gain strength and size, "making the team" is a major concern for many youths, and a boy may spend an excessive amount of time in attempting to perfect athletic skills. The essential bicycle of middle childhood is replaced by the automobile, the symbol of status to the adolescent. If a car cannot be acquired, a motorcycle or motorbike is preferable to walking, riding the bus, or the humiliation of being chauffeured by a parent or sibling. Many boys avidly seek part-time employment, some because of economic necessity.

Girls' leisure interests may also involve sports, and an increased interest in parties and social activities is evident. They may be interested in hobbies and volunteer activities, and many seek part-time jobs through necessity or to purchase more clothes and other teenage "necessities." They are avid conversationalists and spend much of their time in the company of other girls, talking, listening to music, and experimenting with makeup, hairstyles, and clothes. They enjoy shopping for clothes. Many of their thoughts and feelings are confessed in a diary.

Members of both genders enjoy movies, rock concerts, dancing, and other communal activities and entertainment, including "cruising" favorite streets in automobiles and gathering in shopping malls. Movies are often a favorite pastime. With the availability of movies on videotape, adolescents congregate in small groups to watch films on home video players.

Dancing has always occupied a central place in the customs of many cultures. There is delight in physical movement and a feeling of relief that comes from the release of tension in activity. Dancing can also serve as a means of expressing specific sexual and aggressive urges in symbolic form and action. Many of the popular dances have sexual overtones and erotic movements. At the same time the structure of today's teen dances is such that the dancers seldom touch one another. In this way the urges can be expressed without the danger of close physical contact. Conversely, slow dancing provides a socially acceptable mode of close physical contact.

Reading is still a favorite occupation of many teenagers and may serve to satisfy some of their needs for vicarious experiences. Reading is generally more purposeful at this stage than at earlier ages.

Traditional television viewing may decline in adolescence, and many teenagers have a decided preference for music. Teenagers often are avidly addicted to the portable radios and tape or compact disc (CD) players that accompany many of their other activities (e.g., studying, walking, and working). Closely associated with the radio is the stereo, which assumes an important role in teenagers' lives. Much of their money may be spent on recorded media, which are collected in much the same way as books.

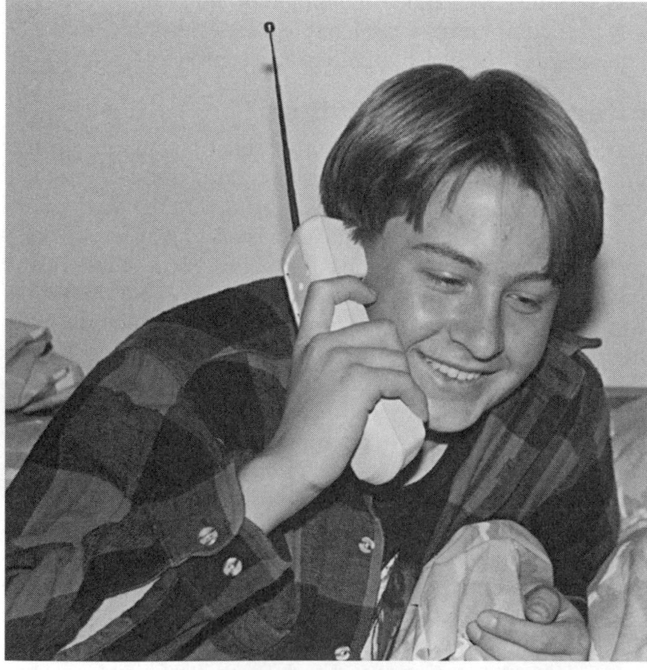

Fig. 37-6 The telephone, especially the portable phone, provides teenagers with hours of conversation with same- and opposite-sex friends.

When they are not engaged in other activities, teenagers enjoy participating in endless conversations in person or on the telephone. The telephone provides that essential link between peers when they are physically removed from one another. It fulfills the need for flight from parents to peers without leaving the home. For boy-girl conversations the telephone provides a way to experience closeness without the fear of complications that physical proximity may engender (Fig. 37-6).

Teenage interests and activities are subject to rapid change. Each succeeding "generation" of teenagers has its own peculiar characteristics, which are evidenced in behavior, vocabulary, dress, and other external manifestations that reflect and establish a clear line of separateness, although superficial, between the peer and the adult cultures. The rapidity with which these external trappings change is often astonishing.

DEVELOPMENT OF SELF-CONCEPT AND BODY IMAGE

The sudden growth that takes place in early adolescence creates feelings of confusion for adolescents. They have lost the security of a familiar body and feel a strangeness about their altered bodies. Consequently, they may try either to hide them or to advertise them, or they may alternate between the two extremes. Teenagers are acutely aware of their appearance as they begin to acquire images of themselves as adults, but they see discrepancies between their ideal and actual skills and abilities.

Adolescents are continually comparing themselves with their peers and making judgments about their own normality based on these observations. Pubertal children feel most comfortable when they are just like their friends and age-mates. Perceived defects or deviations from the group average are threatening to their idealized image. Any blemish is likely to be magnified out of proportion, and any delay of the visible evidence of maturity is cause for worry. Unfortunately, this is also the time when the hormonal effect of the sebaceous glands produces acne, creating problems for many youngsters. To the adolescent, even the most insignificant pimple may be viewed as a gross disfigurement; every blemish is a major catastrophe. The advent of chronic disease or a permanent physical disability has very special significance during adolescence and creates additional stresses for both the youngster with the condition and for health workers.

It has been determined that the body image established during adolescence is the one that individuals retain throughout life. Much of adolescents' search for identity takes place before a mirror as they try to read from the reflected features just who they are and what they look like to other people. Adolescents practice facial expressions and postures, try out hair arrangements, worry about a pimple, and in other ways attempt to assess the best means to achieve a maximum effect —to reveal the "true self."

The self-concept becomes more differentiated as adolescents acquire a more complex picture of themselves, one that takes situational factors into account. The self-concept becomes more individuated and distinct from the concepts of others. Whereas younger children describe themselves in terms of similarities with peers, as adolescence advances, youngsters describe themselves more in terms of their special characteristics.

Boys' Responses to Puberty

The early adolescent increases in height and muscle mass are welcomed by the adolescent boy, whose growth, for several months, has lagged significantly behind that of his female age-mates. Although his more mature physique brings a highly valued increase in strength and more mature athletic skills, this rapid growth is uneven. When bones grow faster than muscles, muscles are taut and respond with quick, jerky movements; when muscles grow faster than bones, they become somewhat loose and sluggish. For a period of time, he is awkward and uncoordinated.

The development of secondary sex characteristics, especially the growth of facial and body hair, has psychologic and social meaning for the adolescent boy. This, more than any other secondary characteristic, is associated with the masculine gender role, and the ritual act of shaving at the slightest evidence of growth is a way for the young boy to validate his identification with this role. Shaving also provides a legitimate excuse to gaze at and admire the broadening shoulders and altered features of his changing body image (Fig. 37-7).

The growth of the penis and testes creates some important problems for the adolescent male. Unlike the reproductive organs in the female, the male reproductive organs are readily visible and provide the boy with concrete evidence of his masculine character. He knows by the sensations localized within these organs that he is maturing. His reproductive organs become sensitive to sexual stimulation. Sexual feelings are directly related to the genitals, desire is urgent, and he seeks rapid relief from pressure and tension through ejaculation.

The maturation of male genital function allows the male to produce seminal fluid. This may be released spontaneously as a **nocturnal emission,** or "wet dream." Spontaneous ejaculations are often puzzling, troublesome, and embarrassing events. Unless he has been prepared in advance for this eventuality, the boy often finds it difficult to seek an explanation from his parents. Therefore he turns to friends or reading material to gain information, or he may puzzle about the meaning in his own mind.

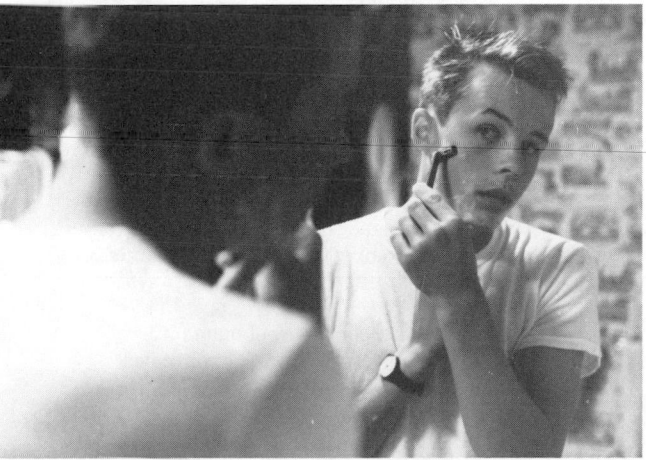

Fig. 37-7 The act of shaving offers the adolescent male the opportunity to study his changing appearance.

The frequency of erections is increased in response to various stimuli, as is the frequency of sexual outlet through masturbation or intercourse. The opportunity for gratification of these genital urges through heterosexual expression is often limited by Western cultural standards; early premarital sexual involvement is fraught with many problems and conflicts. In addition, homosexual activities are not universally accepted by society. As a consequence, the teenage boy resorts to masturbation, manipulating the genitals for the purpose of ejaculation, to relieve himself of the accumulated pressures in his genital organs. Almost every boy masturbates alone or in relation to sexual experimentation with others of the same gender. However, this, too, is often associated with guilt and anxiety. Misconceptions still dominate the feelings of many people who believe masturbation to be evil, unmanly, or "not nice" and who attribute a wide assortment of ills to the practice. Adolescent males need to be reassured that to engage in the practice from time to time is normal and that it temporarily helps provide the young man with important information about how his body works and how adult physical sexuality and reproduction are accomplished.

Girls' Responses to Puberty

As girls begin the pubertal changes, they, too, become very body conscious. Because in girls the onset of puberty is almost 2 years before that in boys, their initial reaction to increased height may be embarrassment as they find themselves towering above their male classmates. They worry about becoming too tall. Adolescent girls often slouch or adopt a hunched posture in an attempt to minimize this increased height—especially early-maturing girls, who are normally of above-average height. The increase in weight and the normal plumping of features with fat deposition are predominant concerns of pubescent girls. They perceive these changes to be evidence of a tendency toward obesity; many attempt to avoid them by strict and rather faddish dieting. This poorly timed strategy can deprive their bodies of essential nutrients during a period of rapid body development.

The young girl is interested in her changing form and feminine curves. The average girl looks on her budding breasts with pleasure as a sign of approaching maturity and evidence of her femininity. She observes and may even measure the progress of her developing breasts and continually compares her own progress with that of her friends and classmates. She begins to wear a bra. Some girls are sensitive about their breast development and attempt to hide it, whereas others are delighted with their new figures and wear tight sweaters and clothes that accentuate their curves.

Development of some of the secondary sex characteristics may be less pleasing to girls than they are to boys, particularly the growth of body hair. The dominant culture in which smooth-skinned females are preferred makes it necessary for the girl to shave her underarms and legs regularly to meet the standards for feminine appearance. The girl becomes increasingly conscious of the feminine ideal and, in an effort to approach this standard, experiments with a variety of cosmetics and hairstyles. Alone and together, she and her friends spend

TABLE 37-1 Growth and development during adolescence

EARLY ADOLESCENCE (11-14 YEARS)	MIDDLE ADOLESCENCE (15-17 YEARS)	LATE ADOLESCENCE (18-20 YEARS)
Growth		
Rapidly accelerating growth Reaches peak velocity Secondary sex characteristics appear	Growth decelerating in girls Stature reaches 95% of adult height Secondary sex characteristics well advanced	Physically mature Structure and reproductive growth almost complete
Cognition		
Explores newfound ability for limited abstract thought Clumsy groping for new values and engeries Comparison of "normality" with peers of same gender	Developing capacity for abstract thinking Enjoys intellectual powers, often in idealistic terms Concern with philosophic, political, and social problems	Established abstract thought Can perceive and act on long-range options Able to view problems comprehensively Intellectual and functional identity established
Identity		
Preoccupied with rapid body changes Tries out various roles Measures attractiveness by acceptance or rejection of peers Conformity to group norms	Modifies body image Very self-centered; increased narcissism Tendency toward inner experience and self-discovery Has a rich fantasy life Idealistic Able to perceive future implications of current behavior and decisions; variable application	Body image and gender role definition nearly secured Mature sexual identity Phase of consolidation of identity Stability of self-esteem Comfortable with physical growth Social roles defined and articulated
Relationships with parents		
Defining independence-dependence boundaries Strong desire to remain dependent on parents while trying to detach No major conflicts over parental control	Major conflicts over independence and control Low point in parent-child relationship Greatest push for emancipation; disengagement Final and irreversible emotional detachment from parents; mourning	Emotional and physical separation from parents completed Independence from family with less conflict Emancipation nearly secured
Relationships with peers		
Seeks peer affiliations to counter instability generated by rapid change Upsurge of close idealized friendships with members of the same gender Struggle for mastery takes place within peer group	Strong need for identity to affirm self-image Behavioral standards set by peer group Acceptance by peers extremely important—fear of rejection Exploration of ability to attract the opposite gender	Peer group recedes in importance in favor of individual friendship Testing of male-female relationships against possibility of permanent alliance Relationships characterized by giving and sharing
Sexuality		
Self-exploration and evaluation Limited dating, usually group Limited intimacy	Multiple plural relationships Decisive turn toward heterosexuality (if is homosexual, knows by this time) Exploration of "sex appeal" Feeling of "being in love" Tentative establishment of relationships	Forms stable relationships and attachment to another Growing capacity for mutuality and reciprocity Dating as a male-female pair Intimacy involves commitment rather than exploration and romanticism
Psychologic health		
Wide mood swings Intense daydreaming Anger outwardly expressed with moodiness, temper outbursts, and verbal insults and name-calling	Tendency toward inner experiences; more introspective Tendency to withdraw when upset or feelings are hurt Vascillation of emotions in time and range Feelings of inadequacy common; difficulty in asking for help	More constancy of emotion Anger more apt to be concealed

endless hours before the mirror posing, applying cosmetics, and combing their hair.

The advent of menstruation, that exclusive feature of female puberty, provides the greatest impetus toward full realization and acceptance of female sexuality. Menstruation is positive evidence of womanhood and the potential for pregnancy and childbearing. Most girls are adequately prepared for the event and take this new function in stride, looking forward to menstruation, feeling satisfaction at its onset, and seeing it as the symbol of their passage from childhood to womanhood. Others find it distressing, frightening, and difficult to accept. Because of its sudden onset, the first menstruation can be a traumatic experience for the girl who has not been taught what to expect.

Unlike the adolescent boy, strong sexual feelings in the adolescent girl are not usually centered in the genital region but are more generalized. Girls' first sexual experiences are likely to be different from and have different meanings than those of boys. Masturbation is less regularly practiced. Adolescent girls are more likely than boys to experience sex for the first time in a perceived close relationship than by masturbation. The changes that occur during the early, middle and late phases of adolescence are summarized in Table 37-1.

Promoting Optimum Health During Adolescence

Adolescents are, on the whole, healthy individuals. The disease level is low during this period, but there is heightened concern about the body (McKay and Diem, 1995). Most of the health problems and the more common illnesses are in some way related to the body changes of puberty or to engaging in high-risk behaviors.

Health promotion in persons in this age group is primarily one of health teaching and guidance. There is a growing consensus that the most effective adolescent health promotion efforts involve multiple systems and address multiple issues (Willard and Schoenborn, 1995). Research suggests that interventions integrating programs and expertise from health care, school, and community-based settings can effectively increase adolescents' prevention skills, improve their access to health care services, build adult motivation and support for adolescent prevention practices, and change physical environments and social norms to support healthy behavior (Pentz, 1993).

Adolescents are able to assume the major responsibility for their own health, including maintaining health practices (e.g., toothbrushing, caring for appliances), taking prescribed medications, keeping appointments, and performing procedures when necessary. Interview approaches should consider the adolescent's increasing independence and responsibility (see the Guidelines box below, left and the Critical Thinking Q & A box below).

Guidelines 

INTERVIEWING ADOLESCENTS

- Ensure confidentiality and privacy; interview adolescent without parents.
- Show concern for adolescent's perspective: "First, I'd like to talk about your main concerns" and "I'd like to know what you think is happening."
- Offer a nonthreatening explanation for the questions you ask: "I'm going to ask a number of questions to help me better understand your health."
- Maintain objectivity; avoid assumptions, judgments, and lectures.
- Ask open-ended questions when possible; move to more directive questions if necessary.
- Begin with less sensitive issues and proceed to more sensitive ones.
- Use language that both the adolescent and you understand.
- Restate: reflect back to adolescents what they have said, along with feelings that may be associated with their descriptions.

Critical Thinking  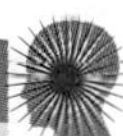

RESPECTING PRIVACY

Jamie, a 17-year-old female, arrives with her mother for a routine history and physical examination for college entrance. As you are taking Jamie to an examination room, her mother whispers, "I need to speak with you in private." Your most appropriate response is:

1. Ask Jamie to undress to prepare for the examination while you take her mother to another room to find out what's on her mind.
2. Say to Jamie's mother in Jamie's presence, "Mrs. S., whatever you have to say to me you need to say in front of Jamie."
3. Say to Jamie and her mother, "I would like to begin by speaking with both of you together, then spend some time just with you, Mrs. S, then just with you, Jamie."
4. Say to Jamie and her mother, "I would like to begin by speaking with both of you together, then spend some time just with you, Jamie, then just with you, Mrs. S."

The most appropriate response is number four. Jamie and her mother need to know ahead of time that they will each have an opportunity to express their concerns in private. Since Jamie is your patient, she will be first. Knowing that her mother will also have an opportunity to express concerns, Jamie will likely be more open and may even say, "I know what my mother will tell you," and address the issue herself. Option one is disrespectful of Jamie and is poor for two additional reasons. First, an explanation of what will occur and of the interview should precede getting undressed for an examination. Second, Jamie likely will be aware that you are speaking with her mother, feel that her privacy is being violated, and become defensive and distrustful of both you and her mother. Option two is disrespectful of Jamie's mother and her concerns. Also, Jamie's parents are legally responsible for her welfare. Although answer number three gives both mother and daughter an opportunity to express concerns, if Mrs. S goes first, Jamie is likely spend a good bit of time trying to draw from you what her mother said and/or become defensive.

IMMUNIZATIONS

An immunization update is an important part of adolescent preventive care. Obtaining a record of the teenager's prior immunizations is important. Adolescents should receive a tetanus-diphtheria (Td) vaccine 10 years after their most recent childhood diphtheria-pertussis-tetanus (DPT) vaccination, which is typically given at 4 to 5 years of age. With the exception of pregnant teens, all adolescents should receive a second measles-mumps-rubella (MMR) vaccine unless they have documentation of two MMR vaccinations during childhood but not before 12 months of age. All adolescents who have not previously received three doses of hepatitis B vaccine should be vaccinated against hepatitis B virus (American Academy of Pediatrics, 1997) (see Immunizations, Chapter 33).

NUTRITION

The rapid and extensive increase in height, weight, muscle mass, and sexual maturity of adolescence is accompanied by greater nutritional requirements. Since nutritional needs are closely related to the increase in body mass, the peak requirements occur in the years of maximum growth, during which time the body mass almost doubles. The caloric and protein requirements during this time are higher than at almost any other time of life. As a result of this increased anabolic need, the adolescent is highly sensitive to caloric restrictions. Adolescents' appetites soar, and they often eat at very frequent intervals.

The nutritional needs of adolescents are difficult to determine because of meager nutritional information on members of this age group. This difficulty is further complicated by the influence of emotional and other stress factors affecting nutrient utilization and the psychologic factors that influence eating habits. In addition, the wide variations in growth rates during adolescence and the equally wide variations in ages at which these changes take place complicate any attempt to set minimum dietary standards for any given age.

Adolescents usually have sufficient intake of protein to meet their needs except in those young people who limit their food intake because of economic problems or in an attempt to lose weight. There is a substantial increase in the need for the minerals calcium, iron, and zinc during periods of rapid growth—calcium for skeletal growth, iron for expansion of muscle mass and blood volume, and zinc for the generation of both skeletal and bone tissue. Girls may be especially susceptible to iron deficiency at menarche.

Maximum bone mass is acquired during adolescence; therefore the calcium deposited during adolescence determines the risk of osteoporosis (Key and Key, 1994). A balanced intake of protein, fats, and carbohydrates is recommended to prevent the chronic degenerative disorders of adulthood (Agostoni et al, 1994). Dietary intervention should promote the regular consumption of breakfast, a balanced intake of animal and vegetable foods, and an increased calcium supply to maximize bone density.

Eating Habits and Behavior

Eating and attitudes toward food are primarily family centered during early and middle childhood, and food habits are largely related to cultural and individual family preferences and patterns. With adolescence and the move toward independence, family influences on the child change. Children's interests, attitudes, and routines are altered as an increasing number of meals are eaten away from home. These changes largely result from the high value that teenagers place on peer acceptability and sociability; therefore their eating habits are easily influenced by their associates.

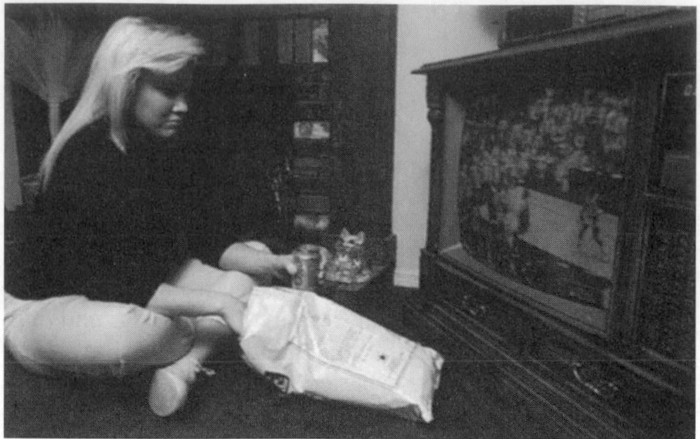

Fig. 37-8 Snacking on empty calories is common among adolescents, especially during inactivity.

Pressure for time and commitments to activities adversely affect the teenager's eating habits. Omitting breakfast or eating a breakfast that is nutritionally poor in quality is also frequently a problem. Snacks, usually selected on the basis of accessibility rather than nutritional merit, become more and more a part of the habitual eating pattern during adolescence (Fig. 37-8). Adolescents characteristically reject or only infrequently eat a sufficient amount of fresh fruits and vegetables, especially those that are rich in ascorbic acid. Milk is usually passed over in favor of soft drinks.

Overeating or undereating during adolescence presents special problems. As they experience the normal increase in weight and fat deposition of the growth spurt, teenage girls often resort to dieting. The desire for the admired slim figure and a fear of becoming "fat" prompt teenage girls to embark on nutritionally inadequate reducing regimens that drain their energy and deprive their growing bodies of essential nutrients. They resort to diets on their own or with peers in an effort to conform. Many adopt the current fad diets and are victims of food misinformation. Boys are less inclined to undereat. They are more concerned about gaining size and strength. However, they tend to eat foods high in calories but low in other essential nutrients.

The number of overweight adolescents is on the rise (Troiano et al, 1995). Along with increased availability of energy-dense foods, the U.S. population has moved toward a sedentary life-style. Although some overweight adolescents lose their excess weight as they mature and develop, many go on to become overweight adults. Because treatment of obesity for adults is largely ineffective and dietary treatment of adolescents is complicated by possible interference with growth, preventing overweight by encouraging increased physical activity may provide the greatest promise.

Nursing Care Management

Healthy dietary habits should be discussed with all adolescents. Adolescents need to learn about the Food Guide Pyramid (see Chapter 44); the relationship between dietary fat, weight status, and health; and food sources of fat, salt, and fiber (Murphy et al, 1994). Their food habits must be considered when planning nutritional education and guidance because they reflect many influences and conditions.

In helping teenagers select a nutritious diet, it is best to begin with their present diet and actively involve them in the process. Teenagers do not respond well to judgmental attitudes and dislike being preached to, but they do respond when their independence is respected and they are given the opportunity to make their own decisions regarding food choices.

In general, adolescents are body conscious and concerned about their appearance. When diet is associated with clear skin, firm flesh, and glossy hair, the teenager is more likely to be receptive to nutritional education. However, helping young persons arrive at a decision for change is more difficult than providing information. They respond best when the counselor provides straightforward information, uses instructional methods that actively involve them, talks with them and not at them, and listens to what they have to say.

SLEEP AND REST

Teenagers vary in their need for sleep and rest. Rapid physical growth, the tendency toward overexertion, and the overall increased activity of this age contribute to fatigue in adolescents. During growth spurts the need for sleep is increased. Their propensity for staying up late makes it very difficult to get out of bed in the morning, and they may sleep late at every opportunity. Adequate sleep and rest at this time are important to a total health regimen.

EXERCISE AND ACTIVITY

Although today's youth are less fit than children 20 years ago, adolescents probably spend more time and energy practicing and participating in sports activities than do members of any other age group. The number of girls and boys participating in youth sports within and outside school settings has increased dramatically in recent years (Ostrum, 1993) (Fig. 37-9). School-based, health-oriented physical education may provide both the immediate effects of the activity and the sustained effects through encouragement of lifelong activity patterns. Unfortunately, games and competitive sports are the mainstays of existing programs instead of moderate-intensity activities that contribute to the public health goal of lifelong activity (Troiano et al, 1995).

Sports, games, and even dancing contribute significantly to growth and development, the education process, and better health. These activities provide exercise for growing muscles, interactions with peers, and socially acceptable means of enjoying stimulation and conflict. In addition, competitive activities help the teenager in the process of self-appraisal, development of self-respect, and concern for others. Because physical fitness appears to be a major influence on one's lifelong health status, children should be encouraged to participate in activities that contribute to lifelong physical fitness. Nurses can encourage participation as an excellent means for health promotion and building of self-esteem. However, youngsters should not be encouraged to engage in physical activity that is beyond their physical or emotional capacity (see also Health Problems Related to Sports Participation, Chapter 36).

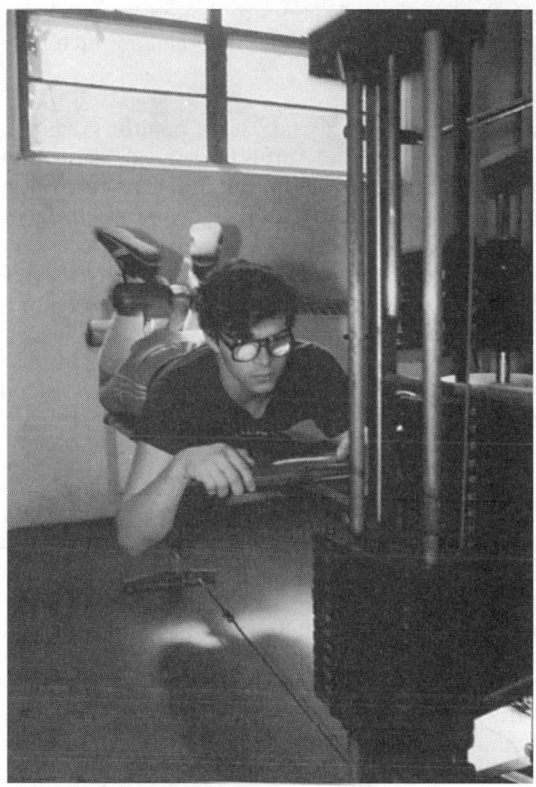

Fig. 37-9 Adolescents should be encouraged to participate in activities that contribute to lifelong physical fitness.

DENTAL HEALTH

Dental health should not be neglected during adolescence, although the rate of caries formation is not as great as it was in childhood. Early adolescence is usually the time when corrective orthodontic appliances are worn, and these are frequently a source of embarrassment and concern to the youngster. Reassurance regarding the temporary nature of the annoyance and anticipation of an improved appearance help to make the inconvenience tolerable. It is also important to reinforce the orthodontist's directions regarding use and care of the appliances and to emphasize careful attention to toothbrushing during this time (see also Chapters 34 and 36).

PERSONAL CARE

The body-conscious teenager is highly amenable to discussion and counseling about personal care and hygiene. Body changes associated with puberty bring with them special needs for cleanliness. The hyperactive sebaceous glands and newly functioning apocrine glands make frequent bathing or showering a necessity, and underarm deodorants assume an important place in personal care. The adolescent will find that hair requires more frequent shampooing, and girls will have questions about hair removal, use of cosmetics, and menstrual hygiene. Many group discussions center around the virtues of particular products or methods. Adolescents are continually bombarded with messages from the media regarding the best means of enhancing their popularity and appeal to the opposite gender. Nurses are in a position to help them evaluate the relative merits of commercial products.

Vision

Regular vision testing is a vital part of health care and supervision during adolescence. At this time the incidence of visual refractive difficulties reaches a peak that is not exceeded until the fifth decade of life. The increased demands of schoolwork make good vision important for academic success. Consequently, teenagers are more likely to be referred for visual evaluation. The need for corrective lenses can create psychologic problems for teenagers if they believe that glasses spoil their appearance or do not fit their body image. For those who can afford them, contact lenses are a preferred solution. For some the impact of a visual defect, no matter how slight, may prove to be a great personal concern.

Hearing

There has been considerable concern regarding current teenage practices that cause possible damage to hearing. Cochlear damage from relatively continuous exposure to the loud sound levels of rock music has been documented. The popularity of portable radios and stereo cassette and CD players with lightweight earphones, which enable the listener to adjust the volume, are of particular concern to health care professionals. When these units are used for extended periods, permanent hearing loss can occur. Appealing to individual youngsters for more judicious use is not always successful, although they should be informed of the risk. Efforts directed toward legislating legal limits to the noise exposure that can be achieved through the sets and widespread education may be possible solutions. (See Chapter 39 for a discussion of noise-related hearing loss.)

Posture

The process of normal development during adolescence may result in altered posture. The rapid skeletal growth that is usually associated with a significant lag in muscular growth leads to weakness, easy fatigability, and awkwardness. This situation predisposes youngsters to slumping and makes them less inclined to stand or sit erect. A reduction in physical activity, which often accompanies the rapid skeletal growth, aggravates the situation, especially in teenage girls. (The adolescent who is routinely engaged in vigorous physical activity appears to have fewer problems with posture.) Carrying heavy backpacks in school may also cause postural problems. Most postural problems resolve as the adolescent matures, and most do not require special attention.

The best approach to counseling teenagers about posture is to show, not tell, them and to serve as a proper model. Good posture can be demonstrated best by having the adolescent stand before a full-length mirror or by taking a photograph of the adolescent's body profile. Postural defects and desired alterations can be pointed out in full view of both the young person and the nurse. A sunken chest, winged scapulas, swayback, protruberant abdomen, and drooping head and shoulders are clearly visible, and the nurse is able to demonstrate the simple corrections that can transform the youngster into a more attractive and, ultimately, healthier person. Adolescents will need reassurance that the fatigue they feel when attempting to maintain correct posture is a transient effect caused by weak muscles, especially those of the back, and that they will soon acquire the strength and endurance to maintain the desired posture. If they concentrate on assuming correct positioning several times each day, with regular practice it will eventually become a permanent aspect of their person.

Serious postural defects detected in the process of a physical assessment require early medical intervention. Scoliosis is usually intensified during adolescence, and tight muscles often produce postural problems that need special attention. Nurses can refer a youngster to the appropriate source, such as the family physician, pediatrician, or health clinic, for evaluation and implementation of corrective therapy (see Scoliosis, Chapter 51).

Body Piercing

The popular trend of ear or, less commonly, nose, nipple, navel, or tongue piercing may sometimes create a health problem in the uninformed teenager. It is a nursing responsibility to caution girls or boys against the practice of having piercing performed by friends, mothers, or themselves. Although in most cases there are few if any serious side effects, there is always a danger of complications such as infection, cyst or keloid formation, bleeding, dermatitis, or metal allergy. Therefore the procedure should be performed by a qualified operator using proper sterile technique. This is especially important if a youngster has a history of diabetes, allergies, or skin disorders. Teenagers need to know that using the same unsterilized needle to pierce body parts of multiple teens presents the same risk of human immunodeficiency virus (HIV) transmission as occurs with other needle-sharing activities.

Suntanning

The continuous quest for an attractive appearance leads many teenagers to excessive sunbathing and artificial means for acquiring a tan skin. However, the practice is not without risks, and the adolescent should be educated regarding the detrimental effects of sunlight on the skin (see Sunburn, Chapter 50). Some long-term effects include premature aging of the skin, increased risk of skin cancer, and, in susceptible individuals, phototoxic reactions.

The increasing popularity of artificial suntanning has prompted concern on the part of health professionals regarding the use of sun lamps and suntanning machines. Because the long-term effects of tanning machines (especially whole-body irradiation) are unknown, dermatologists do not recommend suntanning by this means. Those who insist on using suntanning equipment should be warned that goggles must be worn in tanning booths to prevent serious corneal burning. Education on the use of sunscreens, including hypoallergenic products, with a sun protective factor (SPF) of at least 15 is important health teaching.

STRESS REDUCTION

The multiple changes occurring in adolescence potentially result in a great deal of stress (see Fig. 37-10 and Box 37-2). The adolescent is faced with pressures from peers to conform, which often involve flaunting adult authority and even taking serious health risks. Health risks include pressures for sexual experimentation and use of drugs, alcohol, and tobacco, as well as potentially dangerous physical activities.

Early-maturing girls and late-maturing children are espe-

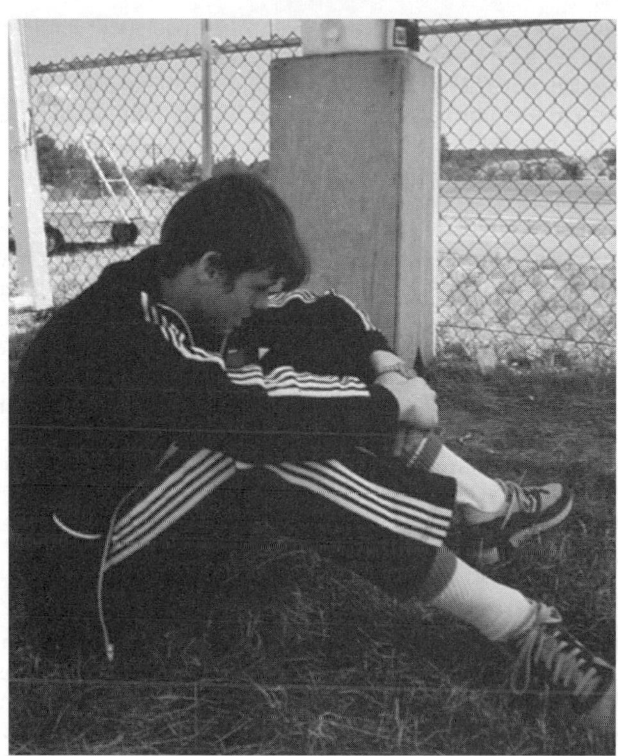

Fig. 37-10 Adolescents may use being alone as a method of coping with stress.

cially sensitive to the stresses of being different from their peers. Many feel intense anxiety over their identity. Both early- and late-maturing children feel out of place among their classmates, but slow-maturing children appear to suffer the most pronounced inner turmoil and may be hesitant to voice their concerns. Slow-maturing youngsters need support and reassurance that they are not abnormal and need only be patient until the time comes when they, too, will develop the characteristics for which they yearn.

SEXUALITY EDUCATION AND GUIDANCE

Contemporary adolescents are constantly exposed to sexual symbolism and erotic stimulation from the mass media. At the same time the development of primary and secondary sex characteristics and the increased sensitivity of the genitals produce thoughts and fantasies about sexual relationships. Young people are at the stage of life when the sexual aspects of interpersonal relationships become particularly important. Societal expectations push them toward dating, and their own inner sex drive urges them toward exploration. Although many adolescents have received sexuality education from parents and school throughout childhood, they are not always adequately prepared for the impact of puberty. A large portion of their knowledge is acquired from peers, television, movies, and magazines. Even information acquired from parents may be inaccurate (McGrory, 1995). Consequently, much of the sexuality information they accumulate is incomplete, inaccurate, riddled with cultural and moral values, and not very helpful.

BOX 37-2
Areas of Stress in Adolescence

Body image
Sexuality conflicts
School pressures
Competitive pressures
Relationships with parents
Relationships with siblings
Relationships with peers
Finances
Decisions about present and future roles
Career planning
Ideologic conflicts

The responsibility for providing sexuality education has been assumed by parents, schools, churches, community agencies such as Planned Parenthood Federation of America, Inc.,* and health professionals, especially nurses. The public perceives nurses as having authoritative information and as willing to take time with patients (Croft and Asmussen, 1993). To be able to discuss the topic with teenagers adequately, nurses must have not only an understanding of the physiologic aspects of sexuality and a knowledge of cultural and societal values, but also an awareness of their own attitudes, feelings, and biases about sexuality.

The most comprehensive approach to sexuality education is offered by the Sexuality Information and Education Council of the United States (SIECUS)† and the Sex Information and Education Council of Canada (SIECCAN),‡ interdisciplinary organizations founded to establish sexuality as a health entity and to dignify it through an open approach, study, and scientific research. SIECUS maintains that every sexuality education program should present the topic from six aspects: biologic, social, health, personal adjustments and attitudes, interpersonal associations, and the establishment of values.

Whether nurses counsel young people on an individual basis, in mixed groups, or in groups segregated by gender makes little difference. Ideally boys and girls should be able to discuss sexuality objectively with one another and in groups, but this is not always possible. The difference in the rate of maturation between boys and girls and between different members of the same gender often makes it desirable to discuss certain aspects of sexuality in segregated groups. As a general rule the need for separate discussion groups diminishes as young people progress toward maturity.

Sexuality education should consist of instruction concerning normal body functions and should be presented in a straightforward manner using correct terminology. When discussing sexuality and sexual activities, nurses should use simple but correct language—not street language, highly scientific terminology, or evasive jargon. Once the meanings of biologic terms such as uterus, testicles, and vagina are understood, most teenagers prefer to use them in their discussions.

*810 Seventh Ave., New York, NY 10019; (212) 541-7800 or (800) 829-7732.
†130 W. 42nd St., Suite 350, New York, NY 10036; (212) 819-9770.
‡850 Coxwell Ave., E. York, Ontario M4C 5R1; (416) 466-5304.

Many girls arrive at menarche with conflicted attitudes, myths, and illogical beliefs. Even girls adequately prepared for menstruation do not always understand its relationship to the total process of reproduction. Many are under the incorrect impression that the "safe" time for sexual intercourse is midway between menstrual periods.

Teenagers' curiosity and desire for information extend beyond the need for anatomic and physiologic knowledge. They need to know more than the mechanics of conception, pregnancy, and birth. Adolescents, girls in particular, want answers to questions such as, "What is it like?" "Does it hurt?" "What happens when . . . ?" and "Is it all right if you . . . . ?" Boys are often concerned about the fallacy that there is a relationship between penis size and sexual function. They need reassurance that masturbation is a normal and common practice, that some degree of homosexuality is not unusual in early adolescence, and that oral-genital relations can be normal substitutes for intercourse.

However, sexuality education cannot end there. Teens need to discuss intercourse, alternative methods of sexual satisfaction, and how to resist peer pressure. With the increased incidence of sexually transmitted diseases, especially AIDS, the topic of "safe sex," especially the use of condoms and abstinence, is essential. Role play can help them learn effective approaches to dealing with difficult situations. Sex and sexuality cannot be taught without discussions on mature decision making, sexual responsibility, and values clarification.

Adolescents need role models and life experiences with delayed gratification. Most importantly, they need problem-solving experience and decision-making skills so that they can anticipate the positive and negative outcomes of a decision. With these types of assistance, teenagers can become sexually responsible young adults.

INJURY PREVENTION

Physical injuries are the greatest single cause of death in the adolescent age group and claim more lives than all other causes combined. The most vulnerable ages are the years 15 to 24, when accidental injuries account for about 60% of deaths in boys and 40% of deaths in girls. The tragedy of this is that these figures remain fairly constant from year to year and that almost all fatal injuries are preventable.

During adolescence, peak physical, sensory, and psychomotor function gives teenagers a feeling of strength and confidence that they have never experienced before, and the physiologic changes of puberty give impetus to many basic instinctual forces. One manifestation of this is an increase in energy that simply must be discharged through action, often at the expense of logical thinking and other control mechanisms. Their propensity for risk-taking behavior plus feelings of indestructibility make adolescents especially prone to injuries. Some of the developmental characteristics of teenagers and the common injuries associated with this age group are outlined in Table 37-2.

Vehicle-Related Injuries

The adolescent's newly acquired ability to drive and the normal developmental need for independence and freedom make the automobile an attractive part of an adolescent's life. Motor vehicle crashes are the single greatest cause of death, accounting for nearly two thirds of fatal injuries among young people (Bearinger and Blum, 1994). The majority of fatal and nonfatal motor vehicle crashes involve alcohol. Adolescents practice other behaviors that may increase their likelihood of death in a motor vehicle. In a survey of high school students, 19.1% reported rarely or never using a seat belt, and 35.3% had ridden within the previous month with a driver who had been drinking alcohol (Kann et al, 1995).

Nonautomotive vehicle injuries. The increasing use of other motorized vehicles, such as motorized bicycles, all terrain vehicles (ATVs), and snowmobiles, has caused an increase in injuries, especially among youngsters below the legal age for driving automobiles. Many adolescents ride bicycles without helmets and without lights at night, and the overwhelming majority of deaths from bicycle injuries (primarily head injuries) involve teenagers. Most motorcycle injuries involve the motorcycle and another vehicle, but burn injuries have been reported from contact with the hot muffler, especially when youngsters are riding double.

Firearms

Improper use of firearms continues to be one of the leading causes of accidental death in the adolescent age group. Most of these deaths occur in or on home premises. Almost half the victims of firearm fatalities are between the ages of 15 and 24 years. Firearms are increasingly a factor in intentional as well as unintentional death for adolescents. The murder rate for teenage boys age 15 to 19 years more than doubled between 1985 and 1991; for African-American males in this age group, the rate nearly tripled (Children's Defense Fund, 1995). Virtually all of this increase (97%) was attributed to the use of guns.

Most accidental injuries can be prevented when proper safety precautions are taken in the use and storage of firearms. For example, loaded guns should never be permitted in or around the home, and guns and ammunition must be stored where only appropriate adults have access to them. Asking families about the presence of a gun in the home and offering these preventive actions if one is present may be the most effective action health professionals can take (American Academy of Pediatrics, Committee on Adolescence, 1992).

Nonpowder firearms. Nonpowder guns (air rifles, BB guns), although viewed as toys by many, account for almost as many injuries as powder guns. The regulations regarding nonpowder guns are relaxed; they can be purchased legally by youngsters and are labeled as suitable for children as young as 8 years. Few states regulate their use. As child advocates, nurses can press for legislation to regulate the sale of these potentially dangerous "toys."

Sports Injuries

Because the degree of physical maturation, size, coordination, and endurance varies greatly among adolescents of the same age, sports competition between young people who differ markedly in strength and agility is unfair and hazardous. Matching candidates for sports should be done relative to physical maturity, height, weight, and physical fitness and skills, particularly in a sport involving rigorous body contact. Age is a less important consideration.

Every sport has some potential for injury—whether one

TABLE 37-2 Injury prevention during adolescence

DEVELOPMENTAL ABILITIES RELATED TO RISK OF INJURY	INJURY PREVENTION
Need for independence and freedom Testing independence Age permitted to drive a motor vehicle (varies) Inclination for risk taking Feeling of indestructibility Need for discharging energy, often at expense of logical thinking and other control mechanisms Strong need for peer approval May attempt hazardous feats Peak incidence for practice and participation in sports Access to more complex tools, objects, and locations Can assume responsibility for own actions	**Motor/nonmotor vehicles** *Pedestrian*—emphasize and encourage safe pedestrian behavior *Passenger*—promote appropriate behavior while riding in a motor vehicle *Driver*—provide competent driver education; encourage judicious use of vehicle, discourage drag racing, "playing chicken"; maintain vehicle in proper condition (brakes, tires, etc.) Teach and promote safety and maintenance of two-wheeled vehicles Promote and encourage wearing of safety apparel such as helmet, long trousers Reinforce the dangers of drugs, including alcohol, when operating a motor vehicle **Drowning** Teach nonswimmer to swim Teach basic rules of water safety Judicious selection of place to swim Sufficient water depth for diving Swimming with companion **Burns** Reinforce proper behavior in areas involving contact with burn hazards (gasoline, electric wires, fires) Advise regarding excessive exposure to natural or artificial sunlight (ultraviolet burn) Discourage smoking Encourage use of sunscreen **Poisoning** Educate in hazards of drug use, including alcohol **Falls** Teach and encourage general safety measures in all activities **Bodily damage** Promote acquisition of proper instruction in sports and use of sports equipment Instruct in safe use of and respect for firearms and other devices with potential danger (e.g., power tools, firecrackers) Provide and encourage use of protective equipment when using potentially hazardous devices Promote access to and/or provision of safe sports and recreational facilities Be alert for signs of depression (potential suicide) Discourage use of and/or availability of hazardous sports equipment (trampoline, surfboards) Instruct regarding proper use of corrective devices such as glasses, contact lenses, hearing aids Encourage and foster judicious application of safety principles and prevention

participates in serious competition or is actively engaged in the activity for pure enjoyment. A large number of severe or fatal injuries occur in persons who are not physically prepared for the activity. The increase in strength and vigor in adolescence may tempt youngsters to overextend themselves, especially boys who are egged on by teammates or are stimulated by the admiration of female observers. The range of injuries sustained in sports or recreational activities can involve any part of the body and extend from relatively minor cuts, bruises, and abrasions to totally incapacitating central nervous system injuries or death.

Nursing Care Management

Injury prevention is an ongoing part of nursing responsibility throughout the childhood years. Anticipatory guidance for parents and children regarding the expected problems and hazards related to growth and development does not end as children approach maturity. They need the same education in basic safety precautions, as well as instruction in skills required in performance of activities such as sports, in skills for handling motor vehicles and firearms, and in proper maintenance of equipment. However, during adolescence, health and safety education and guidance are more effective when the young people are involved directly; parents and health professionals can emphasize the importance of safety during the performance of activities and the proper conditioning and preparation for sports.

Prevention activities can occur on various levels. Safety advocacy, changing public policy, and legislation can curtail injuries. Examples of such approaches are laws that mandate wearing seat belts, mandatory helmet use while driving moving vehicles other than automobiles, keeping the legal drinking age at 21 years, and instituting curfews for teenage drivers. In addition to improving the environment, health education for teenagers and significant adults is essential. Helping adolescents understand their need for engaging in risk behavior, exploring possible negative outcomes, and weighing possible alternatives are critical components of injury prevention.

ANTICIPATORY GUIDANCE—CARE OF FAMILIES

The parents of the adolescent are usually as confused and perplexed about the changes and behavior of this stage of development as the youngster is. Parents also need support and guidance to help them through this trying time. They need to understand the changes taking place and to understand and accept the expected behaviors that accompany the process of detachment, to be prepared to "let go," and to promote the changed relationship from one of dependence to one of mutuality. The Home Care box to the left lists suggestions for anticipatory guidance of parents with an adolescent.

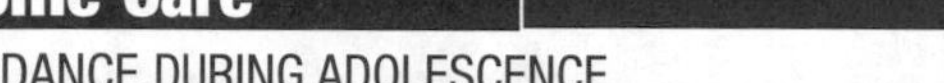

GUIDANCE DURING ADOLESCENCE

Encourage parents to:

- Accept adolescent as a unique individual
- Respect adolescent's ideas, likes and dislikes, wishes
- Be involved with school functions and attend the adolescent's performances, whether it be a sporting event or a school play
- Listen and try to be open to youngster's views, even when they disagree with parental views
- Avoid criticism about no-win topics
- Provide opportunity for choosing options and accept natural consequences of these choices
- Allow youngster to learn by doing, even when choices and methods differ from those of adults
- Provide adolescent with clear, reasonable limits
- Clarify house rules and consequences for breaking them
- Let society's rules and consequences teach responsibility outside the home
- Allow increasing independence within limitations of safety and well-being
- Be available but avoid pressing youngster too far
- Respect adolescent's privacy
- Try to share adolescent's feelings of joy or sorrow
- Respond to feelings as well as words
- Be available to answer questions, give information, and provide companionship
- Try to make communication clear
- Avoid comparisons with siblings
- Assist adolescent in selecting appropriate career goals and preparing for adult role
- Welcome adolescent's friends into the home and treat them with respect
- Provide unconditional love
- Be willing to apologize when mistaken

Be aware that adolescents:

- Are subject to turbulent, unpredictable behavior
- Are struggling for independence
- Are extremely sensitive to feelings and behavior that affect them
- May receive a different message than what was sent
- Consider friends extremely important
- Have a strong need to "belong"

Special Health Problems

DISORDERS RELATED TO THE REPRODUCTIVE SYSTEM

Amenorrhea

It is not unusual for an adolescent girl to skip a menstrual period or two when establishing normal menstrual and ovulatory cycles. Delay in initiation of menstruation is ordinarily a temporary problem resulting from late onset of puberty and requires no intervention. This is of little concern unless it creates undue anxiety on the part of the girl and her parents, which can ordinarily be allayed by explanation and reassurance. Careful examination will reveal any congenital defects of the genital tract (a rare cause).

Primary **amenorrhea** is defined as no menses by age 16 years in the presence of normal secondary sex characteristics, no menses 1 to 2 years after reaching Tanner stage V, or no menses 3 to 5 years after the onset of breast development (see Fig. 37-1). Primary amenorrhea may result from absence or malformation of the female genital structures, the inability of normal structures to respond to hormonal stimulation, or strenuous physical activity. The most common cause of *secondary amenorrhea* (prolonged absence of menstruation for 6 months or more in the first 2 years following menarche or when more than three periods have been missed after menses have become established) is pregnancy. Other factors include immaturity, extreme physical stress, severe emotional stress, sudden environmental change, hyperthyroidism or hypothyroidism, chronic systemic illness, extreme weight loss or gain, anorexia nervosa (even before marked weight loss), ovarian disturbance, and pharmacologic agents (e.g., some prescribed medications, abused substances, hormones).

Exercise-related menstrual dysfunction. Delayed menarche has been associated with girls who engage in strenuous exercise. It is not clear whether exercise delays menarche, or menarcheal delay promotes athletic success. Some attribute delayed menarche and maintenance of regular ovulation to lack of development of body fat. Alterations have also been noted in menstrual bleeding patterns of girls who engage in strenuous exercise. The activities that appear to be associated with delayed or altered menstruation are ballet dancing, running, gymnastics, and swimming. This condition may cause embarrassment and concern to the youngster and her parents, which can be minimized by explanation and reassurance regarding its benign and temporary nature.

Dysmenorrhea

A certain amount of discomfort during the first day or two of the menstrual flow is extremely common. Most girls experience cramping, abdominal pain, backache, and leg ache, but in a few the pain is intolerable and incapacitating. *Primary* **dysmenorrhea** is painful menses not related to any pelvic disease. When the discomfort can be attributed to endometriosis, infection, adhesions from peritonitis, or other pelvic disease, the complaint is termed *secondary dysmenorrhea.*

Primary dysmenorrhea is directly related to the occurrence of prior ovulation. There is also a relationship between uterine contractility and the secretion of prostaglandins. Psychogenic factors such as sexual abuse, familial conditioning, gender-role confusion, and school avoidance may also contribute to dysmenorrhea.

A thorough gynecologic examination is carried out to exclude any pelvic abnormalities, and a careful history is taken regarding the type and duration of pain, its relationship to menstrual flow, and any associated symptoms. These questions not only provide information for the examiner, but also serve to provide the girl with evidence that her problem is being taken seriously. An explanation of the physiology of menstruation helps to give reassurance.

Therapeutic management. The treatment of choice for adolescents is the administration of nonsteroidal antiinflammatory drugs that block the formation of prostaglandins for 2 to 3 days of the menstrual cycle. Cyclic estrogen therapy and the use of oral contraceptives are also effective. Simple exercises, such as pelvic rocking, assuming the knee-chest position, and breathing exercises, may be beneficial. Good hygiene and participation in regular activities are encouraged.

Nursing care management. All young teenagers need reassurance that menstruation is a normal function. The nurse who is sought out for advice regarding menstrual problems has an opportunity to engage in health teaching concerning menstrual physiology and hygiene, as well as the importance of a well-balanced diet, exercise, and general health maintenance. Health teaching can also dispel any myths that may be held in relation to menstruation and femininity. When assessment indicates a potential problem and the need for evaluation, referral to an appropriate practitioner, health service, or clinic may be necessary.

One of the most difficult experiences facing the adolescent girl is the gynecologic examination. Whether it is her first experience or not, she is most likely filled with apprehension. Almost all adolescents are extremely self-conscious about their bodies and the changes taking place. They need continuing support in the form of anticipatory guidance regarding what to expect and suggestions of what to do to help relax during the procedure. Usually the stressful experience of being placed in stirrups for the pelvic examination can be avoided. The young female who is relaxed may be examined in the supine position with hips and knees flexed and legs abducted. If a female nurse is not the examiner, it is essential for her to remain with the patient during the examination to offer support and guidance.

Vaginitis

Vaginitis can be caused by physical, chemical, or infectious agents. Physical causes may include a forgotten tampon or contraceptive sponge. Chemical irritants include bubble bath, douching, and deodorant pads. Removal of the offending material or discontinuing use of the irritating substance is usually all that is necessary to treat physical or chemical vaginitis. Infectious vaginitis can be caused by the *Candida* fungi, *Trichomonas* protozoal parasites, or bacteria. Diagnosis is confirmed with microscopic evaluation of vaginal secretions. Treatment varies, depending on the infectious agent.

Health teaching is important in the prevention and management of all types of vaginitis. Adolescent females must be reassured that increased vaginal mucus can occur at the time of ovulation, before menstruation, or with sexual excitement. Many teenagers mistake these variations as signs of infection. Young females should be taught to wipe front to back after toileting and to realize that vaginitis can result from irritation, foreign objects, and sexual activity. Nurses need to stress the importance of an evaluation to determine the exact cause.

Disorders of the Male Reproductive System

Most obvious anomalies, such as hypospadias, hydrocele, phimosis, and cryptorchidism, have been identified, and corrective measures instituted during early childhood. The most frequent problems related to the reproductive organs in later childhood are (1) infections, such as urethritis (see Urinary Tract Infection, Chapter 47); (2) hematuria; (3) penile problems, such as nonretractable foreskin in uncircumcised males, carcinoma, and trauma; (4) scrotal conditions, such as varicocele (elongation, dilation, and tortuosity of the veins superior to the testicle); and (5) testicular torsion (a condition in which the testicle hangs free from its vascular structures, which can result in partial or complete venous occlusion with rotation). Tumors of the testes are not a common condition, but when manifested in adolescence, they are generally malignant and demand immediate evaluation.

The usual presenting symptom for testicular cancer is a heavy, hard painless mass (either smooth or nodular) that is palpated on the testis. Treatment involves surgical removal of the affected testicle (orchiectomy) and possibly chemotherapy and radiation if metastasis has occurred.

Nursing care management. The adolescent male is extremely self-conscious about his changing body and needs preparation for a genital examination. The most successful approach is to assume a matter-of-fact attitude toward the examination, explain precisely what will take place, and maintain a continuous commentary about what is being done and

Critical Thinking Q & A 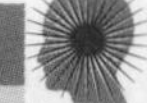

TESTICULAR SELF-EXAMINATION

At a recent faculty meeting the school nurse presented plans for a class on testicular self-examination (TSE) to be delivered to the sophomore boys. Several faculty questioned the value of providing such a class when there is limited time to deliver content relating to "routine academic subjects." Which of the following responses could the nurse use to justify including the TSE class in the curriculum?

1. TSE provides an opportunity for adolescent males to pick up early cases of epididymitis, a common infection in this age group.
2. TSE allows adolescent boys to determine if they have an asymptomatic sexually transmitted disease.
3. TSE permits detection of any tumors of the testes, which are not common in adolescence, but which are often malignant and demand immediate attention when they occur.
4. TSE allows easy identification of malignant testicular tumors that occur in 5% of adolescent males.

The correct response is three. TSE is an easily learned technique that allows the adolescent male to become familiar with his own anatomy and to determine any abnormalities. Although testicular cancer is not common in adolescence, when it does occur the tumors are often malignant and early detection is essential. Although TSE is easily learned by adolescents, the method does not allow the adolescent male to determine if he has a sexually transmitted disease or epididymitis.

the findings at each phase of the examination. The adolescent male is approached as someone important as a person, with the nurse interested in his concerns. To supplement routine health assessment, every adolescent male should be taught frequent testicular self-examination (TSE) to familiarize himself with his own anatomy and to ensure early detection of any abnormality. The normal testicle is a firm organ with a smooth, egg-shaped contour; the epididymis is palpated as a raised swelling on the superior aspect of the testicle and should not be confused as an abnormality (see the Critical Thinking Q & A box above).

Gynecomastia

The male breast, while not strictly part of the male reproductive system, responds to hormonal changes. Some degree of bilateral or unilateral breast enlargement occurs frequently in boys during puberty. It is estimated that approximately half of adolescent boys have transient gynecomastia, usually lasting less than 1 year (Biro et al, 1990), that subsides spontaneously with achievement of male development. Occasionally, however, it is associated with abnormalities such as Klinefelter syndrome or endocrine dysfunction; therefore these possibilities are ruled out by appropriate diagnostic examination.

If the condition persists or is extensive enough to cause embarrassment or to produce doubts about gender identity in the young boy, plastic surgery is indicated for cosmetic and psychologic considerations. Administration of testosterone has no effect on breast development or regression and may even aggravate the condition.

Nursing care management. Treatment usually consists of assurance to the adolescent and his parents that this is a benign and temporary situation. Adolescents who are distressed about physical integrity and masculinity may benefit from the knowledge that it occurs in about 50% of all adolescent males.

EATING DISORDERS

Obesity

Few health problems related to childhood and adolescence are so obvious to others, so difficult to treat, and have such long-term effects on psychologic and physical health status as **obesity.** It is the most common nutritional disturbance of children and one of the most challenging contemporary health problems at all ages.

There is no generally accepted definition of obesity or overweight. Some authorities consider obesity to occur if the child's ideal body weight for height and age is greater than 120%. However, this definition does not take into account the proportion of lean body mass (muscle) to fat. It is possible for two children to have the same height and weight and for one to be obese whereas the other is not.

Regardless of the criteria used to define obesity, the fact is that the number of overweight children in the United States is increasing. The increase parallels the findings of a large increase in the prevalence of overweight adults (Troiano et al, 1995).

Etiology/pathophysiology. Obesity results from a caloric intake that consistently exceeds caloric requirements and expenditure. The causes of this disequilibrium are complex and may involve various influences, including metabolic, hypothalamic, hereditary, social, cultural, and psychologic factors. Less than 5% of cases of childhood obesity can be attributed to an underlying disease such as hypothyroidism, adrenal hypercorticoidism, hyperinsulinism, and dysfunction of or damage to the central nervous system.

The metabolism of glucose plays an important role in the regulation of fat deposition, since excess calories from carbohydrates are stored as fat and a lack of glucose prompts the release of fat as a source of energy. Apparently, people who are obese are able to store fat easily but are unable to release this fat or burn it for energy. People who are obese appear to be more efficient in fat storage and have less heat-producing brown fat than people who are not obese.

Heredity is an important factor in the development of obesity. For example, identical twins reared apart tend to resemble their natural parents to a greater extent than they do their adoptive parents. Obesity can develop in infancy, during childhood, at the onset of puberty, or at any time during adolescence. It is almost impossible to distinguish between hereditary and environmental factors, since both may be operating in any situation when other family members are obese.

Children who are obese are less active than lean children, although it is uncertain whether the inactivity creates the obesity or whether the obesity is responsible for the inactivity. Many people who are obese also demonstrate an overwhelming appetite and often overeat when they are not hungry or have no appetite. They eat more rapidly and tend to ingest more calories at one meal rather than over a period of time.

Adolescents who are obese are characteristically night eaters and often skip meals, particularly breakfast.

Theories that attempt to explain the development of obesity are as follows:

Adipose cell theory—The number of cells in adipose tissue is increased, the size of the fat cells is increased, or a combination of these. It is believed that there are sensitive periods in development when cell numbers increase. Children who are obese have larger cells that stay the same size once they reach a maximum, and their fat cells appear to increase in number during childhood.

Set point theory—Individuals have a predetermined level for body weight that remains relatively stable during adulthood. With increased caloric intake the metabolic rate increases to burn the excess; when intake is reduced, metabolism decreases to conserve energy.

Sociocultural factors also play an important role in weight gain. Patterns of eating are culturally and socially based in most instances, and in some the food preferences of the culture contribute to the development of obesity. Many cultures consider plump children to be a sign of health, and some look on obesity as evidence of well-being and foster weight gain as a desirable feature.

Psychologic factors may provide a basis for eating patterns in childhood. In infancy the child first experiences relief from discomfort through feeding and learns to associate eating with feelings of well-being, security, and the comforting presence of the nurturing person. Soon eating is deeply associated with the feeling of being loved. Many parents use food, such as candy and other "treats," as a positive reinforcer for desired behavior. This practice soon acquires symbolic significance to the extent that the child continues to use food as a reward, a comfort, and a means by which to deal with feelings of depression, hostility, boredom, or loneliness.

Obesity is a serious handicap to the social life of a child and, to an even greater extent, to the social life of a teenager. The common emotional sequelae of obesity in adolescence are defective body image, low self-esteem, social isolation, and feelings of rejection and depression.

Diagnostic evaluation. An obese child looks "too fat." Several tests can be employed to assess obesity (Box 37-3). Skinfold measurements, as well as body fat measurements as determined by bioelectric impedance, computed tomography, or magnetic resonance imaging measurements, may be used for additional data. Appropriate diagnostic tests rule out suspected metabolic and endocrine disorders.

BOX 37-3

Clinical Manifestations of Obesity

Child appears overweight
Weight over established standards
Skinfold thickness greater than established standards
Body fat increased above established standards

Nursing Care Management

Assessment

The presence of obesity is obvious from appearance alone, and a gross determination can be made by a rough comparison of height and weight with standard growth charts. Children who are 20% over the normal for their height and weight should be further evaluated. Evaluation includes height and weight history of the child, parents, and siblings, as well as eating habits, appetite and hunger patterns, and physical activities in which the child is engaged. It is useful to have an estimation of the degree of fatness in order to have some idea of the component of body weight that can be modified. In addition to the foregoing, a psychosocial history is helpful to understand the impact this condition has on the child's life.

Nursing Diagnoses

Based on a thorough assessment of the child or adolescent who is obese, nursing diagnoses become apparent. Although the diagnoses vary according to the needs of the individual child, some of the more prominent ones are outlined in Box 37-4.

Planning

The goals of a weight-loss program include the following:

1. Modify diet to provide loss of fat content without interfering with growth, normal activity, and psychologic well-being
2. Implement a regular exercise program
3. Modify eating behavior
4. Provide psychologic support

Implementation

Motivation to lose weight is the key to success. The reasons behind youngsters' desire to lose weight must be explored with them, but success is rarely achieved unless youngsters are motivated to lose weight and take personal responsibility for their dietary habits and exercise program. Children who are forced by parents to seek help are seldom sufficiently motivated, become rebellious of parental nagging, and are unwilling to control dietary intake. An approach that focuses on healthy eating habits and enjoyable exercise for all members of the family is more likely to be successful.

BOX 37-4

Nursing Diagnoses: The Child Who is Obese

Altered nutrition: more than body requirements related to dysfunctional eating patterns, hereditary factors
Activity intolerance related to sedentary life-style, physical bulk
Ineffective individual coping related to little or no exercise, poor nutrition, personal vulnerability
Self-esteem disturbance related to perception of physical appearance, internalization of negative feedback
Altered family processes related to management of child who is obese

BOX 37-5
Essentials of a Weight-Reduction Dietary Regimen for Children and Adolescents

The diet should provide for:
- Steady slow weight loss
- Lack of metabolic complications
- Lack of hunger
- Preservation of lean body mass
- Absence of psychiatric reactions
- Normal activity
- Growth

Diet. Planning caloric restriction for the adolescent during the rapid growth period requires a careful design (Box 37-5). Since obesity is usually a lifelong problem, it is best to provide the individual with a diet that can be maintained throughout life with the emphasis on restricting calories. The most successful diets are those that use ordinary foods in controlled portions rather than diets that require the avoidance of any specific food. The youngster is taught how to incorporate favorite foods into the diet and how to select satisfying substitutes. The dieting youngster should eat what the rest of the family eats, but less of it, and should be allowed favorite foods in small amounts. There are a multitude of restricted calorie diets available from a number of sources, such as the American Dietetic Association. The caloric values for a wide variety of commercial foods are also available to facilitate meal planning.

For children, especially teenagers, snacking is an integral part of the daily routine, which makes dieting particularly difficult for children who are obese. They have little concept of the caloric content of even the most commonplace snack foods. Vending machines are usually stocked with high-calorie, low-nutrient temptations; they are readily accessible; and children often have pocket money with which to purchase these items. Following pressures from concerned parents and nutritionists, many schools are providing more wholesome "treats," such as fruit, juices, and raw vegetables, in vending machines in school cafeterias. However, the favorite gathering places for children and teens are the fast-food establishments, which are often located near large schools.*

No child or adolescent should be encouraged to initiate a reduction diet without a health assessment and counseling. It is also important to emphasize the undesirable nature of the fad diets and crash programs that continually appear in various publications. Exotic diets have not been successful, and their unbalanced nature makes them potentially dangerous for growing children or adolescents. To be successful from all aspects, a dietary program should be nutritionally sound with sufficient satiety value, produce the desired weight loss, and be accompanied by nutrition education and continued support.

*Information on the nutrient value of name brand foods, including several fast-food restaurants, is available from the Nutrition Coordinating Center, 2221 University Ave., S.E., Suite 310, Minneapolis, MN 55414; (612) 627-4862.

Exercise. Since weight loss will occur only when caloric expenditure is greater than caloric intake, physical activity in the form of regularly scheduled exercise, progressively increased over the child's usual activity, is an integral part of a weight-reduction program. Activities should be those that stress self-improvement rather than competition, and teenagers need continued psychologic support and encouragement to prevent the beginning of the destructive cycle of passivity, withdrawal, and rejection.

Behavioral therapy. Probably the most successful method for treating obesity is diet and exercise combined with behavior modification, which emphasizes identification and elimination of inappropriate eating habits as well as problem-solving techniques to identify solutions to use in situations that encourage overeating. Attention is focused not on food but on the social and behavioral aspects surrounding food consumption.

Group involvement. Some persons on weight-reduction programs find that support and mutual reinforcement provided by a group of persons with a similar problem help them to adjust to the changes needed for successful accomplishment of their goals, including weight loss. Commercial groups, such as Weight Watchers, or diet workshops, composed primarily of adults, may be helpful to a few teenagers; however, a group composed of persons their own age is more effective. Some types of groups for youngsters who are obese include summer camps designed and conducted by health professionals, school groups organized and led by the school nurse, and groups associated with special clinics.

The group is concerned not only with weight loss but also emphasizes the development of a positive self-image. Nutrition education and diet planning are essential elements of the group function, but equally important are discussions centered around better grooming and improvement of social skills. Improvement is measured by positive changes in all aspects of endeavor.

Medical therapies. Little evidence shows that drugs are more effective than diet and exercise in maintaining weight loss. There is also some concern that the use of appetite-suppressing drugs may become a habit for some adolescents. Surgical techniques are available that bypass a substantial portion of the intestine or occlude a large segment of the stomach to produce a marked diet restriction and, hence, weight loss. These shunting techniques are hazardous surgical procedures with many metabolic complications. These metabolic effects need clarification, and this procedure should be restricted to those instances when obesity is life-threatening or when disease states demand weight loss for effective management.

Prevention. Unfortunately, weight-loss programs do not enjoy the successes of therapeutic interventions for most other disorders. The failure rate is dismally high. The most successful treatment of preadolescent obesity that often leads to adult obesity is to treat preschool obesity with programs that include frequent visits (Davis and Christoffel, 1994). The ultimate goal is to prevent obesity in children.

Evaluation

The effectiveness of nursing interventions is determined by continual reassessment based on the following observational guidelines and expected outcomes:

1. Assess weight at regular intervals (usually weekly); discuss with child or teen his or her feelings, reactions, and concerns; analyze daily recordings (log) of activities (eating, behavior, exercise) and feelings.
2. Review exercise program with child or teen.
3. Review log of eating behaviors; discuss observations with child or teen.
4. Interview child or teen about the plan of care and progress toward short-term and long-term goals.

Expected outcomes:

1. Eating patterns lead to weight loss; child or teen expresses feelings and concerns regarding problems.
2. Child or teen engages in preferred exercise and activities regularly.
3. Child or teen demonstrates an understanding of eating patterns.
4. Child or teen evidences a steady weight loss (or weight maintenance in a growing child).

See also Nursing Care Plan: The Child Who Is Obese.*

Anorexia Nervosa

Anorexia nervosa (AN) is an eating disorder characterized by a refusal to maintain a minimally normal body weight and severe weight loss in the absence of obvious physical causes. AN occurs predominantly in adolescent or young adult females, and the incidence is increasing.

The onset of AN generally takes place at or near menarche, but it may begin in preadolescence or in adulthood. The disease has two peaks: between 12 and 14 and between 16 and 17 years of age. Young people who have this disorder are most frequently from the upper or middle socioeconomic groups; are often described as "good children"; are academically high achievers, conforming, and conscientious; and have a high energy level, even with marked emaciation. These adolescents are usually strongly dependent on their parents, and frequently an ambivalent mother-daughter relationship is present for females. Sexual abuse may be a factor in some cases of AN and/or bulimia.

Etiology/pathophysiology. The etiology of the disorder remains unclear. There is a distinct psychologic component, and the diagnosis is based primarily on psychologic and behavioral criteria. Nevertheless, the physical manifestations of anorexia lend support to possible organic factors in the etiology.

Dominating the psychologic aspects of AN are a relentless pursuit of thinness and a fear of fatness, usually preceded by a period of 1 or 2 years of mood disturbances and behavior changes. The weight loss is usually triggered by a typical adolescent crisis such as the onset of menstruation or traumatic interpersonal incidents that precipitate serious dieting that continues out of control.

Frequently there is an exaggerated misinterpretation of the normal fat deposition characteristic of the early adolescent period, or someone may comment that the adolescent girl is putting on weight. The weight loss may be a response to teasing or to some event, such as gymnastic or ballet training, changing schools, or going to college. Youngsters entering the growth phase of puberty, when biologic fat accumulation is normal, are particularly vulnerable. The current emphasis on slimness is a very significant factor. The standard for beauty is often one exemplified by tall, thin models in many forms of media.

In some situations the adolescent is experiencing severe family stress, such as parental separation or divorce. In these and other circumstances in which the youngster perceives having no personal control, the decision to eat or not eat becomes one area where individual control can be exercised.

Diagnostic evaluation. Diagnosis is made on the basis of clinical manifestations (Box 37-6) and conformity to the criteria established by the American Psychiatric Association (1994) (Box 37-7).

BOX 37-6
Clinical Manifestations of Anorexia Nervosa

Severe and profound weight loss
Signs of altered metabolic activity:
- Secondary amenorrhea (if menarche attained)
- Primary amenorrhea (if menarche not attained)
- Bradycardia
- Lowered body temperature
- Decreased blood pressure
- Cold intolerance
- Dry skin and brittle nails
- Appearance of lanugo hair

BOX 37-7
Diagnostic Criteria for Anorexia Nervosa

A. Refusal to maintain body weight over a minimal normal weight for age and height (e.g., weight loss leading to maintenance of body weight less than 85% of that expected) or failure to make expected weight gain during period of growth, leading to body weight less than 85% of expected
B. Intense fear of gaining weight or becoming fat, even though underweight
C. Disturbance in the way in which one's body weight, size, or shape is experienced (e.g., the person claims to "feel fat" even when emaciated or believes that one area of the body is "too fat" even when obviously underweight)
D. In females, absence of at least three consecutive menstrual cycles when otherwise expected to occur (primary or secondary amenorrhea) (A woman is considered to have amenorrhea if her periods occur only after hormone [e.g., estrogen] administration.)

From American Psychiatric Association: *Diagnostic and statistical manual of mental disorders*, ed 4 (DSM-IV), Washington, DC, 1994, The Association.

*In Wong DL: *Wong and Whaley's clinical manual of pediatric nursing*, ed 4, St Louis, 1996, Mosby.

Therapeutic management. The initial goal is to treat the life-threatening malnutrition with strict adherence to dietary requirements, which sometimes necessitates intravenous and tube feedings (although these methods are usually reserved for severe situations). Rapid weight gain should be avoided because it can be medically unsafe and often overwhelms the patient. Many deaths associated with AN occur during rehabilitation as a result of cardiovascular overload. A safe and reasonable target weight is calculated by the physician and dietitian—usually 18% fat.

One treatment approach that has met with varied degrees of success is behavior modification. This requires team involvement with the following essential aspects:

- The health team determines an approach with the patient and adheres to it consistently.
- All team members are involved.
- There is continuity of caregivers (team members).
- There is clear communication among team members and with the patient so that the patient understands precisely what is expected.
- The patient is supported in his or her efforts (e.g., positive feedback for accomplishments).

Individuals whose disorder can be clearly related to a dysfunctional family situation will need intensive family therapy. Many of those whose therapy plan is implemented in the hospital need a continued behavior modification program after discharge to maintain the desired weight.

Family therapy seems to be effective when begun soon after the onset of illness, but it is less successful when the condition has existed for some time. Therapy is directed toward disengagement and redirection of malfunctioning processes in the family. Individual psychotherapy is aimed at helping the young person resolve the adolescent identity crisis, particularly as it relates to a distorted body image.

Nursing care management. The management of AN is directed toward correction of the severe state of malnutrition and resolution of the psychologic dynamics. Because of the psychogenic nature of the disorder, treatment is difficult and lengthy. All of those involved in therapy must keep in mind the adolescent's distorted sense of body image and self-awareness, as well as feelings of self-doubt, ineffectiveness, and helplessness that prompt such self-damaging behavior in order to feel in control.

Nurses must adopt and maintain a kind, supporting, yet firm manner in managing the care of a teen with AN. The child requires sustained support and reassurance to cope with ambivalent feelings related to the body concept and the desire to see oneself as a cooperative and reliable person worthy of receiving kindness. Encouraging the child with education and activities that strengthen self-esteem facilitates the resocialization process and promotes social acceptance among peers.

It is important for nurses to be aware of some of the physical side effects of AN. Patients with AN often limit their fluid intake, leading to urinary tract problems. Ketones and protein may be detected in the urine as a result of breakdown of fat and protein. Vital sign instability can be severe (including orthostatic hypotension). The pulse becomes irregular, and the rate decreases markedly. Bradycardia and hypothermia can result in cardiac arrest (see the Critical Thinking Q & A box above)

Critical Thinking Q & A

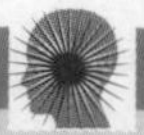

ANOREXIA NERVOSA

Jane is a 13-year-old student whose grades have been excellent and whom the teachers describe as a "model student." Recently, some of Jane's friends have expressed concern to the school nurse practitioner that Jane has begun to "jog" during lunch time and seldom eats with them. Jane has told her friends that she gained weight over the winter months and that she is "jogging" because she wants to qualify for the track team this spring. In addition to severe weight loss, which of the following symptoms of anorexia nervosa is the school nurse practitioner likely to observe when she interviews Jane and performs a sports physical?

1. **Decreased body temperature**
2. **History of dysmenorrhea**
3. **Tachycardia**
4. **Heat intolerance**

The correct answer is one. **Anorexia nervosa is a condition in which several alterations in metabolic activity can occur after excessive weight loss. These alterations include lowered body temperature, bradycardia, secondary amenorrhea, decreased blood pressure, and cold intolerance. When the nutritional status improves and normal body weight has been restored, these metabolic changes are usually reversed.**

Health professionals, patients, and families can find assistance and information from any of the following organizations: The National Eating Disorders Organization,* the National Association of Anorexia Nervosa and Associated Disorders, Inc.,† and the American Anorexia/Bulimia Association, Inc.‡

See also Nursing Care Plan: The Adolescent with Anorexia Nervosa.§

Bulimia

Bulimia is an eating disorder characterized by binge eating. The binge behavior consists of secretive, frenzied consumption of large amounts of high-calorie (or "forbidden") foods during a brief period of time (usually less than 2 hours). The binge is counteracted by various weight-control methods (purging), including self-induced vomiting, diuretic and laxative abuse, and rigorous exercise. The frequency of binging can be anywhere from once a week to seven or eight times a day. These binge/purge cycles are followed by self-deprecating thoughts, a depressed mood, and an awareness that the eating pattern is abnormal.

The disorder is observed more frequently in older adolescent girls and young women. Characteristically, affected persons have been unsuccessful dieters, have low impulse control, and may have been self-conscious about being overweight in childhood. They fall into two categories: (1) those

*445 E. Granville Rd., Worthington, OH 43085, (614) 436-1112.
†Box 7, Highland Park, IL 60035; (708) 831-3438.
‡Regents Hospital, 425 E. 61st St., New York, NY 10021; (212) 891-8686.
§In Wong DL: *Wong and Whaley's clinical manual of pediatric nursing,* ed 4, St Louis, 1996, Mosby.

who consume vast quantities of food followed by purging but who, if unable to purge, still consume large amounts, and (2) those who restrict their caloric intake, especially when unable to purge. Some are of normal weight or (more often) are slightly above normal weight; others become as underweight as anorectic individuals. This condition is called *bulimarexia.*

Diagnostic evaluation. The diagnosis may be first suspected from the presence of complications, including fluid and electrolyte disturbances from gastrointestinal losses, abdominal complaints from laxative abuse, erosion of tooth enamel and increased dental caries from vomited gastric acid, and throat complaints. The diagnosis is established on the basis of criteria established by the American Psychiatric Association (1994) (Box 37-8).

Therapeutic management. Therapy is similar to management of AN. Hospitalization may be required, especially for complications such as potassium depletion and esophageal damage. Intravenous fluids and potassium replacement are essential elements of care, and cardiac monitoring is indicated. Behavior therapy may also be used.

Nursing care management. Nursing care is similar to care of the patient with AN. Acute care also involves careful monitoring of fluid and electrolyte alterations and observation for signs of cardiac complications.

DISORDERS WITH BEHAVIORAL COMPONENTS

Smoking

Seventy percent of children experiment with cigarettes during the course of their childhood, many while in elementary school. Some youngsters then progress to occasional use (on weekends, at parties, on dates). By the end of high school, about 20% to 30% of senior high school boys and 25% to 35% of senior high school girls report having smoked in the past 30 days (Johnston, Bachman, and O'Malley, 1992).

The hazards of smoking at any age are undisputed; however, a preventive approach to teenage smoking is especially important. Smoking almost immediately brings about reduced lung function, "smoker's" cough, and other respiratory difficulties. Most harmful of all is the likelihood of lifelong addiction, since the earlier a person starts smoking, the more difficult it is to quit later in life. Furthermore, research findings indicate a clear association between the use of tobacco, alcohol, and other drugs (Torabi, Bailey, and Majd-Jabbari, 1993).

Etiology. There are various reasons why teenagers begin smoking, such as imitation of adult behavior, peer pressure, and emulation of traits popularly attributed to smokers. Teenagers least likely to smoke are those whose families and friends do not smoke, those who are interested in academics or athletics (particularly high-performance sports, such as basketball, swimming, and track), and those who plan to go on to college (see the Family Focus box below).

Smokeless tobacco. Tobacco products that are placed in the mouth but not ignited (e.g., snuff and chewing tobacco) are referred to as smokeless tobacco. This increasingly popular substitute for cigarettes is now posing a serious hazard to children and adolescents, as well as young adults. These products have been shown to be carcinogenic, and regular use has been reported to cause foul-smelling breath, periodontal disease, and tooth erosion or loss. A 1994 report of the Surgeon

BOX 37-8
Diagnostic Criteria for Bulimia

A. Recurrent episodes of binge eating (rapid consumption of a large amount of food in a discrete period of time)
B. A feeling of lack of control over eating behavior during the eating binges
C. The person regularly engages in either self-induced vomiting, use of laxatives or diuretics, strict dieting or fasting, or vigorous exercise to prevent weight gain
D. A minimum average of two binge eating episodes a week for at least 3 months
E. Persistent overconcern with body shape and weight

From American Psychiatric Association: *Diagnostic and statistical manual of mental disorders,* ed 4 (DSM IV), Washington, DC, 1994, The Association.

Family Focus

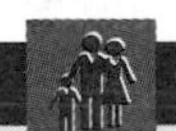

EARLY SEXUAL MATURATION, ALCOHOL, AND CIGARETTES

Cigarette smoking and the drinking of alcohol among adolescents are complex behaviors that cannot be explained by any single causative factor. However, theorists and investigators have looked at the relationship between biologic maturation and these behaviors. In particular, early sexual maturation in girls is related to the earlier onset of cigarette smoking and alcohol use (Wilson et al, 1994). One explanation for this association focuses on the rationale that girls who enter puberty early have a decreased self-image because their bodies are out of synchrony with those of other girls in their age group. Consequently, a young girl who is sexually mature at age 12 years may be attracted to a group of 14- to 16-year-old girls and boys who smoke and drink. If these teens have not been in any motor vehicle accidents while drinking, the young girl reasons that she, too, will be safe if she smokes, drinks, or is in an automobile with friends who are drinking.

Although parents and nurses cannot influence the time of biologic maturation, they can identify young girls who are at risk for the initiation of smoking and drinking because of early puberty. Parents must understand that an early maturing daughter might be uncomfortable with her body, and they should take advantage of all opportunities to build her self-esteem. Parental sensitivity to the importance of peer group acceptance is critical. Parents must be very supportive of a teenage daughter who feels left out or different. School nurses are in an excellent position to provide anticipatory guidance to girls who enter puberty early and to help them role play responses they can use to cope with situations that involve offers to smoke and drink. In addition, school nurses can provide information on the body changes that accompany puberty and emphasize that fact that not all teens enter puberty at the same time.

Wilson DM et al: Timing and rate of sexual maturation and the onset of cigarette and alcohol use among teenage girls, *Arch Pediatr Adolesc Med* 148:789-795, 1994.

General (U.S. Department of Health and Human Services, 1994) concluded that smokeless tobacco is also associated with lesions in oral soft tissue and can lead to cigarette smoking.

Nursing care management. Prevention of regular smoking in teenagers appears to be the most effective way to reduce the overall incidence of smoking. Various methods have been employed to deal with the problem. For the most part, smoking prevention programs that focus on the negative long-term effects of smoking on health have been ineffective. Those emphasizing immediate effects and youth-to-youth programs have been somewhat more effective, but primarily in improving teenagers' attitudes toward smoking. Because smoking and smoking-related behavior function as a key social symbol, antismoking campaigns must be addressed to the norms of the potential smokers without ridicule or threat to the social norms of the group.

Two areas of focus are gaining interest among health advocates: (1) peer-led programming emphasizing social consequences of smoking and (2) use of media, such as videotapes and films, in smoking prevention. If a significant number of influential peers can "sell" their classmates on the idea that the habit is not popular, the followers will imitate their behavior. Short-term rather than long-term consequences are emphasized (e.g., the effects of smoking on personal appearance, such as the unattractive stains on teeth and hands and the unpleasant odor that smoking gives to the breath and clothing). Several strategies are recommended for health professionals (Box 37-9).

Schools are ideal settings for tobacco use prevention programs. The majority of states have mandated that schools incorporate education that relays the adverse effects of smoking to students (Clubb, 1991). Smoking bans in schools also accomplish several goals: (1) they discourage students from starting to smoke; (2) they reinforce knowledge of the health hazards of cigarette smoking and exposure to environmental tobacco smoke; and (3) they promote a smoke-free environment as the norm. There is also pressure from the United States federal government for states to enforce the legal age for buying cigarettes.

BOX 37-9

Recommended Nonsmoking Strategies

- Provide only a cursory mention of long-term health consequences (e.g., cardiovascular and cancer risks)
- Discuss immediate physiologic consequences in some detail (e.g., changes in heart rate and blood pressure, minor respiratory symptoms, and blood carbon monoxide concentrations)
- Mention alternatives to smoking for establishing a self-image that appears tough, independent, mature, or sophisticated (e.g., establishing a weight-lifting regimen, jogging and dancing, joining a Boys' Club or a Girls' Club, engaging in volunteer work for a hospital or political or religious group)
- Mention the negative effects of smoking (e.g., earlier wrinkling of skin, yellow stains on teeth and fingers, tobacco odor on breath and clothing)
- Mention the increasing ostracism of smokers by nonsmokers, both legal and informal, in places of work and public places
- Mention the increasing evidence that second-hand smoke is injurious to the health of nonsmokers who are regularly exposed, especially small children
- Acknowledge that many adults once believed that important social benefits were associated with smoking, but point out that the vast majority of adult smokers would now quit smoking if they could
- Arm the cooperative adolescent with arguments for dealing with peer pressure (e.g., by not smoking, a teenager demonstrates independence and nonconformity, traits normally prized by youth)
- Request posters and pamphlets from local voluntary agencies (e.g., American Cancer Society, American Heart Association, and American Lung Association) to display prominently

Modified from Wong-McCarthy WJ, Gritz ER: Preventing regular teenage cigarette smoking, *Pediatr Ann* 11:683-689, 1982.

Substance Abuse

The use of other substances, primarily drugs, by children and adolescents to produce an altered state of consciousness is believed to reflect the variety of changes taking place in their lives and the stresses engendered by these changes. Experimenting with drugs is widespread during adolescence, but most teenagers do not become high-risk users. Today's youth are much less likely to use illicit drugs (e.g., hallucinogens, heroin, and nonmedical use of psychotherapeutic drugs) than were youths of the 1970s. However, alcohol, tobacco, and marijuana consumption among adolescents remains high, and cocaine use—particularly "crack"—appears to be increasing (National Institute on Drug Abuse, 1991).

Drug abuse is the regular use of drugs for other than the accepted medical purposes and to the extent that it results in physical or psychologic harm to the user and/or is detrimental to society. *Drug abuse, misuse,* and **addiction** are culturally defined and are voluntary behaviors. **Drug tolerance** and *physical dependence* are involuntary behaviors based on physiologic changes. Consequently, an individual can be addicted to a narcotic with or without being physically dependent, whereas a person may be physically dependent on a narcotic without being addicted, such as patients who are experiencing pain. (See discussion on fear of addiction under Pain Assessment, Chapter 41.)

Most drugs to which young people turn induce changes in perception, a feeling of well-being, and a sense of closeness. To most, they provide a feeling of happiness. In the majority of cases, drug use begins with experimentation. The individual may try a drug only once, may use it occasionally, or may make it an integral part of a drug-centered life-style.

Motivation. There are several common motives for drug use. Children and adolescents try drugs out of curiosity, for "kicks." Drugs produce for some persons a dreamy state of altered consciousness and a feeling of power, excitement, heightened acuity, or confidence. Others seek visual hallucinatory experiences and sexual sensation. Many youngsters use drugs not only for the perceptual and sensory experiences, but also for the social aspects. They use drugs because others use them and because they want to "belong." Teenagers are highly influenced by society's fads and fashions, and they are, developmentally, sensation-hungry risk takers. Adolescents are also trying to find a means to cope with the stress of the adult world, its social and technologic concerns, and their powerlessness to change it. Adolescents may seek escape from reality and want to achieve a sense of closeness and intimacy with other people, to escape from distress or decision making, and to feel a sense of insight into the mysteries of life and death.

Types of drugs abused. Any drug can be abused, and most are potentially harmful to youngsters still going through formative life experiences. Although rarely conceived of as drugs by society, the chemically active substances most frequently abused are caffeine and theobromines contained in chocolate and in common beverages such as tea, coffee, and colas. Common analgesics (e.g., Darvon Compound, Fiorinal), ethyl alcohol (ethanol), and nicotine are others that, although recognized as drugs, are sanctioned by society. These drugs can produce mild to moderate euphoric and/or stimulant effects and can lead to physical and psychic dependence. Many of the hazards associated with drug use are also related to adolescents driving a car while under the influence of drugs.

Drugs with mind-altering capacity that are available on the black market and that are of medical and legal concern are the hallucinogenic, narcotic, hypnotic, and stimulant drugs. In addition, those of concern to health professionals are alcohol and various volatile substances, such as antifreeze, plastic model airplane cement, typewriter correction fluid, and organic solvents, which are inhaled to achieve altered sensation in the user. Drugs available on the street are often mixed with other compounds and fillers so that the purity of the drug, its strength, and the nature of additives are highly variable.

Alcohol. Acute or chronic abuse of ethanol, a socially accepted depressant, is responsible for many acts of violence, suicide, accidental injury, and death. It is the most widely accepted drug, can be purchased legally by adults, is relatively inexpensive, is often used as part of a meal (wine and beer), and is approved by adults throughout the world when used in moderation. Youngsters may be afraid of hard drugs but feel comfortable with alcohol, which is increasingly being used by children of elementary school age.

The most noticeable effects of alcohol are on the central nervous system—incoordination, emotional lability, and impaired judgment, memory, and perception. Youthful alcoholics enjoy the effect of the alcohol and look forward to becoming intoxicated. They drink rapidly to obtain a "high" emotional state, often drink alone, and cannot predictably control their use of alcohol. Not all of these characteristics are observed in the alcoholic, but if several of the signs are evident, the youngsters should be considered at risk and detoxification therapy initiated to assure safe and complete withdrawal from the drug. Information about alcohol and answers to questions can be obtained by calling the Alcohol Hotline.*

Cocaine. The use of cocaine by adolescents is increasing more rapidly than any other form of substance abuse. Cocaine is available in two forms: water-soluble cocaine hydrochloride administered by "snorting" and a non-soluble alkaloid (freebase) used primarily for smoking. "Crack" is a purer and more menacing form of the drug; it can be produced cheaply and smoked in either water pipes or mentholated cigarettes. The increased use of cocaine is related to its availability and affordability, the false perception of safety in its use, its association with persons in glamorous occupations, its snob appeal, its reputation as a sexually enhancing drug, and peer pressure.

Cocaine creates a sense of euphoria, or an indefinable high. Withdrawal does not produce the dramatic symptoms observed in withdrawal from other substances. The effects are those more commonly seen in depression, including lack of energy and motivation, irritability, appetite changes, psychomotor retardation, and irregular sleep patterns. More serious symptoms include cardiovascular manifestations and seizures. Withdrawal is not to be confused with the so-called crash after a cocaine high, which consists of a long period of sleep. Answers to questions about health risks of cocaine can be obtained by calling the National Cocaine Hotline.* It also provides referrals to support groups and treatment centers.

Narcotics. Narcotic drugs include opiates such as heroin, morphine, meperidine hydrochloride (Demerol), fentanyl, hydromorphone (Dilaudid), and codeine. They produce a state of euphoria by removing painful feelings and creating a pleasurable experience and a sense of success accompanied by clouding of consciousness and a dreamlike state. Physical signs of narcotic abuse include constricted pupils, respiratory depression, and, often, cyanosis. Needle marks may be visible on the arms or legs in chronic users. Withdrawal from opiates is extremely unpleasant unless controlled with supervised substitution of methadone.

Perhaps more important are the indirect consequences related to the illegal status of narcotic use and the problems associated with securing the drug—time-consuming searches and often illegal methods used to meet the high cost. Health problems result from self-neglect of physical needs (nutrition, cleanliness, dental care), overdose, contamination, and infection, including HIV infection and hepatitis.

Central nervous system depressants. Various hypnotic drugs that produce physical dependence and withdrawal symptoms on abrupt discontinuation may be used by adolescents. They create a feeling of relaxation and sleepiness but impair general functioning. Drugs in this category include both barbiturates and nonbarbiturates (such as methaqualone [Quaalude]), as well as alcohol. Barbiturates combined with alcohol produce a profound depressant effect.

Central nervous system stimulants. Amphetamines and cocaine do not produce strong physical dependence and can be withdrawn without much danger. However, psychologic dependence is strong, and acute intoxication can lead to violent aggressive behavior or psychotic episodes characterized by paranoia, uncontrollable agitation, and restlessness. When combined with barbiturates, the euphoric effects are particularly addictive.

Methamphetamine is gradually assuming an important place in drug abuse. The drug can be snorted, injected, swallowed, or smoked and produces a burst of energy in its users, along with intense, alternating attacks of boldness and paranoia. It provokes excitement far more intense than that caused by crack and cocaine. The drug, with the street names "crank," "meth," and "crystal," is inexpensive and has a

*(800) ALCOHOL.

*(800) COCAINE.

longer period of action than cocaine. Instead of a short (few minutes) high, as achieved with crack, a user can remain "up" for hours on a similar dose of crank.

Mind-altering drugs. Hallucinogens (psychedelic, psychotomimetic, psychotropic, or illusionogenic) are drugs that produce vivid hallucinations and euphoria. These drugs do not produce physical dependence, since they can be abruptly withdrawn without ill effect. However, acute and long-term effects are variable, and in some individuals the dissociative behavior may be unduly prolonged. This category includes cannabis (marijuana, hashish) and lysergic acid diethylamide (LSD).

Inhalants. Glue "sniffing," the inhalation of plastic cement, and inhalation of other volatile substances that youngsters breathe and rebreathe in paper or plastic bags produce euphoria and altered consciousness. These substances are extremely hazardous to the individual, causing rapid loss of consciousness and respiratory arrest. Many persons taking these drugs do not have time to remove the bag from their heads and quickly become asphyxiated.

A new addition to the list of "sniffing" substances is air dusters, cans of pressurized gas used to blow dust from such surfaces as computers and camera lenses. The dusters contain chemical solvents and usually a form of freon, which can cause fatal cardiac dysrhythmias.

Nursing care management. Nurses in almost every setting are increasingly likely to have contact with youthful drug abusers or to be in a position to serve as educator and patient advocate. The nurse most often encounters young drug abusers when they are (1) experiencing overdose symptoms, (2) experiencing withdrawal symptoms, (3) manifesting bizarre behavior or confusion secondary to drug ingestion, (4) worried that they are becoming or will become addicted, or (5) worried about a friend or family member who is addicted.

Drug use may be encountered in relation to other health problems; therefore nurses caring for adolescents who are in the hospital or under treatment for other illnesses need to know if the youngsters use drugs compulsively, since withdrawal phenomena can seriously complicate the illness. Nurses should be able to recognize physical or behavioral clues that indicate the onset of withdrawal or the effects of drugs that might have been brought to the youngster secretly by well-meaning relatives or friends.

Acute care. Adolescents experiencing toxic drug effects or withdrawal symptoms are frequently seen as emergencies. Experienced emergency room personnel are familiar with the management of acute drug toxicosis; the signs, symptoms, and behavioral characteristics of a variety of substances; and differences and similarities among them. Observation or description of the behavior is often more valuable than a report by patients or their friends as to the chemical agent taken.

The treatment for drug toxicity or withdrawal varies according to the drug and the method used. Every effort is made to determine the type and amount of drug taken, the time it was taken, the mode of administration, and factors related to the onset of presenting symptoms. It is helpful to know the individual's pattern of use. For example, if two types of drugs are involved, they may require different treatments. Gastric lavage may be employed when the drug has been ingested recently and the cough reflex is intact, but it would be of little value when the drug has been administered by the intravenous ("mainlined") or intranasal ("sniffed") route. Since the actual content of most street drugs is highly questionable, other pharmaceutical agents are administered with caution, except perhaps naloxone (Narcan) or flumazenil (Mazicon) in cases of suspected opiate or benzodiazepine overdose, respectively. It is also necessary to assess for possible trauma sustained while the patient was under the influence of the drug.

Long-term management. A major factor in the treatment and rehabilitation of young drug users is careful assessment, in the nonacute stage, to determine the function that the drug plays in the youngster's life. Adolescents need help to identify the problem that motivated them to use drugs and to recognize their own role in self-destructive, inappropriate drug-abuse behavior before they can embark on a rehabilitation program.

Rehabilitation begins when youngsters decide, with the help of concerned and supportive adults, that they can and are willing to change. The family is an integral part of the rehabilitation process. Rehabilitation implies not only environmental manipulation and involvement in therapy, but also commitment on the part of the youth to substitute dependency on people for dependency on drugs and to explore alternative mechanisms for problem solving and coping with stress. Persons working with troubled youth must be prepared for recidivism, or the tendency to relapse, and maintain a plan for reentry into the treatment process.

Family support. Organizations that have achieved success in helping others cope with problems of drug abuse are excellent sources for both youngsters and their families. The Tough Love* philosophy first employed by Alcoholics Anonymous and Al-Anon is based on the conviction that parents have the right and responsibility to be the policymakers in the family, set limits on the behavior of their children, and take control of the household from out-of-control youngsters. The premise is that allowing teenagers to experience the negative consequences of their behavior will bring them closer to accepting help and/or changing their behavior.

Another group that provides support and counseling for families experiencing crises with their children is Parents Anonymous,† which maintains crisis counseling on a 24-hour basis. Al-Anon, Ala-Teen, and Ala-Tot are support groups for children and families who have an alcoholic family member. Information can be obtained from Alcoholics Anonymous listings in local telephone directories.

Prevention. Substance abuse in adolescence is both an individual and a community problem, and nurses play an important role in education and legislation, as well as in individual observation, assessment, and therapy. In this drug-oriented society, patterns of drug use may be established through parental models and the influence of the media as an

*Tough Love International, P.O. Box 1069, Doylestown, PA, 18901; (215) 348-7090.

†2230 Hawthorne Blvd., No. 208, Torrance, CA 90505; (800) 352-0386 (California) and (800) 421-0353 (elsewhere). Other sources of information include National Clearinghouse for Alcohol and Drug Information, P.O. Box 2345, Rockville, MD 20847-2345, (800) 729-6686; National Federation of Parents for Drug-Free Youth, (800) 554-KIDS or (301) 585-5437 (Maryland); and Center for Substance Abuse Prevention, 5600 Fishers Lane, Rockville, MD 20857, (301) 443-0365.

effective means to make the user "feel better." Impressionable youth need to be educated regarding appropriate use of chemicals. More important, those associated with adolescents should listen to what they are saying, determine what is bothering them, and try to help them meet these needs through alternative methods before they resort to drugs.

Peer pressure is a powerful tool and can be used effectively in prevention. A group that has had some success in reducing injury from drunk driving is Students Against Driving Drunk (SADD),* an organization designed to help eliminate drunk driving in teenagers. Some of the techniques used by the group include peer counseling, parental guidelines for teenage parties, and community awareness. Nurses can encourage the formation of chapters of SADD in the high schools in their communities.

Researchers have identified specific individual and environmental factors believed to make some children more vulnerable than others to substance abuse. An important predictor is age of initial use. Drug use initiated before the age of 15 years is a major risk factor for serious drug abuse problems (National Institute on Drug Abuse, 1991). Therefore prevention efforts must begin well before children reach adolescence.

The most effective substance abuse prevention strategies are part of a broader, generic prevention effort to promote health and success. Health-compromising behaviors tend to be interconnected and to have common antecedents. Prevention efforts that focus on changing only one behavior (e.g., alcohol and other drug use) are less likely to be successful.

Family Focus 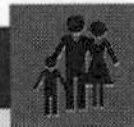

SUICIDE AND HOMOSEXUALITY

Thirty percent of all teen suicides each year occur among homosexual youths. Gay or lesbian adolescents who live in families or communities that do not accept homosexuality are very likely to suffer from low self-esteem and may even internalize the homophobic feelings of their family or community. Such internalization can lead to self-loathing, despair, hopelessness, and eventually suicide. Supportive parents, friends, or relationships serve as protective factors against suicide. However, many gay or lesbian adolescents have no friends and are not supported by their parents or families. Nurses who interact with adolescents must be aware of the association between adolescent homosexuality and suicide. School nurses may be the first individuals to identify and discuss issues of homosexuality with an adolescent. In their professional capacity, nurses can also serve as support persons for adolescents who are homosexual and provide the supportive relationship that will help prevent suicide. Nurses must also capitalize on those opportunities or experiences that promote the healthy development of self-esteem in gay, lesbian, and bisexual youths. One experience might include providing educational programs in the school to raise the level of consciousness about the risk factors for suicide and its warning signs. Another experience could be programs conducted in or outside of school that are designed to foster peer relationships and competency in social skills among high-risk adolescents and young adults.

Suicide

Suicide is the third leading cause of death during the teenage years, surpassed only by death from injury and homicide (see Chapter 27). A striking feature is the rise among people in the younger age groups. During the years 1950 to 1988 the suicide rate quadrupled in adolescents between the ages of 15 and 19 years (*Attempted suicide*, 1991).

Most authorities distinguish between suicidal ideation, gesture, and attempt, and all three must be acknowledged. *Suicidal ideation* involves thoughts about or plans for suicide. A *gesture* is made without any real attempt to cause either serious injury or death but rather to send out a signal that something is wrong. An *attempt*, unlike a gesture, is intended to cause injury or death but is unsuccessful. Teenagers sometimes make a number of gestures to draw attention to the fact that they are unable to cope. If the signals are not detected and responded to promptly, they may escalate in seriousness until they become serious attempts or completed acts. Another category, an *impulsive act*, describes a rage response designed to punish or manipulate a loved person perceived as withdrawing that love. Moreover, many experts believe that numerous "accidental" deaths are actually suicides.

Etiology. Adolescence has always been characterized by turmoil, heightened emotionality, and wide variations in mood. With limited capacities for problem solving and with fewer and less sophisticated resources for resolving difficulties, some teenagers have difficulty coping with critical events, especially a situation that is forced on them, such as the death of a friend, parent, or sibling. Impulsive behavior, characteristic of younger children, places children and adolescents at high risk for unintentional suicide.

Biologic, sociologic, and psychologic factors may be involved. Suicidal youngsters almost invariably come from a disturbed family situation, with economic stresses, family disintegration, medical problems, or psychiatric illness. Divorce, separation, abandonment, alcoholism, and death are highly significant factors that are often noted in the histories of suicidal youth. During a family crisis, youngsters may become suicidal when they feel overwhelmed by the crisis and unable to help the family recover equilibrium. A history of suicide by another family member is a common finding. Suicide risk is greater among youngsters with depression, chemical dependency, or psychosis. Gay and lesbian adolescents are at high risk for suicide, especially if they live in an environment without a support system (see the Family Focus box above). The availability of firearms in the American society has also been identified as a risk factor for adolescent suicide.

Suicidal methods. The outcome of suicidal behavior is influenced to some extent by the method used. Violent methods of destruction used by adults, such as jumping from heights or in front of trains, are less frequently employed by youths. Overdose of drugs is the method of choice for most adolescents who attempt suicide. Drugs used by adolescents include medications prescribed for parents (such as barbiturates and antidepressants), those intended for household use (aspirin or acetaminophen), or solvents. Ingestion of medications and wrist lacerations are the favored methods of females; males use more lethal methods such as knives, guns, and automobiles. Younger children (under 13½ years) are more likely to resort to hanging.

*P.O. Box 800, Malboro, MA 01752; (508) 481-3568.

Motivation. Many youngsters cannot identify a cause for their suicidal ideas. Ambivalence about life and death and hopelessness are common feelings. Most suicidal gestures are impulsive acts committed to force parents or other significant people to pay attention to the youngster's need for help. The attempt usually is the culmination of a behavioral pattern. These youngsters often have a history of attention-getting behaviors that range from minor acts to increasingly dramatic ones. With the ultimate act of attempted suicide, youngsters finally make themselves heard. They seldom actually plan a suicidal act because they really want to die; successful suicides are committed either impulsively or accidentally.

Suicidal ideation is not uncommon in adolescents. It represents numerous fantasies, such as relief from suffering, a means to gain comfort and sympathy, or a means of revenge against those who have hurt them. Adolescents have the erroneous perception that the act of suicide will evoke remorse and pity and that they will be able to return and witness the grief. Some children and younger adolescents desire to punish others who will be grieved by their death. Angry children who are unable to punish directly those who have injured or insulted them will take revenge on those who love them through self-destruction ("They'll be sorry when they find me dead"; "They'll be sorry they were mean to me").

Occasionally there are adolescents who are so severely depressed that suicide seems to be the only means of release from their despair. These youngsters rarely give evidence of their intent, concealing their suicidal thoughts for fear of outside intervention. Most adolescents tell their peers of their suicidal thoughts or plans but avoid telling adults. Sometimes this self-destructive behavior on the part of adolescents is a desire to punish themselves for guilt-filled actions or thoughts. Peer pressure has also convinced many young people that there is something wrong with them if they feel lonely or depressed; therefore they direct these feelings inward to avoid the risk of rejection. Social isolation is the most significant factor in distinguishing adolescents who will kill themselves from those who will not. It is also more characteristic of those who complete suicide than of those who make attempts or threats.

A cluster phenomenon, known as "contagion," has also been observed. Sometimes referred to as a teenage "epidemic," this situation occurs when one suicide appears to trigger several other suicides in a group such as a school or community. Suicide of a public figure sometimes prompts a number of suicides.

BOX 37-10

Clinical Manifestations Associated with Suicide Risk

Mood/Affect

Marked persistent depression
Feelings of hopelessness, helplessness, isolation
Deteriorating schoolwork
Remains distant, sad, remote
Flat affect—has "frozen" facial expression
Persistently looks or sounds sad and unhappy
Describes self as worthless
Feelings of self-hatred or excessive guilt
Feelings of humiliation, often brought on by inadequate performance at school
Sudden cheerfulness following deep depression*
Wish to be punished

Behavior

Changes in physical appearance—a child previously neat and well-groomed who stops bathing and begins to look slovenly
Loss of function as a result of illness or trauma
Loss of energy—loss of interest, listlessness, exhaustion without obvious cause
Sleep disturbances—difficulty going to sleep or sleeping excessively, taking voluntary naps during afternoon or evening
Increased irritability, argumentativeness, or stubbornness
Physical complaints—recurrent stomachaches, headaches
Repeated visits to doctor's office or emergency room for treatment of injuries
Antisocial behavior—engages in drinking, uses drugs, fights, commits acts of vandalism, runs away from home, becomes sexually promiscuous
Preoccupation with death—focuses on morbid thoughts; speaks repeatedly about people getting killed*
May begin referring to own death

School and Interpersonal Relationships

Resists or refuses to go to school
May become truant, cuts classes, does not complete assignments
Social withdrawal from friends, activities, interests that were previously enjoyed
Wants to give away cherished possessions*
Lacks an effective social support system

Coping Skills

Loses reality boundaries
Withdraws and isolates self
No use of support systems
Sees self as totally helpless, a victim of fate

*Absolute "red flags" or danger signals.

Diagnostic evaluation. Depression is a symptom common to adolescents who attempt suicide. Depression is characterized by both subjective symptoms and objective signs that reflect the adolescent's grief. Adolescents describe feelings of sadness, despair, helplessness, hopelessness, boredom, loss of interest, and isolation. They may also feel self-reproach, self-deprecation, and guilt. Subjective symptoms of depression or specific changes in behavior may place an adolescent at risk for suicide (Box 37-10).

Therapeutic management. *Suicidal threats must be taken very seriously.* There has been a general tendency to dismiss a suicide attempt as an impulsive act resulting from a temporary crisis or depression. If this drastic move to gain attention fails to draw attention to their problems or makes them worse, adolescents may conclude that suicide is the only answer to their escalating, unsolvable, and unbearable problems.

Children need to know that someone cares and must be provided with swift and efficient crisis intervention. Although an acute depressive reaction can be managed without difficulty by ordinary practitioners, the youngster who has made a serious attempt or has made a plan for suicide should receive immediate attention and competent psychiatric care.

Nursing care management. Care of the suicidal youngster includes early recognition, management, and prevention. Probably the most important aspect of management is the recognition of warning signs that indicate a youngster is troubled and might attempt suicide. Health professionals must be alert to the signs of depression, and anyone who exhibits such behavior, subtle or overt, should be referred for thorough psychologic assessment. Depression can be manifested in two different ways: young people who feel depressed may talk about suicide and feelings of worthlessness, or they may build themselves a solid defense against such intolerable feelings of depression with behavioral or psychosomatic disturbances.

Nursing ALERT

No threat of suicide should be ignored or challenged in any way. It is a symptom that must be taken seriously. Too often, suicidal threats or minor attempts are confused with bids for attention. It is also a mistake to be lulled into a false sense of security when the adolescent's depression is apparently relieved. The improvement in attitude may very well mean that the youngster has made the decision to carry out the threat.

Peers or other confidants are excellent sources of information and valuable observers. They may not be able to diagnose depression, but they are able to sense when a friend has undergone a marked personality change. It is important to emphasize that the peer who detects any changes in a friend is a potential rescuer and should not remain quiet about the observations. Friendship does not imply collusion. A peer who believes that a friend may be suicidal should alert someone who is in a position to help—a parent, teacher, guidance counselor, school nurse, or other person.

As soon as the youngster who attempts suicide is out of danger from medical problems resulting from the attempt, the data-gathering process should begin. It should include information from several sources to help evaluate the extent to which the child is suffering, the direction for therapy, and the probability of a repeated attempt. The youngster is questioned directly about the depression or suicidal behavior. Clues to a youngster's feelings may be elicited by questions such as the following (Greydanus and Pratt, 1995):

- Do you consider yourself more a happy person, an unhappy person, or somewhere in the middle?
- Have you ever been so unhappy or upset that you felt like being dead?
- Have you ever thought about hurting yourself?
- Have you ever developed a plan to hurt yourself or kill yourself?
- Have you ever attempted to kill yourself?

A prevention strategy is to ask youngsters to give their written word that they will not attempt suicide during an agreed-on period of time (a week, a day, maybe even just 5 minutes) and that they will contact help immediately if they feel that they cannot keep their contract. The length of time a youngster suggests provides valuable information regarding the seriousness of the threat. Furthermore, most teenagers attach significance to signing their name to a document, and, if they sign a no-suicide contract, will usually honor it. Contracts can be extended when the time limit expires.

Since the suicide attempt is frequently an outgrowth of family distress, it is essential to deal with the family as well. Ideally the most effective approach is recognition of susceptible youngsters during the early stages of intra-family distress so that family counseling can be started. This emphasizes again the importance of parent-child relationships and the role of the nurse in assessing family interactions and recognizing disturbed relationships. Prevention efforts must be directed toward improving childrearing practices through support and education of parents and changing societal conditions that generate defeat, despair, and maladaptive behavior.

Follow-up care is of utmost importance. Although confidentiality is the usual approach with adolescent counseling, in the case of self-destructive behaviors this cannot be honored. The suicidal behavior is reported to the family and other professionals, and youngsters are informed that this will be done. Such action conveys an important message to an attempter—that the professionals understand and care.

Some schools have instituted suicide-prevention programs. Most are designed for high school–age youth, but many are attempting to reach elementary school–age children as well. Schools with programs in operation offer services such as drop-in counseling and a peer-counseling telephone line. Information can be obtained from the American Association of Suicidology.*

*2459 S. Ash, Denver, CO 80222.

Key Points

- The pubescent growth spurt that begins around age 10 years in girls and age 12 years in boys signals the beginning of adolescence.
- Biologic development during puberty is characterized by increased activity of the pituitary gland, which results in sexual maturity and the appearance of secondary sex characteristics.
- According to Erikson, the major developmental crisis of adolescence is establishing a sense of identity.
- Cognitive development in adolescence includes abstract thought, thinking beyond the present, logical reasoning, and a sense of idealism.
- Development of body image is closely tied to body changes and social interactions.
- According to Kohlberg's theory of moral development, adolescents begin to question existing moral values and learn to make choices.

- Spiritual development is characterized by the questioning of family values and ideals, a move to more philosophical thinking, and emphasis on personal religion.
- Adolescent relationships with parents may be strained, whereas the influence of the peer group increases and heterosexual relationships assume importance.
- Teenagers demonstrate a wide variety of interests, and their increased physical and cognitive skills allow them to engage in increasingly difficult and complex activities.
- Adolescents' emotions fluctuate.
- Nutritional needs, especially for calcium, zinc, and iron, may not be met by teenagers' eating habits, such as snacking and irregular mealtimes.
- Motor vehicle injuries are the primary cause of death from injury in the adolescent years.
- The rapid changes, growth, and stress accompanying the transition to adulthood may predispose youngsters to faulty problem solving.
- The most frequent health problems related to the female reproductive system involve menstrual dysfunction.
- Eating disorders observed in middle and late childhood are obesity, anorexia nervosa, and bulimia.
- Smoking is a widespread problem among teenagers; reasons for smoking include social pressure, mass media influence, and a need to develop a self-concept.
- The substances abused by children and adolescents are alcohol, marijuana, narcotics, central nervous system depressants, central nervous system stimulants, hydrocarbons and fluorocarbons, and mind-altering drugs.
- Suicide, the deliberate act of self-injury with the intent to kill, may occur because of difficulties coping with stress, disturbed family environment, chemical dependency, or psychoses.

References

Agostoni C et al: Dairy products and adolescent nutrition, *J Int Med Res* 22(2):67-76, 1994.

American Academy of Pediatrics, Committee on Adolescence: Firearms and adolescents, *Pediatrics* 89(4):784-787, 1992.

American Psychiatric Association: *Diagnostic and statistical manual of mental disorders,* ed 4 (DSM-IV), Washington, DC, 1994, The Association.

American Academy of Pediatrics, Committee on Infectious Diseases: Recommended childhood immunization schedule—United States, January-December, 1997, *Pediatrics* 99(1):137-138, 1997.

Attempted suicide among high school students—United States, 1990, *MMWR* 40(37):633-635, 1991.

Bearinger L, Blum R: *Adolescent health care.* In Wallace H, Nelson R, Sweeney P, editors: *Maternal and child health practices,* ed 4, Oakland, Calif, 1994, Third Party.

Biro FM et al: Hormonal studies and physical maturation in adolescent gynecomastia, *J Pediatr* 116:450-455, 1990.

Children's Defense Fund: *The state of America's children yearbook,* Washington, DC, 1995, Children's Defense Fund.

Clubb R: Promoting non-tobacco use in childhood, *Pediatr Nurs* 17(6):566-570, 1991.

Croft C, Asmussen L: A developmental approach to sexuality education: implications for medical practice, *J Adolesc Health* 24(2): 109-114, 1993.

Davis K, Christoffel KK: Obesity in preschool and school-age children: treatment early and often may be best, *Arch Pediatr Adolesc Med* 148(12):1257-1261, 1994.

Erikson EH: *Childhood and society,* ed 2, New York, 1963, WW Norton.

Friedman R, Downey J: Homosexuality; *N Engl J Med* 331(14):923-930, 1994.

Greydanus DE, Pratt HD: *Adolescent health update: emotional and behavioral disorders of adolescence: part 2,* vol 8, no 1, Elk Grove Village, Ill., 1995, American Academy of Pediatrics.

Johnston LD, Bachman JG, O'Malley PM: *Monitoring the future questionnaire responses from the nation's high school seniors 1989,* Ann Arbor, Mich., 1992, Institute for Social Research, University of Michigan.

Kann L et al: Youth risk behavior surveillance—United States, 1993, *MMWR CDC Surveill Summ* 44(1):1-56, 1995.

Key JD, Key LL Jr: Calcium needs of adolescents, *Curr Opin Pediatr* 6(4):379-382, 1994.

McGrory A: Education for the menarche, *Pediatr Nurs* 21(5):439-443, 1995.

McKay L, Diem E: Health concerns of adolescent girls, *J Pediatr Nurs* 10(1):19-27, 1995.

Murphy AS et al: Nutrition education needs and learning preferences of Michigan students in grades 5, 8, and 11, *J Sch Health* 64(7):273-278, 1994.

National Institute on Drug Abuse: *Drug abuse and drug abuse research,* Rockville, Md, 1991, The Institute.

Ostrum G: Sports-related injuries in youths: prevention is the key—and nurses can help! *Pediatr Nurs* 19(4):333-342, 1993.

Pentz M: *Benefits of integrating strategies in different settings.* In Elster A, Panzarine S, Holt K, editors: *American Medical Association state of the art conference on adolescent health promotion: proceedings,* Arlington, Va., 1993, National Center for Education in Maternal and Child Health.

Prothrow-Stith D: *Deadly consequences: how violence is destroying our teenage population and a plan to begin solving the problem,* New York, 1993, HarperCollins.

Seidman S, Rieder R: A review of sexual behavior in the United States, *Am J Psychiatry* 151(3):330-341, 1994.

Torabi MR, Bailey WJ, Majd-Jabbari, M: Cigarette smoking as a predictor of alcohol and other drug use by children and adolescents: evidence of the "gateway drug effect," *J Sch Health* 63:302-306, 1993.

Troiano R, et al: Overweight prevalence and trends for children and adolescents, *Arch Pediatr Adolesc Med* 149(10):1085-1091, 1995.

US Department of Health and Human Services: *Preventing tobacco use among young people: a report of the surgeon general,* Atlanta, 1994, U.S. Department of Health and Human Services, Public Health Service, Centers for Disease Control and Prevention, National Center for Chronic Disease Prevention and Health Promotion, Office on Smoking and Health.

Willard JC, Schoenborn CA: Relationship between cigarette smoking and other unhealthy behaviors among our nation's youth: United States, 1992, *Advance data for vital and health statistics* (No. 263). Hyattsville, Md., 1995, National Center for Health Statistics.

Wilson DM et al: Timing and rate of sexual maturation and the onset of cigarette and alcohol use among teenage girls, *Arch Pediatr Adolesc Med* 148:789-795, 1994.

Bibliography

General

American Medical Association: *Guidelines for adolescent preventive services*, Chicago, 1992, The Association.

Andersen LB: Changes in physical activity are reflected in changes in fitness during late adolescence: a 2-year follow-up study, *J Sports Med Phys Fitness* 34(4):390-397, 1994.

Bearinger L, Gephart J: Interdisciplinary education in adolescent health, *J Pediatr Child Health* 29(suppl 1):S10-S15, 1993.

Bearinger L et al: Nursing competence in adolescent health: anticipating the future needs of youth, *J Prof Nurs* 8(2):80-86, 1992.

Blum RW et al: American Indian-Alaska Native youth health, *JAMA* 267(12):1637-1644, 1992.

Braun BL, Wagenaar AC, Flack JM: Alcohol consumption and physical fitness among young adults, *Alcohol Clin Exp Res* 19(4):1048-1054, 1995.

Fulton RAB, Moore CM: Spiritual care of the school-age child with a chronic condition, *J Pediatr Nurs* 10(4):224-231, 1995.

Groer MW et al: Adolescent stress and coping: a longitudinal study, *Res Nurs Health* 15(3):209-217, 1992.

Grubbs S et al: Self-efficacy in normal adolescents, *Issues Ment Health Nurs* 13:121-128, 1992.

Haggerty R: Care of the poor and underserved in America: older adolescents: a group at special risk, *Am J Dis Child* 145:569-571, 1991.

Hendee W et al: *The health of adolescents*, San Francisco, 1991, Jossey-Bass.

Kollar M et al: Adolescent anger: a developmental study, *J Child Adolesc Psychiatr Ment Health Nurs* 4(1):9-15, 1991.

Millstein S: *A view of health from the adolescent's perspective.* In Millstein S, Petersen A, Nightingale E, editors: *Promoting the health of adolescents: new directions for the twenty-first century*, New York, 1993, Oxford University Press.

Moffit TE et al: Childhood experience and the onset of menarche: a test of a sociobiological model, *Child Dev* 63(1):59-67, 1992.

Piaget J: *The theory of stages in cognitive development*, New York, 1969, McGraw-Hill.

Rosella JD, Albrecht SA: Anticipatory guidance: alcohol, adolescents, and recognizing abuse and dependence, *Issues Compr Pediatr Nurs* 16(4):207-218, 1993.

Schmitt B: Dealing with normal adolescent rebellion, *Contemp Pediatr* 7(7):55-60, 1990.

Slusher IL et al: State of the art of nursing research and theory development in adolescent health, *Issues Compr Pediatr Nurs* 16:1-11, 1993.

Steinberg L et al: Impact of parenting practices on adolescent achievement: authorative parenting, school involvement, and encouragement to succeed,*Child Dev* 63(5):1266-1281, 1992.

Health Promotion

Alderman EM, Fleischman AR: Should adolescents make their own health-care choices? *Contemp Pediatr* 10(1):65-82, 1993.

Availability of comprehensive adolescent health services, *MMWR* 42(26):507-515, 1993.

Blum RW: Global trends in adolescent health, *JAMA* 265(20):2711-2719, 1991.

Council on Scientific Affairs, American Medical Association: Confidential health services for adolescents, *JAMA* 269(11):1420-1424, 1993.

Crockett L, Petersen A: *Adolescent development: health risks and opportunities for health promotion.* In Millstein S, Petersen A, Nightingale E, editors: *Promoting the health of adolescents: new directions for the twenty-first century*, New York, 1993, Oxford University Press.

Cromer BA et al: Compliance with breast self-examination instruction in high school students, *Clin Pediatr* 215-220, 1992.

Glenmark B, Hedberg G, Jansson E: Prediction of physical activity level in adulthood by physical characteristics, physical performance and physical activity in adolescence: an 11-year follow-up study, *Eur J Appl Physiol* 69(6):530-538, 1994.

Isaacs M: *Developing culturally competent strategies for adolescents of color.* In Elster A, Panzarine S, Holt K, editors: *American Medical Association State of the Art Conference on Adolescent Health Promotion: proceedings*, Arlington, Va., 1993, National Center for Education in Maternal and Child Health.

Ranade B: Nutritional recommendations for children and adolescents, *Int J Clin Pharmacol Ther Toxicol* 31(6):285-290, 1993.

Schreiner B, Brondum LA: Nutrition in pediatric primary care: assessment and common problems, *Nurse Pract Forum* 5(1):13-23, 1994.

Sobczk W et al: Health promotion schools of excellence: a model program for Kentucky and the nation, *J Ky Med Assoc* 93(4):142-147, 1995.

VandenBergh MF et al: Physical activity, calcium intake, and bone mineral content in children in The Netherlands, *J Epidemiol Community Health* 49(3):299-304, 1995.

Yarcheski A, Scoloveno A, Mahon N: Social support and well-being in adolescents: the mediating role of hopefulness, *Nurs Res* 43(5):288-292, 1994.

Sexuality and Sexuality Education

American Academy of Pediatrics, Committee on Adolescence: Homosexuality and adolescence, *Pediatrics* 92(4):631-634, 1993.

Flaming D, Morse J: Minimizing embarrassment: boys' experiences of pubertal changes, *Iss Compr Pediatr Nurs* 14(4):211-230, 1991.

Laumann D, et al: *The social organization of sexuality*, Chicago, 1995, University of Chicago Press.

Meeropool E: One of the gang: sexual development of adolescents with physical disabilities, *J Pediatr Nurs* 6(4):243-249, 1991.

Mellanby A, Phelps F, Tripp JH: Teenagers, sex, and risk taking, *Br Med J* 307(6895):25, 1993.

Roth B: Fertility awareness as a component of sexuality education: preliminary research findings with adolescents, *Nurse Pract* 18(3):40, 43, 47-48, 1993.

Taylor BA, Remafedi G: Youth coping with sexual orientation issues, *J Sch Nurs* 9(2):26-39, 1993.

Tucker S: Adolescent patterns of communication about the menstrual cycle, sex, and contraception, *J Pediatr Nurs* 5(6):393-400, 1990.

Woodcock A, Stenner K, Ingham R: "All these contraceptives, videos and that . . . ": young people talking about school sex education, *Health Educ Res* 7(4):517-531, 1992.

Yarber W, Parrillo A: Adolescents and sexually transmitted diseases, *J Sch Health* 62(7):331-338, 1992.

Injury Prevention

Dexheimer Pharris M, editor: *The community responds to youth violence: what works? What doesn't?* Monograph, 1994, Division of General, Pediatric, and Adolescent Health, University of Minnesota Medical School.

Dryfoos J: Preventing high-risk behavior, *Am J Public Health* 81(2):157-158, 1991.

Fingerhut L et al: *Firearm mortality among children, youth, and young adults, 1-34 years of age: trends and current status—United States, 1979-1990*, Washington, DC, 1991, U.S. Government Printing Office.

Garmezy N: Resilience in children's adaptation to negative life events and stressed environments, *Pediatr Ann* 20(9):459-466, 1991.

Meehan PJ, O'Carroll PW: Gangs, drugs, and homicide in Los Angeles, *Am J Dis Child* 146(6):683-687, 1992.

Metcalf J, Roberts S: Strength training and the immature athlete: an overview, *Pediatr Nurs* 19(4):325-332, 1993.

Lawrence HS: Fatal nonpowder firearm wounds: case report and review of the literature, *Pediatrics* 85:177-181, 1990.

Lipp E, Trimble N: Health behaviors of adolescent male football athletes, *Pediatr Nurs* 19(4):395-397; 399, 1993.

Sheley JF, McGee ZT, Wright JD: Gun-related violence in and around inner-city schools, *Am J Dis Child* 146(6):677-682, 1992.

Wilson P, Testani-Dufour L: Bicycle safety programs: targeting injury prevention through education, *Pediatr Nurs* 19(4):343-346, 1993.

Disorders of the Reproductive System

Coupey SM, Ahlstrom P: Common menstrual disorders, *Pediatr Clin North Am* 36:551-571, 1989.

Cumming DC, Cumming CE, Kieren DK: Menstrual mythology and sources of information about menstruation, *Am J Obstet Gynecol* 164:472-476, 1991.

Elvik S: Vaginal discharge in the prepuberal girl, *J Pediatr Health Care* 4(4):181-185, 1990.

Greydanus DE, Shearin RB: *Adolescent sexuality and gynecology*, Philadelphia, 1990, Lea & Febiger.

Higgs D: The patient with testicular cancer: nursing management of chemotherapy, *Clin Rev* 17(2):243-249, 1990.

Klein TF, Berry CC, Felice M: The development of a testicular self-examination instructional booklet, *J Adolesc Health Care* 11:235-239, 1990.

Tuttle J: Menstrual disorders during adolescence, *J Pediatr Health Care* 5(4):197-203, 1991.

Obesity

Alexander MA: Obesity in school children, *Sch Nurse* 7(4):6-10, 1991.

Castiglia PT: Obesity in adolescence, *J Pediatr Health Care* 3:221-223, 1989.

Dietz WH Jr: The overweight child: psychosocial effects and treatment, *Feelings Med Signif* 31(1):1-4, 1989.

Epstein L et al: Growth in obese children treated for obesity, *Am J Dis Child* 14(12):1360-1364, 1990.

Feldman W, Feldman E, Goodman JT: Culture versus biology: children's attitudes toward thinness and fatness, *Pediatrics* 81:190-194, 1988.

Moore DC: Body image and eating behavior in adolescent boys, *Am J Dis Child* 144:475-479, 1990.

Schmitt BD: A weight reduction program for overweight older children and adolescents, *Contemp Pediatr* 8(8):85-91, 1991.

Stunkard A, Berkowitz R: Treatment of obesity in children, *JAMA* 264(19):2550-2551, 1990.

Anorexia Nervosa/Bulimia

Castiglia PT: Anorexia nervosa, *J Pediatr Health Care* 3:105-107, 1989.

Castiglia PT: Bulimia, *J Pediatr Health Care* 3:167-169, 1989.

Comerci GD: Eating disorders in adolescents, *Pediatr Rev* 10:1-6, 1988.

Ferraro AR: Bulimia: a look from within, *Pediatr Nurs* 16:187-191, 1990.

Flood M: Addictive eating disorders, *Nurs Clin North Am* 24:65-69, 1989.

Garner D: Pathogenesis of anorexia nervosa, *Lancet* 431:1631-1634, 1993.

Muscari ME: Effective nursing strategies for adolescents with anorexia nervosa and bulimia nervosa, *Pediatr Nurs* 14:475-482, 1988.

Stewart DE et al: Infertility and eating disorders, *Am J Obstet Gynecol* 163:1196-1199, 1990.

Smoking

American Academy of Pediatrics, Committee on Substance Abuse: "Smokeless cigarettes" and other nicotine delivery devices, *Pediatrics* 87:410-411, 1991.

American Academy of Pediatrics, Committee on Substance Abuse: Tobacco-free environment: an imperative for the health of children and adolescents, *AAP News* 10(4):25-27, 1994.

Cigarette smoking among youth—United States, 1989, *MMWR* 40(41):712-715, 1991.

Davis R, Tollestrup K, Milham S: Trends in teenage smoking during pregnancy, *Am J Dis Child* 144(12):1297-1301, 1990.

Winkelstein M: Adolescent smoking: influential factors, past preventive efforts and future nursing implications, *J Pediatr Nurs* 7:120-127, 1992.

Substance Abuse

Alexander DE, Gwyther RE: Alcoholism in adolescents and their families: family-focused assessment and management, *Pediatr Clin North Am* 42(1):217-234, 1995.

American Academy of Pediatrics, Committee on Adolescence, Committee on Bioethics, and Provisional Committee on Substance Abuse: Screening for drugs of abuse in children and adolescents, *Pediatrics* 84:396-398, 1989.

Bateman DA, Heagarty MC: Passive freebase cocaine ("crack") inhalation by infants and toddlers, *Am J Dis Child* 143:25-27, 1989.

Brown BS and others: Kids and cocaine—a treatment dilemma, *J Subst Abuse Treat* 6:3-8, 1989.

Castiglia PT et al: Influences on children's attitudes toward alcohol consumption, *Pediatr Nurs* 15:263-266, 1989.

Clouet D, Asghar K, Brown R, editors: *Mechanisms of cocaine abuse and toxicity*, NIDA Research Monograph 88, Washington, DC, 1988, U.S. Government Printing Office.

Estroff TW, Schwartz RH, Hoffmann NG: Adolescent cocaine abuse, *Clin Pediatr* 28:550-555, 1989.

Heagarty MC: Crack cocaine: a new danger for children, *Am J Dis Child* 14:756-757, 1990.

Rich J: Action stat! Acute alcohol intoxication, *Nurs 89* 19(9):33, 1989.

Robinson DP, Green JW: The adolescent alcohol and drug problem: a practical approach, *Pediatr Nurs* 14:305-310, 1988.

Schubiner H: Treatment: validating toughlove, *Child Teens Today* 11(4):1-3, 1991.

Washburn P: Identification, assessment, and referral of adolescent drug abusers, *Pediatr Nurs* 17(2):137-40, 1991.

Suicide

American Academy of Pediatrics, Committee on Adolescence: Suicide and suicide attempts in adolescents and young adults, *Pediatrics* 81:322-324, 1988.

Bakkala CF: The role of the school nurse in suicide prevention, *School Nurse* 6(1):13-15, 1990.

Berman AL, Jobes DA: *Adolescent suicide: assessment and intervention*, Washington, DC, 1991, American Psychological Association.

Brent DA et al: Risk factors for adolescent suicide, *Arch Gen Psychiatry* 45:581-588, 1988.

Gemma PB: Coping with suicidal behavior, *Am J Matern Child Nurs* 14:101-103, 1989.

Gyulay JE: What suicide leaves behind, *Issues Compr Pediatr Nurs* 12:103-118, 1989.

Lamb JM: The suicidal adolescent: how you can help, *Nurs 90* 20(5):72-76, 1990.

Pfeffer CR: Spotting the red flags for adolescent suicide, *Contemp Pediatr* 6(2):59-70, 1989.

Reinherz H, Frost A, Pakiz B: Changing faces: correlates of depressive symptoms in late adolescence, *Fam Community Health* 14(3):53-63, 1991.

Reynolds WM: A school-based procedure for the identification of adolescents at risk for suicidal behaviors, *Fam Community Health* 14(3):64-75, 1991.

CHAPTER 38

Chronic Illness, Disability, and Death

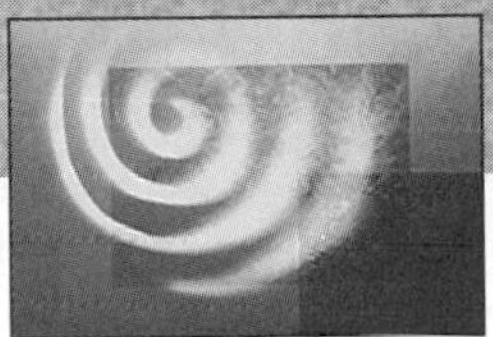

PERSPECTIVES IN THE CARE OF CHILDREN WITH SPECIAL NEEDS, P. 1121

Scope of the problem, p. 1121

Changing trends in care, p. 1121

THE FAMILY OF THE CHILD WITH SPECIAL NEEDS, P. 1123

Reactions of families to a chronic illness or disability, p. 1123

Impact of child's chronic illness or disability on family members, p. 1125

Factors affecting the family's adjustment, p. 1128

Reactions of families to childhood death: the grief process, p. 1128

THE CHILD WITH SPECIAL NEEDS, P. 1129

Impact of chronic illness or disability on the child, p. 1129

Impact of impending death on the child, p. 1132

NURSING CARE OF THE FAMILY AND CHILD WITH SPECIAL NEEDS, P. 1135

NURSING CARE OF THE FAMILY AND CHILD WHO IS TERMINALLY ILL OR DYING, P. 1148

Perspectives in the Care of Children with Special Needs

SCOPE OF THE PROBLEM

Despite the interest and concern for children with special needs, exact definitions and prevalence rates of chronic illness, disability, and terminal illness do not exist. For the purposes of this chapter, see the definitions listed in Box 38-1.

Statistics regarding chronic illness and disability are at best only estimates of the actual prevalence of the problem. In the United States an estimated 20% of children under 18 years of age experienced mild chronic conditions, 9% experienced chronic conditions of moderate severity, and 2% experienced severe chronic conditions (Newacheck, Stoddard, and McManus, 1993). Cancer and mental health problems without physical manifestations are not included in these figures. Asthma and congenital heart defects account for two thirds of all cases of chronic illness in children.

Although there has been little change in the survival patterns for asthma and acquired immune deficiency syndrome (AIDS), there have been improvements in other diseases such as cancer, cystic fibrosis, and spina bifida. In addition, technologic advances have increased survival rates of very low-birth-weight infants. The resulting progress for these children at risk contributes to the growing number of children who have chronic and/or disabling conditions, many of whom remain dependent on technology.

Broadly expanding chronic conditions to include speech, learning, emotional, sensory, and cognitive disorders yields an even greater number of children who have a significant long-term condition. Terminal illness also significantly adds to the number of children with special needs. Cancer is the leading cause of death from disease in children ages 1 through 15 years (Cancer facts, 1994). However, many children survive for long periods and experience problems commonly associated with chronic illness or physical disability. Considering also those who care deeply about the child, the number of individuals intimately affected by these children's illnesses and disabilities is staggering.

CHANGING TRENDS IN CARE

Developmental Focus

One change is in the focus on the child's *developmental age* rather than chronologic age or diagnosis. Using the developmental approach emphasizes the child's abilities and strengths rather than disabilities. Attention is paid to normalizing experiences, environmental adaptations, and promoting coping skills. Nurses often are in vital positions to redirect at-

BOX 38-1

Common Terms Regarding Children with Special Needs

Chronic illness—a condition that interferes with daily functioning for more than 3 months in a year, causes hospitalization of more than 1 month in a year, or (at time of diagnosis) is likely to do either of these

Congenital disability—a disability that has existed since birth but is not necessarily hereditary

Developmental delay—a maturational lag—an abnormal, slower rate of development in which a child demonstrates a functioning level below that observed in normal children of the same age

Developmental disability—any mental and/or physical disability that is manifested before age 22 years and is likely to continue indefinitely

Disability—a functional limitation that interferes with a person's ability, for example, to walk, lift, hear, or learn

Handicap—a condition or barrier imposed by society, the environment, or one's own self; not a synonym for disability

Impairment—a loss or abnormality of structure or function

Technology-dependent child—a child between the ages of birth to 21 years with a chronic disability that requires the routine use of a medical device to compensate for the loss of a life-sustaining body function; daily ongoing care and/or monitoring is required by trained personnel

Data from Research and Training Center on Independent Living (RTC/IL): *Guidelines for reporting and writing about people with disabilities*, ed 3, Lawrence, KS, 1990, The Center; Hobbs N, Perrin J, editors: *Issues in the care of children with chronic illness*, San Francisco, 1985, Jossey-Bass; and *Report to Congress and the Secretary by the Task Force on Technology-Dependent Children: Fostering home and community-based care for technology-dependent children*, vol 2, US Department of Health and Human Services, Health Care Financing Administration, HCFA Pub No 88-02171, 1988, childhood-disability definition created, *AAP News* 11(7):4, 1995.

tention from the pathologic model, with its focus on weaknesses and problems, to the developmental model to meet the unique needs of the child and family.

A developmental focus also considers family development. The life cycle of the family unit reflects changing ages and needs of family members, as well as changing emotional demands. A family member's serious illness or disability can cause significant stress or crisis at any stage of the family life cycle. Just as with individual development, family development may be interrupted or even regress to an earlier level of functioning. Nurses can use the concept of family development to plan meaningful interventions and evaluate care (see Developmental Theory, Chapter 30).

Family-Centered Care

The importance of family-centered care—a philosophy that considers the family as the constant in the child's life—is especially evident in the care of children with special needs (see also Family-Centered Care, Chapter 27). As parents learn about the youngster's health care needs, they often become experts in delivering care. Health care providers, including nurses, are adjuncts to the child's care and need to form partnerships with parents. Collaboration is essential to forming trusting and effective partnerships. Collaborative relationships are characterized by communication, dialogue, active listening, awareness, and acceptance of differences (Bishop, Woll, and Arango, 1993).

Communicating with families. Families whose child is ill react along what health care providers may view as a continuum from the "good" to the "difficult" family stereotype. Nurses readily form relationships with the "good" family, who perceives staff as having power or control and accepts this hierarchy (Satariano and Briggs, 1989). However, this is often not the case with the "difficult" family, who is characterized as being underinvolved or overinvolved in the child's care. Dixon (1993) describes four patterns of involvement in parents' relationships with nurses. *Silent in care* parents choose to have limited involvement with the hospitalized child and nursing staff. These parents do not initiate relationships with nurses and are difficult to engage in decision making. *Recipients of care* believe nurses both know what is best for the child and should be in control. Their level of trust in professionals is very high, whereas their level of need for information is low. Parents who are *monitors of care* keep track of the performance of all hospital staff, seek care from nurses, and request detailed information. Finally, *managers of care* are in control of health-related decisions and use nurses for direct care and consultation. They are frequently involved in providing technologically complex care to their chronically ill child. Nurses should respect families' varying styles of interacting with health care providers and can base strategies for working with families on understanding a family's style (Table 38-1).

Care conferences, especially multidisciplinary meetings that include the family and key health professionals, provide an opportunity for joint sharing of ideas and expression of feelings or concerns. Individual discussions, especially with the case manager, primary nurse, or clinical nurse specialist (advanced nurse practitioner), help establish a consistent and flexible plan of care that can prevent conflicts or deal with them before they become major issues. In family-centered care, the goal is to maintain the integrity of the family, empower family members to assume a leadership role, and support the family during stressful times (Baker, 1994).

Issues of culture, ethnicity, and race affect access to services, use, and follow-through with referrals and recommendations (Newacheck, Stoddard, and McManus, 1993; Huber, Holditch-Davis, and Brandon, 1993). For some ethnic and minority populations, cultural understandings of illness and disability, the structure of family life, social roles for individuals who are disabled, and other factors related to the perception of children may differ from "mainstream" American culture (Groce and Zola, 1993). These factors may affect family needs and family choices regarding the care of their child with special needs. Nurses play an important role in explaining the health care system to the family. Nurses should also listen to the family's understanding, needs, and concerns, and should assist the family in incorporating their cultural preferences and priorities into the plan of care.

Normalization

Another principle that is increasingly used is that of **normalization,** which refers to establishing a normal pattern of living (see the Guidelines box on p. 1140). By applying the prin-

TABLE 38-1 Strategies for managing parent-nurse interaction

PARENT CHARACTERISTICS	STRATEGIES
Silent in care	
Have trust and mistrust	Do not force participation
May not accompany child; prefer to wait outside	Avoid authoritarian stance
Are very uncertain, quiet	Use simple terms and demystify surroundings
Use little verbal communication	Explain what will happen
Visit on limited or irregular basis	Point out how their presence helps child
Recipient of care	
Have total trust	Offer/provide information; elicit feedback to ensure their understanding
Want nurse to make decisions	Allow unlimited contact with child
Offer numerous positive comments	Engage them in gaining child's cooperation
Are easily impressed with information	
Are prone to misunderstandings	
Comply with rules	
Focus on child while visiting	
Monitor of care	
Have high levels of mistrust	Believe that you can build trust
Have attitude that "mistakes can happen"	Negotiate, negotiate, negotiate!
Monitor everyone's performance	Be flexible regarding rules
Involved in all decisions	Avoid issues of control
Want high levels of information	Ask their opinion and use their suggestions
Know agency's hierarchy	
Seek care from nurses	
Ask for rule changes	
Manager of care	
Are similar to monitors, but less angry	Recognize them as experts about their child
Achieve complex coordination of child's chronic care	Recognize need for respite

Developed by Donna M. Dixon, Memorial Medical Center, Springfield, Ill, 1993. Used with permission. Modified from Knafl KA, Cavallari KA, Dixon DM: *Pediatric hospitalization: family and nurse perspectives,* Glenview, Ill, 1988, Scott, Foresman.

ciples of normalization, the environment for the child is "normalized" and "humanized." Normalization principles can be applied to service delivery, as well as to patterns of daily care for the child. Another trend is the earlier discharge of children from acute or chronic care facilities to the family and community. *Home care* represents the return to a system and set of priorities in which family values are as important to the care of a child with a chronic health problem as they are in the care of other children. Home care seeks to achieve goals that are consistent with the developmental model (Stein, 1985):

1. Normalize the life of a child with special needs, including those with technologically complex care, in a family and community context and setting.
2. Minimize the disruptive impact of the child's condition on the family.
3. Foster the child's maximum growth and development.

With appropriate training and support, families provide complex procedures and treatments in the home. Parents are challenged to retain a homelike setting among monitors, ventilators, and other sophisticated equipment. Throughout the text home care is discussed as appropriate for specific conditions. The process of transition from hospital to home is elaborated in Chapter 40.

Paralleling normalization and home care is a trend toward **mainstreaming,** or integrating children with special needs into regular classrooms. Just as the home is the natural environment for children, so school must also be included as an essential component of the children's overall physical, intellectual, and social development. Children who attend school have the advantages of learning and socializing with a wide group of peers. There is an increased focus on individualization as the academic needs of these children are planned along with those of the rest of the students. A variety of supplemental programs have been designed in the school system to accommodate special needs, both at school age and younger, through early intervention programs, thus providing these children with an equal educational opportunity. This change and increasing opportunities for normalization for children with special needs have in great part resulted from the passage of Public Law 94-142 (the Education of All Handicapped Children Act of 1975), its 1990 amendments (PL 101-476), which changed the name of the act to the Individuals with Disabilities Education Act (IDEA), Public Law 99-457 (the Education of the Handicapped Act Amendments of 1986), and the Americans with Disabilities Act (ADA) of 1990 (see also Chapter 27). Nurses can provide parents with information about those laws* and in some cases may participate in the development of Individualized Educational Programs (IEPs) or Individualized Family Service Plans (IFSPs) for children with special needs.†

The Family of the Child with Special Needs

REACTIONS OF FAMILIES TO A CHRONIC ILLNESS OR DISABILITY

When the diagnosis of a disability or chronic illness is made, the family progresses through a fairly predictable sequence of

*The *NICHCY New Digest,* vol. 1, No. 1, 1991, was entirely devoted to the topic "The Education of Children and Youth with Special Needs: What do the Laws Say?" (NICHCY, P.O. Box 1492, Washington, DC 20013).

†The following resource is recommended for developing an IFSP: Johnson B, McGonigel M, and Kaufmann R: *Guidelines and recommended practices for the individualized family service plan,* available from the **Association for the Care of Children's Health,** 7910 Woodmount Ave., Suite 300, Bethesda, MD 20814; (301) 654-6549.

stages, regardless of the actual nature of the condition. Although a number of "stages" have been described, no one set of phases is universally accepted. Not all families experience this process, and each family member varies widely in the time needed to progress through any of the stages and the need to use earlier stages.

The nurse explores family reactions for all possible interpretations, not just negative ones. Too often a parent's angry reaction is attributed to a stage of adjustment or a maladaptive reaction, rather than an appropriate response to, for instance, an insulting remark.

Shock and Denial

The initial stage, or impact, is intensely emotional and is characterized by *shock, disbelief,* and sometimes *denial,* especially if the disorder is not obvious, such as in chronic illness. Denial is probably the least understood and most poorly dealt with reaction. Health professionals tend to label denial as "maladaptive" and may actively attempt to remove it by repeated and sometimes blunt explanations of prognosis. However, denial is often an adaptive approach.

It is a necessary cushion to prevent disintegration and is a normal response to any type of loss. Probably all family members experience various degrees of adaptive denial as they learn of the impact that the diagnosis has on their lives. Denial becomes maladaptive when it prevents recognition of treatment or rehabilitative goals necessary for the child's optimum survival or development.

Shock and denial can last from days to months, sometimes even longer. Examples of denial that may be exhibited at the time of diagnosis include the following: (1) shopping for physicians; (2) attributing the symptoms of the actual illness to a minor condition; (3) refusing to believe the diagnostic tests; (4) delaying agreement to treatment; (5) acting very happy and optimistic, despite the revealed diagnosis; (6) refusing to tell or talk to anyone about the condition; (7) insisting that no one is telling the truth, regardless of others' attempts to do so; (8) denying the reason for admission; and (9) asking no questions about the diagnosis, treatment, or prognosis. Each of these mechanisms allows individuals to distance themselves from the onslaught of a tremendous emotional impact and to collect and mobilize their energies toward goal-directed, problem-solving behaviors.

In some instances, various indicators of denial can be viewed as adaptive. Searching for another professional opinion may mean that parents cannot obtain answers to their questions or that they are looking for a different approach to treatment that better meets the needs of their child and family. When parents discuss their strengths and the benefits they derive from caring for their child with special needs, it does not necessarily reflect refusal to accept their difficult circumstances. Sometimes delay in making decisions or failure to ask questions simply reflects a lack of information.

Partial denial, such as seeking additional professional consultations or occasionally acting as if nothing were wrong, is common for families with children who have life-threatening conditions. Without such a temporary protective mechanism, few people could survive the constant emotional drain of anticipating their own death or the death of a family member. Partial denial allows the child and family to absorb stressful information in amounts they can personally manage at the time.

The importance of children's denial has repeatedly been demonstrated as a factor in their positive coping with the diagnosis. Denial allows an individual to maintain hope in the face of overwhelming odds. Like hope, denial may be an adaptive mechanism for dealing with loss that persists until a family or patient is ready for or needs other responses.

Adjustment

Adjustment gradually follows shock and is usually characterized by an open admission that the condition exists. This stage is manifested by several responses, probably the most universal of which are *guilt* and *anger.* Guilt arises from a human need to find rational causes for events. The concept of cause and effect implies an ability to change future events. It is often greatest when the cause of the disorder is directly traceable to the parent, such as in genetic diseases or from an injury. However, it occurs even without any scientific or realistic basis for parental responsibility. Frequently the guilt stems from a false assumption that the disability is a result of personal failing or wrongdoing, such as drinking alcohol, taking drugs, smoking, not eating correctly, having sex or an affair, or not doing something correctly during pregnancy or the birth. Guilt may also be related to thoughts of wishing the child dead, especially when the demands of care seem overwhelming and unrelenting, and may be associated with religious beliefs, either as a punishment or as a test of faith. Children, too, may interpret their serious illness as retribution for past misbehavior.

Nursing ALERT

Be particularly sensitive to the child who passively accepts all painful procedures. This child may believe that such acts are inflicted as deserved punishment. It is always vital to assure children that what happens to them during diagnosis or treatment is to make them well.

Another common reaction in family members is *anger.* Anger directed inwardly may be evident as self-reproaching or punitive behavior, such as neglecting one's health and verbally degrading oneself. Anger directed outwardly may be manifest in open arguments or withdrawal from communication and may be evident in the person's relationship with any number of individuals such as the spouse, the child, and siblings. Passive anger toward the ill child may be evident in decreased visiting, refusal to believe how sick the child is, or inability to provide comfort. One of the most common targets for parental anger is a staff member.

The child who is sick or disabled and the well siblings are also apt to respond with anger. Affected children are aware of the loss engendered by the illness or disability and may react angrily to the imposed restrictions or the feelings of being different. Siblings also feel anger and resentment toward the ill child and parents for the loss of routine and for decreased parental attention. It is difficult for older children and almost impossible for younger children to comprehend the plight of the affected child. Their perception is of a brother or sister who has the undivided attention of their parents, receives cards and gifts, and is the focus of everyone's concern.

A number of other reactions among family members, especially parents, are typical and include:

Lowered self-esteem, in which parents perceive a defect in their child as a defect in themselves; their life goals may be abruptly and dramatically altered, and they lose the fantasy of immortality through their child

Shame, in which family members anticipate social rejection, pity, or ridicule and related loss of social prestige; may experience social withdrawal

Ambivalence, in which the simultaneous experience of love and hatred normally experienced by parents toward their children is likely to be greatly intensified

Depression, in which parents experience chronic feelings of sorrow; for example, to some parents mental retardation symbolizes the child's death and therefore precipitates a grief reaction.

During the period of adjustment, four types of parental reactions to the child may occur that influence the child's eventual response to the disorder (Box 38-2). The most common initial response, especially among mothers, is **benevolent overreaction.** This is usually a consequence of unresolved guilt or fear, such as ambivalent feelings or not wanting the child during pregnancy, reactivated feelings about a previous death of a loved one, feeling responsible for the disorder, or believing that the child would die at the time of birth or diagnosis. The benevolent overreaction results in a vicious cycle of overprotective, permissive parent and dependent, demanding child. Without early intervention and anticipatory guidance, this pattern might prevent the child from developing self-control, independence, initiative, and self-esteem.

Reintegration and Acknowledgment

For many families a final stage in adjustment is characterized by realistic expectations for the child and reintegration of family life, with the illness or disability in proper perspective. Since a large portion of the adjustment phase is one of grief for a loss, total resolution is not possible until the child dies or leaves home as an independent adult.

This adjustment phase also involves social reintegration, in which the family broadens its activities to include relationships outside of the home, with the child as an acceptable and participating member of the group. This last criterion often differentiates gradual acceptance during the adjustment period from total acceptance or acknowledgment.

Many parents of children with special needs experience **chronic sorrow,** an emotional response that is manifested through the life span of the parent-child interaction (Clubb, 1991). Acceptance is interspersed with periods of intensified sorrow for the loss, especially at certain landmarks of the child's development (e.g., entry into school, the onset of puberty), since each new age traditionally brings new expectations and a reminder of what could have been. Situational stress, such as inability to pay the child's medical bills, may also cause grief to resurface. Consequently, even families who have achieved a high level of adjustment and acceptance are, at predictable times (Box 38-3), in need of support from professionals or other families who have coped successfully with similar experiences.

IMPACT OF CHILD'S CHRONIC ILLNESS OR DISABILITY ON FAMILY MEMBERS

Parents

Besides grieving for the loss of a perfect child, parents may or may not receive positive feedback from transactions with their child. Many parents feel satisfaction and fulfillment from the parenting role. For others, parenting may be a series of unrewarding experiences, which contribute to parental feelings of inadequacy and failure. These responses may be most evident in parents who are responsible for the child's care. For example, parents may become preoccupied with their ability to carry out certain procedures, overlooking the child's personal comfort and satisfaction or failing to offer praise for anything less than perfect cooperation or performance. They may pursue a frustrating activity until they achieve "success"—long after the child has become irritable and uncooperative. As a result, parents can become caught in a pattern of interaction that is mutually unrewarding and minimally productive. For these parents several strategies may be helpful: education regarding what can reasonably be expected of their child, assistance in identifying the child's strengths, praise for a parental job well done, and finding respite care so that the parent can renew his or her own energies.

BOX 38-2
Parental Responses that Influence Child's Response to the Disorder

Overprotection, in which the parents fear letting the child achieve any new skill, avoid all discipline, and cater to the child's every desire so as to prevent frustration

Rejection, in which the parents detach themselves emotionally from the child but usually provide adequate physical care or constantly nag and scold the child

Denial, in which parents act as if the disorder does not exist or attempt to have the child overcompensate for it

Gradual acceptance, in which parents place necessary and realistic restrictions on the child, encourage self-care activities, and promote reasonable physical and social abilities

BOX 38-3
Anticipated Parental Stress Points

Diagnosis of the condition—requires considerable learning, as well as dealing with emotional response

Developmental milestones—times children normally achieve walking, talking, and self-care are delayed or impossible for the child

Start of schooling—particularly stressful are situations in which appropriate schooling will not be in a regular class placement

Reaching the ultimate attainment—situations such as realizing that ambulation will be impossible or that the child will not learn to read must be handled

Adolescence—issues such as sexuality and independence become prominent

Future placement—decisions about placement must be made when the child becomes an adult or when the parents can no longer care for the child

Death of the child

Parental roles. Excessive demands may be placed on parental time, energy, and financial resources. Depending on the roles assumed by each spouse, these responsibilities may be shared or shifted more heavily to one member. In a shared approach, parents often divide tasks in a very specific way, according to their skills or level of comfort. For example, the parent with patience for waiting may be the logical person to take the child for tests, examinations, and procedures. The parent who deals best with the sickness and side effects of treatment can ready the environment for the child's return home. It is important for nurses to realize that the absence of one parent from the hospital or clinic does not necessarily indicate that the shared parent pattern is not in effect (Clements, Copeland, and Loftus, 1990). On the other hand, making efforts to involve both parents in decision making and in learning how to care for the child's special needs can reduce some of the burden of care often placed inadvertently on mothers.

In other families changing sex roles mean added responsibilities for one parent. For example, the working mother may feel the need to continue employment to help defray the expenses, but she also incurs the added burden of additional child/home responsibilities. Marital conflicts can be the result, as one partner views his or her share as unequal.

In addition, the partner who is not included in the caregiving activities may feel neglected, since all the attention is directed toward the child, and resentful that he or she is not sufficiently informed to be competent in the care. Without active participation in the child's care, the parent has little appreciation of the time and energy involved in performing those activities. When the less prepared partner does attempt to participate, the other parent frequently criticizes the less skillful efforts. As a result, communication and support for one another may suffer.

Although marital stress often increases, divorce rates in these families are not substantially higher than those for the general population. Research suggests that families of children with chronic conditions who adjust poorly are those who had problems before the illness. A couple's marital functioning before the birth or diagnosis of a child with special needs may well be the best predictor of long-term marital adjustment.

The nurse can assist the family in avoiding conflict by providing anticipatory guidance early on. Guidance can address the stressors often cited as having an impact on the marriage: (1) the home care program with the burden of care assumed by primarily one parent, (2) the financial burden, (3) the fear of the child dying, (4) pressure from relatives, (5) the hereditary nature of the disease (if applicable), and (6) fear of pregnancy. Other causes of tension may center on the inconveniences associated with care, such as long waiting for appointments, lack of parking near care facilities, or lack of overnight accommodations. Certainly these last stressors are within health professionals' domain to minimize, if not eliminate.

Mother/father differences. Mothers and fathers in the same family often adjust and cope differently as parents of a child with special needs. Some mothers experience a peaks-and-valleys periodic crisis pattern, whereas most fathers tend to experience a steady, gradual recovery.

The father of a child with special needs struggles with issues that may be quite distinct from those of the mother. He may feel that his role of protector is challenged because he does not know how to help and cannot protect the family from the seemingly overwhelming recurring problems. Dreams of lineage, ego fulfillment, and athletic and vocational achievement are threatened and in turn may threaten the father's self-esteem. Because the traditional paternal role, particularly with sons, emphasizes joint reaction over caregiving, fathers seem to have more difficulty adjusting to a son with special needs than to a daughter with special needs. With today's increased emphasis on fathers' involvement in the lives of their children, this loss is felt more profoundly than in the past. The extensive stresses in the family can leave the father feeling depressed, weak, guilty, powerless, isolated, embarrassed, and very angry. Yet, fearful that he will lose control or be viewed as weak or ineffectual, the father will often hide his feelings and display an outward confidence that may lead others to believe that everything is fine. Feelings are further exacerbated by a health care system that frequently excludes and disregards men. Too often the father feels like an afterthought in the care of his child (May, 1990).

Fathers worry about what the future holds for their children, as well as about their ability to manage the increasing financial burden. Some fathers escape in their work as a means for dulling the pain. Others view all of the difficulties of having a child with special needs as challenges to overcome and are not afraid to push limits and be assertive to acquire the needed services for their children (May, 1990).

Single-parent families. Single-parent families are of special concern. The absence of a parent may be due to divorce or death, or the parents may never have married. As the only parent of a child who may require extensive, sophisticated, and lifelong care, the single parent may feel an enormous burden. Available financial and emotional resources may already be stretched to the limit. Nurses must recognize that external sources of support and personal inner strength are particularly crucial for single parents to enable them to care for their child (Clements, Copeland, and Loftus, 1990). A special effort should be made to assist the single parent in finding financial and support services that can ease the burden of care. Nurses can also assist the single parent in identifying helping roles that may be acceptable to relatives and friends.

Siblings

Results of studies on how siblings are affected by having a brother or sister with special needs are inconsistent. Some confirm that brothers and sisters of children with chronic or disabling conditions are at high risk for maladjustment; others report no significant differences between siblings of children with special needs and siblings of children without chronic or disabling conditions; and still others note the absence of effects (Gallo et al, 1992). However, most investigators do agree that brothers and sisters of children with special needs are no more at risk for *severe* psychiatric problems than are siblings of children without chronic or disabling conditions.

Some difficulties for siblings arise from the demands of the child's condition. For example, at diagnosis the child with special needs by necessity becomes the focus of parental attention and concern. Frequent hospitalizations or trips to the physician or clinic disrupt the family routine. Siblings are pushed to the background, often staying at the homes of family and friends. The child's condition may interfere with holiday celebrations, vacations, and other special events. Siblings may resent these intrusions, which frequently demand self-sacrifice. Their parents may be unable to attend their school functions, ball games, or other activities, and at times may be physically and emotionally unavailable for them. The family's financial and emotional resources may be directed toward the child with special needs.

Many of the difficulties siblings encounter are a result of the nature of the sibling relationship itself (see Chapter 30). It is within the sibling relationship that children learn to share, compete, and compromise with others close to them in status. The equality of this relationship is often lost when a brother or sister has special needs. The child with special needs is suddenly "out of tune," unable to contribute to the family or the sibling relationship in his or her usual way. Because identification is another characteristic of sibling relationships, some siblings believe that they, too, will "catch" the condition, a reasonable assumption considering experiences with contagious diseases, such as chickenpox. Identification, combined with a young child's egocentric thinking, may lead a sibling to feel responsible for a brother or sister's condition.

Most brothers and sisters experience mixed and sometimes contradictory feelings. They may feel left out of new family developments and changing roles, guilty that they escaped getting the condition, or sad when their brother or sister is unable to participate in a particular activity or event. Some siblings feel embarrassed and ashamed; having a child in the family who is ill, disfigured, or disabled marks the family as "different." Siblings may actually experience a **courtesy stigma**—a spoiled identity because of a close relationship with someone who is devalued and avoided because he or she is different. These painful feelings may lead to isolation and loneliness.

When parents give the child with special needs preferential treatment, siblings may feel resentful and jealous—feelings that are often distorted by their own sense of loss and concern. Older siblings in particular may resent stepping in as surrogate parents for their younger brothers and sisters. Siblings may be angry at parents for being unable to protect their brother or sister from getting the condition or at insensitive friends and classmates. Some siblings must also deal with anger from the child with special needs who resents them for escaping the experience.

Some siblings develop adjustment or behavior problems, especially younger male or older female siblings. Younger children having difficulty tend to become withdrawn and irritable, whereas older siblings tend to act out. Some typical problems include bed-wetting, headaches, and other physical complaints; changes in school performance; school phobia; sleep problems; proneness to injury; depression; and severe separation anxiety.

Often overlooked is the positive caring between children with special needs and their brothers and sisters. Siblings can experience pride and satisfaction in their own contributions to the family, joy and excitement in their brother or sister's accomplishments, and genuine love. Parents may report an increased closeness among the siblings or an increase in their home responsibilities (Ferrell et al, 1994). Ultimately, most brothers and sisters seem to adapt well, and many demonstrate high levels of self-confidence, independence, maturity, altruism, and tolerance.

BOX 38-4
Anticipated Sibling Stress Points

Birth of another child—may be the sibling with special needs or the subsequent birth of another child
Diagnosis of condition—in certain illnesses times of remission and exacerbations are difficult
When the child is hospitalized—parental time and attention are focused on the child with special needs
Start of schooling—particularly stressful if friends reject the child with special needs
Adolescence—when dating begins, may be embarrassed to bring dates home
Future placement—may worry about responsibility for the sibling with special needs, especially if the parents are ill or die
Death of the child

Certain factors (e.g., family size, age between children) seem to influence sibling adjustment. However, the most important factors appear to be parental feelings, perceptions, and reactions. Siblings are more at risk for adjustment problems when parents are unaccepting of the child with special needs. Also, certain times seem to be more difficult for siblings (Box 38-4).

How siblings react will have an important impact on the child's overall adjustment. When siblings act in a normal fashion, a secure, stable training ground is provided for social relationships for the child with special needs.

Extended Family Members and Society

Two other groups of people may experience the effects of a child's chronic illness or disability: (1) significant nonnuclear family members or friends, and (2) society as a whole. Although extended family relationships are often helpful to parents in rearing a child with special needs, they may also be sources of stress. For example, grandparents or other well-meaning relatives may have more difficulty accepting the diagnosis than the parents themselves do. They may attempt to reassure the parents that the child "will grow out of" his or her slowness at a time when parents are struggling to accept reality.

Most grandparents experience some ambivalence: they love their grandchild and yet feel personal disappointment. They often experience a double grief, both for their grandchild and for their child, the parent. The future is now unpredictable not only for the grandchild, but also for the child's parents. Grandparents do not often acknowledge these emotions and are left to adapt on their own. Support groups for grandparents are uncommon, but they can be beneficial (Burns and Madian, 1992).

Although society's views of individuals with chronic illness or disability are changing toward a more accepting, nonjudgmental, and open attitude, parents, siblings, and the child with special needs frequently are victims of prejudice, ostracism, or criticism. A great deal of this stems from public ignorance and fear, and this remains a crucial area for intervention by health professionals. Other areas in which society could better meet the needs of families of children with chronic illness or disability include the development of support services such as respite care, financing care, and insurance practices that do not discriminate against individuals with chronic illness.

FACTORS AFFECTING THE FAMILY'S ADJUSTMENT

Although it is easy to assume that families of children with the most severe illnesses or disabilities would have the poorest adjustment, the severity of the condition reflects only one part of the overall picture. The family's ability to adjust to having a child with special needs is influenced by factors such as their available support system, perception of the event, coping mechanisms, reactions to the child, available resources, and concurrent stresses within the family (Table 38-3).

A family's level of adjustment is significantly influenced by the functional burden on the individual family (Stein, 1985). This concept considers the issues related to caring for and living with the child in relation to the family's resources and ability to cope. Thus the family of a child who has multiple disabilities and demands complex care (but who has many resources and coping skills) may adjust more successfully to their situation than the family of a child with a less serious condition and fewer resources.

The significant others who are available to individuals for emotional strength during periods of crisis comprise their *support system*. Support systems may be available through a variety of relationships and may consist of one significant other such as a spouse or a group of significant others such as the extended family or the health team.

The source of support is a determining factor in the effectiveness of certain forms of support. For example, expressive support is best provided by individuals with whom one has strong ties and who are like oneself. On the other hand, instrumental support can often be provided by those to whom the family has weaker ties and who can link the family to a broader, more diverse social network. Therefore the most appropriate sources of informational support might include both professionals who have theoretic and practical knowledge and nonprofessionals—parents—whose experience equips them as experts. Parent-to-parent support, in fact, is unique and unobtainable from any other source.* When professionals develop a strong therapeutic relationship with the family, they, too, can be appropriate sources of emotional support (see discussion on therapeutic relationships in Chapter 27).

Although a support system exists, it may not be effective unless the individual is able to use the system through mutual channels of communication. Providing parents with written information they can share with extended family can often help them in reaching out to others during a difficult time.

When necessary, nurses can assist family members to recognize their strengths and use their adaptive *coping mechanisms*—which may include information seeking, using social support networks, drawing on personal strengths or relying on their faith life—in adjusting to and managing chronic illness, disability, or life-threatening illness in a child. At times, nurses can assist family members in developing new coping mechanisms.

REACTIONS OF FAMILIES TO CHILDHOOD DEATH: THE GRIEF PROCESS

No event is more devastating for families than the threatened or actual loss of a child. Families, especially parents, are deprived of the joy and fulfillment of watching a child grow. All family members are affected by the loss, and their needs must be recognized to resolve their grief. Nurses require a basic understanding of the grief process before (if the death is anticipated), at the time of, and after the death to provide guidance and emotional support to the survivors.

In response to any loss there is a grief reaction. **Anticipatory grief** may precede an anticipated death. **Acute grief** develops within hours to days after a death and is characterized by somatic symptoms and intense subjective distress. *Grief work*, or **mourning,** refers to the lengthy process that begins with acute grief and extends into a period of reorganization of psychologic life, with attachment to new people and interests. **Bereavement** often refers to the period of mourning, although grief, mourning, and bereavement are used interchangeably.

In expected death the child and family are generally involved in the plan for intervention both before and after the death. In unexpected death the survivors face the tremendous task of integrating the loss into their lives, with no opportunity for anticipatory grief. In either situation nurses can facilitate the grief process by being aware of expected psychologic and somatic reactions and by dialoguing with family members, ascertaining their needs, and supporting their efforts to cope, adapt, and grieve. The application of principles of family-centered care is as important at this time as any other.

Anticipatory Grief

When death is the expected or possible outcome of a disorder, the child and family members experience behavioral reactions of anticipatory grief. Anticipatory grief may be manifest in varying behaviors and intensities and may include denial, anger, depression and other psychologic and somatic symptoms.

The "stages" of dying described by Kübler-Ross (1969) are not included here, because they were not based on work with children. The importance of the work of Kübler-Ross to the care of children and families lies in its emphasis on recognizing the dying person as being alive and dying itself as a process in which the dying person is engaged. Care providers are most effective when actively engaging those coping with death and empowering them to address their remaining needs (Corr, 1993).

Acute Grief

When death occurs, whether it is expected or unexpected, acute grief develops within hours to days. Acute grief is a definite syndrome with psychologic and somatic symptoms that cause intense distress (Box 38-5). Reactions such as hearing the dead person's voice, feeling distant from others who want to help, or feeling overwhelming guilt for failing to prevent the

*The *Parent Resource Directory* lists over 400 parents of children with chronic illness or disabilities in the United States and Canada, including addresses, phone numbers, the child's condition, and the health facility where the child receives care. It is available from the **Association for the Care of Children's Health,** 7910 Woodmont Ave., Suite 300, Bethesda, MD 20814; (301) 654-6549. Information about self-help groups, as well as books and pamphlets, is available from the **National Self-Help Clearinghouse,** CUNY Graduate Center, 25 W. 43rd St., New York, NY 10036; (212) 642-2944.

BOX 38-5
Characteristics of Normal Grief Reaction

Sensations of somatic distress
Feeling of tightness in the throat
Choking, with shortness of breath
Marked tendency toward sighing
Empty feeling in abdomen
Lack of muscular power
Intense subjective distress described as tension or mental pain

Preoccupation with image of the deceased
Hears, sees, or imagines that the dead person is present
Slight sense of unreality
Feeling of emotional distance from others
Feeling of approaching insanity

Feelings of guilt
Searches for evidence of failure in preventing the death
Accuses self of negligence or exaggerates minor omissions

Feelings of hostility
Loss of warmth toward others
Tendency toward irritability and anger
Wish not to be bothered by friends or relatives

Loss of usual pattern of conduct
Restlessness, inability to sit still, aimless moving about
Continual searching for something to do or thinking about what should be done
Lack of capacity to initiate and maintain organized patterns of activity

Modified from the landmark publication by Lindemann E: Symptomatology and management of acute grief, *Am J Psychiatry* 101:141-143, 1944.

death may make grieving persons fear that they are approaching a mental breakdown. On the contrary, these symptoms are normal, necessary, and expected responses. They signify that survivors are working through the acute grief and will probably satisfactorily resolve the loss and resume or restructure a meaningful role in their social environment.

Although grief symptoms should appear immediately after a crisis, they may be delayed, exaggerated, or apparently absent. In the place of normal grief responses, *distorted reactions* such as excessive hostility, depression with signs of suicide, or overactivity without a sense of loss, may occur. Such distorted reactions can be transformed into normal grief with appropriate intervention, such as by a grief counselor. Nurses working with grieving families should be aware of the symptomatology of normal grief (Box 38-5) to recognize the rare occurrence of morbid grief reactions.

Mourning

After the death the lengthy process of grief work or mourning begins and extends into a period of adjustment to the loss, with attachment to new people and the development of new interests. Contrary to the common belief that mourning is completed in a year, research indicates that resolution of grief may take years and that there may be an *intensification* of grief during the early years.

Shock and disbelief. Shock, numbness, and disbelief are seen during the immediate phase of grief. As one parent described, "We were as prepared for our son's death as anyone could be, but it was a shock when in a moment his life was finished. I just can't get over the rapidity with which life ends." This temporary numbness protects the survivors from the overwhelming pain associated with grief. Often decisions are made automatically, and only certain details are remembered.

Expression of grief. When the numbness fades, there begins a period of intense grief characterized by a yearning and loneliness for the deceased. During this stage many of the signs of acute grief are evident, and physical complaints such as inability to sleep and appetite changes are common. There is a tendency to review the events of the deceased's life and to evaluate the relationship with the loved one. At this time feelings of guilt and anger are common.

Disorganization and despair. During this stage the pain of the loss is replaced primarily by emptiness, apathy, and deep depression. There is a feeling that life has no meaning and that the pain will never end. This is particularly relevant for parents. For example, mothers often comment that they feel they have suffered a double loss—loss of their child and loss of the mothering role. Feelings of estrangement from other loved ones are common, and social isolation may foster the depression.

Reorganization. Reorganization refers to recovery from the loss. During this very gradual process the survivors again find meaning in living, readjust to life without the deceased, develop new or renewed relationships, and learn to live with the memory of the deceased with much less pain. It never means that the loved one is forgotten and the pain is gone. There always remains a deep ache that is never totally replaced with happiness and one that returns more intensely, for example, on holidays or anniversaries (see Post death, p. 1151).

The Child With Special Needs

IMPACT OF CHRONIC ILLNESS OR DISABILITY ON THE CHILD

The child's reaction to chronic illness or disability depends to a great extent on his or her developmental level, temperament, and available coping mechanisms; on the reactions of family members or significant others; and to a lesser extent on the condition itself. A child's conceptual understanding of his or her own illness is based in part on age and developmental level, but also on the duration and type of experience accumulated with the disease (Yoos, 1994). Knowledge of these variables is essential in providing the kind of information and support needed by these children to cope with a sometimes overwhelming situation.

Developmental Aspects

The impact of a chronic illness or disability is influenced by the age at onset. Chronic illness affects children of all ages, but the developmental aspects of each age group dictate particular stresses and risks for the child. The nurse must also recognize that children need to redefine their condition and its implications as they develop and grow. Children's developmental concepts of illness are discussed in Chapter 41. An understanding of these developmental factors facilitates planning care to support the child and minimize the risks.

Infancy. During infancy the child is engaged in the task of developing trust, which necessitates a reciprocal satisfying relationship between the child and parent. When illness or disability occurs, this relationship is potentially affected. For example, a visible defect can retard parent bonding as the parent mourns the loss of the perfect child. In addition, prolonged illness may impose separations that prevent the child and parent from normal attachment and deprive the infant of the nurturing relationship.

The illness itself affects the infant, especially since sensorimotor experiences are critical at this age. Illness and/or disability often impairs the child's motor abilities by confining the child to a crib and lessening contact with the environment. Certainly, the messages transmitted to infants about their bodies are influenced by the amount of pain and discomfort they experience. Associating touch with pain can compromise the infant's ability to give and receive affection. Lack of pleasurable sensations can lead to an irritable and unhappy child. Consequently, parents may interpret the behaviors as evidence that they are not adequately meeting the child's physical and emotional needs, which further affects the parent-child relationship and the acquisition of trust.

Nursing intervention can be important in helping parents work with the irritable child in a way that encourages understanding and caring. Nurses should advocate for policies and practices that will best meet the needs of the infant and family, such as 24-hour visitation in the neonatal intensive care unit and other infant units.

Toddler. The toddler is in the stage of autonomy; the need for mastery of locomotor and language skills is paramount. The child learning to walk and talk progresses toward becoming a separate person, both physically and psychologically. However, illness or disability can hinder mobility and deprive the child of mastery. In addition, overprotective parents can magnify the problem by setting limits on the child's exploration and experimentation for fear of injury or exertion. Even the most basic self-help skills, such as feeding and dressing, may be done for the child. Age-appropriate tasks such as toilet training may be delayed. With such limited opportunities for testing mastery, children soon fear to venture on their own and develop little confidence in their abilities. Over time they may feel defeated and become apathetic, passive, and clinging.

Illness can impose separations that are detrimental to the toddler. Like the infant, separation is the most anxiety-producing event. If the need to preserve the parent-child relationship is not appreciated, the child may become depressed and eventually detach from the parent. Children seem to have a tremendous capacity to withstand stress, provided their attachment to the parent is preserved.

Preschooler. The preschooler is in the stage of initiative; numerous tasks are achieved during this age that can be severely hampered by chronic illness and disability. Impairment can limit the preschooler's learning about the environment, especially in terms of social development. Rather than being encouraged to play with peers and participate in nursery school activities, the preschooler may be confined to the home, where socialization is limited to the secure and tolerant family. Immature behavior may be tolerated because age-appropriate standards and discipline are not enforced. Consequently, when paired with children the same age or placed in school, the child may not know how to act and can easily be criticized by peers and viewed as a "baby." The illness or disability may provoke much less criticism than his or her inappropriate behavior. Faced with such reactions from others, in contrast to the security of the home, the child may gradually choose a life of social isolation and loneliness, especially during the school-age years.

One of the major tasks of this period is establishing sexual identity, and one of the principal methods is through imitation of sex-related activities. However, the sick child may have fewer opportunities to engage in such activity and may view the parent predominantly in the caregiving role, since this may be the focus of their relationship. Some families expect the mother to assume the care of the child while the father provides the financial base by working outside the home. This can limit the child's identification with the male role.

In addition to sexual identity, the child's body image is forming. Children's knowledge of their bodies is limited to what they see, feel, and use. If the child is chronically ill, body awareness is focused on the personal pain and anxiety it causes. The young child may lose control over newly acquired bowel and bladder function and feel embarrassed and inferior. The child with a disability may have difficulty forming a mental image of impaired body parts such as paralyzed extremities. This poorly developed sense of body integrity makes children especially fearful of intrusive or mutilating experiences, which can be frequent during prolonged illness.

One of the more critical influences of chronic illness or disability on preschoolers is the feeling of guilt that they "caused" the condition by a real or imagined misdeed. This is probably less a factor if the child is born with the disorder than if it occurs during the preschool years. Such guilt can greatly affect the child's developing but fragile self-esteem. Unless situations are structured for success, life can become a series of failures—of never being strong enough or good enough to compete with peers.

School-age child. The child of school age is striving to achieve a sense of accomplishment while overcoming a sense of inferiority. Successful mastery of this task depends on the child's ability to cooperate and compete with others. Consequently, physical impairments can greatly affect the ability to achieve and compete. For example, physical disability may hinder participation in sports, and repeated absences from school caused by illness can place the child at an academic disadvantage.

During this age there is a transition from relationships with family members to strong identification with peers. Peers increasingly influence school-age children's views of themselves and their self-esteem. Anything that labels children as "different" can affect their sense of belonging to the group. Many children cope with their "differentness" by retreating from socialization. However, if they are helped to deal with their feelings of being different and to recognize their unique abilities, these children can cope very well. Nurses can help families promote social competence in their children by addressing feelings of inadequacy and assisting children to recognize their unique abilities (Breitmayer et al, 1992). Specific training in social skills may be useful (Turner-Henson et al, 1994; Hills and Lutkenhoff, 1993). Naturally, all children will be unable to master some tasks and will feel some degree of inferiority. If this is stressed to children with physical impairment, the burden to achieve is lessened.

As school-age children identify more with the peer group and authority figures outside the home, there is a concurrent striving for independence from the family. However, the ill child may be forced into an extended period of dependency either from the disorder or from parental overprotectiveness. Attempts to demonstrate independence may be manifested as resentment toward the parents, refusal to comply with treatment, or risk-taking behavior, such as cheating on the special diet. If parents can understand that these behaviors represent a normal phase of development, they may be more tolerant and able to find appropriate outlets for independence (e.g., increasing the child's responsibility for home care or increasing the child's control in nondisease-related activities).

Adolescence. The impact of illness or disability can be most detrimental during adolescence. The major task of the adolescent is to establish a personal identity. Pubertal changes must be integrated into the self-image while the teenager is gaining control and mastery over increased physical capabilities and sexuality. During early adolescence this takes place primarily within the peer group. Illness or injury at this time interferes with teenagers' sense of mastery and control over a changing body. They are different at a stage of development when being different is unacceptable to the peer group, who may view a disability in one member as a threat to the established uniformity by which all are measured. At no time of life is an individual so vulnerable to the emotional stress of biologic impairment. In fact, adolescents with physical differences tend to blame most of their problems on the fact that they have something wrong with them. Appearance, skills, and abilities are highly valued by peers (Fig. 38-1); a teenager who is limited in any of these qualities is subject to rejection. This is especially marked when a physical disability interferes with sexual attractiveness.

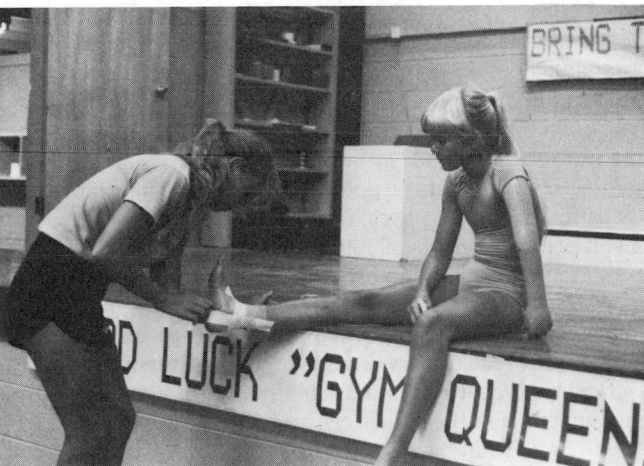

Fig. 38-1 Children with any type of impairment should have the opportunity to develop their skills. Despite her prosthetic left arm, this youngster excels in competitive sports.

Teenagers with special needs are faced with the task of incorporating their disabilities into the changing self-concept. The youngster who develops the illness or acquires the disability during the crucial adolescent years has more difficulty accomplishing this task than has the teenager who has been affected since childhood. It appears that the earlier the onset of a limiting condition, the better the individual is able to adapt to it. The youngster with a newly acquired disorder will have the additional task of grieving for a lost "perfection" while adjusting to the changes taking place as a natural course of events. He or she often feels rejected because of personal appearance or an inability to engage in activities expected of a healthy adolescent. The threat is greatest during middle adolescence, when the teenager has less available energy to cope with illness, since emotional resources are being used to meet the normal demands of this developmental phase.

Adolescence is a time for achieving independence from the family and planning for future goals and responsibilities. Adolescents with long-term chronic illness may be less future directed and less independent than well peers. Enforced dependency caused by physical impairment can exacerbate the parent-child conflicts surrounding independence. Lack of understanding from both parties can result in bitter feelings and intrafamilial turmoil. The tendency toward rebellion may be directed at the disorder and reflected in decreased compliance with treatment, denial of the disorder to preserve a sense of normalcy with peers, and risk-taking behavior that can place the teenager in jeopardy such as driving a car despite a disorder that increases the change of an injury. Such behaviors can further strain an already tense parent-child relationship. On the other hand, parents can promote independence by giving the adolescent a greater role in his or her own treatment regimen, encouraging the adolescent to develop a relationship with the health care team that is not mediated by parents, and promoting normalization principles.

Coping Mechanisms

Children's innate and learned coping mechanisms play an important role in their ability to deal with their disorder. Individual characteristics and the social support afforded the child are critically important influences on the child's ability to cope with stress. The better the family copes, the better the child is able to deal with the stressors imposed by the illness or disability. Individual characteristics associated with positive coping are female sex, early infancy and age older than 4 years, active or easy temperament, high self-esteem, above-average intelligence, and strong social skills (Garmezy, 1991).

Children with chronic conditions tend to use five distinct patterns of coping (Box 38-6). Children with more positive and accepting attitudes about their chronic illness use a more adaptive coping style characterized by optimism, competence, and compliance. They show fewer behavior problems at home and at school. The two maladaptive coping patterns—"Feels different and withdraws" and "Is irritable, moody and acts out"—are associated with poorer adaptation; children using these strategies have poorer self-concepts, more negative attitudes about their conditions, and more behavior problems (Austin, Patterson, and Huberty, 1991).

Well-adapted children gradually learn to accept their physical limitations and find achievement in a variety of compensatory motor and intellectual pursuits. They function well at

BOX 38-6

Coping Patterns Used by Children with Special Needs

Develops competence and optimism—accentuates the positive aspects of the situation and concentrates more on what he or she has or can do rather than on what is missing or what he or she cannot do; is as independent as possible

Feels different and withdraws—sees self as being different from other children because of the chronic health condition; views being different as negative; sees self as less worthy than others; focuses on things he or she cannot do, and sometimes overrestricts activities needlessly

Is irritable, moody, and acts out—uses proactive and self-initiated coping behaviors, although usually counterproductive in that the behaviors are not ego enhancing or socially responsible and do not result in desired outcomes; acts out irritability, which may or may not be associated with condition's symptoms

Complies with treatment—takes necessary medications, treatments; adheres to activity restrictions; also uses behaviors that indicate developing independence (e.g., assumes responsibility for taking medication)

Seeks support—talks with adults, children, physicians, and nurses; develops plans to handle problems as they occur; uses downward comparison (i.e., realizes that others have it worse)

Modified from Austin J, Patterson J, Huberty T: Development of the coping health inventory for children, *J Pediatr Nurs* 6(3):166-174, 1991.

home, at school, and with peers. They have an understanding of their disorder that allows them to accept their limitations, assume responsibility for care, and assist in treatment and rehabilitation regimens. They express appropriate emotions such as sadness, anxiety, and anger at times of exacerbations but confidence and guarded optimism during periods of clinical stability. They are able to identify with other similarly affected individuals, promoting positive self-images and displaying pride and self-confidence in their ability to master a productive, successful life despite the disability.

Responses to Parental Behavior

The parents' behavior toward the child, especially in terms of childrearing, is one of the most important influencing factors in the child's adjustment. For example, children whose parents are overprotective tend to have marked dependency (especially on the mother), fearfulness, inactivity, and lack of outside interests. Children who are raised by overly solicitous and guilt-ridden parents are often overly independent, defiant, and risk takers. Children who are reared by parents who emphasize their deficits and tend to "hide" or isolate them appear as shy and lonely individuals who harbor resentful and hostile attitudes toward unaffected persons. In contrast, children who are reared by parents who establish reasonable limits tend to develop age-appropriate independence and achievement commensurate with their limitations. In addition, family organization and illness-related support and involvement of parents influence the child's adjustment to chronic illness (Savinetti-Rose, 1994). They often display pride and confidence in their ability to cope successfully with the challenges imposed by their disorder. Anticipatory guidance by the nurse and encouragement of normalizing practices may assist parents in facilitating positive adjustment in their children.

Type of Illness or Disability

The type of illness or disability also influences the child's emotional response. Interestingly, children with *more severe* disorders often cope better than those with milder conditions. However, the presence of multiple conditions may place a child at risk for more behavioral problems (Newacheck, McManus, and Fox, 1991). Considering children's cognitive ability and their delay in achieving abstract thinking until adolescence, it is likely that an obvious condition is easier to accept because its limitations are concrete. For example, children who are blind or disabled are constantly reminded of their inability to run. However, children with cardiac defects not only live by rules they do not understand, but also only vaguely and occasionally sense their illness, such as when they try to run and experience dyspnea and fatigue. Therefore some chronic illnesses pose special threats to children.

The onset of a disabling condition may generate a state of confusion for children, who may have trouble differentiating between actual body functions and their image of their bodies. They may also experience problems in identifying themselves and those extensions of self (e.g., wheelchairs, braces, crutches, or other mechanical or prosthetic devices) and may have difficulty in accepting functional aids.

IMPACT OF IMPENDING DEATH ON THE CHILD

Children with life-threatening conditions must face the possibility of death, a realization that can have a profound effect on their lives. However, the impact of impending death is greatly influenced by a number of factors, including the child's developmental age, the child's experience with his or her diagnosis, and the role and reaction of the child's parents.

Developmental Concepts of Death

Children's understanding of death parallels their cognitive and psychosocial development. Exactly how preverbal children view death is a mystery, because there is no way of reliably assessing their views of death. It is quite likely, on the basis of their cognitive abilities, that they have no concept of death. Toddler's egocentricity and vague separation of fact and fantasy make it impossible for them to comprehend absence of life.

Children between 3 and 5 years of age usually have heard the word *death*, and they have some idea of its meaning. They see death as a departure, possibly as a kind of sleep. They may recognize the fact of physical death, but they do not see that it involves the loss of the abilities a person has in life. The dead person in the coffin still breathes, eats, and sleeps. Death is temporary and gradual; life and death can change places with one another. Because of their immature concept of time, there is no real understanding of the universality and inevitability of death. Words such as *forever* and *everyone* have meaning only in the child's egocentric thinking.

Much of what pertains to the preschool period regarding the understanding of death also relates to school-age children, particularly those near 6 or 7 years of age. However, these children have a deeper understanding of death in the

TABLE 38-2 Children's understanding of and reactions to death

CONCEPTS OF DEATH	REACTIONS TO DEATH	INTERVENTIONS
Infants and toddlers		
Death has least significance to children under 6 months After parent-child attachment and the development of trust is established, the loss, even temporary, of the significant person is profound Prolonged separation during the first several years is thought to be more significant in terms of future physical, social, and emotional growth than at any subsequent age Toddlers are egocentric and can only think about events in terms of their own frame of reference—living Their egocentricity and vague separation of fact and fantasy make it impossible for them to comprehend absence of life Instead of understanding death, this age group is affected more by any change in life-style	In the death of someone else, they may continue to act as though the person is alive As children grow older, they will be increasingly able and willing to let go of the dead person Ritualism is important; a change in life-style could be anxiety producing This age group reacts more to the pain and discomfort of a serious illness than to the probable fatal prognosis This age group also reacts to parental anxiety and sadness	Help parents deal with their feelings, allowing them more emotional reserve to meet the needs of their children Encourage parents to remain as near to child as possible, yet be sensitive to parents' needs Maintain as normal an environment as possible to retain ritualism If a parent has died, encourage having consistent caregiver for child Promote primary nursing
Preschool children		
Believe their thoughts are sufficient to cause death; the consequence is the burden of guilt, shame, and punishment Their egocentricity implies a tremendous sense of self-power and omnipotence Usually have some connotation of its meaning Seen as a departure, a kind of sleep May recognize the fact of physical death but do not separate it from living abilities Seen as temporary and gradual; life and death can change places with one another No understanding of the universality and inevitability of death	If they become seriously ill, they conceive of the illness as a punishment for their thoughts or actions May feel guilty and responsible for the death of a sibling Greatest fear concerning death is separation from parents May engage in activities that seem strange or abnormal to adults Because of their fewer defense mechanisms to deal with loss, young children may react to a less significant loss with more outward grief than to the loss of a very significant person The loss is so deep, painful, and threatening that the child must deny it for the present in order to survive its overwhelming impact Behavior reactions such as giggling, joking, attracting attention, or regressing to earlier developmental skills indicate children's need to distance themselves from tremendous loss	Help parents deal with their feelings, allowing them more emotional reserve to meet the needs of their children Help parents to understand behavioral reactions of their children Encourage parents to remain near the child as much as possible, to minimize the child's great fear of separation from parents If a parent has died, encourage having a consistent caregiver for child Promote primary nursing
School-age children		
Still associate misdeeds or bad thoughts with causing death and feel intense guilt and responsibility for the event Because of their higher cognitive abilities, they respond well to logical explanations and comprehend the figurative meaning of words Have a deeper understanding of death in a concrete sense Particularly fear the mutilation and punishment they associate with death Personify death as devil, monster, or bogeyman	Because of their increased ability to comprehend, they may have more fears, for example: The reason for the illness Communicability of the disease to themselves or others Consequences of the disease The process of dying and death itself Their fear of the unknown is greater than that of the known The realization of impending death is a tremendous threat to their sense of security and ego strength	Help parents deal with their feelings, allowing them more emotional reserve to meet the needs of their children Encourage parents to remain near child as much as possible, yet be sensitive to parents' needs Because of children's fear of the unknown, anticipatory preparation is very important

Continued.

TABLE 38-2 Children's understanding of and reactions to death—cont'd

CONCEPTS OF DEATH	REACTIONS TO DEATH	INTERVENTIONS
School-age children—cont'd		
May have naturalistic/physiologic explanations of death By 9 or 10, children have an adult concept of death, realizing that it is inevitable, universal, and irreversible	Likely to exhibit fear through verbal uncooperativeness rather than actual physical aggression Very interested in postdeath services May be inquisitive about what happens to the body	Since the developmental task of this age is industry, helping children maintain control over their bodies and increasing their understanding allows them to achieve independence, self-worth, and self-esteem and avoids a sense of inferiority Encourage children to talk about their feelings and provide aggressive outlets Encourage parents to honestly answer questions about dying rather than avoiding or fabricating euphemisms Encourage parents to share their moments of sorrow with their children Provide preparation for postdeath services
Adolescents		
Have a mature understanding of death Still very much influenced by "remnants" of magical thinking and are subject to guilt and shame Likely to see deviations from accepted behavior as reasons for their illness	Straddle transition from childhood to adulthood Have the most difficulty in coping with death Least likely to accept cessation of life, particularly if it is their own Concern is for the present much more than for the past or the future May consider themselves alienated from their peers and unable to communicate with their parents for emotional support—feeling alone in their struggle Adolescents' orientation to the present compels them to worry about physical changes even more than the prognosis Because of their idealistic view of the world, they may criticize funeral rites as barbaric, money making, and unnecessary	Help parents deal with their feelings, allowing them more emotional reserve to meet the needs of their children Avoid alliances with either parent or child Structure hospital admission to allow for maximum self-control and independence Answer adolescents' questions honestly, treating them as mature individuals and respecting their needs for privacy, solitude, and personal expressions of emotions Help parents understand their child's reactions to death and dying, especially that concern for present crises such as loss of hair may be much greater than for future ones, including possible death

concrete sense. They may attempt to ascribe a more comprehensible meaning to the event by personifying death as a devil, God, a ghost, or a bogeyman. As some of these names imply, children attach a destructive connotation to death that is often associated with fear of mutilation and punishment. Naturalistic and physiologic explanations of death such as, "When you die, your body decays in the ground," are also common.

By 9 or 10 years of age most children have an adult concept of death. They realize that it is inevitable, universal, and irreversible. Their attitudes toward death are greatly influenced by the reactions and attitudes of others, particularly their parents.

Table 38-2 summarizes children's concepts of and reactions to death and outlines supportive interventions for each developmental stage.

Influence of Experience

Although children's concept of death is limited by their cognitive abilities, children develop an appreciation for what is happening to them through their experience with life-threatening illness. As these children acquire information about their situation, they develop different conceptions of themselves, a process that occurs in five stages (Bluebond-Langner, 1989):

Stage 1—Disease is a serious illness. New identity of "sick" child.

Stage 2—Discovery of the relationship of medication and recovery. Learns the taboos of disease and death.

Stage 3—Marked by an understanding of the purposes and implications of special procedures. Sense of well-being begins to fade and child perceives self as different from other children.

Stage 4—Illness is viewed as a permanent condition. Sense of always being sick and never getting better.

Stage 5—Realization that there is only a finite number of medications. Awareness (directly or indirectly) of the fatal prognosis.

The time lapse between stages tends to be the same for all children, regardless of age. Passage from the first stage to the second stage occurs rapidly on relapse. Passage through the second, third, and fourth stages takes somewhat longer, but passage to the fifth stage may take place as soon as the child learns of the death of another, and all knowledge from previous stages is quickly synthesized into a new self-awareness. Since experience, not age or intellectual ability, is the critical factor in passing through these stages, young children who have undergone treatment for several months may know more about their prognosis than adolescents whose disease is newly diagnosed.

Nursing Care of the Family and Child With Special Needs

Assessment

Since the nurse may meet a family during any phase of the adjustment process, several assessment areas are important. Knowledge of the family's available support system is essential and may include the marital relationship, nonmarital partners, extended family, colleagues and co-workers, friends, and professionals. The family's perception of the illness or disability is also an area that influences family adjustment. Assessment questions should focus on members' general knowledge of the condition even before the child's diagnosis was made, the influence of religion on their thinking, imagined causes of the condition, and the effects of the child's disorder on the family.

Since the family's ability to cope with previous stresses influences the current situation, answers to questions about their usual coping skills are enlightening. Knowledge of concurrent stresses, such as financial, marital or nonmarital career, or unemployment, helps identify families who may have fewer resources to cope with the child's needs.

Nursing ALERT

Be aware that many families do not have a telephone, a service most practitioners consider essential for families of children with special needs. Other families may have telephones but are reluctant to reveal the telephone number. To overcome these difficulties, use the following strategies:

Help family identify telephone access close to home (e.g., neighbor's home, nearby store).

Explore methods to obtain telephone service for the family (e.g., social service agencies, charitable organizations).

Be sensitive to family's concern for privacy when asking for a telephone number; explain reason for needing number and to whom it will be given.

Finally, awareness of the family members' reactions to the child and the illness or disability is important. Sample questions that the nurse and family can use to evaluate the support system, perception of the illness, coping mechanisms, resources, and concurrent stresses are listed in Table 38-3. Because factors affecting the family's response may change at any point during the illness, assessment must be a continuous process.

Special challenges exist in assessing the child's feelings about having a disability. Chapter 31 presents several approaches to encourage a child to discuss feelings about the condition. The nurse should use a variety of communication techniques such as drawing and play as assessment tools rather than rely solely on parental reports. Often children are neglected partners in their care, and their unique needs are not identified.

The needs of working parents and siblings also should be assessed, a goal that requires flexibility in scheduling appointments to include these important family members. When working parents know that their input is valuable, they will often change their work schedule to meet with a health professional. Since siblings can be of any age, the use of appropriate communication strategies for assessment must be considered. Nonverbal techniques such as those discussed in Chapter 31 should be considered for these children.

Several instruments can be used to assist the family in assessing their overall functioning and support system (see Chapter 31).

Nursing Diagnoses

A number of nursing diagnoses are prominent in the nursing care of the family and child with special needs. Others specific to individual cases become evident, especially when the child's actual disorder is considered. The most common nursing diagnoses are outlined in the Nursing Care Plan on pp. 1147-1148.

Planning

The nursing plan depends to a large extent on the child's actual illness or disability. However, the following are basic goals for all families and children with special needs:

1. The child and family receive support at time of diagnosis.
2. The family's emotional reactions are accepted.
3. The child and family cope with stresses of situation.
4. The child and family receive appropriate information about the condition.
5. The family establishes an environment of normalization for the child.

Implementation

The main objective in working with the family is to assist them to cope effectively with the stresses imposed by the child's special needs. To achieve this goal, the entire family should be considered in every aspect of the implementation process (see the Family Focus box on p. 1136).

Provide Support at Time of Diagnosis

The time of diagnosis may be experienced as a crisis by some families. The impact of the crisis may occur at the time of birth, following a long period of physical and/or psychologic testing, or immediately after a tragic injury. The impact may begin before the diagnosis is made, when parents are aware that something is wrong with their child, but before medical confirmation (Clements, Copeland, and Loftus, 1990). It is a

TABLE 38-3 Assessment of factors affecting family adjustment

FACTORS AFFECTING ADJUSTMENT	ASSESSMENT QUESTIONS
Available support system	
Status of marital relationship	Whom do you talk to when you have something on your mind? (If answer is not the spouse, ask for the reason.)
Alternate support systems	When something is worrying you, what do you do? What helps you most when you are upset?
Ability to communicate	Does talking seem to help when you feel upset?
Perception of the illness/disability	
Previous knowledge of disorder	Have you ever heard the word (name of diagnosis) before? Tell me about it (if answer is yes).
Influence of religion	Has your religion or faith been of help to you? Tell me how (if answer is yes).
Imagined cause of disorder	What are your thoughts about the causes of the disorder?
Effects of illness or disability on family	How has your child's illness or disability affected you and your family? How has your life-style changed?
Coping mechanisms	
Reactions to previous crises	Tell me one time you've had another crisis (problem, bad time) in your family. How did you solve that problem?
Reactions to the child Childrearing practices Attitudes	Do you find yourself being a little more cautious with this child than with your other children? Do you feel as comfortable disciplining this child compared with your other children? How is this child different from the siblings or other children of similar age? Describe your child's personality. Is it easy, difficult, or in-between? When you think of your child's future, what thoughts come to mind?
Available resources	What parts of your child's care are causing the most difficulty for you and/or your family? What services are available to help? What services do you need that presently are not available?
Concurrent stresses	What other problems are you facing now? (Be specific—ask about financial, marital, sibling, and extended family/friends concerns.)

critical time for parents. Although they may not hear or remember all that is said to them, they frequently sense a certain attitude of acceptance, rejection, hope, or despair that may influence their ability to absorb the shock and begin adapting to the family's altered future.

Parents should be encouraged to be together when they are informed of their child's condition, thus avoiding the problem of one parent having to interpret complex findings and deal with the initial emotional reaction of the other. The informing session should take place in a private, comfortable setting free of distractions and interruptions, in an atmosphere in which the parents feel free to express their emotions (Fig. 38-2). If their feelings can be expressed and acknowledged, the parents can be helped to deal openly with them. Their emotional needs are acknowledged by showing acceptance of such expressions as crying, sadness, anger, and disappointment. Emotional support is offered by having tissues available if a family member cries and demonstrating through facial and bodily language that indeed this is a difficult and painful period. Although touching is a powerful expression of empathy, it must be used wisely. For example, it can prematurely terminate free expression of feelings, especially when combined with statements such as "Everything will be all right." Nurses should also be aware of cultural issues regarding touching (see Chapter 28).

Parents should receive the kind of information they desire. Most parents want a clear, simple explanation of the diagnosis, a prediction of possible futures for the child, advice on what to do next, an opportunity to ask questions, a warm and sympathetic listener, and, most important, time. Clarification of explanations is elicited with such questions as, "Do you see what I mean?" or, "Is this clear to you?" Technical terms are used with simple definitions. If the parents are unaware of the term, they are given written literature or at least a written summary of the diagnosis.

Finally, the informing conference should not end with the presentation of devastating news. Instead, the child's strengths, appealing behaviors, and potential for development are stressed, as well as available rehabilitation efforts or treatment. Parents can be encouraged to view their experiences as

Family Focus

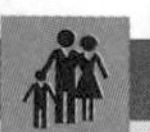

IDENTIFYING FAMILY NEEDS

To ensure an effective plan of care, attention to *family-identified needs and priorities* is essential. For example, a family may have difficulty focusing on treatment issues if their current priority is obtaining enough food to feed their children.

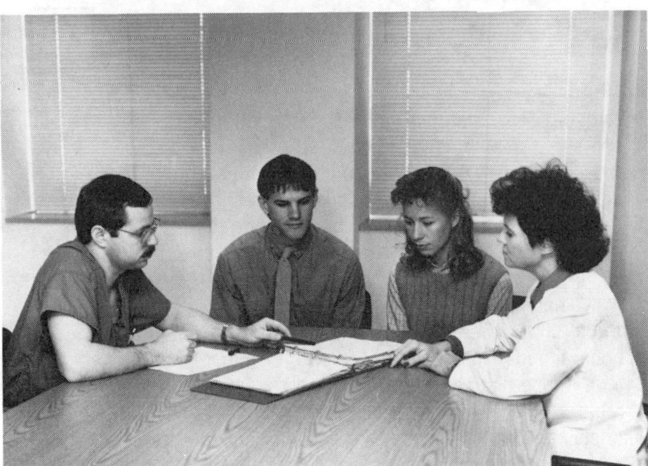

Fig. 38-2 An informing session should take place in a private, comfortable setting free of distractions and interruptions.

Guidelines

ENCOURAGING EXPRESSION OF EMOTION

Describe the behavior: "You seem angry at everyone."
Give evidence of understanding: "Being angry is only natural."
Give evidence of caring: "It must be difficult to endure so many painful procedures."
Help focus on feelings: "Maybe you wonder why this happened to your child."

a series of challenges that they are capable of handling, particularly with available professional feedback. The parents are assured that the nurse will be available to answer questions and to provide further assistance as needed.

The preceding discussion relates primarily to the initial informing interview. However, because of the need for long-term follow-up, it is only one in a series of continuing discussions. In all interactions the family's input is solicited and incorporated into the plan of care. Some situations require consideration of special problems (see the Guidelines box on p. 1138).

Accept Family's Emotional Reactions

One of the most supportive interventions is to accept the family's emotional reactions to the child's condition in as nonjudgmental a manner as possible. Although all families respond differently and in varying degrees of intensity, three responses are so common and often so poorly handled that they deserve special consideration.

Denial. The nurse's response to denial is a critical component of the individual's continuing need for this defense mechanism. The most effective method of support is active listening. Silence neither reinforces nor rejects denial (or any other emotional reaction) but implies a willingness and acceptance of the person's need for this behavior. However, silence alone can be misinterpreted. For example, if the person demonstrates denial, such as by saying, "I am sure the doctors made a mistake," and the nurse responds silently and leaves, the person may infer disapproval, agreement, avoidance, or rejection from this behavior.

To be effective, silence and listening must be accompanied by physical and mental concentration and use of body language to communicate interest and concern. Direct eye contact, touch, physical closeness, and body posture such as sitting and leaning slightly forward demonstrate silent but effective communication. (See also Communication Techniques, Chapter 31.)

Guilt. Since guilt is such a common response and can cause family members tremendous anxiety, they should be told directly that there is no known cause of the disorder (when appropriate) and that they are not to be blamed. Using the third-person technique is valuable in eliciting thoughts of guilt. For example, with children an appropriate statement may be, "When people get sick, they often wonder if they did anything to make themselves sick." This allows children an opportunity to explore any feelings of responsibility they harbor.

If family members are expressing feelings of guilt, it is important to allow them to talk about their feelings rather than quickly trying to dispel them with long "scientific" explanations. Statements such as, "If you believe you are responsible for Johnny's condition, no wonder you feel so bad," acknowledge the family member's feelings. This step is frequently appreciated and necessary before the facts can be presented and absorbed. An effective method in lessening guilt is to *encourage the irrationality of thought.* For example, one mother stated that her son probably developed cancer by sitting too close to the television, which should could have prevented by being more strict. By following her reasoning and talking about how *many* children sit close to the television and how *few* of them ever have cancer, the nurse was able to help the mother realize that this activity was not a cause.

Anger. Anger is one of the more difficult reactions to accept and deal with therapeutically. The responses to anger may be reciprocal anger, fear, acceptance, and/or encouragement. The first two reactions impede communication and express disapproval and rejection of the person. They most commonly occur when the listener views the anger as a personal assault. The last two responses allow the individual to express his or her feelings in an atmosphere of nonjudgmental acceptance. Two basic rules for dealing with the angry person are to avoid losing one's temper and to encourage the person to talk (see the Guidelines box above). One essential element to the successful implementation of this process is to wait for the person to respond to a statement before proceeding to the next step. Since the objective of each statement is for the person to speak freely, the responses should avoid "yes" or "no" types of answers (as in the Guidelines box).

Help Family Cope

For the family to meet the stresses of optimally adjusting to the child's condition, each member must be individually supported so that the family system is strong. Although the family can indefinitely support a member who is in need of assistance, its greatest strength lies in every member supporting

Guidelines

SITUATIONS REQUIRING SPECIAL CONSIDERATION

Congenital anomaly—Tension in delivery room conveys the sense that something is seriously wrong. Communication is often delayed while physician is involved with mother's care. The manner in which the infant is presented36 may well set the tone for the early parent-child relationship.

Clarify role with physician in regard to revealing information, to enable immediate parental support.

Explain to parents briefly in simple language what the defect is and something concerning the immediate prognosis before showing them the infant, when they are more apt to "hear" what is said.

Be aware of nonverbal communication. Parents watch the facial expressions of others for signs of revulsion or rejection.

Present the infant as something precious.

Emphasize the well-formed aspects of the infant's body.

Allow time and opportunity for parents to express their initial response.

Encourage parents to ask questions and provide honest, straightforward answers without undue optimism or pessimism.

Cognitive impairment—Unless cognitive impairment (mental retardation) is associated with other physical problems, it is often easy for parents to miss clues to its presence or to make defensive excuses regarding diagnosis.

Plan situations that help parents become aware of the problem.

Encourage parents to discuss their observations of the child, but withhold diagnostic opinions.

Focus on what the child can do and appropriate interventions to promote progress (e.g., infant stimulation programs), to involve parents in their child's care while helping them gain an awareness of the child's disability.

Physical disability—If loss of motor or sensory ability occurs during childhood, diagnosis is readily apparent. The challenge lies in helping the child and parents over the period of shock and grief and toward the phase of acceptance and reintegration. Institute early rehabilitation (e.g., using a prosthetic limb, learning to read braille, or learning to read lips).

Be aware that physical rehabilitation usually precedes psychologic adjustment.

When the cause of the disability is accidental, avoid implying that parents or child was responsible for the injury, yet allow them the opportunity to discuss feelings of blame.

Encourage expression of feelings (see Communication Techniques, Chapter 31).

Chronic illness—Realization of the true impact may take months or years. Conflict over parent's vs. child's concerns may result in serious problems. When condition is inherited, parents may blame themselves, and/or child may blame parents.

Help each family member gain an appreciation of the other's concerns.

Discuss hereditary aspect of condition with parents at time of diagnosis to lessen guilt and accusatory feelings.

Encourage child to express feelings by using third-person technique (e.g., "Sometimes when a person has an illness that was passed on by the parents, that person feels angry or bitter toward them").

Multiple disabilities—The child or parent may require additional time for the shock phase and may only be able to attend to one diagnosis before hearing significant information regarding other disorders.

Acknowledge parents' understanding and acceptance of all diagnoses, especially when an obvious and more hidden disability coexists.

Appreciate the devastating consequences of more than one disability to a child, especially if they interfere with expressive-receptive abilities.

Terminal illness—Parents require much support to deal with their own feelings and guidance in how to tell the child the diagnosis. They may wish to conceal the diagnosis from the child. They may believe that the child is too young to know, will not be able to cope with the information, or will lose hope and the will to live.

Approach the subject of disclosure in a positive way by asking, "How will you tell your child about the diagnosis?"

Help parents understand the disadvantages of not telling children (e.g., deprives them of the opportunity to openly discuss their feelings and ask questions, incurs the risk of them learning the truth from outside and sometimes less tactful sources, may lessen children's trust and confidence in their parents once they learn the truth).

Guide parents to see the potential problems involved in fostering a conspiracy.

Offer parents guidelines for how and what to tell children about their disease or the possibility of death. Explanations should be tailored to the child's cognitive ability, be based on knowledge child already has, and be honest. Honesty must be tempered with concern for the child's feelings.

Assure parents that telling a child the name of the illness and the reason for treatment instills hope, provides support from others, and serves as a foundation for explaining and understanding subsequent events.

Acknowledge that being honest is not always easy, because the truth may prompt children to ask other distressing questions such as, "Am I going to die?" However, even this difficult question must be answered.

each other. The nurse should bear in mind that the family member in greatest need is not necessarily the affected child but may be a parent or sibling who is dealing with stresses that require intervention.

Parents. The nurse can provide support by being attentive to families' responses to their children. Mothers and fathers need to experience success, joy, and pride in their children to give the support they need. Children, too, require support for their interactions, adjustments, and efforts. They must be reinforced for attempts to get to know their care providers and to communicate their needs to them.

Nurses must examine their attitudes to determine their ability to engage in parent-professional partnerships. An essential characteristic is the belief that parents are equal to professionals and that parents are experts regarding their child. See the Guidelines box on p. 1139.

Since the majority of mothers and fathers of children with special needs have little or no experience with children who have chronic or disabling conditions, the nurse can role model

Guidelines

DEVELOPING SUCCESSFUL PARENT-PROFESSIONAL PARTNERSHIPS

Promote primary nursing; in nonhospital settings designate a case manager.
Acknowledge parents' overall competence and their unique expertise with their child.
Respect parents' time as having equal value to that of other members of child's health care team.
Explain or define any medical, technical, or disciplinary-specific terms.
Tell families, "I am not sure" or, "I don't know" when appropriate.
Facilitate family's effectiveness in team meetings (e.g., provide parents with same information as other participants).

appropriate interactions with the child. Above all, the nurse should ensure that the parents and siblings learn to perceive the child as a child first, with unique and individual needs. The nurse needs to convey a humanistic, accepting approach to the child to enable the parents to observe this acceptance. This attitude of liking, concern for, and acceptance of the child should begin in early infancy and continue throughout the child's life.

Communication among all family members is encouraged. Parent group sessions are helpful in assisting parents to verbalize thoughts and feelings to each other but often do not take into account siblings' or the child's viewpoint. Therefore the nurse may need to set up a family session such as during a home or clinic visit. Although the ideal situation is to have all the members present at once, this is often not possible. However, inviting members to participate at various visits is an appropriate alternative.

Parents can be encouraged to discuss their feelings toward the child, the impact of this event on their marriage, and associated stresses such as financial burdens. For most families, regardless of their income or insurance coverage, financial concerns exist. The costs of caring for a child with special needs can be overwhelming. In addition, the family wage earner may have to sacrifice job opportunities to remain close to a medical facility or to avoid losing insurance benefits.*

The nurse should regard fathers as able, effective parents, competent and capable of coping with the challenges they face. Every effort is made to include the father in visits such as to the nursery, clinic, special school, and stimulation programs. The father should be included in the assessment process, with specific emphasis on having him describe the child's strengths and difficulties. It is not unusual to find two parents who have differing views of the child's abilities, especially in the area of developmental disabilities.*

Numerous volunteer and community resources are available that provide assistance, rehabilitation, equipment, and funding for a variety of health problems.† National and local disease-oriented organizations may provide needed assistance and support to families that qualify. Many of these are discussed elsewhere in the text under the diagnosis. State and federal departments of health, mental health, social service, and labor may be able to help locate appropriate regional resources. For example, state Programs for Children with Special Health Needs (formerly Crippled Children's Services) provide financial assistance for children with many disabling conditions. Local and national sources of respite care and medical day care may be useful to families. Nurses should become acquainted with those in their communities and with vocational programs for special groups.

Although community resources may exist, it is often very difficult for parents to locate suitable services, and coordination among several agencies may be lacking. Fragmented care is one of the chief complaints from families. Consequently, community networking for improved services is essential. Although this topic is beyond the scope of the present discussion, nurses can become key figures in coordinating services.

Parent-to-parent support. The support a parent receives from another parent is unique and unobtainable from any other source. A growing number of hospitals and clinics now have a parent on staff. The services these parents provide are particularly valuable for parents of children with special needs who are likely to experience frequent and lengthy hospitalizations, as well as numerous routine clinic visits.

Just being with another parent who has shared similar experiences is helpful. A parent of a child with the same diagnosis is not always necessary, for parents in the process of adjusting to a child with special needs—or finding respite services, educational or rehabilitative services, special equipment vendors, financial counseling—tread a common path. If the agency does not have a parent staff position, the nurse can contact parent groups, who will often send a representative. Another strategy is ask another parent to talk to the par-

---

*Information regarding financial issues is available from the **Federation for Children with Special Needs,** 95 Berkeley St., Suite 104, Boston, MA 02116; (617) 482-2915. A helpful book for families is: Rosenfeld L: *Your child and health care: A "dollars and sense" guide for families with special needs,* Baltimore, Md, 1994, Paul H. Brookes Publishing. Available from **The Association for the Care of Children's Health,** 7910 Woodmont Ave., Suite 300, Bethesda, MD, 20814, (301) 654-6549.

*Excellent resources on fathers' issues are presented in a training film, *Special Kids, Special Dads: Fathers of Children with Disabilities,* and a monograph, *Fathers of Children with Special Needs: New Horizons,* which are available from the **Association for the Care of Children's Health,** 7910 Woodmont Ave., Suite 300, Bethesda, MD 20814; (301) 654-6549.

†General sources of information are **Clearinghouse for Disability Information,** Room 3132, Switzer Building, C St., S.W., Washington, DC 20202-2524, **National Information Center for Children and Youth with Disabilities,** P.O. Box 1492, Washington, DC 20013, (202) 884-8200 or (800) 695-0285; **National Information Clearinghouse for Infants with Disabilities and Life-Threatening Conditions,** Center for Developmental Disabilities, The University of South Carolina, Benson Building, Columbia, SC 29208, (800) 922-1107, ext. 201 (in SC) or (800) 922-9234, ext. 201; and **National Center for Children with Chronic Illness and Disability,** Box 721-UMHC, Harvard St. at E. River Rd., Minneapolis, MN 55455, (612) 626-4032. A comprehensive list of books and pamphlets for parents and teachers is available from the **National Easter Seal Society,** 230 West Monroe St., Suite 1800, Chicago, IL 60606; (312) 726-6200. In Canada: **Coalition of Provincial Organizations of the Handicapped,** Suite 926, 294 Portage Ave., Winnipeg, Manitoba R3C 0B9, (204) 947-0303; and **Canadian Rehabilitation Council for Disabled,** 45 Sheppard Ave., E., Suite 801, Toronto, Ontario M2N 5W9, (416) 250-7490.

ents.* The nurse should seek out a parent who is a good listener, has a nonjudgmental approach to differences in families, and possesses good advocacy and problem-solving skills.

The parent self-help group is another way to promote parent-to-parent support.† Group members feel less alone and have the opportunity to observe both coping and mastery role modeling from other members. Parents' groups are rich resources for information. Even if parents are unable to attend meetings, they can still benefit from group newsletters and other literature that often accompany membership. The nurse can foster parent participation in self-help groups by serving as a referral agent, a group advisory board member, a resource person, a group member, or an assistant in founding a group. Sometimes all that is required in starting a group is identifying one or two parents as leaders; sharing with them the names, telephone numbers, and addresses of other families who have expressed both an interest and a willingness to release their phone number and address; and guiding them in how to initiate a first meeting.‡

Advocate for empowerment. Nurses can advocate for methods that foster opportunities for parent empowerment. For example, nurses can suggest reimbursement for travel and child care, as well as stipends to enable parents' voices to be heard at meetings and conferences. They can encourage parent membership on staff, committees, and boards. They can keep parents informed of pending legislation on child health issues or take action when parents inform them.

Guidelines

PROMOTING NORMALIZATION

Preparation—Prepare child in advance for changes that may occur from the illness or disability; for example, the child is told in advance of the possible side effects of drug therapy.

Participation—Include child in as many decisions as possible, especially those relating to his or her care regimen; for example, the child is responsible for taking medications or scheduling home treatments.

Sharing—Allow both family members and child's peers to be a part of the care regimen whenever possible; for example, the child is given his or her medication when the other siblings receive their vitamins; the parent cooks the same menu for the whole family; and if the child is invited to another's home, the parent advises the family of the child's dietary restrictions.

Control—Identify areas in which child can be in control so that feelings of uncertainty, passivity, and helplessness are decreased; for example, the child identifies activities that are appropriate to his or her energy level and chooses to rest when fatigued.

Expectation—Apply the same family rules to the child with a chronic illness or disability as to the well siblings or peers; for example, the child is disciplined, expected to fulfill household responsibilities, and attends school in accordance with abilities.

The child. Through ongoing contacts with the child, the nurse (1) observes the child's responses to the disorder, ability to function, and adaptive behaviors within the environment and with significant others; (2) explores the child's own understanding of the nature of his or her illness or condition; and (3) provides support while the child learns to cope with his or her feelings. Children are encouraged to express their concerns rather than allowing others to express them for them.

Parents sometimes convey concern because children cannot express their anxieties. If children cannot or will not talk, they may have to play out their feelings. They can be provided with toys to express threatening or stressful emotions. The nurse may find that children respond best to drawing pictures or telling stories (see Chapter 31). Puppets can also be used. By demonstrating to parents how useful these techniques are, the nurse also helps them learn new ways of communicating with their child. For youngsters with extremely serious handicaps and/or persistent maladjustment, psychiatric evaluation and management may be needed.

One of the most important interventions is alleviating the child's feeling of being different and normalizing his or her life as much as possible. The Guidelines box above contains fundamental steps in implementing the normalizing process. Whenever possible, the nurse should assist the family to assess the child's daily routine for indications of normalizing practices. For example, the child who remains in a bedroom all day is in need of a restructured daily routine to provide activities in different parts of the house, such as eating in the kitchen or dining room with the family. Such children may also be deprived of social, recreational, and academic activities that can be recognized by applying normalization practices. For example, home and out-of-home health-related treatments should be planned at times that least interfere with normal daily activities.

Children who are concerned that their condition detracts from their physical attractiveness need attention focused on the normal aspects of appearance and capabilites. Health professionals must help strengthen and consolidate the self-image by emphasizing the normal, while at the same time allowing children to express anger, isolation, fear of rejection, feelings of sadness, and loneliness. They need positive reinforcement for compliance and any evidence of improvement. Anything that might improve attractiveness and contribute to a positive self-image is used, such as makeup for a teenager with a scar, clothing that disguises a prosthesis, or a hairstyle or wig to cover a deformity or lost hair.

*The *Parent Resource Directory* lists over 400 parents of children with chronic illness or disabilities in the United States and Canada, including addresses, phone numbers, the child's condition, and the health facility where the child receives care. It is available from the **Association for the Care of Children's Health,** 7910 Woodmont Ave., Suite 300, Bethesda, MD 20814; (301) 654-6549.

†Information about self-help groups, as well as books and pamphlets, is available from the **National Self-Help Clearinghouse,** 25 W. 43rd St., Room 620, New York, NY 10036; (212) 642-2944.

‡The following resources are recommended: Minna Newman Nathanson: *Organizing and maintaining support groups for parents of children with chronic illness and handicapping conditions,* available from the **Association for the Care of Children's Health,** 7910 Woodmont Ave., Suite 300, Bethesda, MD 20814, (301) 654-6549; and Madara EJ, Meese A: *The self-help sourcebook: finding and forming mutual aid self-help groups,* available from the **New Jersey Self-Help Clearinghouse,** Saint Clares-Riverside Medical Center, Denville, NJ 07834, (201) 625-9565.

Siblings. The presence of a child with special needs in a family may result in parents paying less attention to the other children. Siblings may respond by developing negative attitudes toward the child or by expressing anger in different forms. The nurse can help by using "anticipatory guidance," questioning the parents about what they believe is the best way to have siblings respond to the child, and guiding them through ways to meet their other children's needs for attention. This questioning should take place before serious negative effects occur.

Siblings may also experience embarrassment associated with courtesy stigma. Parents are then faced with the difficulty of responding to this embarrassment in an understanding and appropriate manner without punishing the siblings for feeling the way they do. Parents should talk with the siblings about how they view their affected sibling. For example, siblings of a child who is retarded may express fears about their ability to bear normal children. Adolescents in particular may not be able to discuss these vital issues with their parents and may prefer to consult with the nurse. Many siblings benefit from sharing their concerns with other young people who are experiencing a similar situation.* Support groups for siblings can help decrease isolation, promote expression of feelings, and provide examples of effective coping skills.

*For information on the **Sibling Information Network**, contact the Information Network, CUAP, 991 Main St., Suite 3A, East Hartford, CT 06108; (203) 282-7050.

Many parents express concern about when and how to inform the other children in the family about a sibling's disability. The answer depends on each child's level of sophistication and understanding. However, it is usually best to inform the siblings before someone else does. Uninformed siblings may fantasize or develop apprehensions that are out of proportion to the child's actual condition. Furthermore, if parents choose to be silent or deceptive about the issue, they are setting a negative precedent for the siblings to follow, rather than encouraging the siblings to cope with the experience in a healthy and nurturing way.

The nurse must be sensitive to the reactions of siblings and whenever possible intervene to promote more positive adjustments. For example, siblings often mention that they are expected to take on additional responsibilities to help the parents care for the child. It is not unusual for them to express a positive reaction to assuming the extra duties but a negative response to feeling unappreciated for doing so. Such feelings can often be minimized by encouraging siblings to discuss this with the parents and by suggesting to parents ways of showing gratitude, such as an increase in allowance, special privileges, and, most significantly, verbal praise (see the Family focus box below).

Extended family members and society. The nurse must also be sensitive to the family's cues regarding sources of stress from extended members such as grandparents. For example, the nurse may encourage the parents to invite the

Family Focus

SUPPORTING SIBLINGS

Promoting healthy sibling relationships

- Value each child individually and avoid comparisons. Remind each child of his or her positive qualities and contribution to other family members.
- Help siblings see the differences and similarities between themselves and a child with special needs. Create a climate in which children can achieve successes without feeling guilty.
- Teach siblings ways to interact with the child.
- Seek to be fair in terms of discipline, attention, and resources; require the affected child to do as much for himself or herself as possible.
- Let siblings settle their own differences; intervene only to prevent siblings from hurting one another.
- Legitimize reasonable anger. Even children with special needs behave badly sometimes.
- Respect a sibling's reluctance to be with or to include the child with special needs in activities.

Help siblings cope

- Listen to siblings to let them know that their thoughts and suggestions are valued.
- Praise siblings when they have been patient, have sacrificed, or have been particularly helpful. Do not expect siblings to always act in this manner.
- Acknowledge the personal strengths siblings have and their ability to cope with stress successfully.
- Provide age-appropriate information about the child's condition, and update when appropriate.
- Let teachers know what is happening so they can be understanding and helpful.
- Recognize special stress times for siblings and plan to minimize negative effects.
- Schedule special time with siblings; have a friend or family member substitute when parent is unavailable.
- Encourage sibling to join or help establish a sibling support group.
- Use the services of professionals when needed. If parent feels that such a service is necessary, it should be provided in as vigorous a manner as a service for the child with special needs.

Involve siblings

- Seek out ways to realistically include siblings in the care and treatment of the child with special needs.
- Limit caregiving responsibilities and give recognition when siblings perform them.
- Develop a library of children's books on special needs.
- Invite siblings to attend meetings to develop plans for the child with special needs.
- Discuss future plans with them.
- Solicit their ideas on treatment and service needs.
- Have them visit professionals who work with the child.
- Help them develop competencies to teach the child new skills.
- Provide opportunities for siblings to advocate for the child.
- Allow siblings to set their own pace for learning and involvement.

Modified from Powell T, Ogle P: *Brothers and sisters—a special part of exceptional families*, Baltimore, 1985, Paul H Brookes; Spokane Washington Deaconess Medical Center Pediatric Oncology Unit: Tips for dealing with siblings, *The Candlelighters Childhood Cancer Foundation Quarterly Newsletter* 11(3, 4):7, 1987; and Carlson J, Leviton A, Mueller M: Services to siblings: An important component of family-centered practice, *The ACCH Advocate* 1(1):53-56, 1993.

grandparents to be present during one of the child's visits to the clinic, during the diagnostic workup, or at a parent conference or to provide appropriate literature. Including grandparents in a discussion in which they can share their concerns may help them deal with their feelings, thus reducing stress on the entire family. Grandparents' feelings of blame and anger, as well as any "cure fantasies" they harbor, can be brought out in the open and discussed if necessary. Grandparents can be helped to understand the effects of their behavior on the family with an appropriate statement, such as, "Your daughter is currently experiencing a great deal of pain and anguish. We realize that this is difficult for you as well as your daughter; however, you can be of tremendous help by being supportive toward her."

Considerable stress can also arise from nonfamilial sources such as friends, neighbors, or strangers. Inability to cope with comments about the disorder or curious stares by others may foster the tendency to isolate and protect the child within the home. The family needs guidance in preparing for these inevitable experiences. One approach is encouraging parents to dress the child as much as possible like other children. Good grooming is very important in minimizing differences in appearance. Through role playing parents can practice responses to comments such as, "Is your child retarded?" or "Has he always been crippled?" Through parent groups family members can share experiences and learn from each other how they successfully deal with probing questions or unkind remarks. Interventions should include the siblings and the affected child, who must also face and deal with these events. Nurses can teach young children about disabilities to familiarize them with the special needs and abilities of these individuals. For example, school nurses can simulate experiences such as having only one leg through role playing, use books or films, or invite community guests with physical limitations to visit the class.

Educate About the Disorder and General Health Care

Educating the family about the disorder is actually an extension of revealing the diagnosis.* Education involves not only supplying technical information, but also discussing how the condition will affect the child. Parents may only be able to digest so much information at a time. It may be helpful to provide essential information and then ask, "What else would you like to know about your child's condition?" Responding to parent's questions and concerns assures them that their information needs are met.

Activities of daily living. Parents also need guidance in how the condition may interfere with or alter activities of daily living such as eating, dressing, sleeping, and toileting. Guidance in normalizing these activities for the child and family and in promoting age-appropriate self-care should be provided (Ahmann and Bond, 1992). One area frequently affected is nutrition. Common problems are undernutrition as a result of food being inappropriately restricted, loss of appetite, vomiting, or motor deficits that interfere with feeding, and overnutrition usually caused by a caloric intake in excess of energy expenditure or boredom and lack of stimulation in other areas. Although the child requires the same basic nutrients as other children, the daily requirements may differ.

Safe transportation. Modifications may also be needed regarding car safety. Children with conditions such as low birth weight or orthopedic, neuromuscular, or respiratory problems often cannot safely use conventional car restraints. Modifications can be made to some commercial models, and for older children a special vest is available that secures the child to the back seat in a lying-down position.*

If a child requires a wheelchair, the family should consult the wheelchair manufacturer for specific instructions regarding safe car transportation. Considerations for wheelchairs used for vehicle transportation must address the security of the wheelchair and the security of the occupant in the wheelchair. Wheelchairs should be secured forward facing with tie downs at four points. The tie-down system should be dynamically crash tested, as should the system that secures the child in the wheelchair. For example, use of trays would not be recommended for transportation. When children must travel with additional medical equipment, this equipment (i.e., oxygen, monitors, ventilators) should be anchored to the floor or underneath the vehicle seat or wheelchair. Soft padding should be added around the equipment to reduce movement. A second adult should be present to monitor the condition of a medically fragile child while traveling.

Primary health care. Children with special needs require all the usual health care recommended for any child. Attention to injury prevention, immunizations, dental health, and regular physical examinations is essential. Nurses can play an important role in reminding parents of these aspects of care that are so often neglected when the concern is focused on the child's specific illness or disability. Specific discussions of nutrition, sleep and activity, dental health, immunizations, and injury prevention are presented in the chapters on health promotion for specific age groups.

Parents also need to be aware of the importance of communicating the child's condition in the event of a medical emergency. Young children are unable to give information about their disorder, and although older children may be reliable sources, after an accident they may be physically unable to speak. Therefore all children with any type of chronic condition that may affect medical care should wear some type of identification such as a Medic-Alert bracelet† or carry a card in their wallet, which lists the medical condition and a phone number for emergency medical records and other personal information.

Children need information about their condition, the therapeutic plan, and how the disease or the therapy might affect their particular situation. Children nearing puberty also need to understand the maturation process and how their disability may alter this event. Information should not be given all at once but be timed appropriately to meet the changing needs of

*See Wong DL: *Wong and Whaley's clinical manual of pediatric nursing*, ed 4, St Louis, 1996, Mosby for home care instruction sheets, which may be copied and given to families.

*Information on car safety restraints for children with special needs is available from **Automotive Safety for Children Program,** Riley Hospital for Children, 702 Barnhill Dr., S-139, Indianapolis, IN 46223; (317) 274-2977 or (800) KID-N-CAR (in Indiana).

†P.O. Box 1009, Turlock, CA 95381-1009; (800) ID-ALERT.

the youngsters, and it should be described and repeated as often as the situation demands. The subject of sexuality related to the effects of the disorder is a prominent concern of adolescents, but they rarely initiate a discussion of this sensitive topic. Any probable interference in sexual function because of the disability should be discussed openly and candidly with the teenager.

Promote Normal Development

Aside from knowledge of the condition and its effect on the child's abilities, the family must be guided toward fostering appropriate development in their child. Although each stage may take longer to achieve, parents are guided to helping the child fully realize potential in preparation for the next developmental stage. See Table 38-4 for developmental aspects of chronic illness or disability and supportive interventions. With appropriate planning and knowledge of strategies to improve the child's functional abilities, most children can live fulfilling and productive lives.

One important aspect of promoting normal development is to encourage the child's self-care abilities in both activities of daily living and the medical regimen. The child's age and physical, emotional, and mental capacities, as well as the supportiveness and structure provided by the family should be considered in determining the appropriate level of self-care in the medical regimen (Savinetti-Rose, 1994). Even toddlers can be involved in their own care by holding supplies for the parent during a procedure. Over time children be encouraged toward greater autonomy in the self-care arena.

Early childhood. During infancy the child is achieving basic *trust* through a satisfying, intimate, consistent relationship with his or her parents. However, the affected child's early existence may be stressful, chaotic, and unsatisfying. Consequently, he or she may need more parental support and expressions of affection to achieve trust. Likewise, the parents require assistance in finding ways to meet the infant's needs, such as how to hold a rigid or flaccid infant, how to feed a child with tongue thrust or episodes of dyspnea, and how to stimulate a child who seems incapable of achieving any skills. If hospitalizations are frequent or prolonged, every effort is made to preserve the parent-child relationship (see also Chapter 41). Hospital policies should promote visitation by and involvement of families.

During early childhood the goal is to achieve separation from parents, autonomy, and initiative. However, the natural parental response to having a sick child is overprotection. Parents need help in realizing the importance of brief separations from the child and from others involved in the child's care and of providing social experiences outside the home whenever possible. Respite care, which provides temporary relief for family members, can be essential in allowing caregivers time away from the daily burdens.

Young children also need the opportunity to develop independence. Frequently the child is able to learn self-help skills such as holding the bottle, finger feeding, and removing simple articles of clothing; but the parent continues to perform the act. The nurse can guide parents to the usual milestones expected from the child.

When the young child has a disability that interferes with motor development, intervention must be based on providing

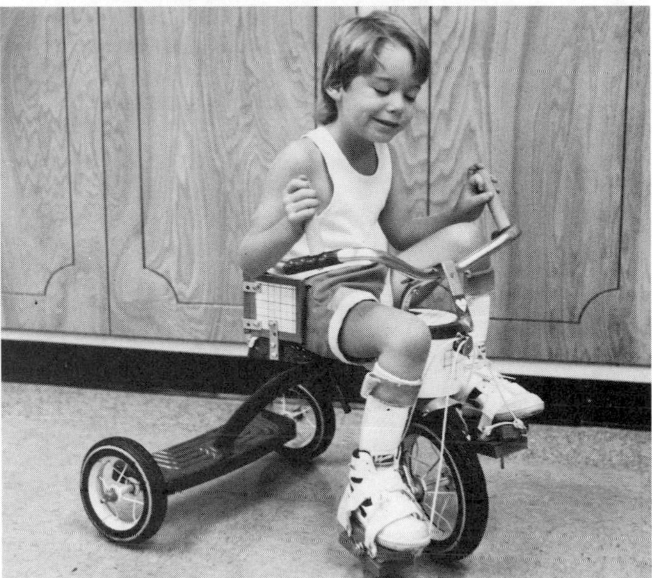

Fig. 38-3 A modified tricycle with block pedals, self-adhesive straps for support, and modified seat and handle bars can help a child with disabilities gain mobility.

activities that allow maximum motor development. Also, the activity must take into account the child's need for social interaction, sense of control over the body, feeling of competence and achievement, and an outlet for aggression.

When a child is unable to perform a skill independently, functional aids should be used. With innovation many adaptations can be implemented in children's environments to increase their mobility and independence and allow them to play like other children their age. For example, with slight modifications, a child with physical limitations may be able to ride a tricycle (Fig. 38-3).

Another critical component for normal child development is discipline. Discipline and guidance serve several purposes: they provide a child with boundaries within which to test their behavior and they also teach children socially acceptable behavior. Resentment and hostility can arise among siblings if different standards are applied to each child. The nurse's responsibility is to help parents learn successful methods of managing a child's behaviors before they become problems (see Chapter 29).

School-age. For school-age children, the major tasks are entry into school and achieving a sense of *industry.* Although the importance of school in the life of all children is well known, school absences are significantly higher among children with chronic illness than among their healthy peers. The more school absences the child experiences, the more difficult it is to resume attendance, and "school phobia" may result. The child should return to school as soon as possible following diagnosis or treatments.

Preparation for entry into or resumption of school is best accomplished through a team approach with the parents, child, schoolteacher, school nurse, and primary nurse in the

TABLE 38-4 Developmental aspects of chronic illness or disability on children

AGE/DEVELOPMENTAL TASKS	POTENTIAL EFFECTS OF CHRONIC ILLNESS OR DISABILITY	SUPPORTIVE INTERVENTIONS
Infancy		
Develop a sense of trust	Multiple caregivers and frequent separations, especially if hospitalized Deprived of consistent nurturing	Encourage consistent caregivers in hospital or other care settings Encourage parental presence, "rooming in" during hospitalization, and participation in care
Bond/attach to parent	Delayed because of separation, parental grief for loss of "dream" child, parental inability to accept the condition, especially a visible defect	Emphasize healthy, perfect qualities of infant Help parents learn special care needs of infant for them to feel competent
Learn through sensorimotor experiences	Increased exposure to painful experiences over pleasurable ones Limited contact with environment from restricted movement or confinement	Expose infant to pleasurable experiences through all senses (touch, hearing, sight, taste, movement) Encourage age-appropriate developmental skills (e.g., holding bottle, finger feeding, crawling)
Begin to develop a sense of separateness from parent	Increased dependency on parent for care Overinvolvement of parent in care	Encourage all family members to participate in care to prevent overinvolvement of one member Encourage periodic respite from demands of care responsibilities
Toddlerhood		
Develop autonomy Master locomotor and language skills Learn through sensorimotor experience, beginning preoperational thought	Increased dependency on parent Limited opportunity to test own abilities and limits Increased exposure to painful experiences	Encourage independence in as many areas as possible (e.g., toileting, dressing, feeding) Provide gross motor skill activity and modification of toys or equipment such as modified swing or rocking horse Give choices to allow simple feeling of control (e.g., choice of what book to look at or what kind of sandwich to eat) Institute age-appropriate discipline and limitsetting Recognize that negative and ritualistic behavior are normal Provide sensory experiences (e.g., water play, sandbox, finger paint)
Preschool		
Develop initiative and purpose Master self-care skills Begin to develop peer relationships	Limited opportunities for success in accomplishing simple tasks or mastering self-care skills Limited opportunities for socialization with peers; may appear "like a baby" to age-mates Protection within tolerant and secure family may cause child to fear criticism and withdraw	Encourage mastery of self-help skills Provide devices that make task easier (e.g., self-dressing) Encourage socialization (e.g., inviting friends to play, day care experience, trips to park) Provide age-appropriate play, especially associative play opportunities Emphasize child's abilities; dress appropriately to enhance desirable appearance
Develop sense of body image and sexual identification	Awareness of body may center on pain, anxiety, and failure Sex role identification focused primarily on mothering skills	Encourage relationships with same-sex and opposite-sex peers and adults Help child with criticisms; realize that too much protection prevents child from realities of world
Learn through preoperational thought (magical thinking)	Guilt (thinking he or she caused the illness/disability or is being punished for wrongdoing)	Clarify that cause of child's illness or disability is not his or her fault or a punishment
School age		
Develop a sense of accomplishment	Limited opportunities to achieve and compete (e.g., many school absences or inability to join regular athletic activities)	Encourage school attendance; schedule medical visits at times other than school; encourage child to make up missed work Educate teachers and classmates about child's condition, abilities, and special needs
Form peer relationships Learn through concrete operations	Limited opportunities for socialization Incomplete comprehension of the imposed physical limitations or treatment of the disorder	Encourage sports activities (e.g., Special Olympics) Encourage socialization (e.g., Girl Scouts, Campfire, Boy Scouts, 4-H Clubs, having a best friend or club membership) Provide child with knowledge about his or her condition Encourage creative activities (e.g., Very Special Arts)

TABLE 38-4 Developmental aspects of chronic illness or disability on children—cont'd

AGE/DEVELOPMENTAL TASKS	POTENTIAL EFFECTS OF CHRONIC ILLNESS OR DISABILITY	SUPPORTIVE INTERVENTIONS
Adolescence		
Develop personal and sexual identity	Increased sense of feeling different from peers and less able to compete with peers in appearance, abilities, special skills	Realize that many of the difficulties the teenager is experiencing are part of normal adolescence (rebelliousness, risk taking, lack of cooperation, hostility toward authority)
Achieve independence from family	Increased dependency on family; limited job/career opportunities	Provide instruction on interpersonal and coping skills Encourage socialization with peers, including peers with special needs and those without special needs
Form heterosexual relationships	Limited opportunities for heterosexual friendships; less opportunity to discuss sexual concerns with peers	Provide instruction on decision making, assertiveness, and other skills necessary to manage personal plans
Learn through abstract thinking	Increased concern with issues such as why did he or she get the disorder, can he or she marry and have a family Decreased opportunity for earlier stages of cognition may impede achieving level of abstract thinking	Encourage increased responsibility for care and management of the disease or condition, (e.g., assuming responsibility for making and keeping appointment [ideally alone], sharing assessment and planning stages of health care delivery, contacting resources) Encourage activities appropriate for age (e.g., attending mixed-sex parties, sports activities, driving a car) Be alert to cues that signal readiness for information regarding implications of condition on sexuality and reproduction Emphasize good appearance and wearing stylish clothes, use of makeup Understand that adolescent has same sexual needs and concerns as any other teenager Discuss planning for future and how condition can affect choices

hospital. Ideally this planning should begin before hospital discharge, provided the child is well enough to resume usual activities. A structured plan should be developed, with attention to those aspects of care that must be continued during school hours, such as administration of medication or other treatments.

Children also need individual preparation before entering or resuming school. Having a tutor in the hospital or home as soon as children are physically able helps them realize that school will continue and gives them time to consider this prospect (Fig. 38-4). They need to investigate possible answers to the many questions others will ask. One method of anticipatory preparation is to role play, with the child as the "returned pupil" and the nurse or parent as "other schoolmates." If the child returns to school with some obvious physical change such as hair loss, amputation, or visible scar, the nurse might also ask questions about these alterations to prompt preparatory responses from the child.

Classroom peers also need preparation; a joint plan of the schoolteacher, nurse, and child is best. At a minimum the classmates should be given a description of the child's condition, prepared for any visible changes in the child, and allowed an opportunity to ask questions. The child should have the option of attending this session. As the child's condition changes, particularly if the illness is potentially fatal, school personnel, including the students, need periodic appraisal of the child's status and preparation for what to expect.

Children with special needs are encouraged to maintain or reestablish relationships with peers and to participate accord-

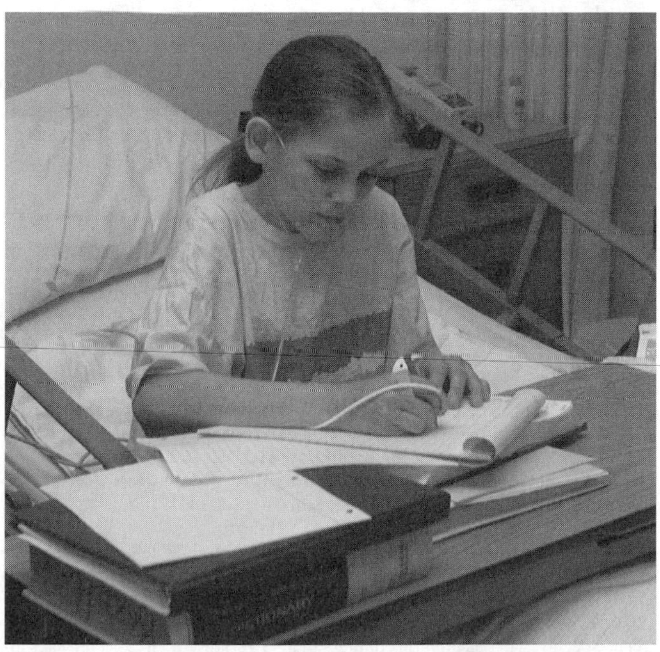

Fig. 38-4 Children with special needs should continue their schooling as soon as their condition permits.

ing to their capabilities in any age-appropriate activities. Alternative activities may be substituted for those that are impossible or that place a strain on the child's condition. Programs such as the Special Olympics* offer children an opportunity to compete with their peers and to achieve athletic skill. Summer camps† allow children to associate with peers and develop a wide variety of skills. Children with special needs can derive enormous benefits from expressive activities such as art, music, poetry, dance, and drama. With adaptive equipment and imagination, children can participate in a variety of activities. Organizations such as Very Special Arts offer children an opportunity to celebrate and share their accomplishments.‡ Children need the opportunity to interact with healthy peers, as well as to engage in activities with groups or clubs composed of similarly affected age-mates.

Adolescence. Adolescence can be a particularly difficult period for the teenager and family. All the needs discussed before apply to this age group as well. Developing *independence* or *autonomy*, however, is a major task for the adolescent as planning for the future becomes a prominent concern. Although the emphasis in the past has been on achieving independence from physical assistance, recent developments in the fields of special education, adolescent development, and family systems suggest redefining autonomy in terms of individuals' capacities to take responsibility for their own behavior, to make decisions regarding their own lives, and to maintain supportive social relationships. Given this understanding, even individuals with severe impairment can be viewed as autonomous if they perceive their own needs and take responsibility for meeting them—either directly or by engaging the assistance of others. As adolescents become more autonomous, the nurse can help them express their needs, participate in developing their own plan of care, and discover and articulate how others can be of greatest assistance.

Physical symptoms are high on the teenager's list of health-related concerns. Because adolescence is a time of enormous physical and emotional changes, it is important for the nurse to make a distinction between body changes that are related to disability and those that are a result of normal body development. It can be a great comfort for teenagers with disabling conditions to know that many of the changes they experience are normal developmental outcomes.

A sense of feeling different from peers can lead to loneliness, isolation, and depression. Participation in groups of teenagers with chronic conditions or disabilities can alleviate feelings of isolation and smooth the transition to a meaningful relationship with one person in adulthood.

*1350 New York Ave., N.W., Suite 500, Washington, DC 20005-1581; (202) 628-3630. Several pamphlets are available from the **National Easter Seal Society,** 70 E. Lake St., Chicago, IL 60601, (312) 726-6200, and the **American Alliance for Health, Physical Education, Recreation and Dance (AAHPERD),** 1900 Association Dr., Reston, VA 22091, (703) 476-3400, on sports and recreation for children with disabilities.

†A directory of camps for children with a variety of chronic illnesses or general physical disabilities is available for a fee from **American Camping Association,** Publications Service, 5000 State Rd., 67 N., Martinsville, IN 46151; (800) 428-CAMP.

‡Very Special Arts has affiliate chapters in all 50 states and in selected sites internationally—yearly festivals are held throughout the world. Information is available from **Very Special Arts,** Education Office, John F. Kennedy Center for the Performing Arts, Washington, DC 20566; (202) 628 2800.

Establish Realistic Future Goals

One of the most difficult adjustments is setting realistic future goals for the child and for those involved in his or her continued care. Sometimes the impact of this decision does not surface until the child finishes school or the parents near retirement, when a crisis can arise because all the family roles and relationships that maintained stability are now disrupted.

Planning for the future should be a gradual process. All along the parents should cultivate realistic vocations for the child. For example, if children have physical disabilities, they are directed to intellectual, artistic, or musical pursuits. Children with developmental disabilities are taught manual skills. In this way the child's development proceeds in the direction of self-support through gainful employment.

With prolonged survival young people with chronic illnesses must deal with new decisions and problems such as marriage, employment, and insurance coverage. With appropriate guidance, gainful employment, marriage, and a family are attainable goals. For those whose conditions are genetic, there is the need for counseling regarding future offspring. Prospective spouses often benefit from an opportunity to discuss their feelings regarding marriage to an individual with continued health needs and possibly a limited life span. Health insurance coverage is a critical issue because some private carriers may no longer insure a young person who leaves home or may be unwilling to reinsure the person who is independent. Life insurance is another dilemma, especially when children have serious defects such as congenital heart anomalies.

Unfortunately vocational pursuits and completely independent living are not realistic goals for all persons. Persons with multiple or severe disabilities may require lifelong care and assistance. In these situations parents must look to the time when they will no longer be able to care for their child. Residential placement may be very difficult unless the family mutually participates in the decision making and planning process. Placement outside the home should not be viewed as abandonment. Frequently it is the only way to preserve the family unit. The nurse should help the family investigate suitable placements, discuss their feelings regarding this decision, and help the family explore measures to maintain meaningful communication between family members.

Evaluation

The effectiveness of nursing interventions is determined by continual reassessment and evaluation of care based on the following observational guidelines and expected outcomes:

1. Observe family members' responses to the diagnosis and the types of questions or concerns that they have.
2. Interview family regarding their knowledge and understanding of the child's condition; observe if they have instituted suggestions such as the use of identification devices for children with certain conditions.
3. Observe the response of professionals to reactions such as denial, guilt, and anger and whether supportive interventions are used with the family.
4. Observe family's communication patterns with each other and their ability to discuss feelings about issues such as the impact of the child's condition on the marriage or additional care responsibilities; investi-

Nursing Care Plan

THE CHILD WITH CHRONIC ILLNESS OR DISABILITY

Nursing Diagnosis: Altered growth and development related to chronic illness, disability, parent overbenevolence, repeated hospitalization

Expected Outcomes: Patient will exhibit appropriate physical, psychosocial and cognitive development for age and abilities.

• **NURSING INTERVENTIONS/*RATIONALES***
See Table 38-4.

Nursing Diagnosis: Altered family processes related to situational crises (child with chronic disease/disability)

Expected Outcomes Family will exhibit adaptation of usual roles and will function to accommodate special needs of child; family will exhibit growth-promoting behaviors.

• **NURSING INTERVENTIONS/*RATIONALES***

Provide opportunity for family to absorb and adjust to diagnosis (i.e., repeat information *to allow time for family to hear and understand;* encourage expression of concerns, fears, and feelings about diagnosis and potential impact *to facilitate adjustment;* and identify support systems *to provide resources for coping*).

Assist family to understand expected treatment, rationale, and implications *to provide a sound basis for decision making.*

Explore family reaction to the child; assist them to achieve a realistic view of child's abilities and limitations; encourage family in attempts to promote child growth and development; have family emphasize what child can do; and explore ways for family to include child in family activities *to help family increase abilities to cope with and incorporate child into family structure.*

Arrange for and participate in family conferences *to provide forum for communication, mutual goal setting and effective strategizing.*

Have parents spend special time with siblings *so that they don't feel neglected or left out.*

Identify additional resource systems (i.e., relatives, friends, church, health care services, community programs) and strategize with family about making good use of these systems *to develop broad base of support.*

Provide a system of ongoing follow up and evaluation to *ensure long-term adaptation to challenges presented to family functioning by a child with chronic disease/disability.*

Nursing Diagnosis: Risk for injury related to physical/developmental limitations

Expected Outcomes: Child will remain free of injury and will exhibit appropriate adaptation to limitations.

• **NURSING INTERVENTIONS/*RATIONALES***

Survey environment for hazards; institute needed safety measures *to decrease risk of injury.*

Encourage use of necessary assistive devices *to enhance safety.*

Help child and parents to identify activities that are appropriate for child's abilities and limitations and encourage participation *to maximize abilities and limit injury.*

Explore limits and rationale for them with child; encourage older child to take responsibility for own safety *to promote involvement of child in care.*

Confer with school nurse, teacher, coach, counselor as needed about special needs *to ensure safe school environment.*

Nursing Diagnosis: Impaired social interaction related to repeated hospitalizations, confinement, activity intolerance

Expected Outcome: Child will engage in appropriate family and peer interactions.

• **NURSING INTERVENTIONS/*RATIONALES***

Encourage regular school attendance and promote peer contacts *to provide opportunity to develop and maintain peer relationships.*

Encourage selection of play activities and recreational outlets *that encourage interaction;* restrict time spent in solo activities *that promote social isolation.*

Encourage contact with peers and siblings by telephone or visit when hospitalized or confined *to maintain social interaction and reduce sense of isolation.*

Plan in specific periods of developmentally appropriate diversional activity suited to child's physical condition and energy level *to decrease feelings of boredom and negative self-absorption.*

Nursing Diagnosis: Self-care deficit related to illness/disability

Expected Outcome: Child will engage in self-care activities commensurate with capabilities.

• **NURSING INTERVENTIONS/*RATIONALES***

Encourage child to assist in self-care activities as age and capabilities permit, and discourage parents from doing it for the child *to foster independence and confidence in abilities.*

Modify environment, introduce use of assistive devices and specialized equipment, and devise alternative methods of completing tasks as needed *to facilitate maximum functioning.*

Use therapeutic play and adapted toys *to increase developmental and functional abilities and encourage cooperation of child.*

Emphasize child's abilities, praise effort and accomplishments, and promote and reinforce successful endeavors *to foster a sense of self-esteem and competence.*

Nursing Diagnosis: Body image/self-esteem disturbances related to perception of illness/disability, feeling of being different

Continued.

Nursing Care Plan

THE CHILD WITH CHRONIC ILLNESS OR DISABILITY—CONT'D

Expected Outcome: Child will demonstrate acceptance of self, physical appearance, and physical and developmental abilities.

• NURSING INTERVENTIONS/*RATIONALES*

Relate to child on appropriate cognitive level conveying an attitude of caring and acceptance *to encourage positive feelings about self;* serve as role model for others *to foster positive attitudes of acceptance toward child.*

Encourage child to verbalize feelings and perceptions about the disease/disability (e.g., repeated treatments and hospitalizations, feelings of being different, implications of functional limits, difficulty in making friends, views of self) *to facilitate coping and open expression of problems, fears, wants, wishes and needs.*

Have child identify strengths, assets, and things he or she likes about self *to increase positive feelings about self and abilities.*

Support positive coping behaviors.

Introduce child to other children who have similar disabilities, and arrange for support groups for child and parents *to increase coping skills.*

Refer child for counseling if needed *to enhance adaptation.*

Encourage use of regular hygiene and grooming practices *to promote positive appearance.*

gate family's use of services, such as self-help groups or other community resources.

5. Perform a developmental screening test on young children and compare the result to expected milestones for the child's abilities; investigate the use of functional aids to assist children in developing to their potential; question family about the child's attendance at school and interaction with peers.
6. Interview family to determine whether their self-identified needs and concerns have been adequately addressed.

Expected outcomes:

See the Nursing Care Plan on pp. 1147-1148.

Nursing Care of the Family and Child Who Is Terminally Ill or Dying

UNEXPECTED CHILDHOOD DEATH

In sudden, unexpected death, the family is deprived of any of the advantages of anticipatory grief. There is no opportunity to prepare oneself or others for the death and no time to complete "unfinished business"; initial denial may be very strong. Because of this lack of time to prepare, many families feel great guilt and remorse for not having done something additional or different with the child. For example, they may berate themselves for depriving the child of some desired material object or privilege or, more painfully, for not having prevented the sudden death in some way. "If only I'd been a better parent" is a common feeling at this time.

Nursing intervention for families who experience the sudden death of a child must be sensitive to the special needs and concerns of these families. Box 38-7 outlines four major areas for intervention with survivors of sudden death. Arriving at the hospital and awaiting news of the child's condition is a vulnerable time. The communication of the child's death must be done with great sensitivity; and the physician or nurse should be prepared to handle feelings of denial, guilt, and anger without judgment. Offering an opportunity to view the body, even if it is disfigured, can be important, since a parent's imagined view of the child is often worse than the reality. Informing the family of what to expect when they view the child can lessen the shock. The need for autopsy and the fact that it will not influence an open viewing at a funeral should be explained. Finally, formal closure and follow-up with the family are important.

Families who experience a child's sudden death may experience recurrent memories of both the child and the death experience and may long grieve over missed opportunities (Kachoyeanos and Selder, 1993). Support and resource groups that may be useful to families include the Sudden Infant Death Syndrome Alliance,* National Sudden Infant Death Syndrome Resource Center,† American Sudden Infant Death Syndrome Institute,‡ Mothers Against Drunk Driving,§ and National Organization of Parents of Murdered Children, Inc.||

ANTICIPATED DEATH

When death is anticipated, a terminal phase, the time of dying before the actual death, presents the opportunity for the family to make plans in advance, such as where the child should spend the last days or what type of funeral arrangements are desired. When death is unexpected, the shock is sufficient to render the survivors incapable of making even simple decisions. Those in attendance at the death and those car-

*10500 Little Patuxent Parkway, Suite 420, Columbia, MD 21044; (800) 221-7437.

†8201 Greensboro Dr., Suite 600, McLean, VA 22102; (703) 821-8955.

‡6065 Roswell Rd., Suite 876, Atlanta, GA 30328; (800) 232-SIDS (in Georgia: [800] 847-SIDS).

§P.O. Box 541688, Dallas, TX 75354-1688; (800) 438-6233.

||100 E. 8th St., Rm. B41, Cincinnati, OH 45202; (513) 721-5683.

BOX 38-7
Strategies for Intervention with Survivors of Sudden Childhood Death

Arrival of the family

Meet the family immediately and escort to a private area.
A health care worker with bereavement training should remain with the family.
Provide information about the extent of illness or injury and treatment efforts.
If the health care worker must leave the family or the family requests privacy, return in 15 minutes so the family does not feel forgotten.
Provide tissues, telephone, coffee, and a Bible.

Pronouncement of death

When available, the family's own physician should inform them of the child's death.
Alternatively, the physician or nurse should introduce themselves and establish calm, reassuring eye contact with the parents.
Honest, clear communication that avoids misinterpretation is essential.
Nonverbal communication such as hugging, touching, or remaining with the family in silence may be most empathetic.
Acknowledge the family's guilt, attempt to alleviate it, and deal openly and nonjudgmentally with anger.
Provide information, answer questions, and offer reassurance that everything possible was done for the child.

Viewing the body

Offer the parents the opportunity to see the body; repeat the offer later if they decline.
Before viewing, inform the parents of bodily changes they should expect (tubes, injuries, cold skin).
A single staff member should accompany the family but remain inconspicuous.
Offer the opportunity to hold the child.
Allow the family as much time as they need.
Offer parents the opportunity for siblings to view the body.

Formal concluding process

Discuss and answer questions concerning autopsy and funeral arrangements; obtain signatures on the body release and autopsy forms.
Provide anticipatory guidance regarding symptoms of grief response and their normalcy.
Provide written materials about grief symptoms.
Escort the family to the exit or to their car if necessary.
Provide a follow-up phone call in 24 to 48 hours to answer questions and provide support.
Provide referrals to local support and resource groups (bereavement groups, bereavement counselors, SIDS groups, Parents of Murdered Children, and Mothers against Drunk Driving are examples).

Modified from Back K: Sudden, unexpected pediatric death: caring for the parents, *Pediatr Nurs* 17(6):571-574, 1991.

ing for the dying child can be instrumental in initiating discussions that may facilitate the grief process.

Especially in the traditional hospital setting, many families are not given the option of terminating treatment when cure is unlikely, and staff may be reluctant to make decisions about "no code" or do not resuscitate (DNR) orders (withholding cardiopulmonary resuscitation in response to cardiac arrest). Some of these situations, such as the dying child's right to refuse additional treatment, often pose difficult ethical questions. Of even greater complexity is the cessation of life-sustaining measures such as artificial ventilation or tube feeding in patients who are in a persistent vegetative state.

As the group of health professionals who are most involved with families, nurses are in an excellent position to ensure that families are given the options available to them at the time of death. The nurse's first responsibility is to explore the family's wishes and empower them to be sure the wishes are met (see the Family Focus box on p. 1150). Statements such as, "Tell me about your thoughts for the kind of care you want your child to receive when he [or she] is dying" or, "Have you considered the kinds of interventions you would like us to use when your child is near death?" can begin discussion of this sensitive but critical aspect of terminal care.

To make an informed decision, the family needs an honest appraisal of the child's prognosis, especially if the condition is a sudden illness or injury. Nurses can also assist the family in the decision-making process by minimizing environmental stressors, providing relevant information, discussing relief of pain the child may experience, and encouraging the family to use formal and informal sources of support (relatives, pastors, professionals) as they face difficult decisions (Rushton and Glover 1990). If parents choose "no code," they are assured that this does not mean "no care" and that everything possible will be done to make the child comfortable. For example, the family may wish that oxygen be given to the child for difficult breathing but not want active resuscitation.

Nursing ALERT

Once a decision to not resuscitate is made, it must be communicated to all members of the health team, including a *written* medical order that specifies the exact nature of the treatments that are to be withheld. DNR orders are reviewed on a regular basis.

Another important option for the family should be the choice of hospice* or hospital care for the terminal stage of illness. *Hospital care* refers to the traditional practices of caring for dying patients in an acute care facility; **hospice** is a concept, not necessarily a facility. Its services are to provide palliative care for the child with no reasonable expectation of cure so that he or she can live life to the fullest without pain,

*Information on hospice services for children is available from the **National Hospice Organization,** 1901 N. Moore St., Arlington, VA 22209; (800) 658-8898. A recommended resource is Moldow D, Martinson I: *Home care for seriously ill children: a manual for parents,* available from **Children's Hospice International,** 901 N. Washington St., 7th Floor, Alexandria, VA 22314; (800) 24-CHILD.

Family Focus

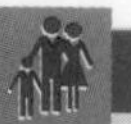

THE FAMILY OF THE DYING CHILD

No matter whether you have a PhD or many children, when your child dies, it is a new experience, and nothing can prepare you for it. Like so many things in life, experience is the best teacher.

Three of our children have died, and by the time the third was dying, we handled many things differently. We learned a lot about dignity and the rights of the child and family. For example, at first we didn't know that we had a right to have our child die at home. We also didn't understand pain medications and that if the child is receiving pain medication and is still in agony, the child has not overdosed.

We learned a lot about case management. With our first two children, lots of different people were making decisions and disagreeing about what was best and what should be done. No one had primary authority. With our third, one doctor took a primary role. Any questions and problems were turfed to one person. I could call him 24 hours a day. It made a lot of difference, and I felt our concerns and needs were better heard and respected.

The nurses caring for our third child at home enabled me to step back and just be his mommy. When I could do this, I realized that we were fighting so hard for his life that we weren't really letting him die. His nurses had worked with him for a long time and really loved him. It was hard for them when we decided to let him die. In his last several days we wanted a lot of family time with our son, and I think the nurses felt left out. Something about their reaction to our increased time with him in the last few days made us feel guilty. If we had all been able to communicate a little more openly, I would have understood that they needed more time with him at the end too. Everyone's needs could have been met.

Jeni Stepanek
Mother
Upper Marlboro, MD

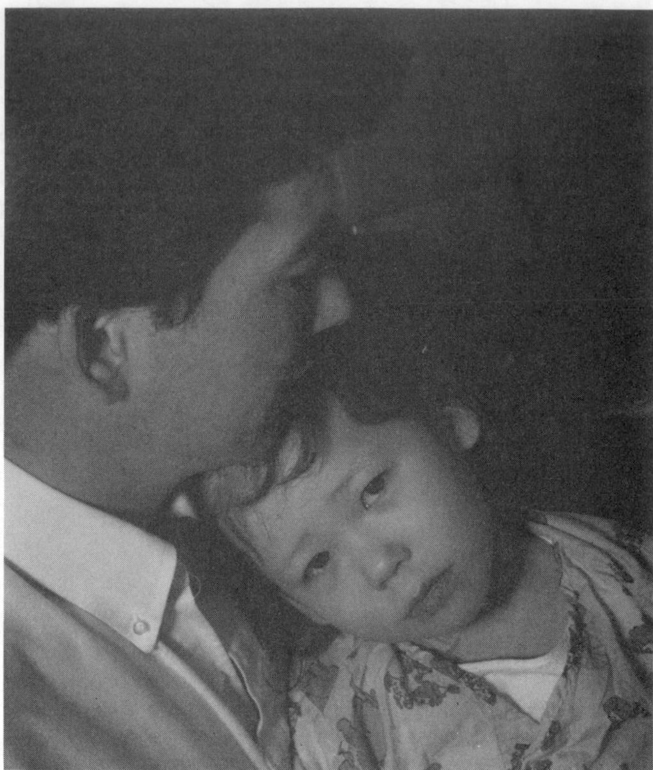

Fig. 38-5 For the dying child there is no greater comfort than the security and closeness of a parent.

with choices and dignity, and with family support (Sumner and Hurula, 1993). The three basic ways of providing hospice care are in a hospice, in a facility that employs the hospice concept, or in the child's home. If the home is chosen, the goal is to enable the child and family to have the best possible quality of life until the time of death. The child may or may not die in the home. Nurses working in hospice settings and with children dying at home are critical members of the health team. They often prepare the family for the home care experience, provide psychologic support for the family, and teach the physical care, especially comfort measures, such as pain control (see Chapter 41).

Regardless of where the child is cared for during the terminal stage, both the child and family commonly experience the following fears: (1) fear of what the actual death will be like, (2) fear of dying alone or not being present when the child dies, and (3) fear of pain. Nurses play a major role in managing care so that each of these fears is lessened. Although no one can predict exactly what the child's death will be like, the nurse can explore the family's expectations, clarify misconceptions, and supply information based on how the death is most likely to occur. Since the child and family have fears of isolation and loneliness, their wishes to be together must be respected (Fig. 38-5). If the family members temporarily leave the child's room, they need reassurance that they will be summoned if the child's condition worsens (see Box 38-8 for signs of approaching death).

All parents want their child's death to be comfortable, and no nursing intervention is more important than control of pain. Pain is managed on a *preventive schedule,* with adjustments made as needed to provide maximum comfort. Optimum pain relief requires using opioid analgesics such as morphine, increasing doses of opioids as needed, decreasing the duration between doses, and changing routes of administration to comply with the child's needs and wishes. Whenever possible, the oral route is preferred, but when that is no longer possible, continuous intravenous or subcutaneous infusion may provide the greatest benefit. Any nonpharmacologic measures that may augment pain relief and promote relaxation are used, such as cutaneous stimulation (e.g., rocking or stroking the skin) or diversion (e.g., reading to the child or playing music). (See also Chapter 41 for a discussion of pain assessment and management.)

The experience of a child with life-threatening illness and/or the child's death has profound effects on the family, including the siblings. Parents may turn to nurses for advice on how to inform siblings of a child's impending death and how to incorporate siblings into the child's final days. When a brother or sister dies, the sibling's reaction will depend on many factors, including the circumstances of the death, the quality of the prior sibling relationship, the age of the child, parental reactions, and family communication patterns (Gibbons, 1992).

Predominant feelings of children when a sibling's diagnosis is potentially fatal, such as serious trauma or a disease such as cancer, include isolation and displacement—the parents devote the majority of their time to caring for the ill or injured child, causing the siblings to feel left out of the parent–sick child partnership and to be regarded as unimportant family members.

Siblings may also express concern for their own health status, recognizing the possibility of death and at times manifesting physical symptoms similar to those of the child. Siblings' knowledge of the ill child's diagnosis is often inadequate, although many children perceive cancer to be the "scariest disease" (Martinson et al, 1990).

Sibling's responses to death arise in part from their cognitive understanding of death. Two common feelings are guilt and shame. Books can be used to help children deal with death (see Bibliography for list of resources).

BOX 38-8

Physical Signs of Approaching Death

Loss of sensation and movement in the lower extremities, progressing toward the upper body
Sensation of heat, although body feels cool
Loss of senses:
- Tactile sensation decreases
- Sensitive to light
- Hearing is last sense to fail

Confusion, loss of consciousness, slurred speech
Muscle weakness
Loss of bowel and bladder control
Decreased appetite/thirst
Difficulty swallowing
Change in respiratory pattern:
- Cheyne-Stokes respirations (waxing and waning of depth of breathing with regular periods of apnea)
- "Death rattle" (noisy chest sounds from accumulation of pulmonary and pharyngeal secretions)

Weak, slow pulse; decreased blood pressure

AT THE TIME OF DEATH

As death approaches, the nurse should both recognize and assist the family to recognize the physical signs (Box 38-8) and institute appropriate care to make the death as peaceful as possible (see Nursing Care Plan, p. 1152). The nurse should explain everything that is being done to make the child comfortable, even if the child does not appear to be coherent. The nurse can offer support to the family by visiting frequently, sitting quietly with them, and attending to their needs such as bringing them some nourishment. Immediately after the death the family is encouraged to stay with the child as long as they wish. Many parents want to hold or rock the child one last time.

A topic that should be considered when a child dies is tissue donation. For some families this may be a meaningful act—one that benefits another human being despite the loss of their child. In centers where transplants are performed, a full-time transplant coordinator is usually available to inform the family about organ donation and to take care of details. If a transplant coordinator's services are not available, the staff needs to decide which members should discuss this topic with the family. Ideally this should be the person who knows the family best, knows when the death is expected, or has the opportunity to spend time with the family when the death is unexpected. Often nurses are in an optimum position to suggest tissue donation after consultation with the attending physician. The request should be made in a private and quiet area of the hospital and should be simple and direct, with questions such as, "Have you ever considered organ donation?" or, "Did [the child's name] ever express such a wish?"* Words such as "options" or "choices" should be used to reiterate that the decision is theirs and that no pressure will be applied. Family members should also be reassured that everything possible has been done or is being done to save their child (Cerney, 1993). Finally, written consent is required. Any number of body tissues or organs can be donated (skin, eyes, bone, kidney, heart, liver, pancreas), and their removal does not mutilate or desecrate the body or cause any suffering. The family may have an open casket, and there is no delay in the funeral. There is no cost to the donor family.

In cases of unexplained death, violent death, or suspected suicide, autopsy is required by law. In other instances it may be optional, and parents should be informed of this choice. The procedure, as well as forms that require signing, should be explained. The family should know that the child can be in an open casket following an autopsy.

At some point the nurse should discuss if the family has made preparations for a burial service and if the staff can help in any way. Parents often have concerns about the funeral, such as siblings' involvement in the death rituals. Although no absolute answers exist regarding the question of siblings attending the funeral or burial services, the general consensus is that the surviving children benefit from being involved in these events. However, children need preparation for postdeath services. They should be told what to expect, particularly how the deceased person will look if the casket is open, allowed their private time to say good-bye, and permitted to stay as long as they wish. Ideally the parents should prepare the siblings. If the parents' grief prevents this communication, a significant family member or friend should substitute.

POSTDEATH

The crisis of loss does not end with the child's death. In many ways it only begins. Unfortunately the child's death often marks the close of the family's contacts with health professionals involved in the care. Consequently, many of these families never receive the support and guidance that could assist them in resolving the loss. Fortunately hospice programs recognize this need and provide regular follow-up after the death. In addition, self-help groups are present in many communities (e.g., The Compassionate Friends,* an international orga-

*Information about being an organ donor is available from **The Living Bank,** P.O. Box 6725, Houston, TX 77265, (800) 528-2971; and **The United Network for Organ Sharing (UNOS),** (800) 24-DONOR.

*P.O. Box 3696, Oak Brook, IL 60522-3696; (708) 990-0010.

Nursing Care Plan

THE CHILD WHO IS TERMINALLY ILL OR DYING

Nursing Diagnosis: Anticipatory grieving related to terminal illness/impending death

Expected Outcomes: **Child will participate in age-appropriate constructive anticipatory grief work and will exhibit free expression of feelings.**

• NURSING INTERVENTIONS/*RATIONALES*

Encourage child to express feelings in own way through play, drawing, or verbalization *to promote free expression in accordance with their specific cognitive and emotional abilities.*

Provide a safe, acceptable outlet for expressions of feelings (e.g., crying, sadness, anger, aggression) *as this is needed part of grieving process.*

Structure the care experience to allow child choices and participation in process within constraints of physical condition *to help child maintain a sense of control and self-esteem.*

Encourage family to remain near child and to stay engaged with child *to provide support and to allay child's fear of being abandoned or no longer being loved.*

Nursing Diagnosis: Pain related to terminal stage of illness

Expected Outcome: **Child will exhibit minimal signs of physical discomfort.**

• NURSING INTERVENTIONS/*RATIONALES*

Provide and encourage family to provide the child's favorite comfort measures (e.g., rocking, stroking, story telling, singing); move and turn carefully; avoid excessive noise or light; use noninvasive care monitoring when possible; limit care to essentials *to minimize discomfort and promote comfort.*

Administer treatments as prescribed (i.e., oxygen *for respiratory distress,* anticonvulsants *for seizures,* analgesics *for pain,* anticholinergics *to decrease secretions) that can cause unpleasant manifestations.*

Talk with child in clear distinct voice *to offer calm reassurance;* avoid whispering or talking about child *to reduce anxiety;* phrase questions to require "yes" or "no" responses *to conserve energy.*

Nursing Diagnosis: Anticipatory grieving related to impending loss of a child

Expected Outcomes: **Family will exhibit evidence of constructive grief process (verbalization/expression of feelings, maintenance of interpersonal relationships, use of support systems and coping mechanisms).**

• NURSING INTERVENTIONS/*RATIONALES*

Spend time with family to listen, answer questions, provide information *as a way to establish trust, demonstrate support and caring.*

Provide opportunities for family to express their emotions and deal with their feelings *as a part of the grieving process.*

Help family to understand the grief process and to accept feelings being experienced (denial, sadness, guilt, anger, relief) as normal part of the process *to enhance understanding and ability to cope.*

Encourage expression and discussion of perceptions of loss and the impact on life of the family *to provide ventilation and reinforcement of reality.*

Keep family informed of child' status, help them interpret child's responses, and encourage their participation in child's care *to allay fears and anxiety and promote involvement.*

Encourage parents to face child's fears and questions about death openly and honestly *to facilitate grief work by child and parents.*

Explore family religious and cultural beliefs related to death (i.e., prayers, rites, rituals) and arrange for appropriate spiritual care if appropriate.

Emphasize family's identified strengths and provide encouragement for decisions that demonstrate effective coping skills *to help reinforce ability to cope.*

When death is imminent, allow the family privacy and time to be with and hold, touch, and/or talk to the child *to facilitate saying goodbye.*

At death, allow family to remain with child's body for as long as they wish, to rock, hold, bathe or talk with child *to facilitate grieving.*

Be physically present with the family, offer nonverbal comfort, touch if appropriate; help them move through the process of leaving the facility (i.e., gathering belongings, checking out) *to provide supportive presence and guidance in next steps.*

Determine support sources (e.g., relatives, friends, church, community) and how they can help with disruptions that occur in life-style (e.g., arrangements, activities of daily living, finances, transportation) *to bolster coping and provide needed support during crisis.*

Refer family to grief counseling if indicated *to aid in coping and to prevent dysfunctional grieving.*

Initiate and maintain contact, attend the funeral, visitation, or memorial service if there was a special closeness with family *to facilitate grief process and termination of therapeutic relationship with caregiver.*

nization for bereaved parents and siblings, and specialty groups such as Parents of Murdered Children†).

Follow-up can help the family understand the process of mourning, particularly its duration and pain, and can provide assistance in making decisions that involve the loss. One especially difficult dilemma faced by many parents is the decision to have additional children. The advisability of having another child soon after the death is controversial. Consequently, the nurse's role is not to give answers but to assist parents in assessing their readiness for another pregnancy through knowledge of the parents' progress through grief and their motivations for conceiving.

At times family members may need assistance in their grieving. (See the Guidelines box to the right.) Mothers in particular often feel a great sense of loneliness and emptiness, and part of resolving their grief is finding a substitute role that is fulfilling and rewarding. Nurses can be instrumental in this process by (1) preparing the mother for anticipating the *normal* feelings of emptiness, loneliness, and sometimes even failure; (2) helping her reevaluate her role as parent and spouse, stressing that giving up the lost child must occur before she can reestablish emotional relationships; (3) encouraging her to explore fulfilling activities that use her special interests, talents, and qualifications; and (4) supporting her as her role changes, particularly assisting with communication between affected family members.

Nurses should also be aware of behaviors that indicate siblings' difficulty with resolving their grief such as persistent blame and guilt, patterns of overactivity with aggressive and destructive outbursts, compulsive caregiving, persistent anxieties (such as fear of another family death or of their own), excessive clinging to the parent, difficulty with forming new relationships, problems at school, or delinquency (such as stealing). Providing anticipatory guidance to parents regarding behaviors to watch for may be helpful. Even siblings as young as 2 years of age can experience survivor guilt (Gibbons, 1992). In these situations professional assistance may be required, and the nurse can provide appropriate referral.

Communication with the bereaved family is essential, but often there is a feeling of not knowing what to say and of helplessness in offering words of comfort. The most supportive approach is to avoid judging the family's reactions or offering advice or rationalizations and to focus on feelings. Perhaps the most valuable supportive measure the nurse can perform for families is to listen (Parkman, 1992). Families understand that no words will relieve their pain; all they want is acceptance, understanding, and respect for their grief. A plan for regular follow-up with bereaved families can be beneficial.

The crisis of loss does not end with the child's death. In many ways it only begins. It is important for families to understand that mourning takes a long time. Whereas acute grief may last only weeks or months, resolving the loss is measured in years. Holidays and anniversaries can be particularly difficult, and people who previously had been supportive may now expect the family to have "adjusted." Consequently, prolonged mourning is often silent and lonely.

Many families never receive the support and guidance that could help them resolve the loss. At a minimum, one follow-up phone call or meeting with the family should be arranged,

†100 E. 8th St., Rm. B41, Cincinnati, OH 45202; (513) 721-5683.

Guidelines

SUPPORTING GRIEVING FAMILIES*

General

Stay with the family; sit quietly if they prefer not to talk; cry with them if desired.

Accept the family's grief reactions; avoid judgmental statements (e.g., "You should be feeling better by now").

Avoid offering rationalizations for the child's death (e.g., "You should be glad your child isn't suffering anymore").

Avoid artificial consolation (e.g., "I know how you feel," or "You are still young enough to have another baby").

Deal opening with feelings such as guilt, anger, and loss of self-esteem.

Focus on feelings by using a feeling word in the statement (e.g., "You're still feeling all the pain of losing a child").

Refer the family to an appropriate self-help group or for professional help if needed.

At the time of death

Reassure the family that everything possible is being done for the child, if they wish lifesaving interventions.

Do everything possible to ensure the child's comfort, especially relieving pain.

Provide the child and family the opportunity to review special experiences or memories in their lives.

Express personal feelings of loss and/or frustrations (e.g., "We will miss him so much," or "We tried everything; we feel so sorry that we couldn't save him").

Provide information that the family requests and be honest.

Respect the emotional needs of family members such as siblings, who may need brief respites from the dying child.

Make every effort to arrange for family members, especially parents, to be with the child at the moment of death, if they wish to be present.

Allow the family to stay with the dead child for as long as they wish and to rock, hold, or bathe the child.

Provide practical help when possible, such as collecting the child's belongings.

Arrange for spiritual support such as clergy; pray with the family if no one else can stay with them.

After the death

Attend the funeral or visitation if there was a special closeness with the family.

Initiate and maintain contact (e.g., sending cards, telephoning, inviting them back to the unit, or making a home visit).

Refer to the dead child by name; discuss shared memories with the family.

Discourage the use of drugs or alcohol as a method of escaping grief.

Encourage all family members to communicate their feelings rather than remaining silent to avoid upsetting another member.

Emphasize that grieving is a painful process that often takes years to resolve.

*"Family" refers to all significant persons involved in the child's life, such as the parents, siblings, grandparents, or other close relatives or friends.

possibly 1 month after the child's death, to give the family time to overcome the phase of shock and disbelief (Jankovic et al, 1989). Families can also be referred to self-help groups. When such groups are not available, nurses can be instrumental in networking families or facilitating parent and sibling groups. Formal bereavement programs or bereavement counseling can be helpful as well.*

NURSES' REACTIONS TO CARING FOR DYING CHILDREN

The death of a patient is one of the most stressful aspects of critical care or oncology nursing (see the Family Focus box to the right). Nurses experience reactions to a fatal illness that are very similar to the responses of family members. These include denial, anger, depression, guilt, and ambivalent feelings.

Strategies that can assist the nurse in maintaining the ability to work effectively in these settings include maintaining good general health, developing well-rounded interests, using distancing techniques such as taking time off when needed, developing and using professional and personal support systems, cultivating the capacity for empathy, focusing on the positive aspects of the caregiver role, and basing nursing interventions on sound theory and empiric observations.

Attending shared remembrance rituals assists some nurses in resolving grief (Zappa and Parks, 1993). Similarly, attending the funeral services can be a supportive act for both the family and the nurse and in no way detracts from the professionalism of care.

Family Focus

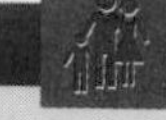

A DYING CHILD—A NURSE'S PERSPECTIVE

Claire was unresponsive with slow, grasping breathing. Her mother asked me what I thought was going on. I replied honestly, "Your baby is dying because of her brain tumor." The mother put her arms around me and cried. We arranged for Claire to be baptized.

Painful as the loss of a child is, my job is to assist the family through this experience. Although I usually wait until a private moment such as driving home, I found tears streaming down my face as family and friends gathered for Claire's baptism. I went into the kitchen to compose myself, only to find several of my colleagues crying. Saying goodbye to a dying child will always be a difficult but shared experience.

Jeanne O'Connor Egan, RN, MSN
Children's Hospital
Washington, DC

*A manual that can be useful in the development of a family-centered bereavement program is: Rose T, Stewart ES (1993): *Whispers of hope: a hospital-based program for bereaved parents and their families,* available from **Duke University Pediatric Brain Tumor Family Support Program,** Durham, NC, 27710; (919) 684-5301.

Key Points

- Trends in the treatment of children with chronic illness or disability have focused on developmental age, the child's strengths and uniqueness, family-centered care, establishment of normalization, early discharge, home care, mainstreaming, and early intervention.
- Families' reactions to disability or chronic illness are manifested in the following stages: shock and denial, adjustment, reintegration and acknowledgment.
- Assessment of the family's adjustment to a child's chronic illness, disability, or death includes the availability of a support system, their perception of the event, their coping mechanisms, concurrent stressors, and their response to the child.
- To help parents cope with their child's chronic illness or disability, nurses must offer attentiveness, humanistic support, solicitation of suggestions for care, facilitation of communication, verbalization of feelings, and referral to volunteer and community agencies.
- Supporting the child involves encouraging self-expression, alleviating feelings of being different, and strengthening self-image.
- Acute grief is a syndrome with intense and distressing psychologic and somatic symptoms that appear at the time of death.
- Mourning is a prolonged, painful process that consists of four phases: shock and disbelief, expression of grief, disorganization and despair, and reorganization.
- In response to the child with chronic illness or disability, parents may be affected by feelings of inadequacy and failure; excessive demands on time, energy, and financial resources; and strain on the marital relationship.
- The child's reaction to illness or disability depends on developmental level, coping mechanisms, others' reactions, and the illness itself.
- Children's concept of death is determined by their cognitive ability and their experience with life-threatening illness.
- Young children see death as temporary and reversible and mainly fear separation.
- School-age children view death as irreversible but not necessarily inevitable and may fear mutilation.
- Children beyond 9 or 10 years realize death is irreversible, universal, and inevitable but may resist the thought of their own death.
- Siblings have special needs, including the need for information, reassurarnce about their own health status, assurance that they are not responsible for the illness or death, and support for their own grieving process.
- Special needs of the family facing the unexpected death of a child include support while awaiting news of the child's status; a sensitive pronouncement of death, acknowledgement of feelings of denial, guilt and anger; an opportunity to view the body; closure; and referrals for support.

- Special decisions at the time of dying and death may involve hospital or hospice care, the child's right to die, visualization of the body, tissue donation/autopsy, and siblings' attendance at the funeral.
- In dealing with stress related to the dying patient, the nurse can cope successfully through self-awareness, consciousness raising, knowledge and practice, available support system, maintaining general good health, and focusing on the positive rewards of involvement with dying children and their families.

References

Ahmann E, Bond NJ: Promoting normal development in school age children and adolescents who are technology dependent: a family centered model, *Pediatr Nurs* 18(4):399-405, 1992

Austin J, Patterson J, Huberty T: Development of the Coping Health Inventory for Children, *J Pediatr Nurs* 6(3):166-174, 1991.

Baker NA: Avoiding collisions with challenging families, *AM J Matern Child Nurs* 19:97-101, 1994.

Bishop KK, Woll J, Arango P: *Family/professional collaboration for children with special health needs,* Burlington, Vt, 1993, Department of Social Work, University of Vermont.

Bluebond-Langner M: Worlds of dying children and their well siblings, *Death Studies* 13:1-16, 1989.

Breitmayer BJ et al: Social competence of school aged children with chronic illnesses, *J Pediatr Nurs* 7(3):181-188, 1992.

Burns C, Madian N: Experiences with a support group for grandparents of children with disabilities, *Pediatr Nurs* 18(1):17-21, 1992.

Cancer facts and figures—1994, Atlanta, 1994, American Cancer Society.

Cerney MS: Solving the organ donor shortage by meeting the bereaved family's needs, *Crit Care Nurs* 13(1):32-36, 1993.

Clements D, Copeland L, Loftus M: Critical times for families with a chronically ill child, *Pediatr Nurs* 16(2):157-161, 224, 1990.

Clubb R: Chronic sorrow: adaptation patterns of parents with chronically ill children, *Pediatr Nurs* 17(5):461-466, 1991.

Corr CA: Coping with dying: lessons that we should and should not learn from the work of Elisabeth Kübler-Ross, *Death Stud* 17(1):69-83, 1993.

Dixon DM: *Parent participation during hospitalization: understanding differences,* Springfield, Ill, 1993, Memorial Medical Center (unpublished manuscript).

Ferrell BR et al: The experience of pediatric cancer pain. Part I, Impact of pain on the family, *J Pediatr Nurs* 9(6):368-379, 1994.

Gallo A et al: Well siblings of children with chronic illness: parents' reports of their psychologic adjustment, *Pediatr Nurs* 18(1):23-27, 1992.

Garmezy N: Resilience in children's adaptation to negative life events and stressed environments, *Pediatr Ann* 20(9):459-466, 1991.

Gibbons M: A child dies, a child survives: the impact of sibling loss, *J Pediatr Health Care* 6(2):65-72, 1992.

Groce NE, Zola IK: Multiculturalism, chronic illness, and disability, *Pediatrics* 91(5):1048-1055, 1993.

Hills RG, Lutkenhoff ML: Social skills group for physically challenged school-age children, *Pediatr Nurs* 19(6):573-577, 1993.

Huber C, Holditch-Davis D, Brandon D: High risk preterm infants at 3 years of age: parental response to the presence of developmental problems, *Child Health Care* 22(2):107, 124, 1993.

Jankovic M et al: Meetings with parents after the death of their child from leukemia, *Pediatr Hematol Oncol* 6:155-160, 1989.

Kachoyeanos MK, Selder FE: Life transitions of parents at the unexpected death of a school age and older child, *J Pediatr Nurs* 8(1):41-49, 1993.

Kübler-Ross E: *On death and dying,* New York, 1969, MacMillan.

Martinson IM et al: Impact of childhood cancer on healthy school-age siblings, *Cancer Nurs* 13(3):183-190, 1990.

May J: *Fathers of children with special needs: new horizons,* Washington, DC, 1990, Association for the Care of Children's Health.

Newacheck PW, Stoddard JJ, McManus M: Ethnocultural variations in the prevalence and impact of childhood chronic conditions, *Pediatrics* 91(5)1031-1039, 1993.

Newacheck PW, McManus MA, Fox HB: Prevalence and impact of chronic illness among adolescents, *Am J Dis Child* 145(12):1367-1373, 1991.

Parkman S: Helping families say good-bye, *MCN* 17(1):14-17, 1992.

Rushton CH, Glover JJ: Involving parents in decisions to forego life-sustaining treatment for critically ill infants and children, *AACN Clin Issues Crit Care Nurs* 1(1):206-214, 1990.

Satariano JH, Briggs NJ: The good family syndrome, *Pediatr Nurs* 15(3):285-286, 1989.

Savinetti-Rose B: Developmental issues in managing children with diabetes, *Pediatr Nurs* 20(1):11-15, 1994.

Stein REK: Home care: a challenging opportunity, *Child Health Care* 14(2):90-95, 1985.

Sumner L, Hurula J: Pediatric hospice nursing: making the most of each moment, *Nursing '93,* August 1993, pp. 50-55.

Turner-Henson A, et al: The experiences of discrimination: challenges for chronically ill children, *Pediatr Nurs* 20(6):571-577, 1994.

Yoos HL: Children's illness concepts: old and new paradigms, *Pediatr Nurs* 20(2):134-140, 1994.

Zappa S, Parks G: A remembrance ceremony to help families and staff work through the grieving process, *J Pediatr Oncol Nurs* 10(2):65-66, 1993. (abstract).

Bibliography

Chronic Illness/Disability

Ahmann E, Lierman C: Promoting normal development in technology-dependent children: an introduction to the issues, *Pediatr Nurs* 18(2):143-148, 1992.

Ahmann E, Lipsi K: Developmental assessment of the technology-dependent infant and young child, *Pediatr Nurs* 18(3):299-305, 1992.

American Academy of Pediatrics, Committee on Children with Disabilities: Pediatric services for infants and children with special health care needs, *Pediatrics* 92(1):163-165, 1993.

Baker NA: Avoiding collisions with challenging families, *MCN* 19:97-101, 1994.

Bluebond-Langner M et al: Children's knowledge of cancer and its treatment: impact of an oncology camp experience, *J Pediatr* 116(2):207-213, 1990.

Bossert E, Martinson I: Kinetic family drawings—revised: a method of determining the impact of cancer on the family as perceived by the child with cancer, *J Pediatr Nurs* 5(3):204-213, 1990.

Bossert E et al: Strategies of normalization used by parents of chronically ill school-age children, *Child Adolesc Psychiatr Ment Health Nurs* 3(2):57-61, 1990.

Brookins GK: Culture, ethnicity, and bicultural competence: implications for children with chronic illness and disability, *Pediatrics* 91(5, Pt 2):1056-1062, 1993.

Burke S, Roberts C: Nursing research and the care of chronically ill and disabled children, *J Pediatr Nurs* 5(5):316-327, 1990.

Cardoso P: Family-centered care, *Child Health Care* 20(4):258-260, 1991.

Chambas K: Sexual concerns of adolescents with cancer, *J Pediatr Oncol Nurs* 8(4):165-172, 1991.

Cooper E: Helping parents cope with the reality of parenting a child with a disabling condition, *Child Health Care* 20(3):189-190, 1991.

Crowley A: Integrating handicapped and chronically ill children into day care centers, *Pediatr Nurs* 16(1):39-44, 1990.

Davis B, Steele S: Case management for young children with special health care needs, *Pediatr Nurs* 17(1):15-19, 1991.

Davis P, May J: Involving fathers in early intervention and family support programs: issues and strategies, *Child Health Care* 20(2):87-92, 1991.

Deatrick JA, Knafl KA: Management behaviors: day-to-day adjustments to childhood chronic conditions, *J Pediatr Nurs* 5(1):15-22, 1990.

Diehl S, Moffitt K, Wade S: Focus group interview with parents of children with medically complex needs: an intimate look at their perceptions and feelings, *Child Health Care* 20(3):170-178, 1991.

Faux S: Sibling relationships in families with congenitally impaired children, *J Pediatr Nurs* 6(3):175-184, 1991.

Fisman S, Wolf L: The handicapped child: psychological effects of parental, marital, and sibling relationships, *Psychiatr Clin North Am* 14(1):199-217, 1991.

Fraley A: Chronic sorrow: a parental response, *J Pediatr Nurs* 5(4):268-273, 1990.

Gallo AM et al: Stigma in childhood chronic illness: a well sibling perspective, *Pediatr Nurs* 17(1):21-25, 1991.

Gallo AM et al: Well siblings of children with chronic illness: parent's reports of their psychologic adjustment, *Pediatr Nurs* 18(1):23-29, 1992.

Heiney SP et al: Lasting impressions: a psychosocial support program for adolescents with cancer and their parents, *Cancer Nurs* 13(1):13-20, 1990.

Hewson M et al: Comprehensive team care, *MCN* 18(4):198-205, 1993.

Hixson D, Stoff E, White P: Parents of children with chronic health impairments: a new approach to advocacy training, *Child Health Care* 21(2):111-115, 1992.

Hockenberry-Eaton M, Minick P: Living with cancer: children with extraordinary courage, *Oncol Nurs Forum* 21(6):1025-1031, 1994.

Jackson B, Finkler D, Robinson C: A case management system for infants with chronic illnesses and developmental disabilities, *Child Health Care* 21(4):224-232, 1992.

Jackson P, Vessey J: *Primary care of the child with a chronic condition*, ed 2, St Louis, 1996, Mosby.

Jellinek MS et al: Coping with the truly difficult parent, *Contemp Pediatr* 8(2):19-49, 1991.

Knafl KA et al: Learning from stories: parents' accounts of the pathway to diagnosis, *Pediatr Nurs* 21(5):411-415, 1995.

Knafl KA et al: Parent's views of health care providers: an exploration of the components of a positive working relationship, *Child Health Care* 21(2):90-95, 1992.

Krahn GL, Hallum A, Kime C: Are there good ways to give bad news? *Pediatrics* 91(3):578-582, 1993.

Liptak GS, Weitzman M: Children with chronic conditions need your help at school, *Contemp Pediatr* 12(9):64-80, 1995.

Meeropol E: One of the gang: sexual development of adolescents with physical disabilities, *J Pediatr Nurs* 6(4):243-250, 1991.

Patterson JM et al: Caring for medically fragile children at home: the parent-professional relationship, *J Pediatr Nurs* 9(2):98-106, 1994.

Selekman J, McIlvain-Simpson G: Sex and sexuality for the adolescent with a chronic condition, *Pediatr Nurs* 17(6):535-538, 1991.

Wells PW et al: Growing up in the hospital. I. Let's focus on the child, *J Pediatr Nurs* 9(2):66-73, 1994.

Whyte DA: A family nursing approach to the care of a child with a chronic illness, *J Adv Nurs* 17(3):317-327, 1992.

Zagorsky ES: Caring for families who follow alternative health practices, *Pediatr Nurs* 19(1):71-75, 1993.

Terminal Illness/Death

American Academy of Pediatrics, Committee on Pediatric Emergency Medicine: Death of a child in the emergency department, *Pediatrics* 93(5):861-862, 1994.

Antonacci M: Sudden death: helping bereaved parents in the PICU, *Crit Care Nurse* 10(4):65-70, 1990.

Black KJ: Sudden, unexpected pediatric death: caring for the parents, *Pediatr Nurs* 17(6):571-575, 1991.

Bosworth T: Leukemia through a teenager's eyes, *MCN* 14(2):93-94, 1989.

Brett AS: Limitations of listing specific medical interventions in advance directives, *JAMA* 266(6):825-828, 1991.

Carlson JAS: The psychologic effects of sudden infant death syndrome on parents, *J Pediatr Health Care* 7(2):77-81, 1993.

Cassidy M: Supportive care and the dying child, *J Home Health Care Pract* 3(1):34-38, 1990.

Davies B, Eng B: Factors influencing nursing care of children who are terminally ill, *Pediatr Nurs* 19(1):9-14, 1993.

Davis FD: Organ procurement and transplantation, *Nurs Clin North Am* 24(4):823-836, 1989.

Dufour DF: Home or hospital care for the child with end-stage cancer: effects on the family, *Issues Compr Pediatr Nurs* 12(5):371-383, 1989.

Dychkowski LB: Caring for the terminally ill child in the school setting, *School Nurse* 6(2):8-10, 12, 1990.

Gary GA: Facing terminal illness in children with AIDS: developing a philosophy of care for patients, families, and caregivers, *Home Healthc Nurse* 10(2):40-43, 1992.

Grogan LB: Grief of an adolescent when a sibling dies, *MCN* 15(1):21-24, 1990.

Hall MD: The way it is . . . caring for dying children, *Am J Nurs* 90(7):86, 1990.

Hammer M et al: A ritual of remembrance . . . grief suffered by nurses themselves, *MCN* 17(6):310-313, 1992.

Hoekstra-Weebers JEH et al: A comparison of parental coping styles following the death of adolescent and preadolescent children, *Death Stud* 15(6):565-575, 1991.

Hogan NS, Balk DE: Adolescent reactions to sibling death: perceptions of mothers, fathers, and teenagers, *Nurs Res* 39(2):103-106, 1990.

Jefidoff A, Gasner R: Helping the parents of the dying child: an Israeli experience, *J Pediatr Nurs* 8(6):413-415, 1993.

Jezewski MA et al: Consenting to DNR: critical care nurses' interactions with patients and family members, *Am J Crit Care* 2(4):302-309, 1993.

Kachoyeanos MK, Selder FE: Life transitions of parents at the unexpected death of a school-age and older child, *J Pediatr Nurs* 8(1):41-49, 1993.

Kahn EC: A comparison of family needs based on the presence or absence of DNR orders, *Dimens Crit Care Nurs* 11(5):286-292, 1992.

Mahon MM: Death of a sibling: primary care intervention, *Pediatr Nurs* 20(3):293-295, 1994.

Martinson IM et al: Impact of childhood cancer on healthy school-age siblings, *Cancer Nurs* 13(3):183-190, 1990.

McCown DE: When children face death in a family, *J Pediatr Health Care* 2(1):14-19, 1988.

Miles A: Caring for families when a child dies, *Pediatr Nurse* 16(4):346-347, 1990.

Pazola KJ, Gerberg AK: Privileged communication—talking with a dying adolescent, *MCN* 15(1):16-21, 1990.

Pengra H, Morgan D, Warren L: Nursing implementation of do not resuscitate policy into home healthcare, *Home Healthc Nurse* 10(2):32-39, 1992.

Perrone J: Adolescents with cancer: are they at risk for suicide? *Pediatr Nurs* 19(1):22-25, 1993.

Redding B: Facilitating grieving. In Smith D et al, editors: *Comprehensive child and family nursing skills*, St Louis, 1991, Mosby.

CHAPTER 39

Cognitive and Sensory Impairment

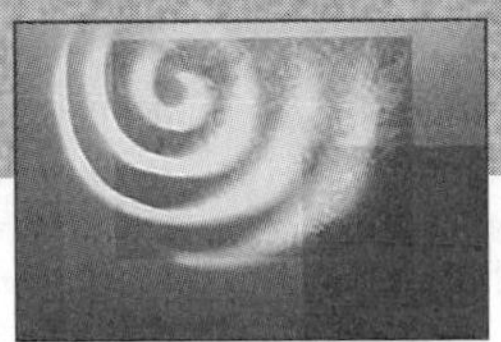

COGNITIVE IMPAIRMENT, P. 1157
General concepts, p. 1157
Nursing care of children with cognitive impairment, p. 1159
Down syndrome, p. 1163
Fragile X syndrome, p. 1167

SENSORY IMPAIRMENT, P. 1168
Hearing impairment, p. 1168
Visual impairment, p. 1175
Conjunctivitis, p. 1181
Deaf-blind children, p. 1182
Retinoblastoma, p. 1182

Cognitive Impairment

GENERAL CONCEPTS

Cognitive impairment is a general term that encompasses any type of mental difficulty or deficiency. In this chapter the term is used synonymously with **mental retardation (MR).** Although the needs and concerns of the family are a primary focus throughout the chapter, the reader is encouraged to review Chapter 38, which details the family's adjustment to disabilities in general.

The classic definition of MR has three components: subaverage intellectual functioning, deficits in adaptive behavior, and onset before 18 years of age (Batshaw, 1993). Recently the American Association on Mental Retardation (AAMR) significantly changed this definition by raising the upper limit of subaverage intellectual functioning from an intellectual quotient (IQ) of 70 to 75 and by defining more clearly the deficit in adaptive behaviors. Adaptive limitations must occur in two or more of the following ten areas: communication, self-care, home living, social skills, leisure, health and safety, self-direction, functional academics, community use, and work (Luckasson, 1992).

It is critical to note that a low IQ is not the sole criterion for MR. For example, individuals with IQ scores near 75 may not be classified as retarded if they are able to adapt to the environment. In addition, if cognitive impairment accompanied by adaptive limitations occurs from injury and disease after age 18, the person is not considered retarded.

The new definition also does not include a classification based on IQ scores as it did previously (Table 39-1). Rather, it emphasizes abilities, environments, supports, and empowerment. The intensity of needed support is classified as intermittent, limited, extensive, or pervasive. The underlying assumption is that with appropriate supports over a prolonged period, the ability of the person with MR to function each day will generally improve.

Diagnosis and Classification

The diagnosis of MR is usually made after a period of suspicion, by professionals or the family, that the child's developmental progress is delayed. In some cases it is confirmed at birth because of the recognition of distinct syndromes such as Down syndrome. At the other extreme, the diagnosis is made after the child begins school, when problems such as speech delays arouse concern. In all cases a high index of suspicion for developmental delay and behavioral signs (Box 39-1) is necessary for early diagnosis, and routine developmental screening (see Chapter 32) can assist in early identification. Delays are commonly seen in gross and fine motor and speech development, but the latter is most predictive.

Results of standardized tests are used in making the diagnosis of MR. The most commonly used IQ tests include the Stanford-Binet Test and Wechsler Intelligence Scale for Children–Revised (WISC-R). Tests for assessing adaptive behaviors include the Vineland Social Maturity Scale and the AAMR Adaptive Behavior Scale. Informal appraisal of adaptive behavior may be made by those fully acquainted with the child (e.g., teachers, parents, or other care providers). These observations commonly lead parents to seek evaluation of the child's development.

TABLE 39-1 Classification of mental retardation

LEVEL (IQ)*	PRESCHOOL (BIRTH-5 YEARS)—MATURATION AND DEVELOPMENT	SCHOOL AGE (6-21 YEARS)—TRAINING AND EDUCATION	ADULT (21 YEARS AND OLDER)—SOCIAL AND VOCATIONAL ADEQUACY
Mild—50-55 to approximately 70	Often not noticed as retarded by casual observer but is slower to walk, feed self, and talk than most children; follows same sequence in development as normal children	Can acquire practical skills and useful reading and arithmetic to a third to sixth grade level with special education; can be guided toward social conformity; achieves mental age of 8 to 12 years	Can usually achieve social and vocational skills adequate to self-maintenance; may need occasional guidance and support when under unusual social or economic stress; can adjust to marriage but not childrearing
Moderate—35-40 to 50-55	Noticeable delays in motor development, especially in speech; responds to training in various self-help activities	Can learn simple communication, elementary health and safety habits, and simple manual skills; does not progress in functional reading or arithmetic; achieves mental age of 3 to 7 years	Can perform simple tasks under sheltered conditions: participates in simple recreation; travels alone in familiar places; usually incapable of self-maintenance
Severe—20-25 to 35-40	Marked delay in motor development; little or no communication skills; may respond to training in elementary self-care (e.g., self-feeding)	Usually walks, barring specific disability; has some understanding of speech and some response; can profit from systematic habit training; achieves mental age of toddler	Can conform to daily routines and repetitive activities; needs continuing direction and supervision in protective environment
Profound—below 20-25	Gross retardation; minimum capacity for functioning in sensorimotor areas; needs total care	Obvious delays in all areas of development; shows basic emotional responses; may respond to skillful training in use of legs, hands, and jaws; needs close supervision; achieves mental age of young infant	May walk; needs complete custodial care; has primitive speech; usually benefits from regular physical activity

*Data from American Psychiatric Association: *Diagnostic and statistical manual of mental disorders (DSM-IV)*, ed 4, Washington, DC, 1994, The Association.

The severity of retardation is based on the IQ scores (see Table 39-1). A more useful approach for clinical application is classification on the basis of educational potential or symptom severity. For educational purposes the terms **educable mentally retarded (EMR)** or **trainable mentally retarded (TMR)** may be used. EMR corresponds to the mildly retarded group, which constitutes approximately 85% of all people with MR. TMR is generally equivalent to children with moderate levels of cognitive impairment and accounts for approximately 10% of the MR population (American Psychiatric Association, 1994). Although nurses may be familiar with the approximate range of IQ for classifying severity, they should refrain from using numbers as the criterion for assessing or evaluating the child's abilities, because numbers are of little value in counseling parents or training these children.

Etiology

The causes of severe mental retardation are primarily genetic, biochemical, and infectious. Although the etiology is unknown in the majority of cases, general categories of events that may lead to retardation include the following (Grossman, 1983):

1. Infection and intoxication, such as congenital rubella, syphilis, maternal drug consumption (such as excessive alcohol), chronic lead ingestion, or kernicterus
2. Trauma or physical agent, namely injury to the brain suffered during the prenatal, perinatal, or postnatal period
3. Inadequate nutrition and metabolic disorders such as phenylketonuria
4. Gross postnatal brain disease such as neurofibromatosis and tuberous sclerosis
5. Unknown prenatal influence, including cerebral and cranial malformations, such as microcephaly and hydrocephalus
6. Gestational disorders, including prematurity, low birth weight, and postmaturity
7. Psychiatric disorders that have their onset during the child's developmental period up to age 18 years, such as autism
8. Environmental influences, including evidence of a deprived environment associated with a history of mental retardation among parents and siblings
9. Chromosomal abnormalities, such as Down syndrome and fragile X syndrome

BOX 39-1
Early Behavioral Signs Suggestive of Cognitive Impairment

Nonresponsiveness to contact
Poor eye contact during feeding
Diminished spontaneous activity
Decreased alertness to voice or movement
Irritability
Slow feeding

From Crocker A, Nelson R: *Mental retardation.* In Levine M et al: *Developmental-behavioral pediatrics*, Philadelphia, 1983, WB Saunders.

NURSING CARE OF CHILDREN WITH COGNITIVE IMPAIRMENT

Assessment

Nurses play a major role in identifying children with cognitive impairment. In the newborn and early infancy period few signs are present, with the exception of Down syndrome (see p. 1163). However, after this age delayed developmental milestones are the major clues to MR. In addition, nurses must have a high index of suspicion for early behavior patterns that may suggest cognitive impairment (Box 39-1) and be aware of stereotypes that may delay diagnosis, such as "retarded children have to look dumb." Parental concerns, such as delayed development as compared with siblings, need to be taken seriously. All children should receive regular developmental assessment, and the nurse is often the person responsible for performing such assessments (see Chapter 32). When delays are found, the nurse must use sensitivity and discretion in revealing this finding to parents.

Nursing Diagnoses

A number of nursing diagnoses are prominent in the nursing care of the child with cognitive impairment and the child's family; other diagnoses specific to individual cases become evident. The most common nursing diagnoses are outlined in the Nursing Care Plan on p. 1164.

Planning

The goals of nursing care for the child with MR and the family are as follows:

1. The child will be educated using effective teaching strategies.
2. The child's optimum development will be promoted.
3. The child will learn self-care skills.
4. The family will plan for future care.
5. The child will be cared for appropriately during hospitalization.

Implementation

Educate child and family. To teach children with cognitive impairment, it is necessary to investigate their learning abilities and deficits. This knowledge is important for the nurse who may be involved in a home care type of program or who may be caring for the child in a health care setting. The nurse who understands how these children learn can effectively teach them basic skills or prepare them for various health-related procedures.

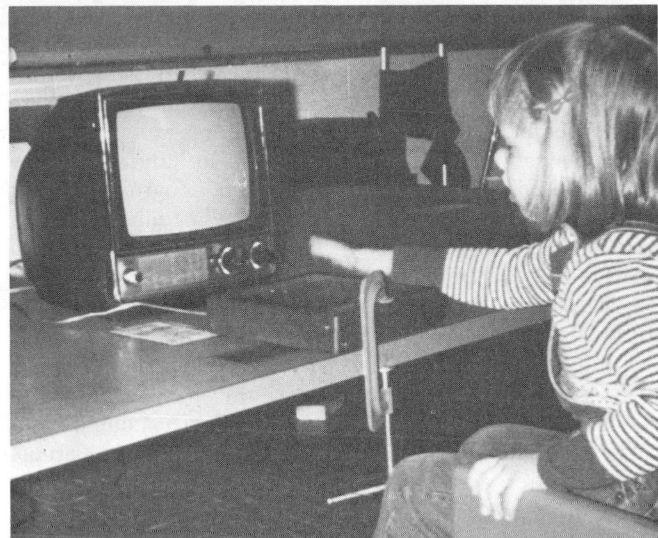

Fig. 39-1 A single push panel allows a child with cognitive impairment to turn a television on and off.

Children with cognitive impairment have a marked deficit in their ability to discriminate between two or more stimuli because of difficulty in recognizing the relevance of specific cues. However, these children can learn to discriminate if the cues are presented in an exaggerated, concrete form and if all extraneous stimuli are eliminated. For example, the use of colors to emphasize visual cues or the use of singing or rhymes to stress auditory cues can help them learn. Their deficit in discrimination also implies that concrete ideas are learned much more effectively than abstract ideas. Therefore demonstration is preferable to verbal explanation, and learning should be directed toward mastering a skill rather than understanding the scientific principles underlying a procedure.

Another cognitive deficit is in short-term memory. Whereas children of average intelligence can remember several words, numbers, or directions at one time, children with cognitive impairment are less able to do so and therefore need simple one-step directions. Learning through a step-by-step process requires a **task analysis**, in which each task is separated into its necessary components and each step is taught completely before proceeding to the next activity.

One critical area of learning that has had a tremendous impact on education for cognitively impaired individuals is motivation. Programs based on the motivational principles of behavior modification, using positive reinforcement for specific tasks or behaviors, have demonstrated marked improvement in children's ability to learn. Advances in technology have greatly aided in providing reinforcement, especially in children who are severely retarded and who may have physical disabilities that limit their range of capabilities. For example, with the use of specially designed switches, children are given control of some event in the environment, such as turning on the television (Fig. 39-1). The television picture becomes reinforcement for activating the switch. Repetitive use of these switches provides an early, simplistic association with a technical device that may progress to increasingly more complex aids.

Early intervention programs have been widely promoted for children with developmental disabilities, and there is considerable evidence that these programs are valuable for cognitively impaired children. Nurses working with these families need to be aware of the types of programs in their community. Under Public Law 101-476, The Individuals with Disabilities Education Act of 1990, states are encouraged to provide full early intervention services and are required to provide educational opportunities for all children with disabilities from 0 to 21 years of age. Services may be provided under state Programs for Children with Special Health Needs (formerly Crippled Children's Program) or by private organizations such as the National Easter Seal Society* and the Association of Retarded Citizens of the United States.† Parents should inquire about these programs by contacting the appropriate agencies. The child's education should begin as soon as possible, not at 5 or 6 years of age. As children grow older, their education should be directed toward vocational training that prepares them for as independent a life-style as possible within their scope of abilities.

Teach child self-care skills. When a child with cognitive impairment is born, parents need assistance in promoting normal developmental skills that are almost automatically learned by other children, including self-care skills such as feeding, toileting, dressing, and grooming. Teaching these skills requires a basic knowledge of the developmental sequence in learning the skills demonstrated by children of average intelligence. For example, children with subaverage intelligence would not be expected to dress themselves as early as unaffected youngsters.

Teaching self-care skills also necessitates a working knowledge of the individual steps needed to master a skill. For example, before beginning a self-feeding program, a task analysis is performed. Following a task analysis, the child is observed in a particular situation, such as eating, to determine what skills are possessed and the child's developmental readiness to learn the task. Family members are included in this process because their "readiness" is as important as the child's. Numerous self-help aids are available to facilitate independence and can be most helpful in eliminating some of the difficulties of learning, such as using a plate with suction cups to prevent accidental spills (Fig. 39-2).

Promote child's optimum development. Optimum development involves more than achieving independence. It requires appropriate guidance for establishing acceptable social behavior and personal feelings of self-esteem, worth, and security. These attributes are not simply learned through a stimulation program. Rather, they must arise from the genuine love and caring that exist among family members. However, families need guidance in providing an environment that fosters optimum development. Often it is the nurse who can provide assistance in these areas of childrearing.

Another important area for promoting optimum development and self-esteem is in ensuring the child's physical well-being. Any congenital defects, such as cardiac, gastrointestinal, or orthopedic anomalies, should be repaired. Plastic surgery may be considered in situations in which the child's appearance may be substantially improved. Dental health is very significant, and orthodontic and restorative procedures can immensely improve facial appearance.

Play/exercise. A child who is cognitively impaired has the same needs for recreation and exercise as other children. However, because of the child's slower development, parents may be less aware of the need to provide such activities. Therefore the nurse guides parents toward the selection of suitable play and exercise activities. Because play has been discussed for children in each age group in earlier chapters, only the exceptions are presented here.

The type of play is based on the child's developmental age, although the need for sensorimotor play may be prolonged for several years. Parents should use every opportunity to expose the child to as many different sounds, sights, and sensations as possible. Appropriate play includes musical mobiles, stuffed

*70 E. Lake St., Chicago, IL 60601; (312) 726-6200 or (800) 221-6827.
†500 East Border, Suite 300, Arlington, TX 76010; (817) 261-6003.
Information on early intervention programs in each state is available from the **National Down Syndrome Society,** 666 Broadway, New York, NY 10012; (212) 460-9330 or (800) 221-4602.

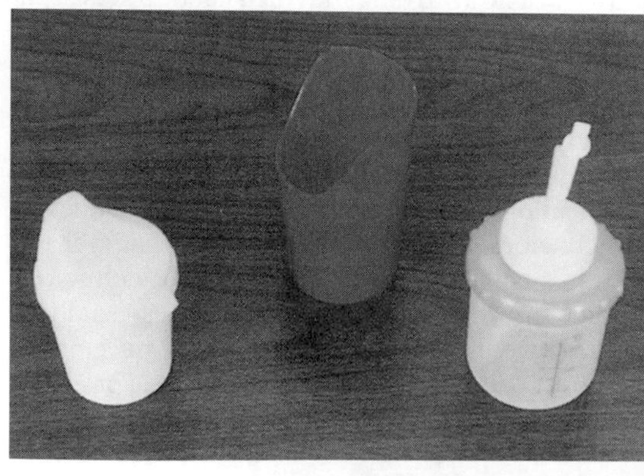

A

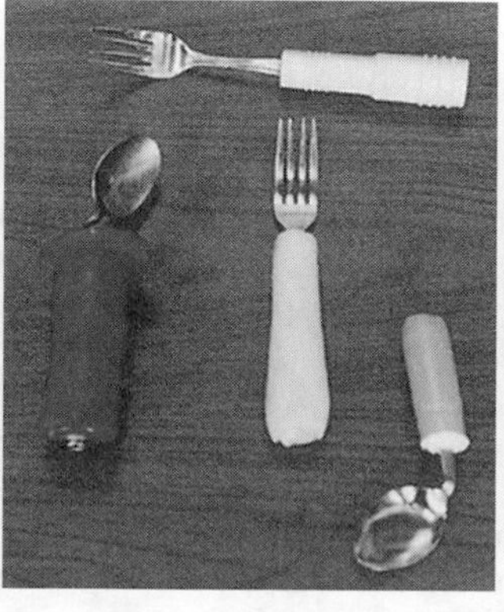

B

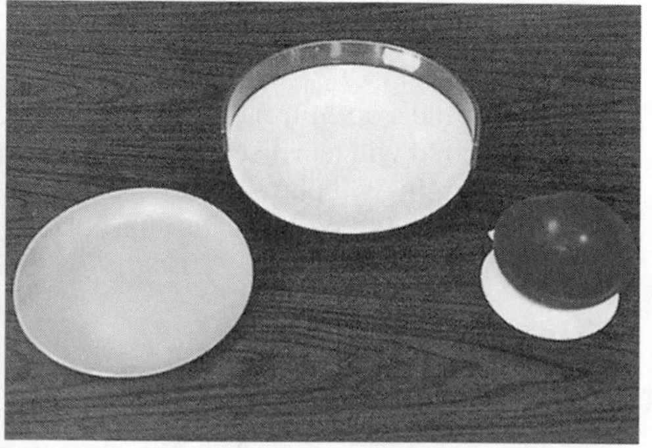

C

Fig. 39-2 Self-help aids for feeding. **A,** Modified drinking cups. **B,** Modified utensils. **C,** Modified dishes.

toys, water play, floating toys, a rocking chair or horse, a swing, bells, and rattles. The child should be taken on outings, such as trips to the grocery store or shopping center. Other people should be encouraged to visit in the home, and the child should be related to directly, such as by cuddling, holding, rocking, talking to the child in the *en face* (face-to-face) position, and giving "rides" on the parents' shoulders.

Toys are selected for their recreational and educational value. For example, a large inflatable beach ball is a good water toy; it encourages interactive play and can be used to learn motor skills such as balance, rocking, kicking, and throwing. A doll with removable clothes and different types of closures can help the child learn dressing skills. Musical toys that mimic animal sounds or respond with social phrases are excellent for encouraging speech. Toys should be simple in design so that the child can learn to manipulate them without help. For children with severe cognitive and physical impairment, electronic switches can be used to allow them to operate toys (Fig. 39-3).

Suitable activities for physical activity are based on the child's size, coordination, physical fitness and maturity, motivation, and health (Fig. 39-4). Some children may have physical problems that prevent participation in certain sports, such as atlantoaxial instability in children with Down syndrome (see pp. 1165-1166). These children often have greater success in individual and dual sports than in team sports and enjoy themselves most with children of the same developmental level. The Special Olympics* provides these children with a unique competitive opportunity.

Safety is a major consideration in selecting recreational and exercise activities. For example, toys that may be appropriate developmentally may present dangers to a child who is strong enough to break them or use them incorrectly.

Communication. Verbal skills are typically delayed more than other physical skills. Speech requires hearing and interpretation **(receptive skills)** and facial muscle coordination **(expressive skills).** Because both types of skills may be impaired, these children need frequent audiometric testing and should be fitted with hearing aids if indicated. In addition, they may need help in learning to control their facial muscles. For example, some children may need tongue exercises to correct the tongue thrust or gentle reminders to keep the lips closed.

Nonverbal communication may be appropriate for some of these children, and various devices are available. For the child without associated physical disabilities, a talking picture board is helpful. For children with physical limitations a number of adaptations or types of communication devices are available to facilitate selection of the appropriate picture or word (Fig. 39-5). Some children may be taught sign language or *Blissymbols*—a highly stylized system of graphic symbols that represent words, ideas, and concepts. Although they require education to learn their meaning, no reading skill is needed. The symbols are usually arranged on a board, and the person points or uses some type of selector to convey a message.

Discipline. Discipline must begin early. Limit-setting measures need to be simple, consistently applied, and appropriate for the child's mental age. Control measures are primarily based on teaching a specific behavior rather than on understanding the reasons behind it. Stressing moral lessons is of little value to a child who lacks the cognitive skills to learn from self criticism or from a lesson based on previous wrongdoing. Behavior modification, especially reinforcement of desired actions, and time-out are appropriate forms of behavior control.

*1350 New York Ave., N.W., Suite 500, Washington, DC 20005-4709; (202) 628-3630. In Canada: **Canadian Special Olympics, Inc.,** 40 St. Clair Ave., W., Suite 209, Toronto, Ontario M4V 1M6.

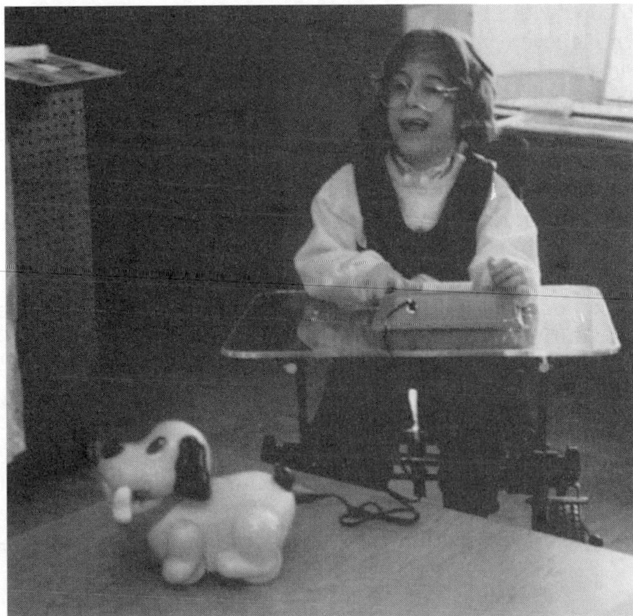

Fig. 39-3 A manual switch allows a child with cognitive impairment to play with a battery-operated toy.

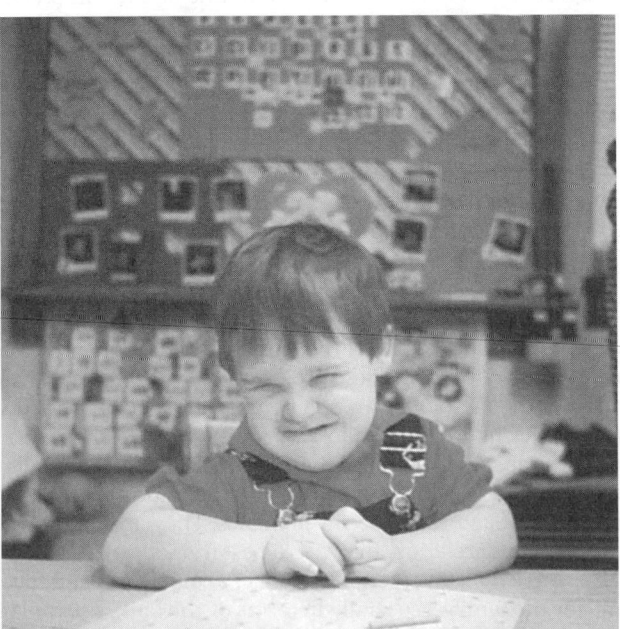

Fig. 39-4 Play activities for children with cognitive impairments need to be appropriate for their abilities.

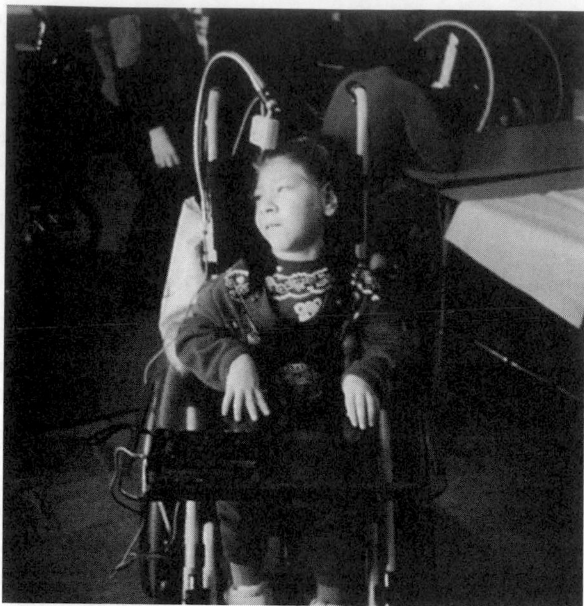

Fig. 39-5 A child with cognitive and physical impairments can play a tape recorder by moving a device near her head.

Socialization. Acquiring social skills and learning self-care procedures are complex tasks. Active rehearsal with role playing and practice sessions and positive reinforcement for desired behavior have been the most successful approaches. Parents should be encouraged early to teach their child socially acceptable behavior—waving goodbye, saying hello and thank you, responding to his or her name, greeting visitors but not being overly affectionate, and sitting modestly. The teaching of socially acceptable sexual behavior is especially important to minimize sexual exploitation. Parents also need to expose the child to strangers so that he or she can practice manners, because there is no automatic transfer of learning from one situation to another.

Dressing and grooming are also important aspects of socialization. A child who is dressed in appropriate-age clothing and is well groomed is much more likely to be accepted and to develop good self-esteem. Clothes should be clean, up-to-date, and well fitted. Many attractive outfits can be adapted with self-adhering fasteners and elastic openings to facilitate self-dressing.

Children of all ages need peer relationships, and children with cognitive impairments are no exception. As soon as possible, parents should enroll the child in appropriate preschool programs. Not only do these programs provide education and training, they also offer an opportunity for social experiences among the children. As children grow older, they should have peer experiences similar to those of other children, including group outings, sports, and organized activities such as Boy Scouts, Girl Scouts, or Special Olympics. They are encouraged to form a close relationship with a best friend.

Sexuality. Adolescence may be a particularly difficult time for the family, especially in terms of the child's sexual behavior, possibility of pregnancy, future plans to marry, and ability to be independent. Often, little anticipatory guidance has been offered to parents to prepare the child for physical and sexual maturation. The nurse can help in this area by providing parents with information about sex education that is geared to the child's developmental level. For example, the adolescent female needs a *simple* explanation of menstruation and instructions on personal hygiene during the menstrual cycle.

These adolescents also need practical sexual information regarding anatomy, physical development, and conception.* Because of their easy persuasion and lack of judgment, they need a well-defined, concrete code of conduct. The subtleties of social sexual behavior are less beneficial than specific instructions for handling certain situations. For example, a girl should be firmly told never to go alone anywhere with any person she does not know well. A boy should be warned about intimate advances from other males. To protect him or her from abusive sexual activities, parents must closely observe their teenager's activities and associates.

The question of contraceptive protection for female retarded adolescents is often a parental concern. Permanent contraception through sterilization is a special dilemma because of moral and ethical questions and the psychologic effects on the adolescent. State laws vary; some allow no sterilization, and others permit review of sterilization requests.

Parents are often very concerned about the advisability of marriage between two individuals with significant cognitive impairment. There is no conclusive answer; each situation must be judged individually. In some instances marriage is possible, but parenthood is usually not desirable because of the complexity of childrearing and the potential problem of perpetuating mental deficiency. The nurse should discuss this topic with parents and with the prospective couple, stressing suitable living accommodations and contraceptive methods to prevent pregnancy. If children are conceived, these parents require specialized assistance in learning to meet the needs of their offspring (Keltner and Tymchuk, 1992).

Help family adjust to future care. Not all families are able to cope with home care of their affected child, especially one who is severely or profoundly retarded and/or multidisabled. Older parents may not be able to assume care responsibilities once they reach retirement or old age. For these parents, the decision regarding residential placement is a difficult one, and the availability of such facilities varies widely. In addition to assisting them in their adjustment to the decision for placement, the nurse working with a family should help investigate and evaluate various programs.

Care for child during hospitalization. Caring for the child during hospitalization can be a special challenge. Nurses are often unfamiliar with children who are cognitively impaired, and they may cope with their feelings of insecurity and fear by ignoring or isolating the child. Not only is this approach nonsupportive, but it may also be destructive for the child's sense of self-esteem and optimum development, and it may hamper the parents' ability to cope with the stress of the experience. One method that successfully avoids this nonther-

*Sources of information on sexuality and conception are the **Association for Retarded Citizens of the United States,** 500 East Border, Suite 300, Arlington, TX 76010, (817) 261-6003; and **Planned Parenthood Federation of America,** 810 7th Ave., New York, NY 10019, (212) 541-7800.

apeutic approach is the use of the mutual participation model in planning the child's care. Parents are encouraged to room with their child but should not be made to feel as if the responsibility is totally theirs.

When the child is admitted, a detailed history is obtained (see Chapter 41), especially in terms of all self-care activity. During the interview the child's developmental age is assessed. It is best to avoid directly asking about IQ levels because doing so may make the parents uncomfortable and often reveals little about the child's actual abilities. Questions are approached positively. For example, rather than asking, "Is your child toilet trained yet?" the nurse may state, "Tell me about your child's toileting habits." The assessment should also focus on any special devices the child uses, effective measures of limit-setting, unusual or favorite routines, and any behaviors that may require intervention. For example, if the parent states that the child engages in self-stimulatory activities, the nurse inquires about events that precipitate them and techniques that the parents use to manage them.

The child's functional level of eating and playing, ability to express needs verbally, progress in toilet training, and relationship with objects, toys, and other children are also assessed. The child is encouraged to be as independent as possible in the hospital.

Realizing that the child may be lonely in the hospital, the nurse makes certain that toys and other activities are provided. The child is placed in a room with other children of approximate developmental age (preferably a room with two beds to avoid overstimulation). The nurse discusses with the other parents the child's abilities and introduces the parents and children to each other. By the nurse's example of treating the child with dignity and respect, others who may be fearful of what they do not understand are encouraged to accept the child.

Procedures are explained to the child through methods of communication that are at the appropriate cognitive level. In general, explanations should be simple, short, and concrete, emphasizing what the child will experience *physically*. Demonstration either through actual practice or with visual aids is always preferable to verbal explanation. The nurse repeats instructions often and evaluates the child's understanding by asking questions such as "What will it feel like?" "What will the doctor look like?" "Show me how you must lie," or "Where will the dressing be?" Parents are included in preprocedural teaching, both for their own learning and to help the nurse learn effective methods of communicating with the child.

During hospitalization the nurse should also focus on growth-promoting experiences for the child. For example, hospitalization may be an excellent opportunity to emphasize to parents any abilities that the child does have but has not had the opportunity to practice, such as self-dressing. It may also be an opportunity for social experiences with peers, group play, or new educational/recreational activities. For example, one child who had the habit of screaming and kicking demonstrated a definite decrease in those behaviors after he learned to pound pegs and use a punching bag. Through social services the parents may become aware of specialized programs for the child. Hospitalization may also offer parents a respite from everyday care responsibilities and an opportunity to discuss their feelings with a concerned professional.

Assist in measures to prevent retardation. Besides having a responsibility to families with a child with MR, nurses also need to be involved in programs aimed at preventing MR. Many of the familial, social, and environmental factors known to cause mild retardation are preventable. Counseling and education can reduce or eliminate such factors (e.g., poor nutrition, cigarette smoking, and chemical abuse, which increase the risk of prematurity and intrauterine growth retardation). Consequently, the major interventions are directed at improving maternal health and educating women regarding the dangers of chemicals, including alcohol, during pregnancy. Other preventive strategies that play an important role include optimum medical care for high-risk newborns; rubella immunization; genetic counseling and prenatal screening, especially in terms of Down or fragile X syndrome; newborn screening for treatable inborn errors of metabolism such as congenital hypothyroidism, phenylketonuria, and galactosemia; and early appropriate therapies and rehabilitation services for children with developmental disabilities.

Evaluation

The effectiveness of nursing interventions is determined by continual reassessment and evaluation of care on the basis of the following observational guidelines and expected outcomes:

1. Observe techniques used to teach child and the success of these techniques in accomplishing education; inquire if child is enrolled in early stimulation program.
2. Interview family regarding provision of appropriate socialization, discipline, and play for child; observe child's ability to communicate with others; if possible, interview child regarding feelings of self-worth.
3. Observe those activities of daily living that child can completely or partially perform.
4. Interview family regarding any plans for future care and their awareness of community services.
5. Check patient record for evidence of nursing admission history, especially for self-help activities; observe parent's involvement in child's care; observe social interaction of child and family with other patients.
6. Investigate community programs aimed at preventing retardation and inquire about nursing involvement in these efforts.

Expected outcomes:
See the Nursing Care Plan on p. 1164.

DOWN SYNDROME

Down syndrome is the most common chromosomal abnormality of a generalized syndrome, occurring in 1 in 800 to 1000 live births. It owes its once common but unacceptable name, *mongolism*, to the particular facial characteristics, which resemble those of the Mongol race.

Etiology

The cause of Down syndrome is not known, but evidence from cytogenetic and epidemiologic studies supports the concept of multiple causality. Approximately 95% of all cases of Down syndrome are attributable to an extra chromosome 21 (group G), hence the name *trisomy 21*. Although children

Nursing Care Plan

CHILD WITH MENTAL RETARDATION

Nursing Diagnosis: Altered growth and development related to impaired cognitive functioning

Expected Outcome: **Child exhibits evidence of appropriate growth and development behaviors for age and abilities.**

• NURSING INTERVENTIONS/*RATIONALES*

Involve child and family in early developmental stimulation and intervention (refer to available programs) *to maximize developmental potential.*

Assess child's developmental progress at regular intervals and note changes in functional abilities *to revise interventions as needed.*

Help family to set realistic goals and determine child's readiness for specific developmental tasks; encourage and reinforce learning of self-care skills *to facilitate development.*

Emphasize to family that this child has needs that are the same as other children (e.g., play, discipline, interaction, approval), and encourage interventions that help child to meet these needs at appropriate times and in appropriate ways (e.g., teaching socially acceptable behavior; encouraging appropriate grooming, hygiene, and dress; providing opportunities for peer interactions such as school, after-school activities, special events; reinforcing positive behaviors and setting limits) *to optimize development and socialization.*

As child matures, counsel child and parents on such issues as sexuality, sexual behavior, birth control, marriage and family, and vocational interests and opportunities *to assist in management of ongoing developmental issues.*

Nursing Diagnosis: Altered family processes related to having a child with mental retardation

Expected Outcome: **Family members demonstrate acceptance of child.**

• NURSING INTERVENTIONS/*RATIONALES*

Inform family of infant problem as soon as possible after birth *to decrease anxiety of unknown.*

Provide opportunity for family to absorb and adjust to diagnosis (i.e., repeat information *to allow time for family to hear and understand;* encourage expression of concerns, fears, and feelings about diagnosis and potential impact *to facilitate adjustment;* identify support systems *to provide resources for coping*).

Provide family written materials about child's condition *for long-term reference;* introduce family to other families with similarly affected children *to enhance support mechanisms.*

Demonstrate acceptance of child through own behavior *to serve as role model for family;* encourage family to participate in care *to form emotional attachments.*

Explore family reaction to the child; assist them to achieve a realistic view of child's abilities and limitations; encourage family in attempts to promote child growth and development; have family emphasize what child can do; explore ways for family to include child in family activities *to help family increase abilities to cope with and incorporate child into family structure.*

Arrange for and participate in family conferences *to provide forum for communication, mutual goal setting, and effective strategizing.*

Assess family resources and coping abilities when discussing care options on discharge *so that family can make realistic choices on the basis of their specific circumstances.*

If family opts for home care, assist them in developing a plan of care for the child, and teach them the skills needed in carrying out that plan *to provide optimum care in which the entire family is involved.*

Identify additional resource systems (e.g., relatives, friends, church, health care services, community programs), and strategize with family about making good use of these systems *to develop broad base of support.*

Provide a system of ongoing follow-up and evaluation *to ensure long-term adaptation to challenges presented to family functioning by a child with mental retardation.*

As child ages, help parents explore decisions about future care options that assist in dealing with behavioral management problems, parent debility, or retirement issues *to facilitate long-term care.*

Make referrals to appropriate social agencies *for needed assistance, support, and continuity of care.*

---

with trisomy 21 are born to parents of all ages, there is a statistically greater risk in older women, particularly those over 35 years of age. For example, in women 30 years of age the incidence of Down syndrome is approximately 1 in 1500 live births, but in women age 40 it is approximately 1 in 100. However, the majority (approximately 80%) of infants with Down Syndrome are born to women under age 35. In less than 5% of cases, paternal age is a factor, especially in men 55 years of age or older (Cooley and Graham, 1991).

Approximately 3% to 4% of the cases may be caused by *translocation* of chromosomes 15 and 21 or 22. This type of genetic aberration is usually hereditary and is not associated with advanced parental age. From 1% to 2% of affected persons demonstrate *mosaicism,* which refers to cells with both normal and abnormal chromosomes. The degree of physical and cognitive impairment is related to the percentage of cells with the abnormal chromosome makeup.

Diagnostic Evaluation

Down syndrome can usually be diagnosed by the clinical manifestations alone (Box 39-2; Fig. 39-6), but a chromosomal analysis should be done to confirm the genetic abnormality.

Several physical problems are associated with Down syndrome. Many of these children have congenital heart malformations, the most common being septal defects. Respiratory

BOX 39-2
Clinical Manifestations of Down Syndrome

Head
*Separated sagittal suture
Brachycephaly
Skull rounded and small
Flat occiput
Enlarged anterior fontanel
Sparse hair (variable)

Face
Flat profile

Eyes
*Oblique palpebral fissures (upward, outward slant)
Inner epicanthal folds
Speckling of iris (Brushfield's spots)
Short, sparse eyelashes
Blepharitis

Nose
*Small
*Depressed nasal bridge (saddle nose)

Ears
Small
Short pinna (vertical ear length)
Overlapping upper helices
Narrow canals

Mouth
*High, arched, narrow palate
Small osseous orbit
Protruding tongue, may be fissured at lip and furrowed on the surface
Hypoplastic mandible
Downward curve (especially noted when crying)
Mouth kept open

Teeth
Delayed eruption
Alignment abnormalities common
Microdontia
Periodontal disease

Chest
Shortened rib cage
12th rib anomalies
Pectus excavatum/carinatum

Neck
*Skin excess and lax
Short and broad

Abdomen
Protruding
Muscles lax and flabby
Diastasis recti
Umbilical hernia

Genitalia
Small penis
Cryptorchidism
Bulbous vulva

Hands
Broad, short
Stubby fingers
Incurved little finger (clinodactyly)
Transverse palmar crease
Characteristic dermal ridge patterns
Distally located axial triradius
Increased ulnar loops on fingers

Feet
*Wide space between big and second toes
*Plantar crease between big and second toes
Broad, stubby, short

Musculoskeleton
*Hyperflexibility
*Muscle weakness
Hypotonia
Atlantoaxial instability

Skin
Dry, cracked, and frequent fissuring
Cutis marmorata (mottling)

Other
Reduced birth weight

*Most common findings (Pueschel, 1992).

tract infections are very prevalent and when combined with cardiac anomalies are the chief cause of death, particularly during the first year of life. Hypotonicity of chest and abdominal muscles and dysfunction of the immune system probably predispose these children to the development of respiratory tract infection. Other physical problems include thyroid dysfunction, especially congenital hypothyroidism, and an increased incidence of leukemia.

Therapeutic Management

Although there is no cure for Down syndrome, a number of therapies are advocated, such as surgery to correct serious congenital anomalies and possibly the physical stigmata, although the latter is controversial. These children also benefit from regular medical care. Evaluation of sight and hearing is essential, and treatment of otitis media is required to prevent auditory loss, which can influence cognitive function. Periodic testing of thyroid function is recommended, especially if growth is severely delayed. Children participating in sports that may involve stress on the head and neck, such as gymnastics, diving, the butterfly stroke in swimming, high jump, and soccer, should be evaluated radiologically for atlantoaxial

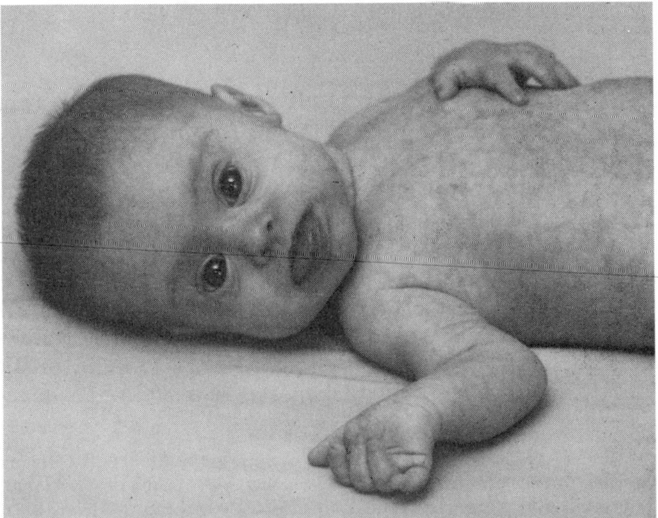

Fig. 39-6 Down syndrome in infant. Note small square head with upward slant to the eyes, flat nasal bridge, protruding tongue, mottled skin, and hypotonia.

instability. Symptoms of the disorder include neck pain, weakness, and torticollis. Affected children are at risk for spinal cord compression.

Nursing ALERT

Report immediately any child with the following signs of spinal cord compression:
- Persistent neck pain
- Loss of established motor skills and bladder/bowel control
- Changes in sensation

Prognosis. Life expectancy has improved in recent years but remains lower than that for the general population. More than 80% survive to age 30 years and beyond. Down syndrome is associated with earlier aging, and virtually all deceased individuals have neurologic changes associated with Alzheimer's disease (Cooley and Graham, 1991).

Nursing Care Management

Support family at time of diagnosis. Because of the unique physical characteristics, the infant with Down syndrome is usually diagnosed at birth, and parents should be informed of the diagnosis at this time. Parents usually prefer that both of them be present during the informing interview so that they can support one another emotionally. They appreciate receiving reading material about the syndrome* and being referred to others for help or advice, such as parent groups or professional counseling.

Once parents are aware of the diagnosis, they are confronted with the crisis of losing their perfect or dream child and grieving for and accepting their reality child. Consequently, the parents' responses to the child may greatly influence decisions regarding future care. Whereas some families willingly wish to take the child home, others consider immediate residential placement. The nurse must carefully answer questions regarding developmental potential. Institutionalization is no longer an option. For families unable or unready to choose taking the newborn home, specialized foster care or adoption are other options. (See the Critical Thinking Q & A box above).

Critical Thinking Q & A

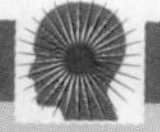

DIAGNOSIS OF DOWN SYNDROME

The parents of Melissa, a newborn diagnosed as having Down syndrome, ask you, "What are we supposed to do with her?" They further state that they already have three other children at home. How should you respond?

1. Encourage the parents to consider placement arrangements.
2. Actively listen to the parents' concerns.
3. Refer the parents to their pediatrician.
4. Ask the social worker to see the parents.

The correct answer is two. The parents of a newborn child who has Down syndrome need time to process information given to them. The best choice for the nurse is to listen and then be able to guide them to appropriate resources, not to give them suggestions that would affect their family's future. Options three and four are appropriate interventions but should not replace the nurse's role with the family.

Assist family in preventing physical problems. Many of the physical characteristics of Down syndrome present nursing problems. The hypotonicity of muscles and hyperextensibility of joints complicate positioning. The limp, flaccid extremities resemble the posture of a rag doll; as a result, holding the infant is difficult and cumbersome. Sometimes parents perceive this lack of molding to their bodies as evidence of inadequate parenting. The extended body position promotes heat loss because more surface area is exposed to the environment. Parents are encouraged to swaddle or wrap the infant tightly in a blanket before picking up the child to provide security and warmth. The nurse also discusses with parents their feelings concerning attachment to the child, emphasizing that the child's lack of clinging or molding is a physical characteristic, not a sign of detachment or rejection.

Decreased muscle tone compromises respiratory expansion. In addition, the underdeveloped nasal bone causes a chronic problem of inadequate drainage of mucus. The constant stuffy nose forces the child to breathe through the mouth, which dries the oropharyngeal membranes and increases the susceptibility to upper respiratory tract infections. Measures to lessen these problems include clearing the nose with a bulb-type syringe,* rinsing the mouth with water after feedings, using a cool-mist vaporizer to keep the mucous membranes moist, changing the child's position frequently, and performing postural drainage and percussion if necessary (practicing good handwashing and proper disposal of soiled articles such as tissues). If antibiotics are ordered, the importance of completing the full course of therapy for successful eradication of the infection and the prevention of growth of resistant organisms is stressed.

Inadequate drainage and pooling of mucus in the nose also interfere with feeding. Because the child breathes by mouth, sucking for any length of time is difficult. When eating solids, the child may gag on the food because of mucus in the oropharynx. Parents are advised to clear the nose before each feeding, to give small, frequent feedings, and to allow opportunities for rest at mealtime.

The protruding tongue also interferes with feeding, especially solid foods. Parents need to know that the tongue thrust is not an indication of refusal to feed but rather a physiologic response. Parents are advised to use a small but long, straight-handled spoon to push the food toward the back and side of the mouth. If food is thrust out, it is refed.

Dietary intake needs supervision. Decreased muscle tone affects gastric motility, predisposing the child to constipation.

*Sources of information include the **Association for Retarded Citizens of the United States,** 500 East Border, Suite 300, Arlington, TX 76010, (817) 261-6003. **American Association on Mental Retardation,** 1719 Kalorama Rd., N.W., Washington, DC 20009, (202) 387-1968 or (800) 424-3688; the **National Down Syndrome Society,** 141 5th Ave., New York, NY 10011, (800) 221-4602; and the **National Down Syndrome Congress,** 1605 Chantilly Dr., Suite 250, Atlanta, GA 30324 (404) 633-1555 or (800) 232-6372.

*Home care instructions on using a bulb syringe are available in Wong DL: *Wong and Whaley's clinical manual of pediatric nursing,* ed 4, St Louis, 1996, Mosby.

Dietary measures such as increased fiber and fluid promote evacuation. The child's eating habits may need careful scrutiny to prevent obesity. Height and weight measurements should be obtained on a serial basis, especially during infancy. Because the growth of these children is slower than trends of the general pediatric population, special growth charts developed for these children should be used (Cronk et al, 1988).

During infancy the child's skin is pliable and soft. However, it gradually becomes rough and dry and is prone to cracking and infection. Skin care involves the minimal use of soap and the application of lubricants. Lip balm is applied to the lips, especially when the child is outdoors, to prevent excessive chapping.

Assist in prenatal diagnosis and genetic counseling. Prenatal diagnosis of Down syndrome is possible through chorionic villus sampling and amniocentesis, because chromosomal analysis of fetal cells can detect the presence of trisomy or translocation. However, analysis will not identify sporadic cases in young women when there is no indication for prenatal testing.

However, testing for low maternal serum α-fetoprotein, high chorionic gonadotropin, and low unconjugated estriol levels may identify affected young women, who can then undergo amniocentesis (American Academy of Pediatrics, 1989; Haddow et al, 1992).

The nurse has a role in genetic counseling of women who are of advanced maternal age or who have a family history of the disorder to discuss the possibility of amniocentesis. If the fetus is affected, the nurse must allow the parents to express their feelings concerning elective abortion and support their decision to terminate or proceed with the pregnancy.

See also Nursing Care Plan: The Child with Down Syndrome.*

FRAGILE X SYNDROME

Fragile X syndrome is the most common inherited cause of MR and the second most common genetic cause of MR after Down syndrome. It has been described in all ethnic groups and races; the incidence of affected males is 1 in 1250; 1 in 2500 females are affected, and 1 in 259 females are carriers. Because its identification as a disorder is relatively new, many health professionals and educators lack the necessary familiarity with the manifestations for appropriate referral and management once it is diagnosed (Hagerman and Cronister, 1996).

The syndrome is caused by an abnormal gene on the lower end of the long arm of the X chromosome. Chromosome analysis may demonstrate a **fragile site** (a region that fails to condense during mitosis and is characterized by a nonstaining gap or narrowing) in the cells of affected males and females and in carrier females. This fragile site has been determined to be caused by a gene mutation that results in excessive repeats of nucleotide in a specific DNA segment of the X chromosome. The number of repeats in a normal individual is between 6 and 50. An individual with 50 to 200 base pair repeats is said to have a *premutation* and is therefore a carrier. When passed from a parent to a child, these base pair repeats can expand from 200 or more, which is termed a *full mutation.* This expansion occurs only when a carrier mother passes the mutation to her offspring; it does not occur when a carrier father passes the mutation to his daughters.

The inheritance pattern has been termed *X-linked dominant with reduced penetrance.* It is in distinct contrast to the classic X-linked recessive pattern in which all carrier females are normal, all affected males have symptoms of the disorder, and no males are carriers. Consequently, genetic counseling of affected families is more complex than that for families with a classic X-linked disorder such as hemophilia. Prenatal diagnosis of the fragile X gene mutation is now possible with direct DNA testing in a family with an established history, by amniocentesis or chorionic villus sampling (Brown et al, 1993). Both affected genders are fertile and therefore capable of transmitting the fragile X disorder.

Clinical Manifestations

The classic trend of physical findings in adult males with fragile X syndrome consists of a long face with a prominent jaw (prognathism); large, protruding ears, and large testes (macroorchidism). However, in prepubertal children these features may be less obvious, and behavioral manifestations may initially suggest the diagnosis (Box 39-3). In carrier females the clinical manifestations are extremely varied.

Therapeutic Management

There is no cure for fragile X syndrome. Medical treatment may include the use of serotonin agents such as carbamazepine (Tegretol) or fluoxetine (Prozac) to control violent temper outbursts and the use of central nervous system (CNS)

BOX 39-3
Clinical Manifestations of Fragile X Syndrome

Physical Features

- Long, wide, and/or protruding ears
- Long, narrow face, with prominent jaw
- In postpubertal males, enlarged testicles
- Long palpebral fissures
- High; arched palate
- Strabismus
- Increased head circumference
- Mitral valve prolapse/aortic root dilation
- Hypotonia
- Hyperextensible finger joints
- Transpalmar crease
- Pes planus (flat feet)

Behavioral Features

- Mild-to-severe MR (occasional normal IQ with learning disabilities)
- Speech delay; speech may be rapid, with stuttering and repetition of words
- Short attention span, hyperactivity
- Mouthing beyond expected age for behavior
- Hypersensitivity to taste, sounds, touch
- Intolerance to change in routine
- Autistic-like behaviors
- May exhibit aggressive behavior

*In Wong DL: *Wong and Whaley's clinical manual of pediatric nursing,* ed 4, St Louis, 1996, Mosby.

stimulants or clonidine (Catapres) to improve attention span and decrease hyperactivity. The use of folic acid, which affects the metabolism of CNS transmitters, is controversial.

All affected children require early speech and language therapy, occupational therapy, and special education assistance. Without appropriate intervention, a progressive decline in IQ can occur.

Prognosis. Individuals with fragile X syndrome are expected to live a normal life span. Their cognitive impairment may be ameliorated by behavioral and educational interventions.

Nursing Care Management

Because cognitive impairment is a fairly consistent finding in individuals with fragile X syndrome, the care given to these families is the same as for any child with MR. Because the disorder is hereditary, genetic counseling is necessary to inform parents and siblings of the risks of transmission. In addition, any male or female with unexplained or nonspecific mental impairment should be referred for genetic testing and, if needed, counseling. Families with a member affected by the disorder should be referred to the National Fragile X Foundation.*

Sensory Impairment

HEARING IMPAIRMENT

Hearing impairment is one of the most common disabilities in the United States. An estimated 1 in 1000 infants are born deaf. For infants admitted to the neonatal intensive care unit, the incidence rises sharply to approximately 1 to 3 per 100 neonates (National Institutes of Health, 1993). There are approximately 1 million hearing-impaired children ranging in age from birth to 21 years in the United States, and almost one third of these children have other disabilities, such as visual or cognitive deficits.

Definition and Classification

Hearing impairment is a general term indicating a disability that may range in severity from mild to profound and includes the subsets of deaf and hard-of-hearing. **Deaf** refers to a person whose hearing disability precludes successful processing of linguistic information through audition, with or without a hearing aid. **Hard-of-hearing** refers to a person who, generally with the use of a hearing aid, has residual hearing sufficient to enable successful processing of linguistic information through audition. Other terms, such as *deaf and dumb, mute,* or *deaf-mute,* are unacceptable. Hearing-impaired persons are not dumb and, if mute, have no physical speech defect other than that caused by the inability to hear.

Hearing defects may be classified according to etiology, pathology, or symptom severity. Each is important in terms of treatment, possible prevention, and rehabilitation.

Etiology. Hearing loss may be caused by a number of prenatal and postnatal conditions. These include a family history of childhood hearing impairment, anatomic malformations of the head or neck, low birth weight, severe perinatal asphyxia, perinatal infection (cytomegalovirus, rubella, herpes, syphilis, toxoplasmosis, and bacterial meningitis), chronic ear infection, cerebral palsy, Down syndrome, or administration of ototoxic drugs.

In addition, high-risk neonates who are surviving formerly fatal prenatal or perinatal conditions may be susceptible to hearing loss from the disorder or its treatment. For example, sensorineural hearing loss may be a result of continuous humming noises or high noise levels associated with incubators, oxygen hoods, or intensive care units, especially when combined with the use of potentially ototoxic antibiotics.

Environmental noise is a special concern. Sounds loud enough to damage sensitive hair cells of the inner ear can produce irreversible hearing loss. Very loud, brief noise, such as gunfire, can cause immediate, severe, and permanent loss of hearing. Longer exposure to less intense but still hazardous sounds, such as music, can also produce hearing loss (Consensus Conference, 1990). The exact sound level that produces hearing loss is unknown.

Pathology. Disorders of hearing are divided according to the location of the defect. *Conductive* or *middle-ear hearing loss* results from interference of transmission of sound to the middle ear. It is the most common of all types of hearing loss and most often is a result of recurrent serous otitis media. Conductive hearing impairment mainly involves interference with loudness of sound.

Sensorineural hearing loss, also called *perceptive* or *nerve deafness,* involves damage to the inner ear structures and/or the auditory nerve. The most common causes are congenital defects of inner ear structures or consequences of acquired conditions, such as kernicterus, infection, administration of ototoxic drugs, or exposure to excessive noise. Sensorineural hearing loss results in distortion of sound and problems in discrimination. Although the child hears some of everything going on around him or her, the sounds are distorted, severely affecting discrimination and comprehension.

Mixed conductive-sensorineural hearing loss results from interference with the transmission of sound in the middle ear and along neural pathways. It often results from recurrent otitis media and its complications.

Central auditory imperception includes all hearing losses that do not demonstrate defects in the conductive or sensorineural structures. They are usually divided into organic or functional losses. In the organic type of central auditory imperception, the defect involves the reception of auditory stimuli along the central pathways and the expression of the message into meaningful communication. Examples are **aphasia,** an inability to express ideas in any form, either written or verbally; **agnosia,** the inability to interpret sound correctly; and **dysacusis,** difficulty in processing details or discrimination among sounds.

In the *functional type* of hearing loss there is no organic lesion to explain a central auditory loss. Examples of functional hearing loss are conversion hysteria (an unconscious withdrawal from hearing to block remembrance of a traumatic event), infantile autism, and childhood schizophrenia.

Symptom severity. Hearing impairment is expressed in terms of a **decibel (dB),** a unit of loudness (Table 39-2); it is

*1441 York St., Suite 303, Denver, CO 80206; (800) 688-8765 or (303) 333-6155 in Colorado.

TABLE 39-2 Intensity of sounds expressed in decibels

DECIBELS (dB)	REPRESENTATIVE SOUND
0	Softest sound normal ear can hear
10	Heartbeat, rustling of leaves
20	Whisper at 1.8 m (5 feet)
30-45	Normal conversation
60	Noise in average restaurant
70-80	Street noises
80	Loud radio in home
90-100	Train
120	Thunder, rock music
140	Jet airplane during departure
>140	Pain threshold

measured at various frequencies such as 500, 1000, and 2000 cycles per second, the critical listening speech range. Hearing impairment can be classified according to **hearing-threshold level** (the measurement of an individual's hearing threshold by means of an audiometer) and the degree of symptom severity as it affects speech (Table 39-3). These classifications offer only general guidelines regarding the effect of the impairment on any individual child because children differ greatly in their ability to use residual hearing.

Therapeutic Management

Treatment of hearing loss depends on the cause and type of hearing impairment. Many conductive hearing defects respond to medical or surgical treatment, such as antibiotic therapy for acute otitis media or insertion of tympanostomy tubes for chronic otitis media. When the conductive loss is permanent, hearing can be improved with the use of a hearing aid to amplify sound.

Treatment for sensorineural hearing loss is much less satisfactory. Because the defect is not one of intensity of sound, hearing aids are of less value in this type of defect. The use of cochlear implants (a surgically implanted prosthetic device) provides hope for some affected children.

Disorders of central auditory imperception depend on the cause. Functional types, such as conversion hysteria, may require psychologic intervention, but others, such as autism, may not respond to any therapy.

Tactile devices are another option for those with profound deafness to improve their speech perception. A vibrotactile or electrotactile signal is used to transmit impulses to a point of stimulation, usually the fingers or hands. This information is then transmitted to the language-processing center in the brain (Sarant et al, 1993).

Nursing Care Management

Assessment

Assessment of children for hearing impairment is a critical nursing responsibility. Discovery of a hearing impairment within the first 6 to 12 months of life is essential to prevent social, physical, and psychologic damage to the child. Assessment involves (1) identifying those children who by virtue of their history are at risk (Box 39-4), (2) observing for behaviors that indicate a hearing loss, and (3) screening all children

TABLE 39-3 Classification of hearing loss based on symptom severity

HEARING LEVEL (dB)	EFFECT
Slight—<30 (hard of hearing)	Has difficulty hearing faint or distant speech Usually is unaware of hearing difficulty Likely to achieve in school but may have problems No speech defects
Mild to moderate—30-55 (hard of hearing)	Understands conversational speech at 3 to 5 feet but has difficulty if speech is faint or if not facing speaker May have speech difficulties
Marked—55-70 (hard of hearing)	Unable to understand conversational speech unless loud Considerable difficulty with group or classroom discussion Requires special speech training
Severe—70-90 (deaf)	May hear a loud voice if nearby May be able to identify loud environmental noises Can distinguish vowels but not most consonants Requires speech training
Profound—>90 (deaf)	May hear only loud sounds Requires extensive speech training

for auditory function. This discussion focuses on developmental/behavioral indices associated with hearing impairment. Auditory testing is presented in Chapter 32.

Infancy. At birth the nurse can observe the neonate's response to auditory stimuli as evidenced by the startle reflex, head turning, eye blinking, and cessation of body movement. The infant may vary in the intensity of the response, depending on the state of alertness. However, a consistent absence of a reaction should lead to suspicion of hearing loss. Other clinical manifestations of hearing impairment in the infant are summarized in Box 39-5.

Childhood. The profoundly deaf child is much more likely to be diagnosed during infancy than the less severely affected one. If the defect is not detected during early childhood, the likelihood is that it will become evident during entry into school, when the child has difficulty in learning. Unfortunately, some of these children are mistakenly placed in special classes for students with learning disabilities or MR. Therefore it is essential that the nurse suspect a hearing impairment in any child who demonstrates the behaviors listed in Box 39-5.

Of primary importance is the effect of hearing impairment on speech development. A child with a mild conductive hearing loss may speak fairly clearly but in a loud, monotone voice. A child with a sensorineural defect usually has difficulty in articulation. For example, inability to hear higher fre-

BOX 39-4

Risk Criteria for Sensorineural Hearing Impairment in Young Children

Neonates (Birth to 28 Days)

1. Family history of congenital or delayed-onset childhood sensorineural impairment
2. Congenital infection known or suspected to be associated with sensorineural hearing impairment such as toxoplasmosis, syphilis, rubella, cytomegalovirus, and herpes
3. Craniofacial anomalies, including morphologic abnormalities of the pinna and ear canal, absent philtrum, low hairline
4. Birth weight less than 1500 g (<3.3 lb)
5. Hyperbilirubinemia at a level exceeding indication for exchange transfusion
6. Ototoxic medications, including but not limited to the aminoglycosides used for more than 5 days (e.g., gentamicin, tobramycin, kanamycin, streptomycin) and loop diuretics used in combination with aminoglycosides
7. Bacterial meningitis
8. Severe depression at birth, which may include infants with Apgar scores of 0 to 3 at 5 minutes and those who fail to initiate spontaneous respiration by 10 minutes or those with hypotonia persisting to 2 hours of age
9. Prolonged mechanical ventilation for a duration equal to or greater than 10 days (e.g., persistent pulmonary hypertension)
10. Stigmata or other findings associated with a syndrome known to include sensorineural hearing loss (e.g., Waardenburg or Usher syndrome)

Infants (29 Days to 2 Years)

1. Parent/caregiver concern regarding hearing, speech, language, and/or developmental delay
2. Bacterial meningitis
3. Neonatal risk factors that may be associated with progressive sensorineural hearing loss (e.g., cytomegalovirus, prolonged mechanical ventilation, and inherited disorders)
4. Head trauma, especially with either a longitudinal or transverse fracture of the temporal bone
5. Stigmata or other findings associated with syndromes known to include sensorineural hearing loss (e.g., Waardenburg or Usher syndrome)
6. Ototoxic medications, including but not limited to the aminoglycosides used for more than 5 days (e.g., gentamicin, tobramycin, kanamycin, streptomycin) and loop diuretics used in combination with aminoglycosides
7. Children with neurodegenerative disorders such as neurofibromatosis, myoclonic epilepsy, Werdnig-Hoffmann disease, Tay-Sachs disease, Niemann-Pick disease, any metachromatic leukodystrophy, or any infantile demyelinating neuropathy
8. Childhood infectious diseases known to be associated with sensorineural hearing loss (e.g., mumps, measles)

From American Speech-Language Hearing Association: Joint Committee on Infant Hearing 1990 position statement, *ASHA* 33(suppl 5):3-6, 1991.

BOX 39-5

Clinical Manifestations of Hearing Impairment

Infants

Lack of startle or blink reflex to a loud sound
Failure to be awakened by loud environmental noises
Failure to localize a source of sound by 6 months of age
Absence of babble or inflections in voice by age 7 months
General indifference to sound
Lack of response to the spoken word; failure to follow verbal directions
Response to loud noises as opposed to the voice

Children

Use of gestures rather than verbalization to express desires, especially after age 15 months
Failure to develop intelligible speech by age 24 months
Monotone quality, unintelligible speech, lessened laughter
Vocal play, head banging, or foot stamping for vibratory sensation
Yelling or screeching to express pleasure, annoyance (tantrums), or need
Asking to have statements repeated or answering them incorrectly
Responding more to facial expression and gestures than to verbal explanation
Avoidance of social interaction; often puzzled and unhappy in such situations; prefer to play alone
Inquiring, sometimes confused facial expression
Suspicious alertness, sometimes interpreted as paranoia, alternating with cooperation
Frequent stubbornness because of lack of comprehension
Irritable at not making themselves understood
Shy, timid, and withdrawn
Often appear "dreamy," "in a world of their own," or markedly inattentive

quencies may result in the word *spoon* being pronounced "poon." Children with articulation problems need to have their hearing tested.

Nursing ALERT

When parents express concern about their child's hearing and speech development, refer the child for a hearing evaluation. The absence of well-formed syllables ("da," "na," "yaya") by 11 months of age should result in immediate referral (Eilers and Oller, 1994).

Nursing Diagnoses

A number of nursing diagnoses are prominent in the nursing care of the child with a hearing impairment and the child's family; other diagnoses specific to individual cases become evident. The most common nursing diagnoses are outlined in the Nursing Care Plan on p. 1174.

Planning

The goals of care for the child with a hearing impairment and the family are as follows:

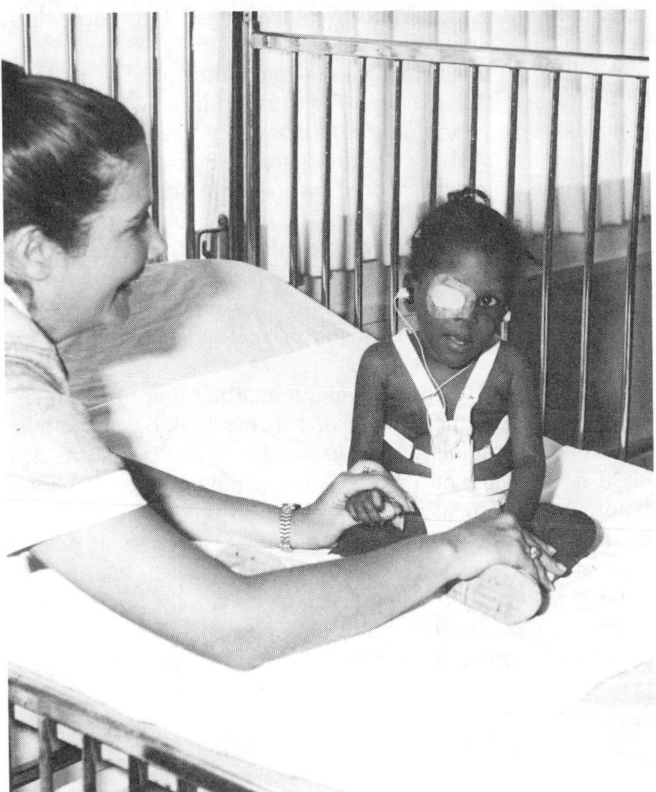

Fig. 39-7 On-the-body hearing aids are convenient for young children, such as this child with severe bilateral hearing loss. Note eye patching for strabismus.

1. The child will achieve optimum development through enhancement of the communication process and socialization.
2. The child and family will receive support.
3. The child will receive appropriate care during hospitalization.

Implementation

Promote communication process. The nurse's initial role in rehabilitation is to encourage the family to participate in an auditory training program.* Rehabilitation training consists of using a hearing aid and learning lipreading (speech reading), sign language, and verbal communication.

Hearing aids. The nurse should be familiar with the types, basic care, and handling of hearing aids, especially when the child is hospitalized.† Types of aids include those worn in or behind the ear, models incorporated into an eyeglass frame, or types worn on the body with a wire connection to the ear (Fig. 39-7). One of the most common problems with a hearing aid is *acoustic feedback,* an annoying whistling sound usually caused by improper fit of the ear mold. Sometimes the whistling may be at a frequency that the child cannot hear but that is annoying to others. In this case, if children are old enough, they are told of the noise and asked to readjust the aid. Whistling can often be reduced or eliminated by reinserting the aid, making certain that no hair is caught between the ear mold and canal, cleaning the ear mold or ear, or lowering the volume of the aid.

As children grow older, they may be self-conscious about the device. Every effort is made to make the aid inconspicuous, such as an appropriate hairstyle to cover behind-the-ear or in-the-ear models, attractive frames for glasses, and placement of the on-the-body type where it is not seen, such as under a blouse or sweater. Children are given responsibility for the care of the device as soon as they are able because fostering independence is a primary goal of rehabilitation.

Guidelines 

FACILITATING LIPREADING

Attract child's attention before speaking; use light touch to signal speaker's presence.
Stand close to child.
Face child directly or move to a 45-degree angle.
Stand still; do not walk back and forth or turn away to point or look elsewhere.
Establish eye contact and show interest.
Speak at eye level and with good lighting on speaker's face.
Be certain nothing interferes with speech patterns, such as chewing food or gum.
Speak clearly and at a slow and even rate.
Use facial expression to assist in conveying messages.
Keep sentences short.
Rephrase message if child does not understand the words.

Nursing ALERT

Stress to parents the importance of storing batteries for hearing aids in a safe location and teaching children or supervising young children not to remove the battery from the hearing aid. Ingestion of batteries is most often of those from hearing aids, including the child's own aid (Litovitz and Schmitz, 1992).

Lipreading. Even though the child may become an expert at lipreading, only approximately 40% of the spoken word is understood, and less if the speaker has an accent, mustache, or beard. Exaggerating pronunciation or speaking in an altered rhythm further lessens comprehension. Parents can help the child understand the spoken word by using the suggestions in the Guidelines box above. The child learns to supplement the spoken word with sensitivity to visual cues, primarily body language and facial expression (e.g., tightening the lips, muscle tension, and eye contact).

*Home training correspondence programs are sponsored by the **John T. Tracy Clinic,** 806 West Adams Blvd., Los Angeles, CA 90007; (213) 748-5481. Other sources of information on several aspects of hearing loss and on the International Parents' Organization are the **Alexander Graham Bell Association for the Deaf,** 3417 Volta Place, N.W., Washington, DC 20007, (202) 337-5220; and Canadian Hearing Society, 271 Spadina Rd., Toronto, Ontario M5R 2V3, (416) 964-9595.

†Information about hearing aids is available from the **National Hearing Aid Society,** 20361 Middlebelt Rd., Livonia, MI 48152; (800) 521-5247 or (313) 478-2610 (in Michigan).

Cued speech. Cued speech is an adjunct to straight lipreading. It uses hand signals to help the hearing-impaired child distinguish between words that look alike when formed by the lips (e.g., "mat," "bat"). It is most commonly used by hearing-impaired children who are using speech rather than those who are nonverbal.

Sign language. Sign language, such as the **American Sign Language (ASL)** or **British Sign Language (BSL),** is a visual-gestural language that uses hand signals that roughly correspond to specific words and concepts in the English language. Family members are encouraged to learn signing because using or watching hands requires much less concentration than lipreading or talking. In addition, a symbol method enables some deaf children to learn more and to learn faster.

Speech therapy. The most formidable task in the education of a deaf child is learning to speak. Speech is learned through a multisensory approach using visual, tactile, kinesthetic, and auditory stimulation. Because the usual mechanism for learning language (imitation and reinforcement) is not available to the deaf child, systematic formal education is required. Parents are encouraged to participate fully in the learning process.

Additional aids. Everyday activities present problems for older children with hearing impairment. For example, they may not be able to hear the telephone, doorbell, or alarm clock. Several commercial devices are available to help them adjust to these dilemmas. Flashing lights can be attached to a telephone or doorbell to signal its ringing. Trained hearing ear dogs can provide great assistance to deaf individuals because they alert the person to sounds, such as someone approaching, a moving car, a signal to wake up, or a child's cry. Special **teletypewriters** or **telecommunications devices for the deaf (TDD)** help deaf people communicate with each other over the telephone; the typed message is conveyed via the telephone lines and displayed on a small screen.*

Any audiovisual medium presents dilemmas for these children, who can see the picture but cannot hear the message. However, with **closed captioning** a special decoding device is attached to the television; the audio portion of a program is translated into subtitles that appear on the screen.†

As deaf children learn to compensate for their lack of hearing, they become extremely perceptive to visual and vibratory changes. They often know when another person wishes to talk to them because the person will walk close by but not pass. They learn to be alert to other people approaching them by seeing their shadows or feeling the vibrations of their footsteps. They are acutely aware of facial expressions and may comprehend the unspoken word more quickly than the spoken word.

Socialization. Because socialization is extremely important to the child's development, the nurse discusses with the family methods of fostering social contact. If children attend a special school for the deaf, they are able to socialize with peers in that setting. Classmates become a potential source of close friendships because they communicate more easily among themselves. Parents are encouraged to promote these relationships whenever possible.

Children with a hearing impairment may need special help in school or social activities. For those children wearing hearing aids, background noise should be kept to a minimum. Because many of these children are able to attend regular classes, the teacher may need assistance in adapting teaching methods for the child's benefit. The school nurse is often in an optimum position to emphasize methods of facilitated communication, such as lipreading (see p. 1171). Because group projects and audiovisual teaching aids may hinder the deaf child's learning, these educational methods should be carefully evaluated.

In a group setting, it is helpful for the other group members to sit in a semicircle in front of the child. Because one of the difficulties in following a group discussion is that the deaf child is unaware of who will speak next, someone should point out each speaker. Speakers can also be given numbers, or their names can be written down as each person talks. If one person writes down the main topic of the discussion, the child is able to follow lipreading more closely. Such suggestions can increase the child's ability to participate in sports, activities such as Boy Scouts or Girl Scouts, and group projects.

Support child and family. Once the diagnosis of hearing impairment has been made, parents need extensive support to adjust to the shock of learning about their child's disability and an opportunity to realize the extent of the hearing loss. If the hearing loss occurs during childhood, the child also requires sensitive, supportive care during the long and often difficult adjustment to this sensory loss. Early rehabilitation is one of the best strategies for fostering adjustment. However, progress in learning communication may not always coincide with emotional adjustment. Depression or anger is common, and such feelings are a normal part of the grieving process. (See also Chapter 38 for an extensive discussion of the emotional support of the child and family.)

Care for child during hospitalization. The needs of the hospitalized deaf child are the same as those of any other child, but the disability presents special challenges to the nurse (see the Critical Thinking Q & A box on p. 1173). For example, verbal explanations must be supplemented with tactile and visual aids, such as books or actual demonstration and practice. The child's understanding of an explanation needs to be constantly reassessed. If verbal skills are poorly developed, the child can answer questions through drawing, writing, or gesturing. For example, if the nurse is attempting to clarify where a spinal tap is done, the child is asked to point to where the procedure will be done on the body. Because deaf children often need more time to grasp the full meaning of an explanation, the nurse needs to be patient and allow ample time for understanding.

When communicating with the child, the nurse should use the same principles as those outlined for facilitating lipreading. Ideally nurses without foreign accents should be assigned to the child. The child's hearing aid is checked to ensure that it is working properly. If it is necessary to awaken the child at night, the nurse gently shakes the child or turns on the hearing aid before arousing him or her. The nurse always

---

*Directory listings stating "TDD only" before a phone number indicate that regular telephone use is not possible; "TDD and voice" indicates that both TDD users and speaking/hearing people can use the telephone number.

†Additional information is available from the National Captioning Institute, Inc., 1900 Gallows Rd., Vienna, VA 22182; (703) 917-7600 or (703) 998-2400 (TDD and Voice).

Critical Thinking Q & A

HEARING IMPAIRMENT

Five-year-old Jason has a severe congenital hearing impairment. You have been assigned to care for him in the day surgery postanesthesia care unit (PACU), where he has just been admitted following a herniorrhaphy. As he emerges from the anesthetic, he becomes more and more agitated. What is the most likely cause for his behavior?

1. This is a normal reaction to anesthesia.
2. He is experiencing separation anxiety.
3. He is unable to communicate properly.
4. He is in pain.

The correct answer is three. Because Jason became increasingly more agitated as he emerged from the anesthetic, his behavior does not suggest the transitory confusion associated with the initial emergence from the anesthetic. Rather, it suggests that as Jason became more aware of his surroundings and tried to communicate with the staff, he became increasingly frustrated. Reasons for this might include (1) not having his hearing aid in place; (2) having his arms restrained by IVs, pulse oximetry monitors, and a blood pressure cuff, thus restricting his use of sign language; (3) being unable to read the nurse's lips from a prone position; or (4) not having a nurse who could understand his speech or know or recognize his attempts to use sign language. Although pain is a possibility and needs to be evaluated, it is common to give regional blocks during the surgery to keep children comfortable until after they are discharged home. It is unlikely that he is having separation anxiety, because this usually occurs in younger children.

makes sure that the child can see him or her before performing any procedures, even routine ones such as changing a diaper or regulating an infusion. It is important to remember that the child may not be aware of anyone's presence until alerted through visual or tactile cues.

Ideally parents are encouraged to room with the child. However, it must be conveyed to them that this is not to serve as a convenience to the nurse but as a benefit to the child. Although the parents' aid can be enlisted in familiarizing the child with the hospital and in explaining procedures, the nurse also talks directly to the youngster, encouraging expression of feelings about the experience. If there is difficulty in understanding the child's speech, an effort is made to become familiar with his or her pronunciation of words. Parents often can be helpful by explaining the child's usual speech habits. Nonvocal communication devices that use pictures or words that the child can point to are also available (see p. 1161). Such boards can also be made up by drawing pictures or writing the words of common needs on cardboard, such as *parent, food, water,* or *toilet.*

The nurse has a special role as child advocate with the deaf and is in a strategic position to alert other health team members and other patients to the child's special needs regarding communication. For example, the nurse should accompany other practitioners on visits to the child's room to ensure that they speak to the child and that the child understands what is said. Caregivers often forget that the child has the ability to perceive and learn despite a hearing loss and consequently communicate only with the parents. As a result, the child's needs and feelings remain unrecognized and unmet.

Because deaf children often have difficulty in forming social relationships with other children, the child is introduced to roommates and encouraged to engage in play activities. The hospital setting can provide growth-promoting opportunities for social relationships. With the assistance of a child-life specialist, the child can learn new recreational activities, experiment with group games, and engage in therapeutic play. The use of puppets, doll-houses, role playing with dress-up clothes, building with a hammer and nails, finger painting, playing with syringes, and water play can help the child express previously suppressed feelings.

Assist in measures to prevent hearing impairment. A primary nursing role is prevention of hearing loss. Because the most common cause of impaired hearing is chronic otitis media, it is essential that appropriate measures be instituted to treat existing infections and prevent recurrences (see Chapter 43). Children with histories of ear or respiratory infections or any other condition known to increase the risk of hearing impairment should receive periodic auditory testing.

To prevent the causes of prenatal and perinatal hearing loss, pregnant women need counseling regarding the necessity of early prenatal care, including genetic counseling for known familial disorders; avoidance of all ototoxic drugs, especially during the first trimester; tests to rule out syphilis, rubella, or blood incompatibility; medical management of maternal diabetes; control of alcoholism; and adequate dietary intake. The necessity of routine immunization during childhood to eliminate the possibility of acquired sensorineural loss from rubella, mumps, or measles (encephalitis) is stressed.

Exposure to excessive noise pollution is a well-established cause of sensorineural hearing loss. The nurse should routinely assess the possibility of environmental noise pollution and advise children and parents of the potential danger. When individuals engage in activities associated with high-intensity noise, such as flying model airplanes, target shooting, or snowmobiling, they should wear ear protection such as earmuffs or earplugs (not ordinary dry cotton). However, any protection is better than none. Even common household equipment, such as lawn mowers, power vacuum cleaners, cordless telephones, and tape and compact disc players can be hazardous.

Nursing ALERT

Suspect hazardous noise if the listener experiences (1) difficulty in communication while hearing the sound, (2) ringing in the ears (tinnitus) after exposure to the sound, or (3) muffled hearing after leaving the sound.

Evaluation

The effectiveness of nursing interventions is determined by continual reassessment and evaluation of care on the basis of the following observational guidelines and expected outcomes:

1. Observe the techniques used to communicate with the child; inquire if child is enrolled in auditory training program; inquire about socialization opportunities

Nursing Care Plan

CHILD WITH HEARING IMPAIRMENT

Nursing Diagnosis: Impaired verbal communication related to conductive and/or sensorineural hearing loss

Expected Outcome: Child is able to communicate with others in the environment.

• NURSING INTERVENTIONS/*RATIONALES*

Explore family's knowledge of hearing loss and of the speech development process *to assess baseline for interventions.*

Explain the relationship between the loss of hearing and speech; discuss how speech develops; discuss alternative methods of communication (gestures, drawing, play, sign language, lip reading) *to increase family's understanding of child's speech impairment and how to cope with the loss.*

Encourage family to pursue appropriate communication interventions (e.g., oral speech classes, signing classes) for their child and family members as dictated by the child's degree of hearing loss and the child's developmental level *to promote successful communication.*

Refer family to appropriate community resources such as American Organization for the Education of the Hearing Impaired and family support groups *to aid in coping and adaptation.*

Nursing Diagnosis: Sensory/perceptual alterations (auditory) related to conductive and/or sensorineural hearing loss

Expected Outcome: Child exhibits use of appropriate mechanisms to compensate for hearing loss (e.g., hearing aid, cochlear implants); child is oriented to and displays interest in external environment.

• NURSING INTERVENTIONS/*RATIONALES*

If appropriate, explore mechanisms *that may enhance hearing abilities* (e.g., hearing aids, visual cues in environment, amplifier devices on telephone, doorbells, cochlear implant surgery).

If hearing aid is used, teach child and family how to use the aid, how to replace batteries, and how to prevent young children from ingesting/aspirating batteries *to promote optimum benefit and safety.*

Use tactile and visual stimuli with child *to enhance sensory stimulation through other modalities.*

Observe child's interaction with and interest in external environment *to assess orientation and function.*

Provide reality orientation *to counteract confusion and disorientation.*

Nursing Diagnosis: Risk for altered growth and development related to hearing loss and impaired communication

Expected Outcome: Child exhibits evidence of appropriate growth and development behaviors for age and abilities.

• NURSING INTERVENTIONS/*RATIONALES*

Involve child and family in early stimulation and intervention exercises (refer to available programs) *to enhance development of remaining senses and maximize overall development.*

Assess child's developmental progress at regular intervals and note changes in functional abilities *to revise interventions as needed.*

Help family to set realistic goals and determine child's readiness for specific developmental tasks; encourage and reinforce learning of self-care skills *to facilitate development.*

Emphasize to family that this child has needs that are the same as other children (e.g., play, discipline, interaction, approval), and encourage interventions that help child to meet these needs (e.g., selecting toys that maximize visual and tactile resources, using close-captioned television, reinforcing positive behaviors and setting limits, participating in group and peer activities, giving positive feedback for successes and good efforts) *to optimize development and socialization.*

Work with school (teachers, nurse, classmates) *to enhance understanding and ensure meeting of educational needs.*

Nursing Diagnosis: Altered family processes related to a diagnosis of deafness of a child

Expected Outcome: Family members demonstrate acceptance of child.

• NURSING INTERVENTIONS/*RATIONALES*

Provide opportunity for family to absorb and adjust to diagnosis (e.g., repeat information *to allow time for family to hear and understand;* encourage expression of concerns, fears, and feelings about diagnosis and potential impact *to facilitate adjustment;* identify support systems *to provide resources for coping).*

Provide family written materials about child's condition *for long-term reference;* introduce family to other families with similarly affected children *to enhance support mechanisms.*

Explore family reaction to the child; assist them to achieve a realistic view of child's abilities and limitations; encourage family in attempts to promote child growth and development; have family emphasize what child can do; explore ways for family to include child in family activities; encourage all family members to learn alternative communication measures *to help family increase abilities to cope with and incorporate child into family structure.*

Arrange for and participate in family conferences *to provide forum for communication, mutual goal setting, and effective strategizing.*

for the child (i.e., who are child's friends, what are his or her extracurricular activities).

2. Interview family regarding their adjustment to the sensory impairment; observe family members' relationship with the child; interview child regarding feelings about the sensory impairment and its effect on activities of daily living (especially important if impairment is recent).
3. Observe types of preparation/communication used to prepare child for hospitalization or procedures; observe parents' involvement in child's care; observe interaction of child and family with other patients.
4. Investigate community programs aimed at preventing or detecting hearing loss and inquire about nursing involvement in these efforts.

Expected outcomes

See the Nursing Care Plan on p. 1174.

VISUAL IMPAIRMENT

Visual impairment is a common problem during childhood. In the United States the prevalence of blindness and serious visual impairment in the pediatric population is estimated to be between 30 and 64 children per 100,000 population. Another 100 children per 100,000 have less serious impairment (Davidson, 1992). The nurse's role is clearly one of assessment, prevention, referral and, in some instances, rehabilitation.

Definition and Classification

Visual impairment is a general term that refers to visual loss that cannot be corrected with regular prescription lenses. However, more useful definitions for classifying visual impairments include the following. **School vision** (also known as partially sighted) refers to visual acuity between 20/70 and 20/200. The child should be able to obtain an education in the usual public school system with the use of normal-sized print. Near vision is almost always better than distance vision. **Legal blindness,** visual acuity of 20/200 or less and/or a visual field of 20 degrees or less in the better eye, is useful only as a legal definition, not as a medical diagnosis. It allows special considerations with regard to taxes, entrance into special schools, eligibility for aid, and other benefits.

Etiology

Visual impairment can be caused by a number of genetic and prenatal or postnatal conditions. These conditions include perinatal infections (herpes, chlamydia, gonococci, rubella, syphilis, or toxoplasmosis), retinopathy of prematurity, trauma, postnatal infections (meningitis), and disorders such as sickle cell disease, juvenile rheumatoid arthritis, Tay-Sachs disease, albinism, and retinoblastoma. In many instances, such as with refractive errors, the cause of the defect is unknown.

Refractive errors are the most common types of visual disorders in children. The term *refraction* means bending and refers to the bending of light rays as they pass through the lens of the eye. Normally, light rays enter the lens and fall directly on the retina. However, in refractive disorders the light rays either fall in front of the retina (myopia) or beyond it (hyperopia). Other eye problems such as strabismus may or may not include refractive errors, but they are very important because they result in blindness from amblyopia if left untreated. These other less common visual disorders are summarized in Box 39-6. In addition to these disorders, other visual problems can be the result of infection or trauma.

Trauma. Trauma is a common cause of blindness in children. Injuries to the eyeball and adnexa (the supporting or ac-

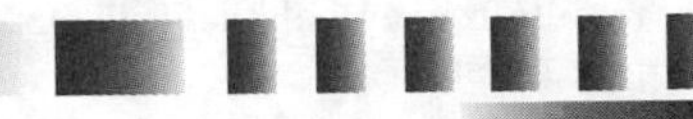

EMERGENCY

EYE INJURIES

Foreign object

Examine eye for presence of a foreign body (evert upper lid to examine upper eye).
Remove a freely movable object with pointed corner of gauze pad lightly moistened with water.
Do not irrigate eye or attempt to remove a penetrating object (see below).
Caution child against rubbing eye.

Chemical burns

Irrigate eye copiously with tap water for 20 minutes.
Evert upper lid to flush thoroughly.
Hold child's head with eye under tap of running lukewarm water.
Take child to emergency room.
Have child rest with eyes closed.
Keep room darkened.

Ultraviolet burns

If skin is burned, patch both eyes (make sure lids are completely closed); secure dressing with Kling bandages wrapped around head rather than tape.
Have child rest with eyes closed.
Refer to an ophthalmologist.

Hematoma ("Black Eye")

Use a flashlight to check for gross **hyphema** (hemorrhage into anterior chamber; visible fluid meniscus across iris; more easily seen in light-colored than in brown eyes).
Apply ice for first 24 hours to reduce swelling if no hyphema is present.
Refer to an ophthalmologist immediately if hyphema is present.
Have child rest with eyes closed.

Penetrating injuries

Take child to emergency room.
Never remove an object that has penetrated eye.
Follow strict aseptic technique in examining eye.
Observe for the following:
- Aqueous or vitreous leaks (fluid leaking from point of penetration)
- Hyphema
- Shape and equality of pupils, reaction to light
- Prolapsed iris (not perfectly circular)

Apply a Fox shield if available (not a regular eye patch), and apply patch over unaffected eye to prevent bilateral movement.
Maintain bed rest with child in 30-degree Fowler position.
Caution child against rubbing eye.

BOX 39-6
TYPES OF VISUAL IMPAIRMENT

REFRACTIVE ERRORS

Myopia

Nearsightedness—Ability to see objects clearly at close range but not at a distance

Pathophysiology

Results from eyeball that is too long, causing image to fall in front of retina

Clinical manifestations

Rubs eyes excessively
Tilts head or thrusts head forward
Has difficulty in reading or other close work
Holds books close to eyes
Writes or colors with head close to table
Clumsy; walks into objects
Blinks more than usual or is irritable when doing close work
Is unable to see objects clearly
Does poorly in school, especially in subjects that require demonstration, such as arithmetic
Dizziness
Headache
Nausea following close work

Treatment

Corrected with biconcave lenses that focus rays on retina

Hyperopia

Farsightedness—Ability to see objects at a distance

Pathophysiology

Results from eyeball that is too short, causing image to focus beyond retina

Clinical manifestations

Because of accommodative ability, child can usually see objects at all ranges
Most children normally hyperopic until approximately 7 years of age

Treatment

If correction is required, use convex lenses to focus rays on retina

Astigmatism

Unequal curvatures in refractive apparatus

Pathophysiology

Results from unequal curvatures in cornea or lens that cause light rays to bend in different directions

Clinical manifestations

Depends on severity of refractive error in each eye
May have clinical manifestations of myopia

Treatment

Corrected with special lenses that compensate for refractive errors

Anisometropia

Different refractive strength in each eye

Pathophysiology

May develop amblyopia as weaker eye is used less

Clinical manifestations

Depends on severity of refractive error in each eye
May have clinical manifestations of myopia

Treatment

Treated with corrective lenses, preferably contact lenses, to improve vision in each eye so they work as a unit

AMBLYOPIA

Lazy eye—Reduced visual acuity in one eye

Pathophysiology

Results when one eye does not receive sufficient stimulation
Each retina receives different images, resulting in diplopia (double vision)
Brain accommodates by suppressing less intense image
Visual cortex eventually does not respond to visual stimulation, with loss of vision in that eye

Clinical manifestations

Poor vision in affected eye

Treatment

Preventable if treatment of primary visual defect, such as anisometropia or strabismus, begins before 6 years of age

STRABISMUS

"Squint" or cross-eye—Malalignment of eyes (Fig. 39-8)
Esotropia—Inward deviation of eye
Exotropia—Outward deviation of eye

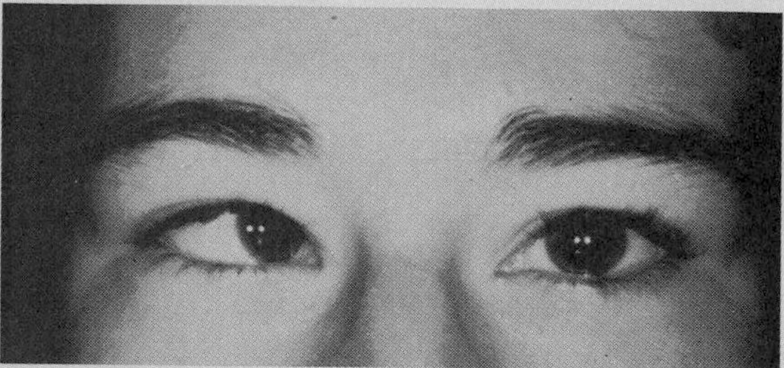

Fig. 39-8 Strabismus (esotropia). Note obvious malalignment of eyes. Light reflections are centered in the left cornea and to the side of the right cornea. (From Havener WH et al: *Nursing care in eye, ear, nose, and throat disorders*, ed 3, St Louis, 1974, Mosby.)

Pathophysiology

May result from muscle imbalance or paralysis, poor vision, or congenital defect
Because visual axes are not parallel, brain receives two images, and amblyopia can result

Clinical manifestations

Squints eyelids together or frowns
Has difficulty in focusing from one distance to another
Inaccurate judgment in picking up objects
Unable to see print or moving objects clearly

BOX 39-6
TYPES OF VISUAL IMPAIRMENT—cont'd

Closes one eye to see
Tilts head to one side
If combined with refractive errors, may see any of the manifestations listed for refractive errors
Diplopia
Photophobia
Dizziness
Headache
Cross-eye

Treatment

Treatment depends on cause of strabismus
May involve occlusion therapy (patching stronger eye) or surgery to increase visual stimulation to weaker eye
Early diagnosis is essential to prevent vision loss

CATARACTS

Opacity of crystalline lens

Pathophysiology

Prevents light rays from entering eye and refracting them on retina

Clinical manifestations

Gradually less able to see objects clearly
May lose peripheral vision
Nystagmus (with complete blindness)
Gray opacities of lens
Strabismus
Absence of red reflex

Treatment

Requires surgery to remove cloudy lens and replace lens (intraocular lens implant, removable contact lens, prescription glasses)
Must be treated early to prevent blindness from amblyopia

GLAUCOMA

Increased intraocular pressure

Pathophysiology

Congenital type results from defective development of some component related to flow of aqueous humor
Increased pressure on optic nerve causes eventual atrophy and blindness

Clinical manifestations

Mostly seen in acquired types—loses peripheral vision
May bump into objects not directly in front
Sees halos around objects
May complain of mild pain or discomfort (severe pain, nausea, vomiting, if sudden rise in pressure)
Redness
Excessive tearing (epiphora)
Photophobia
Spasmodic winking (blepharospasm)
Corneal haziness
Enlargement of eyeball (buphthalmos)

Treatment

Requires surgical treatment (goniotomy) to open outflow tracts
May require more than one procedure

cessory structures, such as eyelids, conjunctivae, and lacrimal glands) can be classified as penetrating or non-penetrating. *Penetrating wounds* are most often a result of sharp instruments such as sticks, knives, or scissors; propulsive objects such as firecrackers, guns, bows and arrows, or slingshots; or a powerful contusion by a blunt object, which may occur during a fight or from a serious car accident. *Nonpenetrating injuries* may be a result of foreign objects in the eyes, lacerations, a blow from a blunt object such as a ball (baseball, softball, basketball, and racquet sports) or fist, or thermal or chemical burns.

Treatment is aimed at preventing further ocular damage and is primarily the responsibility of the ophthalmologist. It involves adequate examination of the injured eye (with the child sedated or anesthetized in severe injuries), appropriate immediate intervention such as removal of the foreign body or suturing of the laceration, and prevention of complications, such as administration of antibiotics or steroids and complete bed rest to allow the eye to heal and blood to reabsorb (see the Emergency box on p. 1175). The prognosis varies according to the type of injury. It is usually guarded in all cases of penetrating wounds because of the high risk of serious complications.

Infections. Infections of the adnexa and the structures of the eyeball or globe are common in children. The most common eye infection is conjunctivitis (see p. 1181). Treatment is usually ophthalmic antibiotics. Severe infections may require systemic antibiotic therapy. Steroids are used cautiously because they exacerbate viral infections such as herpes simplex and increase the risk of damage to the involved structures.

Nursing Care Management

Assessment

Assessment of children for visual impairment is a critical nursing responsibility. Discovery of a visual impairment as early as possible is essential to prevent social, physical, and psychologic damage to the child. Assessment involves (1) identifying those children who by virtue of their history are at risk, (2) observing for behaviors that indicate a vision loss, and (3) screening all children for visual acuity and signs of other ocular disorders, such as strabismus. This discussion focuses on the clinical manifestation of various types of visual problems (see Box 39-6). Vision testing is discussed in Chapter 32.

Infancy. At birth the nurse should observe the neonate's response to visual stimuli, such as following a light or object and cessation of body movement. The infant may vary in the intensity of the response, depending on the state of alertness.

Of special importance in detecting visual impairment during infancy are the parents' concerns regarding visual responsiveness in their child. Their concerns, such as lack of eye contact from the infant, must be taken seriously. During infancy the child should be tested for strabismus. Lack of binocularity after 4 months of age is considered abnormal and must be treated to prevent amblyopia.

Nursing ALERT

Suspect blindness if the infant does not react to light and in a child of any age if parents express concern.

Childhood. Because the most common visual impairments during childhood are refractive errors, testing for visual acuity is essential. The school nurse usually assumes major responsibility for vision testing in schoolchildren. Besides refractive errors, the nurse should be aware of signs and symptoms that indicate other ocular problems. If a referral is made to the family requesting further eye testing, the nurse is responsible for follow-up concerning the recommendation.

Nursing Diagnoses

A number of nursing diagnoses are prominent in the nursing care of the child with visual impairment and the child's family; other diagnoses specific to individual cases become evident.

Planning

The goals of care for the child with visual impairment and the child's family are as follows:

1. The child and family will receive support and education.
2. The parent-child attachment will develop.
3. The child will achieve optimum development.
4. The child will receive appropriate care during hospitalization.

Implementation

Support child and family. The shock of learning that their child is blind or partially sighted is an immense crisis for families. Of all types of disabilities, many people fear loss of sight the most. Vision is involved in almost every activity of daily living. Parents need support during the initial phase of learning about the diagnosis and help to gain a realistic understanding of their child's abilities. The family is encouraged to investigate appropriate stimulation and educational programs for their child as soon as possible. Sources of information include state Commissions for the Blind, local schools for the blind, the American Foundation for the Blind,* National Federation of the Blind,† National Association for Parents of the Visually Impaired, Inc.,* National Association for Visually Handicapped,† and American Council of the Blind.‡

When blindness is not congenital but acquired, newly blind children need a great deal of support to help them adjust to the disability. They are usually frightened and confused by the sudden or progressive loss of sight and benefit from an environment that provides security and familiarity.

Promote parent-child attachment. A crucial time in the life of blind infants is when they and their parents are getting acquainted with each other. Pleasurable patterns of interaction between the infant and parents may be lacking if there is not enough reciprocity. For example, if the parent gazes fondly at the infant's face and seeks eye contact but the infant fails to respond because he or she cannot see the parent, a troubled cycle of responses may occur. The nurse can help parents learn to look for other cues that indicate the infant is responding to them, such as whether the eyelids blink; whether the activity level accelerates or slows; whether respiratory patterns change, such as faster or slower breathing, when the parents come near; and whether the infant makes throaty sounds when they speak to the infant. In time parents learn that the infant has unique ways of relating to them. They are encouraged to show affection using nonvisual methods, such as talking or reading, cuddling, and walking the child.

Promote child's optimum development. Promoting the child's optimum development requires rehabilitation in a number of important areas. These include learning self-help skills and appropriate communication techniques to become independent. Although nurses may not be directly involved in such programs, they can provide direction and guidance to families regarding the availability of programs and the need to promote these activities in their child.

Development and independence. Motor development depends on sight almost as much as verbal communication depends on hearing. From earliest infancy parents are encouraged to expose the infant to as many visual-motor experiences as possible, such as sitting supported in an infant seat or swing and being given opportunities for holding up the head, sitting unsupported, reaching for objects, and crawling.

Despite visual impairment the child can become independent in all aspects of self-care. The same principles used for promoting independence in sighted children apply, with additional emphasis on nonvisual cues. For example, the child may need help in dressing, such as special arrangement of clothing for style coordination and braille tags to distinguish colors and prints.

The blind child also must learn to become independent in navigational skills. The two main techniques are the *tapping method* (use of a cane to survey the environment for direction and to avoid obstacles) and *guides*, such as a human sighted guide or a dog guide such as a Seeing Eye dog. Partially

*11 Penn Plaza, Suite 300, NY 10001; (212) 502-7600.
†1800 Johnson St., Baltimore, MD 21230; (410) 659-9314.

*2180 Linway Dr., Beloit, WI 53511; (800) 562-6265.
†22 W. 21st St., New York, NY 10010; (212) 889-3141.
‡1155 15th St., N.W., Washington, DC 20005; (202) 467-5081 or (800) 424-8666 (afternoons only).
Sources of information in Canada include the **Canadian National Institute for the Blind**, 1931 Bayview Ave., Toronto, Ontario M4G 4C8; **Low Vision Association of Canada**, 145 Adelaide St. West, Toronto, Ontario M5H 3H4; and **Blind Organization of Ontario**, 597 Parliament St., Suite B-3, Toronto, Ontario M4X 1W3.

sighted children may benefit from ocular aids such as a monocular telescope.

Play and socialization. Blind children do not learn to play automatically. Because they cannot imitate others or actively explore the environment as sighted children do, they depend much more on others to stimulate them and teach them how to play. Parents need help in selecting appropriate play material, especially those that encourage fine and gross motor development and stimulate the senses of hearing, touch, and smell. Toys with educational value are especially useful, such as dolls with various clothing closures.

Blind children have the same needs for socialization as sighted children. Because they have little difficulty in learning verbal skills, they are able to communicate with age-mates and participate in suitable activities. The nurse discusses with parents opportunities for socialization outside of the home, especially regular preschools. The trend is to include these children with sighted children to help them adjust to the outside world for eventual independence.

To compensate for inadequate stimulation, these children may develop *blindisms* (self-stimulatory activities, such as body rocking, finger flicking, or arm twirling). Such habits retard the child's social acceptance and are discouraged. Behavior modification is often successful in reducing or eliminating blindisms.

Education. The main obstacle to learning is the child's total dependence on nonvisual cues. Although the child can learn via verbal lecturing, he or she is unable to read the written word or to write without special education. Therefore the child must rely on *braille*, a system that uses raised dots to represent letters and numbers. The child can read the braille with the fingers and can write a message using a braille writer. However, unless others read braille, this system is not useful for communicating with others. A more portable system for written communication is the use of a braille slate and stylus (Fig. 39-9) or a microcassette tape recorder. A recorder is especially helpful for leaving messages for others and for taking notes during classroom lecturing. For mathematic calculations, portable calculators with voice synthesizers are available.*

Records and tapes are significant sources of reading material other than braille books, which are large and cumbersome. The Library of Congress* has talking books, braille books, and a special records program, which are available at many local and state libraries and directly from the Library of Congress. The talking book machine and tape player are provided at no cost to families, and there is no postage fee for returning the materials. Recording for the Blind, Inc.,† also provides texts and tapes of books, which are very helpful for secondary and college students who are blind.

*A catalog of numerous products for people with vision problems is available from the American Foundation for the Blind (see footnote on p. 1178).

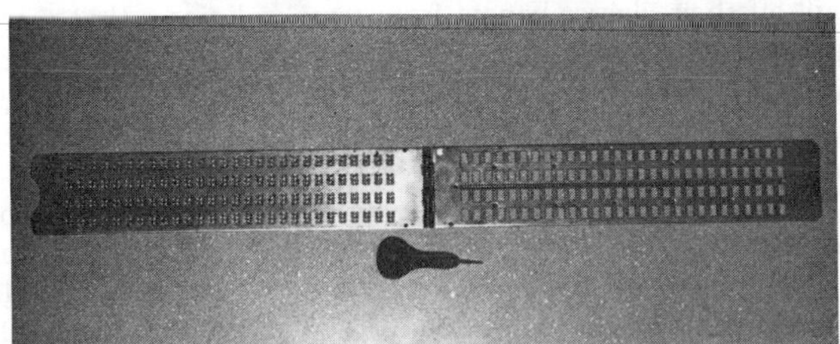

Fig. 39-9 Braille slate and stylus. The hinged slate consists of a series of open rectangles on one side and standard braille cells on the other. The paper is clamped or sandwiched between these two metal bars, and the appropriate dots are punched with the stylus.

Learning to use a regular typewriter is another form of writing, but the blind person is unable to check the accuracy of the typing. Computers eliminate this drawback; a home computer with a voice synthesizer can be adapted to speak each letter or word that has been typed.

The partially sighted child benefits from specialized visual aids that produce a magnified retinal image. The basic devices are accommodation, such as bringing the object closer, special plus lenses, hand-held and stand magnifiers, telescopes, video projection systems, and large print. Special equipment is available to enlarge print. Information about services for the partially sighted is available from the National Association for Visually Handicapped and American Foundation for the Blind (see the footnote on p. 1178 for the addresses). Children with diminished vision often prefer to do close work without their glasses and compensate by bringing the object very near to their eyes. This practice should be allowed. The exception is the child with vision in only one eye, who should always wear glasses for protection.

Care for child during hospitalization. Because nurses are more likely to care for children who are hospitalized for procedures that involve temporary loss of vision than for children who are blind, the following discussion concentrates primarily on the needs of children with temporary blindness. The nursing care objectives in either situation are to (1) reassure the child and family throughout every phase of treatment, (2) orient the child to the surroundings, (3) provide a safe environment, and (4) encourage independence. Whenever possible, the same nurse should care for the child to ensure consistency in the approach. These same principles also apply to a blind child who requires hospitalization.

When sighted children temporarily lose their vision, almost every aspect of the environment becomes bewildering and frightening. They are forced to rely on nonvisual senses for help in adjusting to the blindness without the benefit of any special training. Nurses have a major role in minimizing the effects of temporary vision loss. They need to talk to the child about everything that is occurring, emphasizing aspects of procedures that are felt or heard. They should approach the child by always identifying themselves as soon as they enter the room. Because unfamiliar sounds are especially frightening, they are explained. Parents are encouraged to room with their child and participate in the care. Familiar objects, such as a teddy bear or doll, should be brought from home to help lessen the strangeness of the hospital. As soon as the child is able to be out of bed, he or she is oriented to the immediate surroundings. If the child is able to see on admission, an opportunity is taken to point out significant aspects of the room.

***Division for the Blind and Visually Handicapped,** 1291 Taylor St., N.W., Washington, DC 20542; (202) 707-5100 or (800) 424-8567.
†20 Roszel Rd., Princeton, NJ 08540; (609) 452-0606.

The child is encouraged to practice ambulating with the eyes closed to become accustomed to this experience.

The room is arranged with safety in mind. For example, a stool or chair is placed next to the bed to help the child climb into and out of bed. The furniture is always placed in the same position to prevent collisions. Cleaning personnel are reminded of the need to keep the room in order. If the child has difficulty navigating by feeling the walls, a rope can be attached from the bed to the point of destination, such as the bathroom. Attention to details such as well-fitting slippers or robes that do not hang on the floor is important in preventing tripping. Unlike the child who is blind, children experiencing a temporary loss of vision are not familiar with navigating with a cane.

The child is encouraged to be independent in self-care activities, especially if the vision loss may be prolonged or potentially permanent. For example, during bathing the nurse sets up all the equipment and encourages the child to participate. At mealtime the nurse explains where each food item is on the tray, opens any special containers, and prepares cereal or toast but encourages the child in self-feeding. Favorite finger foods such as sandwiches, hamburgers, hot dogs, or pizza may be good selections. The child is praised for efforts at being cooperative and independent. Any improvements made in self-care, no matter how small, are stressed.

Appropriate recreational activities are provided, and if a child-life specialist is available, such planning is done jointly. Because children with temporary blindness have a wide variety of play experiences, they are encouraged to select activities. For example, if they like to read, they may enjoy being read to. If they prefer manual activity, they may appreciate playing with clay or building blocks or feeling different textures and naming them. If they need an outlet for aggression, activities such as pounding or banging on a drum can be helpful. Simple board and card games can be played with a "seeing partner" or if the opponent helps with the game. They should have familiar toys from home to play with, because familiar items are more easily manipulated than new ones. If parents wish to bring presents, they should be objects that stimulate hearing and touch, such as a radio, music box, or stuffed animal.

Occasionally children who are blind come to the hospital for procedures to restore their vision. Although this is an extremely happy time, it also requires intervention to help them adjust to sight. They need an opportunity to take in all that they see. They should not be bombarded with visual stimuli. They may need to concentrate on people's faces or their own to become accustomed to this experience. They often need to talk about what they see and to compare the visual images with their mental ones. The child may also go through a period of depression, which must be respected and supported. The nurse or parents should refrain from statements such as "How can you be so sad when you can see again?" Instead the child should be encouraged to discuss how it feels to see, especially in terms of seeing himself or herself.

Newly sighted children also need time to adjust to the ability to engage in activities that were impossible before. For example, they may prefer to use braille to read, rather than learning a new "visual approach," because of their familiarity with the touch system. Eventually, as they learn to recognize letters and numbers, they will integrate these new skills into reading and writing. However, parents and teachers must be careful not to push them before they are ready. This applies to social relationships and physical activities, as well as to learning situations.

Assist in measures to prevent visual impairment. An essential nursing goal is to prevent visual impairment. This goal involves many of the same interventions discussed under hearing impairments, namely (1) prenatal screening for pregnant women at risk, such as those with rubella or syphilis infection and family histories of genetic disorders associated with vision loss; (2) adequate prenatal and perinatal care to prevent prematurity and iatrogenic damage from excessive oxygen administration; (3) periodic screening of all children, especially newborns through preschoolers, for congenital blindness and visual impairments caused by refractive errors, strabismus, and other conditions; (4) rubella immunization of all children; and (5) safety counseling regarding the common causes of ocular trauma.

Safety counseling should include safe practices when working with, playing with, or carrying objects such as scissors, knives, and balls.

Nursing ALERT

A face mask and helmet should be required gear for children playing baseball or softball (especially catcher, batter, umpire, and base runner), hockey, or football.

Following detection of eye problems, the nurse has a responsibility to prevent further ocular damage by ensuring that corrective treatment is provided. For the child with strabismus, such treatment often necessitates occlusion patching of the stronger eye. Compliance with the procedure is greatest during the early preschool years. It is more difficult to encourage school-age children to wear the occlusive patch because the poor visual acuity of the uncovered weaker eye interferes with schoolwork and because the patch sets them apart from their peers. In school they benefit from being positioned favorably (closer to the chalkboard) and allowed extra time to read or complete an assignment. If treatment of the eye disorder requires instillation of ophthalmic medication, the family is taught the correct procedure (see Chapter 42).*

For the child with refractive errors, the nurse helps with the adjustment to wearing glasses. Young children who often pull off their glasses benefit from temporal pieces that wrap around the ears or from an elastic strap attached to the frames and around the back of the head to hold the glasses securely. Once children appreciate the value of clear vision, they are more likely to wear the corrective lenses.

Glasses should not interfere with any activity. Special protective guards are available during contact sports to prevent accidental injury, and all corrective lenses should be made from safety glass, which is shatterproof. Corrective lenses often improve visual acuity so dramatically that children are

*Home care instructions on giving eye medications are available in Wong DL: *Wong and Whaley's clinical manual of pediatric nursing*, ed 4, St Louis, 1996, Mosby.

able to compete more effectively in sports. This in itself is a tremendous inducement to continue wearing glasses.

Contact lenses are a popular alternative, especially for adolescents. Several types are available, such as hard lenses, including gas permeable ones, and soft lenses, which may be designed for daily or extended wear. Contact lenses offer several advantages over glasses, such as greater visual acuity, total corrected field of vision, convenience (especially with the disposable type), and optimal cosmetic benefit. Unfortunately, they are usually more expensive and require much more care than glasses, including considerable practice to learn techniques for insertion and removal. If they are prescribed, the nurse can be very helpful in teaching parents or older children how to care for the lenses.

Because trauma is the leading cause of blindness, the nurse has the major responsibility of preventing further eye injury until the specific treatment is instituted. The major principles to follow when caring for an eye injury are outlined in the Emergency box on p. 1175. Because patients with a serious eye injury fear blindness, the nurse should stay with the child and family to provide support and reassurance.

Evaluation

The effectiveness of nursing interventions is determined by continual reassessment and evaluation of care on the basis of the following observational guidelines and expected outcomes:

1. Interview family regarding their adjustment to the sensory impairment; observe family members' relationship with the child; interview child regarding feelings about the sensory impairment and its effect on activities of daily living (especially important if a visual loss).
2. Have parents identify those cues that indicate the infant is responding to them; observe nonvisual behaviors of parents as they respond to infant.
3. Observe the techniques the child uses to read and navigate; inquire if the child is enrolled in a visual training program; inquire about socialization opportunities for the child (i.e., who are the child's friends, what are the child's extracurricular activities).
4. Observe preparation of the room and self-care activities that provide for safety and independence during hospitalization.

Expected outcomes:

1. Parents express their feelings and concerns regarding loss of sight and demonstrate an understanding of child's disability and its implications.
2. Parents demonstrate attachment behaviors.
3. Infant or child engages in appropriate activities for level of development (specify), and child demonstrates an attitude of security in the environment.
4. Child and family receive safe and supportive care during hospitalization.

See also Nursing Care Plan: The Child with Visual Impairment.*

*In Wong DL: *Wong and Whaley's clinical manual of pediatric nursing*, ed 4, St Louis, 1996, Mosby.

CONJUNCTIVITIS

Acute conjunctivitis, inflammation of the conjunctiva, occurs from a variety of causes that are typically age related. In newborns conjunctivitis can occur from infection during birth, most often from *Chlamydia trachomatis* (inclusion conjunctivitis). In infants recurrent conjunctivitis may be a sign of nasolacrimal duct obstruction. In children the usual causes are viral, bacterial, allergic, or related to a foreign body. Bacterial infection accounts for most instances of acute conjunctivitis in children. Diagnosis is made primarily from the clinical manifestations (Box 39-7), although cultures of purulent drainage may be needed to identify the specific cause.

Therapeutic Management

Treatment of conjunctivitis depends on the cause. Viral conjunctivitis is self-limiting, and treatment is limited to removal of the accumulated secretions. Bacterial conjunctivitis is usually treated with topical antibacterial agents. Drops may be used during the day; an ointment may be used at bedtime because the ointment preparation remains in the eye longer. Ointments are usually not used in the daytime because they blur vision.

Nursing Care Management

Nursing goals include keeping the eye clean and properly administering ophthalmic medication. Accumulated secretions are always removed by wiping from the inner canthus downward and outward, away from the opposite eye. Warm, moist compresses, such as a clean washcloth wrung out with hot tap water, are helpful in removing the crusts. Compresses are *not* kept on the eye, because an occlusive covering promotes

BOX 39-7
Clinical Manifestations of Conjunctivitis

Bacterial conjunctivitis ("pink eye")
Purulent drainage
Crusting of eyelids, especially on awakening
Inflamed conjunctiva
Swollen lids
Usually both eyes infected

Viral conjunctivitis
Usually occurs with upper respiratory tract infection
Serous (watery) drainage
Inflamed conjunctiva
Swollen lids
Usually both eyes infected

Allergic conjunctivitis
Itching
Watery to thick, stringy discharge
Inflamed conjunctiva
Swollen lids
Usually both eyes affected

Conjunctivitis caused by foreign body
Tearing
Pain
Inflamed conjunctiva
Usually only one eye affected

bacterial growth. Medication is instilled immediately after the eyes have been cleaned and according to correct procedure (see Chapter 42).

Prevention of infection in other family members is an important consideration with bacterial conjunctivitis. The child's washcloth and towel are kept separate from those used by others. Tissues used to clean the eye are discarded. The child should refrain from rubbing the eye and is instructed in good handwashing.

DEAF-BLIND CHILDREN

The most traumatic sensory impairment is loss of sight and hearing. Obviously, auditory and visual disabilities have profound effects on a child's development. They interfere with the normal sequence of physical, intellectual, and psychosocial growth. Although such children often achieve the usual motor milestones, their rate of development is slower. These children learn communication only with specialized training. Some deaf-blind children, especially those with residual hearing or sight, can learn to speak. Whenever possible, speech is encouraged because it allows communication with other individuals.

The future prospects for deaf-blind children are at best unpredictable. Congenital blindness and/or deafness is commonly accompanied by other physical or neurologic problems, which further lessen the child's learning potential. The most favorable prognosis is for children who have acquired deafness and blindness and have few, if any, associated disabilities. Their learning capacity is greatly potentiated by their developmental progress before the sensory impairments. Although total independence, including gainful vocational training, is the goal, some deaf-blind children are unable to develop to this level. They may require lifelong parental or residential care. The nurse working with such families helps them deal with future goals for the child, including possible alternatives to home care during the parents' advancing years.

RETINOBLASTOMA

Retinoblastoma is a rare congenital malignant tumor arising from the retina. It may be present at birth or may arise in the retina during the first 2 years of life. Retinoblastoma may be hereditary or nonhereditary, and unilateral or bilateral. Hereditary retinoblastomas are transmitted as an autosomal-dominant trait with incomplete penetrance.

Diagnostic Evaluation

Retinoblastoma has few grossly obvious signs (Box 39-8). Typically it is the parent who first observes a whitish "glow" in the pupil. The white reflex or white pupil *(leukokoria)*, known as the *cat's eye reflex*, represents visualization of the tumor as the light momentarily falls on the mass (Fig. 39-10).

BOX 39-8
Clinical Manifestations of Retinoblastoma

Cat's eye reflex (most common sign)
Strabismus (second most common sign)
Red, painful eye, often with glaucoma
Blindness (late sign)

The first step in diagnosis is carefully listening to and recognizing the significance of reports from family members regarding suspected abnormalities within the eye. Because the cat's eye reflex is a momentary sign visualized only under specific conditions, the practitioner must attempt to duplicate those conditions necessary to observe the tumor. Children suspected of having this disorder are referred to an ophthalmologist. Definitive diagnosis is usually based on indirect ophthalmoscopy, which is performed with the patient under general anesthesia with maximum dilation of the pupils.

Therapeutic Management

Treatment of retinoblastoma depends chiefly on the stage of the tumor at the time of diagnosis. Staging includes five groups; group I refers to a small localized tumor(s), whereas group V is reserved for tumors involving more than half the retina and vitreous seeding. In general, early-stage unilateral retinoblastomas are treated with irradiation or other techniques such as cryotherapy, which freezes the tumor. The aim of therapy is to preserve useful vision in the affected eye and eradicate the tumor.

With advanced tumor growth, especially optic nerve involvement, enucleation of the affected eye is the treatment of choice. The use of chemotherapy in advanced disease is controversial but if used may include the drugs vincristine, cyclophosphamide, and doxorubicin (Adriamycin).

With bilateral disease, every attempt is made to preserve useful vision in the least affected eye, with enucleation of the severely diseased eye. When bilateral tumors are found early, radiotherapy or other treatments to both eyes may prevent the need for enucleation.

Prognosis. The overall prognosis for retinoblastoma is very favorable, with a survival rate of nearly 90% for both unilateral and bilateral tumors. Retinoblastoma is one of the tumors that may spontaneously regress.

Of major concern in long-term survivors is the development of secondary tumors, especially osteogenic sarcoma. Children with bilateral disease (hereditary form) are more likely to develop secondary cancers than are children with

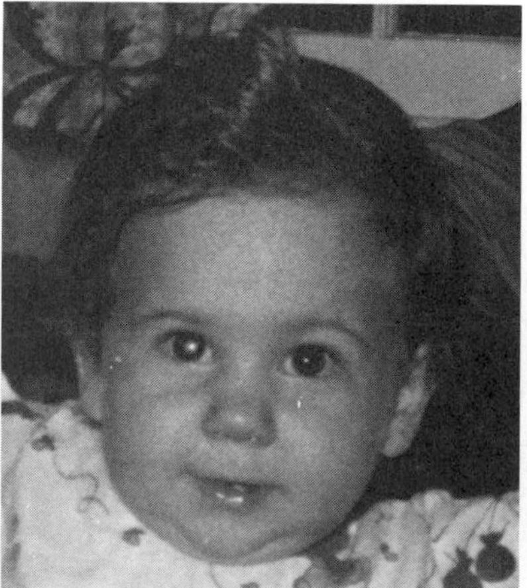

Fig. 39-10 Cat's eye reflex. Whitish appearance of lens is produced as light falls on tumor mass in right eye.

unilateral disease. It is thought that these individuals are predisposed to developing cancer, and radiation increases their risk.

Nursing Care Management

One of the most important nursing goals is to have a high index of suspicion for this rare malignancy. If parents report noticing a strange light in the eye or expression, these concerns must be taken seriously. Families with a history of retinoblastoma require follow-up, and the nurse can be instrumental in reminding parents of appointments.

Because the tumor is usually diagnosed in infants or very young children, most of the preparation for diagnostic tests and treatment involves parents. After indirect ophthalmoscopy, the child may not see very clearly, or the eyes may be sensitive to light because of pupillary dilation. Parents are made aware of these normal reactions before the procedure. They also are informed that a battery of screening tests, such as bone surveys and bone marrow aspiration, may be performed to detect metastasis.

Once the disease is staged, the physician confers with the parents regarding treatment. Unless the diagnosis is made very early, an enucleation is performed. Parents are told about the procedure, as well as about the positive benefits of a prosthesis. Showing them pictures of another child with an artificial eye may be very helpful in their adjustment to the thought of disfigurement (Fig. 39-11).

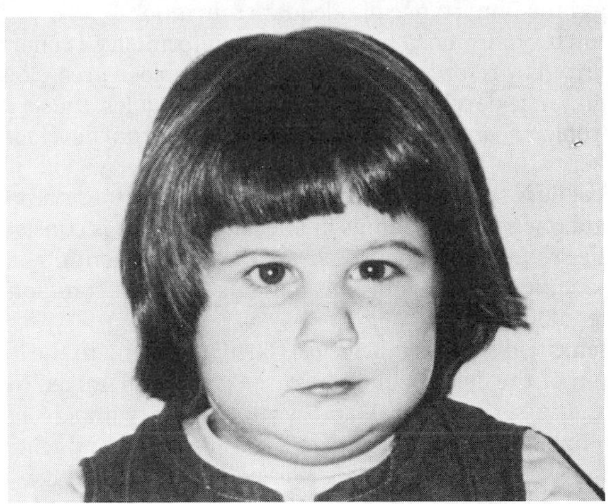

Fig. 39-11 Preschooler with right prosthetic eye.

After surgery the parents are prepared for the child's facial appearance. An eye patch is in place, and the child's face may be edematous or ecchymotic. Parents often fear seeing the surgical site because they imagine a cavity in the skull. On the contrary, the lids are usually closed and the area does not appear sunken because a surgically implanted sphere maintains the shape of the eyeball. The implant is covered with conjunctiva, and when the lids are open the exposed area resembles the mucosal lining of the mouth. Once the child is fitted for a prosthesis (usually within 3 weeks), the facial appearance returns to normal. Initial instructions for care of the prosthesis are given by the ocularist, who fits and manufactures the device.

Care of the socket is minimal and easily accomplished. The wound itself is clean and has little or no drainage. If an antibiotic ointment is prescribed, it is applied in a thin line on the surface of the tissues of the socket. To cleanse the site, an irrigating solution may be ordered and is instilled daily or more frequently if necessary, *before* application of the antibiotic ointment. The dressing consists of an eye pad taped over the surgical site with nonirritating tape; it is changed daily. Once the socket has healed completely, a dressing is no longer necessary, but it is a preventive measure against infection.

A long-term consideration is the survivor's ability to transmit the defective gene to his or her offspring. Parents are encouraged to seek genetic counseling for themselves and for the child during puberty.

Family support. Families with a history of retinoblastoma may feel great guilt for transmitting the defect to their offspring. In families with no history of retinoblastoma, the discovery of the diagnosis is a shock, often complicated by guilt for not having found it sooner. Because parents often are the first to observe the cat's eye reflex, they may feel angry at themselves or others, especially health professionals, for delaying a more thorough examination. The nurse assesses each of these variables in planning care on the basis of understanding the family's emotional reactions and adjustment (see Chapter 38).

See also Nursing Care Plan: The Child with Cancer, Chapter 46.

Key Points

- Mental retardation is the most common developmental disability in the United States, affecting approximately 3% of the population.
- According to the American Association of Mental Deficiencies, mental retardation is a "significantly subaverage general intellectual functioning existing concurrently with deficits in adaptive behavior and manifested during the developmental period."
- Causes of severe mental retardation are primarily genetic, biochemical, viral, and developmental. Mild retardation is associated primarily with familial, social, and environmental causes, whereas severe retardation is more likely to be associated with specific syndromes.
- Education of children with cognitive impairment emphasizes sensory and verbal discrimination, improvement of short-term memory, motivation, and technologic support.
- Promoting optimum development may be achieved through family guidance regarding play, communication, discipline, socialization, and sexuality.
- Prevention efforts regarding mental retardation focus on support for the premature neonate and other high-risk newborns, rubella immunization, genetic counseling, and

maternal education regarding the risks of chemical use and the importance of adequate nutrition.
- Down syndrome, a chromosomal abnormality, is characterized by retarded intelligence of variable degree, slowed language development, congenital anomalies, sensory problems, and diminished growth and sexual development.
- Fragile X syndrome is characterized by mental retardation and phenotypic findings in affected males. It is considered the second leading chromosomal cause of mental retardation after Down syndrome, and it is the most common hereditary cause.
- Hearing disorders may be classified according to the location of the defect: conductive, sensorineural, mixed conductive-sensorineural, and central auditory imperception.
- Rehabilitation for hearing loss involves parent education and support, hearing aids, lipreading, sign language, speech therapy, and promotion of socialization.
- Prevention of hearing loss includes treatment of infection, auditory testing, immunization, pregnancy and genetic counseling, and reduction of noise pollution.
- Visual impairments in childhood include refractive errors, amblyopia, strabismus, cataracts, glaucoma, trauma, and infections.
- Nursing goals in visual rehabilitation include helping the family and child adjust to the child's visual impairment, promoting parent-child attachment, fostering optimum development and independence, providing for play and socialization, and being aware of educational facilities.
- For the child undergoing ocular surgery, nursing care is aimed at reassuring the child and family throughout treatment, orienting the child to the surroundings, providing a safe environment, and encouraging independence.
- Prevention of visual impairment focuses on prenatal screening, prenatal and perinatal care, periodic vision screening, immunization, and safety counseling.
- Conjunctivitis is an infectious disorder common in children.
- Retinoblastoma is a rare congenital malignant tumor; its most common clinical manifestations are cat's eye reflex (white pupil) and strabismus.

References

American Academy of Pediatrics, Committee on Genetics: Prenatal diagnosis for pediatricians, *Pediatrics* 84(4):741-744, 1989.

American Psychiatric Association: *Diagnostic and statistical manual of mental disorders*, ed 4 (DSM-IV), Washington, DC, 1994, The Association.

Batshaw ML: Mental retardation, *Pediatr Clin North Am* 40(3):465-692, 1993.

Brown WT et al: Rapid fragile X carrier screening and prenatal diagnosis using a nonradioactive PCR test, *JAMA* 270(13):1569-1575, 1993.

Consensus Conference: Noise and hearing loss, *JAMA* 263(23):3185-3190, 1990.

Cooley SC, Graham JM: Down syndrome—an update and review for the primary pediatrician, *Clin Pediatr* 30(4):233-253, 1991.

Cronk C et al: Growth charts for children with Down syndrome: 1 month to 18 years of age, *Pediatrics* 81(1):102-110, 1988.

Davidson PW: *Visual impairment and blindness.* In Levine MD, Carey WB, Crocker AC, editors: *Developmental-behavioral pediatrics*, ed 2, Philadelphia, 1992, WB Saunders.

Eilers RE, Oller DK: Infant vocalizations and the early diagnosis of severe hearing impairment, *J Pediatr* 124:199-203, 1994.

Grossman HJ, editor: *Classification in mental retardation*, Washington, DC, 1983, American Association on Mental Retardation.

Haddow JE et al: Prenatal screening for Down's syndrome with use of maternal serum markers, *N Engl J Med* 327:588-593, 1992.

Hagerman RJ, Cronister A: *Fragile X syndrome.* In Jackson PL, Vessey JA: *Primary care of the child with a chronic condition*, ed 2, St Louis, 1996, Mosby.

Keltner BR, Tymchuk AJ: Reaching out to mothers with mental retardation, *MCN* 17(3):136-140, 1992.

Litovitz T, Schmitz BF: Ingestion of cylindrical and button batteries: an analysis of 2382 cases, *Pediatrics* 89:747-757, 1992.

Luckasson R, editor: *Mental retardation: definition, classification and systems of support*, ed 9, Washington, DC, 1992, American Association on Mental Retardation.

National Institutes of Health: *NIH consensus statement: early identification of hearing impairment in infants and young children*, vol 11, no 1, Washington, DC, 1993, NIH.

Pueschel SM: The child with Down syndrome. In Levine MD et al, editors: *Developmental-behavioral pediatrics*, ed 2, Philadelphia, 1992, WB Saunders.

Sarant JZ et al: The effect of handedness in tactile speech perception, *J Rehabil Res* 30:423-435, 1993.

Bibliography

Cognitive Impairment

American Academy of Pediatrics, Committee on Bioethics: Sterilization of women who are mentally handicapped, *Pediatrics* 85(5):868-871, 1990.

American Academy of Pediatrics, Committee on Children With Disabilities: Screening infants and young children for developmental disabilities, *Pediatrics* 93(5):863-865, 1994.

Brizee L, Sophos C, McLaughlin J: Nutrition issues in developmental disabilities, *Inf Young Child* 2(3):10-21, 1990.

Brown FR et al: Intellectual and adaptive functioning in individuals with Down syndrome in relation to age and environmental placement, *Pediatrics* 85:450-452, 1990.

Chomicki S, Wilgosh L: Health care concerns among parents of children with mental retardation, *Child Health Care* 21(4):206-212, 1992.

Cronister AE, Hagerman RJ: Fragile X syndrome, *J Pediatr Health Care* 3(1):9-19, 1989.

Forness SR, Hecht B: Special education for handicapped and disabled children: classification, programs, and trends, *J Pediatr Nurs* 3(2):75-88, 1988.

Friedrich WN, Cohen DS, Wilturner LT: Specific beliefs as moderator variables in maternal coping with mental retardation, *Child Health Care* 17(1):40-44, 1988.

Hayes A, Batshaw ML: Down syndrome, *Pediatr Clin North Am* 40(3):523-535, 1993.

Krais WA: The incompetent developmentally disabled person's right of self-determination, right to die, sterilization and institutionalization, *Am J Law Med* 15(2-3):333-361, 1989.

Oehler JM et al: How to target infants at highest risk for developmental delay, *MCN* 18(1):20-23, 1993.

Steele S: Assessing developmental delays in preschool children, *J Pediatr Health Care* 2(3):141-145, 1988.

Steele S: Fostering potentiality in persons with mental retardation, *Issues Compr Pediatr Nurs* 11:283-290, 1988.

Steele S: Preschool children with developmental delays: nursing intervention, *J Pediatr Health Care* 2(5):215-252, 1988.

Steele S: Down syndrome: nursing interventions, newborn through preschool age years, *Issues Compr Pediatr Nurs* 13(2):111-126, 1990.

Steele S et al: Home management of URI in children with Down syndrome, *Pediatr Nurs* 15(5):484-488, 1989.

Taylor EH: Understanding and helping families with neurodevelopmental and neuropsychiatric special needs, *Pediatr Clin North Am* 42:143-152, 1995.

Taylor MO: Teaching parents about their impaired adolescent's sexuality, *MCN* 14:109-112, 1989.

Vessey JA: Care of the hospitalized child with a cognitive developmental delay, *Holistic Nurs Pract* 2:48-54, 1988.

Vessey JA: *Down syndrome.* In Jackson PL, Vessey JA: *Primary care of the child with a chronic condition,* ed 2, St Louis, 1996, Mosby.

Vessey JA, Swanson MN: Caring for the child with Down syndrome, *J School Nurs* 9(14):20-33, 1993.

Walden BJ: The newborn infant with Down syndrome: realities and possibilities, *J Perinat Neonat Nurs* 2(4):72-82, 1989.

Hearing Impairment

American Academy of Otolaryngology—Head and Neck Surgery Subcommittee on Cochlear Implants, Kveton J, Balkany TJ: Status of cochlear implantation in children, *J Pediatr* 118(25):1-7, 1991.

Badger T, Jones E: Deaf and hearing children's conceptions of the body interior, *Pediatr Nurs* 16(2):201-205, 1990.

Coplan J: Deafness: ever heard of it? Delayed recognition of permanent hearing loss, *Pediatrics* 79(2):206-213, 1987.

Epstein S, Reilly JS: Sensorineural hearing loss, *Pediatr Clin North Am* 36(6):1501-1520, 1989.

Harrison LL: Minimizing barriers when teaching hearing-impaired clients, *MCN* 15(2):113, 1990.

Jackson CB: Primary health care for deaf children, part I, *J Pediatr Health Care* 3(6):316-318, 1989.

Jackson CB: Primary health care for deaf children, part II, *J Pediatr Health Care* 4(1):39-41, 1990.

Kravitz L, Selekman J: Understanding hearing loss in children, *Pediatr Nurs* 18:591-594, 1992.

McGarr N: Research on the use of sensory aids for hearing-impaired people, *Volta Rev* 91(5):1-138, 1989.

Oberklaid F, Harris C, Keir E: Auditory dysfunction in children with school problems, *Clin Pediatr* 28(9):397-403, 1989.

Thomas KA: How the NICU environment sounds to a preterm infant, *MCN* 14:249-251, 1989.

Thompson M, Thompson G: Early identification of hearing loss: listen to parents, *Clin Pediatr* 30(2):77-80, 1991.

Weibley T: Inside the incubator, *MCN* 14(2):96-100, 1989.

Vision Impairment

Bailey C, Buckley R: Ocular prostheses and contact lenses. II. Contact lenses, *Br Med J* 302(6784):1066-1069, 1991.

DeRespinis PA: Cyanoacrylage nail glue mistaken for eye drops, *JAMA* 263(17):2301, 1990.

Donaldson SS, Smith LM: Retinoblastoma: biology, presentation, and current management, *Oncology* 3(4):45-51, 1989.

Dudley N: Aids for visual impairment, *Br Med J* 302(6761):1151-1153, 1990.

Friendly DS: Development of vision in infants and young children, *Pediatr Clin North Am* 40:693-704, 1993.

Kodadek SM, Haylor MJ: Using interpretive methods to understand family caregiving when a child is blind, *J Pediatr Nurs* 5(1):42-49, 1990.

Kovalesky A: *Nurse's guide to children's eyes,* New York, 1985, Grune & Stratton.

Nelson LB, Wilson TW, Jeffers JB: Eye injuries in childhood: demography, etiology, and prevention, *Pediatrics* 84(3):438-441, 1989.

Phillips S, Hartley JT: Developmental differences and interventions for blind children, *Pediatr Nurs* 14(3):201-204, 1988.

Rollins JA: National Library Service for the Blind and Physically Handicapped, *Pediatr Nurs* 14(6):522, 1988.

Schraeder B, McEvoy-Shields K: Visual acuity, binocular vision, and ocular muscle balance in VLBW children, *Pediatr Nurs* 17(1):30-33, 1991.

Servodidio CA, Abramson DH, Romanella A: Retinoblastoma, *Cancer Nurs* 14(2):117-123, 1991.

Tongue AC: Refractive errors in children, *Pediatr Clin North Am* 34(6):1425-1437, 1987.

Conjunctivitis

Bringing pinkeye under control, *Patient Care* 27:47-48, 1993.

Lewis L, Glauser T, Joffie M: Gonococcal conjunctivitis in prepubertal children, *Am J Dis Child* 144(5):546-548, 1990.

Schmitt BD: When your child has an eye infection with pus, *Contemp Pediatr* 10(3):117-118, 1993.

Stanker P et al: Protocol—conjunctivitis, *Sch Nurse* 5(2):34-36, 1989.

Trobe JD: *The physician's guide to eye care,* San Francisco, 1993, American Academy of Ophthalmology.

Weiss A, Brinser JH, Nazar-Stewart V: Acute conjunctivitis in childhood, *J Pediatr* 122(1):10-14, 1993.

Multiple Impairments: Deaf-Blind

Luiselli JK: Training self-feeding skills in children who are deaf and blind, *Behav Mod* 17:457-473, 1993.

Programs for deaf-blind children and adults, *Am Ann Deaf* 138:205-209, 1993.

CHAPTER 40

Family-Centered Home Care

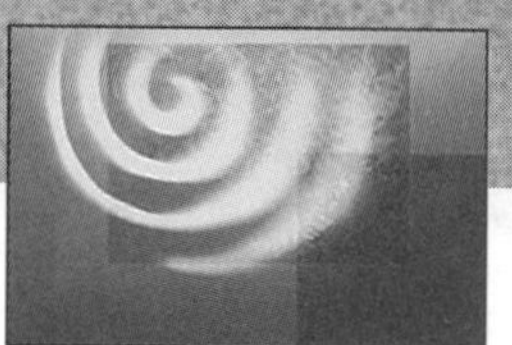

GENERAL CONCEPTS OF HOME CARE, P. 1186

Definition, p. 1186

Impetus for home care, p. 1186

Effectiveness of home care, p. 1187

Discharge planning and selection of a home care agency, p. 1187

Case management, p. 1187

Role of the nurse, training, and standards of care, p. 1188

FAMILY-CENTERED HOME CARE, P. 1188

Respect for diversity, p. 1188

Parent-professional collaboration, p. 1189

The nursing process, p. 1190

Promotion of optimum development, self-care, and education, p. 1191

Safety issues in the home, p. 1192

Family-to-family support, p. 1193

General Concepts of Home Care

DEFINITION

Home care is not a new concept in pediatrics. Over time the term has referred to parents caring for mildly ill children at home, to home visits after children are discharged from the hospital, to hospice care and, more recently, to care at home for children with more serious chronic illness and dependence on medical technology. With insurance companies insisting on earlier hospital discharge for healthy newborns, public and community health nurses may increasingly return to providing parenting education for postpartum women at home.

As discussed in this chapter, **home care** refers to care provided in the family's residence for children with complex health care needs and their families. The purpose of home care services is to promote, maintain, or restore health or to maximize the level of independence while minimizing the effects of disability and illness, including terminal illness. Home care differs from **hospice care,** which is a program of palliative and supportive care services providing physical, psychologic, social, and spiritual care for dying persons, their families, and other loved ones. Hospice services are available both in the home and in inpatient settings.

IMPETUS FOR HOME CARE

The initial impetus for home care for children with complex medical conditions came from parental desire to have their children at home and from professionals' willingness to work with families to achieve this goal. Improving the quality of life for both the child and the family was the driving force in efforts to move technology-dependent children from the hospital to the home setting.

Other factors eventually influenced the shift toward an emphasis on home care for this population: increasing numbers of children requiring long-term complex medical and nursing care, and lower costs for home care as compared with hospital care.

Dramatic advances in medical care over the past two decades have resulted in increased numbers of children requiring long-term complex medical care: improvements in trauma care and the survival of severe trauma victims; increased survival rates for children with leukemia and other cancers, chronic kidney disorders, sickle cell anemia, cystic fibrosis, spina bifida, and cardiac or intestinal malformations; more aggressive care for muscular dystrophy and degenerative neuromuscular disorders; and more children with acquired immunodeficiency syndrome (AIDS).

The cost of care is another critical factor. For third-party payers and the government, the cost of home care is generally less than the cost of hospital care for children who are dependent on medical technology and require substantial and complex care. However, families may absorb many of the costs of home care, including medication, supplies, transportation, shelter, utilities, food, laundry, and housekeeping. In addition, families generally provide at least some portion of the nursing

Portions of this text are modified from Ahmann E: *An overview of issues in pediatric high tech home care.* In Gorski L: *High tech home care manual,* Gaithersburg, Md, 1994, Aspen; and Ahmann E: Family-centered care: shifting our orientation, *Pediatr Nurs* 20(2):113-117, 1994.

care, and some may become unemployed or only partially employed to stay at home. These out-of-pocket expenses and the loss of income can become a financial burden for the family.

EFFECTIVENESS OF HOME CARE

Home care is effective for many children but may not be possible in all circumstances. A number of factors must be present to make it effective. First, the child's condition must be medically stable so that care can be managed in the home setting and supported by available home care equipment. Second, the family must want the child at home and must have the motivation and ability to learn the child's care. Families must also be able to live with the intrusion of the child's equipment, care schedule, and nurses and other providers in their daily life. Third, professionals and the community must be prepared to provide the necessary support to make home care successful, including nursing and other therapeutic services, transportation, accessible emergency facilities, and case management. Fourth, financial support, both public and private, is essential.

Even if home care is initially successful for a child and family, changing factors may influence the plan. Alterations in the child's medical condition, the lack of adequate community resources, depletion of the family's financial resources, high levels of family stress and exhaustion, and disagreements between family members and the health care team can affect the success of home care (Harris, 1988). Changes in the home care plan or short- or long-term residential placement may be alternatives if any of these changes occur.

DISCHARGE PLANNING AND SELECTION OF A HOME CARE AGENCY

Much of the success of home care for the child who is dependent on medical technology depends on careful planning and preparation. Despite the rapid growth of home care for technology-dependent children, negotiation with the insurance company may be required. General principles of discharge planning and transition to home care are addressed in Chapter 41. *Discharge planning must begin early, be a multidisciplinary process, and involve the family.* Early involvement of the home care agency promotes continuity of care and a smooth transition from hospital to home. The home care plan for a child with complex care requirements should address the many health and community services that may be needed. Comprehensive written home care instructions facilitate continuity of care across settings and providers (Box 40-1).*

Video recordings are an excellent way to provide home care instructions. Once the family masters the procedures, consider video recording their performance on tape. Visual learning is most helpful for people who cannot read or who are not fluent in English (Curry and Cullen, 1990).

The plans for transition from hospital to home should include family members (at least two persons) both learning and demonstrating all aspects of the child's care in the hospital. An in-hospital trial period during which parents provide total care for the child is also generally beneficial. After a successful trial, the family may benefit from taking the child home on a brief pass before making final discharge plans. (This step may need to be negotiated with the insurance company.) The home care nurse plays an important role in assessing this experience with the family. Whether or not the child is taken home on a pass, a pre-discharge home visit offers the home care nurse the opportunity to meet the family, help them assess their preparedness and the preparedness of the home environment, discuss plans for arranging the child's equipment at home (Fig. 40-1), reinforce prior discharge teaching, and implement any additional teaching that may be necessary.

* Numerous home care instructions are available in Wong DL: *Wong and Whaley's clinical manual of pediatric nursing,* ed 4, St Louis, 1996, Mosby.

BOX 40-1
Minimum Contents of Written Home Care Instructions

A schedule of routine care needs
Correct settings for any equipment required
A list of signs, symptoms, and parameters (physical and behavioral) that are normal for the individual child
A list of signs, symptoms, and parameters (physical and behavioral) that indicate a problem for the individual child
Guidelines and a list for whom to contact about what problems
An explanation of pertinent emergency procedures

From Ahmann E: *An overview of issues in pediatric high-tech home care.* In Gorski L, editor: *High-tech home care manual,* Gaithersburg, Md, 1994, Aspen.

CASE MANAGEMENT

Parents of children with complex care requirements often experience frustration about the fragmentation of services and desire competent case management. Traditional definitions of **case management** generally focus on cost control, attainment of desired clinical outcomes, and monitoring and evaluation of care provided. However, for optimum home care of the child who is technology dependent, case management—or **care coordination**—should be viewed more broadly.

Care coordination serves several purposes. Its primary goal is to ensure continuity for the child and family across hospital, home, educational, therapeutic, and other settings. Care should be coordinated among multiple providers to reduce the complexity of care for the child, reduce fragmentation of care, and decrease the burden of care for the family. Care coordination should ensure that the medical, nursing, and health maintenance needs of the child are addressed, as well as the financial issues, psychosocial concerns, and educational needs of the child and family.

Although professionals must always see part of their role as ensuring that integrated, coordinated care is provided, care coordination should promote the family's role as primary decision maker and enhance the family's capability to meet the special needs of the child and the family unit (Johnson, Jeppson, and Redburn, 1992). Care coordination is most effective if a single person works with the family to accomplish the many tasks and responsibilities involved. These tasks include assessing needs and resources, planning for comprehensive care, coordinating services and referrals, monitoring and evaluating services, and providing administrative support and advocacy. The American Nurses Association (ANA, 1988)

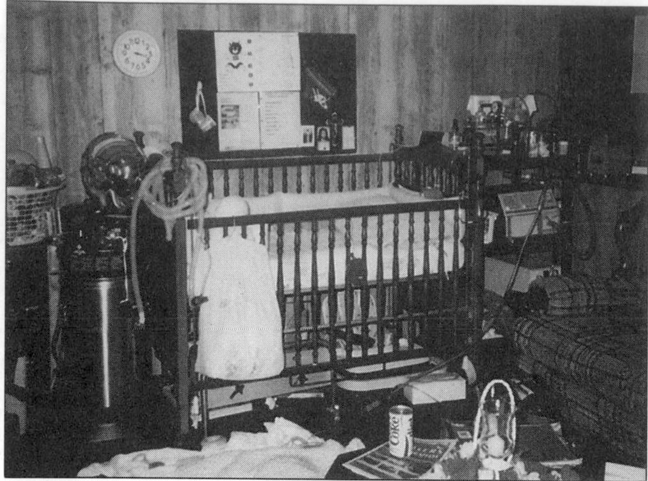

Fig. 40-1 Arranging equipment and supplies is an essential aspect of preparation for home.

recommends that the nurse case manager have a minimum of a baccalaureate degree in nursing and 3 years of experience.

Families may choose to be involved to varying degrees in the tasks involved in coordinating their child's care. Many parents assume increasing responsibility for care coordination over time; they should be encouraged and supported in this role.

ROLE OF THE NURSE, TRAINING, AND STANDARDS OF CARE

The home care nurse must share a level of technical expertise with the critical care nurse while being able to adapt equipment, procedures, and the nursing process to the home setting. (See Chapter 42 for specific technical skills that may be required in home care practice.) The need for technical expertise must be matched by a knowledge of child development and an ability to work creatively with the child who is challenged by chronic illness and technology dependence. When practicing in the home, the nurse must be comfortable making independent nursing judgments and problem solving with no immediate assistance. At the same time, the nurse must have excellent interpersonal skills, an ability to work with other professionals and the family and, most important, an ability to respect family autonomy.

When working with a home care agency, nurses should expect to receive patient placements appropriate to their expertise. They should also expect orientation in the following areas: the individual patient's care plan and equipment needs; the agency's policies and procedures, including procedures for addressing any problems that may occur when care is provided in the home; documentation procedures (reimbursement-driven documentation in home care differs from documentation practices in the hospital setting); and legal liability issues. Supervision of practice, including occasional site visits by a nursing supervisor, should be provided.

Public and private home care agencies that participate in the Medicare or Medicaid programs must be certified by a federally designated state-certifying body and abide by federal and state regulations. Private agencies that do not participate in the federal programs are not mandated to meet the federal standards. The trend is for large, national, private agencies to develop a certifying process that ensures greater credibility and acceptable standards of practice (Klug, 1992). The ANA has developed standards of nursing practice for both community health and home care nurses that should guide practice in the home setting (ANA, 1986a, 1986b). Despite some important differences between pediatric and adult care in the home, as of this writing no national standards specific to pediatric home care practice have been developed.

Family-Centered Home Care

Technology dependence, chronic illness, and complex care requirements cross social, cultural, spiritual, and economic boundaries. No matter what a family's background, family values must be respected in the provision of home care services. *The home is the family's domain,* and the child is at home because the family's central role is to nurture and raise their child. The nurse must respect the family's central role in the care of the child and must work in collaboration with the family in efforts to care for the child. Family-centered nursing practice is essential in the home setting.

The first of the nine key components of **family-centered care** (see Chapter 27) provides the philosophic basis for family-centered practice: recognition that the family is the constant in the child's life, whereas the service systems and personnel within those systems fluctuate (Shelton and Stepanek, 1994). Nurses working with families of children with complex chronic problems must respect the family's central, caring role, their knowledge, and their particular and unique expertise. Families have the most intimate knowledge of the child's strengths and abilities, the challenges of providing care, and the abilities and needs of other family members (Bishop, Woll, and Arango, 1993). *Believing that no one knows the child better than the family is critical* to the success of any health care plan.

RESPECT FOR DIVERSITY

Respect for varied family structures and for racial, ethnic, cultural, spiritual, and socioeconomic diversity among families is essential in home care (see Chapter 28). Nurses work in close relationship with family members and in the family's own domain. The family's background and their life-style choices are respected. Particular attention is given to communication. The meaning of words used and the way in which they are said may affect various cultural groups in different ways. For example, the words "family support" may be interpreted by some families as an implication that they are weak and in need of help (Patterson and Blum, 1993). Families may also differ in their cultural view of children, in childrearing practices, and in their view of illness, its causes, and its meaning. The views of illness may influence the type or level of investment a family makes in the child's care. Families may have beliefs about health care and healing practices that are foreign to the nurse's background and experience. The home care nurse, aware that value systems drive behavior, needs to learn

Family Focus

DEVELOPING A RELATIONSHIP WITH CULTURALLY DIVERSE FAMILIES

I work in the inner city, and my home care patients come from a variety of racial and ethnic backgrounds. I am caucasian and from Australia. When I first visit a family, there often is an initial coolness or apprehension toward me. This reaction is understandable because I am a stranger, and perhaps families think I'll judge them in one way or another. Probably they also have instinctive suspicions based on racial stereotypes. However, by the end of the first visit, there is usually a smile as I leave; by the second visit they often greet me with a smile at the door; and by the third visit we usually have a friendship, a trust, and an ease of communication.

If I'm working on a case for an extended time, I use a holistic nursing approach. This approach involves being aware of how the illness of the child affects the entire family. As I listen over many weeks to their fears and questions and often share faith perspectives, a bond begins to form. I find it a privilege to share in their joys and their pain, and I feel rewarded by the trust that they invest in me.

Julie Edgerton, RN
Home Care Nurse
Children's National Medical Center
Washington, DC

about the family's culture, ask questions without implying judgment, interpret the mainstream medical culture, and help families design interventions that meet their preferences (Stone and Hoffman, 1993) (see the Family Focus box above).

Respect for family diversity and an awareness of both family developmental stages (see Chapter 29) and the stages of a family's adjustment to illness in a child (see Chapter 38) will assist the home care nurse in recognizing and promoting family strengths and in respecting varied coping mechanisms. Labels such as "dysfunctional," "difficult," and "noncompliant" can reinforce negative expectations and shape the behaviors of both parents and professionals (see the Critical Thinking Q & A box above, right). On the other hand, emphasizing, identifying, and building on family strengths and coping mechanisms are strategies that promote a central goal in nursing care of the child and family: family empowerment (see Chapter 27). The nurse working with families should remain flexible and open-minded because new family strengths may emerge over time, and coping mechanisms may wax and wane with the stresses of caring for a child with serious or multiple problems.

PARENT-PROFESSIONAL COLLABORATION

Family-centered nursing practice is built on a foundation of parent-professional collaboration, which represents a shift from the traditional unidirectional relationships between health care providers and families. **Collaborative relationships,** essential in the home care setting, are characterized by several features (Bishop, Woll, and Arango, 1993):

Communication—Including complete and unbiased sharing of information with parents about their child's care and prognosis

Critical Thinking Q & A

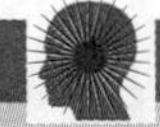

MEDICAL NEGLECT

The home care nurse notes that the family has failed to give a dose of the child's medication. The nurse is responsible for all of the following actions *except:*

1. Educate and counsel the family about the child's medication requirements and schedule
2. Report the family for medical neglect
3. Assess the child's condition
4. Document the missed dose and any corrective measures taken

The correct answer is two. Some behaviors that might be considered medical neglect may result from the family's feeling overwhelmed, not being fully educated about the child's care requirements, or denial. The nurse has a responsibility to address these issues with the family. At the same time, the nurse should be cognizant that home care providers may have legal liability not only for their own actions but even when it is the parents who are "noncompliant" with medical orders. The frequency and severity of "noncompliance" affects the nurses' responsibility. For example, one missed medication dose may be appropriately handled by documentation and counseling. On the other hand, regularly missed doses or one instance of turning off a ventilator alarm requires a more vigorous response. The point at which these instances cross the line into reportable medical neglect depends in part on the definitions of abuse or neglect in the state in which services are provided.

Modified from Ahmann E: Thinking critically about family-centered home care nursing, *Pediatr Nurs* 20(6):588-590, 1994.

Dialogue—Exchanging information and sharing reactions and ideas

Active listening—Listening beyond the words to hear and understand concerns, including checking to be certain that interpretations are correct

Awareness and acceptance of difference—Willingness to examine one's own cultural biases and accept that others may think and act out of different value systems

Negotiation—The process of examining different options, priorities, and preferences to best meet the needs of the child and family

Communication with the family should not be invasive. There is no need to collect information from the family that can be obtained from the child's records. The nurse should explain to the family the reason for questions (particularly those that the family may perceive as intrusive) and should inform families about who will have access to the information. The nurse must also assure families that they have a right to expect confidentiality in regard to the data collected. When working in the home, the nurse must respect the privacy of family members' communications with each other, which might be overheard.

Nursing ALERT

Home care nurses should restrict their communications with other professionals to clinically relevant information about the family.

Communication with family members should include sharing in a supportive manner complete and unbiased information regarding all aspects of the child's condition and care (Shelton and Stepanek, 1994). Parents can feel overwhelming frustration related to obtaining accurate information about their child's illness and its management. Nurses should answer the family's questions in a straightforward manner, including admitting when they do not know the answers. Information should be shared with families in a way that has meaning in their cultural context (Huber, Holditch-Davis, and Brandon, 1993). Many parents report a preference for interactions with professionals that communicate empathy and concern. Although they want accurate information, many parents prefer that providers moderate the amount of information on possible complications and unfavorable prognoses (Knafl et al, 1992). A resource guide for families in which to record pertinent medical information can assist parents in managing their child's care (Lobosco et al, 1991).

Disagreements may arise between parents and nurses regarding proper procedures for care of the child. In any situation that does not pose danger or risk for the child, nurses should respect parental preferences. If disagreements cannot be resolved, a home care supervisor or case manager should be contacted to assist with problem solving (Ahmann and Bond, 1992). If parents wish to alter a plan of treatment that is part of medical orders, the nurse should ask that they negotiate the change with the practitioner, because the nurse must follow the written medical orders (Klug, 1993).

Other options to help resolve conflicts include the following (Ahmann and Bond, 1992):

- Work with the family's priorities and reevaluate over time.
- Provide the family with additional information that may affect their perception of priorities.
- Share the nurse's perception of priorities and rationales without judgment.
- Suggest an additional priority goal if the family agrees.

THE NURSING PROCESS

In the home the family is a partner in each step of the nursing process. The use of formal self-report assessment tools can help families identify needs for information, training, services, and support (Bond, Phillips, and Rollins, 1994). Assessment should also address family strengths and resources (see Family Assessment, Chapter 29). The principles of communication previously discussed guide data collection. The nurse's observations are shared neutrally, without value judgment, and in a way that preserves the family's own role in decision making (Bond, Phillips, and Rollins, 1994).

All of the information gathered as part of the assessment process is shared with the family. The nurse should recognize that the family's perception of their most important need generally guides their behavior and consumes their attention and energy. For this reason, family priorities guide the planning process.

Both short- and long-term goals should be outlined and agreed on by the child, family, and professionals involved. To minimize duplication and consolidate care requirements, the plan of care should integrate the various disciplines that may be involved with the child. Cross-training of professionals and a transdisciplinary mode of treatment can also be useful when a child has multiple and complex care requirements. For example, certain physical or occupational therapy routines may be incorporated into the child's morning nursing procedures, or speech therapy interventions may be conducted by the parent or nurse around eating times so that the entire day is not occupied by procedures. A written schedule of daily routines should be developed and followed by all caregivers.

Goals of care are supported by intervention strategies that reflect normalization (see Chapter 38) and the interests and abilities of the child and family. Nurses can help families explore a range of alternative strategies, services, and resources so that the family can choose the best match for their situation.

Family participation in evaluating a home care plan can occur on several levels. Families and care providers should regularly review the goals of care and update the care plan as required. The nurse can also ask the family open-ended questions at regular intervals to assess their opinions on the effectiveness of care (Bond, Phillips, and Rollins, 1994). As part of the evaluation process, families should be acknowledged for their successes and accomplishments. Finally, families should be given an opportunity to evaluate individual home care services, the home care agency, and other service providers periodically. The evaluation should address the nurses' knowledge, skills, and respect for the family's choices, as well as the agency's handling of the schedule, provision of qualified nurses, and problem-solving abilities (Klug, 1992). The evaluations should be used by the agency to improve quality of care (see the Family Focus box below).

Home care nursing encourages a close and rewarding relationship with the family. One of the most important aspects of this relationship is maintaining professional boundaries and a

Family Focus

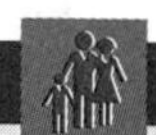

WHAT I LEARNED ABOUT HOME CARE

I learned many things as a result of having home care for four children over 8 years. Two of the major things I learned were families' rights and communication. It took a long time to learn some of what I learned.

Initially, I tried very hard to be sensitive to the professionals and often put aside my own feelings and needs. It took awhile to learn that I could stand up for myself and my family and that my child could continue to receive good care. One area that was important to me was to have nurses withhold judgment on our parenting style, even if they might have parented differently.

Communication needs to be open and two-way. Families and nurses should tell each other what is going well. For example, "Thanks for keeping the room so neat while you're here," can help a nurse see a family's appreciation. There was so little I could do as just "Mommy" that it really meant a lot to me when nurses would say "That's such a cute outfit you picked out for him today." Communicating about little things—even about things as inconsequential as favorite television shows—makes it easier to communicate about bigger things and about problems. Communication must also be open about problems.

Jeni Stepanek
Mother
Upper Marlboro, Md

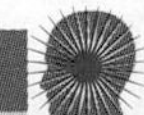

Critical Thinking Q & A

MAINTAINING THERAPEUTIC BOUNDARIES

You are a home care nurse who has been working with a 3-year-old child who is ventilator dependent. You have been visiting the Jones family several days a week for the last 5 months. You notice that the parents are arguing more often. Some of the arguments concern whether Mr. Jones helps enough with the child's care. Mrs. Jones approaches you to complain about her husband. Depending on your relationship with the family, you might do any of the following *except:*

1. Mention that home care can be stressful for a family.
2. Indicate that you can provide referrals for counseling should the parents want them.
3. Agree with Mrs. Jones that her husband is not helping with the child's care.
4. Listen and reflect Mrs. Jones' feelings to her.

The correct answer is three. Therapeutic boundaries are not rigid and fixed. They must be responsive to the relationship preferred by the family and the style with which the family operates. For this reason, options one, two, or four (or a combination) might be most appropriate depending on the family. In any circumstance, it would be inappropriate to agree with Mrs. Jones that her husband is not helping with the child's care. Such an action implies a judgment that is not within the nurse's role to make, and it undermines rather than supports the family system.

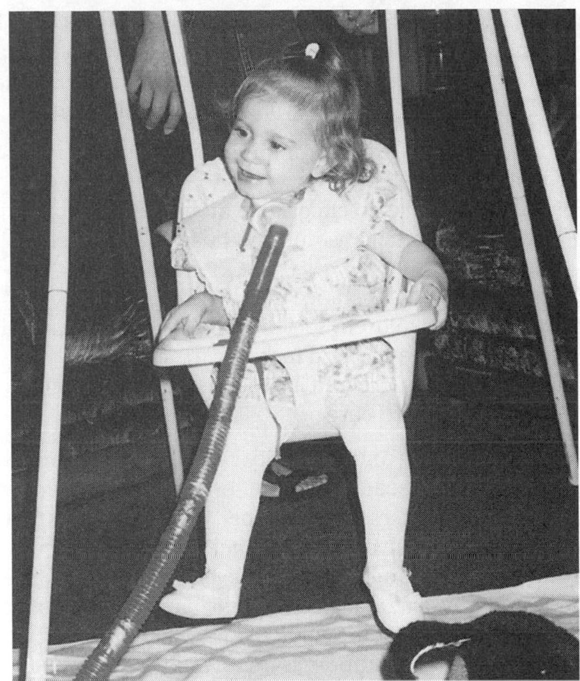

Fig. 40-2 The use of lengthy tubing facilitates freedom of movement.

therapeutic role that is supportive but not intrusive. Some of these issues are discussed under Therapeutic Relationship in Chapter 27 (see the Critical Thinking Q & A box above).

PROMOTION OF OPTIMUM DEVELOPMENT, SELF-CARE, AND EDUCATION

There is little question that living at home offers most children with complex medical problems great social and emotional advantages over living in the hospital or another institutional setting. However, in infancy and throughout the developmental stages, a child's medical condition(s) and the dependence on medical technology can place constraints on and pose challenges to *normal development.* For example, the child may have lengthy and repeated hospitalizations; developmental regression can occur in response to stress; fatigue may result from underlying pathology, the flare of an illness, or medication side effects; and equipment requirements may impede mobility, exploration, and independence. The challenge of providing support for normal development in a child who is chronically ill and technology dependent is to optimize the opportunities for developmentally appropriate experiences within the constraints posed by the medical condition and the equipment requirements.

Home care plans are designed to promote optimum child development through initial and periodic assessment, planning, referrals for further assessment or therapeutic services, and interventions that address **normalization** issues and self-care (see Chapter 38 for a discussion of normalization). General principles for a family-centered assessment and planning process have been addressed earlier in this chapter and are also applied in developmental assessment and planning.

Some parents may not pursue early developmental intervention because they do not view their child as needing the services. In this case professionals need to explain the child's developmental needs to parents in ways that are meaningful from the parents' own cultural and socioeconomic perspectives (Huber, Holditch-Davis, and Brandon, 1993). Only then can parents make truly informed decisions. Developmental goals outlined by the child and family should guide planning and intervention once parents have been fully informed of the child's condition, likely developmental sequelae, and the expected benefits of intervention.

Each family should have an *Individual Family Service Plan (IFSP)* to help ensure early intervention. All states provide agencies that develop IFSP (American Academy of Pediatrics, 1995).

Several principles underlie appropriate developmental intervention plans for children with complex medical problems (Ahmann and Lierman, 1992). First, understanding a child's medical condition ensures that the nurse and family can plan to maximize developmental opportunities at times during which the child has the most energy and endurance and when stress signals that determine the child's tolerance for type, intensity, and duration of activity will be noted (Ahmann and Lipsi, 1991). Second, plans for developmental support must be flexible and tailored to the individual child's abilities, interests, and needs. Third, familiarity with the child's medical equipment facilitates the planning of creative ways to meet the child's developmental needs. For example, the use of lengthy oxygen tubing allows the active toddler freedom of movement during the day (Fig. 40-2); portable equipment of any type facilitates family outings; and mounting a ventilator to a wheelchair allows the adolescent greater independence.

Many developmental aspects of chronic illness or disability in children are discussed in Chapter 38. Some additional factors apply when children are or have been dependent on medical technology and should be considered in developing plans to promote normal development (Ahmann and Lierman, 1992). These special needs may include the following:

For infants, attention to promoting oral-motor development
For toddlers, efforts to encourage mobility and exploration and extra assistance with language development
For preschoolers, assistance in self-care
For school-age children, socialization opportunities and provision of games and tasks for mastery
For adolescents, increased independence in managing their own health care

Promoting coping and capability can buffer stress and contribute to mental health and self-esteem in a child with chronic illness (Patterson and Geber, 1991). The extent to which a child is involved in his or her own care depends on many factors, including the child's developmental age, level of interest, and physical ability, as well as parental comfort and support. *Self-care,* both in activities of daily living and in regard to the medical condition, is important.

The frame of reference for self-care in activities of daily living should be the goal of attaining age-appropriate competence. Some modifications in the environment, medical equipment, or techniques for daily activities may be required to promote and support self-care. Effective teaching for self-care is focused at the child's own level of conceptual understanding and may be augmented by the use of dolls, other models and diagrams, simple explanations, and repetition.

For the school-age child or adolescent who is dependent on medical technology, *educational planning* is important. Despite laws that ensure a "free appropriate public education" for these children, conflict regarding payment for health care services in the school setting has often been an impediment to mainstreaming children with complex medical problems (Walker, 1991). When a child requiring special medical care is to be placed in an educational setting, the parents, child, school health coordinator, educational evaluation team, and education and administrative staff should meet to determine safe and appropriate placement, as well as the necessary services and personnel to enable the child to attend school in the least restrictive environment. Training of educational staff and caregivers is essential to ensuring the child's safety in the educational setting (Haynie, Porter, and Palfrey, 1989; Krier, 1993).* Special assistance can also be beneficial in reintegrating previously schooled children, such as those with cancer, into the school setting. Parents may need assistance in developing the skills necessary to advocate effectively for their child in the educational system (DiGregorio-Hixson, Stoff, and White, 1992).

SAFETY ISSUES IN THE HOME

Safety is an important consideration in pediatric home care and should be addressed in the home care plan. First, emergency preparations must be made before hospital discharge. The home should have a telephone. If the family does not have a telephone, arrangements may be made with the telephone company to supply service. Alternatively, one or two nearby neighbors may agree to let the family use their services. In rural areas a local pharmacy or a police or ranger station may be willing to receive messages and relay them to the family.

The telephone and electric companies (if use of medical equipment requires electricity) are notified that the family needs to be placed on a priority service list so that the family will learn of any anticipated interruptions in service and receive priority in reinstatement of interrupted services. Prior contact with rescue squad and local emergency facility personnel can help ensure prompt and appropriate interventions if required.

Before hospital discharge, emergency protocols are developed and reviewed with both the parents and the professional caregivers. Cardiopulmonary resuscitation (CPR) guidelines, if appropriate, should be posted near the child's bedside or in another accessible location. A list of emergency telephone numbers can be placed near each home telephone and should include those of the rescue squad, emergency room, managing physician(s)/nurse practitioner(s), nursing agency, and equipment vendor(s).

Another aspect of safety relates to the provision of care by appropriately trained individuals. Family members should receive thorough training in the child's care requirements and should have the opportunity to demonstrate knowledge and confidence before the child is discharged from the hospital. Professional staff caring for the child should have the appropriate background and training for the child's particular care needs. Because of the child's body size, special skill and caution are required in both the performance of procedures (e.g., gastrostomy feedings, suctioning) and in monitoring the use of equipment (e.g., ventilator settings, intravenous flow rates, and total fluid volumes) (see Chapter 42).

The activity level and curiosity of young children raise additional safety considerations in the provision of home care. All medications, needles, syringes, and any contaminated materials are securely stored well out of the reach of curious hands. Special attention is paid to childproofing the control panels of ventilators, pumps, monitors, and other equipment. Using clear plastic tape, covers, or panels to cover control knobs or buttons reduces the risk of accidental changes in settings. Electrical cords are kept short and out of reach, and safety covers are used on any open outlets. When not in use, equipment is unplugged, and any wires (e.g., lead wires for an apnea monitor) are stored out of reach.

Care at night poses other safety concerns. Care must be taken to prevent accidental strangulation on apnea, oximeter, or cardiac monitor wires or on lengthy intravenous tubing during sleep. For example, coiling extra tubing and taping it at the exit site, as well as running wires or tubes out the bottoms of pajamas, is a precaution against strangulation. Parents or other caregivers need to be able to clearly hear the monitor, ventilator, or pump alarms at night; an inexpensive intercom system or baby monitor can be used.

Safe transportation is a vitally important concern. Any wheelchairs or equipment may need to be properly secured to the vehicle, including vans and buses. Additional information on car safety and general health supervision is in Chapter 38 (see Educate About the Disorder and General Health Care).

*A thorough discussion of training issues, content, and guidelines for care in the school are provided in Haynie M, Porter SM, Palfrey JS: *Children assisted by medical technology in educational settings: guidelines for care,* Boston, 1989, The Children's Hospital (Project School Care).

FAMILY-TO-FAMILY SUPPORT

Family-to-family support networks can be an important source of emotional and instrumental support, as well as empowerment for families of children with chronic health problems. **Family-to-family support** does not replace professional sources of support but rather is a unique resource promoting family strengths through shared experience (Johnson, Jeppson, and Redburn, 1992). Existing parent support groups may not necessarily meet an individual family's needs; when nurses refer a family to a particular group, they should inform the family of the group's purposes (Betz et al, 1990). The value of informal support networks should not be overlooked. Similarly, the support needs of fathers, grandparents, and siblings may be different from those of mothers and should be acknowledged as part of the plan of care. (Some sources of information and support for families are listed at the end of this chapter.) Peer support for school-age children and adolescents with complex care themselves may also be beneficial.

Key Points

- Effective home care depends on many factors, including the child's relative medical stability; the family's willingness, training, and ability to accommodate the child's care requirements; and professional, financial, and community support.
- Comprehensive, multidisciplinary discharge planning should begin early and should include the family and a home care representative in addition to hospital personnel.
- Thorough training of the family, including a trial of care, a predischarge pass to home, and a predischarge home visit, can ease the transition to home.
- Care coordination ensures continuity of care and reduces fragmentation of services. The family may assume varying degrees of care coordination over time.
- The home care nurse must share a level of technical expertise with the critical care nurse while being able to adapt equipment, procedures, and the nursing process to the home setting.
- Federal standards apply to agencies that participate in Medicare or Medicaid; standards of practice by The American Nurses Association can guide nurses in the home setting.
- Family-centered nursing practice is applied in the home setting; diversity in family structures, cultural backgrounds, strengths, and coping mechanisms is respected.
- Collaborative relationships are characterized by communication, dialogue, active listening, awareness and acceptance of difference, and negotiation.
- The nursing process is adapted to involve the family in each step and to preserve the family's central role in decision making.
- "House rules" agreed on by the nurse and family allow a family to maintain a feeling of control over their own environment when professionals are present.
- Home care plans are designed to promote optimum development of the child and to focus on normalization, self-care, educational needs, and the impact of the child's medical condition and technologic requirements on development.
- Safety in the provision of home care services involves emergency preparations and protocols, appropriate training of family and home care personnel, and the safe use and childproofing of medical equipment.
- Family-to-family support networks can both provide emotional and instrumental support and encourage family empowerment.

References

Ahmann E, Bond NJ: Promoting normal development in school-age children and adolescents who are technology dependent: a family centered model, *Pediatr Nurs* 18:399-405, 1992.

Ahmann E, Lierman C: Promoting normal development in technology-dependent children: an introduction to the issues, *Pediatr Nurs* 18:143-152, 1992.

Ahmann E, Lipsi KA: Early intervention for technology-dependent infants and young children, *Infants Young Child* 3(4):67-77, 1991.

American Academy of Pediatrics: *The medical home and early intervention*, Elk Grove Village, Ill, 1995, The Academy.

American Nurses Association: *Standards of community health nursing practice*, Washington, DC, 1986a, The Association.

American Nurses Association: *Standards of home health nursing practice*, Washington, DC, 1986b, The Association.

American Nurses Association: *Nursing case management*, Washington, DC, 1988, The Association.

Betz CL et al: A survey of self-help groups in California for parents of children with chronic conditions, *Pediatr Nurs* 16(3):293-296, 1990.

Bishop KK, Woll J, Arango P: *Family/professional collaboration*, Burlington, Vt, 1993, Department of Social Work, University of Vermont.

Bond N, Phillips P, Rollins JA: Family-centered care at home for families with children who are technology-dependent, *Pediatr Nurs* 20(2):123-130, 1994.

Curry R, Cullen J: Using videorecordings in pediatric nursing practice, *Pediatr Nurs* 16(5):501-504, 1990.

DiGregorio-Hixson D, Stoff E, White PH: Parents of children with chronic health impairments: a new approach to advocacy training, *Child Health Care* 21(2):111-115, 1992.

Harris PJ: Sometimes pediatric home care doesn't work, *Am J Nurs* 88:851-854, 1988.

Haynie M, Porter SM, Palfrey JS: *Children assisted by medical technology in educational settings: guidelines for care*, Boston, 1989, The Children's Hospital (Project School Care).

Huber C, Holditch-Davis D, Brandon D: High-risk preterm infants at 3 years of age: parental response to the presence of developmental problems, *Child Health Care* 22(2):107-124, 1993.

Johnson BH, Jeppson ES, Redburn L: *Caring for children and families: guidelines for hospitals*, Bethesda, Md, 1992, Association for the Care of Children's Health.

Klug RM: Selecting a home care agency, *Pediatr Nurs* 18:504-507, 1992.

Klug RM: Clarifying roles and expectations in home care, *Pediatr Nurs* 19:374-376, 1993.

Knafl K et al: Parents' view of health care providers: an exploration of the components of a positive working relationship, *Child Health Care* 21(2):90-95, 1992.

Krier JJ: Involvement of educational staff in the health care of medically fragile children, *Pediatr Nurs* 19(3):251-254, 1993.

Lobosco AF et al: Local coalitions for coordinating services to children dependent on technology and their families, *Child Health Care* 20(2):75-86, 1991.

Patterson JM, Blum RW: A conference on culture and chronic illness in childhood: conference summary, *Pediatrics* 91:1025-1030, 1993.

Patterson JM, Gerber G: Preventing mental health problems in children with chronic illness or disability, *Child Health Care* 20(3):150-161, 1991.

Shelton TL, Stepanek JS: *Family-centered care for children needing specialized health and developmental services*, Bethesda, Md, 1994, The Association for the Care of Children's Health.

Stone M, Hoffman R: *Cultural understanding: how far do you go?* Paper presented at the ACCH local conference on Incorporating Cultural Awareness into Pediatric Healthcare, Washington, DC, April 30, 1993.

Walker P: Where there is a way there is not always a will: technology, public policy, and the social integration of children who are technology-assisted, *Child Health Care* 20(2):68-74, 1991.

Bibliography

Aday LA, Aitken MJ, Wegener DH: *Pediatric home care: results of a national evaluation of programs for ventilator-assisted children*, Chicago, 1988, Pluribus Press.

Ahmann E: "Chunky stew": appreciating cultural diversity while providing health care for children, *Pediatr Nurs* 20(3):320-324, 1994.

Ahmann E: Family-centered care: the time has come, *Pediatr Nurs* 20(1):52-53, 1994.

Ahmann E: Thinking critically about family-centered home care nursing, *Pediatr Nurs* 20(6):588-590, 1994.

Ahmann E: *Home care for the high-risk infant: a family-centered approach*, Gaithersburg, Md, 1996, Aspen.

Ahmann E, Lipsi KA: Developmental assessment of the technology-dependent infant and young child, *Pediatr Nurs* 18:299-313, 1992.

American Academy of Pediatrics, Committee on Children with Disabilities: Pediatric services for infants and children with special health care needs, *Pediatrics* 92(1):163-165, 1993.

Britton LJ, Johnston JD: Dependent on technology: a child grows up hospitalized, *Pediatr Nurs* 19(6):579-584, 1993.

Buehler JA, Lee HJ: Exploration of home care resources for rural families with cancer, *Cancer Nurs* 15(4):299-308, 1992.

Burns CE, Madian N: Experiences with a support group for grandparents of children with disabilities, *Pediatr Nurs* 18:17-22, 1992.

Cady C, Yoshioko RS: Using a learning contract to successfully discharge an infant on home total parenteral nutrition, *Pediatr Nurs* 17:67-74, 1991.

Davis BD, Steele S: Case management for young children with special care needs, *Pediatr Nurs* 17:15-19, 1991.

Diehl SF, Moffitt KA, Wade SM: Focus group interview with parents of children with medically complex needs: an intimate look at their perceptions and feelings, *Child Health Care* 20(3):170-178, 1991.

Dunst C, Trivette C, Deal A: *Enabling and empowering families*, Cambridge, Mass, 1988, Brookline Books.

Dunst C et al: Enabling and empowering families of children with health impairments, *Child Health Care* 17(2):71-81, 1988.

Fields A et al: Home care cost-effectiveness for respiratory technology-dependent children, *Am J Dis Child* 145(7):729-733, 1991.

Fleming J et al: Impact on the family of children who are technology-dependent and cared for in the home, *Pediatr Nurs* 20(4):379-388, 1994.

Gallo AM: Stigma in childhood chronic illness: a well-sibling perspective, *Pediatr Nurs* 75:21-25, 1991.

Gallo AM et al: Well siblings of children with chronic illness: parents' reports of their psychological adjustment, *Pediatr Nurs* 18:23-27, 1992.

Grammatica G: Developing a quality home care program for children, *Pediatr Nurs* 15(1):33-35, 1989.

Groce NE, Zola IK: Multiculturalism, chronic illness and disability, *Pediatrics* 91:1048-1055, 1993.

Haas DL: Family-centered, community-based, coordinated care for children with special health care needs, part II, *Issues Compr Pediatr Nurs* 15(2, entire issue), 1992.

Hamilton B, Vessey J: Pediatric discharge planning, *Pediatr Nurs* 18:475-480, 1992.

Hewson M et al: Comprehensive team care, *MCN* 18(4):198-205, 1993.

Hogue E: Liability for premature discharge: an update, *Pediatr Nurs* 17(1):76-78, 1991.

Jackson B, Finkler DE, Robinson C: A case management system for infants with chronic illnesses and developmental disabilities, *Child Health Care* 21(4):224-232, 1992.

Kasprisin C: Home care instructions. In Wong DL: *Wong and Whaley's clinical manual of pediatric nursing*, ed 4, St Louis, 1996, Mosby.

Kaufman J: An overview of public sector financing for pediatric home care, part I, *Pediatr Nurs* 17:280-281, 1991.

Kaufman J: An overview of public sector financing for pediatric home care, part II, *Pediatr Nurs* 17(4):380, 381, 422, 1991.

Klug RM: Understanding private insurance for funding pediatric home care, *Pediatr Nurs* 17:197-198, 1991.

Leff P, Walizer E: *Building the healing partnership*, Cambridge, Mass, 1992, Brookline Books.

Leighton EM, Davis RH, Anderson LJW: An orientation program for high-technology home care nursing, *Pediatr Nurs* 16:182-185, 1990.

Marrelli TM: *Handbook of home health standards and documentation: guidelines for reimbursement*, ed 2, St Louis, 1994, Mosby.

McClowry S: Pediatric nursing psychosocial care: a vision beyond hospitalization, *Pediatr Nurs* 19(2):146-148, 1993.

McClung RL: Considerations for the use of a conceptual model in home health nursing, *Pediatr Nurs* 21(1):68-70, 1995.

Nissam LG, Sten MB: The ventilator-assisted child: a case for empowerment, *Pediatr Nurs* 17:507-511, 1991.

Nugent K et al: A practice model for a parent support group, *Pediatr Nurs* 18:11-16, 1992.

Office of Technology Assessment (OTA), Congress of the United States: *Technology-dependent children: hospital v. home care—a technical memorandum* (OTA-TM-H-38), Washington, DC, 1987, US Government Printing Office.

Parette HP, Bartlett CR, Holder-Brown L: The nurse's role in planning for inclusion of medically fragile and technology-dependent children in public school settings, *Issues Compr Pediatr Nurs* 17(2):61-72, 1994.

Steele S: Nurse and parent collaborative case management in a rural setting, *Pediatr Nurs* 19(6):612-615, 1993.

Stein R, Jessop DJ: Does pediatric home care make a difference for children with chronic illness? Findings from the Pediatric Ambulatory Care Treatment Study, *Pediatrics* 73(6):845-853, 1984.

Stutts AL: Selected outcomes of technology-dependent children receiving home care and prescribed child care services, *Pediatr Nurs* 20(5):501-507, 1994.

Wegener DH, Aday LA: Home care for ventilator-assisted children: predicting family stress, *Pediatr Nurs* 15:371-376, 1989.

Wheeler TW, Lewis CC: Home care for medically fragile children: urban versus rural settings, *Issues Compr Pediatr Nurs* 16:13-30, 1993.

Worthington RC: Effective transitions for families: life beyond the hospital, *Pediatr Nurs* 21(1):86-87, 1995.

Youngblut JM, Brennan PF, Swegart LA: Families with medically fragile children: an exploratory study, *Pediatr Nurs* 20(5):463-468, 1994.

Zagorsky ES: Caring for families who follow alternative health care practices, *Pediatr Nurs* 19(1):71-75, 1993.

Zanoa JS: Beyond the stack of bills: what home care of cancer patients really costs, *Cancer Nurs News* 10(3):13, 1992.

Selected Resources on Home Care

Association for the Care of Children's Health
7910 Woodmont Ave., Suite 300
Bethesda, MD 20814
(301) 654-6549

National Association for Home Care
519 C Street, N.E.
Washington, DC 20002-5809
(202) 547-7424

National Father's Network
The Kindering Center
16120 Northeast 8th St.
Bellevue, WA 98008
(206) 747-4004

National Information Center for Children and Youth with Disabilities
PO Box 1492
Washington, DC 20013
(202) 884-8200 or (800) 695-0285

National Information Clearinghouse for Infants with Disabilities and Life-Threatening Conditions
NIS
CDD/USC
Benson Building
Columbia, SC 29208
(800) 922-9234, ext. 201 (voice or TDD);
in South Carolina: (800) 922 1107

Project Copernicus
(Family-Centered Care)
Kennedy Krieger
Community Resources
2911 E. Biddle St.
Baltimore, MD 21213
(410) 550-9700
(410) 550-9758 (TDD)

Sibling Support Project
Children's Hospital and Medical Center
4800 Sand Point Way, N.E.
Seattle, WA 98105
(206) 368-4911

Skip (Sick Kids Need Involved People, Inc.)
545 Madison Ave., 13th Floor
New York, NY 10022
(212) 421-9160

CHAPTER 41

Reaction to Illness and Hospitalization

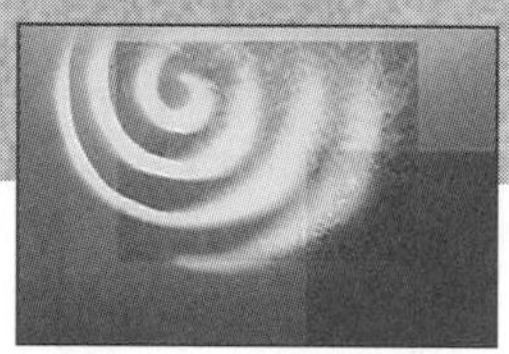

STRESSORS OF HOSPITALIZATION AND CHILDREN'S REACTIONS, P. 1196

Separation anxiety, p. 1196
Loss of control, p. 1198
Bodily injury and pain, p. 1200
Effects of hospitalization on the child, p. 1203

NURSING CARE OF THE CHILD WHO IS HOSPITALIZED, P. 1204

STRESSORS AND REACTIONS IN THE FAMILY OF THE CHILD WHO IS HOSPITALIZED, P. 1236

Parental reactions, p. 1236
Sibling reactions, p. 1236
Altered family roles, p. 1236

NURSING CARE OF THE FAMILY, P. 1237

CARE OF THE CHILD AND FAMILY IN SPECIAL HOSPITAL SITUATIONS, P. 1241

Ambulatory/outpatient setting, p. 1241
Isolation, p. 1242
Emergency admission, p. 1242
Intensive care unit (ICU), p. 1243

Stressors of Hospitalization and Children's Reactions

Often illness and hospitalization are the first crises children must face. Children, especially during the early years, are particularly vulnerable to the crises of illness and hospitalization because (1) stress represents a change from the usual state of health and environmental routine and (2) children have a limited number of coping mechanisms to resolve ***stressors*** (those events that produce stress). Children's reactions to these crises are influenced by their developmental age; previous experience with illness, separation, or hospitalization; innate and acquired coping skills; the seriousness of the diagnosis; and the support system available.

SEPARATION ANXIETY

The major stress from middle infancy throughout the preschool years, especially for children ages 6 to 30 months, is **separation anxiety.** The principal behavioral responses to this stressor during early childhood are summarized in Box 41-1.

During the phase of *protest,* children react aggressively to the separation from the parent. They cry and scream for their parents, refuse the attention of anyone else, and are inconsolable in their grief (Fig. 41-1). During the phase of *despair* the crying stops, and depression is evident. The child is much less active, is uninterested in play or food, and withdraws from others (Fig. 41-2).

The third stage is *detachment,* which is sometimes also called *denial.* Superficially it appears that the child has finally adjusted to the loss. The child becomes more interested in the surroundings, plays with others, and seems to form new relationships. However, this behavior is the result of resignation and is not a sign of contentment. The child detaches from the parent in an effort to escape the emotional pain of desiring the parent's presence and copes by forming shallow relationships with others, becoming increasingly self-centered, and attaching primary importance to material objects. This is the most serious stage in that reversal of the potential adverse effects is less likely to occur once detachment is established. However, in most situations the temporary separations imposed by hospitalization do not cause such prolonged parental absences that the child enters into detachment. In addition, considerable evidence suggests that even with stressors such as separation children are remarkably adaptable and permanent ill effects are rare.

Although progression to the stage of detachment is uncommon, the initial stages are frequently observed even with very brief separations from either parent. Unless health team members understand the meaning of each stage of behavior, they may erroneously label the behaviors as positive or negative. For example, they may see the loud crying of the protest

BOX 41-1
Manifestations of Separation Anxiety in Young Children

Phase of protest

Observed behaviors during later infancy:
- Cries
- Screams
- Searches for parent with eyes
- Clings to parent
- Avoids and rejects contact with strangers

Additional behaviors observed during toddlerhood:
- Verbally attacks strangers (e.g., "Go away")
- Physically attacks strangers (e.g., kicks, bites, hits, pinches)
- Attempts to escape to find parent
- Attempts to physically force parent to stay

Behaviors may last from hours to days

Protest, such as crying, may be continuous, ceasing only with physical exhaustion

Approach of stranger may precipitate increased protest

Phase of despair

Observed behaviors:
- Inactive
- Withdraws from others
- Depressed, sad
- Uninterested in environment
- Uncommunicative
- Regresses to earlier behavior (e.g., thumb-sucking, bedwetting, use of pacifier, use of bottle)

Behaviors may last for variable length of time

Child's physical condition may deteriorate from refusal to eat, drink, or move

Phase of detachment

Observed behaviors:
- Shows increased interest in surroundings
- Interacts with strangers or familiar caregivers
- Forms new but superficial relationships
- Appears happy

Detachment usually occurs after prolonged separation from parent; rarely seen in hospitalized children

Behaviors represent a superficial adjustment to loss

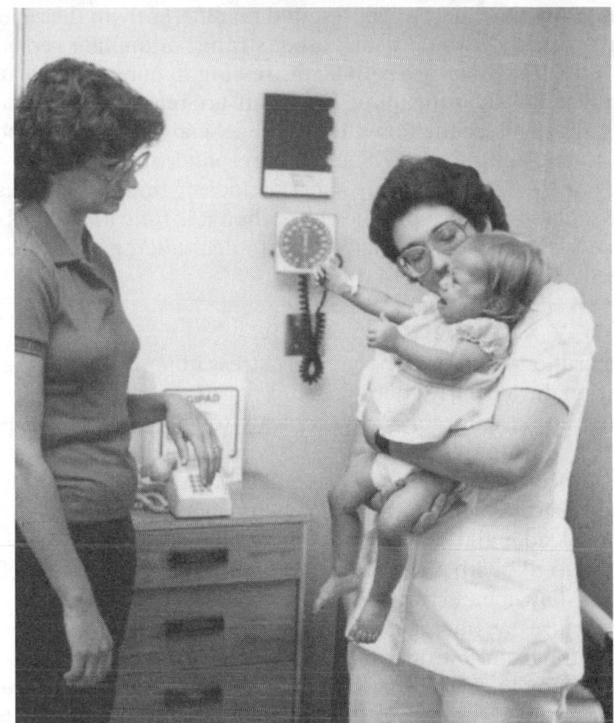

Fig. 41-1 In the protest phase of separation anxiety, children cry loudly and are inconsolable in their grief for the parent.

phase as "bad" behavior. Since the protesting increases when a stranger approaches the child, they may interpret that reaction as meaning they should stay away. During the quiet, withdrawn phase of despair, health team members may think the child is finally "settling in" to the new surroundings, and they may see the detachment behaviors as proof of a "good adjustment." The faster this stage is reached, the more likely it is that the child will be regarded as the "ideal patient."

Since children seem to react "negatively" to visits by their parents, uninformed observers feel justified in restricting parental visiting privileges. For example, during the protest stage, children outwardly do not appear happy to see their parents. In fact, they may even cry louder. If they are depressed, they may reject their parents or begin to protest once more. Often they cling to their parents in an effort to ensure their continued presence. Consequently, such reactions may be regarded as "disturbing" the child's adjustment to the new surroundings. If the separation has progressed to the phase of

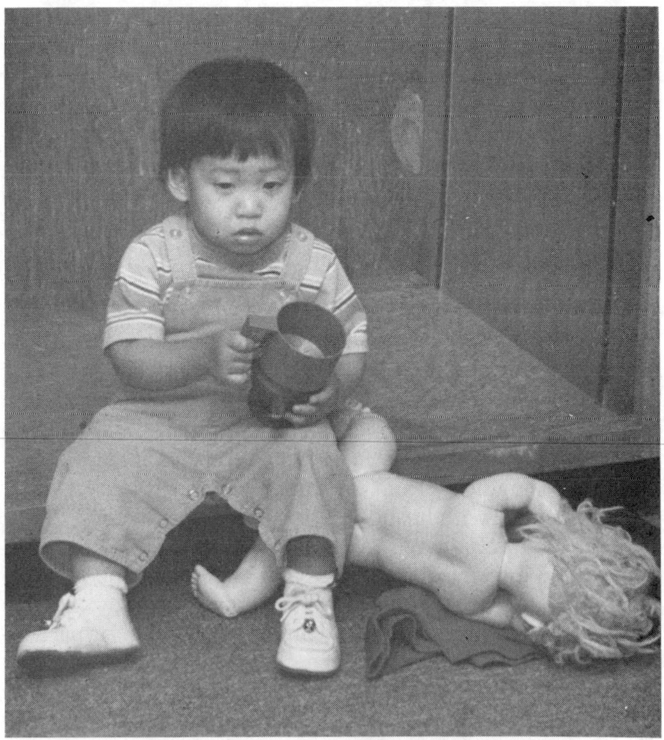

Fig. 41-2 During the despair phase of separation anxiety, children are sad, lonely, and uninterested in play or food.

detachment, children will respond no differently to their parents than they would to any other strange or familiar person.

Such reactions are equally distressing to parents, who are unaware of their meaning. If parents are regarded as intruders, they will see their absence as "beneficial" to the child's adjustment and recovery. They may respond to the child's behavior by staying for only short periods of time, visiting less frequently, or deceiving the child when it is time to leave. The result is a destructive cycle of misunderstanding and unmet needs.

Early Childhood

Separation anxiety is the greatest stress imposed by hospitalization during early childhood. If separation is avoided, young children have a tremendous capacity to withstand any other stress. During this age period the typical reactions previously described are seen. However, children in the toddler stage demonstrate more goal-directed behaviors. For example, they may plead with the parents to stay and physically try to keep the parents with them or try to find parents who have left. They may demonstrate displeasure on the parents' return or departure by having temper tantrums; refusing to comply with the usual routines of mealtime, bedtime, or toileting; or regressing to more primitive levels of development. However, temper tantrums, bed-wetting, or other behaviors may also be expressions of anger or even a physiologic response to stress.

Since preschoolers are more secure interpersonally than toddlers, they can tolerate brief periods of separation from their parents and are more inclined to develop substitute trust in other significant adults. However, the stress of illness usually renders preschoolers less able to cope with separation; as a result, they manifest many of the stage behaviors of separation anxiety, although in general the protest behaviors are more subtle and passive than those seen in younger children. Preschoolers may demonstrate separation anxiety by refusing to eat, experiencing difficulty in sleeping, crying quietly for their parents, continually asking when the parents will visit, or withdrawing from others. They may express anger indirectly by breaking their toys, hitting other children, or refusing to cooperate during usual self-care activities. Nurses need to be sensitive to these less obvious signs of separation anxiety in order to intervene appropriately.

Later Childhood and Adolescence

Previous research, usually based on adult recollections, indicated that the family does not play as important a role for school-age children as it does during the toddler and preschool years. However, in a recent study wherein children were asked about their fears when hospitalized, children ranked "being away from my family" higher than any other fear associated with hospitalization (Hart and Bossert, 1994).

Although school-age children are better able to cope with separation in general, the stress and often accompanying regression imposed by illness or hospitalization may increase their need for parental security and guidance. This is particularly true for young school-age children who have only recently left the safety of the home and are struggling with the crisis of school adjustment. Middle and late school-age children may react more to the separation from their usual activities and peers than to the absence of their parents. These children have a high level of physical and mental activity that frequently finds no suitable outlets in the hospital environment, and even when they dislike school, they admit to missing its routine and worry that they will not be able to compete or "fit in" with their classmates when they return. Feelings of loneliness, boredom, isolation, and depression are common. Such reactions may occur more as a result of separation than from concern over the illness, treatment, or hospital setting.

School-age children may need and desire parental guidance or support from other adult figures but be unable or unwilling to ask for it. Because the goal of attaining independence is so important to them, they are reluctant to seek help directly for fear that they will appear weak, childish, or dependent. Cultural expectations to "act like a man" or to "be brave and strong" bear heavily on these children, especially boys, who tend to react to stress with stoicism, withdrawal, or passive acceptance. Often the need to express hostile, angry, or other negative feelings finds outlets in alternate ways, such as irritability and aggression toward parents, withdrawal from hospital personnel, inability to relate to peers, rejection of siblings, or subsequent behavioral problems in school.

For adolescents, separation from home and parents may be a welcomed and appreciated event. However, loss of peer-group contact may pose a severe emotional threat because of loss of group status, inability to exert group control or leadership, and loss of group acceptance. Deviations within peer groups are poorly tolerated, and, although group members may express concern for the adolescent's illness or need for hospitalization, they continue their group activities, quickly filling the gap of the absent member. During the temporary separation from their usual group, ill adolescents may benefit from group associations with other hospitalized age-mates.

LOSS OF CONTROL

One of the factors influencing the amount of stress imposed by hospitalization is the amount of control that persons perceive themselves as having. Lack of control increases the perception of threat and can affect children's coping skills. Many hospital situations decrease the amount of control a child feels. Because children's needs vary greatly depending on their age, the major areas of loss of control in terms of physical restriction, altered routine or rituals, and dependency are discussed for each age group.

Infants

Infants are developing the most important attribute of a healthy personality—trust. Trust is established through consistent, loving care by a mothering person. Infants attempt to control their environment through emotional expressions, such as crying or smiling. In the hospital setting, cues may be missed or misinterpreted, and routines may be established to meet the hospital staff's needs instead of the infant's needs. Inconsistent care and deviations from the infant's daily routine may lead to mistrust and a decreased sense of control (Wells et al, 1994).

Toddlers

Toddlers are striving for autonomy, and this goal is evident in most of their behaviors—motor skills, play, interpersonal relationships, activities of daily living, and communication. When their egocentric pleasures meet with obstacles, toddlers react with negativism, especially temper tantrums. Any restriction or limitation of movement, such as the simple act of making toddlers lie down, can cause forceful resistance and noncompliance.

Loss of control also results from altered routines and rituals. Toddlers rely on the consistency and familiarity of daily rituals to provide a measure of stability and control in their complex world of growing and developing. The experience of hospitalization or illness severely limits their sense of expectation and predictability, since practically every detail of the hospital environment differs from that of the home.

Toddlers' main areas for rituals include eating, sleeping, bathing, toileting, and play. When the routines are disrupted, difficulties can occur in any or all of these areas. The principal reaction to such change is regression. For example, when mealtime and food choices differ from those at home, toddlers often refuse to eat, demand a bottle, or ask others to feed them. Although regression to earlier forms of behavior may seem to increase toddlers' security and comfort, in reality it is very threatening for them to relinquish their most recently acquired achievements.

Enforced dependency is a chief characteristic of the sick role and accounts for the numerous instances of toddler negativism. For example, rigid schedules, different clothes, altered caregiving activities, unfamiliar surroundings, separation from parents, and medical procedures usurp toddlers' control over their world. Although most toddlers initially react negatively and aggressively to such dependency, prolonged loss of autonomy may result in passive withdrawal from interpersonal relationships and regression in all areas of development. Therefore the effects of the sick role are most severe in instances of chronic, long-term illnesses or in those families in which the sick role is fostered despite the child's improved state of health.

Preschoolers

Preschoolers also suffer from loss of control caused by physical restriction, altered routines, and enforced dependency. However, their specific cognitive abilities, which make them feel omnipotent and all-powerful, also make them feel out of control. This loss of control in the context of their sense of self-power is a critical influencing factor in their perception of and reaction to separation, pain, illness, and hospitalization.

Preschoolers' egocentric and magical thinking limits their ability to understand events because they view all experiences from their own self-referenced (egocentric) perspective. Without adequate preparation for unfamiliar settings or experiences, preschoolers' fantasy explanations for such events are usually more exaggerated, bizarre, and frightening than the actual facts. One typical fantasy to explain the reason for illness or hospitalization is that it represents punishment for real or imagined misdeeds. In response to such thinking the child usually feels shame, guilt, and fear.

Preschoolers' concrete thinking means that explanations are understood only in terms of real events. Purely verbal instructions are often inadequate for them because they are unable to abstract and synthesize beyond what their senses tell them. When combined with their egocentric and magical thinking, this characteristic may lead them to interpret messages according to their particular past experiences. Even with the best preparation for a procedure, they may misconstrue the details.

Transductive reasoning implies that preschoolers deduct from the particular to the particular, rather than from the specific to the general, or vice versa. For example, if preschoolers' concept of nurses is that they inflict pain, preschoolers will think that every nurse (or everyone wearing a similar uniform) will also inflict pain.

School-Age Children

Because of their striving for independence and productivity, school-age children are particularly vulnerable to events that may lessen their feeling of control and power. In particular, altered family roles; physical disability; fears of death, abandonment, or permanent injury; loss of peer acceptance; lack of productivity; and inability to cope with stress according to perceived cultural expectation may result in loss of control.

Because of the nature of the patient role, many routine hospital activities usurp individual power and identity. For school-age children, dependent activities such as enforced bed rest, use of a bedpan, lack of privacy, help with a bed bath, or transport by use of a wheelchair or stretcher can be a direct threat to their security. Although all of these usual hospital procedures seem routine and inconsequential, to children who want to "act grown-up" they allow no freedom of choice. However, when children are allowed to exert a measure of control, regardless of how limited it may be, they generally respond very well to any procedure. For example, some of the most cooperative, satisfied, and contented patients are those school-age children who help make their beds, choose their schedule of activities, assist in procedures, and help the nurses care for the younger children. An increased sense of control is usually an outcome of feeling useful and productive.

Besides the hospital environment, illness also may cause a feeling of loss of control. One of the most significant problems of children in this age group centers on boredom. When physical or enforced limitations curtail their usual abilities to care for themselves or to engage in favorite activities, school-age children generally respond with depression, hostility, or frustration. Keeping a normally active child on bed rest is no small challenge. However, by emphasizing areas of control for the child and capitalizing on quiet activities, particularly hobbies such as building models or collecting specific objects, nurses can promote school-age children's adjustment to physical restriction. Nursing judgment regarding selection of a roommate is one of the most important contributing factors to the overall adjustment of children in this age group to illness and hospitalization.

Adolescents

Adolescents' struggle for independence, self-assertion, and liberation centers on the quest for personal identity. Anything that interferes with this poses a threat to their sense of identity and results in a loss of control. Illness, which limits their physical abilities, and hospitalization, which separates them from their usual support systems, constitute major situational crises.

The patient role fosters dependency and depersonalization. Adolescents may react to dependency with rejection, uncooperativeness, or withdrawal. They may respond to depersonalization with self-assertion, anger, or frustration. Regardless of response, hospital personnel often regard them as difficult, unmanageable patients. Parents may not be a source of help because these behaviors serve to further isolate them from understanding the adolescent. Although peers may visit, they may not be able to offer the kind of support and guidance needed. Sick adolescents often voluntarily isolate themselves from age-mates until they feel they can compete on an equal basis and meet group expectations. As a result, adolescents may be left with virtually no support system.

Loss of control also occurs for many of the reasons discussed for school-age children. However, adolescents are more sensitive to potential instances of loss of control and dependency than are younger children. For example, both groups seek information about their physical status and rely heavily on anticipatory preparation to decrease fear and anxiety. However, adolescents react not only to the kinds of information supplied them, but also to the means by which it is conveyed. They may feel very threatened by others who relate facts in a condescending manner. Adolescents want to know that others can relate to them on their own level. This necessitates a careful assessment of their intellectual abilities, previous knowledge, and present needs.

BODILY INJURY AND PAIN

In caring for children, nurses must have an appreciation of a child's concerns about bodily harm and the reactions to pain at different developmental periods. Developmental considerations related to children's understanding of illness and pain are summarized in Table 41-1. Developmental characteristics of children's reactions to pain are summarized in Box 41-2.

Infants

Research exploring children's development of illness concepts and how their understanding of illness relates to fears of bodily injury includes no findings for preverbal children. Consequently, the following discussion is limited to infants' reactions to pain.

Infants' response to pain after the neonatal period is quite similar to earlier reactions, although there is marked variability in measures of distress, especially initial cry and heart rate, which may decrease in some infants. The most consistent indicator of distress is a facial expression of discomfort (Fig. 41-3). Body movements include squirming, writhing, jerking, and flailing. Some infants may cry loudly after the procedure, whereas others are easily calmed by a gentle hug. It is important to recognize and respect such early signs of individuality and to realize that children who react less intensely may still be experiencing significant discomfort (Broome et al, 1990).

Children's response to pain is increasingly influenced by their prior painful experiences and the emotional reaction of parents during the procedure. Older infants react intensely with physical resistance and uncooperativeness. They may refuse to lie still, attempt to push the person away, or try to escape with whatever motor activity they have achieved. Distraction does little to lessen their immediate reaction to pain, and anticipatory preparation, such as showing them the equipment, can increase their fear and resistance.

Toddlers

Toddlers' concept of body image, particularly the definition of body boundaries, is very poorly developed. Intrusive experiences, such as examining the ears or mouth or checking a rectal temperature, are very anxiety producing. Toddlers may react to such painless procedures as intensely as they do to painful ones.

Toddlers' reactions to pain are similar to those seen during

TABLE 41-1 Children's developmental concepts of illness and pain

CONCEPT OF ILLNESS*	CONCEPT OF PAIN†
Preoperational thought (2 to 7 years)	
Phenomenism: Perceives an external, unrelated, concrete phenomenon as the cause of illness (e.g., "being sick because you don't feel well") ***Contagion:*** Perceives cause of illness as proximity between two events that occurs by "magic" (e.g., "getting a cold because you are near someone who has a cold")	Relates to pain primarily as physical, concrete experience Thinks in terms of magical disappearance of pain May view pain as punishment for wrongdoing Tends to hold someone accountable for own pain and may strike out at person
Concrete operational thought (7 to 10+ years)	
Contamination: Perceives cause as a person, object, or action external to the child that is "bad" or "harmful" to the body (e.g., "getting a cold because you didn't wear a hat") ***Internalization:*** Perceives illness as having an external cause but as being located inside the body (e.g., "getting a cold by breathing in air and bacteria")	Relates to pain physically (e.g., headache, stomachache) Is able to perceive of psychologic pain (e.g., someone dying) Fears bodily harm and annihilation (body destruction and death) May view pain as punishment for wrongdoing
Formal operational thought (13 years and older)	
Physiologic: Perceives cause as malfunctioning or nonfunctioning organ or process; can explain illness in sequence of events ***Psychophysiologic:*** Realizes that psychologic actions and attitudes affect health and illness	Is able to give reason for pain (e.g., fell and hit nerve) Perceives several types of psychologic pain Has limited life experiences to cope with pain as adult might cope despite mature understanding of pain Fears losing control during painful experience

*From Bibace R, Walsh ME: Development of children's concepts of illness, *Pediatrics* 66(6):912-917, 1980.
†From Hurley A, Whelan EG: Cognitive development and children's perception of pain, *Pediatr Nurs* 14(1):21-24, 1988.

BOX 41-2
Developmental Characteristics of Children's Responses to Pain

Young infants

Generalized body response of rigidity or thrashing, possibly with local reflex withdrawal of stimulated area
Loud crying
Facial expression of pain (brows lowered and drawn together, eyes tightly closed, and mouth open and squarish) (Fig. 41-3)
Demonstrates no association between approaching stimulus and subsequent pain

Older infants

Localized body response with deliberate withdrawal of stimulated area
Loud crying
Facial expression of pain and/or anger (same facial characteristics as pain but eyes are open)
Physical resistance, especially pushing the stimulus away *after* it is applied

Young child

Loud crying, screaming
Verbal expressions of "Ow," "Ouch," "It hurts"
Thrashing of arms and legs
Attempts to push stimulus away *before* it is applied
Uncooperative; needs physical restraint
Requests termination of procedure
Clings to parent, nurse, or other significant person
Requests emotional support, such as hugs or other forms of physical comfort
May become restless and irritable with continuing pain
All of these behaviors may be seen in anticipation of actual painful procedure

School-age child

May see all behaviors of young child, especially *during* actual painful procedure but less in anticipatory period
Stalling behavior, such as "Wait a minute" or "I'm not ready"
Muscular rigidity, such as clenched fists, white knuckles, gritted teeth, contracted limbs, body stiffness, closed eyes, wrinkled forehead

Adolescent

Less vocal protest
Less motor activity
More verbal expressions, such as "It hurts" or "You're hurting me"
Increased muscle tension and body control

Data from Craig KD: Developmental changes in infant pain expression during immunization injections, *Soc Sci Med* 19(12):1331-1337, 1984; and Katz ER, Kellerman J, Siegel SE: Behavioral distress in children with cancer undergoing medical procedures: developmental considerations, *J Consult Clin Psychol* 48(3):356-365, 1980.

infancy, except that the number of variables influencing the individual response is highly complex and varied. Memory, physical restraint, separation from parents, emotional reactions of others, and lack of preparation partially determine the intensity of the behavioral response. In general, children in this age group continue to react with intense emotional upset and physical resistance to any actual or perceived painful experience. Behaviors indicating pain include grimacing, clenching their teeth and/or lips, opening their eyes wide, rocking, rubbing, and acting aggressively, such as biting, kicking, hitting, or running away. Unlike adults, who usually decrease their activity when in pain, young children typically become restless and overly active; frequently this response is not recognized as a consequence of pain.

By the end of this age period, toddlers usually are able to communicate about their pain. Although they have not developed the ability to describe the type or intensity of the pain, they usually are able to localize it by pointing to a specific area.

Preschoolers

Concepts of illness begin during the preschool period and are influenced by the cognitive abilities of the preoperational stage. Preschoolers differentiate poorly between themselves and the external world. Their thinking is focused on externally perceived events, and causality is based on the proximity of two events. Consequently, children define illness according to what they are told or are given external evidence of, such as "You are sick because you have a fever." The cause of illness is seen as a concrete action the child does or fails to do, such as

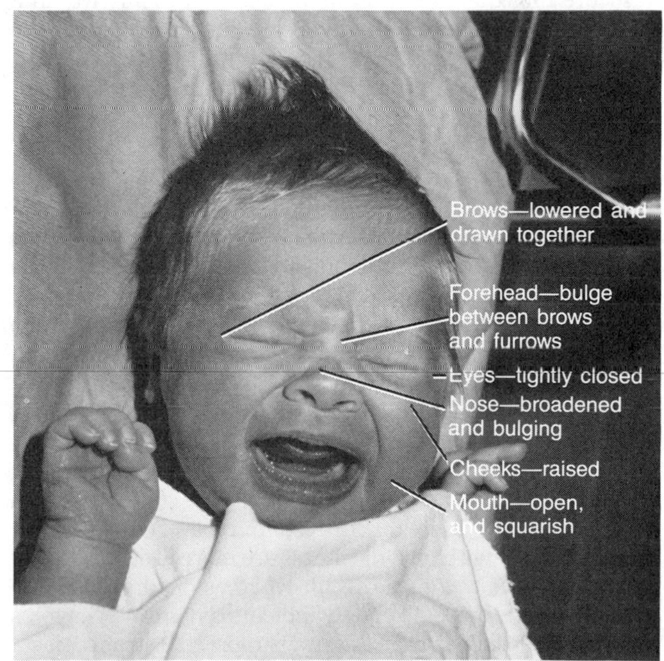

Fig. 41-3 Facial expression of physical distress is the most consistent behavioral indicator of pain in infants.

"Catching a cold because you go out into cold weather"; consequently, it implies a degree of responsibility and self-blame. Another explanation may be based on contagion, that the proximity of two objects or persons causes the illness; for example, "A person gets a cold when someone else with a cold gets near him."

The psychosexual conflicts of children in this age group make them very vulnerable to threats of bodily injury. Intrusive procedures, whether painful or painless, are threatening to preschoolers, whose concept of body integrity is still poorly developed. Preschoolers may react to an injection with as much concern for withdrawal of the needle as for the actual pain. They fear that the intrusion or puncture will not reclose and that their "insides" will leak out.

Concerns of mutilation are paramount during this age period. Loss of any body part is threatening, but preschool boys' fears of castration complicate their understanding of surgical or medical procedures associated with the genital area, such as circumcision, repair of hypospadias or epispadias, cystoscopy, or catheterization. Their limited comprehension of body functioning also increases their difficulty in understanding how or why body parts are "fixed." For example, telling preschoolers that their tonsils are to be removed may be interpreted as "taking out their voice," or having the penis "fixed" may be understood as cutting it off. Words such as "dye," "cut off," "take out," or "draw" (e.g., "draw some blood") are understood literally and can lead to confusion and fear (see the discussion of communicating with children, Chapter 31).

Reactions to pain tend to be similar to those seen during toddlerhood, although some differences become apparent. For example, preschoolers respond more favorably than younger children to preparatory interventions, such as explanation and distraction. Physical and verbal aggression are more specific and goal directed. Instead of showing total body resistance, preschoolers may push the offending person away, try to secure the equipment, or attempt to lock themselves in a safe place. Much more thought is evident in their plan of attack or escape.

Verbal expression in particular demonstrates their advanced development in response to stress. They may verbally abuse the nurse by stating, "Get out of here" or "I hate you." They may also use the more cunning approach of trying to persuade the person to give up the intended activity. A common plea is, "Please don't give me a shot; I'll be good." Some statements are not only attempts to avoid the event but also evidence of children's perceptions about the experience.

Preschoolers can locate their pain and can use appropriate pain scales. Children as young as 3 years can use assessment tools based on facial expressions of pain (Table 41-2, p. 1211).

School-Age Children

Fears concerning the physical nature of the illness surface at this time. School-age children may be less concerned with pain than with disability, uncertain recovery, or possible death. Children with chronic illness are more likely to identify intrusive procedures as stressful, whereas children who are acutely ill are more likely to indicate physical symptoms (Bossert, 1994). Girls tend to express more and stronger fears than boys, and previous hospitalizations may have no effect on the frequency or intensity of these fears. Because of their developing cognitive abilities, school-age children are aware of the significance of different illnesses, the indispensability of certain body parts, potential hazards of treatments, lifelong consequences of permanent injury or loss of function, and the meaning of death. A major concern of school-age children when hospitalized is their fear of being told that something is wrong with them (Hart and Bossert, 1994). They generally take a very active interest in their health or illness. Even those children who rarely ask questions usually reveal detailed knowledge of their condition by attentively listening to all that is said around them. They request factual information and quickly perceive lies or half-truths. Seeking information tends to be one way of coping or maintaining a sense of control despite the stress and uncertainty of the condition.

The school-age child defines illness by a set of multiple concrete symptoms, such as signs of a cold, and views the cause as primarily germs or bacteria. The germs have a powerful, almost magical quality, so that in the child's mind, illness can be prevented by avoiding people with the germs. There is also the notion of contamination, which is similar to that seen in the younger age group; for example, the illness occurs because of physical contact or because the child engaged in a harmful action and became contaminated. Consequently, feelings of self-blame and guilt may be associated with the reason for becoming ill.

School-age children begin to show concern for the potential beneficial and hazardous effects of procedures. Besides wanting to know if a procedure will hurt, they want to know what it is for, how it will make them better, and what injury or harm could result. For example, these children may fear the actual procedure of anesthesia. Unlike preschoolers, who fear the mask and the strange surroundings, school-age children fear what may happen while they are asleep, whether they will wake up, and that they may die. Preadolescents also worry about the procedure itself, particularly if it is one that will result in visible changes in body appearance.

Intrusive procedures of a nonsexual nature, such as routine physical examination of the ears, nose, mouth, and throat, are generally well tolerated. However, concerns for privacy become evident and increasingly significant. Although school-age children may cooperate during examination of, or procedures performed on, the genital area, it is usually very stressful for them, especially for preadolescents who are beginning pubertal changes. Nurses who respect children's need for privacy can provide them with much assurance and support.

By the age of 9 or 10 years, most school-age children show less fright or overt resistance to pain than younger children. They generally have learned coping methods of dealing with discomfort, such as holding rigidly still, clenching their fists or teeth, or trying to act brave by the "grin-and-bear-it" routine. If they do display signs of overt resistance, such as biting, kicking, pulling away, trying to escape, crying, or plea bargaining, they may deny such reactions later, especially to their peers for fear of embarrassment.

School-age children verbally communicate about their pain in respect to its location, intensity, and description. Unlike younger children, who may have difficulty choosing words to describe pain, children 8 years and older use a wide variety of words and phrases, such as hurting, sore, burning, stinging, aching, and "like a sharp knife" (Tesler et al, 1991).

School-age children also use words as a means of controlling their reactions to pain. For example, these children may ask the nurse to talk to them during a procedure. Some prefer to participate in a procedure, whereas others choose to distance themselves by not looking at what is happening. Most appreciate an explanation of the procedure and seem less fearful when they know what to expect. Others try to gain control by attempting to postpone the event. A typical request is, "Give me the shot when I am finished with this." Although the ability to make decisions does increase their sense of control, unlimited procrastination results in heightened anxiety. When choices are allowed, such as selection of the injection site, it is best to structure the number of possible sites and to limit the number of "procrastination" techniques.

Similar to their more passive acceptance of pain is their nondirective request for support or help. School-age children rarely initiate a conversation about their feelings or request someone to stay with them during a lonely or stressful period. Their visible composure, calmness, and acceptance often mask their inner longing for support. It is especially important to be aware of nonverbal clues, such as a serious facial expression, a half-hearted reply of "I am fine," silence, lack of activity, or social isolation, as signs of the need for help. Usually when someone identifies the unspoken messages and offers support, they readily accept it.

Adolescents

Although the development of body image begins at birth, its relevance is paramount during adolescence. Injury, pain, disability, and death are viewed primarily in terms of how each affects adolescents' views of themselves in the present. Any change that differentiates the adolescent from peers is regarded as a major tragedy. For example, diseases such as diabetes mellitus often present a more difficult adjustment period for children in this age group than for younger children because of the necessary changes in the adolescent's life style. Conversely, serious, even life-threatening illnesses that entail no visible body changes or physical restrictions may have less immediate significance for the adolescent. Therefore the nature of bodily injury may be more important in terms of adolescents' perception of the illness than its actual degree of severity.

Adolescents' rapidly changing body image during pubertal development often makes them feel insecure about their bodies. Illness, medical or surgical intervention, and hospitalization increase their existing concerns for normalcy. They may respond to such events by asking numerous questions, withdrawing, rejecting others, or questioning the adequacy of care. Often their fear for loss of control and body image change is demonstrated as overconfidence, conceit, or a "know-it-all" attitude.

Because of sexual changes, adolescents are very concerned about privacy. Lack of respect for this need can cause greater stress than physical pain. In addition, adolescents look for signs that indicate that they are developing normally and according to acceptable standards. When illness occurs, they fear that growth may be retarded, leaving them behind their peers. Although they may not voice this concern, they may demonstrate it by carefully observing others' reactions to them.

Adolescents typically react to pain with much self-control. Physical resistance and aggression are less likely at this age, unless the adolescent is totally unprepared for a procedure. As with older school-age children, adolescents are very concerned with remaining composed and feel embarrassed and ashamed of losing control. They are able to describe their pain experience and to use any of the pain assessment tools developed for adults. However, they may be reluctant to disclose their pain, requiring the nurse to listen closely and observe physical indications, such as limited movement, excessive quiet, or irritability. They may also believe that the nurse knows how they feel; thus they may see no need to ask for analgesia (Favaloro and Touzel, 1990).

EFFECTS OF HOSPITALIZATION ON THE CHILD

Children may react to the stresses of hospitalization before admission, during hospitalization, and after discharge. A child's conception of illness is even more important than age and intellectual maturity in predicting the level of adjustment before hospitalization (Carson, Gravley, and Council, 1992). Although age and intellectual ability are strongly related to children's concepts of illness, research indicates that the duration of a child's medical condition, total hospitalization days, and more life-threatening medical condition are not associated with more sophisticated illness concepts (Kury and Rodrigue, 1995). Therefore nurses should avoid overestimating the illness concepts of children with prior medical experience. Many children, especially those under 4 years of age, demonstrate temporary behavioral changes after discharge (Box 41-3). These changes are a result of (1) separation from significant people, (2) a lack of opportunity to form new attachments, and (3) a strange environment.

BOX 41-3
Posthospital Behaviors in Children

Young Children

Some initial aloofness toward parents; may last from a few minutes (most common) to a few days
Frequently followed by dependency behaviors:
- Tendency to cling to parents
- Demand parents' attention
- Vigorously oppose any separation (e.g., staying at preschool or with a baby-sitter)

Other negative behaviors include:
- New fears (e.g., nightmares)
- Resistance to going to bed, night waking
- Withdrawal and shyness
- Hyperactivity
- Temper tantrums
- Food finickiness
- Attachment to blanket or toy
- Regression in newly learned skills (e.g., self-toileting)

Older Children

Negative behaviors include:
- Emotional coldness, followed by intense, demanding dependence on parents
- Anger toward parents
- Jealousy toward others (e.g., siblings)

BOX 41-4
Risk Factors That Increase Children's Vulnerability to the Stresses of Hospitalization

"Difficult" temperament
Lack of fit between child and parent
Age (especially between 6 months and 5 years)
Male gender
Below-average intelligence
Multiple and continuing stresses (e.g., frequent hospitalizations)

Individual Risk Factors

A number of risk factors make certain children more vulnerable than others to the stresses of hospitalization (Box 41-4). It has also been noted that rural children exhibit significantly greater degrees of psychologic upset than urban children, possibly because urban children have opportunities to become familiar with a local hospital (Gillis, 1990). Perhaps because separation is such an important issue surrounding hospitalization for young children, children who are active and strong willed tend to fare better when hospitalized than youngsters who are passive. Consequently, nurses should be alert to children who passively accept all changes and requests; these children may need more support than the "oppositional" child.

The development of subsequent long-term emotional disturbance may be related to the *length* and *number* of hospital admissions and the type of hospital practices. A single hospitalization of 4 weeks or more and repeated hospital admissions have been associated with later disturbances. However, supportive practices, such as frequent family visiting, may lessen the detrimental effects of such admissions.

Changes in the pediatric population. The pediatric population in hospitals today has changed dramatically over the last two decades. A greater percentage of the children hospitalized today have more serious and complex problems than those hospitalized in the past. Many of these children are fragile newborns and children with severe injuries or disabilities who survived because of incredible technologic advances, yet were left with chronic or disabling conditions that require frequent and lengthy hospital stays. Research suggests that prior experience and familiarity with medical events related to hospitalization do not reduce fears in children (Hart and Bossert, 1994). Rather, prior experience may simply replace fear of the unknown with fear of the known. The nature of their conditions increases the likelihood that they will experience more invasive and traumatic procedures while they are hospitalized. These factors make them more vulnerable to the emotional consequences of hospitalization and result in their needs being significantly different from those of the short-term patients of the past (see Chapter 38 for further discussion on children with special needs). The majority of these children are infants and toddlers, the age group most vulnerable to the effects of hospitalization.

Concern in recent years has focused on the increasing numbers of these children "growing up in hospitals" (Britton and Johnston, 1993). Discharge is prolonged because of complex medical and nursing care, elusive diagnoses, complicated psychosocial issues, and inconsistent community resources (Wells et al, 1994). Without special attention devoted to meeting the child's psychosocial and developmental needs in the "artificial" hospital environment, the detrimental consequences of prolonged hospitalization may be severe.

Beneficial Effects of Hospitalization

While hospitalization can be and usually is stressful for children, it can also be beneficial. The most obvious benefit is the recovery from illness, but hospitalization also can present an opportunity for children to master stress and feel competent in their coping abilities. The hospital environment can provide children with new socialization experiences that can broaden their interpersonal relationships. Sciarillo (1995) suggests that a simple paradigm shift—from "promoting adaptation" to that of "participating in growth"—can be strategic in changing how individuals view illness and hospitalization. By viewing these events as a challenge rather than a problem, children, families, and health care professionals are presented with an opportunity for growing in new ways. The psychologic benefits need to be considered and maximized during hospitalization. Appropriate nursing strategies to achieve this goal are presented in the Nursing Care Plan on p. 1235.

Nursing Care of the Child Who is Hospitalized

Assessment

A number of important areas must be assessed to identify nursing diagnoses and plan care for an individual child. In some instances, such as with elective admission, assessment begins even before the child is hospitalized so that appropriate preadmission preparation can be instituted. At other times, assessment occurs at the time of admission and should be integrated into other admission procedures so that the child's specific needs are recognized *early* in the hospitalization. Another critical area is assessment of pain for implementing appropriate relief of discomfort. Although assessment is discussed under nursing care of the child who is hospitalized, a comprehensive approach must involve the child's parents or other caregivers.

The nurse's primary intent is to provide **atraumatic care** (see Chapter 27). Therefore patient assessment should be individualized and include an evaluation of the child's growth and development, psychosocial needs, educational needs, and the effects of the illness on the child's family or guardian.

Admission Assessment

A nursing admission history should be taken to ensure a systematic collection of data about the child and family that allows the nurse to plan individualized care. The nursing admission history presented in Box 41-5 is organized according to the Functional Health Patterns outlined by Gordon (1994) to facilitate the formulation of nursing diagnoses.

BOX 41-5
Nursing Admission History According to Functional Health Patterns*

Health Perception—Health Management Pattern

Why has your child been admitted?
How has your child's general health been?
What does your child know about this hospitalization?
Ask the child why he or she came to the hospital.
If answer is "For an operation or for tests," ask the child to tell you about what will happen before, during, and after the operation or tests.
Has your child ever been in the hospital before?
How was that hospital experience?
What things were important to you and your child during that hospitalization? How can we be most helpful now?
What medications does your child take at home?
Why are they given?
When are they given?
How are they given (if a liquid, with a spoon; if a tablet, swallowed with water; or other)?
Does your child have any trouble taking medication? If so, what helps?
Is your child allergic to any medications?
What, if any, forms of complementary medicine practices are being used?

Nutrition-Metabolic Pattern

What are the family's usual mealtimes?
Do family members eat together or at separate times?
What are your child's favorite foods, beverages, and snacks?
What are the average amounts consumed or usual size portions?
Are there any special cultural practices, such as family eats only ethnic food?
What foods and beverages does your child dislike?
What are your child's feeding habits (bottle, cup, spoon, eats by self, needs assistance, any special devices)?
How does your child like the food served (warmed, cold, one item at a time)?
How would you describe your child's usual appetite (hearty eater, picky eater)?
Has being sick affected your child's appetite? In what ways?
Are there any known or suspected food allergies?
Is your child on a special diet?
Are there any feeding problems (excessive fussiness, spitting up, colic); any dental or gum problems that affect feeding?
What do you do for these problems?

Elimination Pattern

What are your child's toilet habits (diaper, toilet trained—day only or day and night, use of word to communicate urination or defecation, potty chair, regular toilet, other routines)?
What is your child's usual pattern of elimination (bowel movements)?
Do you have any concerns about elimination (bed-wetting, constipation, diarrhea)?
What do you do for these problems?
Have you ever noticed that your child sweats a lot?

Sleep-Rest Pattern

What is your child's usual hour of sleep and awakening?
What is your child's schedule for naps; length of naps?
Is there a special routine before sleeping (bottle, drink of water, bedtime story, nightlight, favorite blanket or toy, prayers)?
Is there a special routine during sleep time, such as waking to go to the bathroom?
What type of bed does your child sleep in?
Does your child have a separate room or share a room; if shares, with whom?
What are the home sleeping arrangements (alone or with others (e.g., sibling, parent, other person)?
What is your child's favorite sleeping position?
Are there any sleeping problems (falling asleep, waking during night, nightmares, sleep walking)?
Are there any problems in awakening and getting ready in the morning?
What do you do for these problems?

Activity-Exercise Pattern

What is your child's schedule during the day (preschool, daycare center, regular school, extracurricular activities)?
What are your child's favorite activities or toys (both active and quiet interests)?
What is your child's usual television-viewing schedule at home?
What are your child's favorite programs?
Are there any television restrictions?
Does your child have any illness or disabilities that limit activity? If so, how?
What are your child's usual habits and schedule for bathing (bath in tub or shower, sponge bath, shampoo)?
What are your child's dental habits (brushing, flossing, fluoride supplements or rinses, favorite toothpaste); schedule of daily dental care?
Does your child need help with dressing or grooming, such as hair combing?
Are there any problems with the above (dislike of or refusal to bathe, shampoo hair, or brush teeth)?
What do you do for these problems?
Are there special devices that your child requires help in managing (eyeglasses, contact lenses, hearing aid, orthodontic appliances, artificial elimination appliances, orthopedic devices)?
NOTE: Use the following code to assess functional self-care level for feeding, bathing/hygiene, dressing/grooming, toileting:
0: Full self-care
I: Requires use of equipment or device
II: Requires assistance or supervision from another person
III: Requires assistance or supervision from another person and equipment or device
IV: Is dependent and does not participate

Cognitive–Perceptual Pattern

Does your child have any hearing difficulty?
Does the child use a hearing aid?
Have "tubes" been placed in your child's ears?
Does your child have any vision problems?
Does the child wear glasses or contact lenses?
Does your child have any learning difficulties?
What is the child's grade in school?
For information on pain, see box on p. 1214

*The focus of the admission history is the child's psychosocial environment. Most of the questions are worded in terms of parental responses. Depending on the child's age, they should be addressed directly to the child when appropriate.

Continued.

BOX 41-5
Nursing Admission History According to Functional Health Patterns—cont'd

Self-Perception–Self-Concept Pattern

How would you describe your child (e.g., takes time to adjust, settles in easily, shy, friendly, quiet, talkative, serious, playful, stubborn, easygoing)?
What makes your child angry, annoyed, anxious, or sad? What helps?
How does your child act when annoyed or upset?
What have been your child's experiences with and reactions to temporary separation from you (parent)?
Does your child have any fears (places, objects, animals, people, situations)? How do you handle them?
Do you think your child's illness has changed the way he or she thinks about self (e.g., more shy, embarrassed about appearance, less competitive with friends, stays at home more)?

Role-Relationship Pattern

Does your child have a favorite nickname?
What are the names of other family members or others who live in the home (relatives, friends, pets)?
Who usually takes care of your child during the day/night (especially if other than parent, such as baby-sitter, relative)?
What are the parents' occupations and work schedules?
Are there any special family considerations (adoption, foster child, stepparent, divorce, single parent)?
Have any major changes in the family occurred lately (death, divorce, separation, birth of a sibling, loss of a job, financial strain, mother beginning a career, other)? Describe child's reaction.
Who are your child's play companions or social groups (peers, younger or older children, adults, prefers to be alone)?
Do things generally go well for your child in school or with friends?
Does your child have "security" objects at home (pacifier, thumb, bottle, blanket, stuffed animal, or doll)? Did you bring any of these to the hospital?
How do you handle discipline problems at home? Are these methods always effective?
Does your child have any condition that interferes with communication? If so, what are your suggestions for communicating with your child?
Will your child's hospitalization affect the family's financial support or care of other family members (e.g., other children)?
What concerns do you have about your child's illness and hospitalization?
Who will be staying with your child while hospitalized?
How can we contact you or another close family member outside of the hospital?

Sexuality–Reproductive Pattern

(Answer questions that apply to your child's age group.)
Has your child begun puberty (developing physical sexual characteristics, menstruation)? Have you or your child had any concerns?
Does your daughter know how to do breast self-examination?
Does your son know how to do testicular self-examination?
How have you approached topics of sexuality with your child?
Do you feel you might need some help with some topics?
Has your child's illness affected the way he or she feels about being a boy or a girl? If so, how?
Do you have any concerns with behaviors in your child, such as masturbation, asking many questions or talking about sex, not respecting others' privacy, or wanting too much privacy?
Initiate a conversation about an adolescent's sexual concerns with open-ended to more direct questions and using the terms "friends" or "partners" rather than "girlfriend" or "boyfriend":
- Tell me about your social life.
- Who are your closest friends? (If one friend is identified, could ask more about that relationship, such as how much time they spend together, how serious they are about each other, if the relationship is going the way the teenager hoped.)
- Might ask about dating and sexual issues, such as the teenager's views on sex education, "going steady," "living together," or premarital sex.
- Which friends would you like to have visit in the hospital?

Coping–Stress Tolerance Pattern

(Answer questions that apply to your child's age group.)
What does your child do when tired or upset?
- If upset, does your child want a special person or object? If so, explain.

If your child has temper tantrums, what causes them and how do you handle them?
Whom does your child talk to when worried about something?
How does your child usually handle problems or disappointments?
Have there been any big changes or problems in your family recently?
- How have you handled them?

Has your child ever had a problem with drugs or alcohol or tried suicide?
Do you think your child is "accident prone"? If so, explain.

Value–Belief Pattern

What is your religion?
How is religion or faith important in your child's life?
What religious practices would you like continued in the hospital (e.g., prayers before meals/bedtime; visit by minister, priest, or rabbi; prayer group)?

One of the main purposes of the history is to assess the child's usual health habits at home to promote a more normal environment in the hospital. Therefore questions related to activities of daily living in the nutritional-metabolic, elimination, sleep-rest, and activity-exercise patterns are a major part of the assessment.

The questions found under the health perception–health management pattern are directed toward evaluation of the child's preparation for hospitalization and are key factors in determining if additional preparation is needed. The questions included in the self-perception–self-concept and role-relationship patterns offer insight into the child's potential reaction to hospitalization, especially in terms of separation. The nurse should also inquire about the use of any complementary medicine practices (Box 41-6). In a national survey, over a third of adults had used at least one unconventional therapy within the previous year, yet 72% did not inform their medical doctor that they had done so (Eisenberg et al, 1993). It is rea-

BOX 41-6
Complementary Medicine Practices and Examples

Nutrition, diet, and life-style/behavioral health changes—Macrobiotics, megavitamins, diets, life-style modification, health risk reduction/health education, wellness
Mind/body control therapies—Biofeedback, relaxation, prayer therapy, guided imagery, hypnotherapy, music/sound therapy, education therapy
Traditional and ethnomedicine therapies—Acupuncture, ayurvedic medicine, herbal medicine, homeopathic medicine, Native American medicine, natural products, traditional Oriental medicine
Structural manipulation and energetic therapies—Acupressure, chiropractic medicine, massage, reflexology, rolfing, therapeutic touch, Qi Gong
Pharmacologic and biologic therapies—Antioxidants, cell treatment, chelation therapy, metabolic therapy, oxidizing agents
Bioelectromagnetic therapies—Diagnostic and therapeutic application of electromagnetic fields (e.g., transcranial electrostimulation, neuromagnetic stimulation, electroacupuncture)

sonable to expect that many of these adults have children who also use complementary medicine practices (see Critical Thinking Q & A Box to the right).

Once the data are collected, the information must be applied to the nursing process and communicated to other staff. It makes little sense to assess a child's home routine if none of this knowledge is integrated into the plan of care. Most nursing units have provisions for care plans in which specific information about the child's habits and needs are recorded and incorporated in the hospital routine.

Besides taking the nursing admission history, nurses should also perform a physical assessment (see Chapter 32) or obtain the information from the medical examination before planning care. At the very least, the nurse's physical assessment of the child should include observation of the body for any bruises, rashes, signs of neglect, deformities, or physical limitations. The nurse should also listen to the heart and lungs to assess overall physical status. For example, it is impossible to evaluate improvement in respiratory function in a child admitted with pulmonary disease unless there are baseline data with which to compare subsequent findings.

Pain Assessment

Pain assessment is a critical component of the nursing process. Unfortunately, health professionals, including nurses, tend to underestimate pain in children (Box 41-7).

One of the reasons for inadequate management of pain is a lack of understanding of what pain is—a personal phenomenon that *cannot* be experienced by any other individual. Therefore defining pain in terms of another's perceptions is inappropriate and inaccurate. An operational definition that is useful in clinical practice is *pain is whatever the experiencing person says it is, existing whenever the person says it does* (McCaffery and Beebe, 1989). This definition implies a very important attitude toward patients—*that they are believed.* It includes both verbal and nonverbal expressions of pain.

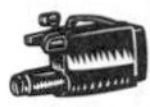
For additional information, please view "Pain Assessment and Management" in *Whaley and Wong's Pediatric Nursing Video Series*, St Louis, 1996, Mosby; (800) 426-4545.

Critical Thinking Q & A
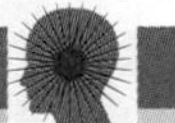
COMPLEMENTARY MEDICINE PRACTICES

Maria, a 10-year-old Hispanic female, has severe nose bleeds. She is admitted to the hospital for a complete workup in an attempt to determine the cause. Her parents and grandparents have gathered around her bed. When you enter her room to begin admitting procedures, you notice an unusual scent. Maria's mother is rubbing the contents from an unfamiliar bottle of liquid on Maria. Meanwhile, the grandmother is rubbing Maria's head. She is startled at your entry and drops something on the floor near your feet. You bend over to pick it up and discover that it is a penny. After introducing yourself and explaining the purpose of your visit, your most appropriate response is:
1. "Here is your penny."
2. "I need to take this bottle and have the lab examine its contents."
3. "Many families tell me that they use certain medicine practices that are traditional in their families. Can you tell me about yours?"
4. "What is going on here?"

The correct answer is three. The third person technique (Chapter 31) gives families permission to share information. What you have probably observed is *Santeria,* the Afro-Caribbean religion that was brought to the New World by slaves from West Africa. Although it is most common among immigrants from Cuba, Puerto Rico, Brazil, and Santo Domingo, it is believed that a majority of Latin immigrants have contact with Santeria at some point in their lives. Answer number one avoids the issue, which could be very important. Although at some point you may need to have the contents of the bottle examined (answer number two), it is an inappropriate initial response. Answer four is confrontive and disrespectful.

Fallacies and facts. Children are undertreated for pain for a number of complex and interrelated reasons, including professionals' misconceptions about pain; the complexities of pain assessment, particularly in nonverbal children; and the lack of information regarding currently available pain reduction techniques. A number of fallacies continue to flourish because of incorrect knowledge about pain in infants and children, despite these fallacies having been disproved by current research on pediatric pain (Box 41-9).

Fear of addiction. A major concern that prevents health professionals from adequately using opioids* to relieve pain is an unwarranted fear of addiction. Studies on addiction rates in patients treated with opioids have found an incidence of less than 1% (Friedman, 1990). The Acute Pain Management Guideline Panel (1992) has made the following statement re-

*The term *opioid* refers to natural or synthetic analgesics with morphinelike actions. It is preferred to the term *narcotic,* which in a legal context refers to any substance that causes psychologic dependence, such as cocaine, which is not an opioid. The word "narcotic" also engenders fears of addiction in older children and parents that are unwarranted when opioids are used for pain control.

BOX 41-7
Undermedication of Pain in Children

Several studies have examined the pattern of pain medication for children as compared with adults and have found remarkably consistent findings—that children have been undermedicated for pain. Eland and Anderson (1977) investigated the incidence of administration of analgesics to 25 hospitalized children for postoperative pain. Twelve of the children received a total of 24 doses of analgesics; the remaining 13 children were never given any medication for pain relief. In contrast, 18 adults with identical diagnoses received 372 opioid analgesic doses and 299 non-opioid analgesic doses for a total of 671 doses. One of the saddest findings was that more than twice as many children had pain medication ordered as received it. This lack of response to the need for pain medication directly relates to the nurses who failed to administer the analgesic.

Another study investigating analgesic prescriptions given to children and adults after open heart surgery found that all of the adults received medication, for a total of 564 doses, but only three fourths of the children were given medication, for a total of 237 doses during the first 3 postoperative days. This difference was even greater on the fifth postoperative day, when 83% of the adults continued to receive analgesics (a total of 136 doses) but only 12% of the children were medicated (a total of 10 doses) (Beyer et al, 1983).

Another study on postoperative pain found that 75% of the children reported pain on the day of surgery and if orders for opioid or nonopioid analgesics were written, the nonopioid was given exclusively. In addition, the doses ordered were usually too small and/or too infrequent to be maximally effective. Most orders were written "PRN," which was often interpreted by nursing staff to mean "as little as possible" (Mather and Mackie, 1983). A review of analgesic use in the emergency department reported significantly low use in children with mild to moderate trauma, including children with painful fractures. Head injury was associated with especially low use of analgesics (Friedland and Kulick, 1994).

The situation is even more serious with infants. One analysis of anesthetic practices with newborns undergoing surgical ligation of patent ductus arteriosus found that 76% of the infants received only nitrous oxide and a paralyzing agent. These infants could not move during surgery but could feel all the pain of a thoracotomy. (Anand and Aynsley-Green, 1985). In a survey of nurses working in neonatal intensive care units, 79% believed that infants were undermedicated for pain. The same study found that more than half of the medications used for pain relief had no analgesic properties (Franck, 1987). A study comparing premedication for procedures, such as arterial line or chest tube placement, found that infants in neonatal intensive care units received no premedication much more often than children in pediatric intensive care units (Bauchner, May, and Coates, 1992).

Fortunately, professionals' response to recognizing and treating pediatric pain has been improving. Studies such as those described have prompted the American Academy of Pediatrics (1987) and the American Society of Anesthesiologists to publish jointly a statement on neonatal anesthesia that encourages the use of local or systemic pharmacologic agents "according to the usual guidelines for the administration of anesthesia to high-risk, potentially unstable patients." If medication is withheld, the decision should be based on the same medical criteria used for older patients, not on the infant's age or perceived degree of cortical maturity.

Guidelines are also available that help practitioners to assess and manage pain using methods based on the published scientific literature. In the United States the Agency for Health Care Policy and Research (AHCPR) has published guidelines developed by pain experts that focus on the issues of postoperative, procedure-related or trauma, and cancer pain. Other national and international organizations have also contributed research-based recommendations that nurses can use to improve pain control (Box 41-8).

In your agency, see if these references are readily available to staff. If not, order them, especially the free AHCPR publications, and distribute them, stressing that they provide state-of-the-art information. As you practice, carry your copy of the guidelines; mark sections, such as those discussing addiction and listing drug dosages, for quick reference. Compare your pain assessment and management interventions with those in the published guidelines, and make a commitment to increase your knowledge. *Remember: to effectively relieve pain, its management must be based on scientific research, not personal opinion or belief.*

garding addiction from opioid use in pain management for children: *"There is no known aspect of childhood development or physiology that indicates any increased risk of physiologic or psychologic dependence from the brief use of opioids for acute pain management."*

Fear of respiratory depression. Although respiratory depression is the most serious side effect of opioids, it is a rare occurrence in children receiving appropriate doses. Evidence suggests that in children over 3 to 6 months of age, opioids cause no greater respiratory depression than in adults. Respiratory depression is most likely to occur when the opioid is administered with other sedating drugs, such as hydroxyzine (Vistaril), promethazine (Phenergan), chlorpromazine (Thorazine), midazolam (Versed), or diazepam (Valium). Unlike many sedatives, opioids have the advantage of the antidote naloxone (Narcan), which rapidly reverses the respiratory depressant effect. Fortunately, the benzodiazepines, such as diazepam and midazolam, have the drug flumazenil (Romazicon) to treat respiratory depression (see also the Guidelines box on p. 1230).

In addition, as tolerance to the analgesic effect of opioids occurs, tolerance to the respiratory depressant effect also occurs. Pain acts as a natural antagonist to the action of opioids. With increased pain a patient can receive increased opioids and, except for constipation, will not experience increased side effects. Respiratory depression is rare in children receiving long-term opioid therapy.

Principles of pain assessment in children. Since pain is both a sensory and an emotional experience, several assessment strategies should be used to gather information about pain. One approach to pain assessment in children is QUESTT:

Question the child.

Use pain rating scales.

BOX 41-8
Selected Resources for Guidelines on Children's Pain

Acute Pain Management: Operative or Medical Procedures and Trauma
Acute Pain Management in Infants, Children and Adolescents: Operative and Medical Procedures
Management of Cancer Pain
Quick reference guide for clinicians: Management of cancer pain: adults
Available at no charge from the Agency for Health Care Policy and Research Publications, P.O. Box 8527, Silver Spring, MD 20907; (800) 358-9295.

Principles of Analgesic Use in the Treatment of Acute Pain and Chronic Cancer Pain
Available from the American Pain Society, 4700 West Lake Ave Glenview, IL 60025; (847) 375-4700.

Management of Acute Pain: A Practical Guide
Available from the International Association for the Study of Pain (IASP), 909 N.E. 43rd St., Suite 306, Seattle, WA 98105-6020; (206) 547-6409.

Handbook of Cancer Pain Management
Available from the Wisconsin Cancer Pain Initiative, 3675 Medical Sciences Center, University of Wisconsin Medical School, 1300 University Ave., Madison, WI 53706; (608) 262-0978.

Report of the Consensus Conference on the Management of Pain in Childhood Cancer
In *Pediatrics* 86(5, suppl):813-834, 1990; available from the American Academy of Pediatrics, P.O. Box 927, Elk Grove Village, IL 60009-0927; (800) 433-9016.

ANA Position Statements on Promotion of Comfort and Relief of Pain in Dying Patients and on the Role of the Registered Nurse in the Management of Patients Receiving IV Conscious Sedation for Short-Term Therapeutic, Diagnostic, or Surgical Procedures
Published in *The American Nurse*, Feb 1992, pp 7-8. May be available from American Nurses' Association Publications Distribution Center, P.O. Box 4100, Kearneysville, WV 25430; (800) 637-0323.

Oncology Nursing Society position paper on cancer pain
By Spross JA, McGuire DB: *Oncol Nurs Forum* 17(5):753, 1990.

Mayday Pain Resource Center
From City of Hope National Medical Center, The Mayday Fund Pain Resource Center, 1500 East Duarte Road, Duarte, CA 91010; (818) 359-8111, ext. 3829; FAX (818) 301-8941.

Whaley and Wong's Pediatric Pain Assessment and Management
Videotape available from Mosby, 11830 Westline Industrial Drive, St. Louis, MO 63146; (800) 426-4545.

Also available for families:

Pain Control After Surgery: A Patient's Guide
Managing Cancer Pain: Patient Guide
Available at no charge from the Agency for Health Care Policy and Research Publications, P.O. Box 8527, Silver Spring, MD 20907; (800) 358-9295.

Children's Cancer Pain Can Be Relieved: A Guide for Parents and Families
Available from Wisconsin Cancer Pain Initiative, 3675 Medical Sciences Center, University of Wisconsin Medical School, 1300 University Ave., Madison, WI 53706; (608) 262-0978.

Pain Relief: How to Say No to Acute, Chronic, and Cancer Pain!
By Jane Cowles, 1993; available from MasterMedia Limited, 17 E. 89th St., New York, NY 10128; (212) 546-7650.

Questions and Answers About Pain Control: A Guide for People with Cancer and their Families
Available at no charge from the Office of Cancer Communications, Bldg. 31, Rm. 10A24, Bethesda, MD 20892, (800) 4-CANCER; and from local branches of the American Cancer Society, or call (800) ACS-2345.

Sickle Cell Related Pain: Assessment and Management—A Guide for Patients and Parents
Available from the New England Regional Genetics Groups (NERGG), P.O. Box 670, Mt Desert, ME 040660; (207) 288-2704; FAX (207) 288-2705.

Evaluate behavior and physiologic changes.
Secure parents' involvement.
Take cause of pain into account.
Take action and evaluate results.

Question child. Children's verbal statements and descriptions of pain are the *most* important factors in assessing pain. However, young children may not know what the word "pain" means and may need help in describing it using familiar language. Therefore using a variety of words to describe pain, such as "owie," "boo-boo," "feel funnys," or "hurts," is necessary. Appropriate foreign language words may also be used; for example, in Spanish, pain is "duele," "dolor," or "ai ai." Older children also benefit from using simple words to describe pain. Suggested questions for obtaining information about children's experiences with pain are presented in the accompanying box. Asking children to locate the pain is also helpful, and play can provide other means for helping children to reveal discomfort. For example, children can show areas on a doll where it "hurts" or "doesn't feel good" (Fig. 41-4).

When asking children about pain, the nurse must remember that they may deny pain because they fear receiving an injectable analgesic or because they believe they deserve to suffer as punishment for some misdeed. They may also deny pain to a stranger but readily admit it to a parent. This behavior should not be interpreted as seeking attention from the parent, but as a valid indication of pain.

Use a pain rating scale. Pain rating scales (tools) provide a quantitative self-report measure of pain. Although various pain scales exist (Table 41-2), not all of them are appropriate for young children. For the most valid and reliable pain intensity rating, a scale is selected that is suitable to the child's age, abilities, and preference. Scales using facial expressions are readily accepted by children and can be used by very young children. There is some evidence that children may prefer a

BOX 41-9
Fallacies and Facts About Children and Pain

Fallacy: Infants do not feel pain.
Fact: Infants demonstrate behavioral, especially facial, and physiologic, including hormonal, indicators of pain. Neonates have the neural mechanisms to transmit noxious stimuli by 20 weeks' gestation.

Fallacy: Children tolerate pain better than adults.
Fact: Children's tolerance for pain actually *increases* with age. Younger children tend to rate procedure-related pain higher than older children.

Fallacy: Children cannot tell you where they hurt.
Fact: By 4 years of age, children can accurately point to the body area or mark the painful site on a drawing; children as young as 3 years old can use pain scales, such as faces.

Fallacy: Children always tell the truth about pain.
Fact: Children may not admit having pain to avoid an injection; because of constant pain, they may not realize how much they are hurting; children may believe that others know how they are feeling and not ask for analgesia.

Fallacy: Children become accustomed to pain or painful procedures.
Fact: Children often demonstrate *increased* behavioral signs of discomfort with repeated painful procedures.

Fallacy: Behavioral manifestations reflect pain intensity.
Fact: Children's developmental level, coping abilities, and temperament, such as activity level and intensity of reaction to pain, influence pain behavior. Children with more active, resisting behaviors may rate pain lower than children with passive, accepting behaviors.

Fallacy: Parents do not want to be involved in their child's pain control.
Fact: Parents do want to be involved. They know their child best and can help in assessing pain and pain relief measures. Since they may not have seen their child in severe pain, they may need guidance in interpreting pain responses.

Fallacy: Narcotics are more dangerous for children than they are for adults.
Fact: Narcotics (opioids) are no more dangerous for children than they are for adults. Addiction to opioids used to treat pain is extremely rare in children. Reports of respiratory depression in children are also uncommon. By 3 to 6 months of age, healthy infants can metabolize opioids similarly to older children.

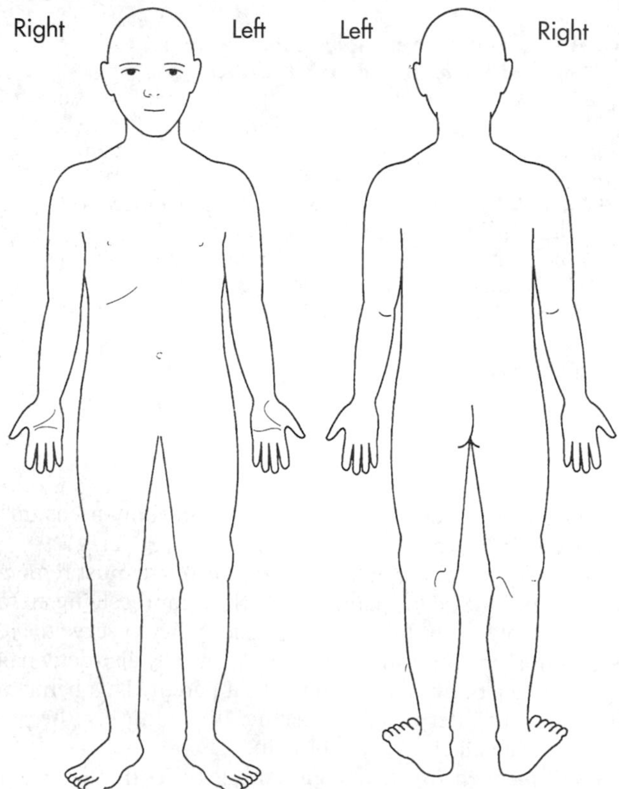

Fig. 41-4 Adolescent pediatric pain tool (APPT): body outlines for pain assessment. Instructions: "Color in the areas on these drawings to show where you have pain. Make the marks as big or as small as the place where the pain is." (From Savedra MC et al: San Francisco, Calif. 1989, 1992, School of Nursing, University of California-San Francisco.)

faces scale to other tools (West et al, 1994; Wong and Baker, 1988).

It is best to use the same scale with children to avoid confusing them with different instructions and to use the pain assessment scale for pain only. Multiple uses of the scale (e.g., as a general measure of the child's feelings) can cause the child to lose interest in the scale. In introducing the pain scale, nurses should explain that this is one way for children to let nurses know how they are feeling. Ideally, children should be taught to use the scale before pain is expected, such as preoperatively. Familiarizing children with the scale facilitates its use when children are actually in pain.

Evaluate behavioral and physiologic changes. Behavioral changes are common indicators of pain and are especially valuable in assessing pain in nonverbal children. Children's behavioral responses to pain change with age and follow a developmental trend (Box 41-2). However, children vary widely in their responses and may exhibit behaviors at one age that are more typically seen at a different age. In addition, temperament affects coping style, and children with more positive moods may appear to be in less pain than they actually are. Children who use passive coping behaviors (offering no resistance, cooperating) may rate pain as more intense than children who use active coping behaviors (resisting, attacking) (Broome et al, 1990). Cultural background may also play a role in children's pain responses, although the influence appears slight (Pfefferbaum, Adams, and Aceves, 1990). Unfortunately, nurses often make judgments about pain based on behavior, which results in some children receiving inadequate pain medication (Wallace, 1989) (see also the Critical Thinking Q & A box on p. 1213).

TABLE 41-2 Pain rating scales for children

PAIN SCALE/DESCRIPTION	INSTRUCTIONS	RECOMMENDED AGE/COMMENTS
FACES pain rating scale* (Wong and Baker, 1988,): Consists of six cartoon faces ranging from smiling face for "no pain" to tearful face for "worst pain"	***Original Instructions:*** Explain to child that each face is for a person who feels happy because there is no pain (hurt) or sad because there is some or a lot of pain. FACE 0 is very happy because there is no hurt. FACE 1 hurts just a little bit. FACE 2 hurts a little more. FACE 3 hurts even more. FACE 4 hurts a whole lot, but FACE 5 hurts as much as you can imagine, although you don't have to be crying to feel this bad. Ask child to choose face that best describes own pain. Record the number under chosen face on pain assessment record.	Children as young as 3 years Using same instructions without affect words, such as *happy* or *sad*, results in same pain rating, probably reflecting child's rating of pain intensity.
	Brief Instructions: Explain to the child that each face is for a person who has no hurt to a lot of hurt. Use the words under each face to describe the amount of pain. Ask child to choose face that best describes own pain. Record the number under chosen face on pain assessment record.  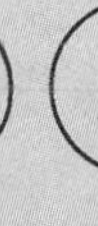  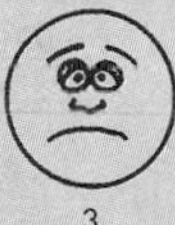   0 No Hurt; 1 Hurts Little Bit; 2 Hurts Little More; 3 Hurts Even More; 4 Hurts Whole Lot; 5 Hurts Worst	Use of the brief instructions is recommended (Lefkowitz. Keller, Wong, and Clutter, 1997).
Oucher† (Beyer et al, 1995): Consists of six photographs of child's face representing "no hurt" to "biggest hurt you could ever have"; also includes a vertical scale with numbers from 0 to 100; scales for African-American and Hispanic children have been developed	***Numeric scale:*** Point to each section of scale to explain variations in pain intensity: "0 means no hurt." "This means little hurts" (pointing to lower part of scale, 1 to 29). "This means middle hurts" (pointing to middle part of scale, 30 to 69). "This means big hurts" (pointing to upper part of scale, 70 to 99). "100 means the biggest hurt you could ever have." Score is actual number stated by child. ***Photographic scale:*** Point to each photograph on Oucher and explain variations in pain intensity using following language: first picture from the bottom is "no hurt," second is "a little hurt," third is "a little more hurt," fourth is "even more hurt than that," fifth is "pretty much or a lot of hurt," and the sixth is the "biggest hurt you could ever have." Score pictures from 0 to 5, with the bottom picture scored as 0. ***General*** Practice using Oucher by recalling and rating previous pain experiences (example: falling off a bike). Child points to number or photograph that describes pain intensity associated with experience. Obtain current pain score from child by asking "How much hurt do you have right now?"	Children 3 to 13 years; use numeric scale if child can count to 100 by ones and identify larger of any two numbers, or by tens. Determine whether child has cognitive ability to use photographic scale; child should be able to seriate six geometric shapes from largest to smallest. Determine which ethnic version of Oucher to use. Allow the child to select a version of Oucher, or use version that most closely matches physical characteristics of child.
Numeric scale Uses straight line with end points identified as "no pain" and "worst pain"; divisions along line are marked in units from 0 to 10 (high number may vary)	Explain to child that at one end of the line is a 0, which means that a person feels no pain (hurt). At the other end is a 10, which means the person feels the worst pain imaginable. The numbers 1 to 9 are for a very little pain to a whole lot of pain. Ask child to choose a number that best describes own pain.	Children as young as 5 years, as long as they can count and have some concept of numbers and their values in relation to other numbers

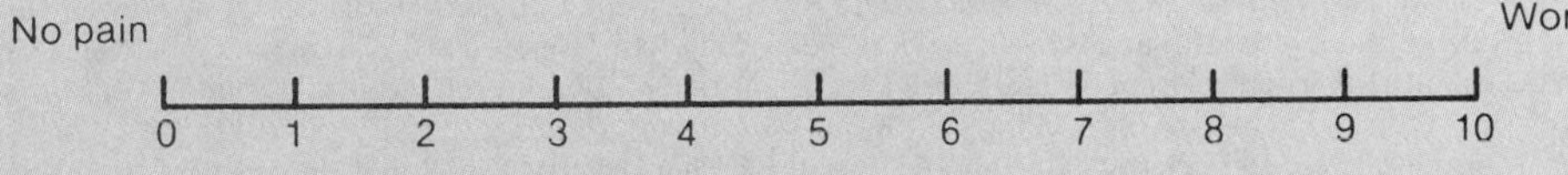

*Several variations of faces scales exist. Wong-Baker FACES Pain Rating Scale is available from Purdue Frederick Co., 100 Connecticut Ave., Norwalk CT 06856; (203) 853-0123, ext. 7236. For translations of FACES, see Appendix. *Reference manual for the Wong-Baker FACES Pain Rating Scale* is also available from the City of Hope National Medical Center, Mayday Fund Pain Resource Center, 1500 East Duarte Road, Duarte, CA 91010; Phone (818) 359-8111 x3829; Fax: (818) 301-8941.

†Oucher is available from Association for the Care of Children's Health, 7910 Woodmont Avenue, Suite 300, Bethesda, MD 20814; (301) 654-6549 or (800) 808-ACCH.

Continued.

TABLE 41-2 Pain rating scales for children—cont'd

PAIN SCALE/DESCRIPTION	INSTRUCTIONS	RECOMMENDED AGE/COMMENTS
Poker chip tool‡		
Uses four red poker chips placed horizontally in front of child (Hester, Foster, and Kristensen, 1990)	Tell child, "These are pieces of hurt." Beginning at the chip nearest child's left side and ending at the one nearest child's right side, point to chips and say, "This [the first chip] is a little bit of hurt and this [the fourth chip] is the most hurt you could ever have." For a young child or for any child who does not comprehend the instructions, clarify by saying, "That means this [the first chip] is just a little hurt; this [the second chip] is a little more hurt; this [the third chip] is more hurt; and this [the fourth chip] is the most hurt you could ever have." Ask child, "How many pieces of hurt do you have right now?" Children without pain will say they don't have any. Clarify child's answer by words such as, "Oh, you have a little hurt? Tell me about the hurt." Elicit descriptors, location, and cause. Ask the child, "What would you like me to do for you?" Record number of chips selected. *Spanish Instructions:* Follow English instructions, substituting the following words. Tell parent, if present: "Estas fichas son una manera de medir dolor. Usamos cuatro fichas." Say to child: "Estas son pedazos de dolor: una es un poquito de dolor y cuatro son el dolor maximo que tu puedes sentir. Cuantos pedazos de dolor tienes?"	Children as young as 4 to $4^1/_2$ years, provided they can count and have some concept of numbers
Word graphic rating scale‡§		
(Tesler et al, 1991): Uses descriptive words (may vary in other scales) to denote varying intensities of pain	Explain to child, "This is a line with words to describe how much pain you may have. This side of the line means no pain and over here the line means worst possible pain." (Point with your finger where "no pain," is, and run your finger along the line to "worst possible pain," as you say it.) "If you have no pain, you would mark like this." (Show example.) "If you have some pain, you would mark somewhere along the line, depending on how much pain you have." (Show example.) "The more pain you have, the closer to worst pain you would mark. The worst pain possible is marked like this." (Show example.) "Show me how much pain you have right now by marking with a straight, up-and-down line anywhere along the line to show how much pain you have right now." With a millimeter rule, measure from the "no pain" end to the mark and record this measurement as the pain score.	Children ages 4 to 17 years
	No pain — Little pain — Medium pain — Large pain — Worst possible pain	
Visual analogue scale		
Uses 10-cm horizontal line with end points marked "no pain" and "worst pain"	Ask child to place a mark on line that best describes amount of own pain. With a centimeter ruler, measure from the "no pain" end to the mark and record this measurement as the pain score.	Children as young as $4^1/_2$ years; vertical or horizontal scale may be used

‡Instructions for Poker Chip Tool and Word Graphic Rating Scale from Acute Pain Management Guideline Panel: *Acute pain management in infants, children, and adolescents: operative and medical procedures; quick reference guide for clinicians,* AHCPR Pub No 92-0020, Rockville, MD, 1992, Agency for Health Care Policy and Research, Public Health Service, US Department of Health and Human Services. Poker Chip Tool developed in 1975 by Nancy O. Hester, University of Colorado Health Sciences Center, Denver, CO. Spanish instructions from Jordan-Marsh M et al: *The Harbor–UCLA Medical Center Humor Project for Children,* Los Angeles, 1990, Harbor–UCLA Medical Center.

§Word Graphic Rating Scale is part of the Adolescent Pediatric Pain Tool and is available from Pediatric Pain Study, University of California, School of Nursing, Department of Family Health Care Nursing, San Francisco, CA 94143-0606; (415) 476-4040.

TABLE 41-2 Pain rating scales for children—cont'd

PAIN SCALE/DESCRIPTION	INSTRUCTIONS	RECOMMENDED AGE/COMMENTS
Color tool (Eland, 1993): Uses markers for child to construct own scale that is used with body outline	Present eight markers to child in a random order. Ask child, "Of these colors, which color is like . . . ?" (the event identified by the child as having hurt the most). Place the marker away from the other markers. (Represents severe pain.) Ask child, "Which color is like a hurt, but not quite as much as . . . ?" (the event identified by the child as having hurt the most). Place the marker with the marker chosen to represent severe pain. Ask child, "Which color is like something that hurts just a little?" Place the marker with the other colors. Ask child, "Which color is like no hurt at all?" Show the four marker choices to child in order from the worst to the no-hurt color. Ask child to show on the body outlines where they hurt, using the markers they have chosen. After child has colored the hurts, ask if they are current hurts or hurts from the past. Ask if child knows why the area hurts if it is not clear to you why it does.	Children as young as 4 years, provided they know their colors, are not color blind, and are able to construct the scale if in pain

Nursing ALERT

If children's behaviors appear to differ from their rating of pain, believe their pain rating.

Depending on the type and location of pain, children may display behaviors that indicate local body pain, such as pulling the ears for ear pain, rolling the head from side to side for head and ear pain, lying on the side with legs flexed for abdominal pain, limping for leg or foot pain, and refusing to move a body part. Children who experience chronic or repeated pain often develop effective behavioral coping strategies, such as squeezing a hand, talking, counting, relaxing, or thinking about pleasant events. Once these coping skills are identified, the child is encouraged to use them in future experiences with pain.

Critical Thinking Q & A

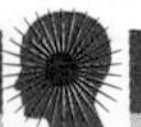

PAIN ASSESSMENT

Stacy is 14 years old, and this is her second day after abdominal surgery. As you enter her room, she smiles at you and continues to talk and joke with her visitor. Stacy rates her pain a 4 on a scale of 0 to 5, no to worst pain, respectively. Her roommate, Jill, is 12 years old, and this is her third day after scoliosis surgery. She does not smile and is lying very still in bed. Jill rates her pain a 4 on the same scale. Based on your assessment, you write the following in their charts (choose two items):

1. Stacy: In no acute distress and appears comfortable, talking and joking with a visitor.
2. Jill: Rates her surgical pain a 4 on a 0 to 5 scale and is unable to move because of pain; she appears depressed.
3. Stacy: Rates her surgical pain a 4 on a 0 to 5 scale.
4. Jill: Rates her surgical pain a 4 on a 0 to 5 scale.

The correct answers are three and four. The best estimate of pain is the person's self-report. Responses one and two are based on subjective impressions. In response one the adolescent's report of pain is totally disregarded. In response two there are no assessment data to support that Jill's behavior indicates inability to move or depression.

Physiologic responses indicating pain include flushing of the skin; increases in sweating, blood pressure, pulse, and respiration; restlessness; and dilation of the pupils. However, these signs vary considerably—for example, heart rate may actually decrease—and they may be produced by emotions such as fear, anger, or anxiety. They occur primarily in acute pain from stimulation of the sympathetic nervous system. If pain persists, the body begins to adapt and these responses decrease or stabilize. Consequently, if nurses rely primarily on observing these physiologic indications or expecting "pain" behaviors before believing that pain exists, many instances of pain will go unrecognized.

One of the most valuable clues to pain is a change in behavior and vital signs after administration of an analgesic. Behaviors such as less irritability or cessation of crying, and decreased pulse, respirations, and blood pressure provide important evidence for pain. Often the change in vital signs is attributed to the depressant effect of opioids, when in reality the return to more normal physiologic functioning is due to pain relief.

Secure parents' involvement. Parents know their child, are sensitive to changes in their child's behavior, and typically want to be involved in their child's pain relief. Parents' ability to recognize pain in their children varies. Some parents may never have seen their child in severe pain and may equate certain responses, such as irritability or withdrawal, with discomfort. However, others are aware that certain behaviors signal pain because the child has acted similarly during previous painful events. In addition, parents usually know what

BOX 41-10
Pain Experience Inventory

Questions for parents

Describe any pain your child has had before.
How does your child usually react to pain?
Does your child tell you or others when he or she is hurting?
How do you know when your child is in pain?
What do you do to ease discomfort for your child when your child is hurting?
What does your child do to get relief when hurting?
Which of these actions work best to decrease or take away your child's pain?
Is there anything special that you would like me to know about your child and pain? (If yes, have parent[s] describe.)

Questions for child

Tell me what pain is.
Tell me about the hurt you have had before.
What do you do when you hurt?
Do you tell others when you hurt?
What do you want others to do for you when you hurt?
What don't you want others to do for you when you hurt?
What helps the most to take away your hurt?
Is there anything special that you want me to know about you when you hurt? (If yes, have child describe.)

From Hester N, Barcus C: *Assessment and management of pain in children.* In *Pediatrics: Nursing Update* 1(14):3, Princeton, NJ, 1986, Continuing Professional Education Center.

comforts their child, such as rocking, stroking, or talking. They are the most consistent persons caring for the child and want to be involved in pain relief (Watt-Watson, Everden, and Lawson, 1990). Encouraging their participation gives them control and a sense of helping.

To better assess the child's pain the nurse can interview the parents about their child's previous pain experiences (Box 41-10). Ideally, this questioning should occur before the child is in pain, such as on admission to the hospital. Parents must realize that their knowledge of their child is important in providing care. Parents sometimes leave the assessment of pain up to the nurse because "nurses are more experienced," and consequently parents do not report pain. Parents need to be taught nonverbal pain behaviors in children and encouraged to inform the staff when they occur.

Take cause of pain into account. When children exhibit behaviors or other clues that suggest pain, reasons for discomfort should be investigated. Pathology may give clues to the expected intensity and type of pain. For example, pain associated with vasoocclusive crises in sickle cell disease is severe. Pain caused by bone marrow puncture is typically greater than the discomfort associated with a venipuncture. However, it is a mistake to believe that certain conditions or procedures always produce a standard amount of pain. For example, sore throat pain may be mild or severe—only the child knows the intensity.

Nursing ALERT

A golden rule to follow in pain assessment is as follows: Whatever is painful to an adult is painful to an infant or child until proved otherwise.

Take action and evaluate results. The reason for assessing pain is to relieve it (see p. 1219). Total pain relief should be the goal, with the combined use of pharmacologic and nonpharmacologic interventions. However, complete relief may not be possible. When children are able, they can tell the nurse what level of pain is acceptable to them.

Regardless of the type of pain intervention, *evaluation of the results is essential.* No one pain reduction technique is effective for all children. Therefore a pain assessment record is used to monitor the effectiveness of the interventions (Fig. 41-5). With nonverbal children, behavioral and physiologic signs are evaluated for evidence of pain relief. With verbal children, their statements about pain relief and pain ratings are also recorded. Changes in the medication regimen are made as needed to provide the maximum pain relief with the minimum side effects. Family members are often excellent partners in keeping a pain assessment record for the nurse.

Nursing ALERT

Presenting practitioners with objective documentation of pain, rather than opinion, is more likely to lead to a favorable change in analgesic disorders (Walker and Wong, 1991).

Nursing Diagnoses

A number of nursing diagnoses are prominent in the nursing care of children who are ill and/or hospitalized. Other nursing diagnoses specific to individual cases may become evident in addition to those outlined in the Nursing Care Plan on pp. 1235.

Planning

An effective plan of care for the child who is hospitalized is based on patient- and family-identified needs, as well as those identified by the nurse. Family members and the child should play active roles in developing the plan whenever possible.

The main goals for the child who is ill and/or hospitalized are as follows:

1. The child will be prepared for hospitalization.
2. The child will experience little or no separation.
3. The child will maintain a sense of control.
4. The child will exhibit decreased fear of bodily injury.
5. The child will experience reduction of pain that is acceptable to child.
6. The child will have opportunities to participate in developmentally appropriate diversional activities.
7. The child will experience maximum benefits from hospitalization.

Implementation

Prepare Child for Hospitalization

The rationale for preparing children for the hospital experience and related procedures is based on the principle that fear of the unknown (fantasy) exceeds fear of the known. Therefore decreasing the elements of the unknown results in less fear. When children do not have paralyzing fear to cope with, they are able to direct their energies toward dealing with the other, unavoidable stresses of hospitalization and to benefit optimally from the growth potential of the experience.

PAIN ASSESSMENT RECORD

Directions for each column:

1. Record date and time of administering analgesic; assess analgesic effect ______ minutes later and then ______ .
2. Use a pain rating scale if child understands its use. Name of scale ______ .
   Ratings: No pain = ______ . Worst pain = ______ . Acceptable pain rating ______ .
3. Record analgesic, dose, and route.
4. Record possible indications or effects of pain, such as shallow breathing due to incisional pain, parental request for pain relief; record indications or effects of pain relief, such as "moves easily, playing."
5. Record level of arousal, using sedation scale in box. Also, record any other side effects (e.g., nausea, itching).
6. R = respiratory function. Record breaths per minute and/or other observations of respiratory status (e.g., depth of respiration, change in color of skin).
7. Signature or initials of person recording information.

SEDATION SCALE

S = Sleeping, easily aroused.*
1 = Awake and alert.*
2 = Occasionally drowsy, easy to arouse.*
3 = Frequently drowsy, arousable, drifts off to sleep during conversation.†
4 = Somnolent, minimal or no response to stimuli.†

* Requires no action.
† Notify practitioner.

1 Date/ time	2 Pain rating	3 Analgesic	4 Possible effects/indications of pain or relief of pain	5 Arousal/ side effects	6 R	7 Signature

Fig. 41-5 Pain assessment record.

The preparation process may be elaborate, with tours, puppet shows, and playtime with miniature hospital equipment; it may involve the use of books (see p. 1249) and/or films; or it may be limited to a brief description of the major aspects of any hospital stay. No firm consensus exists on the timing of the event. Some authorities recommend preparing children 4 to 7 years of age about 1 week in advance so they can assimilate the information and ask questions. For older children the time may be longer. However, for young children, who may begin to fantasize about what they observed, 1 or 2 days before admission is sufficient time for anticipatory preparation (Petrillo and Sanger, 1980). Children ages 5 to 12 years prefer to know about impending hospitalization from several weeks to a few minutes before the event. Because standardized programs cannot adequately meet the needs of the full age range of pediatric patients, some hospitals have developed preparation programs that target a specific age group, such as toddlers or adolescents (Johnson, Jeppson, and Redburn, 1992). The length of the session should be suited to the children's attention span—the younger the child, the shorter the program. The optimum approach is one that is individualized for each child and family. Regardless of the specific type of program, all children, even those who have been hospitalized before, benefit from an introduction to the environment and routine of the unit.

In many hospitals *child-life specialists*, health care professionals with extensive knowledge of child growth and development, as well as the special psychosocial needs of children who are hospitalized and their families, help prepare children for hospitalization, surgery, and procedures. A *collaborative effort* between the nurse, child-life specialist, and other members of the child's health care team helps ensure the best possible hospital experience for the child and family.

Hospital admission. The preparation that children require on the day of admission depends on the kind of prehospital counseling they have received. However, prehospital counseling does not preclude the need for support during procedures such as obtaining blood specimens, x-ray tests, or physical examination. For example, undressing young children before

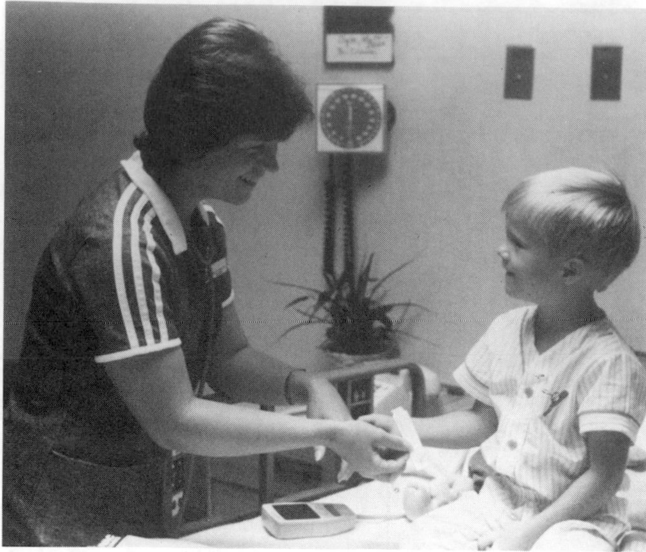

Fig. 41-6 The initial admission procedures give the nurse an opportunity to get to know the child and to assess the child's understanding of the hospital experience. (Courtesy St. Louis Children's Hospital.)

Guidelines

ADMISSION

Preadmission

Assign a room based on developmental age, seriousness of diagnosis, communicability of illness, and projected length of stay.
Prepare roommate(s) for the arrival of a new patient; when children are too young to benefit from this consideration, prepare parents.
Prepare room for child and family, with admission forms and equipment nearby to eliminate need to leave child.

Admission

Introduce primary nurse to child and family.
Orient child and family to inpatient facilities, especially to assigned room and unit; emphasize positive areas of pediatric unit.
- Room: explain call light, bed controls, television, bathroom, telephone, etc.
- Unit: Direct to playroom, desk, dining area, or other areas

Introduce family to roommate and his or her parents.
Apply identification band to child's wrist, ankle, or both (if not done).
Explain hospital regulations and schedules (e.g., visiting hours, mealtimes, bedtime, limitations [give written information if available]).
Perform nursing admission history (see box on pp. 1205-1206).
Take vital signs, blood pressure, height, and weight.
Obtain specimens as needed and order needed laboratory work.
Support child and assist practitioner with physical examination (for purposes of nursing assessment).

they feel comfortable in their new surroundings can be very upsetting. Causing needless anxiety and fear during admission may adversely affect the nurse's establishment of trust with these children. Therefore nursing assistance during the admission procedure is vital, regardless of how well prepared any child is for the experience of hospitalization. In addition, spending this time with the child gives the nurse an opportunity to evaluate the child's understanding of subsequent procedures (Fig. 41-6). Ideally, a primary nurse is assigned whenever possible to allow for individualized care and to provide a substitute support person for the child (see Chapter 27).

When a child is admitted, nurses follow several fairly universal admission procedures, which are outlined in the Guidelines box to the right. One particularly important decision is room assignment. The minimum considerations for room assignment are age, sex, and nature of the illness. Ideally, however, room selection should be based on a variety of developmental and psychobiologic needs. Determining compatible roommates, both for the children and for rooming-in parents, greatly influences the growth potential from the hospital experience.

No absolute rules govern room selection, but in general, placing children of the same age group and with similar types of illness in the same room is both psychologically and medically advantageous. However, there are many exceptions. For example, a school-age child may thrive on the responsibility of caring for a younger child. A child in traction may be very therapeutic for another child confined to bed because of a serious illness. A child who is very independent despite physical disabilities may help another child with similar or different limitations, and the parents of the child with disabilities may achieve deeper insight and acceptance of their child's disorder.

Age grouping is especially important for adolescents. Many hospitals make an effort to place teenagers on their own unit or in a separate designated section of the pediatric or general unit whenever possible.

Prevent or Minimize Separation

A primary nursing goal is to prevent separation, particularly in children under 5 years of age. Changes in hospitals' policies over recent years reflect a changed attitude toward parents; many hospitals no longer consider parents "visitors" and welcome their presence at all times throughout the child's hospitalization. Today most hospitals offer unrestricted visiting hours for parents on general pediatric units. Limitations on visitation result primarily from hospital policy or nursing judgment (Whitis, 1994). Many provide facilities such as a chair or bed for at least one person per child, unit kitchen privileges, and other amenities that create a welcoming atmosphere for parents. However, not all hospitals provide such an invitation, and parents' own schedules may prevent rooming-in. In such instances, strategies to minimize the effects of separation must be implemented.

As previously mentioned, ideally a primary nurse, along with associates, is assigned to meet the child's needs. A thorough, detailed nursing history (Box 41-5) specifically identifies the child's established daily routine. Usual daily activities such as food preparation and method of feeding help establish a complementary schedule of caregiving practices. Incorporating these normal activities also helps the parents feel that they are participating in the child's care, even if through another person. A consistent staff member can be designated to keep the family informed of the child's condition and to support the family's concerns and priorities without being judgmental (Stepanek and Ahmann, 1995).

Nurses must have an appreciation of the child's separation behaviors. As discussed earlier, the phases of protest and despair are normal. The child is allowed to cry. Even if the child rejects strangers, the nurse provides support through physical presence. *Presence* is defined as spending time being physically close to the child while using a quiet tone of voice, appropriate choice of words, eye contact, and touch in ways that establish rapport and communicate empathy (Pederson, 1993). If behaviors of detachment are evident, the nurse maintains the child's contact with the parents by frequently talking about them, encouraging the child to remember them, and stressing the significance of their visits, telephone calls, or letters.

Separation may be equally as difficult for parents, especially when they do not understand the behaviors of separation anxiety. To avoid the immediate protest, parents may sneak out or lie to the child about leaving. As a result, the child does not learn that absence is associated with a guaranteed return, but that absence means loss of parents. Helping parents recognize that separation behaviors are normal and expected can decrease the parents' anxiety and may ease their fears about leaving without telling the child. Explaining to parents how the child reacts after they leave may also be helpful. Many parents imagine that the child cries for hours after they leave, whereas in reality the child may cry for a few minutes but settle down when comforted by someone else.

Toddlers and preschoolers have a very limited concept of time. The young child's question, "Will my mommy come yesterday?" symbolizes a lack of understanding for usual measurements of time, such as days, hours, and weeks. Time is measured in associations, such as eating dinner "when Daddy comes home." Therefore when helping parents with their fears of separation, nurses should suggest ways of explaining leaving and returning. For example, if parents must leave to go to work or to make meals for the other family members, they should tell the child the reason for leaving. They also need to convey the expected time of return in terms of anticipated events. For example, if the parents will return in the morning, they can say to the child, "We'll see you after the sun comes up" or "We'll come back when (a favorite program) is on television."

The young child's ability to tolerate parental absence is very limited. Therefore parental visits should be frequent (e.g., visiting 3 times a day for short periods rather than once a day for an extended time). This may necessitate that each parent visit at different times to lessen the length of separation. When parents cannot visit, the presence of other significant people can be most comforting for the child.

If parents leave after the child is asleep, they still need to communicate their absence. The parents of a 5-year-old boy solved this problem by devising a sign; on one side they drew a picture of a telephone, and on the other they drew a hamburger. Before they left, they turned the sign to the appropriate side to tell the child when he awoke that they were out using the telephone or eating.

Older children who know how to tell time may find it helpful to have a clock or watch. However, these children have the same need for honesty from their parents regarding visiting schedules. Because their peer groups are important, adolescents often appreciate planning visiting hours with their parents to ensure that the patient has some private time for friends.

Familiar surroundings also increase the child's adjustment to separation. If parents cannot room-in, they should leave favorite home articles with the child, such as a blanket, toy, bottle, feeding utensil, or article of clothing. Since young children associate such inanimate objects with significant people, they gain comfort and reassurance from these possessions. They make the association that if the parents left this, the parents will surely return. Placing an identification band on the toy lessens the chances of its being misplaced and provides a symbol that the toy is experiencing the same needs as the child. Other mementos of home include photographs and audiotape or videocassette recordings of family members reading a story, singing a song, or relating events at home. The tapes can be played at lonely times, such as on awakening or before sleeping. Some units allow pets to visit, which can have therapeutic benefits for a child. Animals should be carefully screened for medical or behavioral problems, and patients should be screened for allergies.

Older children also appreciate familiar articles from home, particularly photographs, a radio, a favorite toy or game, and the usual pajamas. Often the importance of treasured objects to school-age children is overlooked or criticized. However, many school-age children have a special object to which they formed an attachment in early childhood. Therefore such treasured or transitional objects can help even older children feel more comfortable in a strange environment.

The strange sights, smells, and sounds in the hospital that are commonplace for the nurse can be frightening and confusing for children. It is important for the nurse to try to evaluate stimuli in the environment from the child's point of view (considering also what the child may see or hear happening to other patients) and to make every effort to protect the child from frightening and unfamiliar sights, sounds, and equipment. The nurse should offer explanations or prepare the child for those experiences that are unavoidable. Combining familiar or comforting sights with the unfamiliar can relieve much of the harshness of medical equipment.

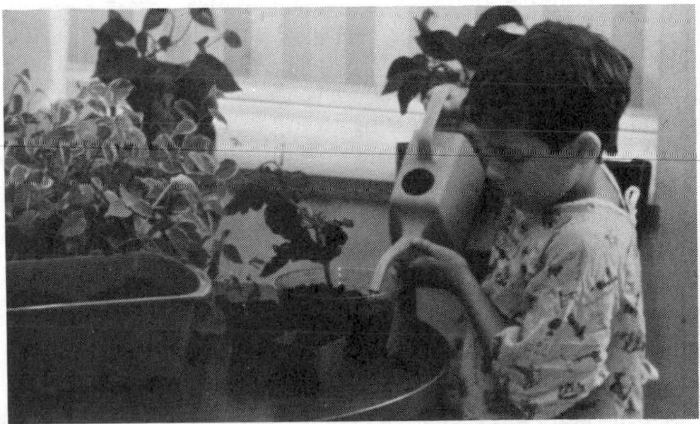

Fig. 41-7 For extended hospitalizations, children enjoy having projects to occupy time, such as caring for plants. (Courtesy St. Louis Children's Hospital.)

Helping children maintain their usual nonhome contacts also minimizes the effects of separation imposed by hospitalization. This includes continuing school lessons during the illness and confinement, visiting with friends either directly or through letter writing or telephone calls, and participating in stimulating projects whenever possible (Fig. 41-7). For extended hospitalizations, youngsters enjoy personalizing the hospital room to make it "home" by decorating the walls with posters and cards, rearranging the furniture (when possible), and displaying a collection or hobby.

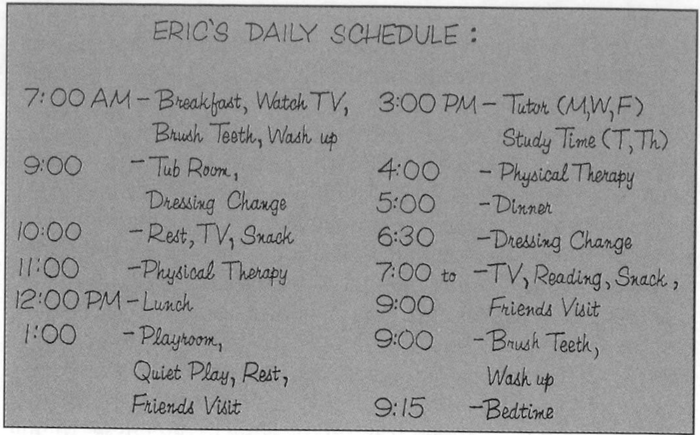

Fig. 41-8 Time structuring is an effective strategy for normalizing the hospital environment and increasing the child's sense of control.

Minimize Loss of Control

Feelings of loss of control result from separation, physical restriction, changed routines, enforced dependency, and magical thinking. Although some of these cannot be prevented, most can be minimized through individualized planning of nursing care.

Promote freedom of movement. Younger children react most strenuously to any type of physical restriction or immobilization. Although some restraint, such as immobilizing an extremity for insertion of an intravenous line is frequently necessary, most physical restriction can be prevented if the nurse gains the child's cooperation.

For young children, particularly infants and toddlers, preserving parent-child contact is the best means of decreasing the need for or stress of restraint. For example, almost the entire physical examination can be done in a parent's lap, with the parent hugging the child for procedures such as otoscopy. For painful procedures the parents' preferences for assisting, observing, or waiting outside the room are assessed (see also Parental Support, Chapter 42).

Environmental factors also influence the need for physical restraint. Keeping children in cribs or playpens may not represent immobilization in a concrete sense, but it certainly limits sensory stimulation. Increasing mobility by transporting children in carriages, wheelchairs, carts, wagons, or on stretchers or beds provides them with mechanical freedom.

Maintain child's routine. Altered daily schedules and loss of rituals are particularly stressful for toddlers and early preschoolers and may increase the stress of separation. The nursing admission history provides a baseline for planning care around the child's usual home activities.

A frequently neglected aspect of altered routines is the change in the child's daily activities. A nonhospitalized child's day, especially during the school years, is structured with specific times for eating, dressing, going to school, playing, and sleeping. However, this time structure vanishes when the child is hospitalized. Although the nurses have a set schedule, the child is frequently unaware of it; new schedules are imposed that may be rigid or flexible. For example, some units have uniform nap and bedtimes for all children, whereas others allow children to stay up very late. Many children obtain significantly less sleep in the hospital than at home; the primary causes are delay in sleep onset and early termination of sleep because of hospital routines. Not only are hours of sleep disrupted, but waking hours are spent in passive activities. For example, few institutions impose any regulation on the amount of time the child spends watching television.

One technique that can minimize the disruption in the child's routine is *time structuring*. This approach is most suitable for the noncritically ill school-age and adolescent child who has mastered the concept of time. It involves scheduling the child's day to include all those activities that are important to the child and nurse, such as treatment procedures, schoolwork, exercise, television, playroom, and hobbies. Together the nurse, parent, and child then plan a daily schedule with times and activities written down (Fig. 41-8). This is left in the child's room, and a clock or watch is available for the child's use. Whenever possible, a calendar is also constructed with special events marked, such as favorite television programs, visits by friends or relatives, events in the playroom, and holidays or birthdays. If specific changes in treatment are expected (e.g., "beginning physical therapy in 2 days"), these are added.

Encourage independence. The dependent role of the hospitalized patient imposes tremendous feelings of loss on older children. Principal interventions should focus on respect for individuality and the opportunity for decision making. Although these sound simple, their efficacy lies with nurses who are flexible, tolerant, and personally secure. The last is particularly important because when decision making is geared toward the patient, nurses can feel threatened by a sense of lessened control.

Promoting children's control involves maintaining independence, and the concept of self-care can be most beneficial. *Self-care* refers to the practice of activities that individuals personally initiate and perform on their own behalf in maintaining life, health, and well-being (Orem, 1995). Although self-care is limited by the child's age and physical condition, most children beyond infancy can perform some activities with little or no help. Whenever possible, these activities are encouraged in the hospital. Other approaches include jointly planning care; time structuring; wearing street clothes; making choices in food selections, bedtime, and so on; continuing school activities; and rooming with an appropriate age-mate.

Promote understanding. Loss of control can occur from feelings of having too little influence on one's destiny, as well

BOX 41-11
Bill of Rights for Children and Teens

In this hospital you and your family have the right to:
- Respect and personal dignity
- Care that supports you and your family
- Information you can understand
- Quality health care
- Emotional support
- Care that respects your need to grow, play, and learn
- Make choices and decisions

From Association for the Care of Children's Health: *A pediatric bill of rights, Bethesda*, MD, 1991, The Association. A detailed explanation of each right plus a separate "Bill of Rights for Parents" is available for a fee from the Association for the Care of Children's Health, 7910 Woodmont Ave., Suite 300, Bethesda, MD 20814; (301) 654-6549, (800) 808-ACCH.

as from sensing overwhelming control or power over fate. Although preschoolers' cognitive abilities predispose them most to magical thinking and self-power, all children are vulnerable to misinterpreting causes for stresses such as illness and hospitalization.

Most children feel more in control when they know what to expect because the element of fear is reduced. Anticipatory preparation and providing information help greatly to lessen stress and prevent lack of understanding (see the discussion of Preparation for Procedures, Chapter 42).

Informing children of their rights while hospitalized fosters greater understanding and may relieve some of the feelings of powerlessness they typically experience. Hospitals providing services to children should have a hospital-wide policy on the rights and responsibilities of these patients and of their parents and/or guardians. An increasing number of hospitals and organizations have developed a "Bill of Rights" that is prominently displayed throughout the hospital or is presented to children and their families on admission (Box 41-11).

Prevent or Minimize Bodily Injury

Beyond early infancy, all children fear bodily injury from mutilation, bodily intrusion, body image change, disability, or death. In general, preparation of children for painful procedures decreases their fears. Manipulating procedural techniques for children in each age group also minimizes fear of bodily injury. For example, since toddlers and young preschoolers are traumatized by insertion of a rectal thermometer, axillary temperatures or temperatures taken with electronic or tympanic membrane devices can effectively be substituted. Whenever procedures are performed on young children, the most supportive intervention is to do the procedure as quickly as possible while maintaining parent-child contact.

Because of young children's poorly defined body boundaries, the use of bandages may be particularly helpful. For example, telling children that the bleeding will stop after the needle is removed does little to relieve their fears, whereas applying a small Band-Aid usually provides much reassurance. The size of bandages is also significant to children in this age group; the larger the bandage, the more importance is attached to the wound. Watching their surgical dressings get successively smaller is one way young children can measure healing and improvement. Prematurely removing a dressing may cause these children considerable concern for their well-being.

For children who fear mutilation of body parts, it is essential that the nurse repeatedly stress the reason for a procedure and evaluate the child's understanding. For example, explaining cast removal to preschoolers may seem simple enough, but children's comprehension of the details may vary considerably from the explanation. Asking them to draw a picture of what they think will happen presents substantial evidence of the perceived events.

Children may fear bodily injury from a great variety of sources. X-ray machines, use of strange equipment for examination, unfamiliar rooms, or awkward positions can be perceived as potentially hazardous. In addition, thoughts and actions can be imagined sources of bodily damage. For older children, masturbation or sex play may be perceived as powerful weapons of potential destruction. Therefore it is important to investigate imagined reasons, particularly of a sexual nature, for illness. Since children may fear revealing such thoughts, using projective techniques such as drawing or doll play may elicit previously undisclosed misconceptions.

Older children fear bodily injury of both internal and external origins. For example, school-age children are aware of the significance of the heart and may fear the actual operation as much as the pain, the stitches, and the possible scar. Adolescents may express concern about the actual procedure but be much more anxious over the resulting scar. An appreciation of each child's special concerns helps nurses focus on critical areas during preparation for procedures or when giving explanations of the disease processes.

Children can grasp information only if it is presented on or close to their level of cognitive development. This necessitates an awareness of the words used to describe events or processes. For example, young children told that they are going to have a "CAT scan" may wonder, "Will there be cats? Or something that scratches?" It is clearer to describe the procedure in simple terms and explain what the letters of the common name stand for (Gaynard et al, 1990). When children are upset about their illness, their perception can be changed by (1) providing a somewhat different and less negative account of the disease or (2) offering an explanation that is characteristic of the next stage of cognitive development. An example of the first strategy is reassuring a preschooler who fears that after a tonsillectomy, another sore throat means a second operation. Explaining that once tonsils are "fixed" they do not need fixing again can help relieve the fear. An example of the latter strategy is to explain that germs made the tonsils sick and even though germs can cause another sore throat, they cannot cause the tonsils to ever be sick again. This higher-level explanation is based on the school-age child's concept of germs as a cause of disease.

Provide Pain Management

Relief of pain is a basic need and right of all children. Effective pain management requires that health professionals be willing to try a number of interventions to achieve optimum results. Basically, pain-reducing methods can be grouped into two categories: nonpharmacologic and pharmacologic. Whenever possible, both should be used; however, nonpharmacologic measures are not substitutes for analgesics.

Guidelines

NONPHARMACOLOGIC PAIN MANAGEMENT

General strategies

Form a trusting relationship with child and family.
- Express concern regarding their reports of pain.
- Take an active role in seeking effective pain management strategies.

Use general guidelines to prepare child for procedure (see Chapter 42)

Prepare child before potentially painful procedures but avoid "planting" the idea of pain. For example, instead of saying, "This is going to (or may) hurt," say, "Sometimes this feels like pushing, sticking, or pinching, and sometimes it doesn't bother people. Tell me what it feels like to you."
- Use "nonpain" descriptors when possible (e.g., "It feels like intense heat" rather than "It's a burning pain").
- This allows for variation in sensory perception, avoids suggesting pain, and gives child control in describing reactions.

Avoid evaluative statements or descriptions (e.g., "This is a terrible procedure" or "It really will hurt a lot").

Stay with child during a painful procedure.

Encourage parents to stay with child if child and parent desire; encourage parent to talk softly to child and to remain near child's head.

Involve parents in learning specific nonpharmacologic strategies and assisting child in their use.

Educate child about the pain, especially when explanation may lessen anxiety (e.g., that child's pain is expected after surgery and does not indicate something is wrong; reassure that child is not responsible for the pain).

For long-term pain control, give child a doll, which becomes "the patient," and allow child to do everything to the doll that is done to the child; pain control can be emphasized through the doll by stating, "Dolly feels better after the medicine."

Teach procedures to child and family for later use.

Specific strategies

Distraction

Involve parent and child in identifying strong distractors.

Involve child in play; use radio, tape recorder, record player; have child sing or use rhythmic breathing.

Have child take a deep breath and blow it out until told to stop (French, Painter, and Courty, 1994).

Have child blow bubbles to "blow the hurt away."

Have child concentrate on yelling or saying "ouch" by focusing on "yelling loud or soft as you feel it hurt: that way I know what's happening."

Have child look through kaleidoscope (type with glitter suspended in fluid-filled tube) and encourage to concentrate by asking, "Do you see the different designs? (Vessey, Carlson, and McGill, 1994)

Use humor, such as watching cartoons, telling jokes or funny stories, or acting silly with child.

Have child read, play games, or visit with friends.

Relaxation

With an infant or young child:
- Hold in a comfortable, well-supported position, such as vertically against the chest and shoulder.
- Rock in a wide, rhythmic arc in a rocking chair or sway back and forth, rather than bouncing child.
- Repeat one or two words softly, such as "Mommy's here."

With a slightly older child:
- Ask child to take a deep breath and "go limp as a rag doll" while exhaling slowly, then ask child to yawn (demonstrate if needed).
- Help child assume a comfortable position (e.g., pillow under neck and knees).
- Begin progressive relaxation: starting with the toes, systematically instruct child to let each body part "go limp" or "feel heavy"; if child has difficulty with relaxing, instruct child to tense or tighten each body part and then relax it.
- Allow child to keep eyes open, since children may respond better if eyes are open rather than closed during relaxation.

Guided imagery

Have child identify some highly pleasurable real or pretend experience.

Have child describe details of the event, including as many senses as possible (e.g., "feel the cool breezes," "see the beautiful colors," "hear the pleasant music").

Have child write down or record script.

Encourage child to concentrate only on the pleasurable event during the painful time; enhance the image by recalling specific details, such as reading the script or playing the record.

Combine with relaxation.

Positive self-talk

Teach child positive statements to say when in pain (e.g., "I will be feeling better soon," "When I go home, I will feel better," "Relaxing will make me hurt less").

Thought stopping

Identify positive facts about the painful event (e.g., "It does not last long").

Identify reassuring information (e.g., "If I think about something else, it does not hurt as much").

Condense positive and reassuring facts into a set of brief statements, and have child memorize them (e.g.: "Short procedure, good veins, little hurt, nice nurse, go home").

Have child repeat the memorized statements whenever thinking about or experiencing the painful event.

Cutaneous stimulation

Includes simple rhythmic rubbing; use of pressure, electric vibrator; massage with hand lotion, powder, or menthol cream; application of heat or cold, such as an ice cube on the site before giving injection or application of ice to the site opposite the painful area (e.g., if right knee hurts, place ice on left knee).

A more sophisticated method is transcutaneous electrical nerve stimulation (TENS) (use of controlled low-voltage electricity to the body via electrodes placed on the skin).

Behavioral contracting

Informal—May be used with children as young as 4 or 5 years of age:
- Use stars or tokens as rewards.
- Give uncooperative or procrastinating children (during a procedure) a limited time (measured by a visible timer) to complete the procedure.
- Proceed as needed if child is unable to comply.
- Reinforce cooperation with a reward if the procedure is accomplished within specified time.

Formal—Use written contract, which includes the following:
- Realistic (seems possible) goal or desired behavior
- Measurable behavior (e.g., agrees not to hit anyone during procedures)
- Contract written, dated, and signed by all persons involved in any of the agreements
- Identified rewards or consequences are reinforcing
- Goals can be evaluated

Nonpharmacologic management. A number of nonpharmacologic techniques exist for lessening the perception of pain and, when used with analgesics, can enhance these drugs' effectiveness. However, nonpharmacologic strategies can also produce a cooperative child who continues to suffer "in silence." Therefore nurses must carefully evaluate the effectiveness of the intervention in truly reducing pain and avoid setting an expectation of passive acceptance. Aside from this risk, nonpharmacologic methods are extremely safe and most are independent nursing functions.

Nonpharmacologic interventions include *general strategies* that are effective with most children, especially those who can benefit from explanations. However, *specific* ***nonpharmacologic strategies*** are more effective with certain children than with others (see the Guidelines box on p. 1220). Experimentation with several strategies that are suitable to the child's age, pain intensity, and abilities is often necessary to determine the most effective approach.

Nursing ALERT

Most specific nonpharmacologic strategies require children's understanding and cooperation. Therefore try to match the strategy with the pain severity. Children in severe pain may not be able to expend the effort necessary to learn the technique, and those with very mild symptoms may not be motivated to learn. Therefore these strategies may be most useful with mid-range pain.

In the selection of a pain reducer, it is best to use a strategy familiar to the child or to describe several strategies and let the child select the most appealing one. Parents should be involved in the selection process; they may be familiar with the child's usual coping skills and can help identify potentially successful strategies. Involving parents also encourages their participation in learning the skill with the child and acting as coach. If the parent cannot assist the child, other appropriate persons may include a grandparent, older sibling, nurse, or child-life specialist.

Children should learn a specific strategy *before* pain occurs or before it becomes severe. To reduce the child's effort, instructions for a strategy, such as distraction or relaxation, can be audiotaped and played during a period of discomfort.

Pharmacologic management. Using pharmacologic methods to control pain requires attention to four "rights": right drug, right dose, right route, and right time. Although nurses may not prescribe the medication, knowledge of these essential principles assists in optimally implementing analgesic orders and discussing with other practitioners possible strategies to improve pain control.

Right drug. Nonopioids, including acetaminophen (Tylenol, paracetamol) and nonsteroidal antiinflammatory drugs (NSAIDs), are suitable for mild to moderate pain; opioids are needed for moderate to severe pain. A combination of the two analgesics attacks pain on two levels: nonopioids at the peripheral nervous system and opioids at the central nervous system. This approach provides increased analgesia without increased side effects. Several commercially available combinations, such as Tylenol with Codeine, may have increasing

BOX 41-12

Selected Combination Opioid and Nonopioid Oral Analgesics

Product	Contents
Nonaspirin Products	
Darvocet-N 50	50 mg propoxyphene napsylate 325 mg actaminophen
Darvocet-N 100	100 mg propoxyphene napsylate 650 mg acetaminophen
Lortab	2.5, 5, or 7.5 mg hydrocodone bitartrate 500 mg acetaminophen
Lortab Liquid (each 5 ml)	2.5 mg hydrocodone bitartrate 120 mg acetaminophen
Percocet-5*	5 mg oxycodone HC1 325 mg acetaminophen
Tylenol with Codeine No. 1	7.5 mg codeine 300 mg acetaminophen
Tylenol with Codeine No. 2	15 mg codeine 300 mg acetaminophen
Tylenol with Codeine No. 3	30 mg codeine 300 mg acetaminophen
Tylenol with Codeine No. 4	60 mg codeine 300 mg acetaminophen
Tylenol and Codeine Elixir (each 5 ml)	12 mg codeine 120 mg acetaminophen 7% alcohol
Tylox*	5 mg oxycodon HCl 500 mg acetaminophen
Vicodin	5 mg hydrocodone 500 mg acetaminophen
Aspirin Products†	
Darvon Compound	32 mg propoxyphene HCl 389 mg aspirin 32.4 mg caffeine
Darvon Compound-65	65 mg propoxyphene HC1 389 mg aspirin 32.4 mg caffeine
Darvon with A.S.A.	65 mg propoxyphene HC1 325 mg aspirin
Darvon-N with A.S.A.	100 mg propoxyphene napsylate 325 mg aspirin
Percodan*	4.5 mg oxycodone HC1 0.38 mg oxycodone terephthalate 325 mg aspirin
Percodan-Demi*	2.25 mg oxycodone HC1 0.19 mg oxycodone terephthalate 325 mg aspirin

*All medications require a prescription, but these are classified as schedule II drugs (like morphine), and each filling requires a written prescription that includes the patient's name and address, the practitioner's Drug Enforcement Agency (DEA) number, and the date. The prescription must be filled within 5 days.

†Aspirin is not recommended for children because of its possible association with Reye syndrome.

doses of the opioid but a constant dose of the nonopioid (Box 41-12). Therefore before increasing the opioid, it may be preferable to increase the nonopioid component, for example, adding one plain Tylenol (300 mg) to Tylenol with Codeine No. 3 before advancing to Tylenol with Codeine No. 4. However, if this approach is not successful, the pain most likely requires a stronger opioid.

The action of various opioids differs. Morphine is considered the drug of choice. When morphine is not a suitable opioid, drugs such as hydromorphone (Dilaudid) and fentanyl (Sublimaze) are effective substitutes. Although fentanyl is used as an anesthetic in the operating room, it is classified as an analgesic. It can be safely administered by nurses (Willens, 1994).

Meperidine (Demerol, pethidine) is not recommended for chronic use (or for more than 48 hours at a time), such as for postoperative pain control, because of the accumulation of its metabolite, *normeperidine.* Normeperidine is a central nervous system stimulant that can produce anxiety, tremors, myoclonus, and generalized seizures. Normeperidine's half-life is 15 to 20 hours, compared with 3 hours for meperidine, and the central nervous system excitation is not reversed with naloxone. According to the Acute Pain Management Guideline Panel (1992), "meperidine should be reserved for very brief courses in otherwise healthy patients who have demonstrated an unusual reaction (e.g., local histamine release at the infusion site) or allergic response during treatment with other opioids such as morphine or hydromorphone."

Nursing ALERT

Assess the child at least every 8 hours for early signs of normeperidine toxicity, such as tremors in the outstretched hand, episodes of twitching or jerking, or increased agitation or excitability (may be upset easily). If toxicity is suspected, discontinue the meperidine immediately and notify the practitioner (Love, 1994). The pharmacist should complete an adverse drug reaction report to MedWatch*

*The FDA Medical Products Reporting Program, Food and Drug Administration, 5600 Fishers Lane, Rockville, MD 20852-9787; (800) FDA-1088, Fax (800) FDA-0178.

Opioids are often combined with other drugs that are considered "potentiators." However, there is little evidence that any drug potentiates the analgesic effect of opioids: rather, drugs that produce sedation are erroneously equated with producing analgesia. One common drug combination—*meperidine (pethidine [Demerol]), promethazine (Phenergan),* and *chlorpromazine (Thorazine),* known as *DPT* or *lytic cocktail*—is used for conscious sedation for procedures (see the discussion of preoperative care, Chapter 42). Meperidine, a short-acting analgesic, provides pain relief for 2 to 3 hours but is irritating to the tissues. Promethazine has antianalgesic properties, produces excessive sedation, and can cause extrapyramidal reactions (spasms of neck, face, tongue, and back; fixed eyeballs). All these drugs cause respiratory depression and lower the seizure threshold, a particular risk to those with a convulsive disorder. In addition, the "cocktail" is usually administered intramuscularly, causing additional pain. For these reasons, DPT is not recommended for general use and should be used only in exceptional circumstances (Acute Pain Management Guideline Panel, 1992). Appropriate drugs for conscious sedation are listed in Box 41-13.

BOX 41-13

Effective Medications for Conscious Sedation

Opioids*

Morphine sulfate, 0.05 to 0.10 mg/kg IV over 1 to 2 minutes given 5 minutes before procedure

Fentanyl, 1 to 2 μg/kg (0.001 to 0.002 mg/kg) IV 3 minutes before procedure,

Fentanyl Oralet, 5 to 15 μg/kg, maximum to 400 μg, orally 20 to 40 minutes before procedure†

Meperidine (if morphine sulfate or fentanyl is not available), 0.5 to 1.0 mg/kg IV over 1 to 2 minutes given 2 to 5 minutes before procedure or 1.5 mg/kg orally 45 to 60 minutes before procedure

Sedatives‡

Diazepam (Valium), 0.2 to 0.3 mg/kg, maximum of 10 mg orally 45 to 60 minutes before procedure

Midazolam (Versed), 0.2 to 0.4 mg/kg, maximum to 15 mg (IV solution) orally 30 to 45 minutes or 0.05 mg/kg IV 3 minutes before procedure

Pentobarbital (Nembutal), 1 to 3 mg/kg IV boluses to a maximum of 100 mg until asleep

Chloral hydrate, 20 to 75 mg/kg to a maximum dose of 100 mg/kg or 2.0 g given orally or rectally 60 minutes before procedure

Modified from Zeltzer LK et al: Report of the subcommittee on the management of pain associated with procedures in children with cancer, *Pediatrics* 86(suppl):826-831, 1990; and Coté CJ: Sedation for the pediatric patient, *Pediatr Clin North Am* 41(1):31-58, 1994.

*Provide analgesia and sedation.

†Not recommended for children less than 15 kg. Lozenge should be sucked, not chewed and swallowed. If chewed, drug is less effective because part of it is metabolized by liver before entering bloodstream. Swallowing drug rapidly does not increase risk of respiratory depression during first 15 to 30 minutes, period of greatest risk for decreased respiration.

‡Provide sedation but no analgesia.

Several drugs, known as *adjuvant analgesics,* may be used alone or with opioids to control pain symptoms, although they may or may not have analgesic properties. Commonly used drugs to relieve anxiety, cause sedation, and provide amnesia are diazepam (Valium) and midazolam (Versed); however, they are not analgesics. Other adjuvants include tricyclic antidepressants (i.e., amitriptyline, imiprimine) and antiepileptics for neuropathic pain (brief, lancinating pain); steroids for inflammation and bone pain; and dextroamphetamine and caffeine for increased analgesia and decreased sedation (McCaffery, 1996).

At times, health professionals question whether pain really exists and administer *placebos* to "see if the pain is real." This practice is unjustified and unethical; a positive response to a placebo, such as a saline injection, is common in patients who have a documented organic basis for pain. Therefore the deceptive use of placebos does not provide useful information about the presence or severity of pain. In addition, the use of placebos can cause side effects similar to those of opioids, can destroy the client's trust in the health care staff, and raises serious ethical and legal questions (Hinnant, 1995). Therefore the use of placebos should be avoided (American Pain Society, 1992).

Right Dosage. The optimum dosage is one that controls pain without causing severe side effects. This usually requires *titration*, the gradual adjustment of drug dosage (usually by increasing the dose) until optimum pain relief without excessive sedation is achieved. Dosage recommendations, such as those in Tables 41-3 and 41-4, are only safe initial dosages, not optimum dosages. Children (except infants younger than about 3 to 6 months of age) metabolize drugs more rapidly than adults; younger children may require higher doses of opioids to achieve the same analgesic effect. Therefore the therapeutic effect and duration of analgesia vary. Children's dosages are usually calculated according to body weight, except in children who weigh 50 kg (110 lb) or more, where the weight formula may exceed the average adult dose. In this case the adult dose is used.

A reasonable starting dose of opioid for the neonate who is *not* mechanically ventilated is one fourth to one third of the recommended starting dose for older children. The infant is monitored very closely for signs of pain relief and respiratory depression. The dose is titrated to effect. Since tolerance can develop rapidly, very large opioid doses may be needed for continued severe pain (American Pain Society, 1992).

If pain relief is inadequate, the initial dosage is increased (usually by 50% if pain is moderate or by 100% if pain is severe) to provide greater analgesic effectiveness. Decreasing the interval between doses may also provide more continuous pain relief. A major difference between opioids and nonopioids is that nonopioids have a *ceiling effect*, which means that doses higher than the recommended dose will not produce greater pain relief. Opioids do not have a ceiling effect other than that imposed by side effects; therefore larger dosages can be given safely for increasing severity of pain (see the Critical Thinking Q & A box on p. 1225).

Nursing ALERT

A frequent error in attempts to improve pain control is to change to another analgesic. If an opioid, such as morphine, hydromorphone, or fentanyl, is used, rarely is the problem one of drug choice. Rather, the problem is usually one of inadequate dosage. If changing to another analgesic is warranted because of adverse side effects, the new drug should be at least equal in potency to the original analgesic.

TABLE 41-3 Nonopiod analgesic drugs approved for children*

DRUG (TRADE NAME)	DOSE	COMMENTS
Acetaminophen (paracetamol; Tylenol and other brands)	10-20 mg/kg/dose every 4-6 hours not to exceed five doses in 24 hours	Available in drops (80 mg/0.8 ml), elixir (160 mg/5 ml), tablets (80 mg), swallowable caplets (160 mg), and rectal suppositories (several dosages) Nonprescription Higher dosage range may provide increased analgesia
Choline magnesium trisalicylate (Trilisate)	Children 37 kg or less: 50 mg/kg/day divided into two doses Children over 37 kg: 2250 mg/day divided into two doses	Available in elixir 500 mg/5 ml Prescription
Ibuprofen		
Children's Motrin	Children 6 months to 12 years: 5-10 mg/kg/dose every 6-8 hours not to exceed 40 mg/kg/day for fever Children over 12 years: 200-400 mg/dose every 6-8 hours	Available in suspension 100 mg/5 ml Nonprescription Recommended for fever reduction in children age 6 months to 12 years, but also indicated for juvenile rheumatoid arthritis and mild to moderate pain in children over 12 years of age
Children's Advil	Children 6 months and older: 5-10 mg/kg/dose every 6-8 hours not to exceed 40 mg/kg/day for fever	Available in suspension 100 mg/5 ml Prescription Dosage recommendation is for juvenile rheumatoid arthritis and fever
Naproxen (Naprosyn)	Children over 2 years: 10 mg/kg/day divided into two doses	Available in elixir 125 mg/5 ml Prescription
Tolmetin (Tolectin)	Children over 2 years: 20 mg/kg/day divided into three or four doses	Available in scored 200 mg tablets Prescription

*All drugs except aceptaminophen are nonsteroidal antiinflammatory drugs (NSAIDS).
Acetylsalicylic acid (aspirin) is also an NSAID but is not recommended for children because of its possible association with Reye syndrome. The NSAIDs in the table have no known association with Reye syndrome. However, caution should be exercised in prescribing any salicylate-containing drug (e.g., Trilisate) for children with known or suspected viral infection.
Ketorolac (Toradol) is the only NSAID that can be given intravenously. Although it is not approved for patients less than 16 years of age, it is used in children.
Side effects of ibuprofen, naproxen, and tolmetin include nausea, vomiting, diarrhea, constipation, gastric ulceration, bleeding nephritis, and fluid retention.
Acetaminophen and choline magnesium trisalicylate are well tolerated in the gastrointestinal tract and do not interfere with platelet function. NSAIDs except acetaminophen should not be given to patients with allergic reactions to salicylates. All the NSAIDs should be used cautiously in patients with renal impairment.

TABLE 41-4 Dosage of selected opioids for children

DRUG	APPROXIMATE EQUIANALGESIC ORAL DOSE	APPROXIMATE EQUIANALGESIC PARENTERAL DOSE	RECOMMENDED STARTING DOSE (CHILDREN LESS THAN 50 KG BODY WEIGHT)*	
			ORAL	PARENTERAL†
Morphine‡	30 mg every 3-4 hours (around-the-clock dosing) 60 mg every 3-4 hours (single dose or intermittent dosing)	10 mg every 3-4 hours	0.2-0.4 mg/kg oral every 3-4 hours 0.3-0.6 mg/kg oral time released every 12 hours	0.1-0.2 mg/kg IM every 3-4 hours 0.02-0.1 mg/kg IV bolus every 2 hours 0.015 mg/kg every 8 minutes PCA 0.01-0.02 mg/kg/hr IV infusion (neonates) 0.01-0.06 mg/kg/hr IV infusion (child)
Fentanyl (Sublimaze) (oral mucosal form—Fentanyl Oralet)§	Not available	0.1 mg IV	5-15 μg/kg maximum dose = 400 μg	0.5-1.5 μg/kg IV bolus every 0.5 hours 1-2 μg/hr IV infusion
Codeine||	130 mg every 3-4 hours	75 mg every 3-4 hours	1 mg/kg every 3-4 hours	Not recommended
Hydromorphone‡ (Dilaudid)	75 mg every 3-4 hours	1.5 mg every 3-4 hours	0.04-0.1 mg/kg oral every 4-6 hours	0.02-0.1 mg/kg IM every 3-4 hours 0.005-0.2 mg/kg IV bolus every 2 hours
Hydrocodone (in **Lorcet, Lortab, Vicodin,** others)	30 mg every 3-4 hours	Not available	0.2 mg/kg every 3-4 hours¶	Not available
Levorphanol (Levo-Dromoran)	4 mg every 6-8 hours	2 mg every 6-8 hours	0.04 mg/kg every 6-8 hours	0.02 mg/kg every 6-8 hours
Meperidine (Demerol)**	300 mg every 2-3 hours	100 mg every 3 hours	Not recommended	0.75 mg/kg every 2-3 hours
Methadone (Dolophine, others)	20 mg every 6-8 hours	10 mg every 6-8 hours	0.2 mg/kg every 6-8 hours	0.1 mg/kg every 6-8 hours
Oxycodone (Roxicodone, also in **Percocet, Percodan, Tylox,** others)	30 mg every 3-4 hours	Not available	0.2 mg/kg every 3-4 hours¶	Not available

Data from Acute Pain Management Guideline Panel: *Acute pain management: operative or medical procedures and trauma: clinical practice guideline,* AHCPR Pub No 92-0032, Rockville, Md, 1992, Agency for Health Care Policy and Research, Public Health Service, US Department of Health and Human Services; and Berde C et al: Report of the subcommittee on disease-related pain in childhood cancer, *Pediatrics* 86(5, pt 2):820, 1990.

IV, Intravenous; *IM,* intramuscular; *SC,* subcutaneous; *PO,* oral; *PCA,* patient-controlled analgesia.

note: Published tables vary in the suggested doses that are equianalgesic to morphine. Clinical response is the criterion that must be applied for each patient; titration to clinical response is necessary. Because there is not complete cross-tolerance among these drugs, it is usually necessary to use a lower than equianalgesic dose when changing drugs and to retitrate to response. **CAUTION:** Recommended doses do not apply to patients with renal or hepatic insufficiency or other conditions affecting drug metabolism and kinetics.

***CAUTION:** Doses listed for patients with body weight less than 50 kg cannot be used as initial starting doses in infants less than 6 months of age. For nonventilated infants under 6 months of age, the initial opioid dose should be about one fourth to one third of the dose recommended for older infants and children. For example, morphine could be used at a dose of 0.03 mg/kg instead of the traditional 0.1 mg/kg.

†IM injections should not be used.

‡For morphine, hydromorphone, and oxymorphone, rectal administration is an alternate route for patients unable to take oral medications, but equianalgesic doses may differ from oral and parenteral doses because of pharmacokinetic differences.

§Fentanyl Oralet is indicated for use in a hospital setting only (1) as an anesthetic premedication in the operating room setting or (2) to induce conscious sedation before a diagnostic or therapeutic procedure in other monitored anesthesia care settings in the hospital; is contraindicated in children who weigh less than 15 kg (33 lb).

||**CAUTION:** Codeine doses above 65 mg often are not appropriate because of diminishing incremental analgesia with increasing doses but continually increasing constipation and other side effects.

¶**CAUTION:** Doses of aspirin and acetaminophen in combination with opioid/NSAID preparations must also be adjusted to the patient's body weight.

**Meperidine is not recommended for continuous pain control, i.e., postoperatively, because of risk of normeperidine toxicity (see the Nursing Alert on p. 1222).

Parenteral and oral dosages of opioids are not the same. Because of the *first-pass effect*, an oral opioid is rapidly absorbed from the gastrointestinal tract and enters the portal circulation, where it is partially metabolized before reaching the central circulation. Therefore oral dosages must be larger to compensate for the partial loss of analgesic potency to achieve *equianalgesia* (equal analgesic effect). Conversion factors for selected opioids, when a change is made from intramuscular (IM) or intravenous (IV) to oral, are listed in Tables 41-4 and 41-5. Immediate conversion from IM or IV to the suggested equianalgesic oral dose may result in a substantial error in the individual child. For example, the dose may be significantly more or less than what the child requires. Small changes ensure small errors.

Right Route. Several routes of administration exist (Box 41-14). Children should not have to endure pain, as from IM injections, to achieve pain relief. Therefore the most effective and least traumatic route of administration should be selected.

A significant advance in the administration of IV or subcutaneous [SC] analgesics is the use of *patient-controlled analgesia (PCA)*. As the name implies, the patient controls the amount and frequency of the analgesic, which is typically delivered through a special infusion device. Children who are physically able to "push a button" and who can understand the concept of "pushing a button" to obtain pain relief (usually during later preschool age) can use PCA (Gureno and Reisinger, 1991). Although it is controversial, parents and nurses have used the PCA system for the child (Ruble and Billet, 1993; Webb, Paarlberg, and Sussman, 1991). Nurses can efficiently use the infusion device on any-age child to administer analgesics without the need for signing for and preparing opioid injections every time one is needed. When used as "nurse"- or "parent"-controlled analgesia, the concept of patient control is negated and may lead to excessive dosing.

PCA infusion devices typically allow for three methods or modes of drug administration to be used alone or in combination:

1. Patient-administered boluses that can only be infused according to the preset amount and lockout interval (time between doses); more frequent "pushing of the button" means no drug is delivered, but the patient may need the dose and time adjusted for better pain control
2. *Nurse-administered boluses* that are typically used to given an initial loading dose to increase blood levels rapidly and to relieve breakthrough pain (pain not relieved with the usual programmed dose)
3. *Continuous basal or background infusion* that delivers a constant amount of analgesic and prevents pain from returning during those times, such as sleep, when the patient cannot control the infusion; may decrease safety of PCA

At present the optimum use of these three modes is under investigation. However, as with any type of analgesic management plan, continued assessment of the child's pain relief is essential for the greatest benefit from PCA (see the Critical Thinking Q & A box below). Typical uses of PCA are for con-

TABLE 41-5 Selected analgesics (equianalgesia)

TRADE (GENERIC) DRUG*	EQUAL TO ORAL MORPHINE (mg)	EQUAL TO IM/IV MORPHINE (mg)
Propoxyphene hydrochloride (Darvon) 65 mg	4.8	1.6
Propoxyphene napsylate + acetaminophen (Darvocet-N 50)	4.8	1.6
30 mg codeine + 300 mg acetaminophen (Tylenol No. 3)	7.2	2.4
Oxycodone 5 mg + 325 mg acetaminophen (Percocet)	7.2	2.4
Oxycodone 5 mg + 325 mg aspirin (Percodan)	7.2	2.4
Hydrocodone 5 mg + 500 mg acetaminophen (Vicodin)	9	3
Oxycodone 5 mg + 500 mg acetaminophen (Tylox)	9	3
Acetaminophen (Tylenol Extra Strength) 500 mg	4	1.3
Transdermal fentanyl patch (Duragesic) (based on 25 μg patch applied q 3 days = 50 mg oral morphine q 24 hrs or divided into six doses = 8.3 mg)	8.3	2.77

Table by Betty R. Ferrell, PhD, FAAN, 1994.
*Oral medication with exception of Fentanyl.

Critical Thinking Q & A 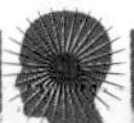

PAIN MANAGEMENT

Juan, 9 years old, is hospitalized for a fractured pelvis and multiple other trauma as a result of a motor vehicle injury. Since admission he has been receiving PCA ordered as "morphine, 2.0 to 2.5 mg/hr, lock-out 10 minutes; bolus dose 1.5 mg, not to exceed one dose per hour." In assessing his pain, you note that he rates the pain a 4 on a scale of 0 to 5, no to worst pain, respectively, and he has been pushing the PCA button an average of 15 times an hour. The first action you take is to:

1. Tell Juan that he is pushing the button too often; he should wait 10 minutes before using the PCA machine.
2. Administer the bolus dose of morphine and reassess pain in 10 minutes.
3. Increase the hourly dose of morphine from 2.0 to 2.5 mg and reassess pain in 1 hour.
4. Contact the surgeon about Juan's inadequate pain management.

The correct answer is two. Juan's pain is inadequately treated, and your first intervention is to give the ordered bolus dose. If the bolus dose relieves the pain to an acceptable level for Juan, the next step is to increase the hourly dose to 2.5 mg. Since the PCA order allows titrating (adjusting) the dosage upward, this action precedes calling the surgeon. It is absolutely inappropriate to tell Juan to push the PCA button less often; this response disregards his need for improved pain control and eliminates a valuable assessment parameter, the number of PCA uses.

BOX 41-14
Routes and Methods of Analgesic Drug Administration

Oral

Preferred because of convenience, cost, and relatively steady blood levels
Higher dosages of oral form of opioids required for equivalent parenteral analgesia
Peak drug effect occurs after $1^1/_2$ to 2 hours for most analgesics
Delay in onset is disadvantage when rapid control of severe pain or fluctuating pain is desired

Sublingual/buccal/transmucosal

Tablet or liquid placed between cheek and gum (buccal) or under tongue (sublingual)
Highly desirable because more rapid onset than oral
Avoids first-pass effect through liver, which normally reduces analgesia from oral opioids (unless sublingual/buccal form swallowed, which occurs often in children)
Few drugs commercially available in this form
Many drugs can be compounded into a sublingual troche or lozenge*

Fentanyl oralet—Fentanyl in hard confection base on a plastic holder used for preoperative or preprocedural sedation/analgesia

Intravenous (IV) (bolus)

Preferred for rapid control of severe pain
Provides most rapid onset of effect, usually in about 5 minutes
Advantage for acute pain, procedural pain, and breakthrough pain
Initial bolus dose is controversial; one recommendation is one-half IM dose
Must be repeated hourly for continuous pain control
Drugs with short half-life (morphine, fentanyl, hydromorphone) are preferred, to avoid toxic accumulation of drug

Intravenous (IV) (continuous)

Preferred over bolus and IM for maintaining control of pain
Provides steady blood levels
Easy to titrate dosage
Suggested initial dose is controversial; one approach to calculating hourly infusion rate is to divide IM dose by drug's expected duration for IM route
Full peak effect is delayed; best if combined with initial IV bolus dose

Subcutaneous (SC) (continuous)

Used when oral and IV routes not available
Provides equivalent blood levels to continuous IV infusion
Suggested initial bolus dose to equal 2-hour IV dose; total -24 -hour dose usually equal to total IV or IM 24-hour dose.

Patient-controlled analgesia (PAC)

Generally refers to self-administration of drugs, regardless of route
Typically uses programmable infusion pump (IV or SC) that permits self-administration of boluses of medication at preset dose and time interval (*lockout interval* is time between doses)
Best pain control may be achieved with initial bolus and continuous (basal or background) infusion of opioid
Optimum lockout interval not known, but must be at least as long as time needed for onset of drug
Should effectively control pain during movement or procedures
Longer lockout requires larger dose
May be used as a convenient analgesic delivery system for neonates; nurse pushes button for increased pain control

Intramuscular (IM)

Available in many opioid preparations
Painful administration (hated by children)
Some drugs (e.g., meperidine) can cause tissue damage
Wide fluctuation in absorption of drug from muscle
Faster absorption from deltoid than gluteal sites
Shorter duration and more expensive than oral drugs
Time consuming for staff

Intranasal

Midazolam (Versed) has been used as nasal spray
Although effective, may be traumatic route for children
Available commercially as Stadol NS (butorphanol); approved for those over 18 years of age; should not be used in patient receiving morphine-like drugs because butorphanol is partial antagonist

Intradermal

Used primarily for skin anesthesia (e.g., for lumbar puncture, bone marrow aspiration, arterial puncture, skin biopsy)
Local anesthetics (lidocaine) cause stinging, burning sensation
Duration of stinging may depend on type of "caine" used
To avoid stinging sensation associated with lidocaine:
Buffer the solution by adding 1 part of sodium bicarbonate (1 mEq/ml) to 10 parts of 1% or 2% lidocaine (see the Guidelines box on p. 1229)

Topical/transdermal

EMLA (eutectic mixture of local anesthetics [lidocaine/prilocaine]) cream
Eliminates or reduces pain from most procedures involving skin puncture
Must be placed over puncture site under occlusive dressing for 1 hour or more before procedure (see Guidelines box on p. 1228)

TAC (tetracaine/adrenalin/cocaine) or ***TC (without adrenalin)*** or ***LAT*** (lidocaine/adrenaline/tetracaine)
Provides skin anesthesia about 15 minutes after application
Gel (preferably) or liquid placed on wounds for suturing (nonintact skin)
Must not be used on mucous membranes and denuded areas because of the risk of systemic absorption and toxicity
Adrenalin must not be used on end arterioles (fingers, toes, tip of nose, penis, earlobes) because of vasoconstriction
LAT is safer and less expensive

Data primarily from American Pain Society: *Principles of analgesic use in the treatment of acute pain or chronic cancer pain*, ed 2, Skokie, Ill, 1992, The Society; and McCaffery M, Beebe A: *Pain: clinical manual for nursing practice*, St Louis, 1989, Mosby.
*For further information about compounding drugs in troches or suppositories, contact Technical Staff, Professional Compounding Centers of America, P.O. Box 368, Sugarland, TX 77487; (800) 331-2498.

BOX 41-14
Routes and Methods of Analgesic Drug Administration—cont'd

Transdermal fentanyl (Duragesic)

Available as "patch" for continuous cancer pain control
Safety and efficacy not established in children under 12 years
Not appropriate for initial relief of acute pain because of long interval to peak effect (from 12 to 24 hours)
Orders for "rescue doses" of an opioid should be available for pain that "breaks through"
Has duration of up to 72 hours for prolonged pain relief
If respiratory depression occurs, several doses of naloxone may be needed

Rectal

Alternative to oral or parenteral routes
Variable absorption rate
Generally disliked by children, but often preferred over IM injection
Acceptance may be culturally influenced
Many drugs can be compounded into rectal suppositories

Regional nerve block

Use of long-acting anesthetic (bupivacaine) injected into site, usually at end of surgery
Provides prolonged analgesia postoperatively, such as after inguinal herniorrhaphy
May be used to provide local anesthesia for surgery, such as dorsal penile nerve block for circumcision

Inhalation

Use of anesthetics, such as nitrous oxide or halothane, to produce partial or complete analgesia for painful procedures
Occupational exposure to high levels of nitrous oxide may cause side effects

Epidural/intrathecal

Involves catheter placed into epidural or intrathecal space for continuous drip or intermittent administration of opioid (with or without a long-acting anesthetic, e.g., bupivacaine)
Analgesia primarily from drug's direct effect on opiate receptors in spinal canal
Provides steady drug levels and long-lasting analgesia
Respiratory depression is very rare but may have slow and delayed onset; can be prevented by checking level of consciousness and respiratory rate and depth hourly for initial 24 hours
Nausea, itching, and urinary retention are common dose-related side effects

trolling pain from surgery, sickle cell crisis, trauma, and cancer.

Morphine is the drug of choice for PCA and is usually prepared in a concentration of 1 mg/ml. Other options are hydromorphone and fentanyl. Because PCA is typically used for continuous and extended pain control, meperidine should not be administered (see p. 1222). Another risk of using meperidine is confusion between its concentration (10 mg/ml) and that of morphine when the PCA pump is programmed, which can result in undermedication or overmedication.

Another advance is the use of the *epidural* or *intrathecal route,* primarily postoperatively or in selected cases of terminal care. A catheter is placed into the epidural or intrathecal space of the spinal column. An opioid (usually fentanyl or preservative-free morphine), often with a long-acting local anesthetic (usually bupivacaine), is instilled via continuous-drip or intermittent administration. Analgesia results primarily from the drug's direct effect on opiate receptors in the spinal cord, rather than in the brain, which is responsible for undesirable effects (e.g., sedation and respiratory depression) Respiratory depression is rare, but if it occurs, it develops slowly and is evident several hours after the infusion.

Nursing ALERT

When the epidural or intrathecal route is used, check the child's level of consciousness and respiratory rate and depth hourly for the first 24 hours to detect delayed-onset respiratory depression (American Pain Society, 1992).

Other routes that have benefited from new products for pain control are the *oral transmucosal* and *transdermal routes.* Oral transmucosal *fentanyl* (Fentanyl Oralet) provides nontraumatic preoperative oral sedation. Fentanyl is also available as a transdermal patch (Duragesic). It may be used for older children and adolescents who have chronic cancer pain.

One of the most significant improvements in the ability to provide atraumatic care to children is the anesthetic cream, EMLA,* a eutectic mixture of local anesthetics (lidocaine 2.5% and prilocaine 2.5%). The eutectic mixture, whose melting point is lower than that of the two anesthetics alone, permits effective concentrations of the drug to penetrate *intact* skin. A thick layer of cream is applied under an occlusive transparent dressing for 1 hour or more before procedures, such as lumbar, venous, arterial, finger, heel, or earlobe punctures; implanted port access; insertion of peripherally inserted central catheters (PICC lines); superficial biopsy; skin graft; laser treatment of port wine stains; removal of epicardial (pacing) wires, chest tubes, or hair (electrolysis); bone marrow examination; allergy testing; and IM or SC injections. For deeper pain, such as IM injections, the application time should be extended up to 2 hours (see the Guidelines box on p. 1228). The duration of anesthesia is up to 4 hours.

EMLA is approved for children over 1 month of age but has been used safely on newborns for circumcision and in preterm neonates for heel punctures (Benini et al, 1993; Taddio et al, 1995). It should be used cautiously on infants between the

*For additional information about EMLA, contact Astra Pharmaceuticals, (800) 228-EMLA.

Guidelines

USING EMLA (EUTECTIC MIXTURE OF LOCAL ANESTHETICS-LIDOCAINE 2.5% AND PRILOCAINE 2.5%)

Explain to child that EMLA is like a "magic cream that takes hurt away." Tap or lightly scratch site of procedure to show child that "skin is now awake."

Apply thick layer (dollop) of EMLA over normal intact skin to anesthetize site (about ½ of 5-gram tube; can use ⅓ of tube if puncture site is localized and superficial, e.g., intradermal injection or heel/finger puncture).

For venous access, apply to two sites; place enough cream on antecubital fossa to cover medial and lateral veins. Do not rub.

Place transparent adhesive dressing (e.g., Tegaderm) over EMLA. Make sure cream remains dollop. A piece of plastic film (e.g., Saran Wrap) with tape to seal the edges can be used. Use only as much adhesive as needed to prevent leakage.

To make the dressing less accessible, cover it with a self-adhering Ace-type bandage, such as *Coban,* or an IV protector, such as *I.V. House.** Label the dressing with "EMLA applied," the date, and the time to distinguish it from other types of dressings. Instruct older children not to disturb the dressing. (Covering the dressing with an opaque material may reduce the attraction and discourage "fingering.") Supervise younger or cognitively compromised children throughout the application time.

Leave EMLA on skin for at least 60 minutes for superficial puncture and 120 minutes for deep penetration, for example, IM injection or biopsy. EMLA may be applied at home and may need to be kept on longer in persons with dark and/or thicker skin. Anesthesia may last up to 3 hours after EMLA is removed.

Remove dressing before procedure and wipe cream from skin. With transparent adhesive, grasp opposite sides, and while holding dressing *parallel* to skin, pull sides away from each other to stretch and loosen dressing. An adhesive remover may be used.

Observe skin reaction, either blanched or reddened. If there is no obvious skin reaction, EMLA may not have penetrated adequately; test skin sensitivity and, if needed, reapply.

Repeat tapping or lightly scratching skin to show child that "skin is asleep" so that "it cannot feel a needle either."

After procedure, assess behavioral response. If child was upset, use pain scale, such as FACES, to help child distinguish between pain and fear.

In the United States, EMLA is not approved for use in infants under 1 month of age.† It should not be used in those rare patients with congenital or idiopathic *methemoglobinemia* and in infants under the age of 12 months who are receiving treatment with methemoglobin-inducing agents, for example, sulfonamides, phenytoin (Dilantin), phenobarbital, and acetaminophen (Tylenol). *Methemoglobin,* a dysfunctional form of hemoglobin, reduces the blood's oxygen-carrying capacity, causing cyanosis and hypoxemia. The use of intravenous methylene blue promptly eliminates the methemoglobinemia.

NOTE: EMLA is contraindicated in anyone with a known history of sensitivity or allergy to amide-type local anesthetics (lidocaine, prilocaine, mepivacaine, bupivacaine, etidocaine) or to any other component of the product.

EMLA cream maximum recommended application area to intact skin for infants and children

Body weight (kg)	Maximum application area (cm^2)
Up to 10 kg	100
10 to 20 kg	600
Above 20 kg	2000

These are broad guidelines for avoiding systemic toxicity in applying EMLA to patients with normal, intact skin and with normal renal function and hepatic function.

For more individualized calculation of how much lidocaine and prilocaine may be absorbed, practitioners can use the following estimates of lidocaine and prilocaine absorption for children and adults:

The estimated mean (+SD) absorption of lidocaine is 0.045 (+0.016) $mg/cm^2/hr$.

The estimated mean (+SD) absorption of prilocaine is 0.077 (+0.036) $mg/cm^2/hr$.

Modified from Wong DL: Overcoming 'needle phobia' with EMLA, *Am J Nurs* 65(2):24, 1995.
*For more information, contact I.V. House, 7400 Foxmont Dr., Hazelwood, MO 63042-2198; 800-530-0400; Fax 314-831-3683.
†In Canada, EMLA is not approved for use in infants under 6 months of age.

ages of 1 and 12 months who are receiving treatment with methemoglobin-inducing agents, such as sulfonamides, phenytoin (Dilantin), and acetaminophen (Tylenol). However, the use of these drugs is not a contraindication for applying EMLA, and there are no published reports of methemoglobinemia caused by EMLA when an infant received acetaminophen. Because of their diminished levels of erythrocyte-methemoglobin reductase, infants less than 3 months old are more susceptible to prilocaine-induced *methemoglobinemia,* a very rare and reversible side effect. *Methemoglobin* is a dysfunctional form of hemoglobin that reduces the oxygen-carrying capacity of the blood, causing cyanosis and hypoxemia. The use of intravenous methylene blue promptly eliminates the methemoglobinemia (Farrington, 1993). Other side effects are very mild and include pallor or erythema or edema at the application site.

The *intradermal route* is often used to inject a local anesthetic, typically lidocaine (Zylocaine), into the skin to reduce the pain from a lumbar puncture, bone marrow aspiration, suturing, or venous or arterial access. One problem with the use of lidocaine is the stinging and burning that initially occur. However, the use of *buffered lidocaine* reduces the stinging sensation (Orlinsky et al, 1992) (see the Guidelines box on p. 1229). Warming the lidocaine to 37° C (98.6° F) may also accomplish the same effect (Davidson and Boom, 1992).

Right time. The right timing for administering analgesics depends on the type of pain. For continuous pain control, such as for postoperative or cancer pain, a preventive schedule of medication *around the clock (ATC)* is effective. The ATC schedule avoids the low plasma concentrations that permit breakthrough pain. If analgesics are administered only when pain returns (a typical use of the PRN, or "as needed," order), pain relief may take several hours. This may require higher doses, leading to a cycle of undermedication of pain alternating with periods of overmedication and drug toxicity. This cycle of erratic pain control also promotes "clock watching,"

Guidelines

USING BUFFERED LIDOCAINE (BL)

Supplies: 8.4% sodium bicarbonate (1 mEq/ml), 1% to 2% lidocaine with or without epinephrine, syringe with removable needle, and a 30-gauge needle

Instructions:

Use 1 part sodium bicarbonate to 10 parts lidocaine (i.e., draw up 1 ml of lidocaine and 0.1 ml of sodium bicarbonate).

Change needle used to withdraw BL to 30-gauge needle for intradermal injection.

For venipuncture or port access, inject 0.1 ml or less BL intradermally directly over intended puncture site; anesthesia occurs almost immediately.

Suggested maximum dose of lidocaine for local anesthesia is 4.5 mg/kg.

If buffering lidocaine vial (e.g., 20 ml lidocaine with 2 ml sodium bicarbonate), use solution for 7 days or less and preferably when freshly prepared.

which may be erroneously equated with "addiction." Nurses can effectively use PRN orders by giving the drug at regular intervals, since "as needed" can be interpreted to mean "as needed to prevent return of pain."

Preventive pain control is best provided through continuous IV infusion rather than intermittent boluses. If intermittent boluses are given, the intervals between doses should not exceed the drug's expected duration of effectiveness. For extended pain control with fewer administration times, drugs that provide longer duration of action (e.g., some NSAIDs, time-release morphine, methadone, levorphanol) can be used.

Nursing ALERT

Since breakthrough pain can occur even with optimum ATC scheduling, there should be an order for PRN "rescue" doses of an analgesic.

Continuous analgesia is not always appropriate because not all pain is continuous. Frequently, temporary pain control is needed to provide analgesia before a scheduled procedure. When pain can be predicted, the drug's peak effect should be timed to coincide with the painful event. For example, with opioids the peak effect is approximately ½ to 1 hour for the IM or SC route (considerably less for the IV route); with nonopioids the peak effect occurs about 2 hours after oral administration. For rapid onset and peak of action, opioids that quickly penetrate the blood-brain barrier (e.g., IV fentanyl) provide excellent pain control.

Observe for side effects. Both NSAIDs and opioids have side effects, although the major concern is with those from opioids (Box 41-15). Respiratory depression is the most serious complication and is most likely to occur in sedated patients. The respiratory rate may decrease gradually or cease abruptly; lower limits of normal are not established for children, but any significant change from a previous rate calls for increased vigilance. A slower respiratory rate does not necessarily reflect decreased arterial oxygenation; an increased depth of ventilation may compensate for the altered rate (Rowbotham et al, 1989). If respiratory depression or arrest occurs, the nurse must be prepared to intervene quickly (Pasero and McCaffery, 1994) (see the Guidelines box on p. 1230).

Although respiratory depression is the most feared side effect, constipation is a common and sometimes serious side effect of opioids, which decrease peristaltic activity and increase anal sphincter tone. Prevention with stool softeners and laxatives is more effective than treatment once constipation occurs. Dietary treatment, such as increased fiber, is usually not sufficient to promote regular bowel evacuation. However, dietary measures, such as increased fluid, fruit, and bran intake, as well as activity, are encouraged.

Pruritus from epidural or intrathecal infusion can be treated with low doses of naloxone infused slowly or with IV nalbuphine. Pruritus from IV infusion usually responds to oral antihistamines. Nausea, vomiting, and sedation usually subside after 2 days of opioid administration, although oral or rectal antiemetics may be necessary.

Both tolerance and physical dependence can occur with prolonged use of opioids. Treatment of tolerance involves increasing the dose or decreasing the duration between doses. Treatment of physical dependence involves gradually reducing the dose over several days to prevent the occurrence of withdrawal symptoms (similar to tapering of steroid dosages after chronic steroid therapy). The following are suggested guidelines for treating physical dependence (American Pain Society, 1992):

- Gradually reduce dose (similar to tapering of steroids): Give one half of previous daily dose in q 6 hr doses for first 2 days.
  Then reduce dose by 25% every 2 days.
- Continue this schedule until total daily dose of 0.6 mg/kg/day of morphine (or equivalent) is reached.

BOX 41-15

Side Effects of Opioids

General

Constipation (possibly severe)
Respiratory depression
Sedation
Nausea and vomiting
Agitation, euphoria
Mental clouding
Hallucinations
Orthostatic hypotension
Pruritus
Urticaria
Sweating
Miosis (may be sign of toxicity)
Anaphylaxis (rare)

Signs of tolerance

Decreasing pain relief
Decreasing duration of pain relief

Signs of physical dependence

Initial signs of withdrawal:
- Lacrimation
- Rhinorrhea
- Yawning
- Sweating

Later signs:
- Restlessness
- Irritability
- Tremors
- Anorexia
- Dilated pupils
- Gooseflesh

Guidelines

MANAGING OPIOID-INDUCED RESPIRATORY DEPRESSION

If respirations are depressed:
- Reduce infusion by 25% when possible.
- Stimulate patient (shake gently, call by name, ask to breathe).
- Administer oxygen (consider naloxone).

If patient cannot be aroused or is apneic (American Pain Society, 1992):

Administer naloxone (Narcan):
- For children less than 40 kg: dilute 0.1 mg of naloxone in 10 ml of sterile saline solution to make 10 μg/ml solution and give 0.5 μg/kg.
- For children over 40 kg: dilute 0.4 mg ampule in 10 ml of sterile saline solution and give 0.5 ml.
- Administer bolus IV push every 2 minutes until effect is obtained.

Closely monitor patient. Naloxone's duration of antagonist action may be shorter than that of opioid, requiring repeated doses of naloxone.

NOTE: Respiratory depression due to benzodiazepines (e.g., diazepam [Valium] or midazolam [Versed]) can be reversed with flumazenil (Romazicon). Pediatric dosing experience suggests 0.01 mg/kg (0.1 ml/kg) as loading dose followed by 0.005 mg/kg/min (0.05 ml/kg/min) until awake or to a maximum of 1 mg (10 ml) (Jones et al, 1991). The recommended initial dose for children 20 kg or more is 0.2 mg (2 ml) IV over 15 seconds; if no response after 45 seconds, administer same dose and repeat as needed at 60-second intervals for maximum dose of 1 mg (10 ml).

- After 2 days on this dose, discontinue opioid.
- May also switch to oral methadone, using one fourth of equianalgesic dose as initial weaning dose and proceeding as described above.

Use supportive statements when administering analgesics. The effectiveness of analgesics can be enhanced by a supportive attitude toward the child. By reinforcing the cause and effect of the medication and analgesia, the nurse can condition the child to expect pain relief, provided the regimen is likely to be effective. Although IM injections should *not* be given, when they are, children need to understand that the "little hurt from the needle will take away the bigger hurt for a long time."

Parents and older children may have concerns about the use of opioids because of fear of addiction. These concerns should be addressed with assurance that any such risk is extremely low. It may be helpful to ask the question, "If you did not have this pain, would you want to take this medicine?" The answer is invariably no, which reinforces the solely therapeutic nature of the drug. It is also important to avoid making statements to the family such as "We don't want you to get used to this medicine" or "By now you shouldn't need this medicine," which may reinforce the fear of becoming addicted.

Provide Developmentally Appropriate Activities

A primary goal of nursing care for the child who is hospitalized is to minimize threats to the child's development. Many strategies (e.g., minimizing separation) have been discussed and may be all that the short-term patient requires. However, children who experience prolonged or repeated hospitalization are at greater risk for developmental delays or regression. The nurse who provides opportunities for the child to participate in developmentally appropriate activities further normalizes the child's environment and helps reduce interference with the child's ongoing development (see Normalization, Chapter 38).

Play is the "work" of children of all ages and assumes a critical role in their development. Because of its other important purposes in the hospital setting, play is the focus of a separate discussion.

Perhaps at no other age is the concept of interference with normal development more crucial than when it is applied to the rapidly developing infant and toddler. The nurse plays a primary role in identifying children at risk and helping to plan, implement, and evaluate developmental intervention (see Chapters 33 and 34).

School is an integral part of the school-age child's and adolescent's development. Accreditation standards for hospitals serving children consider access to appropriate educational services a key factor in the accreditation decision process when a child's treatment requires a significant absence from school. The nurse can encourage children to resume schoolwork as quickly as their condition permits, help them schedule and protect a selected time for studies, and help the family coordinate hospital educational services with their children's schools. Children should have the opportunity to "keep up" with art and music classes, as well as their academic subjects.

To meet the unique developmental needs of adolescents, special units have been developed that provide privacy, increased socialization, and appropriate activities for these young people. Typically these units are set apart from the general pediatric facility so that the teenagers do not share space with younger children, who are often perceived as a threat to their maturity. When adolescents must share a common activity room with younger patients, referring to the area as the "activity" room rather than the "playroom" may entice them to visit the room and participate in activities.

These units also provide more flexible routines and activities, such as more group activity, wearing of street clothes, provisions to leave the adolescent unit temporarily, and access to the items so critical to teenagers—telephones, compact disc and tape players, videocassette recorders (VCRs), computers, and televisions. Because adolescents' food habits are rarely limited to the three traditional meals a day, a ready supply of snacks should be available. However, the most important benefit of these units is increased socialization with peers. In addition, staff members usually enjoy working with this age group and are well suited to establishing the trust so essential for communication.

Provide Opportunities for Play/Expressive Activities

Play is one of the most important aspects of a child's life and one of the most effective tools for managing stress. Since ill-

BOX 41-16
Functions of Play in the Hospital

- Provides diversion and brings about relaxation
- Helps the child feel more secure in a strange environment
- Helps to lessen the stress of separation and the feelings of homesickness
- Provides a means for release of tension and expression of feelings
- Encourages interaction and development of positive attitudes toward others
- Provides an expressive outlet for creative ideas and interests
- Provides a means for accomplishing therapeutic goals (see the discussion of use of play in procedures, Chapter 42)
- Places child in active role and provides opportunity to make choices and be in control

Critical Thinking Q & A 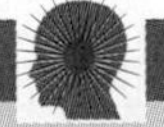

THE PLAYROOM

Seven-year-old Hannah is playing a board game with her brother, sister, and several other children in the playroom. A laboratory technician enters the playroom and says, "Hannah, I need to take some blood. I can see that you are playing a game, so I'll just do it while you play. It will just take a minute." Your most appropriate response would be:

1. "Go right ahead. It's silly to have to interrupt her game."
2. "Let me help you so that you can finish sooner."
3. "Hannah, is this okay with you?"
4. "We don't allow any procedures in the playroom."

Number four is the best response. The playroom should be considered a safe place—a sanctuary—and therefore off-limits for procedures. In many hospitals the child's bed is accorded the same status; children are taken to a treatment room. Even if it is okay with Hannah (number three), it is important to consider its possible impact on the other children in the room who may be confused about even a simple procedure (such as checking blood pressure) or the sanctuary status of the playroom for themselves.

An exception is sometimes made when all of the children present are older and the procedure is a quick painless one (such as checking blood pressure or giving oral medication) that all of the children present have experienced. In such cases the patient and the other children are asked if it is okay and give permission before the procedure is undertaken.

ness and hospitalization constitute crises in the life of a child, and since these situations are often fraught with overwhelming stresses, children need to play out their fears and anxieties as a means of coping with these stresses.

Play is essential to children's mental, emotional, and social well-being, and, like their developmental needs, the need for play does not stop when children are ill or in the hospital. On the contrary, play in the hospital serves many functions (Box 41-16).

Engaging in such activities puts children in charge, removing them for a time from the usual passive role of recipients of a constant stream of "things" being done to them. In the hospital environment, most decisions are made for the child; play and other expressive activities offer the child much-needed opportunities to make choices. Even if a child chooses not to participate in a particular activity, the nurse has offered the child a choice, perhaps one of the few real choices the child has had that day (Rollins, 1993).

Of all hospital facilities, probably no room does more to alleviate the stressors of hospitalization than the playroom or activity room. In this room, children temporarily distance themselves from the fears of separation, loss of control, and bodily injury. They can work through their feelings in a nonthreatening, comfortable atmosphere and in the manner that is most natural for them. They also know that the boundaries of this room are safe from intrusive or painful procedures and probing questions (see the Critical Thinking Q & A box above, right).

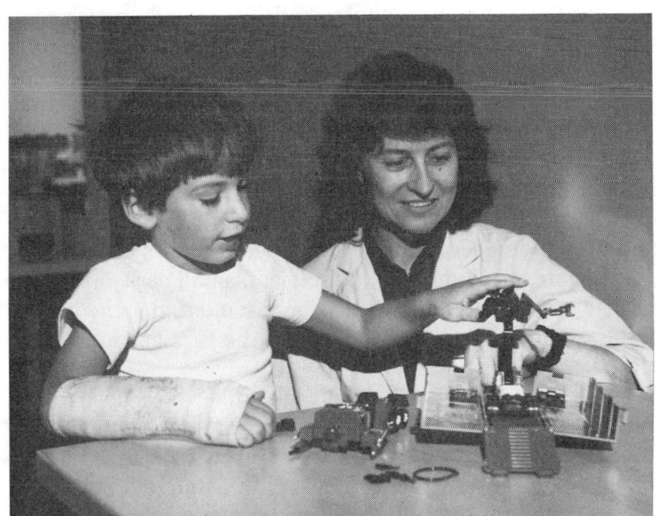

Fig. 41-9 Play materials for children in the hospital need to be appropriate for their age, interests, and limitations.

Diversional activities. Almost any form of play can be used for diversion and recreation, but the activity should be selected on the basis of the child's age, interests, and limitations (Fig. 41-9). Children do not necessarily need special direction for using play materials. All they require is the raw materials with which to work and adult approval and supervision to help keep their natural enthusiasm or expression of feelings from getting out of control. Small children enjoy a variety of small, colorful toys that they can play with in bed or in their room, or more elaborate play equipment, such as playhouses, sandboxes, rhythm instruments, or large boxes and blocks, that may be a part of the hospital playroom.

Games that can be played alone or with another child or an adult are popular with older children, as are puzzles; reading material; quiet, individual activities, such as sewing, stringing beads, and weaving; and Lego blocks and other building materials. Assembling models is an excellent pasttime, but it is a good idea to make certain that all pieces and necessary materials are included in the package. It is disappointing to the child to be ready to begin a project only to find that an essential item, such as glue, is missing from the set.

Well-selected books are of infinite value to the child. Children never tire of stories; having someone read aloud gives them endless hours of pleasure and is of special value to the child who has limited energy to expend in play. A radio, VCR, electronic games, and television, included among most hospital room equipment, are useful tools for entertaining a child, but parents and nurses should monitor program selection and the time spent using these devices so they don't become a substitute for social interaction or therapeutic play.

When supervising play for ill or convalescent children, it is best to select activities that are simpler than would normally be chosen according to the specific developmental level of the child. These children usually do not have the energy to cope with more challenging activities. Other limitations also influence the type of activities. Special consideration must be given to the child who is confined in terms of movement, has a restricted extremity, or is isolated. Toys for isolated children may need to be disinfected before and/or after use.

Toys. Parents of hospitalized children often ask nurses about the types of toys that would be best to bring for their child. It is wise to assure the parents that although it is natural to want to provide new toys for their child, it is often better to wait awhile to bring new things, especially in the case of younger children. Small children need the comfort and reassurance of familiar things, such as the stuffed animal the child hugs for comfort and takes to bed at night. These familiar items are a link with home and the world outside the hospital.

Large numbers of toys often confuse and frustrate a small child. A few small, well-chosen toys are usually preferred to one large, expensive one. Children who are hospitalized for an extended time benefit from changes. Rather than a confusing accumulation of toys, older toys should be replaced periodically as interest wanes.

Children love putting things in and taking things out of a larger container. Many simple items, such as a small magnifying glass, a magnet, grooming aids, a small mirror, crayons and drawing paper, colorful paper with scissors and paste, a magic slate, small dolls or toy soldiers, small cars, and beads to string, afford endless hours of amusement. It is the nurse's responsibility to assess the safety of the toys brought to the child.

A highly successful diversion for a child who is hospitalized for a length of time and whose parents are unable to visit frequently is having the parents bring a box with seven small, inexpensive, brightly wrapped items with a different day of the week printed on the outside of each package. The child will eagerly anticipate the time for opening each one. When the parents know when their next visit will be, they can provide the number of packages that corresponds to the days between visits. In this way the child knows that the diminishing packages also represent the anticipated visit from the parent.

Expressive activities. Play and other expressive activities provide one of the best opportunities for encouraging emotional expression, including the safe release of anger and hostility. Nondirective play that allows children freedom for expression can be tremendously therapeutic. Therapeutic play, however, should not be confused with **play therapy,** a psychologic technique reserved for use by trained and qualified therapists as an interpretative method with emotionally disturbed children. **Therapeutic play,** on the other hand, is a very effective, nondirective modality for helping children deal with their concerns and fears, whereas at the same time it often helps the nurse gain insights into children's needs and feelings.

Tension release can be facilitated through almost any activity, and with younger ambulatory children large-muscle activity such as use of tricycles and wagons is especially beneficial. A great deal of aggression can be safely directed into pounding and throwing games and activities. Beanbags are often thrown at a target or open receptable with surprising vigor and hostility. A pounding board is employed with enthusiasm by young children; clay and playdough are marvelous media for use at any age.

Creative expression. Although all children derive physical, social, emotional, and cognitive benefits from engaging in art or other creative activities, when children are hospitalized their need for such activities is intensified (Rollins, 1993). Children are more at ease expressing their thoughts and feelings through art, since humans think first in images and later learn to translate these images into words. A child's drawing before surgery, for example, will often reveal unvoiced concerns about mutilation, body changes, and loss of self-control (O'Malley and McNamara, 1993). Drawing and painting are excellent media for expression. The child needs only to be supplied with the raw materials, such as crayons and paper; pots of bright poster color, large brushes, and an ample supply of newsprint supported on easels; or materials for finger painting (Fig. 41-10). Children can work individually or collaborate on a group project, such as a mural painted on a long piece of paper. For children confined to bed, an old sheet (acquired from

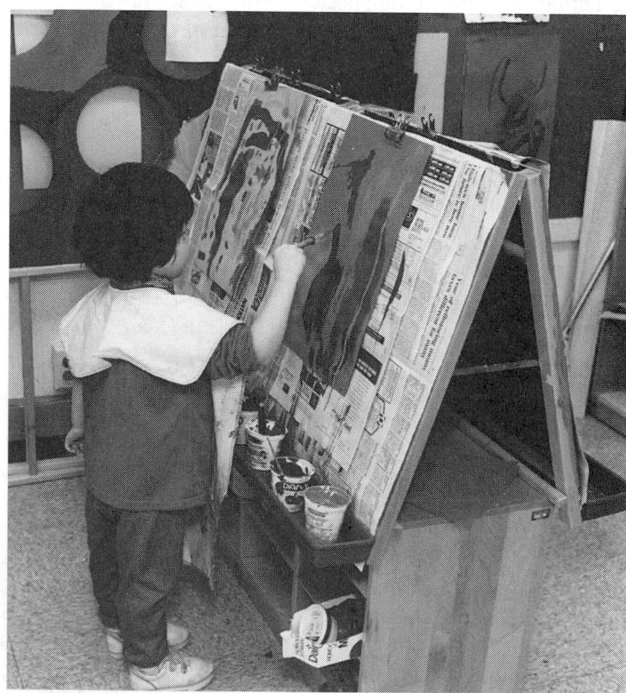

Fig. 41-10 Drawing and painting are excellent media for expression.

the laundry) spread over the bed and a large gown that extends down over the bedclothes to cover the child's own gown provide protection for clean linen.

While interpretation of children's drawing requires special training, observing changes in a series of the child's drawings over time can be helpful in assessing psychosocial adjustment and coping (Rae, 1991). The nurse can use children's drawings, stories, poetry, and other products of creative expression as a springboard for discussion of thoughts, fears, and understanding of concepts or events (see the discussion of communication techniques, Chapter 31).

Nurses can incorporate opportunities for musical expression into routine nursing care. For example, simple musical instruments, such as bracelets with bells, can be placed on infants' legs for them to shake to accompany mealtime music or dressing changes. Dance/movement suggestions may encourage a child to ambulate. Holidays provide stimulus and direction for unlimited creative projects. Children can participate in decorating the pediatric unit, and making pictures and decorations for their rooms gives the children a sense of pride and accomplishment. This is especially beneficial for children who are immobilized and isolated. Making gifts for someone at home helps to maintain interpersonal ties.

Dramatic play. Dramatic play is a well-recognized technique for emotional release, allowing children to reenact frightening or puzzling hospital experiences. Through use of puppets, replicas of hospital equipment, or some actual hospital equipment, children can play out the situations that are a part of their hospital experience. Dramatic play enables children to learn about procedures and events that will concern them and to assume the roles of the adults in the hospital environment.

Puppets are universally effective for communicating with children. Most children see them as peers and readily communicate with them. Children will relate to the puppet feelings that they hesitate to express to adults. Puppets can share children's own experiences and help them to find solutions to their problems. Puppets dressed to represent figures in the child's environment—for example, a physician, nurse, child patient, therapist, and members of the child's own family—are especially useful (Fig. 41-11). Small, appropriately attired dolls are equally effective in encouraging the child to play out situations, although puppets are usually best for direct conversation.

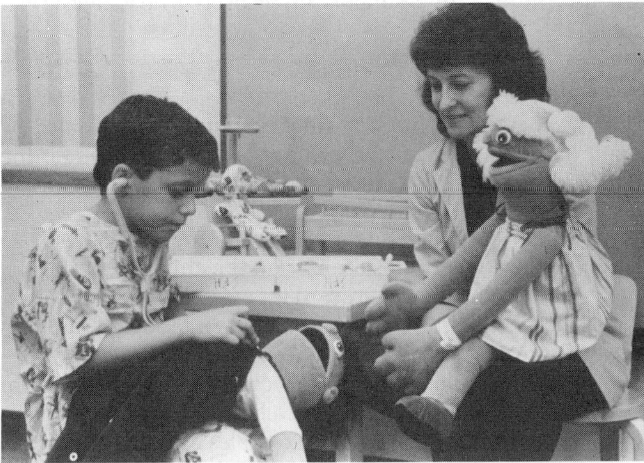

Fig. 41-11 Playing with miniature hospital equipment and puppets allows children to safely explore feelings and concerns. (Courtesy St. Louis Children's Hospital.)

Play must consider medical needs, yet at times a procedure can be postponed for a short time to allow the child to complete a special activity (see the Critical Thinking Q & A box below). Play must consider any limitations imposed by the child's condition. For example, it is not uncommon for small children to eat paste and other creative media; therefore a child who is allergic to wheat should not be given finger paint made from wallpaper paste or playdough made with flour. A child on a restricted salt intake should not play with modeling dough, since salt is one of its major constituents. At home the play program can be planned around the therapy regimen. However, play can be satisfactorily incorporated into the child's care if the nurse and others involved allow some flexibility and use creativity in planning for play.

Maximize Potential Benefits of Hospitalization

Foster parent-child relationships. The crisis of illness and/or hospitalization can mobilize parents into more acute awareness of the needs of their children. For example, one school-age child who was diagnosed with a serious physical condition commented to the nurse that he "enjoyed" the hospital because it was the first time that he had seen so much of his parents. He expressed concern over discharge because he anticipated the loss of the intensified love and attention. The nurse was able to discuss these feelings with the parents and to increase their awareness of their child's need for them.

Critical Thinking Q & A

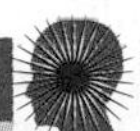

SCHEDULING PROCEDURES

Robert, 5 years old, is recovering from abdominal surgery. You enter his room to check his dressing. His mother is reading him a story. Your most appropriate response is:

1. To Robert's mother: "I need to check Robert's dressing."
2. "Robert, I need to check your dressing, but I can see that you are in the middle of a story right now. I'll check back in about 5 minutes and do it then."
3. "It's time to check your dressing, Robert. Let's get started."
4. "Robert, I need to check your dressing. It should take about 5 minutes. Would you like me to check it now, or to come back in about 10 minutes when you have finished hearing the story?"

Your best response would be number four, although number two would also be acceptable. Number four not only indicates that you value and respect the activity Robert is engaged in, but also offers him an opportunity to make a choice—to interrupt the story and get the procedure completed, or to finish the story and wait for your return. If, because of your own schedule, you are unable to offer such choices, express your desire to come back later, but explain that this time it is impossible. Number one ignores Robert's presence; number three fosters a passive role.

Hospitalization provides opportunities for parents to learn more about their children's growth and development. When parents are helped to understand children's usual reactions to stress, such as regression or aggression, they are not only better able to support the child through the hospital experience but also may extend their insights into childrearing practices after discharge.

Difficulties in parent-child relationships that may result in feeding problems, negative behavior, and sleep disturbances may decrease during hospitalization. The temporary cessation of such problems sometimes alerts parents to the role they may be playing in propagating the negative behavior. With assistance from health professionals, parents can restructure ways of relating to their children to foster more positive behavior.

Hospitalization may also represent a temporary reprieve or refuge from a disturbed home. Typically, abused or neglected children's dramatic physical and social improvement during hospitalization is proof of the growth potential of this experience. Hospitalized children temporarily are able to seek support, reassurance, and security from new relationships, particularly with nurses and hospitalized peers.

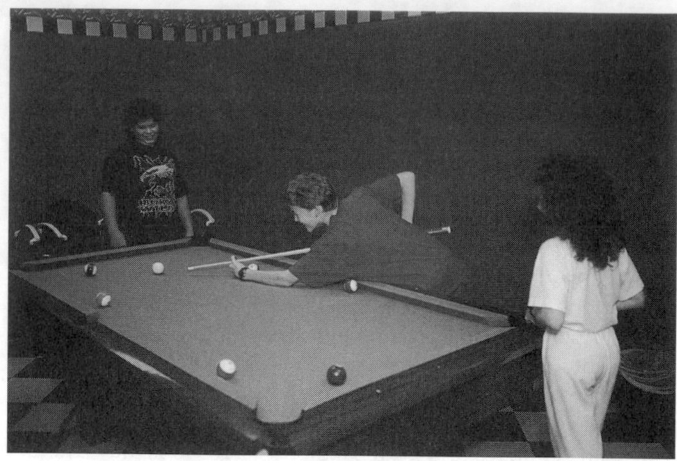

Fig. 41-12 The hospital environment can present an opportunity for forming new friendships and an accepting peer group for children.

Provide educational opportunities. Illness and hospitalization represent excellent opportunities for children and other family members to learn more about their bodies, each other, and the health professions. For example, during a hospital admission for a diabetic crisis, the child may learn about the disease; the parents may learn about the child's needs for independence, normalcy, and appropriate limits; and each of them may find a new support system in the hospital staff.

The special tutoring that children may receive during extended hospitalizations can help them advance their studies and concentrate on subjects that were difficult. The child's relationship with a tutor can foster a more positive attitude toward school and learning.

Illness or hospitalization can also help older children in choosing a vocation. Frequently children have impressions of physicians or nurses that are disproportionately glorified or horrified. Actual experience with different health professionals can influence their attitude about health professionals and even a decision regarding a health career.

Promote self-mastery. The experience of facing a crisis such as illness or hospitalization, coping successfully with it, and maturing as a result of it constitutes an opportunity for self-mastery. Younger children have the chance to test fantasy vs reality fears. They realize that they were not abandoned, mutilated, castrated, or punished. In fact, they were loved, cared for, and treated with respect for their individual concerns. It is not unusual for children who have undergone hospitalization or surgery to tell others that "it was nothing" or to proudly display their scars or bandages. For older children, hospitalization may represent an opportunity for decision making, independence, and self-reliance. They are proud of having survived the experience and may feel a genuine self-respect for their achievements. Nurses can facilitate such feelings of self-mastery by emphasizing aspects of personal competence in the child and not focusing on uncooperative or negative behavior.

Provide socialization. Hospitalization may offer children a special opportunity for social acceptance. Lonely, asocial, sometimes delinquent children find a sympathetic environment in the hospital. Children who are physically deformed or in some other way "different" from their age-mates may find an accepting social peer group (Fig. 41-12). Although this does not always spontaneously occur, nurses can structure the environment to foster a supportive child group. Forming relationships with significant members of the health care team, such as the physician, nurse, child-life specialist, or minister, can greatly enhance children's adjustment in many areas of life.

Parents may also encounter a new social group in other parents who have similar problems. The waiting room or hallway "self-help" groups are inherent to every institution. Nurses can capitalize on this informal gathering by encouraging parents to collectively discuss their concerns and feelings. Nurses can also refer parents to organized parent groups or can use the help and support of recovered hospitalized patients.

Evaluation

The effectiveness of nursing interventions is determined by continual reassessment and evaluation of care based on the following observational guidelines and expected outcomes:

1. Interview child and parents regarding the type of preparation for hospitalization the child received.
2. Review the medical record for evidence of parental visitation; interview parents and child regarding strategies used to minimize separation.
3. Observe child's hospital schedule and compare it with the schedule the child typically follows at home; interview child and family for examples of when they were allowed choices in the child's care.
4. Review the medical record for evidence of pain assessment and administration of analgesics or nonphar-

Nursing Care Plan

CHILD IN THE HOSPITAL

Nursing Diagnosis: Anxiety/fear related to disruption of familiar routine, unfamiliar environment, distressing events and procedures

Expected Outcome: Patient will exhibit minimal signs of emotional or physical distress (i.e., is calm, relaxed, cooperative; engages in nonnutritive sucking, appropriate play).

• NURSING INTERVENTIONS/*RATIONALES*

Acknowledge child's fear and help child *to identify sources of that fear to facilitate identification and use of coping strategies.*

Orient the child to hospital sights and sounds; provide child with accurate information about condition, procedures, and treatments; spend time with child *to promote trust and dispel fear.*

Encourage frequent family visitation with active participation in care *to prevent distress from separation.*

Use frequent touch, holding, and talking as appropriate *to provide comfort.*

Provide diversion and sensory stimulation appropriate to the child's developmental level and physical condition.

Instruct family in importance of comfort measures and in their active participation in care *to ease child's fears.*

Prepare child for procedures using developmentally appropriate approaches (therapeutic play) *to reduce fear and promote cooperation.*

Allow child choices when possible *to give child some measure of control.*

Work with parents to create a routine similar to the child's usual routine at home *to increase comfort with environment.*

Nursing Diagnosis: Diversional activity deficit related to illness and confinement to hospital

Expected Outcome: Child will engage in activities that are developmentally appropriate and within physical and environmental limitations.

• NURSING INTERVENTIONS/*RATIONALES*

Schedule therapies and rest periods *to allow time for play activities.* Time play periods when child may be feeling particularly vulnerable or alone *to provide needed distraction.*

Arrange for social interactions with others *to promote socialization.*

Interview parents and child to discover the child's favorite activities and games; adapt these activities to the child's physical limitations *to provide optimum diversions.*

Have parents bring in treasured toys or objects, decorate room with familiar pictures and drawings *to familiarize an unfamiliar environment.*

Nursing Diagnosis: Activity intolerance related to illness and generalized weakness

Expected Outcome: Patient's vital signs will remain within prescribed limits during activity, and child will tolerate increasing levels of activity.

• NURSING INTERVENTIONS/*RATIONALES*

Monitor child's vital signs *to assess level of physical tolerance;* monitor child's behavior and look for signs of irritability, shortened attention span, fussiness *that are indicative of a need for rest.*

Balance rest and activity, match play activities with tolerance levels *to conserve energy and prevent intolerance.*

Administer analgesics and sedatives per physician order *to decrease pain and restlessness.*

Remove stimulation and provide a quiet and calm environment during rest periods *to enhance rest and sleep.*

Nursing Diagnosis: Risk for injury related to unfamiliar environment, therapies, hazardous equipment

Expected Outcome: Patient will exhibit no evidence of injury.

• NURSING INTERVENTIONS/*RATIONALES*

Employ environmental safety measures (i.e., use of side rails; bed in low position; avoidance of hazards; keeping small, sharp and breakable items out of reach) *to prevent injury.*

Transport children using age-appropriate equipment and use of locks and safety belts *to minimize risk of injury.*

Maintain vigilance during trips to bathroom, use of bathtub or shower, performance of procedures *to minimize risk of injury.*

Identify specific motor/sensory deficits and provide appropriate assistive devices *to promote function and enhance safety.*

Instruct family in standard safety practices *to promote safety.*

Nursing Diagnosis: Self-care deficit: toileting, bathing/hygiene, dressing/grooming, dressing, feeding related to illness, physical restrictions, emotional regression

Expected Outcome: Patient will exhibit self-care activities within current physical and psychologic capacities.

• NURSING INTERVENTIONS/*RATIONALES*

Teach parents that some regression is expected when a child is ill *so behavior can be anticipated and viewed as normal part of disease process.*

Identify the level of regression and use developmental strategies appropriate to that level *to facilitate care.*

Involve child in planning and initiating daily routines as appropriate *to foster a sense of control.*

Assist child in performing activities of daily living as indicated, *allowing needed dependency and provision of support.*

Encourage child to perform activities within abilities *to promote self-confidence and independence.*

macologic pain reducers. Compare child's behavior and pain scores before and after administration of pain reducers for evidence of pain relief.

5. Interview child regarding the types of play and other activities that were introduced by the nurses or child-life specialist and the times the child visited the playroom. For preverbal child, observe child's use of play materials.
6. Interview child and parents regarding their perception of any beneficial aspects of the hospitalization. Observe behaviors that indicate benefits, such as the formation of new friendships.

Expected outcomes:

See the Nursing Care Plan on p. 1235.

Stressors and Reactions in the Family of the Child Who is Hospitalized

PARENTAL REACTIONS

Parents' reactions to illness in their child depend on a variety of influencing factors. Although which factors are most likely to influence their response cannot be predicted, a number of variables have been identified (Box 41-17). (See also Chapter 38.)

Almost all parents respond to their child's illness and hospitalization with remarkably consistent reactions. Initially, parents may react with *disbelief*, especially if the illness is sudden and serious. Following the realization of illness, parents react with *anger, guilt*, or both. They may blame themselves for the child's illness or become angry at others for some wrongdoing. Even in the mildest of illnesses, parents question their adequacy as caregivers and review any actions or omissions that could have prevented or caused the illness. When hospitalization is indicated, parental guilt is intensified because the parents feel helpless in alleviating the child's physical and emotional pain.

Fear, anxiety, and *frustration* are common feelings expressed by parents. Fear and anxiety may be related to the seriousness of the illness and the type of medical procedures involved. Often a great deal of anxiety is related to the trauma and pain inflicted on the child. Feelings of frustration are often related to lack of information about procedures and treatments, unfamiliarity with hospital rules and regulations, a sense of unwelcomeness from the staff, or fear of asking questions. Much frustration can be alleviated in a pediatric unit when parents are aware of what to expect and what is expected of them, are encouraged to participate in their child's care, and are regarded as the most significant contributors to the child's total health.

Parents eventually may react with some degree of *depression*. The depression usually occurs when the acute crisis is over, such as after hospital discharge or complete recovery. Mothers often comment on their feeling of physical and mental exhaustion after all the other family members have adapted to the crisis. Parents may also worry about and miss their other children, who may be left in the care of family, friends, or neighbors. Other reasons for anxiety and depression are related to concerns for the child's future well-being, including negative effects produced by the hospitalization and any financial burden incurred from the hospitalization.

BOX 41-17
Factors Affecting Parents' Reactions to Their Child's Illness

Seriousness of the threat to the child
Previous experience with illness or hospitalization
Medical procedures involved in diagnosis and treatment
Available support systems
Personal ego strengths
Previous coping abilities
Additional stresses on the family system
Cultural and religious beliefs
Communication patterns among family members

SIBLING REACTIONS

Siblings' reactions to a sister's or brother's illness or hospitalization are discussed in Chapter 38 and differ little when a child becomes temporarily ill. They experience loneliness, fear, and worry, as well as anger, resentment, jealousy, and guilt. Various factors have been identified that influence the effects of the child's hospitalization on siblings. Although these factors are similar to those seen when a child has a chronic illness, Craft (1993) reported that the following are related specifically to the hospital experience and have been found to increase the effects on the sibling:

- Younger and experiencing many changes
- Cared for outside the home by care providers who are not relatives
- Received little information about their ill brother or sister
- Perceived their parents to be treating them differently as compared with before their sibling's hospitalization

Simon (1993) asked 45 siblings of children who were hospitalized their perceptions of the stress of the hospitalization of a brother or sister. The siblings' perceptions of the stress they experienced were equal to the level of stress of hospitalized children.

Parents are often unaware of the number of effects that siblings experience during the sick child's hospitalization and of the benefit of simple interventions to minimize such effects, such as explicit explanations about the illness, sibling visitation, and provisions for the siblings to remain at home.

ALTERED FAMILY ROLES

In addition to the effects of separation on family roles, loss of parenting, sibling, and offspring roles may affect each family member differently. One of the most common reactions of parents is specialized and intensified attention toward the sick child. The other siblings usually regard this as unfair and interpret the parents' attitude toward them as rejection. Although such responses are usually unconscious and unintended, they place unique burdens on ill children. For example, the ill child may feel obligated to play the sick role in order to meet parents' expectations, especially children who have had limited physical ability and regain normal health status, such as following corrective heart surgery. Parents, as well, may be unable to perceive the child's recovery and therefore need to continue the pattern of overprotection and indulgent attention.

Ill children may also feel jealousy and resentment from other siblings. Because of their singular position in the family, they may be denied the companionship of their brothers and sisters. Rivalry between siblings tends to be greatest in the sibling who is nearest in age to the ill child. Without an understanding of the interpersonal dynamics between siblings, parents are likely to blame the well children for antisocial behavior. Illness may also result in children's loss of status within either their family or social group. For example, illness in the oldest child may temporarily terminate special privileges as "big" brother or sister.

Nursing Care of the Family

Assessment

Assessment involves those factors that are most likely to influence the family's responses to the child's illness and/or hospitalization. Although it is not possible to predict exactly which factors are most likely to have an effect on the family's reactions, the areas discussed in Table 38-2 should be included in the assessment process. Other important variables are (1) the seriousness of the child's illness, (2) the family's previous experience with hospitalization, and (3) the medical procedures involved in the diagnosis and treatment. Important information is also obtained in the nursing admission history (Box 41-5).

Discharge Assessment

Throughout the hospitalization the nurse should be aware of the need for discharge planning and those assessment factors that affect the family's ability to provide home care. Discharge planning must begin early in the hospital admission to permit sufficient time to assess the family's ability to perform care at home and to institute needed teaching. With the current concern for cost containment and recognition of children's emotional needs, home care for children with technologically complex care, such as youngsters on ventilators, has become increasingly common.

In terms of home care for children with complex care, a thorough assessment of the family and home environment should be performed to ensure that the family's emotional and physical resources are sufficient to manage the tasks of home care. (For a discussion of family and home assessment strategies, see Chapter 31. See also Chapter 40 on home care.) In addition to adequate family resources, an investigation of community services, including respite care, is needed to ensure that appropriate support agencies are available, such as emergency facilities, home health agencies, and equipment vendors. Financial resources may also be a consideration. To coordinate the immense task of assessment and to plan implementation, a case coordinator or manager should be appointed early in the discharge program.

Discharge planning is also concerned with those skills that parents or children are expected to continue at home. Assessment for planning appropriate teaching includes knowledge of (1) the actual and perceived complexity of the skill, (2) the parents' or child's ability to learn the skill, and (3) the parents' or child's previous or present experience with such procedures.

Nursing Diagnoses

A number of nursing diagnoses are prominent in the nursing care of the family of the hospitalized child, and others specific to individual cases become evident. The most common nursing diagnoses are outlined in the Nursing Care Plan on p. 1241.

Planning

The main goals for the family are as follows:

1. The family will participate in child's care to the extent they desire.
2. The family will receive support.
3. The family will be informed of child's care.
4. The family will be prepared for discharge and home care.

Implementation

Encourage Parent Participation

Preventing or minimizing separation is a key nursing goal with the child who is hospitalized, but maintaining parent-child contact is also beneficial for the family. One of the best approaches is encouraging parents to stay with their child and to participate in the care whenever possible. Although some health facilities provide special accommodations for parents, the concept of "rooming-in" can be instituted anywhere. The first requirement is the staff's positive attitude toward parents. When hospital staff genuinely appreciate the importance of continued parent-child attachment, they foster an environment that encourages parents to stay. When parents are included in the care planning and understand that they are a contributing factor to the child's recovery, they are more inclined to remain with their child and have more emotional reserves to support themselves and the child through the crisis. An empowerment model of helping allows the nurse to focus on parents' strengths and seek ways to promote growth and family functioning so that the parents become empowered in caring for their child (Fig. 41-13).

Since the mother tends to be the usual family caregiver, she usually spends more time in the hospital than the father. However, not all mothers (or fathers) feel equally comfortable in assuming responsibility for their child's care. Some may be under such great emotional stress that they need a temporary reprieve from total participation in caregiving activities. Others may feel insecure in participating in specialized areas of care, such as bathing the child after surgery. On the other hand, some mothers may feel a great need to have control of their child's care. This seems particularly true of young mothers who have more recently established their role as a parent, mothers of children too young to verbalize their needs, and ethnic minority mothers when the hospital setting is predominantly staffed by nonminority personnel (Schepp, 1992). Individual assessment of each parent's preferred involvement is necessary in order to prevent the effects of separation while supporting parents in their needs as well. Both underinvolve-

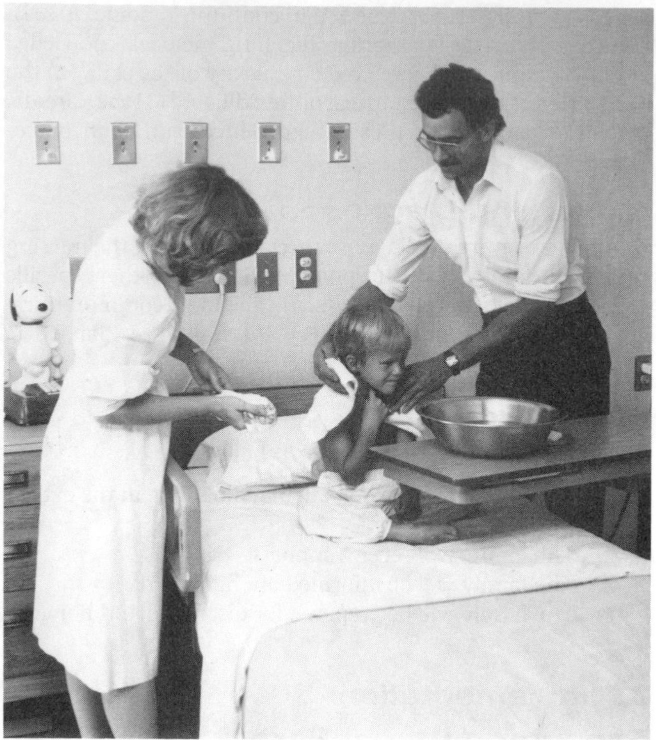

Fig. 41-13 Parental presence during hospitalization, including during procedures, provides emotional support for the child and increases the parent's sense of empowerment in the caregiver role. (Courtesy St. Louis Children's Hospital.)

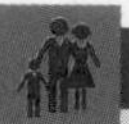

Family Focus

PARENTS' RELUCTANCE TO LEAVE THEIR CHILDREN UNATTENDED

Parents are often very reluctant to leave their children or to ask the nurse to watch their children while they take a break. In his research on the experiences of nurses and parents when parents room in, Darbyshire (1994) found that many parents did not eat properly, or in some cases, at all. The following are two mothers' experiences:

> I just about starved to death the first couple of days . . . just . . . I mean, it was my own fault really, 'cos I wouldn't leave the wee one. There was always going to be something else happening and I thought . . . if he gets upset I'd better be there when it finishes.
>
> There was one day I couldn't get any of the visitors to look after the wee chap so I could go for something to eat and it was about six o'clock at night and nurse said, "You look awful, are you OK?" and I said, "No, actually I feel awful and I think I'm going to pass out," and she said, "Oh, you've just gone a funny colour," and I said, "What time is it?" and I said, "It's OK, it's just because I haven't eaten all day"—because none of my family had come to take the child from me, and I didn't think to say to a nurse, "Could you watch him till I go for something to eat?"

From Darbyshire P: *Living with a sick child in hospital,* London, 1994, Chapman & Hall.

ment and overinvolvement of parents in the child's care can be detrimental; therefore every effort is extended to help parents identify moderate amounts of visiting and participation.

With life-styles and sex roles changing, fathers may assume all or some of the usual mothering roles in the household. In this case, it may be the father-child relationship that requires preservation. Fathers need to be included in the plan of care and respected for their parental role. For some fathers the child's hospitalization may represent an opportunity to alter their usual caregiving role and increase their involvement. In single-parent families the caregiver may not be a parent but an extended family member, such as a grandparent or aunt.

One of the potential problems with continuous parent rooming-in is neglect of the parent's need for sleep, nutrition, and relaxation (see the Family Focus box above). Often the sleeping accommodations are limited to a chair, and sleep is disrupted by nursing procedures. Encouraging the parents to leave for brief periods, arranging for sleeping quarters on the unit but outside the child's room, and planning a schedule of alternating visiting with another family member can minimize the stresses for the parent. If parents are reluctant to leave the hospital, sometimes it is possible for them to have a remote "beeper" that can provide immediate communication regardless of their location.

All too often, nurses respond to parent participation by abandoning their patient responsibilities. Nurses need to restructure their roles to complement and augment the caregiving functions of parents. Even in units structured to provide care by parents, parents frequently feel anxiety in their caregiving responsibilities; those more involved in direct care may feel more anxiety than those less involved in direct care. Therefore 24-hour responsibility may be too much for some parents. Assistance and relief by nursing personnel should always be available to these families, and nurses must often work diligently to establish the strong bond of trust some parents need to take advantage of these opportunities.

Support Family Members

Support involves the willingness to stay and listen to parents' verbal and nonverbal messages. Sometimes the nurse does not give this support directly. For example, the nurse may offer to stay with the child to allow the parents time alone or may discuss with other family members the parents' need for extra relief. Often relatives and friends want to help but do not know how. Suggesting ways, such as baby-sitting, preparing meals, tending the garden or home, doing laundry, or transporting the siblings to school, can prompt others to help lessen the responsibilities that burden parents. An ongoing parent support group held on the pediatric unit during the children's traditional nap time has also proved effective in helping parents share emotions and concerns related to hospitalization (Nugent et al, 1992).

Support may also be provided through the clergy. Parents with deep religious beliefs may appreciate the counsel of a clergy member, but because of their stress they may not have sufficient energy to initiate the contact. Nurses can be supportive by arranging for clergy to visit, upholding parents' religious beliefs, and respecting the individual meaning and significance of those beliefs.

Support involves an acceptance of cultural, socioeconomic, and ethnic values. For example, health and illness are defined differently by various ethnic groups. For some a disorder that has few outward manifestations of illness, such as diabetes, hypertension, or cardiac problems, is not a sickness. Consequently, following a prescribed treatment may be seen as unnecessary. Nurses who appreciate the influences of culture are more likely to intervene therapeutically (see also Chapter 28 for an extensive discussion of cultural and religious influences on health care).

Parents need help in accepting their own feelings toward the ill child. If given the opportunity, parents often disclose their feelings of loss of control, anger, and guilt. They often resist admitting to such feelings because they expect others to disapprove of behavior that is less than perfect. Unfortunately, health personnel, including nurses, sometimes do exercise little tolerance for deviation from the expected norm. This only increases the psychologic impact of a child's illness on family members. Helping parents identify the specific reason for such feelings and emphasizing that each is a normal, expected, and healthy response to stress provides the parents with an opportunity to lessen their emotional burden.

Support may also involve preparing siblings for hospital visits, assessing their adjustment, and providing appropriate interventions or referrals when needed. The nurse can invite visiting siblings to participate in playroom activities or other unit events. Siblings' needs are often neglected as parents and health personnel focus attention on the child who is hospitalized.

Provide Information

One of the most important nursing interventions is providing information about (1) the disease, its treatment, prognosis, and home care; (2) the child's emotional, as well as physical, reaction to illness and hospitalization; and (3) the probable emotional reactions of family members to the crisis.

For many families the child's illness is the first contact they have with the hospital experience. Often parents are not prepared for the child's behavioral reactions to hospitalization, such as separation behaviors, regression, aggression, and hostility. Providing the parents with information about these normal and expected behavioral responses can lessen the parents' anxiety during the hospital admission. The family is equally unfamiliar with hospital rules, which often adds to feelings of confusion and anxiety. Therefore the family needs clear explanations about what to expect and what is expected of them.

Parents also must be aware of the effects of illness on the family and strategies that prevent negative changes. Specifically, parents should keep the family well informed and communicating as much as possible. They should treat all the children as equally and as normally as before the illness occurred. Discipline, which initially may be lessened for the ill child, should be continued to provide a measure of security and predictability. When ill children know that their parents expect certain standards of conduct from them, they feel certain that they will recover. Conversely, when all limits are removed, they fear that something catastrophic will happen.

Nurses should help parents understand and accept the meaning of posthospitalization behaviors so that the parents can tolerate and support such behaviors. Consequently, parents should be forewarned of the usual continuance of such reactions after discharge (Box 41-3). Parents who do not expect such reactions may misinterpret them as evidence of the child's "being spoiled" and demand perfect behavior at a time when the child is still reacting to the stress of illness and hospitalization. If the behaviors, especially the demand for attention, are dealt with in a supportive manner, most children are able to relinquish them and assume precrisis levels of functioning.

Nurses should also forewarn parents of the reactions of siblings—particularly anger, jealousy, and resentment. Older siblings may deny such reactions because they provoke feelings of guilt. However, everyone needs outlets for emotions, and the repressed feelings may surface as problems in school, with age-mates, as psychosomatic illnesses, or in delinquent behavior.

Probably one of the most neglected areas involves giving information to siblings. Frequently age becomes the only factor that leads to an awareness of this problem because older children may begin to ask questions or request explanations. However, even in this situation the information may be seriously inadequate. Children in every age group deserve some explanation of the sibling's illness or hospitalization. Although the exact wording may differ, the explanation should focus on the following concerns: (1) "Will I get sick and have to go to the hospital?" (2) "Did I cause the illness?" (for actual or imagined reasons), and (3) "Will my parents abandon me if my brother or sister doesn't recover?" If parents or nurses address the explanations to these three questions, the siblings' own fears of illness, guilt, and abandonment are minimized. See the Home Care box on p. 1240 for ways parents can support siblings during hospitalization.

Prepare for Discharge and Home Care

Most hospitalizations necessitate some type of discharge preparation. Often this involves education of the family for continued care and follow-up in the home. Depending on the diagnosis, this may be relatively simple or highly complex. Preparing the family for home care demands a high degree of competence in planning and implementing discharge instructions. Although this is usually a team effort, nurses are often key individuals in initiating the process and collaborating with others in the planning and implementing stages.

Nurses frequently are responsible for all or some of the teaching as well. The teaching plan incorporates levels of learning, such as observing, participating with assistance, and, finally, acting without help or guidance. The skill is divided into discrete steps, and each step is taught to the family member until it is learned. Return demonstration of the skill is requested before new skills are introduced. A record of teaching and performance provides an efficient checklist for evaluation. All families need to receive detailed *written* instructions about home care,* with telephone numbers for assistance, before they leave the hospital (see the Critical Thinking Q & A box on p. 1240).

Videocassette recordings offer another excellent vehicle for

*Home care instructions for a wide variety of technical skills are available in Wong DL: *Wong and Whaley's clinical manual of pediatric nursing*, ed 4, St Louis, 1996, Mosby. Home modifications for numerous technical skills are available in Smith DP et al, editors: *Comprehensive child and family nursing skills*, St Louis, 1991, Mosby.

Home Care

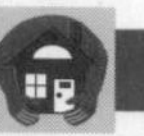

SUPPORTING SIBLINGS DURING HOSPITALIZATION

Trade off staying at the hospital with spouse or have a parent surrogate who knows the siblings well stay in the home.

Offer information about the child's condition to young siblings, as well as older siblings; respect the sibling who avoids information as a means of coping with the situation.

Arrange for children to visit their brother or sister in the hospital if possible.

Encourage phone visits and mail between brothers and sisters; provide children with phone numbers, writing supplies, and stamps.

Help each sibling identify an extended family member or friend to be their support person and provide extra attention during parental absence.

Make or buy inexpensive toys or trinkets for siblings, one gift for each day the child will be hospitalized.

- Wrap each gift separately and place in a basket, box, or other container at each child's bedside.
- Instruct siblings to open one gift each night at bedtime and to remember that he or she is in the parent's thoughts.

If the child's condition is stable and distance is not prohibitive, plan a special time at home with the siblings or have spouse or another relative or friend bring the children to meet parent(s) at a restaurant or other location near the hospital.

- Have extended family members or friends schedule a visit to the child in the hospital during parental absence.
- Arrange a pass for the child to leave the hospital to join the family if the child's condition permits.

Modified from Craft M, Craft J: Perceived changes in siblings of hospitalized children: a comparison of sibling and parent reports, *Child Health Care* 18(1):42-48, 1989; and Rollins J: *Brothers and sisters: a discussion guide for families,* Landover, Md, 1992, Epilepsy Foundation of America.

Critical Thinking Q & A

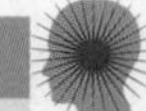

DISCHARGE PLANNING AND HOME CARE

Two-year-old Rhonda comes from a rural home 150 miles from the medical center. Last month she suffered a severe case of meningitis that left her profoundly cognitively impaired. During her hospitalization her parents have called infrequently and have never visited because they do not have a telephone or car as a result of their low income. Rhonda is now ready to be discharged from the tertiary care center. As the primary nurse who is responsible for Rhonda's discharge planning, you initiate which of the following activities:

1. Arrange for Rhonda to be institutionalized because her family will be unable to care for her.
2. Give a list of local services with an encouraging note about the importance of arranging follow-up care to the transport team to give to her parents.
3. Call and arrange for the public health nurse from Rhonda's district to make a home visit shortly after her return.
4. Arrange for a multidisciplinary case conference to discuss Rhonda's discharge.

The correct answer is four. A multidisciplinary case conference including the parents can be arranged with some planning. The public health department can be asked to either escort Rhonda's parents to the medical center or arrange for them to participate over a speaker phone. The public health nurse from Rhonda's district also will be able to advise the team of the services available in Rhonda's community. Since Rhonda will need care from a variety of professionals, this conference will help ensure that there are no gaps or overlaps in services.

Providing Rhonda's parents with a list of agencies is inappropriate. First, they do not own their own phone. Second, the parents are not in the position of knowing what services they will need. Third, dealing with professional agencies is often an arduous task and one that parents should not be expected to do while adjusting to the child's disability. Although contacting the local public health nurse is a good idea, this should be done well in advance of discharge. This way the nurse could do a home assessment to help arrange for appropriate services. Institutionalization of children with mental retardation is considered a last resort. All other options should be explored first.

home teaching. The actual teaching session in the hospital can be recorded and played for the family as often as needed. If the family has a VCR at home, the filmed instructions serve as a refresher when parents have questions about the procedure.

Once the family is competent in performing the skill, they are given responsibility for the care. Whenever possible, the family should have a transition or trial period to assume care with minimum supervision. This may be arranged on the unit, during a home pass, or in a facility, such as a motel, near the hospital. Such transitions provide a safe practice period for the family, with assistance readily available when needed, and are especially valuable when the family lives at a distance from the treating center.

In many instances, parents need only simple instructions and understanding of follow-up care. However, the often overwhelming care assumed by some families coupled with other stressors families may be experiencing necessitates continued professional support after discharge. A follow-up home visit or telephone call gives the nurse a better opportunity to individualize care and provide information in perhaps a less stressful learning environment than the hospital (Snowdon and Kane, 1995). Appropriate referrals and resources may include visiting nurse or home health agencies, private nurse services, the school system, physical therapist, mental health counselor, social worker, or any number of community agencies, including special organizations, such as SKIP.* Sharing the important issues surrounding the child's and family's needs is essential. Referral summaries should be concise, specific, and factual. When numerous support services are involved, periodic collaboration among the professionals involved and the family is an excellent strategy to ensure efficient usage and comprehensive delivery of services.

Evaluation

The effectiveness of nursing interventions is determined by continual reassessment and evaluation of care based on the following observational guidelines and expected outcomes:

*__SKIP (Sick Kids need Involved People)__ serves as an educational, support, and resource agency that provides assistance to families who have chosen home care for their child with complex medical needs. The address of the national headquarters is 545 Madison Ave, 13th floor, New York, NY 10022; (212) 421-9160.

1. Observe schedule of parental presence and amount of participation in child's care; observe their willingness and ability to take care of their own needs, such as regular breaks to eat, sleep, and care for the family's needs at home.
2. Interview family regarding their concerns; observe support offered by others, such as relatives, friends, and clergy; observe if special cultural practices (if applicable) are respected in the hospital.
3. Interview family regarding their knowledge of the child's illness, the child's expected reactions to the hospitalization experience, and the emotional needs of the other family members, especially siblings. Observe frequency of siblings' visits and interview siblings regarding their understanding of the ill child's condition.
4. Observe family's performance of skills and determine their understanding of other aspects of home care before discharge; interview family and/or resource persons regarding the family's use of appropriate referral services.

Expected outcomes:

See the Nursing Care Plan below.

Care of the Child and Family in Special Hospital Situations

AMBULATORY/OUTPATIENT SETTING

The ambulatory or outpatient setting provides needed medical services for the child while eliminating the necessity of overnight admission. Among the benefits of ambulatory care are (1) minimization of the stressors of hospitalization, especially separation from the family; (2) reduced chance of infection; and (3) cost savings. Admission to the day hospital usually is for surgical or diagnostic procedures, such as insertion of tympanostomy tubes, hernia repair, tonsillectomy, cystoscopy, or bronchoscopy.

Because of the limited contact with the child, nursing admission procedures are extremely important. Ideally, each child and family should receive preadmission counseling, including a tour of the facility and a review of the expected day's procedures. When this is not possible, surgery should be scheduled to allow time for children to become acquainted with their surroundings and for nurses to assess, plan, and implement appropriate teaching.

Nursing Care Plan

FAMILY OF ILL/HOSPITALIZED CHILD

Nursing Diagnosis: Altered family processes and/or ineffective family coping related to situational crisis, threat to role functioning, change in environment

Expected Outcome: **Family will exhibit use of appropriate coping mechanisms, and stress levels are reduced.**

• **NURSING INTERVENTIONS/*RATIONALES***

Explore family background, structure, normal roles and functions, usual coping mechanisms *to identify family strengths and weaknesses and assist in meeting needs.*

Help family arrange a schedule that balances needs of hospitalized child with functions of home and work *to help family manage stress and adapt to the situation.*

Help family prioritize needs, explore options, make decisions *to reduce stress and increase coping.*

Encourage use of available support systems (i.e., extended family, friends, church, community) and make referrals to appropriate social service agencies *to increase support and enhance available resources.*

Keep family informed about child's condition, procedures, and treatments *to reduce anxiety about the unknown.*

Give family members specific suggestions as to what each can contribute to help the child during the hospital stay and recovery *to provide for concrete family contributions and involvement.*

Provide a ready outlet for family to vent feelings, fears, and frustrations *to promote coping.*

Encourage family to take care of their own needs for rest, nutrition, relaxation, and respite *to promote coping.*

Nursing Diagnosis: Powerlessness related to health care environment

Expected Outcome: **Family will exhibit a sense of control within the environment.**

• **NURSING INTERVENTIONS/*RATIONALES***

Encourage family to identify feelings about having a child in the hospital *to enhance trust, communication, and ventilation.*

Help family identify specific modifications and adjustments that can be made within the environment (i.e., participation in child's care, decision making, scheduling; rearranging and personalizing environmental space; provision of privacy, ready access to specifically identified personnel) *to enhance feelings of control.*

Incorporate family suggestions, needs into plan of care *to enhance sense of contribution and control.*

Keep family informed about child's condition, progress; educate about treatments and procedures *to enhance knowledge.*

Discharge instructions must also be explicit (see the discussion of preparation for discharge and home care, p. 1239). Parents need guidelines on when to call their practitioner regarding a change in the child's condition. It is helpful for the nurse to make a follow-up telephone call or to specify a time for the family to report on the child's progress. Even hints for taking the child home in the car are appreciated. For example, it may be helpful to have a blanket and pillow in the car and a basin or plastic bag in case of vomiting.

ISOLATION

Admission to an isolation room increases all the stressors typically associated with hospitalization. There is further separation from familiar persons, additional loss of control, and added environmental changes, such as sensory deprivation and the strange appearance of visitors. Children may feel depersonalized from reduced interaction with the environment and the people in it (Hart et al, 1992). Their orientation to time and place is affected. These stressors are compounded by children's limited understanding of isolation. Preschool children have difficulty understanding the rationale for isolation because they cannot comprehend the cause-and-effect relationship between germs and illness. They are likely to view isolation as punishment. Older children understand the causality better but still require information to decrease fantasizing or misinterpretation.

When a child is placed in isolation, preparation is essential for the child to feel in control. With young children the best approach is a simple explanation, such as "You need to be in this room to help you get better. This is a special place to make all the germs go away. The germs made you sick, and you could not help that."

All children, but especially younger ones, need preparation in terms of what they will see, hear, or feel in isolation. Therefore they are shown the mask, gloves, and gown and are encouraged to "dress up" in them. Playing with the strange apparel lessens the fear of seeing "ghost-like" people walk into the room. Before entering the room, nurses and other health personnel should introduce themselves and let the child see their face before donning a mask. In this way the child associates them with significant experiences and gains a sense of familiarity in an otherwise strange and lonely environment.

When the child's condition improves, appropriate play activities are provided to minimize boredom, stimulate the senses, provide a real or perceived sense of movement, orient the child to time and place, provide social interaction, and reduce depersonalization.* For example, the environment can be manipulated to increase sensory freedom by moving the bed toward the door or window. Opening window shades; providing musical, visual, or tactile toys; and increasing interpersonal contact can substitute mental mobility for the limitations of physical movement. Rather than dwelling on the negative aspects of isolation, the child can be encouraged to view this experience as challenging and positive. For example, the nurse can help the child look at isolation as a method of keeping others out and letting only special people in. Children often think of intriguing signs for their doors, such as "Enter at your own risk" or "Many have entered but few have left." These signs also encourage people "on the outside" to talk with the child about the ominous greetings.

*An excellent resource for activities for children in isolation is: Hart et al: *Therapeutic play activities for hospitalized children*, St Louis, 1992, Mosby.

EMERGENCY ADMISSION

One of the most traumatic hospital experiences for the child and parents is an emergency admission. The sudden onset of an illness or the occurrence of an injury leaves little time for preparation and explanation. Sometimes the emergency admission is compounded by admission to an intensive care unit or the need for immediate surgery. However, even in those instances requiring only outpatient treatment, the child is exposed to a strange, frightening environment and to people who often inflict pain. Thus every medical emergency requires psychologic intervention to reduce the fear and anxiety frequently associated with the experience.

Lengthy preparatory admission procedures are often inappropriate for emergency situations. In such instances, nurses must focus their nursing interventions on the essential components of admission counseling (Box 41-18) and complete the process as soon as the child's condition is stabilized.

Unless an emergency is life-threatening, children need to participate in their care to maintain a sense of control. Because emergency rooms are frequently hectic, there is a tendency to rush through procedures in order to save time. However, the extra few minutes needed to allow children to participate may save many more minutes of useless resistance and uncooperativeness during subsequent procedures. Other supportive measures include ensuring privacy, accepting various emotional responses to fear or pain, preserving parent-child contact, explaining all events before or as they occur, and personally remaining calm.

At times, because of the child's physical condition, little or no preparatory counseling for emergency hospitalization can be done. In such situations the implementation of *postvention*, or counseling subsequent to the event, has therapeutic value. The process of postvention involves evaluating children's thoughts regarding admission and related procedures. It is similar to precounseling techniques; however, instead of supplying information, the nurse listens to the explanations offered by the child. Projective techniques such as drawing, doll play, or story-telling are especially effective. The nurse then bases additional information on what has already been revealed.

BOX 41-18
Essential Components of Emergency Admissions Counseling

- Appropriate introduction to the family
- Use of child's name, not terms such as "honey" or "dear"
- Determination of child's age and some judgment made about developmental age (if the child is of school age, asking about the grade level will offer some evidence for concurrent intellectual ability)
- Information about the chief complaint from both the parents and the child
- Information about child's general state of health, any problems that may interfere with medical treatment, such as sensitivity to medication, and previous experience with hospital facilities

Family Focus

ARTISTS AS PARTNERS IN CARE

A teenage boy with a rare genetic disorder, having made steady progress after awakening from a coma, relapsed and seemed very depressed. When told that the musician was on the pediatric intensive care unit (PICU), he immediately perked up and asked to have his room lights turned on. He whispered endless song requests to the musician. Family members and staff were treated to some of his first smiles in days; his biggest came when the musician held his hand and guided it across the guitar strings while they sang together at the boy's request, "Born to Be Wild." His dad was misty-eyed as he thanked the musician for the visit.

A few weeks later the boy's condition worsened and he again lapsed into a coma. There was nothing more to be done. His parents began the necessary preparations to take their son home to die.

We continued to visit our friend and his family, offering a song, a story, or just simply to say hello. I hold a vivid picture of our final visit. We stood around the boy's bed with his parents singing together songs they remembered from their youth, from more carefree times. Song and laughter filled the boy's room.

Perhaps the boy heard his parents' laughter and knew then that they would be okay. He died a few days later on the morning he was to have been discharged.

Judy Rollins, MS, RN
Washington, DC

Modified from Rollins J: *Placed in our keeping,* 1995, unpublished.

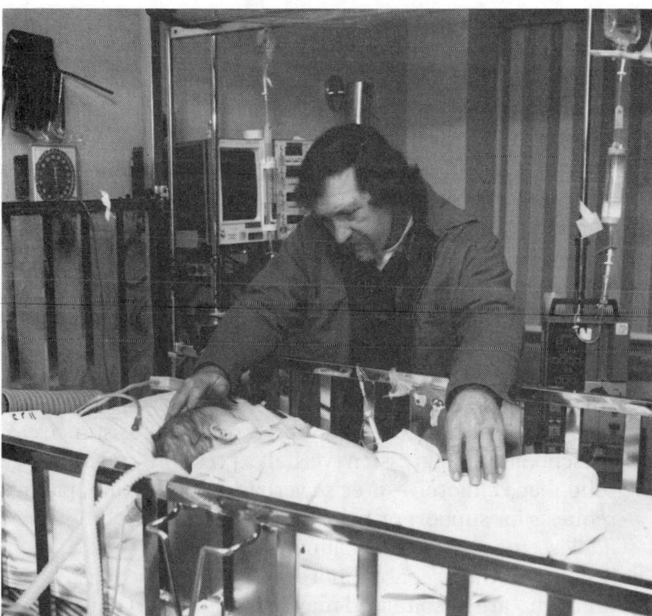

Fig. 41-14 Parents can be overwhelmed when their child is critically ill and requires care in an ICU.

INTENSIVE CARE UNIT (ICU)

Admission to an ICU can be a particularly traumatic event for both the child and the parents (Fig. 41-14). The nature and severity of the illness and the circumstances surrounding the admission are major factors, especially for parents. Parents experience significantly more stress when the admission is unexpected than expected. Stressors for the child and parent are described in Box 41-19. Although several studies have described what parents perceive as most stressful, the most effective strategy may be to simply ask parents what is stressful and what they are doing to cope with the stressors they identify (Hughes et al, 1994). Assessment should be repeated periodically to account for changes in perceptions over time.

The emotional needs of the family are paramount when a child is admitted to an ICU. While the same interventions that were discussed earlier for the stressors of separation, loss of control, and bodily injury and pain apply here, additional interventions may also benefit the family and child (see the Guidelines box on p. 1244 and the Family Focus box at left).

BOX 41-19
Neonatal/Pediatric ICU Stressors for the Child and Family

Physical Stressors

Pain and discomfort (e.g., injections, intubation, suctioning, dressing changes, other invasive procedures)
Immobility (e.g., use of restraints, bed rest)
Sleep deprivation
Inability to eat or drink
Changes in elimination habits

Environmental Stressors

Unfamiliar surroundings (e.g., crowding)
Unfamiliar sounds
  Equipment noise (e.g., monitors, telephone, suctioning, computer printout)
  Human sounds (e.g., talking, laughing, crying, coughing, moaning, retching, walking)
Unfamiliar people (e.g., health care professionals, patients, visitors)
Unfamiliar and unpleasant smells (e.g., alcohol, adhesive remover, body odors)
Constant lights (disturb day/night rhythms)
Activity related to other patients
Sense of urgency among staff
Unkind or thoughtless comments from staff

Psychologic Stressors

Lack of privacy
Inability to communicate (if intubated)
Inadequate knowledge and understanding of situation
Severity of illness
Parental behavior (expression of concern)

Social Stressors

Disrupted relationships (especially with family and friends)
Concern with missing school/work
Play deprivation

Data from Tichy AM et al: Stressors in pediatric intensive care units, *Pediatr Nurs* 14(1):40-42, 1988.

Guidelines

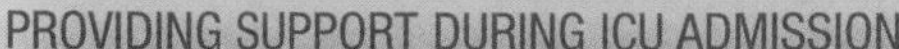

PROVIDING SUPPORT DURING ICU ADMISSION

- Prepare child and parents for elective ICU admission, such as for postoperative care after cardiac surgery.
- Prepare child and parents for unanticipated ICU admission by focusing primarily on the sensory aspects of the experience and on usual family concerns (e.g., persons in charge of child's care, schedule for visiting, area where family can stay).
- Prepare parents regarding child's appearance and behavior when they first visit child in ICU.
- Accompany family to bedside to provide emotional support and answer questions.
- Prepare siblings for their visit; plan length of time for sibling visitation; monitor siblings' reactions during visit to prevent them from becoming overwhelmed.
- Encourage parents to stay with their child:
  - If visiting hours are limited, allow flexibility in schedule to accommodate parental needs.
  - Give family members a written schedule of visiting times.
  - If visiting hours are liberal, be aware of family members' needs and suggest periodic respites.
  - Assure family they can call the unit at any time.
- Prepare parents for expected role changes and identify ways for parents to participate in child's care without overwhelming them with responsibilities:
  - Help with bath or feeding.
  - Touch and talk to child.
  - Help with procedures.
- Provide information about child's condition in understandable language:
  - Repeat information often.
  - Seek clarification of understanding.
  - During bedside conferences, interpret information for family members and child or, if appropriate, conduct report outside room.
- Prepare child for procedures, even if this involves explanation while procedure is performed.
- Assess and manage pain; recognize that a child who cannot talk, such as an infant or child in a coma or on a ventilator, can be in pain.
- Establish a routine that maintains some similarity to daily events in child's life whenever possible:
  - Organize care during normal waking hours.
  - Keep regular bedtime schedules, including quiet times when television or radio is lowered or turned off.
  - Provide uninterrupted sleep cycles (60 minutes for infant, 90 minutes for older child).
  - Close and open drapes and dim lights to allow for day/night.
  - Place curtain around bed for privacy.
  - Orient child to day and time; have clocks or calendars in easy view for older children.
- Schedule a time when child is left undisturbed (e.g., during naps, visit with family, playtime, or favorite program).
- Reduce stimulation in environment:
  - Refrain from loud talking or laughing.
  - Keep equipment noise to a minimum:
    - Turn alarms as low as safely possible.
    - Perform treatments requiring equipment at one time.
    - Turn off bedside equipment that is not in use, such as suction and oxygen.
    - Avoid loud, abrupt noises, such as clattering bedpans or toilets flushing.

Critically ill children become the focus of the parents' lives, and parents' most pressing need is for information (Fisher, 1994). They want to know if their child will live and, if so, whether the child will be the same as before. They need to know why things are being done for the child, that the child is being treated for pain and/or is comfortable, and that the child may be able to hear them even though not awake.

Despite the stresses normally associated with ICU admission, a special security develops from being carefully monitored and receiving individualized care. Therefore planning for transition to the regular unit is essential and should include (1) assignment of a primary nurse on the regular unit who visits before the transfer, (2) continued visits by the ICU staff to assess the child's and parents' adjustment and to act as a temporary liaison with the nursing staff, (3) explanation of the differences between the two units and the rationale for the change to less intense monitoring of the child's physical condition, and (4) selection of an appropriate room, such as one that is close to the nursing station, and a compatible roommate.

Key Points

- Children are particularly vulnerable to the stresses of illness and hospitalization because stress represents a change from the usual state of health and routine and because they possess limited coping mechanisms.
- The three phases of separation anxiety are protest, despair, and detachment.
- Feelings of loss of control are caused by unfamiliar environmental stimuli, physical restriction, altered routine, and dependency.
- Fear of bodily pain may be manifested in the following ways: infants—facial expressions, body movements; toddlers—intense emotional upset, physical resistance; preschoolers—aggression, verbal expression, dependency; school-age children—precise verbalization of pain, passive requests for support or help, procrastination technique; adolescents—self-control, limited movement.
- Because of their separation from significant people, children who are hospitalized may lack the opportunity to form new attachments in the strange environment of the hospital and exhibit negative behaviors after discharge.

- Nursing care of the child in the hospital is aimed at preventing or minimizing separation, decreasing loss of control, minimizing bodily injury and pain, promoting normal development, using play/expressive activities to lessen stress, and maximizing the potential benefits of hospitalization.
- Pain assessment includes questioning the child, using pain rating scales, evaluating behavior, securing parents' involvement, taking the cause of the pain into account, and taking action. Pain management should incorporate both pharmacologic and nonpharmacologic methods.
- The nurse can maximize the potential benefits of hospitalization by fostering parent-child relations, providing educational opportunities, promoting self-mastery, and encouraging socialization.
- Family reactions are influenced by the seriousness of the illness; experience with illness or hospitalization and diagnostic or therapeutic procedures; available support systems; personal ego strengths; coping abilities; presence of additional stresses; cultural and religious beliefs; and family communication patterns.
- Fear of contracting illness, their younger age, a close relationship with the ill sibling, substitute child care, minimum explanation of the illness, and perceived changes in parenting all increase the deleterious effects of a brother's or sister's illness and hospitalization on siblings.
- Nursing care of the family involves listening to parents' verbal and nonverbal messages; providing clergy support; accepting cultural, socioeconomic, and ethnic values; giving information to families and siblings; and preparing for discharge and home care.
- Admission to an outpatient setting, emergency department, isolation room, or intensive care unit requires additional intervention strategies to meet the child's and family's needs.

References

Acute Pain Management Guideline Panel: *Acute pain management in infants, children, and adolescents: operative and medical procedures: quick reference guide for clinicians,* AHCPR Pub No 92-0020, Rockville, Md, 1992, Agency for Health Care Policy and Research, Public Health Service, US Department of Health and Human Services.

American Academy of Pediatrics: Neonatal anesthesia, *Pediatrics* 80(3):446, 1987.

American Pain Society: *Principles of analgesic use in the treatment of acute pain and chronic cancer pain,* ed 3, Skokie, Ill, 1992, The Society.

Anand K, Aynsley-Green A: Metabolic and endocrine effects of surgical ligation of patent ductus arteriosus in the human preterm neonate: are there implications for further improvement of postoperative outcome? *Mod Probl Paediatr* 23:143-157, 1985.

Bauchner H, May A, Coates E: Use of analgesic agents for invasive medical procedures in pediatric and neonatal intensive care units, *J Pediatr* 121(4):647-649, 1992.

Benini F et al: Topical anesthesia during circumcision in newborn infants, *JAMA* 270(7):850-853, 1993.

Beyer JE et al: Patterns of postoperative analgesic use with adults and children following cardiac surgery, *Pain* 17:71-81, 1983.

Beyer JE et al: *The Oucher: a user's manual and technical report,* Bethesda, Md, 1995, Association for the Care of Children's Health.

Bossert E: Stress appraisals of hospitalized school-age children, *Child Health Care* 23(1):33-49, 1994.

Britton LJ, Johnston JD: Dependent on technology: a child grows up hospitalized, *Pediatr Nurs* 19(6):579, 1993.

Broome M et al: Children's medical fears, coping behaviors, and pain perceptions during a lumbar puncture, *Oncol Nurs Forum* 17(3):361-367, 1990.

Carson D, Gravley J, Council J: Children's prehospitalization conceptions of illness, cognitive development, and personal adjustment, *Child Health Care* 21(2):103-110, 1992.

Craft M: Siblings of hospitalized children: assessment and intervention, *J Pediatr Nurs* 8(5):289-297, 1993.

Darbyshire P: *Living with a sick child in hospital,* London, 1994, Chapman & Hall.

Davidson JAH, Boom SJ: Warming lidocaine to reduce pain associated with injection, *Br Med J* 305:617-618, 1992.

Eisenberg DM et al: Unconventional medicine in the United States: prevalence, costs, and patterns of use, *N Engl J Med* 328(4):246-252, 1993.

Eland J: *Children with pain.* In Jackson OB, Saunders RB: *Child health nursing,* Philadelphia, 1993, JB Lippincott.

Eland J, Anderson JE: *The experience of pain in children.* In Jacox A, editor: *Pain: a source book for nurses and other health professionals,* Boston, 1977, Little, Brown.

Farrington E: Lidocaine 2.5%/prilocaine 2.5% EMLA Cream, *Pediatr Nurs* 19(5):484-486, 488, 1993.

Favaloro R, Touzel B: A comparison of adolescents' and nurses' postoperative pain ratings and perceptions, *Pediatr Nurs* 16(4):414-417, 424, 1990.

Fisher M: Identified needs of parents in a pediatric intensive care unit, *Crit Care Nurse* 14(3):82-90, 1994.

Franck L: A national survey of the assessment and treatment of pain and agitation in the neonatal intensive care unit, *J Obstet Gynecol Neonatal Nurs* 16:387-393, 1987.

French GM, Painter EC, Courty DL: Blowing away shot pain: a technique for pain management during immunization, *Pediatrics* 93(3):384-388, 1994.

Friedland LR, Kulick RM: Emergency department analgesic use in pediatric trauma victims with fractures, *Ann Emerg Med* 23(2):203-207, 1994.

Friedman DP: Perspectives on the medical use of drugs of abuse, *J Pain Symptom Manage* 5(1):52-55, 1990.

Gaynard L et al: *Psychosocial care of children in hospitals,* Bethesda, Md, 1990, Association for the Care of Children's Health.

Gordon M: *Nursing diagnosis: process and application,* ed 3, St Louis, 1994, Mosby.

Gordon M: *Manual of nursing diagnosis: 1995-1996,* St Louis, 1995, Mosby.

Gillis A: Hospital preparation: the children's story, *Child Health Care* 19(1):19-27, 1990.

Gureno MA, Reisinger CL: Patient-controlled analgesia for the young pediatric patient, *Pediatr Nurs* 1991.

Hart D, Bossert E: Self-reported fears of hospitalized school-age children, *J Pediatr Nurs* 9(2):83-90, 1994.

Hart RH et al: *Therapeutic play activities for hospitalized children,* St Louis, 1992, Mosby.

Hester NO, Foster RL, Kristensen K: *Measurement of pain in children: generalizability and validity of the pain ladder and poker chip tool.* In Tyler D, Krane E, editors: *Advances in pain research and therapy: pediatric pain 15,* New York, 1990, Raven Press.

Hinnant DC: Reality check on placebos, *Am J Nurs* 95(8):20, 1995.
Hughes M, et al: How parents cope with the experience of neonatal intensive care, *Child Health Care* 23(1):1-14, 1994.
Johnson BH, Jeppson ES, Redburn L: *Caring for children and families: guidelines for hospitals*, ed 1, Bethesda, Md, 1992, Association for the Care of Children's Health.
Jones RDM et al: Antagonism of the hypnotic effect of midazolam in children: a randomized double-blind study of placebo and flumazenil administered after midazolam-induced anesthesia, *Brit J Anaesthesia* 66:660-666, 1991.
Kury S, Rodrigue J: Concepts of illness causality in a pediatric sample: relationship to illness duration, frequency of hospitalization, and degree of life-threat, *Clin Pediatrics* 34(4):178-184, 1995.
Lefkowicz AB, Keller V, Wong DL, Clutter LB: Young children's pain rating using the FACES Pain Rating Scale with original vs abbreviated word instructions. Part 2. In Wong DL, Baker CM: Reference manual for the Wong-Baker FACES Pain Rating Scale, Duarte, CA, 1997 (revised).
Love G: The dangers of normepederine toxicity, *Am J Nurs* 94(6):14, 1994.
Mather L, Mackie J: The incidence of postoperative pain in children, *Pain* 15:271-282, 1983.
McCaffery M: Analgesics: mapping out pain relief, *Nurs 96* 26(1):41-46, 1996.
McCaffery M, Beebe A: *Pain: clinical manual for nursing practice*, St Louis, 1989, Mosby.
Nugent K et al: A practice model for a parent support group, *Pediatr Nurs* 18(1):11-16, 1992.
O'Malley M, McNamara S: Children's drawings: a preoperative assessment tool, *AORN J* 57(5):1074-1089, 1993.
Orem D: *Nursing: concepts of practice*, ed 5, St Louis, 1995, Mosby.
Orlinsky M et al: Pain comparison of unbuffered versus buffered lidocaine in local wound infiltration, *J Emerg Med* 10:411-415, 1992.
Pasero CL, McCaffery M: Avoiding opioid-induced respiratory depression, *Am J Nurs* 94(4):25-31, 1994.
Pederson C: Presence as a nursing intervention with hospitalized children, *Matern Child Nurs J* 21(3):75-81, 1993.
Petrillo M, Sanger S: *Emotional care of hospitalized children*, ed 2, Philadelphia, 1980, JB Lippincott.
Pfefferbaum B, Adams J, Aceves, J: The influence of culture on pain in Anglo and Hispanic children with cancer, *J Am Acad Child Adolesc Psychiatry* 29(4):642-647, 1990.
Rae W: Analyzing drawings of children who are physically ill or hospitalized using the Ipsative method, *Child Health Care* 20(4):198-207, 1991.
Rollins J: Medical students as facilitators of the arts for children in hospitals, *Int J Arts Med* 2(1):7-13, 1993.
Rollins J: Art: helping children meet the challenges of hospitalization, *Interacta* 15(3):36-41, 1995.
Rowbothan D et al: Transdermal fentanyl for the relief of pain after upper abdominal surgery, Br J Anaesth 63:56-59, 1989.
Ruble K, Billett C: Innovative pain management for toddlers: parent-controlled analgesia, *Oncol Nurse Forum* 20(2):321, 1993.
Schepp K: Correlates of mothers who prefer control over their hospitalized child's care, *J Pediatr Nurs* 7(2):83-89, 1992.
Sciarillo W: Humanizing health care for children and families: revitalizing the spirit of our work, *ACCH Advocate* 2(11):4-8, 1995.
Simon K: Perceived stress of nonhospitalized children during the hospitalization of a sibling, *J Pediatr Nurs* 8(5):298-304, 1993.
Snowdon A, Dane D: Parental needs following the discharge of the hospitalized child, *Pediatr Nurs* 21(5):425-428, 1995.
Stepanek JS, Ahmann E: Parent-professional collaboration when hospital visits are infrequent, *Pediatr Nurs* 21(5):466-468, 1995.
Taddio A et al: Safety of lidocaine-prilocaine cream in the treatment of preterm neonates, *J Pediatr* 127(6):1002-1005, 1995.
Tesler M et al: The word-graphic rating scale as a measure of children's and adolescents' pain intensity, *Res Nurs Health* 14:361-371, 1991.
Vessey JA, Carlson KL, McGill J: Use of distraction with children during an acute pain experience, *Nurs Res* 43(6):369, 1994.
Walker M, Wong DL: A battle plan for patients in pain, *Am J Nurs* 91(6):32-36, 1991.
Wallace M: Temperament: a variable in children's pain management, *Pediatr Nurs* 15(2):118-121, 1989.
Watt-Watson JH, Evernden C, Lawson C: Parents' perceptions of their child's acute pain experience, *J Pediatr Nurs* 5(5):344-349, 1990.
Webb C, Paarlberg J, Sussman M: The use of a PCA device by parents or nurses for postoperative pain in children with cerebral palsy, *J Pain Symptom Manage* 6(3):160, 1991.
Wells P et al: Growing up in the hospital. I. Let's focus on the child, *J Pediatr Nurs* 9(2):66-73, 1994.
West N et al: Measuring pain in pediatric patients in the ICU, *J Pediatr Oncol Nurs* 11(2):64-68, 1994.
Whitis G: Visiting hospitalized patients, *J Adv Nurs* 19(1):85-88, 1994.
Willens JS: Giving fentanyl for pain outside the OR, *Am J Nurs* 94(2):24-28, 1994.
Wong D, Baker C: Pain in children: comparison of assessment scales, *Pediatr Nurs* 14(1):9-17, 1988.
Wong D, Baker C: *Reference manual for the Wong-Baker FACES Pain Rating Scale*, Tulsa, Okla, 1996, Wong & Baker.

Bibliography

Hospitalization: The Child and Family

Adams H: Humor: strong medicine ... in a children's burn unit in a hospital in Tallinn, Estonia, *IJAM* 2(2):22-23, 1993.
American Academy of Pediatrics, Committee on Hospital Care: Staffing patterns for patient care and support personnel in a general pediatric unit, *Pediatrics* 93(5):850-854, 1994.
Baker N: Avoiding collisions with challenging families, *Am J Matern Child Nurs* 19(2):97-101, 1994.
Banks E: Concepts of health and sickness of preschool- and school-aged children, *Child Health Care* 19(1):43-48, 1990.
Balayewich C, Gasson A: Oh, Suzanna! A nursing challenge, *Axone* 15(1):9-12, 1993.
Biddinger L: Bruner's theory of instruction and preprocedural anxiety in the pediatric population, *Issues Compr Pediatr Nurs* 16(3):147-154, 1993.
Biehler B: Impact of role-sets on implementing self-care theory with children, *Pediatr Nurs* 18(1):30-34, 1992.
Bolig R, Brown R, Kuo J: A comparison of never-hospitalized and previously hospitalized adolescents: self-esteem and locus of control, *Adolescence* 27(105):227-234, 1992.
Bossert E: Factors influencing the coping of hospitalized school-age children, *J Pediatr Nurs* 9(5):299-306, 1994.
Britton L et al: Dependent on technology: a child grows up hospitalized, *Pediatr Nurs* 19(6):579-584, 1993.
Brown J, Ritchie JA: Nurses' perceptions of parent and nurse roles in caring for hospitalized children, *Child Health Care* 19(1):28-36, 1990.
Burke SO et al: Hazardous secrets and reluctantly taking charge: parenting a child with repeated hospitalizations, *Image J Nurs Sch* 23(1):39-45, 1991.
Chambers M: Play as therapy for the hospitalized child, *J Clin Nurs* 2(6):349-353, 1993.
Coffman S, Levitt MJ, Guacci-Franco N: Mothers' stress and close relationships: correlates with infant health status, *Pediatr Nurs* 19(2):135-140, 1993.
Coyne I: Partnership in care: parents' views of participation in their hospitalized child's care, *J Clin Nurs* 4(2):71-79, 1995.

Curley MA, Wallace J: Effects of the nursing Mutual Participation Model of Care on parental stress in the pediatric intensive care unit: a replication, *J Pediatr Nurs* 7(6):377-385, 1992.

Curtin L: There's no place like home, *Nurs Manag* 26(1):26-29, 1995.

Darbyshire P: Parents, nurses and paediatric nursing: a critical review, *J Adv Nurs* 18(11):1670-1680, 1993.

Darbyshire P: Parents in paediatrics, *Paediatr Nurs* 7(1):8-9, 1995.

Denholm CJ: Memories of adolescent hospitalization: results from a 4-year follow-up study, *Child Health Care* 19(2):101-105, 1990.

Dixon DM: Parent and nurse interaction during acute care, pediatric hospitalization, *Capsules Comments Pediatr Nurs* 2(2):91-99, 1995.

Evans M: An investigation into the feasibility of parental participation in the nursing care of their children, *J Adv Nurs* 20(3):477-482, 1994.

Gaynard L, Goldberger J, Laidley L: The use of stuffed body-outline dolls with hospitalized children and adolescents, *Child Health Care* 20(4):216-224, 1991.

Glendon K et al: Using a personal storybook and Mr. Potato Head toy as a creative approach to individualized teaching, *ACCH Advocate* 1(12):49-51, 1993.

Goodill S et al: The role of dance/movement therapy with medically involved children, *IJAM* 2(2):24-27, 1993.

Graves JK, Ware ME: Parents' and health professionals' perceptions concerning parental stress during a child's hospitalization, *Child Health Care* 19(10):37-42, 1990.

Greenberg LA: Teaching children who are learning disabled about illness and hospitalization, *Am J Matern Child Nurs* 16(5):260-263, 1991.

Grey M: Stressors and children's health, *J Pediatr Nurs* 8(2):85-91, 1993.

Grimm DL, Pefley PT: Opening doors for the child "inside," *Pediatr Nurs* 16(4):368-369, 1990.

Jones D: Effect of parental participation on hospitalized child behavior, *Issues Compr Pediatr Nurs* 17(2):81-92, 1994.

Kennedy C, Gyr P, Garst K: A nursing tool to assess children upon hospital admission, *Am J Matern Child Nurs* 16(2):78-82, 1991.

Kristjansdottir G: A study of the needs of parents of hospitalized 2 to 6 year-old children, *Issues Compr Pediatr Nurs* 14(1):49-64, 1991.

Lau C: Parents in partnership: a family centered care program, *Paediatr Nurs* 6(2):11-15, 1993.

Levi R: Childhood illness through a child's eyes, *ACCH Advocate* 2(1):43-45, 1995.

LeVieux-Anglin L et al: Incorporating play interventions into nursing care, *Pediatr Nurs* 19(5):459-463, 1993.

Lipsi K, Clements-Shafer K, Rushton C: Developmental rounds: an intervention strategy for hospitalized infants, *Pediatr Nurs* 17(5):433-437, 468, 1991.

Lloyd J et al: Screening for psychosocial dysfunction in pediatric inpatients, *Clin Pediatrics* 34(1):18-24, 1995.

Logsdon DA: Conceptions of health and health behaviors of preschool children, *J Pediatr Nurs* 6(6):396-406, 1991.

Mabe P, Treiber F, Riley W: Examining emotional distress during pediatric hospitalization for school-aged children, *Child Health Care* 20(3):162-169, 1991.

McBurney BH, Schultz C: Defining quality services in a general pediatric unit, *J Nurs Care Qual* 7(3):51-60, 1993.

McClowry SG: The relationship of temperament to pre- and posthospitalization behavioral responses of school-age children, *Nurs Res* 39(1):30-35, 1990.

McClowry SG: Behavioral disturbances among medically hospitalized school-age children, *J Child Adolesc Psychiatr Ment Health Nurs* 4(2):62-67, 1991.

McClowry SG, McLeod SM: The psychosocial responses of school-age children to hospitalization, *Child Health Care* 19(3):155-161, 1990.

McLeod SM, McClowry SG: Using temperament theory to individualize the psychosocial care of hospitalized children, *Child Health Care* 19(2):79-85, 1990.

Merkens MJ: A pediatric chronic illness transition unit, *Child Health Care* 19(1):4-9, 1990.

Miron J: What children think about hospitals, *Can Nurs* 86(3):23-25, 1990.

Nelson-Smith J: Programs for play . . . real benefits of computers for children in hospital, *Nurs Times* 87(42):55-57, 1991.

Nix KS: *Children and the health care system.* In Smith DP et al, editors: *Comprehensive child and family nursing skills,* St Louis, 1991, Mosby.

Palmer S: Care of sick children by parents: a meaningful role, *J Adv Nurs* 18(2):185-191, 1993.

Porter CP, Villarruel AM: Socialization and caring for hospitalized African- and Mexican-American children, *Issues Compr Pediatr Nurs* 14(1):1-16, 1991.

Price S: The special needs of children, *J Adv Nurs* 20(2):227-232, 1994.

Rape R, Bush J: Psychological preparation for pediatric oncology patients undergoing painful procedures: a methodological critique of the research, *Child Health Care* 23(1):51-67, 1994.

Rikard-Bell C: The impact of critical incidents in paediatric hospitals: a review, *Aust J Adv Nurs* 12(1):29-35, 1994.

Schepp KG: Factors influencing the coping effort of mothers of hospitalized children, *Nurs Res* 40(1):42-46, 1991.

Slusher IL, McClure MJ: Infant stimulation during hospitalization, *J Pediatr Nurs* 7(4):276-279, 1992.

Strachan R: Emotional responses to paediatric hospitalisation, *Nurs Times* 89(46):45-49, 1993.

Thomas S: Child's play? . . . physical and emotional needs of sick children, *Nurs Times* 90(3):42-44, 1994.

Tiedman M, Clatworthy S: Anxiety responses of 5- and 11-year-old children during and after hospitalization, *J Pediatr Nurs* 5(5):334-343, 1990.

Tye V et al: Children's distress during magnetic resonance imaging procedures, *Child Health Care* 24(1):5-19, 1995.

Vessey J, Mahon M: Therapeutic play and the hospitalized child, *J Pediatr Nurs* 5(5):328-333, 1990.

Wells P et al: Growing up in the hospital: nurturing the philosophy of family-centered care. II, *J Pediatr Nurs* 9(3):141-149, 1994.

While A: The contribution of nurses to children's well-being in hospital: a selective review of the literature, *J Clin Nurs* 1(3):117-121, 1992.

White MA et al: Sleep onset latency and distress in hospitalized children, *Nurs Res* 39(3):134-139, 1990.

Wilson C: Use of children's artwork to evaluate the effectiveness of a hospital preparation program, *Child Health Care* 20(2):120-121, 1991.

Wright MC: Behavioral effects of hospitalization in children, *J Paediatr Child Health* 31:165-167, 1995.

Yoos HL: Children's illness concepts: old and new paradigms, *Pediatr Nurs* 20(2):134-140, 145, 1994.

Young J: Changing attitudes towards families of hospitalized children from 1935 to 1975: a case study, *J Adv Nurs* 17(12):1422-1429, 1992.

Ziegler D et al: Preparation for surgery and adjustment to hospitalization, *Nurs Clin North Am* 29(4):655-669, 1994.

Special Hospital Situations

Bernardo LM, Conway K, Bove M: The ABC method of emotional assessment and intervention: a new approach in pediatric emergency care, *J Emerg Nurs* 16(2):70-76, 1990.

Braun R et al: Transitional family care: PICU to pediatrics, *Crit Care Nurse* 14(4):65-68, 1994.

Brunnquell D, Kohen D: Emotions in pediatric emergencies: what we know, what we can do, *Child Health Care* 20(4):240-247, 1991.

Curley MAQ: Caring for parents of critically ill children, *Crit Care Med* 21(9, suppl):S386-S387, 1993.

Doll-Speck L, Miller B, Rohrs K: Sibling education: implementing a program for the NICU, *Neonatal Network* 12(4)P:49-52, 1993.

Gillis AJ: Hospital preparation: the children's story, *Child Health Care* 19(1):19-27, 1990.

Heuer L: Parental stressors in a pediatric intensive care unit, *Pediatr Nurs* 19(2):128-131, 1993.

LaMontagne L et al: Psychophysiological responses of parents to pediatric critical care stress, *Clin Nurs Res* 3(2):104-118, 1994.

LaMontagne L, Pawlak R: Stress and coping of parents of children in a pediatric intensive care unit, *Heart Lung* 19(4):416-421, 1990.

Lynch M: Preparing children for day surgery, *Child Health Care* 23(3):78-85, 1994.

Melnyk B: Coping with unplanned childhood hospitalization: effects of informational interventions on mothers and children, *Nurs Res* 43(1):50-55, 1994.

Miles MS, Funk SG, Carelson J: Parental stressor scale: neonatal intensive care unit, *Nurs Res* 42(3):148-152, 1993.

Miles M, Mathes M: Preparation of parents for the ICU experience: what are we missing? *Child Health Care* 20(3):132-137, 1991.

Page N et al: Visitation in the pediatric intensive care unit: controversy and compromise, *AACN Clin Issues Crit Care Nurs* 5(3):289-295, 1994.

Pawlak R, Chiafery M: Parental coping and activities during pediatric critical care, *Am J Crit Care* 1(2):76-80, 1992.

Prudhoe C, Peters, D: Social support of parents and grandparents in the neonatal intensive care unit, *Pediatr Nurs* 21(2):140-146, 1995.

Rushton CH: Family-centered care in the critical care setting: myth or reality? *Child Health Care* 19(2):68-78, 1990a.

Rushton CH: Strategies for family-centered care in the critical care setting, *Pediatr Nurs* 16(2):195-199, 1990b.

Rushton CH: Child/family advocacy: ethical issues, practical strategies, *Crit Care Med* 21(9, suppl):S387, 1993.

Saunders, A: Changing nurses' attitudes toward parenting in the NICU, *Pediatr Nurs* 20(4):392-394, 1994.

Small M, Engler A, Rushton C: Saying goodbye in the intensive care unit: helping caregivers grieve, *Pediatr Nurs* 17(1):103-105, 1991.

Stern HP et al: Communication, decision making, and perception of nursing roles in a pediatric intensive care unit, *Crit Care Nurs Q* 14(3):56-68, 1991.

Thomas DO: How to deal with children in the emergency department, *J Emerg Nurs* 17(1):49-50, 1991.

Todres ID: Communication between physician, patient, and family in the pediatric intensive care unit, *Crit Care Med* 21(9, suppl):S383-S385, 1993.

Tughan L: Visiting in the PICU: a study of the perceptions of patients, parents, and staff members, *Crit Care Nurs Q* 15(1):57-68, 1992.

Vessey J, Farley J, Risom L: Iatrogenic developmental effects of pediatric intensive care, *Pediatr Nurs* 17(3):229-232, 1991.

Voepel-Lewis T, Andrea CM, Magee SS: Parent perceptions of pediatric ambulatory surgery: using family feedback for program evaluation, *J Post Anesth Nurs* 7(2):106-114, 1992.

Youngblut JM, Shiao SP: Child and family reactions during and after pediatric ICU hospitalization: a pilot study, *Heart Lung*, 22, 46-53, 1993.

While A, Wilcox, V: Paediatric day surgery: day-case unit admission compared with general paediatric ward admission, *J Adv Nurs* 19(1):52-57, 1994.

Pain Assessment

Beard J: Pain control: when your patient can't speak, *Am J Nurs* 94(4):22-23, 1994.

Beyer JE, Denyes MJ, Villarruel AM: The creation, validation and continuing development of the Oucher: a measure of pain intensity in children, *J Pediatr Nurs* 7(5):335-346, 1992.

Beyer JE, Knapp TR: Methodologic issues in the measurement of children's pain, *Child Health Care* 14(4):233-241, 1986.

Beyer JE, McGrath PJ, Berde CB: Discordance between self-report and behavioral pain measures in children aged 3-7 years after surgery, *J Pain Symptom Manag* 5(6):350-356, 1990.

Beyer JE, Wells N: The assessment of pain in children, *Pediatr Clin North Am* 36(4):837-854, 1989.

Bieri D et al: The Faces Pain Scale for the self-assessment of the severity of pain experienced by children: development, initial validation, and preliminary investigation for ratio scale properties, *Pain* 41(2):139-150, 1990.

Broome M: Measurement of pain: self-report strategies, *J Pediatr Oncol Nurs* 8(3):131-133, 1991.

Eland JM, Banner W: *Assessment and management of pain in children.* In Hazinski MF: *Nursing care of the critically ill child,* ed 2, St Louis, 1992, Mosby.

Gujol MC: A survey of pain assessment and management practices among critical care nurses, *Am J Crit Care* 3(2):123-128, 1994.

Harbeck C, Peterson L: Elephants dancing in my head: a developmental approach to children's concepts of specific pains, *Child Dev* 63:138-149, 1992.

Hester NO: *Pain in children.* In Fitzpatrick JJ, Stevenson JS, editors: *Annual review of nursing research,* vol 11, New York, 1993, Springer.

Jordan-Marsh M et al: Alternate Oucher form testing gender ethnicity and age variations, *Res Nurs Health* 17:111-118, 1994.

Knott C et al: Using the Oucher: developmental approach to pain assessment in children, *Am J Matern Child Nurs* 19(6):314-320, 1994.

Kuttner L, LePage T: Face scales for the assessment of pediatric pain: a critical review, *Can J Behav Sci* 21(2) 198-209, 1989.

LaMontagne LL et al: Children's ratings of postoperative pain compared to ratings by nurses and physicians, *Issues Compr Pediatr Nurs* 14(4):241-247, 1991.

Lincoln LM: Children's response to acute pain: a developmental approach, *J Am Acad Nurse Practitioners* 4(4):139-141, 1992.

Mackey D, Jordan-Marsh M: Innovative assessment of children's pain, *J Emerg Nurs* 17(4):205-215, 1991.

McCaffery M: How reliable is your patient's pain assessment? *Nursing 94* 24(1):19, 1994.

McCaffery M, Ferrel B: Opioid analgesics: nurses' knowledge of doses and psychological dependence, *J Nurs Staff Dev* 8(2):77-84, 1992.

McGrath PA: Evaluating a child's pain, *J Pain Symptom Manag* 4(4):198-214, 1989.

McGrath PJ, Craig KD: Developmental and psychological factors in children's pain, *Pediatr Clin North Am* 36(4):823-836, 1989.

Pasero CL: The right tool for the job, *Am J Nurs* 94(2):22, 1994.

Savedra MC et al: Assessment of postoperative pain in children and adolescents using the Adolescent Pediatric Pain tool, *Nurs Res* 42(1):5-9, 1993.

Schechter NL: The undertreatment of pain in children: an overview, *Pediatr Clin North Am* 36(4):781-794, 1989.

Schmidt K, Eland J, Weiler K: Pediatric cancer pain management: a survey of nurses' knowledge, *J Pediatr Oncol Nurs* 11(1):4-12, 1994.

Stevens B: Development and testing of a pediatric pain management sheet, *Pediatr Nurs* 16(6):543-548, 1990.

Van Cleve L, Savedra M: Pain location: validity and reliability of body outline markings for 4- to 7-year-old children who are hospitalized, *Pediatr Nurs* 19(3):217-220, 1993.

Wilkie DJ et al: Measuring pain quality: validity and reliability of children's and adolescents' pain language, *Pain* 41:151-159, 1990.

Wong DL: Pediatric pain assessment scales: where do we go from here? *J Pediatr Oncol Nurs* 11(2):69-70, 1994.

Wong DL: The FACES pain rating scale, *Home Health Focus* 2(8):63, 1996.

Wong DL, Baker C: The school nurse and the child in pain, *Sch Nurs* 5(2):14-28, 1989.

Pain Management

Bonadio W, Wagner V: Adrenaline—cocaine gel topical anesthetic for dermal laceration repair in children, *Ann Emerg Med* 21(12):1435-1438, 1992.

Bostrom B, McCormick P, Hooke C: Painless procedures with propofol, *J Pediatr Oncol Nurs* 10(2):64-65, 1993.

Broome M, Lillis P, Smith MC: Pain management with children: a meta-analysis of the research, *Nurs Res* 2:154-158, 1989.

Engebo D: Safe and effective use of tetracaine, adrenaline, and cocaine (TAC) solution anesthetic for anesthetizing of lacerations, *J Emerg Nurs* 16(2):100-101, 1990.

French JP, Nocera M: Drug withdrawal symptoms in children after continuous infusions of fentanyl, *J Pediatr Nurs* 9(2):107-113, 1994.
Fox AE: Confronting the use of placebos for pain, *Am J Nurs* 9(9):42-46, 1994.
Goode IA, Betcher DL: EMLA, *J Pediatr Oncol Nurs* 11(1):38-41, 1994.
Gordon D: Hydroxyzine doesn't 'help' opioids, *Am J Nurs* 95(8):20, 1995.
Heiney S: Helping children through painful procedures, *Am J Nurs* 1(11):20-24, 1991.
Howe CJ: A new standard of care for pediatric pain management, *Am J Matern Child Nurs* 18(6):325-329, 1993.
Leaby S, Hockenberry-Eaton M, Sigler-Price K: Clinical management of pain in children with cancer: selected approaches and innovative strategies, *Cancer Pract* 2(1):37-45, 1994.
Pederson C: Ways to feel comfortable: teaching aids to promote children's comfort, *Issues Compr Pediatr Nurs* 17(1):37-46, 1994.
Position statement in the role of the RN in the management of patients receiving IV conscious sedation for short-term therapeutic, diagnostic, or surgical procedures, *AORN J* 55:207-208, 1992.
Proudfoot J: Analgesia, anesthesia, and conscious sedation, *Emerg Med Clin North Am* 13(2):357-379, 1995.
Sacchetti A et al: Pediatric analgesia and sedation, *Ann Emerg Med* 23:237-250, 1994.
Schechter NL, Altman A, Weisman S: Report of the Consensus Conference on the Management of Pain in Childhood Cancer, *Pediatrics* 86(5, suppl):813-834, 1990.
Schechter NL et al: The use of oral transmucosal fentanyl citrate for painful procedures in children, *Pediatrics* 95(3):335-339, 1995.
Selbst SM, Clark M: Analgesic use in the emergency department, *Ann Emerg Med* 19:1010-1013, 1990.
Steward DJ: Management of childhood pain: new approaches to procedure-related pain, *J Pediatr* 122(5, pt 2):entire issue, 1993.
Taddio A et al: Use of lidocaine-prilocaine cream for vaccination pain in infants, *J Pediatr* 124(4):643-648, 1994.
Tobias JD: Indications and applications of epidural anesthesia in a pediatric population outside the perioperative period, *Clin Pediatr* 32(2):81-85, 1993.
Tobias JD, Rasmussen GE: Pain management and sedation in the pediatric intensive care unit, *Pediatr Clin North Am* 41(6):1269-1292, 1994.
Tobias JD et al: Oral ketamine premedication to alleviate the distress of invasive procedures in pediatric oncology patients, *Pediatrics* 90(4):537-541, 1992.
Tyler DC: Pharmacology of pain management, *Pediatr Clin North Am* 41(1):59, 1994.
Valente S: Using hypnosis with children for pain management, *Oncol Nurs Forum*, 18(4):699-704, 1991.
Weisman SJ, Schechter NL: The management of pain in children, *Pediatr Rev* 12(8):237-243, 1991.
Wong DL: *Managing pain.* In Smith DP et al, editors: *Comprehensive child and family nursing skills,* St Louis, 1991, Mosby.
Wong DL: DPT pedi-cocktail: not a good mix, *Am J Nurs* 94(6):14-15, 1994.
Wong DL: Overcoming 'needle phobia' with EMLA, *Am J Nurs* 65(2):24, 1995.
Yaster M: Pain relief, *Pediatrics* 95(3):427-428, 1995.
Yaster M et al: Local anesthetics in the management of acute pain in children, *J Pediatr* 124(2):165-176, 1994.
Zajac J: Pediatric pain management, *Crit Care Nurse Q* 15(2):35-51, 1992.

Discharge Planning and Home Care

Cady C, Yoshioka R: Using a learning contract to successfully discharge an infant on home total parenteral nutrition, *Pediatr Nurs* 17(1):67-71, 74, 1991.
Crummette B, Boatwright D: Case management in inpatient pediatric nursing, *Pediatr Nurs* 17(5):469-473, 1991.
Curry R, Cullen J: Using videorecordings in pediatric nursing practice, *Pediatr Nurs* 16(5):501-504, 1990.
DeWitt P et al: Obstacles to discharge of ventilator-assisted children from the hospital to home, *Chest* 103(5):1560-1565, 1993.
Hill DS: Coordinating a multidisciplinary discharge for the technology-dependent child based on parental needs, *Issues Compr Pediatr Nurs* 16(4):229-237, 1993.
Hogue E: Liability for premature discharge: an update, *Pediatr Nurs* 17(1):76, 78, 1991.
Isaacman DJ et al: Standardized instructions: do they improve communication of discharge information from the emergency department? *Pediatrics* 89(6):1204-1208, 1992.
Kasprisin C: *Home care instructions.* In Wong DL: *Wong and Whaley's clinical manual of pediatric nursing,* ed 4, St Louis, 1996, Mosby.
McClowry SG: Pediatric nursing psychosocial care: a vision beyond hospitalization, *Pediatr Nurs* 19(2):146-148, 1993.
Nuttall P, Nicholes P: Cystic fibrosis: adolescent and maternal concerns about hospital and home care, *Issues Compr Pediatr Nurs* 15(3):199-213, 1992.
Scharer K et al: Evaluating written discharge instructions in a pediatric setting, *J Nurs Qual Assur* 4(4):63-71, 1990.
Sheikh L, O'Brien M, McCluskey-Fawcett K: Parent preparation for the NICU-to-home transition: staff and parent perceptions, *Child Health Care* 22(3):227-239, 1993.
Siarkowski-Amer K, Piegeon V: Documentation of discharge teaching before and after use of a discharge teaching tool, *J Pediatr Nurs* 6(5):296-301, 1991.
While AE: Consumer views of health care: a comparison of hospital and home care, *Child Care Health Dev* 18(2):107-116, 1992.
Wong DL: Transition from hospital to home for children with complex medical care, *J Pediatr Oncol Nurs* 8(1):3-9, 1991.
Worthington R: Family matters. Effective transitions for families: life beyond the hospital, *Pediatr Nurs* 21(1):86-87, 1995.

Selected Books for Children

Banks A: *Hospital journal: a kid's guide to a strange place,* New York, 1989, Viking Penguin.
Chase F, Coleman L: *A visit to the hospital,* New York, 1974, Grosset & Dunlap.
Clark B: *Going to the hospital,* New York, 1970, Random House (pop-up book).
Collier J: *Danny goes to the hospital,* New York, 1970, WW Norton.
Drescher, J: *The moon balloon,* Bethesda, Md, 1996, Association for the Care of Children's Health.
Howe J: *The hospital book,* New York, 1981, Crown.
Moore A: *Broken Arrow boy,* Kansas City, Mo, 1990, Landmark Editions.
Rey M, Rey H: *Curious George goes to the hospital,* New York, 1966, Houghton Mifflin.
Stein S: *A hospital story,* New York, 1974, Walker.
Weber A: *Elizabeth gets well,* New York, 1970, Thomas Y Crowell.

Other Resources

Association for Care of Children's Health, 7910 Woodmont Ave., Suite 300, Bethesda, MD 20814; (301) 654-6549.
Centering Corporation, 1531 N. Saddle Creek Rd., Omaha, NE 68104; (402) 555-1200.
Talks About the Hospital, a series written by Fred Rogers, is available from Family Communications, Inc., 4802 Fifth Ave., Pittsburgh, PA 15213; (412) 687-2990.

CHAPTER 42

Pediatric Nursing Interventions

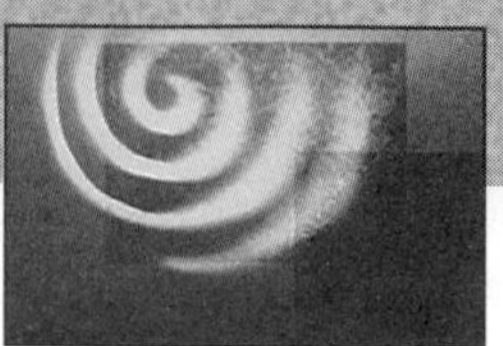

GENERAL CONCEPTS RELATED TO PEDIATRIC PROCEDURES, P. 1250

Informed consent, p. 1250
Preparation for procedures, p. 1252
Surgical procedures, p. 1257
Compliance, p. 1262

GENERAL HYGIENE AND CARE, P. 1264

Maintaining healthy skin, p. 1264
Bathing, p. 1266
Oral hygiene, p. 1266
Hair care, p. 1267
Feeding the sick child, p. 1268
Controlling elevated temperatures, p. 1268
Family teaching and home care, p. 1271

SAFETY, P. 1271

Infection control, p. 1272
Environmental factors, p. 1274
Limit-setting, p. 1275
Transporting infants and children, p. 1275
Restraints, p. 1276
Positioning for procedures, p. 1278

COLLECTION OF SPECIMENS, P. 1280

Urine specimens, p. 1280
Stool specimens, p. 1282
Blood specimens, p. 1282
Respiratory secretion/throat specimens, p. 1284

ADMINISTRATION OF MEDICATION, P. 1284

Preparation for safe administration, p. 1284
Oral administration, p. 1286
Intramuscular (IM) administration, p. 1288
Subcutaneous and intradermal administration, p. 1292
Intravenous (IV) administration, p. 1293
Nasogastric, orogastric, or gastrostomy administration, p. 1296
Rectal administration, p. 1296
Optic, otic, and nasal administration, p. 1297
Family teaching and home care, p. 1298

PROCEDURES RELATED TO MAINTAINING FLUID BALANCE, P. 1299

Measurement of intake and output (I & O), p. 1299
Parenteral fluid therapy, p. 1299
Family teaching and home care, p. 1302

PROCEDURES FOR MAINTAINING RESPIRATORY FUNCTION, P. 1302

Inhalation therapy, p. 1302
Bronchial (postural) drainage, p. 1305
Chest physiotherapy (CPT), p. 1305
Artificial ventilation, p. 1305
Family teaching and home care, p. 1310

PROCEDURES RELATED TO ALTERNATIVE FEEDING TECHNIQUES, P. 1311

Gavage feeding, p. 1311
Gastrostomy feeding, p. 1313
Total parenteral nutrition (TPN), p. 1314
Family teaching and home care, p. 1314

PROCEDURES RELATED TO ELIMINATION, P. 1315

Enema, p. 1315
Ostomies, p. 1315
Family teaching and home care, p. 1316

General Concepts Related to Pediatric Procedures

INFORMED CONSENT

Informed consent refers to the legal and ethical requirement that the patient clearly, fully, and completely understand the proposed medical treatment to be performed, including significant risks associated with the treatment. The patient must also be informed of alternative treatments that could be offered, including their benefits and risks and risks of nontreatment before giving informed consent. To obtain valid informed consent, three conditions must be met (Hogue, 1988):

1. The person must be capable of giving consent; he or she must be over the age of majority and must be considered competent (i.e., possess the mental capacity to make choices and understand their consequences).
2. The person must receive the information needed to make an intelligent decision.
3. The person must act voluntarily when exercising freedom of choice without force, fraud, deceit, duress, or other forms of constraint or coercion.

Because of the numerous variations of the laws and institutional policies within the United States, the following discussion of informed consent is presented in general terms and is not to be interpreted as legal advice. Although informing patients of the risks, benefits, and alternatives of a procedure is the physician's responsibility, nurses are often responsible for securing the person's signature on a written consent form. In caring for children, special dilemmas may arise regarding who may sign the consent for treatment when parental consent is not available. The age of majority is especially important when caring for adolescents, and competence is a key issue in decisions involving minors who are retarded. Also, the judicial system may intervene in cases where the parents' views and the child's best interests conflict (Nix, 1991). Consequently, nurses need to be familiar with the issues involved in this highly significant and complex subject and must keep current on legal aspects of practice within their community.

Requirements for Obtaining Informed Consent

Written informed consent of the parent or legal guardian is usually required for medical or surgical treatment, including many diagnostic procedures. One blanket consent is not sufficient. Separate informed permissions must be obtained for each surgical or diagnostic procedure, including:

1. Major surgery
2. Minor surgery (e.g., cutdown, biopsy, dental extraction, suturing a laceration [especially one that may have a cosmetic effect], removal of a cyst, closed reduction of a fracture)
3. Diagnostic tests with an element of risk (e.g., bronchoscopy, needle biopsy, angiography, electroencephalogram, lumbar puncture, cardiac catheterization, ventriculography, bone marrow aspiration)
4. Medical treatments with an element of risk (e.g., blood transfusion, thoracentesis or paracentesis, radiation therapy, shock therapies)

In addition, there are certain situations, such as the following, that are not directly related to medical treatment but that require parental consent:

1. Taking photographs for medical, educational, or other public use
2. Removal of the child from health care institutions against the advice of the physician
3. Postmortem examinations, except in unexplained deaths, such as sudden infant death, violent death, or suspected suicide
4. Examination of medical records by unauthorized persons, such as attorneys or insurance representatives (family members have legal right to medical records)

The need for informed consent is also an issue with proposed treatments or research involving children with a mental age of 7 years or older. *Assent* (usually verbal agreement) requires that the child be informed about the proposed treatment or research and agree or concur with the decisions made by the person(s) who can give informed consent. Including children in the decision-making process and gaining their acceptance ensures that children are treated with respect. Assent is not a legal requirement but an ethical one to protect the rights of children.

Eligibility for Giving Informed Consent

In most situations the parent or legal guardian gives informed consent. However, problems may arise when parents are not available to give informed consent, the child is a borderline or emancipated minor, or the parents neglect or refuse care for their minor children.

Informed consent of parents or legal guardians. Parents have full responsibility for the care and rearing of their minor children, including legal control over them. Therefore as long as children are minors, their parents or legal guardians are required to give informed consent before medical treatment is rendered or any procedure is performed on them. Parents also have a right to withdraw consent later.

Evidence of consent. A signed consent form is only evidence that the process of informed consent has occurred; it is not legally required, although it may be an institutional policy. Verbal consent is also evidence of the process (Cushing, 1991). For example, when parents are unavailable to sign consent forms, verbal consent may be obtained via telephone. Verbal consent may also be obtained from parents who are unable to sign (e.g., because of injury). It is good risk management to have a witness to a parent's or guardian's verbal consent. Another nurse may be present or listening on a telephone extension. Both nurses record that informed consent was given and the name, address, and relationship of the person giving consent, together with their signatures, indicating that they witnessed the consent.

Informed consent of mature and emancipated minors. State laws differ with regard to the so-called age of majority. Although some variation still exists, children become adults on their eighteenth birthday in most states. Competent adults can give informed consent on their own behalf. Nonetheless, some courts have permitted minors to consent to their treatment on the basis of the **mature minors' doctrine,** which permits minors to give consent even though they are not technically adults as long as they understand the consequences of their decisions (Brent, 1991). For example, statutes in many states permit minors to give consent on their own behalf to certain treatments, such as for sexually transmitted diseases, contraceptive services, pregnancy, or drug or alcohol abuse.

An **emancipated minor** is one who is legally under the age of majority but is recognized as having the legal capacity of an adult under circumstances prescribed by state law, such as pregnancy, marriage, high school graduation, living independently, or military service. Consent to abortion is more complex. The issue of parental notification before or after an abortion is still undecided, although several states have enacted laws stating that minors seeking abortions must involve their parents or obtain court permission (Johannsen, 1995).

Treatment without parental consent. Exceptions to requiring parental consent before treating minor children occur in situations in which children need prompt medical or surgical treatment and a parent is not readily available to give consent or refuses to give consent. In the absence of parents or legal guardians, some providers permit persons in charge of the child to give informed consent for treatment. In emergencies, consent is not needed; it is implied according to the law (Hogue, 1988). Emergencies include danger to life or possibility of permanent injury.

Refusal to give consent can occur when the treatment, such as blood transfusions, conflicts with the parents' religious beliefs. All states recognize such exceptions and have statutory procedures to permit treatment if the life or health of such a minor is in jeopardy or if delayed treatment would create a risk to the health of the minor. The state is also able to intervene in situations that jeopardize the health and welfare of children, as in cases in which parents neglect or impose excessive or improper punishment on a child. In most communities there are procedures by which custody of the child can be transferred to a governmental or a private agency when parental neglect or abuse can be proved.

PREPARATION FOR PROCEDURES

For most procedures no special physical preparation is needed and the focus of care is psychologic preparation of the child and family (see next section). However, some procedures require specific physical preparation, such as cleansing and shaving of the skin before surgery. One area of special concern is the administration of appropriate sedation and/or analgesia before stressful procedures (see p. 1261). The drug is given before the procedure to allow time for the medication to reach its peak effect. Whenever possible, the intravenous (through an existing infusion), oral, or rectal route is used rather than the intramuscular route because children dislike injections. Some institutions are using short-acting anesthetics, such as ketamine, or potent analgesics, such as fentanyl, to eliminate the pain and trauma associated with treatments, such as bone marrow tests, lumbar punctures, burn débridement, and suturing. (See also Pain Management, Chapter 41).

Psychologic Preparation

Preparing children for procedures decreases their anxiety, promotes their cooperation, supports their coping skills and may teach them new ones, and facilitates a feeling of mastery in experiencing a potentially stressful event. Preparatory methods may be formal, such as group preparation for hospitalization. Most preparation strategies used by nurses are informal, focus on providing information about the experience, and are directed at stressful and/or painful procedures. In general, young children respond better to play materials, and older youngsters benefit more from viewing peer-modeling films (Bates and Broome, 1986). Especially for painful procedures, the most effective preparation includes providing sensory-procedural information and helping the child develop coping skills, such as imagery or relaxation (Broome, 1990).

General guidelines for preparing children for procedures are described in Box 42-1, and age-specific guidelines that consider children's developmental needs and cognitive abilities are presented in Box 42-2. In addition to these suggestions, nurses should consider the child's temperament, existing coping strategies, and previous experiences in individualizing the preparatory process. Children who are distractible and highly active, as well as those who are "slow to warm up," may need individualized sessions that are shorter for the active child but more slowly paced for the shy child. Youngsters who tend to cope well may need more emphasis on using their present skills, whereas those who appear to cope less adequately can benefit from more time devoted to simple coping strategies, such as relaxing, breathing, counting, squeezing a hand, or singing. Children also are different in their "information-seeking dimension"; some want and actively solicit information about the intended procedure, whereas others characteristically avoid information.

The exact timing of the preparation for a procedure varies with the child's age and the type of procedure. There are no exact guidelines to govern timing, but in general the younger the child, the closer the explanation should be to the actual procedure to prevent undue fantasizing and worrying. With complex procedures more time may be needed for assimilation of information, especially with older children. For example, the explanation for an injection can immediately precede the procedure for all ages, but preparation for surgery may begin the day before for young children and a few days before for older children, although older children's preferences should be elicited (see Prepare Child for Hospitalization, Chapter 41).

Establish trust and provide support. The nurse who has spent time with and who has established a positive relationship with a child will usually find it easier to gain the child's cooperation. If the relationship is based on trust, the child will associate the nurse with caregiving activities that provide comfort and pleasure most of the time and not regard the nurse as someone who causes discomfort and stress. If the nurse does not know the child, it is best that the nurse be introduced by another staff person whom the child trusts. The first visit with the child should not include any painful procedure and ideally should focus on the child first, then on the explanation of the procedure. When talking with the child, the nurse uses the same guidelines for communicating with children that are discussed in Chapter 31.

Parental support. Children need support during procedures, and for young children the greatest source of comfort is the parents. However, controversy exists regarding the role parents should assume during procedures, especially if discomfort is involved. Nurses need to consider the issues in deciding whether parental presence is beneficial. The parents' preferences for assisting, observing, or waiting outside the room should be assessed, as well as the child's preference for parental presence. The child's choice should be respected. Parents who wish to stay should be educated, since they do not automatically know what to do, where to be, and what to say to help their child through the procedure (Acute Pain Management Guideline Panel, 1992). Simple instructions such as clarifying where parents can stay in the room and positioning them where they have eye contact with the child provide support and lessen anxiety. Parents who do not wish to be present or participate are supported in their decision and encouraged to remain close by so that they can be available to console the child immediately after the procedure. Parents should also know that someone will be with their child to provide support. Ideally this person should inform the parents after the procedure about how the child did.

Provide an explanation. Children need an explanation for anything that involves them directly. Before performing a procedure, the nurse explains to children what is to be done and

BOX 42-1
General Guidelines for Preparing Children for Procedures

Determine details of exact procedure to be performed.
Review parents' and child's present level of understanding.
Plan actual teaching based on child's developmental age and existing level of knowledge.
Incorporate parents in the teaching if they desire, and especially if they plan to participate in care.
Inform parents of their role during procedure, such as standing near child's head or in line of vision and talking softly to child.
While preparing child and family, allow for ample discussion to prevent information overload and ensure adequate feedback.
Use concrete, not abstract, terms and visual aids to describe procedure. For example, use a simple line drawing of a boy or girl (Fig. 42-1), and mark the body part that will be involved in the procedure.
Emphasize that no other body part will be involved.
If the body part is associated with a specific function, stress the change or noninvolvement of that ability (e.g., after tonsillectomy, child can still speak).
Use words appropriate to child's level of understanding (a rule of thumb for number of words is age in years plus 1).
Avoid words/phrases with dual meanings (see the Guidelines box on p. 1256) unless child understands such words.
Clarify all unfamiliar words (e.g., "Anesthesia is a *special* sleep").
Emphasize sensory aspects of procedure—what child will feel, see, smell, and touch and what child can do during procedure (e.g., lie still, count out loud, squeeze a hand, hug a doll).
Allow child to practice those procedures that will require cooperation (e.g., turning, deep breathing, using an incentive spirometer or mask).
Introduce anxiety-laden information (e.g., the preoperative injection) last.
Be honest with child about unpleasant aspects of a procedure but avoid creating undue concern. When discussing that a procedure may be uncomfortable, state that it feels different to different people and have child describe how it felt.
Emphasize end of procedure and any pleasurable events afterward (e.g., going home, seeing the parent).
Stress positive benefits of procedure (e.g., "After your tonsils are fixed, you won't have as many sore throats").

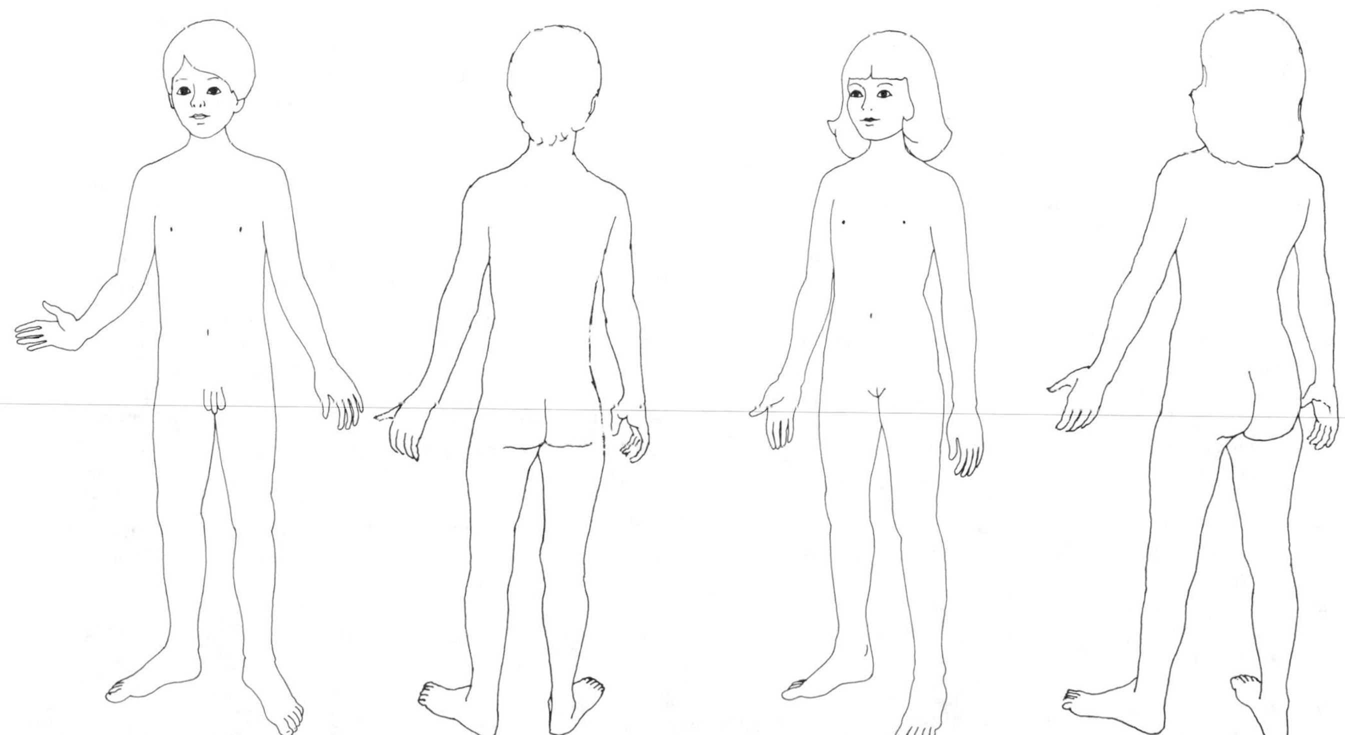

Fig. 42-1 Examples of line drawings to be used in preparing child for procedures.

BOX 42-2
Age-Specific Guidelines for Preparing Children for Procedures Based on Developmental Characteristics

Infancy: developing a sense of trust and sensorimotor thought

Attachment to parent

*Involve parent in procedure if desired.
Keep parent in infant's line of vision.
If parent is unable to be with infant, place familiar object with infant (e.g., stuffed toy).

Stranger anxiety

*Have usual caregivers perform or assist with procedure.
Make advances slowly and in nonthreatening manner.
*Limit number of strangers entering room during procedure.

Sensorimotor phase of learning

During procedure use sensory soothing measures (e.g., stroking skin, talking softly, giving pacifier).
*Use analgesics (e.g., local anesthetic, intravenous opioid) to control discomfort.
Cuddle and hug child after stressful procedure; encourage parent to comfort child.

Increased muscle control

Expect older infants to resist.
Restrain adequately.
Keep harmful objects out of reach.

Memory for past experiences

Realize that older infants may associate objects, places, or persons with prior painful experiences and will cry and resist at the sight of them.
*Keep frightening objects out of view.
*Perform painful procedures in a separate room, not in crib (or bed).
*Use nonintrusive procedures whenever possible (e.g., axillary or tympanic temperatures and oral medications).

Imitation of gestures

Model desired behavior (e.g., opening mouth).

Toddler: developing a sense of autonomy and sensorimotor to preoperational thought

Use same approaches as for infant in addition to the following:

Egocentric thought

Explain procedure in relation to what child will see, hear, taste, smell, and feel.
Emphasize those aspects of procedure that require cooperation (e.g., lying still).
Tell child it's okay to cry, yell, or use other means to express discomfort verbally.

Negative behavior

Expect treatments to be resisted; child may try to run away.
Use firm, direct approach.
Ignore temper tantrums.
Use distraction techniques (e.g., singing a song *with* a child).
Restrain adequately.

Animism

Keep frightening objects out of view (young children believe objects have lifelike qualities and can harm them).

Limited language skills

Communicate using behaviors.
Use few, simple terms familiar to child.
Give one direction at a time (e.g., "Lie down," then "Hold my hand").
Use small replicas of equipment; allow child to handle equipment.
Use play; demonstrate on doll but avoid child's favorite doll, since child may think doll is really "feeling" procedure.
Prepare parents separately to prevent child's misinterpreting words.

Limited concept of time

Prepare child shortly or immediately before procedure.
Keeping teaching sessions short (about 5 to 10 minutes).
Have preparations completed before involving child in procedure.
Have extra equipment nearby (e.g., alcohol swabs, new needle, Band-Aids) to prevent delays.
Tell child when procedure is completed.

Striving for independence

Allow choices whenever possible but realize that child may still be resistant and negative.
Allow child to participate in care and to help whenever possible (e.g., drink medicine from a cup, hold a dressing).

Preschooler: developing a sense of initiative and preoperational thought

Egocentric

Explain procedure in simple terms and in relation to how it affects child (as with toddler, stress sensory aspects).
Demonstrate use of equipment.
Allow child to play with miniature or actual equipment.
Encourage "playing out" experience on a doll both before and after procedure to clarify misconceptions.
Use neutral words to describe the procedure (see box p. 1256).

Increased language skills

Use verbal explanation but avoid overestimating child's comprehension of words.
Encourage child to verbalize ideas and feelings.

Concept of time and frustration tolerance still limited

Implement same approaches as for toddler but may plan longer teaching session (10 to 15 minutes); may divide information into more than one session.

Illness and hospitalization may be viewed as punishment

Clarify why each procedure is performed; a child will find it difficult to understand how medicine can make him or her feel better and can taste bad at the same time.
Ask child thoughts regarding why a procedure is performed.
State directly that procedures are never a form of punishment.

Animism

Keep equipment out of sight, except when shown to or used on child.

*Applies to any age.

BOX 42-2

Age-Specific Guidelines for Preparing Children for Procedures Based on Developmental Characteristics—cont'd

Fears of bodily harm, intrusion, and castration

Point out on drawing, doll, or child where procedure is performed.
Emphasize that no other body part will be involved.
Use nonintrusive procedures whenever possible (e.g., axillary temperatures, oral medication).
Apply a Band-Aid over puncture site.
Encourage parental presence.
Realize that procedures involving genitals provoke anxiety.
Allow child to wear underpants with gown.
Explain unfamiliar situations, especially noises or lights.

Striving for initiative

Involve child in care whenever possible (e.g., hold equipment, remove dressing).
Give choices whenever possible but prevent excessive delays.
Praise child for helping and attempting to cooperate; never shame child for lack of cooperation.

School-age child: developing a sense of industry and concrete thought

Increased language skills; interest in acquiring knowledge

Explain procedures using correct scientific/medical terminology.
Explain reason for procedure using simple diagrams of anatomic and physiologic features.
Explain function and operation of equipment in concrete terms.
Allow child to manipulate equipment; use doll or another person as model to practice using equipment whenever possible (doll play may be considered childish by older school-age child).
Allow time before and after procedure for questions and discussion.

Improved concept of time

Plan for longer teaching sessions (about 20 minutes).
Prepare for procedure.

Increased self-control

Gain child's cooperation.
Tell child what is expected.
Suggest ways of maintaining control (e.g., deep breathing, relaxation, counting).

Striving for industry

Allow responsibility for simple tasks (e.g., collecting specimens).
Include in decision making (e.g., time of day to perform procedure, preferred site).
Encourage active participation (e.g., removing dressings, handling equipment, opening packages).

Developing relationships with peers

May prepare two or more children for same procedure or encourage one to help prepare another peer.
Provide privacy from peers during procedure to maintain self-esteem.

Adolescent: developing a sense of identity and abstract thought

Increasingly capable of abstract thought and reasoning

Supplement explanations with reasons why procedure is necessary or beneficial.
Explain long term consequences of procedures.
Realize that adolescent may fear death, disability, or other potential risks.
Encourage questioning regarding fears, options, and alternatives.

Conscious of appearance

Provide privacy.
Discuss how procedure may affect appearance (e.g., scar) and what can be done to minimize it.
Emphasize any physical benefits of procedure.

Concerned more with present than with future

Realize that immediate effects of procedure are more significant than future benefits.

Striving for independence

Involve in decision making and planning (e.g., choice of time; place; individuals present during procedure, such as parents; clothing to wear).
Impose as few restrictions as possible.
Suggest methods of maintaining control.
Accept regression to more childish methods of coping.
Realize that adolescent may have difficulty in accepting new authority figures and may resist complying with procedures.

Developing peer relationships and group identity

Same as for school-age child but assumes even greater significance.
Allow adolescents to talk with other adolescents who have had the same procedure.

what is expected of them. The explanation should be short, simple, and appropriate to the child's level of comprehension. Long explanations are not necessary and may only increase anxiety in a small child. This is especially true regarding painful procedures. When explaining the procedure to parents with the child present, the nurse uses language appropriate to the child because unfamiliar words can be misunderstood (see the Guidelines box on p. 1256). If the parents need additional preparation, this is done in an area away from the child. Teaching sessions are planned at times most conducive to the child's learning (e.g., after a rest period) and for the usual span of attention.

Special equipment is not necessary for preparing a child, but for young children who cannot yet think in concepts, using objects to supplement verbal explanation is important. Allowing children to handle actual items that will be used in their care, such as a stethoscope, sphygmomanometer, or oxygen mask, helps them to develop familiarity with these items and to reduce the threat often associated with their use. Miniature versions of hospital items such as gurneys and x-ray and intravenous equipment can be used to explain what the children can expect and permit them to safely experience situations that are unfamiliar and potentially frightening. Photographs of children in different areas of the hospital

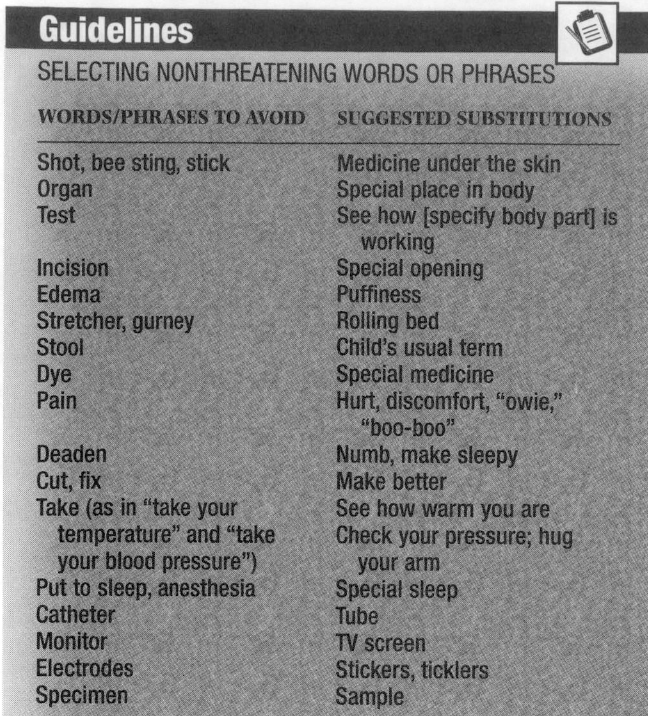

Guidelines

SELECTING NONTHREATENING WORDS OR PHRASES

WORDS/PHRASES TO AVOID	SUGGESTED SUBSTITUTIONS
Shot, bee sting, stick	Medicine under the skin
Organ	Special place in body
Test	See how [specify body part] is working
Incision	Special opening
Edema	Puffiness
Stretcher, gurney	Rolling bed
Stool	Child's usual term
Dye	Special medicine
Pain	Hurt, discomfort, "owie," "boo-boo"
Deaden	Numb, make sleepy
Cut, fix	Make better
Take (as in "take your temperature" and "take your blood pressure")	See how warm you are Check your pressure; hug your arm
Put to sleep, anesthesia	Special sleep
Catheter	Tube
Monitor	TV screen
Electrodes	Stickers, ticklers
Specimen	Sample

(e.g., radiology department, operating room) can be used to give children a more realistic idea of equipment they may encounter. Written and illustrated materials are also valuable aids to preparation.*

Performance of the Procedure

Supportive care continues during the procedure and can be a major factor in a child's ability to cooperate and achieve mastery. Before the procedure is begun, all equipment is assembled and the room is readied to prevent unnecessary delays and interruptions that only serve to increase the child's anxiety. If at all possible, procedures are performed in a special treatment room rather than the child's hospital room. Traumatic procedures should never be performed in "safe" areas, such as the playroom. If the procedure is lengthy, conversation that could be misinterpreted by the child is avoided. As the procedure is nearing completion, the nurse should inform the child that it is almost over in language that the child understands.

Expect success. Nurses who approach children with confidence and who convey the impression that they expect to be successful are less likely to encounter difficulty. It is best to approach children as though cooperation is expected. Children sense anxiety in another and may respond to a perceived threat by striking out or resisting actively. Although some children will still exhibit such behavior, the firm approach and positive attitude of the nurse tend to convey a feeling of security to most children.

Involve child. As in any other aspect of care, involving children helps to gain their cooperation. Permitting them to make choices gives them some measure of control. However, a choice is given only in situations in which one is available. Asking children, "Do you want to take your medicine now?" or "I'm going to give you an injection now, okay?" leads them to believe that there is an option and provides them with the opportunity to refuse to delay the medication legitimately. This places the nurse in an awkward, if not impossible, position. It is much better to state firmly, "It's time to drink your medicine now." Children usually like to make choices, but the choice must be one that they may have (e.g., "It's time for your medicine. Do you want to drink it plain or with a little water?").

Many children respond to tactics that appeal to their maturity or courage. This approach also gives them a sense of participation and achievement. For example, preschool children will be proud that they can hold the dressing during the procedure or remove the tape. The same is true for school-age children, who often cooperate with minimal resistance.

Provide distraction. When children are occupied with some activity that interests them, they are less likely to focus on the procedure. For example, when an injection is given, it is helpful to give the child something to do or something on which to focus attention. For example, asking the child to point the toes inward and wiggle them not only helps relax the gluteal muscles but provides a diversion. Other strategies for diverting attention are to have the child tightly squeeze the hands of a parent or an assistant, count aloud, sing a familiar song such as a nursery rhyme, or verbally express discomfort. It is helpful to have the child select and practice a coping technique before it is needed. (For other interventions that may lessen discomfort, see Pain Management, Chapter 41.)

Allow expression of feelings. The child is allowed to express feelings of anger, anxiety, fear, frustration, or any other emotion. It is natural for children to strike out in frustration or to try to avoid stress-provoking situations. The child needs to know that it is all right to cry. Behavior is children's primary means of communication and coping and should be permitted unless it inflicts harm on them or those caring for them.

Postprocedural Support

After the procedure the child continues to need reassurance that he or she performed well and is accepted and loved. If the parents did not participate, the child is united with them as soon as possible so that they can provide comfort.

Encourage expression of feelings. Planned activity after the procedure is helpful in encouraging constructive expression of feelings. For verbal children, reviewing the details of the procedure can help clarify misconceptions and provide feedback for improving the nurse's preparatory strategies. Play is an excellent activity for all children. Infants and young children are given the opportunity for gross motor movement. Older children can vent their anger and frustration in accept-

*Sources of preparatory materials are the *You're Gonna Do What?* series of diagnosis and treatment procedures, available from Arkansas Children's Hospital, Attn: Barbara Widell, 800 Marshall St., Little Rock, AR 72202, (501) 320-1199; *Talks About the Hospital Series* by Fred Rogers, available from Family Communications, Inc., Attn: Marketing Department, 4802 Fifth Ave., Pittsburgh, PA 15213, (412) 687-2990; *Hospital Friends*, available from the Centering Corp., 1531 N. Saddle Creek Rd., Omaha, NE 68104, (402) 553-1200.

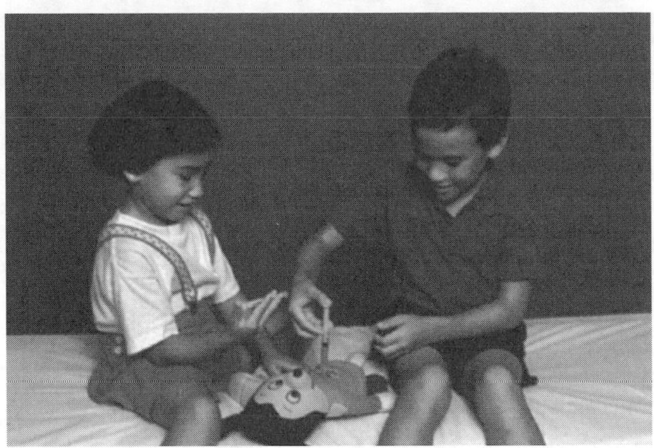

Fig. 42-2 Playing with syringes provides children with the opportunity to play out fears and concerns.

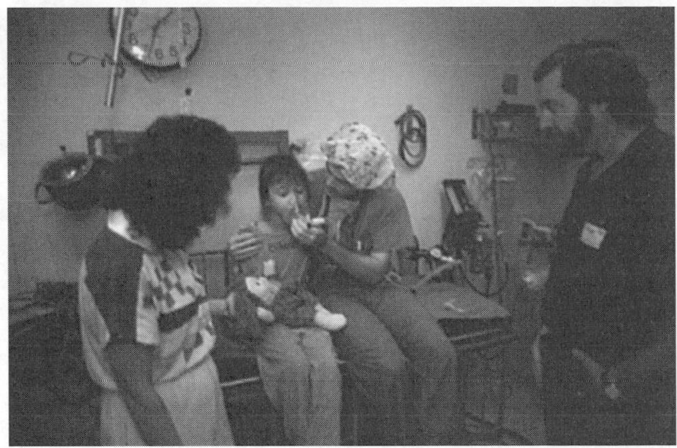

Fig. 42-3 Parental presence during induction of anesthesia can minimize the child's and parents' anxiety during the preoperative period.

able pounding or throwing activities. Claylike material (Playdough) is a remarkably versatile medium for pounding and shaping. Dramatic play provides an outlet for anger and places the child in a position of control, in contrast to the position of helplessness in the real situation. Puppets may also be used to allow the child to communicate in a nonthreatening way. One of the most effective interventions is therapeutic play, which includes activities such as permitting the child to give an injection to a doll or stuffed toy to reduce the stress of injections (Fig. 42-2).

Praise child. Children need to hear from adults that they know that the youngsters did the best they could in the situation—no matter how they behaved. It is important for children to know that their worth is not being judged on the basis of their behavior in a stressful situation. Reward systems, such as earning stars or tokens or saving the empty medicine cup as evidence of achievement, are often helpful. Children who require unpleasant-tasting medications or injections over time can look with pride on a series of stars or stickers on a calendar, especially if an accumulated number represents a special privilege or reward.

Returning to the child a short while after the procedure helps the nurse to strengthen a supportive relationship. Relating with the child in a relaxed and nonstressful period allows him or her to see the nurse not only as someone associated with stressful situations, but as someone with whom to share pleasurable experiences as well.

Use of Play in Procedures

The use of play is an integral part of relationships with children. As such, its value in specific situations is discussed throughout this book, such as in Chapter 41 in relation to hospitalization. Nurses can easily include play activities as part of nursing care. Play can be used for teaching, for expression of feelings, or as a method to achieve a therapeutic goal. Consequently, it should be included in preparing children for and encouraging their cooperation during procedures. Play sessions after procedures can be structured, such as those directed toward playing with syringes, or general, with a wide variety of equipment available for children to play with. Suggestions for incorporating play into nursing procedures and activities for the hospitalized child that facilitate learning and adjustment to a new situation are described in Box 42-3.

Play can also be spontaneous at the bedside and does not always require many supplies or much nursing time. For example, small items, such as finger puppets or a small bottle of bubbles, can be kept in the nurse's pocket for immediate use.

SURGICAL PROCEDURES

Preoperative Care

Children experiencing surgical procedures require both psychologic and physical preparation. In general, psychologic preparation is similar to that discussed for any procedure and may employ many of the same techniques used in preparing a child for hospitalization, such as films, books, play, and tours. However, some important differences exist. Even though children are asleep for the actual surgical intervention, they are subjected to numerous preoperative and postoperative procedures, which require a series of preparatory sessions to prevent overstressing the child with too much information.

Psychologic intervention consisting of systematic preparation, rehearsal of the forthcoming events, and supportive care at times of stress, such as admission, has been shown to be more effective than a single-session preparation or consistent supportive care without systematic preparation and rehearsal. Play is always an effective strategy in preparing children, and increased familiarity with medical procedures decreases anxiety.

Although fear of anesthesia is thought to be a major concern among children, little evidence for this exists. One study of school-age children found that the most feared events were the injection and the mask on the face.

Parental presence during induction is becoming a more common practice, although few institutions endorse the policy (Fig. 42-3). Reports from parents who attend the induction are very favorable. Even though some may become anxious, most parents can control their anxiety, do not disrupt the induction, and support the child (Hall et al, 1995; LaRosa-Nash

BOX 42-3
Play Activities for Specific Procedures

Fluid intake

Make freezer pops using child's favorite juice.
Cut gelatin into fun shapes.
Make game of taking sip when turning page of book or in games such as "Simon Says."
Use small medicine cups; decorate the cups.
Color water with food coloring or powdered drink mix.
Have tea party; pour at small table.
Let child fill a syringe and squirt it into mouth or use it to fill small decorated cups.
Cut straws in half and place in small container (much easier for child to suck liquid).
Decorate straw: cut out small design with two holes and pass straw through; place small sticker on straw.
Use a "crazy" straw.
Make a "progress poster"; give rewards for drinking a predetermined quantity.

Deep breathing

Blow bubbles with bubble blower.
Blow bubbles with straw (no soap).
Blow on pinwheel, feathers, whistle, harmonica, balloons, toy horns, party blowers.
Practice band instruments.
Have blowing contest using balloons,* boats, cotton balls, feathers, marbles, Ping-Pong balls, pieces of paper; blow such objects on a tabletop over a goal line, over water, through an obstacle course, up in the air, against an opponent, or up and down a string.
Suck paper or cloth from one container to another using a straw.
Use blow bottles with colored water to transfer water from one side to the other.
Dramatize stories, such as "I'll huff and puff and blow your house down" from "The Three Little Pigs."
Do straw-blowing painting.
Take a deep breath and "blow out the candles" on a birthday cake.
Use a little paint brush to "paint" nails with water and blow nails dry.

Range of motion and use of extremities

Throw beanbags at fixed or movable target, wadded paper into wastebasket.
Touch or kick Mylar balloons held or hung in different positions (if child is in traction, hang balloon from trapeze).
Play "tickle toes"; wiggle them on request.
Play Twister game or "Simon Says."
Play pretend and guess games (e.g., imitate a bird, butterfly, horse).
Have tricycle or wheelchair races in safe area.
Play kickball or throw ball with soft foam ball in safe area.
Position bed so that child must turn to view television or doorway.
Climb wall like a "spider."
Pretend to teach "aerobic" dancing or exercises; encourage parents to participate.
Encourage swimming if feasible.
Play video games or pinball (fine motor movement).
Play "hide and seek" game: hide toy somewhere in bed (or room if ambulatory) and have child find it using specified hand or foot.
Provide clay to mold with fingers.
Paint or draw on large sheets of paper placed on floor or wall.
Encourage combing own hair; play "beauty shop" with "customer" in different positions.

Soaks

Play with small toys or objects (cups, syringes, soap dishes) in water.
Wash dolls or toys.
Bubbles may be added to bath water if permissible; move bubbles to create shapes or "monsters."
Pick up marbles or pennies* from bottom of bath container.
Make designs with coins on bottom of container.
Pretend a boat is a submarine by keeping it immersed.
Read to child during soaks, sing with child, or play game, such as cards, checkers, or other board game (if both hands are immersed, move the board pieces for the child).
Sitz bath: give child something to listen to (music, stories) or look at (Viewmaster, book).
Punch holes in bottom of plastic cup, fill with water, and let it "rain" on child.

Injections

Let child handle syringe, vial, alcohol swab and give an injection to doll or stuffed animal.
Use syringes to decorate cookies with frosting, squirt paint, or target shoot into a container.
Draw a "magic circle" on area before injection; draw smiling face in circle after injection, but avoid drawing on puncture site.
Allow child to have a "collection" of syringes (without needles); make "wild" creative objects with syringes.
If multiple injections or venipunctures, make a "progress poster"; give rewards for predetermined number of injections.
Have child count to 10 or 15 during injection.

Ambulation

Give child something to push.
- Toddler: push-pull toy
- School-age child: wagon or decorated IV stand
- Adolescent: a baby in a stroller or wheelchair

Have a parade; make hats, drums, etc.

Extending environment (patients in traction, etc.)

Make bed into a pirate ship or airplane with decorations.
Put up mirrors so patient can see around room.
Move patient's bed frequently, especially to playroom, hallway, or outside.

*Small objects such as marbles or coins, as well as gloves or balloons, are unsafe for young children because of possible aspiration.

et al, 1995). There is some concern regarding the appropriateness of this practice for all parents. A few parents are visibly upset by the rapid succession of induction events, observing their child becoming limp, and leaving the child in the care of strangers (Vessey, Caserza, and Bogetz, 1990).

However, on the basis of the parents' favorable response to the practice and most children's desire to have parents with them during any stressful procedure, a policy of offering parents the option of attending the induction, combined with a program that prepares them for what to expect and what is expected of them, is recommended. When parents choose not to or are not allowed to attend this induction, leaving a favorite possession with the child and uniting the child and parents as soon as possible after surgery (preferably in the postanesthesia care unit [PACU]) are important interventions. During surgery the family should have a designated place to wait and needs to be kept informed of the child's progress. Family members also should know where and when they can visit the child after surgery.

Aside from possibly being separated from the parents before and after surgery, children may be cared for by a number of unfamiliar practitioners. Although the same supportive nurse should remain with the child through as many of the procedures as possible, the child may have other nurses, especially if the patient returns to a special care unit postoperatively. Many hospitals have surgical tours for children and parents to familiarize them with the strange environment and to introduce them to other individuals who will be involved in their care.

Guidelines

PREOPERATIVE CHECKLIST

- ☐ Signed informed consent on chart and properly witnessed.
- ☐ Child NPO for appropriate length of time.
- ☐ Child's medication orders changed as needed because of NPO status.
- ☐ Results of laboratory tests and vital signs reviewed for abnormal findings, such as elevated temperature, and reported to practitioner.
- ☐ Any specific physical preparation of surgical area, such as shaving or administration of enemas, performed.
- ☐ Child appropriately attired and any personal items (e.g., underwear or favorite toy) labeled.
- ☐ Dental appliances (e.g., retainers) contact lenses, prosthesis, hearing aid, nail polish, and makeup removed.
- ☐ Loose teeth and appliances remaining with child noted on chart.
- ☐ Child voided before preoperative sedation administered.
- ☐ Child wearing correct patient identification.
- ☐ Child's identification charge card on chart.
- ☐ Child and family adequately prepared for surgery experience (i.e., where family can wait for surgeon's report; whether parents can accompany the child to perioperative suite, induction area, or PACU).
- ☐ Any special circumstances, such as allergies,* skin problems, respiratory or cardiac conditions, paralysis, or family history of malignant hyperthermia, clearly displayed on front of chart.
- ☐ History and physical examination, including child's weight, and laboratory test results, indicated on chart.

*For a discussion of latex allergy, see Spina Bifida, Chapter 52.

In addition to psychologic preparation, children usually require various types of physical care before surgery such as those listed in the Nursing Care Plan on pp. 1260-1261 and in the preoperative checklist (see the Guidelines box below, left). An important concern is restriction of food and fluids before surgery to prevent aspiration during anesthesia. Before fluids are restricted, children are encouraged to drink to promote hydration and minimize the dryness and thirst they experience. Infants require special attention to fluid needs. They should not be without oral fluids for an extended period preoperatively, to prevent glycogen depletion and dehydration (see the Guidelines box below). Typical recommendations for food or fluids before anesthesia induction are no milk or solids after midnight before scheduled procedures and no clear liquids from 4 to 8 hours before the procedure. However, research indicates that clear liquids up to 2 hours before surgery for children at any age pose no additional risk for pulmonary aspiration during elective surgery (Schreiner, 1994).

Although most preoperative care procedures are routine, nurses should keep in mind that they can be anxiety-provoking for children and parents. For example, for young children, having to wear a loose-fitting hospital gown without the security of underpants or pajama bottoms can be traumatic. Therefore these articles of clothing should be allowed.

The most upsetting event for children is generally the preoperative injection. Unfortunately, little research has been done on the value of this practice. If children have no preoperative pain, are well prepared psychologically for surgery, and have their parents nearby, preanesthetic medication may be unnecessary. When drugs are used, they should be "atraumatic," administered by oral, existing intravenous, or rectal routes.

Numerous preanesthetic drug regimens are used with children, and no consensus exists on the optimal method. Drugs used should achieve five goals (American Academy of Pediatrics, 1992): (1) to guard the patient's safety and welfare; (2) to minimize physical discomfort or pain; (3) to minimize negative psychologic responses to treatment by providing analgesia, and to maximize the potential for anesthesia; (4) to control behavior; and (5) to return the patient to a state in which safe discharge, as determined by recognized criteria, is possible.

Guidelines

RECOMMENDED PREOPERATIVE FEEDING

At 8 PM or midnight the evening before surgery, **stop all food,** including:
- Solid food, candy,* and chewing gum*
- Milk, milk products, and formulas†
- Orange juice and juice containing pulp

Breastfeeding may continue until **3 hours** before surgery.
Clear fluids may be continued until **2 hours** before surgery.
Clear fluids include water, apple juice, clear juice drinks, plain gelatin, clear broth, Pedialyte, and ice pops.

Modified from Schreiner MS: Preoperative and postoperative fasting in children, *Pediatr Clin North Am* 41(1):111-120, 1994.
*Hard sucking candy is probably of little concern, and a variety of opinions exist regarding the significance of gum chewing.
†The duration for fasting after formulas is uncertain at present, and shorter intervals may be appropriate.

Nursing Care Plan

CHILD UNDERGOING SURGERY

Nursing Diagnosis: Risk for injury related to surgical procedure, anesthesia

Expected Outcome: Child shows no evidence of injury.

• NURSING INTERVENTIONS/*RATIONALES*

Carry out preoperative preparations such as: NPO, anticholinergic medications as ordered *to prevent aspiration;* bathing, cleansing of operative site, antibiotics as ordered *to prevent infection;* emptying of bowel and bladder, insertion of catheter as ordered, cleansing enemas as ordered *to prevent distention and incontinence;* checking vital signs, lab values for systematic abnormality *that may complicate surgery* (i.e., elevated temperature, white blood cells [WBCs] *for signs of infection,* hemoglobin [Hb] and hematocrit [Hct] *for anemia,* platelets, clotting times *for bleeding tendencies*); clearly delineate allergies *to prevent reactions or complications;* removal of jewelry, prosthetic devices *to prevent injury;* removal of makeup, nail polish *to improve monitoring for cyanosis;* start IV per order *to provide route for fluids and medications;* dress in attire for operating room (OR) *to provide easy access to surgical site.*

Transport to surgical holding area using safety belt and side rails on stretcher *to prevent falls;* check identification and chart with surgical personnel *to ensure correct identity and completion of all preoperative preparations.*

Carry out intraoperative preparations such as: Transfer and proper securing to surgical table *to prevent falls;* check identification *to ensure correct identity;* check chart *to ensure correct surgical procedure at correct site;* talk/play with child before anesthesia administered *to keep anxiety, fear minimal;* after child is anesthetized, careful alignment and positioning *to prevent injury to joints or pressure spots to skin;* apply restraints *to prevent falls;* place on warming blanket per order *to prevent hypothermia;* place grounding plate if electrocautery is to be used *to prevent injury;* cleanse and drape surgical site *to prevent infection;* check expiration dates on all sterile packages before use *to maintain integrity of sterile field;* monitor sterile field and institute immediate corrective measures for technique breaks *to prevent contamination of wound;* ensure correct instrument and sponge count *to prevent loss of foreign substances in wound;* dress surgical site *to prevent infection;* transfer to recovery bed, raise side rails, and transport to recovery room *for postoperative monitoring.*

Carry out recovery room procedures such as: Monitor vital signs frequently *to assess for signs of infection, hemorrhage, aspiration;* suction as needed *to prevent aspiration, infection;* monitor neurologic status, gag and swallow reflex, cough *to assess recovery from anesthesia;* monitor intake and output, skin tone and turgor *to assess hydration status;* monitor for signs of sensory overload; orient frequently as child is waking *to prevent overload and confusion;* monitor incision site *for hemorrhage.*

Carry out postoperative procedures such as: Employ careful wound care and good handwashing techniques *to prevent infection;* monitor vital signs *to assess for signs of infection, hemorrhage, aspiration;* turn, cough, and deep breathe *to prevent respiratory infection;* encourage graduated nutritious oral intake after bowel sounds heard *to prevent intestinal complications and promote wound healing;* ambulate per physician order *to decrease complications of immobility;* monitor intake and output, skin turgor *to assess hydration status;* monitor and maintain bedside equipment (i.e., IVs, IV pumps, nasogastric [NG] tubes, suction machines, wound drains, chest tubes, catheters) *to ensure function and safe operation.*

Nursing Diagnosis: Anxiety/fear related to surgery, separation from support system

Expected Outcome: Child exhibits reduced signs of fear and anxiety.

• NURSING INTERVENTIONS/*RATIONALES*

Preoperatively: Teach child (using developmentally appropriate approach) what to expect before, during, and after surgery; explain where parents will be during surgery *to reduce fear of unknown;* administer preoperative medications as ordered *to provide relaxation and sleep;* encourage parents to stay with child as long as possible and to touch or hold child until asleep *to reduce fear and feelings of abandonment;* allow child to take a favorite toy to the surgical holding area *to establish a sense of security.*

Postoperatively: Orient child as he/she awakes, explain what is happening as it happens, be calm and reassuring *to reduce anxieties;* encourage parental presence as soon as feasible *to decrease separation anxiety.*

Nursing Diagnosis: Pain related to surgical incision

Expected Outcome: Child exhibits minimal evidence of pain.

• NURSING INTERVENTIONS/*RATIONALES*

Administer postoperative pain medications as ordered before expression of pain *to prevent pain from occurring.*

Splint operative site when coughing or deep breathing; turn and position gently; avoid palpation of surgical site unless necessary *to reduce pain.*

Insert rectal tube as needed *to relieve discomfort from gas.*

Monitor bladder for fullness and encourage voiding *to prevent pain from bladder distention.*

Administer comfort measures (i.e., mouth care, lubrication of eyes if irritated, lubrication of nostril if nasogastric (NG) tube present, massage of back) *to reduce discomfort.*

Coordinate nursing activities and procedures with administration of analgesia *to decrease pain and increase effectiveness of activity.*

Administer analgesics, antiemetics per physician order and monitor effectiveness of medications in *pain and nausea relief.*

Nursing Diagnosis: Risk for fluid volume deficit related to NPO status, operative losses, vomiting, loss of appetite

Expected Outcome: Child exhibits no signs of dehydration.

• NURSING INTERVENTIONS/*RATIONALES*

Monitor intake and output, IV infusion rate and patency, skin turgor, mucous membranes *to evaluate hydration status.*

Offer oral fluids as ordered and tolerated; use favorite fluids *to establish oral intake after surgery.*

Nursing Care Plan

CHILD UNDERGOING SURGERY—CONT'D

Nursing Diagnosis: Risk for infection related to break in skin integrity, anesthesia, immobility, presence of pathogens in environment

Expected Outcome: Lungs remain clear; surgical incision site is clean.

- NURSING INTERVENTIONS/*RATIONALES*

Turn, cough, deep breathe, use incentive spirometer or blow bottle *to promote movement and clearing of lung secretions.*

Suction secretions as needed *to keep airway clear.*

Monitor respirations, auscultate breath sounds *to assess respiratory status.*

Ambulate as early as permitted *to promote increased circulation and improved gas exchange.*

Keep surgical site dressed, using careful wound care and handwashing techniques *to prevent infection.*

Monitor temperature; inspect wound for redness, swelling, pus *indicative of infection.*

Nursing Diagnosis: Altered family process related to surgical procedure

Expected Outcome: Family demonstrates understanding of surgery and related processes; family complies with directives.

- NURSING INTERVENTIONS/*RATIONALES*

Teach family about surgical procedure and related tests and procedures; outline the preoperative, operative, and postoperative processes *to provide understanding of what will happen and prepare family for what is to occur;* allow time for questions; get feedback *to evaluate level of understanding.*

Be available to family *to provide support;* explore family's feelings *to offer needed emotional support.*

Let family know where to wait and whom to talk to while surgery occurring; give them an expected time frame for the procedure; let them know when they can see child after surgery *to provide support.*

Explain child's expected appearance, equipment and attached apparatus after surgery *to prepare family and reduce fear.*

Explain care after surgery; encourage family to participate in child's care as they feel able *to facilitate a sense of control and ability to cope.*

See also Nursing Care Plan: Family of Ill or Hospitalized Child p. 1241.

The use of sedating drugs for procedures has serious associated risks, such as hypoventilation, apnea, airway obstruction, and cardiopulmonary impairment. They produce *conscious sedation*—a medically controlled state of depressed consciousness that (1) allows protective reflexes to be maintained; (2) retains the patient's ability to maintain a patent airway independently and continuously; and (3) permits appropriate response by the patient to physical stimulation or verbal command (e.g., "Open your eyes").

The American Academy of Pediatrics (1992) has developed policies that provide guidelines for conscious sedation. These guidelines include provision of emergency equipment, such as a positive-pressure oxygen delivery system, airway management and breathing equipment, and an emergency cart. The patient's level of consciousness and responsiveness, heart rate, blood pressure, respiratory rate, and oxygen saturation (via pulse oximetry) must be monitored during the procedure by an individual present for this purpose. In all cases the patient's condition after the procedure is also documented.

Children may also fear induction of anesthesia by mask. Practices that can minimize anxiety related to inhalation anesthesia are (1) disguising the unpleasant odor of anesthetic gases by applying a pleasant-smelling substance on the mask; (2) using a transparent plastic mask rather than an opaque black mask and gradually moving it toward the face; (3) directing a stream of gas toward the child's face from the bare tube until the child becomes drowsy, then using the mask; and (4) allowing the child to sit up rather than lie down for anesthesia induction.

Postoperative Care

After surgical procedures, various psychologic and physical interventions and observations are required to prevent or minimize possible untoward effects from anesthesia and the surgical procedure (see the Nursing Care Plan on pp. 1260-1261 and the Guidelines box on p. 1262). Although most of these interventions are prescribed by physicians, it is the nurse's responsibility to exercise judgment in their implementation. For example, vital signs are taken as frequently as necessary until they are stable. Simply recording temperature, pulse, respiration, and blood pressure without comparing the present readings with previous ones is a useless technical function. Each vital sign is evaluated in terms of side effects from anesthesia and signs of impending shock, respiratory compromise, or pain. The nurse should also be alert for the development of malignant hyperthermia, a potentially lethal genetic myopathy. In susceptible children certain anesthetic agents trigger the disorder, producing elevated temperature, muscle rigidity, hypermetabolism, and muscle cell destruction. The symptoms may or may not occur during surgery; therefore, alert observation in the PACU and regular care unit is essential (Wlody, 1991). Early signs of the disorder include tachycardia, rising blood pressure, tachypnea, mottled skin, and muscle rigidity.

Nursing ALERT

When taking the preoperative history, ask the family whether any relatives have had anesthetic difficulties suggesting malignant hyperthermia; report findings immediately.

Guidelines

POSTOPERATIVE CARE

Ensure that preparations are made to receive child.
- Bed or crib is ready.
- Intravenous equipment, such as pumps, and any other relevant equipment, such as suction apparatus, oxygen flow meter, or Gomco suction, is at bedside.

Obtain baseline information:
- Take vital signs, including blood pressure (BP); keep BP cuff in place, deflated in order to lessen amount of disturbance to child.
- Take and record more frequently if any value fluctuates.
- Inspect operative area.
- Check dressing if present.
- Outline any bleeding area on dressing or cast with pen.
- Reinforce, but do not remove, loose dressing.
- Observe areas below surgical site for blood that may have drained toward bed.

Assess for bleeding and other symptoms in areas not covered with a dressing, such as throat after tonsillectomy.

Assess skin color and characteristics.

Assess level of consciousness, activity.

Notify physician of any irregularities in child's condition.

Assess for evidence of pain (see Pain Assessment, Chapter 41).

Review surgeon's orders after completing initial assessment, and check that any preoperative orders, such as seizure or cardiac medications, have been reordered and can be given by available routes (oral preparations may be contraindicated).

Monitor vital signs as ordered and more often if indicated.

Check dressings for bleeding or other abnormalities.

Check bowel sounds.

Observe for signs of shock, abdominal distention, bleeding.

Assess for bladder distention.

Observe for signs of dehydration.

Detect presence of infection:
- Take vital signs every 2-4 hours, as ordered.
- Collect or request needed specimens.
- Inspect wound for signs of infection—redness, swelling, heat, pain, purulent drainage.

Providing comfort is a major nursing responsibility after surgery. Pain is assessed and analgesics are administered to provide comfort and to facilitate the child's cooperation with postoperative procedures, such as ambulating and deep breathing. Routinely scheduled intravenous analgesics and the use of patient-controlled analgesia (PCA), rather than PRN (as necessary) orders, afford more satisfactory pain control (see Pain Management, Chapter 41). Mouth care is another important aspect of care, because most children are allowed nothing orally until bowel sounds return (see p. 1266).

Since respiratory infections are a potential complication, every effort is taken to aerate the lungs and remove secretions. The lungs are auscultated regularly to identify abnormal sounds or any areas of diminished or absent breath sounds. To prevent hypostatic pneumonia, respiratory movement can be encouraged with incentive spirometers or other motivating activities (see p. 1258). If these measures are presented as games, the child is more likely to comply. The child's position is changed every 2 hours, and deep breathing is encouraged.

Nursing ALERT

Early signs of respiratory involvement are abnormal rate, shallow depth, and cough. These findings are reported immediately.

Because deep breathing is usually painful after surgery, premedicate the child for pain and have the child splint the operative site (depending on its location) by hugging a small pillow or a favorite stuffed animal.

During the recovery period some time should be spent with children to assess their perception of surgery. Play, drawing, and storytelling are excellent methods of discovering their thoughts. With such information the nurse can support or correct their perceptions and assist children in feeling a sense of mastery for having gone through a stressful procedure.

COMPLIANCE

The extent to which the patient's behavior in terms of taking medication, following diets, or executing other life-style changes coincides with the prescribed regimen is known as *compliance* (or *adherence*). Reviews of compliance rates in children and adolescents with chronic diseases estimate that the rate of noncompliance ranges from 36% to more than 80% (Pidgeon, 1989). Since nurses are frequently responsible for teaching families about treatment protocols, they must have knowledge of factors that influence compliance, methods to measure compliance, and strategies to enhance adherence to prescribed treatment.

Assessment of Compliance

In developing strategies to provide compliance, the nurse must first assess factors that influence compliance in the patient. Since many children are too young to assume partial or total responsibility for their care, parents are usually the primary caregivers in terms of home management. Consequently, the nurse needs to assess their ability to carry out instructions. The first approach to assessment is knowledge of those factors that influence compliance and the second is application of methods to assess compliance more objectively.

Several factors influence compliance (Box 42-4), although no typical characteristics of noncompliers exist, and even education is not correlated with compliance (Rosenstock, 1988). Basically, any aspect of the health care environment that increases the family's satisfaction with the care they are receiving positively influences adherence to the treatment regimen. However, the more complex, expensive, inconvenient, and disruptive the treatment protocol, the less likely the family is to comply. During long-term conditions that involve multiple treatments and considerable rearrangement of life-style, compliance is severely affected.

Although it is helpful to know those factors that influence compliance, assessment must include more direct measurement techniques. A number of methods exist, although no

BOX 42-4
Factors That Positively Influence Compliance

Individual/family factors
High self-esteem
Positive body image
High degree of autonomy (increased locus of control)
Supportive and well-adjusted family
Effective family communication
Family expectation for successful completion of therapy

Care-setting factors
Perceived satisfaction with care
Positive interactions with practitioners
Continuity of care
Individualized care
Minimum waiting time for appointments
Convenient care setting

Treatment factors
Simple regimen
Minimum disruption in usual life-style
Short duration
Inexpensiveness
Visible benefits
Tolerable side effects

one method is totally reliable. The most successful approach combines at least two of the following methods:

Clinical judgment—The nurse judges family compliance. This is a very poor method that is subject to bias and inaccuracy unless the nurse carefully evaluates the criteria used in evaluation.

Self-reporting—The family is asked about their ability to carry out the prescribed treatments, although most people overestimate their compliance by about 20% even when they admit to lapses in treatment.

Direct observation—The nurse directly observes the patient or family performing the treatment. This method is difficult to employ outside the health care setting, and the family's awareness of being observed frequently affects their performance.

Monitoring appointments—The family's attendance at scheduled appointments is recorded, although this method only indirectly indicates compliance with the prescribed care.

Monitoring therapeutic response—The child's response in terms of benefit from treatment is monitored and preferably recorded on a graph or chart. Unfortunately, few treatments yield directly measurable results.

Pill counts—The nurse counts the number of pills remaining in the original container and compares the amount missing with the number of days the medication should have been taken. Although this is a simple method, families may forget to bring the container or deliberately alter the number of pills to prevent detection. This method is also poorly suited to liquid medication, which is commonly prescribed in pediatrics. Another strategy is to call the pharmacy and check on number of refills for a prescription given for a chronic condition.

Chemical assay.—For certain drugs, such as digoxin and phenytoin, measurement of plasma drug levels provides information on the amount of drug recently ingested. However, this method is expensive, indicates only short-term compliance, and requires precise timing of the assay for accurate results.

Strategies to Enhance Compliance

Organizational strategies are those interventions that are concerned with the care setting and the therapeutic plan. They include employing the factors listed in Box 42-4 that are known to affect compliance positively. Depending on the individual situation, this may involve increasing the frequency of appointments, designating a primary practitioner, reducing the cost of medication by purchasing generic brands, reducing the treatment's disruption of the family's life-style, and using "cues" to minimize forgetting. Numerous devices are available commercially or can be improvised for cueing, such as pill dispensers; watches with alarms; charts to record completed therapy; reminders, such as messages on the refrigerator or morning coffee pot; and treatment schedules that incorporate the treatment plan into the daily routine, such as physical therapy after the evening bath.

Educational strategies are concerned with instructing the family about the treatment plan. Although education is an important component in enhancing compliance and patients who are more knowledgeable about their condition are more likely to comply, education alone does not ensure compliant behavior. Also, for education to be effective it must incorporate teaching principles known to enhance understanding and retention of material (see the Guidelines box on p. 1264). Written materials are essential, especially in any regimen requiring multiple or complex treatments, and need to be understandable to the average individual, who reads at about the fourth-grade level. Including the culturally significant decision maker (e.g., maternal grandmother) in teaching sessions will help improve compliance (Faber, 1986).

Treatment strategies are related to the child's refusal or inability to take the prescribed medication. The family may also have difficulty following a prescribed treatment regimen. They may remember and understand the instructions but may not be able to give the medicine as prescribed. It is essential to assess the reason for refusal. For example, the child may not be able to swallow pills. In this case, perhaps they can be crushed or a liquid medication substituted. The opposite also may occur; the child is having difficulty drinking a liquid medication but is able to swallow pills.

Also assess the treatment/medication schedule to determine whether it is reasonable for a home situation. Whereas an every-6-hour or every-8-hour schedule is reasonable for hospitals, a parent would have difficulty getting up one or two times in the night when a medication could be given during the day at times that would be easy to remember (see the Critical Thinking Q & A box on p. 1264).

Behavioral strategies encompass those interventions designed to modify behavior directly. Several strategies are effective in encouraging the desired behavior and are very useful with children. Also, positive reinforcement may be employed

Guidelines

EFFECTIVE TEACHING OF FAMILY MEMBERS

Establish rapport; reduce anxiety and fear.
Assess what family knows and expects to learn, especially if they have concerns, and address their concerns before beginning teaching.
Assess family's learning style; ask whether they like to have everything explained in detail or prefer knowing only the major facts.
Use a variety of teaching materials (lecture, demonstration, video or slide presentation, written material).
Speak family's language, avoid jargon, and clarify all terms.
Be specific when giving information.
Divide the information into small steps.
Keep information short, simple, and concrete.
Introduce most important information first.
Use verbal headings to organize information, such as "There are two things you need to learn: how to give the medicine and what side effects to look for. First, how to give . . . . Second, what side effects . . . "
Stress how important the instructions are and the expected benefits; explain the detrimental effects of inadequate treatment but do not use fear tactics.
Evaluate the teaching by eliciting feedback to ensure that the family understands the information.
Repeat information as needed.
Reward the family for learning through verbal praise.
Use "teachable moments"—times when family is most likely to accept new information (e.g., when member asks a question or when symptoms are present).
Use "hands on" demonstration and return demonstration to encourage mastery of skills and retention of information.

Critical Thinking Q & A

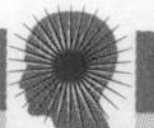

DISCHARGE INSTRUCTIONS

Ms. Jordan is getting ready to take 2-month-old Brittany home from the hospital after a 4-day admission for a severe ear infection and eye infection. Brittany will be going home taking an antibiotic that you have been giving every 8 hours and eye drops that you have been giving every 6 hours. The infant is fed about every 4 hours. Choose the appropriate home schedule.

1. 12 AM—Feed and give antibiotic and eye drops
   4 AM—Feed
   6 AM—Give eye drops
   8 AM—Feed and give antibiotic
   12 PM—Feed and give eye drops
   4 PM—Feed and give antibiotic
   6 PM—Give eye drops
   8 PM—Feed
2. 12 AM—Feed and give antibiotic
   4 AM—Feed
   8 AM—Feed and give antibiotic and eye drops
   12 PM—Feed and give eye drops
   4 PM—Feed and give antibiotic and eye drops
   8 PM—Feed and give eye drops
3. 12 AM—Feed and give antibiotic and eye drops
   6 AM—Feed and give antibiotic and eye drops
   10 AM—Feed and give eye drops
   2 PM—Feed and give antibiotic
   6 PM—Feed and give eye drops
   9 PM—Feed

The best answer is two. Even though you followed the every-6-hour schedule for the eye drops in the hospital, it is unlikely that the parent could manage this at home. It is sometimes difficult getting eye drops into an infant's eyes, and giving the parent a schedule in which they must be given twice during the night would be difficult. Reducing the number of times the parent and infant must awaken during the night decreases the likelihood of a missed dose because the parent forgot to get up.

If this were an older child, the antibiotic schedule could also be altered to waking hours only so the child and parent would not have to awaken in the night for medication.

Although not every medication can be given on a more flexible schedule, most can. Ask the practitioner whether the medication can be given 3 times a day instead of every 8 hours or 4 times a day instead of every 6 hours, etc. Medications or treatments given at unusual times are more likely to be missed. Discharge instructions should always take into account the parent's ability to be compliant with them.

to strengthen the behavior; this may consist of earning stars or tokens, to gain a special privilege or gift. A more formal method is the use of contracting (see Limit-setting and Discipline, Chapter 29). However, at times techniques such as time out for young children or withholding of privileges for older children may be needed to reduce noncompliance.

General Hygiene and Care

MAINTAINING HEALTHY SKIN

Skin, the largest organ of the body, is not merely a covering but also a complex structure that serves many functions, the most important of which is to protect the tissues that it encloses and to protect itself. Many routine nursing activities—maintaining an intravenous line, removing a dressing, positioning a child in bed, changing a diaper, using electrode patches, or maintaining restraints—have the potential to contribute to skin injury. Skin care must go beyond the daily bath and become a part of each nursing intervention. General guidelines for skin care are listed in the Guidelines box on p. 1265. Specific guidelines for skin care of neonates are provided in Chapter 23.

Assessment of the skin is most easily accomplished during the bath, but often the nurse is not the one who bathes the child. In this case the nurse needs to plan a time to observe the child's skin and to request feedback from the caregiver. The skin is examined for any early signs of injury, especially in the child who is at risk. Risk factors include impaired mobility, protein malnutrition, edema, incontinence, sensory loss, anemia, and infection. Identification of risk factors helps to determine those children who need more thorough skin assessment.

When capillary blood flow is interrupted by pressure, the blood flows back into the tissue when the pressure is relieved. As the body attempts to reoxygenate the area, a bright-red flush appears. This *reactive hyperemia,* or flush, may be present one-half to three-fourths as long as the time the pressure occluded the blood flow to the area.

Guidelines

SKIN CARE

Cleanse skin with gentle soap (e.g., Dove) or cleanser (e.g., Cetaphil). Rinse well with plain warm water.

Provide daily cleansing of eyes, oral, and diaper or perianal areas and any areas of skin breakdown.

Apply moisturizing agents after cleansing to retain moisture and rehydrate skin; however, cleanse skin of any old cream before adding a new layer.

Use minimum tape/adhesive. On very sensitive skin, use a protective pectin-based or hydrocolloid skin barrier between skin and tape/adhesives.

Use water or possibly adhesive remover (if skin is not fragile) when removing tape/adhesives.

Place pectin-based or hydrocolloid skin barriers directly over excoriated skin. Leave barrier undisturbed until it begins to peel off. With wet, oozing excoriations, place a small amount of stoma powder (as used in ostomy care) on site, remove excess powder, and apply skin barrier. Hold barrier in place for several minutes to allow barrier to soften and mold to skin surface.

Alternate electrode placement and thoroughly assess skin underneath electrodes at least every 24 hours.

Be certain fingers or toes are visible whenever extremity is used for IV or arterial line.

Reduce friction by keeping skin dry (may apply absorbent powder, such as cornstarch) and using soft, smooth bed linen and clothes.

Use a draw sheet to move a child in bed or onto a gurney to reduce friction and shearing injuries; do not drag the child from under the arms.

Identify children who are risk for skin breakdown before it occurs. Employ measures, such as pressure-reducing or relieving devices, to prevent breakdown.

Do not massage reddened bony prominences because it can cause deep tissue damage; provide pressure relief to those areas instead.

Keep skin free of excess moisture (i.e., urine or fecal incontinence, wound drainage, excessive perspiration).

Routinely assess the child's nutritional status. A child who is NPO for several days and is only receiving IV fluid is nutritionally at risk; that risk can also affect the skin's ability to maintain its integrity. Hyperalimentation should be considered for these children before they are at risk.

Nursing ALERT

If the redness persists, this may be the first sign of skin breakdown, including the possibility of more extensive damage below the skin.

Staging of pressure ulcers is used to classify the amount of tissue damage that has occurred. The tissue in the wound must be visible in order to be staged; it is difficult to assess a wound that is covered with necrotic tissue or a scab. Accurate documentation of redness or obvious skin breakdown is essential. Color, size (diameter and depth), location, presence of sinus tracts, odor, exudate, and response to treatment are observed and recorded at least daily. (For treatment of wounds, see Chapter 50; see also the Critical Thinking Q & A box above.)

Critical Thinking Q & A

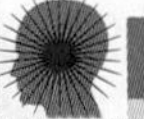

RISK OF SKIN BREAKDOWN

You work on a pediatric surgical unit. In a recent continuous quality improvement report, it was noted that in 10% of the patients some type of skin breakdown developed, most often stage II wounds. Which of the following variables identified about this patient population should be investigated further?

1. Average age of the child is 6 years and sex is more often male.
2. Major reason for surgery is orthopedic repair, especially as a result of trauma.
3. Average length of surgery is 4 hours, and average duration until appearance of wound is 24 to 48 hours.
4. All children received adequate pain medication.

The correct answer is three. During prolonged surgery, patients are often placed on an inadequately padded surface. The excessive pressure on bony prominences causes redness and deeper tissue damage that may not be apparent until hours or days later. The fact that these children are most likely to need orthopaedic surgery (this age group and gender are at risk for injuries) may also be a risk factor if mobility is impaired. However, with good pain control, these children should be able to move quite easily. If pressure ulcers develop postoperatively from immobility, they are most likely to appear after the first 2 days.

The nurse must also have an understanding of the types of mechanical damage that can occur, such as pressure, friction, shearing, and epidermal stripping. When a combination of risk factors and mechanical injury is present, skin breakdown can occur (Hagelgans, 1993).

When a child is identified as at risk for skin breakdown, nursing interventions are directed toward prevention of mechanical injury. Wounds caused by pressure can be prevented by using current technology and resources (Bryant, 1992). *Pressure ulcers* can develop when the pressure on the skin and underlying tissues is greater than the capillary closing pressure, causing capillary occlusion. If the pressure remains unrelieved, vessels can collapse, resulting in tissue anoxia and cellular death. Pressure ulcers most often occur over bony prominences. These lesions are usually very deep (stage IV), extending into subcutaneous tissue or even deeper into muscle, tendon, or bone. Prevention of pressure ulcers includes measures that reduce or relieve pressure.

A *pressure reduction device* reduces pressure more than would usually occur on a regular hospital bed or chair. These products do not prevent pressure from causing capillary closing; therefore turning and repositioning are always included

Nursing ALERT

Convoluted foam mattress pads with a base of 5 cm (2 inches) (measured from where the convolutions begin, not the peak of the convolution) and soft padding, such as sheepskin, do not significantly reduce pressure when compared with a regular hospital mattress (Krouskop et al, 1985).

when using these devices. Most of these items are overlays that are placed on top of the regular mattress. A *pressure-relief device* maintains pressure below that which would cause capillary closing. These devices are usually high-technology beds that are used for patients who have multiple problems and cannot be turned effectively.

Friction and shear both contribute to pressure ulcers. *Friction* occurs when the surface of the skin rubs against another surface, such as the sheets on the bed. The skin may have the appearance of an abrasion. The skin damage is usually limited to the epidermal and upper layers. It most often occurs over the elbows or heels. Prevention of friction injury includes the use of protective sheepskin over the elbows or heels, moisturizing agents, transparent dressings over susceptible areas, and soft, smooth bed linen and clothing. By itself, friction does not cause tissue necrosis, but when it acts with gravity, it results in shear injury.

Shear is the result of the force of gravity pushing down on the body and friction of the body against a surface, such as the bed or chair. For example, when a patient is in the semi-Fowler position and begins to slide to the foot of the bed, the skin over the sacral area remains in the same place because of the resistance of the bed surface. The blood vessels in the area are stretched and may cause small vessel thrombosis and tissue death (Bryant, 1992). The same type of damage can occur when a patient is pulled up in the bed if the skin does not move with the patient. Prevention of shear injury includes using "lift sheets" when repositioning a patient, elevating the bed no more than 30 degrees for short periods, and using the knee gatch to interrupt the pull of gravity on the body toward the foot of the bed.

Epidermal stripping results when the epidermis is unintentionally removed with tape removal. These lesions are usually shallow and irregularly shaped. Prevention of epidermal stripping includes recognizing fragile skin, such as in neonates; using minimum tape; using solid-wafer skin barriers, transparent dressings, or laced binders to secure dressings (Montgomery straps) on areas in which tape must be changed frequently; using skin sealants under adhesives unless skin is fragile; and using porous tapes. Tape is placed so there is no tension, traction, or wrinkle on the skin. To remove tape, slowly peel the tape away while stabilizing the underlying skin. Adhesive remover may be used to break the adhesive bond but may be drying to the skin (Bryant, 1992). Wetting the tape with water may facilitate removal.

Chemical factors can also lead to skin damage. Fecal incontinence, especially when mixed with urine; wound drainage; or gastric drainage around gastrostomy tubes can erode epidermis. The skin can very quickly progress from redness to denudement if exposure continues. Moisture barriers, gentle cleansing as soon after exposure as possible, and skin barriers can be used to prevent damage caused by chemical factors (see also Diaper Dermatitis, Chapter 50).

BATHING

Unless contraindicated, most infants and children can be bathed in a tub at the bedside, on the bed, or in a standard bathtub or shower located on the unit, which is often conveniently adapted for pediatric use. For infants and young children confined to bed, the towel method can be used. Two towels are immersed in a dilute soap solution and wrung damp. With the child lying supine on a dry towel, one damp towel is placed on top of the child and used to gently clean the body. This towel is discarded, and the child is dried and turned prone. The procedure is repeated using the second damp towel.

Infants and small children are *never* left unattended in a bathtub, and infants who are unable to sit alone are securely held with one hand during the bath. The infant's head is supported securely with one hand, or the farther arm is firmly grasped in the nurse's hand while the head rests comfortably on the nurse's wrist or arm. This hold provides secure control of the infant while the other hand is free to wash the infant's body (Fig. 42-4). Infants or children who are able to sit without assistance need only close supervision and a pad placed in the bottom of the tub to prevent slipping and loss of balance, which could result in a bumped head or submersion of the face.

Older children may enjoy a shower if it is available. School-age children may be reluctant to bathe, and many are not accustomed to a daily bath. However, most children who feel well require little encouragement to participate in their daily care. Nurses will need to use judgment regarding the amount of supervision the child requires. Some can be trusted to assume this responsibility unaided, whereas others will need someone in constant attendance. Children with mental or physical limitations and suicidal or psychotic children (who may cause bodily harm) require close supervision.

Areas that require special attention during bed baths and when children perform their own care are the ears, between skinfolds, the neck, the back, and the genital area. The genital area should be carefully cleansed and dried with particular care to skinfolds, and in uncircumcised boys, usually those over 3 years of age, the foreskin should be gently retracted and the exposed surfaces cleansed and then the foreskin replaced. Do not attempt to retract the foreskin in newborns. If the condition of the glans indicates inadequate cleaning, such as accumulated smegma, inflammation, phimosis, or foreskin adhesions, teaching proper hygiene is indicated. In the Vietnamese and Cambodian cultures the foreskin is traditionally not retracted until adulthood (Krueger and Osborn, 1986). Older children have the tendency to avoid these areas; therefore they may need a gentle reminder.

Children who are ill or debilitated will need more extensive assistance with bathing and other aspects of hygienic care, but they should be encouraged to perform as much as they can without overtaxing their energies. Increasing involvement can be expected with improved strength and endurance. Children with limited capacity for self-care but no other contraindications benefit greatly from tub baths. They can be transported to the tub and, with the aid of lifting devices and/or an appropriate number of persons to assist, gain the advantages of a tub bath.

ORAL HYGIENE

Mouth care is an integral part of daily hygiene and should be continued in the hospital. Infants and debilitated children will require the nurse to perform mouth care. Although young children can manage a toothbrush and should be encouraged to use it, most will need assistance to perform a satisfactory job. Older children, although capable of brushing and flossing without assistance, sometimes need to be reminded that this is

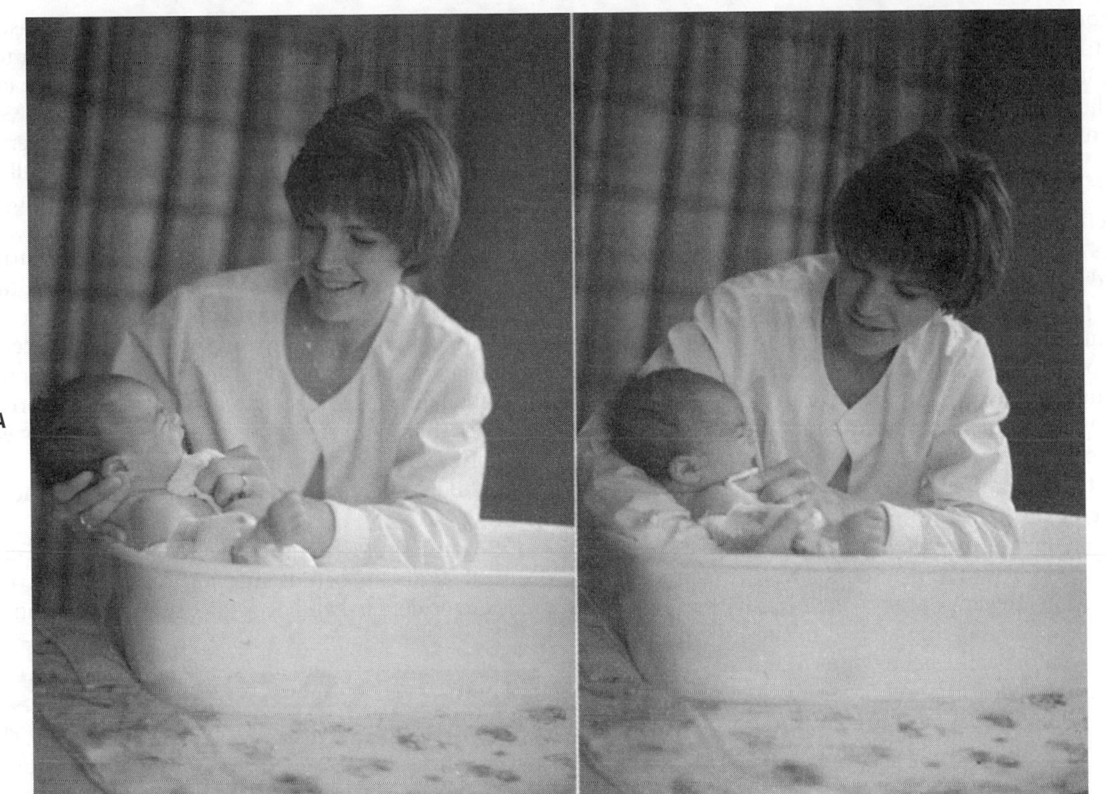

Fig. 42-4 Two methods of supporting infant during tub bath. **A**, Using hand to support neck and head. **B**, Using arm to support neck and head.

a part of their hygienic care. Most hospitals have equipment available for those children who do not have a toothbrush or toothpaste of their own. (See Dental Health, Chapters 33 and 34, for specific oral hygiene techniques; mouth care of children with mucosal ulcers is discussed under nursing care of the child with leukemia in Chapter 46).

HAIR CARE

Brushing and combing hair are a part of the daily care for all persons in the hospital, including infants and children. If the child does not have a brush or comb, many hospitals provide one as part of the usual admission kit. If not, the parents should be asked to supply hair care equipment for the child's use. Both boys and girls should be helped to comb or brush their hair, or it should be done for them, at least once daily. The hair is styled for comfort and in a manner pleasing to the child and parents. A satisfactory style for girls with longer hair is braiding. The hair should not be cut without parental permission, although shaving hair to provide access to a scalp vein for intravenous needle insertion may be necessary.

If children are hospitalized for more than a few days, the hair may need shampooing. Infants' hair may be washed during the daily bath or less frequently. For most children washing the hair and scalp once or twice weekly is sufficient, unless there is an indication to wash it more frequently, such as after a high fever and profuse sweating. Some hospitals have shampoo basins, but almost any child can be conveniently transported by a gurney to an accessible sink or washbasin for shampooing. Those who are unable to be transported can receive a shampoo in their bed with adequate protection and/or specially adapted equipment or positioning. A convenient method involves positioning the child near the edge of the bed, placing towels under the shoulders, and draping a large plastic garbage bag at the edge of the bed with one open side under the shoulders and the other side opened away from the head so that the hair is inside the opening. Water can be transported in a basin or placed in a clean enema bag. The bag is hung from an intravenous pole and the clamp on the bag's tubing is used to adjust the flow of water.

Teenagers, who normally have increased oily sebaceous secretions, are particularly in need of frequent hair care and usually require more frequent shampoos. Commercial no-rinse products also may prove useful on a short-term basis.

African-American children require special hair care, and this need is frequently neglected or inadequately managed. For the child with kinky hair, most standard combs are inadequate and may cause hair breakage and discomfort to the child. If a special comb with widely spaced teeth is not available on the unit, the parent can be reminded to supply a comb, if possible, for the child's use. It is also much easier to comb the hair after shampooing when it is wet. This type of hair also requires a special hair dressing or pomade, which usually has a coconut oil base. The preparation is rubbed on the hands and then transferred to the hair to make it more pliable and manageable. The child's parents should be consulted regarding the preparation they wish to be used on their child's hair, and they should be asked whether they can provide some for use during the child's hospitalization. Petroleum jelly should *not* be used. If braiding or plaiting the hair is desired, the hair should be damp and loosely woven. The hair tightens as it dries; tension folliculitis can result (Joyner, 1988).

FEEDING THE SICK CHILD

Loss of appetite is a symptom common to most childhood illnesses and is frequently the initial evidence of illness, preceding fever and other overt signs of infection. In most cases children can be permitted to determine their own need for food. Since an acute illness is usually short, the nutritional state is seldom compromised. In fact, urging foods on the sick child may precipitate nausea and vomiting and in some cases even cause an aversion to the feeding situation that can extend into the convalescent period and beyond.

Refusing to eat may also be one way children can exert power and control in an otherwise helpless situation. For young children, loss of appetite may be related to the depression of separation from their parents and their natural tendency toward negativism. Parents' concern with eating can intensify the problem. Forcing a child to eat only meets with rebellion and reinforces the behavior as a control mechanism. Parents are encouraged to relax any pressure during the period of acute illness. Although it is best to encourage high-quality nutritious foods, the child may desire foods and liquids that contain mostly calories. Some well-tolerated foods include gelatin, clear soups, carbonated drinks, flavored ice pops, dry toast, crackers, and hard candy. Even though these substances are not nutritious, they can provide necessary fluid and calories.

Dehydration is always a hazard when children are febrile or anorexic, especially when this state is accompanied by vomiting or diarrhea. An adequate fluid intake is encouraged by offering small amounts of favored fluids at frequent intervals and by offering salty foods (which increase thirst) if allowed. If diarrhea is present, high-carbohydrate liquids (e.g., carbonated beverages, gelatin, flavored ice pops) are avoided because they may aggravate the diarrhea by an osmotic effect. Also, replacing abnormal losses with plain water or undiluted broth, which may worsen the electrolyte imbalance, is not advocated. Fluids should not be forced, and the child should not be wakened from rest to take fluids. Forcing fluids may create the same difficulties as urging unwanted food. Gentle persuasion with preferred beverages will usually meet with success. Using play techniques can also be very effective (Box 42-3).

When children are placed on special diets, such as clear liquids after surgery or during episodes of diarrhea, assessment of their intake and readiness to advance to more complex foods is essential.

Nursing ALERT

Evidence of lack of readiness to advance the diet includes:
Vomiting or diarrhea
Decrease in appetite
Abdominal cramping or distention
Absence of bowel sounds
Dehydration or weight loss

Once the child is feeling better, the appetite usually begins to improve. It is best to take advantage of any hungry period by serving high-quality foods and snacks. If the child still refuses to eat, nutritious fluids, such as prepared breakfast drinks, should be encouraged. Parents can be very helpful by supplying favorite food items from home, especially if the family's cultural eating habits differ from the hospital's food service menus.

In general, hot dogs, hamburgers, peanut butter and jelly sandwiches, fruit yogurt, milkshakes, spaghetti, tacos, macaroni and cheese, and pizza are favorite foods of most children. Although alone they may not typify well-balanced diets, they can be adjusted to include sufficient amounts from the different food groups. It is better to work with preferred food choices than with selections that children rarely eat. A number of creative approaches to food preparation can increase the child's interest in eating (see the Guidelines box on p. 1269).

Regardless of the type of diet, charting of the amount consumed is an important nursing responsibility. Descriptions need to be detailed and accurate, such as "4 ounces of orange juice, one pancake, no bacon, and 8 ounces of milk." Comments such as "ate well" or "ate poorly" are inadequate. Charting the percentage of the meal eaten is also inadequate unless food is measured before serving.

Nursing ALERT

Ask the parent whether the child ate all of the food from the tray. Occasionally, a parent may eat something from the tray because the child did not eat or want it. The fact that a family member has eaten some of the food makes a marked difference in the report of how much the child ate.

If parents are involved in the child's care, they are encouraged to keep a list of everything eaten. Using a premeasured cup for fluids ensures a more accurate estimate of intake. A comparison of the intake at meals can isolate food deficiencies, such as insufficient intake of meat or vegetables. Behaviors associated with mealtime also identify possible factors influencing appetite. For example, the observation "Child eats well when with other children but plays with food if left alone in room" helps the nurse plan mealtime activities that stimulate the appetite.

CONTROLLING ELEVATED TEMPERATURES

An elevated temperature, most frequently resulting from fever but occasionally caused by hyperthermia, is one of the most common symptoms of illness in children. This manifestation is frequently misunderstood and of great, but often unnecessary, concern to parents. To facilitate an understanding of fever, the following terms are defined:

Set point—the temperature around which body temperature is regulated by a thermostatlike mechanism in the hypothalamus

Fever—an elevation in set point such that body temperature is regulated at a higher level; may be arbitrarily defined as temperature above 38° C (100° F)

Guidelines

FEEDING THE SICK CHILD

Take a dietary history (see Chapter 31) and use information to make eating time as homelike as possible.
Encourage parents or other family members to feed child or to be present at mealtimes.
Have children eat at tables in groups; take nonambulatory children to eating area in wheelchairs, beds, strollers, gurneys, or wagons.
Use familiar eating utensils, such as a favorite plate, cup, or bottle for small children.
Make mealtimes pleasant; avoid any procedures immediately before or after eating; make sure child is rested and pain-free.
Have a nurse present at mealtimes to offer assistance, prevent disruptions, and praise children for their eating.
Serve small, frequent meals rather than three large meals or serve three meals and nutritious between-meal snacks.
Supply foods from home, especially if food preparation is very different from hospital's; consider cultural differences.
Provide finger foods for young children.
Involve children in food selection and preparation whenever possible.
Serve small portions, and serve each course separately, such as soup first, followed by meat, potatoes, and vegetables, and ending with dessert; with young children camouflage size of food by cutting meat thicker so less appears on plate or by folding a cheese slice in half; offer second helpings; ensure a variety of foods, textures, and colors.
Provide food selections that are favorites of most children, such as peanut butter and jelly sandwiches, hot dogs, hamburgers, macaroni and cheese, pizza, spaghetti, tacos, fried chicken, corn on the cob, and fruit yogurt.
Avoid foods that are highly seasoned, have strong odors, are served hot, or are all mixed together, unless typical of cultural practices.
Provide fluid selections that are favorites of most children, such as fruit punch, cola, ginger ale, sweetened tea, ice pops, sherbet, ice cream, milk and milkshakes, eggnog, pudding, gelatin, clear broth, or creamed soups. (See also Box 42-3 on p. 1258).
Offer nutritious snacks, such as frozen yogurt or pudding, ice cream, oatmeal or peanut butter cookies, hot cocoa, cheese slices or "kisses," pieces of raw vegetable or fruit, and dried fruit or cereal.
Make food attractive and different, for example:
- Serve a "picnic lunch" in a paper bag.
- Pack food in a Chinese-food container; decorate container.
- Put a "face" or a "flower" on a hamburger or sandwich with pieces of vegetable.
- Use a cookie cutter to shape a sandwich.
- Serve pudding, yogurt, or juice frozen as an ice pop.
- Make slurpies or snow cones by pouring flavored syrup on crushed ice.
- Add vegetable coloring to water or milk.
- Serve fluids through brightly colored or unusually shaped straws.
- Make "bowtie" sandwiches by cutting them in triangles and placing two points together.
- Slice sandwiches into "fingers."
- Grate mounds of cheese.
- Cut apples horizontally to make circles.
- Put a banana on a hot dog bun and spread with peanut butter.
- Break uncooked spaghetti into toothpick lengths and skewer cheese, cold meat, vegetables, or fruit chunks.

Praise children for what they do eat.
Do *not* punish children for not eating by removing their dessert or putting them to bed.

Hyperthermia—a situation in which body temperature exceeds the set point, which usually results when the body or external conditions create more heat than the body can eliminate, such as in heat stroke, aspirin toxicity, seizures, or hyperthyroidism

Body temperature is regulated by a thermostatlike mechanism in the hypothalamus. This mechanism receives input from centrally and peripherally located receptors. When temperature changes occur, these receptors relay the information to the thermostat, which either increases or decreases heat production to maintain a constant set point temperature. However, during an infection, pyrogenic substances cause an increase in the body's normal set point, a process that is mediated by prostaglandins. Consequently the hypothalamus increases heat production until the core (internal) temperature reaches the new set point.

Most fevers in children are of viral origin, are of relatively brief duration, and have limited consequences. In addition, fever probably plays a role in enhancing the development of both specific and nonspecific immunity and in aiding recovery and survival from infection. Contrary to popular belief, neither the rise in temperature nor its response to antipyretics indicates the severity or cause of infection; this fact casts doubt on the value of using fever as a diagnostic or prognostic indicator.

Measures to Reduce Elevated Temperature

Treatment of elevated temperature depends on whether it is due to a fever or to hyperthermia. Because the set point is normal in hyperthermia, but increased in fever, different approaches must be used to lower body temperature successfully.

Fever. The principal reason for treating fever is the relief of discomfort; there is no specific degree of fever that requires treatment. Relief measures include pharmacologic and/or environmental intervention. The most effective intervention is the use of antipyretics to lower the set point.

Antipyretic drugs include acetaminophen, aspirin, and nonsteroidal antiinflammtory drugs (NSAIDs). Acetaminophen is the preferred drug; aspirin should not be given to children because of the association between aspirin use in children with influenza virus or chickenpox and Reye syndrome. One nonprescription NSAID, ibuprofen (Children's Motrin and Children's Advil), is approved for fever reduction in chil-

TABLE 42-1 Dosage recommendations for acetaminophen (Tylenol)*

AGE	WEIGHT (POUNDS)	DOSE (mg)	FORM†
Under 3 months	6-11	40	½ dropper
4-11 months	12-17	80	1 dropper or ½ tsp elixir
12-23 months	18-23	120	1½ dropper or ¾ tsp elixir or 1½ chewable tablet (80 mg)
2-3 years	24-35	160	2 droppers or 1 tsp elixir or 2 chewable tablets (80 mg)
4-5 years	36-47	240	1½ tsp elixir or 3 chewable tablets (80 mg)
6-8 years	48-59	320	2 tsp elixir or 4 chewable tablets (80 mg) or 2 swallowable tablets
9-10 years	60-71	400	2½ tsp elixir or 5 chewable tablets (80 mg) or 2½ swallowable tablets
11 years	72-95	480	3 tsp elixir or 6 chewable tablets (80 mg) or 3 swallowable tablets
12 years and above	96+	640	4 swallowable tablets

*Doses should be administered four or five times daily, but not to exceed five doses in 24 hours.

†1 dropper = 80 mg/0.8 ml; elixir = 160 mg/5 ml; chewable tablet = 80 mg each; junior strength chewable tablets = 160 mg each; junior strength swallowable tablets = 160 mg each. Rectal suppositories and sprinkle caps acetaminophen (Feverall) are also available from Upsher-Smith Laboratories, Inc, 14905 23rd Ave N, Minneapolis, MN 55447; (800) 328-3344.

dren as young as 6 months of age. Dosage is based on the initial temperature level: 5 mg/kg of body weight for temperatures less than 39.1° C (102.5° F) or 10 mg/kg for temperatures greater than 39.1° C (102.5° F). The duration of fever reduction is generally 6 to 8 hours and is longer with the higher dose (Simon, 1996). Nonprescription ibuprofen (Advil, Nuprin, Motrin IB, Medipren) is not approved for use in children under 12 years of age. The recommended dosages of acetaminophen are listed in Table 42-1. It may be given every 4 hours but no more than five times in 24 hours. Since body temperature normally decreases at night, three to four doses in 24 hours are usually sufficient to control most fevers. The temperature is usually retaken 30 minutes after the antipyretic is given to assess its effect but should not be repeatedly measured; the child's level of discomfort is the best indication for continued treatment.

Environmental measures to reduce fever may be used if they are tolerated by the child and do not induce shivering. Shivering is the body's way of maintaining the elevated set point by producing heat. Compensatory shivering greatly increases metabolic requirements above those already caused by the fever.

Nursing ALERT

Treatment of shivering is directed at modifying or interfering with the rate of heat loss by warming the body with increased clothing (especially on the extremities), higher environmental temperature, and warm baths (Holtzclaw, 1990).

Traditional cooling measures, such as dressing in minimum clothing, exposing the skin to the air, reducing room temperature, increasing air circulation, and applying cool moist compresses to the skin (e.g., the forehead), are effective if employed approximately 1 hour *after* an antipyretic is given so that the set point is lowered. Cooling procedures such as sponging or tepid baths are ineffective in treating febrile children either when used alone or in combination with antipyretics, and they cause considerable discomfort (Newman, 1985).

Seizures associated with a fever occur in 3% to 4% of all children, usually in those between 3 months and 5 years of age. Although most children never have febrile seizures after the first occurrence, a younger age at onset and a family history of febrile seizures are associated with recurring episodes. For children who have febrile seizures, administration of antipyretics does not prevent recurrences.

Hyperthermia. Unlike with fever, antipyretics are of no value in hyperthermia, because the set point is already normal. Consequently, cooling measures are used. Cool applications to the skin help to reduce the core temperature. Cooled blood from the skin surface is conducted to inner organs and tissues, and warm blood is circulated to the surface, where it is cooled and recirculated. The surface blood vessels dilate as the body attempts to dissipate heat to the environment and facilitate this cooling process.

Commercial cooling devices, such as cooling blankets or mattresses, are available to reduce body temperature. They are placed on the bed and covered with a sheet or lightweight blanket. Frequent temperature monitoring is essential to prevent excessive cooling of the body.

Traditionally, cool compresses have been used to decrease high temperature. However, no particular temperature of water is agreed on as optimal. For tepid tub baths, it is usually best to start with warm water and gradually add cool water until the desired temperature of 37° C (98.6° F) is reached to accustom the child to the lower temperature. Generally, the temperature of the water only has to be 1° to 2° (usually a warm temperature) less than the child's temperature to be effective (Kinmonth, Fulton, and Campbell, 1992). The child is placed directly into the tub of tepid water for 20 to 30 minutes while water is gently squeezed from a washcloth over the back and chest or gently sprayed over the body from a sprayer. In the bed or crib, cool washcloths or towels are used, exposing only one area of the body at a time. The sponging is continued for approximately 30 minutes.

Nursing ALERT

Isopropyl alcohol should never be used for sponging; neurotoxic effects such as stupor, coma, and even death have been reported (Arditi and Killner, 1987).

After the tub or sponge bath, the child is dried and dressed in lightweight pajamas, nightgown, or diaper and placed in a dry bed. The child is dried by gently rubbing the skin surface with a towel to stimulate circulation. The temperature is taken again 30 minutes after the tub bath or sponge bath. The tub or sponge bath should not be continued or restarted until the skin surface is warm or when the child feels chilled. Chilling causes vasoconstriction, which defeats the purpose of the cool applications. In this condition little blood is carried to the skin surface; the blood remains primarily in the viscera to become heated.

Whether a temperature elevation in the critically ill child is caused by fever or hyperthermia, it should be treated more aggressively. The metabolic rate increases 10% for every 1° C increase in temperature and three to five times during shivering, increasing oxygen, fluid, and caloric requirements. If the child's cardiovascular or neurologic system is already compromised, these increased needs are especially hazardous (Bruce and Grove, 1992). In all children with elevated temperature, attention to adequate hydration is essential. Most children's needs can be met through additional oral fluids.

FAMILY TEACHING AND HOME CARE

Nurses have a unique opportunity for teaching the family about health care practices while the child is hospitalized. Although most children have learned self-care and hygiene in the home or at school, many have not. For some young children this is their first introduction to the use of a toothbrush. Much health teaching can be accomplished even when the child is hospitalized for only a short time. The daily bath, handwashing before meals and after bowel and bladder evacuation, and conscientious dental hygiene are taught by example during routine care. Clean hair, nails, and clothing, as well as good grooming, are emphasized as essential to a pleasing appearance. Positive reinforcement of good hygiene practices helps to create a positive body image, promote the development of self-esteem, and prevent health problems (e.g., teaching girls to wipe the genital area from front to back after toileting).

Although sick children's appetites may be poor and not characteristic of their home eating habits, the hospital stay provides numerous opportunities for nurses to assess the family's knowledge of good nutrition and to implement teaching as needed to improve nutritional intake.

Parental education about elevated temperatures is essential, since many parents are unaware of what constitutes a fever, have unrealistic fears about the dangers of fever, and are likely to over- or undermedicate the febrile child. Parents also need to know that sponging is indicated for elevated temperatures from hyperthermia rather than fever and that ice water and alcohol are inappropriate, potentially dangerous solutions. Parents should know how to take the child's temperature, read the thermometer accurately, and have guidelines for seeking professional care (see the Home Care Box above).* Some of the newer temperature-measuring devices, such as tympanic membrane sensors, plastic strips, or digital thermometers, may be better suited for home use, since many parents are unable to read a mercury thermometer or calculate the correct decimal point (see Temperature, Chapter 32).

If the use of acetaminophen is indicated, the parents need instruction in administering the drug.* It is important to emphasize accuracy in both the amount of drug given and the intervals at which it is administered. Since many forms of acetaminophen are available, the nurse must be certain of the type being used in the home when discussing dosage. For example, the chewable tablets are available in *two* strengths (80 mg and 160 mg), and the specially coated swallowable tablets for older children are 160 mg. Alert the parents to this because the tablets for older children may contain *twice* the amount of drug as the lower-dose chewable ones. If parents switch from infant drops to elixir, they are cautioned against using the dropper to measure the elixir, which is much less concentrated than the drops. Also, as children grow, the dosage needs to be recalculated. To ensure the correct dose, it is recommended that a dose for a small child be calculated on the basis of 15 mg/kg/dose rather than 10 mg/kg/dose (Gribetz and Cronley, 1987).

Home Care

THE CHILD WITH FEVER

Call immediately if:
- Child is <2 months of age.
- Fever is >40.5° C (105° F).
- Child is crying inconsolably.
- Child is difficult to awaken.
- Child is confused or delirious.
- Child has had a seizure.
- Child has a stiff neck.
- Child has purple spots on the skin.
- Breathing is difficult, and child does not feel better after nose is cleared.
- Child is acting very sick.
- Child has an underlying risk factor for serious infection (e.g., sickle cell disease).

Call during office hours if:
- Child is 2 to 4 months old (unless fever is due to a diphtheria-pertussis-tetanus [DPT] vaccination).
- Fever is 40° to 40.5° C (104° to 105° F), especially if child is <2 years old.
- Burning or pain occurs with urination.
- Fever has been present for >72 hours.
- Fever has been present for >24 hours without an obvious cause or location of infection.
- Fever disappeared for >24 hours and then returned.
- Child has a history of febrile seizures.

Modified from Schmitt BD: Fever in childhood, *Pediatrics* 74(5, Suppl):934, 1984.

Safety

Safety is an essential component of any patient's care, but children have special characteristics that require an even greater concern for safety. Since small children are separated

*Home care instructions on measuring temperature and giving medications are available in Wong DL: *Wong and Whaley's clinical manual of pediatric nursing*, ed 4, St Louis, 1996, Mosby.

from their usual environment and do not possess the capacity for abstract thinking and reasoning, it is the responsibility of everyone in contact with them to maintain protective measures throughout their hospital stay. Nurses need to understand the age level at which each child is operating and plan for safety accordingly.

Name bands, a part of hospital safety practices, are particularly important for children in the pediatric age group. Infants and unconscious patients are unable to tell or respond to their names. Toddlers may answer to any name or to a nickname only. Older children may exchange places, give an erroneous name, or choose not to respond to their own name as a joke, unaware of the hazards of such practices.

INFECTION CONTROL

The use of medical asepsis and appropriate barrier precautions to reduce the risk of nosocomial (hospital-acquired) infections is essential in caring for children. Children are infected frequently with organisms, such as varicella (chickenpox), that are transmissible and may be dangerous to others, especially immunocompromised patients. In addition, children may not have developed good hygiene habits, such as handwashing after toileting. Young children are especially at risk for infection because of their high oral activity. Children in diapers present infection risks if caregivers do not practice meticulous cleaning and disposal techniques.

To assist hospitals in maintaining up-to-date isolation practices, the Centers for Disease Control and Prevention (CDC) and the Hospital Infection Control Practices Advisory Committee (HICPAC) have revised the "CDC Guideline for Isolation Precautions in Hospitals," which was published in 1983. The guideline was revised to meet the following objectives: (1) to be epidemiologically sound; (2) to recognize the importance of all body fluids, secretions, and excretions in the transmission of nosocomial pathogens; (3) to contain adequate precautions for infections transmitted by the airborne, droplet, and contact routes of transmission; (4) to be as simple and user friendly as possible; and (5) to use new terms to prevent confusion with existing infection control and isolation systems.*

The revised guideline contains two levels of precautions. In the first, and most important level are those precautions designed for the care of all patients in hospitals regardless of their diagnosis or presumed infection status. Implementation of these "Standard Precautions" is the primary strategy for successful nosocomial infection control. In the second level are precautions designed only for the care of specified patients. These additional "Transmission-Based Precautions" are used for patients known or suspected to be infected or colonized with epidemiologically important pathogens that can be transmitted by airborne or droplet transmission or by contact with dry skin or contaminated surfaces.

Standard Precautions synthesize the major features of Universal (Blood and Body Fluid) Precautions (UP) (designed to reduce the risk of transmission of bloodborne pathogens) and Body Substance Isolation (BSI) (designed to reduce the risk of transmission of pathogens from moist body substances). Standard Precautions apply to (1) blood; (2) all body fluids, secretions, and excretions *except sweat*, regardless of whether or not they contain visible blood; (3) nonintact skin; and, (4) mucous membranes. Standard Precautions are designed to reduce the risk of transmission of microorganisms from both recognized and unrecognized sources of infection in hospitals.

Transmission-Based Precautions are designed for patients documented or suspected to be infected or colonized with highly transmissible or epidemiologically important pathogens for which additional precautions beyond Standard Precautions are needed to interrupt transmission in hospitals. There are three types of Transmission-Based Precautions: Airborne Precautions, Droplet Precautions, and Contact Precautions. They may be combined for diseases that have multiple routes of transmission (Box 42-5). When used either alone or in combination, they are to be used in addition to Standard Precautions.

Airborne Precautions are designed to reduce the risk of airborne transmission of infectious agents. Airborne transmission occurs by dissemination of either airborne droplet nuclei (small-particle residue [5 μm or smaller in size] of evaporated droplets that may remain suspended in the air for long periods) or dust particles containing the infectious agent. Microorganisms carried in this manner can be dispersed widely by air currents and may be inhaled by or deposited on a susceptible host within the same room or over a longer distance from the source patient, depending on environmental factors; therefore, *special air handling* and *ventilation* are required to prevent airborne transmission. Airborne Precautions apply to patients known or suspected to be infected with epidemiologically important pathogens that can be transmitted by the airborne route. Examples of such illnesses include measles, varicella (chickenpox), and tuberculosis.

Droplet Precautions are designed to reduce the risk of droplet transmission of infectious agents. Droplet transmission involves contact of the conjunctivae or the mucous membranes of the nose or mouth of a susceptible person with large-particle droplets (larger than 5 μm in size) containing microorganisms generated from a person who has a clinical disease or who is a carrier of the microorganism. Droplets are generated from the source person primarily during coughing, sneezing, or talking and during the performance of certain procedures such as suctioning and bronchoscopy. Transmission via large-particle droplets requires close contact between source and recipient persons, because droplets do not remain suspended in the air and generally travel only short distances, usually 1 m (3 feet) or less, through the air. Because droplets do not remain suspended in the air, special air handling and ventilation are not required to prevent droplet transmission. Droplet Precautions apply to any patient known or suspected to be infected with epidemiologically important pathogens that can be transmitted by infectious droplets (Box 42-5).

Contact Precautions are designed to reduce the risk of transmission of epidemiologically important microorganisms by direct or indirect contact. *Direct-contact transmission* involves skin-to-skin contact and physical transfer of microorganisms to a susceptible host from an infected or colonized person, such as occurs when personnel turn patients, bathe patients, or perform other patient-care activities that require physical contact. Direct-contact transmission also can occur between two patients (e.g., by hand contact), with one serving

*This section is from Garner JS: Guidelines for isolation precautions in hospitals, *Infection Control Hosp Epidemiol* 17(1):54-80, 1996.

BOX 42-5
Summary of Types of Precautions and Patients Requiring Them

Standard precautions

Use Standard Precautions for the care of all patients

Airborne precautions

In addition to Standard Precautions, use Airborne Precautions for patients known or suspected to have serious illnesses transmitted by airborne droplet nuclei. Examples of such illnesses include measles, varicella (including disseminated zoster), and tuberculosis

Droplet precautions

In addition to Standard Precautions, use Droplet Precautions for patients known or suspected to have serious illnesses transmitted by large particle droplets. Examples of such illnesses include the following:

Invasive *Haemophilus influenzae* type b disease, including meningitis, pneumonia, epiglottitis, and sepsis

Invasive *Neisseria meningitidis* disease, including meningitis, pneumonia, and sepsis

Other serious bacterial respiratory infections spread by droplet transmission, including diphtheria (pharyngeal), Mycoplasma pneumonia, pertussis, pneumonic plague, streptococcal pharyngitis, pneumonia, or scarlet fever in infants and young children

Serious viral infections spread by droplet transmission, including adenovirus, influenza, mumps, parvovirus B19, rubella

Contact precautions

In addition to Standard Precautions, use Contact Precautions for patients known or suspected to have serious illnesses easily transmitted by direct patient contact or by contact with items in the patient's environment. Examples of such illnesses include the following:

Gastrointestinal, respiratory, skin, or wound infections or colonization with multidrug-resistant bacteria judged by the infection control program, based on current state, regional, or national recommendations, to be of special clinical and epidemiologic significance

Enteric infections with a low infectious dose or prolonged environmental survival, including *Clostridium difficile*. For diapered or incontinent patients: enterohemorrhagic *Escherichia coli* O157:H7, *Shigella*, hepatitis A, or rotavirus

Respiratory syncytial virus, parainfluenza virus, or enteroviral infections in infants and young children

Skin infections that are highly contagious or that may occur on dry skin, including diphtheria (cutaneous), herpes simplex virus (neonatal or mucocutaneous), impetigo, major (noncontained) abscesses, cellulitis, or decubiti , pediculosis, scabies, staphylococcal furunculosis in infants and young children, zoster (disseminated or in the immunocompromised host)

Viral/hemorrhagic conjunctivitis

Viral hemorrhagic infections (Ebola, Lassa, or Marburg)

From Garner JS: Guidelines for isolation precautions in hospitals, *Infection Control Hosp Epidemiol* 17(1):66, 1996.

as the source of infectious microorganisms and the other as a susceptible host. *Indirect-contact transmission* involves contact of a susceptible host with a contaminated intermediate object, usually inanimate, in the patient's environment. Contact Precautions apply to specified patients known or suspected to be infected or colonized (presence of microorganism in or on patient but without clinical signs and symptoms of infection) with epidemiologically important microorganisms that can be transmitted by direct or indirect contact.

Nurses caring for young children are frequently in contact with body substances, especially urine, feces, and vomitus. Nurses need to exercise judgment for those situations when gloves, gowns, or masks are necessary. For example, gloves and possibly gowns should be worn for changing diapers when there are loose or explosive stools. Otherwise, the plastic lining of disposable diapers provides a sufficient barrier between the hands and body substances. The type of diaper may be an important aspect of infection control. Superabsorbent disposable diapers with elastic legs contain urine and feces better than cloth diapers, and their use can reduce fecal contamination in the environment (Van et al, 1991).

Nursing ALERT

Handwashing is the most critical infection control practice.

During feedings, gowns should be worn if the child is likely to vomit or spit up, as often occurs during burping. If aprons with minimal shoulder protection are worn, the child should be sitting on the nurse's lap, not upright against the shoulder, when the child is bubbled. When gloves are worn, the hands are washed thoroughly after removing the gloves, because both latex and vinyl gloves fail to provide complete protection. The absence of visible leaks does not indicate that gloves are intact. In addition, glove leaks occur more frequently with vinyl than with latex gloves (Olsen et al, 1993). An additional consideration is that some people are allergic to latex (see Spina Bifida, Chapter 52).

Nursing ALERT

Patients and staff may be sensitive to latex and demonstrate allergic reactions ranging from hives, wheezing, and localized swelling to anaphylaxis. Latex is present in numerous health care products, including gloves, tourniquets, airway equipment, catheters, IV supplies, and dressings.

Another essential practice of infection control is that all needles (uncapped and unbroken) are disposed of in a rigid, puncture-resistant container located near the site of use. Consequently, these containers are installed in patients' rooms. Since children are naturally curious, extra attention is needed in selecting a suitable type of container and a location that discourages access to the disposed needles (Fig. 42-5). The use of needleless systems allows secure syringe or IV tubing attachment to vascular access devices without the risk of needle stick injury to the child or nurse. These devices also help maintain IV line integrity.

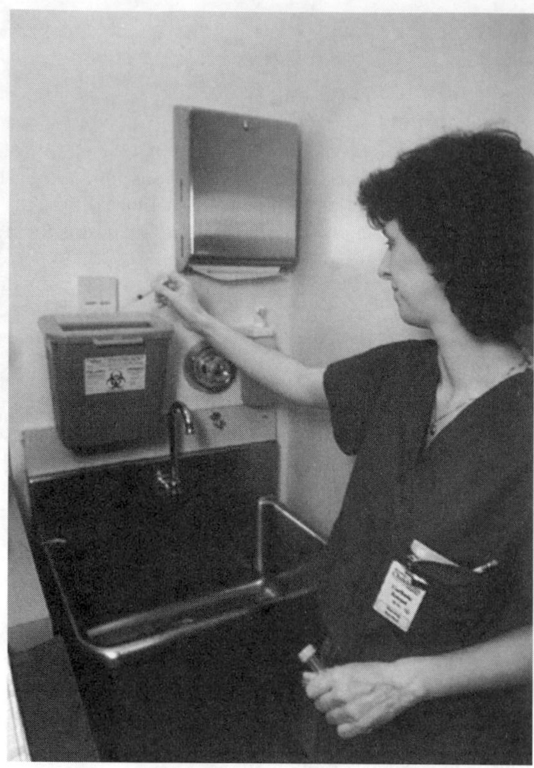

Fig. 42-5 To prevent needle-stick injuries, used needles (and other sharp instruments) are not capped or broken and are disposed of in a rigid, puncture-resistant container located near the site of use. Note placement of the container to prevent children's access to the contents.

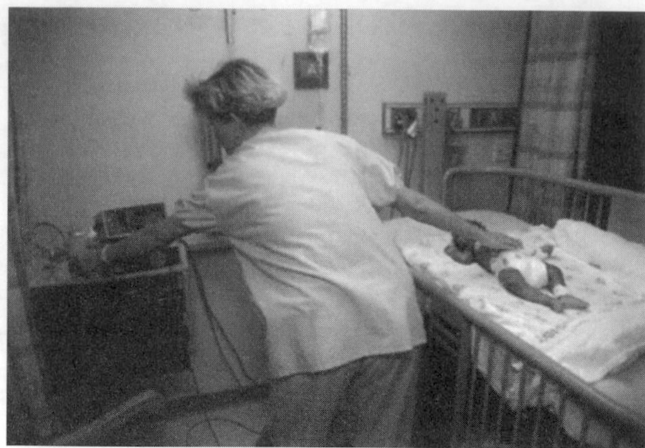

Fig. 42-6 Nurse maintains hand contact when back is turned.

ENVIRONMENTAL FACTORS

All the environmental safety measures in operation for the protection of adults apply to children as well, such as good illumination; floors clear of fluid or objects that might contribute to falls; nonskid surfaces in showers and tubs; electrical equipment that is maintained in good working order, is operated only by personnel familiar with its use, and is not in contact with moisture or near tubs, where it could prove to be a shock hazard; beds of ambulatory patients locked in place and at a height that allows easy access to the floor (a special hazard for children is the danger of entrapment under an electronically controlled bed when it is activated to descend); proper care and disposal of small breakable items such as thermometers and bottles; and a well-organized fire plan known to all staff members.

All windows should be securely screened and elevators and stairways made safe. Ideally, electrical outlets should be provided with covers to prevent burns of small children whose exploratory activities may extend to inserting objects into the small openings. Bathwater is carefully checked before placing the child into it, and children must never be left alone in a bathtub. Infants are helpless in water, and small children (and some older ones) may turn on the hot water faucet and be severely burned.

Furniture is safest when it is scaled to the child's proportions, is sturdy, and is well balanced to prevent its being easily tipped. Infants and small children must be securely strapped into infant seats, feeding chairs, and strollers. Use of baby walkers should be discouraged because they provide access to hazards, resulting in burns, falls, and poisonings. Infants, young children, and those who are weak, paralyzed, agitated, confused, sedated, or cognitively impaired are never left unattended on treatment tables, on scales, or in treatment areas. Even premature infants are capable of surprising mobility; therefore portholes in incubators must be securely fastened when not in use. Beds of ambulatory patients should remain locked in place and at a height that allows easy access to the floor.

Crib sides should be elevated and fastened securely unless an adult is at the bedside. It is safer to leave crib sides up, regardless of the child's ability to get out and even when the crib is unoccupied, to prevent the temptation to climb in. Anyone attending an infant or small child in a crib with the sides down should never turn away without maintaining hand contact with the child; that is, one hand should be kept on the child's back or abdomen to prevent the child from rolling, crawling, or jumping from the open crib (Fig. 42-6). A child who is likely to or has demonstrated the inclination to climb over the sides of the crib is safest when placed in a specially constructed crib with a cover or one that has a safety net placed over the top. If the net is used, it must be tied to the frame in such a manner that there is ready access to the child in case of emergency. Nets are never tied to the movable crib sides, and the knots should be tied in a manner that permits quick release. Cribs are not placed within reach of heating units, appliances, dangling cords, or other objects that can be grabbed by curious hands, and toys are not tied to or across crib rails once children are old enough to reach them.

Toys. Toys play a vital role in the everyday life of children, and they are no less important in the hospital setting. However, it is up to nurses to assess the safety of toys taken to the hospital by well-meaning parents and friends. Toys and gifts should be appropriate to the child's age, condition, and treatment. For example, if the child is in an oxygen tent, electrical or friction toys cannot be placed in the tent. Toys are inspected to make certain that they are nonallergenic, washable, and unbreakable and that they have no small, removable parts that can be aspirated or swallowed or that can in other ways inflict injury on a child.

Nursing ALERT

Plants and flowers harbor gram-negative bacteria and molds that may be of risk to the immunocompromised child. These items may also pose the danger of poisoning to curious toddlers.

LIMIT-SETTING

Setting limits is essential to a child's safety. Children must understand where they are permitted to go and what they are permitted to do in the hospital. These limitations should be made clear to them, consistently enforced, and repeated as frequently as necessary to make certain that they are understood. The nurse is responsible for a child's whereabouts at all times. Children can easily wander off unnoticed, and their access to tubs, laundry chutes, medication rooms/carts, and elevators must be prevented. Normally active older children often become restless when their activity is restricted and may resort to pillow fights, water fights, and other rough play that may endanger the safety of the involved children or other children, staff, or visitors. Children in the hospital require supervision, and appropriate tension-reducing activities can be planned and supervised by nurses and/or by the play therapist. A useful discipline technique is time-out (see Limit-setting and Discipline, Chapter 29).

TRANSPORTING INFANTS AND CHILDREN

In the course of a hospital stay, infants and children usually need to be transported within the unit and to areas outside the pediatric unit. Infants and small children can be carried for

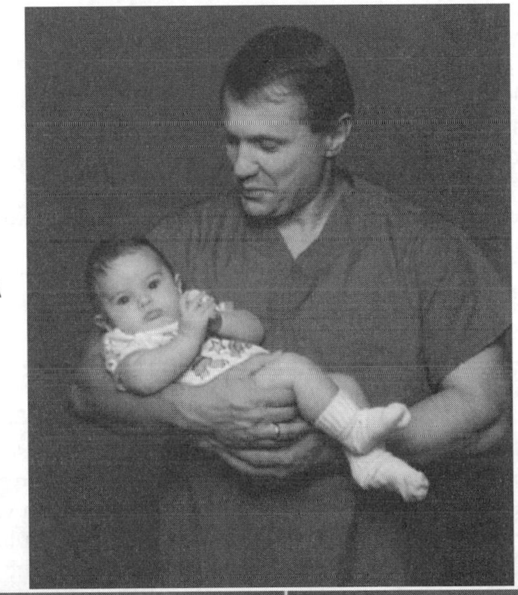

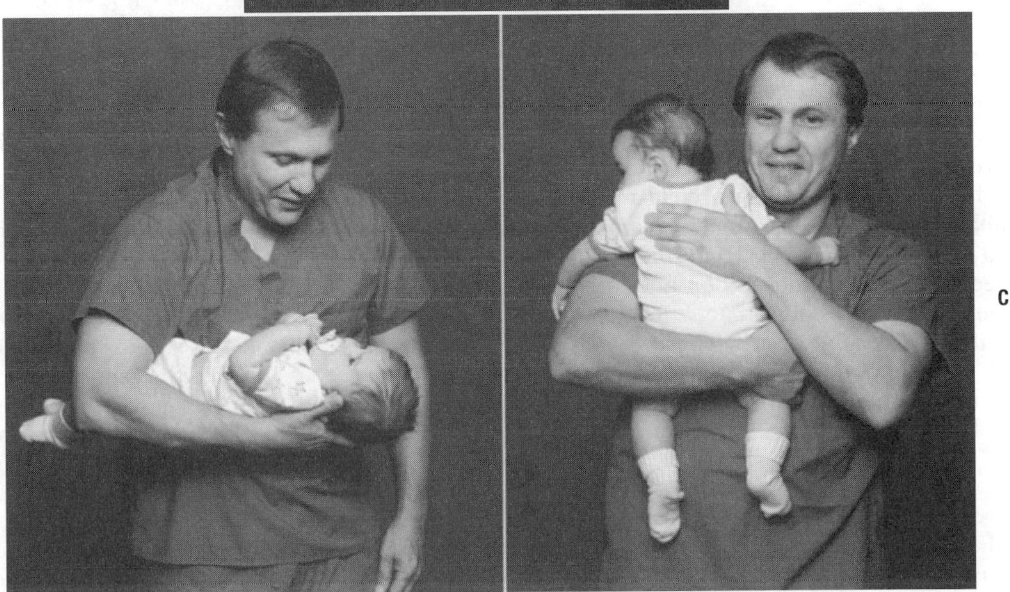

Fig. 42-7 Transporting infants. **A,** Infant's thigh firmly grasped in nurse's hand. **B,** Football hold. **C,** Back supported.

short distances within the unit, but for more extended trips they should be securely transported in a suitable conveyance.

Small infants can be held or carried in the horizontal position with the back supported and the thigh grasped firmly by the carrying arm (Fig. 42-7, *A*). In the football hold the infant is carried on the nurse's arm with the head supported by the hand and the body held securely between the nurse's body and elbow (Fig. 42-7, *B*). Both of these holds leave the nurse's other arm free for activity. The infant can be held in the upright position with the buttocks on the nurse's forearm and the front of the body resting against the nurse's chest. The infant's head and shoulders are supported by the nurse's other arm to allow for any sudden movement by the infant (Fig. 42-7, *C*). Older infants are able to hold the head erect but can still make sudden movements.

Infants can be transported to other areas, such as the radiography department, in their bassinets or cribs. Baby carriages are sometimes used for infants who are not likely to stand up. Strollers and wheeled feeding chairs or tables are also convenient transporters in some situations, such as trips to the playroom or nurse's station.

The method of transporting children is determined by their age, condition, and destination. Most older children are safe in wheelchairs or on gurneys. A younger child can be transported in a crib, on a gurney, in a wagon with raised sides, or in a wheelchair with a safety belt. Gurneys should be equipped with high sides and a safety belt, both of which are secured during transport.

RESTRAINTS

Frequently some method of restraint is needed to ensure a child's safety or comfort, to facilitate examination, or to carry out procedures. Restraint can be accomplished manually or with physical devices. Restraining the child manually provides an element of human contact that is lacking in restraint by mechanical means (Fig. 42-8). A physician's order and parental consent are required for restraints used for reasons other than procedures. These requirements are controversial, and nurses should be aware of their agencies' policies. These requirements originated from some concerns in elderly persons. Restraints can often be avoided with adequate preparation of the child, parental or staff supervision of the child, and adequate protection of a vulnerable site, such as an infusion device.

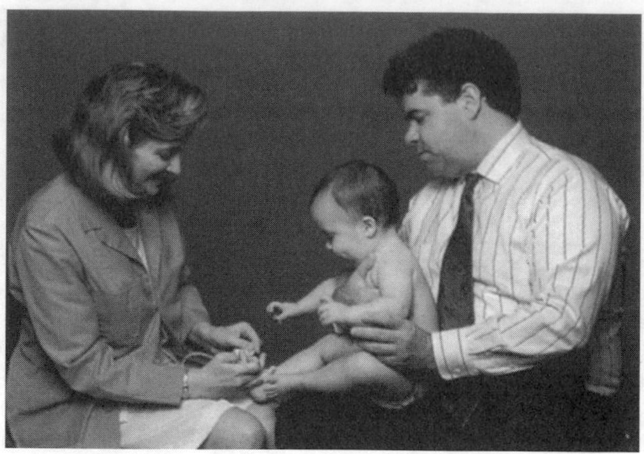

Fig. 42-8 Parent provides comfort and security to infant while nurse carries out procedure.

Mechanical restraints are never used as a punishment or as a substitute for observation. When a child must be restrained, the child and parents need a simple explanation, and if the restraint is applied for an extended time, the explanation must be repeated often to gain cooperation and to help the child understand that it is not a punishment. Restraining devices are not without risk and must be checked and documented every 1 to 2 hours to ensure that they are accomplishing their purpose, that they are applied correctly, and that they do not impair circulation, sensation, or skin integrity.

Parents need to know the purpose of restraints, techniques to remove and reapply them, and the signs of complications from their use. Parents are sometimes upset when their child must be restrained and need to understand how they can help ensure the maximum benefit and minimize the stress related to the use of restraints. Children, too, should be prepared for the procedure or the circumstance for which the restraint is required.

Removing restraints whenever possible (at least every 2 hours when children are awake) is an essential part of nursing care of children who are restrained for treatments or other purposes. Alternate methods may be devised to replace the need for passive restraints. Holding children for periods is a pleasant alternative, as is restraining them in a high chair where they can observe the surrounding activities. If feasible, distraction techniques such as play and reading to the child should be employed to gain cooperation without resorting to restraints. Parental participation is always encouraged.

Jacket Restraint

A jacket restraint is sometimes used as an alternative to the crib net to prevent the child from climbing out of the crib or to keep the child safe in various chairs. The jacket is put on the child with the ties in back so that the child is unable to manipulate them, and the long tapes, secured to the understructure of the crib, keep the child inside the crib. The jacket restraint is also useful as a means to maintain the child in a desired horizontal position. A Posey belt scaled to fit the child is an alternative device. The jacket-type restraint has been associated with accidental strangulation deaths in elderly persons.

Mummy Restraint

When an infant or small child requires short-term restraint for examination or treatment that involves the head and neck—such as venipuncture, throat examination, and gavage feeding—the mummy device effectively controls the child's movements. A blanket or sheet is opened on the bed or crib with one corner folded to the center. The infant is placed on the blanket with shoulders at the fold and feet toward the opposite corner (Fig. 42-9, *A*). With the infant's right arm straight down against the body, the right side of the blanket is pulled firmly across the infant's right shoulder and chest and secured beneath the left side of the body (Fig. 42-9, *B*). The left arm is placed straight against the child's side, and the left side of the blanket is drawn across the shoulder and chest and locked beneath the child's body on the right side. The lower corner is folded and pulled over the body and tucked or fas-

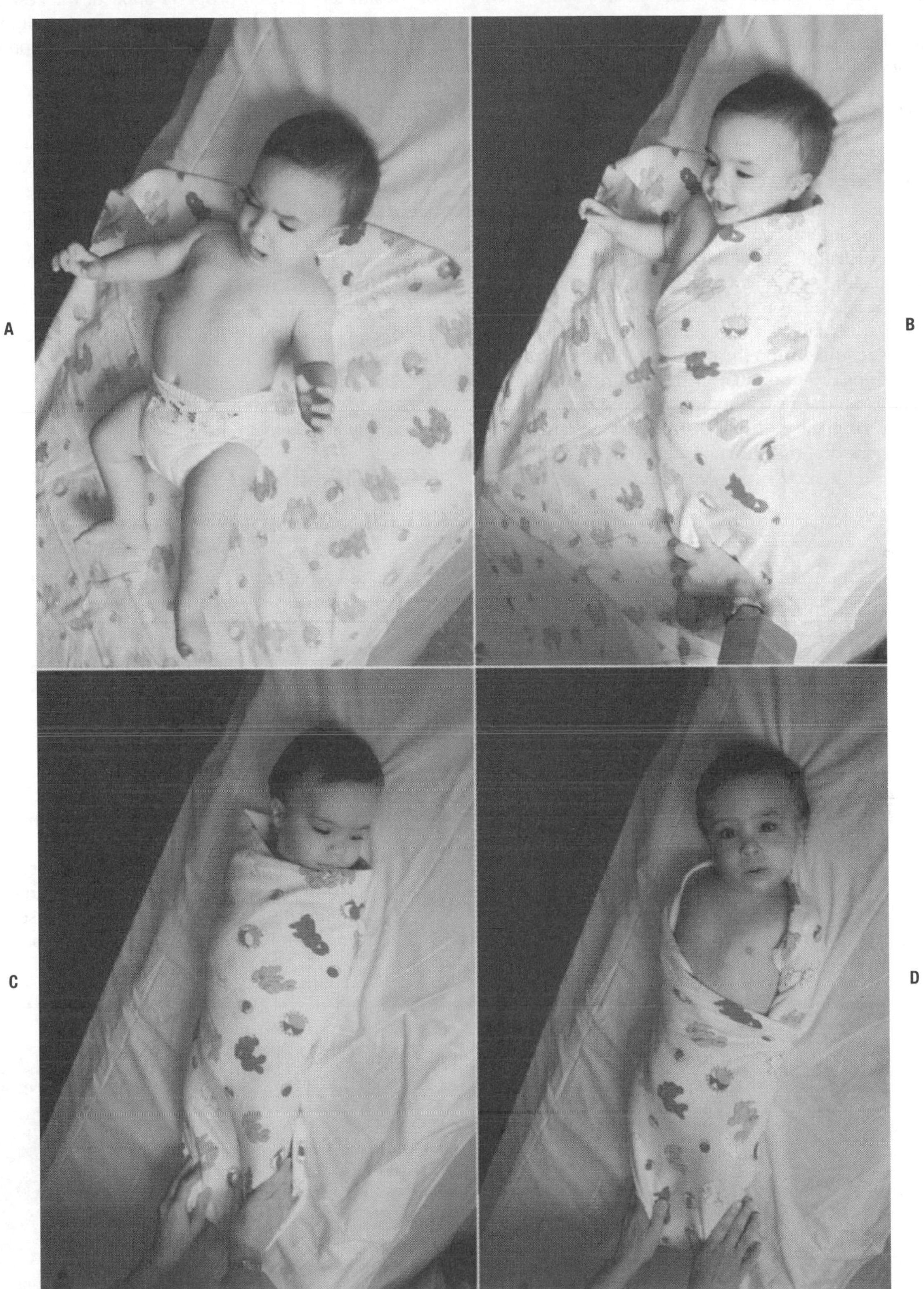

Fig. 42-9 Application of mummy restraint. **A,** Infant placed on folded corner of blanket. **B,** One corner of blanket drawn across body and secured beneath body. **C,** Second corner drawn across body and secured, and lower corner folded and tucked or pinned in place. **D,** Modified mummy restraint with chest uncovered.

tened securely with safety pins (Fig. 42-9, *C*). Safety pins can be used to fasten the blanket in place at any step in the process.

To modify the mummy restraint for chest examination, the folded edge of the blanket is drawn over each arm and under the back, after which the loose edge is folded over and secured at a point below the chest to allow visualization and access to the chest (Fig. 42-9, *D*).

Arm and Leg Restraints

Occasionally one or more extremities must be restrained or limited in motion. Several commercial restraining devices are available, or a restraint can be fashioned from gauze tape, muslin strips, or a length of narrow stockinette. When this type of restraint is used, it must be appropriate to the size of the child; it must be padded to prevent undue pressure, constriction, or tissue injury; and the extremity must be observed frequently for signs of irritation and/or impairment of circulation. The ends of the restraints are never tied to the crib rails, since lowering the rail will disturb the extremity, frequently with a jerk that may hurt or injure the child.

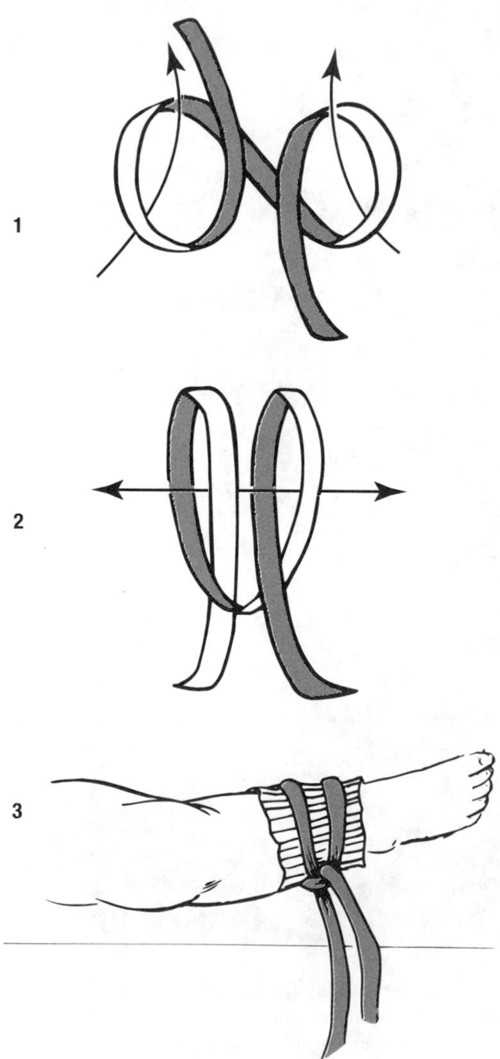

Fig. 42-10 Clove hitch restraint.

The *clove hitch restraint* is fashioned from a length of gauze or muslin tape. When properly applied, the restraint should provide a snug fit with minimum danger of pulling too tightly. Fig. 42-10 illustrates the method of tying and applying a clove hitch restraint.

Elbow Restraint

Sometimes it is important to prevent the child from reaching the head or face (e.g., after lip surgery, when a scalp vein infusion is in place, or for prevention of scratching in skin disorders). For this purpose, elbow restraints fashioned from a variety of materials function very well. The most common form of elbow restraint consists of a piece of muslin long enough to reach comfortably from just below the axilla to the wrist with a number of vertical pockets into which tongue depressors are inserted. The restraint is wrapped around the arm and secured with tapes or pins. It may be necessary to pin the top of the restraint to the undershirt sleeve to prevent the restraint from slipping. Similar restraints are sometimes made from commonly available products.

POSITIONING FOR PROCEDURES

Jugular Venipuncture

The large, superficial external jugular vein may be used to obtain blood specimens from infants and young children. For easy access to the vein, the child is first placed in a mummy restraint in which the top edge of the restraint is low enough to permit access to the vein. The child is placed so that the head and shoulders extend over the edge of a table or a small pillow with the neck extended and the head turned sharply to the side (Fig. 42-11). One alternate method for restraining arms and legs is with the nurse holding the child's arms and legs at the same time that the child's head is restrained and positioned. It is important for the nurse holding the infant to maintain control of the infant's head without interfering with the practitioner's approach to the vein. The infant's crying during the procedure increases intravenous pressure, which facilitates visualization of the vein. After venipuncture, digital pressure is applied to the site with a dry gauze square for 3 to 5 minutes or until bleeding stops. Care must be taken not to

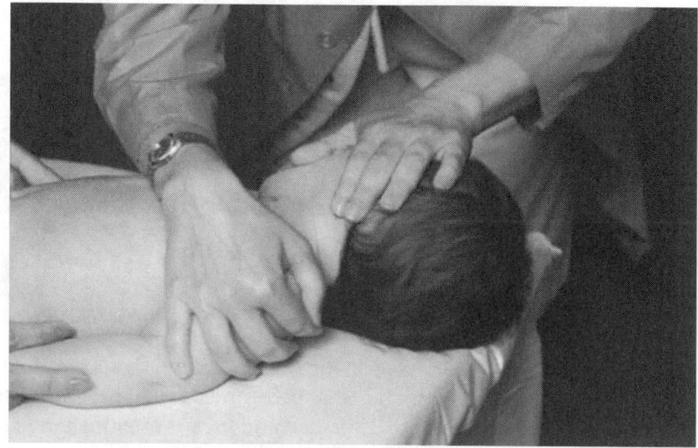

Fig. 42-11 Restraining child for jugular vein puncture.

apply excessive pressure that might compromise circulation or breathing during or after the procedure.

Femoral Venipuncture

Other commonly used sites for venipuncture are the large femoral veins. The nurse restrains the infant by placing the child supine with the legs in a frog position to provide extensive exposure of the groin area. Both the arms and the legs of the infant can be effectively controlled by the nurse's forearms and hands (Fig. 42-12). Only the side used for the venipuncture is uncovered, so that the practitioner is protected should the child urinate during the procedure. Pressure is applied to the site after the withdrawal of blood to prevent oozing from the site.

Extremity Venipuncture

The most common sites of venipuncture are the veins of the extremities, especially the arm and hand. A convenient position for restraint is having one person on either side of the bed. The child's outstretched arm is partially stabilized by the technician drawing the blood. The other person leans across the child's upper body, preventing its movement, and uses an arm to immobilize the venipuncture site. This type of restraint also comforts the child because of the close body contact and allows each person to maintain eye contact (Fig. 42-13).

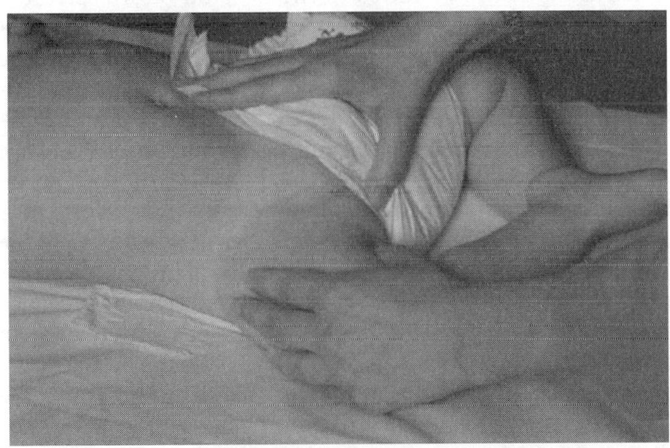

Fig. 42-12 Restraining infant for femoral vein puncture.

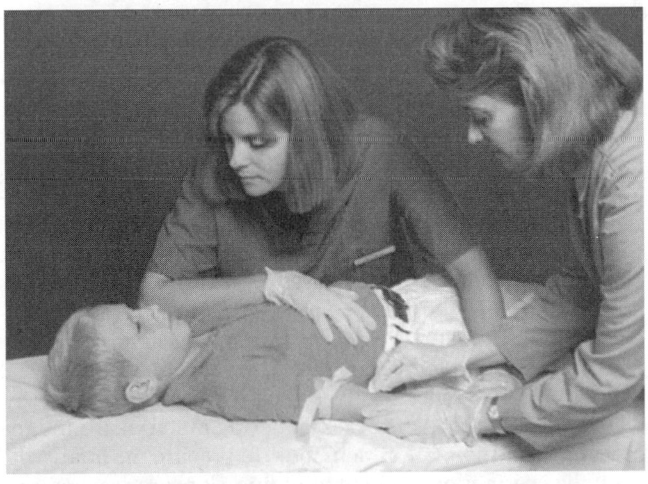

Fig. 42-13 Restraining child for extremity vein puncture.

Lumbar Puncture

The technique for lumbar puncture in infants and children is similar to that in the adult, although modifications are suggested in neonates, who have less distress in a side-lying position with modified neck extension than in flexion or a sitting position (Fig. 42-14, *A*). Neonates tend to have more cardiorespiratory changes during a lumbar puncture than do older infants regardless of positioning; therefore oximetry and heart rate monitoring are advisable (Lehmann et al, 1990). Pediatric lumbar puncture sets contain smaller spinal needles,

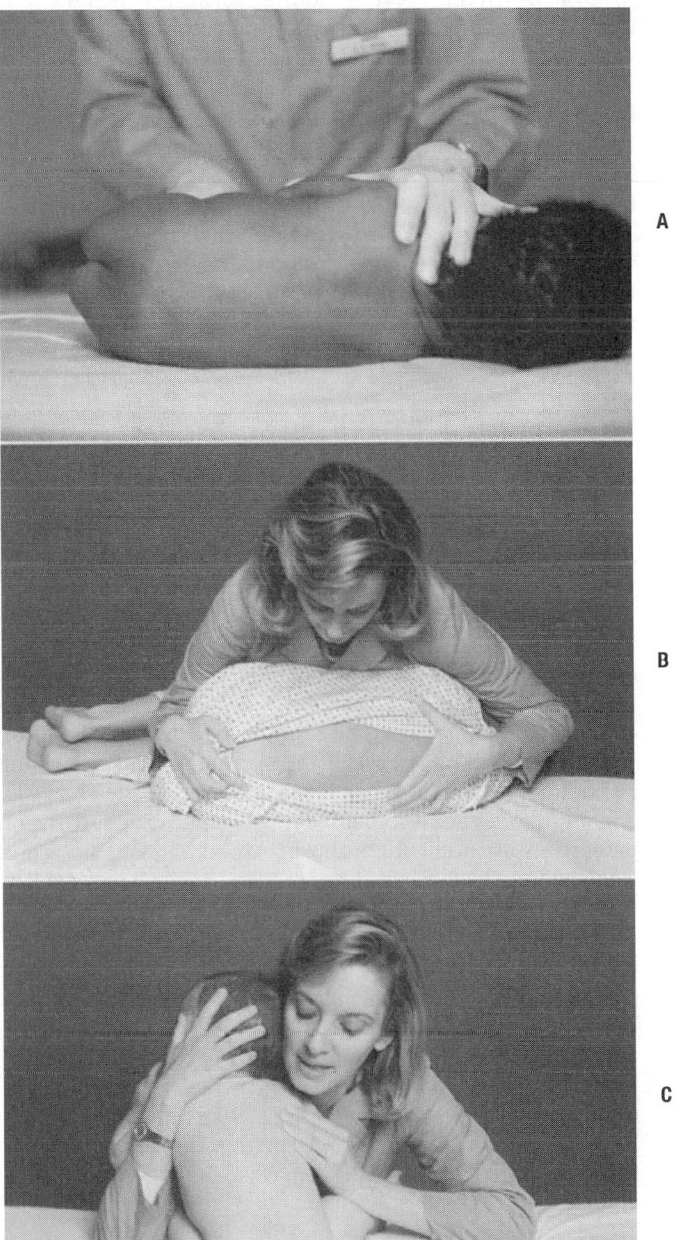

Fig. 42-14 **A,** Modified side-lying position for lumbar puncture. **B,** Older child in side-lying position. **C,** Infant sitting position allows for flexion of lumbar spine.

but sometimes the practitioner will specify a particular size or type of needle that the nurse should make certain is placed on the tray.

Children are usually controlled best in the side-lying position, with the head flexed and the knees drawn up toward the chest. Even cooperative children need to be restrained to prevent possible trauma from unexpected, involuntary movement. They can be reassured that although they are trusted, the restraint will serve as a reminder to maintain the desired position. It also provides a measure of support and reassurance to them.

The child is placed on the side with the back close to the edge of the examining table on the side from which the practitioner is working. The nurse maintains the child's spine in a flexed position by holding the child with one arm behind the neck and the other behind the thighs (Fig. 42-14, *B*). The flexed position enlarges the spaces between the lumbar vertebral spines, facilitating access to the spinal fluid space. It is helpful to wrap the legs before positioning to decrease leg movement.

An alternate position used with small infants and some older children is the sitting position. The child is placed with the buttocks at the edge of the table and with the neck flexed so that the chin rests on the chest. The infant's arms and legs are immobilized by the nurse's hands (Fig. 42-14, *C*).

Nursing ALERT

The sitting position may interfere with chest expansion and diaphragm excursion, and in infants the soft, pliable trachea may collapse. Therefore observe the child for difficulty with breathing.

Another position that employs close and comforting contact for the child involves holding the child upright against the nurse's (or parent's) chest with the child's legs wrapped around the adult's waist. The adult's arms are used to hug and restrain the child. For ease of the examiner, the adult should be standing. A small pillow is placed between the child's abdomen and the adult to help arch the child's back. If the pillow proves unsuccessful, a third person can place an arm in this space to achieve the desired position. Care should be taken that excessive pressure does not compromise circulation or breathing and that the nose and mouth are not covered by the restrainer's body.

Specimens and spinal fluid pressure are obtained, measured, and sent for analysis in the same manner as for the adult patient. Vital signs are taken as ordered, and the child is observed for any changes in level of consciousness, motor activity, or other neurologic signs. Postlumbar puncture headache may occur and is related to postural changes; it is less severe when the child lies flat. Headache is seen much less often in young children than in adolescents.

Bone Marrow Aspiration/Biopsy

Positioning for a bone marrow aspiration or biopsy depends on the location of the chosen site. In children the posterior or anterior iliac crest is most commonly used, although in infants the tibia may be selected because of easy access to the site and restraint of the child.

If the posterior iliac crest is used, the child is positioned prone. Sometimes a small pillow or folded blanket is placed under the hips to facilitate obtaining the bone marrow specimen. In children who have not received adequate analgesia or anesthesia, restraint is needed and is best applied by two people—one person to immobilize the upper body and a second person to immobilize the lower extremities. If the other sites are used, the child is placed supine and restraint is applied in a similar manner with modifications made for access to the tibia or anterior iliac crest.

Other Procedures

For subdural puncture through a fontanel or burr hole, the infant is wrapped in a mummy restraint and placed in the supine position with the head accessible to the examiner. To control the head, the nurse uses a firm hold on each side of it. Procedures for immobilizing the head for examining the ears, nose, or throat are discussed in Chapter 32.

Collection of Specimens

URINE SPECIMENS

When children are admitted to the hospital or are seen in a clinic or office, a urine specimen may be needed. Older children and adolescents can use a bedpan or urinal or can be trusted to follow directions for collection in the bathroom. Attention to their special needs and concerns is warranted, however. School-age children are cooperative but curious and are likely to ask questions regarding the disposition of their specimen and what one expects to discover from it. Self-conscious adolescents may be reluctant to carry a specimen bottle through a hallway or waiting room and appreciate a paper bag or other means for disguising the container. The presence of menses is sometimes an embarrassment or a concern to teenage girls; therefore, it is a good idea to ask whether they are menstruating and to make adjustments as necessary. The specimen can be delayed or a notation made on the laboratory slip to explain the presence of red blood cells.

Preschoolers and toddlers are usually unable to void on request. It is often best to offer them water or other liquids that they enjoy and wait about 30 minutes until they are ready to void voluntarily or to set a timer to alert them that they need to void shortly. The child will better understand what is expected if the nurse uses familiar terms, such as "pee-pee" or "tinkle." Some children will have difficulty voiding in an unfamiliar receptacle. Potty-chairs or a potty hat placed on the toilet will usually prove satisfactory. Toddlers who have recently acquired bladder control may be especially reluctant, since they undoubtedly have been admonished for "going" in places other than those approved by parents. A useful approach is to enlist the help of parents; they are likely to be successful, and this helps them feel a part of the child's care.

For infants and toddlers who are not toilet trained, special urine collection devices may be used. These devices are clear plastic single-use bags with self-adhering material around the opening at the point of attachment. To prepare the infant, the genitalia, perineum, and surrounding skin are washed and dried thoroughly, since the adhesive will not stick to a moist,

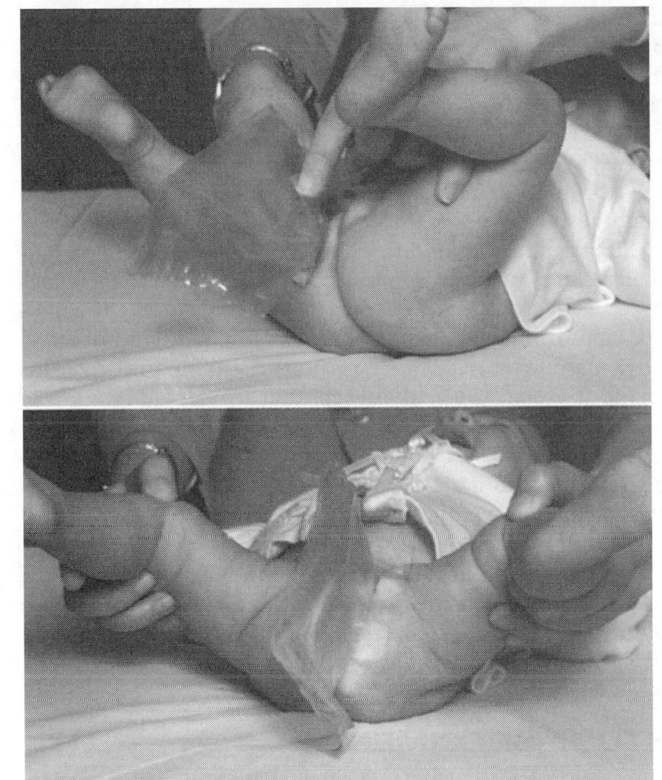

Fig. 42-15 Application of urine collection bag. **A,** On female infants adhesive portion is applied to exposed and dried perineum first. **B,** Bag adheres firmly around perineal area to prevent urine leakage.

powdered, or oily skin surface. The collection bag is easiest to apply if attached first to the perineum, progressing to the symphysis (Fig. 42-15). With little girls the perineum is stretched taut during application to that area to ensure a leak-proof fit. With small boys the penis and scrotum are placed inside the bag. The adhesive portion of the bag must be firmly applied to the skin all around the genital area to prevent possible leakage. For low-birth-weight infants small bags with adhesive that is gentle to the skin are available.* Anatomically correct urine collection bags are also available.†

The diaper is carefully replaced. The bag is checked frequently and removed as soon as the specimen is available, since the moist bag may become loosened on an active child. When urine is collected for culture, the bag is removed immediately. If the urine is not tested within 30 minutes, the specimen is refrigerated or placed in a sterile container with a preservative.

To obtain small amounts of urine, a syringe without a needle is used to aspirate urine directly from the diaper; if diapers with absorbent gelling material that trap urine are used, a small gauze dressing, some cotton balls, or a urine collection device* can be placed inside the diaper to collect urine and aspirate the urine with a syringe.

The abdomen can be wiped with an alcohol pad and fanned dry; cooling effect often causes voiding within 2 minutes (Ellis, 1989). Pressure can be applied over the suprapubic area or paraspinal muscles stroked (along the spine) to elicit the Perez reflex; in infants 4 to 6 months of age, the reflex causes crying, extension of the back, flexion of extremities, and urination.

Urine obtained from disposable diapers can be tested accurately for glucose, ketones, protein, blood, bilirubin, urobilinogen, nitrates, potassium, creatinine, and urea. Erythrocyte and leukocyte counts may be low. Superabsorbent disposable diapers may produce a false crystalluria. Specific gravity measurements are accurate for up to 4 hours provided that the disposable diapers are kept folded. The accuracy of these tests performed on urine obtained from cloth diapers is unknown (Wong et al, 1992).

Traditionally, specific gravity refractometers have been used on nursing units to measure specific gravity. However, current regulations have limited the refractometer's use to the laboratory. Urine dipsticks can be used on the nursing unit with reasonable accuracy.

At times parents may be requested to take a urine sample to a health care facility for examination, especially when infants are unable to void during an outpatient visit. In this instance parents need instruction on applying the collection device and storing the specimen.† Ideally, the specimen should be taken to the designated place as soon as possible; if there is a delay, the sample is refrigerated and the lapsed time reported to the examiner.

Clean-Catch Specimens

The term *clean-catch specimen* traditionally refers to a urine sample obtained for culture after the urethral meatus is cleaned and the first few milliliters of urine is voided before the urine is collected (midstream specimen). The procedure consists of cleaning the perineum or tip of the penis with a soap or antiseptic-soaked sterile pad, and in females wiping from front to back only once with each pad. This is repeated at least two times. The area may be wiped with sterile water to prevent accidental contamination of the urine with a solution that may destroy the pathogens, although minute amounts of antiseptic such as iodine do not alter bacterial counts.

Although this traditional cleansing procedure is often practiced, studies have found that it does not significantly reduce contamination rates in infants, circumcised or uncircumcised males, or toilet-trained prepubertal children. Also, midstream collection does not significantly reduce contamination rates when compared with those of nonmidstream specimens (Lohr, Donowitz, and Dudley, 1989; Saez-Llorens et al, 1989).

Twenty-Four-Hour Collection

Collection of urine voided over a 24-hour period creates a special challenge in infants and children. Collection bags and

*Available from Hollister, Inc., 2000 Hollister Dr., Libertyville, IL 60048; (800) 323-4060.

†Available from ConvaTec, CN 5254, Princeton, NJ 08543-5254; (800) 422-8811.

*The Bard Sure Catch is available from Bard Urological Division, C. R. Bard, Inc., Covington, GA 30209; (707) 784-7754.

†Home care instructions on obtaining a urine sample are available in Wong DL: *Wong and Whaley's clinical manual of pediatric nursing*, ed 4, St Louis, 1996 Mosby.

sometimes restraining methods are required to collect specimens from infants and small children. Older children require special instruction about notifying someone when they need to void or have a bowel movement so that urine can be collected separately and not discarded. Some older school-age children and adolescents can be trusted to take responsibility for collection of their own 24-hour specimens. They can keep output records and transfer each voiding to the 24-hour collection container if this is permitted.

As in any 24-hour urine collection, the collection period always starts and ends with an empty bladder. At the time the collection begins, the child is instructed to void and the specimen is discarded. All urine voided in the subsequent 24 hours is saved in a container with a preservative or is placed on ice. Twenty-four hours from the time the precollection specimen was discarded, the child is again instructed to void, the specimen is added to the container, and the entire collection is taken to the laboratory for examination.

Infants and small children who need a 24-hour urine collection will require a special collection bag; frequent removal and replacement of adhesive collection devices can produce skin irritation. A thin coating of sealant (such as Skin-Prep), applied to the skin helps to protect it and aids adhesion unless its use is contraindicated, such as in a premature infant or a child with irritated skin. Plastic collection bags with collection tubes attached are ideal when the container must be left in place for a time. These can be connected to a collecting device or emptied periodically by aspiration with a syringe. When such devices are not available, a regular bag with a feeding tube inserted through a puncture hole at the top of the bag serves as a satisfactory substitute. However, care must be taken to empty the bag as soon as the infant urinates to prevent leakage and loss of contents. An indwelling catheter may also be placed for the collection period.

Special Techniques

Catheterization or suprapubic aspiration is employed when a specimen is urgently needed or when the child is unable to void or otherwise provide an adequate specimen. *Catheterization* is most often used when urethral obstruction or anuria caused by renal failure is believed to be the cause of the child's failure to void. *Suprapubic aspiration* is useful in clarifying the diagnosis of suspected urinary tract infection in acutely ill infants.

Catheterizing a child requires aseptic technique, good light, and gentle, thorough cleansing of the vulva or glans penis. Most children, including female infants, accommodate a size 8 or 10 French catheter, but in male infants or when the larger catheters cannot be passed, a smaller, soft plastic feeding tube may be needed. Most children are frightened of this procedure, and few small children can be cooperative; therefore even when the procedure is adequately explained, an assistant is needed to help restrain and reassure the child (see also the Family Focus box below, left). Special care must be exercised when catheterizing young males to prevent trauma to the ductal and glandular openings into the urethra, which might result in sterility.

Suprapubic aspiration, which is performed by a practitioner skilled in the procedure, involves aspirating bladder contents by inserting a 20- or 21-gauge needle into the midline approximately 1 cm above the symphysis and directed vertically downward. The skin is prepared as for any needle insertion, but the bladder should contain an adequate volume of urine. This can be assumed if the infant has not voided for at least 1 hour or the bladder can be palpated above the symphysis. This technique is especially useful for obtaining clean specimens from young infants. The bladder is an abdominal organ at this time and is easily accessible.

Suprapubic aspiration is painful and has a higher failure rate than urethral catheterization; also, success depends more on the volume of urine in the bladder (Pollack, Pollack, and Andrew, 1994). (See the Atraumatic Care and Family Focus boxes below.)

STOOL SPECIMENS

Stool specimens are often collected in children to identify parasites and other organisms that cause diarrhea, to assess gastrointestinal function, and to check for occult (hidden) blood. Ideally, stool should be collected without contamination with urine, but in children wearing diapers this is difficult unless a urine bag is applied. Children who are toilet trained should urinate first, flush the toilet, then defecate in the toilet or in a bedpan (preferably one that is placed on the toilet to prevent embarrassment) or a commercial potty hat. Stool specimens should be large enough to obtain an ample sampling, not merely a fecal fragment. Specimens are placed in an appropriate container, which is covered and labeled. If several specimens are needed, the containers are marked with the date and time and kept in a specimen refrigerator. Special care is exercised in handling the specimen because of the risk of contamination.

BLOOD SPECIMENS

Although most blood specimens are obtained by the laboratory staff, nurses are increasingly responsible for specimen collection, especially if the child has an arterial or venous device. Whether the specimen is collected by the nurse or others, the nurse is responsible for making certain that specimens, such as serial examinations and fasting specimens, are col-

Family Focus

BLADDER CATHETERIZATION

Parents may be upset when their child is catheterized. Aside from the trauma the child experiences, some parents, especially those from different cultures, may fear that the procedure affects the daughter's virginity. To correct this misconception, the family needs a detailed explanation of the genitourinary anatomy, preferably with a model that shows the separate vaginal and urethral openings.

Atraumatic Care

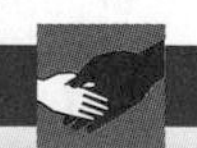

BLADDER CATHETERIZATION OR SUPRAPUBIC ASPIRATION

Use distraction to help the child relax (blowing bubbles, deep breathing, singing a song, etc.).

Use a water-soluble jelly to lubricate the catheter. Lidocaine jelly can be used to anesthetize the area before insertion.

lected on time and that the proper equipment, such as correct collection tubes and ice for blood gas samples, is available.

Venous blood samples can be obtained by venipuncture or by aspiration from a *peripheral* or *central access device.* Withdrawing blood specimens through peripheral lock devices in small peripheral veins has met with varying degrees of success. Although it eliminates the need for an additional venipuncture for the child, attempting to aspirate blood from the peripheral lock may shorten the life of the device. When using an intravenous infusion site for specimen collection, it is important to consider the type of fluid being infused. For example, a specimen collected for glucose determination would be inaccurate if removed from a catheter through which glucose-containing solution was being administered.

A blood specimen can be obtained from a central venous line or peripheral lock when the infusion solution may interfere with test results by first aspirating a quantity of blood equal to the volume of fluid in the catheter and discarding it; then the blood sample is aspirated.

For a blood culture the first sample of blood is used since organisms are most likely to collect within the catheter itself (Schreiner, 1987).

Nursing ALERT

For small or anemic children, keep track of the amount of blood drawn and discarded over time. Frequent taking of blood specimens can rapidly decrease a child's blood count. Coordinate blood samples as much as possible to reduce the frequency.

Arterial blood samples are sometimes needed for blood gas measurement, although noninvasive techniques, such as transcutaneous oxygen/carbon dioxide monitoring and pulse oximetry, are used frequently. Arterial samples may be obtained by arteriopuncture by the radial, brachial, or femoral arteries; by deep heel puncture; or from indwelling arterial catheters. Adequate circulation should be assessed prior to arterial puncture by observing capillary refill or performing the *Allen test,* a procedure that assesses the circulation of the radial, ulnar, or brachial arteries. Since unclotted blood is required, only heparinized collection tubes are used. In addition, no air bubbles should enter the tube, since they can alter blood gas concentration. Crying, fear, and agitation also affect blood gas values; therefore every effort is made to comfort the child. The blood samples are packed in ice to reduce blood cell metabolism and are taken to the laboratory for immediate analysis.

Capillary blood samples are taken from children by finger or earlobe stick methods, just as in the adult patient. The best method for taking peripheral blood samples from infants is by a heel stick. Before the blood sample is taken, the heel is warmed with warm, moist compresses for 5 to 10 minutes in order to dilate the vessels in the area. The area is cleansed with alcohol, and with the infant's foot firmly restrained with the free hand, the heel is punctured with a blade or an automatic lancet device. An automatic device (such as Tenderfoot*) delivers a more precise puncture depth (and possibly a less painful puncture) than that achieved with a blade or lance. Although obtaining capillary blood gases is a common practice, these measures may not accurately reflect arterial values (Courtney et al, 1990).

The most serious complication of infant heel puncture is necrotizing osteochondritis from lancet penetration of the underlying calcaneus bone. To prevent this, the puncture should be no deeper than 2.4 mm and should be made at the outer aspect of the heel. The boundaries of the calcaneus can be marked by an imaginary line extending posteriorly from a point between the fourth and fifth toes and running parallel to the lateral aspect of the heel and another line extending posteriorly from the middle of the great toe and running parallel to the medial aspect of the heel (Fig. 42-16).

The needed specimens are collected quickly, and then pressure is applied to the puncture site with a dry gauze square until bleeding stops. The arm is kept extended, not flexed, and pressure is applied for a few minutes after venipuncture in the antecubital fossa to reduce bruising. The site is then covered with a Band-Aid. In young children, Band-Aids pose an aspiration hazard; their use should be avoided or they should be removed as soon as bleeding stops. Applying warm compresses to ecchymotic areas increases circulation, helps remove extravasated blood, and decreases pain.

No matter how or by whom the specimen is collected, children, even some older ones, fear the loss of their blood. This is particularly true for children whose condition requires frequent blood specimens. They mistakenly believe that blood removal from their bodies is a threat to their lives. Explaining to them that their blood is continually being produced by their bodies provides them with a measure of reassurance regarding this aspect of the stress-provoking procedure. When the blood is drawn, a simple comment such as "Just look how red it is. You're really making a lot of nice red blood" confirms this information and affords them an opportunity to express their concern. A Band-Aid gives them added assurance that the vital fluids will not leak out through the puncture site.

Children also dislike the discomfort associated with ve-

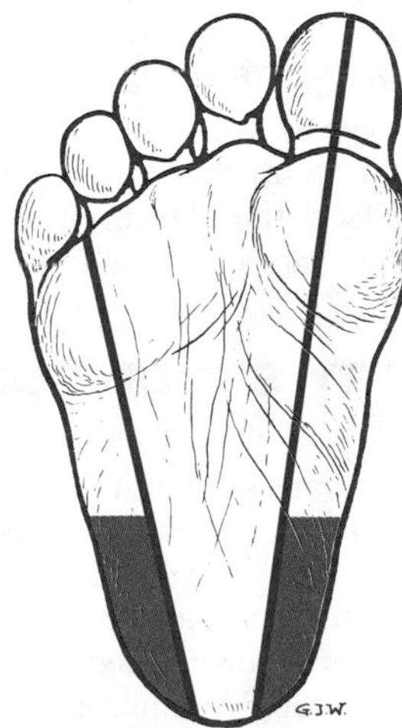

Fig. 42-16 Puncture site *(colored stippled area)* on sole of infant's foot.

*Available from International Technidyne Corp., 23 Nevsky St., Edison, NJ 08820; (908) 548-5700 or (800) 631-5945.

Atraumatic Care

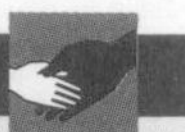

SKIN/VESSEL PUNCTURES AND MULTIPLE BLOOD SAMPLES

To reduce the pain and distress associated with heel, finger, venous, or arterial punctures:

1. Apply EMLA topically over the site if time permits (at least 60 minutes) or use buffered lidocaine (injected intradermally near vein with 30-gauge needle) to numb the skin.
2. Use nonpharmacologic methods of pain and anxiety control (e.g., ask child to take a deep breath when the needle is inserted and again when the needle is withdrawn; ask child to count slowly and then faster and louder if pain is felt).
3. Emphasize that blood entry into syringe or tube does not hurt.
4. Reassure young children that you did not "take their blood" away and that they have a lot more inside.
5. Keep arm extended, not flexed, while applying pressure for a few minutes after venipuncture in the antecubital fossa to reduce bruising (Dyson and Bogod, 1987).
6. Place *small* bandage over puncture site to make removal easy and less painful and to reassure young children that their blood will not leak out.

For multiple blood samples:

1. Use an intermittent infusion device to collect additional samples from existing intravenous line; consider peripherally inserted central catheters (PICCs) early, not as a last resort.
2. Coordinate care to allow several tests to be performed on one blood sample using micromethods of testing.
3. Anticipate tests (i.e., type and cross-match for blood transfusion) and ask laboratory to save blood for additional testing.

Contrary to popular belief, a study of children ages 3 to 6 years found that asking them not to look at the "finger stick" to avoid the sight of blood or applying a decorated bandage did not lessen their rating of pain intensity (Johnston, Stevens, and Arbess, 1993).

nous, arterial, or capillary punctures. In fact, children have identified these procedures as the ones most frequently causing pain during hospitalization and arterial punctures as being one of the most painful of all procedures experienced (Wong and Baker, 1988). Consequently, nurses need to institute pain reduction techniques to lessen the discomfort of these procedures (see the Atraumatic Care box above). Younger children are more distressed by venipuncture than older children.

RESPIRATORY SECRETION/THROAT SPECIMENS

Collection of sputum or nasal discharge is sometimes required for diagnosis of respiratory infections, especially tuberculosis and respiratory syncytial viruses (RSVs). Older children and adolescents are able to cough as directed and supply sputum specimens when given proper directions. It must be made clear to them that a coughed specimen, not mucus that is cleared from the throat, is needed. It is helpful to demonstrate a deep cough so that communication is clear. Infants and small children are unable to follow directions to cough and will swallow any sputum produced; therefore gastric washings (lavage) may be used to collect a sputum specimen. Sometimes it is possible to get a satisfactory specimen by using a suction device such as a mucus trap if the catheter is inserted into the trachea and the cough reflex is elicited. A catheter that is inserted into the back of the throat is not sufficient. For children with a tracheostomy, a specimen is easily aspirated from the trachea or major bronchi by attaching a collecting device to the suction apparatus.

Nasal washings are usually obtained to diagnose an infection of RSV. The child is placed supine, and from 1 to 3 ml of sterile normal saline solution is instilled with a sterile syringe (without needle) into one nostril. The contents are aspirated by a small, sterile bulb syringe and are placed into a sterile container. To prevent any additional discomfort to the child, all the equipment should be ready before the procedure is begun.

Other respiratory secretion collection methods include nasopharyngeal swabs to diagnose *Bordetella pertussis* and throat cultures. The nurse swabs both the tonsils and posterior pharynx when obtaining a throat culture. The swab stick is inserted into the culture tube. Some culture kits require squeezing an ampule to release the culture medium.

Nursing ALERT

Do not attempt to obtain a throat culture if acute epiglottitis is suspected. The trauma from the swab may increase edema, possibly occluding the airway.

Administration of Medication

PREPARATION FOR SAFE ADMINISTRATION

The safe administration of medication to children presents a number of problems that are not encountered when giving medication to adult patients. Children vary widely in age, weight, body surface area, and ability to absorb, metabolize, and excrete medications. Nurses must be particularly alert when computing and administering drugs to infants and children.

Determination of Drug Dosage

It is the physician's responsibility to prescribe drugs in the correct dosage to achieve the desired effect without endangering the health of the child. However, nurses must have an understanding of the safe dosage of medications they administer to children, as well as the expected action, possible side effects, and signs of toxicity. Unlike with adult medications, there are few standardized pediatric dosage ranges, and with a few exceptions drugs are prepared and packaged in average adult-dosage strengths.

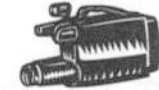

For additional information, please view "Medications and Injections" in *Whaley and Wong's Pediatric Nursing Video Series*, St. Louis, 1996, Mosby; (800) 426-4545.

Factors related to growth and maturation significantly alter an individual's capacity to metabolize and excrete drugs, and deficiencies associated with immaturity become more important with decreasing age. Immaturity or defects in any or all of the important processes of absorption, distribution, biotransformation, or excretion can significantly alter the effects of a drug. Newborn and premature infants with immature enzyme systems in the liver (where most drugs are broken down and detoxified), lower plasma concentrations of protein for binding with drugs, and immaturely functioning kidneys (where most drugs are excreted) are particularly vulnerable to the harmful effects of drugs. Beyond the newborn period, many drugs are metabolized more rapidly by the liver, necessitating larger doses or more frequent administration. This is particularly important in pain control, when the dosage may need to be increased or the interval between administering analgesics may need to be decreased.

Various formulas involving age, weight, and body surface area as the basis for calculations have been devised to determine children's drug dosage from a standard adult dose. Since the administration of medication is a nursing responsibility, nurses need not only a knowledge of drug action and patient responses, but also some resources for estimating safe dosages for children. The method most often used to determine children's dosage is based on a specific dose per kilograms of body weight, such as 0.1 mg/kg.

Another method for determining children's dosage is to calculate the proportional amount of *body surface area (BSA)*

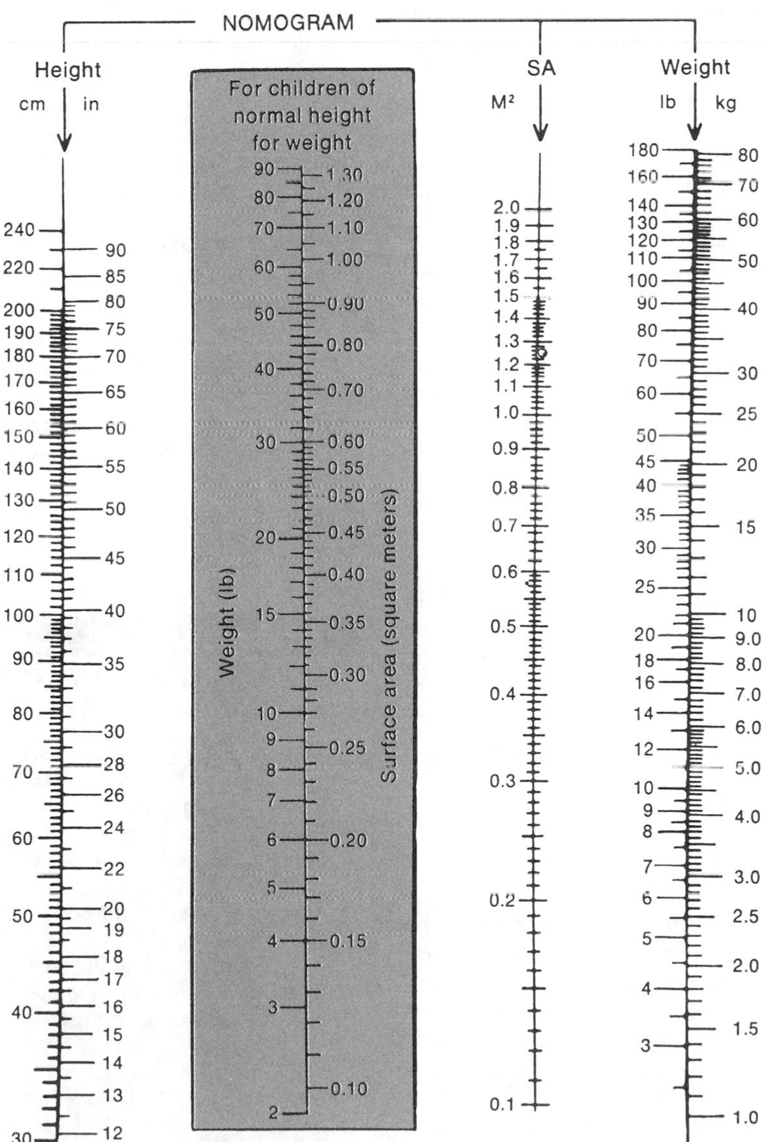

Fig. 42-17 West nomogram (for estimation of surface areas). Surface area is indicated where a straight line connecting height and weight intersects surface area *(SA)* column or, if patient is of roughly normal proportion, from weight alone *(colored area)*. (Nomogram modified from data of E. Boyd by C. D. West; from Behrman RE, Vaughan VC, editors: *Nelson textbook of pediatrics*, ed 14, Philadelphia, 1992, WB Saunders.)

to body weight. The ratio of BSA to weight varies inversely with length; therefore the infant who is shorter and weighs less than an older child or adult has relatively more surface area than would be expected from the weight. The usual determination of BSA requires the use of the West Nomogram (Fig. 42-17). The BSA is estimated from the height and weight of the child.

Checking dosage. Administering the correct dosage of a drug is a shared responsibility of the practitioner who orders the drug and the nurse who carries out that order. Children react with unexpectedly severe symptoms to some drugs, and ill children are especially sensitive. Therefore checking the dose if there is any doubt about its accuracy is a professional duty. When a dose is ordered that is outside the usual range or if there is some question regarding the preparation or the route of administration, the nurse should always check with the prescribing practitioner before proceeding with the administration, since the nurse is legally liable for any drug administered.

Administering some medications requires added safeguards. Even when it has been determined that the dosage is correct for a particular child, there are many drugs that are potentially hazardous or lethal. Most hospital units or other facilities where medications are given to children have regulations requiring that specified drugs be double-checked by another nurse before they are given to the child. Among those drugs that require such safeguards are digoxin, heparin, chemotherapeutic agents, and insulin. Others that are frequently included are epinephrine, opioids, and sedatives. Even if this precaution is not mandatory, nurses would be wise to take such precautions for their own sense of security. Errors in decimal point placement may easily occur and may result in a tenfold or greater dosage error.

Identification

Before the administration of any medication, the child must be correctly identified, since children are not totally reliable in giving correct names on request. Infants are unable to give their name, a toddler or preschooler may admit to any name, and school-age children may deny their identity in an attempt to avoid the medication. Children sometimes exchange beds during play. Parents may be present to identify their child, but the only safe method for identifying children is to check their hospital identification band with the labeled medication or medication card.

Family Aspects

Parents can be useful sources of information regarding the child and his or her capabilities. Nearly all parents have given some kind of medication to their child and can describe approaches that they have found to be successful. In some cases it is less traumatic for the child if a parent gives the medication, provided that the nurse prepares it and supervises its administration and the practice is consistent with hospital or unit policy. Children being given daily medications at home are accustomed to the parent's functioning in this capacity and are less likely to object than they would if the medication were administered by a stranger.

Every child requires psychologic preparation for parenteral administration of medication and supportive care during the procedure (see Box 42-2 on p. 1254). Even if children have received several injections, they rarely become accustomed to the discomfort and have as much right as any other child to understanding and patience from those involved in giving the injection. Safe administration of any drug requires meticulous attention to the safeguards discussed here.

ORAL ADMINISTRATION

The oral route is preferred for administering medications to children whenever possible. Because of the ease of administration of oral medications, most are dissolved or suspended in liquid preparations. Although some children are able to swallow or chew solid medications at an early age, solid preparations are not recommended for young children because of the danger of aspiration.

Most pediatric medications are available in palatable and colorful preparations for added ease of administration. However, some have a slightly unpleasant aftertaste. The nurse should taste a minute amount of an oral preparation to ascertain whether it is palatable or bitter. In this way legitimate complaints of dislike from the child can be accepted and the taste camouflaged whenever possible. Most pediatric units have preparations available for this purpose (see the Atraumatic Care box below).

Preparation

Selecting a method to measure and administer a medication requires careful consideration. The devices available to measure medicines are not always sufficiently accurate for the small amounts needed in pediatric nursing practice (Fig. 42-18). Disposable plastic calibrated cups offer reasonable accuracy in measuring moderate doses of liquids. However, the personal interpretation of a given measure is highly variable, and considerable amounts of thick medication may remain in the cup. Measures of less than a teaspoon are impossible to determine accurately with a cup.

Atraumatic Care

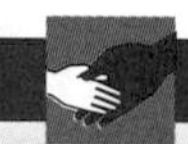

ENCOURAGING A CHILD'S ACCEPTANCE OF ORAL MEDICATION

Give the child an ice pop or small ice cube to suck to numb the tongue before giving the drug.

Mix the drug with a small amount (about 1 tsp) of sweet-tasting substance, such as honey (except in infants because of the risk of botulism), flavored syrups, jam, fruit purees, sherbet, or ice cream; avoid essential food items, because the child may later refuse to eat them.

Give a "chaser" of water, juice, a soft drink, or an ice pop or frozen juice bar after the drug.

If nausea is a problem, give a carbonated beverage poured over finely crushed ice before or immediately after the medication.

When medication has an unpleasant taste, have the child pinch the nose and drink the medicine through a straw. Much of what we taste is associated with smell.

Another alternative is to have the pharmacist prepare the drug in a flavored, chewable troche or lozenge.*

*For information about compounding drugs in troches or suppositories, contact Technical Staff, Professional Compounding Centers of America (PCCA), P.O. Box 368, Sugarland, TX 77487, 800-331-2498.

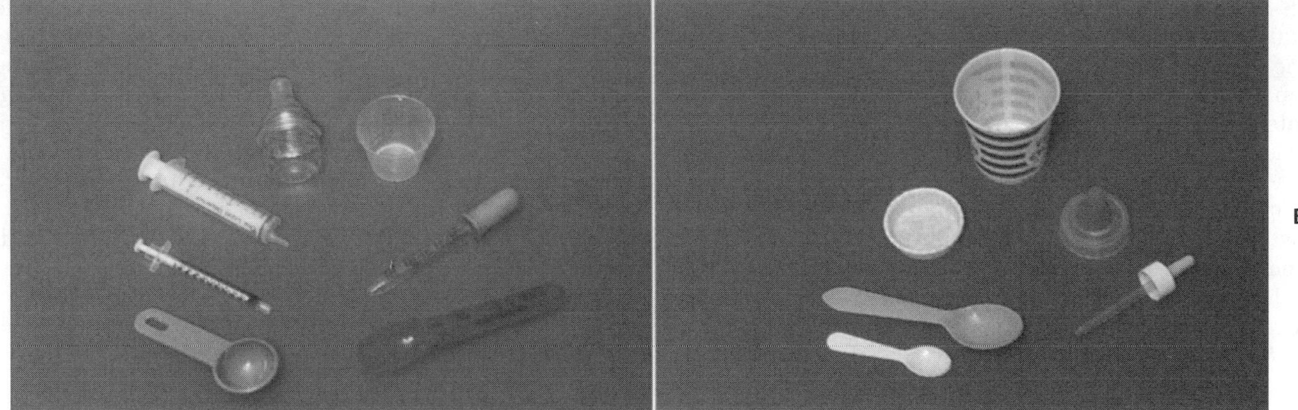

Fig. 42-18 **A,** Acceptable devices for measuring and administering oral medication to children *(clockwise)*: measuring spoon, plastic syringes, calibrated nipple, plastic medicine cup, calibrated dropper, hollow-handled medicine spoon. **B,** Acceptable devices only for administering premeasured oral medication *(clockwise)*: household teaspoons, paper cups, nipple, uncalibrated dropper.

Many liquid preparations are prescribed in measurements of teaspoons. However, the teaspoon is an inaccurate measuring device and is subject to error from a number of variables. For example, household teaspoons vary greatly in capacity, and different persons using the same spoon will pour different amounts. Therefore a drug ordered in teaspoons should be measured in milliliters—the established standard is 5 ml per teaspoon. A convenient hollow-handled medicine spoon is available to measure and administer the drug accurately (Fig. 42-18). Household *measuring* spoons can also be used when other devices are not available.

Another unreliable device for measuring liquids is the dropper, which varies to a greater extent than the teaspoon or measuring cup. Droppers are available in numerous sizes, but, even with the standard USP dropper, the volume of a drop will vary according to the viscosity of the liquid measured; viscid fluids produce much larger drops than thin liquids. Many medications are supplied with caps or droppers designed for measuring each specific preparation. These are accurate when used to measure that specific medication but are not reliable for measuring other liquids. Emptying dropper contents into a medicine cup invites additional error; since some of the liquid clings to the sides of the cup, a significant amount of the drug can be lost.

The most accurate means for measuring small amounts of medication is the plastic disposable (never glass) syringe, especially the tuberculin syringe for volumes of less than 1 ml. Not only does the syringe provide a reliable measure, it also serves as a convenient means for transporting and administering the medication. The medication can be placed directly into the child's mouth from the syringe. For added safety, a short length of flexible tubing can be placed on the tip of the syringe to prevent injury to the mouth, although the tubing must be completely emptied of medication.

Nursing ALERT

Many pediatric medications are given by drops or dropper. A misunderstanding of these terms by parents can result in a potential overdose. In addition, many droppers that come with medications are marked in tenths of cubic centimeters. A parent who used a syringe instead of the dropper might think that 0.4 cc is the same as 4 cc. Provide education to parents on correct methods for giving medication. Demonstrate the technique (Rudy, 1992).

Young children and some older children as well have difficulty swallowing tablets or pills. Since a number of drugs are not available in pediatric preparations, the tablet will need to be crushed before it can be given to these children. Commercial devices* are available, or simple methods can be employed, such as crushing tablets between two spoons. The crushed medication is mixed with a palatable substance.

Not all drugs can be crushed (e.g., medication with an enteric or protective coating or medication formulated for slow release). For some children it may be possible to encourage swallowing the tablet or capsule by using a special glass designed with a shelf that holds the drug. The child drinks normally, and the tablet is carried to the back of the throat. For children who must take solid oral medication for an extended period, training sessions using progressively larger candy to teach the child to swallow can be beneficial (Funk, Mullins, and Olson, 1984).

Since pediatric doses often require dividing adult preparations of medication, the nurse may be faced with the dilemma of accurate dosage. With tablets, only those that are scored can be halved or quartered accurately. If the medication is soluble, the tablet or contents of a capsule can be mixed in a small, premeasured amount of liquid and the appropriate portion given. If half a dose is required, the tablet is dissolved in 5 ml of water or flavored liquid and 2.5 ml is given.

*Trademark Medical manufactures a pill crusher and has compiled a list of more than 190 medications that should not be crushed or chewed. Both are available from Trademark Medical, 1053 Headquarters Park, Fenton, MO 63026-2033; (800) 325-9044.

Administration

Although administering liquids to infants is relatively easy, the nurse must be careful to prevent aspiration. With the infant held in a semireclining position, the medication is placed into the mouth from a spoon, plastic cup, plastic dropper, or plastic syringe (without needle). The dropper or syringe is best placed along the side of the infant's tongue, with the contents administered slowly in small amounts, allowing the child to swallow between deposits. In infants up to 11 months of age and children with neurologic impairments, blowing a small puff of air in the face frequently elicits a swallow reflex (Orenstein and others, 1988).

Medicine cups can be used effectively for older infants who are able to drink from a cup. Because of the natural outward tongue thrust in infancy, medications may need to be retrieved from the lips or chin and refed. Allowing the infant to suck medication that has been placed in an empty nipple or inserting the syringe or dropper into the side of the mouth, parallel to the nipple while the infant nurses, are other convenient methods for giving liquid medications to infants. Medication is not added to the infant's formula feeding. Dispose of any plastic covers that may be on the ends of syringes. These covers are small enough to be aspirated by young children.

The small child who refuses to cooperate or resists consistently despite explanation and encouragement may require mild physical coercion. If so, it is carried out quickly and carefully. Every effort is made to determine why the child resists, and the reasons for the coercion are explained to the child in such a way that the child will know that it is being carried out for his or her well-being and is not a form of punishment. There is always a risk in using even mild forceful techniques. A crying child can aspirate a medication, particularly when lying on the back. If the nurse holds the child in the lap with the child's right arm behind the nurse, the left hand firmly grasped by the nurse's left hand, and the head securely restrained between the nurse's arm and body, the medication can be slowly poured into the mouth (Fig. 42-19).

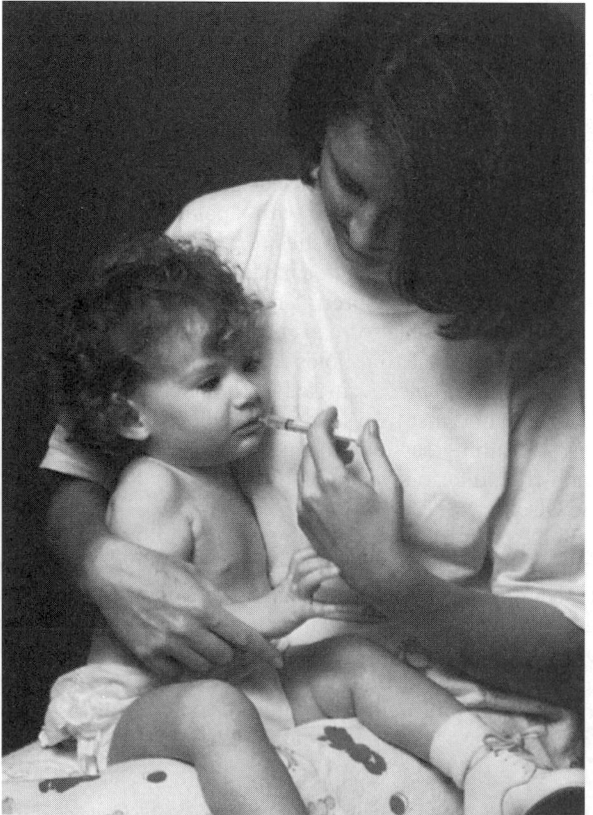

Fig. 42-19 Nurse partially restrains child for easy and comfortable administration of oral medication.

INTRAMUSCULAR (IM) ADMINISTRATION

Selecting the Syringe and Needle

The volume of medication prescribed for small children and the small amount of tissue for injection require that a syringe be selected that can measure very small amounts of solution. For volumes of less than 1 ml the tuberculin syringe, calibrated in one-hundredth increments, is appropriate. Very minute doses may require the use of a 0.5-ml, low-dose syringe. These syringes with specially constructed needles minimize the possibility of inadvertently administering incorrect amounts of a drug because of dead space, which allows fluid to remain in the syringe and needle after the plunger is pushed completely forward. A minimum of 0.2 ml of solution remains in a standard needle hub; therefore when very small amounts of two drugs are combined in the syringe, such as mixtures of insulin, the ratio of the two drugs can be altered significantly. Measures that minimize the effect of dead space follow: (1) when two drugs are combined in the syringe, always draw them up in the same order to maintain a consistent ratio between the drugs; (2) use the same brand of syringe (dead space may vary); and (3) use one-piece syringe units (needle permanently attached to the syringe).

Dead space is also an important factor to consider when injecting medication, since flushing the syringe with an air bubble or parenteral fluid adds medication to the prescribed dose. This can be hazardous when very small amounts of a drug are given. For example, a tuberculin syringe filled to the 0.05-ml mark can deliver *more than twice* the calculated dose of medication when it is flushed with parenteral fluid from an intravenous line. Consequently, flushing is not advisable, especially when less than 1 ml of medication is given. Syringes are calibrated to deliver a prescribed drug dose, and the amount of medication left in the hub and needle is not part of the syringe barrel calibrations. However, the air-bubble technique (drawing up about 0.2 ml of air into the syringe after withdrawing the medication) may be beneficial with certain drugs, such as iron dextran and diphtheria and tetanus toxoid, to prevent tracking the drug through the tissue. Other techniques to minimize tracking include changing the needle after withdrawing the fluid from the vial (not always effective) and using the Z track method.

The needle length must be sufficient to penetrate the subcutaneous tissue and deposit the medication in the body of the muscle. Although research is limited on adequate needle length for children, one study found that a 1-inch needle is necessary to penetrate the vastus lateralis muscle adequately in 4-month-old infants and probably is needed for 2-month-old infants (Hicks et al, 1989).

To estimate the needle length for intramuscular (IM) injection, first the lateralis or deltoid muscle is grasped and a needle length is chosen that is approximately half the distance between the thumb and the index finger. With the ventrogluteal or dorsogluteal site, only subcutaneous tissue is grasped, so a needle length is selected that is slightly more than half the distance. A final needle length is chosen that allows for a small portion of the needle to be exposed at the skin surface as a precaution if the needle should break off from the hub.

Smaller-diameter (25- to 30-gauge) needles cause the least discomfort, but larger diameters are needed for viscous medication and prevention of accidental bending of longer needles.

Determining the Site

Factors that are considered when selecting a site for an IM injection on an infant or child include:

1. The amount and character of the medication to be injected
2. The amount and general condition of the muscle mass
3. The frequency or number of injections to be given during the course of treatment
4. The type of medication being given
5. Factors that may impede access to or cause contamination of the site
6. The ability of the child to assume the required position safely

Older children and adolescents usually pose few problems in selecting a suitable site for intramuscular injections, but infants, with their small and underdeveloped muscles, have fewer available sites. It is sometimes difficult to assess the amount of fluid that can be safely injected into a single site. Usually 1 ml is the maximum volume that should be administered in a single site to small children and older infants. The muscles of small infants may not tolerate more than 0.5 ml. As the child approaches adult size, volumes approaching those given to adults may be used. However, the larger the amount of solution, the larger the muscle into which it is injected must be.

Injections must be placed in muscles large enough to accommodate the medication; yet major nerves and blood vessels must be avoided. There is no universal agreement regarding the best intramuscular injection site for children. The preferred site for infants is the vastus lateralis. A general recommendation for using the gluteal sites is to wait until after the child has been walking (length of suggested time varies), since the muscle develops with locomotion. Unfortunately, this recommendation is often applied to the ventrogluteal muscle site, as well as the dorsogluteal site. However, there are significant differences between these two sites. The ventrogluteal site is relatively free of major nerves and blood vessels, is a relatively large muscle with less subcutaneous tissue than the dorsal site, has well-defined landmarks for safe site location, is less painful than the vastus lateralis, and is easily accessible in several positions (Beecroft and Redick, 1990). Because of these advantages it is preferred to the dorsogluteal muscle, challenging the recommendation that the ventrogluteal site not be used until children have been walking. Although there are published recommendations regarding age, in clinical practice this site has been used in children as young as newborns. Table 42-2 summarizes the four major injection sites and illustrates the location of the preferred intramuscular injection sites for children.

Administration

Although injections that are executed with care are relatively safe, there have been reports of serious disability related to IM injections in children. Repeated use of a single site has been associated with fibrosis of the muscle with subsequent muscle contracture, and injections close to large nerves, such as the sciatic nerve, have been responsible for permanent disability, especially when potentially neurotoxic drugs are administered. There are several reports of tissue damage from penicillin; one of the difficulties in administering the opaque preparations, such as Bicillin, is that aspirated blood cannot be detected at the bottom of the syringe, thus increasing the risk of injecting into a blood vessel. When such drugs are injected, great care must be used in locating the correct site. When aspirating, the nurse should look for blood at the *top* of the syringe near the plunger, since blood may be drawn up through the column of penicillin (Stoller and Losey, 1985).

A reported potential hazard with medication in glass ampules is the presence of glass particles in the ampule after the container is broken. When the medication is withdrawn into the syringe, the glass particles may also be withdrawn and subsequently injected into the patient. As a precaution, medication from glass ampules should be drawn up only through a needle with a filter or injected intravenously through a site in the tubing that is distal to an intravenous filter. Other precautions related to needle use and disposal are on p. 1273.

Children may be unpredictable and cannot be expected to cooperate totally when receiving an injection. Even children who appear to be relaxed and constrained can lose control under the stress of the procedure. It is advisable to have someone available to help restrain the child if needed. Since children often jerk or pull away unexpectedly, it is a good idea to carry an extra needle to exchange for a contaminated one so that there is a minimum of delay. The child, even a small one, is told that he or she is getting an injection (preferably using a phrase such as "putting medicine under the skin"), and then the procedure is carried out as quickly and skillfully as possible to prevent prolonging the stressful experience. Delay caused by lengthy explanations, attempts to hide the syringe from sight, or efforts to soothe the child will only serve to increase the anxiety. It must be kept in mind that intrusive procedures such as injections are especially anxiety-provoking in preschool children and that small children usually associate any assault to the "behind" area with punishment. Since injections are painful, the nurse should employ excellent injection technique and effective pain-reduction measures to reduce discomfort (see the Guidelines box on p. 1292).

Small infants offer little resistance to injections. Although they squirm and may be difficult to hold in position, they can usually be restrained without assistance. The body of a larger infant can be securely restrained between the nurse's elbow and body (Fig. 42-20). To inject into the body of the muscle, the muscle mass is firmly grasped between the thumb and fingers to isolate and stabilize the site. However, in obese children it is preferable first to spread the skin with the thumb and in-

TABLE 42-2 Intramuscular injection sites in children

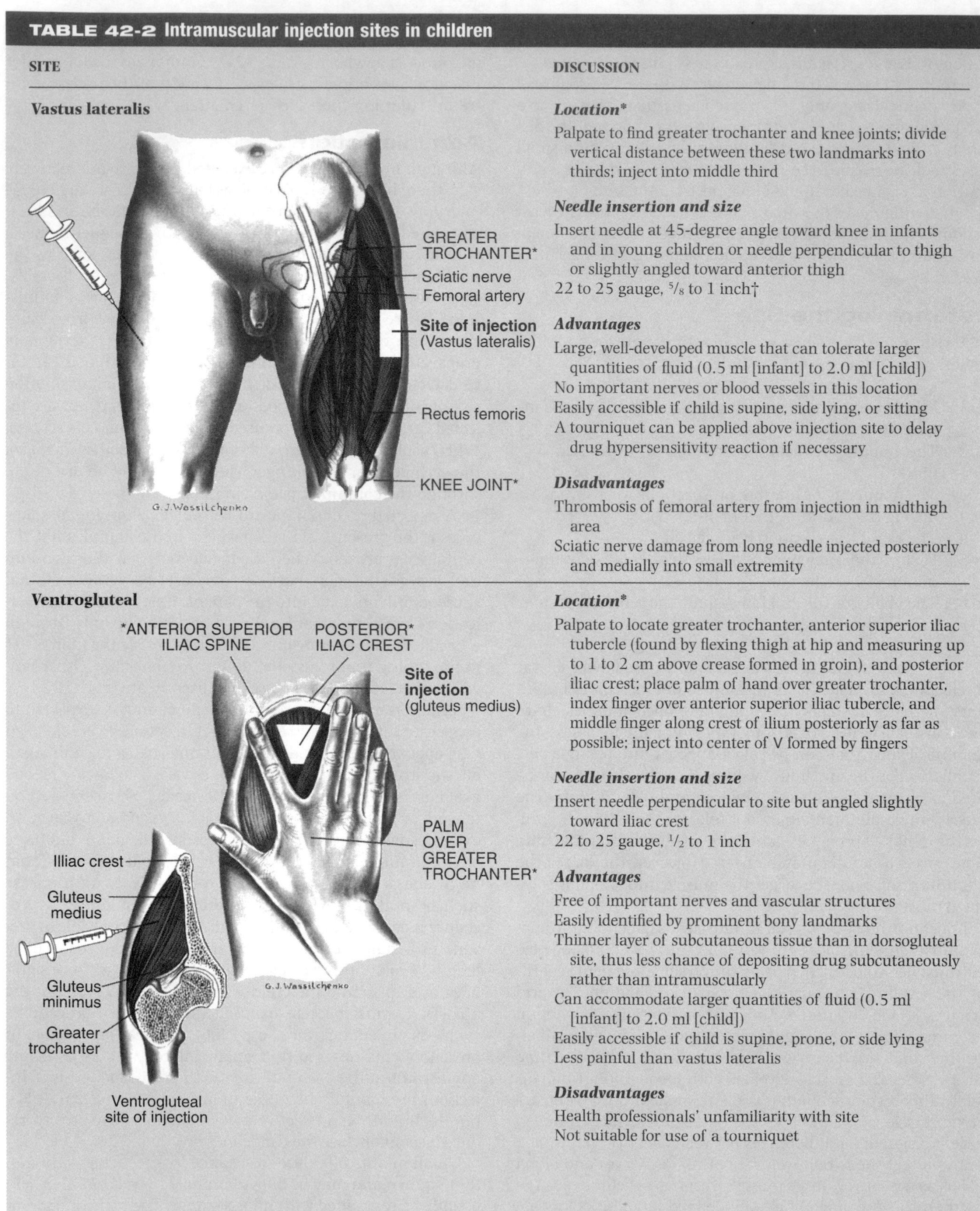

SITE	DISCUSSION
Vastus lateralis	***Location**** Palpate to find greater trochanter and knee joints; divide vertical distance between these two landmarks into thirds; inject into middle third ***Needle insertion and size*** Insert needle at 45-degree angle toward knee in infants and in young children or needle perpendicular to thigh or slightly angled toward anterior thigh 22 to 25 gauge, 5/8 to 1 inch† ***Advantages*** Large, well-developed muscle that can tolerate larger quantities of fluid (0.5 ml [infant] to 2.0 ml [child]) No important nerves or blood vessels in this location Easily accessible if child is supine, side lying, or sitting A tourniquet can be applied above injection site to delay drug hypersensitivity reaction if necessary ***Disadvantages*** Thrombosis of femoral artery from injection in midthigh area Sciatic nerve damage from long needle injected posteriorly and medially into small extremity
Ventrogluteal	***Location**** Palpate to locate greater trochanter, anterior superior iliac tubercle (found by flexing thigh at hip and measuring up to 1 to 2 cm above crease formed in groin), and posterior iliac crest; place palm of hand over greater trochanter, index finger over anterior superior iliac tubercle, and middle finger along crest of ilium posteriorly as far as possible; inject into center of V formed by fingers ***Needle insertion and size*** Insert needle perpendicular to site but angled slightly toward iliac crest 22 to 25 gauge, 1/2 to 1 inch ***Advantages*** Free of important nerves and vascular structures Easily identified by prominent bony landmarks Thinner layer of subcutaneous tissue than in dorsogluteal site, thus less chance of depositing drug subcutaneously rather than intramuscularly Can accommodate larger quantities of fluid (0.5 ml [infant] to 2.0 ml [child]) Easily accessible if child is supine, prone, or side lying Less painful than vastus lateralis ***Disadvantages*** Health professionals' unfamiliarity with site Not suitable for use of a tourniquet

*Locations are indicated by asterisks on illustrations.
†Research has shown that a 1-inch needle is needed for adequate muscle penetration in infants 4 months old and possibly in infants as young as 2 months (Hicks and others, 1989). Other recommendations for needle size and volume of fluid are based on traditional practice and have not been verified by research.

TABLE 42-2 Intramuscular injection sites in children—cont'd

SITE	DISCUSSION
Dorsogluteal 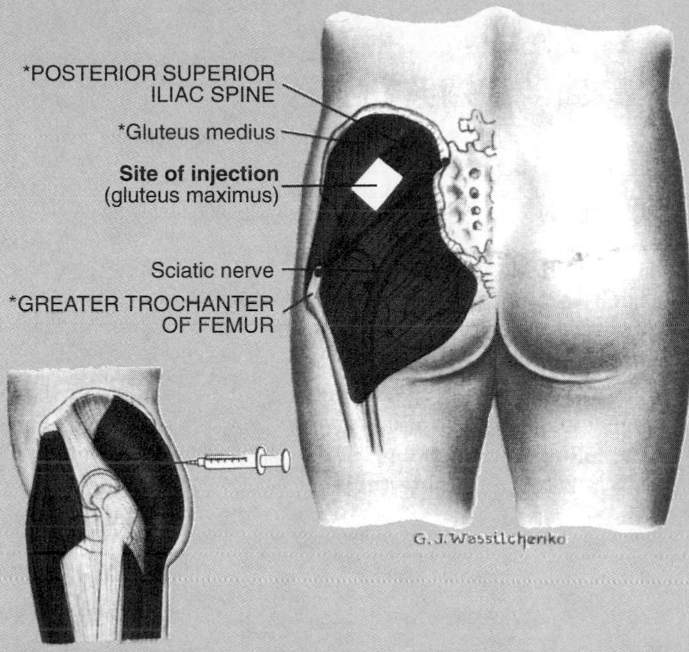	***Location**** Locate greater trochanter and posterior superior iliac spine; draw imaginary line between these two points and inject lateral and superior to line into gluteus maximus or medius muscle ***Needle insertion and size*** Insert needle perpendicular to surface on which child is lying when prone 20 to 25 gauge, $^{1}/_{2}$ to $1^{1}/_{2}$ inches ***Advantages*** In older child, large muscle mass; well-developed muscle can tolerate greater volume of fluid (up to 2.0 ml) Child does not see needle and syringe Easily accessible if child is prone or side lying ***Disadvantages*** Contraindicated in children who have not been walking for at least 1 year Danger of injury to sciatic nerve Thick, subcutaneous fat, predisposing to deposition of drug subcutaneously rather than intramuscularly Not suitable for use of a tourniquet Inaccessible if child is supine Exposure of site may cause embarrassment in older child
Deltoid	***Location**** Locate acromion process; inject only into upper third of muscle that begins about 2 fingerbreadths below acromion ***Needle insertion and size*** Insert needle perpendicular to site but angled slightly toward shoulder 22 to 25 gauge, $^{1}/_{2}$ to 1 inch ***Advantages*** Faster absorption rates than gluteal sites Tourniquet can be applied above injection site Easily accessible with minimum removal of clothing Less pain and fewer local side effects from vaccines as compared with vastus lateralis ***Disadvantages*** Small muscle mass; only limited amounts of drug can be injected (0.5 to 1.0 ml) Small margins of safety with possible damage to radial nerve and axillary nerve (not shown, lies under deltoid at head of humerus)

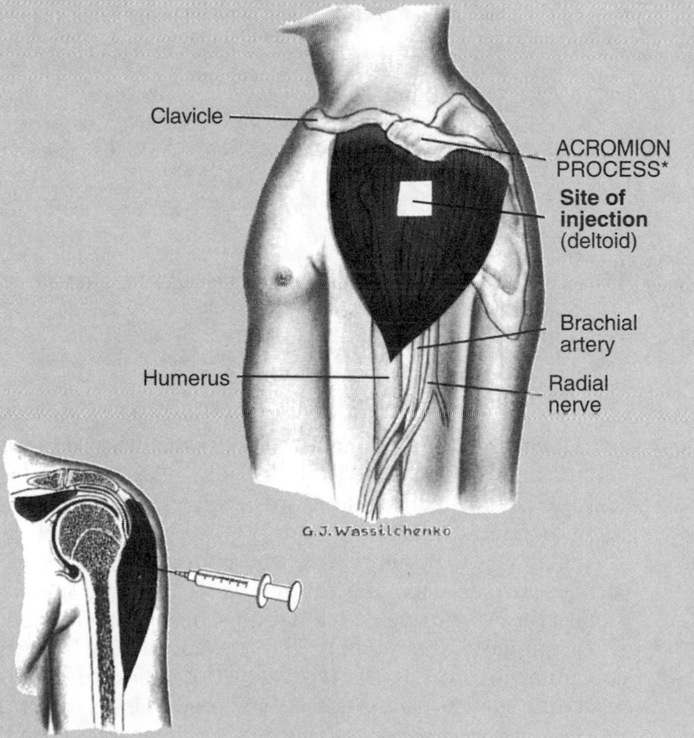

*Locations are indicated by asterisks on illustrations.

Guidelines

INTRAMUSCULAR ADMINISTRATION OF MEDICATION

- Use safety precautions in administering medication (e.g., check child's identification).
- Prepare medication.
  - Select needle and syringe appropriate to the following:
    - Amount of fluid to be administered (syringe size)
    - Viscosity of fluid to be administered (needle gauge)
    - Amount of tissue to be penetrated (needle length)
  - Maximum volume to be administered in a single site is 1 ml for older infants and small children.
- Determine the site of injection (see Table 42-2); make certain muscle is large enough to accommodate volume and type of medication.
  - Older children: select site as with adult patient; allow child some choice of site, if feasible.
  - Following are acceptable sites for infants and small or debilitated children:
    - Vastus lateralis muscle
    - Ventrogluteal muscle
  - Dorsogluteal muscle is insufficiently developed to be a safe site for infants and small children.
- Administer medication.
  - Provide for sufficient help in restraining child; children are often uncooperative, and their behavior is usually unpredictable.
  - Explain briefly what is to be done and, if appropriate, what child can do to help.
  - Expose injection area for unobstructed view of landmarks.
  - Select a site where skin is free of irritation and danger of infection; palpate for and avoid sensitive or hardened areas. With multiple injections, rotate sites.
  - Place child in a lying or sitting position; child is not allowed to stand because:
    - Landmarks are more difficult to assess.
    - Restraint is more difficult.
    - Child may faint and fall.
  - Use a new, sharp needle with smallest diameter that permits free flow of the medication.
  - Grasp muscle firmly between thumb and fingers to isolate and stabilize muscle for deposition of drug in its deepest part; in obese children, spread skin with thumb and index finger to displace subcutaneous tissue and grasp muscle deeply on each side.
  - Allow skin preparation to dry completely before skin is penetrated.
  - Have medication at room temperature.
- Decrease perception of pain:
  - Distract child with conversation.
  - Give child something on which to concentrate (e.g., squeezing a hand or bed rail, pinching own nose, humming, counting, yelling "Ouch!").
  - Place a cold compress or wrapped ice cube on site about a minute before injection, or apply cold to contralateral site.
  - Say to child, "If you feel this, tell me to take it out, please."
  - Have child hold a small Band-Aid and place it on puncture site after IM injection is given.
  - Apply EMLA topically over the site if time permits (at least 60 minutes, preferably 2 to 2½ hours for IM injection) (see Pain management, Chapter 41).
- Insert needle quickly, using a dartlike motion.
  - Use new needle, not one that has pierced rubber stopper on vial.
- Avoid tracking any medication through superficial tissues:
  - Replace needle after withdrawing medication, or wipe medication from needle with sterile gauze.
  - If withdrawing medication from an ampule, use a needle equipped with a filter that removes glass particles; then use a new, nonfilter needle for injection.
  - Use the Z track and/or air-bubble technique as indicated.
  - Avoid any depression of the plunger during insertion of the needle.
- Aspirate for blood.
  - If blood is found, remove syringe from site, change needle, and reinsert into new location.
  - If no blood is found, inject into a relaxed muscle:
    - Dorsogluteal—place child on abdomen with legs and toes rotated inward.
    - Ventrogluteal—place child on side with upper leg flexed and placed in front of lower leg.
  - Inject medication slowly.
  - Remove needle quickly; hold gauze sponge firmly against skin near needle when removing it to avoid pulling on tissue.
  - Apply firm pressure to site after injection; massage site to hasten absorption unless contraindicated, as with irritating drugs and heparin.
  - Place a small Band-Aid on puncture site; with young children decorate Band-Aid by drawing a smiling face or other symbol of acceptance.
  - Hold and cuddle young child and encourage parents to comfort child; praise older child.
  - Allow expression of feelings.
- Discard syringe and uncapped, uncut needle in puncture-resistant container located near site of use.
- Record time of injection, drug, dose, and injection site.

dex finger to displace subcutaneous tissue and then grasp the muscle deeply on each side.

The nurse should not try to administer an injection to a sleeping child, even though it may seem to be easier than waking the youngster. This practice can cause the child to fear going to sleep. When awakened first, the child knows that nothing will be done unless he or she is forewarned.

SUBCUTANEOUS AND INTRADERMAL ADMINISTRATION

Subcutaneous and intradermal injections are commonly administered to children, but the technique differs little from the method used with adults. Examples of subcutaneous injections include insulin, hormone replacement, allergy desensitization, and some vaccines. Tuberculin (TB) testing, local anesthesia, and allergy testing are examples of frequently administered intradermal injections.

Techniques to minimize the pain associated with these injections include changing the needle if it pierced a rubber stopper on a vial, using 26- to 30-gauge needles, and injecting small volumes (up to 0.5 ml). The angle of the needle for the subcutaneous injection is typically 90 degrees. In children with little subcutaneous tissue, some practitioners insert the needle at a 45-degree angle. However, the benefit of using the 45-degree angle rather than the 90-degree angle remains controversial.

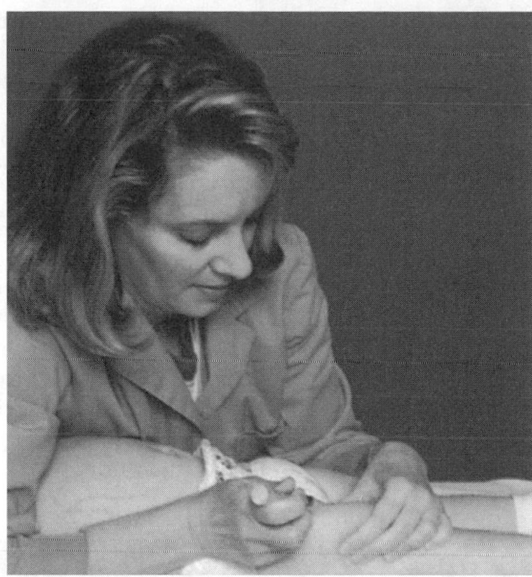

Fig. 42-20 Restraining small child for intramuscular injection. Note how nurse isolates and stabilizes muscle.

Although *subcutaneous injections* can be given anywhere there is subcutaneous tissue, common sites include the center third of the lateral aspect of the upper arm, the abdomen, and the center third of the anterior thigh. Some practitioners believe it is not necessary to aspirate before injecting subcutaneously; however, this idea is not universally accepted. Automatic injector devices do not aspirate before injecting.

When giving an intradermal injection into the volar surface of the forearm, the nurse should avoid the medial side of the arm, where the skin is more sensitive. Families often need to learn subcutaneous injection technique to administer medications, such as insulin, at home. Teaching is begun as early as possible to allow the family the maximum amount of practice time possible.*

INTRAVENOUS (IV) ADMINISTRATION

The IV route for administering medications has gained widespread use in pediatric therapy. For some important drugs it is the only effective route of administration. This method is used for giving drugs to children who have poor absorption as a result of diarrhea, dehydration, or peripheral vascular collapse; children who need a high serum concentration of a drug; children with resistant infections that require parenteral medication over an extended time; children who need continuous pain relief; and children who require emergency treatment.

Insertion sites and observation of the IV infusion are discussed on p.1299. However, several factors need to be considered in relation to IV medication. When a drug is administered intravenously, the effect is almost instantaneous and further control is limited. Most drugs for IV administration require a specified minimum dilution and/or rate of flow, and many are highly irritating or toxic to tissues outside the vascular system. In addition to the precautions and nursing observations related to IV therapy, factors to consider when preparing and administering drugs to infants and children by the IV route include:

1. Amount of drug to be administered
2. Minimum dilution of drug and whether child is fluid-restricted
3. Type of solution in which drug can be diluted
4. Length of time over which drug can be safely administered
5. Rate of infusion that child and vessels can tolerate safely
6. Time that this or another drug is to be administered
7. Compatibility of all drugs that child is receiving intravenously

Before any IV infusion, the site of insertion is checked for patency. Medications are never administered with blood products. Only one antibiotic should be administered at a time.

IV infusion is suitable for children who can tolerate the necessary infusion rate and the extra fluid needed to administer the medication. For the very small infant or fluid-restricted child who is not able to tolerate the increased rate or fluids, other IV methods available are the direct technique and the retrograde technique. Although the medication must still be minimally diluted as recommended, the dose is administered closer to the child's vein, eliminating the need to also infuse the tubing volume.

In the *direct technique*, appropriately diluted medication is injected into the tubing at the site of the Y connection or through a stopcock in the direction of the child. A syringe pump may be used for a controlled rate. As syringe pumps become increasingly available, this method is being used more often for pediatric patients because of convenience, greater control over administration time, and the need to flush with less fluid when administering medications.

In the *retrograde technique*, appropriately diluted medication is injected into the IV tubing at the site of the Y connection or a stopcock, in the direction away from (retrograde to) the child. The tubing is clamped, or the stopcock to the child is turned off. After the medication is injected, the tubing is unclamped or the stopcock opened, and the infusion resumes, with subsequent administration of the medication. The rate may still need to be adjusted to deliver the medication in the specified time. This method does result in displacement of the fluid in the IV tubing, since the diluted medication is injected retrogradely. This fluid (but not more than 3 ml) can be accommodated by an empty drip chamber or by an empty syringe connected to an upper Y site or stopcock, which will accept the displaced fluid for discard. If the empty syringe method is used, the tubing volume between the two Y sites or stopcocks must be greater than the amount of diluted medication volume injected to prevent the medication from reaching the discard syringe.

Nursing ALERT

An often unrecognized source of contamination of vascular access lines (peripheral and central) is stopcock ports. Unaccessed ports should be covered at all times with a sterile cap or syringe, which is changed if contaminated during access for medication administration or blood collection (Brosnan et al, 1988).

---

*Home care instructions on giving subcutaneous injections are available in Wong DL: *Wong and Whaley's clinical manual of pediatric nursing*, ed 4, St Louis, 1996, Mosby.

Peripheral Venous Access Devices (VADs)

The *peripheral lock,* also known as an *intermittent infusion device, PRN adapter,* and *saline* or *heparin lock,* is used as an alternative for a keep-open infusion when extended access to a vein is required without the need for continuous fluid. It is most frequently employed for intermittent infusion of medication into a peripheral venous route. A short, flexible catheter (or occasionally a steel butterfly needle) is used as the lock device, and a site is selected where there will be minimum movement, such as the forearm. The needle/catheter is inserted and secured in the same manner as any IV infusion device, but the hub is occluded with a stopper.

The type of device used may vary among medical establishments, and the care and use of the peripheral lock are carried out according to the specific protocol of the institution or unit. However, the general concept is the same. The needle or catheter remains in place and is flushed with saline or heparin solution (1:10 units/ml) after infusion of the medication. Either solution prevents blood from clotting in the device between infusions.

Heparin is incompatible with many drugs, so the peripheral lock must be flushed with saline solution before and after administering medication. Many studies show saline to be as effective in maintaining patency as heparin solution and to cause less pain during infusion (McMullen et al, 1993; Robertson, 1994).

Using a positive-pressure technique in which the flush syringe is slowly withdrawn from the peripheral lock as the last 0.5 ml of flush is being injected may prevent backflow of blood into the infusion device, thus preventing clot formation in the catheter.

Children may be discharged with a peripheral lock in place in order to continue receiving medications without hospitalization; if so, this is usually reserved for children who require medications on a short-term basis and are referred to a home-based infusion company. Those with chronic illnesses who require repeated blood sampling or medications, long-term chemotherapy, or frequent hyperalimentation or antibiotic therapy are best managed with a central venous catheter.

Central Venous Access Devices

Central VADs have several different characteristics. The practitioner has to consider the best type of catheter for the individual patient's needs. Factors that can influence the decision include the reason for placement of the catheter (diagnosis), length of therapy, risk to the patient in placement of the catheter, and availability of resources to assist the family in maintaining the catheter (Camp-Sorrell, 1990).

Short-term or *nontunneled catheters* are used in acute, emergency, and intensive care units. These catheters are made of polyurethane and are placed in large veins such as the subclavian, femoral, or jugular. A chest x-ray film should be taken to verify placement of the catheter tip before administration of fluids or medications.

Peripherally inserted central catheters (PICCs) can be used for short-term to moderate-length therapy. These catheters consist of silicone or polymer material and are placed by specially trained nurses (Brown, 1989). The most common insertion site is the antecubital area, using the median, cephalic, or basilic vein. The catheter is threaded either with or without a guidewire into the superior vena cava. PICCs can be trimmed before insertion, and the catheter can be inserted "midline," between the insertion site and the head of the clavicle (Meares, 1992). If the catheter is threaded midline, total parenteral nutrition (TPN) should not be administered since the high concentration of glucose makes it irritating to the vessel; TPN should be infused through a central catheter.

The decision to insert a PICC needs to be made before several attempts at IV lines or blood sampling by phlebotomy. Once the antecubital veins have been punctured repeatedly, they are not considered to be suitable for this type of catheter. Since this catheter is the least costly and has less chance of complications than other central VADs, it is an excellent choice for many pediatric patients. This catheter is also usually inserted either at the child's bedside or, more appropriately when available, in the unit's treatment room.

Nursing ALERT

Most PICC lines are not sutured into place, so care must be maintained when changing the dressing.

Long-term central VADs include tunneled and implanted infusion ports. They may have single, double, or triple lumens. Several lumens (multilumen catheters) allow more than one therapy to be administered at the same time (Table 42-3). Reasons to use multilumen catheters include repeated blood sampling, TPN, administration of blood products or infusion of large quantities and/or concentrations of fluids, ability to administer incompatible drugs or fluids at the same time (through different lumens), and central venous pressure (CVP) monitoring.

With any of the central venous catheters, instilling medication through the injection cap is easily accomplished. With the implanted device, the port must be palpated for placement and stabilized, the overlying skin cleansed, and only special noncoring Huber needles used to pierce the port's diaphragm on the top or side, depending on the style. To prevent repeated skin punctures, a special infusion set with a Huber needle and extension tubing with Luer connection can be used (Fig. 42-21). With this attached, the injection procedure is the same as for the heparin device or venous catheter. To prevent infection, meticulous aseptic technique must be used anytime the devices are entered, including during instillation of heparin or saline solution to prevent clotting.

The children and parents are taught the procedure for care of the VAD before discharge from the hospital, including preparation and injection of the prescribed medication, the flush, and dressing changes. A protective device may be recommended for some active children to prevent their accidentally dislodging the needle. Many children take responsibility for preparing and administering medications. Both verbal and written step-by-step instructions* are provided for the learners.

The use of a spandex-nylon bodysuit on active toddlers has

*Home care instructions for caring for an intermittent infusion device are available in Wong DL: *Wong and Whaley's clinical manual of pediatric nursing,* ed 4, St Louis, 1996, Mosby.

TABLE 42-3 Comparison of long-term central venous access devices

DESCRIPTION	BENEFITS	CARE CONSIDERATIONS
Tunneled catheter (e.g., Hickman/Broviac catheter)		
Silicone, radiopaque, flexible catheter with open ends One or two Dacron Cuffs or Vitacuffs (biosynthetic material impregnated with silver ions) on catheter(s) enhances tissue ingrowth May have more than one lumen	Reduced risk of bacterial migration after tissue adheres to Dacron cuff or Vitacuff Easy to use for self-administered infusions Removal requires pulling catheter from site (nonsurgical procedure)	Requires daily heparin flushes Must be clamped or have clamp nearby at all times Must keep exit site dry Heavy activity restricted until tissue adheres to cuff Risk of infection still present Protrudes outside body; susceptible to damage from sharp instruments and may be pulled out; may affect body image More difficult to repair Patient/family must learn catheter care
Groshong catheter		
Clear, flexible, silicone, radiopaque catheter with closed tip and two-way valve at proximal end Dacron cuff or Vitacuff on catheter enhances tissue ingrowth May have more than one lumen	Reduced time and cost for maintenance care; no heparin flushes needed Reduced catheter damage—no clamping needed because of two-way valve Increased patient safety because of minimum potential for blood backflow or air embolism Reduced risk of bacterial migration after tissue adheres to Dacron cuff or Vitacuff Easily repaired Easy to use for self-administered IV infusions	Requires weekly irrigation with normal saline solution Must keep exit site dry Heavy activity restricted until tissue adheres to cuff Risk of infection still present Protrudes outside body; susceptible to damage from sharp instruments and may be pulled out; can affect body image Patient/family must learn catheter care
Implanted ports (Port-A-Cath, Infus-A-Port, Mediport, Norport, Groshong port)		
Totally implantable metal or plastic device that consists of self-sealing injection port with top or side access with preconnected or attachable silicone catheter that is placed in large blood vessel	Reduced risk of infection Placed completely under the skin; therefore cannot be pulled out or damaged No maintenance care and reduced cost for family Heparinized monthly and after each infusion to maintain patency (Groshong port only requires saline solution) No limitations on regular physical activity, including swimming Dressing only needed when port accessed with Huber needle that is not removed No or only slight change in body appearance (slight bulge on chest)	Must pierce skin for access; pain with insertion of needle; can use local anesthetic (EMLA) or intradermal buffered lidocaine before accessing port Special noncoring needle (Huber) with straight or angled design must be used to inject into port Skin preparation needed before injection Hard to manipulate for self-administered infusions Catheter may dislodge from port, especially if child "plays" with port site (twiddler syndrome) Vigorous contact sports generally not allowed Removal requires surgical procedure

successfully maintained central lines. The line could not be removed by the toddler and the bodysuit fit snugly over the catheter, its exit site, and its connections. The cost of two bodysuits per child—one worn while the other is being cleaned—is less than the costs and the risks of repeated central line insertions. (Janik, Wayne, and Janik, 1995). A pocket sewn on the inside of a T-shirt provides a place in which to coil the catheter line while the child is at play if a dressing is not used.

Infection and an occluded catheter are two of the most common complications of central venous catheters. Although neither is an emergency, both require treatment: antibiotics for infection and a fibrinolytic agent, such as urokinase, for clots. Uncapping can be prevented by taping the cap securely to the catheter and the clamped line to the dressing. Leaks can be prevented by using a smooth-edged clamp only. Parents are cautioned to keep scissors away from the child to prevent accidental cutting of the catheter. If the catheter leaks, they are instructed to tape it above the leak and then clamp the catheter at the taped site. The child should be taken to the practitioner as soon as possible to prevent infection or clotting after a catheter leak.

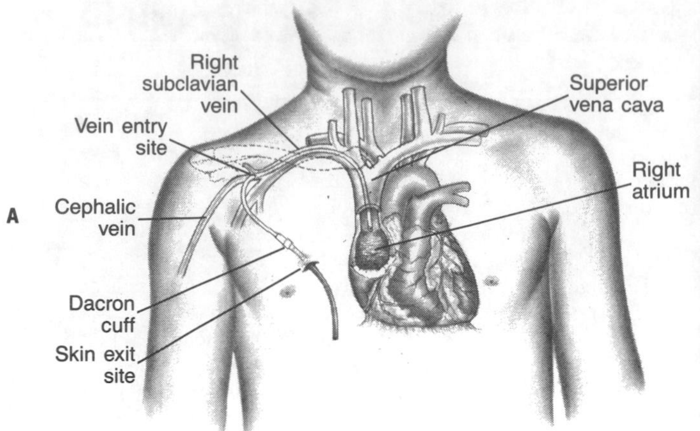

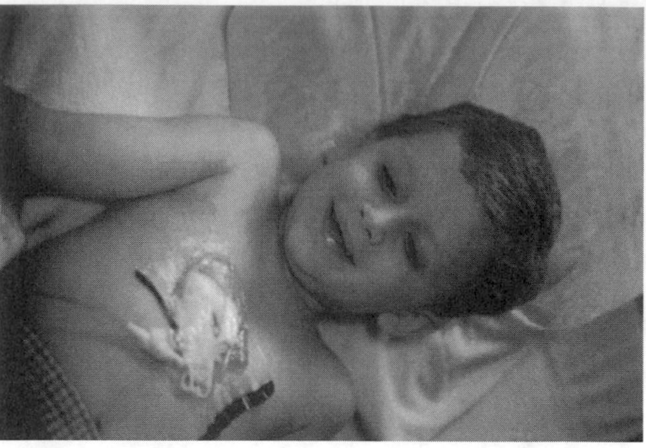

Fig. 42-21 Venous access devices. **A,** Central venous catheter insertion and exit site. **B,** Child receiving medication by way of an implantable port. Note needle and extension tubing inserted into port and secured with gauze dressings and a transparent dressing.

Guidelines

NASOGASTRIC, OROGASTRIC, OR GASTROSTOMY MEDICATION ADMINISTRATION IN CHILDREN

- Use elixir or suspension (rather than tablet) preparations of medication whenever possible.
- Dilute viscous medication or syrup if possible with a small amount of water.
- If administering tablets, crush tablet to a very fine powder and dissolve drug in a small amount of warm water.
  - Never crush enteric-coated or sustained-release tablets or capsules.
- Avoid oily medications because they tend to cling to side of tube.
- Do not mix medication with enteral formula unless fluid is restricted. If adding a drug:
  - Check with pharmacist for compatibility.
  - Shake formula well and observe for any physical reaction (e.g., separation, precipitation).
  - Label formula container with name of medication, dosage, date, and time infusion started.
- Have medication at room temperature.
- Measure medication in calibrated cup or syringe.
- Check for correct placement of nasogastric or orogastric tube.
- Attach syringe (with adaptable tip but without plunger) to tube.
- Pour medication into syringe.
- Unclamp tube and allow medication to flow by gravity.
- Adjust height of container to achieve desired flow rate (e.g., increase height for faster flow).
- As soon as syringe is empty, pour in water to flush tubing.
  - Amount of water depends on length and gauge of tubing.
  - Determine amount before administering any medication by using a syringe to fill an unused nasogastric or orogastric tube completely with water. The amount of flush solution is usually $1\frac{1}{2}$ times this volume.
  - For certain drug preparations (e.g., suspensions) more fluid may be needed.
- If administering more than one drug at the same time, flush tube between each medication with clear water.

Nursing ALERT

If a central venous catheter is accidentally removed, apply pressure to the *entry* site to the vein, not the exit site on the skin (Marcoux, Fisher, and Wong, 1990).

NASOGASTRIC, OROGASTRIC, OR GASTROSTOMY ADMINISTRATION

When a child has an indwelling feeding tube or a gastrostomy, oral medications are usually given via that route. An advantage of this method is the ability to administer oral medications around the clock without disturbing the child. A disadvantage is the risk of occluding or "clogging" the tube, especially when giving viscous solutions through small-bore feeding tubes. The most important preventive measure is adequate flushing after the medication is instilled. The Guidelines box to the left discusses administration.

Nursing ALERT

Sprinkle-type medication should be avoided. However, if there is no other option and the tube is large-gauge (18 French or greater), but usually not a Foley catheter, it may be given by mixing the sprinkles with a small amount of pureed fruit and thinning with water. The fruit keeps the sprinkles suspended so they do not float to the top. Flush well. This procedure is not recommended for skin-level gastrostomy devices.

RECTAL ADMINISTRATION

The rectal route of administration is less reliable but is sometimes used when the oral route is difficult or contraindicated. Some of the drugs available in suppository form are aspirin, sedatives, analgesics (morphine), and antiemetics. The difficulty in using the rectal route is that unless the rectal ampulla is empty at the time of insertion, the absorption of the drug may be delayed, diminished, or prevented by the presence of feces. Sometimes the drug is later evacuated, securely surrounded by stool. However, the rectal route is used most often in children who are unable to take anything by mouth and are unlikely to have large amounts of stool. It is also used when oral preparations are unsuitable to control vomiting.

To insert a suppository, the wrapper is removed and the suppository is lubricated with water-soluble jelly or warm water. A gloved finger is used to place the suppository quickly but gently into the rectum, beyond both of the rectal sphincters. The buttocks are then held or taped together firmly to relieve pressure on the anal sphincter until the urge to expel the suppository has passed—5 to 10 minutes. Sometimes the amount of drug ordered is less than the dosage available. The irregular shape of most suppositories makes the process of dividing them into a desired dose difficult if not dangerous. If the suppository must be halved, it should be cut lengthwise. However, there is no guarantee that the drug will be evenly dispersed throughout the petrolatum base.

Rectal suppositories are usually inserted with the apex (pointed end) foremost. One study demonstrated easier insertion and a lower expulsion rate when the suppository was inserted with the base (blunt end) first. Reverse contractions or the pressure gradient of the anal canal may help the suppository to slip higher into the canal (Abd-El-Maeboud et al, 1991). This study, however, did not consider the issue of comfort on insertion.

If medication is administered via a retention enema, the same procedure is used. Drugs given by enema are diluted in the smallest amount of solution possible to minimize the likelihood of being evacuated.

OPTIC, OTIC, AND NASAL ADMINISTRATION

There are few differences in administering eye, ear, and nose medication to children or to adults. The major difficulty is in gaining children's cooperation or employing restraining techniques. The infant or young child's head is immobilized in the same manner as described in Fig. 32-22, *B*. Older children need only explanation and direction. Although the administration of optic, otic, and nasal medication is not painful, these drugs can cause unpleasant sensations that can be eliminated with various techniques:

- **Eye**—Apply finger pressure to the lacrimal punctum at the inner aspect of the lid for 1 minute to prevent drainage of medication to the nasopharynx and the unpleasant "tasting" of the drug.
- **Ear**—Allow medications stored in the refrigerator to warm to room temperature before instillation.
- **Nose**—Position the child with the head hyperextended to prevent strangling sensations caused by medication trickling into the throat rather than up into the nasal passages.

To instill eye medication, the child is placed supine or sitting with the head extended and is asked to look up. One hand is used to pull the lower lid downward; the hand that holds the dropper rests on the head so that it may move synchronously with the child's head, thus reducing the possibility of trauma to a struggling child or of dropping medication onto the face

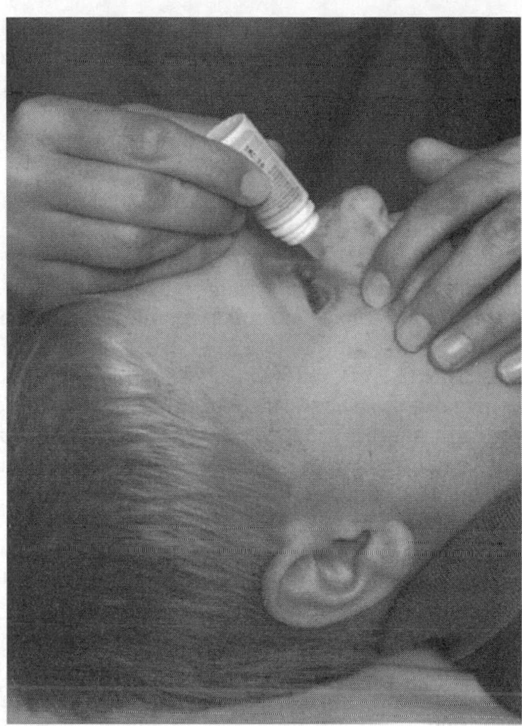

Fig. 42-22 Administering eye drops.

(Fig. 42- 22). As the lower lid is pulled down, a small conjunctival sac is formed; the solution or ointment is applied to this area, never directly onto the eyeball. Another effective technique is to pull the lower lid down and out to form a cup, into which the medication is dropped. The lids are gently closed to prevent expression of the medication, and the child is asked to look in all directions to enhance even distribution of the preparation. Excess medication is wiped from the inner canthus outward to prevent contamination to the contralateral eye.

Instilling eye drops in infants can be most difficult, since they often clench the lids tightly closed. One approach is to place the drops in the nasal corner where the lids meet. The medication pools in this area, and when the child opens the lids, the medication flows onto the conjunctiva. For young children, playing a game can be helpful, for example, instructing the child to keep the eyes closed until the count of 3, then to open them, at which time the drops are quickly instilled. Ointment can be applied when the child is sleeping by gently pulling down the lower lid and placing the ointment in the lower conjunctival sac.

Nursing ALERT

If both eye ointment and drops are ordered, give drops first, wait 3 minutes, then apply the ointment to allow each drug to work. When possible, administer eye ointments before bedtime or naptime, since the child's vision will be blurred temporarily.

Ear drops are instilled with the child restrained in the supine position and the head turned to the appropriate side. For children younger than 3 years of age, the external auditory canal is straightened by gently pulling the pinna downward and straight back. The pinna is pulled upward and back in children older than 3 years of age (see Fig. 32-19). To place the drops deep into the ear canal without contaminating the tip of the dropper, place a disposable ear speculum in the canal and administer the drops through the speculum. After instillation, the child should remain lying on the unaffected side for a few minutes. Gentle massage of the area immediately anterior to the ear facilitates the entry of drops into the ear canal. The use of cotton pledgets prevents medication from flowing out of the external canal. However, the pledgets should be loose enough to allow any discharge to exit from the ear. Premoistening the cotton with a few drops of medication prevents the wicking action from absorbing the medication instilled in the ear.

Nose drops are instilled in the same manner as in the adult patient. Unpleasant sensations associated with medicated nose drops are minimized when care is taken to position the child with the head extended well over the edge of the bed or a pillow (Fig. 42-23). Depending on size, the infant can be positioned in the football hold (see Fig. 42-7, *B*), in the nurse's arm with the head extended and stabilized between the nurse's body and elbow and the arms and hands immobilized with the nurse's hands, or as in Fig. 42-23. After instillation of the drops, the child should remain in position for 1 minute to allow the drops to come in contact with the nasal surfaces.

Nasal sprays are inserted into the nose vertically then angled nasally to prevent trauma to the septum and to direct medication toward the inferior turbinate.

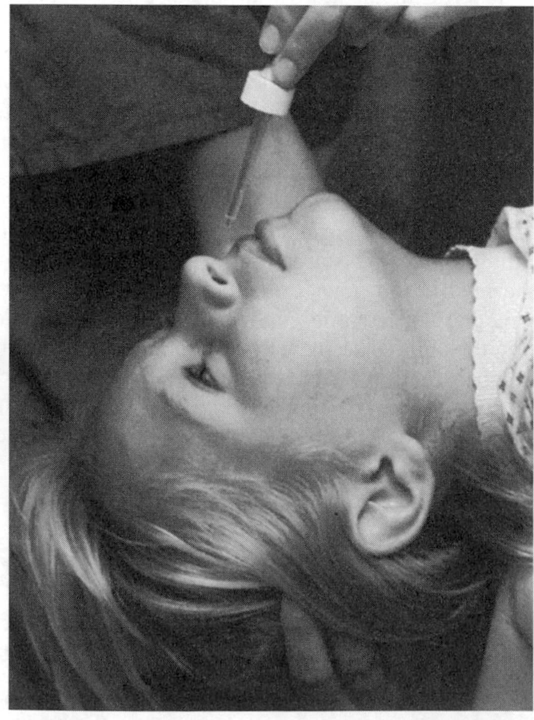

Fig. 42-23 Proper position for instilling nose drops.

FAMILY TEACHING AND HOME CARE

It is usually the nurse who assumes the responsibility for preparing families to administer medications at home. The family should have an understanding of why the child is receiving the medication and the effects that might be expected, as well as the amount, frequency, and length of time the drug is to be administered. Instruction should be carried out in an unhurried, relaxed manner, preferably in an area away from busy ward or office routine, following the same guidelines for teaching as outlined in the Guidelines box on p. 1264.

The caregiver is carefully instructed regarding the correct dosage, and it is the nurse's responsibility to prepare parents for the specifics of the task. Some persons have difficulty understanding or interpreting terminology from the pharmacy, and if they nod or otherwise indicate an understanding, it cannot be assumed that the message is clear. It is important to ascertain their interpretation of a teaspoon, for example, and to be certain they have acceptable devices for measuring the drug. If the drug is packaged with a dropper, syringe, or plastic cup, the nurse should show the point on the device that indicates the prescribed dose and demonstrate how the dose is drawn up into a dropper or syringe and measured and the bubbles are eliminated. Also, the nurse must be certain that families understand that a prescription ordered in drops means single drops, not dropperfuls, a potential source of administration error (see the Nursing Alert on p. 1287). If the nurse has any doubts about the parent's ability to administer the correct dose, the parent should be asked to give a return demonstration. This verification is especially important when the drug has potentially serious consequences from incorrect dosage, such as insulin or digoxin, or when more complex administration is required, such as parenteral injections. When a parent is taught to give an injection, adequate time for instruction and practice must be allotted.

Home modifications are often necessary, because the availability of equipment or assistance can differ from that of the hospital setting. For example, restraint is often necessary when giving medications to children, and the parent may need guidance in devising methods that allow for one person to restrain the child and safely give the drug. One successful method is to use the following procedure:

- Place child supine on flat surface (bed, couch, floor)
- Sit facing child so that his or her head is between operator's thighs and his or her arms are under operator's legs
- Place lower legs over child's legs to restrain lower body, if necessary.
- To administer oral medication, place small pillow under child's head to reduce risk of aspiration.
- To administer nasal medication, place small pillow under child's shoulders to aid flow of liquid through nasal passages.

The time that the drug is to be administered is clarified with the parent. For instance, when a drug is prescribed in association with meals, the number of meals that the family is accustomed to eating influences the amount of drug the child receives; do they have meals twice a day or five times a day? When a drug is to be given several times during the day, together the nurse and parents can work out a schedule that accommodates the family's routine. This is particularly significant if the drug must be given at equal intervals throughout a 24-hour period. For example, telling parents that the child needs 1 teaspoon of medicine 4 times a day is subject to misinterpretation, since parents may routinely schedule the doses at incorrect times. Instead, a preplanned schedule based on 6-hour intervals should be set up with the number of days required for therapeutic dosage listed. Written instruction should accompany all drug prescriptions.* If parents have difficulty reading or understanding English, colors can be used to convey instructions. For example, each drug is marked with a color and the appropriate color is placed on a calendar chart or on a drawing of a clock to identify when the drug needs to be given. If a liquid medication and syringe are used, the syringe is also marked at the place the plunger needs to be with color-coded tape.

Procedures Related to Maintaining Fluid Balance

MEASUREMENT OF INTAKE AND OUTPUT (I & O)

One of the most important roles of the nurse in maintaining fluid balance is accurate measurement of fluid balance. Although the physician usually indicates when I & O are to be recorded, it is a nursing responsibility to keep an accurate I & O record on patients in the following situations:

- After major surgery
- Intravenous, diuretic, or corticosteroid therapy
- Severe thermal burns or injuries
- Renal disease or damage
- Congestive heart failure
- Dehydration (vomiting and diarrhea)
- Diabetes mellitus
- Oliguria
- 2 years of age or younger

Infants or small children who are unable to use a bedpan or those who have bowel movements with every voiding will require the application of a collecting device (p. 1280). If collecting bags are not used, wet diapers or pads are carefully weighed to ascertain the amount of fluid lost. This includes liquid stool, vomitus, and other losses. The volume of fluid in milliliters is equivalent to the weight of the fluid measured in grams. The specific gravity as a measure of osmolality is determined with a urinometer or a refractometer and assists in assessing the degree of hydration.

The weighed diaper method of fluid measurement has disadvantages, including (1) inability to differentiate one type of loss from another because of admixture, (2) loss of urine or liquid stool from leakage or evaporation (especially if the infant is under a radiant warmer), and (3) additional fluid in diaper (superabsorbent disposable type) from absorption of atmospheric moisture (from high-humidity incubators). However, when several types of diapers, including cloth, conventional disposable, and superabsorbent disposable diapers, were compared for accuracy in terms of evaporative effects, closed superabsorbent disposable diapers followed by open superabsorbent disposable diapers were affected least (Fox, 1992). To prevent the problem of evaporative losses and leakage of excreta, diapers should be weighed as soon as possible after becoming soiled.

It is important to measure and record all intake—oral and parenteral —and output from all sources, including urine, stool, emesis, drainage tubes, fistulas, and wounds from which appreciable amounts of fluid are lost.

Special Needs When the Child Is NPO

Infants or children who are unable or not permitted to take fluids by mouth (NPO) have special needs. To ensure that they do not receive fluids, a sign can be placed in some obvious place, such as over their beds or on their shirts, to alert others to their status. To prevent temptation to drink, fluids should not be left at the bedside.

Oral hygiene, a part of routine hygienic care, is especially important when fluids are restricted or withheld (see p. 1266). For the young child who cannot brush the teeth or rinse the mouth without swallowing fluid, the nurse can institute oral hygiene by wiping the teeth, gums, and tongue with a cloth moistened with saline solution. To keep the mouth feeling moist when the child is NPO, ice chips are given (if this is permitted by the practitioner) or the mouth is sprayed with a fine mist of cool water from a spray bottle. The lips are kept moist with petrolatum (Vaseline) or another commercial lip aid. Lemon-glycerin swabs are avoided because they dry the skin, irritate open lesions, and can decay the teeth. To meet the need to suck, the infant is provided with a pacifier.

The child who is fluid-restricted presents an equal challenge. Limiting of fluids is often more difficult for the child than NPO, especially when IV fluids are also eliminated. To make certain the child does not drink the entire amount allowed early in the day, the daily allotment is calculated to provide fluids at periodic intervals throughout the child's waking hours. Serving the fluids in small containers gives the illusion of larger servings. No extra liquid is left at the bedside if compliance is a problem.

PARENTERAL FLUID THERAPY

Site/Equipment

The site selected for IV infusion depends on accessibility and convenience. In older children any accessible vein may be used. In small infants a scalp vein or a superficial vein of the wrist, hand, foot, or arm is usually most convenient and most easily stabilized (Fig. 42-24). Since superficial veins of the scalp have no valves, insertion is easier, and they can be used in infants up to about 9 months of age. For veins in the extremities, it is best to start with the most distal sites and to use the nondominant hand.

For most IV infusions in children, an over-the-needle 20- to 24-gauge catheter or a scalp-vein size 21 or 23 needle with flexible winged tabs is used. In situations in which fluids are urgently needed and there is difficulty in entering a vein, a catheter inserted by the surgical cutdown procedure may be necessary. The vein of choice for this alternative is the internal

*Home care instructions on giving medications to children are available in Wong DL: *Wong and Whaley's clinical manual of pediatric nursing*, ed 4, St Louis, 1996, Mosby.

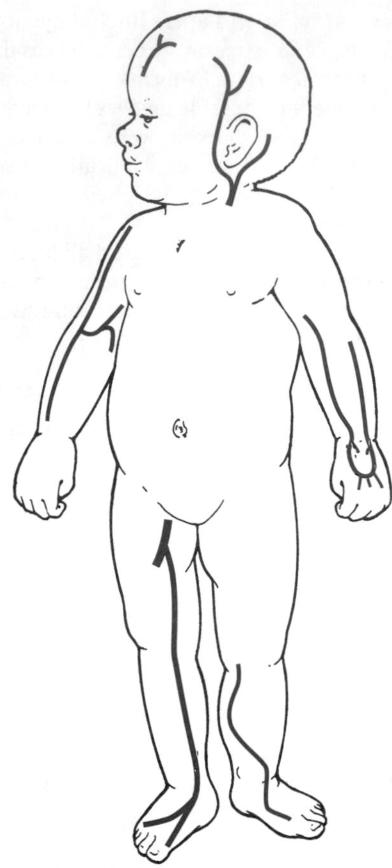

Fig. 42-24 Preferred sites for venous access in infants. (From Smith DP et al, editors: *Comprehensive child and family nursing skills*, St Louis, 1991, Mosby.)

saphenous vein, located just anterior to the medial malleolus of the tibia. For long-term IV therapy a number of other devices may be used (see p. 1294).

Other equipment needed includes an antiseptic swab to clean the site, a tourniquet, an appropriately sized padded armboard (when an extremity is used), rolled towels or small blankets for maintaining position of the head or extremity, tape (or dressing and bacteriostatic ointment if the hospital dictates), and a device to protect the IV site after insertion. The prescribed solution, tubing, filter, and infusion pump are prepared in advance, ready to connect to the needle after insertion.

Selection of a scalp vein as the venipuncture site requires shaving the area around the site to visualize the vein better and provide a smooth surface on which to tape the tubing. A rubber band slipped onto the head from brow to occiput will usually suffice as a tourniquet. Shaving off a portion of the infant's hair is very upsetting to parents; therefore they should be told what to expect and reassured that the hair will grow in again rapidly.

Situations may occur in which rapid establishment of a systemic access is vital and venous access may be hampered by peripheral circulatory collapse, cardiopulmonary arrest, burns, or other conditions. *Intraosseous infusion* provides an alternate route for administration of fluids and medications until intravascular access can be attained. A large-bore needle, such as a bone marrow needle, is inserted into the medullary cavity of a long bone, most often the distal femur, proximal tibia, or distal tibia. This procedure is usually reserved for children under 3 years of age who are unconscious or are receiving analgesics, because the procedure is painful.

There are several modifications in equipment used for IV infusion for children. A gravity drainage apparatus used for children is much the same as that for adults except that it is designed to deliver a reduced drop size (60 drops/ml) and contains a calibrated volume control chamber (e.g., a Buretrol or Solu-set) that regulates the amount of fluid that can be infused. A microdropper greatly facilitates calculation of flow rate because a prescribed number of milliliters per hour equals the number of drops per minute. For example, if the solution is to infuse at a rate of 30 ml per hour, the infusion is regulated to deliver 30 drops per minute.

A variety of infusion pumps that are available infuse a programmed amount of fluid from a bag hanging above the machine or from a syringe placed in the machine. Infusion devices are widely used in pediatrics because they can accurately infuse fluids, especially the syringe pumps, which infuse very small amounts of fluid. It is an important nursing responsibility to calculate the amount to be infused in a given length of time, set the infusion rate, and monitor the apparatus frequently (at least every 1 to 2 hours) to make certain that the desired rate is maintained, the integrity of the system remains intact, the site remains intact (free of infiltration or irritation), and the infusion does not stop.

Continuous infusion pumps, although convenient and efficient, are not without risks. Overreliance on the accuracy of the machine can cause either too much or too little fluid to be infused; therefore careful periodic assessment is essential. Excess pressure can build up if the machine is set at a rate faster than the vein is able to accommodate (or continues to pump when the needle is out of the lumen). This is especially true in very small infants and when circumstances necessitate the use of a capillary. No matter what device is used, a thorough understanding of the apparatus is essential for safe fluid administration.

Special Care Considerations

To maintain the integrity of the IV site, adequate protection will be required for the child. An attempt is made to position the extremity in a natural anatomic position with the use of gauze pads or rolls as needed. To prevent trauma to the skin from removal of tape, gauze or a barrier such as transparent film can be placed between the skin and the adhesive. Sometimes a covered board is taped to the extremities to prevent flexion of a foot, hand, or arm.

After insertion, the catheter or needle is firmly secured at the puncture site with nonallergenic tape and protected from becoming dislodged by immobilization of the extremity. The insertion site and about 1 inch of skin beyond the site are left uncovered for early detection of infiltration. Clear plastic dressings are ideal because they allow ready visualization of the insertion site. Some finger or toe areas are left unoccluded by dressings or tape to allow for assessment of circulation. The thumb is never immobilized because of the danger of contractures with limited movement later on. A commercial device (such as I.V. House*) or an improvised device, such as a plastic or wax paper cup that is cut in half (with the rigid edges covered with tape) can be applied directly over the needle site for further protection. Some needle containers make excellent protective covers. A colorful and interesting sticker can be applied to the armboard or protecting device to add a positive note to the procedure.

Older children who are alert and cooperative can usually be trusted to protect the IV site. An IV infusion is not always a deterrent to mobility. When the child is feeling well and the insertion site is well secured, the child can be held or be walked, but precautions must be observed to preserve the integrity of the IV system.

Infants, small children, and uncooperative children require varying degrees of immobilization, and on rare occasions, complete restriction of movement may be needed to prevent removal of the IV infusion. The affected extremity is secured to the bed, and the remaining extremities that might be used to dislodge the needle are restrained. This includes feet, as well as hands, since most infants will attempt to brush away the offending attachment by rubbing it against another extremity or body part. Whenever possible, the infant or child should be held and cuddled to help meet emotional needs during this trying time (Fig. 42-25).

When it comes time to discontinue an IV infusion, many children are distressed by the thought of needle removal. Therefore they need a careful explanation of the process and suggestions for helping. One way is to allow children to remove or help remove the tape from the site. This provides them with a measure of control and often encourages their cooperation. The procedure consists of turning off any pump apparatus, occluding the IV tubing, removing the tape, and pulling the needle or catheter out of the vessel while exerting firm pressure at the site. A dry dressing (adhesive bandage strip) is placed over the puncture site. If a catheter was used for the IV infusion, the tip is inspected to make certain the catheter is intact and no portion remains in the vein.

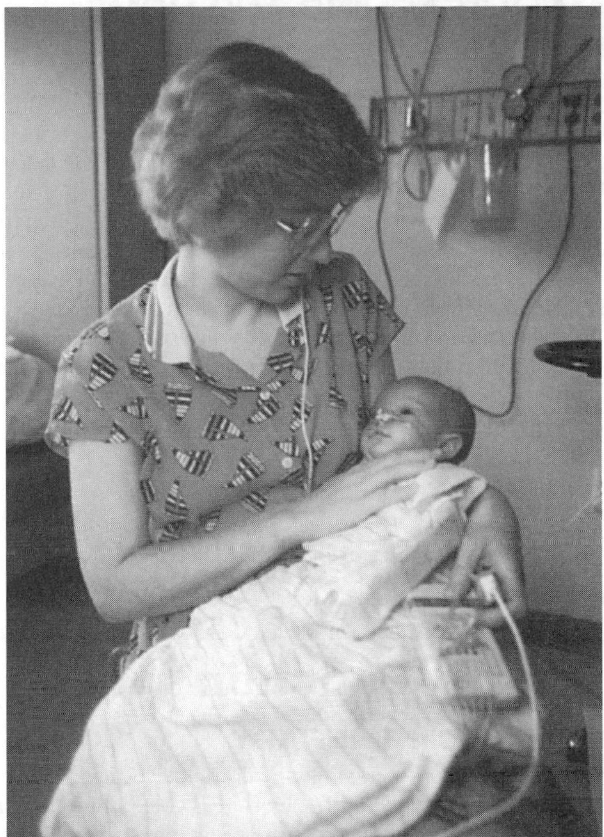

Fig. 42-25 Intravenous infusion, as well as other equipment, does not prevent infant from being picked up and cuddled.

Complications. The same precautions regarding maintenance of asepsis, prevention of infection, and observation for infiltration are carried out with patients of any age. However, infiltration is more difficult to detect in infants and small children than it is in adults. The increased amount of subcutaneous fat and the amount of tape used to secure the needle often obscure the signs of early infiltration. When the fluid appears to be infusing too slowly or ceases, the usual assessment for obstruction within the apparatus—kinks, screw clamps, shutoff valve, and positioning interference (e.g., a bent elbow)—often locates the difficulty. When these actions fail to detect the problem, it may be necessary to carefully remove some of the tape and other material that obscure a clear view of the venipuncture site. Dependent areas, such as the palm and undersides of the extremity or the occiput and the area behind the ears, are examined.

Whenever possible, the IV infusion should be placed in an extremity to which the identification band (or bracelet) is not attached. Serious circulatory impairment can result from infiltrated solution distal to the band, which acts as a tourniquet preventing adequate venous return. To check for return blood flow through the needle, the bottle is lowered below the level of the infusion site. If the tubing is connected to an infusion pump, it must be removed from the pump before lowering.

Drugs are available to diffuse extravasated fluid or neutralize the extravasated medication. Hyaluronidase is used in severe cases to diffuse extravasated fluids rapidly through the tissue and increase the absorption rate. When it is used, the IV infusion is discontinued, and with the needle still in place, the drug is injected into the site. If the catheter is removed, the drug is then injected (as prescribed) into the area surrounding the insertion site. Assessment and documentation of the site continue until the infiltration has completely resolved. Staging of IV infiltrates may be performed to evaluate treatment options (Flemmer and Chan, 1993).

Prevention of infection is a major nursing function during IV therapy. The infusion site is protected from trauma and entry of bacteria. When an IV infusion continues for several days or longer, the tubing and bottle are changed at regular intervals according to hospital policy. Frequency ranges from every 24 to every 72 hours—most often every 48 hours. To ensure that the equipment is changed regularly, it is labeled with the date and time that the new bottle and tubing are attached. Any signs of inflammation, such as redness or pain, should be reported immediately. This usually requires removing the infusion and restarting it at another site.

*Available from I.V. House, 7400 Foxmont Dr., Hazelwood, MO 63042; (800) 530-0400; FAX (314) 831-3863.

FAMILY TEACHING AND HOME CARE

Since maintaining fluid balance is critical, especially in young children, families may need to continue some procedures, such as measuring intake, output, and daily weight, at home. Although these are simple skills, families require time to learn and practice them before discharge. With the widespread use of superabsorbent disposable diapers, parents are advised that the diaper may be wet but still feel dry. Placing some cotton balls or tissues in the diaper facilitates checking for wetness. Also, the wet diaper may feel "doughy" and heavy.

IV therapy for fluid replacement is rarely carried out in the home, although parenteral administration of drugs or hyperalimentation is becoming more common. Home care of the child with home hyperalimentation is discussed on p. 1314.

Procedures for Maintaining Respiratory Function

INHALATION THERAPY

The term *inhalation therapy* is an all-inclusive term that encompasses a variety of therapies that involve changing the composition, volume, or pressure of inspired gases. These therapies include primarily increasing the oxygen concentration of inspired gas (oxygen therapy), increasing the water vapor content of inspired gas (humidification), adding airborne particles with beneficial properties (aerosol therapy), and employing various means for controlling or assisting respiration (artificial ventilation, continuous positive airway pressure).

Oxygen Therapy

Oxygen therapy is primarily carried out in the hospital, although increasing numbers of children are receiving oxygen in the home. Oxygen delivered to the infant via the incubator is satisfactory when lower levels are adequate to prevent cyanosis, but the highest concentration (almost 100%) is supplied by way of a *plastic hood* (Fig. 42-26). The gas is not allowed to blow directly into the infant's face, and the hood should not rub against the infant's neck, chin, or shoulder. Older cooperative children can use a *nasal cannula* or *prongs*, which can supply a concentration of about 50%. A *mask* is not well tolerated by children.

For children beyond early infancy, the *oxygen tent* is a satisfactory means for administration of oxygen (Fig. 42-27). A tent does not require any device to come into direct contact with the face, but the concentration of oxygen within the tent is difficult to control and to maintain above 30% to 50%. A major difficulty with the use of the tent is keeping the tent closed so that oxygen concentration is maintained.

To reduce oxygen loss, nursing care is planned carefully so that the tent is opened as little as possible. Since oxygen is heavier than air, loss will be greater at the bottom of the tent; therefore the tent is tucked in snugly without open edges. The bottom of the tent should be examined more often when the child is restless and fussy and likely to pull the covers loose. Some tents are open at the top. Because of the rapid diffusing qualities of carbon dioxide, the levels of the gas do not build up within these enclosures.

After the tent has been opened for an extended period, it is flushed with oxygen by increasing the flow meter for a few minutes to raise the oxygen and mist concentration quickly. The flow meter is then reset to the prescribed number of liters.

The enclosed tent becomes very warm; therefore some type of cooling mechanism is provided. The temperature inside the tent must be checked periodically to be certain that it is maintained at the desired level. It is important to make certain that the child is kept warm and dry. Since oxygen is drying to the tissues, the gas is humidified, causing moisture to condense on the tent walls.

Nursing ALERT

Keep the child warm and dry by checking the temperature inside the tent and the child's bedding and clothing frequently. Adjust the temperature and change clothing as often as needed.

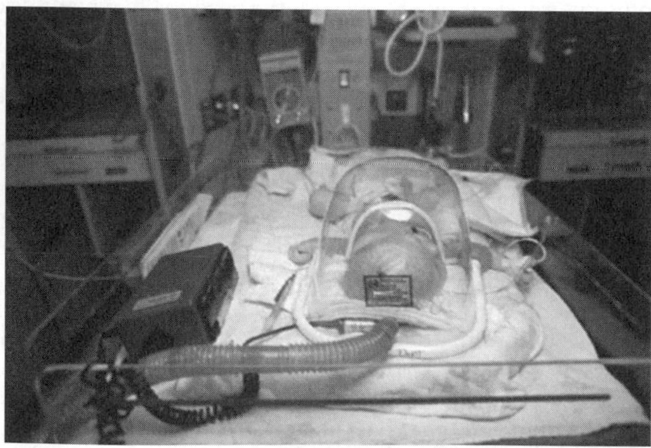

Fig. 42-26 Oxygen administered to infant by means of a plastic hood. Note oxygen analyzer *(machine on left)*.

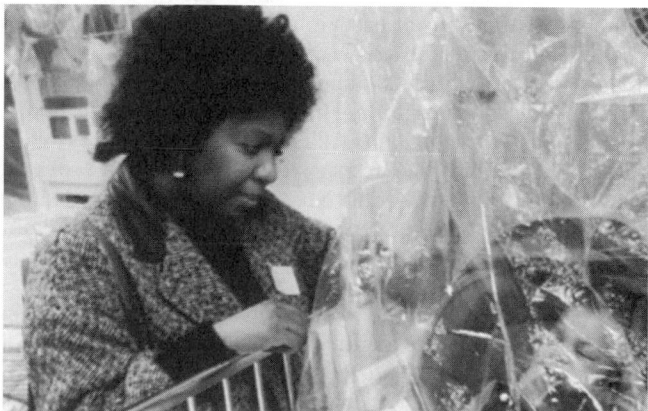

Fig. 42-27 The tent provides a comfortable method for oxygen administration.

The reactions of children to the oxygen tent are variable. Some, especially older children, feel comfortable in the tent and like the cozy, close privacy it affords. Others, more often younger children, may be frightened by the forced enclosure. The plastic walls distort their view of the world and constitute a barrier between them and their source of comfort, their parent. Their distress can be minimized if they are able to see someone nearby and are reassured that they will not be left alone. A favorite toy or object can accompany the child inside the tent. However, all toys should be inspected for safety and suitability. Other familiar items can be placed at the foot of the bed or otherwise in view.

Nursing ALERT

Inspect all toys for safety and suitability (e.g., vinyl or plastic—not stuffed items that absorb moisture and are difficult to keep dry). The high O_2 environment makes any source of sparks (such as mechanical or electrical toys) a potential fire hazard.

In most instances the child can be removed from the oxygen tent for activities such as feeding and bathing, whereas in other cases the child is placed in the tent only during periods of rest. Still other children may require oxygen continuously and can be removed from the tent or incubator only if an oxygen source is held close to the child's face. Any change in color, increased respiratory effort, or restlessness is an indication to return the child to the oxygen tent.

Oxygen toxicity. Oxygen is essential to life and a valuable therapeutic aid. However, prolonged exposure to high oxygen tensions can be damaging to some body tissues and functions. The organs most vulnerable to the adverse effects of excessive oxygenation are the retina of the premature infant and the lungs of persons at any age.

Oxygen-induced carbon dioxide narcosis is a physiologic hazard of oxygen therapy that may occur in persons with chronic pulmonary disease, such as cystic fibrosis. These children have chronic alveolar hypoventilation with concomitant chronic carbon dioxide retention and hypoxemia. In these patients the respiratory center has adapted to the continuously higher arterial carbon dioxide ($Paco_2$) levels, and therefore hypoxia becomes the more powerful stimulus for respiration. When the arterial oxygen (Pao_2) level is elevated during oxygen administration, the hypoxic drive is removed, causing progressive hypoventilation and increased $Paco_2$ levels, and the child rapidly becomes unconscious.

Monitoring Oxygen Therapy

Pulse oximetry is a simple, continuous, noninvasive method of determining oxygen saturation (Sao_2) to guide oxygen therapy. A sensor comprising a light-emitting diode (LED) and a photodetector is placed in opposition around a foot, hand, finger, toe, or earlobe, with the LED placed on top of the nail when digits are used (Fig. 42-28). The diode emits red and infrared lights that pass through the skin to the photodetector. The photodetector measures the amount of each type of light absorbed by functional hemoglobins. Hemoglobin saturated with oxygen (oxyhemoglobin) absorbs more infrared light than does hemoglobin not saturated with oxygen (deoxyhemoglobin). Therefore pulsatile blood flow is the primary physiologic factor that influences accuracy of the pulse oximeter.

Another noninvasive method is **transcutaneous monitoring (TCM),** which provides continual monitoring of transcutaneous partial pressure of oxygen in arterial blood ($tcPao_2$) and, with some devices, of carbon dioxide in arterial blood ($tcPaco_2$). An electrode is attached to the warmed skin to facilitate arterialization of cutaneous capillaries. The site of the electrode must be changed every 3 to 4 hours to prevent burning of the skin, and the machine must be calibrated with every site change. This monitoring is used frequently in neonatal intensive care units, but it may not reflect Pao_2 in infants with impaired local circulation or in older infants whose skin is thicker.

The Pao_2 can be correlated with the Sao_2 by means of the oxyhemoglobin dissociation curve (Fig. 42-29). Most important, changes in Pao_2 do not cause identical changes in Sao_2. Rather, in the steep portion of the curve, small changes in Pao_2. result in large changes in Sao_2. In the flat portion of the curve, large changes in Pao_2 result in only small changes in Sao_2 A quick formula for calculating correlation of Pao_2 with Sao_2 is the 30-60, 60-90 rule. Assuming a normal pH, $Paco_2$, and body temperature, this rule can apply: when Pao_2 = 30 mm Hg, Sao_2 = 60%; when Pao_2 = 60 mm Hg, Sao_2 = 90%.

Oximetry is insensitive to hyperoxia because hemoglobin approaches 100% saturation for all Pao_2 readings above approximately 100 mm Hg, creating a dangerous situation for the premature infant at risk for developing retinopathy of prematurity (see Chapter 25). Therefore the premature infant being monitored with oximetry should have upper limits identified, such as 90% to 95%, and a protocol established for decreasing O_2 when saturations are high.

The degree to which O_2 combines with hemoglobin is affected by several factors. A shift of the curve to the left causes an increased affinity of hemoglobin for O_2, but the O_2 is not easily released to the tissues. This represents an increase in the Sao_2 if it is measured against the same Pao_2 of the normal oxyhemoblobin dissociation curve. This left shift can be

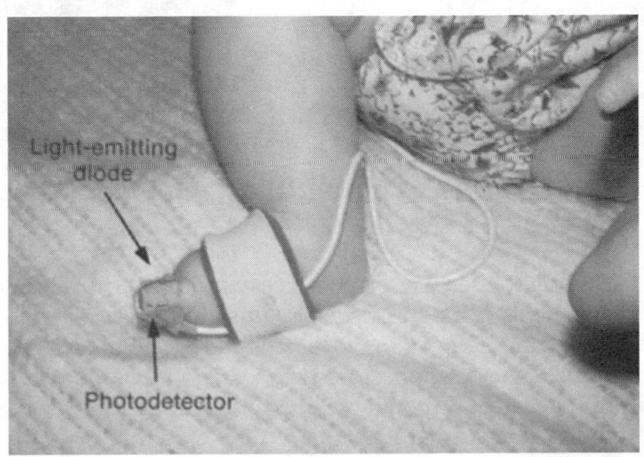

Fig. 42-28 Oximeter sensor on great toe. Note that sensor is positioned with light-emitting diode opposite photodetector. Cord is secured to foot to minimize movement of sensor.

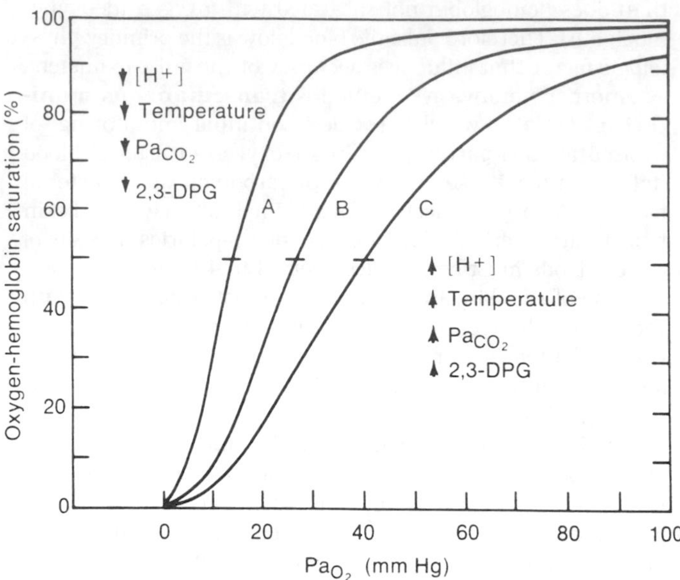

Fig. 42-29 Oxyhemoglobin dissociation curve.

caused by an increase in blood pH or a decrease in arterial carbon dioxide pressure ($Paco_2$), body temperature, or 2,3-diphosphoglycerate (2,3-DPG), a substance in the red blood cells.

A shift of the curve to the right causes a decreased affinity of hemoglobin for O_2, but improved O_2 release to the tissues. This represents a lower Sao_2 if measured against the same Pao_2 of the normal oxyhemoglobin dissociation curve. This right shift can be caused by a decrease in blood pH or an increase in $Paco_2$, body temperature, or 2,3-DPG.

Oximetry offers several advantages over TCM: it (1) does not require heating the skin, thus reducing the risk of burns; (2) eliminates a delay period for transducer equilibration; and (3) maintains an accurate measurement regardless of the patient's age or skin characteristics or the presence of lung disease.

Nursing ALERT

It is important to make certain that sensory connectors and oximeters are compatible. Wiring that is incompatible can generate considerable heat at the tip of the sensor, causing second- and third-degree burns under the sensors. Pressure necrosis can also occur from sensors attached too tightly. Therefore inspect the skin under the sensor frequently.

Applying the sensor correctly is essential for accurate Sao_2 measurements. Since the sensor must identify every pulse beat to calculate the Sao_2, movement can interfere with sensing. Some devices synchronize the oxygen saturation reading with the heartbeat, thereby reducing the interference caused by motion. Sensors are not placed on extremities used for blood pressure monitoring or with indwelling arterial catheters, since pulsatile blood flow can be affected.

When applying the sensor to infants, the sensor is taped securely to the great toe, and the wire is taped to the sole of the foot (or a commercial holder is used that fastens with a self-adhering closure). A snugly fitting sock is then placed over the foot. In children, the sensor is taped securely to the index finger and the wire to the back of the hand. A self-adhering Ace-type wrap (e.g., Coban) is used around the finger and/or hand to secure the sensor and wire further.

Ambient light from ceiling lights and phototherapy, as well as high-intensity heat and light from radiant warmers, can interfere with readings. Therefore the sensor should be covered to block these light sources. Intravenous dyes; green, purple, or black nail polish; nonopaque synthetic nails; and possibly ink used for footprinting can also cause inaccurate Sao_2 measurements. The dyes should be removed or, in the case of porcelain nails, a different area used for the sensor. Skin color, thickness, and edema do not affect the readings.

Aerosol Therapy

Aerosol therapy can be effective in depositing medication directly into the airway. This route of administration can be useful in preventing the systemic side effects of certain drugs and in reducing the amount of drug necessary to achieve the desired effect. Bronchodilators, steroids, and antibiotics can be suspended in particulate form and then inhaled so that the medication reaches the small airways. The use of aerosol therapy is particularly challenging in children who are too young to cooperate with controlling the rate and depth of breathing. Administration of this therapy requires skill, patience, and creativity.

The value of aerosolized water or "mist therapy" is controversial. Continuous administration of mist, or aerosolized water, for the treatment of inflammatory conditions of the airways is a common practice that has no proven benefit (Alderson and Warren, 1984), although clinical improvement has been noted in some cases (e.g., the use of a mist tent or a very humid environment, such as a steamy bathroom, for the treatment of croup). For other pathologic conditions, however, mist therapy can be detrimental. For example, bronchoconstriction in children with asthma can be exacerbated by mist therapy.

The notion that inhaled mist can influence the viscosity of mucus in dehydrated children is erroneous; inhaled mist does not affect the water content of expectorated mucus. If dehydration is evident, oral or parenteral rehydration will normalize the water content of respiratory mucus.

Medications can be aerosolized or nebulized with air or with oxygen-enriched gas. *Hand-held nebulizers* are the most commonly used equipment. The medicated "mist" is discharged into a small plastic mask, which the child holds over the nose and mouth. In order to prevent particle deposition in the nose and pharynx, the child is instructed to take slow, deep breaths through an open mouth during the treatment. For home use, an air compressor is necessary to force air through the liquid medication to form the aerosol. Fairly compact, portable units can be rented from health equipment companies. The *metered dose inhaler (MDI)* is a self-contained, hand-held device that allows for intermittent delivery of a specified amount of medication. Many bronchodilators are available in this form and are successfully used by children with asthma. For children under the age of 5 or 6 years, a spacer device attached to the MDI can help with coordination of breathing and aerosol delivery. It allows the aerosolized particles to remain in suspension longer (see also Asthma, Chapter 43).

A major nursing responsibility during aerosol therapy is to assess the effectiveness of the treatment and the patient's tolerance of the procedure. Assessments of breath sounds and work of breathing should be done before and after treatments. Small children who become upset with having a mask held close to the face may become fatigued with fighting the procedure and may actually appear worse during and immediately after the therapy. Careful assessment by the nurse and practitioner is necessary to determine whether the treatment is worthwhile. It may be necessary to spend a few minutes calming the child after the procedure, and allowing the vital signs to return to baseline, in order to assess changes in breath sounds and work of breathing accurately.

BRONCHIAL (POSTURAL) DRAINAGE

Bronchial drainage is indicated whenever excessive fluid or mucus in the bronchi is not being removed by normal ciliary activity and cough. Positioning the child to take maximum advantage of gravity facilitates removal of secretions. The effect is sometimes dramatic in children with chronic lung disease characterized by thick mucous secretions, such as asthma and cystic fibrosis.

Postural drainage is carried out 3 to 4 times daily and is more effective when it follows other respiratory therapy, such as bronchodilator and/or nebulization medication. Bronchial drainage is generally performed before meals (or 1 to $1^1/_2$ hours after meals) to minimize the chance of vomiting and is repeated at bedtime. The length and duration of treatment depend on the child's condition and tolerance level—usually 20 to 30 minutes. There are positions to facilitate drainage from all major lung segments (Fig. 42-30), but all positions are not employed at each session. Children will usually cooperate for four to six positions, but more than six tend to exceed their limits of tolerance. Older children can be expected to tolerate longer periods.

In the hospital an older child can be positioned over an elevated knee rest. Small children and infants can be positioned with pillows or on the therapist's lap and legs (Fig. 42-31). Infants should not be placed in the Trendelenburg position, because they do not have an autonomic regulation of blood flow to the head. Special modifications of the techniques are required in children whose conditions contraindicate the standard positioning, such as head injuries, some types of surgical incisions or burns, and casts or traction. At home, small children can be positioned on a padded ironing board.* Children who require postural drainage over months or years may benefit from specially constructed tables padded and adjusted to their individual needs. The position used and the frequency and duration of treatment are individualized.

CHEST PHYSIOTHERAPY (CPT)

CPT usually refers to the use of postural drainage in combination with adjunctive techniques that are thought to enhance the clearance of mucus from the airway. These techniques include manual percussion, vibration, and squeezing of the chest; cough; forceful expiration; and breathing exercises. The efficacies of these techniques, both individually and combined, are controversial, however. Postural drainage in combination with forced expiration has been shown to be beneficial, but the benefit of the other techniques has yet to be demonstrated.

The most common technique used in association with postural drainage is manual percussion of the chest wall. Nurses are often responsible for this maneuver if a respiratory therapist is not available, so they should be skilled in the technique. The patient is dressed in a lightweight shirt and placed in a postural drainage position; then the nurse gently but firmly strikes the chest wall with a cupped hand (Fig. 42-32, *A*). For infants, special devices are available for percussing small areas (Fig. 42-32, *B*). A "popping," hollow sound should be the result, not a slapping sound. The procedure should be done over the rib cage only and should be painless. Percussion can be performed with a soft circular mask (adapted to maintain air trapping) or a percussion cup marketed especially for the purpose of aiding the loosening of secretions.

CPT is contraindicated when patients have pulmonary hemorrhage, pulmonary embolism, end-stage renal disease, increased intracranial pressure, osteogenesis imperfecta, or minimal cardiac reserves.

CPT should be used for patients who have increased sputum production. It is probably of no value to the uncomplicated postoperative patient or the patient with pneumonia. Forced expiration combined with postural drainage is more effective than cough alone, but percussion and vibration have no proven value. Appropriate use of bronchodilators before chest physiotherapy will enhance mucus clearance.

ARTIFICIAL VENTILATION

Artificial Airways

An artificial airway is usually used in association with artificial ventilation and in children with upper airway obstruction. Endotracheal intubation can be accomplished by the nasal (nasotracheal), oral (orotracheal), or direct tracheal (tracheostomy) route. Although it is more difficult to place, nasotracheal intubation is preferred to orotracheal intubation because it facilitates oral hygiene and provides more stable fixation, which reduces the complication of tracheal erosion and the danger of accidental extubation. Uncuffed endotracheal tubes are almost always used with infants and children. Cuffed tubes may be used with adolescents to help provide an airtight seal. Air or gas delivered directly to the trachea must be humidified as in tracheostomy.

Tracheostomy

A tracheostomy is a surgical opening in the trachea; the procedure may be done on an emergency basis or it may be an elective one, and it may be combined with mechanical ventilation.

Pediatric tracheostomy tubes are usually made of plastic or Silastic. These tubes are constructed with a more acute angle than adult tubes, and they soften at body temperature, conforming to the contours of the trachea. Since these materials resist the formation of crusted respiratory secretions, they are made without an inner cannula. Some children require a

*Home care instructions on performing postural drainage are available in Wong DL: *Wong and Whaley's clinical manual of pediatric nursing*, ed 4, St Louis, 1996, Mosby.

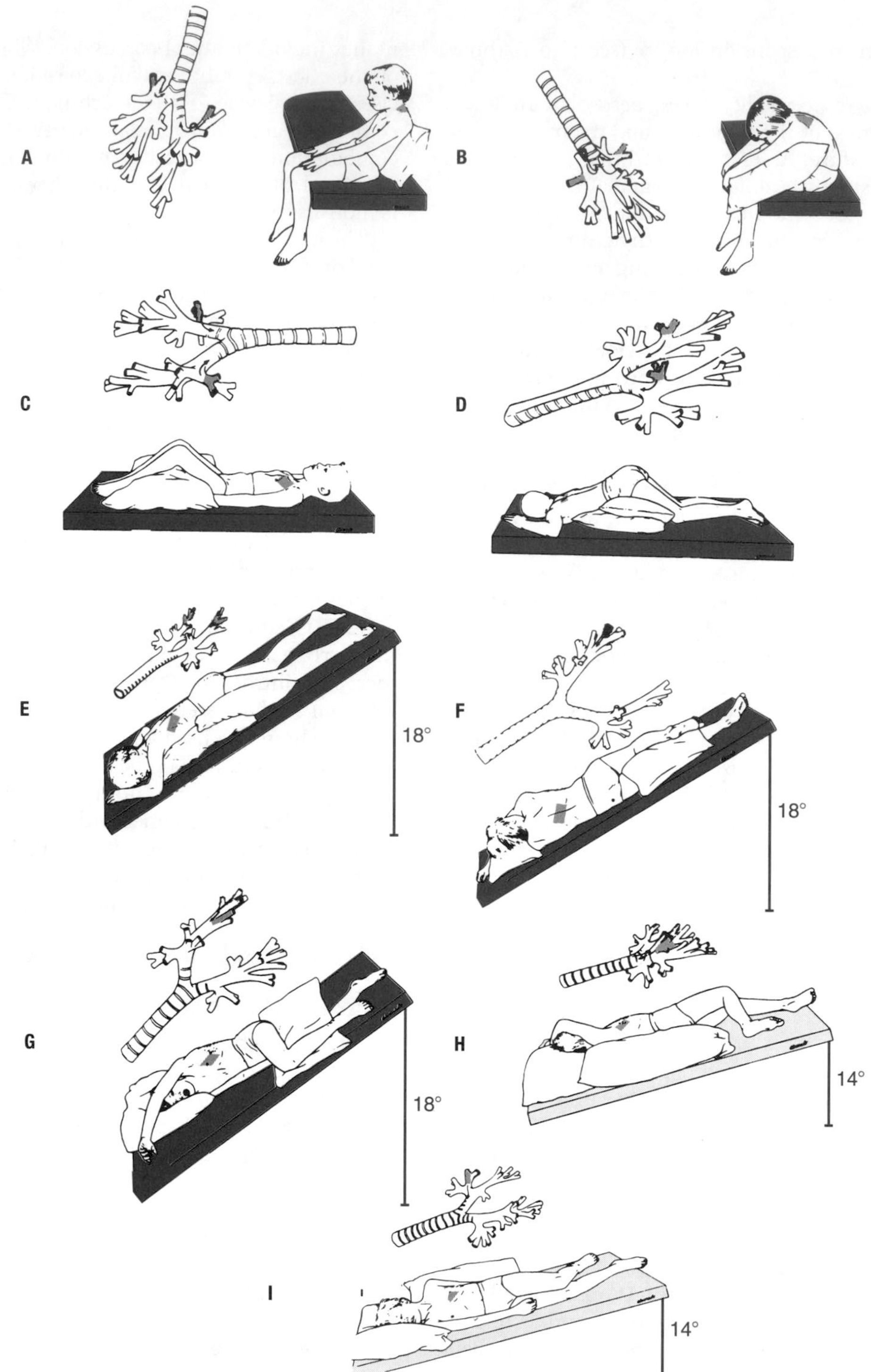

Fig. 42-30 Bronchial drainage positions for all major segments of child. For each position, model of tracheobronchial tree is projected beside child to show segmental bronchus *(striped)* being drained and pathway *(arrow)* of secretions out of bronchus. Drainage platform is horizontal unless otherwise noted. Colored area on child indicates area to be cupped or vibrated by therapist. **A,** Apical segment of right upper lobe and apical subsegment of apical-posterior segment of left upper lobe. **B,** Posterior segment of right upper lobe and posterior subsegment of apical-posterior segment of left upper lobe. **C,** Anterior segments of both upper lobes; child should be rotated slightly away from side being drained. **D,** Superior segments of both lower lobes. **E,** Posterior basal segments of both lower lobes. **F,** Lateral basal segments of right lower lobe; left lateral basal segment would be drained by mirror image of this position *(right side down)*. **G,** Anterior basal segment of left lower lobe; right anterior basal segment would be drained by mirror image of this position *(left side down)*. **H,** Medial and lateral segments of right middle lobe. **I,** Lingular segments *(superior and inferior)* of left upper lobe *(homologue of right middle lobe)*. (From Chernick V, editor: *Kendig's disorders of the respiratory tract of children*, ed 5, Philadelphia, 1990, WB Saunders.)

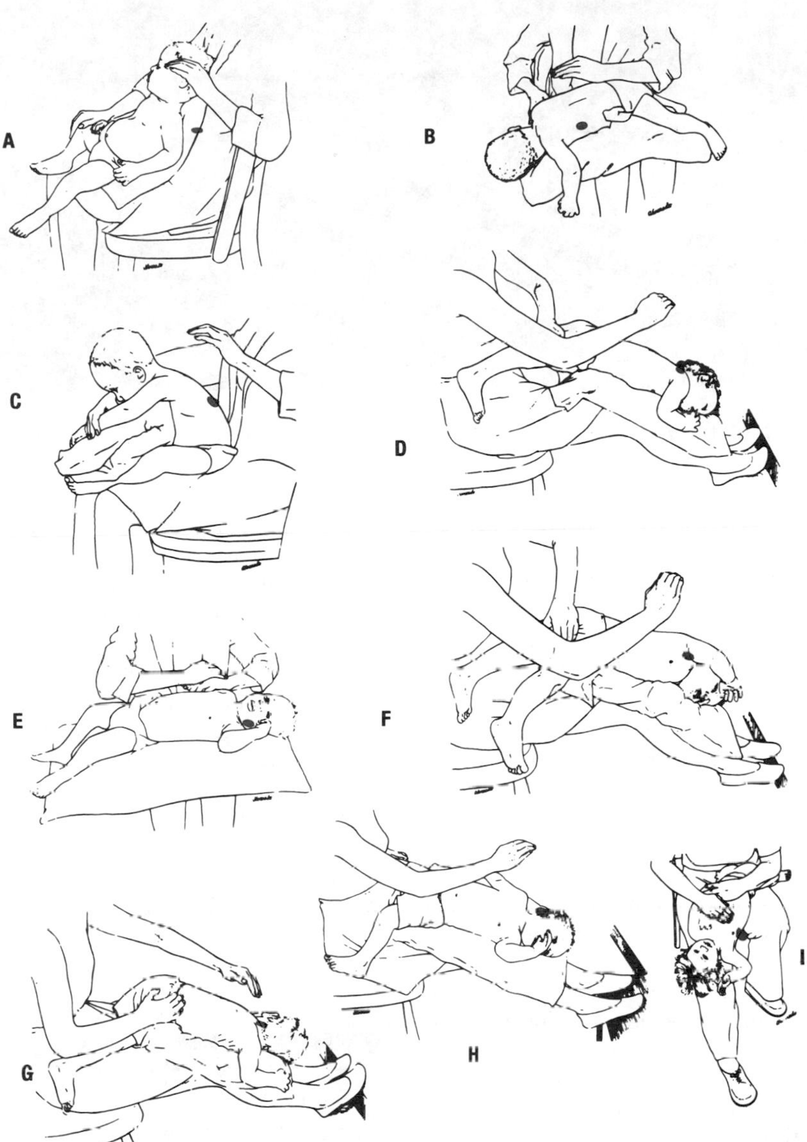

Fig. 42-31 Bronchial drainage positions for major segments of all lobes in infant. Procedure is most easily carried out in therapist's lap. Therapist's hand on chest indicates area to be cupped or vibrated. **A,** Apical segment of left upper lobe. **B,** Posterior segment of left upper lobe. **C,** Anterior segment of left upper lobe. **D,** Superior segment of right lower lobe. **E,** Posterior basal segment of right lower lobe. **F,** Lateral basal segment of right lower lobe. **G,** Anterior basal segment of right lower lobe. **H,** Medial and lateral segments of right middle lobe. **I,** Lingular segments *(superior and inferior)* of left upper lobe. (Modified from Cystic Fibrosis Foundation: *Infant segmental bronchial drainage,* Rockville, Md, The Foundation.)

metal tracheostomy tube (usually made of sterling silver or stainless steel), which contains an inner cannula.

Children who have undergone a tracheostomy require a 7- to 10-day hospital stay. During this time the child is closely monitored for the development of complications such as hemorrhage, edema, aspiration, and the entrance of free air into the pleural cavity. The focus of postoperative nursing care is maintaining a patent airway, facilitating the removal of pulmonary secretions, providing humidified air or O_2, cleansing the stoma, monitoring the child's ability to swallow, and teaching while preventing complications (the most dangerous being related to accidental decannulation and tube obstruction). Since the child may be unable to signal for help, direct observation and use of respiratory and cardiac monitors are essential. Respiratory assessments include breath sounds and work of breathing, vital signs, and tightness of the tracheostomy ties, and the type and amount of secretions. Large amounts of bloody secretions are also uncommon and should be considered a sign of hemorrhage. The practitioner should be notified immediately if they are present.

The child is positioned with the head of the bed raised, or in the position most comfortable to him or her, with the call

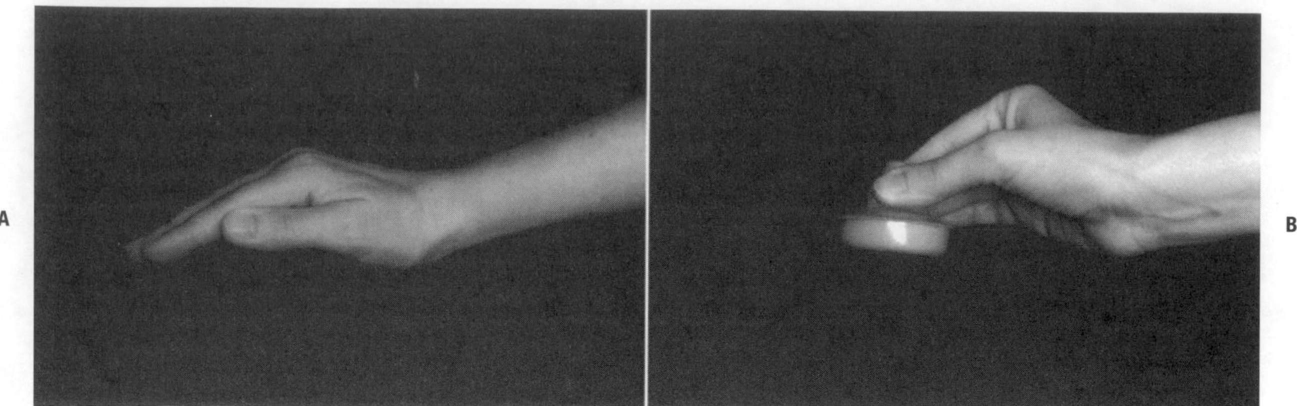

Fig. 42-32 **A,** Cupped hand position for percussion. **B,** Device for infant percussion.

light easily available. Suction catheters, suction source, gloves, sterile saline solution, sterile gauze for wiping away secretions, scissors, an extra tracheostomy tube of the same size with ties already attached, another tracheostomy tube one size smaller, and the obturator are kept at the bedside. A source of humidification is provided, since the normal humidification and filtering functions of the airway have been bypassed. Intravenous fluids ensure adequate hydration until the child is able to swallow sufficient amounts of fluids.

Suctioning. The airway must remain patent and requires frequent suctioning during the first few hours after a tracheostomy to remove mucous plugs and excessive secretions. Proper vacuum pressure and suction catheter size are important to prevent atelectasis and decrease hypoxia from the suctioning procedure. Vacuum pressure should range from 60 to 100 mm Hg and from 40 to 60 mm Hg for premature infants. Unless secretions are thick and tenacious, the lower range of negative pressure is recommended. Tracheal suction catheters are available in a variety of sizes. The catheter selected should have a diameter one half the diameter of the tracheostomy tube. If the catheter is too large, it can block the airway. The catheter is constructed with a side port so that it can be introduced without suction and removed while intermittent suction is applied by covering the port with the thumb (Fig. 42-33). The catheter is inserted to 0.5 cm beyond or just to the end of the tracheostomy tube. Traditional technique for suctioning endotracheal (ET) or tracheostomy tubes recommends advancing a suction catheter into the tube until it meets resistance, then withdrawing it slightly and applying suction. However, studies indicate that this approach causes trauma to the tracheobronchial wall. This trauma can be prevented by inserting the catheter and advancing it to the premeasured depth of just to the tip (especially in infants) or no more than 0.5 cm beyond the tube (Kleiber, Krutzfield, and Rose, 1988).

Calibrated catheters are easier to use for premeasured suctioning technique, but unmarked catheters can also be used. To measure the length for catheter insertion, the catheter is placed near a sample ET or tracheostomy tube (same size as child's tube) with the end of the catheter at the correct position. The catheter is grasped with a sterile-gloved hand to mark the length and insert the catheter until the hand reaches the stoma.

A small amount of sterile isotonic saline solution (a few drops to 0.5 to 2 ml, depending on the child's size) injected into the tube may help loosen secretions and crusts for easier aspiration. However, this technique may contribute to the problems of lower airway colonization and nosocomial pneumonia through repeated washing of organisms from the tube's surface into the lower airway (Hagler and Traver, 1994). Also, the use of saline solution has been shown to *decrease* the oxygen saturation (Sao_2) more than when it is not used in adults (Ackerman, 1993). In infants, saline solution did not cause a significant change in Sao_2 (Shorten, Byrne, and Jones, 1991). More research is needed to demonstrate the value of instilling saline solution in the tube.

Nursing ALERT

Suctioning should require no more than 5 seconds (Chandra and Hazinski, 1994).

Counting 1—one thousand, 2—one thousand, 3—one thousand, and so on while suctioning is a simple means for monitoring the time. Without a safeguard the airway may be obstructed for too long. Hyperventilating the child with 100% O_2 before and after suctioning (using a bag-valve-mask or increasing the Fio_2 ventilator setting) is also performed to prevent hypoxia. Closed tracheal suctioning systems that allow for uninterrupted O_2 delivery may also be used.

Nursing ALERT

Suctioning carried out *only as often as needed* to keep the tube patent. Signs of mucus partially occluding the airway include an increased heart rate, a rise in respiratory effort, a drop in O_2 saturation, cyanosis, or an increase in the positive inspiratory pressure (PIP) on the ventilator (Musser, 1992).

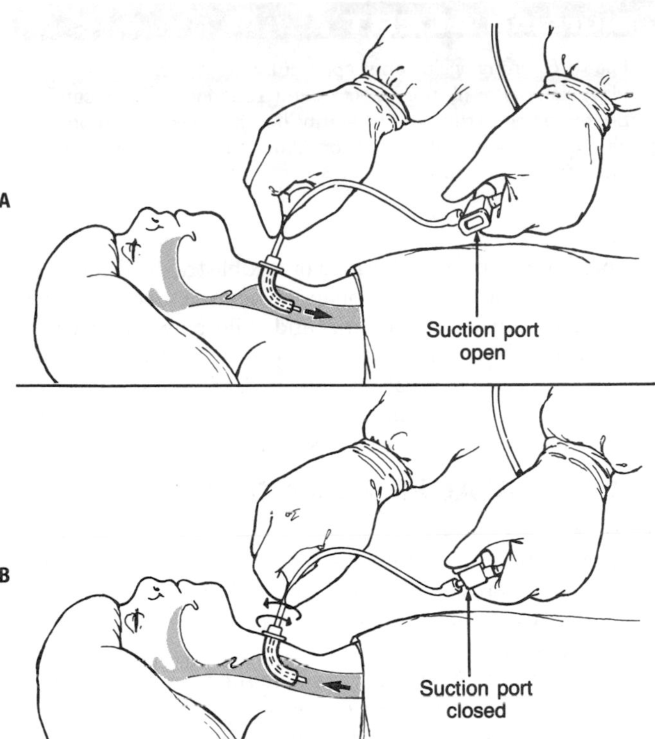

Fig. 42-33 Tracheostomy suctioning. **A,** Insertion, port open. **B,** Withdrawal, port occluded. Note that catheter is inserted just slightly beyond end of tracheostomy tube.

The child is allowed to rest for 30 to 60 seconds after each aspiration to allow O_2 tension to return to normal; then the process is repeated until the trachea is clear. Suctioning should be limited to about three aspirations in one period. Oximetry is used to monitor suctioning and prevent hypoxia.

In the acute care setting, aseptic technique is used during care of the tracheostomy. Secondary infection is a major concern, since the air entering the lower airway bypasses the natural defenses of the upper airway. Gloves are worn during the aspiration procedure, although a sterile glove is needed only on the hand touching the catheter. A new tube, gloves, and sterile saline solution are used each time (see the Critical Thinking Q & A box to the right).

Routine Care. The tracheostomy stoma requires daily care. Assessments of the stoma area include observations for signs of infection and breakdown of the skin. The skin is kept clean and dry, and secretions around the stoma may be gently removed with half-strength hydrogen peroxide. Hydrogen peroxide should not be used with sterling silver tracheostomy tubes, because it tends to pit and stain the silver surface. The nurse should be aware of wet tracheostomy dressings, which can predispose the peristomal area to skin breakdown. Several products are available to prevent or treat excoriation. The Allevyn tracheostomy dressing is a hydrophilic sponge with a polyurethane back that is highly absorptive. Other possible barriers to help maintain skin integrity include the use of hydrocolloid wafers (such as Duoderm CGF and Hollister Restore) under the tracheostomy flanges, as well as use of extra-thin hydrocolloid wafers under the chin.

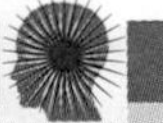

Critical Thinking Q & A

PLANNING FOR HOME TRACHEOSTOMY CARE

Jose, 18 months old, has been ventilator-dependent since birth. He is presently hospitalized with pneumonia that has responded well to antibiotic therapy. You are discussing plans for discharge and home care with the family. Jose lives with his mother and her parents. Home nursing support is available only during the day. The family does not want to take Jose home, because he is frequently suctioned at night. Your initial intervention is to:

1. Talk with the night nurses about their suctioning program.
2. Design a plan for the family that allows them to each assume responsibility for night care with scheduled suctioning times.
3. Arrange with social service to request additional financial support for the family.
4. Suggest that Jose stay in the hospital until he needs less frequent suctioning.

The correct answer is one. If the family managed with daytime nursing assistance before this hospitalization and the pneumonia has resolved, the child should not require intensive suctioning. In talking with the night staff, you find that the nurses suction anytime they walk past the room and hear Jose "gurgling." They also do not use premeasured suctioning technique. You discuss with them a program of premeasured suctioning only as needed to reduce the production of secretion that may be from tracheal irritation.

The other three responses assume that the frequent suctioning is needed and are not appropriate initial interventions. Suctioning should not be performed on a set schedule, but only as needed. Seeking additional financial support for nighttime nurses will not help the family return to the prehospital home care arrangements. Jose should be discharged as soon as possible to avoid nosocomial infection, promote normalization for a toddler, and contain health care costs. In this case changing the suctioning regimen decreased the frequency to a minimum of once or twice a night—a level of care the family was able to manage.

The tracheostomy tube is held in place with tracheostomy ties made of a durable, nonfraying material. The ties are changed daily and when soiled. New ties are looped through the flanges and tied snugly in a triple knot at the side of the neck *before* the soiled ties are cut and removed. Some nurses have found that threading the ties through a piece of $^1/_4$-inch surgical tubing cushions the ties; others have found the tubing to be irritating to the skin. The ties should be tight enough to allow just a fingertip to be inserted between the ties and the neck (Fig. 42-34). It is easier to ensure a snug fit if the child's head is flexed rather than extended while ties are being secured. Ties fastened with self-adhering closures are also available. These devices, such as the Dale tracheostomy tube holder, are made of a soft, cushioning, and slightly stretchy material that is very comfortable. They are becoming increasingly popular because of their ease of use and ability to maintain better skin integrity. One should still be aware, however, of the safety factor and use them on children who are unlikely to pull and undo the fastener.

Routine tracheostomy tube changes are usually carried out weekly after a tract has been formed to minimize formation of granulation tissue. The first change is usually performed by the surgeon; subsequent changes are performed by

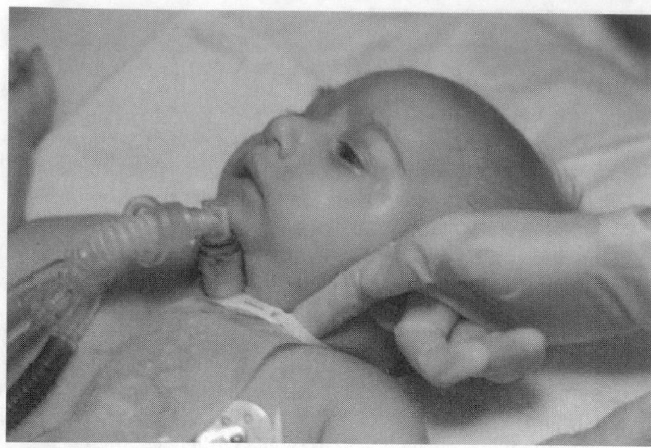

Fig. 42-34 Tracheostomy ties are snug but allow one finger to be inserted.

the nurse and, if the child is discharged home with the tracheostomy, by either a parent or a visiting nurse. Ideally two caregivers participate in the procedure to assist with positioning the child.

Changing the tracheostomy tube is accomplished by using sterile technique. The new, sterile tube is prepared by inserting the obturator and attaching new ties. The child is suctioned before the procedure to minimize secretions, then restrained and positioned with the neck slightly extended. One caregiver cuts the old ties and removes the tube from the stoma. The new tube is inserted gently into the stoma (using a downward and forward motion that follows the curve of the trachea), the obturator is removed, and the ties are secured. The adequacy of ventilation must be assessed after a tube change because the tube can be inserted into the soft tissue surrounding the trachea; therefore breath sounds and respiratory effort are carefully monitored.

Supplemental O_2 is always delivered with a humidification system to prevent drying of the respiratory mucosa. Humidification of room air for an established tracheostomy can be intermittent if secretions remain thin enough to be coughed or suctioned from the tracheostomy. Direct humidification via tracheostomy mask can be provided during naps and at night so that the child is able to be up and around unencumbered during much of the day. Room humidifiers are also used successfully.

The inner cannula, if used, should be removed with each suctioning, cleaned with sterile saline solution and pipe cleaners to remove crusted material, dried thoroughly, and reinserted.

Emergency care: tube occlusion and accidental decannulation. Occlusion of the tracheostomy tube is life-threatening, and infants and children are at greater risk than adults because of the smaller diameter of the tube. Maintaining patency of the tube is accomplished with suctioning and routine tube changes to prevent formation of crusts that can occlude the tube.

Accidental decannulation also requires immediate tube replacement. Some children have a fairly rigid trachea, so that the airway remains partially open when the tube is removed.

> **Nursing ALERT**
>
> Life-threatening occlusion is apparent when the child displays signs of respiratory distress and a suction catheter cannot be passed to the end of the tube despite several attempts and instillation of saline solution. This situation requires an immediate tube change.

However, others have malformed or flexible tracheal cartilage, which causes the airway to collapse when the tube is removed or dislodged. Since many infants and children with upper airway problems have little airway reserve, if replacement of the dislodged tube is impossible, a smaller-sized tube should be inserted. If the stoma cannot be cannulated with another tracheostomy tube, oral intubation should be performed.

FAMILY TEACHING AND HOME CARE

Some of the treatments families need to continue at home are often related to respiratory procedures. Some of these treatments, such as postural drainage, require less preparation than others, such as tracheostomy care. Regardless of the home therapy, the family needs ample time to learn the skills and demonstrate them before discharge. Therefore instruction should begin as soon as it is determined that the child will go home with a tracheostomy. The more comfortable they are with all the aspects of care, the more confident and less anxious they will be when faced with total care of the child at home. For example, the family may require many practice sessions before they feel comfortable with suctioning, cleaning, and changing a tracheostomy tube and performing cardiopulmonary resuscitation (CPR) in case of an emergency. Teaching sessions should be short, and written material must accompany instructions to reinforce what is being taught.* To facilitate the family's adjustment, supplies identical to the ones to which they are accustomed should be available in the home. In the event of substitution, parents need to be reassured that the unfamiliar equipment is safe to use on their child. The home should be properly equipped with all supplies and equipment needed before the child arrives.

A nurse from the public health department or other home care service should be available to the family and should periodically assess the family's ability to carry out the activities needed in care of the child. The parents may find it helpful to talk to other parents of children with similar needs. They also need to know whom to call and where they can get help and support in times of uncertainty or in an emergency.

To prepare for any emergency, the family must be taught infant or child CPR. The local utilities company and local emergency medical service (EMS) should be notified of the child's condition and the equipment used in the home. Prior notification allows for a quicker response if help is needed.

When a child has a tracheostomy, parents are encouraged to provide as normal a life as possible for their child and other family members. The child who is physically able (e.g., a child with a a tracheostomy without respiratory disability such as

*Home care instructions for tracheostomy care, postural drainage, and cardiopulmonary resuscitation are available in Wong DL: *Wong and Whaley's clinical manual of pediatric nursing*, ed 4, St Louis, 1996, Mosby.

recurrent laryngeal polyps) can usually be allowed to engage in most activities that are appropriate for the child's age. The child may play outdoors with a scarf or other protection to cover the tracheostomy stoma loosely. Both child and parents must be cautioned regarding play near any body of water, such as a swimming pool or stream, and informed about safety precautions in the bathtub. The child should not be exposed to noxious fumes (e.g., paint, varnish, hair spray) or talc (baby powder). Young children who may spill food near the stoma should wear a fabric bib (without plastic lining) or other device to prevent dribbled food or crumbs from being aspirated. The family should have a bag with routine and emergency supplies to take with the child at all times.

Procedures Related to Alternative Feeding Techniques

Some children are unable to take nourishment by mouth because of conditions such as anomalies of the throat, esophagus, or bowel; impaired swallowing capacity; severe debilitation; respiratory distress; or unconsciousness. These children are frequently fed by way of a tube inserted orally or nasally into the stomach (*orogastric* or *nasogastric gavage*) or duodenum/jejunum (*enteral gavage*) or by a tube inserted directly into the stomach (*gastrostomy*) or jejunum (*jejunostomy*). Such feedings may be intermittent or by continuous drip. At times the entire alimentary tract must be bypassed, using intravenous feeding (TPN). Because enteral feedings are used less often than gastric or IV feedings, the following discussion is limited to gastric gavage, gastrostomy, and TPN.

Feeding resistance is a problem that may result from any long-term feeding method that bypasses the mouth. During nonoral feedings, infants are given a pacifier; nonnutritive sucking has several advantages, such as increased weight gain and decreased crying. However, to prevent the possibility of aspiration, only pacifiers with a safe design may be used. Using improvised pacifiers made from bottle nipples is not a safe practice.

Nursing ALERT

When a child is concurrently receiving continuous-drip gastric or enteral feedings and parenteral (IV) therapy, the potential exists for inadvertent administration of the enteral formula through the circulatory system, especially when the parenteral solution is a fat emulsion, which looks milky. Safeguards to prevent this potentially serious error include (Garvin and Franck, 1989):

Using a separate, specifically designed enteral feeding pump mounted on a separate pole for continuous-feeding solutions.

Labeling all tubing for continuous enteral feeding with brightly colored tape or labels.

Using specifically designed continuous-feeding bags to contain the solutions instead of parenteral equipment, such as a burette.

GAVAGE FEEDING

Infants and children can be fed simply and safely by a tube passed into the stomach through either the nares or the mouth. The tube can be left in place or inserted and removed with each feeding. In older children it is usually less traumatic to tape the tube securely in place between feedings. When this alternative is used, the tube should be removed and replaced with a new tube according to hospital policy, specific orders, and the type of tube used. Meticulous handwashing is practiced during the procedure to prevent bacterial contamination of the feeding, especially during continuous-drip feedings.

Preparation

The equipment needed for gavage feeding includes:

- A suitable tube selected according to the size of the child and the viscosity of the solution being fed. Feeding tubes are available in silicone rubber, polyurethane, polyethylene, and polyvinylchloride. Polyurethane and silicone rubber tubes are smaller in diameter and more flexible than the others and are often referred to as small-bore tubes.
- A receptacle for the fluid; for small amounts a 10- to 30-ml syringe barrel or Asepto syringe is satisfactory; for larger amounts a 50-ml syringe with a catheter tip is more convenient.
- A syringe to aspirate stomach contents and/or to inject air-after the tube has been placed.
- Water or water-soluble lubricant to lubricate the tube; sterile water is used for infants.
- Paper or nonallergenic tape to mark the tube and to attach the tube to the infant's or child's cheek (and nose, if placed through the nares).
- A stethoscope to determine the correct placement in the stomach.
- The solution for feeding.

Not all feeding tubes are the same. Polyethylene and polyvinylchloride types lose their flexibility and need to be replaced frequently, usually every 3 to 4 days. The polyurethane and silicone rubber tubes are indwelling and remain flexible so that they can remain in place longer and afford more patient comfort. Use of these small-bore tubes for continuous feeding has greatly reduced the incidence of complications, such as pharyngitis, otitis media, and incompetence of the lower esophageal sphincter. Although the increased softness and flexibility of the tubes are advantages, they also cause disadvantages, such as difficult insertion (may require a stylet, or metal guide wire), collapse of the tube during aspiration of gastric contents to test for correct placement, dislodgment during forceful coughing, and unsuitability for thick feedings. Traditional methods for verifying placement are less reliable with the small-bore tubes.

Procedure

Infants will be easier to control if they are first wrapped in a mummy restraint (see Fig. 42-9). Even tiny infants with random movements can grasp and dislodge the tube. Premature infants do not ordinarily require restraint, but if they do, a small towel folded across the chest and secured beneath the shoulders is usually sufficient. Care must be taken so that breathing is not compromised.

Guidelines

NASOGASTRIC TUBE FEEDINGS IN CHILDREN

Place the child supine with head slightly hyperflexed or in a sniffing position (nose pointed toward ceiling).

Measure the tube for approximate length of insertion, and mark the point with a small piece of tape.

Insert the tube that has been lubricated with sterile water or water-soluble lubricant through either the mouth or one of the nares to the predetermined mark. Since most young infants are obligatory nose breathers, insertion through the mouth causes less distress and helps to stimulate sucking. In older infants and children the tube is passed through the nose and alternated between nostrils. An indwelling tube is almost always placed through the nose.

- When using the nose, slip the tube along the base of the nose and direct it straight back toward the occiput.
- When entering through the mouth, direct the tube toward the back of the throat (Fig. 42-35, *B*).
- If the child is able to swallow on command, synchronize passing the tube with swallowing.

Check the position of the tube by using *both* the following:

- Attach the syringe to the feeding tube and apply negative pressure. Aspiration of stomach contents indicates proper placement, but aspiration of respiratory secretions may be mistaken for stomach contents. However, absence of fluid is not necessarily evidence of improper placement. The stomach may be empty, the tube may not be in contact with stomach contents, or a small-bore flexible tube may collapse. Note the amount and character of any fluid aspirated and return the fluid to the stomach.
- With the syringe, inject a small amount of air (0.5 to 1 ml in premature or very small infants to 5 ml in larger children) into the tube while simultaneously listening with a stethoscope over the stomach area. Sounds of gurgling or growling will be heard if the tube is properly situated in the stomach, although it is possible to hear the air entering the stomach even when the tube is positioned above the gastroesophageal sphincter.
- Stabilize the tube by holding or taping it to the cheek, not to the forehead, because of possible damage to the nostril. To maintain correct placement, measure and record the amount of tubing extending from the nose or mouth to the distal port when the tube is first positioned. Recheck this measurement before each feeding.

Warm the formula to room temperature. Pour formula into the barrel of the syringe attached to the feeding tube. To start the flow, give a gentle push with the plunger, but then remove the plunger and allow the fluid to flow into the stomach by gravity. The rate of flow should not exceed 5 ml every 5 to 10 minutes in premature and very small infants and 10 ml/min in older infants and children to prevent nausea and regurgitation. The rate is determined by the diameter of the tubing and the height of the reservoir containing the feeding and is regulated by adjusting the height of the syringe. A usual feeding may take from 15 to 30 minutes to complete.

Flush the tube with sterile water (1 or 2 ml for small tubes to 5 to 15 ml or more for large ones) to clear it of formula.

Cap or clamp indwelling tubes to prevent loss of feeding. If the tube is to be removed, first pinch it firmly to prevent escape of fluid as the tube is withdrawn. Withdraw the tube quickly.

Position the child on the right side or abdomen for at least 1 hour in the same manner as after any infant feeding to minimize the possibility of regurgitation and aspiration. If the child's condition permits, bubble the youngster after the feeding.

Record the feeding, including the type and amount of residual, the type and amount of formula, and how it was tolerated. For most infant feedings, any amount of residual fluid aspirated from the stomach is refed to prevent electrolyte imbalance, and the amount is subtracted from the prescribed amount of feeding. For example, if the infant is to receive 30 ml and 10 ml is aspirated from the stomach before the feeding, the 10 ml of aspirated stomach contents is refed plus 20 ml of feeding. Another method can be used in children. If residual is more than one-fourth of the last feeding, return the aspirate and recheck in 30 to 60 minutes. When residual is less than one-fourth of the last feeding, give scheduled feeding. If high aspirates persist and the child is due for another feeding, notify the practitioner.

Whenever possible, the infant should be held during the procedure to associate the comfort of physical contact with the feeding. When this is not possible, gavage feeding is carried out with the infant or child on the back or toward the right side and the head and chest elevated. Feeding the child in a sitting position helps maintain the placement of the tube in the lowest position, thus increasing the likelihood of correct placement in the stomach.

The feeding tube can be passed through either the nose (nasogastric) or the mouth (orogastric). Since most young infants are obligatory nose breathers, insertion through the mouth causes less distress and helps to stimulate sucking. A tube passed through one of the nares in older infants and children is satisfactory once the tube is in place. An indwelling tube is almost always placed through the nose; the tube is alternated between nares with each insertion to minimize irritation, chance of infection, and possible breakdown of mucous membranes from pressure that occurs over time. The procedure for gavage feeding is described in the Guidelines box above.

Two standard methods of measuring tube length for insertion are (1) measuring from the nose to the bottom of the earlobe and then to the end of the xiphoid process or (2) measuring from the nose to the earlobe and then to a point midway between the xiphoid process and the umbilicus (Fig. 42-35, *A*). However, research on using these methods in infants and children has cast serious doubt on their accuracy (Weibley et al, 1987). Studies have shown that height as a predictor of gastric tube insertion distance may provide a more valid measurement method (Ellett et al, 1992). For very-low-birth-weight infants, daily weight can be used to predict insertion length (Table 42-4).

Unfortunately, "bedside" methods used to verify the placement of the tube have serious shortcomings (see the Guidelines box above). The only accurate method for testing tube placement is radiography, but this practice is not feasible be-

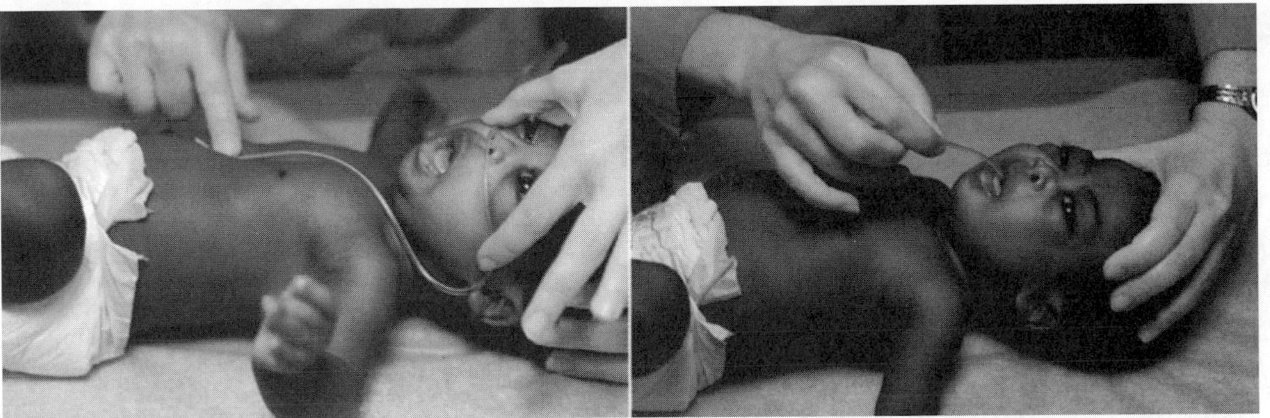

Fig. 42-35 Gavage feeding. **A,** Measuring tube for orogastric feeding from tip of nose to earlobe and to midpoint between end of xiphoid process and umbilicus. **B,** Inserting tube.

fore each feeding. One method that appears promising is pH testing of aspirated fluid, since respiratory, gastric, and intestinal fluids have different pH values (Metheny et al, 1989). Until pH is studied further, especially in children, nurses need to use the traditional methods with an awareness of their limitations. If doubt exists regarding correct placement, the practitioner should be consulted.

GASTROSTOMY FEEDING

Feeding by way of a gastrostomy tube is a variation of tube feeding that is often used for children in whom passage of a tube through the mouth, pharynx, esophagus, and cardiac sphincter of the stomach is contraindicated or impossible. It is also used to prevent the constant irritation of a gastric tube in children who require tube feeding over an extended period. Placement of a gastrostomy tube may be performed with the patient under general anesthesia or percutaneously using an endoscope with the patient sedated and under local anesthesia. The tube is inserted through the abdominal wall into the stomach about midway along the greater curvature and when surgically placed secured by a purse-string suture. The stomach is anchored to the peritoneum at the operative site. The tube used can be a Foley, wing-tip, or mushroom catheter.

Immediately after surgery the catheter is left open and attached to gravity drainage for 24 hours or more. Postoperative care of the wound site is directed toward prevention of infection and irritation. The area is cleansed at least daily or as often as needed to keep the area free of drainage. After healing takes place, meticulous care is needed to keep the area surrounding the tube clean and dry to prevent excoriation and infection. Daily applications of antibiotic ointment or other preparations may be prescribed to aid in healing and prevention of irritation. Care is exercised to prevent excessive pull on the catheter that might cause widening of the opening and subsequent leakage of highly irritating gastric juices.

For children on long-term gastrostomy feeding, a skin level device (MIC-KEY, Bard Button, Gastroport) offers several advantages. The small, flexible silicone device protrudes slightly from the abdomen, is cosmetically pleasing in appearance, affords increased comfort and mobility to the child, is easy to care for, and is fully immersible in water. The one-way valve at the proximal end minimizes reflux and eliminates the need for clamping. However, the button requires a well-established gastrostomy site and is more expensive than the conventional tube. In addition, the valve may become clogged. When functioning, the valve prevents air from escaping; therefore the child may require frequent bubbling. With some devices, during feedings the child must remain fairly still, since the tubing easily disconnects from the opening if the child moves. With other devices extension tubing can be securely attached to the opening (Fig. 42-36). The feeding is instilled at the other end of the tubing in a manner similar to that for a regular gastrostomy. The extension tubing may also have a separate medication port. Both the feeding and the medication ports have plugs attached. Some skin level devices require a special tube to allow one to decompress the stomach (to check residual or decompress air).

Positioning and feeding of water, formula, or pureed foods are carried out in the same manner and rate as in gavage feeding. After feedings the infant or child is positioned on the right side or in the Fowler position, and the tube may be clamped or left open and suspended between feedings, depending on the child's condition. A clamped tube allows more mobility but is appropriate only if the child can tolerate intermittent feedings without vomiting or prolonged backup of feeding into the tube. Sometimes a Y tube is used to allow for simultaneous decompression during feeding. If a Foley catheter is used as the

TABLE 42-4 Recommended minimum insertion lengths for orogastric tubes in very-low-birth-weight infants

	DAILY WEIGHT (G)			
	<750	750-999	1000-1249	1250-1499
Insertion length (cm)	13	15	16	17

From Gallaher KJ et al: Orogastric tube insertion length in very-low-birth-weight infants (< 1500 grams), *J Perinatol* 13(2):128-131, 1993.

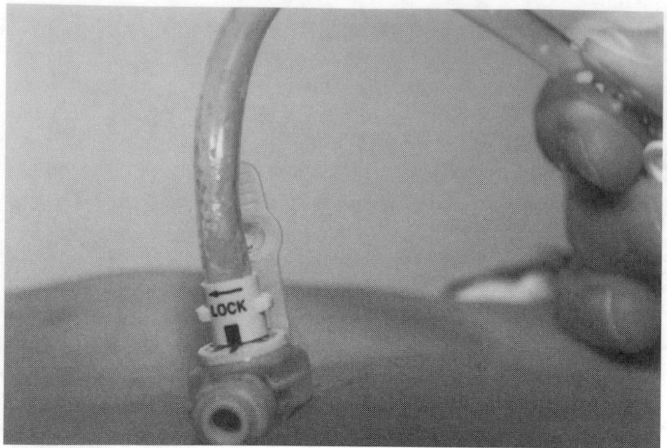

Fig. 42-36 Child with skin level gastrostomy device (MIC-KEY), which provides for secure attachment of extension tubing to gastrostomy opening.

gastrostomy tube, very slight tension is applied and the tube is securely taped to maintain the balloon at the gastrostomy opening and to prevent leakage of gastric contents and the tube's progression toward the pyloric sphincter, where it may occlude the stomach outlet. As a precaution, the length of the tube should be measured postoperatively and then remeasured each shift to be sure it has not slipped. A mark can be made above the skin level to further ensure its placement. When the gastrostomy tube is no longer needed, it is removed; the skin opening usually closes spontaneously by contracture.

TOTAL PARENTERAL NUTRITION (TPN)

Total parenteral nutrition (TPN), also known as IV alimentation or hyperalimentation, provides for the total nutritional needs of infants or children whose lives are threatened because feeding by way of the gastrointestinal tract is impossible, inadequate, or hazardous.

Hyperalimentation therapy involves IV infusion of highly concentrated solutions of protein, glucose, and other nutrients. The hyperalimentation solution is infused through conventional tubing with a special filter attached to remove particulate matter or microorganisms that may have contaminated the solution. The highly concentrated solutions require infusion into a vessel with sufficient volume and turbulence to allow for rapid dilution. The wide-diameter vessels selected are the superior vena cava and innominate or intrathoracic subclavian veins approached by way of the external or internal jugular veins. The highly irritating nature of concentrated glucose precludes the use of the small peripheral veins in most instances. However, dilute glucose-protein hydrolysates that are appropriate for infusing into peripheral veins are being used with increasing frequency. When peripheral veins are used, intralipid becomes the major calorie source. For long-term alimentation, VADs are usually used (see p. 1294).

The major nursing responsibilities are the same as for any IV therapy: control of sepsis, monitoring of the infusion rate, and continuous observations. The TPN solution must be prepared under rigid aseptic conditions best accomplished by specially trained technicians. The solution and tubing are changed and the infusion site redressed by specially trained nurses using meticulous aseptic precautions. In some institutions this may be a nursing responsibility. If so, the procedure is carried out according to hospital protocol.

The infusion is maintained at a slow, uniform rate by means of a constant infusion pump to ensure the proper concentrations of glucose and amino acids. Accurate calculation of the rate is required to deliver a measured amount in a given length of time. Since alterations in flow rate are relatively common, the drip should be checked frequently to ensure an even, continuous infusion. The hyperalimentation infusion rate should not be increased or decreased without the practitioner being made aware, since alterations can cause hyperglycemia or hypoglycemia.

General assessments, such as vital signs, intake and output measurements, and checking of results of laboratory tests, facilitate early detection of infection or fluid and electrolyte imbalance. Additional amounts of potassium and sodium chloride are often required in hyperalimentation; therefore observation for signs of potassium or sodium deficit or excess is part of nursing care. This is rarely a problem except in children with reduced renal function or metabolic defects. Hyperglycemia may occur during the first day or two, as the child adapts to the high-glucose load of the hyperalimentation solution. Infrequently insulin may be required to assist the body's adjustment to the hyperglycemia. When this occurs, nursing responsibilities include blood glucose testing. To prevent hypoglycemia at the time the hyperalimentation is disconnected, the rate of the infusion and the amount of insulin are decreased gradually.

In addition to children's physical needs, their developmental needs must also be considered during the often long-term use of TPN. Regular assessment of development should be performed to assess the child's progress, and appropriate interventions should be instituted to encourage expected milestones. Delays in the areas of gross motor and language skills are found most often; therefore special attention should be directed to these areas.

FAMILY TEACHING AND HOME CARE

When alternative feedings are needed for an extended period, the family may need to learn how to feed the child with a nasogastric, gastrostomy, or TPN feeding regimen. The same principles discussed earlier in this chapter for compliance, especially in terms of education (see p. 1264), and in Chapter 40 for discharge planning and home care are applied.* Because of the numerous skills the family must learn for home TPN, ample time must be planned for the family to learn and perform the procedures under supervision before assuming full responsibility for the child's care.

The family may be referred to community agencies that provide support and practical assistance. The Oley Foundation† is a nonprofit research and education organization that assists persons receiving enteral nutrition and home TPN.

*Home care instructions for gavage and gastrostomy feeding are available in Wong DL: *Wong and Whaley's clinical manual of pediatric nursing*, ed 4, St Louis, 1996, Mosby.

†214 Hun Memorial, A23, Albany Medical Center, Albany, NY 12208; (800) 776-OLEY.

Procedures Related to Elimination

ENEMA

The procedure for giving an enema to an infant or child does not differ essentially from that for an adult, except for the type and amount of fluid administered and the distance for inserting the tube into the rectum. Depending on the volume, use a syringe with rubber tubing, enema bottle, or enema bag (see the Guidelines box below).

Nursing ALERT

Proper insertion of the catheter tip, especially in infants, is essential to prevent rectal damage and perforation (see Fig. 32-7, *B*). If insertion of the enema tip causes discomfort, remove the tip and notify the practitioner.

An isotonic solution is used in children. Plain water is not used because, being hypotonic, it can cause rapid fluid shift and fluid overload. The Fleet enema (pediatric or adult sized) is not advised for children because of the harsh action of its ingredients (sodium biphosphate and sodium phosphate). Commercial enemas can be dangerous to patients with megacolon and to dehydrated or azotemic children. The osmotic effect of the Fleet enema may produce diarrhea, which can lead to metabolic acidosis. Other potential complications are extreme hyperphosphatemia, hypernatremia, and hypocalcemia, which may lead to neuromuscular irritability and coma (McCabe, Sibert, and Routledge, 1991). If prepared saline solution is not available, it can be made by adding 1 tsp table salt to 500 ml (1 pint) tap water.

Since infants and young children are unable to retain the solution after it is administered, the buttocks must be held together for a short time to retain the fluid. The enema is administered and expelled while the child is lying with the buttocks over the bedpan and with the head and back supported by pillows. Older children are ordinarily able to hold the solution if they understand what to do and if they are not expected to hold it for too long. The nurse should have the bedpan handy or, for the ambulatory child, ensure that the bathroom is readily available before beginning the procedure. An enema is an intrusive procedure and thus threatening to the preschool child; therefore a careful explanation is especially important to ease possible fear.

A preoperative bowel preparation solution given orally or through a nasogastric tube is increasingly being used instead of an enema. The polyethylene glycol–electrolyte lavage solution (Golytely) mechanically flushes the bowel without significant absorption, thereby preventing potential fluid and electrolyte imbalances (Konings, 1989).*

Guidelines

ADMINISTRATION OF ENEMAS TO CHILDREN

Age	Amount (ml)	Insertion Distance (cm/inches)
Infant	120-240	2.5 (1 inch)
2-4 years	240-360	5.0 (2 inches)
4-10 years	360-480	7.5 (3 inches)
11 years	480-720	10.0 (4 inches)

OSTOMIES

Children may require stomas for various health problems. The most frequent causes are necrotizing enterocolitis and imperforate anus in the infant (less often, Hirschsprung disease). In older children the most common causes are inflammatory bowel disease and ureterostomies for distal ureter or bladder defects.

Care and management of ostomies in the older child differ little from the care of ostomies in the adult patient. The major emphases in pediatric care are the preparation of the child for the procedure and teaching care of the ostomy to the child and family. The basic principles of preparation are the same as for any procedure (see p. 1253). Simple, straightforward language is most effective, together with the use of illustrations and a replica model (e.g., drawing a picture of a child with a stoma on the abdomen and explaining it as "another opening where bowel movements [or any other term the child uses] will come out"). At another time the nurse can draw a pouch over the opening to demonstrate how the contents are collected. Using a doll to demonstrate the process is an excellent teaching strategy, and special books are available.†

All children with ileostomies are fitted immediately after surgery with an appliance to protect the skin from the proteolytic enzymes in the liquid stool. Parents are usually given a choice of caring for the colostomy with or without an appliance. Pediatric appliances are available in a variety of sizes to ensure an adequate fit.‡

Ostomy equipment consists of a one- or two-piece system with a hypoallergenic skin barrier to maintain peristomal skin integrity. The pouch should be large enough to contain a moderate amount of stool and flatus but not so large as to overwhelm the infant or child. A backing helps minimize the risk of skin breakdown from moisture trapped between the skin and pouch. Small clips or rubber bands should be avoided to prevent choking in the young child. Granulation tissue may grow around an ostomy site. This moist, beefy red tissue is not a sign of infection. However, if it continues to grow, the excess moisture can cause irritation of the surrounding skin.

Protection of the peristomal skin is a major aspect of stoma care. Well-fitting appliances are important to prevent leakage of contents. Before the appliance is applied, the skin is prepared with a skin sealant that is allowed to dry. Then stoma paste is applied around the base of the stoma. The sealant and paste work together to prevent peristomal breakdown.

In infants with a colostomy left unpouched, skin care is similar to that of any diapered child. However, the peristomal skin is protected with a wafer barrier, such as a hydrocolloid dressing (e.g., Duoderm) or a barrier substance (e.g., zinc oxide ointment [Desitin], karaya products, or a mixture of the

*Home care instructions for giving an enema are available in Wong DL: *Wong and Whaley's clinical manual of pediatric nursing*, ed 4, St Louis, 1996, Mosby.

†*Chris Has an Ostomy* is available from United Ostomy Association, Inc., 36 Executive Park, Suite 120, Irvine, CA 92714-6744; (800) 826-0826.

‡Little Ones Ostomy Products, ConvaTec, CN 5254, Princeton, NJ 08543-5254; (800) 422-8811.

zinc oxide ointment and karaya powder). If the skin becomes inflamed, denuded, or infected, the care is similar to the interventions used for diaper dermatitis (see Chapter 50). A product that helps protect healthy skin, heal excoriated skin, and minimize pain associated with skin breakdown is Ilex Dermalytc Protective Barrier Ointment.* The ointment adheres to denuded weeping skin. It can be applied over topical antifungal and antibacterial agents if infection is present. If the infant is diapered, a coating of petrolatum is applied over the Ilex to prevent the gluteal creases and diaper from adhering to the ointment. When the area is cleaned, only the petrolatum is wiped off and reapplied. The Ilex is left intact to minimize trauma to the irritated skin. If Ilex is used under an appliance, an adhesive spray is applied over the ointment to help the appliance adhere.

With young children, protection of the pouch from being pulled off is also an important consideration. One-piece outfits prevent exploring hands from reaching the pouch, and the loose waist prevents any pressure on the appliance. Keeping the child occupied with toys during the pouch change is also helpful. As children mature, their participation in ostomy care is encouraged. Even preschoolers can assist by holding supplies, pulling paper backings from the appliance, and helping clean the stoma area. Toilet training for bladder control needs to begin at the appropriate time as for any other child.

*Available from MEDCON Products, Inc., 50 Brigham Hill Rd., Grafton, MA 01519; (800) 443-6332.

Older children and adolescents should eventually have total responsibility for ostomy care just as they would for usual bowel function. During adolescence, concerns for body image and the ostomy's impact on intimacy and sexuality emerge. The nurse should stress to teenagers that the presence of a stoma need not interfere with their activities. These youngsters can choose which ostomy equipment is best suited to their needs. Attractively designed and decorated pouch covers are well liked by teenagers.

FAMILY TEACHING AND HOME CARE

Since children with an ostomy are almost always discharged with a functioning colostomy, preparation of the family should begin as early as possible in the hospital. The family is instructed in the application of the device (if used), care of the skin, and instructions regarding appropriate action in case skin problems develop. Early evidence of skin breakdown or stomal complications, such as ribbonlike stools, excessive diarrhea, bleeding, prolapse, or failure to pass flatus or stool, is called to the attention of the physician, the nurse, or the stoma specialist. The same principles are applied as discussed earlier in this chapter for compliance, especially in terms of education (see p. 1264) and in Chapter 41 for discharge planning and home care.*

*Home care instructions on caring for a colostomy are available in Wong DL: *Wong and Whaley's clinical manual of pediatric nursing*, ed 4, St Louis, 1996, Mosby.

Key Points

- Informed consent is valid when the person is capable of giving consent (is over the age of majority and is competent), is supplied with information needed to make an intelligent decision, and acts voluntarily when exercising freedom of choice.
- Informed consent is needed for major surgery, minor surgery, and diagnostic tests and medical treatments with an element of risk.
- The major principles in psychologic preparation of the child for procedures are to establish trust, provide support, and give an explanation in easy-to-understand terms.
- In the performance of a procedure the nurse should expect success, involve the child when possible in the procedure, provide distraction, and allow for expression of feelings.
- In giving postprocedural support, the nurse should encourage the child to express feelings and praise the youngster for completion of the procedure.
- Assessment of compliance entails measuring factors that affect compliance through self-reporting, direct observation, monitoring appointments and therapeutic response, taking pill counts, and performing chemical assay.
- Compliance strategies may be classified as organizational, educational, and behavioral.
- Knowledge of the sick child's eating habits and favorite foods can help in maintaining adequate nutrition.
- Control of fever may be accomplished by pharmacologic means (administration of antipyretics); hyperthermia is controlled by environmental means (minimum clothing, increased air circulation, or cool compresses).
- Infection control may be based on one of three basic systems: category-specific isolation precautions, disease-specific isolation precautions, or universal precautions. Only the system of universal precautions, especially body substance isolation, provides protection when the infected person is undiagnosed.
- Ensuring safety in the hospital setting is a major concern and can be achieved through environmental measures, limit-setting, and safe transportation.
- Common types of physical restraints for children are jacket, mummy, arm and leg, and elbow restraints.
- Factors that affect drug dosage determination are growth and maturation, difficulty in evaluating drug response, and body surface area.
- The preferred sites for intramuscular injection in children are the vastus lateralis and ventrogluteal areas.
- Intermittent venous access is accomplished by intermittent infusion devices, central venous catheters, peripherally inserted catheters, or implanted ports.
- Nursing assessment of fluid and electrolyte disturbances entails observation of general appearance, vital signs, and intake and output measurement.

- Oxygen can be administered by plastic hood, mask, nasal cannula, incubator, or oxygen tent.
- Tracheostomy suctioning involves premeasured insertion of the catheter, application of suction for seconds when withdrawing the catheter, and supplemental oxygen before and after suctioning.
- Alternative forms of feeding include gavage feeding, gastrostomy feeding, and total parenteral nutrition.
- In the care of children with ostomies, nurses play an important role in family support and instruction in care of the stoma site.

References

Abd-El-Maeboud K et al: Rectal suppository: commonsense and mode of insertion, *Lancet* 338(8770):798-800, 1991.

Ackerman MH: The effect of saline lavage prior to suctioning, *Am J Crit Care* 2(4):326-330, 1993.

Acute Pain Management Guideline Panel: *Acute pain management: operative or medical procedures and trauma: clinical practice guideline,* AHCPR Pub No 92-0032, Rockville, Md, 1992, Agency for Health Care Policy and Research, Public Health Service, US Department of Health and Human Services.

Alderson SH, Warren RH: Pediatric aerosol therapy guidelines, *Clin Pediatr* 23(10):553-557, 1984.

American Academy of Pediatrics, Committee on Drugs: Guidelines for monitoring and management of pediatric patients during and after sedation for diagnostic and therapeutic procedures, *Pediatrics* 86(6):1110-1115, 1992.

Arditi M, Killner M: Coma following use of rubbing alcohol for fever control, *Am J Dis Child* 141(3):237-238, 1987.

Bates T, Broome M: Preparation of children for hospitalization and surgery: a review of the literature, *J Pediatr Nurs* 1(4):230-234, 1986.

Beecroft P, Redick S: Intramuscular injection practices of pediatric nurses: site selection, *Nurse Educ* 15(4):23-28, 1990.

Brent NJ: The pediatric patient and consent for treatment, *Home Healthcare Nurse* 9(5):10-12, 1991.

Broome ME: Preparation of children for painful procedures, *Pediatr Nurs* 16(6):537-541, 1990.

Brosnan KM et al: Contamination stopcock, *Am J Nurs* 88(3):320-323, 1988.

Brown JM: Peripherally inserted central catheters—use in home care, *J Intravenous Nurs* 12(3):144-150, 1989.

Bruce JL, Grove SK: Fever: pathology and treatment, *Crit Care Nurs* 12(1):40-55, 1992.

Bryant RA, editor: *Acute and chronic wounds: nursing management,* St Louis, 1992, Mosby.

Camp-Sorrell D: Advanced central venous access: selection, catheters, devices, and nursing management, *J Intravenous Nurs* 13(6):361-370, 1990.

Chandra NC, Hazinski MF, editors: *Textbook of basic life support for healthcare providers,* Dallas, 1994, American Heart Association.

Courtney SE et al: Capillary blood gases in the neonate: a reassessment and review of the literature, *Am J Dis Child* 144:168-172, 1990.

Cushing M: Demystifying informed consent, *Am J Nurs* 17-19, 1991.

Dyson A, Bogod D: Minimizing bruising in the antecubital fossa after venipuncture, *Br Med J* 294(6588):1659, 1987.

Ellett M et al: Predicting the distance for gavage tube placement in children using regression on height, *Pediatr Nurs* 18(2):119-121, 127, 1992.

Ellis R: Once more into the void, *Contemp Pediatr* 6(8):164, 1989.

Faber MM: A review of efforts to protect children from injury in crashes, *Fam Community Health* 4(3):25-41, 1986.

Fox MD: Measurement of urine output volume: accuracy of diaper weights in neonatal environments, *Neonatal Network* 11(3):11-18, 1992.

Flemmer L, Chan JSL: A pediatric protocol for management of extravasation injuries, *Pediatr Nurs* 19(4):355-368, 1993.

Funk MJ, Mullins LL, Olson RA: Teaching children to swallow pills: a case study, *Child Health Care* 13(1):20-23, 1984.

Garvin G, Franck L: Preventing delivery of enteral formula via parenteral route, *Pediatr Nurs* 15(1):17-18, 1989.

Gribetz B, Cronley S: Underdosing of acetaminophen by parents, *Pediatrics* 80(5):630-633, 1987.

Hagelgans NA: Pediatric skin care issues for the home care nurse, *Pediatr Nurs* 19(5):499-507, 1993.

Hagler DA, Traver GA: Endotracheal saline and suction catheters: sources of lower airway contamination, *Am J Crit Care* 3(6):444-447, 1994.

Hall PA et al: Parents in the recovery room: survey of parental and staff attitudes, *Br Med J* 310(6973):163-164, 1995.

Heiney SP: Helping children through painful procedures, *Am J Nurs* 20-24, 1991.

Hicks JF et al: Optimum needle length for diphtheria-inoculation of infants, *Pediatrics* 84(1):136 137, 1989.

Hogue EE: Informed consent: implications for critical care nurses, *Pediatr Nurs* 14(4):315-316, 1988.

Holtzclaw BJ: Control of febrile shivering during amphotericin B therapy, *Oncol Nurs Forum* 17(4):521-524, 1990.

Janik JP, Wayne ER, Janik JS: Securing central lines in rambunctious toddlers, *Pediatrics* 96(3):523-524, 1995.

Johannsen L: Adolescent abortion and mandated parental involvement, *Pediatr Nurs* 21(1):82-84, 1995.

Johnston CC, Stevens B, Arbess G: The effect of the sight of blood and use of decorative adhesive bandages on pain intensity ratings by preschool children, *J Pediatr Nurs* 8(3):147-151, 1993.

Joyner M: Hair care in the black patient, *J Pediatr Health Care* 2(6):281-287, 1988.

Kinmouth AL, Fulton Y, Campbell MJ: Management of feverish children at home, *Br Med J* 305(6862):1134-1136, 1992.

Kleiber C, Krutzfield N, Rose EF: Acute histologic changes in tracheobronchial tree associated with different suction catheter insertion techniques, *Heart Lung* 17:10-14, 1988.

Konings K: Preop use of Golytely in pediatrics, *Pediatr Nurs* 15(5):473-474, 1989.

Krouskop TA et al: Effectiveness of mattress overlays in reducing interface pressures during recumbency, *J Rehabil Res Dev* 22(3):7-10, 1985.

Krueger H, Osborn L: Effects of hygiene among the uncircumcised, *J Fam Pract* 22(4):353-355, 1986.

LaRosa-Nash PA et al: Implementing a parent-present induction program, *AORN J* 61(3):526-531, 1995.

Lehmann M et al: Upright or lying down: is one better for doing a lumbar puncture (LP)? *Am J Dis Child* 144:427, 1990.

Lohr J, Donowitz L, Dudley S: Bacterial contamination rates in voided urine collections in girls, *J Pediatr* 114(1):91-93, 1989.

Marcoux C, Fisher S, Wong D: Central venous access devices in children, *Pediatric Nurs* 16(2) 123-133, 1990.

McCabe M, Sibert JR, Routledge PA: Phosphate enemas in childhood: cause for concern, *Br Med J* 302(6784):1074, 1991.

McMullen A et al: Heparinized saline or normal saline: as a flush solution in intermittent intravenous lines in infants and children, *MCN Am J Matern Child Nurs* 18:78-85, 1993.

Meares C: PICC and MLC lines: options worth exploring, *Nursing 92* 22(10):52-55, 1992.

Metheny N et al: Effectiveness of pH measurements in predicting feeding tube placement, *Nurs Res* 38(5):280-285, 1989.

Musser V: How do you use shallow-suction technique in children? *Am J Nurs* 92(5):79-83, 1992.

Newman J: Evaluation of sponging to reduce body temperature in febrile children, *Can Med Assoc J* 132:641-642, 1985.

Nix KS: *Obtaining informed consent.* In Smith DP et al: editors: *Comprehensive child and family nursing skills,* St Louis, 1991, Mosby.

Olsen RJ et al: Examination gloves as barriers to hand contamination in clinical practice, *JAMA* 270(3):350-353, 1993.

Orenstein S et al: The Santmyer swallow: a new and useful infant reflex, *Lancet* 1(8581):345-346, 1988.

Pidgeon V: Compliance with chronic illness regimens: school-aged children and adolescents, *J Pediatr Nurs* 4(1):36-47, 1989.

Pollack CV, Pollack ES, Andrew ME: Suprapubic bladder aspiration versus urethral catheterization in ill infants: success, efficiency, and complication rates, *Ann Emerg Med* 23(2):225-230, 1994.

Robertson J: Intermittent intravenous therapy: a comparison of two flushing solutions, *Contemporary Nurse* 3(4):174-179, 1994.

Rosenstock IM: Enhancing patient compliance with health recommendations, *J Pediatr Health Care* 2(2):67-72, 1988.

Rudy C: A drop or a dropper: the risk of overdose, *J Pediatr Health Care,* 6(1):40, 1992.

Saez-Llorens X et al: Bacterial contamination rates for nonclean catch and clean catch midstream urine collections in uncircumcised boys, *J Pediatr* 114(1):93-95, 1989.

Schreiner MS: Preoperative and postoperative fasting in children, *Pediatr Clin North Am* 41(1):111-120, 1994.

Schreiner V: Don't discard this specimen, *Nursing 87* 17(10):5, 1987.

Shorten DR, Byrne PJ, Jones RL: Infant responses to saline instillations and endotracheal suctioning, *J Obstet Gynecol Neonatal Nurs* 20(6):464-469, 1991.

Simon RE: Ibuprofen suspension: pediatric antipyretic, *Pediatr Nurs* 22(2):118-120, 1996.

Stoller KP, Losey R: Inadvertent intra-arterial injection of penicillin: an unseen danger, *Pediatrics* 75(4)785-786, 1985.

Van R et al: The effect of diaper type and overclothing on fecal contamination in day-care centers, *JAMA* 265(14):1840-1844, 1991.

Vessey J, Caserza L, Bogetz M: In my opinion . . . another Pandora's box? Parental participation in anesthetic induction, *Child Health Care* 19(2):116-118, 1990.

Weibley TT and others: Gavage tube insertion in the premature infant, *MCN Am J Matern Child Nurs* 12:24-27, 1987.

Wlody GS: Malignant hyperthermia, *Crit Care Nurs Clin North Am* 3(1):129-134, 1991.

Wong DL, Baker CM: Pain in children: comparison of assessment scales, *Pediatr Nurs* 14(1):9-17, 1988.

Wong DL et al: Diapering choices: a critical review of the issues, *Pediatr Nurs* 18(1):41-54, 1992.

Bibliography

Informed Consent

Allen A: Informed consent: how far must it go? *J Post Anesth Nurs* 5(6):425-426, 1990.

Broome ME, Stieglitz KA: The consent process and children, *Res Nurs Health* 15(2):147-152, 1992.

Erlen JA: The child's choice: an essential component in treatment decisions, *Child Health Care* 15(3):156-160, 1987.

Hogue EE: Consent for minors, *Pediatr Nurs* 15(4):404, 1989.

Horton R: The context of consent, *Lancet* 344(8917):211-212, 1994.

Leikin S: A proposal concerning decisions to forgo life-sustaining treatment for young people, *J Pediatr* 115(1):17-22, 1989.

Rhodes AM: Consent for medical treatment, *MCN Am J Matern Child Nurs* 12(2):133, 1987a.

Rhodes AM: Obtaining consent to treat minors, *MCN Am J Matern Child Nurs* 12(3):209, 1987b.

Rhodes AM: When parents refuse to consent, *MCN Am J Matern Child Nurs* 12(4):289, 1987c.

Rhodes AM: The rights of minors, *MCN Am J Matern Child Nurs* 13(4):281, 1988.

Rhodes AM: A minor's refusal of treatment, *MCN Am J Matern Child Nurs* 15(4):261, 1990.

Ruccione K et al: Informed consent for treatment of childhood cancer: factors affecting parents' decision making, *J Pediatr Oncol Nurs* 8(3):112-121, 1991.

Preparation for Procedures/Use of Play

Azarnoff P: Teaching materials for pediatric health professionals, *J Pediatr Health Care* 4(6):282-289, 1990.

Bauchner H, Vinci R, Waring C: Pediatric procedures: do parents want to watch? *Pediatrics* 84(5):907-909, 1989.

Cook BA et al: Sedation of children for technical procedures: current standard of practice, *Clin Pediatr* 31(3):137-142, 1992.

Cote CJ: Sedation for the pediatric patient: a review, *Pediatr Clin North Am* 41(1):31-58, 1994.

Emergency Nurses Association Position Statement: *Family presence at the bedside during invasive procedures and/or resuscitation,* Park Ridge, Ill, 1994, Emergency Nurses Association.

Goldberger J, Wolfer J: Helping children cope with health-care procedures, *Contemp Pediatr* 7(3): 141-162, 1990.

LeVieux-Anglin L et al: Incorporating play interventions into nursing care, *Pediatr Nurs* 19(5):459-463, 1993.

Rollins J, Brantly D: *Preparing the child for procedures.* In Smith DP et al: editors: *Comprehensive child and family nursing skills,* St Louis, 1991, Mosby.

Zeltzer LK, Jay SM, Fisher DM: The management of pain associated with pediatric procedures, *Pediatr Clin North Am* 36(4):941-964, 1989.

Surgical Procedures

Ashby D: Malignant hyperthermia: a potential crisis in the postanesthesia care unit, *J Post Anesth Nurs* 5(4):279-281, 1990.

Avigne G, Phillips TL: Pediatric preoperative tours, *AORN J* 53(6):1458-1465, 1991.

Bender LH, Weaver K, Edwards K: Postoperative patient-controlled analgesia in children, *Pediatr Nurs* 16(6):549-554, 1990.

Cehaich K: Preparing the pediatric patient for surgery, *Plast Surg Nurs* 14(2):105-107, 1994.

Cote CJ: NPO after midnight for children—a reappraisal, *Anesthesiology* 72(4):589-592, 1990.

Davis JL et al: Perioperative care of the pediatric trauma patient, *AORN J* 60(4):599, 561, 563-565, 1994.

Ellerton ML: Preparing kids and parents for surgery, *Can Nurs* 10(10):25-27, 1994.

Hannallah, RS: Who benefits when parents are present during anaesthesia induction in their children? *Can J Anaesth 41*(4):271-275, 1994.

Heffline MS: A comparative study of pharmacological versus nursing interventions in the treatment of postanesthesia shivering, *J Post Anesth Nurs* 6(5):311-320, 1991.

Jones JG: Memory of intraoperative events, *Br Med J* 309(6960):967-968, 1994.

Kennedy CM, Riddle II: The influence of the timing of preparation on the anxiety of preschool children experiencing surgery, *Matern Child Nurs J* 18(2):117-132, 1989.

McIlvaine WB: Perioperative pain management in children: a review. *J Pain Symptom Manage* 4(4):215-229, 1989.

Meyer-Pahoulis E: Pediatric postanesthesia care, *Plast Surg Nurs* 14(2):92-98, 1994.

Moyer S, Howe C: Pediatric pain intervention in the PACU, *Crit Care Nurs Clin North Am* 3(1):49-57, 1991.

Noonan AT et al: Family-centered nursing in the postanesthesia care unit: the evaluation of practice, *J Post Anesth Nurs* 6(1):13-16, 1991.

Ogilvie L: Hospitalization of children for surgery: the parents' view, *Child Health Care* 19(1):49-56, 1990.

Pierce LA: Safety and care of children during surgery, *Plast Surg Nurs* 14(2):99-100, 1994.

Rivera WB: Practical points in the assessment and management of post-operative pediatric pain, *J Post Anesth Nurs* 6(1):40-42, 1991.

Tobias JD et al: Postoperative analgesia: use of intrathecal morphine in children, *Clin Pediatr* 29:44-48, 1990.

Vessey JA et al: Parental upset associated with participation in induction of anaesthesia in children, *Can J Anaesth 41*(4):276-280, 1994.

Compliance

Burckhardt CS: Ethical issues in compliance, *Top Clin Nurs* 7(4):9-16, 1986.

Clark SR: Compliance and health behaviors, *Top Clin Nurs* 7(4):39-46, 1986.

Connaway N: My patient won't follow the medical plan treatment. What should I do to protect myself—legally? . . . home health care, *Home Healthcare Nurse* 3(4):6-8, 1985.

DiFlorio IA, Duncan PA: Design for successful patient teaching, *MCN Am J Matern Child Nurs* 11:246-249, 1986.

Friedman IM, Litt IF: Promoting adolescents' compliance with therapeutic regimens, *Pediatr Clin North Am* 33(4):955-973, 1986.

Gibson L: Patient education: effects of two teaching methods upon parental retention of infant feeding practices, *Pediatr Nurs* 21(1):78-80, 1995.

Kelloway JS et al: Comparison of patients' compliance with prescribed oral and inhaled asthma medications, *Arch Intern Med* 154:1349-1352, 1994.

Littlefield LC: Therapeutic drug monitoring in ambulatory pediatrics, *J Pediatr Health Care* 1(2):113-116, 1987.

McCord MA: Compliance: self-care or compromise? *Top Clin Nurs* 7(4):1-8, 1986.

McHatton M: A theory for timely teaching, *Am J Nurs* 85(7):798-800, 1985.

Miller A: When is the time ripe for teaching? *Am J Nurs* 85(7):801-804, 1985.

Padrick KP: Compliance: myths and motivators, *Top Clin Nurs* 7(4):17-22, 1986.

Sallis JF: Improving adherence to pediatric therapeutic regimens, *Pediatr Nurs* 11(2):118-120, 1985.

Spicher CM, Yund C: Effects of preadmission preparation on compliance with home care instructions, *J Pediatr Nurs* 4(4):255-262, 1989.

Stang H: Compliance: get parents in on the diagnosis, *Contemp Pediatr* 7(3):170, 1990.

Wright EC: A lesson in noncompliance, *Lancet* 343(8908):27, 1994.

General Hygiene and Care/Fever

American College of Emergency Physicians: Clinical policy for the initial approach to children under the age of 2 years presenting with fever, *Ann Emerg Med* 22:628-637, 1993.

Baraff LJ et al: Practice guideline for the management of infants and children 0 to 36 months of age with fever without source, *Ann Emerg Med* 22(7):108-120, 1993.

Barnett RI, Ablarde JA: Skin vascular reaction to standard patient positioning on a hospital mattress, *Adv Wound Care* 7(1):58-65, 1994.

Bedi A: A tool to fill the gap: developing a wound risk assessment chart for children, *Prof Nurs* 9(2), 1993.

Gildea JH: When fever becomes an enemy, *Pediatr Nurs* 18(2):165-167, 1992.

Gould KE et al: Therapeutic beds: the Trojan horses of the 1990s? *Lancet* 433(8914):65-66, 1994.

Herzog LW, Coyne LJ: What is fever? Normal temperature in infants less than 3 months old, *Clin Pediatr* 32(4):142-146, 1993.

Kleiman MB: Feverish children, frightened parents, *Contemp Pediatr* 6(3):161-167, 1989.

Marchand AC, Lidowski H: Reassessment of the use of genuine sheep-skin for pressure ulcer prevention and treatment, *Decubitus* 6(1):44-47, 1993.

Reeves-Swift R: Rational management of a child's acute fever, *MCN Am J Matern Child Nurs* 15(2):82-85, 1990.

Singer L: When a sick child won't—or can't—eat, *Contemp Pediatr* 7(12):60-76, 1990.

Thurgood G: Nurse maintenance of oral hygiene, *Br J Nurs* 3(7):332-353, 1994.

Safety/Collection of Specimens/Infection Control

Amir J et al: The reliability of midstream urine culture from circumcised male infants, *Am J Dis Child* 147.969-970, 1993.

Blain-Lewis N: Comparative studies of bruising and healing after heel-stick, *Neonatal Intensive Care* 5(5):18-21, 1992.

Brantly DK: *Applying and maintaining restraints and restraining for procedures.* In Smith DP et al, editors: *Comprehensive child and family nursing skills,* St Louis, 1991, Mosby.

Dennehy P: Heel blood sampling on older infants, *Neonatal Intensive Care* 5(5):21-23, 1992.

Fleischman AR: Clinical considerations for infant heel blood sampling, *Neonatal Intensive Care* 5(3):62-68, 1992.

Gleeson RM: Use of non-latex gloves for children with latex allergies, *J Pediatr Nurs* 10(1):64-65, 1995.

Jackson MM: Infection prevention and control for HIV and other infectious agents in obstetric, gynecologic and neonatal settings, *Clin Issues Perinat Women's Health Nurs* 1(1):115-121, 1990.

Jackson MM: *Infection prevention and control.* In Swearingen PL, Keen JH, editors: *Manual of critical care nursing,* ed 3, St Louis, 1995, Mosby.

Korniewicz D, Kirwin M, Larson E: Do your gloves fit the task? *Am J Nurs* 91(6):38-40, 1991.

Larson E: Handwashing: it's essential—even when you use gloves, *Am J Nurs* 89(7):934-939, 1989.

Preusser BA et al: Quantifying the minimum discard sample required for accurate arterial blood gases, *Nurs Res* 38:276-279, 1989.

Schmitt BD: Protecting your child from infections, *Contemp Pediatr* 12(9):83-84, 1995.

Selekman J, Snyder B: Nursing perceptions of using physical restraints on hospitalized children, *Pediatr Nurs* 21(5):460-464, 1995.

Suri S: Simplifying urine collection from infants and children without losing accuracy, *MCN Am J Matern Child Nurs* 13(12):438-441, 1988.

Vernon S et al: Urine collection on sanitary towels, *Lancet* 344:612, 1994.

Weatherly KS, Young S, Andresky J: Needle stick injury in pediatric hospitals, *Pediatr Nurs* 17(1):95-99, 1991.

Whitehall J, Shvartzman P, Miller MA: A novel method for isolating and quantifying urine pathogens collected from gel-based diapers, *J Fam Pract* 40(5):476-479, 1995.

Administration of Medication

Beecroft PC, Redick S: Possible complications of intramuscular injections on the pediatric unit, *Pediatr Nurs* 15(4):333-376, 1989.

Beyea SC, Nicoll LH: Back to basics: administering IM injections the right way, *Am J Nurs* 96(1):34-35, 1996.

Bosserman G et al: Multidisciplinary management of vascular access devices, *Oncol Nurs Forum* 17(6):879-886, 1990.

Botash SA: Syringe caps: an aspiration hazard, *Pediatrics* 90(1):92-93, 1992.

Buckley T, Dudley SM, Donowitz LG: Defining unnecessary disinfection procedures for single-dose and multiple-dose vials, *Am J Crit Care* 3(6):448-451, 1994.

Dennis-Smithart R: Taking medication: the last straw, *Contemp Pediatr* 10(3):5, 1993.

Gahart BL: *Intravenous medications: a handbook for nurses and other allied health personnel,* ed 10, St Louis, 1994, Mosby.

Glassman SK, Measel CP: A makeshift mini-bottle: accurate small volume fluid or oral medication administration to infants, *Neonatal Network* 7(4):29-31, 1989.

Halperin D et al: Topical skin anesthesia for venous, subcutaneous drug reservoir and lumbar puncture in children, *Pediatrics* 84:281-284, 1989.

Intramuscular injections: a guide to sites and techniques, Philadelphia, 1985, Wyeth Laboratories.

Losek JD, Gyuro J: Pediatric intramuscular injections: do you know the procedure and complications? *Pediatr Emerg Care* 8(2):79-81, 1992.

Penatzer M et al: Common pediatric IV meds at a glance, *Pediatr Nurs* 14(1):56-58, 1988.

Raju TN et al: Medication errors in neonatal and paediatric intensive-care units, *Lancet* 2(8659):374-376, 1989.

Smith SE: Eyedrop instillation for reluctant children, *Br J Opthalmol* 75:480-481, 1991.

Thigpen J: Minimizing medication errors, *Neonatal Network* 14(2):85-86, 1995.

Wink DM: Giving infants and children drugs: precision + caution = safety. *MCN Am J Matern Child Nurs* 16(6):317-321, 1991.

Parenteral Therapy and Fluid Balance

Banta C: Hyaluronidase, *Neonatal Network* 11(6):103-105, 1992.

Baranowski L: Central venous access devices: current technologies, uses, and management strategies, *J Intravenous Nurs* 16(3):167-194, 1993.

Danek GD, Noris EM: Pediatric IV catheters: efficacy of saline flush, *Pediatr Nurs* 18(2):111-113, 1992.

Dick M et al: How to boost the odds of a painless IV start, *Am J Nurs* 92(6):49-50, 1992.

Gyr P et al: Double blind comparison of heparin and saline flush solutions in maintenance of peripheral infusion devices, *Pediatr Nurs* 21(4):383-389,366, 1995.

Hanrahan KS, Kleiber C, Fagan C: Evaluation of saline for IV locks in children, *Pediatr Nurs* 20(6):549-552, 1994.

Hastings-Tolsma MT et al: Effect of warm and cold applications on the resolution of IV infiltrations, *Res Nurs Health* 16(3):171-178, 1993.

Hodler C, Alexander J: A new and improved guide to IV therapy: protocols for intravenous therapy, *Am J Nurs* 90(2):43-47, 1990.

Kelly C et al: A change in flushing protocols of central venous catheters, *Oncol Nurs Forum* 19(4):599-605, 1992.

Kleiber C et al: Heparin vs. saline for peripheral IV locks in children, *Pediatr Nurs* 19:405-409, 1993.

Marcoux C, Fisher S, Wong D: Central venous access devices in children, *Pediatr Nurs* 16(2):123-133, 1991.

Moss JR, Craft MJ: Accurate assessment of infant emesis volume, *Pediatr Nurs* 16(5):455-457, 1990.

O'Brien R: Starting intravenous lines in children, *J Emerg Nurs* 17(4):225-231, 1991.

Orlowski JP: Emergency alternatives to intravenous access, *Pediatr Clin North Am* 41(6):1183-1199, 1994.

Pettit J, Hughes K: Intravenous extravasation: mechanisms, management, and prevention, *J Perinat Neonatal Nurs* 6(4):69-79, 1993.

Ryder MA: Peripherally inserted central venous catheters, *Nurs Clin North Am* 28(4):937-971, 1993.

Tidwell B Jr, Parks BR Jr: Intraosseous infusions, *Pediatr Nurs* 17(1):56-57, 1991.

Tietjen SD: Starting an infant's IV, *Am J Nurs* 90:44-47, 1990.

Wilson D: Neonatal IVs: practical tips, *Neonatal Nurs* 11(2):49-53, 1992.

Zimerman E: The Landry vein light: increasing venipuncture success rates, *J Pediatr Nurs* 6(1):64-66, 1991.

Respiratory Therapy

AARC Clinical Practice Guideline: Endotracheal suctioning of mechanically ventilated adults and children with artificial airways, *Respir Care* 38(5):500-504, 1993.

Brown KA, Sauve RS: Evaluation of a caregiver education program: home oxygen therapy for infants, *J Obstet Gynecol Neonatal Nurs* 23(5):429-435, 1994.

Comer DM: Pulse oximetry: implications for practice, *J Obstet Gynecol Neonatal Nurs* 21(1):35-41, 1992.

Fitton CM: Nursing management of the child with a tracheotomy, *Pediatr Clin North Am* 41(3):513-523, 1994.

Giganti AW: Lifesaving tubes, lifetime scars? *MCN Am J Matern Child Nurs* 20:192-197, 1995.

Hodge D: Endotracheal suctioning and the infant: a nursing care protocol to decrease complications, *Neonatal Network* 9(5):7-15, 1991.

Noll ML, Hix C, Scott G: Closed tracheal suction systems: effectiveness and nursing complications, *AACN Clin Issues Crit Care Nurs* 1(2):327-328, 1990.

Ronczy NM, Beddome M: Preparing the family for home tracheotomy care, *AACN Clin Issues Crit Care Nurs* 1(2):367-377, 1990.

Runton N: Suctioning artificial airways in children: appropriate technique, *Pediatr Nurs* 18(2):115-118, 1992.

Russell R, Helms P: Comparative accuracy of pulse oximetry and transcutaneous oxygen in assessing arterial saturation in pediatric intensive care, *Neonatal Intensive Care* 5(1):38-40, 1992.

Salyer J, Lewis D: Pulse oximetry: application in the pediatric and neonatal critical care unit, *AACN Clin Issues Crit Care Nurs* 1(2):339-347, 1990.

Sobel DB: Burning of a neonate due to a pulse oximeter: arterial saturation monitoring, *Pediatrics* 89(1):154-155, 1992.

Stoneham MD, Saville GM, Wilson IH: Knowledge about pulse oximetry among medical and nursing staff, *Lancet* 334(8933):1339-1342, 1994.

Tolles CL, Stone KS: National survey of neonatal endotracheal suctioning practices, *Neonatal Network* 9(2):7-14, 1990.

Turner BS: Maintaining the artificial airway: current concepts, *Pediatr Nurs* 16(5):487-493, 1990.

Withiam-Wilson MJ: Accidental breathing circuit disconnections in the neonatal or pediatric critical care setting, *Pediatr Nurs* 17(3):283-286, 293, 1991.

Alternative Feeding Techniques/Elimination

Boarini JH: Principles of stoma care for infants, *J Enterostom Ther* 16(1):21-25, 1989.

Bockus S: Troubleshooting your tube feedings, *Am J Nurs* 91(5):24-28, 1991.

Cady C, Yoshioka R: Using a learning contract to successfully discharge an infant on home total parenteral nutrition, *Pediatr Nurs* 17(1):67-71, 74, 1991.

Embon CM: Ostomy care for the infant with necrotizing enterocolitis: nursing considerations, *J Perinat Neonat Nurs* 4(3):56-63, 1990.

Ferraro AR, Huddleston KC: Safe administration of small-volume enteral feedings: an alternative to intravenous pumps, *J Pediatr Nurs* 6(5):352-354, 1991.

Garvin G: Caring for children with ostomies, *Nurs Clin North Am* 29(4):645-655, 1994.

Metheny N: Measures to test placement of nasogastrointestinal feeding tubes: a review, *Nurs Res* 37(6):324-329 1988.

Metheny N et al: Visual characteristics of aspirates from feeding tubes as a method for predicting tube location, *Nurs Res* 43(5):282-287, 1994.

Steele NF: The button: replacement gastrostomy device, *J Pediatr Nurs* 6(6):421-424, 1991.

Van Niel J: What's wrong with this peristomal skin? *Am J Nurs* 91(12):44-45, 1991.

Young RJ, Murray ND: Adapting intravenous pumps for enteral feeding, *MCN Am J Matern Child Nurs* 16:212-216, 1991.

CHAPTER 43

Respiratory Dysfunction

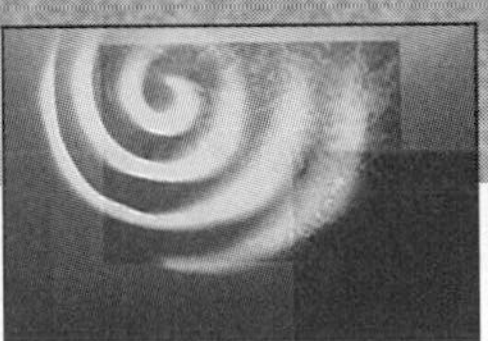

RESPIRATORY INFECTION, P. 1321

General aspects of respiratory infections, p. 1321

UPPER RESPIRATORY TRACT INFECTIONS (URIs), P. 1326

Nasopharyngitis, p. 1326
Pharyngitis, p. 1327
Tonsillitis, p. 1328
Infectious mononucleosis, p. 1330
Influenza, p. 1331
Otitis media (OM), p. 1331

CROUP SYNDROMES, P. 1334

Acute epiglottitis, p. 1334
Acute laryngitis, p. 1335
Acute laryngotracheobronchitis (LTB), p. 1335
Acute spasmodic laryngitis, p. 1337
Bacterial tracheitis, p. 1337

INFECTIONS OF THE LOWER AIRWAYS, P. 1337

Bronchitis, p. 1337
Respiratory syncytial virus (RSV)/bronchiolitis, p. 1337
Pneumonias, p. 1339

OTHER INFECTIONS OF THE RESPIRATORY TRACT, P. 1341

Pertussis (whooping cough), p. 1341
Tuberculosis (TB), p. 1341

PULMONARY DYSFUNCTION CAUSED BY NONINFECTIOUS IRRITANTS, P. 1344

Foreign body (FB) aspiration, p. 1344
Aspiration pneumonia, p. 1345
Adult respiratory distress syndrome (ARDS), p. 1345
Inhalation injury: smoke and carbon monoxide, p. 1345
Passive smoking, p. 1346

LONG-TERM RESPIRATORY DYSFUNCTION, P. 1347

Asthma, p. 1347
Cystic fibrosis, p. 1356

RESPIRATORY EMERGENCY, P. 1361

Respiratory failure, p. 1361
Cardiopulmonary resuscitation (CPR), p. 1362
Airway obstruction, p. 1365

Respiratory Infection

GENERAL ASPECTS OF RESPIRATORY INFECTIONS

Infections of the respiratory tract are described in a number of different ways according to the general areas of involvement in the more common infections. The *upper respiratory tract*, or *upper airway*, consists primarily of the nose and pharynx. The *lower respiratory tract* consists of the bronchi and bronchioles (which constitute the reactive portion of the airway because of their smooth muscle content and ability to constrict) and the alveoli. Authorities disagree about the designation for the structurally stable portion of the airway (including the epiglottis, larynx, and trachea). For this discussion, the trachea is considered with lower tract disorders, and infections of the epiglottis and larynx are categorized as croup syndromes. Respiratory infections seldom fall neatly into discrete anatomic areas. Infections tend to spread from one structure to another because of the contiguous nature of the mucous membrane lining the entire tract. Consequently, infections of the respiratory tract involve several areas rather than a single structure, although the effect on one may predominate in any given illness.

Etiology and Characteristics

Respiratory infections account for a large majority of acute illnesses in children. The cause and course of these infections are influenced by a number of factors, including the age of the child, season, living conditions, and preexisting medical problems.

Infectious agents. The respiratory tract is subject to a wide variety of infective organisms, but the largest percentage of infections are caused by viruses, particularly in the upper respiratory passages. These infections account for a large majority of acute illnesses in children. Other agents that may be involved in primary or secondary invasion include group A β-hemolytic streptococci, staphylococci, *Haemophilus influenzae, Chlamydia trachomatis, Mycoplasma*, and pneumococci.

Age. The pattern of respiratory infection varies considerably with the age of the child. Infants under age 3 months have a lower infection rate, presumably because of the protective function of maternal antibodies. The infection rate soars from age 3 to 6 months, the time between the disappearance of maternal antibodies and the infant's own antibody production. The viral infection rate continues to be high during the toddler and preschool years but drops steadily. By the time the child reaches 5 years of age, viral respiratory infections are much less frequent, but the incidence of *Mycoplasma pneumoniae* and group A β-streptococcal infections increases.

Some of the viral agents produce a mild illness in older children but cause severe lower respiratory tract illness or croup in infants. The amount of lymphoid tissue increases throughout middle childhood, and repeated exposure to organisms confers increasing immunity as the child grows older; thus older children have a greater resistance to most organisms. Whooping cough is a relatively harmless tracheobronchitis in childhood but a serious disease in infancy.

Size. Anatomic differences influence the degree to which children respond to respiratory tract infections. The diameter of the airways is smaller in young children than in older children and is therefore subject to considerable narrowing from edematous mucous membranes and increased production of secretions. In addition, the distance between structures within the tract is shorter anatomically in the young child; therefore organisms move more rapidly down the respiratory

BOX 43-1
Signs and Symptoms Associated with Respiratory Infections in Infants and Small Children

Fever

May be absent in newborn infants, who may be hypothermic
Greatest at ages 6 months to 3 years
- Temperature may reach 39.5° to 40.5° C (103° to 105° F) even with mild infections

Often appears as first sign of infection
May be listless and irritable or somewhat euphoric and more active than normal, temporarily; some children talk with unaccustomed rapidity
Tendency to have high temperatures with infection in certain families
- May precipitate febrile seizures (see Chapter 48)
- Febrile seizures uncommon after 3 or 4 years of age

Meningismus

Meningeal signs without infection of the meninges
Occurs with abrupt onset of fever
Accompanied by:
- Headache
- Pain and stiffness in the back and neck
- Presence of Kernig and Brudzinski signs

Subsides as the temperature decreases

Anorexia

Common with most childhood illnesses
Frequently the initial evidence of illness
Almost invariably accompanies acute infections in small children
Persists to a greater or lesser degree throughout febrile stage of illness; often extends into convalescence

Vomiting

Small children vomit readily with illness
A clue to the onset of infection
May precede other signs by several hours
Usually short-lived, but may persist during the illness

Diarrhea

Usually mild, transient diarrhea but may become severe
Often accompanies respiratory infections, especially viral infections
Frequent cause of dehydration

Abdominal pain

Common complaint
Sometimes indistinguishable from pain of appendicitis
Mesenteric lymphadenitis may be cause
Muscle spasms from vomiting may be a factor, especially in nervous, tense child

Nasal blockage

Small nasal passages of infants easily blocked by mucosal swelling and exudation
Can interfere with respiration and feeding in infants
May contribute to the development of otitis media and sinusitis

Nasal discharge

Frequently accompanies respiratory infections
May be thin and watery (rhinorrhea) or thick and purulent
Depends on the type and/or stage of infection
Associated with itching
May irritate upper lip and skin surrounding the nose

Cough

Common feature of respiratory disease
May be evident only during the acute phase
May persist several months after a disease

Respiratory sounds

Sounds associated with respiratory disease:
- Cough
- Hoarseness
- Grunting
- Stridor

Auscultation:
- Wheezing
- Crackles
- Absence of air movement

Sore throat

Frequent complaint of older children
Young children (unable to describe symptoms) may not complain even when throat is highly inflamed
Child will often refuse to take oral fluids or solids

tract, producing more extensive involvement. The relatively short and open eustachian tube in infants and young children allows pathogens easy access to the middle ear.

Resistance. The ability to resist invading organisms depends on several factors. Deficiencies of the immune system place the child at risk for any infectious process. The general conditions that appear to decrease resistance to infection are malnutrition, anemia, fatigue, and chilling of the body. Conditions affecting the respiratory tract that weaken its defenses and predispose to infection include allergies (e.g., allergic rhinitis), asthma, cardiac anomalies that have a tendency to cause pulmonary congestion, and cystic fibrosis. Day-care attendance, especially if the caregivers smoke, also increases the likelihood of infection (Holberg, Wright, and Martinez, 1993).

Seasonal variations. The most common respiratory tract pathogens appear in epidemics during the winter and spring months, but mycoplasma infections occur more often in autumn and early winter. Infection-related asthma (e.g., asthmatic bronchitis) occurs more frequently during cold weather.

Clinical Manifestations

Infants and young children, especially those between 6 months and 3 years of age, react more severely to acute respiratory tract infection than older children, and they are often more ill than their local manifestations would indicate. Young children display a number of generalized signs and symptoms, as well as local manifestations, that differ from those seen in older children and adults. An infant or child may display any or all of the signs and symptoms listed in Box 43-1.

Nursing Care Management

Assessment

The general assessment of the respiratory system follows the guidelines described in Chapter 32 (for nose, mouth and throat, chest, and lungs), and normal vital signs can be found in the Appendix. In addition, special attention is given to the specific observations outlined in Box 43-2.

Nursing Diagnoses

After a thorough assessment, a number of nursing diagnoses may be identified. The most likely diagnoses are outlined and discussed in the Nursing Care Plan on p. 1325. Others may be apparent in individual cases.

Planning

The goals for the child with an acute respiratory infection and the family are as follows:

1. The child will exhibit normal respiratory efforts.
2. The child will receive adequate rest.
3. The child will remain comfortable.
4. The child will not spread primary infection to others.
5. The child's temperature will remain within normal limits.
6. The child will maintain normal hydration and adequate nutrition.
7. The child will experience no complications as a result of treatments/care.
8. The child and family will receive information, especially for home care, and support.

BOX 43-2
Components for Assessing Respiratory Function

Respirations

The pattern of respirations is observed for rate, depth, ease, and rhythm of breathing:

Rate—Rapid (tachypnea), normal, or slow for the particular child

Depth—Normal depth, too shallow (hypopnea), too deep (hyperpnea); usually estimated from the amplitude of thoracic and abdominal excursion

Ease—Effortless, labored (dyspnea); orthopnea (difficult breathing except in upright position); associated with intercostal and/or substernal retractions (inspiratory "sinking in" of soft tissues in relation to the cartilaginous and bony thorax); pulsus paradoxus (blood pressure falls with inspiration and rises with expiration); flaring nares; head bobbing (head of sleeping child with suboccipital area supported on caregiver's forearm bobs forward in synchrony with each inspiration); grunting; wheezing

Labored breathing—Continuous, intermittent, becoming steadily worse, sudden onset, at rest or on exertion, associated with wheezing or grunting, associated with pain

Rhythm—Variation in rate and depth of respirations

Other Observations

In addition to respirations, particular attention is addressed to the following:

Evidence of infection—Check for elevated temperature, enlarged cervical lymph nodes, inflamed mucous membranes, and purulent discharges from the nose, ears, or lungs (sputum)

Cough—Observe the characteristics of the cough (if present); for example, under what circumstances the cough is heard (e.g., night only, on arising), the nature of the cough (paroxysmal with or without wheeze, "croupy" or "brassy"), frequency of cough, association with swallowing or other activity, character of the cough (moist and dry), productivity

Wheeze—Expiratory or inspiratory, high-pitched or musical, prolonged, slowly progressive or sudden, associated with labored breathing

Cyanosis—Note distribution (peripheral, perioral, facial, trunk as well as face), degree, duration, association with activity

Chest pain—May be a complaint of older children. Note location and circumstances: localized or generalized, referred to base of neck or abdomen, dull or sharp, deep or superficial, associated with rapid, shallow respirations or grunting

Sputum—Older children may provide sputum sample by coughing, whereas young children may need use of bulb suction to provide a sample. Note volume, color, viscosity, and odor

Bad breath—May be associated with some lung infections

Implementation

Ease respiratory efforts. Most acute respiratory infections are mild and cause few distressing symptoms. Although children may feel uncomfortable and have a "stuffy" nose and some mucosal swelling, respiratory distress is uncommon. The interventions described in the remainder of the discussion are usually sufficient to relieve most minor discomfort and ease respiratory efforts. However, in children with croup or epiglottitis sufficient swelling may develop to obstruct the airway. These children are hospitalized for observation and therapy (see discussions of specific disorders). Positioning for optimum respiration and observation for signs of respiratory distress are primary nursing interventions.

Warm or cool mist has been a common therapeutic measure for symptomatic relief of respiratory discomfort. The moisture soothes inflamed membranes and seems to be especially beneficial when there is hoarseness or any laryngeal involvement. However, use of steam vaporizers in the home should be discouraged because of the hazards related to their use and the little evidence to support their efficacy. Shallow pans with wide surface areas for evaporation increase humidity but should be placed where they do not pose a safety hazard.

A time-honored method of producing warm mist is the shower. Running a shower of hot water into the empty bathtub or open shower stall with the bathroom door closed produces a quick source of steam. Keeping a child in this environment for 10 to 15 minutes offers the same advantages as the mist tent without the fear and restraint often associated with the confines of a tent. A small child can be held on the lap of a parent or other adult. Older children can sit in the bathroom under the supervision of an adult.

Promote rest. Children who have an acute febrile illness should be placed on bed rest. This is usually not difficult while the temperature is elevated but may be difficult when children, particularly young children, feel fairly well. When parents take the advice seriously and consistently keep them in bed, most children learn to cooperate during illness. Often children are more likely to comply if they are allowed to lie quietly on a couch where they can watch television or participate in an alternate quiet activity. If children are unreasoning and expend an inordinate amount of energy in protest, allowing them to play quietly on the floor serves the purpose of rest better than allowing them to cry excessively in bed. A number of entertainment devices, based on individual interests and developmental stage, can be used to keep children quiet.

Promote comfort. Older children are usually able to manage nasal secretions with little difficulty. Parents are instructed about the correct administration of nose drops and throat irrigations, if ordered. For very young infants, who normally breathe through their noses, an infant nasal aspirator or a rubber ear syringe is helpful in removing nasal secretions before feeding. This practice in conjunction with the instillation of saline nose drops, may be all that is necessary to clear nasal passages and promote feeding. Saline nose drops can be prepared at home by dissolving 1 teaspoon of salt in 1 pint of warm water.*

For older infants and children who can better tolerate decongestants, vasoconstrictive nose drops may be administered 15 to 20 minutes before feeding and at bedtime. Two drops are instilled, and since this shrinks only the anterior mucous membranes, 2 more drops are instilled 5 to 10 minutes later. Phenylephrine (Neo-Synephrine) 0.25% is the usual choice of decongestant nose drops, although others, such as ephedrine 1%, may be prescribed. Older cooperative children often prefer nasal sprays. They are taught to compress the plastic container at the moment of inspiration to gain relief. Spray bottles and bottles of nose drops should be used for one child only and only for one illness, since they readily become contaminated with bacteria. Medicated nose drops or sprays should not be administered for more than 3 days, to prevent rebound congestion.

Hot or cold applications sometimes provide relief for other children with painful cervical adenitis. An ice bag or heating pad applied to the neck may decrease the discomfort, but safety precautions must be observed to prevent burns. The ice bag or heating device must be covered, and the heating pad should not be set at high ranges.

Prevent spread of infection. Careful handwashing should be carried out when caring for children with respiratory infections. Children and families are taught the correct disposal of respiratory secretions and proper behavior related to airborne droplets (coughing and sneezing). They are taught to use a tissue or their hand to cover their nose and mouth when they cough or sneeze and to dispose of the tissues properly, as well as wash their hands.

Nursing ALERT

To prevent contamination with respiratory viruses, wash hands and do not touch your eyes, nose, or mouth.

Every endeavor should be made to remove affected children from contact with other children. Parents are encouraged to keep affected children out of school and day-care settings to prevent the spread of infection. Ideally, ill children should be isolated in a separate bedroom at the first sign of illness. This is seldom a problem with an only child but is often difficult when living arrangements are crowded and there are several children in the family. If no separate bedroom is available, the other children perhaps could sleep on a couch or cot, or with relatives or friends. An effort should be made to teach well children to stay away from ill children if the living conditions allow for separation, although this recommendation may be difficult or impossible to enforce.

Reduce temperature. If the child has a significantly elevated temperature, controlling the fever becomes a major nursing task. The parent should know how to take a child's temperature and read the thermometer accurately. Most parents are able to do this, but nurses cannot make this assumption. An assessment of the parents' learning needs precedes teaching for measures such as taking the child's temperature.*

*Home care instructions for administration of nose drops and nasal aspiration are available in Wong DL: *Wong and Whaley's clinical manual of pediatric nursing,* ed 4, St Louis, 1996, Mosby.

*Home care instructions for measuring temperature and administration of medication are available in Wong DL: *Wong and Whaley's clinical manual of pediatric nursing,* ed 4, St Louis, 1996, Mosby.

If the practitioner has prescribed an antipyretic, parents may need help administering the drug. Most parents can read the label and calculate the desired dose, but some have difficulty and will require careful instruction or precise direction. It is important to emphasize accuracy in both the amount of drug given and the intervals at which the drug is administered in order to prevent accumulation effects. Cool liquids are encouraged to help reduce the temperature and to minimize the chances of dehydration. (See Controlling Elevated Temperatures, Chapter 42).

Promote hydration. Dehydration is always a hazard when children are febrile or anorexic, especially when vomiting or diarrhea is also present. Adequate fluid intake should be encouraged by offering small amounts of favorite fluids at frequent intervals. High-calorie liquids, such as colas, fruit

Nursing Care Plan

THE CHILD WITH ACUTE RESPIRATORY INFECTION

Nursing Diagnosis: Ineffective breathing pattern related to the inflammatory process

Expected Outcome: Respiration patterns are within normal limits.

- **NURSING INTERVENTIONS/*RATIONALES***

Position and reposition child as needed (i.e., elevate head of bed, tripod or upright sitting position, use of support pillows and wedges) *to maintain open airway, to allow maximum use of accessory muscles, and to allow maximum lung and diaphragm expansion for ventilation and comfort.*

Avoid constrictive clothing or bedding *that may interfere with breathing.*

Provide increased humidity and supplemental oxygen per physician order *to aid in oxygenation and breathing.*

Suction airway as needed *to remove secretions.*

Alternate rest and activity cycles *to reduce oxygen demands.*

Administer bronchodilators and other medications as prescribed *to assist with ventilation.*

Nursing Diagnosis: Ineffective airway clearance related to inflammation, increased secretions, obstruction

Expected Outcome: Airway is patent.

- **NURSING INTERVENTIONS/*RATIONALES***

Position child (prone, side lying, sitting) using proper body alignment *for maximum ventilation and prevention of aspiration of secretions.*

Ensure adequate fluid intake *to keep secretions liquid* and provide humidified environment *to keep mucous membranes moist.*

Administer chest physiotherapy (percussion, vibration postural drainage) *to promote loosening and drainage of lung secretions.*

Assist child to cough and expectorate effectively using suctioning if needed *to clear accumulated secretions.*

Administer expectorants, nebulizer treatments and bronchodilators as prescribed *to facilitate liquefaction and clearance of secretions.*

Administer prescribed pain medications and provide splinting during coughing *to minimize discomfort and increase effectiveness of coughing.*

Nursing Diagnosis: Risk for spread of infection related to presence of infective organisms

Expected Outcomes: Child shows no signs of secondary infection, and there are no signs of infection in others in environment.

- **NURSING INTERVENTIONS/*RATIONALES***

Maintain aeseptic environment, use good handwashing techniques, use isolation techniques and universal precautions as needed *to prevent spread of infection and avoid cross contamination and nosocomial infection.*

Administer antibiotics per physician *to treat or prevent infection.*

Instruct child and family in appropriate precautions (i.e., handwashing, tissue disposal) *to prevent spread of infection.*

Nursing Diagnosis: Activity intolerance related to inflammatory process, imbalance between oxygen supply and demand

Expected Outcomes: Child shows no signs increased respiratory distress; child's activity tolerance is appropriate for age and abilities.

- **NURSING INTERVENTIONS/*RATIONALES***

Schedule activities, treatments, visits and play around child's needs and energy levels *to maximize rest and minimize fatigue.*

Implement measures (quiet, darkened room) *to ensure sleep.*

Encourage frequent rest periods *to balance energy needs.*

Administer pain medications and sedatives per physician order *for restlessness and pain.*

Monitor vital signs *for signs of oxygen lack.*

Nursing Diagnosis: Fear/anxiety related to difficulty breathing

Expected Outcome: Child exhibits reduced signs of fear and anxiety.

- **NURSING INTERVENTIONS/*RATIONALES***

Acknowledge child's fear and help child identify sources of that fear *to facilitate identification and use of coping strategies.*

Explain respiratory treatments and procedures to child in developmentally appropriate terms *to allay fear of unknown.*

Show child how coughing and deep breathing help aid breathing *to allay fears and give child a measure of control.*

See also Nursing Care Plans: Ill or Hospitalized Child and Family of Ill or Hospitalized Child, Chapter 41.

juices, water flavored and sweetened with corn syrup, or similar drinks, help prevent catabolism and dehydration but should be avoided if diarrhea is present. Oral rehydration solutions, such as Infalyte or Pedialyte, should then be considered for infants, and sports drinks such as Gatorade should be considered for older children. Fluids should not be forced, and children should not be awakened to take fluids. Forcing fluids may create the same difficulties as urging unwanted food. Gentle persuasion with preferred beverages will usually be successful.

Parents should know how to assess their child's level of hydration (see Chapter 49). They are advised to observe the frequency of voiding and notify the nurse or practitioner if there appears to be insufficient voiding.

Provide nutrition. Loss of appetite is characteristic of children with acute infections, and in most cases, children can be permitted to determine their own need for food. Many children show no decrease in appetite, and others respond well to certain foods, such as gelatin, soup, and puddings (see also Feeding the Sick Child, Chapter 42). Since the illness is relatively short, the nutritional state is seldom compromised. In fact, urging foods on anorexic children may precipitate nausea and vomiting and in some cases even cause an aversion to the feeding situation that can extend into the convalescent period and beyond.

Family support and home care. Small children with respiratory infections are irritable and often difficult to comfort. Therefore the family needs support, encouragement, and practical suggestions for care. Since most care involves comfort measures and administration of medication, a primary goal of education is related to these activities.

In addition to antipyretics and nose drops, the child may require antibiotic therapy. It is usually the nurse who instructs the parents about continuing medication begun in the hospital or initiating medications at home, especially antibiotics. Parents of children who are sent home with oral antibiotics need to understand the importance of regular administration and continuation of the drug for the prescribed length of time, regardless of whether the child appears to be ill.

Parents are also cautioned against giving the child any medications that are not approved by the health practitioner. Adverse effects have been noted in children who have received some preparations intended for adults (e.g., some long-acting nose drops [Neo-Synephrine II] and dextromethorphan cough squares [mistaken for candy]). They are also cautioned about giving the child unprescribed antibiotics left over from a previous illness. Self-medication with nonprescribed antibiotics is a significant problem. It should be emphasized that some drugs interact with others to produce serious side effects, and such a likelihood is increased when medications are administered to children without consultation with the practitioner. The nurse is in an excellent position to provide drug information to families. (See Chapter 42 for administration of medications and teaching parents.)

Evaluation

The effectiveness of nursing interventions is determined by continual reassessment and evaluation of care based on the following observational guidelines and expected outcomes:

1. Observe child's respiratory effort and movement.
2. Observe signs and symptoms for progress toward health status before illness.
3. Observe child's behavior and activity.
4. Observe other family members and contacts for evidence of infection.
5. Take temperature.
6. Observe for signs of adequate hydration.
7. Observe eating behavior.
8. Assess child for evidence of complications, such as dehydration, weight loss, or spread of infection to other areas of the body.
9. Observe family's behavior and interview members regarding their feelings and concerns.

Expected outcomes:
See the Nursing Care Plan on p. 1325.

Upper Respiratory Tract Infections (URIs)

NASOPHARYNGITIS

Acute nasopharyngitis (the equivalent of the "common cold") is caused by any of a number of different viruses, usually rhinoviruses, respiratory syncytial virus (RSV), adenovirus, influenza virus, or parainfluenza virus.

Clinical Manifestations

Symptoms of nasopharyngitis are more severe in infants and children than in adults. Fever is common, especially in young children. Older children have low-grade fevers, which appear early in the process. Other clinical manifestations are listed in Box 43-3.

Therapeutic Management

Children with nasopharyngitis are managed at home. There is no specific treatment, and effective vaccines are not available. Antipyretics are usually prescribed for mild fever and discomfort (see Chapter 42 for management of fever). Decongestants may be prescribed for children and infants over 6 months of age in an effort to shrink swollen nasal passages. The decongestants that exert their effect by vasoconstriction are usually less effective when taken orally than when applied topically as nose drops. Since these drugs affect *all* vascular beds, they should be given with caution to children with diabetes.

Cough suppressants containing dextromethorphan may be prescribed for a dry, hacking cough. Some preparations contain up to 22% alcohol; they should not be administered to young children continuously and must be stored securely away from children.

Antihistamines are largely ineffective in treatment of nasopharyngitis. The drugs have a weak atropinelike effect that tends to dry secretions, but they can cause drowsiness and, paradoxically, have a stimulatory effect on children. There is no support for the usefulness of expectorants, and antibiotics are usually contraindicated because they can sensitize a child, who may need the drugs in a severe illness.

BOX 43-3
Clinical Manifestations of Nasopharyngitis and Pharyngitis

Nasopharyngitis

Younger child

Fever
Irritability, restlessness
Sneezing
Vomiting and/or diarrhea, sometimes

Older child

Dryness and irritation of nose and throat
Sneezing, chilly sensation
Muscular aches
Cough, sometimes

Physical signs

Edema and vasodilation of mucosa

Pharyngitis

Younger child

Fever
General malaise
Anorexia
Moderate sore throat
Headache

Older child

Fever (may reach 40° C [104° F])
Headache
Anorexia
Dysphagia
Abdominal pain
Vomiting

Physical signs

Younger child

Mild to moderate hyperemia

Older Child

Mild to fiery red, edematous pharynx
Hyperemia of tonsils and pharynx; may extend to soft palate and uvula
Often abundant follicular exudate that spreads and coalesces to form pseudomembrane on tonsils

Prevention. Nasopharyngitis is so widespread in the general population that it is difficult to prevent. In addition, children are more susceptible to colds because their resistance to many types of viruses has not yet developed. Very young infants are subject to relatively serious complications; therefore some attempt should be made to protect them from exposure. Rest is recommended until the child is afebrile for at least 1 day.

Nursing Care Management

A cold is often the parents' first introduction to an illness in their infants. Parents are assisted in managing the infant or child as described for general care. Most of the distress of nasopharyngitis is related to the nasal obstruction, especially in small infants. Placing the child in a prone position (unless respirations are compromised) and elevating the head of bed (assists with drainage of secretions), suctioning, and vaporization may help provide relief. Saline nose drops and gentle suction with a bulb syringe, particularly before feeding, are sometimes useful.

Maintaining adequate fluid intake is essential during any infectious process. Although a child's appetite for solid foods is usually diminished for several days, it is important to offer favorite fluids to prevent dehydration. Fluids can be cool or warm, depending on individual preference.

BOX 43-4
Early Evidence of Respiratory Complications

Parents are instructed to notify the health professional if any of the following is noted:

Evidence of earache (see p. 1331)
Respirations faster than 50 to 60 per minute
Fever over 38.3° C (101° F)
Listlessness
Increasing irritability with or without fever
Persistent cough 2 days or more
Wheezing
Crying
Refusal to eat
Restlessness and poor sleep patterns

Modified from National Association of Pediatric Nurse Associates and Practitioners (NAPNAP): *Baby's first cold,* New York, 1989, Winthrop Consumer Products. Copies available from NAPNAP, 1101 Kings Hwy., N., No. 206, Cherry Hill, NJ 08034; (609) 667-1773.

Because nasopharyngitis is spread from secretions, the best means for prevention is avoidance of contact with affected persons. This goal is difficult in places where large numbers of people are confined in a small area for a long time, such as classrooms and day-care centers. Family members with a cold should try to "keep it to themselves" by carefully disposing of tissues; not sharing towels, glasses, or eating utensils; covering the mouth and nose with tissues when coughing or sneezing; and washing the hands thoroughly after nose blowing or sneezing. The most frequent carriers of infection are the human hands, which deposit viruses on doorknobs, faucets, and other everyday objects. Therefore children should be taught to wash their hands thoroughly before putting them near their eyes, nose, or mouth.

Family support. Support and reassurance are important elements of care for families of young children with recurrent URIs. Because URIs are common in children less than 3 years of age, families may feel they are on an endless roller coaster of illness. They can be reassured that frequent colds are a normal part of childhood and that by 5 years of age, their children will have immunity to many viruses. Parents who work outside the home should expect to have to take time off to care for ill children during the fall and winter months. If the children are cared for routinely in day-care centers, the infection rate will be higher than if they were being cared for in the home. Parents should know the signs of respiratory complications and be counseled to notify a health professional if any signs of complications appear or if the child does not improve within 2 or 3 days (Box 43-4).

PHARYNGITIS

Group A β-hemolytic streptococcus (GABHS) infection of the upper airway (strep throat) is not in itself a serious disease, but affected children are at risk for serious sequelae: acute rheumatic fever (ARF), an inflammatory disease of heart, joints, and central nervous system (see Chapter 45), and acute glomerulonephritis, an acute kidney infection (see Chapter 47). Permanent damage can result from these sequelae, especially ARF.

Clinical Manifestations

GABHS is generally a relatively brief illness that varies greatly in severity from subclinical (no symptoms) to comparatively severe toxicity. The onset is generally abrupt and characterized by pharyngitis, headache, fever, and (especially in small children) abdominal pain. The tonsils and pharynx may be inflamed and covered with exudate, which usually appears by the second day of illness. Anterior cervical lymphadenopathy (30% to 50% of cases) usually occurs early, and the nodes are often tender. Pain can be relatively mild to severe enough to make swallowing difficult. Clinical manifestations usually subside in 3 to 5 days unless complicated by sinusitis or parapharyngeal, peritonsillar, or retropharyngeal abscess. Nonsuppurative complications may appear after the onset of GABHS—acute nephritis in about 10 days and rheumatic fever in an average of 18 days.

Diagnostic Evaluation

Clinical diagnosis of GABHS infection can present difficulties. Although 80% to 90% of all cases of acute pharyngitis are viral, a throat culture should be performed to rule out GABHS and (in some cases) *Corynebacterium diphtheriae.* Because some children normally harbor streptococci in the throat, a positive culture result is not always conclusive evidence of active disease. Since most streptococcal infections are short-term illnesses, antibody (antistreptolysin O) responses do not appear until relatively late and are useful only for retrospective diagnosis.

Rapid identification of GABHS is possible with diagnostic test kits that can be used in the office or clinic setting. However, because of their questionable sensitivity, they are not yet considered to be a substitute for culture, especially if the organism is endemic in the community.

Therapeutic Management

If streptococcal sore throat infection is present, oral penicillin is prescribed in a dose sufficient to control the acute local manifestations and to maintain an adequate level for at least 10 days to eliminate any organisms that may remain to initiate rheumatic fever symptoms. Penicillin does not appear to prevent the development of acute glomerulonephritis in susceptible children; however, it may prevent the spread of a nephrogenic strain of GABHS to others in the family. Penicillin usually produces a prompt response within 24 hours. Occasionally patients require retreatment if the organism is not eradicated.

A combination of penicillin and rifampin is more effective in eradicating GABHS than penicillin alone and is recommended for carriers and persons resistant to penicillin. Erythromycin or a cephalosporin may be used for children who are sensitive to penicillin. Clinical manifestations are treated symptomatically.

Nursing Care Management

The nurse is often the person who performs a throat smear for culture and instructs the parents about administering penicillin and analgesics as prescribed. Most children prefer to remain in bed during the acute phase of the illness. Cold or warm compresses to the neck may provide relief. In children old enough to cooperate, warm saline gargles offer some relief of throat discomfort. Pain may interfere with oral intake, and the child should not be forced to eat. Cool liquids or ice chips are usually more acceptable than solids and are encouraged.

Special emphasis is placed on correct administration of oral medication and completing the course of antibiotic therapy (see Administration of Medication and Compliance, Chapter 42). If injections are required, they must be administered deep into a large muscle mass (e.g., the vastus lateralis or gluteus muscle). Parents need to be aware of the residual tenderness, which may cause the child to limp for a day or two. Local applications of heat are helpful in relieving some of the discomfort.

TONSILLITIS

The tonsils are masses of lymphoid tissue located in the pharyngeal cavity. Their function is to filter and protect the respiratory and alimentary tracts from invasion by pathogenic organisms. They also may have a role in antibody formation. Although the size of tonsils varies, children generally have much larger tonsils than adolescents or adults. This difference is thought to be a protective mechanism at a time when young children are especially susceptible to URI.

Pathophysiology

Several pairs of tonsils are part of a mass of lymphoid tissue encircling the nasal and oral pharynx, known as the *Waldeyer tonsillar ring* (Fig. 43-1). The *palatine,* or *faucial, tonsils* are located on either side of the oropharynx, behind and below the pillars of the fauces (opening from the mouth). A free surface of the palatine tonsils is usually visible during oral examination. The palatine tonsils are those removed during tonsillectomy. The *pharyngeal tonsils,* also known as the *adenoids,* are located above the palatine tonsils on the posterior wall of the nasopharynx. Their proximity to the nares and eustachian tubes causes difficulties in instances of inflammation. The *lingual tonsils* are located at the base of the tongue and only rarely are removed. The *tubal tonsils,* found near the posterior nasopharyngeal opening of the eustachian tubes, are not part of the Waldeyer tonsillar ring.

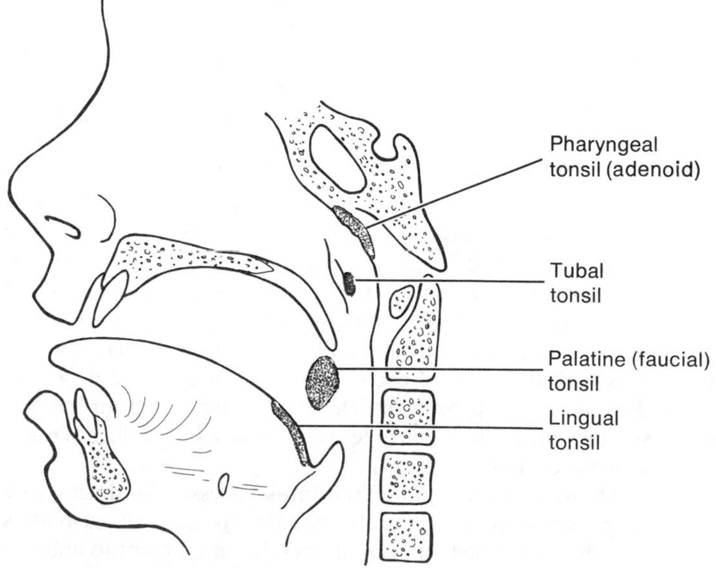

Fig. 43-1 Location of the various tonsillar masses.

Etiology

Tonsillitis usually occurs in association with pharyngitis. Because of the abundant lymphoid tissue and the frequency of URIs, tonsillitis is a very common cause of morbidity in young children. The causative agent may be viral or bacterial.

Clinical Manifestations

The manifestations of tonsillitis are chiefly caused by inflammation. As the palatine tonsils enlarge from edema, they may meet in the midline (kissing tonsils), obstructing the passage of air or food. The child has difficulty swallowing and breathing. When enlargement of the adenoids occurs, the space behind the posterior nares may become blocked, making it difficult or impossible for air to pass from the nose to the throat. As a result, the child breathes through the mouth.

Therapeutic Management

Since the illness is self-limiting, treatment of viral pharyngitis is symptomatic. Throat cultures with results positive for GABHS infection warrant antibiotic treatment. It is important to differentiate between viral and streptococcal infection in febrile exudative tonsillitis. Since the majority of infections are of viral origin, early rapid tests can eliminate unnecessary antibiotic administration. *Tonsillectomy* (removal of the palatine tonsils) is indicated for massive hypertrophy that results in difficulty breathing or eating (Derkay, Darrow, and LeFebvre, 1994). Absolute indications are malignancy and obstruction of the airway. *Adenoidectomy* (removal of the adenoids) is recommended for those children in whom hypertrophied adenoids obstruct nasal breathing. Their removal may be warranted in the child under 3 years of age and should be performed without a tonsillectomy. Contraindications to either tonsillectomy or adenoidectomy are (1) cleft palate, since both tonsils help minimize escape of air during speech; (2) acute infections at the time of surgery, since the locally inflamed tissues increase the risk of bleeding; and (3) uncontrolled systemic diseases or blood dyscrasias.

Nursing Care Management

Nursing care of the child with tonsillitis mainly involves providing comfort and minimizing activities or interventions that may precipitate bleeding. A soft to liquid diet is generally preferred. A cool-mist vaporizer helps keep the mucous membranes moist during periods of mouth breathing. Warm saltwater gargles, throat lozenges, and analgesic/antipyretic drugs such as acetaminophen (Tylenol) and codeine are useful to promote comfort.

If surgery is needed, the child requires the same psychologic preparation and physical care as for any other procedure (see Chapters 41 and 42). The following discussion focuses on postoperative nursing care for tonsillectomy and adenoidectomy (T & A), although both procedures may not be performed.

Until they are fully awake, children are placed on the abdomen or side to facilitate drainage of secretions, and any needed suctioning is performed carefully to prevent trauma to the oropharynx. When alert, children may prefer sitting up, although they should remain in bed for the remainder of the day. They are discouraged from coughing frequently, clearing their throat, and blowing their nose, activities that may aggravate the operative site.

Some secretions are common, particularly dried blood from surgery. All secretions and vomitus are inspected for evidence of fresh bleeding (some blood-tinged mucus is expected). Dark-brown (old) blood is usually present in the emesis, as well as in the nose and between the teeth. If parents do not expect this, they may be frightened at a time when they need to be calm and reassuring for their children.

The throat is very sore after surgery. An ice collar may provide relief, but many children find it bothersome and prefer not to have it. Most children experience considerable pain after a T and/or A and should receive pain medication for at least the first 24 hours. Analgesics are ordered but may need to be given rectally or intravenously to avoid the oral route. Older children may find liquid medications easier to swallow than tablets or capsules. Since pain is continuous, pain control should be continuous or administered at regular intervals (see Pain Management, Chapter 41). Irritable children may require mild sedation to lessen crying, which irritates the operative site, increasing the chance of bleeding.

Food and fluid are restricted until children are fully alert and there are no signs of hemorrhage. Cool water, crushed ice, flavored ice pops, or dilute fruit juice is given first, although fluids with a red or brown color are avoided to distinguish fresh or old blood in emesis from the ingested liquid. Citrus juice may cause discomfort and is usually poorly tolerated. Milk, ice cream, or pudding is not offered until clear fluids are retained, because milk products coat the mouth and throat, causing the child to clear the throat more often, potentially initiating bleeding. Soft foods, particularly gelatin, cooked fruits, sherbet, soup, and mashed potatoes, are started on the first or second postoperative day or as the child tolerates feeding. The pain from surgery often inhibits intake, reinforcing the need for adequate pain control.

Postoperative hemorrhage is unusual but can occur. Therefore the nurse observes the throat directly for evidence of bleeding, using a good source of light and, if necessary, carefully inserting a tongue depressor. Other signs of hemorrhage are increased pulse (greater than 120 beats/min), pallor, frequent clearing of the throat or swallowing by a younger child, and vomiting of bright-red blood. Restlessness, an indication of hemorrhage, may be difficult to differentiate from general discomfort after surgery. Decreasing blood pressure is a much later sign of shock.

Nursing ALERT

The most obvious early sign of bleeding is the child's continuous swallowing of the trickling blood. While the child is sleeping, note the frequency of swallowing. If continuous bleeding is suspected, notify the surgeon immediately.

Family support and home care. Discharge instructions include (1) avoiding foods that are irritating or highly seasoned, (2) avoiding the use of gargles or vigorous toothbrushing, (3) discouraging the child from coughing or clearing the throat or putting objects in the mouth, (4) using mild analgesics or an ice collar for pain, and (5) limiting activity to decrease the potential for bleeding. Hemorrhage may occur up to 10 days after surgery as a result of tissue sloughing from the healing process. Any sign of bleeding warrants immediate medical attention.

INFECTIOUS MONONUCLEOSIS

Infectious mononucleosis is an acute, self-limiting infectious disease that is common among young persons up to 25 years of age. The disease is characterized by an increase in the mononuclear elements of the blood and by general symptoms of an infectious process. The course is usually mild but occasionally can be severe or, rarely, accompanied by serious complications. Although not a respiratory condition, infectious mononucleosis is discussed here because its principal areas of involvement include the lymph glands, such as the tonsils, in the neck.

Etiology/Pathophysiology

The herpeslike Epstein-Barr virus is the principal cause of infectious mononucleosis. It appears in both sporadic and epidemic forms; the sporadic cases are more common. The mechanism of spread has not been proved, although it is believed to be transmitted by direct intimate contact with oral secretions. It also appears to be only mildly contagious, and the period of communicability is unknown. The incubation period following exposure is 4 to 6 weeks.

Diagnostic Tests

The onset of symptoms may be acute or insidious. The common presenting symptoms vary greatly in type, severity, and duration (Box 43-5). The leukocyte count may be normal or low, but usually lymphocytic leukocytosis develops. There is also an increase in atypical leukocytes in the peripheral blood smear. The heterophil antibody test determines the extent to which the patient's serum will agglutinate sheep red blood cells. In infectious mononucleosis, a titer of 1:160 is considered diagnostic, although a rising titer during the earlier stages is the best indicator.

The "spot test" (Monospot), a slide test of high specificity, is rapid, sensitive, inexpensive, and easy to perform and has the advantage that it can detect significant agglutinins at lower levels, thus permitting earlier diagnosis. Blood is usually obtained for the test by finger puncture.

BOX 43-5

Clinical Manifestations of Infectious Mononucleosis

Early signs

Headache
Malaise
Fatigue
Chilliness
Low-grade fever
Loss of appetite
Puffy eyes

Full-blown disease

Cardinal features

Fever
Sore throat
Cervical adenopathy

Common features

Splenomegaly (may persist for several months)
Palatine petechiae
Macular eruption (especially on trunk)
Exudative pharyngitis/tonsillitis
Hepatic involvement to some degree, often associated with jaundice

Therapeutic Management

There is no specific treatment for infectious mononucleosis. Common symptoms are ordinarily relieved by simple remedies. A mild analgesic is usually sufficient to relieve the bothersome symptoms of headache, fever, and malaise. Bed rest is encouraged for fatigue but is not imposed for any specified period. Affected youngsters are instructed to regulate activities according to their own tolerance unless complicating factors are present. If the spleen is enlarged, activities in which children may receive a blow to the abdomen or chest are avoided.

A short course of oral penicillin is sometimes prescribed for sore throat, especially if β-hemolytic streptococci are present. Administration of ampicillin frequently precipitates a maculopapular rash in affected persons; therefore its use is contraindicated. Sore throat, which can be severe, can be relieved by gargles, hot drinks, analgesic troches, or analgesics, including opioids. The use of corticosteroids has demonstrated effectiveness in reducing respiratory distress from tonsillar hypertrophy, hemolytic anemia, thrombocytopenia, and neurologic complications. Although steroids can shorten the course of the illness, their use is reserved for complicated cases.

Prognosis. The course of infectious mononucleosis is self-limiting and usually uncomplicated. Acute symptoms usually disappear within 7 to 10 days, and the persistent fatigue subsides within 2 to 4 weeks. A number of affected youngsters may need to restrict activities for 2 to 3 months; the disease rarely extends for longer periods. Complications are uncommon but can be serious and require appropriate management.

Nursing ALERT

Advise family to seek medical evaluation of the youngster if:
Breathing becomes difficult
Abdominal pain develops
Sore throat pain is so severe that the child is unable to eat or drink

Nursing Care Management

Nursing responsibilities are directed toward providing comfort measures to relieve the symptoms and helping affected youngsters and their families determine appropriate activities according to the stage of the disease and their interests. They may need diet counseling to select foods that contain sufficient calories to meet growth and energy needs but are easy to swallow. Every effort should be made to prevent a secondary infection; therefore the adolescent is counseled to limit exposure to persons outside the family, especially during the acute phase of illness.

The illness and its associated weakness and fatigue can

cause depression and resentment in usually vigorous, active teenagers. It is important to spend time with youngsters to listen to their concerns and to allow them to express their feelings and vent their anger. Adolescents need reassurance that the limitations are only temporary, that social activities—so essential at this stage of development—can be resumed after the acute phase, and that they will have sufficient autonomy to determine the extent of their capabilities and the rate of resumption of activities.

INFLUENZA

Influenza, or "flu," is caused by different viruses that may undergo significant changes from time to time. The disease is spread from one individual to another by direct contact (large-droplet infection) or by articles recently contaminated by nasopharyngeal secretions. There is no predilection for a specific age-group, but attack rates are highest in young children who have not had previous contact with a strain. It is frequently most severe in infants. During epidemics, infection among school-age children is believed to be a major source of transmission in a community. Influenza is more common during the winter months. The disease has a 1- to 3-day incubation period, and affected persons are most infectious for 24 hours before and after onset of symptoms.

Clinical Manifestations

The manifestations of influenza may be subclinical, mild, moderate, or severe. In most cases of overt illness, the throat and nasal mucosa are dry, and there are a dry cough and a tendency toward hoarseness. A sudden onset of fever and chills is accompanied by flushed face, photophobia, myalgia, hyperesthesia, and sometimes prostration. Subglottal croup is common, especially in infants. The symptoms last for 4 to 5 days. Complications include severe viral pneumonia (often hemorrhagic), encephalitis, and secondary bacterial infections, such as otitis media, sinusitis, or pneumonia.

Therapeutic Management

Uncomplicated influenza in children usually requires only symptomatic treatment: acetaminophen for fever, dextromethorphan for cough (if needed), and sufficient fluids to maintain hydration. Amantadine hydrochloride (Symmetrel) has been effective in reducing symptoms associated with type A disease if administered within 24 to 48 hours after onset. It is ineffective against type B or C influenza or other viral diseases. It should not be given to children under 1 year of age but is recommended for unvaccinated high-risk children. Children with influenza (or other similar viruses) should not receive aspirin because of its possible link with Reye syndrome.

Prevention. Inactivated influenza viral vaccines are safe and effective for prevention of influenza provided the antigens in the vaccine correlate with circulating influenza viruses. For information on immunization, see Chapter 33.

Nursing Care Management

Nursing care is the same as for any child with a URI, including helping the family to implement measures to relieve symptoms. The greatest danger to affected children is development of a secondary infection.

Nursing ALERT

Prolonged fever or appearance of fever during early convalescence is a sign of secondary bacterial infection and should be reported to the practitioner for antibiotic therapy.

OTITIS MEDIA (OM)

OM is one of the most prevalent diseases of early childhood. The incidence is highest in children ages 6 months to 2 years; it then gradually decreases with age, except for a small increase at age 5 or 6 years, the time of school entry. OM occurs infrequently in children over 7 years of age. Boys are affected more frequently than girls in children less than school age; later the sexes are affected equally. The incidence of acute otitis media (AOM) is highest in the winter months. Children living in households with many members (especially smokers) are more likely to have OM than those living with fewer persons, and children with siblings or parents who have a history of chronic OM have a higher incidence than those who do not.

OM has been defined in a variety of ways. The standard terminology that has been established to describe OM is outlined in Box 43-6.

Etiology

AOM is most frequently caused by *Streptococcus pneumoniae* and *Haemophilus influenzae.* The cause of the noninfectious type is unknown, although it is frequently the result of blocked eustachian tubes from the edema of URIs, allergic rhinitis, or hypertrophic adenoids. OME is frequently an extension of an acute episode. Passive smoking has been established as a significant factor in the development of OM. Tobacco smoke inhalation may increase the risk of a blocked eustachian tube by impairing mucociliary function, causing congestion of soft nasopharyngeal tissues, or predisposing patients to URI. Day-care attendance is also a risk factor for OM (Alho et al, 1993).

Infants fed breast milk have a lower incidence of OM than formula-fed infants. Breastfeeding may protect infants against respiratory viruses and allergy by the presence of increased secretory immunoglobulin A (IgA) and limits the exposure of the eustachian tube and middle ear mucosa to microbial pathogens and foreign proteins. Also, reflux of milk up the eustachian tubes is less likely in breastfed infants because of the semivertical positioning during breastfeeding compared with

BOX 43-6
Standard Terminology for Otitis Media

Otitis media (OM)—An inflammation of the middle ear without reference to etiology or pathogenesis
Acute otitis media (AOM)—A rapid and short onset of signs and symptoms lasting approximately 3 weeks
Otitis media with effusion (OME)—An inflammation of the middle ear in which a collection of fluid is present in the middle ear space
Chronic otitis media with effusion—Middle ear effusion that persists beyond 3 months

bottle-feeding. There is a definite link between the supine position during feeding and the reflux of fluid into the middle ear (Tully, Bar-Haim, and Bradley, 1995).

OM is primarily the result of dysfunctioning eustachian tubes. The eustachian tube, which connects the middle ear to the nasopharynx, is normally closed and flat, preventing organisms from the pharyngeal cavity from entering the middle ear. It opens to allow drainage of secretions produced by the middle ear mucosa and to equalize air pressure between the middle ear and outside environment. Impaired drainage causes retention of secretions in the middle ear. Air, unable to escape through the obstructed tubes, is absorbed into the circulation, causing negative pressure within the middle ear. If the tube opens, this difference in pressure causes bacteria to be swept into the middle ear chamber, where the organisms quickly proliferate and invade the mucosa.

Diagnostic Evaluation

In AOM otoscopy reveals an intact membrane that appears bright red and bulging, with no visible bony landmarks or light reflex. In OME otoscopic findings may include a slightly injected, dull gray membrane; obscured landmarks; and a visible fluid level or meniscus behind the eardrum if air is present above the fluid. Diagnosis is usually based on clinical manifestations (Box 43-7) and confirmed with **tympanometry,** which measures the change in air pressure in the external auditory canal from movement of the eardrum. The presence of fluid in the middle ear decreases membrane movement or compliance. **Pneumatic otoscopy** also allows an assessment of typanic membrane mobility. If purulent discharge is present, it should be cultured and a specific antibiotic selected for that organism. Hearing evaluation is recommended for a child who has had bilateral OME for a total of 3 months.

BOX 43-7
Clinical Manifestations of Otitis Media

Acute otitis media
Follows an upper respiratory infection
Otalgia (earache)
Purulent otorrhea may be present
Fever
Purulent discharge may or may not be present

Infant or very young child
Crying
Fussy, restless, irritable
Tendency to rub, hold, or pull affected ear
Rolls head side to side
Difficulty comforting child
Loss of appetite

Older child
Crying and/or verbalizes feelings of discomfort
Irritability
Lethargy
Loss of appetite

Chronic otitis media
Hearing loss
Difficulty communicating
Feeling of fullness, tinnitus, vertigo may be present

Therapeutic Management

Treatment of AOM is the administration of antibiotics, such as ampicillin, amoxicillin, sulfonamides, trimethoprim-sulfamethoxazole (Bactrim, Septra), erythromycin-sulfisoxazole (Pediazole), and the cephalosporins. With appropriate therapy most children improve within 48 to 72 hours. *Myringotomy* (surgical incision of the eardrum) may be required to relieve the symptoms in some children, especially those with acute suppuration who are in severe pain. Children with AOM should be seen after antibiotic therapy is complete to evaluate the effectiveness of the treatment and to identify potential complications, such as effusion or hearing impairment. Analgesic/antipyretic drugs are used to alleviate discomfort and reduce an elevated temperature.

The major goals in the management of OME are to establish and maintain an aerated middle ear that is free of fluid and with a normal mucosa and to achieve normal hearing. A trial of antibiotic therapy or simply observing of the child may be tried first. The use of steroids, decongestants, and antihistamines to shrink the mucous membranes and increase eustachian tube function is not recommended. Surgical treatment involves tympanoplasty or insertion of ventilating tubes. Tympanostomy tubes (pressure-equalizer [PE] tubes or grommets) facilitate continued drainage of fluid and allow ventilation of the middle ear.

Myringotomy with or without insertion of tympanostomy tubes should *not* be performed for initial management of OME in an otherwise healthy child. Adenoidectomy is not recommended for treatment of OME in a child age 1 year through 3 years, in the absence of specific adenoid abnormality. Tonsillectomy should not be performed, either alone or with adenoidectomy, for the treatment of OME in a child of any age (Stool et al, 1994).

Although the insertion of *tympanostomy* or *pressure-equilizing (PE) tubes* is the most common operation performed in pediatrics, its use is highly controversial and considered unnecessary by many authorities. In a study done to assess the appropriateness of using PE tubes, only about 40% of the proposed PE tube placements were defined as appropriate (Kleinman et al, 1994). Although nurses do not make the decision regarding surgical intervention for OM, they do play an important role in counseling families about proposed treatments and assessing whether parents are fully informed. The Agency for Health Care Planning and Research (AHCPR) has released federal guidelines for the treatment of OME. Nurses should be familiar with this publication, which may become accepted as the standard of care.*

Nursing Care Management

Assessment

Examination of the external auditory canal is an integral part of the physical assessment (see Chapter 32). Nurses should be alert to any child recovering from a URI who displays evidence of hearing difficulty (see Chapter 39).

*The *Managing Otitis Media with Effusion in Young Children* guidelines include an overview (AHCPR Pub. No. 94-0620), a quick reference guide (94-0623), and a parent guide (94-0624) that are available in English and Spanish from the AHCPR Publications Clearinghouse, OME/AAP, PO Box 8547, Silver Spring, Md, 20907, (800) 358-9295.

BOX 43-8

Nursing Diagnoses: The Child With Acute Otitis Media

Pain related to pressure caused by inflammatory process
Risk for impaired skin integrity related to drainage
Altered family processes related to ill child

Nursing Diagnoses

On the basis of a careful assessment, several nursing diagnoses become evident (Box 43-8). Others may apply in specific situations and in the case of chronic OM or OME.

Planning

Goals for the care of the child with acute OM and the family include the following:

1. The child will experience no pain or a reduction of pain/discomfort to level acceptable to child.
2. The child will not experience recurrence of infection.
3. The child will not experience complications from illness or treatment modalities.
4. The family will receive adequate support and education.

Implementation

Analgesics/antipyretics, such as acetaminophen, are helpful in reducing the severe earache and fever. The application of heat with a heating pad on low setting and wrapped in a towel may reduce the discomfort. Local heat should be placed over the ear with the child lying on the affected side. This position also facilitates drainage of the exudate if the eardrum has ruptured or if myringotomy was performed. An ice bag placed over the affected ear may also be beneficial, since it reduces edema and pressure. If the child is cooperative, either procedure can be tried to determine which offers greater relief.

If the ear is draining, the external canal may be cleaned with sterile cotton swabs or pledgets soaked in hydrogen peroxide. If ear wicks or lightly rolled sterile gauze packs are placed in the ear after surgical treatment, they should be loose enough to allow accumulated drainage to flow out of the ear; otherwise the infection may be transferred to the mastoid process. The wicks need to stay dry during shampoos or baths. Occasionally drainage is so profuse that the auricle and the skin surrounding the ear become excoriated from the exudate. This is prevented by frequent cleansing and application of various moisture barriers (e.g., Aloe Vesta, Proshield Plus) or petrolatum jelly (e.g., Vaseline).

Parents require anticipatory guidance regarding temporary hearing loss that accompanies OM. The nurse should caution parents not to assume that the child is ignoring them, but to realize that the child may be unaware of being spoken to. Parents are instructed to speak louder, at closer proximity, and facing the child. Persistent difficulty in hearing beyond the acute stage is evaluated.

A concern presented with the use of myringotomy tubes is the possibility that water will enter the middle ear and introduce bacteria. Recommendations for the use of ear plugs are inconsistent, but research indicates that swimming without earplugs poses no increased risk of infection. The question of whether or not bathwater is harmful remains unanswered. Bath and shampoo water should be kept out of the ear, if possible, since soap reduces the surface tension of water, facilitating entry through the tube.

Parents should be aware of the appearance of a grommet (usually a tiny, white, plastic spool-shaped tube) so that they can observe if it falls out. They are reassured that this is normal and requires no immediate intervention, although they should notify the practitioner.

Prevention of recurrence requires adequate parent education regarding antibiotic therapy. Since the symptoms of pain and fever usually subside within 24 to 48 hours, nurses must emphasize that although the child appears well, the infection is not completely eradicated until all the prescribed medication is taken. Parents should be aware of the potential complications of OM that can occur with inadequate treatment, such as (1) conductive hearing loss; (2) a perforated and scarred eardrum; (3) mastoiditis, an inflammation of the mastoid air cell system; (4) cholesteatoma, a cystlike lesion that can invade and destroy surrounding auditory structures; and (5) intracranial infections, such as meningitis.

Nurses need to take an active role in teaching parents about the possibility that otitis media will result from the supine feeding position when the infant does not sit or walk afterward. During bottle- and breastfeeding the child should be semiupright. Propping bottles is discouraged both to avoid the supine position and to ensure human contact during feeding. Since infants have difficulty expressing themselves verbally, parents should be taught that some initial signs of otitis media may be irritability and ear pulling. Eliminating tobacco smoke and known allergens is also recommended.

Evaluation

The efficacy of nursing intervention is determined by the following observational guidelines and expected outcomes:

1. Observe behaviors that indicate pain relief; seek verbal confirmation.
2. Observe skin in and around the external auditory canal.
3. Interview family regarding practices that prevent recurrence of infection.
4. Observe and interview family regarding their understanding of OM and therapies.
5. Interview family regarding their feelings and concerns.

Expected outcomes:

1. The child sleeps and rests quietly and exhibits no signs of discomfort.
2. The child exhibits no evidence of excoriated skin.
3. The child remains free of complications.
4. The family demonstrates the ability to care for child's condition.
5. The family and child express their feelings and concerns.

See also Nursing Care Plan: The Child with Acute Otitis Media.*

*In Wong DL: *Wong and Whaley's clinical manual of pediatric nursing*, ed 4, St Louis, 1996, Mosby.

Croup Syndromes

Croup is a general term applied to a symptom complex characterized by hoarseness, a resonant cough described as "barking" or "brassy" (croupy), varying degrees of inspiratory stridor, and varying degrees of respiratory distress resulting from swelling or obstruction in the region of the larynx. Acute infections of the larynx are of greater importance in infants and small children than they are in older children, in part because of the increased incidence in children in this age group and the smaller diameter of the airway, which renders it subject to significantly greater narrowing with the same degree of inflammation.

Acute respiratory infections of the nonreactive airway involve all areas to some extent and are seldom restricted to one area. Croup syndromes affect to varying degrees the larynx, trachea, and bronchi. However, laryngeal involvement often dominates the clinical picture because of the severe effects on the voice and breathing. Croup syndromes are usually described according to the primary anatomic area affected (i.e., epiglottitis [or supraglottitis], laryngitis, laryngotracheobronchitis [LTB], and tracheitis). In general, LTB tends to occur in very young children, whereas epiglottitis is more characteristic of older children (see Table 43-1 for a comparison of croup syndromes).

ACUTE EPIGLOTTITIS

Acute epiglottitis, or acute supraglottitis, is a serious obstructive inflammatory process that occurs principally in children between 2 and 5 years of age, but can occur from infancy to adulthood. The disorder requires immediate attention. The obstruction is supraglottic, as opposed to the subglottic obstruction of laryngitis. The responsible organism is usually *H. influenzae;* LTB and epiglottitis do not occur together.

Clinical Manifestations

The onset of epiglottitis is abrupt, often preceded by a sore throat, and rapidly progressive to severe respiratory distress. The child usually goes to bed asymptomatic to awaken later, complaining of sore throat and pain on swallowing. The child has a fever, appears toxic out of proportion to the clinical findings, and presents a classic picture; the child generally insists on sitting upright and leaning forward, with chin thrust out, mouth open, and tongue protruding *(tripod position).* Drooling of saliva is common because of the difficulty or pain on swallowing and excessive secretions.

Nursing ALERT

Three clinical observations that indicate epiglottitis are absence of spontaneous cough, presence of drooling, and agitation.

The child is irritable and markedly restless and has an anxious, apprehensive, and frightened expression. The voice is thick and muffled, with a froglike croaking sound on inspiration. The child is not hoarse. Suprasternal and substernal retractions may be visible. The child seldom struggles to breathe, and slow, quiet breathing provides better air exchange. The sallow color of mild hypoxia may progress to frank cyanosis. The throat is red and inflamed, and a distinctive large, cherry-red edematous epiglottis is visible on careful throat inspection. *Throat inspection should be attempted only when immediate intubation can be performed if needed.*

Therapeutic Management

The course of epiglottitis may be fulminant, with respiratory obstruction appearing suddenly. Progressive obstruction leads

TABLE 43-1 Comparison of croup syndromes

	ACUTE EPIGLOTTITIS (SUPRAGLOTTITIS)	ACUTE LARYNGOTRACHEOBRONCHITIS	ACUTE SPASMODIC LARYNGITIS (SPASMODIC CROUP)	ACUTE TRACHEITIS
Age-group affected	1-8 years	3 months–8 years	3 months–3 years	1 month–6 years
Etiologic agent	Bacterial, usually *H. influenzae*	Viral	Viral with allergic component	Bacterial, usually *S. aureus*
Onset	Rapidly progressive	Slowly progressive	Sudden; at night	Moderately progressive
Major symptoms	Dysphagia Stridor aggravated when supine Drooling High fever Toxic appearance Rapid pulse and respirations	URI Stridor Brassy cough Hoarseness Dyspnea Restlessness Irritability Low-grade fever Nontoxic appearance	URI Croupy cough Stridor Hoarseness Dyspnea Restlessness Symptoms waken child Symptoms disappear during day Tends to recur	URI Croupy cough Stridor Purulent secretions High fever No response to LTB therapy
Treatment	Antibiotics Airway protection	Humidity Racemic epinephrine	Humidity	Antibiotics

to hypoxia, hypercapnia, and acidosis followed by decreased muscular tone, reduced level of consciousness, and, when obstruction becomes more or less complete, a rather sudden death. A presumptive diagnosis of epiglottitis constitutes an emergency.

The child suspected of having epiglottitis should be examined where facilities are available for coping with this type of emergency. Examination of the throat with a tongue depressor is contraindicated until properly experienced personnel and equipment are at hand to proceed with immediate intubation or tracheostomy in the event that the examination precipitates further or complete obstruction.

If a lateral neck film is indicated, the same experienced personnel should accompany the child to the radiology department. Most practitioners prefer that the child not be transported but remain on the parent's lap in the examination area during portable radiology.

Endotracheal intubation or tracheostomy is usually considered for *H. influenzae* epiglottitis with severe respiratory distress. Whether or not there is an artificial airway, the child requires intensive observation by experienced personnel. The epiglottal swelling usually decreases after 24 hours of antibiotic therapy, and the epiglottis is near normal by the third day. Intubated children are generally extubated at this time.

Children with suspected bacterial epiglottitis are given antibiotics intravenously, followed by oral administration to complete a 7- to 10-day course. The use of corticosteroids for reducing edema may be beneficial during the early hours of treatment. Most intubated children will have had a course of corticosteroids for 24 hours before extubation.

Prevention. The American Academy of Pediatrics, Committee on Infectious Diseases (1996b) recommends that beginning at 2 months of age all children receive the *H. influenzae* type B conjugate vaccine. Since administration of the vaccine has become a routine part of the regular immunization schedule, a decline in the incidence of epiglottitis has occurred. Patients now tend to be older and have disease caused by other organisms. (See also Immunizations, Chapter 33.)

Nursing Care Management

Epiglottitis is a serious and frightening disease for the child and family. It is important to act quickly but calmly and provide support without unduly increasing anxiety. The child is allowed to remain in the position that provides the most comfort and security, and parents are reassured that everything possible is being done to obtain relief for their child.

Nursing ALERT

A nurse who suspects epiglottitis should not attempt to visualize the epiglottis directly with a tongue depressor or take a throat culture but should refer the child for medical evaluation immediately. (See Critical Thinking Q & A box above).

Acute care of the child is the same as that described for the child with laryngotracheobronchitis (see p. 1336). Continuous monitoring of respiratory status, including pulse oximetry and blood gases, is part of nursing observations, and the intravenous infusion is maintained as described in Chapter 42.

Critical Thinking Q & A

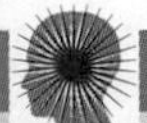

CROUP SYNDROME

Kim, 4 years old, is admitted to the emergency department with a sore throat, pain on swallowing, drooling, and a fever of 39° C (102.2° F). She looks ill, is agitated, and prefers to sit up and lean over. Which of the following medical orders should you question?

1. Obtain a complete blood count (CBC) and throat culture STAT.
2. Place child on oxygen saturation monitor.
3. Start an intravenous (IV) line of 5% dextrose in normal saline solution to run at 30 ml/hr.
4. Have pediatric-size tracheostomy tray available.

The correct answer is one. This child's symptoms suggest epiglottitis. The nurse should question the order for a throat culture because the procedure can precipitate obstruction of the airway. The CBC and other interventions are appropriate.

ACUTE LARYNGITIS

Acute infectious laryngitis is a common illness in older children and adolescents. Infants and smaller children experience more generalized involvement (see following section on laryngotracheobronchitis). Viruses are the usual causative agents, and the principal complaint is hoarseness, which may be accompanied by other upper respiratory symptoms (e.g., coryza, sore throat, nasal congestion) and systemic manifestations (e.g., fever, headache, myalgia, malaise). Associated complaints vary with the infecting virus. Adenoviruses and influenza viruses are responsible for more systemic involvement; parainfluenza viruses, rhinoviruses, and RSV cause more mild illness.

Therapeutic and Nursing Care Management

The disease is almost always self-limited without long-term sequelae. Treatment is symptomatic with fluids and humidified air (see the Nursing Care Plan on p. 1325).

ACUTE LARYNGOTRACHEOBRONCHITIS (LTB)

LTB is the most common of the croup syndromes and primarily affects children younger than 5 years of age. Organisms usually responsible for LTB are the parainfluenza virus RSV, *H. influenzae* type B, and *Mycoplasma pneumoniae.* The disease is usually preceded by an upper respiratory infection, which gradually descends to adjacent structures. It is characterized by gradual onset of low- grade fever.

Inflammation of the mucosa lining the larynx and trachea causes a narrowing of the airway. When the airway is significantly narrowed, the child struggles to inhale air past the obstruction and into the lungs, producing the characteristic inspiratory stridor and suprasternal retractions. The typical child with LTB is a toddler who has the classic barking or seal-like cough and stridor after several days of coryza. When the child is unable to inhale a sufficient volume of air, symptoms of hypoxia become evident. Obstruction that is severe enough to prevent adequate exhalation of carbon dioxide causes res-

BOX 43-9
Progression of Symptoms in Laryngotracheobronchitis

Stage 1
Fear
Hoarseness
Croupy cough
Inspiratory stridor when disturbed

Stage II
Continuous respiratory stridor
Lower rib retraction
Retraction of soft tissue of neck
Use of accessory muscles of respiration
Labored respiration

Stage III
Signs of anoxia and carbon dioxide retention
Restlessness
Anxiety
Pallor
Sweating
Rapid respiration

Stage IV
Intermittent cyanosis
Permanent cyanosis
Cessation of breathing

As described by Forbes. From Krugman S and others: *Infectious diseases of children*, ed 9, St Louis, 1992, Mosby.

piratory acidosis, and eventually the child experiences respiratory failure. (See the progression of symptoms outlined in Box 43-9.)

Therapeutic Management

The major objectives in medical management of infectious LTB are maintaining an airway and providing for adequate respiratory exchange. Children with mild croup (no stridor at rest) are managed at home. Parents are taught the signs of respiratory distress so that professional help can be summoned early if needed. Children who progress to serious respiratory symptoms should receive medical attention, usually with hospitalization.

High humidity with cool mist provides relief for most children. A cool air vaporizer or a steamy bathroom can be used at home. In the hospital setting, hoods for infants or tents for toddlers are sometimes used to provide increased humidity and supplemental oxygen.

Nebulized epinephrine (racemic epinephrine) is often used in children with more severe disease, stridor at rest, retractions, or difficulty in breathing. The α-adrenergic effects cause mucosal vasoconstriction and subsequent decreased subglottic edema. The onset of action is rapid, with detectable clinical improvement within 10 to 15 minutes, although symptoms frequently reappear—typically called "relapse"—within 2 hours. In a significant number of children, however, improvement persists and additional treatments are not necessary.

The use of corticosteroids is beneficial because the antiinflammatory effects decrease subglottic edema. The onset of action is clinically detectable as early as 6 hours after administration, with continued improvement over 12 to 24 hours.

It is essential to allow children with mild croup to continue to drink beverages they like and to encourage parents to try whatever comforting measures work best with their child (e.g., being held, rocked, walked, sung to). If the child is unable to take oral fluids, intravenous fluid therapy may be indicated.

Nursing ALERT

Children with severe respiratory distress (traditionally, for infants with a respiratory rate >60 breaths/min) should not be given anything by mouth to prevent aspiration and decrease the work of breathing.

Nursing Care Management

The most important nursing functions in the care of children with croup are continuous vigilant observation and accurate assessment of respiratory status. Cardiac, respiratory, and noninvasive blood gas monitoring equipment supplement visual observations. Changes in therapy are frequently based on nurses' observations and assessment of a child's status, response to therapy, and tolerance of procedures. The trend away from early intubation of children with LTB emphasizes the importance of nursing observation and the ability to recognize impending respiratory failure so that intubation can be implemented without delay. Intubation equipment should be readily accessible and taken with the child during transport to other areas (e.g., radiology, operating room).

Nursing ALERT

Early signs of impending airway obstruction include increased pulse and respiratory rate; substernal, suprasternal, and intercostal retractions; flaring nares; and increased restlessness.

To conserve energy, children are given every opportunity to rest. Infants or small children find that being enclosed within a tent, coughing, having laryngeal spasms, and needing intravenous therapy are additional sources of distress. Infants and small children prefer sitting upright, and most want to be held. Children need the security of the parent's presence. Since crying increases respiratory distress and hypoxia, a child's individual tolerance for these therapies must be assessed. An extremely fussy child may do better when held in the parent's lap with cool mist directed toward the child's face.

The rapid progression of croup, the alarming sound of the cough and stridor, and the child's apprehensive behavior and ill appearance combine to create a very frightening experience for the parents. They need reassurance regarding the child's progress and an explanation of treatments. They may feel guilty for not having suspected the seriousness of the condition sooner. The family should be allowed to remain with their child as much as possible, especially when this decreases the child's distress.

The nurse can provide the parents with an opportunity to express their feelings, thus minimizing any blame or guilt. They need frequent reassurance provided in a calm, quiet manner and education regarding what they can do to make their child more comfortable. Fortunately, as the crisis subsides and the child responds to therapy, breathing becomes easier and recovery is generally prompt. Home care after discharge includes continued humidity, adequate hydration, and nourishment. Parents are encouraged to ask questions about home care and preparation for discharge. Referral to a public health agency for follow-up care may be advisable.

ACUTE SPASMODIC LARYNGITIS

Acute spasmodic laryngitis (spasmodic croup, "midnight croup," or "twilight croup") is distinct from laryngitis and LTB and is characterized by paroxysmal attacks of laryngeal obstruction that occur chiefly at night. Signs of inflammation are absent or mild, and there is frequently a history of previous attacks lasting 2 to 5 days, followed by uneventful recovery. It usually affects children ages 1 to 3 years. Some children appear to be predisposed to the condition; allergy and psychogenic factors are implicated in some cases.

The child goes to bed well or with some very mild respiratory symptoms but awakes suddenly with characteristic barking, metallic cough, hoarseness, noisy inspirations, and restlessness. The child appears anxious, frightened, and prostrated. Dyspnea is aggravated by excitement, but there is no fever, the attack subsides in a few hours, and the child appears well the next day.

Therapeutic and Nursing Care Management

Children with spasmodic croup are managed at home with cool mist recommended for the child's room. Warm mist provided by steam from hot running water in a closed bathroom may be helpful. Sometimes the spasm is relieved by sudden exposure to cold air (as when the child is taken out into the night air to see the practitioner). Parents are usually advised to have the child sleep in humidified air until the cough has subsided so that subsequent episodes may be prevented. Children with moderately severe symptoms may be hospitalized for observation and therapy with cool mist and racemic epinephrine, as for LTB. Patients may respond to corticosteroid therapy. The disease is usually self-limited.

BACTERIAL TRACHEITIS

Bacterial tracheitis, an infection of the mucosa of the upper trachea, is a distinct entity with features of both croup and epiglottitis. The disease is seen in children ages 1 month to 6 years and may be a serious cause of airway obstruction—severe enough to cause respiratory arrest. It is believed to be a complication of LTB, and although *S. aureus* is the most frequent organism responsible, group A β-hemolytic streptococci and *H. influenzae* have also been implicated.

Many of the manifestations of bacterial tracheitis are similar to those of LTB but are unresponsive to LTB therapy. There is a history of previous upper respiratory infection with croupy cough, stridor unaffected by position, toxicity, and high fever. A prominent manifestation is the production of thick, purulent tracheal secretions. Respiratory difficulties are secondary to these copious secretions.

Therapeutic and Nursing Care Management

Bacterial tracheitis requires vigorous management. Humidified oxygen, antipyretics, and antibiotics are prescribed. Most children require endotracheal intubation and frequent tracheal suctioning to prevent airway obstruction. The emphasis in this disorder is early recognition in order to prevent catastrophic airway obstruction.

Infections of the Lower Airways

The *reactive portion* of the lower respiratory tract includes the bronchi and bronchioles in children. Cartilaginous support of the large airway is not fully developed until adolescence. Consequently, the smooth muscle in these structures represents a major factor in the constriction of the airway, particularly in the bronchioles, that portion that extends from the bronchi to the alveoli. Table 43-2 compares some of the major features of bronchial and bronchiolar infections.

BRONCHITIS

Bronchitis (sometimes referred to as tracheobronchitis) is inflammation of large airways (trachea and bronchi), which is almost invariably associated with an upper respiratory infection. Viral agents are the primary cause of the disease, although *Mycoplasma pneumoniae* is a common cause in children older than 6 years of age. The condition is characterized by a dry, hacking, and nonproductive cough that is worse at night and becomes productive in 2 to 3 days.

Bronchitis is a mild self-limiting disease that requires only symptomatic treatment, including analgesics, antipyretics, and humidity. Cough suppressants may be useful to allow rest but can interfere with clearance of secretions. Most patients recover uneventfully in 5 to 10 days.

RESPIRATORY SYNCYTIAL VIRUS (RSV)/BRONCHIOLITIS

Bronchiolitis is an acute viral infection with maximum effect at the bronchiolar level. The infection occurs primarily in winter and spring and is rare in children over 2 years of age. Although few children with bronchiolitis require hospitalization, it can be a serious disease. RSV is responsible for over half of all episodes of bronchiolitis. It is estimated that RSV is responsible for 90,000 hospitalizations and 4500 deaths in infants and young children each year in United States. Adenoviruses and parainfluenza viruses may also cause acute bronchiolitis. The virus becomes epidemic in communities during the late fall and winter months and is easily spread by hand-to-nose or eye transmission.

Pathophysiology

Bronchiole mucosa is swollen, and lumina are filled with mucus and exudate; the walls of the bronchi and bronchioles are infiltrated with inflammatory cells; peribronchiolar interstitial pneumonitis is usually present. The variable degrees of obstruction produced in small air passages by these changes lead to hyperinflation, obstructive emphysema resulting from

TABLE 43-2 Comparison of conditions affecting the bronchi

	VIRAL-INDUCED ASTHMA*	BRONCHITIS	RESPIRATORY SYNCYTIAL VIRUS (RSV), BRONCHIOLITIS
Description	Exaggerated response of bronchi to infection Bronchospasm, exudation, and edema of bronchi	Usually occurs in association with URI Seldom an isolated entity	A more common infectious disease of lower airways Maximum obstructive impact at bronchiolar level
Age-group affected	Late infancy and early childhood	Affects children in first 4 years of life	Usually children 2-12 months of age; rare after age 2 Peak incidence at approximately age 6 months
Etiologic agents	Most often viruses but may be any of a variety of URI pathogens	Usually viral Other agents (e.g., bacteria, fungi, allergic disorders, airborne irritants) can trigger symptoms	Viruses, predominantly respiratory syncytial viruses; also adenoviruses, parainfluenza viruses, and *Mycoplasma pneumoniae*
Predominant characteristics	Wheezing, productive cough	Persistent dry, hacking cough (worse at night) becoming productive in 2-3 days	Dyspnea, paroxysmal nonproductive cough, tachypnea with retractions and flaring nares, emphysema, may be wheezing
Treatment	Bronchodilators	Cough suppressants if needed	Oxygen mist Ribavirin if severe or in high-risk population

*See Asthma, p. 1347.

partial obstruction, and patchy areas of atelectasis. Dilation of bronchial passages on inspiration allows sufficient space for intake of air, but narrowing of the passages on expiration prevents air from leaving the lungs. Thus air is trapped distal to the obstruction and causes progressive overinflation *(emphysema)*.

Diagnostic Evaluation

Diagnosis of bronchiolitis is made on the basis of clinical findings, child's age, season, and epidemiology of the community. Bronchiolitis begins as a simple URI with serous nasal discharge that may be accompanied by mild fever. Increasing respiratory distress gradually develops with tachypnea, paroxysmal cough, and irritability. There may be wheezing. Chest radiographs show hyperaeration and areas of consolidation that are difficult to differentiate from bacterial pneumonia. Children may have considerable dyspnea but do not have the toxic appearance of children with bacterial infections. See Box 43-10 for signs and symptoms of RSV.

Apnea may be the first recognized indicator of RSV infection in very young infants. Severe disease may be followed by a rise in arterial carbon dioxide tension ($Paco_2$) (hypercapnia), leading to respiratory acidosis and hypoxemia. Positive identification of RSV is accomplished by enzyme-linked immunosorbent assay (ELISA) or rapid immunofluorescent antibody (IFA) from direct aspiration of nasal secretions or nasopharyngeal washings (see Respiratory Secretions Specimens, Chapter 42).

Therapeutic Management

Bronchiolitis is treated symptomatically with high humidity, adequate fluid intake, and rest. Most children with bronchiolitis can be managed at home. Hospitalization is usually recommended for children with complicating conditions, such as underlying lung or heart disease, associated debilitated states, or questionable adequacy of caregiver. The child should also be admitted who is tachypneic, has marked retractions, seems listless, or has a history of poor fluid intake. Mist therapy is generally combined with oxygen by hood or tent in concentrations sufficient to alleviate dyspnea and hypoxia, after

BOX 43-10

Signs and Symptoms of Respiratory Syncytial Virus

Initial

Rhinorrhea
Pharyngitis
Coughing/sneezing
Wheezing
Possible ear infection or eye drainage
Fever

With progression of illness

Increased coughing and wheezing
Air hunger
Tachypnea and retractions
Cyanosis

Severe illness

Tachypnea >70 breaths/min
Listlessness
Apneic spells
Poor air exchange; poor breath sounds

which mist alone is continued for mild dyspnea. Fluids by mouth may be contraindicated because of tachypnea, weakness, and fatigue; therefore intravenous fluids are preferred until the acute crisis of the disease has passed.

Clinical assessments, noninvasive oxygen monitoring, and blood gas values guide therapy. Medical therapy for bronchiolitis is controversial. Bronchodilators, corticosteroids, cough suppressants, and antibiotics have not proved to be effective in uncomplicated disease and are not recommended for routine use. Corticosteroids, theophylline, and furosemide have all been used for intubated and ventilated infants and children.

Ribavirin, an antiviral agent, may be used to treat RSV infection. The drug is delivered via hood, tent, or mask. Since the use of the drug is controversial, infection with RSV is usually self-limiting, the drug is very expensive, and recent studies failed to show a significant decrease in mortality when ribavirin was used; the Committee on Infectious Diseases of the American Academy of Pediatrics (1996A) now recommends that ribavirin aerosol therapy be considered for:

1. Infants at high risk for severe or complicated RSV infection (i.e., infants with complicated congenital heart disease, bronchopulmonary dysplasia, cystic fibrosis, and other chronic lung disease. Some preterm infants (less than 37 weeks); and infants younger than 6 weeks of age
2. Infants hospitalized with RSV lower respiratory tract disease who are severely ill with or without mechanical ventilation
3. Infants hospitalized with lower respiratory tract disease that is not initially severe, but who may be at some increased risk of progressing to a more complicated course (e.g., less than 6 weeks of age or those in whom prolonged illness might be particularly detrimental, such as multiple congenital anomalies, or neurologic or metabolic disease)
4. Infants with underlying immunosuppressive diseases or therapy such as acquired immunodeficiency syndrome, severe combined immunodeficiency disease, or organ transplantation who have a high mortality rate and/or prolonged RSV illness

Prognosis. The disease lasts about 3 to 10 days, and the prognosis is generally good. Although most infants with RSV bronchiolitis appear to recover completely, severe disease is associated with recurrent pulmonary infection and bronchospasm. Infants with preexisting cardiopulmonary disease may have an increased incidence of death related to RSV infection. The recent development and use of an RSV immune globulin in combination with ribavirin have the potential for significantly decreasing RSV morbidity and mortality rates.

Nursing Care Management

Children admitted to the hospital with suspected RSV infection may be assigned separate rooms or grouped with other RSV-infection children over age 2 years. A variety of infection control procedures have been employed over the years, the most important of which are consistent handwashing and not touching the nasal mucosa or conjunctiva. The routine use of gowns and masks has not been shown to be of additional benefit, although gowns may help diminish the potential for fomite spread during close contact when infectious secretions may contaminate clothing. Other isolation procedures of potential benefit are those aimed at diminishing the number of hospital personnel, visitors, and uninfected patients in contact with the child. Another measure includes making patient assignments so that nurses assigned to children with RSV are not taking care of other patients who may be considered high risk.

Patient care sometimes warrants opening the tent while the small-particle aerosol generator (SPAG) is still running; in these cases it is recommended that one first shut off the machine and wait a few moments before opening the tent. Gloves and gowns are not essential, since dermal absorption appears to be negligible. Scavenger devices are commercially available to help decrease the escape of aerosolized ribavirin.

Nursing ALERT

Pregnant health care providers should avoid caring for a child receiving ribavirin.

PNEUMONIAS

Pneumonia, inflammation of the pulmonary parenchyma, is common throughout childhood but occurs more frequently in infancy and early childhood. Clinically, pneumonia may occur either as a primary disease or as a complication of some other illness. Morphologically, pneumonias are recognized as follows:

Lobar pneumonia—all or a large segment of one or more pulmonary lobes is involved. When both lungs are affected, it is known as bilateral or "double" pneumonia.

Bronchopneumonia—begins in the terminal bronchioles, which become clogged with mucopurulent exudate to form consolidated patches in nearby lobules; also called lobular pneumonia.

Interstitial pneumonia—the inflammatory process is more or less confined within the alveolar walls (interstitium) and the peribronchial and interlobular tissues.

Pneumonitis is a localized acute inflammation of the lung without the toxemia associated with lobar pneumonia.

The pneumonias are more often classified according to morphological characteristics, clinical form, and causative agent: viral, atypical (mycoplasma), bacterial, or aspiration of foreign substances (see p. 1345). Less often pneumonia may be caused by histomycosis, coccidioidomycosis, and other fungi. The causative agent is identified largely from the clinical history, the child's age, the general health history, the physical examination, radiography, and the laboratory examination.

Viral Pneumonia

Viral pneumonias occur more frequently than bacterial pneumonias and are seen in children of all age groups. They are often associated with viral URIs, and RSV accounts for the largest percentage in infants. There are few clinical symptoms to distinguish between the responsible organisms, and differentiations between viruses can be made only by laboratory examination. See Box 43-11 for clinical manifestations.

The prognosis is generally good, although viral infections

BOX 43-11

Clinical Manifestations of Viral and Atypical Pneumonias

Viral pneumonia	Atypical pneumonia
May be acute or insidious Symptoms variable *Mild:* low-grade fever, slight cough, malaise *Severe:* high fever, severe cough, prostration Cough usually unproductive early in disease A few wheezes or crackles heard on auscultation	May be sudden or insidious General systemic symptoms: Fever Chills (older children) Headache Malaise Anorexia Myalgia Followed by: Rhinitis Sore throat Dry, hacking cough Nonproductive early, then seromucoid sputum, to mucopurulent or blood streaked Fine crepitant rales over various lung areas

of the respiratory tract render the affected child more susceptible to secondary bacterial invasion, especially when there is denuded bronchial mucosa. Treatment is usually symptomatic and includes measures to promote oxygenation and comfort, such as oxygen administration with cool mist, chest physiotherapy and postural drainage, antipyretics for fever management, fluid intake, and family support. Although some authorities recommend antimicrobial therapy in the hope of reducing or preventing secondary bacterial infection, it is usually reserved for children in whom the presence of such infection is demonstrated by appropriate cultures.

Primary Atypical Pneumonia

Approximately 10% to 20% of hospital admissions of children with pneumonia are caused by *M. pneumoniae.* It occurs principally in the fall and winter months and is more prevalent where there are crowded living conditions. See Box 43-11 for outline of clinical manifestations.

Most affected people recover from acute illness in 7 to 10 days with symptomatic treatment followed by a week of convalescence. Hospitalization is rarely necessary.

Bacterial Pneumonia

In children beyond the neonatal period, bacterial pneumonias display distinct clinical patterns that facilitate their differentiation from other forms of pneumonia, and individual microorganisms produce a distinct clinical picture. Onset is abrupt and is generally preceded by a viral infection that disturbs the natural defense mechanisms of the upper respiratory tract and allows the pathogenic bacteria normally harbored in the upper passages to increase in number.

Children with bacterial pneumonia appear ill and exhibit both general and localized physical findings. Symptoms and signs include fever, malaise, rapid and shallow respirations, cough, and chest pain that is often exaggerated by deep breathing. The pain may be referred to the abdomen and confused with appendicitis. Chills frequently occur, and meningeal symptoms (meningism) are also common. Pleural reactions and effusions often accompany the disease, and the consolidation process usually proceeds rapidly.

The majority of older children with pneumococcal pneumonia can be treated at home, especially if the condition is recognized and treatment initiated early. Antibiotic therapy, bed rest, liberal oral intake of fluid, and administration of an antipyretic for fever and an antitussive for dry, hacking cough constitute the principal therapeutic measures. Hospitalization is indicated when pleural effusion or empyema accompanies the disease and is mandatory for children with staphylococcal pneumonia. Pneumonia in the infant or young child is best treated in the hospital, since the course of illness is more variable and complications are more common in very young patients. Fluids are usually given intravenously, and oxygen therapy may be required if the child is in respiratory distress.

At the present time the classic features and clinical course of pneumonia are rarely seen because of early and vigorous antibiotic and supportive therapy. However, in a large number of children, especially infants, with staphylococcal pneumonia, empyema, pyopneumothorax, or tension pneumothorax develops. Pleural effusion is not uncommon in children with lobar (pneumococcal) pneumonia. A thoracentesis may be performed to remove fluid in the pleural cavity, to obtain a culture of the fluid, and to instill antibiotics directly into the pleural space. Nonpurulent effusions, such as occur in pneumococcal pneumonia, do not require surgical drainage. Continuous closed-chest drainage is instituted when purulent fluid is aspirated, a frequent finding in staphylococcal infections.

Prognosis. The prognosis for pneumococcal infections is generally good, with rapid recovery when they are recognized and treated early. Streptococcal infections vary in duration but usually resolve spontaneously. The course of staphylococcal pneumonia is generally prolonged. The prognosis varies with the length of illness before treatment is begun, although early recognition and treatment are usually effective. Complications of bacterial pneumonia include pleural effusion, empyema, and tension pneumothorax.

Prevention. Use of pneumococcal polysaccharide vaccine is recommended for selected individuals such as children over age 2 years who are at risk of acquiring pneumococcal infection or are at risk of serious disease. (See Immunizations, Chapter 33). The infant or child with recurrent pneumonias should be further evaluated for cystic fibrosis.

Nursing Care Management

Nursing care of the child with pneumonia is primarily supportive and symptomatic but necessitates thorough respiratory assessment and administration of oxygen and antibiotics. The child's respiratory rate and status, as well as general disposition and level of activity, are frequently assessed.

Isolation procedures are instituted according to hospital policy; rest and conservation of energy are encouraged by relief of physical and psychologic stress. The child is disturbed as little as possible by clustering care to encourage the child's regular sleep cycle. If the cough is disturbing, judicious use of antitussives, especially before rest times and meals, is often helpful. To prevent dehydration, fluids are frequently administered intravenously during the acute phase. Oral fluids, if allowed, are given cautiously to prevent aspiration and to decrease the possibility of aggravating a fatiguing cough.

Children may be placed in a mist tent with oxygen. Cool mist moistens the airways and provides a cool atmosphere that aids in temperature reduction. Children often require frequent clothing and linen changes to prevent chilling in the damp atmosphere. They are usually more comfortable in a semierect position but should be allowed to determine the position of comfort. Lying on the affected side (if pneumonia is unilateral) splints the chest on that side and reduces the pleural rubbing that often causes discomfort. Fever is usually controlled by administration of antipyretic drugs as prescribed, and temperature is monitored regularly.

Vital signs and breath sounds are monitored to assess the progress of the disease and to detect early signs of complications. Children with ineffectual cough or those with difficulty handling secretions, especially infants, will require suctioning to maintain a patent airway. A simple bulb syringe is usually sufficient for clearing the nares and nasopharynx of infants, but mechanical suction should be readily available if needed. Older children can usually handle secretions without assistance. Postural drainage and chest physiotherapy are generally prescribed every 4 hours or more often, depending on the child's condition.

The hospitalized child is apprehensive, and many of the treatments and tests are frightening and stress producing. Reducing anxiety and apprehension reduces psychologic distress in the child, and when the child is more relaxed, the respiratory efforts are lessened. Easing respiratory efforts makes the child less apprehensive, and encouraging the presence of the caregiver provides the child with a customary source of comfort and support.

The family also needs support. The child's dry, hacking cough can be tiring for the parents because it often disturbs the child's and family's sleep. Parents are kept informed of the child's progress and taught appropriate home care, such as use of a nasal aspirator and administration of antibiotics.*

Other Infections of the Respiratory Tract

PERTUSSIS (WHOOPING COUGH)

Pertussis (whooping cough) is an acute respiratory infection caused by *Bordetella pertussis* that occurs chiefly in children younger than 4 years of age who have not been immunized. It is highly contagious and is particularly threatening in young infants, in whom there are higher morbidity and mortality rates. (See Table 35-2 for signs, symptoms, and management of pertussis and Chapter 33 for immunization.) The incidence is highest in the spring and summer months, and a single attack confers lifetime immunity. Pertussis vaccine is effective, but the immunity diminishes with time after the initial infection or immunization. In a small number of immunized adolescents an asymptomatic case of pertussis may develop.

*Home care instructions for administration of medication and nasal aspiration are available in Wong DL: *Wong and Whaley's clinical manual of pediatric nursing*, ed 4, St Louis, 1996, Mosby.

TUBERCULOSIS (TB)

TB is an ancient disease that, although controlled in most developed countries, remains a health hazard and a leading cause of death throughout many parts of the world. After decades of steady decline in the United States, the incidence of TB is increasing. The age-group affected most is adults between ages 25 and 44, but the disease has also increased significantly in children (Jackson, 1993). The increases are attributed in part to the interaction of foreign-born persons emigrating to the United States, the rise in homelessness, and the human immunodeficiency virus (HIV) epidemic (Hoffman, Kelly, and Futterman, 1996).

TB is caused by *Mycobacterium tuberculosis.* Children are susceptible to both the human *(M. tuberculosis)* and the bovine (*M. bovis*) organisms, and in parts of the world where tuberculosis in cattle is not controlled or pasteurization of milk is not practiced, the bovine type is a common source of infection in children. Although the causative agent is the tubercle bacillus, other factors influence the degree to which the organism is able to produce an altered state in the host, including heredity (resistance to the infection may be genetically transmitted), sex (higher in adolescent girls), age (lower resistance in infants; higher incidence during adolescence), stress (emotional or physical), nutritional state, and intercurrent infection (especially measles and pertussis). Currently, infection with HIV is the most important risk factor for TB infection progression to active disease.

The source of infection in children is, in most situations, an infected adult or a teenager, usually a member of the household. It can also be a baby-sitter, domestic worker, or frequent visitor to the household. The lung is the usual portal of entry in human beings; the organism enters less often by ingestion. In the lungs a proliferation of epithelial cells surround and encapsulate the multiplying bacilli in an attempt to wall off the invading organisms, thus forming the typical tubercle. Extension of the primary lesion at the original site causes progressive tissue destruction as it spreads within the lung, discharges material from foci to other areas of the lungs (e.g., bronchi or pleura), or produces pneumonia. Erosion of blood vessels by the primary lesion can cause widespread dissemination of the tubercle bacillus to near and distant sites (miliary tuberculosis). Areas that are frequently affected include lymph nodes, meninges, and bone.

Diagnostic Evaluation

Several tests and procedures are used to establish a diagnosis. Diagnosis is based on information derived from physical examination, history, reaction to tuberculin tests, radiographic examinations, and organism cultures (Box 43-12). In addition, it must be determined whether or not the lesion is in the active, quiescent, or healed stage.

The **tuberculin test** is the most important test to determine whether a child has been infected with the tubercle bacillus. The recommended procedure is the **Mantoux test,** which uses purified protein derivative (PPD).

The standard dose is 5 tuberculin units in 0.1 ml of solution, injected intradermally. Recommendations for TB skin

BOX 43-12
Clinical Manifestations of Tuberculosis

Extremely variable
May be asymptomatic or produce a broad range of symptoms:
- Fever
- Malaise
- Anorexia
- Weight loss
- Cough may or may not be present (progresses slowly over weeks to months)
- Aching pain and tightness in the chest
- Hemoptysis (rare)

With progression:
- Respiratory rate increases
- Poor expansion of lung on the affected side
- Diminished breath sounds and rales
- Dullness to percussion
- Fever persists
- Generalized symptoms are manifested
- Development of pallor, anemia, weakness, and weight loss

testing of children are listed in Box 43-13. Routine testing of children with no risk factors residing in communities with a low prevalence of TB is not indicated (American Academy of Pediatrics, 1996c).

A *positive reaction* indicates that the individual has been infected and a sensitivity to the protein of the tubercle bacillus has developed; however, it does not confirm the presence of active disease. Once individuals have a positive reaction, they will always have a positive reaction. A previously negative reaction that becomes positive indicates that the person has been infected since the last test. Guidelines for interpreting the Mantoux skin test are listed in Box 43-14.

Nursing ALERT

The American Academy of Pediatrics (1996c) recommends that Mantoux skin test results be read by health care professionals.

Therapeutic Management

Medical management of tuberculous lesions in children consists of adequate nutrition, chemotherapy, general supportive measures, prevention of unnecessary exposure to other infections that further compromise the body's defenses, prevention

BOX 43-13
Revised Tuberculin Skin Test Recommendations*

Children for whom immediate skin testing is indicated
- Contacts of persons with confirmed or suspected infectious tuberculosis (contact investigation); this includes children identified as contacts of family members or associates in jail or prison in the last 5 y
- Children with radiographic or clinical findings suggesting tuberculosis
- Children immigrating from endemic countries (eg, Asia, Middle East, Africa, Latin America)
- Children with history of travel to endemic countries and/or significant contact with indigenous persons from such countries

Children who should be tested annually for tuberculosis†
- Children infected with HIV
- Incarcerated adolescents

Children who should be tested every 2-3 y†
- Children exposed to the following individuals: HIV infected, homeless, residents of nursing homes, institutionalized adolescents or adults, users of illicit drugs, incarcerated adolescents or adults, and migrant farm workers; this would include foster children with exposure to adults in the high-risk groups

Children who should be considered for tuberculin skin testing at ages 4-6 and 11-16 y
- Children whose parents immigrated (with unknown tuberculin skin test status) from regions of the world with high prevalence of tuberculosis; continued potential exposure by travel to the endemic areas and/or household contact with persons from the endemic areas (with unknown tuberculin skin test status) should be an indication for repeat tuberculin skin testing
- Children without specific risk factors who reside in high-prevalence areas; in general, a high-risk neighborhood or community does not mean an entire city is at high risk; it is recognized that rates in any area of the city may vary by neighborhood, or even from block to block; physicians should be aware of these patterns in determining the likelihood of exposure; public health officials or local tuberculosis experts should help clinicians identify areas that have appreciable tuberculosis rates

Risk for progression to disease
- Children with other medical risk factors, including diabetes mellitus, chronic renal failure, malnutrition, and congenital or acquired immunodeficiencies deserve special consideration; without recent exposure, these persons are not at increased risk of acquiring tuberculous infection; underlying immune deficiencies associated with these conditions theoretically would enhance the possibility for progression to severe disease; initial histories of potential exposure to tuberculosis should be included on all of these patients; if these histories or local epidemiologic factors suggest a possibility of exposure, immediate and periodic tuberculin skin testing should be considered in these patients; an initial Mantoux tuberculin skin test should be performed before initiation of immunosuppressive therapy in any child with an underlying condition that necessitates immunosuppressive therapy

From American Academy of Pediatrics, Committee on Infectious Diseases; Update on tuberculosis skin testing of children, *Pediatrics* 97(2):282-284, 1996.
*Bacille Calmette-Guérin (BCG) immunization is not a contraindication to tuberculin skin testing.
†Initial tuberculin skin testing initiated at the time of diagnosis or circumstance.

BOX 43-14

Definition of Positive Mantoux Skin Test (5 TU-PPD) in Children*

Reaction ≥5 mm

Children in close contact with persons who have known or suspected infectious cases of tuberculosis
- Households with active or previously active cases if (1) treatment cannot be verified as adequate before exposure, (2) treatment was initiated after period of child's contact, or (3) reactivation is suspected

Children suspected to have tuberculosis disease
- Chest roentgenogram consistent with active or previously active tuberculosis
- Clinical evidence of tuberculosis

Children with immunosuppressive conditions† or HIV infection

Reaction ≥10 mm

Children at increased risk of dissemination
- Young age: less than 4 years of age
- Other medical risk factors, including Hodgkin disease, lymphoma, diabetes mellitus, chronic renal failure, and malnutrition

Children with increased environmental exposure
- Born, or whose parents were born, in regions of the world where tuberculosis is highly prevalent
- Frequently exposed to adults who are HIV infected, homeless, users of intravenous and other street drugs, poor and medically indigent city dwellers, residents of nursing homes, incarcerated or institutionalized persons, and migrant farm workers

Reaction ≥ 15mm

Children 4 years of age or older without any risk factors

From American Academy of Pediatrics, Committee on Infectious Diseases: Update on tuberculin skin testing of children, *Pediatrics* 97(2):282-284, 1996.
*These recommendations should apply regardless of whether Bacille Calmette-Guérin (BCG) has been previously administered.
†Including immunosuppressive doses of corticosteroids.

of reinfection, and sometimes surgical procedures. Hospitalization, except in acute illness, is usually only required for diagnostic tests, to obtain culture material, to ascertain tolerance and compliance with medication, to investigate household contacts for exposure, to identify and initiate treatment for the index case, and to remove active sources from the environment before returning the child to the home.

Chemotherapy. Chemotherapy is the most important therapeutic modality available for management of tuberculosis. A variety of chemical agents can be employed, and a regimen involving two or more drugs simultaneously has been found to be effective and is usually the mode of choice. The most commonly used combinations of drugs are isoniazid (INH) and rifampin, with the optional addition of pyrazinamide (PZA). Either a 6-month or a 9-month treatment regimen may be used. In either regimen, INH and rifampin are continued for at least 6 months after conversion of cultures. The HIV-infected child may require drug therapy for up to 12 months.

Surgical procedures. Surgery may be required to remove the source of infection in tissues that are inaccessible to chemotherapy or that are destroyed by the disease. Orthopaedic operations for correction of bone deformities, bronchoscopy for removal of a tuberculous granulomatous polyp, or resection of a portion of a diseased lung may also be performed.

Prognosis. Most children recover from primary tuberculosis infection and are often unaware of its presence. However, very young children have a higher incidence of disseminated disease. It is a serious disease during the first 2 years of life , during adolescence, and in children who are HIV-positive. Except in cases of tuberculous meningitis, death seldom occurs in treated children. Antibiotic therapy has decreased the death rate and the hematogenous spread from primary lesions.

Prevention. The only certain means to prevent TB is to avoid contact with the tubercle bacillus. Maintaining an optimum state of health with adequate nutrition and avoidance of fatigue and debilitating infections promotes natural resistance but does not prevent infection.

Limited immunity can be produced by administration of the only successful vaccine to date, *bacillus Calmette-Guérin (BCG)*, a vaccine containing bovine bacilli with reduced virulence. The freshly prepared vaccine, injected intradermally, produces definite although incomplete (about 50%) protection against tuberculosis. The distribution of the vaccine is controlled by local or state health departments, but the vaccine is not used extensively, even in areas with a high prevalence of disease. Greater protection is afforded by daily prophylactic administration of INH. The drug is given to children with a positive tuberculin test result but no evidence of active disease.

Nursing Care Management

Most children with pulmonary TB almost always have noninfectious disease; therefore they seldom need to be isolated. There are few bacilli in the sputum, the amount of sputum produced is quite small, and sputum is swallowed rather than expectorated. Hospitalization is seldom necessary except for needed diagnostic tests; most children are managed satisfactorily at home. Therefore the major nursing care of children with TB is administered in ambulatory settings—outpatient departments, schools, and especially public health agencies.

Asymptomatic children are able to lead an essentially unrestricted life. They can, and should, attend school (or preschool), but older children are restricted from vigorous activities such as competitive games and contact sports during the active stage of primary tuberculosis. They should be protected from stresses, including parental anxieties, the tendency toward overprotection, and pressures regarding nutritional intake. The regular immunization schedule should be continued. Care should be exerted to maintain an optimum health status with proper diet, adequate rest, and avoidance of infection.

Nurses assume several important roles in management of the disease, including assisting with radiographic examinations, performing skin tests, and obtaining specimens for laboratory examination. Sputum specimens are difficult or impossible to obtain in an infant or young child, since they swallow any mucus coughed from the lower respiratory tract.

Therefore the best means for obtaining material for smears or culture is gastric washing (i.e., aspiration of lavaged contents from the fasting stomach). The procedure is carried out and the specimen obtained early in the morning before the customary breakfast time. Because the success of therapy depends on compliance with the drug regimen, parents are instructed regarding the importance of giving the medication as often and for as long as it is ordered (see Compliance, Chapter 42).

Pulmonary Dysfunction Caused by Noninfectious Irritants

FOREIGN BODY (FB) ASPIRATION

Small children characteristically explore matter with their mouths and are therefore particularly prone to aspirate an FB into the air passages. Aspiration of an FB can occur at any age but is most commonly seen in children under 3 years of age. The signs and changes produced depend on the degree of obstruction and the nature of the foreign body. For example, dry vegetable matter, such as a seed, nut, or piece of carrot or popcorn, that does not dissolve and that may swell when wet creates a particularly difficult problem. The high fat content of potato chips and peanuts may cause the added risk of lipoid pneumonia. "Fun foods" of any kind are among the worst offenders. Offending foods in the order of frequency of aspiration are as follows: hot dog, round candy, peanut or other nut, grape, cookie or biscuit, other meat, carrot, apple, and peanut butter.

Round foods are the most frequent offenders. The first four items together contribute more than 40% of all specified food items. A sharp or irritating object produces irritation and edema. A round, pliable object that does not readily break apart is more likely to occlude an airway than an object with a different shape. Balloons are especially hazardous. A small object may cause little if any pathologic change, whereas an object of sufficient size to obstruct a passage can produce various changes, including atelectasis, emphysema, inflammation, and abscess.

Diagnostic Evaluation

The diagnosis of FB aspiration is usually suspected on the basis of the history and physical signs. Initially a foreign body in the air passages produces choking, gagging, wheezing, or coughing. After the initial period there is often an interval of hours, days, or even weeks without symptoms. Secondary symptoms are related to the anatomic area in which the object is lodged and are usually caused by a persistent respiratory infection focused distal to the obstruction. An FB is always a possibility in acute or chronic pulmonary lesions. Often, by the time secondary symptoms appear, the parents have forgotten the initial episode of coughing and gagging.

The most common symptoms observed in children brought to medical attention are stridor, wheezing, sternal retraction, and cough. When the object is lodged in the larynx, there is inability to speak or breathe. An object in the bronchi produces cough, decreased airway entry, wheezing, and dyspnea. A nonobstructive, nonirritating object may cause few symptoms; an obstructive object quickly produces pathologic changes; a slight obstruction may be evidenced only by a wheeze.

Radiographic examination reveals opaque FBs but may be of limited use in localizing vegetable matter. Bronchoscopy is usually required for definitive diagnosis of an object in the larynx and trachea. Fluoroscopic examination is a valuable aid in detecting and localizing an object in the bronchi.

Therapeutic Management

FB aspiration may result in life-threatening airway obstruction, especially in infants because of the small diameters of their airways. Current recommendations for the emergency treatment of the choking child include the use of abdominal thrusts for children over 1 year of age and back blows and chest thrusts for children less than 1 year of age (see Cardiopulmonary Resuscitation, p. 1362).

An FB is rarely coughed up spontaneously; therefore it must be removed instrumentally by direct laryngoscopy or bronchoscopy. This should be carried out as soon as possible, since the progressive local inflammatory process triggered by the foreign material hampers removal, a chemical pneumonia soon develops, and vegetable matter begins to macerate within a few days, causing it to be even more difficult to remove. After removal of the FB, the child is placed in a high-humidity atmosphere and any secondary infection is treated with appropriate antibiotics.

Nursing Care Management

A major role of nurses caring for a child who has aspirated an FB is to recognize the signs of FB aspiration and implement immediate measures to relieve the obstruction.

All persons working with children should be prepared to deal effectively with aspiration of an FB. Choking on food or other material should not be fatal. Two very simple procedures, back blows and the Heimlich maneuver, which can be used by both health professionals and lay persons, can save lives. It is the obligation of nurses to learn the techniques and teach them to parents and other groups. (Fig. 43-6, *I-K*).

To aid a child who is choking, nurses need to recognize the signs of distress. Not every child who gags or coughs while eating is truly choking.

Nursing ALERT

The child in distress (1) *cannot speak*, (2) *becomes cyanotic*, and (3) *collapses*. These three signs indicate that the child is truly choking and requires immediate and quick action. The child can die within 4 minutes. Follow-up care after the foreign body is removed includes chest physiotherapy as indicated, monitoring for respiratory distress, and education of the parents.

Prevention. Small children should not be allowed access to enticing small objects that they might place in the mouth. Rubber balloons are high-risk items for children; Mylar balloons are the only safe variety for children. Unlikely items (foil tabs from soft drink containers, Band-Aids applied to fingers of infants or very small children, plastic tabs from protective coverings on containers and from price tags on clothing) can be hazardous. Peanut butter, a staple in the diet of children, should never be given to a child unless it is spread thinly on bread or a cracker. A spoonful of peanut butter can obstruct the airway and stick to mucous membranes, becoming difficult or impossible for the child to dislodge.

Nurses, as child advocates, are in a position to teach prevention in a variety of settings. They can educate parents singly or in groups about hazards of aspiration in relation to the developmental level of their children and encourage them to teach their children safety. Parents teach by example; therefore, they should be cautioned about behaviors that their children might imitate, for example, holding foreign objects, such as pins, nails, and toothpicks, in their lips or mouth. Prevention based on the child's age is discussed in Chapters 33 and 34.

ASPIRATION PNEUMONIA

Aspiration of fluid or food substances is a particular hazard in the child who has difficulty with swallowing or is unable to swallow because of paralysis, weakness, debility, congenital anomalies, or absent cough reflex, or who is force fed, especially while crying or breathing rapidly. In addition to fluids, food, vomitus, and nasopharyngeal secretions, other substances that cause pneumonia are hydrocarbons, lipids, talcum powder, and barium.

Nursing Care Management

Care of the child with aspiration pneumonia is the same as that described for the child with pneumonia from other causes. However, the major thrust of nursing care is aimed at prevention of aspiration. Proper feeding techniques should be carried out for weak, debilitated, and uncooperative children, and preventive measures are used to prevent aspiration of any material that might enter the nasopharynx.

Oily nose drops and oil-based vitamin preparations are not appropriate for infants and small children. Solvents, lighter fluid, and other hydrocarbon substances should be kept away from older infants and small children, who are likely to put anything in their mouths and who may be attracted by the slightly sweet smell. Talcum powder should not be used; if it is used, careful application (placing it on the caregiver's hand and then the child's skin) and proper storage are essential.

Infants and debilitated children should be positioned on the abdomen or the right side after feedings to minimize the possibility of aspirating vomitus or regurgitated feeding. Nurses play a major role in education for injury prevention (see Injury Prevention, Chapters 33 and 34).

ADULT RESPIRATORY DISTRESS SYNDROME (ARDS)

ARDS is now recognized in children as well as in adults and poses a major threat to a child recovering from a primary insult. It is characterized by respiratory distress and hypoxemia that occur within 72 hours of a serious injury or surgery in a person with previously normal lungs. It is a syndrome and not a disease; shock is the most common event associated with the onset of the syndrome.

The hallmark of ARDS is increased permeability of the alveolar-capillary membrane that results in pulmonary edema. The lungs become stiff, gas diffusion is impaired, and eventually bronchiolar mucosal swelling and congestive atelectasis occur. Surfactant secretion is reduced, and the atelectasis and fluid-filled alveoli provide an excellent medium for bacterial growth. The criteria for diagnosis of ARDS in children are an acute antecedent illness or injury, acute respiratory distress or failure, no evidence of prior cardiopulmonary disease, and diffuse bilateral infiltrates evidenced on chest radiography.

Treatment involves general supportive measures, such as prevention of infection, maintenance of vascular pressure and cardiac output, adequate nutrition, comfort measures, positioning to improve functional residual capacity, and psychologic support. Definitive therapy is primarily directed toward improvement of oxygenation. Recent developments in the treatment of ARDS include (1) medications to interrupt the formation or activation of mediators contributing to progression of intrapulmonary shunting and lung injury, such as nonsteroidal antiinflammatory drugs (NSAIDs); (2) immunotherapy with monocolonal antibodies that work against the specific toxins causing the lung injury; and (3) human and artificial surfactant to reduce the severity of and sequelae from RDS which may be useful in treating lung disease associated with ARDS and near-drowning.

The prognosis for ARDS varies. Some children recover completely, whereas others are left with varying degrees of pulmonary dysfunction.

Nursing care involves careful monitoring of cardiac output, heart rate, perfusion, capillary filling, and urine output, as well as assessment of respiratory status. Blood gas analysis and pulse oximetry are important evaluation tools. Respiratory distress is a frightening situation for both the child and the parents, and attention to their psychologic needs is a major element in the care of these children.

INHALATION INJURY: SMOKE AND CARBON MONOXIDE

A number of noxious substances that may be inhaled are toxic to humans. They are primarily products of incomplete combustion and are believed to cause more deaths from fires than do flame injuries. The severity of the injury depends on the nature of the substances generated by the material being burned and whether the victim is confined in a closed space. Inhaled substances produce injuries (1) locally by irritation, inflammation, and damage to pulmonary tissues or (2) systemically.

Local Injury

A wide variety of gases may be generated during the combustion of materials such as clothing, furniture, and floor coverings. The synthetic materials are especially toxic. Irritant gases such as nitrous oxide or carbon dioxide combine with water in the lungs to form corrosive acids; aldehydes cause denaturation of proteins, cellular damage, and edema of pulmonary tissues.

Possible inhalation injury is suspected when there is a history of flames in a closed space whether burns are present or not. Sooty material around the nose or in the sputum, singed nasal hairs, or mucosal burns of the nose, lips, mouth, or throat are all signs that the affected person demands observation for possible pulmonary injury from inhalants. A hoarse voice and cough, inspiratory and expiratory stridor, and signs of respiratory distress are further evidence of airway involvement.

Systemic Injury

Gases that are nontoxic to the airways (e.g., carbon monoxide [CO] and hydrogen cyanide) can cause injury and death by interfering with or inhibiting cellular respiration. CO is an extremely dangerous gas and is responsible for more than half of all fatal inhalation poisonings in the United States. It is a colorless, odorless gas with an affinity for hemoglobin (Hb) 230 times greater than that of oxygen. When it enters the bloodstream, CO combines readily with hemoglobin to form carboxyhemoglobin but is released less readily. Therefore tissue hypoxia reaches dangerous levels before oxygen is available to meet tissue needs.

Nursing ALERT

The oxygen saturation (Sao_2) obtained by pulse oximetry will be normal because the device measures only oxygenated and deoxygenated hemoglobin; it does not measure dysfunctional hemoglobin, such as COHb.

Accidental carbon monoxide poisoning is most often the result of exposure to fumes of heaters or smoke from structural fires, although poorly ventilated recreational vehicles with improperly operated or maintained gas lamps or stoves and cooking in underventilated areas with charcoal grills or hibachis are also frequent causes. CO is produced by incomplete combustion of carbon or carbonaceous material such as wood or charcoal.

The signs and symptoms of CO poisoning are secondary to tissue hypoxia and vary with the level of carboxyhemoglobin. Mild manifestations may produce headache, visual disturbances, irritability, and nausea, whereas more severe intoxication causes confusion, hallucinations, ataxia, and coma. The bright, cherry-red lips and skin often described are less often observed; pallor and cyanosis are seen more frequently.

Therapeutic Management

When smoke inhalation injury is suspected, the patient is given humidified 100% oxygen by mask, and blood is drawn to determine baseline arterial blood gases and COHb levels. Surprisingly, arterial oxygen partial pressure may be within normal limits unless there is marked respiratory depression. If CO poisoning is confirmed, 100% oxygen is continued until COHb levels fall to the nontoxic range of about 10%, and artificial ventilation may be implemented in selected cases. Where a hyperbaric oxygen chamber is available, the breakdown of the CO-hemoglobin bond is greatly accelerated.

Respiratory distress may occur early in the course of smoke inhalation as a result of hypoxia, or patients who are breathing well on admission may later experience sudden respiratory distress. Therefore intubation and/or tracheostomy equipment should be available at the bedside. More often distress is related to transient edema of the airways, which can occur at any level in the tracheobronchial tree. Assessment and localization of the obstruction should be accomplished before severe swelling of the head, neck, or oropharynx occurs. Intubation is often necessary when (1) severe burns in the area of the nose, mouth, and face increase the likelihood of development of oropharyngeal edema and obstruction; (2) vocal cord edema causes obstruction; (3) the patient has difficulty handling secretions; and (4) progressive respiratory distress requires artificial ventilation. There is a good deal of controversy regarding tracheostomy, but many prefer this procedure when the obstruction is proximal to the larynx and reserve nasotracheal intubation for lower tract involvement.

Use of corticosteroids, although controversial, may be of value in reducing edema, and bronchodilators (usually isoproterenol) are often given intravenously or by nebulizer. A broad-spectrum antibiotic is sometimes administered prophylactically, but this, too, is controversial.

Nursing Care Management

Nursing care of the child with inhalation injury is the same as that for any child with respiratory distress. Vital signs and other respiratory assessments are performed frequently, and the pulmonary status is carefully observed and maintained. Pulmonary physiotherapy is usually part of the therapeutic program, as is mechanical ventilation if needed.

In addition to the observation and management of the physical aspects of inhalation injury, the nurse deals with the psychologic needs of a frightened child and distraught parents. As with any accidental injury, the parents feel overwhelming guilt, even when the injury occurred through no fault of their own. More often, however, the injury could have been prevented, and that fact compounds their guilt feelings. They need a great deal of support, reassurance, and information regarding the child's condition, treatment, and progress.

PASSIVE SMOKING

Numerous researchers have investigated the effects of environmental pollution on children's health and have determined that the worst pollutant is parental smoking, especially maternal smoking. Children exposed to environmental tobacco smoke have an increased number of respiratory illnesses and may have reduced performance on pulmonary function tests. When they are compared with children of nonsmoking parents, the number of illnesses is positively correlated with the number of cigarettes smoked.

Maternal cigarette smoking is associated with increases in the rates of respiratory illnesses such as bronchitis, asthma, otitis media, decreased fetal growth, increased stillbirth and preterm deliveries, and incidences of sudden infant death syndrome (SIDS). Parental smoking may have a deleterious effect on children's growth, a finding that has important implications in disorders such as cystic fibrosis. The American Academy of Pediatrics has renewed its statement on hazards of **passive smoking** (American Academy of Pediatrics, 1994a). The report states: "The dangers to children of both active and passive tobacco exposure, including smokeless forms, are so well established that pediatricians should make the elimination of this threat a major issue as they pursue the goal of a tobacco-free generation by the year 2000."

Nursing Care Management

Passive smoking during childhood may well be the most important precursor of chronic lung disease in the adult. Nurses

Home Care

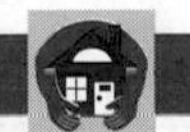

HOUSE RULES FOR SMOKING HOUSEHOLDS

Do not smoke in same room with children.
Restrict smoking to an isolated, preferably outdoor, area.
Do not smoke in motor vehicles with children.
Do not smoke in rooms children use.

and other health professionals need to be aware of the problem and include this information in all health assessments of children, especially those with respiratory and allergic illnesses. In families where smokers refuse to quit, house rules should be established for reducing smoke in the child's environment (see the Home Care box above). Nurses should also inform caregivers of the health hazards of children's exposure to environments of tobacco smoke, set an example for children and families, and become advocates for "no smoking" ordinances in public places, prohibition of advertising tobacco products in the media, and inclusion of health warnings of sidestream smoke on tobacco products.

BOX 43-15
Triggers Tending to Precipitate and/or Aggravate Asthmatic Exacerbations

Allergens
- *Outdoor:* Trees, shrubs, weeds, grasses, molds, pollens, air pollution, spores
- *Indoor:* Dust and/or dust mites, mold, cockroach antigen

Irritants: tobacco smoke, wood smoke, odors, sprays
Exposure to occupational chemicals
Exercise
Cold air
Changes in weather or temperature
Environmental change: moving to new home, starting new school, etc.
Colds and infections
Animals: cats, dogs, rodents, horses
Medications: aspirin, nonsteroidal antiinflammatory drugs (NSAIDs), antibiotics, beta blockers
Strong emotions: fear, anger, laughing, crying
Conditions: gastroesophageal reflux, tracheoesophageal fistula
Food additives: sulfite preservatives
Foods: nuts, milk/dairy products
Endocrine factors: menses, pregnancy, thyroid disease

Long-Term Respiratory Dysfunction

ASTHMA

Asthma is defined as "airway obstruction or a narrowing that is characterized by bronchial irritability after exposure to various stimuli" and that is reversible either spontaneously or with treatment. When the symptoms (shortness of breath, wheezing, and/or chest tightness) become worse, either abruptly or progressively, the child is experiencing an **exacerbation** (American Academy of Pediatrics, 1994b). Asthma can be *intermittent,* in which the child is symptom-free for extended periods without medication, or *chronic,* in which the child requires frequent or continuous medical therapy.

The incidence, severity, and mortality rate associated with asthma have risen steadily throughout the world. The increasing numbers may result from increasing air pollution, poor access to medical care, and/or underdiagnosis and undertreatment. Asthma is the most common chronic disease of childhood, is the primary cause of school absences, and is responsible for a major proportion of pediatric admissions to emergency rooms and hospitals.

Etiology

Although the exact etiology of asthma remains equivocal, evidence suggests that the disease results from hypersensitivity to environmental substances that trigger an allergic reaction. A strong relationship exists between viral infections and asthma induction in infants, with **allergens** playing a less important role in this age group because of the time needed for allergic sensitivity to develop. Studies in children with asthma suggest, however, that allergy influences the persistence and severity of the disease. Important triggers that tend to induce exacerbations are listed in Box 43-15. There tends to be a family predisposition toward hyperactivity of the airways, but this relationship remains just one variable as a potential cause of asthma.

Although allergy does provide an explanation for triggering asthma, there are instances where no allergic process can be detected. Theories that attempt to explain the airway reaction include (1) a basic defect in the β-adrenergic receptors on leukocytes and (2) increased cholinergic activity in the airways (Duff and Platts-Mills, 1992). Asthma is an extremely complex disorder involving biochemical, immunologic, infectious, endocrine, and psychologic factors.

Pathophysiology

There is general agreement that heightened airway reactivity is characteristic of children with asthma. The reasons for this are less clear, and most theories do not explain all types and causes of asthma. However, the mechanisms responsible for the obstructive symptoms of asthma are (Fig. 43-2) as follows:

1. Inflammation and edema of the mucous membranes
2. Accumulation of tenacious secretions from mucous glands
3. Spasm of the smooth muscle of the bronchi and bronchioles, which decreases the caliber of the bronchioles

The role that each of these mechanisms plays varies from patient to patient and during the course of the disease in a given patient. In some patients smooth muscle contraction is the major factor early in the episode, followed by mucosal inflammation and increased mucous secretion. In others the sequence of the responses is reversed.

Bronchial constriction is a normal reaction to foreign stimuli, but in the child with asthma it is abnormally severe, producing impaired respiratory function. The smooth muscle, arranged in spiral bundles around the airway, causes narrow-

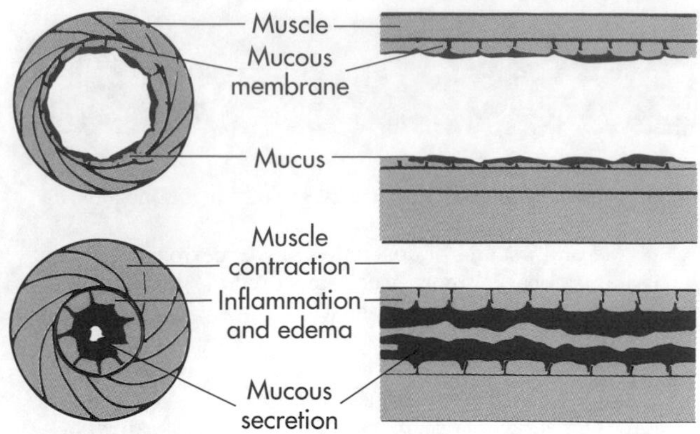

Fig. 43-2 Mechanisms of obstruction in asthma.

ing and shortening of the airway, which significantly increase airway resistance to airflow. Since the bronchi normally dilate and elongate during inspiration and contract and shorten on expiration, the respiratory difficulty is more pronounced during the expiratory phase of respiration. After the initial bronchial constrictions, an inflammatory process begins that causes the airways to obstruct and become more hyperresponsive to allergens. Recognition of the importance of this inflammatory response has made the use of antiinflammatory agents, especially inhaled steroids, a key component of treatment.

Increased resistance in the airway causes forced expiration through the narrowed lumen. The volume of air trapped in the lungs increases as airways are functionally closed at a point between the alveoli and the lobar bronchi by the combined mechanisms just described. This trapping of gas forces the individual to breathe at higher and higher lung volumes. Consequently, the person with asthma fights to inspire sufficient air. This expenditure of effort for breathing causes fatigue, decreased respiratory effectiveness, and increased oxygen consumption. Also, the inspiration occurring at higher lung volumes hyperinflates the alveoli and reduces the effectiveness of the cough. As the severity of obstruction increases, there is a reduced alveolar ventilation with carbon dioxide (CO_2) retention, hypoxemia, respiratory acidosis, and, eventually, respiratory failure.

Diagnostic Evaluation

Children with asthma may show signs and experience symptoms that range from acute episodes of shortness of breath, wheezing, and cough followed by a quiet period to a relatively continuous pattern of chronic symptoms that fluctuate in severity (Box 43-16). An attack may develop gradually or appear abruptly and may be preceded by a URI. The age of the child is often a significant factor, since the first attack in most cases occurs between ages 3 and 8 years. In infancy an attack usually follows a respiratory infection. Some children may experience a prodromal itching at the front of the neck or over the upper part of the back just before an attack.

The diagnosis is determined primarily on the basis of clinical manifestations, history, physical examination, and, to a lesser extent, laboratory tests. Radiographic examinations are used primarily to rule out other diseases and to evaluate coexisting disease. Generally, chronic cough in the absence of infection or diffuse wheezing during the expiratory phase of respiration is sufficient to establish a diagnosis.

BOX 43-16
Clinical Manifestations of Asthma

Cough

Hacking, paroxysmal, irritative, and nonproductive
Becomes rattling and productive of frothy, clear, gelatinous sputum in later stages

Respiration-related signs

Shortness of breath
Prolonged expiratory phase
Audible wheeze
May have a malar flush and red ears
Lips deep, dark red color
May progress to cyanosis of nail beds, and/or circumoral cyanosis
Restlessness
Apprehension
Sweating may be prominent as the attack progresses
Older children may sit upright with shoulders in a hunched-over position, hands on the bed or chair, and arms braced
Speaks with short, panting, broken phrases

Chest

Hyperresonance on percussion
Coarse, loud breath sounds
Wheezes throughout the lung fields
Prolonged expiration
Crackles
Generalized inspiratory and expiratory wheezing; increasingly high pitched

With repeated episodes

Barrel chest
Elevated shoulders
Use of accessory muscles of respiration
Facial appearance—flattened malar bones, circles beneath the eyes, narrow nose, prominent upper teeth

Pulmonary function tests (PFTs) provide an objective and reproducible method of evaluating the presence and degree of lung disease, as well as the response to therapy. Spirometry can generally be performed reliably on children by the age of 5 or 6 years, by using either the traditional and simple mechanical spirometer often used in clinics, offices, and the home or the new computerized versions. One of the key measurements is the **peak expiratory flow rate (PEFR),** or the greatest flow velocity that can be obtained during a forced expiration by using a *peak expiratory flow meter (PEFM)*. Three zones of measurement are typically used to interpret PEFR. The zone system is adapted to a traffic light so that the categories are easier to use and remember (see the Guidelines box on p. 1349). Each child needs to establish his or her *personal best value.* A personal best value can be established during a 2- to 3-week period during which the child records PEFR at least twice a day. The present PEFR is then compared with the personal best (National Heart, Lung, and Blood Institute, 1991).

Skin testing is useful in identifying specific allergens, and those obtained by the puncture technique correlate better than intracutaneous tests with symptoms and measurements of specific IgE antibody (see the Atraumatic Care box on p. 1349). *Provocative testing,* direct exposure of the mucous

Guidelines

INTERPRETING PEAK EXPIRATORY FLOW RATES*

- *Green (80% to 100% of personal best)* signals all clear. Asthma is under reasonably good control. No symptoms are present, and the routine treatment plan for maintaining control can be followed.
- *Yellow (50% to 80% of personal best)* signals caution. Asthma is not well controlled. An acute exacerbation may be present. Maintenance therapy may need to be increased. Call the practitioner if the child stays in this zone.
- *Red (below 50% of personal best)* signals a medical alert. Severe airway narrowing may be occurring. An immediate bronchodilator should be taken. Notify the practitioner if the PEFR measure does not return immediately and stay in yellow or green zones.

*These zones are guidelines only. Specific zones and management may be individualized for each child by the practitioner.

membranes to a suspected antigen in increasing concentrations, helps to identify inhaled allergens. The Radioallergosorbent Test (RAST) helps identify antigens against various foods and is often useful in determining appropriate therapy.

Therapeutic Management

The overall goal of asthma management is to prevent disability and to minimize physical and psychologic morbidity—to help the child live as normal and happy a life as possible. This includes facilitating the child's social adjustments in the family, school, and community and normal participation in recreational activities and sports. To accomplish these goals, efforts are directed toward recognizing acute episodes early and implementing appropriate therapy, identifying and eliminating irritant and allergic factors from the child's environment, educating parents to the long-term nature of the disease and how to manage exacerbations, and helping the child to deal constructively with the disease. Compliance with the prescribed regimen is essential to successful management.

Allergen control. The goals of nonpharmacologic therapy are prevention and reduction of the child's exposure to airborne allergens and irritants. *House dust mites* and other components of house dust are the agents identified most often in children allergic to inhalants. The most important method to eliminate dust mites is to keep the humidity in the house under 50%, the level below which dust mites do not survive. Other recommendations for controlling allergens are in the Home Care box on p. 1352.

Specific allergens are identified by skin testing, and steps are taken to eliminate or avoid the offending allergens. Often, simply removing the offending environmental factors will decrease the frequency of asthma episodes, for example, removal of a dog or cat from the home of a child sensitive to animal dander. Nonspecific factors that may trigger an episode, such as extremes of temperature, are sometimes controlled by dehumidifiers or air conditioners.

Drug therapy. Most children do not require continuous medication. The goal is to control the acute exacerbation; therefore, early recognition and treatment at the onset are most important. Rapid relief of the bronchospasm reduces the need for drastic measures and increases the likelihood that relief will be complete. Several drugs are prescribed, often in combination, to reverse or prevent bronchospasm. Many of the medications are given by inhalation with a nebulizer or metered-dose inhaler (MDI). The MDI may have a spacing unit or reservoir attached, which makes it easier for young children to use. Children who have difficulty using the MDI can obtain effective relief with nebulization. The medication is mixed with saline solution and then nebulized with compressed air. Children are instructed to breathe normally with the mouth open to provide a direct route to the trachea.

Atraumatic Care

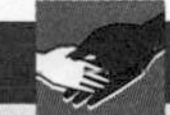

SKIN TESTING

To help allay children's fears of skin tests, they need a careful and thorough explanation of what is to be done and how many "pricks" are involved (about 30 tests). Very young, anxious patients may benefit from one prick on the arm to demonstrate how it feels. The skin is pierced with a stylet rather than a regular needle and syringe; then a drop of allergen is placed on the site. A helpful strategy is to have the child count off the number of pricks with the nurse as a distraction. For intradermal skin injection, eutectic mixture of local anesthetics (EMLA), a topical anesthetic, reduces or eliminates pain without altering test results (Wolf et al, 1994).

Corticosteroids. Corticosteroids are the most effective antiinflammatory drugs for the treatment of reversible airflow obstruction and are highly effective in controlling symptoms and reducing bronchial hyperreactivity in chronic asthma. Corticosteroids may be administered parenterally, orally, or by aerosol. Oral medications are metabolized slowly, with an onset of action up to 3 hours after administration and peak effectiveness occurring within 6 to 12 hours. Acute short-term therapy is typically begun with high dosages, which can be maintained for 5 to 10 days. Long-term use is limited by the risk of significant adverse effects, such as osteoporosis, hypertension, Cushing syndrome, impaired immune mechanisms, and hypothalamic-pituitary-adrenal suppression (National Heart, Lung, and Blood Institute, 1991).

Inhaled corticosteroids should be attempted to determine whether oral corticosteroid treatment can be reduced or eliminated. Their use appears to result in few side effects, such as oral or nasal irritation.

Cromolyn sodium. Cromolyn sodium is a nonsteroidal antiinflammatory drug for asthma. Although the exact mechanism of how it works is not known, it appears to act superficially to inhibit mast cell degranulation in both early-phase and late-phase allergen-induced airway narrowing and acute airway narrowing after exposure to exercise, cold dry air, and sulfur dioxide. There is no way to predict reliably whether a child will respond to the drug. Cromolyn sodium produces only minimal side effects, such as occasional coughing on inhalation of the powder formulation, and may be given via nebulizer or MDI. Another drug, *nedocromil sodium,* has both antiallergic and antiinflammatory properties. It is also being used with children.

β-Adrenergic agents. β-Adrenergic agonists (primarily albuterol, metaproterenol, and terbutaline) are the medications of choice for treatment of acute exacerbations of asthma and for the prevention of exercise-induced asthma. They can be given via inhalation or as oral or parenteral preparations. The inhaled drug has a more rapid onset of action than the oral form but is more costly. Inhalation also reduces troublesome systemic side effects: irritability, tremor, nervousness, and insomnia.

Inhaled β-adrenergics can be taken two to four times daily for acute symptoms. *Salmeterol* (Serevent) is a long-acting bronchodilator that is used two times per day. Children with exercise-induced bronchospasm are advised to use the drug prophylactically 10 to 15 minutes before exercise.

Methylxanthines. Methylxanthines, principally theophylline, have been used for decades to relieve symptoms and prevent asthma attacks. Theophylline, however, is now considered as a third-line agent and perhaps even unnecessary for treating asthma exacerbations.

When theophylline is used, it may be taken intravenously, intramuscularly, orally, or rectally (seldom used). The drug is also available in sustained-release form for oral ingestion. In addition to its bronchodilator effect, theophylline is a central respiratory stimulant and increases respiratory muscle contractility.

Monitoring serum concentrations is an important component of both acute care and long-term management. Monitoring is required for children who fail to exhibit the expected bronchodilator effect, as well as for those who experience adverse effects on the usual dose. Although theophylline has been accepted to have a therapeutic level of 10 to 20 μg/ml, a more conservative approach would be to aim for levels of 5 to 15 μg/ml (National Heart, Lung, and Blood Institute, 1991). The signs and symptoms of theophylline intoxication involve many different organ systems, with gastrointestinal symptoms—nausea and vomiting—the most common early events. Cardiopulmonary effects include tachycardia, dysrhythmias, and stimulation of the respiratory center (tachypnea), with diuresis, irritability, and even seizures possible. There have been reports that theophylline may cause behavior problems and poor school performance, but most research does not support these findings (Milgrom and Bender, 1995).

Exercise. Airway obstruction often develops in children with asthma. *Exercise-induced bronchospasm,* or *exercise-induced asthma (EIA),* does not represent a unique syndrome but rather an example of the airway hyperactivity common to all persons with asthma. EIA is an acute, reversible, usually self-terminating airway obstruction that develops 5 to 15 minutes after strenuous exercise and lasts 15 to 60 minutes after the onset. Usually the episode subsides spontaneously in ½ to 1 hour. The severity of an attack increases as the exercise becomes increasingly strenuous. Patients with a history of EIA often have normal pulmonary function test results and are only symptomatic with exercise.

The problem is rare in activities that require only short bursts of energy (such as baseball, sprints, gymnastics, skiing) rather than those that involve endurance exercise (e.g., soccer, basketball, distance running). Swimming, even long-distance swimming, is well tolerated by children with EIA, partly because they are breathing air fully saturated with moisture, but the type of breathing required may also play a role. Exhaling under water is of benefit because it prolongs each expiration and increases the end-expiratory pressure within the respiratory tree (essentially pursed-lip breathing).

Children with asthma are often excluded from exercise by parents, teachers, and practitioners, as well as by the children themselves because they are reluctant to provoke an attack. This can seriously hamper peer interaction. Moderate or even strenuous exercise is advantageous for children with asthma. These children can participate in activities at school and in sports with minimum difficulty, provided that the asthma is under control. Participation should be evaluated on an individual basis in terms of tolerance for duration and intensity of effort. Appropriate prophylactic treatment with β-adrenergic agents or cromolyn sodium before exercise will usually permit full participation in strenuous exertion. Restrictions are invoked only when the child's condition makes them necessary.

Chest physiotherapy. Chest physiotherapy (CPT), a standard adjunct to treatment of chronic asthma, includes breathing exercises, physical training, and inhalation therapy. These therapies help produce physical and mental relaxation, improve posture, strengthen respiratory musculature, and develop more efficient patterns of breathing. For the motivated child, breathing exercises and controlled breathing are of value in preventing overinflation and improving the strength of respiratory muscles and the efficiency of the cough. Stretch exercises sometimes help increase the flexibility of the ribs. Sit-ups and leg exercises strengthen abdominal muscles and aid expiration.

Hyposensitization. The role of hyposensitization in childhood asthma has not been clarified. In many cases the child demonstrates multiple sensitivities, which make such therapy impractical. Moreover, the injections can be expensive and uncomfortable. When the allergen can be defined and cannot be avoided or controlled satisfactorily by drugs, specific hyposensitization is seriously considered.

Injection therapy is usually limited to clinically significant allergens, such as house dust, pollens, and molds. The initial dose of the offending allergen(s), based on the size of the skin reaction, is injected subcutaneously. The amount is increased at weekly intervals until a maximum tolerance is reached, after which a maintenance dose is given at 4-week intervals. This may be extended to 5- or 6-week intervals during the off-season for seasonal allergens. Successful treatment is continued for a minimum of 3 years and then stopped. If no symptoms appear, acquired immunity is said to be retained; if symptoms recur, treatment is reinstituted.

Nursing ALERT

Hyposensitization injections should only be administered with emergency equipment and medications readily available in the event of an anaphylactic reaction.

Prognosis. The outlook for children with asthma varies widely. Many children lose their symptoms at puberty, but there is no factor that can predict which children will "outgrow" their asthma. Some have other forms of allergy in adulthood—most commonly involving the nose.

The prognosis for control of or disappearance of symptoms will differ in children who have rare and infrequent attacks and in those who are constantly wheezing or who are subject to status asthmaticus. In general, the more severe and numerous the symptoms, the longer they have been present, and when there is a family history of allergy, the poorer is the prog-

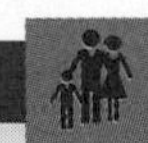

Family Focus

ASTHMA: FACTORS AFFECTING PROGNOSIS

Psychologic factors play an important role in children who die during an asthmatic episode. Those who die tend to have significant psychologic problems, such as extreme reactions to separation or loss, a history of family turmoil, and expressed hopelessness or despair that leads to depression. Their families are less likely to recognize the severity of the asthma and the need to comply with therapy. In this situation appropriate family education concerning the risks of the child's disease if treatment is inconsistent can be lifesaving (Klinnert, Miller, and Mrazek, 1990).

nosis for improvement. Many who outgrow their symptoms are subject to exercise-induced asthma as adults, and the associated disorders, such as growth impairment, chest deformity, and airway obstruction, are maintained throughout life.

Although death from asthma is rare, the death rate has increased 46% from 1980 to 1989 despite advances in therapy (American Academy of Pediatrics, 1994b). The adolescent age group appears to be the most vulnerable, with the greatest increase occurring in ages 10 to 14. No reliable data explain this increase. Factors that have been postulated include exposure of atopic persons to more allergens, change in severity of the disease, abuse of drug therapy (toxicity), failure of families and practitioners to recognize severity of asthma, and psychologic factors, such as denial or refusal to accept the disease. Risk factors for asthma deaths appear to be onset at an early age, frequent attacks, difficult-to-manage disease, adolescence, history of respiratory failure, psychologic problems (refusal to take medications), dependency on or misuse of drugs (high use), presence of physical stigmata (barrel chest, intercostal retractions), and abnormal pulmonary function test results (see the Family Focus box above).

Status asthmaticus. Children who continue to display respiratory distress despite vigorous therapeutic measures, especially sympathomimetics, are considered to be in status asthmaticus. The condition may develop gradually or rapidly, often coincident with complicating conditions (such as pneumonia) that can influence the duration and treatment of the attack. These children are acutely ill and require hospitalization, preferably where pediatric intensive care is available. They need continuous nursing attendance with cardiorespiratory monitoring and vigilant observation.

Nursing ALERT

Status asthmaticus is a medical emergency that can result in respiratory failure and death if untreated. The child who sweats profusely, remains sitting upright, and refuses to lie down is in severe respiratory distress. The child who suddenly becomes agitated or the agitated child who suddenly becomes quiet and listless may be seriously hypoxic and requires immediate intervention.

Therapy for status asthmaticus is directed toward improvement of ventilation, correction of dehydration and acidosis, and treatment of any concurrent infection. Bronchospasm is relieved by giving nebulized albuterol (either intermittent or continuous) along with corticosteroids (either oral or intravenous). For the child not responding to either of these therapies, subcutaneous epinephrine (1:1000) at a dose of 0.01 ml/kg with a maximum dose of 0.3 ml or subcutaneous terbutaline is administered.

The child is given intravenous fluids and nothing by mouth except liquids if the condition persists. The intravenous infusion provides a means for hydration and administering medications. The correction of dehydration, acidosis, hypoxia, and electrolyte derangements is guided by frequent determination of oxygenation (pulse oximetry), blood gases, and serum electrolytes. Humidified oxygen is administered by tent, face mask, or cannula to maintain satisfactory oxygenation. Since oxygen is a stimulus for respiration, high levels may significantly depress respirations.

Administration of antibiotics is frequently advisable in therapy, since infection may be masked or may not always be evident and is always a threatening complication. As the attack subsides, fluids and medication are given orally and discharge plans are initiated, especially for follow-up care.

Nursing Care Management

Assessment

Physical assessment of asthma involves the same observations and techniques described in the general discussion of assessment of respiratory infection (Box 43-2) and physical assessment of the chest (see Chapter 32). In addition, some physical characteristics of chronic respiratory involvement are noted and evaluated. These include chest configuration, posturing, and type of breathing. The chest of a child with chronic obstructive respiratory disease often assumes a barrel shape from chronic hyperinflation.

Psychologic assessment consists of assessing the degree to which the disorder interferes with everyday activities, the child and the family cope with the condition, the disorder alters the child's self-concept, and the child and family comply with the therapeutic management.

Nursing Diagnoses

On the basis of a thorough assessment, several nursing diagnoses are identified. The more common diagnoses for the child with asthma are included in the Nursing Care Plan on p. 1355). Others may apply in specific situations.

Planning

The goals for a child with asthma and the family include the following:

1. The child will not experience an asthmatic episode.
2. The child will exhibit improved ventilatory capacity.
3. The child will maintain optimum health.
4. The child will not have complications.
5. The child will engage in normal activities for age.
6. The child and family will receive appropriate support and education regarding the disease and its management.

Implementation

Avoid allergens. The primary goal of asthma management is avoidance of an exacerbation. Parents need to know the nature of the disease and, when the allergens are determined, how they can prevent and/or relieve asthmatic episodes by

Home Care

"ALLERGY-PROOFING" THE HOME

- Keep humidity between 40% and 50%; use dehumidifier if available.
- Have carpets cleaned professionally frequently or remove them, including carpeting on concrete.
  - Avoid vacuuming carpets, which sends allergens into the air, although it does remove waste particles of dust mites.
  - If available, use central vacuum cleaner with collecting bag outside home or use cleaner filters (e.g., high-efficiency particulate air [HEPA] filters).
- Use chemical agents to kill mites or alter antigens in house.
  - Treating carpet with 3% tannic acid solution or benzylbenzoate (available in foam for mattresses and furniture and in powder for carpets) kills dust mites; keep child away from treated areas during and several hours after chemical application.*
- If possible, use an air-cleaning device, such as electrostatic precipitator or with a HEPA filter; approximate-size units can be used in child's room.
- Have air and heat ducts professionally cleaned annually; change or clean filters monthly.
- Place airtight plastic, vinyl, or hypoallergenic covers on mattress, box spring, and pillows.*
- Use foam rubber mattress and pillows or Dacron pillows and synthetic blankets.
- Launder blankets and sheets in hot water (over 48.8° C).
- Store nothing under bed; keep closets and storage areas uncluttered.
- Use washable shades rather than blinds or curtains.
- Use child's bedroom for sleeping, not playing.
- Remove from room unnecessary furniture, rugs, stuffed or real animals, toys, books, upholstered furniture, plants, aquariums, wall hangings, etc.
- Cover or replace upholstered furniture; avoid rattan or wicker furniture.
- Cover walls with washable paint or wallpaper.
- Limit child's exposure to animals.
- Change child's clothes after play outdoors; wash hair nightly if outside and pollen count is high.
- Keep child indoors while lawn in being mowed, bushes/trees are being trimmed, or pollen count is high.
- Keep windows and doors closed during pollen season; use air conditioner if available.
- Cover heating vents with filter material (e.g., cheesecloth) to prevent circulation of dust, especially when heat is turned on after summer.
- Use smooth cotton or synthetic fabric for bedcovers, curtains, and scatter rugs and launder weekly.
- Wet mop bare floors weekly.
- Wet dust (or use Endust) and clean room weekly; child should not be present during housecleaning activities.
- Encase wool or feather items in nonallergenic coverings.*
- Limit or avoid child's exposure to tobacco and wood smoke.
- Avoid odors or sprays (e.g., perfumes, talcum powder, room deodorizers, fresh paint).
- Avoid cellar (basement) as play area and use dehumidifier in damp cellar.
- Clean showers and tile areas; spray with antimold agent (e.g., Lysol).
- Keep vaporizers and air conditioners (including automobile air conditioner) clean and free of mold.

*A source of information is Allergy Control Products, Inc., 96 Danbury Rd, Ridgefield, CT 06877; (800) 422-DUST.

modifying the environment to reduce contact with the offending allergen(s) (see the Home Care box above). The parents are cautioned to avoid exposing a sensitive child to excessive cold, wind, or other extremes of weather; smoke; sprays; or other irritants. Passive smoking has been associated with exacerbation of symptoms in children with hyperresponsive airways, especially in boys and older children.

Since approximately 2% to 6% of children with asthma are sensitive to aspirin, acetaminophen is recommended. Those children with aspirin-induced asthma may also be sensitive to nonsteroidal antiinflammatory drugs and tartrazine (yellow dye number 5, a common food coloring).

Relieve bronchospasm. Parents and other children need to learn how to use the medications prescribed to relieve bronchospasm. They are taught to recognize early signs and symptoms of an impending attack so that it can be controlled before symptoms become distressing. Most children can recognize prodromal symptoms well before an attack (about 6 hours) so that preventive therapy can be implemented. Some objective signs that parents may observe include rhinorrhea, cough, low-grade fever, irritability, itching (especially in front of neck and chest), apathy, anxiety, sleep disturbance, abdominal discomfort, and loss of appetite. A variety of easy-to-use, inexpensive PEFMs are available for use in the home to help assess the extent of the child's symptoms (see the Home Care box to the right).

Home Care

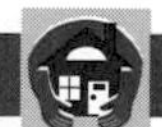

USE OF A PEAK EXPIRATORY FLOW METER (PEFM)

1. Before each use, make sure the sliding marker or arrow on the PEFM is at the bottom of the numbered scale.
2. Stand up straight.
3. Remove gum or any food from the mouth.
4. Close your lips tightly around the mouthpiece. Be sure to keep your tongue away from the mouthpiece.
5. Blow out as hard and as quickly as you can, a "fast hard puff."
6. Note the number by the marker on the numbered scale.
7. Repeat entire routine three times.
8. Record the *highest* of the three readings, not the average.
9. Measure your peak expiratory flow rate (PEFR) close to the same time and same way each day (i.e., morning and evening; before and/or 15 minutes after taking medication).
10. Keep a chart of your PEFRs.

Nursing ALERT

Long-acting β-adrenergic inhalers (Serevent) should be used only as directed (usually every 12 hours) and not more frequently. They are not intended to relieve acute asthmatic symptoms.

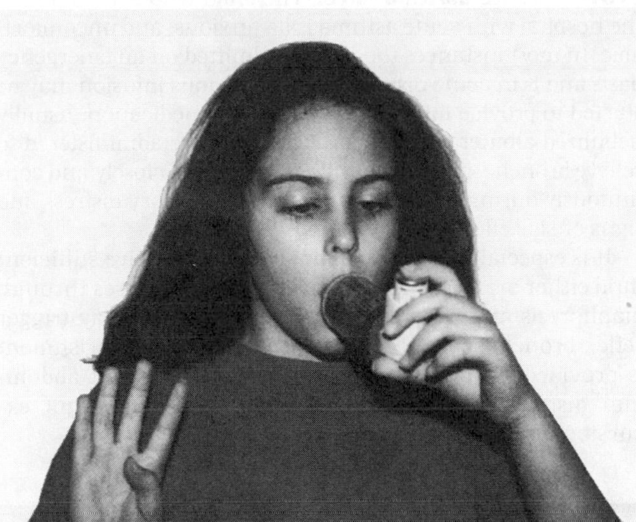

Fig. 43-3 Child using metered-dose inhaler with spacer. Fingers are used for counting to 10 seconds.

Older children who use a nebulizer or aerosol device to deliver adrenergic drugs need to learn how to use the device correctly. The MDI (Fig. 43-3) combines portability with a rapid and reliable dose for patients managed at home. The objective of the device is to distribute the prescribed medication directly to the narrowed airways. It is important that the child learn to breathe slowly and deeply for better distribution to narrowed airways (see the Home Care box to the right).

Young children and those who are otherwise unable to manipulate the device or coordinate breathing with activation of the MDI are able to use special chambers called *spacers*. These permit an operator to deliver the medication from the MDI into the spacer from which the child inhales (see the Critical Thinking Q & A to the right).

The child and parents also need to be cautioned about the adverse effects of prescribed drugs and the dangers of overuse. They should know that it is important to use them when needed but not indiscriminately or as a substitute for avoiding the symptom-provoking allergen.

Nursing ALERT

Side effects from theophylline include nausea, headache, irritability, and insomnia. Early signs of toxicity are nausea, tachycardia, and irritability; seizures and dysrhythmias occur at blood theophylline levels over 30 μg/ml.

The family can acquire a peak flow meter that measures the maximum peak expiratory flow rate to predict an acute exacerbation. This provides information for adjusting medication dosage.

The parents are cautioned to avoid exposing the child to excessive cold, wind, or other extremes of weather and to smoke, sprays, or other irritants. Although foods are an unusual cause of asthma, foods known to provoke symptoms should be eliminated from the diet. The foods most commonly allergenic are eggs, milk, grains, peanuts, and chocolate. Par-

Home Care

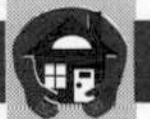

USE OF A METERED-DOSE INHALER*

Steps for checking how much medicine is in the canister

1. If the canister is new, it is full.
2. If the canister has been used repeatedly, it may be empty. (Check product label to see how many inhalations should be in each canister.)
3. To check how much medicine is left in the canister, put the canister (not the mouthpiece) into a cup of water.
   a. If the canister sinks to the bottom, it is full.
   b. If the canister floats sideways on the surface, it is empty.

Steps for using the inhaler

1. Remove the cap and hold inhaler upright.
2. Shake the inhaler.
3. Tilt the head back slightly and breathe out.
4. With the inhaler in an upright position, insert the mouthpiece:
   a. About 3 to 4 cm from the mouth *or*
   b. Into an aerochamber *or*
   c. Into the mouth, forming an airtight seal between the lips and the mouthpiece.
5. At the end of a normal expiration, depress the top of the inhaler canister firmly to release the medication (into either the aerochamber or the mouth), and breathe in slowly (about 3-5 seconds). Relax the pressure on the top of the canister.
6. Hold the breath for at least 5 to 10 seconds to allow the aerosol medication to reach deeply into the lungs.
7. Remove the inhaler and breathe out slowly through the nose.
8. Wait 1 minute between puffs (if additional one is needed).
9. To determine whether child is using an inhaler properly, have child use the device in front of a mirror. If vapor does not appear on the mirror, the inhaler is being used correctly.

Modified from National Heart, Lung, and Blood Institute, National Institutes of Health: *Guidelines for the diagnosis and management of asthma,* Pub No 91-3042, Bethesda, MD, 1991, The Institute.

*NOTE: Inhaled dry powder capsules require a different inhalation technique. To use a dry powder inhaler, it is important to close the mouth tightly around the mouthpiece of the inhaler and inhale rapidly.

Critical Thinking Q & A

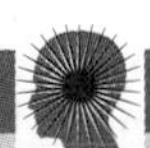

ASTHMA

Traditional thinking about the pathophysiologic characteristics of asthma has changed in recent years. Which one of the following treatments reflects this better understanding of the mechanisms involved in an asthmatic episode?

1. Peak expiratory flow meter (PEFM)
2. Metered-dose inhaler (MDI)
3. Allergy hyposensitization
4. Chest physiotherapy

The correct answer is two. Inflammation of the bronchial airways is now recognized as a critical component in the pathophysiologic characteristics of asthma. MDIs are used to deliver corticosteroids to decrease the inflammation. The PEFM is an assessment device; the other two choices have been used traditionally.

ents are advised to read labels on prepared foods and snacks to determine the presence of allergens. For example, a number of foods contain sodium caseinate or dried milk products. Since approximately 2% to 6% of these children are sensitive to aspirin, nurses caution the parents to use other analgesic/antipyretic drugs for discomfort or fever.

The child should be protected from a respiratory infection that can trigger an attack or aggravate the asthmatic state, especially in young children. Their airways are mechanically smaller and more reactive; therefore edema from infection causes wheezing and other signs of respiratory obstruction. Also, the equipment used for the child, such as nebulizers, must be kept absolutely clean to decrease the chances of contamination with bacteria and fungi.

Breathing exercises and controlled breathing are taught and encouraged for motivated youngsters, and the nurse can help them select activities suitable to their capacity. Anything that promotes proper diaphragmatic breathing, side expansion, and generally improved mobility of the chest wall is encouraged. Play techniques that can be employed for younger children to extend their expiratory time and increase expiratory pressure include blowing cotton balls or a Ping-Pong ball on a table, blowing a pinwheel or bubbles, or preventing a tissue from falling by blowing it against the wall. If the child requires postural drainage and percussion, someone in the family must assume responsibility for carrying out the procedure. It is the responsibility of the physical therapist or the nurse to teach the parent the proper technique.

Self-care is a hallmark of effective asthma management, and self-management programs are important in helping the child and family cope with the disease. The principles that are conveyed are the following:

1. Asthma is a very common disease, and having asthma is annoying but not disgraceful.
2. Persons with asthma are able to live full and active lives.
3. It is much easier to prevent than to treat an asthmatic attack.
4. Individuals do not become addicted to asthma medication, but they do prefer to breathe more freely whenever possible.

Asthma camps have become popular in recent years as a means of encouraging physical activity in a more homogeneous, more controlled, and less competitive environment. Although not all persons subscribe to this practice, some support the benefits, which are primarily that the denominator of asthma is removed as a factor. Everyone at the camp has asthma; therefore, no child is different from the others.

Several organizations provide education and services for health professionals and families of children with asthma.* Asthma education and awareness are important aspects of asthma management. Although the principles of self-management are very general and the programs are designed for general use, each child and family has special needs that require individualized care and attention.

*__Asthma and Allergy Foundation of America (AAFA),__ 1125 15th St. N.W., Washington, DC 20005, (202) 466-7643; **American Lung Association,** 1740 Broadway, New York, NY 10019, (212) 315-8700; **Canadian Lung Association,** 75 Albert St., Suite 908, Ottawa, Ontario K1P 5E7, (613) 237-1208; **The Lung Association,** 573 King St. East, Suite 201, Toronto, Ontario M5A 4L3, (416) 922-9440.

Provide acute asthma care. The child who is admitted to the hospital with acute asthma is ill, anxious, and uncomfortable. In most instances the child is admitted on an emergency basis and is in acute distress. An intravenous infusion may be started to provide immediate access, and medication, usually nebulized albuterol and a corticosteroid, are administered to relieve bronchospasm. The child is monitored closely and continuously during therapy for relief of respiratory distress and signs of side effects.

It is especially important that the child receive sufficient fluid either orally or intravenously to replace losses through diaphoresis and hyperventilation. Cold liquids may trigger reflex bronchospasm and should be avoided. Nourishment is provided in small, frequent feedings to prevent abdominal distention that may interfere with diaphragm excursion.

Nursing ALERT

Dehydration should be corrected slowly; overhydration can increase the accumulation of interstitial pulmonary fluid to exacerbate small airway obstruction.

Older children usually prefer the high-Fowler position, although they may be more comfortable sitting upright or leaning slightly forward. When possible, the nurse communicates in such a way that a child need only reply in a few words to prevent fatigue. Shortness of breath makes talking difficult. Oxygen is indicated for relief of dyspnea and cyanosis; however, it is not administered indiscriminately but regulated according to the blood gas analysis, pulse oximetry, and objective observation of color, respiratory effort, and sensorium. Associated treatments such as intermittent positive-pressure breathing or postural drainage and tests (e.g., blood gases, PFTs) may be performed by specialized personnel or may be the nurse's responsibility.

Children with acute asthma are apprehensive and anxious. The calm, efficient presence of a nurse helps reassure them that they are safe and will be cared for during this stressful period. It is important to assure children that they will not be left alone and that their parents are allowed to be near and available when they need them.

Parents need reassurance, too. They want to be informed of their child's condition and the therapies being employed. Often they feel that they may have in some way contributed to the child's condition or could have prevented the attack. Reassurance regarding their efforts expended on the child's behalf and their parenting capabilities can help alleviate their stress. All efforts to reduce parental apprehension will, in turn, help reduce the child's distress. Anxiety is easily communicated to the child by parents and members of the staff.

Child and family support. The nurse working with children with asthma can provide them with support in a number of ways. Many children voice frustration about the ways their exacerbations interfere with their goal achievements and social lives. They need education about their disease, including what to do to prevent an episode and what to do during one. These children need reassurance from the health team and reinforcement of their coping mechanisms.

Nursing ALERT

Be aware of children, especially adolescents, who are depressed and may not comply with therapy as a means of passive suicide. Refer these youngsters for psychologic support.

Both short- and long-term adaptation of affected children to the disease depends to a great extent on the family's acceptance of the disorder and compliance with therapy. The task of living day-to-day with affected children involves the family continually. There are periodic crises and the ever-present threat of a crisis, requiring parental vigilance, sleepless nights, frequent emergency trips to the hospital, and often overwhelming medical expenses. Throughout these stresses, parents are expected and encouraged to promote as normal a life as possible for their children without neglecting the needs of siblings.

Evaluation

The effectiveness of nursing interventions is determined by continual assessment and evaluation of care based on the following observational guidelines and expected outcomes:

1. Interview family about removal or avoidance of known allergens.
2. Observe child for evidence of respiratory symptoms.
3. Assess child's general health.
4. Observe child and interview family about any infections or other complications.

Nursing Care Plan

THE CHILD WITH ASTHMA

Nursing Diagnosis: Risk for suffocation related to interaction of child with allergens

Expected Outcome: Asthmatic episodes are reduced or eliminated.

• NURSING INTERVENTIONS/*RATIONALES*

Make an inventory of allergens that trigger reactions or asthmatic episodes *to establish a baseline for prevention.*

Teach child and family how to avoid, limit exposure to, modify or eliminate conditions that trigger allergy attacks and asthmatic episodes.

Teach child and family to recognize early signs *so an impending asthmatic episode can be treated early.*

Instruct child and family in correct use of prescribed bronchodilators, antiinflammatants and other asthma medications *to avoid underuse or overuse of the drugs.*

Instruct child and family in correct use of equipment (e.g., inhalers, nebulizers, peak flow meters) *to ensure correct use and optimum benefit.*

Encourage sound health practices (good nutrition, adequate rest, appropriate exercise, good hygiene) *to support body's natural defenses.*

Encourage child and family to prevent exposure to respiratory infections *since they can serve as triggers for asthma attacks.*

Nursing Diagnosis: Ineffective airway clearance related to allergenic response and inflamed bronchial tree

Expected Outcome: The patient will exhibit evidence of improved ventilatory capacity (i.e., absence of dyspnea, respiration rate and rhythm within normal limits).

• NURSING INTERVENTIONS/*RATIONALES*

Implement breathing exercises and controlled breathing *to improve chest wall mobility and diaphragmatic expansion.*

Use developmentally appropriate play techniques *to increase expiratory pressure and extend expiratory time.*

Use coughing, percussion, and postural drainage as needed *to clear secretions.*

Supervise use of equipment (e.g., inhalers, nebulizers, peak flow meters) *to evaluate use patterns and optimum benefit.*

Administer medications as ordered *to decrease inflammatory response and improve breathing.*

Nursing Diagnosis: Activity intolerance related to imbalance between oxygen supply and demand

Expected Outcome: The patient's activity level will be within normal limits.

• NURSING INTERVENTIONS/*RATIONALES*

Balance rest and physical activity, increasing activity levels as tolerated *to regain balance between oxygen supply and demand.*

Nursing Diagnosis: Altered family processes related to having a child with chronic health problem

Expected Outcome: Family exhibits positive adaptive behaviors to child's condition.

• NURSING INTERVENTIONS/*RATIONALES*

Identify and praise positive coping mechanisms of child and family members *to reinforce long-term use.*

Explore child's and family's understanding of the disease and treatment process *to evaluate family's ability to carry out preventive and emergency intervention.*

Reinforce need for consistent use of preventive measures and need for early response to signs of impending attack *to prevent severe exacerbation.*

Be alert to signs of maladaptation (e.g., parental rejection or overprotection, nonadherence to treatment regimen, lack of alterations in environment or life-style, sporadic health care follow up).

Encourage family to work with school *to develop a consistent plan of care in the school setting.*

Refer family to appropriate support groups and community resources *to provide ongoing support.*

See also the Nursing Care Plan: The Child with Chronic Illness or Disability, Ch. 38.

5. Interview child about daily activities.
6. Determine the degree to which the family and child understand the child's condition and the extent to which the therapies are carried out.

Expected outcomes:
See the Nursing Care Plan on p. 1355.

CYSTIC FIBROSIS

Cystic fibrosis (CF) is inherited as an autosomal recessive trait; the affected child inherits the defective gene from both parents, with an overall incidence of 1:4. The mutated gene responsible for CF is located on the long arm of chromosome 7, along with its protein product, *cystic fibrosis transmembrane regulator (CFTR).* Almost 300 alterations that diverge from the original sequence of the gene have been reported; the ΔF508 is the most common alteration, found in about 70% of all known CF chromosomes (Tizzano and Buchwald, 1993).

Pathophysiology

With the discovery of the CFTR gene, research is continuing to determine its multisystem effects on the body. CF is characterized by several apparently unrelated clinical features: increased viscosity of mucous gland secretions, striking elevation of sweat electrolytes, increase in several organic and enzymatic constituents of saliva, and abnormalities in autonomic nervous system function. Although both sodium and chloride are affected, the defect appears to be primarily a result of abnormal chloride movement; the CFTR appears to function as a chloride channel. Further evidence indicates that ΔF508 is closely related to pancreatic insufficiency. The role of CFTR, however, is not definitive.

The primary factor, and the one that is responsible for the multiple clinical manifestations of the disease, is mechanical obstruction caused by the increased viscosity of mucous gland secretions (Fig. 43-4). Instead of forming a thin, freely flowing secretion, the mucous glands produce a thick, inspissated mucoprotein that accumulates and dilates them. Small passages in organs such as the pancreas and bronchioles become obstructed as secretions precipitate or coagulate to form concretions in glands and ducts. The earliest manifestation of cystic fibrosis is **meconium ileus** in the newborn, in which the small intestine is blocked with thick, puttylike, tenacious, mucilaginous meconium.

In the pancreas the thick secretions block the ducts, eventually causing *pancreatic fibrosis.* This blockage prevents essential pancreatic enzymes from reaching the duodenum, causing marked impairment in the digestion and absorption of nutrients. The disturbed function is reflected in bulky stools that are frothy from undigested fat and foul smelling from putrified protein. The islands of Langerhans may decrease in number as pancreatic fibrosis progresses, and in the liver localized biliary obstruction and fibrosis are common and become more extensive with time.

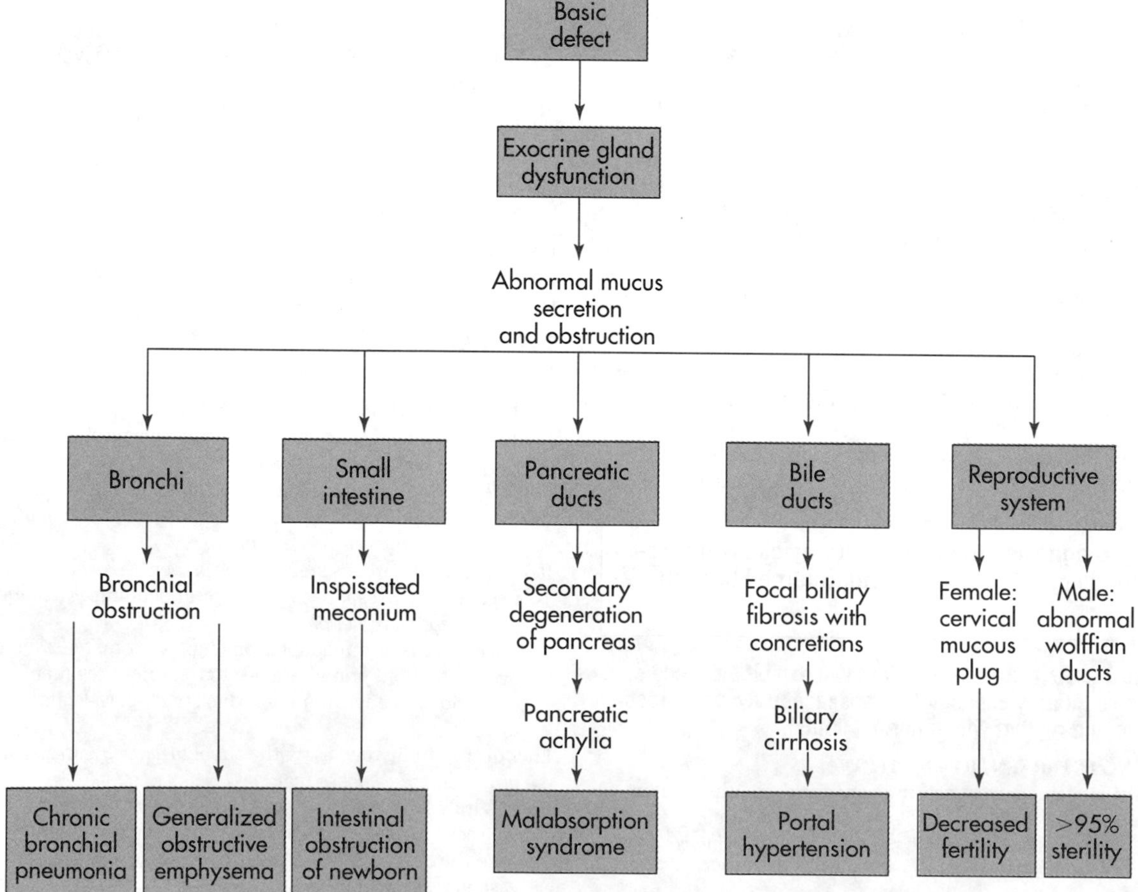

Fig. 43-4 Various effects of exocrine gland dysfunction in cystic fibrosis.

The most common gastrointestinal complication associated with CF is *prolapse of the rectum*, which occurs most often in infancy and childhood. Affected children of all ages are subject to intestinal obstruction from inspissated or impacted feces.

Pulmonary complications are present in almost all children with CF and constitute the most serious threat to life. However, the time of appearance is variable. The majority of children show evidence before 1 year of age; others may not have symptoms for weeks, months, or years. Bronchial and bronchiolar obstruction by the abnormally thick, tenacious mucus causes patchy atelectasis with hyperinflation. The child is unable to expectorate the mucus because of its increased viscosity. This retained mucus serves as an excellent medium for any bacterial growth. Reduced oxgyen–carbon dioxide exchange causes variable degrees of hypoxia, hypercapnia, and acidosis.

Diagnostic Evaluation

An initial evaluation is conducted with general appraisal in the areas of general activity, physical findings, nutritional status, and findings on chest radiograms (Box 43-17). The diagnosis of CF is established on the basis of (1) a history of the disease in the family, (2) absence of pancreatic enzymes, (3) increase in electrolyte concentration of sweat, and (4) chronic pulmonary involvement.

The consistent finding of abnormally high sodium and chloride concentrations in the sweat is a unique characteristic of CF. Parents often observe that their infants taste "salty" when they kiss them. For diagnostic purposes the quantitative sweat chloride test is performed on sweat obtained by iontophoresis of pilocarpine. Normally the sweat chloride content is less than 40 mEq/L; a chloride concentration greater than 60 mEq/L is diagnostic of CF.

Chest radiography reveals characteristic patchy atelectasis and obstructive emphysema. Pulmonary function tests are sensitive indexes of lung function, providing evidence of abnormal small airway function in CF. Other diagnostic tools that may aid in diagnosis include stool fat and/or enzyme analysis. Stool analysis requires a 72-hour sample with accurate recording of food intake during that time. Radiographs, including barium enema, are used for diagnosis of meconium ileus.

Therapeutic Management

The improved survival rate of patients with CF during the past two decades is attributable largely to antibiotic therapy and improved nutritional management. Goals of therapy, therefore, include the following: (1) to prevent or minimize pulmonary complications; (2) to ensure adequate nutrition for growth; and (3) to assist the child and family in adapting to a chronic disorder. In attempting to attain these, there is a multisystem approach to treatment modalities.

Management of pulmonary problems. Management of pulmonary problems is directed toward prevention and treatment of pulmonary infection by improving aeration, removing mucopurulent secretions, and administering antimicrobial agents. Most children will exhibit respiratory symptoms by 3 years of age. Young children normally have small airways and are predisposed to frequent viral infections. The large amounts and viscosity of respiratory secretions in children with CF contribute to the likelihood of infection. Once infection becomes established in relatively defenseless lungs, it is difficult to eradicate.

Prevention of infection involves a daily routine of *chest physiotherapy (CPT)* to maintain pulmonary hygiene (see Chapter 42).

CPT is usually performed twice daily (on rising and in the evening) and more often if needed, especially during pulmonary infection. A new device, the *flutter mucus clearance device,** is a small hand-held plastic pipe with a stainless steel ball on the inside, which facilitates removal of mucus. It has the advantage of increasing sputum expectoration and being usable without assistance (Davis, 1994).

*Manufactured by Scandipharm, Inc., 22 Inverness Center Parkway, Birmingham, AL 35242; (205) 991-8085.

BOX 43-17
Clinical Manifestations of Cystic Fibrosis

Meconium ileus*
Abdominal distention
Vomiting
Failure to pass stools
Rapid development of dehydration

Gastrointestinal manifestations
Large, bulky, loose, frothy, extremely foul-smelling stools
Voracious appetite (early in disease)
Loss of appetite (later in disease)
Weight loss
Marked tissue wasting
Failure to grow
Distended abdomen
Thin extremities
Sallow skin
Evidence of deficiency of fat-soluble vitamins A, D, E, K
Anemia

Pulmonary manifestations
Initial signs:
- Wheezy respirations
- Dry, nonproductive cough

Eventually:
- Increased dyspnea
- Paroxysmal cough
- Evidence of obstructive emphysema and patchy areas of atelectasis

Progressive involvement:
- Overinflated, barrel-shaped chest
- Cyanosis
- Clubbing of fingers and toes
- Repeated episodes of bronchitis and bronchopneumonia

*In about 10% of cases.

Bronchodilator medication delivered in an aerosol helps open bronchi for easier expectoration and is administered before CPT when the patient exhibits evidence of reactive airway disease and/or wheezing.

Another form of aerosolized medication is *recombinant human deoxyribonuclease* (*rhDNase,* known generically as dornase alpha [Pulmozyme]), which decreases the viscosity of mucus. It is well tolerated and has no major adverse effects; minor reactions are voice alteration and laryngitis. The drug causes slight improvement in results of pulmonary function tests and perceptions of well-being and dyspnea (Fuchs et al, 1994). However, its high cost may limit its use.

Physical exercise is an important adjunct to daily CPT. Exercise not only stimulates mucus secretion, it also provides a sense of well-being and increased self-esteem. In some instances, exercise can be substituted for CPT. Any aerobic exercise that is enjoyed by the patient should be encouraged. The ultimate aim of exercise is to establish a good habitual breathing pattern.

Pulmonary infections are treated as soon as they are recognized. Some practitioners prefer to prescribe oral antibiotics prophylactically at the time of diagnosis; others begin therapy when pulmonary symptoms arise. Sputum culture and sensitivity guide the choice of antibiotic.

Intravenous antibiotics are often administered at home as an alternative to hospitalization. Most children have central venous access devices for home administration of intravenous medications. When pulmonary function does not improve with outpatient management, hospitalization may be recommended for continued antibiotic therapy and vigorous CPT.

Oxygen administration is usually recommended for children with acute episodes, but since many of these children have chronic CO_2 retention, the unsupervised use of O_2 can be harmful (see Oxygen Toxicity, Chapter 41).

Pneumothorax is most often caused by rupture of subpleural blebs through the visceral pleura and usually occurs in patients with more advanced disease.

Nursing ALERT

Signs of a pneumothorax are usually nonspecific. They include tachypnea, tachycardia, dyspnea, pallor, and cyanosis.

Management of gastrointestinal problems. The principal treatment for pancreatic insufficiency is replacement pancreatic enzymes, which are administered with meals and snacks to ensure that digestive enzymes are mixed with food in the duodenum. Enteric-coated products prevent the neutralization of enzymes by gastric acids, thus allowing activation to occur in the alkaline environment of the small bowel. The amount of enzymes depends on the severity of the insufficiency, the response of the child to enzyme replacement, and the philosophy of the practitioner. Usually one to five capsules are administered with a meal, and a smaller amount is taken with snacks. Capsules can be swallowed whole or taken apart and the contents sprinkled on a small amount of food to be taken at the beginning of the meal. The amount of enzyme is adjusted to achieve normal growth and a decrease in the number of stools to one or two per day.

Children with CF require a well-balanced, high-protein, high-calorie diet (high calorie because of the impaired intestinal absorption). In fact, they often require up to 150% of the recommended daily allowances to meet their needs for growth. Breastfeeding with enzyme supplementation should be continued whenever possible for parents who prefer this method and, when necessary, supplemented with a higher-calorie-per-ounce formula. For formula-fed infants, commercial cow's milk formulas are usually adequate, although commonly a hydrolysate formula with medium-chain triglycerides (e.g., Pregestimil or Alimentum) may be recommended. Enzymes are mixed into cereal or fruit, such as applesauce. Since the uptake of fat-soluble vitamins is decreased, water-miscible forms of these vitamins (A, D, E, K) are given, along with multivitamins and the enzymes. When high-fat foods are eaten, the child is encouraged to add extra enzymes. Occasionally patients will be placed on supplemental tube feedings or parenteral alimentation in an effort to build up nutritional reserves if there has been a history of inability to maintain weight.

Prognosis. Despite more than 40 years of progress and a recent surge in new treatment modalities, CF remains a progressive and incurable disease. The pulmonary involvement ultimately determines the patient's outcome, since pancreatic enzyme deficiency is less of a problem if adequate nutrition is ensured. With advances in technology, parents and adolescents are now being challenged to set future goals that may include college, careers, social relationships, and marriage. Concurrently, they are faced with increasing morbidity and higher rates of CF complications as they grow older.

Screening. The impact of genetic discoveries on understanding the cause and treatment of CF is steadily unfolding at the same time that approaches to detection are changing to reflect new technologies. Although the standard method of diagnosis relies on detection of abnormal chloride secretions in sweat, genetic testing is now able to confirm the diagnosis. Carrier screening is available and reliable for siblings and family members of a child with CF.

Nursing Care Management

Assessment

Assessment of the child with CF involves both pulmonary and gastrointestinal (GI) observations. Pulmonary assessment is the same as that described for respiratory function (Box 43-2), with special attention to lung sounds, observation of cough, and evidence or degree of finger clubbing. GI assessment primarily involves observing the frequency and nature of the stools and abdominal distention. The observer is also alert to evidence of failure to thrive (e.g., weight loss, wasting, pallor, fatigue). Family members are interviewed to determine the child's eating and eliminating habits, to observe salty perspiration, and to confirm a history of frequent respiratory infections or bowel obstruction in infancy.

On initial contact, often in the hospital setting, nurses are involved in performing or assisting with diagnostic tests, primarily sweat for laboratory analysis of chloride content and, less often, stool specimens for trypsin and fat.

Nursing Diagnoses

After a careful assessment numerous nursing diagnoses will become evident. The degree of both pulmonary and gastrointestinal involvement varies among affected children; therefore, nursing diagnoses will also vary according to the individual case. See Box 43-18 for the most common nursing diagnoses.

Planning

The plan of care for the child with CF involves both the child and the family. Major goals include, but are not limited to, the following:

1. The child will demonstrate signs of adequate gas exchange.
2. The child will expectorate mucus.
3. The child will exhibit signs of adequate digestion.
4. The child will experience few or no complications.
5. The child will demonstrate adequate growth and development.
6. The child and family will receive adequate education about the disease and its management.
7. The child and family will receive adequate support.

Implementation

Hospital care. When the child is hospitalized for confirmation of the diagnosis or for pulmonary complications, aerosol therapy is instituted or continued. Respiratory therapy is usually initiated and supervised by a trained respiratory therapist or physiotherapist. Institutions with large support staffs may provide all treatments. Otherwise, it becomes the responsibility of the nurse to perform the prescribed aerosol therapy and CPT and to teach supervised breathing exercises. CPT should not be performed before or immediately after meals. Planning the activity so that it does not coincide with meals is difficult in the hospital. However, it is very important and is often overlooked by nursing personnel.

BOX 43-18

Nursing Diagnoses: The Child with Cystic Fibrosis

Ineffective airway clearance related to secretion of thick, tenacious mucus
Impaired gas exchange related to airway obstruction
Ineffective breathing pattern related to tracheobronchial obstruction
Altered nutrition: less than body requirements related to inability to digest nutrients, loss of appetite (advanced disease)
Altered growth and development related to inadequate digestion of nutrients
Risk for infection related to impaired body defenses, presence of mucus as medium for growth of organisms
Activity intolerance related to imbalance between oxygen supply and demand
Altered family processes related to situational crises
Impaired social interaction related to frequent hospitalizations, confinement to home, fatigue
Anticipatory grieving related to perceived potential loss of child

Oxygen is cautiously administered to a child in respiratory distress, and the child requires frequent assessment. The hazard of oxygen narcosis is a constant threat in children with long-standing disease who receive oxygen (see Chapter 42). The child requires close observation to assist with cough and expectoration.

The diet is implemented for the newly diagnosed child or continued for the child who is hospitalized for pulmonary disease. Children in the early stages of the disease maintain a good appetite, and some will eat excessively. With infection and increased lung involvement, however, the appetite diminishes. Eventually it becomes a challenge to tempt failing appetites (see Feeding the Sick Child, Chapter 42). Some younger children may object to the extra fluids that are encouraged to prevent dehydration. Food is considered therapy for these patients. The caloric intake should be increased significantly. Pancreatic enzymes are supplied for each meal or snack, and adequate salt is provided, especially for febrile children.

Frequent skin care is carried out to prevent irritation and skin breakdown over bony prominences. Particular attention is necessary after use of the bedpan or when the diaper is changed. Careful cleansing helps to reduce irritation and odor from offensive stools, and the use of moisture barriers will protect the skin.

The child will need support for the many treatments and tests that are a necessary part of the hospital therapy. Intravenous fluids and blood tests are almost always a part of the treatment, and the child soon associates hospitalization with these stress-provoking procedures. Because these children are usually quite thin with little muscle mass, careful selection of injection sites is required.

Support of both child and family is a vital part of nursing care. The progressive nature of the disease makes each illness requiring hospitalization a potentially life-threatening event. Skilled nursing care and sympathetic attention to the emotional needs of the child and family help them cope with the stresses associated with repeated respiratory infections and hospitalization.

Home care. After the diagnosis is confirmed and a treatment program determined, preparation for home care is implemented. The plan of care should be flexible enough so that family activities are disrupted as little as possible. Parents will need help finding inhalation equipment available for home use that best meets their needs. They will need opportunities to learn about and practice the use of the equipment, as well as understanding some of the problems they may encounter.

They need to learn about the preferred diet of nutritious meals with tolerated fat and ample protein and carbohydrate and the administration of pancreatic enzymes. Children usually adjust well to taking pancreatic enzymes. For infants and young children, the enzymes can be mixed with pureed fruit, such as applesauce, and fed with a spoon. Capsules are suitable for older children. It is important to stress to parents that the enzymes, in the amount regulated to the child's needs, should be administered about 30 minutes before all meals and snacks. They are cautioned about not restricting salt, especially during hot weather, and ensuring an adequate fluid intake, since dehydration aggravates the thick mucus secretions. Oral hygiene is important because of interference with salivation and the increased susceptibility to oral infections.

One of the most important aspects of educating parents for home care is teaching CPT and breathing exercises. The success of a therapy program depends on conscientious regular performance of these treatments as prescribed. The number of times these therapies are performed each day is determined on an individual basis, and often parents readily learn to adjust the number and intensity of the treatments to the child's needs. When additional respiratory exercises are introduced to established routines, the family will need to be reeducated in new techniques, such as "huffing."

Postural drainage can be achieved with simple activities that are fun, such as hanging by the knees from a bar or low-hanging trapeze that can be easily built in the backyard (or indoors), turning somersaults, or playing "wheelbarrow" with the child suspended head down and propelling with the hands while the adult holds onto the feet. Most children respond to a challenge, such as, "How long can you stand on your head?" Small children can "stand on their heads" on the cushion of a large chair with or without an adult holding onto their feet. Parents soon learn to respond to cues from their children and incorporate spontaneous activities into the treatment regimen.

The nurse can assist the family in contacting resources that provide help to families with affected children. The various special child health services, many local clinics, private agencies, service clubs, and other community groups often offer equipment and medications either free or at reduced rates. The Cystic Fibrosis Foundation* has chapters throughout the United States to provide education and services to families and professionals.

Family support. One of the most important and difficult aspects of providing care for the family of a child with CF is coping with the emotional needs of the child and family. The diagnosis, treatment, and prognosis are fraught with many problems, frustrations, and feelings. The diagnosis with all its implications evokes feelings of guilt and self-recrimination in parents. These feelings may be particularly marked if the newly diagnosed child is the second affected child in the family, and the parents had been counseled about the 1:4 risk of such an event.

The long-range problems are those encountered in the care of a child with a chronic illness (see Chapter 38). Both the child and the family must make many adjustments, the success of which depends on their abiilty to cope and also on the quality and quantity of support they receive from outside sources. Combined efforts of a variety of health professionals offer the most comprehensive services to families. It is often the responsibility of the nurse to organize and coordinate these services, to assess the home situation, and to collect the data needed to evaluate the effectiveness of the services in meeting the family's needs.

The persistent need for treatment several times daily also places a strain on the family. Someone must perform the procedures, such as percussion and vibration, even on older children who are able to assume responsibility for their own exercises and respiratory therapy. Children often balk at the treatments, and the parents are placed in the position of insisting on compliance. Sometimes the stress and anxiety related to this continual routine generate feelings of resentment, which are frequently focused on one aspect of the regimen, such as the diet or equipment. When possible, occasional trusted respite care should be made available to the parent or parents to allow them the opportunity to leave the situation for short periods without undue anxiety about the child's welfare.

The affected child may also become resentful about the disease, its relentless routine of therapy, and the necessary curtailment it places on activities and relationships. The child's activities are interrupted or built around treatment, medications, and diet that impose hardships (such as carrying medication to school and other places where the child may eat away from home), and the growth retardation associated with most chronic illnesses may be trying. Any of these aspects of the disease may be the cause of ridicule by other children. However, the child should be encouraged to attend school and join age-appropriate groups, such as scouting, to foster a life that is as normal and productive as possible.

Families afflicted with CF have psychologic hurdles similar to those of all families coping with a child with a chronic illness, and a constant source of anxiety for both parents and child is the ever-present fear of death.

As the disease progresses, however, family stress should be expected, and the patient may become angry and noncompliant. It is important for the nurse to recognize the changing needs of the family. Families should be made aware of sources for counseling as stressful setbacks occur. Patients need to be guided into activities that enable them to express anger, sorrow, and fear without guilt.

As life expectancy continues to rise for children with CF, issues related to marriage, childbearing, and career choice become more pressing. Men must be informed at some point that they will be unable to produce offspring. It is important that the distinction be made between sterility and impotence. Normal sexual relationships can be expected. Female patients may be able to bear children but must be made aware of the possible deleterious effects on the respiratory system created by the burden of pregnancy. They need to know that their children will be carriers of the CF gene.

Life as an independent adult, the goal that most families have for their children, should be encouraged for children with CF. From the time that children can take partial responsibility for their own care (e.g., CPT and taking enzymes), independence and accountability should be fostered. Although the prognosis for these children has improved, many do not survive through the second decade of life. Anticipatory grieving and other aspects related to care of a child with a terminal illness are part of nursing care (see Chapter 38).

*6931 Arlington Rd., Bethesda, MD 20814-3205; (800) FIGHT CF or (301) 951-4422. In Canada: Canadian Cystic Fibrosis Foundation, 586 Eglinton Ave., E., Suite 204, Toronto, Ontario M4P 1P2. Two excellent publications available from the Cystic Fibrosis Foundation are *What Everyone Should Know About Cystic Fibrosis* and *Cystic Fibrosis: A Summary of Symptoms, Diagnosis, and Treatment.* For information about specialized medications, especially Pulmozyne, and equipment for CF and other pulmonary diseases, contact Cystic Fibrosis Pharmacy, Inc., H.H.C.S. Pharmacy Services, 633 E. Colonial Drive, Orlando, FL 32803; (800) 741-4427.

Evaluation

The efficacy of nursing management can be evaluated by application of observational guidelines, which may include the following:

1. Monitor vital signs, especially respiratory parameters.
2. Monitor chest physiotherapy and other procedures to assess the expected outcomes (e.g., expectoration of secretions, increased lung expansion).
3. Monitor meals to ensure that enzymes are taken.
4. Monitor child for evidence of respiratory infection, gastrointestinal dysfunction, and other complications.
5. Observe nutritional intake. For the child at home, interview the family regarding child's intake or have child maintain a log of nutritional intake. Obtain regular measurements of growth, and interview child and family regarding school attendance, interaction with peers, and participation in sports and other activities.
6. Explore family's understanding of the disease and its therapies and the family's ability to carry out the treatment plan.
7. Maintain contact with family (if feasible) at follow-up evaluations and during home care. Observe for readmissions. Interview child and family regarding involvement with agencies and services for children with CF.

Expected outcomes include the following:

1. Child breathes easily and without dyspnea.
2. Child manages secretions with minimum distress.
3. Child takes pancreatic enzymes as prescribed.
4. Child displays no evidence of an infective process.
5. Child is well nourished, exhibits satisfactory weight gain, and engages in appropriate activities.
6. Child and family demonstrate an understanding of the disease and comply with the therapeutic regimen (specify knowledge and method of demonstration).
7. Family maintains contact with health care providers.

See also the Nursing Care Plan: The Child With Cystic Fibrosis.*

Respiratory Emergency

Nurses must be prepared to deal effectively with respiratory emergencies. Although the interventions are similar to those used for adults, there are some variations for infants and children.

RESPIRATORY FAILURE

In general, the term **respiratory insufficiency** is applied to two conditions: (1) increased work of breathing but with gas exchange function near normal (ventilatory insufficiency) and (2) inability to maintain normal blood gas tensions and development of hypoxemia and acidosis as a result of CO_2 retention.

Respiratory failure is defined as the inability of the respiratory apparatus to maintain adequate oxygenation of the blood, with or without CO_2 retention. **Respiratory arrest** is the cessation of respiration. **Apnea** is the absence of airflow (breathing).

Effective pulmonary gas exchange requires clear airways, normal lungs and chest wall, and adequate pulmonary circulation. Anything that affects these functions or their relationships can compromise respiration.

Diagnostic Evaluation

Respiratory failure that occurs as a result of acute obstruction of a major airway or cardiac arrest is sudden and readily apparent. Gradual or progressive deterioration of respiratory function is less easily recognized. Therefore, nursing observation and judgment are vital to the recognition and early management of respiratory failure. Nurses must be able to assess a situation and initiate appropriate action within moments. Signs of respiratory failure are listed in Box 43-19.

Therapeutic Management

The interventions used in the management of respiratory failure are often dramatic, requiring special skills, and are often

BOX 43-19
Clinical Manifestations of Respiratory Failure

Cardinal signs
Restlessness
Tachypnea
Tachycardia
Diaphoresis

Early but less obvious signs
Mood changes, such as euphoria or depression
Headache
Altered depth and pattern of respirations
Hypertension
Exertional dyspnea
Anorexia
Increased cardiac output and renal output
Central nervous system symptoms (decreased efficiency, impaired judgment, anxiety, confusion, restlessness, and irritability)
Flaring nares
Chest wall retractions
Expiratory grunt
Wheezing and/or prolonged expiration

Signs of more severe hypoxia
Hypotension or hypertension
Dimness of vision
Somnolence
Stupor
Coma
Dyspnea
Depressed respirations
Bradycardia
Cyanosis, peripheral or central

*In Wong DL: *Wong and Whaley's clinical manual of pediatric nursing*, ed 4, St Louis, 1996, Mosby.

Family Focus

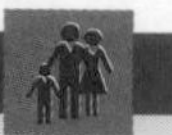

PARENTAL PRESENCE DURING CPR

Few acute care facilities allow parents to stay during CPR or a "code." Health professionals' reasons for this decision include believing the experience is too upsetting for the family, fearing the family will need care that will interfere with the staff's resuscitation efforts, experiencing discomfort being "watched" by the family, and fearing increased legal liability if the family knows what has been done or not done.

In reality, when parents do observe their child's CPR, these reasons are not supported. One study found that parents who were given the choice of staying during the code unanimously stated that they would choose this option again. Parents did not interfere with the resuscitation, they were assured that everything was done for their child, and they considered being present one of the most important memories of this difficult experience (Villarreal, 1992).

Of family members who stayed during CPR of an adult patient, 76% said their adjustment to death was easier and 64% felt their presence was beneficial to the dying person; 71% of staff members endorsed the policy (Hanson and Strawser, 1992). Also, the Emergency Nurses Association (1994) supports the option of family presence during invasive procedures and/or resuscitation efforts.

On the basis of these findings, we need to question the wisdom of excluding parents during CPR. All may not choose to be present, but shouldn't they be given the opportunity? Whose benefit is served by family exclusion? If the main reason is the staff's own fears and anxieties about being observed and possibly judged on their performance, is depriving the family of their wishes justified? Consider out-of-hospital arrests; EMS personnel routinely perform CPR with family and strangers watching. Why is this public rescue attempt considered acceptable but an inhospital code considered a private event?

emergency procedures. Some of the techniques employed to assist ventilation include artificial ventilation, artificial airway, and cardiopulmonary resuscitation.

Artificial ventilation. There are a variety of methods for controlling or assisting ventilation. Temporary assistance can be provided by a manual self-inflating ventilation bag with a mask and nonreturnable valve to prevent rebreathing. With the mask placed over the child's nose and mouth (an open airway is established by correct positioning with the chin forward and the neck extended to the "sniffing" position), the bag is rhythmically compressed, forcing the gas from the bag into the child's lungs.

For more prolonged assistance, mechanical ventilation is employed to replace the bellows function of the diaphragm and thoracic wall muscles. The lungs are inflated by the application of either positive or negative pressure. The positive-pressure machine inflates the lung by increasing airway pressure above atmospheric pressure, and a negative-pressure ventilator creates a subatmospheric pressure around the chest wall, whereas airway pressure remains atmospheric. Application of positive pressure by mechanical means usually improves the distribution of gas within the lung and often reinflates partially collapsed lung segments. The overall effect is the improvement of gas exchange.

Nursing Care Management

For those families whose child experiences a respiratory arrest, support focuses on keeping the family informed of the child's status and helping them cope with a near-death experience or an actual death (see Chapter 38). Knowing that their child requires CPR is a frightening and often overwhelming experience for parents. Uncertainty regarding outcome—both mortality and morbidity—is a primary concern. Traditionally, family members are not allowed to be present during resuscitation efforts (see the Family Focus box to the left). Nurses can serve as the family's advocate by either being present with them or making sure a support person, such as a member of the clergy, is present. After the child's recovery or death, the family needs continued support and thorough medical information regarding lifesaving measures, the prognosis if the child survives, and the cause of death if the child dies.

CARDIOPULMONARY RESUSCITATION (CPR)

Cardiac arrest in the pediatric population is less often of cardiac origin than from prolonged hypoxemia secondary to inadequate oxygenation, ventilation, and circulation (shock). Some causes include injuries, suffocation (e.g., foreign body aspiration), smoke inhalation, sudden infant death syndrome (SIDS), or infection. Respiratory arrest has been associated with a better survival than cardiac arrest. Once cardiac arrest occurs, the outcome of resuscitative efforts is poor.

Complete apnea signals the need for rapid and vigorous action to prevent cardiac arrest. In such situations nurses must be prepared to initiate action immediately. Neurologically intact survival has occurred only in those children who receive immediate resuscitation and respond promptly. In the hospital, emergency equipment should be readily available in patient care centers, and the status of this resuscitation equipment should be checked at least once daily. Regardless of the cause of the arrest, some very basic procedures are carried out, modified somewhat according to the child's size.

Nursing ALERT

Rescuers who have infections that may be transmitted by blood or saliva should not perform mouth-to-mouth resuscitation if the circumstances allow other immediate or effective methods of ventilation.

Outside the hospital, the first action in an emergency is to assess quickly the extent of any injury and determine whether the child is unconscious. A child who is struggling to breathe but conscious should be transported immediately to an *advanced life support (ALS)* facility, with the child maintaining whatever position affords the most comfort. However, attempting to transport a child by automobile wastes valuable time in obtaining help; transport by an *emergency medical service (EMS)* is recommended or preferable. Services in larger communities can institute ALS immediately or en route to a medical facility.

An unconscious child is managed with care to prevent additional trauma if a head or spinal cord injury has been sustained. The circumstances in which the child is found offer some clues to a possible injury. For example, a child who has been thrown from a bicycle or fallen from a tree is more likely to sustain trauma than a child who is discovered in bed. The child should be turned as a unit with firm support provided to the head and neck to prevent rolling, twisting, or tilting backward or forward.

Resuscitation Procedure

For effective CPR the victim is placed on the back on a firm flat surface, employing appropriate precautions (Fig. 43-5). With loss of consciousness the tongue, which is attached to the lower jaw, relaxes and falls back, obstructing the airway. To open the airway, the head is positioned with either the head tilt/chin lift or jaw thrust maneuver. Health professionals should be able to use both maneuvers. *Head tilt* is accomplished by placing one hand on the victim's forehead and ap-

One-rescuer CPR

		ACTIONS		
	Objectives	**Adult (over 8 yr)**	**Child (1 to 8 yr)**	**Infant (under 1 yr)**
A. AIRWAY	1. Assessment: determine unresponsiveness.	Tap or gently shake shoulder.		
		Say, "Are you okay?"		Speak loudly.
	2. Get help.	Activate EMS.	Shout for help. If second rescuer available, have person activate EMS.	
	3. Position the victim.	Turn on back as a unit, supporting head and neck if necessary (4-10 seconds).		
	4. Open the airway.	Head-tilt/chin-lift.		
B. BREATHING	5. Assessment: determine breathlessness.	Maintain open airway. Place ear over mouth, observing chest. Look, listen, feel for breathing (3-5 seconds).*		
	6. Give 2 rescue breaths.	Maintain open airway.		
		Seal mouth to mouth.		Mouth to nose/mouth.
		Give 2 slow breaths. Observe chest rise. Allow lung deflation between breaths.		
		1½ to 2 seconds each	1 to 1½ seconds each	
	7. Option for obstructed airway.	a. Reposition victim's head. Try again to give rescue breaths.		
			b. Activate EMS.	
		c. Give 5 subdiaphragmatic abdominal thrusts (the Heimlich maneuver).		c. Give 5 back blows.
				c. Give 5 chest thrusts.
		d. Tongue-jaw lift and finger sweep.	d. Tongue-jaw lift, but finger sweep only if you see a foreign object.	
		If unsuccessful, repeat a, c, and d until successful.		
C. CIRCULATION	8. Assessment: determine pulselessness.	Feel for carotid pulse with one hand; maintain head-tilt with the other (5-10 seconds).		Feel for brachial pulse: keep head-tilt.
CPR	Pulse absent: begin chest compressions. 9. Landmark check.	Run middle finger along bottom edge of rib cage to notch at center (top of sternum).		Imagine a line drawn between the nipples.
	10. Hand position.	Place index finger next to finger on notch:		Place 2-3 fingers on sternum. 1 finger's width below line. Depress ½-1 in.
		Two hands next to index finger. Depress 1½-2 in.	Heel of one hand next to index finger. Depress 1-1½ in.	
	11. Compression rate.	80-100 per minute	100 per minute	At least 100 per minute
	12. Compressions to breaths.	2 breaths to every 15 compressions	1 breath to every 5 compressions	
	13. Number of cycles.	4	20 (approximately 1 minute)	
	14. Reassessment.	Feel for carotid pulse.		Feel for brachial pulse.
		If no pulse, resume CPR, starting with compressions.	If alone, activate EMS. If no pulse, resume CPR, starting with compressions.	
	Pulse present; not breathing: Begin rescue breathing.	1 breath every 5 seconds (12 per minute)	1 breath every 3 seconds (20 per minute)	

Fig. 43-5 One-rescuer CPR. (Modified from Chandra NC, Hazinski MF, eds: *Textbook of basic life support for healthcare providers*, Dallas, 1994, American Heart Association.)

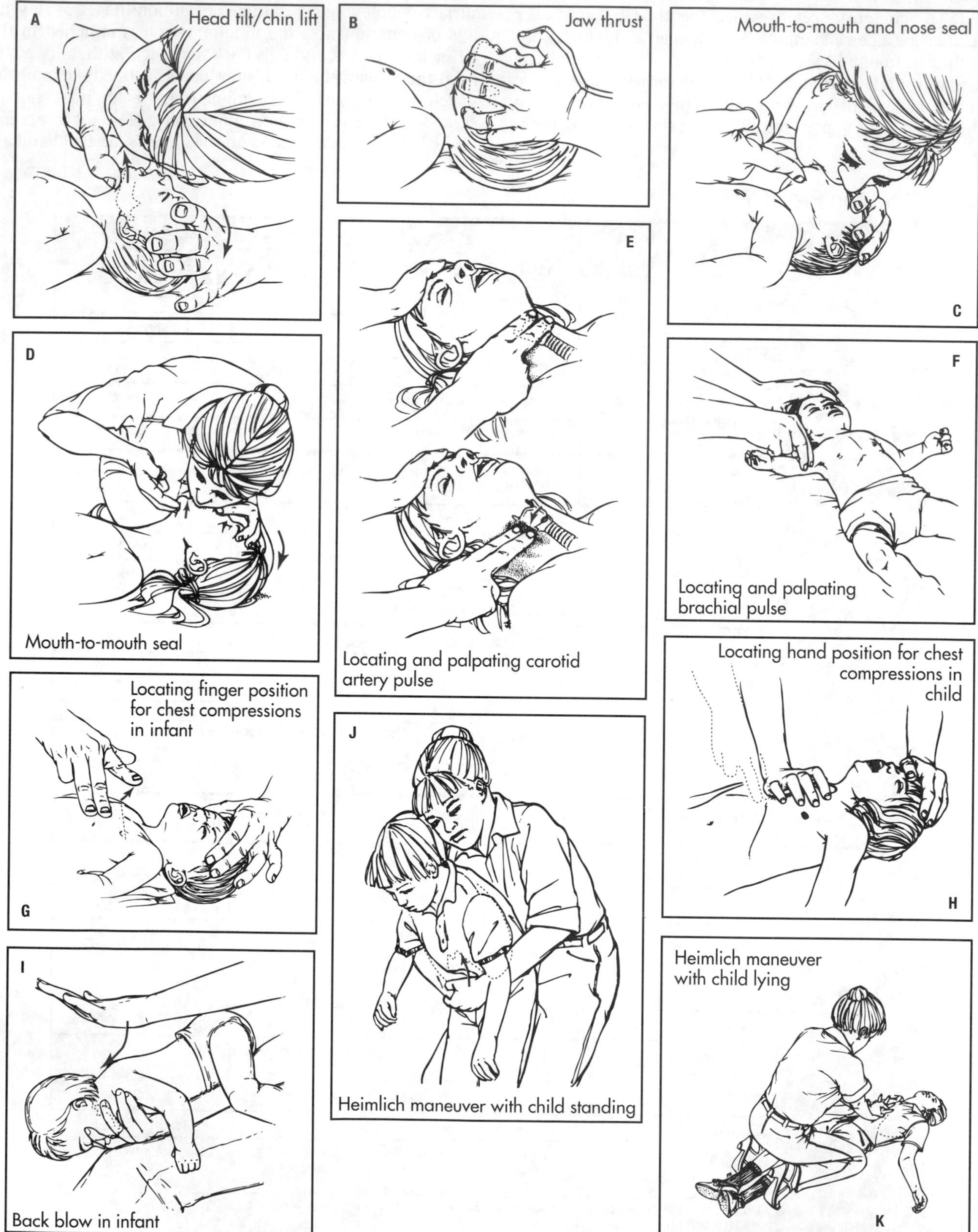

Fig. 43-6 Procedures for cardiopulmonary resuscitation, **A** to **H**, and airway obstruction, **I** to **K.** (From Chandra NC, Hazinski MF, eds: *Textbook of basic life support for healthcare providers*, Dallas, 1994, American Heart Association.)

plying firm, backward pressure with the palm to tilt the head back. The fingers of the free hand are placed under the bony portion of the lower jaw near the chin to lift and bring the chin forward *(chin lift)*. This supports the jaw and helps tilt the head back (Fig. 43-6, *A*).

The *jaw thrust* is accomplished by grasping the angles of the victim's lower jaw and lifting with both hands, one on each side, displacing the mandible upward and outward (Fig. 43-6, *B*). In suspected neck injuries, the jaw thrust method should be used while the cervical spine is completely immobilized. After restoration of a patent airway by removal of foreign material and secretions (if indicated), and if the child is not breathing, continuation of the airway is maintained and rescue breathing is initiated. To ventilate the lungs in the infant (birth to 1 year of age), the operator's mouth is placed in such a way that both the mouth and the nostrils are covered (Fig. 43-6, *C*). Children (over 1 year of age) are ventilated through the mouth while the nostrils are firmly pinched for airtight contact (Fig. 43-6, *D*).

When a child requires CPR, consider the size, not just the age, of the child, since the guidelines for infants and for children ages 1 to 8 years may not always apply. For example, the volume of air in an infant's lungs is small and the air passages are considerably smaller, with resistance to flow potentially higher than in adults. Therefore small puffs of air are delivered. Also, young children who can be placed on the rescuer's thigh should receive infant CPR. Since many older children with severe chronic illness or disability remain small in size, pediatric, not adult CPR, may be appropriate.

If air enters freely and the chest rises, the airway is assumed to be clear. Volume must be provided without causing abdominal distention. Gastric distention, which interferes with diaphragmatic excursion, commonly occurs when more volume than necessary is delivered and the breaths are delivered too rapidly.

After the initial two breaths, the pulse is palpated to ascertain the presence of a heartbeat. The carotid is the most central and accessible artery in children over 1 year of age (Fig. 43-6, *E*). However, the very short and often fat neck of the infant renders the carotid pulse difficult to palpate. Therefore it is preferable to use the brachial pulse in the infant, which is located on the inner side of the upper arm midway between the elbow and shoulder (Fig. 43-6, *F*). Absence of a carotid or brachial pulse is considered sufficient indication to begin external cardiac massage.

Chest compression. External chest compression consists of serial, rhythmic compressions of the chest to maintain circulation to vital organs until the child achieves spontaneous vital signs or ALS can be provided. *Chest compressions are always interposed with ventilation of the lungs.* For optimum compressions, it is essential that the child's spine be supported on a firm surface during compressions of the sternum, and sternal pressure must be forceful but not traumatic. For an infant the hard surface can be the rescuer's hand or forearm, with the palm supporting the infant's back. The child's head is positioned for optimum airway opening using the head tilt/chin lift maneuver. It is essential to prevent overextension of the head of small infants, since this tends to close the flexible trachea.

The placement of the fingers for compression in infants is at a point on the lower sterum, one fingerbreadth below the intersection of the sternum and an imaginary line drawn between the nipples (Fig. 43-6, *G*). Compressions on the child 1 to 8 years of age are applied to the lower sternum two fingerbreadths above the sternal notch (Fig. 43-6, *H*). Sternal compression to infants is applied with two fingers on the sternum exerting a firm downward thrust; for children pressure is applied with the heel of one hand. The depth of compression is also adapted to the child's size. The location, rate, and depth for children over 8 years of age are the same as for adults.

CPR is continued at the appropriate ratio of breaths/compressions for age until signs of recovery appear. These are evidenced by palpable peripheral pulses, return of pupils to normal size, disappearance of mottling and cyanosis, and possibly return of spontaneous respiration.

Medications. Medications are an important adjunct to resuscitation, especially cardiac arrest, and are used during and after resuscitation in children. Appropriate fluid therapy is initiated immediately to children in the hospital or by EMS personnel during transport (see Parenteral Fluid Therapy, Chapter 42, and Shock, Chapter 45). A complete supply of emergency medications is kept and maintained in all EMS vehicles and on all hospital units. The supply is checked on a regular basis (usually once on each 8-hour shift). Resuscitation medications are listed in Table 43-3.

Nursing ALERT

When administering drugs during CPR (or a "code"), use a saline solution flush between medications to prevent drug interactions. Document all drugs, dosages, and time and route of administration.

AIRWAY OBSTRUCTION

Attempts at clearing the airway should be considered for (1) children in whom a foreign body aspiration is witnessed or strongly suspected, and (2) unconscious, nonbreathing children whose airways remain obstructed despite the usual maneuvers to open them. When foreign body aspiration is strongly suspected, the child is encouraged to continue coughing as long as the cough remains forceful. If the cough becomes ineffective, mechanical maneuvers should be used in an attempt to dislodge the object.

Nursing ALERT

In a conscious choking child attempt to relieve the obstruction only if:
The child is unable to make any sounds
The cough becomes ineffective
There is increasing respiratory difficulty with stridor

Blind finger sweeps are avoided in both infants and children. A combination of back blows (over the spine between the shoulder blades) and chest thrusts (on sternum, same location as chest compressions) are recommended to relieve foreign body obstruction in infants.

TABLE 43-3 Drugs for pediatric cardiopulmonary resuscitation

DRUG/DOSE	ACTION	IMPLICATIONS
Epinephrine HCl		
IV/IO: 0.01 mg/kg (1:10,000)* ET: 0.1 mg/kg (1:1000)*	Adrenergic Acts on both alpha- and beta-receptor sites, especially heart and vascular and other smooth muscle	Most useful drug in cardiac arrest Disappears rapidly from bloodstream after injection May produce renal vessel constriction and decreased urine formation
Sodium bicarbonate		
1 mEq/kg	Alkalinizer Buffers pH	Infuse slowly and only when ventilation is adequate
Atropine sulfate		
0.02 mg/kg/dose Minimum dose: 0.1 mg Maximum single dose: infants and children, 0.5 mg; adolescents, 1.0 mg	Anticholinergic-parasympatholytic Increases cardiac output, heart rate by blocking vagal stimulation in heart	Used to treat bradycardia after ventilatory assessment
Calcium chloride 10%		
20 mg/kg	Electrolyte replacement Needed for maintenance of normal cardiac contractility	Used only for hypocalcemia, calcium blocker overdose, hyperkalemia, or hypermagnesemia Administer slowly
Lidocaine HCl		
1 mg/kg	Antidysrhythmic Inhibits nerve impulses from sensory nerves	Used for ventricular dysrhythmias only
Bretylium		
5 mg/kg; may be increased to 10 mg/kg	Antidysrhythmic Inhibits release of norepinephrine in postganglionic nerve endings that control ventricular tachycardia	Used if lidocaine is not effective Administer rapidly
Adenosine		
0.1 to 0.2 mg/kg Maximum single dose: 12 mg	Antidysrhythmic Causes a temporary block through the atrioventricular (AV) node and interrupts the reentry circuits	Administer rapidly Very effective Minimal side effects
Infusions		
Epinephrine HCl infusion		
0.1-1.0 μg/kg/min	Adrenergic See above	Titrated to desired hemodynamic effect
Dopamine HCl infusion		
2-20 μg/kg/min	Agonist Acts on alpha receptors, causing vasoconstriction Increases cardiac output	Titrated to desired hemodynamic response
Dobutamine HCl infusion		
2-20 μg/kg/min	Adrenergic direct-acting $beta_1$-agonist Increases contractility and heart rate	Titrated to desired hemodynamic response Little vasoconstriction, even at high rates
Lidocaine HCl infusion		
20-50 μg/kg/min	Antidysrhythmic Increases electrical stimulation threshold of ventricle	See above Lower infusion dose used in shock Used for ventricular tachycardia

**IV,* Intravenous route; *IO,* intraosseous route; *ET,* endotracheal route.

Signs of life-threatening obstruction

The truly choking child *cannot speak, becomes cyanotic,* and *collapses*				
		Actions		
	Objectives	Adult (over 8 yr)	Child (1 to 8 yr)	Infant (under 1 yr)
CONSCIOUS VICTIM	1. Assessment: determine airway obstruction.	Ask, "Are you choking?" Determine if victim can cough or speak.		Observe breathing difficulty, ineffective cough, no strong cry.
	2. Act to relieve obstruction.	Perform up to 5 subdiaphragmatic abdominal thrusts (Heimlich maneuver).		Give 5 back blows.
				Give 5 chest thrusts.
	Be persistent.	Repeat Step 2 until obstruction is relieved or victim becomes unconscious.		
VICTIM WHO BECOMES UNCONSCIOUS	3. Position the victim: call for help.	Turn on back as a unit, supporting head and neck, face up, arms by sides. Call out, "Help!" Activate EMS. If second rescuer available, have person activate EMS.		
	4. Check for foreign body.	Perform tongue-jaw lift and finger sweep.	Perform tongue-jaw lift. Remove foreign object only if you actually see it.	
	5. Give rescue breaths.	Open the airway with head tilt/chin lift. Try to give rescue breaths. If airway is obstructed, reposition head and try to ventilate again.		
	6. Act to relieve obstruction.	Perform up to 5 subdiaphragmatic abdominal thrusts (Heimlich maneuver).		Give 5 back blows.
				Give 5 chest thrusts.
	7. Be persistent.	Repeat steps 4-6 until obstruction is relieved.		
UNCONSCIOUS VICTIM	1. Assessment: determine unresponsiveness.	Tap or gently shake shoulder. Shout, "Are you okay?"	Tap or gently shake shoulder.	
		If unresponsive, activate EMS.		
	2. Call for help: position the victim.	Turn on back as a unit, supporting head and neck, face up, arms by sides.		
			Call out for help.	
	3. Open the airway.	Head-tilt/chin-lift.		Head-tilt/chin-lift, but do not tilt too far.
	4. Assessment: determine breathlessness.	Maintain an open airway. Ear over mouth; observe chest. Look, listen, feel for breathing. (3-5 seconds)		
	5. Give rescue breaths.	Make mouth-to-mouth seal.		Make mouth-to-nose-and-mouth seal.
		Try to give rescue breaths.		
	6. If chest is not rising, try again to give rescue breaths.	Reposition head. Try rescue breaths again.		
	7. Activate the EMS system.		If airway obstruction not relieved after about 1 minute, activate EMS as rapidly as possible.	
	8. Act to relieve obstruction.	Perform up to 5 subdiaphragmatic abdominal thrusts (Heimlich maneuver).		Give 5 back blows.
				Give 5 chest thrusts.
	9. Check for foreign body.	Perform tongue-jaw lift and finger sweep.	Perform tongue-jaw lift. Remove foreign object only if you actually see it.	
	10. Rescue breaths.	Open the airway with head-tilt/chin-lift. Try again to give rescue breaths. If airway is obstructed, reposition head and try to ventilate again.		
	11. Be persistent.	Repeat steps 8-10 until obstruction is relieved.		

Fig. 43-7 Foreign body airway obstruction management. (Modified from Chandra NC, Hazinski MF, eds: *Textbook of basic life support for healthcare providers,* Dallas, 1994, American Heart Association.)

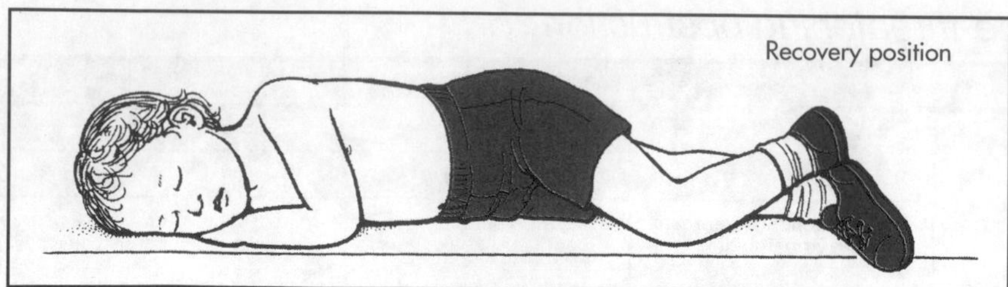

Fig. 43-8 Recovery position.

Infants

A choking infant is placed face down over the rescuer's arm with the head lower than the trunk and the head supported (Fig. 43-6, *I*). For additional support the rescuer should support the arm firmly against the thigh. Up to five quick, sharp, back blows are delivered between the infant's shoulder blades with the heel of the rescuer's hand. Less force is required than would be applied to an adult. After delivery of the back blows, the rescuer's free hand is placed flat on the infant's back so that the infant is "sandwiched" between the two hands, making certain the neck and chin are well supported. While the rescuer maintains support with the infant's head lower than the trunk, the infant is turned and placed supine on the rescuer's thigh, where up to five quick downward chest thrusts are applied in rapid succession in the same location as external chest compressions described for CPR. Back blows and chest thrusts are continued until the object is removed or the infant becomes unconscious.

Children

The **Heimlich manuever**, a series of *subdiaphragmatic abdominal thrusts*, is recommended for children over 1 year of age. The maneuver creates an artificial cough that forces air, and with it the foreign body, out of the airway. The procedure is carried out with the child in a standing, sitting, or lying position (Fig. 43-6, *J* and *K*). In the conscious choking child, upward thrusts are delivered to the upper abdomen with the fisted hand at a point just below the rib cage (Fig. 43-7). To prevent damage to the internal organs, the rescuer's hands should not touch the xiphoid process of the sternum or the lower margins of the ribs. Five thrusts are repeated in rapid succession until the foreign body is expelled.

It is neither necessary nor desirable to squeeze or compress the arms during the procedure. It is not a punch or a bear hug. The child may vomit after relief of the obstruction and should be positioned to prevent aspiration. After breathing is restored, the child should receive medical attention and be assessed for complications.

The success of the technique is primarily a result of the obstruction's occurring at the end of a maximum respiration. The victim is most likely to choke on food during inspiration; therefore the tidal volume plus expiratory reserve volume is present in the lungs. When pressure is exerted on the diaphragm by the maneuver, the food bolus is ejected with considerable force by this trapped air.

Nursing ALERT

If victim is breathing or resumes effective breathing after emergency interventions, place in recovery position: (1) move head, shoulders, and torso simultaneously; (2) turn onto side; and (3) leg not in contact with ground may be bent and knee moved forward to stabilize victim (Fig. 43-8). Victim should not be moved in any way if trauma is suspected and should not be placed in recovery position if rescue breathing or CPR is required.

Key Points

- Acute infection of the respiratory tract is the most common cause of illness in infancy and childhood.
- The incidence and severity of respiratory tract infections are influenced by the infectious agents involved, the child's age, and the child's natural defenses.
- Common respiratory tract infections of childhood include acute nasopharyngitis, acute pharyngitis (including tonsillitis), influenza, and otitis media.
- Croup syndromes involve acute inflammation and variable degrees of obstruction of the epiglottis, larynx, and/or trachea.
- The primary goals in the care of children with croup are observation for signs of respiratory distress and relief of laryngeal obstruction.
- Common infections of the lower airways are bacterial tracheitis, asthmatic bronchitis, bronchitis, and bronchiolitis.
- Pneumonias are classified according to site (lobar, bronchial, or interstitial) or by etiologic agent (viruses, bacteria, mycoplasms, or associated with aspiration of foreign material).
- In tuberculosis, susceptibility to the bacillus can be influenced by heredity, age, stress, poor nutrition, and intercurrent infection.
- Passive inhalation of cigarette smoke is one of the primary environmental pollutants contributing to respiratory disease in children.
- Asthma is the leading cause of chronic illness in children.
- General therapeutic management of asthma includes allergen control, drug therapy, controlled exercise, physical therapy, and hyposensitization.
- Support for the family of the child with asthma includes education about the disease and its therapy and facilitation of self-management.

- Cystic fibrosis is the most common inherited disease in children.
- The diagnosis of cystic fibrosis is based on the family history, increased sweat electrolyte content, absent pancreatic enzymes, and chronic pulmonary involvement.
- Choking and respiratory failure are respiratory emergencies that necessitate immediate intervention.
- The Heimlich maneuver is reserved for children in whom foreign body aspiration is witnessed or strongly suspected. A combination of back blows and chest thrusts is used for infants with foreign body aspiration.
- In a conscious choking child attempts to relieve the obstruction are used only if the child is unable to make any sounds; the cough becomes ineffective; or there is increasing respiratory difficulty with stridor.

References

Alho OP et al: Control of the temporal aspect when considering risk factors for acute otitis media, *Arch Otolaryngeal Head Neck Surg* 119:444-449, 1993.

American Academy of Pediatrics, Committee on Infectious Diseases: Reassessment of the indications for ribavirin therapy in respiratory syncitial virus infections, *Pediatrics* 97(1):137-140, 1996a.

American Academy of Pediatrics, Committee on Infectious Diseases: The recommended childhood immunization schedule for 1996, *Pediatrics* 97(1):143, 1996b.

American Academy of Pediatrics, Committee on Infectious Diseases: Update on tuberculin skin testing of children, *Pediatrics* 97(2):282-284, 1996c.

American Academy of Pediatrics, Committee on Substance Abuse: Tobacco-free environment: an imperative for the health of children and adolescents, *Pediatrics* 93(5):866-868, 1994a.

American Academy of Pediatrics, Provisional Committee on Quality Improvement: Practice parameter: the office management of acute exacerbations of asthma in children, *Pediatrics* 93(1):119-126, 1994b.

Colditz GA et al: Efficacy of BCG vaccine in the prevention of tuberculosis, *JAMA* 271(9):698-702, 1994.

Collins F: Cystic fibrosis: molecular biology and therapeutic implications, *Science* 256:774-779, 1992.

Davis PB: Evolution of therapy for cystic fibrosis, *NEJM* 331(10)672-675, 1994.

Derkay CS, Darrow D, LeFebvre S: Pediatric tonsillectomy and adenoidectomy procedures, *AORN J* 62(6):887-904, 1995.

Duff A, Platts-Mills T: Allergens and asthma, *Pediatr Clin North Am* 39(6):1277-1291, 1992.

Emergency Nurses Association Position Statement: *Family presence at the bedside during invasive procedures and/or resuscitation*, Park Ridge, Ill, 1994, Emergency Nurses Association.

Fuchs HJ et al: Effect of aerosolized recombinant human D Nase on exacerbations of respiratory symptoms and on pulmonary function in patients with cystic fibrosis, *NEJM* 331(10):637-642, 1994.

Hanson C, Strawser D: Family presence during cardiopulmonary resuscitation: Foote Hospital emergency department's nine-year perspective, *J Emerg Nurs* 18(2):104-106, 1992.

Hoffman N, Kelly C, Futterman D: Tuberculosis infection in human immunodeficiency virus-positive adolescents and young adults: a New York city cohort, *Pediatrics* 97(2):198-203, 1996.

Holberg CJ, Wright AL, Martinez FD: Child day care, smoking by caregivers, and lower respiratory tract illness in the first 3 years of life, *Pediatrics* 91:885-892, 1993.

Jackson M: Tuberculosis in infants, children, and adolescents: new dilemmas with an old disease, *Pediatr Nurs* 19(5):437-442, 1993.

Kleinman LC et al: The medical appropriateness of tympanostomy tubes proposed for children younger than 16 years in the United States, *JAMA* 271(16):1250-1255, 1994.

Klinnert M, Miller B, Mrazek D: Asthma failures: who's at risk? *Contemp Pediatr* 7(11):81-98, 1990.

Milgram H, Berder B: Behavioral side effects of medications used to treat asthma and allergic rhinitis, *Pediatr Rev* 16(9):333-335, 1995.

National Heart, Lung, and Blood Institute, National Institutes of Health: *Guidelines for the diagnosis and management of asthma*, Pub No 91-3402, Bethesda, Md, Aug 1991.

Ott MJ, Horn M, McLaughlin D: Pediatric TB in the 1990s, *MCN Am J Matern Child Nurs* 20(1):16-20, 1995.

Stool SE et al: *Managing otitis media with effusion in young children: quick reference guide for clinicians*, AHCPR Publication No 94-0623, Rockville, Md; July 1994, Agency for Health Care Policy and Research, Public Health Service, U.S. Department of Health and Human Services.

Tizzano E, Buchwald M: Recent advances in cystic fibrosis research, *J Pediatr* 122(6):985-988, 1993.

Tully SB, Bar-Haim Y, Bradley RL: Abnormal tympanography after supine bottle feeding, *J Pediatr* 126:S105-111, 1995.

Villarreal P: Personal communication, University of Texas, San Antonio, 1992.

Wolf SI et al: EMLA cream for painless skin testing: a preliminary report, *Ann Allergy* 73(1):40-42, 1994.

Bibliography

Respiratory Infection

American Academy of Pediatrics, Committee on Rheumatic Fever, Endocarditis, and Kwashiorkor Disease of the Council on Cardiovascular Disease in the young, The American Heart Association. *Pediatrics* 96(4):758-764, 1995.

Buttaro TM, Ezell B, Gray V: A care plan for children with tuberculosis, *Public Health Nurs* 12(3):181-188, 1995.

Clark G: Childhood tuberculosis cases escalate: disease makes comeback, new strains develop, *AAP News* 10(5):1, 8-9, 11, 1994.

Feldstein TJ et al: Ribavirin therapy: implementation of hospital guidelines and effect on usage and cost of therapy, *Pediatrics* 96(1):14-17, 1995.

Groothius JR et al: Prophylactic administration of respiratory syncytial virus immune globulin to high-risk infants and young children, *N Engl J Med* 329:1524-1530, 1993.

Hurwitz ES and others: Risk of respiratory illness associated with daycare attendance: a nationwide study, *Pediatrics* 87:62-69, 1991.

Jackson M: Tuberculosis in infants, children, and adolescents: new dilemmas with an old disease, *Pediatr News* 19(5):437-442, 1993.

Kitchens GG: Relationship of environmental tobacco smoke to otitis media in young children, *Laryngoscope* 105(5)(Pt 2 Suppl 69):1-13, 1995.

Petree CA: Sputum testing for TB: getting good specimens, *Am J Nurs* 96(2):14, 1996.

Pichichero ME, Pichichero CL: Persistent acute otitis media. I. Causative pathogens, *Pediatric Infect Dis J* 14(3):178-183, 1995.

Pichichero ME, Pichichero CL: Persistent acute otitis media. II. Antimicrobial treatment, *Pediatr Infect Dis J* 14(3):183-188, 1995.

Prows CA et al: Nature and prevalence of Ribavirin aerosol administration in U.S. pediatric hospitals, *J Pediatr Nurs* 8(6):370-375, 1993.

Stamos JK, Rowley AH: Pediatric tuberculosis: an update, *Curr Probl Pediatr* 25(4):131-136, 1995.

Sumaya CA: *Infectious mononucleosis and Epstein-Barr virus.* In Hoekelman RA et al, editors: *Primary pediatric care,* ed 2, St Louis, 1992, Mosby.

Swanson DS, Starke JR: Drug-resistant tuberculosis in pediatrics, *Pediatr Clin North Am* 42(3):553-569, 1995.

Turcios NL: Gauging the severity of bronchiolitis, *J Respir Dis* 15(10):875-888, 1994.

Wolf SI et al: EMLA cream for painless skin testing: a preliminary report, *Ann Allergy* 73(1):40-42, 1994.

Otitis Media

Barnett ED, Klein JO: The problem of resistant bacteria for the management of acute otitis media, *Pediatr Clin North Am* 42(3):509-517, 1995.

Casselbrant M et al: Efficacy of antimicrobial prophylaxis and of tympanostomy tube insertion for prevention of recurrent acute otitis media, *Pediatr Infect Dis J* 11:278-286, 1992.

Duncan B et al: Exclusive breast-feeding for at least 4 months protects against otitis media, *Pediatrics* 91(5):867-872, 1993.

Etzel R et al: Passive smoking and middle ear effusion among children in day care, *Pediatrics* 90(2):228-232, 1992.

Heikkinen T, Ruuskanen O: Signs and symptoms predicting acute otitis media, *Arch Pediatr Adolesc Med* 149(1):26-29, 1995.

Mandel E et al: Antibiotic therapy for otitis media with effusion, *JAMA* 269(4):516-517, 1993.

Shurin P et al: Bacterial polysaccharide immune globulin for prophylaxis of acute otitis media in high-risk children, *J Pediatr* 123:801-810, 1993.

Williams R et al: Use of antibiotics in preventing recurrent acute otitis media and in treating otitis media with effusion, *JAMA* 270(11):1344-1351, 1993.

Zeisei SA et al: Prospective surveillance for otitis media with effusion among black infants in group child care, *J Pediatr* 127:875-880, 1995.

Noninfectious Irritants

Bakoula CG et al: Objective passive-smoking indicators and respiratory morbidity in young children, *Lancet* 346(8970):280-281, 1995.

Eliopoulos C et al: Hair concentrations of nicotine and cotinine in women and their newborn infants, *JAMA* 271:621-623, 1994.

Espeland K: Identifying the manifestations of inhalant abuse, *Nurse Pract* 20(5):49-50, 53, 1995.

Fitzpatrick JC, Cioffi WG Jr: Inhalation injury, *Trauma Q* 11(2):114-126, 1994.

Huston CJ: Carbon monoxide poisoning, *Am J Nurs* 96(1):48, 1996.

Mitchell A et al: Acute organophosphate pesticide poisoning in children, *MCN Am J Matern Child Nurs* 20(5):261-268, 1995.

Ruddy RM: Smoke inhalation injury, *Peadiatr Clin North Am* 41(2):317-336, 1994.

Asthma

Bechler-Karsch A: Assessment and management of status asthmaticus, *Pediatric Nurs* 20(3):217-223, 238-239, 1994.

Buist AS, Vollmer WM: Preventing deaths from asthma, *N Engl J Med* 331(23):1584-1585, 1994 (editorial).

Capen CL et al: The team approach to pediatric asthma education, *Pediatr Nurs* 20(3):231-237, 1994.

Chou KJ, Cunningham SJ, Crain EF: Metered-dose inhalers with spacers vs. nebulizers pediatric asthma, *Arch Pediatr Adolesc Med* 149(2):201-205, 1995.

Clark NK, Gotsch A, Rosenstock I: Patient, professional and public education on behavioral aspects of asthma: a review of strategies for change and needed research, *J Asthma* 39(4):241-255, 1993.

DiGiullo G et al: Hospital treatment of asthma: lack of benefit from theophylline given in addition to nebulized albuterol and intravenously administered corticosteroid, *J Pediatr* 122(3):464-466, 1993.

Ferrante S, Painter E: Continuous nebulization: a treatment modality for pediatric asthma patients, *Pediatr Nurs* 21(4):327-331, 1995.

Fitzpatrick MF et al: Effect of therapeutic theophylline levels on the sleep quality and daytime cognitive performance of normal subjects, *Am Rev Respir Dis* 145:1355-1358, 1992.

Karsch AB: Assessment and management of status asthmaticus, *Pediatr Nurs* 20(3):217-223, 1994.

Larter N, Kieckhefer G: *Asthma.* In Jackson P, Vessey J, editors: *Primary care of the child with a chronic condition,* ed 2, St Louis, 1996, Mosby.

Morray B, Redding G: Factors associated with prolonged hospitalization of children with asthma, *Arch Pediatr Adolesc Med* 149(3):276-279, 1995.

Murphy S, Kelly W: Asthma, inflammation, and airway hyperresponsiveness in children, *Curr Opin Pediatr* 5:255-265, 1993.

Peter JFM et al: Long-term effect of inhaled corticosteroids on growth rate in adolescents with asthma, *Pediatrics* 91(3):1121-1126, 1993.

Racheletsy G et al: An update on the diagnosis and management of pediatric asthma: based on the National Heart, Lung, and Blood Institute Expert Panel report, *Nurse Practitioner* 18(2):51-52+, 1993.

Ryan-Wenger N, Walsh M: Children's perspectives on coping with asthma, *Pediatr Nurs* 20(3):224-228, 1994.

Strauss RE et al: Aminophylline therapy does not improve outcome and increases adverse effects in children hospitalized with acute asthmatic exacerbations, *Pediatrics* 93(2):205-206, 1994.

Wenger NMR, Walsh M: Children's perspectives on coping with asthma, *Pediatr Nurs* 20(3):224, 1994.

Whatling J: Childhood asthma and passive smoking, *Nurs Standard* 8(46):25-27, 1994.

Cystic Fibrosis

Fulginiti V, Lewy J: Pediatrics: update on cystic fibrosis, *JAMA* 270(2):246-248, 1993.

Geller G; Cystic fibrosis and the pediatric caregiver: benefits and burdens of technology, *Pediatr Nurs* 21(1):57-61, 1995.

Gutteridge C, Kuhn RJ: Pulmozyme—dornase alfa, *Pediatr Nurs* 20(3):278-279, 1994.

Jedlicka-Köhler I, Gotz M, Eichler I: Parents' recollection of the initial communication of the diagnosis of cystic fibrosis, *Pediatrics* 97(2):204-209, 1996.

Loutzenhiser JL, Clark R: Physical activity and exercise in children with cystic fibrosis, *J Pediatr Nurs* 8(2):112-119, 1993.

Maynard LC: Pediatric heart-lung transplant for cystic fibrosis, *Heart-Lung* 23(4):279-284, 1994.

McMullen AH: *Cystic fibrosis.* In Jackson PL, Vessey JA, editors: *Primary care of the child with a chronic condition,* ed 2, St Louis, 1996, Mosby.

Rosenstein BJ: Molecular basis, diagnosis, and treatment of cystic fibrosis, *Pediatr Rounds* 4(2):5-8, 1995.

Sawyer SM et al: The self-image of adolescents with cystic fibrosis, *J Adolesc Health* 16(3):204-208, 1995.

Tizzano E, Buchwald M: Recent advances in cystic fibrosis research, *J Pediatr* 122(6):985-988, 1993.

White K, Munro CL, Pickler R: Therapeutic implications of recent advances in cystic fibrosis, *MCN Am J Matern Child Nurs* 20(6):304-308, 1995.

Williams JK: Genetics and cystic fibrosis: a focus on carrier testing. *Pediatr Nurs* 21(5):444-448, 1995.

Respiratory Emergencies

Bledsoe BE: Pediatric respiratory emergencies, *J Emerg Med Serv* 19(2):38-41, 43-49, 1994.

Eichhorn DJ, Meyers TA, Guzzetta CE: Family presence during resuscitation: it is time to open the door, *Crit Care Nurs* 3(1): 8-13, 1995.

Kabbani M, Goodwin SR: Traumatic epiglottitis following blind finger sweep to remove a pharyngeal foreign body, *Clin Pediatr* 34(9):495-497, 1995.

Leuthner SR, Jansen RD, Hageman JR: Cardiopulmonary resuscitation of the newborn, *Pediatr Clin North Am* 41(5):893-907, 1994.

Malinowski C: Neonatal resuscitation program and pediatric advanced life support, *Respir Care* 40(5):575-587, 1995.

Paediatric Life Support Working Party of the European Resuscitation Council: Guidelines for paediatric life support, *Br Med J* 308:1349-1355, 1994.

Poole SR, Chetham M, Anderson M: Grunting respirations in infants and children, *Pediatr Emerg Care* 11(3):158-161, 1995.

Schroeder LL, Knapp JF: Recognition and emergency management of infectious causes of upper airway obstruction in children, *Semin Respir Infect* 10(1):21-30, 1995.

Walsh E, Ioli J: Childhood near-drowning: nursing care and primary prevention, *Pediatr Nurs* 20(3):265-269, 1994.

CHAPTER 44

Gastrointestinal Dysfunction

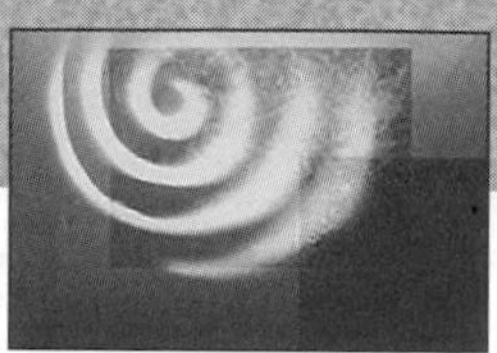

NUTRITIONAL DISTURBANCES, P. 1372

Vitamin disturbances, p. 1372
Mineral disturbances, p. 1377
Vegetarian diets, p. 1382
Protein and energy malnutrition (PEM), p. 1384
Kwashiorkor, p. 1384
Marasmus, p. 1384
Food sensitivity, p. 1384
Cow's milk allergy, p. 1385
Lactose intolerance, p. 1386

GASTROINTESTINAL (GI) DYSFUNCTION, P. 1386

Dehydration, p. 1386

DISORDERS OF MOTILITY, P. 1390

Acute diarrhea, p. 1390
Acute infectious diarrhea, p. 1393
Constipation, p. 1395
Hirschsprung disease, p. 1399
Vomiting, p. 1401
Gastroesophageal reflux (GER), p. 1401

INTESTINAL PARASITIC DISEASES, P. 1403

General nursing considerations, p. 1403
Giardiasis, p. 1403
Enterobiasis (pinworms), p. 1405

INFLAMMATORY DISORDERS, P. 1406

Stomatitis, p. 1406
Acute appendicitis, p. 1406
Meckel diverticulum, p. 1409
Inflammatory bowel disease (IBD), p. 1409
Peptic ulcer, p. 1412

HEPATIC DISORDERS, P. 1414

Acute hepatitis, p. 1414
Cirrhosis, p. 1416
Biliary atresia, p. 1417

STRUCTURAL DEFECTS, P. 1418

Cleft lip (CL) and/or cleft palate (CP), p. 1418
Esophageal atresia (EA) and tracheoesophageal fistula (TEF), p. 1422
Hernias, p. 1425

OBSTRUCTIVE DISORDERS, P. 1425

Hypertrophic pyloric stenosis (HPS), p. 1426
Intussusception, p. 1429
Anorectal malformations, p. 1431

MALABSORPTION SYNDROMES, P. 1432

Celiac disease (CD), p. 1432
Short bowel syndrome (SBS), p. 1433

INGESTION OF INJURIOUS AGENTS, P. 1434

Principles of emergency treatment, p. 1435
Heavy metal poisoning, p. 1439
Lead poisoning, p. 1440

Nutritional Disturbances

VITAMIN DISTURBANCES

True **vitamin** disturbances are rare in the United States, but subclinical deficiencies are commonly seen, especially in lower socioeconomic groups, where dietary intake may be unbalanced. Vitamin deficiencies of the fat-soluble vitamins A and D may occur in malabsorptive disorders. Certain groups are at risk for vitamin D–deficient rickets: (1) children born of and breastfed by mothers who are vitamin D–deficient; (2) individuals who are exposed to minimal sunlight because of clothing, housing in areas of high pollution, or dark skin pigmentation; (3) individuals who adhere to vegetarian diets that are low in sources of vitamin D; and (4) those who use milk products, such as yogurt or unpasteurized cow's milk, that are not supplemented with vitamin D, as the primary source of milk. Children may also be at risk secondary to disorders or their treatment. For example, children receiving high doses of salicylates as therapy for rheumatoid arthritis may have impaired vitamin C storage. Recent studies indicate that vitamin A deficiency correlates with increased morbidity and mortality in children with measles. Complications from diarrhea and infections were increased, as was morbidity, in infants and children with vitamin A deficiency (Fawzi and others, 1993).

Of equal if not greater concern is the overuse of vitamins. An excessive dose of a vitamin is generally defined as 10 or more times the recommended dietary allowances (RDA), although the fat-soluble vitamins, especially A and D, tend to cause toxic reactions at lower doses. With the addition of vitamins to commercially packaged foods, the potential for hypervitaminosis has escalated, especially when vitamin supplements are used injudiciously. Hypervitaminoses of A and D present the greatest problems, because the fat-soluble vitamins are stored in the body and a much lower excess dose causes toxicity. However, it is now well documented that the water-soluble vitamins, B complex and C, can also cause toxicity.

Text continued on p. 1377.

TABLE 44-1 Vitamins and their nutritional significance

PHYSIOLOGIC FUNCTIONS/SOURCES	RESULTS OF DEFICIENCY OR EXCESS	NURSING CONSIDERATIONS
Vitamin A (retinol)*		
Functions Necessary component in formation of pigment rhodopsin (visual purple) Formation and maintenance of epithelial tissue Normal bone growth and tooth development Needed for growth and spermatogenesis Involved in thyroxine formation Antioxidant	***Deficiency*** Night blindness Keratinization (hardening and scaling) of epithelium Xerophthalmia (hardening and scaling of cornea and conjunctiva) Phrynoderma (toad skin) Drying of respiratory, gastrointestinal, and genitourinary tracts Defective tooth enamel Retarded growth Impaired bone formation Decreased thyroxine formation	Encourage foods rich in vitamin A, such as whole cow's milk As milk consumption decreases, encourage foods rich in vitamin A Ensure adequate intake in preterm infants Advise parents of safe use of supplements in child with measles
Sources ***Natural form***—liver, kidney, fish oils, milk and nonskimmed milk products, egg yolk ***Provitamin A (carotene)***—carrots, sweet potatoes, squash, apricots, spinach, collards, broccoli, cabbage, artichoke	***Excess*** ***Early signs***—irritability, anorexia, pruritus, fissures at corners of nose and lips ***Later signs***—hepatomegaly, jaundice, retarded growth, poor weight gain, thickening of the cortex of long bones with pain and fragility, hard tender lumps in extremities and occiput of the skull May cause birth defects from excessive maternal intake NOTE: Overdose results from ingestion of large quantities of the vitamin only, not the provitamin; large amounts of carotene (carotenemia) cause yellow or orange discoloration of the skin (not the sclera, urine, or feces as in jaundice), but none of the specified symptoms	Emphasize correct use of vitamin supplements and potential hazards of excess Investigate child's dietary habits to calculate approximate intake; if excessive, remove supplemental source (e.g., daily feeding of liver) Advise parents of the benign nature of carotenemia; treatment is avoidance of excess pigmented fruits or vegetables, especially carrots; skin color returns to normal in 2 to 6 weeks
Vitamin B_1 (thiamin)†		
Functions Coenzyme (with phosphorus) in carbohydrate metabolism Needed for healthy nervous system ***Sources*** Pork, beef, liver, legumes, nuts, whole or enriched grains and cereals, green vegetables, fruits, milk, brown rice	***Deficiency*** ***Gastrointestinal***—anorexia, constipation, indigestion ***Neurologic***—apathy, fatigue, emotional instability, polyneuritis, tenderness of calf muscles, partial anesthesia, muscle weakness, paresthesia, hyperesthesia, decreased or absent tendon reflexes, convulsions, and coma (in infants) ***Cardiovascular***—palpitations, cardiac failure, peripheral vasodilation, edema ***Excess*** Headache Irritability Insomnia Rapid pulse Weakness	***Vitamin B complex*** Encourage foods rich in B vitamins Stress proper cooking and storage techniques to preserve potency, such as minimum cooking of vegetables in small amount of liquid; storage of milk in opaque container Advise against fad diets that severely restrict groups of food, such as vegetarianism (vegans or macrobiotics) Explore need for vitamin supplements when dieting or when using goat milk exclusively for infant feeding (deficient in folic acid) or when the breastfeeding mother is a strict vegetarian (vitamin B_{12}) Emphasize correct use of vitamin supplements and potential hazards of excesses

*Fat soluble.
†Water soluble.

Continued.

TABLE 44-1 Vitamins and their nutritional significance—cont'd

PHYSIOLOGIC FUNCTIONS/SOURCES	RESULTS OF DEFICIENCY OR EXCESS	NURSING CONSIDERATIONS
Vitamin B_2 (riboflavin)†		
Functions Coenzyme (with phosphorus) in carbohydrate, protein, and fat metabolism Maintenance of healthy skin, especially around mouth, nose, and eyes ***Sources*** Milk and its products, eggs, organ meat (liver, kidney, and heart), enriched cereals, some green leafy vegetables,‡ legumes	***Deficiency*** Ariboflavinosis ***Lips***—cheilosis (fissures at corners of lips), perlèche (inflammation at corners of lips) ***Tongue***—glossitis ***Nose***—irritation and cracks at nasal angle ***Eyes***—burning, itching, tearing, photophobia, corneal vascularization, cataracts ***Skin***—seborrheic dermatitis, delayed wound healing and tissue repair ***Excess*** Paresthesia, pruritus	Same as vitamin B complex
Niacin (nicotinic acid, nicotinamide)†		
Functions Coenzyme (with riboflavin) in protein and fat metabolism Needed for healthy nervous system, skin, and normal digestion May lower cholesterol ***Sources*** Meat, poultry, fish, peanuts, beans, peas, whole or enriched grains except corn and rice Milk and its products are sources of tryptophan (60 mg of tryptophan = 1 mg of niacin)	***Deficiency*** Pellagra Oral—stomatitis, glossitis Cutaneous—scaly dermatitis on exposed areas Gastrointestinal—anorexia, weight loss, diarrhea, fatigue Neurologic—apathy, anxiety, confusion, depression, dementia Death ***Excess*** Release of vasodilator, histamine (flushing, decreased blood pressure, increased cerebral blood flow; aggravates asthma) Dermatologic problems (pruritus, rash, hyperkeratosis, acanthosis nigricans) Increased gastric acidity (aggravates peptic ulcer disease) Hepatotoxicity Increased serum uric acid levels Elevated plasma glucose levels Certain cardiac dysrhythmias	Same as vitamin B complex If used as hypolipidemic agent, stress safe dosage to prevent child's accidental ingestion
Vitamin B_6 (pyridoxine)†		
Functions Coenzyme in protein and fat metabolism Needed for formation of antibodies, hemoglobin Needed for utilization of copper and iron Aids in conversion of tryptophan to niacin ***Sources*** Meats, especially liver and kidney; cereal grains (wheat and corn); yeast; soybeans; peanuts; tuna; chicken; salmon	***Deficiency*** Scaly dermatitis, weight loss, anemia, retarded growth, irritability, convulsions, peripheral neuritis ***Excess*** Peripheral nervous system toxicity (unsteady gait, numb feet and hands, clumsiness of hands, sometimes perioral numbness) May cause peptic ulcer disease or seizures	Same as vitamin B complex Stress proper cooking and storing techniques to preserve potency Cook food covered in small amount of water Do not soak food in water Store in light-resistant container

†Water-soluble.
‡Green leafy vegetables include spinach, broccoli, kale, turnip greens, mustard greens, collards, dandelion greens, and beet greens.

TABLE 44-1 Vitamins and their nutritional significance—cont'd

PHYSIOLOGIC FUNCTIONS/SOURCES	RESULTS OF DEFICIENCY OR EXCESS	NURSING CONSIDERATIONS
Folic acid (folacin; reduced form is called folinic acid or citrovorum factor)†		
Functions Coenzyme for single-carbon transfer (purines, thymine, hemoglobin) Necessary for formation of red blood cells ***Sources*** Green leafy vegetables, cabbage, asparagus, liver, kidneys, nuts, eggs, whole grain cereals, legumes, bananas	***Deficiency*** Macrocytic anemia, bone marrow depression, glossitis, intestinal malabsorption ***Excess*** Rare because megadoses not available over the counter May cause insomnia and irritability	Same as vitamin B complex Stress proper cooking and storing techniques to preserve potency Cook food covered in small amount of water Do not soak food in water Store in light-resistant container Women of childbearing age should supplement to prevent neural tube defects
Vitamin B_{12} (cobalamin)†		
Functions Coenzyme in protein synthesis; indirect effect on formation of red blood cells (particularly on formation of nucleic acids and folic acid metabolism) Needed for normal functioning of nervous tissue ***Sources*** Meat, liver, kidney, fish, shellfish, poultry, milk, eggs, cheese, nutritional yeast, sea vegetables	***Deficiency*** Pernicious anemia (One form of deficiency from absence of intrinsic factor in gastric secretions) General signs of severe anemia Lemon-yellow tinge to skin Spinal cord degeneration Delayed brain growth ***Excess*** Excess is rare	Same as vitamin B complex
Biotin		
Functions Coenzyme in carbohydrate, protein, and fat metabolism Interrelated with functions of other B vitamins ***Sources*** Liver, kidney, egg yolk, tomatoes, legumes, nuts	***Deficiency*** Deficiency is uncommon because synthesized by bacterial flora ***Excess*** Unknown	Same as vitamin B complex
Pantothenic acid†		
Functions Coenzyme in carbohydrate, protein, and fat metabolism Synthesis of amino acids, fatty acids, and steroids ***Sources*** Liver, kidney, heart, salmon, eggs, vegetables, legumes, whole grains	***Deficiency*** Deficiency is uncommon because of its multiple food sources and synthesis by bacterial flora ***Excess*** Minimum toxicity (occasional diarrhea and water retention)	Same as vitamin B complex
Vitamin C (ascorbic acid)†		
Functions Essential for collagen formation Increases absorption of iron for hemoglobin formation Enhances conversion of folid acid to folinic acid Affects cholesterol synthesis and conversion of proline to hydroxyproline	***Deficiency*** Scurvy ***Skin***—dry, rough, petechiae, perifollicular hyperkeratotic papules (raised areas around hair follicles) ***Musculoskeletal***—bleeding muscles and joints, pseudoparalysis from pain, swelling of joints, costochondral beading (scorbutic rosary)	Encourage foods rich in vitamin C Investigate infant's diet for sources of vitamin, especially when cow's milk is principal source of nutrition Stress proper cooking and storing techniques to preserve potency Wash vegetables quickly; do not soak in water

†Water-soluble.

Continued.

TABLE 44-1 Vitamins and their nutritional significance—cont'd

PHYSIOLOGIC FUNCTIONS/SOURCES	RESULTS OF DEFICIENCY OR EXCESS	NURSING CONSIDERATIONS
Vitamin C (ascorbic acid)†—cont'd		
Probably a coenzyme in metabolism of tyrosine and phenylalanine May play role in hydroxylation of adrenal steroids May have stimulating effect on phagocytic activity of leukocytes and formation of antibodies Antioxidant agent ***Sources*** Citrus fruits, strawberries, tomatoes, potatoes, melon, cabbage, broccoli, cauliflower, spinach, papaya, mango	***Gums***—spongy, friable, swollen, bleed easily, bluish red or black color, teeth loosen and fall out ***General disposition***—irritable, anorexic, apprehensive, in pain, refuses to move, assumes semifroglike position when supine (scorbutic pose) Signs of anemia Decreased wound healing Increased susceptibility to infection ***Excess*** Diarrhea Increased excretion of uric acid and acidification of urine (may cause urate precipitation and formation of oxalate stones) Hemolysis Impaired leukocytosis activity Damage to beta cells of pancreas and decreased insulin production Reproductive failure "Rebound scurvy" from withdrawal of large amounts	Cook vegetables in covered pot with minimum water and for short time; avoid copper or cast iron cookware Do not add baking soda to cooking water Use fresh fruits and vegetables as soon as possible; store in refrigerator Store juice in airtight, opaque container Wrap cut fruit or eat soon after exposing to air In caring for child with scurvy: Position for comfort and rest Handle very gently and minimally Administer analgesics as needed Prevent infection Provide good oral care Provide soft, bland diet Emphasize rapid recovery when vitamin is replaced Emphasize correct use of vitamin supplement and potential hazards of excess Identify groups at risk for vitamin C supplements: those with thalassemia; those on anticoagulant or aminoglycoside antibiotic therapy
Vitamin D_2 (ergocalciferol) and D_3 (cholecalciferol)*		
Functions Absorption of calcium and phosphorus and decreased renal excretion of phosphorus ***Sources*** Direct sunlight Cod liver oil, herring, mackerel, salmon, tuna, sardines ***Enriched food sources***—milk, milk products, enriched cereals, margarine, breads, many breakfast drinks	***Deficiency*** Rickets ***Head***—craniotabes (softening of cranial bones, prominence of frontal bones), deformed shape (skull flat and depressed toward middle), delayed closure of fontanels ***Chest***—rachitic rosary (enlargement of costochondral junction of ribs), Harrison groove (horizontal depression in lower portion of rib cage), pigeon chest (sharp protrusion of sternum) ***Spine***—kyphosis, scoliosis, lordosis ***Abdomen***—potbelly, constipation ***Extremities***—bowing of arms and legs, knock-knee, saber shins, instability of hip joints, pelvic deformity, enlargement of epiphysis at ends of long bones ***Teeth***—delayed calcification, especially of permanent teeth ***Rachitic tetany***—seizures	Encourage foods rich in vitamin D, especially fortified cow's milk In breastfed infants encourage use of vitamin D supplements if maternal diet inadequate or infant exposed to minimal sunlight In caring for child with rickets: Maintain good body alignment Reposition frequently to prevent decubiti and respiratory infection Handle very gently and minimally Prevent infection Institute seizure precautions Have 10% calcium gluconate available in case of tetany Observe for possibility of overdose from supplements If prescribed, supervise proper use of orthopedic splints or braces
	Excess ***Acute***—vomiting, dehydration, fever, abdominal cramps, bone pain, convulsions, and coma ***Chronic***—lassitude, mental slowness, anorexia, failure to thrive, thirst, urinary urgency, polyuria, vomiting, diarrhea, abdominal cramps, bone pain, pathologic fractures	Same as vitamin A; may include low-calcium diet during initial therapy

*Fat-soluble.
†Water-soluble.

TABLE 44-1 Vitamins and their nutritional significance—cont'd

PHYSIOLOGIC FUNCTIONS/SOURCES	RESULTS OF DEFICIENCY OR EXCESS	NURSING CONSIDERATIONS
Vitamin D_2 (ergocalciferol) and D_3 (cholecalciferol)*		
	Calcification of soft tissue—kidneys, lungs, adrenal glands, vessels (hypertension), heart, gastric lining, tympanic membrane (deafness) Osteoporosis of long bones Elevated serum levels of calcium and phosphorus	
Vitamin E (tocopherol)*		
Functions Production of red blood cells and protection from hemolysis Muscle and liver integrity Coenzyme factor in tissue respiration Minimizes oxidation of polyunsaturated fatty acids and vitamins A and C in intestinal tract and tissues Possible role in treatment and prevention of bronchopulmonary dysplasia and retinopathy of prematurity is under investigation ***Sources*** Vegetable oils, wheat germ oil, milk, egg yolk, muscle meats, fish, whole grains, nuts, legumes, spinach, broccoli	***Deficiency*** Hemolytic anemia from hemolysis caused by shortened life of red blood cells, especially in premature infants, and focal necrosis of tissues Causes infertility in rats, but not in humans (does *not* increase human male virility or potency) ***Excess*** Little is known; less toxic than other fat-soluble vitamins	Initiate early feeding in premature infants; may need supplementation
Vitamin K*		
Functions Catalyst for production of prothrombin and blood-clotting factors II, VII, IX, and X by the liver ***Sources*** Pork, liver, green leafy vegetables (spinach, kale, cabbage)‡, tomatoes, egg yolk, cheese	***Deficiency*** Hemorrhage ***Excess*** Hemolytic anemia in individuals who are deficient in glucose-6-phosphate dehydrogenase	Administer prophylactically to all newborns Other indications include intestinal disease, lack of bile, prolonged antibiotic therapy; may be used in management of blood-clotting time when anticoagulants such as warfarin (Coumadin) and dicumarol (bishydroxycoumarin), which are vitamin K antagonists, are used

*Fat-soluble.
‡Green leafy vegetables include spinach, broccoli, kale, turnip greens, mustard greens, collards, dandelion greens, and beet greens.

Deficiencies and excesses of vitamins A, B complex, C, D, E, and K are summarized in Table 44-1. General nursing considerations are discussed later, and specific interventions are presented in the table.

MINERAL DISTURBANCES

A number of minerals are essential nutrients. **Macrominerals** are those with daily requirements greater than 100 mg and include calcium, phosphorus, magnesium, sodium, potassium, chloride, and sulfur. **Microminerals,** or *trace elements,* have daily requirements less than 100 mg and include several essential minerals and those whose exact role in nutrition is still unclear. The greatest concern with minerals is deficiency, especially iron, calcium, and zinc.

The regulation of mineral balance in the body is a complex process. Dietary extremes of mineral intake can cause a number of mineral interactions that can result in unexpected deficiencies or excesses. For example, excessive amounts of one mineral, such as zinc, can result in a deficiency of another mineral, such as copper, even if sufficient amounts of copper are ingested. Deficiencies can also occur when various substances in the diet interact with minerals. For example, iron, zinc, and calcium can form insoluble complexes with phytates and/or oxalates (found in plant proteins), which impair the bioavailability of the mineral. This type of interaction is important in vegetarian diets because plant foods, such as soy, are high in phytates. An example is spinach, which is not a rich source of iron or calcium, as commonly believed, because of its oxalate content.

Deficiencies and excesses of selected macrominerals and microminerals are summarized in Table 44-2. General nursing considerations are discussed later, and specific interventions are presented in the table.

Text continued on p. 1382.

TABLE 44-2 Minerals and their nutritional significance

PHYSIOLOGIC FUNCTIONS/SOURCES	RESULTS OF DEFICIENCY OR EXCESS	NURSING CONSIDERATIONS
Calcium*		
Functions Bone and tooth development and maintenance (in combination with phosphorus) Muscle contractions, especially the heart Blood clotting Absorption of vitamin B_{12} Enzyme activation Nerve conduction Integrity of intracellular cement substances and various membranes ***Sources*** Dairy products, egg yolk, sardines, canned salmon with bones, dark green leafy vegetables (except spinach), soybeans, dried beans, and peas	***Deficiency*** Rickets Tetany Impaired growth, especially of bones and teeth ***Excess*** Drowsiness, extreme lethargy Impaired absorption of other minerals (iron, zinc, manganese) Calcium deposits in tissues (renal failure)	Encourage foods rich in calcium, especially dairy products Caution that oxalates in leafy vegetables (spinach), oxalates in chocolates, and high phosphorus intake (especially from carbonated beverages) can decrease calcium absorption Discourage use of whole cow's milk in newborns because the phosphorus-to-calcium ratio favors excretion of calcium Advise against fad diets, especially those that restrict dairy products Emphasize correct use of calcium supplement, especially the possible interaction between megadoses of calcium and resulting deficiency states of other minerals
Chloride*		
Functions Acid-base and fluid balance Enzyme activation in saliva Component of hydrochloric acid in stomach ***Sources*** Salt, meat, eggs, dairy products, many prepared and preserved foods	***Deficiency*** Acid-base disturbances (hypochloremic alkalosis, dehydration); occurs mostly in combination with sodium loss ***Excess*** Acid-base disturbance	Deficiency and excess are unusual; most diets supply adequate chloride (usually in combination with sodium) Disease states such as excessive vomiting can necessitate chloride replacement
Chromium†		
Functions Involved in glucose metabolism and energy production ***Sources*** Meat, cheese, whole-grain breads and cereals, legumes, peanuts, brewer's yeast, vegetable oils	***Deficiency*** Possible abnormal glucose metabolism ***Excess*** Unknown	No specific recommendations are needed
Copper†		
Functions Production of hemoglobin Essential component of several enzyme systems ***Sources*** Organ meats, oysters, nuts, seeds, legumes, corn oil margarine	***Deficiency*** Anemia, leukopenia, neutropenia ***Excess*** Severe vomiting and diarrhea Hemolytic anemia	Deficiency from inadequate food sources is less likely than from excess intake of other minerals, especially zinc and possibly iron; therefore emphasize the correct use of any vitamin supplement Caution against cooking acid foods in unlined copper pots (can lead to chronic and toxic accumulation of copper)

*Macrominerals—required intake >100 mg/day.
†Microminerals or trace elements—required intake <100 mg/day.

TABLE 44-2 Minerals and their nutritional significance—cont'd

PHYSIOLOGIC FUNCTIONS/SOURCES	RESULTS OF DEFICIENCY OR EXCESS	NURSING CONSIDERATIONS
Fluorine†		
Functions Formation of caries-resistant teeth Strong bone development ***Sources*** Fluoridated water and foods or beverages prepared with fluoridated water; fish, tea, commercially prepared chicken for infants	***Deficiency*** Increased susceptibility to tooth decay ***Excess*** Fluorosis (mottling and/or pitting of enamel) Severe bone deformities	In areas with optimally fluoridated water, encourage sufficient intake to supply recommended amount of fluoride (see p. 1005) In areas of unfluoridated water or when ready-to-use formula, bottled water, or breast milk is used, stress the importance of fluoride supplements In areas with excess fluoride in the water, consider the use of bottled water in drinking and possibly cooking to reduce the fluoride intake to safe levels Fluorine has the narrowest range of safe and adequate intake; therefore stress the importance of storing supplements in a safe area
Iodine†		
Functions Production of thyroid hormone Normal reproduction ***Sources*** Seafood, kelp, iodized salt, sea salt, enriched bread, milk (from dairy processing)	***Deficiency*** Goiter (enlarged thyroid from decreased thyroxine formation) ***Excess*** Unknown from food sources; may result from ingestion of iodine preparations, such as saturated solutions of potassium iodide (SSKI)	Encourage use of iodized salt for individuals living far from the sea If iodine preparations are in the home, stress the importance of safe storage
Iron†		
Functions Formation of hemoglobin and myoglobin Essential part of several enzymes and proteins	***Deficiency*** Anemia (see Chapter 46)	Encourage foods rich in iron Discourage excessive milk consumption, especially more than 1 L per day (milk is a very poor source of iron) If iron supplements are prescribed, teach parents factors that affect absorption (see Box 44-1)

BOX 44-1
Factors That Affect Iron Absorption

Increase

Acidity (low pH)—Administer iron between meals (gastric hydrochloric acid)
Ascorbic acid (vitamin C)—Administer iron with juice, fruit, or multivitamin preparation
Vitamin A
Calcium
Tissue need
Meat, fish, poultry
Cooking in cast iron pots

Decrease

Alkalinity (high pH)—Avoid any antacid preparation
Phosphates—Milk is unfavorable vehicle for iron administration
Phytates—Found in cereals
Oxalates—Found in many fruits and vegetables (plums, currants, green beans, spinach, sweet potatoes, tomatoes)
Tannins—Found in tea, coffee
Tissue saturation
Malabsorptive disorders
Disturbances that cause diarrhea or steatorrhea
Infection

†Microminerals or trace elements—required intake <100 mg/day.

Continued.

TABLE 44-2 Minerals and their nutritional significance—cont'd

PHYSIOLOGIC FUNCTIONS/SOURCES	RESULTS OF DEFICIENCY OR EXCESS	NURSING CONSIDERATIONS
Iron—con'd		
Sources	***Excess***	
Liver, especially pork, followed by calf, beef, and chicken; kidney, red meat, poultry, shellfish, whole grains, iron-enriched infant formula and cereal, enriched cereals and bread, legumes, nuts, seeds, green leafy vegetables (except spinach), dried fruits, potatoes, molasses	Hemosiderosis (excess iron storage in various tissues of the body, especially the spleen, liver, lymph glands, heart, and pancreas) Hemochromatosis (excess iron storage with cellular damage)	Stress the importance of storing iron supplements in a safe area
Magnesium*		
Functions	***Deficiency***	
Bone and tooth formation Production of proteins Nerve conduction to muscles Activation of enzymes needed for carbohydrate and protein metabolism	Tremors, spasm Irregular heartbeat Muscular weakness Lower extremity cramps Convulsions, delirium	Deficiency and excess are unusual, except in disease states such as prolonged vomiting or diarrhea or kidney dysfunction, where replacement may be needed
Sources	***Excess***	
Whole grains, nuts, soybeans, meat, green leafy vegetables (uncooked), tea, cocoa, raisins	Nervous system disturbances due to imbalance in calcium-to-magnesium ratio	
Manganese†		
Functions	***Deficiency***	
Activation of enzymes involved in reproduction, growth, and fat metabolism Normal bone structure Nervous system functioning	Unknown ***Excess*** Unknown	No specific recommendations are needed
Sources		
Nuts, whole grains, legumes, green vegetables, fruit		
Molybdenum†		
Functions	***Deficiency***	
Essential component of several oxidative enzymes	Very rare; diagnosed in patients on complete total parenteral alimentation	No specific recommendations are needed
Sources	***Excess***	
Legumes, whole grains, organ meats, some dark green vegetables	Produces secondary copper deficiency (growth failure, anemia, and disturbed bone development)	
Phosphorus*		
Functions	***Deficiency***	
Bone and tooth development (in combination with calcium) Involved in numerous chemical reactions, including protein, carbohydrate, and fat metabolism Acid-base balance	Weakness, anorexia, malaise, bone pain	Dietary deficiency is uncommon, although prolonged use of antacids can produce deficiency, in which case supplementation is recommended
Sources	***Excess***	
Dairy products, eggs, meat, poultry, legumes, carbonated beverages	Produces secondary calcium deficiency from disturbed calcium-to-phosphorus ratio	To preserve calcium-to-phosphorus ratio in newborns, discourage use of whole cow's milk

*Macrominerals—required intake >100 mg/day.
†Microminerals or trace elements—required intake <100 mg/day.

TABLE 44-2 Minerals and their nutritional significance—cont'd

PHYSIOLOGIC FUNCTIONS/SOURCES	RESULTS OF DEFICIENCY OR EXCESS	NURSING CONSIDERATIONS
Potassium*		
Functions Acid-base and fluid balance (major extracellular fluid areas) Nerve conduction Muscular contraction, especially the heart Release of energy ***Sources*** Bananas, citrus fruit, dried fruits, meat, fish, bran, legumes, peanut butter, potatoes, coffee, tea, cocoa	***Deficiency*** Cardiac arrhythmias Muscular weakness Lethargy Kidney and respiratory failure Heart failure ***Excess*** Cardiac dysrhythmias Respiratory failure Mental confusion Numbness of extremities	Dietary deficiency and excess are unlikely, although disease states such as prolonged nausea and vomiting or the use of diuretics can result in hypokalemia; in such instances encourage replacement with supplements of rich food sources, such as bananas
Selenium†		
Functions Antioxidant, especially protective of vitamin E Protects against toxicity of heavy metals Associated with fat metabolism ***Sources*** Seafood, organ meats, egg yolk, whole grains; chicken, meat, tomatoes, cabbage, garlic, mushrooms, milk	***Deficiency*** Keshan disease (cardiomyopathy in children; occurs in China) ***Excess*** Eye, nose, and throat irritation Increased dental caries Liver and kidney degeneration	Deficiency and excess are uncommon in North America, although selenium deficiency can occur in patients on prolonged total parenteral alimentation; in these instances supplementation is required
Sodium*		
Functions Acid-base and fluid balance (major extracellular fluid cation) Cell permeability; absorption of glucose Muscle contraction ***Sources*** Table salt, seafood, meat, poultry, numerous prepared foods	***Deficiency*** Dehydration Hypotension Convulsions Muscle cramps ***Excess*** Edema Hypertension Intracranial hemorrhage	Deficiency intake is very rare, although losses secondary to nausea, vomiting, excessive sweating, and use of diuretics can occur and require replacement Encourage parents to limit excessive use of salt in preparing foods and to limit commercial foods with high sodium content, such as smoked meats
Sulfur*		
Functions Essential component of cell protein, especially of hair and skin Enzyme activation Associated with energy metabolism Detoxification of certain chemical reactions ***Sources*** Dairy products, eggs, meat, fish, nuts, legumes	***Deficiency*** Unknown ***Excess*** Unknown	No specific recommendations are needed

*Macrominerals—required intake >100 mg/day.
†Microminerals or trace elements—required intake <100 mg/day.

Continued.

TABLE 44-2 Minerals and their nutritional significance—cont'd

PHYSIOLOGIC FUNCTIONS/SOURCES	RESULTS OF DEFICIENCY OR EXCESS	NURSING CONSIDERATIONS
Zinc†		
Functions	***Deficiency***	
Component of about 100 enzymes Synthesis of nucleic acids and protein in immune system and coagulation Release of vitamin A from liver Improved wound healing with vitamin C ***Sources*** Seafood (especially oysters), meat, poultry, eggs, wheat, legumes	Loss of appetite Diminished taste sensation Delayed healing ***Skin lesions***—erythematous, crusted lesions around body orifices Alopecia Diarrhea Growth failure Retarded sexual maturity ***Excess*** Vomiting and diarrhea Malaise, dizziness Anemia, gastric bleeding Impaired absorption of calcium and copper	Encourage food sources rich in zinc, especially protein Caution that fiber, phytates, oxalates, tannins (in tea or coffee), iron, and calcium adversely affect zinc absorption Recognize groups at risk for zinc deficiency, such as vegetarians and Mexican-Americans, whose diets may have restricted or low meat content and high fiber, phytate content; and patients with malabsorption syndromes Emphasize correct use of zinc supplements and the possible interaction with other minerals

†Microminerals or trace elements—required intake <100 mg/day.

VEGETARIAN DIETS

Vegetarian diets can potentially cause nutritional deficiencies in children. The stricter the vegetarian diet, the more difficult it becomes to ensure adequate nutrition for infants and children. The major types of **vegetarianism** are the following:

- **Lactoovovegetarianism,** which excludes meat from the diet but includes milk and eggs and sometimes fish
- **Lactovegetarianism,** which excludes meat and eggs but includes milk
- **Pure vegetarianism (veganism),** which eliminates any food of animal origin, including milk and eggs
- **Zen macrobiotics,** which is even more restrictive than pure vegetarianism in that cereals, especially brown rice, are the mainstay of the diet

Many individuals who are concerned about healthful diets subscribe to vegetarian diets that are not typified by the preceding categories. Therefore during nutritional assessment it is necessary to list clearly exactly what the diet includes and excludes.

The lactoovovegetarian diet is associated with the least deficiencies, although protein intake needs to be monitored. The lactovegetarian diet may also be low in protein, as well as iron. The major deficiencies in the stricter vegetarian diets are inadequate protein for growth; inadequate calories for energy and growth; poor digestibility of many of the natural, unprocessed foods, especially for infants; and deficiencies of vitamin B_{12}, niacin, thiamine, riboflavin, vitamin D, iron, calcium, and zinc. In the United States strict vegetarian diets are common among members of Black Muslim and Seventh Day Adventist faiths.

Nursing Care Management

Identification of nutrient imbalance (or the potential for imbalance) is the initial nursing goal and requires assessment based on a dietary history and physical examination for signs of deficiency or excess (see Nutritional Assessment, Chapter 31). Once assessment data are collected, this information is evaluated against standard intakes to identify areas of concern. The most widely used standard is the **Recommended Dietary Allowances (RDAs),** developed by the National Academy of Sciences, Food and Nutrition Board. The RDAs are not average requirements but recommendations intended to meet the physiologic needs of almost every healthy person. To meet the needs of those with the highest requirements, the RDAs will exceed most people's requirements. Therefore children consuming less than the RDAs are not necessarily consuming an inadequate diet, but they are more likely at risk for deficiency than those who are consuming nutrients in amounts equal to the RDAs.

Several organizations have published dietary advice for the public. Most well-known are the Dietary Guidelines for Americans, which encourage eating a variety of foods, maintaining ideal body weight, consuming adequate starch and fiber, and limiting intake of fat, cholesterol, sugar, salt, and alcohol. Another source is the *Food Guide Pyramid* (Fig. 44-1), which replaces the basic four food groups that have traditionally been used to convey nutrition information to the public and applies to children as young as 2 years of age.

The number of servings and serving sizes are important components of the Food Guide Pyramid. Suggested serving sizes for the five food groups are listed in Box 44-2. Young children need the same variety of foods as older children but may need less than the 1600 calories provided by the suggested minimum number of servings in each food group. To meet their caloric needs, adjustments are made by using the minimum number of servings and smaller serving sizes. However, it is important that children have the equivalent of at least 2 cups of milk a day. Adolescents, who require increased calories for growth, should have 3 cups of milk a day and may require the maximum number of suggested servings. Current recommendations for fat intake for children over 2 years of

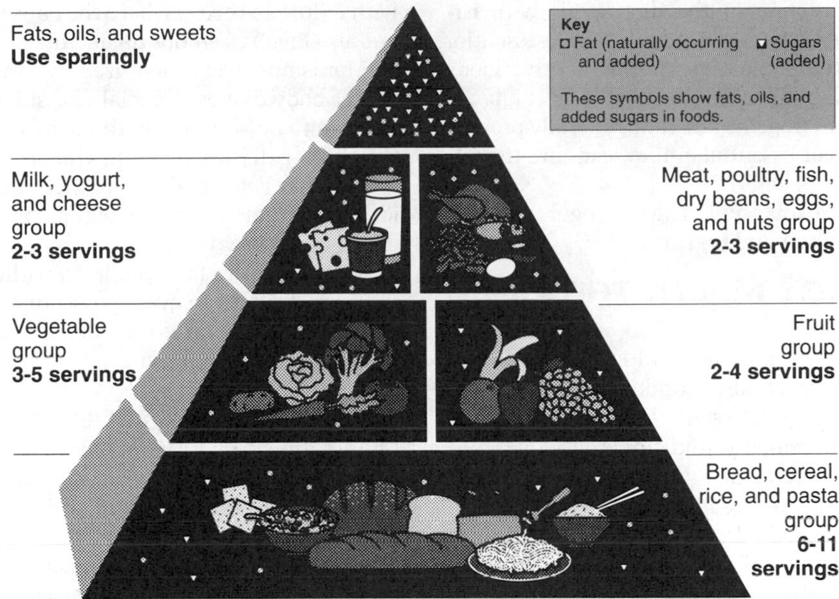

Fig. 44-1 Food Guide Pyramid: a guide to daily food choices. (Courtesy U.S. Department of Agriculture, 1992).

age are that no more than 30% of calories should be from fat and the remainder from carbohydrates and protein (see also Hyperlipidemia [Hypercholesterolemia], Chapter 45).

Since one of the best assurances of nutritional adequacy is eating a variety of foods, families need guidelines for selecting foods that provide essential nutrients without exceeding energy requirements. With a varied and well-balanced diet most children do not need vitamin or mineral supplements. Unfortunately there are no restrictions on the availability of toxic doses of vitamins or minerals. Nurses need to inform families of the potential dangers from excess vitamins or minerals. The idea that "more is better" is probably best dispelled by a simple explanation of the body's inability to use more than the needed requirement.

Achieving a nutritionally adequate vegetarian diet (with the exception of the strictest diets) is not difficult, but it requires careful planning and knowledge of nutrient sources. For children the lactoovovegetarian diet is nutritionally adequate; however, the vegan diet requires supplementation with vitamins D and B_{12} for children ages 2 to 12 years. Most authorities indicate that human breast milk or iron-fortified modified cow's milk (formula) is adequate for the first 6 months; breastfeeding may continue up to 1 year of age. Although not required to meet nutritional requirements, iron-fortified rice cereal may be introduced after 4 months. The introduction of other solids is nutritionally unnecessary until 12 months and each should only be introduced one at a time. Iron-fortified cereal, in combination with breast milk or formula, is an adequate source of nutrition in the first year of life. The use of vitamin C juices with foods high in iron will further improve iron absorption. However breast milk from vegetarian mothers can be deficient in vitamin B_{12}; supplementation of both mother and child is advisable. If cow's or human milk or commercial infant formula is not given, fortified soy milk is recommended. A variety of foods should be gradually introduced during the early years to ensure a more well-balanced intake.

BOX 44-2
Food Guide Pyramid: Sample Serving Sizes

Bread, cereal, rice, and pasta group
1 slice of bread
1 ounce of ready-to-eat cereal
1/2 cup of cooked cereal, rice, or pasta

Vegetable group
1 cup of raw leafy vegetable
1/2 cup of other vegetable, cooked or chopped raw
3/4 cup of vegetable juice

Fruit group
1 medium apple, banana, or orange
1/2 cup of chopped, cooked, or canned fruit
3/4 cup of fruit juice

Milk, yogurt, and cheese group
1 cup of milk or yogurt
1 1/2 ounces of natural cheese
2 ounces of processed cheese

Meat, poultry, fish, dry beans, eggs, and nuts group
2-3 ounces of cooked lean meat, poultry, or fish
1/2 cup of cooked dry beans, 1 egg, or 2 tablespoons of peanut butter count as 1 ounce of lean meat

Nursing ALERT

When solid foods are introduced, the safety and digestibility of the selections must be considered. Raw fruits with seeds, vegetables, and nuts are hazardous for young children because of the danger of aspiration. Beans, grain cereals, and vegetables should be served well cooked and mashed during infancy.

To ensure sufficient protein in the diet, foods with **incomplete proteins** (those that do not have all the essential amino acids) must be eaten at the same meal with other foods that supply the missing amino acids. The two basic combinations of foods consumed by vegetarians that generally provide the appropriate amounts of essential amino acids are the following:

Grains and **milk products** (milk, cheese, yogurt)
Seeds (sesame, sunflower) and **legumes**

PROTEIN ENERGY MALNUTRITION (PEM)

Malnutrition continues to be a major health problem in the world today, particularly in children under 5 years of age. The lack of food, however, is not always the primary cause of malnutrition. In many developing and underdeveloped nations diarrhea is a major factor in malnutrition. Additional factors are bottle feeding (in poor sanitary conditions), inadequate knowledge of proper child care practices; parental illiteracy; economic and political factors, and lack of food (David and Lobo, 1995a). The most extreme forms of malnutrition, or protein energy malnutrition, are kwashiorkor and marasmus.

Kwashiorkor

Kwashiorkor is a severe deficiency of energy with an adequate supply of calories. Taken from the Ghan language, the word means "the sickness the older child gets when displaced from the breast by another child" and aptly describes the syndrome that develops in the first child, usually between 1 and 4 years of age. A diet consisting mainly of starch grains or tubers provides adequate calories in the form of carbohydrates but an inadequate amount of high-quality proteins.

The child with kwashiorkor has thin, wasted extremities and a prominent abdomen caused by edema (ascites). The edema often masks the severe muscular atrophy, making the child appear less debilitated than he or she actually is. The skin is scaly and dry and has areas of depigmentation. Several dermatoses may be evident, partly resulting from the vitamin deficiencies. Permanent blindness often results from the severe lack of vitamin A. Mineral deficiencies are common, especially of iron, calcium, and zinc. The hair is thin, dry, coarse, and dull; and patchy alopecia may occur.

Diarrhea frequently occurs as a result of lowered resistance to infection and subsequent gastroenteritis, anorexia, and malabsorption. Gastrointestinal disturbances include reversible fatty infiltration of the liver and atrophy of the acinar cells of the pancreas. Behavioral changes are evident as the child grows progressively irritable, lethargic, withdrawn, and apathetic. Fatal deterioration may be caused by recurrent diarrhea, infection, or circulatory failure.

Marasmus

Marasmus results from a low intake of both calories and protein. It is a common occurrence in underdeveloped countries during times of drought, especially in cultures where adults eat first; the remaining food is often insufficient in quality and quantity for the children.

Marasmus is usually a syndrome of physical and emotional deprivation and is not confined to geographic areas where food supplies are inadequate. It may be seen in children with failure to thrive, where the cause is not solely nutritional but also involves emotional factors.

Marasmus is characterized by gradual wasting and atrophy of body tissues, especially of subcutaneous fat. The child appears to be very old, with flabby and wrinkled skin, unlike the child with kwashiorkor, who appears more rounded from the edema. Fat metabolism is less impaired than in kwashiorkor, so that deficiency of fat-soluble vitamins is usually minimal or absent.

The child is fretful, apathetic, withdrawn, and so lethargic that prostration frequently occurs. Intercurrent infection with debilitating diseases, such as tuberculosis, parasitosis, and dysentery, is common.

Therapeutic Management

The treatment of PEM includes providing a diet with high-quality proteins, carbohydrates, vitamins, and minerals. When PEM occurs as a result of diarrhea, three management goals are identified: (1) rehydration with an oral rehydration solution (ORS) that also replaces electrolytes; (2) medications such as antibiotics and antidiarrheals; and (3) provision of adequate nutrition either by breastfeeding or proper weaning diet. When the child is too ill to tolerate oral fluids, intravenous administration of fluids and electrolytes will be required to prevent death (David and Lobo, 1995b).

Nursing Care Management

Provision of essential physiologic needs, such as rest, individually tailored activity, and protection from infection, is paramount. Since children are usually weak and withdrawn, they depend on others for feeding. Hygiene may be distressing because of the poor integrity of the skin, and decubiti are a constant threat. Appropriate developmental stimulation should be provided also.

The larger problem is the prevention of these conditions through education concerning the importance of proper nutrition, whether breastfeeding or bottle-feeding, when the child is being weaned to semisolid foods. Since children with marasmus may suffer from emotional starvation as well, care should be consistent with care of the child with failure to thrive (see Chapter 33).

FOOD SENSITIVITY

Food sensitivity is a general term that includes any type of adverse reaction to food or food additives. Food sensitivities can be divided into two broad categories:

Food allergy or hypersensitivity—reactions involving immunologic mechanisms, usually immunoglobulin E (IgE); the reactions may be immediate or delayed and mild or severe, such as anaphylactic reactions

Food intolerance—reactions involving known or unknown nonimmunologic mechanisms; lactose intolerance is an example of a reaction that looks like allergy but is due to deficiency of the enzyme lactase

Food allergy is caused by exposure to **allergens,** usually proteins (but not the smaller amino acids) that are capable of inducing IgE antibody formation ("sensitization") when ingested. **Sensitization** is the initial exposure of an individual to an allergen, resulting in an immune response; subsequent exposure induces a much stronger response that is clinically apparent. Consequently food hypersensitivity typically occurs after the food has been ingested one or more times, but it can occur at the first ingestion because of transplacental sensitization in utero or because of sensitization to the substance passed through breast milk (Wilson, Self, and Hamburger, 1990). The most common food allergens are listed in Box 44-3.

Food allergies can develop at any time but are common during infancy, because the immature intestinal tract is more permeable to proteins than the mature intestinal tract, thus increasing the likelihood of an immune response. Allergies in general demonstrate a genetic component: children who have one parent with allergy have a 50% or greater risk of development of allergy; children who have both parents with allergy have up to a 100% risk of development of allergy. Allergy with a hereditary tendency is referred to as *atopy.*

Although the reason is unknown, many children "outgrow" their food allergies. Children with several food allergies may acquire tolerance to each food at different times. The most common allergens, such as soy, are outgrown less readily than other food allergens. Because of the tendency to lose the hypersensitivity, allergic foods should be reintroduced into the diet after a period of abstinence (usually a year or more) to evaluate whether the food can be safely added to the diet. Because of the incidence and severity of peanut allergy, it is recommended that children under 3 years of age not ingest peanuts or peanut products.

BOX 44-3
Hyperallergenic Foods/Sources

Milk*: Ice cream, butter, margarine (if it contains dairy products), yogurt, cheese, pudding, baked goods, wieners, bologna, canned creamed soups, instant breakfast drinks, powdered milk drinks, milk chocolate
Eggs*: Mayonnaise, creamy salad dressing, baked goods, egg noodles, some cake icing, meringue, custard, pancakes, French toast, root beer
Wheat*: Almost all baked goods, wieners, bologna, pressed or chopped cold cuts, gravy, pasta, some canned soups
Legumes: Peanuts,* peanut butter or oil, beans, peas, lentils
Nuts*: Some chocolates, candy, baked goods, cherry soda (may be flavored with a nut extract), walnut oil
Fish or shellfish*: Cod liver oil, pizza with anchovies, Caesar salad dressing, any food fried in same oil as fish
Soy*: Soy sauce, teriyaki or worcestershire sauce, tofu, baked goods using soy flour or oil, soy nuts, soy infant formulas or milk, soybean paste, tuna packed in vegetable oil, many margarines
Chocolate: Cola beverages, cocoa, chocolate-flavored drinks
Buckwheat: Some cereals, pancakes
Pork, chicken: Bacon, wieners, sausage, pork fat, chicken broth
Strawberries, melon, pineapple: Gelatin, syrups
Corn: Popcorn, cereal, muffins, cornstarch, corn meal, corn bread, corn tortilla
Citrus fruits: Orange, lemon, lime, grapefruit; any of these in drinks, gelatin, juice, or medicines
Tomatoes: Juice, some vegetable soups, spaghetti, pizza sauce, and catsup
Spices: Chili, pepper, vinegar, cinnamon

*Most common allergens.

There is evidence that food allergies can be prevented. The protective role of exclusive breastfeeding and avoidance of hyperallergenic foods is controversial, but most authorities often recommend such interventions with a family history of allergy.

Cow's Milk Allergy

Cow's milk allergy is a multifaceted disorder representing adverse systemic and local gastrointestinal reactions to cow's milk protein (Box 44-4). The diagnosis is initially made from the history, although the practitioner needs to be highly suspicious, since the timing and type of clinical manifestations vary greatly. Cow's milk allergy may be manifested as colic (see Chapter 33) or sleeplessness in an otherwise healthy infant.

Diagnostic evaluation. A number of diagnostic tests may be performed, including stool analysis for blood (both frank and occult bleeding can occur from the colitis), serum IgE levels, skin-prick testing, and radioallergosorbent test (RAST) (measures IgE antibodies to specific allergens in serum by radioimmunoassay). Both skin testing and RAST help identify the offending food, but the results are not always conclusive.

The most definitive diagnostic strategy is elimination of milk, followed by challenge testing after improvement of symptoms. Challenge testing involves reintroducing small quantities of milk in the diet to detect resurgence of symptoms; at times challenge testing involves the use of a placebo so that the parent is unaware of or "blind" to the timing of allergen ingestion.

Nursing ALERT

Careful observation of the child is required during a challenge test because of the possibility of anaphylactic reaction.

BOX 44-4
Common Clinical Manifestations of Cow's Milk Sensitivity

Gastrointestinal
Diarrhea
Vomiting
Colic
Abdominal pain

Respiratory
Rhinitis
Bronchitis
Asthma
Wheezing
Sneezing
Coughing
Chronic nasal discharge

Other signs and symptoms
Eczema
Excessive crying
Pallor (from anemia secondary to chronic blood loss in gastrointestinal tract)

Therapeutic management. Treatment of cow's milk allergy is elimination of all dairy products. For infants fed cow's milk formula, this primarily involves changing the formula to a casein or whey hydrolysate milk formula, in which the protein has been broken down (or "predigested") into its amino acids through enzymatic hydrolysis. Soy-based formula is not recommended, because as many as 20% of infants who are allergic to cow's milk are also allergic to soy. Goat's milk is not an acceptable substitute, since it cross-reacts with cow's milk protein and is deficient in folic acid. Infants who are breastfed but have symptoms of cow's milk hypersensitivity are treated by eliminating all dairy products from the lactating mother's diet. These women will require vitamin D and calcium supplementation to prevent deficiency. Infants are maintained on the dairy-free diet for 1 or 2 years, at which time very small quantities of milk are reintroduced.

Nursing care management. The principal nursing objectives are identification of potential milk allergy and appropriate counseling of parents regarding substitute formulas. The protein hydrolysate formulas are less palatable than milk-based formulas. Consequently reluctance to accept the new formula may be a problem. This can be overcome by introducing the formula gradually over a few days using 1 ounce of new formula to 7 ounces of old formula, then 2 to 6 ounces, then 3 to 4, and as needed. Parents also need to be reassured that the infant will receive complete nutrition from the new formula and will suffer no ill effects from the absence of cow's milk.

Once solid foods are started, parents need guidance in avoiding all associated milk products (Box 44-3). Carefully reading all food labels helps prevent use of prepared foods containing milk products.

Lactose Intolerance

Lactose intolerance entails at least two different entities that involve a deficiency of the enzyme lactase, which is needed for the digestion of lactose. *Congenital lactose intolerance* appears soon after birth when the diet contains lactose from milk. Causes of lactose intolerance are attributed to disorders such as human immunodeficiency virus (HIV) or gastrointestinal infections, such as rotavirus and giardiasis. *Late-onset lactose intolerance* is similar to the congenital type but is manifested later in life. Ethnic groups with a high incidence of lactose intolerance include Orientals, southern Europeans, Arabs, Jews, and blacks. The principal manifestations include diarrhea, abdominal pain, distention, and flatus shortly after ingesting milk products.

In older children lactose intolerance may be diagnosed on the basis of the history and improvement with a lactose-free diet. In infants the hydrogen-breath test is frequently used. Undigested carbohydrate, such as lactose, in the colon causes gas production by bacteria. Breath samples are analyzed for the amount of hydrogen.

Treatment of lactose intolerance is elimination of offending dairy products or the use of enzyme replacement. In infants soy-based formula can be substituted for cow's milk formula or human milk. Some children are able to tolerate small amounts of lactose. Pretreated milk (with microbial-derived lactase) may improve lactose absorption. Since dairy products are a major source of calcium and vitamin D, supplementation of these nutrients is needed to prevent deficiency. Yogurt contains inactive lactase enzyme, which is activated by the temperature and pH of the duodenum; this lactase activity substitutes for the lack of endogenous lactase. Fresh yogurt may be tolerated better than frozen yogurt.

Home Care

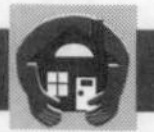

CONTROLLING SYMPTOMS OF LACTOSE INTOLERANCE

- In infants substitute soy-based formula for cow's milk formula or human milk.
- Limit milk consumption to one glass at a time.
- Drink milk with other foods rather than alone.
- Eat hard cheese, cottage cheese, or yogurt instead of drinking milk.
- Use enzyme tablets (Lactaid, Lactrase, Dairy Ease) to predigest the lactose in milk or supplement the body's own lactase (add tablets to milk or sprinkle on dairy products such as ice cream).
- Eat small amounts of dairy foods daily to help colonic bacteria adapt to ingested lactose.

Nursing care management. Nursing care is similar to the interventions discussed for cow's milk allergy: explaining the dietary restrictions to the family; identifying alternate sources of calcium, such as yogurt, and ways of controlling the symptoms (see the Home Care box above); stressing the importance of calcium and vitamin D supplementation; and discussing hidden sources of lactose, such as its use as a bulk agent in certain medications. Parents are advised to check with the pharmacist regarding this possibility when obtaining medication.

Gastrointestinal (GI) Dysfunction

The extensive surface area of the GI tract and its digestive function represent the major means of exchange between the human organism and the environment. Inflammatory and malabsorptive disorders impair the functional integrity of the GI tract. In addition, since the immune system and mucosal barrier continue to mature after birth, the intestine of infants is extremely vulnerable to infection. Acute infectious diarrhea can cause significant alterations in fluid and electrolyte balance in infants and children.

Numerous general observations provide possible clues to specific gastrointestinal problems (Box 44-5). In any disorder that involves GI losses, particularly large amounts of fluid, dehydration poses a serious threat to life and demands immediate attention.

DEHYDRATION

Dehydration is a common body fluid disturbance in infants and children and occurs whenever the total output of fluid exceeds the total intake, regardless of the underlying cause. Dehydration may result from a number of diseases that cause insensible losses through the skin and respiratory tract, through increased renal excretion, and through the GI tract. Although dehydration can result from lack of oral intake (especially in elevated environmental temperatures), more often it is a result of abnormal losses, such as those that occur in vomiting or diarrhea, when oral intake only partially compensates for the abnormal losses. Other significant causes of dehydration are diabetic ketoacidosis and extensive burns.

Water Balance in Infants

As a result of several characteristics, infants and young children have a greater need for water and are more vulnerable to alterations in fluid and electrolyte balance. Compared with older children and adults, they have a greater fluid intake and output relative to size. Water and electrolyte disturbances occur more frequently and more rapidly, and children adjust less promptly to these alterations.

The fluid compartments in the infant vary significantly from those in the adult, primarily because of an expanded extracellular compartment. The **extracellular fluid (ECF)** compartment constitutes over half of the total body water at birth and has a greater relative content of extracellular sodium and chloride. The infant loses a large amount of fluid at birth and still maintains a larger amount of extracellular fluid than the adult until about 2 years of age. This contributes to greater and more rapid water loss during this age period.

Fluid losses create compartment deficits that reflect the duration of dehydration. In general, approximately 60% of fluid is lost from the extracellular fluid, and the remaining 40% comes from the **intracellular fluid (ICF).** The amount of fluid lost from the ECF increases with acute illness and decreases with chronic loss.

Fluid losses may be divided into insensible, urinary, and fecal losses and vary with the patient's age. Approximately two thirds of insensible losses occur through the skin, and the remaining one third is lost through the respiratory tract. Insensible fluid loss is influenced by heat and humidity, body temperature, and respiratory rate. Infants and children have a much greater tendency to become highly febrile than do adults. Fever increases insensible water loss by approximately 7 ml/kg/24 hours for each degree rise in temperature above 99° F (37.2°C). Fever and increased surface area relative to volume are both factors that contribute to greater insensible fluid losses in young patients.

Surface area. The infant's relatively greater body surface area (BSA) allows larger quantities of fluid to be lost in insensible perspiration through the skin. It is estimated that the BSA of the premature neonate is five times as great, and that of the newborn is two to three times as great, as that of the older child or adult. The proportionately longer GI tract in infancy is also a source of relatively greater fluid loss, especially from diarrhea.

Metabolic rate. The rate of metabolism in infancy is significantly higher than in adulthood because of the larger BSA in relation to the mass of active tissue. Consequently, there is a greater production of metabolic wastes that must be excreted by the kidneys. Any condition that increases metabolism causes greater heat production, with its concomitant insensi-

BOX 44-5

Clinical Manifestations of Gastrointestinal Dysfunction in Children

Failure to thrive—Deceleration from established growth pattern or consistently below the fifth percentile for height and weight on standard growth charts; sometimes accompanied by developmental delays

Spitting up or regurgitation—Passive transfer of gastric contents into the esophagus or mouth

Vomiting—Forceful ejection of gastric contents; involves a complex process under central nervous system control that causes salivation, pallor, sweating, and tachycardia; usually accompanied by nausea

- ***Projectile vomiting***—Vomiting accompanied by vigorous peristaltic waves and typically associated with pyloric stenosis or pylorospasm

Nausea—Unpleasant sensation vaguely referred to the throat or abdomen with an inclination to vomit

Constipation—Passage of firm or hard stools or infrequent passage of stool with associated symptoms such as difficulty expelling the stools, blood-streaked stools, and abdominal discomfort

Encopresis—Overflow of incontinent stool causing soiling; often due to fecal retention or impaction

Diarrhea—Increase in the number of stools with an increased water content as a result of alterations of water and electrolyte transport by the GI tract; may be acute or chronic

Hypoactive, hyperactive, or absent bowel sounds—Evidence of intestinal motility problems that may be caused by inflammation or obstruction

Abdominal distention—protuberant contour of the abdomen that may be caused by delayed gastric emptying, accumulation of gas or stool, inflammation, or obstruction

Abdominal pain—Pain associated with the abdomen that may be localized or diffuse, acute or chronic; often caused by inflammation, obstruction, or hemorrhage

Gastrointestinal bleeding—May be from an upper or lower GI source and may be acute or chronic

- ***Hematemesis***—Vomiting of bright red blood or denatured blood that results from bleeding in the upper GI tract or from swallowed blood from the nose or oropharynx
- ***Hematochezia***—Passage of bright red blood per rectum, usually indicating lower GI tract bleeding
- ***Melena***—Passage of dark-colored, "tarry" stools due to denatured blood, suggesting upper GI tract bleeding or bleeding from the right colon

Jaundice—Yellow coloration of the skin and sclerae associated with liver dysfunction

Dysphagia—Difficulty swallowing caused by abnormalities in the neuromuscular function of the pharynx or upper esophageal sphincter or by disorders of the esophagus

Dysfunctional swallowing—Impaired swallowing due to central nervous system defects or structural defects of the oral cavity, pharynx, or esophagus; can cause feeding problems or aspiration

Fever—Common manifestation of illness in children with GI disorders; usually associated with dehydration, infection, or inflammation

TABLE 44-3 Daily maintenance fluid requirements

1. Calculate weight of child in kilograms:

$$\frac{\text{Weight of child (in pounds)}}{2.2 \text{ lb/kg}} = \text{Weight in kilograms}$$

2. Allow 100 ml per kilogram for first 10 kg.
3. Allow 50 ml per kilogram for second 10 kg.
4. Allow 20 ml per kilogram for remainder of weight in kilograms.
5. Divide total amount by 24 hours to obtain rate in milliliters per hour.

ble fluid loss and an increased need for water for excretion. The basal metabolic rate (BMR) in infants and children is higher to support growth.

Kidney function. The kidneys of the infant are functionally immature at birth and are therefore inefficient in excreting waste products of metabolism. Of particular importance for fluid balance is the inability of the infant's kidneys to concentrate or dilute urine, to conserve or excrete sodium, and to acidify urine. Therefore the infant is less able to handle large quantities of solute-free water than is the older child and is more likely to become dehydrated when given concentrated formulas or overhydrated when given excessive water or dilute formula.

Fluid requirements. As a result of these characteristics, infants ingest and excrete a greater amount of fluid per kilogram of body weight than do older children. Since electrolytes are excreted with water and the infant has limited ability for conservation, maintenance requirements include both water and electrolytes. The daily exchange of extracellular fluid in the infant is much greater than that of older children, leaving the infant little fluid volume reserve in dehydrated states. Fluid requirements depend on hydration status, size, environmental factors, and underlying disease. Daily maintenance fluid requirements are outlined in Table 44-3.

Types of Dehydration

The pathophysiologic characteristics of dehydration can best be understood by recognizing that the distribution of water between the extracellular and intracellular spaces depends on active transport of potassium into and sodium out of cells by energy-requiring processes. Sodium is the chief solute in ECF and thus is the primary determinant of ECF volume. Potassium is primarily intracellular. When ECF volume is reduced in acute dehydration, the total body sodium content is almost always reduced as well, regardless of serum sodium measurements. Replacement of fluid volume should therefore be accompanied by sodium repletion. Sodium depletion in diarrhea occurs in two ways: out of the body in stool and into the intracellular compartment to replace potassium to maintain electrical equilibrium.

Dehydration is classified into three categories on the basis of osmolality and depends primarily on the serum sodium concentration: (1) isotonic, (2) hypotonic, and (3) hypertonic.

Isotonic (isosmotic or *isonatremic) dehydration,* the most common form, occurs in conditions in which the electrolyte and water deficits are present in approximately balanced proportion; that is, salt and water are lost in equal amounts. Shock is the greatest threat to life in isotonic dehydration, and the child displays the symptoms characteristic of hypovolemic shock. Serum sodium remains within normal limits, between 130 and 150 mEq/L.

Hypotonic (hyposmotic or *hyponatremic) dehydration* occurs when the electrolyte deficit exceeds the water deficit, leaving the serum hypotonic. Since ICF is more concentrated than ECF in hypotonic dehydration, water moves from the ECF to the ICF to establish osmotic equilibrium. Therefore this further increases the ECF volume loss, and shock is a frequent result. Since there is a greater proportional loss of ECF in hypotonic dehydration, the physical signs tend to be more severe with smaller fluid losses than with isotonic or hypertonic dehydration. Serum sodium concentration is less than 130 mEq/L.

Hypertonic (hyperosmotic or *hypernatremic) dehydration* results from water loss in excess of electrolyte loss and is usually caused by a proportionately larger loss of water and/or a larger intake of electrolytes. This sometimes occurs in infants with diarrhea who are given fluids by mouth that contain large amounts of solute, such as those receiving high-protein nasogastric tube feedings. In hypertonic dehydration, fluid shifts from the lesser concentration of the ICF to the ECF. Serum sodium concentration is greater than 150 mEq/L. Since the ECF volume is proportionately larger, hypertonic dehydration has a larger degree of water loss for the same intensity of physical signs. Shock is less apparent in hypertonic dehydration. However neurologic disturbances, such as seizures, are more likely to occur. Cerebral changes are serious and may result in permanent damage.

Diagnostic Evaluation

Diagnosis of the type and degree of dehydration is made on the basis of clinical manifestations (Table 44-4). In infants isotonic dehydration is usually described as 5% (mild), 10% (moderate), or 15% (severe). A more accurate means of describing dehydration is to reflect acute loss (over 48 hours or less) in milliliters per kilogram of body weight (Finberg, 1990). Older children and adolescents, with proportionately less total body water, display smaller proportional losses; therefore the estimates of 3%, 6%, and 9% more nearly describe mild, moderate, and severe dehydration, respectively, in these age groups (Table 44-5).

Shock is a common feature of severe depletion of ECF volume with tachycardia and very low blood pressure (see Shock, Chapter 46). Delayed capillary refill, cold extremities, acidosis, and coma are additional signs of severe dehydration, and in infants the anterior fontanel is depressed.

Therapeutic Management

See the discussion on therapeutic management of diarrhea, p. 1391.

Nursing Care Management

Nursing observation and intervention are essential to the detection and therapeutic management of dehydration. There are a wide variety of circumstances in which fluid loss may be

TABLE 44-4 Clinical manifestations of dehydration

	ISOTONIC (LOSS OF WATER AND SALT)	HYPOTONIC (LOSS OF SALT IN EXCESS OF WATER)	HYPERTONIC (LOSS OF WATER IN EXCESS OF SALT)
Skin			
Color	Gray	Gray	Gray
Temperature	Cold	Cold	Cold or hot
Turgor	Poor	Very poor	Fair
Feel	Dry	Clammy	Thickened, doughy
Mucous membranes	Dry	Slightly moist	Parched
Tearing and salivation	Absent	Absent	Absent
Eyeball	Sunken	Sunken	Sunken
Fontanel	Sunken	Sunken	Sunken
Body temperature	Subnormal or elevated	Subnormal or elevated	Subnormal or elevated
Pulse	Rapid	Very rapid	Moderately rapid
Respirations	Rapid	Rapid	Rapid
Behavior	Irritable to lethargic	Lethargic to comatose; convulsions	Marked lethargy with extreme hyperirritability on stimulation

TABLE 44-5 Intensity of clinical signs associated with varying degrees of isotonic dehydration in infants

	DEGREE OF DEHYDRATION		
	MILD	MODERATE	SEVERE
Fluid volume loss	<50 ml/kg	50-90 ml/kg	≥100 ml/kg
Skin color	Pale	Gray	Mottled
Skin elasticity	Decreased	Poor	Very poor
Mucous membranes	Dry	Very dry	Parched
Urine output	Decreased	Oliguria	Marked oliguria and azotemia
Blood pressure	Normal	Normal or lowered	Lowered
Pulse	Normal or increased	Increased	Rapid and thready
Capillary filling time	<2 seconds	2-3 seconds	>3 seconds

precipitated, especially in infants, and changes can take place in a very short time. Therefore an important nursing responsibility is perceptive observation for any signs of dehydration. Conditions in which changes can develop with surprising rapidity in young children include diarrhea; vomiting; sweating; fever; disorders such as diabetes, renal disease, and cardiac anomalies; administration of certain drugs, such as diuretics and steroids; and trauma, such as major surgery, burns, and other types of extensive injury.

The nursing assessment of suspected or potential fluid loss begins with the observation of general appearance and then proceeds with specific observations.

Intake and output. Accurate measurements of fluid intake and output are vital to the assessment of dehydration. This includes oral and parenteral intake and losses from urine, stools, vomiting, fistulas, nasogastric suction, sweat, and wound drainage.

Urine—assess frequency, volume, color, and consistency of urine
Stools—assess frequency, volume, and consistency of stools
Vomitus—assess for volume, frequency, and type of vomitus
Sweating—can be only estimated from frequency of clothing and linen changes

Other observations. In addition to fluid intake and output, the following observations assist in assessment of dehydration:

Vital signs—temperature (normal, elevated, or lowered depending on degree of dehydration), pulse (tachycardia), respirations (tachypnea), and blood pressure (hypotension).
Skin—assess for color, temperature, turgor, presence or absence of edema, and capillary refill
Mucous membranes—assess for moisture, color, and presence of and consistency of secretions
Body weight—decreased in relation to degree of dehydration
Fontanel (infants)—sunken, soft, normal
Sensory alterations—presence of thirst

For nursing interventions, see the discussion of specific disorders.

Disorders of Motility

ACUTE DIARRHEA

Diarrhea is a symptom that can result from disorders involving digestive, absorptive, and secretory functions. There are wide variations in colonic function among different individuals; therefore a precise definition and identification of what constitutes diarrhea pose a problem in terms of number or consistency of stools. For example, one infant may have one firm stool every second or third day, whereas another normally passes from five to eight small, soft stools daily. Important considerations are (1) a noticeable or sudden increase in the number of stools, (2) a change in their consistency with an increase in fluid content, and (3) a tendency for the stools to be greenish in color and contain mucus or blood.

Diarrhea may be acute or chronic, and inflammatory or noninflammatory; the physiologic consequences vary considerably in relation to its severity, duration, associated symptoms, the age of the child, and the child's nutritional status before the onset of diarrhea. Diarrhea related to an inflammatory process is usually described as gastroenteritis, and the terms are often used interchangeably.

Etiology

Diarrhea can be attributed to a large number of specific causes, mechanisms, and predisposing factors. Factors that predispose a child to diarrhea and its physiologic consequences include the following: (1) the younger the child, the greater the susceptibility to diarrhea and the more severe the diarrhea is likely to be; (2) children who are malnourished or debilitated from disease are more susceptible to diarrhea, as are children who have an immune deficiency; and (3) lack of clean water and insufficient understanding of hygiene contribute to contamination, as do crowding and poor sanitation with inadequate facilities for food preparation and refrigeration.

Specific causes. A variety of factors can produce diarrhea in the infant or child either as the presenting symptom or as an associated symptom. Often a specific etiologic diagnosis is lacking. *Acute* diarrhea is a leading cause of illness in children younger than 5 years of age; the dehydration that it causes is fatal for approximately 400 of these children a year in the United States (Kleinman, 1992). The sudden change in the frequency and consistency of stools is more often caused by an inflammatory process of infectious origin but may also be the result of a toxic reaction to ingestion of poisons, dietary indiscretions, or infection outside the GI tract (e.g., communicable diseases, infections of the respiratory or urinary tracts, and emotional tension). Most are self-limited and will ultimately subside without specific treatment if dehydration does not create a serious complication. Antibiotic therapy is also a common cause of diarrhea in children.

Chronic diarrhea, the passage of loose stools with increased frequency that lasts for more than 2 weeks, is more likely to be associated with disorders of malabsorption, anatomic defects, abnormal bowel motility, hypersensitivity (allergic) reaction, or a long-term inflammatory response.

Diarrheal disturbances can involve the stomach and intestine *(gastroenteritis),* the small intestine *(enteritis),* the colon *(colitis),* or the colon and intestine *(enterocolitis). Dysentery,* intestinal inflammation, especially of the colon, is accompanied by cramping abdominal pain and watery stools containing blood and mucus. Infectious organisms are frequent causes of diarrhea in infancy and childhood and are further discussed in relation to gastroenteritis.

Common causes of diarrhea are dietary indiscretions (e.g., eating green apples or other fruits and drinking fruit juices in large amounts), food sensitivities, and use of concentrated formulas. In some children apple juice has been repeatedly demonstrated to cause or perpetuate nonspecific diarrhea. Studies indicate that "cloudy" apple juice, which is freshly pressed and unprocessed, is less likely to cause diarrhea than the more "clear" juice, which is processed (Hoekstra and others, 1995). Also, sorbitol, the sweetener used in some "sugar-free" gum and other products, is poorly absorbed in the GI tract and may produce osmotic diarrhea if ingested in large amounts.

Pathophysiology

Invasion of the gastrointestinal tract by pathogens produces diarrhea by (1) production of enterotoxins that stimulate secretion of water and electrolytes, (2) direct invasion and destruction of intestinal epithelial cells, and (3) local inflammation and systemic invasion by the organisms. However, the most serious and immediate physiologic disturbances associated with severe diarrheal disease are (1) dehydration, (2) acid-base imbalance with acidosis, and (3) shock that occurs when dehydration progresses to the point that circulatory status is seriously impaired.

Diagnostic Evaluation

The history provides valuable information regarding exposure to infectious agents, personal contact, travel, or probable contact with contaminated foods. Allergic and dietary history may indicate food intolerances or allergies. Crowding and close person-to-person contact make epidemics of any enteric pathogen more likely.

The age of the child provides clues to the cause of diarrheal disturbances. For example, milk allergy or intolerance of other formula constituents is suspected in early infancy. In later infancy new foods added to the diet are frequent offenders. Most acute, inflammatory diarrheas are infectious, and the type of stools and the symptoms associated with the diarrhea provide clues to the organism (Table 44-6).

The clinical manifestations of diarrhea are outlined in Box 44-6. Manifestations of severe diarrhea are primarily those of dehydration (see Table 44-4). Although vomiting may occur in all infectious diarrheas, it is not a major feature.

Although the child may not gain weight or may even show a slight loss in mild diarrhea, signs of dehydration are usually absent. If the diarrhea persists, if the child loses weight, if there is blood in the stools, or if the child exhibits associated signs such as deep breathing, listlessness, or reduced urinary output that may signal complications, the child should be medically evaluated.

Laboratory examination. Extensive laboratory evaluation is not indicated in a child with uncomplicated diarrhea and no evidence of dehydration. Laboratory tests are indicated when a child is moderately to severely dehydrated. Many cases of diarrhea are self-limiting, regardless of the cause.

BOX 44-6
Clinical Manifestations of Diarrhea

Mild diarrhea—a few loose stools each day without other evidence of illness
Moderate diarrhea—several loose or watery stools daily
- Normal or elevated temperature
- Vomiting
- Fretfulness and irritability
- Signs of dehydration usually absent, although may not gain weight or may even show weight loss

Severe diarrhea—numerous to continuous stools
- Signs of moderate to severe dehydration evident (see Table 44-4)
- Drawn, flaccid expressions
- Cry lacks vigor, is often whining and higher pitched than usual
- Irritable
- Seeks comfort and attention of parent
- Displays purposeless movements and inappropriate responses to people and familiar things
- May become lethargic, moribund, or comatose

Stool specimens should be examined in all children with diarrhea that persists for more than a few days. Examination of the stool for polymorphonuclear leukocytes ("polys") is the most widely used test to differentiate bacterial infections from viral ones. Cultures of the stool should be performed when blood or mucus is present in the stool, when abdominal cramps are severe, when there is a history of travel to a developing country, and when polys are found in the stool (indicating bacterial infection).

The stool should also be examined for ova and parasites when bacterial and viral culture findings are negative and the diarrhea persists for more than a few days. Stool specimens to be tested for ova and parasites need to be preserved in a special solution to minimize false results. If there is a history of recent antibiotic use, the stool should be tested for the presence of *Clostridium difficile* toxin, and a sigmoidoscopy evaluation for pseudomembranous colitis may be indicated. A stool pH of less than 6 and the presence of reducing substances (determined with a Clinitest tablet and a small specimen of stool) suggest carbohydrate malabsorption or secondary lactase deficiency.

The urine specific gravity should be determined if dehydration is suspected. A complete blood count, serum electrolytes, and creatinine and blood urea nitrogen (BUN) values should be obtained in the child who requires hospitalization. The hemoglobin, hematocrit, creatinine, and BUN levels are usually elevated in acute diarrhea and should also normalize with rehydration.

Therapeutic Management

Therapeutic management is directed at correcting the fluid imbalance and treating the underlying cause. Initial and regular ongoing evaluations are carried out to assess the patient's progress toward equilibrium and the effectiveness of therapy.

Mild or moderate diarrhea. Mild or moderate diarrhea is usually managed by simple measures and seldom requires hospitalization. When the moderate diarrhea becomes worse or does not respond to simple measures, hospitalization is indicated.

The major goals in the management of acute diarrhea include (1) assessment of the fluid and electrolyte imbalance, (2) rehydration, (3) maintenance fluid therapy, and (4) reintroduction of adequate diet. Infants and children with acute diarrhea and dehydration should be treated first with ***oral rehydration therapy (ORT)*** or, in the few cases where this is not possible, with parenteral fluid therapy. ORT is effective, safer, less painful, and less costly than intravenous rehydration. ORT is one of the major worldwide health care advances of the past decade in underdeveloped, or Third World, countries. In developed countries, however, oral rehydration has not been widely used because of the relative ease of access to intravenous fluids and entrenched patterns of care.

Oral rehydration solutions (ORSs) are successful in treating infants with isotonic, hypotonic, and hypertonic dehydration. In a child with mild to moderate dehydration 60 to 80 ml/kg should be administered over a 2-hour period (Johnson, 1993). After rehydration, ORS may be used during maintenance fluid therapy by alternating the solution with a low-sodium fluid such as water, breast milk, lactose-free formula, or half-strength lactose-containing formula. For older children, ORS can be given and a regular diet continued. Ongoing stool losses should be replaced on a 1:1 basis with ORS. If the stool output is not known, approximately 10 ml/kg or ½ to 1 cup of ORS should be given for each diarrheal stool.

Infants without clinical signs of dehydration do not need ORT. They should, however, receive the same fluids recommended for infants with signs of dehydration in the maintenance phase and for ongoing stool losses.

An ORS is useful in most cases of dehydration, and vomiting is not a contraindication. A child who is vomiting should be given ORS frequently in small amounts. The fluid may be given with a spoon or small syringe in 5- to 10-ml increments every 1 to 5 minutes by the child's caregiver. ORS may also be given through a nasogastric tube. In the United States, commercially prepared solutions such as Pedialyte, Lytren, Ricelyte, and Resol are used almost exclusively for oral rehydration.

Nursing ALERT

Diarrhea is not managed by encouraging intake of clear fluids by mouth, such as fruit juices, carbonated soft drinks, and gelatin. These fluids usually have a high carbohydrate content, a very low electrolyte content, and high osmolality (Avery and Snyder, 1990). Caffeinated soda is avoided, because caffeine is a mild diuretic and may lead to increased loss of water and sodium. Chicken or beef broth is not given, because it contains excessive sodium and inadequate carbohydrate.

Glucose-mediated enhanced sodium absorption forms the physiologic basis for the composition of ORS. Recent studies have evaluated the effectiveness of rice-based ORS. Results demonstrate that these nutrient-based solutions markedly reduced vomiting, decreased diarrhea volume loss, and shortened the duration of the disease (Santosham and Greenough, 1991).

Early reintroduction of normal nutrients is desirable and is gaining more widespread acceptance. Controversy still exists, however, regarding the best method of reintroducing feeding during recovery from diarrhea. Recent studies indicate that early reintroduction of normal diet is beneficial because of its nutritional advantage and may reduce the number of stools, reduce weight loss, and shorten the duration of illness (Brown, 1991; Margolis and others, 1990). Continued feeding may protect against starvation-induced intestinal mucosal atrophy and enhance more rapid mucosal recovery following infectious diarrhea.

Breastfeeding, if being done, should be continued as a supplement to the ORS. Available evidence indicates that continued human milk feeding during diarrheal illness results in reduced severity and duration of the illness (Brown, 1991). Tolerance to human milk may be due to its lower osmolality and its antimicrobial, enzymatic, and hormonal factors.

The use of nonhuman milk for infants and children with diarrhea remains controversial. This milk is of concern because maldigestion of lactose can occur in children with infectious diarrhea. However, there is evidence that well-hydrated infants may resume full nonhuman milk feeding immediately without adverse reactions (Brown, Peerson, and Fontaine, 1994; Chew et al, 1993).

Many infants and children can be safely managed with a milk diet. Some practitioners advocate the use of a lactose-free formula only if milk or regular formula is not tolerated.

For older children a regular diet can generally be offered once rehydration has occurred. Bland foods may be better tolerated by some children. It is important to consider that recommendations to restrict infants' diets may be associated with significant noncompliance.

Parenteral fluid therapy is initiated whenever the child is unable to ingest sufficient amounts of fluid and electrolytes to (1) meet ongoing daily physiologic losses, (2) replace previous deficits, and (3) replace ongoing abnormal losses. Patients who usually require intravenous fluids are those with severe dehydration, those with uncontrollable vomiting, those who are unable to drink for any reason (such as extreme fatigue or coma), and those with severe gastric distention.

Severe diarrhea. Severe diarrhea is largely a problem of infants and very young children, and regardless of the cause, successful management relies primarily on appropriate treatment of physiologic disturbances and is only secondarily concerned with specific treatment of the causative agent. Severe diarrhea warrants hospitalization, comprehensive evaluation, and parenteral fluid therapy. Fluid therapy is directed toward replacement of (1) the fluid deficit, as determined by weight loss and clinical signs; (2) ongoing normal losses from urine, lungs, and sweat; and (3) continued abnormal GI losses.

Intravenous administration of fluid is begun immediately, and the solution is selected on the basis of what is known regarding the probable type and cause of the dehydration—usually a saline solution containing 5% dextrose in water. Sodium bicarbonate may be added, since acidosis is usually associated with severe dehydration. Although the initial phase of fluid replacement is rapid in both isotonic and hypotonic dehydration, it is contraindicated in hypertonic dehydration because of the risk of water intoxication, especially in the brain cells.

Once the severe effects of dehydration are under control, specific diagnostic and therapeutic measures are begun to detect and treat the cause of the diarrhea. This includes antimicrobial therapy where indicated and treatment of secondary effects of the illness or its therapy. For example, secondary bacterial growth may be countered with a short course of non absorbable antibiotics.

Nursing Care Management

Assessment

The nursing assessment of diarrhea begins with observation of the infant's or child's general appearance and behavior. The physical assessment includes all the parameters described for assessment of dehydration (p. 1389). A history provides valuable information regarding probable etiologic agents, such as introduction of a new food, exposure to infectious agents, travel to an area of high susceptibility, contact with foods that might be contaminated, and contact with pets that are known to be sources of enteric infections. An allergy, drug, and dietary history may indicate food allergies.

Nursing Diagnoses

Several nursing diagnoses become apparent on the basis of a thorough physical assessment. The major diagnoses appropriate for the infant or child are described in the Nursing Care Plan on p. 1394. Other diagnoses will be evident, depending on the child's age and condition, and the cause of the diarrhea.

Planning

The goals for the dehydrated infant or child and for the family are as follows:

1. Infant or child will maintain adequate hydration.
2. Infant or child will maintain appropriate nutrition for age.
3. Infant or child will not spread infection (if etiologic agent) to others.
4. Family will receive appropriate support and education, especially regarding home care.

Implementation

Mild or moderate diarrhea is usually managed at home under the supervision of the nurse. The parents are allowed to give fluids to the child. Fluids are usually tolerated best at room temperature, and the parent is cautioned against giving fluids other than those prescribed by the practitioner. The ORS is usually well accepted by infants, but older children find these solutions unpalatable. However, flavored solutions may be better accepted (see the Critical Thinking Q & A box, on p. 1393).

Severe diarrhea. The infant or child admitted to the hospital with diarrhea is usually isolated from children who do not have diarrhea, and appropriate precautions are implemented to prevent possible spread to other patients and personnel. Most infections that cause diarrhea are spread by the fecal-oral route or through contaminated food. Strict attention to disposal of soiled diapers, hygienic food preparation, not sharing toys, and proper handwashing will minimize transmission. The containment of feces is a key factor in infection control. Research indicates that superabsorbent paper diapers with elastic legs permit less fecal leakage than cloth diapers

Critical Thinking Q & A

ACUTE DIARRHEA

An 8-month-old infant is evaluated in the primary care clinic because of fever, vomiting, and diarrhea of 12 hours duration. The caregivers report that the infant had three times as many stools as usual, and the stools are watery in consistency. After the initial examination of the infant, it is apparent that the child is mildly dehydrated as a result of stool losses secondary to acute infectious diarrhea. Which of the following interventions would be indicated in this situation?

1. Recommendations to offer fruit juice only and delay reintroduction of food for 48 hours.
2. Administration of antidiarrheal medications.
3. Education of the infant's caregivers regarding administration of oral rehydration solution (ORS).
4. Administration of intravenous fluids and provision of nothing by mouth for several hours.

The correct answer is three. The goals of management of acute diarrhea include assessment of hydration, provision of fluids for rehydration and maintenance, and reintroduction of an adequate diet. In this case since the infant is mildly dehydrated, oral rehydration therapy (ORT) should be attempted. ORT is effective, and is safer, less painful, and less costly than intravenous rehydration. If ORS is administered at frequent intervals, vomiting can be minimized and intravenous hydration can likely be prevented.

Early reintroduction of normal nutrients is desirable, and delayed introduction of food may be harmful in terms of nutritional status and duration of illness. Breastfeeding should generally be continued, and most infants who receive cow's milk formulas may resume their usual feedings as soon as they are rehydrated. Occasionally a soy formula will be recommended after an episode of acute infectious diarrhea if the infant demonstrates evidence of lactose malabsorption. Use of antidiarrheal medications should not be recommended for acute infectious diarrhea. These drugs may be harmful, since adverse effects such as slowed motility and ileus may result from their use.

with plastic coverings (Kubiak et al, 1993). Each hospital has a policy regarding necessary precautions (see Infection Control, Chapter 42).

The child is weighed on admission and frequently during the initial rehydration period. Accurate intake and output measurement is imperative, and (if needed) a urine collection bag is placed to determine the volume of output, to measure specific gravity, and to determine whether the renal blood flow is sufficient to permit administration of potassium. Unless urine is separated from stool, this essential information cannot be obtained.

Children who are sufficiently ill to require hospitalization may be placed on parenteral fluid therapy with nothing by mouth for 12 to 48 hours. Monitoring the intravenous infusion is a primary nursing function, with careful attention given to ascertain that the correct fluid and electrolyte concentration is infused, the flow rate is adjusted to deliver the desired volume in a given period of time, and the intravenous site is maintained.

The nurse is responsible for examination of stools and collection of specimens for laboratory examination. Care should be exerted in obtaining and transporting stools to prevent possible spread of infection. Stool specimens should be transported to the laboratory in appropriate containers and media according to hospital policy. A clean tongue depressor can be used to obtain specimens for laboratory examination when a larger volume is needed or as an applicator for transfer to a culture medium. Tests for pH, blood, and reducing substance can be done on the nursing unit (see Collection of Specimens, Chapter 42).

Since diarrheal stools are highly irritating to the skin, extra care is needed to protect the skin of the diaper region from becoming excoriated (see Diaper Dermatitis, Chapter 50). Rectal temperatures are avoided, because they can stimulate the bowel, increasing passage of stool.

Support for the child and family involves the same care and consideration as for all hospitalized children (see Chapter 41). Parents are kept informed of the child's progress and instructed in special care behaviors, such as handwashing and proper disposal of soiled diapers, clothes, and bed linen. Everyone caring for the child must be aware of "clean" areas and "dirty" areas, especially in the hospital, where the sink in the child's room is used for many purposes. For example, food, eating and drinking utensils, toothbrushes, pacifiers, toys, and other personal items are stored away from the sink, diaper-changing surface, and scale used to weigh diapers (1 g wet diaper weight = 1 ml urine). Soiled diapers and linen should be discarded in receptacles close to the bedside.

Evaluation

The effectiveness of nursing interventions is determined by continued reassessment according to the following observational guidelines and expected outcomes:

1. Monitor fluid losses with careful intake and output measurements and daily weights.
2. Monitor food intake, especially calories.
3. Observe for evidence of complications from underlying disease (specify) and/or therapy.
4. Observe and interview family to determine extent and effectiveness of care.

Expected outcomes:

See the Nursing Care Plan on p. 1394.

ACUTE INFECTIOUS DIARRHEA

Acute infectious diarrhea (infectious gastroenteritis) is caused by a wide variety of viral, bacterial, and parasitic pathogens. In the United States the incidence of acute infectious diarrhea is approximately $2^1/_2$ episodes per person per year (Cohen, 1991). Infants and young children are at a high risk for the development of dehydration and malnutrition, the two major consequences of diarrhea.

Etiology/Epidemiology

Most organisms that cause diarrhea are spread by the fecal-oral route. Some are transmitted by direct person-to-person contact, especially where groups are in direct contact, such as in day-care centers. Viral disease is more frequent in winter months; bacterial disorders are more prevalent during summer and fall. Although acute gastroenteritis affects all age groups, there is a greater frequency of diarrheal disease in younger children.

In young children in the United States and in other industrialized countries most episodes of diarrhea are due to viral pathogens.

Nursing Care Plan

THE CHILD WITH ACUTE DIARRHEA (GASTROENTERITIS)

Nursing Diagnosis: Fluid volume deficit related to excessive GI losses from diarrhea/emesis

Expected Outcome: **Patient exhibits signs of adequate hydration (i.e., skin—normal turgor, moist mucous membranes; vital signs within normal limits [WNL]; balanced intake and output [I & O]; no thirst; blood—electrolytes, hemoglobin/hematocrit, and osmolality WNL; urine—appearance, specific gravity, and osmolality WNL; clear mental processes).**

• **NURSING INTERVENTIONS/*RATIONALES***

Administer prescribed oral rehydration solutions (ORS) and/or intravenous (IV) solutions alternated with small amounts of low-sodium fluids such as water, breast milk, or lactose-reduced formula *for rehydration and replacement.* **(Avoid fluids with high-carbohydrate, low-electrolyte values such as carbonated drinks, fruit juices, and gelatin.)**

Monitor thirst, skin turgor, capillary refill, mucous membranes, mental status, intake and output, vital signs, appropriate blood and urine lab results *to assess hydration status.*

Describe all episodes of diarrhea/emesis *to evaluate for continuing fluid loss.*

Instruct family about appropriate administration of fluids, maintenance of I & O records, signs and symptoms of continuing dehydration *to optimize compliance.*

Nursing Diagnosis: Altered nutrition: less than body requirements related to diarrheal losses, inadequate intake

Expected Outcome: **Patient exhibits adequate intake of appropriate nourishment and satisfactory gain of any lost weight.**

• **NURSING INTERVENTIONS/*RATIONALES***

After rehydration begin refeeding by reintroducing foods from a normal diet as tolerated *to reduce number of stools and weight loss and shorten duration of illness.* **(Avoid bananas, rice, apples, and toast or tea [BRAT] diet as it is low in protein, electrolytes, and energy and too high in carbohydrates).**

Observe and record response to feedings *to assess feeding tolerance.*

Weigh *to monitor weight status.*

Instruct family about appropriate foods **to optimize compliance**; instruct breastfeeding mothers to continue breastfeeding **as it reduces duration and severity of the illness.**

Nursing Diagnosis: Risk for transmitting infection related to invasion of the GI tract by microorganisms

Expected Outcome: **Patient shows no evidence of transmission of infection to patient contacts.**

• **NURSING INTERVENTIONS/*RATIONALES***

Implement appropriate standard precautions, careful handwashing techniques, use of snug-fitting and superabsorbent disposable diapers *to reduce likelihood of fecal transmission.*

Instruct all members in the environment in isolation procedures and handwashing techniques *to optimize compliance and reduce spread of organisms.*

Nursing Diagnosis: Impaired skin integrity related to irritation caused by frequent, loose stools

Expected Outcome: **Patient's skin is intact.**

• **NURSING INTERVENTIONS/*RATIONALES***

Keep skin clean and dry through frequent diaper changes, use of superabsorbant disposable diapers, and use of gentle nonalkaline soap and water solution *to protect skin from irritation.* **(Avoid commercial baby wipes that contain alcohol as they add to the irritation).**

Inspect skin for redness and excoriation; expose reddened areas to air *to promote healing;* use a moisture barrier ointment or cream *to protect excoriated areas.*

Inspect perineum and buttocks *for signs of infection such as fungal growth or Candida* and treat with appropriate medication as prescribed.

Instruct family about skin inspection *for early detection of skin problems.*

Nursing Diagnosis: Anxiety/fear related to separation from parents, unfamiliar environment, distressing procedures

Expected Outcome: **Patient exhibits minimal signs of emotional or physical distress (i.e., is calm, relaxed, cooperative; engages in nonnutritive sucking, appropriate play).**

• **NURSING INTERVENTIONS/*RATIONALES***

Encourage frequent family visitation with active participation in care *to prevent distress from separation.*

Use frequent touch, holding, and talking *to provide comfort;* use pacifier and mouth care for infants who are on nothing by mouth (NPO) status.

Provide diversion and sensory stimulation appropriate to the child's developmental level and physical condition.

Instruct family in importance of comfort measures and in their active participation in care *to ease child's fears.*

Rotavirus is the most important cause of dehydrating diarrhea in young children throughout the world. Its symptoms may range from no manifestations to death from dehydration. Rotavirus infection accounts for the majority of hospitalizations for severe diarrhea in young children and is a significant nosocomial (hospital-acquired) pathogen. As of this writing an oral vaccine that has been highly effective against very severe rotavirus gastroenteritis is being tested (Rennels and others, 1996). *Salmonella, Shigella,* and *Campylobacter* are the most frequently isolated bacterial pathogens, and *Giardia* and *Cryptosporidium* are the parasites that most commonly produce acute, infectious diarrhea (Table 44-6).

Diagnostic Evaluation

Infectious diarrheas have some features in common, such as vomiting, and frequently there is abdominal discomfort. Bacterial infections and some viral infections are accompanied by fever. The manifestations and severity are variable among the various forms (Table 44-4). Laboratory confirmation of the specific organism confirms the diagnosis and serves as a guideline for appropriate therapeutic management.

Therapeutic Management

The primary concerns in infectious gastroenteritis, as in all conditions in which fluid is lost in large amounts, are dehydration and the attendant physical deterioration. Fluid replacement, nutritional therapy, and monitoring of electrolyte status with replacement are the same as for any diarrheal disorder.

Treatment for acute infectious diarrhea should begin with effective preventive measures. Because spread of most of these organisms is fecal-oral, personal hygiene, water supplies, sewage control, and food preparation are important considerations (see Infection Control, Chapter 42).

Enteric infections are generally self-limited conditions. Antimicrobial therapy is not indicated in the majority of children with acute diarrhea. Specific antimicrobial therapy is indicated only for culture-proven bacterial or parasitic infections in which this therapy can reduce the duration of the illness, severity of symptoms, shedding of organisms, and secondary spread of organisms (see also Intestinal Parasitic Diseases, p. 1403). Effective antimicrobial therapy is not available for enteric viruses. Indiscriminate use of antibiotics may lead to pseudomembranous colitis and worsen the existing diarrhea.

Antidiarrheal drug therapy is usually not indicated in acute infectious diarrhea. Adverse side effects may occur, such as worsening of the diarrhea because of slowing of motility or prevention of absorption of medicines or nutrients in the intestine.

Nursing Care Management

Basic nursing care for the infant or child with infectious gastroenteritis is the same as for any diarrheal disease. However, appropriate isolation precautions are carried out to prevent the spread of the infection to others.

It may be necessary to obtain stool specimens from the child and other family members who are affected or suspected of being carriers of infectious organisms. The parents are provided with specimen containers and instructed in collection and disposition of stool samples.

There are some medications that appear to be safe for adults in preventing traveler's diarrhea; however, parents should be cautioned against giving any drugs to children. Until vaccines or other prophylactic measures are proved safe for children, the best prevention during travel to areas where the water supply may be contaminated is to allow children to drink only bottled water and carbonated beverages (from the container through a straw supply brought from home). Tap water, ice, unpasteurized dairy products, raw vegetables, and unpeeled fruits are avoided. Meats and seafoods may be risky as well, and are best avoided or eaten fully cooked.

Nursing ALERT

To reduce the risk of bacteria transmitted via food, encourage parents to:

Quickly freeze or refrigerate all ground meat and other perishable foods.

Never thaw food on the counter or let it sit out of the refrigerator for more than 2 hours.

Wash hands, utensils, and work areas with hot soapy water after contact with raw meat to prevent bacteria from spreading.

Check meat with a fork to make sure no pink is showing beofre taking a bite.

Cook all dishes made with ground meat until brown or gray inside, or to an internal temperature of 71° C (160° F).

CONSTIPATION

Constipation is the infrequent passage of firm or hard stools or of small, hard masses with associated symptoms such as difficulty in expulsion of the stools, blood-streaked bowel movements, and abdominal discomfort. The frequency of bowel movements is not considered a diagnostic criterion, because it varies widely among children.

Constipation may arise secondary to a variety of organic disorders of the GI tract or in association with a wide range of systemic disorders. Structural disorders of the intestine may be found in association with constipation, such as strictures, ectopic anus, and Hirschsprung disease. A wide range of systemic disorders may be associated with constipation. Hypothyroidism disorders associated with hypercalcemia, such as hyperparathyroidism and vitamin D excess, are commonly associated with chronic constipation in childhood. Chronic high-level lead poisoning may cause anorexia, vomiting, abdominal pain, and constipation. Constipation may also be associated with a wide range of drugs, such as antacids, diuretics, phenytoin (Dilantin), antihistamines, and opioids (narcotics), and with iron supplementation. Spinal cord lesions may produce loss of rectal tone and sensation. These patients are therefore prone to chronic fecal retention and overflow incontinence. Having extremely long intervals between defecation is termed **obstipation.** Constipation with fecal soiling is called **encopresis.**

In the majority of children with chronic constipation, no underlying cause can be clearly identified. These children have idiopathic or functional constipation. Chronic constipation may be initiated by environmental or psychosocial factors. Transient illness, overzealous toilet-training attempts, personality, and emotional factors may play a role in causing constipation.

TABLE 44-6 Infectious causes of acute diarrhea

ORGANISM	PATHOLOGIC FEATURES	CHARACTERISTICS	COMMENTS
Viral agents			
Rotavirus Incubation period: 1-3 days	Invade epithelium of small bowel mucosa Severely distorted mucosal architecture with atrophic mucosa and severe inflammatory changes Absorption of salt and water is decreased	Abrupt onset Fever (38° C [100.4° F] or above) lasting approximately 48 hours Nausea/vomiting Abdominal pain Associated upper respiratory tract infection Diarrhea may persist for more than a week	Incidence higher in cool weather (80% in winter) Affects all age groups; 6- to 24-month-old infants more vulnerable Usually mild and self-limited Important cause of nosocomial infections in hospitals and gastroenteritis in children attending daycare centers
Norwalk-like organisms Incubation period: 1-3 days	Mechanism of effect unknown Blunting of villi and inflammatory changes in lamina propria Reduced enzymes	Fever Loss of appetite Nausea/vomiting Abdominal pain Diarrhea Malaise	Source of infection: drinking water, recreation water, food (including shellfish) Affects all ages Self-limited (2-3 days)
Bacterial agents			
Pathogenic *Escherichia coli* Incubation period: highly variable; depends on strain	Usually caused by enterotoxin production (small bowel) Reduces absorption and increases secretion of fluids and electrolytes	Onset gradual or abrupt Variable clinical manifestations Most—green, watery diarrhea with blood and mucus; becomes explosive Vomiting may be present from onset Abdominal distention Diarrhea Fever, appears toxic	Incidence higher in summer Usually interpersonal transmission but may transmit via inanimate objects and undercooked meat, especially chopped beef A cause of nursery epidemics With symptomatic treatment only, may continue for weeks Full breastfeeding has a protective effect Symptoms generally subside in 3-7 days Relapse rate approximately 20%
Salmonella groups (nontyphoidal)—gram-negative, nonencapsulated, nonsporulating Incubation period: 6-72 hours for gastroenteritis (usually less than 24); 3-60 days for enteric fever (usually 7-14)	Penetration of lamina propria (small bowel and colon) Local inflammation—no extensive destruction Stimulation of intestinal fluid excretion Systemic invasion of other sites	Rapid onset Variable symptoms—mild to severe Nausea, vomiting, and colicky abdominal pain followed by diarrhea, occasionally with blood and mucus Fever Hyperactive peristalsis and mild abdominal tenderness Symptoms usually subside within 5 days May have headache and cerebral manifestations (e.g., drowsiness, confusion, meningismus, or seizures) Infants may be afebrile and nontoxic May result in life-threatening septicemia and meningitis	Two thirds of patients are younger than 20 years of age; highest incidence in children younger than age 5 years, especially infants Highest incidence occurs from July through October, lowest from January through April Transmission primarily via contaminated food and drink—most from animal sources, including fowl, mammals, reptiles, and insects Most common sources are poultry and eggs In children—pets (e.g., dogs, cats, hamsters, and especially pet turtles) Communicable as long as organisms are excreted.
S. typhi	Rapid invasion of bloodstream from minor sites of inflammation Marked inflammation and necrosis of intestinal mucosa and lymphatics	Variable in infants Older children—irregular fever, headache, malaise, lethargy Diarrhea occurs in 50% at early stage Cough is common In a few days fever rises and is consistent; fatigue, cough, abdominal pain, anorexia, and weight	Decreased incidence in last decade Acute symptoms may persist for a week or more Transmitted by contaminated food or water (primary), infected animals (e.g., pet turtles)

TABLE 44-6 Infectious causes of acute diarrhea—cont'd

ORGANISM	PATHOLOGIC FEATURES	CHARACTERISTICS	COMMENTS
Shigella groups—gram-negative, nonmotile anaerobic bacilli Incubation period: 1-7 days, usually 2-4	Enterotoxin Stimulates loss of fluids and electrolytes Invasion of epithelium with superficial mucosal ulcerations *S. dysenteriae* forms exotoxin	Onset variable but usually abrupt Fever and cramping abdominal pain initially Fever—may reach 40.5° C (105° F) Convulsions in about 10%—usually associated with fever Patient appears sick Headache, nuchal rigidity, delirium Watery diarrhea with mucus and pus starts about 12-48 hours after onset Stools preceded by abdominal cramps; tenesmus and straining follow Symptoms usually subside in 5-10 days	Approximately 60% of cases in children younger than age 9 years with more than one third between ages 1 and 4 years Peak incidence in late summer Transmitted directly or indirectly from infected persons Communicable for 1-4 weeks Self-limited disease Treat with antibiotics Severe dehydration and collapse can affect all patients Acute symptoms may persist for a week or more
Yersinia enterocolitica Incubation period: dose-dependent; 1-3 weeks		Diarrhea—may be bloody Fever (>38.7° C [102° F]) Abdominal pain in right lower quadrant (RLQ) Vomiting, diarrhea	Seen more frequently in winter Majority in first 3 years of life Transmitted by food and pets Can resemble appendicitis May be relapsing and last for weeks
Campylobacter jejuni Incubation period: 1-7 days or longer	Precise mechanism unclear Jejunum, ileum, and colon involvement Extensive ulceration with hemorrhagic ileitis Broadening and flattening of mucosa	Fever Abdominal pain—often severe, cramping, periumbilical Watery, profuse, foul-smelling diarrhea with blood Vomiting	Person-to-person transmission May be transmitted by pets (e.g., cat, dog, hamster) Food (especially chicken) and water-borne transmission Relapse possible Most patients recover spontaneously Antibiotics may speed recovery Peak incidence in summer
Vibrio cholerae (cholera) groups Incubation period: usually 2-3 days; range from few hours to 5 days	Enterotoxin causes increased secretion of chloride and possibly bicarbonate Intestinal mucosa congested with enlarged lymph follicles Intact mucosal surface	Sudden onset of profuse, watery diarrhea without cramping, tenesmus, or anal irritation, although children may complain of cramping Stools are intermittent at first, then almost continuous Stools are bloody with mucus	Rare in infants younger than 1 year old Mortality high in both treated and untreated infants and small children Transmitted via contaminated food and water Attack confers immunity
Clostridium difficile	Toxin stimulates colonic secretion by damaging epithelium	Diarrhea with blood in stools	May cause pseudomembranous colitis Follows antibiotic therapy
Food poisoning			
Staphylococcus Incubation period: 4-6 hours	Produce heat-stable enterotoxin	Nausea, vomiting Severe abdominal cramps Profuse diarrhea Shock may occur in severe cases May be a mild fever	Transferred via contaminated food—inadequately cooked or refrigerated (e.g., custards, mayonnaise, cream-filled or cream-topped desserts) Self-limited; improvement apparent within 24 hours Excellent prognosis
Clostridium perfringens Incubation period: 8-24 hours, usually 8-12	Produces heat-resistant and heat-sensitive toxins	Moderate to severe crampy, mid-epigastric pain	Self-limited illness Transmission by commercial food products, most often meat and poultry
Clostridium botulinum Incubation period: 12-26 hours (range, 6 hours to 8 days)	Highly potent neurotoxin	Nausea, vomiting Diarrhea Central nervous system (CNS) symptoms with curare-like effect Dry mouth, dysphagia	Transmitted by contaminated food products Variable severity—mild symptoms to rapidly fatal within a few hours Antitoxin administration

Newborn Period

Normally the newborn infant passes a first **meconium** stool within 24 to 36 hours of birth. Any infant who does not do so is assessed for evidence of intestinal atresia or stenosis, Hirschsprung disease (congenital aganglionic megacolon), hypothyroidism, meconium plug, or meconium ileus. A *meconium plug* is caused by meconium that has reduced water content and is usually evacuated after digital rectal examination but may require irrigations of normal saline solution or iodinated contrast medium.

Meconium ileus, often the initial manifestation of cystic fibrosis, is the luminal obstruction of the distal small intestine by meconium. Treatment is based on the cause of the ileus.

Infancy

The onset of constipation frequently occurs during infancy and is often related to dietary practices. It is almost unknown in breastfed infants. Constipation may accompany a change from human milk or modified cow's milk to whole cow's milk. Simple measures ordinarily correct the problem, such as adding or increasing the amount of cereal, vegetables, and fruit in the diet of the older infant. Stool-withholding behavior may begin at this age in response to pain on defecation (see the Critical Thinking Q & A box below).

Childhood

Children between 1 and 3 years of age are most likely to have constipation, usually as a result of environmental changes. It may be a result of some medications (e.g., iron or calcium supplements, diuretics, antacids, opioids, or anticonvulsant agents). If there are associated manifestations, such as vomiting, abdominal distention or pain, and evidence of growth failure, the condition merits further investigation.

The management of simple constipation consists of a plan to keep the bowel relatively empty of stool and dietary management to prevent further constipation. There is not total agreement on the most effective means to clean the bowel, although most agree that the use of laxatives is not usually recommended because of their tendency to create dependency. Enemas are sometimes used to empty the bowel and repeated if voluntary evacuation does not occur within 48 hours. Treatment may also include the use of bisacadyl (Dulcolax) suppositories. Occasionally a polyethylene glycol-electrolyte solution (Golytely) by oral or nasogastric administration is necessary for severe fecal impaction.

Increasing the intake of fluids and implementing a high-fiber diet are advised. Any foods known to be constipating are eliminated. Sometimes a stool softener such as dioctyl sodium sulfosuccinate or mineral oil is of benefit.

Effective counseling is an essential element of the treatment plan for children with chronic constipation. Bowel function, the purpose of interventions, and the need for persistence should be explained to the child and family. Erroneous concepts concerning this condition need to be corrected. A child who has experienced discomfort during bowel movements may deliberately try to withhold stool. The rectum accommodates the stool accumulation, and the urge to defecate passes. When bowel contents are ultimately evacuated, the accumulated feces are passed with even greater pain, reinforcing the desire to withhold stool.

Retraining therapy involves habit training, reinforcement for toilet sitting and defecation, and emotional support. A regular toilet time is established once or twice a day, preferably after a meal. A reasonable amount of time (5 to 10 minutes) should be spent attempting to defecate completely. Biofeedback may be indicated as a form of behavioral modification. Children with chronic constipation and encopresis frequently experience inappropriate external anal sphincter contraction during defecation. Rectal biofeedback can teach children to relax the anal sphincter during defecation.

Constipation in *school-age children* may represent an ongoing chronic problem or may develop for the first time. The onset of constipation at this age is often due to environmental changes, stresses, and changes in toileting patterns. A common cause of new-onset constipation at school entry is fear of using school bathrooms, which are noted for their lack of privacy. Also, early and hurried departure for school immediately after breakfast may impede bathroom use. Most schools will liberalize bathroom rules for individual children who have been identified and have a parent or health professional intervene on their behalf. Encopresis often causes additional emotional stress for the school-age child (see Chapter 36).

Critical Thinking Q & A

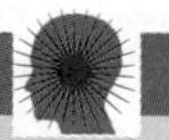

CONSTIPATION

A 6-month-old infant is referred to a pediatric gastroenterologist because of concerns about constipation. Every 4-5 days the infant usually has one hard stool, which causes discomfort when it is passed. Abdominal distention and vomiting are not common occurrences, and growth has been normal. The infant's diet consists of cow's milk formula only. The infant's caregivers report that the infrequent passage of hard stools began approximately 1 month ago. It is determined that this infant likely has functional constipation because no underlying cause can be clearly identified. All of the following early interventions would be indicated in this situation except:

1. Education of the infant's caregivers concerning normal bowel habits.
2. Administration of two or three mineral oil enemas to cleanse the bowel.
3. Recommendation to introduce food and fruit juice into the infant's diet.
4. Use of several medications daily to maintain a loose consistency of stools.

The correct answer is four. The management of an infant with functional constipation should initially include education of the caregivers, simple measures to keep the bowel relatively empty of stool, and diet management to prevent further constipation. The caregivers should be educated that short periods of constipation are not uncommon and usually resolve as solid food is introduced into the diet. One or two offerings of fruit juice each day may be beneficial in preventing further constipation. If hard stools or anal fissures persist after initial bowel cleansing and diet management, medications such as malt extract or lactulose may be required.

Nursing Care Management

Constipation unfortunately tends to be self-perpetuating. A child who has difficulty or discomfort when attempting to evacuate the bowels has a tendency to retain the bowel contents, and thus begins a vicious cycle. Nursing assessment begins with an accurate history of bowel habits; diet; events that

BOX 44-7
High-Fiber Foods

Bread, grains
Whole-grain bread or rolls
Whole-grain cereals
Bran
Pancakes, waffles, and muffins with fruit or bran
Unrefined (brown) rice

Vegetables
Raw vegetables, especially broccoli, cabbage, carrots, cauliflower, celery, lettuce, and spinach
Cooked vegetables, such as those listed above, and asparagus, beans, brussels sprouts, corn, potatoes, rhubarb, squash, string beans, and turnips

Fruits
Raw fruits, especially those with skins or seeds, other than ripe banana or avocado
Raisins, prunes, or other dried fruits

Miscellaneous
Nuts, seeds, legumes, popcorn
High-fiber snack bars

may be associated with the onset of constipation; drugs or other substances that the child may be taking; and consistency, color, frequency, and other characteristics of the stool. If there is no evidence of a pathologic condition that requires further investigation, the major task of the nurse is to educate the parents regarding normal stool patterns and to participate in the education and treatment of the child.

Dietary modifications are usually essential in preventing constipation. During infancy simply increasing the carbohydrate (sugar or corn syrup) in the infant's formula will often relieve the problem. During childhood the diet should contain increased amounts of fiber and fluid. Parents benefit from guidance in dietary planning, especially regarding foods that facilitate bowel movements (Box 44-7). They need reassurance concerning the benign nature of the condition. It is important to discuss with them their attitudes and expectations regarding toilet habits.

HIRSCHSPRUNG DISEASE

Hirschsprung disease (congenital aganglionic megacolon) is a mechanical obstruction caused by inadequate motility of part of the large intestine. It accounts for about one fourth of all cases of neonatal intestinal obstruction, although it may not be diagnosed until later in infancy or childhood. It is four times more common in males than in females, follows a familial pattern in a small number of cases, and is considerably more common in children with Down syndrome. The incidence is 1 in 5000 live births. Depending on its presentation, it may be an acute, life-threatening condition or a chronic disorder.

Pathophysiology

Hirschsprung disease results from failure of ganglion cells to migrate craniocaudally along the GI tract during gestation.

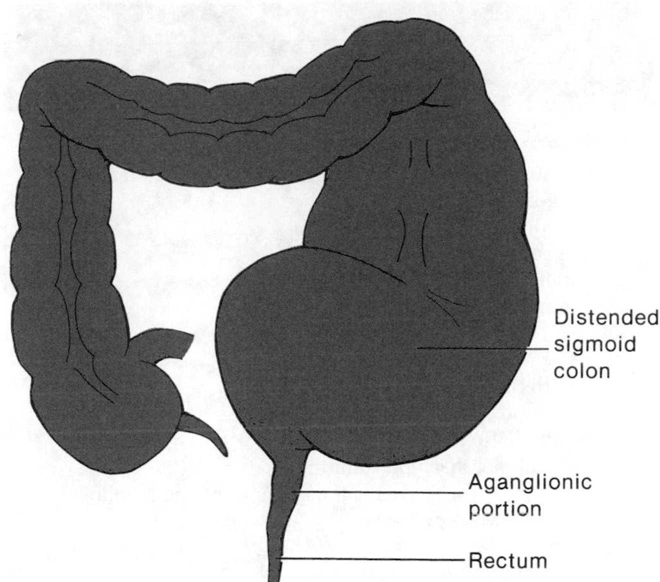

Fig. 44-2 Hirschsprung disease.

The aganglionic segment almost always includes the rectum and a proximal portion of the large intestine. Rarely, "skip segments" or total intestinal aganglionosis may occur. Absence of propulsive movements (peristalsis) in the aganglionic bowel causes accumulation of intestinal contents and distention of the bowel proximal to the defect, hence the term **megacolon,** or large colon. In addition, the internal rectal sphincter fails to relax, preventing evacuation of solids, liquids, and gas, and thus contributing to the manifestations of obstruction (Fig. 44-2). Intestinal distention and ischemia may occur as a result of distention of the bowel wall, which contributes to the development of *enterocolitis* (inflammation of the small bowel and colon), the leading cause of death in children with Hirschsprung disease (Kirschner, 1991).

Diagnostic Evaluation

Clinical manifestations vary according to the age when symptoms are first recognized and the presence of complications, such as enterocolitis (Box 44-8). In the neonate, diagnosis is usually made on the basis of clinical signs of intestinal obstruction and failure to pass meconium. Radiographs, barium enema, and anorectal manometric examinations assist in the differential diagnosis, which is then confirmed by histologic examination of a full-thickness rectal biopsy demonstrating absence of ganglion cells in the myenteric and submucosal plexus.

Therapeutic Management

Treatment is primarily surgical to remove the aganglionic portion of the bowel in order to permit normal bowel motility and establish continence by improved functioning of the internal anal sphincter. In most cases this is accomplished in two stages. First, a temporary ostomy proximal to the aganglionic segment is performed to allow the normal bowel time to rest and resume its normal caliber and tonicity. Second, complete correction is accomplished with a pull-through procedure of the bowel, which consists of "pulling" the end of

BOX 44-8
Clinical Manifestations of Hirschsprung Disease

Newborn period
- Failure to pass meconium within 24 to 48 hours after birth
- Spitting-up
- Poor feeding
- Visible bowel loops
- Bile-stained vomitus
- Abdominal distention

Infancy
- Failure to thrive
- Constipation
- Abdominal distention
- Episodes of diarrhea and vomiting
- Ominous signs (often signify the presence of enterocolitis)
  - Explosive, watery diarrhea
  - Fever
  - Severe prostration

Childhood*
- Constipation
- Ribbonlike, foul-smelling stools
- Abdominal distention
- Visible peristalsis
- Fecal masses easily palpable
- Child usually poorly nourished and anemic

*Symptoms are more chronic.

functioning ganglionated bowel down through the muscular sleeve of the rectum. This procedure is referred to as the *Soave endorectal pull-through procedure.* The ostomy is usually closed at the time of the pull-through procedure. This surgery is typically delayed until the child weighs approximately 20 pounds. Other definitive procedures that can be performed include the Swenson, Duhamel, and Boley procedures.

Prognosis. Most children with Hirschsprung disease require surgery rather than medical therapy. Once the condition of the patient is stabilized with fluid and electrolyte replacement, if needed, the temporary colostomy is performed with a high rate of success. After the later pull-through procedure, anal stricture and incontinence are potential complications, requiring further therapy, including dilation or bowel-retraining therapy.

Nursing Care Management

Many of the nursing concerns depend on the child's age and the type of treatment. If the disorder is diagnosed during the neonatal period, the main objectives are (1) to help the parents adjust to a congenital defect in their child, (2) to foster infant-parent bonding, (3) to prepare them for the medical/surgical intervention, and (4) to assist them in colostomy care after discharge.

Preoperative care. Much of the child's preoperative care depends on the age and clinical condition. A child who is malnourished may not be able to withstand surgery until the physical status improves. Often this involves symptomatic treatment with enemas; a low-fiber, high-calorie, and high-protein diet; and, in severe situations, the use of total parenteral nutrition (TPN).

Physical preoperative preparation entails the same measures that are common to any surgery (see Surgical Procedures, Chapter 42). In the newborn, whose bowel is sterile, no additional preparation is necessary. However, in other children, in preparation for the pull-through procedure, emptying the bowel with repeated saline solution enemas and decreasing bacterial flora with systemic antibiotics and colonic irrigations using antibiotic solution are usually ordered. Oral antibiotics may also be prescribed.

Since progressive distention of the abdomen is a serious sign, the nurse measures abdominal circumference with a paper tape measure, usually at the level of the umbilicus or at the widest part of the abdomen. The point of measurement is marked with a pen to ensure reliability of subsequent measurements. Abdominal measurement can be performed at the same time that vital signs are taken, and is recorded in serial order so that a change is readily apparent. To reduce any stress to the acutely ill child when frequent measurements of abdominal circumference are needed, the tape measure can be left in place beneath the child, rather than removed each time.

The age of the child dictates the type and extent of psychologic preparation necessary for child and parents. Since a colostomy is usually performed, the child who is of at least preschool age is told about the procedure in concrete terms, with the use of visual aids (see Chapter 42 for preparing a child for a colostomy). It is important to time explanations appropriately to prevent the anxiety and confusion that can result from too much information.

It is important to stress to parents and older children that the colostomy for Hirschsprung disease is temporary, unless so much bowel is involved that a permanent ileostomy must be performed. In most instances the extent of bowel resection prior to surgery is known, although the nurse should be aware of those instances when there is doubt concerning repair. The nurse should also keep in mind that although a temporary colostomy is favorable in terms of future health and adjustment, it also requires additional surgery, which may be very stressful to parents and children.

Postoperative care. Postoperative care is the same as for any child or infant with abdominal surgery (see Surgical Procedures, Chapter 42). When a colostomy is part of the corrective procedure, stomal care becomes a major nursing task (see Ostomies, Chapter 42). To prevent contamination of the abdominal wound with urine in the infant, the diaper should be pinned below the dressing. Sometimes a Foley catheter is used in the immediate postoperative period to divert the flow of urine away from the abdomen.

Discharge care. Postoperatively parents need instruction concerning colostomy care. Even a preschooler can be included in the care by handing articles to the parent, rolling up the colostomy pouch after it is emptied, or applying barrier preparations to the surrounding skin. Although diagnosis of Hirschsprung disease is less frequent in school-age children or adolescents, if it is discovered in older children, they should be involved in colostomy care to the point of total responsibility.

Referral to a home health care agency establishes continuity of care, especially in relation to colostomy care and dietary management. The community nurse can also assist parents and children in anticipating subsequent surgery. Sometimes families require financial assistance and additional psychologic support. Therefore a referral to a social worker or other service agency may be necessary. *

See also the Nursing Care Plan: The Child with Hirschsprung Disease (Megacolon).†

VOMITING

Vomiting, the forceful ejection of gastric contents through the mouth, is a well-defined, complex, coordinated process under nervous system control. Often it is of a minor and temporary nature, but when vomiting is persistent and prolonged, the complications for the infant or child can be serious. Vomiting in childhood can be caused by numerous intrinsic and extrinsic factors but is usually the result of infections or psychologic causes.

Therapeutic Management

Management is directed toward detection and treatment of the cause of the vomiting and prevention of complications from the loss of fluid. Fluids are administered in the same manner and in a similar electrolyte composition to those administered in diarrhea (see p. 1391). Although most children respond well to these measures, antiemetic drugs may be needed. The specific antiemetic may block the receptors in the chemoreceptor trigger zone (ondansetron [Zofran] or trimethobenzamide [Tigan]); enhance gastroduodenal peristalsis (metoclopramide [Reglan]); or compete for H_1-receptor sites (promethazine [Phenergan]). For children who are prone to motion sickness it is often helpful to administer an appropriate dose of dimenhydrinate (Dramamine) before a trip.

Nursing Care Management

The major emphasis of nursing care of the vomiting infant or child is on observation and reporting of vomiting behavior and associated symptoms, and on implementation of measures to reduce the vomiting. Accurate assessment of the type of vomiting, the appearance of the vomitus, and the child's behavior in association with the vomiting greatly aids in establishing a diagnosis of disorders that have vomiting as a clinical feature.

Nursing interventions are determined by the cause of the vomiting. When the vomiting is identified as a manifestation of improper feeding methods, establishing proper techniques through teaching and example will ordinarily correct the situation. If the vomiting is assessed as a probable sign of a GI obstruction, food is usually withheld and intravenous (IV) therapy implemented. In situations in which vomiting is related to concurrent infection, dietary indiscretion, or emotional factors, efforts are directed toward maintaining hydration or preventing dehydration.

The thirst mechanism is the most sensitive guide to fluid needs, and ad libitum administration of a glucose-electrolyte solution to an alert child will restore water and electrolytes satisfactorily. It is important to include carbohydrate to spare body protein and to prevent ketosis resulting from exhaustion of glycogen stores. Once vomiting has abated, more liberal amounts of fluids can be offered, followed by simple foods such as gelatin, crackers, clear broth, and buttered toast in small portions, when the child desires, followed by gradual resumption of the regular diet.

The vomiting infant or child is positioned to prevent aspiration and observed for evidence of dehydration. It is important to emphasize the need for the child to brush the teeth or rinse the mouth after vomiting to dilute hydrochloric acid that comes in contact with the teeth. A flavored mouthwash or brushing also helps freshen the mouth. Careful monitoring of fluid and electrolyte status must be exercised to prevent possible electrolyte disturbance.

GASTROESOPHAGEAL REFLUX (GER)

GER can best be defined as the transfer of gastric contents into the esophagus. GER occurs in everyone; it is the frequency and persistence that make it abnormal. Approximately 1 in 300 to 1 in 1000 children has a significant problem. Earlier a great emphasis was placed on the resting or baseline *lower esophageal sphincter (LES) pressure;* however, studies have been unable to show a relationship between baseline LES pressure and abnormal reflux. GER most likely occurs during transient and inappropriate relaxations of the LES. The exact cause is not known, but potential causes of this inappropriate relaxation of the LES may be related to the central nervous system or to a developmentally exaggerated enteric reflex (Hillemeier, 1991). Several factors that cause the LES pressure to vary include gastric distention, increased abdominal pressure caused by coughing, central nervous system disease, delayed gastric emptying, hiatal hernia, and gastrostomy placement.

Some children are especially prone to development of GER. This condition is not uncommon in children who have had tracheoesophageal or esophageal atresia repair, neurologic disorders, scoliosis, asthma, and cystic fibrosis, and in preterm infants.

Reflux of stomach contents to the esophagus predisposes to aspiration and development of respiratory symptoms, particularly pneumonia. A particular concern is the association of life-threatening apnea with GER. Repeated irritation of the esophageal lining with gastric acid can lead to esophagitis and

BOX 44-9
Clinical Manifestations of Gastroesophageal Reflux

- Spitting up
- Vomiting—can be quite forceful
- Weight loss
- Gagging, choking at end of feeding
- Respiratory problems
- Hematemesis
- Melena
- Anemia
- Heartburn/irritability
- Apnea/acute life-threatening episode

*Home care instructions on caring for the child with a colostomy are available in Wong DL: *Wong and Whaley's clinical manual of pediatric nursing,* ed 4, St Louis, 1996, Mosby.

†In Wong DL: *Wong and Whaley's clinical manual of pediatric nursing,* ed 4, St Louis, 1996, Mosby.

subsequent bleeding. Blood loss produces anemia and is seen as hematemesis or melena (blood in stools). Heartburn is also a frequent symptom in older children who are able to describe it, but it may be unrecognized in infants. For a summary of clinical manifestations, see Box 44-9.

Diagnostic Evaluation

In addition to the history, several tests are available to establish the presence of reflux: observation of reflux after a barium swallow; 8-, 12-, or 24-hour pH probe study; upper endoscopy; and scintigraphy (detects radioactive substances in the esophagus after a feeding of the compound and assesses gastric emptying).

Therapeutic Management

Therapeutic management of GER depends on its severity. No therapy may be required for the infant who is thriving and has no respiratory complications. Some children require modification of feeding with small, frequent feedings of thickened formula and positioning therapy, which may help minimize the symptoms until the child grows and a normal physiologic barrier to reflux develops.

There are controversies regarding thickened feedings as a treatment for GER. Small, frequent feedings and frequent burping are generally accepted as reasonable strategies to minimize reflux. Constant nasogastric feedings may be necessary for the infant with severe reflux and failure to thrive. Feedings thickened with 1 teaspoon to 1 tablespoon of rice cereal per ounce of formula may be recommended as an initial measure to manage GER. The added calories may benefit the infant.

Several studies have examined the effectiveness of positioning therapy for infants with GER. Traditionally the upright position in an infant seat was recommended for infants with GER. Later a head-elevated prone position maintained by use of an upper body harness was found to be superior. However, another study found no significant differences between the flat prone and head-elevated prone positions and concluded that the head-elevated prone position is probably not worth the extra effort required to maintain this position (Orenstein, 1990). At this time the available information suggests that either the flat prone or head-elevated prone position after feeding and at night is a reasonable measure for treating infants with GER. The supine position is not used because GER worsens when the infant lies on the back. This is an exception to the recommended supine sleep position for healthy infants to decrease the risk of sudden infant death syndrome (SIDS) (see Chapter 33) (Orenstein, 1994).

Pharmacologic therapy is sometimes used as an adjunct therapy to treat infants and children with GER. H_2 antagonists, such as cimetidine (Tagamet), ranitidine (Zantac), or famotidine (Pepcid), have proved effective in reducing the amount of acid present in gastric contents and may prevent esophagitis. Omeprazole (Prilosec) more completely suppresses gastric acid secretions than do H_2 blockers; however, the long-term effects are not known. Metoclopramide (Reglan) has been found to increase resting LES pressure mildly and to increase rates of gastric emptying. However, side effects, including restlessness, drowsiness, and extrapyramidal reaction, may occur, and metoclopramide may in some cases actually increase the number of reflux episodes.

Cisapride (Propulsid) increases LES pressure, promotes gastric emptying, and has fewer central nervous system side effects than metoclopramide. It is often the preferred medication for GER (Orenstein, 1992). Bethanechol has also been shown to increase LES pressure greatly, but it has not been proved to decrease reflux by pH probe studies. Bethanechol also has side effects, including respiratory symptoms such as wheezing.

Surgical management as a treatment for GER is selected for children with severe complications, such as recurrent aspiration pneumonia, apnea, and severe esophagitis, in whom medical therapy has failed. The *Nissen fundoplication*, which involves a 360-degree wrap of the fundus of the stomach around the distal esophagus, is the most common surgical procedure. Fundoplication combined with pyloroplasty may be performed in children with GER who also have delayed gastric emptying. Unfortunately complications can occur after fundoplication; therefore the decision to perform this procedure should be carefully considered. Postoperative problems include small bowel obstruction, retching, gas-bloat syndrome, and dumping syndrome. For children with neurologic impairment who are continuously tube-fed, an alternative to fundoplication with gastrostomy tube placement is a nonsurgical percutaneous gastrojejunostomy with placement of a jejunostomy tube (Albanese et al, 1993).

Prognosis. The majority of infants with GER have a mild problem that generally improves by about 1 year of age and requires only medical therapy. If GER is severe and unsuccessfully treated, multiple complications can occur. Esophageal strictures caused by persistent esophagitis with scarring are among the most significant complications. Recurrent respiratory distress with aspiration pneumonia is another serious complication that is an indication for surgery. Failure to thrive caused by GER can often be managed with medical therapy and nutritional support.

Nursing Care Management

Nursing care is directed at (1) identifying children with symptoms that suggest GER; (2) educating parents regarding home care, including feeding, positioning, and medications when indicated; and (3) if appropriate, providing care for the child undergoing surgical repair (see Surgical Procedures, Chapter 42).

To help parents cope with the inconvenience of dealing with a child who vomits frequently, simple measures such as using bibs and protective cloths during and after feeding are beneficial. The greatest challenge lies in maintaining the desired position for the child and adhering to a frequent feeding schedule. The 30-degree angle can be provided by elevating the head of the infant's crib with extra bedding, a wood or metal frame, or a wedge constructed from a cardboard box. An alternative is a specially constructed frame that can be moved about to allow the child a change of environment with minimum disturbance. The child is suspended from the head of the crib or frame in a prepared or improvised harness.

When the infant is older and more mobile, maintaining correct positioning becomes increasingly difficult. An alternative frame that has been described consists of a cradle bed, bassinet, or board with a firm wooden base and a wooden spindle or large dowel that protrudes through the center of the mattress. To prevent undue pressure on areas such as the infant's knees and elbows, the mattress is covered with a sheepskin or soft blanket, and pressure areas are inspected for signs of redness.

Early in the treatment program both parents and other available family members should be encouraged to participate in the feeding regimen, especially with alternate night shifts. Nurses need to be sensitive to the demands placed on the family and recognize those situations when hospitalization may be required to ensure continued treatment.

Intestinal Parasitic Diseases

Intestinal parasitic diseases, including helminths (worms) and protozoa, constitute the most common infections in the world. In the United States the incidence of intestinal parasitic disease, especially giardiasis, has increased among young children who are attending day-care centers.

Intestinal parasitic diseases in humans are caused by various infecting organisms. This discussion is limited to the two most common parasitic infections among children in the United States: giardiasis and pinworms. Table 44-7 describes the outstanding features of selected helminths that belong to the family of nematodes.

GENERAL NURSING CONSIDERATIONS

Nursing responsibilities related to intestinal parasitic infections involve assistance with identification of the parasite, treatment of the infection, and prevention of initial infection or reinfection. Identification of the organism is accomplished by laboratory examination of substances containing the worm, its larvae, or ova. Most are identified by examining feces smears from the stools of persons suspected of harboring the parasite. Fresh specimens are best for revealing parasites or larvae; therefore collected specimens should be taken directly to the laboratory for examination. If this is not feasible, the specimen is placed in a container with a preservative (see Stool Specimens, Chapter 42).

In most parasitic infections examination of other family members, especially children, may be carried out to identify those who are similarly affected. Nurses frequently assume the responsibility for directing and instructing families in the collection and disposition of specimens. Parents need clear written instructions on obtaining an adequate sample and the number of samples required.

Once the diagnosis is confirmed and an appropriate treatment regimen is planned, parents need further explanation and reinforcement. Compliance in terms of drug therapy and any other measures, such as thorough handwashing, are essential for eradication of the parasite. The family needs to understand the nature of transmission and to comprehend that in some cases the medication must be repeated in 2 weeks to 1 month to kill organisms hatched since initial treatment.

The nurse's most important function in relation to these parasites is preventive education of children and families regarding good hygiene and health habits. Thorough handwashing before eating or handling food and after using the toilet is the most important precautionary method. Other preventive practices are listed in the Home Care box above.

Home Care 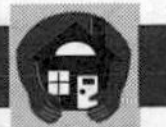

PREVENTING INTESTINAL PARASITIC DISEASE

- Always wash hands and fingernails with soap and water before eating and handling food and after toileting.
- Avoid placing fingers in mouth and biting nails.
- Discourage children from scratching bare anal area.
- Use superabsorbent disposable diapers to prevent leakage.
- Change diapers as soon as soiled and dispose of diapers in closed receptable out of children's reach.
- Do not rinse diapers in toilet.
- Disinfect toilet seats and diaper changing areas; use dilute household bleach (10% solution) or Lysol and wipe clean with paper towels.
- Drink water that is specially treated, especially if camping.
- Wash all raw fruits and vegetables, or food that has fallen on the floor.
- Avoid growing foods in soil fertilized with human excreta.
- Teach children to defecate only in a toilet, not on the ground.
- Keep dogs and cats away from playgrounds or sandboxes.
- Avoid swimming in pools frequented by diapered children.
- Wear shoes outside.

GIARDIASIS

Giardiasis is caused by the protozoan *Giardia lamblia* (also called *G. intestinalis, G. duodenalis,* and *Lamblia intestinalis*). It is the most common intestinal parasitic pathogen in the United States, and its prevalence among children in day-care centers may range from 17% to over 50% during outbreaks (Bartlett et al, 1991). Breastfed infants exposed to *Giardia* have much less diarrhea but are not protected from becoming infected (Walterspiel et al, 1994).

The potential for transmission is great, since the cysts, the nonmotile stage of the protozoa, can survive in the environment for months. Chief modes of transmission are person-to-person; water (especially mountain lakes, streams, and pools frequented by diapered infants); food; and animals, especially puppies. In children, person-to-person transmission is the most likely cause.

Diagnostic Evaluation

Although individuals infected with giardiasis may be asymptomatic, young children, especially infants, usually manifest symptoms at any early stage (Box 44-10). Unlike most other intestinal parasites, *G. lamblia* is not easily diagnosed from stool specimens. Since *Giardia* organisms are excreted in a highly variable pattern, six or more stool specimens collected over several weeks may be necessary to identify the trophozoites (active parasites) or cysts.

Since the organism lives in the upper intestine, aspiration or biopsy of the duodenum or upper jejunum may be performed. The *string test* may be used to aspirate duodenal fluid directly. A nylon string is attached to a gelatin capsule, which is swallowed; several hours later the string is withdrawn and the contents are examined microscopically for trophozoites.

TABLE 44-7 Selected intestinal parasites

CLINICAL MANIFESTATIONS	COMMENTS
Ascariasis—*ascaris lumbricoides* (common roundworm)	
Light infections: asymptomatic Heavy infections: anorexia, irritability, nervousness, enlarged abdomen, weight loss, fever, intestinal colic Severe infections: intestinal obstruction, appendicitis, perforation of intestine with peritonitis, obstructive jaundice, lung involvement—pneumonitis	Transferred to mouth by way of contaminated food, fingers, or toys Largest of the intestinal helminths Affects principally young children 1-4 years of age Prevalent in warm climates
Hookworm disease—*necator americanus*	
Light infections in well-nourished individuals: no problems Heavier infections: mild to severe anemia, malnutrition May be itching and burning ("ground itch") followed by erythema and a papular eruption in areas to which the organism migrates	Transmitted by discharging eggs on the soil and in turn picked up infection from direct skin contact with contaminated soil Wearing shoes is recommended, although children playing in contaminated soil expose many skin surfaces
Strongyloidiasis—*strongyloides stercoralis* (threadworm)	
Light infection: asymptomatic Heavy infection: respiratory signs and symptoms; abdominal pain, distention; nausea and vomiting; diarrhea—large, pale stools, often with mucus Threat to life in children with weakened immunologic defenses	Transmission is same as for hookworm except autoinfection common Older children and adults affected more often than young children Severe infections may lead to severe nutritional deficiency
Visceral larva migrans—*toxocara canis* (dogs); *intestinal toxocariasis—toxocara cati* (cats)	
Depends on reactivity of infected individual May be asymptomatic except for eosinophilia Specific diagnosis difficult	Transmitted by direct contamination of hands from contact with dog, cat, or objects; or ingestion of soil Dogs and cats should be kept away from areas where children play; sandboxes are especially important transmission areas Periodic deworming of diagnosed dogs and cats Control of dog and cat population Continued education and laws to prevent indiscriminate canine and feline defecation
Trichuriasis—*trichuris trichura* (whipworm)	
Light infections: asymptomatic Heavy infections: abdominal pain and distention, diarrhea	Transmitted from contaminated soil, vegetables, toys, and other objects Most frequent in warm, moist climates Occurs most often in undernourished children living in unsanitary conditions

However, the string test is being used less often because other tests that detect *Giardia* antigen in the stool, such as counterimmunoelectrophoresis (CIE) and enzyme-linked immunosorbent assay (ELISA), are available.

Therapeutic Management

The drugs available for treatment of giardiasis are quinacrine (Atabrine), furazolidone (Furoxone), and metronidazole (Flagyl). The drug of choice is furazolidone, unless cost is a factor, in which case quinacrine is substituted. Quinacrine is less than one tenth the cost of furazolidone, and its long-term safety is established over the use of metronidazole. For pregnant women who need treatment, paromomycin may be used first, followed by metronidazole if the initial treatment is unsuccessful (Hill, 1993). Unfortunately quinacrine has the highest frequency of side effects, especially nausea and vomiting; causes temporary yellow staining of the skin, sclera, and urine; and has a very bitter taste.

Nursing Care Management

The most important nursing consideration is prevention of giardiasis, especially among children and staff of day-care centers. Attention to meticulous sanitary practices, especially during diaper changes, is essential (see the Home Care box on p. 1403 and Fig. 44-3). Nurses can play an important role in educating day-care staff regarding appropriate sanitation practices (see Preschool or Day Care Experience, Chapter 35).

Once children are infected, family education regarding administration of the drug is essential. Parents often need suggestions for encouraging the child to take quinacrine. If other household members are infected, the nurse should inquire about their understanding and management of the disease.

BOX 44-10
Clinical Manifestations of Giardiasis

Infants and young children:
- Diarrhea
- Vomiting
- Anorexia
- Poor weight gain

Children over 5 years of age:
- Abdominal cramps
- Intermittent loose stools
- Constipation
- Stools may be malodorous, watery, pale, and greasy

Most infections resolve spontaneously in 4 to 6 weeks

Rarely, chronic form occurs:
- Intermittent loose, foul-smelling stools
- Possibility of abdominal bloating, flatulence, sulfur-tasting belches, epigastric pain, vomiting, headache, and weight loss
- Failure to thrive

BOX 44-11
Clinical Manifestations of Pinworms

Intense perianal itching (principal symptom); evidence of itching in young children includes:
- General irritability
- Restlessness
- Poor sleep
- Bed-wetting
- Distractibility
- Short attention span

Perianal dermatitis and excoriation secondary to itching

If worms migrate, possible vaginal and urethral infection

To decrease the side effects of quinacrine and increase its palatability:

- Administer the drug with or after meals.
- Crush tablets and mix with a strong flavoring, such as jam or syrup.

ENTEROBIASIS (PINWORMS)

Enterobiasis (or pinworms) caused by the nematode *Enterobius vermicularis,* is the most common helminthic infection in the United States. It is universally present in temperate climatic zones and may infect over 30% of all children at any one time. Crowded conditions, such as in classrooms and day-care centers, favor transmission.

Since the eggs float in the air, they are also easily inhaled. The movement of the worms on skin and mucous membrane surfaces causes intense itching. As the child scratches, eggs are deposited on the hands and under the fingernails. The typical hand-to-mouth activity of youngsters makes them especially prone to continual reinfection. Pinworm eggs also persist in the home to contaminate anything they contact, such as toilet seats, doorknobs, bed linen, underwear, and food.

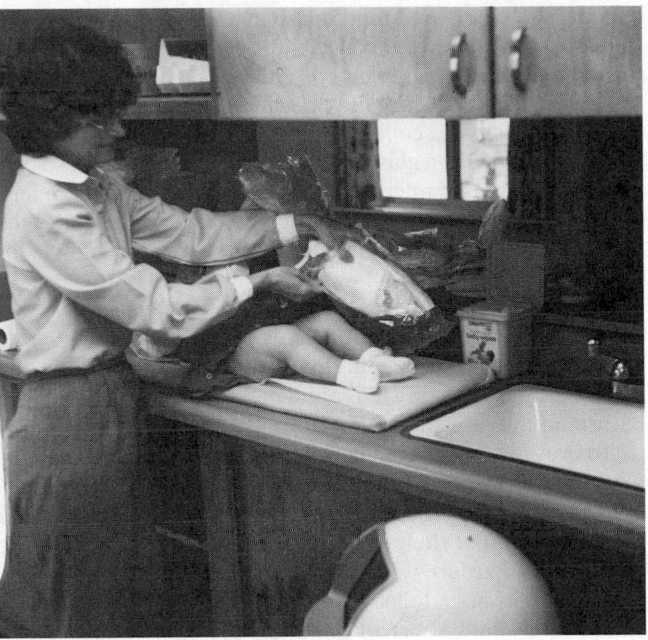

Fig. 44-3 Prevention of giardiasis, especially in day-care centers, requires sanitary practices during diaper changes, such as discarding paper diapers in a covered receptacle, changing paper covers on the diaper-changing surface, and having facilities for handwashing nearby. *Note:* Soiled cloth diapers and clothing should be stored in a plastic bag for transport home.

Diagnostic Evaluation

Except for the intense rectal itching associated with pinworms, the clinical manifestations (Box 44-11) are nonspecific. Diagnosis is most commonly made from the tape test (see Nursing Care Management). Repeated tests to collect eggs may be necessary, and if there is a possibility that other family members may be infected, a tape test should be performed on them.

Therapeutic Management

The drugs available for treatment of pinworms include mebendazole (Vermox), pyrantel pamoate (Antiminth), piperazine phosphate, and pyrvinium pamoate (Povan). The drug of choice is mebendazole, which is safe, effective, and convenient, with few side effects. However, it is not recommended for children under 2 years of age. If pyrvinium pamoate is prescribed, parents are advised that the drug stains stool and vomitus bright red, as well as clothing or skin that comes in contact with the drug. Since pinworms are easily transmitted, all household members are treated. The drugs may be repeated in 2 weeks to prevent reinfection.

Nursing Care Management

Nursing care is directed at identifying the parasite, eradicating the organism, and preventing reinfection. Parents need clear, detailed instructions for the *tape test.* A loop of transparent (not "frosted" or "magic") tape, sticky side out, is placed around the end of a tongue depressor, which is then firmly pressed against the child's perianal area. A convenient commercially prepared tape is also available for this purpose. Pinworm specimens are collected in the morning as soon as the child awakens and *before* the child has a bowel movement or bathes. The procedure may need to be repeated more than once before eggs are collected. Parents are instructed to place the tongue blade in a glass jar or loosely in a plastic bag so that it can be taken for microscopic examination. For specimens collected in the hospital, practitioner's office, or clinic, the tape is placed smoothly on a glass slide, sticky side down, for examination.

Compliance with the drug regimen is usually excellent, because the duration of treatment is typically only one dose. However, the family is reminded of the need to take a second dose in 2 weeks. Posting a reminder on the refrigerator door or bathroom mirror is helpful.

To prevent reinfection, certain cleaning practices, such as washing all clothes and bed linen in hot water and vacuuming the house, may be recommended. However, there is little documentation of their effectiveness, since pinworms survive on so many surfaces. Suggestions that are helpful include handwashing after toileting and before eating, keeping the child's fingernails short to minimize the chance of ova collecting under the nails, dressing children in one-piece sleeping outfits, and showering rather than tub bathing daily.

Inflammatory Disorders

STOMATITIS

Stomatitis is inflammation of the oral mucosa, which may include the buccal (cheek) and labial (lip) mucosa, tongue, gingiva, palate, and floor of the mouth. It may be infectious or noninfectious and may be due to local or systemic factors. In children, aphthous stomatitis and herpetic stomatitis are typically seen.

Aphthous stomatitis (aphthous ulcer, canker sore) is a benign but painful condition whose cause is unknown. Its onset is usually associated with mild traumatic injury (biting the cheek, hitting the mucosa with a toothbrush, or rubbing of a mouth appliance on the mucosa), allergy, and emotional stress. The lesions are painful, small, whitish ulcerations surrounded by a red border. They are distinguished from other types of stomatitis by healthy adjacent tissues, absence of vesicles, and absence of systemic illness. The ulcers persist for 4 to 12 days and heal uneventfully.

Herpetic gingivostomatitis (HGS) is caused by the herpes simplex virus (HSV), most often type 1, and may occur as a primary infection or recur in a less severe form known as recurrent herpes labialis (commonly called "cold sores" or "fever blisters"). The primary infection usually begins with a fever; the pharynx becomes edematous and erythematous; and vesicles erupt on the mucosa, causing severe pain. Cervical lymphadenitis often occurs, and the breath has a distinctly foul odor. The disease can last 5 to 14 days with varying degrees of severity.

Therapeutic Management

Treatment for both types of stomatitis is aimed at relief of symptoms, primarily pain. Acetaminophen is usually sufficient for mild cases, but with more severe HGS, stronger analgesics such as codeine may be needed. Topical anesthetics are helpful and include over-the-counter preparations, such as Orabase, Anbesol, and Kanka, or prescription formulas, such as viscous xylocaine. Specific treatment for children with severe cases of HGS is the use of acyclovir (Zovirax).

Nursing Care Management

The chief nursing goals for children with stomatitis are relief of pain and prevention of spread of the herpes virus. Analgesics and topical anesthetics are used as needed to provide relief, especially before meals, to encourage food and fluid intake. Drinking bland fluids through a straw is helpful in avoiding the painful lesions. An oral dressing (Orahesive)* that adheres to the mucosa can provide a barrier over the lesions. Mouth care is encouraged; the use of a very soft bristle toothbrush or disposable foam-tipped toothbrush provides gentle cleaning near ulcerated areas.

Careful handwashing is essential when caring for children with HGS. Since the infection is autoinoculable, children should keep their fingers out of the mouth; contaminated hands also can infect other body parts. Very young children may need elbow restraints to ensure compliance. All articles placed in the mouth are cleaned thoroughly. Newborns and individuals with immunosuppression should not be exposed to infected children.

Nursing ALERT

When examining herpetic lesions, wear gloves. The virus easily enters breaks in the skin and can cause herpetic whitlow of the fingers.

Because herpes infection is often associated with sexual transmission, the nurse should explain to parents and older children that HGS is usually caused by type 1 HSV, the type not associated with sexual activity.

ACUTE APPENDICITIS

Appendicitis, inflammation of the *vermiform appendix* (blind sac at the end of the cecum), is the most common condition requiring abdominal surgery during childhood. Although uncommon in children younger than 2 years of age, it is associated with increased complications and mortality in this age group. Primarily an acute condition, appendicitis rapidly progresses to perforation and peritonitis if it remains undiagnosed. It is a significant pediatric problem, because early diagnosis is frequently delayed as a result of the child's inability to verbalize symptoms; also the clinical signs may be mistaken for other illnesses.

Etiology

The exact cause of appendicitis is poorly understood, but it is almost always a result of obstruction of the lumen, usually by a *fecalith* (a hard fecal material). Sometimes a fold of peritoneum causes the appendix to adhere to the cecum, resulting in an obstructive kink. Other causes include lymphoid hyperplasia, fibrous stenosis from an earlier inflammation, and tumors. Parasites and microorganisms are potential etiologic

*Manufactured by Convatec, Princeton, NJ.

agents. Pinworms have not been shown to be a cause of appendicitis. Dietary habits may play a role. Children with high-fiber diets have a lower incidence of appendicitis than those whose fiber intake is low (Shandling, 1991). Fiber increases the bulk and softness of the stool—a factor that minimizes the chance of obstruction and promotes evacuation.

Pathophysiology

With acute obstruction the outflow of mucous secretions is blocked and pressure builds within the lumen, resulting in compression of blood vessels. The resulting ischemia is followed by ulceration of the epithelial lining and bacterial invasion. Subsequent necrosis causes perforation or rupture with fecal and bacterial contamination of the peritoneal cavity. The resulting inflammation spreads rapidly throughout the abdomen *(peritonitis)*—especially in young children who are unable to localize infection. Progressive peritoneal inflammation results in functional intestinal obstruction of the small bowel *(ileus)*, since intense GI reflexes severely inhibit bowel motility. Since the peritoneum represents a major portion of total body surface, the loss of extracellular fluid to the peritoneal cavity leads to electrolyte imbalance and hypovolemic shock.

Diagnostic Evaluation

Diagnosis is based primarily on the history and physical examination (Box 44-12). The total white blood cell count and the percentage of neutrophils are usually elevated. The white blood cell count is seldom higher than 15,000 to 20,000/mm^3, and radiographic studies of the abdomen may reveal possible contributing causes of appendicitis, such as fecaliths or a foreign body.

Pain, the cardinal feature, is initially generalized (usually periumbilical); however, it usually descends to the lower right quadrant. The most intense site of pain may be at the *McBurney point*, located midway between the anterior superior iliac crest and the umbilicus. Rebound tenderness is not a reliable sign and is extremely painful to the child. Referred pain, elicited by light percussion around the perimeter of the abdomen, indicates the presence of peritoneal irritation. Movement, such as riding over bumps in an automobile or gurney, aggravates the pain. In addition to pain, probably the most significant clinical manifestations are a change in behavior, anorexia, and vomiting.

BOX 44-12

Clinical Manifestations of Appendicitis

Right lower quadrant abdominal pain
Fever
Rigid abdomen
Decreased or absent bowel sounds
Vomiting (commonly follows onset of pain)
Constipation or diarrhea possible
Anorexia
Tachycardia, rapid shallow breathing
Pallor
Lethargy
Irritability
Stooped posture

Abdominal radiographs may aid in the diagnosis of appendicitis. Ultrasonography should be used to aid in the differentiation of pediatric abdominal pain from other causes. Findings such as visualization of the appendix and presence of fluid around the appendix are important sonographic signs `(Borowski, 1994).

Numerous infectious processes have features in common. For example, fever, vomiting, abdominal pain, and an elevated blood count are associated with inflammatory bowel disease, pelvic inflammatory disease, gastroenteritis, urinary tract infection, right lower lobe pneumonia, constipation, mesenteric adenitis, Meckel diverticulum, and intussusception. Fever is usually present, varying from 37.5° to 38.5° C (99.5° to 101.5° F). If the temperature is greater than 39° C (102.2° F), a viral illness or perforation is likely. Prolonged symptoms and delayed diagnosis are not uncommon in preschool children, most likely because of their inability to verbalize their complaints clearly. Consequently the risk of perforation is greater.

Nursing ALERT

Signs of peritonitis in addition to fever include sudden relief from pain after perforation; subsequent increase in pain, which is usually diffuse and accompanied by rigid guarding of the abdomen; progressive abdominal distention; tachycardia; rapid shallow breathing; pallor; chills; and irritability.

Therapeutic Management

The definitive treatment of appendicitis before perforation is surgical removal of the appendix *(appendectomy)*. However, fluid and electrolyte imbalances need to be corrected before surgery, since the child is likely to be dehydrated as a result of the marked anorexia characteristic of appendicitis. Recovery is rapid, and, if there are no complications, the child is discharged within 2 or 3 days.

Ruptured appendix. Management of the child diagnosed with peritonitis caused by a ruptured appendix often begins preoperatively with intravenous administration of fluid and electrolytes, systemic antibiotics, and nasogastric suction. Postoperative management includes intravenous fluids, continued administration of antibiotics, and nasogastric (NG) suction for abdominal decompression until intestinal activity returns. The child with peritonitis is given antibiotics, including ampicillin, gentamicin, and clindamycin, for 7 to 10 days.

In some instances the wound is closed after irrigation of the peritoneal cavity. Many surgeons, however, leave the wound open (delayed closure) to prevent wound infection. A Penrose drain may be used to permit transperitoneal drainage. When delayed closure is used, wound irrigations and wet-to-dry dressings are a routine part of postoperative care.

Prognosis. Complications are uncommon after a simple appendectomy, and recovery is usually rapid and complete. The mortality rate from perforating appendicitis has improved from nearly certain death a century ago to 1% or less at the present time. Wound infection and intraabdominal abscess may complicate a perforated appendix. The key to reducing complications from appendicitis is early recognition of the illness.

Nursing Care Management

Assessment

Since abdominal pain is the most common childhood complaint, the nurse needs to make some preliminary evaluation of the severity of pain (see Chapter 41 for assessment of pain). One of the most reliable estimates is the degree of change in behavior. For example, a child who stays home from school and voluntarily lies down or refuses to play is much more likely to have considerable discomfort than the child who is absent from school but plays contentedly at home. The younger, nonverbal child will assume a rigid, motionless, side-lying posture with the knees flexed on the abdomen, and there is decreased range of motion of the right hip. Older children may exhibit all of these behaviors while complaining of abdominal pain. They can always indicate a point at which the pain is worse than at any other location.

Nursing Diagnoses

On the basis of a thorough assessment, a number of nursing diagnoses become evident. The more likely diagnoses are listed in Box 44-13. Others will be apparent in specific circumstances.

Planning

The goals of care for the child with a simple appendectomy include the following:

1. Child and family will be prepared for surgical intervention.
2. Child will receive postoperative care as described for the child undergoing surgery in Chapter 42.
3. Child with peritonitis will not experience postoperative complications, such as spread of infection.
4. Child and family will receive support and education.

Implementation

Physical preparation of the child with appendicitis is the same as that for any child undergoing surgery.

Nursing ALERT

In any instance when severe abdominal pain is expected, be aware of the danger of administering laxatives or enemas, or of applying heat to the area. Such measures stimulate bowel motility and increase the risk of perforation.

Postoperative care. Postoperative care for the nonperforated appendix is the same as for most abdominal operations. The child with a ruptured appendix and peritonitis requires more complex care, and the course of recovery is considerably longer.

The child is maintained on intravenous fluids, allowed nothing by mouth, and kept on low continuous gastric decompression until there is evidence of intestinal activity. Listening for bowel sounds and observing for other signs of bowel activity (such as passage of stool) are part of the routine assessment. Management of intravenous therapy is the same as for any child receiving fluids and parenteral antibiotics.

BOX 44-13
Nursing Diagnoses: The Child With Appendicitis

Pain related to inflamed appendix
Risk for fluid volume deficit related to decreased intake and losses secondary to loss of appetite, vomiting
Risk for infection related to possibility of rupture
Altered family processes related to illness and hospitalization of a child

Frequent dressing changes are usually needed, as well as meticulous skin care to prevent excoriation of the area surrounding the surgical site. Often wound care includes irrigation with antibacterial solution.

Psychologic care of the child and parents is similar to that used in other emergency situations (see Emergency Admission, Chapter 41). Parents and older children need an opportunity to express their feelings and concerns regarding the events surrounding the illness and hospitalization. The nurse can provide important education and psychosocial support to promote adequate coping, with alleviation of anxiety for both the child and the family.

Evaluation

The effectiveness of nursing interventions is determined by continual reassessment and evaluation of care based on the following observational guidelines:

1. Observe child preoperatively for reaction to the situation and compliance with care.
2. Observe for documentation regarding child's emotional and physical needs, especially assessment of pain and administration of analgesics.
3. Monitor child for evidence of infection.
4. Interview and observe child and family for evidence of their understanding of the condition, especially its sudden onset and the need for surgery.

Expected outcomes:

1. Child complies with directives and exhibits evidence of understanding the rationale for care appropriate to his or her age and developmental level (specify).
2. Child is relaxed and exhibits no evidence of distress (specify expected behaviors related to the characteristics of the child).
3. Child exhibits no evidence of dehydration.
4. Child exhibits no evidence of infection at other body sites.
5. Child and family readily express feelings and concerns and appear relaxed within the limitations imposed by the hospitalization (specify behaviors identified for specific case).

See also the Nursing Care Plan: The Child with Appendicitis.*

*In Wong DL: *Wong and Whaley's clinical manual of pediatric nursing*, ed 4, St Louis, 1996, Mosby.

MECKEL DIVERTICULUM

Meckel diverticulum is a remnant of the fetal omphalomesenteric duct that connects the yolk sac with the primitive midgut during fetal life. Normally this structure is obliterated by the seventh to eighth week of gestation when the placenta replaces the yolk sac as the source of nutrition for the fetus. Failure of obliteration may result in an *omphalomesenteric fistula* (a fibrous band connecting the small intestine to the umbilicus, known as Meckel diverticulum).

Meckel diverticulum is a true diverticulum because it arises from the antimesenteric border of the small intestine, and all layers of the intestinal wall are present. The diverticulum is usually found within 100 cm of the ileocecal valve and averages 1 to 10 cm in length (Turgeon and Barnett, 1990).

Meckel diverticulum is the most common congenital malformation of the gastrointestinal tract and is present in 1% to 3% of the population. It is twice as common in males as in females, and complications are several times more frequent in males. Most symptomatic cases are seen in childhood.

BOX 44-14
Clinical Manifestations of Meckel Diverticulum

Abdominal pain
Similar to appendicitis
May be vague and recurrent

Bloody stools*
Painless
Bright or dark red with mucus ("currant jelly" stool)
In infants, bleeding may be accompanied by pain

Sometimes
Severe anemia
Shock

*Often a presenting sign.

Pathophysiology

The symptomatic complications of Meckel diverticulum are caused by bleeding, obstruction, or inflammation. Gastric mucosa is the most common ectopic tissue found in Meckel diverticulum. Bleeding, which is the most common problem in children, is caused by peptic ulceration or perforation because of the unbuffered acidic secretion. Several mechanisms may cause obstruction. Intussusception may be led by the diverticulum. Obstruction may also be caused by entanglement of the small intestine around a fibrous cord, trapping of a loop of intestine under the band, incarceration within a hernia sac, or volvulus of the intestinal segment containing the diverticulum. Diverticulitis occurs when peptic ulceration or obstruction leads to inflammation.

Diagnostic Evaluation

Diagnosis is ordinarily based on the history, physical examination, and radiographic studies. The signs and symptoms reflect the pathologic process, for example, intestinal obstruction. Acute diverticulitis presents the same clinical picture as acute appendicitis, although the pain may be vague and recurrent (Box 44-14). In the pediatric population bleeding most commonly appears as dark red or "currant jelly" stools and is frequently severe enough to require transfusion. Abdominal radiographs, barium enema, and arteriography have generally been unsuccessful as aids to diagnosis. A specific nuclear scintigraphic study, which detects the presence of gastric mucosa, is the most sensitive and specific noninvasive test for Meckel diverticulum, with an overall diagnostic accuracy of 90% (Turgeon and Barnett, 1990). Blood studies are usually part of the general laboratory workup to rule out any bleeding disorders and to evaluate the severity of the anemia.

Therapeutic Management

The standard treatment is surgical removal of the diverticulum. In instances in which severe hemorrhage increases the surgical risk, medical intervention to correct hypovolemic shock, such as blood replacement, intravenous fluids, and oxygen, may be necessary. In diverticulitis, antibiotics may be used preoperatively to control infection. If intestinal obstruction has occurred, appropriate preoperative measures are used to reverse electrolyte imbalances and prevent abdominal distention.

Prognosis. If Meckel diverticulum is diagnosed and treated early, full recovery is likely. The mortality rate of untreated Meckel diverticulum has been reported to range from 2.5% to 15%. The serious complications of untreated Meckel diverticulum include GI hemorrhage and bowel obstruction.

Nursing Care Management

Nursing objectives are the same as for any child undergoing surgery (see Chapter 42). Since the onset is usually rapid, psychologic support parallels that for other conditions, such as appendicitis. It is important to remember that the massive intestinal bleeding is most often traumatic to both the child and the parent and may significantly affect their emotional reaction to hospitalization and surgery.

Specific preoperative considerations when intestinal bleeding is present include (1) frequently monitoring vital signs and blood pressure for shock, (2) keeping the child on bed rest, and (3) recording the approximate amount of blood lost in stools. In the absence of frank hemorrhage the nurse tests the stools for occult blood.

INFLAMMATORY BOWEL DISEASE (IBD)

The general term *inflammatory bowel disease* is used to designate two chronic intestinal disorders *ulcerative colitis (UC)* and *Crohn disease (CD)*. Although these two diseases are classified as IBD because of their similar epidemiologic, immunologic, and clinical features, they are two distinct conditions with significant differences (Table 44-8). The most important reason for differentiating between the two is the prognosis. Crohn disease is considered the more serious and disabling disorder, and medical/surgical treatment is less effective than in ulcerative colitis. Growth failure is a unique and important feature of IBD in the pediatric population.

Crohn disease is now more common than ulcerative colitis. Between 25% and 40% of patients with Crohn disease and 15% and 40% of patients with ulcerative colitis are diagnosed in childhood and adolescence.

TABLE 44-8 Clinical manifestations of inflammatory bowel diseases

CHARACTERISTICS	ULCERATIVE COLITIS	CROHN DISEASE
Rectal bleeding	Common	Uncommon
Diarrhea	Often severe	Moderate to absent
Pain	Less frequent	Common
Anorexia	Mild or moderate	Can be severe
Weight loss	Moderate	Severe
Growth retardation	Usually mild	Often marked
Anal and perianal lesions	Rare	Common
Fistulas and strictures	Rare	Common
Rashes	Mild	Mild
Joint pain	Mild to moderate	Mild to moderate

Etiology

The cause of IBD is unknown, although there is evidence for a multifactorial etiology. The current hypothesis is that IBD is the result of a genetically determined susceptibility that may be promoted by one or more environmental influences. The inflammatory response is probably immunologically mediated. A primary role for psychologic factors in the pathogenesis of IBD has not been supported by evidence, although psychologic problems may occur secondary to IBD, and may intensify symptoms and influence the course of the disease.

Several genetic and environmental factors influence the incidence of IBD: (1) there is a familial tendency in about 20% to 25% of the cases; (2) more whites than nonwhites are affected; (3) the incidence is several times greater in Jews living in Europe and North America than in the general population; and (4) there is a higher occurrence of the disease in children living in urban settings than in those living in rural areas.

Pathophysiology: Ulcerative Colitis

The inflammation in ulcerative colitis is limited to the colon and rectum. The distal colon and rectum are often most severely affected, producing bloody diarrhea or occult fecal blood, abdominal pain, and varying degrees of systemic manifestations and growth abnormalities (Jackson and Grand, 1991). Inflammation usually is limited to the mucosa and involves continuous segments along the length of the bowel, with varying degrees of ulceration, bleeding, and edema. In long-standing disease the bowel becomes narrowed, smooth, and inflexible, with thin or absent mucosa heavily infiltrated by scar tissue.

Pathophysiology: Crohn Disease

Crohn disease is a chronic inflammatory process that may involve any part of the GI tract from mouth to anus but most commonly affects the terminal ileum. The disease characteristically involves all layers of the bowel wall (transmural). Acute edema and inflammation eventually progress to deep, transverse, or longitudinal ulcerations often associated with fissure formation. The inflammation may result in ulcerations, fibrosis, adhesions, stiffening of the bowel wall, stricture formation, and fistulas to other loops of bowel, bladder, vagina, or skin.

Diagnostic Evaluation

Diagnosis is suspected on the basis of the history and physical examination and is usually confirmed by endoscopic examination. A barium enema and small bowel series are often helpful, and mucosal biopsy is useful in demonstrating characteristic bowel changes. Stool examination is performed to rule out infections. Blood tests are completed and include a complete blood count with differential, serum iron, total protein, albumin, and erythrocyte sedimentation rate (ESR).

Therapeutic Management

The goals of therapy are as follows: (1) control the inflammatory process in order to reduce or eliminate the symptoms, (2) obtain long-term remission, (3) promote normal growth and development, and (4) allow as normal a life-style as possible. Treatment must be individualized and managed according to the severity of the disease, its location, and the response to therapy.

Medical treatment. The drug sulfasalazine has proved useful in decreasing the frequency of recurrences in patients with mild cases of IBD. Because it interferes with the absorption and utilization of folic acid, daily supplements of folic acid are prescribed. Side effects of sulfasalazine include headache, nausea, vomiting, neutropenia, and oligospermia. Sulfasalazine is a combination of 5-aminosalicylate and sulfapyridine. Since many of the side effects are caused primarily by the sulfapyridine, alternative nonabsorbable salicylate drugs are being studied.

Corticosteroids are the most important and effective drugs for treating moderate and severe IBD. Among the newer corticosteroids, budesonide (Rhinocort) has emerged as the most promising (Sachar, 1994). High doses are administered for acute episodes and are then tapered according to the clinical response. Although high doses of corticosteroids can also interfere with growth, significant growth can be achieved with judicious management and maintenance of optimal nutrition. Sometimes steroid enemas are helpful in reducing the need for systemic administration for children with rectosigmoid involvement. Hospitalization and administration of intravenous corticosteroids are prescribed for severe disease. Some of the complications of high-dose steroid therapy include hypertension, osteoporosis, glaucoma, cataracts, hirsutism, diabetes, and altered body composition.

Other drugs include metronidazole for treatment of perianal Crohn disease; antispasmodic agents, which sometimes help relieve the discomfort of diarrhea and cramping; and immunosuppressive agents, which are efficacious in patients on high-dose corticosteroids. 6-Mercaptopurine, azathioprine, and cyclosporine A have been used with success in selected patients with IBD. The major risks of these drugs include immunosuppression and bone marrow suppression, which can cause leukopenia and opportunistic infections.

Nutritional support. Increasing evidence supports the importance of nutritional therapy as an adjunctive, if not primary, therapy in children with IBD. Malnutrition is a common feature of IBD. The major complications of malnutrition in children and adolescents are alteration in body composition and disturbance in growth and sexual maturation. Nutritional deficiency is characterized by protein-energy malnutrition and multiple vitamin (vitamins B and D) and mineral (calcium, magnesium, iron, and zinc) deficiencies. Growth failure is characterized by weight deficits, alteration in body composition, linear growth retardation, and delayed sexual maturation. Growth failure affects approximately one third of pediatric patients with IBD and is significantly more common in children with Crohn disease than in those with ulcerative colitis.

The cause of malnutrition is multifactorial and includes inadequate dietary intake, excessive GI losses, malabsorption, and increased nutritional requirements. Inadequate dietary intake results from the anorexia associated with chronic illness and episodes of increased inflammatory activity. Excessive losses of nutrients occur secondary to intestinal mucosal inflammation and diarrhea. Stool losses include protein, blood, electrolytes, and minerals. Malabsorption is common with IBD, particularly in Crohn disease, because of mucosal injury and bacterial overgrowth. Carbohydrate, lactose, fat, vitamin, and mineral malabsorption can occur. Vitamin B_{12} and folic acid deficiencies are common in patients with disease or resection of the terminal ileum. Nutritional requirements are increased with increased inflammatory activity, fever, and fistulas and during periods of rapid growth such as adolescence.

The goals of nutritional support include (1) correction of specific nutrient deficits and replacement of ongoing losses, (2) provision of adequate energy and protein for healing, and (3) provision of adequate nutrients to promote normal growth. Nutritional support may include both enteral and parenteral nutrition. A well-balanced, high-protein, high-calorie diet is recommended for children whose symptoms do not prohibit an adequate oral intake. There is little evidence that avoiding specific foods influences the severity of the disease. Supplementation with multivitamins, iron, and folic acid is generally recommended.

Special enteral formulas, given either by mouth or by continuous nasogastric infusion (often at night), may be required. Elemental formulas have been used successfully to improve nutritional status, as well as to induce remission in children and adolescents with Crohn disease. Elemental formulas are completely absorbed in the small intestine with almost no residue. Several studies have demonstrated that a diet consisting only of elemental formula not only improved nutritional status but also induced disease remission, either without steroids or with a diminished dosage of steroids required. An elemental diet is a safe and potentially effective primary therapy for patients with Crohn disease.

TPN has been shown to improve nutritional status in patients with IBD. Short-term remissions have been achieved after TPN, although complete bowel rest has not been proved to reduce inflammation or to add to the benefits of improved nutrition by TPN (Jackson and Grand, 1991). Nutritional support in patients with ulcerative colitis is less likely to induce a remission than it is in patients with Crohn disease. Improvement of nutritional status is important, however, in preventing deterioration of the patient's health status and in preparing the patient for surgery.

Surgical treatment. Ulcerative colitis can be cured by performance of a total colectomy. Surgery is indicated when medical and nutritional therapies fail to prevent significant complications. Surgical options include a *subtotal colectomy* and *ileostomy*, which leaves a rectal stump as a blind pouch; the *J-pouch* or *Kock pouch*, consisting of terminal ileum, which aids in continence; and an *ileoanal pull-through*, which preserves the normal pathway for defecation.

Surgery is required by children with Crohn disease when complications cannot be controlled by medical and nutritional therapy. Local resection is not curative, however, since the disease tends to recur, and further surgery may be needed. Removing the colon *(total colectomy)* is curative.

Prognosis. IBD is a chronic incurable disease. Relatively long periods of quiescent disease may follow exacerbations. The outcome of the disease process is influenced by the regions and severity of GI involvement, as well as by appropriate therapeutic management. Malnutrition, growth failure, and GI bleeding are serious complications of the disease. The overall prognosis for ulcerative colitis is good.

The development of carcinoma of the colon is a long-term complication of IBD. In ulcerative colitis removal of the diseased bowel prevents development of carcinoma. However, in Crohn disease surgical removal of the affected bowel does not prevent bowel cancer; therefore routine screening of stool specimens is needed for early detection.

Nursing Care Management

Many of the nursing considerations relate directly to the therapeutic management in treating IBD colitis. However the scope of nursing responsibilities extends beyond the immediate period of hospitalization and involves (1) providing continued guidance to families in terms of dietary management, (2) coping with those factors that increase stress and emotional lability, (3) adjusting to a disease of remissions and exacerbations or one of chronic ill health, and (4) when indicated, preparing the child and parents for the possibility of diversionary bowel surgery.

Since diet therapy is very important, the nurse and nutritionist should collaborate to provide dietary counseling for the child and family members. Encouraging the anorexic child to consume sufficient quantities of this diet is of primary importance and is frequently a nursing challenge. An approach that is more likely to meet with success involves including the child in meal planning; encouraging small, frequent meals or snacks rather than three large meals a day; serving meals around medication schedules when diarrhea, mouth pain, and intestinal spasm are controlled; and preparing high-protein, high-calorie foods, such as eggnog, milk shakes, cream soups, puddings, or custard (if lactose is tolerated) (see also Feeding the Sick Child, Chapter 41). Foods that are known to aggravate the condition are avoided. The routine practice of using bran or a high-fiber diet for IBD is currently being questioned. Bran, even in small amounts, has been shown to worsen the patient's condition (Francis and Whorwell, 1994). Occasionally the occurrence of aphthous stomatitis further complicates adherence to dietary management. Good mouth care before eating and the selection of bland foods help relieve the discomfort of mouth sores.

Nurses have an important role in preparing children and

Critical Thinking Q & A 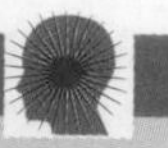

INFLAMMATORY BOWEL DISEASE

A 13-year-old girl is admitted to the hospital because of bloody diarrhea, abdominal pain, and weight loss. After a thorough evaluation including laboratory tests, radiographic studies, and gastrointestinal endoscopy procedures, the diagnosis of Crohn disease is made. Medical treatment including corticosteroid drugs and nutritional support is initiated in the hospital. Enteral formula administered by continuous nighttime nasogastric tube infusion and vitamin and mineral supplements will need to be continued at home after the hospitalization. All of the following interventions are important preparations for successful home care *except:*

1. Education of the adolescent and family regarding the disease process.
2. Education of the adolescent and family regarding medication therapy and administration of nasogastric tube feedings.
3. Provision of psychosocial support to aid in the adjustment to a chronic disease of remissions and exacerbations.
4. Restriction of school attendance and extracurricular activities for the duration of home therapy.

The correct answer is four. School absences or inability to compete with peers in some activities may occur during exacerbations of the disease, but self-esteem, positive school performance, and social interactions can be enhanced through support and guidance by the family and health care providers. Once the acute disease exacerbation is under control, the adolescent should be encouraged to resume school attendance and participation with peers in activities of interest. Important nursing responsibilities include educating the adolescent and her family regarding the disease process and therapeutic management and promoting adjustment to the chronic nature of the disease. The importance of continued drug therapy as prescribed despite remission of symptoms should be emphasized. The purpose and expected outcomes of nutrition support therapy should be explained thoroughly. The adolescent and her family members should be given adequate time to demonstrate skills necessary to continue therapy at home. Referral to a home health agency to ensure continuity of care is often beneficial.

families to administer nasogastric feedings or TPN when indicated. The purpose and the expected outcomes of these therapies should be carefully explained. The child's and family members' anxieties should be acknowledged, and they should be given adequate time to demonstrate the skills necessary to continue the therapy at home if needed.* (See the Critical Thinking Q & A above).

The importance of continued drug therapy despite remission of symptoms must be stressed to the parents and child. Failure to adhere to the pharmacologic regimen can result in exacerbation of the disease process (see Chapter 42 for a discussion of compliance).

Family support. Attending to the emotional components of a chronic disease requires a thorough assessment of those stress factors that are disease related. Frequently the nurse can be instrumental in helping these children adjust to the problems of growth retardation, delayed sexual maturation, dietary restrictions, feelings of being "different" or "sickly," inability to compete with peers, and necessary absence from school during exacerbations of the illness (see Chapter 38).

In the event that a permanent colectomy/ileostomy is required, the nurse can assist the child and family in accepting and adjusting to the change by teaching them how to care for the ileostomy; by emphasizing the positive aspects of surgery, particularly accelerated growth and sexual development, permanent recovery, and eliminated risk of colonic cancer in ulcerative colitis; and by stressing the normality of life despite bowel diversion. Introducing the child and parents to other ostomy patients, especially those of the child's age, can be the most effective therapeutic measure in fostering eventual acceptance. Whenever possible, the newer continent ostomies should be offered as options to the child, although they are not performed in all centers throughout the United States.

Because of the chronic and often lifelong nature of the disease, families benefit from many of the services provided by organizations such as the Crohn's and Colitis Foundation of America, Inc (CCFA),* which has branches in many major communities and provides education regarding the management of inflammatory bowel disease. If diversionary bowel surgery is indicated, the United Ostomy Association,† and the Wound and Ostomy Continence Nurse Society‡ are available to assist with ileostomy care and provide important psychologic support through their self-help groups. Adolescents often benefit by participating in peer-support groups, which are sponsored in some areas by the CCFA.

See also the Nursing Care Plan: The Child with Inflammatory Bowel Disease.§

PEPTIC ULCER

A peptic ulcer, or peptic ulcer disease (PUD), is an erosion of the mucosal wall of the stomach, pylorus, or duodenum. *Gastric ulcers* affect the lining of the stomach, whereas *duodenal ulcers* involve the pylorus or duodenum. Although peptic ulcers are more common in adults, they are also a significant pediatric problem, occurring at any age.

Ulcers are described as either primary or secondary. *Primary ulcers* occur in the absence of a predisposing factor. *Secondary ulcers,* or *stress ulcers,* result from the stress of a severe underlying disease or injury (e.g., severe burns, sepsis, multisystem organ failure) or ingestion of an ulcerogenic drug (e.g., salicylates, nonsteroidal antiinflammatory agents, ferrous sulfate). Stress ulcers occur more often in infancy and early childhood. In older children and adolescents the majority of ulcers are primary. The incidence of ulcers in boys is two to three times greater than in girls, although this difference is less in very young children.

*Home care instructions on caring for a central venous catheter are available in Wong DL: *Wong and Whaley's clinical manual of pediatric nursing,* ed 4, St Louis, 1996, Mosby.

*444 Park Ave., South, New York, NY 10016; (212) 679-1570.

†36 Executive Park, Suite 120, Irvine, CA 92714-6744; (714) 660-8624.

‡2755 Bristol St., Suite 110, Costa Mesa, CA 92626; (714) 476-0268. In Canada: **Canadian Foundation for Ileitis and Colitis,** 21 St. Clair Ave., East, Suite 301, Toronto, Ontario M4TL 1L9, (416) 920-5035; **United Ostomy Association, Canada,** 5 Hamilton Ave., Hamilton, Ontario L8V 2L3, (416) 389-8822.

§In Wong DL: *Wong and Whaley's clinical manual of pediatric nursing,* ed, 4, St Louis, 1996, Mosby.

Etiology

The exact cause of peptic ulcer is not always known, although infectious, genetic, and environmental factors are important causative factors. A strong relationship exists between *Helicobacter pylori* (formerly *Campylobacter pylori*) and upper gastrointestinal disease. Nearly all patients with duodenal ulcers have *H. pylori* gastritis. Therefore infection with the organism may be a prerequisite for the occurrence of almost all duodenal ulcers in the absence of other precipitating factors (NIH Consensus Conference, 1994). This organism may cause ulcers by weakening the gastric mucosal barrier and allowing acid to damage the mucosa. Genetic factors play a role in causing PUD, and a positive relationship to blood group O exists. Several drugs are known to contribute to ulcer formation, including aspirin, nonsteroidal antiinflammatory agents, steroids, and alcohol. Smoking has also been associated with PUD. Psychologic factors may also play a role in the development of PUD. Stressful life events, dependency, passiveness, and hostility have all been implicated as contributing factors in PUD.

Pathophysiology

Most likely the pathogenesis of PUD is due to an imbalance between destructive factors that promote the formation of peptic ulcers and protective factors that guard against ulcer formation (Ziller and Netchvolodoff, 1993). The gastroduodenal epithelium secretes a water-insoluble mucous gel that serves as a protective barrier. It is a barrier to hydrogen ions, which are neutralized by the bicarbonate within the mucous gel. Prostaglandins appear to play a role in mucosal defense because they stimulate both mucous and alkali secretion. Abnormalities of the mucous-bicarbonate barrier are likely to contribute to ulcer formation. As a result of either of these two conditions the gastric mucosa is highly vulnerable to the digestive effects of gastric juice. Prolonged contact with the highly acidic contents of the stomach and duodenum causes an erosion of the mucosal wall, especially in those areas least protected, such as the cardiac and lesser curve of the stomach and the area immediately beyond the pylorus.

Diagnostic Evaluation

Diagnosis is based on the history (pattern of pain) (Box 44-15), physical examination, and diagnostic testing such as radiographs and barium studies. Upper endoscopy is the most reliable tool to diagnose PUD. Other tests include blood studies (anemia), stool samples (occult blood), and occasionally gastric acid measurements (to identify hypersecretion).

Therapeutic Management

The objectives of therapy for children with peptic ulcers are to relieve discomfort, promote healing, and prevent complications and recurrence. The management of ulcers is primarily medical and consists of administration of medications that reduce or neutralize gastric acid secretion and, when possible, implementation of measures to eliminate or reduce stresses.

Antacids may be used in the initial treatment of peptic ulcers. The antacid of choice, usually a liquid aluminum or magnesium preparation, is administered every 1 and 3 hours after each meal and at bedtime. The dosage is determined by the size of the child. As healing progresses, the frequency of administration is gradually reduced but not usually discontinued for several weeks. Diarrhea may be a side effect of large amounts of magnesium-containing antacids.

One of the histamine (H_2) receptor antagonists—cimetidine (Tagamet), ranitidine (Zantac), or famotidine (Pepcid)—is usually prescribed for the treatment of PUD. Omeprazole is an extremely potent gastric acid antisecretory agent. The general course of therapy is 4 to 6 weeks. A nightly maintenance dose may be given for 6 months. Each of these drugs suppresses pepsin and gastric acid secretion and provides for greater compliance because of the reduced frequency of administration compared with antacids.

Sucralfate, an aluminum salt of sucrose octasulfate, forms a protective barrier for ulcerated mucosa against acid and pepsin. Sucralfate is not available in liquid form, although the pill can be mixed with water and given with a syringe or spoon. This drug may be given four times per day for 6 weeks. Bismuth compounds are sometimes prescribed for the relief of ulcers. The mechanism of their activity is poorly understood, but they do have an effect on inhibiting the growth of microorganisms. Bismuth demonstrates activity against *H. pylori*, and the eradication of *H. pylori* from GI tissue has been associated with improved healing of ulcers. Bismuth does not eradicate the organism in all cases, and antiinfectives may be used.

The child is provided with a nutritious diet but advised to avoid caffeine and alcohol. Since aspirin is known to have a damaging effect on gastric mucosa, acetaminophen is recommended as a substitute. Psychologic assistance may be required for children with overlying anxiety problems.

BOX 44-15
Clinical Manifestations of Peptic Ulcer

Neonates (usually gastric)
- Usually perforation
- Often massive hemorrhage
- Almost the same as seen in stress ulcers

Infants to 2-year-old children (gastric or duodenal, primary or secondary)
- Poor eating, vomiting, crying spells after feeding, abdominal distention, tarry stools, melena
- Vague discomfort
- Irritability
- Usually bleed rather than perforate

2- to 6-year-old children (gastric or duodenal)
- May have vomiting related to eating, generalized or periumbilical pain, melena, hematemesis
- Wake at night or early morning, crying with pain
- Perforation more likely in secondary ulcers

6- to 9-year-old children (usually duodenal and primary)
- Pain—burning or gnawing sensation in epigastrium related to fasting state, melena, hematemesis, vomiting
- Often with obstruction

Over 9 years (usually duodenal)
- Same as above
- More typical of adult type.

A child with an acute ulcer who has complications, such as massive hemorrhage, requires emergency care. Administration of intravenous fluids, blood, or plasma depends on the amount of blood loss. Blood replacement with whole blood or packed cells may be necessary for significant loss.

Surgical intervention may be required in the management of complications of PUD, such as hemorrhage, perforation, or gastric outlet obstruction. Ligation of the source of bleeding or closure of a perforation may be performed. A vagotomy and pylorosplasty may be indicated in children with ulcers that recur despite aggressive medical treatment.

Prognosis. The long-term prognosis for PUD is variable. Many ulcers can be successfully treated with medical therapy; however, primary duodenal peptic ulcers frequently recur. A high incidence of complications, such as GI bleeding, can occur and extend into adult life. The effect of maintenance drug therapy on long-term morbidity remains to be established with further studies.

Nursing Care Management

The main nursing objective is to promote healing of the ulcer through compliance with the medication regimen. The diet is usually quite liberal, with avoidance of any food that causes the child discomfort. Substances that may irritate the gastric wall are avoided, such as alcohol, tobacco, tea, coffee, and aspirin. Use of alcohol and tobacco may be an issue for adolescents with ulcers.

Drug compliance is essential and can be a problem with frequent administration of antacids. Therefore strategies to improve compliance are instituted early in the course of therapy (see Chapter 41). When traveling and during school the use of antacid tablets rather than liquid is more convenient.

Although the exact role stress plays in the pathogenesis of ulcers in children is unclear, especially since many ulcers occur secondary to other conditions, the nurse should be aware of those family and environmental conditions that may have precipitated or may aggravate the condition. Children may benefit from psychologic counseling and from learning how to cope more constructively with stresses in their lives.

See also the Nursing Care Plan: The Child with Peptic Ulcer Disease.*

Hepatic Disorders

ACUTE HEPATITIS

Hepatitis, or inflammation of the liver, is rapidly emerging as one of the major causes of morbidity and a significant cause of mortality in children. The discussion that follows is focused primarily on acute hepatitis, although the chronic disease may involve many of the same mechanisms.

Etiology

Hepatitis in children may be caused by a virus, a chemical or drug reaction, or some other disease process. The majority (90%) of cases of viral hepatitis are caused by five viruses:

- Hepatitis A virus (HAV, previously designated infectious hepatitis)
- Hepatitis B virus (HBV, previously designated serum hepatitis)
- Hepatitis C virus (HCV, previously designated parenterally transmitted non-A, non-B hepatitis virus [PT-NANB])
- Hepatitis D virus (HDV, delta agent)
- Hepatitis E virus (enterically transmitted non-A, non-B hepatitis virus [ET-NANB])

In addition, cytomegalovirus (CMV), Epstein-Barr virus (EBV), and HSV may occasionally cause hepatitis. The clinical symptoms of these viruses are similar. Epidemiologic features and serologic testing are used to differentiate the causes. Table 44-9 compares the features of HAV, HBV, and HCV.

Hepatitis A. HAV is highly contagious and is transmitted from one person to another primarily by the fecal-oral route, usually from ingestion of contaminated food or water. This includes eating shellfish caught in contaminated water and swimming in this water. Hepatitis A is usually an acute and mild illness. There is no known carrier state. HAV can affect individuals at any age but often is found in children under 15 years of age. Additional sources for children are day-care centers (especially those that have children in diapers) and custodial care facilities. School contacts are considered a relatively low risk. The incubation period is approximately 4 weeks.

Hepatitis B. HBV can cause a wide spectrum of acute and chronic infection, ranging from asymptomatic limited infection to fatal fulminant hepatitis. Transmission is usually via the parenteral route through the exchange of blood or any bodily secretion or fluid. Intimate physical contact and spread from mother to infant are potential sources of infection. Contaminated fluids splashed into the mouth or eyes can cause infection. HBV infection from blood transfusion has been reduced as a result of blood product–screening procedures. Transplanted organs can also serve as a source of HBV. Adults whose occupations are associated with considerable exposure to blood or blood products, such as health care workers, are at an increased risk of exposure and may choose to receive HBV vaccination. HBV infection occurs in children and adolescents in specific high-risk situations: (1) infants of mothers who are chronic carriers, (2) children with hemophilia and others who have received multiple transfusions, (3) children involved in intravenous drug abuse, (4) institutionalized children, and (5) preschool children in endemic areas. The incubation period ranges from 50 to 180 days.

Most HBV in children is acquired perinatally. Newborn infants are at risk for hepatitis if the mother is infected with HBV or was a carrier of HBV during pregnancy. Possible routes of maternal-fetal (infant) transmission include (1) leakage of virus across the placenta late in pregnancy or during labor, (2) ingestion of amniotic fluid or maternal blood, and (3) breastfeeding, especially if the mother has cracked nipples.

Hepatitis C. Hepatitis C has been called "non-A, non-B hepatitis" because of the absence of HAV and HBV serologic markers of infection. HCV transmission appears to be largely

*In Wong DL: *Wong and Whaley's clinical manual of pediatric nursing,* ed 4, St Louis, 1996, Mosby.

TABLE 44-9 Clinical manifestations of types A, B, and C hepatitis

CHARACTERISTICS	TYPE A	TYPE B	TYPE C
Onset	Usually rapid, acute	More insidious	Usually insidious
Fever	Common and early	Less frequent	Less frequent
Anorexia	Common	Mild to moderate	Mild to moderate
Nausea and vomiting	Common	Less common	Mild to moderate
Rash	Rare	Common	Sometimes present
Arthralgia	Rare	Common	Rare
Pruritus	Rare	Sometimes present	Sometimes present
Jaundice	Sometimes present	Present	Present

parenteral, although other routes may occasionally be responsible (Carey and Patel, 1992). HCV is the primary cause of posttransfusion hepatitis, and before heat treatment of clotting factor concentrates, patients with hemophilia who needed replacement therapy were at risk for acquiring hepatitis C (Kanesaki et al, 1993). The clinical course is variable. The incubation period ranges from 14 days to 6 months. Some children may be asymptomatic, but hepatitis C often becomes a chronic condition and can cause cirrhosis and hepatocellular carcinoma. In about 50% of individuals infected with HCV chronic disease develops (Carey and Patel, 1992). Although aplastic anemia is a rare complication of all forms of viral hepatitis, it is more common with hepatitis C.

Hepatitis D. HDV infection occurs in patients already infected with HBV. HDV, which can result in chronic hepatitis, is a defective ribonucleic acid (RNA) virus that requires the function of HBV. HDV infection occurs primarily in hemophiliacs and intravenous drug abusers. Usually more severe than hepatitis B, HDV infection can lead to cirrhosis and death. The incubation period is most likely several weeks.

Hepatitis E. Hepatitis E is epidemic or enterally transmitted non-A, non-B hepatitis. Transmission may occur via contaminated water. This illness is not chronic, and there is no carrier state. However it can be a devastating disease among pregnant women, with a mortality rate of 10% to 20% (Krugman, 1992).

Pathophysiology

The pathologic changes occur primarily in the parenchymal cells of the liver and result in variable degrees of swelling, infiltration of liver cells by mononuclear cells, subsequent degeneration, necrosis, and autolysis. Structural changes within the hepatocyte are thought to account for altered liver functions.

Hepatitis can be self-limited, and complete regeneration of liver cells without scarring may occur within 2 to 3 months. However some forms of hepatitis do not result in complete return of liver function. These include *fulminant hepatitis,* which is characterized by a severe, acute course with hepatic necrosis and death frequently occurring within 1 to 2 weeks, and *subacute or chronic active hepatitis,* which is characterized by progressive liver destruction and uncertain regeneration with the possibility of scarring.

The initial *anicteric (absence of jaundice) phase* symptoms include nausea and vomiting, extreme anorexia, malaise, easy fatigability, and slight to moderate fever. The child may have abdominal pain (especially epigastric or upper right quadrant); usually acts ill, preferring to rest in bed; and is fretful or irritable. This phase usually lasts 5 to 7 days and may be mistaken for influenza.

The *icteric (jaundice) phase* begins with darkening of the urine and the presence of light-colored stools, followed by yellowing of the sclera and skin. As jaundice worsens, the child usually begins to feel better, with improved appetite and behavior and the absence of nausea, vomiting, and fever, although pruritus can be a bothersome symptom. The icteric phase commonly lasts less than 4 weeks. Complete recovery with return of normal liver function and a feeling of well-being with absence of fatigue or malaise may take 1 to 3 months.

Diagnostic Evaluation

The clinical manifestations of most types of viral hepatitis are similar except for a more rapid, acute onset in type A and a slower, more insidious onset in type B (Table 44-9). Types A and B may present with flulike symptoms. Some may never be recognized as actual cases of hepatitis.

Diagnosis of hepatitis is based on the history (especially regarding possible exposure to a hepatitis virus), physical examination, serologic markers, and liver function tests. The diagnosis is confirmed by detection of antibodies or antigens formed in response to the specific virus, such as HBsAg (the hepatitis B surface antigen). During the initial infective period anti-HAV of the immunoglobulin M (IgM) class is present, but after about 3 to 6 months this antibody declines and anti-HAV of the IgG class increases. Therefore detection of anti-HAV IgM indicates active infection, and anti-HAV IgG indicates past infection and immunity (Krugman, 1992). Antibodies to different HCV antigens can also be detected (Kanesaki et al, 1993).

No liver function test is specific for hepatitis. Serum aminotransferase (AST, ALT) levels are markedly elevated. Serum bilirubin levels peak 5 to 10 days after clinical jaundice appears.

Therapeutic Management

There is no specific treatment for viral hepatitis. Management primarily includes treatment of symptoms. The value of bed rest in promoting overall recovery is controversial. Since children feel ill and tired in the anicteric phase, they usually choose to stay in bed. However, once improvement of physical complaints begins, children usually prefer to resume normal activity gradually. The best approach is probably to allow them to regulate their own pace. Precautionary measures are implemented to prevent spread of the infection.

Children are allowed to choose foods they prefer, especially during the initial stage when anorexia is severe. A special diet is generally not of value. Hospitalization is required if coagulopathy or fulminant hepatitis develops.

Steroid therapy should not be used. Human alpha-interferon has been used with some success in the treatment of chronic hepatitis B and chronic hepatitis C infections (Bacon, 1991). Antiviral drugs are currently being studied.

Prevention. Proper handwashing and standard isolation precautions can prevent spread of hepatitis. Prophylactic use of standard immune globulin (Ig) is effective in preventing HAV infection in situations of preexposure (such as anticipated travel to areas where HAV is prevalent) or in situations of postexposure during the early part of the incubation period. Hepatitis B immune globulin (HBIg) is effective in preventing HBV infection after exposure. Immune globulins must be administered less than 2 weeks after exposure.

Active immunizations are not available against the non-A, non-B viruses. However, vaccines have been developed to prevent HBV and HAV infection. HBV vaccination is recommended for all newborns and adolescents not previously immunized (see Immunizations, Chapter 33). It is possible to prevent hepatitis D by preventing hepatitis B (Lisanti and Talotta, 1992).

Prognosis. The prognosis for children with hepatitis is variable and depends on the type of virus causing the disease. HAV usually causes a mild and brief illness with no carrier state. HBV can cause a wide spectrum of acute and chronic illness. Chronic HBV infection leads to cirrhosis in 25% to 30% of cases (Ergun and Miskovitz, 1990). Hepatocellular carcinoma is a potentially fatal complication of HBV infection. HCV infection frequently becomes chronic, and cirrhosis may develop in as many as 20% of these patients. Fulminant hepatic failure occurs in approximately 1% to 2% of cases of viral hepatitis, regardless of the cause, and is associated with a mortality rate of 60% to 90%, with higher mortality in older children (Krugman, 1992).

Nursing Care Management

Nursing objectives depend largely on the severity of the hepatitis, the medical management, and factors influencing the control and transmission of the disease. Since children with benign viral hepatitis are frequently cared for at home, the responsibility of explaining any medical therapies and control measures is frequently left to the clinic or office nurse. In instances in which further assistance is needed for parents to comply with such instructions, a public health nursing referral may be necessary.

The emphasis is on encouraging a well-balanced diet and a realistic schedule of rest and activity adjusted to the child's condition. Since hepatitis A is not infectious within a week or so after the onset of jaundice, the child may feel well enough to resume school shortly thereafter. The parents are also cautioned about administering any medication to the child, since normal doses of many drugs may become dangerous because of the liver's inability to detoxify and excrete them.

Handwashing is the single most critical measure in reducing risk of hepatitis transmission in any setting. The nurse should explain to parents and children the usual ways in which HAV (oral-fecal route) and HBV (parenteral route) are spread.

Children who are hospitalized are not usually isolated in a separate room unless they are fecally incontinent or their toys and other items might become contaminated with feces. They are discouraged from sharing their toys. For further discussion see Infection Control, Chapter 41.

When children with HBV infection have a known or suspected history of illicit drug use, the nurse has the additional responsibility of helping them realize the associated dangers of drug abuse, stressing the parenteral mode of transmission of hepatitis, and encouraging them to seek counseling through a drug program.

See also Nursing Care Plan: The Child with Acute Hepatitis.*

CIRRHOSIS

Cirrhosis occurs as the end stage of many chronic liver diseases. Liver damage can be caused by infectious, autoimmune, toxic, or structural factors. Cirrhosis results from cell injury, tissue repair, and regeneration. A cirrhotic liver is irreversibly damaged.

Clinical manifestations of cirrhosis develop from the features commonly seen with all chronic liver disorders. Children with cirrhosis often exhibit jaundice, poor growth, anorexia, muscle weakness, and lethargy. Ascites, edema, GI bleeding, anemia, and abdominal pain may be present in children with impaired intrahepatic blood flow. Pulmonary function may be impaired in children with cirrhosis because of pressure against the diaphragm caused by hepatosplenomegaly and ascites. Dyspnea and cyanosis may occur, especially on exertion. Intrapulmonary arteriovenous shunts, which can also cause hypoxemia, may develop. Spider angiomas and prominent blood vessels on the upper torso are often present.

Therapeutic Management

Therapy is directed primarily toward (1) frequent assessment of liver status with physical examination and liver function tests and (2) management of specific complications. The only successful treatment for end-stage liver disease and liver failure may be liver transplantation, which has improved the prognosis substantially for many children with cirrhosis. Average 4-year survival rates are about 64% after orthotopic liver transplantation (Lloyd-Still, 1991). Unfortunately many children die while waiting for a suitable donor.

Prognosis. The success of liver transplantation has revolutionized the approach to liver cirrhosis. Liver failure and cirrhosis are currently indications for transplantation. Liver transplantation reflects the failure of other medical and surgical measures to prevent or treat cirrhosis. Careful monitoring of the child's condition and quality of life are necessary in order to evaluate the need for and timing of transplantation (see the Family Focus box on p. 1417).

*In Wong DL: *Wong and Whaley's clinical manual of pediatric nursing*, ed 4, St Louis, 1996, Mosby.

Family Focus

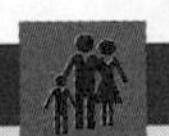

END-STAGE LIVER DISEASE

In many cases the child and family must cope with an uncertain progression of the disease. The only hope for long-term survival may be liver transplantation. Transplantation can be very successful, but the waiting period may be long, and there are many more children in need of organs than there are donors. The nurse should recognize the unique stresses of coping with end-stage liver disease and waiting for transplantation, and should assist the family in coping with these stressors. The assistance of social workers and support from other parents can be very beneficial.

Nursing Care Management

Nursing objectives in caring for the child with cirrhosis depend on several factors, including the precipitating cause of the cirrhosis, the severity of complications, and the prognosis. Overall the last factor has the greatest impact, because the prognosis for life is poor unless successful liver transplantation can be performed. Therefore nursing care of this child is similar to that for any child with a life-threatening illness (Chapter 38). Hospitalization is usually required when complications occur.

BILIARY ATRESIA

Biliary atresia, now referred to as *extrahepatic biliary atresia (EHBA)*, is the atresia or absence of the bile ducts outside the liver. This disease is a progressive inflammatory process that causes both intrahepatic and extrahepatic bile duct fibrosis, resulting in eventual ductal obstruction. The incidence of biliary atresia is between 1 in 10,000 and 1 in 25,000 live births. There does not seem to be a racial or genetic predilection, although there is a female predominance of 1.4:1 (Karrer et al, 1990). Associated malformations include polysplenia, intestinal atresia, and malrotation of the intestine. Biliary atresia, if untreated, usually leads to cirrhosis, liver failure, and death in the first 2 years of life. EHBA is categorized as either correctable or noncorrectable, depending on the anatomy of the extrahepatic biliary system. Correctable lesions involve distal atresia with a patent proximal portion of the extrahepatic duct or patency of the gallbladder, cystic duct, and common bile duct. Noncorrectable EHBA involves obstruction at the porta hepatis. The majority of cases of EHBA are noncorrectable.

Etiology/Pathophysiology

EHBA is a progressive obliterative process. The pathologic process may occur in fetal life or early in the postnatal period. Reports have indicated that biliary atresia is not seen in the fetus or the stillborn or newborn infant (Fanaroff and Martin, 1992). The exact cause is unknown, although immune mechanisms or viral injury may be responsible. Inflammation is progressive, causing both intrahepatic and extrahepatic bile duct fibrosis and obstruction. Surgery to obtain effective bile drainage must be achieved within 2 to 3 months after birth to diminish progressive liver damage.

Little is known regarding the development and maintenance of intrahepatic bile ducts; therefore the exact cause of intrahepatic biliary disease is unknown. Intralobular ducts are lost over a period of months or years. Varying degrees of cholestasis occur. Cirrhosis may or may not occur. Irritants and toxins, such as bile acids, are retained, often causing severe pruritus. There may be a marked hypercholesterolemia.

BOX 44-16
Clinical Manifestations of Biliary Atresia

- Jaundice
  - Earliest manifestation and most striking feature of disorder
  - First observed in sclera
  - May be present at birth
  - Usually not apparent until age 2 to 3 weeks
- Urine dark and stains diaper
- Stools lighter than expected or white or tan
- Hepatomegaly and abdominal distention common
- Splenomegaly occurs later
- Poor fat metabolism results in
  - Poor weight gain
  - General failure to thrive
- Pruritis
- Irritability
- Difficulty in comforting infant

Diagnostic Evaluation

Diagnosis of biliary disease is based on the history, physical examination, and a variety of tests. Growth parameters and nutritional status should be assessed, since many of these infants and children have nutritional deficiencies and poor growth. The disease is suspected on the basis of clinical signs (Box 44-16). Blood tests, including complete blood count and levels of electrolytes, bilirubin, and liver enzymes, are obtained. Additional laboratory analyses, including alpha-1-antitrypsin level, TORCHS titers, hepatitis serology, urine cytomegalovirus, and a sweat test, may be indicated to rule out other conditions that cause persistent cholestasis and jaundice. Abdominal ultrasonography allows evaluation of the liver and biliary system. Biliary patency can be determined with hepatobiliary scintigraphy. Liver biopsy evaluates hepatic abnormality. Definitive diagnosis of EHBA is obtained during an exploratory laparotomy and an intraoperative cholangiogram.

Therapeutic Management

The major hope in care of these children is that the condition will benefit from surgery. Although successful surgical correction is possible in only a few cases of EHBA, surgery is most successful when performed early; therefore diagnosis is urgent. The surgical procedure for EHBA is *hepatoportoenterostomy (Kasai procedure)*, in which a segment of intestine is anastomosed to the resected porta hepatis to attempt bile drainage. There are several variations of this procedure. In approximately 80% to 90% of infants with biliary atresia who are operated on when younger than 10 weeks of age, bile drainage is achieved (Ryckman et al, 1993). However, progressive cirrhosis still occurs in many children, and up to 80% may eventually require liver transplantation (Laurent et al, 1990).

Therapeutic management is primarily supportive. It is the method of choice for intrahepatic disease and supplemental to surgical therapy in EHBA. Medical management consists of a high-calorie formula containing fats that can be digested without bile (Pregestimil), as well as water-soluble vitamins. Phenobarbital may be given to promote bile flow. A low-salt diet and diuretics may reduce ascites formation. Ursodeoxycholic acid has been used successfully to treat pruritis and hypercholesterolemia in children with liver disease. Prophylactic antibiotics are given after the Kasai procedure to prevent ascending cholangitis.

Prognosis. Untreated EHBA results in progressive cirrhosis and death in all children at a mean age of 19 months. The Kasai procedure does improve the prognosis, but it is not a cure. Biliary drainage can be achieved if the surgery is done before the intrahepatic bile ducts are destroyed, usually by 8 weeks of age. Long-term survival has been reported in children who received the Kasai procedure (Toyosaka et al, 1993). In spite of successful bile drainage, many children ultimately experience liver failure.

Pediatric liver disorders can be cured with successful liver transplantation. The advances in surgical techniques and the development of cyclosporine A and other antirejection drugs have significantly improved the success of transplantation. The 1- to 4-year survival rate of pediatric liver transplantation is now 70% to 88% in most centers (Ryckman et al, 1993). The major obstacle remains the shortage of donor livers. Success with segmental size reduction of adult donor livers and increased public awareness may improve the availability of donor organs for children in the future.

Nursing Care Management

Nursing care of the infant with biliary atresia is primarily supportive. Initially the infant is not uncomfortable and requires care suited to any infant of the same age. As the disease progresses, the accumulation of toxic products causes the child to become irritable, restless, and difficult to comfort. Efforts are extended to allow as much sleep and rest as possible. The child is cared for when he or she awakes and is provided with comfort measures.

During the diagnostic phase of the illness the nurse assists with tests and procedures as ordered. The child who has undergone exploratory or corrective surgery is given the same care as any infant who has had abdominal surgery. Parental teaching includes administration of antibiotics and observation for signs of cholangitis. Families of children with liver disease can get help from the Children's Liver Foundation,* which provides educational materials, programs, and support systems for these families, who require special psychosocial support. The uncertain prognosis, discomfort, and waiting for transplantation can all produce considerable stress. In addition, as with any chronic illness, extended hospitalizations plus pharmacologic and nutritional therapy can impose significant financial burdens on the family. Parent support groups can be very helpful.

Early recognition and monitoring of the clinical signs of biliary disease are important nursing responsibilities. Nutritional support is an important task for the nurse and family. In cases of severe malnutrition and malabsorption, continuous nasogastric feedings or parenteral nutrition may be needed. The family should be educated about the purpose of these therapies and prepared to continue nutritional support at home if indicated.

*76 South Orange Ave., Suite 202, South Orange, NJ 07079.

Structural Defects

CLEFT LIP (CL) AND/OR CLEFT PALATE (CP)

Clefts of the lip and palate are facial malformations that occur during embryonic development, are common to all human populations, and can constitute a severe disability to the affected individual. They may appear separately or, more commonly, together. CL results from failure of the maxillary and median nasal processes to fuse; CP is a midline fissure of the palate that results from failure of the two sides to fuse. This discussion is concerned primarily with cleft lip and palate (CL/P).

CL may vary from a small notch to a complete cleft extending into the base of the nose (Fig. 44-4). Clefts can be unilateral or bilateral. Deformed dental structures are associated with CL. CP alone occurs in the midline and may involve the soft and hard palates. When associated with CL, the defect may involve the midline and extend into the soft palate on one or both sides.

The incidence of CL with or without CP is approximately 1 in 800 live births. The incidence of CP alone is 1 in 2000 live births. CL with or without CP is more common in males, and CP alone is more common in females. The defect appears more often in Orientals and certain tribes of Native Americans than in whites and less frequently in blacks.

Etiology

The majority of cases appear to be consistent with the concept of multifactorial inheritance, as evidenced by an increased incidence in relatives and a higher concordance in monozygotic twins than in dizygotic twins. Many recognized syndromes include these defects as a feature and are the result of chromosomal abnormalities; environmental factors or teratogens may be responsible for clefts at a critical point in embryonic development.

Pathophysiology

CL/P results from failure of the maxillary and premaxillary processes to come in contact during early embryonic life. Although often appearing together, CL and CP are distinct malformations embryologically, occurring at different times during the developmental process. Merging of the upper lip at the midline is completed between the seventh and eighth weeks of gestation. Fusion of the secondary palate (hard and soft palate) takes place later in development, between the seventh and twelfth weeks of gestation. In the process of migrating to a horizontal position they are, for a short time, separated by the tongue.

If there is delay in this movement or if the tongue fails to descend soon enough, the remainder of development proceeds but the palate never fuses.

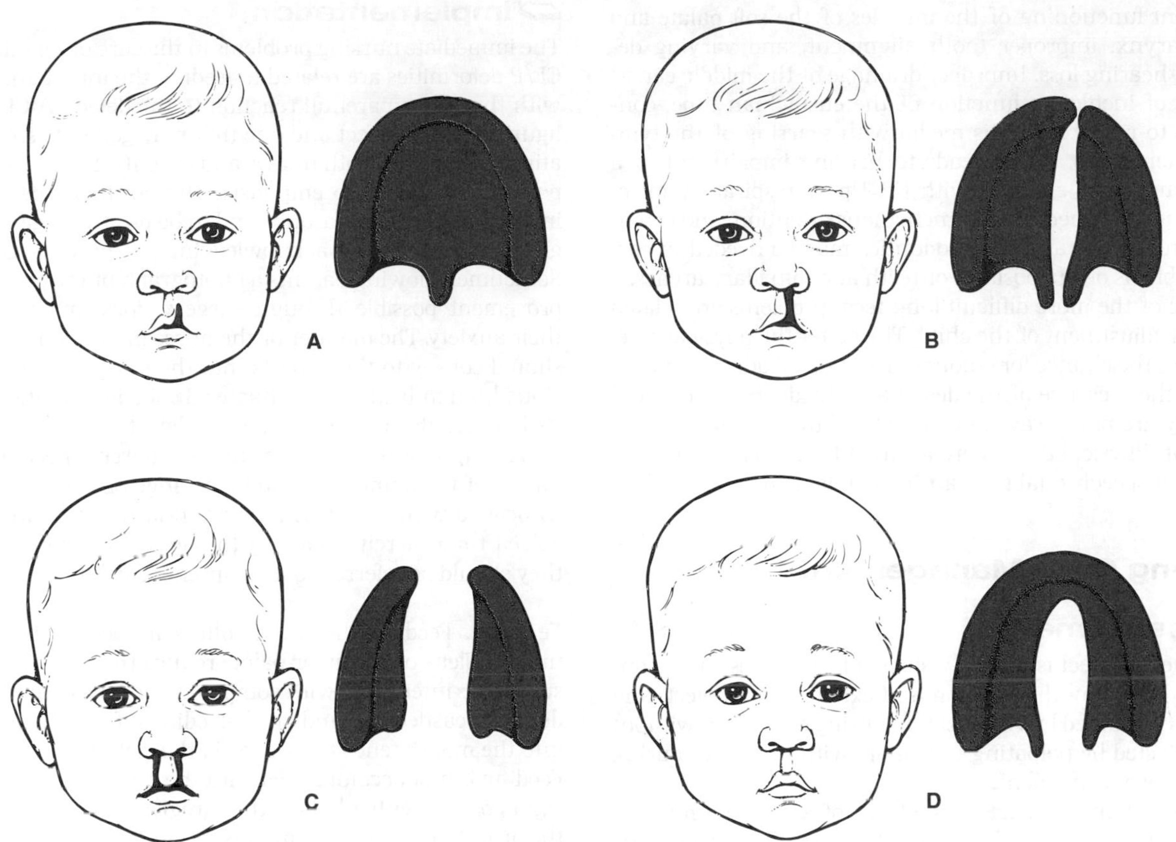

Fig. 44-4 Variations in clefts of lip and palate at birth. **A,** Notch in vermilion border. **B,** Unilateral cleft lip and palate. **C,** Bilateral cleft lip and palate. **D,** Cleft palate.

Diagnostic Evaluation

CL with or without CP is readily apparent at birth and is a defect that elicits severe emotional reactions in parents. Varying degrees of nasal distortion usually accompany CL with or without CP. CP may occur as an isolated defect or in association with CL. Less obvious than CL, the defect may not be detected without a thorough assessment of the mouth. The deformity can be identified by placing the examiner's fingers directly on the palate. Clefts of the hard palate form a continuous opening between the mouth and the nasal cavity. The severity of the CP has an impact on feeding; the infant is unable to generate negative pressure and create suction in the oral cavity. This impairs feeding even though in most cases the infant's ability to swallow is normal.

Therapeutic Management

Treatment of the child with CL/P involves the collaborative efforts of a number of specialists—pediatrician, nurses, plastic surgeon, orthodontist, prosthodontist, otolaryngologist, speech therapist, and, sometimes, a mental health professional. Medical management is directed toward closure of the cleft(s), prevention of complications, and facilitation of normal growth and development of the child.

Surgical correction: CL. Closure of the lip defect precedes that of the palate, usually at 6 to 12 weeks of age. Surgical correction is performed when the infant is free of any oral, respiratory, or systemic infection. The method of repair of the CL involves one of several staggered suture lines (Z-plasty) to minimize notching of the lip from retraction of scar tissue.

Immediately after surgery the suture line is protected from tension and trauma by a thin, arched metal device (the Logan bow) taped to the cheeks or by a butterfly-type adhesive restraint, and the arms are restrained at the elbows to prevent the infant from rubbing the incision with the hands. In the absence of infection or trauma, healing takes place with little scar formation.

Surgical correction: CP. CP repair is generally postponed until the infant is 12 to 18 months of age in order to take advantage of palatal changes that take place with normal growth. Most surgeons prefer to close the cleft at this time, before the child develops faulty speech habits.

Prognosis. Even with good anatomic closure the majority of children with CL/P have some degree of speech impairment that requires speech therapy. Physical problems result from inefficient functioning of the muscles of the soft palate and nasopharynx, improper tooth alignment, and varying degrees of hearing loss. Improper drainage of the middle ear, as a result of inefficient function of the eustachian tube, contributes to recurrent otitis media with scarring of the tympanic membrane, which leads to hearing impairment in a large number of children with CP. Upper respiratory infections require immediate and meticulous attention, and extensive orthodontics and prosthodontics may be needed to correct problems of malposition of teeth and maxillary arches.

Some of the more difficult long-term problems are related to social adjustment of the child. The better the physical care, the better the chance for emotional and social adjustment, although the presence of the defect and the degree of residual disability are not always directly related to a satisfactory adjustment. Physical defects are a threat to the self-image, and abnormal speech quality is an impediment to social expression.

Nursing Care Management

Assessment

Since the lip defect is readily visible at birth, assessment consists of describing the location and extent of the defect, and the CP is estimated by visualization during crying. CP without CL is detected by palpating the palate with the finger during the newborn assessment.

The emotional impact of the birth of a child with a cosmetic, as well as a functional, disability is especially traumatic to the family. Consequently the nursing assessment is also concerned with the emotional reaction of the family to the child and the defect.

Nursing Diagnoses

On the basis of a thorough physical assessment a number of nursing diagnoses are evident. These are described in the Nursing Care Plan on p. 1423.

Planning

The goals of care for the infant with CL and CP are related to preoperative care, short-term postoperative care, and long-term management. The major goals of care for the infant and family include the following:

Preoperative care

1. Family will cope with the impact of an infant with a defect.
2. Infant will receive optimum nutrition.
3. Infant will be prepared for surgery.

Postoperative care

1. Infant will experience no trauma and minimal or no pain.
2. Infant will receive optimum nutrition.
3. Infant will experience no complications.
4. Infant and family will receive adequate support.
5. Family will be prepared for care at home and long-term needs of a child with CP.

Implementation

The immediate nursing problems in the care of an infant with CL/P deformities are related to feeding the infant and dealing with the severe parental reaction to the defect. A CL is a disfiguring visible defect and one that may generate strong negative responses in both nurses and parents. It is especially important for nurses to emphasize the positive aspects of the infant's physical appearance and to be positive regarding surgical correction after acknowledging the parents' concerns. Sometimes showing parents a photograph of the cosmetic improvement possible through surgery does much to relieve their anxiety. The manner of the nurse in handling the infant should convey to the parents that the infant is indeed a precious human being. (See Chapter 38 for interventions in assisting parents in accepting a birth defect.)

Throughout the course of therapy parents need an explanation of the immediate and long-range problems frequently associated with CP. Often they are unaware that more is involved than merely repairing the defect. Whenever possible they should be referred to a comprehensive CP team.

Feeding. Feeding the infant offers a special challenge to nurses. Clefts of the lip or palate reduce the infant's ability to suck, thus interfering with compression of the areola and rendering breastfeeding and bottle-feeding difficult. Liquid taken into the mouth tends to escape via the cleft through the nose. Feeding is best accomplished with the infant's head in an upright position, either held in the caregiver's hand or cradled in the arm. Normal nipples are unsuitable for these infants, who are unable to generate the suction required; therefore special nipples or other feeding devices are needed. A variety of special "cleft palate" nipples have been devised and used with some success. However, large, soft nipples with large holes; Nursettes; or the long, soft lamb's nipples appear to offer the best means for nipple feeding (Fig. 44-5). The newer "gravity flow" nipple* attached to a squeezable plastic bottle allows formula to be deposited directly into the mouth in much the same manner as with a bulb syringe. Success has also been achieved by the modification of a standard nipple. A single small slit or cross-cut is made in the end of the nipple with a sharp surgical blade or a pair of scissors with sharp, thin blades. This allows the infant to swallow the formula easily, thereby bypassing the suction problem (Richard, 1991). The size of the slit is adjusted to the needs of the infant.

Using these various types of nipples for feeding also has the advantage of helping to meet the infant's sucking needs. Muscle development is especially important for later development of speech. The nipple is positioned in such a way that it is compressed by the infant's tongue and existing palate. If a single-slit nipple is used, the slit is placed vertically so that the infant will be able to produce and stop a flow of milk by alternately opening and closing the opening. No matter which type of nipple is used, gentle, steady pressure on the base of the bottle reduces the chance of choking or coughing, and the person feeding should resist the temptation to remove the nipple because of the noise the infant makes or for fear that the infant will choke. Since these infants have a tendency to swallow excessive amounts of air, they require frequent burping.

*Ross Laboratories, Columbus, OH 43216.

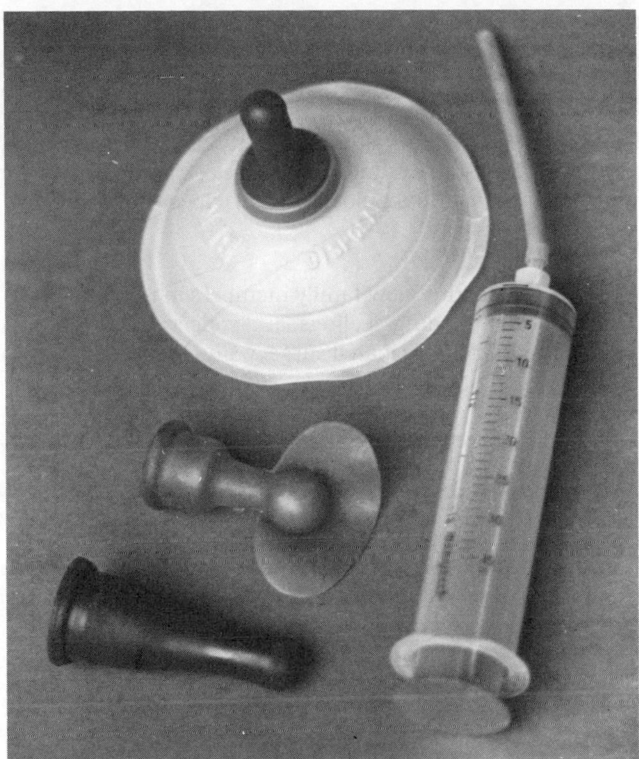

Fig. 44-5 Some devices used to feed an infant with a cleft lip and palate. *Counterclockwise:* Lamb's nipple, flanged nipple, special nurser, and syringe with rubber tubing (Breck feeder).

When the infant has trouble with nipple feeding, a rubber-tipped medicine dropper, Asepto syringe, or Breck feeder (a large syringe with soft rubber tubing) often provides an efficient, safe feeding device. The rubber extension should be sufficiently long to extend well back into the mouth to reduce the likelihood of regurgitation through the nose. The formula is deposited on the back of the tongue and the flow controlled by bulb or syringe compression that is adjusted to the infant's needs. For some infants spoon feeding works best, especially if the formula is slightly thickened with cereal. After feeding, the infant is given water to rinse the mouth.

Breastfeeding is also an option. The nipple is positioned and stabilized well back in the oral cavity so that tongue action facilitates milk expression. However, the suction required to stimulate milk may be absent initially; therefore a breast pump may be useful before nursing to stimulate the let-down reflex.

Regardless of the feeding method used, the mother should begin to feed the infant as soon as possible, preferably after the initial nursery feeding. In this way she is able to help determine the method best suited to her and the infant and to become adept in the technique before they are discharged from the hospital.

Preoperative care. In preparation for surgical repair the parent is frequently instructed to accustom the infant to some of the needs of the early postoperative period, particularly if surgery is delayed for several months. Since it is mandatory for the infant to be positioned on the back or side postoperatively, it is helpful to train the infant to lie in these positions a great deal of the time to reduce the irritability and resistance associated with any change in routine. It is also helpful to place the infant or child in arm restraints periodically prior to admission and, after admission, to feed him or her with a rubber-tipped Asepto syringe or other device in the manner to be used postoperatively.

Postoperative care: CL. The major efforts in the postoperative period are directed to protecting the operative site. After CL repair *(cheiloplasty)*, a metal appliance or adhesive strips are securely taped to the cheeks to relax the operative site and prevent tension on the suture line caused by crying or other facial movement. Elbow restraints are needed to prevent the infant from rubbing or otherwise disturbing the suture line and are usually applied immediately after surgery. It is advisable to pin the cuff of the restraints to the infant's clothing to keep the restraints in place. The older infant who is able to roll over will require a jacket restraint in addition to restricting arm movement to prevent rolling on the abdomen and rubbing the face on the sheet, especially if the repair involves the lip. It is important to remove the restraints periodically to exercise the arms, to provide relief from restrictions, and to observe the skin for signs of irritation. It is advisable to release the restraints one at a time, especially in a very vigorous, active infant. Removing restraints also offers an opportunity for cuddling and body contact. Sitting the infant in an infant seat provides a change of position and a different perspective of the environment. Sedation and appropriate analgesic medication are sometimes needed for a very restless, anxious infant. Rooming-in is always encouraged because preserving parent contact greatly increases the child's comfort.

Clear liquids are offered when the infant has fully recovered from the anesthesia, and formula feeding is usually resumed when tolerated. The Breck feeder is preferred in most cases. Care is taken to slip the rubber tip in from the side of the mouth to avoid the operative area and to prevent the infant from sucking on the tubing. This method is continued until the lip is well healed, after which bottle-feeding can be resumed if it has been the infant's mode of feeding. The mouth is rinsed with water after each feeding. The suture site is carefully cleansed of formula or serosanguineous drainage as needed with a cotton-tipped swab dipped in saline solution. A thin layer of antibiotic ointment is then applied to the suture line. Meticulous care of the suture line is a nursing responsibility, since inflammation or sloughing will interfere with optimal healing and the ultimate cosmetic effect of the surgical repair.

Gentle aspiration of mouth and nasopharyngeal secretions may be necessary to prevent aspiration and respiratory complications. An upright or infant seat position is helpful for the infant in the immediate postoperative period and for one who has difficulty in handling secretions.

Postoperative care: CP. The child with a cleft palate repair *(palatoplasty)* is allowed to lie on the abdomen, especially immediately postoperatively. Fluids are best taken from a cup. Young children are not given a pacifier and children old enough to understand are cautioned against rubbing the tongue against the roof of the mouth. A blenderized diet is given postoperatively.

Nursing ALERT

Avoid the use of suction or other objects in the mouth, such as tongue depressors, thermometers, spoons, or straws.

Usually oral packing is secured to the palate after palatoplasty and is left in place for 2 to 3 days. As with cleft lip repair the elbows are immobilized to keep the hands away from the mouth, and the parents are instructed to continue this precaution at home until the palate is healed. They are instructed to remove the restraints (usually one at a time) at frequent intervals to allow the child to exercise the arms. It is important to stress that the child should be closely supervised during this time.

The child is generally discharged on a blenderized or soft diet, which parents are instructed to continue until the surgeon directs them otherwise. They are cautioned against allowing the child to eat hard items such as toast, hard cookies, and potato chips, which can damage the newly repaired palate. The nurse might suggest that the parents not offer the child any food harder than mashed potatoes.

Occasionally the child will have difficulty in breathing after surgery, especially the child with CP repair who must alter an established pattern of breathing and adjust to breathing through the nose. This is frustrating but seldom requires more than positioning and support. Sometimes the infant or child is placed in a mist tent for a short period after surgery.

The infant or child should be assessed for pain postoperatively. Opioids may be prescribed for the first 24 hours or more postoperatively and acetaminophen with or without codeine thereafter.

Long-term care. Children with CL/P often require a variety of services during the process of recovery. Secondary palate surgery may be required, including a pharyngeal flap procedure or palate bone grafting. Families of these children need support and encouragement by health professionals and guidance in activities that facilitate the most normal outcome for their children. With the combined efforts of the family and the health team the majority of these children achieve a satisfactory outcome. Many children with CL/P have surgical correction that creates a near-normal-appearing lip and permits good function. Parents need to understand the function of therapy and the purpose and care of any appliance, as well as the importance of establishing good mouth care and proper brushing habits.

Throughout the child's development an important goal is the development of a healthy personality and self-esteem. Many local areas have CP parents' groups who offer help and support to families. Several agencies provide services and information for children with CL/P and their families. These include the American Cleft Palate Association and the Cleft Palate Foundation,* the March of Dimes—Birth Defects Foundation,* and state Program for Children with Special Health Needs (formerly Crippled Children's Services).

Evaluation

The effectiveness of nursing interventions is determined by continual reassessment and evaluation of care based on the following observational guidelines and expected outcomes:

Preoperative care

1. Observe and interview family members in relation to their understanding, feelings, and concerns regarding the defect and anticipated surgery, and the interactions with the infant.
2. Observe infant during feeding.
3. Complete preoperative checklist.

Postoperative care

1. Inspect operative site, including the protective device.
2. Observe for behavioral and physiologic indicators of pain and response to analgesics.
3. Observe infant during feeding, measure intake and output, and weigh infant daily.
4. Observe operative site for evidence of infection, bleeding, sloughing, or irritation.
5. Observe and interview family regarding their understanding and concerns about the infant, including long-term needs.

Expected outcomes:

See the Nursing Care Plan on p. 1423.

ESOPHAGEAL ATRESIA (EA) AND TRACHEOESOPHAGEAL FISTULA (TEF)

Congenital atresia of the esophagus and TEF are rare malformations that represent a failure of the esophagus to develop as a continuous passage. These defects may occur as separate entities or in combination (Fig. 44-6) and without early diagnosis and treatment are rapidly fatal.

Etiology

The cause of EA and TEF is not known. The incidence has been estimated to be from 1 in 3000 to 1 in 3500 live births. There appears to be an equal sex incidence, but the birth weight of most affected infants is significantly lower than average and there is an unusually high incidence of prematurity in infants with EA. Other congenital anomalies occur frequently. *VATER syndrome* is the combination of vertebral, anorectal, and renal anomalies in addition to TEF.

Pathophysiology

The most commonly encountered form of EA and TEF (80% to 95% of cases) is one in which the proximal esophageal segment terminates in a blind pouch and the distal segment is connected to the trachea or primary bronchus by a short fistula at or near the bifurcation (Fig. 44-6, *C*). The second most common variety (5% to 8%) consists of a blind pouch at each end, widely separated and with no communication to the tra-

*1218 Grandview Ave., Pittsburgh, PA 15211; (800) 24-CLEFT or (412) 418-1376.

*1275 Mamaroneck Ave., White Plains, NY 10605; (914) 428-7100. In Canada: **Canadian Cleft Lip and Palate Family Association,** 170 Elizabeth St., Toronto, Ontario, Canada M5G 1E8; and **Aboutface,** 123 Edward St., Suite 1405, Toronto, Ontario, Canada M5G 1E2, (416) 928-0888.

Nursing Care Plan

CHILD WITH CLEFT LIP AND/OR PALATE

Nursing Diagnosis: Altered nutrition less than body requirements, related to physical defect of oral cavity

Expected Outcome: Patient exhibits signs of adequate nutritional intake (i.e., appropriate weight gain).

• NURSING INTERVENTIONS/*RATIONALES*

Administer diet appropriate for age and nutritional needs *to ensure adequate nutritional content.*

If infant is breastfeeding, teach mother to stimulate let-down reflex prior to feeding with a breast pump or manually *as required suction from infant may be lacking.*

Have mother position and stabilize nipple well back in infant's oral cavity against existing palate *to facilitate expression of milk.*

Hold child in upright position to feed *to prevent aspiration* and burp frequently *as infant takes in excess amounts of air.*

If child is unable to maintain adequate suction on a nipple, try using alternative feeding appliances (i.e., Breck feeder, Aesepto syringe) *to facilitate feeding.*

Postoperatively, administer prescribed intravenous fluids *to ensure adequate hydration.*

Maintain feeding records and weigh regularly *to assess adequacy of intake.*

Nursing Diagnosis: Potential for altered parenting related to having child with highly visible physical defect

Expected Outcome: Parents demonstrate acceptance of the infant.

• NURSING INTERVENTIONS/*RATIONALES*

Allow parents to express feelings, fears *to facilitate coping.*

Convey attitudes and behaviors of acceptance of infant *to serve as a role model for parents.*

Describe results of surgical correction of defect with photos of satisfactory results *to alleviate fears of the unknown and foster hope.*

Arrange for parents to meet with others who have experienced and successfully coped with similar situations *to provide ongoing support.*

Nursing Diagnosis: Risk for trauma of surgical site related to position of site

Expected Outcome: Operative site is undamaged.

• NURSING INTERVENTIONS/*RATIONALES*

For cleft lip repair, use a lip protective device; position on back or side *to protect suture line.*

For cleft palate repair, prevent sustained crying, placement of objects in mouth *to protect suture line.*

Restrain infant at elbows *to prevent access to operative site;* use jacket restraints on older infants *to prevent rolling onto abdomen and rubbing of suture line on bedding.*

Cleanse suture line after feeding *to reduce presence of foreign materials that may irritate suture line.*

Teach restraint and cleansing techniques to parents *to minimize complications after discharge.*

Nursing Diagnosis: Pain related to surgical procedure

Expected Outcome: Infant is resting comfortably.

• NURSING INTERVENTIONS/*RATIONALES*

Administer pain medications per physician order *to prevent or minimize pain.*

Remove restraints periodically under careful supervision *to exercise arms and provide relief from restrictions.*

Monitor vital signs and behavior *for evidence of pain or discomfort.*

See also the Nursing Care Plan: Child Undergoing Surgery, p. 1260.

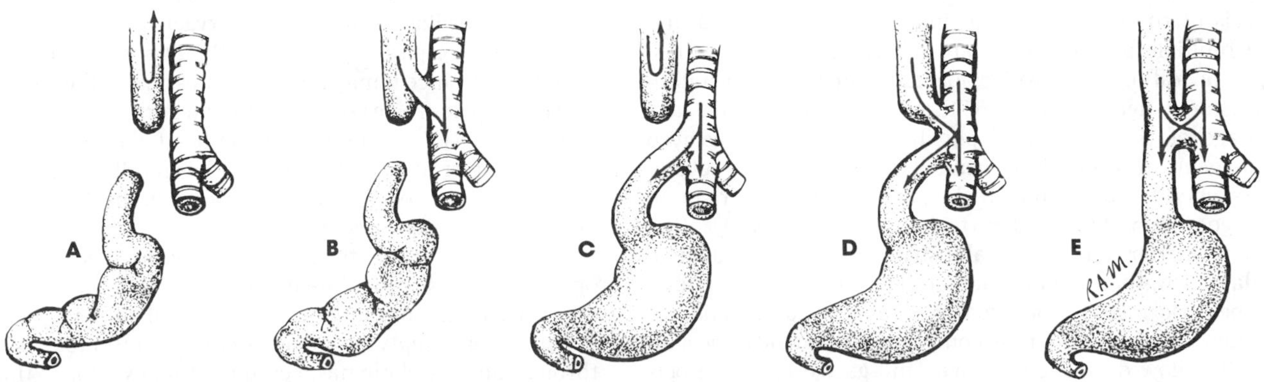

Fig. 44-6 Five most common types of esophageal atresia and tracheoesophageal fistula.

BOX 44-17
Clinical Manifestations of Tracheoesophageal Fistula

Excessive salivation and drooling
Three Cs of TEF:
- Coughing
- Choking
- Cyanosis

Apnea
Increased respiratory distress after feeding
Abdominal distention

chea (Fig. 44-6, *A*). Less frequently an otherwise normal trachea and esophagus are connected by a common fistula (Fig. 44-6, *E*). Extremely rare anomalies involve a fistula from the trachea to the upper esophageal segment (Fig. 44-6, *B*) or to both the upper and lower segments (Fig. 44-6, *D*).

Diagnostic Evaluation

The disorder is suspected on the basis of clinical manifestations (Box 44-17). Although the diagnosis is established on the basis of clinical signs and symptoms, the exact type of anomaly is determined by radiographic studies. A radiopaque catheter is inserted into the hypopharynx and advanced until it encounters an obstruction. Chest films are taken to ascertain esophageal patency or the presence and level of a blind pouch. Sometimes fistulas are not patent, making their presence more difficult to diagnose. Complete absence of air in the GI tract indicates EA without TEF.

Therapeutic Management

The treatment of EA and TEF consists of prevention of pneumonia and surgical repair of the anomaly. When a TEF is suspected, the infant is immediately deprived of oral intake, started on intravenous fluids, and placed in the position least likely to cause aspiration of either mouth or stomach secretions. Removal of secretions from the mouth and upper pouch requires frequent or continuous suction. Since aspiration pneumonia is almost inevitable and appears early, broad-spectrum antibiotic therapy is instituted.

Primary surgical correction consists of a thoracotomy with division and ligation of the TEF and an end-to-end anastomosis of the esophagus. For infants who are premature, have multiple anomalies, or are in very poor condition, a staged operation that involves palliative measures including gastrostomy, ligation of the TEF, and provision of constant drainage of the esophageal pouch is preferred. A delayed esophageal anastomosis is usually attempted after several weeks when the upper pouch elongates and the lower pouch undergoes hypertrophy. The technique of *bougienage* (the process whereby a blunt metal instrument is used to dilate a fistula or lengthen membranous tissue) of the upper pouch may be performed to elongate this segment. If an esophageal anastomosis still cannot be accomplished, a *cervical esophagostomy* (to allow drainage of saliva) and gastrostomy are performed.

There are rare instances in which a primary anastomosis cannot be accomplished because of insufficient length of the two segments of esophagus. In these cases the defect must be bridged with a colon interposition, gastric tube, or gastric interposition procedure. This esophageal replacement is usually deferred until the child is 16 to 24 months old. Endotracheal intubation may be required, since many of these infants may also have *tracheomalacia*, a weakness in the tracheal wall that occurs when a dilated proximal pouch compresses the trachea from early in fetal life or when the trachea does not develop normally because of a loss of intratracheal pressure.

Complications of a primary repair include an anastomotic leak, strictures caused by tension or ischemia, esophageal motility disorders causing dysphagia, and gastroesophageal reflux. Motility disorders are common after EA or TEF repair.

Prognosis. The prognosis for infants with EA or TEF is related to the birth weight, associated congenital anomalies, and time of diagnosis. The survival rate is nearly 100% in full-term infants without severe respiratory distress or other anomalies. In premature low-birth-weight infants with associated anomalies the incidence of complications is high. The overall mortality rate is 10% to 15% (Wright, 1991).

Nursing Care Management

Nursing responsibility for detection of this serious malformation begins *immediately* after birth. Ideally the condition is diagnosed before the initial feeding, but often it is not. If fed, the infant swallows normally but suddenly coughs and struggles, and the fluid is aspirated or returns through the nose and mouth. For this reason it is customary for the nurse to give the infant the first feeding of plain water or to be present when a parent feeds the child in order to observe the infant's response.

Nursing ALERT

Any infant who has an excessive amount of frothy saliva in the mouth or difficulty with secretions and unexplained episodes of cyanosis should be suspected of having a TEF.

Cyanosis is usually the result of laryngospasm caused by overflow of saliva into the larynx from the proximal esophageal pouch, and it normally clears after removal of the secretions from the oropharynx by suctioning. Any such suspicion is reported immediately. The infant is placed in an incubator or under a radiant warmer, and oxygen is administered to help relieve respiratory distress. Positive pressure is contraindicated, since it may add to air pressure in the stomach.

The most desirable position for a newborn who is suspected of having a TEF is supine with the head elevated on an inclined plane of at least 30 degrees. This positioning serves to minimize the reflux of gastric secretions up the distal esophagus into the trachea and bronchi.

It is imperative that the source of aspiration be removed at once. Oral fluids are withheld and the infant's fluid needs are met parenterally or via gastrostomy. Until surgery the blind pouch is kept empty by intermittent or continuous suction through an indwelling nasal catheter that extends to the end of the pouch. The catheter needs attention, since it has a tendency to become clogged with mucus. It is usually replaced daily by the physician. In the event that a staged repair is performed, the gastrostomy tube is inserted and left open so that air entering the stomach through the fistula can escape, thus minimizing the danger that gastric contents will be regurgitated into the trachea. The tube empties by gravity drainage. It is imperative that any secretions that can be a source of aspiration be removed at once.

Postoperative care. Postoperative care of these infants is essentially the same as the care of any high-risk newborn (see Nursing Care of the High-Risk Newborn and Family, Chapter 25). The infant is returned to the warm incubator, and the gastrostomy tube is returned to gravity drainage until the infant can tolerate feedings, usually by the fifth to seventh postoperative day. At this time the tube is elevated and secured at a point above the level of the stomach. This allows gastric secretions to pass to the duodenum, whereas swallowed air can escape through the open tube. If tolerated, gastrostomy feedings are continued until the esophageal anastomosis is healed, on about the tenth to fourteenth day, after which oral feedings are initiated.

The initial attempt at oral feeding must be carefully observed to make certain that the infant is able to swallow without choking. Until the infant is able to take a sufficient amount by mouth, oral intake may need to be supplemented by gastrostomy feedings or parenteral nutrition. Ordinarily infants are not discharged until they are taking oral fluids well and the gastrostomy tube has been removed. However, the infant who has undergone palliative surgery will be discharged with the gastrostomy tube in place. The nurse is responsible for making certain that the caregiver is educated and practiced in the care of the gastrostomy (see Chapter 42).*

Special problems. Upper respiratory complications are a threat to life in both the preoperative and postoperative period. In addition to pneumonia there is a constant danger of respiratory distress resulting from atelectasis, pneumothorax, and laryngeal edema. Any persistent respiratory difficulty after removal of secretions is reported to the surgeon immediately. The infant is monitored for anastomotic leaks as evidenced by purulent chest tube drainage, increased white blood cell count, and temperature instability.

In the infant awaiting esophageal replacement surgery, the catheter is removed and the upper esophageal segment is drained through a cervical esophagostomy. This is a source of annoyance, since the skin may become irritated by moisture from the continual discharge of saliva. Frequent removal of drainage and application of a layer of protective ointment are usually sufficient treatment. A dressing or ostomy appliance may need to be applied to collect the drainage. An enterostomal therapist may provide helpful guidance in the prevention and/or treatment of skin breakdown.

Meeting the oral needs of infants who are unable to suck on a bottle should not be overlooked. A pacifier offered periodically is an acceptable substitute until oral feedings are instituted. The child who has corrective surgery delayed until 16 to 24 months of age may have a different problem. Children who have not been able to go through the process of eating in the normal manner often have difficulty with this new task and require patient guidance in learning the techniques of taking food into the mouth and swallowing. It is important to provide oral desensitization therapy to minimize this problem while the child is deprived of oral feeding.

As with any congenital anomaly, parents need support in adjusting to the child's condition (see Chapter 38). One of the difficulties in TEF is the immediate transfer of the sick newborn to the intensive care unit and sometimes lengthy hospitalization. The attachment process is facilitated by encouraging parents to visit the infant, participate in his or her care where appropriate, and express their feelings regarding the infant's condition. The nurse in the intensive care unit should assume responsibility for ensuring that the parents are kept fully informed of the infant's progress.

See also the Nursing Care Plan: The Child with Esophageal Atresia and Tracheoesophageal Fistula.*

HERNIAS

A hernia is a protrusion of a portion of an organ or organs through an abnormal opening. The danger from herniation arises when the organ protruding through the opening is constricted to the extent that circulation is impaired or when the protruding organs encroach on and impair the function of other structures. A hernia that cannot be reduced easily is called an *incarcerated hernia.* A *strangulated hernia* is one in which the blood supply to the herniated organ is impaired. The herniations of concern are those that protrude through the diaphragm, the abdominal wall, or the inguinal canal (see also Genitourinary Tract Disorders/Defects, Chapter 47). The other hernias of significance to the pediatric age groups are outlined in Table 44-10.

Obstructive Disorders

Obstruction of the bowel occurs when the passage of intestinal contents is mechanically impeded by a constricted or occluded lumen or when there is interference with normal muscular contraction. The latter, commonly called *paralytic ileus,* occurs when there is motor dysfunction of the intestine. Intestinal obstruction from any cause is characterized by similar signs and symptoms (Box 44-18), although the progression may vary greatly. For example in acute conditions, such as intussusception, the clinical manifestations are apparent within a few hours of the onset of the disorder. In other conditions, such as pyloric stenosis, the signs and symptoms usually develop more gradually and can be missed in the early stages.

Mechanical obstructions may be congenital or acquired. Congenital obstructions, such as duodenal, jejunal, or ileal atresia, usually appear in the neonatal period. Malrotation, duodenal web, and Hirschsprung disease often appear after the first few weeks of life.

*Home care instructions on gastrostomy feedings and caring for a central venous catheter (for TPN) are available in Wong DL: *Wong and Whaley's clinical manual of pediatric nursing,* ed 4, St Louis, 1996, Mosby.

*In Wong DL: *Wong and Whaley's clinical manual of pediatric nursing,* ed 4, St Louis, 1996, Mosby.

TABLE 44-10 Summary outline of diaphragmatic and abdominal hernias

TYPE	MANIFESTATIONS/DIAGNOSTIC EVALUATION	MANAGEMENT
Diaphragmatic		
Through foramen of Bochdalek: protrusion of part of the abdominal organs through an opening in the diaphragm	Symptoms—mild to severe respiratory distress within a few hours after birth; tachypnea, cyanosis, dyspnea, and severe acidosis Breath sounds absent in affected area; bowel sounds may be present Vomiting, abdominal pain Rarely asymptomatic Diagnosis made by radiographic study	Therapeutic: Supportive treatment of respiratory distress and correction of acidosis; possible use of extracorporeal membrane oxygenation (ECMO) Prophylactic antibiotic administration Surgical reduction of hernia and repair of defect Nursing: Preoperative Maintain suction, oxygen, and intravenous fluids Place in semi-Fowler position Assist with diagnostic and preoperative procedures Administer medications Postoperative Carry out routine postoperative care and observation Use comfort measures Support parents since child is seriously ill
Hiatal		
Sliding: Protrusion of an abdominal structure (usually the stomach) through the esophageal hiatus	Symptoms—dysphagia, failure to thrive, vomiting, neck contortions, frequent unexplained respiratory problems, bleeding Diagnosis made by fluoroscopy	Therapeutic: Surgical repair of defect Nursing: Be alert to significant signs Carry out routine postoperative care
Abdominal		
Umbilical: Soft skin-covered protrusion of intestine and omentum through a weakness in the abdominal wall around the umbilicus	Inspection and palpation of abdomen High incidence in black infants Spontaneous closure by age 1 to 2 years	Therapeutic: No treatment of small defects Operative repair if persists to age 2 to 5 years Strangulation requires immediate attention Nursing: Discourage use of home remedies (e.g., belly bands, coins) Reassure parents
Omphalocele: Protrusion of intraabdominal viscera into the base of the umbilical cord; the sac is covered with peritoneum without skin *Gastroschisis:* Protrusion of intraabdominal contents through a defect in the abdominal wall lateral to the umbilical ring; there is never a peritoneal sac	Obvious on inspection Observation for other malformations	Therapeutic: Surgical repair of defect Preoperative Large lesions—gradual reduction of abdominal contents Prophylactic antibiotic administration Nursing (preoperative): Keep sac or viscera moist with saline-solution–soaked pads Use overhead warming unit Carry out routine care of intravenous line, nasogastric suction Give nothing by mouth Use comfort measures

HYPERTROPHIC PYLORIC STENOSIS (HPS)

HPS (obstruction at the pyloric sphincter by hypertrophy of the circular muscle of the pylorus) is one of the most common surgical disorders of early infancy. This functional anomaly is seen soon after birth with vomiting that becomes progressively more severe and projectile. It is five times more common in male infants than in female infants, affecting approximately 5 of every 1000 males and only 1 of every 1000 females. It is seen less frequently in black and Asian infants than in white infants. It is more likely to affect a full-term infant than a premature infant.

BOX 44-18
Clinical Manifestations of Mechanical/Paralytic Intestinal Obstruction

Colicky abdominal pain—from peristalsis attempting to overcome the obstruction
Abdominal distention—as a result of accumulation of gas and fluid above the level of the obstruction
Vomiting—often the earliest sign of a high obstruction; a later sign of lower obstruction (may be bilious or feculent)
Constipation and obstipation—early signs of low obstructions; later signs of higher obstructions
Dehydration—from losses of large quantities of fluid and electrolytes into the intestine
Rigid and boardlike abdomen—from increased distention
Bowel sounds—gradually diminish and cease
Respiratory distress—occurs as the diaphragm is pushed up into the pleural cavity
Shock—plasma volume diminishes as fluids and electrolytes are lost from the bloodstream into the intestinal lumen
Sepsis—caused by bacterial proliferation with invasion into the circulation

The cause of the increased size of the pyloric musculature is unknown. There is a genetic predisposition, and siblings and offspring of affected persons are at increased risk of development of HPS.

Pathophysiology

The circular muscle of the pylorus is grossly enlarged as a result of both hypertrophy (increased size) and hyperplasia (increased mass). This produces severe narrowing of the pyloric canal between the stomach and the duodenum. Consequently the lumen at this point is partially obstructed. Over time, inflammation and edema further reduce the size of the opening until the partial obstruction may progress to complete obstruction. The muscle is thickened to as much as twice its usual size—2 to 3 cm long—and is almost cartilaginous in consistency. The distal portion ends abruptly and is externally distinct and easily palpated, but the proximal end merges into the gastric antrum. The stomach is usually dilated (Fig. 44-7, *A*).

Evidence suggests that local innervation is involved in the pathogenesis. In most cases this is an isolated lesion; however, it may be associated with intestinal malrotation, esophageal and duodenal atresia, and anorectal anomalies.

Diagnostic Evaluation

The age of onset and pattern of vomiting are variable. Typically, infants with HPS are well during the first weeks of life. Initially there is only regurgitation or occasional nonprojectile vomiting that begins about the second to the fourth week after birth, although in a few infants symptoms begin at birth. Others do well for the first few weeks and then suddenly experience projectile vomiting that rapidly leads to dehydration. The projectile vomiting usually develops within a week and may lead to complete obstruction by 4 to 6 weeks. The emesis usually contains stale milk and is not bile-stained. Often these infants become dehydrated and lethargic and appear significantly malnourished.

If the diagnosis is inconclusive from the history and physical signs (Box 44-19), upper GI radiographic studies will reveal delayed gastric emptying and an elongated, threadlike pyloric channel. Ultrasound is accurate and less traumatic for diagnosis of HPS. Laboratory findings reflect the metabolic alterations created by severe depletion of both fluid and electrolytes from extensive and prolonged vomiting. There are decreased serum levels of both sodium and potassium, although these may be masked by the hemoconcentration from extracellular fluid depletion. Of greater diagnostic value are a decrease in serum chloride levels and increases in pH and bicarbonate (carbon dioxide content) characteristic of metabolic alkalosis.

Therapeutic Management

Surgical relief of the pyloric obstruction by *pyloromyotomy*, sometimes called *Fredt-Ramstedt procedure*, is the standard

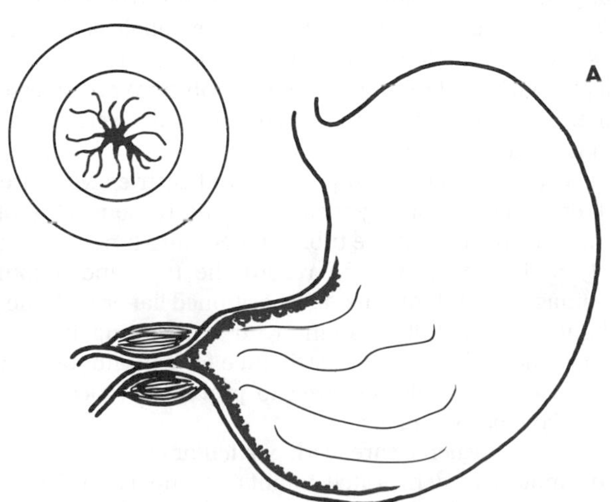

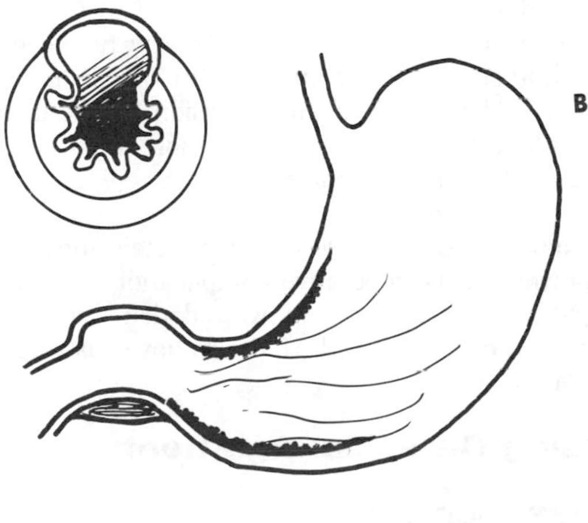

Fig. 44-7 Hypertrophic pyloric stenosis. **A,** Enlarged muscular area nearly obliterates pyloric channel. **B,** Longitudinal surgical division of muscle down to submucosa establishes adequate passageway.

BOX 44-19
Clinical Manifestations of Hypertrophic Pyloric Stenosis

Projectile vomiting
- May be ejected 3 to 4 feet from the child when in a side-lying position, 1 foot or more when in a back-lying position
- Occurs shortly after a feeding (may not occur for several hours)
- May follow each feeding or appear intermittently
- Nonbilious vomitus; may be blood-tinged

Infant hungry, avid nurser; eagerly accepts a second feeding after vomiting episode
No evidence of pain or discomfort except that of chronic hunger
Weight loss
Signs of dehydration
Distended upper abdomen
Readily palpable olive-shaped tumor in the epigastrium just to the right of the umbilicus
Visible gastric peristaltic waves that move from left to right across the epigastrium

treatment for this disorder. The surgical procedure is performed through a right upper quadrant incision (laparotomy) and consists of a longitudinal incision through the circular muscle fibers of the pylorus down to, but not including, the submucosa (Fig. 44-7, *B*). The procedure has a very high success rate when infants receive careful preoperative preparation to correct fluid and electrolyte imbalances.

Feedings are usually begun 4 to 6 hours postoperatively, beginning with small, frequent feedings of glucose water or electrolyte solutions. If clear fluids are retained, formula is started about 24 hours after surgery in the same stepwise increments, with the amount and interval between feedings gradually increased until a full feeding schedule is reinstated, usually in about 48 hours. The infant is ready to be discharged from the hospital by about the second or third postoperative day.

Recently another procedure, *laparoscopy*, has been found to be safe and successful for infants with HPS (Najmaldin and Tan, 1995.) The use of a small incision for the laparoscope may result in a shorter surgical time, more rapid postoperative feeding, and quicker discharge.

Prognosis. Most infants recover completely and rapidly after pyloromyotomy. Postoperative complications include persistent pyloric obstruction and wound dehiscence. Approximately 15% of infants with HPS also have gastroesophageal reflux (Milla, 1991).

Nursing Care Management

Assessment

HPS should be considered as a possibility in the very young infant who appears alert but fails to gain weight and has a history of vomiting after feedings. Assessment is based on observation of eating behaviors and evidence of other characteristic clinical manifestations.

BOX 44-20
Nursing Diagnoses: The Infant with Hypertrophic Pyloric Stenosis

High risk for fluid volume deficit related to persistent vomiting
Altered nutrition: less than body requirements related to persistent vomiting
Altered family processes related to hospitalization of infant

Nursing Diagnoses

On the basis of a thorough assessment, a number of nursing diagnoses are evident. The most typical are those listed in Box 44-20.

Planning

The goals of care for the child with HPS are primarily related to presurgical and postsurgical care of the infant. These include the following:

1. Child will consume sufficient amount of formula.
2. Infant will retain feedings.
3. Child will experience no complications.
4. Family will receive adequate support and education.

Implementation

Preoperatively the emphasis is placed on restoring hydration and electrolyte balance. These infants are usually given no oral feedings and receive intravenous fluids with glucose and electrolyte replacement based on laboratory serum electrolyte values. Careful monitoring of the intravenous infusion and diligent attention to intake, output, and urine-specific gravity measurements are important to the success of fluid replacement. Any vomiting, as well as the number and character of stools, is observed and recorded accurately.

Observations include assessment of vital signs, particularly those that might indicate fluid or electrolyte imbalances. These infants are especially prone to metabolic alkalosis from loss of hydrogen ions and to potassium, sodium, and chloride depletion. The skin and mucous membranes are assessed for alterations in hydration status, and daily weight provides added clues to water gain or loss.

When stomach decompression and gastric lavage are part of preoperative management, it is the responsibility of the nurse to ensure that the tube is patent and functioning properly and to measure and record the type and amount of drainage. The infant is usually positioned flat or with the head slightly elevated. The infant who is receiving intravenous fluids and/or has a nasogastric tube for continuous drainage must be adequately observed to prevent the needle and/or tube from becoming dislodged.

General hygienic care, with particular attention to the skin and mouth in dehydrated infants, is important. Protection from infection is also important, since infants with impaired nutritional status are even more susceptible than normal newborn infants. Parental involvement is encouraged and promoted.

Postoperative care. Postoperative vomiting is not uncommon, and most infants, even with successful surgery, exhibit some vomiting during the first 24 to 48 hours. Intravenous fluids are administered until the infant is taking and retaining adequate amounts by mouth. Therefore much of the same care that was instituted prior to surgery is continued postoperatively (i.e., observation of physical signs, monitoring of intravenous fluids, and careful observation and recording of intake and output). In addition, the infant is observed for responses to the stress of surgery and for evidence of pain. Appropriate analgesics are given. The nasogastric tube may be maintained after surgery for a variable length of time.

Feedings are usually instituted relatively soon, beginning with clear liquids containing glucose and electrolytes. They are offered slowly, in small amounts, and at frequent intervals as ordered by the practitioner. If the infant has been breastfed, breast milk, expressed by the mother, is given by bottle when the infant is able to tolerate feedings, and breastfeeding is resumed as soon as feasible. Observation and recording of feedings and the infant's responses to feedings and feeding techniques are vital parts of postoperative care. Positioning with the head elevated is usually continued postoperatively. Care of the operative site consists of observation for any drainage or signs of inflammation and care of the incision as directed by the surgeon.

As with any child in the hospital, parents are encouraged to remain with the child and become involved in the child's care. Vomiting of a projectile nature is frightening to parents, and they often believe that they may have done something wrong or that surgery was not successful. Most parents need support and reassurance that the condition is caused by a structural problem and is in no way a reflection on their parenting skills and capacities.

Evaluation

The effectiveness of nursing interventions is determined by reassessment based on the following observational guidelines and expected outcomes:

1. Observe feeding behavior, especially vomiting episodes.
2. Weigh infant daily.
3. Observe for evidence of complications.
4. Observe and interview family regarding feelings, understanding, and concerns.

Expected outcomes:

1. Infant will consume a sufficient amount of formula.
2. Infant will take and retain feedings.
3. Infant will recover with no evidence of complications.
4. Family members will express their feelings and concerns, demonstrate an understanding of infant's condition, and be actively involved in infant's care.

See also the Nursing Care Plan: The Child with Hypertrophic Pyloric Stenosis.*

INTUSSUSCEPTION

Intussusception is one of the most common causes of intestinal obstruction in children generally between the ages of 3 months and 5 years. Half of the cases occur in children younger than age 1 year; more commonly intussusception occurs in children between 3 and 12 months of age, and most of the other cases occur during the second year. Intussusception is twice as common in males as in females and in children with cystic fibrosis. Although specific intestinal lesions can be found in a small percentage of these children, generally the cause is not known. More than 90% of intussusceptions do not have a pathologic lead point, such as a polyp, lymphoma, or Meckel diverticulum. The idiopathic cases are most likely a result of hypertrophy of intestinal lymphoid tissue secondary to viral infection.

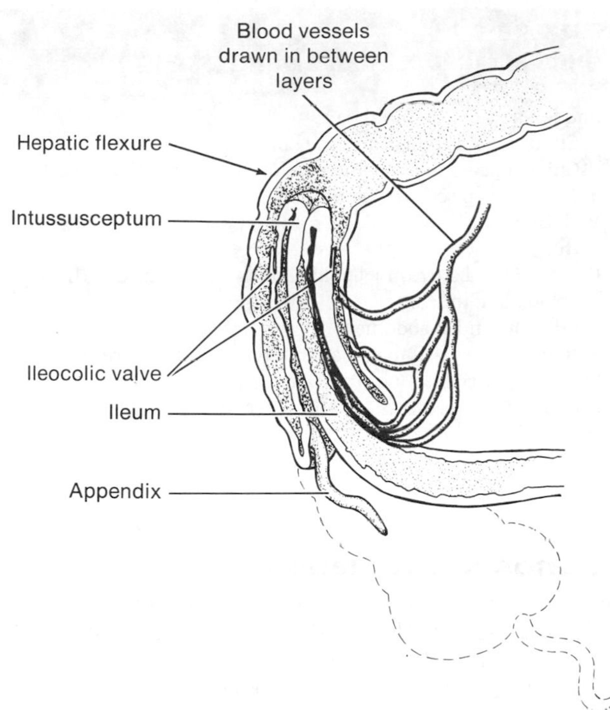

Fig. 44-8 Ileocolic intussusception.

Pathophysiology

Intussusception is an invagination or telescoping of one portion of the intestine into another. The most common site is the *ileocecal valve,* where the ileum invaginates into the cecum and colon (Fig. 44-8), producing an obstruction to the passage of intestinal contents beyond the defect. In addition, the two walls of the intestine press against each other, causing inflammation, edema, and eventually decreased blood flow. Because fecal material is unable to move beyond the obstruction, the stools primarily contain blood and mucus, resulting in the "currant jelly" stools characteristic of the disorder. Ischemia, perforation, peritonitis, and shock are serious complications of intussusception. If left untreated, this condition is incompatible with life.

Nursing ALERT

A report of severe colicky abdominal pain in a child with vomiting and currant jelly–like stools is a significant clue to intussusception.

*In Wong DL: *Wong and Whaley's clinical manual of pediatric nursing,* ed 4, St Louis, 1996, Mosby.

BOX 44-21
Clinical Manifestations of Intussusception

Sudden acute abdominal pain
- Child screams and draws the knees onto the chest
- Child appears normal and comfortable during intervals between episodes of pain

Vomiting
Lethargy
Passage of red currant jelly–like stools (stool mixed with blood and mucus)
Tender, distended abdomen
Palpable sausage-shaped mass in upper right quadrant
Empty lower right quadrant (Dance sign)
Eventual fever, prostration, and other signs of peritonitis

Diagnostic Evaluation

Frequently the diagnosis can be made on subjective findings alone (Box 44-21). The classic presentation of intussusception is a healthy, thriving child, usually between 3 and 12 months of age, who suddenly has an episode of acute abdominal pain, vomiting, bloody stool, and a palpable abdominal mass. Definitive diagnosis is based on a barium enema, which clearly demonstrates the obstruction to the flow of barium. Initially, however, an abdominal radiograph is obtained to detect intraperitoneal air, which would contraindicate a barium enema. A rectal examination reveals mucus, blood, and, occasionally, a low intussusception itself. In atypical cases lethargy may be the primary presenting symptom (Hickey, Sodhi, and Johnson, 1990).

Therapeutic Management

In most cases the initial treatment of choice is nonsurgical hydrostatic reduction by barium enema at the time of diagnostic testing. The force exerted by the flowing barium is usually sufficient to push the invaginated portion of the bowel into its original position, similarly to pushing an inverted "finger" out of a glove. This procedure is not recommended if there are clinical signs of shock or perforation. The use of barium as the contrast agent is becoming less routine. Presently a high percentage of radiologists use water-soluble contrast and air pressure to reduce intussusceptions (Meyer, 1992). Since this procedure may not always reduce the intussusception, the child is prepared for surgery. Fluid resuscitation, nasogastric decompression, and antibiotic therapy are often given before hydrostatic reduction attempts are made. Surgical intervention consists of reducing the invagination manually and, where indicated, resecting any nonviable intestine.

Prognosis. Many patients with intussusception can be successfully treated by hydrostatic reduction. Surgery is required for patients in whom the reduction was unsuccessful. If untreated, approximately 10% of children will have spontaneous reduction or chronic intussusception. The other 90% of untreated patients will worsen or die of complications such as perforation, peritonitis, and sepsis. With early diagnosis and treatment, serious complications and death are uncommon.

Nursing Care Management

The nurse can help establish a diagnosis by carefully listening to the parent's description of the child's physical and behavioral symptoms. Parents are astute in detecting that something is wrong with their child, and it is not unusual for parents to express that they felt something was seriously wrong before others shared their concerns. The description of the child's severe colicky abdominal pain combined with vomiting is a significant sign of intussusception.

As soon as a possible diagnosis of intussusception is made, the nurse begins to prepare the parents for the immediate need for hospitalization, the usual nonsurgical technique of hydrostatic reduction, and the possibility of surgery. It is important at this time to explain the basic defect of intussusception.

Since this hospitalization may be the child's first separation from the parents, it is especially important to preserve the parent-child relationship by encouraging rooming-in or extended visiting. It may also be the parents' first experience with hospital care for their child, necessitating their preparation for procedures such as intravenous therapy, frequent vital sign and blood pressure monitoring, dressings, and special orders, such as nothing by mouth. Because of the rapidity of the onset, diagnosis, and treatment, parents may be left with the feeling of stunned numbness. They may ask few questions, or they may constantly make inquiries, sometimes the same ones several times. If the nurse realizes the circumstances surrounding this condition, the parents' reactions are more likely to be understood and accepted.

Physical care of the child with intussusception differs little from that for any child undergoing abdominal surgery. Even though nonsurgical intervention may be successful, the usual preoperative procedures, such as withholding of fluids by mouth, routine laboratory testing (complete blood count and urinalysis), signed parental consent, and preanesthetic sedation, are carried out. For the child with signs of electrolyte imbalance, hemorrhage, or peritonitis, additional medical preparation such as replacement fluids, whole blood or plasma, and nasogastric suctioning may be performed. Before surgery the nurse monitors all stools.

Nursing ALERT

Passage of a normal brown stool usually indicates that the intussusception has reduced itself. This is immediately reported to the physician, who may choose to alter the diagnostic/therapeutic plan of care.

Postprocedural care includes the usual postoperative observations, such as vital signs, blood pressure, intact sutures and dressing, and return of bowel sounds. In the case of hydrostatic reduction or autoreduction the nurse observes for passage of barium or water-soluble contrast material and the stool patterns, since there may be recurrences of the intussusception. Children may be admitted to the hospital or monitored closely on an outpatient basis. A recurrence of intussusception is usually treated with hydrostatic reduction. A laparotomy is considered for multiple recurrences.

See also the Nursing Care Plan: The Child with Intussusception.*

ANORECTAL MALFORMATIONS

Malformations in the anorectal region of the GI tract are among the more common congenital malformations caused by abnormal development. The incidence is approximately 1 in 5000 live births. All are classified as *imperforate anus*. However distinguishing among these categories is important for planning therapy and determining a prognosis.

Clinically, anorectal malformations can be divided into three categories according to the relationship of the rectum to the puborectalis muscle:

Low anomalies—The rectum has descended normally through the puborectalis muscle, the internal and external sphincters are present and well developed with normal function, and there is no connection to the genitourinary tract (Fig. 44-9, *A* or *B*).

Intermediate anomalies—The rectum is at or below the level of the puborectalis muscle; the anal dimple and external sphincter are positioned normally.

High anomalies—The rectum ends above the puborectalis muscle, and there is absence of the internal sphincter. This is usually associated with a genitourinary fistula—rectourethral (male) or rectovaginal (female) (Fig. 44-9, *F*).

Cloacal exstrophy is a rare form of imperforate anus. The bowel and the bladder open into the lower abdominal wall, and the common mucosa is composed of bladder epithelium and intestinal epithelium. The genitalia are ambiguous, and most of these children are raised as females.

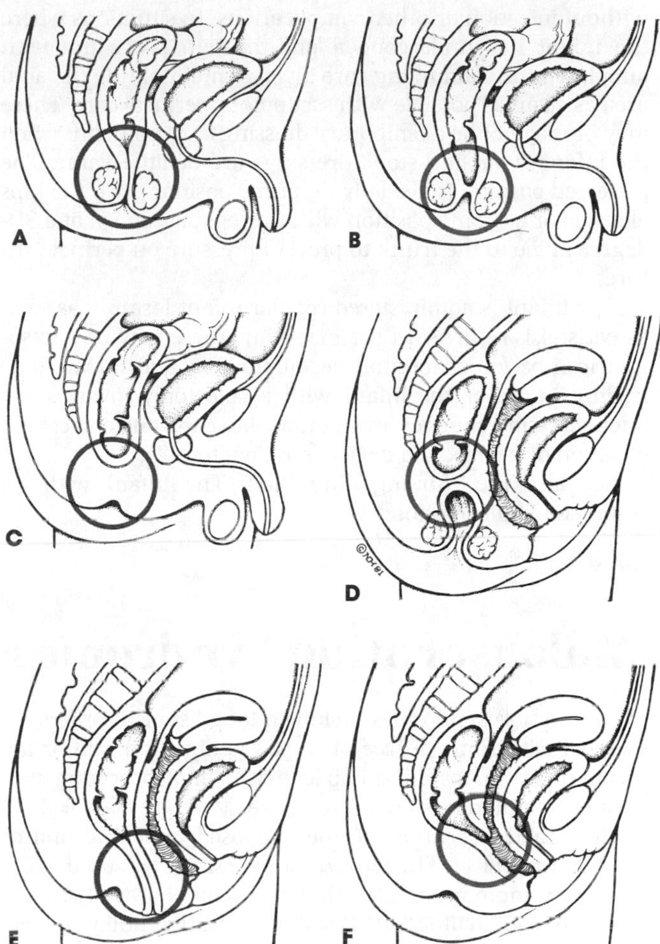

Fig. 44-9 Anorectal stenosis and imperforate anus. **A,** Congenital anal stenosis. **B,** Anal membrane atresia. **C,** Anal agenesis. **D,** Rectal atresia. **E,** Rectoperitoneal fistula. **F,** Rectovaginal fistula.

Diagnostic Evaluation

Inspection of the perineal area and checking for patency of the anus and rectum, as well as observation or inquiries regarding the passage of meconium, are a routine part of the newborn assessment. Failure to pass meconium is cause for investigation. Digital and endoscopic examinations identify constriction or the blind pouch of rectal atresia. Stenosis may not become apparent until 1 year of age or older, when the child has a history of difficult defecation, abdominal distention, and ribbonlike stools.

Fistulas associated with types B and C anomalies are not usually apparent at birth, but as peristalsis gradually forces the meconium through the fistula, they can be identified by careful examination. With a rectourinary fistula meconium appears in the urine.

Definitive diagnosis of the extent and location of the rectal pouch is made by radiographic examination. With the infant inverted and an opaque marker at the anal dimple, air ascending into the rectum and lower bowel will outline the location of the pouch in relation to the anal depression.

Therapeutic Management

Successful treatment for anal stenosis is generally accomplished by manual dilations. The procedure, begun by the physician, is repeated on a regular basis by the nurses in the hospital and is continued at home by the parents after they are carefully instructed in the technique. An imperforate anal membrane is excised and followed by daily anal dilations.

Reconstruction of an anus in the proper position is the goal of surgical treatment of other anorectal malformations. Malformations of the lower rectum often can be corrected in the neonatal period by way of simple dilation or a minor perineal operation. Infants with higher anomalies require a temporary colostomy in the newborn period. Final correction of higher defects is usually postponed for a year, when a pull-through procedure with *anorectoplasty* is performed.

Nursing Care Management

The first nursing responsibility is identification of undetected anorectal malformations. A newborn who does not pass a stool within 24 to 36 hours of birth requires further assessment, and meconium that appears at an inappropriate orifice on the perineum is reported.

Postoperative nursing care ordinarily presents few problems and is primarily directed toward healing of the anoplasty

*In Wong DL: *Wong and Whaley's clinical manual of pediatric nursing,* ed 4, St Louis, 1996, Mosby.

without infection or other complications. In situations where the infant has undergone a pull-through procedure with anoplasty, special nursing care involves maintaining the anal area as clean as possible with scrupulous perineal care. There may or may not be a temporary dressing and drain, but when the infant is passing stool, dressings are of little value. The preferred position is a side-lying prone position with the hips elevated or a supine position with the legs suspended at a 90-degree angle to the trunk to prevent pressure on perineal sutures.

The infant is administered regular infant formula as soon as peristalsis returns. In the meantime there may be a nasogastric tube for abdominal decompression and intravenous feedings. Care of the infant with a colostomy involves frequent dressing changes, meticulous skin care, and correct application of a collection device (see Chapter 42).

See also the Nursing Care Plan: The Infant with an Anorectal Malformation.*

Malabsorption Syndromes

Malabsorption syndromes include a long list of disorders associated with some degree of impaired digestion and/or absorption. An important complication of malabsorption syndromes in children is failure to thrive. Most are classified according to the location of the supposed anatomic and/or biochemical defect. The term *celiac disease* is often used to describe a symptom complex that has four characteristics in common: (1) steatorrhea (fatty, foul, frothy, bulky stools), (2) general malnutrition, (3) abdominal distention, and (4) secondary vitamin deficiencies.

Digestive defects primarily are conditions in which the enzymes necessary for digestion are diminished or absent, such as (1) cystic fibrosis, in which pancreatic enzymes are absent; (2) biliary or liver disease, in which bile flow is affected; or (3) lactase deficiency, in which there is congenital or secondary lactose intolerance.

Absorptive defects are conditions in which the intestinal mucosal transport system is impaired. It may be caused by a primary defect (such as in celiac disease) or secondary to inflammatory disease of the bowel that results in impaired absorption because bowel motility is accelerated (such as ulcerative colitis). Obstructive disorders (such as Hirschsprung disease) can also cause secondary malabsorption from enterocolitis.

Anatomic defects, such as extensive resection of the bowel or "short bowel syndrome," affect digestion by decreasing the transit time of substances and affect absorption by severely compromising the absorptive surface.

CELIAC DISEASE (CD)

CD, also known as gluten-induced enteropathy, gluten-sensitive enteropathy (GSE), and celiac sprue, is second only to cystic fibrosis as a cause of malabsorption in children. The incidence is highly variable, being reported as 1 in 300 to 1 in 4000, and appears to be declining—possibly in relation to environmental factors. It is seen more frequently in Europe than in America and is rarely reported in Asians or blacks. The exact cause of CD is not known, but there appears to be an inherited predisposition with an influence by environmental factors.

*In Wong DL: *Wong and Whaley's clinical manual of pediatric nursing,* ed 4, St Louis, 1996, Mosby.

Pathophysiology

The disease is characterized by an intolerance for *gluten,* one of the proteins found in wheat, barley, rye, and oats. Gluten consists of two factions: glutenin and gliadin. Although the pathologic process is still obscure, susceptible individuals are unable to digest the gliadin faction, resulting in an accumulation of a toxic substance that is damaging to the mucosal cells. Eventually villi atrophy, reducing the absorptive surface of the small intestine. There are two main theories regarding the damaging effect of gluten in CD: (1) the biochemical theory that there is a specific enzyme deficiency and (2) the theory that the primary cause of the disease is an immunologic abnormality (Walker-Smith, 1991).

Diagnostic Evaluation

Symptoms of CD are first noted about 3 to 6 months after the introduction of gluten-containing grains into the diet, typically at 9 to 18 months of age, although it may not be evident until early childhood (Box 44-22). The clinical manifestations are usually insidious and chronic. The first evidence of the disease may be failure to thrive and diarrhea.

A definitive diagnosis is based on a jejunal biopsy, which demonstrates the atrophic changes in the mucosa of the small intestine. This procedure is performed by passing an endoscope through the mouth along the alimentary tract to the jejunum.

BOX 44-22
Clinical Manifestations of Celiac Disease

Impaired fat absorption

Steatorrhea (excessively large, pale, oily, frothy stools)
Exceedingly foul smelling stools

Impaired absorption of nutrients

Malnutrition
Muscle wasting (especially prominent in legs and buttocks)
Anemia
Anorexia
Abdominal distention

Behavioral changes

Irritability
Fretfulness
Uncooperativeness
Apathy

Celiac Crisis*

Acute, severe episodes of profuse watery diarrhea and vomiting
May be precipitated by:
- Infections (especially gastrointestinal)
- Prolonged fluid and electrolyte depletion
- Emotional disturbance

*In very young children.

Another essential criterion of diagnosis is dramatic clinical improvement after adherence to a gluten-free diet. Within a day or two after instituting the diet, most children with CD demonstrate a favorable personality change. Weight gain, improved appetite, and disappearance of diarrhea and steatorrhea usually do not occur for several days or weeks. Diagnostic criteria for CD also usually include a histologic and/or clinical relapse after gluten reintroduction.

Therapeutic Management

Treatment of chronic CD is primarily dietary management. Although the diet is called "gluten-free," it is in reality low in gluten, since it is impossible to remove every source of this protein. Also, studies demonstrate that most patients are able to tolerate restricted amounts of gluten. Because gluten is found primarily in the grains of wheat and rye, but also in smaller quantities in barley and oats, these four foods are eliminated. Corn and rice become substitute grain foods.

In children with severe malnutrition, specific deficiencies may be treated with supplemental vitamins, iron, and calories.

Prognosis. CD is generally regarded as a chronic disease. The extent of the disease varies a great deal among children. The most severe symptoms usually occur in early childhood and again in adult life. Strict dietary avoidance of gluten can prevent symptoms and may minimize the risk of development of lymphoma, one of the most serious complications of the disease.

Nursing Care Management

The main nursing consideration is helping the parents and child adhere to the prescribed diet. A considerable amount of time is involved in explaining the disease process, the specific role of gluten in aggravating the pathologic condition, and those foods that must be restricted. Although the chief source of grain is cereal and baked goods, grains are frequently added to processed foods as thickeners or fillers. To add to the difficulty, gluten is added to many foods but is obscurely listed on the label as "hydrolyzed vegetable protein." The nurse must advise parents to read all ingredients on labels carefully in order to avoid hidden sources of gluten. Many of the gluten-containing products can be eliminated from the infant's or young child's diet fairly easily, but monitoring the diet of a school-age child or adolescent is a much more difficult situation. Many favorite foods, such as hot dogs, pizza, and spaghetti, are chief offenders. Luncheon preparation away from home is particularly difficult, since bread, luncheon meats, and instant soups are not allowed.

In addition to restricting gluten, other dietary alterations may be necessary in the beginning. For example in some children who have more severe mucosal damage, the digestion of disaccharides is impaired, especially in relation to lactose. Therefore these children often need a temporary lactose-free diet, which necessitates eliminating all milk products.

Generally management includes a diet high in calories and proteins, with simple carbohydrates, such as fruits and vegetables, but low in fats. Since the bowel is usually inflamed as a result of the pathologic processes in absorption, high-fiber foods, such as nuts, raisins, raw vegetables, and raw fruits with skin, are avoided until inflammation has subsided.

It is frequently recommended that the child continue the diet indefinitely. This is especially difficult for parents and children to understand when there have been no symptoms of the disease for an extended period and occasional dietary indiscretions, probably the result of increased tolerance to glutens, have not caused untoward effects. However, evidence demonstrates that the majority of individuals who relax their diet will experience a relapse of their disease and possibly exhibit growth retardation, anemia, or osteomalacia. There is also the risk of development of malignant lymphoma of the small intestine or other GI malignancies.

Several resources are available to assist parents in all aspects of coping with CD. The American Celiac Society* and the Celiac Sprue Association/United States of America† are organizations that provide support and guidance to families and supply educational materials concerning gluten-free diet, food sources, and recipes, and travel information.‡

See also the Nursing Care Plan: The Child with Celiac Disease.§

SHORT BOWEL SYNDROME (SBS)

SBS is a condition in which there is a loss of intestine resulting in a diminished ability to digest and absorb a regular diet normally. The most common causes of SBS in children include congenital anomalies (jejunal and ileal atresia, gastroschisis), ischemia (necrotizing enterocolitis), and trauma or vascular injury (volvulus [twisting of bowel on itself]). SBS occurs when a large part of gangrenous or atretic small intestine is resected.

Both the amount and the location of bowel lost are important in determining the severity of the condition. Preservation of the distal ileum and the ileocecal valve appears to be a factor important to the survival of the infant. Up to 50% of the intestine can be lost without affecting the health of the child, unless the loss includes the distal ileum. A loss of greater than 70% of the small bowel results in severe malabsorption. However, the remaining intestine and stomach may adapt to the loss through compensatory growth, provided that the child is kept alive with special nutritional support.

The small intestine has significant capacity for adaptation after resection. During the *adaptation process* the villus height increases (villus hyperplasia), which is the primary compensatory mechanism of the bowel. The cell number and absorptive surface area are also increased. A small amount of dilation and lengthening of the small bowel occur as well. As villus length and the number of enterocytes available for absorption per centimeter of bowel increase, nutrient absorption increases. Atrophy of the absorptive surface of the bowel occurs with nonuse (no enteral intake), even if nutrients are provided intravenously. Intraluminal enteral feedings stimulate the adaptation process and maintain the structural and functional integrity of the small intestine.

---

*Dept. N83, 45 Gifford Ave., Jersey City, NJ 07304.

†3213 Rocklyn Dr., Des Moines, IA 50322. In Canada: **Canadian Celiac Association, Inc.,** L5N IA6; (905) 567-7195; Mississauga, Ontario.

‡A booklet, *Pointers for Parents: Coping with Celiac Sprue,* which provides information on shopping, cooking, and living with an affected child, is available from Clinical Dietetics Dept., Children's Memorial Hospital, 2300 Children's Plaza, Chicago, IL 60614; (312) 880-4000.

§In Wong DL: *Wong and Whaley's clinical manual of pediatric nursing,* ed 4, St. Louis, 1996, Mosby.

Therapeutic Management

The goals of treatment are (1) to preserve as much length of bowel as possible during surgery, (2) to maintain the child's nutritional status until adaptation to the altered bowel takes place, and (3) to stimulate the adaptation process of the bowel. For the severely affected child total parenteral nutrition (TPN) is initially used with gradually increasing amounts of enteral feedings.

Enteral nutrition stimulates bowel adaptation. Elemental formulas are better tolerated than traditional infant formulas. Glucose or glucose polymers, medium-chain triglycerides, and hydrolyzed proteins require less digestion. Usually these formulas are better tolerated if provided by continuous slow infusion by either nasogastric tube or gastrostomy. The transition to completely enteral feedings may take months or years. Home enteral and parenteral nutrition should be considered if it is anticipated that nutritional support will be required on a long-term basis.

There are numerous complications associated with SBS and long-term TPN (see Chapter 42). Infectious, metabolic, and technical complications can occur secondary to TPN. Catheter sepsis can follow improper care of the catheter. The GI tract can also be a source of microbial seeding of the catheter in children with SBS. Bowel atrophy may foster increased intestinal permeability of bacteria. A lack of adequate sites for central lines may become a significant problem for the child in need of long-term TPN. Hepatic dysfunction is also one of the common complications of TPN. Hepatomegaly with abnormal liver function tests and cholestasis may occur.

Chronic *bacterial overgrowth* is a common problem associated with SBS, which exacerbates malabsorption. Bacterial overgrowth often occurs when the ileocecal valve is absent, when a partial obstruction is present, or when a dilated segment of bowel with poor motility exists. These patients may respond to intermittent broad-spectrum antimicrobial therapy.

Many surgical interventions, including intestinal valves, antiperistaltic segments, recirculating loops, and intestinal lengthening procedures, have been attempted in order to delay intestinal transit time or increase absorptive surface area. None of these surgical procedures is sufficiently safe and successful to be used routinely (Thompson, 1993). Transplantation of the small intestine may become a treatment option for selected children with SBS in the future. This procedure has recently been completed with success in children; however, the experience is limited, and the long-term results are unknown. Advancements in antirejection drugs have improved the outlook for this procedure. However, only children with severe disease and complications would be considered candidates for transplantation.

Prognosis. The prognosis for infants with SBS has improved with advances in parenteral nutrition and with the understanding of the importance of intraluminal nutrition. Establishment of the prognosis depends in part on the length of the residual small intestine. An intact ileocecal valve improves the prognosis.

Nursing Care Management

Nursing care is directed toward maintaining adequate nutrition. Once the child has reached the enteral feeding goal, transition is made to bolus or oral feedings if possible. Aversion to oral feedings can be a problem for children fed for an extended period with TPN or tube feedings. It has been suggested that lack of oral stimulation at the critical period of 6 to 12 months of age results in difficulty in eating solid food (Tuchman, 1991). In addition, there may be an extreme sensitivity to anything placed in the mouth. An extensive training program with behavioral modification, using the expertise of speech-language and occupational therapists, may be necessary. To minimize later food aversion, early oral stimulation and nonnutritive sucking should be provided. In addition to a pacifier, occasionally it is acceptable to offer a few drops or tastes of liquids by mouth.

Every effort is made to prevent complications such as infection, especially in central venous access devices. When long-term parenteral nutrition is required, preparing the family for home care of the child is a major nursing responsibility that should be initiated early, whenever possible, to prevent a lengthy hospitalization with subsequent problems such as family dysfunction and developmental delays.* Many infants and children can be successfully cared for at home with enteral and parenteral nutrition if the family is thoroughly prepared and provided with adequate support services. Careful follow-up care by a multidisciplinary nutritional support service is essential. The nurse can have an active and important role in the success of a home nutrition program. Home infusion companies now provide portable equipment, which enables the child and family to maintain a more normal lifestyle.

When hospitalization is prolonged, the child's developmental and emotional needs must be met as well. This often requires special planning to promote normal family adjustment and adaptation of the hospital routines.

Ingestion of Injurious Agents

Since the passage of the Poison Prevention Packaging Act of 1970, which provides that certain potentially hazardous drugs and household products be sold in child-resistant containers, the incidence of poisonings in children has decreased dramatically. However, despite these advances, poisoning remains a significant health concern, with most cases occurring in children under 6 years of age. Children are poisoned by a variety of substances. Although the reported incidence of ingested substances varies, the most frequently ingested poisons are the following (Litovitz et al, 1993):

- Cosmetics/personal care products (perfume, cologne, aftershave)†
- Cleaning products (hypochlorite ["household"] bleach, pine oil disinfectant)

*Home care instructions on caring for a central venous catheter are available in Wong DL: *Wong and Whaley's clinical manual of pediatric nursing*, ed 4, St Louis, 1996, Mosby.

†Most common substances in each category are in parentheses. Substances ingested are not necessarily most toxic but often represent ready availability.

BOX 44-23
Poisonous and Nonpoisonous Plants

Poisonous plants	Toxic parts	Nonpoisonous plants
Apple	Leaves, seeds	African violet
Apricot	Leaves, stem, seed pits	Aluminum plant
		Asparagus fern
Azalea	Foliage and flowers	Begonia
Buttercup	All parts	Boston fern
Cherry (wild or cultivated	Twigs, seeds, foliage	Christmas cactus
		Coleus
Daffodil	Bulbs	Gardenia
Dumb cane, dieffenbachia	All parts	Grape ivy
		Jade plant
Elephant ear	All parts	Marigolds
English ivy	All parts	Piggyback begonia
Fox glove	Leaves, seeds, flowers	Piggyback plant
		Poinsettia†
Holly	Berries	Prayer plant
Hyacinth	Bulbs	Rubber tree
Ivy	Leaves	Snake plant
Mistletoe*	Berries, leaves	Spider plant
Oak tree	Acorn, foliage	Swedish ivy
Philodendron	All parts	Wax plant
Plum	Pit	Weeping fig
Poison ivy, poison oak	Leaves, fruit, stems, smoke from burning plants	Zebra plant
Pothos	All parts	
Rhubarb	Leaves	
Tulip	Bulbs	
Water hemlock	All parts	
Wisteria	Seeds, pods	
Yew	All parts	

- Plants (nontoxic gastrointestinal irritants, oxalates) (Box 44-23).
- Foreign bodies/toys/miscellaneous (desiccants, thermometer, bubble-blowing solutions)
- Hydrocarbons (gasoline)

Over 90% of poisonings occur in the home, although a significant number take place elsewhere, such as in a grandparent's or friend's home, in a school, or in a health care facility.

Nursing ALERT

The following five commonly used and readily available drugs (first four are over-the-counter) can cause serious or fatal consequences if as little as 1/4 teaspoon or 1/2 tablet is ingested: methyl salicylate, camphor, topical imidazolines (sympathomimetics such as those contained in Visine, Afrin, Otrivin, and Clear Eyes), benzocaine, and diphenoxylate-atropine (Lomotil and others). Stress to parents the importance of keeping such drugs away from children. If these agents are ingested, advise parents to seek medical treatment immediately. Emesis is not induced for significant camphor, topical imidazolines, or Lomotil ingestions (Liebelt and Shannon, 1993).

Critical Thinking Q & A

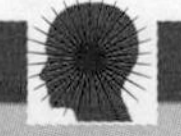

POISONING

Mrs. Berry, a neighbor, calls you. She is very upset because her 2-year-old son has eaten several chewable multivitamins with iron. She asks you whether she should give syrup of ipecac. You advise her to :

1. First call the Poison Control Center.
2. Give the antiemetic.
3. Dilute the poison with several glasses of water.
4. Wait to see if the child develops symptoms.

The correct action for the mother is one: first call the Poison Control Center, where they will advise her of home treatment, such as using ipecac. The goal is to remove the poison, not dilute it, making option three inappropriate. The most toxic ingredient in the drug is iron, which produces symptoms after several hours. Treatment, if needed, should begin long before symptoms appear.

The developmental characteristics of young children predispose them to poisoning by ingestion. Infants and toddlers explore their environment through oral experimentation. Since the sense of taste is less discriminatory at this age, many unpalatable substances are ingested. In addition, toddlers and preschoolers are developing autonomy and initiative, which increase their curiosity and noncompliant behavior. Imitation is also a powerful motivator, especially when combined with lack of awareness of danger.

This section is primarily concerned with the immediate emergency treatment of ingestion of injurious agents. Specific management of corrosive, hydrocarbon, acetaminophen, salicylate, plant, and iron poisoning is summarized in Box 44-24. Because of the importance of lead poisoning among young children, ingestion of lead is discussed separately. Appropriate suggestions for poison prevention are discussed on p. 1439 and in Chapter 34.

PRINCIPLES OF EMERGENCY TREATMENT

A poisoning may or may not require emergency intervention, but in every instance medical evaluation is necessary to initiate appropriate action. Parents are advised to call the Poison Control Center (PCC) *before* initiating any intervention. The local PCC telephone number (usually listed in the front of the telephone directory) should be posted near each phone in the house.* There is some evidence that the information given by Poison Control Centers is more accurate than instructions given by hospital emergency departments (see the Critical Thinking Q & A box above).

On the basis of the initial telephone assessment the PCC counsels the parents to begin treatment at home and/or to take the child to an emergency facility. When a call is taken, the name and telephone number of the caller are recorded to reestablish contact if the connection is interrupted. Since most poisonings are managed in the home, expert advice is essential in minimizing adverse effects. When the exact quantity or type of ingested toxin is not known, admission to a hospital

*Also available by calling (800) 555-1212 for any state in the United States.

BOX 44-24
Selected Poisonings in Children

Corrosives (strong acids or alkali)

Drain, toilet, or oven cleaners
Electric dishwasher detergent (liquid, because of higher pH, is more hazardous than granular)
Mildew remover
Batteries
Clinitest tablets
Denture cleaners

Clinical manifestations

Severe burning pain in mouth, throat and stomach
White, swollen mucous membranes, edema of lips, tongue, and pharynx (respiratory obstruction)
Violent vomiting (hemoptysis)
Drooling and inability to clear secretions
Signs of shock
Anxiety and agitation

Comments

Household bleach is a frequently ingested corrosive but rarely causes serious damage
Liquid preparations cause more damage than granular preparations

Treatment

Inducing emesis is contraindicated (vomiting redamages the mucosa)
Dilute corrosive with water (usually no more than 120 ml [4 oz]), not milk (coats membranes, making assessment difficult) unless vomiting occurs
Provide patent airway if needed
Administer analgesics
Do not allow oral intake
Esophageal stricture may require repeated dilations and/or surgery

Hydrocarbons

Gasoline
Kerosene
Lamp oil
Mineral seal oil (found in furniture polish)
Lighter fluid
Turpentine
Paint thinner and remover (some types)

Clinical manifestations

Gagging, choking, and coughing
Nausea
Vomiting
Alterations in sensorium, such as lethargy
Weakness
Respiratory symptoms of pulmonary involvement
- Tachypnea
- Cyanosis
- Retractions
- Grunting

Comments

Immediate danger is aspiration (even small amounts can cause bronchitis and chemical pneumonia)
Gasoline, kerosene, lighter fluid, mineral seal oil, and turpentine cause severe pneumonia

Treatment (controversial):

Inducing emesis is generally contraindicated
Gastric lavage may be used
Symptomatic treatment of chemical pneumonia includes high humidity, oxygen, hydration, and antibiotics for secondary infection

Acetaminophen

Clinical manifestations

Occurs in four stages

1. Initial period (2 to 4 hours after ingestion)
   Nausea
   Vomiting
   Sweating
   Pallor
2. Latent period (24 to 36 hours)
   Patient improves
3. Hepatic involvement (may last up to 7 days and be permanent)
   Pain in right upper quadrant
   Jaundice
   Confusion
   Stupor
   Coagulation abnormalities
4. Patients who do not die in hepatic stage gradually recover

Comments

Most common drug poisoning in children
Occurs from acute ingestion
Toxic dose is 150 mg/kg or greater in children
Toxicity from chronic therapeutic use is rare but may occur with ingestion of approximately 150 mg/kg/day, or about double the recommended maximum therapeutic dose (90 mg/kg/day) of acetaminophen, for several days (Douidar, Al-Khalil, and Habersang, 1994); toxicity is more likely in children with hepatic dysfunction (Cheung, Potts, and Meyer, 1994)

Treatment

Emesis, lavage, activated charcoal
Antidote *N*-acetylcysteine (NAC) is given, usually by nasogastric tube because of the antidote's offensive odor (smells like rotten eggs)
Given as one loading dose and usually 17 maintenance doses in different dosages
May be given intravenously, but use is investigational

Aspirin (ASA)

Clinical manifestations

Acute poisoning
- Nausea
- Disorientation
- Vomiting
- Dehydration
- Diaphoresis
- Hyperpnea
- Hyperpyrexia
- Oliguria
- Tinnitus

BOX 44-24
Selected Poisonings in Children—cont'd

Coma
Convulsions
Chronic poisoning
Same as above but subtle onset (often confused with illness being treated)
Dehydration, coma, and seizures may be more severe
Bleeding tendencies

Comments

May be caused by acute ingestion (severe toxicity occurs with 300 to 500 mg/kg [4 to 7 g/kg])
May be caused by chronic ingestion (i.e., more than 100 mg/kg/day for 2 or more days); can be more serious than acute ingestion
Time to peak serum salicylate can vary with enteric aspirin or the presence of concretions (bezoars)

Treatment

Home use of ipecac for moderate toxicity
Hospitalization for severe toxicity
Emesis, lavage, activated charcoal, and/or cathartic
Lavage will not remove concretions of ASA
Activated charcoal is important early in ASA toxicity
Sodium bicarbonate transfusions to correct metabolic acidosis and urinary alkalinization is effective in enhancing elimination
External cooling for hyperpyrexia
Diazepam for seizures
Oxygen and ventilation for respiratory depression
Vitamin K for bleeding
In extreme cases, hemodialysis (not peritoneal dialysis) may be used

Iron

Mineral supplement or vitamin containing iron

Clinical manifestations

Occurs in five stages
1. Initial period ($^1/_2$ to 6 hours after ingestion) (if child does not have gastrointestinal symptoms in 6 hours, toxicity is unlikely)
   Vomiting
   Hematemesis
   Diarrhea
   Hematochezia (bloody stools)
   Gastric pain
2. Latency (2 to 12 hours)
   Patient improves
3. Systemic toxicity (4 to 24 hours after ingestion)
   Metabolic acidosis
   Fever
   Hyperglycemia
   Bleeding
   Shock
   Death (may occur)
4. Hepatic injury (48 to 96 hours)
   Seizures
   Coma
5. Rarely pyloric stenosis develops at 2 to 5 weeks

Comments

Factors related to frequency of iron poisoning include:
Widespread availability
Packaging of large quantities in individual containers
Lack of parental awareness of iron toxicity
Resemblance of iron tablets to candy (e.g., M & Ms)
Toxic dose is based on the amount of elemental iron in various salts (sulfate, gluconate, fumarate), which ranges from 20% to 33%; ingestions of 60 mg/kg are considered dangerous

Treatment

Emesis or lavage
Lavage for all chewable tablets or liquids if spontaneous vomiting has not occurred
Chelation therapy with deferoxamine in severe intoxication (turns urine a red to orange color)
If intravenous deferoxamine is given too rapidly, hypotension, facial flushing, rash, urticaria, tachycardia, and shock may occur; stop the infusion, maintain the intravenous line with normal saline, and notify the practitioner immediately

Plants

See Box 44-23 on p. 1435

Clinical manifestations

Depends on type of plant ingested
May cause local irritation of oropharynx and entire gastrointestinal tract
May cause respiratory, renal, and central nervous system symptoms
Topical contact with plants can cause dermatitis

Comments

Some of most frequently ingested substances
Rarely cause serious problems, although some plant ingestions can be fatal
Can also cause choking and allergic reactions

Treatment

Remove plant parts (emesis)
Wash from skin or eyes
Supportive care as needed

for laboratory evaluation and surveillance is critical during the postingestion period.

General guidelines for emergency treatment of poisoning are listed on p. 1438. Selected interventions, especially those that require professional intervention, are discussed next.

Assessment

The first and most important principle in dealing with a poisoning is to treat the child first, not the poison. This necessitates an immediate concern for life support; vital signs are taken and respiratory and/or circulatory support instituted as needed. The victim's condition is routinely reevaluated. Since shock is a complication of several types of household poisons, particularly corrosives, measures to reduce the effects of shock, such as elevation of the legs and head to the level of the heart to promote venous drainage and provision of warmth and rest, are important. Maintenance of respiratory function may require insertion of an airway and/or mechanical ventilation.

The emergency room nurse's responsibility is to be prepared for immediate intervention with any of the necessary equipment. Since time and speed are critical factors in recovery from serious poisonings, anticipation of potential problems and complications may mean the difference between life and death.

Gastric Decontamination

In general the immediate treatment is to remove the ingested poison by inducing vomiting. The preferred method for use at home is to administer *ipecac syrup*, an emetic that exerts its action by direct stimulation of the vomiting center and through an irritant effect on the gastric mucosa.

Nursing ALERT

The use of an emetic is generally contraindicated in conditions that increase the risk of aspiration and when emesis of the poison, such as a corrosive, redamages the mucosa of the esophagus and pharynx. Emesis is also contraindicated in cases where there is existing or potential rapid onset of central nervous system depression, dystonias (unusual muscle tone or movements), or seizures.

EMERGENCY

POISONING

1. Assess the victim:
   a. Take vital signs; reevaluate routinely.
   b. Initiate cardiorespiratory support if needed.
   c. Treat other symptoms, such as seizures.
2. Terminate exposure:
   a. Empty mouth of pills, plant parts, or other material.
   b. Flush eyes continuously with normal saline solution (room-temperature tap water at home) for 15 to 20 minutes.
   c. Flush skin and wash with soap and a soft cloth; remove contaminated clothes, especially if a pesticide, acid, alkali, or hydrocarbon is involved.
   d. Bring victim of an inhalation poisoning into fresh air.
   e. Give one sip of water to dilute ingested poison.
3. Identify the poison:
   a. Question the victim and witnesses.
   b. Look for environmental cues (empty container, nearby spill, odor on breath) and save all evidence of poison (container, vomitus, urine).
   c. Be alert to signs and symptoms of potential poisoning in absence of other evidence, including symptoms of ocular or dermal exposure.
   d. Call Poison Control Center or other competent emergency facility for immediate advice regarding treatment.
4. Remove poison and prevent absorption:
   a. Induce vomiting; administer ipecac if ordered:
      —6 to 12 months: 10 ml; do not repeat.*
      —1 to 12 years: 15 ml; repeat dosage *once* if vomiting has not occurred within 20 minutes.
      —Over 12 years: 30 ml; repeat dosage *once* if vomiting has not occurred within 20 minutes.
      —Give 10 to 20 ml/kg of clear fluids after ipecac.
   b. Do not induce vomiting if:
      —Victim is comatose, in severe shock, or convulsing, or has lost the gag reflex.
      —Poison is a low-viscosity hydrocarbon (unless it contains a more toxic substance [e.g., pesticide or heavy metal] or a strong acid or alkali).
   c. Place child in side-lying, sitting, or kneeling position with head below chest to prevent aspiration.
   d. Administer activated charcoal with cathartic (unless used repeatedly; usual dose 1 g/kg unless amount of toxin is know) 30 to 60 minutes *after* vomiting from ipecac, if ordered.

*Emesis of children at home is generally contraindicated between ages 6 to 10 months. Ipecac can only be administered safely in a health care facility because of the high risk of aspiration.

Proper administration of ipecac is essential (see the Emergency box on the right). Ipecac is available in 1-ounce (30-ml) vials. However, the label information does not include directions for a second dose if the child fails to vomit after the first dose. Therefore parents need clear instructions for proper use and dose. As a precaution parents are advised to have full doses of ipecac for *each child* in the home, to carry the emetic when traveling, and to be certain that other caregivers (babysitters or relatives) have the emetic available. Because children share activities, it is not uncommon for more than one child to ingest the toxic substance. In an emergency ipecac can be obtained from an all-night pharmacy, convenience store, emergency squad, or emergency department. It is inexpensive. Although out-of-date ipecac may be used in a dire emergency, the family is encouraged to replace the expired bottle. Since neither milk, fluid volume, food, nor activity level alters ipecac's effectiveness, the common suggestions of forcing fluids and encouraging movement are unnecessary. If given, clear liquids are preferred for better visualization of white pill fragments. For maximum benefit in removing the poison, ipecac should be administered within 1 hour of a toxic ingestion.

If the child is admitted to an emergency facility, *gastric lavage* may also be done to empty the stomach of the toxic agent. Lavage is indicated for young infants in whom ipecac is contraindicated; if the patient is comatose or convulsing, or requires a protected airway; or if the ingested poison is rapidly absorbed (strychnine or cyanide). The use of lavage in petroleum distillate poisoning remains controversial because of the danger of aspiration. When lavage is performed, the largest-diameter tube that can be inserted is used to facilitate passage of gastric contents.

Another method of decontaminating the stomach is the use of *activated charcoal*, an odorless, tasteless, fine black powder that adsorbs many compounds, creating a stable complex. It is used within 1 hour of the poisoning but *after* giving an emetic, to prevent the charcoal from also adsorbing the emetic and preventing its pharmacologic effect. It is mixed with water or a saline solution to form a slurry. Slurries are neither gritty nor distasteful but resemble black mud. Sorbitol, an artificial sweetener, is added to many commercial preparations (Actidose) as a flavoring and a cathartic. However, concentrated amounts of sorbitol have been known to cause severe dehydration in infants. Cathartics, such as sodium or magnesium, may be administered to stimulate evacuation of the bowel, thus decreasing systemic absorption of the poison and aiding in removal of the charcoal. However, the use of cathartics is controversial. To increase the child's acceptance of activated charcoal, it can be mixed with flavoring or a sweetener

Family Focus

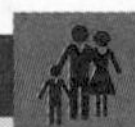

POISONING

A poisoning is more than a physical emergency for the child. It usually represents an emotional crisis for the parents, particularly in terms of guilt, self-reproach, and insecurity in the parenting role. The emergency room is no place to admonish the family for negligence, lack of appropriate supervision, or failure to safe-proof the home. Rather, it is a time to calm and support the child and parents while unaccusingly exploring the circumstances of the injury. If the nurse prematurely attempts to discuss ways of preventing such an incident from recurring, the parents' anxiety will block out any suggestions or offered guidance. Therefore it is preferable for the nurse to delay the discussion until the child's condition is stabilized or, if the child is discharged immediately after emergency treatment, to make a public health referral or send a packet of information (Woolf, Saperstein, and Forjuoh, 1992).

and served through a straw and in an opaque glass with a cover, such as a disposable coffee cup and lid or an ordinary cup covered with aluminum foil or placed inside a small paper bag.

In a minority of poisonings specific *antidotes* are available to counteract the poison. They are highly effective and should be available in all emergency facilities. The supply of antidotes should be checked routinely and replaced as used or according to expiration dates. Among the more commonly employed antidotes are N-acetylcysteine for acetaminophen poisoning, oxygen for carbon monoxide inhalation, naloxone for opioid overdose, flumazenil (Mazicon) for benzodiazepine (Valium, Versed) overdose, Digibind for digoxin toxicity, and antivenin for certain poisonous bites.

Prevention of Recurrence

The ultimate objective is to prevent poisonings from occurring or recurring. One effective counseling method is first to discuss the difficulties of constantly watching and safeguarding young children (see the Family Focus box above). In this way the challenging task of raising children can lead to a discussion of injury prevention as one part of the parental role. This approach also incorporates other contributory causes for the incident, such as inadequate support systems, marital discord, discipline techniques (especially use of physical punishment), and maternal distress. A visit to the home, especially after a repeat poisoning situation, is recommended as part of the follow-up care to assess hazards, including family factors, and to evaluate appropriate safe-proofing measures. One method of identifying risk areas is to ask specific questions or to have the parent complete a questionnaire designed to isolate factors that predispose children to poisoning. Parents are encouraged to bend down to the child's eye level and survey the home environment for potential hazards. Having the parents try to open cabinets and reach shelves to access poisons can also be helpful.

Passive measures (those that do not require active participation) have been the most successful in preventing poisoning and include child-resistant closures and limiting the number of tablets in one container. However, these measures alone are not sufficient to prevent poisoning, since the majority of toxic agents in the home do not have safety closures. Therefore *active measures* (those that require participation) are essential. Guidelines for preventing the occurrence or recurrence of a poisoning are listed in the Guidelines box above.

See also the Nursing Care Plan: The Child with Poisoning.*

Guidelines

POISON PREVENTION

Assess possible contributing factors in occurrence of injury, such as discipline, parent-child relationship, developmental ability, environmental factors, and behavior problems.
Institute anticipatory guidance for possible future injuries based on child's age and maturational level.
Refer to visiting nurse agency to evaluate home environment and need for safe-proofing measures.
Provide assistance with environmental manipulation when necessary, such as lead removal.
Educate parents regarding safe storage of toxic substances.
Advise parents to take drugs out of sight of children.
Advise parents to return *immediately* all toxic substances to safe storage.
Teach children the hazards of ingesting nonfood items without supervision.
Advise parents against using plants for teas or medicine.
Discuss problems of discipline and children's noncompliance and offer strategies for effective discipline (see Limit-Setting and Discipline, Chapter 29).
Instruct parents regarding correct administration of drugs for therapeutic purposes and to discontinue drug if there is evidence of mild toxicity.
Have syrup of ipecac available—two doses for each child in the family—but to use only if advised to do so by poison control center or practitioner.
Encourage grandparents or other frequent caregivers to keep syrup of ipecac in home.
Post number of local poison control center with emergency phone list by telephone.
Include by the telephone the home address with nearest cross street in case an ambulance is needed. (In an emergency family members may not remember the house address, and baby-sitters may not be aware of the information.)

HEAVY METAL POISONING

Heavy metal poisoning can occur from the ingestion of a variety of substances, the most common being lead. Other sources that are important in terms of children are iron (Box 44-24) and mercury. *Mercury toxicity*, a rare form of heavy metal poisoning, has occurred in children from a variety of sources, such as broken thermometers or thermostats, broken fluorescent lights, and use of interior latex house paint. Elemental mercury (also called metallic mercury or quicksilver) is nontoxic if ingested and the gastrointestinal tract is healthy (e.g., has no fistulas). However, mercury is volatile at room temperature and enters the bloodstream after it is inhaled, causing toxicity (tremors, memory loss, insomnia, gingivitis, diarrhea, anorexia, weight loss). The classic form of mercury poisoning is called *acrodynia* (or "painful extremities").

*In Wong DL: *Wong and Whaley's clinical manual of pediatric nursing*, ed 4, St Louis, 1996, Mosby.

Nursing ALERT

To prevent inhalation, spilled mercury must be cleaned up quickly, using disposable towels and rubber gloves and washing the hands well after removing the spill.

Heavy metals have an affinity for certain essential tissue chemicals, which must remain free for adequate cell functioning. When metals are bound to these substances, cellular enzyme systems are inactivated. Treatment involves *chelation*, use of a chemical compound that combines with the metal for rapid and safe excretion.

LEAD POISONING

Lead poisoning (sometimes termed *plumbism*) is a prevalent, significant, and preventable pediatric problem. Although lead poisoning associated life-threatening encephalopathy is rarely seen today, many young children have lead levels sufficiently elevated to cause neurologic and intellectual damage. As the detrimental effects of low levels of lead on the developing central nervous system have been identified, blood lead levels indicating toxicity have decreased. For example, in 1991 the lower level of blood lead concentration was set at <10 μg/dl, a reduction from the 1985 level of <25 μg/dl (Centers for Disease Control, 1991).

Factors Related to Lead Ingestion

The most important contributing factor to lead poisoning is the availability of lead in the environment. Lead enters the system either by ingestion or inhalation. In an unborn fetus lead can enter the body transplacentally if the mother is exposed. The major environmental sources of lead are deteriorating lead-based paint, which contaminates household dust and soil; drinking water contaminated by exposed lead solder or old lead pipes; occupations and hobbies where parents or others in the house bring home lead on clothes, shoes, and skin; and for some children, folk remedies or cosmetics, as well as the use of lead-containing pottery or leaded dishes for food storage. Lead-based paint from old housing remains the most frequent source of lead poisoning in children.

Most lead poisoning results from ingestion of lead dust during normal hand-to-mouth activity. A number of children have been known to actually eat loose lead paint chips. Some children are poisoned during renovation of their home. As mentioned earlier, sanding, scraping, and burning can release large amounts of lead into the air. In 1978 the U.S. Consumer Product Safety Commission banned the addition of lead to paints for residential use, but substantial amounts of lead remain on the painted interior and exterior surfaces of older homes. Although the child's home environment is usually the source of lead, other buildings, such as preschools or day-care centers, as well as a friend or relative's home, can contribute to lead exposure.

Other significant sources of lead in the child's environment are dust, soil, and air that become contaminated by emissions from lead smelters. Fortunately, the use of deleaded gasoline has significantly reduced the level of lead in the air and the incidence of severe lead poisoning in children (Piomelli, 1994). Lead-soldered cans for food products, which have been outlawed in the United States, may still be found with imported products. Leaded containers, such as some water fountains and liquids stored in lead crystal, can also contribute to ingested sources of the heavy metal. Use of lead-contaminated water to prepare formula is a major source of poisoning in infants (Shannon and Graef, 1992).*

Some sources of lead are listed in Box 44-25. Some ethnic groups, especially Hispanics, use improperly fired ceramic pottery and ethnic remedies that include lead (see the Cultural Considerations box above).

Developmentally, young children are at risk for lead poisoning because of their high level of oral activity. Particularly during late infancy and toddlerhood children explore their environment by putting objects in their mouth. This normal hand-to-mouth activity contributes to the amount of lead they ingest in dust and dirt. Because of their size, young children inhale air that is closer to the ground, which is more heavily contaminated with lead. In addition, the child who ingests lead often practices *pica*, the habitual, purposeful, and compulsive ingestion of nonfood substances. Children under the age of 6 are also most at risk for lead poisoning because of their developing nervous system. In addition, three to five times more lead is absorbed in children than in adults. Diets deficient in iron and calcium and diets high in fats, such as those containing many fried foods, also increase the exposure risk for children living in leaded environments. These conditions make it possible for lead to be more quickly and readily absorbed. The greatest risk appears to be from iron deficiency, even in the absence of anemia (Wasserman et al, 1992).

Cultural Considerations 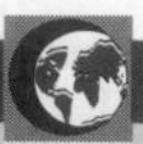

SOURCES OF LEAD

In some cultures the use of traditional ethnic remedies may contain lead and increase children's risk of lead poisoning. These remedies include:

Azarcon (Mexico)—For digestive problems; a bright orange powder; usual dose is ¼-1 teaspoon, often mixed with oil, milk, or sugar, or sometimes given as a tea; sometimes a pinch is added to a baby bottle or tortilla dough for preventive purposes

Greta (Mexico)—A yellow-orange powder, used in the same way as azarcon

Paylooah (Southeast Asia)—used for rash or fever; an orange-red powder given as ½ teaspoon straight or in a tea

Surma (India)—black powder applied to the inner lower eyelid that is used as a cosmetic to improve eyesight

Unknown ayurvedic (Tibet)—Small, gray-brown balls used to improve slow development; two balls are given orally three times a day.

Modified from Lead poisoning associated with use of traditional ethnic remedies—California, 1991-1992 *MMWR* 42(27):521-524, 1993.

Pathophysiology and Clinical Manifestations

Normally, ingested lead is very slowly excreted via the kidneys, alimentary tract, and, to a small extent, sweat. Retained lead

*A suggested resource for families is *Lead in Your Drinking Water*, available from the U.S. Environmental Protection Agency, P.O. Box 42419, Cincinnati, OH 45242.

BOX 44-25
Potential Sources of Lead

Ingested	Inhaled
Lead-based paint Interior: walls, window sills, floors, furniture Exterior: door frames, fences, porches, siding Plaster, caulking Unglazed pottery Cigarette butts and ashes Water from leaded pipes Foods or liquids from cans soldered with lead Household dust Soil, especially along heavily trafficked roadways Food grown in contaminated soil Urban playgrounds Folk remedies Hobby materials, e.g., leaded paint or solder for stained glass windows Lead containing dishware: pottery, ceramics, lead crystal Some antique pewterware Some dyes used in items such as papers, magazines, and wrappers Leaded objects: curtain weights, fishing sinkers, bullets	Sanding and scraping of lead-based painted surfaces Burning of leaded objects Automobile batteries Newspaper logs of colored paper Leaded gasoline (automobile exhaust) Sniffing leaded gasoline Dust Poorly cleaned urban housing Contaminated clothing and skin of household members working in smelting factories, in lead abatement projects, or as urban police Lead-based insecticides

is stored chiefly in the bone and teeth, where it is inert. However, with chronic ingestion the rate of absorption exceeds the rate of excretion, and excess lead is deposited in the tissues and circulatory system, with about 90% attached to the erythrocytes. Even when the chronic ingestion stops, it takes the body twice as long to excrete the stored lead as it did to accumulate it. As a result, several body systems continue to be affected after the environmental removal of the poison (Fig. 44-10).

Central nervous system. The most serious and irreversible side effects of lead intoxication are on the nervous system. Initially, membrane permeability increases, with a shift of fluid into the interstitial spaces of the brain. As a result, increased intracranial pressure causes cortical atrophy and *lead encephalopathy* (convulsions, mental retardation, paralysis, blindness, and ultimately coma and death), which is almost always associated with a blood lead concentration of >100 μg/dl.

However, before lead encephalopathy occurs, low-dose exposure to lead causes neurologic and intellectual deficits that may or may not be reversible. Hyperactivity, aggression, impulsiveness, decreased interest in play, lethargy, irritability, hearing impairment, learning difficulties, short attention span, and distractibility are common signs of low levels of lead poisoning. Studies demonstrate that as prenatal and postnatal lead levels increase, the child's intelligence quotient decreases (Bellinger, Stiles, and Needleman, 1992). Such manifestations of behavioral disturbance are important clues to the identification of children with early poisoning.

Hematologic system. Lead is extremely toxic to the biosynthesis of heme, preventing the formation of hemoglobin and causing its precursors, especially erythrocyte protoporphyrin, coproporphyrin, and delta-aminolevulinic acid (ALA), to increase in the body. The level of *erythrocyte protoporphorin (EP)* is elevated in the blood when the blood lead concentration is moderately increased but is not a sensitive indicator for low lead exposure. Reduction of the heme molecule in the red blood cell results in anemia. However, with low levels of lead toxicity, anemia may not be present.

Renal system. Lead damages the cells of the proximal tubules, resulting in abnormal excretion of glucose, protein, amino acids, and phosphate and in interference with the synthesis of vitamin D. With adequate treatment, kidney damage is usually reversible. Severe irreversible lead nephropathy is probably limited to prolonged childhood plumbism.

Other manifestations. Other vague symptoms of plumbism are acute crampy abdominal pain, vomiting, constipation, anorexia, headache, and fever. Some evidence suggests that in young children lead impairs growth, especially in infants with elevated prenatal and postnatal blood lead levels.

Diagnostic Evaluation

Diagnosis is made on measurement of blood lead levels. Since virtually all children are at risk for lead poisoning, universal screening is recommended. Priority for screening is given to children ages 6 to 72 months who are at highest risk: (1) those who live in or frequent deteriorated housing or such housing during remodeling, (2) those whose siblings or other close peers have lead poisoning, and (3) those whose household members have lead-related occupations or hobbies, or who live near lead-related industries (Centers for Disease Control, 1991).

Screening tests are usually done on blood collected by finger or heel puncture. However, blood collected by venipuncture is needed to confirm the diagnosis. Other tests that are helpful in determining the presence of lead in the body are (1) radiographs of the long bones for "lead lines," caused by deposition of lead, and of the abdomen for the presence of recently ingested lead; (2) blood studies for evidence of anemia; and (3) a lead mobilization test to help predict the amount of lead that may be removed by chelation.

Therapeutic Management

The child's blood lead level determines the degree of risk and the type of intervention (Table 44-11). The objective of treatment is to remove lead in the body and prevent further accumulation of the metal. Therapeutic modalities include removing the source of lead, improving nutrition, and using chelation therapy. With emphasis on early detection of low blood lead levels, removing sources of lead in the environment is the major goal (see the Home Care box on p. 1443).

Chelation therapy is reserved for children with high blood

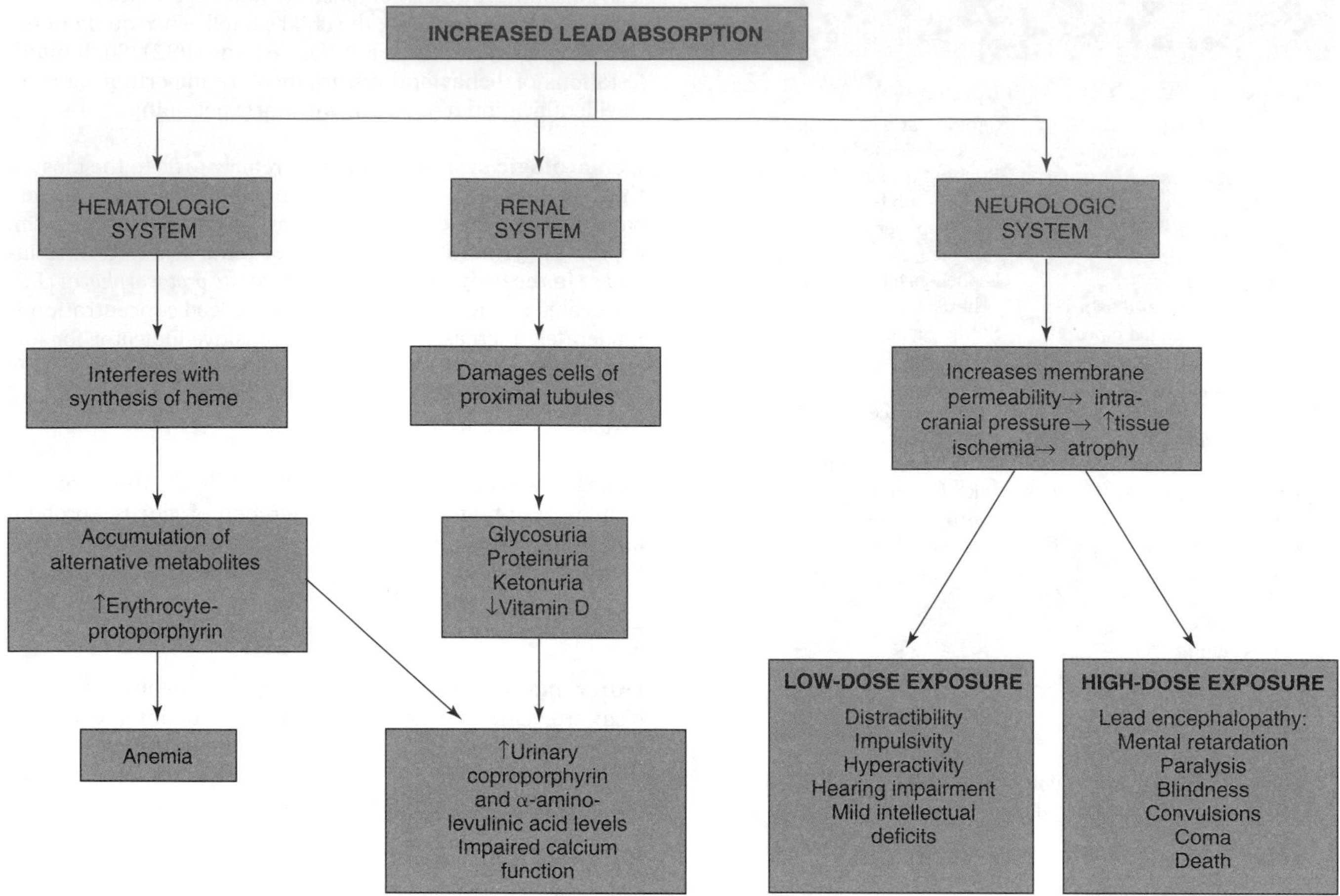

Fig. 44-10 Main effects of lead on body systems.

lead levels. Drugs that may be used are calcium disodium edetate ($CaNa_2$ EDTA), dimercaprol (also called BAL [British antilewisite]), penicillamine (Cuprimine, Depen), or succimer (Chemet).

The exact course of therapy depends on the severity of the child's condition and the practitioner's preference. $CaNa_2$EDTA is given preferably intravenously; intramuscular injections are very painful. BAL (prepared in peanut oil) is given only intramuscularly and is also a very painful injection. D-Penicillamine and succimer are administered orally.

Nursing ALERT

Children with allergy to peanuts or penicillin cannot receive BAL or D-penicillamine, respectively.

Symptomatic treatment during chelation therapy involves observing for and controlling seizures for which the child is at risk and taking measures to reduce the side effects of some of the medications, such as the nausea that can occur with BAL. Depending on the drug being used, serum electrolyte levels should be taken at prescribed intervals, urine specimens analyzed, and fluid intake and output measured. If numerous paint chips are visible in the gastrointestinal tract on radiologic examination, cleansing enemas or a cathartic may be ordered. Every effort is made to prevent infection and maintain adequate hydration. When succimer is given, adequate fluid intake is especially important, as is close monitoring of the absolute neutrophil count. Neutropenia can occur during drug therapy. If nutritional deficiencies coexist, they are treated appropriately, such as with administration of supplemental iron for iron-deficiency anemia. Iron should not be given during chelation, however, especially with BAL because of possible interactive effects.

Prognosis. Although most of the pathophysiologic effects of lead are reversible, the most serious consequences of both high and low lead exposure are the effects on the central nervous system. In children with lead encephalopathy, permanent brain damage results in mental retardation, behavior changes, possible paralysis, and seizures. However, low-dose exposure may also cause permanent neurologic deficits.

Nursing Care Management

The primary nursing goal in lead poisoning is to prevent the child's initial or further exposure to lead. For children with low-level exposure, this often requires identifying the sources of lead in the environment. Careful history taking is one of the most useful and valuable tools and should concentrate on the areas listed in the Guidelines box on p. 1443, especially

TABLE 44-11 Classification of risk and treatment for lead poisoning

BLOOD LEAD CONCENTRATION (μg/dl)	INTERVENTION
≤9	Child is not considered to be lead poisoned.
10-14	Many children with blood lead levels in this range should trigger community-wide childhood lead poisoning prevention activities. Children may need to be rescreened more frequently.
15-19	Child should receive nutritional and educational interventions and more frequent screening. If blood lead level persists in this range, environmental investigation and intervention should be done.
20-44	Child should receive environmental evaluation and remediation and a medical evaluation; may need pharmacologic treatment of lead poisoning.
45-69	Child will need both medical and environmental interventions, including chelation therapy.
≥70	Child's condition is a medical emergency; medical and environmental management must begin immediately.

Modified from Centers for Disease Control and Prevention: *Preventing lead poisoning in young children,* Atlanta, 1991, Centers for Disease Control.

Guidelines

ASSESSING POTENTIAL FOR LEAD POISONING

Does your child:

1. Live in a house or regularly visit a day-care center, preschool, home of a baby-sitter or relative, or other house built before 1960 that has peeling or chipping paint?
2. Live in or regularly visit a house built before 1960 with recent, ongoing, or planned renovation or remodeling?
3. Have a brother or sister, housemate, or playmate being followed up or treated for lead poisoning (i.e., blood level ≥15 mg/dl)?
4. Live with an adult whose job, hobby , or use of ethnic remedies involves exposure to lead?
5. Live near an active lead smelter, battery recycling plant, or other industry likely to release lead?

Modified from Centers for Disease Control and Prevention: *Preventing lead poisoning in young children,* Atlanta, 1991, Centers for Disease Control and Prevention.

Home Care

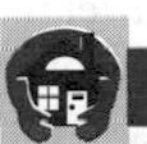

REDUCING BLOOD LEAD LEVELS

Make sure child does not have access to peeling paint or chewable surfaces painted with lead-based paint, especially window sills and wells.

If a house was built before 1960 (possibly before 1980) and has hard-surface floors, wet mop them at least once a week with a high-phosphate solution (e.g., trisodium phosphate [available in hardware stores]). Wipe other hard surfaces (such as window sills and baseboards) with the same kind of solution. If there are loose paint chips in an area, such as a window well, use a disposable cloth soaked with the high phosphate (5% to 8%) solution to pick up and discard them. Do not vacuum hard-surfaced floors or window sills or wells, since this spreads dust. Use vacuum cleaners with agitaors to remove dust from rugs rather than vacuum cleaners with suction only. If a rug is known to contain lead dust and cannot be washed, it should be discarded.

Wash and dry child's hands and face frequently, especially before eating.

Wash toys and pacifiers frequently.

If soil around home is or is likely to be contaminated with lead (e.g., if home was built before 1960 or is near a major highway), plant grass or other ground cover; plant bushes around outside of house so that child cannot play there.

During remodeling of older homes, be sure to follow correct procedures. Be certain children and pregnant women are not in the home, day or night, until process is completed. Following deleading, thoroughly clean house using high-phosphate cleaning solution to damp mop and dust before inhabitants return.

In areas where lead content of water exceeds the drinking water standard, run cold water until it is as cold as it will get before using it for drinking, cooking, and making formula; may use first-flush water for other purposes.

Do not store food in open cans, particularly if cans are imported.

Do not use pottery or ceramic ware that was inadequately fired or is meant for decorative use for food storage or service. Do not store drinks or food in lead crystal.

Avoid folk remedies or cosmetics that contain lead.

Make sure that home exposure is not occurring from parental occupations or hobbies. Household members employed in occupations such as lead smelting should shower and change into clean clothing before leaving work. Construction and abatement workers may also bring home lead contaminants.

Make sure child eats regular meals, since more lead is absorbed on an empty stomach.

Make sure child's diet contains plenty of iron and calcium and not too much fat.

Modified from Centers for Disease Control and Prevention: *Preventing lead poisoning in young children,* Atlanta, 1991, Centers for Disease Control and Prevention.

Critical Thinking Q & A

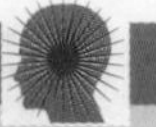

LEAD POISONING

The clinic in which you practice has received funds to begin a program to reduce lead poisoning in children. As a member of the planning committee, which of the following initial projects is effective and easy to implement?

1. Screening for blood lead levels by heel or finger puncture in all children under age 6 years
2. Questioning parents about the age and condition of their home(s) since the child's birth, including recent renovations
3. Screening for blood lead levels by venipuncture in all children under age 6 years who are at risk for lead exposure
4. Questioning parents about hobbies, occupations, and ethnic remedies that may expose the child to lead

The correct answer is two. Asking about the family's dwelling to identify instances where lead, especially on painted surfaces, could be present is the single most important screening procedure. Although asking about hobbies, occupations, and ethnic remedies should be considered, option four is not the priority question. Screening for blood lead levels is expensive and time consuming. Option three is incorrect because collection of blood by venipuncture is not a recommended screening procedure, and all children, regardless of risk, should be screened.

those related to the home environment (Nordin, Rolnick, and Griffin, 1994) (see the Critical Thinking Q & A box above). Suggestions for reducing lead in the child's environment are listed in the Home Care box on p. 1443.

Children who must undergo chelation therapy are prepared for the injections and allowed to express their pain and anger. Playing with syringes and aggressive play, such as pounding clay or throwing beanbags, provide an excellent outlet for their frustrations. Children also deserve an explanation of the need for the treatment, particularly that it is not a punishment for eating lead or paint. During home oral chelation therapy, parents need to understand the importance of giving the drug as prescribed.

Atraumatic Care

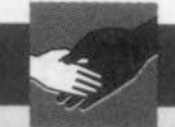

LEAD CHELATION THERAPY

To lesson pain from $CaNa_2EDTA$, the local anesthetic procaine is injected with the drug. Apply EMLA cream over the puncture site $2^1/_2$ hours before injection.

Chelating agents are administered deeply into a large muscle mass (see the Atraumatic Care box above). Rotation of sites is essential to prevent the formation of painful areas of fibrotic tissue. Since $CaNa_2EDTA$ and lead are toxic to the kidneys, records are kept of intake and output, and the results of urinalysis are assessed to monitor renal functioning. Because of the risk of seizures, appropriate precautions are instituted at the bedside of children with high blood lead levels.

Nursing ALERT

$CaNa_2EDTA$ is never given in the absence of an adequate urinary output. Children receiving the drug intramuscularly must be able to maintain adequate oral intake of fluids.

As in any situational crisis, parents need support and understanding if their child is treated for lead poisoning. Many of the families at highest risk for lead poisoning have the fewest resources to comply with measures such as relocation or deleading the home. Appropriate referrals are essential in locating assistance for parents (see also the Nursing Care Plan: The Child with Lead Poisoning*).

*In Wong DL: *Wong and Whaley's clinical manual of pediatric nursing,* ed 4, St Louis, 1996, Mosby.

Key Points

- Common nutritional disturbances of infancy may result from vitamin and mineral deficiency or excess, some types of vegetarian diets, protein and calorie malnutrition, and food intolerance.
- Malnutrition is poor or inadequate nutrition and may result from undernutrition or overnutrition. Common manifestations of undernutrition in the infant include iron-deficiency anemia, vitamin deficiencies, and failure to thrive. Manifestations of overnutrition are hypervitaminosis and obesity.
- Mineral disturbances may be caused by mineral-mineral interactions and mineral-diet interactions.
- Vegetarians may be classified into four groups: lactoovovegetarians, lactovegetarians, pure vegetarians, and zen macrobiotics.
- Protein-energy malnutrition may occur as a complication of underlying disease or as a result of fad diets, lack of parental education about infant nutrition, inappropriate management of food allergy, or incorrect preparation of formula.
- Food intolerance encompasses food allergies and food sensitivities, the most serious of which are cow's milk allergy and lactose intolerance.
- Infants are subject to fluid depletion because of their greater surface area relative to body mass, high rate of metabolism, and immature kidney function.
- Dehydration can be classified as isotonic, hypotonic, and hypertonic.
- Vomiting and diarrhea account for significant fluid depletion, especially in infants and small children.
- The amount, frequency, and characteristics of stool and vomitus are important nursing observations.
- Acute diarrhea can be caused by an inflammatory process of infectious origin, a toxic reaction to ingestion of poisonous substances, or dietary indiscretions, or it can be associated with infections outside the alimentary tract. The

primary treatment of diarrhea is the use of oral rehydrating solution.

- Postoperative care of the child with abdominal surgery involves assessing the abdomen; providing hydration, nutrition, and intravenous fluids; proper positioning; wound care; and psychologic support.
- Surgical correction in Hirschsprung disease is a two-stage approach: a temporary colostomy and reanastomosis at 8 months to 1 year of age with closure of the colostomy.
- Nursing care of gastrointestinal reflux is aimed at identifying children with suggestive symptoms, helping parents with home care feeding and positioning, and caring for the child undergoing surgical intervention.
- Stomatitis is an infectious disorder common in children.
- Although the cause of appendicitis is poorly understood, it is commonly a result of obstruction of the lumen, usually by a fecalith. Common signs and symptoms are right lower quadrant abdominal pain, tenderness, and fever.
- Meckel diverticulum, the most common congenital malformation of the GI tract, is characterized by bloody stools.
- Inflammatory bowel disease refers to ulcerative colitis and Crohn disease, of which persistent and recurring diarrhea is the most common feature. It is treated by dietary management and medication, although surgery is needed in a number of cases.
- Peptic ulcers are poorly understood, but one of two mechanisms probably reflects the basic defect: an increase in the rate of production of gastric juice or interference with the normal protective mechanisms of the mucosal lining.
- Viral hepatitis is caused by at least five types of virus: hepatitis A virus, hepatitis B virus, hepatitis D virus, and hepatitis C and E viruses (non-A, non-B viruses).
- Hepatitis A virus is spread by the fecal-oral route, whereas hepatitis B virus is transmitted primarily by the parenteral route. The most effective measures in prevention and control of hepatitis in any setting are handwashing and universal precautions.
- Structural disorders of the GI tract include cleft lip, cleft palate, esophageal atresia with tracheoesophageal fistula, anorectal malformations, and biliary atresia.
- Biliary atresia is a serious disorder, often causing progressive liver failure, which is an indication for liver transplantation.
- Cleft lip and palate, the most common facial malformation, may involve nutritional, dental, and speech problems.
- Hernias related to the GI tract can be minor (umbilical hernia) or life-threatening (hiatal, diaphragmatic, gastroschisis, omphalocele).
- General signs of obstruction include colicky abdominal pain, nausea and vomiting, abdominal distention, and decreased stool output.
- Hypertrophic pyloric stenosis is recognized by characteristic projectile vomiting, malnutrition, dehydration, and a palpable mass in the epigastrium and is relieved by pyloromyotomy.
- Intussusception is one of the most common causes of intestinal obstruction during infancy and is characterized by abdominal pain and blood in stools. Treatment is either nonsurgical hydrostatic reduction or surgical reduction.
- Malabsorption syndromes are disorders associated with some degree of impaired digestion and/or absorption. They include digestive defects, absorptive defects, and anatomic defects.
- Celiac disease, the second leading cause of malabsorption in children, is characterized by an intolerance for gluten. It is thought to be either an inborn error of metabolism or an immunologic response.
- Short bowel syndrome is characterized by a loss of intestine resulting in a diminished ability to digest and absorb a regular diet normally. Specialized enteral and parenteral nutrition is a major element of care for these children.
- Intestinal parasitic diseases constitute the most common infections in the world; giardiasis and enterobiasis are the most widespread parasitic infections among children in the United States.
- Although the incidence of poisoning has decreased in the last 30 years as a result of more stringent packaging regulations, childhoood poisoning remains a serious health concern.
- The major principles of emergency treatment for poisoning are assessment, supportive measures, gastric decontamination, family support, and prevention of recurrence.
- Ipecac is an effective and safe emetic for home use in poisonings but is contraindicated in situations that increase the risk of aspiration and that involve ingestion of corrosives, wherein vomiting redamages the mucosa.
- Three simple measures that can reduce the severity of a poisoning are knowing the telephone number of the Poison Control Center, having ipecac in the home (two doses per child), and administering it correctly.
- Acetaminophen poisoning is the most common drug poisoning among children and occurs primarily from acute overdose.
- The most important factor contributing to lead poisoning is its availability in the child's environment. Lead-based paint is the most common and toxic source of lead.
- With increasing awareness of the detrimental effects of low levels of lead on the developing nervous system, acceptable blood lead levels have been decreasing and now are at <10 μg/dl.

References

Albanese CT et al: Percutaneous gastrojejunostomy versus Nissen fundoplication for enteral feeding of the neurologically impaired child with gastroesophageal reflux, *J Pediatr* 123:371-375, 1993.

Avery M, Snyder J: Oral therapy for acute diarrhea: the underused simple solution, *N Engl J Med* 323(13):891-894, 1990.

Bacon B: managing chronic hepatitis, *Postgrad Med* 90(5):103-112, 1991.

Bartlett AV et al: Controlled trial of *Giardia lamblia:* control strategies in day care centers, *Am J Public Health* 81(6):1001-1006, 1991.

Bellinger DC, Stiles KM, Needleman HL: Low-level lead exposure, intelligence and academic achievement: a long-term follow-up study, *Pediatrics* 90(6):855-861, 1992.

Borowski S: Common pediatric surgical problems, *Nurs Clin North Am* 29(4):551-562, 1994.

Brown K: Dietary management of acute childhood diarrhea: optimal timing of feeding and appropriate use of milks and mixed diets, *J Pediatr* 118(4):S92-S98, 1991.

Brown KH, Peerson JM, Fontaine O: Use of nonhuman milks in the dietary management of young children with acute diarrhea: a meta-analysis of clinical trials, *Pediatrics* 93(1):17-27, 1994.

Carey W, Patel G: Viral hepatitis in the 1990's. III. Hepatitis C, hepatitis E, and other viruses, *Cleve Clin J Med* 59(6):595-601, 1992.

Centers for Disease Control and Prevention: *Preventing lead poisoning in young children,* Atlanta, 1991, Centers for Disease Control and Prevention.

Cheung L, Potts R, Meyer K: Acetaminophen treatment nomogram, *N Engl J Med* 330(26):1907-1908, 1994.

Chew F et al: Is dilution of cows' milk formula necessary for dietary management of acute diarrhoea in infants aged less than 6 months? *Lancet* 341:194-197, 1993.

Cohen M: Etiology and mechanisms of acute infectious diarrhea in infants in the United States, *J Pediatr* 118(4):S34-S39, 1991.

David S, Lobo ML: Childhood diarrhea and malnutrition in Pakistan. I. Incidence and prevalence, *J Pediatr Nurs* 10(2):131-137, 1995a.

David S, Lobo ML: Childhood diarrhea and malnutrition in Pakistan. II. Treatment and malnutrition, *J Pediatr Nurs* 10(3):204-209, 1995b.

Douidar SM, Al-Khalil I, Habersang RW: Severe hepatoxicity, acute renal failure, and pancytopenia in a young child after repeated acetominophen overdosing, *Clin Pediatr* 33(1):42-45, 1994.

Ergun G, Miskovitz P: Viral hepatitis, *Postgrad Med* 88(5):69-76, 1990.

Fanaroff AA, Martin RJ: *Jaundice and liver disease.* In Fanaroff AA, Martin RJ, editors: *Neonatal-perinatal medicine: diseases of the fetus and infant,* St Louis, 1992, Mosby.

Fawzi WW et al: Vitamin A supplementation and child mortality: a meta-analysis, *JAMA* 269(7):898-903, 1993.

Finberg L: Assessing the clinical clues to dehydration, *Contemp Pediatr* 7(4):45-57, 1990.

Francis CY, Whorwell PJ: Bran and irritable bowel syndrome: time for reappraisal, *Lancet* 344(8914):39-40, 1994.

Hickey R, Sodhi S, Johnson W: Two children with lethargy and intussusception, *Ann Emerg Med* 19(4):390-392, 1990.

Hill DR: Giardiasis: issues in diagnosis and management, *Infect Dis Clin North Am* 7(3): 503-525, 1993.

Hillemeier A: *Reflux and esophagitis.* In Walker W et al: editors: *Pediatric gastrointestinal disease,* Philadelphia, 1991, BC Decker.

Hoekstra JH et al: Fluid intake and industrial processing in apple juice induced chronic non-specific diarrhoea, *Arch Dis Child* 73(2):126-30, 1995.

Jackson W, Grand R: *Crohn's disease.* In Walker W et al, editors: *Pediatric gastrointestinal disease,* Philadelphia, 1991, BC Decker.

Kanesaki T et al, Hepatitis C virus infection in children with hemophilia: characterization of antibody response to four different antigens and relationship of antibody response, viremia, and hepatic dysfunction, *J Pediatr* 123:381-387, 1993.

Karrer F et al: Congenital biliary tract disease, *Surg Clin North Am* 70(6):1403-1418, 1990.

Kirschner B: *Hirschsprung's disease.* In Walker W et al, editors: *Pediatric gastrointestinal disease,* Philadelphia, 1991, BC Decker.

Kleinman RE: We have the solution: now what's the problem? *Pediatrics* 90(1):113-115, 1992.

Krugman S: Viral hepatitis: A, B, C, D and E—infection, *Pediatr Rev* 13(6):203-212, 1992.

Kubiak M et al: Comparison of stool containment in cloth and single-use diapers using a simulated infant feces, *Pediatrics* 91(3):632-636, 1993.

Laurent J et al: Long-term outcome after surgery for biliary atresia, *Gastroenterology* 99(6):1793-1797, 1990.

Liebelt EL, Shannon MW: Small doses, big problems: a selected review of highly toxic common medications, *Pediatr Emerg Care* 9(5):292-297, 1993.

Lisanti P, Talotta D: Hepatitis update: the delta virus, *AORN J* 55(3):790-800, 1992.

Litovitz T et al: 1992 annual report of the American Association of Poison Control Centers Toxic Exposure Surveillance System, *Am J Emerg Med* 11(5):494-555, 1993.

Lloyd-Still JD: Impact of orthotopic liver transplantation on mortality from pediatric liver disease, *J Pediatr Gastroenterol Nutr* 12:305-309, 1991.

Margolis P et al: Effects of unrestricted diet on mild infantile diarrhea, *Am J Dis Child* 144:162-164, 1990.

Meyer J: The current radiologic management of intussusception: a survey and review, *Pediatr Radiol* 22:323-325, 1992.

Milla P: *Motor disorders including pyloric stenosis.* In Walker W et al, editors: *Pediatric gastrointestinal disease,* Philadelphia, 1991, BC Decker.

Najmaldin A, Tan HL: Early experience with laparoscopic pyloromyotomy for infantile hypertrophic pyloric stenosis, *J Pediatr Surg* 30(1):37-38, 1995.

NIH Consensus Development Panel on *Helicobacter pylori* in peptic ulcer disease: *Helicobacter pylori* in peptic ulcer disease, *JAMA* 272(1):65-69, 1994.

Nordin JD, Rolnick SJ, Griffin JM: Prevalence of excess lead absorption and associated risk factors in children enrolled in a midwestern health maintenance organization, *Pediatrics* 93(4):508-5510, 1994

Orenstein S: Prone positioning in infant gastroesophageal reflux: is elevation of the head worth the trouble? *J Pediatr* 117(2):184-187, 1990.

Orenstein SR: The prone alternative, *Pediatrics* 94(1):104-105, 1994.

Piomelli S: Childhood lead poisoning in the '90's, *Pediatrics* 93(4):508-510, 1994.

Rennels MB et al: Safety and efficacy of high-dose rhesus-human reassortant rotavirus vaccines—Report of the National Multicenter Trial, *Pediatrics* 97(1):7-13, 1996.

Richard M: Feeding the newborn with cleft lip and/or palate: the enlargement, stimulate, swallow rest (ESSR) method, *J Pediatr Nurs* 6(5):317-321, 1991.

Ryckman F et al: Improved survival in biliary atresia patients in the present era of liver transplantation, *J Pediatr Surg* 28(3):382-386, 1993.

Sachar DB: Budesonide for inflammatory bowel disease: is it a magic bullet? *New Engl J Med* 331(13):873-874, 1994.

Santosham M, Greenough W: Oral rehydration therapy: a global perspective, *J Pediatr* 118(4):S44-S51, 1991.

Shandling B: *Appendicitis.* In Walker W et al, editors: *Pediatric gastrointestinal disease,* Philadelphia, 1991, BC Decker.

Shannon M, Graef I: Lead intoxication in infancy, *Pediatrics* 89(1):87-90, 1992.

Siegel MJ, Carel C, Surratt S: Ultrasonography of acute abdominal pain in children, *JAMA* 266:1987-1989, 1991.

Thompson J: Surgical considerations in the short bowel syndrome, *Surg Gynecol Obstet* 176:89-101, 1993.

Toyosaka A et al: Outcome of 21 patients with biliary atresia living more than 10 years, *J Pediatr Surg* 28:1498-1501, 1993.

Tuchman D: *Disorders of deglutition.* In Walker W et al, editors: *Pediatric gastrointestinal disease,* Philadelphia, 1991, BC Decker.

Turgeon D, Barnett J: Meckel's diverticulum, *Am J Gastroenterol* 85(7):777-781, 1990.

Walker-Smith J: *Celiac disease.* In Walker W et al, editors: *Pediatric gastrointestinal disease,* Philadelphia, 1991, BC Decker.

Walterspiel JN et al: Secretory antigiardia lamblia antibodies in human milk: protective effect against diarrhea, *Pediatrics* 93(1):28-31, 1994.

Wasserman G et al: Independent effects of lead exposure and iron deficiency anemia on developmental outcome at age 2 years, *J Pediatr* 121(5):695-703, 1992.

Wilson N, Self T, Hamburger R: Severe cow milk induced colitis in an exclusively breast fed neonate, *Clin Pediatr* 29(2):77-80, 1990.

Woolf AD, Saperstein A, Forjuoh S: Poisoning prevention knowledge and practices of parents after a childhood poisoning incident, *Pediatrics* 90(6):867-870, 1992.

Wright V: *The esophagus: congenital anomalies.* In Walker W et al: editors: *Pediatric gastrointestinal disease,* Philadelphia, 1991, BC Decker.

Ziller S, Netchvolodoff C: Uncomplicated peptic ulcer disease, *Postgrad Med* 93(4):126-138, 1993.

Bibliography

Vitamin and Mineral Disturbances/Protein Energy Malnutrition

Graham SM, Arvela OM, Wise GA: Long-term neurologic consequences of nutritional vitamin B_{12} deficiency in infants, *J Pediatr* 121(5):710-714, 1992.

Hendrickse RG: Kwashiorkor: the hypothesis that incriminates aflatoxins, *Pediatrics* 88(2):376-379, 1991.

Herrera MG et al: Vitamin A supplementation and child survival, *Lancet* 340:267-271, 1992.

Jelliffe DB, Jelliffe EFP: Causation of kwashiorkor: toward a multifactorial consensus, *Pediatrics* 90(1):110-113, 1992.

NIIH Concensus Development Panel on Optimal Calcium Intake, *JAMA* 272(24):1942-1948, 1994.

Raiha NCR, Axelsson IE: Protein nutrition during infancy: an update, *Pediatr Clin North Am* 42(4):745-761, 1995.

Sills IN et al: Vitamin D deficiency rickets: reports of its demise are exaggerated, *Clin Pediatr* 33:491-493, 1994.

Udall JN Jr, Greene HL: Vitamin update, *Pediatr Rev* 13(5):185-194, 1992.

Vegetarian Diets

Dagnelie P et al: High prevalence of rickets in infants on macrobiotic diets, *Am J Clin Nutr* 51:202-208, 1990.

O'Connell J et al: Growth of vegetarian children: the farm study, *Pediatrics* 84(3):475-481, 1989.

Trahms CM: *Vegetarian diets for children.* In Pipes PL, Trahms CM, editors: *Nutrition in infancy and childhood,* ed 5, St Louis, 1993, Mosby.

Food Sensitivity

Bock SA, Sampson HA: Food allergy in infancy, *Pediatr Clin North Am* 41(5):1047-1067, 1994.

Castiglia PT: Lactose intolerance, *J Pediatr Health Care* 8(1):36-8, 1994.

Preventing food allergy fatalities, *Emerg Med* 25(7):119-123, 1993.

Sampson HA et al: Anaphylactic reactions to foods, *N Engl J Med* 327:380-384, 1992.

Disorders of Motility

Booth IW: Dietary management of acute diarrhoea in childhood, *Lancet* 341(8851):996, 1993.

Clayden G: Management of chronic constipation, *Arch Dis Child* 67:340-344, 1992.

Dipalma J: Metoclopramide: a dopamine receptor antagonist, *Am Fam Physician* 41(3):919-921, 1990.

Ellett ML: Constipation/encopresis: a nursing perspective, *J Pediatr Health Care* 4(3):141-146, 1990.

Evans K: Pediatric management problems...chronic constipation, *Pediatr Nurs* 16(6):590-591, 1990.

Foster P, Cowan G, Wrenn E: Twenty-five years' experience with Hirschsprung's disease, *J Pediatr Surg* 25(5):531-534, 1990.

Hlusko D, McMurray J: Gastroesophageal reflux: treatment and nursing care, *Neonatal Network* 9(5):33-36, 1991.

Konings, K: Preop use of Golytely in pediatrics, *Pediatr Nurs* 15:473-474, 1989.

Lifshitz F, Ament M: Role of juice carbohydrate malabsorption in chronic nonspecific diarrhea in children, *J Pediatr* 120(5):825-829, 1992.

Loening-Baucke V: Constipation in children, *Curr Opin Pediatr* 6:556-561, 1994.

Margolis P et al: Effects of unrestricted diet on mild infantile diarrhea, *Am J Dis Child* 144:162-164, 1990.

Orenstein SR et al: Reliability and validity of an infant gastroesophageal reflux questionnaire, *Clin Pediatr* 32(8):472-484, 1993.

Orenstein ST: Gastroesophageal reflux disease, *Semin Gastrointest Dis* 5(1):2-14, 1994.

Say B, Smith DP: Midline field defects and Hirschsprung disease, *Am J Med Genetics* 61:293-294, 1996 (letter to editor).

Sterling C, Schaffer S, Jolley S: Home management related to medical treatment for childhood gastroesophageal reflux, *Pediatr Nurs* 19(2):167-173, 1993.

Sterling C et al: Nursing responsibility in the diagnosis, care, and treatment of the child with gastroesophageal reflux, *J Pediatr Nurs* 6(6):435-440, 1991.

Thorye SM: Mothers' internal working models with infants with gastroesophageal reflux, *Maternal-Child Nurs J* 22(2):39-48, 1994.

Intestinal Parasitic Diseases

Addiss DG, Juranek DD, Spencer HC: Treatment of children with asymptomatic and nondiarrheal *Giardia* infection, *Pediatr Infect Dis J* 10(11):843-846, 1991.

Glickman LT, Magnaval JF: Zoonotic roundworm infections, *Infect Dis Clin North Am* 7(3):717-732, 1993.

Gratz RR, Boulton P: Health considerations for pregnant child care staff, *J Pediatr Health Care* 8:18-26, 1994.

Korman S: The duodenal string test, *Am J Dis Child* 144(7):803-805, 1990.

Kuhls TL: Protozoal infections of the intestinal tract in children, *Adv Pediatr Infect Dis* 8:177-202, 1993.

Inflammatory Disorders

Anderson ML: *Helicobacter pylori infection, Postgrad Med* 96(6):40-50, 1994.

Andersson R et al: Indications for operation in suspected appendicitis and incidence of perforation, *Br Med J* 308(6921):107-110, 1994.

Christie PM, Hill GI: Effect of intravenous nutrition on nutrition and function in acute attacks of inflammatory bowel disease, *Gastroenterology* 99:730-736, 1990.

Cooke D: Inflammatory bowel disease: primary health care management of ulcerative colitis and Crohn's disease, *Nurse Pract* 16(8):27-39, 1991.

De Giacomo C et al: Omeprazole treatment of severe peptic disease associated with antral G cell hyperfunction and hyperpepsinogenemia I in an infant, *J Pediatr* 117(6):989-993, 1990.

Dunlap C, Barker B, Lowe J: 10 oral lesions you should know, *Contemp Pediatr* 8(12):16-28, 1991.
Feagan BG et al: Low-dose cyclosporine for the treatment of Crohn's disease, *New Engl J Med* 330(26):1846-1851, 1994.
Ferguson A: Ulcerative colitis and Crohn's disease, *Br Med J* 309(6951): 355-356, 1994.
Gamal R, Moore TC: Appendicitis in children aged 13 years and younger, *Am J Surg* 159:589-592, 1990.
Garretson DC, Frederich DO, Frederich ME: Meckel's diverticulum, *Am Fam Physician* 42(1):115-119, 1990.
Greenberger NJ, Miner PB: Is maintenance therapy effective in Crohn's disease? *Lancet* 344(8927):900-901, 1994.
Kisumoto et al: Complications and diagnosis of Meckel's diverticulum in 776 patients, *Am J Surg* 164:382-383, 1992.
Lichtiger S et al: Cyclosporine in severe ulcerative colitis refractory to steroid therapy, *New Engl J Med* 330(26):1841-1845, 1994.
McKenna CJ: Gastrointestinal bleeding in children: implications for nursing, *Nurs Clin North Am* 29(4):599-598, 1994.
Perrone VE: *Inflammatory bowel disease*. In Jackson PL, Vessey JA: *Primary care of the child with a chronic condition*, ed 2, St Louis, 1996, Mosby.
Rothrock et al: Clinical features of misdiagnosed appendicitis in children, *Ann Emerg Med* 20(1):45-50, 1991.
Scully C, Porter S: Recurrent aphthous stomatitis: current concepts of etiology, pathogenesis and management, *J Oral Pathol Med* 18(1):21-27, 1989.
Sherman PM: Peptic ulcer disease in children, *Gastroenterol Clin North Am* 23(4):707-725, 1994.

Hepatic Disorders

A-Kader HH: Hepatitis C virus: Implications to pediatric practice, *Pediatr Infect Dis J* 12(10):853-866, 1993.
Beath S et al: Liver transplantation in babies and children with extrahepatic biliary atresia, *J Pediatr Surg* 28(8):1044-1047, 1993.
Beath SV et al: Successful liver transplantation in babies under 1 year, *Br Med J* 307:825-828, 1993.
Bodenhorn K: Hepatitis B: the challenge for nurses, *J Pediatr Health Care* 6(1):41-42, 1992.
Carey W, Patel G: Viral hepatitis in the 1990's. I. Current principles of management, *Cleve Clin J Med* 59(4):317-325, 1992.
Carey W, Patel G: Viral hepatitis in the 1990's. II. Hepatitis B and delta virus, *Cleve Clin J Med* 59(4):393-401, 1992.
Karrer FM et al: Congenital biliary tract disease, *Surg Clin North Am* 70(6):1403-1418, 1990.
Nowicki M, Balistreri W: Hepatitis A to E: building up the alphabet, *Contemp Pediatr* 9(11):118-128, 1992.
Pasquale M, Cerra F: Sengstaken-Blakemore tube placement, *Crit Care Clin* 8(4):743-753, 1992.
Smith J: Hepatitis C: a major public health problem, *J Adv Nurs* 18:503-506, 1993.

Structural Defects

Borkowski S: Common pediatric surgical problems, *Nurs Clin North Am* 29(4):551-562, 1994.
Curtin G: The infant with cleft lip or palate: more than a surgical problem, *J Perinat Neonat Nurs* 3(3):80-89, 1990.
Dado DV: Experience with the functional cleft lip repair, *Plast Reconstr Surg* 86(5):872-881, 1990.
Eliason MJ: Cleft lip and palate: developmental effects, *J Pediatr Nurs* 6(2):107, 1991.
Filston HC: Fluid and electrolyte management in the pediatric surgical patient, *Surg Clin North Am* 72(6):1189-1200, 1992.
Kaufman FL: Managing the cleft lip and palate patient, *Pediatr Clin North Am* 38(5):1127-1147, 1991.
Kent PA, Curley MA: Challenges in nursing: infants with congenital diaphragmatic hernia, *Heart Lung* 21(4):381-389, 1992.
Laurent J et al: Long-term outcome after surgery for biliary atresia, *Gastroenterology* 99:1793-1797, 1990.
Levine AH: Fetal surgery: in utero repair of congenital diaphragmatic hernia, *AORN J* 54(1):16, 1991.
MacDonald CA: Biliary atresia, *J Pediatr Nurs* 6(6):374-383, 1991.
Moreno CN, Iovanne BA: Congenital diaphragmatic hernia. I. *Neonatal Network* 12(1):19, 1993.
Nyhus LM et al: Inguinal hernia repairs, *AORN* 52(2):292-304, 1990.
Puntis JW et al: Growth and feeding problems after repair of esophageal atresia, *Arch Dis Child* 65:84-88, 1990.
Ricketts R et al: Modern treatment of cloacal exstrophy, *J Pediatr Surg* 26(4):444-450, 1991.
Skinner M, Grosfeld J: Inguinal and umbilical hernia repair in infants and children, *Surg Clin North Am* 73(3):439-449, 1993.
Theorell CJ: Congenital diaphragmatic hernia: a physiologic approach to management, *J Perinat Neonat Nurs* 3(3):66-79, 1990.
Torfs C, Curry C, Roeper P: Gastroschisis, *J Pediatr* 116:1-6, 1990.
Van Meurs KP et al: Effect of extracorporeal membrane oxygenation on survival of infants with congenital diaphragmatic hernia, *J Pediatr* 117(6):954-960, 1990.

Obstructive Disorders/Malabsorption Syndromes

Anson O, Weizman Z, Zeevi N: Celiac disease: parental knowledge and attitudes of dietary compliance, *Pediatrics* 85:98-103, 1990.
Champoux AN, Beccaro MA, Nazar-Stewart V: Recurrent intussusception: risks and features, *Arch Pediatr Adolesc-Med*, 148(5):474-478, 1994.
Deluca S: Hypertrophic pyloric stenosis, *Am Fam Physician* 47(8):1771-1773, 1993.
Edes TE: Clinical management of short-bowel syndrome, *Postgrad Med* 88(4):91-95, 1990.
Horman SH: Pica as a presenting symptom in childhood celiac disease, *Am J Clin Nutr* 51:139-141, 1990.
Saunderlin G: Celiac disease: a review, *Gastroenterol Nurs* 17(3):100-105, 1994.
Skipper R, Boeckman C, Klein R: Childhood intussusception, *Surg Gynecol Obstet* 171:151-153, 1990.
Trier J: Diagnosis and treatment of celiac sprue, *Hosp Pract* 30:41-54, 1993.
Wise B: Neonatal short bowel syndrome, *Neonatal Network* 11(7):9-15, 1992.
Zahr LK et al: The short bowel syndrome: an update and a case study, *J Pediatr Nurs* 7(3):189-195, 1992.

Ingestion of Injurious Agents

Beware the hazards of activated charcoal, *Am J Nurs* 94(12): 10, 1994.
Birkland P: International update: alternative treatment for common but dangerous acetaminophen overdoses, *J Emerg Nurs* 19(2):32A-33A, 1993.
Fine JS, Goldfrank LR: Update in medical toxicology, *Pediatr Emerg Med* 39(5):1031-1051, 1992.
Henretig F et al: Repeated acetaminophen overdosing causing hepatotoxicity in children, *Clin Pediatr* 28(11):525-528, 1989.
Kulig K: Initial management of ingestions of toxic substances, *N Engl J Med* 326(25):1677-1681, 1992.
Lewis RK, Paloucek FP: Assessment and treatment of acetaminophen overdose, *Clin Pharm* 10:765-774, 1991.
Lovejoy FH Jr: Diagnosis of the unknown poison, *Pediatr Rev* 13(7):273-274, 1992.
Mack R: Hydrocarbon ingestion—to Eyre is human, *Contemp Pediatr* 8(12):47-64, 1991.
Mack RB: Dishwasher detergent toxicity—here's looking at you, kid, *Contemp Pediatr* 10(11):49-58, 1993.
Manoguerra AS: Pediatric poisoning, *Emergency* 24(10):19-24, 1992.
Preventing strictures after caustic ingestion, *Emerg Med* 25(6):48, 1993.
Rogers GC, Matyunas NJ: *Handbook of common poisonings in children*, ed 3, Elk Grove Village, Ill, 1994, American Academy of Pediatrics.
Vertrees J, McWilliams B, Kelly H: Repeated oral administration of activated charcoal for treating aspirin overdose in young children, *Pediatrics* 85(4):594-598, 1990.

Wigder HN et al: Emergency department poison advice telephone calls, *Ann Emerg Med* 25(3):349-352, 1995.

Heavy Metal Poisoning

Binder S: Childhood lead poisoning: the impact of prevention, *JAMA* 269(13):1679-1681, 1993.

Brown M, Bellinger D, Matthews J: In utero lead exposure, *MCN Am J Matern Child Nurs* 15(2):94-96, 1990.

Castiglia PT: Pica, *J Pediatr Health Care* 7(4):174-176, 1993.

Cummins SK, Goldman LR: Even advantaged children show cognitive deficits from low-level lead toxicity, *Pediatrics* 90(6):995-997, 1992.

DeRienzo-DeVivio S: Childhood lead poisoning: shifting to primary prevention, *Pediatr Nurs* 18(6):565-567, 1992.

Goldman LR: Childhood lead poisoning in 1994, *JAMA* 272(4):315-316, 1994 (editorial).

Kimbrough RD, LeVois M, Webb DR: Management of children with slightly elevated blood lead levels, *Pediatrics* 93(2):188-191, 1994.

Mahaffey KR: Exposure to lead in childhood: the importance of prevention, *N Engl J Med* 327(18):1308-1309, 1992.

Matte TD et al: Acute high-dose lead exposure from beverage contaminated by traditional Mexican pottery, *Lancet* 344(8928):1064-1065, 1994.

Needham DD: Diagnosis and management of lead-poisoned children: the pediatric nurse practitioner in a specialty program, *J Pediatr Health Care* 8(6):268-273, 1994.

Pirkle JL et al: The decline in blood lead levels in the United States, *JAMA* 272(4):284-291, 1994.

Swindell SL et al: Home abatement and blood lead changes in children with class III lead poisoning, *Clin Pediatr* 33(9):536-541, 1994.

Update: iron poisonings—so tragic, so preventable, *Contemp Pediatr* 10(4):123, 1993.

Weitzman M, Glotzer D: Lead poisoning, *Pediatr Rev* 13(12):461-468, 1992.

Weitzman M et al: Lead-contaminated soil abatement and urban children's blood lead levels, *JAMA* 269(13):1647-1654, 1993.

Zelman M et al: Toxicity from vacuumed mercury: a household hazard, *Clin Pediatr* 30(2):121-123, 1991.

CHAPTER 45

Cardiovascular Dysfunction

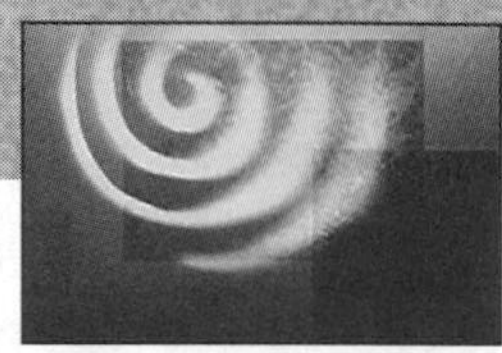

CARDIOVASCULAR DYSFUNCTION, P. 1450

Assessment of cardiac function, p. 1450
Cardiac catheterization, p. 1451

CONGENITAL HEART DISEASE, P. 1453

General concepts, p. 1453
Classification of defects, p. 1454

DEFECTS WITH INCREASED PULMONARY BLOOD FLOW, P. 1455

Atrial septal defect (ASD), p. 1456
Ventricular septal defect (VSD), p. 1456
Atrioventricular canal (AVC) defect, p. 1457
Patent ductus arteriosus (PDA), p. 1458

OBSTRUCTIVE DEFECTS, P. 1455

Coarctation of the aorta (COA), p. 1458
Aortic stenosis (AS), p. 1459
Pulmonic stenosis (PS), p. 1460

DEFECTS WITH DECREASED PULMONARY BLOOD FLOW, P. 1457

Tetralogy of Fallot (TOF), p. 1460
Tricuspid atresia, p. 1461

MIXED DEFECTS, P. 1465

Transposition of the great arteries (TGA) or transposition of the great vessels (TGV), p. 1462
Total anomalous pulmonary venous connection (TAPVC), p. 1462
Truncus arteriosus (TA), p. 1463
Hypoplastic left heart syndrome (HLHS), p. 1464

CLINICAL CONSEQUENCES OF CONGENITAL HEART DISEASE, P. 1465

Congestive heart failure (CHF), p. 1465
Hypoxemia, p. 1472

NURSING CARE OF THE FAMILY AND CHILD WITH CONGENITAL HEART DISEASE, P. 1474

ACQUIRED CARDIOVASCULAR DISORDERS, P. 1481

Bacterial (infective) endocarditis (BE), p. 1481
Rheumatic fever (RF), p. 1482
Hyperlipidemia (hypercholesterolemia), p. 1483
Cardiac dysrhythmias, p. 1484

VASCULAR DYSFUNCTION, P. 1486

Systemic hypertension, p. 1486
Kawasaki disease (KD) (mucocutaneous lymph node syndrome), p. 1487
Shock, p. 1489
Anaphylaxis, p. 1491
Toxic shock syndrome (TSS), p. 1492
Henoch-Schönlein purpura (HSP), p. 1493

HEART TRANSPLANTATION, P. 1494

Cardiovascular Dysfunction

Cardiovascular disorders in children are divided into two major groups, congenital heart disease and acquired heart disorders. **Congenital heart disease** includes primarily anatomic abnormalities present at birth that result in abnormal cardiac function. The clinical consequences of congenital heart defects fall into two broad categories, congestive heart failure and hypoxemia. **Acquired cardiac disorders** refer to disease processes or abnormalities that occur after birth and can be seen in the normal heart or in the presence of congenital heart defects. They result from various factors, including infection, autoimmune responses, environmental factors, and familial tendencies.

ASSESSMENT OF CARDIAC FUNCTION

History and Physical Examination

Nursing assessment of children for evidence of cardiac dysfunction begins with a careful history to elicit information regarding possible causes of heart disease: (1) history of heart disease in other family members, such as a parent or sibling; (2) contact with known teratogens, such as rubella, during pregnancy; (3) presence of chromosomal abnormalities such as Down syndrome; (4) poor weight gain and/or feeding behavior; (5) frequent respiratory infections; (6) prior murmurs; (7) respiratory difficulties such as tachypnea, dyspnea, shortness of breath; or (8) recent streptococcal infection in the child. Exercise intolerance and fatigue (such as during feeding in the infant) are characteristic features of heart disease.

The physical assessment of suspected cardiac disease begins with observation of general appearance, then proceeds with more specific observations. The following are supplementary to the general assessment techniques described for physical assessment of the chest and heart in Chapter 32.

Inspection

Nutritional state—failure to thrive, or poor weight gain, is associated with heart disease

Color—cyanosis is a common feature of congenital heart disease, and pallor is associated with poor perfusion

Chest deformities—an enlarged heart sometimes distorts the chest configuration

Unusual pulsations—visible pulsations of the neck veins are seen in some patients

Respiratory excursion—the ease or difficulty of respiration (e.g., tachypnea, dyspnea, presence of expiratory grunt)

Clubbing of fingers—is associated with cyanosis

Palpation and percussion

Chest—helps discern heart size and other characteristics (such as thrills) associated with heart disease

Abdomen—hepatomegaly and/or splenomegaly may be evident

Peripheral pulses—rate, regularity, and amplitude (strength) may reveal discrepancies

Auscultation

Heart rate and rhythm—listen for fast heart rates **(tachycardia)**, slow heart rates **(bradycardia)**, or irregular rhythms

Character of heart sounds—distinct or muffled, murmurs, additional heart sounds

Diagnostic Evaluation

A variety of invasive and noninvasive tests may be used in the diagnosis of heart disease (Table 45-1). Cardiac catheterization, which generates more anxiety than any other cardiac test, is discussed in detail.

CARDIAC CATHETERIZATION

Cardiac catheterization is a diagnostic procedure in which a radiopaque catheter is inserted through a peripheral blood vessel into the heart. The catheter is usually introduced through a cutdown procedure, in which a small incision is made to expose the vessel, or through a percutaneous technique, in which the catheter is threaded through a large-bore needle that is inserted into the vein. The catheter is guided through the heart with the aid of fluoroscopy. Once the tip of the catheter is within a heart chamber, contrast material is injected, and films are taken of the dilution and circulation of the material *(angiography)*.

Types of cardiac catherizations include the following:

1. **Diagnostic catheterizations**—used to diagnose congenital cardiac defects, particularly in symptomatic infants and before surgical repair. These are divided into right-sided catheterizations, in which the catheter is introduced through a vein (usually the femoral vein) and threaded to the right atrium (most common), and left-sided catheterizations, in which the catheter is threaded through an artery into the aorta and into the heart.

TABLE 45-1 Procedures for cardiac diagnosis

PROCEDURE	DESCRIPTION
Chest radiograph (x-ray)	Provides information on heart size and pulmonary blood flow patterns
Electrocardiography (ECG)	Graphic measure of the electrical activity of the heart
Holter monitor	24-Hour continuous ECG recording used to assess dysrhythmias
Echocardiography	Use of high-frequency sound waves obtained by a transducer to produce an image of cardiac structures
Transthoracic	Done with transducer on chest
M-Mode	One-dimensional graphic view used to estimate ventricular size and function
Two-dimensional (2-D)	Real-time, cross-sectional views of heart used to identify cardiac structures and cardiac anatomy
Doppler	Identifies blood flow patterns and pressure gradients across structures
Fetal	Imaging fetal heart in utero
Transesophageal (TEE)	Transducer placed in esophagus behind the heart to obtain images of posterior heart structures or in patients with poor images from chest approach
Cardiac catheterization	Imaging study using radiopaque catheters placed in a peripheral blood vessel and advanced into heart to measure pressures and oxygen levels in heart chambers and visualize heart structures and blood flow patterns
Hemodynamics	Measures pressures and oxygen saturations in heart chambers
Angiography	Use of contrast material to illuminate heart structures and blood flow patterns
Biopsy	Use of special catheter to remove tiny samples of heart muscle for microscopic evaluation; used in assessing infection, inflammation, or muscle dysfunction disorders; also to evaluate for rejection after heart transplantation
Electrophysiology (EPS)	Employ special catheters with electrodes to record electrical activity from within heart; used to diagnose rhythm disturbances
Exercise stress test	Monitoring of heart rate, blood pressure, ECG, and oxygen consumption at rest and during progressive exercise on a treadmill or bicycle

2. **Interventional catheterizations (therapeutic catheterizations)**—a balloon catheter or other device is used to alter the cardiac anatomic characteristics. Examples include dilating stenotic valves or vessels and closing abnormal connections.
3. **Electrophysiology studies**—catheters with tiny electrodes that record the impulses of the heart directly from the conduction system are used to evaluate dysrhythmias and sometimes destroy accessory pathways that cause some tachydysrhythmias.

Nursing Care Management

Cardiac catheterization has become a routine diagnostic procedure and may be done on an outpatient basis. However, it is not without risks, especially in neonates and seriously ill infants and children. Typical reactions include acute hemorrhage from the entry site (more likely with interventional procedures because larger catheters are used), low-grade fever, nausea, vomiting, loss of pulse in the catheterized extremity (usually transient, resulting from a clot, hematoma, or intimal tear), and transient dysrhythmias (generally catheter-induced).

Preprocedural care. A complete nursing assessment is necessary to ensure a safe procedure with minimum complications. This assessment should include accurate height (essential to correct catheter selection) and weight. Obtaining a history of allergic reactions is important since some of the contrast agents are iodine-based. Specific attention to signs and symptoms of infection is crucial. Severe diaper rash may be a reason to cancel the procedure if femoral access is required. Since assessment of pedal pulses is important after catheterization, the nurse should assess and mark pulses (dorsalis pedis, posterior tibial) before the child goes to the catheterization room. The presence and quality of pulses in both feet are clearly documented. Baseline oxygen saturation using pulse oximetry in children with cyanosis is also recorded.

Preparing the child and family for the procedure is the joint responsibility of the physician and nurse. The cardiologist usually explains the procedure to the parents, but nurses can reinforce and clarify the information. Many parents and older children who undergo both cardiac catheterization and cardiac surgery say, in retrospect, that they were more anxious about cardiac catheterization than about the surgery. Preparation for cardiac catheterization requires the same attention to the principles of preparation for procedures described in Chapter 42.

It is important to describe the catheterization ("cath") room because the x-ray machinery can appear frightening. Other aspects of the procedure that should be explained (using words the child understands) include, specifically, that (1) the groin (or sometimes the antecubital fossa) is cleansed with a special brown solution; (2) the child will receive some medicine (lidocaine) in that area so that the skin will go to sleep; (3) a tube will be placed in a blood vessel, and the child may feel a little pushing at times; (4) when a special "medicine" (referring to the contrast material) is put into the tubing, the child may feel warm for a few seconds; and (5) as soon as the medicine is put in, the lights will go off and a machine will begin to take pictures. The last point is important to stress because younger children may associate the lights going off with "causing" the warm feeling from the contrast agent. As a result, they may become fearful of the dark and the noise from the machines.

Atraumatic Care

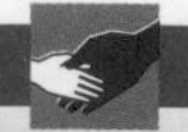

CARDIAC CATHETERIZATION

To reduce the pain of the catheter insertion, apply eutectic mixture of local anesthetics (EMLA) topically to site for 60 minutes or use buffered lidocaine and 30-gauge needle for intradermal injection (see Pain Management, Chapter 41).

Methods of sedation vary among institutions and may include oral or intravenous medications (see the Atraumatic Care box above). The child's age, heart defect, clinical status, and type of catheterization procedure planned are considered when sedation is determined. Children are allowed nothing by mouth (NPO) for 2 or more hours before the procedure, and infants and patients with polycythemia may need intravenous fluids to prevent dehydration and hypoglycemia.

Postprocedural care. Essentially the care following cardiac catheterization is the same as general postoperative care. However, since children are not anesthetized during the procedure, they usually return directly to their room. Patients are usually placed on a cardiac monitor and a pulse oximeter for the first few hours of recovery. The most important nursing responsibility is observation of the following for signs of complications:

- Pulses, especially below the catheterization site, for equality and symmetry (pulse distal to the site may be weaker for the first few hours after catheterization but should gradually increase in strength)
- Temperature and color of the affected extremity, since coolness or blanching may indicate arterial obstruction
- Vital signs, which are taken as frequently as every 15 minutes, with special emphasis on heart rate, which is counted for 1 full minute for evidence of dysrhythmias or bradycardia
- Blood pressure, especially for hypotension, which may indicate hemorrhage from cardiac perforation or bleeding at the site of initial catheterization
- Dressing, for evidence of bleeding or hematoma formation in the femoral or antecubital area
- Fluid intake, both intravenous and oral, to ensure adequate hydration. (Blood loss in the catheterization laboratory, the child's NPO status, and diuretic actions of dyes used during the procedure put children at risk for hypovolemia and dehydration.)
- Hypoglycemia, especially in infants who should receive dextrose containing intravenous (IV) fluids; blood glucose levels should be checked

Nursing ALERT

If bleeding occurs, direct continuous pressure is applied 2.5 cm (1 inch) above the percutaneous skin site to localize pressure over the vessel puncture (Agamalian, 1986).

Critical Thinking Q & A 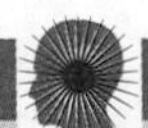

CARDIAC CATHETERIZATION

David, a 4-year-old with tetralogy of Fallot, has just returned from the catheterization laboratory. He has vomited, and his mother calls you to the bedside to tell you that he is bleeding. You arrive to find David crying and sitting up in a puddle of blood. The first thing you do is:

1. Increase the rate of his intravenous fluids.
2. Give an antiemetic and keep David on nothing by mouth (NPO) status.
3. Call the cardiologist.
4. Lay David down, remove the dressing, and apply direct pressure above the catheterization site.

The correct answer is four. This may be an arterial bleed, and David is at risk for losing a large amount of blood in a short time. Your first priority should be to control the bleeding. Pressure is applied above the visible catheterization site where the vessel was entered. Placing the child flat decreases the effect of gravity on the rate of bleeding and is the appropriate position in case of shock. When this is done, you can notify the practitioner and replace fluids and control emesis as ordered.

Home Care 

FOLLOWING CARDIAC CATHETERIZATION

Remove pressure dressing the day after catheterization. Cover site with an adhesive bandage strip for several days.
Keep site clean and dry. Avoid tub baths for several days; may shower.
Observe site for redness, swelling, drainage, and bleeding. Monitor for fever. Notify practitioner if these occur.
Avoid strenuous exercise for several days. May attend school.
Resume regular diet without restrictions.
Use acetaminophen or ibuprofen for pain.
Keep follow-up appointments per practitioner's instruction.

Modified from Children's Hospital (Boston) Cardiovascular Program, 1994.

Depending on hospital policy the child may be kept in bed with the affected extremity maintained straight for 4 to 6 hours after venous catheterization and 6 to 8 hours after arterial catheterization to facilitate healing of the cannulated vessel. If younger children have difficulty complying, they can be held in the parent's lap with the leg maintained in the correct position. The child's usual diet can be resumed as soon as tolerated, beginning with sips of clear liquids and advancing as the condition allows. The child is encouraged to void to clear the contrast material from the blood. Generally there is only slight discomfort at the percutaneous site. To prevent infection, the catheterization area is protected from possible contamination. If the child wears diapers, the dressing can be kept dry by covering it with a piece of plastic film and sealing the edges of the film to the skin with tape. However, the nurse must be careful to continue to observe the site for any evidence of bleeding. (See also the Critical Thinking Q & A and Home Care boxes above).

See also Nursing Care Plan: The Child Who Undergoes Cardiac Catheterization.*

Congenital Heart Disease

GENERAL CONCEPTS

The incidence of congenital heart disease (CHD) in children is generally believed to be 4 to 10 per 1000 live births, and CHD is the major cause of death in the first year (other than prematurity). The sexes are affected differently, depending on the defect. Children with CHD are also more likely to have extracardiac defects, such as tracheoesophageal fistula, renal agenesis, and diaphragmatic hernias.

The cause of most congenital heart defects is not known. However, several factors are associated with a higher-than-normal incidence of the disease. These include prenatal factors such as (1) maternal rubella during pregnancy, (2) maternal alcoholism, (3) maternal age over 40 years, and (4) maternal insulin-dependent diabetes. Several genetic factors are also implicated, although the influence is multifactorial. For example, there is an increased risk of CHD in the child who (1) has a sibling with a heart defect; (2) has a parent with CHD; (3) has a chromosomal aberration, such as Down syndrome; or (4) is born with other, noncardiac congenital anomalies.

Circulatory Changes at Birth

During fetal life, blood carrying oxygen and nutritive materials from the placenta enters the fetal system through the umbilicus via the large umbilical vein. Oxygenated blood enters the heart by way of the inferior vena cava. Because of the higher pressure of blood entering the right atrium, it is directed posteriorly in a straight pathway across the right atrium and through the *foramen ovale* to the left atrium. In this way the better-oxygenated blood enters the left atrium and ventricle, to be pumped through the aorta to the head and upper extremities. Blood from the head and upper extremities entering the right atrium from the superior vena cava is directed downward through the tricuspid valve into the right ventricle. From here it is pumped through the pulmonary artery, where the major portion is shunted to the descending aorta via the *ductus arteriosus*. Only a small amount flows to and from the nonfunctioning fetal lungs (Fig. 45-1, *A*).

Before birth the high pulmonary vascular resistance created by the collapsed fetal lung causes greater pressures in the right side of the heart and the pulmonary arteries. At the same time the free-flowing placental circulation and the ductus arteriosus produce a low vascular resistance in the remainder of the fetal vascular system. With the cessation of placental blood flow from clamping of the umbilical cord and the expansion of the lungs at birth, the hemodynamic characteristics of the fetal vascular system undergo pronounced and abrupt changes (Fig. 45-1, *B*).

With the first breath, the lungs are expanded, and increased oxygen causes pulmonary vasodilation. Pulmonary pressures start to fall as systemic pressures, given the removal of the placenta, start to rise. Normally the foramen ovale closes as the pressure in the left atrium exceeds the pressure in

*In Wong DL: *Wong and Whaley's clinical manual of pediatric nursing*, ed 4, St Louis, 1996, Mosby.

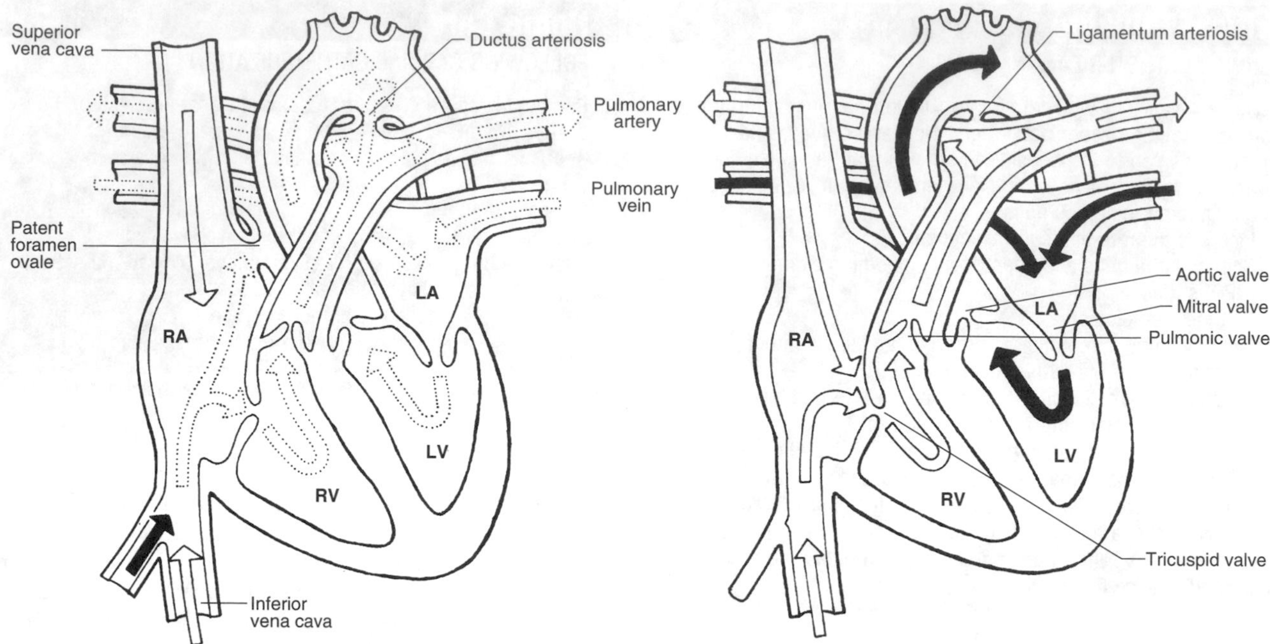

Fig. 45-1 Changes in circulation at birth. **A,** Prenatal circulation. **B,** Postnatal circulation. *Arrows* indicate direction of blood flow. Although four pulmonary veins enter the LA, for simplicity this diagram shows only two. *RA,* Right atrium; *LA,* left atrium; *RV,* right ventricle; *LV,* left ventricle.

the right atrium. The ductus arteriosus starts to close in the presence of increased oxygen concentration in the blood and other factors.

Altered Hemodynamics

To appreciate the physiology of heart defects, it is necessary to understand the role of pressure gradients, flow, and resistance within the circulation. Like any fluid, blood flows from an area of high pressure to one of lower pressure and toward the path of least resistance in response to the pumping action of the heart. In general, the higher the pressure gradient, the greater the rate of flow; the higher the resistance, the less the rate of flow.

Normally the pressure on the right side of the heart is lower than that on the left side, and the resistance in the pulmonary circulation is less than that in the systemic circulation. Vessels entering or exiting these chambers have corresponding pressures. Therefore if there is an abnormal connection between the heart chambers (such as a septal defect), blood will necessarily flow from an area of higher pressure (left side) to one of lower pressure (right side). Such a flow of blood is termed a *left-to-right shunt.*

Anomalies that cause cyanosis may result from a change in pressure so that the blood is shunted from the right to the left side of the heart *(right-to-left shunt)* because of either increased pulmonary vascular resistance or obstruction to blood flow through the pulmonic valve and artery. Cyanosis may also result from a defect that allows mixing of oxygenated and deoxygenated blood within the heart chambers or great arteries, such as occurs in truncus arteriosus.

CLASSIFICATION OF DEFECTS

Congenital heart defects have been divided into two categories. Traditionally, a physical characteristic, cyanosis, has been used as the distinguishing feature, dividing the anomalies into *acyanotic* and *cyanotic* defects. In clinical practice this system is problematic because cyanosis may develop in children with acyanotic defects. Also, more often, those with cyanotic defects may be pink and have more clinical signs of congestive heart failure (CHF).

Another classification system, based on *hemodynamic characteristics,* also is used. The defining characteristic is blood flow patterns: (1) increased pulmonary blood flow, (2) decreased pulmonary blood flow, (3) obstruction to blood flow out of the heart, and (4) mixed blood flow, in which saturated and desaturated blood mix within the heart or great arteries. As a comparison, both classification systems are outlined in Fig. 45-2.

With the hemodynamic classification system, the clinical manifestations of each group are more uniform and predictable. Defects that allow blood flow from the high-pressure left side of the heart to the lower-pressure right side (left-to-right shunt) result in increased pulmonary blood flow and cause CHF. Obstructive defects impede blood flow out of the ventricles; obstruction on the left side of the heart results in CHF, whereas severe obstruction on the right side causes cyanosis. Defects that cause decreased pulmonary blood flow result in cyanosis. Mixed lesions present a variable clinical picture based on degree of mixing and amount of pulmonary blood flow; hypoxemia (with or without cyanosis) and CHF usually occur together. This system is used in the following discussion.

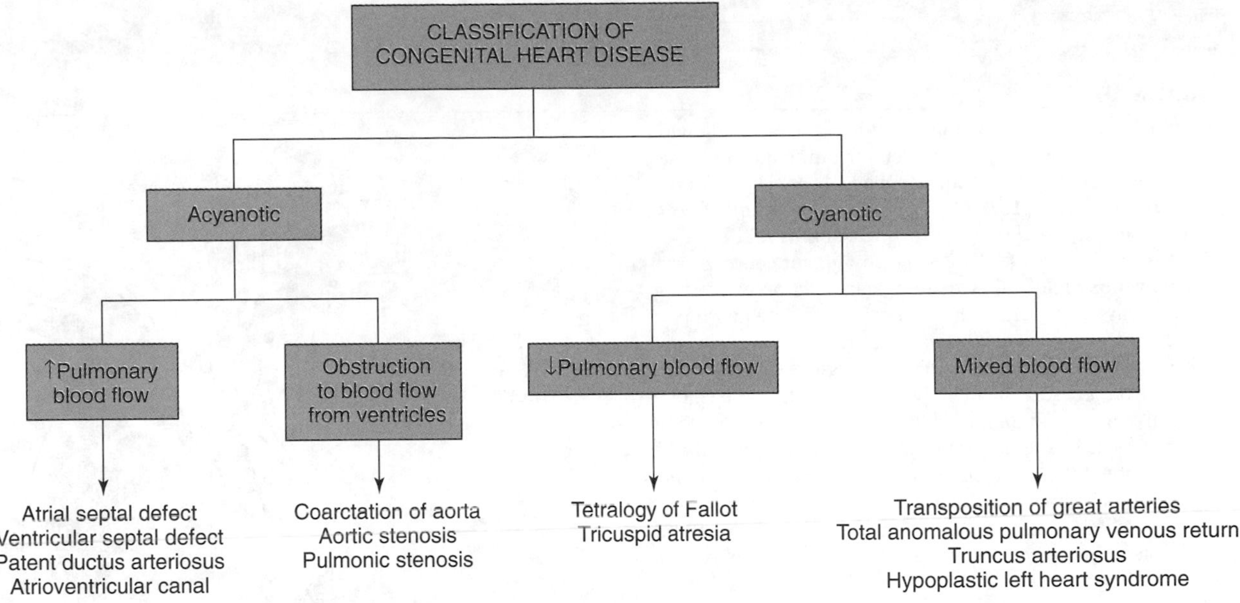

Fig. 45-2 Comparison of acyanotic-cyanotic and hemodynamic classification systems of congenital heart disease.

Defects With Increased Pulmonary Blood Flow

In the group of cardiac defects characterized by increased pulmonary blood flow, intracardiac communications along the septum or an abnormal connection between the great arteries allows blood to flow from the high-pressure left side of the heart to the lower-pressure right side of the heart (Fig. 45-3). Increased blood volume on the right side of the heart increases pulmonary blood flow at the expense of systemic blood flow. Clinically patients demonstrate signs and symptoms of CHF. Atrial and ventricular septal defects and patent ductus arteriosus are typical anomalies in this group (Box 45-1).

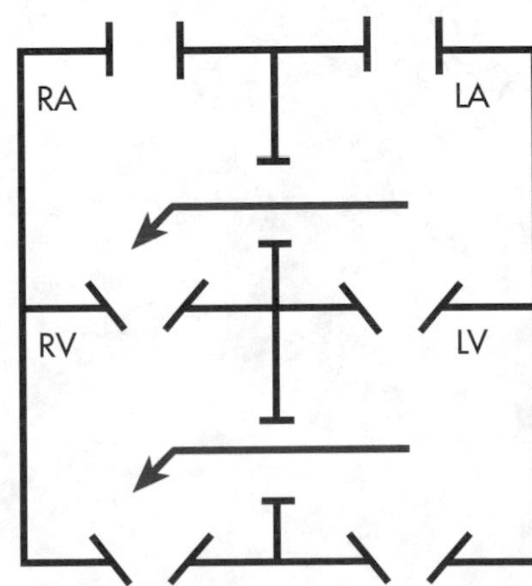

Fig. 45-3 Hemodynamics in defects with increased pulmonary blood flow.

Obstructive Defects

Obstructive defects are those in which blood exiting the heart meets an area of anatomic narrowing (stenosis), causing obstruction to blood flow. The pressure in the ventricle and in the great artery before the obstruction is increased, and the pressure in the area beyond the obstruction is decreased. The location of the narrowing is usually near the valve (Fig. 45-4):

Valvular—At the site of the valve itself
Subvalvular—Narrowing in the ventricle below the valve (also referred to as the *ventricular outflow tract*)

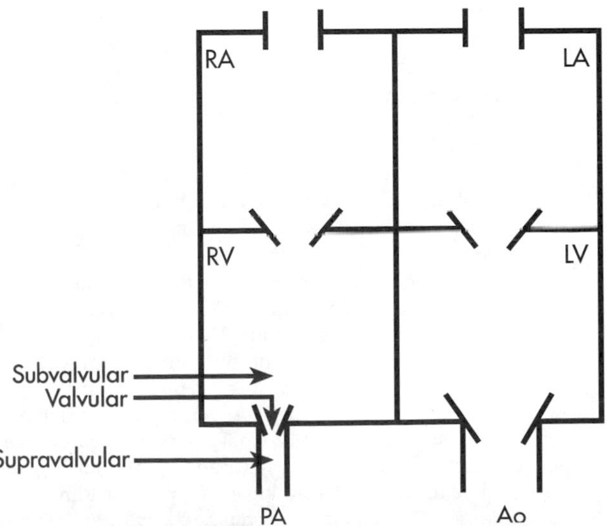

Fig. 45-4 Obstruction to ventricular ejection can occur at the valvular level *(shown)*, below the valve *(subvalvular)*, or above the valve *(supravalvular)*. Pulmonary stenosis is shown here.

BOX 45-1
Defects With Increased Pulmonary Blood Flow

ATRIAL SEPTAL DEFECT (ASD)

Description: Abnormal opening between the atria, allowing blood from the higher-pressure left atrium to flow into the lower-pressure right atrium. There are three types:

Ostium primum (ASD 1)—Opening at lower end of septum; may be associated with mitral valve abnormalities

Ostium secundum (ASD 2)—Opening near center of septum

Sinus venosus defect—Opening near junction of superior vena cava and right atrium; may be associated with partial anomalous pulmonary venous connection

Pathophysiology: Because left atrial pressure slightly exceeds right atrial pressure, blood flows from the left to the right atrium, causing an increased flow of oxygenated blood into the right side of the heart. Despite the low pressure difference, a high rate of flow can still occur because of low pulmonary vascular resistance and the greater distensibility of the right atrium, which further reduces flow resistance. This volume is well tolerated by the right ventricle because it is delivered under much lower pressure than in a ventricular septal defect. Although there is right atrial and ventricular enlargement, cardiac failure is unusual in an uncomplicated atrial septal defect. Pulmonary vascular changes usually occur only after several decades if the defect is unrepaired.

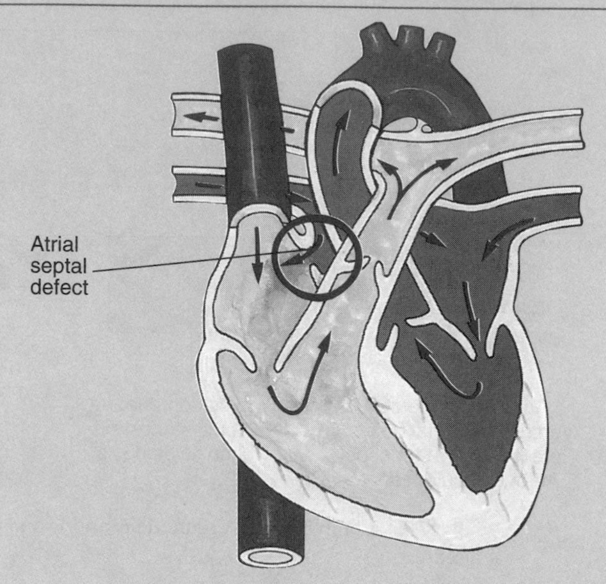

Clinical manifestations: Patients may be asymptomatic. Congestive heart failure (CHF) may develop. There is a characteristic murmur. Patients are at risk for atrial dysrhythmias (probably caused by atrial enlargement and stretching of conduction fibers) and pulmonary vascular obstructive disease and emboli formation later in life from chronic increased pulmonary blood flow.

Surgical treatment: Surgical (Dacron) patch closure of moderate to large defects similar to closure of ventricular septal defects. Open repair with cardiopulmonary bypass is usually performed before school age. In addition, the sinus venosus defect requires patch placement, so the anomalous right pulmonary venous return is directed to the left atrium with a baffle. The ASD 1 may require repair or, rarely, replacement of the mitral valve.

Nonsurgical treatment: ASD 2 may also be closed using devices during cardiac catheterization. This technique is in clinical trials in some centers.

Prognosis: Very low operative mortality rate, less than 1%.

VENTRICULAR SEPTAL DEFECT (VSD)

Description: Abnormal opening between the right and left ventricles. May be classified according to location: membranous (accounting for 80%) or muscular. May vary in size from a small pinhole to absence of the septum, resulting in a common ventricle. Frequently associated with other defects, such as pulmonary stenosis, transposition of the great vessels, patent ductus arteriosus, atrial defects, and coarctation of the aorta. Many VSDs, especially those in infants with small defects, close spontaneously. Spontaneous closure is most likely to occur during the first year of life in children having small or moderate defects. A left-to-right shunt is caused by the flow of blood from the higher-pressure left ventricle to the lower-pressure right ventricle.

Pathophysiology: Because of the higher pressure within the left ventricle and because the systemic arterial circulation offers more resistance than the pulmonary circulation, blood flows through the defect into the pulmonary artery. The increased blood volume is pumped into the lungs; increased pulmonary vascular resistance may eventually result. Increased pressure in the right ventricle as a result of left-to-right shunting and pulmonary resistance causes the muscle to hypertrophy. If the right ventricle is unable to accommodate the increased workload, the right atrium may also enlarge as it attempts to overcome the resistance offered by incomplete right ventricular emptying. In severe defects Eisenmenger syndrome may develop.

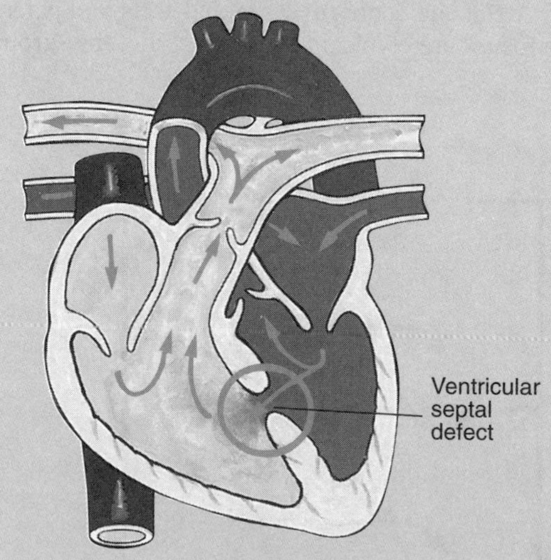

BOX 45-1
Defects With Increased Pulmonary Blood Flow—cont'd

Clinical manifestations: CHF is common. There is a characteristic murmur. Patients are at risk for bacterial endocarditis and pulmonary vascular obstructive disease. In severe defects, Eisenmenger syndrome may develop.

Surgical treatment:

Palliative: Pulmonary banding in symptomatic infants. Although palliation using a pulmonary artery band is done in some institutions, data suggest that complete primary repair can be performed without an increased risk during the first year of life. Age alone has little influence on the outcome of the repair, although younger infants are frequently sicker in the postoperative period.

Complete repair: Small defects are repaired with a purse-string approach. Large defects usually require a knitted patch (Dacron) sewn over the opening. Both procedures are performed via cardiopulmonary bypass. The repair is generally approached through the right atrium and the tricuspid valve. Postoperative complications include residual VSD and conduction disturbances.

Nonsurgical treatment: Device closure during cardiac catheterization is under clinical trials in some centers for closure of muscular defects that carry a high operative risk.

Prognosis: Risks depend on the location of the defect, number of defects, and other associated cardiac defects. Single membranous defects have a low mortality rate (less than 5%); multiple muscular defects can have a risk of more than 20%.

ATRIOVENTRICULAR CANAL (AVC) DEFECT

Description: Incomplete fusion of endocardial cushions. Consists of a low atrial septal defect that is continuous with a high ventricular septal defect and clefts of the mitral and tricuspid valves, creating a large central atrioventricular valve that allows blood to flow between all four chambers of the heart. The directions and pathways of flow are determined by pulmonary and systemic resistance, left and right ventricular pressures, and the compliance of each chamber, although flow is generally from left to right. It is the most common cardiac defect in children with Down syndrome.

Pathophysiology: The alterations in the hemodynamics depend on the defect's severity and the child's pulmonary vascular resistance. Immediately after birth, while the newborn's pulmonary vascular resistance is high, there is minimum shunting of blood through the defect. Once this resistance falls, left-to-right shunting occurs and pulmonary blood flow increases. The resultant pulmonary vascular engorgement predisposes to development of CHF.

Clinical manifestations: Patients usually have moderate to severe CHF. There is a characteristic murmur. There may be mild cyanosis that increases with crying. Patients are at high risk for development of pulmonary vascular obstructive disease.

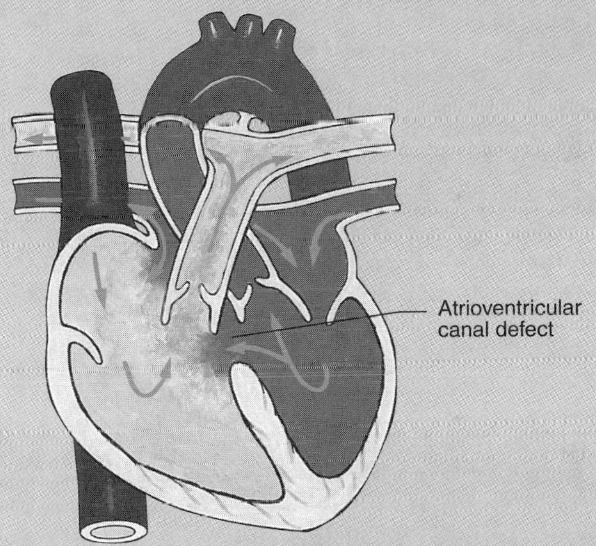

Surgical treatment:

Palliative: Pulmonary artery banding is done for infants with severe symptoms that are caused by increased pulmonary blood flow in some centers. Other centers believe complete repair can be performed in infants.

Complete repair: Surgical repair consists of patch closure of the septal defects and reconstruction of the (AV) valve tissue (either repair of the mitral valve cleft or fashioning of two AV valves). If the mitral valve defect is severe, a valve replacement may be needed. Postoperative complications include heart block, CHF, mitral regurgitation, dysrhythmias, and pulmonary hypertension.

Prognosis: Operative mortality rate is about 10%. Potential later problem is mitral regurgitation, which may require valve replacement.

Continued.

Supravalvular—Narrowing in the great artery above the valve

Coarctation of the aorta (narrowing of the aortic arch), aortic stenosis, and pulmonic stenosis are typical defects in this group (Box 45-2). Hemodynamically there is a pressure load on the ventricle and decreased cardiac output. Clinically infants and children exhibit signs of CHF. Children with mild obstruction may be asymptomatic. Rarely, as in severe pulmonic stenosis, hypoxemia may be seen.

Defects With Decreased Pulmonary Blood Flow

In the group of defects characterized by decreased pulmonary blood flow, there is obstruction of pulmonary blood flow and an anatomic defect (ASD or VSD) between the right and left sides of the heart (Fig. 45-5). Because blood has difficulty exiting the right side of the heart via the pulmonary artery, pres-

Text continued on p. 1465.

BOX 45-1
Defects With Increased Pulmonary Blood Flow—cont'd

PATENT DUCTUS ARTERIOSUS (PDA)

Description: Failure of the fetal ductus arteriosus (artery connecting the aorta and pulmonary artery) to close within the first weeks of life. The continued patency of this vessel allows blood to flow from the higher-pressure aorta to the lower-pressure pulmonary artery, causing a left-to-right shunt.

Pathophysiology: The hemodynamic consequences of PDA depend on the size of the ductus and the pulmonary vascular resistance. At birth the resistance is almost identical in the pulmonary and systemic circulations, thus equalizing the resistance in the aorta and pulmonary artery. As the systemic pressure exceeds the pulmonary pressure, blood begins to shunt from the aorta, across the duct, to the pulmonary artery (left-to-right shunt).

The additional blood is recirculated through the lungs and returned to the left atrium and left ventricle. The effects of this altered circulation are increased workload on the left side of the heart, increased pulmonary vascular congestion and possibly resistance, and potentially increased right ventricular pressure and hypertrophy.

Clinical manifestations: Patients may be asymptomatic or show signs of CHF. There is a characteristic machinery-like murmur. A widened pulse pressure and bounding pulses result from runoff of blood from the aorta to the pulmonary artery. Patients are at risk for bacterial endocarditis and pulmonary vascular obstructive disease in later life from chronic excessive pulmonary blood flow.

Medical management: Administration of indomethacin (prostaglandin inhibitor) has proved successful in closing a patent ductus in premature infants and some newborns.

Surgical treatment: Surgical division or ligation of the patent vessel via a left thoracotomy. A newer technique, visual assisted thoracoscopic surgery (VATS), uses a thoracoscope and instruments placed through three small incisions on the left side of the chest to place a clip on the ductus. It is used in some centers and eliminates the need for a thoracotomy, thereby speeding postoperative recovery.

Nonsurgical treatment: Closure with placement of an occluder device during cardiac catheterization is done in some institutions.

Prognosis: Both procedures can be done at low risk with less than 1% mortality rate.

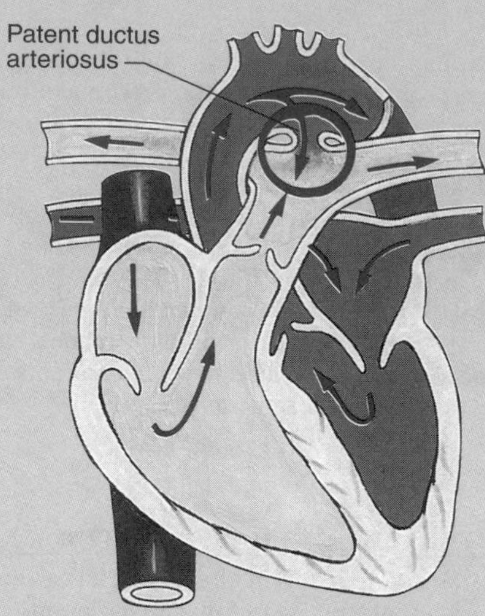

BOX 45-2
Obstructive Defects

COARCTATION OF THE AORTA (COA)

Description: Localized narrowing near the insertion of the ductus arteriosus, resulting in increased pressure proximal to the defect (head and upper extremities) and decreased pressure distal to the obstruction (body and lower extremities).

Pathophysiology: The effects of a narrowing within the aorta are increased pressure proximal to the defect and decreased pressure distal to it. In the preductal type of COA the lower half of the body is supplied with blood by the right ventricle through the ductus arteriosus. In the postductal type, right ventricular outflow cannot maintain blood flow to the descending aorta. Therefore collateral circulation develops during fetal life to maintain flow from the ascending to the descending aorta.

Clinical manifestations: There may be high blood pressure and bounding pulses in arms, weak or absent femoral pulses, and cool lower extremities with lower blood pressure. There are signs of CHF in infants. Often these patients' hemodynamic condition deteriorates rapidly, and they are admitted to the intensive care unit near death, usually severely acidotic and hypotensive. Mechanical ventilation and inotropic support are often necessary before surgery. Older children may experience dizziness, headaches, fainting, and epistaxis resulting from hypertension. Patients are at risk for hypertension, ruptured aorta, aortic aneurysm, or cerebrovascular accident (stroke).

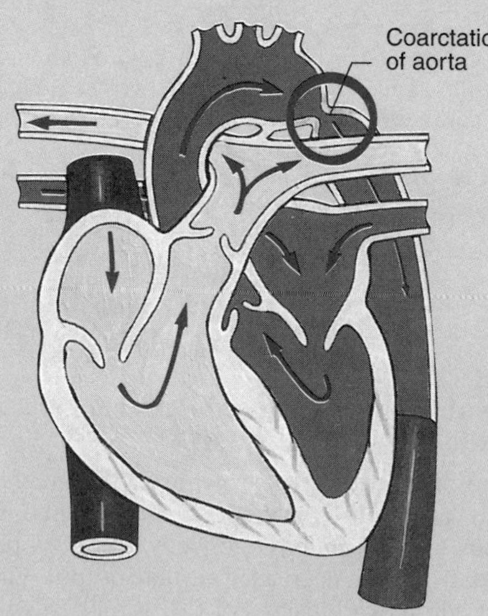

BOX 45-2
Obstructive Defects

Surgical treatment: Either resection of the coarcted portion with an end-to-end anastomosis of the aorta or enlargement of the constricted section using a graft of prosthetic material or a portion of the left subclavian artery. Because this defect is outside the heart and pericardium, cardiopulmonary bypass is not required and a thoracotomy incision is used. Postoperative hypertension (greater than 160 mm Hg) is treated with intravenous sodium nitroprusside or amrinone, followed by oral medications, such as captopril, hydralazine, and/or propranolol. Residual permanent hypertension after repair of COA seems to be related to age and time of repair. To prevent both hypertension at rest and exercise-provoked systemic hypertension after repair, elective surgery for COA is advised within the first 2 years of life. There is a small risk of recurrent narrowing in patients who underwent surgical repair as infants. Percutaneous balloon angioplasty techniques have proved very effective in relieving residual postoperative coarctation gradients.

Nonsurgical treatment: Balloon angioplasty as a primary intervention for COA is being performed in some centers, but concerns about inadequate relief of gradients, risk of aneurysm formation, and restenosis have limited its widespread use. More clinical experience and longer follow-up evaluation are needed (Friedman, 1992).

Prognosis: Less than 5% mortality rate in patients with isolated coarctation; increased risk in infants with other complex cardiac defects.

AORTIC STENOSIS (AS)

Description: Narrowing or stricture of the aortic valve, causing resistance to blood flow in the left ventricle, decreased cardiac output, left ventricular hypertrophy, and pulmonary vascular congestion. The prominent anatomic consequence of AS is the hypertrophy of the left ventricular wall, which eventually will lead to increased end-diastolic pressure, resulting in pulmonary venous and pulmonary arterial hypertension. Left ventricular hypertrophy also interferes with coronary artery perfusion and may result in myocardial infarction or scarring of the papillary muscles of the left ventricle, causing mitral insufficiency. ***Valvular stenosis,*** the most common type, is usually caused by malformed cusps resulting in a bicuspid rather than tricuspid valve or fusion of the cusps. ***Subvalvular stenosis*** is a stricture caused by a fibrous ring below a normal valve. ***Supravalvular stenosis*** occurs infrequently. Valvular AS is a serious defect for the following reasons: (1) the obstruction tends to be progressive; (2) sudden episodes of myocardial ischemia, or low cardiac output, can result in sudden death; and (3) surgical repair rarely results in a normal valve. This is one of the rare instances in which strenuous physical activity may be curtailed because of the cardiac condition.

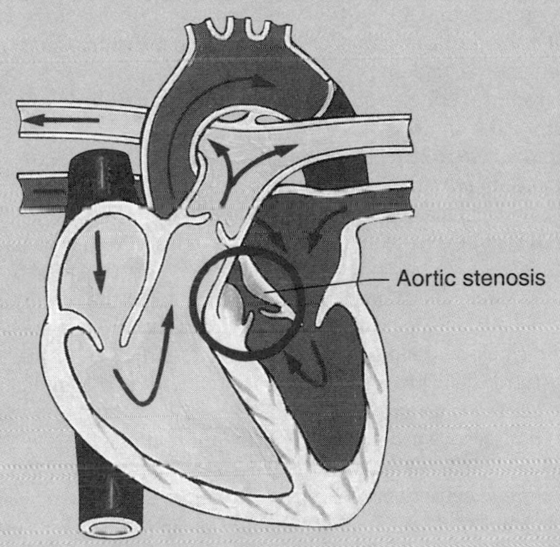

Pathophysiology: A stricture in the aortic outflow tract causes resistance to ejection of blood from the left ventricle. The extra workload on the left ventricle causes hypertrophy. If left ventricular failure develops, left atrial pressure will increase; this causes increased pressure in the pulmonary veins, resulting in pulmonary vascular congestion (pulmonary edema).

Clinical manifestations: Infants with severe defects demonstrate signs of decreased cardiac output with faint pulses, hypotension, tachycardia, and poor feeding. Children show signs of exercise intolerance, chest pain, and dizziness when standing for long periods. There is a characteristic murmur. Patients are at risk for bacterial endocarditis, coronary insufficiency, and ventricular dysfunction.

Valvular aortic stenosis

Surgical treatment: Aortic valvotomy under inflow occlusion.

Prognosis: Aortic valvotomy in critically ill neonates and infants still carries a mortality rate of 10% to 20% in major medical centers. Results of aortic valvotomy in older children are very good, with mortality rate close to 0%. However, aortic valvotomy remains a palliative procedure, and approximately 25% of patients require additional surgery within 10 years for recurrent stenosis. A valve replacement may be required at the second procedure.

Nonsurgical treatment: Dilating narrowed valve with balloon angioplasty in the catheterization laboratory.

Prognosis: The incidence of side effects and complications, including aortic insufficiency or valvular regurgitation, tearing of the valve leaflets, loss of pulse in the catheterized limb, or serious dysrhythmias, is about 40%. In critically ill neonates the mortality rate is similar to that of surgery.

Subvalvular aortic stenosis

Surgical treatment: May involve incising a membrane if one exists or cutting the fibromuscular ring. If the obstruction results from narrowing of the left ventricular outflow tract and a small aortic valve annulus, a patch may be required to enlarge the entire left ventricular outflow tract and annulus and replace the aortic valve, an approach known as the ***Konno*** procedure. An aortic homograft with a valve may also be used ***(extended aortic root replacement)*** or the pulmonary valve may be moved to the aortic position and replaced with a homograft valve (***Ross*** procedure).

Prognosis: Mortality rate from surgical repairs of subvalvular AS is less than 2% in major centers; however, in about 10% of these patients recurrent subaortic stenosis develops and requires additional surgery. All procedures to replace the aortic root and enlarge the left ventricular outflow tract require further evaluation.

Continued.

BOX 45-2
Obstructive Defects—cont'd

PULMONIC STENOSIS (PS)

Description: Narrowing at the entrance to the pulmonary artery. Resistance to blood flow causes right ventricular hypertrophy and decreased pulmonary blood flow. ***Pulmonary atresia*** is the extreme form of PS in that there is total fusion of the commissures and no blood flows to the lungs. The right ventricle may be hypoplastic.

Pathophysiology: When PS is present, resistance to blood flow causes right ventricular hypertrophy. If right ventricular failure develops, right atrial pressure will increase and this may result in reopening of the foramen ovale, shunting of unoxygenated blood into the left atrium, and systemic cyanosis. If PS is severe, CHF occurs, and systemic venous engorgement will be noted. An associated defect such as a PDA partially compensates for the obstruction by shunting blood from the aorta to the pulmonary artery and into the lungs.

Clinical manifestations: Patients may be asymptomatic; some have mild cyanosis or CHF. Newborns with severe narrowing will be cyanotic. There is a characteristic murmur. Cardiomegaly is evident on chest x-ray film. Patients are at risk for bacterial endocarditis, with progressive narrowing causing increased symptoms.

Surgical treatment: In infants, transventricular (closed) valvotomy *(Brock procedure)*. In children, pulmonary valvotomy with cardiopulmonary bypass.

Nonsurgical treatment: Balloon angioplasty in the cardiac catheterization laboratory to dilate valve. A catheter is inserted across the stenotic pulmonic valve into the pulmonary artery, and a balloon at the end of the catheter is inflated and rapidly passed through the narrowed opening (see figure below, right). The procedure is associated with few complications and has proved highly effective, with a significant reduction in pressure gradient across the pulmonic valve and a low rate of complications. It is the treatment of choice for discrete PS in most centers and can be done safely in neonates.

Prognosis: Low risk for both procedures; less than 2% mortality. Both balloon dilation and surgical valvotomy leave the pulmonic valve incompetent because they involve opening the fused valve leaflets; however, these patients are clinically asymptomatic. Long-term problems with restenosis or valve incompetence may occur.

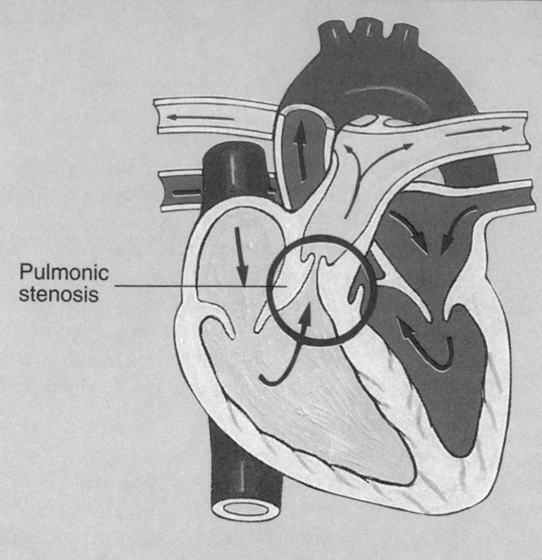

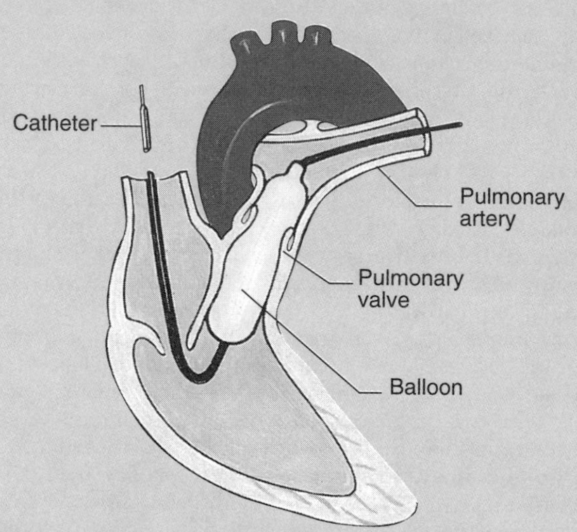

BOX 45-3
Defects With Decreased Pulmonary Blood Flow

TETRALOGY OF FALLOT (TOF)

Description: The classic form includes four defects: (1) ventricular septal defect (VSD), (2) pulmonic stenosis (PS), (3) overriding aorta, and (4) right ventricular hypertrophy.

Pathophysiology: The altered hemodynamic features vary widely, depending primarily on the degree of PS, but also on the size of the VSD and the pulmonary and systemic resistance to flow. Because the VSD is usually large, pressures may be equal in the right and left ventricles. Therefore the shunt direction depends on the difference between pulmonary and systemic vascular resistance. If pulmonary vascular resistance is higher than systemic resistance, the shunt is from right to left. If systemic resistance is higher than pulmonary resistance, the shunt is from left to right. PS decreases blood flow to the lungs and, consequently, the amount of oxygenated blood that returns to the left heart. Depending on the position of the aorta, blood from both ventricles may be distributed systemically.

Clinical manifestations:

Infants: Some infants may be acutely cyanotic at birth; others have mild cyanosis that progresses over the first year of life as the PS worsens. There is a characteristic murmur. There are acute episodes of cyanosis and hypoxia, called blue spells or tet spells. Anoxic spells occur when the infant's oxygen requirements exceed the blood supply, usually during crying or after feeding.

Children: With increasing cyanosis, there may be clubbing of the fingers, squatting, and poor growth.

Patients are at risk for emboli, cerebrovascular disease, brain abscess, seizures, and loss of consciousness or sudden death after an anoxic spell.

Surgical treatment:

Palliative shunt: In infants who cannot undergo primary repair, a palliative procedure to increase pulmonary blood flow and increase oxygen saturation may be performed. The preferred procedure is the *modified Blalock-Taussig*

BOX 45-3
Defects With Decreased Pulmonary Blood Flow—cont'd

TETRALOGY OF FALLOT (TOF)

shunt, which provides blood flow to the pulmonary arteries from the left or right subclavian artery (see Table 45-3). In general, however, shunts are avoided because they may result in pulmonary artery distortion.

Complete repair: Elective repair is usually performed in the first year of life. Indications for repair include increasing cyanosis and development of hypercyanotic spells. Complete repair involves closure of the VSD and resection of the infundibular stenosis, with a pericardial patch to enlarge the right ventricular outflow tract. The procedure requires a median sternotomy and the use of cardiopulmonary bypass.

Prognosis: The operative mortality rate for total correction of TOF is less than 5%. With improved surgical techniques there are a lower incidence of dysrhythmias and sudden death; surgical heart block is rare. CHF may occur postoperatively.

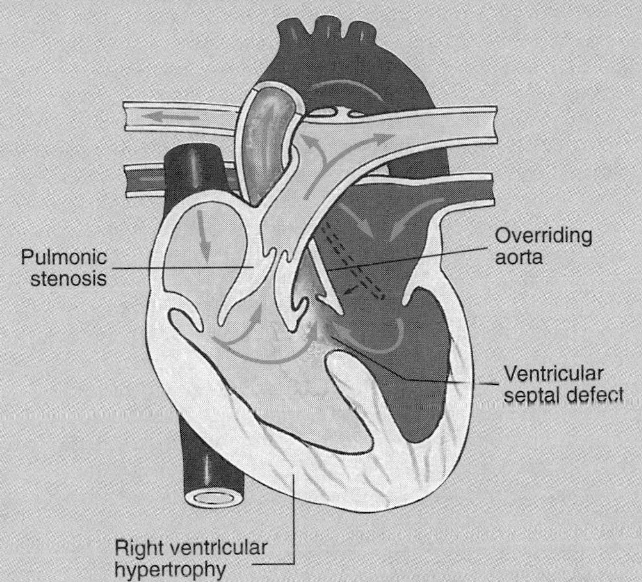

TRICUSPID ATRESIA

Description: Failure of the tricuspid valve to develop, consequently no communication from right atrium to right ventricle. Blood flows through an atrial septal defect (ASD) or a patent foramen ovale to the left side of the heart and through a VSD to the right ventricle and out to the lungs. It is often associated with PS and transposition of the great arteries. There is complete mixing of unoxygenated and oxygenated blood in the left side of the heart, resulting in systemic desaturation and varying amounts of pulmonary obstruction, causing decreased pulmonary blood flow.

Pathophysiology: At birth the presence of a patent foramen ovale (or other atrial septal opening) is required to permit blood flow across the septum into the left atrium; the PDA allows blood flow to the pulmonary artery into the lungs for oxygenation. A VSD allows a modest amount of blood to enter the right ventricle and pulmonary artery for oxygenation. Pulmonary blood flow usually is diminished.

Clinical manifestations: Cyanosis is usually seen in the newborn period. There may be tachycardia and dyspnea. Older children have signs of chronic hypoxemia with clubbing. Patients are at risk for bacterial endocarditis, brain abscess, and stroke.

Therapeutic management: For the neonate whose pulmonary blood flow depends on the patency of the ductus arteriosus, a continuous infusion of prostaglandin E_1 is started until surgical intervention can be arranged.

Surgical treatment: *Palliative* treatment is the placement of a shunt (*systemic-to-pulmonary artery*) to increase blood flow to the lungs. If the ASD is small, an atrial septostomy is done during cardiac catheterization. Some children have increased pulmonary blood flow and require *pulmonary artery banding* to lessen the volume of blood to the lungs. A *bidirectional Glenn shunt* (cavopulmonary anastomosis) may be performed at 6 to 9 months as a second stage (see Table 45-3).

Modified Fontan procedure—Systemic venous return is directed to the lungs without a ventricular pump through surgical connections between the right atrium and the pulmonary artery. A fenestration (opening) in the right atrial baffle is sometimes done to relieve pressure. Patient must have normal ventricular function and a low pulmonary vascular resistance for the procedure to be successful. The modified Fontan procedure separates oxygenated and unoxygenated blood inside the heart and eliminates the excess volume load on the ventricle but does not restore normal anatomy or hemodynamics.

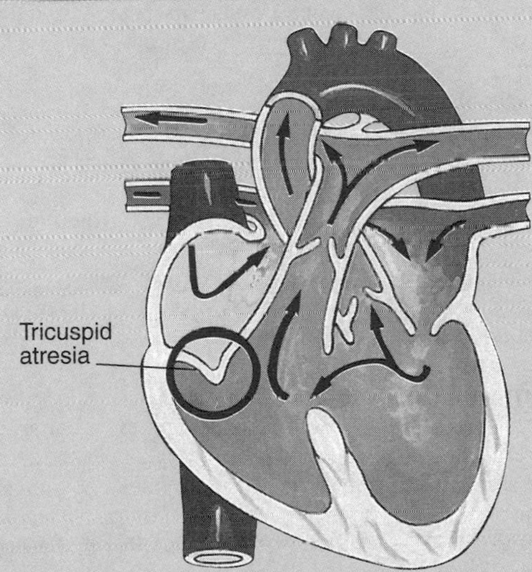

Prognosis: Surgical mortality rate is greater than 10%. Postoperative complications include dysrhythmias, systemic venous hypertension, pleural and pericardial effusions, elevated pulmonary vascular resistance, and ventricular dysfunction. Although initial results have been encouraging, long-term survival and morbidity rates must await future studies.

BOX 45-4
Mixed Defects

TRANSPOSITION OF THE GREAT ARTERIES (TGA) OR TRANSPOSITION OF THE GREAT VESSELS (TGV)

Description: The pulmonary artery leaves the left ventricle, and the aorta exits from the right ventricle, with no communication between the systemic and pulmonary circulations.

Pathophysiology: Associated defects such as septal defects or patent ductus arteriosus (PDA) must be present to permit blood to enter the systemic circulation and/or the pulmonary circulation for mixing of saturated and desaturated blood. The most common defect associated with TGA is a patent foramen ovale. At birth there is also a PDA, although in most instances this closes after the neonatal period. Another associated anomaly may be VSD. Presence of these defects increases the risk of CHF, since they often produce high pulmonary blood flow under high pressure. For example, a large VSD permits blood to flow from the right to the left ventricle, into the pulmonary artery, and finally to the lungs. However, it also produces high pulmonary blood flow under high pressure, which can result in pulmonary vascular resistance. The same series of events occurs with a large PDA, since blood directly from the aorta flows under high pressure into the pulmonary artery and lungs.

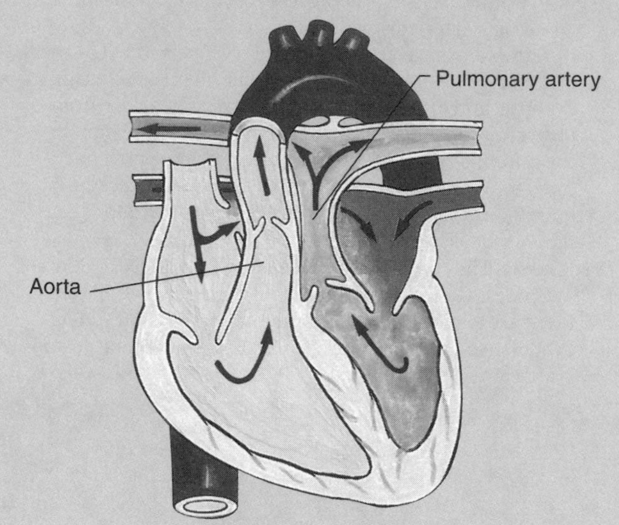

Clinical manifestations: Depend on the type and size of the associated defects. Children with minimum communication are severely cyanotic and depressed at birth. Those with large septal defects or a PDA may be less severely cyanotic but may have symptoms of CHF. Heart sounds vary according to the type of defect present. Cardiomegaly is usually evident a few weeks after birth.

Therapeutic Management:

To provide intracardiac mixing: The administration of intravenous prostaglandin E_1 may be initiated to increase blood mixing temporarily if systemic and pulmonary mixing is inadequate to provide an oxygen saturation of 75% or to maintain cardiac output. During cardiac catheterization a balloon atrial septostomy *(Rashkind procedure)* may also be performed to increase mixing and maintain cardiac output over a longer period.

Surgical treatment:

Arterial switch procedure: Procedure of choice performed in first weeks of life. Involves transecting the great arteries and anastomosing the main pulmonary artery to the proximal aorta (just above the aortic valve) and anastomosing the ascending aorta to the proximal pulmonary artery. The coronary arteries are switched from the proximal aorta to the proximal pulmonary artery, creating a new aorta. Reimplantation of the coronary arteries is critical to the infant's survival, and they must be reattached without torsion or kinking to provide the heart with its supply of oxygen. The advantage of the arterial switch procedure is the reestablishment of normal circulation, with the left ventricle acting as the systemic pump. Potential complications of the arterial switch include narrowing at the great artery anastomoses and coronary artery insufficiency.

Creation of an intraatrial baffle to divert venous blood to the mitral valve and pulmonary venous blood to the tricuspid valve using the patient's atrial septum *(Senning procedure)* or a prosthetic material *(Mustard procedure)*. Performed in first year of life. Disadvantages are the continuing role of the right ventricle as the systemic pump and the late development of right ventricular failure and rhythm disturbances. Other potential postoperative complications include loss of normal sinus rhythm, baffle leaks, and ventricular dysfunction.

Rastelli procedure: Operative choice in infants with TGA, VSD, and severe PS. It involves closure of the VSD with a baffle, directing left ventricular blood through the VSD into the aorta. The pulmonic valve is then closed, and a conduit is placed from the right ventricle to the pulmonary artery, creating physiologically normal circulation. Unfortunately, this procedure requires multiple conduit replacements as the child grows.

Prognosis: Operative mortality rate is about 5% to 10% with all procedures; with atrial level repairs there is a later risk of dysrhythmias and ventricular dysfunction.

TOTAL ANOMALOUS PULMONARY VENOUS CONNECTION (TAPVC)

Description: Rare defect characterized by failure of the pulmonary veins to join the left atrium. Instead, the pulmonary veins are abnormally connected to the systemic venous circuit via the right atrium or various veins draining toward the right atrium, such as the superior vena cava. The abnormal attachment causes mixed blood to be returned to the right atrium and shunted from the right to the left through an ASD. The type of TAPVC is classified according to the pulmonary venous point of attachment as:

Supracardiac—Attachment above the diaphragm, such as to the superior vena cava (most common form)

Cardiac—Direct attachment to the heart, such as to the right atrium or coronary sinus

Infracardiac—Attachment below the diaphragm, such as to the inferior vena cava (most severe form)

TAPVC is also called *total anomalous pulmonary venous return (TAPVR)* or *total anomalous pulmonary venous drainage (TAPVD)*.

BOX 45-4
Mixed Defects—cont'd

TOTAL ANOMALOUS PULMONARY VENOUS CONNECTION (TAPVC)—cont'd

Pathophysiology: The right atrium receives all the blood that normally would flow into the left atrium. As a result, the right side of the heart hypertrophies, whereas the left side, especially the left atrium, may remain small. An associated ASD or patient foramen ovale allows systemic venous blood to shunt from the higher-pressure right atrium to the left atrium and into the left side of the heart. As a result, the oxygen saturation of the blood is the same in both sides of the heart (and ultimately, in the systemic arterial circulation). If the pulmonary blood flow is large, pulmonary venous return is also large and the amount of saturated blood is relatively high. However, if there is obstruction to pulmonary venous drainage, pulmonary venous return is impeded, pulmonary venous pressure rises, and pulmonary interstitial edema develops and eventually contributes to CHF. Infracardiac TAPVC is often associated with obstruction to pulmonary venous drainage and is a surgical emergency.

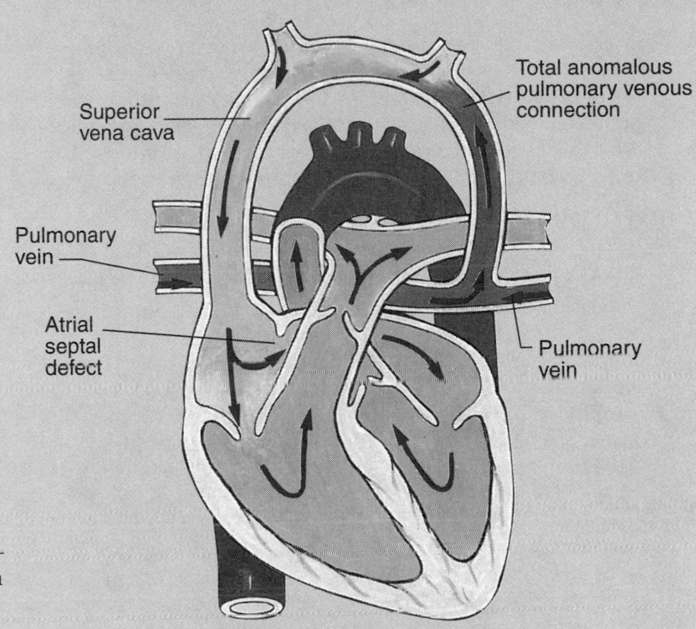

Clinical manifestations: In most infants cyanosis develops early in life. The degree of cyanosis is inversely related to the amount of pulmonary blood flow—the more pulmonary blood, the less cyanosis. Children with unobstructed TAPVC may be asymptomatic until pulmonary vascular resistance decreases during infancy, increasing pulmonary blood flow, with resulting signs of CHF. Cyanosis becomes worse with pulmonary vein obstruction; once obstruction occurs, the infant's condition usually deteriorates rapidly. Without intervention, cardiac failure will progress to death.

Surgical treatment: Corrective repair in early infancy. The surgical approach varies with the anatomic defect. In general, however, the common pulmonary vein is anastomosed to the left atrium, the ASD is closed, and the anomalous pulmonary venous connection is ligated. The cardiac type is most easily repaired; the infracardiac type has the highest morbidity and mortality rates because of the higher incidence of pulmonary vein obstruction. Potential postoperative complications include reobstruction; bleeding; dysrhythmias, particularly heart block; pulmonary artery hypertension; and persistent heart failure.

Prognosis: The cardiac type has a surgical mortality rate of less than 5%; the incidence of morbidity is greater with the other types and increases with the presence of pulmonary vein obstruction.

TRUNCUS ARTERIOSUS (TA)

Description: Failure of normal septation and division of the embryonic bulbar trunk into the pulmonary artery and the aorta, resulting in a single vessel that overrides both ventricles. Blood from both ventricles mixes in the common great artery, causing desaturation and hypoxemia. Blood ejected from the heart flows preferentially to the lower-pressure pulmonary arteries, causing increased pulmonary blood flow and reduced systemic blood flow. There are three types:

- ***Type I***—A single pulmonary trunk arises near the base of the truncus and divides into the left and right pulmonary arteries.
- ***Type II***—The left and right pulmonary arteries arise separately from the posterior aspect of the truncus.
- ***Type III***—The pulmonary arteries arise independently from the lateral aspect of the truncus.

Pathophysiology: Blood ejected from the left and right ventricles enters the common trunk, mixing pulmonary and systemic circulations. Blood flow is distributed to the pulmonary and systemic circulations according to the relative resistances of each system. The amount of pulmonary blood flow depends on the size of the pulmonary arteries and the pulmonary vascular resistance. Generally, resistance to pulmonary blood flow is less than systemic vascular resistance, resulting in preferential blood flow to the lungs. Pulmonary vascular disease develops at an early age in patients with truncus arteriosus.

Clinical manifestations: Most infants are symptomatic with moderate to severe CHF and variable cyanosis, poor growth, and activity intolerance. There is a characteristic murmur. Patients are at risk for brain abscess and bacterial endocarditis.

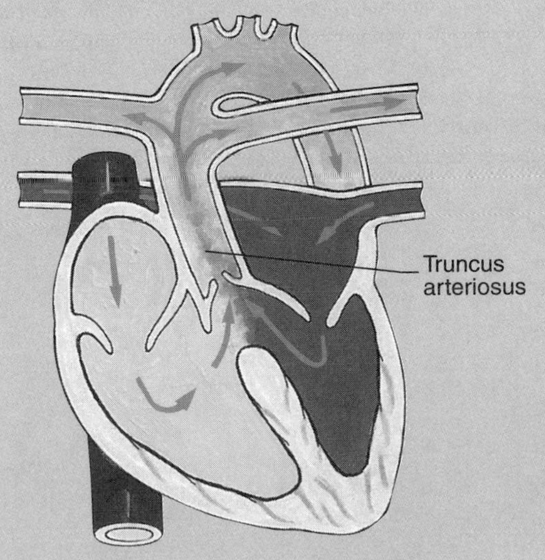

BOX 45-4
Mixed Defects—cont'd

TRUNCUS ARTERIOSUS (TA)—cont'd

Surgical treatment: Early repair in the first few months of life. Corrective repair involves closing the VSD so that the truncus arteriosus receives the outflow from the left ventricle, excising the pulmonary arteries from the aorta, and attaching them to the right ventricle by means of a homograft. Currently, homografts (segments of cadaver aorta and pulmonary artery that are treated with antibiotics and cryopreserved) are preferred to synthetic conduits to establish continuity between the right ventricle and pulmonary artery. Homografts are more flexible and easier to use during the procedure and appear less prone to obstruction. Postoperative complications include persistent heart failure, bleeding, pulmonary artery hypertension, dysrhythmias, and residual VSD.

Prognosis: Mortality rate is greater than 10%; future operations are required to replace the conduits.

HYPOPLASTIC LEFT HEART SYNDROME (HLHS)

Description: Underdevelopment of the left side of the heart, resulting in a hypoplastic left ventricle and aortic atresia. Most blood from the left atrium flows across the patent foramen ovale to the right atrium, to the right ventricle, and out the pulmonary artery. The descending aorta receives blood from the patent ductus arteriosus supplying systemic blood flow.

Pathophysiology: An ASD or patent foramen ovale allows saturated blood from the left atrium to mix with desaturated blood from the right atrium and to flow through the right ventricle and out into the pulmonary artery. From the pulmonary artery the blood flows to the lungs, then through the ductus arteriosus into the aorta, and out to the body. The amount of blood flow to the pulmonary and systemic circulations depends on the relationship between the pulmonary and systemic vascular resistances. The coronary and cerebral vessels receive blood by retrograde flow through the hypoplastic ascending aorta.

Clinical manifestations: There are mild cyanosis and signs of CHF until the PDA closes, then progressive deterioration with cyanosis and decreased cardiac output, leading to cardiovascular collapse. It is usually fatal in the first months of life without intervention.

Therapeutic management: Neonates require stabilization with mechanical ventilation and inotropic support preoperatively. A prostaglandin E_1 infusion is needed to maintain ductal patency, ensuring adequate systemic blood flow.

Surgical treatment: Several-staged approach: First stage is ***Norwood procedure***—anastomosis of the main pulmonary artery to the aorta to create a new aorta, shunting to provide pulmonary blood flow, and creation of a large ASD. Postoperative complications include imbalance of systemic and pulmonary blood flow, bleeding, low cardiac output, and persistent heart failure. Second stage is often a ***bidirectional Glenn shunt*** (Table 45-3) done at 6 to 9 months of age to relieve cyanosis and reduce the volume load on the right ventricle. The final repair is a ***modified Fontan procedure*** (see Tricuspid Atresia in Box 45-3).

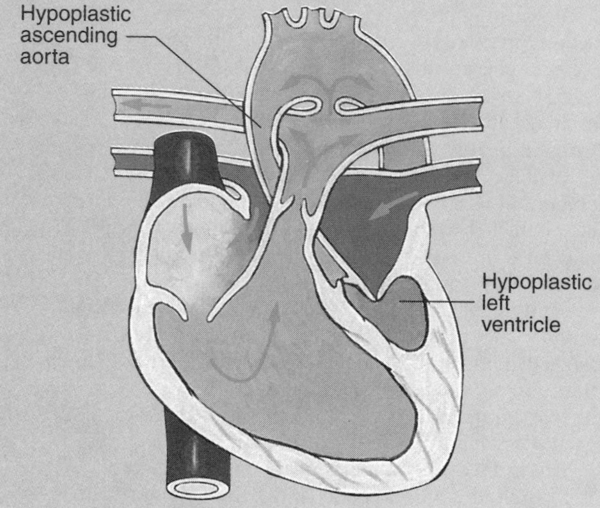

Transplantation: Some programs believe that heart transplantation in the newborn period is the best option for these infants. Problems include the shortage of newborn organ donors, risk of rejection, long-term problems with chronic immunosuppression, and infection.

Prognosis: Mortality rate above 25% with both surgery and transplantation. Because of the high-risk nature of both surgical palliation and neonatal heart transplantation, some cardiologists continue to recommend no treatment for this defect.

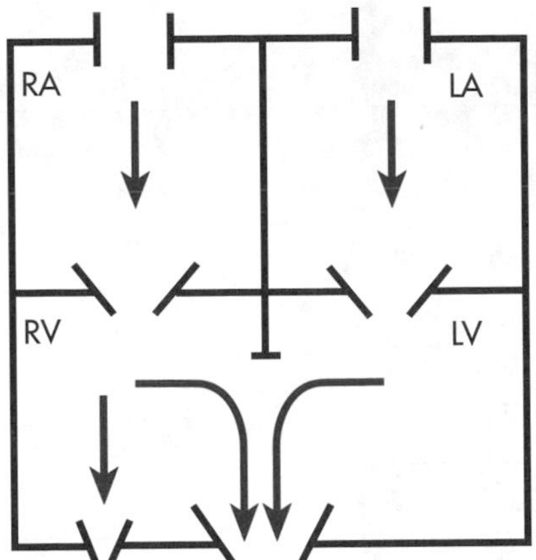

Fig. 45-5 Hemodynamic defects with decreased pulmonary blood flow. For abbreviations, see Fig. 45-1.

sure on the right side increases, exceeding left-sided pressure. This allows desaturated blood to shunt right to left, causing desaturation in the left side of the heart and in the systemic circulation. Clinically these patients are hypoxemic and usually appear cyanotic. Tetralogy of Fallot and tricuspid atresia are the more common defects in this group (Box 45-3).

Mixed Defects

Many complex cardiac anomalies are classified together in the *mixed* category (Box 45-4) because survival in the postnatal period depends on mixing of blood from the pulmonary and systemic circulations within the heart chambers. Hemodynamically, fully saturated systemic blood flow mixes with the desaturated pulmonary blood flow, causing a relative desaturation of the systemic blood flow. Pulmonary congestion occurs because the differences in pulmonary artery pressure and aortic pressure favor pulmonary blood flow. Cardiac output decreases because of a volume load on the ventricle. Clinically, these patients have a variable picture that combines some degree of desaturation (although cyanosis is not always visible) and signs of CHF. Some defects, such as transposition of the great arteries, cause severe cyanosis in the first days of life and later cause CHF. Others, such as truncus arteriosus, cause severe CHF in the first weeks of life and mild desaturation.

Clinical Consequences of Congenital Heart Disease

CONGESTIVE HEART FAILURE

Congestive heart failure (CHF) is the inability of the heart to pump an adequate amount of blood to the systemic circulation to meet the metabolic demands of the body. In children CHF most commonly occurs secondary to structural abnormalities that result in increased blood volume and pressure. CHF is a symptom caused by an underlying cardiac defect, not a disease in itself, since it is usually the result of an excessive work load imposed on a normal myocardium. CHF is most common in infants.

Pathophysiology

Heart failure is often separated into two categories, right-sided and left-sided failure. In *right-sided failure* the right ventricle is unable to pump blood effectively into the pulmonary artery, resulting in increased pressure in the right atrium and systemic venous circulation. Systemic venous hypertension causes hepatosplenomegaly and occasionally edema. In *left-sided failure* the left ventricle is unable to pump blood into the systemic circulation, resulting in increased pressure in the left atrium and pulmonary veins. The lungs become congested with blood, causing elevated pulmonary pressures and pulmonary edema.

Although each type of heart failure produces different signs and symptoms, clinically it is unusual to observe solely right- or left-sided failure in children. Since each side of the heart depends on adequate function of the other side, failure of one chamber causes a reciprocal change in the opposite chamber.

If the abnormalities precipitating heart failure are not corrected, the heart muscle becomes damaged. Despite compensatory mechanisms, the heart is unable to maintain an adequate cardiac output. Decreased blood flow to the kidneys continues to stimulate sodium and water reabsorption, leading to hypervolemia, increased workload on the heart, and congestion in the pulmonary and systemic circulations (Fig. 45-6).

The signs and symptoms of CHF can be divided into three groups: (1) impaired myocardial function, (2) pulmonary congestion, and (3) systemic venous congestion (Box 45-5). Because these hemodynamic changes result from different causes and at differing times, the clinical presentation may vary among children.

Diagnostic Evaluation

Diagnosis is made on the basis of clinical manifestations (Box 45-5). A chest x-ray film demonstrates cardiomegaly and increased pulmonary vascular markings that result from increased pulmonary blood flow. Ventricular hypertrophy appears on the electrocardiogram (ECG).

Therapeutic Management

The goals of treatment are to (1) improve cardiac function, (2) remove accumulated fluid and sodium, (3) decrease cardiac demands, and (4) improve tissue oxygenation and decrease oxygen consumption.

Improve cardiac function. Myocardial efficiency is improved through administration of digitalis glycosides. The beneficial effects are increased cardiac output, decreased heart size, decreased venous pressure, and relief of edema. In pediatrics, *digoxin (Lanoxin)* is used almost exclusively, because of its rapid onset. It is available as an elixir (0.05 mg/ml) for oral administration. For infants the dose is calculated in micrograms (1000 μg = 1 mg).

Treatment consists of a digitalizing dose, given orally or in-

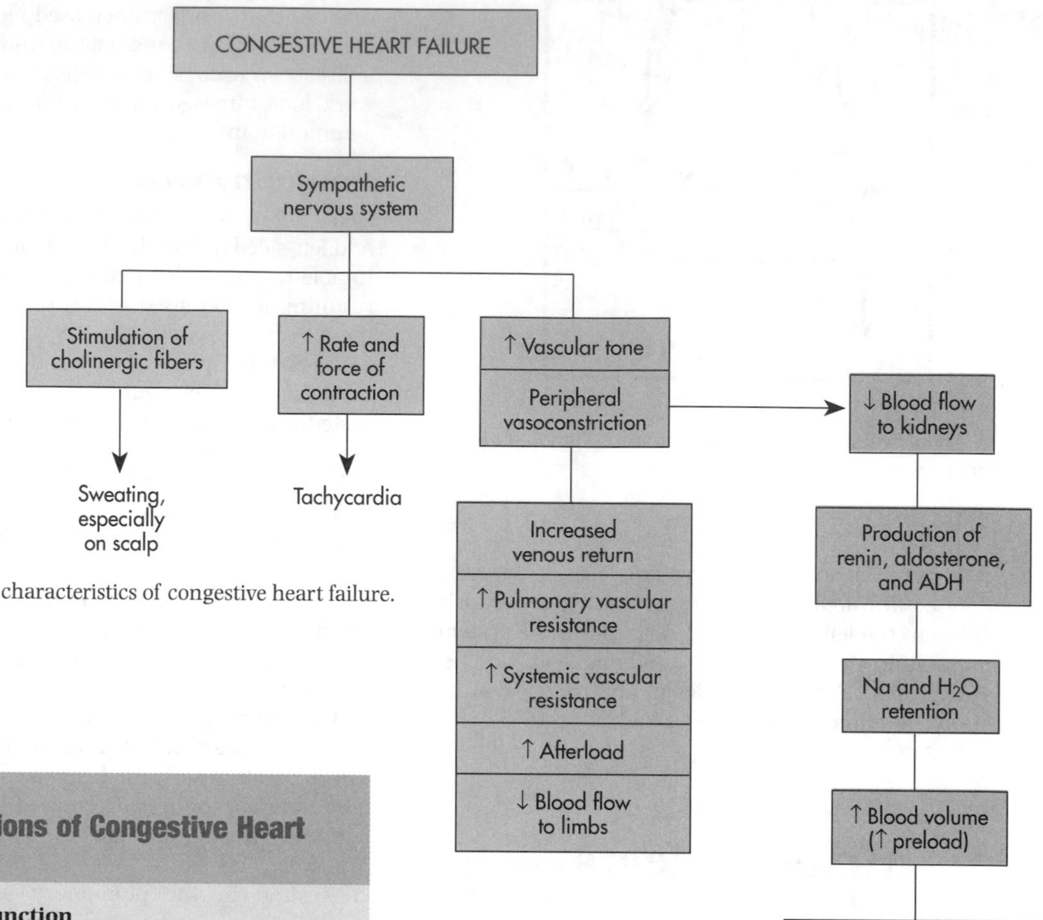

Fig. 45-6 Pathophysiologic characteristics of congestive heart failure.

BOX 45-5

Clinical Manifestations of Congestive Heart Failure

Impaired myocardial function
Tachycardia
Sweating (inappropriate)
Decreased urine output
Fatigue
Weakness
Restlessness
Anorexia
Pale, cool extremities
Weak peripheral pulses
Decreased blood pressure
Gallop rhythm
Cardiomegaly

Pulmonary congestion
Tachypnea
Dyspnea
Retractions (infants)
Flaring nares
Exercise intolerance
Orthopnea
Cough, hoarseness
Cyanosis
Wheezing
Grunting

Systemic venous congestion
Weight gain
Hepatomegaly
Peripheral edema, especially periorbital
Ascites
Neck vein distention (children)

travenously in divided doses over 24 hours to produce optimal cardiac effects, and a maintenance dose, given orally twice a day to maintain blood levels. During digitalization the child is monitored by means of an ECG to observe for the desired effects (prolonged P-R interval and reduced ventricular rate) and detect side effects, especially dysrhythmias.

Nursing ALERT

Therapeutic serum digoxin levels range from 0.8 to 2.0 μ/L.

A newer group of drugs used in the treatment of CHF are the *angiotensin-converting enzyme (ACE) inhibitors.* As their name implies, these drugs inhibit the normal function of the renin-angiotensin system in the kidney. The ACE inhibitors block the conversion of angiotensin I to angiotensin II so that instead of vasoconstriction, vasodilation occurs. Vasodilation results in decreased pulmonary and systemic vascular resistance, decreased blood pressure, and a reduction in afterload. Two ACE inhibitors are currently used in pediatrics: *captopril (Capoten),* given three times a day, and *enalapril (Vasotec),* given twice a day. Captopril is used in infants and young children because it can be given in smaller doses; its principal side effects are hypotension, renal dysfunction, and cough.

TABLE 45-2 Diuretics used in congestive heart failure

ACTION	COMMENTS	NURSING CONSIDERATIONS
Furosemide (lasix) Blocks reabsorption of sodium and water in proximal renal tubule and interferes with reabsorption of sodium	Drug of choice in severe CHF Causes excretion of chloride and potassium (hypokalemia may precipitate digitalis toxicity)	Begin to record output as soon as drug is given Observe for dehydration caused by profound diuresis Observe for side effects (nausea and vomiting, diarrhea, ototoxicity, hypokalemia, dermatitis, postural hypotension) Encourage foods high in potassium and/or give potassium supplements Monitor chloride and acid-base balance with long term therapy Observe for signs of digoxin toxicity
Chlorothiazide (diuril) Acts directly on distal tubules to decrease sodium, water, potassium, chloride, and bicarbonate absorption	Less frequently used drug Causes hypokalemia, acidosis from large doses May be given on alternate days or for 4 or 5 days and stopped for 2 days to allow for reabsorption of potassium	Observe for side effects (nausea, weakness, dizziness, paresthesia, muscle cramps, skin eruptions, hypokalemia, acidosis) Encourage foods high in potassium and/or give potassium supplements
Spironolactone (aldactone) Blocks action of aldosterone, which promotes retention of sodium and excretion of potassium	Weak diuretic Has potassium-sparing effect; frequently used with thiazides, furosemide Poorly absorbed from gastrointestinal tract Takes several days to achieve maximum actions	Observe for side effects (skin rash, drowsiness, ataxia, hyperkalemia) Do not administer potassium supplements

Nursing ALERT

Because ACE inhibitors also block the action of aldosterone, the addition of potassium supplements or spironolactone (Aldactone) to the drug regimen of patients taking diuretics is usually not needed and may cause hyperkalemia.

Remove accumulated fluid and sodium. Treatment consists of diuretics, possible fluid restriction, and possible sodium restriction. Diuretics are the mainstay of therapy to eliminate excess water and salt to prevent reaccumulation. The most commonly used agents are *furosemide (Lasix)*, the *thiazides (chlorothiazide suspension* or *hydrochlorothiazide tablets)*, and *spironolactone* (Table 45-2). Since furosemide and the thiazides are potassium-losing diuretics, potassium supplements may be prescribed, and rich sources of the electrolyte are encouraged in the diet.

Nursing ALERT

A fall in the serum potassium level enhances the effects of digitalis, increasing the risk of digoxin toxicity. Therefore serum potassium levels must be carefully monitored.

Fluid restriction may be required in the acute states of CHF and must be carefully calculated to prevent dehydrating the child, especially if cyanotic CHD and significant polycythemia are present. Infants rarely need fluid restrictions because CHF makes feeding so difficult that they struggle to take maintenance fluids.

Sodium-restricted diets are used less often in children than in adults to control CHF, because of their potential negative effects on appetite. If salt intake is restricted, the diet usually consists of avoiding additional table salt and highly salted foods.

Decrease cardiac demands. The workload on the heart is reduced when metabolic needs are kept to a minimum. This is accomplished by limiting physical activity (bed rest), preserving body temperature, treating any infections, reducing the effort of breathing (semi-Fowler position), and using medication to sedate an irritable child.

Improve tissue oxygenation and decrease oxygen consumption. All of the preceding measures serve to increase tissue oxygenation, either by improving myocardial function or by lessening tissue oxygen demands. Supplemental cool humidified oxygen is usually provided to increase the amount of available oxygen during inspiration. Oxygen is a vasodilator that decreases pulmonary vascular resistance. The amount of cool humidity is carefully regulated to prevent chilling.

Nursing ALERT

Oxygen is a drug and is only administered with an appropriate order. There are some uncommon circumstances in patients with complex hemodynamics in which oxygen can be detrimental.

Nursing Care Management

The infant or child with CHF is usually admitted to the hospital, where intensive nursing care is available. The child is positioned for optimal ventilation and administered oxygen by the most effective means, an intravenous access is established, and cardiac and respiratory function is monitored continuously using a cardiac monitor and pulse oximeter to monitor oxygen saturation. Urinary output and serum electrolytes are evaluated frequently.

Assessment

Nurses need to be alert to signs of CHF in infants and children with suspected or known congenital defects. Signs of CHF indicate a worsening clinical condition; the earlier they are detected, the sooner treatment can be started.

Nursing ALERT

The early signs of CHF are:
Tachycardia, especially during rest and slight exertion
Tachypnea
Profuse scalp sweating, especially in infants
Fatigue and irritability
Sudden weight gain
Respiratory distress

Nursing Diagnoses

A number of nursing diagnoses are identified after a thorough assessment. Some of these are included in the Nursing Care Plan on p. 1471. Others may become apparent in special circumstances and with children in different age groups.

Planning

The goals for the infant or child with CHF and the family are as follows:

1. Child will exhibit improved cardiac output.
2. Child will experience decreased cardiac demands.
3. Child will exhibit improved respiratory function.
4. Child will maintain adequate nutritional status.
5. Child will exhibit no evidence of fluid excess.
6. Child and family will receive adequate support and education.

Implementation

Although the objectives of nursing care are the same, the interventions differ, depending on the child's age. Interventions for infants are quite different from those for older children.

Assist in measures to improve cardiac function. The nurse's responsibility in administering digoxin includes observing for signs of toxicity, calculating and administering the correct dosage, and instituting parental teaching regarding drug administration at home. The child's apical pulse is always checked before administering digoxin. As a general rule the drug is not given if the pulse is below 90 to 110 beats/min in infants and young children or below 70 beats/min in older children (the cutoff point for adults is 60). However, since the pulse rate varies in children in different age groups, the written drug order should specify at what heart rate the drug is withheld. The nurse should also use judgment in evaluating the pulse rate. If it is significantly lower than the previous recording, the dose should be withheld until the practitioner is notified.

The apical rate is taken because a pulse deficit (radial pulse rate lower than apical) may be present with decreased cardiac output. It is auscultated for 1 full minute to evaluate alterations in rhythm. If the child is monitored by means of an ECG, a rhythm strip is obtained and attached to the chart for rate and rhythm analysis, such as abnormal lengthening of the P-R interval (more than a 50% increase over predigitalization interval) and dysrhythmias.

Digoxin is a potentially dangerous drug because the margin of safety of therapeutic, toxic, and lethal doses is very narrow. Many toxic responses are extensions of its therapeutic effects. Therefore the nurse must maintain a high index of suspicion for signs of toxicity when administering digoxin (Box 45-6).

Since digoxin toxicity can result from accidental overdose, great care must be taken in properly calculating and measuring the dosage. When converting milligrams to micrograms to milliliters, the nurse carefully checks the placement of the decimal point, since an error causes a significant change in dosage. For example, 0.1 mg is 10 times the dosage of 0.01 mg.

Nursing ALERT

Infants rarely receive more than 1 ml (50 μg or 0.05 mg) in one dose; a higher dose is an immediate warning of a dosage error. To ensure safety, compare the calculation with another staff member before giving the drug.

These same principles are taught to parents in preparation for discharge, although the correct dose in milliliters is usually specified on the container, thus reducing the potential for errors in calculation. The nurse observes the parent measure the elixir in the dropper and stresses the level mark as the meniscus of the fluid that is observed at eye level. Other instructions for administering digoxin are listed in the Home Care box and the Critical Thinking Q & A box on p. 1469.

BOX 45-6
Common Signs of Digoxin Toxicity in Children

Gastrointestinal	Cardiac
Nausea	Bradycardia
Vomiting	Dysrhythmias
Anorexia	

Home Care 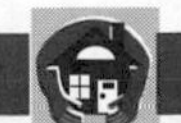

ADMINISTERING DIGOXIN

Give digoxin at regular intervals, usually every 12 hours, such as 8 AM and 8 PM.
Plan the times so that the drug is given *1 hour before* or *2 hours after* feedings.
Use a calendar to mark off each dose that is given or post a reminder, such as a sign on the refrigerator.
Have the prescription refilled *before* the medication is completely used.
Administer the drug carefully by slowly directing it on the side and back of the mouth.
Do not mix it with other foods or fluids, since refusal to consume these results in inaccurate intake of the drug.
If the child has teeth, give water after administering the drug; whenever possible, brush the teeth to prevent tooth decay from the sweetened liquid.
If a dose is missed and more than 4 hours has elapsed, withhold the dose and give the next dose at the regular time; if less than 4 hours has elapsed, give the missed dose.
If the child vomits, do not give a second dose.
If more than two consecutive doses have been missed, notify the practitioner.
Do not increase or double the dose for missed doses.
If the child becomes ill, notify the practitioner immediately.
Keep digoxin in a safe place, preferably a locked cabinet.
In case of accidental overdose of digoxin, call the nearest poison control center immediately; the number is usually listed in the front of the telephone directory.

Parents are also advised of the signs of toxicity. According to the practitioner's preference, they may be taught to take the pulse before giving the drug. A return demonstration of the procedure from both parents or other principal caregiver is included as part of the teaching plan. Their level of anxiety in counting the pulse is assessed, since overconcern about the heart rate may result in excessive withholding of the drug.

Afterload reduction. For patients receiving ACE inhibitors for afterload reduction, the nurse should carefully monitor blood pressure before and after dose administration, observe for symptoms of hypotension, and notify the practitioner if blood pressure is low. Numerous medications affecting the kidney can potentiate renal dysfunction, so children who are taking multiple diuretics along with an ACE inhibitor require careful assessment of serum electrolyte levels and renal function.

Decrease cardiac demands. The infant requires rest and conservation of energy for feeding. Every effort is made to organize nursing activities to allow for uninterrupted periods of sleep. Whenever possible, parents are encouraged to stay with their infant to provide the holding, rocking, and cuddling that help children sleep more soundly. To minimize disturbing the infant, changing bed linen and complete bathing are done only when necessary. Feeding is planned to accommodate the infant's sleep and wake patterns. The child is fed when hungry, such as when sucking on fists rather than when crying for a bottle, since the stress of crying exhausts the limited energy supply. Since infants with CHF tire easily and may sleep through feedings, smaller feedings every 3 hours may be helpful. Gavage feedings may be instituted to provide adequate nutrition and allow the infant to rest.

Critical Thinking 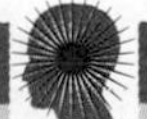

DIGOXIN TOXICITY

You are visiting a 3-month-old infant at home who was begun on digoxin and Lasix 5 days ago for management of CHF. The infant seems well. The mother mentions that the infant vomited several times yesterday and again this morning. Your assessment reveals an irregular heartbeat at 104 beats/min. You should:

1. Give the digoxin and instruct the mother to call the practioner in a few days if the vomiting persists.
2. Explain that vomiting and a slow heart rate are common side effects of digoxin.
3. Calm the infant and check the heart rate again.
4. Notify the practitioner of your findings before giving digoxin.

The correct answer is four. A slow and irregular heartbeat and intermittent vomiting are common signs of possible digoxin toxicity in infants. This medication was only started 5 days ago. The practitioner should be notified for further assessment and management. The margin of safety for digoxin blood levels is narrow. Continuing to give the digoxin can cause a fatal toxic reaction. Calming the infant is inappropriate in the context of the data given. If the infant were crying, soothing measures would produce an even slower heart rate.

Every effort is made to minimize unnecessary stress. Older children need an explanation of what is happening to them to decrease anxiety about their illness and necessary treatments such as cardiac monitoring, oxygen administration, and medications. Outlining a plan for the day, preparing for tests and procedures, providing quiet activities, and allowing for adequate rest periods are all helpful interventions with older children. Some infants and children require sedation during the acute phase of illness to allow them to rest.

Temperature is carefully monitored because hyperthermia or hypothermia increases the need for oxygen. Febrile states are reported to the physician, since infection must be promptly treated. Maintaining body temperature is of special importance in children who are receiving cool, humidified oxygen and in infants who tend to be diaphoretic and lose heat by way of evaporation.

Skin breakdown from edema is prevented with change of position every 2 hours (from side to side while in semi-Fowler position) and use of pressure-relieving mattress or bed. The skin, especially over the sacrum, is checked for evidence of redness from pressure.

Reduce respiratory distress. Careful assessment, positioning, and oxygen administration can reduce respiratory distress. Respirations are counted for 1 full minute during a resting state. Any evidence of increased respiratory distress is reported, since this may indicate worsening CHF.

Infants are positioned to encourage maximum chest expansion, with the head of the bed elevated; they should sit up in an infant seat or be held at a 45-degree angle. Children prefer to sleep on several pillows and remain in a semi-Fowler or high Fowler position during waking hours. Shirts and diapers are pinned loosely to allow maximum chest expansion. Safety restraints, such as those used with infant seats, are applied low on the abdomen and loosely enough to provide both safety and maximum expansion.

The infant or child is often given humidified supplemental oxygen via oxygen hood or tent, nasal cannula, or mask. The child's response to oxygen therapy is carefully evaluated by noting respiratory rate, ease of respiration, color, and especially oxygen saturations, as measured by oximetry.

Respiratory infections can exacerbate CHF and should be appropriately treated and prevented if possible. The child should be protected from persons with respiratory infections and have a noninfectious roommate. With an older child, it is advantageous to choose a roommate who is also confined to bed and relatively quiet in order to promote a restful environment. Good handwashing is practiced before and after caring for any hospitalized child. Antibiotics may be given to combat respiratory infection. The nurse ensures that the drug is given at equally divided times over a 24-hour schedule to maintain high blood levels of the antibiotic.

Maintain nutritional status. Meeting the nutritional needs of infants with CHF or serious cardiac defects is a nursing challenge. The metabolic rate of these infants is greater because of poor cardiac function and increased heart and respiratory rates. Their caloric needs are greater than those of the average infant because of their increased metabolic rate, yet their ability to take in adequate calories is hampered by their fatigue. Feeding for a fragile infant with serious CHD is similar to exercise in an adult, and they often do not have the energy or cardiac reserve to do extra work. The nurse seeks measures to enable the infant to feed easily without excess fatigue and to increase the caloric density of the formula.

The infant should be well rested before feeding and fed soon after awakening so as not to expend energy on crying. A 3-hour feeding schedule works well for many infants. (Feeding every 2 hours does not provide enough rest in between feedings, and a 4-hour schedule requires an increased volume of feeding, which many infants are unable to take.) The feeding schedule should be individualized to the infant's needs. A soft preemie nipple or a slit in a regular nipple to enlarge the opening decreases the energy expenditure of the infant while sucking. Infants should be well supported and fed in a semi-upright position. The infant may need to rest frequently and may need to have the jaw and cheeks stroked to encourage sucking. Generally, giving an infant about a half hour to complete a feeding is reasonable. Prolonging the feeding time can exhaust the infant and decrease the rest period between feedings.

Infants with feeding difficulties are often gavage-fed by using a nasogastric tube to supplement their oral intake and ensure adequate calories. If they are very stressed and fatigued, in respiratory distress, or tachypneic to 80 to 100 breaths/min, oral feedings may be withheld and all nutrition given by gavage feedings. Gavage feedings are usually a temporary measure until the infant's medical status improves and nutritional needs can be met through oral feedings. Some infants with severe CHF, neurologic deficits, or significant gastroesophageal reflux may need placement of a gastrostomy tube to allow adequate nutrition.

Increasing the caloric density of formulas by concentration and then adding corn, medium-chain triglycerides (MCT Oil), or polycose is frequently done. Infant formulas provide 20 calories per ounce, and the use of additives can increase the calories to 30 calories or more per ounce. This allows the infant to obtain more calories despite a smaller volume intake of formula. The caloric density of the formula needs to be increased slowly (by 2 calories per ounce per day) to prevent diarrhea or formula intolerance. Breastfeeding mothers are encouraged to provide the infant with alternating feedings of breast milk and high-calorie formulas. Some lactating mothers will prefer to feed the child expressed breast milk that has been fortified with nutritional formula (Similac or Enfamil) powder, polycose, or corn oil to increase caloric intake. A supplemental nurser may also be helpful. A diet plan specific to the individual infant's needs is calculated and prescribed by the nutritionist in collaboration with the other health personnel. The nurse needs to reinforce this information with the parents as necessary.

Assist in measures to promote fluid loss. When diuretics are given, the nurse records fluid intake and output and monitors body weight at the same time each day to evaluate benefit from the drug. Since profound diuresis may cause dehydration and electrolyte imbalance (loss of sodium, potassium, chloride, bicarbonate), the nurse observes for signs indicating either complication, as well as signs and symptoms suggesting reactions to the drugs. Diuretics should be given early in the day to children who are toilet-trained to eliminate the need to urinate at night. If potassium-losing diuretics are given, the nurse encourages foods high in potassium, such as bananas, oranges, whole grains, legumes, and leafy vegetables, and administers prescribed supplements. When giving potassium supplements, mix the elixir with fruit juice (red punch or grape juice works well) to disguise the bitter taste and to prevent intestinal irritation from a concentrated solution. Serum potassium levels are checked frequently.

Fluid restriction is rarely necessary in infants because of their difficulty in feeding. However, if fluids are restricted, the nurse plans fluid intake schedules for a 24-hour period, allowing for ingestion of most fluids during waking hours. With toddlers and preschoolers give small amounts of liquid in small cups so the containers appear full. Suitable utensils are decorated medicine cups, paper cups, doll-sized teacups, and measuring cups. It is also important not to leave extra fluids at the bedside, since older children may help themselves to additional servings. Older children's cooperation is gained by placing them in charge of recording fluid intake.

If salt is limited, the nurse discusses food sources of sodium with the family and discourages them from giving salt-containing treats to the child. At mealtime the child's tray is checked to make sure the appropriate diet is given.

Support child and family. CHF is a serious complication of heart disease. Parents and older children are usually acutely aware of the critical nature of the condition. Since stress places additional demands on cardiac function, the nurse should focus on reducing anxiety through anticipatory preparation, frequent communication with the parent regarding the child's progress, and constant reassurance that everything possible is being done.

Home care involves many of the same interventions dis-

Nursing Care Plan

THE CHILD WITH CONGESTIVE HEART FAILURE

Nursing Diagnosis: Decreased cardiac output related to structural defect, myocardial dysfunction

Expected Outcome: Patient exhibits signs of improved cardiac output (i.e., strong, regular pulse with rates within normal limits [WNL]; blood pressure WNL; absence of pallor, adequate capillary refill).

• **NURSING INTERVENTIONS/*RATIONALES***

Administer diagoxin (lanoxin) per physician order *to improve myocardial efficiency;* make certain dosage is within safe limits; count pulse for 1 minute before giving drug and withhold if too slow; monitor for adverse or toxic effects. Ensure adequate intake of potassium and monitor potassium levels, *since decreased levels enhance toxicity of digoxin.*

Administer medications to decrease afterload as ordered; monitor for hypotension and electrolyte levels.

Administer oxygen per physician order *to increase supply to myocardium.*

Monitor apical and radial pulses frequently for rate and rhythm *to detect presence of arrythmias;* monitor skin color, temperature, capillary refill, vital signs *to assess for status of cardiac output.*

Plan child's care and activities to prevent overexertion, *which increases myocardial oxygen demand.*

Administer stool softeners as ordered *to prevent straining at stool and resultant bradycardia.*

Nursing Diagnosis: Ineffective breathing pattern related to pulmonary congestion

Expected Outcome: Patient exhibits signs of improved respiratory function (i.e., regular, even respirations with rates WNL; good color; adequate oxygen saturations; decreased restlessness).

• **NURSING INTERVENTIONS/*RATIONALES***

Place in inclined posture of 30 to 45 degrees and avoid constrictive clothing or restraints around abdomen or chest *to encourage maximum chest expansion.*

Administer humidified oxygen as ordered *to reduce hypoxia.*

Monitor respiratory rate, rhythm, ease of breathing, skin color, oxygen saturations by oximetry, breath sounds, restlessness *to assess pulmonary status.*

Suction airway as needed *to remove secretions.*

Plan child's care and activities with adequate rest *to prevent fatigue and reduce oxygen demand.*

Nursing Diagnosis: Fluid volume excess related to pulmonary congestion and fluid accumulation

Expected Outcome: Patient exhibits evidence of fluid loss (i.e., increased urine output, weight loss, reduction of edema).

• **NURSING INTERVENTIONS/*RATIONALES***

Administer diuretics as prescribed *to induce diuresis.*

Monitor weight, intake and output, level of edema, urine specific gravity, electrolytes *to assess fluid status;* blood urea nitrogen, creatinine levels *to assess renal function.*

Monitor intravenous and oral intake carefully *to prevent further fluid overload.*

Provide skin care and reposition frequently when edematous *to prevent skin breakdown;* provide oral care *to prevent drying of mucous membranes.*

Monitor skin turgor *to assess for dehydration.*

Nursing Diagnosis: Activity intolerance related to oxygen imbalance

Expected Outcome: Patient's activity level is within normal limits.

• **NURSING INTERVENTIONS/*RATIONALES***

Maintain neutral thermal environment *to decrease oxygen demands.*

Feed small volumes at frequent intervals using soft nipple with moderately large opening *to decrease fatigue;* implement gavage feeding if necessary *to prevent fatigue and ensure adequate intake.*

Implement measures to reduce anxiety, crying, signs of distress, *which increase demand for oxygen.*

Perform only necessary functions *to reduce fatigue and energy expenditure.*

Balance rest and physical activity, increasing activity levels as tolerated *to regain balance between oxygen supply and demand.*

See also the Nursing Care Plan: Family of Ill or Hospitalized Child, Chapter 41.

---

cussed under Plan for Discharge and Home Care (see p. 1479). The nurse teaches the family about the medications that need to be administered and alerts them to the signs of worsening CHF that require medical attention, such as increased sweating, decreased urine output (noted in fewer wet diapers or infrequent use of the toilet), or poor feeding. Compliance is a major issue, and every effort is extended to improve the family's adherence to the medication schedule (see Chapter 42). Written instructions regarding correct administration of digoxin are essential (see the Home Care box on p. 1469), including an explanation of signs of toxicity.

If CHF is the end stage of a severe heart defect, the nurse cares for this child as for any child who is terminally ill, using the principles discussed in Chapter 38.

Evaluation

The effectiveness of nursing interventions for the family and the child with CHF is determined by continual reassessment and evaluation of care based on the following observational guidelines and expected outcomes:

1. Monitor heart rate and quality, respiratory rate and efforts, and color and observe behaviors that provide clues to expended effort.
2. Observe nutritional intake, feeding behaviors, and weight.
3. Monitor intake, output, and weight.
4. Interview and observe behaviors of family.

Expected outcomes:

See the Nursing Care Plan above.

HYPOXEMIA

Hypoxemia refers to an arterial oxygen tension (or pressure, Pao_2) that is less than normal and can be identified by a decreased arterial saturation or a decreased Pao_2. **Hypoxia** is a reduction in tissue oxygenation that results from low oxygen saturations and Pao_2 and results in impaired cellular processes. **Cyanosis** is a blue discoloration in the mucous membranes, skin, and nail beds of the child with reduced oxygen saturation. It results from the presence of deoxygenated hemoglobin (hemoglobin not bound to oxygen) in a concentration of 5 g/dl of blood or more. Cyanosis is usually apparent when arterial oxygen saturations are 80% to 85%. Determination of cyanosis is subjective, depending on skin pigment, quality of light, color of the room, or clothing worn by the child. The presence of cyanosis may not accurately reflect arterial hypoxemia because both oxygen saturation and amount of circulating hemoglobin are involved. Children with severe anemia may not be cyanotic despite severe hypoxemia because the hemoglobin level may be too low to produce the characteristic blue color. Conversely patients with polycythemia may appear cyanotic despite a near-normal Pao_2. Heart defects that cause hypoxemia and cyanosis result from desaturated venous blood (blue blood) that enters the systemic circulation without passing through the lungs.

Adolescents and young adults may become cyanotic because of unrepaired septal defects in which the increased pulmonary blood flow over many years results in pulmonary vascular changes. *Eisenmenger complex (syndrome)* is the clinical situation in which a left-to-right shunt becomes a right-to-left shunt because of a progressive increase in pulmonary vascular resistance. With increasing pulmonary vascular thickening, the resistance in the pulmonary circulation can exceed or equal that in the systemic circulation, causing a reversal of blood flow from the right to the left ventricle.

Clinical Manifestations

Over time, two physiologic changes occur in the body in response to chronic hypoxemia: polycythemia and clubbing. **Polycythemia,** an increased number of red blood cells, increases the oxygen-carrying capacity of the blood. However, anemia may result if iron is not readily available for the formation of hemoglobin. Polycythemia increases the viscosity of the blood and crowds out clotting factors. **Clubbing,** a thickening and flattening of the tips of the fingers and toes, is thought to be the result of chronic tissue hypoxemia and polycythemia (Fig. 45-7). Infants with mild hypoxemia may be asymptomatic except for cyanosis and exhibit near-normal growth and development. Those with more severe hypoxemia may exhibit fatigue with feeding, poor weight gain, tachypnea, and dyspnea. Severe hypoxemia resulting in tissue hypoxia is manifested by clinical deterioration and signs of poor perfusion.

Squatting, most characteristic of children with tetralogy of Fallot, is seen in toddlers and older children as an unconscious attempt to relieve chronic hypoxia, especially during exercise. Because of early surgical intervention during infancy, squatting is rarely seen.

Hypercyanotic spells, also referred to as ***blue spells*** or ***"tet" spells*** because they are often seen in infants with tetralogy of Fallot, may occur in any child whose heart defect includes obstruction to pulmonary blood flow and communication between the ventricles. The infant becomes acutely cyanotic and hyperpneic because sudden infundibular spasm decreases pulmonary blood flow and increases right-to-left shunting (the proposed mechanism in tetralogy of Fallot). Spells, rarely seen before 2 months of age, occur most frequently in the first year of life. They occur more often in the morning and may be preceded by feeding, crying, defecation, or stressful procedures (see the Critical Thinking Q & A box on p. 1473). Because profound hypoxemia causes cerebral hypoxia, hypercyanotic spells require prompt assessment and treatment to prevent brain damage or possible death.

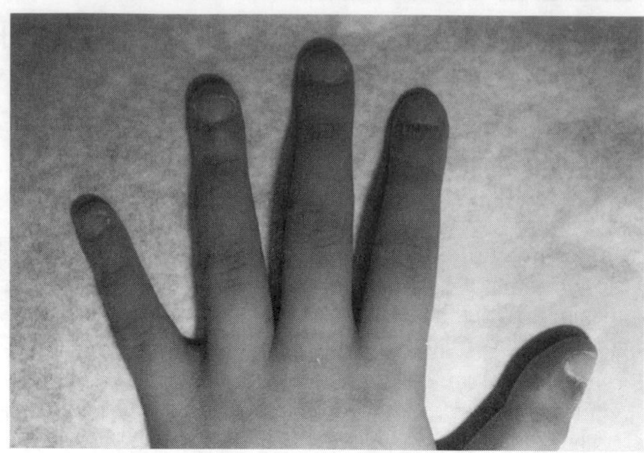

Fig. 45-7 Clubbing of fingers.

Persistent cyanosis as a result of cyanotic cardiac defects places the child at risk for significant ***neurologic complications.*** Cerebrovascular accident (CVA, stroke), brain abscess, and developmental delays, especially in motor and cognitive development, may result from chronic hypoxia.

Therapeutic Management

Hypercyanotic spells occur suddenly, and prompt recognition and treatment are essential. In the hospital setting spells are often seen during blood drawing or intravenous insertion, when the child is highly agitated, or after cardiac catheterization. Treatment of a hypercyanotic spell is outlined in the Guidelines box on p. 1473. Morphine, administered subcutaneously or through an existing intravenous line, helps to reduce infundibular spasm. Generally, a spell indicates the need for prompt surgical treatment if possible (Driscoll, 1990). In infants with defects not amenable to surgical repair, a shunt may be created surgically to increase blood flow to the lungs. Currently used types of shunts are described in Table 45-3.

The cyanotic infant and child are well hydrated to keep the hematocrit and blood viscosity within acceptable limits to reduce the risk of CVAs. Fevers are carefully evaluated because bacteremia can result in bacterial endocarditis. The infant is monitored closely for anemia because of the risk of CVAs and the reduced arterial oxygen-carrying capacity that occurs. Iron supplementation and possibly blood transfusion are used as needed.

Respiratory infections or reduced pulmonary function from any cause can worsen hypoxemia in the cyanotic child. Aggressive pulmonary hygiene, chest physiotherapy, administration of antibiotics, and use of oxygen to improve arterial saturations are important interventions.

Critical Thinking Q & A

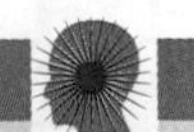

HYPERCYANOTIC SPELL

A 4-month-old infant known to have tetralogy of Fallot is seen in the emergency department because of a 2-day history of diarrhea, low-grade fever, and poor oral intake. When blood tests are done, he becomes acutely cyanotic with rapid shallow respirations. You would:

1. Begin cardiopulmonary resuscitation (CPR).
2. Calm the infant, place in the knee-chest position, administer blowby oxygen, and call for assistance.
3. Continue the procedure; this is expected for an infant with tetralogy of Fallot.
4. Stop the procedure and wait for color to improve before completing the blood test.

The correct answer is two. The infant is having a hypercyanotic or "tet" spell and the first actions should be to calm the infant, place the infant in the knee-chest position, and give supplemental oxygen. A hypercyanotic spell will likely worsen without intervention so prompt action is needed. CPR is inappropriate at this time because the infant has an adequate heart rate and effective respirations. A severe hypercyanotic spell may require intravenous medications, hydration, and resuscitative measures to stabilize the condition of the infant.

Guidelines

TREATING HYPERCYANOTIC SPELLS

Place infant in knee-chest position.
Employ calm, comforting approach.
Administer 100% oxygen by face mask.
Give morphine subcutaneously or through existing intravenous line.
Begin intravenous fluid replacement and volume expansion if needed.
Repeat morphine administration.

Nursing Care Management

The general appearance of infants and children with significant cyanosis poses unique concerns. Blue lips and fingernails are obvious signs of their hidden cardiac defect. Clubbing and small, thin stature in older children further indicate severe heart disease. Adolescents are especially concerned about their body image; children with cyanosis are often teased about their appearance and singled out as different. Many children, when asked what surgery will do, reply, "Make me pink." Their joy and excitement after surgery are evident when they see their pink fingers. Accentuating the normal and positive and being careful not to call attention to their cyanosis are helpful interventions. Meeting other children who are cyanotic in the clinic or hospital reassures them that they are not the only ones who are blue.

Parents are often fearful of their child's bluish color, since cyanosis is usually associated with lack of oxygen and severe illness. They also must deal with comments from relatives, friends, and strangers about their child's abnormal color. They need a simple explanation of hypoxemia and cyanosis and reassurance that cyanosis does not imply a lack of oxygen to the brain. Their questions and fears need to be addressed in a calm, supportive manner, and positive aspects of their child's growth and development are emphasized. They are taught the treatment for hypercyanotic spells (see the Guidelines box at left).

Dehydration must be prevented in hypoxemic children because it potentiates the risk of CVAs. Fluid status is carefully monitored, with accurate intake and output and daily weight measurements. Maintenance fluid therapy is the minimum requirement, supplemental fluids should be readily available, and gavage feeding or intravenous hydration is given to children unable to take adequate oral fluids. Fever, vomiting, and diarrhea can cause dehydration and require prompt treatment. Parents are instructed in the importance of adequate fluid intake and measures to prevent dehydration. An oral

TABLE 45-3 Selected shunt procedures for children with cardiac defects

TYPE OF SHUNT/LOCATION	COMMENTS
Modified Blalock-Taussig (BT) Subclavian artery to pulmonary artery using Gore-Tex or Impra tube graft	Shunt flow sometimes excessive, requiring use of diuretics Possibility of thrombosis; antiplatelet therapy may be used postoperatively Easy to ligate at time of definitive correction Shunt size fixed and may become too small as child grows
Central Ascending aorta to main pulmonary aorta using Gore-Tex graft	Length of shunt acts to restrict blood flow, limiting symptoms of CHF; may require diuretics Uncommon; used when modified BT shunt cannot be done Easy to perform and remove at time of repair
Glenn Superior vena cava to side of right pulmonary artery, which is ligated from main pulmonary artery Blood flow to right lung only	Used as a second shunt procedure if complete repair not possible High mortality rate in infants under age 6 months Superior vena cava syndrome may occur Pulmonary arteriovenous fistulas may occur many years later Difficult to take down at time of definitive repair
Bidirectional Glenn (cavopulmonary anastomosis) Superior vena cava to side of right pulmonary artery Blood flow to both lungs	Done as a second shunt; often as a staging step to a Fontan procedure Can be incorporated into eventual modified Fontan procedure Relieves cyanosis and decreases volume overload on ventricle

electrolyte solution should be available at home in the event the infant is unable to tolerate the usual formula. The practitioner should be notified of fever, vomiting, diarrhea, or other problems.

Preventive measures and accurate assessment of respiratory infection are important nursing considerations. Any compromise in pulmonary function will increase the infant's hypoxemia. Good handwashing and protection from individuals with an obvious respiratory infection are important. Aggressive pulmonary hygiene, treatment with antibiotics or antiviral agents as indicated, and supplemental oxygen to decrease hypoxemia are necessary measures. Infants may need to be gavage-fed or given parenteral hydration if respiratory distress prevents oral feeding.

Nursing ALERT

Intracardiac shunting of blood from the right side (desaturated) to the left side of the heart allows air in the venous system to go directly to the brain, resulting in an air embolism. Therefore all intravenous lines should have filters in place to prevent air from entering the system, the entire tubing should be checked for air, all connections should be taped securely, and any air should be removed.

BOX 45-7
Clinical Manifestations of Congenital Heart Disease

Infants

Cyanosis—generalized, especially mucous membranes, lips and tongue, conjunctiva; highly vascularized areas
Cyanosis during exertion such as crying, feeding, straining, or when immersed in water; peripheral or central
Dyspnea, especially after physical effort such as feeding, crying, straining
Fatigue
Poor growth and development (failure to thrive)
Frequent respiratory tract infections
Feeding difficulties
Hypotonia
Excessive sweating
Syncopal attacks such as paroxysmal hyperpnea, anoxic spells

Older children

Impaired growth
Delicate, frail body build
Fatigue
Effort dyspnea
Orthopnea
Digital clubbing
Squatting for relief of dyspnea
Headache
Epistaxis
Leg fatigue

Nursing Care of the Family and Child With Congenital Heart Disease

Assessment

Nursing care of the child with CHD begins as soon as the diagnosis is suspected. However, in many instances symptoms that suggest a cardiac anomaly are not present at birth or, if manifest, are so subtle that they are easily overlooked (Box 45-7).

Many heart defects are not evident until the child's growth and/or energy expenditure exceeds the ability of the heart to supply oxygenated blood. Since the onset is gradual, the child may curtail activity so that the signs of exercise intolerance are less obvious.

A vital component of nursing assessment is related to the impact of the disorder on the family, especially the parents. Therefore the reactions, coping, and concerns of the family are also included in the assessment process (see Chapter 38).

Nursing Diagnoses

Many nursing diagnoses are apparent after a thorough assessment of the child and family. Some of these are developed in the Nursing Care Plan on p. 1480. Others will be evident on the basis of assessment of individual cases.

Planning

The goals for the infant with CHD and the family include the following:

1. Family and child (if appropriate) will adjust to the diagnosis.
2. Family will be knowledgeable regarding symptoms of the disease and their management.
3. Family will cope with effects of the disorder.
4. Child (if appropriate) and family will be prepared for surgical repair of a defect.
5. Child undergoing cardiac surgery will receive appropriate care.
6. Family will receive adequate emotional support.
7. Family will be prepared for home care.

Implementation

Help Family Adjust to the Disorder

Once parents learn of the heart defect, whether it is soon after the child's birth or at a later period in life, they are initially in a period of shock, followed by high anxiety, especially fear of the child's death. The family needs time to grieve before it can assimilate the meaning of the defect. Unfortunately the demands for medical treatment may not allow this, necessitating that the parents immediately give informed consent for diagnostic/therapeutic procedures. The nurse can be instrumental in supporting parents in their loss, assessing their level of understanding, supplying information as needed, and helping other members of the health team to understand the parents' reactions (see the Family Focus box on p. 1475).

Severely distressed newborns usually remain in the hospital. This can seriously affect parent-infant attachment unless parents are encouraged to hold, touch, and look at their child.

Family Focus

THE DIAGNOSIS OF HEART DISEASE

Remember, we don't have your experience. We don't see children everyday who have heart disease. We would have been upset finding out our child had to have his tonsils out. How could we ever be prepared for this? Please remember, we only know people who have trivial heart murmurs. How could we ever expect this to happen? And to us, this is the worst problem we've ever heard of.

We still fear most what we don't know and understand. Be honest with us. If you don't know either, tell us. But at least don't leave us wondering about what you know and we don't. Not knowing anything really can be worse than knowing something bad. Be honest, but don't strip us of hope.

Please, remember we are trying to learn complex information in a moment of time. And trying to learn it in a context of great pain and emotional investment. This is our lives you're talking about. Please be thorough, but keep it simple. Tell us again, maybe even again and again, when we can hear better.

From: Schrey C, Schrey M: A parents' perspective: our needs and our message, *Critical Care Nurs Clin North Am* 6(1):113-121, 1994.

Every effort must be made by health personnel to foster attachment.

The effect of a child with a serious heart defect on the family is complex. No member, regardless of the degree of positive adjustment, is unaffected. Mothers frequently feel inadequate in their mothering ability because they gave birth to a child with a defect and are unable to keep the child well. They often feel constantly exhausted from the pressures of caring for these children and the other family members. Fathers and siblings may feel neglected and resentful, a reaction similar to the feelings of family members toward other chronic conditions (see Chapter 38). Often parents do not feel confident leaving the child in another's care. This often sets up a trap for parents, especially mothers, who become locked into the child's care with no relief. Although the fears are justified, they can be minimized by gradually teaching someone (a reliable relative or neighbor) how to care for the child.

The need to maintain discipline and set consistent limits cannot be overemphasized. Using behavior modification techniques, in the form of either concrete awards (e.g., a favorite activity) or social reinforcement (e.g., approval), can be effective. However, it is most beneficial if employed *before* the child learns to control the family. Therefore it is necessary to indicate to parents the need for discipline while the child is in infancy to prevent later problems. Use of behavior modification techniques also teaches these children how to tolerate frustration and delayed gratification (this ability often is lacking because all of their needs are satisfied immediately).

Another issue that may develop within family relationships is the child's overdependency. This is often the result of parental fear that the child may die. The best approach to dealing with this dilemma is prevention. Parents need guidance to recognize the eventual hazards of continuing dependency and protectiveness as the child grows older, and the nurse can assist parents in learning ways to foster optimal development. Unless parents are shown what activities the child can do, they may focus on physical limitations and encourage dependency.

The child also needs opportunities for social development. These children do not need to be prevented from playing with other children because of concern regarding overexertion. Such practices foster increased dependency in the home environment. Parents need to be encouraged to seek appropriate social activity, especially before kindergarten.

CHD may constitute a long-term family crisis. Frequently the continuing unremitting stresses of care—physical exhaustion, financial costs, emotional upset, fear of death, and concern for the child's future—are not fully appreciated by those caring for the family. Even when the child's condition is stabilized or corrected, the family may need to make new adjustments in their lifestyle. Introducing them to other families with similarly affected children can help them adjust to the daily stresses.*

Educate Family About the Disorder

Once parents are ready to hear about the heart condition, it is essential that they be given a clear explanation based on their level of understanding. Lack of familiarity with the cardiovascular system may be a major reason for lack of parental understanding, and it is usually helpful to review the basic structure and function of the heart before describing the defect. A simple diagram, pictures, or a model of the heart can be most helpful in visualizing the heart and the congenital defect. Parents appreciate receiving written information about the specific condition.† Parents also require information on the treatment options for the cardiac condition and the prognosis.

Another fact to remember is that different health personnel may convey the same information using different diagrams and medical terms. To prevent this from becoming a problem, as often happens when several health team members work with a family, the same type of diagram should be used, and the parents should write down any unclear terms or ask for clarification. Sometimes it is helpful to provide the family with a glossary of frequently used words for reference.

Infants and children with CHD require good nutrition. Providing infants with adequate nutrition is especially difficult because of their high caloric requirements and inability to suck effectively because of fatigue and tachypnea. Instructing parents in feeding methods that decrease the work of the infant and giving high-calorie formula are important interventions. (See p. 1470 for a discussion on feeding the infant with CHF.)

Children with severe cardiac defects are often anorexic. Encouraging them to eat can be a tremendous challenge. Because of the parents' concern about eating, children learn early to manipulate parents, for example, making unrealistic demands for foods that are not available. The nurse advises parents of this potential problem, since prevention yields greater success than intervention. For example, the child should be given a choice of available high-quality foods. Suggestions for feeding sick children are discussed in Chapter 42.

The family also needs to be knowledgeable regarding the

*Some local chapters of the **American Heart Association** have organized parent groups.

†A booklet that can be given to parents is *If Your Child Has a Congenital Heart Defect: A Guide for Parents,* available from the American Heart Association, 7272 Greenville Ave., Dallas, TX 75231; (214) 373-6300.

therapeutic management of the disorder, especially in terms of the medications that the child is receiving. Parents are taught the correct procedure for giving drugs* and cautioned to keep them in a safe area to prevent accidental ingestion (see the Home Care box on p. 1469).

Children of various ages have different ideas about their heart. Children between ages 4 and 6 years have heard about the heart, know its approximate anatomic location in the chest or back, illustrate it as valentine-shaped, and characterize it by sounds such as *tick-tock* and *thump.* Children ages 7 to 10 have a clearer concept of the heart, realizing that it is not shaped like a valentine and that it has vital functions, such as, "It makes you live." However, their knowledge of its integrated functions to pump blood through a system of vessels to all parts of the body is still hazy. By the age of 10 or 11 children have a much more complex concept of the heart, with knowledge of veins, valves, pumping action, and circulation. They are beginning to appreciate why death occurs when the heart stops.

Information given to the child must be tailored to the child's developmental age. As the child matures, the level of information is revised to meet the child's new cognitive level. Preschoolers need basic information about what they will experience more than what is actually occurring physiologically. School-age children benefit from a concrete explanation of the defect. Preadolescents and adolescents often appreciate a more detailed description of how the defect affects their heart. Children of all ages need to express their feelings concerning the diagnosis.

Help Family Cope with Effects of the Disorder

Parents also need an explanation regarding the symptoms of the disease. Many children have few symptoms but may develop CHF. Therefore parents should be aware of early signs of worsening physical status, such as sweating, sudden weight gain, decreased exercise tolerance, poor feeding, and increased breathing effort. These symptoms need medical evaluation, but the family is assured that the symptoms usually respond quickly to therapeutic intervention.

Another area of parental concern is the child's level of physical activity. Children do not need to restrict activity, and the best approach is to treat the child normally and allow self-limited activity. Deliberately attempting to prevent crying should be avoided because it can establish a maladaptive parental pattern of relating to the infant. Exceptions to self-determined activity primarily involve strenuous recreational and competitive sports.

Prepare Child and Family for Surgery

Few surgical procedures demand as much planning for preoperative preparation and postoperative care as heart surgery. The reader is urged to review the general principles for preparing children for procedures, such as surgery, discussed in Chapter 42. This discussion focuses on those measures specific to cardiovascular procedures. The child is usually admitted to the hospital 1 day before surgery or the day of surgery. Preoperative preparation is often done in the outpatient setting.

Introduce child and family to the environment. Ideally, when the child is admitted, a plan should be made to provide consistent caregivers. In some institutions the nurse who will care for the child postoperatively in the intensive care unit is also assigned to the child at admission to facilitate forming a relationship with the family and to share preoperative teaching, such as introduction to the recovery room and intensive care unit. To increase familiarity, all nurses should call the child and parents by name and refer to themselves by name. Wearing a name tag reinforces this policy. Postoperatively the family will feel more at ease recognizing familiar names, faces, and voices.

If a visit to the recovery room and/or intensive care unit is planned, it should take place when there is least activity in the area, the parents can accompany the child, and the child is well rested. Usually a day before surgery is ample time to allow the child to ask questions and to prevent undue fantasizing about the experience. If a visit is not included in the teaching plan, the nurse can use a book, preferably with pictures or photographs of the actual rooms, to explain the environment to the child.

During the visit to the intensive care unit the child and parents should experience everything that directly affects the child's care, such as the sounds of ECG monitors, oxygen tents, and placement of the bed. All positive, nonfrightening aspects of the environment are emphasized, such as the play area, visitors' section, pictures or mobiles in the room, or television. If it is a pediatric intensive care unit, the nurse can introduce the family to other children who may be recovering from surgery. The child should be protected from the frightening sights in the unit, and equipment not in view postoperatively, such as that located behind or below the bed, needs less attention. The child and parents are encouraged to ask questions or to explore further any equipment in the room, but they should not be pushed to assimilate more information than they appear to be tolerating.

Familiarize child and family with equipment. Some of the equipment, such as the stethoscope, blood pressure apparatus, and thermometer, will already be familiar to the child and parents. However, the nurse emphasizes that procedures involving such equipment will be done more frequently. If monitoring devices, such as those for blood pressure or oximetry, are used, the child is told about the placement of the sensor on the skin.

Types of equipment new to many families are the oxygen mask, suction, chest tubes, endotracheal tubes, incentive spirometers, nasogastric tube, and intravenous tubing. Each of these is shown and demonstrated either on the child or on a doll, if he or she appears ready. With a younger child, miniaturized equipment suitable for use with a doll or puppet is often less anxiety-producing than the actual samples. If other children in the unit have an intravenous infusion or are in oxygen tents, the older child may benefit from seeing them, but this visit must be planned carefully to prevent frightening the child.

Several intravenous lines are inserted perioperatively: (1) an ordinary line for infusion of fluids, inserted in a periph-

*Home care instructions on giving medications to children are available in Wong DL; *Wong and Whaley's clinical manual of pediatric nursing,* ed 4, St Louis, 1996, Mosby.

eral vein; (2) a venous pressure line, inserted into the right subclavian or jugular vein; and (3) an arterial line for direct measurement of arterial pressure. Younger children need only know the location of each tubing. Older children may appreciate knowing the reason for each infusion. Since the lines are inserted during surgery, they are not painful; they only cause discomfort because movement is restricted.

The type and size of incision the child will have after surgery are discussed and can be shown on a doll. Usually one of two types of incisions is made: a ***median sternotomy,*** which splits the sternum, or a ***lateral thoracotomy,*** which extends from the midaxillary line to the scapula. Frequently no sutures are visible because subcuticular, absorbable sutures may be used. If this is done, it should be pointed out to the child and parents, who may fear the incision will open.

The child may be told about chest tubes and their purpose in draining fluid from around the heart and lungs. An endotracheal (ET) tube is inserted during surgery and may be left in place for ventilatory assistance and tracheobronchial suctioning. However, it may be best to prepare older children for the ET tube only if *prolonged* ventilatory support is planned. The ET tube can be presented as a "breathing tube" that is placed in the nose or mouth. The nurse explains that while the tube is in, the child will feel it in the throat and will not be able to talk, but nothing is wrong. The child can express desires by pointing or using a picture communication board. At this point communicating the amount of discomfort from the surgery can also be discussed, especially using measurement tools such as numbers or faces (see Pain Assessment, Chapter 41). The nurse stresses that the tube will be removed as soon as possible, often during the first postoperative day.

Preoperative physical care differs little, if any, from that for any other surgery and is discussed in Chapter 42. The child should be assured that the parents will be there when he or she wakes up; parents should be allowed to accompany their child as far as possible to the operating suite. After all the equipment and procedures have been explained, it is important to talk about "getting well" and going home. If a doll was used during the preparatory session, the tubes can be removed, and the doll can be dressed in regular clothes in anticipation of discharge.

Provide Postoperative Care

Immediate postoperative care is usually provided by specially trained nurses in intensive care units. Many of the procedures, such as arterial pressure and central venous pressure (CVP) monitoring and the observations related to vital functions, require advanced educational training (the reader should refer to critical care texts for further information). However, nurses caring for the child before surgery and during the convalescent period need to be familiar with the major principles of care. Selected complications that may occur postoperatively are described in Box 45-8.

Observe vital signs. Vital signs and blood pressure are recorded frequently until stable. Heart rate and respirations are counted for 1 full minute, compared with the ECG monitor, and recorded with activity. The heart rate is normally increased after surgery. The nurse observes cardiac rhythm and notifies the practitioner of any changes in regularity. Dysrhythmias may occur postoperatively secondary to anesthetics, acid-base and electrolyte imbalance, hypoxia, surgical intervention, or trauma to conduction pathways (see also p. 1484).

At least hourly the lungs are auscultated for breath sounds. Diminished or absent sounds most likely indicate an area of atelectasis, which necessitates further medical assessment.

Temperature changes are typical during the early postoperative period. Hypothermia is expected immediately after surgery from hypothermia procedures, effects of anesthesia, and loss of body heat to the cool environment. During this period the child is kept warm to prevent additional heat loss. Infants may be placed under radiant heat warmers. During the next 24 to 48 hours the body temperature may rise to 37.7° C (100° F) or slightly higher as part of the inflammatory response to tissue trauma. After this period an elevated temperature is most likely a sign of infection and warrants immediate investigation for probable cause.

Maintain respiratory status. The child is generally maintained on mechanical ventilation in the immediate postopera-

BOX 45-8

Selected Complications After Cardiac Surgery and Treatment Approaches

Cardiac

Congestive heart failure—digoxin, diuretics, etc. (see p. 1465)
Low cardiac output—intravenous inotropes (see shock, p. 1489)
Dysrhythmias—identification, drug treatment, possible pacing, cardioversion (see p. 1484)
Tamponade (blood or fluid in the pericardial space constricting the heart)—prompt removal of fluid by pericardiocentesis

Respiratory

Atelectasis—chest physiotherapy, coughing, deep breathing, ambulation
Pulmonary edema—diuretics
Pleural effusions—diuretics, possible chest tube drainage
Pneumothorax—possible chest tube drainage

Neurologic

Seizures—assessment, antiepileptic drugs
Stroke, cerebral edema, neurologic deficits—assessment and treatment

Infectious disease

Infections (especially wound, pneumonia, otitis media, and sepsis)—antibiotics

Hematologic

Anemia—iron supplementation, possible transfusion
Postoperative bleeding—initially give clotting factors, blood products; may need repeat surgery to locate and ligate source of bleeding

Other

Postpericardiotomy syndrome (syndrome of fever, leukocytosis, friction rub, pericardial and pleural effusions, lethargy seen about 7-21 days after cardiac surgery, possible viral or autoimmune cause)—antipyretics, diuretics, antiinflammatory medications

tive period. When weaning and extubation are completed, humidified oxygen is delivered by mask or hood. The child is kept warm and dry, since excessive chilling from wet linens causes an increased metabolic need and consequent increased cardiac demand. The child is encouraged to turn and deep breathe at least hourly. Every measure is used to enhance ventilation and decrease pain, such as splinting of the operative site and judicious use of analgesics.

Nursing ALERT

During suctioning observe for signs and symptoms of respiratory distress, such as tachypnea, use of accessory muscles for breathing, restlessness, and changes in oxygen saturation on the pulse oximeter.

Suctioning is performed *only* as needed and maintained for no more than 5 seconds at a time to prevent depleting the oxygen supply. Supplemental oxygen is administered with a manual resuscitation bag before and after the procedure to prevent hypoxia. Heart rate is monitored after suctioning to detect changes in rhythm or rate, especially bradycardia. The child should be positioned facing the nurse to permit assessment of the child's color and tolerance to the procedure.

Drainage from chest tubes is checked hourly for color and quantity. Immediately after surgery the drainage may be bright red, but afterward it should be serous. The largest volume of drainage occurs in the first 12 to 24 hours and is greater in extensive heart surgery.

Nursing ALERT

Chest tube drainage greater than 3 ml/kg/hour for more than 3 consecutive hours is excessive and may indicate postoperative hemorrhage (Hazinski, 1992). The surgeon is notified immediately, since cardiac tamponade can develop rapidly and is life-threatening.

Chest tubes are usually removed on the first to third postoperative day. Removal of chest tubes is a painful, frightening experience. Analgesics such as morphine sulfate, often combined with midazolam (Versed), should be given before the procedure. Older children are forewarned that they will feel a sharp, momentary pain. After the suture is cut, the tubes are quickly pulled out at the end of full inspiration to prevent intake of air into the pleural cavity. A purse-string suture (placed when the tubes were inserted) is pulled tight to close the opening. A petrolatum-covered gauze dressing is immediately applied over the wound and securely taped to the skin on all four sides so that an airtight seal is formed. The dressing is checked for signs of drainage and any evidence of infection.

Monitor fluids. Intake and output of all fluids must be accurately calculated. Intake is primarily intravenous fluids; however, a record of fluid used to flush the arterial and central venous pressure lines or to dilute medications is also kept. Output includes hourly recordings of urine (usually a Foley catheter is inserted and attached to a closed collecting device), drainage from chest and nasogastric tubes, and blood drawn for analysis. Urine is analyzed for specific gravity to assess the concentrating ability of the kidneys and to assess approximately the body's degree of hydration. Renal failure is a potential risk from a transient period of low cardiac output.

Nursing ALERT

The signs of renal failure are decreased urine output (less than 1 ml/kg/hour) and elevated levels of blood urea nitrogen and serum creatinine.

Fluids are restricted during the immediate postoperative period to prevent hypervolemia, which places additional demands on the myocardium, predisposing to cardiac failure. To monitor fluid retention, the child is weighed daily, and the same scale is used at approximately the same time each day to prevent errors in measurement. The child is usually given nothing by mouth for the first 24 hours. If an ET tube is inserted, oral fluids are usually withheld until the child is extubated. Fluid restriction may be imposed even when oral fluids are given. The nurse calculates the distribution over a 24-hour period based on the child's preoperative weight and drinking habits. The distribution should allow for the majority of fluid to be given during the child's most wakeful and active periods.

Provide rest and progressive activity. After heart surgery rest should be provided to decrease the work load of the heart and promote healing. The simplest way to ensure individualized, efficient, high-quality care is to plan at the beginning of the shift the nursing procedures to be done, with periods of rest identified. The schedule should be shared with parents to allow them to visit at the most advantageous times, such as after a rest period when no special treatments are anticipated.

A progressive schedule of ambulation and activity, based on the child's preoperative activity patterns and postoperative cardiovascular and pulmonary function, is planned. Ambulation is initiated early, usually by the second postoperative day, when chest tubes, arterial lines, and assisted ventilatory equipment may be removed. Activity progresses from sitting on the edge of the bed and dangling the legs to standing up and to sitting in a chair. Heart rate and respirations are carefully monitored to assess the degree of cardiac demand imposed by each activity. Tachycardia, dyspnea, cyanosis, desaturation, progressive fatigue, or dysrhythmias indicate the need to limit further energy expenditure.

Provide comfort and emotional support. Heart surgery is both painful and frightening for children, and comfort is a primary nursing concern. Recent improvements have been made in the management of pain after cardiac surgery. Continuous intravenous opioid infusions, particularly morphine and fentanyl, are safe and effective analgesics (Maguire and Maloney, 1988). Patient-controlled analgesia may be used with children old enough to understand the concept. Nonsteroidal antiinflammatory drugs such as Keterolac (Toradol) may be used intravenously. Epidural morphine may be another option, since it affords very good pain control when a thoracotomy is performed. Paralyzing agents such as pancuronium (Pavulon) or metocurine (Metubine) may also be used with the analgesics for children who are very agitated or hemodynamically unstable.

Most patients need intravenous analgesics for pain control during the immediate postoperative period. After extubation and removal of lines and tubes, pain can be satisfactorily controlled with oral medications such as ibuprofen, codeine with acetaminophen (Tylenol), or oxycodone and acetaminophen (Tylox). Acetaminophen alone provides adequate pain relief for most children at discharge. Sternotomy incisions are usually well tolerated, with some discomfort when walking and coughing. Thoracotomy incisions are usually more painful because the incision is through muscle; a more aggressive pain management plan with round-the-clock medications for several days is often necessary to allow for adequate rest, ambulation, and pulmonary hygiene.

In addition to pharmacologic pain control, every effort is made to minimize the discomfort of procedures, such as using a firm pillow or favorite stuffed animal placed against the chest incision during movement and performing treatments *after* pain medication is given, preferably at a time that coincides with the drug's peak effect. Nonpharmacologic measures are used to lessen the perception of pain, and parents are encouraged to comfort their child as much as possible. (See also Pain Assessment; Pain Management, Chapter 41).

Children may also be angry and uncooperative after surgery as a response to the physical pain and to the loss of control imposed by the surgery and treatments. They need an opportunity to express feelings, either verbally or through activity. Children also may express feelings of anger or rejection toward parents. The nurse must reassure parents that this is normal and that with continued support the anger will subside.

The nurse can support the parents by being available for information and explaining all the procedures to them. The first few postoperative days are particularly difficult because parents see their child in pain and realize the potential risks from surgery. They often are overwhelmed by the physical environment of the intensive care unit and feel useless because they can do so little for their child. The importance of their presence in making the child feel more secure is stressed, even if they do not provide physical care.

Plan for Discharge and Home Care

Ideally discharge planning begins on admission for cardiac surgery and includes an assessment of the parents' adjustment to the child's altered state of health. As mentioned earlier, one of the most common parental reactions is overprotection, and the nurse needs to be aware of times when the family may need help in recognizing the child's improved health status. With surgical correction of heart anomalies occurring during infancy, there is less likelihood this pattern of overdependency will develop.

The family will need both verbal and written instructions on medication, nutrition, activity restrictions, subacute bacterial endocarditis, return to school, wound care, and signs and symptoms of infection or complications (see the Home Care box above). Referrals to community agencies may be warranted to assist parents in the transition from hospital to home and to reinforce the teaching.

Home Care

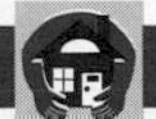

TOPICS TO INCLUDE IN DISCHARGE TEACHING AFTER CARDIAC SURGERY

- Medication teaching (for digoxin, see p. 1469)
- Activity restrictions
- Diet and nutrition
- Wound care (include dressings if any; suture removal; bathing)
- Bacterial endocarditis prophylaxis (see p. 1481)
- Follow-up appointments (cardiologist, primary care provider)
- Community agencies as needed (visiting nurse service, early developmental intervention)
- When to call practitioner; signs and symptoms of postoperative problems
- Review of cardiac defect and surgical repair

The parents will also need clear instructions on when to seek medical care, such as for a change in the child's behavior or an unexplained fever. Follow-up evaluation with the cardiologist is also arranged before discharge. Appropriate identification, such as a medical alert device, is indicated for children with a pacemaker or heart transplantation and for those receiving anticoagulation therapy or antidysrhythmic medication.

The nurse also discusses common behavior disturbances that may occur after discharge, such as nightmares, sleep disturbances, separation anxiety, and overdependence. A supportive, consistent response is essential to allow the child to overcome the surgical experience. The child should be encouraged to work out feelings and fears through therapeutic play.

Although surgical correction of heart defects has improved dramatically, it is still not possible to reverse many of the complex anomalies totally. For many children repeat procedures are required to replace conduits or grafts or to manage complications, such as restenosis. Consequently the long-term prognosis is uncertain, and full recovery is not always possible. For these families medical follow-up care and continued emotional support are essential. The nurse can often serve as an important primary health professional and as a resource for referrals when needed.

Evaluation

The effectiveness of nursing interventions for the family and the child with CHD is determined by continual reassessment and evaluation of care based on the following observational guidelines and expected outcomes:

1. Interview family and observe their behavior with infant or child.
2. Encourage family to discuss their feelings and concerns; observe their response to education.
3. Interview child and observe his or her behavior and concerns; encourage verbal child to express feelings.
4. Interview family and observe family interactions and relationships.
5. Interview family regarding their understanding of the condition and the proposed surgery.
6. Monitor and observe infant or child and family preoperatively and postoperatively.

Nursing Care Plan

THE CHILD WITH CONGENITAL HEART DISEASE

Nursing Diagnosis: Potential for decreased cardiac output related to structural defect

Expected Outcome: **Patient exhibits signs of adequate cardiac output (i.e., strong, regular pulse with rates within normal limits [WNL]; blood pressure WNL; absence of pallor, adequate capillary refill).**

• NURSING INTERVENTIONS/*RATIONALES*

Administer digoxin per physician order using established precautons *to prevent toxicity* (see pp. 1468-1469) monitor for adverse or toxic effects. Ensure adequate intake of potassium and monitor potassium levels, *as decreased levels enhance toxicity of digoxin.*

Administer diuretics as ordered (see p. 1467).

Administer aferload reduction medications as ordered (see p. 1469).

Monitor apical and radial pulses frequently for rate and rhythm *to detect presence of arrhythmias;* monitor skin color, temperature, capillary refill, vital signs *to assess for status of cardiac output.*

Plan child's care and activities to prevent overexertion, *which increases myocardial oxygen demand.*

Nursing Diagnosis: Activity intolerance related to oxygen imbalance

Expected Outcome: **Patient's activity level is within normal limits for physical condition.**

• NURSING INTERVENTIONS/*RATIONALES*

Prevent temperature extremes, *which can increase oxygen demands.*

Implement measures to reduce anxiety and signs of distress, *which can increase oxygen demands.*

Balance rest and physical activity, increasing activity levels as tolerated *to maintain balance between oxygen supply and demand.* Help child to select activities appropriate to age, physical condition, and capabilities.

Nursing Diagnosis: Altered growth and development related to inadequate oxygenation of tissues; social isolation

Expected Outcomes: **Patient exhibits height, weight gains that follow growth curve; Patient exhibits gross and fine motor abilities, language abilities, and social skills that are within normal limits (WNL) for age.**

• NURSING INTERVENTIONS/*RATIONALES*

Provide well-balanced, highly nutritious diet *to promote adequate growth.*

Monitor height and weight using growth charts *to plot growth trends.*

Administer iron supplements as ordered *to correct or prevent anemia.*

Encourage age-appropriate activity *to build gross and fine motor skills.*

Plan regular storytelling or reading sessions *to enhance verbal abilities.*

Encourage interaction with other children *to promote social interaction.*

Test child's developmental level periodically *to evaluate for developmental delay.*

Nursing Diagnosis: Potential infection related to debilitated physical status

Expected Outcome: **Patient exhibits no signs of infection.**

• NURSING INTERVENTIONS/*RATIONALES*

Avoid high-exposure social settings such as nursery schools, day care, crowds, *which increase risk of infection.*

Screen visitors and playmates and prevent contact with infected persons *to decrease infection risk.*

Provide for adequate rest and nutrition *to support body's natural defenses.*

Have family and child practice good hygiene and handwashing techniques *to contain germ spread.*

Nursing Diagnosis: Potential for injury (complications) related to cardiac status and therapies

Expected Outcome: **Signs of cardiac complications are absent or detected in a timely fashion.**

• NURSING INTERVENTIONS/*RATIONALES*

Teach family to recognize early signs of congestive heart failure (i.e., tachycardia, tachypnea, profuse scalp sweating, fatigue and irritability, sudden weight gain, respiratory distress); hypoxemia (i.e., cyanosis, restlessness); digoxin toxicity (i.e., nausea, vomiting, anorexia, bradycardia, dysrhythmias) *to ensure timely intervention.*

Give family written instructions about what to do and whom to call if any of the signs occurs *to ensure timely intervention.*

Nursing Diagnosis: Altered family processes related to having child with heart condition

See the Nursing Care Plan: Child with Chronic Illness or Disability, Chapter 38.

7. Observe and interview child and family regarding their understanding of home care needs, ability to carry out care, and compliance with the plan of care.

Expected outcomes:

See the Nursing Care Plan on p. 1480.

Acquired Cardiovascular Disorders

BACTERIAL (INFECTIVE) ENDOCARDITIS (BE)

BE, or infective endocarditis (IE), also referred to as *subacute bacterial endocarditis (SBE)*, is an infection of the valves and inner lining of the heart. Although it can occur without underlying heart disease, it most often is a sequela of bacteremia in the child with acquired or congenital anomalies of the heart or great vessels. It especially affects children with valvular abnormalities, prosthetic valves, recent cardiac surgery with invasive lines, and rheumatic heart disease with valve involvement. In addition a growing problem is endocarditis associated with drug abuse (Dajani and Taubert, 1995). The most common causative agent is *Streptococcus viridans;* other causative agents are *Staphylococcus aureus*, gram-negative bacteria, and fungi such as *Candida albicans*.

Pathophysiology

Organisms may enter the bloodstream from any site of localized infection. The most common portals of entry are oral from dental work *(S. viridans);* urinary tract, such as from urinary tract infection after catheterization (gram-negative bacilli); heart, from cardiac surgery, especially if synthetic material is used (valves, patches, conduits); and the bloodstream from long-term indwelling catheters. The microorganisms grow on the endocardium, forming vegetations (verrucae), deposits of fibrin, and platelet thrombi. The lesion may invade adjacent tissues, such as aortic and mitral valves, and may break off and embolize elsewhere, especially in the spleen, kidney, and central nervous system.

Diagnostic Evaluation

The diagnosis is suspected on the basis of clinical manifestations (Box 45-9). Several laboratory findings may suggest infective endocarditis, for example, electrocardiographic changes (prolonged P-R interval), radiographic evidence of cardiomegaly, anemia, elevated erythrocyte sedimentation rate, leukocytosis, and microscopic hematuria. Vegetations on the valve and abnormal valve function can often be visualized by echocardiography. Definitive diagnosis rests on growth and identification of the causative agent in the blood.

Therapeutic Management

Treatment should be instituted immediately and consists of administration of high doses of appropriate antibiotics intravenously and/or intramuscularly for at least 4 weeks. Blood cultures are taken periodically to evaluate response to antibiotic therapy.

Infective endocarditis in susceptible children is prevented by administering prophylactic antibiotic therapy both before and for a short period after procedures known to increase the risk of entry of organisms, including dental work and any manipulation of the respiratory, genitourinary, or gastrointestinal tract. In female adolescents this includes childbirth (Box 45-10).

BOX 45-9
Clinical Manifestations of Infective Endocarditis

Onset usually insidious
Unexplained fever (low grade and intermittent)
Anorexia
Malaise
Weight loss
Characteristic findings caused by extracardiac emboli formation:
- Splinter hemorrhages (thin black lines) under the nails
- Osler nodes (red, painful intradermal nodes found on pads of phalanges)
- Janeway lesions (painless hemorrhagic areas on palms and soles)
- Petechiae on oral mucous membranes

May be present:
- Congestive heart failure
- Cardiac dysrhythmias
- New murmur or change in previously existing one

BOX 45-10
Procedures Requiring Prophylaxis for Bacterial Endocarditis

All dental procedures likely to induce gingival or mucosal bleeding, including professional teeth cleaning (not simple adjustment of orthodontic appliances or shedding of deciduous teeth)
Tonsillectomy and/or adenoidectomy
Surgical procedures or biopsy involving respiratory or intestinal mucosa
Bronchoscopy with a rigid bronchoscope
Incision and drainage of infected tissue
Genitourinary and gastrointestinal procedures, including most diagnostic and therapeutic procedures that are invasive (sclerotherapy for esophageal varices, esophageal dilation, cystoscopy, urethral dilation, urethral catheterization or surgery if urinary tract infection is present, prostatic surgery, vaginal hysterectomy, and vaginal delivery in presence of infection)

Data from Dajani AS and others: Prevention of bacterial endocarditis: recommendations by the American Heart Association, *JAMA* 264(22):2919-2922, 1990.

Nursing Care Management

Ideally the objective of nursing care is prevention through counseling parents of high-risk children about the need for prophylactic antibiotic therapy before procedures such as dental work. Unless parents are aware of the risk inherent in exposing their child to these procedures, they may not be in-

Guidelines

THE DIAGNOSIS OF INITIAL ATTACK OF RHEUMATIC FEVER (JONES CRITERIA, 1992 UPDATE)*

Minor manifestations

Clinical findings
- Arthralgia
- Fever

Laboratory findings
- Elevated acute-phase reactants
  - Erythrocyte sedimentation rate
  - C-reactive protein

Major manifestations

Carditis

Tachycardia out of proportion to degree of fever
Cardiomegaly
New murmurs or change in preexisting murmurs
Muffled heart sounds
Precardial friction rub
Precordial pain
Changes in ECG (especially prolonged P-R interval)

Polyarthritis

Swollen, hot, red, painful joint(s)
After 1 to 2 days affects different joint(s)
Favors large joints—knees, elbows, hips, shoulders, wrists

Erythema marginatum

Erythematous macules with clear center and wavy, well-demarcated border
Transitory
Nonpruritic
Primarily affects trunk and extremities (inner surfaces)

Chorea (St. Vitus Dance, Sydenham Chorea)

Sudden aimless, irregular movements of extremities
Involuntary facial grimaces
Speech disturbances
Emotional lability
Muscle weakness (can be profound)
Muscle movements exaggerated by anxiety and attempts at fine motor activity; relieved by rest

Subcutaneous nodes

Nontender swelling
Located over bony prominences
May persist for some time, then gradually resolve

Supporting evidence of antecedent group A streptococcal infection

Positive throat culture or rapid streptococcal antigen test result
Elevated or rising streptococcal antibody titer

From Special Writing Group of the Committee on Rheumatic Fever, Endocarditis, and Kawasaki Disease of the Council on the Cardiovascular Disease in the Young of the American Heart Association: Guidelines for the diagnosis of rheumatic fever: Jones Criteria, 1992 (update), *JAMA* 268:2069-2073, 1992.

*If supported by evidence of preceding group A streptococcal infection, the presence of two major manifestations or of one major and two minor manifestations indicates a high probability of acute rheumatic fever.

clined to seek medical treatment beforehand. The family's regular dentist should be advised of existing cardiac problems in the child as an added precaution and to ensure that preventive treatment is carried out.

Treatment requires parenteral drug therapy. Nursing goals during this period are (1) preparation of the child for continuous intravenous infusion, possibly for several venipunctures for blood cultures; (2) observation for side effects of antibiotics; and (3) observation for complications, especially from embolism, and the possibility of heart failure. For specific interventions see the Nursing Care Plan: The Child with Congestive Heart Failure, p. 1471.

RHEUMATIC FEVER (RF)

RF, or acute RF, is an inflammatory disease affecting the heart, joints, central nervous system, and subcutaneous tissue. It derives its name from involvement of joints and presence of fever in the acute stage. The most significant sequela of RF is ***rheumatic heart disease,*** especially damage to and scarring of the mitral valve. Although the disease has declined during the past 30 years, recent outbreaks have been reported in several areas, causing concern among health professionals.

Etiology

Strong evidence supports a relationship between upper respiratory infection with group A streptococci and subsequent development of RF (usually within 2 to 6 weeks). In almost all cases of RF a previous infection with group A streptococci can be documented by laboratory evidence of rising antibody titers. Prevention or treatment of group A streptococcal infection prevents RF.

Diagnostic Evaluation

Diagnosis is based on a set of guidelines recommended by the American Heart Association. These guidelines, known as modifications of the Jones criteria, suggest that the presence of two major manifestations or one major and two minor manifestations, such as fever and arthralgia, with supportive evidence of recent streptococcal infection, indicates a high probability of RF (see the Guidelines box to the left).

Children suspected of having RF are tested for streptococcal antibodies. The most reliable and best standardized test is an elevated or rising *antistreptolysin-O (ASO* or *ASLO)* titer, which occurs in 80% of children with RF. Others include anti-DNAse B and anti-DPNase tests, erythrocyte sedimentation rate (ESR), and C-reactive protein. Electrocardiographs and radiographs are obtained to detect any evidence of heart involvement.

Therapeutic Management

The goals of medical management are (1) eradication of hemolytic streptococci, (2) prevention of permanent cardiac damage, (3) palliation of the other symptoms, and (4) prevention of recurrences of RF. Penicillin is the drug of choice, with erythromycin as a substitute in penicillin-sensitive children. Salicylates are used to control the inflammatory process, especially in the joints, and reduce the fever and discomfort. Bed rest is recommended during the acute febrile phase but need not be strict.

Prophylactic treatment against recurrence of RF is started after the acute therapy and involves monthly intramuscular injections of benzathine penicillin G (1.2 million U), two daily oral doses of penicillin (200,000 U), or one daily dose of sulfadiazine (1 g). The duration of long-term prophylaxis is uncertain. Because of the risk of BE in rheumatic heart disease the same prophylaxis discussed earlier is implemented. The antibiotic regimens used to prevent recurrences of RF are inadequate for the prevention of BE.

Children who have had acute RF are susceptible to recurrent RF for the rest of their lives and should be followed medically for at least 5 years. Children and families must be aware of the need for continuing antibiotic prophylaxis for dental work, infection, and invasive procedures.

Nursing Care Management

The objectives of nursing care for the child with RF are to (1) encourage compliance with drug regimens, (2) facilitate recovery from the illness, (3) provide emotional support, and (4) prevent the disease. Since compliance is a major concern in long-term drug therapy, every effort is made to encourage adherence to the therapeutic plan (see Compliance, Chapter 42). When compliance is poor, monthly injections may be substituted for daily oral administration of antibiotics, and children need preparation for this often dreaded procedure.

Interventions during home care are primarily concerned with providing rest and adequate nutrition. Usually once the febrile stage is over, children can resume moderate activity, and their appetite improves. If carditis is present, the family must be aware of any activity restrictions and may need help in choosing less strenuous activities for the child.

One of the most disturbing and frustrating manifestations of the disease is chorea. The onset is gradual and may occur weeks to months after the illness; it sometimes even occurs in children who have not been diagnosed with RF. It may be mistaken for nervousness, clumsiness, behavioral changes, inattentiveness, and learning disability. It is usually a source of great frustration to the child because the movements, incoordination, and weakness severely limit physical ability. The child needs an opportunity to verbalize feelings. Of utmost importance is stressing to parents and schoolteachers that movements are involuntary and sudden; that the chorea is transitory; and that all manifestations eventually disappear.

Nurses also have a role in prevention, primarily in screening school-age children for sore throats caused by group A streptococci. This may involve actively participating in throat culture screening programs or in referring children with a possible streptococcal infection for testing.

See also the Nursing Care Plan: The Child with Rheumatic Fever.*

HYPERLIPIDEMIA (HYPERCHOLESTEROLEMIA)

Hyperlipidemia is a general term for excessive lipids (fat and fatlike substances); **hypercholesterolemia** refers to excessive cholesterol in the blood. High lipid or cholesterol levels are believed to play an important role in producing *atherosclerosis* (fatty plaques on the arteries), which eventually can lead to coronary artery disease, a primary cause of morbidity and mortality in the adult population. Current research indicates that a presymptomatic phase of atherosclerosis begins in childhood.

Cholesterol is part of the lipoprotein complex in plasma that is essential for cellular metabolism. Triglycerides, natural fats synthesized from carbohydrates, are used for energy. Both are major lipids transported on ***lipoproteins,*** a combination of lipids and proteins, which include the following:

Low-density lipoproteins (LDLs)—contain low concentrations of triglycerides, high levels of cholesterol, and moderate levels of protein. LDL is the major carrier of cholesterol to the cells. Cells use cholesterol for synthesis of membranes and steroid production. Elevated circulating LDL level is a strong risk factor in cardiovascular disease.

High-density lipoproteins (HDLs)—contain very low concentrations of triglycerides, relatively little cholesterol, and high levels of protein. They transport free cholesterol to the liver for excretion in the bile. High levels of HDL are thought to protect against cardiovascular disease.

Diagnostic Evaluation

Hyperlipidemia is diagnosed on the basis of analysis of blood for a full lipid profile. Two samples drawn in the fasting state (12 hours) should be analyzed, and the average of the values used for diagnosis. Blood samples should be collected after having the child sit for 5 minutes, and the tourniquet should be applied immediately before the needle puncture, since posture and vascular stasis may affect results. Diagnostic values for acceptable, borderline, and high total cholesterol and LDL cholesterol levels are listed in Table 45-4.

Screening children for hypercholesterolemia is a controversial issue; some authorities advocate universal screening and others propose selective screening. Current guidelines recommended by the National Cholesterol Education Program (NCEP) (1992) recommend a strategy that combines two complementary approaches: (1) a population approach that aims to lower the average levels of blood cholesterol among all American children through populationwide changes in nutrient intake and eating patterns and (2) an individualized approach that targets children and adolescents for screening who have a family history of premature cardiovascular disease or at least one parent with high blood cholesterol level (240 mg/dl or higher). For the present, nurses play an important

TABLE 45-4 Classification of total and low-density lipoprotein (LDL) cholesterol levels in children and adolescents from families with hypercholesterolemia or premature cardiovascular disease

CATEGORY	TOTAL CHOLESTEROL, mg/dl	LDL CHOLESTEROL, mg/dl
Acceptable	<170	<110
Borderline	170-199	110-129
High	≥200	≥130

From National Cholesterol Education Program: Report of the Expert Panel on Blood Cholesterol Levels in children and adolescents, *Pediatrics* 89(3, pt 2): 527, 1992.

*In Wong DL: *Wong and Whaley's clinical manual of pediatric nursing,* ed 4, St Louis, 1996, Mosby.

role in identifying children who meet the criteria for selective screening.

Therapeutic Management

Treatment of high cholesterol level is primarily dietary. Children with borderline LDL cholesterol are advised to follow the same nutrient intake recommended for the general population (i.e., less than 10% of total calories from saturated fatty acids, no more than 30% of calories from total fat, less than 300 mg/day of cholesterol, and adequate calories to support growth and development and to reach or maintain desirable body weight). Children with high LDL cholesterol levels initially are placed on this diet. If these dietary modifications fail to achieve satisfactory levels of LDL after 3 months of therapy, dietary restrictions include a further reduction of saturated fatty acid intake to 7% of calories and of cholesterol intake to less than 200 mg/day.

Nursing ALERT

The Report of the Expert Panel on Blood Cholesterol Levels in Children and Adolescents regarding recommendations for fat intake are not intended for infants from birth to 2 years of age, whose fast growth requires a higher percentage of calories from fat. Toddlers 2 to 3 years of age may safely make the transition to the recommended eating pattern as they begin to eat with the family. No treatment recommendations are made for any child younger than 2 years of age.

For children with severe hypercholesterolemia who do not respond to dietary modifications, drug therapy may be necessary. Two drugs recommended for treatment are the bile acid sequestrants *cholestyramine* and *colestipol.* These two drugs act by binding bile acids in the intestinal lumen. Because they are not absorbed by the intestine, they do not produce systemic toxicity and are safe for children. Cholestyramine and colestipol are both powders that are mixed with water or juice just before ingestion. The most common side effects of the bile acid sequestrants are gastrointestinal symptoms, such as constipation, nausea, bloating, epigastric fullness, and flatulence. The bile acid sequestrants may also prevent absorption of fats, fat-soluble vitamins, and folic acid. Therefore in addition to monitoring children's height and weight during therapy attention should be paid to a sufficient intake of fat-soluble vitamins and folic acid to prevent deficiencies.

Niacin (nicotinic acid), a B vitamin, may be given in therapeutic doses to older children. Although available without a prescription, niacin is treated as a prescription medicine in children. Its use is monitored closely by a health care professional with clinical and laboratory monitoring, especially liver function tests (Colletti and others, 1993).

Nursing Care Management

Nurses play an important role in the screening, education, and support of children with hyperlipidemia and their families. When a child is referred to a lipid clinic, it is essential that the family be adequately prepared for the first visit. Generally the parents will be asked to keep a dietary history of the child before this visit. Sometimes they will need to complete a questionnaire regarding the child's normal dietary habits over the preceding year. Families should be instructed to keep their child fasting for at least 12 hours before screening. Therefore it is important to schedule the blood test early in the morning and to arrange for nourishment immediately thereafter. At the visit a full family history should be taken, including the health of both parents and all first-degree relatives. Specific questions should be asked regarding early heart disease, hypertension, strokes (CVAs), sudden death, hyperlipidemia, diabetes, and endocrine abnormalities. Nurses may also uncover risk factors when obtaining a health history for other purposes; it is therefore important that they be familiar with current screening practices and the availability of resources for children with positive family histories.

Parents and extended families should be informed about cholesterol and hyperlipidemia. This education should include a brief introduction to the different lipoprotein categories, including cholesterol, HDL, LDL, and triglycerides. Also, behavioral risk factors for heart disease, such as smoking and exercise, should be reviewed. For management to be effective, parents need to understand the rationale for dietary and/or pharmacologic intervention. The key is prevention of future cardiovascular disease.

Stringent dietary guidelines may become an issue of control and a source of great stress for many families. Children should not be viewed as having a disease. Rather the positive aspects of healthy eating, regular exercise, and avoiding smoking should be emphasized. Basic dietary changes should be encouraged for the whole family so that the affected sibling is not singled out. Cultural differences must be considered, and recommendations individualized. Substitution rather than elimination needs to be emphasized. Visual aids are often helpful, especially for children (e.g., test tubes depicting the amount of fat in a hot dog). Diets should be flexible and individually tailored by a nutritionist experienced in combining recommendations that meet both the nutritional demands of the growing child and lipid modifications. Parents are encouraged to participate in dietary and educational sessions, ask questions, and share ideas and experiences.

Parents often feel guilty about the hereditary component of hyperlipidemia. Many also believe they have failed if the diet alone is not making a significant difference in their child's lipid profile. They need to be reassured that a dietary approach alone is often not sufficient, especially for children with LDL values greater than 130 mg/dl.

Parents of children who require pharmacologic therapy need to understand the purpose, dosage, and possible side effects of the various drugs. Medication schedules should remain flexible and should not interfere with the child's daily activities. For example, children of elementary school age may have better compliance if they take a resin-binding agent (e.g., cholestyramine, colestipol) twice a day (i.e., before school and at night) rather than the standard three times a day. Follow-up phone calls by the nurse between visits allow parents to discuss their concerns and ask any questions that have arisen.

CARDIAC DYSRHYTHMIAS

Cardiac *dysrhythmias,* or abnormal heart rhythms, occur less frequently in children than in adults. However, they are not rare and the incidence is rising. The survival rate of children undergoing complex cardiac surgical procedures is higher, and conduction system damage may be a complication. Practitioners are also more aware that certain cardiac dysrhythmias in otherwise normal children are important.

The basic diagnostic procedure is the ECG, including 24-hour Holter monitoring. *Electrophysiologic cardiac catheterization* allows for identification of the conduction disturbance and immediate investigation of drugs that may control the dysrhythmia. Another procedure that may be employed is *transesophageal recording.* An electrode catheter is passed to the lower esophagus and, when in position at a point proximal to the heart, is used to stimulate and record dysrhythmias.

Classification

Dysrhythmias can be classified according to various criteria, such as effect on heart rate and rhythm:

Bradydysrhythmias—abnormally slow rate
Tachydysrhythmias—abnormally rapid rate
Conduction disturbances—irregular heart rate

Before classifying an infant or child with an abnormal rate, nurses must be familiar with the standards of normal heart rate for the particular age group (see the Appendix). Heart rate variations considered normal for a particular child can vary tremendously.

Bradydysrhythmias. The most common bradydysrhythmia in children is *complete atrioventricular block (A-V block),* also referred to as *complete heart block.* This can be either congenital or acquired, as seen in postoperative patients after surgery in the area of the A-V valves and ventricular septum.

Sinus bradycardia in children can be caused by the influence of the autonomic nervous system, as with hypervagal tone, or in response to hypoxia and hypotension. *Junctional* or *nodal rhythms* are common in the postoperative patient. The impulse for these rhythms originates farther down the conduction system, in the A-V node. Identification is marked by absence of P waves on the ECG, and often little change occurs in the heart rate or cardiac output. If there is no significant compromise to the patient's cardiac status, no treatment is necessary.

Tachydysrhythmias. *Sinus tachycardia* caused by fever, anxiety, pain, anemia, dehydration, or any other factor requiring increased cardiac output should be ruled out first before diagnosing an increased heart rate as pathologic. *Supraventricular tachycardia (SVT),* a rapid regular heart rate of 200 to 300 beats/min, is one of the most common dysrhythmias found in children. The onset of SVT is often sudden, and the duration is variable. Infants and young children with SVT may be unable to communicate the rapid heart rate, and the clinical course can progress to CHF. Important signs in the infant and young child are poor feeding, extreme irritability, and pallor.

Conduction disturbances. Most rhythm disturbances are seen postoperatively in the child undergoing cardiac surgery and are of little significance. A-V blocks are most often related to edema around the conduction system and resolve without treatment. Temporary epicardial wires are placed in most patients at surgery; if a rhythm disturbance occurs, temporary pacing can be employed. Just before discharge the health practitioner removes the wires by pulling slowly and deliberately down on them from the site of insertion.

Premature contractions can result from an atrial, ventricular, or junctional focus. Their significance depends on the degree of compromise and the presence or absence of underlying CHD.

Therapeutic Management

Treatment of dysrhythmias depends on the cause and severity. Whenever possible, the underlying cause is treated. However, in some cases it is necessary to use antidysrhythmic drugs, with the goal being control, not cure. A permanent ***pacemaker*** may be needed in some children, such as those with postsurgical A-V block or, less frequently, congenital A-V block. The pacemaker takes over or assists in the conduction function of the heart. The surgical implantation of a pacemaker is usually a low-risk procedure. Once the wire has been introduced, a small incision is made, and a pocket formed under the muscle to house and protect the generator. Continuous ECG monitoring is necessary during the recovery phase to assess pacemaker function. The nurse should be aware of the programmed rate and expected individual generator variations. A baseline ECG strip should be documented for future comparison.

The treatment of SVT depends on the degree of compromise imposed by the dysrhythmia. In some instances, **vagal maneuvers,** such as applying ice to the face, massaging the carotid artery (on *one* side of the neck only), or having an older child perform a Valsalva maneuver (e.g., exhaling against a closed glottis, blowing on the thumb as if it were a trumpet for 30 to 60 seconds), have reversed the SVT. When vagal maneuvers fail, adenosine may be used to end the episode of SVT by impairing A-V node conduction. If the infant or child is minimally symptomatic, digitalization should be undertaken, with careful monitoring of vital signs and patient response to the intervention. If cardiac output is significantly compromised or signs of CHF exist, esophageal overdrive pacing or synchronized cardioversion can be employed in the intensive care setting.

Nursing Care Management

An initial nursing responsibility is recognition of an abnormal heartbeat, in either rate or rhythm. When a dysrhythmia is suspected, the apical rate is counted for 1 full minute and compared with the radial rate. Consistently high or low heart rates should be regarded as suspicious. Accurate nursing assessment, especially in regard to cardiac output, is essential.

The onset and diagnosis of a cardiac dysrhythmia are frightening experiences for parents and the older child. Sometimes the dysrhythmia rapidly leads to heart failure and an emergency medical crisis. In this situation parents need much support to express their feelings, understand the diagnosis, and comply with home therapy, such as daily drug administration. Often an unspoken fear of potential death exists even if the dysrhythmia is benign, and repeated explanations are needed to allay the anxiety.

A primary focus of nursing care is education of the family regarding the specific treatment of the dysrhythmia. After the first episode of SVT, parents should be taught to take a pulse for 1 full minute. If medication is prescribed, instructions regarding the accurate dosage and the importance of administering the correct dose at specified intervals are stressed.

When a pacemaker is implanted, the education of the parents and child includes an explanation of the device, a description of the component parts and the surgical procedure, and discharge teaching. For example, discharge teaching includes information about the signs and symptoms of infection, general wound care, and any specific limitations to activity. Instructions for telephone transmission of ECG readings are also given. Children with pacemakers should wear a medical alert device, and their parents should have a pacer identification card with specific pacer data in case of an emergency.

Vascular Dysfunction

SYSTEMIC HYPERTENSION

Hypertension is the consistent elevation of blood pressure (BP) beyond values considered to be the upper limits of normal. The National Heart, Lung, and Blood Institute: Report of the Second Task Force on blood pressure control in Children (1987) defines BP as follows:

Normal BP—systolic and diastolic pressure below the 90th percentile for age and sex

Normal high BP—average systolic and/or average diastolic BP between 90th and 95th percentiles for age and sex

High BP—average systolic and/or average diastolic BP at or greater than the 95th percentile for age and sex, with measurements obtained on at least three occasions

The two major categories of hypertension are *essential hypertension* (no identifiable cause) and *secondary hypertension* (subsequent to an identifiable cause). Hypertension is a primary risk for CVAs and a major risk factor for myocardial infarction in adults. In recent years there has been increasing interest in this disorder as it occurs in adolescents and children, particularly in terms of prevention of later morbidity and mortality.

Routine BP measurements of children have detected hypertension with surprising frequency in asymptomatic children, especially teenagers. Although the prevalence of the condition in adolescents is difficult to evaluate, evidence is accumulating to indicate that the essential hypertension of adulthood may have its origin in childhood; thus its early detection has significance for prevention and treatment.

Etiology

Most instances of hypertension observed in young children are secondary to a structural abnormality or an underlying pathologic process, although this is being challenged by screening programs of relatively healthy children. The most common cause of secondary hypertension is renal disease, followed by cardiovascular, endocrine, and some neurologic disorders.

The causes of essential hypertension are undetermined, but there is evidence to indicate that both genetic and environmental factors play a role. The incidence of hypertension has been shown to be higher in children whose parents are hypertensive. American blacks have a higher incidence of hypertension than whites, and in these persons it develops earlier, is frequently more severe, and results in mortality at an earlier age. Environmental factors that contribute to the risk of development of hypertension include obesity, salt ingestion, smoking, and stress.

Diagnostic Evaluation

From the increasing numbers of hypertensive or potentially hypertensive children and adolescents being identified, a BP determination should be a routine part of annual assessment in children. Although clinical manifestations associated with hypertension depend largely on the underlying cause, there are some observations that can provide clues to the examiner that an elevated BP may be a factor (Box 45-11). In infants and very young children who cannot communicate symptoms, observation of behavior provides clues, although gross behavioral changes may not be apparent until complications are present.

No definitive cutoff values are used in the diagnosis of hypertension in the pediatric patient. The suggested classification is in Table 45-5. *Significant hypertension* is a BP persistently between the 95th and 99th percentiles for age and sex. *Severe hypertension* is a BP persistently at or above the 99th percentile for age and sex. It is important to note that a child who is large for age may normally have a higher BP than a child who is of average size. Before a diagnosis is made, BP should be measured on at least three separate occasions.

In children with suspected primary hypertension, initial laboratory data are also obtained, generally including urinalysis; renal function studies, such as creatinine and blood urea nitrogen levels; a lipid profile; complete blood count; and electrolytes. More intensive tests may be indicated for those with probable secondary hypertension.

Therapeutic Management

Therapy for secondary hypertension involves diagnosis and treatment of the underlying cause. In cases amenable to surgical repair, the nature of the condition, the type of surgery, and the age of the child are all important considerations. Children or adolescents with consistently elevated BP readings with no known cause or those with secondary hypertension not amenable to surgical correction may be treated with a combination of nonpharmacologic and pharmacologic interventions. Dietary practices and life-style changes are important in the control of hypertension both for children and for adults. Nonpharmacologic measures, such as limitation of di-

BOX 45-11
Clinical Manifestations of Hypertension

Adolescents and older children
Frequent headaches
Dizziness
Changes in vision

Infants or young children
Irritability
Head banging or head rubbing
May wake up screaming in the night

TABLE 45-5 Classification of hypertension by age group

AGE GROUP	SIGNIFICANT HYPERTENSION (mm Hg)	SEVERE HYPERTENSION (mm Hg)
Newborn (7 d)	Systolic BP ≥96	Systolic BP ≥106
(8-30 d)	Systolic BP ≥104	Systolic BP ≥110
Infant (<2 yr)	Systolic BP ≥112 Diastolic BP ≥74	Systolic BP ≥118 Diastolic BP ≥82
Children (3-5 yr)	Systolic BP ≥116 Diastolic BP ≥76	Systolic BP ≥124 Diastolic BP ≥84
Children (6-9 yr)	Systolic BP ≥122 Diastolic BP ≥78	Systolic BP ≥130 Diastolic BP ≥86
Children (10-12 yr)	Systolic BP ≥126 Diastolic BP ≥82	Systolic BP ≥134 Diastolic BP ≥90
Adolescents (13-15 yr)	Systolic BP ≥136 Diastolic BP ≥86	Systolic BP ≥144 Diastolic BP ≥92
Adolescents (16-18 yr)	Systolic BP ≥142 Diastolic BP ≥92	Systolic BP ≥150 Diastolic BP ≥98

From National Heart, Lung, and Blood Institute: Report of the Second Task Force on Blood Pressure Control in Children, 1987, *Pediatrics* 79(1):1-25, 1987.

etary salt, weight control, increased exercise, and avoidance of stress and smoking, carry no risk and should be instituted first, except in severe cases. Since the long-term effects of antihypertensive agents on children are not known, drug treatment of asymptomatic children with mild or borderline hypertension is not recommended.

Drug therapy is instituted with caution in children with significant elevations of BP resistant to nonpharmacologic intervention. The treatment should begin with one drug and should add other drugs only if control is not obtained. Compliance with antihypertensive drug regimens is extremely difficult. The oral antihypertensive drugs used most often in children include the beta blockers (propranolol), ACE inhibitors, diuretics, and occasionally a vasodilator (hydralazine). The goal is to achieve a normotensive state throughout the day without accompanying drug side effects.

Nursing Care Management

The nurse is active in detection, diagnosis, and therapy in many settings. Nurses are frequently the persons who operate well-child care and follow up units and are usually the primary contact between health services and the child and family.

BP measurement should always be a part of the routine assessment of infants and children. To obtain an accurate reading, care is taken to quiet the child or relax the adolescent while the measurement is recorded to prevent false readings caused by excitement. The chief cause of falsely elevated BP readings is the use of improperly fitting, narrow cuffs. Therefore attention to correct measurement technique is essential (see Blood Pressure, Chapter 32).

Nursing counseling and guidance of affected children are challenges. Education aimed at understanding hypertension and its implications over the life span is essential in promoting patient and family compliance with both nonpharmacologic and pharmacologic therapies (see Compliance, Chapter 42).

Home BP measurements can facilitate surveillance in youngsters with chronic hypertension and can document effectiveness of therapy. A family member can be instructed in how to take and record accurate BP measurements, thus decreasing the number of trips to a health care facility. This individual needs to understand when to contact the practitioner regarding elevated values. The school nurse can often be a valuable resource in monitoring BPs.

The nurse plays an important role in assessing individual families and providing targeted information regarding nonpharmacologic modes of intervention, such as diet, weight loss, smoking, and exercise programs. If extensive dietary counseling is required, the child should be referred to a nutritionist with expertise in working with children and adolescents. Exercise regimens should be individualized. Schoolchildren and young adolescents generally prefer team sports rather than individual training, which they may view as a burden rather than an enjoyable activity. If peers and family members can be encouraged to participate in any of the management strategies, the child's compliance is likely to be greater.

Young hypertensive women should avoid oral contraceptives because of their pressor effects. Other options need to be presented before this form of birth control is discontinued.

If drug therapy is prescribed, the nurse needs to provide information to the family regarding the reasons for it, how the drug works, and possible side effects. General instructions for all the antihypertensive drugs include the following:

- Rise slowly from a horizontal position and avoid sudden position changes.
- Take drug as prescribed.
- Notify practitioner if unpleasant side effects occur, but do not discontinue drug.
- Avoid alcohol and stay on prescribed diet.

The need for follow-up evaluation is stressed, especially since antihypertensive therapy can sometimes be safely discontinued if BP remains under control over time.

KAWASAKI DISEASE (KD) (MUCOCUTANEOUS LYMPH NODE SYNDROME)

KD is an acute systemic vasculitis. It is seen in every racial group, and about 80% of the cases occur in children under the age of 5 years, with peak incidence in the toddler age group. The acute disease is self-limited. Without treatment, however, in approximately one in five children cardiac sequelae develop. Infants less than 1 year of age are most seriously affected by KD and are at the greatest risk for heart involvement.

The cause of KD remains unconfirmed. Although it is not spread by person-to-person contact, several factors support infectious etiologic factors. It is often seen in geographic and seasonal outbreaks, with most cases reported in the late winter and early spring.

Pathophysiology

The principal area of involvement is the cardiovascular system. During the initial stage of the illness there is extensive in-

BOX 45-12
Diagnostic Criteria For Kawasaki Disease

The child must exhibit five of the following six criteria, including fever:

1. Fever for 5 or more days (often diagnosed with shorter duration of fever if other symptoms are present)
2. Bilateral conjunctival injection (inflammation) without exudation
3. Changes in the oral mucous membranes, such as erythema, dryness, and fissuring of the lips; oropharyngeal reddening; or "strawberry tongue" (large papillae are exposed)
4. Changes in the extremities, such as peripheral edema, erythema of the palms and soles, and periungual desquamation (peeling) of the hands and feet
5. Polymorphous rash
6. Cervical lymphadenopathy (one lymph node >1.5 cm)

flammation of the arterioles, the venules, and the capillaries, which later progresses to the formation of coronary artery aneurysms in some children. When death occurs, it is usually the result of coronary thrombosis or severe scar formation and stenosis of the main coronary artery.

Clinical Manifestations

Since no specific diagnostic test exists for KD, the diagnosis is established on the basis of clinical findings and associated laboratory results (Box 45-12). KD manifests in three phases: acute, subacute, and convalescent. The *acute phase* begins with the abrupt onset of high fever that is unresponsive to antibiotics and antipyretics. The child then experiences the remaining diagnostic symptoms. During this stage the child is typically *very* irritable. The *subacute phase* begins with resolution of the fever and lasts until all clinical signs of KD have disappeared. During this phase the child is at greatest risk for the development of coronary artery aneurysms. Echocardiograms are used to monitor myocardial and coronary artery status. A baseline echocardiogram should be obtained at the time of diagnosis for comparison with future studies. Irritability persists during this phase. In the *convalescent phase* all the clinical signs of KD have resolved, but the laboratory values have not returned to normal. This phase is complete when all blood values are normal (6 to 8 weeks after onset). At the end of this stage the child has regained his or her usual temperament, energy, and appetite.

Therapeutic Management

The current treatment of KD includes high-dose intravenous gamma globulin along with salicylate therapy. Gamma globulin has been demonstrated to be effective at reducing the incidence of coronary artery abnormalities when given within the first 10 days of the illness. A single large infusion of 2 g/kg over 8 to 12 hours is safe and effective in reducing fever and aneurysm formation (Newburger and others, 1991).

Aspirin is given initially in an antiinflammatory dose (80 to 100 mg/kg/day in divided doses every 6 hours) to control fever and symptoms of inflammation. Once fever has subsided, aspirin is continued at an antiplatelet dose (3 to 5 mg/kg/day). Low-dose aspirin is continued in patients without echocardiographic evidence of coronary abnormalities until the platelet count has returned to normal (6 to 8 weeks). If coronary abnormalities develop, salicylate therapy is continued indefinitely. Additional anticoagulation with coumadin may be indicated in children with giant aneurysms.

Prognosis. Most children with KD recover fully after treatment. However, when cardiovascular complications occur, serious morbidity may result. Death occurs rarely and almost always results from coronary thrombosis.

Nursing Care Management

In the initial phase the nurse must monitor the child's cardiac status carefully. Intake and output and daily weight measurements are recorded. Although the child may be reluctant to eat and therefore may be partially dehydrated, fluids need to be administered with care because of the usual finding of myocarditis. The child should be assessed frequently for signs of CHF, including decreased urinary output, gallop rhythm (an additional heart sound), tachycardia, and respiratory distress.

The administration of gamma globulin should follow the same guidelines as for any blood product, with frequent monitoring of vital signs. Patients must be watched for allergic reactions (see Table 46-4). Cardiac status must be monitored because of the large volume being administered to patients with myocarditis and diminished left ventricular function.

Most nursing care focuses on symptomatic relief. To minimize skin discomfort cool cloths, nonscented lotions, and soft, loose clothing are helpful. During the acute phase mouth care, including lubricating ointment to the lips, is important for the mucosal inflammation. Clear liquids and soft foods can be offered.

Patient irritability is perhaps the most challenging problem. These children need to be placed in a quiet environment that promotes adequate rest. Their parents need to be supported in their efforts to comfort an often inconsolable child. They may need time away from their child, and nurses can often provide respite care for the family. Parents need to understand that irritability is a hallmark of KD and that they need not feel guilty or embarrassed about their child's behavior.

Discharge teaching. Parents need accurate information about the progression of KD, including the importance of follow-up monitoring and circumstances in which they should contact their practitioner. Irritability is likely to persist for up to 2 months after the onset of symptoms. Peeling of the hands and feet is painless and occurs primarily in the second and third weeks. Arthritis, especially of the larger weight-bearing joints, may persist for several weeks. Children are typically most stiff in the mornings, during cold weather, and after naps. Passive range of motion in the bathtub is often helpful in increasing flexibility. Any live immunizations (e.g., measles-mumps-rubella) should be deferred for 3 months after the administration of gamma globulin, since the body may not produce the appropriate amount of antibodies. The decision to give the varicella (chickenpox) vaccination to the child or aspirin therapy is made individually by the practitioner.

Temperature should be recorded after discharge until the child has been afebrile for several days.*

All parents should understand the unlikely but real possibility of myocardial infarction as well as the signs and symptoms of cardiac ischemia in a child. At discharge the ultimate cardiac sequela is generally not known, since changes occur up to a month after the onset of KD. In addition the parents of children with known severe coronary artery sequelae may be taught cardiopulmonary resuscitation.*

SHOCK

Shock, or circulatory failure, is a complex clinical syndrome characterized by inadequate tissue perfusion to meet the metabolic demands of the body, resulting in cellular dysfunction and eventual organ failure. Although the causes differ, the physiologic consequences are the same: hypotension, tissue hypoxia, and metabolic acidosis. Circulatory failure in children is the result of hypovolemia, altered peripheral vascular resistance, or pump failure. Types of shock are outlined in Box 45-13.

Pathophysiology

A healthy child's circulatory system is able to transport oxygen and metabolic substrates to body tissues, which require a constant source of these essential needs. The cardiac output and distribution to the various body tissues can change very rapidly in response to intrinsic (myocardial and intravascular) or extrinsic (neuronal) control mechanisms. In shock states these mechanisms are altered or challenged.

Reduced blood flow, as in hypovolemic shock, causes diminished venous return to the heart, low central venous pressure, low cardiac output, and hypotension. Vasomotor centers in the medulla are signaled, causing a compensatory increase in the force and rate of cardiac contraction and constriction of arterioles and veins, thereby increasing peripheral vascular resistance. Simultaneously the lowered blood volume leads to the release of large amounts of catecholamines, antidiuretic hormone, adrenocorticosteroids, and aldosterone in an effort to conserve body fluids. This causes reduced blood flow to the skin, kidneys, muscles, and viscera in order to shunt the available blood to the brain and heart. Consequently the skin feels cold and clammy, there is poor capillary filling, and glomerular filtration and urine output are significantly reduced.

As a result of impaired perfusion oxygen is depleted in the tissue cells, causing them to revert to anaerobic metabolism, producing lactic acidosis. The acidosis places an extra burden on the lungs as they attempt to compensate for the metabolic acidosis by increased respiratory rate to remove excess carbon dioxide. Prolonged vasoconstriction results in fatigue and atony of the peripheral arterioles, which lead to vessel dilation. Venules, less sensitive to vasodilator substances, remain constricted for a time, causing massive pooling in the capillary and venular beds, which further depletes blood volume.

Complications of shock create further hazards. Central nervous system (CNS) hypoperfusion may eventually lead to cerebral edema, cortical infarction, or intraventricular hemorrhage. Renal hypoperfusion causes renal ischemia with possible tubular or glomerular necrosis and renal vein thrombosis. Reduced blood flow to the lungs can interfere with surfactant secretion and result in adult respiratory syndrome (ARDS). It is characterized by sudden pulmonary congestion and atelectasis with formation of a hyaline membrane. Gastrointestinal tract bleeding and perforation are always possibilities after splanchnic ischemia and necrosis of intestinal mucosa. Metabolic complications of shock may include hypoglycemia, hypocalcemia, and other electrolyte disturbances.

BOX 45-13
Types of Shock

Hypovolemic shock

Characteristics

Reduction in size of vascular compartment
Falling blood pressure
Poor capillary filling
Low central venous pressure (CVP)

Most frequent causes

Blood loss (hemorrhagic shock)—trauma, gastrointestinal (GI) bleeding, intracranial hemorrhage
Plasma loss—increased capillary permeability associated with sepsis and acidosis, hypoproteinemia, burns, peritonitis
Extracellular fluid loss—vomiting, diarrhea, glycosuric diuresis, sunstroke

Distributive shock

Characteristics

Reduction in peripheral vascular resistance
Profound inadequacies in tissue perfusion
Increased venous capacity and pooling
Acute reduction in return blood flow to the heart
Diminished cardiac output

Most frequent causes

Anaphylaxis (anaphylactic shock)—extreme allergy or hypersensitivity to a foreign substance
Sepsis (septic shock, bacteremic shock, endotoxic shock)—overwhelming sepsis and circulating bacterial toxins
Loss of neuronal control (neurogenic shock)—interruption of neuronal transmission (spinal cord injury)
Myocardial depression and peripheral dilation—exposure to anesthesia or ingestion of barbiturates, tranquilizers, narcotics, antihypertensive agents, or ganglionic blocking agents

Cardiogenic shock

Characteristic

Decreased cardiac output

Most frequent causes

After surgery for congenital heart disease
Primary pump failure—myocarditis, myocardial trauma, biochemical derangements, congestive heart failure
Dysrhythmias—paroxysmal atrial tachycardia, atrioventricular block, and ventricular dysrhythmias; secondary to myocarditis or biochemical abnormalities (occasionally)

Diagnostic Evaluation

The cause of shock can be discerned from the history and the physical examination. The severity of the shock is determined

*Home care instructions for measuring a child's temperature and for infant and child cardiopulmonary resuscitation are available in Wong DL: *Wong and Whaley's clinical manual of pediatric nursing*, ed 4, St Louis, 1996, Mosby.

BOX 45-14
Clinical Manifestations of Shock

Compensated
Apprehensiveness
Irritability
Unexplained tachycardia
Normal blood pressure
Narrowing pulse pressure
Thirst
Pallor
Diminished urinary output
Reduced perfusion of extremities

Uncompensated
Confusion and somnolence
Tachypnea
Moderate metabolic acidosis
Oliguria
Cool, pale extremities
Decreased skin turgor
Poor capillary filling

Irreversible
Thready, weak pulse
Hypotension
Periodic breathing or apnea
Anuria
Stupor or coma

by measurements of vital signs, including central venous pressure and capillary filling (Box 45-14). Shock can be regarded as a form of compensation for circulatory failure. Because of the progressive nature of shock it can be divided into three stages or phases:

Compensated shock—Vital organ function is maintained by intrinsic compensatory mechanisms; blood flow is usually normal or increased but generally uneven or maldistributed in the microcirculation.

Nursing ALERT

Unexplained mild tachycardia and a decrease in perfusion of the hands and feet are differentiating features of compensated shock.

Uncompensated shock—Efficiency of the cardiovascular system gradually diminishes, until perfusion in the microcirculation becomes marginal despite compensatory adjustments. The outcomes of circulatory failure that progress beyond the limits of compensation are tissue hypoxia, metabolic acidosis, and eventual dysfunction of all organ systems.

Nursing ALERT

Tachycardia is pronounced; BP is maintained, but pulse pressure (difference between systolic and diastolic BP) becomes narrowed; there is poor capillary filling; and the child in uncompensated shock exhibits decreased responsiveness, confusion, and sleepiness.

Irreversible, or terminal, shock—Damage to vital organs, such as the heart or brain, of such magnitude that the entire organism will be disrupted regardless of therapeutic intervention. Death occurs even if cardiovascular measurements return to normal levels with therapy.

At all stages the principal differentiating signs are observed in the (1) degree of tachycardia and perfusion to extremities, (2) level of consciousness, and (3) BP. Additional signs or modifications of these more universal signs may be present, depending on the type and cause of the shock. Initially the child's ability to compensate is effective; therefore early signs are subtle. As the shock state advances, signs are more obvious and indicate early decompensation.

Additional signs may be present, depending on the type and cause of the shock. In early septic shock there are chills, fever, and vasodilation, with increased cardiac output that results in warm, flushed skin (hyperdynamic or "hot" shock). A later and ominous development is disseminated intravascular coagulation (see Chapter 46), the major hematologic complication of septic shock. Anaphylactic shock is frequently accompanied by urticaria and angioneurotic edema, which is life-threatening when it involves the respiratory passages (see p. 1491).

Laboratory tests that assist in assessment are blood gas measurements, pH, and sometimes liver function tests. Coagulation tests are evaluated when there is evidence of bleeding, such as oozing from a venipuncture site, bleeding from any orifice, or petechiae. Cultures of blood and other sites are indicated when there is a high suspicion of sepsis. Renal function tests are performed when impaired renal function is evident.

Therapeutic Management

Treatment of shock consists of three major thrusts: (1) ventilation, (2) fluid administration, and (3) improvement of the pumping action of the heart (vasopressor support). The first priority is to establish an airway and administer oxygen. Once the airway is assured, circulatory stabilization is the major concern.

Ventilatory support. The lung is the organ most sensitive to shock. Decreased or redistributed blood flow to respiratory muscles plus the increased work of breathing can rapidly lead to respiratory failure. Critically ill patients are unable to maintain an adequate airway. To place the lung at rest and improve ventilation, tracheal intubation is initiated early with positive-pressure ventilation. Supplemental oxygen is always given as soon as possible. Blood gases and pH are monitored frequently.

Increased extravascular lung water caused by edema contributes to the development of respiratory complications. Therapy is directed to maintaining normal arterial blood gas measurements, acid-base balance, and circulation. Efforts are made to remove fluid and prevent its accumulation with the use of diuretics.

Cardiovascular support. In most cases rapid restoration of blood volume is all that is needed for resuscitation of the child in shock. An isotonic crystalloid solution (normal saline or Ringer's lactated solution) is the fluid of choice; colloids such as albumin are also used. Successful resuscitation will be reflected by an increase in blood pressure and a reduction in heart rate; increased cardiac output will result in improved capillary circulation and skin color. Central venous pressure measurements of right atrial pressure help guide fluid therapy, and urinary output measurement is an important indicator of adequacy of circulation. Correction of acidosis, hypoxemia, and any metabolic derangements is mandatory.

Temporary pharmacologic support may be required to enhance myocardial contractility, to reverse metabolic or respiratory acidosis, and/or to maintain arterial pressure. The principal agents used to improve cardiac output and circulation are the sympathetic amines administered by constant infusion pump. Those given most often are catecholamines, such as dopamine (Intropin), epinephrine (Adrenalin), and isoproterenol (Isuprel). Vasodilators that are sometimes used include nitroprusside (Nipride) and hydralazine (Apresoline).

Acidosis is corrected with adequate ventilatory support, including oxygen, and the administration of sodium bicarbonate. Calcium chloride may be administered to improve cardiac function. Appropriate antibiotics are administered to patients with septic shock. In cases of septic shock caused by gram-negative organisms, corticosteroids are of value. Other complicating disorders are treated appropriately.

Nursing Care Management

When shock is a likely complication, the child is observed carefully for any early signs, which are reported immediately for further medical evaluation.

Nursing ALERT

Early clinical signs include apprehension, irritability, normal blood pressure, narrowing pulse pressure (difference between diastolic and systolic blood pressures), thirst, pallor, diminished urinary output, unexplained mild tachycardia, and a decrease in perfusion of the hands and feet.

The child who is in shock requires intensive observation and care. *The initial action is to ensure adequate tissue oxygenation.* The nurse should be prepared to administer oxygen by the appropriate route and to assist with any intubation and ventilatory procedures indicated. Other procedures and activities that require immediate attention are establishing an intravenous line, weighing the child, obtaining baseline vital signs, placing an indwelling catheter, obtaining blood gas and other measurements, and administering medications as indicated. The child is best positioned flat with the legs elevated.

The nurse's responsibilities are to monitor the intravenous infusion, intake and output, vital signs (including central venous pressure), and general systems assessments on a routine basis. Intravenous medications are titrated according to patient responses, and vital signs are taken every 15 minutes during the critical periods and thereafter as needed. Urine output is measured hourly; blood gases, hematocrit, pH, and electrolytes are monitored frequently to assess the status of the child and the efficacy of therapy. An apnea and cardiac monitor is attached and monitored continuously. In the initial

EMERGENCY

SHOCK

Ventilation

Establish airway—be prepared for intubation.
Administer oxygen, usually 100% by mask.

Fluid administration

Restore blood or fluid volume as ordered.

Cardiovascular support

Administer vasopressors, especially epinephrine, in dose of 0.01 mg/kg until maximum dose of 0.5 ml of 1:1000 dilution subcutaneously; may repeat in 30 minutes.

General support

Keep child flat with legs raised above level of heart.
Keep child warm and calm.

In addition:

Septic shock: Administer broad-spectrum antibiotics intravenously.
Anaphylaxis: Remove allergen if possible; may place tourniquet above site of injection.

stages of acute shock the care of the child often requires the attendance of more than one nurse in order to manage all the necessary activities that must be carried out simultaneously (see the Emergency box above).

Throughout the intense activity the family must not be overlooked. Someone should contact family members at frequent intervals to inform them about what is being done and whether there is any progress. Ideally someone should remain with the parents to serve as liaison between them and the intensive care team. However, this is not always feasible in such a critical situation. As soon as possible they should be allowed to see the child. A member of the clergy may be called to help provide comfort and support.

See also Nursing Care Plan: The Child in Circulatory Failure (Shock).*

ANAPHYLAXIS

Anaphylaxis is the acute clinical syndrome resulting from the interaction of an allergen and a patient who is hypersensitive. When the antigen enters the circulatory system, a generalized reaction rapidly takes place. Vasoactive amines (principally histamine or a histamine-like substance) are released and cause vasodilation, bronchoconstriction, and increased capillary permeability.

Severe reactions are immediate in onset, are often life-threatening, and frequently involve multiple systems, primarily the cardiovascular, respiratory, gastrointestinal, and integumentary. Exposure to the antigen can be by ingestion, inhalation, skin contact, or injection. Examples of common allergens associated with anaphylaxis include drugs (such as antibiotics, chemotherapeutic agents, or radiologic contrast

---

*In Wong DL: *Wong and Whaley's clinical manual of pediatric nursing,* ed 4, St Louis, 1996, Mosby.

media), latex, foods, venoms from bees or snakes, and biologic agents (antisera, enzymes, hormones, and blood products).

Nursing ALERT

Penicillin allergy is associated with an immediate-onset (within an hour of administration) or accelerated-onset (1 to 72 hours after administration) of skin eruption, especially a urticarial rash, or more serious symptoms such as laryngeal edema or anaphylactic shock.

Clinical Manifestations

The onset of clinical symptoms usually occurs within seconds or minutes of exposure to the antigen, and the rapidity of the reaction is directly related to its intensity—the sooner the onset, the more severe the reaction. The reaction may be preceded by symptoms of uneasiness, restlessness, irritability, severe anxiety, headache, dizziness, paresthesia, and disorientation. The patient may lose consciousness. Cutaneous signs of flushing and urticaria are common early signs, followed by angioedema, most notable in the eyelids, lips, tongue, hands, feet, and genitalia.

Bronchiolar constriction may follow, causing narrowing of the airway; pulmonary edema and hemorrhage may occur also. Laryngeal edema with severe acute upper airway obstruction may be life-threatening and requires rapid intervention. Shock occurs as a result of mediator-induced vasodilation, which causes capillary permeability and loss of intravascular fluid into the interstitial space. Sudden hypotension and impaired cardiac output with poor perfusion are seen.

Therapeutic Management

Successful outcome of anaphylactic reactions depends on rapid recognition and institution of treatment. The goals of treatment are to provide ventilation, restore adequate circulation, and prevent further exposure by identifying and removing the cause when possible.

A mild reaction with no evidence of respiratory distress or cardiovascular compromise can be managed with subcutaneous administration of antihistamines, such as diphenhydramine (Benadryl) and epinephrine.

Moderate or severe distress presents a potentially life-threatening emergency. Establishing an airway is the first concern, as with all shock states. Epinephrine is given subcutaneously or intravenously as an antihistamine and to support the cardiovascular system and increase blood pressure. Other routes for giving epinephrine are intramuscular and via the airway, either nebulized or injected through the endotracheal tube. In severe anaphylaxis epinephrine by any route is better than none (Fisher, 1992). Fluids are given to restore blood volume. Additional vasopressors may be given to improve cardiac output. Children with serious anaphylaxis should be hospitalized and monitored for at least 24 hours, since relapses may occur (Bochner and Lichtenstein, 1991).

Prevention of a reaction is preferable. Preventing exposure is more easily accomplished in children known to be at risk, including those with (1) a history of previous allergic reaction to specific antigen, (2) a history of atopy, (3) a history of severe reactions in immediate family members, and (4) a reaction to a skin test, although skin tests are not available for all allergens. Desensitization may be recommended in certain cases.

Nursing Care Management

The major nursing responsibility in anaphylaxis is anticipating which children are likely to have a reaction, recognizing the early signs, and intervening appropriately. When an anaphylactic reaction is suspected, both immediate intervention and preparation for medical therapy are nursing responsibilities. Ventilation is assured by placing the child in a head-elevated position, unless contraindicated by hypotension, to facilitate breathing and administer oxygen. If the child is not breathing, cardiopulmonary resuscitation is initiated, and emergency medical services are summoned.

If the cause can be determined, measures are implemented to slow the spread of the offending substance. For example, a tourniquet is applied above the point of entry (e.g., sting, injection), or intravenous medication or dye infusion is discontinued. An intravenous infusion is established immediately. Emergency medications are given intravenously whenever possible; however, epinephrine may be given subcutaneously (see the Emergency box on p. 1491). Vital signs and urine output are monitored frequently. Medications are administered as prescribed with regular assessment to monitor effectiveness and to detect signs of side effects of medication and fluid overload.

To prevent an anaphylactic reaction, parents are always asked about possible allergic responses to foods, latex, medications, and environmental conditions (see Guidelines for Taking an Allergy History, Chapter 31). These are displayed prominently on the patient's chart. The specific allergen is noted, as well as the type and severity of the reaction. Parents are excellent historians, especially when the child has displayed a pronounced reaction to a substance. Drugs, including related drugs (e.g., penicillin, nafcillin), and other items, such as latex, that have produced a reaction previously are *never* used. If the child is allergic to insect venom, the family is instructed to purchase an emergency kit to be kept with the child at all times. Both the family and the child, if the child is old enough, are taught how to use the equipment. Medical identification should be carried by the patient at all times.

TOXIC SHOCK SYNDROME (TSS)

TSS is a relatively rare disease that occurs predominantly (but not exclusively) in previously healthy young women during their menstrual periods. The organism implicated is the phage group 1 *Staphylococcus aureus*, which is believed to produce an epidermal toxin. The disease has been observed primarily in women who use tampons during a menstrual period. The tampons may carry the organism from the fingers or the vulva into the vagina during insertion, the tampon may traumatize the vaginal wall and provide a focus of infection, or the tampon itself may provide a favorable environment for growth of the organism or elaboration of its toxin.

Diagnostic Evaluation

Diagnosis is established on the basis of the criteria established by the Centers for Disease Control's toxic case definition (Box 45-15). A history of tampon use contributes to the diagnosis. Additional laboratory tests include cultures from blood,

BOX 45-15
Case Definition of Toxic Shock Syndrome

1. Fever (temperature at or above 38.9° C [102° F])
2. Rash (diffuse macular erythroderma)
3. Desquamation 1 to 2 weeks after onset of illness, particularly of the palms and soles
4. Hypotension (systolic blood pressure at or below 90 mm Hg for adults or below the fifth percentile for age for children younger than 16 years of age, or orthostatic syncope)
5. Involvement of three or more of the following organ systems:
   a. Gastrointestinal (vomiting or diarrhea at onset of illness)
   b. Muscular (severe myalgia or creatine phosphokinase level above two times the upper limits of normal)
   c. Mucous membrane (vagina, oropharyngeal, or conjunctival hyperemia)
   d. Renal (blood urea nitrogen or creatinine levels above two times the upper limits of normal or above 5 white blood cells per high-power field—in the absence of a urinary tract infection)
   e. Hepatic (total bilirubin, serum glutamic oxaloacetic transaminase [SGOT], or serum glutamic pyruvic transaminase [SGPT] above two times the upper limits of normal)
   f. Hematologic (platelets below 100,000/mm^3)
   g. Central nervous system (disorientation or alterations in consciousness without focal neurologic signs when fever and hypotension are absent)
6. Negative results on the following tests, if obtained:
   a. Blood, throat, or cerebrospinal fluid cultures
   b. Serologic tests for Rocky Mountain spotted fever, leptospirosis, or measles

From Centers for Disease Control *MMWR* 29:442, 1980.

vagina, cervix, and any discharge. Other laboratory tests are those that facilitate the management of shock.

Therapeutic Management

The management of toxic shock syndrome is the same as management of shock of any origin and may involve supportive care in mild cases to hospitalization and intensive care in severe cases. Appropriate parenteral antibiotics are usually administered after cultures are obtained.

Nursing Care Management

Nursing care and observation of the acutely ill patient are the same as those described for shock of any cause. Since the disease is relatively rare, the major efforts of nursing are directed to prevention. The association between the disease and the use of tampons provides some direction for education. Avoiding the use of tampons offers the most certain preventive measure, although this approach is probably unacceptable to most adolescent girls, who prefer the freedom, comfort, and inconspicuousness that tampons afford.

Adolescent girls who use tampons can be taught general hygiene measures, such as handwashing before insertion of the tampon and not using a tampon that has been dropped or otherwise soiled. Tampons should be inserted carefully to prevent vaginal abrasion. Also it is wise to modify their use. For example tampons may be used intermittently during the menstrual cycle, alternating with sanitary napkins—perhaps using the napkins during the night, when at home during the day, and when flow is slight. Young girls are advised not to use superabsorbent tampons and not to leave any tampon in the body for more than 4 to 6 hours.

Patients who use tampons need to understand that they should remove the tampon and consult their health professional if they experience sudden high fever, vomiting, diarrhea, muscle pain, dizziness, fainting or near fainting when standing up, or rash that resembles a sunburn.

HENOCH-SCHÖNLEIN PURPURA (HSP)

HSP (Schönlein-Henoch vasculitis, allergic purpura, anaphylactoid purpura) is a relatively common acquired disorder in children characterized by a nonthrombocytopenic purpura and variable joint and visceral abnormalities. The cause is unknown, but the disease often follows an upper respiratory infection, and allergy or drug sensitivity play a role in some instances. The disease occurs in children ages 6 months to 16 years but more frequently in children between ages 2 to 8 years. It is observed more often in white children, and in boys three times more often than in girls.

Pathophysiology

The disease is characterized by inflammation of small blood vessels, and the manifestations observed are influenced by the size and distribution of the affected vessels. A generalized vasculitis of dermal capillaries (and to a lesser extent small arterioles and veins) causing extravasation of red blood cells produces the petechial skin lesions. Inflammation and hemorrhage may also occur in the gastrointestinal tract, synovium, glomeruli, and central nervous system.

Diagnostic Evaluation

Diagnosis is usually established on the basis of clinical manifestations (Box 45-16). The onset of the disease may be abrupt, with simultaneous appearance of several manifestations, or gradual, with sequential appearance of different manifestations. Laboratory tests are used to assess gastrointestinal and renal involvement and to determine adequacy of hematostatic function.

Therapeutic Management

Management is primarily supportive, with close observation for signs of renal or gastrointestinal manifestations. Edema, rash, malaise, and arthralgia are usually managed with appropriate analgesics, such as acetaminophen, and mild sedation if necessary. Corticosteroids may be prescribed for relief of more severe edema, arthralgia, and colicky abdominal pain but are not warranted in all cases.

Prognosis. Most children recover without the need for hospitalization, and in most instances a single acute episode clears spontaneously within a month. Others may have periodic recurrences for as long as 2 to 3 years before permanent remission from symptoms. Rarely death results from severe gastrointestinal complications, acute renal failure, or central nervous system involvement.

BOX 45-16

Clinical Manifestations of Henoch-Schönlein Purpura

Primary feature: symmetric purpura
- Involves buttocks and lower extremities
- May extend to include extensor surfaces of upper extremities; less commonly, upper trunk and face
- May be associated with maculopapular lesions and variable elements of urticaria and erythema
- Often marked edema of scalp, eyelids, lips, ears, and dorsal surfaces of hands and feet—especially in infants and younger children

Arthritic effects (two thirds of affected children)
- Asymptomatic swelling around a single joint
- Painful tender swelling of several joints, most often the knees and ankles

Gastrointestinal involvement (two thirds of affected children)
- Recurrent colicky midabdominal pain
- Often associated with nausea and vomiting
- Stools contain gross or occult blood and mucus

Renal involvement (up to one half of affected children)
- Hematuria
- Casts
- Proteinuria

Nursing Care Management

Nursing care of the child hospitalized with HSP is primarily supportive, with vigilant observation for signs of complications. Vital signs are taken and recorded at regular intervals, specimens obtained for laboratory examination, and medication administered as prescribed. Urine and stools are carefully observed for fresh and occult blood.

If the child suffers from joint pain positioning, careful movement and administration of analgesics help reduce discomfort. Analgesics also relieve the discomfort of fever and malaise. More severe involvement such as gastrointestinal symptoms and nephritis are managed as for any such disorder.

Concern about the unsightly appearance of the rash is common. The child and parents are reassured that it is only a temporary phenomenon, and the child can be encouraged to wear clothing that helps to hide the rash, such as long sleeves, pants, and robe. Emphasizing good grooming and attractive apparel helps promote a more positive self-image.

Heart Transplantation

Heart transplantation has become a treatment option for infants and children with worsening heart failure and a limited life expectancy despite maximum medical and surgical management. Indications for cardiac transplantation in children are cardiomyopathy and end-stage congenital heart disease. An important and controversial group of patients with congenital heart disease are infants with hypoplastic left heart syndrome who undergo heart transplantation as their initial treatment.

Most heart transplantations have been performed in infants and children less than 10 years of age, the majority in infants. In a study of infants from 3 hours to 12 months of age the overall survival was 83%, with the best results in very young infants (Bailey et al, 1993). In the short term after successful transplantation, children are able to return to full participation in age-appropriate activities and appear to adapt well to their new life-style. The long-term prognosis is unknown.

The heart transplantation procedure may be orthotopic or heterotopic. **Orthotopic heart transplantation** entails removing the recipient's own heart and implanting a new heart from a donor who has had brain death but a healthy heart. The donor and recipient are matched by weight and blood type. **Heterotopic heart transplantation** involves leaving the recipient's own heart in place and implanting a new heart to act as an additional pump or "piggyback" heart; this type of transplantation is rarely done in children.

Before transplantation potential recipients are carefully evaluated to identify problems in other organ systems that might preclude or increase the risk of transplantation. A psychosocial evaluation of the patient and family is done to identify possible problems in complying with the complex medical regimen that follows transplantation and in providing needed support systems. Patients are listed on a national computer network organized by the United Network for Organ Sharing (UNOS) to match donors and recipients. Because of the limited donor supply, some infants waiting for heart transplantation will die before receiving a donor heart (see also Tissue Donation/Autopsy, Chapter 38).

Nursing Care Management

Nursing care after transplantation is demanding and complex, with careful attention to both the physical needs of the child and the emotional needs of the child and family. Successful care of a child after heart transplantation requires the expertise and dedication of many members of the health care team. Nurses play vital roles in assessment, coordination of care, psychosocial support, and patient and family education.

Transplantation raises a number of ethical issues, including the use of newborns with anencephaly as organ donors, use of animal hearts in human transplantation, scarcity of donors, and donor allocation issues. Other factors, often unique to pediatrics, involve the patient's status as a minor, specifically issues of informed consent and parental responsibility and authority.

Key Points

- Congenital heart disease (CHD) is the most common form of cardiac disease in children.
- Major categories to investigate in the cardiac history are poor weight gain, poor feeding habits, and fatigue during feeding; frequent respiratory infections and difficulties; and evidence of exercise intolerance.
- The most common tests used in assessing cardiac function are radiography, electrocardiography, echocardiography, and cardiac catheterization.
- Cardiac catheterization procedures can be divided into three groups: (1) diagnostic procedures, including angiography, that measure pressures and saturations to establish cardiac diagnosis; (2) interventional procedures, in which catheters or balloon devices are used to correct cardiac defects; and (3) electrophysiology studies, in which catheters with electrodes are used to evaluate dysrhythmias.
- Diagnostic cardiac catheterization provides important information about oxygen saturation of blood within the chambers and great vessels, pressure changes, changes in cardiac output or stroke volume, and anatomic abnormalities.
- Several prenatal factors may predispose children to congenital heart disease: maternal rubella during pregnancy, maternal alcoholism, maternal age above 40 years, and maternal insulin-dependent diabetes.
- Congenital heart defects can be divided into four main groups, as determined by hemodynamic patterns: (1) defects that result in increased pulmonary blood flow, (2) obstructive defects, (3) defects that result in decreased pulmonary blood flow, and (4) mixed defects.
- Clinical consequences of congenital heart defects include congestive heart failure (CHF) and hypoxemia. A child can have both hypoxemia and CHF, although usually they occur independently.
- Clinical manifestations of CHF are impaired myocardial function (tachycardia, cardiomegaly), pulmonary congestion (dyspnea, tachypnea, orthopnea, cyanosis), and systemic congestion (hepatosplenomegaly, edema, distended veins).
- Nursing measures in the care of a child with CHF are to assist in improving cardiac function, decrease cardiac demands, reduce respiratory distress, maintain nutritional status, promote fluid loss, and provide family support.
- Clinical manifestations of hypoxemia are cyanosis, polycythemia, clubbing, and delayed growth and development. The child is at increased risk for hypercyanotic spells, cerebrovascular accidents, brain abscess, and bacterial endocarditis.
- Caring for the child with CHD and the family requires helping them to adjust to the disorder and to cope with the effects of the defect and fostering growth-promoting family relationships.
- Preoperative care of the child with a congenital heart defect involves introducing the child and family to the hospital and preparing them for preoperative and postoperative procedures.
- Providing postoperative care includes observing vital signs and arterial/venous pressures, maintaining respiratory status, allowing maximum rest, providing comfort, monitoring fluids, planning for progressive activities, giving emotional support, observing for complications of surgery, and planning for discharge and home care.
- Acquired cardiovascular disorders include bacterial endocarditis, rheumatic fever, hyperlipidemia (hypercholesterolemia), and cardiac dysrhythmias.
- Prevention of bacterial endocarditis in certain children with CHD involves administration of prophylactic antibiotics when specific procedures are performed.
- Acute rheumatic fever is a systemic inflammatory disease that can damage the cardiac valves and is associated with previous group A streptococcal infection. Its incidence has increased in some areas of the United States.
- Cholesterol screening in children is controversial; currently, children with known risk factors for hyperlipidemia are screened and treated as needed. The influence of childhood cholesterol levels on later development of coronary artery disease is under investigation.
- Common dysrhythmias in children include slow rhythms (bradycardias, heart block) and fast rhythms (sinus tachycardia, supraventricular tachycardia).
- Education of the child with hypertension and the family focuses on drug therapy, diet control, and appropriate exercise.
- Kawasaki disease is an extensive inflammation of small vessels and capillaries that may progress to involve the coronary arteries, causing aneurysm formation. The administration of gamma globulin is an important aspect of treatment.
- Emergency treatment for shock includes ensuring ventilation; administering vasopressors, fluids/blood, and antibiotics as needed; and providing supportive measures, such as correct positioning, warmth, and psychologic reassurance to the child and family.
- Persons at risk for anaphylaxis may be identified by a history of previous allergic reaction, history of atopy, history of severe reactions in family, and positive skin test to the allergen.
- Nursing management of the patient with toxic shock syndrome focuses on prevention primarily through education concerning safe tampon use.
- Henoch-Schönlein purpura is characterized by a nonthrombocytic purpura and variable joint and visceral abnormalities. Nursing care is primarily supportive, with observation for complications and provision of comfort being key nursing goals.
- Heart transplantation has been extended to infants and children with cardiomyopathy and complex congenital heart defects involving ventricular dysfunction, such as hypoplastic left heart syndrome.

References

Agamalian B: Pediatric cardiac catheterization, *J Pediatr Nurs* 1(2):73-79, 1986.

Bailey LL et al: Bless the babies: one hundred fifteen late survivors of heart transplantation during the first year of life, *J Thorac Cardiovasc Surg* 105(5):805-815, 1993.

Bochner BS, Lichtenstein LM: Anaphylaxis, *N Engl J Med* 324(25):1785-1790, 1991.

Colletti RB et al: Niacin treatment of hypercholesterolemia in children, *Pediatrics* 92(1):78-82, 1993.

Dajani AS, Taubert RA: Infective endocarditis. In Emmanulides GC, and others, editors: *Moss and Adams heart disease in infants, children, and adolescents,* ed 5, Baltimore, 1995, Williams & Wilkins.

Driscoll DJ: Evaluation of the cyanotic newborn, *Pediatr Clin North Am* 37(1):1-23, 1990.

Fisher M: Treating anaphylaxis with sympathomimetic drugs, *Br Med J* 305:1107-1108, 1992.

Friedman WF: *Congenital heart disease in infancy and childhood.* In Braunwald E, editor: *Heart disease: a textbook of cardiovascular medicine,* ed 4, Philadelphia, 1992, WB Saunders.

Hazinski MF: *Cardiovascular disorders.* In Hazinski MF, editor *Nursing care of the critically ill child,* ed 2, St Louis, 1992, Mosby.

Maquire DP, Maloney P: A comparison of fentanyl and morphine use in neonates, *Neonatal Network* 7(1):27-35, 1988.

National Cholesterol Education Program: Report of the expert panel on blood cholesterol levels in children and adolescents, *Pediatrics* 89(3, pt 2):525-584, 1992.

National Heart, Lung and Blood Institute: Report of the Second Task Force on Blood Pressure Control in Children—1987, *Pediatrics* 79:1-25, 1987.

Newburger J et al: A single intravenous infusion of gammaglobulin as compared with four infusions in the treatment of acute Kawasaki syndrome, *N Engl J Med* 324(23):1623-1639, 1991.

Bibliography

Cardiac Diagnosis

Apple S, Thurkauf GE: Preparing for and understanding transesophageal echocardiography, *Crit Care Nurse* 12:29-34, 1992.

Driscoll DJ: Evaluation of the cyanotic newborn, *Pediatr Clin North Am* 37(1):1-23, 1990.

Fabius DB: Understanding heart sounds: solving the mystery of heart murmurs, *Nursing 1994* 24(7):39-44, 1994.

Fabius DB: Understanding heart sounds: uncovering the secrets of snaps, rubs, and clicks, *Nursing 1994* 24(7):45-50, 1994.

Gardner RM, Hujes M: Fundamentals of physiologic monitoring, *AACN Clin Issues Crit Care Nurs* 4(1):11-24, 1993.

Monett Z, Moynihan P: Cardiovascular assessment of the neonatal heart, *J Perinat Neonat Nurs* 5(2):50-59, 1991.

Monett Z, Roberts P: Patient care for interventional cardiac catheterization, *Nurs Clin North Am* 29(2):333-346, 1995.

Pederson C: Children's and adolescents' experiences while undergoing cardiac catheterization, *Matern Child Nurs J* 23(1):15-25, 1995.

Radtke W, Lock JE: Balloon dilation, *Pediatr Clin North Am* 37(1):193-214, 1990.

Roberts PJ: Caring for patients undergoing therapeutic cardiac catheterization, *Crit Care Nurs Clin North Am* 1(2):275-288, 1989.

Sondheimer HM: Cardiac catheterization—a new role in the 90s, *Contemp Pediatr* 7(3):91-106, 1990.

Vargo L: Evaluation of cardiac size on the neonatal chest x-ray, *Neonatal Network* 12(3):65-67, 1993.

Webster H, Chellis MJ: Physiologic monitoring of infants and children, *AACN Clin Issues Crit Care Nurs* 4(1):180-197, 1993.

Congenital Heart Disease

Abbott K: Therapeutic use of play in the psychological preparation of preschool children undergoing cardiac surgery, *Issues Compr Pediatr Nurs* 13(4):265-277, 1990.

Cardiovascular health and disease in children: current status, *Circulation* 89(2):923-930, 1994.

Combs VL, Marino BL: A comparison of growth patterns in breast and bottle fed infants with congenital heart disease, *Pediatr Nurs* 19(2):175-179, 1993.

Craig J: The postoperative cardiac infant: physiologic basis for neonatal nursing interventions, *J Perinat Neonatal Nurs* 5(2):60-70, 1991.

Cullen S, Celermajer DS, Deanfield JE: Exercise in congenital heart disease, *Cardiol Young* 1(2):129-135, 1991.

Johnson AB, Davis JS: Treatment options for the neonate with hypoplastic left heart syndrome, *J Perinat Neonatal Nurs* 5(2):84-92, 1991.

Kulik L et al: Pharmacologic interventions for the neonate with compromised cardiac function, *J Perinat Neonatal Nurs* 5(2):71-84, 1991.

Lobo ML: Parent infant interactions during feeding with infants with congenital heart defects, *J Pediatr Nurs* 7(2):97-105, 1992.

Moynihan P, Naclerio L, Kiley K: Parent participation, *Nurs Clin North Am* 29(2):231-242, 1995.

Norris MKG, editor: Pediatric and neonatal cardiology, *Crit Care Nurs Clin North Am* 9(2):111-236, 1994.

Norris MKG, Hill CS: Nutritional issues in infants and children with congenital heart disease, *Crit Care Nurs Clin North Am* 9(2):153-164, 1994.

O'Brien P, Boisvert JT: Discharge planning for children with heart disease, *Crit Care Nurs Clin North Am* 1(2):297-305, 1989.

Smith JB, Vernon-Levett P: Care of infants with HLHS, *AACN Clin Issues Crit Care Nurs* 4(2):329-339, 1993.

Swanson LT: Treatment options for hypoplastic left heart syndrome: a mother's perspective, *Crit Care Nurse* 15(3):70-79 1995.

Tong E, Sparacino P: Special management issues for adolescents and young adults with congenital heart disease, *Crit Care Nurs Clin North Am,* 9(2):199-214, 1994.

Uzark K: Counseling adolescents with congenital heart disease, *J Cardiovasc Nurs* 6(3):65-73, 1992.

Congestive Heart Failure/Hypoxemia

Brown KK: Boosting the failing heart with inotropic drugs, *Nursing 93* 23(6):34-44, 1993.

Dahlmann AR: Captopril, *Neonatal Network* 7(5):41-43, 1989.

Delgizzi LJ, Ueda JN: Using inotropic and vasodilating agents in pediatric patients with cardiac disease, *AACN Clin Issues Crit Care Nurs* 1(1):131-147, 1990.

Hagedorn MI, Gardner SL: Physiologic sequelae of prematurity: the nurse practitioner's role, part III, *J Pediatr Health* 4(5):229-236, 1990.

Kaplan S: New drug approaches to the treatment of heart failure in infants and children, *Drugs* 39(3):388-393, 1990.

Kohr L, O'Brien P: Current management of congestive heart failure in infants and children, *Nurs Clin North Am* 29(2):261-290, 1995.

Noerr B: Captopril, *Neonatal Network* 9(5):69-71, 1991.

O'Brien P, Smith P: Chronic hypoxemia in children with cyanotic heart disease, *Crit Care Nurs Clin North Am* 9(2):215-226, 1994.

Werner NP: Congestive heart failure: pathophysiology and management throughout infancy, *J Perinat Neonatal Nurs* 7(3):59-76, 1993.

Cardiac Surgery

Callow LB: Current strategies in the nursing care of infants with HLHS undergoing 1st stage palliation with the Norwood procedure, *Heart Lung* 21(5):463-470, 1992.

Callow LB: Postoperative nursing management of the infant with TAPVC, *DCCN* 10(3):140-149, 1991.

Cohen DM: Surgical management of congenital heart disease in the 1990's, *Am J Dis Child* 146:1447-1452, 1992.

Craig J: The postoperative cardiac infant: physiologic basis for neonatal nursing interventions, *J Perinat Neonatal Nurs* 5(2):60-70, 1991.

Jensen CA: Nursing care of a child following an arterial switch procedure for transposition of the great arteries, *Crit Care Nurs* 12(8):51-57, 1992.

Johnston J: Cardiac transplant in early infancy, *Crit Care Nurs Clin North Am* 4(3):521-535, 1992.

Ludwick F et al: Examining management of pain for infants following cardiac surgery, *DCCN* 14(3):136-143, 1995.

Medicus L et al: Preventing pulmonary hypertensive crisis in the pediatric patient after cardiac surgery, *Am J Crit Care* 4(1):49-55, 1995.

Muirhead J: Heart transplantation in children: indications, complications, and management, *J Cardiovasc Nurs* 6(3):44-55, 1992.

Noonan DM et al: Nursing considerations for neonates awaiting heart transplant for HLHS, *J Pediatr Nurs* 6(5):327-330, 1991.

O'Brien P, Elixson M: The child following the Fontan procedure: nursing strategies, *Clin Issues Crit Care Nurs* 1(1):46-58, 1990.

O'Brien P, Hanley FH: New directions in pediatric heart transplantation, *Crit Care Nurs Clin North Am* 4:193-203, 1992.

Rotondi P, editor: Neonatal and pediatric cardiovascular nursing, *Crit Care Nurs Clin North Am* 1(2):195-305, 1989.

Stinson J et al: Mother's information needs related to caring for infants at home following cardiac surgery, *J Pediatr Nurs* 10(1):48-57, 1995.

Tong E: An overview of artificial heart valve replacement in infants and children, *J Cardiovasc Nurs* 6(3):30-43, 1992.

Uzark K: Caring for families of pediatric transplant recipients: psychosocial implications, *Crit Care Nurs Clin North Am* 4:255-263, 1992.

Bacterial Endocarditis

Dajani AS et al: Prevention of bacterial endocarditis: recommendations by the American Heart Association, *JAMA* 264(22):2919-2911, 1990.

Kaplan EL: Bacterial endocarditis prophylaxis, *Pediatr Ann* 21(4):249-255, 1992.

Saiman L, Prince A, Gersony W: Pediatric infective endocarditis in the modern era, *J Pediatr* 122(6):847-853, 1993.

Scrima DA: Infective endocarditis: nursing considerations, *Crit Care Nurse* 7:47-56, 1987.

Snelson C, Cline BA, Luby C: Infective endocarditis: a challenging diagnosis, *Dimens Crit Care Nurs* 12(1):4-16, 1993.

Rheumatic Fever

Bisno AL: Group A streptococcal infections and acute rheumatic fever, *N Engl J Med* 325(11):783-793, 1991.

Forster J, editor: Rheumatic fever: keeping up with the Jones criteria, *Contemp Pediatr* 10:51-60, 1993.

Freund B et al: Acute rheumatic fever revisited, *J Pediatr Nurs* 8:167-176, 1993.

Griffiths SP: *Rheumatic fever.* In Hoekelman RA and others, editors: *Primary pediatric care*, ed 2, St Louis, 1992, Mosby.

Grimes DE, Woolbert LF: Facts and fallacies about streptococcal infection and rheumatic fever, *J Pediatr Health Care* 4(4):186-192, 1990.

Special Writing Group of the Committee on Rheumatic Fever, Endocarditis, and Kawasaki Disease of the Council on the Cardiovascular Disease in the Young of the American Heart Association: Guidelines for the diagnosis of rheumatic fever: Jones Criteria, 1992 (update), *JAMA* 268:2069-2073, 1992.

Veasy LG, Tani LY, Hill HR: Persistence of acute rheumatic fever in the intermountain area of the United States, *J Pediatr* 124:9-16, 1994.

Hyperlipidemia (Hypercholesterolemia)

Baker A, Roberts C, Gothing C: Dyslipidemias in childhood: an overview, *Nurs Clin North Am* 29(2):243-260, 1995.

Davidson DM, Smith RM, Qaqundah PY: Cholesterol screening in children during office visits, *J Pediatr Health Care* 4(1):11-17, 1990.

Gillman MW: Screening for familial hypercholesterolemia in childhood, *Am J Dis Child* 147(4):393-396, 1993.

Neufeld EJ, Newburger JW: How should children with hypercholesterolemia be managed? *Choices Cardiol* 7:233-236, 1993.

Nolan R: Child hypercholesterolemia: implications for nurse practitioners, *Pediatr Nurs* 20(11):46-50, 1994.

Cardiac Dysrhythmias

Alpern D, Uzark K, Dick M: Psychosocial responses of children to cardiac pacemakers, *J Pediatr* 114(3):494-501, 1989.

Boisvert J, Reidy S, Lulu J: Overview of pediatric arrhythmias, *Nurs Clin North Am* 29(2):345-380, 1995.

Cox DM: Complete heart block in the pediatric patient, *J Emerg Nurs* 18(6):497-500, 1992.

Farrington E: Adenosine, *Pediatr Nurs* 17(6):590, 1991.

Hanisch DG et al: Complex dysrhythmias in infants and children, *AACN Clin Issues Crit Care Nurs* 3(1):255-269, 1992.

Moulton L et al: Radiofrequency catheter ablation for supraventricular tachycardia, *Heart Lung* 22:3-14, 1993.

Philich LM et al: A pediatric case study: use of adenosine in the treatment of SVT, *Am J Crit Care* 3(3):228-231, 1994.

Suddaby E, Riker S: Defibrillation and cardioversion in children, *Pediatr Nurs* 17(5):477-481, 1991.

Zeigler V: Adenosine in the pediatric population: nursing implications, *Pediatr Nurs* 17(6):600-602, 1991.

Zeigler V: Postoperative rhythm disturbances, *Crit Care Nurs Clin North Am* 9(2):227-236, 1994.

Systemic Hypertension

Carmon M et al: Cardiovascular screening programs: implications for school nurses, *Pediatr Nurs* 16(5):509-511, 1990.

Daniels SR: Primary hypertension in childhood and adolescence, *Pediatr Ann* 21(4):224-234, 1992.

Falkner B: Essential hypertension in children, *Curr Opin Pediatr* 1(1):131-134, 1989.

Gillman MW et al: Identifying children at high risk for the development of essential hypertension, *J Pediatr* 122:837-846, 1993.

Jung FF, Ingelfinger JR: Hypertension in childhood and adolescence, *Pediatr Rev* 14(5):169-179, 1993.

Rocchini A, editor: Childhood hypertension, *Pediatr Clin North Am* 40(1):entire issue, 1993.

Kawasaki Disease

American Academy of Pediatrics, Committee on Infectious Diseases: Intravenous γ-globulin use in children with Kawasaki disease, *Pediatrics* 82(1):122, 1988.

Baker A: Acquired heart disease in infants and children, *Crit Care Nurs Clin North Am* 9(2):175-186, 1994.

Fujita Y et al: Kawasaki disease in families, *Pediatrics* 84(4):666-669, 1989.

Gersony WM: Long-term issues in Kawasaki disease, *J Pediatr* 121(5):731-733, 1992.

Shreve B: Kawasaki disease: early treatment/positive results, *Pediatr Nurs* 19(6):607-610, 1993.

Shock

Barry W et al: Intravenous immunoglobulin therapy for toxic shock syndrome, *JAMA* 267(24):3315-3316, 1992.

Berro EA, Bechler-Karsch A: A closer look at septic shock, *Pediatr Nurs* 19:289-297, 1993.

Brown KK: Septic shock: how to stop the deadly cascade, part 1, *Am J Nurs* 94(9):20-27, 1994.

Brown KK: Critical interventions in septic shock, part 2, *Am J Nurs* 94(10):20-26, 1994.

Pamillo JE: Pathogenetic mechanisms of septic shock, *N Engl J Med* 328:1471-1477, 1993.

Rice V: Shock, a clinical syndrome: an update, part 1, *Crit Care Nurse* 11:20-27, 1991.

Rice V: Shock, a clinical syndrome: an update, part 2, *Crit Care Nurse* 11:74-82, 1991.

Rice V: Shock, a clinical syndrome, an update, part 3, *Crit Care Nurse* 11:34-39, 1991.

Rice V: Shock, a clinical syndrome, an update, part 4, *Crit Care Nurse* 11:28-32, 35-43, 1991.

Strodtbeck F, Joyce B: Shock in newborns and children, *Crit Care Nurs Q* 11:75-83, 1988.

Wynn SR: Anaphylaxis at school, *J School Nurs* 9:5-11, 1993.

CHAPTER 46

Hematologic and Immunologic Dysfunction

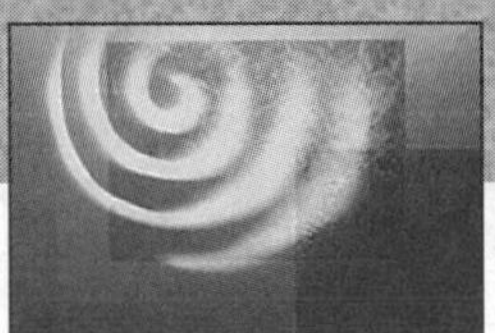

HEMATOLOGIC AND IMMUNOLOGIC DYSFUNCTION, P. 1499

Assessment of hematologic function, p. 1499

RED BLOOD CELL (RBC) DISORDERS, P. 1499

Anemia, p. 1499
Iron deficiency anemia, p. 1503
Sickle cell anemia (SCA), p. 1505
β-Thalassemia (Cooley anemia), p. 1510
Aplastic anemia, p. 1511

DEFECTS IN HEMOSTASIS, P. 1512

Hemophilia, p. 1512
Idiopathic thrombocytopenic purpura (ITP), p. 1515
Disseminated intravascular coagulation (DIC), p. 1516
Epistaxis (nosebleeding), p. 1516

NEOPLASTIC DISORDERS, P. 1517

Leukemias, p. 1517
Lymphomas, p. 1528
Hodgkin disease, p. 1528
Non-Hodgkin lymphoma (NHL), p. 1530

IMMUNOLOGIC DEFICIENCY DISORDERS, P. 1530

Mechanisms involved in immunity, p. 1530
Acquired immunodeficiency syndrome (AIDS), p. 1531
Severe combined immunodeficiency disease (SCID), p. 1533
Wiskott-Aldrich syndrome, p. 1534

TECHNOLOGIC MANAGEMENT OF HEMATOLOGIC AND IMMUNOLOGIC DISORDERS, P. 1534

Blood transfusion therapy, p. 1534
Bone marrow transplantation (BMT), p. 1536
Apheresis, p. 1537

Hematologic and Immunologic Dysfunction

ASSESSMENT OF HEMATOLOGIC FUNCTION

Several tests can be performed to assess hematologic function, including additional procedures to identify the cause of the dysfunction. The following discussion is limited to a description of the most common and one of the most valuable tests, the *complete blood count (CBC)*. Other procedures, such as those related to iron, coagulation, and immune status, are discussed throughout the chapter as appropriate. The nurse should be familiar with the significance of the findings from the CBC (Table 46-1) and aware of normal values for age, which are listed in the Appendix.

As with any disorder, the history and physical examination are essential to the identification of hematologic dysfunction, and the nurse is often the first person to suspect a problem based on information from these sources. Comments by the parent regarding the child's lack of energy, food diary of poor sources of iron, frequent infections, and bleeding that is difficult to control offer clues to the more common disorders affecting the blood. A careful physical appraisal, especially of the skin, can reveal findings such as pallor, petechiae, or bruising that may indicate minor or serious hematologic conditions. Nurses must be aware of the clinical manifestations of blood diseases in order to assist in recognizing symptoms and establishing a diagnosis.

Red Blood Cell (RBC) Disorders

ANEMIA

The term **anemia** describes a condition in which the number of RBCs and/or the hemoglobin (Hgb or Hb) concentration is reduced below normal. As a result of this decrease, the oxygen-carrying capacity of the blood is diminished, causing a reduction in the oxygen available to the tissues. Anemia is the most common hematologic disorder of infancy and childhood and is not a disease itself but an indication or manifestation of an underlying pathologic process.

TABLE 46-1 Tests performed as part of the CBC

TEST (AVERAGE VALUE)*	DESCRIPTION/COMMENTS
RBC count (4.5 to 5.5 million/mm³)	Number of RBCs/mm³ of blood Indirectly estimates Hgb content of blood Reflects function of bone marrow
Hemoglobin (Hgb) determination (11.5 to 15.5 g/dl)	Amount of Hgb/dl of whole blood Total blood Hgb primarily depends on number of circulating RBCs, but also on amount of Hgb in each cell
Hematocrit (Hct) (35% to 45%)	Percentage or volume of packed RBCs to whole blood Indirectly measures Hgb content Is approximately three times Hgb content
RBC indices	MCV and MCH depend on accurate counts of RBCs, whereas MCHC does not; therefore MCHC is often more reliable All indices depend on *average* cell measurements and do not show anisocytosis (individual RBC variations)
Mean corpuscular volume (MCV) (77 to 95 μm³)	Average of mean volume (size) of a single RBC MCV values expressed as cubic microns (μm³) or femtoliters (fl)
Mean corpuscular hemoglobin (MCH) (25 to 33 pg/cell)	Average or mean quantity (weight) of Hgb of a single RBC MCH values expressed as picograms (pg) or micromicrograms (μμg)
Mean corpuscular hemoglobin concentration (MCHC) (31% to 37% Hgb [g]/dl RBC)	Average concentration of Hgb in a single RBC MCHC values expressed as % Hgb (g)/cell or Hgb (g)/dl RBC
RBC volume distribution width (RDW) 13.4% ± 1.2%	Average size of RBCs
Reticulocyte count (0.5% to 1.5% erythrocytes)	% Reticulocytes to RBCs Index of production of mature RBCs by red bone marrow Decreased count indicates depressed bone marrow function Increased count indicates erythrogenesis in response to some stimulus When reticulocyte count is extremely high, other forms of immature RBCs (normoblasts, even erythroblasts) may be present Indirectly estimates hypochromic anemia Usually elevated in patients with chronic hemolytic anemia
White blood cell (WBC) count (4.5 to 13.5 × 10³ cells/mm³)	Number of WBCs/mm³ of blood Total number of WBCs less important than differential count
Differential WBC count	Inspection and quantification of WBC types present in peripheral blood Values are expressed as percentages; to obtain absolute number of any type of WBCs, multiply its respective percentage by total number of WBCs
Neutrophils (polys) (54% to 62%) (3.0 to 5.8 × 10³ cells/mm³)	Primary defense in bacterial infection; capable of phagocytizing and killing bacteria
Bands (3% to 5%) (0.15 to 0.4 × 10³ cells/mm³)	Immature neutrophil Increased numbers in bacterial infection Also capable of phagocytosis and killing
Eosinophils (1% to 3%) (0.05 to 0.25 × 10³ cells/mm³)	Named for their staining characteristics with eosin dye Increased in allergic disorders, parasitic diseases, certain neoplasms, and other diseases
Basophils (0.075%) (0.015 to 0.030 cells/mm³)	Named for their characteristic basophilic stippling Contain histamine, heparin, serotonin; believed to cause increased blood flow to injured tissues while preventing excessive clotting
Lymphocytes (25% to 33%) (1.5 to 3.0 × 10³ cells/mm³)	Involved in development of antibody and delayed hypersensitivity
Monocytes (3% to 7%)	Large phagocytic cells that are involved in early stage of inflammatory reaction
Absolute neutrophil count (ANC) (>1000)	% neutrophils × WBCs Indicates body's ability to handle bacterial infections
Platelet count (150 to 400 × 10³/mm³)	Cellular fragments that are necessary for clotting to occur
Stained peripheral blood smear	Visual estimation of amount of Hgb in RBCs and overall size, shape, and structure of RBCs Various staining properties of RBC structures may be evidence of immature forms of erythrocyte Shows variation in size and shape of RBCs—microcytic, macrocytic, poikilocytic (variable shapes)

*See the Appendix for normal values according to ages.

Classification

Anemias are classified in relation to (1) *etiology* or *physiology*, manifested by erythrocyte and/or Hgb depletion, and (2) *morphology*, the characteristic changes in RBC size, shape, and/or color. Although the morphologic classification is more useful in terms of laboratory evaluation of anemia, the etiologic approach provides direction for planning nursing care. For example, anemia with reduced hemoglobin concentration may be caused by a dietary depletion of iron, and the principal intervention is replenishing iron stores. Etiologic factors responsible for anemia are described in Box 46-1.

Consequences of Anemia

The basic physiologic defect caused by anemia is a decrease in the oxygen-carrying capacity of blood and consequently a reduction in the amount of oxygen available to the cells. When the anemia has developed slowly, the child usually adapts to the declining hemoglobin level, and most children seem to have a remarkable ability to function quite well despite low levels of hemoglobin.

The effects of anemia on the circulatory system can be profound. Because the viscosity of blood depends almost entirely on the concentration of RBCs, the resulting hemodilution of severe anemia decreases peripheral resistance, causing greater quantities of blood to return to the heart. The increased circulation and turbulence within the heart may produce a murmur. Since the cardiac work load is markedly increased (especially during exercise, infection, or emotional stress), cardiac failure may ensue.

As just noted, children seem to have a remarkable ability to function quite well despite low levels of hemoglobin. Cyanosis (the result of the quantity of deoxygenated hemoglobin in arterial blood) is typically not evident. Growth retardation, resulting from decreased cellular metabolism and coexisting anorexia, is a common finding in chronic severe anemia and is frequently accompanied by delayed sexual maturation in the older child.

Diagnostic Evaluation

In general, anemia may be suspected from findings on the history and physical examination, such as lack of energy, easy fatigability, and pallor, but unless the anemia is severe, the first clue to the disorder may be alterations in the CBC, such as decreased RBCs, and decreased Hgb and hematocrit (Hct) levels (Box 46-2). Although anemia is sometimes defined as an Hgb value below 10 or 11 g/dl, this arbitrary cutoff is inappropriate for all children because hemoglobin levels normally vary with age (Table 46-1 and the Appendix).

Other tests specific to a particular type of anemia are employed to determine the underlying cause of anemia. These are discussed in relation to the particular disorder.

Therapeutic Management

The objective of medical management is to reverse the anemia by treating the underlying cause and to make up for any deficiency of blood, blood component, or substance the blood needs for normal functioning. For example, blood or blood cells are replaced after hemorrhage; in nutritional anemias the specific deficiency is addressed.

In cases of severe anemia, supportive medical care may include oxygen therapy, bed rest, and replacement of intravascular volume with intravenous fluids. Table 46-2 gives the

BOX 46-1
Classification of Anemia

Etiology/pathophysiology

Excessive blood loss—from acute or chronic hemorrhage (internal or external); until stores are replaced, there is usually a normocytic (normal size), normochromic (normal color) anemia, provided that there are sufficient iron stores for hemoglobin synthesis

Destruction (hemolysis) of erythrocytes—as a result of an intracorpuscular defect within the RBC (such as sickle cell anemia) or an extracorpuscular factor (such as infectious agents, chemicals, or immune mechanisms) that causes destruction to outpace production

Decreased or impaired production of erythrocytes or their components—as a result of bone marrow failure (caused by factors such as neoplastic diseases, irradiation, chemicals, or disease) or deficiency of essential nutrients (such as iron)

Morphology

Size—cell size; for example, **normocytes** (normal), **microcytes** (smaller than normal), or **macrocytes** (larger than normal)

Shape—irregularly shaped RBCs; for example, **poikilocytes** (irregularly shaped cells), **spherocytes** (globular cells), and **drepanocytes** (sickle cells)

Staining characteristics or color—reflects the hemoglobin concentration; for example, **normochromic** (sufficient or normal amount) or **hypochromic** (reduced amount)

BOX 46-2
Clinical Manifestations of Anemia

General manifestations

Muscle weakness
Easy fatigability
- Frequent resting
- Shortness of breath
- Poor sucking (infants)

Pale skin
- Waxy pallor seen in severe anemia

Pica—eating clay, ice, paste

Central nervous system manifestations

Headache
Dizziness
Lightheadedness
Irritability
Slowed thought processes
Decreased attention span
Apathy
Depression

Shock (blood loss anemia)

Poor peripheral perfusion
Skin moist and cool
Low blood pressure and central venous pressure
Increased heart rate

TABLE 46-2 Management of selected anemias

TYPE OF ANEMIA	DESCRIPTION	MANAGEMENT
Blood loss anemia	Until 20% or more of blood volume is lost with normal vital signs	No therapy needed
	Altered vital signs with losses of 30% to 40% of blood volume and signs of shock	Blood replacement Plasma or plasma protein product given until blood is available
Iron deficiency anemia	Decreased RBC production	See discussion in text
Anemia of renal disease	Usually not until symptomatic and Hb is less than 7 to 8 mg/dl	Transfusion of packed RBCs
Hemolytic anemias Spherocytosis Elliptocytosis	Shortened survival of RBCs	Splenectomy
Sickle cell anemia	Shortened survival of RBCs	See discussion in text
Thalassemia	Shortened survival of RBCs	See discussion in text

medical management of selected anemias. The prognosis for anemia depends on the correction of the cause.

Nursing Care Management

Assessment

The assessment of anemia includes the basic techniques that are applicable to any condition. The age of the infant or child provides some clues regarding the possible etiology of the anemia. For example, iron deficiency anemia occurs more frequently in infants between 6 and 24 months of age and during the growth spurt of adolescence.

Racial or ethnic background is significant. For example, the anemias related to abnormal hemoglobins are found in Southeast Asians and persons of African or Mediterranean ancestry. These same groups may be genetically deficient in the enzyme lactase after infancy. Affected individuals are unable to tolerate lactose in the diet, with consequent intestinal irritation and chronic blood loss.

Special emphasis is placed on a careful history to elicit any information that might help identify the cause of the anemia. For example, a statement such as "The baby drinks lots of milk" is a frequent finding in the histories of infants with iron deficiency anemia. An episode of diarrhea may have precipitated a temporary lactose intolerance in the infant.

Stool examination for occult (invisible) blood (Hemacult test) can identify chronic intestinal bleeding that results from a primary or secondary lactase deficiency. It is also important to understand the significance of various blood tests. Blood loss from overt hemorrhage may be manifested as shock.

Nursing Diagnoses

A variety of nursing diagnoses may be evident after the assessment of anemia. Some of the general aspects of nursing management are included in the Nursing Care Plan on p. 1504. Others become apparent in specific situations.

Planning

The goals of care for the infant or child with anemia depend on the severity of the condition and the cause. Most children tolerate mild anemia well, and a priority goal is preparing them for diagnostic tests and possible blood transfusion (p. 1534). Other goals of care are the following:

1. Child and family will receive adequate support and education.
2. Child will exhibit minimal physical or emotional exertion.
3. Child will experience no complications from anemia or its treatment.

Implementation

Prepare child and family for laboratory tests. Usually several blood tests are ordered, but since they are generally done sequentially rather than all at one time, the child is subjected to multiple finger or heel punctures and/or venipunctures. Laboratory technicians frequently are not aware of the trauma that repeated punctures represent to a child. However, these invasive procedures need not be painful (see the discussion of blood specimens, Chapter 42). For example, the topical application of eutectic mixture of local anesthetics (EMLA) before needle punctures can eliminate any pain (see Pain Management, Chapter 41). Therefore the nurse is responsible for preparing the child and family for the tests by (1) explaining the significance of each test, particularly why the tests are not done at one time; (2) encouraging parents or another supportive person to be with the child during the procedure; and (3) allowing the child to play with the equipment on a doll and/or participate in the actual procedure (e.g., by cleansing the finger with an alcohol swab). Older children may appreciate the opportunity to observe the blood cells under a microscope or in photographs. This experience is an especially important consideration if a serious blood disorder, such as leukemia, is suspected, since it serves as a foundation for explaining the pathophysiology of the disorder.

Bone marrow aspiration is not a routine hematologic test but is essential for the definitive diagnosis of the leukemias, lymphomas, and certain anemias. Suggested explanations for teaching children about blood components are as follows:

Red blood cells—Carry the oxygen you breathe from your lungs to all parts of your body.
White blood cells—Help keep germs from causing infection.
Platelets—Small parts of cells that help to make bleeding stop; platelets help your body stop bleeding by forming a clot (scab) over the hurt area.
Plasma—The liquid portion of blood; has clotting factors that help make the bleeding stop.

Decrease tissue oxygen needs. Since the basic pathology in anemia is a decrease in oxygen-carrying capacity, an important nursing responsibility is to assess the child's energy level and minimize excess demands. The child's level of tolerance for activities of daily living and play is assessed, and adjustments are made to allow as much self-care as possible without undue exertion. During periods of rest the nurse takes vital signs and observes behavior to establish a baseline of nonexertion energy expenditure. During periods of activity the nurse repeats these measurements and observations to compare them with resting values.

Nursing ALERT

Signs of exertion include tachycardia, palpitations, tachypnea, dyspnea, shortness of breath, hyperpnea, breathlessness, dizziness, lightheadedness, diaphoresis, and change in skin color. The child looks fatigued (sagging, limp posture; slow, strained movements; inability to tolerate additional activity).

Diversional activities are planned that promote rest but prevent boredom and withdrawal. Since short attention span, irritability, and restlessness are common in anemia and increase stress demands on the body, appropriate activities are planned, such as listening to music; using a tape recorder; watching television; reading or listening to stories or comics; continuing a favorite hobby, such as stamp collecting, coloring, or drawing; playing board and card games; or being wheeled in a carriage or chair. Choosing the appropriate roommate, such as a child of similar age with a diagnosis that also requires restricted activity, is a helpful intervention.

If infants or young children are hospitalized, the importance of preventing separation from parents must be considered. Crying and fretfulness place increased stress demands on the body, which increases oxygen needs. Parents need help in understanding the importance of their presence, even though the child may be less responsive than usual. The nurse also explains the reason for mood changes and the necessity of allowing the child's dependency.

Prevent complications. Children who are so severely anemic that they are hospitalized may require oxygen to prevent or reduce tissue hypoxia. Since these children are susceptible to infection, every effort is expended to prevent exposure to infectious agents. All the usual precautions are taken to prevent infection, such as practicing thorough handwashing, selecting an appropriate room in a noninfectious area, restricting visitors or hospital personnel with active infection, and maintaining adequate nutrition. The nurse also observes for signs of infection, particularly temperature elevation and leukocytosis.

Family support. See Nursing Care Plan on p. 1504 for other supportive and educational strategies.

Evaluation

The effectiveness of nursing interventions is determined by continual reassessment and evaluation of care based on the following observational guidelines and expected outcomes:

1. Interview the child and family regarding their understanding of diagnostic procedures and the blood disorder, as well as regarding their feelings and concerns.
2. Monitor therapeutic interventions and the child's tolerance for activity.
3. Assess the child for evidence of complications of therapies.

Expected outcomes:

See the Nursing Care Plan on p. 1504

IRON DEFICIENCY ANEMIA

Anemia caused by an inadequate supply of dietary iron is the most prevalent nutritional disorder in the United States and the most common mineral disturbance. Almost 16% of lower-income children 6 to 24 months of age are anemic (Wimberly and Parks, 1991). However, the prevalence has decreased, probably in part because of families' participation in the Women, Infants, and Children (WIC) program, which provides iron-fortified formula for the first year of life (Oski, 1993). Premature infants are especially at risk because of their reduced fetal iron supply. Adolescents are also at risk because of their rapid growth rate combined with poor eating habits.

Pathophysiology

Iron deficiency anemia can be caused by any number of factors that decrease the supply of iron, impair its absorption, increase the body's need for iron, or affect the synthesis of hemoglobin. Although the clinical manifestations and diagnostic evaluation are quite similar regardless of the cause, the therapeutic and nursing considerations depend on the specific reason for the iron deficiency. The following discussion is limited to iron deficiency anemia resulting from inadequate iron in the diet.

During the last trimester of pregnancy, iron is transferred from mother to fetus. Most of the iron is stored in the circulating erythrocytes of the fetus, with the remainder stored in the fetal liver, spleen, and bone marrow. These iron stores are usually adequate for the first 5 to 6 months in a full-term infant but for only 2 to 3 months in premature infants or multiple births. If dietary iron is not supplied to meet the infant's growth demands once the fetal iron stores are depleted, then iron deficiency anemia results.

Although the majority of infants with iron deficiency anemia are underweight, many are overweight because of excessive milk ingestion (known as *milk babies*). These children become anemic for two reasons. Milk, a poor source of iron, is given almost to the exclusion of solid foods, and some infants fed cow's milk have an increased fecal loss of blood.

Therapeutic Management

Once the diagnosis of iron deficiency anemia is made, therapeutic management focuses on increasing the amount of supplemental iron the child receives. This is usually done through dietary counseling and the administration of oral iron supplements.

In formula-fed infants the most convenient and best sources of supplemental iron are iron-fortified commercial formula and iron-fortified infant cereal. Iron-fortified formula provides a relatively constant and predictable amount of iron and is not associated with an increased incidence of gastrointestinal symptoms, such as colic, diarrhea, or constipation. Infants under 12 months of age should not be given fresh cow milk to decrease the possibility of iron deficiency from gas-

Nursing Care Plan

THE CHILD WITH ANEMIA

Nursing Diagnosis: Anxiety/fear related to diagnostic procedures, transfusions

Expected Outcome: Child and family will exhibit minimal signs of fear or anxiety.

• NURSING INTERVENTIONS/*RATIONALES*

Prepare child and family for tests and procedures using a developmentally appropriate approach (i.e., demonstration of procedure using dolls) *to relieve fear of unknown.*

Explain purpose of tests, procedures, and interventions such as transfusions to child and family *to increase understanding and relieve anxiety.*

Remain with child during tests and procedures and provide comfort measures *to provide support.*

Encourage a parent to remain *to minimize separation anxiety.*

Enlist the child's and parent's help during procedure, giving them very specific tasks and a range of choices as appropriate *to provide a measure of control.*

Nursing Diagnosis: Activity intolerance related to generalized weakness, diminished oxygen delivery to tissues

Expected Outcome: Child's activity level is within normal limits for his or her physical condition.

• NURSING INTERVENTIONS/*RATIONALES*

Observe for signs of physical exertion (i.e., tachycardia, palpitations, tachypnea, shortness of breath, dizziness, sweating, fatigue) *to assess need for rest.*

Balance rest and activity when planning nursing and medical interventions and play *to diminish exertion.*

Provide quiet diversional activities *that promote rest and prevent boredom.*

Administer oxygen as ordered *to increase oxygenation of tissues.*

Administer blood products as ordered *to replace lost blood and stimulate new blood cell formation;* observe child carefully during and after transfusion *for possible side effects and complications.*

Nursing Diagnosis: Altered nutrition: less than body requirements related to inadequate iron intake

Expected Outcome: Child receives minimum daily requirements of iron.

• NURSING INTERVENTIONS/*RATIONALES*

Teach caregiver what iron does, what the minimum daily requirements of iron are, and what foods are iron-rich *to promote adequate iron intake in child's diet.*

Administer iron preparations as prescribed *to replenish depleted iron stores.*

Instruct family regarding correct administration of iron preparation (i.e., give between meals *for maximum absorption*, give with fruit juice or multivitamin preparation *because vitamin C appears to increase absorption*, do not give with milk or antacids *since they decrease absorption*).

Observe stools *as adequate dosages of oral iron turn stools a tarry green.*

---

trointestinal blood loss occurring as a result of allergy to the milk protein. Dietary addition of iron-rich foods is usually inadequate as the sole treatment of iron deficiency anemia because the iron is poorly absorbed and provides insufficient supplemental quantities of iron. If dietary sources of iron cannot replace body stores, oral iron supplements are prescribed for approximately 3 months. Ferrous iron, more readily absorbed than ferric iron, results in higher hemoglobin levels. Ascorbic acid (vitamin C) appears to facilitate the absorption of iron and may be prescribed in addition to the iron preparation.

If the hemoglobin level is very low or if levels fail to rise after 1 month of oral therapy, intramuscular or intravenous iron is administered. Transfusions are indicated for the most severe anemia and in cases of serious infection, cardiac dysfunction, or surgical emergency where anesthesia is required. Packed RBCs, not whole blood, is used to minimize the chance of circulatory overload. Supplemental oxygen is administered when tissue hypoxia is severe.

Prognosis. The prognosis for a child with this condition is very good. However, there is some evidence that if the iron deficiency anemia is long-standing, mild cognitive impairment may result (Idjradinata and Pollitt, 1993).

Nursing Care Management

An essential nursing responsibility is instructing parents in the administration of iron. Oral iron should be given as prescribed in three divided doses between meals, when the presence of free hydrochloric acid is greatest, because more iron is absorbed in the acidic environment of the upper gastrointestinal tract. A citrus fruit or juice taken with the medication aids in absorption.

An adequate dosage of oral iron turns the stools a tarry green color. The nurse advises parents of this normally expected change and inquires about its occurrence on follow-up visits. Absence of the greenish black stool may be a clue to poor administration of iron, either in schedule or in dosage. Vomiting and/or diarrhea can occur with iron therapy. If the parents report these symptoms, the iron can be given with meals and the dosage reduced and then gradually increased until tolerated.

Liquid preparations of iron may temporarily stain the teeth. If possible, the medication should be taken through a straw or given through a syringe or medicine dropper placed toward the back of the mouth. Brushing the teeth after administration of the drug lessens the discoloration.

If parenteral iron preparations are prescribed, iron dextran must be injected deeply into a large muscle mass using the Z-tract method. The injection site is *not* massaged after injection to minimize skin staining and irritation. Since no more than 1 ml should be given in one site, the intravenous route should be considered to avoid multiple injections. Careful observation is required because of the risk of adverse reactions, such as anaphylaxis with intravenous administration. A test dose is recommended before routine use.

Diet. A primary nursing objective is to prevent nutritional anemia through family education. The nurse discusses with parents the importance of using iron-fortified formula and the introduction of solid foods at the appropriate age. The best solid food source of iron is commercial infant cereals. It may be difficult at first to teach the infant to accept foods other than milk. The same principles are applied as those for introducing new foods (see the discussion of nutrition, Chapter 33), especially feeding the solid food before the milk. Predominantly milk-fed infants rebel against solid foods, and parents are cautioned about this and the need to be firm in not relinquishing control to the child. It may require intense problem solving on the part of both the family and the nurse to overcome the child's resistance.

A difficulty encountered in discouraging the parents from feeding milk to the exclusion of other foods is dispelling the popular myth that milk is a "perfect food." Many parents believe that milk is best for the infant and equate the weight gain with a "healthy child" and "good mothering." They are not concerned about providing other foods as long as the child continues to take milk. The nurse can also stress that overweight is not synonymous with good health.

Diet education of teenagers is especially difficult, especially since teenage girls are particularly prone to following weight-reduction diets. Emphasizing the effect of anemia on appearance (pallor) and energy level (difficulty maintaining popular activities) may be useful. (See Chapter 44, Mineral Disturbances, and Table 44-2 for sources of iron-rich foods.)

SICKLE CELL ANEMIA (SCA)

SCA is one of a group of diseases collectively termed *hemoglobinopathies,* in which normal adult hemoglobin (hemoglobin A [HbA]) is partly or completely replaced by abnormal sickle hemoglobin (HbS). *Sickle cell disease (SCD)* includes all those hereditary disorders whose clinical, hematologic, and pathologic features are related to the presence of HbS. Even though SCD is sometimes used to refer to SCA, this use is incorrect. Other correct terms for SCA are *SS* and *homozygous sickle cell disease.*

In the United States the most common forms of SCD are as follows:

- Sickle cell trait, the heterozygous form of the disease (HbA and HbS, HbAS or SA)
- Sickle cell anemia, the homozygous form of the disease (HbSS or SS)
- Sickle cell–C disease, a heterozygous variant of SCD, including both HbS and HbC (SC)
- Sickle cell–hemoglobin E disease, a variant of SCD in which glutamic acid has been substituted for lysine in the number 26 position of the β chain (SE)
- Sickle thalassemia disease, a combination of sickle cell trait and β-thalassemia trait (SβThal)

Of the SCDs, SCA is the most common form in African Americans, followed by sickle cell–C disease and sickle β-thalassemia.

SCA infrequently affects Caucasians, especially those of Mediterranean descent. The incidence of the disease varies in different geographic locations. Among African Americans the incidence of sickle cell trait is about 8%. In West Africa the incidence is reported to be as high as 40% among native blacks. The high incidence of sickle cell trait in West Africans is believed by some to be the result of selective protection afforded trait carriers against one type of malaria.

The gene that determines the production of HbS is situated on an autosome and, when present, is always detectable and therefore dominant. Heterozygous persons who have hemoglobin containing both normal HbA and abnormal HbS are said to have **sickle cell trait.** Persons who are homozygous have predominantly HbS and have **sickle cell anemia.** The inheritance pattern is essentially that of an autosomal recessive disorder. Therefore, when both parents have sickle cell trait, there is a 25% chance of their producing an offspring with SCA.

Although the defect is inherited, the sickling phenomenon is usually not apparent until later in infancy because of the presence of fetal hemoglobin (HbF). As long as HbF persists, sickling does not occur because there is HbS present. The newborn has from 60% to 80% HbF, but this rapidly decreases during the first year, so that the child is at risk for sickle cell–related complications (Sickle Cell Disease Guideline Panel, 1993).

Pathophysiology

The clinical features of SCA are primarily the result of (1) *obstruction* caused by the sickled RBCs and (2) increased RBC *destruction* (Fig. 46-1). The entanglement and enmeshing of rigid sickle-shaped cells with one another intermittently block the microcirculation, causing vaso-occlusion. The resultant absence of blood flow to adjacent tissues causes local hypoxia, leading to tissue ischemia and infarction (cellular death). Most of the complications seen in SCA can be traced to this process and its impact on various organs of the body.

The effect of sickling and infarction on organ structures occurs in the following sequence (see also consequences in Box 46-3):

1. Stasis with enlargement
2. Infarction with ischemia and destruction
3. Replacement with fibrous tissue (scarring)

Clinical Manifestations

The clinical manifestations of SCA vary markedly in severity and frequency (Box 46-3). The most acute symptoms of the disease occur during periods of exacerbation called *crises.* The crises may occur individually or concomitantly with one or more other crises. The episode may be a *vasoocclusive crisis,* preferably called a "painful episode," characterized by distal ischemia and pain; *sequestration crisis,* a pooling of blood in liver and spleen with decreased blood volume and shock;

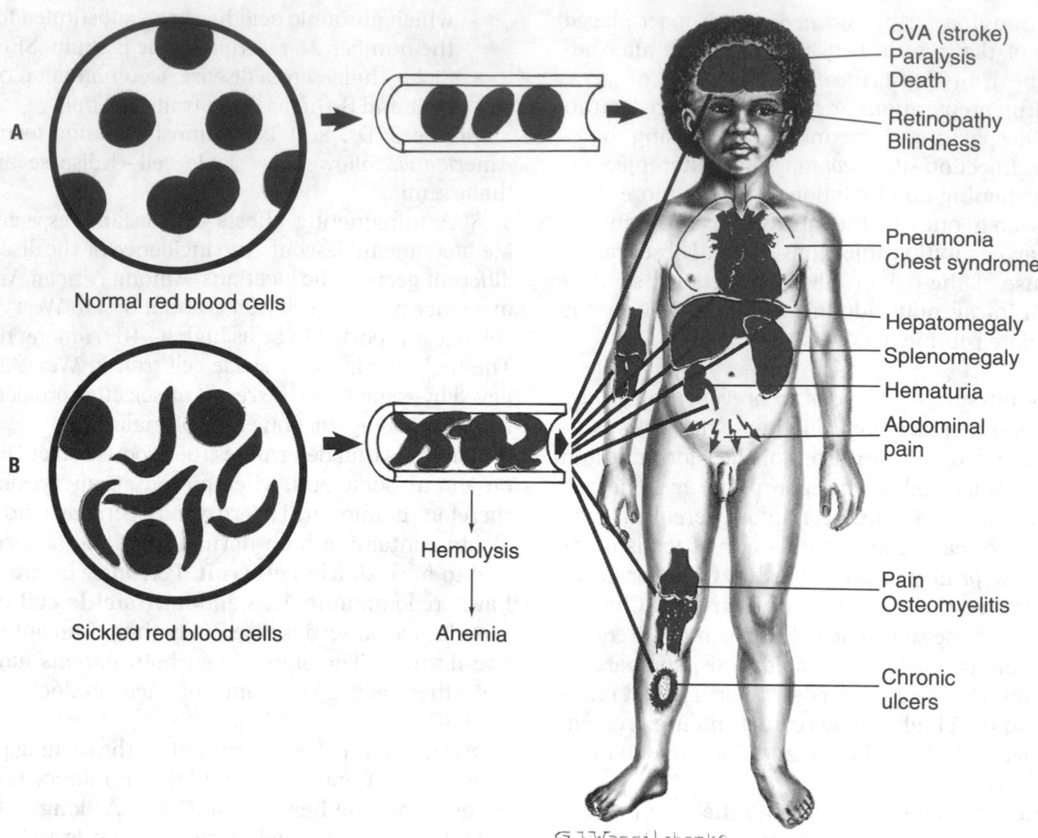

Fig. 46-1 Differences between normal and sickled blood cells.

aplastic crisis, diminished RBC production resulting in profound anemia; and *hyperhemolytic crisis,* an accelerated rate of RBC destruction characterized by anemia, jaundice, and reticulocytosis. This complication frequently suggests other coexisting conditions, such as viral illness, or glucose-6-dehydrogenase (G6PD) deficiency, which is also common in African Americans.

Another serious complication is *chest syndrome,* which is clinically similar to pneumonia. It is associated with chest pain, fever, pneumonia-like cough, and associated anemia. A cerebrovascular accident (*CVA, stroke*) is a sudden and severe complication, often with no related illnesses. Sickled cells block the major blood vessels in the brain, resulting in cerebral infarction, which causes variable degrees of neurologic impairment. Repeat strokes causing progressively greater brain damage occur in 60% of children who have already experienced one stroke.

Diagnostic Evaluation

Newborn screening for SCA is mandatory in most of the United States, so infants can be identified before symptoms occur. At birth the infant has up to 80% of HbF, which does not carry the defect. During the first months of life the infant begins production of RBCs with HbA and HbS if the gene is present. At this point the child may become symptomatic. Since levels of HbS are low at birth, hemoglobin electrophoresis or other tests that measure HgB concentrations are indicated. Early diagnosis (before 3 months of age) enables the initiation of appropriate interventions to minimize complications. The family is taught to administer prophylactic antibiotics and identify early signs of infection in order to seek medical therapy as soon as possible.

If SCA is not diagnosed in early infancy, it is likely to show symptoms during the toddler and preschool years. SCA is occasionally first diagnosed during a crisis that follows an acute respiratory or gastrointestinal infection. Routine hematologic tests are done to evaluate the anemia. Several specific tests detect the presence of the abnormal hemoglobin in the heterozygote and/or the homozygote. For screening purposes the *sickle-turbidity test (Sickledex)* is commonly used because it can be performed on blood from a finger stick and yields accurate results in 3 minutes. However, if the test is positive, hemoglobin electrophoresis is necessary to distinguish between those children with the trait and those with the disease. *Hemoglobin electrophoresis* ("fingerprinting" of the protein) is an accurate, rapid, and specific test for detecting the homozygous and heterozygous forms of the disease, as well as the percentages of the various hemoglobins.

Therapeutic Management

There is no cure for SCA. The aims of therapy are (1) to prevent conditions that enhance the sickling phenomena, which are responsible for the pathologic sequelae, and (2) to treat the medical emergencies of sickle cell crisis. Prevention consists of

BOX 46-3
Clinical Manifestations of SCA

General
Possible growth retardation
Chronic anemia (hemoglobin 6 to 9 g/dl)
Possible delayed sexual maturation
Marked susceptibility to sepsis

Vasoocclusive crisis
Pain in area(s) of involvement
Manifestations related to ischemia of involved areas:
- Extremities: painful swelling of hands and feet (sickle cell dactylitis, or "hand-foot syndrome"), painful joints
- Abdomen: severe pain resembling acute surgical condition
- Cerebrum: stroke, visual disturbances
- Chest: symptoms resembling pneumonia, protracted episodes of pulmonary disease
- Liver: obstructive jaundice, hepatic coma
- Kidney: hematuria
- Genital: priapism (painful constant penile erection)

Sequestration crisis
Pooling of large amounts of blood:
- Hepatomegaly
- Splenomegaly
- Circulatory collapse

Effects of chronic vasoocclusive phenomena
Heart: cardiomegaly, systolic murmurs
Lungs: altered pulmonary function, susceptibility to infections, pulmonary insufficiency
Kidneys: inability to concentrate urine, progressive renal failure, enuresis
Liver: hepatomegaly, cirrhosis, intrahepatic cholestasis
Spleen: splenomegaly, susceptibility to infection, functional reduction in splenic activity progressing to autosplenectomy
Eyes: intraocular abnormalities with visual disturbances, sometimes progressive retinal detachment and blindness
Extremities: skeletal deformities, especially lordosis and kyphosis, chronic leg ulcers, susceptibility to osteomyelitis
Central nervous system: hemiparesis, seizures (acute, not chronic)

maintaining hemodilution. The successful implementation of this goal depends more often on nursing interventions than on medical therapies.

Medical management of a crisis is usually directed at supportive and symptomatic treatment. The main objectives are to provide (1) bed rest to minimize energy expenditure and oxygen use, (2) hydration through oral and intravenous therapy, (3) electrolyte replacement, (4) analgesics for the severe abdominal and joint pain, (5) blood replacement to treat anemia, and (6) antibiotics to treat any existing infection.

Administration of pneumococcal and meningococcal vaccines beginning at 2 years of age is recommended for these children because of their susceptibility to infection as a result of functional asplenia. With the likelihood of transfusion therapy for individuals with SCA, hepatitis B vaccine is recommended for those children who have not received it as part of their routine immunization schedule (see Immunizations, Chapter 33.) Oral penicillin prophylaxis is also recommended twice daily (Sickle Cell Disease Guideline Panel, 1993).

Short-term oxygen therapy may be helpful if a child has symptoms of respiratory difficulty. Severe hypoxia must be prevented because this causes massive systemic sickling that can be fatal. Although oxygen may prevent more sickling, it usually is not effective in reversing sickling because the oxygen is unable to reach the enmeshed sickled erythrocytes in clogged vessels. In addition, prolonged administration can depress bone marrow, further aggravating the anemia.

Exchange transfusion, which reduces the number of circulating sickle cells and slows down the vicious cycle of hypoxia, thrombosis, tissue ischemia, and injury, has been successful. The procedure is sometimes advocated as a possible preventive technique. However, multiple transfusions carry the risk of hepatitis, hemosiderosis, and transfusion reactions. Once a stroke has occurred, blood transfusions are usually given every 4 to 5 weeks to help prevent a repeat stroke. To reduce iron overload, home subcutaneous chelation therapy may be started (see p. 1441).

In children with recurrent splenic sequestration, splenectomy may be a lifesaving measure. However, since the spleen usually atrophies on its own through progressive fibrotic changes (*functional asplenia*), routine splenectomy is not recommended. Any procedure that requires anesthesia has increased risk for these children. *Painful priapism (continual erection)* may be treated by aspiration of the corpora cavernosum. This complication is particularly frequent in vasoocclusive crises.

The most frequent problem for patients with SCA is vasoocclusive pain. The chronic nature of this pain can greatly affect the child's development. A multidisciplinary approach is best for its management. When mild to moderate pain is reported, ibuprofen or acetaminophen is used initially. If these drugs are not effective alone, codeine can be added. The dosages of both drugs are titrated (adjusted) to a therapeutic level. Opioids such as immediate- and sustained-release morphine, oxycodone, hydromorphone (Dilaudid), and methadone are administered intravenously or orally for severe pain and are administered around the clock. Patient-controlled analgesia (PCA) has been used successfully for sickle cell–related pain. PCA reinforces the patient's role and responsibility in managing the pain, and provides flexibility for pain, which may vary in severity over time. The use of high-dose intravenous methylprednisolone has decreased the duration of severe pain in children (Griffin, McIntire, and Buchanan, 1994). (See Pain Management, Chapter 41.)

Nursing ALERT

Meperidine (pethidine [Demerol]) is not recommended. Normeperidine, a metabolite of meperidine, is a central nervous system stimulant that produces anxiety, tremors, myoclonus, and generalized seizures when it accumulates with repetitive dosing. Patients with sickle cell disease are particularly at risk for normeperidine-induced seizures (American Pain Society, 1992).

Prognosis. The prognosis varies. Most of the time, children are without symptoms and participate in normal activities without restrictions. The greatest risk is usually in children between 1 and 3 years of age, and the majority of deaths in these children and individuals under age 20, are caused by overwhelming infection. Consequently, SCA is a chronic illness with a potentially terminal outcome.

Individuals with low levels of HbF are more likely to die earlier than those with higher levels (Platt et al, 1994). Research is investigating hydroxyurea and erythropoietin, which may increase the concentration of HbF and ultimately reduce complications (Charache, 1994). Bone marrow transplant may be a possible cure for SCD (Johnson et al, 1994; Vermylen and Cornu, 1994) (see p. 1536).

Nursing Care Management

Assessment

Many nurses are involved in screening programs for SCA to identify persons with the abnormal hemoglobin in order to implement therapy for homozygotes and provide genetic counseling for heterozygotes. Young children from families of at-risk racial or geographic origins who exhibit any of the signs previously described are advised to seek medical attention immediately.

Assessment of the child in sickle cell crisis involves all areas and systems that can be affected by circulatory obstruction, including vital signs, neurologic signs and vision and hearing assessment, as well as assessment of the respiratory, gastrointestinal, renal, and musculoskeletal systems. It is also important to assess the location and intensity of pain (see Pain Assessment, Chapter 41).

Nursing Diagnoses

Nursing diagnoses are derived from observation and assessment of children with the disease or those in crisis (Box 46-4). Others will be apparent depending on the state of the child's health, the organs involved, and the individual needs of the child and family.

Planning

The primary goals are as follows:

1. The family and child (when appropriate) will receive education regarding the sickling phenomenon and possible consequences and early recognition of crises and infection.
2. The child will receive supportive therapies during crises.
3. The child and parents will adjust to a lifelong, potentially fatal hereditary disease.
4. Family members will receive genetic counseling.

BOX 46-4
Nursing Diagnoses: The Child with SCA

Risk for infection related to decreased or absent splenic function
Impaired physical mobility related to tissue ischemia, generalized weakness
Altered family processes related to child with a chronic condition

Sickle cell crisis

Pain related to tissue ischemia (sickle cell crisis)
Altered tissue perfusion related to impaired arterial blood flow

Implementation

Educate family and child. Family education begins with an explanation of the disease and its consequences. Following this explanation, the most important things to teach are (1) seek early intervention for problems, such as a fever of 38.5° C (101.5° F) or greater, (2) give penicillin as ordered, (3) recognize signs and symptoms of splenic sequestration as well as respiratory problems that can lead to hypoxia, and (4) treat the child normally. Families should be told that the child is normal but can get sick in ways that other children cannot.

The nurse can demonstrate the effect of sickling by rolling rounded objects, such as marbles or beads, through a tube to simulate normal circulation and then rolling pointed objects, such as screws or jacks, through the tube. The effect of sickling and clumping of the pointed objects is especially noticeable at a bend or slight narrowing of the tube. This same idea can be expanded to discuss the importance of increased fluid in keeping the pointed objects suspended away from each other to prevent concentration.

The nurse emphasizes the importance of adequate hydration to prevent sickling and to delay the stasis-thrombosis-ischemia cycle in a crisis. It is not sufficient to advise parents to "force fluids" or "encourage drinking." They need specific instructions on how many daily glasses or bottles of fluid are required. Many foods are also a source of fluid, particularly soups, popsicles, ice cream, sherbert, gelatin, and puddings.

Nursing ALERT

Advise parents to be particularly alert to situations where dehydration may be a possibility, such as hot weather, and to recognize early signs of reduced intake, such as decreased urine output (e.g., fewer wet diapers) and increased thirst.

Increased fluids combined with impaired kidney function result in the problem of *enuresis.* Parents who are unaware of this fact frequently employ the usual measures to discourage bed-wetting, such as limiting fluids at night, and may resort to punishment and shame to force bladder control. Enuresis is treated as a complication of the disease, such as joint pain or some other symptom, in order to alleviate parental pressure on the child.

Promote supportive therapies during crises. The success of many of the medical therapies relies heavily on nursing implementation. Management of pain is an especially difficult problem and often involves experimenting with various analgesics, including opioids, and schedules before relief is achieved. Unfortunately, these children tend to be undermedicated, resulting in "clock watching" and demands for additional doses sooner than might be expected. Often this incorrectly raises suspicions of drug addiction, when in fact the problem is one of improper dosage (see the Family Focus box

Family Focus

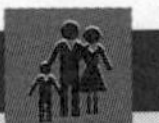

FEAR OF ADDICTION

Although pain is usually severe and opioids are warranted, many families fear that their child will become addicted to the narcotic. Unfortunately, misinformed health professionals may foster this unfounded fear, resulting in needless suffering. Few, if any, children who receive opioids for severe pain become behaviorally addicted to the drug (Morrison, 1991). Families and older children, especially adolescents, must be reassured that opioids are medically indicated, high doses may be needed, and addiction is rare.

above). In choosing and scheduling analgesics the goal should be *prevention* of pain.

Any pain program should be combined with psychologic support to help the child deal with the depression, anxiety, and fear that may accompany the disease. This includes regular visits with the child to discuss any concerns during the hospitalization and positive reinforcement of coping skills, such as successful methods of dealing with the pain and compliance with treatment prescriptions.

Frequently, heat to the affected area is soothing. Cold compresses are not applied to the area because this enhances sickling and vasoconstriction. Bed rest is usually well tolerated during a crisis, although actual rest depends a great deal on pain alleviation and organized schedules of nursing care. Some activity, particularly passive range-of-motion exercises, is beneficial to promote circulation. Usually the best course of action is to let children dictate their activity tolerance.

If blood transfusions or exchange transfusions are given, the nurse is responsible for observing for signs of transfusion reaction (Table 46-4). Since hypervolemia from too rapid transfusion can increase the work load of the heart, the nurse is also alert to signs of cardiac failure.

In splenic sequestration the size of the spleen is gently measured by abdominal palpation (see the discussion of the abdomen, Chapter 32). The nurse should be aware of spleen size because an increasing splenomegaly is an ominous sign. A decreasing spleen size denotes response to therapy. Vital signs and blood pressure are also closely monitored for impending shock. Anemia is typically not a presenting complication in vasoocclusive crises but is a critical problem in other types of crises. The nurse monitors for evidence of increasing anemia and institutes appropriate nursing intervention (see p. 1504). If oxygen is ordered, pulse oximetry values for blood oxygen saturation are monitored for evidence of the oxygen's benefit. No improvement in oxygen saturation is especially important to report. The drug oxygen can have side effects, such as decreasing RBC production.

Intake, especially of intravenous fluids, and output are recorded. The child's weight should be taken on admission, since it serves as a baseline for evaluating hydration. Since diuresis can result in electrolyte loss, the nurse also observes for signs of hypokalemia and should be familiar with normal serum electrolyte values to report changes.

Recognize other complications. Nurses also need to be aware of the signs of chest syndrome and CVA, both potentially fatal complications.

Nursing ALERT

Report signs of the following immediately:

Chest syndrome:

- Severe chest pain, sometimes spreading to abdomen
- Fever of 38.8° C (102° F) or higher
- Very congested cough
- Dyspnea, tachypnea
- Retractions
- Declining oxygen saturation (oximetry)

Cerebrovascular accident (CVA, stroke):

- Jerking or twitching of the face, legs, or arms
- Convulsions or seizures
- Strange, abnormal behavior
- Inability to move an arm and/or a leg
- Stagger or an unsteady walk
- Stutter or slurred speech
- Weakness in the hands, feet, or legs
- Changes in vision
- Severe, unrelieved headaches
- Severe vomiting

Support family. Families need the opportunity to discuss their feelings regarding transmitting a potentially fatal, chronic illness to their child. Because of the widely publicized prognosis for children with SCA, many parents express their prevalent fear of the child's death. Since there is no way to predict which child will follow a favorable course, nursing care for the family should be the same as for any family with a child who has a life-threatening illness. Particular emphasis is placed on the siblings' reactions, the stress on the marital relationship, and the childrearing attitudes displayed toward the child (see Chapter 38). Several resources are available to the family who has a child with a sickling disorder.*

The nurse advises parents to inform all treating personnel of the child's condition. The use of medical identification, such as a bracelet, is another way of ensuring awareness of the disease.

If family members have the sickle cell disease trait and/or SCA, genetic counseling is necessary. A primary goal is informing parents who carry the trait of the one-in-four risk of having a child with the disease in language they can understand.

Evaluation

The effectiveness of nursing interventions is determined by continual reassessment and evaluation of care based on the following observational guidelines and expected outcomes:

1. Interview family regarding their understanding of the disease, the sickling phenomena, its consequences, and early recognition of complications.

*A Sickle Cell Home Study Kit For Families is available from the **National Association for Sickle Cell Disease, Inc.,** 3345 Wilshire Blvd., Suite 1106, Los Angeles, CA 90010-1880; (800) 421-8453. Additional resources are **Howard University, Center for Sickle Cell Disease,** 2121 Georgia Ave., N.W., Washington, DC 20059, (202) 806-7930; **National Sickle Cell Disease Program, National Heart, Lung, and Blood Institute,** Bldg 31, Room 4A-21, Rockville Pike, Bethesda, MD 20205, (301) 496-4236; and **Sickle Cell Association of Ontario,** 1076 Bathurst St., Suite 305, Toronto, Ontario M5R 3G9, (416) 789-2855.

2. Observe child for any evidence of sickling; monitor preventive strategies and therapies, especially pain assessment and management.
3. Interview and observe child and family regarding the way the disease has affected their lives.
4. Interview the family to determine their understanding of the risk of having another child with SCA.
5. Medical attention is sought appropriately.

Expected outcomes:

1. The family demonstrates an understanding of the disease and its consequences and verbalizes symptoms to report (specify knowledge and method of demonstration).
2. The family gives antibiotic on a consistent basis.
3. The child exhibits few episodes of sickling; pain is effectively controlled.
4. The family takes advantage of genetic counseling services and medical care.
5. The child and family express their feelings and concerns regarding the disease.

See also Nursing Care Plan: The Child with Sickle Cell Disease.*

β-THALASSEMIA (COOLEY ANEMIA)

The term *thalassemia,* which is derived from the Greek word *thalassa,* meaning *sea,* is applied to a variety of inherited blood disorders characterized by deficiencies in the rate of production of specific globin chains in hemoglobin. The name appropriately refers to descendants of or those people living near the Mediterranean Sea who have the highest incidence of the disease, namely, Italians, Greeks, and Syrians. There is evidence to suggest that the high incidence of the disorders among these groups is a result of selective advantage of the trait to malaria, as is postulated in sickle cell disease.

β-Thalassemia is the most common of the thalassemias and occurs in three forms: a heterozygous form, *thalassemia minor* or *thalassemia trait,* which produces a mild microcytic anemia; *thalassemia intermedia,* which is manifested as splenomegaly and moderate to severe anemia; and a homozygous form, *thalassemia major* (also known as *Cooley anemia*), which results in a severe anemia that would lead to cardiac failure and death in early childhood without transfusion support.

Pathophysiology

Normal postnatal hemoglobin is composed of 2 α- and 2 β-polypeptide chains. In β-thalassemia there is a partial or complete deficiency in the synthesis of the β-chain of the hemoglobin molecule. Consequently, there is a compensatory increase in the synthesis of α-chains, and γ-chain production remains activated, resulting in defective hemoglobin formation. This unbalanced polypeptide unit is very unstable; when it disintegrates, it damages RBCs, causing severe anemia.

To compensate for the hemolytic process, an overabundance of erythrocytes is formed unless the bone marrow is suppressed by transfusion therapy. Excess iron from hemolysis of supplemental RBCs in transfusions and from the rapid destruction of defective cells is stored in various organs (*hemosiderosis*).

*In Wong DL: *Wong and Whaley's clinical manual of pediatric nursing,* ed 4, St Louis, 1996, Mosby.

BOX 46-5
Clinical Manifestations of β-Thalassemia

Anemia—before diagnosis
Unexplained fever
Poor feeding
Markedly enlarged spleen

With progressive anemia
Signs of chronic hypoxia
- Headache
- Precordial and bone pain
- Decreased exercise tolerance
- Listlessness
- Anorexia

Other features
Small stature
Delayed sexual maturation
Bronzed, freckled complexion (if not chelated)

Bone changes (older children if untreated)
Enlarged head
Prominent frontal and parietal bosses
Prominent malar eminences
Flat or depressed bridge of the nose
Enlarged maxilla
Protrusion of the lip and upper central incisors and eventual malocclusion
Oriental appearance of eyes

Diagnostic Evaluation

The onset of thalassemia major may be insidious and not recognized until the latter half of infancy. The clinical effects of thalassemia major are primarily attributable to (1) defective synthesis of HbA, (2) structurally impaired RBCs, and (3) shortened life span of erythrocytes (Box 46-5).

Hematologic studies reveal the characteristic changes in RBCs and immature erythrocytes. Low hemoglobin and hematocrit levels are seen in severe anemia, although they are typically lower than the reduction in RBC count because of the proliferation of immature erythrocytes. Hemoglobin electrophoresis confirms the diagnosis, and radiographs of involved bones reveal characteristic findings.

Therapeutic Management

The objective of supportive therapy is to maintain sufficient hemoglobin levels to prevent bone marrow expansion and the resulting bony deformities, as well as to provide sufficient RBCs to support normal growth and normal physical activity. Transfusions are the foundation of medical management. Recent studies have evaluated the benefits of maintaining the child's hemoglobin level above 10 g/dl, a goal that may require transfusions as often as every 3 weeks. The advantages of this therapy include (1) improved physical and psychologic well-being because of the ability to participate in normal activities, (2) decreased cardiomegaly and hepatosplenomegaly,

(3) fewer bone changes, and (4) normal or near-normal growth and development until puberty.

One of the potential complications of frequent blood transfusions is iron overload. Since the body has no effective means of eliminating the excess iron, the mineral is deposited in body tissues. To minimize the development of hemosiderosis, deferoxamine (Desferal), an iron-chelating agent, is given with small oral supplements of vitamin C. Deferoxamine is given intravenously or subcutaneously, often at home using a portable infusion pump over 8 to 24 hours on a daily basis. Creative strategies such as behavioral contracting have been used to assist the child in complying with the deferoxamine regimen (Koch et al, 1993).

In some children with severe splenomegaly who demonstrate increased transfusion requirements, a splenectomy may be necessary. Over time the spleen may accelerate the rate of RBC destruction and thus increase transfusion requirements. After a splenectomy, children generally require fewer transfusions, although the basic defect in hemoglobin synthesis remains unaffected. A major postsplenectomy complication is severe and overwhelming infection. Therefore these children are kept on prophylactic antibiotics with close medical supervision for many years and should receive the pneumococcal and meningococcal vaccines (see Immunizations, Chapter 33).

Nursing ALERT

Ensure the family and patient understand the need to notify the health professional of all fevers of 38.5°C (101.5° F) or greater because of the risk of sepsis in a child with asplenia.

Prognosis. Most children treated with blood transfusion and early chelation therapy survive well into adulthood. The most common cause of death is iron-induced heart disease, followed by infection, liver disease, and malignancy (Zurlo et al, 1989). A promising treatment for some children is bone marrow transplantation (see p. 1536). In one study, children under 16 years of age who underwent allogeneic bone marrow transplantation had a 59% to 98% rate of complication-free survival (Lucarelli et al, 1990).

Nursing Care Management

The objectives of nursing care are to (1) promote compliance with transfusion and chelation therapy, (2) assist the child in coping with the anxiety-provoking treatments and the effects of the illness, and (3) foster the child's and family's adjustment to a chronic illness. Basic to each of these goals is explaining to parents and older children the defect responsible for the disorder, its effect on RBCs, and the potential effects of untreated iron overload, such as diabetes and heart disease. Since the prevalence of this condition is high among families of Mediterranean descent, the nurse also inquires about the family's previous knowledge about thalassemia. All families who have a child with thalassemia should be tested for the trait and referred for genetic counseling.

As with any chronic illness, the needs of the family must be met for optimum adjustment to the stresses imposed by the disorder. These needs are discussed in Chapter 38. One source of information for the family is the *Cooley's Anemia Foundation.** Genetic counseling for the parents and fertile offspring is mandatory, and both prenatal diagnosis using amniocentesis at 10 weeks' gestation or fetal blood sampling at 20 weeks and screening for thalassemia trait are available.

See also Nursing Care Plan: The Child with Beta-Thalassemia (Cooley Anemia).†

APLASTIC ANEMIA

Aplastic anemia refers to a condition in which all formed elements of the blood are simultaneously depressed. The peripheral blood smear demonstrates pancytopenia or the triad of profound anemia, leukopenia, and thombocytopenia. *Hypoplastic anemia* is characterized by a profound depression of erythrocytes but normal or slightly decreased WBCs and platelets.

Etiology

Aplastic anemia can be *primary (congenital)* or *secondary (acquired)*. The best-known congenital disorder of which aplastic anemia is an outstanding feature is *Fanconi syndrome,* a rare hereditary disorder characterized by pancytopenia, hypoplasia of the bone marrow, and patchy brown discoloration of the skin as a result of melanin deposits and associated with multiple congenital anomalies of the musculoskeletal and genitourinary systems. The syndrome appears to be inherited as an autosomal recessive trait with varying penetrance; therefore affected siblings may demonstrate several different combinations of defects.

Several factors contribute to the development of acquired hypoplastic anemia. The most common causes of acquired aplastic anemia are listed in Box 46-6. The following discussion focuses on acquired aplastic anemia, which carries a poorer prognosis and follows a more rapidly fatal course than do the primary types.

Diagnostic Evaluation

The onset of clinical manifestations, which include anemia, leukopenia, and decreased platelet count, is usually insidious, not unlike that seen in leukemia. Definitive diagnosis is determined from bone marrow aspiration, which demonstrates the conversion of red bone marrow to yellow, fatty bone marrow.

Therapeutic Management

The objectives of treatment are based on the recognition that the underlying disease process is failure of the bone marrow to carry out its hematopoietic functions. Therefore therapy is directed at restoring function to the marrow and involves two main approaches: (1) immunosuppressive therapy to remove the presumed immunologic functions that prolong aplasia and/or (2) replacement of the bone marrow through transplantation. Bone marrow transplantation is the treatment of choice for severe aplastic anemia when a suitable donor exists.

Currently, antilymphocyte globulin (ALG) or antithymocyte globulin (ATG) is the principal drug treatment for aplastic anemia. The rationale for using ATG is based on the theory that aplastic anemia may be the result of autoimmunity. ATG

*129-09 26th Ave., Flushing, NY 11354; (718) 321-2873 or (800) 522-7222.

†In Wong DL: *Wong and Whaley's clinical manual of pediatric nursing,* ed 4. St Louis, 1996, Mosby.

BOX 46-6
Common Causes of Acquired Aplastic Anemia

Infection with the human parvovirus (HPV), hepatitis, or overwhelming infection
Irradiation
Drugs such as the chemotherapeutic agents and several antibiotics, one of the most notable being chloramphenicol
Industrial and household chemicals, including benzene and its derivatives, which are found in petroleum products, dyes, paint remover, shellac, and lacquers
Infiltration and replacement of myeloid elements, such as in leukemia or the lymphomas
Idiopathic, in which no identifiable precipitating cause can be found

suppresses T-cell-dependent autoimmune responses but does not cause bone marrow suppression. The optimum schedule for ATG administration is still under investigation. It is usually given intravenously over 12 to 16 hours, after a test dose to check for hypersensitivity. Subsequent doses are given depending on the reduction in circulating lymphocytes.

Colony-stimulating factors (CSFs), given parenterally, may be used to enhance bone marrow production. Androgens may be used with ATG to stimulate erythropoiesis, although the exact mechanism of erythropoietic action is unclear. Cyclosporine may also be administered in children who fail to respond to ATG, and success has also been achieved using high-dose methylprednisolone. Intravenous immunoglobulin has been used with success in aplastic anemia of infectious origin (Dwyer, 1992).

Because of the relatively poor prognosis in aplastic anemia treated with drug therapy, bone marrow transplantation should be considered *early* in the course of the disease if a compatible donor can be found. Transplantation is more successful when performed before multiple transfusions have sensitized the child to leukocyte and HLA antigens. Bone marrow transplantation is associated with a 63% 5-year survival rate (Pinkel, 1993; Sanders et al, 1994).

Nursing Care Management

The care of the child with aplastic anemia is similar to that of the child with leukemia (p. 1517)—specifically, preparing the child and family for the diagnostic and therapeutic procedures, preventing complications from the severe pancytopenia, and emotionally supporting them in terms of a potentially fatal outcome. Since each of these nursing considerations is discussed in the section on leukemia, only the exceptions are presented here.

The drug ATG is usually administered by way of a central vein. If not, vigilant care must be directed to the intravenous infusion to prevent extravasation. Meticulous care of the venous access is essential because of the child's susceptibility to infection. CSFs are usually given by subcutaneous injection over several days. The topical anesthetic cream, EMLA, minimizes the puncture pain.

Testosterone produces several undesirable effects that, when combined with the effects of steroid therapy, such as moon face, result in dramatic body image alterations. The virilizing effects of testosterone include deepening of the voice, hirsutism, growth of pubic hair, enlargement of the penis in males, flushing of the skin, and acne. Potentially, testosterone can cause muscular and skeletal maturation, resulting in severely retarded height in a young child. Not only are these changes difficult to accept, they are especially difficult to explain to children not approaching puberty. Parents may feel embarrassed because they are unprepared for the sexual changes. Information and support is available from the Aplastic Anemia Foundation of America.*

Since chemotherapeutic agents may be used, many of the reactions, such as nausea and vomiting, alopecia, and painful mucosal ulceration can be encountered. In addition, extensive ecchymotic areas of the oral mucosa that result from thrombocytopenia require meticulous mouth care to prevent breakdown, bleeding, and infection. Local anesthetics are usually not necessary, but anorexia is still a consequence because of the edematous nature of the lesions. Liquid, bland, and soft diets are usually tolerated best (see Feeding the Sick Child, Chapter 42). Specialized care is required for children who have a bone marrow transplant (see p. 1536).

Defects in Hemostasis

Hemostasis is the process that stops bleeding when a blood vessel is injured. Vascular and plasma clotting factors, as well as platelets, are required. A complex system of clotting, anticlotting, and clot breakdown *(fibrinolysis)* exists in equilibrium to ensure clot formation only in the presence of blood vessel injury and to limit the clotting process to the site of vessel wall injury. Dysfunction in these systems will lead to bleeding or abnormal clotting. Although the coagulation process is complex, clotting depends on three factors: (1) vascular influence, (2) platelet role, and (3) clotting factors.

HEMOPHILIA

The term *hemophilia* refers to a group of bleeding disorders in which there is a deficiency of one of the factors necessary for coagulation of the blood. Although the symptomatology is similar regardless of which clotting factor is deficient, the identification of specific factor deficiencies allows definitive treatment with replacement agents.

In about 80% of all cases of hemophilia the inheritance pattern is demonstrated as X-linked recessive. The two most common forms of the disorder are *factor VIII deficiency (hemophilia A* or *classic hemophilia)*, and *factor IX deficiency (hemophilia B* or *Christmas disease)*. The following discussion is primarily concerned with factor VIII deficiency, which accounts for about 75% of all cases.

Pathophysiology

The basic defect of hemophilia A is a deficiency of *factor VIII (antihemophilic factor [AHF])*. AHF is produced by the liver and is necessary for the formation of thromboplastin in phase I of blood coagulation. The less antihemophilic factor found in the blood, the more severe the disease. Individuals with he-

*P.O. Box 22689, Baltimore, MD 21203; (800) 747-2820.

mophilia have two of the three factors required for coagulation, vascular influence, and platelets. Therefore they may bleed for longer periods of time, but not at a faster rate.

Bleeding into tissue can occur anywhere, but hemorrhaging into joint cavities and muscles is the most frequent type of internal bleeding. Bony changes and crippling deformities occur after repeated bleeding episodes over a period of several years. Bleeding in the neck, mouth, or thorax is serious, since the airway can become obstructed. Intracranial hemorrhage can be fatal. Hemorrhage anywhere along the gastrointestinal tract can lead to anemia, and hematomas in the spinal cord can cause paralysis.

Diagnostic Evaluation

Overt, prolonged hemorrhage is readily apparent; bleeding into tissues is less apparent (Box 46-7). The diagnosis is usually based on a history of bleeding episodes, evidence of X-linked inheritance (only one third of the cases are new mutations), and laboratory findings. The tests specific for hemophilia are those that depend on specific plasma factors for a reaction to occur, such as the partial thromboplastin time (PTT). Specific determination of factor deficiencies requires assay procedures normally performed in specialized laboratories.

Therapeutic Management

The primary therapy for hemophilia is replacement of the missing clotting factor. The products currently available are (1) *factor VIII concentrate* from pooled plasma or genetically engineered recombinant, to be reconstituted with sterile water immediately before use; (2) *cryoprecipitate*, a concentrated form of AHF plus fibrinogen; and (3) *1-deamino-8-D-arginine vasopressin (DDAVP)*, a synthetic form of vasopressin that may be the treatment of choice in mild hemophilia if the child shows an appropriate response. Vigorous therapy is instituted to prevent chronic crippling effects from joint bleeding.

Other drugs may be included in the therapy plan, depending on the source of the hemorrhage. Corticosteroids are used judiciously to treat inflammation in the joints. Nonsteroidal antiinflammatory drugs (NSAIDs), such as aspirin, indomethacin (Indocin), and phenylbutazone (Butazolidin), should not be used because they inhibit platelet function. Ibuprofen (Motrin, Advil, or Nuprin) has been demonstrated to be safe despite its antiplatelet aggregation effect. Oral administration and/or local application of epsilon-aminocaproic acid (Amicar) prevents clot destruction; however, its use is limited to mouth or trauma surgery.

A regular program of exercise and physical therapy is an important aspect of management. Physical activity within reasonable limits strengthens muscles around joints, which will help retard or confine bleeding in the area.

Treatment without delay results in more rapid recovery and a decreased likelihood of complications; therefore most children are treated at home. The family is taught the technique of venipuncture and to administer the AHF to children over 3 years of age. The child learns the procedure for self-administration at 9 to 12 years of age. Home treatment is highly successful, and the rewards, in addition to the immediacy, are less disruption of family life, fewer school or work days missed, and enhancement of the child's self-esteem.

Prognosis. Although there is no cure for hemophilia, its symptoms can be controlled and its potentially crippling deformities markedly reduced or even avoided. Today many children with hemophilia function with minimal or no joint damage. They are normal children with an average life expectancy in every respect but one: they have a tendency to bleed, which is a significant inconvenience but not necessarily a life-threatening event.

Unfortunately, those individuals with hemophilia who were treated before current purification techniques for factor VIII concentrate may have been exposed to human immunodeficiency virus (HIV). One estimate is that 70% to 90% of these patients have seroconverted to HIV positive and a significant number have acquired immunodeficiency syndrome (AIDS). As these individuals become sexually active, the issue of sexual transmission of HIV becomes increasingly important. The adolescent must be knowledgeable regarding high-risk sexual behavior. Individuals with hemophilia diagnosed and treated with factor concentrates since 1985 are at virtually no risk for developing HIV infection. Current manufacturing techniques have also greatly reduced the risk of hepatitis transmission.

Nursing Care Management

Assessment

The earlier a bleeding episode is recognized, the more effectively it can be treated. Signs that indicate internal bleeding are especially important to recognize. Children are aware of internal bleeding and are very reliable in telling the examiner where the internal bleeding is. In addition to the manifestations described (Box 46-7), the nurse maintains a high level of suspicion when a child with hemophilia demonstrates unlikely signs, such as headache, slurred speech, loss of consciousness (from cerebral bleeding), and black tarry stools (from gastrointestinal bleeding).

Nursing Diagnoses

Nursing diagnoses for the child with hemophilia include but are not limited to the diagnoses listed in Box 46-8.

Planning

The objectives of care can be divided into immediate needs and long-term goals. The patient and family goals for nursing care include the following:

1. The family and child will receive education regarding

BOX 46-7
Clinical Manifestations of Hemophilia

Prolonged bleeding anywhere from or in the body
Hemorrhage from any trauma—loss of deciduous teeth, circumcision, cuts, epistaxis, injections
Excessive bruising—even from a slight injury, such as a fall
Subcutaneous and intramuscular hemorrhages
Hemarthrosis (bleeding into the joint cavities), especially the knees, ankles, and elbows
Hematomas—pain, swelling, and limited motion
Spontaneous hematuria

BOX 46-8
Nursing Diagnoses: The Child with Hemophilia

Risk for injury (trauma)
Pain related to bleeding into tissues
Impaired physical mobility related to hemorrhaging into joints and other tissues
Altered family processes related to child with a chronic illness

hemophilia and early recognition of bleeding episodes.
2. Bleeding episodes will be recognized and controlled and the child will receive supportive therapy.
3. The child and parents will adjust to a chronic hereditary disease.
4. Family members will receive genetic counseling.

Implementation

Prevent bleeding. The goal of prevention of bleeding episodes is directed toward decreasing the risk of injury. Prophylactic administration of factor VIII concentrates is reserved for troublesome target joints in an effort to break the bleeding cycle. The cost of the factor concentrate is prohibitive for routine administration. Prevention of bleeding episodes is geared mostly toward appropriate exercises to strengthen muscles and joints and to allow age-appropriate activity. During infancy and toddlerhood the normal acquisition of motor skills creates innumerable opportunities for falls, bruises, and minor wounds. Restraining the child from mastering motor development can herald more serious long-term problems than allowing the behavior. However, the environment should be made as safe as possible, with close supervision maintained during playtime to minimize incidental injuries.

For older children the family usually needs assistance in preparing for school. A nurse who knows the family can be instrumental in discussing the situation with the school nurse and in jointly planning an appropriate schedule of activity. Since almost all persons with hemophilia are boys, the physical limitations with regard to active sports may be a difficult adjustment, and activity restrictions must be tempered with sensitivity to the child's emotional, as well as physical, needs. Use of protective equipment, such as padding and helmets, is particularly important, and noncontact sports, especially swimming, are encouraged.

To prevent oral bleeding, some readjustment in terms of dental hygiene may be needed to minimize trauma to the gums, such as use of a water irrigating device, softening the toothbrush in warm water before brushing, or using a sponge-tipped disposable toothbrush. A regular toothbrush should be small and soft bristled.

Since any trauma can lead to a bleeding episode, all persons caring for these children must be aware of their disorder. These children should wear medical identification, and older children should be encouraged to recognize situations in which disclosing their condition is important, such as during dental extraction or injections. Health personnel must take special precautions to prevent the use of procedures that may cause bleeding, such as intramuscular injections or venipunctures. The intravenous and subcutaneous routes are substituted for intramuscular injections whenever possible. Neither aspirin nor any aspirin-containing compound should be used. Acetaminophen (Tylenol) is a suitable aspirin substitute, especially for use for pain control at home.

Recognize and control bleeding. The earlier a bleeding episode is recognized, the more effectively it can be treated. Factor replacement therapy should be instituted according to established medical protocol, and supportive measures may be implemented, such as (1) applying pressure to the area for at least 10 to 15 minutes to allow clot formation, (2) immobilizing and elevating the area above the level of the heart to decrease blood flow, and (3) applying cold to promote vasoconstriction. When parents and older children are taught such measures beforehand, they can be prepared to initiate immediate treatment. Plastic bags of ice or cold packs should be kept in the freezer for such emergencies. However, such measures do not take the place of factor replacement.

Prevent crippling effects of bleeding. As a result of repeated episodes of hemarthrosis, incompletely absorbed blood in the joints, and limitation of motion, bone and muscle changes occur that result in flexion contractures and joint fixation. During bleeding episodes the joint is elevated and immobilized. Active range-of-motion exercises are usually instituted after the acute episode. This allows the child to control the degree of exercise and discomfort. If an exercise program is instituted in the home, a physical therapist or public health nurse may need to supervise compliance with the regimen. Diet is also an important consideration, since excessive body weight can increase the strain on affected joints, especially the knees, and predispose to hemarthrosis. Consequently, calories must be supplied in accordance with energy requirements.

Support family and prepare for home care. Genetic counseling is essential as soon as possible after diagnosis. Unlike many other disorders in which both parents carry the trait, the feeling of responsibility for this condition usually rests with the mother. Without an opportunity to discuss her feelings, the marital relationship can suffer. Technology is now available to identify carriers in approximately 80% of cases and may reduce the anxiety regarding childbearing in females who may be at risk of carrying the defective gene, such as sisters or maternal aunts of an affected male.

The discovery of factor concentrates has greatly changed the outlook for these children. Bleeding can be minimized, and the child can live a much more normal, unrestricted life. Children are taught to take responsibility for their disease at an early age. They learn their limitations and other preventive measures, as well as self-administration of the prophylactic AHF.

The needs of families who have children with hemophilia are best met through a comprehensive team approach of physicians (pediatrician, hematologist, orthopedist), nurse, social worker, and physical therapist. Parent-group discussions are beneficial in meeting those needs often best met by similarly affected families. For example, with the improved prognosis for these children, parents and adolescents with hemophilia are faced with vocational and financial problems, in addition to concern over future childbearing. Once children reach 21 years of age, many insurance companies will no longer carry them. This can be disastrous in terms of the cost of treatment. The National Hemophilia Foundation* and the Canadian Hemophilia Society† provide numerous services and publications for both health providers and families. Financial support is particularly important. A person with severe hemophilia may require factor replacement therapy and other medical treatments that cost in excess of $70,000 to $90,000 a year.

Children who have become infected with HIV through transfusions and factor replacement products are faced with the consequences of this dreaded disease. Consequently, they need the support of health professionals, especially in the area of public education, regarding AIDS and ways to deal with public reactions to persons who have AIDS (see p. 1531 for a discussion of AIDS).

Evaluation

The effectiveness of nursing interventions is determined by continual reassessment and evaluation of care based on the following observational guidelines and expected outcomes:

1. Interview the child and family regarding preventive measures implemented and any bleeding episodes the child suffers.
2. Observe the child for evidence of bleeding episodes; monitor preventive strategies and therapies, especially pain assessment and management.
3. Observe and interview the family regarding treatments and the schedule for prophylactic administration of antihemophilic factor.
4. Interview the family and/or consult the genetic counseling service regarding the carrier status of other members of the family.

Expected outcomes:

1. The child exhibits no evidence of bleeding.
2. The child exhibits no evidence of tissue damage.
3. The child and family discuss their feelings and concerns and demonstrate an understanding of the disease and its therapy (specify knowledge and method of demonstration).
4. The family seeks genetic counseling.

See also Nursing Care Plan: The Child with Hemophilia.‡

IDIOPATHIC THROMBOCYTOPENIC PURPURA (ITP)

ITP is an acquired hemorrhagic disorder that is characterized by (1) *thrombocytopenia,* excessive destruction of platelets and (2) *purpura,* a discoloration caused by petechiae beneath the skin. Although the cause is unknown, it is believed to be an autoimmune response to disease-related antigens. It is the most frequently occurring thrombocytopenia of childhood.

The disease occurs in one of two forms: an acute, self-limiting course or a chronic condition interspersed with remissions. The acute form is most commonly seen after upper respiratory infections or after the childhood diseases measles, rubella, mumps, and chickenpox.

BOX 46-9
Clinical Manifestations of ITP

- Easy bruising
  - Petechiae
  - Ecchymoses
  - Most commonly over bony prominences
- Bleeding from mucous membranes
  - Epistaxis
  - Bleeding gums
  - Internal hemorrhage evidenced by:
    - Hematuria
    - Hematemesis
    - Melena
    - Hemarthrosis
    - Menorrhagia
- Hematomas over lower extremities

Diagnostic Evaluation

The diagnosis is suspected on the basis of clinical manifestations (Box 46-9). In ITP the platelet count is reduced to below 20,000 mm^3; therefore tests that depend on platelet function are abnormal, such as the tourniquet test, bleeding time, and clot retraction. Although there is no definitive test on which to establish a diagnosis of ITP, several are usually performed to rule out other disorders in which thrombocytopenia is a manifestation, such as systemic lupus erythematosus, lymphoma, or leukemia.

Therapeutic Management

Management is primarily supportive, since the course of the disease is self-limited in the majority of cases. Activity is restricted at the onset while the platelet count is low and while active bleeding or progression of lesions is occurring. This restriction is most easily accomplished in the hospital. Corticosteroids are employed for children with the highest risk for serious bleeding, for chronic cases with increased bleeding tendencies, as an adjunct to life-threatening hemorrhage, or before splenectomy to decrease the risk of surgical bleeding. Administration of intravenous gamma globulin has proved successful in increasing the platelet count of children with chronic disease. Children with chronic ITP have also experienced and sustained a rise in platelet count when treated with ascorbate (a product of ascorbic acid [vitamin C]) (Cohen et al, 1993). Splenectomy is reserved for symptomatic children with chronic disease or as an emergency measure in the event of life-threatening hemorrhage. Packed RBCs may be given to replace blood lost in symptomatic children. Platelets are seldom administered.

Prognosis. The majority of children have a self-limited course without major complications. Some children will develop chronic ITP and require ongoing therapy. A splenectomy may modify the disease process, and the child will be asymptomatic.

*110 Green St., Room 303, New York, NY 10012; (212) 219-8180 or (800) 42HANDI.

†1450 City Councillors, Bureau 840, Montreal, Quebec H3A 2E6; (514) 848-0503.

‡In Wong DL: *Wong and Whaley's clinical manual of pediatric nursing,* ed 4, St Louis, 1996, Mosby.

Nursing Care Management

Nursing care is largely supportive. Children and parents need careful explanations of the rationale behind the therapies employed and support in their efforts to comply. The nursing considerations of controlling bleeding and preventing bruising are similar to those discussed in the section on leukemia. The harmful effects of using aspirin and NSAIDs to control pain are critical for these children; therefore substitutes such as acetaminophen (paracetamol) are used.

DISSEMINATED INTRAVASCULAR COAGULATION (DIC)

DIC, also known as *consumption coagulopathy,* is a secondary disorder of coagulation that occurs as a complication of a number of pathologic processes, such as hypoxia, acidosis, shock, and endothelial damage. It can result from many severe systemic diseases, such as congenital heart disease, necrotizing enterocolitis, gram-negative bacterial sepsis, rickettsial infections, and some severe viral infections. The disorder is characterized by inappropriate systemic activation and acceleration of the normal clotting mechanism.

Pathophysiology

DIC occurs when the first stage of the coagulation process is abnormally stimulated. Although there is no well-defined sequence of events, two distinct phases can be identified. First, when the clotting mechanism is triggered in the circulation, thrombin is generated in greater amounts than can be neutralized by the body. Consequently, there is rapid conversion of fibrinogen to fibrin with aggregation and destruction of platelets. If local and widespread fibrin deposition in blood vessels takes place, obstruction and eventual necrosis of tissues occur. Second, the fibrinolytic mechanism is activated, causing extensive destruction of clotting factors. With a deficiency of clotting factors the child is vulnerable to uncontrollable hemorrhage into vital organs. An additional complication is damage and hemolysis of RBCs (Fig. 46-2).

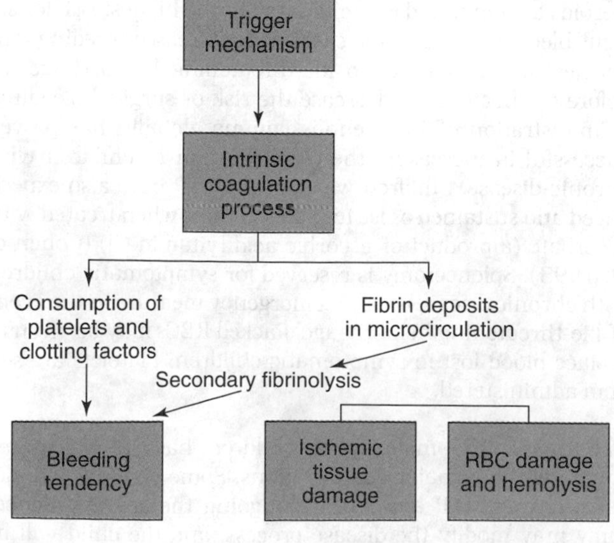

Fig. 46-2 Effects of DIC.

Diagnostic Evaluation

DIC is suspected when there is an increased tendency to bleed (Box 46-10). Hematologic findings include prolonged prothrombin (PT), partial PTT, and thrombin times. There is a profoundly depressed platelet count, fragmented RBCs, and depleted fibrinogen.

Therapeutic Management

Treatment of DIC is directed toward control of the underlying or initiating cause, which in most instances stops the coagulation problem spontaneously. Platelets and fresh frozen plasma may be needed to replace lost plasma components, especially in the child whose underlying disease remains uncontrolled. The extremely ill newborn may require exchange transfusion with fresh blood. The intravenous administration of heparin to inhibit thrombin formation is most often restricted to severe cases.

Nursing Care Management

The goals of nursing care are to be aware of the possibility of DIC in the severely ill child and to recognize signs that might indicate its presence. The skills needed to monitor intravenous infusion and blood transfusions and to administer heparin are the same as for any child receiving these therapies (see p. 1534). See Chapter 38 for care of the child with a life-threatening illness.

EPISTAXIS (NOSEBLEEDING)

Isolated and transient episodes of **epistaxis,** or nosebleeding, are common in childhood. The nose, especially the septum, is a highly vascular structure, and bleeding usually results from direct trauma, including blows to the nose, foreign bodies, and nose picking, or from mucosal inflammation associated with allergic rhinitis and upper respiratory infections. The bleeding ordinarily stops spontaneously or with minimum pressure and requires no medical evaluation or therapy.

Recurrent epistaxis and severe bleeding may indicate an underlying disease, particularly vascular abnormalities, leukemia, thrombocytopenia, and clotting factor deficiency diseases, such as hemophilia and von Willebrand disease. Nosebleeds are sometimes associated with the administration of aspirin, even in normal amounts. Persistent episodes of epistaxis require medical evaluation.

Nursing Care Management

In the event of a nosebleed an essential intervention is to remain calm. Otherwise the child will become more agitated,

BOX 46-10
Clinical Manifestations of DIC

- Petechiae
- Purpura
- Bleeding from openings in the skin
  - Venipuncture site
  - Surgical incision
- Bleeding from umbilicus, trachea (newborn)
- Evidence of gastrointestinal bleeding
- Hypotension
- Organ dysfunction from infarction and ischemia

EMERGENCY

EPISTAXIS

Have child sit up and lean forward (not lying down).
Apply continuous pressure to nose with thumb and forefinger for at least 10 minutes.
Insert cotton or wadded tissue into each nostril and apply ice or cold cloth to bridge of nose if bleeding persists.
Keep child calm and quiet.

the blood pressure will increase, and the child will not cooperate. Although in most instances a nosebleed is not serious, it can be very upsetting to family members as well. They need reassurance that the loss of blood is not serious and that the bleeding usually stops within 10 to 15 minutes.

To control the bleeding the child is instructed to sit up and lean forward (not to lie down) to avoid aspiration of blood. Most of the nosebleeding originates in the anterior part of the nasal septum and can be controlled by applying pressure to the soft lower portion of the nose with the thumb and forefinger (see the Emergency box above). During this time the child breathes through the mouth.

If hemorrhage continues, the child should be evaluated by a practitioner, who may pack the nose with epinephrine-soaked gauze. After a nosebleed, petroleum or water-soluble jelly can be inserted into each nostril to prevent crusting of old blood and to lessen the likelihood of the child's picking at the nose and restarting the hemorrhage. If a child has numerous nosebleeds, factors believed to increase the likelihood of bleeding are eliminated, such as discouraging nose picking or altering the household humidity by placing a cool-mist humidifier in the child's room. Repeated bleeding episodes may be an indication to refer the child for evaluation for the possibility of a bleeding disorder.

Neoplastic Disorders

Neoplastic disorders are the leading cause of death from disease in children past infancy, and almost half of all childhood cancers involve the blood or blood-forming organs. Leukemias and lymphomas are discussed here. Malignant solid tumors of childhood are discussed elsewhere in relation to the tissues or organs involved.

LEUKEMIAS

Leukemia, cancer of the blood-forming tissues, is the most common form of childhood cancer. The annual incidence is 4.2 per 100,000 in white children under 15 years of age and 2.4 per 100,000 in black children (Poplack, 1993). It occurs more frequently in males than in females after age 1 year, and the peak onset is between 2 and 6 years of age. It is one of the forms of cancer that has demonstrated dramatic improvements in survival rates. Current 4-year survival rates for children with acute lymphoid leukemia exceed 80% in major research centers, and a majority of these children may be cured (Pediatric Oncology Group, 1992). (See also Prognosis, p. 1519.)

Classification

Leukemia is a broad term given to a group of malignant diseases of the bone marrow and lymphatic system. Current research has revealed that it is a complex disease of varying heterogeneity. Consequently, classification has become increasingly complex, sophisticated, and essential, since identification of the subtype of leukemia has therapeutic and prognostic implications (see pp. 1518-1519). The following is a brief overview of the major classification systems currently being used.

Morphology. Leukemia is classified according to its predominant cell type and level of maturity, as described by the following:

- **Lympho**—for leukemias involving the lymphoid or lymphatic system
- **Myelo**—for those of myeloid (bone marrow) origin
- **Blastic and acute**—for those involving immature cells
- **Cytic and chronic**—for those involving mature cells

In children, two forms are generally recognized: *acute lymphoid leukemia (ALL)* and *acute nonlymphoid (myelogenous) leukemia (ANLL or AML)*. Synonyms for ALL include lymphatic, lymphocytic, lymphoblastic, and lymphoblastoid leukemia. Usually the terms *stem cell* or *blast cell leukemia* also refer to the lymphoid type of leukemia. Synonyms for the AML type include granulocytic, myelocytic, monocytic, myelogenous, monoblastic, and monomyeloblastic. There are also much rarer forms of leukemia that are named for the specific cell involved, such as basophilic or eosinophilic leukemia.

Cytochemical markers. Leukemic cells demonstrate different reactions when they are exposed to certain chemicals. For example, terminal deoxynucleotidyl transferase is able to provide excellent differentiation between ALL and AML.

Chromosomal studies. Chromosomal analysis has become an important tool in the diagnosis of ALL. For example, children with trisomy 21 have 15 times the risk of other children for developing ALL (Poplack, 1993).

Children who are hyperdiploid (more chromosomes) have a better prognosis. Translocation of chromosomes 4 and 10 is also associated with a better prognosis (Poplack, 1993).

Cell-surface immunologic markers. Cell-surface antigens have permitted differentiation of ALL into three broad classes: non-T, non-B-cell ALL (also called early pre-B-cell), B-cell ALL, and T-cell ALL. Children with non-T, non-B-cell ALL have the best prognosis, especially if they have the common ALL antigen, known as CALLA positive, on their cell surfaces (Poplack, 1993).

Pathophysiology

Leukemia is an unrestricted proliferation of immature WBCs in the blood-forming tissues of the body. Although not a "tumor" as such, the leukemic cells demonstrate the same neoplastic properties as solid cancers. Therefore the resulting pathologic condition and clinical manifestations are caused by infiltration and replacement of any tissue of the body with nonfunctional leukemic cells. Highly vascular organs, such as the spleen and liver, are the most severely affected.

To understand the pathophysiology of the leukemic process, it is important to clarify two common misconceptions. First, although leukemia is an overproduction of WBCs, most often in the acute form the leukocyte count is low (hence, the term *leukemia*). Second, these immature cells do not deliberately attack and destroy the normal blood cells or vascular tissues. Cellular destruction takes place by infiltration and subsequent competition for metabolic elements (Table 46-3).

In all types of leukemia the proliferating cells depress the production of formed elements of the blood in bone marrow by competing for and depriving the normal cells of the essential nutrients for metabolism. The most frequent presenting signs and symptoms of leukemia are a result of infiltration of the bone marrow. The three main consequences are (1) *anemia* from decreased erythrocytes, (2) *infection* from neutropenia, and (3) *bleeding tendencies* from decreased platelet production. The invasion of the bone marrow with leukemic cells gradually causes a weakening of the bone and a tendency toward fractures. As leukemic cells invade the periosteum, increasing pressure causes severe pain.

The spleen, liver, and lymph glands demonstrate marked infiltration, enlargement, and eventually fibrosis. Hepatosplenomegaly is typically more common than lymphadenopathy. The next most important site of involvement is the central nervous system. The usual effect of leukemic infiltration is increased intracranial pressure, which causes the signs and symptoms normally associated with this condition. Cranial nerves may also be involved, and the signs and symptoms observed reflect the area affected.

Leukemic cells may also invade the testes, kidneys, prostate, ovaries, gastrointestinal tract, and lungs. With long-term survivors becoming more common, such sites of leukemia invasion, especially the testes, are becoming more important clinically.

The immense metabolic needs of proliferating leukemic cells eventually deprive all body cells of nutrients necessary for survival. Obviously, in addition to the risk of death from infection and hemorrhage, uncontrolled growth of leukemic cells can also terminate in metabolic starvation.

TABLE 46-3 Pathology and related clinical manifestations of leukemia

ORGAN OR TISSUE	CONSEQUENCES	MANIFESTATIONS
Bone marrow dysfunction	Decreased RBCs—anemia	Pallor, fatigue
	Neutropenia—infection	Fever
	Decreased platelets—bleeding tendencies	Hemorrhage (petechiae)
	Invasion of bone marrow—bone weakness; invasion of periosteum	Tendency toward fractures Pain
Liver Spleen Lymph glands	Infiltration, enlargement, eventual fibrosis	Hepatomegaly Splenomegaly Lymphadenopathy
Central nervous system		
Meninges	Increased intracranial pressure, ventricular enlargement Meningeal irritation	Severe headache Vomiting Irritability, lethargy Papilledema Eventual coma Pain Stiff neck and back
Hypermetabolism	Cell deprivation of nutrients by invading cells	Muscle wasting Weight loss Anorexia Fatigue

Diagnostic Evaluation

Leukemia is usually suspected by the history, physical manifestations (Table 46-3), and a peripheral blood smear that contains immature forms of leukocytes, frequently combined with low blood counts. Definitive diagnosis is based on bone marrow aspiration or biopsy. Typically the bone marrow is hypercellular, with primarily blast cells. Once the diagnosis is confirmed, a lumbar puncture is performed to determine if there is any central nervous system involvement, although a very small number of children have such involvement at the time of diagnosis, and most are asymptomatic.

Therapeutic Management

Treatment of leukemia involves the use of chemotherapeutic agents with or without cranial irradiation in three phases: (1) *induction therapy*, which achieves a complete remission or disappearance of leukemic cells; (2) *central nervous system prophylactic therapy*, which prevents leukemic cells from invading the central nervous system; and (3) *maintenance with intensification therapy* (consolidation), which serves to maintain the remission phase. Although the combination of drugs and radiation may vary according to institutions, the prognostic or risk characteristics of the patient, and the type of leukemia being treated, the following general principles for each phase are employed quite consistently.

Remission induction. Almost immediately after confirmation of the diagnosis, induction therapy is begun and lasts for 4 to 6 weeks. The principal drugs used for induction in ALL are corticosteroids (especially prednisone), vincristine, and L-asparaginase, with or without doxorubicin. Drug therapy for AML includes doxorubicin or daunomycin and cytosine arabinoside; various other drugs may be used.

Since many of the drugs also cause myelosuppression of normal blood elements, the period immediately after a remission can be critical. The body is defenseless against and highly susceptible to infection and spontaneous hemorrhage. Consequently, supportive therapy during this time is essential.

Central nervous system prophylactic therapy. Treatment of the central nervous system consists of intrathecal chemotherapy with methotrexate, cytarabine, and hydrocortisone. Because of the concern regarding late effects of cranial irradiation, this treatment is reserved for high-risk patients and/or those with central nervous system disease.

Once complete remission is obtained, a period of intensified treatment is administered to further reduce the leukemia burden. Drugs commonly used during consolidation include methotrexate, cytosine arabinoside, and L-asparaginase.

Maintenance therapy. Maintenance therapy is begun after completion of successful induction and consolidation therapy to preserve the remission and further lessen the number of leukemic cells. As with induction therapy, combined drug regimens have been more successful in maintaining remissions and preventing drug resistance. Also, during maintenance therapy, weekly CBCs are taken to evaluate the marrow's response to the drugs.

Reinduction following relapse. When the presence of leukemic cells are observed in the bone marrow, central nervous system, or testes, the child has relapsed. Therapy for the child who has relapsed includes reinduction with prednisone and vincristine, along with a combination of other drugs not previously used. Once remission occurs, central nervous system preventive therapy and maintenance therapy follow as outlined before.

Bone marrow transplantation. Bone marrow transplants have been used successfully for treating children who have ALL and AML. Bone marrow transplantation is not recommended for children with ALL during the first remission because of the excellent results possible with chemotherapy. Because of the poorer prognosis in children with AML, transplantation may be considered during the first remission (Johnson, 1991).

A small number of hematopoietic stem cells circulate in the peripheral blood. These peripheral blood stem cells (PBSCs) are capable of differentiating into the specialized cells of the hematologic system including RBCs, WBCs, and platelets. PBSC transplantation may be used either as an alternative to or in conjunction with bone marrow transplantation to restore bone marrow function after myeloablative therapy (Hooper and Santas, 1994). Patients receiving PBSC transplantation are hospitalized for a shorter period of time because engraftment occurs much sooner. This therapy is undergoing research to learn more about its usefulness.

Prognosis. The most important prognostic factors for determining long-term survival for children with ALL (in addition to treatment) are (1) the initial WBC count, (2) the child's age at the time of diagnosis, (3) the type of cell involved, (4) the sex of the child, and (5) karyotype analysis. Children with a normal or low WBC count and who have non-T, non-B-cell ALL and are CALLA positive have a much better prognosis than those with a high count or other cell types. Children diagnosed between 2 and 9 years of age have consistently demonstrated a better outlook than those diagnosed before 2 or after 10 years of age, and females appear to have a more favorable prognosis than males. Children with a deoxyribonucleic acid (DNA) index greater than 1.16 (hyperdiploid) and translocation of chromosomes 4 and 10 have a better prognosis (Poplack, 1993). In addition, it appears that the more rapid the induction of a remission in AML, the better the chance for an ultimate long-term continuous remission.

Late effects of treatment. While vigorous treatment of childhood cancers has resulted in dramatically improved survival rates, there is increasing concern regarding late effects—adverse changes related to treatment modalities—and recurrence of the disease process. Almost no organ is exempt, and almost every antineoplastic agent, including and especially irradiation, is responsible for some adverse effect. There is a substantially increased risk of developing secondary cancers.

In children with leukemia, impairment caused by treatment with cranial irradiation and intrathecal chemotherapy is of particular concern, especially the risk of developing central nervous system tumors (Allen, 1993). In addition, intellectual and motor function may be impaired because of interference with neural development before maturation of the brain is complete. Children under the age of 5 years are at the highest risk for these complications.

Nursing Care Management

Nursing care of the child with leukemia is directly related to the regimen of therapy. General psychologic interventions during each phase of therapy are discussed in Chapter 38.

Assessment

The history and physical examination often yield the first clues to the presence of neoplastic disease. Vague complaints, such as fatigue, pain in a limb, night sweating, lack of appetite, headache, and general malaise, may be the earliest clues and must be taken seriously. Most children have a great deal of energy and if sick with a cold or other childhood affliction recover quickly and completely. Any evidence of a lingering disorder is often the first sign of leukemia.

Nursing Diagnoses

A number of nursing diagnoses become apparent following an assessment of the child with leukemia and the family. Some are considered in the Nursing Care Plan on pp. 1526-1528. Others will be identified in specific situations.

Planning

The goals of nursing care for the child with leukemia and the family include the following:

1. The child will receive appropriate primary health care.
2. The child and family will be prepared for diagnostic and therapeutic procedures.
3. The child will experience minimal complications of myelosuppression.
4. Problems of irradiation and drug toxicity will be managed.
5. The child and family will receive adequate support and education.

Implementation

Nursing care of the child with leukemia is directly related to the regimen of therapy. Nurses working with families of children with cancer have a significant supportive role in helping them understand the various therapies, preventing or managing expected side effects or toxicities, observing for late effects of treatment, and helping the child and family live as normal a life as possible and cope with the emotional aspects of the disease. Education is a constant feature of the nursing role, especially in terms of new treatments, clinical trials, and home care.

Because of the anxiety generated by the diagnosis of leukemia, some families may resort to unproven methods of therapy that are frequently referred to as "cancer quackery." These unorthodox approaches are a threat to every cancer family. Nurses can be instrumental in working against cancer quackery by being aware of factors that increase a family's likelihood of seeking unproven remedies, communicating effectively with families about the diagnosis and forms of therapy, and providing all possible support and reassurance during treatment.

Prepare child and family for diagnostic and therapeutic procedures. From the time before diagnosis to cessation of therapy, children must undergo several tests, the most traumatic of which are bone marrow aspiration or biopsy and lumbar punctures. Multiple finger punctures and venipunctures for blood analysis and drug infusion are common occurrences for several years after the diagnosis. Therefore the child needs an explanation of why each procedure is done and what can be expected. In addition, effective pharmacologic, including conscious and unconscious sedation, and nonpharmacologic strategies are used to reduce discomfort associated with these painful procedures.

Relieve pain. The effective use of analgesia is especially important when the malignant process is uncontrolled and causes pain. Bone pain is particularly acute. Dosages of opioids (narcotics) are adjusted or *titrated to the child's needs* and administered *around the clock* for optimum pain control. Nonpharmacologic strategies should be implemented as needed but are not substitutes for pharmacologic management. The reader is encouraged to review the principles of pain assessment and management presented in Chapter 41 and preparation for procedures in Chapter 42 when caring for a child with leukemia.

Prevent complications of myelosuppression. The leukemic process and most of the chemotherapeutic agents cause myelosuppression. The reduced numbers of blood cells result in secondary problems of infection, bleeding tendencies, and anemia. Supportive care involves both medical and nursing management. Because they are so closely linked, they are discussed together rather than separately.

Infection. A frequent complication of treatment for childhood cancer is overwhelming infection secondary to neutropenia. The child is most susceptible to overwhelming infection during three phases of the disease: (1) at the time of diagnosis and relapse when the leukemic process has replaced normal leukocytes, (2) during immunosuppressive therapy, and (3) after prolonged antibiotic therapy that predisposes to the growth of resistant organisms. However, the use of granulocyte colony stimulating factor (GCSF) has reduced the incidence and duration of infection in children receiving treatment for cancer.

The first defense against infection is prevention. When the child is hospitalized, the nurse employs all measures to control transfer of infection. These typically include the use of a private room, restriction of all visitors and health personnel with active infection, and strict handwashing technique with an antiseptic solution. In some research centers, special germ-free environments are available during complete myelosuppression from intensive chemotherapy or for bone marrow transplant.

Nursing ALERT

Because the usual viral infections of childhood are particularly dangerous, the child is *not* immunized against these diseases (measles, rubella, mumps, and polio) until the immune system is capable of responding appropriately to the vaccine. If given when the immune system is depressed, the attenuated virus can result in an overwhelming infection. The child can receive the Salk (inactivated) vaccine for poliomyelitis. The varicella (chickenpox) vaccine is being given to certain children with ALL (see Immunizations, Chapter 33).

The child is evaluated for potential sites of infection (e.g., mucosal ulceration, skin abrasion or tear, such as a hangnail) and observed for any elevation in temperature. To identify the source of infection, chest radiographs and blood, stool, urine, and nasopharyngeal cultures are taken. Intravenous antibiotics are administered, and if this therapy is prolonged a venous access device, such as a peripherally inserted central catheter (PICC), or intermittent infusion device (saline lock or PRN adaptor), or implanted infusion port, is used to maintain an intravenous access.

Prevention of infection continues to be a priority after discharge from the hospital. Ordinarily the child is allowed to return to school when the WBC count is at a satisfactory level, usually an absolute neutrophil count (ANC) greater than $500/mm^3$. At all times, family members are encouraged to practice good handwashing to avoid introducing pathogens into the home. The child may need to be isolated from school contacts in the event of an outbreak of a childhood disease, especially chickenpox.

Nutrition is another important component of infection prevention. An adequate protein-caloric intake provides the child with better host defenses against infection and increased tolerance to chemotherapy and irradiation. However, providing optimum nutrition during periods of anorexia and vomiting from chemotherapy is a tremendous challenge (see Feeding the Sick Child, Chapter 42).

Hemorrhage. Before the use of transfused platelets, hemorrhage was a leading cause of death in leukemia. Now most bleeding episodes can be prevented or controlled with the administration of platelet concentrates or platelet-rich plasma.

Since infection increases the tendency toward hemorrhage, and since bleeding sites become more easily infected, skin punctures are avoided whenever possible. When finger sticks, venipunctures, intramuscular injections, and bone marrow aspirations are performed, aseptic technique must be employed, as well as continued observation for bleeding. Meticulous mouth care is essential, since gingival bleeding with resultant mucositis is a frequent problem. Because the rectal area is prone to ulceration from various drugs, feces and urine are removed immediately and the perianal area is washed. Rectal temperatures are avoided to prevent trauma. Children are advised to avoid activities that might cause injury or bleeding, such as riding bicycles or skateboards, climbing trees or playground equipment, and playing contact sports.

Platelet transfusions are generally reserved for active bleeding episodes that do not respond to local treatment and that may occur during induction or relapse therapy. Epistaxis and gingival bleeding are the most common. The nurse teaches parents and older children measures to control nosebleeding (see p. 1517). Pressure at the site without disturbing clot formation is the general rule.

During bleeding episodes the parents and child need much emotional support. The sight of oozing blood is very upsetting. Often parents will request a platelet transfusion, unaware of the need for trying local measures first. The nurse can be instrumental in allaying anxiety by acknowledging the feelings of the child and family and explaining the reason for delaying a platelet transfusion until absolutely necessary.

Anemia. Initially anemia may be profound from complete replacement of the bone marrow by leukemic cells. During induction therapy, blood transfusions with packed RBCs may be necessary to raise the hemoglobin to levels approaching 10 g/dl. The usual precautions in caring for the child with anemia are instituted (see p. 1504).

Use precautions in administering and handling chemotherapeutic agents. Many chemotherapeutic agents are vesicants (sclerosing agents) that can cause severe cellular damage if even minute amounts of the drug infiltrate surrounding tissue. Only nurses experienced with chemotherapeutic agents should administer vesicants. Guidelines are available* and must be followed exactly to prevent tissue damage to patients. Interventions for extravasation vary, but each nurse should be aware of the institution's policies and implement them at once.

Nursing ALERT

Chemotherapeutic drugs must be given through a free-flowing intravenous line. The infusion is stopped *immediately* if any sign of infiltration (pain, stinging, swelling, or redness at the insertion site) occurs.

In addition to extravasation, a potentially fatal complication is anaphylaxis, especially from L-asparaginase, teniposide (VM-26), etoposide VP-16), bleomycin, and cisplatin. Nursing responsibilities include prevention of, recognition of, and preparation for serious reactions. Prevention begins with a careful history for known allergy.

Cancer Chemotherapy Guidelines can be obtained from the Oncology Nursing Society, 501 Holiday Dr., Pittsburgh, PA 15220-2749; (412) 921-7373.

Nursing ALERT

When chemotherapeutic and immunologic agents are given, the child must be observed for 20 minutes after the infusion for signs of anaphylaxis (cyanosis, hypotension, wheezing, severe urticaria). Emergency equipment (especially blood pressure monitor and bag-valve-mask) and emergency drugs (especially oxygen, epinephrine, antihistamine, aminophylline, corticosteroids, and vasopressors) must be available. If a reaction is suspected, the drug is discontinued, the intravenous line is flushed with saline solution, and the child's vital signs and subsequent responses are monitored.

In addition to the many responsibilities nurses must have in regard to the child and family, they must also use safeguards to protect themselves. Handling chemotherapeutic agents may present risks to handlers and to their offspring, although the exact degree of risk is not known.

Some children have a venous access device, which facilitates administration of intravenous drugs. During treatment and remission, many drugs are taken orally at home. Compliance with the medication schedule is essential, and nurses play an important role in educating the family about the drugs and encouraging adherence to the plan.*

Manage problems of drug toxicity. Chemotherapy presents several nursing challenges. The complexity of the treatment protocols are often overwhelming to families. In addition, each therapy is associated with a number of predictable side effects. Nurses must be aware of these side effects and use judgment in recognizing which are normal reactions and which indicate toxicity (Box 46-11).

Nausea and vomiting. The nausea and vomiting that occur shortly after administration of several of the drugs and as a result of cranial or abdominal radiation can be profound.

The serotonin-receptor antagonists (e.g., ondansetron [Zofran]) are effective in the control of nausea and vomiting occurring after emetogenic chemotherapy and radiation therapy. When combined with dexamethasone, these agents are the treatment of choice in the prevention of cisplatin-induced emesis (Tonato et al, 1994).

The most beneficial regimen for antiemetic control has been the administration of the antiemetic *before* the chemotherapy begins. The goal is to prevent the child from ever experiencing nausea or vomiting, thus preventing development of anticipatory symptoms (the conditioned response of developing nausea and vomiting before receiving the drug) (Hockenberry-Eaton and Benner, 1990).

Anorexia. Loss of appetite is a direct consequence of the chemotherapy and/or irradiation. It is a major problem for parents because it is the one area they feel responsible for, particularly when so many other facets of care are outside their control. There are no universally successful techniques for encouraging a sick child to eat. However, the guidelines in Chapter 42 can be helpful during the anorexic period and can prevent additional problems during the remission.

*Home care instructions on caring for a venous access device and administering medications to children are available in Wong DL: *Wong and Whaley's clinical manual of pediatric nursing*, ed 4, St Louis, 1996, Mosby.

BOX 46-11

Summary of Selected Chemotherapeutic Agents Used in the Treatment of Childhood Leukemias and Lymphomas*

Bleomycin (Blenoxane)

Administration

IV, IM, SC†

Side effects and toxicity

Allergic reaction—fever, chills, hypotension, anaphylaxis
Fever (nonallergic)
N/V (mild)‡
Stomatitis
Cumulative dose effects include:
Skin—rash, hyperpigmentation, thickening, ulceration, peeling, nail changes, alopecia
Lungs—pneumonitis with infiltrate that can progress to fatal fibrosis

Comments and specific nursing considerations

Should give test dose (SC) before therapeutic dose administered
Have emergency drugs at bedside
Hypersensitivity occurs with first one to two doses
May give acetaminophen before drug to reduce likelihood of fever
Concentration of drug in skin and lungs accounts for toxic effects

Corticosteroids (Prednisone)

Administration

PO; IM or IV rarely used

Side effects and toxicity, short-term

For short-term use, no acute toxicity
Usual side effects are mild: moon face, fluid retention, weight gain, mood changes, increased appetite, gastric irritation, insomnia, susceptibility to infection

Comments and specific nursing considerations

Explain expected effects, especially in terms of body image, increased appetite, and personality changes
Monitor weight gain
Recommend moderate salt restriction
Administer with antacid and early in morning (sometimes given every other day to minimize side effects)
May need to disguise bitter taste (crush tablet and mix with syrup, jam, ice cream, or other highly flavored substance; use ice to numb tongue before administration; place tablet in gelatin capsule if child can swallow it)
Observe for potential infection sites; usual inflammatory response and fever are absent

Side effects and toxicity, long-term

Long-term effects of chronic steroid administration are mood changes, hirsutism, trunk obesity (buffalo hump), thin extremities, muscle wasting and weakness, osteoporosis, poor wound healing, bruising, potassium loss, gastric bleeding, hypertension, diabetes mellitus, growth retardation

Comments and specific nursing considerations

Same as for short-term use; in addition, encourage foods high in potassium (bananas, raisins, prunes, coffee, chocolate)
Test stools for occult blood
Monitor blood pressure
Test blood for sugar and urine for acetone
Observe for signs of abrupt steroid withdrawal: flulike symptoms, hypotension, hypoglycemia, shock

Daunorubicin (Daunomycin, Rubidomycin) and Doxorubicin (Adriamycin, Doxyrubicin)

Administration

IV

Side effects and toxicity

N/V (moderate)
Stomatitis
BMD§ (7 to 14 days later)
Fever, chills
Local phlebitis
Alopecia
Cumulative-dose toxicity includes:
Cardiac abnormalities
Electrocardiographic (ECG) changes
Heart failure

Comments and specific nursing considerations

Vesicant|| (extravasation may *not* cause pain)
Use only sterile distilled water as a diluent
Observe for any changes in heart rate or rhythm and signs of failure
Cumulative dose must not exceed 400 mg/m^2
Warn parents that drug causes urine to turn red (for up to 12 days after administration); this is normal, not hematuria

L-Asparaginase (Elspar)

Administration

IM, IV

Side effects and toxicity

Allergic reactions (including anaphylactic shock)
Fever
N/V (mild)
Anorexia
Weight loss
Arthralgia
Toxicity:
Liver dysfunction
Hyperglycemia
Renal failure
Pancreatitis

Comments and specific nursing considerations

Have emergency drugs at bedside
Record signs of allergic reaction, such as urticaria, facial edema, hypotension, or abdominal cramps
Check weight daily
Normally, blood urea nitrogen (BUN) and ammonia levels rise as a result of drug; not evidence of liver damage
Check urine for sugar and blood amylase

Mechlorethamine (Nitrogen Mustard, Mustargen)

Administration

IV, IT

Side effects and toxicity

N/V ($^1/_2$-8 hours later) (severe)
BMD (2-3 weeks later)
Alopecia
Local phlebitis

Comments and specific nursing considerations

Vesicant

*Includes principal drugs used in the treatment of childhood leukemias and lymphomas. Several other conventional and investigational chemotherapeutic agents may be employed in the treatment regimen.

BOX 46-11

Summary of Selected Chemotherapeutic Agents Used in the Treatment of Childhood Leukemias and Lymphomas—cont'd

Mercaptopurine (6-MP, Purinethol)

Administration

PO

Side effects and toxicity

N/V (mild)
Diarrhea
Anorexia
Stomatitis
BMD (4 to 6 weeks later)
Immunosuppression
Dermatitis
Less commonly may be hepatic dysfunction

Comments and specific nursing considerations

6-MP is an analog of xanthine; therefore allopurinol (Zyloprim) delays its metabolism and increases its potency, necessitating a lower dose (1/3 to 1/4) of 6-MP

Methotrexate (MTX, Amethopterin)

Administration

PO, IV, IM, IT
May be given in conventional doses (mg/m^2) or high doses (g/m^2)

Side effects and toxicity

N/V (severe at high doses)
Diarrhea
Mucosal ulceration (2 to 5 days later)
BMD (10 days later)
Immunosuppression
Dermatitis
Photosensitivity
Alopecia (uncommon)
Toxic effects include:
- Hepatitis (fibrosis)
- Osteoporosis
- Nephropathy
- Pneumonitis (fibrosis)

Neurologic toxicity with IT use—pain at injection site, meningismus (signs of meningitis without actual inflammation), especially fever and headache; potential sequelae—transient or permanent hemiparesis, convulsions, dementia, death

Comments and specific nursing considerations

Side effects and toxicity are dose related
Potency and toxicity are increased by reduced renal function, salicylates, sulfonamides, and aminobenzoic acid; avoid use of these substances, such as aspirin
Avoid exposure to sun
High-dose therapy:
- Citrovorum factor (folinic acid or leucovorin) decreases cytotoxic action of MTX; used as an antidote for overdose and to enhance normal cell recovery after high-dose therapy; avoid use of vitamins containing folic acid during MTX therapy unless prescribed by physician

IT therapy:
- Drug *must* be mixed with preservative-free diluent
- Report signs of neurotoxicity immediately

Procarbazine (Matulane)

Administration

PO

Side effects and toxicity

N/V (moderate)
BMD (3 to 4 weeks later)
Lethargy
Dermatitis
Myalgia
Arthralgia
Less commonly:
- Stomatitis
- Neuropathy
- Alopecia
- Diarrhea

Comments and specific nursing considerations

Central nervous system (CNS) depressants (phenothiazines, barbiturates) enhance CNS symptoms
Monoamine oxidase (MAO) inhibition sometimes occurs; therefore all other drugs are avoided unless medically approved; red wine, fava beans, and broad bean pods are avoided

Vincristine (Oncovin) and Vinblastine (Velban)

Administration

IV

Side effects and toxicity

Neurotoxicity (less severe with vinblastine)—paresthesia (numbness); ataxia; weakness; footdrop; hyporeflexia; constipation (dynamic ileus); hoarseness (vocal cord paralysis); abdominal, chest, and jaw pain; mental depression
Fever
N/V (mild)
BMD (minimal; 7 to 14 days later)
Alopecia

Comments and specific nursing considerations

Vesicant
Report signs of neurotoxicity because may necessitate cessation of drug
Individuals with underlying neurologic problems may be more prone to neurotoxicity
Monitor stool patterns closely; administer stool softener
Excreted primarily by liver into biliary system; administer cautiously to anyone with biliary disease

Cytosine Arabinoside (Ara-C, Cytosar, Cytarabine, Arabinosyl Cytosine)

Administration

IV, IM, SC, IT

Side effects and toxicity

N/V (mild)
BMD (7 to 14 days later)
Mucosal ulceration
Immunosuppression
Hepatitis (usually subclinical)

Comments and specific nursing considerations

Crosses blood-brain barrier
Use with caution in patients with hepatic dysfunction

†*IV,* Intravenous; *IT,* intrathecal; *PO,* by mouth, *IM,* intramuscular; *SC,* subcutaneous.

Continued.

‡*N/V,* Nausea and vomiting. Mild = <20% incidence; moderate = 20% to 70% incidence; severe = >75% incidence.
§*BMD,* Bone marrow depression.
| |Vesicants (sclerosing agents) can cause severe cellular damage if even minute amounts of the drug infiltrate surrounding tissue.

BOX 46-11

Summary of Selected Chemotherapeutic Agents Used in the Treatment of Childhood Leukemias and Lymphomas*—cont'd

Cyclophosphamide (Cytoxan, CTX, Neosar)
Administration

PO, IV, IM

Side effects and toxicity

N/V (3 to 4 hours later) (severe at high doses)
BMD (10 to 14 days later)
Alopecia
Hemorrhagic cystitis
Severe immunosuppression
Stomatitis (rare)
Hyperpigmentation
Transverse ridging of nails
Infertility

Comments and specific nursing considerations

BMD has platelet-sparing effect
Give dose early in day to allow adequate fluids afterward
Force fluids before administering drug and for 2 days after to prevent chemical cystitis; encourage frequent voiding even during night
Warn parents to report signs of burning on urination or hematuria to practitioner

Dacarbazine (DTIC-Dome)
Administration

IV

Side effects and toxicity

N/V (especially after first dose) (severe)
BMD (7 to 14 days later)
Alopecia
Flulike syndrome
Burning sensation in vein during infusion (not extravasation)

Comments and specific nursing considerations

Vesicant (less sclerosive)
Must be given cautiously in patients with renal dysfunction
Decrease IV rate or use warm moist towels on IV site to decrease burning

Some children still do not eat despite these approaches. When loss of appetite and weight persist, the nurse should investigate the family situation to determine if there are any factors (such as conditioned aversion to food, environmental stress related to eating, controlling behavior, or anger) that might be contributing to the problem. Nasogastric (NG) tube feedings or total parenteral nutrition may be implemented for children with significant nutritional problems.

Mucosal ulceration. One of the most distressing side effects of several drugs is gastrointestinal mucosal cell damage, which can produce ulcers anywhere along the alimentary tract. Oral ulcers greatly compound anorexia because eating is extremely uncomfortable, but the following interventions may be helpful: (1) provide a bland, moist, soft diet appropriate for the child's age and preferences; (2) use a soft sponge toothbrush (Toothettes)* or cotton-tipped applicator; (3) provide frequent mouthwashes with normal saline solution (using a solution of 1 teaspoon of table salt and 1 pint of water) or sodium bicarbonate mouthrinses (using a solution of 1 teaspoon of baking soda in 1 quart of water); and (4) use local anesthetics such as Chloraseptic lozenges or nonprescription preparations without alcohol, such as Orabase or Ulcerase. Although local anesthetics are effective in temporarily relieving the pain, many children dislike the taste and numb feeling they produce.

Other preparations that may be used to prevent or treat mucositis include chlorhexidine gluconate (Peridex) because of its dual effectiveness against candidal as well as bacterial, infections, antifungal troches (lozenges) or mouthwash, and lip balm, such as Aquaphor, to keep the lips moist. Agents that should not be used are lemon glycerine swabs (irritate eroded tissue and can decay teeth), hydrogen peroxide (delays healing by breaking down protein), and milk of magnesia (dries mucosa) (Galbraith et al, 1991).

Nursing ALERT

Viscous lidocaine is not recommended for young children; if applied to the pharynx, it may depress the gag reflex, increasing the risk of aspiration. Seizures have been rarely associated with the use of oral viscous lidocaine (Hess and Walson, 1988).

Stomatitis may cause such difficulty with eating that the child may require hospitalization for hydration, parenteral nutrition, and pain control (often with intravenous morphine). The child will usually choose the foods that are best tolerated, and the nurse should encourage parents to relax any eating pressures. Since the stomatitis is a temporary condition, once the ulcers heal the child can resume good food habits. Dental hygiene can become a serious problem for children with orthodontic appliances. Sometimes it may be necessary to remove the braces to allow chemotherapy to continue.

Rectal ulcers are managed by meticulous toilet hygiene, and use of an occlusive ointment or dressing applied to the ulcerated area to promote epithelialization. Exposing the denuded skin to air, heat, or supplemental oxygen delays healing (see Process of Wound Healing, Chapter 50). Parents are advised to record bowel movements, since the child may voluntarily avoid defecation to prevent discomfort. Rectal temperatures and suppositories are contraindicated because the thermometer may further traumatize the area.

*Manufactured by Halbrand, Inc., Willoughby, Ohio.

Neuropathy. Vincristine and, to a lesser extent, vinblastine can cause various neurotoxic effects. Nursing interventions for management of these effects include (1) administering stool softeners or laxatives for severe constipation caused by decreased bowel innervation; (2) maintaining good body alignment and, if on bed rest, using a footboard or high-top shoes to minimize or prevent footdrop; (3) carrying out safety measures during ambulation because of weakness and numbing of the extremities, which may cause difficulty in walking or fine hand movement; and (4) providing a soft or liquid diet for severe jaw pain.

Hemorrhagic cystitis. Sterile hemorrhagic cystitis, a side effect of chemical irritation to the bladder from cyclophosphamide, can be decreased and often prevented by (1) a liberal fluid intake (at least one and a half times the recommended daily fluid requirement); (2) frequent voiding immediately after feeling the urge, before bed, and after arising; (3) administering the drug early in the day to allow for sufficient oral intake and voiding; and (4) administering mesna as ordered, an agent that provides protection to the bladder. If oral home administration is prescribed, the family needs *specific* instructions regarding exactly how much fluid the child must have.

Nursing ALERT

If signs of cystitis occur, such as burning on urination, prompt medical evaluation is needed.

Alopecia. Hair loss is a common side effect of several chemotherapeutic drugs and cranial irradiation, although not all children lose their hair during drug therapy. It is better to warn children and parents of this side effect than to allow them to think that it is only a remote possibility. A soft cotton cap is the most comfortable head wear for children. Polyester increases perspiration and causes itching. Other options include scarves, hats, or a wig. If the child chooses to wear a wig, encouraging the child to select one similar to his or her own hairstyle and color before the hair falls out is helpful in fostering later adjustment to hair loss. The nurse should also inform the family that hair regrows in 3 to 6 months and may be of a different color and texture. Frequently the hair is darker, thicker, and curlier than before. If the child chooses not to wear a wig, attention to some type of head covering, especially in cold climates and during exposure to sun, and scalp hygiene are important. The scalp should be washed like any other body part.

Moon face. Short-term steroid therapy provokes no acute toxicities and produces two beneficial reactions—increased appetite and a sense of well-being. However, it does produce alterations in body image, which, although not clinically significant, can be extremely distressing to older children. One of these is moon face, in which the child's face becomes rounded and puffy. It is not unusual for other children to make fun of the child with such remarks as "Miss Piggy," or "fat face." It is helpful to reassure children who experience such name-calling that after cessation of the drug the facial changes will return to normal. Unlike hair loss, little can be done to camouflage this obvious change. If the child resumes activity early in the course of treatment, the change may be less noticeable to peers than after a long absence.

Mood changes. Shortly after beginning steroid therapy, children experience a number of mood changes that range from feelings of well-being and euphoria to depression and irritability. If parents are unaware of these drug-induced changes, they may become unduly concerned. Therefore the nurse should warn them of the reactions and encourage them to discuss the behavioral changes with each other and with the child.

Provide continued physical care and emotional support. Because of the improved survival of these children, continued monitoring of physical and intellectual growth and development is essential. Nurses should stress the importance of regular follow-up care.

An important aspect of continued emotional support involves the prognosis. Although leukemia is no longer invariably fatal, it must be remembered that survival statistics are only average estimates and apply to those children treated with the latest protocols since diagnosis. For the low-risk child the chances may be better, but for the high-risk child they may be significantly poorer. Of those who do survive after discontinuing therapy, a portion will relapse. Therefore at present only the passage of time is positive confirmation of the child's being ultimately "cured" of the disease. Remission, even in excess of 5 years, cannot be equated with a cure. With increasing concern regarding late effects of treatment, continued surveillance of the child's health status is needed. The nurse who is working with family members must individualize information regarding the "numbers" and the potential risks. An understanding of each member's emotional needs, as well as competent care of physical ones, is essential to the positive, growth-promoting support of the family. Comprehensive emotional support for the family of the child with a potentially fatal illness is discussed in Chapter 38.

Evaluation

The effectiveness of nursing interventions is determined by continual reassessment and evaluation of care based on the following observational guidelines and expected outcomes:

1. Compare number of visits for primary health with recommended schedule of health supervision.
2. Monitor growth, development, and other aspects of regular health assessment; check mouth for adequacy of dental hygiene; review immunization record for age-appropriate vaccines and use of non–live virus preparations.
3. Interview child and family regarding their understanding of treatments and diagnostic tests.
4. Employ pain assessment techniques for procedural pain.
5. Make careful observations of physical status:
   Take vital signs regularly.
   Observe for evidence of bleeding, infection, neuropathy, cystitis, and mucosal ulceration.
   Observe and record intake and output.
6. Interview child and family and observe behaviors as a result of complications of therapies.
7. Interview child and family and observe behaviors that

Nursing Care Plan

THE CHILD WITH CANCER

Nursing Diagnosis: Risk for injury related to malignant process and treatment

Expected Outcome: Complications from chemotherapy are minimized, and the child exhibits signs of complete or partial remission.

• **NURSING INTERVENTIONS/*RATIONALES***

Administer chemotherapeutic agents per physician order and monitor IV site closely for signs of infiltration *to prevent severe tissue damage.*

Obtain allergy history *to prevent anaphylaxis.*

Observe child for at least 20 minutes after chemotherapy infusion *for signs of anaphylaxis* (cyanosis, wheezing, hypotension, urticaria); stop infusion and flush IV line reaction suspected *to minimize reaction;* have emergency equipment and drugs readily available *to prevent delay in treatment of anaphylactic reaction.*

Nursing Diagnosis: Risk for injury (hemorrhage, hemorrhagic cystitis) related to interference with cell proliferation

Expected Outcome: The child exhibits no evidence of bleeding or hematuria.

• **NURSING INTERVENTIONS/*RATIONALES***

Monitor platelet counts and administer platelets per physician order *to raise platelet count and minimize bleeding tendencies.*

Avoid aspirin products *as they interfere with platelet function.*

Teach child and family to limit activity when platelet count drops *to minimize chances of accidental injury.*

Use care in the administration of therapy (i.e., avoid grabbing with fingers and friction with clothing and bedclothes when turning; keep skin clean and dry and sheets clean and wrinkle free; use soft sponge for oral care) *to reduce bruising and injury.*

Turn and reposition frequently, use pressure-relieving mattresses *to prevent pressure ulcers.*

Implement only essential skin puncturing procedures; monitor puncture site carefully; apply gentle pressure, ice to bleeding sites *to minimize bleeding.*

Teach child and parents how to manage nosebleeds *to reduce blood loss.*

Administer ordered drugs that are irritating to the bladder mucosa early in day *to allow sufficient fluid intake and voiding for flushing of irritants.*

Ensure increased oral intake as ordered and encourage frequent voiding *to flush metabolites from system and prevent irritation.*

Observe for and report signs of cystitis (burning and pain on urination) *to ensure prompt medical treatment.*

Nursing Diagnosis: Risk for infection related to depressed body defenses

Expected Outcome: The child exhibits no evidence of infection.

• **NURSING INTERVENTIONS/*RATIONALES***

Place child in private room and screen all visitors and staff for signs of infection *to minimize exposure to infective organisms.*

Teach child and family about good hygiene and careful handwashing techniques *to prevent spread of infection.*

Use good handwashing for all contacts with child and scrupulous aseptic technique for all invasive procedures *to minimize exposure to infection.*

Encourage a nutritionally complete diet *to support body's natural defenses.*

Administer antibiotics and GCSF per physician order *to prevent infection.*

Monitor vital signs and observe skin and mucosa *to detect signs of infection.*

Avoid administration of live attenuated virus vaccines (i.e., measles-mumps-rubella, oral polio, varicella zoster) to child with depressed immune system *to prevent overwhelming the system and introducing an infectious disease;* use inactivated virus vaccines as prescribed (i.e., chickenpox, Salk polio, influenza) *to prevent common childhood illnesses.*

Nursing Diagnosis: Risk for fluid volume deficit related to chemotherapy-induced nausea and vomiting

Expected Outcome: The child is adequately hydrated.

• **NURSING INTERVENTIONS/*RATIONALES***

Administer initial dose of antiemetic before starting chemotherapy *to reduce incidence of nausea and vomiting.*

Administer regular doses of antiemetic as ordered for the duration of expected cycle of nausea and vomiting *to decrease or prevent nausea and vomiting episodes.*

Administer IV fluids as ordered *to maintain hydration;* encourage oral fluids and foods in small amounts *to increase toleration.*

Monitor child's response to antiemetic *as reactions are idiosyncratic and adjustments in drugs or dose may be needed.*

Monitor intake and output *to ensure adequate hydration.*

Avoid foods with strong odors *that may induce nausea and vomiting.*

Encourage frequent intake of fluids in small amounts *since small portions are usually better tolerated.*

Nursing Diagnosis: Altered mucous membranes related to administration of chemotherapeutic agents

Expected Outcome: The child exhibits no evidence of oral mucositis or rectal ulceration.

• **NURSING INTERVENTIONS/*RATIONALES***

Institute meticulous oral hygiene (i.e., soft sponge toothbrush *to avoid trauma;* frequent mouthwashes *to promote healing;* lip balm *to keep lips moist).* **Avoid use of lemon glycerin swabs, *which irritate eroded tissue and induce tooth decay,* hydrogen peroxide, *which delays healing of ulcers,* and milk of magnesia, *which dries oral mucosa.***

Nursing Care Plan

THE CHILD WITH CANCER—CONT'D

Inspect oral mucosa daily for ulcers and report immediately *to ensure early treatment.*

Apply local anesthetics as ordered to ulcerated areas before meals *to relieve pain and increase food intake.* **Avoid use of viscous lidocaine in young children *as it may depress gag reflex.***

Serve a bland, moist soft diet, avoid juices with ascorbic acid, use a straw for fluids, avoid oral and rectal temperature taking *to decrease pain and injury to ulcerated areas.*

Administer prescribed antiinfective agents *to prevent or treat mucositis,* analgesics *to control pain.*

Wash perianal area after stools *to lessen irritation.*

Use warm sitz baths *to ease pain and promote healing.*

Expose reddened mucosal areas to air; apply protective skin barriers to perianal area *to protect mucosa and promote healing.*

Use stool softeners, bulk laxatives *to prevent constipation.*

Track frequency and description of bowel movements *to assess for constipation.*

Nursing Diagnosis: Altered nutrition: less than body requirements related to chemotherapeutically induced loss of appetite

Expected Outcome: Nutritional intake is adequate.

• NURSING INTERVENTIONS/*RATIONALES*

Allow child any food tolerated, fortify foods with supplements, use small frequent feedings, make food appealing, involve child in selection and preparation *to increase intake and tolerance.*

Take family history *to assess any food issues that may require intervention* (i.e., use of food as control mechanism or reward and punishment).

Nursing Diagnosis: Impaired skin integrity related to administration of chemotherapy, radiotherapy, immobility

Expected Outcome: Skin is clean and intact.

• NURSING INTERVENTIONS/*RATIONALES*

Provide meticulous skin care, turn and reposition frequently *to prevent skin breakdown.*

Inspect skin frequently *to assess for areas of impending breakdown.*

Encourage adequate caloric-protein intake *to prevent negative nitrogen balance.*

Nursing Diagnosis: Impaired physical mobility related to neuromuscular impairment (neuropathy)

Expected Outcomes: The child is as mobile as condition permits, and signs of neuropathy are minimal.

• NURSING INTERVENTIONS/*RATIONALES*

Match activity level to physical condition and abilities *to prevent overexertion and injury.*

If bedridden, perform passive range of motion *to retain full range of motion;* use a footboard or high-top shoes *to prevent foot-drop;* position body in correct alignment with adequate support *to prevent pain and contractures.*

Nursing Diagnosis: Pain related to cancer and treatments

Expected Outcome: The child exhibits no signs of discomfort.

• NURSING INTERVENTIONS/*RATIONALES*

Be judicious in caregiving and handling *to minimize pain.*

Administer analgesics as prescribed on a regular schedule *to prevent start or recurrence of pain.*

Implement appropriate nonpharmacologic pain reduction techniques *as an adjunct to analgesics.*

Monitor child for vital signs, signs of irritability, restlessness *to assess need for and effectiveness of pain management techniques.*

Nursing Diagnosis: Fear related to diagnosis, prognosis, treatment procedure

Expected Outcome: The child exhibits signs of reduced fear.

• NURSING INTERVENTIONS/*RATIONALES*

Acknowledge child's fear and help child to identify sources of that fear *to facilitate identification and use of coping strategies.*

Orient child to hospital sights and sounds; provide child with accurate information about condition, procedures, and treatments; spend time with child *to promote trust and dispel fear.*

Encourage frequent family visitation with active participation in care *to prevent distress from separation.*

Use frequent touch, holding, and talking as appropriate *to provide comfort.*

Provide diversion and sensory stimulation appropriate to the child's developmental level and physical condition.

Instruct family in importance of comfort measures and in their active participation in care *to ease child's fears.*

Prepare child for procedures using developmentally appropriate approaches (therapeutic play) *to reduce fear and promote cooperation.*

Allow child choices when possible *to give child some measure of control.*

Work with parents to create a routine that is similar to the child's usual routine at home *to increase comfort with environment.*

Nursing Diagnosis: Altered family processes related to situational crises (child with life-threatening disease), treatment approaches

Expected Outcomes: The family exhibits adaptation of their usual roles, functions to accommodate special needs of child, and exhibits growth-promoting behaviors.

Continued.

Nursing Care Plan

THE CHILD WITH CANCER—CONT'D

• **NURSING INTERVENTIONS/*RATIONALES***

Provide opportunity for family to absorb and adjust to diagnosis (i.e., repeat information *to allow time for family to hear and understand;* encourage expression of concerns, fears, and feelings about diagnosis and potential impact *to facilitate adjustment;* identify support systems *to provide resources for coping*).

Assist family to understand expected treatment, rationale, and implications *to provide a sound basis for decision making.*

Teach family about expected side effects and toxicities of treatment *to prevent surprises and prepare them for what will happen.*

Explore family reaction to the child; assist them to achieve a realistic view of child's condition; have family emphasize what child can do; explore ways for family to include child in family activities *to help family increase abilities to cope with child's illness and to help child remain a part of the family structure.*

Arrange for and participate in family conferences *to provide forum for communication, mutual goal setting, and effective strategizing.*

Have parents spend special time with siblings *so that they do not feel neglected or left out.*

Identify additional resource systems (i.e., relatives, friends, church, health care services, community programs) and strategize with family about making good use of these systems *to develop broad base of support.*

Nursing Diagnosis: Anticipatory grieving related to impending loss of a child

See the Nursing Care Plan: the Child Who Is Terminally Ill or Dying, Chapter 38.

---

provide clues to their response to the disease, its therapy, and nursing interventions.

Expected outcomes:

See the Nursing Care Plan on pp. 1526-1528.

LYMPHOMAS

The lymphomas are a group of neoplastic diseases that arise from the lymphoid and hemopoietic systems. They are usually divided into Hodgkin disease and non-Hodgkin lymphoma (NHL) and subdivided according to tissue type and extent of disease (staging). Before adolescence, NHL is more common than Hodgkin disease.

HODGKIN DISEASE

Hodgkin disease is a neoplastic disease that originates in the lymphoid system and primarily involves the lymph nodes. Although Hodgkin disease is extremely rare before 5 years of age, there is a striking increase in children 15 to 19 years of age, when it occurs with almost the same frequency as leukemia. The malignancy originates in the lymphoid system and primarily involves the lymph nodes. It predictably metastasizes to nonnodal or extralymphatic sites, especially the spleen, liver, bone marrow, and lungs, although no tissue is exempt from involvement (Fig. 46-3).

The disease is usually classified according to four histologic types: (1) lymphocytic predominance, (2) nodular sclerosis, (3) mixed cellularity, and (4) lymphocytic depletion. Accurate staging of the extent of disease is the basis for treatment protocols and expected prognoses. The specific classification for each patient is derived from the history, physical examination, radiographic studies, laboratory tests, and biopsy findings. The staging system proceeds from stages I to IV, or from most to least favorable prognosis, respectively.

Diagnostic Evaluation

The diagnosis is often suspected on the basis of clinical manifestations and detection of enlarged lymph nodes during a physical examination (Box 46-12). Because of the multiple organs that can become involved, diagnosis consists of several tests to confirm the presence of Hodgkin disease and to assess the extent of involvement for accurate staging. Tests include complete blood count, uric acid levels, liver function tests, urinalysis, and erythrocyte sedimentation rate. Computed tomography (CT) of the chest, liver, and spleen, and bone scans are performed to detect metastasis.

Although used less frequently, *lymphangiography* may be performed. This is the visualization of lymphatic circulation of the lower extremities, groin, ileopelvic and abdominal-aortic regions, and the thoracic duct by way of a radiopaque medium injected in the feet or hands.

Lymph node biopsy is essential to diagnosis and staging. A bone marrow aspiration or biopsy is also performed. A laparotomy is recommended for definitive pathologic staging, and the spleen is removed, although this remains a controversial practice because of the risk of overwhelming infections from asplenia.

Therapeutic Management

The primary modalities of therapy are radiation and chemotherapy. Each may be used alone or in combination based on the clinical staging. Radiation may involve only the involved field (IF), an extended field (EF) (involved areas plus adjacent nodes), or total nodal irradiation (TNI), depending on the extent of involvement. The most widely used chemotherapeutic regimen is *MOPP (mechlorethamine [Mustargen], vincristine [Oncovin], prednisone, and procarbazine)*, which is alternated with *adriamycin, bleomycin, vinblastine, and dacarbazine, (ABVD).*

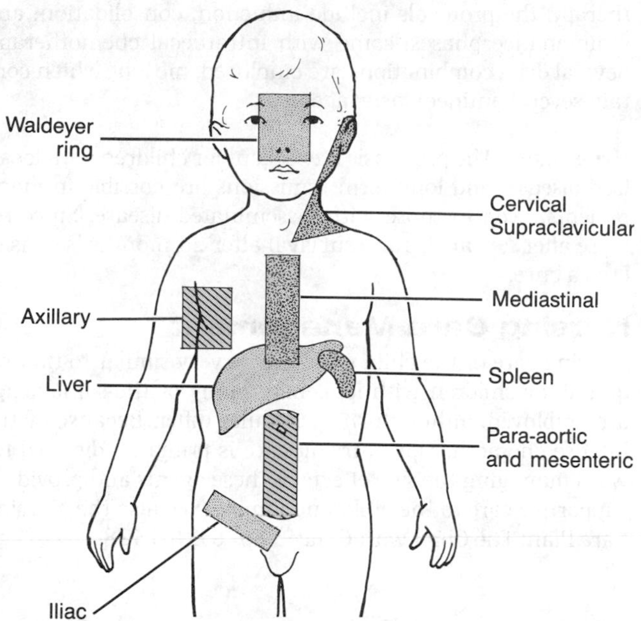

Fig. 46-3 Main areas of lymphadenopathy and organ involvement in Hodgkin disease.

Follow-up care of children no longer receiving therapy is essential to identify relapse and secondary cancers. In children with asplenia, prophylactic antibiotics are administered for an indefinite period, and immunizations against pneumococci and meningococci are recommended.

Prognosis. Long-term survival for all stages of Hodgkin disease is excellent. Early-stage disease can have survival rates greater than 90%, with advanced stages having rates between 65% and 75%. The most serious consequence of curative therapy is the development of secondary cancer, especially leukemia (AML) and solid tumors (Urba and Longo, 1992).

Nursing Care Management

Nursing care involves the same objectives as for patients with other types of cancer—specifically (1) preparation for diagnostic and operative procedures, (2) explanation of treatment side effects (Box 46-11), and (3) child and family support (see Chapter 38). Since this is most often a disease of adolescents and young adults, the nurse must have an appreciation of their psychologic needs and reactions during the diagnostic and treatment phases. (See also the Nursing Care Plan: The Child with Cancer, pp. 1526-1528.)

Once the child is hospitalized for suspected Hodgkin disease, a battery of diagnostic tests is ordered. The family needs an explanation of why each test is performed, since many of them, such as bone marrow aspiration, are not routine. The one test that deserves special explanation is *lymphangiography.*

The child must be prepared for the lymphangiogram and particularly told that the length of the procedure frequently averages 4 to 5 hours. Although the feet or hands are anesthetized, the initial injections are painful. The use of EMLA cream and/or buffered lidocaine reduces or eliminates the pain (see Pain Management, Chapter 41). Immobilization of the feet or hands during lymphatic vessel catheterization may be uncomfortable and tiresome, especially since the child must remain still for long periods. Whenever possible, the child is encouraged to sleep, or diversions should be provided, such as listening to music, reading, or talking. Ideally, a family member should be allowed to accompany the child. Fluids and food are not necessarily restricted. If allowed, provisions are made for the child to have a favorite drink or snack.

The procedure is not without complications, the most serious of which is pulmonary embolism from the oil-based contrast media.

BOX 46-12
Clinical Manifestations of Hodgkin Disease

Painless enlargement of the lymph nodes:
- Enlarged, firm, nontender, movable nodes in the cervical area are most common
- "Sentinel" node located near the left clavicle may be first enlarged node
- Axillary and inguinal lymph nodes less frequently

Other signs and symptoms of lymphadenopathy:
- Enlarged mediastinal nodes cause persistent nonproductive cough
- Enlarged retroperitoneal nodes produce unexplained abdominal pain

Systemic symptoms (usually indicate advanced involvement):
- Low-grade and/or intermittent fever
- Anorexia
- Nausea
- Weight loss
- Night sweats
- Pruritus

Nursing ALERT

Signs of pulmonary embolism include apprehension, cyanosis, distended neck veins, hypotension, liver tenderness, and edema in the lower extremities from increased venous resistance. Emergency medical treatment usually involves supplemental oxygen and antihypotensive drugs.

The child and family need considerable reassurance. The contrast medium also turns the urine and skin of the feet and/or hands bluish green. Although the urine clears rapidly, the discoloration of the skin may last for months. Adolescents may be very self-conscious about the staining, especially in the hands.

The most common side effect of irradiation is fatigue, which may last for a year after treatment. This is particularly difficult for active, outgoing school-age children and adolescents, because it prevents them from keeping up with their peers. Sometimes adolescents will push themselves to the point of physical exhaustion rather than admit and succumb to the decreased activity tolerance. The nurse cautions parents to observe for such behavior, such as extreme fatigue at the end of the day, falling asleep at the dinner table, inability to concentrate on homework, or an increased susceptibility to infection. A regular bedtime and scheduled rest periods are important for these children, especially during chemotherapy, when myelosuppression increases the risk of infection and debilitation. Before discharge the nurse should discuss a feasible school schedule with the parents and child.

An area of concern for adolescents is the high risk of sterility from irradiation and chemotherapy. Both irradiation to the gonads and drugs, particularly procarbazine and alkylating agents, can lead to infertility. Adolescents should be informed of these side effects early in the course of the diagnosis and treatment. Sperm banking is now offered at many cancer centers before the initiation of treatment in adolescent males. Sexual function is not altered, although the appearance of secondary sexual characteristics and menstruation may be delayed in the pubescent child. Delayed sexual maturation may be an extremely sensitive and stressful issue for children (see Chapter 37). It is important for the nurse to respect their concern and refrain from casually placating them with expressions such as "You'll catch up someday."

NON-HODGKIN LYMPHOMA (NHL)

NHL in children is strikingly different from Hodgkin disease and adult NHL in several aspects (Sandlund, Hutchison, and Crist, 1991):

1. The disease is usually diffuse rather than nodular.
2. The cell type is either undifferentiated or poorly differentiated.
3. Dissemination occurs early, more often, and rapidly.
4. Mediastinal involvement and invasion of meninges are common.

NHL exhibits a variety of morphologic, cytochemical, and immunologic features, not unlike the diversity seen in leukemia. Classification is based on the histologic pattern: (1) lymphoblastic; (2) Burkitt or non-Burkitt; or (3) large-cell (Huizdala, 1991). Immunologically these cells are also classified as T-cells, B-cells, or null cells (lacking immunologic properties).

The clinical staging system used in Hodgkin disease is of little value in NHL, although it has been modified and other systems have been developed.

Diagnostic Evaluation

Because the clinical presentation of most children with NHL is widespread disseminated disease, thorough pathologic staging is unnecessary. Clinical manifestations depend on the anatomic site and extent of involvement. These manifestations include many of those seen in Hodgkin disease and leukemia, as well as organ symptoms related to pressure from enlargement of adjacent lymph nodes, such as intestinal or airway obstruction, cranial nerve palsies, and spinal paralysis.

Current recommendations for staging include a surgical biopsy of an enlarged node, histopathologic confirmation of disease with cytochemical and immunologic evaluation, bone marrow examination, radiographic studies (especially tomograms of the lungs and gastrointestinal organs), and lumbar puncture.

Therapeutic Management

The present treatment protocols for NHL include aggressive use of irradiation and chemotherapy. Similar to leukemic therapy, the protocols include induction, consolidation, and maintenance phases, some with intrathecal chemotherapy. Several drug combinations are employed, most of which contain several antineoplastic agents.

Prognosis. The prognosis is excellent for children with localized disease, and long-term remissions are possible in many patients, even in those with disseminated disease. Since relapse after 2 years is rare, survival after 24 months is considered a cure.

Nursing Care Management

Nursing care of the child with NHL is very similar to that required for children with leukemia. Many of the same drugs are employed, although the schedules differ. Because of the intense chemotherapy, nursing care is primarily directed toward managing the side effects of these agents and providing supportive care to the child and family. (See also the Nursing Care Plan: The Child with Cancer, pp. 1526-1528.)

Immunologic Deficiency Disorders

A number of disorders can cause profound, often life-threatening alterations within the body's immune system. The most serious are those conditions that completely depress immunity, such as severe combined immunodeficiency disease. However, the one disorder that generates the most anxiety, within both the family and the community at large, is acquired immunodeficiency syndrome (AIDS).

Several classifications of immune dysfunction exist. *AIDS, severe combined immunodeficiency syndrome (SCIDS),* and *Wiskott-Aldrich syndrome* are syndromes wherein the body is unable to mount an immune response. The immune response can also be misdirected. In *autoimmune disorders,* antibodies, macrophages, and lymphocytes attack healthy cells.

MECHANISMS INVOLVED IN IMMUNITY

In simple terms, the function of the immune system is to recognize "self" from "nonself" and to initiate responses to eliminate the nonself or the foreign substance known as *antigen.* However, the specific processes involved in this function are complex and interrelated, and advances in the understanding of immunologic mechanisms are helping to further explain the complexities of this system.

Intact skin serves as the first line of protection for the body. Body secretions such as mucus, saliva, sweat, and tears contain chemicals that can kill many organisms. The stomach contains acids that can destroy swallowed pathogens as they adhere to the mucus of the nose and mouth. Organisms trapped in these areas are expelled by sneezing or coughing. If the foreign substance has penetrated these barriers, cellular elements are mobilized to provide further protection.

The immune system includes the primary lymphoid organs (thymus, bone marrow, and probably liver) and the secondary lymphoid organs (lymph nodes, spleen, and gut-associated lymphoid tissue [GALT]). The functions of the immune system are basically of two types: nonspecific and specific. *Nonspecific immune defenses* are activated on exposure to any foreign substance but react similarly regardless of the type of antigen; they are unable to identify the antigen, except to know that it is "nonself." The principal activity of this system is *phagocytosis,* the process of ingesting and digesting foreign substances. Phagocytic cells include neutrophils and monocytes.

Specific (adaptive) defenses are those that have the ability to recognize the antigen and respond selectively. Adaptive immunity consists of (1) *humoral immunity,* which includes antibodies in the form of immunoglobulin (Ig) and which is concerned primarily with response to foreign antigens, and (2) *cell-mediated immunity,* which provides protection against most invading organisms. Conditions that cause interference with any or all of these protective mechanisms leave the body vulnerable to disease.

ACQUIRED IMMUNODEFICIENCY SYNDROME (AIDS)

AIDS is a disorder that has generated intense medical investigation and even greater public concern and fear. *Human immunodeficiency virus (HIV)* causes AIDS. The virus has been found in blood and almost all body fluids (semen, saliva, vaginal secretions, urine, breast milk, and tears), but the evidence to date is that the virus is transmitted primarily through direct contact with blood or blood products, including sharing of intravenous needles for drug use and intimate sexual contact. There is no evidence that *casual* contact between affected and unaffected individuals can spread the virus (Caldwell and Rogers, 1991).

People with AIDS (PWA) make up a diverse group. In the pediatric age group, three populations are primarily affected—children who are exposed in utero to an infected mother (referred to as "vertical transmission"; maternal transmission can also occur at delivery or through breastfeeding); children who have received blood products, such as children with hemophilia; and adolescents who are infected because of sexual activity with an infected partner and other high-risk behaviors. Each group has unique needs relative to the origin of the infection. The majority of children with AIDS are less than 2 years of age and constitute a small percentage of the total AIDS population.

BOX 46-13 Risk Factors for AIDS in Children

Maternal factors

Intravenous drug use
Maternal promiscuity
Diagnosis of AIDS in mother
Haitian or sub-Saharan African origin

High-risk groups

Intravenous drug abusers
Sexual partners of risk-group
Sexually active homosexual males
Bisexual males
Disadvantaged, out-of-school youth, especially females

Diagnostic Evaluation

HIV infection has spread beyond the previously identified risk groups and geographic areas (Box 46-13). With the prevalence of the virus, the American Academy of Pediatrics, Provisional Committee on Pediatric Aids (1995) recommends maternal and/or newborn HIV testing. Perinatal transmission of the HIV virus has been significantly reduced in those pregnant women with HIV who take zidovudine during pregnancy. The current testing enables 50% of affected infants to be identified at birth and 95% can be diagnosed by 1 to 3 months of age. This allows prophylaxis for *Pneumocystis carinii* pneumonia (PCP), the most frequent opportunistic infection associated with HIV, to begin within the first few months of life. Clinical manifestations of AIDS in children are presented in Box 46-14.

Therapeutic Management

There is currently no cure for pediatric HIV disease. Treatment is primarily supportive, although some drugs have increased the life span for these children. AZT (zidovudine) and DDI (dideoxyinosine) are the current drugs used to treat pediatric HIV disease. A combination of these drugs is effective in delaying symptoms of AIDS. These children also receive prophylaxis for PCP infection with trimethoprim sulfamethoxazole (TMP/SMZ).

Disease prevention is of great importance for these children, and immunization against common childhood illnesses is recommended for all children with HIV infection. The only change in the schedule is the avoidance of varicella (chickenpox) vaccine and the use of inactivated poliovirus (IPV) rather than oral poliovirus (OPV) for these children and their close contacts (American Academy of Pediatrics, 1995). For children with AIDS, the pneumococcal and influenza vaccines are recommended. These children must be evaluated for their response to the immunizations.

Prognosis. Early recognition and improved medical care have changed HIV disease from a rapidly fatal to a chronic, but terminal, disease of childhood. The ultimate prognosis for perinatal HIV infection depends on the age of the child at di-

BOX 46-14 Clinical Manifestations of AIDS in Children

All

Failure to thrive
Hepatosplenomegaly
Chronic interstitial pneumonitis

Infants

Oral candidiasis
Failure to thrive
Hepatosplenomegaly
Respiratory distress secondary to *Pneumocystis carinii* pneumonia (PCP)

Toddlers

Parotitis
Generalized lymphadenopathy
Recurrent bacterial infections
Neurologic disease
Developmental abnormalities

agnosis and the types of secondary diseases. Children diagnosed with AIDS in early infancy are more likely to die at an earlier age. Secondary diseases that are associated with more rapid death include severe bacterial infections, progressive encephalopathy, anemia, fever, and diarrhea. Children with recurrent respiratory tract infections, hepatosplenomegaly, lymphadenopathy, parotitis, and skin diseases have a better prognosis (Tovo et al, 1992). However, most develop progressive encephalopathy, which is manifested by delayed development or loss of milestones in infants (Joshi, 1991) and by progressive cognitive impairment in older children (Spiegel and Mayers, 1991). A serious issue for AIDS patients is pain management. These individuals report significant pain that is often undertreated (see Pain Management, Chapter 41).

Nursing Care Plan

THE CHILD WITH HIV INFECTION

Nursing Diagnosis: Risk for infection related to impaired body defenses

Expected Outcomes: The child exhibits no evidence of infection and no evidence of spread of the HIV virus.

• NURSING INTERVENTIONS/*RATIONALES*

Place child in private room and screen all visitors and staff for signs of infection *to minimize exposure to infective organisms.*

Teach child and family about good hygiene and careful handwashing techniques *to prevent spread of infection.*

Use good handwashing for all contacts with child and scrupulous aeseptic technique for all invasive procedures *to minimize exposure to infection.*

Encourage a nutritionally complete diet *to support body's natural defenses.*

Administer prescribed antibiotics *to prevent infection,* antiretroviral drugs *to increase lymphocyte production,* trimethoprim sulfamethoxazole tablets *to prevent Pneumocystis pneumonia,* Rifabutin *to prevent mycobacterium avium.*

Monitor vital signs and observe skin and mucosa, auscultate lungs *to detect signs of infection.*

Avoid administration of live attenuated virus vaccines (i.e., MMR, oral polio, varicella zoster) to child with depressed immune system *to prevent overwhelming the system and introducing an infectious disease;* use inactivated virus vaccines as prescribed (i.e., Salk polio, influenza) *to prevent common childhood illnesses.*

Instruct child and family about protective methods (i.e., handwashing after using bathroom, avoidance of blood and body fluids by others; avoidance of biting, scratching behaviors) *to prevent spread of virus.*

Use appropriate universal precautions when administering care and performing invasive procedures *to prevent spread of HIV virus.*

Nursing Diagnosis: Altered nutrition: less than body requirements related to recurrent illness, diarrhea, loss of appetite, oral thrush

Expected Outcome: The child's nutritional intake is adequate.

• NURSING INTERVENTIONS/*RATIONALES*

Provide high-calorie, high-protein diet *to meet body requirements for metabolism and growth;* fortify foods with nutritional supplements *to maximize quality of intake.*

Involve child in selection and preparation *to increase intake and tolerance.*

Use creativity to encourage child to eat (see Feeding the Sick Child, Chapter 42).

Monitor height and weight *to assess for slowed growth or weight loss.*

Administer antifungal medications as ordered *to prevent or treat thrush.*

Nursing Diagnosis: Impaired social interaction related to recurrent illness, social stigma of HIV

Expected Outcome: The child is involved in age-appropriate peer group and family activities.

• NURSING INTERVENTIONS/*RATIONALES*

Assist child to identify personal strengths *to facilitate coping.*

Educate school personnel and classmates about HIV *so child is not unnecessarily isolated.*

Encourage family to plan activities that include child as a participating member *to increase family interaction.*

Encourage child to maintain phone contact with friends during hospitalization *to reduce feelings of isolation.*

Introduce child to other children with HIV *to provide mutual support system.*

Nursing Diagnosis: Altered sexuality pattern related to risk of disease transmission

Expected Outcomes: The adolescent displays appropriate sexual behavior and exhibits positive sexual identity.

• NURSING INTERVENTIONS/*RATIONALES*

Educate adolescent about sexual transmission risks, perinatal infection risks, avoidance of high-risk behavior, abstinence/use of condoms *so adolescent can make informed decisions about safe and healthy expressions of sexuality.*

Encourage adolescent to talk about feelings and concerns related to sexuality *to facilitate coping.*

Nursing Diagnosis: Altered family processes related to situational crises (child with life-threatening disease) and treatment approaches

See the Nursing Care Plan: The Child with Cancer, pp. 1526-1528 and the Nursing Care Plan: The Child Who Is Terminally Ill or Dying, Chapter 38

Nursing Care Management

Nursing considerations are primarily directed at caring for the child with AIDS, preventing the transmission of the virus, and educating the public regarding the *realistic* concerns in terms of communicability of the virus. Recommendations for preventing spread of the virus consist of the use of universal precautions (see Infection Control, Chapter 42, and the Nursing Care Plan, p. 1532).*

The nurse's role is central to the child and family. The nurse serves as educator, direct care provider, case manager, and advocate. As with all chronic illnesses, these children will have a great deal of involvement with the health care system. The physiologic care of the AIDS patient is directed at minimum exposure to infections, nutritional support, comfort measures, and assessment and recognition of changes in status that may indicate impending sepsis or other complications. The psychologic interventions will vary with the unique circumstances of the child and family.

The family of the child with perinatal transmission usually is faced with multiple problems, since the mother is infected. The nurse must encourage the pregnant mother to be tested for HIV and to receive regular health care. Assistance should be offered to help them parent a child with a chronic illness (see the Family Focus box below). Grandparents or other relatives may have to assume responsibility for the care of the child. These surrogate parents should be given support for their role. If no extended family is available, the child may be placed in a foster home or group home.

Since these children are frequently ill, they may have multiple hospitalizations (Boland and Santacroce, 1994). Foster care is difficult to arrange because of the nature of the illness and the fear of disease transmission. These children have many symptoms, including diarrhea, lung infections, failure to thrive, and encephalopathy. They are often irritable, with a

*Home care instructions on preventing HIV and hepatitis infection are available in Wong DL: *Wong and Whaley's clinical manual of pediatric nursing*, ed 4, St Louis, 1996, Mosby.

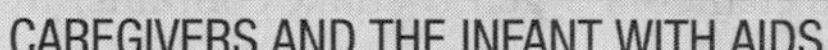

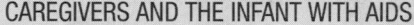

Family Focus

CAREGIVERS AND THE INFANT WITH AIDS

Unlike other fatal pediatric diseases, AIDS is associated with special family alterations. The infant infected in utero faces multiple physical and parental problems. Because the mother is infected, she may be ill or dying and therefore unable to care for the child. If possible, grandparents or other relatives may assume care. Foster care is often difficult to arrange because of the nature of the disease, especially in relation to the social stigma and the child's multiple medical needs. When extended family members or foster care is not available, the child may become a ward of the state or a "boarder" in an acute care hospital. Because these children are frequently ill, they may spend most of their lives in the hospital. When children remain in the hospital, the importance of consistent caregivers, especially primary nurses, who attend to the youngsters' physical, developmental, and emotional needs cannot be overemphasized. However, primary nurses may face the risk of overinvolvement and must be aware of the boundaries of a therapeutic relationship.

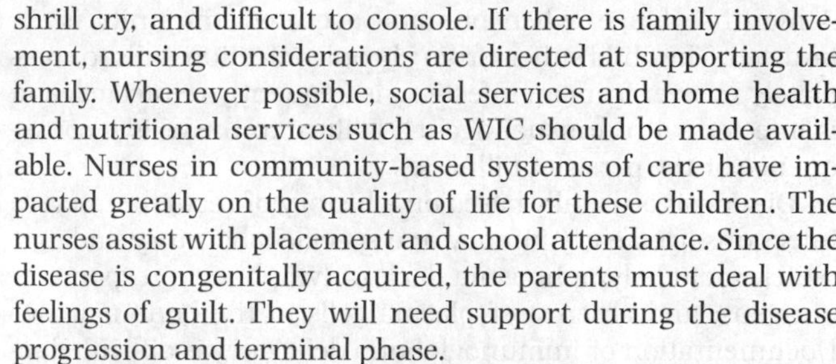

shrill cry, and difficult to console. If there is family involvement, nursing considerations are directed at supporting the family. Whenever possible, social services and home health and nutritional services such as WIC should be made available. Nurses in community-based systems of care have impacted greatly on the quality of life for these children. The nurses assist with placement and school attendance. Since the disease is congenitally acquired, the parents must deal with feelings of guilt. They will need support during the disease progression and terminal phase.

Another group of individuals increasingly infected with HIV is adolescents. As young people engage in the high-risk behaviors associated with AIDS, the possibility of infection increases. Adolescents must be taught about the risk factors, including injection drug use and high-risk sexual practices, such as anal intercourse and sex with multiple partners. Numerous AIDS educational materials are available.*

One of the most pressing concerns in caring for PWA is protection for the caregiver. Although children with HIV infection can be held, cuddled, and fed safely, universal precautions (Chapter 42) must be used in caring for all patients. Unfortunately, the public is very fearful of contracting the disease from AIDS victims, and criticism and ostracism of the child and family are common. In an effort to protect the child and deal with the community's fear, the family may keep the child at home in an atmosphere of overprotection. While certain precautions are justified in limiting exposure to sources of infection, they must be tempered with concern for the child's normal developmental needs. Both the family and the community need education about HIV to dispel many of the myths that have been perpetuated by the uninformed.

Of major concern for both family and community has been school attendance for children with AIDS. Both the Centers for Disease Control (1985) and the American Academy of Pediatrics (1986) have published guidelines regarding school attendance, which include the following:

- Unrestricted school attendance for most school-age children and adolescents, including children with AIDS or who have antibody to the virus, with the approval of their personal physician, is recommended.
- Students who do not have control of their bodily secretions, who display behaviors such as biting, or who have open sores that cannot be covered may present a greater risk and should be given a more restricted school environment until more is known about the disease.

SEVERE COMBINED IMMUNODEFICIENCY DISEASE (SCID)

SCID is a defect characterized by absence of both humoral and cell-mediated immunity. The terms *Swiss-type lymphopenic agammaglobulinemia,* an autosomal-recessive form of the disease, and *X-linked lymphopenic agammaglobulinemia* have been used to describe this disorder, which, as the names imply, can follow either mode of inheritance.

Susceptibility to infection occurs early in life, most often by

*Information is available from the AIDS hotline: (800) 342-2437 (AIDS); and from the National Pediatric HIV Resource Center, 15 S. 9th St., Newark, NJ 07107; (201) 268-8251 or (800) 362-0071.

3 months of age, when prenatal acquired immunity is exhausted. The child suffers from chronic infection, fails to completely recover from an infection, is frequently reinfected, and is infected with unusual agents. Failure to thrive is a consequence of the persistent illnesses.

Diagnosis is usually based on a history of recurrent, severe infections from early infancy and specific laboratory findings, which include lymphopenia, lack of lymphocyte response to antigens, and absence of plasma cells in the bone marrow. Documentation of immunoglobulin deficiency is difficult during infancy because of the normally delayed response of infants to producing their own immunoglobulins and material transfer of IgG.

Therapeutic Management

The only definitive treatment for SCID is a bone marrow transplant from a histocompatible donor, usually a sibling. If a compatible sibling is not available, a parent's marrow can be used after the T lymphocytes have been depleted. Intravenous Ig can be used to augment the humoral immunity until the transplant is performed.

Nursing Care Management

Nursing care focuses on the prevention of infection and supporting the child and family. If bone marrow transplantation is attempted, the care is consistent with that needed for bone marrow transplantation for any condition (p. 1536). Since the prognosis for SCID is very poor if a compatible bone marrow donor is not available, nursing care is directed at supporting the family in caring for a child with a life-threatening illness (Chapter 38). Genetic counseling is essential because of the modes of transmission in either form of the disorder.

WISKOTT-ALDRICH SYNDROME

Wiskott-Aldrich syndrome is an X-linked recessive disorder characterized by a triad of abnormalities: (1) thrombocytopenia, (2) eczema, and (3) immunodeficiency of selective functions of B- and T-lymphocytes. At birth the major effect of the disorder is bleeding as a result of the thrombocytopenia. As the child grows older, recurrent infection and eczema become more severe, and the bleeding becomes less frequent.

Eczema is typical of the allergic type and easily becomes superinfected. Chronic infection with herpes simplex is a frequent problem and may lead to chronic keratitis of the eye with loss of vision. Chronic pulmonary disease, sinusitis, and otitis media result from repeated infections. In those children who survive the bleeding episodes and overwhelming infections, malignancy presents an additional risk to survival.

Specific tests for immunologic function confirm the diagnosis. Medical treatment involves (1) counteracting the bleeding tendencies with platelet transfusions, (2) providing gamma globulin to provide passive immunity, and (3) administering prophylactic antibiotics to prevent and control infection. Bone marrow transplants have been attempted but, even if successful, do not reverse all the defects of this disorder.

Nursing Care Management

Because of the grave prognosis for these children, the main nursing consideration is supporting the family in the care of a fatally ill child (Chapter 38). Physical care is directed at controlling the problems imposed by the disorder. The measures used to control bleeding are similar to those for hemophilia. Another major goal is prevention or control of infection. Since eczema is a troublesome problem, nursing measures specific to this condition are especially important (Chapter 50). The genetic implications of this X-linked recessive disorder differ little from those of any other X-linked disorder.

Technologic Management of Hematologic and Immunologic Disorders

BLOOD TRANSFUSION THERAPY

Technologic advances in blood banking and transfusion medicine enable the administration of only the blood component needed by the child, such as packed RBCs in anemia or platelets for bleeding disorders. However, regardless of the blood component infused, all transfusions have some risks. Therefore nurses must be aware of the possible complications and the appropriate interventions. Table 46-4 summarizes the major hazards of transfusions, the signs and symptoms commonly associated with each, and nursing responsibilities. General guidelines that apply to all transfusions include the following:

- Take vital signs, including blood pressure, *before* administering blood to establish baseline data for intratransfusion and posttransfusion comparison, then every 15 minutes for 1 hour while blood is infusing.
- Check the identification of the recipient with the donor's blood group and type, regardless of the blood product used.
- Administer the first 50 ml of blood or ⅕ volume (whichever is smaller) *slowly* and stay with the child.
- Administer with normal saline solution on a piggyback setup.
- Administer blood through an appropriate filter to eliminate particles in the blood and prevent the precipitation of formed elements—gently shake container frequently.
- Use blood within 30 minutes of its arrival from the blood bank; if it is not used, return to blood bank—do not store in regular unit refrigerator.
- Infuse a unit of blood (or the specified amount) within 4 hours. If the infusion will exceed this time, the blood should be divided into appropriate-size quantities by the blood bank and the unused portion refrigerated under controlled conditions.
- If a reaction of any type is suspected, take vital signs, stop the transfusion, maintain a patent intravenous line with normal saline solution and new tubing, notify the physician, and do not restart the transfusion until the child's condition has been evaluated medically.

Although hemolytic reactions are rare, ABO incompatibility remains the most common cause of death from blood transfusion, and human error is usually responsible (administration of the wrong type to the patient or mislabeling of the

TABLE 46-4 Nursing care of the child receiving blood transfusions

COMPLICATION	SIGNS/SYMPTOMS	PRECAUTIONS/NURSING RESPONSIBILITIES
Immediate reactions		
Hemolytic reactions		
Most severe type, but rare Incompatible blood Intradonor incompatibility in multiple transfusions	Chills Shaking Fever Pain at needle site and along venous tract Nausea/vomiting Sensation of tightness in chest Red or black urine Headache Flank pain Progressive signs of shock and/or renal failure	Identify donor and recipient blood types and groups before transfusion is begun; verify with another nurse or practitioner Transfuse blood slowly for first 15 to 20 minutes and/or initial 1/5 volume of blood; remain with patient Stop transfusion immediately in event of signs or symptoms, maintain patent intravenous line, and notify practitioner Save donor blood to re-crossmatch with patient's blood Monitor for evidence of shock Insert urinary catheter and monitor hourly outputs Send sample of patient's blood and urine to laboratory for presence of hemoglobin (indicates intravascular hemolysis) Observe for signs of hemorrhage resulting from DIC Support medical therapies to reverse shock
Febrile reactions		
Leukocyte or platelet antibodies Plasma protein antibodies	Fever Chills	May give acetaminophen for prophylaxis Leukocyte-poor RBCs are less likely to cause reaction Stop transfusion immediately; report to practitioner for evaluation
Allergic reactions		
Recipient reacts to allergens in donor's blood	Urticaria Flushing Asthmatic wheezing Laryngeal edema	Give antihistamines for prophylaxis to children with tendency toward allergic reactions Stop transfusions immediately Administer epinephrine for wheezing or anaphylactic reaction
Circulatory overload		
Too rapid transfusion (even a small quantity) Excessive quantity of blood transfused (even slowly)	Precordial pain Dyspnea Rales Cyanosis Dry cough Distended neck veins	Transfuse blood slowly Prevent overload by using packed RBCs or administering divided amounts of blood Use infusion pump to regulate and maintain flow rate Stop transfusion immediately if signs of overload Place child upright with feet in dependent position to increase venous resistance
Air emboli		
May occur when blood is transfused under pressure	Sudden difficulty breathing Sharp pain in chest Apprehension	Normalize pressure before container is empty when infusing blood under pressure Clear tubing of air by aspirating air with syringe at nearest Y connector if air is observed in tubing; disconnect tubing and allow blood to flow until air has escaped only if a Y connector is not available
Hypothermia	Chills Low temperature Irregular heart rate Possible cardiac arrests	Allow blood to warm at room temperature (less than 1 hour) Use approved mechanical blood warmer or electric warming coil to rapidly warm blood; never use microwave oven Take temperature if patient complains of chills; if subnormal, stop transfusion

Continued.

TABLE 46-4 Nursing care of the child receiving blood transfusions—cont'd

COMPLICATION	SIGNS/SYMPTOMS	PRECAUTIONS/NURSING RESPONSIBILITIES
Immediate reactions—cont'd		
Electrolyte disturbances		
Hyperkalemia (in massive transfusions or in patients with renal problems)	Nausea, diarrhea Muscular weakness Flaccid paralysis Paresthesia of extremities Bradycardia Apprehension Cardiac arrest	Use washed RBCs or fresh blood if patient is at risk
Delayed reactions		
Transmission of infection		
Hepatitis AIDS Malaria Syphilis Bacteria or viruses Other	Signs of infection (e.g., jaundice) Toxic reaction: high fever, severe headache or substernal pain, hypotension, intense flushing, vomiting/diarrhea	Blood is tested for antibodies to HIV, hepatitis C virus, (HCV), hepatitis B core antigen (HBcAg); in addition, blood is tested for hepatitis B surface antigen (HBsAg), alanine aminotransferase (ALT), and a serology test is performed for syphilis; positive units are destroyed; individuals at risk for carrying certain viruses are deferred from donation Report any sign of infection and, if occurring during transfusion, stop transfusion immediately, send sample for culture and sensitivity tests, and notify physician
Alloimmunization		
(Antibody formation) Occurs in patients receiving multiple transfusions	Increased risk of hemolytic, febrile, and allergic reactions	Use limited number of donors Observe carefully for signs of reactions
Delayed hemolytic reaction	Destruction of RBCs and fever 5 to 10 days after transfusion	Observe for posttransfusion anemia and decreasing benefit from successive transfusion

blood product). Hemolysis can also cause the release of large quantities of phospholipids, which are capable of stimulating DIC. Acute kidney shutdown and eventual renal failure result from renal vasoconstriction caused by antigen-antibody complexes derived from the RBC surface.

Blood is usually administered to children by infusion pump; therefore the usual precautions and management related to pumps apply. When the blood is started with a standard transfusion set, the filter chamber is filled to allow the total filter to be used. The drip chamber is partially filled with blood to permit counting of the drops. In adjusting the flow rate, it is important to remember that blood administration sets do not use microdrops (60 drops/ml) but regular drops (usually 10 or 15 drops/ml). Therefore this must be considered when calculating the flow rate.

BONE MARROW TRANSPLANTATION (BMT)

Advances in the selection of bone marrow donors and prevention of posttransplant complications have offered the hope of a cure to children with a variety of sometimes fatal disorders. BMT may be used to replace nonfunctioning marrow (aplastic anemia), dysfunctioning marrow (sickle cell disease or thalassemia), or malignant marrow (leukemia, lymphoma).

Presently three types of BMT may be done:

Allogeneic, which involves the matching of a histocompatible donor, usually a sibling, with the recipient; may also involve an unmatched donor

Autologous, which uses the patient's own marrow that was collected from disease-free tissue and frozen or stem cells that were collected from peripheral blood through apheresis (also referred to as peripheral blood cell transplantation)

Syngeneic, which uses marrow from an identical twin

The most common type of bone marrow transplantation is allogeneic. Finding a suitable donor involves matching antigens from the **human leukocyte antigen (HLA)** system. Siblings have a 25% chance of being a match.

The importance of HLA matching is to prevent the serious complication known as *graft-versus-host disease (GVHD)*, which is characterized by a hardening of organ tissues and drying of the mucous membranes. The donor's marrow may contain antigens not matched to the recipient's antigens, which begin attacking body cells. The more closely the HLA systems match, the less likely GVHD is to develop. However, it can occur even with a perfect HLA match because there are as

Family Focus

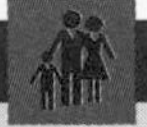

THE DECISION FOR A BONE MARROW TRANSPLANT

The family's decision for a child to undergo a bone marrow transplant is one with special issues. Often the child is facing certain death from aplastic anemia, a severe genetic disease, or a malignancy. The preparation of the child for the transplant also places the patient at great medical risk.

Once the preparatory regimen is begun and the child's immune system is destroyed, there is no turning back. Unlike kidney transplantation, BMT does not have a "rescue" procedure, such as dialysis, for supportive therapy. If the donor is a sibling, the issue of his or her marrow "saving" the brother or sister is a concern, especially if the transplant fails. Parents often must leave the home to stay at the transplant center and encounter additional stressors such as arranging child care, taking a leave from work, and managing finances. The patient faces the greatest stress—fear of BMT failure or life-threatening complications.

yet unidentified and thus unmatched antigens. GVHD is not a complication in autologous BMT.

The pretransplant procedure depends on the reason for the BMT. In most instances, lethal doses of chemotherapy, often combined with total-body radiotherapy, are given to kill malignant cells, prepare the host marrow cavity for donor engraftment, and reduce the risk of rejection. The actual transplant procedure involves harvesting several bone marrow specimens from the donor (which is done with the patient under general anesthesia) and administering diluted marrow intravenously to the recipient.

The posttransplant period involves a long stay in a protected environment. Before the marrow begins to function (engrafts), the child is extremely susceptible to infections, as well as to the risk of GVHD. During the posttransplant period the child's and family's emotional needs are equally important. Nurses can offer a great deal of support and encouragement to the family through the stages of the transplant (see the Family Focus box above).

APHERESIS

Apheresis is the removal of blood from an individual, the separation of the blood into its components, the retention of one or more of these components and the remainder of the blood reinfused into the individual. Apheresis is most commonly used to remove large quantities of platelets from healthy adult donors. These transfusion products have greatly prolonged the survival of patients with hematologic and oncologic diseases.

This technique is used to remove peripheral blood stem cells (PBSCs) from children before they receive BMTs or high-dose chemotherapy/radiation therapy that is severely toxic to the bone marrow. These PBSCs can then be used to restore the child's bone marrow. Apheresis is also used as a therapeutic modality. The blood component that is diseased or toxic is separated from the blood, and the remainder is returned to the individual. Therapeutic apheresis is considered part of standard therapy for many diseases. Plasma is selectively removed from individuals with hyperviscosity, life-threatening complications of myasthenia gravis, Guillain-Barré syndrome, thrombotic thrombocytopenic purpura, and certain drug overdoses. WBCs are removed from individuals with high-white-count leukemia.

Nursing Care Management

Difficult venous access and small blood volume can limit the ability to use this therapy in the infant and young child. Education of the family and child focuses on the purposes of the therapy, in addition, to the technology.

Specially trained individuals perform the apheresis procedure. Attention is focused on rate of removal, blood component separation, and the reinfusion of blood into the child. Vital signs are monitored, and the child is continuously observed for any adverse reactions secondary to the circulatory volume changes and/or the anticoagulant used.

When apheresis components are infused, nursing measures will differ if the product is autologous (blood component from the child) or allogeneic (blood component from another individual). Autologous components are the child's own blood; therefore major precaution is proper identification to ensure it is the correct component. The rate of infusion should be adjusted to the child's tolerance. If the product is allogeneic product, all precautions for blood transfusions apply.

Key Points

- Anemia is defined as reduction of red blood cell volume or hemoglobin concentration to levels below normal; disorders are classified either by etiology/physiology or by morphology.
- The role of the nurse in treatment of anemia is to assist in establishing a diagnosis, prepare the child for laboratory tests, administer prescribed medications, decrease tissue oxygen needs, implement safety precautions, and observe for complications.
- The main nursing goal in prevention of nutritional anemia is parent education regarding optimum feeding practices to ensure adequate sources of iron.
- Sickle cell anemia is a hereditary hemoglobinopathy affecting primarily African-Americans.
- Nursing care of the child with sickle cell anemia is aimed at teaching the family how to prevent and recognize sickling, managing pain during crises, and helping the child and parents adjust to a lifelong, potentially fatal disease.
- Nursing care of the child with thalassemia involves observing for complications of multiple blood transfusions, assisting the child in coping with the effects of illness, and fostering parent-child adjustment to long-term illness.
- Causes of acquired aplastic anemia include irradiation, drugs, industrial and household chemicals, infections, infiltration and replacement of myeloid elements, and idiopathic conditions.

- The human body controls bleeding through three processes: vascular spasm, platelet aggregation, and coagulation and clot formation.
- Nursing care of the child with hemophilia involves preventing bleeding by decreasing the risk of injury, recognizing and managing bleeding with factor replacement, preventing the crippling effects of joint degeneration, and preparing and supporting the child and family for home care.
- Goals in the care of the child with leukemia are to prepare the family for diagnostic and therapeutic procedures, prevent complications of myelosuppression, manage problems of irradiation and drug toxicity, and provide continued emotional support.
- The lymphomas include Hodgkin and non-Hodgkin lymphoma and are disorders involving the lymph glands.
- Immunodeficiency disorders are those that in some way render the affected individual unable to fight infectious organisms.
- Pediatric AIDS is acquired primarily from a parent with AIDS and in adolescents from engaging in high-risk behaviors. Blood transfusions are no longer a source of HIV infection but were responsible for AIDS in children treated with multiple blood transfusions, especially those with hemophilia.
- Blood transfusions supply needed blood components.
- Bone marrow transplantation replaces the diseased or malfunctioning bone marrow with viable blood stem cells.
- Apheresis is the selective removal of a blood component. It can be used to supply cellular elements needed for therapy (i.e., platelets or stem cells) or to remove diseased components.

References

Allen JC: What we learn from infants with brain tumors, *N Engl J Med* 328(24):1780-1781, 1993.

American Academy of Pediatrics, Committee on Infectious Diseases: Recommendations for the use of live attenuated varicella vaccine, *Pediatrics* 95:791-796, 1995.

American Academy of Pediatrics, Committee on School Health, Committee on Infectious Disease: School attendance of children and adolescents with human T-lymphotropic virus III/lymphadenopathy-associated virus infection, *Pediatrics* 77:430-432, 1986.

American Academy of Pediatrics, Provisional Committee on Pediatric AIDS: Perinatal Human Immunodeficiency Virus Testing, *Pediatrics* 95:303-307, 1995.

American Pain Society: *Principles of analgesic use in the treatment of acute pain and chronic cancer pain,* ed 3, Skokie, IL, 1992, The Society.

Boland MG, Santacroce SJ: *Case management: nursing care roles in the care of the child and family.* In Pizzo PA, Wilfert CM: *Pediatric AIDS: the challenge of HIV infection in infants, children, and adolescents,* ed 2, Baltimore, 1994, Williams & Wilkins.

Caldwell MB, Rogers MF: Epidemiology of pediatric HIV infection, *Pediatr Clin North Am* 38(1):1-16, 1991.

Centers for Disease Control: Education and foster care of children infected with human T-lymphotropic virus type III/lymphadenopathy-associated virus, *MMWR* 34:517-521, 1985.

Charache S: Experimental therapy of sickle cell disease, *Am J Pediatr Hematol Oncol* 16(1):62-66, 1994.

Cohen HA et al: Treatment of chronic idiopathic thrombocytopenic purpura with ascorbate, *Clin Pediatr* 32(5):300, 1993.

Dwyer JM: Manipulating the immune system with immune globulin, *N Engl J Med* 326(2):107-116, 1992.

Galbraith LK et al: Treatment for alteration in oral mucosa related to chemotherapy, *Pediatr Nurs* 17(3):233-236, 1991.

Griffin TC, McIntire D, Buchanan GR: High-dose intravenous methylprednisolone therapy for pain in children and adolescents with sickle cell disease, *N Engl J Med* 330(11):733-737, 1994.

Hess G, Walson P: Seizures secondary to oral viscous lidocaine, *Ann Emerg Med* 17:725-727, 1988.

Hockenberry-Eaton M, Benner A: Patterns of nausea and vomiting in children: assessment and intervention, *Oncol Nurs Forum* 17(4):574-584, 1990.

Hooper PJ, Santas ED: Peripheral blood stem cell transplantation, *Oncol Nurs Forum* 20:1215-1220, 1994.

Huizdala EV: Nonlymphoblastic lymphoma in children, *J Clin Oncol* 9:1189-1195, 1991.

Idjradinata P, Pollitt E: Reversal of developmental delays in iron-deficient anaemic infants treated with iron, *Lancet* 341:1-4, 1993.

Johnson FL: *Bone marrow transplantation.* In Fernbach DJ, Vietti TJ, editors: *Clinical pediatric oncology,* ed 4, St Louis, 1991, Mosby.

Johnson FL et al: Bone marrow transplantation for sickle cell disease: the United States experience, *Am J Pediatr Hematol Oncol* 16(1):22-26, 1994.

Joshi VV: Pathology of childhood AIDS, *Pediatr Clin North Am* 38(1):97-120, 1991.

Koch DA et al: Behavioral contracting to improve adherence in patients with thalassemia, *J Pediatr Nurs* 8(2):106-111, 1993.

Lucarelli G et al: Bone marrow transplantation in patients with thalassemia, *N Engl J Med* 322(7):417-421, 1990.

Morrison R: Update on sickle cell disease: incidence of addiction and choice of opioid in pain management, *Pediatr Nurs* 17(5):503, 1991.

Oski FA: Iron deficiency in infancy and childhood, *N Engl J Med* 329(3):190-193, 1993.

Pediatric Oncology Group: Progress against childhood cancer: the Pediatric Oncology Group experience, *Pediatrics* 89(4):597-600, 1992.

Pinkel D: Bone marrow transplantation in children, *J Pediatr* 122(3):331, 1993.

Platt, OS et al: Mortality in sickle cell disease-life expectancy and risk factors for early death, *N Engl J Med* 330(23):1639-1644, 1994.

Poplack DHG: *Acute lymphoblastic leukemia.* In Pizzo PA, Poplack DG: *Principles and practice of pediatric oncology,* ed 2, Philadelphia, 1993, Lippincott.

Sanders JE et al: Marrow transplant experience for children with severe aplastic anemia, *Am J Pediatr Hematol Oncol* 16(1):43-49, 1994.

Sandlund JT, Hutchison RE, Crist WM: *Non-Hodgkin's lymphoma.* In Fernback DJ, Vietti TJ, editors: *Clinical pediatric oncology,* ed 4, St Louis, 1991, Mosby.

Sickle Cell Disease Guideline Panel, Agency for Health Care Policy and Research: *Sickle cell disease: screening, diagnosis, management, and counselling in newborns and infants,* AHCPR Publication No. 93-0562, Rockville, MD, April 1993, The Agency.

Spiegel L, Mayers A: Psychosocial aspects of AIDS in children and adolescents, *Pediatr Clin North Am* 38(1):153-168, 1991.

Tonato M, Roila F, Del Favero A: Are there differences among the serotonin antagonists? *Support Care Cancer* 2(5):293-296, 1994.

Tovo PA et al: Prognostic factors and survival in children with perinatal HIV-1 infection, *Lancet* 339:1249-1253, 1992.

Urba WJ, Longo DL: Hodgkin's disease, *N Engl J Med* 326(10):678-687, 1992.

Vermylen C, Cornu G: Bone marrow transplantation for sickle cell disease: the European experience, *Am J Pediatr Hematol Oncol* 16(1):18-21, 1994.

Wimburly TH, Parks BR: Iron preparations: it's elementary, my dear, *Pediatr Nurs* 17:274-275, 1991.

Zurlo MG et al: Survival and causes of death in thalassemia major, *Lancet* 1(8653):27-29, 1989.

Bibliography

Anemia/Iron Deficiency Anemia

Francis EE, Williams D, Yarandi H: Anemia as an indicator of nutrition in children enrolled in a Head Start program, *J Pediatr Health Care* 7:156-160, 1993.

Fuchs G et al: Gastrointestinal blood loss in older infants: impact of cow milk versus formula, *J Pediatr Gastroenterol Nutr* 16(1):4-9, 1993.

Furman WL, Crist WM: Biology and clinical applications of hemopoietins in pediatric practice, *Pediatrics* 90(5):716, 1992.

Gavin MW, McCarthy DM, Garry PJ: Evidence that iron stores regulate iron absorption—a setpoint theory, *Am J Clin Nutr* 59:1376-1380, 1994.

Idjradinata P, Pollitt E: Reversal of developmental delays in iron-deficient anaemic infants treated with iron, *Lancet* 341:1-4, 1994.

Idjradinata P, Watkins WE, Pollitt E: Adverse effect of iron supplementation on weight gain of iron-replete young children, *Lancet* 343:1252-1254, 1994.

Lozoff B, Jimenez E, Wolf AW: Long-term developmental outcome of infants with iron deficiency, *N Engl J Med* 325:687-694, 1991.

Raunikar RA, Sabio H: Anemia in the adolescent athlete, *Am J Dis Child* 146(10):1201-S, 1992.

Shannon KM: Recombinant erythropoietin in pediatrics: a clinical perspective. *Pediatr Ann* 19(3):197-206, 1990.

Walter T et al: Effectiveness of iron-fortified infant cereal in prevention of iron deficiency anemia, *Pediatrics* 91:976-982, 1993.

Wimberley TH, Parks BR: Iron preparations it's elementary, my dear, *Pediatr Nurs* 17:274-275, 1991.

Sickle Cell Disease

Balkaran B et al: Stroke in a cohort of patients with homozygous sickle cell disease, *J Pediatr* 120(3):360-366, 1992.

Bray GL et al: Assessing clinical severity in children with sickle cell disease: preliminary results from a cooperative study, *Am J Pediatr Hematol Oncol* 16(1):50-54, 1994.

Carroll BA: Sickle cell disease. In Jackson PL, Vessey JA: *Primary care of the child with a chronic condition* ed 2, St Louis, 1996, Mosby.

Cohen AR et al: Increased blood requirements during long-term transfusion therapy for sickle cell disease, *J Pediatr* 118(3):405-407, 1991.

Day S, Brunson G, Wang W: A successful education program for parents of infants with newly diagnosed sickle cell disease, *J Pediatr Nurs* 17(1):52-57, 1992.

Day S et al: Iron overload? In sickle cell disease? *Am J Matern Child Nurs* 18:330, 1993.

Evans JPM, Rogers DW: Sickle cell disease and thalassemia, *Curr Opin Pediatr* 2(1):121-123, 1990.

Howard RJ, Lillis C, Tuck SM: Contraceptives, counselling, and pregnancy in women with sickle cell disease, *Br Med J* 306:1735-1737, 1993.

Mankad VN: Growth and development in sickle hemoglobinopathies, *Am J Pediatr Hematol Oncol* 14(4):283-284, 1992 (editorial).

Mentzer WB et al: Availability of related donors for bone marrow transplantation in sickle cell anemia, *Am J Pediatr Hematol Oncol* 16(1):27-29, 1994.

Milne RIG: Assessment of care of children with sickle cell disease: implications for neonatal screening programmes, *Br Med J* 300:371-374, 1990.

Resar LM, Oski FA: Cold water exposure and vaso-occlusive crises in sickle cell anemia, *J Pediatr* 118(3):407-409, 1991.

Vichinsky, E: A comparison of conservative and aggressive transfusion regimens in perioperative management of sickle cell disease, *N Engl J Med* 333(4):206-213, 1995.

Wang WC et al: High risk of recurrent stroke after discontinuance of five to twelve years of transfusion therapy in patients with sickle cell disease, *J Pediatr* 118(3):377-382, 1991.

Ware RF, Filston HC: Surgical management of children with hemoglobinopathies, *Surg Clin North Am* 72(6):1223-1231, 1992.

Zipursky A et al: Oxygen therapy in sickle cell disease, *Am J Pediatr Hematol Oncol* 14(3):222-228, 1992.

Thalassemia

Bhambhani K, Aronow R: Lead poisoning and thalassemia trait or iron deficiency, *Am J Dis Child* 144(11):1231-1233, 1990.

Brittenham GM et al: Efficacy of deferoxamine in preventing complications of iron overload in patients with thalassemia major, *N Engl J Med* 331(9):557-573, 1994.

Butler RB et al: β-Thalassemia major and sickle cell disease, *NAACOG Clin Issues Perinat Women's Health Nurs* 2(3):345-356, 1991.

Esposito NW: Thalassemias: simple screening for hereditary anemias, *Nurse Pract* 17(2):50, 53-56, 61, 1992.

Giardina PJ, Hilgartner MW: Update on thalassemia, *Pediatr Rev* 13(2):55-62, 1992.

Giardini C: Bone marrow transplantation for thalassemia: experience in Pesaro, Italy, *Am J Pediatr Hematol Oncol* 16(1):6-10, 1994.

Lucarelli G et al: Bone marrow transplantation in patients with thalassemia, *N Engl J Med* 322(7):417-421, 1990.

Martin MB, Butler RB: Understanding the basics of β-thalassemia major, *Pediatr Nurs* 19(2):143-145, 1993.

Olivieri, N et al: Survival in medically treated patients with homozygous beta thalassemia, *N Engl J Med* 331(9):574-578, 1994.

Uysal Z et al: Desferrioxamine and urinary zinc excretion in β-thalassemia major, *Pediatr Hematol Oncol* 10:257-260, 1993.

Walters MC, Thomas ED: Bone marrow transplantation for thalassemia: the USA experience, *Am J Pediatr Hematol Oncol* 16(1):11-17, 1994.

Aplastic Anemia

Glader BE: Red blood aplasias in children, *Pediatr Ann* (19)3:168-176, 1990.

Sanders JE et al: Marrow transplant experience for children with severe aplastic anemia, *Am J Pediatr Hematol Oncol* 16(1):43-49, 1994.

Werner EJ et al: Immunosuppressive therapy versus bone marrow transplantation for children with aplastic anemia, *Pediatrics* 83(1):61-65, 1989.

Defects in Hemostasis

Aledort LM: New approaches to management of bleeding disorders, *Hosp Pract* 24(2):207-226, 1989.

Brubaker DB, Simpson MB, editors: *Dynamics of hemostasis and thrombosis*, Bethesda, Md, 1995, American Association of Blood Banks.

Bussel JB: Thrombocytopenia in newborns, infants, and children, *Pediatr Ann* 19(3):181-193, 1990.

Conway JH, Hilgartner MW: Initial presentations of pediatric hemophiliacs, *Arch Pediatr Adolesc Med* 148:589-594, 1994.

Dragone MA, Karp S: Bleeding disorders. In Jackson PL, Vessey JA: *Primary care of the child with a chronic condition*, ed 2, St Louis, 1996, Mosby.

Dwyer JM: Manipulating the immune system with immune globulin, *N Engl J Med* 326(2):107-116, 1992.

George JN, El-Harake MA, Raskob GE: Chronic idiopathic thrombocytopenic purpura, *N Engl J Med* 331(18):1207-1211, 1994.

Lusher JM et al: Recombinant factor VIII for the treatment of previously untreated patients with hemophilia A: safety, efficacy, and development of inhibitors, *N Engl J Med* 328:453-459, 1993.

Manno CS: Difficult pediatric diagnoses: bruising and bleeding, *Pediatr Clin North Am* 38(3):637, 1991.

Spitzer A: Children's knowledge of illness and treatment experiences in hemophilia, *J Pediatr Nurs* 7(1):43-51, 1992.

Leukemias/Lymphomas

Boice J, Linet M: Chernobyl, childhood cancer, and chromosome 21, *Br Med J* (8917)309:139-140, 1994.

Bucholtz J: Issues concerning the sedation of children for radiation therapy, *Oncol Nurs Forum* 19(4):649-655, 1992.

Cooley ME et al: Cisplatin: a clinical review. Current uses of cisplatin and administration guidelines, *Cancer Nurs* 17(3):173-184,1994.

Cooley ME et al: Cisplatin: a clinical review. II. Nursing assessment and management of side effects of cisplatin, *Cancer Nurs* 17(4):283-293, 1994.

Frankiewicz V, Farrington E: Ondansetron HCL (Zofran), *Pediatr Nurs* 18(4):385-386, 1992.

Galbraith L et al: Treatment for alteration in oral mucosa related to chemotherapy, *Pediatr Nurs* 17(3):233-236, 1991.

General recommendations on immunization: recommendations of the Advisory Committee on Immunization Practices (ACIP), *MMWR* 43(RR-1):22, 1994.

Jankovic M et al: Association of 1800 cGy cranial irradiation with intellectual function in children with acute lymphoblastic leukaemia, *Lancet* 344:224-227, 1994.

Kapelushnik J et al: Evaluating the efficacy of EMLA in alleviating pain associated with lumbar puncture: comparison of open and double-blinded protocols in children, *Pain* 41:31-34, 1990.

Kennedy BJ: Hodgkin's disease, *CA Cancer J Clin* 43(6):325-326, 1993.

Mack TM et al: Concordance for Hodgkin's disease in identical twins suggesting genetic susceptibility to the young adult form of the disease, *N Engl J Med* 332(7):413-418, 1995.

McCalla JL, Santacroce SJ, Woolery-Antill M: *Nursing support of the child with cancer.* In Pizzo PA, Poplack DG, editors: *Principles and practice of pediatric oncology,* ed 2, Philadelphia, 1993, Lippincott.

Moore BD III et al: Cognitive deficits in long-term survivors of childhood cancer, *Arch Neurol* 49:809-817, 1992.

Mulvihill J: *Clinical genetics of pediatric oncology.* In Pizzo PA, Poplack DG: *Principles and practice of pediatric oncology,* ed 2, Philadelphia, 1993, Lippincott.

National Cancer Institute: Bone marrow transplantation, NIH Publ No 92-1178, Bethesda, Md, April 1991, National Institutes of Health.

Pui CH: Medical progress: childhood leukemia, *N Engl J Med* 332(24):1618-1630, 1995.

Ramsay NK: *Bone marrow transplantation in pediatric oncology.* In Pizzo PA, Poplack DG: *Principles and practice of pediatric oncology,* ed 2, Philadelphia, 1993, Lippincott.

Rivera GK et al: Treatment of acute lymphoblastic leukemia, *N Engl J Med* 329(18):1289-1295, 1993.

Robertson CM, Hawkins MM, Kingston JE: Late deaths and survival after childhood cancer: implications for cure, *Br Med J* 309(6948):162-166, 1994.

Schecter N, Altman A, Weisman S: Report of the consensus conference on the management of pain in childhood cancer, *Pediatrics* 86(5):entire issue, 1990.

Smith MC, Holcombe JK, Stullenbarger E: A meta-analysis of intervention effectiveness for symptom management in oncology nursing research, *Oncdol* Nurs *forum* 21(7):1201-1210, 1994.

Immunologic Deficiency Disorders

American Academy of Pediatrics: Guidelines for human immunodeficiency virus (HIV)–infected children and their foster families, *Pediatrics* 89(4):681-683, 1992.

Armstrong FD, Seidel JF, Swales TP: Pediatric HIV infection: a neuropsychological and educational challenge, *J Learn Disabil* 26(2):92-103, 1993.

Bale JF: The neurologic complications of AIDS in infants and young children, *Inf Young Child* 3(2):15-23, 1990.

Boland MJ, Conviser R: *Nursing care of the child.* In Pizzo PA, Wilfert CM: *Pediatric AIDS: the challenge of HIV infection in infants, children, and adolescents,* Baltimore, 1991, Williams & Wilkins.

Butz AM et al: Care of HIV-risk infants: nursing outreach by PNPs, *J Pediatr Health Care* 6(3):138-145, 1992.

Chaisson RE, Keruly JC, Moore RD: Race, sex, drug use, and progression of human immunodeficiency virus disease, *N Engl J Med* 333(12):751-756, 1995.

Cohen DG: Similarities between the nursing care needs of children with cancer and children with human immunodeficiency virus infection, *J Pediatr Oncol Nurs* 7(4):149-153, 1990.

Connor EM et al: Reduction of maternal-infant transmission of human immunodeficiency virus type 1 with zidovudine treatment, *N Engl J Med* 331(18):1173-1180, 1994.

Czarniecki L, Oleske J: Pain in children with HIV infection, *J Pain Symptom Manage* 6(3):177, 1991.

Edelson PJ, editor: Childhood AIDS, *Pediatr Clin North Am* 38(1):entire issue, 1991.

Edlin BR et al: Intersecting epidemics—crack cocaine use and HIV infection among inner-city young adults, *N Engl J Med* 331(21):1422-1427, 1994.

Fahrner R, Benson M: *Pediatric HIV infection and AIDS.* In Jackson PL, Vessey JA: *Primary care of the child with a chronic condition,* ed 2, St Louis, 1996, Mosby.

Flaskerud JH: *AIDS/HIV infection: a reference guide for nursing professionals,* Philadelphia, 1989, WB Saunders.

Fry-Revere S: A bioethics consultant's thoughts on caring for pediatric patients with HIV, *Pediatr Nurs* 20(2):177-180, 1994.

Graham BS, Wright PF: Drug therapy: candidate AIDS vaccines, *N Engl J Med* 333(20):1331-1339, 1995.

Greene WC: AIDS and the immune system, *Sci Am* 269(3):99-105, 1993.

Guidelines for prevention of transmission of human immunodeficiency virus and hepatitis B virus to health-care and public-safety workers, *MMWR* 38(S-6),June 23, 1989.

Hutto C et al: A hospital-based prospective study of perinatal infection with human immunodeficiency virus type I, *J Pediatr* 118(3):347-353, 1991.

Janeway Jr CA: How the immune system recognizes invaders, *Sci Am* 269(3):73-79, 1993.

Majer LS: HIV-infected students in school: who really "needs to know"? *J School Health* 62(6):243, 1992.

Marrack P, Kappler JW: How the immune system recognizes the body, *Sci Am* 269(3):81-89, 1993.

Mugrditchian L et al: The nutrition of the HIV infected child. II. Care management. *Top Clin Nutr* 7(2):11-20, 1992.

Murphy JM, Famolare NE: Caring for pediatric patients with HIV: personal concerns and ethical dilemmas, *Pediatr Nurs* 20(2):171-176, 180, 1994.

National Pediatric HIV Resource Center in cooperation with the Region II Head Start Resource Center: *Getting a head start on HIV: a resource manual for enhancing services to HIV-affected children in Head Start,* Newark, NJ, 1992, National Pediatric HIV Resource Center.

Nicholas SW: Management of the HIV-positive child with fever, *J Pediatr* 119(1):21-24, 1991.

1993 revised classification system for HIV infection and expanded surveillance case definition for AIDS among adolescents and adults, *MMWR* 41(RR-17):2, 1992.

Nossal GJV: Life, death and the immune system, *Sci Am* 269(3):53-62, 1993.

Pantaleo G, Graziosi C, Fauci AS: The immunopathogenesis of human immunodeficiency virus infection, *N Engl J Med* 328(5):327-335, 1993.

Pekham C, Gibb D: Mother to child transmission of the immunodeficiency virus, *N Engl J Med* 333(5):298-306, 1995.

Peterson K: Iatrogenic immune suppression, *Pediatr Nurs* 21(1):11-26, 98, 1995.

Projections of the number of persons diagnosed with AIDS and the number of immunosuppressed HIV-infected persons—United States, 1992-1994, *MMWR* 41(RR-18):1-29, 1992.

Recommendations for HIV testing services for inpatients and outpatients in acute-care hospital settings and technical guidance on HIV counseling, *MMWR* 42(RR-2):1-6, 1993.

Santelli JS, Birn AE, Linde J: School placement for human immunodeficiency virus–infected children: the Baltimore City experience, *Pediatrics* 89:843-848, 1992.

Schvaneveldt JD: Children's understanding of AIDS: a developmental viewpoint, *Fam Relations* 39(3):330-335, 1990.

Spector SA et al: A controlled trial of intravenous immune globulin for the prevention of serious bacterial infections in children receiving zidovudine for advanced human immunodeficiency virus infection, *N Engl J Med* 331(18):1181-1187, 1994.

St Louis ME et al: Human immunodeficiency virus infection in disadvantaged adolescents, *JAMA* 266(17):2387-2391, 1991.

Stiehm ER, Vink P: Transmission of human immunodeficiency virus infection by breast-feeding, *J Pediatr* 118(3):410-412, 1991.

Task Force on Pediatric AIDS: Adolescents and human immunodeficiency virus infection: the role of the pediatrician in prevention and intervention, *Pediatrics* 92(4):626-630, 1993.

Todd J: A most intimate foe: how the immune system can betray the body it defends, *Science* 30(2):20-27, 1990.

Turner BJ et al: Survival experience of 789 children with the acquired immunodeficiency syndrome, *Pediatr Infect Dis J* 12(4):310-320, 1993.

US Public Health Service Task Force on anti-Pneumocystis Prophylaxis for Patients with Human Immunodeficiency Virus Infection: Recommendations for prophylaxis against *Pneumocystis carinii* pneumonia for adults and adolescents infected with human immunodeficiency virus, *MMWR* 41(4), 1992.

Weissman IL, Cooper MD: How the immune system develops, *Sci Am* 269(3):65-71, 1993.

Wiener L, Fair C, Pizzo PA: *Care for the child with HIV infection and AIDS*. Pediatric Branch National Cancer Institute and Social Work Department, Bethseda, Md, 1993, The Clinical Center, National Institutes of Health.

Wigzell H: The immune system as a therapeutic agent, *Sci Am* 269(3):127-134, 1993.

Working Group on Antiretroviral Therapy: National Pediatric HIV Resource Center: Antiretroviral therapy and medical management of the human immunodeficiency virus–infected child, *Pediatr Infect Dis J* 12:513-522, 1993.

Blood Transfusion/Bone Marrow Transplantation (General)

Armstrong TS: Stomatitis in the bone marrow transplant patient—an overview and proposed oral care protocol, *Cancer Nurs* 17(5):403-410, 1994.

Finfer S et al: Managing patients who refuse blood transfusions: an ethical dilemma, *Br Med J* 308:1423-1426, 1994.

Ford REN: Psychosocial and ethical issues in bone marrow transplantation. In Kasprisin CA, Snyder EL, editors: *Bone marrow transplantation: a nursing perspective,* Arlington, Va, 1990, American Association of Blood Banks.

Holyoake TL: Bone marrow transplants from periperal blood, *Br Med J* 309:6946-6947, 1994.

Hooper PF, Santas EJ: Periperal blood stem cell transplantation, *Oncol Nurs Forum* 20(8):1215-1223, 1993.

Jassak PF, Riley MB: Autologous stem cell transplant, *Cancer Pract* 2(2):141-145, 1995.

Lasky LC et al: Collection and use of peripheral blood stem cells in very small children, *Bone Marrow Transplant* 7(4):281-284, 1991.

Leibundgut K et al: Autotransplants with peripheral blood stem cells and clinical results obtained in children: a review, *European J Pediatr* 152(7):546-554, 1993.

Linden JV, Paul B, Dressler KP: A report of 104 transfusion errors in New York State, *Transfusion* 32:601-606, 1992.

Quintero C: Blood administration in pediatric Jehovah's Witnesses, *Pediatr Nurs* 19(1):46-48, 1993.

Rockwood MT, Graham-Pole J: Development of an art program on a bone marrow transplant unit, *Cancer Nurs* 17(3):185-192, 1994.

Secundy MG: Psychosocial issues: unanswered questions in the use of bone marrow transplantation for treatment of hemoglobinopathies, *Am J Pediatr Hematol Oncol* 16(1):76-79, 1994.

Tong MJ et al: Clinical outcomes after transfusion associated hepatitis C, *N Engl J Med* 332:1463-1466, 1995.

Walker F et al: Guiding patients and their families through periperal stem cell transplantation with the help of a teaching booklet, *Oncol Nurs Forum* 21(3):585-591, 1994.

Walker F et al: An overview of the rationale, process, and nursing implications of peripheral blood stem cell transplantation, *Cancer Nurs* 17(2):141-148, 1994.

Winters G et al: Provisional practice: the nature of psychosocial bone marrow transplant nursing, *Oncol Nurs Forum* 21(7):1147-1154, 1994.

CHAPTER 47

Genitourinary Dysfunction

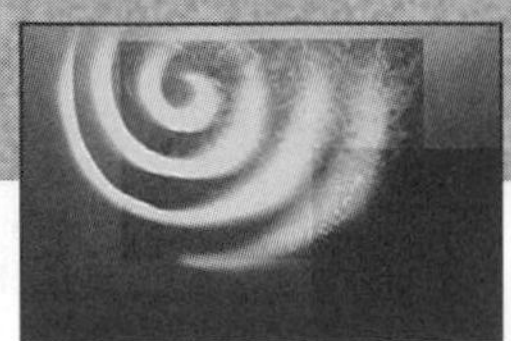

GENITOURINARY DYSFUNCTION, P. 1542
Assessment of renal function, p. 1542

GENITOURINARY TRACT DISORDERS/DEFECTS, P. 1545
Urinary tract infection (UTI), p. 1545
Obstructive uropathy, p. 1549
External defects, p. 1550

GLOMERULAR DISEASE, P. 1551
Nephrotic syndrome, p. 1551
Acute glomerulonephritis (AGN), p. 1556

MISCELLANEOUS RENAL DISORDERS, P. 1558
Hemolytic-uremic syndrome (HUS), p. 1558
Wilms tumor, p. 1559

RENAL FAILURE, P. 1560
Acute renal failure (ARF), p. 1560
Chronic renal failure (CRF), p. 1563

TECHNOLOGIC MANAGEMENT OF RENAL FAILURE, P. 1568
Dialysis, p. 1568
Transplantation, p. 1569

Genitourinary Dysfunction

ASSESSMENT OF RENAL FUNCTION

Assessment of kidney and urinary tract integrity and diagnosis of renal or urinary tract disease are based on several evaluative tools. Physical examination, history taking, and observation of symptoms are the initial procedures. In suspected urinary tract diseases or disorders, further assessment by laboratory, radiologic, and other evaluative methods is carried out.

Clinical Manifestations

As in most disorders of childhood, the incidence and type of kidney or urinary tract dysfunction change with the age and maturation of the child. In addition, the presenting complaints and the significance of these complaints vary with maturation. For example, a complaint of enuresis has greater significance at age 8 years than at age 4. In the newborn, urinary tract disorders are associated with a number of obvious malformations of other body systems, including the curious and unexplained but common association between malformed or low-set ears and urinary tract anomalies.

Many of the clinical manifestations of renal disease are common to a variety of childhood disorders, but their presence is an indication to obtain further information from the past history, family history, and laboratory studies as part of a complete physical examination. Suspected renal disease can be further evaluated by means of radiographic studies and renal biopsy (Table 47-1).

Laboratory Tests

Both urine and blood studies contribute vital information for the detection of renal problems. The single most important test is probably routine urinalysis. Specific urine and blood tests provide additional information. Because nurses are usually the persons who collect the specimens for examination and who often perform many of the screening tests, they should be familiar with the test, its function, and factors that can alter or distort the results. The major urine and blood tests are outlined in Tables 47-2 and 47-3.

Nursing Care Management

Nursing responsibilities in the assessment of genitourinary disorders and/or diseases begin with observation of the child for any manifestations that might indicate dysfunction. Many conditions have specific characteristics that distinguish them from other disorders. These characteristics are discussed as appropriate throughout the chapter.

The nurse is generally the one responsible for preparing infants, children, and parents for tests and for collection of urine and (sometimes) blood specimens (see Preparation for Procedures, Chapter 42, and Collection of Specimens, Chapter 42) for observation and laboratory analysis. An important nursing responsibility is to maintain careful *intake* and *output* and *blood pressure* measurements on most children with genitourinary dysfunction and on those who might be at risk for developing renal complications (e.g., children in shock, postoperative patients). For example, any significant degree of re-

TABLE 47-1 Radiologic and other tests of urinary system function

TEST	PROCEDURE	PURPOSE	COMMENTS AND NURSING RESPONSIBILITIES
Renal biopsy	Removal of kidney tissue by open or percutaneous technique for study by light, electron, or immunofluorescent microscopy	Yields histologic and microscopic information about glomeruli and tubules; helps to distinguish between types of nephrotic syndromes Distinguishes other renal disorders	Give nothing orally 4-6 hours before test* Premedicate as ordered Prepare setup for procedure Assist with procedure Obtain vital signs Apply pressure to area with pressure dressing and, if feasible, a sandbag Bed rest for 24 hours Observe for abdominal pain, tenderness Monitor input and output; surgical incision may be required in infants
Renal/bladder ultrasound	Transmission of ultrasonic waves through renal parenchyma, along ureteral course, and over bladder	Allows visualization of renal parenchyma, renal pelvis without exposure to external beam radiation or radioactive isotopes Visualization of dilated ureters and bladder wall also possible	Noninvasive procedure
Testicular (scrotal) ultrasound	Transmission of ultrasonic waves through scrotal contents and testis	Allows visualization of scrotal contents, including testis Testicular ultrasound is used to identify masses, and Doppler-enhanced ultrasound is used to differentiate hyperemia of epididymo-orchitis from ischemia of torsion	Noninvasive procedure
Computed tomography (CT)	Narrow-beam x-rays and computer analysis provide precise reconstruction of area	Visualizes vertical or horizontal cross section of kidney Especially valuable to distinguish tumors and cysts	Noncontrast scan is noninvasive Contrast-enhanced CT scan preparation is similar to intravenous pyelogram (IVP)
Urine culture and sensitivity	Collection of sterile specimen	Determines presence of pathogens and the drugs to which they are sensitive	Does not require specific parental permission Send specimen to laboratory immediately after collection Catheterization, clean-catch, or suprapubic specimen
Urodynamics	Set of tests designed to measure bladder filling, storage, and evacuation functions *Uroflowmetry* is a test to determine efficiency of urination *Cystometrogram* is a graphic comparison of bladder pressure as a function of volume *Sphincter electromyogram* (EMG) is a test of pelvic muscle function during bladder filling and evacuation *Voiding pressure study* is a comparison of detrusor contraction pressure, sphincter EMG, and urinary flow	Determine characteristics of voiding dysfunction Used to identify type (cause) of incontinence or urinary retention Especially valuable for voiding dysfunction complicated by urinary infection, urinary retention, or neurogenic bladder dysfunction	Prepare child for catheterization Insertion of a rectal tube will produce feelings of rectal fullness or pressure Insertion of needles may be required for sphincter EMG
Whitaker perfusion test	Injection of contrast material through renal pelvis and ureters Pressures are measured in renal pelvis and urinary bladder	Determine presence of obstruction causing upper urinary tract dilation	Prepare child for insertion of a spinal needle or perfusion catheter in renal pelvis (anesthetic is often required)

*Current research supports oral intake of clear fluids up to 2 hours before test.

TABLE 47-2 Urine tests of renal function

TEST	NORMAL RANGE	DEVIATIONS	SIGNIFICANCE OF DEVIATIONS
Physical tests			
Volume	Age related	Polyuria	Osmotic factors (urinary glucose level in diabetes mellitus)
		Oliguria	Retention caused by obstructive disease
			Inadequate bladder emptying caused by neurogenic bladder or obstructive disorder
		Anuria	Obstruction of urinary tract; acute renal failure
Specific gravity	With normal fluid intake: 1.016-1.022 Newborn: 1.001-1.020	High	Dehydration Presence of protein or glucose Presence of radiopaque contrast medium after radiologic examinations
	Others: 1.001-1.030	Low	Excessive fluid intake Distal tubular dysfunction Insufficient antidiuretic hormone Diuresis
		Fixed at 1.010	Chronic glomerular disease
Osmolality	Newborn: 50-600 mOsm/L Thereafter: 50-1400 mOsm/L	High or low	Same as for specific gravity More sensitive index than specific gravity
Appearance	Clear pale yellow to deep gold	Cloudy	Contains sediment
		Cloudy reddish pink to reddish brown	Blood from trauma or disease Myoglobin following severe muscle destruction
		Light	Dilute
		Dark	Concentrated
		Red	Trauma
Chemical tests			
pH	Newborn: 5-7 Thereafter: 4.8-7.8 Average: 6	Weak acid or neutral	If associated with metabolic acidosis, suggests tubular acidosis If associated with metabolic alkalosis, suggests potassium deficiency Urinary infection Metabolic alkalosis
		Alkaline	Metabolic alkalosis
Protein level	Absent	Present	Abnormal glomerular permeability (e.g., glomerular disease, changes in blood pressure) Most kidney disease Orthostatic in some individuals
Glucose level	Absent	Present	Diabetes mellitus Infusion of concentrated glucose-containing fluids Glomerulonephritis Impaired tubular reabsorption
Ketone levels	Absent	Present	Conditions of acute metabolic demand (stress) Diabetic ketoacidosis
Leukocyte esterase	Absent	Present	Can identify both lysed and intact white blood cells via enzyme detection
Nitrites	Absent	Present	Most species of bacteria convert nitrates to nitrites in the urine

TABLE 47-2 Urine tests of renal function—cont'd

TEST	NORMAL RANGE	DEVIATIONS	SIGNIFICANCE OF DEVIATIONS
Microscopic tests			
White blood cell count	Less than 1 or 2	More than 5 polymorphonuclear leukocytes/field	Urinary tract inflammatory process
		Lymphocytes	Allograft rejection Malignancy
Red blood cell count	Less than 1 or 2	4-6/field in centrifuged specimen	Trauma Stones Glomerular injury Infection Neoplasms
Presence of bacteria	Absent to a few	More than 100,000 organisms/ml in centrifuged specimen	Urinary tract infection
Presence of casts	Occasional	Granular casts	Tubular or glomerular disorders Degenerative process in advanced renal disease
		Cellular casts White blood cell Red blood cell Hyaline casts	Pyelonephritis Glomerulonephritis Proteinuria; usually transient

TABLE 47-3 Blood tests of renal function

TEST	NORMAL RANGE (mg/dl)	DEVIATIONS	SIGNIFICANCE OF DEVIATIONS
Blood urea nitrogen (BUN)	Newborn: 4-18 Infant, child: 5-18	Elevated	Renal disease—acute or chronic (the higher the BUN, the more severe the disease) Increased protein catabolism Dehydration Hemorrhage High protein intake Corticosteroid therapy
Uric acid	Child: 2.0-5.5	Increased	Severe renal disease
Creatinine	Infant: 0.2-0.4 Child: 0.3-0.7 Adolescent: 0.5-1.0	Increased	Severe renal impairment

nal disease can diminish the glomerular filtration rate, a measure of the amount of plasma from which a given substance is totally cleared in 1 minute. A number of substances can be used, but the most useful clinical estimation of glomerular filtration is the clearance of *creatinine*, an end product of protein metabolism in muscle and a substance that is freely filtered by the glomerulus and secreted by renal tubular cells. The nurse's responsibility in this test is the collection of urine, usually a 12- or 24-hour specimen.

Genitourinary Tract Disorders/Defects

URINARY TRACT INFECTION (UTI)

Infection of the genitourinary tract (UTI) is one of the most common conditions of childhood. UTIs may involve the urethra, bladder (lower urinary tract), and/or the ureters, renal pelvis, calyces, and renal parenchyma (upper urinary tract). Because it is often impossible to localize the infection, the broad designation of UTI is applied to the presence of significant numbers of microorganisms anywhere within the urinary tract (except the distal one third of the urethra, which is usually colonized with bacteria). The peak incidence of UTIs not caused by structural anomalies occurs between 2 and 6 years of age, and except for the neonatal period, females have 10 to 30 times the risk of males for developing UTI. An increased incidence of UTIs is observed in adolescents, especially those who are sexually active.

Classification

Infection of the urinary tract may be present with or without clinical symptoms. As a result, the site of infection is often difficult to pinpoint with any degree of accuracy. Various terms used to describe urinary tract disorders include the following:

Bacteriuria—Presence of bacteria in the urine
Asymptomatic bacteriuria—Significant bacteriuria with no evidence of clinical infection (usually defined as greater than 100,000 colony-forming units [CFU])
Symptomatic bacteriuria—Bacteriuria accompanied by physical signs of urinary infection (dysuria, suprapubic discomfort, hematuria, fever)
Recurrent UTI—Repeated episode of bacteriuria or symptomatic UTI
Persistent UTI—Persistence of bacteriuria despite antibiotic treatment
Febrile UTI—Bacteriuria accompanied by fever and other physical signs of urinary infection; presence of a fever typically implies a pyelonephritis
Cystitis—Inflammation of the bladder
Urethritis—Inflammation of the urethra
Pyelonephritis—Inflammation of the upper urinary tract and kidneys
Urosepsis—Febrile UTI coexisting with systemic signs of bacterial illness; blood culture reveals presence of urinary pathogen

Etiology

A variety of organisms can be responsible for UTI. *Escherichia coli* (80% of cases) and other gram-negative enteric organisms are most commonly implicated; these organisms are usually found in the anal and perineal region. Other organisms associated with UTI include *Proteus, Pseudomonas, Klebsiella, Staphylococcus aureus, Haemophilus,* and coagulase-negative *Staphylococcus.* Several factors contribute to the development of UTI in childhood.

Anatomic and physical factors. The structure of the lower urinary tract is believed to account for the increased incidence of bacteriuria in females. The short urethra, which measures approximately 2 cm ($^3/_4$ inch) in young girls and 4 cm ($1^1/_2$ inches) in mature women, provides a ready pathway for invasion of organisms. In addition, the closure of the urethra at the end of micturition may return contaminated bacteria to the bladder. The longer male urethra (as long as 20 cm [8 inches] in an adult) and the antibacterial properties of prostatic secretions inhibit the entry and growth of pathogens. Considerable evidence suggests that there is a higher incidence of UTI in uncircumcised male infants than in circumcised male infants (Wiswell and Hachey, 1993; Craig et al, 1996). However, other research suggests that the uncircumcised male infant is not at increased risk for UTI (Fleiss, 1995).

The single most important host factor influencing the occurrence of UTI is *urinary stasis.* Ordinarily, urine is sterile, but at 37° C (98.6° F) it provides an excellent culture medium. Under normal conditions the act of completely and repeatedly emptying the bladder flushes away any organisms before they have an opportunity to multiply and invade surrounding tissue. However, urine that remains in the bladder allows bacteria from the urethra to rapidly become established in the rich medium. Incomplete bladder emptying (stasis) may result from *reflux* (see p. 1547), anatomic abnormalities (especially those involving the ureters), dysfunction of the voiding mechanism, or extrinsic ureteral or bladder compression that may be caused by constipation.

Altered urine and bladder chemistry. Several mechanical and chemical characteristics of the urine and bladder mucosa help maintain urinary sterility. An increased fluid intake promotes flushing of the normal bladder and lowers the concentration of organisms in the infected bladder. Diuresis also seems to enhance the antibacterial properties of the renal medulla.

Most pathogens favor an alkaline medium. Normally urine is slightly acidic, but it can be made more acidic by diet (apple juice, cranberry juice, and large amounts of ascorbic acid) or acid-forming drugs. A urine pH of approximately 5 hampers bacterial multiplication, although the acidification rarely eliminates the bacteriuria. However, it may enhance the therapeutic effectiveness of drugs and the natural defense mechanisms and may help relieve some of the symptoms.

Diagnostic Evaluation

The clinical manifestations of UTIs depend on the age of the child (Box 47-1). Diagnosis of UTI is confirmed by detection of bacteriuria in urine culture, but urine collection is often difficult, especially in infants and very small children. Several factors may alter a urine specimen, and contamination of a specimen by organisms from sources other than the urine, such as perineal and perianal flora in bag specimens, is the most common cause of false-positive results. Unless the specimen is a first morning sample, a recent high fluid intake may indicate a falsely low organism count. Therefore children should not be encouraged to drink large volumes of water in an attempt to obtain a specimen quickly.

More accurate estimates of bacterial content are obtained from *suprapubic aspiration* (in children younger than 2 years of age) and properly performed bladder catheterization (as long as the first few milliliters are excluded from collection). The specimen should be taken directly to the laboratory for culture immediately.

Tests to detect bacteriuria are being used with increased frequency in screening for UTI. The dipstick tests that test for leukocyte esterase or nitrite are quick and inexpensive methods for detecting infection before obtaining final culture results.

Localization of the infection site may involve more specific tests, including ureteral catheterization and bladder washout procedures. Other tests such as ultrasonography, voiding cystourethrogram (VCUG), intravenous pyelogram (IVP), and dimercaptosuccinic acid (DSMA) scan may be performed after the infection subsides to identify anatomic abnormalities contributing to the development of infection and existing kidney changes from recurrent infection.

Therapeutic Management

The objectives of treatment of children with UTI are (1) to eliminate current infection, (2) to identify contributing factors to reduce the risk of recurrence, (3) to prevent systemic spread of the infection, and (4) to preserve renal function. Antibiotic therapy should be initiated on the basis of identification of the pathogen, the child's history of antibiotic use, and the location of the infection. A variety of antimicrobial drugs are available for treating UTI, but all of them can occasionally be ineffective because of resistance of organisms. Common antiinfective agents used for UTI include the penicillins, sul-

BOX 47-1

Signs and Symptoms of Urinary Tract Disorders or Disease at Different Ages

Neonatal period (birth to 1 month)

Poor feeding
Vomiting
Failure to gain weight
Rapid respiration (acidosis)
Respiratory distress
Spontaneous pneumothorax or pneumomediastinum
Frequent urination
Screaming on urination
Poor urinary stream
Jaundice
Seizures
Dehydration
Other anomalies or stigmata
Enlarged kidneys or bladder

Infancy (1 to 24 months)

Poor feeding
Vomiting
Failure to gain weight
Excessive thirst
Frequent urination
Straining or screaming on urination
Foul-smelling urine
Pallor
Fever
Persistent diaper rash
Seizures (with or without fever)
Dehydration
Enlarged kidneys or bladder

Childhood (2 to 14 years)

Poor appetite
Vomiting
Growth failure
Excessive thirst
Enuresis, incontinence, frequent urination
Painful urination
Swelling of face
Seizures
Pallor
Fatigue
Blood in urine
Abdominal or back pain
Edema
Hypertension
Tetany

fonamide (including trimethoprim and sulfisoxazole in combination), the cephalosporins, nitrofurantoin, and the tetracyclines. All antibiotics may cause side effects or may prove ineffective because of bacterial resistance.

If anatomic defects such as primary reflux or bladder neck obstruction are present, surgical correction may be necessary to prevent recurrent infection. Follow-up study is an important component of medical management, because the relapse rate is high and recurrent infection tends to occur 1 to 2 months after termination of treatment. The aim of therapy and careful follow-up is to reduce the chance of renal scarring.

Renal damage is rare if no anatomic abnormalities complicate the condition. However, recurrent infection of the urinary bladder predisposes the individual to transient episodes of vesicoureteral reflux.

Vesicoureteral reflux. Vesicoureteral reflux (VUR) refers to the retrograde flow of bladder urine into the ureters. During voiding, urine is swept up the ureters and flows back into the empty bladder, where it acts as a reservoir for bacterial growth until the next void. Therefore reflux increases the chances for and perpetuates infection. *Primary reflux* results from congenitally abnormal insertion of ureters into the bladder; *secondary reflux* occurs as a result of an acquired condition.

VUR is managed conservatively with low-dose antibacterial therapy and frequent urine cultures and requires a motivated, reliable, and cooperative family. Indications for surgical intervention include significant anatomic abnormality at the ureterovesical junction, recurrent UTIs, severe forms of VUR, noncompliance with medical therapy, intolerance to antibiotics, and VUR after puberty in females.

Prognosis. With prompt and adequate treatment at the time of diagnosis, the long-term prognosis for UTIs is usually excellent. However, the hazard of progressive renal injury is greatest when infection occurs in young children (especially under 2 years of age) and is associated with congenital renal malformations and reflux. Therefore early diagnosis of children at risk is particularly important during infancy and toddlerhood.

Nursing Care Management

Assessment

Because children are not a captive population, mass screening is difficult. However, annual health examinations should include a routine urinalysis. In addition, nurses should instruct parents to observe regularly for clues suggesting UTI. Unfortunately, the signs of UTI are not as evident as those of upper respiratory tract infection. Therefore many cases go undetected because no one thought to investigate this very common problem.

Nursing ALERT

A child who exhibits the following should be evaluated for UTI:
Incontinence in a toilet-trained child
Strong-smelling urine
Frequency and/or urgency

Because infants and young children are unable to express their feelings and sensations verbally, it is difficult to detect discomfort they may be experiencing from dysuria. A careful history regarding voiding habits, stooling pattern, and episodes of unexplained irritability may assist in detecting less obvious cases of UTI. Consequently, parents should be cautioned to observe for specific clues of UTI in suspected cases.

For example, it may be helpful if parents check the young child's diaper every ½ hour, which increases the opportunity for observing the stream for such findings as straining or fretting before voiding begins, signs of discomfort before and during urinating, starting and stopping the stream intermittently, and frequent dripping of small amounts of urine.

Collecting an appropriate specimen is essential when infection is suspected. It is the nurse's responsibility to take every precaution to obtain acceptable clean-voided specimens to avoid the use of other collecting procedures except when absolutely indicated.

Nursing Diagnoses

A number of nursing diagnoses become evident following a thorough assessment. These diagnoses include but are not limited to those listed in Box 47-2.

Planning

The goals of care for the child with UTI and the family are as follows:

1. Child and family will be prepared properly for needed tests and procedures.
2. Parents and child will receive appropriate education regarding prevention and treatment of infection.

Implementation

Additional tests are often performed to detect anatomic defects. Children are prepared for these tests as appropriate for their age, including an explanation of the procedure, its purpose, and what the children will experience (see Chapter 42). Sometimes a simple description of the urinary system is helpful. Especially for preschool children, the nurse must clarify that the urinary tract is separate from any sexual function and that the test is for a problem that they did not cause. It is not uncommon for children to associate blame for perceived wrongdoing (e.g., masturbation) or unacceptable thoughts with the reason for the illness or the tests. With children under 3 or 4 years of age, the procedure can be explained on a doll. With older children, a simple drawing of the bladder, urethra, ureters, and kidneys makes the explanation more understandable.

For some procedures children may be treated as outpatients to avoid overnight separation from home. In such cases nurses must be careful not to overlook the need for adequate preparation. If surgery is subsequently indicated, the child will be able to encounter the impending operation with facts and understanding of the procedures, which will help to decrease his or her fear and anxiety concerning more extensive medical-surgical intervention.

BOX 47-2

Nursing Diagnoses: The Child With Urinary Tract Infection

Risk for injury related to possibility of kidney damage from chronic infection
Anxiety related to unfamiliar procedures
Altered family processes related to illness of a child

Since antibacterial drugs are indicated in UTI, the nurse advises parents of proper dosage and administration. When antiseptics such as nitrofurantoin are used for prolonged therapy to maintain urine sterility, parents need an explanation of the continued necessity of the drug when no signs of infection are present.* An adequate or increased fluid intake is encouraged for all children.

Prevention. Prevention is the most important goal in both primary and recurrent infection, and most preventive measures are simple hygienic habits that should be a routine part of daily care (see the Guidelines box below). For example, parents are taught to cleanse their infant's genital areas from front to back to avoid contaminating the urethral area with fecal organisms. Female children are taught to wipe from front to back after voiding or defecating. Children should void as soon as they feel the urge (see the Critical Thinking Q & A box on p. 1549).

Sexually active adolescent females are advised to urinate as soon as possible after intercourse to flush out bacteria introduced during sexual activity. Children with disabilities involving the bladder are often on a prophylactic regimen such as acidifying agents and prescribed fluid intake. The nurse should reinforce the importance of compliance to parents and responsible children.

*Home care instructions for giving medications to children and collecting a urine sample are available in Wong DL: *Wong and Whaley's clinical manual of pediatric nursing*, ed 4, St Louis, 1996, Mosby.

Guidelines

PREVENTION OF URINARY TRACT INFECTION

Factors predisposing to development	Measures of prevention
Short female urethra close to vagina and anus	Perineal hygiene—wipe from front to back Avoid tight clothing or diapers; wear cotton panties rather than nylon Check for vaginitis or pinworms, especially if child scratches between legs
Incomplete emptying (reflux) and overdistention of bladder	Avoid "holding" urine; encourage child to void frequently, especially before a long trip or other circumstances in which toilet facilities are not available Empty bladder completely with each void Avoid straining during defecation, and avoid constipation
Concentrated and alkaline urine	Encourage generous fluid intake Acidify urine with juices such as cranberry and a diet high in animal protein

Evaluation

The effectiveness of nursing interventions is determined by continual reassessment and evaluation of care on the basis of the following observational guidelines and expected outcomes:

1. Question children and families regarding their understanding of the disease and the diagnostic measures required for identifying the presence of infection or physical abnormalities.
2. Observe and interview family and child regarding preventive practices, and observe laboratory reports of urinalyses and cultures for evidence of treatment efficacy.

Expected outcomes

1. Child and family demonstrate an understanding of the illness and diagnostic tests (specify knowledge and means of demonstration).
2. Child and family demonstrate an understanding of preventive practices (specify means of demonstration).

Critical Thinking Q & A

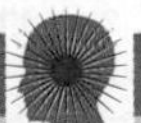

RECURRENT URINARY TRACT INFECTIONS

Joyce is 10 years old and has been hospitalized for acute pyelonephritis. She has a history of UTI and VUR. As the nurse assigned to Joyce, you are obtaining a detailed history of Joyce's voiding pattern and fluid intake. Her mother reports that when she does laundry, Joyce's underwear smells strongly of urine. The mother denies any problem with enuresis or accidental urination. When describing Joyce's fluid intake, both Joyce and her mother agree on her consumption of 8-10 oz of juice after school each day, 8 oz of milk with the evening meal, and 8 oz of water or juice in the evening. Joyce eats both breakfast and lunch at school. On Saturday and Sunday, she routinely consumes 46 oz of fluid per day. Joyce's weight is 26 kg.

In continuing this interaction, you should do which of the following?

1) Ask about Joyce's bowel elimination pattern.
2) Develop an intervention strategy to increase Joyce's fluid intake to 54 oz per day.
3) Develop an intervention strategy to decrease fluid intake in the evening.
4) Develop a line of inquiry about Joyce's fluid and elimination pattern at school.

The correct answer is number four. All of the actions are appropriate except number three. The relationship of chronic constipation to recurrent UTIs is well documented. Joyce's calculated fluid requirement per day is 54 ounces; decreasing her fluid intake is not warranted. However, currently of most concern is the information related to Joyce's behavior at school. It is not unusual for both boys and girls to avoid using the rest-rooms at school. Some children are known to omit drinking during the daytime to avoid needing to use the school restroom. They sometimes lose small amounts of urine into their underwear as they attempt to "hold" their urine until they get home. This fact may or may not be true for Joyce, but your inquiry should elicit school behavior before changing lines of inquiry or moving to interventions.

See also the Nursing Care Plan: The Child with Urinary Tract Infection.*

OBSTRUCTIVE UROPATHY

Structural or functional abnormalities of the urinary system that obstruct the normal flow of urine can produce renal disorders. When there is interference with urine flow, the back up of urine above the obstruction causes **hydronephrosis** (the collection of urine in the renal pelvis to the point of cyst formation from the distention) with eventual pressure destruction to renal parenchyma, although the dilating ureters form a reservoir that reduces the effect on the kidneys for a long time.

Obstruction may be congenital or acquired, unilateral or bilateral, and complete or incomplete, and the manifestations may be acute or chronic. The obstruction can occur at any level of the upper or lower urinary tract (Fig. 47-1). Partial obstruction may not be symptomatic unless there is a water or solute diuresis. Boys are affected more commonly than girls, and malformations should be suspected when patients have other congenital defects (e.g., prune belly syndrome, chromosome anomalies, hypospadias, anorectal malformations, or defects of the pinna of the ear).

Damage to distal nephrons in chronic uropathy alters the ability to concentrate urine, which contributes to the increased urine flow and metabolic acidosis that results from decreased excretion of acid secondary to impaired ability of the

*In Wong DL: *Wong and Whaley's clinical manual of pediatric nursing*, ed 4, St Louis, 1996, Mosby.

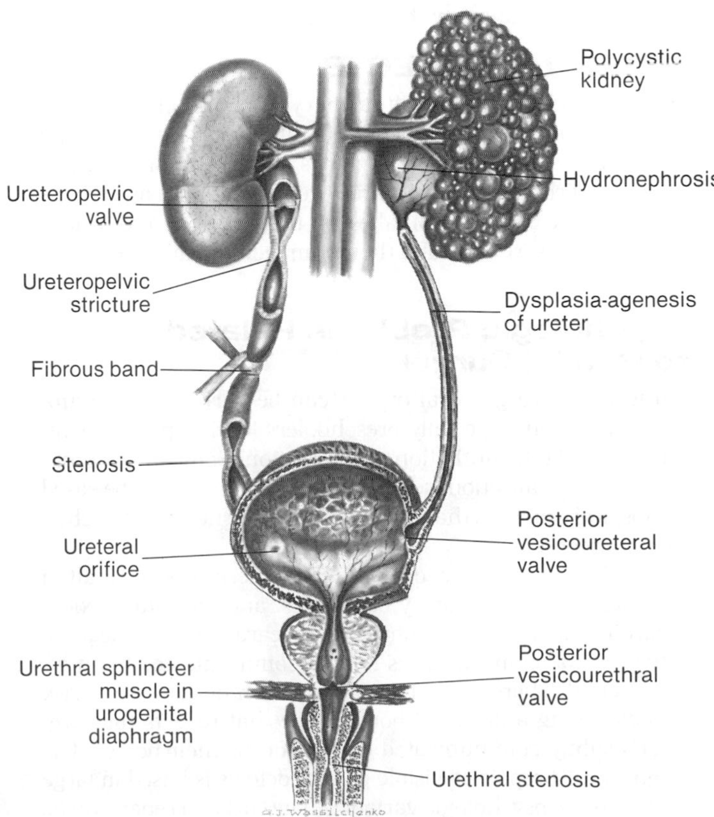

Fig. 47-1 Major sites of urinary tract obstruction.

distal nephron to secrete hydrogen ions. Partial obstruction results in progressive loss of renal function as a result of irreversible damage to the nephrons. Pooled urine serves as a medium for bacterial growth; therefore UTIs further increase the extent of renal damage.

Early diagnosis and surgical correction or procedures that divert the flow of urine to bypass the obstruction, such as *ileal conduit* or *cutaneous ureterostomy*, are essential to prevent progressive renal damage. Medical complications of acute or chronic renal failure or infection are managed as described for those disorders.

Nursing Care Management

Nursing goals in urinary tract obstruction include helping to identify cases, assisting with diagnostic procedures, and caring for children with complications. Preparing parents and children for procedures is a major nursing responsibility. Preparation for urinary diversion procedures is of special importance (see Preparation for Procedures, Chapter 42).

Parents and children need emotional support and counseling during the lengthy management of these disorders. Many children are discharged with ureteral drainage systems in place that must be protected from damage, and the danger of infection is a constant concern. Parents are taught to care for the equipment and recognize the signs of possible obstruction or infection within the system.

Children with external diversional systems need psychologic support and guidance, especially as they reach adolescence and body image concerns assume more prominence. Those with progressive renal deterioration may face the prospect of dialysis and/or transplantation and the emotional aspects that accompany these procedures.

EXTERNAL DEFECTS

Defects of the external genitourinary tract are serious conditions primarily because of the psychologic impact on the child. Satisfactory surgical repair is successful for the more common disorders and is carried out or initiated as early as possible. The major anomalies of the lower genitourinary tract, their description, and their management are outlined in Table 47-4.

Psychologic Problems Related to Genital Surgery

Surgery involving sexual organs can be particularly disruptive to children, especially preschoolers fearing punishment, retaliation, body mutilation, or castration. Some of the problems of hospitalization, separation, and anxiety can be eased by hospital practices that are sensitive to the needs of the child (see Chapter 41).

The body image of a child is largely derived as a result of feedback from the primary caregivers, and parental anxiety regarding an acceptable physical appearance and adequate future sexual competency is readily communicated to an affected child. Therefore children with birth defects are at risk for developing a distorted body image that reflects the caregiver's subtly communicated evaluation of their bodies. The trend toward repair of visible genital defects is based in large part on these psychologic variables. The earlier a repair can be achieved, the more likely the possibility that the child will develop a normal body image.

Critical Thinking Q & A

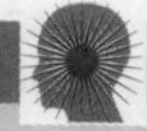

URINARY TRACT SURGERY

Mr. and Mrs. Scott are receiving preoperative instructions before their son David's surgery for reimplantation of the ureters. David is 4 ½ years old. The nurse includes a significant discussion of postoperative pain management with the parents. In addition to pain management and an explanation of what tubes and dressings to expect, the most significant other topic for presentation is which of the following?

1) The need to reassure David that his genitalia are intact and will function when the catheters have been removed
2) The importance of monitoring the urine drainage from ureteral stents and urethral catheter
3) The need to assess the surgical site for bleeding or excessive drainage
4) The home care regimen that can be anticipated after David's discharge from the hospital

The correct answer is one. Monitoring urine drainage and assessing the surgical site are postoperative priorities for the nurse. Parents, when present, will often notify the nurse of their observations. Parents need to learn about the anticipated home care and follow-up regimens. David's concern about his genitalia being intact is the parents' higher priority. He is most concerned about the possibility of mutilation, castration, and punishment for wrongdoing, which in his case may include accidental urination. His parents are the most appropriate persons to reassure him, and they need to know that this is a priority for both them and David.

Between 3 and 6 years of age, the phallic-oedipal period, children show a strong interest and concern about the genital area, gender differences, and genital normality or its lack. It is also a time when children are frightened of what they perceive to be threats to their body and bodily function. They also view any untoward happening as a punishment for real or imagined wrongdoing or unacceptable sexual feelings, such as masturbation, sex play, or erotic feelings. Surgical repair is recommended before these fears and anxieties develop (see the Critical Thinking Q & A box above).

Nursing Care Management

Preparing children and their families for diagnostic and surgical procedures (see Preparation for Procedures, Chapter 42) and for home care are major nursing functions. Most postoperative care involves care of the surgical site. Tub baths are discouraged for 1 week following simple surgeries, and the surgical site is kept clean and otherwise protected from infection and is inspected for signs of infection. Dressings, if any, are inspected regularly. More complex surgeries require additional care and observation (e.g., catheter care for urethral reconstruction and care of urinary diversion stomas and collection devices).

Some older children's activities such as pushing, lifting, playing with straddle toys, playing in sandboxes, swimming, and rough activities may be restricted for some types of surgical repairs. Precise restrictions depend on the specific type of surgery. Activities of infants and toddlers are not limited.

In most cases the results of surgery are quite satisfactory. However, additional emotional interventions may be needed for some of the more severe defects such as exstrophy and

TABLE 47-4 Defects of the genitourinary tract

DEFECT	THERAPEUTIC MANAGEMENT
Inguinal hernia Protrusion of abdominal contents through inguinal canal into scrotum	Detected as painless inguinal swelling of variable size Surgical closure of inguinal defect
Hydrocele Fluid in scrotum	Surgical repair indicated if spontaneous resolution not accomplished in 1 year
Phimosis Narrowing or stenosis of preputial opening of foreskin	Mild cases: manual retraction of foreskin and proper cleansing of area Severe cases: circumcision or vertical division and transverse suturing of foreskin
Hypospadias Urethral opening located behind glans penis or anywhere along ventral surface of penile shaft	Objectives of surgical correction: Enable child to void in standing position and direct stream voluntarily in usual manner Improve physical appearance of genitalia Produce a sexually adequate organ
Chordee Ventral curvature of penis, often associated with hypospadias	Surgical release of fibrous band causing the deformity
Epispadias Meatal opening located on dorsal surface of penis	Surgical correction, usually including penile and urethral lengthening and bladder neck reconstruction (if necessary)
Cryptorchidism Failure of one or both testes to descend normally through inguinal canal	Detected by inability to palpate testes within scrotum Medical: administration of human chorionic gonadotropin (older child) Surgical: orchiopexy Objectives of therapy: Prevent damage to undescended testicle Decrease incidence of malignant tumor formation Avoid trauma and torsion Close inguinal canal Prevent cosmetic and psychologic disability from empty scrotum
Exstrophy of bladder Eversion of posterior bladder through anterior bladder wall and lower abdominal wall; associated with open pubic arch (a severe defect)	Potential objectives of surgical correction: Preserve renal function Attain urinary control Adequate reconstructive repair Improve sexual function (especially in males)
Ambiguous genitalia Types:	Assignment of gender Surgical correction if needed:
Masculinized female (female pseudohermaphrodite)	gender assignment—female
Incompletely masculinized male (male pseudohermaphrodite)	Gender assignment—female
True hermaphrodite (both ovaries and testes)	Gender assignment depends on predominant characteristics
Mixed gonadal dysgenesis	Gender assignment depends on predominant characteristics

those defects that require stomas. A major concern of parents and children is related to surgery that directly affects the genitalia. Concerns about penile size, appearance of the genitalia, potential ability to procreate, and rejection by peers (especially the opposite gender) are potential fears that require psychologic adjustment, particularly during adolescence.

Glomerular Disease

NEPHROTIC SYNDROME

Nephrotic syndrome is a clinical state that includes massive proteinuria, hypoalbuminemia, hyperlipemia, and edema. The disorder can occur as (1) a primary disease known as *idiopathic nephrosis, childhood nephrosis,* or *minimal-change nephrotic syndrome (MCNS)*; (2) a secondary disorder that occurs as a clinical manifestation after or in association with glomerular damage of known or presumed etiology; or (3) a congenital form inherited as an autosomal recessive disorder. The disorder is characterized by increased glomerular permeability to plasma protein, which results in massive urinary protein loss. The glomerulus is responsible for the initial step in the formation of urine; filtration rate depends on an intact glomerular membrane. This discussion is devoted to MCNS because it constitutes 80% of nephrotic syndrome cases.

Pathophysiology

The onset of MCNS can occur at any age but predominantly occurs in children between 2 and 7 years of age. It is rare in children younger than 6 months of age, uncommon in infants

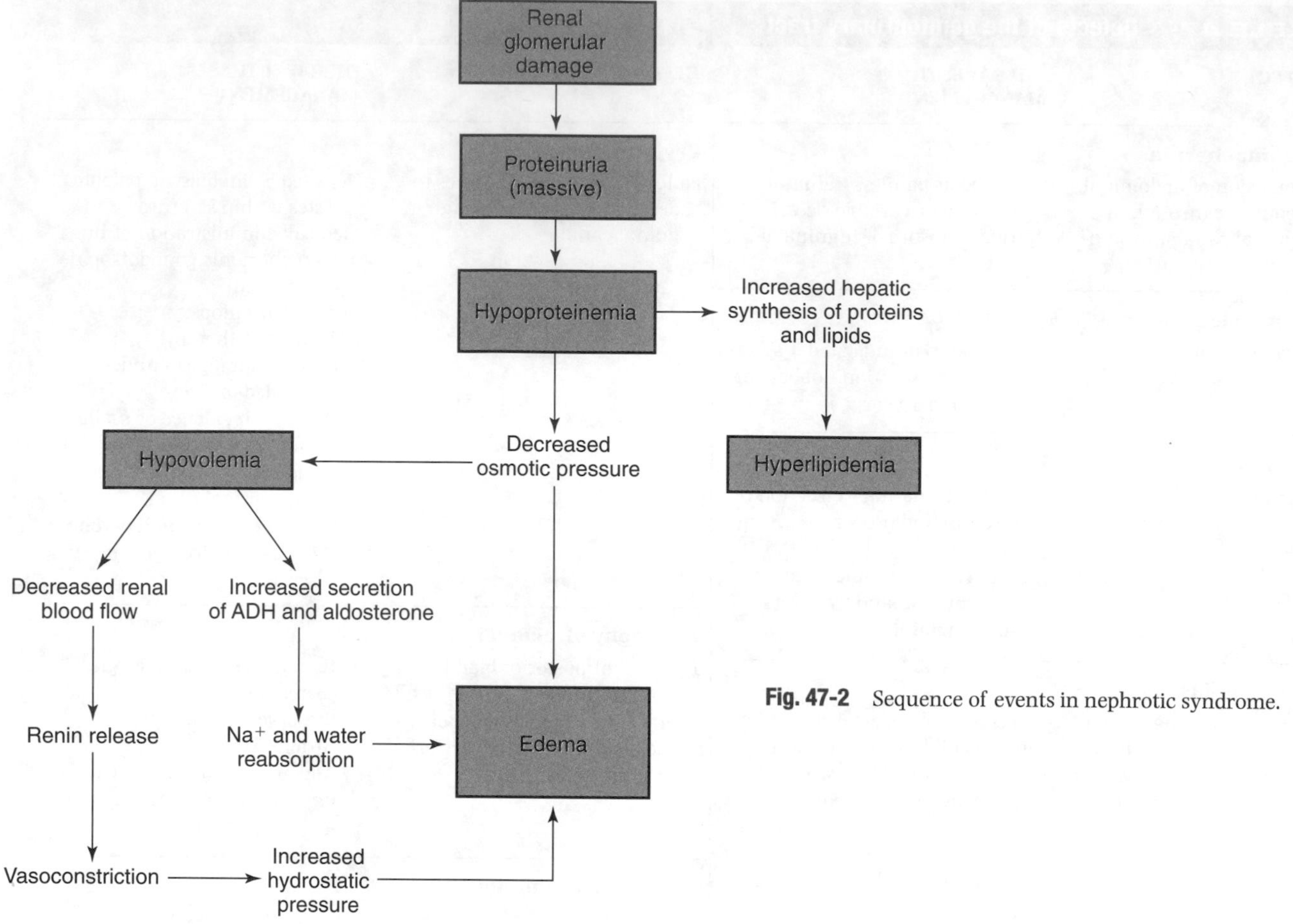

Fig. 47-2 Sequence of events in nephrotic syndrome.

younger than 1 year of age, and unusual after 8 years of age.

The pathogenesis of MCNS is not understood. There may be a metabolic, biochemical, physiochemical, or immune-mediated disturbance that causes the basement membrane of the glomeruli to become increasingly permeable to protein, but the cause and mechanisms are only speculative.

With MCNS, the glomerular membrane, which is normally impermeable to albumin and other proteins, becomes permeable to proteins, especially albumin, which leak through the membrane and are lost in urine **(hyperalbuminuria).** This loss reduces the serum albumin level **(hypoalbuminemia),** decreasing the colloidal osmotic pressure in the capillaries. As a result, the vascular hydrostatic pressure exceeds the pull of the colloidal osmotic pressure, causing fluid to accumulate in the interstitial spaces **(edema)** and body cavities, particularly in the abdominal cavity (**ascites**). The shift of fluid from the plasma to the interstitial spaces reduces the vascular fluid volume **(hypovolemia),** which in turn stimulates the renin-angiotensin system and the secretion of antidiuretic hormone and aldosterone. Tubular reabsorption of sodium and water is increased in an attempt to increase intravascular volume. The elevation of serum lipids is unexplained. The sequence of events in nephrotic syndrome is diagrammed in Fig. 47-2.

Diagnostic Evaluation

MCNS is suspected on the basis of clinical manifestations (Box 47-3), especially when weight gain in a previously well child increases slowly over a period of days or weeks. The generalized edema may develop rapidly or gradually but eventually prompts the family to seek medical attention. Parents usually give a history of the child being well but steadily gaining weight and then becoming anorexic, irritable, and less active.

Nursing ALERT

A child who exhibits the following should be evaluated for the possibility of nephrotic syndrome:

Weight gain over that expected on the basis of previous patterns

Parent observation that the child's clothes fit tightly

Decreased urine output

Pallor, fatigue

The diagnosis of MCNS is made on the basis of the history and clinical manifestations (edema, proteinuria, hypoalbuminemia, and hypercholesterolemia in the absence of hematuria and hypertension) in children between 2 and 8 years of age.

Massive proteinuria is reflected in urinary excretion of protein, with high specific gravity proportionate to the concentration of protein. Hyaline casts, fat bodies, and a few red blood cells can be found in the urine of most affected children, but there is seldom gross hematuria. The glomerular filtration

BOX 47-3
Clinical Manifestations of Nephrotic Syndrome

Weight gain
Edema
Puffiness of face
- Especially around the eyes
- Apparent on arising in the morning
- Subsides during the day

Abdominal swelling (ascites)
Respiratory difficulty (pleural effusion)
Labial or scrotal swelling
Edema of intestinal mucosa causes the following:
- Diarrhea
- Anorexia
- Poor intestinal absorption

Extreme skin pallor (often)
Irritability
Easily fatigued
Lethargic
Blood pressure normal or slightly decreased
Susceptibility to infection
Urine alterations
- Decreased volume
- Darkly opalescent
- Frothy

rate is usually normal if hypovolemia is not significant and if the child is well hydrated.

Total serum protein concentrations are lowered, with the albumin fractions significantly reduced and plasma lipids elevated. Hemoglobin and hematocrit are usually normal or elevated and the platelet count is high as a result of hemoconcentration. Serum sodium concentration is usually low.

A renal biopsy may be performed to distinguish between types of nephrotic syndrome to predict the probable disease course and response to drugs. The biopsy of children with MCNS is remarkable for fusion of the foot processes of the basement membrane and otherwise normal kidney tissue.

Therapeutic Management

Objectives of therapeutic management include (1) reducing excretion of urinary protein, (2) reducing fluid retention in the tissues, (3) preventing infection, and (4) minimizing complications related to therapies. Ambulation is encouraged if edema is not incapacitating. Dietary restrictions include a *low-salt diet* during periods of generalized edema. If complications of edema develop (severe gastrointestinal upset, ascites, or respiratory distress), diuretic therapy, including plasma expanders, may be initiated to provide temporary relief from edema. Acute and intercurrent infections are treated with appropriate antibiotics, and efforts are made to eliminate possible infection.

Corticosteroids have been found to have therapeutic value in treating MCNS, but the success of the treatment depends on the individual child's response to the medication (*prednisone*). In most children this response occurs within 7 to 21 days. The medication is tapered over several weeks and eventually stopped if the child remains asymptomatic. A relapse in which proteinuria returns requires immediate repeated

Critical Thinking Q & A

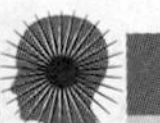

NEPHROTIC SYNDROME

Jerome is an 8-year-old boy with relapsing nephrotic syndrome who has become steroid dependent. During your initial assessment in the outpatient clinic you identify the following: (1) weight has increased 2 kg in the last 2 weeks; (2) blood pressure is 100/70; (3) mother reports that Jerome is not urinating very much and that she does not know how much he has been drinking; (4) while you are measuring Jerome's abdominal girth, he guards his abdomen and complains of stomachache; (5) his temperature is 38° C (100.4° F) orally. Of the following correct actions, you should first do which of the following?

1. Examine Jerome's abdomen more thoroughly while eliciting a 24-hour recall of illness symptoms from his mother.
2. Elicit a 24-hour recall of food and fluid intake from Jerome and his mother together.
3. Obtain a clean-catch urine specimen. Divide the specimen so that you can perform a dipstick analysis immediately and retain the other specimen for possible urinalysis and culture after consultation with the primary health practitioner.
4. Explore the mother's understanding of Jerome's illness and its relationship to his current condition to begin outlining your teaching plan for this family.

The correct response is one. One of the complications of severe nephrotic syndrome is peritonitis, which can occur secondary to migration of intestinal bacteria across the bowel wall and into the protein-rich acidic fluid. Jerome's mother has already said that she does not know what he has been drinking. Therefore your only possibility of assessing his intake is to elicit the recall while they are together. Although his weight gain and reduced urine output are major concerns, they are secondary to peritonitis. (It should be recognized that children on strict fluid restrictions are prone to obtain fluids from unauthorized sources.) Obtaining a urine specimen for dipstick analysis is part of the initial assessment for Jerome. In this instance the fever and abdominal pain are the first priority. As with option three, the fourth choice must be addressed (along with evaluation of the current stress level in the home) after the fever and pain have been addressed.

courses of high-dose steroid therapy. Side effects of the medication include rounding of the face, increased appetite, abdominal distention, hirsutism, growth retardation, cataracts, hypertension, gastrointestinal bleeding, bone demineralization, infection, and hyperglycemia. Children who do not respond to steroid therapy, those who have frequent relapses, and those in whom the side effects threaten their growth and general health may be considered for a course of therapy using other immunosuppressant medications (cyclophosphamide, chorambucil, or cyclosporine).

Complications of nephrotic syndrome include relapse, infection, circulatory insufficiency secondary to hypovolemia, and thromboembolism. Relapses can be triggered by many factors such as viruses, allergies, bacterial infections and, occasionally, immunizations. Relapses in children with MCNS occur two to four times per year and continue over many years. Infections that may be seen in children with nephrotic syndrome include peritonitis, cellulitis, and pneumonia and require prompt recognition and vigorous treatment with appropriate antibiotic therapy (see the Critical Thinking Q & A box above).

Prognosis. The prognosis for ultimate recovery in most cases is good. MCNS is a self-limiting disease, and in children who respond to steroid therapy the tendency to relapse decreases with time. With early detection and prompt implementation of therapy to eradicate proteinuria, progressive basement membrane damage is minimized, so that when the tendency for exacerbations is past, renal function is usually normal or near normal. It is estimated that approximately 80% of affected children have this favorable prognosis, although half the children have relapses even after 5 years.

Nursing Care Management

Assessment

Continuous monitoring of fluid retention or excretion is an important nursing function. Strict intake and output records are essential but may be difficult to obtain from very young children. Application of collection bags is highly irritating to edematous skin that is readily subject to breakdown. Applying diapers or weighing wet pads may be necessary. Other methods of monitoring progress include urine examination for specific gravity and albumin, daily weight, and measurement of abdominal girth. Assessment of edema (such as increased or decreased swelling around the eyes and dependent areas), the degree of pitting (if noted), and the color and texture of skin are part of nursing care. Vital signs are monitored to detect any early signs of complications such as shock or an infective process.

Nursing Diagnoses

Constant reassessment and evaluation reveal a number of nursing diagnoses that are relevant to the care of these children and their families (see the Nursing Care Plan on p. 1555). Others will be apparent in specific situations.

Planning

The goals of nursing care of the child with nephrotic syndrome and the family are as follows:

1. Child will exhibit no evidence of fluid accumulation.
2. Child will exhibit no evidence of skin breakdown or infection.
3. Child will receive optimum nutrition.
4. Child and family will express feelings and concerns.

Implementation

Children hospitalized with MCNS may be placed on bed rest during the edema phase of the disease. They seldom offer resistance because they are usually lethargic and easily fatigued, and their cumbersome edematous bulk is not conducive to movement.

Reducing the excretion of urinary protein primarily involves the administration of corticosteroids. Nurses must be aware of the problems associated with these drugs and be alert to complications from their use.

Infection is a constant source of danger to edematous children and those receiving corticosteroid therapy. These children are particularly vulnerable to upper respiratory infection; therefore they must be kept warm and dry, turned frequently, and protected from contact with infected roommates, visitors, and personnel. Vital signs are monitored to detect any early signs of an infective process.

The loss of appetite that accompanies active nephrosis creates a perplexing problem for nurses. During this time the combined efforts of the nurse, dietitian, parents, and child are needed to formulate a nutritionally adequate and attractive diet. Salt is usually restricted (but not eliminated) during the edema phase, and fluid restriction (if prescribed) is limited to short-term use during massive edema. Every effort should be made to serve attractive meals with preferred foods and a minimum of fuss, but it usually requires a considerable amount of ingenuity and enticement to get the child to eat (see Feeding the Sick Child, Chapter 42).

As the edema subsides, children are allowed increased activity. Although easily fatigued, children usually adjust activities according to their tolerance level. However, they may require guidance in selecting play activities. Suitable recreational and diversional activities are an important part of their care. Once edema fluid has been lost, children are allowed to resume their usual activities with discretion. Irritability and mood swings that accompany the inactivity, disease process, and steroid therapy are not unusual manifestations in these children, and they create an additional challenge to the nurse and the family.

Family support and home care. Continuous support of the child and family is one of the major nursing considerations. Many children are treated at home during exacerbations. Parents are taught to detect signs of relapse and to bring the child for treatment at the earliest indications. Home care is preferred unless the edema and proteinuria are severe or the parents, for some reason, are unable to care for the ill child. Parents are instructed in testing urine for albumin, administration of medications, and general care. Parents are also instructed regarding avoiding contact with infected playmates, but the child should attend school.

The prolonged course of the relapsing form of nephrotic syndrome is taxing to both the child and the family. The up-and-down course of remissions and exacerbations with periodic disruption of family life by hospitalization places a severe strain on the child and the family, both psychologically and financially. Parents and children older than 5 or 6 years of age need reassurance regarding this characteristic of the course of the disease, with emphasis on the importance of long-term care to gain their cooperation. A satisfactory response is more likely when relapses are detected and therapy is instituted early, and remissions are prolonged when instructions are carried out faithfully. Continuous support of the child and family is one of the major nursing considerations (see Chapter 38).

Evaluation

The effectiveness of nursing interventions is determined by continual reassessment and evaluation of care on the basis of the following observational guidelines and expected outcomes:

1. Measure intake and output and examine urine for albumin.
2. Monitor vital signs and assess the skin for evidence of breakdown or infection.
3. Assess appetite and eating behaviors.

Nursing Care Plan

THE CHILD WITH NEPHROTIC SYNDROME

Nursing Diagnosis: Fluid volume excess (total body) related to fluid accumulation in tissues and third spaces

Expected Outcome: Child exhibits no or minimal evidence of fluid accumulation.

- **NURSING INTERVENTIONS/*RATIONALES***

Monitor intake and output, weigh daily, and monitor changes in edema of abdomen, around eyes, and in dependent areas *to assess fluid retention.*

Monitor urine for specific gravity and albumin *to assess presence of hyperalbuminuria.*

Limit fluids as indicated and regulate oral and intravenous fluid intake carefully *so fluid restrictions are maintained.*

Keep mouth moist and lips lubricated *to prevent dryness and cracking.*

Administer diuretics and corticosteroids as ordered *to reduce edema and lower excretion of urinary protein.*

Nursing Diagnosis: Risk for fluid volume deficit (intravascular) related to protein and fluid loss, edema

Expected Outcome: Child exhibits no evidence of intravascular fluid loss or hypovolemic shock.

- **NURSING INTERVENTIONS/*RATIONALES***

Monitor vital signs (e.g., weak, rapid pulse; tachypnea; hyperventilation, decreased blood pressure); monitor for rising Hbg or Hct; note condition of skin (e.g., cold, moist, cyanotic, pale); note signs of confusion and lethargy *to detect evidence of depletion and impending shock.*

Report any suspected signs of impending shock promptly *to ensure rapid treatment.*

Administer salt-poor albumin per physician's order *to serve as a plasma expander.*

Nursing Diagnosis: Risk for infection related to lowered body defenses, fluid overload

Expected Outcome: Child exhibits no evidence of infection.

- **NURSING INTERVENTIONS/*RATIONALES***

Place child in private room and screen all visitors and staff for signs of infection *to minimize exposure to infective organisms.*

Teach child and family about good hygiene and careful handwashing techniques *to prevent spread of infection.*

Observe medical aesepsis *to prevent spread of infection.*

Encourage a nutritionally complete diet *to support body's natural defenses.*

Monitor vital signs, observe skin, and auscultate lungs *to detect signs of infection.*

Nursing Diagnosis: Altered nutrition: less than body requirements related to loss of appetite

Expected Outcome: Nutritional intake is adequate.

- **NURSING INTERVENTIONS/*RATIONALES***

Provide balanced, sodium-restricted diet *to meet body requirements for metabolism and growth;* fortify foods with vitamin and iron supplements as ordered *to maximize quality of intake.*

Involve child in selection and preparation *to increase intake and tolerance.*

Serve meals in small, attractively arranged quantities and in a relaxed atmosphere *to increase appetite.*

See also Feeding the Sick Child, Chapter 42.

Nursing Diagnosis: Risk for impaired skin integrity related to edema and lowered body defenses

Expected Outcome: Skin is clean and intact.

- **NURSING INTERVENTIONS/*RATIONALES***

Provide meticulous skin care, turn and reposition frequently and align correctly *to prevent skin breakdown.*

Avoid restrictive clothing, support edematous organs, use pressure-reducing mattresses *to prevent skin breakdown.*

Inspect skin frequently *to assess for areas of impending breakdown.*

Nursing Diagnosis: Activity intolerance related to fatigue

Expected Outcome: Child appears rested.

- **NURSING INTERVENTIONS/*RATIONALES***

Maintain initial bedrest with severe edema and provide quiet in-bed activities *to reduce energy expenditure.*

Balance rest and activity, monitoring child's fatigue level *so that needed rest periods can be provided.*

Allow for periods of uninterrupted sleep *to restore energy levels.*

Nursing Diagnosis: Body image disturbance related to change in appearance

Expected Outcome: Child exhibits signs of acceptance of alteration in appearance.

- **NURSING INTERVENTIONS/*RATIONALES***

Explore feelings and concerns about appearance and emphasize temporary nature of the change *to facilitate coping.*

Involve child in edema measures *so they can monitor results of edema decline.*

Encourage social interaction by telephone with peers and siblings *to prevent feelings of isolation.*

Nursing Diagnosis: Altered family processes related to situational crises (child with serious illness)

See the Nursing Care Plan: The Family of the Ill or Hospitalized Child, Chapter 41.

4. Observe and interview child and family regarding their understanding of the disease, therapies, and compliance with the prescribed regimen.

Expected outcomes:

See the Nursing Care Plan box on p. 1555.

ACUTE GLOMERULONEPHRITIS (AGN)

Acute glomerulonephritis (AGN) may be a primary event or a manifestation of a systemic disorder that can range from minimal to severe. Common features include oliguria, edema, hypertension and circulatory congestion, hematuria, and proteinuria. Most cases are postinfectious and have been associated with pneumococcal, streptococcal, and viral infections. *Acute poststreptococcal glomerulonephritis (APSGN)* is the most common of the postinfectious, associated renal diseases in childhood and is the one for which a cause can be established in the majority of cases. APSGN can occur at any age but primarily affects early school-age children, with a peak age of onset of 6 to 7 years. It is uncommon in children younger than 2 years of age, and males out-number females 2:1.

Etiology

APSGN is an immune-complex disease that occurs as a byproduct of an antecedent streptococcal infection with certain strains of the group A β-hemolytic streptococcus. Most streptococcal infections *do not* cause APSGN. A latent period of 10 to 14 days occurs between the streptococcal infection and the onset of clinical manifestations. The peak incidence of disease corresponds to the incidence of streptococcal infection. Disease secondary to streptococcal pharyngitis is more common in the winter or spring, but when it is associated with pyoderma (principally *impetigo*) it may be more prevalent in late summer or early fall, especially in warmer climates. Multiple cases tend to occur in families. Second episodes of AGN are rare.

Pathophysiology

The mechanism by which the reaction takes place is still speculative; one explanation is that the streptococcal infection is followed by the release of a membranelike material from the specific organism into the circulation. Because it is antigenic, an antibody is formed, and an immune-complex reaction occurs after the appropriate amount of time. The glomeruli become edematous and infiltrated with polymorphonuclear leukocytes, which occlude the capillary lumen. The resulting decrease in plasma filtration results in an excessive accumulation of water and retention of sodium that expands plasma and interstitial fluid volumes, leading to circulatory congestion and edema. It is unclear whether the decreased glomerular filtration rate, increased capillary permeability, or vascular spasm is responsible for these various manifestations. The cause of the hypertension associated with AGN is also unexplained.

Diagnostic Evaluation

Typically, affected children are in good health until they experience the streptococcal infection. In some instances there is no history of an infection, or it is described only as a mild cold. The onset of nephritis appears after an average latent period of approximately 10 days (Box 47-4). Because the child appears to be well during this time, the association is not recognized by the parents. The edema is relatively moderate and may not be appreciated by someone unfamiliar with the child's normal appearance.

Urinalysis during the acute phase characteristically shows hematuria, proteinuria, and increased specific gravity. The specific gravity is moderately elevated and seldom exceeds 1.02. Proteinuria generally parallels the hematuria, and the content usually shows 3+ or 4+ but is not the massive proteinuria seen in nephrotic syndrome. Gross discoloration of the urine reflects its red blood cell and hemoglobin content. Microscopic examination of the sediment shows many red blood cells, leukocytes, epithelial cells, and granular and red blood cell casts. Bacteria are not seen, and urine cultures are negative.

Azotemia that results from impaired glomerular filtration is reflected in elevated blood urea nitrogen and creatinine levels in at least 50% of cases. When proteinuria is excessive, there may be changes associated with nephrotic syndrome (e.g., transient hypoproteinemia and hyperlipidemia).

Cultures of the pharynx are positive for streptococci in only a few cases, and the numbers are not significantly greater than the normal carrier incidence in many communities. Positive cultures help to establish a diagnosis. Cultures should be obtained from other household members, and persons positive for group A streptococci should receive a course of antistreptococcal therapy.

BOX 47-4
Clinical Manifestations of Acute Poststreptococcal Glomerulonephritis

- Edema
  - Especially periorbital
  - Facial edema more prominent in the morning
  - Spreads during the day to involve extremities and abdomen
- Anorexia
- Urine
  - Cloudy, smoky brown (resembles tea or cola)
  - Severely reduced volume
- Pallor
- Irritability
- Lethargy
- Child appears ill
- Child seldom expresses specific complaints
- Older children may complain of the following:
  - Headaches
  - Abdominal discomfort
  - Dysuria
- Vomiting possible
- Mild to moderately elevated blood pressure

Nursing ALERT

A child who exhibits the following should be evaluated for possible AGN:

Orbital edema, which parents report is worse in the morning
- Loss of appetite
- Decreased output
- Dark-colored urine
- Antecedent streptococcal infection

Some serologic tests may help in the diagnosis of AGN. The *antistreptolysin O (ASO) titer* is the most familiar and readily available test for streptococcal infection. It is used to detect the presence of antibodies, which documents a recent infection, especially a rising titer in two samples obtained 1 week apart. Other serologic tests that may aid in diagnosis following streptococcal skin infections are elevated antihyaluronidase (AHase), antideoxyribonuclease-B (ADNase-B), and antinicotyladenine dinucleotidase (ANADase) titers.

Because AGN is an immune-complex disease, there is reduced total serum complement activity in the early stages. Rising complement levels (C3, C4) are used as a guide to indicate improvement of the disease. Other studies that are used include a chest x-ray examination, which shows characteristic generalized cardiac enlargement, pulmonary congestion, and pleural effusion during the edematous phase of acute disease. Renal biopsy for diagnostic purposes is seldom required but may be useful in the diagnosis of atypical cases.

Therapeutic Management

Management consists of general supportive measures and early recognition and treatment of complications. Children who have normal blood pressure and a satisfactory urine output can generally be treated at home. Those with substantial edema, hypertension, gross hematuria, and/or significant oliguria should be hospitalized because of the unpredictability of complications.

Bed rest may be recommended during the acute phase, but ambulation does not seem to have an adverse effect on the course of the disease once the symptoms have resolved. Dietary restrictions depend on the stage and severity of the disease, especially the extent of edema. Moderate sodium restriction is usually instituted for children with hypertension and edema. Foods with substantial amounts of potassium are generally restricted during the period of oliguria.

Regular measurement of vital signs, body weight, and intake and output is essential to monitor the progress of the disease and to detect complications that may appear at any time during the course of the disease. *A record of daily weight is the most useful means for assessing fluid balance.* Children with AGN rarely develop acute renal failure with oliguria that significantly alters the fluid and electrolyte balance (resulting in hyperkalemia, acidosis, hypocalcemia, and/or hyperphosphatemia). These children require careful management that may include peritoneal dialysis or hemodialysis.

Acute hypertension must be anticipated and identified early. Blood pressure measurements are taken every 4 to 6 hours. A variety of antihypertensive medications and diuretics are used to control mild-to-moderate hypertension. Seizure activity associated with hypertensive encephalopathy requires anticonvulsant therapy and antihypertensive agents.

Antibiotic therapy is indicated only for those children with evidence of persistent streptococcal infections. It is used to prevent transmission of nephritogenic streptococci to other family members.

Prognosis. Almost all children correctly diagnosed as having APSGN recover completely. Subsequent recurrences are uncommon because specific immunity is conferred. Deaths from complications still occur but fortunately are rare. A few of these children may develop chronic disease, but many of these cases are believed to be (probably) different glomerular diseases misdiagnosed as poststreptococcal disease.

Nursing Care Management

Assessment

Vital signs provide clues to the severity of the disease and early signs of complications. They are carefully measured, and any deviations are reported and recorded. The volume and character of urine are noted, and the child is weighed daily. Children with restricted fluid intake, especially those who are not severely edematous or those who have lost weight, are observed for signs of dehydration.

Assessment of the child's appearance for signs of cerebral complications is an important nursing function because the severity of the acute phase is variable and unpredictable. The child with edema, hypertension, and gross hematuria may be subject to complications, and anticipatory preparations such as seizure precautions and intravenous equipment are included in the nursing care plan.

Nursing Diagnoses

Several nursing diagnoses become obvious on the basis of assessment (Box 47-5). Others may be evident in specific situations.

Planning

The goals of care for the child with AGN and the family include the following:

1. Child will receive optimum rest.
2. Child will receive sufficient nutrition.
3. Child will exhibit no evidence of complications.
4. Child and family will receive appropriate support and education regarding child's condition.

Implementation

During the acute phase children are generally quite content to lie in bed. Activities should be those that require little expenditure of energy. Because they are generally listless and experience fatigue and malaise, most children voluntarily restrict their activities during the most active phase of the disease. As they begin to feel better and as their symptoms subside, activities are planned to allow for frequent rest periods and avoidance of fatigue.

For most children a regular diet is allowed, but it should contain no added salt. Foods high in sodium and salted treats are eliminated, and parents and friends are advised not to bring items such as potato chips or pretzels. However, the total amount of salt ingested is usually less than prescribed because

BOX 47-5
Nursing Diagnoses: The Child With Acute Glomerulonephritis

Fluid volume excess related to decreased plasma filtration
Activity intolerance related to fatigue
Altered patterns of urinary elimination related to fluid retention and impaired glomerular filtration
Altered family processes related to the child with a renal disorder

of the child's poor appetite. Fluid restriction, if prescribed, is more difficult, and the amount permitted should be evenly divided throughout the waking hours and served in small cups to give the illusion of larger servings. Meal preparation and service require special attention because the child is indifferent to meals during the acute phase. Again, collaboration with parents and the dietitian and special consideration for food preferences facilitate meal planning.

Children who have mild edema and no hypertension, as well as convalescent children who are being treated at home, need follow-up care. Parents are instructed regarding general measures, including activity, diet, and prevention of infection. Strenuous activity is usually restricted until there is no evidence of proteinuria or macroscopic hematuria, which may persist for months.

Health supervision is continued with weekly, followed by monthly, visits for evaluation and urinalysis. Parent education and support in preparation for discharge and home care include education in home management and the need for follow-up care and health supervision.

Evaluation

The effectiveness of nursing interventions is determined by continual reassessment and evaluation of care on the basis of the following observational guidelines and expected outcomes:

1. Observe child's behavior.
2. Monitor dietary and fluid intake; interview family regarding child's diet and appetite.
3. Monitor vital signs, intake and output, and observe for signs of complications such as hypertension, increased intracranial pressure, and infection.
4. Observe behaviors and interview child and family regarding reaction to the disease and therapies.

Expected outcomes

1. Child plays and rests quietly.
2. Child consumes a sufficient amount of appropriate foods.
3. Child exhibits no evidence of complications.
4. Child and family demonstrate an understanding of the disease and its therapy (specify learning and methods of demonstration), and they express their feelings and concerns.

See also Nursing Care Plan: The Child with Acute Poststreptoccocal Glomerulonephritis.*

Miscellaneous Renal Disorders

HEMOLYTIC-UREMIC SYNDROME (HUS)

Hemolytic-uremic syndrome (HUS) is an uncommon, acute renal disease that occurs primarily in infants and small children between the ages of 6 months and 5 years. It occurs worldwide but is recognized predominantly in white children. HUS is the most common cause of acquired acute renal failure in children (Brandt et al, 1994). The clinical features of the disease include acquired hemolytic anemia, thrombocytopenia, renal injury, and central nervous system symptoms. The etiology of HUS is thought to be associated with bacterial toxins, chemicals, and viruses. The appearance of the disease has been associated with *Rickettsia,* viruses (especially coxsackie virus, echovirus, and adenovirus), *E. coli,* pneumococci, *Shigella,* and *Salmonella* and may represent an unusual response to these infections. Multiple cases of HUS caused by enteric infection of the *E. coli* 0157:H7 serotype have been traced to undercooked meat. The clinical presentation is usually a history of a prodromal illness (most often gastroenteritis or an upper respiratory infection) followed by the sudden onset of hemolysis and renal failure.

Pathophysiology

The primary site of injury appears to be the endothelial lining of the small glomerular arterioles, which become swollen and occluded with deposits of platelets and fibrin clots (intravascular coagulation). Red blood cells are damaged as they attempt to move through the partially occluded blood vessels. These damaged cells are removed by the spleen, causing acute hemolytic anemia. The platelet aggregation within the damaged blood vessels or the damage and removal of platelets produce the characteristic thrombocytopenia.

Diagnostic Evaluation

The triad of anemia, thrombocytopenia, and renal failure is sufficient for diagnosis (Box 47-6). Renal involvement is evidenced by proteinuria, hematuria, and the presence of urinary casts; blood urea nitrogen and serum creatinine levels are elevated. A low hemoglobin and hematocrit, and a high reticulocyte count confirm the hemolytic nature of the anemia.

Therapeutic Management

The goals of therapy are early diagnosis and aggressive, supportive care of the acute renal failure and hemolytic anemia. The most consistently effective treatment of HUS is hemodial-

BOX 47-6
Clinical Manifestations of Hemolytic-Uremic Syndrome

- Vomiting
- Irritability
- Lethargy
- Marked pallor
- Hemorrhagic manifestations
  - Bruising
  - Petechiae
  - Jaundice
  - Bloody diarrhea
- Oliguria or anuria
- Central nervous system involvement
  - Convulsions
  - Stupor/coma
- Signs of acute heart failure (sometimes)

*In Wong DL: *Wong and Whaley's clinical manual of pediatric nursing,* ed 4, St Louis, 1996, Mosby.

ysis or peritoneal dialysis, which is instituted in any child who has been anuric for 24 hours or who demonstrates oliguria with uremia or hypertension and seizures. Other treatments include the use of pharmacologic agents, fresh frozen plasma, and plasma pheresis. Blood transfusions with fresh, washed packed cells are administered for severe anemia but are used with caution to prevent circulatory overload from added volume.

Prognosis. With prompt treatment the recovery rate is approximately 95%, but residual renal impairment ranges from 10% to 50% in various areas. Long-term complications include chronic renal failure, hypertension, and central nervous system disorders. Death is usually caused by residual renal impairment or central nervous system injury.

Nursing Care Management

Nursing care is the same as that provided in acute renal failure and, for children with continued impairment, includes management of chronic disease.

WILMS TUMOR

Wilms tumor, or nephroblastoma, is the most common primary malignant tumor of the kidney in children. Its frequency is estimated to be 1 per 125,000 Caucasian children less than 15 years of age. Wilms tumor occurs approximately three times more often in African-Americans than in East Asians in the United States. The peak age at diagnosis is approximately 3 years; and occurrence is slightly more common in boys than in girls. Wilms tumor is one of the childhood cancers that may be genetically inherited. Unfortunately, there is currently no method of identifying gene carriers.

Etiology

Wilms tumor probably arises from a malignant, undifferentiated cluster of primordial cells capable of initiating the regeneration of an abnormal structure. Its occurrence slightly favors the left kidney, which is advantageous because surgically this kidney is easier to manipulate and remove. In approximately 10% of cases both kidneys are involved. Although the tumor may become quite large, it remains encapsulated for an extended period of time. Studies have shown that development of Wilms tumor involves both genetic and somatic mosaicism, not germ-line mutation (Green et al, 1996).

Diagnostic Evaluation

In a child suspected of having Wilms tumor, special emphasis is placed on the history and physical examination for the presence of congenital anomalies, a family history of cancer, and signs of malignancy such as weight loss, size of liver and spleen, indications of anemia, and lymphadenopathy. Most children with Wilms tumor are brought to the practitioner because of abdominal swelling or an abdominal mass (Box 47-7). Specific tests include radiographic studies, including abdominal ultrasound, computerized tomography, hematologic studies (polycythemia is sometimes present if the tumor secretes excess erythropoietin), biochemical studies, and urinalysis. Studies to demonstrate the relationship of the tumor to the ipsilateral kidney and the presence of a normal functioning kidney on the contralateral side are essential. If a large tumor is present, an inferior venacavogram is necessary to demonstrate possible tumor involvement adjacent to the vena cava. A bone marrow aspiration may be performed to rule out metastasis, which is rare in children with Wilms tumor.

BOX 47-7
Clinical Manifestations of Wilms Tumor

- Abdominal swelling or mass
  - Firm
  - Nontender
  - Confined to one side
- Hematuria (less than ¼ of cases)
- Fatigue/malaise
- Hypertension (occasionally)
- Weight loss
- Fever
- Manifestations resulting from compression of tumor mass
- Secondary metabolic alterations from tumor or metastasis
- If metastasis, symptoms of lung involvement
  - Dyspnea
  - Cough
  - Shortness of breath
  - Chest pain (sometimes)

Therapeutic Management

Combined treatment of surgery and chemotherapy with or without radiation is based on the clinical stage and histologic pattern.

Surgery is scheduled as soon as possible after confirmation of a renal mass, usually within 24 to 48 hours of admission. A large transabdominal incision is performed for optimum visualization of the abdominal cavity. The tumor, affected kidney, and adjacent adrenal gland are removed. Great care is taken to keep the encapsulated tumor intact, because rupture can seed cancer cells throughout the abdomen, lymph channel, and bloodstream. The contralateral kidney is carefully inspected for evidence of disease or dysfunction. Regional lymph nodes are inspected, and a biopsy is performed when indicated. Any involved structures, such as part of the colon, diaphragm, or vena cava, are removed. Metal clips are placed around the tumor site for exact marking during radiotherapy.

If both kidneys are involved, the child may be treated with radiotherapy and/or chemotherapy before surgery to decrease the size of the tumor and allow more conservative surgery. It may be possible to perform a partial nephrectomy on the less affected kidney, with a total nephrectomy on the opposite side. When a transplant is feasible, such as from a twin, sibling, or parent, bilateral nephrectomy is considered.

Postoperative radiation therapy is indicated for children with large tumors, metastasis, residual postoperative disease, unfavorable histology, or recurrence.

Chemotherapy is indicated for all stages. The most effective agents for treating Wilms tumor are actinomycin D (dactinomycin), vincristine, and doxorubicin (Adriamycin). The duration of therapy varies, ranging from 6 to 15 months. Wilms tumor may recur, especially in the lungs.

Prognosis. Survival rates for Wilms tumor are the highest among all childhood cancers. Children with a localized tumor (stages I and II) have a 90% chance of cure with multimodal therapy. Factors that favorably affect the success of further therapy include initial treatment with only vincristine and dactinomycin, relapse to the lungs only, relapse in the abdomen of a patient who received no prior abdominal irradiation, and relapse more than 12 months after diagnosis. Both chemotherapy and radiation therapy can induce second tumors, usually in areas that have been irradiated (Green et al, 1996).

Nursing Care Management

Nursing care of the child with Wilms tumor is similar to that of children with other cancers treated with surgery, irradiation, and chemotherapy. However, there are some significant differences; these are discussed for each phase of nursing intervention.

Preoperative care. The preoperative period is one of swift diagnosis. The nurse is faced with the challenge of preparing the child and parents for all laboratory and operative procedures. Because of the little time available, explanations are kept simple, focused on what the child will experience, and repeated often. In addition to the usual preoperative observations, blood pressure is monitored because hypertension from excess renin production is a possibility.

There are several special preoperative concerns, the most important of which is that the *tumor is not palpated unless absolutely necessary,* because manipulation of the mass may cause dissemination of cancer cells to adjacent and distant sites.

Nursing ALERT

To reinforce the need for caution, it may be necessary to post a sign on the bed that reads "DO NOT PALPATE ABDOMEN." Careful bathing and handling are also important in preventing trauma to the tumor site.

Since radiotherapy and chemotherapy are usually begun immediately after surgery, parents need an explanation of what to expect, such as major benefits and side effects. The timing of the information should be considered to avoid overwhelming the family. Ideally, the nurse should be present during physician-parent conferences to answer questions as they arise. It is usually better to reserve telling the child about these side effects until after surgery. Alopecia, usually of most concern to older children, does not occur until 2 weeks after the initial treatment regimen. Therefore the child can be prepared for the hair loss postoperatively.

Postoperative care. Despite the extensive surgical intervention necessary in many children with Wilms tumor, the recovery is usually rapid. The major nursing responsibilities are the same as those following any abdominal surgery (see Surgical Procedures, Chapter 42). Gastrointestinal activity such as bowel movements, bowel sounds, distention, vomiting, and pain are carefully monitored because these children are at risk for intestinal obstruction from vincristine-induced adynamic ileus, radiation-induced edema, and postsurgical adhesion formation.

The nurse also monitors blood pressure for a possible drop after removal of the tumor, urine output to assess functioning of the remaining kidney, and signs of infection, especially during chemotherapy. Because of the myelosuppression from the drugs, pulmonary hygiene measures are instituted in the immediate postoperative period to prevent lung involvement.

Nursing ALERT

Because the child is left with one kidney, certain precautions, such as avoiding contact sports, are recommended to prevent injury to the remaining organ. Prompt detection and treatment of any genitourinary signs or symptoms is mandatory.

Family support. The postoperative period is often difficult for parents. The shock of seeing their child immediately after surgery may be the first realization of the seriousness of the diagnosis. It also marks the confirmation of the stage of the tumor. Again, during this period, the nurse should be with the parents to assure them of the child's recovery after surgery and to assess the parents' understanding of the operative report. They need an opportunity to express their feelings and to realize that their feelings are normal and realistic. The same emotional care discussed in Chapter 38 for families who have a child with a life-threatening disorder is applied to these individuals.

Older children need an opportunity to deal with their feelings concerning the many procedures to which they have been subjected in rapid succession. Play therapy with dolls or puppets or through drawing can be extremely beneficial in helping them adjust to the surgery and hair loss. It is not unusual for children to feel angry because they were not adequately prepared for the extent of surgery, the need for additional therapy, or the seriousness of the disorder.

Renal Failure

Renal failure is the inability of the kidneys to excrete waste material, concentrate urine, and conserve electrolytes. It can occur suddenly *(acute renal failure)* in response to inadequate perfusion, kidney disease, or urinary tract obstruction, or it can develop slowly *(chronic renal failure)* as a result of long-standing kidney disease or an anomaly.

Azotemia and uremia are terms often used in relation to renal failure. **Azotemia** is the accumulation of nitrogenous waste within the blood. **Uremia** is a more advanced condition in which retention of nitrogenous products produces toxic symptoms. Azotemia is not life threatening, whereas uremia is a serious condition that often involves other body systems.

ACUTE RENAL FAILURE (ARF)

Acute renal failure (ARF) is said to exist when the kidneys suddenly are unable to regulate the volume and composition of urine appropriately in response to food and fluid intake and the needs of the organism. The principal feature of ARF is oliguria* associated with azotemia, metabolic acidosis, and diverse electrolyte disturbances. ARF is not common in childhood, but the outcome depends on the cause, associated findings, and prompt recognition and treatment.

The pathologic conditions that produce ARF caused by glomerulonephritis and HUS have been discussed in relation to those disorders. ARF can also develop as a result of a large number of related or unrelated clinical conditions—poor renal perfusion, urinary tract obstruction, acute renal injury, or the final expression of chronic, irreversible renal disease. The most common cause in children is transient renal failure resulting from severe dehydration or other causes of poor perfusion that may respond to restoration of fluid volume.

BOX 47-8
Clinical Manifestations of Acute Renal Failure

Specific
- Oliguria
- Anuria uncommon (except in obstructive disorders)

Nonspecific (may develop)
- Nausea
- Vomiting
- Drowsiness
- Edema
- Hypertension

Manifestations of underlying disorder or pathologic condition

Pathophysiology

ARF is usually reversible, but the deviations of physiologic function can be extreme, and mortality in the pediatric age group remains high. There is severe reduction in the glomerular filtration rate, an elevated blood urea nitrogen level, and a significant reduction in renal blood flow.

The clinical course is variable and depends on the cause. In reversible ARF there is a period of severe oliguria, or a low-output phase, followed by an abrupt onset of diuresis, or a high-output phase, and then a gradual return to, or toward, normal urine volumes.

Diagnostic Evaluation

In many instances of ARF the infant or child is already critically ill with the precipitating disorder, and the explanation for development of oliguria may or may not be readily apparent (Box 47-8). When a previously well child develops ARF without obvious cause, a careful history is taken to reveal symptoms that may be related to glomerulonephritis or obstructive uropathy or exposure to nephrotoxic chemicals such as ingestion of heavy metals or inhalation of carbon tetrachloride or other organic solvents or drugs known to be toxic to the kidneys. Significant laboratory measurements during renal shutdown that serve as a guide for therapy are blood urea nitrogen, serum creatinine pH, sodium, potassium, and calcium.

Therapeutic Management

Treatment of ARF is directed toward (1) treatment of the underlying cause, (2) management of the complications of renal failure, and (3) provision of supportive therapy within the constraints imposed by the renal failure.

Treatment of poor perfusion resulting from dehydration consists of volume restoration as described in Chapter 44 in treatment of dehydration. If oliguria persists after restoration of fluid volume or if the renal failure is caused by intrinsic renal damage, the physiologic and biochemical abnormalities that have resulted from kidney dysfunction must be corrected or controlled. Initially a Foley catheter is inserted to rule out urine retention, to collect available urine for analysis, and to monitor results of diuretic administration. The catheter may or may not be removed.

The amount of exogenous water provided should not exceed the amount needed to maintain zero water balance. It is calculated on the basis of estimated endogenous water formation and losses from sensible (primarily gastrointestinal) and insensible sources. No allotment is calculated for urine as long as oliguria persists.

When the output begins to increase, either spontaneously or in response to diuretic therapy, the intake of fluid, potassium, and sodium must be monitored and adequate replacement provided to prevent depletion and its consequences. Some patients pass enormous amounts of electrolyte-rich urine.

Complications. The child with ARF has a tendency to develop water intoxication and hyponatremia, which make it difficult to provide calories in sufficient amounts to meet the needs of the child and reduce the tissue catabolism, metabolic acidosis, hyperkalemia, and uremia. If the child is able to tolerate oral foods, food sources high in concentrated carbohydrate and fat but low in protein, potassium, and sodium may be provided. However, many children have functional disturbances of the gastrointestinal tract, such as nausea and vomiting; therefore the intravenous route is generally preferred and usually consists of essential amino acids or a combination of essential and nonessential amino acids administered by the central venous route.

Control of water balance in these patients requires careful monitoring of feedback information, such as accurate intake and output, body weight, and electrolyte measurements. In general, no sodium, chloride, or potassium is given during the oliguric phase unless there are other large, ongoing losses. Regular measurement of plasma electrolyte, pH, blood urea nitrogen, and creatinine levels is required to assess the adequacy of fluid therapy and to anticipate complications that require specific treatment.

Hyperkalemia is the most immediate threat to the life of the child with ARF. **Hyperkalemia** can be minimized and sometimes avoided by eliminating potassium from all food and fluid, by reducing tissue catabolism, and by correcting acidosis. Measures used for the reduction of serum potassium levels are oral or rectal administration of an ion-exchange resin such as sodium polystyrene sulfonate (Kayexalate) and peritoneal dialysis or hemodialysis (see p. 1568). The resin produces its effect by exchange of its sodium for the potassium, thus binding potassium for removal from the body. This increased sodium concentration may contribute to fluid overload, hypertension, and cardiac failure. Dialysis removes

*The definition of oliguria varies extensively in the literature, from 1.8 to 4 dl/m²/24 hours.

potassium and other waste products from the serum by diffusion through a semipermeable membrane.

Nursing ALERT

Any of the following signs of hyperkalemia constitute an emergency and are reported immediately:
Serum potassium concentrations in excess of 7 mEq/L
Presence of electrocardiogram abnormalities, such as prolonged QRS complex, depressed ST segment, high peaked T waves, bradycardia, or heart block

Hypertension is a common and serious complication of ARF; to detect it early, blood pressure measurements are obtained every 4 to 6 hours. The most common cause of hypertension in ARF is overexpansion of extra-cellular fluid and plasma volume together with activation of the renin-angiotensin system. Hypertension is controlled with antihypertensive drugs. Other measures that may be used include limiting fluids and salt.

Anemia is commonly associated with ARF, but transfusion is not recommended unless the hemoglobin drops below 6 g/dl. Transfusions, if used, consist of fresh, packed red blood cells given slowly to reduce the likelihood of increasing blood volume, hypertension, and hyperkalemia.

Seizures occur rather often when renal failure progresses to uremia and are also related to hypertension, hyponatremia, and hypocalcemia. Treatment is directed to the specific cause when known. More obscure causes are managed with antiepileptic drugs.

Cardiac failure with pulmonary edema is almost always associated with hypervolemia. Treatment is directed toward reduction of fluid volume, with water and sodium restriction and administration of diuretics.

Prognosis. The prognosis of ARF depends largely on the nature and severity of the causative factor or precipitating event and the promptness and competence of management. The outcome is least favorable in children with rapidly progressive nephritis and cortical necrosis. Children in whom ARF is a result of HUS or AGN may recover completely, but residual renal impairment or hypertension is more often the rule. Complete recovery is usually expected in children whose renal failure is a result of dehydration, nephrotoxins, or ischemia. ARF following cardiac surgery is less favorable. It is often impossible to assess the extent of recovery for several months.

Nursing Care Management

Assessment

Meticulous attention to fluid intake and output is mandatory and includes all the physical measurements discussed previously in relation to problems of fluid balance. Monitoring fluid balance and vital signs is a continuous process, and observers are constantly on the alert for signs of complications so that appropriate interventions can be implemented. Because children with ARF require intensive observation and often specialized treatment such as dialysis, they are usually admitted to an intensive care unit, in which needed equipment and trained personnel are available.

Nursing ALERT

Diminished urine output and lethargy in a child who is dehydrated, in shock, or recently postoperative should be evaluated for possible acute kidney failure.

Nursing Diagnoses

A number of nursing diagnoses are evident following a thorough assessment of the child with ARF (Box 47-9). Others will be noted depending on the age of the child, the cause of the renal failure, and any concomitant complications.

Planning

The major goals for the child with ARF and the family are as follows:

1. Child will maintain appropriate fluid volume.
2. Child will maintain normal electrolyte levels.
3. Child will maintain blood pressure within acceptable limits.
4. Child will experience minimized risk of infection.
5. Child and family will receive adequate support.

Implementation

The major nursing task in the care of the infant or child with ARF is monitoring and assessing fluid and electrolyte balance. Limiting fluid intake requires ingenuity on the part of caregivers to cope with the child who is thirsty. One strategy involves rationing the daily intake in small amounts of fluid served in containers that give the impression of larger volumes. Older children who understand the rationale of fluid limits can help determine how their daily ration should be distributed.

Meeting nutritional needs is sometimes a problem; the child may be nauseated, and encouraging concentrated foods without fluids may be difficult. When nourishment is provided intravenously, careful monitoring is essential to prevent fluid overload. In addition, nursing measures such as maintaining an optimum thermal environment, reducing any elevation of body temperature, and reducing restlessness and anxiety are used to decrease the rate of tissue catabolism.

The nurse must be continually alert for changes in behavior that indicate the onset of complications. Infection from reduced resistance, anemia, and general morbidity is a constant threat. Fluid overload and electrolyte disturbances can precip-

BOX 47-9
Nursing Diagnoses: The Child With Acute Renal Failure

Fluid volume excess related to failure of or compromised renal regulatory mechanisms
Risk for injury related to accumulated electrolytes and waste products
Risk for infection related to lowered body defenses, fluid overload
Altered family processes related to a child with a serious disorder

Critical Thinking Q & A

ASSESSMENT AND THE CHILD IN ACUTE RENAL FAILURE

Jackie is a 7-year-old boy in ARF secondary to HUS. His blood pressure is 180/94. When you call the physician for orders to treat the blood pressure, what additional information should be readily available?

1) The results of most recent laboratory studies: CBC, platelets, and electrolytes
2) Jackie's morning weight and current intake and output (I & O) status
3) The current antibiotics in Jackie's peritoneal dialysis solution
4) The amount of decrease in blood pressure Jackie experienced with his last antihypertensive medication

The correct answer is two. To respond to the hypertension the child is currently experiencing, the status of his fluid balance is most essential and probably reflected in the weight and I & O. Laboratory values, current antibiotics, and responsiveness to medications are other important pieces of information in designing Jackie's treatment regimen.

itate cardiovascular complications such as hypertension and cardiac failure. Fluid and electrolyte imbalances, acidosis, and accumulation of nitrogenous waste products can produce neurologic involvement manifested by coma, seizures, or alterations in sensorium (see the Critical Thinking Q & A box above).

Although children with ARF are usually quite ill and voluntarily diminish their activity, infants may become restless and irritable, and children are often anxious and frightened. There are frequent, painful, and stress-producing treatments and tests that must be performed. The presence of a supportive, empathetic nurse can provide comfort and stability in a threatening and unnatural environment.

Family support. Providing support and reassurance to parents is among the major nursing responsibilities. The seriousness and emergency nature of ARF are stressful to parents, and most feel some degree of guilt regarding the child's condition, especially when the illness is the result of ingestion of a toxic substance, dehydration, or a genetic disease. They need reassurance and a sympathetic listener. They also need to be kept informed of the child's progress and provided with explanations regarding the therapeutic regimen. The equipment and the child's behavior are sometimes frightening and anxiety provoking. Nurses can do much to help parents comprehend and deal with the stresses of the situation.

Evaluation

The effectiveness of nursing interventions is determined by continual reassessment and evaluation of care on the basis of the following observational guidelines and expected outcomes:

1. Carry out frequent assessment of vital signs and behaviors.
2. Observe eating behaviors and energy expenditure; monitor intake of protein and calories; carefully monitor intake and output; weigh daily or more often as prescribed.
3. Monitor vital signs, sensorium, and other neurologic signs; evaluate laboratory results and observe for signs of electrolyte imbalance.
4. Observe and interview child and family regarding their understanding of the disease and therapies; encourage child and family to express feelings and concerns.

Expected outcomes

1. Alterations in vital signs and behavior are detected.
2. Child consumes a sufficient amount of appropriate nutrients without evidence of fluid gain or waste product accumulation.
3. Child exhibits no evidence of infection.
4. Evidence of complications is detected early, and appropriate interventions are implemented.
5. Child and family express their feelings and concerns and demonstrate their understanding of the condition and the therapies (specify knowledge and method of demonstration).

See also Nursing Care Plan: The Child with Acute Renal Failure.*

CHRONIC RENAL FAILURE (CRF)

The kidneys are able to maintain the chemical composition of fluids within normal limits until more than 50% of functional renal capacity is destroyed by disease or injury. Chronic renal insufficiency or failure begins when the diseased kidneys can no longer maintain the normal chemical structure of body fluids under normal conditions. Progressive deterioration over months or years produces a variety of clinical and biochemical disturbances that eventually culminate in the clinical syndrome known as **uremia.**

A variety of diseases and disorders can result in CRF. The most common causes are congenital renal and urinary tract malformations, VUR associated with recurrent UTI, chronic pyelonephritis, hereditary disorders, chronic glomerulonephritis, and glomerulonephropathy associated with systemic diseases such as anaphylactoid purpura and lupus erythematosus.

Pathophysiology

Early in the course of progressive nephrotic destruction, the child remains asymptomatic with only minimal biochemical abnormalities. Unless the presence of CRF is detected in the process of routine assessment, signs and symptoms that indicate advanced renal damage often emerge only late in the course of the disease. Midway in the disease process, increasing numbers of nephrons are totally destroyed, and as most others are damaged in varying degree, the few that remain intact are hypertrophied but functional. These few normal nephrons are able to make sufficient adjustments to stresses to maintain reasonable degrees of fluid and electrolyte balance. Definitive biochemical examination at this time reveals restricted tolerance to excesses or restrictions. As the disease progresses to the end stage, the kidneys are no longer able to maintain fluid and electrolyte balance because of a severe re-

*In Wong DL: *Wong and Whaley's clinical manual of pediatric nursing,* ed 4, St Louis, 1996, Mosby.

duction in the number of functioning nephrons, and the features of uremic syndrome appear.

The accumulation of various biochemical substances in the blood, those that result from diminished renal function, produces complications such as the following:

1. Retention of waste products, especially the blood urea nitrogen and creatinine
2. Water and sodium retention, which contributes to edema and vascular congestion
3. Hyperkalemia of dangerous levels
4. Metabolic acidosis of a sustained nature because of continual hydrogen ion retention and bicarbonate loss
5. Calcium and phosphorus disturbances, resulting in altered bone metabolism, which in turn causes growth arrest or retardation, bone pain, and deformities known as *renal osteodystrophy*
6. Anemia caused by hematologic dysfunction, including shortened life span of red blood cells, impaired red blood cell production related to decreased production of erythropoietin, prolonged bleeding time, and nutritional anemia
7. Growth disturbance, probably caused by factors such as renal osteodystrophy, poor nutrition associated with dietary restrictions and loss of appetite, and biochemical abnormalities

Children with CRF seem to be more susceptible to infection, especially pneumonia, UTI, and septicemia, although the reason for this susceptibility is unclear. These children become extraordinarily sensitive to changes in vascular volume that may cause pulmonary overload, central nervous system symptoms, hypertension, and cardiac failure.

Diagnostic Evaluation

The diagnosis of CRF is usually suspected on the basis of any number of clinical manifestations, a history of prior renal disease, and/or biochemical findings. The onset is usually gradual, and the initial signs and symptoms are vague and nonspecific (Box 47-10).

Laboratory and other diagnostic tools and tests are of value in assessing the extent of renal damage, biochemical disturbances, and related physical dysfunction (Tables 47-1, 47-2, and 47-3). Often they can help establish the nature of the underlying disease and differentiate between other disease processes and the pathologic consequences of renal dysfunction.

Therapeutic Management

In irreversible renal failure the goals of medical management are (1) to promote maximal renal function, (2) to maintain body fluid and electrolyte balance within safe biochemical limits, (3) to treat systemic complications, and (4) to promote as active and normal a life as possible for the child for as long as possible. The child is allowed unrestricted activity and is allowed to set his or her own limits regarding rest and extent of exertion. School attendance is encouraged as long as the child is able. When the effort is too great, home tutoring is arranged.

Diet regulation is the most effective means short of dialysis for reducing the quantity of materials that require renal excretion. The goal of the diet in renal failure is to provide sufficient calories and protein for growth while limiting the excretory demands made on the kidney, to minimize metabolic bone disease *(osteodystrophy)*, and to minimize fluid and electrolyte disturbances. Dietary protein intake is limited only to the recommended daily allowance (RDA) for the child's age. Restriction of protein intake below the RDA is believed to negatively impact growth and neurodevelopment (Raymond et al, 1990).

BOX 47-10

Clinical Manifestations of Chronic Renal Failure

- Early signs
  - Loss of normal energy
  - Increased fatigue on exertion
  - Pallor, subtle (may not be noticed)
  - Elevated blood pressure (sometimes)
- As the disease progresses
  - Decreased appetite (especially at breakfast)
  - Less interest in normal activities
  - Increased or decreased urinary output with compensatory intake of fluid
  - Pallor more evident
  - Sallow, muddy appearance of skin
- Child may complain of the following:
  - Headache
  - Muscle cramps
  - Nausea
- Other signs and symptoms
  - Weight loss
  - Facial edema
  - Malaise
  - Bone or joint pain
  - Growth retardation
  - Dryness or itching of the skin
  - Bruised skin
  - Sensory or motor loss (sometimes)
  - Amenorrhea (common in adolescent girls)
- Uremic syndrome (untreated)
  - Gastrointestinal symptoms
    - Anorexia
    - Nausea and vomiting
  - Bleeding tendencies
    - Bruises
    - Bloody diarrheal stools
    - Stomatitis
    - Bleeding from lips and mouth
  - Intractable itching
  - Uremic frost (deposits of urea crystals on skin)
  - Unpleasant "uremic" breath odor
  - Deep respirations
  - Hypertension
  - Congestive heart failure
  - Pulmonary edema
  - Neurologic involvement
    - Progressive confusion
    - Dulled sensorium
    - Coma (ultimately)
    - Tremors
    - Muscular twitching
    - Seizures

Sodium and water are not usually limited unless there is evidence of edema or hypertension, and potassium is not usually restricted. However, restrictions of any or all of these substances may be imposed in later stages or at any time that abnormal serum concentrations are evident.

Dietary phosphorus is controlled to prevent or correct the calcium/phosphorus imbalance by the reduction of protein and milk intake. Phosphorus levels can be further reduced by oral administration of calcium carbonate preparations that combine with the phosphorus to decrease gastrointestinal absorption and thus the serum levels of phosphate. At the same time serum calcium levels are increased from the calcium carbonate, vitamin D therapy is begun to increase calcium absorption.

Metabolic acidosis is alleviated through administration of alkalizing agents such as sodium bicarbonate or a combination of sodium and potassium citrate.

Growth failure is one major consequence of CRF, especially in the preadolescent. Children with CRF grow poorly both before and after the initiation of hemodialysis. The use of recombinant human growth hormone to accelerate growth in children with growth retardation secondary to CRF has been successful (Hokken-Koelega et al, 1994). *Osseous deformities* that result from renal osteodystrophy, especially those related to ambulation, are troublesome and require correction if they occur. *Dental defects* are common in children with CRF, and the earlier the onset of the disease, the more severe are the dental manifestations (including hypoplasia, hypomineralization, tooth discoloration, alteration in size and shape of teeth, malocclusion, and ulcerative stomatitis). Therefore regular dental care is especially important in these children.

Anemia in children with CRF is related to decreased production of erythropoietin. Recombinant human erythropoietin (rHuEPO) is being offered to these children as thrice-weekly or weekly subcutaneous injections and is replacing the need for frequent blood transfusions. This drug corrects the anemia and in turn increases appetite, activity, and general well-being in the children who receive it.

Hypertension of advanced renal disease may be managed initially by cautious use of a low-sodium diet, fluid restriction, and perhaps diuretics such as hydrochlorothiazide or furosemide. Severe hypertension requires the use of antihypertensive agents either by themselves or in combinations.

Intercurrent infections are treated with appropriate antimicrobials at the first sign of infection; however, any drug eliminated through the kidneys is administered with caution. Other complications are treated symptomatically (e.g., central-acting antiemetics for *nausea,* antiepileptics for *seizures,* and diphenhydramine [Benadryl] for *pruritus*).

Once evidence of *end-stage renal disease (ESRD)* appears in a child, the disease runs its relentless course and results in death in a few weeks unless waste products and toxins are removed from body fluids by dialysis and/or kidney transplantation. Since these techniques have been adapted for infants and small children, these alternatives have been implemented in most cases of renal failure once conservative management is no longer effective (see p. 1568).

Prognosis. Dialysis and transplantation are the only treatments currently available for children with ESRD. Although children may survive on dialysis, it is not an ideal long-term modality. Complications include infection of access sites, growth failure, and disruption of normal socialization. Many pediatric centers encourage families of children with ESRD to consider renal transplantation. The overall graft survival rate for kidneys from living related donors is 89% at 1 year and 80% at 3 years. For cadaver kidneys the graft survival rate is 74% at 1 year and 62% at 3 years (McEnery et al, 1992). Post-transplant complications include infection, hypertension, steroid toxicity, hyperlipidemia, aseptic necrosis, malignancy, and growth retardation (Suthanthiran and Strom, 1994). Long-term graft survival is not guaranteed, and many children require a second or third transplant. Successful renal transplantation does improve rehabilitation of children with CRF, both educationally and psychologically. Increasing use of primary or preemptive renal transplant without a prior course of dialysis is being recommended in many pediatric centers (Fine, Tejani, and Sullivan, 1994).

Nursing Care Management

Assessment

Assessment of the child with CRF is primarily one of observation for signs of complications and evidence of improvement through therapy. Some of the first changes observed are growth failure, developmental delay, bone disease, and hypertension.

Nursing Diagnoses

A number of nursing diagnoses become evident on assessment of the child. The most relevant in the majority of cases are outlined in the Nursing Care Plan on pp. 1566-1567. Others will be appropriate for individual children and their families.

Planning

The goals of care for the child with CRF, especially one in ESRD, and the family are the following:

1. The child will receive encouragement in his or her normal growth and development, minimizing the impact of the disease process.
2. The child will remain free of complications.
3. The child and family will receive appropriate support, guidance, and education.

Implementation

The multiple complications of ESRD are managed according to medical protocols prescribed for the care of those specific problems. However, progressive disease places a number of stresses on the child and family, including those of a potentially fatal illness (see Chapter 38). There is a continuing need for repeated examinations that often entail painful procedures, side effects, and frequent hospitalizations. Diet therapy becomes progressively more restricted and intense, and the child is required to take a variety of medications. Ever present in all aspects of the treatment regimen is the agonizing realization that without treatment, death is inevitable.

Some specific stresses related to ESRD and its treatment are predictable. When it first becomes apparent that ESRD is inevitable, both parents and child experience depression and anxiety. Acceptance is particularly difficult if renal failure progresses rapidly after diagnosis. Denial and disbelief are

Nursing Care Plan

THE CHILD WITH CHRONIC RENAL FAILURE

Nursing Diagnosis: Risk for injury related to accumulated electrolytes and waste products

Expected Outcomes: Child exhibits no evidence of accumulation of waste products and no evidence of injury.

• **NURSING INTERVENTIONS/*RATIONALES***

Provide diet low in protein, potassium, sodium, and phosphorous; high in calories and calcium; and supplemented with essential amino acids as ordered *to reduce excretory demand on kidneys.*

Assist and monitor renal or peritoneal dialysis as prescribed *to maintain excretory function.*

Administer potassium-removing resins as prescribed *to reduce potassium levels;* antihypertensives *for hypertension;* diuretics *for edema;* phosphate binders *for hyperphosphatemia;* antiinfectives *for infection;* and antipruritics *for itching.*

Monitor for signs of accumulating waste products (i.e., elevated BUN, creatinine; hyperkalemia, hyperphosphatemia; muscle twitching; muscle cramps; anorexia, nausea, vomiting; hypertension; pruritis; yellowing skin; confusion, lethargy) *to ensure prompt treatment.*

Balance activity and rest and plan appropriate activities *to reduce fatigue and chances of injury.*

Provide meticulous skin care and avoid shearing and frictional forces *to reduce injury to skin.*

Nursing Diagnosis: Fluid volume excess related to failure of renal regulatory mechanisms

Expected Outcome: Child exhibits no evidence of increase in fluid accumulation.

• **NURSING INTERVENTIONS/*RATIONALES***

Instruct child and family about fluid restrictions and strategize ways to maintain those restrictions (e.g., keeping mouth moist with hard candies, gum, ice chips; keeping lips lubricated; divide fluids into small, even quantities throughout day) *to decrease chances of fluid overload.*

Monitor I & O, weight changes, girth measurements *to track fluid accumulation.*

Nursing Diagnosis: Altered nutrition: less than body requirements related to restricted diet and loss of appetite

Expected Outcome: Child exhibits adequate and appropriate food intake.

• **NURSING INTERVENTIONS/*RATIONALES***

Provide dietary instructions for child and family, including allowed foods, recipes, and menus *to increase successful use of restrictive diet and to reduce excretory demand on kidneys.*

Nursing Diagnosis: Body image/self-esteem disturbance related to altered appearance, chronic illness, frequent treatments, feelings of being different

Expected Outcomes: Child exhibits signs of acceptance of self and of alteration in appearance; child exhibits signs of coping with disease process.

• **NURSING INTERVENTIONS/*RATIONALES***

Relate to child on appropriate cognitive level, conveying an attitude of caring and acceptance *to encourage positive feelings about self;* serve as role model for others *to foster positive attitudes of acceptance toward child.*

Encourage child to verbalize feelings and perceptions about CRF (e.g., repeated treatments and hospitalizations, feelings of differentness, implications of functional limits, difficulty in making friends, views of self) *to facilitate coping and open expression of problems, fears, wants, wishes, and needs.*

Have child identify strengths, assets, and things he or she likes about self *to increase positive feelings about self and abilities.*

Support positive coping behaviors.

Involve child in care and management of disease *to promote a sense of control, independence, and self-esteem.*

Introduce child to other children who have similar disabilities; arrange for support groups for child and parents *to increase coping skills.*

Refer child for counseling if needed *to enhance adaptation.*

Encourage use of regular hygiene and grooming practices *to promote positive appearance.*

Nursing Diagnosis: Impaired social interaction related to repeated hospitalizations, confinement, activity intolerance

Expected Outcome: Child engages in appropriate family and peer interactions.

• **NURSING INTERVENTIONS/*RATIONALES***

Encourage regular school attendance and promote peer contacts *to provide opportunity to develop and maintain peer relationships.*

Encourage selection of play activities and recreational outlets *that encourage interaction;* restrict time spent in solo activities *that promote social isolation.*

Encourage contact with peers and siblings by telephone or visit when hospitalized or confined *to maintain social interaction and reduce sense of isolation.*

Plan specific periods of developmentally appropriate diversional activity suited to child's physical condition and energy level *to decrease feelings of boredom and negative self-absorption.*

Nursing Care Plan

THE CHILD WITH CHRONIC RENAL FAILURE - cont'd

Nursing Diagnosis: Altered family processes related to child with chronic illness

Expected Outcomes: Family exhibits adaptation of usual roles and functions to accommodate special needs of child; family exhibits growth-promoting behaviors.

• NURSING INTERVENTIONS/*RATIONALES*

Provide opportunity for family to absorb and adjust to diagnosis (e.g., repeat information *to allow time for family to hear and understand;* encourage expression of concerns, fears, and feelings about diagnosis and potential impact *to facilitate adjustment;* identify support systems *to provide resources for coping*).

Assist family to understand expected treatment, rationales, and implications *to provide a sound basis for decision making.*

Explore family reaction to the child, assist them to achieve a realistic view of child's abilities and limitations, encourage family in attempts to promote child growth and development, have family emphasize what child can do, and explore ways for family to include child in family activities *to help family increase abilities to cope with and incorporate child into family structure.*

Arrange for and participate in family conferences *to provide forum for communication, mutual goal setting, and effective strategizing.*

Have parents spend special time with siblings *so that they do not feel neglected or left out.*

Identify additional resource systems (e.g., relatives, friends, church, health care services, community programs), and strategize with family about making good use of these systems *to develop broad base of support.*

Provide a system of ongoing follow-up and evaluation *to ensure long-term adaptation to challenges presented to family functioning by a child with chronic disease.*

usually pronounced, especially among the parents. Once the kidney failure is established and symptoms become progressively more distressing, the initiation of hemodialysis is usually perceived as a positive experience, and after experiencing initial concerns regarding the treatment, the child begins to feel better, and parental anxiety is relieved for a time.

Initiating a hemodialysis regimen is a traumatic and anxiety-provoking experience for most children because it involves surgery for implantation of a graft, fistula, or peritoneal catheter. The initial experience with the dialysis procedure is frightening to most children. They need reassurance about the nature of the preparations for hemodialysis and the conduct of the treatment.

Both the graft and the fistula require needle insertions at each dialysis. The goal is to perform pain-free venipuncture. One method involves using buffered lidocaine or one of the more rapid onset novacaines (e.g., procaine) with a small-gauge needle (30 gauge) to anesthetize the area before venipuncture of the graft/fistula. Another approach involves using an anesthetizing topical preparation such as EMLA (eutetic mixture of local anesthetics [lidocaine and prilocaine]) 1 hour before venipuncture.

External dual lumen venous access devices eliminate the need for needles but are more prone to infection and other central-line complications.

Adolescents, with their increased need for independence and their urge for rebellion, usually adapt less well. They resent the control and enforced dependence imposed by the rigorous and unrelenting therapy program. They resent being dependent on hemodialysis technology, their parents, and the professional staff. Depression and/or hostility are common in adolescents undergoing hemodialysis.

The availability of home dialysis has offered a greater degree of freedom for persons undergoing long-term dialysis. The nurse is responsible for teaching the family about (1) the disease, its implications, and the therapeutic plan; (2) the possible psychologic effects of the disease and the treatment; and (3) the technical aspects of the procedure. The family learns to manage the various aspects of the dialysis procedure, how to maintain accurate records, and how to observe for signs of complications that need to be reported to the proper persons.

Body changes related to the disease process, such as skin color, growth retardation, and lack of sexual maturation, are stress provoking. Dietary restrictions are particularly burdensome for both children and parents. Children feel deprived when they are unable to eat foods they previously enjoyed and that are unrestricted for other family members. Consequently, failure to cooperate may occur. Diet restrictions may be interpreted as punishment. Some children, unable to fully under-

Family Focus

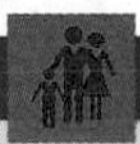

FAMILY PRIORITIES

Families who have children with long-term chronic illnesses, such as ESRD, spend much time in hospitals, outpatient clinics, and primary health care facilities. When they miss appointments or respond less quickly than anticipated, they are sometimes quickly labeled "noncompliant." It is important to remember that families need to develop priorities for the unit as a whole. Sometimes the family may decide that it is more important for the parent to go to work or to attend a sibling's school performance than to attend an appointment scheduled for them by health care personnel. The chronically ill child cannot and should not always be the number one priority for the family. The professional staff who works with the family can help the parents prioritize the needs of the ill child within the needs of the family constellation.

Teresa Hall, MS, RN
Hathaway Children's Services
Sylmar, California

stand the purpose of restrictions, will sneak forbidden food items at every opportunity. Allowing children, especially adolescents, maximum participation in and responsibility for their own treatment program is helpful.

After months or years of dialysis, the parents and child feel anxiety associated with the prognosis and continued pressures of the treatment. The relentless need for treatment interferes with family plans. The time spent in transportation to and from the dialysis unit and the time spent undergoing dialysis treatments cut into time for outside activities, including school. Graft and fistula problems, as well as peritoneal catheter exit site infections, may develop and present a common source of aggravation (see the Family Focus box on p. 1567).

The possibility of renal transplantation often provides hope for relief from the rigors of hemodialysis and peritoneal dialysis. Most children and families respond well to a kidney transplant, and most children can be successfully rehabilitated.

The National Kidney Foundation* and other agencies provide a number of services and information for families of children with renal disease.

Evaluation

The effectiveness of nursing interventions is determined by continual reassessment and evaluation of care on the basis of the following observational guidelines and expected outcomes:

1. Observe and interview family regarding their compliance with the medical and dietary regimen.
2. Monitor vital signs, growth measurements, laboratory reports, behavior, and appearance.
3. Observe and interview child and family regarding their feelings, concerns, and fears; observe reactions to therapies and prognosis.

Expected outcomes
See the Nursing Care Plan on pp. 1566-1567.

Technologic Management of Renal Failure

DIALYSIS

Dialysis is the process of separating colloids and crystalline substances in solution by the difference in their rate of diffusion through a semipermeable membrane. Methods of dialysis currently available for clinical management of renal failure are **peritoneal dialysis,** wherein the abdominal cavity acts as a semipermeable membrane through which water and solutes of small molecular size move by osmosis and diffusion according to their respective concentrations on either side of the membrane, and **hemodialysis,** in which blood is circulated outside the body through artificial membranes that permit a similar passage of water and solutes. A third type of dialysis is **hemofiltration,** in which blood filtrate is circulated outside the body by hydrostatic pressure exerted across a semipermeable membrane with simultaneous infusion of a replacement solution. Types of hemofiltration include *continuous arteriovenous hemofiltration (CAVH), continuous arteriovenous hemodialysis (CAVHD)* and *continuous veno venous hemofiltration (CVVH).* CAVH, CAVHD, and CVVH are used primarily in acute conditions, such as to remove fluid overload, rather than in ESRD.

Peritoneal dialysis is the preferred form of dialysis for children/parents who wish to remain independent, families who live a long distance from the medical center, and children who prefer fewer dietary restrictions and a gentler form of dialysis. Chronic peritoneal dialysis is most often performed at home. The two types of peritoneal dialysis are *continuous ambulatory peritoneal dialysis (CAPD)* and *continuous cycling peritoneal dialysis (CCPD).* In both methods, commercially available sterile dialysate is instilled into the peritoneal cavity through a surgically implanted indwelling catheter that is tunneled subcutaneously and sutured into place. The warmed solution is allowed to enter the peritoneal cavity by gravity and remains a variable length of time according to the procedure used. The care and management of the procedure is the responsibility of the parents of young children. Use of home health nurses to give parents respite from care has been initiated in some centers. (Cascio et al, 1994). Older children and adolescents can carry out the procedure themselves, which provides them with some control and less dependency. This is especially important for adolescents.

Nursing ALERT

Observe for changes in the color of the dialysate draining from the child. The solution should be straw-colored. If the solution is pink, bright yellow, brown, or cloudy, notify the physician immediately.

Hemodialysis requires the creation of a vascular access and the use of special dialysis equipment—the hemodialyzer, or so-called artificial kidney. Vascular access may be one of three types: fistulas, grafts, or external vascular access devices. An *atriovenous fistula* is an access in which a vein and artery are connected surgically. The preferred site is the radial artery and a forearm vein. An alternative is the creation of a subcutaneous (internal) *arteriovenous graft* by anastomosing a segment of a saphenous vein autograft or a bovine arterial xenograft to the brachial artery and brachiocephalic vein, which produces dilation and thickening of the superficial vessels of the forearm to provide easy access for repeated venipuncture. Both the graft and the fistula require needle insertions at each dialysis.

For external vascular access devices, percutaneous catheters are inserted in the femoral, subclavian, or internal jugular veins, even in very small children. A more permanent form of external access is available via a central catheter inserted surgically into the subclavian vein or internal jugular vein. This catheter has a dual lumen, which allows differenti-

*30 E. 33rd St., New York, NY 10016; (212) 889-2210 or (800) 622-9010. In Canada: the **Kidney Foundation of Canada,** 5160 Boulevard Decarle, Bureau 780, Montreal, Quebec H3X 2H9; (514) 369-4806.

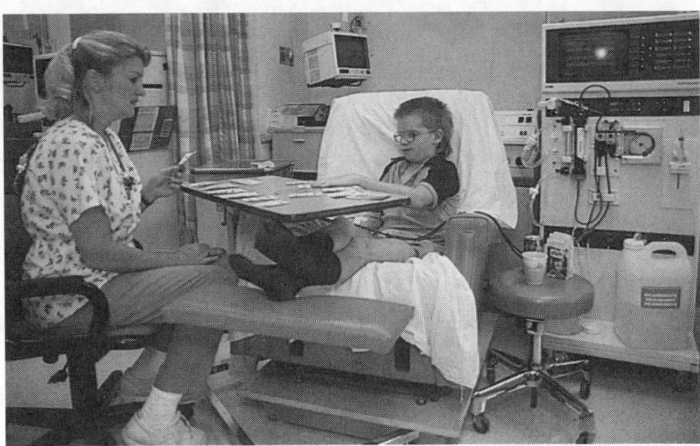

Fig. 47-3 Diversional activities help lessen the boredom that children can experience during hemodialysis.

ation between arterial and venous blood. Catheters eliminate the need for skin punctures but require some home care.*

Hemodialysis is best suited to children who do not have someone in the family who is capable of learning to perform home dialysis and to those who live close to a dialysis center. The procedure is usually performed three times a week for 4 to 6 hours, depending on the size of the child. Hemodialysis achieves rapid correction of fluid and electrolyte abnormalities but can cause problems in association with this rapid change, such as muscle cramping and hypotension. Disadvantages include school absence during dialysis and strict fluid and dietary restrictions between dialysis sessions. Boredom for the child and family is often a problem during dialysis, and planned quiet activities should be introduced (Fig. 47-3).

Most children show rapid clinical improvement with the implementation of dialysis, although it is directly related to the duration of uremia before dialysis and the extent to which dietary regulations are followed. Growth rate and skeletal maturation improve, but recovery of normal growth occurs infrequently. In many cases sexual development, although delayed, progresses to completion.

*Home care instructions on central venous catheters are available in Wong DL: *Wong and Whaley's clinical manual of pediatric nursing,* ed 4, St Louis, 1996, Mosby.

TRANSPLANTATION

Renal transplantation is now an acceptable and effective means of therapy in the pediatric age group. Although peritoneal dialysis and hemodialysis are life preserving, both require major alterations in life-style. Transplantation offers the opportunity for a relatively normal life and is the preferred form of treatment for children with CRF. Primary or preemptive transplants maintain the greatest amount of normalcy in the family's life.

Kidneys for transplant are available from two sources: a *living related donor (LRD),* usually a parent or a sibling, or a *cadaver donor (CAD),* wherein the family of a dead or brain-dead patient consents to donation of a healthy kidney. The criteria for selection of kidney recipients are quite liberal, with no limit regarding age. Retransplantation occurs often.

The primary goal in transplantation is the long-term survival of grafted tissue by securing tissue that is antigenically similar to that of the recipient and by suppressing the recipient's immune mechanism. The immunosuppressant therapy of choice has been corticosteroids (prednisone) in conjunction with cyclosporine and azathioprine. Other therapies include antilymphoblast globulin or monoclonal antibodies. New immunosuppressant medications are rapidly coming into clinical trials and into use in large transplant centers. It is important for the nurse to learn about the medications used in the antirejection protocol(s), as well as their side effects. Because the immunosuppressant medications are taken indefinitely, transplant patients experience many side effects of the drugs, including hypertension, growth retardation, cataracts, risk of infection, obesity, characteristics of Cushing syndrome, and hirsutism.

Rejection of the transplanted kidney is the most common cause of transplant failure. Rejection is treated aggressively with immunosuppressant medications and can often be reversed. Some patients do not respond to treatment of acute rejection or develop chronic rejection and must eventually return to dialysis or undergo another kidney transplant.

Nursing ALERT

The child with a recent kidney transplant (a few days) or one who was grafted approximately 6 months previously who exhibits any of the following should be evaluated immediately for possible rejection:
Fever
Swelling and tenderness over graft area
Diminished urine output
Elevated blood pressure

Key Points

- Common inflammatory disorders of the genitourinary tract include urinary tract infection, nephrotic syndrome, and acute glomerulonephritis.
- Management of urinary tract infections is directed at eliminating infection, detecting and correcting functional or anatomic abnormalities, preventing recurrences, and preserving renal function.
- Vesicoureteral reflux is the retrograde flow of bladder urine into the ureters.
- Obstructive uropathy is a result of structural or functional abnormalities of the urinary system that obstruct the normal flow of urine.
- The more common defects of the genitourinary tract include phimosis, cryptorchidism, inguinal hernia, hydrocele, and hypospadias.
- Body image concerns and castration anxiety are particularly intense in children with defects in the genital area.
- Nephrotic syndrome is characterized by increased

glomerular permeability to protein, with massive urinary loss of protein resulting in hypoproteinemia and edema.

- Management of nephrotic syndrome is aimed at reducing excretion of protein, reducing or preventing fluid retention by tissues, and preventing infection and other complications.
- Common features of acute glomerulonephritis are oliguria, edema, hypertension, circulatory congestion, hematuria, and proteinuria.
- Therapeutic management of acute glomerulonephritis is maintenance of fluid balance, treatment of hypertension, and antibiotic therapy.
- Management of hemolytic-uremic syndrome is aimed at control of complications and hematologic manifestations of renal failure.
- Wilms tumor is the most common malignant neoplasm of the kidney in infants and children.
- In acute renal failure, management is directed at determining treatment of the underlying cause, management of complications of renal failure, and supportive therapy.
- Abnormalities in chronic renal failure are waste product retention, water and sodium retention, hyperkalemia, acidosis, calcium and phosphorus disturbance, anemia, and growth disturbances.
- The types of dialysis used in end-stage renal disease are peritoneal dialysis and hemodialysis.
- When the child needs home dialysis, the nurse educates the family on the disease, its implications, the therapeutic plan, possible psychologic effects of the disease, and the treatment and technical aspects of the procedure.
- The major concerns in renal transplantation are tissue matching and prevention of rejection; psychologic concerns involve self-image as related to possible body changes as a result of the effects of corticosteroid therapy.

References

Brandt JR et al: More on *E. coli*–induced hemolytic-uremic syndrome, *J Pediatr* 125(41):519-526, 1994.

Cascio C et al: Use of private duty nurses for daily CCPD and family relief in pediatric PD patients, *Adv Perit Dial* 10:304-306, 1994.

Craig JC et al: Effect of circumcision on incidence of urinary tract infection in preschool boys, *J Pediatr* 128(1):23-27, 1996.

Fine RN, Tejani A, Sullivan EK: Preemptive renal transplantation in children: report of the North American Pediatric Renal Transplant Cooperative Study, *Clin Transplant* 8(5):474-478, 1994.

Fleiss PM: Explanation for false-positive urine cultures obtained by bag technique, *Arch Pediatr Adolesc Med* 149(9):1041-1042, 1995.

Green DM et al: Wilms tumor, *CA Cancer J Clin* 46:46-63, 1996.

Hokken-Koelega ACS et al: Growth hormone treatment in growth-retarded adolescents after renal transplant, *Lancet* 343:1313-1317, 1994.

McEnery PT et al: Renal transplantation in children, *N Engl J Med* 326(26):1727-1732, 1992.

Raymond NG et al: An approach to protein restriction in children with renal insufficiency, *Pediatr Nephrol* 4:145-148, 1990.

Suthanthiran M, Strom TB: Renal transplantation, *N Engl J Med* 331(6):365-376, 1994.

Wiswell TE, Hachey W: Urinary tract infections and the uncircumcised state: an update, *Clin Pediatr* 32(4):130-134, 1993.

Bibliography

General

Collecting a 24-hour urine sample, *Patient Care* 24(17):99, 1990.

Gibbs T: Genitourinary embryology and congenital malformations: the kidneys and ureters, part I, *Urol Nurs* 10(3):16-24, 1990.

Gillenwater JY et al, editors: Adult and pediatric urology, ed 3, vol 3, St Louis, 1996, Mosby.

Gray ML: *Genitourinary disorders*, St Louis, 1992, Mosby.

Jacobson H, Striker GE, Klahr S, editors: *The principles and practice of nephrology*, ed 2, St Louis, 1995, Mosby.

Kaplan WE: Summary of the urologic section, *Pediatrics* 93(5):845-849, 1994.

Kelalis PP, King LR, Belman AB, editors: *Clinical pediatric urology*, Philadelphia, 1992, WB Saunders.

Kenner C, Brueggemeyer A: *Assessment and management of genitourinary dysfunction*. In Kenner C et al, editors: *Comprehensive neonatal nursing: a physiologic perspective*, Philadelphia, 1993, WB Saunders.

Perelstein EM: Renal tubular acidosis, *Int Pediatr* 8(3):326-333, 1993.

Raymond NG et al: An approach to protein restriction in children with renal insufficiency, *Pediatr Nephrol* 4:145-148, 1990.

Rowe PC et al: Epidemiology of hemolytic-uremic syndrome in Canadian children from 1986-1988, *J Pediatr* 119(2):218-224, 1994.

Urinary Tract Infection/Reflux

Andrich MP, Majd M: Diagnostic imaging in the evaluation of the first urinary tract infection in infants and young children, *Pediatrics* 90(3):436-441, 1992.

Avorn J et al: Reduction of bacteriuria and pyuria after ingestion of cranberry juice, *JAMA* 271(10):751-754, 1994.

Brindle M: Urinary tract infection in children, *Br Med J* 309(6954):609, 1994.

Cepero-Akselrad A, Ramirez-Seijas F, Castaneda A: Urinary tract infection in children, *Int Pediatr* 8(3):314-325, 1993.

Conway JJ, Cohn RA: Evolving role of nuclear medicine for the diagnosis and management of urinary tract infection, *J Pediatr* 124(1):87-90, 1994.

Dick PT, Feldman W: Routine diagnostic imaging for childhood urinary tract infections: a systematic overview, *J Pediatr* 128(1):15-22, 1996.

Edelmann CM Jr: Urinary tract infection and vesicoureteral reflux, *Pediatr Ann* 17:568-582, 1988.

Heldrich FJ: UTI diagnosis: getting it right the first time, *Contemp Pediatr* 12(2):110-133, 1995.

Kramer SA: *Vesicoureteral reflux*. In Kelalis PP, King LR, Belman AB, editors: *Clinical pediatric urology*, Philadelphia, 1992, WB Saunders.

Rosenfeld DL et al: Current recommendations for children with urinary tract infections, *Clin Pediatr* pp.261-264, 1995.

Schlager TA et al: Explanation for false-positive urine cultures obtained by bag technique, *Arch Pediatr Adolesc Med* 149:170-173, 1995.

Todd JK: Management of urinary tract infections: children are different, *Pediatr Rev* 16(5):190-196, 1995.

When to rely on the urine dipstick in children, *Emerg Med* 24(2):224-225, 1992.

Winberg J: What hygiene measures are advisable to prevent recurrent urinary tract infection and what evidence is there to support this advice? *Pediatr Nephrol* 8(6):652, 1994.

Wiswell TE, Geschke DW: Risks from circumcision during the first month of life compared with those for uncircumcised boys, *Pediatrics* 83:1011-1015, 1989.

Structural Defects of the Urinary Tract

Castiglia PT: Ambiguous genitalia, *J Pediatr Health Care* 3(6):319-321, 1989.

Forest-Lalande L: Teaching nonsterile intermittent catheterization in a pediatric setting, *CAET J* 9(6):7-10, 1990.

Horton H et al: Hypospadius: when baby boys need surgery, *RN* 53(6):48-52, 1990.

Rajput A, Gauderer MWL, Hack M: Inguinal hernias in very low–birth-weight infants: incidence and timing of repair, *J Pediatr Surg* 27(10):1322-1324, 1992.

Skinner M, Grosfeld J: Inguinal and umbilical hernia repair in infants and children, *Surg Clin North Am* 73(3):439-449, 1993.

Smoyer WE: Urinary tract obstruction in children, *Clin Pediatr* 31(2):109-119, 1992.

Steele BT, De Maria J: A new perspective on the natural history of vesicoureteric reflux, *Pediatrics* 90(1):30-32, 1992.

Stylianos L, Jacir NN, Harris BH: Incarceration of inguinal hernia in infants prior to elective repair, *J Pediatr Surg* 28(4):582-583, 1993.

Van Gool JD et al: Historical clues to the complex of dysfunctional voiding, urinary tract infection and vesicoureteral reflux, *J Urol* 148:1699-1702, 1992.

Renal Diseases and Tumors

Andrews PE, Kelalis PP, Haase GM: Extrarenal Wilms' tumor: results of the National Wilms' Tumor Study, *J Pediatr Surg* 27(9):1181-1184, 1992.

Brodeur FA, Brodeur GM: Abdominal masses in children: neuroblastoma, Wilms tumor and other considerations, *Pediatr Rev* 12(7):196-207, 1991.

Canpolat C, Pearson P, Jaffe N: Cisplatin-associated hemolytic-uremic syndrome, *Cancer* 74(11):3059-3062, 1994.

D'Anglo G et al: Wilms' tumor: status report, *J Clin Oncol* 9:877-887, 1991.

Haws RM, Baum M: Efficacy of albumin and diuretic therapy in children with nephrotic syndrome, *Pediatrics* 91(6):1142-1146, 1993.

Kelsch RC, Sedman AB: Nephrotic syndrome, *Pediatr Rev* 14(1):30-38, 1993.

Klee KM, AcAfee N, Greefleaf K: Pediatric case study: hemolytic-uremic syndrome, *ANNA J* 20(4):505-506, 1993.

Ruccione KS: Wilms' tumor: a paradigm, a parallel, and a puzzle, *Semin Oncol Nurs* 8(4):241-251, 1992.

Sakarcan A, Timmons C, Seikaly MG: Reversible idiopathic acute renal failure in children with primary nephrotic syndrome, *J Pediatr* 125(5):723-727, 1994.

Renal Failure

Doolittle RF: Biotechnology: the enormous cost of success, *N Engl J Med* 324(19):1360-1362, 1991.

Frauman A et al: Care of the family of the child with end stage renal disease, *ANNA J* 17(5):383-396, 1990.

Kling PJ et al: Pharmacogenetics and pharmacodynamics of erythropoietin during therapy in an infant with renal failure, *J Pediatr* 121(5):822-825, 1992.

Obrecht JA, Gallo AM, Knafl KA: A case of illustration of family management style in childhood end stage renal disease, *ANNA J* 19(3):255-260, 1992.

Dialysis/Transplantation

Alexander SR, Honda, M: Continuous peritoneal dialysis for children: a decade of worldwide growth and development, *Kidney Int Suppl* 40:S65-S74, 1993.

Avner ED et al: Renal transplantation and chronic dialysis in children and adolescents: the 1993 annual report of the North American Pediatric Renal Transplant Cooperative Study, *Pediatr Nephrol* 9(1):61-73, 1995.

Bunchman TE et al: Continuous venovenous hemodiafiltration in infants and children, *Am J Kidney Dis* 25(1):17-21, 1995.

Cohen B et al: Children's compliance to dialysis, *Pediatr Nurs* 17(4):359-365, 420, 1991.

Currier H: Ethical issues in the neonatal patient with end-stage renal disease, *J Perinat Neonat Nurs* 8(1):74-78, 1994.

Doyle CL, Flanigan MJ, Mabe C: Tidal peritoneal dialysis vs continuous cyclic peritoneal dialysis: children's preference, *ANNA J* 19(3):249-254, 1992.

Ellis D et al: Comparison of FK-506 and cyclosporine regimens in pediatric renal transplantation *Pediatr Nephrol* 8(2):193-200, 1994.

Gorynski L, Knight F: A peer group for adolescent dialysis patients, *ANNA J* 19(3):262-264, 1992.

Gutch CF, Stoner MH, Corea AL: *Review of hemodialysis for nurses and dialysis personnel*, ed 5, St Louis, 1992, Mosby.

Hendrix B: Dialysis therapies in critically ill children, *ACCN Clin Issues Crit Care Nurs* 3(3):605-613, 1992.

Knight F, Gorynski L, Bentson M, Harmon WE: Hemodialysis of the infant or small child with chronic renal failure, *ANNA J* 20(3):315-323, 1993.

Kurtin PS, Landgraf JM, Abetz L: Patient-based health status measurements in pediatric dialyasis: expanding the assessment of outcome, *Am J Kidney Dis* 24(2):376-382, 1994.

Miller D: Immunosuppression in pediatric transplant patients, *Pediatr Nurs* 21(1):21-26, 1995.

Peterson K: Iatrogenic immune suppression, *Pediatr Nurs* 21(1):11-15, 1995.

Suddaby EC, Bell SB, Murphy KJ: Continuous hemofiltration in infants and children, *Pediatr Nurs* 16:79-82, 1990.

Tejani A, Fine RN: Cadaver renal transplantation in children, *Clin Pediatr* 32(4):194-202, 1993.

Tejani A et al: Factors predictive of sustained growth in children after renal transplantation, *J Pediatr* 122(3):397-402, 1993.

Tejani A et al: Analysis of rejection outcomes and implications—a report of the North American Pediatric Renal Transplant Cooperative Study, *Transplantation* 59(4):500-504, 1995.

Uzark K: Caring for families of pediatric transplant recipients: psychosocial implications, *Crit Care Nurs Clin North Am* 4(2):255-261, 1992.

Weichler NK: Caretakers' informational needs after their children's renal or liver transplant, *ANNA J* 20(2):135-139, 1993.

Wise BV: Advances in pediatric solid organ transplantation, *Nurs Clin North Am* 29(4):615-629, 1994.

CHAPTER 48

Cerebral Dysfunction

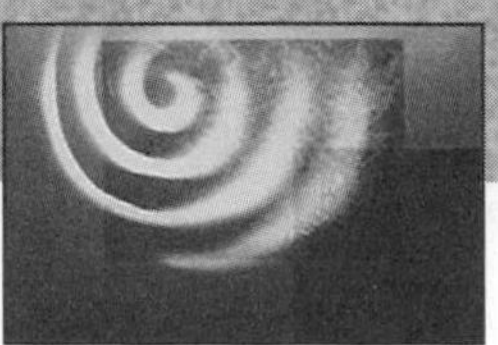

CEREBRAL DYSFUNCTION, P. 1572
Assessment of cerebral function, p. 1572

NURSING CARE OF THE UNCONSCIOUS CHILD, P. 1578

CEREBRAL TRAUMA, P. 1585
Head injury, p. 1585
Near-drowning, p. 1593

CENTRAL NERVOUS SYSTEM TUMORS, P. 1594
Brain tumors, p. 1594
Neuroblastoma, p. 1599

INTRACRANIAL INFECTIONS, P. 1600
Bacterial meningitis, p. 1600
Nonbacterial (aseptic) meningitis, p. 1602
Encephalitis, p. 1603
Reye syndrome (RS), p. 1603
Human immunodeficiency virus (HIV) encephalopathy, p. 1604
Rabies, p. 1604

SEIZURE DISORDERS, P. 1605
Epilepsy, p. 1605
Febrile seizures, p. 1614

CEREBRAL MALFORMATIONS, P. 1615
Cranial deformities, p. 1615
Hydrocephalus, p. 1615

Cerebral Dysfunction

ASSESSMENT OF CEREBRAL FUNCTION

Most of the information about the status of the brain is obtained by indirect measurements. Some of these measurements are discussed in relation to numerous aspects of child care (e.g., as part of assessments of health [Chapter 32], newborn status [Chapter 22], mental retardation [Chapter 39], hypoxic injury [cerebral palsy, Chapter 52], and attainment of developmental milestones at each stage of development). Since increased intracranial pressure and altered states of consciousness have such prominent places in neurologic dysfunction, they are described here, followed by techniques for neurologic assessment and diagnostic tests.

General Aspects

Children younger than 2 years of age require special evaluation, since they are unable to respond to directions designed to elicit specific responses in infants neurologically. Early neurologic responses in infants are primarily reflexive; these responses are gradually replaced by meaningful movement in the characteristic cephalocaudal direction of development. This evidence of progressive maturation reflects more extensive myelinization and changes in neurochemical and electrophysiologic properties.

Most information about infants and small children is gained by observing their spontaneous and elicited reflex responses as they develop increasingly complex locomotor and fine motor skills and by eliciting progressively sophisticated communicative and adaptive behaviors. Delay or deviation from expected milestones helps identify high-risk children. Persistence or reappearance of reflexes that normally disappear indicates the presence of a disorder. In evaluating the infant or young child, it is also important to obtain the pregnancy and birth history to determine the possible effect of intrauterine environmental influences known to affect the orderly maturation of the central nervous system (CNS). These influences include maternal infections, chemicals, trauma, and metabolic insults.

General aspects of assessment that provide clues to the cause of dysfunction include:

Family history—sometimes offers clues regarding possible genetic disorders with neurologic manifestations

Health history—may provide valuable clues regarding the cause of dysfunction (e.g., an injury, short febrile illness, encounter with an animal or insect, ingestion of neurotoxic substances, inhalation of chemicals, past illness, or known diabetes mellitus)

Physical evaluation of infants—includes observation of:

Size and shape of the head

- Spontaneous activity and postural reflex activity
- Sensory responses
- Attitude—normal flexed posture, extreme extension, opisthotonos, hypotonia
- Symmetry in movement of extremities
- Excessive tremulousness or frequent twitching movements
- Altered expiratory cycle:
  - Prolonged apnea
  - Ataxic breathing
  - Paradoxic chest movement
  - Hyperventilation
- Skin and hair texture
- Distinctive facial features
- Presence of a high-pitched, piercing cry
- Abnormal eye movements
- Inability to suck or swallow
- Lip smacking
- Asymmetric contraction of facial muscles
- Yawning (may indicate cranial nerve involvement)
- Muscular activity and coordination
- Level of development

Increased Intracranial Pressure (ICP)

The brain, tightly enclosed in the solid bony cranium, is well protected but highly vulnerable to pressure that may accumulate within the enclosure. Its total volume—brain, cerebrospinal fluid (CSF), and blood—must remain approximately the same at all times. A change in the proportional volume of one of these components (e.g., increase or decrease in intracranial blood) must be accompanied by a compensatory change in another. In this way the volume and pressure normally remain constant. Examples of compensatory changes are reduction in blood volume, decrease in CSF production, increase in CSF absorption, or shrinkage of brain mass by displacement of intracellular and extracellular fluid. Children with open fontanels compensate by skull expansion and widened sutures. However, at any age the capacity for spatial compensation is limited. An increase in ICP may be caused by tumors or other space-occupying lesions, accumulation of fluid within the ventricular system, bleeding, or edema of cerebral tissues. Once compensation is exhausted, any further increase in volume will result in a rapid rise in ICP.

Early signs and symptoms of increased ICP are often subtle and assume many patterns (Box 48-1). As pressure increases, signs and symptoms become more pronounced and the level of consciousness deteriorates.

BOX 48-1
Clinical Manifestations of Increased Intracranial Pressure in Infants and Children

Infants

- Tense, bulging fontanel; lack of normal pulsations
- Separated cranial sutures
- Macewen (cracked-pot) sign
- Irritability
- High-pitched cry
- Increased occipital-frontal circumference
- Distended scalp veins
- Changes in feeding
- Crying when held or rocked
- "Setting sun" sign

Children

- Headache
- Nausea
- Vomiting—often without nausea
- Diplopia, blurred vision
- Seizures

Personality and behavior signs

- Irritability (toddlers), restlessness
- Indifference, drowsiness, or lack of interest
- Decline in school performance
- Diminished physical activity and motor performance
- Increased complaints of fatigue, tiredness; increased time devoted to sleep
- Significant weight loss possible from anorexia and vomiting
- Memory loss if pressure is markedly increased
- Inability to follow simple commands
- Progression to lethargy and drowsiness

Late signs

- Lowered level of consciousness
- Decreased motor response to command
- Decreased sensory response to painful stimuli
- Alterations in pupil size and reactivity
- Sometimes decerebrate or decorticate posturing
- Cheyne-Stokes respirations
- Papilledema

Altered States of Consciousness

Consciousness implies awareness—the ability to respond to sensory stimuli and have subjective experiences. There are two components of consciousness: **alertness,** an arousal-waking state including the ability to respond to stimuli, and **cognitive power,** including the ability to process stimuli and produce verbal and motor responses.

An altered state of consciousness usually refers to varying states of unconsciousness that may be momentary or may extend for hours, days, or indefinitely. **Unconsciousness** is depressed cerebral function—the inability to respond to sensory stimuli and have subjective experiences. **Coma** is defined as a state of unconsciousness from which the patient cannot be aroused even with powerful stimuli.

Level of consciousness. Assessment of **level of consciousness (LOC)** remains the earliest indicator of improvement or deterioration in neurologic status. LOC is determined by observations of the child's responses to the environment. Other diagnostic tests, such as motor activity, reflexes, and vital signs, are more variable and do not necessarily directly parallel the depth of the comatose state. The most consistently used terms are described in Box 48-2.

Coma assessment. Several scales have been devised in an attempt to standardize the description and interpretation of the degree of depressed consciousness. The most popular of these is the *Glasgow Coma Scale (GCS),* which consists of a three-part assessment: eye opening, verbal response, and motor response (Fig 48-1). When LOC is being assessed in young children, it is often useful to have a parent present to help elicit a desired response. An infant or child may not respond in an

BOX 48-2
Levels of Consciousness

Full consciousness—awake and alert, oriented to time, place, and person—behavior appropriate for age
Confusion—impaired decision making
Disorientation—disorientation to time, place, decreased level of consciousness
Lethargy—limited spontaneous movement, sluggish speech
Obtundation—arousable with stimulation
Stupor—remains in a deep sleep, responsive only to vigorous and repeated stimulation
Coma—no motor or verbal response to noxious (painful) stimuli
Persistent vegetative state (PVS)—the permanently lost function of the cerebral cortex—eyes follow objects only by reflex or when attracted to the direction of loud sounds; all four limbs are spastic but can withdraw from painful stimuli; hands show reflexive grasping and groping; the face can grimace, some food may be swallowed, and the child may groan or cry but utter no words

Modified from Hazinski MF, editor: *Care of the critically ill child,* ed 2, St Louis, 1992, Mosby.

unfamiliar environment or to unfamiliar voices. Children over 3 years of age should be able to give their name, although they may not be cognizant of place or time.

Numeric values are assigned to the levels of response in each category, and the sum of these numeric values provides an objective measure of the patient's LOC. The lower the score, the deeper the coma. A person with an unaltered LOC would score the highest, 15; a score of 7 or below is generally accepted as a definition of coma; the lowest score, 3, indicates deep coma. In cases of irreversible coma, the Task Force for the Determination of Brain Death in Children has established physical examination criteria.

Nursing ALERT

Lack of response to painful stimuli is abnormal and is reported immediately.

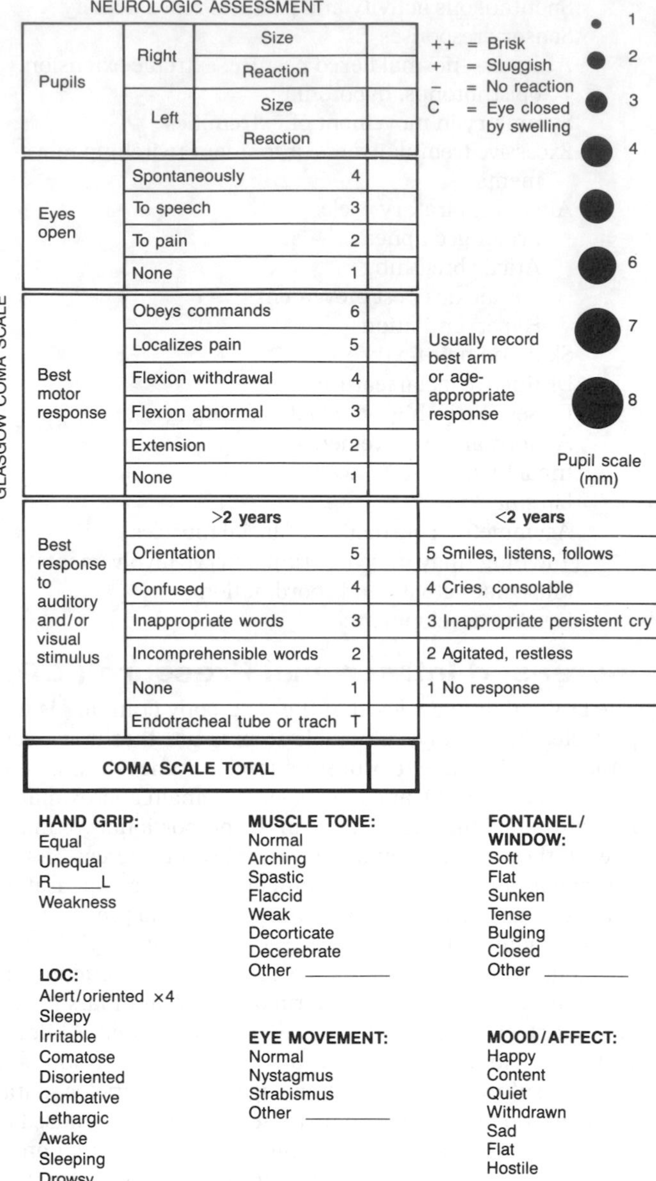
NEUROLOGIC ASSESSMENT

Pupils	Right	Size	
		Reaction	
	Left	Size	
		Reaction	

++ = Brisk
\+ = Sluggish
− = No reaction
C = Eye closed by swelling

Pupil scale (mm): 1, 2, 3, 4, 5, 6, 7, 8

GLASGOW COMA SCALE

Eyes open	Spontaneously	4	
	To speech	3	
	To pain	2	
	None	1	
Best motor response	Obeys commands	6	
	Localizes pain	5	
	Flexion withdrawal	4	
	Flexion abnormal	3	
	Extension	2	
	None	1	

Usually record best arm or age-appropriate response

	>2 years			<2 years
Best response to auditory and/or visual stimulus	Orientation	5		5 Smiles, listens, follows
	Confused	4		4 Cries, consolable
	Inappropriate words	3		3 Inappropriate persistent cry
	Incomprehensible words	2		2 Agitated, restless
	None	1		1 No response
	Endotracheal tube or trach	T		
COMA SCALE TOTAL				

HAND GRIP: Equal, Unequal, R_____L, Weakness

MUSCLE TONE: Normal, Arching, Spastic, Flaccid, Weak, Decorticate, Decerebrate, Other ________

FONTANEL/WINDOW: Soft, Flat, Sunken, Tense, Bulging, Closed, Other ________

LOC: Alert/oriented ×4, Sleepy, Irritable, Comatose, Disoriented, Combative, Lethargic, Awake, Sleeping, Drowsy, Agitated

EYE MOVEMENT: Normal, Nystagmus, Strabismus, Other ________

MOOD/AFFECT: Happy, Content, Quiet, Withdrawn, Sad, Flat, Hostile

Fig. 48-1 Pediatric coma scale.

Neurologic Examination

The purpose of the neurologic examination is to establish an accurate, objective baseline of neurologic information. It is essential that the neurologic examination be documented in a fashion that can be reproduced by others. Descriptions of behaviors should be simple, objective, and easily interpreted: "Drowsy but awake and conversationally rational/oriented"; "Sleepy but arousable with vigorous physical stimuli. Pressure to nail base of right hand results in upper extremity flexion/lower extremity extension."

Vital signs. Pulse, respiration, and blood pressure provide information regarding the adequacy of circulation and the possible underlying cause of altered consciousness. Autonomic activity is most intensively disturbed in deep coma and in brainstem lesions.

Body temperature is often elevated, and sometimes the elevation may be extreme. Coma of a toxic origin may produce hypothermia. High temperature is most frequently a sign of an acute infectious process or heat stroke but may be caused by ingestion of some drugs (especially salicylates, alcohol, and barbiturates) or intracranial bleeding, especially subarachnoid hemorrhage. A fever sometimes follows a cerebral seizure.

The *pulse* is variable and may be rapid, slow and bounding, or feeble. *Blood pressure* may be normal, elevated, or at shock levels. The Cushing reflex or pressor response, which causes a slowing of the pulse and an increase in blood pressure, is uncommon in children; when it occurs, it is a very late sign. Vital signs are also affected by medications. For assessment purposes *changes* in pulse and blood pressure are more important than direction.

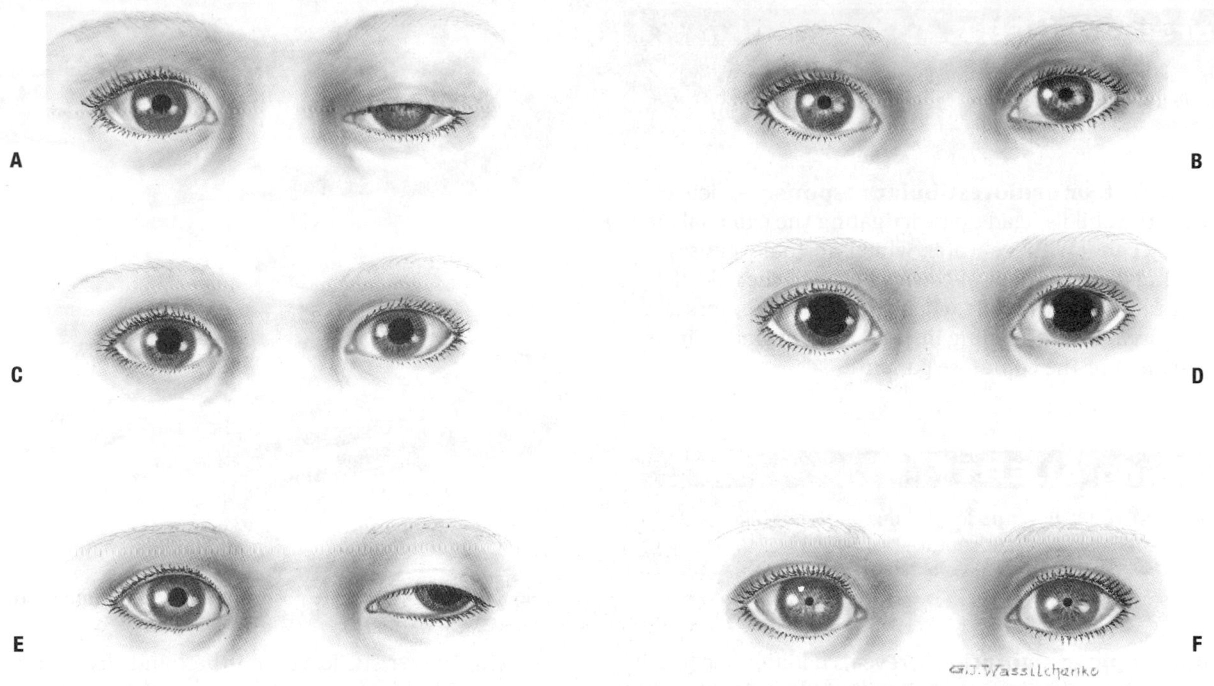

A B C D E F

G.J.Wassilchenko

Fig. 48-2 Variations in pupil size with altered states of consciousness. **A,** Ipsilateral pupillary constriction with slight ptosis; **B,** bilateral small pupils; **C,** midposition, light fixed to all stimuli; **D,** bilateral dilated and fixed pupils; **E,** dilated pupil, left eye abducted with ptosis; **F,** pinpoint pupils.

Respirations are often slow, deep, and irregular. Slow, deep breathing is often seen in the heavy sleep caused by sedatives, after seizures, or in cerebral infections. Slow, shallow breathing may result from sedatives or opioids (narcotics). Hyperventilation (deep and rapid respirations) is usually the result of metabolic acidosis or abnormal stimulation of the respiratory center in the medulla caused by salicylate poisoning, hepatic coma, or Reye syndrome.

Breathing patterns have been described with a number of terms (e.g., apneustic, cluster, ataxic, Cheyne-Stokes). However, it is better to describe what is being observed rather than placing a label on it. The terms are often used and interpreted incorrectly. Periodic or irregular breathing is an ominous sign of brainstem (especially medullary) dysfunction that often precedes complete apnea. The *odor* of the breath may provide additional clues (e.g., the fruity, acetone odor of ketosis; the foul odor of uremia; the fetid odor of hepatic failure; or the odor of alcohol).

Skin. The skin may offer clues to the cause of unconsciousness. The body surface should be examined for the presence of injury, needle marks, petechiae, bites, and ticks. Evidence of toxic substances may be found on the hands, face, mouth, and clothing—especially in small children.

Eyes. Pupil size and reactivity are assessed (Figs. 48-1 and 48-2). Pinpoint pupils are commonly observed in poisoning, such as opiate or barbiturate poisoning, or in brainstem dysfunction. Widely dilated and reactive pupils are often seen after seizures and may involve only one side. Dilated pupils may also be caused by eye trauma. Widely dilated and fixed pupils suggest paralysis of cranial nerve III secondary to pressure from herniation of the brain through the tentorium. A unilateral fixed pupil usually suggests a lesion on the same side. Bilateral fixed pupils usually imply brainstem damage if present for more than 5 minutes. Dilated and unreactive pupils are also seen in hypothermia, anoxia, ischemia, poisoning with atropine-like substances, or prior instillation of mydriatic drugs.

Nursing ALERT

The sudden appearance of a fixed and dilated pupil is a neurosurgical emergency.

The description of eye movements should indicate whether one or both eyes are involved and how the reaction was elicited. The parents should be asked about preexisting strabismus, which will cause the eyes to appear normal under compromise. A posttraumatic strabismus indicates cranial nerve VI damage.

Special tests, usually performed by qualified persons, include the following:

Doll's head maneuver—the child's head is rotated quickly to one side and then to the other. Conjugate (paired or working together) movement of the eyes in the direction opposite to the head rotation is normal. Absence of this response suggests dysfunction of the brainstem or oculomotor nerve (cranial nerve III).

Nursing ALERT

This assessment is not attempted until cervical spine injury has been ruled out.

Caloric test, or oculovestibular response—elicited with the child's head up by irrigating the external auditory canal with ice water, which normally causes conjugate movement of the eyes toward the side of stimulation. This is lost when the pontine centers are impaired, thus providing important information in assessment of the comatose patient.

Nursing ALERT

This painful test is never performed on the awake child or if the tympanic membrane is ruptured.

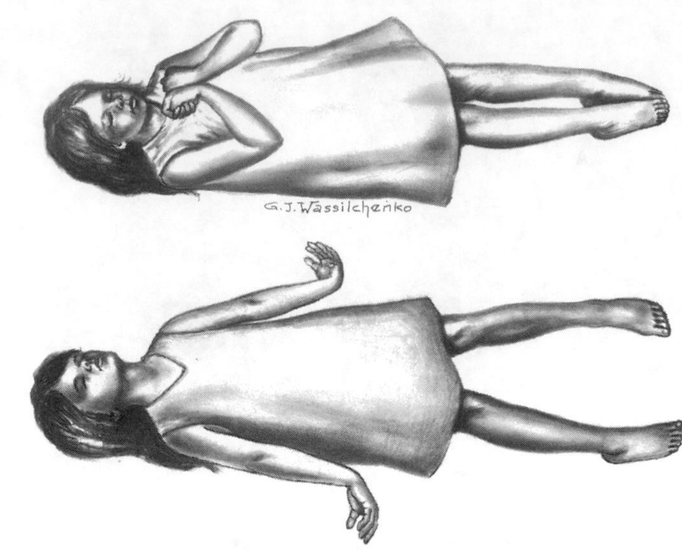

Fig. 48-3 **A,** Decorticate posturing. **B,** Decerebrate posturing.

Funduscopic examination—reveals additional clues. If papilledema develops at all, it will not be evident early in the course of unconsciousness because it takes 24 to 48 hours to develop. The presence of preretinal (subhyaloid) hemorrhages in children is almost invariably the result of acute trauma with intracranial bleeding, usually subarachnoid or subdural hemorrhage.

Motor function. Observing spontaneous activity, posture, and response to painful stimuli provides clues to the location and extent of cerebral dysfunction. Even subtle movements (e.g., the outward rotation of a hip) should be noted, and the child observed for other signs. Asymmetric movements of the limbs or absence of movement suggests paralysis. In hemiplegia the affected limb lies in external rotation and will fall uncontrollably when lifted and allowed to drop. These observations should be described rather than labeled.

In the deeper comatose states there is little or no spontaneous movement, and the musculature tends to be flaccid. There is considerable variability in the motor behavior in lesser degrees of coma. For example, the child may be relatively immobile or restless and hyperkinetic; muscle tone may be increased or decreased. Tremors, twitching, and spasms of muscles are common observations. The patient may display purposeless plucking or tossing movements. Combative or negativistic behavior is not uncommon. Hyperactivity is more common in acute febrile and toxic states than in cases of increased ICP. Convulsions are common in children and may be present in coma from any cause. Any repetitive or convulsive movements should be described.

Posturing. Since cortical control over motor function is lost in brain dysfunction, primitive postural reflexes emerge. These are evident in posturing and motor movements directly related to the area of the brain involved. **Decorticate posturing** (Fig. 48-3, *A*) is seen when there is severe dysfunction of the cerebral cortex. Typical decorticate posturing includes adduction of arms at the shoulders, flexion of the arms on the chest with the wrists flexed and the hands fisted, and extension and adduction of the lower extremities. **Decerebrate posturing** (Fig. 48-3, *B*), a sign of dysfunction at the level of the midbrain, is characterized by rigid extension and pronation of the arms and legs. The posturing may not be evident when the child is quiet but can usually be elicited by applying painful stimuli, such as pressure of a blunt object on the base of the nail.

Reflexes. Testing of some reflexes may be of limited value. In general, the corneal, pupillary, muscle-stretch, superficial, and plantar reflexes tend to be absent in deep coma. The state of reflexes is variable in lighter grades of unconsciousness and depends on the underlying pathologic process and the location of the lesion. Absence of corneal reflexes and presence of a tonic neck reflex are associated with severe brain damage. The Babinski reflex (see Extremities, Chapter 32) may be of value if it is found to be present consistently in children older than 18 months. A positive Babinski reflex finding is significant in assessment of pyramidal tract lesions when it is unilateral and associated with other pyramidal signs.

Nursing ALERT

Three key reflexes that demonstrate neurologic health in young infants are the Moro, tonic neck, and withdrawal reflexes.

Special Diagnostic Procedures

Numerous diagnostic procedures are used for assessment of cerebral function. Laboratory tests that may help determine the cause of unconsciousness include blood glucose, urea nitrogen, and electrolyte (pH, sodium, potassium, chloride, calcium, and bicarbonate) tests; clotting studies, hematocrit, and a complete blood count; liver function tests; blood cultures if there is fever; and sometimes studies to detect lead or other toxic substances, such as drugs.

BOX 48-3
Procedures Used in Cerebral Assessment

Lumbar puncture (LP)

Diagnostic—measures spinal fluid pressure, obtains CSF for visualization and laboratory analysis

Subdural tap

Helps rule out subdural effusions
Relieves ICP

Electroencephalography (EEG)

Measures electric activity of cerebral cortex
Detects electric abnormalities—diagnosis of seizures
Used to determine brain death

Video EEG

Split-screen simultaneous visualization of whole body, facial, and EEG recording

Computed tomography (CT) scan

Visualizes horizontal and vertical cross sections of brain at any axis
Distinguishes density of various intracranial tissues and structures—congenital abnormalities, hemorrhage, tumors, and demyelinating and inflammatory processes

Nuclear brain scan

Test material accumulates in areas where blood-brain barrier is defective
Identifies focal brain lesions (e.g., tumors, abscesses)
Positive uptake of material with encephalitis and subdural hematoma
Visualizes CSF pathways

Transillumination

Varying degrees of localized glowing may be seen in abnormal fluid accumulation in various areas of head

Echoencephalography

Identifies shifts in midline structures from their normal positions as a result of intracranial lesions
May show ventricular dilation

Radiography

Shows fractures, dislocations, spreading suture lines, and craniostenosis
Shows degenerative changes, bone erosion, and calcifications

Magnetic resonance imaging (MRI)

Permits visualization of morphologic features of target structures
Permits tissue discrimination unavailable with many techniques

Positron emission transaxial tomography (PETT) or Positron emission tomography (PET)

Detects and measures such functions as blood volume and flow in brain, metabolic activity, and biochemical changes within tissues

Real-time ultrasonography (RTUS)

Allows high-resolution anatomic visualization in variety of imaging planes

Digital subtraction angiography (DSA)

Visualizes vasculature of target tissue
Visualizes finite vascular abnormalities

Highly sophisticated tests are carried out with specialized equipment by skilled personnel. Most of these tests are outlined in Box 48-3. Because such tests can be threatening to children, a child will need preparation for, and support and reassurance during, them (see also Preparation for Procedures, Chapter 42).

Children who are old enough to understand require careful explanation of the procedure, why it is being done, what they will experience, and how they can help. School-age children usually appreciate a more detailed description of why contrast material is injected. The importance of lying still for tests, particularly tomography, needs to be stressed. Children unfamiliar with the machines can be shown a picture beforehand. Although radiographic examinations are not painful, the machinery is often so frightening in appearance that children protest because of anxiety.

Tests such as computed tomography (CT) and magnetic resonance imaging (MRI) require that children be immobilized. Chin and cheek pads are sometimes used to prevent the slightest head movement, and straps are applied to the body to prevent a slight change in body position. The nurse can explain these events to a frightened child by comparing them to an astronaut's preparation for a space flight. It is very important to emphasize to the child that at no time is the procedure painful.

Because of developmental limitations, the nurse should not expect cooperation from a young child. **Conscious sedation** will be required. Drugs commonly used are intravenous pentobarbital and oral chloral hydrate. Chloral hydrate may be the drug of choice for children under 2 years of age. The suggested oral dosage is the following (Barkovich, 1990):

- <10 kg: 75 to 100 mg/kg
- >10 kg: 75 to 100 mg/kg plus 50 mg/kg for each 1 kg of weight >10 kg (to a maximum dose of 2 g)
- If child is still awake after 20 minutes, supplementary doses may be given up to a total dose of 2 g.
- The drug should be given 35 to 45 minutes before the anticipated imaging time.

It is helpful for nurses to become acquainted with the equipment and the general environment in which the test will take place so that they can better explain the procedure to children at their level of understanding. Equipment is often strange and ominous to a child and may be perceived as a frightening monster. They need constant reassurance from a trusted companion. Since children are particularly frightened of needles, they need to be informed of any medication or contrast medium to be administered intravenously.

Physical preparation may involve administering a sedative or providing intravenous access for infusion of contrast material. If so, children should be helped through the preparation and administration and assured that someone will remain with them (if this is possible). Children will need continual support and reinforcement during procedures in which they remain conscious. Vital signs and physiologic response to the procedure are monitored throughout. Conscious sedation records become part of the child's chart. Many diagnostic procedures performed on an outpatient basis require sedation, and children need recovery time and observation. Written instructions should be reviewed with parents if the child is discharged to the home after a procedure (see the Critical Thinking Q & A on p. 1578).

Critical Thinking Q & A 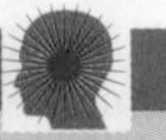

CONSCIOUS SEDATION

Brian, 4 weeks old, is returned to his room after a CT scan to evaluate a seizure episode. On examination you find a sleepy infant who is arousable with vigorous stimulation and has pale, dusky colored skin and mucous membranes. The vital signs are temperature of 35.8° C (96.4° F), pulse of 110, respiratory rate of 20, and blood pressure of 82/40; the oxygen saturation is 89% to 92%. His weight is 5 kg, and he received 500 mg of chloral hydrate (<10 kg: 75-100 mg/kg dosage) as ordered before leaving for the CT. During report the CT nurse reviews the conscious sedation record, and you note that it does not include the infant's temperature. An additional dosage of 250 mg of chloral hydrate was administered in CT to achieve sleep for Brian. The best intervention is to:

1. Monitor the vital signs and cover the infant
2. Place a radiant warmer over the infant and notify the physician
3. Fill out a medication error report
4. Allow the infant to sleep

The correct answer is two. Brian is experiencing thermoregulation problems compounded by administration of too much chloral hydrate for conscious sedation. A maximum dosage of sedation was exceeded for this infant. Conscious sedation flow sheets to record vital signs often do not include temperature measurement, an essential observation in infants because of their inability to maintain body temperature.

Children who have undergone a procedure while under general anesthesia require postanesthesia care, including positioning to prevent aspiration of secretions and frequent assessment of vital signs and LOC. In addition, other neurologic functions, such as pupillary responses, motor strength, and movement, are tested at regular intervals. Any surgical wound resulting from the test is checked for bleeding, CSF leakage, and other complications. Children who undergo repeated subdural taps should have the hematocrit measured daily to detect any blood loss from the procedure.

Children's emotional reactions to procedures are also considered. They should be allowed to express their feelings about their experiences through verbal expression and the use of therapeutic play. Parents also seek and are entitled to an explanation of results of tests and procedures performed on their children. Nurses are in a unique position to provide support and education to parents regarding procedures.

Nursing Care of the Unconscious Child

The unconscious child requires continuous nursing attendance with observation, recording, and evaluation of changes in objective signs. These observations provide valuable information regarding the patient's progress. Often they serve as a guide to diagnosis and treatment. Therefore careful and detailed observations are essential for the patient's welfare. In addition, vital functions must be maintained, and complications prevented through conscientious and meticulous nursing care. The outcome of unconsciousness may be early with complete recovery, death within a few hours or days, persistent and permanent unconsciousness, or recovery with varying degrees of residual mental and/or physical disability. The outcome and recovery of the unconscious child may depend on the level of nursing care and observational skills.

Emergency measures are directed toward ensuring a patent airway, treating shock, and reducing ICP (if present). Delayed treatment often leads to increased damage. As soon as emergency measures have been implemented—in many cases concurrently—therapies for specific causes are begun. Because nursing care is closely related to medical management, both are considered here.

Assessment

Continual observation of LOC, pupillary reaction, and vital signs is essential to management of CNS disorders. Regular assessment of neurologic signs is a vital part of nursing comatose children. Vital signs are taken and recorded regularly. The frequency depends on the cause of coma, the status, and the progression of cerebral involvement. Intervals may be as frequent as every 15 minutes or as long as every 2 hours. Significant alterations are reported immediately. Temperature is taken every 2 to 4 hours, depending on the patient's condition.

An elevated temperature may occur in children with CNS dysfunction; therefore a light covering is sufficient. Vigorous efforts, such as tepid sponge baths or application of a hypothermia blanket, are needed to prevent brain damage if temperature exceeds 40° C (104° F) rectally.

The LOC is assessed periodically, including size, equality, and reaction of pupils to light and signs of meningeal irritation, such as nuchal rigidity. Response to vocal commands, spontaneous behavior, resistance to care, and response to painful stimuli are included in this assessment. Motions of any type, changes in muscle tone or strength, and body position are noted. Seizure activity is described according to the type and length of seizure and body areas involved (Box 48-14).

Pain management for the comatose child requires astute nursing observation and management. Signs of pain include changes in behavior (e.g., increased agitation and rigidity, and alterations in physiologic parameters); usually increased heart rate, respiratory rate, and blood pressure; and decreased oxygen saturation. Since these findings are not specific for pain, the nurse should observe for their appearance during times of induced or suspected pain and their disappearance after the inciting procedure or the administration of analgesia. A pain assessment record should be used to document indications of pain and the effectiveness of interventions (see Pain Assessment, Chapter 41).

The use of opioids, such as morphine, to relieve pain is controversial because they may mask signs of altered consciousness or depress respirations. However, unrelieved pain activates the stress response, which can elevate ICP. To block the stress response, some authorities advocate the use of analgesics, sedatives, and, in some cases such as head injury, paralyzing agents via continuous intravenous infusion. A frequently used combination is fentanyl, midazolam (Versed), and vecuronium. If there are concerns about assessing the LOC or respiratory depression, naloxone can be used to reverse the opioid effects. Acetaminophen and codeine may also be effective analgesics for mild to moderate pain. Regardless of the drugs used, adequate dosage and regular administration are essential to providing optimal pain relief.

Other measures to relieve discomfort include providing a quiet, dimly lit environment; limiting visitors to a minimum; preventing any sudden jarring movement, such as banging into the bed; and preventing an increase in ICP. The last is most effectively achieved by proper positioning and prevention of straining, such as during coughing, vomiting, or defecating (see Pain Management, Chapter 41).

Nursing ALERT

When opioids are used, bowel elimination must be closely monitored because of their constipating effect. A stool softener should be given regularly with laxatives as needed to prevent constipation.

Antiepileptic drugs, such as phenytoin (Dilantin) or phenobarbital, are ordered for control of seizure activity.

Nursing Diagnoses

On the basis of a thorough assessment, several nursing diagnoses are identified. The more common diagnoses for the unconscious child are included in the Nursing Care Plan on pp. 1584-1585. Others may apply in specific situations.

Planning

Goals for the unconscious child and family include the following:

1. Child will maintain respiratory integrity.
2. Child will not experience increasing ICP.
3. Child will have basic needs (hygiene, nutrition, hydration, elimination) met.
4. Child will not experience complications of immobility.
5. Family will receive adequate support and education.

Implementation

Respiratory Management

Respiratory effectiveness is the primary concern in care of the unconscious child, and establishment of an adequate airway is *always* the first priority. Carbon dioxide has a potent vasodilating effect and will increase cerebral blood flow (CBF) and ICP. Cerebral hypoxia that lasts longer than 4 minutes nearly always causes irreversible brain damage.

Nursing ALERT

Respiratory obstruction leads to cardiac arrest. Always maintain an adequate airway.

Children in lighter states of coma may be able to cough and swallow, but those in deeper states are unable to handle secretions, which tend to pool in the throat and pharynx. Dysfunction of cranial nerves IX and X place the child at risk for aspiration and cardiac arrest; therefore the child is positioned to prevent aspiration of secretions, and the stomach is emptied to reduce the likelihood of vomiting. In infants blockage of air passages from secretions can happen in seconds. In addition, upper airway obstruction from laryngospasm is a frequent complication in comatose children.

An oral airway can be used for the child who is suffering a temporary loss of consciousness, such as after a contusion, seizure, or anesthesia. For children who remain unconscious for a time, a nasotracheal or orotracheal tube is inserted to maintain the open airway and facilitate removal of secretions. A tracheostomy is performed in cases in which laryngoscopy for introduction of an endotracheal tube would be difficult or dangerous. Suctioning is used only as needed to clear the airway, exerting care to prevent increasing ICP. Respiratory status is observed and evaluated regularly. Signs of respiratory embarrassment may be an indication for ventilatory assistance.

When the respiratory center is involved, mechanical ventilation is usually indicated (see Chapter 42). Blood gas analysis is performed regularly, and oxygen is administered when indicated. Moderately severe hypoxia and respiratory acidosis are often present but not always evident in clinical manifestations. Hyperventilation often accompanies unconsciousness and may lead to respiratory alkalosis, or it may represent the body's attempt to compensate for metabolic acidosis. Therefore blood gas and pH determinations are essential guides for electrolyte therapy. Chest physiotherapy is carried out on a regular basis, and the child's position is changed at least every 2 hours to prevent pulmonary complications.

Increased ICP Monitoring

Management of the child with increased ICP is possibly the most formidable task and the most controversial subject in pediatric critical care. It appears that the outcome in pediatric neurologic injury may reflect the initial cerebral damage more than subsequent intracranial hypertension.

When increased ICP is the result of accumulation of CSF from obstruction of CSF flow, a ventricular tap will provide re-

Critical Thinking Q & A 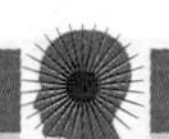

HYDROCEPHALUS

Three-year-old Emma is five days post operative for removal of a posterior fossa tumor. Although an EVD was placed to treat her hydrocephalus, she continues to demonstrate signs of ICP, including holding the back of her head, anorexia, crying when moved or strangers enter room, and lethargy. On examination, fluid drainage is noted on the mother's clothes, and Emma is experiencing repetitive, rapid eyelid blinking. The best intervention is to:

1. Lower the EVD drain
2. Check the EVD dressing site, do a neurologic examination and notify the practitioner
3. Change the dressing to a transparent adhesive
4. Request a CT scan

The correct answer is two. The EVD is not draining properly but is taking the path of least resistance through the insertion site. Lowering the EVD may cause rapid drainage of the CSF, resulting in subdural complications. The dressing may need changing to a clear adhesive so the site can be observed. A CT may be required, but the priority is to stabilize the patient's condition, because Emma is demonstrating signs of increased ICP and cranial neuropathy.

lief quickly and effectively. Evacuation of a hematoma reduces pressure from this source. Indications for inserting an ICP monitor are (1) Glasgow Coma Scale evaluation of less than 7, (2) Glasgow Coma Scale evaluation of less than 8 with respiratory assistance, (3) deterioration of condition, and (4) subjective judgment of clinical appearance and response.

Four major types of ICP monitors are (1) intraventricular catheter with fibroscopic sensors attached to a monitoring system, (2) subarachnoid bolt (Richmond screw), (3) epidural sensor, and (4) anterior fontanel pressure monitor. Transducers for both ventricular and subarachnoid monitoring should be set up without the use of a flush device. Direct ventricular pressure measurement remains the gold standard of ICP monitoring.

The catheter method involves introduction of a catheter into the lateral ventricle on the nondominant side, if known, or placement in the subdural space. The catheter has the advantage of providing a means of extraventricular (or continuous) drainage to reduce pressure. A drainage bag attached to the system is kept at the level of the ventricles and can be lowered to decrease ICP (see the Critical Thinking Q & A box on p. 1579).

Nursing ALERT

If the external ventricular drain (EVD) is unclamped for CSF drainage, carefully monitor the level of the collection container. If the container is too low, improper CSF decompression could lower ICP too rapidly, causing bleeding and pain.

In the bolt method the end of the bolt is placed into the subarachnoid space. The bolt cannot be adequately secured in a small child's pliant skull, although special modifications have been developed for children under 6 years of age.

Nursing ALERT

The bolt is stabilized with dressings, but these are not changed or disturbed, even to check the site.

The placement of the bolt is not adjusted by anyone except the neurosurgeon who placed the device. The neurosurgeon is notified if a satisfactory wave form is not observed.

An epidural sensor can be placed between the dura and the skull through a burr hole and connected to a stopcock assembly and a transducer, which provides a readout of the pressure. Correlation of pressure readings is less invasive but may be inconsistent. In infants a fontanel transducer can be used to detect impulses from a pressure sensor and convert them to electrical energy. The electrical energy is then converted to visible waves or numeric readings on an oscilloscope. ICP measurement from the anterior fontanel is noninvasive but may prove to be inaccurate if the equipment is poorly placed or inconsistently recalibrated. The intraparenchymal pressure monitoring device (e.g., Camino) is a result of fiberoptic technology and performs reliably.

ICP can be increased by instillation of solutions; therefore antibiotics are administered systemically if a positive CSF culture result is obtained. However, intravenous ICP monitoring rarely causes infection. Since CSF is a body fluid, isolation precautions may be implemented according to hospital policy (see Infection Control, Chapter 42).

Nurses caring for patients with intracranial monitoring devices must be acquainted with the system, assist with insertion, interpret the monitor readings, and be able to distinguish between danger signals and mechanical dysfunction.

For increased ICP resulting from cerebral edema several medical measures are available. Osmotic diuretics may provide rapid relief in emergencies; although their effect is transient, lasting only about 6 hours, they can be lifesaving. These substances are rapidly excreted by the kidneys and carry with them large quantities of sodium and water. Mannitol (or sometimes urea) administered intravenously is the drug most often used for rapid reduction. The infusion is generally given slowly but may be pushed rapidly if there is herniation or impending herniation. Because of the profound diuretic effect of the drug, an indwelling catheter is inserted to ensure bladder emptying. Adrenocorticosteroids are not recommended for cerebral edema secondary to head trauma. $Paco_2$ should be maintained at 25 to 30 mm Hg to produce vasoconstriction, which reduces CBF, thereby decreasing ICP.

Nursing activities. In cases of high levels of increased ICP, nursing procedures tend to trigger reactive pressure waves in many patients. For example, increased intrathoracic or abdominal pressure will be transmitted to the cranium. Particular care should be taken in positioning these patients to prevent neck vein compression, which may further increase ICP by interfering with venous return.

Nursing ALERT

The head of the bed is elevated 15 to 30 degrees, and the child is positioned so that the head is maintained in midline to facilitate venous drainage and prevent jugular compression. Turning side to side is contraindicated because of the risk of jugular compression.

The child can be propped to one side or the other, and the use of an alternating-pressure mattress reduces the chance of prolonged pressure to vulnerable areas. Frequent clinical assessment of the child cannot be replaced by an ICP monitoring device.

It is important to eliminate activities that may increase ICP by causing pain, emotional stress, or crying, or those that might trigger a convulsive seizure. Gentle range-of-motion exercises can be carried out but should not be performed vigorously. Nontherapeutic touch can cause an increase in ICP. Any disturbing procedures to be performed should be scheduled to take advantage of therapies that reduce ICP, such as osmotherapy and sedation. Efforts are taken to minimize or eliminate environmental noise. Assessment and intervention to relieve pain are important nursing functions to decrease ICP.

Suctioning. Suctioning and percussion are poorly tolerated and are therefore contraindicated unless there are concurrent respiratory problems. Hypoxia and the Valsalva maneuver associated with cough both acutely elevate ICP. Vibration, which does not increase ICP, accomplishes excellent results and should be tried first if treatment is needed. If suctioning is necessary, it should be brief and preceded by hyperventilation with 100% oxygen, which can be monitored during suctioning with a pulse oxygen sensor reading to determine oxygen saturation.

Nutrition and Hydration

Fluids and calories are supplied initially by the intravenous route (see Chapter 42). An intravenous infusion is started early, and the type of fluid administered is determined by the general condition of the patient. Fluid therapy requires careful monitoring and adjustment based on neurologic signs and electrolyte determinations. Often comatose children are unable to cope with the same amounts of fluid they could tolerate at other times, and overhydration must be avoided to prevent fatal cerebral edema.

Later, nutrition is provided in a balanced formula given by nasogastric or gastrostomy tube. The nasogastric tube is usually taped in place with care to prevent pressure on the nares. Most children have continuous feedings, but if bolus feedings are used, the tube is rinsed with water after each feeding. Tubes are replaced according to unit policy. Nostrils are alternated with each replacement to prevent nasal irritation and pressure. Overfeeding should be avoided to prevent vomiting with its attendant danger of aspiration. Stomach contents are aspirated and measured before feeding to ascertain the amount remaining in the stomach. If the residual volume is excessive (depending on the size of the child), the dietitian and physician should be consulted regarding alteration of the formula composition to provide the needed calories and nutrients in a smaller volume. The aspirated contents should always be refed.

Hydration is maintained in the same manner. When cerebral edema is a threat, fluids may be restricted to reduce the chance of fluid overload. Skin and mucous membranes are examined for signs of dehydration. Observation for signs of altered fluid balance related to abnormal pituitary secretions is a part of nursing care.

Altered pituitary secretion. An altered ability to handle fluid loads is attributed in part to the syndrome of inappropriate antidiuretic hormone (SIADH) and diabetes insipidus (DI) resulting from hypothalamic dysfunction (see Chapter 49). SIADH frequently accompanies CNS disorders such as head injury, meningitis, encephalitis, brain abscess, brain tumor, and subarachnoid hemorrhage. In the patient with SIADH, scant quantities of urine are excreted, electrolyte analysis reveals hyponatremia and hyposmolality, and manifestations of overhydration are evident. It is important to evaluate all parameters, since the reduced urine output might be erroneously interpreted as a sign of dehydration.

The treatment of SIADH consists of restriction of fluids until serum electrolytes and osmolality return to normal levels. Since SIADH frequently accompanies meningitis in children, fluid restriction is often prescribed. Likewise, DI may follow intracranial trauma. There are increased urine volume and the accompanying danger of dehydration (see Table 48-1 for comparison of fluid changes in SIADH and DI). Adequate replacement of fluids is essential, and observation of electrolyte balance is necessary to detect signs of hypernatremia and hyperosmolality. Exogenous vasopressin may be administered.

TABLE 48-1 Effects of altered pituitary secretion

MEASUREMENT	DI	SIADH
Urine output	Increased	Decreased
Specific gravity	Decreased	Increased
Serum sodium	Increased (hypernatremia)	Decreased (hyponatremia)

Medications

The cause of unconsciousness determines specific drug therapies. Children with infectious processes are given antibiotics appropriate to the disease and the infecting organism, and corticosteroids are prescribed for inflammatory conditions and edema. Cerebral edema is an indication for osmotherapy with osmotic diuretics. Sedatives or antiepileptics are prescribed for seizure activity. Sedation in the combative child provides amnesic and anxiolytic properties in conjunction with a paralytic agent. The combination decreases ICP and allows treatment of cerebral edema. Usual drugs include morphine, midazolam (Versed), and pancuronium. Midazolam is attractive because of its short half-life.

Nursing ALERT

When used for seizures, phenytoin should be administered slowly by direct IV push at a rate not to exceed 50 mg/min. Since phenytoin precipitates in the presence of glucose, only normal saline solution is used for flushing the needle or catheter.

Deep coma, induced by administration of barbiturates, is controversial in the management of ICP. Barbiturates are currently reserved for the reduction of increased ICP when all else has failed. They decrease the cerebral metabolic rate for oxygen and protect the brain during times of reduced CPP. Barbiturate coma requires extensive monitoring, cardiovascular and respiratory support, and ICP monitoring to assess response to therapy. Paralyzing agents, such as pancuronium (Pavulon), also may be needed to aid in performing diagnostic tests, improving effectiveness of therapy, and reducing risks of secondary complications. Elevation of ICP and/or heart rate of patients who are being given paralyzing agents or are under sedation may indicate the need for another dose of either or both medications.

Thermoregulation

Hyperthermia often accompanies cerebral dysfunction; if it is present, measures are implemented to reduce the temperature to prevent brain damage and to reduce metabolic demands generated by the increased body temperature. Antipyretics are the method of choice for fever reduction; cooling devices are used for hyperthermia. Laboratory tests and other methods are used in an attempt to determine the cause, if any, of the hyperthermia. Shivering responses triggered by a cooling blanket can often be alleviated by keeping the child warm. Treatment with hypothermia and barbiturates increases the risk of iatrogenic complications.

Elimination

A retention catheter is usually inserted in the acute phase, although diapers may be used and weighed to record urinary output. The child who formerly had bowel and bladder control is generally incontinent. If the child remains comatose for a long period, the indwelling catheter may be removed and periodic bladder emptying accomplished by intermittent catheterization. Stool softeners are usually sufficient to maintain bowel function, but suppositories or enemas may be needed occasionally for adequate elimination and prevention of impaction. The passage of liquid stool after a period of no bowel activity is usually a sign of an impaction. To avoid this preventable problem, daily recording of bowel activity is essential.

Hygienic Care

Routine measures for cleansing and maintaining skin integrity are an integral part of nursing care of the unconscious child. Skinfolds require special attention to prevent excoriation. The child who is unable to move is prone to development of tissue breakdown and pressure necrosis; therefore the child may be placed on a pressure-reducing or pressure-relieving device to prevent pressure on prominent areas of the body. The goal is prevention by regular change of position and inspection of vulnerable areas, such as the ankle, trochanter, and shoulder. Since unconscious children undergo numerous invasive procedures, these skin sites require special assessment and intervention to promote healing and to prevent infection. Bed linen and any clothing are kept dry and free of wrinkles. If the child requires surgery or radiography, the nurse checks all dressings, bony sites, catheters, and intravenous access lines (see also Maintaining Healthy Skin, Chapter 42).

Mouth care is performed at least twice daily, since the mouth tends to become dry or coated with mucus. The teeth are carefully brushed with a soft toothbrush or cleaned with gauze saturated with saline solution. Commercially prepared cleansing devices (such as Toothettes) are convenient for cleansing the mouth and teeth. Lips are coated with ointment or other preparations to protect them from drying, cracking, or blistering.

The deeply comatose child is also prone to eye irritation. The corneal reflexes are absent; therefore the eyes are easily irritated or damaged by linen, dust, or other substances that may come in contact with them. Excessive dryness is a result of decreased secretions, especially if the child is undergoing osmotherapy to reduce or prevent brain edema, and incomplete closure of the eyes may occur.

Nursing ALERT

The eyes should be examined regularly and carefully for early signs of irritation or inflammation. Artificial tears (methylcellulose) are placed in the eyes every 1 to 2 hours. Sometimes eye dressings may be needed to protect the eyes from possible damage.

The hair is combed and styled neatly. Long hair is usually braided and secured with rubber bands. The scalp should be kept clean with dry or wet shampoos as needed. The child's head may be shaved for tests or surgical procedures. If so, the hair is saved if possible and given to the family.

Positioning and Exercise

The unconscious child is positioned to prevent aspiration of saliva, nasogastric secretions, and vomitus and to minimize ICP. The head of the bed is elevated, and the child is placed in a side-lying or semiprone position. A small, firm pillow is placed under the head, and the uppermost limbs are flexed and supported with pillows. The weight of the body should not rest on the dependent arm. In the semiprone position the child lies with the dependent arm at the side behind the body, the opposite side supported on pillows, and the uppermost arm and leg flexed and resting on the pillows. This position prevents undue pressure on the dependent extremities. The dependent position of the face encourages drainage of secretions and prevents the flaccid tongue from obstructing the airway.

Normal range-of-motion exercises help maintain function and prevent contractures of joints. Exercises should be done gently and with full range of motion. A small rolled pad can be placed in the palms to help maintain proper position of fingers; footboards or boots can be used to help prevent footdrop; and splinting may be needed to prevent severe contractures of wrist, knee, or ankle in decerebrate children.

Stimulation

Sensory stimulation is important in the care of the unconscious child, just as it is in the care of the alert child. For the temporarily unconscious or semiconscious child, sensory stimulation helps arouse the child to the conscious state and orient the child in terms of time and place. Auditory and tactile stimulation are especially valuable. Tactile stimulation is not appropriate for the child in whom it may elicit an undesirable response. However, for other children tactile contact often has a relaxing and calming effect. When the child's condition permits, holding or rocking has a soothing effect and provides the body contact needed by young children.

The auditory sense is often present in a state of coma. Hearing is the last sense to be lost and the first to be regained; therefore the child should be spoken to as any other child. Conversation around the child should not include thoughtless or derogatory remarks. A radio playing soft music, a music box, or a record player is frequently used to provide auditory stimulation. Singing the child's favorite songs or reading a favorite story is a tactic used to maintain the child's contact with a familiar world. Having parents tape songs or stories provides a continuous source of familiar stimulation. Above all it is important to remember that this is a child who has all the needs of any ill child.

Regaining consciousness. Awakening from a coma is a gradual process; however, sometimes children regain consciousness within a short time. Regaining orientation involves knowing person, place, and time, in that order.

Certain behaviors have been observed when children awaken from the unconscious state. The stress and anxiety they appear to feel in a strange and unfamiliar environment are consistently expressed in silent and withdrawn behavior. Children respond to basic questioning but usually do not display their prehospitalization personality and social behavior until they are transferred from the critical care area.

Family Support

Helping parents of an unconscious child cope with the situation is especially difficult. They may demonstrate all the guilt, fear, hostility, and anxiety of any parent of a seriously ill child (see Chapter 38). In addition, these parents are faced with the uncertain outcome of the cerebral dysfunction. The fear of death, mental retardation, or other permanent disability is present. Nursing intervention with parents depends on the nature of the pathologic condition, the personality of the parents, and the parent-child relationship before injury or illness.

The child may regain consciousness within a short time. If there is little or no residual effect, the child will be dismissed to home care fairly soon. The parents need the most intensive nursing intervention during the period of crisis and uncertainty. During the recovery phase they are given information, information is clarified, and they are encouraged to become involved in the child's care. Often the child's hospitalization is brief; however, some children require extended hospitalization for intensive therapy and rehabilitation.

The parents of children who die within hours or days require the support and guidance that the parents of any dying child would need in coping with the reality of the death and resolving their grief (see Chapter 38).

Probably the most difficult situations are those that involve children who are unconscious permanently or for an indefinite period. Unlike parents who lose a child through death, the finality is lacking for these parents; they are often left in a state of suspended grief. The presence of the child renders the parents unable to resolve the loss. Like parents of dying children, parents of the comatose child search for any signs of hope. Well-meaning friends and relatives relate instances of miraculous recoveries. The parents seek confirmation and support for such possibilities and assign erroneous meanings to any sign in the child, such as reflexive muscle contractions, that might be interpreted as evidence of recovery.

At these times nurses need to respond with compassion and gentle honesty. They can acknowledge that miraculous recoveries do occur, but they are rare. The important point is to maintain open communication with the family.

Like parents who lose a child through death, the parents of the child lost to their world attempt to reconstitute a representation of the child. They bring items that belong to the child, such as favorite toys, music, and other objects cherished by the child. This is interpreted as an attempt to provide stimulation for the child in the hope of eliciting a response, to let the hospital staff know the child as the unique individual he or she was so that the parents' distress can be better appreciated, and to reconstitute an image of the child "lost" to them and for whom they mourn. An awareness of these behaviors and coping mechanisms provides nurses with the understanding that helps them support the parents in their grief process.

Superimposed on the process of grieving for the "lost" child, parents may be faced with difficult decisions. When the child's brain is so severely damaged that vital functions must be maintained by artificial means, the parents must make the final decision to remove life-support systems. Since the decision is difficult for parents, the practitioner is frequently placed in a position of making the decision indirectly. After providing the parents with all the information, the practitioner will suggest that the child be removed from the life support to "see whether the child can make it without help." The approach relieves the parents of the decision and can be effective, but it is based on an evaluation of the parents' intellectual level and emotional state. Sometimes parents may even choose to refuse treatment if they believe it to be best for the child and the family (informed dissent). At other times parents request that "everything possible" be done for the child.

The nurses can be instrumental in providing guidance and clarifying information—a valued but demanding undertaking. It is not unusual for the family to ask the same questions and to compare responses elicited from different staff members. A child's death is an intensely personal issue that deserves direct involvement by the nurse and auxiliary support systems.

When the child has survived the illness or injury that produced the brain damage but is left unconscious permanently, the parents must decide whether to place the child in a chronic care facility or make arrangements to care for the child at home. The nurse can listen to the parents' discussions regarding alternatives, provide information where appropriate, and support the family in their decision. The nurse can help the family prepare for the transfer of the child and make referrals to persons or agencies that can provide additional assistance.

When the child has survived the cerebral insult and is not comatose, but physical and/or mental capacity is limited, either minimally or severely, families must cope with the long and tedious rehabilitation process and uncertain outcome. The drain on financial, emotional, and social resources can be enormous.

For parents who choose to care for their child at home, planning for home care begins early in the process of recovery. The family should become involved with the care of the child as soon as they indicate an interest and ability to do so. They need education and support in learning to care for the child, regular follow-up observation and assessment of the home management, and planning for some respite care of the child. Parents need to understand that it is important to plan for periodic relief from the continual care of the child (see Prepare for Discharge and Home Care, Chapter 41, and Home Care, Chapter 40).

Evaluation

The effectiveness of nursing interventions for the unconscious child is determined by continual reassessment and evaluation of care based on the following observational guidelines and expected outcomes:

1. Monitor child's neurologic signs, vital signs, and behavior.
2. Observe child's response to nursing activities, therapies, and diagnostic procedures; monitor ICP.
3. Observe child's color, position, and motor activity; measure fluid and nutritional intake and output.
4. Monitor status of child's respiratory, renal, and gastrointestinal systems and skin.

Nursing Care Plan

THE UNCONSCIOUS CHILD

Nursing Diagnosis: Risk for suffocation (aspiration) related to ineffective airway clearance secondary to depressed sensorium, impaired motor function

Expected Outcomes: Patent airway is maintained; no signs of cerebral hypoxia are present.

• NURSING INTERVENTIONS/*RATIONALES*

Position semiprone or side-lying with neck slightly extended, nose in "sniffing" position *to provide optimal ventilation and prevent aspiration.* **Avoid neck hyperextension, which can block airway.**

Insert oral airway if indicated *to promote ventilation.*

Remove pooled secretions promptly *to prevent aspiration.*

Have emergency equipment available for insertion of endotracheal tube or tracheostomy *to prevent delay in treatment response to blocked airway.*

Administer oxygen, hyperventilate as ordered *to increase oxygenation to tissues.*

Monitor vital signs, blood gases, and pH *for evidence of hypoxia.*

Nursing Diagnosis: Risk for infection (respiratory) related to coma, immobility, pooling or respiratory secretions

Expected Outcomes: Patient exhibits no evidence of infection; lungs are clear.

• NURSING INTERVENTIONS/*RATIONALES*

Place child in private room and screen all visitors and staff for signs of infection *to minimize exposure to infective organisms.*

Teach family about good hygiene and careful handwashing techniques *to prevent spread of infection.*

Observe careful asepsis in all procedures *to prevent spread of infection.*

Remove nasal and oral secretions as they form and provide good oral hygiene *to remove medium for growth of microorganisms.*

Monitor vital signs, auscultate lungs *to detect signs of infection.*

Nursing Diagnosis: Risk for injury related to depressed sensorium, intracranial abnormality

Expected Outcomes: Child exhibits no evidence of injury (i.e., no increased ICP, cerebral edema, seizure activity).

• NURSING INTERVENTIONS/*RATIONALES*

Elevate head of bed 15 to 30 degrees with child's head in midline position *to facilitate venous drainage and prevent jugular compression.*

Prevent constipation, excessive stimuli in environment, painful stimuli, vigorous suctioning, or percussing, *as these activities can lead to increased ICP and seizure activity.*

Use stool softeners as ordered; monitor bowel movements *to prevent constipation and Valsalva maneuver.*

Keep room darkened, quiet; play soothing background music; place earphones over child's ears; use touching and calm, soothing voice to talk with child when performing care *to reduce environmental stimuli.*

Use sedation as ordered *for episodes of agitation or restlessness.*

Observe child for signs of pain (i.e., agitation, increases in pulse, blood pressure) and medicate with analgesic or paralyzing agents as ordered *to reduce pain.*

Arrange painful procedures to occur after sedation or analgesic administration *to decrease chances of increasing ICP.*

Administer antiseizure medication as ordered *to prevent seizure activity.*

Monitor neurologic vital signs *to assess neurosensory status.*

Nursing Diagnosis: Ineffective thermoregulation related to intracranial abnormality, CNS dysfunction

Expected Outcome: Child maintains body temperature at normothermic levels.

• NURSING INTERVENTIONS/*RATIONALES*

Monitor and record body temperature frequently *to assess status of thermoregulatory system and effectiveness of interventions.*

Administer antipyretics as ordered *for fever.*

Remove blankets, administer tepid sponge bath, use hypothermia blankets *to reduce hyperthermia.*

Maintain adequate hydration *to reduce or prevent fever.*

Use blankets, bed warmers *to reduce hypothermia.*

Prevent shivering, *which can increase ICP and metabolic rate.*

Monitor blood urea nitrogen (BUN), pH, electrolyte, glucose levels, *as they may be affected by thermal instability.*

Nursing Diagnosis: Risk for disuse syndrome related to coma, prolonged immobility

Expected Outcomes: Child maintains full range of motion; muscle tone (no contractures, foot drop); skin integrity (no skin redness, irritation, breakdown, decubiti); normal patterns of elimination (no constipation, renal retention, renal calculi); normal circulatory function (no thrombus formation, venous stasis); adequate dietary intake (no weight loss, muscle wasting).

• NURSING INTERVENTIONS/*RATIONALES*

Turn and reposition every 2 hours *to promote circulation and prevent skin breakdown* (align properly, provide positional supports, use handrolls or splints *to position hands in functional position;* use footboard or hightop tennis shoes *to prevent foot drop*); perform passive range of motion frequently *to maintain full range in all joints and prevent contracture formation;* seat in chair *to improve circulation;* place on tilt table *to prevent loss of bone density to long bones.*

Use pressure reduction mattress overlay *to prevent pressure necrosis;* use foam pads on ankles, heels, elbows *to protect bony prominences;* massage skin with lotion regularly *to stimulate circulation and prevent friction and shearing effects;* keep bedclothes clean, dry, and wrinkle-free *to prevent skin irritation;*

Nursing Care Plan
UNCONSCIOUS CHILD—CONT'D

lubricate lips *to prevent drying and cracking;* lubricate eyes and keep them closed *to prevent drying and corneal irritation;* cleanse skin, mucous membranes of mouth and perianal area regularly *to prevent irritation and breakdown;* keep skin folds clean and dry *to prevent excoriation;* inspect skin, mucous membranes, corneas regularly *to assess for early signs of irritation or breakdown.*

Ensure adequate fluid intake, administer stool softeners *to maintain urinary output, prevent calculi, and aid bowel elimination;* monitor intake and output (I & O), hydration status, electrolytes, BUN, creatinine, urine characteristics *to assess for adequate hydration.*

Apply elastic stockings as indicated *to promote venous return, prevent stasis.*

Provide tube feedings that are adequate *to support the nutritional and metabolic needs of child (i.e., increased fiber, protein, vitamin C; decreased calcium);* monitor weight daily *to assess nutritional adequacy.*

Nursing Diagnosis: Altered family processes related to situational crises (child in coma)

Expected Outcomes: **Family exhibits adaptation of usual roles and functions to accommodate special needs of child; family exhibits growth-promoting behaviors.**

• **NURSING INTERVENTIONS/*RATIONALES***

Provide opportunity for family to absorb and adjust to diagnosis (i.e., repeat information *to allow time for family to hear and understand;* encourage expression of concerns, fears, and feelings about diagnosis and potential impact *to facilitate adjustment;* identify support systems *to provide resources for coping).*

Keep family informed of child's status, assist family to understand expected treatment, *to promote trust and provide a sound basis for decision making.*

Explore parents' reaction to the child, involve them in child's daily care routines, have them touch and hold child *to provide some measure of control.*

Have parents spend special time with siblings *so they don't feel neglected or left out.*

Identify additional resource systems (i.e., relatives, friends, church, health care services, community programs) and strategize with family about making good use of these systems *to develop broad base of support.*

Provide a system of ongoing follow-up observation and evaluation *to ensure long-term adaptation to challenges presented to family functioning by a child who is in a long-term comatose state.*

5. Observe family behaviors and interview members regarding their understandings and their feelings and concerns.

Expected outcomes:

See the Nursing Care Plan on pp. 1584-1585.

Cerebral Trauma

HEAD INJURY

Head injury is a pathologic process involving the scalp, skull, meninges, or brain as a result of mechanical force. According to national statistics and the Safe Kids Campaign,* injuries are the number one health risk for children and the leading cause of death in children older than 1 year of age. Yearly, one child in four in the United States will suffer an injury serious enough to require medical attention. Tragically, 8000 children are killed every year by injuries. It has been estimated that 300 per 100,000 children per year have a traumatic brain injury and that 10 per 100,000 children per year die as a result of the brain injury. Studies indicate that as many as three fourths of the childhood deaths caused by mechanical trauma are the direct result of a brain injury.

*SAFE KIDS, 111 Michigan Ave., N.W., Washington, DC 20010-2970; (202) 884-4993.

Etiology

The three major causes of brain damage in childhood in order of importance are falls, motor vehicle injuries, and bicycle injuries. Neurologic injury accounts for the highest mortality rate, with boys usually affected twice as often as girls. In motor vehicle accidents, children younger than 2 years of age are almost exclusively injured as passengers, whereas older children may also be injured as pedestrians or cyclists. The majority of deaths from brain trauma caused by bicycle injuries occur between the ages of 5 and 15 years. With the advent of bike helmet laws this should be a decreasing trend.

The exposed nature of the head renders it particularly vulnerable to external violence, and many of the physical characteristics of children predispose them to craniocerebral trauma. For example, infants may be left unattended on beds, in high chairs, and in other places from which they can fall. Because the head of an infant or toddler is proportionately large and heavy in relation to other body parts, it is the most likely to be injured. Incomplete motor development contributes to falls at young ages, and the natural curiosity and exuberance of children increase their risk of an injury.

Pathophysiology

The pathology of brain injury is directly related to the force of impact. Intracranial contents (brain, blood, CSF) are damaged because the force is too great to be absorbed by the skull and musculoligamentous support of the head. The elastic, pliable skulls of infants and young children absorb much of the direct energy of physical impact to the head and afford some protection to intracranial structures. Although nervous tissue is delicate, it usually requires a severe blow to cause significant damage.

A child's response to head injury is different from that of adults. The larger head size and insufficient musculoskeletal support render the very young child particularly vulnerable to acceleration-deceleration injuries. The surface area of the child's scalp is large with remarkable vascularity; therefore a child can bleed to death from a severe scalp laceration.

Primary head injuries are those that occur at a time of trauma; they include skull fracture, contusions, intracranial hematoma, and diffuse injury. Subsequent complications include hypoxic brain damage, ICP, infection, and cerebral edema. The predominant feature of a child's brain injury is the diffuse amount of swelling that occurs. Hypoxia and hypercapnia threaten the energy requirements of the brain and increase cerebral blood flow (CBF). The added volume across the blood-brain barrier plus the loss of autoregulation exacerbate cerebral edema. Pressure inside the skull greater than arterial pressure results in inadequate perfusion.

Cerebral hyperemia occurs more often in children, and this volume expansion may account for their tendency to develop intracranial hypertension (Ward, 1994). However, because the cranium of very young children has the ability to expand and the thin skull is more compliant, they may tolerate increases in ICP better than older children and adults. Children have a significantly higher percentage of good outcomes and a lower mortality rate, as well as a lower incidence of surgical mass lesions after severe head trauma. However, their thinner, softer brain may sustain greater long-term damage than previously suggested.

Physical forces act on the head through *acceleration, deceleration,* or *deformation.* Acceleration or deceleration is more descriptive of the circumstances responsible for most head injuries. When the stationary head receives a blow, the sudden acceleration causes deformation of the skull and mass movement of the brain. Continued movement of the intracranial contents allows the brain to strike parts of the skull (e.g., the sharp edges of the sphenoid or the irregular surface of the anterior fossa) or the edges of the tentorium.

Although the brain volume remains unchanged, significant distortion takes place as the brain changes shape in response to the force of impact to the skull. This movement can cause bruising at the point of impact (*coup*) and/or at a distance as the brain collides with the unyielding surfaces far removed from the point of impact (*contrecoup*) (Fig. 48-4). Thus a blow to the occipital region can cause severe injury to the frontal and temporal areas of the brain. Sudden deceleration, such as takes place during a fall, causes the greatest cerebral injury at the point of impact.

Children with an acceleration-deceleration injury demonstrate diffuse generalized cerebral swelling produced by increased blood volume or a redistribution of cerebral blood volume (cerebral hyperemia) rather than by increased water content (edema), as seen in adults.

Another effect of brain movement is shearing stresses, which may tear small arteries and cause subdural hemorrhages. Another source of damage occurs when severe compression of the skull causes the brain to be forced through the tentorial opening. This can produce irreparable damage to the brainstem (Figs. 48-5 and 48-6).

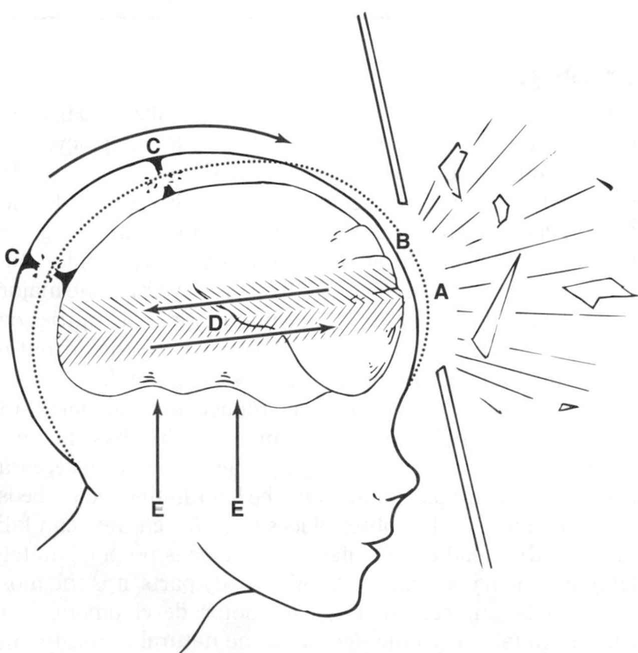

Fig. 48-4 Mechanical distortions of cranium during closed head injury. *A,* Preinjury contour of skull; *B,* immediate post-injury contour of skull; *C,* torn subdural vessels; *D,* shearing forces; *E,* trauma from contact with floor of cranium. (Redrawn from Grubb RL, Coxe WS: *Central nervous system trauma: cranial.* In Eliasson SG, Prensky AL, Hardin WB Jr, editors: *Neurological pathophysiology,* New York, 1974, Oxford University Press.)

Concussion. The most common head injury is **concussion,** a transient and reversible neuronal dysfunction, with instantaneous loss of awareness and responsiveness, that results from trauma to the head and persists for a relatively short time, usually minutes or hours. It is generally followed by amnesia for the moment of the injury and a variable period before the injury. The common misconception that loss of consciousness is the hallmark of concussion is not true, especially for children. Concussion is correctly defined as "a traumati-

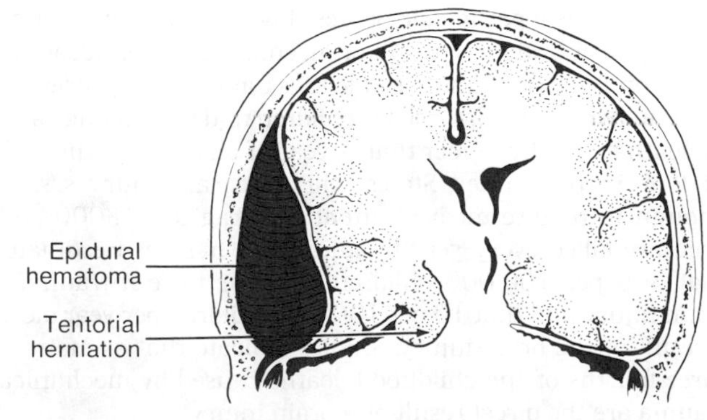

Fig. 48-5 Epidural (extradural) hematoma and compression of portion of temporal lobe through tentorial hiatus.

cally induced alteration in mental status." Confusion and amnesia after head impact are the hallmarks of concussion.

The pathogenesis of concussion is still unclear; it may be a result of shearing forces that cause stretching, compression, and tearing of nerve fibers, particularly in the area of the central brainstem, the seat of the reticular activating system. It has also been suggested that the anatomic alterations of nerve fibers cause the release of large quantities of acetylcholine into the CSF and a reduction in oxygen consumption with increased lactate production.

Contusion and laceration. The terms *contusion* and *laceration* are used to describe visible bruising and tearing of cerebral tissue. Contusions represent petechial hemorrhages along the superficial aspects of the brain at the site of impact (coup injury) and/or a lesion remote from the site of direct trauma (contrecoup injury). In serious accidents there may be multiple sites of injury.

The major areas of the brain susceptible to contusion or laceration are the occipital, frontal, and temporal lobes. The irregular surfaces of the anterior and middle fossae at the base of the skull are also capable of producing bruises or lacerations on forceful impact. Contusions may cause focal disturbances in strength, sensation, or visual awareness. The degree of brain damage in the contused areas varies according to the extent of vascular injury. Signs will vary from mild, transient weakness of a limb to prolonged unconsciousness and paralysis. However, the signs and symptoms may be clinically indistinguishable from those of concussion.

The lower incidence of cerebral contusion in infancy has been attributed to the infant's pliable skull, which has fewer convolutional markings of the inner space between brain tissue and bone. The infant's brain tissue also has a softer consistency, which also reduces surface injury. However, infants who are roughly shaken (shaken baby syndrome) can sustain profound neurologic impairment, seizures, retinal hemorrhages, and intracranial subarachnoid or subdural hemorrhages. In addition to these classic injuries, high cervical spinal cord hemorrhages and contusions can occur.

Cerebral lacerations are generally associated with penetrating or depressed skull fractures. However, they may occur without fracture in small children. When brain tissue is actually torn, with bleeding into and around the tear, usually more severe and prolonged unconsciousness and paralysis occur, leaving permanent scarring and some degree of disability.

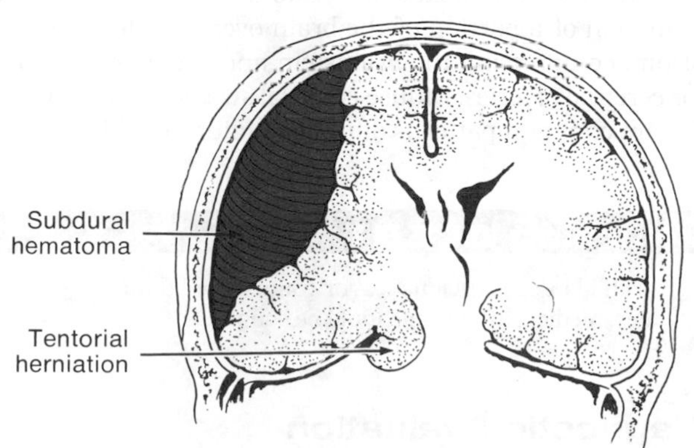

Fig. 48-6 Subdural hematoma.

Fractures. Because of its flexibility the immature skull is able to sustain a greater degree of deformation than the adult skull before it incurs a fracture. A great deal of force is required to produce a fracture in the skull of an infant. However, the undersurface of the skull contains grooves in which the meningeal arteries lie. A fracture that runs through one of these grooves may tear the artery and produce severe and damaging hemorrhage. Hypovolemic hypotension can occur in infants with skull fractures. A fracture may occur with little or no brain damage, or severe and fatal brain injury can take place without fracture.

The types of fractures that occur are as follows:

Linear fractures are those in which the lines of the fracture are predetermined by the site and velocity of the impact, as well as by the strength of the bone. These are uncommon before 2 to 3 years of age but constitute the majority of childhood skull fractures.

Depressed fractures are those in which the bone is locally broken, usually into several irregular fragments that are pushed inward, causing pressure on the brain. The inner portion of the bone is more extensively fragmented than the outer portion, which almost invariably produces tears in the dura. These are uncommon before 2 to 3 years of age. In infants and very young children the soft, malleable bone may become dented in a peculiar rounded or Ping-Pong ball depression, without laceration of either skin or dura.

Compound fractures consist of laceration of skin that extends to the site of the bony fracture, which can be linear, depressed, or comminuted.

Basilar fractures involve the basilar portion of the frontal, ethmoid, sphenoid, temporal, or occipital bones. Because of the proximity of the fracture line to structures surrounding the brainstem, this is a serious head injury.

Diastatic fractures are traumatic separations of cranial sutures. These most frequently affect the lambdoid suture and are rarely seen beyond the first 4 years of life. They require no specific treatment but should be observed for "growing fractures," development of fluid-filled cysts.

Complications

The major complications of trauma to the head are hemorrhage, infection, edema, and herniation through the tentorium. Infection is always a hazard in open injuries, and edema is related to tissue trauma. Vascular rupture may occur even in minor head injuries, causing hemorrhage between the skull and cerebral surfaces. Compression of the underlying brain produces effects that can be rapidly fatal or insidiously progressive.

Nursing ALERT

Posttraumatic meningitis should be suspected in children with increasing drowsiness and fever who also have basilar skull fractures.

Epidural hemorrhage. The blood accumulates between the dura and the skull to form a hematoma, which, because of the difficulty with which dura is stripped from bone, forces the underlying brain contents downward and inward as the brain expands (see Fig. 48-5). Since bleeding is generally arterial, brain compression occurs rapidly. Most often the expanding hematoma is located in the parietotemporal region, forcing the medial portion of the temporal lobe under the edge of the tentorium, where it causes pressure on nerves and blood vessels. The lower incidence of epidural hematoma in childhood has been attributed to the fact that the middle meningeal artery is not embedded in the bone surface of the skull until approximately 2 years of age. Therefore a fracture of the temporal bone is less likely to lacerate the artery. Second, the dura closely adheres to the inner table of the skull, especially at the level of the sutures, making separation from bleeding less likely.

However, a child's skull can be indented with sufficient force to tear the middle meningeal artery and the rebound intact without causing a fracture. Hemorrhage can also derive from dural veins or the dural sinuses, especially in infants and small children, in whom fracture is less likely to occur. In 20% to 40% of children a skull fracture is not detectable.

The classic clinical picture of epidural hemorrhage (momentary unconsciousness followed by a normal period, then lethargy or coma) is seldom evident in children (Box 48-4). The period of impaired consciousness is frequently lacking, and the symptom-free period is atypical because of nonspecific complaints such as irritability, headache, and vomiting. The symptom-free period frequently lasts longer than 48 hours. Clinically significant epidural hematomas are uncommon in children younger than 4 years of age. These differences may be caused by the decreased tendency of the resilient skull to fracture; the ability of blood to escape through widened sutures, an open fontanel, or a fracture; bleeding from smaller vessels with less rapid and massive bleeding; lower systolic blood pressure in children; and possibly decreased susceptibility of the child's brain to pressure changes.

BOX 48-4

Clinical Manifestations of Acute Head Injury

Minor injury

May or may not lose consciousness
Transient period of confusion
Somnolence
Listlessness
Irritability
Pallor
Vomiting (one or more episodes)

Signs of progression

Altered mental status (e.g., difficulty in rousing child)
Mounting agitation
Development of focal lateral neurologic signs
Marked changes in vital signs

Severe injury

Signs of increased ICP (Box 48-1)
- Increased head size (infant)
- Bulging fontanel (infant)

Retinal hemorrhage
Extraocular palsies (especially cranial nerve VI)
Hemiparesis
Quadriplegia
Elevated temperature (sometimes)
Unsteady gait (older child)
Papilledema (older child)

Associated signs

Skin injury (to area of head sustaining injury)
Other injuries (e.g., to extremities)

Subdural hemorrhage. A subdural hemorrhage is bleeding between the dura and the cerebrum, usually as a result of rupture of cortical veins that bridge the subdural space (Fig. 48-6).

Subdural hematomas are 10 times more common than epidural hematomas, occurring most often in infancy, with a peak incidence at 6 months.

Unlike epidural hemorrhage, which develops inwardly against the less resistant brain tissue, subdural hemorrhage tends to develop more slowly and spreads thinly and widely until it is limited by the dural barriers—the falx and tentorium. Subdural hematoma is fairly common in infants, frequently as a result of birth trauma, falls, assaults, or violent shaking. The small subdural space and dura firmly attached to the skull in this area are highly vulnerable to increased ICP.

Nursing ALERT

Children with a subdural hematoma and retinal hemorrhages should be evaluated for the possibility of child abuse, especially shaken baby syndrome (SBS).

Repeated subdural taps often provide relief in the infant, as revealed by follow-up CT scans, improved neurologic status, and a flat anterior fontanel. Surgical evacuation of the hematoma is the treatment of choice in the older child and is frequently required in infants.

Cerebral edema. Some degree of brain edema is expected, especially 24 to 72 hours after craniocerebral trauma. Cerebral edema caused by direct cellular injury or vascular injury induces vascular stasis, anoxia, and further vasodilation. If the progression continues unchecked, ICP exceeds arterial pressure and fatal anoxia ensues, and/or the pressure causes herniation of a portion of the brain over the edge of the tentorium, compressing the brainstem and occluding the posterior cerebral arteries. Diffuse cerebral swelling and changes in CBF are common patterns after head injury in children.

Nursing ALERT

If a child loses consciousness or vomits more than three times, medical attention should be sought.

Diagnostic Evaluation

A detailed history, especially a health history, both past and present, is essential in evaluating the child with craniocerebral trauma. Certain disorders, such as drug allergies, hemophilia, diabetes mellitus, or epilepsy, may produce similar symptoms. Furthermore, even minor traumatic injury can aggravate a preexisting disease process. Events surrounding the injury often supply significant data. It must be determined whether the infant or child exhibited alterations in consciousness, and any other signs and behaviors exhibited by the child must be noted. Since head injuries are frequently accompanied by injuries in other areas, the examination is performed with care to prevent further damage.

Nursing ALERT

Stabilize a child's spine after head injury until a spinal cord injury is confirmed or ruled out.

Initial assessment. Priorities in the initial phase in the care of a child with a head injury include assessment of the ABCs (airway, breathing, circulation); evaluation for shock; a neurologic examination, especially LOC; pupillary symmetry and response to light; and seizures. The assessment is carried out quickly in relation to vital signs (see the Emergency box at right). Excited and irritable children may have a rapid pulse, hyperventilate, appear pale, and feel clammy shortly after an injury.

Nursing ALERT

Deep, rapid, periodic, or intermittent and gasping respirations; wide fluctuations or noticeable slowing of the pulse; and widening pulse pressure or extreme fluctuations in blood pressure are signs of brainstem involvement. It is important to note that marked hypotension may represent internal injuries.

Ocular signs such as fixed and dilated pupils, fixed and constricted pupils, and pupils that are poorly reactive or unreactive to light and accommodation indicate increased ICP or brainstem involvement. It is important to remain with the child who demonstrates fixed and dilated pupils, since these are ominous signs, with the probability of respiratory arrest. Dilated, nonpulsating blood vessels indicate increased ICP before the appearance of papilledema. Retinal hemorrhages are seen in acute head injuries.

Nursing ALERT

Observation of asymmetric pupils or one dilated, unreactive pupil in a comatose child is a neurosurgical emergency that may require evacuation of an epidural hematoma.

Less urgent but important additional assessments include examination of the scalp for lacerations and palpation for other abnormalities. However, a significant amount of blood loss can occur from scalp lacerations.

EMERGENCY

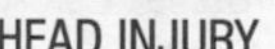

HEAD INJURY

Assess child:
- A—airway
- B—bleeding
- C—circulation
- Stabilize neck and spine

Clean any abrasions with soap and water.
- Apply clean dressing.
- If bleeding, apply ice for 1 hour to relieve pain and swelling.

Give only clear liquids until no vomiting for at least 6 hours.

Assess pain.

Check pupil reaction every 4 hours (including twice during night) for 48 hours.

Awaken two times during night to check level of consciousness.

Seek medical attention if there is any of the following:
- Injury sustained
  - —at high speed (e.g., auto)
  - —fall from a significant distance (e.g., roof, tree)
  - —from great force (e.g., baseball bat)
  - —under suspicious circumstances
- Child younger than 6 months of age
- Unconscious more than 5 seconds
- Discomfort (crying) more than 10 minutes after injury
- Headache that is severe, worsening, interferes with sleep
- Vomiting three or more times
- Swelling in front of or above earlobe or swelling that increases in size
- Confused or not behaving normally
- Difficult to rouse from sleep
- Difficulty with speaking
- Blurring of vision or seeing double
- Unsteady gait
- Difficulty using upper extremities
- Neck pain
- Pupils dilated or fixed
- Infant with bulging fontanel

Nursing ALERT

Bleeding from the nose or ears necessitates further evaluation, and a watery discharge from the nose (rhinorrhea) that is a positive finding of glucose (as tested with Dextrostix) suggests leaking of CSF from a skull fracture.

An accurate assessment of clinical signs provides baseline information (Box 48-4). Serial evaluations, preferably by a single observer, help detect changes in the neurologic status. Alterations in mental status, evidenced by increased difficulty in rousing the child, mounting agitation, development of focal lateral neurologic signs, or marked changes in vital signs, usually indicate extension or progression of the basic pathologic process.

Special tests. After a thorough clinical examination a variety of diagnostic tests are helpful in providing a more definitive diagnosis of the type and extent of the trauma. The severity of a head injury may not be apparent on clinical examination of a child, but it will be detectable on a CT scan. Whenever the child has a history consistent with a serious head injury (unrestrained occupant in a severe motor vehicle accident or a fall from a significant height), it is important that a scan be performed even if the child initially appears alert and oriented. All children with head injuries who have any alteration of consciousness, headache, vomiting, skull fracture, seizure, or a predisposing medical condition should also undergo CT scanning.

MRI and neurobehavioral assessment after early head injury may be useful in documenting cognitive impairment in relation to structural alterations in the young brain. MRI provides details of soft tissues better than any other noninvasive technique. Electroencephalography is not particularly helpful for early diagnosis but is useful for definition of seizure activity or focal destructive lesions after the acute phase of illness. Lumbar puncture is rarely used in craniocerebral trauma and is contraindicated in the presence of increased ICP. In some centers monitoring ICP is part of the assessment.

Posttraumatic syndromes. Posttraumatic syndromes can be clinically manifested because of structural complications resulting from a head injury and through the signs and symptoms demonstrated by the child. Structural complications can include hydrocephalus and focal deficits such as optic atrophy, cranial nerve palsies, motor deficits, diabetes insipidus, aphasia, and seizures. Behavioral disturbances include sleep disturbances, phobias, emotional lability, altered school performance, and changes related to aggressiveness or withdrawal. *Postconcussion syndrome* is a common sequela to brain injury and occurs within minutes to an hour after a minimum head injury. The manifestations vary with the age of the child. The syndrome occurs very frequently in children under 1 year of age. In adolescents it is similar to that in adults. The duration of manifestations can vary from several days to several months. Death from concussion is preventable unless overwhelming secondary brain injury has occurred (Bruce, 1993).

Posttraumatic seizures occur in a number of children who survive a head injury. The onset may be in the first 24 hours, usually within the first year, and in most cases within 2 years of the injury. *Structural complications* may occur, and the type of residual effect depends on the location and nature of the trauma. True mental retardation occurs only after severe injuries.

Therapeutic Management

The majority of children with mild to moderate concussion who have not lost consciousness can be cared for and observed at home after careful examination reveals no serious intracranial injury. Nurses should provide parents with clear explanations and instructions and should encourage them to ask questions both before and after leaving the medical facility if clarification is needed (see the Family Focus box above). The parents are instructed to check the child every 2 hours to determine any changes in responsiveness. The sleeping child should be wakened to see whether he or she can be roused normally. Parents are advised to maintain contact with the health professional, who usually wishes to examine the child again in 1 or 2 days. The manifestations of epidural hematoma in children do not generally appear until 24 hours or more after injury.

Family Focus

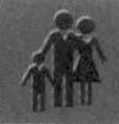

MAINTAINING CONTACT

Maintaining contact with parents for continued observation and reevaluation of the child, when indicated, facilitates early diagnosis and treatment of possible complications from head injury, such as hematoma, hydrocephalus, cysts, and posttraumatic seizures. Children are generally hospitalized for 24 to 48 hours' observation if their family lives far from medical facilities or lacks transportation or a telephone that would provide access to immediate help. Other circumstances, such as language or other communication barriers, or even emotional trauma, may hinder learning and make it difficult for families to feel confident in caring for their child at home.

Children with severe injuries, those who have lost consciousness for more than a few minutes, and those with prolonged and continued seizures or other focal or diffuse neurologic signs must be hospitalized until their condition is stable and their neurologic signs have diminished.

The child is maintained on nothing by mouth or restricted to clear liquids, if able to take fluids by mouth, until it is determined that vomiting will not occur. Intravenous fluids are indicated in the child who is comatose or displays dulled sensorium and/or in the child with persistent vomiting. Fluid balance is closely monitored by daily weights, accurate intake and output measurements, and serum osmolality to detect early signs of water retention, excessive dehydration, and states of hypertonicity or hypotonicity.

The volume of intravenous fluid is carefully monitored to prevent aggravating any cerebral edema and to minimize the possibility of overhydration in case of SIADH. However, damage to the hypothalamus or pituitary gland may produce diabetes insipidus with its accompanying hypertonicity and dehydration.

Restlessness can be satisfactorily managed, if necessary, with mild sedation, and headache is usually controlled with acetaminophen (Tylenol). Antiepileptics are used for seizure control and frequently in cases of suspected contusion or laceration. Antibiotics may be administered if there are lacerations, CSF leakage, or excessive cerebral tissue damage. Prophylactic tetanus toxoid is given as appropriate. Cerebral edema is managed as described for the unconscious child. Hyperthermia is controlled with tepid sponges or a hypothermia blanket.

Surgical therapy. Scalp lacerations are sutured or stapled after the underlying bone is carefully examined (see the Atraumatic Care box on p. 1591). Depressed fractures require surgical reduction and removal of bone fragments. Torn dura is sutured. "Ping-Pong ball" skull fractures in very young infants ordinarily correct themselves within a few weeks and do not require specific treatment, although they can be reduced by pressure against the bone.

Prognosis. The outcome of craniocerebral trauma depends on the extent of injury and complications. However, the out-

Atraumatic Care 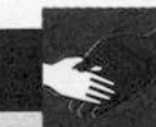

NONINVASIVE LOCAL ANESTHESIA

The use of topical lidocaine, adrenalin, and tetracaine (LAT) adrenaline and cocaine (TC), or TC with tetracaine (TAC) provides noninvasive anesthesia for suturing of lacerations (Bonadio and Wagner, 1992; Ernst and others, 1995).

look is generally more favorable for children than for adults. Over 90% of children with concussions or simple linear fractures recover without symptoms after the initial period. The incidence of fatalities and neurologic sequelae is lower in children, even in those with severe head injuries. The prognosis for recovery is primarily related to the duration of coma and the degree of injury. The combination of impaired consciousness and skull fracture carries the highest risk of complication.

The concern regarding outcome is increasingly focused on potential cognitive, emotional, and/or mental problems. Recent studies indicate that children experience a higher frequency of psychologic disturbances after head injury than adults, who are more prone to complaints of a physical nature.

Children may be more vulnerable than adults to long-term cognitive and behavioral dysfunction after diffuse brain injury. Even with recovery the effects of brain injury on a child's potential can never be known.

True coma (not obeying commands, eyes closed, and not speaking) usually does not last more than 2 weeks. A child's eventual outcome can range from brain death to a persistent vegetative state to complete recovery. However, even the best recovery may be associated with personality changes, including mood lability and loss of confidence, impaired short-term memory, headaches, and subtle cognitive impairments. Many children are left with significant disabilities after head injury that appear months later as learning difficulties, behavioral changes, or emotional disturbances (Reynolds, 1992). Generally within 6 months to 1 year after the injury, 90% of the long-term neurologic outcome has been achieved.

Nursing Care Management

The hospitalized child requires careful neurologic assessment and evaluation (including vital signs) repeated at frequent intervals to provide information needed to establish a correct diagnosis, to reveal signs and symptoms of increased ICP, to determine clinical management, to prevent many complications, and to provide support to the child and family during the recovery phases.

The child is placed on bed rest, usually with the head of the bed elevated slightly, and appropriate safety measures, such as siderails kept up for older children and seizure precautions for children of all ages, are implemented. For the extremely restless child, hard surfaces may have to be padded and restraint used to prevent the possibility of further injury. Care is individualized according to the specific needs of the child. The unconscious child is managed as described in the previous section, but most childhood head injuries are those causing momentary stunning or temporary unconsciousness. Children may be restless and irritable, but more often their reaction is to fall asleep when left undisturbed. A quiet environment helps reduce the restlessness and irritability. Shining bright lights directly into the child's face is irritating and often makes checking the ocular responses more difficult to perform and more aggravating to the child.

Frequent examinations of vital signs, neurologic signs, and LOC are extremely important nursing observations. When possible they should be performed by a single observer to ensure better detection of subtle changes that may indicate worsening of neurologic status. Pupils are checked for size, equality, reaction to light, and accommodation. After the initial elevations usually seen after injury, the vital signs generally return to normal unless there is brainstem involvement. An axillary measurement of temperature is the safest method, since seizures are not uncommon and vomiting is a frequent response in children, especially when they are disturbed.

The most important nursing observation is assessment of the child's LOC. Alterations in consciousness appear earlier in the progression of an injury than alterations of vital signs or focal neurologic signs. Some expected responses may be misinterpreted as deviations from the normal. Frequent examinations of alertness are fatiguing to the child; therefore the child often desires to fall asleep, and that desire may be confused with depressed consciousness. When left alone, the child promptly dozes. It is not uncommon to observe ocular divergence through the partially closed eyelids.

A key nursing role is to provide sedation and analgesia for the child. The conflict between the need to promote comfort and relieve anxiety in the child versus the need to be able to assess for neurologic changes presents a dilemma. However, both goals can be achieved with close observation of the child's LOC and response to analgesics, using a pain assessment record, and effective communication with the practitioner. To differentiate between sedation from an opioid and that from the injury, naloxone (Narcan) can be given slowly to reverse the opioid's sedative effect. Decreasing restlessness after administration of an analgesic most likely reflects pain control rather than a decreasing LOC.

Observations of position and movement provide additional information. Any abnormal posturing is noted, as well as whether or not it occurs continuously or intermittently. Are the child's handgrips strong and equal in strength? Are there any signs of decerebrate or decorticate posturing? What is the child's response to stimulation? Is movement purposeful, random, or absent? Are movement and/or sensation equal on both sides or restricted to one side only?

The child may complain of headache or other discomfort. The child who is too young to describe a headache will be fussy and resist being handled. The child who suffers from vertigo will often assume a position and vigorously resist efforts to be moved. Forcible movement causes the child to vomit and display spontaneous nystagmus. Seizures, relatively common in children with craniocerebral trauma, may be of any type but are more often generalized, regardless of the type of injury. Any seizure activity should be carefully observed and described in detail. Children in postictal (postseizure) states are more lethargic, with sluggish pupils.

Drainage from any orifice is noted. Bleeding from the ear suggests the possibility of a basal skull fracture. The amount and characteristics of the drainage are observed, and since the auditory canal may be a source of infection, dry, sterile cotton can be placed loosely at the orifice and changed when soiled.

Nursing ALERT

Suctioning through the nares or passing a nasogastric tube is contraindicated because of the high risk of secondary infection and the probability of the catheter entering the brain substance through the fracture.

Head trauma is frequently accompanied by other undetected injuries; therefore any bruises, lacerations, or evidence of internal injuries or fractures of the extremities is noted and reported. Associated injuries are evaluated and treated appropriately.

The child with normal LOC is usually allowed clear liquids unless fluid is restricted. If the child has an intravenous infusion, it is maintained as prescribed. The diet is advanced to that appropriate for the child's age as soon as the condition permits. Intake and output are measured and recorded, and any incontinence of bowel or bladder is noted in the child who has been toilet-trained.

The child should be observed for any unusual behavior, but behavior should be interpreted in relation to the child's normal behavior. For example, urinary incontinence during sleep would be of no consequence in a child who routinely wets the bed but would be highly significant for one who is always dry. In addition, a child who is subject to nightmares might cry out and demonstrate agitated behavior at night. Parents are valuable resources. Information obtained from parents at or shortly after admission is helpful in evaluating the child's behavior, for example, the ease with which the child is roused normally, the usual sleeping position, how much the child sleeps during the day, motor activity the child is capable of (rolling over, sitting up, climbing), hearing and visual acuity, appetite, and manner of eating (spoon, bottle, cup). There would be less concern about a child who falls asleep several times during the day if this particular type of behavior is consistent with the child's usual behavior.

Family support. The emotional and educational support of the family of children who have suffered head injury presents a formidable, challenging aspect to nursing care. Witnessing the parents' ordeal of grief and helplessness on seeing their child in an intensive care unit connected to monitoring equipment in an altered state evokes empathy. The nurse can encourage the family to be involved in the child's care, to bring in familiar belongings, or to make a tape recording of familiar voices and sounds. Parents may need a demonstration on how to touch or cuddle their child and may want to talk about their grief. The nurse can listen attentively, reinforce what is being done to assist the child, and direct parents toward signs and symptoms of recovery to instill hope without promises. A common phenomenon is for families to seek information from all health care providers, asking, "What will be? What do you know?" as they search for some clue that the child is recovering. Honesty and kindness, along with competent care, distinguish excellent nursing abilities.

When the child is discharged, the parents are advised of probable posttraumatic symptoms that may be expected, such as behavioral changes, sleep disturbances, phobias, and seizures. They should understand observations that should be made and the way to contact the physician, nurse, or health facility in case any unusual signs or symptoms develop. The importance of follow-up evaluation should be emphasized. It is often advisable to refer the family to a public health agency for home follow-through to be certain that the child receives posthospital evaluation.

Rehabilitation. The rehabilitation and management of the child with permanent brain injury are essential aspects of care. Rehabilitation of brain-injured children is begun as soon as feasible and usually involves the family and a rehabilitation team. Careful assessment of the child's capabilities, limitations, and probable potential is made as early as possible and appropriate interventions are implemented to maximize the residual capacities. The National Head Injury Foundation* "arose from the mutual frustration and sense of hopelessness experienced by families in their search for appropriate facilities and support to return head-injured loved ones to their maximum functioning potential." It provides information and listings of rehabilitation services and support groups throughout the country.

Pediatric trauma rehabilitation is a national concern. Coordinating care and services for early rehabilitation involves identifying the child and family's response to the traumatic injury and disability, securing available resources, and recognizing the parental role in the process.

The child with a disability resulting from head trauma requires assessment on the physical, cognitive, emotional, and social levels. The child has experienced separation, pain, sensory deprivation, and overload; changes in circadian cycle; and fear of the unknown. Recovery and transition require new coping strategies at the same time that regressive and acting-out behavior may start. Parents and children need honest communication for decision making. Rehabilitation is advocated when the child is making progress beyond what can be provided in a hospital setting. The Rancho Los Amigos Scale provides a systematic assessment of the progress a child with a severe head injury may achieve.

Prevention. Tremendous strides have been taken in the prevention of cerebral damage after head injury in children. New developments requiring research point to the prevention of cellular injury or the primary insult. However, the greatest benefit lies in prevention of head injuries. Nurses can exert a valuable influence on behalf of children through education. The reason injuries remain preventable is that unnecessary risks are unchecked. Inadequate supervision combined with a child's natural sense of indestructibility and exploration can lead to lethal results. Nurses are in the unique position of influencing caregivers in terms of growth and development. Banning the use of infant walkers is an example. This equipment does not help develop motor skills but places infants at risk for head and neck injuries from falls, especially down steps. Public education, coupled with legislative support, can prevent childhood injuries.

*1140 Connecticut Ave., N.W., Suite 812, Washington, DC 20036; (202) 296-6443 or (800) 444-6443 (Family Helpline).

For extensive discussions of childhood injuries, see the discussions on injury prevention in Chapters 33, 34, 35, 36, and 37; see also Childhood Mortality, Chapter 27; and the Nursing Care Plan: The Child with a Head Injury*).

NEAR-DROWNING

Drowning ranks second as a cause of accidental death in children. Most cases of drowning are accidental, usually involving children who are helpless in water, such as inadequately attended children in or near swimming pools or infants in bathtubs; small children who fall into ponds, streams, and flooded excavations, usually near home; occupants of pleasure boats who fail to wear life preservers; children who have diving accidents; and children who are able to swim but overestimate their endurance. Accidental drowning occurs five times more often in boys than in girls, 50% of children are under the age of 4, and 90% drown in private swimming pools (Kyriacou, Arcinve, and Peek, 1994).

Drowning can take place in any body of water, including such unlikely places as a pail of water. Top-heavy toddlers fall head first into a pail of water, their arms become trapped, and they are unable to free themselves. Hot tubs and whirlpool spas have been implicated in childhood drowning injury. The suction created at the outlet is strong enough to trap even larger children underwater. Drowning as a form of fatal child abuse has also been recognized as a problem. Homicidal drownings are not witnessed, they usually occur in the home, and the victims are either infants or toddlers. However, with expeditious treatment many children can be and are being saved. For purposes of this discussion, two terms need clarification:

Drowning—death from asphyxia while submerged, regardless of whether fluid has entered the lungs

Near-drowning—survival at least 24 hours after submersion in a fluid medium

Pathophysiology

The major pulmonary changes that occur in drowning are directly related to the length of submersion (regardless of the type and amount of fluid aspirated), the physiologic response of the victim, and the development and degree of immersion hypothermia. In addition, cerebral recovery depends on the effectiveness of initial resuscitation and subsequent critical care measures to support cerebral salvage.

Physiologic factors that influence the extent of damage from immersion include resistance to asphyxia and anoxia, which shows some individual variation. There is greater resistance with diminishing age; young children can withstand longer periods of submersion. More important is the drowning, or diving, reflex. This neurologic response is triggered by immersion of the face in cold water. Blood is shunted away from the periphery, and the flow is concentrated to the brain and heart predominantly.

The problems created by near-drowning are (1) hypoxia and asphyxiation, (2) aspiration, and (3) hypothermia (except near-drowning in hot tubs). Cardiopulmonary arrest is secondary to asphyxia.

Hypoxia is the primary problem because it results in global cell damage, and different cells tolerate variable lengths of anoxia. Neurons, especially cerebral cells, sustain irreversible damage after 4 to 6 minutes of submersion. The heart and lungs can survive up to 30 minutes. Regardless of the amount of water aspirated, arterial hypoxemia (resulting from atelectasis with shunting of blood through the nonventilated alveoli) and a combined respiratory acidosis (resulting from retained carbon dioxide) and metabolic acidosis (caused by buildup of acid metabolites caused by anaerobic metabolism) occur. The pathologic events are directly related to the duration of submersion. The major difficulty is acute ventilatory insufficiency. Approximately 10% of drowning victims die without aspirating fluid but succumb from acute asphyxia as a result of prolonged reflex laryngospasm.

Aspiration of fluid occurs in the majority of drownings. The aspirated fluid causes pulmonary edema, atelectasis, airway spasm, and pneumonitis, all of which aggravate the hypoxia. It was previously thought that submersion in salt water or fresh water altered the physiologic response to near-drowning. However, there is no clinically significant difference in the response of human survivors, and the submersion does not alter the therapy or outcome.

Hypothermia occurs rapidly in infants and children partly because of their large surface area relative to body mass and partly as a result of the cold water itself. Water is an excellent heat conductor, and the contact with the skin is increased by struggling. Hypothermia may make resumption or maintenance of cardiac function possible if body temperature is less than 30° C (86° F). Profound hypothermia is usually evidence of lengthy submersion.

Therapeutic Management

Resuscitative measures should begin at the scene of a drowning, and the victim should be transported to the hospital with maximum ventilatory and circulatory support. Many victims need care for some time after aspiration of fluid. In the hospital, intensive pulmonary care is implemented and continued according to the needs of the patient.

In general the management of the near-drowning victim is based on the degree of cerebral insult (Box 48-5). The first priority is to restore oxygen delivery to the cells and prevent further hypoxic damage. A spontaneously breathing child will do well in an oxygen-enriched atmosphere; the more severely affected child will require endotracheal intubation and mechanical ventilation. Blood gases and pH are monitored frequently as a guide to oxygen, fluid, and electrolyte therapies.

Nursing ALERT

All children who experience near-drowning should be admitted to the hospital for observation. Complications of respiratory distress and cerebral edema may occur 24 hours after the incident.

Aspiration pneumonia is a frequent complication that occurs about 48 to 72 hours after the episode. Bronchospasm, alveolar-capillary membrane damage, atelectasis, abscess formation, and hyaline membrane disease are other complications that occur after aspiration of fluid.

*In Wong DL: *Wong and Whaley's clinical manual of pediatric nursing*, ed 4, St Louis, 1996, Mosby.

BOX 48-5
Clinical Manifestations of Near-Drowning

Directly related to the degree of consciousness following rescue and resuscitation:

Category A: Awake (minimum injury)
- Fully conscious
- May have mild hypothermia
- Mild chest radiographic changes
- Mild arterial blood gas abnormalities

Category B: Blunted sensorium (moderate injury)
- Obtunded
- Stuporous
- Purposeful response to painful stimuli
- Mild to moderate hypothermia
- Respiratory distress (frequently)
- Chest radiographs abnormal
- Arterial blood gas abnormalities

Category C: Comatose (severe anoxia)
- Patient unarousable
- Abnormal response to pain
- Abnormal respiratory pattern
- Seizures
- Shock
- Marked arterial blood gas abnormalities
- Abnormal chest radiographs
- Dysrhythmias
- Metabolic acidosis
- Hyperkalemia, hyperglycemia
- Disseminated intravascular coagulation

Also:
- **C1:** Decorticate, Cheyne-Stokes respirations
- **C2:** Decerebrate, central hyperventilation
- **C3:** Flaccid, apneustic or cluster breathing
- **C4:** Flaccid, apneic, no detectable circulation

Prognosis. Studies report that the best predictors of a good outcome were length of submersion in nonicy water (>5° C [41° F]) for less than 5 minutes and the presence of sinus rhythm, reactive pupils, and neurologic responsiveness at the scene. The worst prognoses—for death or severe neurologic impairment—were in children submerged for more than 10 minutes and not responding to advanced life support within 25 minutes. All children without spontaneous, purposeful movement and normal brainstem function 24 hours after near-drowning suffered severe neurologic deficits or death (Bratton, Jardine, and Morray, 1994).

Nursing Care Management

Nursing care depends on the condition of the child. A child who survives may need intensive respiratory nursing care with attention to vital signs, mechanical ventilation and/or tracheostomy, blood gas determination, chest therapy, and intravenous infusion. Frequently the child is comatose for an indefinite period and requires the same care as an unconscious child.

A difficult aspect of the care of the child victim of near-drowning is helping the parents cope with severe guilt reactions. The magnitude of the event is so great that efforts to provide comfort and support have only limited success. Parents need to hear that everything possible is being done to treat the child, and this message needs to be repeated often.

The parents of the child who is saved from death are also faced with the anxiety of not knowing what the outcome will be, and sometimes they wish for the death of the child. Because their situation generates such intense feelings of loneliness, it is important for families to know that they are not alone. They need to be reminded frequently that there are caring people to assist them both during the crisis and later. Additional sources of support that can be recommended are psychiatric and social work consultants, community services, and religious support. Self-help groups are excellent if these are available in the community.

Nurses often have difficulty relating to the parents if obvious neglect has precipitated the accident and subsequent problems; therefore it is important for those who care for these children and their families to assess their own feelings about the situation, as well as the coping abilities and resources of the family. Caring for near-drowning victims and their families requires nurses to be sensitive to the needs of the child and the family and to recognize their own reactions and emotions.

Prevention. Most drownings, particularly of infants or small children, can be prevented with adequate supervision. Water safety and survival training should be required for all school-age children, and nurses can be active advocates in their communities. Nurses are also in a position to emphasize the importance of adequate adult supervision when children are in the water. Young children should never be left unattended when in or near the water. Parents with pools and hot tubs should know cardiopulmonary resuscitation (CPR) techniques.* See also Injury Prevention, Chapters 33, 34, 35, 36, and 37.

Central Nervous System Tumors

Two major forms of childhood cancer—brain tumors and neuroblastomas—are derived from neural tissue. Both of these tumors have proved difficult to treat and have not demonstrated the dramatic improvements in survival rate seen in many other forms of childhood cancer. Neuroblastomas, tumors that usually arise in the autonomic nervous system or adrenal medulla, are not cerebral tumors but are discussed here for convenience.

BRAIN TUMORS

Brain tumors are the most common solid tumors that occur in children and are second only to leukemia as a form of cancer. They may be benign or malignant. The majority of tumors (about 60%) are **infratentorial** (below the tentorium cerebelli). They occur in the posterior third of the brain, primarily in the cerebellum or brainstem. This anatomic distribution accounts for the frequency of symptoms resulting from in-

*Home care instructions for CPR are in Wong DL: *Wong and Whaley's clinical manual of pediatric nursing*, ed 4, St Louis, 1996, Mosby.

creased ICP. A smaller number are **supratentorial**, or within the anterior two thirds of the brain, mainly the cerebrum.

Neoplasms can arise from any cell within the cranium, and the type of cell in which the tumor has its origin provides a histologic classification for major tumors. The major infratentorial tumors of childhood are medulloblastoma, cerebellar astrocytoma, brainstem glioma, and ependymomas. Gliomas, arising from glial cells (the supporting structures of the brain), are the most common brain tumors in children. Astrocytoma, the most common glial tumor, arises from astrocytes, cells that form most of the supportive tissues for the neurons.

Diagnostic Evaluation

The signs and symptoms of brain tumors are those of increased ICP and are directly related to their anatomic location and size and to some extent the age of the child. In infants, whose cranial sutures are still open, virtually no early detectable symptoms develop. It is not until spinal fluid obstruction causes markedly increased head size that a lesion may be suspected. Even in older children, clinical manifestations are nonspecific. However, the most common symptoms are headache, especially on awakening, and vomiting that is not related to feeding. The common clinical manifestations of brain tumors are presented in Box 48-6.

Diagnosis of a brain tumor is based subjectively on presenting clinical signs (Box 48-6) and objectively on results of neurologic tests. Because the signs and symptoms are vague and easily overlooked, early diagnosis necessitates suspicion during history taking. A number of tests may be used in the neurologic evaluation, but the most common diagnostic procedure is MRI, which determines the location and extent of the tumor. Other tests that may be used include CT, angiography, electroencephalography, and lumbar puncture, although lumbar puncture is dangerous in the presence of increased ICP because of the possibility of brain stem herniation after a sudden release of pressure.

Therapeutic Management

Treatment may involve the use of surgery, radiotherapy, and chemotherapy. All three may or may not be used, depending on the type of tumor. The treatment of choice is total removal of the tumor without residual neurologic damage. Patients with the most complete tumor removal have the greatest chance of survival. Radiotherapy is used to treat most tumors and to shrink the size of the tumor before attempting surgical removal. Chemotherapy is being used with increased frequency and is helpful in delaying the timing of radiation (Duffner et al, 1993).

Prognosis. The prognosis for the child with a brain tumor depends on the type of brain tumor, the size of the tumor, the extent of the disease, and the age of the child. Problems associated with treatment and relatively poor prognosis, primarily in infants and young children, are compounded by serious late effects of therapy (Duffner and Cohen, 1991). A decline in incidence of children with medulloblastoma has been significantly linked with a protective effect of maternal folate, iron, and multivitamin supplementation. The introduction of periconceptional multivitamin supplementation in the 1980s may have caused this significant decline of medulloblastoma (Thorne, Pearson, and Nicoll, 1994).

BOX 48-6
Clinical Manifestations of Brain Tumors

Headache

Recurrent and progressive
In frontal or occipital areas
Worse on arising, less severe during day
Intensified by lowering head and straining, such as during bowel movement, coughing, sneezing

Vomiting

With or without nausea or feeding
Progressively more projectile
More severe in morning
Relieved by moving about and changing position

Neuromuscular changes

Incoordination or clumsiness
Loss of balance (use of wide-based stance, falling, tripping, banging into objects)
Poor fine motor control
Weakness
Hyporeflexia or hyperreflexia
Positive Babinski sign
Spasticity (in child older than 1 year of age)
Paralysis

Behavioral changes

Irritability
Decreased appetite
Failure to thrive
Fatigue (frequent naps)
Lethargy
Coma

Cranial nerve neuropathy

Cranial nerve involvement varies according to tumor location
Most common signs
- Head tilt
- Visual defects (nystagmus, diplopia, strabismus, episodic "graying out" of vision, and visual field defects)

Vital sign disturbances

Decreased pulse and respiration
Increased blood pressure
Widened pulse pressure
Hypothermia or hyperthermia

Other signs

Seizures
Cranial enlargement*
Tense, bulging fontanel at rest*
Nuchal ridigity
Papilledema (edema of optic nerve)

*Present only in infants and young children.

Nursing Care Management

Assessment

A child admitted to the hospital with neurologic dysfunction is often suspected of having a brain tumor, although the actual diagnosis is as yet unconfirmed. Establishing a baseline of data on which to compare preoperative and postoperative changes is an essential step toward planning physical care and preventing complications. It also allows the nurse to assess the degree of physical incapacity and the family's emotional reaction to the diagnosis.

Vital signs, including blood pressure and pulse pressure (the difference between systolic and diastolic pressures), are taken routinely and more often when any change is noted. Any sudden variations are reported immediately. It is especially important to note a change in vital signs during or after diagnostic procedures. A routine neurologic assessment is also performed at the same time as vital signs, and head circumference is measured on infants and very young children.

The child is observed for evidence of headache, vomiting, and any seizure activity. The location, severity, and duration of the headache are noted, as well as its relationship to activity and time of day. Behaviors such as lying flat and facing away from light or refusing to engage in play are clues to discomfort in the nonverbal child. The child's gait is observed at least once daily. Head tilt and other changes in posturing are always noted.

Nursing Diagnoses

A number of nursing diagnoses will be evident after a thorough assessment of the child and family. Some of these are outlined in Box 48-7. Others may be determined in individual cases.

Planning

The goals of care for the child with a brain tumor are as follows:

1. Child and family will be prepared for diagnostic/operative procedures.
2. Child will experience no postoperative complications.
3. Child and family will receive adequate support.
4. Child will return to normal functioning.

Implementation

The suspected diagnosis of a brain tumor is always a crisis event. Despite the fact that some tumors are removed with excellent results, the physician can rarely give definitive answers regarding prognosis until after surgery. Therefore parents and older children require much emotional support to face the diagnostic procedures and a craniotomy.

Prepare the child and family for diagnostic/operative procedures. How children are prepared for the diagnostic tests depends on their age and previous experience. Since most of the tests involve radiographic equipment, the child may be familiar with the procedure. By the time most children are late preschoolers, they know that the head and brain are important parts of the body. It may be helpful to have them draw their concept of the brain in order to clarify misconceptions and base the explanation on their level of understanding.

Although the temptation is to justify the need for surgery by stating that removing the tumor will take away various symptoms, the nurse should refrain from emphasizing this point too strenuously. Postsurgery headaches and cerebellar symptoms, such as ataxia, may be aggravated rather than improved. Surgery may not improve vision. With optic gliomas the child will be blind in one eye. Finally, surgical removal of the mass may be impossible, and after surgery there may be temporary deterioration of functioning. Being honest before surgery most often makes honesty after the operation easier because no false hopes are created.

However, honesty does not negate instilling hope. A truthful explanation regarding the operation is "The surgeon will see exactly where the tumor is. If it is small and in one place, it will be removed. If it is large, as much of it as possible will be removed so that some of your symptoms will go away." It is best to deliver information in small amounts to let the child pursue additional answers. For example, some children will ask about what happens when part of the tumor is left in. An honest reply is that, after surgery, a special radiation machine and/or drugs may be used to make the tumor smaller. A further explanation of radiation or chemotherapy should be delayed until a decision regarding these treatments is made.

The hair is shaved in the operating room just before surgery, or in the child's room, usually the night before surgery. When shaving is done with the child awake, the procedure is approached in a sensitive, positive way. If the child's hair is long, it should be braided so that the long swatch can be saved. Showing children how they look at different stages of the process helps them prepare for the final appearance.

Once the hair is clipped very short or shaved, the child can be given a cap or scarf to wear to camouflage the baldness. Every precaution is taken to provide privacy during the procedure and to protect the child from teasing or ridicule by other children before surgery. It is also emphasized that the hair will regrow shortly after surgery. Depending on the child's immediate adjustment to the hair loss, the nurse may introduce the idea of wearing a wig until the hair is grown in, particularly if additional irradiation or chemotherapy is anticipated.

The child is also told about the size of the dressing. Usually the entire scalp is covered to maintain a tight wound closure, even if a small incision is made. Infratentorial head dressings may be attached to the upper back and extend forward on the neck to maintain slight extension and alignment as a precaution against wound rupture. Applying a similar dressing or "special hat" to a doll is often a less traumatic way of demonstrating the physical appearance.

The child also needs a brief explanation of how he or she will feel after surgery and where he or she will be. Ordinarily children will return to a special intensive care unit, which they may visit beforehand, depending on hospital policy. The child should be aware that he or she may be sleepy for some time after surgery and that a headache is likely, although it should last only a few days.

BOX 48-7

Nursing Diagnoses: the Child with a Brain Tumor

Sensory/perceptual alterations (visual, auditory, kinesthetic, gustatory, tactile, olfactory related to altered sensory reception, transmission, and/or integration)
Pain related to increased ICP
Altered family processes related to situational crisis (child with a serious illness)
Anxiety related to diagnosis, diagnostic and treatment procedures
Anticipatory grieving related to potential loss of child

Parents need similar explanations before surgery, especially in terms of special equipment used in the intensive care unit, dressings, and their child's behavior. For example, they should know that it is not unusual for the child to be comatose or lethargic for a few days after surgery. The nurse may wish to encourage less frequent visiting during this period so that parents can rest and be able to support their child when he or she awakens.

It is also advisable for the nurse to participate in preoperative conferences with the physician and parents. The nurse needs to know what information the parents have been given in order to be able to give further explanations or emotional support when necessary.

Prevent postoperative complications. Usually the surgeon will prescribe specific orders for vital signs, neurologic checks, positioning, fluid regulation, and medication. These vary somewhat, depending on the location of the craniotomy. The following are general principles of care for infratentorial or supratentorial surgery. Additional aspects of care that are discussed elsewhere may include care of the child with seizures and care of the unconscious child in terms of neurologic assessment.

Vital signs are taken as frequently as every 15 to 30 minutes until stable. Temperature measurement is particularly important because of hyperthermia resulting from surgical intervention in the hypothalamus or brainstem and from some types of general anesthesia. To prepare for this reaction a cooling blanket should be placed on the bed *before* the child returns to the unit so that it is ready for use when needed. The temperature is monitored carefully when any cooling measures are taken because hypothermia can occur suddenly. Observations for signs of other complications include increased ICP, meningitis, and respiratory tract infection.

Nursing ALERT

When temperature is elevated, an infectious process must always be suspected, particularly if the febrile state occurs 1 to 2 days after surgery.

Neurologic checks are an essential aspect of care; they include pupillary reaction to light, LOC, sleep patterns, and response to stimuli. Although children may be comatose for a few days, once they regain consciousness there should be a steady increase in alertness. Regression to a lethargic, irritable state indicates increasing pressure, possibly caused by meningitis or cerebral edema.

Nursing ALERT

Sluggish, dilated, or unequal pupils are reported immediately because they may indicate increased ICP and potential brainstem herniation, a medical emergency.

Observations for function are not instituted until the child regains consciousness. However, as soon as possible the nurse should begin testing reflexes, handgrip, and functioning of the cranial nerves. Muscle strength is usually diminished as a result of general weakness after surgery but should improve daily. Ataxia may be significantly worse with cerebellar intervention, but it will slowly improve. Edema near the cranial nerves may depress important functions such as the gag, blink, or swallowing reflex.

Dressings are observed for evidence of drainage. If soiled, the dressing is not removed but reinforced with dry sterile gauze. The approximate amount of drainage is estimated and recorded. A drain may be placed in the operative site.

Nursing ALERT

To keep an accurate account of drainage, the soiled area is circled with a pen every hour or so. In this way continuous bleeding is easily recognized. The presence of colorless drainage is reported immediately, since it most likely is CSF from the incisional area. A foul odor from the dressing may indicate an infection. Such a finding is reported, and a culture is taken.

Once the younger child is alert, the arms may need to be restrained to preserve the dressing. Even a child who has been cooperative before surgery must be closely supervised during the initial stages of regaining consciousness, when disorientation and restlessness are common. Correct positioning after surgery is critical to prevent pressure against the operative site, reduce ICP, and prevent aspiration. If a large tumor was removed, the child is not placed on the operative site, since the brain may suddenly shift to that cavity, causing trauma to the blood vessels, linings, and the brain itself. The nurse confers with the surgeon to be certain of the correct position, including degree of neck flexion. The first 24 to 48 hours after brain surgery are critical. If position is restricted, notice of this is posted above the head of the bed. When the child is turned, every precaution is used to prevent jarring or malalignment in order to prevent undue strain on the sutures. Two nurses, one supporting the head and the other the body, are needed. The use of a turning sheet may facilitate turning a heavy child.

The child with an infratentorial procedure is usually positioned flat and on either side. Pillows should be placed against the child's back, not the head, to maintain the desired position. Ordinarily the head and neck are kept in midline with the body and slightly extended. In a supratentorial craniotomy the head is usually elevated above the heart to facilitate CSF drainage and decrease excessive blood flow to the brain to prevent hemorrhage.

Nursing ALERT

The Trendelenburg position is contraindicated in both infratentorial and supratentorial surgeries because it increases ICP and the risk of hemorrhage. If shock is impending, the practitioner is notified immediately, before the head is lowered.

With an infratentorial craniotomy the child is allowed nothing by mouth for at least 24 hours, or longer if the gag and swallowing reflexes are depressed or the child is comatose. After a supratentorial operation, feeding may be resumed soon after the child is alert, sometimes within 24 hours. If the child vomits, oral liquids are stopped. Vomiting not only predisposes to aspiration, but increases intracranial pressure and potential for incisional rupture.

The child should be fed to conserve energy and minimize movement. If there is any sign of facial paralysis, the child is fed slowly to prevent choking or aspiration. Sometimes gavage feeding is necessary when bodily functions are too depressed to permit safe oral feedings or when the child refuses to eat or drink. Intravenous fluids are continued until fluids are well tolerated. Because of postoperative cerebral edema and danger of increased ICP, fluids are carefully monitored.

Headache may be severe and is largely the result of cerebral edema. Measures to relieve some of the discomfort include providing a quiet, dimly lit environment; restricting visitors to a minimum; preventing any sudden jarring movement, such as banging into the bed; and preventing an increase in ICP. The last is most effectively achieved by proper positioning and prevention of straining, such as during coughing, vomiting, or defecating. The use of opioids, such as morphine, to relieve pain is controversial because it is thought that they may mask signs of altered consciousness or depress respirations. However, they can be given safely, since naloxone can be used to reverse opioid effects, such as sedation or respiratory depression. Acetaminophen and codeine are also effective analgesics for mild to moderate pain. Regardless of the drugs used, adequate dosage and regular administration are essential to providing optimal pain relief (see also Pain Assessment; Pain Management, Chapter 41).

Bowel movements are monitored to prevent constipation. Stool softeners may be given as soon as liquids are tolerated to facilitate easy passage of stool. Placing an ice bag on the forehead may also provide some headache relief, especially if facial edema is severe. Saline drops, or artificial tears, may be needed if the eyelids do not close completely, to prevent corneal ulceration.

Support child and family. The emotional needs of the family are great when the diagnosis is a brain tumor, and feelings are influenced by the extent of surgery, any neurologic deficits, expected prognosis, and additional therapy. Since few definitive answers can be given before surgery, the surgeon's report is a significant finding that can vary from a completely benign, resected neoplasm to a highly malignant, invasive, and only partially removed tumor. Although parents try to prepare themselves for a potentially fatal diagnosis, it is a shock for them.

Ideally a nurse should be with the family when the physician visits to discuss the expected prognosis and plan of therapy with them. Although parents may hear only a fraction of what they are told, they can begin to put the future into perspective. Although some children will be cured, those with residual tumor may die within a relatively short period or live for several years. Regardless of the future prospects, the parents' thinking must be directed toward helping the child recover and resume a normal life to his or her maximum potential.

It is also a time to encourage parents to verbalize their feelings about the diagnosis. Often they express tremendous guilt for attributing the insidious onset of symptoms, such as ataxia, visual difficulty, or headache, to "minor complaints" by the child. Any comments that insinuate that the parents should have sought medical advice sooner are avoided, since such remarks only add to their guilt feelings.

During this period the nurse should also discuss with parents what they plan to tell the child. If the child was prepared honestly, the diagnosis can be expressed in a similar manner, such as "The physician removed most of the tumor; the rest will be treated with special medicine and x-ray treatments." As the child improves, additional explanation of the treatment (similar to that discussed for leukemia), as well as the reason for any residual neurologic effects, such as ataxia or blindness, may be needed.

Promote return to optimal functioning. The ultimate goal is a cured child who has maximum functioning. As soon as possible the child should resume usual activities within tolerable limits, especially returning to school.* Until the skull is completely healed, the child may need to wear a helmet when engaging in any active sport. The school nurse and teacher should confer with the parents to discuss activity restrictions, such as physical education and the reactions of schoolmates to the child's appearance. Since children often equate brain surgery with "going crazy," it is important to prepare the child for possible remarks to this effect. As one child told a classmate, "It's *your* head they should have fixed, because you're crazy. Can't you see that I'm all better?"

After discharge the family needs continuing medical and emotional support from health personnel. Children who are long-term survivors after treatment for a brain tumor may have residual disabilities, such as growth retardation; cranial nerve palsies; sensory defects; motor abnormalities, especially ataxia; intellectual deficits; memory loss; dysphagia; dysgraphia; and behavioral problems. The high frequency of late effects requires follow-up care despite successful treatment of the tumor (Heideman et al, 1993).

Evaluation

The effectiveness of nursing interventions is determined by continual reassessment and evaluation of care based on the following observational guidelines and expected outcomes:

1. Interview child and family regarding their understanding of scheduled tests and procedures; observe child's behavior during procedures.
2. Monitor child's vital signs, neurologic signs, and dressing.
3. Interview child and family and observe their behaviors during hospitalization and recovery.
4. Interview child and family regarding activities and interests.

Expected outcomes:

1. Child is able to demonstrate an understanding of the tests and procedures and copes with a minimum of stress.
2. Child exhibits no evidence of complications.

*Excellent publications, including the pamphlet *When Your Child is Ready to Return to School*, are available from the Association for Brain Tumor Research, 3725 N. Talman Ave., Chicago, IL 60618; (312) 684-1400.

3. Child and family demonstrate evidence of healthy coping.
4. Family devises and carries out a realistic activity schedule, and child attends school with reasonable regularity (specify).

See also the Nursing Care Plan: The Child with Cancer, Chapter 46; and the Nursing Care Plan: The Child with a Brain Tumor.*

NEUROBLASTOMA

Neuroblastomas are the most common malignant tumors of infancy and are second only to brain tumors as the type of solid malignancy seen during the first 10 years. They occur in about 1 per 10,000 live births, with a slightly higher incidence in males. About half the cases occur in children under 2 years of age, and another fourth occur in children under age 4 years. These tumors originate from embryonic neural crest cells that normally give rise to the adrenal medulla and the sympathetic ganglia. Consequently the majority of tumors develop in the adrenal gland or the retroperitoneal sympathetic chain. Other sites may be in the head, neck, chest, or pelvis.

Neuroblastoma is a "silent" tumor. In more than 70% of cases, diagnosis is made after metastasis occurs, with the first signs caused by involvement in the nonprimary site, usually the lymph nodes, bone marrow, skeletal system, skin, or liver.

Diagnostic Evaluation

The objective of diagnosis is to locate the primary site and areas of metastasis. The signs and symptoms of neuroblastoma depend on the location and stage of the disease. Most presenting signs are caused by compression of adjacent structures (Box 48-8). Skeletal survey; skull, neck, chest, abdominal, and bone CT scans; and a bone marrow test are used to locate a tumor mass and/or metastasis. An intravenous pyelogram may provide evidence of renal involvement.

Urinary excretion of catecholamines is increased in children with adrenal or sympathetic tumors. A 24-hour urine collection analyzed for breakdown products of catecholamine metabolism permits detection of a suspected tumor both before and after therapeutic intervention.

In recent years considerable controversy has developed about the use of mass screening for neuroblastoma in infants by measuring catecholamine metabolites (vanillymandelic acid [VMA] and homovanillic acid [HVA]). However, the effectiveness of mass screening in terms of reducing mortality rate from the tumor remains unproved (Murphy et al, 1991).

Therapeutic Management

Accurate clinical staging is important for establishing initial treatment. Therefore surgery is used both to remove as much of the tumor as possible and to obtain biopsy specimens. In early stages, complete surgical removal of the tumor is the treatment of choice. If the tumors are large, partial resection is attempted, with a course of postoperative irradiation to shrink the tumor in the hope of complete removal at a later date. Radiation therapy also offers palliation for metastatic lesions in bones, lung, liver, or brain. Chemotherapy, administered in a variety of combinations, is the mainstay of therapy for extensive local or disseminated disease.

BOX 48-8
Clinical Manifestations of Neuroblastoma

Abdominal tumors

Firm, nontender, irregular mass
Crosses the midline
Compression of kidney, ureter, or bladder may cause urinary frequency or retention

Distant metastasis

Ocular:
- Supraorbital ecchymosis
- Periorbital edema
- Proptosis (exophthalmos) from invasion of retrobulbar soft tissue

Lymphadenopathy, especially cervical and supraclavicular
Skeletal: bone pain may or may not be present
Intracranial: neurologic impairment
Thoracic: respiratory obstruction
Spinal cord: varying degrees of paralysis
Adrenal:
- Increased catecholamine excretion
- Flushing
- Hypertension
- Tachycardia
- Diaphoresis

Widespread metastasis—vague symptoms

Pallor
Weakness
Irritability
Anorexia
Weight loss

Prognosis. Because of the frequency of invasiveness the prognosis for neuroblastoma is poor. Generally the younger the child at diagnosis (especially under 1 year of age), the better the survival rates. Also, neuroblastoma is one of the few tumors that demonstrates spontaneous regression, possibly as a result of maturity of the embryonic cell or the development of an active immune system.

Nursing Care Management

Nursing considerations are similar to those discussed for leukemia and brain tumors, including psychologic and physical preparation for diagnostic and operative procedures; prevention of postoperative complications for abdominal, thoracic, or cranial surgery; and explanation of chemotherapy and radiotherapy and their side effects.

Since this tumor carries a poor prognosis for many children, every consideration must be given the family in terms of coping with a life-threatening illness (see Chapter 38). Because of the high degree of metastasis at the time of diagnosis, many parents suffer much guilt for not having recognized signs earlier. Often the guilt is expressed as anger toward practitioners for not diagnosing it sooner. Parents need much support in dealing with these feelings and expressing them to the appropriate people.

*In Wong DL: *Wong and Whaley's clinical manual of pediatric nursing*, ed 4, St Louis, 1996, Mosby.

Intracranial Infections

The nervous system and its coverings are subject to infection by the same organisms that affect other organs of the body. However, the nervous system is limited in the ways in which it responds to injury. Infectious processes share virtually the same clinical and pathologic features. They differ primarily in the growth and virulence of the specific organism. It is generally difficult to distinguish between the various causative agents by looking at clinical manifestations. Laboratory studies are needed to identify the causative agent. The inflammatory process can affect the meninges (*meningitis*), the brain (*encephalitis*), or the spinal cord (*myelitis*).

The most common infection of the CNS is meningitis. It can be caused by a variety of organisms; the three main types are the following:

1. **Bacterial,** or pyogenic, caused by pus-forming bacteria, especially the meningococcus, pneumococcus, and influenza bacillus
2. **Tuberculous,** caused by the tubercle bacillus
3. **Viral,** caused by a wide variety of viral agents

BACTERIAL MENINGITIS

Bacterial meningitis is a potentially fatal disease, and although the advent of antimicrobial therapy has had a marked effect on the course and prognosis, it remains a significant cause of illness in the pediatric age group. Its importance lies primarily in the frequency with which it occurs in infancy and childhood and the unnecessarily high death rates and residual damage caused by undiagnosed and untreated or inadequately treated cases. Ninety percent of all cases appear before 5 years of age; infants demonstrate the greatest risk (Booy and Kroll, 1994).

Bacterial meningitis can be caused by any of a variety of bacterial agents. *Haemophilus influenzae* (type B), *Streptococcus pneumoniae,* and *Neisseria meningitidis* (meningococcal) organisms are responsible for bacterial meningitis in 95% of children older than 2 months of age. The leading causes of neonatal meningitis are the group B streptococci and *Escherichia coli* organisms. *E. coli* infection is seldom seen beyond infancy. Meningococcic (epidemic cerebrospinal) meningitis occurs in epidemic form and is the only form readily transmitted to others. It is transmitted by droplet infection from nasopharyngeal secretions. Although it may develop at any age, the risk of meningococcal infection increases with the number of contacts; therefore it occurs predominantly in school-age children and adolescents.

Pathophysiology

Meningitis appears to occur as an extension of a variety of bacterial infections, probably as a result of the lack of acquired resistance to the various causative organisms. The most common route of infection is vascular dissemination from a focus of infection elsewhere. Organisms also gain entry by direct implantation after penetrating wounds, skull fractures that provide an opening into the skin or sinuses, lumbar puncture or surgical procedures, anatomic abnormalities such as spina bifida, or foreign bodies such as a ventricular shunt. Once implanted, the organisms spread into the CSF, which serves as a conduit for spread of infection throughout the subarachnoid space.

The infective process is that seen in any bacterial infection —inflammation, exudation, white blood cell accumulation, and varying degrees of tissue damage. The brain becomes hyperemic and edematous, and the entire surface of the brain is covered with a layer of purulent exudate. As infection extends to the ventricles, thick pus, fibrin, or adhesions may occlude the narrow passages, obstructing the flow of CSF.

Nursing ALERT

Any child who is acutely ill and has a purpuric rash (petechiae and ecchymoses) must receive medical evaluation immediately for the possibility of fulminant (overwhelming) meningococcemia (Box 48-9).

Diagnostic Evaluation

A lumbar puncture (LP) is the definitive diagnostic test. The fluid pressure is measured, and samples are obtained for culture, Gram stain, blood cell count, and determination of glucose and protein content. The findings are usually diagnostic. Culture and stain are needed to identify the causative organism. Spinal fluid pressure is usually elevated, but interpretation is often difficult when the child is crying. Sedation with meperidine (Demerol) or fentanyl and midazolam (Versed) can alleviate the child's pain and the fear associated with this procedure. Eeutectic mixture of local anesthetics (EMLA), a cream applied topically to the spinal area 1 hour before LP, reduces pain for children undergoing this procedure. The site of application is usually at lumbar vertebrae 2 and 3. There is generally an elevated white blood cell count, predominantly polymorphonuclear leukocytes, but it may be extremely variable. The glucose level is reduced, generally in proportion to the duration and severity of the infection.

A blood culture is advisable for all children suspected of having meningitis and occasionally has a positive result when results of CSF culture are negative. Nose and throat cultures may provide helpful information in some cases.

Therapeutic Management

Acute bacterial meningitis is a medical emergency that requires early recognition and immediate institution of therapy to prevent death and residual disabilities. The initial therapeutic management includes:

- Isolation precautions
- Initiation of antimicrobial therapy
- Maintenance of optimal hydration
- Maintenance of ventilation
- Reduction of increased ICP
- Management of bacterial shock
- Control of seizures
- Control of extremes of temperature
- Correction of anemia
- Treatment of complications

The child is isolated from other children, usually in an intensive care unit for close observation. An intravenous infusion is started as soon as the lumbar puncture has been completed in order to facilitate the administration of antimicrobial agents, fluids, anticonvulsant drugs, and blood if needed. The child is placed on a cardiac monitor.

BOX 48-9
Clinical Manifestations of Bacterial Meningitis

Children and adolescents
Usually abrupt onset
Fever
Chills
Headache
Vomiting
Alterations in sensorium
Seizures (often the initial sign)
Irritability
Agitation
May exhibit:
- Photophobia
- Delirium
- Hallucinations
- Aggressive or maniacal behavior
- Drowsiness
- Stupor
- Coma

Nuchal rigidity
- May progress to opisthotonos

Positive Kernig and Brudzinski signs
Hyperactive but variable reflex responses
Signs and symptoms peculiar to individual organisms:
- Petechial or purpuric rashes (meningococcal infection), especially when associated with a shocklike state
- Joint involvement (meningococcal and *H. influenzae* infection)
- Chronically draining ear (pneumococcal meningitis)

Infants and young children
Classic picture rarely seen in children between 3 months and 2 years of age
Fever
Poor feeding
Vomiting
Marked irritability
Frequent seizures (often accompanied by a high-pitched cry)
Bulging fontanel
Nuchal rigidity may or may not be present
Brudzinski and Kernig signs are not helpful in diagnosis
- Difficult to elicit and evaluate in this age group

Subdural empyhema (*H. influenzae* infection)

Neonates: specific signs
Extremely difficult to diagnose
Manifestations vague and nonspecific
Well at birth but within a few days begins to look unwell and behave poorly
Refuses feedings
Poor sucking ability
Vomiting or diarrhea
Poor tone
Lack of movement
Poor cry
Full, tense, and bulging fontanel may appear late in course of illness
Neck usually supple

Neonates: nonspecific signs that may be present
Hypothermia or fever (depending on the maturity of the infant)
Jaundice
Irritability
Drowsiness
Seizures
Respiratory irregularities or apnea
Cyanosis
Weight loss

Until the causative organism is identified, antibiotics such as chloramphenicol, ampicillin, ceftriaxone, gentamycin, or tobramycin may be used. Afterward, the choice of antibiotic is based on the known sensitivity of the organism. Except under special circumstances the drugs are administered intravenously throughout the course of treatment. They are given in large doses, and the period of therapy is determined by CSF findings (normal glucose level and negative culture result) and the child's clinical condition. Appropriate antibiotics are administered after identification of the causative organism. The use of dexamethasone as an antiinflammatory agent to reduce hearing loss and/or neurologic sequelae is controversial (Wald et al, 1995).

Maintaining hydration is a prime concern, and the decision to administer intravenous fluids and the type and amount of fluid are determined by the patient's condition. Optimal hydration involves correction of any fluid deficits followed by maintenance of low levels to prevent cerebral edema. Cerebral edema and electrolyte disturbances are complications associated with poor neurologic outcomes (Brown and Feigin, 1994). If indicated, measures are taken to reduce ICP as described previously (see p. 1579).

Complications are treated appropriately, such as aspiration of subdural effusion in infants and heparin therapy for children who have disseminated intravascular coagulation syndrome. If shock occurs, it is managed by restoration of blood volume and maintenance of electrolyte balance. Seizures, which occur in a large number of children, are controlled with anticonvulsants.

Lumbar puncture is carried out as needed to determine the effectiveness of therapy. The patient is evaluated neurologically during the convalescent period and at regular intervals during the succeeding year.

Prognosis. The age of the child, the type of organism, the severity of the infection, the duration of the illness before the onset of therapy, and the sensitivity of the organism to antimicrobial drugs are important factors in determining the prognosis. Sequelae are most commonly seen when the disease occurs in the first 2 months of life and least often in children with meningococcal meningitis. The residual deficits in infants are primarily a result of communicating hydrocephalus and the greater effects of cerebritis on the immature brain. In older children the residual effects are related to the inflammatory process itself or result from vasculitis associated with the disease. Evaluation of cranial nerve VIII is needed for at least a 6-month follow-up period to assess for possible hearing loss.

Prevention. Vaccines are available for types A, C, Y, and W-135 meningococci and *H. influenzae* type b. Routine meningococcal vaccination of children is not recommended. However, routine vaccinations for *H. influenzae* type b are recommended for all children beginning at 2 months of age (see Immunizations, Chapter 33). A declining incidence of *H. influenzae* type b disease has occurred since the introduction of the Hib vaccination (Murphy et al, 1993).

Nursing Care Management

Nurses should take necessary precautions to protect themselves and others from possible infection. Parents are taught the proper procedures and supervised in their application.

Nursing ALERT

The first priority of nursing care of a child suspected of having meningitis is to administer the antibiotic as soon as it is ordered. The child is also placed on respiratory isolation for at least 24 hours after implementation of antimicrobial therapy.

The room should be kept as quiet as possible, and environmental stimuli kept at a minimum, since most affected children are sensitive to noise, bright lights, and other external stimuli. Most children are more comfortable without a pillow and with the head of the bed slightly elevated. A side-lying position is more often assumed because of nuchal rigidity. The nurse should avoid actions, such as lifting the child's head, that cause pain or increase discomfort. Measures are taken to ensure safety, since the child is often restless and subject to seizures.

The nursing care of the child with meningitis is determined by the child's symptoms and treatment. Observation of vital signs, neurologic signs, LOC, urine output, and other pertinent data is carried out at frequent intervals. The child who is unconscious is managed as described previously (see p. 1578), and all children are observed carefully for signs of complications just described, especially increased ICP, shock, or respiratory distress. Head circumference is measured on the infant because subdural effusions and obstructive hydrocephalus can develop as a complication of meningitis.

Fluids and nourishment are determined by the child's status. The child with dulled sensorium is usually given nothing by mouth. Other children are allowed clear liquids initially and progress to a diet suitable for their age. Careful monitoring and recording of intake and output are needed to determine deviations that might indicate impending shock or increasing fluid accumulation, such as cerebral edema or subdural effusion.

One of the problems in nursing care of children with meningitis is maintaining the intravenous infusion for the time needed to provide adequate antimicrobial therapy (usually 10 days). Since continuous intravenous fluids are usually not necessary, an intermittent infusion device is used. In some cases, children who are recovering uneventfully are sent home with the device, and parents are taught intravenous drug administration.*

*Home care instructions for caring for an intermittent infusion lock are available in Wong DL: *Wong and Whaley's clinical manual of pediatric nursing,* ed 4, St Louis, 1996, Mosby.

Family Focus

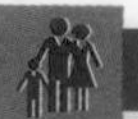

PREVENTING BACTERIAL MENINGITIS

With the change in immunization schedules calling for administration of Hib vaccine to infants at 2 months of age, parents should be encouraged to bring their child to a health facility so that the full series of inoculations is completed. With the high mortality associated with bacterial meningitis, early immunization can prevent families from experiencing the tragic death of a child. Nurses play a significant role in educating families regarding preventive measures, such as early Hib vaccination.

See also the Nursing Care Plan: The Child with Acute Bacterial Meningitis.*

Family support. The sudden nature of the illness makes emotional support of the child and parents extremely important. Parents are very upset and concerned about their child's condition and frequently feel guilty for not having suspected the seriousness of the illness sooner. They need much reassurance that the natural onset of meningitis is sudden and that they acted responsibly in seeking medical assistance when they did. The nurse encourages them to discuss their feelings openly to minimize blame and guilt. They also are kept informed of the child's progress and of all procedures and treatments. In the event that the child's condition worsens, they need the same psychologic care as parents facing the possible death of their child (see Chapter 38; see also the Family Focus box above).

NONBACTERIAL (ASEPTIC) MENINGITIS

Aseptic meningitis is caused by a number of agents, principally viruses, and is frequently associated with other diseases, such as measles, mumps, herpes, and leukemia. Enteroviruses and mumps viruses account for a large number of cases.

The onset may be abrupt or gradual. The initial manifestations are headache, fever, malaise, gastrointestinal symptoms, and signs of meningeal irritation that develop a day or two after the onset of illness. Abdominal pain and nausea and vomiting are common; back and leg pain, sore throat, chest pain, photophobia, and generalized muscular aches or pains are found occasionally. There may be a maculopapular rash. These symptoms usually subside spontaneously and rapidly, and the child is well in 3 to 10 days with no residual effects.

Diagnosis is based on clinical features and CSF findings, which include increased lymphocytes, predominantly mononuclear cells. It is important to differentiate this self-limited disorder from the more serious form of meningitis and to diagnose and treat any disease of which it is a manifestation.

Treatment is primarily symptomatic, such as acetaminophen for headache and muscle pain and positioning for comfort. Antimicrobial agents may be administered and isolation enforced until a definitive diagnosis is made as a precaution against the possibility that the disease may be of bacterial origin.

*In Wong DL: *Wong and Whaley's clinical manual of pediatric nursing,* ed 4, St Louis, 1996, Mosby.

Nursing care is similar to nursing care of the child with bacterial meningitis.

ENCEPHALITIS

Encephalitis is an inflammatory process of the CNS producing altered function of various portions of the brain and spinal cord. Encephalitis can be caused by a variety of organisms, including bacteria, spirochetes, fungi, protozoa, helminths, and viruses. Most infections are associated with viruses, and this discussion will be limited to these causative agents.

Etiology

Encephalitis can occur as a result of (1) direct invasion of the CNS by a virus or (2) postinfectious involvement of the CNS after a viral disease. Often the specific type of encephalitis in a particular child may not be identified for some time or at all. The majority of cases of known cause are associated with the childhood viral diseases. Most other viral infections are those involved with arthropod vectors and those associated with hemorrhagic fevers. The vector reservoir for most agents pathogenic for humans and detected in the United States are mosquitoes and ticks; therefore most cases of encephalitis appear during the hot summer months.

Herpes simplex encephalitis is an uncommon disease, but 30% of cases involve children. The initial clinical findings are nonspecific (fever, altered mental status), but most cases evolve to demonstrate focal neurologic signs and symptoms. Children may experience focal seizures. The CSF is abnormal in most cases. Because of a rise in the number of children with herpes simplex virus encephalitis, suspected cases require prompt attention, especially since the diagnosis can be difficult. The clinical diagnosis can be confirmed by the rapid appearance of immunoglobulin M (IgM) antibody to herpes simplex virus type 1 in CSF and serum. The early use of intravenous acyclovir reduces mortality and morbidity rates.

Diagnostic Evaluation

The clinical features are similar, regardless of the agent involved. Manifestations can range from a mild, benign form that resembles aseptic meningitis, lasting a few days and followed by rapid and complete recovery, to a fulminating encephalitis with severe CNS involvement (Box 48-10).

The diagnosis is made on the basis of clinical findings, circumstances associated with the disease, and (where possible) identification of the specific virus. A diagnostic evaluation of encephalitis may include a brain biopsy, usually from the temporal lobe area. Togaviruses (some of which were formerly labeled arboviruses) are rarely detected in the blood or spinal fluid, but herpes, mumps, and measles viruses and enteroviruses may be found in CSF. Serologic diagnosis may be reached by means of a variety of antibody tests. The first should be drawn as soon after onset as possible, and the second 2 or 3 weeks later. Laboratory detection of herpes simplex virus deoxyribonucleic acid (DNA) in CSF may be used to expedite diagnosis of herpes simplex encephalitis.

BOX 48-10
Clinical Manifestations of Encephalitis

Onset: sudden or gradual	Severe cases
Malaise	High fever
Fever	Stupor
Headache	Seizures
Dizziness	Disorientation
Apathy	Spasticity
Neck stiffness	Coma (may proceed to death)
Nausea and vomiting	Ocular palsies (may occur)
Ataxia	Paralysis (may occur)
Tremors	
Hyperactivity	
Speech difficulties	

Therapeutic Management

Patients suspected of having encephalitis are hospitalized promptly for skilled nursing care and observation. Treatment is primarily supportive, including conscientious nursing care, control of cerebral manifestations, and adequate nutrition and hydration, with observations and management as for other disorders involving cerebral injury. Follow-up care and periodic reevaluation and rehabilitation are important requisites to survival with residual effects of the disease.

Prognosis. The prognosis for the child afflicted with encephalitis depends on the child's age, the type of organism, and residual neurologic damage. Very young children, younger than 2 years of age, may exhibit increased neurologic disability, including learning difficulties and seizure disorders.

Nursing Care Management

Nursing care of the child with encephalitis is the same as for any unconscious child and the child with meningitis. Neurologic monitoring, administration of medications, and support to the child and parents are the major aspects of care.

REYE SYNDROME (RS)

RS is a disorder defined as toxic encephalopathy associated with other characteristic organ involvement. It is characterized by fever, profoundly impaired consciousness, and disordered hepatic function. The cause of the disorder is obscure, but most cases of RS follow a common viral illness, most frequently influenza or varicella. The link between aspirin and RS is possible but has not been firmly established as a cause-and-effect relationship. However, use of aspirin and nonsteroidal antiinflammatory drugs (NSAIDs), such as ibuprofen, is not recommended for children with varicella or those suspected of having influenza.

Pathophysiology

RS has been defined by the Centers for Disease Control and Prevention as an acute noninflammatory encephalopathy and hepatopathy, with no reasonable explanation for the cerebral and hepatic abnormalities. The pathologic mechanism of RS is a mitochondrial insult induced by different viruses, drugs, exogenous toxins, and genetic factors.

Diagnostic Evaluation

Elevated ammonia levels tend to correlate with the clinical manifestations and prognosis. Definitive diagnosis is established by liver biopsy (Box 48-11). Children who in the past would have been diagnosed with RS are now given other di-

BOX 48-11
Staging Criteria for Reye Syndrome

Stage I	Vomiting, lethargy, and drowsiness; liver dysfunction; type I EEG, follows commands, pupillary reaction brisk
Stage II	Disorientation, combativeness, delirium, hyperventilation, hyperactive reflexes, appropriate responses to painful stimuli; evidence of liver dysfunction; type I EEG, pupillary reaction sluggish
Stage III	Obtunded, coma, hyperventilation, decorticate rigidity, preservation of pupillary light reaction and oculovestibular reflexes (although sluggish); type II EEG
Stage IV	Deepening coma, decerebrate rigidity, loss of oculocephalic reflexes, large and fixed pupils, loss of doll's eye reflex, loss of corneal reflexes; minimum liver dysfunction; type III or IV EEG, evidence of brainstem dysfunction
Stage V	Seizures, loss of deep tendon reflexes, respiratory arrest, flaccidity; type IV EEG; usually no evidence of liver dysfunction

agnoses such as metabolic disorders, as a result of improved diagnostic techniques.

Therapeutic Management

The most important aspects of successful management of the child with RS are early diagnosis and aggressive therapy. Rapid progression through coma stages and high peak ammonia concentrations are associated with a more serious prognosis. Cerebral edema with increased ICP represents the most immediate threat to life. Recovery from RS is rapid and usually without sequelae if there has been early diagnosis and implementation of therapy.

Prognosis. Although the incidence of Reye syndrome is declining, survivors may have subtle neuropsychologic deficits. Generally recovery is good, given the gravity of the disease (Quam, 1994).

Nursing Care Management

The child who is acutely ill with RS requires continuous and intensive nursing care. In addition to an appraisal of vital functions and neurologic status the nurse assists with a lumbar puncture, obtains blood for laboratory examination, and inserts various intravenous lines such as peripheral, arterial, and central venous pressure. A retention catheter and a nasogastric tube are inserted, and when respirations are compromised, an endotracheal tube is inserted and attached to a respirator for controlled respirations.

Care and observations are implemented as for any child with an altered state of consciousness (see p. 1578) and increasing ICP. Accurate and frequent monitoring of intake and output is essential for adjusting fluid volumes to prevent both dehydration and cerebral edema. The child who is paralyzed and in a drug-induced coma is totally dependent on the caregivers, and meticulous vigilance and attention to all biologic needs are mandatory. Since hypovolemic shock is a constant danger in children with controlled fluid intake and osmotic diuresis, vital signs, including central venous pressure and/or cardiac output (Swan-Ganz catheter), are monitored frequently. Because of related liver dysfunction, the nurse must observe for signs of impaired coagulation such as prolonged bleeding time.

Family support. Parents of children with RS need a great deal of emotional support. They are usually frightened by the child's appearance, the treatment, and the life-threatening severity and suddenness of the illness. Their distress is increased if they believe that their actions may have contributed to a delay in diagnosis. They need to be kept informed of the child's progress, to have diagnostic procedures and therapeutic management explained, and to be given concerned and sympathetic support.

The National Reye's Syndrome Foundation* has been established by the parents of a child who died of this disease in hope of encouraging research on the disease and of educating parents and health professionals.

HUMAN IMMUNODEFICIENCY VIRUS (HIV) ENCEPHALOPATHY

About 2000 infants are born each year with HIV. It is the seventh leading killer of young children. Documented routine HIV education and routine testing with consent for all pregnant women in the United States are recommended (American Academy of Pediatrics, 1995). The use of zidovudine (ZDV) by HIV-infected pregnant women significantly reduces the chance a mother will infect the infant.

Children with HIV encephalopathy, a complication of acquired immunodeficiency syndrome (AIDS), present a nursing challenge. Progressive encephalopathy occurs in 30% to 50% of infants and children infected with HIV; 82% are younger than 5 years of age.

Neurologic manifestations in children suggest that the progressive encephalopathy is the result of primary and persistent infection of the brain with the virus. Unexplained neurodevelopmental regression and focal seizures are the dominant clinical features of the disorder. Others include progressive motor dysfunction and atypical CNS infections. These manifestations indicate a poor prognosis and, almost invariably, a fatal outcome. However, earlier implementation of therapies for AIDS may allow for slower progression of these neurologic complications.

Appropriate precautions are practiced by nurses when caring for these children. Careful handling of the child is a hallmark of excellent nursing, since these children may experience pain, isolation, social stigma, susceptibility to infection, and abandonment resulting in less than minimum sensorimotor stimulation. Nursing assessment and intervention warrant planning time to meet developmental needs, especially holding, rocking, and comforting the child. (See Chapter 46 for a more extensive discussion of AIDS.)

RABIES

Rabies is an acute infection of the nervous system caused by a virus that is almost invariably fatal if untreated. It is transmitted to humans by the saliva of an infected mammal intro-

*P.O. Box 829, Bryan, OH 43506; (419) 636-2679.

duced through a bite or skin abrasion. After entry into a new host the virus multiplies in muscle cells and is spread through neural pathways without stimulating a protective host immune response.

Approximately 88% of rabies cases occur among wild animals, and 12% in domestic animals. Cats are now the most common domestic animals and should be the target of rabies vaccination programs. Carnivorous wild animals (especially raccoons, skunks, and foxes) and bats are the animals most often infected with rabies and the cause of most indigenous cases of human rabies in the United States (Raccoon rabies, 1994). The likelihood of human exposure to a rabid domestic animal has decreased greatly. The circumstances of a biting incident are important. An unprovoked attack is more likely to indicate a rabid animal than a provoked attack. Bites inflicted on a child attempting to feed or handle an apparently healthy animal can generally be regarded as provoked. Any child bitten by a wild animal is assumed to be exposed to rabies.

Nursing ALERT

Unusual behavior in an animal is cause for suspicion; children should be warned to beware of wild animals that appear friendly.

The disease is uncommon in humans; the highest incidence occurs in children under 15 years of age. The incubation period usually ranges from 1 to 3 months but may be as short as 10 days or as long as 8 months. The disease develops in only 10% to 15% of persons bitten, but once symptoms are present, rabies progresses inexorably to a fatal outcome. Diagnosis is made on the basis of the history and clinical features (Box 48-12). Although treatment is of little avail once symptoms appear, the long incubation period allows time for induction of active and passive immunity before the onset of illness.

BOX 48-12
Clinical Manifestations of Rabies

Initial signs
General malaise
Fever
Sore throat

Excitement phase
Hypersensitivity
Increased reaction to external stimuli
Convulsions
Maniacal behavior
Choking

Severe spasm of respiratory muscles*
Apnea
Cyanosis
Anoxia

*From attempts at swallowing (characteristics from which the term "hydrophobia" was derived).

Therapeutic Management

Two types of immunizing products are available for use in humans: (1) the *inactivated rabies vaccines*, which induce an active immune response, and (2) the *globulins*, which contain preformed antibodies. The two types of products should be used concurrently for rabies postexposure treatment when prophylaxis is indicated.

The current therapy for a rabid animal bite consists of thorough cleansing of the wound and passive immunization with *human rabies immune globulin (HRIG)* as soon as possible after exposure to provide rapid, short-term passive immunity (Baevsky and Bartfield, 1993).

Postexposure active immunity is conferred by administration of the *human diploid cell rabies vaccine (HDCV)*. The first dose of the vaccine is given at the same time as the immune globulin and followed by intramuscular injections at 3, 7, 14, and 28 days after the first dose. An additional dose in 90 days is recommended by the World Health Organization. Before antirabies prophylaxis is initiated, the local or state health department is consulted.

Nursing Care Management

Both parents and children are frightened by the urgency and seriousness of the situation. They need anticipatory guidance for the therapy and support and reassurance about the efficacy of the preventive measures for this dreaded disease. EMLA cream, a topical anesthetic, can be placed on the injection site 2 hours before the procedure to reduce the pain.

Mass immunization is unnecessary and unlikely to be implemented. Certain circumstances may warrant vaccination, such as when a child is being taken to an area of the world where rabies in stray dogs is still a problem.

Seizure Disorders

Seizures are brief malfunctions of the brain's electrical system resulting from cortical neuronal discharge. The manifestations of seizures are determined by the site of origin and may include unconsciousness or altered consciousness, involuntary movements, and changes in perception, behaviors, sensations, and posture. Seizures are the most frequently observed neurologic dysfunction in children and can occur with a wide variety of conditions involving the CNS.

EPILEPSY

Seizures result from paroxysmal discharges in cortical neurons and are symptoms of abnormal brain function. They are considered to be a symptom of an underlying disease process. Once it is determined that the child has had a seizure, it is important to distinguish whether the episode was epileptic or nonepileptic. Seizures are the indispensable characteristic of epilepsy; however, not every seizure is epileptic. Epilepsy is a chronic seizure disorder with recurrent and unprovoked seizures.

Etiology

Seizure disorders have numerous and varied causes (e.g., tumors, infections, neoplasms). Most are *idiopathic*. Although the cause of idiopathic epilepsy is unknown, genetic factors may in some way alter the seizure threshold to influence neuronal discharge. A seizure disorder also can be *acquired* as a result of brain injury during the prenatal, perinatal, or postnatal periods. This injury may be caused by trauma, hypoxia, infections, exogenous or endogenous toxins, and a variety of other factors. Biochemical events (e.g., hypoglycemia, hypocalcemia, and certain nutritional deficiencies) produce seizure activity.

The incidence of causative factors associated with childhood seizures is frequently related to the age of the child. Seizures are more common during the first 2 years of life than during any other period of childhood. In very young infants the most frequent causes are birth injuries, such as intracranial trauma, hemorrhage, or anoxia, and congenital defects of the brain. Acute infections are a frequent cause of seizures in late infancy and early childhood but become an infrequent cause in middle childhood. In children older than 3 years of age the most common factor is idiopathic epilepsy.

Seizure activity is believed to be caused by spontaneous electric discharge initiated by a group of hyperexcitable cells referred to as the *epileptogenic focus.* These cells display in-

BOX 48-13

Classification and Clinical Manifestations of Seizures

Partial seizures

Simple partial seizures with motor signs

Characterized by:
- Localized motor symptoms
- Somatosensory, psychic, autonomic symptoms
- Combination of these
- Abnormal discharges remain unilateral

Manifestations:
- Aversive seizure (most common motor seizure in children)
  - Eye or eyes and head turn away from the side of the focus
  - Awareness of movement or loss of consciousness
- Rolandic (sylvan) seizure
  - Tonic-clonic movements involving the face
  - Salivation
  - Arrested speech
  - Most common during sleep
- Jacksonian march (rare in children)
  - Orderly, sequential progression of clonic movements beginning in a foot, hand, or face and moving or "marching" to adjacent body parts

Simple partial seizures with sensory signs

Characterized by various sensations, including:
- Numbness, tingling, prickling, paresthesia, or pain originating in one area (e.g., face or extremities) and spreading to other parts of the body
- Visual sensations or formed images
- Motor phenomena such as posturing or hypertonia
- Uncommon in children under 8 years of age

Complex partial seizures (psychomotor seizures)

Observed more often in children from 3 years through adolescence

Characterized by:
- Period of altered behavior
- Amnesia for event (no recollection of behavior)
- Inability to respond to environment
- Impaired consciousness during event
- Drowsiness or sleep usually follows seizure
- Confusion and amnesia may be prolonged
- Complex sensory phenomena (aura)
  - Most frequent sensation—strange feeling in the pit of the stomach that rises toward the throat
  - Often accompanied by:
    - Odd or unpleasant odors or tastes
    - Complex auditory or visual hallucinations
    - Ill-defined feelings of elation or strangeness (e.g., deja vu, a feeling of familiarity in a strange environment)
  - May be strong feelings of fear and anxiety, distorted sense of time and self
  - Small children may emit a cry or attempt to run for help

Patterns of motor behavior:
- Stereotypic
- Similar with each subsequent seizure
- May suddenly cease activity, appear dazed, stare into space, become confused and apathetic, and become limp or stiff or display some form of posturing
- May be confused
- May perform purposeless, complicated activities in a repetitive manner (automatisms), such as walking, running, kicking, laughing, or speaking incoherently, most often followed by postictal confusion or sleep
- May be oropharyngeal activities, such as smacking, chewing, drooling, swallowing, and nausea or abdominal pain followed by stiffness, a fall, and postictal sleep
- Rarely manifests auras such as rage or temper tantrums
- Aggressive acts uncommon during seizure

Atonic and akinetic seizures (also known as drop attacks)

Characterized by:
- Onset usually between 2 and 5 years of age
- Sudden, momentary loss of muscle tone and postural control
- Events recur frequently during the day, particularly in the morning hours and shortly after awakening

Manifestations:
- Loss of tone causes child to fall to floor violently
  - Unable to break fall by putting out hand
  - May incur a serious injury to the face, head, or shoulder
- Loss of consciousness only momentary

Myoclonic seizures

A variety of convulsive episodes

May be isolated as benign essential myoclonus

May occur in association with other seizure forms

Characterized by:
- Sudden, brief contractures of a muscle or group of muscles
- Occur singly or repetitively
- No postictal state
- May or may not be symmetric
- May or may not be loss of consciousness

creased electric excitability in response to any of a variety of physiologic stimuli, such as cellular dehydration, abnormal blood sugar levels, electrolyte imbalance, fatigue, emotional stress, and endocrine changes. When neuronal excitation from the epileptogenic focus spreads to the brainstem, a generalized seizure develops. Seizures are designated as *focal, (localized), focal with rapid generalization,* and *generalized,* on the basis of the characteristic neuronal discharges. In a large proportion of children focal seizures spread to other areas, ultimately becoming generalized with loss of consciousness.

Classification

There are many different types of epileptic seizures, and each has unique characteristics. The onset of a seizure is abrupt, paroxysmal, and transitory, and signs are highly variable. The current classification system divides seizures into two major categories: partial and generalized seizures (Box 48-13). Some of these are described in the following segment.

Partial seizures are caused by abnormal electric discharges from epileptogenic foci limited to a more or less circumscribed region of the cerebral cortex. Focal seizures may arise from

BOX 48-13
Classification and Clinical Manifestations of Seizures—Cont'd

Generalized seizures

Tonic-clonic seizures (formerly known as grand mal)

Most common and most dramatic of all seizure manifestations
Occur without warning
Tonic phase: lasts approximately 10 to 20 seconds
Manifestations:
- Eyes roll upward
- Immediate loss of consciousness
- If standing, falls to floor or ground
- Stiffens in generalized, symmetric tonic contraction of entire body musculature
- Arms usually flexed
- Legs, head, and neck extended
- May utter a peculiar piercing cry
- Apneic, may become cyanotic
- Increased salivation and loss of swallowing reflex

Clonic phase: lasts about 30 seconds but can vary from only a few seconds to a half hour or longer
Manifestations:
- Violent jerking movements as the trunk and extremities undergo rhythmic contraction and relaxation
- May foam at the mouth
- May be incontinent of urine and feces

As event ends, movements become less intense, occur at longer intervals, then cease entirely
Status epilepticus: series of seizures at intervals too brief to allow the child to regain consciousness between the time one event ends and the next begins
- Requires emergency intervention
- Can lead to exhaustion, respiratory failure, and death

Postictal state:
- Appears to relax
- May remain semiconscious and difficult to rouse
- May awaken in a few minutes
- Remains confused for several hours
- Poor coordination
- Mild impairment of fine motor movements
- May have visual and speech difficulties
- May vomit or complain of severe headache
- When left alone, usually sleeps for several hours
- On awakening is fully conscious
- Usually feels tired and complains of sore muscles and headache
- No recollection of entire event

Absence seizures (formerly called petit mal or lapses)

Characterized by:
- Onset usually between 4 and 12 years of age
- More common in girls than in boys
- Usually cease at puberty
- Brief loss of consciousness
- Minimal or no alteration in muscle tone
- May be unrecognized because little change in child's behavior
- Abrupt onset; suddenly develops 20 or more events daily
- Event often mistaken for inattentiveness or daydreaming
- Events can be precipitated by hyperventilation, hypoglycemia, stresses (emotional and physiologic), fatigue, or sleeplessness

Manifestations:
- Brief loss of consciousness
- Appear without warning or aura
- Usually last about 5 to 10 seconds
- Slight loss of muscle tone may cause child to drop objects
- Able to maintain postural control; seldom falls
- Minor movements such as lip smacking, twitching of eyelids or face, or slight hand movements
- Not accompanied by incontinence
- Amnesia for episode
- May need to reorient self to previous activity

Infantile spasms

Also called: infantile myoclonus, massive spasms, hypsarrhythmia, salaam episodes or infantile myoclonic spasms
Most commonly occur during the first 6 to 8 months of life
Twice as common in males as in females
Child may have numerous seizures during the day without postictal drowsiness or sleep
Outlook for normal intelligence poor
Manifestations:
- Possible series of sudden, brief, symmetric, muscular contractions
- Head flexed, arms extended, and legs drawn up
- Eyes may roll upward or inward
- May be preceded or followed by a cry or giggling
- May or may not be loss of consciousness
- Sometimes flushing, pallor, or cyanosis

Infants who are able to sit but not stand:
- Sudden dropping forward of the head and neck with trunk flexed forward and knees drawn up—the "salaam" or "jackknife" seizure

Less often: alternate clinical forms observed
- Extensor spasms rather than flexion of arms, legs, and trunk and head nodding
- Lightning events involving a single, momentary, shocklike contraction of the entire body

any area of the cereberal cortex, but the frontal, temporal, and parietal lobes are the ones most often affected. The area of cerebral involvement is reflected by clinical manifestations. Partial seizures are subdivided into three types.

Simple partial seizures have elementary or simple symptoms and no alteration of consciousness (also called an aura).

Complex partial seizures involve complex symptoms and impairment of consciousness. These seizures may begin with an *aura,* a simple partial seizure that is usually a sensation or sensory phenomenon that reflects the complicated connections and integrative functions of that area of the brain. The aura is part of the seizure event and is associated with EEG changes (Van Donselaar, Geerts, and Schimscheimer 1990).

Simple or complex seizures secondarily generalized develop into generalized seizures, usually a tonic-clonic event.

Generalized seizures without a focal onset appear to arise in the reticular formation, and the clinical observations indicate that the initial involvement is from both hemispheres. Frequently, loss of consciousness occurs and is the initial clinical manifestation. Unlike partial seizures that become generalized, there is no aura. Episodes occur at any time, day or night, and the interval between episodes may be minutes, hours, weeks, or even years. Most affected persons first experience seizures in childhood, and children whose seizures begin before age 4 years have mental retardation and behavioral and learning problems more frequently than those whose seizures begin after age 4.

Diagnostic Evaluation

Up to 20% of children have been misdiagnosed as having epilepsy (Sagraves, 1990). The careful diagnosis of epilepsy should be made and substantiated with clinical evidence because of the important prognostic and therapeutic implications, which also involve the identification and treatment of the cause.

Establishing a diagnosis is critical. The process of diagnosis in a child with a seizure disorder has two major foci: (1) to ascertain the type of seizure the child has experienced and (2) to attempt to understand the cause of the events. The assessment and diagnosis rely heavily on a thorough history, skilled observation, and use of several diagnostic tests.

During the assessment process it is unusual to observe the child having a seizure; therefore a complete, accurate, and detailed history should be obtained from a reliable and knowledgeable informant. This history involves prenatal, perinatal, and neonatal periods, including any instances of infection, apnea, colic, or poor feeding, and information regarding any previous accidents or serious illnesses.

History of the seizure(s) should be equally detailed, including the type of seizure or description of the child's behavior during the event, the age at onset, and the time at which the seizure occurs (i.e., early morning, before meals, while awake, or during sleep). Any factors that may have precipitated the seizure are important, including fever, infection, falls that may have caused trauma to the head, anxiety, fatigue, activity (e.g., hyperventilation), and environmental events (exposure to strong stimuli such as bright, flashing lights or loud noises). If the child can describe any sensory phenomena, these are recorded. The duration and progression of the seizure (if any) and the postictal feelings and behavior, such as confusion, inability to speak, amnesia, headache, and sleep, are recorded. The ability to identify seizure types accurately has resulted from the technologic advances in video recording and long-term electroencephalogram (EEG) monitoring.

A complete physical and neurologic examination, including developmental assessment of language, learning, behavior, and motor abilities, often provides clues to neurologic disturbances. A family history can offer clues to paroxysmal disorders such as migraine, breath-holding spells, and febrile seizures or neurologic diseases that may be related to the seizure disorder.

Laboratory studies that may prove to be of value include a complete blood cell count (for evidence of lead poisoning) and white blood cell count (for signs of infection). Blood and CSF glucose may give evidence of hypoglycemic episodes; serum electrolytes, blood urea nitrogen, calcium, and other blood studies may indicate metabolic disturbances. Lumbar puncture can confirm a suspected diagnosis of cerebrospinal infection or trauma.

Skull radiographs, CT scans, echoencephalograms, brain scans, and other studies help to identify skull abnormalities, separation of sutures, and intracranial calcifications. Focal seizures in children younger than 1 year of age are indications for a diagnostic CT scan to rule out supratentorial tumor. The EEG is obtained for all children with seizure manifestations and is the most useful tool for evaluating seizure disorders. The EEG is carried out under varying conditions—with the child asleep, awake, awake with provocative stimulation (flashing lights, noise), and hyperventilating. Stimulation elicits abnormal electrical activity, which is recorded on the EEG.

Variations of the EEG are video recordings and simultaneous polygraphs of the patient during waking and/or sleeping. These techniques can be used concurrently and are especially valuable in differentiating epileptic activity from paroxysmal behavior or nonepileptic motor events. *MRI* can identify skull abnormalities, separation of sutures, and intracranial calcifications.

Therapeutic Management

The objectives of treatment of seizure disorders are to (1) control the seizures or reduce their frequency, (2) discover and correct the cause when possible, and (3) help the child who has recurrent seizures to live as normal a life as possible. Seizures of a recurrent nature are treated as soon as the diagnosis is established. If the seizure activity is a manifestation of an infectious, traumatic, or metabolic process, the seizure therapy is instituted as a part of the general therapeutic regimen. Seizure control is considered to prevent secondary brain cell injury from the neuronal discharge and hypoxia.

It is known that persons predisposed to epilepsy have seizures when their basal level of neuronal excitability exceeds a critical point or threshold; no event occurs if the excitability is maintained below this threshold. The administration of antiepileptic drugs serves to raise this threshold and prevent seizures. Consequently the primary therapy for seizure disorders is the administration of the appropriate antiepileptic drug or combination of drugs in a dosage that provides the desired effect without causing undesirable side effects or toxic reactions.

Numerous drugs are available for control of seizures. The primary drugs prescribed for partial seizures and/or generalized tonic-clonic seizures are carbamazepine (Tegretol), phenytoin (Dilantin), and valproic acid (Depakote or Depakene). The drugs of choice for absence seizures are ethosuximide (Zarontin) and valproic acid. The dosage is determined by monitoring serum drug levels. Complete control can be achieved in only 50% to 75% of affected children, however, even with careful attention to details of therapy.

A present breakthrough in drug management is the realization that polypharmacy confers no benefit over monotherapy in about 90% of individuals with epilepsy (Brodie, 1990). There is increasing evidence that diminishing polypharmacy can bring about a better quality of life; therefore single-drug therapy is recommended. Several new drugs have also increased seizure control for many children. These include gabapentin, lamotrigine, and felbamate. The use of felbamate is controversial because of the side effects: aplastic anemia and hepatic failure.

Once seizures are controlled, the drug or drugs are continued for a prolonged time. However, periodic reevaluation of the drug is important to assess the continued effectiveness and to alter the dosage if indicated. The dosage will need to be increased as the child grows.

Withdrawal of antiepileptic therapy follows a predesigned protocol, usually begun when the child has been seizure-free for at least 2 years with a normal EEG finding. Relapse in children may be related to factors such as neurologic deficit or a positive family history for epilepsy. Recurrence is most likely within the first year after discontinuance of the medication. When a medication is discontinued, the dosage should be reduced gradually over 1 to 2 weeks. Sudden withdrawal can cause an increase in the number and severity of seizures, often precipitating status epilepticus. If the time for reducing the medication coincides with puberty or, in younger children, occurs during periods when the child is subject to frequent infections, the drug is continued for a longer period. Repeat EEGs are generally obtained every 6 months to 2 years.

When seizure activity is determined to be caused by a hematoma, tumor, or other progressive cerebral lesion, surgical removal is the treatment. Surgery also may be indicated for those who suffer from repetitive, incapacitating seizures that are caused by a focal brain abnormality, if removal of the lesion does not result in significant loss of vital functions, such as speech and movement. The risks of brain surgery cannot be underestimated. Also, the costs of surgical interventions must be taken into consideration, as well as the numerous tests necessary to assess the child before surgery.

Status epilepticus. Status epilepticus is a continuous seizure that lasts more than 30 minutes or a series of seizures from which the child does not regain a premorbid level of consciousness. The initial treatment is directed toward support and maintenance of vital functions, including maintenance of an adequate airway, administration of oxygen, and hydration, and followed by intravenous administration of either diazepam (Valium) or phenobarbital. Rectal diazepam is a simple, effective, and safe treatment for prehospital management (Dieckmann, 1994). Lorazepam (Ativan) may be replacing intravenous diazepam as the drug of choice. It has a longer duration of action and causes less respiratory distress in children over 2 years of age.

Nursing ALERT

Status epilepticus is a medical emergency requiring immediate intervention to prevent permanent injury to the brain, exhaustion, respiratory failure, and death.

The child must be closely monitored during administration to detect early alterations in vital signs that may indicate impending cardiac arrest or respiratory depression. When diazepam is ineffective, phenobarbital, often in extremely high levels that may require respiratory support, is given intravenously as the initial medication. Patients who do not respond to drug therapy may require the use of intravenous lidocaine, general anesthesia, or a potent skeletal muscle relaxant such as curare. This should be administered by an anesthesiologist.

Nursing ALERT

Diazepam is incompatible with many drugs. To give intravenously, inject slowly directly into the vein or through tubing as close as possible to the vein insertion site. To decrease the burning sensation, dilute with normal saline solution.

Equally imperative to halting the tonic-clonic movement is correct diagnosis of the underlying problem. The outcome is related to the cause and duration of the status epilepticus.

Prognosis. The course and prognosis for children who have seizures depend on the cause, type of seizure, age at onset, and family and medical histories. In one study of children with epilepsy (excluding those with generalized absence, myoclonus, akinetic, atonic, and infantile seizures), 55% "outgrew" the disorder and remained seizure-free without medication during an average 7-year follow-up period. At diagnosis the best predictors of remission were age under 12 years at onset, normal intelligence, no prior neonatal seizures, and fewer than 21 seizures before treatment (Camfield and Camfield, 1993).

Risk factors associated with recurrence of epilepsy include being 16 years of age or older, taking more than one antiepileptic drug, having seizures after starting drug treatment, having a history of primarily or secondarily generalized tonic-clonic seizures or an EEG showing myoclonic seizures; and having an abnormal EEG. The risk of seizure recurrence decreases with increasing time without seizures (Medical Research Council, 1993).

The prognosis after treatment for status epilepticus is more favorable than previously reported. The majority of children will probably have no intellectual impairment. Those who do have cognitive deficits or who die are likely to have preceding developmental delay, neurologic abnormality, or concurrent serious illness (Verity, Ross, and Golding, 1993).

BOX 48-14
Assessment of the Child During Tonic-Clonic Seizure

Observe seizure

Describe

Only what is actually observed
Order of events
Duration of seizure

Onset

Significant preseizure events—bright lights, noise, excitement, emotional outbursts
Behavior
- Change in facial expression, such as of fear
- Cry or other sound
- Stereotyped or automatous movements
- Random activity

Position of head, body, extremities
- Unilateral or bilateral posturing of one or more extremities
- Body deviation to side

Time of onset

Movement

Change of position, if any
Site of commencement—hand, thumb, mouth, generalized
Tonic phase, if present—length, parts of body involved
Clonic phase—twitching or jerking movements, parts of body involved, sequence of parts involved, generalized, change in character of movements
Lack of movement of any extremity

Face

Color change—pallor, cyanosis, flushing
Perspiration
Mouth—position, deviation to one side, teeth clenched, tongue bitten, frothing at mouth, flecks of blood or bleeding

Eyes

Position—straight ahead, deviation upward, deviation outward, conjugate or divergent
Pupils (if able to assess)—change in size, equality, reaction to light and accommodation

Respiratory effort

Presence and length of apnea
Presence of stertor

Other

Involuntary urination
Involuntary defecation

Observe postictally

Method of termination
State of consciousness—unresponsiveness, drowsiness, confusion
Orientation to time, place, persons, and so on
Sleeping but able to be aroused
Record length of postictal sleep
Motor ability
- Any change in motor power
- Ability to move all extremities
- Any paresis or weakness
- Ability to whistle (if appropriate to age)

Speech—changes, peculiarities, type and extent of any difficulties
Sensations
- Complaint of discomfort or pain
- Any sensory impairment of hearing, vision
- Recollection of preseizure sensations, warning of event
- Awareness that event was beginning

Nursing Care Management

Assessment

An important nursing function during a seizure is observing the seizure and describing its pertinent features. Any alterations in behavior and characteristics of the seizure, such as sensory-hallucinatory phenomena (e.g., an aura), motor effects (e.g., eye movements, muscular contractions, laterality, and complex activities), alterations in consciousness, and postictal state, are noted and recorded (Box 48-14).

Generalized seizures and others with dramatic manifestations are easily detected, but absences may be more difficult to detect. They are easily misinterpreted as inattention. Any unusual behavior, even seemingly inconsequential behavior such as a momentary interruption of activity, staring, or mental blankness, should be described. The more detailed these descriptions, the more valuable they are for assessment. The nurse notes the time that the seizure began and times its length. This is especially important if the child becomes cyanotic.

History taking is a vital tool for helping to identify factors that are valuable in establishing a cause of the seizures. Interviewing the child and family helps to elicit problems related to the psychologic impact of the disorder on their lives.

Nursing Diagnoses

Several nursing diagnoses that become apparent after an assessment of the child with a seizure disorder are listed in Box 48-15. Others may be identified in specific cases.

Planning

The goals for the child with a seizure disorder and the family include the following:

1. Child will be protected during a seizure.
2. Child will experience as few seizures as possible.
3. Child and family will cope with the challenges associated with the disorder.
4. Child will develop a positive self-image.
5. Child and family will identify triggering factors.

BOX 48-15
Nursing Diagnoses: The Child with Epilepsy

Risk for injury related to sudden and unexpected loss of consciousness
Body image disturbance related to perception of seizure disorder
Altered family processes related to chronic disease of a child

Implementation

When they first witness a child in a generalized cerebral seizure, nurses are often frightened, puzzled, and immobilized. These reactions are normal but can reduce the effectiveness of care for the child and interfere with observations of the event. The child must be protected from injury during the seizure, and nursing observations made during the event provide valuable information for diagnosis and management of the disorder (see the Emergency box below).

It is impossible to halt a seizure once it has begun, and no attempt should be made to do so. The nurse must remain calm, stay with the child, and prevent the child from sustaining any harm during the seizure. If possible the child should be isolated from the view of others by closing a door or pulling screens. A seizure can be very upsetting to the child, other visitors, and their families. If other people are present, they should be assured that everything is being done for the child. After the seizure they can be given a simple explanation about the event as needed.

Nursing ALERT

Do not move or forcefully restrain the child during a tonic-clonic seizure and do not place a solid object between the teeth.

If the nurse is able to reach the child in time, a child who is standing or is seated in a chair (including a wheelchair) is eased to the floor immediately. During and sometimes after the tonic-clonic seizure the swallowing reflex is lost, salivation increases, and the tongue is hypotonic. Therefore the child is at risk for aspiration and airway occlusion. Placing the child on the side facilitates drainage and helps to maintain a patent airway. After the seizure the child is kept on the side in bed or a similar place to allow the youngster to sleep. If the child is at school or away from home, the child is allowed to rest. When feasible the child is integrated into the environment as soon as

EMERGENCY

SEIZURES

Tonic-Clonic Seizure

During the Seizure

Time seizure episode.
Approach calmly.
If child is standing or seated, ease child down.
Place pillow or folded blanket under child's head. If no bedding is available, place own hands under child's head.
Do not:
 Attempt to restrain child or use force.
 Put anything in child's mouth.
 Give any food or liquids.
Loosen restrictive clothing.
Remove eyeglasses.
Clear area of any hazards or hard objects.
Allow seizure to end without interference.
If vomiting occurs, try to turn child to one side as a unit.

After the seizure

Time postictal period.
Check for breathing. Check position of head and tongue.
 Reposition if head is hyperextended. If breathing is not present, give rescue breathing and call emergency medical service (EMS).
Check around mouth for evidence of burns or suspicious substances that might indicate poisoning.
Keep child on side.
Remain with child until full recovery.
Do not give food or liquids until fully alert and swallowing reflex has returned.
Call EMS when necessary.
Look for medical identification and determine what incidents occurred before onset of seizure and which may have been triggering factors.
Check head and body for possible injuries and fractures.
 Check inside of mouth to see whether tongue or lips have been bitten.

Complex partial seizure

During the seizure

Do not restrain unless in danger.
Remove harmful objects from path.
Redirect to safe area.
Do not agitate; instead, talk in calm, reassuring manner.
Do not expect child to follow instructions.
Watch to see whether seizure generalizes to tonic-clonic type.

After the seizure

Stay with child and reassure until fully conscious.

Call emergency medical service if:

Child stops breathing.
There is evidence of injury or youngster is diabetic or pregnant.
Seizure lasts for more than 5 minutes (unless duration is typically longer than 5 minutes as specified by medical orders).
Status epilepticus occurs.
Pupils are not equal in size after seizure.
Child vomits continuously 30 minutes after seizure has ended (sign of possible acute problem).
Child cannot be awakened and is unresponsive to pain after seizure has ended.
Seizure occurs in water (shock and aspiration may be delayed).
This is child's first seizure.

Modified from *Seizure recognition and first aid,* Landover, Md, 1989, Epilepsy Foundation of America.

BOX 48-16
Seizure Precautions

Extent of precautions depends on type, severity, and frequency of seizures

May include:

- Siderails raised when child is sleeping or resting
- Siderails and other hard objects padded
- Waterproof mattress/pad on bed/crib
- Appropriate precautions during potentially hazardous activities:
  - Swimming with a companion
  - Use of protective helmet and padding during bicycle riding, skate-boarding, in-line skating
  - Supervision during use of hazardous machinery/equipment

Have child carry or wear medical identification

Alert other caregivers to need for any special precautions

Identify and avoid triggering factors whenever possible

possible. Sending a child with a chronic seizure disorder home is not necessary, unless the parents request this.

Children who are known to have seizures or who are under observation for seizures will require some precautions. The extent of these measures depends on the type and frequency of the seizure (Box 48-16).

Long-term care. Care of the child with a recurrent convulsive disorder involves physical care and instruction regarding the importance of the drug therapy and, probably more significant, the problems related to the emotional aspects of the disorder. There are few diseases that generate as much anxiety among relatives as epilepsy. Fears and misconceptions about the disease and its treatment abound in the lay person's mind. For many it represents the archetype of severe hereditary affliction. Therefore the foci of nursing care are directed toward helping the child and the family to deal with the psychologic and sociologic problems related to the disorder and educating the child, the family, peers, and the public toward a more realistic and liberal view of the disease.

Children subject to seizures are placed on some type of drug therapy. The nurse can help the parents plan the administration of the medication at convenient times to minimize disruption to the family routine. The most convenient times for administration seem to be with meals or at bedtime. Although the antiepileptic drugs are available in liquid extracts or emulsions, the tablet form is preferred by neurologists. The unequal distribution of the drug in the solute and the increased likelihood of inaccurate measurements make liquid medication less desirable. For small children the tablet of the proper dosage can be crushed and administered in syrup, jelly, or other palatable substances.

Nursing ALERT

Children who are taking phenobarbital and/or phenytoin should receive adequate vitamin D and folic acid, since deficiencies of both have been associated with these anticonvulsants. Phenytoin should not be taken with milk.

It is important to impress on the family the need to continue the medication regularly without interruption for as long as required. The parents and the child will need to know the common side effects of the drug prescribed and observe for signs that might indicate unfavorable reactions.

Parents need to be warned of possible behavioral changes as the seizures are controlled in children who are taking primidone, phenobarbital, or phenytoin. Changes in personality, indifference to school activities and family, hyperactivity, or even psychotic behavior may sometimes be observed. The potential effects of antiepileptics on learning and behavior should be considered. Progressive intellectual deterioration in a child with epilepsy requires investigation of present medication plus the role of the underlying cerebral pathologic condition. Parents should notify the health professional if the child has an illness, including vomiting or fever. Vomiting can interfere with drug absorption; fever may increase metabolic requirements. Both can precipitate seizure activity.

Rectal preparations of some medications are highly useful and effective when a child is unable to take oral medications because of repeated vomiting, gastrointestinal surgery, or status epilepticus. Administration of rectal drugs can be learned by parents for home treatment during a seizure.* Rectal Ativan is useful adjunctive home treatment for children at risk for prolonged seizures. Hospitalization is minimized, and parental confidence enhanced (Camfield et al, 1989).

The degree to which activities are restricted is individualized for each child and depends on the type, frequency, and severity of the seizures; the child's response to therapy; and the length of time the seizures have been controlled. Normal healthy activities are encouraged for children, and participation in competitive sports is determined on an individual basis. With encouragement most older children can accept the restrictions placed on activities. Only essential restrictions regarding sports, automobile driving, and peer activity should be placed on children to reduce the likelihood of needlessly accentuating differences.

Because the child is encouraged to attend school, camp, and other normal activities, the school nurse and the teacher should be made aware of the child's condition and therapy. They can help to ensure regularity of medication and any special care the child may need. Teachers, child care providers, camp counselors, youth organization leaders, coaches, and other adults who assume responsibility for children should be instructed about care of the child during a seizure so that they can act in a calm manner to promote the welfare of the child and to influence the attitude of the child's peers.†

Triggering factors. Careful and detailed documentation of seizures over time may reveal a pattern. When this occurs the nurse or responsible adult may intervene to identify the triggering factors and make changes in the environment that may prevent seizures or decrease their frequency. Frequently the necessary changes are very simple and cost-free but can

*Home care instructions for administering oral and rectal medications are available in Wong DL: *Wong and Whaley's clinical manual of pediatric nursing*, ed 4, St Louis, 1996, Mosby.

†An excellent resource is *Students with seizures: a manual for school nurses* by N. Santilli, W.E. Dodson, and A.V. Walton (1991, Epilepsy Foundation of America).

Critical Thinking Q & A

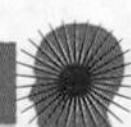

SEIZURES

Since age 2, Jane has had epilepsy that is well controlled with medication. However, now that she has begun elementary school, her seizures have returned. On the way home Jane usually has a seizure on the bus; however, on weekends and holidays she is seizure-free. As the school nurse, you advise Jane's parents to:

1. Take her for medical reevaluation.
2. Increase her antiepileptic medication.
3. Drive her home from school.
4. Ride with her on the school bus.

The correct answer is four. Your first priority is to help the family identify triggering events. At your suggestion Mrs. Little rode the school bus home with Jane. As the child began to seize, the mother noted that they had just passed a white picket fence, the triggering factor. Once the child was seated on the other side of the bus, the seizure episodes stopped.

With the consistent pattern and abrupt onset of the seizures, seeking medical reevaluation should be advised only if no triggering event is identified. It is not within the scope of nursing practice for you to change the dosage of the medication. Even if the child rides home in a car, the seizures may occur if Jane sits in the same position as on the school bus.

make an enormous difference in the child's and family's lives (see the Critical Thinking Q & A box above).

Factors that may trigger seizures in children include changes in dark-light patterns, such as those that occur with a flash on a camera, automobile headlights, walking by a picket fence, reflections of light on snow or water, or rotating blades on a fan; sudden loud noises; specific voices, songs, or nursery rhymes; startling or sudden movements; extreme or drastic changes in temperature; dehydration; fatigue; hyperventilation; hypoglycemia; caffeine; and insufficient protein in the diet (protein is needed to metabolize some antiepileptic drugs). Although there have been reports of seizures triggered by flashing video games, this relationship has not been confirmed by controlled studies. Seizures may be due to the length of playing time, which may cause sleep deprivation, fatigue, excitement, or photosensitivity (Ferrie et al, 1994). On the basis of current knowledge, the overwhelming majority of children with seizures can play video games without the risk of seizures.*

If a child is photosensitive, avoiding such things as wallpaper with stripes, a ceiling fan, and blinking lights and viewing the television screen from a distance of at least 2 meters, and covering one eye may be necessary.

Family support. Parental attitudes and management of a child with a seizure disorder are as varied as those of other parents of children with a chronic disorder, and they are subject to the same long-term problems (see Chapter 38). Whether the seizures result from illness, injury, or an unknown cause, the parents may feel guilt, anxiety, and often humiliation. They want to know whether the disorder will affect the child's mental capacities. To many persons epilepsy is erroneously associated with mental deficiency. Seizures do frequently accompany other manifestations of severe brain damage from disease or injury, but the majority of children with seizures, like any population of healthy children, display a wide range of intelligence.

Parents also wonder how the illness will affect the child's future and need reassurance that it will not shorten the life of the child and that the child can attend school, marry, and elect to have children. The child will need vocational guidance, and the parents should become familiar with the laws in their state regarding any limitations that might be imposed on the child because of the disorder. It should be emphasized that seizures can be controlled or greatly reduced in the majority of children and that new studies hold the promise of progress in future treatment. Parents also need reassurance that in this enlightened day and age there is less stigma attached to the disease than there was in the past.

It is important to encourage a healthy attitude toward the child and the disease and to help the parents feel competent in their ability to meet their responsibilities. The child should be reared as any normal child, with natural concern tempered by the understanding of the need not to be overprotective. Many parents refrain from correcting or punishing the child, especially if they have witnessed a seizure precipitated by such emotional stress. The child must not be made to feel different in any way. Parents should be encouraged to be honest and open about the disorder with the child and others. Some parents are tempted to conceal the nature of the child's illness because of their belief that the disorder is shameful or a disgrace to the family.

Restrictions on the child's activities will be necessary for safety, but this area can be approached in a positive way in terms of what the child *can* do rather than what the child cannot do. Sometimes parents curtail the child's activities more than necessary. The child needs to experience the maturing influences of play and work. The Epilepsy Foundation of America* is a national organization that works toward and for the welfare of persons with epilepsy and their families, helps with employment and legal problems, and provides education to patients, families, and communities.

The child with epilepsy. The child who is provided the security of a loving family, rewards and punishments no different from those of other children, and support in acquiring self-esteem is more likely to have a positive attitude toward the disease. Children derive their self-concept and self-esteem from observations of others' reactions to them and their own perception of their capabilities. The suddenness and unpredictability of seizures and the reactions of others further influence their feelings. When others consider children to be different, inferior, or objects of ridicule, they come to view themselves as different, inferior, and incapable.

Behavioral problems are common in children with epilepsy and can become more serious than the seizures. Much of the behavior difficulty, especially aggressive or delinquent behavior, has been attributed to the child's reaction to parental re-

*For more information on video games and epilepsy, contact the **Epilepsy Foundation of America**.

*4351 Garden City Drive, Landover, MD 20785; (301) 459-3700. In Canada: **Epilepsy Canada,** 1470 Peel St., Suite 745, Montreal, Quebec H3A 1T1; (514) 845-7855.

jection. Feelings of guilt, frustration, depression, and self-negation can contribute to antisocial behaviors.

Behavioral problems and school difficulties, such as dependency and underachievement, are common in children with epilepsy and can become more serious than the seizures (Vining, 1990). Children with epilepsy need to learn about their disease and the role that the medication plays in contributing to their prolonged well-being. As soon as they are old enough, children should assume responsibility for taking their own medication and be advised to carry medical identification with pertinent information about their condition. Planning activities with children and emphasizing those in which they can engage rather than those in which they cannot participate help them succeed and gain satisfaction in their achievements. They should be offered opportunities and encouraged to exercise judgment in their daily lives.

The adolescent period may prove to be a trying time for the child with epilepsy. Limits imposed on the young person's activities at a time when freedom and independence are desired may bring the disability into sharp focus. For example, some states do not allow persons with epilepsy to obtain a driver's license, even when the disease is controlled; in others there are restrictions on employment insurance.

Epilepsy should not be a severe impairment to most youngsters, and the nurse, by assuming the role of patient advocate, helping to educate the public about the disease, working toward making opportunities available to persons with the disorder, and lobbying for legislation that recognizes the needs of the individual with a seizure disorder, can help to erase the stigma that remains regarding the disease.

Evaluation

The effectiveness of nursing interventions for the child with epilepsy is determined by continual reassessment and evaluation of care based on the following observational guidelines and expected outcomes:

1. Observe child's behavior for evidence of seizure activity and assess the environment for situations that could cause injury to child in the event of a seizure; interview family regarding management of child during a seizure.
2. Interview child and family regarding compliance with the medication regimen and identification of triggering factors.
3. Observe and interview family regarding their feelings and concerns and their understanding of child's condition.
4. Observe child's interactions with others and interview child about any feelings or concerns about own health.

Expected outcomes:

1. Child exhibits no evidence of physical injury.
2. Family complies with instructions; child remains free of seizure activity.
3. Child exhibits no or minimal complications from medication.
4. Child and family identify triggering factors and make adjustments that diminish the frequency of seizure episodes.
5. Child expresses feelings and concerns and has a positive self-image.
6. Child and family demonstrate a healthy view of the disorder and alterations in life-style that it imposes.

See also the Nursing Care Plan: The Child with Epilepsy.*

FEBRILE SEIZURES

Febrile seizures are transient disorders of children that occur in association with a fever. They are one of the most common neurologic disorders of childhood, affecting about 4% of children. Most febrile seizures occur after 6 months of age and usually before age 3 years, with increased frequency in children younger than 18 months. They are unusual after 5 years of age. Boys are affected about twice as often as girls, and there is an increased susceptibility in families, indicating a possible genetic predisposition. Most febrile seizures are generalized and last less than 5 minutes (Farwell et al, 1994). About 30% to 40% of children will have one recurrence.

The cause of febrile seizures is still uncertain. In most children the height but not the rapidity of the temperature elevation seems to be a factor. The fever usually exceeds 38.8° C (101.8° F) and occurs during the temperature rise rather than after a prolonged elevation. Sometimes it constitutes the dramatic beginning of an illness. Febrile seizures usually accompany an upper respiratory or gastrointestinal infection. Although pertussis vaccine does not cause febrile seizures, this immunization is a precipitating factor in initial episodes of febrile seizures in children prone to having seizures (Cherry et al, 1993).

Most febrile seizures have stopped by the time the child is taken to a medical facility. However, if the seizure continues, treatment consists of controlling it with diazepam (Valium) and reducing the temperature by administration of acetaminophen. Antiepileptic prophylaxis may be considered for children who are experiencing a focal or prolonged seizure, neurologic abnormalities, afebrile seizures in a first-degree relative; whose age is younger than 1 year; and who are experiencing multiple seizures that occur within 24 hours. The febrile seizure tendency may be a fundamental marker of an individual's seizure threshold (Camfield, Camfield, and Gordon, 1994). Little risk of neurologic deficit, epilepsy, mental retardation, or altered behavior has been observed as a sequela of febrile seizures.

Parents need reassurance of the *benign* nature of febrile seizures (almost 95% of children with febrile seizures will not develop epilepsy or any neurologic damage). They should be told that their child is in no danger of dying during a febrile seizure. They also need education regarding protecting the child from harm and observing exactly what happens to the child during the event. Attempts to lower the temperature with acetaminophen or to use diazepam to prevent a seizure are of no benefit in most children (Uhari et al, 1995). Tepid sponge baths are ineffective in significantly lowering the temperature; the shivering effect further increases metabolic output; and cooling causes discomfort in the child.

*In Wong DL: *Wong and Whaley's clinical manual of pediatric nursing,* ed 4, St Louis, 1996, Mosby.

Nursing ALERT

If a febrile seizure lasts more than 10 minutes, parents should seek medical attention right away. Encourage them to drive carefully; a few extra minutes will not make any significant difference (Camfield and Camfield, 1993).

Cerebral Malformations

CRANIAL DEFORMITIES

In the normal newborn the cranial sutures are separated by membranous seams several millimeters wide. For the first few hours to 1 to 2 days after birth the cranial bones are highly mobile, allowing them to mold and slide over one another, adjusting the circumference of the head to accommodate to the changing shape and character of the birth canal. The principal sutures in the infant's skull are the sagittal, coronal, and lambdoidal sutures, and the major soft areas at the juncture of these sutures are the anterior and posterior fontanels.

After birth, growth of the skull bones occurs in a direction *perpendicular* to the line of the suture, and normal closure occurs in a regular and predictable order. Although there are wide variations in the age at which closure takes place in individual children, normally all sutures and fontanels are ossified by the following ages:

8 weeks—Posterior fontanel closed
6 months—Fibrous union of suture lines and interlocking of serrated edges
18 months—Anterior fontanel closed
12 years—Sutures unable to be separated by increased ICP

Solid union of all sutures is not completed until very late childhood.

Closure of a suture before the expected time inhibits the perpendicular growth. Since normal increase in brain volume requires expansion, the skull is forced to grow in a direction *parallel* to the fused suture. This alteration in skull growth always produces a distortion of the head shape when the underlying brain growth is normal. The small head with closed and normal shape is the result of deficient brain growth; the suture closure is secondary to this brain growth failure. Failure of brain growth is not secondary to suture closure.

Various types of cranial deformities are encountered in early infancy. These include the enlarged head with frontal protrusion (bossing) characteristic of hydrocephalus, the parietal bossing that is seen in chronic subdural hematoma, the small head, and a variety of skull deformities (Box 48-17). Some occur during prenatal development; in others, head circumference is usually within normal limits at birth, and the deviation from normal development becomes apparent with advancing age.

Prognosis. The majority of infants who have craniosynostosis have normal brain development. The exceptions are those genetic disorders that involve brain abnormality.

BOX 48-17
Cranial Deformities

Microcephaly—head circumference more than 2 standard deviations below average for age, sex, and gestation; caused by failure of brain development
Management—no treatment available
Craniosynostosis—premature closure of single or multiple sutures of the cranial vault, face, and base of skull
Scaphocephaly—premature closure of sagittal suture causes skull to become elongated in an anteroposterior direction with a high cranial vault and a subnormal transverse diameter
Brachycephaly—premature closure of the coronal sutures causes skull to become shortened in an anteroposterior direction with flattening of occiput and forehead
Oxycephaly—premature closure of both coronal and sagittal sutures causes an excessively high and narrow skull that tapers upward on all sides
Plagiocephaly—unilateral closure of one coronal or lambdoidal suture causes skull to become asymmetric
Craniofacial dysostosis (Crouzon disease)—premature closure of any or all cranial sutures, most frequently the coronal, and a typical facial deformity (widely spaced eyes, hypoplastic maxilla, and beaklike nose; tongue appears large and protruding; frequently with exophthalmos)
Management—surgical release of closed sutures; Crouzon disease—surgical correction of major facial deformities

Nursing Care Management

Nursing care of families in which there is a child with a cranial defect involves identifying children with deformities and referring them for evaluation. Since there is no therapy available for children with microcephaly, nursing care is directed toward helping parents adjust to rearing a child with brain damage (see Chapter 39).

The care for infants who benefit from surgery requires special emphasis on observation for signs of decreased hematocrit and hemoglobin because of the large blood loss during surgery (see the Family Focus box on p. 1616). A cardiac monitor may demonstrate a resting heart rate of 200. Nursing care includes observation for signs of hemorrhage, infection, pain, and swelling and parental education for suture care and safety. Surgical sutures should remain dry and intact. Parents need to observe for any signs of redness, drainage, or swelling and report any temperature greater than 38.4° C (101° F).

Early surgical management of craniosynostosis allows proper expansion of the brain and the creation of an acceptable appearance. Parents require special support and education during this time, especially from other parents whose infants have undergone similar operations (Richards, 1994). The nurse can serve as a liaison for this type of parental support.

HYDROCEPHALUS

Hydrocephalus is a condition caused by an imbalance in the production and absorption of CSF in the ventricular system. When production is greater than absorption, CSF accumu-

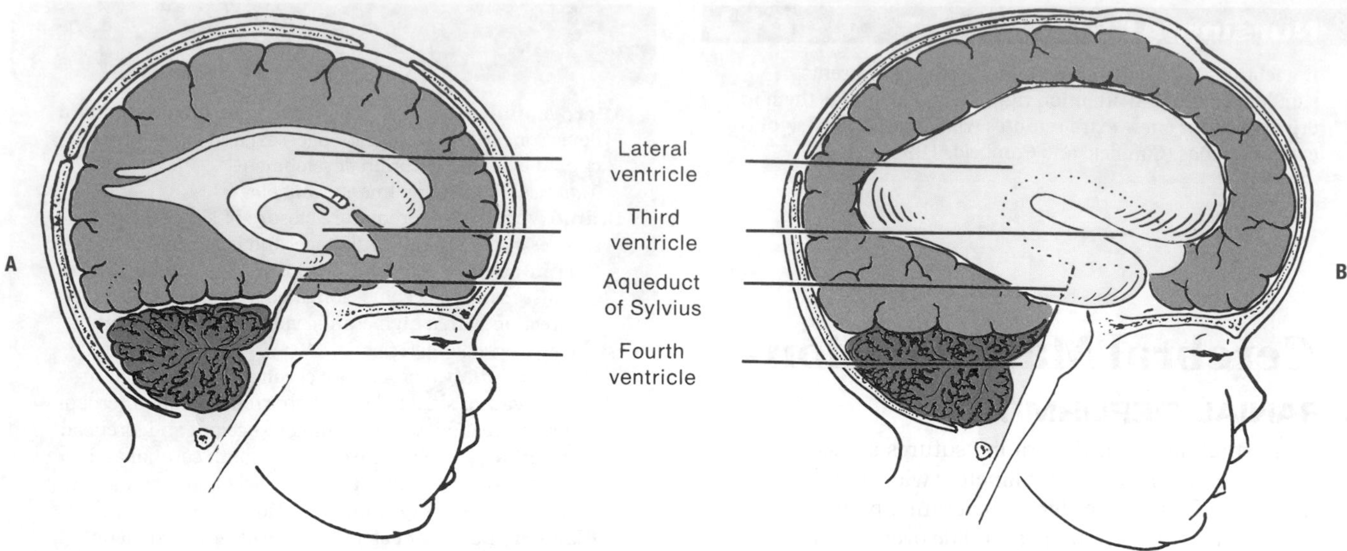

Fig. 48-7 Hydrocephalus: a block in the flow of CSF. **A,** Patent cerebrospinal fluid circulation; **B,** enlarged lateral and third ventricle caused by obstruction of circulation—stenosis of the aqueduct of Sylvius.

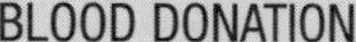

Family Focus

BLOOD DONATION

Parents may wish to provide a compatible blood donor for their infant who is undergoing a planned surgical correction for craniosynostosis. Nurses need to inform and guide parents through this blood bank procedure.

lates within the ventricular system, usually under increased pressure, producing passive dilation of the ventricles.

Pathophysiology

The two mechanisms by which CSF is formed include secretion by the choroid plexuses and lymphatic-like drainage by the extracellular fluid of the brain. CSF circulates throughout the ventricular system, then is absorbed within the subarachnoid spaces by a mechanism that is not entirely clear. Prenatal diagnosis is undoubtedly having an impact on the current prevalence at birth of hydrocephalus. The advent of MRI and CT scanning has provided valuable information about the pathophysiologic characteristics of various diseases. The cause may be either a congenital (maldevelopment or intrauterine infection) or acquired (neoplasm, hemorrhage, or infection) condition.

Hydrocephalus is a symptom of an underlying brain abnormality resulting in either (1) impaired absorption of CSF within the subarachnoid space (ventricles communicate: communicating hydrocephalus) or (2) obstruction to the flow of CSF within the ventricles (ventricles do not communicate: noncommunicating hydrocephalus). Any imbalance of secretion and absorption causes an increased accumulation of CSF in the ventricles, which become dilated and compress the brain substance against the surrounding rigid bony cranium. When this occurs before fusion of the cranial sutures, it produces enlargement of the skull, as well as dilation of the ventricles (Fig. 48-7). In children under 10 to 12 years of age, previously closed suture lines, especially the sagittal suture, may become diastatic or opened (Swaiman, 1994).

Most cases of noncommunicating hydrocephalus are a result of developmental malformations. Although the defect usually is apparent in early infancy, it may become evident at any time from the prenatal period to late childhood or early adulthood. Other causes include neoplasms, infections, and trauma. An obstruction to the normal flow can occur at any point in the CSF pathway to produce increased pressure and dilation of the pathways proximal to the site of obstruction.

Developmental defects—for example, Arnold-Chiari malformations (ACMs), aqueduct stenosis, aqueduct gliosis, and atresia of the foramina of Luschka and Magendie (Dandy-Walker syndrome)—account for most cases of hydrocephalus from birth to 2 years of age. Hydrocephalus is so often associated with myelomeningocele that all such infants should be observed for its development. In the remainder of cases there is a history of intrauterine infection, perinatal hemorrhage, and neonatal meningoencephalitis. In older children hydrocephalus is most often the result of space-occupying lesions, intracranial infections, hemorrhage, or preexisting developmental defects, such as aqueduct stenosis or the *Arnold-Chiari malformation* (a congenital anomaly in which the cerebellum and medulla oblongata extend down through the foramen magnum).

Diagnostic Evaluation

The two factors that influence the clinical picture in hydrocephalus are the time of onset and the presence of preexisting structural lesions. In infancy, before closure of the cranial sutures, head enlargement is the predominant sign, whereas in

BOX 48-18
Clinical Manifestations of Hydrocephalus

Infancy, early

Abnormally rapid head growth
Bulging fontanels (especially anterior) sometimes without head enlargement:
- Tense
- Nonpulsatile

Dilated scalp veins
Separated sutures
Macewen sign ("cracked-pot" sound) on percussion
Thinning of skull bones

Infancy, later

Frontal enlargement or "bossing"
Depressed eyes
"Setting sun" sign (sclera visible above the iris)
Pupils sluggish, with unequal response to light

Infancy, general

Irritability
Lethargy
Infant cries when picked up or rocked and quiets when allowed to lie still
Early infantile reflex acts may persist
Normally expected responses fail to appear
May display:
- Change in level of consciousness
- Opisthotonos (often extreme)
- Lower extremity spasticity

Advanced cases:
- Difficulty in sucking and feeding
- Shrill, brief, high-pitched cry
- Cardiopulmonary embarrassment

Childhood

Headache on awakening; improvement after emesis or upright posture
Papilledema
Strabismus
Extrapyramidal tract signs (e.g., ataxia)
Irritability
Lethargy
Apathy
Confusion
Often incoherence

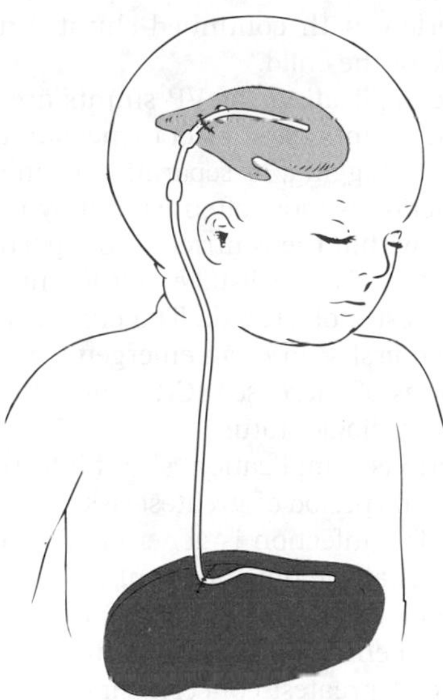

Fig. 48-8 Ventricular peritoneal shunt. Catheter is threaded subcutaneously from small incisions at the sites of ventricular and peritoneal insertions.

older infants and children the lesions responsible for hydrocephalus produce other neurologic signs through pressure on adjacent structures before causing CSF obstruction (Box 48-18).

In infancy the diagnosis of hydrocephalus is based on head circumference that crosses one or more grid lines on the measurement chart within a period of 2 to 4 weeks and on associated neurologic signs that are present and progressive. However, other diagnostic studies are needed to localize the site of CSF obstruction. Routine daily head circumference measurements are carried out in infants with myelomeningocele and intracranial infections. In evaluation of a premature infant, specially adapted head circumference charts are consulted to distinguish abnormal head growth from rapid head growth that takes place normally.

The signs and symptoms in early to late childhood are caused by increased ICP, and specific manifestations are related to the focal lesion. Most commonly resulting from posterior fossa neoplasms and aqueduct stenosis, the clinical manifestations are primarily those associated with space-occupying lesions.

The primary diagnostic tools for detecting hydrocephalus are CT and MRI. Sedation is required, since the child must remain absolutely still for an accurate picture to be produced. Diagnostic evaluation of children who have symptoms of hydrocephalus after infancy is similar to that used in those with suspected intracranial tumor. In the neonate echoencephalography is useful in comparing the ratio of lateral ventricle to cortex.

Therapeutic Management

The treatment of hydrocephalus is directed toward (1) relief of the hydrocephalus, (2) treatment of complications, and (3) management of problems related to the effect of the disorder on psychomotor development. The treatment is, with few exceptions, surgical. This is accomplished by direct removal of an obstruction (such as a tumor) or a shunt procedure that provides primary drainage of the CSF from the ventricles to an extracranial compartment, usually the peritoneum (ventricular peritoneal [VP] shunt) (Fig. 48-8).

Most shunt systems consist of a ventricular catheter, a flush pump, a unidirectional flow valve, and a distal catheter. In all models the valves are designed to open at a predetermined intraventricular pressure and close when the pressure falls below that level, thus preventing backflow of secretions.

The initial shunt is placed when necessary to relieve CSF obstruction, and revisions are needed when there are signs of malfunction. In all mechanisms the initial success rate is relatively high; however, shunts are associated with complications that interfere with continued shunt function or that threaten the life of the child.

The major complications of VP shunts are infection and malfunction. All shunts are subject to mechanical difficulties, such as kinking, plugging, or separation or migration of the tubing. Malfunction is most often caused by mechanical obstruction either within the ventricles from particulate matter (tissue or exudate) or at the distal end from thrombosis or displacement as a result of growth. The child with a shunt obstruction is often first seen in an emergency room with clinical manifestations of increased ICP, frequently accompanied by worsening neurologic status.

The most serious complication, shunt infection, can occur at any time, but the period of greatest risk is 1 to 2 months after placement. The infection is generally the result of intercurrent infections at the time of shunt placement. Infections include septicemia, bacterial endocarditis, wound infection, shunt nephritis, meningitis, and ventriculitis. Meningitis and ventriculitis are of greatest concern, since any complicating CNS infection is a significant predictor of intellectual outcome. Infection is treated with massive doses of antibiotics administered by the intravenous route. A persistent infection requires removal of the shunt until the infection is controlled. EVD is used until CSF is sterile.

Prognosis. The prognosis of children with treated hydrocephalus depends largely on the rate at which hydrocephalus develops, the duration of raised ICP, the frequency of complications, and the cause of the hydrocephalus. For example, malignant tumors may have a high mortality rate regardless of other complicating factors.

Surgically treated hydrocephalus with continued neurosurgical and medical management has a survival rate of about 80%, with the highest incidence of mortality occurring within the first year of treatment. Of the surviving children approximately one third are both intellectually and neurologically normal, and one half have neurologic disabilities.

Nursing Care Management

Assessment

Preoperatively the infant with diagnosed or suspected hydrocephalus is observed carefully for signs of increasing ICP. In infants the head is measured daily at the point of largest measurement—the occipitofrontal circumference (OFC) (see Head Circumference, Chapter 22, for technique). Fontanels and suture lines are gently palpated for size, signs of bulging, tenseness, and separation. An infant with normal ICP will display bulging under certain circumstances such as straining or crying; therefore such accompanying behavior should be noted. Irritability, lethargy, or seizure activity, as well as altered vital signs and feeding behavior, may indicate an advancing pathologic condition.

In older children, who are usually admitted to the hospital for elective or emergency shunt revision, the most valuable indicator of increasing ICP is an alteration in the child's LOC and the way in which the child interacts with the environment. Changes are identified by observation and by comparison of present behavior with customary behavior, sleep patterns, developmental capabilities, and habits, all obtained through a detailed history and a baseline assessment. This baseline information serves as a guide for postoperative assessment and evaluation of shunt function.

BOX 48-19
Nursing Diagnoses: The Child With Hydrocephalus

Risk for altered neurologic function related to increased ICP
Risk for infection related to presence of mechanical drainage system
Risk for impaired skin integrity related to pressure areas, paralysis, relaxed anal sphincter
Altered family processes related to situational crisis (child with a physical defect)

Nursing Diagnoses

After a thorough assessment, nursing diagnoses become apparent. These include, but are not limited to, those listed in Box 48-19.

Planning

The goals of care of the child with hydrocephalus and family include the following:

1. Child will experience no complications of hydrocephalus and/or corrective surgery.
2. The family will receive adequate education and emotional support.

Implementation

General nursing care of the infant with hydrocephalus may present special problems. Maintaining adequate nutrition often requires flexible feeding schedules to accommodate diagnostic procedures, since feeding before or after handling can precipitate an episode of vomiting. Small feedings at more frequent intervals are often better tolerated than are larger ones spaced further apart. These infants are often difficult to feed and require extra time and innovation.

The nurse is responsible for preparing the child for diagnostic tests such as tomography and for assisting the physician with procedures such as a ventricular tap, which is often performed to relieve excessive pressure during the preoperative period and for CSF examination. Sedation is required, since the child must remain absolutely still during diagnostic testing. Intravenous pentobarbital or oral chloral hydrate is commonly used for these procedures. (See Chapter 42 for preparing children for procedures.)

Nursing ALERT

If surgery is anticipated, intravenous infusions should not be placed in a scalp vein on a child with hydrocephalus.

Fortunately, almost all affected children are recognized, and treatment is begun early. For those children with significant head enlargement, care must be exercised to see that the head is well supported when the infant is fed or moved to prevent extra strain on the infant's neck, and measures must be taken to prevent development of pressure areas. As the hydrocephalus progresses, untreated children become increasingly helpless and prone to the multiple problems of immobility (e.g., pressure sores and contracture deformities). Not infrequently infants with irreversible brain damage or with severe developmental defects such as hydranencephaly, in which both cerebral hemispheres fail to develop and are replaced with a membranous sac filled with cerebrospinal fluid, are placed in long-term facilities for care.

Postoperative care. Routine postoperative care and observation are instituted. In addition, the infant or child is positioned carefully on the unoperated side to prevent pressure on the shunt valve and pressure areas. The child is kept flat to help avert complications resulting from too rapid reduction of intracranial fluid. When the ventricular size is reduced too rapidly, the cerebral cortex may pull away from the dura and tear the small interlacing veins, producing a subdural hematoma. This is not a problem in children with elective shunt revision, since their intraventricular size and pressure have been normal. The surgeon indicates the position to be maintained and the extent of activity allowed. If there is increased ICP, the surgeon will prescribe elevation of the head of the bed and/or that the child be allowed to sit up to enhance gravity flow through the shunt. Pain management can usually be achieved with acetaminophen with or without codeine for mild to moderate pain and opioids for severe pain (see Chapter 41 for pain management).

Observation for signs of increased ICP, which indicates obstruction of the shunt, is continued. Neurologic assessment includes evaluation of pupil dilation (pressure causes compression or stretching of the oculomotor nerve, producing dilation on the same side as the pressure) and blood pressure (hypoxia to the brainstem causes variability in these vital signs).

Nursing ALERT

Never pump the shunt to assess function, because this may pull choroid plexuses into the ventricular slits, resulting in blockage; cause headache by decreasing CSF; or obstruct the peritoneal end of the catheter.

The child is also observed for abdominal distention, because CSF may cause peritonitis or a postoperative ileus as a complication of distal catheter placement. In addition, intake and output are carefully monitored. Children may be placed on fluid restriction with nothing by mouth (NPO) for 24 hours. The intravenous infusion is closely monitored to prevent fluid overload. Routine feeding is resumed after the prescribed NPO period, but the presence of bowel sounds is determined before feeding children with VP shunts.

Since infection is the greatest hazard of the postoperative period, nurses are continually on the alert for the usual manifestations of CSF infection, which may include elevated vital signs, poor feeding, vomiting, decreased responsiveness, and seizure activity. There may be signs of local inflammation at the operative sites and along the shunt tract. The child's diaper should be kept off the peritoneal dressing site or suture line. Antibiotics are administered by the intravenous route as ordered, and the nurse may also need to assist the physician with intraventricular instillation. The incision site is inspected for leakage, and any suspected drainage is tested for glucose, an indication of cerebrospinal fluid.

Meticulous skin care is continued postoperatively, with extra care taken to prevent tissue damage from pressure. A pressure-reducing mattress or overlay pad underneath the child helps prevent pressure on prominent areas. Skin is inspected regularly for any signs of pressure, irritation, or infection.

Family support. Specific needs and concerns of parents during periods of hospitalization are related to the reason for the child's hospitalization (shunt revision, infection, diagnosis) and the diagnostic and/or surgical procedures to which the child must be subjected. Often parents have very little understanding of anatomy; therefore they need further exploration and reinforcement of information that was given to them by the physician and neurosurgeon, as well as information about what they can expect. They are especially frightened of any procedure that involves the brain, and the fear of retardation or brain damage is very real and pervasive. Nurses can do much to allay their anxiety by explaining the rationale underlying the various nursing and medical activities such as positioning or testing, and by simply being available and willing to listen to their concerns.

To prepare for the child's discharge and home care, the parents are instructed on how to recognize signs that indicate shunt malfunction or infection and how to pump the shunt, if necessary. Active children may have accidents, such as a fall, that can damage the shunt, and the tubing may pull out of the distal insertion site or become disconnected during normal growth.

Safe transportation is an essential issue to discuss with parents. The tendency for the enlarged head to fall forward and to turn to the side, combined with poor head control, influences the type of child restraint system needed. Small infants can be restrained reclining in an approved car restraint bed.*

The management of hydrocephalus in a child is a demanding task for both family and health professionals, and helping a family cope with the child is an important nursing responsibility. It is important to emphasize that hydrocephalus is a lifelong problem and that the child will require evaluation on a regular basis. The overall aim is to establish realistic goals and an appropriate educational program that will assist the child to achieve his or her optimal potential.

Anticipatory guidance will prepare parents for possible problems and help them to avoid being overprotective of the child. There need be few restrictions (mainly contact sports) placed on the child's activities, and the child should be encouraged to live as would any other child of the same age and abilities. Parents need support and encouragement in coping with the child and with problems the child may encounter in relationships with peers and others. Reactions of other children when the child has a noticeably enlarged head or re-

*Information on restraints for children with special needs is available from **Automotive Safety for Children Program,** Riley Hospital for Children, 534 N. Clinical Dr., Rm. 118, Indianapolis, IN 46202-5109; (317) 274-2977 or (800) KID-N-CAR (in Indiana).

quires shaving at the times of revision are stressful for both child and parents (see Chapter 38 for a discussion on problems and coping with the child with a disability).

Families can be referred to community agencies for support and guidance. The National Hydrocephalus Foundation (NHF)* provides information on the condition for families and assists interested groups in establishing local organizations. Helpful booklets are available from this and other sources.

Evaluation

The effectiveness of nursing interventions is determined by continual reassessment and evaluation of care based on the following:

*Route 1, River Rd., Box 210 A, Joliet, IL 60436; (800) 431-8093.

Observational guidelines:

1. Monitor child's neurologic status (physical signs and behavior), take temperature, examine skin at points of pressure.
2. Interview family regarding their feelings and concerns.

Expected outcomes:

1. Child remains free from complications of the disorder and surgical correction.
2. Family discusses their feelings and concerns regarding child's condition.

See also the Nursing Care Plan: The Child with Hydrocephalus.*

*In Wong DL: *Wong and Whaley's clinical manual of pediatric nursing,* ed 4, St Louis, 1996, Mosby

Key Points

- Level of consciousness (LOC) is the most important indicator of neurologic health; altered levels include full consciousness, confusion, disorientation, lethargy, obtundation, stupor, coma, and persistent vegetative state.
- Complete neurologic examination includes LOC; posture; motor, sensory, cranial nerve, and reflex testing; and vital signs.
- Nursing care of the unconscious child focuses on respiratory management, neurologic assessment, intracranial pressure (ICP) monitoring, adequate nutrition and hydration, drug therapy, promotion of elimination, hygienic care, positioning and exercise, stimulation, and family support.
- Fractures resulting from head injuries may be classified as depressed, compound, basilar, and diastatic.
- Primary head injury involves features that occur at the time of trauma, including fractured skull, contusions, intracranial hematoma, and diffuse injury. Secondary complications include hypoxic brain damage, increased ICP, infection, cerebral edema, and posttraumatic syndromes.
- The young child's response to head injury is different because of the following features: larger head size, expandable skull, larger amount of blood volume to the brain, small subdural spaces, and thinner, softer brain tissue.
- Problems resulting from near-drowning include hypoxia and asphyxiation, aspiration, and hypothermia.
- Nursing care of the child with a brain tumor includes observing for signs and symptoms related to the tumor, preparing the child and family for diagnostic tests and operative procedures, preventing postoperative complications, planning for discharge, and promoting a return to optimal health.
- Nursing care of the child with meningitis includes administration of antibiotics, prevention of self-infection, removal of environmental stimuli, correct positioning, vital sign monitoring, intravenous therapy, and promotion of fluid, nutritional status, and supportive care of the family.
- Routine immunization of infants against *H. influenzae* type B infection has reduced the incidence of bacterial meningitis.
- Encephalitis may result from direct invasion of the central nervous system by a virus or from involvement of the central nervous system after viral disease.
- A seizure is a symptom of underlying abnormality and may be manifest by sensory-hallucinatory phenomena, motor effects, sensorimotor effects, and loss of consciousness.
- Partial seizures are categorized as simple (without associated impairment of consciousness) or complex (with impaired consciousness); both types may become generalized.
- Generalized seizures are categorized as tonic-clonic (convulsive), absence, atonic and akinetic, myoclonic, and infantile spasms.
- Long-term care of the child with recurrent seizure disorders includes physical care and education regarding the importance of drug therapy and problems related to emotional aspects of the disorder.
- Febrile seizures are frightening to parents but are usually benign events that do not require antipyretic or antiepileptic therapy.
- Many cranial deformities are amenable to surgical correction.
- Hydrocephalus is a symptom of an underlying brain abnormality, demonstrated by impaired absorption of cerebrospinal fluid (CSF) or obstruction to the flow of CSF within the ventricles.
- Therapy for hydrocephalus involves relief of the hydrocephalus, treatment of the underlying brain abnormality if possible, prevention and/or treatment of complications, and management of problems related to psychomotor development.

References

American Academy of Pediatrics: Perinatal human immunodeficiency virus testing, *Pediatrics* 95(2):303-307, 1995.

Baevsky RH, Bartfield JM: Human rabies: a review, *Am J Emerg Med* 11(3):279-286, 1993.

Barkovich AJ: *Techniques and methods in pediatric imaging.* In Barkovich AJ editor: *Pediatric neuroimaging,* New York, 1990, Raven Press.

Bonadio W, Wagner V: Adrenaline-cocaine gel topical anesthetic for dermal laceration repair in children, *Ann Emerg Med* 21(12):1435-1438, 1992.

Booy R, Kroll S: Bacterial meningitis in children, *Curr Opin Pediatr* 6(1):29-35, 1994.

Bratton SL, Jardine DS, Morray JP: Serial neurological examinations after near drowning and outcome, *Arch Pediatr* 148(2):167-70, 1994.

Brodie MJ: Established anticonvulsants and treatment of refractory epilepsy, *Lancet* 336(8711):350-354, 1990.

Brown LW, Feigin RD: Bacterial meningitis: fluid balance and therapy, *Pediatr Ann* 23(2):93-98, 1994.

Bruce D: *Head trauma.* In Eichelberger, editor: *Pediatric trauma: prevention, acute care, rehabilitation,* St Louis, 1993, Mosby.

Camfield CS et al: Home use of rectal diazepam to prevent status epilepticus in children with convulsive disorders, *J Child Neurol* 4:125-126, 1989.

Camfield CS, Camfield PR: Febrile seizures: an Rx for parent fears and anxiety, *Contemp Pediatr* 10(4):26-44, 1993.

Camfield PR, Camfield CS, Gordon K: What types of epilepsy are preceded by febrile seizures, *Dev Med Child Neurol* 36(10):887-892, 1994.

Cherry JD et al: Pertussis immunization and characteristics related to first seizures in infants and children, *J Pediatr* 122(6):900-903, 1993.

Dieckmann RA: Rectal diazepam for prehospital pediatric status epilepticus, *Ann Emerg Med* 23:216-224, 1994.

Duffner PK, Cohen ME: The long-term effects of CNS therapy on children with brain tumors, *Neurol Clin* 9:479-495, 1991.

Duffner PK et al: Postoperative chemotherapy and delayed radiation in children less than three years of age with malignant brain tumors, *N Engl J Med* 328:1725-1733, 1993.

Ernst AA et al: Lidocaine adrenaline tetracaine gel versus tetracaine adrenaline cocaine gel for topical anesthesia in linear scalp and facial lacerations in children aged 5 to 17 years, *Pediatrics* 95(2):255-258, 1995.

Farwell JR et al: First febrile seizures: characteristics of the child, the seizure, and the illness, *Clin Pediatr* 33(5):263-267, 1994.

Ferrie CD et al: Video-game epilepsy, *Lancet* 344(8938):1710-1711, 1994.

Heideman RL et al: *Tumors of the central nervous system.* In Pizzo PA, Poplack DG, editor: *Principles and practice of pediatric oncology,* ed 2, Philadelphia, 1993, JP Lippincott.

Kyriacou DN, Arcinue EL, Peek C: Effects of immediate resuscitation on children with submersion injury, *Pediatrics* 123:137-142, 1994.

Medical Research Council Antiepileptic Drug Withdrawal Study Group: Prognostic index for recurrence of seizures after remission of epilepsy, *Br Med J* 306:1374-1378, 1993.

Murphy SB et al: Consensus statement from the American Cancer Society Workshop on Neuroblastoma Screening: Do children benefit from mass screening for neuroblastoma? *CA* 41(4):227-230, 1991.

Murphy TV et al: Declining incidence of *Haemophilus influenzae* type b disease since introduction of vaccination, *JAMA* 269(2):246-248, 1993.

Quam DA: Recognizing a case of Reye's syndrome, *Am Fam Physician* 15(7):1491-1496, 1994.

Raccoon rabies epizootic-United States, 1993, *MMWR* 43(15):269-270, 1994.

Reynolds E: Controversies in caring for the child with a head injury, *Am J Matern Care Nurs* 17:246-251, 1992.

Richards MD: Common pediatric craniofacial reconstructions, *Nurs Clin North Am* 29(4):791-799, 1994.

Sagraves R: Antiepileptic drug therapy for pediatric generalized tonic-clonic seizures, *J Pediatr Health Care* 4(6):314-319, 1990.

Swaiman KF: *Pediatric neurology: principles and practice,* ed 2, St Louis, 1994, Mosby.

Thorne RN, Pearson AD, Nicoll JA: Decline in incidence of medulloblastoma in children, *Cancer* 74(12):4350-4354, 1994.

Uhari M et al: Effect of acetaminophen and of low intermittent doses of diazepam on prevention of recurrences of febrile seizures, *J Pediatr* 126(6):991-995, 1995.

van Donselaar CA, Geerts AT, Schimscheimer RJ: Usefulness of an aura for classification of a first generalized seizure, *Epilepsia* 31(5):529-535, 1990.

Verity CM, Ross EM, Golding J: Outcome of childhood status epilepticus and lengthy febrile convulsions: findings of national cohort study, *Br Med J* 307:225-228, 1993.

Vining E: The psychosocial impact of epilepsy in children and their families, *Int Pediatr* 5(2):186-188, 1990.

Wald E et al: Dexamethasone therapy for children with bacterial meningitis, *Pediatrics* 95(1):21-28, 1995.

Bibliography

General

Ashwal S, Eyman RK, Call TL: Life expectancy of children in a persistent vegetative state, *Pediatr Neurol* 10(1):27-33, 1994.

Blevins SH, Benson S: A better way to get kids through scans, *RN* 55(10):40-44, 1992.

Fields AI, Coble DH, Pollack MM: Outcomes of children in a persistent vegetative state, *Crit Care Med* 21(12):1890-1894, 1993.

Hollman GA, Elderbrook MK, VanDenLangenberg B: Results of a pediatric sedation program on head MRI scan success rates and procedure duration times, *Clinical Pediatr* 34:300-305, 1995.

Multi-Society Task Force on PVS: Medical aspects of the persistent vegetative state, *N Engl J Med* 330(22):1572-1579, 1994.

Rushton CH, Hogue EE: When parents demand everything, *Pediatr Nurs* 19(2):180-183, 1993.

Sips HJ, Catsman-Berrevoets CE, van Dongen HR: Measuring right-hemisphere dysfunction in children, *Dev Med Child Neurol* 36(1):57-63, 1994.

Increased Intracranial Pressure

Cotton MR, Donald PR, Schoeman JF: Raised intracranial pressure, the syndrome of inappropriate ADH, *Childs Nerv Syst* 9(1):10-15, 1993.

Gambardella G, Zaccone C, Cardia E: Intracranial pressure monitoring in children: comparison of external ventricular device with fiberoptic system, *Childs Nerv Syst* 9(8):470-473, 1993.

Longatti PL, Carteri A: Active singling out of shunt independence, *Childs Nerv Syst* 10(5):334-336, 1994.

Shankaran S, Woldt E, Bedard MP: Feasibility of invasive monitoring of intracranial pressure, *Brain Dev* 16(2):121-125, 1994.

Bibliography

Taylor GA, Phillips MD, Ichord RN: Intracranial compliance in infants, *Radiology* 191(3):787-791, 1994.

Zaritsky A: Outcome of pediatric cardiopulmonary resuscitation, *Crit Care Med* 21(9):325-327, 1993.

Head Injury

Appleton R: Head injury rehabilitation of children, *Nurs Times* 90(22):39-41, 1994.

Brown JK, Minns RA: Non-accidental head injury, *Dev Med Child Neurol* 35(10):849-869, 1993.

Davis RL, Mullen N, Makela M: Cranial CT scans in children after minimal head injury with loss of consciousness, *Ann Emerg Med* 24(4):640-645, 1994.

Greenspan AI, MacKenzie EJ: Functional outcome after pediatric head injury, *Pediatrics* 94(4):425-432, 1994.

Hoekelman RA: A pediatrician's view: why deaths from head injuries are on the decline, *Pediatr Ann* 23(1):8-10, 1994.

Kaufman BA, Dacey RG: Acute care management of closed head injury in childhood, *Pediatr Ann* 23(1):18-20, 1994.

Kaufman PM, Fletcher JM, Levin HS: Attentional disturbance after pediatric closed head injury, *J Child Neurol* 8(4):348-353, 1993.

Nazarian LF: When parents become critical observers, *Pediatr Rev* 14(8):299-301, 1993.

Weiss BS: Bicycle-related head injuries, *Clin Sports Med* 13(1):99-112, 1994.

Near-Drowning

Fredrickson JM, Fauer W, Arellano D: Emergency nurses' perceived knowledge and comfort levels regarding pediatric patients, *J Emerg Nurs* 20(1):13-17, 1994.

Kallas HJ, O'Rourke PP: Drowning and immersion injuries in children, *Curr Opin Pediatr* 5(3):295-302, 1993.

Kemp AM, Mott Am, Sibert JR: Accidents and child abuse in bathtub submersions, *Arch Dis Child* 70(5):435-438, 1994.

Kriel RL, Krach LE, Luxenberg MG: Outcome of severe anoxic - ischemic brain injury in children, *Pediatr Neurol* 10(3):207-212, 1994.

Lavell JM, Shaw KN: Near drowning, *Crit Care Med* 21(3):368-373, 1993.

Norris MK: Pediatric near drowning, *Nursing* 23(5):33, 1993.

Walsh EA, Ioli JG: Childhood near-drowning: nursing care and primary prevention, *Pediatr Nurs* 20(3):265-269, 292, 1994.

Central Nervous System Tumors

Allen JC: What we learn from infants with brain tumors, *N Engl J Med* 328(24):1780-1781, 1993.

Bucholtz J: Issues concerning the sedation of children for radiation therapy, *Oncol Nurs Forum* 19(4):649-655, 1992.

Cullen PM: Pharmacologic supportive care of children with central nervous system tumors, *J Pediatr Oncol Nurs* 12(4):230-232, 1995.

Green DM, D'Angio GJ: Late effects of treatment for childhood cancer, *J Pediatr Oncol Nurs* 10(1):40-42, 1993.

Lew CM, LaVally B: The role of stereotactic radiation therapy in the management of children with brain tumors, *J Pediatr Oncol Nurs* 12(4):212-222, 1995.

Moore IM: Central nervous system toxicity of cancer therapy in children, *J Pediatr Oncol Nurs* 12(4):203-210, 1995.

Shiminski-Maher T, Shields M: Pediatric brain tumors: diagnosis and management, *J Pediatr Oncol Nurs* 12(4):188-198, 1995.

Intracranial Infections

American Academy of Pediatrics, Committee on Infectious Disease: Dexamethasone therapy for bacterial meningitis in infants and children, *Pediatrics* 86(1):130-133, 1990.

Ashwal S, Perkin RM, Thompson JR: Bacterial meningitis in children, *Adv Pediatr* 40:185-215,1993.

Carno M: Meningococcemia: recognizing and reducing complications in pediatric patients, *AACN Clin Iss Crit Care Nurs* 5(3):278-288, 1994.

Dodge PR: Neurological sequelae of acute bacterial meningitis, *Pediatr Ann* 23(2):101-106, 1994.

Green PA, Singh KV, Murray BE: Recurrent group B streptococcal infections in infants, *J Pediatr* 125(6):931-938, 1994.

Jenkins T: Fulminant meningococcemia in pediatric patients: nursing considerations, *Pediatr Nurs* 18:629-634, 1992.

Klein JO: Antimicrobial treatment and prevention of meningitis, *Pediatr Ann* 23(2):76-81, 1994.

Oliver LG, Harwood-Nuss AL: Bacterial meningitis in infants and children: a review, *J Emerg Med* 11(5):555-564, 1993.

Pavlakis SG, Frank Y, Nocyze M: Acquired immunodeficiency syndrome and the developing nervous system, *Adv Pediatr* 41:427-451, 1994.

Poss WB, Vernon DD, Dean JM: A reemergence of Reye's syndrome, *Arch Pediatr Adolesc Med* 148(8):879-882, 1994.

Epilepsy

Austin JK: Predicting parental anticonvulsant medication compliance, *J Pediatr Nurs* 4:88-95, 1989.

Austin JK, McDermott N: Parental attitude and coping behavior in families of children with epilepsy, *J Neurosci Nurs* 20:174-179, 1988.

Carter JR: The use of new antiepileptic medications in pediatric patients with epilepsy, *J Pediatr Health Care* 8(6):277-282, 1994.

Commission on Classification and Terminology of the International League Against Epilepsy, *Epilepsia* 30:389-399, 1989.

Maytal J et al: Low morbidity and mortality of status epilepticus in children, *Pediatrics* 83:323-331, 1989.

Meldrum BS: Anatomy, physiology, and pathology of epilepsy, *Lancet* 336:231-234, 1990.

Bibliography

National Institutes of Health Consensus Conference: Surgery for epilepsy, *JAMA* 264(6):729-733, 1990.

Pellock JM: Efficacy and adverse effects of antiepileptic drugs, *Pediatr Clin North Am* 36:435-448, 1989.

Pellock JM: Recent advances concerning status epilepticus, *Int Pediatr* 5(2):189-196, 1990.

Santilli N, Dodson WE, Walton AV: *Students with seizures: a manual for school nurses*, Landover, Md, 1991, Epilepsy Foundation of America.

Scheuer ML, Pedley TA: The evaluation and treatment of seizures, *N Engl J Med* 323(21):1468-1474, 1990.

Shorvon SD: Epidemiology, classification, natural history, and genetics of epilepsy, *Lancet* 336:93-96, 1990.

Status epilepticus—the first hour is critical, *Emerg Med* 24(8):181-184, 1992.

Vining EP: Educational, social, and life-long effects of epilepsy, *Pediatr Clin North Am* 36:449-461, 1989.

Ziemba SK: Seizures, *Am J Nurs* 95(2):32-33, 1995.

Febrile Seizures

Berg AT: Are febrile seizures provoked by a rapid rise in temperature? *Am J Dis Child* 147:1101-1103, 1993.

Camfield PR et al: Prevention of recurrent febrile seizures, *J Pediatr* 126(6):929-930, 1995.

Farwell JR, Blackner G, Sulzbacher S: First febrile seizures, *Clin Pediatr* 33(5):263-267, 1994.

Offringa M, Bossuyt PM, Lubsen J: Risk factors for seizure recurrence in children with febrile seizures, *J Pediatr* 124(4):574-584, 1994.

Smith MC: Febrile seizures: recognition and management, *Drugs* 47(6):933-944, 1994.

Stenklyft PH, Carmona M: Febrile seizures, *Emerg Med Clin North Am* 12(4):989-999, 1994.

Van-Esch A, Steyerberg EW, Berger MY: Family history and recurrence of febrile seizures, *Arch Dis Child* 70(5):395-399, 1994.

Cranial Deformities/Hydrocephalus

Bragg CL, Edwards-Beckett J, Eckle N: Shunt dysfunction and constipation, *J Neurosci Nurs* 26(2):91-94, 1994.

Hockley AD: Craniosynostosis, *Lancet* 342(8865):189-190, 1993.

Jackson PL: Primary care needs of children with hydrocephalus, *J Pediatr Health Care*, 4:59-71, 1990.

Kontny U, Hofling B, Gutjahr P: CSF shunt infections in children, *Infection* 21(2):89-92, 1993.

Lee M, Wisofff JH, Abbot R: Management of hydrocephalus in children with medulloblastoma, *Pediatr Neurosurg* 20(4):240-247, 1994.

McCallum JE, Turbeville D: Cost and outcome in a series of shunted premature infants with intraventricular hemorrhage, *Pediatr Neurosurg* 20(1):63-67, 1994.

Richard ME: Common pediatric craniofacial reconstructions, *Nurs Clin North Am* 29(4):791-799, 1994.

Ryan JA, Shiminski-Maher T: Hydrocephalus and shunts in children with brain tumors, *J Pediatr Oncol Nurs* 12(4):223-229, 1995.

Sainte-Rose C: Shunt obstruction: a preventable complication? *Pediatr Neurosurg* 19(3):156-164, 1993.

Scheinblum DT, Hammond M: The treatment of children with shunt infections: extraventricular drainage system care, *Pediatr Nurs* 16:139-143, 1990.

Sloan ES: Face value: trends and advances in craniofacial surgery, *Todays OR Nurse* 12:17-22, 1990.

Tilem D, Greenberg CS: Nursing care of the child with a ventriculostomy, *J Pediatr Nurs* 3:188-193, 1988.

CHAPTER 49

Endocrine Dysfunction

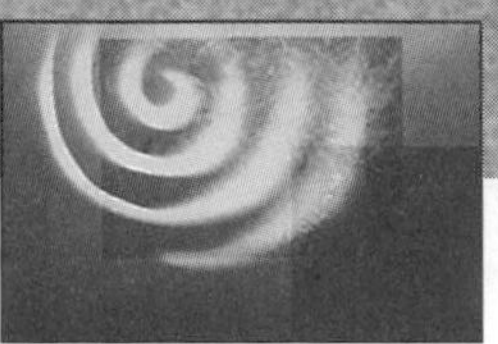

DISORDERS OF PITUITARY FUNCTION, P. 1624
Hypopituitarism: growth hormone (GH) deficiency, p. 1624
Pituitary hyperfunction, p. 1627
Precocious puberty, p. 1627
Diabetes insipidus (DI), p. 1628
Syndrome of inappropriate antidiuretic hormone secretion (SIADH), p. 1629

DISORDERS OF THYROID FUNCTION, P. 1629
Juvenile hypothyroidism, p. 1629
Goiter, p. 1630
Lymphocytic thyroiditis, p. 1631
Hyperthyroidism (Graves disease), p. 1631

DISORDERS OF PARATHYROID FUNCTION, P. 1633
Hypoparathyroidism, p. 1633
Hyperparathyroidism, p. 1634

DISORDERS OF ADRENAL FUNCTION, P. 1634
Acute adrenocortical insufficiency, p. 1634
Chronic adrenocortical insufficiency (Addison disease), p. 1635
Cushing syndrome, p. 1636
Congenital adrenogenital hyperplasia (CAH), p. 1637
Hyperaldosteronism, p. 1639
Pheochromocytoma, p. 1639

DISORDERS OF PANCREATIC HORMONE FUNCTION, P. 1640
Diabetes mellitus (DM), p. 1640

Disorders of Pituitary Function

The *pituitary gland,* or *hypophysis,* is often referred to as the *master gland* because of its role in regulating other endocrine glands. Under the influence of secretions from the hypothalamus, the anterior lobe of the pituitary (adenohypophysis) releases or withholds seven hormones (Table 49-1). These hormones control the secretion of hormones from other endocrine glands and influence somatic and sexual development. Because of this relationship, a dysfunction observed in target tissues can be the result of malfunctions of the hypothalamus, the pituitary gland, or the target gland. If the tropic hormones are involved, the resulting disorder reflects the altered stimulus to the target gland. For example, if thyroid-stimulating hormone is deficient, thyroid hormone is also deficient, and the child displays the manifestations of hypothyroidism. Overproduction of pituitary hormone is thought to be caused by hyperplasia of the pituitary cells or by a primary hypothalamic defect that results in excess production of the hormone's releasing factor.

Deficiencies of the anterior pituitary hormones may be the result of organic defects or of idiopathic cause and may occur as a single hormonal problem or in combination with other hormonal deficiencies. The clinical manifestations depend on the hormones involved and the age of onset. This discussion is limited to dysfunction related primarily to the secretion of growth hormone.

Nursing ALERT

Children with panhypopituitarism should wear medical identification such as a bracelet.

HYPOPITUITARISM: GROWTH HORMONE (GH) DEFICIENCY

Hypopituitarism is primarily a disorder associated with deficient secretion of *GH (somatotropin).* It may be caused by a variety of conditions: developmental defects; destructive lesions such as tumors, trauma, vascular abnormalities, or surgery; certain hereditary disorders; or functional disorders such as anorexia nervosa or psychosocial dwarfism. In more than half of children with hypopituitarism no lesion is evident and the cause is unknown—*idiopathic hypopituitarism* or *idiopathic pituitary growth factor.*

GH deficiency inhibits somatic growth in all body cells (Fig. 49-1). The primary site of dysfunction in the syndrome ap-

TABLE 49-1 Endocrine glands and their function

GLAND/HORMONE	PRIMARY EFFECT
Adenohypophysis (anterior pituitary)	
Growth hormone (GH)	Promotes growth of bone and soft tissues
Thyroid-stimulating hormone (TSH)	Stimulates thyroid hormone secretion
Adrenocorticotropic hormone (ACTH)	Stimulates adrenal cortex to secrete glucocorticoids and androgens
Gonadotropins Follicle-stimulating hormone (FSH) Luteinizing hormone (LH)	Stimulate gonads to mature and produce sex hormones and germ cells
Prolactin	Stimulates milk secretion
Melanocyte-stimulating hormone (MSH)	Promotes pigmentation of skin
Neurohypophysis (posterior pituitary)	
Antidiuretic hormone (ADH)	Acts on kidney tubules to reabsorb water
Oxytocin	Stimulates uterine contractions Causes milk-ejection reflex
Thyroid gland	
Thyroid hormones	Regulate metabolic rate Control rate of body cell growth
Thyrocalcitonin	Influences ossification and development of bone
Parathyroid glands	
Parathyroid hormone (PTH)	Regulates calcium metabolism
Adrenal cortex	
Aldosterone	Regulates sodium retention and excretion
Sex hormones	Influence development of bones, reproductive organs, and secondary sex characteristics
Glucocorticoids	Promote metabolism Mobilize body defenses during stress Suppress inflammatory reaction
Adrenal medulla	
Catecholamines	Produce a sympathetic response Increase blood pressure and blood glucose levels
Islands of Langerhans of pancreas	
Insulin	Promotes utilization of glucose by cells; decreases blood glucose levels
Glucagon	Increases blood glucose levels Accelerates glyconeogenesis
Somatostatin	Inhibits secretion of insulin and glucagon
Ovaries	
Estrogen	Stimulates ripening of ova Produces female secondary sex characteristics Promotes epiphyseal closure of bones
Progesterone	Prepares uterus for fertilization
Testes	
Testosterone	Stimulates spermatogenesis Produces male secondary sex characteristics Promotes epiphyseal closure of bones

pears to be in the hypothalamus. The extent of idiopathic GH deficiency may be complete or partial, but the cause is unknown. It is frequently associated with other pituitary hormone deficiencies and is treated more frequently in boys than in girls.

Diagnostic Evaluation

Only a small number of children with delayed growth or short stature have hypopituitary dwarfism. In the majority of instances the cause is constitutional delay (see Chapter 37). Although children with hypopituitarism are normal at birth, they show growth patterns that progressively deviate from the normal growth rate, often beginning in infancy. The chief complaint in most instances is short stature (Box 49-1).

A complete diagnostic evaluation should include a family history, a history of the child's growth patterns and previous health status, physical examination, radiographic surveys, and endocrine studies. Definitive diagnosis is based on ra-

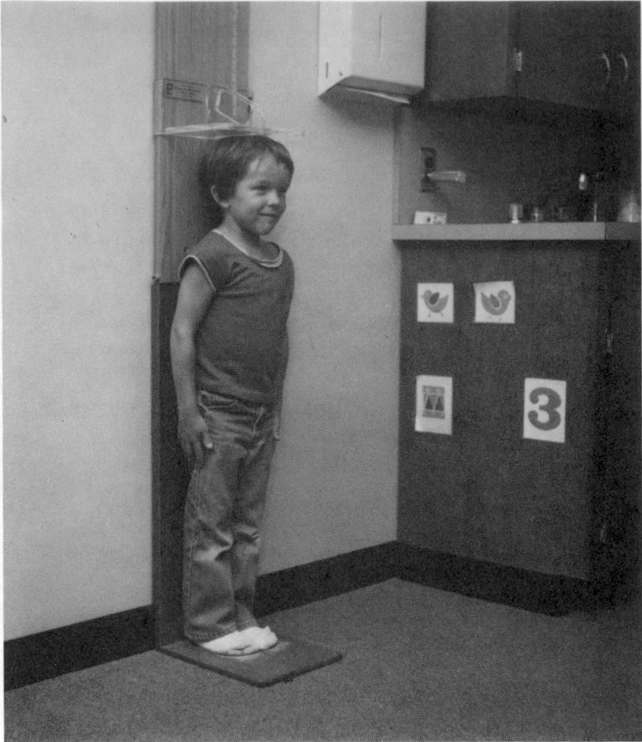

Fig. 49-1 Ten-year-old child with growth hormone deficiency. Height is 42.5 in.

BOX 49-1
Clinical Manifestations of Hypopituitarism

Presenting complaint—short stature
- Usually normal growth first year
- Growth during second year drops below established percentile
- Growth measurements below 5th percentile

Premature aging common in later life
Height may be retarded more than weight
Well-nourished appearance
Skeletal proportions normal
Tendency to be relatively inactive
Less likely to participate in aggressive, sporting-type activities
Bone age nearly always retarded but closely related to height age
Appearance of primary teeth usually at expected age; eruption of permanent teeth delayed
Teeth overcrowded and malpositioned (because of underdeveloped jaw)
Sexual development usually delayed but normal

dioimmunoassay of plasma GH levels stimulated pharmacologically with two or more agents. GH levels below 10 ng/ml after two provocative tests establish the diagnosis.

Radiographic examination of the hand and wrist for centers of ossification is an important procedure in evaluating growth. Endocrine studies to detect tropic hormone deficiencies are also performed if there is evidence of hypothyroidism, hypersecretion of cortisol, or gonadal aplasia.

Therapeutic Management

Treatment of GH deficiency caused by organic lesions is directed toward correction of the underlying disease process (e.g., surgical removal or irradiation of a tumor). The definitive treatment of GH deficiency is replacement of GH. *Biosynthetic GH* prepared by recombinant deoxyribonucleic acid (DNA) technology is the therapy of choice. Children with other hormone deficiencies require replacement therapy to correct the specific disorders. This may involve administration of thyroid extract, cortisone, testosterone, or estrogens and progesterone. The sex hormones are usually begun during adolescence to promote normal sexual maturation.

Prognosis. GH replacement is successful in 80% of affected children. Children who respond to therapy typically increase their growth rate from 3.5 to 4 cm/year before treatment to 8 to 10 cm/year during the first year of therapy. Young children, obese children, and severely GH-deficient children respond best. Although treated children display initial rapid catch-up growth, treatment does not appear to make up a deficit in the *prognosis* of eventual height that is already present at diagnosis, indicating that the dosage of GH is not sufficient to override genetic predisposition (Moore et al, 1992). Therefore early diagnosis is important to successful therapy.

Creutzfeldt-Jakob disease (CJD), a rare neurodegenerative condition, was reported in some patients after administration of the cadaver-derived human growth hormone (HGH) but does not occur with the use of biosynthetic GH. Circumstances make it likely that HGH contaminated with CJD, a slow-growing, viruslike particle, may have been responsible for fatalities in patients treated with HGH. Blood banks do not accept donations from former HGH recipients because of the inability to test for infection with CJD (Zekauskas et al, 1990). Currently much controversy exists over the use of GH in children who are short but not GH-deficient.

Nursing Care Management

Nursing care is primarily directed toward assisting in establishing the diagnosis and providing emotional support to the child and family. Since these children appear younger than their chronologic age, others frequently relate to them in childish ways. Parents and teachers benefit from guidance directed toward realistic expectations of the child based on age and abilities (Stabler, 1993).

Children undergoing hormone replacement require additional support, such as preparation for daily subcutaneous injections* and education for self-management during the school-age years (see the Critical Thinking Q & A box on p. 1627).

Even when hormone replacement is successful, these children attain their eventual adult height at a slower rate than their peers; thus they need assistance in setting realistic expectations regarding improvement. Professionals and families

*Home care instructions on giving subcutaneous injections are available in Wong DL: *Wong and Whaley's clinical manual of pediatric nursing*, ed 4, St Louis, 1996, Mosby.

Critical Thinking 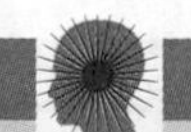

GROWTH HORMONE DEFICIENCY

Kevin, an 11-year-old male, is being treated for GH deficiency. A work-up was initiated after Kevin's mother noticed that his pants size had not changed in 2 years and that his 8-year-old brother was rapidly becoming taller than Kevin. Kevin has become increasingly hostile to his brother and is refusing to attend school on a regular basis. Kevin's mother is administering the daily injections of GH. Which of the following interventions should be initiated first to allow Kevin to regain feelings of mastery and control over his environment?

1. Preparation for home schooling.
2. Family counseling related to sibling rivalry.
3. Education and support related to self-administration of GH.
4. Encouragement and assurance that the therapy is temporary and will maximize his adult height.

The correct answer is three. Children with GH deficiency may develop behaviors related to feelings of inadequacy and loss of control. Often families, teachers, and peers relate to the child in terms of his short height rather than his chronologic age. A child of 11 years is competent to draw up and administer daily injections of GH, which will allow increased control over the environment and a feeling of being responsible for treatment of the growth deficit.

Option one is incorrect; these children must remain in regular school. At this point option two is probably not necessary, since increasing Kevin's control may reduce his hostility. Although option four is always appropriate, it does not address the principle issue—that Kevin should be independently responsible for his therapy.

may find education and support from the Human Growth Foundation.* The treatment is expensive—up to $20,000 to $30,000 per year, depending on dosage.

Nursing ALERT

Injections are given at bedtime to most closely approximate physiologic release of GH.

PITUITARY HYPERFUNCTION

Excess GH before closure of the epiphyseal shafts results in proportional overgrowth of long bones until the individual reaches a height of 8 feet or more. Vertical growth is accompanied by rapid and increased development of muscles and viscera. Weight is increased but is usually in proportion to height. Proportional enlargement of the head circumference also occurs and may result in delayed closure of the fontanels. Children with a pituitary-secreting tumor may also demonstrate signs of increasing intracranial pressure, especially headache.

If hypersecretion of GH occurs after epiphyseal closure, growth is in the transverse direction, producing a condition known as **acromegaly.** Typical facial features include overgrowth of the head, lips, nose, tongue, jaw, and paranasal and mastoid sinuses; separation and malocclusion of the teeth in the enlarged jaw; disproportion of the face to the cerebral division of the skull; increased facial hair; and thickened, deeply creased skin.

Diagnostic Evaluation

Diagnosis is based on a history of excessive growth during childhood and evidence of increased levels of GH. Radiologic studies may reveal a tumor in an enlarged sella turcica; normal bone age; enlargement of bones, such as the paranasal sinuses; and evidence of joint changes. Endocrine studies to confirm excess of other hormones, such as cortisol and sex hormones, are also included in the differential diagnosis.

Therapeutic Management

If a lesion is present, surgical treatment, including cryosurgery or hypophysectomy, may be warranted to remove the tumor whenever feasible. Other therapies that destroy pituitary tissue include external irradiation and radioactive implantation. Depending on the extent of surgical extirpation and the degree of pituitary insufficiency, hormone replacement with thyroid extract, cortisone, and sex hormones may be necessary.

Nursing Care Management

The primary nursing consideration is early identification of children with excessive growth rates. Although medical management does not diminish the height already attained, it can retard further growth. The earlier the treatment is begun, the better the chance to attain a normal adult height.

Children with excessive growth rates require as much emotional support as those with short stature. However, girls may suffer from the effects of excessive height much more than boys, who may find it an asset when pursuing sports such as basketball. A compassionate nurse can be very supportive to these children, especially before adolescence, when they are larger than their peers. The nurse can emphasize to a tall girl that as boys grow older, they become taller and she will not always be looking down at them. Since early adolescence is a time of idol worship, the nurse can point out marriages of celebrities in which the woman is taller than the man to help the girl gain a perspective that not all heterosexual relationships must follow stereotypic models.

PRECOCIOUS PUBERTY

Manifestations of sexual development before age 9 years in boys or age 8 years in girls are considered precocious and should be investigated. Early sexual development can have a number of causes and may result from a disorder of the gonad, the adrenal gland, or the hypothalamic-pituitary gonadol axis. The disorder occurs far more frequently in girls than in boys. No causative factor can be found in 80% to 90% of girls and 50% of boys with the condition (DiGeorge, 1992).

True, or complete, **precocious puberty** is always isosexual and results from premature activation of the hypothalamic pituitary-gonadal axis, which produces early maturation and development of the gonads with secretion of sex hormones, development of secondary sex characteristics, and sometimes production of mature sperm or ova. Precocious puberty is explained only as an unusually early activation of the maturation process regarded as a normal course of events

*7777 Leesburg Pike, Falls Church, VA 22043; (800) 451-6434.

at a later age. There is early acceleration of linear growth with early epiphyseal fusion and ultimate height less than what would have been anticipated with later pubertal onset. Precocious pseudopuberty, or incomplete puberty, differs from true sexual precocity in that there is no early secretion of gonadotropin. Most cases result from early overproduction of sex hormone, usually caused by a tumor of the ovary or testis, a tumor or hyperplasia of the adrenal gland, or exogenous sources of androgens or estrogens.

Therapeutic Management

Treatment of precocious pseudopuberty is directed to the specific cause when known. Precocious puberty of central origin is managed with monthly subcutaneous injections of a synthetic analog of *luteinizing hormone-releasing hormone (LHRH, [Lupron])*, which regulates pituitary secretions. This therapy slows the prepubertal growth to normal rates in affected children. Treatment is discontinued at a chronologically appropriate time, allowing pubertal changes to resume.

Nursing Care Management

Psychologic support and guidance of the child and family are the most important aspects of management. Parents need a more detailed explanation and reassurance of the benign nature of the condition. Dress and activities for the physically precocious child should be appropriate to the chronologic age.

Despite the early sexual development, maturation of the gonads and appearance of secondary sexual characteristics proceed in the usual order. After puberty, physical differences from peers are no longer present. Although the child's heterosexual behavior is appropriate for the chronologic age, the nurse should emphasize to parents that the child is fertile. No form of contraception is necessary, however, unless the child is sexually active.

Children who are receiving LHRH therapy need preparation for the subcutaneous injections. Both parents and children should be taught the injection procedure.*

DIABETES INSIPIDUS (DI)

The principle disorder of posterior pituitary hypofunction is DI, also known as *neurogenic DI*. The disease is the result of hyposecretion of *antidiuretic hormone (ADH)*, or *vasopressin*, which produces a state of uncontrolled diuresis. Primary causes are familial or idiopathic; secondary causes include trauma (accidental or surgical), tumors, granulomatous disease, infections (meningitis or encephalitis), or vascular anomalies (aneurysm). The disorder is not to be confused with nephrogenic DI, a rare hereditary disorder caused by unresponsiveness of the renal tubules to the hormone.

Clinical Manifestations

The cardinal signs of DI are **polyuria** and **polydipsia.** In the older child excessive urination accompanied by a compensatory insatiable thirst may be so intense that the child does little other than drink fluids and void. Not infrequently, the first sign is enuresis. In the infant the initial symptom is irritability that is relieved with feedings of water but not milk.

*Home care instructions on giving subcutaneous injections are available in Wong DL: *Wong and Whaley's clinical manual of pediatric nursing*, ed 4, St Louis, 1996, Mosby.

Nursing ALERT

The child with DI complicated by congenital absence of the thirst center must be encouraged to drink sufficient quantities of liquid to prevent electrolyte imbalance.

The infant is also prone to dehydration, electrolyte imbalance, hyperthermia, azotemia, and potential circulatory collapse.

Diagnostic Evaluation

The simplest test used to diagnose this condition is restriction of oral fluids and observation of consequent changes in urine volume and concentration. In DI fluid restriction has little or no effect on urine formation but causes weight loss from dehydration. If the result of this test is positive, the child should be given a test dose of injected *aqueous vasopressin (Pitressin)*, which should alleviate the polyuria and polydipsia. Unresponsiveness to exogenous vasopressin usually indicates nephrogenic DI.

Nursing ALERT

Small children require close observation during fluid restriction to prevent them from drinking even from toilet bowls, plants, or other unlikely sources of fluid.

Therapeutic Management

The usual treatment is hormone replacement with either an intramuscular or a subcutaneous injection of *vasopressin tannate* in peanut oil or via *aqueous vasopressin* nasal spray. The injectable form has the advantage of lasting 48 to 72 hours, affording the child a full night's sleep. However, it has the disadvantages of requiring frequent injections and proper preparation of the drug.

Desmopressin acetate (DDAVP) is available and administered intranasally by way of a flexible tube to achieve adequate control. It is usually administered twice daily. The response pattern of the child is variable, with duration ranging from 8 to 20 hours (Gildea, 1993). Children who are receiving DDAVP need to be observed for a possible overdose of the drug. The signs of overdosage are those of water intoxication and are similar to manifestations of inappropriate secretion of antidiuretic hormone.

Nursing Care Management

The initial objective of care is identification of the disorder. After confirmation of the diagnosis, parents need a thorough explanation of the condition, with special emphasis on distinguishing the difference between DI and diabetes mellitus. The parents must realize that treatment is lifelong. If the child is to receive the injectable vasopressin, ideally both parents, as well as children who are over 7 years of age, should be taught the correct procedure for preparation and administration of the drug.* Once children are old enough, they should be encouraged to assume full responsibility for care.

*Home care instructions on giving subcutaneous injections are available in Wong DL: *Wong and Whaley's clinical manual of pediatric nursing*, ed 4, St Louis, 1996, Mosby.

Nursing ALERT

To be effective vasopressin must be thoroughly resuspended in the oil by being held under warm running water for 10 to 15 minutes and shaken vigorously before being drawn into the syringe. If this is not done, the oil may be injected without the antidiuretic hormone. Small brown particles, which indicate drug dispersion, must be seen in the suspension.

For emergency purposes these children should wear medical alert identification. Older children are advised to carry the nasal vasopressin spray with them for temporary relief of symptoms. School personnel should be made aware of the problem so that the child is granted unrestricted use of the lavatory and drinking water. Failure to permit this may result in embarrassing accidents that often result in the child's unwillingness to attend school.

SYNDROME OF INAPPROPRIATE ANTIDIURETIC HORMONE SECRETION (SIADH)

Hypersecretion of the posterior pituitary *antidiuretic hormone (ADH, vasopressin)* produces the disorder known as the syndrome of inappropriate ADH secretion (SIADH). SIADH is observed with increased frequency in a variety of conditions, especially those involving infections, tumors, and trauma of the central nervous system.

The manifestations observed are directly related to fluid retention and hypotonicity. Increased secretion of ADH causes the kidneys to reabsorb water, increasing fluid volume and decreasing serum osmolality. When serum sodium levels are lowered to 120 mEq/L, the child displays anorexia, nausea (sometimes vomiting), stomach cramps, irritability, and personality changes. With progressive reduction in sodium, other neurologic signs such as stupor and seizures may be evident. The symptoms disappear when the underlying disorder is corrected. Immediate management consists of restricting fluids.

Nursing Care Management

The first goal of nursing management is recognizing the presence of SIADH from symptoms described in patients at risk. Accurately measuring intake, output, and daily weight, and observing for signs of fluid overload are primary nursing functions, especially in the child receiving intravenous fluids.

Nursing ALERT

Children with SIADH have an expanded circulatory volume but not edema, which is an excess of both water and sodium (Gildea, 1993).

Seizure precautions are implemented, and the child and family need education regarding the rationale for fluid restriction. The rare child with chronic SIADH will be placed on a long-term regimen of ADH-antagonizing medication, and the family will require instructions for its administration.

Disorders of Thyroid Function

The thyroid gland secretes two types of hormones: *thyroid hormone*, which consists of the hormones *thyroxine (T4)* and *triiodothyronine (T3)*, and *thyrocalcitonin*. The secretion of thyroid hormones is controlled by *thyroid-stimulating hormone (TSH)* from the anterior pituitary. Hypothyroidism or hyperthyroidism may result from a defect in the target gland or from a disturbance in secretion of TSH or its releasing factor in the hypothalamus.

Since the functions of T_3 and T_4 are qualitatively the same, the term *thyroid hormone (TH)* is used throughout this discussion.

The synthesis of TH depends on available sources of dietary iodine and tyrosine. The thyroid is the only endocrine gland capable of storing excess amounts of hormones for release as needed. The main physiologic action of TH is to regulate the basal metabolic rate and thereby control the processes of growth and tissue differentiation.

Thyrocalcitonin helps maintain blood calcium levels by decreasing the calcium concentration. Its effect is the opposite of that of parathormone; it inhibits skeletal demineralization and promotes calcium deposition in the bone.

JUVENILE HYPOTHYROIDISM

Hypothyroidism is one of the most common endocrine problems of childhood. It may be either congenital or acquired and represents a deficiency in secretion of TH. Hypothyroidism that results from dietary insufficiency of iodine is rare in the United States because iodized salt is a readily available source of the nutrient. This discussion is limited to the juvenile form of hypothyroidism.

Beyond infancy, primary hypothyroidism may be caused by a number of defects. For example, a congenital hypoplastic thyroid gland may provide sufficient amounts of TH during the first year or two but be inadequate when rapid body growth increases demands on the gland. A partial or complete thyroidectomy for cancer or thyrotoxicosis can leave insufficient thyroid tissue to furnish hormones for body requirements. Irradiation for Hodgkin disease or other malignancies or infectious processes may be a cause of hypothyroidism. A high risk for thyroid disease, including thyroid cancer and Graves disease, persists for more than 25 years after patients have received radiation therapy (Hancock, Cox, and McDougall, 1991).

Clinical manifestations depend on the extent of dysfunction and the age of the child at the onset (Box 49-2). Since brain growth is nearly complete by 2 to 3 years of age, mental retardation or neurologic sequelae are not associated with juvenile hypothyroidism.

Therapy is oral TH replacement, the same as for hypothyroidism in the infant, although the prompt treatment needed in the infant is not required in the child. In children with severe symptoms, the restoration of euthyroidism is achieved more gradually, with administration of increasing amounts of L-thyroxine over 4 to 8 weeks to prevent symptoms of hyperthyroidism that can occur with treatment of chronic hypothyroidism.

BOX 49-2
Clinical Manifestations of Juvenile Hypothyroidism

Decelerated growth
- Less when acquired at later age

Myxedematous skin changes
- Dry skin
- Puffiness around eyes
- Sparse hair

Constipation
Sleepiness
Mental decline

Nursing Care Management

Early recognition in the infant is important. Cessation or retardation of growth in a child whose growth has previously been normal should alert the observer to the possibility of hypothyroidism. After diagnosis and implementation of thyroxine therapy, the importance of compliance and periodic monitoring of the response to therapy should be stressed to the parents. Children should learn to take responsibility for their health as soon as they are old enough, about 9 to 10 years of age.

GOITER

A goiter is an enlargement or hypertrophy of the thyroid gland. It can be congenital or acquired. Congenital disease usually occurs as a result of antithyroid drugs and/or iodides administered to the mother during pregnancy. The acquired disease can result from increased secretion of pituitary thyrotropic hormone in response to decreased circulating levels of TH, neoplastic or inflammatory processes, or dietary iodine deficiency.

Enlargement of the thyroid gland may be mild and noticeable only when there is an increased demand for TH (e.g., during periods of rapid growth). Enlargement of the thyroid at birth can be sufficient to cause severe respiratory distress. TH replacement is necessary to treat the hypothyroidism and reverse the TSH effect on the gland.

Nursing Care Management

Large goiters are identified by their obvious appearance. Smaller nodules may be evident only on palpation. Nurses in ambulatory settings need to be aware of the possibility of goiters and report such findings.

Nursing ALERT

If an infant is born with a goiter, immediate precautions are instituted for emergency ventilation, such as supplemental oxygen and a tracheostomy set. Positioning the child with the neck hyperextended often facilitates breathing.

Immediate surgery to remove part of the gland may be lifesaving. When thyroid replacement is necessary, parents have the same needs regarding its administration as parents of children who have congenital hypothroidism.

BOX 49-3
Clinical Manifestations of Lymphocytic Thyroiditis

Enlarged Thyroid Gland
- Usually symmetric
- Firm
- Freely movable
- Nontender

Tracheal Compression
- Sense of fullness
- Hoarseness
- Dysphagia

Hyperthyroidism (Possible)
- Nervousness
- Irritability
- Increased sweating
- Hyperactivity

LYMPHOCYTIC THYROIDITIS

Lymphocytic thyroiditis *(Hashimoto disease, juvenile autoimmune thyroiditis)* is the most common cause of thyroid disease in children and adolescents, and it accounts for the largest percentage of juvenile hypothyroidism. It also accounts for many of the enlarged thyroid glands formerly designated as thyroid hyperplasia of adolescence, or "adolescent goiter." The disease is more common in girls than in boys and in white persons than in black persons. It occurs more frequently after age 6, reaching a peak incidence at adolescence. There is evidence that the disease is self-limited.

Pathophysiology

There is a strong genetic predisposition to the development of autoimmune thyroiditis, although no mode of inheritance has been delineated and the basic stimulus or autoimmune defect is unknown. The disease is characterized by lymphocytic infiltration of the gland, inflammation, and, in many patients, replacement with fibrous tissue. In the early stages there may be only hyperplasia.

Diagnostic Evaluation

The enlarged thryoid gland may be detected by the practitioner during a routine examination, although it may be noted by parents when the youngster swallows. Most children are euthyroid, but some display symptoms of hypothyroidism. Others have signs that suggest hyperthyroidism (Box 49-3).

Thyroid function tests are usually normal, although TSH levels may be slightly or moderately elevated. With progressive disease the T_4 decreases, followed by a decrease in T_3 and an increase in TSH. A variety of abnormalities in radioactive iodine uptake may be noted. The majority of children have serum antibody titers to thyroid antigens, but fewer children have a positive red blood cell hemagglutination test finding. When both tests are used, almost all children with thyroid autoimmunity are detected.

Therapeutic Management

In many cases the goiter is transient and asymptomatic and regresses spontaneously within a year or two. Therapy of nontoxic diffuse goiter is usually simple, uncomplicated, and effective. Oral administration of TH depresses TSH, thus decreasing the size of the gland significantly. Surgery is contraindicated in this disorder.

Nursing Care Management

Nursing care consists of identifying the youngster with thyroid enlargement, reassuring the child that the condition is probably only temporary, and reinforcing instructions for thyroid therapy.

HYPERTHYROIDISM (GRAVES DISEASE)

The largest percentage of hyperthyroidism in childhood is caused by Graves disease, which is usually associated with an enlarged thyroid gland and **exophthalmos.** The peak incidence of the disease occurs between 12 and 14 years of age, but it may be present at birth in children of thyrotoxic mothers. The incidence is five times higher in girls than in boys. The disease is apparently caused by a serum thyroid-stimulating immunoglobulin, but no specific cause has been identified. There is definitive evidence for familial association; a large number of persons with the disease possess the histocompatibility antigen HLA-B8.

Diagnostic Evaluation

The development of manifestations is highly variable (Box 49-4). Manifestations develop gradually with an interval between onset and diagnosis of approximately 6 to 12 months. Diagnosis is established on the basis of increased levels of T_4 and T_3. Thyrotropin (TSH) is suppressed to unmeasurable levels. Other tests are rarely indicated.

BOX 49-4

Clinical Manifestations of Hyperthyroidism (Graves Disease)

Cardinal Signs

Emotional lability
Physical restlessness, characteristically at rest
Decline in school performance
Voracious appetite with weight loss in 50% of cases
Fatigue

Physical Signs

Tachycardia
Widened pulse pressure
Dyspnea on exertion
Exophthalmos (protruding eyeballs)
Wide-eyed, staring expression with lid lag
Tremor
Goiter (hypertrophy and hyperplasia)
Warm, moist skin
Accelerated linear growth
Heat intolerance (may be severe)
Hair fine and unable to hold a curl
Systolic murmurs

Thyroid Storm

Acute onset
- Severe irritability and restlessness
- Vomiting
- Diarrhea
- Hyperthermia
- Hypertension
- Severe tachycardia
- Prostration

May progress rapidly to:
- Delirium
- Coma
- Death

Therapeutic Management

Therapy for hyperthyroidism is controversial, but all methods are directed toward retarding the rate of hormone secretion. The three acceptable modes available are (1) the antithyroid drugs, which interfere with the biosynthesis of TH, including propylthiouracil (PTU) and methimazole (MTZ, Tapazole); (2) subtotal thyroidectomy; and (3) ablation with radioiodine (^{131}I-iodide). While affected children exhibit signs and symptoms of hyperthyroidism, their activity should be limited. Vigorous exercise is restricted until thyroid levels are decreased to normal or near-normal values.

Thyrotoxicosis. Thyroid "crisis" or thyroid "storm" may result from sudden release of the hormone. Although it is unusual in children, a crisis can be life-threatening. A crisis may be precipitated by acute infection, surgical emergencies, or discontinuation of antithyroid therapy. Treatment, in addition to antithyroid drugs, is administration of β-adrenergic blocking agents (propranolol), which provide relief from the disturbing side effects of the reaction.

Nursing Care Management

The initial nursing objective is identification of children with hyperthyroidism. Since the clinical manifestations often appear gradually, the goiter and ophthalmic changes may not be noticed, and the excessive activity may be attributed to behavioral problems. Nurses in ambulatory settings, particularly those caring for children in school, need to be alert to signs that suggest this disorder, especially weight loss despite an excellent appetite, academic difficulties resulting from a short attention span and inability to sit still, unexplained fatigue, and sleeplessness, and difficulty with fine motor skills, such as writing. Exophthalmos may develop long before the onset of signs and symptoms of hyperthyroidism and may be the only presenting sign (Tallstedt et al, 1992).

Much of the care during diagnosis and initial medical therapy is related to the physical symptoms. The child needs a quiet, unstimulating environment that is conducive to rest, and sometimes hospitalization is necessary during the immediate treatment phase. A regular routine is beneficial and should include frequent rest periods, minimizing the stress of coping with unexpected demands, and meeting the child's needs promptly. Physical activity is restricted; for example, school physical education classes are discontinued. Despite the excessive activity of these children, they tire easily, experience muscle weakness, and are unable to relax to recoup their strength.

Emotional lability is often manifested by sudden episodes of crying or elation. Such behavior, together with irritability, disrupts interpersonal relationships, creating difficulties within and outside the home. Heat intolerance may produce considerable family conflict. Since a cooler environment is preferred, the child is likely to open windows, complain about the heat, wear minimum clothing, and kick off blankets while sleeping. Hygiene should be stressed because of excessive sweating.

Dietary requirements are regulated to meet the child's increased metabolic rate. Although the need for calories is increased, these should be provided in wholesome foods rather than "junk" foods. Vitamin supplements may be needed to meet daily requirements. Rather than by three large meals, the child's appetite may be better satisfied by five or six moderate meals throughout the day.

Once therapy is instituted, the nurse explains the drug regimen, emphasizing the importance of observing for side effects of antithyroid drugs. Untoward effects of propylthiouracil and related compounds include skin rash, drug fever, enlargement of the salivary and cervical lymph glands, diminished sense of taste, hepatitis, and edema of the lower extremities (see the Critical Thinking Q & A box below).

Critical Thinking Q & A

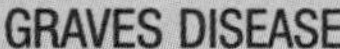

GRAVES DISEASE

Susie, 15 years old, has noticed that she has a racing pulse, ravenous appetite with continued weight loss, heat intolerance, emotional lability, and eyes that appear to be bulging from their sockets. After a diagnosis of Graves disease, Susie is started on a therapeutic dose of propylthiouracil. Because of tachycardia, Susie is cautioned to participate in sedentary activities only and to discontinue school physical education classes. Environmental temperature and appropriate dress related to heat sensitivity, as well as dietary adjustments to meet increased metabolic needs, are addressed by the nurse. Susie is shown that exophthalmos can be minimized with artful application of cosmetics. Episodic emotional lability is discussed with Susie and her family. The drug regimen is explained with special emphasis on side effects. After 6 weeks of treatment Susie has a sore throat and fever. Which of the following interventions is most appropriate?

1. Immediate follow-up by the practitioner.
2. Further instruction related to heat sensitivity.
3. Instruction related to symptomatic relief of the common cold.
4. Psychosocial interventions related to somatization of emotional lability.

The correct answer is one. Therapeutic levels of propylthiouracil can be accompanied by the grave complication of leukocytopenia. Any indication of infection must be promptly evaluated and appropriate therapy instituted. All other options do not address the immediate problem.

Nursing ALERT

Children who are being treated with propylthiouracil must be carefully monitored for side effects of the drug. Since sore throat and fever accompany the grave complication of leukopenia, these children should be seen by a practitioner if such symptoms occur. Parents and children should be taught to recognize and report symptoms immediately.

Parents should also be aware of the signs of hypothyroidism, which can result from overdose of the drugs. The most common indications are lethargy and somnolence.

Surgical care. If surgery is anticipated, iodine is usually administered for a few weeks before the procedure. Since oral iodine preparations are unpalatable, they should be mixed with a strong-tasting fruit juice, such as grape juice or punch, and be given through a straw. Compliance with iodine therapy is essential to prevent the danger of thyroid crisis after sudden discontinuation.

Psychologic preparation of children for thyroidectomy is similar to that for any other surgical procedure (see Chapter 42). However, of special consideration is the site of the incision. The fear of having the throat cut is very real and in older children is associated with death. The nurse should explain that the throat is not cut—only the skin is, to allow for removal of the gland. Showing children a picture of the anatomic location of the thyroid around the trachea is often helpful. Children should be prepared for the dressing around the neck and the possibility of having an endotracheal or "breathing" tube after surgery.

Postoperative care involves positioning with the neck slightly flexed to prevent strain on the sutures and observation for bleeding and complications. Children are taught to support the neck in this position when they sit up. Damage to the recurrent laryngeal nerve is evidenced by severe stridor and/or hoarseness, although some hoarseness is expected. Observation for signs of hypoparathyroidism, which causes hypocalcemia, should be implemented in the immediate postoperative period.

Nursing ALERT

The earliest indications of hypoparathyroidism may be anxiety and mental depression, followed by paresthesia and evidence of heightened neuromuscular excitability, such as

Chvostek sign—facial muscle spasm elicited by tapping the facial nerve in the region of the parotid gland

Trousseau sign—carpal spasm elicited by pressure applied to nerves of the upper arm

Tetany—carpopedal spasm (sharp flexion of wrist and ankle joints), muscle twitching, cramps, seizures, and sometimes stridor

Disorders of Parathyroid Function

The parathyroid glands secrete *parathormone (PTH)*, whose main function, like that of vitamin D, is to maintain homeostasis of blood calcium concentration. PTH exerts its effect by (1) increasing the release of calcium and phosphate from the bone (bone demineralization), (2) increasing the absorption of calcium and excretion of phosphate in the kidneys, and (3) promoting calcium absorption in the gastrointestinal tract. The net result of these actions is to increase the plasma calcium concentration while lowering the plasma phosphate concentration.

HYPOPARATHYROIDISM

Two classic forms of hypoparathyroidism are observed during childhood. *Autoimmune hypoparathyroidism*, in which there is deficient production of PTH, may occur as a component of multiglandular failure, usually in relation to autoimmune phenomena. Familial hypoparathyroidism is inherited as an autosomal recessive trait, with early onset, usually in the first month of life. In *pseudohypoparathyroidism* production of PTH is increased but end-organ responsiveness is also thought to be inherited as an X-linked dominant trait with variable expressivity. Transient hypoparathyroidism may also be observed in infants born to mothers with the disease or in infants fed a milk formula with a high phosphate/calcium ratio.

Diagnostic Evaluation

The diagnosis of hypoparathyroidism is made on the basis of clinical manifestations associated with *decreased serum calcium* and *increased serum phosphorus levels* (Box 49-5). Levels of plasma PTH are low in idiopathic hypoparathyroidism but high in pseudohypoparathyroidism. End-organ responsiveness is tested by the administration of PTH with measurement of urinary cyclic adenosine monophosphate (AMP). Kidney function tests are included in the differential diagnosis to rule out renal insufficiency. Although bone radiograph findings are usually normal, they may demonstrate increased bone density and suppressed growth.

BOX 49-5
Clinical Manifestations of Hypoparathyroidism

Pseudohypoparathyroidism

Short stature
Round face
Short, thick neck
Short, stubby fingers and toes
Dimpling of skin over knuckles
Subcutaneous soft tissue calcifications
Mental retardation a prominent feature

Idiopathic Hypoparathyroidism

None of the specified physical characteristics observed
Papilledema may be seen
May be mental retardation

Both Types

Dry, scaly, coarse skin with eruptions
Hair often brittle
Nails thin and brittle with characteristic transverse grooves
Dental and enamel hypoplasia
Muscle contractions:
- Tetany
- Carpopedal spasm
- Laryngospasm (laryngeal stridor)
- Muscle cramps and twitching
- Positive Chvostek and/or Trousseau sign (see p. 1632)

Paresthesias, tingling
Neurologic:
- Headache
- Seizures (generalized, absences, or focal)
- Swings of emotion
- Loss of memory
- Depression
- Confusion can occur

Gastrointestinal:
- Muscle cramps
- Diarrhea
- Vomiting

Retarded skeletal growth

Therapeutic Management

The objective of treatment is to maintain normal serum calcium and phosphate levels with minimum complications. Acute or severe tetany is corrected immediately by intravenous or oral administration of calcium gluconate and follow-up daily doses to achieve normal levels. When the diagnosis is confirmed, *vitamin D therapy* is begun. Long-term management consists of administration of massive doses of vitamin D; oral calcium supplementation may be useful, although it is not essential.

Nursing Care Management

The initial objective is recognition of hypocalcemia. Unexplained seizures, irritability (especially to external stimuli), gastrointestinal symptoms (e.g., diarrhea, vomiting, abdominal cramps), and positive signs of tetany should lead the nurse to suspect this disorder. Much of the initial nursing care is related to the physical manifestations and includes institution of seizure and safety precautions, reduction of environmental stimuli (e.g., sudden noises or movements, bright lights), and observation for signs of laryngospasm.

Nursing ALERT

Signs of *laryngospasm* are stridor, hoarseness, and a feeling of tightness in the throat. A tracheostomy set and injectable calcium gluconate should be placed near the bedside for emergency use. The intravenous administration of calcium gluconate requires precautions against extravasation of the drug and tissue destruction.

After initiation of treatment the nurse discusses with the parents the need for continuous daily administration of calcium salts and vitamin D. Because vitamin D toxicity can be a serious consequence of therapy, parents are advised to watch for signs, which include weakness, fatigue, lassitude, headache, nausea, vomiting, and diarrhea. Early renal impairment is manifested by polyuria, polydipsia, and nocturia.

HYPERPARATHYROIDISM

Hyperparathyroidism is rare in childhood but can be primary or secondary. The most common cause of primary hyperparathyroidism is adenoma of the gland. The most common causes of secondary hyperparathyroidism are chronic renal disease, renal osteodystrophy, and congenital anomalies of the urinary tract. The common factor is hypercalcemia.

Diagnostic Evaluation

Blood studies to confirm the presence of *elevated calcium* and *lowered phosphorus levels* are routinely performed. Measurement of PTH, as well as several tests to isolate the cause of the hypercalcemia, such as renal function studies, should be included. Other procedures employed to substantiate the physiologic consequences of the disorder include electrocardiography and radiographic bone surveys (Box 49-6).

BOX 49-6
Clinical Manifestations of Hyperparathyroidism

Gastrointestinal
Nausea
Vomiting
Abdominal discomfort
Constipation

Central Nervous System
Delusions
Confusion
Hallucinations
Impaired memory
Lack of interest and initiative
Depression
Varying levels of consciousness

Neuromuscular
Weakness
Easy fatigability
Muscle atrophy (especially proximal muscles of lower limbs)
Tongue twitching
Paresthesias in extremities

Skeletal
Vague bone pain
Subperiosteal resorption of phalanges
Spontaneous fractures
Absence of lamina dura around teeth

Renal
Polyuria
Polydipsia
Renal colic
Hypertension

Therapeutic Management

Treatment depends on the cause. The treatment of primary hyperparathyroidism is surgical removal of the tumor or hyperplastic tissue. Treatment of secondary hyperparathyroidism is directed at the underlying contributing cause, thus subsequently restoring the serum calcium balance. However, in some instances the underlying disorder is irreversible, such as in chronic renal failure (see Chapter 47). In this instance treatment is the same as the treatment for renal osteodystrophy.

Nursing Care Management

Since surgical exploration is the major treatment modality, nursing care is similar to that discussed for the child with hyperthyroidism (see p. 1631). Since hypocalcemia is a potential complication, observation for signs of tetany, institution of seizure precautions, and availability of calcium gluconate for emergency use are included in nursing care.

Disorders of Adrenal Function

The *adrenal cortex* secretes three main groups of hormones collectively called *steroids* and classified according to their biologic activity: (1) *glucocorticoids* (cortisol, corticosterone), (2) *mineralocorticoids* (aldosterone), and (3) *sex steroids* (androgens, estrogens, and progestins). Alterations in the levels of these hormones produce significant dysfunction in a variety of body tissues and organs. Since the adrenocortical cells are capable of producing any of the steroids, pathologic conditions may result in a deficiency or an excess of more than one type of hormone. However, most are rare in children.

The *adrenal medulla* secretes the *catecholamines epinephrine* and *norepinephrine.* Both hormones have essentially the same effects on various organs as those caused by direct sympathetic stimulation, except that the hormonal effects last several times longer. Catecholamine-secreting tumors are the primary cause of adrenal medullary hyperfunction.

ACUTE ADRENOCORTICAL INSUFFICIENCY

The acute form of adrenocortical insufficiency *(adrenal crisis)* may result from a number of causes during childhood. Although it is a rare disorder, some of the more common causative factors are hemorrhage into the gland from trauma, which may be caused by a prolonged, difficult labor; fulminating infections, such as meningococcemia, which result in hemorrhage and necrosis (Waterhouse-Friederichsen syndrome); abrupt withdrawal of exogenous sources of cortisone or failure to increase exogenous supplies during stress; or congenital adrenogenital hyperplasia of the salt-losing type.

Diagnostic Evaluation

There is no rapid, definitive test for confirmation of acute adrenocortical insufficiency. Routine procedures such as measurement of plasma cortisol levels are too time-consuming to be practical. Therefore diagnosis is usually based on clinical

BOX 49-7
Clinical Manifestations of Acute Adrenocortical Insufficiency

Early Symptoms
Increased irritability
Headache
Diffuse abdominal pain
Weakness
Nausea and vomiting
Diarrhea

Generalized Hemorrhagic Manifestations (Waterhouse-Friederichsen Syndrome)
Fever—increases as condition worsens
Central nervous system signs
- Nuchal rigidity
- Seizures
- Stupor
- Coma

Shocklike State
Weak, rapid pulse
Decreased blood pressure
Shallow respirations
Cold, clammy skin
Cyanosis
Circulatory collapse (terminal event)

Newborn
Hyperpyrexia
Tachypnea
Cyanosis
Seizures
Gland may be evident as palpable retroperitoneal mass (hemorrhagic)

symptoms (Box 49-7). Improvement with cortisol therapy confirms the diagnosis.

Therapeutic Management

Treatment involves replacement of cortisol, replacement of body fluids to correct dehydration and hypovolemia, administration of glucose solutions to correct hypoglycemia, and specific antibiotic therapy in the presence of infection. If hemorrhage has been severe, whole blood may be replaced. In the event that these measures do not reverse the circulatory collapse, vasopressors are used for immediate vasoconstriction and elevation of blood pressure. Once the child's condition is stabilized, oral doses of cortisone, fluids, and salt are given, similar to the regimen used for chronic adrenal insufficiency.

Nursing Care Management

Because of the abrupt onset and potentially fatal outcome of this condition, prompt recognition is essential. Vital signs and blood pressure are measured often to monitor the hyperpyrexia and shocklike state. Seizure precautions are instituted, since seizures that result from the elevated temperature are not uncommon. As soon as therapy is instituted, the nurse monitors the child's response to fluid and cortisol replacement, being alert to too rapid administration of fluids and drugs. Overtreatment with cortisol and sodium chloride can precipitate complications, such as an ascending flaccid paralysis. The nurse should observe for signs of hypokalemia and evaluate serum electroyte levels.

Nursing ALERT

Monitor serum electrolyte levels and observe for signs of hypokalemia or hyperkalemia (e.g., weakness, poor muscle control, paralysis, cardiac dysrhythmias, and apnea).

The condition is rapidly corrected with intravenous and oral potassium replacement. When the oral preparation is given, it should be mixed with a small amount of strongly flavored fruit juice to disguise its bitter taste. Intake and urinary output are measured and recorded.

The sudden, severe nature of this disorder requires considerable emotional support for the child and family. The child is usually in an intensive care unit, where the surroundings are strange and frightening. Since recovery within 24 hours is often dramatic, the nurse should keep the parents apprised of the child's condition, emphasizing signs of improvement, such as a lowered temperature and elevated blood pressure. If paralysis occurs, the nurse should assure them that this condition is temporary and quickly reversed.

CHRONIC ADRENOCORTICAL INSUFFICIENCY (ADDISON DISEASE)

Chronic adrenocortical insufficiency is rare in children. When it does occur, it is usually caused by a destructive lesion of the adrenal glands or a neoplasm, or it has an idiopathic cause.

Evidence of this disorder is usually gradual in onset, since 90% of adrenal tissue must be nonfunctional before signs of insufficiency are manifested (Box 49-8). However, during periods of stress, when demands for additional cortisol are increased, symptoms of acute insufficiency may appear in a previously well child (Box 49-7).

Definitive diagnosis is based on measurements of functional cortisol reserve. The cortisol and urinary 17-hydroxycorticosteroid levels are low and fail to rise, whereas plasma adrenocorticotropic hormone (ACTH) levels are elevated with corticotropin stimulation, the definitive test for the disease.

Therapeutic Management

Treatment involves replacement of *glucocorticoids (cortisol)* and *mineralocorticoids (aldosterone)*. Some children are able to be maintained solely on oral supplements of cortisol (cortisone or hydrocortisone preparations) with a liberal intake of salt. Other forms of therapy include monthly injections of desoxycorticosterone acetate or implantation of desoxycorticosterone acetate pellets subcutaneously every 9 to 12 months. During stressful situations, such as infection, emotional upset, or surgery, the dosage must be tripled to accommodate the body's increased need for glucocorticoids. Failure to meet this requirement will precipitate an acute crisis. Overdosage produces cushingoid signs (Fig. 49-2).

Nursing Care Management

Once the disorder is diagnosed, parents need guidance concerning drug therapy. They must be aware of the continuous

BOX 49-8
Clinical Manifestations of Chronic Adrenocortical Insufficiency

Neurologic Symptoms
Muscular weakness
Mental fatigue
Irritability, apathy, and negativism

Pigmentary Changes
Previous scars
Palmar creases
Mucous membranes
Hair
Hyperpigmentation over pressure points (elbows, knees, or waist)
Less frequently, vitiligo (loss of pigmentation)

Gastrointestinal Symptoms
Dehydration
Anorexia
Weight loss

Hypotension and Small Heart Size
Dizziness
Syncopal (fainting) attacks

Hypoglycemia
Headache
Hunger
Weakness
Trembling
Sweating

Other Signs (Seen in Some Children)
Recurrent, unexplained seizures
Intense craving for salt
Acute abdominal pain

need for cortisol replacement. Sudden termination of the drug because of inadequate supplies or inability to ingest the oral form because of vomiting places the child in danger of an acute adrenal crisis. Ideally, the parents should have a prefilled syringe of hydrocortisone in the home and should be taught the proper technique for intramuscular administration of the drug in case of a crisis.* Unnecessary administration of cortisone will not harm the child but, if needed, may be lifesaving. Any evidence of acute insufficiency is reported to the practitioner immediately.

Since the body cannot supply endogenous sources of cortical hormones during times of stress, the home environment should be stable and relatively unstressful. Parents need to be aware that during periods of emotional or physical crisis the child requires additional hormone replacement. The child should wear a medical alert identification tag to permit medical personnel to adjust the requirements during emergency care.

*Home care instructions on giving intramuscular injections are available in Wong DL: *Wong and Whaley's clinical manual of pediatric nursing*, ed 4, St Louis, 1996, Mosby.

CUSHING SYNDROME

Cushing syndrome is a characteristic group of manifestations caused by excessive circulating free cortisol. It can result from a variety of causes, which generally fall into one of four categories:

Pituitary, with adrenal hyperplasia, usually attributed to an excess of ACTH
Adrenal, with hypersecretion of glucocorticoids, generally the result of adrenocortical neoplasms
Ectopic, with autonomous secretion of ACTH, most often caused by extrapituitary neoplasms
Iatrogenic, frequently the result of administration of large amounts of exogenous corticosteroids
Food-dependent, inappropriate sensitivity of adrenal glands to normal postprandial increases in secretion of gastric inhibitory polypeptide (Bertagna, 1992)

Cushing syndrome is uncommon in children. When seen, it is often caused by excessive or prolonged steroid therapy, which produces a cushingoid appearance (Box 49-9 and Fig. 49-2). This condition is reversible once steroids are discontinued. Abrupt withdrawal may precipitate acute adrenal insufficiency; gradual withdrawal of exogenous supplies is necessary to allow the anterior pituitary an opportunity to secrete increasing amounts of ACTH to stimulate the adrenals to produce cortisol.

Diagnostic Evaluation

Several tests are helpful in confirming excess cortisol levels. These include fasting blood glucose levels for hyperglycemia, serum electrolyte levels for hypokalemia and alkalosis, 24-hour urinary levels of elevated 17-hydroxycorticoids and 17-ketosteroids, and radiographic studies of bone for evidence of osteoporosis and of the skull for enlargement of the sella turcica. Administration of an exogenous supply of cortisone normally suppresses ACTH production. However, in individuals with Cushing syndrome, cortisol levels remain elevated. This test is helpful in differentiating between children who are obese and those who appear to have cushingoid features.

Therapeutic Management

Treatment depends on the cause. In most cases surgical intervention involves bilateral adrenalectomy and postoperative replacement of the cortical hormones (the therapy for this is the same as that outlined for chronic adrenal insufficiency). If a pituitary tumor is found, surgical extirpation or irradiation may be chosen. In either of these instances treatment of panhypopituitarism with replacement of growth hormone, thyroid extract, antidiuretic hormone, gonadotropins, and steroids may be necessary for an indefinite period.

Nursing Care Management

Nursing care also depends on the cause. When cushingoid features are caused by steroid therapy, the effects may be lessened with administration of the drug early in the morning and on an alternate-day basis. Giving the drug early in the day maintains the normal diurnal pattern of cortisol secretion. If given during the evening, the drug is more likely to produce symptoms, because endogenous cortisol levels are already low and the additional supply exerts more pronounced effects. An alternate-day schedule gives the anterior pituitary

BOX 49-9
Clinical Manifestations of Cushing Syndrome

- Centripetal fat distribution
  - Truncal obesity
  - Supraclavicular fat pads
  - Fat pads on neck and back ("buffalo hump")
- Rounded or "moon" face
- Muscular wasting
  - Thin extremities
  - Pendulous abdomen
  - Muscle weakness
- Thin skin and subcutaneous tissue
- Poor wound healing
- Increased susceptibility to infection
- Decreased inflammatory response
- Excessive bruising
- Petechial hemorrhages
- Facial plethora ("red cheeks")
- Reddish purple abdominal striae
- Hypertension
- Hypokalemia
- Alkalosis
- Osteoporosis
  - Compression fractures of vertebrae
  - Kyphosis
  - Backache
  - Retarded linear growth
- Hypercalciuria-renal calculi
- Psychoses
  - Irritability
  - Insomnia
  - Euphoria
  - Depression
  - Frank psychoses
- Peptic ulcer
- Hyperglycemia
  - Glycosuria
  - Latent or overt diabetes
- Virilization
  - Hirsutism (excessive body hair)
  - Acne
  - Deepening of voice
  - Clitoral enlargement
  - Tendency toward male physique in female
- Amenorrhea
- Impotence

an opportunity to maintain more normal hypothalamic-pituitary-adrenal control mechanisms.

If an organic cause is found, nursing care is related to the treatment regimen. Although a bilateral adrenalectomy permanently solves one condition, it also produces another syndrome. Before surgery, parents need to be adequately informed of the operative benefits and disadvantages. Postoperative teaching regarding drug replacement is a nursing function.

Nursing ALERT

Postoperative complications of adrenalectomy are related to the sudden withdrawal of cortisol. Observe for signs of a shocklike state, especially hypotension and hyperpyrexia.

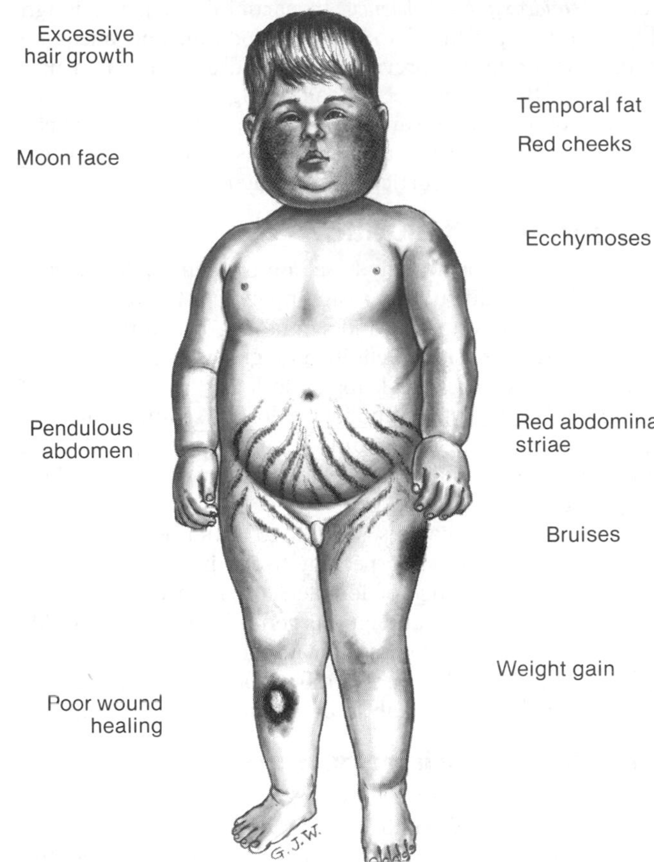

Fig. 49-2 Characteristics of Cushing syndrome.

CONGENITAL ADRENOGENITAL HYPERPLASIA (CAH)

Disorders caused by excessive secretion of androgens by the adrenal cortex are known variously as *congenital adrenogenital hyperplasia (CAH), adrenocortical hyperplasia (ACH), adrenogenital syndrome (AGS),* and *congenital adrenocortical hyperplasia (CAH).* Although hyperfunction of the adrenal gland can result from a number of cases, such as a virilizing adrenal tumor, in children the most common cause is CAH, an inborn deficiency of various enzymes necessary for the biosynthesis of cortisol. CAH is inherited as an autosomal-recessive disorder or may result from a tumor or maternal ingestion of steroids.

Pathophysiology

Interference in the biosynthesis of cortisol during fetal life results in an increased production of ACTH, which stimulates hyperplasia of the adrenal gland. Depending on the enzymatic defect, increased quantities of cortisol precursors and androgens are secreted. There are six major types of biochemical defects. In each there is excess production of androgens, which causes ambiguous genitalia in females and precocious genital development in males. Other forms of CAH do not result in excess production of androgens but cause various degrees of hypoaldosteronism or hyperaldosteronism.

The most common biochemical defect is partial or complete *21-hydroxylase deficiency*. In partial deficiency, enough aldosterone is produced to preserve sodium, and adequate cortisol is produced to prevent signs of adrenocortical insufficiency. In the complete or salt-losing form, insufficient amounts of aldosterone and cortisol are produced, so that circulatory collapse occurs unless there is immediate replacement of the mineralocorticoids and glucocorticoids.

Diagnostic Evaluation

Clinical diagnosis is initially based on congenital abnormalities that lead to difficulty in assigning gender to the newborn (Box 49-10) and on signs and symptoms of adrenal insufficiency or hypertension. Definitive diagnosis is confirmed by evidence of increased 17-ketosteroid levels in most types of CAH. Blood electrolytes demonstrate loss of sodium and chloride and elevation of potassium. A karyotype for positive sex determination should always be done in any case of ambiguous genitalia.

Ultrasonography can also be used to visualize the presence of pelvic structures. It is especially useful in CAH to identify the absence or presence of female reproductive organs in a newborn or child with ambiguous genitalia. Because it yields immediate results, it has the advantage of determining the child's gender long before the more complex laboratory results for chromosomal analysis or steroid levels are available.

Therapeutic Management

The initial medical objective is to confirm the diagnosis and assign a gender to the child, usually according to the genotype. In both sexes cortisone is administered to suppress the abnormally high secretions of ACTH. Cortisone depresses the secretion of ACTH by the adenohypophysis, which in turn inhibits the secretion of adrenocorticosteroids, which stems the progressive virilization. If cortisol is given early enough, the signs and symptoms of masculinization in the female gradually disappear, and excessive early linear growth is slowed. Puberty occurs normally at the appropriate age.

Since these children are unable to produce cortisol in response to stress, the dosage is increased during episodes of infection, fever, or other stresses. Acute emergencies require immediate intravenous or intramuscular administration. Children with the salt-losing type of CAH require aldosterone replacement and supplementary dietary salt.

Depending on the degree of masculinization in the female, reconstructive surgery may be required to reduce the size of the clitoris, separate the labia, and create a vaginal orifice. This should be done after the infant is physically able to tolerate the procedure and before she is old enough to be aware of the abnormal genitalia. Plastic surgery is generally done in stages and yields excellent cosmetic results. The capacity for orgasm and sexual gratification is not necessarily impaired.

Unfortunately not all children who have CAH are diagnosed at birth and raised in accordance with their genetic sex. Particularly in the case of affected females, masculinization of the external genitalia may have led to sex assignment as a male. In these situations it is advisable to continue rearing the child as a male in accordance with the assigned sex and phenotype. Hormone replacement may be required to permit linear growth and to initiate male pubertal changes. Surgery is usually indicated to remove the female organs and reconstruct the phallus for satisfactory sexual relations. These individuals are not fertile. In males, diagnosis is usually delayed until early childhood, when signs of virilism appear.

BOX 49-10
Clinical Manifestations of Adrenogenital Hyperplasia

Female: Masculinization
- Enlarged clitoris (appears as small phallus)
- Fusion of labia (saclike structure resembling a scrotum)
- Vaginal orifice usually closed by fused labia

Male: Precocious genital development
- Genital enlargement (macrogenitosomia precox)
- Frequent erections

Untreated: Early sexual maturation
- Enlargement of external sexual organs
- Development of axillary, pubic, and facial hair
- Deepening of voice
- Acne
- Marked increase in musculature (changes toward an adult male physique)
- Accelerated linear growth
- Premature epiphyseal closure (short stature by end of puberty)
- Female:
  - No breast development
  - Females remain amenorrheic and infertile
- Male:
  - Testes remain small

Nursing Care Management

The nursing care of the child with CAH and family is concerned primarily with identifying the condition and providing support and assistance. Of major importance is recognition of ambiguous genitalia in newborns. If there is any question regarding assignment of sex, the parents need to be told immediately to prevent the embarrassing situation of informing family members of the child's sex and then having to change the announcement (see the Family Focus box on p. 1639). As with any congenital defect, the parents require an adequate explanation of the condition and a period to grieve for the loss of perfection. Parents need an explanation regarding this disorder that facilitates their explaining it to others. The external genitalia are referred to as sex organs, and the similarity between the penis/clitoris and scrotum/labia during fetal development is emphasized to help parents understand that too much male hormone secretion caused some organs to overdevelop. Using a correct vocabulary allows parents to explain the abnormalities to others in a straightforward manner, just as if the defect involved the heart or an extremity.

As soon as the sex is determined, parents are informed of the findings and encouraged to choose an appropriate name, and the child is identified as a male or female, with no reference to ambiguous sex. If the appearance of the enlarged genitalia in a female child concerns the parents, they are encouraged to discuss their feelings.

Nursing considerations regarding cortisol and aldosterone replacement are the same as those for chronic adrenocortical insufficiency. A follow-up visit by a public health nurse may be desirable to ensure that parents understand and comply with the treatment regimen. Likewise, nurses in well-child

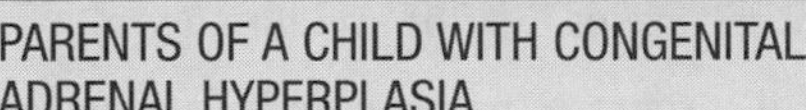

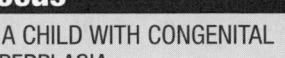

PARENTS OF A CHILD WITH CONGENITAL ADRENAL HYPERPLASIA

The first question parents of a newborn are asked is "Is it a boy or a girl?" For the parents of a child born with ambiguous genitalia, the answer "We are not sure" can be extremely upsetting. It is important for the nurse to keep in mind the social stigmata the parents of a child with CAH face. Parents need to be told immediately of the diagnosis and given an adequate explanation of the condition. Chromosome typing for positive sex determination is always done and can facilitate acceptance of the child's true gender. The nurse should refer to the infant as "child" or "baby" until identification of gender is known. Suggestions of ways to prevent questions from visitors, such as diapering the child in a separate room, are also helpful. If surgery is anticipated, showing parents pictures of reconstruction may reinforce a positive acceptance of the child.

Families can be creative in how they handle questions of gender. One family told only their close relatives that the newborn's sex was unclear until tests were done. To others they stated that they had twins—a boy and a girl. When the gender was confirmed, they said that the opposite-sex twin had died. As nurses, we must be sensitive to parents' and other family members' difficulty in revealing the diagnosis and respect their ways of coping.

facilities should assume responsibility for guidance and supervision in this aspect of care during each visit.

Since these infants are especially prone to dehydration and salt-losing crises, parents need to be aware of signs of dehydration and the urgency of immediate medical intervention to stabilize the child's condition. Parents, and later the child, need to understand that the medical regimen must be a lifelong commitment; therefore they should be provided with the education and counseling that are most likely to ensure informed and willing compliance. They also need to know that growth retardation that may have occurred before therapy cannot be overcome and that normal stature is not a realistic expectation, even though growth velocity may improve with medication. The parents are also taught to give necessary injections (see Chapter 42).*

In the unfortunate situation in which the gender is erroneously assigned and the correct sex determined later, parents need a great deal of help in understanding the reason for the incorrect sex identification and the options for sex reassignment and/or medical/surgical intervention. Since children become aware of their sexual identity by 18 months to 2 years of age, it is believed that any reassignment after this period can cause tremendous psychologic conflicts in the child. Therefore sex rearing should be continued as previously established with medical/surgical intervention as required.

Nursing ALERT

The parents should be advised that there is no physical harm in treating for suspected adrenal insufficiency that is not present, whereas the consequence of not treating acute adrenal insufficiency can be fatal (Ruble, 1992).

A dilemma often arises regarding what these children should know about their condition, especially concerning gender identification. Because the knowledge that one has been reared opposite to the genetic gender can initiate profound psychologic problems, it is recommended that children not be told this fact but rather be given an explanation of their physical disabilities, such as infertility, and the need for hormone replacement and plastic surgery. Parents, in turn, must believe that these children have been raised according to their "true sex," which is absolutely honest, since sex is not solely a biologic entity but an expression of multiple environmental influences.

Since the hereditary form of adrenogenital hyperplasia is an autosomal-recessive disorder, parents should be referred for genetic counseling before conceiving another child. Affected offspring also require genetic counseling, since both sexes are generally able to reproduce.

HYPERALDOSTERONISM

Excessive secretion of aldosterone may be caused by an adrenal tumor; also in some types of adrenogenital syndromes, symptoms are caused by increased sodium levels, water retention, and potassium loss. The clinical diagnosis is suspected when there are findings of hypertension, hypokalemia, and polyuria that fail to respond to antidiuretic hormone administration.

Therapeutic Management

Temporary treatment of the disorder involves replacement of potassium and administration of spironolactone (Aldactone), a diuretic that blocks the effects of aldosterone.

Nursing Care Management

An important nursing consideration is recognition of the syndrome, particularly in children who demonstrate high blood pressure. After the diagnosis, nursing care is related to the treatment regimen, such as education about the diuretic and potassium supplements. Parents need to be aware of the signs of hypokalemia and hyperkalemia (see the Nursing Alert on p. 1635).

PHEOCHROMOCYTOMA

Pheochromocytoma is an adrenal tumor characterized by secretion of catecholamines. In children this type of tumor is most frequently bilateral or multiple and is generally benign. Often there is a familial transmission of the condition as an autosomal-dominant trait that tends to favor males. The clinical manifestations of pheochromocytoma are caused by an increased production of catecholamines, and they mimic those of other disorders, such as hyperthyroidism, diabetes mellitus, or functional hyperventilation (Box 49-11).

Therapeutic Management

Definitive treatment consists of surgical removal of the tumor. In children the tumors may be bilateral, requiring a bilateral adrenalectomy and lifelong glucocorticoid and mineralocorticoid therapy.

*Home care instructions for giving injections are available in Wong DL: *Wong and Whaley's clinical manual of pediatric nursing*, ed 4, St Louis, 1996, Mosby.

BOX 49-11
Clinical Manifestations of Pheochromocytoma

Hypertension	Polyuria
Tachycardia	Polydipsia
Headache	Hyperventilation
Decreased gastrointestinal activity	Nervousness
Resultant constipation	Diaphoresis
Anorexia	Signs of congestive heart failure in severe cases
Weight loss	
Hyperglycemia	

Nursing Care Management

An initial nursing objective is identification of children with this disorder. Outstanding clues are hypertension and hypertensive attacks. Preoperative nursing care involves frequent monitoring of vital signs and observing for evidence of hypertensive attacks and congestive heart failure. Urine should be tested at least daily for sugar and ketones. Any signs of hyperglycemia are noted and reported immediately.

Nursing ALERT

Do not palpate mass. Preoperative palpation may facilitate release of catecholamines, which can stimulate severe hypertension and tachyarrythmias.

The environment should be conducive to rest and free of emotional stress. This requires adequate preparation during hospital admission and before surgery. Parents are encouraged to room-in with their child and to participate in the care. Play activities need to be tailored to the child's energy level but should not be overly strenuous or challenging, since these can increase the metabolic rate and promote frustration and anxiety.

After surgery the child is observed for signs of shock from removal of excess catecholamines. If a bilateral adrenalectomy was performed, the nursing interventions are those discussed for chronic adrenocortical insufficiency.

Disorders of Pancreatic Hormone Function

The islands of Langerhans of the pancreas have three major functioning cells:

1. The *alpha cells* produce *glucagon*, which increases the blood glucose levels by stimulating the liver and other cells to release stored glucose (glycogenolysis).
2. The *beta cells* produce *insulin*, which lowers blood glucose levels by facilitating the entrance of glucose into the cells for metabolism.
3. The *delta cells* produce *somatostatin*, which is believed to regulate the release of insulin and glucagon.

The discussion of disorders of pancreatic hormone secretion is limited to diabetes mellitus.

DIABETES MELLITUS (DM)

DM is a disease of metabolism characterized by total or partial deficiency of the hormone *insulin*, resulting in a metabolic adjustment or physiologic change in almost all areas of the body. It is the most frequent endocrine disorder of childhood, with a peak incidence reached during early adolescence.

DM can be classified into three major groups:

Insulin-dependent (IDDM), or **type I**—characterized by catabolism and the development of ketosis in the absence of insulin replacement therapy; onset is typically in childhood and adolescence but can occur at any age

Non–insulin-dependent (NIDDM), or **type II**—appears to involve resistance in insulin action and defective glucose-mediated insulin secretion; onset is usually after age 40, and there appears to be considerable heterogeneity; affected persons may or may not require daily insulin injections

Maturity-onset diabetes of youth (MODY)—transmitted as an autosomal-dominant disorder in which there is formation of structurally abnormal insulin that has decreased biologic activity

Because DM of childhood is, with few exceptions, the IDDM form, the remainder of this discussion is devoted to this important cause of long-term health problems. However, NIDDM is included as is appropriate for comparison throughout. Native American children tend to have NIDDM rather than IDDM, even when diagnosed in childhood.

Etiology

The clinical syndrome of DM results from a large variety of etiologic and pathogenic mechanisms. IDDM is now believed to be an autoimmune disease that arises when a person with a genetic predisposition is exposed to a precipitating event, such as a viral infection.

Genetic factors. IDDM is not inherited, but heredity is unquestionably a prominent factor in the cause. A variety of genetic mechanisms have been proposed, but most authorities favor a multifactorial inheritance or a recessive gene somehow linked to the human lymphocyte antigen (HLA). However, the genetic influence in NIDDM and IDDM appears to differ in several ways. Studies of NIDDM in identical twins demonstrate a 100% concordance throughout the life span, whereas studies of IDDM in identical twins demonstrate a 30% to 50% concordance rate. The lower rate suggests that environmental and genetic factors are important in the genesis of IDDM (Winters, Chichara, and Schatz, 1993).

Autoimmune mechanisms. An autoimmune process is involved in development of IDDM. The current theory is that the presence of the HLA genes causes a defect in the immune system that renders the possessor susceptible to a trigger event, which may be a dietary source, a virus, bacteria, or a chemical irritant. The predisposing event initiates an autoimmune process that gradually destroys beta cells. Without beta cells no insulin can be produced. There is also a strong association between IDDM and other autoimmune endocrine disorders, such as thyroiditis and Addison disease.

Pathophysiology

Insulin is needed to support the metabolism of carbohydrates, fats, and proteins, primarily by facilitating the entry of these substances into the cell, with the exception of nerve cells and vascular tissue. When there is a deficiency of insulin, glucose is unable to enter the cell, and its concentration in the bloodstream increases *(hyperglycemia)*. The increased concentration of glucose produces an osmotic gradient that causes the movement of body fluid from the intracellular space to the extracellular space; from there the body fluid is excreted by the kidneys. When the serum glucose level exceeds the renal threshold (±180 mg/dl), glucose "spills" into the urine **(glycosuria)**, along with an osmotic diversion of water *(polyuria)*, a cardinal sign of diabetes. The urinary fluid losses cause the excessive thirst *(polydipsia)* observed in diabetes. As might be expected, this water washout results in a depletion of other essential chemicals.

Protein is also wasted during insulin deficiency. Since glucose is unable to enter the cells, protein is broken down and converted to glucose by the liver *(glucogenesis)*; this glucose then contributes to the hyperglycemia. Without the use of carbohydrates for energy, fat and protein stores are depleted as the body attempts to meet its energy needs. The hunger mechanism is triggered, but the increased food intake *(polyphagia)* enhances the problem by further elevating the blood glucose level.

Ketoacidosis. When insulin is absent, glucose is unavailable for cellular metabolism and the body chooses alternate sources of energy, principally fat. Consequently fats break down into fatty acids, and glycerol in fat cells and liver is converted to ketone bodies (β-hydroxybutyric acid, acetoacetic acid, acetone). The ketone bodies can be used as an alternative source of fuel for glucose, but they are used in the cells at a limited rate. Any excess is eliminated in the urine **(ketonuria)** or the lungs (acetone breath). The ketone bodies in the blood *(ketonemia)* are strong acids that lower serum pH, producing **ketoacidosis.** The respiratory system attempts to eliminate the excess carbon dioxide by increased depth and rate—**Kussmaul respirations,** the hyperventilation characteristic of metabolic acidosis.

With cellular death, potassium is released from the cell into the interstitial spaces and then into the bloodstream. It is then excreted by the kidney, where the loss is accelerated by osmotic diuresis. The total body potassium is then decreased, even though the serum potassium level may be elevated as a result of the decreased fluid volume in which it circulates. Alteration in serum and tissue potassium can make cardiac arrest a potential problem.

If these conditions are not reversed by insulin therapy in combination with correction of the fluid deficiency and electrolyte imbalance, progressive deterioration occurs, with dehydration, electrolyte imbalance, acidosis, coma, and death. Diabetic ketoacidosis should be diagnosed promptly and therapy instituted.

Long-term complications. Long-term complications of DM involve the small, as well as large, blood vessels. The principal microvascular complications are *nephropathy* and *retinopathy*. The process appears to be one of *glycosylation*, wherein proteins from the blood become deposited in the basement membrane of small vessels (e.g., glomeruli, retina), where they become trapped by "sticky" glucose compounds (glycosyl radicals). The buildup of these substances over time causes narrowing of the vessels with subsequent interference with microcirculation to the affected areas. With poor control, vascular changes appear as early as 2½ to 3 years after diagnosis; with good control changes have been postponed for 20 or more years.

Neuropathy appears to be an identical process, but glycosylation occurs on the sheath of nerves, interrupting neurotransmission of stimuli. Macrovascular disease develops after 25 years of DM and creates the predominant complications in patients with NIDDM. Intensive insulin therapy appears to delay the onset and slow the progression of clinically important retinopathy, including vision loss, nephropathy, and neuropathy, by 35% to more than 70% (Nathan, 1993).

Mild diabetes. Although most childhood diabetes is recognized during the rapid initial deterioration in carbohydrate metabolism, other cases with more benign disease are being identified with increasing frequency. A few are detected accidentally by urinalysis before overt symptoms are observed. MODY is sometimes seen in obese teenagers. This type, like NIDDM, can often be controlled with diet restriction. Diabetes is a great imitator; influenza, gastroenteritis, and appendicitis are the conditions most often diagnosed.

Nursing ALERT

Recurrent urinary tract infections and vaginal infections, especially with *Candida albicans*, are often an early sign of IDDM, especially in adolescents.

Diagnostic Evaluation

Three groups of children who should be considered as possibly diabetic are (1) those who have glycosuria, polyuria, and a history of weight loss or failure to gain despite a hearty appetite; (2) those with transient or persistent glycosuria; and (3) those who display manifestations of metabolic acidosis, with or without stupor or coma. Clinical manifestations of IDDM are outlined in Box 49-12.

Diagnosis is based on *serum glucose levels*. A fasting blood glucose level of >140 mg/dl or a random blood glucose level of ≥200 mg/dl accompanied by classic signs of IDDM is almost certain to be caused by diabetes. Postprandial blood glucose determinations and the traditional oral glucose tolerance tests are not usually necessary for establishing a diagnosis. Serum insulin levels may be normal or moderately elevated at the onset of diabetes; delayed insulin response to glucose indicates the presence of prediabetes.

Ketoacidosis must be differentiated from other causes of acidosis or coma, including hypoglycemia, uremia, gastroenteritis with metabolic acidosis, salicylate intoxication, encephalitis, and other intracranial conditions. *Diabetic ketoacidosis*

BOX 49-12
Clinical Manifestations of Insulin-Dependent Diabetes Mellitus

Polyphagia
Polyuria
Polydipsia
Weight loss
Child may start bed-wetting
Irritability and "not himself" or "not herself"
Shortened attention span
Lowered frustration tolerance
Appears overly tired
Dry skin
Blurred vision
Sores that are slow to heal
Flushed skin
Headache
Frequent infections
Hyperglycemia:
- Elevated blood glucose levels
- Glucosuria

Diabetic ketosis:
- Ketones as well as glucose in urine
- No noticeable dehydration

Diabetic ketoacidosis:
- Dehydration
- Electrolyte imbalance
- Acidosis

(DKA), is determined by the presence of **hyperglycemia** (blood glucose measurement of ≥300 mg/dl), ketonemia (strongly positive), acidosis (pH of <7.30 and bicarbonate of <15 mEq/L), glycosuria, and ketonuria. Tests used to determine glycosuria and ketonuria are the glucose oxidase tapes (Tes-Tape and Clinistix) or Clinitest tablets.

Therapeutic Management

The management of the child with IDDM consists of a multidisciplinary approach involving the family, the child (when appropriate), and professionals, including a pediatric endocrinologist diabetes nurse educator, and nutritionist, as well as an exercise physiologist. Often psychologic support from a mental health professional is also needed. Communication among the team members is essential and extends to other individuals in the child's life, such as teachers, the school nurse, school guidance counselor, and coach.

The definitive treatment is replacement of insulin. However, insulin needs are affected by nutritional intake, activity, emotions, and other life events, such as illnesses and puberty. Medical and nutritional guidance is primary, but management also includes continuing diabetes education, family guidance, and emotional support.

Insulin therapy. Insulin is available in highly purified beef, pork, or beef-pork preparations and in human insulin manufactured by biosynthesis. Most clinicians consider human insulin the treatment of choice. It is available in rapid-, intermediate-, and long-acting preparations, and all are packaged in the strength of 100 units/ml. (Other dosages are available for situations in which extraordinarily large or small dosages are required.)

The precise dose of insulin needed cannot be predicted. Therefore a regimen of total dosage and the percentage of regular- to intermediate-acting insulin are determined for each child. The amount of insulin is based on capillary blood glucose levels, which the child or family member tests by means of a drop of blood on a chemically treated test strip with the aid of a color chart or a glucose monitor.

Daily insulin is administered subcutaneously by twice-daily injections, by multiple-dose injections, or by a portable pump. Diabetes can be controlled satisfactorily in most children with a *twice-daily insulin* regimen consisting of a combination of *rapid-acting (regular)* and *intermediate-acting (NPH or Lente)* insulin given in the same syringe before breakfast and before the evening meal. The amount of insulin is determined by measurements of the blood glucose level after the peak effect of the insulin has occurred. For example, the amount of regular insulin at breakfast is determined by the previous late-morning blood glucose measurement. Regular insulin is best given at least 30 minutes before meals to allow sufficient time for absorption. Some children require more frequent administration of insulin. This includes children with difficult-to-control diabetes and those experiencing an adolescent growth spurt. A *multiple daily injection* (MDI) program has been shown to reduce microvascular complications in young, healthy patients who have IDDM (Diabetes control, 1993; Reasner, 1994).

The *insulin pump* is designed to deliver fixed amounts of regular insulin continuously, thereby more closely imitating the release of the hormone by the islet cells. The system consists of a syringe to hold the insulin, a plunger, and a mechanism to drive the plunger. The insulin flows from the syringe through a catheter to a needle inserted into subcutaneous tissue (the abdomen or thigh), and the lightweight device is worn on a belt or a shoulder holster. The needle and catheter are changed every 48 hours by the child or parent, using aseptic technique, and taped in place.

Although the pump provides more even insulin release, it has disadvantages. It cannot be removed for more than 1 hour; therefore it may limit some activities, such as bathing and swimming, although some water-safe models are now available; reactions to the needle are common; and, like any other mechanical device, it is subject to malfunction. However, the pumps are equipped with alarms that signal problems that may arise, such as run-down batteries, blocked needle or tubing, or a malfunction that allows uncontrollable insulin delivery.

Researchers are experimenting with *intranasal insulin administration.* Specially prepared insulin combined with bile salts can be administered by means of an aerosol pump. The insulin is able to cross the nasal mucosa to increase serum levels. The duration of action is not long enough to be a total replacement for injections but may be of value as insulin supplementation at mealtime.

Islet cell or whole pancreas transplantation may offer hope to patients in the future. Viable insulin-producing cells have been injected into the portal vein, where they take root in the liver and eventually produce up to two thirds of the needed insulin. The major use of transplantation has been in persons who have serious complications, particularly those whose deteriorating kidneys have required renal transplantation and who are receiving immunosuppression therapy. However, islet cell and pancreatic transplantations tend not to be sustainable over time despite continuation of therapy. The use of nonhuman islets encapsulated in immunoprotective, semipermeable membranes may have a future in the treatment of IDDM (Brouhard and Rogers, 1993).

Monitoring. *Home blood glucose monitoring (HBGM)* has improved diabetes management and is used successfully by children from the onset of their diabetes. By testing their own blood, children are able to change their insulin regimen to maintain their glucose level in the euglycemic (normal) range of 80 to 120 mg/dl. Diabetes management depends to a great extent on HBGM.

Laboratory measurement of *glycosylated hemoglobin (hemoglobin A1c)* levels reflects the average blood glucose levels during the previous 3 months and is of value in assessing glucose control in any person with diabetes. As red blood cells circulate in the bloodstream, glucose molecules gradually attach to the hemoglobin A molecules and remain there for the lifetime of the red blood cell, approximately 120 days.

Urine testing for glucose is no longer used for diabetic management; there is poor correlation between simultaneous glycosuria and blood glucose concentrations. However, urine testing can be carried out to detect evidence of ketonuria.

Nursing ALERT

It is recommended that urine be tested for ketones during an illness and whenever blood glucose level is 250 mg/dl or higher when measured twice in a span of 4 to 6 hours.

Nutrition. Essentially the nutritional needs of children with diabetes are no different from those of unaffected children, except for deletion of concentration sugars. Children with diabetes require no special foods or supplements. They need sufficient calories to balance daily expenditure for energy and to satisfy the requirement for growth and development.

Normally insulin is secreted in response to food intake. However, subcutaneously injected insulin has a relatively predictable time of onset, peak effect, duration of action, and absorption rate, depending on the type of insulin used. Consequently the timing of food consumption is regulated to correspond to the time and action of the insulin prescribed. Meals and snacks must be eaten at the same times each day, and the total number of calories and proportions of basic nutrients must be consistent from day to day. The distribution of calories is determined to fit the activity pattern of each child. Alterations in food intake are made so that food, insulin, and exercise are balanced. Extra food is needed for extra activity.

The food intake is based on a balanced diet that incorporates six basic food groups: milk, meat, vegetables, fat, fruit, and bread. The family may follow the exchange system approved by the American Diabetes Association (ADA) or the point system, based on 75 kcal equaling 1 point. The exchange system indicates the amount (portion size) of each food by volume or weight and is prescribed in terms of the number of exchanges from each food group that constitutes each meal and snack. This ensures day-to-day consistency in total calories, protein, fat, and carbohydrate while allowing a choice among a wide variety of foods. Fiber is important in dietary planning because of its influence on digestion, absorption, and metabolism of many nutrients; it diminishes the rise in the blood glucose level after meals.

Exercise. Exercise is encouraged and never restricted unless indicated by other health conditions, because it lowers blood glucose levels. It is included in diabetic management and is planned around the child's interests and capabilities. However, in most instances children's activities are unplanned, and the resulting decrease in the blood glucose level can be compensated for by providing extra snacks before (and, if prolonged, during) the activity. Besides providing a feeling of well-being, regular exercise aids in the body's use of food and often decreases insulin requirements.

Hypoglycemia. Even a child with well-controlled diabetes may often experience mild symptoms of hypoglycemia, but if the signs and symptoms are recognized early (Table 49-2) and relieved promptly by appropriate therapy, the child's activity should not be interrupted for more than a few minutes.

Nursing ALERT

Children on split-mixed insulin dosage schedules tend to experience hypoglycemic episodes at 11:30 AM and 2:30 AM as peaking of insulin occurs.

The most common causes of **hypoglycemia,** or *insulin reaction* are bursts of physical activity without additional food, or delayed, omitted, or incompletely consumed meals. Reglycosylation of muscles may occur over the ensuing 24 hours. Therefore particular vigilance related to hypoglycemia may be necessary during the night after vigorous exertion.

In the majority of cases simple concentrated sugar, such as honey, that can be held in the mouth for a short time will elevate the blood glucose level and alleviate the symptoms. The simpler the carbohydrate, the more rapidly it will be absorbed. For a mild reaction milk is a good food to use in children. It supplies them with lactose or milk sugar, as well as providing more prolonged action of the protein and fat (aids in decreased absorption). All children with diabetes should carry with them a source of glucose, such as glucose tablets (Instaglucose), candy (Life Savers), or sugar cubes. The rapid-releasing sugar is followed by a complex carbohydrate and protein, such as a slice of bread or a cracker spread with peanut butter.

Glucagon is sometimes prescribed for home treatment of hypoglycemia. It is available in a premixed syringe and is administered intramuscularly or subcutaneously. It functions by releasing stored glycogen from the liver and requires about 15 to 20 minutes to elevate the blood glucose level. Once the child is responsive, the lost glycogen stores are replaced by small amounts of sugar-containing fluid administered frequently until the child feels comfortable about trying solid foods.

Nursing ALERT

Vomiting may occur after administration of glucagon; therefore precautions against aspiration must be taken, such as placing the child on the side, because the child will be unconscious.

The *somogyi effect* should be recognized as a separate response from hypoglycemia. This phenomenon occurs when the blood glucose level decreases to the point where stress hormones (epinephrine, growth hormone, and corticosteroids) are released, causing a rebound hyperglycemia. Treatment consists of increasing the amount of food eaten and/or decreasing the insulin.

Illness management. Illness alters diabetes management, and maintaining control is usually related to the seriousness of the illness. As the illness runs its course, the goal of diabetes management is to maintain some euglycemia while recognizing and treating urinary ketones. Some hyperglycemia and ketonuria are expected in most illnesses, even with diminished food intake, and indicate the need for increased insulin. Insulin should never be omitted during an illness, although dosage requirements may increase, decrease, or remain unchanged, depending on the severity of the illness and the child's appetite. Insulin dosage based on a sliding scale according to ABGM should be implemented by using regular insulin only in place of, not in addition to, prescribed insulin.

Management of diabetic ketoacidosis. DKA, the most complete state of insulin deficiency, is a life-threatening situation. The child is admitted to an intensive care facility for management, which consists of rapid assessment, supply of adequate insulin to reduce the elevated blood glucose level, fluids to overcome dehydration, and electrolyte (especially potassium) replacement. The preferred method for administering insulin to the child with ketoacidosis is a continuous infusion of low-dose regular insulin.

Nursing ALERT

Since insulin can chemically bind to plastic tubing and in-line filters, thereby reducing the amount of the medication reaching the bloodstream, an insulin mixture is run through the tubing to saturate the insulin binding sites before the infusion is begun.

Current trends suggest cautious fluid managment to reduce risk of cerebral edema. The fluid deficit is replaced evenly over 24 to 48 hours. Serum potassium levels may be normal on admission, but rapid return of potassium to cells after initiation of fluid and insulin can seriously deplete serum levels, with the attendant risk of cardiac arrhythmias. A cardiac monitor is employed as a guide to therapy and for determination of changes that may indicate alterations in potassium concentration.

Nursing ALERT

Potassium must never be given until the serum potassium level is known to be normal or low and voiding is observed. All intravenous (IV) fluids should include 20 to 40 mEq/L of potassium. Never give potassium as a rapid IV bolus; cardiac arrest may result.

When the critical period is over, the task of regulating insulin dosage to diet and activity is begun. Children should be actively involved in their own care and are given responsibility according to their ability and guidance of the nurse.

Nursing Care Management

Assessment

Daily monitoring of blood glucose levels, periodic urine analysis for ketones, and observation for signs of hypoglycemia, hyperglycemia, or other complications are part of the daily life of the child with diabetes and the family. Diabetes should be suspected in any child who exhibits the manifestations outlined in Box 49-12, and the child should be referred for further assessment and appropriate testing.

The signs and symptoms of hypoglycemia are caused by both increased adrenergic activity and impaired brain function, and it is often difficult to distinguish between hyper-

TABLE 49-2 Comparison of manifestations of hypoglycemia and hyperglycemia

VARIABLE	HYPOGLYCEMIA	HYPERGLYCEMIA
Onset	Rapid (minutes)	Gradual (days)
Mood	Labile, irritable, nervous, weepy	Lethargic
Mental status	Difficulty concentrating, speaking, focusing, coordinating	Dulled sensorium Confused
Inward feeling	Shaky feeling, hunger Headache Dizziness	Thirst Weakness Nausea/vomiting Abdominal pain
Skin	Pallor Sweating	Flushed Signs of dehydration
Mucous membranes	Normal	Dry, crusty
Respirations	Shallow	Deep, rapid (Kussmaul)
Pulse	Tachycardia	Less rapid, weak
Breath odor	Normal	Fruity, acetone
Neurologic	Tremors Late: hyperflexia, dilated pupils, convulsion	Diminished reflexes Paresthesia
Ominous signs	Shock, coma	Acidosis, coma
Blood:		
Glucose	Low: below 60 mg/dl	High: 250 mg/dl or more
Ketones	Negative	High/large
Osmolarity	Normal	High
pH	Normal	Low (7.25 or less)
Hematocrit	Normal	High
HCO_3	Normal	Less than 20 mEq/L
Urine:		
Output	Normal	Polyuria (early) to oliguria (late)
Sugar	Negative	High
Ketones	Negative/trace	High

glycemia and a hypoglycemic reaction (Table 49-2). Since the symptoms are similar and usually begin with changes in behavior, the simplest way to differentiate between the two is to test the blood glucose level (low in hypoglycemia; elevated in hyperglycemia).

The nurse should also be alert to evidence of complications, although these are usually not manifested until adulthood. Assessment of skin for evidence of breakdown is important in order that appropriate care can be implemented to facilitate healing and prevent infection. Because illnesses, such as respiratory infections or gastrointestinal upsets, complicate diabetes management, they should be detected early.

Education is the cornerstone of diabetes management and the major responsibility in diabetes nursing care. Whether teaching is conducted on an outpatient basis or in a preparatory, in-depth manner on an inpatient basis, the ability of the individuals involved to learn must be accurately assessed. This includes assessment of the educational background and emotional stability of the individual(s) involved and the use of appropriate measurement tools, such as a pretest or an objective assessment of the learner's educational level and literacy.

Nursing Diagnoses

A number of nursing diagnoses are prominent in the nursing management of IDDM, and others specific to individual cases become evident. The most common are outlined in the Nursing Care Plan on p. 1651).

Planning

The goals of care for the child with IDDM and family are as follows:

1. Child and family will be educated about the disease, assessment techniques, and therapy.
2. Child will experience a minimum of complications of diabetes.
3. Child will develop a positive self-image.
4. Child and family will receive adequate support.

Implementation

Once the child with diabetes is diagnosed and insulin therapy initiated, the major nursing responsibilities are education of the family and reinforcement of information. The parents must supervise and manage the child's therapeutic program, but the child should assume responsibility for self-management as soon as he or she is capable. Children can learn to collect their own blood for glucose testing at a relatively young age (4 to 5 years), and most are able to check their blood glucose level and administer insulin at about 9 years of age. In situations in which the parents are inconsistent and/or unreliable, the child is taught self-care at an earlier age.

The first 3 or 4 days after diagnosis is not an optimal time for learning. Therefore the family should be given only essential, or survival, information first and intense information later. A child learns best when sessions are kept short, no more than 15 to 20 minutes. The parents do best in periods of 45 to 60 minutes and often longer if they are inquisitive. Education should involve all the senses, and although visual aids are valuable tools, participation is the most effective method for learning. For example, to teach blood testing, the technique is explained; the procedure is demonstrated; the learner is allowed to perform the procedure (followed by a review of the material by visual aids); and the learning is validated by some testing method that includes feedback. Varying the presentation with a number of audiovisual materials, including videotapes, slide-tape programs, and books, stimulates the senses and helps the individual to learn.

Several organizations are prepared to assist with education and dissemination of knowledge about diabetes. The American Diabetes Association, Inc.,* Canadian Diabetes Association,† Juvenile Diabetes Foundation International,‡ Juvenile Diabetes Foundation—Canada,§ and American Association of Diabetes Educators|| are valuable resources for a wide variety of educational materials. The National Diabetes Information Clearinghouse,¶ publishes a number of comprehensive annotated bibliographies, including *Educational Materials for and about Young People with Diabetes,* a compilation of resource materials for children, siblings, parents, teachers, and health professionals, and *Sports and Exercise for People with Diabetes.*

Self-management, the ultimate goal for the child with diabetes, is more likely to occur when the child understands the disease and the care it requires. Properly educated, any family should be able to follow a program of regulated control satisfactorily. The following information will allow the family to manage the daily aspects of care.

Identification. One of the first issues that should be called to the attention of parents is the need for the child to wear a medical alert bracelet for identification. This essential and immediate information can save the child's life.

Nature of diabetes. The better the parents understand the pathophysiologic characteristics of diabetes and the function and action of insulin and glucagon in relation to caloric intake and exercise, the better their understanding of the disease and its effect on the child. Parents need answers to a number of questions (voiced or unvoiced), because those answers will provide them with an increased feeling of security in coping with the disease.

Meal planning. Normal nutrition is a major aspect of the family education program. Diet instruction is usually conducted by the nutritionist, with reinforcement and guidance from the nurse (Fig. 49-3). Learning about foods with specific food groups helps in making choices. Weights and measures of foods, used as eye-training devices in defining food volumes, should be practiced repeatedly, with gradual conversion to estimating foods. Members of the family are also guided in reading labels for the nutritional value of foods and food contents. Meals and snacks are modified around the child and the present food menu, preserving cultural patterns and preferences as much as possible.

Lists of popular fast-food items and items served at the ma-

---

*1660 Duke St., Alexandria, VA 22314; (800) 232-3472.
†15 Toronto St. Suite 800, Toronto, Ontario, Canada, M5C 2E3, (416) 363-3373.
‡432 Park Ave., S., New York, NY 10016; (800) 223-1138.
§89 Granton Dr., Richmond Hill, Ontario, Canada L4B 2N5; (800) 668-0274.
|| 500 N. Michigan Ave., Chicago, IL 60611; (800) 338-3633.
¶Box NDIC, 9000 Rockville Pike, Bethesda, MD 20892.

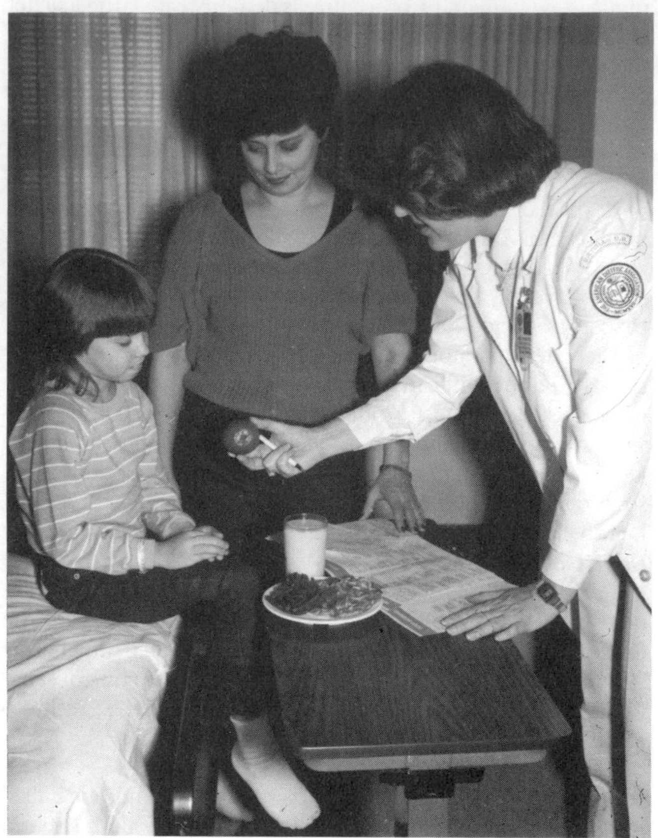

Fig. 49-3 Nutritionist instructs child, using food to explain food exchanges.

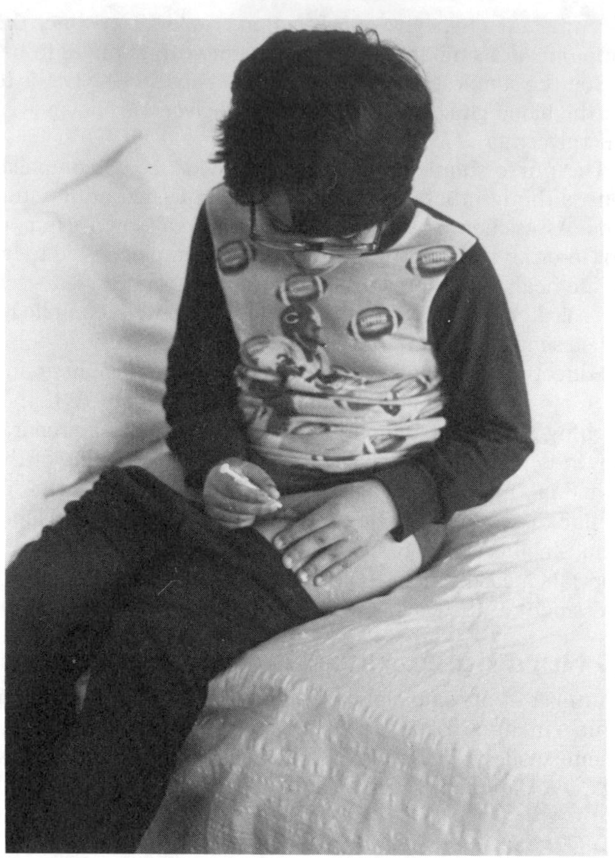

Fig. 49-4 School-age children are able to administer their own insulin.

jor fast-food chains can be obtained from the ADA to help guide food selections. Children are advised to use sugar substitutes with moderation in items such as soft drinks. "Sugar-free" chewing gum and candies made with sorbitol are not usually recommended for children with diabetes. Sorbitol is metabolized to fructose and then to glucose, and large amounts can cause an osmotic diarrhea. Dietetic foods that contain sorbitol are more expensive than regular foods, and the caloric content of the food is the same or even greater.

Insulin. Families need to understand the treatment method and the insulin prescribed, including the effective duration, onset, and peak action. They also need to know the characteristics of the various types of insulins, the proper mixing and dilution of insulins, and how to substitute another type when their usual brand is not available (insulin is a nonprescription drug). Insulin need not be refrigerated but should be maintained at a temperature above freezing and below 29.4° C (85° F). An extra supply can be kept in the refrigerator. Freezing renders insulin inactive.

Injection procedure. Learning to give the insulin injections is a source of anxiety for the family and the child. It is helpful for the learner to know that this important aspect of care will become as routine as brushing the teeth. First the basic injection technique is taught, using an orange or similar item and normal saline solution for practice.* To gain the confidence of the child, the nurse demonstrates the technique by giving a skillful injection to the parent, who then returns the demonstration by giving the nurse an injection. With practice family members soon are able to give the insulin injection to the child. Both parents should participate, and as little time as possible should elapse between instruction and the actual injection, especially with parents and the teenage learner.

Insulin can be injected into any area in which there is skin over muscle with fatty tissue in between (Fig. 49-4). The drug is injected at a 90-degree angle. If the child is especially thin or debilitated, a 45-degree angle can be used. Newly diagnosed children may have lost adipose tissue, and care should be exercised not to inject into the muscle or blood vessel. Usually the smaller the child, the thinner the skin. The pinch technique is the most effective method for obtaining skin tightness to allow easy entrance of the needle into subcutaneous tissues in children. The site selected will sometimes depend on whether the child or parent administers the insulin. The upper arms, thighs, hips, and abdomen are usual injection sites for insulin. The child can reach the thighs, abdomen, and part

*Home care instructions on subcutaneous injection are available in Wong DL: *Wong and Whaley's clinical manual of pediatric nursing*, ed 4, St Louis, 1996, Mosby.

TABLE 49-3 Onset and duration of action related to injection site

	SITE OF INJECTION			
	ABDOMEN	ARM	LEG	BUTTOCK
Rate	Very fast	Fast	Slow	Very slow
Duration	Very short	Short	Long	Very long

From Albisser AM, Sperlich M: Adjusting insulins, *Diabetes Educator* 18(3):211-218, 1992.

of the hip and arm easily but may require help to inject other sites. For example, a parent can pinch a loose fold of skin on the arm while the child injects the insulin.

Injections are rotated to various areas of the body to enhance absorption, since insulin absorption is slowed by the fat pads that develop in overused areas of injection. The parents and child are helped to work out a rotation pattern, which involves giving about four to six injections in one area (each injection about 1 inch, or the diameter of the insulin vial, from the previous injection) and then moving to another area. In this way injection sites for an entire month can be planned in advance on a simple chart or illustration, such as an outline of a body or a teddy bear. It is a good idea for the parents each to give one or two injections a week in the areas that are difficult to reach in order to keep in practice.

It is important to remember that the absorption rate varies in different parts of the body (Table 49-3). Methodically using one anatomic area and then moving to another minimizes variation in absorption rates. Injecting *small* doses of insulin also minimizes changes in plasma glucose levels. Absorption is also altered by vigorous exercise, which enhances absorption from exercised muscles. Therefore it is recommended that excess exercise be avoided during the time the insulin is expected to peak or that other sites be used.

Teaching includes the proper way to equalize pressure in the bottle by injecting an amount of air equal to the amount of solution withdrawn and to remove air bubbles from the syringe. When insulin dosages are small, an air bubble in the syringe can displace a significant amount of medication. Since the introduction of the $^{5}/_{10}$ ml and $^{3}/_{10}$ ml syringes, the risk of incorrect dosage has diminished. However, insulin injections of less than 2 units of U100 have an unacceptably large error. Diluted insulin should be used if the prescribed dose is less than 2 units (Casella et al, 1993). Aspiration for blood before injecting the insulin is not routinely done.

Insulin syringes should be compared for accuracy, comfort, and strength. The family and/or child should be able to choose both "their" insulin and "their" syringe from a variety of samples. Use of the same type of syringe (even during hospitalization) is recommended to prevent errors in dosage caused by varying amounts of dead space among syringes.

Occasionally children are taught to use a syringe-loaded injector *(Injectease)*, especially those who are fearful of puncturing their skin. With the device, puncture is always automatic. Adolescents respond well to a self-contained and compact device resembling a fountain pen (e.g., *NovoPen**), which eliminates conventional vials and syringes. Preloaded pens may also cause less pain, because the needle is not blunted by piercing the rubber top of the insulin vial (Chantelau et at, 1991).

*Squibb-Novo, Inc., Princeton, NJ.

When the child's dosage requires the injection of both short- and intermediate-acting insulin at the same time, most families prefer to mix the two and use a single injection. However, there are some problems associated with this accepted practice, and the family should understand what happens when insulins are mixed. Longer-acting insulins contain ingredients that bind to insulin, allowing for gradual release after injection. Some brands contain extra binding compounds that can bind with regular insulin, converting it to the long-acting type and altering the effect on blood glucose. The degree of alteration depends on the type of longer-acting insulin, the ratio of short- to long-acting insulin, and the time the mixture is allowed to stand before injection. The mixture should be injected less than 5 minutes after mixing (before the zinc content of the long-acting insulin affects the action time of the regular or short-acting insulin) or longer than 15 minutes after mixing (to allow the insulins to recover their long-acting and short-acting properties).

To obtain the maximum benefit from mixing insulins, the recommended practice is as follows:

1. Inject the measured amount of air (equivalent to the dosage) into the longer-acting insulin.
2. Inject the measured amount of air into the regular insulin.
3. Withdraw the regular insulin.
4. Insert the needle (already containing the regular insulin) into the longer-acting insulin and withdraw the desired amount.

Nursing ALERT

When mixing types of insulin always withdraw regular insulin first, then the longer-acting insulin next to prevent contamination of the regular or short-acting insulin with longer-acting insulin.

It has become acceptable practice to reuse disposable needles and syringes for up to 7 days. Bacteria counts are unaffected, and there is a considerable cost saving. If this method is approved, it is important to stress the importance of vigorous handwashing before handling any equipment, as well as capping the syringe immediately after use and storing it in the refrigerator to decrease the growth of organisms.

Nurses should also teach proper disposal of equipment after use in the home. Although it is not standard practice in the hospital, at-home use of a needle clipper is recommended to safely remove and house the used needle. In addition, the syringe plunger can be broken before disposal. An excellent means for syringe disposal is use of an opaque, puncture-resistant container, such as an empty coffee can, bleach bottle, or milk carton. The container is labeled "biohazardous waste" and discarded with similar material only, not with household refuse.

Some children are considered candidates for continuous subcutaneous insulin infusion with a portable insulin pump. The child and parents are taught to operate the device, including the mechanics of the pump, battery changes, and alarm systems. They learn how to load the syringe, insert the catheter, adjust the insulin flow for routine needs and for illnesses, and connect and disconnect the catheter. Nurses who work where the pumps are part of the therapeutic regimen should become familiar with the operation of the specific device being used and the protocol of the regimen.

Glucose monitoring. Nurses should also be prepared to teach and supervise blood glucose monitoring. Blood for testing can be obtained by two different methods: manually or with a spring-loaded puncturing device. The automatic puncture device is recommended because its precise puncture depth produces better blood flow and less pain. However, the child and family should learn to use both methods in the event of mechanical failure. Several lancet devices are available from which to choose, and each provides a means for obtaining an adequate drop of blood for testing (Fig. 49-5).

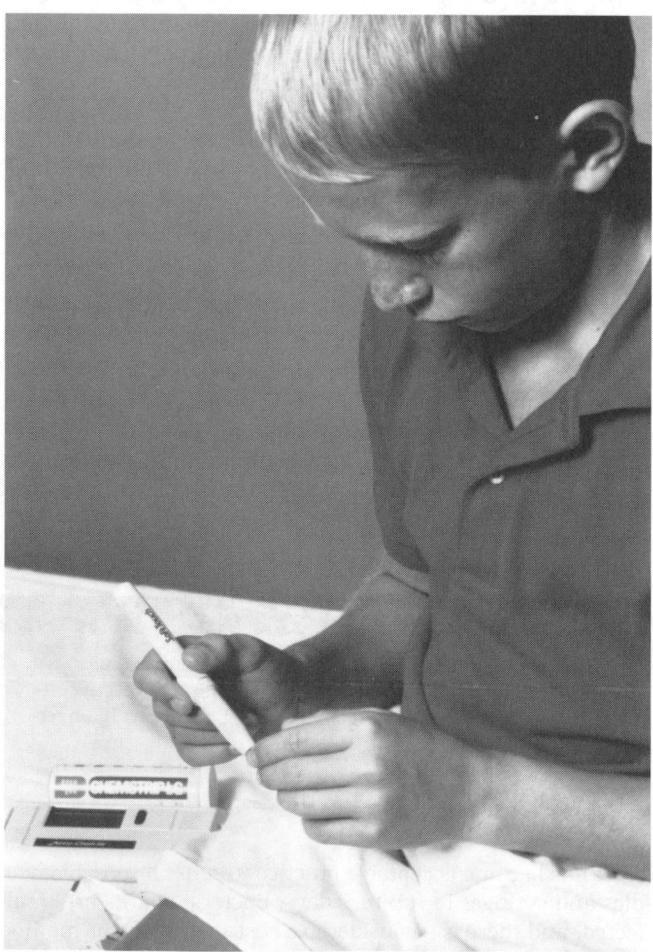

Fig. 49-5 Child using automatic puncture or "finger-stick" device to obtain blood sample. Blood glucose monitor and reagent strips are nearby.

Nursing ALERT

Caution children not to allow anyone else to use their lancet because of the danger of contracting hepatitis B virus or human immunodeficiency virus (HIV).

Repeated finger punctures can be painful, but most children become accustomed to the procedure (see the Atraumatic Care box below). However, persistent signs of redness and soreness at the puncture site should be investigated. It may be evidence of poor technique or poor skin healing relative to poor control.

The least expensive testing method uses a reagent strip to which blood is applied. After blotting, the color change is compared with a color scale for an estimation of the blood glucose level. The strips can be cut in half (although this is not recommended by all professionals) to obtain two readings per strip. This method may be ideal for use at school, where expensive equipment can be lost or broken.

Many types of glucose monitors are available for home use. The family should be shown features of several meters, including advantages and disadvantages, and allowed to choose equipment that best meets their needs. One important consideration is the amount of blood needed. Choosing devices that require small amounts may prevent repunctures.

Urine testing. Urine testing is easily taught and should include all methods, not just the test to be used for the particular child. Testing for ketones is recommended during times of illness or when glucose readings are high. Since moisture will cause changes to take place in both glucose and ketone strips,

Atraumatic Care

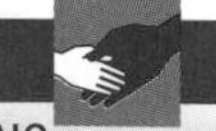

MINIMIZING PAIN OF BLOOD GLUCOSE MONITORING

To enhance blood flow to the finger, hold it under warm water for a few seconds before the puncture.
When obtaining blood samples, use the ring finger or thumb (blood flows more easily to these areas), and puncture the finger just to the side of the finger pad (more blood vessels and fewer nerve endings).
To prevent a deep puncture, press the platform of the lancet device lightly against the skin and avoid steadying the finger against a hard surface.
Use preloaded insulin devices (e.g., NovoPen).
Use glucose monitors that require very small blood samples to prevent repunctures (e.g., Glucometer Elite).
Apply EMLA to puncture site, especially when child is newly diagnosed and skin is still very sensitive (see Pain Management, Chapter 41).

families are instructed to discard strips that are discolored, that have been open for a specified time, or after an expiration date. Test strips are available for testing both glucose and ketones.

Hyperglycemia and hypoglycemia. Severe hyperglycemia is most often caused by illness, growth, or emotional upset. With careful glucose monitoring, any elevation can be managed by adjustment of insulin or food intake. The family should understand how to adjust food, activity, and insulin at the time of illness or when the child is treated for an illness with a medication known to raise the blood glucose level, such as cough syrup or steroids. The hyperglycemia is managed by increasing insulin soon after the increased glucose is noted.

Hypoglycemia is caused by imbalances of food intake, insulin, and activity. Ideally hypoglycemia should be prevented, and parents need to be prepared to prevent, recognize, and treat the problem. They should be familiar with the signs of hypoglycemia and instructed in treatment, including care of the child with seizures (see Chapter 48). Hypoglycemia can be managed effectively as outlined in the Emergency box below.

Exercise. Exercise should be planned (as may be necessary for the sedentary teenager) or observed (as in most active children). If the child is more active at one time of the day than at another, food and/or insulin can be altered to meet the activity pattern of the individual. Food should be increased in the summer, when children tend to be more active. Decreased activity on return to school may require a decrease in food intake. The child who is active in team sports will need an additional snack on the days of activity about ½ hour before the anticipated activity. Races or other competition may call for a slightly higher food intake than practice times.

EMERGENCY

HYPOGLYCEMIA

Mild reaction: adrenergic symptoms

Give child 10 to 15 g simple, high carbohydrate (preferably liquid, e.g., 3 to 6 oz milk).
Follow with starch-protein snack.

Moderate reaction: neuroglycopenic symptoms

Give child 10 to 15 g simple carbohydrate as above.
Repeat in 10 to 15 minutes if symptoms persist.
Follow with larger snack.
Watch child closely.

Severe reaction: unresponsive, unconscious, and/or seizures

Administer glucagon as prescribed.
Watch child closely for seizures and vomiting (glucagon may take up to 15 minutes to have an effect).
Follow with planned meal or snack when child is able to eat, or add a snack of 10% of daily calories.

Nocturnal reaction

Give child 10 to 15 g simple carbohydrate.
Follow with snack of 10% of daily calories.

Food will usually need to be repeated for prolonged activity periods, often as frequently as every 45 minutes to 1 hour. Families should be informed that if increased food is not tolerated, decreased insulin is the next course of action. If the blood glucose level is elevated (240 mg/dl or higher) before planned exercise, the activity should be postponed until the blood glucose level is controlled.

Record keeping. Recording information about food, insulin, blood glucose measurements, and ketonuria is useful to the practitioner, as well as to the family. Insulin reactions are noted, including the time, severity, treatment, and response to treatment. Dietary variations are noted so that an increased blood glucose level can be analyzed in relation to insulin dose, food intake, and activity level.

Self-management. Self-management is the key to close control. Being able to make changes at the time they are needed rather than waiting until the next contact with health professionals is important for self-management and gives the individual and family the feeling that they have control over the disease. As children grow and assume more and more responsibility for self-management, they develop confidence in their ability to manage their disease and in themselves as persons. Self-management techniques to be mastered are the testing of blood and urine and adjustment of insulin and diet with alterations in day-to-day activities and unusual occurrences.

Hygiene. All aspects of personal hygiene are emphasized for the child with diabetes. The child should be cautioned against wearing shoes without socks, wearing sandals, or walking barefoot. The correct method of nail and extremity care instituted for each particular child (with the guidance of a podiatrist) can begin health practices that last a lifetime. Eyes should be checked once a year, unless the child wears glasses, and then as directed by the ophthalmologist. Regular dental care is emphasized, and cuts and scratches should be treated with plain soap and water unless otherwise indicated.

Acute care. Children with diabetes may be admitted to the hospital at the time of their initial diagnosis, during illness or surgery, or during episodes of DKA—especially the small number who exhibit a degree of metabolic lability or who have repeated episodes of DKA. Most children with diabetes are able to keep the disease under control with periodic assessment and adjustment of insulin, diet, and activity as needed under health practitioner supervision.

The child with DKA requires intensive nursing care. On admission to the hospital, usually an intensive care unit, an intravenous infusion is started immediately to hydrate the child and to administer insulin, usually as a continuous infusion (see Management of DKA p.1644). The blood glucose level is monitored at regular intervals, and the insulin administered as ordered.

Sodium, potassium, and bicarbonate levels are monitored and replaced as indicated. Since potassium and sodium reenter the cells rapidly after administration of insulin, depletion of these electrolytes can be a serious consequence. The child is attached to a cardiac monitor for continual assessment of cardiac status, especially when potassium levels are markedly altered.

Careful and accurate records are maintained, including vital signs, blood pressure, intravenous fluids, electrolytes, insulin, blood glucose level, and intake and output. A urine collection device or retention catheter is used to obtain the urine measurements, which include volume, specific gravity, and glucose and ketone values. The volume relative to the glucose content is important, since 5% glucose in a 300 ml sample is a significantly greater amount than a similar reading from a 75 ml sample. A diabetic flow sheet maintained at the bedside provides an ongoing record of the vital signs, urine and blood tests, amount of insulin given, and intake and output of the patient. The level of consciousness is assessed and recorded at frequent intervals. The comatose child generally regains consciousness fairly soon after initiation of therapy but is managed as is any unconscious child during that time.

Family support. In any educational program the psychologic needs of the child are just as important as the physical needs. Adjustment to a chronic illness is difficult and follows the grief process (see Chapter 38). A noticeable adjustment cycle occurs during the week-long education course. First there is interest and perhaps some anger and doubt, followed by denial and accompanied by the overwhelming feeling of "Why me?" There are doubts regarding the ability to absorb so much essential information. Then there are the acceptance and synthesis of material, as the learners realize that they are able to state and demonstrate their understanding of the material.

Children in the years before adolescence tend to accept their condition most easily. However, challenges exist, such as providing regular feedings to the sick infant or to the negative toddler. With toddlers and preschoolers insulin injections and

Family Focus

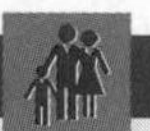

THE ADOLESCENT WITH IDDM

As a nurse caring for adolescents with IDDM I am constantly aware of the wide range of adolescent behaviors that affect the course of this disease. Education of the child and the parents can often make the difference between a disease in control of the teen and a teen in control of the disease.

I have cared for many adolescent females who have episodes of hyperglycemia at the time of menstruation that can result in DKA. I have found that education regarding a sick day protocol with sliding-scale regular insulin instituted at the first sign of hyperglycemia, which may occur 1 to 2 days before onset of menses, can keep the adolescent girl out of the ICU and in control of her diabetes.

Eating disorders, such as bulimia or anorexia nervosa, in the teenager with IDDM pose a serious health hazard. Insulin manipulation or omission has been identified as a weight loss method used by some female adolescents (Rodin, Craven, and Daneman, 1989). Nurses working with these adolescents, especially females, must be aware of the hazards and openly discuss the risks with the young person. A referral for specialized intervention may be needed.

Another group of adolescents with diabetes who are at risk are those who drink alcohol. I have found that confusion about the effects of alcohol on blood glucose is common. Teens may believe that alcohol will increase blood glucose levels, although in fact it has the opposite effect. Ingestion of alcohol inhibits the release of glycogen from the liver, therefore resulting in hypoglycemia. Teens with diabetes who drink alcohol may become hypoglycemic but be treated as if they were inebriated (drunk). Behaviors may be similar, such as shakiness, combativeness, slurred speech, and loss of consciousness. Education regarding the effects of alcohol is important and must be included in a teaching plan. If teens insist on drinking alcohol, they can be cautioned to use sweetened mixers or eat snacks when consuming alcoholic beverages.

Episodes of hyperglycemia or hypoglycemia may become a serious issue for adolescents who are leaving home for the first time. One teenager confided that her mother always recognized her combative, antisocial behavior as impending hypoglycemia and treated her with the appropriate intervention. The teen feared that a college roommate might be offended by the behavior and leave her alone with impending hypoglycemia.

One young man realized he could not live alone when he "took a nap because of feeling tired" and woke up 4 days later in the hospital. Fortunately his family realized he was in a coma and summoned emergency medical service. The fatigue signaled the beginning of a viral infection, which led to a blood glucose level of 410 mg/dl. Nurses need to address these fears openly and facilitate ways in which the teen can enlist the aid of significant peers who may be available during hyperglycemic or hypoglycemic episodes.

Susan Zekauskas, RN, MSN, PNP

Critical Thinking

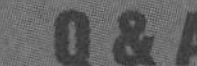

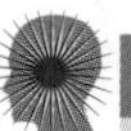

INSULIN-DEPENDENT DIABETES MELLITUS

Rebecca, 15 years old, has a 3-year history of IDDM and has been admitted to the pediatric intensive care unit for treatment of diabetic ketoacidosis (DKA). This is her fifth admission for DKA in 1 year. Rebecca's parents are divorced and she has four younger siblings. Rebecca's mother has maintained two jobs for the past 5 years and frequently leaves Rebecca in charge of the household. In anticipation of her discharge you plan a teaching plan for Rebecca and her mother. Areas of diabetes management that must be stressed are the need for careful management of her diet, an exercise program, the requirement of conscientious self-testing of blood glucose with appropriate administration of daily insulin, the use of sliding-scale insulin therapy as prescribed, urine ketone testing when blood glucose levels are high, and methods to handle emotional stressors. Of the following issues that may be influencing the recurrent episodes of DKA, which one should you address first?

1. The responsibility Rebecca feels for the care of her four younger siblings
2. Fluctuation of blood glucose levels around the time of menses with inadequate insulin coverage
3. Stress related to the absence of Rebecca's mother and the loss of the close relationship Rebecca shared with her father
4. Adolescent issues, such as seeking independence, feeling different because of IDDM, and alcohol use

The correct answer is two. The nurse should concentrate first on those situations directly related to hyperglycemia. Adolescent families with diabetes tend to experience frequent fluctuation of blood glucose levels, especially increased blood glucose immediately before, during, or after menses. Emotional stress related to increased responsibilities, personal loss from divorce, and normal developmental tasks of adolescence can also precipitate a stress response and elevate blood glucose levels. The nurse should address these issues as time for teaching permits or make a referral for special support ser-

glucose testing may be difficult at first. However, they usually accept the procedures when the parents use a matter-of-fact approach without calling attention to a "hurt" and treat the procedure like any other routine part of a child's life. Some special and positive attention, such as reading, talking, or other pleasant activity, after an injection is one way to convert children who initially refuse injections to those who accept them.

School-age children can understand the basic concepts related to their disease and its treatment. They are able to test blood glucose and urine, recognize food groups, give injections, keep records, and distinguish among feelings of fear, excitement, and hypoglycemia. They understand how to recognize, prevent, and treat hypoglycemia. However, they still need considerable parental involvement.

Adolescents appear to have the most difficulty in adjusting. Adolescence is a time when there is much stress on being "perfect" and being like peers and, no matter what others say, having diabetes is being different. Some youngsters are more upset about not being able to have a candy bar than about injections, diet, and other aspects of management. If children can accept the differences as a part of life, in other words, that each person is different in some way, then with adequate family support they should be able to adjust well (see the Family Focus box and the Critical Thinking Q & A box on p. 1651).

For all families, daily compliance with numerous procedures and structured living schedules is difficult. Maintaining good blood glucose control requires ongoing motivation. Nurses can encourage families to adhere to treatment regimens and life-style adjustments by emphasizing the benefits of preventing complications such as hypoglycemia. However,

Nursing Care Plan

THE CHILD WITH DIABETES MELLITUS

Nursing Diagnosis: Risk for injury related to hypoglycemia or hyperglycemia

Expected Outcome: Child demonstrates normal blood glucose levels.

• NURSING INTERVENTIONS/*RATIONALES*

Obtain blood glucose level *to determine appropriate insulin dose and monitor glucose level.*

Administer insulin as ordered *to maintain normal glucose level.*

Make sure nutritional intake is appropriate, timely, and adequate *to maintain blood glucose level.*

Monitor for signs of hypoglycemia (i.e., sweating, shaky nervousness, faintness, fatigue, palpitations, confusion) and hyperglycemia (nausea, urinary frequency, thirst, hunger, tiredness, fruity breath) and correct appropriately (i.e., readily absorbed carbohydrates followed by complex carbohydrate and protein for hypoglycemia; insulin for hyperglycemia) *to maintain glucose balance and prevent long-term complications.*

Nursing Diagnosis: Knowledge deficit related to new health condition (diabetes mellitus)

Expected Outcomes: Child and family delineate plan of care for management of diabetes; child and family exhibit evidence of incorporation of care behaviors into daily routine.

• NURSING INTERVENTIONS/*RATIONALES*

Ascertain family's general knowledge of diabetes *to assess baseline knowledge.* Set up an environment conducive to learning (i.e., teaching methods appropriate to age of child and family; use of written materials, pictures, audiovisuals; use of short repetitive teaching sessions with ongoing reinforcement of information and feedback; encouragement of questions; clarification of misconceptions) *to maximize learning.*

Discuss the pathology and potential sequelae of diabetes, the function and actions of insulin in relation to eating and exercise, the need for careful adherence to the plan of care, and the importance of regular health care *to ensure adequate understanding and promote compliance.*

Help family understand diabetic diet and dietary exchanges and to plan any needed dietary changes within family cultural and food preferences; help with menus, recipes, shopping strategies (refer to dietitian if available) *to promote successful adaptation of dietary practices.*

Teach family the importance of careful blood glucose monitoring *to maintain consistent blood glucose levels and prevent ketoacidosis.*

Teach family about importance of judicious exercise and the need for glucose monitoring after vigorous exercise *to prevent hypoglycemia.*

Teach family about need for careful oral and body hygiene; prompt treatment of cuts and scrapes; careful foot care; regular visits to the dentist, ophthalmologist, and endocrinologist *to prevent or detect early signs of complications.*

Teach family how to use and interpret glucose monitoring equipment; how to store, draw up, and administer insulin; how to rotate injection sites; use of any other needed supplies or equipment by using a demonstration return demonstration technique *to ensure comfort and ability to perform needed procedures and handle equipment.*

Have child wear a medical identification device (bracelet, necklace) at all times *to ensure prompt and proper emergency care if needed.*

Increase child's role in self-management of disease by using age-appropriate guidelines *to move child into a long-term role as independent manager of the disease process and associated treatments.*

Nursing Diagnosis: Altered family processes related to situational crises (child with chronic disease/disability)

See the Nursing Care Plan: The Child with Chronic Illness, Disability, Chapter 38.

complications can have a favorable impact. Once parents experience the child's having a severe insulin reaction with a seizure or the adolescent has one in a public place, the desire to maintain better control is reinforced. They must understand how to prevent problems and how to handle problems calmly if they occur. (See Compliance, Chapter 42.)

Parents develop guilt feelings when they have a child with any chronic disease, especially one with a hereditary component. They cope with these feelings in a number of ways. For example, they may be either overprotective or neglectful. Parents may blame themselves for the disease, consciously or subconsciously. Nevertheless they must come to realize, through education and counseling, that there was nothing they could have done to prevent the disease and that it was not their fault, since environmental, as well as hereditary, factors may be involved in the development of the disease.

Problems in the parental response provide a challenge for the nurse to assist through counseling or, if the problems are severe enough, to refer the parents to appropriate resources designed to help them alter their behavior. Times should be set aside during the child's health visit or afterward to meet the needs of the parents. Parents should also be included in special sessions to keep them abreast of the child's management, to help them continue to participate in the child's care, and to provide them with an opportunity to express their own feelings concerning their own or their child's adjustment to the disease. The amount of information that they offer at this time can give clues to their level of support of the child and help assist in decisions concerning the therapeutic management of the child.

Camps for children with diabetes and other special groups are very useful. In the special camp these children learn that they are not alone. As a result most children become more independent and resourceful outside the camp setting. Camp time also provides parents a respite from the child's daily regimen. Information about such camps and organizations can be obtained from the American Diabetes Association. A free list of accredited camps specifically for children and teens with diabetes is also available.*

Evaluation

The effectiveness of nursing interventions is determined by continual reassessment and evaluation of care based on the following observational guidelines and expected outcomes:

1. Interview family to determine their understanding of the disease; have child and family demonstrate and discuss the needed assessment and therapeutic techniques.
2. Interview family regarding their understanding of tight control; analyze and evaluate management records.
3. Discuss child's disease with him or her.
4. Interview family and child regarding their feelings and concerns about the disease.

Expected outcomes:

See the Nursing Care Plan on p. 1651.

*Camp Directory, 1660 Duke St., Alexandria, VA 22314; (800) 232-3472.

Key Points

- The endocrine system has three components: the cell, which sends a chemical message via a hormone; target cells, which receive the message; and the environment through which the chemical is transported from the site of synthesis to the sites of cellular action.
- Pituitary dysfunction is manifested primarily by growth disturbance.
- The main physiologic action of thyroid hormone is to regulate the basal metabolic rate and control the processes of growth and tissue differentiation.
- Disorders of thyroid function include hypothyroidism, autoimmune thyroiditis, goiter, and hyperthyroidism.
- Therapy for hyperthyroidism is directed at retarding the rate of hormone secretion and may include drug therapy, thyroidectomy, or radioiodine therapy.
- Classic forms of hypoparathyroidism in childhood are idiopathic—deficient production of PTH—and pseudohypoparathyroidism—increased PTH production with end-organ unresponsiveness to PTH.
- The adrenal cortex secretes three important groups of hormones: glucocorticoids, mineralocorticoids, and sex steroids.
- Disorders of adrenal function include acute adrenocortical insufficiency, chronic adrenocortical insufficiency, Cushing syndrome, congenital adrenogenital hyperplasia, and hyperaldosteronism.
- Four categories of Cushing syndrome are pituitary, adrenal, ectopic, and iatrogenic.
- Management of congenital adrenogenital hyperplasia includes assignment of a sex according to genotype, administration of cortisone, and possibly, reconstructive surgery.
- Diabetes mellitus is categorized as insulin-dependent diabetes, non-insulin-dependent diabetes, and maturity-onset diabetes of youth.
- The focus of insulin-dependent diabetes management is insulin replacement, diet, and exercise.
- Education of families includes explanation of diabetes, meal planning, administering insulin injection, monitoring, general hygienic practices, promoting exercise, keeping records, and observing for complications.

References

Albisser AM, Sperlich M: Adjusting insulins, *Diabetes Educator* 18(3):211-218, 1992.

Bertagna X: New causes of Cushing's syndrome, *N Engl J Med* 327(14):1024-1025, 1992.

Brouhard B, Rogers G: Pancreatic and islet replacement therapy for insulin-dependent diabetes mellitus, *Clin Pediatr* 32(5):258-263, 1993.

Casella S et al: Accuracy and precision of low-dose insulin administration, *Pediatrics* 91(6):1155-1157, 1993.

Chantelau E et al: What makes insulin injections painful? *Br Med J* 303(6793):26-27, 1991.

Diabetes Control and Complications Trial Research Group: the effect of intensive treatment of diabetes on the development and progression of long-term complications in insulin-dependent diabetes mellitus, *N Engl J Med* 329(14):977-986, 1993.

DiGeorge AM: *The endocrine system*. In Behrman RE, Vaughan VC III, editors: *Textbook of pediatrics*, ed 14, Philadelphia, 1992, WB Saunders.

Gildea J: High and dry—low and wet: the key to DI and SIADH, *Pediatr Nurs* 19(5):478-481, 1993.

Hancock SL, Cox RS, McDougall R: Thyroid diseases after treatment of Hodgkin's disease, *N Engl J Med* 325(9):599-605, 1991.

Moore KC et al: Clinical diagnoses of children with extremely short stature and their response to growth hormone, *J Pediatr* 122(5):687-692, 1992.

Nathan DM: Long-term complications of diabetes mellitus, *N Engl J Med* 328(23):1678-1685, 1993.

Reasner II C: Clinical implications of the DCCT trial, *Contemp Intern Med* 6(2):5-8, 1994.

Rodin G, Craven J, Daneman D: Eating disorders and insulin manipulation in adolescent females with insulin-dependent diabetes mellitus, *Psychosom Med* 51:244-266, 1989.

Ruble JA: *Congenital adrenal hyperplasia*. In Jackson PL, Vessey JA, editors: *Primary care of the child with a chronic condition*, St Louis, 1992, Mosby.

Stabler B: Psychosocial outcomes of short stature, *Pediatr Rounds* 2(1):5-7, 1993.

Tallstedt L and others: Occurrence of ophthalmopathy after treatment for Graves; hyperthyroidism, *N Engl J Med* 326(26):1733-1738, 1992.

Winters WE, Chihara T, Schatz D. The genetics of autoimmune diabetes, *Am J Dis Child* 147(12):1282-1290, 1993.

Zekauskas S et al: Human growth hormones and Creutzfeldt-Jakob disease, *J Okla State Med Assoc* 83(9):446-449, 1990.

Bibliography

Pituitary Dysfunction

Connaughty MS: Accelerated growth in children, *J Pediatr Health Care* 6(5):316-324, 1992.

Giordano BP: The impact of genetic syndromes on children's growth, *J Pediatr Health Care* 6(5):309-315, 1992.

Henry JJ: Routine growth monitoring and assessment of growth disorders, *J Pediatr Health Care* 6(5, pt 2):291-301, 1992.

Jackson PL, Ott MJ: Precocious puberty: the role of the school nurse, *Sch Nurse* 6(1):16-18, 1990.

Kaplowitz P, Webb J: Diagnostic evaluation of short children with height 3 SD or more below the mean, *Clin Pediatr* 33(19):530-535, 1994.

Reiser PA: Educational psychologic, and social aspects of short stature, *J Pediatr Health Care* 6(5):325-332, 1992.

Schwartz JD, Root AW: Puberty in girls: early, incomplete, or precocious? *Contemp Pediatr* 7(1):147-156, 1990.

Disorders of Thyroid Function/Disorders of the Parathyroid Gland/Adrenal Dysfunction

Burrow GN, Fisher DA, Larsen PR: Maternal and fetal thyroid function, *N Engl J Med* 331(16):1072-1078, 1994.

Darland NW: Congenital adrenocortical hyperplasia: supportive nursing interventions, *J Pediatr Nurs* 1(2):117-123, 1986.

Farnklyn JA: The management of hyperthyroidism, *N Engl J Med* 330(24):1731-1738, 1994.

Mack R: Thyroid medication—don't overdose on conformity, *Contemp Pediatr* 10(3):105-114, 1993.

Magiakou MA et al: Cushing's syndrome in children and adolescents, *N Engl J Med* 331(10):629-636, 1994.

Page J: The newborn with ambiguous genitalia, *Neonat Net* 13(5):15-21, 1994.

Diabetes Mellitus

Bailie MD: Heading off the complications of diabetes, *Contemp Pediatr* 6(1):87-102, 1989.

Chase HP et al: Cyclosporine A for the treatment of new-onset insulin-dependent diabetes mellitus, *Pediatrics* 85:241-245, 1990.

Chase HP et al: Diabetic ketoacidosis in children and the role of outpatient management, *Pediatr Rev* 11(10):297-304, 1990.

Chase HP et al: Prediction of the course of pre–type I diabetes, *J Pediatr* 118(6):838-841, 1991.

Clark LM, Plotnick LP: Insulin pumps in children with diabetes, *J Pediatr Health Care* 4:3-10, 1990.

Dashiff CJ: Parents' perceptions of diabetes in adolescent daughters and its impact on the family, *J Pediatr Nurs* 8(6):361-369, 1993.

Faro B: Students with diabetes: implications of the diabetes control and complications trial for the school setting, *J School Nurs* 11(1):16-21, 1995.

Gallo AM: Family management style in juvenile diabetes: a case illustration, *J Pediatr Nurs* 5:23-32, 1990.

Grey M et al: Initial adaptation in children with newly diagnosed diabetes and healthy children, *Pediatr Nurs* 21(1):17-22, 1994.

Hanna KM, Jacobs PM, Guthrie D: Exploring the concept of health among adolescents with diabetes using photography, *J Pediatr Nurs* 10(5):321-327, 1995.

Henry L, Johnson A, Villarosa L: The black health library guide to diabetes, New York, 1993, Henry Holt.

Kittler MS, Sucher D: Diet counseling in a multicultural society, *Diabetes Educator* 16(2):127-131, 1990.

Lipman TH et al: A developmental approach to diabetes in children: birth through preschool, *Am J Matern Care Nurs* 14:255-259, 1989.

Lipman TH et al: A developmental approach to diabetes in children: school age—adolescence, *Am J Matern Care Nurs* 14:330-332, 1989.

Martin R et al: The infant with diabetes mellitus: a case study, *Pediatr Nurs* 20(1):27-34, 1994.

McNabb WL et al: Increasing children's responsibility for diabetes self-care: in control study, *Diabetes Educator* 20(2):121-124, 1994.

Miller-Johnson S et al: Parent-child relationships and the management of insulin-dependent diabetes mellitus, *J Consult Clin Psychol* 62:603-610, 1994.

Rodrique JR et al: Parenting satisfaction and efficacy among caregivers of children with diabetes, *Child Health Care* 23:181-191, 1994.

Savinetti-Rose B: Developmental issues in managing children with diabetes, *Pediatr Nurs* 20(1):11-15, 1994.

Snyder AL, Clarke WL: The diabetes control and complications trial: new challenges for the school nurse, *J School Nurs* 11(1):22-25, 1995.

CHAPTER 50

Integumentary Dysfunction

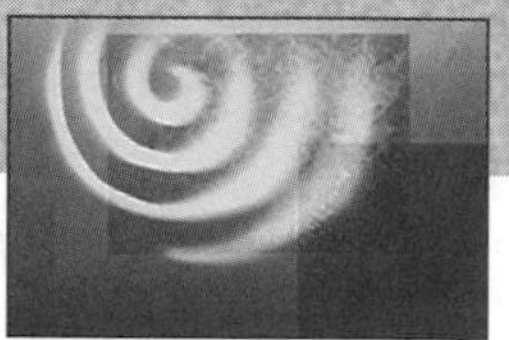

INTEGUMENTARY DYSFUNCTION, P. 1654

Skin lesions, p. 1654

Wounds, p. 1655

General therapeutic management, p. 1660

Nursing care of the child with a skin disorder, p. 1662

INFECTIONS OF THE SKIN, P. 1664

Bacterial infections, p. 1664

Viral infections, p. 1667

Dermatophytoses (fungal infections), p. 1669

Systemic mycotic (fungal) infections, p. 1669

SKIN DISORDERS RELATED TO CHEMICAL OR PHYSICAL CONTACTS, P. 1671

Contact dermatitis, p. 1671

Poison ivy, oak, and sumac, p. 1671

Drug reactions, p. 1672

Foreign bodies, p. 1672

SKIN DISORDERS RELATED TO INSECT AND ANIMAL CONTACTS, P. 1673

Scabies, p. 1673

Pediculosis capitis, p. 1673

Arthropod bites and stings, p. 1674

Infections transmitted by arthropods, p. 1677

Animal bites, p. 1677

Human bites, p. 1678

Cat scratch disease (CSD), p. 1679

MISCELLANEOUS SKIN DISORDERS, P. 1679

SKIN DISORDERS ASSOCIATED WITH SPECIFIC AGE GROUPS, P. 1679

Diaper dermatitis, p. 1679

Atopic dermatitis (AD) (eczema), p. 1682

Seborrheic dermatitis, p. 1685

Acne, p. 1685

THERMAL INJURY, P. 1687

Burns, p. 1687

Sunburn, p. 1700

Cold injury, p. 1703

Integumentary Dysfunction

SKIN LESIONS

Lesions of the skin or disorders with skin manifestations can result from a wide variety of specific etiologic factors. In general, skin lesions originate from (1) contact with injurious agents, such as infective organisms, toxic chemicals, and physical trauma, (2) hereditary factors; or (3) a systemic disease of which the lesions are a cutaneous manifestation (e.g., measles, lupus erythematosus, nutritional deficiency diseases) or some external factor that produces a reaction in the skin (e.g., allergens). In the case of external factors the damage is caused by the body's response to the agent rather than by the agent itself. Such responses are highly individualized. An agent that may be harmless to one individual may be damaging to another, and a single agent may produce various types of responses in different individuals.

Among other factors involved in the etiology of skin manifestations is the age of the child. For example, infants are subject to "birthmark" malformations and atopic dermatitis that appear early in life; the school-age child is susceptible to ringworm of the scalp; and acne is a characteristic skin disorder of puberty. Contact dermatitis, such as poison ivy, is seen only where the noxious agent is a feature of the area. Similarly, reactions to insect bites are associated with life cycle and seasonal activities. Although less common in children, tension and anxiety may produce, modify, or prolong many skin conditions.

Skin of Younger Children

In the infant and small child the epidermis is still loosely bound to the dermis. This poor adherence causes the layers to separate readily during an inflammatory process to form blisters. This is especially true in preterm infants, who have an even greater propensity to blister formation and separation during careless handling (such as removal of adhesive tape). The skin is thinner than in older children, and the cells of all strata are more compressed.

Several characteristics influence skin responses in infants and young children. Their skin is far more susceptible to superficial bacterial infection. They are more likely to have associated systemic symptoms with some infections and are more apt to react to a primary irritant than to a sensitizing allergen. Infants and young children are more frequently affected by chronic atopic dermatitis (eczema). The infant's skin is much more prone to develop a toxic erythema as a result of skin eruptions or drug reactions and is subject to maceration, infection, and the moisture retention associated with diaper rash.

Pathophysiology of Dermatitis

Over half of dermatologic problems are various forms of dermatitis. This implies a sequence of inflammatory changes in the skin that are grossly and microscopically similar but diverse in course and causation. Acute responses produce intercellular and intracellular edema, the formation of intradermal vesicles, and an initial minimum infiltration of inflammatory cells into the epidermis. In the dermis there is edema, vascular dilation, and early perivascular cellular infiltration. The location and manner of these reactions produce the lesions characteristic of each disorder. The changes are reversible, and the skin ordinarily recovers without blemish and completely intact unless complicating factors such as ulceration from the primary irritant, scratching, and infection are introduced or underlying vascular disease develops. In chronic conditions, permanent effects are seen that vary according to the disorder, the general condition of the affected individual, and available therapy.

Diagnostic Evaluation

Although the history and subjective symptoms are explored first, objective findings are often noted simultaneously. One of the more advantageous aspects of skin lesions is that often the diagnosis is readily established after simple, careful inspection.

History and subjective symptoms. Many cutaneous lesions are associated with local symptoms, the most common of which is itching **(pruritus)** that varies in kind and intensity. Pain or tenderness often accompanies some skin lesions, and other sensations may be described as burning, prickling, stinging, or crawling. Alterations in local feeling or sensation include absence of sensation **(anesthesia)**, excessive sensitiveness **(hyperesthesia)**, diminished sensation (*hypesthesia* or **hypoesthesia**) or abnormal sensation, such as burning or prickling **(paresthesia)**. These symptoms may remain localized or migrate, may be constant or intermittent, and may be aggravated by a specific activity or circumstance, such as exposure to sunlight.

It is also important to determine whether the child has had an allergic condition such as asthma or hay fever or has had previous skin disease. Atopic dermatitis, often associated with allergies, frequently begins in infancy. It should be determined when the lesion or symptom first became apparent, as well as whether it is related to ingestion of a food or other substance, including any medication the child might be taking. It should be kept in mind that the condition may be related to an activity such as contact with plants, insects, or chemicals.

Objective findings. Much can be determined by the distribution, size, morphology, and arrangement of the lesions. Extrinsic causes usually result from physical, chemical, or allergic irritants or from an infectious agent such as bacteria, fungi, viruses, or animal parasites. Skin manifestations can be produced by such intrinsic causes as a specific infection (such as measles or chickenpox), drug sensitization, or other allergic phenomena. Other diagnostic tools are subjective symptoms, the history, and medical and laboratory studies.

Lesion. According to the nature of the pathologic process, lesions assume more or less distinct characteristics. Names that have been applied to these lesions are important for descriptive purposes in the processes of record keeping and communication. Nurses should also become familiar with the more common terms used to describe skin lesions seen in dermatologic conditions:

Erythema—a reddened area caused by increased amounts of oxygenated blood in the dermal vasculature

Ecchymoses (bruises)—localized red or purple discolorations caused by extravasation of blood into dermis and subcutaneous tissues

Petechiae—pinpoint, tiny, and sharp circumscribed spots in the superficial layers of the epidermis

Primary lesions—skin changes produced by some causative factor; common primary lesions in pediatric skin disorders are macules, papules, and vesicles (Fig. 50-1)

Secondary lesions—changes that result from alteration in the primary lesions, such as those caused by rubbing, scratching, medication, or involution and healing (Fig. 50-2)

Distribution pattern—the pattern in which lesions are distributed over the body, whether local or generalized, and specific areas associated with the lesions

Configuration and arrangement—the size, shape, and arrangement of a lesion or groups of lesions (e.g., *discrete, clustered, diffuse,* or *confluent*)

Laboratory studies. When it is suspected that a skin problem might be related to a systemic disease, such as one of the collagen diseases or immunodeficiency disease, studies are needed to rule out these possibilities. Diagnostic modalities include microscopic examination, cultures, skin scrapings or biopsy, cytodiagnosis, patch testing, and Wood light examination. Allergic skin testing and various other laboratory tests (blood count, sedimentation rate) are used when indicated.

WOUNDS

Wounds are structural or physiologic disruptions of the integument that call for normal or abnormal tissue repair responses. All wounds can be classified as acute or chronic. *Acute wounds* are those that heal uneventfully within the usual time frame. *Chronic wounds* are those that do not heal in the expected time frame or are associated with many complications. In children, most wounds are acute and can be prevented from becoming chronic through appropriate nursing care. Wounds are classified in the same manner as burns: partial-thickness, full-thickness, and complex wounds that include muscle and/or bone.

Epidermal Injuries

Abrasions are the most common epidermal wounds of childhood, usually in the form of a skinned knee or elbow. In most

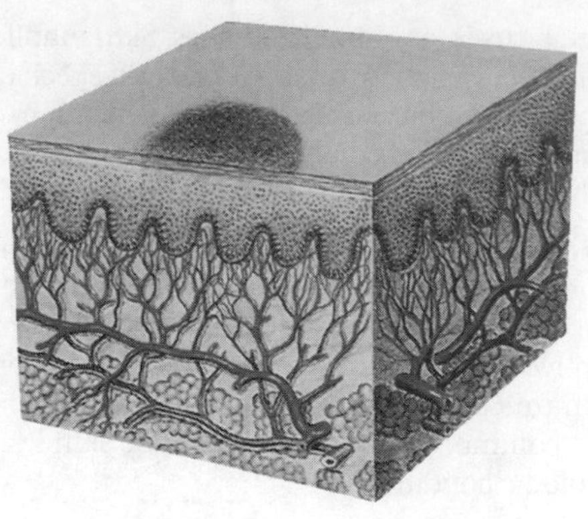

Macule—flat; nonpalpable; circumscribed; less than 1 cm in diameter; brown, red, purple, white, or tan in color
Examples: Freckles; flat moles; rubella; rubeola

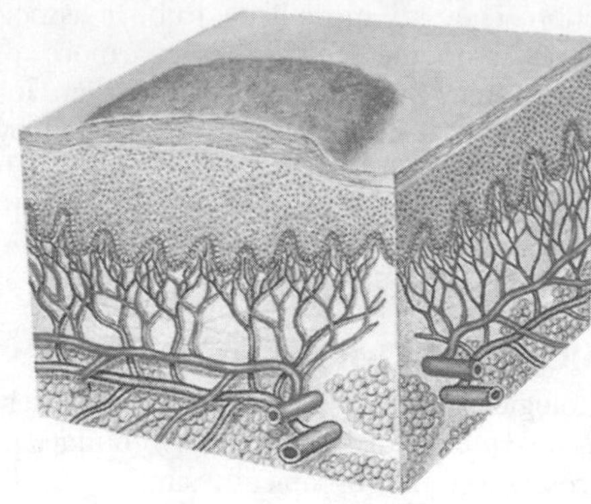

Plaque—elevated; flat topped; firm; rough; superficial papule greater than 1 cm in diameter; may be coalesced papules
Examples: Psoriasis; seborrheic and actinic keratoses

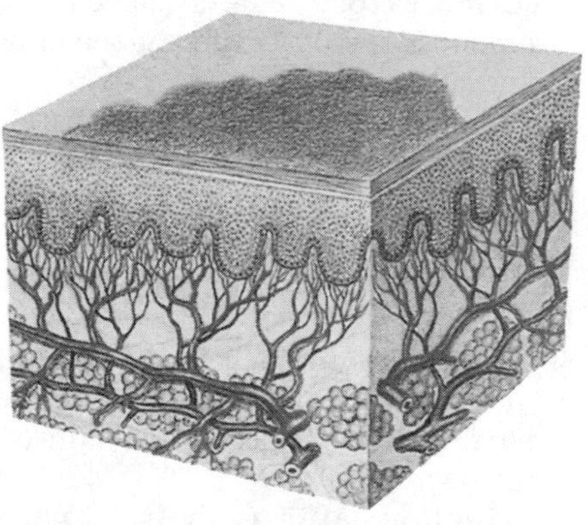

Patch—flat; nonpalpable; irregular in shape; macule that is greater than 1 cm in diameter
Examples: Vitiligo; port-wine marks

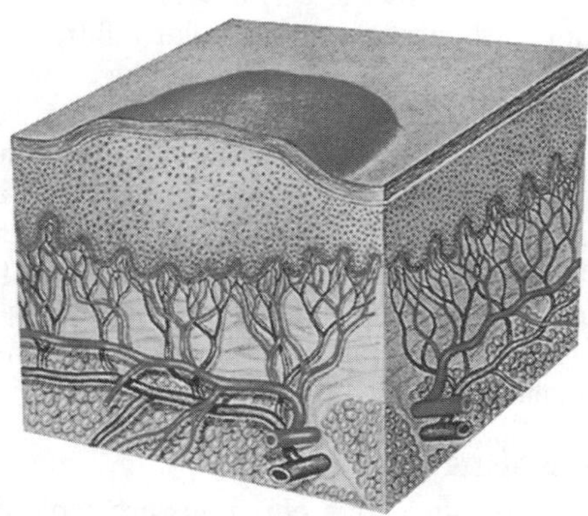

Wheal—elevated, irregular-shaped area of cutaneous edema; solid, transient, changing, variable diameter; pale pink with lighter center
Examples: Urticaria; insect bites

Fig. 50-1 Primary skin lesions. (From Seidel HM et al: *Mosby's guide to physical examination,* ed 3, St Louis, 1995, Mosby.)

injuries the margins of the abraded area are superficial, involving only the outer layers of epidermis, although the central portion may extend into the dermis. Initially the defect is filled by a blood clot and necrotic debris, which subsequently dehydrate to form a scab. Epithelial tissue is composed of *labile cells,* which are constantly destroyed and replaced throughout life. Injury to these tissues results in *regeneration* (i.e., rapid replacement by similar cells).

The epithelial wound heals by migration and proliferation of epithelial cells from the wound margin and from cells surviving in transected skin appendages. This response begins within 24 to 48 hours after the wound is incurred. Cell migration ceases when migrating cells make contact with epithelial cells migrating from all other sites. Fixed basal cells adjacent to the wound edge and in skin appendages begin to divide rapidly to replace the migrated cells. As resurfacing is accomplished, the migrated cells begin to divide and thicken the new epithelial layer.

Epithelial cells advance over the wound surface by "flowing." The first cell advances, anchors, and then moves no more. Instead, a cell from behind advances over it, anchors, and subsequently is overridden by other cells that advance over both the primary cells—similar to a leapfrog movement. Epithelial cells move most rapidly in moist environments, and the rate of epithelization depends on various elements, particularly the amount of oxygen supplied to the wound (Hunt, 1990).

Injury to Deeper Tissues

Tissues composed of *permanent cells,* such as muscle and nerve cells, are unable to regenerate. Therefore these tissues repair themselves by substituting fibrous connective tissue for the injured tissue. This fibrous tissue, or **scar** serves as a patch to preserve or restore the continuity of the tissue. Wounds involving permanent cells include surgical incisions, lacerations, ulcers, evulsions, and full-thickness burns. Injured cells of glandular organs and bones, composed of *stable* cells, multiply less vigorously and heal more slowly.

Process of Wound Healing

The nonspecific repair mechanism of wound healing with scar formation involves the processes of inflammation, fibroplasia, contraction, and scar maturation. The initial response at the site of injury is **inflammation,** a vascular and cellular response, which prepares the tissues for the subsequent repair process. There is a transient constriction of transected blood vessels, lasting 5 to 10 minutes, followed by active vasodilation of all local small vessels and increased blood flow to the area. This is accompanied by increased permeability of small venules, allowing plasma to leak into surrounding tissues

Papule—elevated; palpable; firm; circumscribed; less than 1 cm in diameter; brown, red, pink, tan, or bluish red in color
Examples: Warts; drug-related eruptions; pigmented nevi

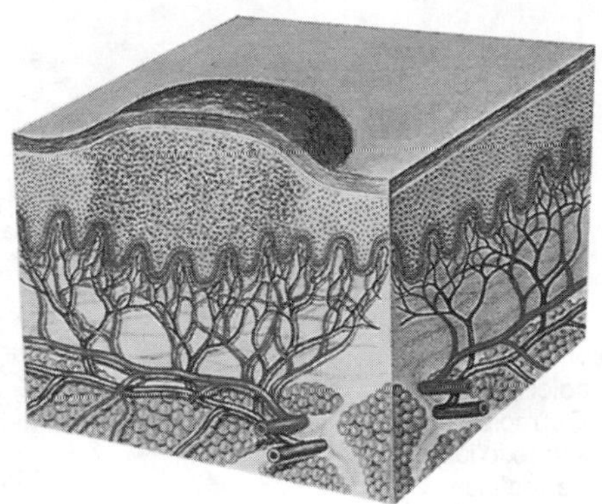

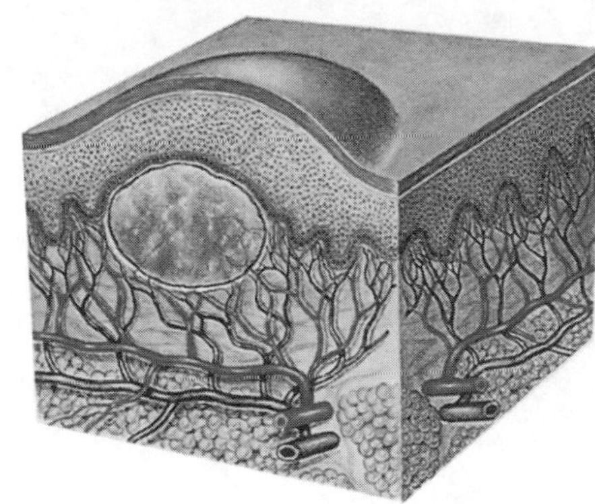

Nodule—elevated; firm; circumscribed; palpable; deeper in dermis than papule; 1 to 2 cm in diameter
Examples: Erythema nodosum; lipomas

Vesicle—elevated; circumscribed; superficial; filled with serous fluid; less than 1 cm in diameter
Examples: Blister; varicella

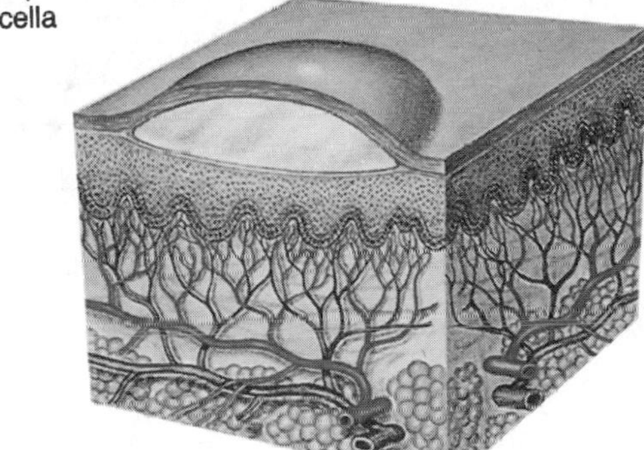

Pustule—elevated; superficial; similar to vesicle but filled with purulent fluid
Examples: Impetigo; acne; variola

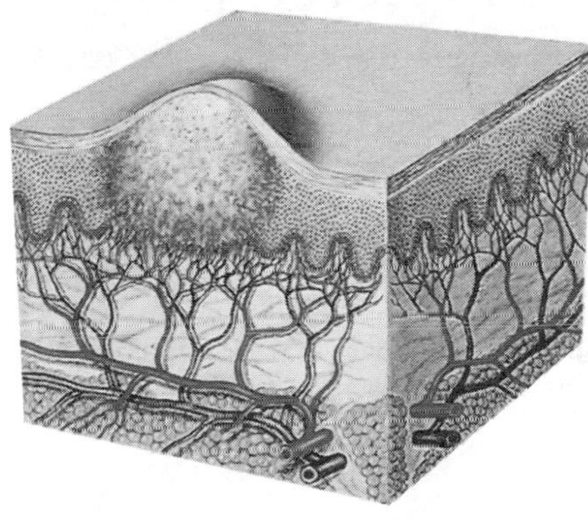

Bulla—vesicle greater than 1 cm in diameter
Examples: Blister; pemphigus vulgaris

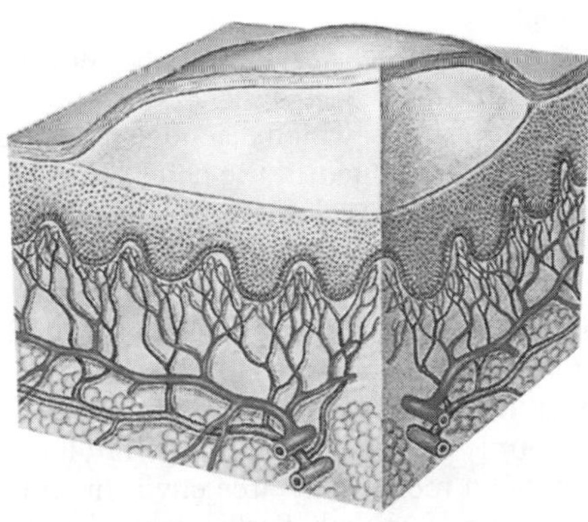

Cyst—elevated; circumscribed; palpable; encapsulated; filled with liquid or semisolid material
Example: Sebaceous cyst

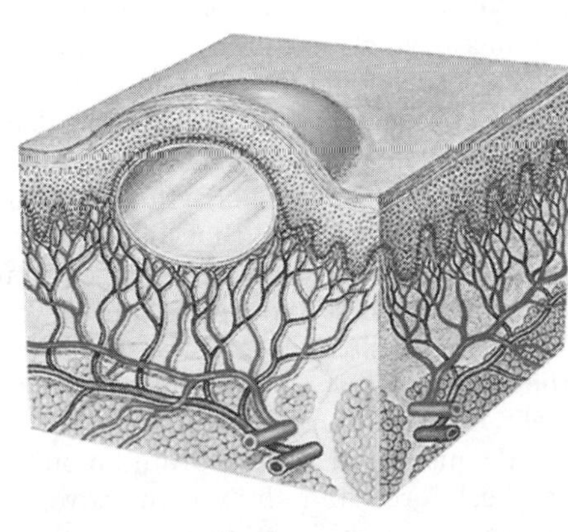

Fig. 50-1, cont'd Primary skin lesions.

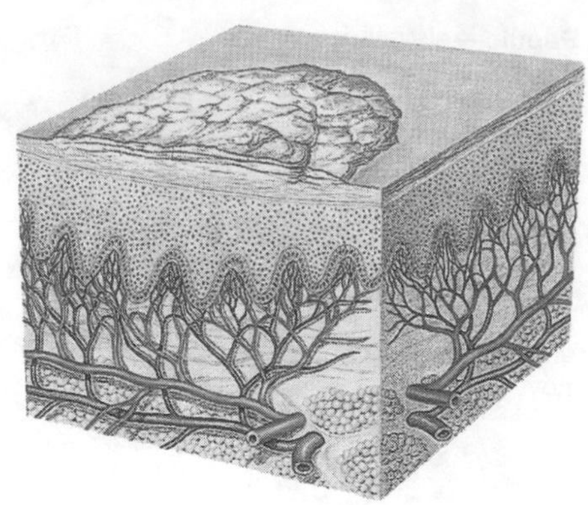

Scale—heaped-up keratinized cells; flaky exfoliation; irregular; thick or thin; dry or oily; varied size; silver, white, or tan in color
Examples: Psoriasis; exfoliative dermatitis

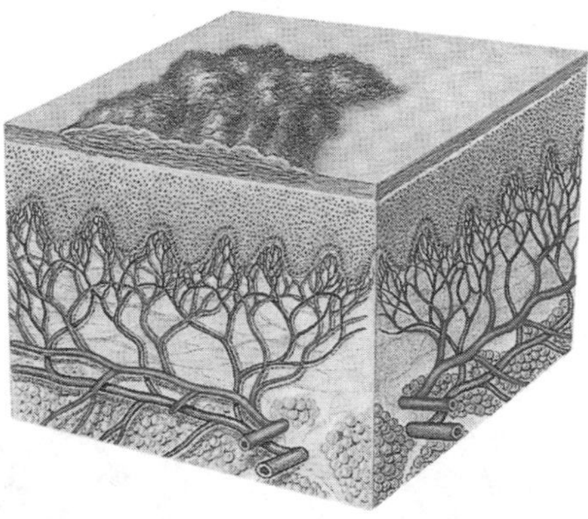

Crust—dried serum, blood, or purulent exudate; slightly elevated; size varies; brown, red, black, tan, or straw in color
Examples: Scab on abrasion; eczema

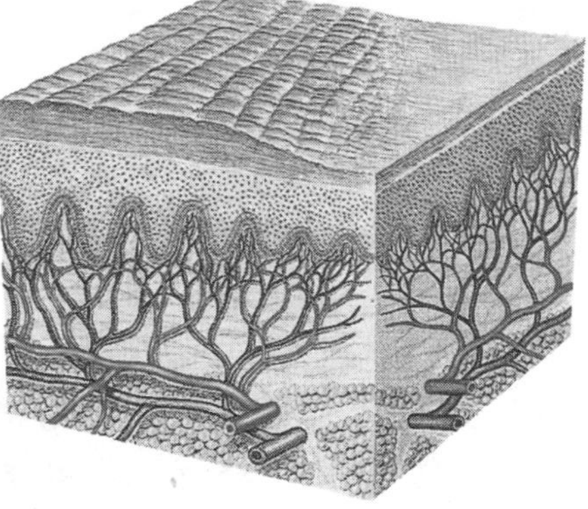

Lichenification—rough, thickened epidermis; accentuated skin markings caused by rubbing or irritation; often involves flexor aspect of extremity
Example: Chronic dermatitis

Fig. 50-2 Secondary skin lesions. (From Seidel HM et al: *Mosby's guide to physical examination*, ed 3, St Louis, 1995, Mosby.)

(edema). A blood clot is formed along wound edges, creating a framework for future growth of capillaries **(angiogenesis)** and epithelial cells.

At the same time, vessel walls become lined with leukocytes, primarily neutrophils, which pass through the walls and concentrate at the injured site, where they ingest bacteria and debris **(phagocytosis).** The presence of neutrophils is superseded by macrophages, which continue phagocytosis, and also by growth factors needed for skin repair and angiogenesis. Fibroblasts attracted to the area from blood vessels deposit fibrin throughout the clot. Adjacent capillaries begin to form buds that stretch across the supporting fibrin threads, and epithelial cells secrete a fibrolytic enzyme that allows their advancement across the wound. This initial phase of wound healing takes place during the first 3 to 5 days after injury.

Fibroplasia *(granulation or proliferation)*, the second phase of healing, lasts from 5 days to 4 weeks. Fibroblasts, immature connective tissue cells, migrate to the healing site and begin to secrete collagen into the meshwork spaces. Granulation tissue is highly vascular, "beefy" red and shiny connective tissue that organizes and restructures, forming thicker, stronger fibers arranged in orderly layers. A thin layer of epithelial tissue is regenerated over the surface of the wound, and leukocytes gradually *disappear from the area.*

During **contraction** and **maturation,** the third and fourth phases of wound healing, collagen continues to be deposited and organized into layers, compressing the new blood vessels and gradually blocking blood flow across the wound. Fibroblasts disappear as the wound becomes stronger. Fibroblast movement causes contraction of the healing area, helping to bring wound edges closer together. A mature scar is then formed. The maturation process may continue for years, and the extent to which the scar remodels and matures varies among individuals.

Children heal aggressively with abundant scar tissue, especially during growth spurts. The highly elastic quality of children's skin pulls on wounds, which defend against the pull by aggressive scarring. Consequently, the child's skin heals with more scar tissue than the less elastic skin of the adult.

Factors That Influence Healing

During the last two decades, understanding of wound healing has revolutionized the interventions used to promote healing. Emphasis has shifted from interventions directed at maintaining a dry environment that promoted **eschar** formation to those that promote a moist, crust-free environment that enhances the migration of epithelial cells across the wound and facilitates resurfacing. An acute full-thickness wound kept in

Scar—thin to thick fibrous tissue replacing injured dermis; irregular; pink, red, or white in color; may be atrophic or hypertrophic
Example: Healed wound or surgical incision

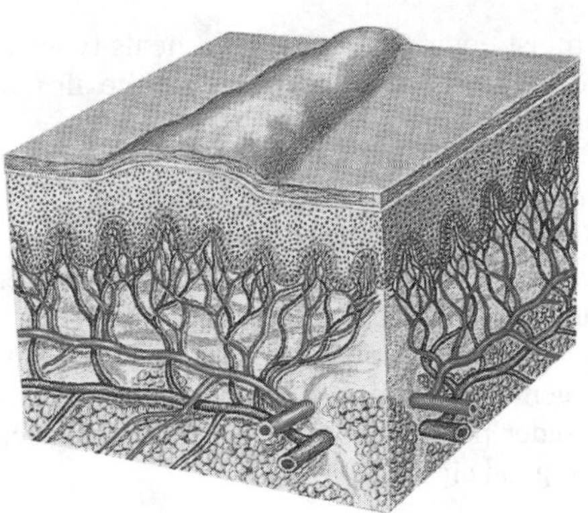

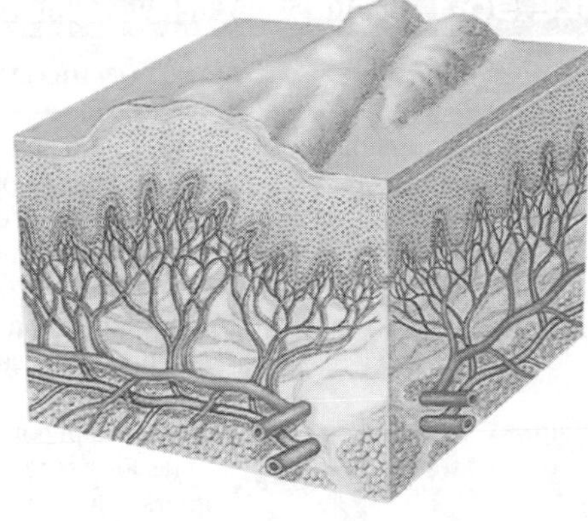

Keloid–irregularly shaped, olovated, progressively enlarging scar; grows beyond boundaries of wound; caused by excessive collagen formation during healing
Example: Keloid from ear piercing or burn scar

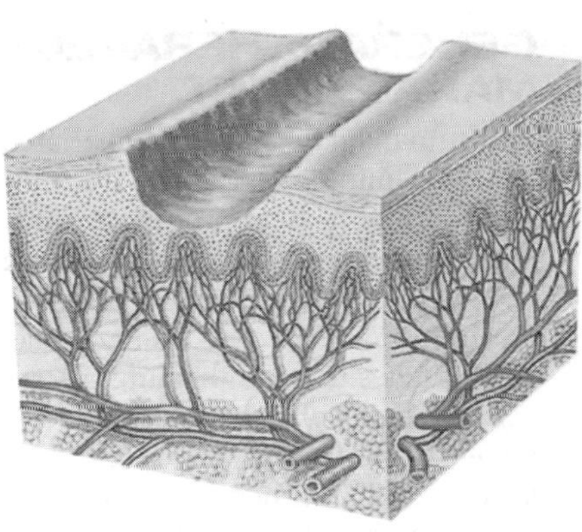

Excoriation–loss of epidermis; linear or hollowed-out crusted area; dermis exposed
Examples: Abrasion; scratch

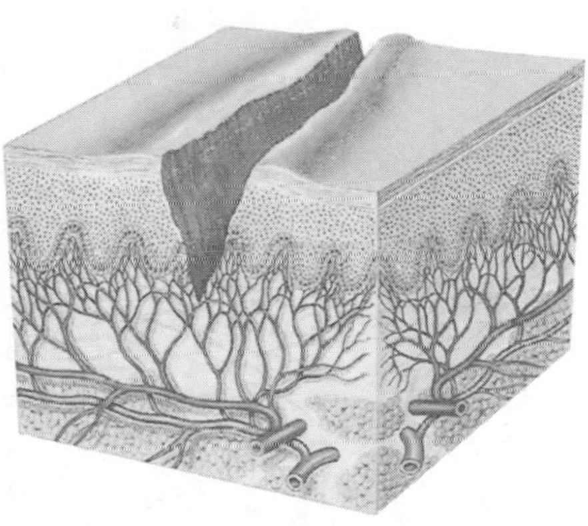

Fissure—linear crack or break from epidermis to dermis; small; deep; red
Examples: Athlete's foot: cheilosis

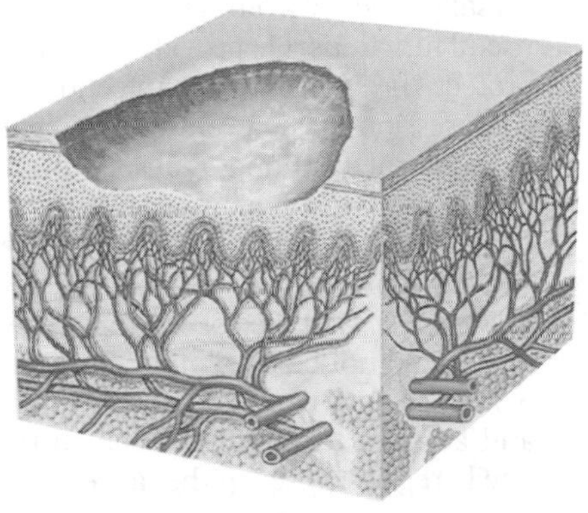

Erosion–loss of all or part of epidermis; depressed; moist; glistening; follows rupture of vesicle or bulla; larger than fissure
Examples: Varicella; variola following rupture

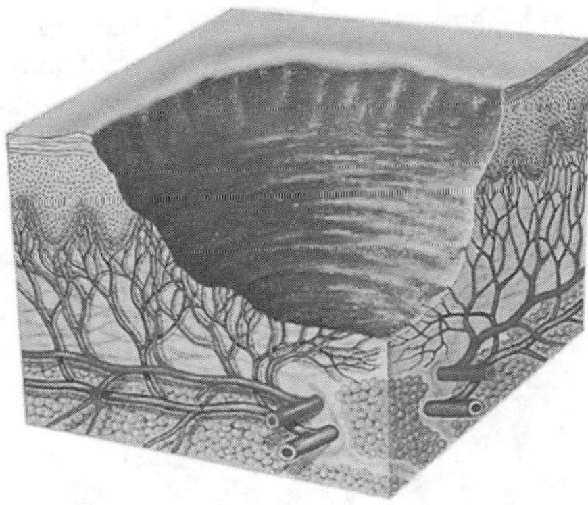

Ulcer—loss of epidermis and dermis; concave; varies in size; exudative; red or reddish blue
Examples: Decubiti; stasis ulcers

Fig. 50-2, cont'd Secondary skin lesions.

TABLE 50-1 Factors that delay wound healing

FACTOR	EFFECT ON HEALING
Dry wound environment	Allows epithelial cells to dry out and die; impairs migration of epithelial cells across the wound surface
Nutritional deficiencies	
Vitamin C	Inhibits formation of collagen fibers and capillary development
Protein	Reduces supply of amino acids for tissue repair
Zinc	Impairs epithelialization
Impaired circulation	Reduces supply of nutrients to wound area Inhibits inflammatory response and removal of debris from wound area
Stress (pain, poor sleep)	Releases catecholamines that cause vasoconstriction
Antiseptics	
Hydrogen peroxide	Toxic to fibroblasts; can cause subcutaneous gas formation (mimics gas-forming infection)
Povidone-iodine	Toxic to white and red blood cells and fibroblasts
Chlorhexidine	Toxic to white blood cells
Corticosteroids	Impair phagocytosis Inhibit fibroblast proliferation Depress formation of granulation tissue Inhibit wound contraction
Foreign bodies	Inhibit wound closure Increase inflammatory response
Infection	Increases inflammatory response Increases tissue destruction
Mechanical friction	Damages or destroys granulation tissue
Fluid accumulation	Accumulation in area inhibits tissues from approximating
Radiation	Inhibits fibroblastic activity and capillary formation May cause tissue necrosis
Diseases	
Diabetes mellitus	Inhibits collagen synthesis Impairs circulation and capillary growth Hyperglycemia impairs phagocytosis
Anemia	Reduces oxygen supply to tissues

a moist environment usually heals twice as fast as the same wound heals when kept open to the air (Alvarez, Rozint, and Meehan, 1990).

In addition to knowing what promotes healing, numerous factors have been identified that delay healing (Table 50-1). Many traditional practices, such as the use of antiseptics (hydrogen peroxide and povidone-iodine [Betadine] solutions), thought to prevent infection, actually have a cytotoxic effect on healthy cells and minimal effect on controlling infections. In general, wounds in children heal more rapidly than those in older persons because of children's increased metabolism and good circulation.

Nursing ALERT

Do not put anything in a wound that one would not put in the eye. The safest solution is normal saline.

GENERAL THERAPEUTIC MANAGEMENT

The human body tends to heal; therefore treatment is directed toward eliminating or ameliorating influences that interfere with normal healing processes. Some disorders may demand aggressive therapy, but by and large the major aim of any treatment is to prevent further damage, eliminate the cause, prevent complications, and provide relief from discomfort while tissues undergo healing. Factors that contribute to the dermatitis and prolong the course of the disease must be eliminated when possible. The most common offenders in pediatrics are environmental factors (such as soaps, bubble baths, shampoos, rough or tight clothing, wet diapers, blankets, and toys) and the natural elements (such as dirt, sand, heat, cold, moisture, and wind). Dermatitis can also be aggravated by home remedies and medications.

Dressings

Dressings are frequently applied to skin lesions and are universally used for wound management. Dressings serve several useful functions: (1) provide a moist healing environment, (2) protect the wound from infection and trauma, (3) provide compression in the event of anticipated bleeding or swelling, (4) apply medication, (5) absorb drainage, (6) debride necrotic tissue, (7) reduce pain, and (8) control odor. To provide a moist environment, open wounds are covered with an occlusive ointment or dressing (Table 50-2). No one dressing meets the needs of all types of wounds. The traditional gauze dressing should not be used on open wounds because it allows the wound surface to dry, does little to prevent bacterial invasion, and adheres to the dried scab so that removal disturbs the newly regenerating epithelial cells.

Topical Therapy

Various agents and methods are available for the treatment of dermatologic problems. In selecting a therapeutic program the practitioner considers (1) a choice of active ingredient, (2) a proper vehicle or base, (3) the cosmetic effect, (4) the cost, and (5) instructions for its use. In addition, several basic concepts are kept in mind. Overtreatment is avoided. For example,

TABLE 50-2 Properties of commonly used occlusive dressings

EXAMPLES	INDICATIONS	ADVANTAGES	DISADVANTAGES	CONSIDERATIONS
Polyurethane films				
Op-Site, Tegaderm, Bioclusive, Blister-film, Ensure-it, Accuderm, Uniflex, Opraflex	Protection of partial-thickness red wounds Cover dressing for hydrophilic preparations and hydrogels	Transparent; good adhesion; waterproof; reduces pain; minimizes friction forces to wound; time-saving; easy to store	Adhesive injury to intact and new skin; nonabsorbent; some products difficult to apply; variable barrier function; can promote wound infection	Protect wound margins; avoid in wounds with infection, copius drainage, or tracts; change only if dressing leaks
Hydrocolloids				
DuoDerm, J & J, Ulcer Dr., Comfeel, Restore, Intact, Intrasite, Tegasorb	Protection of superficial and small, deep red wounds Autolytic debridement of small, noninfected yellow wounds*	Absorbent: nonadhesive to healing tissue; good barrier; waterproof; reduces pain; easy to apply; time-saving; easy to store	Nontransparent; may soften and lose shape with heat or friction; odor and brown drainage on removal (melted dressing material)	Frequency of changes depends on amount of exudate (change as needed for leakage); avoid in wounds with infection
Hydrogel sheets				
Vigilon, Geliperm, Elastogel, Cutinova	Protection of superficial and moderately deep red wounds Autolytic debridement of small, noninfected yellow or black wounds* Delivery system for topical antimicrobial creams (increases penetration)	Absorbent; nonadhesive; reduces pain; compatible with topicals; good conformity; easy to store	Poor barrier; semitransparent; requires cover dressing to secure; can promote growth of *Pseudomonas* and yeast; expensive	Avoid in infected wounds; change every 8 hr or as needed for leakage

Modified from Cuzzell JZ: Choosing a wound dressing: a systematic approach, *AACN Clin Issues Crit Care Nurs* 1(3):566-577, 1990.
*NOTE: Uses should read package inserts for any contraindications to the use of these products. Some dressings, such as Duoderm CGF, have recently been approved for application to infected wounds, provided the wound is cultured and treated for the infection. However, Duoderm CGF should not be used on third-degree burns.

when the dermatitis is acute, the applications should be mild and bland to avoid further irritation. Broken or inflamed skin, especially in children, is more absorbent than intact skin, and chemicals that are nonirritating to intact skin may be quite irritating to inflamed skin.

Topical applications may be applied to treat the disorder, reduce the itching associated with many diseases, decrease external stimuli, or apply external heat or cold. The emollient action of soaks, baths, and lotions provides a soothing film over the skin surface that reduces external stimuli. Ordinarily lukewarm, tepid, or cool applications offer the greatest relief.

Nursing ALERT

Application of heat tends to aggravate most conditions, and its use is usually reserved for reducing specific inflammatory processes, such as folliculitis and cellulitis.

Topical corticosteroid therapy. The glucocorticoids are the therapeutic agents used most widely for skin disorders. Their local antiinflammatory effects are merely palliative so that the medication must be applied until the disease state undergoes a remission or the causative agent is eliminated. Corticosteroids are applied directly to the affected area, and, because they are essentially nonsensitizing and have only minor side effects, they can be applied over prolonged periods with continuing effectiveness. As with the use of any steroids, their use in large amounts may mask signs of infection, and symptoms may be exacerbated after termination of the drug. Families are cautioned that the medication cannot be used for all skin disorders. The concentrations available without prescription are not adequate for some stubborn conditions (e.g., psoriasis) and may cause worsening of inflammation caused by fungus or bacteria. It has also been found that users apply too much topical hydrocortisone; therefore they are counseled that it is both effective and economical to apply only a thin film and massage it into the skin.

Other topical therapies. Other topical treatments include chemical cautery (especially useful for warts), cryosurgery, electrodesiccation (chiefly used for warts, granulomas, and nevi), ultraviolet therapy (primarily used in psoriasis and acne), laser therapy (especially for birthmarks), and special acne therapies such as dermabrasion and chemical peels.

Systemic Therapy

Therapeutic agents are often used as an adjunct to topical therapy in dermatologic disorders, and those most frequently used therapeutically are the corticosteroids and the antibiotics. The corticosteroid hormones with their capacity to inhibit inflammatory and allergic reactions are valuable in the treatment of severe skin disorders. Dosage is carefully adjusted and gradually tapered to the minimum that is effective and tolerated. In infants and children, dosage is larger than is usually calculated from body-weight ratios. However, prolonged use may temporarily suppress growth.

Antibiotics, which interfere with the growth of microorganisms, are used in severe or widespread skin infections. However, because they tend to produce a hypersensitivity in the patient, they are used with caution. Antifungal agents are the only means for treating systemic fungal infections.

NURSING CARE OF THE CHILD WITH A SKIN DISORDER

Assessment

To help establish a diagnosis, it is important for nurses to accurately describe any deviation in the character of the skin, using both inspection and palpation. The color, shape, and distribution of the lesions or wounds are noted. The individual lesions are described according to the accepted terminology and may involve more than one type, such as a maculopapular rash. Wounds are assessed for depth of tissue damage, evidence of healing, and signs of infection.

Nursing ALERT

Signs of wound infection are as follows:

Increased erythema, especially beyond the wound margin
Edema
Purulent exudate
Pain
Increased temperature

To confirm or amplify the findings made by inspection, the skin is gently palpated to detect characteristics such as temperature, moisture, texture, elasticity, and the presence of edema. It should be indicated whether the findings are restricted to the area of the lesion(s) or are generalized.

The child's subjective symptoms provide additional information. Older children are able to describe the condition as painful, itching, or tingling or in other descriptive terms. However, much can be determined by observing the younger child's behavior and the parents' account of these reactions. Does the child scratch? Is the child restless or irritable? Does the child favor or avoid using a part? A careful history may provide clues. Has the child had access to chemicals or been in the woods or around a woodpile? Has the child eaten a new food? Is the child taking medication? Has the child any known allergy? Do any playmates have a similar lesion? A doubtful diagnosis is frequently confirmed on the basis of history.

Nursing Diagnoses

Nursing diagnoses are determined after an assessment of the child and the skin lesions. The major diagnosis identified for the child with a skin disorder are outlined in the Nursing Care Plan on p. 1665.

Planning

The goals for the child with a skin condition and the family are as follows:

1. The child will exhibit signs of wound healing.
2. The child will not experience secondary damage, such as from infection, to the lesion.
3. The child will demonstrate an acceptable level of comfort, especially if pain or itching exist.
4. The child and family will receive appropriate education and support.

Implementation

Therapeutic programs are usually designed to provide general measures such as rest, protection, and relief of discomfort and specific treatments such as a definitive medication or physical technique. Since only a few skin diseases are contagious, it is usually not necessary to isolate the affected child unless there is a danger of acquiring a secondary infection (e.g., the child who is receiving large doses of corticosteroids or other immunosuppressant drugs or the child with an immunologic deficiency disorder). If the skin manifestation is caused by a viral exanthem, such as measles or chickenpox, the child is prevented from exposing other susceptible children.

Wound Care

Small wounds to the skin are managed by the parents at home. The parents are instructed to wash their hands, then wash the wound gently with mild soap and water for several minutes, followed by thorough rinsing. Open wounds are covered with a dressing, such as a commercial adhesive bandage, although larger wounds may benefit from the use of occlusive dressings (see Table 50-2). If occlusive dressings are applied, the parents are instructed concerning their correct application and removal. For example, hydrocolloid dressings adhere best if a wide margin is left around the wound and the dressing is pressed against intact skin until it adheres.* The edges of the dressing can be secured to the skin with waterproof tape. They are removed if leakage occurs or after a specific time interval, usually 7 days. Dressings are removed carefully to protect intact skin from damage and the epithelial surface of the

Nursing ALERT

Advise parents that the yellow gel forming under hydrocolloid dressings may look like pus and has a distinct odor (somewhat fruity) but is normal leakage.

*Information on the use of the hydrocolloid dressing Duoderm is available from ConvaTec Professional Services; (800) 422-8811.

wound. To remove transparent or hydrocolloid dressings, one edge of the dressing is raised and pull exerted *parallel* to the skin to loosen the adhesive. The longer the dressings are left on, the easier they are to remove.

Lacerations present a special challenge. The injured child and family are usually very distressed by the bleeding and are in variable degrees of shock; parental guilt usually accompanies the injury. Because scalp lacerations bleed so profusely, they are especially frightening. The initial nursing intervention is to apply pressure to the area and attempt to calm the child before further examination. Unless there is bleeding from a severed artery, the wound can be cleansed with a forced jet of sterile tepid water or saline solution (via syringe) and examined for extent, depth, and presence of foreign material such as dirt, glass, or fabric fragments.

Nursing ALERT

Hydrogen peroxide and povidone-iodine are contraindicated for cleaning fresh open wounds. Hydrogen peroxide can cause the formation of subcutaneous gas when applied under pressure.

The location of the wound also dictates assessment. For example, wounds over bony areas may contain bone chips, and clear fluid seeping from severe head wounds may indicate cerebrospinal fluid. A pressure dressing is applied for transfer to medical care; the child in a medical facility is prepared for suturing (see the Atraumatic Care box above).

Puncture wounds that do not require a tetanus booster are soaked in hot water and soap for several minutes. Causing the wound to rebleed may be helpful. An adhesive bandage can be applied if desired. Puncture wounds of the head, chest, or abdomen or those that could still contain a portion of the puncturing object must be evaluated.

Parents are cautioned against opening blisters or kissing a wound "to make it better." The wound can easily become contaminated from germs in the human mouth. If scabs form, they are allowed to slough off without assistance; picking or early removal may cause scarring. Parents are advised to seek medical help if there is evidence of infection.

Relief of Symptoms

Most of the therapeutic regimens for skin lesions are directed toward relief of pruritus, the most common subjective complaint. Cooling the affected area and increasing the skin pH with measures such as cool baths or compresses to reduce external stimuli to the area and alkaline applications (e.g., baking soda baths) to increase skin pH help to prevent scratching. Clothing and bed linen should be soft and lightweight to decrease the irritation from friction and stimulation.

During any type of treatment, both affected and unaffected skin is protected from damage and secondary infection. Preventing scratching is of primary importance. Older children usually cooperate, although they may need to be reminded to stop scratching or rubbing; but in smaller and uncooperative children the use of techniques and devices such as mittens (especially during sleep) or special coverings is required. Keeping fingernails short, well-trimmed, and clean helps reduce the chance of secondary infection.

Atraumatic Care 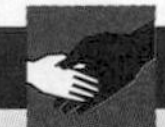

PAINLESS SUTURING AND WOUND CLEANSING

The topical application of lidocaine, adrenaline, and tetracaine (LAT); bupivacaine and norepinephrine; tetracaine, adrenaline, and cocaine (TAC); or AC (without tetracaine) gel to wounds, especially on the head, scalp, and face, provides anesthesia in 10 to 15 minutes (Smith et al, 1996). If further anesthesia is required or if TAC is not available, using *buffered* lidocaine reduces the stinging and burning of the injection (see Pain Management, Chapter 41). The use of a noninvasive tissue adhesive (Histoacryl blue) provides a faster and less painful method of facial laceration repair (Osmond, Klassen, and Quinn, 1995).

Antipruritic medications, such as diphenhydramine (Benadryl) or hydroxyzine (Atarax), may be prescribed for severe itching, especially if it disturbs the child's rest. Pain and discomfort are usually managed with nonpharmacologic measures and mild analgesia; severe pain may require more potent medication. Occlusive dressings over wounds reduce pain. For suturing wounds a topical anesthetic or intradermal buffered lidocaine can be used (See Pain Management, Chapter 41).

Topical Therapy

Therapy usually involves some type of topical treatment, and the mode of application depends on the nature and location of the lesion being treated. It is especially important to wash the hands before and after applying topical therapies. The skin is assessed before the treatment or application of medication and reassessed after the treatment is completed. Any observed changes are noted and described.

Wet compresses or *dressings* cool the skin by evaporation, relieve itching and inflammation, and cleanse the area by loosening and removing crusts and debris. Any of a variety of ingredients, such as plain water or Burow solution (available without a prescription), can be applied on Kerlix gauze, plain gauze, or (preferably) soft cotton cloths such as freshly laundered handkerchiefs or strips from diaper, sheeting, or pillowcase material.

Dressings immersed in the desired solution are wrung out slightly and applied to the affected area wet but not dripping. They are applied flat and smooth and in such a way that motion is not totally restricted—fingers are wrapped separately, and arms and legs are wrapped so that elbows and knees can bend. Dressings are kept in place by Kerlix or other cotton wrap, tubular stockinette, mittens, and socks (two pair—one to hold the dressings in place, the other to take up movement) but are left uncovered. When evaporation begins to dry them, the dressings are removed, rewet in the solution, and reapplied to the area using aseptic technique. The solution is not poured or syringed directly over the dressings. As fluid evaporates, the solution becomes increasingly concentrated and thus stronger, which may be damaging to sensitive lesions.

Fresh solution at room temperature is applied at 2-, 3-, or 4-hour intervals and is allowed to remain on the lesion from 30 minutes to $1^1/_2$ hours. Wet dressings are seldom continued after about 48 hours. The child must be guarded against chilling during treatment, and no more than 20% of the body should be covered at one time to avoid the risk of hypothermia. After treatment the skin is dried thoroughly by patting with a towel. Application of lotion or other medication may be ordered at this time.

When children are uncooperative in the use of wet dressings, *soaks* are often used for removal of crusts and for their mild astringent action, with the same solution as for wet compresses. Gaining young children's cooperation for hand or foot soaks is difficult unless the procedure is made attractive to them through play. For example, washing dishes, cars, dolls, or doll clothes will occupy many children for quite some time. The older child is able to cooperate but may need something to do during the procedure, such as listening to music or a story or watching television.

Baths are especially useful in the treatment of widespread dermatitis by evenly distributing the soothing antipruritic and antiinflammatory effects of the solution, usually oatmeal or mineral oil preparations. The solution is added to a tub of lukewarm water. The temperature of the bath is tepid, and the treatment usually lasts 15 to 30 minutes. Therapeutic baths are always more interesting when the child is accompanied by toy boats or other items for water play.

Topical applications are applied to skin lesions to ease discomfort, prevent further injury, and facilitate healing. Most preparations are placed directly on the skin and left uncovered; others may be applied under an occlusive dressing. A thin application of the ointment or cream is covered with plastic film and anchored with adhesive or covered with a commercial transparent dressing. Occlusive dressings promote moisture retention and nonevaporation of the preparation, which increases the penetration of the medication. Regardless of the type of preparation used, parents need detailed information on how to apply it and how long the preparation should remain on the skin or under an occlusive dressing.

Nursing ALERT

Provide written instructions and demonstrate to parents the correct amount of topical medication to apply (e.g., size of a pea; thin film to cover). If more than one preparation is applied, mark the containers 1 and 2 for patients to remember the correct order. Stress that more is not necessarily better with some medications, such as steroids.

Home Care and Family Support

Dermatologic conditions always involve the family. Since few situations require hospitalization and children who are hospitalized will complete a therapy program at home, the family must carry out the treatment plan; therefore their cooperation is essential. Regimens that are simple to accomplish in the hospital or office may be frustrating and baffling at home. The family often needs assistance in adapting equipment available in the home to the therapy.

It is important that the child and family be given as detailed explanations as possible about both the expected and the unexpected results of treatment, including any ill effects that might occur. If unexplained reactions do develop, the family is directed to discontinue treatment and report the reactions to the appropriate person(s). The use of over-the-counter medicines is discouraged unless they have first been discussed with the attending practitioner and received approval.

Since the skin is the most visible portion of the body, defects in its surface that alter its appearance are sometimes a source of distress to the child and of revulsion and rejection to others. Parents of other children may fear that their children will "catch" the disorder. Occasionally the affected child's own family members will reduce their interaction with him or her, especially close physical contact, or otherwise demonstrate a distaste for the condition, which the child may interpret as rejection. This is seldom a difficulty with dermatitis of short duration, but chronic conditions can create problems in development of a positive self-concept.

Evaluation

The effectiveness of nursing interventions is determined by continual reassessment and evaluation of care based on the following observational guidelines and expected outcomes:

1. Observe if reasonable care is used in performing nursing activities, and observe lesions and child's reactions to therapies.
2. Observe signs of wound healing.
3. Use assessment techniques to identify relief of discomfort as described in Chapter 41.
4. Reassess skin lesions; observe and interview child and family regarding compliance with therapy.

Expected outcomes:
See the Nursing Care Plan on p. 1665.

Infections of the Skin

BACTERIAL INFECTIONS

Normally the skin harbors a variety of bacterial flora, including the major pathogenic varieties of staphylococci and streptococci. The degree of their pathogenicity depends on the invasiveness and toxigenicity of the specific organism, the integrity of the skin, the barrier of the host, and the immune and cellular defenses of the host. Children with immunodeficiency, such as infants, children with congenital immune deficiency disorders, children in a debilitated condition, those taking immunosuppressive therapy, and those with a generalized malignancy such as leukemia or lymphoma, are at risk for developing bacterial infections.

Because of the characteristic "walling-off" process of the inflammatory reaction (abscess formation), staphylococci are more difficult to attack, and the local infected area is associated with an increase in numbers of bacteria all over the skin surface that serve as a source of continuing infection. Staphylococcal infections occur most often in children in the younger age groups, and the incidence decreases with advancing age. All of these factors emphasize the importance of careful handwashing and cleanliness when caring for infected children and their lesions to prevent spread of the infection and as an essential prophylactic measure when caring for infants and small children. Common bacterial skin disorders are outlined in Table 50-3.

Nursing Care Plan
THE CHILD WITH A SKIN DISORDER

Nursing Diagnosis: Impaired skin integrity related to environmental agents, somatic factors, immunologic deficit

Expected Outcome: The child exhibits signs of skin healing, intact skin remains free of irritation or secondary infection, and there is no evidence of recurring lesions.

• **NURSING INTERVENTIONS/*RATIONALES***

Provide moist environment for lesions (dressing, ointment) *to provide optimum healing of wounds.*

Administer topical and systemic medications as ordered *to aid healing and prevent infection.*

Keep lesions, surrounding skin, clothing, and linens clean and dry *to promote healing and prevent secondary infection and mechanical trauma.*

Use good handwashing technique before and after administration of care *to prevent infection;* teach child and family about importance of handwashing and hygiene measures *to prevent spread of infection.*

Use methods as appropriate (i.e., short nails, mittens, elbow splints, clothing that covers lesions) *to prevent child from touching or scratching lesions and prevent autoinoculation and secondary infection.*

Teach child and family to recognize and avoid contact with agents/allergens known to precipitate skin reaction *to prevent recurrence of lesions.*

Observe skin frequently for signs of spread, secondary infection, irritation, or breakdown *so appropriate treatment measures can be instituted.*

Nursing Diagnosis: Risk for infection related to presence of infective organisms

Expected Outcome: Infection is confined to primary site.

• **NURSING INTERVENTIONS/*RATIONALEs***

Implement universal precautions, use careful handwashing, avoid unnecessary close contact during infective stage *to prevent spread of infection.*

Implement isolation techniques as appropriate, including proper disposal of all items that come in contact with infective lesions *to prevent spread of infection.*

Teach child and family about handwashing and hygiene techniques *to reduce risk of spread of infection.*

Nursing Diagnosis: Pain related to itching, trauma of skin lesions

Expected Outcomes: The child exhibits signs of comfort, and there is no evidence of scratching.

• **NURSING INTERVENTIONS/*RATIONALES***

Administer topical and systemic agents as ordered *to reduce pain and itching.*

Implement nonpharmacologic pain reduction techniques as appropriate (i.e., distraction, relaxation, guided imagery, positive self-talk, cutaneous stimulation) *to relieve pain.*

Advocate for child regarding approriate anesthesia for wound suturing *to prevent unnecessary pain and emotional trauma.*

Nursing Diagnosis: Body-image disturbance related to appearance altered by skin lesions

Expected Outcome: The child demonstrates a positive body image.

• **NURSING INTERVENTIONS/*RATIONALES***

Encourage child to express feelings and ask questions about appearance and perceived reactions of others *to facilitate coping.*

Discuss with child and family the expected progression of the skin lesions and healing process *to provide a sense of hope and control.*

Have child participate in care and maintain usual routine and activities as much as possible *to promote a sense of normalcy and adequacy.*

Nursing Care Management

The major nursing functions related to bacterial skin infections are to prevent the spread of infection and complications. Handwashing is mandatory before and after contact with an affected child. Handwashing is also emphasized to both the child and the family, and the child should be provided with towels separate from those of other family members. Impetigo contagiosa is easily spread by self-inoculation; therefore the child must be cautioned against touching the involved area. This is difficult to accomplish; distraction or reminders are useful but are not helpful when the child is alone, as at bedtime.

Children and parents are often tempted to squeeze follicular lesions. They must be warned that squeezing will not hasten the resolution of the infection and that there is a risk of making the lesion worse or spreading the infection. No attempt should be made to puncture the surface of the pustule with a needle or sharp instrument. A child with a sty may waken with the eyelids of the affected eye sealed shut with exudate. The child or the parents are instructed to gently wipe the lid with clear warm water and a clean washcloth until the exudate has been removed.

The child with limited cellulitis of an extremity is usually managed at home on a regimen of oral antibiotics and warm

TABLE 50-3 Bacterial infections

DISORDER/ORGANISM	MANIFESTATIONS	MANAGEMENT	COMMENTS
Impetigo contagiosa (Fig. 50-3)—*Staphylococcus*	Begins as a reddish macule Becomes vesicular Ruptures easily, leaving superficial, moist erosion Tends to spread peripherally in sharply marginated irregular outlines Exudate dries to form heavy, honey-colored crusts Pruritus common Systemic effects: minimal or asymptomatic	Careful removal of undermined skin, crusts, and debris by softening with 1:20 Burow solution compresses Topical application of bactericidal ointment Systemic administration of oral or parenteral antibiotics (penicillin) in severe or extensive lesions	Tends to heal without scarring unless secondary infection Autoinoculable and contagious Very common in toddler, preschooler
Pyoderma—*Staphylococcus, Streptococcus*	Deeper extension of infection into dermis Tissue reaction more severe Systemic effects: fever, lymphangitis	Soap and water cleansing Wet compresses Bathing with antibacterial soap as prescribed	Autoinoculable and contagious May heal with or without scarring
Folliculitis (pimple), furuncle (boil), carbuncle (multiple boils)—*Staphylococcus aureus*	Folliculitis: infection of hair follicle Furuncle: larger lesion with more redness and swelling at a single follicle Carbuncle: more extensive lesion with widespread inflammation and "pointing" at several follicular orifices Systemic effects: malaise, if severe	Skin cleanliness Local warm, moist compresses Topical application of antibiotic agents Systemic antibiotics in severe cases Incision and drainage of severe lesions, followed by wound irrigations with antibiotics or suitable drain implantation	Autoinoculable and contagious Furuncle and carbuncle tend to heal with scar formation A lesion should *never* be squeezed
Cellulitis—*Streptotoccus, Staphylococcus, Haemophilus influenzae* (Fig. 50-4)	Inflammation of skin and subcutaneous tissues with intense redness, swelling, and firm infiltration Lymphangitis "streaking" frequently seen Involvement of regional lymph nodes common May progress to abscess formation Systemic effects: fever, malaise	Oral or parenteral antibiotics Rest and immobilization of both affected area and child Hot moist compresses to area	Hospitalization may be necessary for child with systemic symptoms Otitis media may be associated with facial cellulitis
Staphylococcal scalded skin syndrome—*S. aureus*	Macular erythema with "sandpaper" texture of involved skin Epidermis becomes wrinkled (in 2 days or less) and large bullae appear	Systemic administration of antibiotics Gentle cleansing with saline solution, Burow solution, or 0.25% silver nitrate compresses	Infant subject to fluid loss, impaired body temperature regulation, and secondary infection, such as pneumonia, cellulitis, and septicemia Heals without scarring

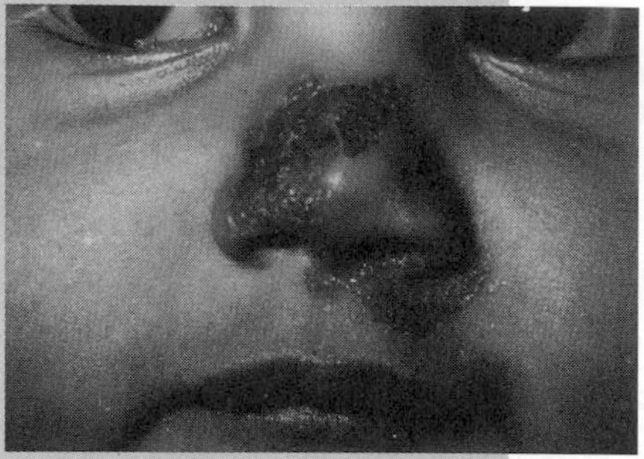

Fig. 50-3 Impetigo contagiosa. (From Weston WL, Lane AT: *Color textbook of pediatric dermatology*, St Louis, 1991, Mosby.)

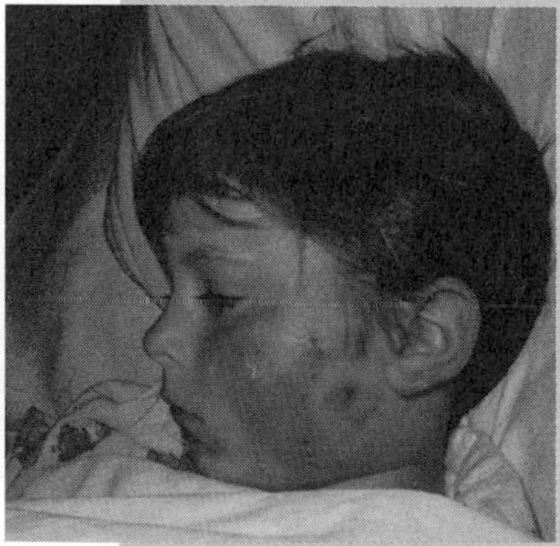

Fig. 50-4 Cellulitis of cheek from puncture wound. (From Weston WL, Lane AT: *Color textbook of pediatric dermatology*, St Louis, 1991, Mosby.)

compresses. The parents are taught the procedures and instructed in how to administer the medication. Children with more extensive cellulitis, especially around a joint with lymphadenitis or on the face, are usually admitted to the hospital for parenteral antibiotics. Nurses are responsible for administering the medication, applying compresses, and maintaining the intravenous infusion.

VIRAL INFECTIONS

Viruses are intracellular parasites that produce their effect by using the intracellular substances of the host cells. Composed of only a DNA or RNA core enclosed in an antigenic protein shell, viruses are unable to provide for their own metabolic needs or to reproduce themselves. After a virus penetrates a cell of the host organism, it sheds the outer shell and disap-

TABLE 50-4 Viral infections

DISEASE	MANIFESTATIONS	MANAGEMENT	COMMENTS
Verruca (warts) Cause: human papillomavirus (various types)	Small, benign tumors Usually well-circumscribed, gray or brown, elevated firm papules with a roughened, finely papillomatous texture Occur anywhere, but usually appear on exposed areas such as fingers, hands, face, and soles May be single or multiple Asymptomatic	Not uniformly successful Local destructive therapy, individualized according to location, type, and number—surgical removal, electrocautery, curettage, cryotherapy (liquid nitrogen), caustic solutions (lactic acid and salicylic acid in flexible collodion, retinoic acid, salicyclic acid plasters), x-ray treatment	Common in children Tend to disappear spontaneously Course unpredictable Most destructive techniques tend to leave scars Autoinoculable Repeated irritation will cause to enlarge
Verruca plantaris (plantar wart)	Located on plantar surface of feet and, because of pressure, are practically flat; may be surrounded by a collar of hyperkeratosis	Apply caustic solution to wart, wear foam insole with hole cut to relieve pressure on wart; soak 20 min after 2 or 3 days; repeat until wart comes out	Destructive techniques tend to leave scars, which may cause problems with walking
Herpes simplex virus Type I (cold sore, fever blister) Type II (genital)	Grouped, burning, and itching vesicles on inflammatory base, usually on or near mucocutaneous junctions (lips, nose, genitals, buttocks) Vesicles dry, forming a crust, followed by exfoliation and spontaneous healing in 8 to 10 days May be accompanied by regional lymphadenopathy	Avoidance of secondary infection Burow solution compresses during weeping stages Topical therapy has proved to have effect on recurrences Oral antiviral (Acyclovir) for initial infection or to reduce severity in recurrence	Heal without scarring unless secondary infection Aggravated by corticosteroids Positive psychologic effect from treatment May be fatal in children with depressed immunity
Varicella zoster virus (herpes zoster; shingles)	Caused by same virus that causes varicella (chickenpox) Virus has affinity for posterior root ganglia, posterior horn of spinal cord, and skin; crops of vesicles usually confined to dermatome following along course of affected nerve Usually preceded by neuralgic pain, hyperesthesias, or itching May be accompanied by constitutional symptoms	Symptomatic Analgesics for pain Mild sedation sometimes helpful Local moist compresses Drying lotions may be helpful Ophthalmic variety: systemic corticotropin (ACTH) and/or corticosteroids Acyclovir	Pain in children usually minimal Postherpetic pain does not occur in children Chickenpox may follow exposure; isolate affected child from other children in a hospital or school May occur in children with depressed immunity; can be fatal
Molluscum contagiosum Cause: poxvirus	Flesh-colored papules with a central caseous plug (umbilicated) Usually asymptomatic	Cases in well children resolve spontaneously in about 18 months Treatment reserved for troublesome cases Curettage or cryotherapy	Common in school-age children Spread by skin-to-skin contact, including autoinoculation and fomite-to-skin contact

TABLE 50-5 Dermatophytoses (fungal infections)

DISEASE/ORGANISM	MANIFESTATIONS	MANAGEMENT	COMMENTS
Tinea capitis—*Trichophyton tonsurans, Microsporum audouini, Microsporum canis* (Fig. 50-5, *A*)	Lesions in scalp but may extend to hairline or neck Characteristic configuration of scaly, circumscribed patches and/or patchy, scaling areas of alopecia Generally asymptomatic, but severe, deep inflammatory reaction may occur that manifests as boggy, encrusted lesions (kerions) Pruritic Microscopic examination of scales is diagnostic	Oral griseofulvin Oral ketoconazole for difficult cases Selenium sulfide shampoos Topical antifungal agents (e.g., clotrimazole, haloprogin, miconazole)	Person-to-person transmission Animal-to-person transmission Rarely, permanent loss of hair *M. audouini* transmitted from one human being to another directly or from personal items; *M. canis* usually contracted from household pets, especially cats Atopic individuals more susceptible
Tinea corporis—*Trichophyton rubrum, Trichophyton mentagrophytes, M. canis, Epidermophyton* (see Fig. 50-5, *B*)	Generally round or oval, erythematous scaling patch that spreads peripherally and clears centrally; may involve nails (tinea unguium) Diagnosis: direct microscopic examination of scales Usually unilateral	Oral griseofulvin Local application of antifungal preparation such as tolnaftate, haloprogin, miconazole, clotrimazole; apply 1 inch beyond periphery of lesion; continual application 1 to 2 weeks after no sign of lesion	Usually of animal origin from infected pets Majority of infections in children caused by *M. canis* and *M. audouini*
Tinea cruris ("jock itch")—*Epidermophyton floccosum, T. rubrum, T. mentagrophytes*	Skin response similar to tinea corporis Localized to medial proximal aspect of thigh and crural fold; may involve scrotum in males Pruritic Diagnosis: same as for tinea corporis	Local application of tolnaftate liquid Wet compresses or sitz baths may be soothing	Rare in preadolescent children Health education regarding personal hygiene

A
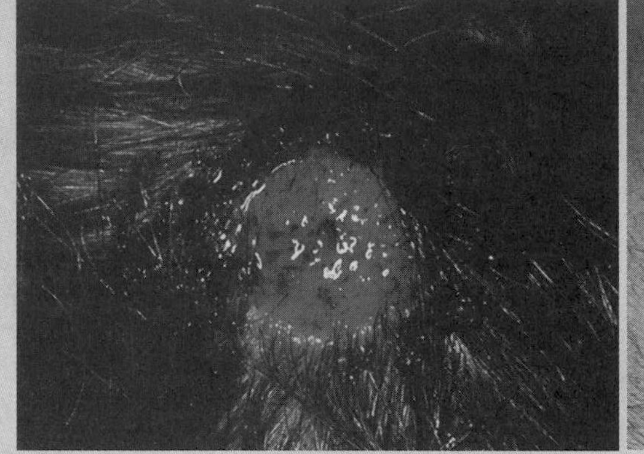
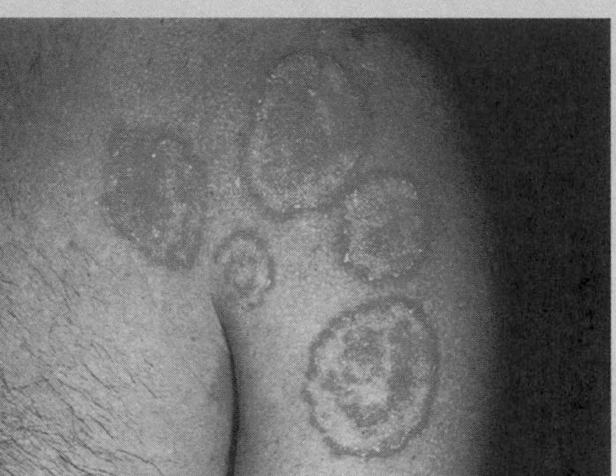
B

Fig. 50-5 **A,** Tinea capitis. **B,** Tinea corporis. Both infections are caused by *Microsporum canis*, the "kitten" or "puppy" fungus. (From Habif TP: *Clinical dermatology: a color guide to diagnosis and therapy*, ed 2, St Louis, 1990, Mosby.)

TABLE 50-5 Dermatophytoses (fungal infections)—cont'd

DISEASE/ORGANISM	MANIFESTATIONS	MANAGEMENT	COMMENTS
Tinea pedis ("athlete's foot")—*T. rubrum, Trichophyton interdigitale, E. floccosum*	On intertriginous areas between toes or on plantar surface of feet Lesions vary: Maceration and fissuring between toes Patches with pinhead-sized vesicles on plantar surface Pruritic Diagnosis: direct microscopic examination of scrapings	Oral griseofulvin Local applications of tolnaftate liquid and antifungal powder containing tolnaftate Acute infections: compresses or soaks followed by application of glucocortocoid cream Elimination of conditions of heat and perspiration by clean, light socks, and well-ventilated shoes; avoidance of occlusive shoes	Most frequent in adolescents and adults; rare in children, but occurrence increases with wearing of plastic shoes Transmission to other individuals rare despite general opinion to contrary Ointments not successful
Candidiasis (moniliasis)—*Candida albicans*	Grows in chronically moist areas Inflamed areas with white exudate, peeling, and easy bleeding Pruritic Diagnosis: characteristic appearance	Amphotericin B, nystatin ointment, or other antifungal preparations to affected areas	Common form of diaper dermatitis (see Fig. 50-12) Oral form common in infants May be disseminated in immunosuppressed children

pears within the cell, where the nucleic acid core stimulates the host cell to form more virus material from its intracellular substance. In a viral infection the epidermal cells react with inflammation and vesiculation (as in herpes simplex) or by proliferating to form growths (warts).

Most of the communicable diseases of childhood are associated with rashes, and each rash is characteristic. The type of lesion and the configuration of the viral exanthems of rubeola, rubella, and chickenpox are described in Table 35-2. Other common viral disorders of the skin are outlined in Table 50-4.

DERMATOPHYTOSES (FUNGAL INFECTIONS)

The dermatophytoses (ringworm) are infections caused by a group of closely related filamentous fungi that invade primarily the stratum corneum, hair, and nails. These are superficial infections that live on, not in, the skin. They are confined to the dead keratin layers and are unable to survive in the deeper layers. Since the keratin is being desquamated constantly, the fungus must multiply at a rate that equals the rate of keratin production to maintain itself; otherwise the infection would be shed with the discarded skin cells. Common dermatophytoses are outlined in Table 50-5.

Dermatophytoses are designated by the Latin word *tinea,* with further designation related to the area of the body where they are found (e.g., tinea capitis [ringworm of the scalp]). Dermatophyte infections are most often transmitted from one person to another or from infected animals to humans. Diagnosis is made from microscopic examination of scrapings taken from the advancing periphery of the lesion, which almost always produces scale.

Nursing Care Management

When teaching families regarding the care of children with ringworm, the nurse should emphasize good health and hygiene. Because of the infectious nature of the disease, several basic hygienic measures are particularly pertinent. Affected children are not to exchange with other children any grooming items, headgear, scarves, or other articles of apparel that have been in proximity to the infected area. Affected children are provided with their own towels and directed to wear protective caps at night to avoid transmitting the fungus to bedding, especially if they sleep with another person. Since the infection can be acquired by animal-to-human transmission, all household pets should be examined for the presence of the disorder. Other sources of infection are seats with headrests, such as theater seats or seats in public transportation.

Treatment with the drug griseofulvin frequently lasts for weeks or months, and, because subjective symptoms subside, children or parents may be tempted to decrease or discontinue the drug. The nurse should impress on members of the family the importance of maintaining the prescribed dosage schedule. They are also instructed regarding the possibility of side effects from the drug such as headache, gastrointestinal upset, fatigue, insomnia, and photosensitivity. For children who take the drug over many months, periodic testing is required to monitor leukopenia and assess liver and renal function.

SYSTEMIC MYCOTIC (FUNGAL) INFECTIONS

Mycotic (systemic or deep fungal) infections have the capacity to invade the viscera as well as the skin. The best known of these infections are primarily lung diseases, which are usually acquired by inhalation of fungal spores. The fungi produce a

TABLE 50-6 Systemic mycoses

DISORDER/ ORGANISM	SKIN MANIFESTATIONS	SYSTEMIC MANIFESTATIONS	TREATMENT	COMMENTS
North American blastomycosis—*Blastomyces dermatitidis*	Chronic granulomatous lesions and microabscesses in any part of body Initial lesion is a papule; undergoes ulceration and peripheral spread	Pulmonary symptoms, such as cough, chest pain, weakness, and weight loss May have skeletal involvement, with bone destruction and formation of cutaneous abscesses	Intravenous administration of amphotericin B	Usual portal of entry is lungs Source of infection unknown Noninfectious Pulmonary infections may be mild and self-limiting and require no treatment Progressive disease often fatal
Cryptococcosis—*Cryptococcus neoformans (Torula histolytica)*	Usually on face; acneiform, firm, nodular, painless eruption	Central nervous system (CNS) manifestations; headache, dizziness, stiff neck, and signs of increased intracranial pressure Low-grade fever, mild cough, lung infiltration	Intravenous amphotericin B; may be administered intrathecally for CNS involvement 5-Fluorocytosine for meningitis Excision and drainage of local lesions	Acquired by inhalation of dust but may enter through skin Prognosis serious Noninfectious Increased incidence in persons receiving corticosteroids with lymphoreticular malignancies, or type II diabetes
Histoplasmosis—*Histoplasma capsulatum*	Not distinctive or uniform but most appear as punched-out or granulomatous ulcers	General systemic symptoms may include pallor, diarrhea, vomiting, irregular spiking temperature, hepatosplenomegaly, and pulmonary symptoms Any tissue of body may be involved with related symptoms	Intravenous amphotericin B for severe cases Oral ketoconazole	Organism cultured from soil, especially where contaminated with fowl droppings Fungus enters through skin or mucous membranes of mouth and respiratory tract Endemic in Mississippi and Ohio River valleys Disseminated diseases most common in infants and children
Coccidioidomycosis (valley fever)—*Coccidioides immitis*	Erythema nodosum Erythema multiforme Erythematous maculopapular rash	Primary lung disease usually asymptomatic May be sign of acute febrile illness Disseminated disease is very serious	Intravenous amphotericin B Intravenous miconazole (synthetic imidazole) Intraventricular miconazole plus oral ketoconazole for CNS involvement Surgical resection of persistent pulmonary cavities	Inhalation of aerospores from soil Endemic in southwestern United States Usually resolves spontaneously Increased incidence in dark-skinned races (Filipino, black, Mexican, Asian)

variable spectrum of disease, and some are quite common in certain geographic areas. They are not transmitted from person to person but appear to reside in the soil, from which their spores are airborne. The cutaneous lesions caused by deep fungal infections are granulomatous and appear as ulcers, plaques, nodules, fungating masses, and abscesses. The course of deep fungal diseases is chronic with slow progression that favors sensitization (Table 50-6).

Skin Disorders Related to Chemical or Physical Contacts

CONTACT DERMATITIS

Contact dermatitis is an inflammatory reaction of the skin to chemical substances, natural or synthetic, that evoke a hypersensitivity response or to those agents that cause direct irritation. The initial reaction occurs in an exposed region, most commonly the face and neck, backs of the hands, forearms, male genitalia, and lower legs. There is characteristically a sharp delineation between inflamed and normal skin early in the reaction that ranges from a faint, transient erythema to massive bullae on an erythematous swollen base. Itching is a constant symptom.

The cause may be a primary irritant or a sensitizing agent. A *primary irritant* is one that irritates any skin. A *sensitizing agent* produces an irritation on those who have met the irritant or something chemically related to it, have undergone an immunologic change, and have become sensitized. Prior exposure is not necessarily a factor in the reaction. A sensitizer irritates in relatively low concentrations only persons who are allergic to it. Sometimes with repeated exposure and reactions the skin loses its capacity to return to normal, or secondary factors become predominant to produce a chronic inflammatory process.

The major goal in treatment is to prevent further exposure of the skin to the offending substance. Provided there is no further irritation, the normal recuperative powers of the skin will produce satisfactory results without treatment. The most frequent offenders are plant and animal irritants, the prototype of which is poison ivy.

The most common contact dermatitis in infants occurs on the convex surfaces of the diaper area (see Diaper Dermatitis, p. 1679). Other agents that frequently produce dermatologic responses from contact are animal irritants such as wool, feathers, and furs; vegetable irritants such as oleoresins, oils, and turpentine; and chemicals of all kinds, including synthetic fabrics, dyes, metals, cosmetics, perfumes, and soaps (including bubble baths). The list is endless.

Nursing Care Management

Nurses frequently detect evidence of contact dermatitis during routine physical assessments. Skin manifestations in specific areas suggest limited contact, such as around the eyes (mascara), areas of the body covered by clothing but not protected by undergarments (wool), or areas of the body not covered by clothing (ultraviolet injury). Generalized involvement is more likely to be caused by bubble bath or soap. Often nurses are able to determine the offending agent and counsel families regarding management. However, if the lesions persist, are extensive, or show evidence of infection, medical evaluation is indicated.

POISON IVY, OAK, AND SUMAC

The prototype of plant offenders is poison ivy (also poison oak and sumac) (Fig. 50-6). Contact with the dry or succulent portions of the plant produces localized, streaked or spotty, oozing, and painful impetiginous lesions. The offending substance in these plants is an oil, *urushiol*, that is extremely potent. Sensitivity to urushiol is not inborn but is developed after one or two exposures and may change over a lifetime. All parts of the plants contain the oil, so dried leaves and stems contain the irritant. Even smoke from burning brush piles can produce a reaction.

Animals do not seem to be affected by the oil; however, dogs or other animals that have run or played in the plants may carry the sap on their fur, and animals who eat the plants can transfer the oil in saliva. Shoes, tools, and toys can transfer the oil. Golf balls that have been in the rough also are sources of contact.

Urushiol takes effect as soon as it touches the skin. It penetrates through the epidermis and bonds with the dermal layer, where it initiates an immune response. The full-blown reaction is evident after about 2 days, with redness, swelling, and itching at the site of contact. Several days later, streaked or spotty blisters oozing serum from damaged cells produce the characteristic impetiginous lesions (Fig. 50-7). The lesions dry and heal spontaneously, and itching stops by 10 to 14 days.

Therapeutic Management

Treatment of the lesions includes calamine lotion, soothing Burow solution compresses, and/or Aveeno baths to relieve discomfort. Topical corticosteroid gel is very effective for prevention or relief of inflammation, especially when applied before blisters form. Oral corticosteroids may be needed for se-

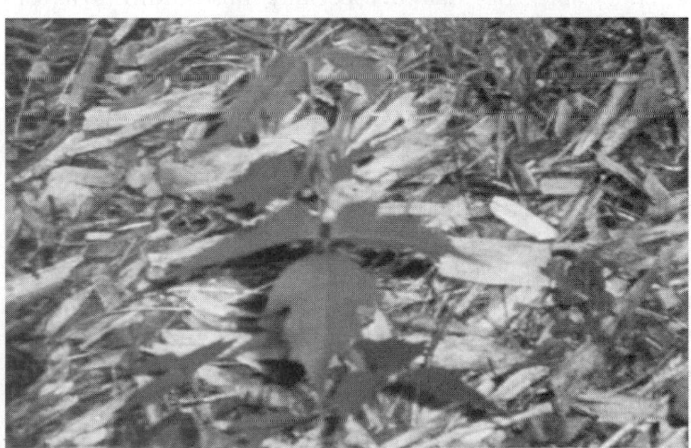

Fig. 50-6 Poison ivy.

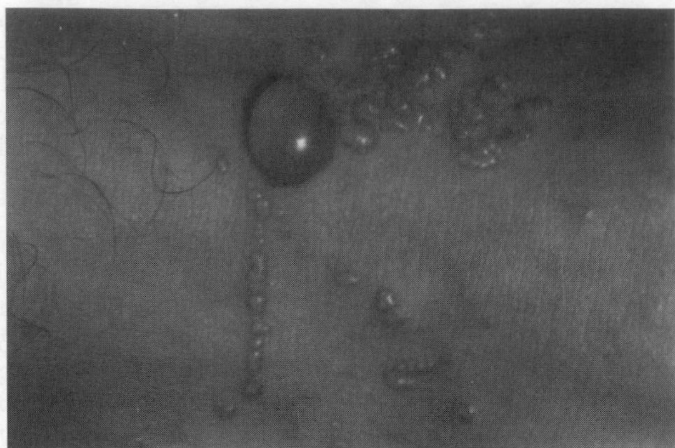

Fig. 50-7 Poison ivy. Note "streaked" blisters surrounding one large blister. (From Habif TP: *Clinical dermatology: a color guide to diagnosis and therapy*, ed 2, St Louis, 1990, Mosby.)

vere reactions, and a sedative such as diphenhydramine (Benadryl) may be ordered.

Nursing Care Management

When it is known that the child has made contact with the plant, the area is immediately flushed (preferably within 15 minutes) with *cold* running water to neutralize the urushiol not yet bonded to the skin. If there is a stream nearby, an effective method is to have the child enter the water (clothes and all) and allow the water to rinse the oil from both skin and clothing. Harsh soap is contraindicated because it removes protective skin oils and dilutes the urushiol, allowing it to spread; also, hard scrubbing irritates the skin. All clothing that has come in contact with the plant is removed with care and thoroughly laundered in hot water and detergent. Every effort is made to prevent the child from scratching the lesions. Although the lesions do not spread by contact with the blister serum or from scratching, they can become secondarily infected.

Prevention. Prevention is best accomplished by avoidance of contact and removal of the plant from the environment when feasible. All children, especially those known to be sensitive, should be taught to recognize the plant. Information regarding means for destroying plants can be obtained from the U.S. Department of Agriculture or Forestry Service. An example of a cream that helps protect exposed skin from poison oak and ivy is Stokogard.*

DRUG REACTIONS

Adverse reactions to drugs are seen more often in the skin than in any other organ, although any organ of the body can be affected. The reaction may be a result of toxicity related to drug concentration, individual intolerance to the average dosage of the drug, or an allergic or idiosyncratic response. The manifestations may be associated with side effects or secondary effects of a drug, either of which are unrelated to its primary pharmacologic actions.

Although any drug is capable of producing almost any form of reaction in the susceptible individual, some have a tendency to produce a particular reaction consistently, and some are more likely than others to produce an untoward effect. Many are allergic responses following a prior administration of the drug, even a topical application. Other factors influence a drug response in a particular individual. For example, the incidence increases with the number and amount of drugs being given, and intravenous drugs are more likely to cause a reaction than are oral drugs.

Manifestations of drug reactions may be delayed or immediate. Seven days are usually required for a child to develop sensitivity to a drug that has never been administered previously. With prior sensitivity the manifestations appear almost immediately. Rashes are the most common manifestation of adverse drug reactions in children. However, individual drug reactions may vary from a single lesion to extensive, generalized epidermal necrosis, such as occurs in Stevens-Johnson syndrome (Table 50-9). Cutaneous manifestations can resemble almost any skin disease and can be seen in almost any degree of severity. With few exceptions, the distribution of a drug eruption is widespread, since it results from a circulating agent, appears as an inflammatory response with itching, is sudden in onset, and may be associated with constitutional symptoms such as fever, malaise, gastrointestinal upsets, anemia, or liver and kidney damage.

In most cases, treatment for simple cutaneous reactions consists of discontinuing the drug. Sometimes a decision is made to continue the drug (such as an antibiotic in an infant or small child) until the cause of the rash is clearly indicated. In urticarial-type eruptions, antihistamines may be ordered, and for widespread and severe lesions, corticosteroids are beneficial. Severe anaphylactic reactions are a medical emergency (see the discussion of anaphylaxis, Chapter 45).

Nursing Care Management

The most effective means of management is prevention. Parents always remember a severe reaction. A careful history will elicit evidence of a previous drug reaction. The history should include the name of the drug, nature of the reaction, drug dose, and how soon after administration the reaction occurred (Chapter 31).

Nurses who suspect that a rash is caused by a medication should withhold any further dose and report the eruption to the practitioner. Frequent offenders in drug reactions are penicillin and sulfonamides, and nurses must be alert to this possibility. However, even commonplace drugs, including aspirin, barbiturates, chemical agents in a number of foods, flavoring agents, and preservatives, can produce an undesired response. Persons who have severe reactions should wear an identification bracelet or chain in case of emergency or inadvertent administration of the offending drug.

FOREIGN BODIES

Small wooden splinters can be removed by parents with a needle and tweezers that have been sterilized with alcohol or a flame. The area around the sliver is washed with soap and water before removal is attempted. The sliver is exposed with the needle, then grasped firmly by the tweezers and pulled out.

*Distributed in the USA by Stockhausen, Inc., Greensboro, NC 27406; (800) 334-0242.

Suggestions for removing cactus spines are as follows:

- Apply a thin layer of household glue and cover with gauze. When glue dries, peel off gauze (Martinez et al, 1987).
- Apply commercial hair removal wax or body sugar (Aplon*), let dry, and remove (Hennes, 1988).
- Place cellophane tape, sticky side down, over the spines and lift off (Cooper, 1988).

Some foreign bodies, such as a fishhook, a piece of glass or other difficult-to-see object, or a deeply embedded object, such as a needle in a foot or near a joint, may need medical evaluation.

Skin Disorders Related to Insect and Animal Contacts

SCABIES

Scabies is an endemic infestation produced by the scabies mite, *Sarcoptes scabiei.* The lesions are created as the impregnated female burrows into the stratum corneum of the epidermis (never into living tissue) to bury her eggs. The inflammatory response and itching occur after the host becomes sensitized to the mite, approximately 30 to 60 days following initial contact. After this time, anywhere the mite has traveled will begin to itch and develop the characteristic eruption (Box 50-1). Consequently, mites will not necessarily be located at all sites of eruption. The picture is often confusing in infants, who often develop an eczematous eruption; therefore the observer must look for discrete papules, burrows, or vesicles.

Nursing Care Management

The treatment of scabies is the application of a scabicide, such as 1% lindane (Kwell, Scavene) in a vanishing cream base. However, crotamiton (Eurax) or permethrin 5% cream (Elimite) is often used to avoid the risk of neurotoxicity from lindane (Taplin et al, 1990). Nurses instructing families in the use of the scabicide should emphasize the importance of following the directions accurately. Lindane is applied to cool, dry skin—not following a hot bath—and left on for the recommended time, usually 4 hours for infants and 6 hours for older children and adults. Permethrin is applied for 8 to 14 hours. One liberal application is sufficient, but all persons in the family (including baby-sitters and others who have close contact with the child) should be treated. Families need to know that although the mite will be killed, the rash and the itch will not be eliminated until the stratum corneum is replaced, which takes approximately 2 to 3 weeks. Soothing ointments or lotions can be applied for itching. Antibiotics may be given for secondary infection.

*Distributed by Corsa, Ltd, Conshohocken, PA 19428.

BOX 50-1
Clinical Manifestations of Scabies

Lesion

Children—minute grayish brown, threadlike (mite burrows), pruritic
Black dot at end of burrow (mite)
Infants—eczematous eruption, pruritic

Distribution

Generally in intertriginous areas—interdigital, axillary-cubital, popliteal, inguinal
Children over 2 years of age—primarily hands and wrists
Children younger than 2 years—primarily feet and ankles

PEDICULOSIS CAPITIS

Pediculosis capitis (head lice, or "cooties") is an infestation of the scalp by *Pediculus humanus capitis,* a very common parasite, especially in school-age children. The adult louse lives only about 48 hours when away from a human host, and the life span of the average female is 1 month. The female lays eggs at the junction of a hair shaft and close to the skin because they need a warm environment. The **nits,** or eggs hatch in approximately 7 to 10 days; the egg is thus about 4 mm (1/4 inch) from the scalp (but may be farther) at the time of hatching.

Diagnostic Evaluation

Diagnosis is made by observation of the white eggs (nits) firmly attached to the base of the hair shafts (Box 50-2). Because of their brief life span and mobility, adult lice are more difficult to locate. Nits must be differentiated from dandruff, lint, hair spray, and other items of similar size and shape. Scratch marks and/or inflammatory papules, caused by secondary infection, may also be found on the scalp in the vulnerable areas.

Therapeutic Management

Treatment consists of the application of pediculocides and manual removal of nit cases. A number of effective products are available. Permethrin 1% creme rinse (Nix) kills both lice and nits after one application. This product and preparations of pyrethrin with piperonyl butoxide (RID or A-200 pyrinate) can be obtained without a prescription and are more effective and safer than lindane. In fact, in a study comparing these pediculicides and other products, as well as their nit-removal combs, Nix (and its comb) was found to be the most effective product (Clore and Longyear, 1993).

Nursing Care Management

Nurses should be aware of several things to successfully manage or assist parents in coping with pediculosis. It should be emphasized that *anyone* can get pediculosis; it has no respect for age, socioeconomic level, or cleanliness. The louse does not jump or fly, but it can be transmitted from one person to another on personal items. Therefore children are cautioned against sharing combs, hats, caps, scarves, coats, and other items used on or near the hair. Children who share lockers are more likely to contract an infestation, and slumbar parties place children at risk. Lice are not carried or transmitted by pets.

BOX 50-2
Clinical Manifestations of Pediculosis

Pruritus (caused by crawling insect and insect saliva on skin)
Nits observable on hair shaft (Fig. 50-8)

Distribution

Occipital area
Behind ears
Nape of neck
Eyebrows and eyelashes (occasionally) (caused by pubic lice)

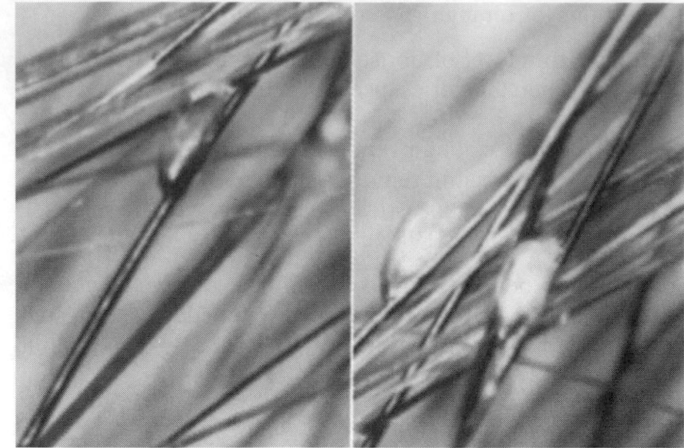

Fig. 50-8 **A,** Empty nit case. **B,** Viable nits. (From *The contemporary approach to the control of head lice in schools and communities,* Pittsburgh, 1991, SmithKline Beecham.)

When a child scratches the head more than usual, nurses or parents should carefully inspect the head for bite marks, redness, and nits. The hair is systematically spread with two flat-sided sticks or tongue depressors, and the scalp observed for any movement that indicates a louse. Nurses should wear gloves when examining the hair. Lice are small and grayish tan, have no wings, and are visible to the naked eye. The nits, or eggs, appear as tiny whitish oval specks adhering to the hair shaft about 4 mm from the scalp. The adherent nature of the nits distinguishes them from dandruff, which falls off readily. *Empty nit cases,* indicating hatched lice, are translucent rather than white and are located more than 4 mm from the scalp (Fig. 50-8).

If evidence of infestation is found, it is important to perform the treatment according to the directions described on the label of the pediculicide. Parents are advised to read the directions carefully before beginning treatment. Instructions on the labels indicate that dead lice and remaining nits are removed with an extra-fine–toothed comb. Most preparations include a comb to dislodge the firmly adhered nits. A commercial product of formic acid solution (Step 2 or Clear) may be used to loosen attached nits for removal. However, if the comb is ineffective in removing the nit cases, they must be removed with tweezers or between the fingernails.

The child is made as comfortable as possible during the application process because the pediculicide must remain on the scalp and hair for several minutes. If eye irritation occurs, the eyes must be flushed with tepid water.

Live lice survive for up to 48 hours away from the host, but nits are shed into the environment and are capable of hatching in 7 to 10 days. Therefore measures must be taken to prevent further infestation (see the Home Care box to the right). Spraying with insecticide is not recommended because of the danger to children and animals. Families also are advised that the pediculicide is relatively costly, especially when several members of the household require treatment.

The psychologic effects of lice infestations can be highly stressful to children. They are influenced by the reactions of others, including their parents, and may be made to feel ashamed or guilty. Parents are strongly cautioned against cutting a child's hair or, worse, shaving a child's head. Lice infest short hair as readily as long hair, and these actions only compound the child's distress and serve as a continual reminder to peers, who are always ready to taunt another with something out of the ordinary.

Home Care

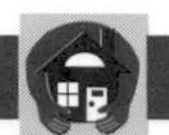

PREVENTING THE SPREAD AND RECURRENCE OF PEDICULOSIS

Machine wash all washable clothing, towels, and bed linens in hot water and dry in a hot dryer for at least 20 minutes. Dry-clean nonwashable items.
Thoroughly vacuum carpets, car seats, pillows, stuffed animals, rugs, mattresses, and upholstered furniture.
Seal nonwashable items in plastic bags for 14 days if unable to dry-clean or vacuum.
Soak combs, brushes, and hair accessories in lice-killing products for 1 hour or in boiling water for 10 minutes.

From Clore ER: Dispelling the common myths about pediculosis, *J Pediatr Health Care* 3:28-33, 1989.

Prevention. The increasing incidence of pediculosis in schoolchildren has become a serious concern for school nurses, parents, and community health agencies. School nurses are usually on the coordinate school-community prevention control programs for pediculosis. The National Pediculosis Association* offers education and advocates a "no nits" policy for treated children's reentry to school.

ARTHROPOD BITES AND STINGS

Bites and stings account for a significant incidence of mild to moderate discomfort, and most are managed by simple symptomatic measures, such as compresses, calamine lotion, and prevention of secondary infection.

Arthropods include insects and arachnids, such as mites, ticks, spiders, and scorpions. The major offending creatures, their manifestations, and management are outlined in Table 50-7.

When an insect stings, its stinger often remains embedded in the skin. For example, bees have barbed stingers that penetrate the skin, and any pressure on the venom sac at the tip of

*P.O. Box 149, Newton, MA 02161; (617) 449-6487 or (800) 446-4NPA.

TABLE 50-7 Skin lesions caused by arthropods

MECHANISM/CHARACTERISTICS	MANIFESTATIONS	MANAGEMENT
Insect bites—flies, gnats, mosquitoes, fleas		
Mechanism: Foreign protein in insects' saliva introduced when skin penetrated for a blood-sucking meal Distribution: Almost everywhere—fleas, mosquitoes, ants Suburbs and rural areas—bees Urban areas—hornets, wasps, yellow jackets	Hypersensitivity reaction Papular urticaria Firm papules; may be capped by vesicles or excoriated Little or no reaction in nonsensitized person	Treatment: Use antipruritic agents and baths Administer antihistamines Prevent secondary infection Prevention: Avoid contact Remove focus, such as treating furniture, mattresses, carpets, and pets, where insects may live Apply insect repellent when exposure is anticipated
Chiggers—harvest mite		
Mechanism: Creeps into skin pores and hair follicles to feed Manifestations: Erythematous papules Intense itching	Same as insect bites Favor warm areas of body, especially in tertriginous areas and areas covered with clothing	Avoid contact, especially in areas of tall grass and underbrush Apply insect repellant when exposure is anticipated May require systemic steroids for extensive bites
Hymenopteran stings—bees, wasps, hornets, yellow jackets, fire ants		
Mechanism: Injection of venom through stinging apparatus Venon contains histamine, allergenic proteins, and often a spreading factor, hyaluronidase Severe reactions caused by hypersensitivity and/or multiple stings	Local reaction: small red area, wheal, itching, and heat Systemic reactions: may be mild to severe, including generalized edema, pain, nausea and vomiting, confusion, respiratory embarrassment, and shock	Treatment: Carefully scrape off stinger if present Cleanse with soap and water Apply cool compresses Apply common household product (e.g., lemon juice, paste made with aspirin, baking soda, or Adolph's Meat Tenderizer) Administer antihistamines Severe reactions: administer epinephrine, corticosteroids; treat for shock Prevention: Teach child to wear shoes, to avoid wearing bright clothing, flowery prints, shiny jewelry, or perfumed grooming products (cologne, scented hairspray) that might attract the insect, and to avoid places where the insect may be contacted Hypersensitive children should wear identifying tag to indicate allergy and therapy needed; family should keep emergency medication and be taught its administration
Black widow spider		
Mechanism: Venom injected through a clawlike appendage; has neurotoxic action Characteristics: Spider is shiny black, with a body about 1.25 cm (0.5 inches) long and a red or orange hourglass-shaped marking on underside Avoids light and bites in self-defense	Mild sting at time of bite Area becomes swollen, painful, and erythematous Dizziness, weakness, and abdominal pain May produce delirium, paralysis, convulsions, and (if large amount of venom absorbed) death	Treatment: Cleanse wound with antiseptic Apply cool compresses Administer antivenin Administer muscle relaxant, such as calcium gluconate; analgesics and/or sedatives; hydrocortisone or diazepam IV Prevention: Teach children to avoid places that harbor the spider (e.g., woodpiles)

Continued.

TABLE 50-7 Skin lesions caused by arthropods—cont'd

MECHANISM/CHARACTERISTICS	MANIFESTATIONS	MANAGEMENT
Brown recluse spider		
Mechanism: Venom injected via fangs Venom contains powerful necrotoxin Characteristics: Spider is slender, long-legged, with body length of 1 to 2 cm; color is fawn to dark brown and recognized by fiddle-shaped mark on head Shy; bites only when annoyed or surprised Prefers dark areas where seldom disturbed	Mild sting at time of bite Transient erythema followed by bleb or blister; mild to severe pain in 2 to 8 hours; purple, star-shaped area in 3 to 4 days; necrotic ulceration in 7 to 14 days (Fig. 50-9) Systemic reactions may include fever, malaise, restlessness, nausea and vomiting, and joint pain Generalized petechial eruption Wounds heal with scar formation	Treatment: Apply cool compresses locally Administer antibiotics, corticosteroids Relieve pain Wound may require skin graft Prevention: Teach children to avoid possible nesting sites

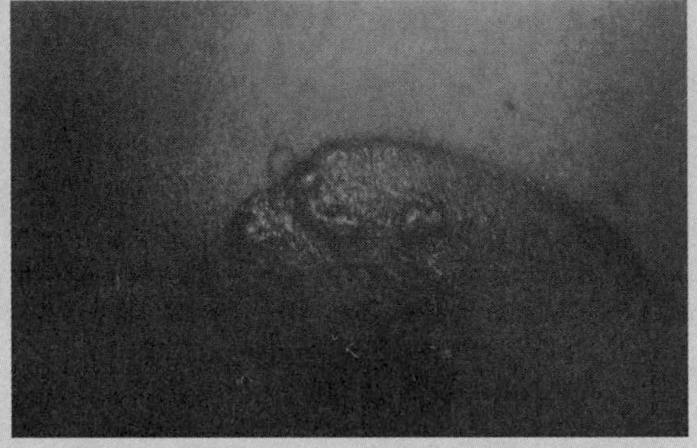

Fig. 50-9 Brown recluse spider bite. Note central necrosis surrounded by purplish areas and blisters. (From Weston WL, Lane AT: *Color textbook of pediatric dermatology*, St Louis, 1991, Mosby.)

MECHANISM/CHARACTERISTICS	MANIFESTATIONS	MANAGEMENT
Scorpions		
Mechanism: Sting by means of a hooked caudal stinger that discharges venom Venom of more venomous species contains hemolysins, endotheliolysins, and neurotoxins Characteristics: Usual habitat is southwestern United States	Intense local pain, erythema, numbness, burning, restlessness, vomiting Ascending motor paralysis with convulsions, weakness, rapid pulse, excessive salivation, thirst, dysuria, pulmonary edema, coma, and death Some species produce only local tissue reaction with swelling at puncture site (distinctive) Symptoms subside in a few hours Deaths occur among children under 4 years of age, usually in first 24 hours	Treatment: Delay absorption of venom by keeping child quiet; place involved area in dependent position Administer antivenin Relieve pain Admit to pediatric intensive care unit for surveillance Prevention: Teach children to avoid possible nesting sites
Ticks		
Mechanism: In process of sucking blood, head and mouth parts are buried in skin Characteristics: Feed on blood of mammals Significant in humans because of pathologic organism carried May be vectors of various infectious diseases, such as Rocky Mountain spotted fever, Q fever, tularemia, relapsing fever, Lyme disease, tick paralysis Must attach and feed 1 to 2 hours to transmit disease Usual habitat is very wooded area	Tick usually attached to skin, head embedded Produce firm, discrete, intensely pruritic nodules at site of attachment May cause urticaria or persistent localized edema	Treatment: Grasp tick with tweezers (forceps) as close as possible to point of attachment Pull straight up with steady, even pressure; if bare hands touch tick during removal, wash hands thoroughly with soap and water Remove any remaining part (e.g., head) with sterile needle Cleanse wounds with soap and disinfectant Prevention: Teach children to avoid areas where prevalent Inspect skin (especially scalp) after being in wooded areas

the barb pushes more venom into the skin. Children who have become sensitized to hymenopteran bites may demonstrate a severe systemic response that can be life-threatening. One sting can produce generalized urticaria, respiratory difficulty (from laryngeal edema), hypotension, and death within 1 hour. Intramuscular administration of epinephrine provides immediate relief and must be available for emergency use.

For hypertensive children a kit must be available that contains epinephrine and a hypodermic syringe; they also should wear a medical identification device. Families are reminded to check the expiration date on the kit and to replace an outdated one. They should determine if a nurse is available at the school and the school policy regarding administration of drugs. If a school nurse is not present, someone at the school should be designated to inject the epinephrine in case of an emergency.

Most arthropods in the United States are relatively harmless, including tarantulas. Although all spiders produce venom that is injected via fangs, some species are unable to pierce the skin; others produce a venom that is insufficiently toxic to be harmful. Only scorpions and two species of spiders—the brown recluse and the black widow—inject venom deadly enough to require immediate attention. Children bitten by these arachnids must receive medical attention as soon as possible.

INFECTIONS TRANSMITTED BY ARTHROPODS

The organisms responsible for a number of disorders are transmitted to human beings via arthropods (Table 50-8). Rickettsiae are intracellular parasites, similar in size to bacteria, that inhabit the alimentary tract of a wide range of natural hosts. Mammals become infected only through the bites of infected lice, fleas, ticks, and mites, all of which serve as both infectors and reservoirs. Rickettsial diseases are more common in temperate and tropical climates and in areas where humans live in association with arthropods. Infection in humans is incidental (except epidemic typhus) and not necessary for the survival of the rickettsial species. However, once the organism invades a human, it causes a disease that varies in intensity from a benign, self-limiting illness to a fulminating and frequently fatal one.

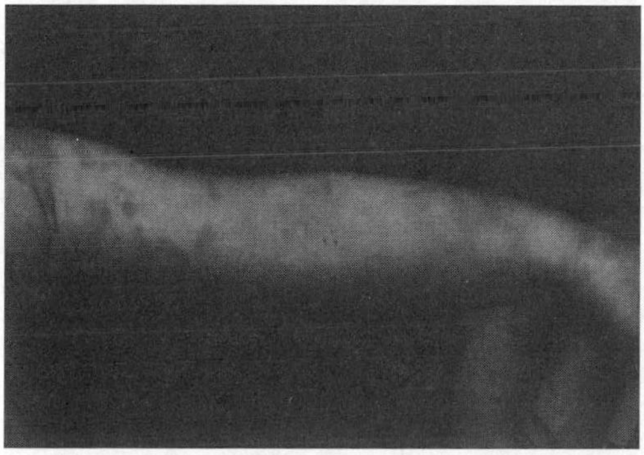

Fig. 50-10 Lyme disease. Note annular red rings in erythema chronicum migrans. (From Weston WL, Lane AT: *Color textbook of pediatric dermatology*, St Louis, 1991, Mosby.)

Lyme disease is a relatively recently recognized disorder caused by a spirochete transmitted by ticks. The disease may first be seen in any of three stages: (1) the tick bite at the time of inoculation, followed in 3 to 32 days by the development of *erythema chronicum migrans (ECH)* at the site of the bite (Fig. 50-10); (2) the most serious stage of the disease—involvement of the neurologic, cardiac, and musculoskeletal systems that appears several weeks after the cutaneous phase is completed; and (3) musculoskeletal pains involving the tendons, bursae, muscles, and synovia may develop. Arthritis may occur; late neurologic problems may include deafness and chronic encephalopathy.

ANIMAL BITES

Contrary to accepted belief, children are bitten more often by animals belonging to the family or to neighbors than by stray animals. Over half of the victims of dog bites are younger than 4 years of age. Boys are bitten more often than girls. Most dog or cat injuries are to the upper extremities. However, small children are more likely to be bitten or scratched on the head, face, and neck because they tend to put their heads near the animal's head and to flail their arms rather than protecting their heads. The injuries vary from small puncture wounds to complete evulsion of tissue and can be associated with significant crush injury.

Therapeutic Management

General wound care consists of rinsing the wound with large amounts of saline or Ringer's lactate solution under pressure (syringe) and washing the surrounding skin with mild soap. A clean pressure dressing is applied, and the extremity is elevated if the wound is bleeding. Medical evaluation is advised, since there is danger of tetanus and rabies, although dogs in most urban areas are required to be immunized against rabies. Bites from wild animals, such as squirrels, bats, and raccoons, are potentially dangerous.

Prophylactic antibiotics are indicated for puncture wounds and wounds in areas that may prove to be cosmetically or functionally impaired if infected. Extensive lacerations are debrided and loosely sutured. Tetanus toxoid is administered according to standard guidelines (see Immunizations, Chapter 33), and rabies protocol is followed (see the discussion of rabies, Chapter 48). Cat bites become infected more easily than dog bites but no more so than lacerations from other causes. Injuries to poorly vascularized areas such as the hands are more likely to become infected than those in more vascularized areas such as the face; puncture wounds are more apt to become infected than lacerations.

Nursing Care Management

The most important aspect related to animal bites is prevention. Children should understand animal behavior and develop a respect for animals. Parents should monitor their children's behavior with a dog and instruct them not to tease or surprise a dog, invade its territory, interfere with its feeding or sleeping, take its toy, or interact with a sick or injured dog or a dog with pups (Riegger and Guntzelman, 1990). Parents who are contemplating getting a pet, especially a dog, for themselves or their children should receive some advice about the dog that is least likely to be a danger to their children. A categorization of dogs related to their potential interaction

TABLE 50-8 Disorders transmitted by arthropods

DISORDER/ORGANISM/HOST	MANIFESTATIONS	MANAGEMENT	COMMENTS
Rocky Mountain spotted fever—*Rickettsia rickettsii* Arthropod: tick Transmission: tick bite Mammal source: wild rodents; dogs	Gradual onset: fever, malaise, anorexia, myalgia Abrupt onset: rapid temperature elevation, chills, vomiting, myalgia, severe headache Maculopapular or petechial rash primarily on extremities (ankles and wrists) but may spread to other areas, characteristically to palms and soles	Control: protection from tick bite by proper wearing apparel, tick repellent Treatment: Tetracycline or chloramphenicol Vigorous supportive therapy	Usually self-limited in children Onset in children may resemble any infectious disease Severe disease rare in children Children and dogs should be inspected regularly if they play in wooded areas See Table 50-7 for management of ticks
Epidemic typhus—*R. prowazekii* Arthropod: body louse Transmission: infected feces into broken skin Mammal source: humans	Abrupt onset of chills, fever, diffuse myalgia, headache, malaise Maculopapular rash becomes petechial 4 to 7 days later, spreading from trunk outward	Control: immediate destruction of vectors Treatment: Tetracycline or chloramphenicol Supportive	Patient should be isolated until deloused See discussion on p. 1673 for management of pediculosis Excreta from infected lice also in dust—disinfect patient's clothing, bedding, and possessions and wash in hot water
Endemic typhus—*R. typhi* Arthropod: rat fleas or body lice Transmission: flea bite; inhaling or ingesting flea excreta Mammal source: rats	Headache, arthralgia, backache followed by fever; may last 9 to 14 days Maculopapular rash after 1 to 8 days of fever; begins in trunk and spreads to periphery; rarely involves face, palms, soles	Control: eliminate rat reservoir, insect vectors, or both Treatment: Tetracycline or chloramphenicol Supportive	Fairly common in United States Shorter duration than epidemic typhus Mild, seldom fatal illness Difficult to distinguish from epidemic typhus
Rickettsialpox—*R. akari* Arthropod: mouse mite Transmission: mite Mammal source: house mouse	Maculopapular rash following primary lesion; eschar at site of bite, fever, chills, headache	Control: eradication of rodent reservoir and mite vector Treatment: Tetracycline or chloramphenicol Supportive	Self-limited nonfatal disease Endemic in New York City Found in many cities in United States
Lyme disease—spirochete *Borrelia burgdorferi* Arthropod: tick Transmission: tick bite Mammal source: rodents, deer	Stage 1: tick bite Stage 2: erythema chronicum migrans; papule at bite site progresses to large circumferential ring with a raised edematous doughnut-like border (see Fig. 50-10) Stage 3: systemic involvement —cardiac, neurologic, musculoskeletal	Control: protection from tick bite by proper wearing apparel, tick repellent Treatment: Tetracycline or penicillin Supportive	Regional distribution: Northeast (Massachusetts, Connecticut, Rhode Island, New York, New Jersey, Pennsylvania, Maryland); Midwest (Wisconsin, Minnesota); West (California, Oregon), but becoming more widespread

with children can be found in the publication *The Right Dog for You.**

HUMAN BITES

Children often acquire lacerations from the teeth of other humans in rough play, during fights, or as victims of child abuse. Many preschool children bite others out of frustration or anger. Because human dental plaque and gingiva harbor pathogenic organisms, all human bites should receive attention.

If the laceration is less than 4 mm in length, the wound can be treated at home. The wound is washed thoroughly with soap and water, and a pressure dressing is applied to stop bleeding. Ice applications minimize discomfort and swelling. Increased pain or redness at the wound site is an indication that the child should receive medical attention for antibiotic

*Tortora DF: *The right dog for you,* New York, 1983, Simon & Schuster.

therapy. Tetanus toxoid is needed if the child is insufficiently immunized. Larger wounds should receive medical attention.

CAT SCRATCH DISEASE (CSD)

CSD is described as a subacute regional adenitis that follows the scratch or bite of an animal, especially a cat (99% of cases). The disease is usually a benign, self-limiting illness that resolves spontaneously in about 2 to 4 months. The diagnosis is made on the basis of three of the following: (1) contact (usually a kitten) and regional inoculation lesion, (2) lymphadenopathy, (3) a positive CSD skin test, and (4) biopsy of lymph node with histopathology compatible with CSD (Margileth and Hadfield, 1990). The disease may persist for several months before gradual resolution. In some children, especially those who are immunocompromised, the adenitis may progress to suppuration and serious complications. Treatment is primarily supportive.

Miscellaneous Skin Disorders

A number of skin lesions are caused by extrinsic or intrinsic factors. Some of these are listed in Table 50-9. There are a number of congenital skin disorders, usually inherited as an autosomal-dominant trait. *Ichthyoses* are a heterogenous group of disorders characterized by scaling that create a challenging problem in treatment. These disorders are not discussed in detail because of their wide variability.

Skin Disorders Associated with Specific Age Groups

Several common and important dermatologic conditions are confined primarily to children in specific age groups. These conditions include atopic, seborrheic, and diaper dermatitis and the acne of adolescence. The treatment modalities include those previously described. However, some special needs and therapies are involved with these disorders.

DIAPER DERMATITIS

Diaper dermatitis, one of the most common dermatoses in infants, is one of several acute inflammatory skin disorders caused either directly or indirectly by the wearing of diapers. The peak age of occurrence is 9 to 12 months of age, and the incidence is generally reported as greater in bottle-fed infants than in breast-fed infants.

Pathophysiology and Clinical Manifestations

Diaper dermatitis is caused by prolonged and repetitive contact with an irritant, principally urine, feces, soaps, detergents, ointments, and friction. Although the obvious irritant in the majority of incidences is urine and feces, the specific components that contribute to irritation include a combination of factors.

Prolonged contact of the skin with diaper wetness affects several skin properties. It produces higher friction, greater abrasion damage, increased transepidermal permeability, and increased microbial counts. Therefore healthy skin becomes less resistant to potential irritants.

Although ammonia was once thought to cause diaper rash because of the association between the strong odor on diapers and dermatitis, ammonia alone is not sufficient. The important function of urine is related to an increase in pH from the breakdown of urea in the presence of fetal urease. The increased pH promotes the activity of fecal enzymes, principally proteases and lipases, which act as irritants. Fecal enzymes also increase the permeability of skin to bile salts, another potential irritant in feces.

The eruption of diaper dermatitis can be manifested primarily on convex surfaces or in the folds, and the lesions can represent a variety of types and configurations. Eruptions involving the skin in most intimate contact with the diaper (e.g., the convex surfaces of buttocks, inner thighs, mons pubis, and scrotum) but sparing the fold are likely to be caused by chemical irritants, especially from urine and feces (Fig. 50-11). Other causes are detergents or soaps from inadequately rinsed cloth diapers or the fragrance added to some diapers or

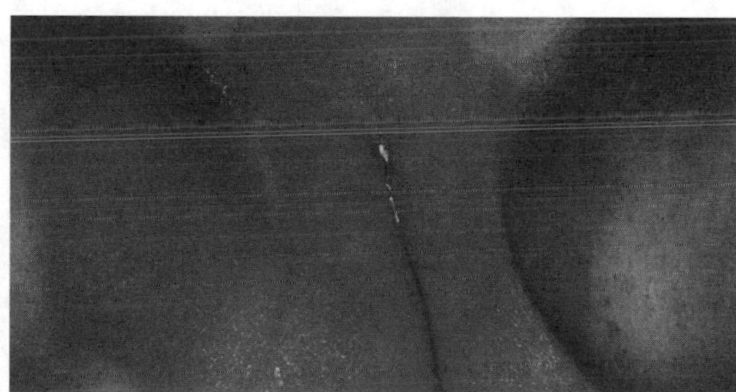

Fig. 50-11 Irritant diaper dermatitis. Note sharply demarcated edges. (From Habif TP: *Clinical dermatology: a color guide to diagnosis and therapy*, ed 2, St Louis, 1990, Mosby.)

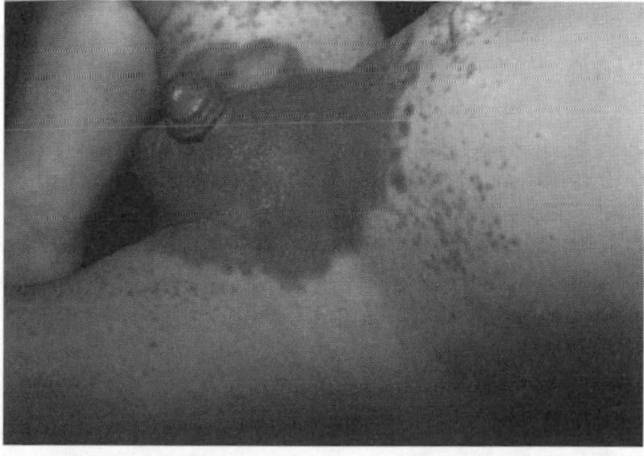

Fig. 50-12 Candidiasis of diaper area. Note beefy-red central erythema with satellite pustules. (From Weston WL, Lane AT: *Color textbook of pediatric dermatology*, St Louis, 1991, Mosby.)

TABLE 50-9 Miscellaneous skin disorders

DISEASE/CAUSATIVE AGENT	LOCAL MANIFESTATIONS	MANAGEMENT	COMMENTS
Urticaria—usually allergic response to drugs or infection	Development of wheals Vary in size and configuration and tend to appear quickly, spread irregularly, and fade within a few hours May be constant or intermittent, sparse or profuse, small or large, discrete or confluent May be acute, chronic, or recurrent in acute attacks	Local soothing and antipruritic applications Antihistamines Epinephrine or ephedrine Cortisone or corticotropin (ACTH) in severe cases Severe upper respiratory involvement may require tracheostomy	Known etiology agents should be avoided May be accompanied by malaise, fever, lymphadenopathy Severe cases may involve mucous membranes, internal organs, and joints Obstruction to air passages constitutes medical emergency (see Chapter 45)
Intertrigo—mechanical trauma and aggravating factors of excessive heat, moisture, and sweat retention	Red, inflamed, moist, partially denuded, marginated areas, the shape of which is determined by location Appears where opposing skin surfaces rub together, such as intergluteal folds, groin, neck, and axilla Excessive moisture and obesity are often factors	Affected areas kept clean and dry Skin folds kept separated with a generous supply of nonmedicated powder Expose to air and light Remove excess clothing	A form of diaper irritation Prevent recurrence by keeping susceptible areas clean and dry Frequently associated with overheating from too much clothing
Psoriasis—unknown; hereditary predisposition; may be triggered by stress	Round, thick, dry, reddish patches covered with coarse, silvery scales over trunk and extremities; first lesions commonly appear in scalp; facial lesions more common in children than adults Affected cells proliferate at a much more rapid rate than normal cells	Exposure to sunlight, ultraviolet light Topical corticosteroids Tar derivatives Trihydroxyanthracine Keratolytic agents (salicylic acid) Psoralin—ultraviolet A (PUVA)* Emollients may provide relief	Uncommon in children under age 6 years Persons are otherwise healthy individuals Coal tar and psoralin act synergistically with ultraviolet light Keratolytic agents enhance absorption of corticosteroids Humidifiers may help in winter
Alopecia			
Alopecia areata	Sudden onset of asymptomatic, noninflammatory, round, bald patches in hairy parts of body	Psychologic support Inducement of allergic contact dermatitis to stimulate growth of hair Minoxidil (peripheral vasodilator)	Family history in 10% to 26% of cases Some concern regarding drug therapy safety Refer to support groups†
Traumatic alopecia	Traction alopecia around scalp margins from tight hair styles (e.g., braids, pony tails, corn rows)	Counseling regarding hair styling, use of hair cosmetics, hot combs, rollers	More prevalent in black children and adolescents Prolonged traction can produce fibrosis of hair root and permanent loss
Trichotillomania	Compulsive hair pulling	Determine and treat cause	Chronic hair pulling may require psychologic therapy
Tinea capitis	See Table 50-5	See Table 50-5	See Table 50-5

*Still considered investigational.
†*National Alopecia Areata Foundation*, 710 C St, Suite 11, San Rafael CA 94901; (415) 456-4644.

TABLE 50-9 Miscellaneous skin disorders—cont'd

DISEASE/CAUSATIVE AGENT	LOCAL MANIFESTATIONS	MANAGEMENT	COMMENTS
Erythema multiforme (Stevens-Johnson syndrome)—unknown; associated with ingestion of some drugs; often follows upper respiratory infection	Erythematous papular rash Lesions enlarge by peripheral expansion; develop central vesicle Involves most skin surfaces except scalp May extend to mucous membranes, especially oral, ocular, and urethral	Symptomatic and supportive Maintain adequate fluid intake (oral or IV), calorie, and protein Cutaneous hygiene Appropriate treatment of complications Diligent monitoring of urine volume and specific gravity, hemoglobin and hematocrit, serum electrolyte levels, total body weight	Rash often preceded by fever and malaise Complications include renal failure and severe eye disease Respiratory involvement in a number of cases Self-limiting, but recovery may extend for weeks; skin lesions subside without scarring; mucous membrane lesions may persist for months Recurrence rate 20%; mortality as high as 10%
Neurofibromatosis—inherited disorder	Café-au-lait spots, pigmented nevi, axillary freckling Slow-growing cutaneous and subcutaneous neurofibromas	Symptomatic treatment of associated manifestations (e.g., speech defects, seizures, skeletal defects such as scoliosis, kyphosis), learning disabilities Surgical removal of troublesome tumors	Autosomal-dominant inheritance pattern High mutation rate Refer to support groups‡

‡*National Neurofibromatosis Foundation, Inc.*, 95 Pine St., 16th Floor, New York, NY 10005; (800) 323-7938, (212) 460-8980.

disposable wipes. Perianal involvement is usually the result of chemical irritation from feces, especially diarrheal stools. *Candida albicans* infection produces perianal inflammation with satellite lesions (Fig. 50-12).

Nursing Care Management

Nursing interventions are aimed at altering the three factors considered to produce dermatitis—wetness, pH, and fecal irritants. The most significant factor amenable to intervention is the moist environment created in the diaper area. Changing the diaper as soon as it becomes wet eliminates a large part of the problem, and removing the diaper to expose healthy skin to air facilitates drying.

Nursing ALERT

A heat lamp, hairdryer, or source of oxygen is not used on very reddened or denuded skin because these interventions dry the skin and retard healing. Instead, occlusive ointments are applied to provide a moist healing environment.

Diaper construction has a significant impact on the incidence and severity of diaper dermatitis. Superabsorbent disposable paper diapers have been shown to reduce diaper dermatitis. They contain an absorbent gelling material. The gel binds water tightly to decrease skin wetness, maintains pH control by providing a buffering capacity, and decreases skin irritation by preventing mixing of urine and feces in the diaper (Wong et al, 1992).

Home Care 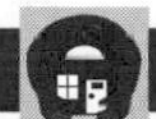

CONTROLLING DIAPER RASH

Keep skin dry
- Use superabsorbent disposable diapers to reduce skin wetness
- If using cloth diapers, use only overwraps that allow air to circulate; avoid rubber pants.
- Change diapers as soon as soiled, especially with stool, whenever possible, preferably once during the night.
- Expose healthy or only slightly irritated skin to air, not heat, to dry completely.

Apply ointment, such as zinc oxide or petrolatum, to protect skin, especially if skin is very red or has moist, open areas.
- When soiled, wipe off top layer of ointment and reapply.
- To completely remove ointment, especially zinc oxide, use mineral oil; do not wash vigorously.

Avoid overwashing the skin, especially with perfumed soaps or commercial wipes that may be irritating.
- May use a moisturizer or nonsoap cleanser, such as cold cream or Cetaphil, to wipe urine from skin.
- Gently wipe stool from skin using water and mild soap, such as Dove.

NOTE: Powder helps keep the skin dry, but talc is very dangerous if breathed into the lungs. Plain cornstarch or cornstarch-based powder is safer. When using any powder product, shake it first into your hand, then apply it to the diaper area. Store the container away from the infant's reach; keep container closed when not in use.

Guidelines for controlling diaper rash are presented in the Home Care box on p. 1681.* A common misconception about using cornstarch on skin is that it promotes the growth of *Candida albicans.* A study comparing cornstarch and talc found that neither product supports growth of the fungi under conditions normally found in the diaper area. Cornstarch is also more effective in reducing friction and tends to cake less than talc when the skin is wet (Leyden, 1984). On the basis of these properties and its safety in terms of inhalation injury, cornstarch is the preferred product.

*Pamphlets describing the development and treatment of diaper rash are *Diaper Rash* from the American Academy of Pediatrics, 141 Northwest Point Blvd., P.O. Box 927, Elk Grove Village, IL 60007, (800) 433-9016; and *An Information Guide for Parents About Diaper Rash* from NAP-NAP Diaper Rash Brochure, 718 Main St., Cincinnati, OH 45202-2137.

ATOPIC DERMATITIS (AD) (ECZEMA)

Eczema or eczematous inflammation of the skin refers to a descriptive category of dermatologic diseases and not to a specific etiology. AD is a type of pruritic eczema that usually begins during infancy and is associated with allergy with a hereditary tendency **(atopy).** AD presents in three forms based on the age of the child and the distribution of lesions:

- **Infantile (infantile eczema)**—usually begins at 2 to 6 months of age and generally undergoes spontaneous remission by 3 years of age.
- **Childhood**—may follow the infantile form; it occurs at 2 to 3 years of age, and 90% of the children will manifest the disease by age 5 years.
- **Preadolescent and adolescent**—begins at about 12 years of age and may continue into the early adult years or indefinitely.

The diagnosis of AD is based on a combination of history and morphologic findings (Box 50-3). Children with the disease have a lower threshold for cutaneous itching, and many authorities believe the dermatologic manifestations appear subsequent to scratching of the intense pruritus. For example, infants will rub their faces against bed linen, and crawling (a form of scratching) results in irritation of knees and elbows. Lesions will disappear if the scratching is stopped.

The majority of children with infantile AD have a family history of eczema, asthma, or allergic rhinitis, which strongly supports a genetic predisposition. The cause is unknown but appears to be related to abnormal function of the skin, including alterations in sweating, peripheral vascular function, and heat tolerance. The symptoms are better in humid climates and worse in fall and winter, when homes are heated and environmental humidity is lower. The disorder can be controlled but not cured.

BOX 50-3 Clinical Manifestations of Atopic Dermatitis

Distribution of lesions

Infantile form—generalized, especially cheeks, scalp, trunk and extensor surfaces of extremities (Fig. 50-13)

Childhood form—flexural areas (antecubital and popliteal fossae, neck), wrists, ankles, and feet

Preadolescent and adolescent form—face, sides of neck, hands, feet, face, and antecubital and popliteal fossae (to a lesser extent)

Appearance of lesions

Infantile form
- Erythema
- Vesicles
- Papules
- Weeping
- Oozing
- Crusting
- Scaling
- Often symmetric

Childhood form
- Symmetric involvement
- Clusters of small erythematous or flesh-colored papules or minimally scaling patches
- Dry and may be hyperpigmented
- Lichenification (thickened skin with accentuation of creases)
- Keratosis pilaris (follicular hyperkeratosis) common

Adolescent/adult form
- Same as childhood manifestations
- Dry, thick lesions (lichenified plaques) common
- Confluent papules

Other physical manifestations

Intense itching
Unaffected skin dry and rough
African-American children likely to exhibit more papular and/or follicular lesions than white children
May exhibit one or more of the following:
Lymphadenopathy, especially near affected sites
Increased palmar creases (many cases)
Atopic pleats (extra line or groove of the lower eyelid)
Prone to cold hands
Pityriasis alba (small, poorly defined areas of hypopigmentation)
Facial pallor (especially around nose, mouth, and ears)
Bluish discoloration beneath eyes ("allergic shiners")
Increased susceptibility to unusual cutaneous infections (especially viral)

Therapeutic Management

The major goals of management are to (1) relieve pruritus, (2) hydrate the skin, (3) reduce inflammation, and (4) prevent or

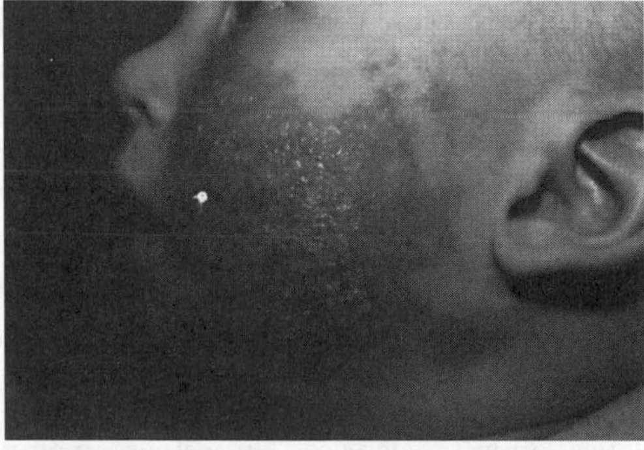

Fig. 50-13 Infantile atopic dermatitis with oozing and crusting of lesions. (From Weston WL, Lane AT: *Color textbook of pediatric dermatology*, St Louis, 1991, Mosby.)

control secondary infection. Most of the general measures for managing AD serve to reduce pruritus as well as other aspects of the disease. General management includes avoiding exposure to skin irritants, avoiding overheating, improving skin hydration, and administration of medications such as antihistamines, topical steroids, and (sometimes) mild sedatives as indicated.

Differing philosophies regarding cleansing and hydrating the skin of the child with AD generally embrace two methods—the wet and the dry methods. In the *dry method,* baths are infrequent and skin is cleansed with a nonlipid, hydrophilic agent such as Cetaphil. The *wet method* consists of frequent baths (up to four times per day) followed immediately by the application of a lubricant (while the skin is still damp) to trap moisture in the skin. No soap or a very mild, nonperfumed soap (such as Dove, Lowila, or Neutrogena) is used. Some advocate oil or oilated oatmeal baths with light drying so that a protective, oily film remains on the skin. Showers are accepted as long as a moisturizer is applied within 3 minutes to prevent drying and damaging the skin (Hanifin, 1991).

Enhancing skin hydration can be accomplished by applying preparations that occlude the skin to prevent evaporation and retain moisture in the upper skin layers and/or by replacement of natural moisturizing substances in the skin. A variety of emollients containing petrolatum or lanolin have occlusive properties and are prescribed according to the degree of occlusion desired. For the majority of patients, lotions applied twice or three times daily maintain satisfactory hydration. The frequency may be increased if greater hydration is required. Creams or ointments provide more occlusion, and those that contain urea or lactic acid improve the binding of water in the skin and prevent evaporation of moisture.

Sometimes colloid baths, such as the addition of 2 cups of cornstarch to a tub of warm water, provide temporary relief of itching and may help the child sleep if given before bedtime. Cool wet compresses are soothing to the skin and provide antiseptic protection.

Moderate or severe pruritus is usually relieved by the administration of oral antihistamine drugs (hydroxyzine [Atarax] or diphenhydramine [Benadryl]); the amount is tailored to the individual child. Since pruritus increases at night, a mild sedative may be needed.

Occasional flare-ups require the use of topical steroids to diminish inflammation. Low-, moderate-, or high-potency topical corticosteroids are prescribed, depending on the degree of involvement, the area of the body to be treated, the age of the child, and the type of vehicle to be used (e.g., cream, lotion, ointment). Secondary infection is managed with appropriate antibiotic therapy.

The prevention of AD by limiting exposure of the fetus and child to allergens is controversial. However, the precautions in the Guidelines box to the left may be recommended.

Guidelines 

PREVENTING ATOPY IN CHILDREN

Identify children at risk

Family history of allergy
Increased IgE in cord blood and postnatal serum

Prenatal precautions (last trimester)

Avoid any known food allergens
Avoid milk and other dairy products, peanuts, and eggs
Minimize ingestion of other hyperallergenic foods

Postnatal precautions

Breast milk or casein/whey hydrolysate formula (e.g., Nutramigen, Pregestimil, Alimentum) exclusively for at least 6 months
No solid food for 6 months
No cow's milk or soy formula for 12 months
No egg, fish, corn, citrus, peanuts, nuts, or chocolate for 12 months
One new food added at 5-day intervals to identify possible reaction

Environmental control

Limited exposure to dust, molds, animals, and cigarette smoke

Data from Johnstone D: Strategy for intervention of food allergy in infants, *Int Pediatr* 4(4):319-325, 1989; and Zeiger R et al: Effectiveness of dietary manipulation in the prevention of food allergy in infants, part 2, *J Allergy Clin Immunol* 78(1, pt 2): 224-238, 1986.

Prognosis. The majority of affected children (90%) "outgrow" AD by adolescence. Some continue to have chronic AD in adulthood.

Nursing Care Management

Assessment

Assessment of the child with AD includes a family history for evidence of atopy, a history of previous involvement, and any environmental or dietary factors associated with the present and previous exacerbations. The skin lesions are examined for type, distribution, and evidence of secondary infection. The parents are interviewed regarding the child's behavior, especially in relation to the child's scratching, irritability, and sleeping patterns. The interview should also include exploration of the family's feelings and methods of coping with the situation.

Nursing Diagnoses

A number of nursing diagnoses identified for the child with AD are outlined in Box 50-4. Others will be apparent in individual cases.

Planning

The objectives for nursing care of the child with AD and the family are as follows:

1. The child will experience no or minimal pruritis.
2. The child will receive appropriate treatment for skin hydration.
3. The child will experience no complications.
4. The child and family will receive adequate support.

Implementation

The child with AD presents a nursing challenge. Controlling the intense pruritus is imperative if the disorder is to be successfully managed, since scratching leads to the formation of new lesions and may cause secondary infection. In addition to

BOX 50-4
Nursing Diagnoses: The Child with Atopic Dermatitis

Impaired skin integrity related to eczematous lesions
Risk for infection related to risk of secondary infection of primary lesions
Altered family processes related to child's discomfort and lengthy therapy

the medical regimen, other measures can be taken to prevent or minimize the scratching. Fingernails and toenails are cut short, kept clean, and filed frequently to prevent sharp edges. Gloves or cotton stockings may have to be placed over the hands and pinned to shirt-sleeves. To prevent any contact with the skin, elbow restraints are sometimes necessary. One-piece outfits with long sleeves and long pants also decrease direct contact with the skin. Whether gloves or restraints are used, the child needs time to be free from such restrictions. An excellent time to remove any protective devices is during the bath or after receiving sedative or antipruritic medication.

Nursing ALERT

Do not remove elbow restraints during sleep because of the likelihood that the child will scratch while asleep.

Conditions that increase itching are eliminated when possible. Woolen clothes or blankets, rough fabrics, and furry stuffed animals should be removed. Since heat and humidity cause perspiration, which intensifies the itching, proper dress for climatic conditions is essential. Pruritus is often precipitated by exposure to the irritant effects of certain components of common products such as soaps, detergents, fabric softeners, perfumes, and powders. Most children experience less itching when soft cotton fabrics are worn next to the skin. During cold months, synthetic fabrics (not wool) should be used for overcoats, hats, gloves, and snowsuits.

Clothes and sheets are laundered in a mild detergent and rinsed thoroughly in clear water (without fabric softeners and antistatic chemicals). Putting the clothes through a second complete wash cycle without using detergent reduces the amount of residue remaining in the fabric.

Preventing infection is usually secondary to preventing scratching. Personal hygiene is accomplished as described previously. Baths are given as prescribed, the water kept tepid, and soaps (except as indicated) and bubble baths are avoided, as well as the use of oils or powders. Skinfolds and diaper areas need frequent cleansing with plain water.

A room humidifier or vaporizer may benefit children with extremely dry skin.

Nursing ALERT

If the child is being treated with frequent baths for hydration, it is imperative that the emollient preparation be applied immediately following bathing (while the skin is still slightly moist) to prevent drying.

Soaks and compresses are applied, and medications for pruritus or infection are administered as directed. The family is given explicit instructions on the preparation and use of soaks, special baths, and topical medications, including the order of application if more than one is prescribed. If children have difficulty remaining still for a 10- or 15-minute soak, bath, or dressing application, these can be carried out at naptime or when the child is engrossed in television, a story, or playing with tub toys.

Since adequate rest is also important for these children, who are usually fretful and irritable, planning meals, baths, medications, and treatments during awake periods is paramount. Sleepy, tired children are normally cranky, and such behavior only intensifies the urge to scratch. During periods of irritability these children tend to have a poor appetite, which is worsened by restriction of their usual foods.

Diet modification is another source of frustration to parents. When a hypoallergenic diet is prescribed, parents need help in understanding the reason for the diet and guidelines for following it. Since hypoallergenic diets take time before visible effects are apparent, parents need reassurance that results may not be seen immediately.

Family support. Parents can be assured that the lesions will not produce scarring (unless secondarily infected) and that the disease is not contagious. However, the child will be subject to repeated exacerbations and remissions.

During periods of acute exacerbation the emotional stress can become intense for the family. They need time to discuss negative feelings and to be reassured that these feelings are normal and acceptable. During acute phases, relieving as much anxiety as possible in both parents and child has a beneficial emotional and physical effect, since stress tends to aggravate the severity of the condition.

Evaluation

The effectiveness of nursing interventions is determined by continual reassessment and evaluation of care based on the following observational guidelines and expected outcomes:

1. Observe child's behavior, clothing, and activities.
2. Examine skin for evidence of dryness.
3. Examine skin lesions for evidence of secondary infection.
4. Interview aspects of family and encourage dialogue regarding the child and aspects of care.

Expected outcomes:

1. Child does not scratch and rests or plays quietly.
2. Skin appears well hydrated.
3. There is no evidence of secondary infection.
4. Family members comply with the therapeutic regimen, freely discuss their feelings and concerns, and appear to be coping with the inconveniences imposed by the disorder (specify).

See also Nursing Care Plan: The Child with Atopic Dermatitis (Eczema).*

*In Wong DL: *Wong and Whaley's clinical manual of pediatric nursing*, ed 4, St Louis, 1996, Mosby.

SEBORRHEIC DERMATITIS

Seborrheic dermatitis is a chronic, recurrent, inflammatory reaction of the skin. It occurs most commonly on the scalp (cradle cap) but may involve the eyelids (blepharitis), external ear canal (otitis externa), nasolabial folds, and inguinal region. The cause is unknown, although it is more common in early infancy, when sebum production is increased. The lesions are characteristically thick, adherent, yellowish, scaly, oily patches that may or may not be mildly pruritic. Unlike atopic dermatitis, seborrheic dermatitis is not associated with a positive family history for allergy and is very common in infants shortly after birth and after puberty. Diagnosis is made primarily by the appearance and location of the crusts or scales.

Nursing Care Management

Cradle cap may be prevented with adequate scalp hygiene. Not infrequently, parents omit shampooing the infant's hair for fear of damaging the "soft spots," or fontanels. It is important to discuss how to shampoo the infant's hair and to emphasize that the fontanel is like skin anywhere else on the body—it does not puncture or tear with mild pressure.

When seborrheic lesions are present, the treatment is mainly directed at removing the crusts. Parents are taught the appropriate procedure to clean the scalp, which may require a demonstration. Shampooing should be done daily with a mild soap or commercial baby shampoo; medicated shampoos are not necessary, but an antiseborrheic shampoo containing sulfur and salicyclic acid may be used (Hurwitz, 1993). Shampoo is applied to the scalp and allowed to penetrate and soften the crusts, and then the scalp is thoroughly rinsed. Using a fine-toothed comb or a soft facial brush after shampooing helps remove the loosened crusts from the strands of hair.

ACNE

There is one skin disorder that, although not limited to the adolescent age group, appears predominantly at this time—*acne vulgaris.* Acne is an almost universal occurrence during these years and involves anatomic, physiologic, biochemical, genetic, immunologic, and psychologic factors of significant import.

It is estimated that about 85% of the population will have had acne by the end of the teenage years. Although the disorder can appear before this time, the peak incidence is in late adolescence, at about age 16 to 17 in girls and 17 to 18 years in boys. It is more common in males than in females. The degree to which an individual is affected may range from nothing more than a few isolated comedones to a severe inflammatory reaction. Although the disease is self-limited and not life-threatening, its significance to the adolescent is great, and it is a mistake to underestimate the impact it can have on young persons.

The etiology of acne is still unclear, although a number of factors appear to be related to its development. Its distribution in families and a high degree of concordance in identical twins suggest that hereditary factors predipose to susceptibility to acne. Androgens are implicated, and the disorder seems to be aggravated by emotional stress; a hot, humid environment; and the premenstrual period in families. There is no positive evidence that any specific foods are factors, except perhaps on an individual basis.

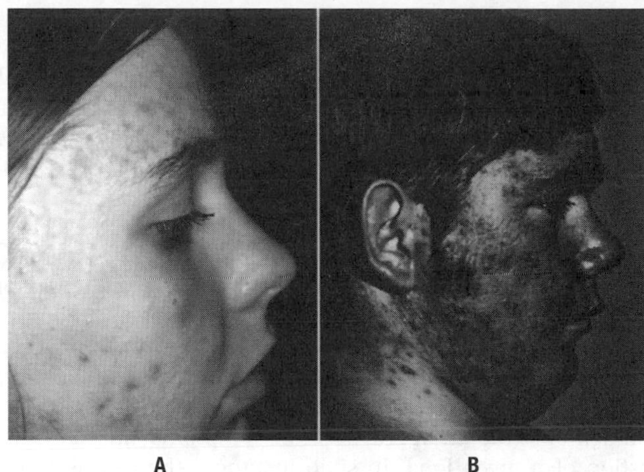

Fig. 50-14 Acne vulgaris. **A,** Comedones with a few inflammatory pustules. **B,** Papulopustular acne. (From Weston WL, Lane AT. *Color textbook of pediatric dermatology,* St Louis, 1991, Mosby.)

Pathophysiology

Acne is a disease that involves the *pilosebaceous follicles* (the hair follicle and sebaceous gland complex) of the face, neck, shoulders, back, and upper chest—the so-called flush areas of the skin. There are two basic types of lesions seen in acne (Fig. 50-14):

- *Noninflamed lesions,* called **comedones,** consisting of compact masses of keratin, lipids, fatty acids, and bacteria that dilate the follicular duct, which may be plugged (*closed comedones,* or whiteheads, with no visible opening) or open (*open comedones,* or blackheads, with visible dilated openings that are discolored as fatty acids are oxidized by air)
- *Inflamed lesions,* which result when the follicular wall ruptures to produce papules, pustules, nodules, and cysts; responsible for the destructiveness and propensity for scarring

A normally harmless bacterium, *Propionibacterium acnes (P. acnes),* is present in larger amounts in persons with acne. Polymorphonuclear leukocytes enter the sebaceous follicle to ingest the bacteria. Hydrolytic enzymes and free fatty acids are released as a by-product. These fatty acids are the major tissue irritants in the sebum and initiate the inflammatory process. Adolescents' concern about their appearance tempts them to pick, finger, squeeze, and otherwise manipulate the lesions; this plays an important role in the perpetuation of acne and possible secondary infection and scarring. In addition to the precipitating factors mentioned previously, the application of creams and oils including some suntanning and sunscreen preparations, and some heavy makeup bases that add to the plugging of the follicles may aggravate acne.

Therapeutic Management

There is little evidence that treatment shortens the duration of the entire course of the disease. However, treatment can bolster self-esteem and prevent unnecessary scarring. No single therapeutic agent is effective in the management of acne, except in a few mild cases. It is usually more effective to use a combination of therapies. The treatment most commonly consists of measures directed toward improving the general health of the person, removing comedones, preventing their formation, controlling excessive sebaceous gland activity, controlling infection, and preventing scar formation.

General measures. Improvement of the adolescent's overall health status is part of the general management. Adequate rest, moderate exercise, a well-balanced diet, reduction of emotional stress, and elimination of any foci of infection are all part of general health promotion. There is no convincing evidence to implicate any single dietary item or combination of foods in the exacerbation of acne. Occasionally a youngster will demonstrate an aggravation of symptoms after each ingestion of a given food. In such instances the food is eliminated for a period of time to assess its influence on the condition.

Medication. There is a wide range of types and combinations of topical agents for the treatment of acne, with selection depending on the type and severity of the lesions. *Tretinoin (retinoic acid, Retin-A)* is the only drug that effectively interrupts the abnormal follicular keratinization that produces microcomedones, precursors of visible comedones. It takes at least 2 to 3 months for significant improvement to be apparent. *Topical* tretinoin is not associated with an increased risk of birth defects. Topical *benzoyl peroxide* kills *P. acnes* organisms. The most effective therapy involves the use of benzoyl peroxide, tretinoin, or a combination of these. Both agents can cause redness and peeling early in their use; therefore the treatment usually begins with graded increases in concentration and/or frequency of application according to the patient's tolerance. Because of these effects, adolescents may be tempted to discontinue their use. The two drugs should not be applied together, since the benzoyl peroxide may oxidize the retinoic acid and render it impotent. The adolescent can be advised that side effects may be minimized by delaying application of medication until the skin is completely dry (20 to 30 minutes after cleansing).

Systemic antibiotic therapy may be needed for some patients who do not respond to topical therapy. *Isotretinoin 13-cis retinoic acid (Accutane)*, a very potent and effective oral agent, is reserved for severe cystic acne. Since the drug is teratogenic and therefore unsuitable for pregnant women, practitioners must follow strict guidelines when prescribing the drug for female patients. All sexually active females should be identified before treatment, and the drug should be given only if they use an effective form of contraception during treatment and have received oral and written warning of the reproductive hazards of the drug (American Academy of Pediatrics, 1992).

Cleansing. Gentle cleansing with a mild cleanser once or twice daily is usually sufficient. Antibacterial soaps are ineffective and may be too drying in combination with topical acne medications. For some adolescents hygiene of the hair and scalp appears to be related to the clinical activity of the acne. In these persons, acne of the forehead can be improved by brushing the hair away from the forehead and shampooing more frequently.

Prognosis. Acne will resolve spontaneously over a variable amount of time, depending on the individual.

Nursing Care Management

Because acne is so common and its appearance may seem so mild, the health care provider may underestimate the relative importance of this phenomenon to the adolescent. The nurse should assess the individual adolescent's level of distress, current management, and perceived success of any regimen before initiating a referral. If adolescents do not perceive the acne to be a problem, they will not be motivated to follow the daily routine necessary to treat the acne.

Teenagers need a supportive, caring individual to help them maintain the persistence required to deal with the disorder over such an extended period of time. The adolescent needs education regarding the disease process and instruction in the prescribed therapy. Instruction should be definite and as specific as practical for each individual youngster. A written instruction sheet that describes the etiology and therapeutic regimen is often helpful, and parents should be cautioned against nagging. Adolescents should assume responsibility for following through on the instructions. They are cautioned against damaging the skin through too vigorous scrubbing. Several points are emphasized as particularly important: using only those preparations prescribed for their particular needs; carrying out associated directions, such as hairstyling and shampooing; and not leaving cosmetics on the face overnight.

Teenagers are subject to the influence of commercial advertising from a variety of media. Washing with a mild, nonabrasive cleanser, such as Dove (unscented) is adequate for cleansing. Most cosmetics do not cause acne, and contrary

Critical Thinking 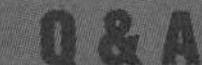 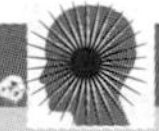

ACNE

Kim, who is 16 years old, recently started "breaking out." During her visit to the dermatologist, she was diagnosed as having a mild form of acne and was told to cleanse her face twice a day and apply Retin-A and benzoyl peroxide daily. Which instructions describe the correct skin care schedule?

1. Use a mild facial scrub in the morning and apply the Retin-A; at night use an astringent to remove makeup and apply benzoyl peroxide.
2. Wash the face with soap in the morning and at night; wait 30 minutes after the night cleaning to apply Retin-A, followed by benzoyl peroxide.
3. Wash the face with soap in the morning and apply benzoyl peroxide; wash the face before bedtime and apply Retin-A.
4. Wash the face with soap in the morning and apply benzoyl peroxide; wash the face in the evening and apply Retin-A about 30 minutes later.

The correct answer is four. The most important aspects of the skin care regimen are to apply the topical preparation at different times of the day because they are less effective when applied close together. Also, the face should be completely dry before applying Retin-A to reduce skin irritation. Although either preparation can be used first, it is preferable to suggest applying Retin-A at night, when the teenager has time to wait after cleansing the skin. Facial scrubs and astringents are not used because they increase skin dryness.

to once-popular belief, it does not make a difference if a cosmetic is oil-free or not (Bikowski, 1992). Cosmetics that do not cause acne are labeled *noncomedogenic.* Certain acne preparations, such as retinoic acid, tetracycline, and Accutane, can cause photosensitivity. Adolescents should be advised to apply the medication at night and use a sunscreen with a sun protective factor of at least 15 in the daytime. Other measures that minimize sun exposure, such as wearing a tightly woven, wide-brimmed hat or sun visor, are encouraged. Teenagers should be advised not to expect any visible improvement for 4 to 6 weeks after the initiation of therapy. Acne may appear to worsen initially. Medications often cause erythema, peeling, itching, burning, and drying when first applied. The use of comedone extractors to remove blackheads is not recommended because this procedure can cause increased scarring. Females taking oral contraceptive pills and oral antibiotics should be instructed to use an additional form of contraception.

During conversations with teenagers, the nurse can dispel the common myths often associated with acne and allow youngsters to discuss any feelings related to the disorder, such as self-consciousness or anxieties regarding relationships with others. Sometimes the nurse also can help teenagers explore job or other after-school interests. The acne lesions need not become an excuse to avoid social contacts and activities (see the Critical Thinking Q & A box on p. 1686).

See also the Nursing Care Plan: The Adolescent with Acne.*

Thermal Injury

BURNS

Minor burn injuries are experienced by everyone in day-to-day living and are relatively commonplace in nursing practice. Extensive burns, on the other hand, are relatively uncommon; however, they account for some of the most difficult nursing problems encountered in the pediatric age group. Serious burn injury accounts for a very large number of children who must undergo prolonged, painful, and restrictive hospitalization. The following discussion of burns focuses on the burn wound; burn prevention is discussed in Chapters 33, 34, 35, and 36.

Burns are caused by thermal, chemical, electrical, or, rarely, radioactive agents. Thermal injuries are the most common, followed by chemical and electrical, respectively. When burns are characterized by patients' age and type of injury, the following pattern arises (Adams, Hunt, and Purdue, 1991): (1) toddlers sustain hot water scalds most frequently, and older children are most likely to have received flame-related burns; (2) 10% of all pediatric admissions can be attributed to child abuse; and (3) the most frequent mode of injury is by submersion in hot water.

The extent of tissue destruction is determined by considering the intensity of the heat source, duration of contact or exposure, conductivity of the tissue involved, and the rate at which the heat energy is dissipated by the skin. A brief exposure to high-intensity heat from a flame can produce burn injuries similar to those induced by long exposure to less intense heat in hot water.

Chemical burns can be serious injuries, but with effective emergency treatment the extent of the injury can be minimized. Chemical agents continue to cauterize the tissues until treated.

Electrical burns can be deceptive, since, although cutaneous injury may be minimal, most of the damage can lie beneath the skin in the tissues of muscle and bone that cannot be seen and initially may be hard to diagnose. Electrical burns are often full-thickness burns involving the muscle and bone (fourth degree burns). Extremities can become mummified, with black, charred eschar present.

Characteristics of Burn Injury

The physiologic responses, therapy, prognosis, and disposition of the injured child are all directly related to the *amount of tissue destroyed;* therefore the severity of the burn injury is assessed on the basis of the percentage of surface burned and the depth of the burn. Also important in determining the seriousness of the injury are the location of the wounds, the age of the child, the causative agent, the presence of respiratory involvement, the general health of the child, and the presence of any associated injury or condition.

Extent of injury. The extent of a burn is expressed as a percentage of *total body surface area (TBSA).* This is most accurately estimated by using specially designed age-related charts (Fig. 50-15). It is generally more efficient to use any of a variety of charts designed to assign body proportions to children of different ages.

Depth of injury. A thermal injury is a three-dimensional wound and therefore is also assessed in relation to depth of injury. Traditionally the terms *first-, second-,* and *third-degree* have been used to describe the depth of tissue injury. However, with the current emphasis on wound healing, these are gradually being replaced by more descriptive terms based on the extent of destruction to the epithelializing elements of the skin (Fig. 50-16).

Superficial (first-degree) burns are usually of minor significance. There is frequently a latent period followed by erythema. Tissue damage is minimal, protective functions remain intact, and systemic effects are rare. Pain is the predominant symptom, and the burn will heal without scarring in 5 to 10 days.

Partial-thickness (second-degree) injuries involve the epidermis and varying degrees of the dermis. These wounds are painful, moist, red, and blistered. *Superficial partial thickness burns* involve the epidermis and part of the dermis. Dermal elements are left intact, and the wound should heal in approximately 14 days with variable amounts of scarring (Fig. 50-17). *Deep dermal burns,* although classified as second-degree or partial-thickness burns, in many respects resemble full-thickness injuries (Fig. 50-18). The difference is that sweat glands and hair follicles are left intact. Although these wounds can heal spontaneously in about 30 days with variable amounts of scarring, they can convert into a full-thickness burn if they become infected.

*In Wong DL: *Wong and Whaley's clinical manual of pediatric nursing,* ed 4, St Louis, 1996, Mosby.

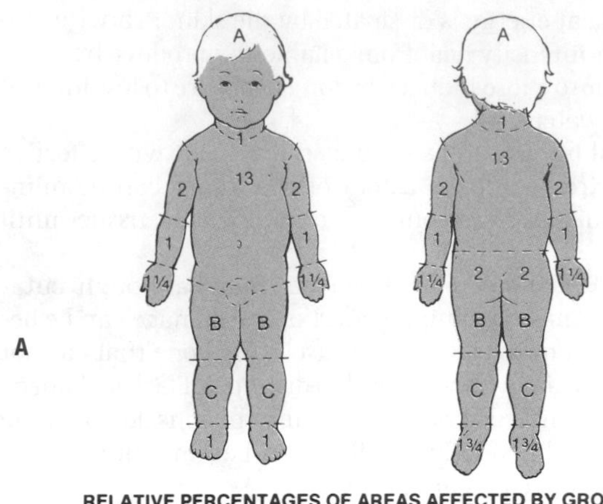

RELATIVE PERCENTAGES OF AREAS AFFECTED BY GROWTH

AREA	BIRTH	AGE 1 YR	AGE 5 YR
A = ½ of head	9½	8½	6½
B = ½ of one thigh	2¾	3¼	4
C = ½ of one leg	2½	2½	2¾

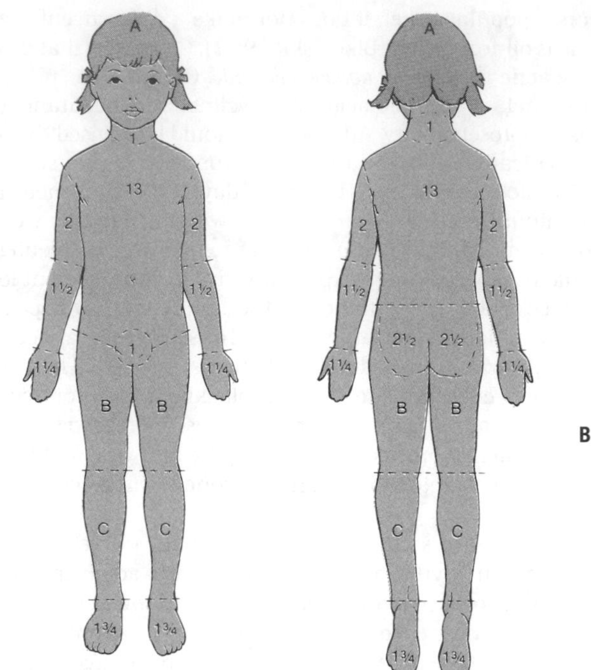

RELATIVE PERCENTAGES OF AREAS AFFECTED BY GROWTH

AREA	AGE 10 YR	AGE 15 YR	ADULT
A = ½ of head	5½	4½	3½
B = ½ of one thigh	4½	4½	4¾
C = ½ of one leg	3	3¼	3½

Fig. 50-15 Estimation of distribution of burns in children. **A,** Children from birth to age 5 years. **B,** Older children.

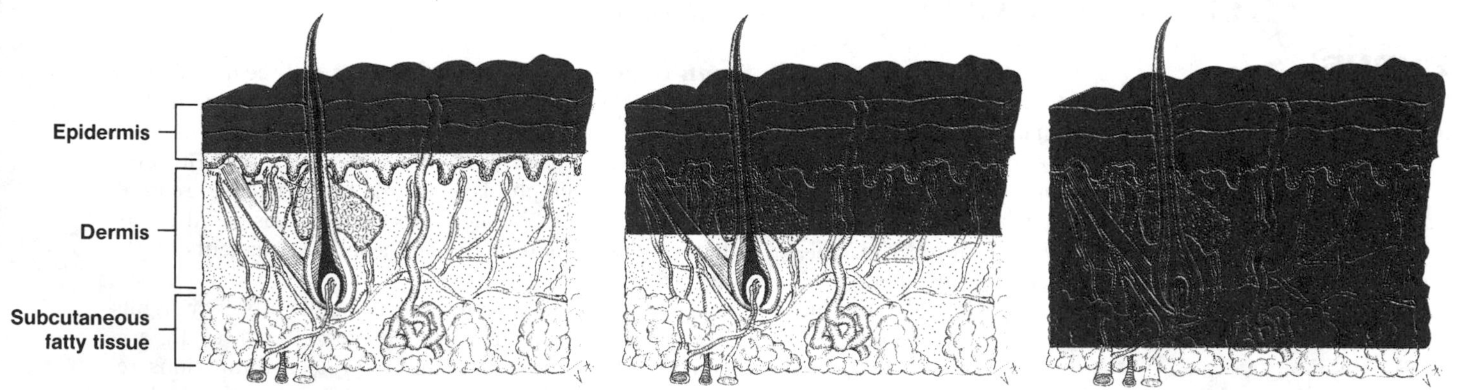

	Superficial (first degree)	Partial-thickness (second degree)	Full-thickness (third degree)
Type of burn	Sunburn; low-intensity flash; brief scald	Scalds; flash flame	Fire; contact with hot objects
Appearance	Dry surface; red; blanches on pressure and refills	Blistered; moist; mottled pink or red, reddened; blanches on pressure and refills	Tough, leathery; brown, tan, black, or red; does not blanch on pressure; dull, dry
Sensation	Painful	Very painful	Variable pain, often severe

Fig. 50-16 Classification of burn depth. Blue screen indicates depth of burn. (Modified from Potter PA, Perry AG: *Basic nursing: theory and practice,* ed 2, St Louis, 1991, Mosby.)

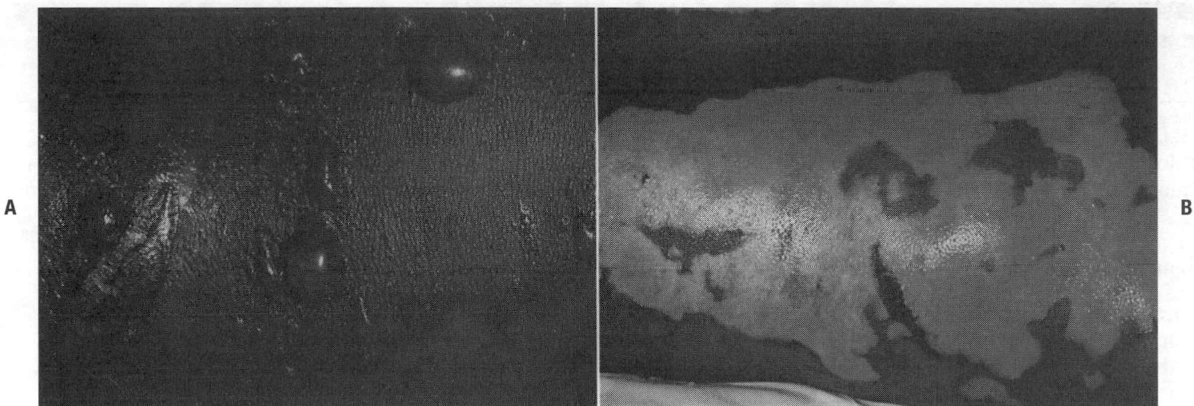

Fig. 50-17 Superficial partial-thickness burns on black child. **A,** Blisters intact. **B,** Blisters removed. (Courtesy Hillcrest Medical Center, Tulsa, Okla.)

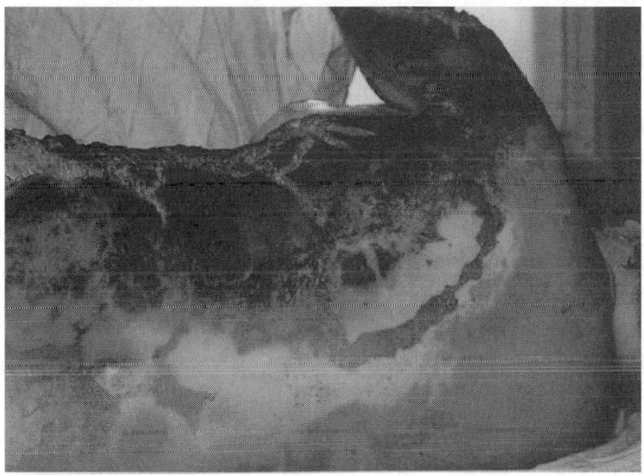

Fig. 50-18 *From bottom to top:* Deep partial-thickness burn *(lower area);* full-thickness burn *(white area);* full-thickness burn with eschar *(dark area).* (Courtesy Hillcrest Medical Center, Tulsa, Okla.)

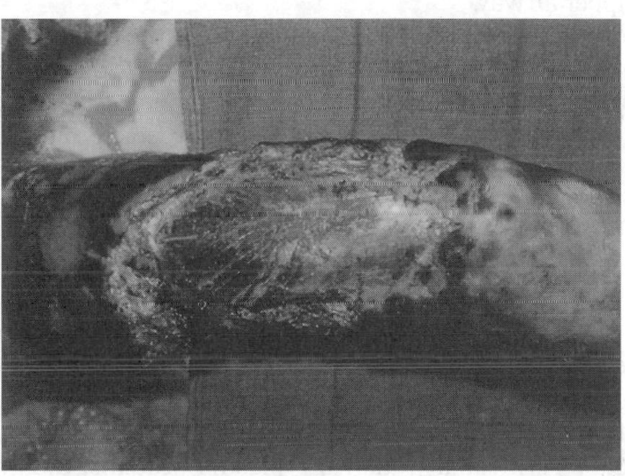

Fig. 50-19 Full-thickness burn with muscle and fascia involved. (Courtesy Hillcrest Medical Center, Tulsa, Okla.)

Full-thickness (third-degree) burns are serious injuries in which all layers of the skin, epidermis, and dermis, are destroyed, and the underlying subcutaneous tissue is affected (Fig. 50-18). Burns extending into the fascia, muscle, and bone are sometimes referred to as *fourth-degree burns* (Fig. 50-19). A full-thickness burn requires surgical excision of burn eschar and grafting to obtain a permanent coverage for the wound. Less scarring occurs with a full-thickness burn that has had surgical excision of the eschar and grafting than with a deep partial-thickness burn allowed to heal spontaneously.

Theoretically, with a full-thickness burn the nerve endings have been destroyed, and no pain should be associated with this type of injury. However, most full-thickness burns occur with superficial and partial-thickness burns in which nerve endings are intact and exposed. Also, excised eschar and donor sites cause exposed nerve fibers. Finally, as peripheral fibers regenerate, painful sensation returns. Consequently, children often experience severe pain that is related to the size and depth of the burn (Atchison et al, 1991). Even when nerve endings are destroyed, children may develop phantom skin pain.

Severity of injury. Burns are also assessed on the basis of their severity, which is useful in determining the disposition and management of the patient. Burned patients can usually be distinguished as (1) those with a major burn injury who require the services and equipment of a special burn unit, (2) those with moderate burns who may be treated in any hospital unit, and (3) those with minor burns who are unable to be treated on an outpatient basis. (See the grading system for burn severity in Table 50-10.) Because infants' skin is so thin, it is likely to sustain deeper injuries. Children younger than 2 years of age, especially 6 months or younger, have a significantly higher mortality rate than older children with burns of similar magnitude. Acute or chronic illnesses or superimposed injuries also complicate burn care and response to treatment.

TABLE 50-10 Severity grading system adopted by the American Burn Association

	MINOR*	MODERATE	MAJOR
Partial-thickness burns	<10% of TBSA	10% to 20% of TBSA	>20% of TBSA
Full-thickness burns			All
Treatment	Usually outpatient; may require 1- or 2-day admission	Admission to hospital, preferably one with expertise in burn care	Admission to a burn center

From Vaccaro P, Trofino RB: *Care of the patient with minor to moderate burns.* In Trofino RB, editor: *Nursing care of the burn-injured patient,* Philadelphia, 1991, FA Davis.

*Minor burns exclude any burn involving the face, hands, feet, perineum, or crossing joints; electrical burns; any injury complicated by the presence of inhalation injury or concomitant trauma; children with psychosocial factors impacting the injury.

Other factors. Regardless of the amount of tissue destroyed, if inhalation injury is suspected, there is risk of airway obstruction. There are two classifications of airway injury: upper airway and lower airway. A patient can have upper airway injury, lower airway injury, or both. Facial edema may endanger the upper airway.

Lower airway injury to the lungs is not the result of direct thermal injury because the upper airway can cool the heated air before it reaches the lung. Steam is the exception to this rule. Damage to the lung may also be caused by a bronchoscopy.

Pathophysiology

Thermal injuries produce both local and systemic effects that are directly related to the extent of tissue destruction. In superficial burns the tissue damage is minimal. In partial-thickness burns there is considerable edema and more severe capillary damage. With a major burn greater than 30% of total TBSA, there is a systemic response involving an increase in capillary permeability, allowing plasma proteins, fluids, and electrolytes to be lost. Maximum edema formation in small wounds occurs about 8 to 12 hours after injury. After a larger injury, hypovolemia, associated with this phenomenon, will slow the rate of edema formation, with maximum effect at 18 to 24 hours.

Another systemic response is anemia, caused by direct heat destruction of red blood cells, hemolysis of injured red blood cells, and trapping of red cells in the microvascular thrombi of damaged cells. A long-term decrease in the number of red blood cells may result in diminished red blood cell life span. Initially there is an increased blood flow to the heart, brain, and kidneys, with decreased blood flow to the gastrointestinal tract. There is an increase in metabolism to maintain body heat, providing for the increased energy needs of the body.

Complications. Thermally injured children are subject to a number of serious complications, both from the wound and from systemic alterations resulting from the injury. The immediate threat to life is related to airway compromise and profound shock. A less apparent respiratory injury is inhalation of carbon monoxide. Carbon monoxide has a greater affinity for hemoglobin than does oxygen, thereby depriving peripheral tissues and oxygen-dependent organs (such as the heart and brain) of the oxygen needed for survival. Treatment for either of these two problems is 100% oxygen, which reverses the situation rapidly. The child must also be observed for signs of local and generalized sepsis complications.

Pulmonary problems persist as a major cause of fatality in children with either thermal burns or injuries/complications in the respiratory tract. A full range of respiratory insufficiency can occur, including inhalation injuries, aspiration in unconscious patients, bacterial pneumonia, pulmonary edema, pulmonary embolus, and posttraumatic pulmonary insufficiency. The most common causative factor in respiratory failure in the pediatric age group is bacterial pneumonia, which requires prolonged intubation and sometimes necessitates a tracheostomy. Because tracheostomies increase the incidence of serious complications, including pneumonia, they are only performed in extreme cases.

Sepsis is the most critical problem in the treatment of burns, and it is an ever-present threat after the shock phase. Initially burns are relatively pathogen free, unless the wound is contaminated with potentially infectious material, such as dirt or polluted water. However, dead tissue and exudate provide a fertile field for bacterial growth. Early colonization of the wound surface by a preponderance of gram-positive organisms (primarily staphylococci) changes on about the third postburn day to predominantly gram-negative organisms, particularly *Pseudomonas aeruginosa.* By the fifth postburn day the bacterial invasion is well under way beneath the surface of the wound. Early surgical excision of eschar along with placement of autograft has reduced the incidence of sepsis today.

Superficial mucosal erosion, *Curling ulcers,* which causes recurrent or intermittent gastrointestinal bleeding, can be a major complication of burns. Prophylactic administration of antacids, histamine H_2-antagonists, or sucralfate, as well as the early initiation of enteral support, usually prevents the development of serious bleeding.

Therapeutic Management: Emergency Care

The first priority is to stop the burning process (see the Emergency box on p. 1691). The child should then be transported immediately to the nearest medical facility for definitive treatment and evaluation for transfer to a burn center. The child and family will be extremely frightened and anxious; sensitivity to their emotional state will provide reassurance during the transport process.

Stop the burning process. The chief aim of rescue in flame burns is to smother the fire, not fan it. Children tend to panic

EMERGENCY

BURNS

Minor burns

Stop the burning process:
- Apply cool water to the burn or hold the burned area under cool running water.

Do not disturb any blisters that form.
Do not apply anything to the wound.
Cover with a clean cloth if risk of damage or contamination.
Remove burned clothing and jewelry.

Major burns

Stop the burning process:
- Flame burns—smother the fire.
- Place victim in the horizontal position.
- Roll victim in a blanket or similar object; avoid covering the head.

Assess for an adequate airway and breathing.
If not breathing, begin mouth-to-mouth resuscitation.
Remove burned clothing and jewelry.
Cover wound with a clean cloth.
Transport to medical aid.
Begin IV and oxygen therapy as prescribed.

and run, which only serves to spread the flames and make assistance more difficult. The injured child should be placed in a horizontal position and rolled in a blanket, rug, or similar article, with care taken not to cover the head and face because of the danger of inhaling toxic fumes. If nothing is available, the victim should lie down and roll over slowly to extinguish the flames. Remaining in the vertical position may cause the hair to ignite or promote the inhalation of flames, heat, or smoke.

Major burns with large amounts of denuded skin should not be cooled. Heat is rapidly lost from burned areas, and additional cooling leads to a drop in core body temperature and potential circulatory collapse. Wet dressings also promote vasoconstriction because of cooling, resulting in impaired circulation to the burned area and increased tissue damage. Chemical burns present special circumstances and require continuous flushing with large amounts of water during transport to a medical facility. The use of neutralizing agents on the skin is contraindicated, since a chemical reaction is initiated and further injury may result. If the chemical is in powder form, the addition of water may spread the caustic agent. The powder should be brushed off if possible.

Burned clothing is removed to prevent further damage from smoldering fabric and hot beads of melted synthetic materials. Any jewelry is also removed to eliminate the transfer of heat from the metal and constriction caused by edema formation. This also provides better access to the wound and precludes more painful removal later on.

Assess the victim's condition. As soon as the flames are extinguished, the condition of the victim is assessed. Airway, breathing, and circulation are the priority concerns. Cardiopulmonary and cerebral emergencies are always a consideration after trauma. Cardiopulmonary complications may result from exposure to electrical current, inhalation of toxic fumes and smoke, hypovolemia, and shock. Emergency measures are instituted as appropriate.

Cover the burn. The burn wound should be covered with a clean cloth to prevent contamination and decrease pain by eliminating air contact. The child with extensive burns is covered to prevent hypothermia. No attempt should be made to treat the burn. Application of topical ointments, oils, or other home remedies is contraindicated.

Transport the child to medical aid. The child with an extensive burn is not given anything by mouth to avoid aspiration in the presence of paralytic ileus and upper airway edema and to prevent water intoxication. The child is transported to the nearest medical facility. If this cannot be accomplished within a relatively short period of time, intravenous access should be established if possible with a large-bore catheter. Oxygen is administered if available at 100%. A report of the initial assessment and any interventions implemented is given to the medical facility assuming responsibility for the care of the child.

Provide reassurance. Providing reassurance and psychologic support to both the family and the child helps immeasurably during postinjury crisis. Reducing anxiety helps to conserve energy needed to cope with the physiologic and emotional stress of a traumatic injury.

Therapeutic Management: Minor Burns

Treatment of burns classified as minor can usually be managed adequately on an outpatient basis when it is determined that the parent can be relied on to carry out instructions for care and observation. Patients with less than optimal circumstances may require close follow-up to ensure compliance with the treatment program.

The wound is cleansed with a mild soap and tepid water. Debridement of the wound includes removal of any embedded debris, chemicals, and devitalized tissue. Removal of intact blisters remains controversial. Some argue that blisters provide a barrier against infection; others maintain that blister fluid is an effective medium for the growth of microorganisms (Peate, 1992). Most practitioners favor covering the wound with an antimicrobial ointment to reduce the risk of infection and to provide some form of pain relief. The dressing consists of a fine-mesh gauze placed over the ointment and a light wrap of gauze dressing that avoids interference with movement. This helps to keep the wound clean and protect it from trauma. The caregiver is instructed to wash the wound twice a day, reapply the dressing, and return the child to the office or clinic as directed for wound observation.

Other practitioners prefer an occlusive dressing, such as a hydrocolloid, which is placed over the wound after cleansing. The dressing is changed once leakage occurs or at regular intervals, usually every 7 days. This method provides a moist healing environment and eliminates the discomfort associated with frequent dressing changes but impairs visualization of the wound surface.

If there is a high probability of infection or other complications or if there is doubt about the ability to carry out instructions, the parents may be directed to return daily for dressing changes and inspection, or a nurse may be assigned to make a home visit for that purpose. Frequent removal of the dressing is an effective mode of debridement. Soaking the dressing in tepid water before removal will help loosen the dressing and debris and reduce discomfort. Burns of the face are usually treated by exposure. The wound is washed and debrided in the same manner, and a thin film of antimicrobial ointment is applied twice a day.

A tetanus history is obtained on admission. When there is no history of immunization or more than 5 years have passed since the last immunization, tetanus prophylaxis is administered. Adminstration of antibiotics for minor burns is controversial. A mild analgesic, such as acetaminophen, is usually sufficient to relieve discomfort; the antipyretic effect of the drug also alleviates the sensation of heat.

Prognosis. Most minor burns heal without difficulty, but if the wound margin becomes erythematous, gross purulence is noted, or the child develops evidence of systemic reaction, such as fever or tachycardia, hospitalization is indicated. The child should also be evaluated for functional impairment, and the caregiver should be instructed in the exercise and ambulation program. After the wound heals, an evaluation of scar maturation and range of motion will indicate any need for further therapy.

Therapeutic Management: Major Burns

Establishment of an adequate airway. The first priority of care is airway maintenance. If there is evidence of respiratory involvement, 100% oxygen is administered; and blood gases, including carbon monoxide, are quickly determined. If the child exhibits air hunger or otherwise appears in critical condition, an endotracheal tube is inserted to maintain the airway. Since early edema subsides within 24 to 48 hours and many have been managed successfully for longer periods of time without significant damage with nasotracheal intubation, tracheostomy is rarely used because of the increased risk of complications.

Frequently, placing the child in a tent or under an oxygen hood with a high flow of oxygen and maximum humidity is sufficient to reduce reflex bronchospasm produced by trauma to the bronchial mucosa. When the child has a facial burn, the bed is elevated 80 to 90 degrees to reduce swelling and the risk of upper airway obstruction.

Fluid replacement therapy. The objectives of fluid therapy are to (1) compensate for water and sodium lost to traumatized areas and interstitial spaces, (2) replenish sodium deficits, (3) restore plasma volume, (4) obtain adequate perfusion, (5) correct acidosis, and (6) improve renal function.

Fluid replacement is required during the first 24 hours because of fluid shifts that are occurring. There are many formulas used to calculate these needs, and the one adopted depends on practitioner preference. Crystalloid solutions are used during this initial phase of therapy. Adequacy of fluid resuscitation is determined by several parameters, such as vital signs (especially heart rate), urine output volume, adequacy of capillary filling, and state of sensorium.

After the initial 24-hour period, theoretically there is a capillary seal, and capillary permeability is restored. Colloid solutions such as albumin, plasmalyte, or fresh frozen plasma are useful in maintaining plasma volume.

Oral fluids are usually withheld in the early resuscitative phase but may be administered in 24 to 48 hours. Fluid balance may continue to be a problem throughout the course of treatment, especially during the periods in which there may be considerable evaporative loss from the wound.

Nutrition. The enhanced metabolic requirements and catabolism in severe burns make nutritional needs of paramount importance and often difficult to provide. The diet must provide sufficient calories to meet the increased metabolic needs and protein to avoid protein breakdown.

Many burn patients are able to eat; a high-protein, high-calorie diet is encouraged as soon as possible after resolution of paralytic ileus. However, many of these children have poor appetites and are unable to meet energy requirements solely by oral feeding. Most children with burns in excess of 25% of the TBSA require supplementation with tube feeding. Absence of bowel sounds does not preclude enteral nutrition. Since the small bowel maintains motility and absorptive capabilities, the placement of a small-bore feeding tube into the duodenum allows for the safe delivery of enteral nutrition during periods of paralytic ileus associated with trauma, sepsis, and anesthesia (Jenkins, Gottschlich, and Warden, 1994). Protection from aspiration is achieved by means of a nasogastric tube to decompress the stomach.

If nutritional requirements cannot be met entirely by the enteral route, parenteral hyperalimentation can be used to supplement intake. However, enteral nutrition is preferred because it eliminates the risk of catheter-related sepsis, maintains intestinal integrity and function, and allows more efficient utilization of nutrients, especially protein.

To facilitate the growth and proliferation of epithelial cells, vitamins A and C are administered early in the postburn period. Zinc is also supplemented because of its important role in wound healing and epithelialization.

Medication. Controversy also exists regarding the use of antibiotics during the first few days after injury. Antibiotics are not generally given prophylactically but are administered to treat specific infections. When a patient has elevated temperature, it is appropriate to obtain blood, sputum, and urine cultures to isolate the source of the infection. Otitis media must not be overlooked as a source of fever. When the source and particular organism are identified, appropriate antibiotics can be administered.

Some form of sedation and analgesia is required in the care of burned children. Morphine sulfate is the drug of choice for severe burn injuries. Morphine has extensive distribution, although it is eliminated rapidly; continuous infusion or frequent administration is needed for pain management in burns. Morphine is administered intravenously and titrated to individual need. The unstable circulatory status and edema formation preclude intramuscular or subcutaneous administration. The addition of scheduled methadone to intermittent morphine administration for painful procedures has proved effective in managing burn pain in some children. Nonopioid/opioid combinations, such as acetaminophen with codeine, are often effective for less severe injuries.

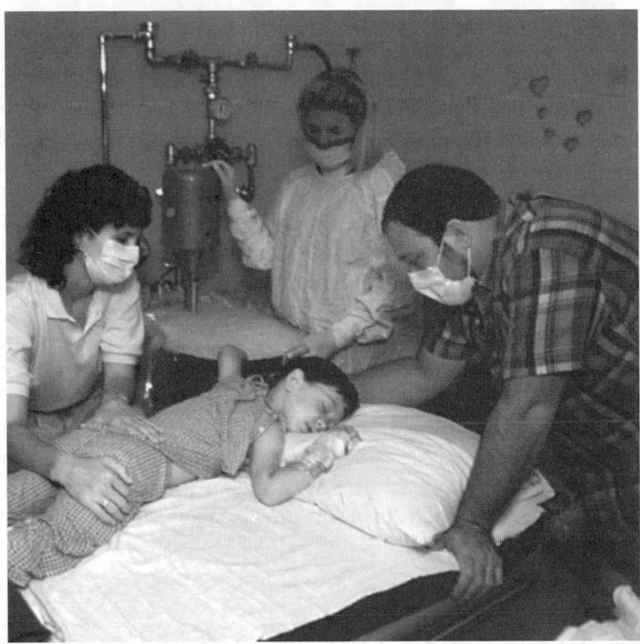

Fig. 50-20 Pain control during burn care. Child is well sedated with oral ketamine and midazolam.

The use of short-acting anesthetic agents, such as ketamine, propofol, and nitrous oxide, has proved beneficial in eliminating procedural pain (Fig. 50-20). Ketamine is a dissociative anesthetic agent that can be administered orally, intravenously, or intramuscularly. Unconsciousness after intravenous administration occurs within 30 seconds and lasts approximately 10 minutes (Groeneveld and Inkson, 1992). Pharyngeal reflexes remain intact, thus ensuring a patent airway. Propofol (Deprivan) is an intravenous sedative hypnotic agent that produces sedation in less than 1 minute and lasts only a few minutes.

Nitronox is a useful short-term analgesic mixture of gases on a fixed ratio of 50% nitrous oxide and 50% oxygen. Initiation of action is approximately 1 minute, with peak effect reached in 3 to 5 minutes. Nitronox is useful to alleviate anxiety and raise the threshold of pain during procedures. The child must be able to follow instructions and may self-administer the Nitronox with assistance (Selbst, 1993). For any conscious or unconscious sedation, the child is monitored continuously during the procedure (see Preoperative Care, Chapter 42 and Chapter 41 for a discussion of pain assessment and management).

Care of burn wounds. After the initial period of shock and the restoration of fluid balance, the primary concern is the burn wound. The objectives of wound management include the prevention of infection, removal of devitalized tissue, and closure of the wound. The application of dressings and topical antimicrobial therapy reduce pain by minimizing the exposure to air.

Primary excision. In children with large, full-thickness burn wounds, excision is performed as soon as the patient is hemodynamically stable after initial resuscitation. Since the burn wound is precipitating the exaggerated physiologic response, many associated complications do not resolve until the eschar is excised and the wound is closed (Finkelstein et al, 1992). Early excision of deep partial-thickness and full-thickness burns has reduced the incidence of infection and the threat of sepsis.

Debridement. Hydrotherapy is employed to cleanse the wound and involves soaking in a tub or showering once or twice a day for no more than 20 minutes. Hydrotherapy helps cleanse not only the wound but the entire body and also aids in maintaining range of motion.

Partial-thickness wounds require debridement of devitalized tissue to promote healing. Debridement is very painful and requires some type of analgesia before the procedure. The water acts to loosen and remove sloughing tissue, exudate, and topical medications. Mesh gauze serves to entrap the exudative slough and is readily removed during hydrotherapy. Any loose tissue is carefully trimmed away before the wound is redressed.

Topical antimicrobial agents. Methods used for managing the burn wound are as follows:

- **Exposure**—Wounds are left open to air; crust forms on partial-thickness wounds, and eschar forms on full-thickness burns.
- **Open**—Topical antimicrobial agent is applied directly to the wound surface, and the wound is left uncovered.
- **Modified**—Antimicrobial is applied directly or impregnated into thin gauze and applied to the wound; gauze or net secures the area.
- **Occlusive**—Antimicrobial is impregnated in gauze or applied directly to the wound; multiple layers of bulky gauze are placed over the primary layer and secured with gauze or net.

All meet the objective of preparation for permanent wound coverage, and all employ some type of topical agent.

Topical agents do not eliminate organisms from the wound but can effectively inhibit bacterial growth. To be effective, a topical application must be nontoxic, capable of diffusing through eschar, harmless to viable tissue, inexpensive, and easy to apply. It should not encourage the development of resistent strains of bacteria and should produce minimum electrolyte derangement. A comparison of commonly used agents are summarized in Table 50-11.

Biologic skin coverings. Temporary closure of the burn wound by the use of material other than the patient's own skin has become commonplace. Biologic dressings are used during the acute phase of therapy to cover the wound surface, protect the wound from bacterial contamination, reduce fluid and protein loss, increase the rate of epithelialization, reduce pain, and facilitate movement of joints to retain range of motion.

Allograft (homograft) skin is obtained from human cadavers that are screened for communicable diseases. Homograft is particularly useful in the coverage of surgically excised deep partial-thickness and full-thickness wounds in extensive burns when available donor sites are limited. Severe immunosuppression occurs in massively burned children, and the allograft becomes adherent. The homograft can remain in place until suitable donor sites become available. Typically, rejection

TABLE 50-11 Comparison of common topical preparations

ADVANTAGES	DISADVANTAGES
Silver nitrate 0.5% ($AgNO_3$)	
Greatly reduces evaporative losses; does not interfere with wound healing; bacteriostatic action against major burn flora, including *Pseudomonas* and *Staphylococcus;* inexpensive	Does not penetrate eschar; ineffective on established burn wound infections; little effect on *Klebsiella* and *Aerobacter* groups; stains skin, clothing, linens; makes assessment of the wound difficult because of staining; hypotonicity pulls electrolytes from the wound, depleting sodium, potassium, chloride, and magnesium; stings on application
Silver sulfadiazine 1% (AgSD) (Silvadene)	
Little pain on application; bactericidal by altering DNA and cell metabolism; effective against gram-positive and gram-negative bacteria; easy to apply; nontoxic	Transient neutropenia; does not penetrate eschar; forms proteinaceous gel on wound surface that is painful to remove; occasional rashes and pruritus; decreases granulocyte formation
Mafenide acetate 10% (Sulfamylon)	
Penetrates eschar and diffuses rapidly into burn wound and underlying tissues; effective in deep flame, electrical, and infected wounds; biostatic against many gram-positive and gram-negative organisms, including *Pseudomonas* and *Clostridium*	Difficult and painful to remove cream; pain on application; metabolic acidosis, hypercapnia, and carbonic anhydrase inhibition; inhibits wound healing; hypersensitivity in some patients
Povidone-iodine (Betadine ointment)	
Microbicidal against gram-positive, gram-negative organisms, yeast, fungi, and viruses; ease of application	Painful on application; elevation of protein-bound iodine may result in metabolic acidosis; stains clothes, linens, and the wound, making evaluation difficult; allergic reaction to iodine
Bacitracin	
Bactericidal and bacteriostatic against gram-positive organisms; low toxicity; painless application; ease of application	Limited activity against gram-negative organisms; allergic reaction to sensitive individuals

is seen approximately 14 days after application. The use of homograft is limited by the availability of tissue banks and a supply of suitable donors.

Xenograft from a variety of species, most notably pigs, is commercially available. Split-thickness pigskin adheres less than allografts and is replaced daily or every 2 to 3 days. Xenograft is particularly effective in children with partial-thickness scald burns of the hands and feet, since it allows relatively pain-free movement, which reduces contracture formation and has the added benefit of improving appetite and morale.

When applied early to a superficial partial-thickness injury, biologic dressings create an environment at the wound surface that is conducive to epithelial growth and faster wound healing. Biologic dressings must be applied to clean wounds. If the dressing covers areas of heavy microbial contamination, infection occurs beneath the dressing. In the case of partial-thickness burns, such infection may convert the wound to a full-thickness injury.

Nursing ALERT

Observe the wound daily for any sign of an infectious process, such as purulence, erythema, or cellulitis around the wound edges or temperature elevation.

Synthetic skin coverings. Skin substitutes are available for the management of partial-thickness burn wounds. Ideally the dressing should provide many of the properties of human skin: adherence, elasticity, durability, and hemostasis. Synthetic skin substitutes are readily available, have an indefinite shelf life, and are relatively inexpensive.

Synthetic dressings, composed of a variety of materials, can be used very successfully in the management of superficial partial-thickness burns and donor sites. Examples include adherent elastic films, hydroactive materials, or colloidal suspensions that are usually permeable to air, vapor, and fluids. Another product that consists of a nylon fabric bonded to a silicone rubber membrane is used by many burn centers. Calcium alginate is gaining popularity for the treatment of donor sites with both patients and staff because of its significant reduction in discomfort. As with biologic dressings, it is important that the wound be free of debris before the dressing is applied.

Permanent skin coverings. Permanent coverage of deep partial-thickness and full thickness burns is usually accomplished with a split-thickness skin graft. This graft consists of the epidermis and a portion of the dermis removed from an intact area of skin by a special instrument, the *dermatome* (Fig. 50-21) (see the Atraumatic Care box on p. 1695).

With extensive burns, it is often difficult to find enough viable skin to cover the wounds; therefore available donor sites are used to the best advantage by special techniques. The various types of split-thickness skin grafts are as follows:

- **Sheet graft**—A sheet of skin, removed from the donor site, is placed intact over the recipient site and sutured in place; used in areas where cosmetic results are most visible (Fig. 50-22).

Atraumatic Care

SKIN GRAFTING

The removal of skin with a dermatome is a very painful procedure. The child should be given conscious or unconscious sedation in combination with the use of the topical anesthetic, EMLA, placed on the donor site 2 hours before the procedure.

- **Mesh graft**—A sheet of skin is removed from the donor site and passed through a mesher, which produces tiny slits in the skin that allow the skin to cover $1\frac{1}{2}$ to 9 times the area of the sheet graft; results in a less desirable cosmetic and functional outcome (Fig. 50-23).

The donor site is dressed with synethetic wound coverings or fine-mesh gauze until the dressing separates at 10 to 14 days when the wound is healed. Dressings are not changed on donor sites to avoid damage to newly healed, delicate epithelium. Healed donor sites are available for reharvesting in patients with extensive burns and limited undamaged skin, but the quality of skin is decreased when multiple grafts are taken.

Cultured epithelium. When burns are extensive and donor sites for split-thickness skin grafting are limited, it is possible to culture cells from a full-thickness skin biopsy and produce coherent sheets that can be applied to clean, excised full-thickness wounds. Some children have been successfully treated with this autologous cultured epithelium (Boyce et al, 1993). Long-term follow-up studies are currently being conducted to determine pathologic changes and functional properties. Epithelial cell culture grafts offer the possibility of an unlimited source of autographs in patients with extensive burns.

Prognosis. Children differ from adults in their responses to thermal injury, and the mortality rates in young children are significantly higher than those in older children and adults. Mortality is greatest for children younger than 48 months of age (Erickson et al, 1991). Among those children who do survive, many have long-term functional and cosmetic impairments.

Nursing Care Management

Assessment

Initial assessment of the burned child includes the wound assessment described on p. 1687, as well as a comprehensive assessment of the child's general condition and behavior. The child with severe and/or extensive burns requires constant observation and assessment, with special attention to signs of complications. Each major phase of care has areas of greatest threat: fluid and electrolyte disturbances (especially shock) in the acute phase, infection in the management phase, and healing and functional disturbances from scar formation in the rehabilitative phase. Respiratory, cardiac, and renal complications may appear early in the postburn period.

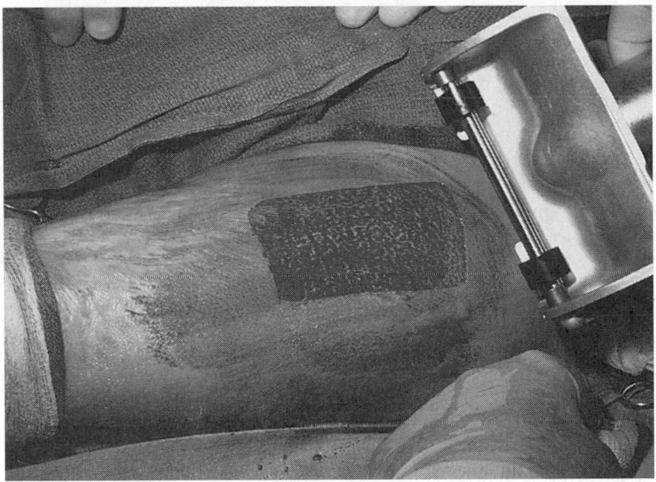

Fig. 50-21 Removal of split-thickness skin graft with a dermatome.

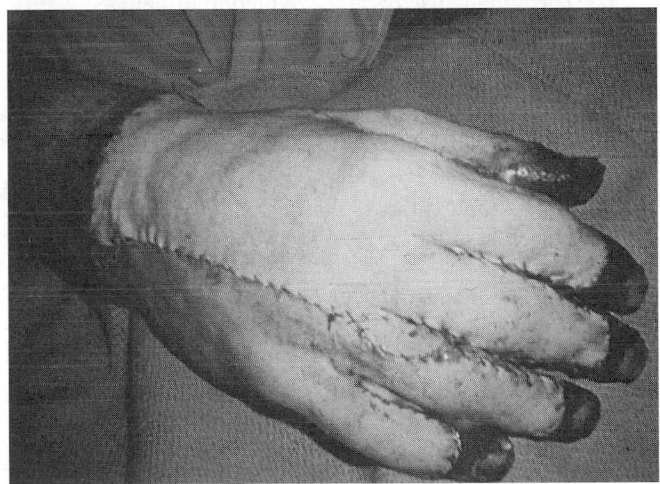

Fig. 50-22 Sheet graft.

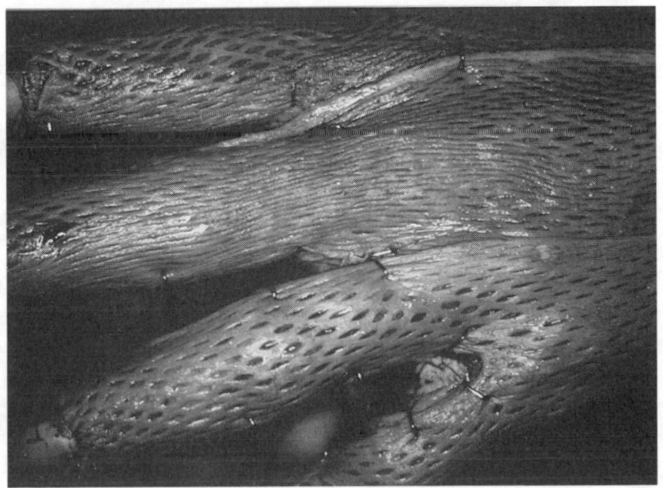

Fig. 50-23 Mesh graft.

Nursing ALERT

Disorientation in the burned patient is one of the first signs of overwhelming sepsis. A spiking fever and diminished bowel sounds accompanied by paralytic ileus are noted and progressively increase over 48 to 72 hours, after which the temperature falls to subnormal limits. At this time the wound deteriorates, the white blood cell count is depressed, and septic shock becomes manifest.

Nursing Diagnoses

Nursing diagnoses identified for the child with severe or extensive burns are included in the Nursing Care Plan on pp. 1701-1702. Additional diagnoses may be ascertained for individual children.

Planning

The goals for the child with a burn injury and the family are as follows:

1. The child will experience reduction of pain.
2. The child will exhibit evidence of wound healing.
3. The child will receive adequate nutrition and will achieve reduction in metabolic losses.
4. The child will not experience acute complications during management phase.
5. The child will not experience long-term complications during rehabilitative phase.
6. The child and family will receive emotional support.

Implementation

Prevent acute complications. The primary emphasis during the initial phases of burn care is on the prevention of burn shock. Checking vital signs, monitoring the intravenous infusion, and measuring urine output are ongoing nursing activities in the hours immediately after injury. The intravenous infusion is started immediately by intracatheter or cutdown and is regulated according to urine output and specific gravity, laboratory data, and objective signs of adequate hydration. Urine volume, measured at least every hour, should be 1 to 2 ml/kg/hr.

Nursing ALERT

Monitor the child's urine for the presence of pigmented myoglobin, a by-product of muscle breakdown, to prevent kidney damage. Testing can be done at the bedside using a reagent strip (Hemastix).

Dextrosticks should be used at least every 4 hours for the first 24 to 48 hours to monitor the blood glucose level. Careful monitoring of the child's serum sodium levels and accurate intake and output records are indicated. A complication associated with hyponatremia is the possibility of seizures.

Children with major burns should initially have nothing by mouth. Placement of a nasogastric tube to a low wall suction is indicated to prevent paralytic ileus during the first 24 hours.

Edema formation in a burned extremity with full-thickness burns must be observed closely for signs of circulatory impairment (i.e., loss of sensation, deep throbbing pain, and loss of pulse—a late sign).

Nursing ALERT

Evaluate the extremity and check the pulse every hour. If unable to palpate, use Doppler to ascertain loss of circulation and pulse. If the pulse is lost, escharotomy may be necessary to relieve the edema causing pressure on blood vessels and thereby restore adequate circulation.

The burn wound is treated according to the protocol of the specific burn facility. Extensive wounds may require the use of special beds and other equipment, such as CircOelectric beds, flotation beds, alternating pressure mattresses, and many other devices, depending on the extent and location of the wound.

The course of treatment is often long and emotion-laden for the child, the family, and the nursing staff. The severe pain of the wound and the therapies, the anxiety generated by these experiences, and the conscious and unconscious interpretations of traumatic events contribute to the psychologic reactions frequently observed in burned children. Much of the difficulty encountered in managing burned children is related to these factors. Soon after hospitalization, many burned children become irritable, depressed, hostile, and aggressive toward the members of the health team. In their helplessness, children often resort to angry outbursts against anything and anybody.

Relieve pain. The burn pain is overwhelming, engulfing, and irrepressible. Consequently, the pain causes anxiety and a feeling of profound helplessness in the child and can produce reactions of confusion, fear, and panic. Compounding the pain is the child's interpretation of it and of the procedures; this is closely related to the developmental level of the child. Many burned children believe their pain is punishment for past misdeeds and therefore deserved. There are often feelings of anger, guilt, and depression and, as in all illness, regressive behavior. When children appear to accept their pain and show little or no aggressive behavior, psychologic consultation is usually in order.

It is always difficult to deal with a child in pain, and to inflict pain on a helpless child is contrary to the empathic nature of nursing. Adequate management of pain is essential to reduce the discomfort of the burn and the necessary therapeutic procedures. Management of pain consists of (1) choosing the correct analgesic, (2) using a sufficient dosage, and (3) observing appropriate timing. To relieve pain adequately, the *onset* of action of the drug must be considered so that the peak effect occurs when the treatment is performed. To relieve pain effectively during burn treatments, IV narcotics are administered immediately before the procedure, but oral nonnarcotics are administered 1 hour before the procedure. Management of pain follows the principles described in Chapter 41.

Facilitate wound healing. The nurse has the major responsibility for cleansing, debriding, and applying topical medication and dressings to the burn wound. Because dressing removal is a painful procedure, children should receive adequate analgesia before the scheduled tubbing. It should be administered so that the peak effect of the drug coincides with the procedure. Both nurses and children must recognize it for exactly what it is—a dreadful but absolutely necessary procedure.

Research has demonstrated that children are more cooperative and demonstrate less anxiety and depression when they are allowed to be active participants in their care (Kavanaugh et al, 1991). Predictability and controllability are promoted during dressing changes. Predictability is increased by providing cues (nurses wearing specific clothing for dressing changes), focusing the patient on the procedure, and providing children with information about physical sensations they are likely to experience (e.g., pulling, stinging, pressure) before they experience them. Controllability is enhanced by providing children with as many choices as possible during the burn care and encouraging active participation. These strategies are unlike the traditional approaches of distraction and passivity. "Learned helplessness" is most intense when the outcomes are unpleasant and the situation is perceived to be unchangeable (see the Guidelines box below).

Outer dressings (if any) are removed before the child is placed in the shower, but adherent dressings are more easily removed after soaking with the water. Loose or easily detached tissue is also removed during hydrotherapy, and children are encouraged to move about as much as possible to exercise muscles and reduce contracture formation. They need to be encouraged and made aware of every little bit of healing as evidence that they are getting better. Merely saying that they are better is insufficient as they gaze at unsightly wounds. In dressing the wound, it is important that all areas be cleansed, that medication is amply applied, and that no two burned surfaces touch each other, such as fingers or toes, or the ears touching the head; to avoid this, a 4 × 4-inch gauze pad can be placed between fingers and toes.

Application of the medication can be a painful experience also, especially when mafenide acetate (Sulfamylon) cream is the agent used. This is used on electrical and fourth-degree burns because of its ability to penetrate eschar, but it can cause metabolic acidosis. Both the nurse and the child must understand that a painful sensation often described as "burning" may have special significance for burned children. They must be reassured that the medication is not inflicting further injury and that the sensation is only a transient discomfort.

When occlusive dressings are applied, elastic (Ace) bandages are worn over dressings to prevent epithelial breakdown and edema, stimulate circulation, and make mobility easier. This is especially important when the child is ambulatory.

Guidelines

REDUCING STRESS OF BURN CARE PROCEDURES

- Establish a consistent signal to alert child to time for burn care (e.g., nurse wears different "scrub" for dressing procedure, same time each day, i.e., after breakfast).
- Establish ground rules with child before beginning burn care, such as allotted time for dressing change or if there is any part of procedure nurse will have to do.
- Give child as many choices as possible before and during dressing change and burn care.
- Tell child first before doing anything.
- When explaining what will be happening, include description of sensations that will be felt, as well as what child can do to cope with them.
- Avoid using emotional words, such as "pain," "scream," or "hurt"; use "pressure," "pulling," and "sticking."
- Encourage child to maintain focus on burn care via running commentary about burns and what nurse is doing, by asking child questions such as what he or she is feeling, how child thinks burns look, and what physical sensations he or she experiences.
- Encourage child to help with dressing change.
- If child cannot help, suggest child count to 10 or 20 as fast as he or she wants. When child completes count, stop working for prearranged, defined "rest period" (e.g., another count of 20).
- Do not use such words as "done" and "finished" until dressing change and burn care are completed.
- If child refuses to focus on dressing change or burn care or refuses to actively participate in it in some way, continue to try to get child's cooperation. Reinforce all focusing on and active participation in burn care with praise, and gradually increase expectations for child's role in it.

From Kavanagh CK et al: *Learned helplessness and the pediatric burn patient: dressing change behavior and serum cortisol and β-endorphin.* In Barness LA, editor: *Advances in pediatrics,* vol 38, St Louis, 1991, Mosby.

Provide nutrition. After the initial phase of care, children are usually allowed oral feedings (unless paralytic ileus persists). Because children frequently lack an appetite, a great deal of encouragement, help, and patience is required on the part of the nursing staff. Consultation with the parents and the dietitian is arranged to determine the best way to provide needed nutrients in foods the child will be more likely to eat. Children who are old enough to participate should be included in the planning.

Nourishing snacks (high-protein milkshakes and enriched supplements such as Pedi-Ensure) are provided between regularly scheduled mealtimes, and if children eat better at a time other than a scheduled mealtime, that is the time to feed them. Most important, meals should not be scheduled immediately after a dressing change. Most children are too physically exhausted and too emotionally upset to eat at this time. If they will not eat, a 72-hour calorie count is taken to determine if tube feeding is necessary, and every effort should be made to encourage oral intake. (See Chapter 42 for suggestions for feeding the sick child.)

Prevent long-term complications. The chief dangers in this phase of burn care are wound infection, generalized sepsis, and bacterial pneumonia. Most burn patients are treated in a protected environment. Children are placed in burn units or private rooms in general units. Staff typically change into "scrub" clothing, and visitors change into gowns, wash their hands, and wear gloves before entering the child's room. In some burn centers, wearing masks and caps is an additional requirement.

The value of strict isolation in preventing infection in the burn wound is controversial. Studies have found that less strict isolation procedures, such as handwashing and wearing gloves, caps, masks, and nonpermeable aprons when providing direct patient contact or when in contact with body secretions, were actually more effective than strict isolation procedures. The use of a simplified isolation protocol can effectively reduce the nosocomial transmission of organisms, increase the compliance with isolation technique, and decrease cost (Lee et al, 1990).

It is important to make accurate ongoing assessments. Wound cultures are obtained at least three times a week, and a blood culture is indicated in any child with a rectal temperature of 39.5° C (103° F) or higher. Urine and sputum cultures may be helpful in isolating the source(s) of infection.

Nursing ALERT

Signs and symptoms of sepsis are (1) disorientation, (2) tachypnea, (3) temperature above 39.5° C (103° F), (4) hypothermia, and (5) distention of the abdomen or development of intestinal ileus.

To reduce metabolic expenditure as much as possible, the ambient temperature of the environment is maintained between 28° and 33° C (82.4° to 91.4° F) to avoid both overheating and underheating. An overhead warming unit may be provided to maintain body heat. Heat is often provided by means of a heat cradle over the child, but if used, the heat source should be situated well away from the child's body. Other methods include using electric heaters, which should be situated 4 to 5 feet away to avoid overheating, and maintaining the room temperature sufficiently elevated to reduce evaporative loss.

Antacids are usually administered prophylactically to prevent or minimize the effect of Curling (stress) ulcer, a frequent complication of severe burns, but nurses must be alert for any signs of bleeding.

Because the child is reluctant to move and doing so causes pain or discomfort, stiffness and joint contracture develop easily. In an effort to prevent this complication, the child is encouraged to move whenever feasible, and active physiotherapy is included as an essential aspect of burn care. When the child is resting or sleeping, contracture is prevented by proper splinting. Frog-legging, where the hips rotate outward and the knees are bent, can be prevented by placing a roll on either side of the legs to promote proper positioning. Children have a natural tendency to be active, and they will usually move spontaneously unless the pain is severe.

Care for skin graft. Effort in the care of children with skin grafts is directed toward facilitating a "take." Trauma, infection, and bleeding must be avoided for a successful transplantation to occur. When the grafted area is left exposed, the child must be immobilized to prevent the graft from becoming dislodged. Flat surfaces usually pose few problems, but grafts over irregular or mobile areas may require special techniques, such as splints or bulky surgical dressings.

The grafted areas have sutures to anchor the graft over the excised area. These are removed about 5 to 7 days after surgery. When the surgical dressings are removed, on approximately the fourth day after surgery, a dressing of fine mesh gauze impregnated with a topical antibiotic ointment (e.g., neomycin) is placed over the new graft and wrapped with Kling to help secure it in place. After the graft is completely healed, it may be left exposed (Fig. 50-24). The child may resume activities after the surgical dressings are removed, with the exception of grafts on the legs, which require bed rest for 7 to 10 days.

Wound contraction and scar tissue formation are normal parts of wound healing. Scar tissue is metabolically active tissue that continually rearranges itself; as a result, disabling contractures, deformity, and disfigurement are ever-present possibilities. Physical therapy, splints, and other methods are used to minimize these long-term effects. Pressure splints and elastic bandages or elasticized (Jobst) garments help reduce scar hypertrophy and may be worn for months to 2 years after hospitalization (Fig. 50-25).

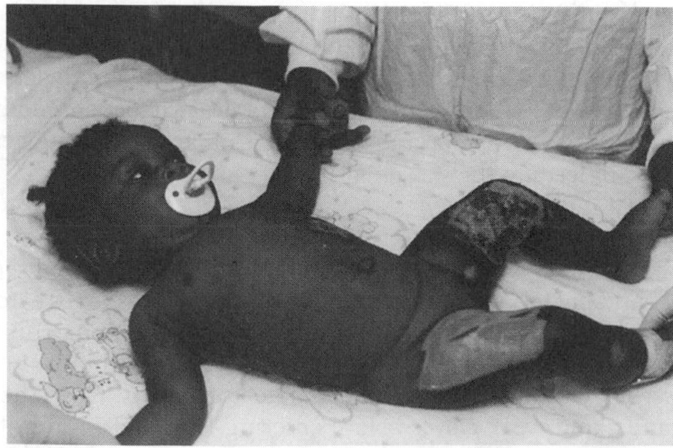

Fig. 50-24 Appearance of donor (right leg) and graft (left leg) sites 9 days after grafting. Dark areas on graft site are engrafted skin.

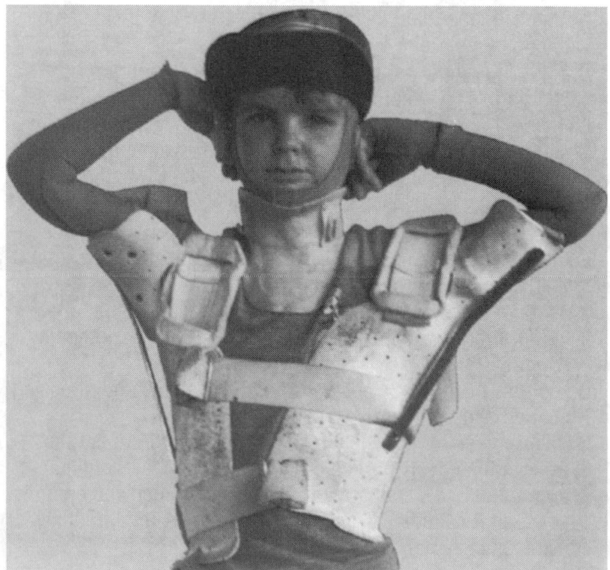

Fig. 50-25 Child in elasticized garment (Jobst) and "airplane" splints.

Scar tissue has some properties that are significant, particularly for growing children. Intense itching occurs in healing burn wounds and scar tissue (especially on the legs and arms, but not the face). It is usually treated with the administration of hydroxyzine (Atarax) or diphenhydramine (Benadryl) and frequent application of a moisturizer such as Eucerin cream, cocoa butter, or Nivea. Because scar tissue has no sweat glands, children with extensive scarring may have difficulty during hot weather or when they develop a fever. Parents must be informed of this characteristic so that they can be prepared to find alternative cooling methods when indicated.

Severely burned children must return to the hospital periodically for additional skin grafts and scar revisions, especially to release contractures over joint spaces and for cosmetic considerations. Achievement of optimum results frequently requires years. In the meantime, burn scars are unsightly, and although improvements can be made, hope should not be extended to the parents and child for complete cosmetic and functional repair.

Support child and family. A critical component of burn care is support for the child and family. Throughout the acute phase of care the child's emotional needs must not be overlooked. Children are frightened, uncomfortable, and often confused. They are isolated from familiar persons and surroundings, and the often overwhelming physical needs at this time are the primary focus of the staff and parents. Children need reassurance that they are all right and that they will get better.

The child is encouraged to participate in as many aspects of care as possible. With illness, children always regress to the developmental level that allows them to deal with the stress. As their condition permits, children can be expected to do things that they were capable of doing for themselves before they were burned, such as oral hygiene, face washing, feeding themselves, and playing. Allowing children to make choices and to help make decisions about the time of their care and recreational activities makes them feel a part of the team and provides them with a measure of control. Children will probably require assistance; however, as they see themselves contributing to their care, they gain confidence and self-esteem.

The psychologic pain and sequelae of severe burn trauma are as intense as the physical trauma. Each burned child goes through a tremendous amount of pain, often continuous for varying periods, and is often separated from the family for extended periods. In addition, there is a continual barrage of painful therapeutic and diagnostic procedures that are inflicted by others. They wonder why this has happened to *them*—what they have done that they should have be punished so. Past experiences cannot serve them in this crisis. They do not understand the "ugliness" and disfigurement they see as their body.

The impact of such severe injury taxes the capabilities of children at all ages, but young children who suffer acutely from separation anxiety and adolescents who are developing an identity are probably most affected psychologically. Toddlers cannot begin to comprehend why the parents whom they love and who have protected them from hurt can leave them in such a dreadful place and allow others to inflict such painful indignities on them.

Adolescents in the process of achieving independence from their parents and seeking to find out who they are in the world find themselves in a dependent position with a damaged body. Being different from others at a time when conformity and being like one's peers are so important is difficult to accept. These children need understanding adults to help them deal with the struggles concerning resentment and other feelings generated by such a catastrophe.

Members of the family, as well as the child, feel the impact of severe burn injury. They are concerned about the child's survival, recovery, and future appearance. Nurses are in the most opportune position to assist parents in coping with the stresses of the child's illness and their feelings of guilt and helplessness. The parents need to be informed of the child's progress and helped in their efforts to cope with their feelings while providing support to the child (Fig. 50-26). The nurse is the person who can help them understand that it is not selfish to look after themselves and their own needs so that they can better meet the needs of the child. For parents whose response to the illness is too severe or whose response to stress is manifested in destructive behavior, professional help may be needed.

Additional information on burn care and prevention can be obtained from the American Burn Association.* The Alisa Ann Ruch California Burn Foundation† provides assistance to burn victims and burn centers, supports research to improve burn care and treatment, and promotes public education in fire and burn prevention. The Shriners Burns Institutes are staffed to treat patients with acute burns and patients needing plastic or reconstructive surgery as a result of healed burns, with severe scarring resulting in contractures or interference of proper limb mobility, or with scarring and deformity of the face. Applications can be obtained through the Shrine Temple, Shrine Club, or Shriners Hospitals or by contacting the International Shrine Headquarters.‡

*New York-Cornell Medical Center, 525 E. 68th St., Room L-706, New York, NY 10021; (800) 548-BURN.
†20944 Sherman Way, Suite 115, Canoga Park, CA 91303; (818) 883-7700.
‡2900 Rocky Point Dr., Tampa, FL 33607; (800) 237-5055 (in Florida [800] 282-9161).

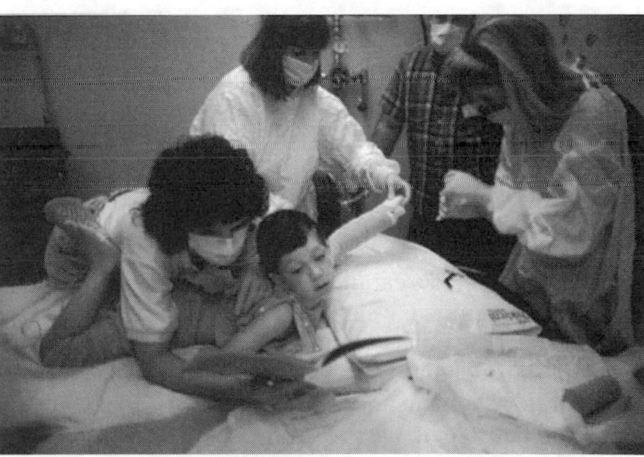

Fig. 50-26 Parents play a critical role in helping their child cope with the burn injury. Here a parent uses distraction by reading her child a book during burn care.

Prepare for discharge and home care. In most burn centers the nurse participates as part of an interdisciplinary discharge team that includes physicians, social workers, physical and occupational therapists, and child development specialists who plan with the patient and family for dismissal. The family's willingness to assume responsibility and their ability to administer care effectively are assessed. Home, school, and other environmental settings are explored; financial concerns and available community resources are discussed; and a specific plan of care for the child with an anticipated follow-up program is developed.

Because the family and/or other caregivers play a vital role in the successful reintroduction of burned children into the social and educational system, health education by the nurse is essential. The parents should observe wound care and at least two to five dressing changes until they feel comfortable in performing the procedure. It is recommended that the parents actually perform at least one dressing change before discharge so that the nurse can determine their knowledge and ability in accomplishing the task successfully. The parents must also be able to explain signs and symptoms of infection to the nurse.

Arrangements with the family for discharge medications and supplies for dressing changes are provided. If the parents are unable to perform wound care and dressing changes, it is important to ensure that the prescribed care will be maintained. This may be accomplished by designating caregivers other than parents to perform the procedures or by requiring daily visits to a clinic.

Some burn centers have a back-to-school reentry program for school-age burn patients to assist the child in returning to a classroom of peers. The program provides information about burn wound care, scarring, and rehabilitation therapy to help the child's classmates understand what the child has experienced and what the child must anticipate. It is hoped that sharing the child's experiences will help the other students appreciate the obstacles the child must overcome to return to normal childhood activities. The intent of the reentry program is to gain peer support for the burned child and allow peers to empathize and understand the needs of the burned child.

Evaluation

The effectiveness of nursing interventions is determined by continual reassessment and evaluation of care based on the following observational guidelines and expected outcomes:

1. Observe child's behavior during all aspects of care; listen to verbal cues; use a pain assessment record to evaluate the effectiveness of analgesia.
2. Observe the burn wound and child's general condition.
3. Observe child's eating behavior and the amount of food consumed; weigh daily or as indicated.
4. Inspect the burn wound for signs of infection; take vital signs; observe for evidence of gastric bleeding, respiratory complications, weight loss, hemoglobin level, and neurologic signs.
5. Observe for evidence of healing and scar formation; assess effectiveness of physical therapy and appliances (splints, pressure garments).
6. Observe child's and family's behaviors; interview child and family regarding their feelings and concerns.

Expected outcomes:

See the Nursing Care Plan on pp. 1701-1702.

SUNBURN

Sunburn is a very common skin injury caused by overexposure to ultraviolet light waves. The sun emits a continuous spectrum of visible and nonvisible light rays that range in length from very short to very long. The shorter, higher-frequency waves are more damaging than longer wavelengths, but much of the light is filtered out as it travels through the atmosphere. Of the light that does filter through, *ultraviolet A (UVA) waves* are the longest and cause only minimum burning, but they potentiate *ultraviolet B (UVB)* effects and play a significant role in photosensitive and photoallergic reactions and premature aging. UVB waves are shorter and responsible for tanning, burning, and most of the harmful effects attributed to sunlight, especially skin cancer.

Numerous factors influence the amount of UVB exposure. Maximum exposure occurs at midday (10 AM to 3 PM), when the distance from the sun to a given spot on the earth is shortest. There is more exposure at higher altitudes, less when the sky is hazy (although the amount of ultraviolet radiation that does penetrate is easily underestimated); window glass effectively screens out UVB but not UVA rays. Fresh snow and water reflect ultraviolet rays, especially when the sun is directly overhead; some rays are reflected by sand.

Nursing Care Management

Protection from sunburn is the major goal of medical and nursing management, and the harmful effects of the sun on the delicate skin of infants and children is receiving increased attention. To protect skin exposed to the sun for extended periods, skin should be covered with clothing, and FDA-approved sun protective agents should be applied.

Two types of products are available for sun protection: *topical sunscreens,* which partially absorb ultraviolet light, and *sun blockers,* which block out ultraviolet rays by reflecting sunlight. The most frequently recommended sun blockers are zinc oxide and titanium dioxide ointments. Sunscreens are products containing a *sun protection factor (SPF)* based on the evaluation of effectiveness against ultraviolet rays. The SPF is indicated by a number, such as 15, which indicates that if individuals normally burn in 10 minutes without a sunscreen, use of a sunscreen with SPF 15 allows them to remain in the sun 15×10 or 150 minutes ($2\frac{1}{2}$ hours) before burning to the same degree. The most effective sunscreens against UVB are *p-aminobenzoic acid (PABA)* and *PABA-esters.* Claims such as "broad-spectrum" or "UVA-UVB sunblock" are usually unsubstantiated. One product that affords protection against UVA is *Parsol 1789,* found in Photoplex and UVA Guard.

Sunscreens are applied evenly to all exposed areas, with special attention to skinfolds and areas that might become exposed as clothing shifts. Parents are directed to read labels of sunscreen products carefully for the SPF and follow the manufacturer's directions for application.

Nursing ALERT

Sunscreens are not recommended for infants under 6 months of age. Infants should be kept out of the sun or physically shaded from it. Dry fabric with a tight weave, such as cotton, and in a darker color, offers good protection (Stanford et al, 1995).

Nursing Care Plan

THE CHILD WITH A FULL-THICKNESS BURN MORE THAN 25% TBSA

Nursing Diagnosis: Impaired skin integrity related to thermal injury

Expected Outcomes: The child exhibits signs of wound healing, and skin grafts remain intact.

• **NURSING INTERVENTIONS/*RATIONALES***

Thoroughly cleanse wound and debride devitalized skin *to decrease infection and promote healing.*

Apply topical and systemic bacterial agents to wounds as ordered *to decrease chances of infection.*

Dress wounds as ordered *to protect against infection and fluid loss.*

Monitor serum electrolytes and blood gases *for potential adverse affects of topical agents.*

Monitor wound appearance for signs of infection or healing *to guide ongoing treatment.*

Monitor grafts for evidence of hematoma/fluid collection; aspirate or express fluids *to maintain graft contact with base of site.*

Use appropriate measures (i.e., splints, dressings, restraints) *to prevent child from touching or picking at wound and graft sites.*

Offer high calorie, high protein meals and snacks *to meet nutritional requirements caused by increased metabolism and catabolism.*

Administer supplemental vitamins A, B, C, iron, and zinc *to facilitate wound healing and epithelialization.*

Nursing Diagnosis: Fluid volume deficit related to active loss of body fluids secondary to thermal injury

Expected Outcome: The child exhibits signs adequate fluid volume and electrolyte balance.

• **NURSING INTERVENTIONS/*RATIONALES***

Administer intravenous fluids with sodium as ordered *to prevent burn shock and maintain perfusion.*

Monitor vital signs, skin turgor, mucous membranes *for signs of fluid volume/electrolyte balance.*

Monitor intake and output (including wound drainage, urinary output) *to assess fluid balance and circulatory status.*

Monitor electrolytes, blood gases, specific gravity *to assess hydration, electrolyte balance.*

Nursing Diagnosis: Risk for fluid volume excess related to retention of fluids and sodium secondary to intravenous therapy, edema formation

Expected Outcome: The child exhibits signs of adequate fluid volume and electrolyte balance.

• **NURSING INTERVENTIONS/*RATIONALES***

Discontinue intravenous fluids as ordered when an established rate of urinary output is reached and adequate circulatory volume is restored *to prevent fluid overload.*

Monitor respiratory status *for signs of fluid accumulation in lungs;* tissue pressures *for signs of edema that may cause permanent injury to underlying nerves and muscles.*

Nursing Diagnosis: Risk for infection related to denuded or absence of skin, presence of pathogenic organisms, and altered immune response

Expected Outcome: The child exhibits no evidence of infection.

• **NURSING INTERVENTIONS/*RATIONALES***

Place child in appropriate protective environment (i.e., laminar air flow, isolation, private room) and screen all visitors and staff for signs of infection *to minimize exposure to infective organisms.*

Teach child and family about good hygiene and careful handwashing techniques *to prevent spread of infection.*

Use good handwashing for all contacts with child and scrupulous aseptic technique with gown, cap, mask, and gloves for all wound care procedures *to minimize exposure to infection.*

Cleanse and debride eschar, crust, and blisters *to remove infection reservoir.*

Administer prescribed topical antimicrobials and cover wound with dry dressings per protocol *to provide a barrier to organisms.*

Encourage a nutritionally complete diet (high-calorie, high-protein) *to support body's natural defenses.*

Monitor vital signs, observe wounds, and obtain wound cultures *to detect signs of infection.*

Nursing Diagnosis: Anxiety/pain related to trauma from burns and debridement therapy and other treatments

Expected Outcome: The child exhibits a reduced level of pain and/or anxiety.

• **NURSING INTERVENTIONS/*RATIONALES***

Monitor closely for pain relief needs and administer medications as ordered *to decrease pain;* anticipate need and administer medication before onset of severe pain and at regular intervals *to better manage pain levels;* medicate before procedures such as debridement, hydrotherapy, dressing changes *to better manage pain levels.*

Administer medications as prescribed, apply lotions *for the relief of itching of scar tissue.*

Prepare child and family for procedures and allow the child to make active choices during procedures (i.e., testing temperature of water for hydrotherapy, selecting which site to start debridement, saying when to stop procedure for a rest, helping with the procedure) *to promote sense of control and cooperation.*

Implement nonpharmacologic pain reduction techniques as appropriate (i.e., distraction, relaxation, guided imagery, positive self-talk, cutaneous stimulation) *to relieve pain.*

Continued.

Nursing Care Plan

THE CHILD WITH A FULL-THICKNESS BURN MORE THAN 25% TBSA—CONT'D

Nursing Diagnosis: Impaired physical mobility related to pain, scar formation, joint contracture

Expected Outcome: The child exhibits a reduced level of pain and/or anxiety.

• **NURSING INTERVENTIONS/*RATIONALES***

Implement active/passive range of motion *to prevent contractures, keep joints mobile, minimize pain.*

Use positioning techniques, splinting, conformers, pressure garments *to prevent flexion and scar contractures.*

Ambulate as soon as possible, promote self-help activities, encourage play *to maintain mobility.*

Use lotion and massage healed areas *to soften scars and promote relaxation.*

Administer analgesic before painful activity (e.g., physical therapy) *so that child is more likely to cooperate and be mobile.*

Nursing Diagnosis: Ineffective thermoregulation related to loss of skin surface, sweat glands

Expected Outcome: The child exhibits tolerance to the environment.

• **NURSING INTERVENTIONS/*RATIONALES***

Carefully control and monitor temperature in environment, limit exposure to temperature extremes *to prevent hypothermia or hyperthermia.*

Avoid vigorous physical activity *that may lead to heat prostration.*

Monitor temperature *to assess for hypothermia or hyperthermia.*

Nursing Diagnosis: Body-image/self-esteem disturbance related to scar formation, alterations in appearance and function

Expected Outcomes: The child demonstrates an acceptance of self, his or her own physical appearance, and physical abilities.

• **NURSING INTERVENTIONS/*RATIONALES***

Relate to child, conveying an attitude of caring and acceptance *to encourage positive feelings about self;* serve as role model for others *to foster positive attitudes of acceptance toward child.*

Encourage child to verbalize feelings and perceptions about the burn incident, wounds and scarring (i.e., nightmares, fears of fire, pain of therapy, multiple treatments and prolonged and multiple hospitalizations, feelings of differentness, implications of functional limits, difficulty in making friends, views of self) *to facilitate coping and open expression of problems, fears, wants, wishes, and needs.*

Have child identify strengths, assets, things he or she likes about self *to increase postive feelings about self and abilities.*

Support positive coping behaviors.

Introduce child to other children who have had similar experiences, arrange for support groups for child and parents *to increase coping skills.*

Refer child and family for counseling as needed *to enhance adaptation.*

Encourage use of regular hygiene and grooming practices, use of accessories (i.e., wigs, concealing makeup, concealing clothing) *to promote positive appearance.*

Prepare peers for child's appearance *to encourage acceptance and support.*

Nursing Diagnosis: Altered family processes related to situational crises (child with scarring, altered appearance and function)

Expected Outcomes: Family members exhibit adaptation of usual roles and functions to accommodate special needs of the child and exhibit growth-promoting behaviors.

• **NURSING INTERVENTIONS/*RATIONALES***

Provide opportunity for family to absorb and adjust to diagnosis (i.e., repeat information *to allow time for family to hear and understand;* encourage expression of concerns, fears, and feelings about diagnosis and potential impact *to facilitate adjustment;* identify support systems *to provide resources for coping*).

Assist family to understand expected treatment, rationale, and implications *to provide a sound basis for decision making.*

Explore family's reaction to the child; assist them to achieve a realistic view of child's abilities and limitations; encourage family in attempts to promote child's growth and development; have family emphasize what child can do; explore ways for family to include child in family activities *to help family increase abilities to cope with and incorporate child into family structure.*

Arrange for and participate in family conferences *to provide forum for communication, mutual goal setting, and effective strategizing.*

Have parents spend special time with siblings *so they do not feel neglected or left out.*

Identify additional resource systems (i.e., relatives, friends, church, health care services, community programs) and strategize with family about making good use of these systems *to develop broad base of support.*

Provide a system of ongoing follow-up and evaluation *to ensure long-term adaptation to challenges presented in family functioning by a child with severely altered appearance and scarring.*

Sunburn is usually an epidermal burn, although severe sunburn can be a partial-thickness burn with blister formation. Treatment involves stopping the burning process, decreasing the inflammatory response, and rehydrating the skin. Local application of cool tap water soaks, or immersion in a tepid water bath for 20 minutes or until the skin is cool limits tissue destruction and relieves the discomfort. Moisturizing lotion is then applied. Partial-thickness burns are treated the same as those from any heat source (see the earlier discussion of burns).

COLD INJURY

Cold injuries are most commonly seen in very cold regions. The nature of the heat-regulating mechanisms of the body are such that the inner portion of the body, or core, produces heat and the periphery, or outer area, conserves or dissipates heat. When the body attempts to conserve heat, the outer tissues are subjected to low temperatures, and local trauma may result.

Chilblain, redness and swelling of the skin, occurs when extremities, usually the hands, are exposed intermittently to temperatures of −1.1° to 15.5° C (30° to 60° F). The response may vary but is characterized by intense vasodilation that increases the temperature of involved tissues above that of unaffected tissue and produces edematous, reddish blue patches that itch and burn. As warming takes place, the sensations become more intense but ordinarily subside in a few days.

Frostbite results from sufficient exposure that heat loss to local tissues allows small ice crystals to form in tissues, resulting in variable degrees of tissue loss and function. The frostbitten part appears white or blanched, feels solid, and is without sensation. Rapid rewarming produces a flush (sometimes deep purple) and a return of sensation, which is extremely painful. In 24 to 48 hours after rewarming, large blisters appear, which begin to reabsorb within 5 to 10 days, followed by the formation of a hard black eschar. Superficial injury often heals without incident. Rewarming is accomplished by immersing the part in well-agitated water at 100° to 108° F. Discomfort is managed with analgesics and sedatives. Care of blistered skin is similar to that described for burns. It is seldom possible to estimate the extent of tissue loss until new skin layers are revealed after the eschar layer separates.

Key Points

- Therapeutic management of skin disorders includes a variety of methods and agents to cool, soothe, and reduce the irritating effects of external stimuli.
- A moist environment promotes healing of wounds.
- Skin infections can be caused by bacteria, viruses, or fungi.
- Some diseases manifested in the skin are transmitted by arthropod vectors, especially ticks.
- The most common skin infestations of childhood—scabies and pediculosis capitis—can affect children of any age and from any social class.
- Contact dermatitis may involve a primary irritant or a sensitizing agent.
- Adverse reactions to drugs are manifested more often in the skin than in any other body organ.
- The most common skin disorders of infancy are diaper dermatitis, seborrheic dermatitis, and atopic dermatitis.
- Acne, a disorder affecting a large proportion of adolescents, is related to maturation of pilosebaceous follicles and increased androgen secretion.
- Noninflammatory acne is predominantly an obstructive disease characterized by open and closed comedones; lesions of inflammatory acne consist of papules, pustules, nodules, and cysts.
- Burns are caused by thermal, chemical, electrical, or radioactive agents.
- Burns are assessed on the extent, depth, and severity of the wound.
- Essentials of emergency care of burn injury include stopping the burning process, covering the burn, transporting the injured child to medical aid, and providing reassurance to the child and family.
- Management of minor burns consists of facilitating wound healing, relieving discomfort, and preventing complications.
- Management of major burns consists of facilitating wound healing, relieving discomfort, replacing destroyed skin, preventing and/or treating complications, and providing rehabilitation.
- Sunscreen is recommended for use when the skin is exposed to the damaging effects of the sun's rays.
- Thermal injuries to the skin can result from exposure to extreme cold.

References

Adams LE, Hunt JL, Purdue GH: Tap water scald burns: awareness is not the problem, *J Burn Care Rehabil* 12(1):91-95, 1991.

Alvarez O, Rozint J, Meehan M: *Principles of moist wound healing: indications for chronic wounds.* In Krasner D, editor: *Chronic wound care: a clinical source book for health care professionals,* King of Prussia, Penn, 1990, Health Management.

American Academy of Pediatrics, Committee on Drugs: Retinoid therapy for severe dermatological disorders, *Pediatrics* 90:119-120, 1992.

Atchison NE et al: Pain during burn dressing change in children: relationship to burn area, depth and analgesic regimens, *Pain* 47:41-45, 1991.

Bikowski J: Effectively treating acne vulgaris, *Phys Sports Med* 20:100-107, 1992.

Boyce ST et al: Skin anatomy and antigen expression after burn wound closure with composite grafts of cultures, skin cells and biopolymers, *Plast Reconstr Surg* 91:632-641, 1993.

Clore ER, Longyear LA: A comparative study of seven pediculides and their packaged nit removal combs, *J Pediatr Health Care* 7(2):55-60, 1993.

Cooper LI: Removing cactus spines, *Am J Dis Child* 142:1140, 1988 (letter).

Erickson EJ et al: Differences in mortality from thermal injury between pediatric and adult patients, *J Pediatr Surg* 26(7):821-825, 1991.

Finkelstein JL et al: Pediatric burns: an overview, *Pediatr Clin North Am* 39:1145-1163, 1992.

Groeneveld A, Inkson T: Ketamine: a solution to procedural pain in burned children, *Can Nurse* 88(8):28-31, 1992.

Hanifin JM: Atopic dermatitis in infants and children, *Pediatr Clin North Am* 38(4):763-790, 1991.

Hennes H: Removal of cactus spines from the skin, *Am J Dis Child* 142:587, 1988.

Hunt TK: Basic principles of wound healing, *J Trauma* 30(12, suppl):S122-S128, 1990.

Hurwitz S et al: Skin lesions in the first year of life, *Contemp Pediatr* 10(1):110-128, 1993.

Jenkins M, Gottschlich M, Warden G: Enteral support during operative procedures, *J Burn Care Rehabil* 15:199-205, 1994.

Kavanagh CK et al: *Learned helplessness and the pediatric burn patient: dressing change behavior and serum cortisol and β-endorphin.* In Barness LA, editor: *Advances in pediatrics*, vol 38, St Louis, 1991, Mosby.

Lee JJ et al: Infection control in a burn center, *J Burn Care Rehabil* 11(6):575-580, 1990.

Leyden JJ: Cornstarch, Candida albicans, and diaper rash, *Pediatr Dermatol* 1(4):322-325, 1984.

Margileth A, Hadfield T: A new look at old cat-scratch, *Contemp Pediatr* 7(12):25-48, 1990.

Martinez TT et al: Removal of cactus spines from the skin, *Am J Dis Child* 141:1291-1292, 1987.

Osmond MH, Klassen TP, Quinn JV: Economic comparison of a tissue adhesive and suturing in the repair of pediatric facial lacerations, *J Pediatr* 126(6):892-895, 1995.

Peate WF: Outpatient management of burns, *Am Fam Physician* 45:1321-1330, 1992.

Riegger M, Guntzelman J: Prevention and amelioration of stress and consequences of interaction between children and dogs, *JAMA* 196(11):1781-1785, 1990.

Selbst SM: *Pain management in the emergency department.* In Schechter N, Berde C, Yaster M: *Pain in infants, children, and adolescents*, Baltimore, 1993, Williams & Wilkins.

Smith GA et al: Comparison of topical anesthetics without cocaine to tetracaine-adrenaline-cocaine and lidocaine infiltration during repair of lacerations: bupivacine-norepinephrine is an effective new topical anesthetic agent, *Pediatrics* 97(3):301-307, 1996.

Stanford DG et al: Sun protection by a summer weight garment: the effects of washing and wearing, *Med J Aust* 162(8):422-425, 1995.

Taplin D et al: Comparison of crotamiton 10% cream (Eurax) and permethrin 5% cream (Elimite) for the treatment of scabies in children, *Pediatr Dermatol* 7(1):67-73, 1990.

Wong DL et al: Diapering choices: a critical review of the issues, *Pediatr Nurs* 18(1):41-54, 1992.

Bibliography

Skin Disorders: General

Bolton L, Rijswijk LV: Wound dressings: meeting clinical and biological needs, *Dermatol Nurs* 3(1):146-161, 1991.

Carney M: A suture nurse program in a pediatric emergency department, *J Emerg Nurs* 20:517-520, 1994.

Ching D, Mell D: Use of adhesive dressings in skin care: DuoDerm Extra Thin, *J Pediatr Health Care* 4(3):155-156, 1990.

Cuzzell JZ, Stotts NA: Trial and error yields to knowledge, *Am J Nurs* 90(10):53-63, 1990.

Engebo DA: Safe and effective use of tetracaine, adrenaline, and cocaine (TAC) solution anesthetic for anesthetizing of lacerations, *J Emerg Nurs* 16:100-101, 1990.

Ernst AA et al: Lidocaine adrenaline tetracaine gel versus tetracaine adrenaline cocaine gel for topical anesthesia in linear scalp and facial lacerations in children aged 5 to 17 years, *Pediatrics* 95(2):255-258, 1995.

Hagelgans NA: Pediatric skin care issues for the home care nurse, *Pediatr Nurs* 19(3):499-507, 1993.

Hurwitz S: *Clinical pediatric dermatology: a textbook of skin disorders of childhood and adolescence*, ed 2, Philadelphia, 1993, WB Saunders.

Schilling CG et al: Tetracaine, epinephrine (adrenalin), and cocaine (TAC) versus lidocaine, epinephrine, and tetracaine (LET) for anesthesia of lacerations in children, *Ann Emerg Med* 25:203-208, 1995.

Smith DP, Kemper JY: *Skin therapy.* In Smith DP et al, editors: *Comprehensive child and family nursing skills*, St Louis, 1991, Mosby.

Wounds

Bryant RA, editor: *Acute and chronic wounds: nursing management*, St Louis, 1992, Mosby.

Cuzzell JZ, Stotts NA: Wound care: trial and error yields to knowledge, *Am J Nurs* 90(10):53-63, 1990.

Garvin G: Wound healing in pediatrics, *Nurs Clin North Am* 25(1):181-192, 1990.

Harding KG: Wound care: putting theory into clinical practice, *Wounds* 2(1):21-32, 1990.

Norris S, Provo B, Stotts N: Physiology of wound healing and risk factors that impede the healing process, *AACN Clin Issues Crit Care Nurs* 1(3):545-552, 1990.

Oberg MS, Lindsey D: Do not put hydrogen peroxide or povidone-iodine into wounds! *Am J Dis Child* 141(1):27-28, 1987.

O'Hanlon-Nichols T: Commonly asked questions about wound healing, *Am J Nurs* 95(4):22-24, 1995.

Ratner MH: A short course in wound care for children, *Contemp Pediatr* 8(8):22-38, 1991.

Rodeheaver G et al: Wound healing and wound management: focus on debridement, *Adv Wound Care* 7(1):22-39, 1994.

Infections/Infestations

Brimhall CL, Esterly NB: Uninvited guests: skin infestations of childhood, *Contemp Pediatr* 7(1):18-57, 1990.

Brozena SJ: Scabies: update on diagnosis and treatment, *J Sch Nurs* 8(4):15-19, 1992.

Clore ER: Head-lice screening, *Sch Health Watch* 5(2):2, 1994.

Halpern JS: Recognition and treatment of pediculosis (head lice) in the emergency department, *J Emerg Nurs* 20(2):130-133, 1994.

Krugman S et al: *Infectious diseases of children*, ed 9, St Louis, 1992, Mosby.

Molinaro F: Treatment of pediculosis and scabies, *Pediatr Nurs* 18(6):600-602, 1992.

Rasmussen JE: Cutaneous fungus infections in children, *Pediatr Rev* 13(4):152-156, 1992a.

Rasmussen JE: Impetigo: changing bacteria, changing therapies, *Contemp Pediatr* 9(2):14-22, 1992b.

Sokoloff F: Identification and management of pediculosis, *Nurs Pract* 19(8):62-64, 1994.

Walker DH, Dumler JS: Emerging and reemerging rickettsial diseases, *N Engl J Med* 331(24):1651-1652, 1994.

Age-Related Skin Disorders

Casimar GJA et al: Atopic dermatitis: role of food and house dust mite allergens, *Pediatrics* 92(2):252-256, 1993.

Castiglia PT: Acne, *J Pediatr Health Care* 3:259-261, 1989.

Farrington E: Diaper dermatitis, *Pediatr Nurs* 18(1):81-82, 1992.

Garvin G: Skin care considerations in the neonate for the ET nurse, *J Enterostom Ther* 17(6):225-230, 1990.

Holaday B et al: Diaper type and fecal contamination in child day care, *J Pediatr Health Care* 9(2):67-74, 1995.

Holaday B et al: Fecal contamination in child day care centers: cloth vs paper, *Am J Public Health* 85(1):30-33, 1995.

Jick SS et al: First trimester topical tretinoin and congenital disorders, *Lancet* 341:1181-1182, 1993.

Kubiak M et al: Comparison of stool containment in cloth and single-use diapers using a simulated infant feces, *Pediatrics* 91(3):632-636, 1993.

Lane A, Rehder P, Helm K: Evaluations of diapers containing absorbent gelling material with conventional disposable diapers in newborn infants, *Am J Dis Child* 144(3):315-318, 1990.

Novick NL: Diaper rashes, *Pharmacol Times* 57(5):41-47, 1991.

Novotny J: Adolescents, acne, and the side-effects of Accutane, *Pediatr Nurs* 15:247-248, 1989.

Pairaudeau P et al: Inhalation of baby powder: an unappreciated hazard, *Br Med J* 302:1200-1201, 1991.

Rothman KF, Lucky AW: Acne vulgaris, *Adv Dermatol* 8:347-374, 1993.

White KH: *Diapering and skin care.* In Smith DP et al, editors: *Comprehensive child and family nursing skills,* St Louis, 1991, Mosby.

Bites, Stings, and Other Animal-Related Disorders

Adamski DB: Assessment and treatment of allergic response to stinging insects, *J Emerg Nurs* 16:77-80, 1990.

Agre F, Schwartz R: The value of early treatment of deer tick bites for the prevention of Lyme disease, *Am J Dis Child* 147:945-947, 1993.

Carithers H, Margileth A: Cat-scratch disease: acute encephalopathy and other neurologic manifestations, *Am J Dis Child* 145(1):98-101, 1991.

Collipp PJ: Cat-scratch disease: therapy with trimethoprim-sulfamethoxazole, *Am J Dis Child* 146(4):397-399, 1992.

Distinguishing Lyme disease from its look-alikes, *Emerg Med* 24(11):28-50, 1992.

Guin JD, Kligman AM, Maibach HI: Managing the poison-plant rashes, *Patient Care* 26(8):63-66, 70-72, 1992.

Hibel JA, Clore ER: Prevention and primary care treatment of stings from imported fire ants, *Nurse Practitioner* 17(6):65-71, 1992.

Koehler JE: Progress in cat scratch disease, *JAMA* 271:531, 1994.

Protecting yourself from poison ivy, oak, and sumac, *Patient Care* 26(8):77-78, 1992.

Shewell PC, Nancarrow JD: Dogs that bite, *Br Med J* 303(6816):1512-1513, 1991.

Slota M, O'Connor K: Recognizing and treating cat scratch disease with encephalopathy in children, *Crit Care Nurse* 12(6):39-42, 1992.

Sofer S, Shahak E, Gueron M: Scorpion envenomation and antivenom therapy, *J Pediatr* 124:973-978, 1994.

Stafford CT, Moffitt JE, Yates AB: Insect sting anaphylaxis referral is imperative, *Emerg Med* 24(11):230-231, 1992.

Walker DH: Rocky Mountain spotted fever: a seasonal alert, *Clin Infect Dis* 20(5):1111-1117, 1995.

Miscellaneous Skin Disorders

Ansell BM, Falcini F, Woo P: Scleroderma in childhood, *Clin Dermatol* 12:299-307, 1994.

Castiglia PT: Alopecia, *J Pediatr Health Care* 5(1):44-46, 1991.

Hofman KJ et al: Neurofibromatosis type 1: the cognitive phenotype, *J Pediatr* 124(4):S1-S8, 1994.

Kaminester LH: The many guises of psoriasis, *J Emerg Med* 25(7):27-41, 1993.

Korf BR: Diagnostic outcome in children with multiple café au lait spots, *Pediatrics* 90(6):924-927, 1992.

Mackreth B: Poison ivy, don't rub it the wrong way, *Patient Care* 16(8):21-25, 1991.

New retinoid gel studied for psoriasis, *Dermatol Nurs* 7(1):65, 1995.

Nigro JF, Esterly NB: Psoriasis—chronic but controllable, *Contemp Pediatr* 10(10):114-128, 1993.

Rasmussen JE: Erythema multiforme, Stevens-Johnson syndrome, and toxic epidermal necrolysis, *Dermatol Nurs* 7(1):37-43, 1995.

Thermal Injuries

Adler R: Burns are different: the child psychiatrist on the pediatric burns ward, *J Burn Care Rehabil* 13(1):28-32, 1992.

Bargoil SC, Erdman LK: Safe tan, an oxymoron, *Cancer Nurs* 16(2):139-144, 1993.

Carr DB, Osgood PF, Szyfelbein SK: *Treatment of pain in acutely burned children.* In Schechter N, Berde C, Yaster M: *Pain in infants, children, and adolescents,* Baltimore, 1993, Williams & Wilkins.

Faldmo L, Kravits M: Management of acute burns and burn shock resuscitation, *AACN Clin Issues* 4:351-366, 1993.

Gottschlich MM, Alexander JW, Bower RH: *Enteral nutrition in patients with burns or trauma.* In Rombeau JL, Caldwell MD, editors: *Enteral and tube feeding,* Philadelphia, 1990, WB Saunders.

Harrell D, Hoelker L, Maley MS: Community burn prevention, *Proc Am Burn Assoc* 26:66, 1994.

Helvig E: Pediatric burn injuries, *AACN Clin Issues* 4:433-442, 1993.

Hendricks L et al: Subanesthetic ketamine for painful nonoperative procedures in pediatric burn patients, *Proc Am Burn Assoc* 23:52, 1991.

Herndon DN, Rutan RL, Rutan TC: Management of the pediatric patient with burns, *J Burn Care Rehabil* 14:3-8, 1993.

Holaday M, Blakeney P: A comparison of psychologic functioning in children and adolescents with severe burns on the Rorschach and the child behavior checklist, *J Burn Care Rehab* 15(5):412-415, 1994.

Housinger TA, Hills J, Warden GD: Management of pediatric facial burns, *J Burn Care Rehab* 15(5):408-411, 1994.

Jessee PO: Perception of body image in children with burns, five years after burn injury, *J Burn Care Rehabil* 13(1):33-38, 1992.

Kinner MA, Daly WL: Skin transplantation, *Crit Care Nurs Clin North Am* 4:173-178, 1992.

Maley M: Scald in the kitchen, *Information Exchange* 9:1-5, 1993.

Martinez S: Ambulatory management of burns in children, *J Pediatr Health Care* 6(1):32-37, 1992.

Munster AM: *Severe burns: a family guide to medical and emotional recovery,* Baltimore, 1993, Johns Hopkins University Press.

Osgood PF, Szyfelbein SK: Management of burn pain in children, *Pediatr Clin North Am* 36:1001-1013, 1989.

Patterson DR: Practical applications of psychological techniques in controlling burn pain, *J Burn Care Rehabil* 13(1):13-18, 1992.

Rieg LS, Jenkins M: Burn injuries in children, *Crit Care Clin North Am* 3:457-470, 1991.

Rumsfield J: Sunscreen: what you and your patients should know, *Dermatol Nurs* 2(3):139-147, 1990.

Sheridan RL et al: Midazolam infusion in pediatric patients with burns who are undergoing mechanical ventilation, *J Burn Care Rehab* 15(6):515-518, 1994.

Sullivan SA: How severe is this frostbite? *Am J Nurs* 93(2):59-64, 1993.

Taking the bite out of frostbite, *Emerg Med* 24(2):121-138, 1992.

Truhan AP: Sun protection in childhood, *Clin Pediatr* 30(7):412-421, 1991.

Vitale M, Fields-Blache C, Luterman A: Severe itching in the patient with burns, *J Burn Care Rehabil* 12(4):330-333, 1991.

Zingg BM: Managing burns in children: an intraoperative nursing care plan, *AORN J* 54:568-575, 1991.

CHAPTER **51**

Musculoskeletal and Articular Dysfunction

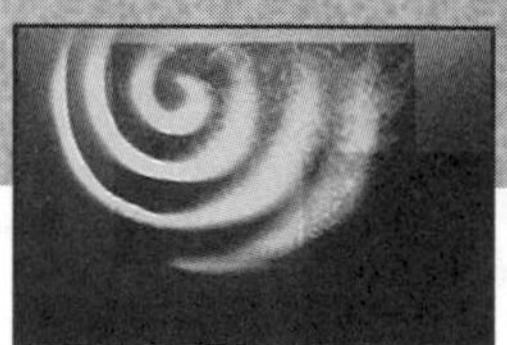

THE IMMOBILIZED CHILD, P. 1706

Immobilization, p. 1706

TRAUMATIC INJURY, P. 1709

Soft tissue injury, p. 1709
Fractures, p. 1711
The child in a cast, p. 1714
The child in traction, p. 1716
Distraction, p. 1720
Amputation, p. 1720

CONGENITAL DEFECTS, P. 1721

Developmental dysplasia of the hip (DDH), p. 1721
Congenital clubfoot, p. 1725
Metatarsus adductus (varus), p. 1726
Skeletal limb deficiency, p. 1727
Osteogenesis imperfecta (OI), p. 1727

ACQUIRED DEFECTS, P. 1728

Legg-Calvé-Perthes disease, p. 1728
Slipped femoral capital epiphysis, p. 1729
Kyphosis and lordosis, p. 1729
Scoliosis, p. 1730

INFECTIONS OF BONES AND JOINTS, P. 1733

Osteomyelitis, p. 1733
Septic (suppurative, pyogenic, purulent) arthritis, p. 1734
Tuberculosis, p. 1734

BONE AND SOFT TISSUE TUMORS, P. 1735

General concepts: bone tumors, p. 1735
Osteogenic sarcoma, p. 1735
Ewing sarcoma, p. 1737
Rhabdomyosarcoma, p. 1737

DISORDERS OF JOINTS, P. 1738

Juvenile rheumatoid arthritis (JRA), p. 1738
Systemic lupus erythematosus (SLE), p. 1741

The Immobilized Child

IMMOBILIZATION

One of the most difficult aspects of illness is the immobility it often imposes on a child. Children's natural tendency to be mobile influences all elements of growth and development—physical, social, psychologic, and emotional. Immobility restricts expression and causes anxiety and frustration. For these reasons children are immobilized only when necessary and for the shortest time possible.

Physiologic Effects of Immobilization

Functional and metabolic responses to restricted movement can be noted in most of the body systems, all of which have a direct influence on the child's growth and development, because homeostatic mechanisms thrive on normal use and need feedback to maintain dynamic equilibrium. Most of the pathologic changes that take place during immobilization arise from decreased muscle strength and mass, decreased metabolism, and bone demineralization, which are closely interrelated. Some results of immobilization are primary and produce a direct effect; others seem to be more indirect, or secondary, and affect more than one body system.

The major effects of immobilization are outlined briefly in Table 51-1. They are related directly or indirectly to decreased muscle activity, which produces numerous primary changes in both muscular and bone structure with secondary alterations in the cardiovascular, respiratory, metabolic, and renal systems. The major consequences are:

1. Significant loss of muscle strength, endurance, and muscle mass (atrophy)
2. Bone demineralization leading to osteoporosis
3. Loss of joint mobility and contractures

The larger the portion of the body immobilized and the longer the immobilization, the greater the hazards of immobility.

Psychologic Effects of Immobilization

Throughout childhood, physical activity is an integral part of daily life and is essential for physical growth and development. The activity helps children deal with a variety of feelings and impulses and provides a mechanism by which they can exert control over inner tensions. Children respond to anxiety with increased activity. Removal of this capacity deprives them of necessary input and a natural outlet for their feelings and fantasies.

TABLE 51-1 Summary of physical effects of immobilization*

PRIMARY EFFECTS	SECONDARY EFFECTS
Muscular system	
Decreased muscle strength, tone, and endurance	Decreased venous return and decreased cardiac output
	Decreased metabolism and need for oxygen
	Decreased exercise tolerance
	Bone demineralization
Disuse atrophy and loss of muscle mass	Catabolism
	Loss of strength
Loss of joint mobility	Contractures, ankylosis of joints
Weak back muscles	Secondary spinal deformities
Weak abdominal muscles	Impaired respiration
Skeletal system	
Bone demineralization—osteoporosis, hypercalcemia	Negative calcium balance
	Pathologic fractures
	Calcium deposits
	Extraosseous bone formation, especially at hip, knee, elbow, and shoulder
	Renal calculi
Negative calcium balance	Life-threatening electrolyte imbalance
Metabolism	
Decreased metabolic rate	Slowing of all systems
	Decreased food intake
Negative nitrogen balance	Decline in nutritional state
	Impaired healing
Hypercalcemia	Electrolyte imbalance
Decreased production of stress hormones	Decreased physical and emotional coping capacity
Cardiovascular system	
Decreased efficiency of orthostatic neurovascular reflexes	Inability to adapt readily to upright position
	Pooling of blood in extremities in upright posture
Diminished vasopressor mechanism	Orthostatic hypotension with syncope—hypotension, decreased cerebral blood flow, tachycardia
Altered distribution of blood volume	Decreased cardiac workload
	Decreased exercise tolerance
Venous stasis	Pulmonary emboli and/or thrombi
Dependent edema	Tissue breakdown and susceptibility to infection
Respiratory system	
Decreased need for oxygen	Altered oxygen–carbon dioxide exchange and metabolism
Decreased chest expansion and diminished vital capacity	Diminished oxygen intake
	Dyspnea and inadequate arterial oxygen saturation; acidosis
Poor abdominal tone and distention	Interference with diaphragmatic excursion
Mechanical or biochemical secretion retention	Hypostatic pneumonia
	Bacterial and viral pneumonia
	Atelectasis
Loss of respiratory muscle strength	Poor cough
	Upper respiratory infection
Gastrointestinal system	
Distention caused by poor abdominal muscle tone	Interference with respiratory movements
No specific primary effect	Difficulty in feeding in prone position; gravitation effect on feces through ascending colon or weakened smooth muscle tone may cause constipation
	Anorexia
Urinary system	
Alteration of gravitational force	Difficulty in voiding in prone position
Impaired ureteral peristalsis	Urinary retention in calyces and bladder
	Infection
	Renal calculi
Integumentary system	
No specific primary effect	Decreased circulation and pressure leading to tissue injury and decreased healing capacity
	Difficulty with personal hygiene

*Not all problems will apply in every situation.

When children are immobilized by disease or as part of a treatment regimen, they experience diminished environmental stimuli with a loss of tactile input and an altered perception of themselves and their environment. Sudden or gradual immobilization narrows the amount and variety of environmental stimuli children receive by means of all of their senses: touch, site, hearing, taste, smell, and proprioception—a feeling of where they are in their environment. This sensory deprivation frequently leads to feelings of isolation and boredom, and of being forgotten, especially by peers. The immobilized child may be labeled as "different," and over time this perception may result in a loss of self-esteem.

Physical interference with the activity of infants and young children gives them a feeling of helplessness. Even speech and language skills require sensorimotor activity and experience. Children who are restrained by casts, splints, or straps during the first 3 years of life may have more difficulty with language than those whose activities are unrestricted.

For the toddler, exploration and imitative behaviors are essential to developing a sense of autonomy; the preschooler's expression of initiative is evidenced by the need for vigorous physical activity; the school-age child's development is strongly influenced by physical achievement and competition; and the adolescent relies on mobility to achieve independence. The quest for mastery at every stage of development is related to mobility.

The monotony of immobilization can lead to sluggish intellectual and psychomotor responses, decreased communication skills, increased fantasizing, and even hallucinations and disorientation. Children are likely to become depressed over loss of ability to function or the marked changes in body image. They may seek the attention of others by reverting to earlier developmental behaviors, such as a desire to be fed, bedwetting, and baby talk.

Limbs in casts or traction transmit less than normal sensory data. Children who have limited ability to feel others touching them not only experience less tactile stimuli in a physical sense but are also deprived of warm, loving feelings that arise from being touched. The loss of feeling deprived from touch can further add to their sense of being isolated and unwanted.

Children may react to immobility by active protest, anger, and aggressive behavior, or they may become quiet, passive, and submissive. Children should be allowed to discharge their anger, but it should be within the limits of safety to their self-esteem and not damaging to the integrity of others. For example, providing an object to attack rather than a person or a valued possession is safe and therapeutic. When children are unable to express anger, aggression is often displayed inappropriately through regressive behavior and outbursts of crying or temper tantrums.

Effect on Families

Brief periods of immobilization have few effects on the family; however, catastrophic illness or disability may severely tax their resources.

The family's needs often must be met by the services of a multidisciplinary team, and nurses play a key role in anticipating the services they will need and in coordinating conferences to plan care. In preparation for discharge, home visits are advisable, and home management is frequently planned weeks in advance of the actual discharge, including special considerations for cultural, economic, physical, and psychologic needs. A child with a severe disability is very dependent, and caregivers need rest periods to revitalize themselves. Individual and group counseling is beneficial for preproblem-solving situations and provides an emotional support system. Parent groups are also helpful and often allow nonthreatening social contact. The families of children with permanent disabilities need long-term resources, since some of the most difficult problems arise as they try to sustain high-quality care for many years (see Chapter 38).

Nursing Care Management

Assessment

Assessment of the child who is immobilized as a result of an injury or a degenerative disease includes not only the injured part, such as a fracture or damaged joint, but also the functioning of other systems that may be affected secondarily—the circulatory, renal, respiratory, muscular, and gastrointestinal systems. In long-term immobilization there may also be neurologic impairment and metabolic changes in electrolyte levels (especially calcium), nitrogen balance, and general metabolic rate.

Nursing assessment includes psychosocial data, as well as physical manifestations, since long-term immobilization has a profound effect on the child and family. Nursing approaches are evaluated frequently and continued, discontinued, or modified to meet the changing problems and goals.

Nursing Diagnoses

Nursing diagnoses for the immobilized child are outlined in the Nursing Care Plan on p. 1710. Others will be identified in specific cases.

Planning

The general goals of care for the immobilized child and family include the following:

1. Child will experience no physical injury.
2. Child will experience no psychologic complications.
3. Child will engage in appropriate diversional activities.
4. Child and family will receive adequate support.

Implementation

Frequent position changes help to prevent dependent edema and fluid movement and to stimulate circulation, respiratory function, gastrointestinal motility, and neurologic sensations. The use of an antiembolitic stocking or Ace wraps may minimize or prevent dependent edema and fluid shifts to third spaces. Metabolism is increased by activity within the limitations of the disability and capabilities of the child. High-protein, high-calorie foods are encouraged for correction of negative nitrogen balance, which may be difficult to correct by diet, especially if there is loss of appetite. Stimulating the appetite with small servings of attractively arranged, preferred foods may be sufficient (see Feeding the Sick Child, Ch. 42). Sometimes supplementary nasogastric feedings, gastrostomy feedings, or total parenteral nutrition may be needed.*

Nursing ALERT

Lying in a prone position during feeding increases the risk of aspiration. Therefore suction is kept nearby.

Adequate hydration promotes bowel and kidney function and helps prevent complications in these systems. It is also a primary measure for managing hypercalcemia, in addition to restricting high-calcium foods.

Children are encouraged to be as active as their condition and restrictive devices allow. This poses few problems for children, whose innate ingenuity and natural inclination toward mobility provide them with the impetus for physical activity.

*Home care instructions on giving nasogastric tube feedings and gastrostomy tube feedings are available in Wong DL: *Wong and Whaley's clinical manual of pediatric nursing*, ed 4, St Louis, 1996, Mosby.

They need the opportunity, the materials or objects to stimulate activity, and the encouragement and participation of others. Those who are unable to move need passive exercise and movement.

Whenever possible, transporting the child by stretcher, stroller, or wagon outside the confines of the room increases environmental stimuli and provides social contact with others. While hospitalized, children benefit from frequent visitors, clocks and calendars, and a program of diversional therapy, all of which help them function in a more normal way. As soon as possible they should wear "street clothes" and resume school and preinjury hobbies. The use of play (see Chapter 41) and any activity that is tolerated (e.g., turning in bed or changing the position of a bed in the room) help to alter the monotony of immobilization and decrease tension and frustration.

Using dolls to illustrate and explain the restraining method is a valuable tool for small children. Placing a cast, tubing, or other restraining equipment on the doll offers the child a nonthreatening opportunity to express, through the doll, feelings concerning the restrictions and feelings toward the nurse and other health providers. It also provides a means for anticipatory teaching and explanation of needed restraining devices.

One of the most useful interventions to help children cope with immobility is participation in their own care. Self-care to the maximum extent is usually well received by children. They can help plan their daily routine, select their diet (when possible), and choose the clothes they are to wear, including innovative adornment, such as a baseball cap, brightly colored stockings, or other items of apparel that express each child's autonomy and individuality. They are encouraged to do as much for themselves as they are able in order to keep muscles active and their interest alive. If feasible, they should be placed where they can benefit from the company of other children who are immobilized, to assure them that they are not singled out for this treatment.

It is important for children to understand behavioral limitations or rules, and their questions should be answered. For example, they need to know the reasons for medical, nursing, occupational, and physical therapy and to understand that schedules are necessary. In some areas they have a choice; in others they do not. They may or may not be permitted to sleep late, but they can choose their own clothing. Most of children's activity of daily living is play; therefore therapies that incorporate this concept are more likely to gain their cooperation.

Visits from significant persons, such as family members and friends, offer occasions for emotional support and also provide opportunities for learning how to care for the child. Some privacy is needed, particularly by the teenager, and most long-term health care facilities recognize that rooms shared by two to four youngsters are better environments for habilitation or rehabilitation than large wards. Selecting roommates according to age and companionship gives each child the chance to test out thoughts and feelings safely with others. If a traumatic incident caused the child's disability, guilt feelings may be displayed overtly or masked behind regressive or aggressive behavior. The feeling that "I must have been bad for this to happen" is common, and honest feedback stating, "It just happened—it was an accident," needs to be repeated many times.

For a child with greatly restricted movement (e.g., the quadriplegic child or the child with a large bilateral hip spica cast), nursing care is a challenge. These situations require long-term care either in the hospital or at home; wherever the care occurs, consistent planning and coordination of activities with professionals and significant others are vital nursing functions.

Family support and home care. The needs of a child with severe disabilities can be very complex, and family members require time to assimilate the teachings and demonstrations needed to understand the child's situation and care. Even the child who is confined on a short-term basis can be a challenge for the family, who are usually unprepared for the problems imposed by the child's special needs. Home modification is usually required for facilitating care, especially when it involves traction, large casts, or extended confinement. Suitable child care may be needed for times when all family members work.

Just as in the hospital, the child at home is encouraged to be as independent as possible and to follow a schedule that approximates his or her normal life-style as nearly as possible, such as continuing school lessons, regular bedtime, and suitable recreational activities.

Evaluation

The effectiveness of nursing interventions is determined by continual reassessment and evaluation of care based on the following observational guidelines and expected outcomes:

1. Observe vital signs, neurologic signs, and respiratory, gastrointestinal, and renal functioning; inspect skin; observe effects of correct functioning of equipment and appliances (restraints, traction, cast, braces).
2. Observe child's behavior; engage in dialogue to elicit feelings, concerns, and interests.
3. Observe child's activities and interests.
4. Interview child and family regarding their feelings and concerns; observe family interaction at home, if possible.

Expected outcomes:

See the Nursing Care Plan on p. 1710.

Traumatic Injury

SOFT TISSUE INJURY

Injuries to the muscles, ligaments, and tendons are common in children (Fig. 51-1). In young children soft tissue injury usually results from mishaps during play. In older children and adolescents, participation in sports is the more common cause.

Contusions

A contusion is damage to the soft tissue, subcutaneous structures, and muscle. The tearing of these tissues and small blood vessels and the inflammatory response lead to hemorrhage, edema, and associated pain when the child attempts to move the injured part. The escape of blood into the tissues is observed as **ecchymosis,** a black-and-blue discoloration. Immediate treatment consists of cold application, as in the treat-

Nursing Care Plan

THE CHILD WHO IS IMMOBILIZED

Nursing Diagnosis: Impaired physical mobility related to mechanical restrictions, physical disability

Expected Outcome: Child engages in activities appropriate to physical limitations.

• NURSING INTERVENTIONS/*RATIONALES*

Arrange for appropriate transport (i.e., wheelchair, stretcher, crutches, stroller) *to maintain mobility;* plan trips outside confines of room *to prevent isolation.*

Rearrange furniture in room when child is confined for long term *to break monotony and provide variety.*

Encourage mobility, freedom of movement, independence in activities of daily living and play within physical limits *to maintain sense of autonomy and control.*

Encourage child to make choices about daily routine, food, clothing, play within physical limits *to maintain sense of control.*

Nursing Diagnosis: Risk for impaired skin integrity related to immobility, therapeutic devices

Expected Outcome: Skin is clean, dry, and intact.

• NURSING INTERVENTIONS/*RATIONALES*

Turn and reposition every 2 hours *to promote circulation and prevent skin breakdown* (align properly, provide positional supports; use handrolls or splints *to position hands in functional position;* use footboard or hightop tennis shoes *to prevent footdrop*); perform passive range of motion frequently *to maintain full range in all joints and prevent contracture formation;* seat child in chair *to improve circulation;* place on tilt table *to prevent loss of bone density to long bones.*

Use pressure reduction mattress overlay *to prevent pressure necrosis;* use foam pads on ankles, heels, elbows *to protect bony prominences;* massage skin with lotion regularly *to stimulate circulation and prevent friction and shearing effects;* keep bedclothes clean, dry, and wrinkle-free *to prevent skin irritation;* cleanse skin, mucous membranes of mouth and perianal area regularly *to prevent irritation and breakdown;* keep skinfolds clean and dry *to prevent excoriation;* inspect skin, mucous membranes, corneas regularly *to assess for early signs of irritation or breakdown.*

Nursing Diagnosis: Risk for injury related to impaired mobility

Expected Outcome: Child exhibits no evidence of injury.

• NURSING INTERVENTIONS/*RATIONALES*

Promote and teach child and family proper transfer techniques, use of mobilizing devices (i.e., wheelchairs, crutches, walkers, braces) *to enhance safety.*

Modify environment as appropriate (i.e., place call bell in easy reach, remove hazards and barriers, clear traffic areas) *to enhance safety.*

Nursing Diagnosis: Diversional activity deficit related to mobility impairment and confinement

Expected Outcome: Child engages in activities that are developmentally appropriate and within physical and environmental limitations.

• NURSING INTERVENTIONS/*RATIONALES*

Schedule therapies and rest periods *to allow time for play activities.* Time play periods when child may be feeling particularly vulnerable or alone *to provide needed distraction.*

Arrange for social interactions with others *to promote socialization.*

Interview parents and child to discover the child's favorite activities and games; adapt activities to the child's physical limitations *to provide optimal diversions.*

Have parents bring in treasured toys or objects; decorate room with familiar pictures and drawings *to familiarize child with an unfamiliar environment.*

---

ment of sprains described below. Return to participation is allowed when the strength and range of motion of the affected extremity are equal to those of the opposite extremity.

Related to contusions are crush injuries that occur in children when they slam their fingers (in doors, folding chairs, or equipment) or hit their fingers (as when hammering a nail). A severe crush injury involves the bone, with swelling and bleeding beneath the nail (subungual) and sometimes laceration of the pulp of the distal phalanx. The subungual hematoma can be released by drilling holes at the proximal end of the nail. The time-honored method of applying a heated paper clip or needle to melt or puncture a small hole in the nail is highly effective and causes few problems. However, any procedure should be performed with aseptic technique. If the bone is fractured, any communication with the skin essentially renders it an open fracture.

Dislocations

Long bones are held in approximation to one another at the joint by ligaments. A dislocation occurs when the force of stress on the ligament is so great as to displace the normal position of the opposing bone ends or the bone end to its socket. The predominant symptom is pain that increases with attempted passive or active movement of the extremity. In dislocations there may be an obvious deformity and inability to move the joint. Temporary restriction of the joint, such as a

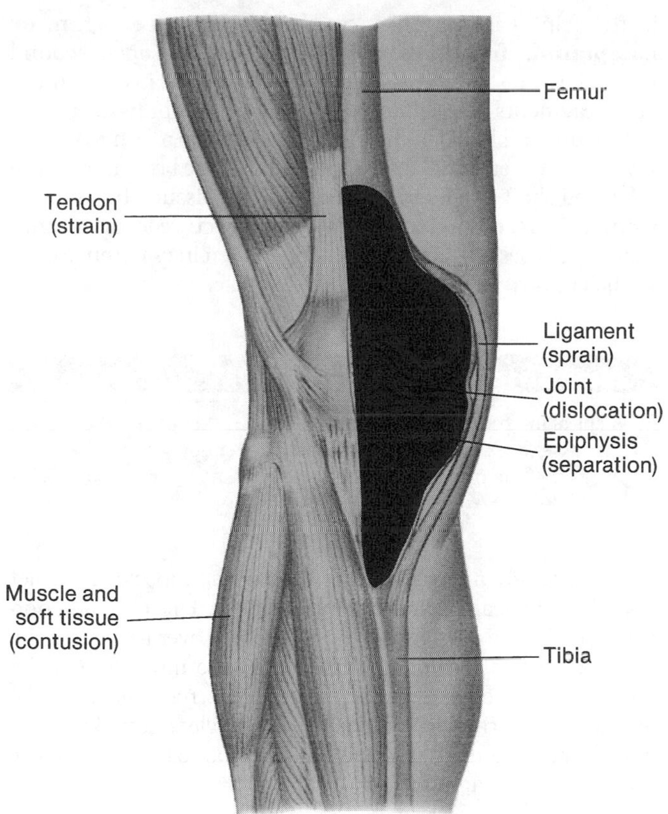

Fig. 51-1 Sites of injuries to bones, joints, and soft tissues.

sling or bandage that secures the arm to the chest in a shoulder dislocation, provides sufficient comfort and immobilization until the child can receive medical help.

Simple dislocations should be reduced as soon as possible with the child under conscious sedation and often local anesthesia. Anesthetics, such as nitrous oxide, parenteral or oral ketamine, or intravenous propofol, can be used to produce partial or complete analgesia (Bostrom, McCormick, and Hooke, 1993; Tobias et al, 1992; Wattenmaker, Kasser, and McGravey, 1990). An unreduced dislocation will be complicated by increased swelling, making reduction difficult and increasing the risk of neurovascular problems. Reduction is accomplished by simple traction and slight flexion, followed by immobilization in a splint for 10 to 16 days or up to 3 weeks or more for healing of torn ligaments.

Sprains

A sprain occurs when trauma to a joint is so severe that a ligament is partially or completely torn or stretched by the force created as a joint is twisted or wrenched, often accompanied by damage to associated blood vessels, muscles, tendons, and nerves.

The presence of joint laxity is the most valid indicator of the severity of a sprain. In a severe injury the child complains of the joint's "feeling loose" or as if "something is coming apart" and may describe hearing a "snap," "pop," or "tearing." Pain is seldom the principal subjective symptom. There is a rapid onset with swelling, often diffuse, accompanied by immediate disability and appreciable reluctance to use the injured joint.

Strains

A strain is a microscopic tear to the musculotendinous unit and has features in common with sprains. The area is painful to touch and swollen. Most strains are incurred over time rather than suddenly, and the rapidity of the appearance provides clues regarding severity. In general the more rapidly the strain occurs, the more severe the injury. When the strain involves the muscular portion, there is more bleeding, often palpable soon after injury and before edema obscures the hematoma.

Therapeutic Management

The first 6 to 12 hours is the most critical period for virtually all soft tissue injuries. Basic principles of managing sprains and other soft tissue injuries are summarized in the acronyms RICE or ICES:

R—rest	**I**—ice
I—ice	**C**—compression
C—compression	**E**—elevation
E—elevation	**S**—support

Soft tissue injuries should be iced immediately. This is best accomplished with crushed ice wrapped in a towel or encased in a screw-top ice bag or resealable storage bag. Another method is to use a plastic bag of frozen vegetables, such as peas, as a convenient ice pack. It is clean, watertight, and easily molded to the injured part. When available, snow placed in a plastic bag works well also. A wet elastic wrap, which transfers cold better than dry wrap, is applied to provide compression and to keep the ice pack in place. Ice has a rapid cooling effect on tissues that reduces the pain threshold. However, ice should never be applied for more than 30 minutes at a time.

Elevating the extremity uses gravity to facilitate venous return and reduce edema formation in the damaged area. The point of injury should be kept several inches above the level of the heart for therapy to be effectve. Several pillows can be used effectively for elevation. Allowing the extremity to be dependent causes excessive fluid accumulation in the area of injury, delaying healing and causing painful swelling.

Torn ligaments, especially those in the knee, are usually treated by immobilization with a cast for 3 to 4 weeks or strapping of the joint with adhesive or Elastoplast bandage. Passive leg exercises, gradually increased to active exercises, are begun as soon as sufficient healing has taken place. Parents and children are cautioned against using any form of liniment or other heat-producing preparation before examination. If the injury requires casting or splinting, the heat generated in the enclosed space can cause extreme discomfort and may even cause tissue damage.

FRACTURES

Bones fracture when the resistance of bone against the stress being exerted yields to the stress force. Fractures are a common injury at any age but are more likely to occur in children and older adults. Because of the characteristics of the child's skeleton, the pattern of fractures, problems of diagnosis, and methods of treatment differ in the child and the adult.

Fracture injuries in children are a result of traumatic incidents at home, at school, in a motor vehicle, or in association with recreational activities. Children's everyday activities include vigorous play that predisposes them to injury—climbing, falling down, running into immovable objects, and receiving blows to any part of their bodies.

Aside from automobile accidents true injuries that cause fractures rarely occur in infancy; therefore bone injury in children of that age group warrants further investigation. In any small child radiographic evidence of fractures at various stages of healing are, with few exceptions, the result of physical abuse. Fractures in school-age children are often the result of bicycle-automobile or skateboard injuries. Adolescents are vulnerable to multiple and severe trauma, because they are mobile on bikes, on motorcycles, and in active sports. Speed and congested surroundings often intensify the impact. Young children and teenagers usually do not calculate risks as they learn to manipulate their environment and achieve developmental goals. Therefore injuries are a part of most childhood experience.

Types of Fractures

A fractured bone consists of fragments—the fragment closer to the midline, or the proximal fragment, and the fragment farther from the midline, or the distal fragment. When fracture fragments are separated, the fracture is *complete;* when fragments remain attached, the fracture is *incomplete.* The fracture line can be any of the following:

Transverse—crosswise, at right angles to the long axis of the bone
Oblique—slanting but straight, between a horizontal and a perpendicular direction
Spiral—slanting and circular, twisting around the bone shaft

The twisting of an extremity while the bone is breaking results in a spiral break. If the fracture does not produce a break in the skin, it is a **simple, or closed, fracture. Open, or compound, fractures** are those with an open wound through which the bone is protruding or has protruded. If the bone fragments cause damage to other organs or tissues (such as the lung or bladder), the injury is said to be a **complicated fracture.** When small fragments of bone are broken from the fractured shaft and lie in the surrounding tissue, the injury is a **comminuted fracture.** This type of fracture is rare in children. The types of fractures seen most often in children are described in Box 51-1 and in Fig. 51-2.

Nursing ALERT

A spiral fracture in children may indicate child abuse. Further assessment and immediate involvement of interdisciplinary team members, such as a social worker, are necessary.

Immediately after a fracture occurs the muscles contract and physiologically splint the injured area. This phenomenon accounts for the muscle tightness observed over a fracture site and the deformity that is produced as the muscles pull the bone ends out of alignment. This muscle response must be overcome by traction or complete muscle relaxation (i.e., anesthesia) in order to realign the distal bone fragment to the proximal bone fragment.

Bone Healing and Remodeling

Bone healing is characteristically rapid in children because of the thickened periosteum and generous blood supply. When there is a break in the continuity of bone, the osteoblasts are

BOX 51-1
Types of Fractures in Children

Bends—occurs when the bone is bent but not broken. A child's flexible bone can be bent 45 degrees or more before breaking. However, if bent, the bone will straighten slowly, but not completely, to produce some deformity but without the angulation seen when the bone breaks. Bends occur most commonly in the ulna and fibula, often in association with fractures of the radius and tibia.

Buckle, or torus, fracture—produced by compression of the porous bone; appears as a raised or bulging projection at the fracture site. These fractures occur in the most porous portion of the bone near the metaphysis (the portion of the bone shaft adjacent to the epiphysis) and are more common in young children.

Green-stick fracture—occurs when a bone is angulated beyond the limits of bending. The compressed side bends, and the tension side fails, causing an incomplete fracture similar to the break observed when a green stick is broken.

Complete fracture—divides the bone fragments. These fragments often remain attached by a periosteal hinge, which can aid or hinder reduction.

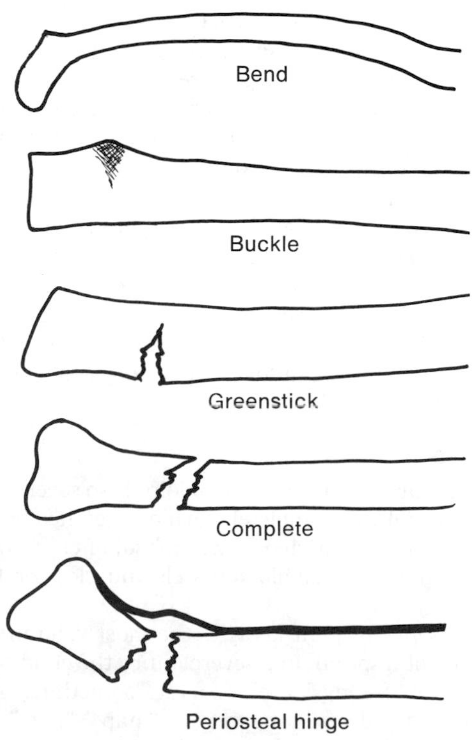

Fig. 51-2 Types of fractures in children.

stimulated to maximum activity. New bone cells are formed in immense numbers almost immediately after the injury and, in time, are evidenced by a bulging growth of new bone tissue between the fractured bone fragments. This is followed by deposition of calcium salts to form a *callus*.

Fractures heal in less time in children than in adults. The approximate healing times for a femoral shaft are:

- Neonatal period—2 to 3 weeks
- Early childhood—4 weeks
- Later childhood—6 to 8 weeks
- Adolescence—8 to 12 weeks

Diagnostic Evaluation

A history is often lacking in childhood injuries. Infants are unable to communicate, and older children seldom volunteer information (even under direct questioning) when the injury occurred during forbidden activities. Unless they are witnesses to the injury, parents may misinterpret what the child is trying to say. In cases of child abuse, parents may give false information to protect themselves.

The child exhibits the same manifestations seen in adults (Box 51-2). However, often a fracture is remarkably stable because of intact periosteum. The child may even be able to use an affected arm or walk on a fractured leg.

Nursing ALERT

A fracture should be strongly suspected when a small child refuses to walk or move an upper extremity.

Radiographic examination is the most useful diagnostic tool for assessing skeletal trauma. The calcium deposits in bone make the entire structure radiopaque. Radiographic films are taken after fracture reduction and, in some cases, may be taken during the healing process to determine satisfactory progress.

Therapeutic Management

The majority of children's fractures heal well, and nonunion is rare. Most fractures are readily reduced by simple traction and immobilization until healing takes place. However, the position of the bone fragments in relation to one another influences the rapidity of healing and the residual deformity. Healing is prompt and complete with end-to-end apposition, but a gap between fragments delays (or prevents) healing. The goals of fracture management are:

1. To regain alignment and length of the bony fragments (reduction)
2. To retain alignment and length (immobilization)
3. To restore function to the injured parts

In children the bone fragments are usually realigned and immobilized by traction or by closed manipulation and casting until adequate callus is formed. Weight bearing on lower extremity fractures and active movement for the purpose of regaining function can begin after the fracture site is stable. The child's natural tendency to be active is usually sufficient to restore normal mobility, and physical therapy is rarely needed. In most cases children's fractures can be managed by closed reduction and plaster immobilization, most often provided on an outpatient basis with reevaluation in 7 to 10 days.

Children are most frequently hospitalized for fractures of the femur and the supracondylar area of the distal humerus. If simple reductions cannot be achieved or if a neurovascular problem is detected after injury, observation in a hospital is indicated. Severe contusions with profound swelling cannot be treated with a cast, which would act as a tourniquet on the extremity. A badly malaligned fracture requires traction for a time before a cast is applied.

The major methods for immobilizing a fracture, casting and traction, are described in the following section in relation to the nursing care involved.

Nursing Care Management

Nurses are frequently the persons who make the initial assessment of a child with a suspected fracture (see the Emergency box below). The child and parents are frightened and upset, the child is in pain, and since most fractures are obvi-

BOX 51-2
Clinical Manifestations of a Fracture

Signs of injury
- Generalized swelling
- Pain or tenderness
- Diminished functional use of affected part

May be
- Bruising
- Severe muscular rigidity
- Crepitus (grating sensation at fracture site)

EMERGENCY

FRACTURE

Assess extent of injury—5 "P's":
- *P*ain and point of tenderness
- *P*ulse—distal to the fracture site
- *P*allor
- *P*aresthesia—sensation distal to the fracture site
- *P*aralysis–movement distal to the fracture site

Determine the mechanism of injury.
Move injured part as little as possible.
Cover open wounds with sterile or clean dressing.
Immobilize the limb, including joints above and below the fracture site; do not attempt to reduce fracture or push protruding bone under the skin.
- Soft splint (pillow or folded towel)
- Rigid splint (rolled newspaper or magazine)
- Uninjured leg can serve as splint for leg fracture if no splint available.

Reassess neurovascular status.
Apply traction if circulatory compromise is present.
Elevate the injured limb if possible.
Apply cold to the injured area.
Call emergency medical service or transport to medical facility

ous, the parents and (frequently) the child are already convinced of the diagnosis. Therefore if the child is alert and there is no evidence of hemorrhage, the initial nursing interventions are directed toward calming and reassuring the child and parents so that a more extensive assessment can be more easily accomplished.

While remaining calm and speaking in a quiet voice, the nurse can ask the parents and older child to describe what happened and how they feel about it. Since the child usually arrives with the limb supported in some manner, this time does not delay or endanger the treatment. Initially it is best not to touch the child but to ask him or her to point to the painful area and to wiggle the fingers or toes. By this time the child usually feels relatively safe and will allow someone to gently touch the area just enough to feel the pulse and test for sensation. A child's anxiety is greatly influenced by previous experiences with injury and with health personnel. However, he or she needs to be told what will happen and what to do to help. The affected limb need not be palpated, and it should not be moved unless properly splinted. If the child is at home or if the practitioner is not present to examine the child, some type of splint is applied carefully for transport to the medical facility.

THE CHILD IN A CAST

The completeness of the fracture, the type of bone involved, and the amount of weight bearing influence how much of the extremity must be included in the cast to immobilize the fracture site completely. In most cases the joints above and below the fracture are immobilized to eliminate the possibility of movement that might cause displacement at the fracture site. Four major categories of casts are used for fractures: *upper extremity* to immobilize the wrist and/or elbow, *lower extremity* to immobilize the ankle and/or knee, *spinal* and *cervical* to immobilize the spine, and *spica casts* to immobilize the hip and knee.

The Cast

When a cast is to be applied, the nurse often must set up the cast materials and hold the extremity in alignment. In most instances only the cast material is required; however, special cast tables that hold the child's body are used for applying large hip spica casts. If possible children should be allowed to play with a doll that has a cast so that they understand what will be done.

Before the cast is applied, the extremities are checked for any abrasions, cuts, or other alterations in the skin surface and for the presence of rings or other items that may cause constriction from swelling; such objects are removed. Identification bands are placed on a noninjured extremity if hospitalization is anticipated.

Casts are constructed from gauze strips and bandages impregnated with plaster of paris or, more commonly, from synthetic lighter-weight and water-resistant materials (e.g., fiberglass and polyurethane resin). With plaster of paris, a heat-producing chemical reaction occurs between the plaster and water as the plaster becomes a crystalline gypsum; the drying process takes 10 to 72 hours, depending on the size of the cast. Synthetic materials dry in 5 to 30 minutes, depending on the type of cast.

A tube of stockinette is stretched over the area to be casted, and bony prominences are padded with soft cotton sheeting. Dry rolls of casting material are immersed in a pail of water. The wet rolls are put on in a bandage fashion and molded to the extremity. During application the underlying stockinette is pulled over the raw edges of the cast and secured with a layer of wet plaster ½ to 1 inch below the rim to form a smooth, padded edge to protect the skin.

If the operator does not form such a protective edge with stockinette, the raw edges of the cast can be protected by a "petaled" edge. Small pieces approximately 2 to 3 inches long are cut from 1- or 1½-inch-wide adhesive tape. The edges are rounded with scissors, and these "petals" are placed over the edge of the cast, with each petal slightly overlapping the previous petal to form a smooth, neat edge. It is easier to apply the petal to the underside of the cast first and then draw the unadhered edge to the front, pressing firmly so that the edges remain securely attached. Adhesive bandages can be used instead of the tape petals for quicker preparation and a slightly padded cast edge.

Nursing Care Management

The complete evaporation of the water from a hip spica cast can take 24 to 48 hours when older types of plaster materials are used. Drying occurs within minutes with new quick-drying substances. The cast must remain uncovered to allow it to dry from the inside out. Turning the child in a plaster cast at least every 2 hours will help dry a body cast evenly and prevent complications related to immobility. A regular fan or cool-air hairdryer to circulate air may be helpful when the humidity is high.

Nursing ALERT

Heated fans or dryers are not used, since they cause the cast to dry on the outside and remain wet beneath or cause burns from heat conduction by way of the cast to the underlying tissue.

A wet cast should be supported by a pillow that is covered with plastic and handled by the palms of the hands to prevent indentation of the cast, which can create pressure areas. A dry plaster of paris cast produces a hollow sound when it is tapped with the finger. If "hot spots" are felt on the cast surface (usually indicating infection beneath the area), they should be reported so that a window can be made in the cast to observe the site.

During the first few hours after a cast is applied the chief concern is that the extremity may continue to swell to the extent that the cast becomes a tourniquet, shutting off circulation and producing neurovascular complications. To reduce the likelihood of this potential problem the body part can be elevated, thereby increasing venous return. If edema is excessive, casts are bivalved (i.e., cut to make anterior and posterior halves that are held together with an elastic bandage). The cast and the involved extremity are observed frequently for neurovascular integrity and signs of compromise.

Nursing ALERT

Observations such as pain, swelling, discoloration (pallor or cyanosis) of the exposed portions, lack of pulsation and warmth, or inability to move the exposed part(s) are reported immediately.

When casting an extremity that has sustained an open fracture, a window is often left over the wound area to allow observation and dressing of the wound. A surgical reduction is usually casted as for a closed fracture. For the first few hours after surgery there may be substantial bleeding that will soak through the cast. Periodically the circumscribed blood-stained area should be outlined with a ballpoint pen or pencil, and the time indicated to provide a guide for assessing the amount of bleeding.

Usually the child is discharged to home care after a cast is applied in the emergency room or clinic. Parents need instructions on drying and caring for the cast and checking for signs and symptoms that indicate the cast is too tight (see the Home Care box below). They should also be told to take the child to the health professional for attention if the cast becomes too loose, since a loose cast no longer serves its purpose. A cast is a badge of honor for the child and serves as visible evidence of an otherwise invisible injury.

Home Care

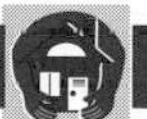

CAST CARE

Keep the casted extremity elevated on pillows or similar support for the first day, or as directed by the health professional.

Avoid indenting the cast while still wet to prevent creation of pressure points.

Observe the extremities (fingers or toes) for any evidence of swelling or discoloration (darker or lighter than a comparable extremity) and contact the health professional if noted.

Check movement and sensation of the visible extremities frequently.

Follow health professional's orders regarding any restriction of activities.

Restrict strenuous activities for the first few days.
- Engage in quiet activities but encourage use of muscles.
- Move the joints above and below the cast on the affected extremity.

Encourage frequent rest for a few days, keeping the injured extremity elevated while resting.

Avoid allowing the affected limb to hang down for any length of time.
- Keep an injured upper extremity elevated (e.g., in a sling) while upright.
- Elevate a lower limb when sitting and avoid standing for too long.

Do not allow the child to put anything inside the cast.
- Keep small items that might be placed inside the cast away from small children

Keep a clear path for ambulation.
- Remove toys, hazardous floor rugs, pets, or other items over which the child might stumble.

Use crutches appropriately if lower limb fracture.
- The crutches should fit properly, have a soft rubber tip to prevent slipping, and be well padded at the axilla.

Cast removal. Cutting the cast to remove it or to relieve tightness is frequently a frightening experience for children. They fear the sound of the cast cutter and are terrified that their flesh, as well as the cast, will be cut. Since it works by vibration, the cast cutter cuts only the hard surface of the cast. This can be demonstrated on the nurse or person removing the cast. The oscillating blade vibrates very rapidly back and forth and will not cut when placed lightly on the skin. Children have described it as producing a "tickly" sensation. The vibration also generates heat that may be felt by the child. Both these feelings should be explained.

Preparation for the procedure will help reduce anxiety, especially if a trusting relationship has been established between the child and the nurse. Many young children come to regard the cast as part of themselves, intensifying their fear of removal (Fig. 51-3). Using the analogy of having fingernails or hair cut sometimes helps reduce their anxiety. They need continual reassurance that all is going well and that their behavior is accepted.

Nurses can help families adapt the child's home environment to meet the temporary encumbrance of a cast. Home care creates problems of various magnitude, especially for children in large casts (e.g., a hip spica). Commonplace situations become problematic, (e.g., returning the child home safely and comfortably). Standard seat belts and car seats are not readily adapted for use by children in casts (see p. 1725 and Fig. 51-15). Sitting can be impossible in a spica cast, and leg casts require extra space.

Children in spica casts usually find the prone position easier for self-feeding from a small table placed next to the dining

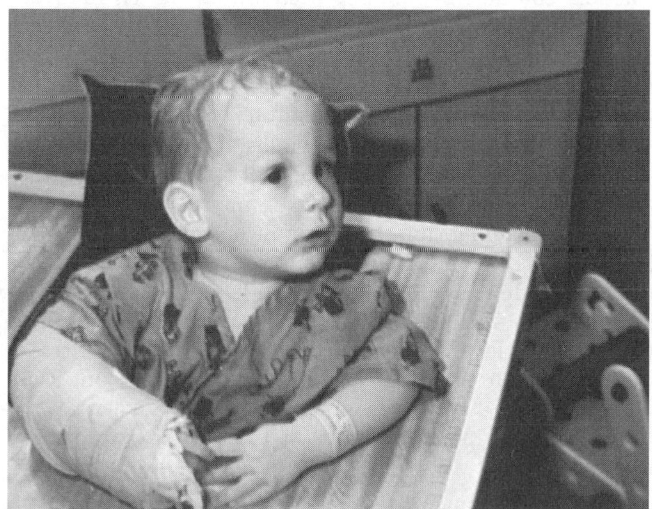

Fig. 51-3 Young children come to regard a cast as part of their body. They usually adapt well but may fear its removal. (Courtesy St. Louis Children's Hospital.)

table. The use of a conventional toilet is almost impossible. Small bedpans or other containers offer alternatives for elimination. The nurse may suggest waterproofing methods, by devising plastic wraps, for elimination and showers. Baths are possible only if the plaster cast is kept out of the water and covered to prevent it from becoming wet from splashes. Synthetic casts can be immersed in water if a special type of cast liner is used.

After the cast is removed, the skin surface will be caked with desquamated skin and sebaceous secretions. Simple soaking in a bathtub is usually sufficient for their removal, but a period of several days may be required to eliminate the accumulation completely. Application of olive oil or lotion may provide comfort. The parents and child should be instructed not to pull or forcibly remove this material with vigorous scrubbing, because it may cause excoriation and bleeding.

See also the Nursing Care Plans: The Child with a Fracture.*

THE CHILD IN TRACTION

Bone fragments that cannot be aligned initially by simple traction and stabilization with a cast require the extended pulling force by continuous traction. Traction may be used for other purposes also:

- To provide rest for an extremity
- To help prevent or improve contracture deformity
- To correct a deformity
- To treat a dislocation
- To allow preoperative or postoperative positioning and alignment
- To provide immobilization of specific areas of the body
- To reduce muscle spasms (rare in children)

In most of these cases the traction is often applied at night and intermittently during the day. Muscle relaxants may be administered for muscle spasms.

Purposes of Traction

The three essential components of traction management are traction, countertraction, and friction (Fig. 51-4). To reduce or realign a fracture site, **traction** (forward force) is produced by attaching weight to the distal bone fragment; body weight provides **countertraction** (backward force); and the patient's contact with the bed constitutes the **frictional** force. These forces are used to align the distal and proximal bone fragments by adjusting the line of pull upward or downward and adducting or abducting the extremity.

To attain equilibrium the amount of forward force is adjusted by adding weight to or subtracting weight from the traction, and/or countertraction can be increased by elevating the foot of the bed to create a greater gravitational pull to the backward force. A bed board placed under the mattress of heavy children prevents sagging, which might otherwise change the direction of the forces applied to the fracture.

The three primary purposes of traction for reduction of fractures are:

1. To fatigue the involved muscle and reduce muscle spasm so that bones can be realigned
2. To position the distal and proximal bone ends in desired realignment to promote satisfactory bone healing
3. To immobilize the fracture site until realignment has been achieved and sufficient healing has taken place to permit casting or splinting

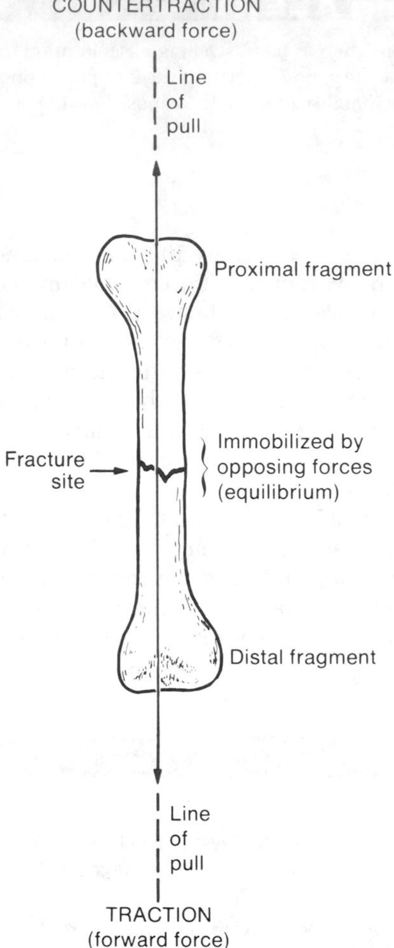

Fig. 51-4 Application of traction for maintaining equilibrium.

The *all-or-none law,* characteristic of muscle contractability, influences the complete relaxation. When muscle is stretched, muscle spasm ceases and permits the realignment of the bone ends. The continuous maintenance of traction is important during this phase because releasing the traction allows the normal contracting ability of the muscle to again cause a malpositioning of the bone ends.

The realignment of the fragments is a gradual process that is achieved more rapidly in infants, who have limited muscle tone, than in muscular teenagers. The desired line of pull and callus formation are checked periodically by radiographic examination. The traction pull to some degree immobilizes the fracture site; however, adjunctive immobilizing devices such as splints or casts are sometimes used with skeletal traction. In injuries in which there is severe soft tissue swelling or vascular and nerve damage, it is customary to use traction until these complications have been resolved and it is safe to apply

*In Wong DL: *Wong and Whaley's clinical manual of pediatric nursing,* ed 4, St Louis, 1996, Mosby.

BOX 51-3
Types of Traction

Manual traction—applied to the body part by the hand placed distally to the fracture site. Nurses frequently provide manual traction during cast application.

Skin traction—applied directly to the skin surface and indirectly to the skeletal structures. The pulling mechanism is attached to the skin with adhesive material or an elastic bandage. Both types are applied over soft, foam-backed traction straps to distribute the traction pull.

Skeletal traction—applied directly to the skeletal structure by a pin, wire, or tongs inserted into or through the diameter of the bone distal to the fracture.

a cast. Immobilization with traction will be maintained until the bone ends are in satisfactory realignment, after which a less-confining type of immobilization, usually a cast, will be applied.

Types of Traction (General)

The pull needed for traction can be applied to the distal bone fragment in several ways (Box 51-3). **Manual traction** is used in uncomplicated arm or leg fractures in which there are little overriding of the bones and minimal muscle pull to overcome. Manual traction is used to realign bone fragments for immediate cast replication. **Skin traction** is applied when there are minimal displacement and little muscle spasticity, but it is contraindicated when there is associated skin damage. Skin traction has specific limits of weight that it can pull without causing tissue breakdown. **Skeletal traction** is used when significant traction pull must be applied to achieve realignment and immobilization. By inserting a pin or wire into the bone, the stress is placed on the bone and not on the surrounding tissue.

The type of traction applied is determined primarily by the age of the child, the condition of the soft tissues, and the type and degree of displacement of the fracture. Fractures most commonly treated by application of traction are those involving the humerus, femur, and vertebrae. The major types of traction for specific fractures are discussed in the following sections.

Upper Extremity Traction

Treatment of fractures of the humerus by traction is accomplished by (1) overhead suspension, in which the arm, bent at the elbow, is suspended vertically by skin or skeletal attachment and traction is applied to the distal end of the humerus, or (2) Dunlop traction. With *Dunlop traction* (Fig. 51-5), the arm is suspended horizontally, using either skin or skeletal attachment. A skeletal wire placed in the upper arm to allow additional weight may be applied in certain instances, such as a supracondylar fracture. When skin traction is used, straps are placed on the lower and upper arm with the arm flexed to accomplish pull in two directions: one along the longitudinal direction of the upper arm and one to maintain vertical alignment of the lower arm.

Fractures of the humerus, which usually result from a fall with the arm in extension, frequently involve the supracondylar portion. These fractures especially place the patient at risk for nerve damage and angulation deformities; therefore they must be reduced carefully, sometimes with the patient under anesthesia. Because of the danger of complications, children with closed reduction of supracondylar fractures are often hospitalized for observation. In severely malaligned fractures, closed reduction with the patient under anesthesia is followed by application of skeletal traction for 2 to 3 weeks, after which a long arm cast is applied for an additional 2 to 3 weeks.

Lower Extremity Traction

The severity of the fracturing force and the ability of the muscles to hold the fracture out of alignment will determine the degree of bone fragment displacement. A fracture in the middle third of the shaft results in significant overriding but minimal displacement. In a fracture in the lower one third of the shaft, the pull of the gastrocnemius muscle causes the distal fragments to become downwardly displaced.

Fractures of the femur can often be reduced with immediate application of a hip spica cast in young children. When traction is required, several types may be used, depending on the initial assessment.

Bryant traction, a type of running traction in which the pull is only in one direction, is not recommended because of the gravitational vascular draining of the elevated extremities, the possible tourniquet effect of the bandages, and the effect of the traction, which can trigger vasospasms and avascular necrosis.

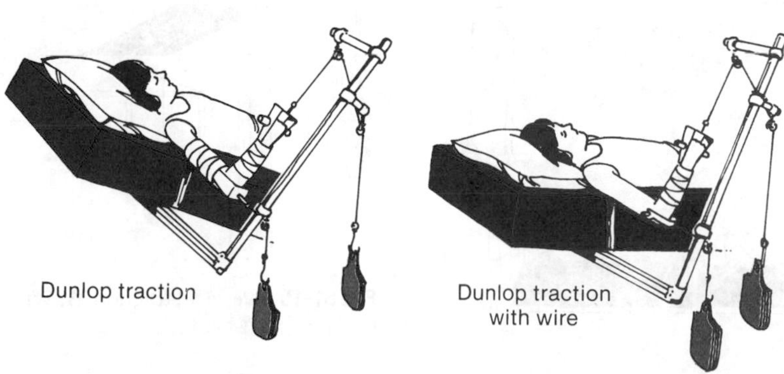

Fig. 51-5 Dunlop traction.

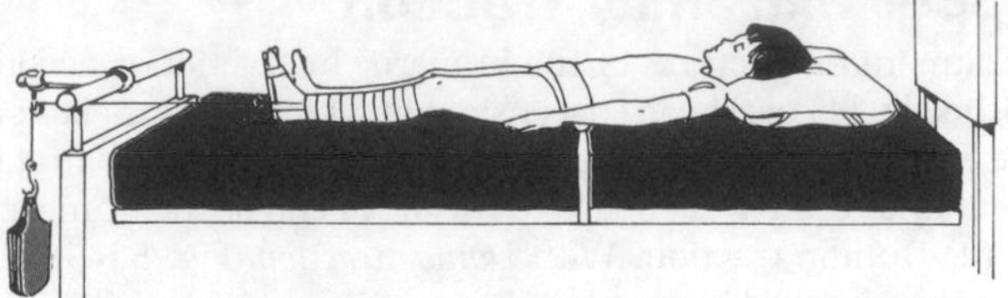

Fig. 51-6 Buck extension traction.

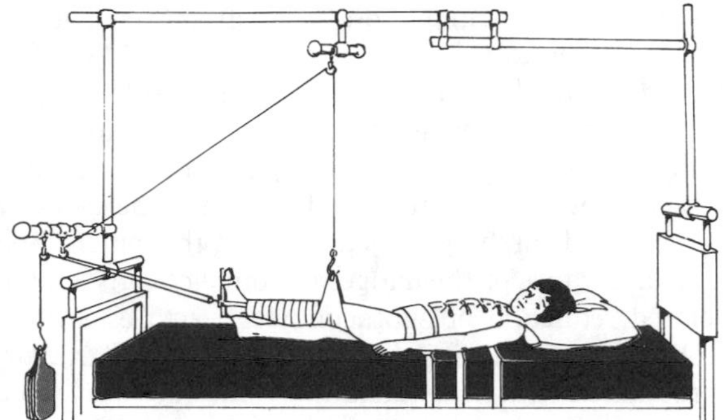

Fig. 51-7 Russell traction.

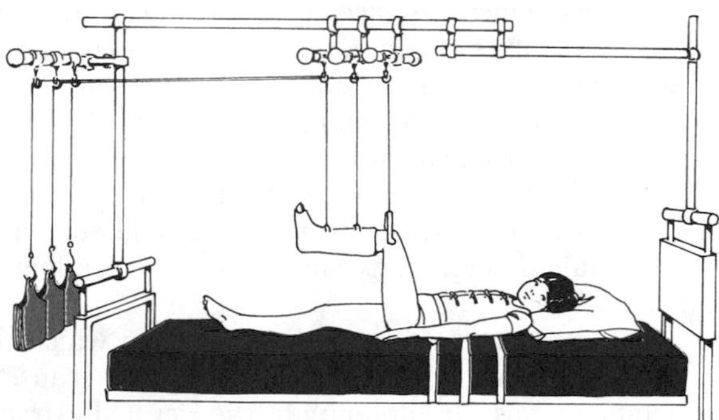

Fig. 51-8 Ninety-degree–ninety-degree traction.

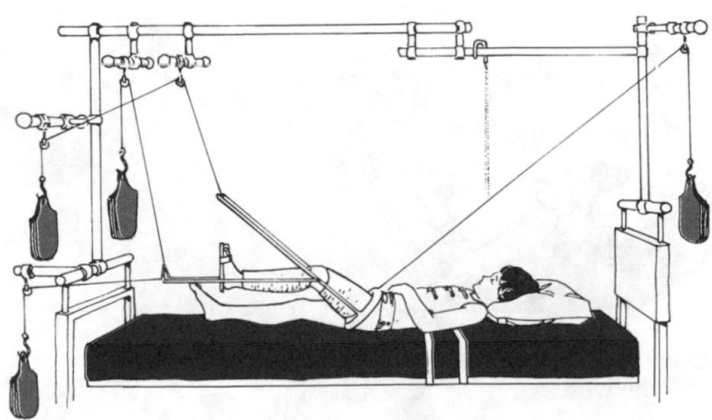

Fig. 51-9 Balance suspension with Thomas ring splint and Pearson attachment.

Buck extension (Fig. 51-6) is a type of skin traction with the legs in an extended position. Except for fracture cases, turning from side to side with care is permitted, to maintain the involved leg alignment. Buck extension is used primarily for short-term immobilization, preoperatively with dislocated hips, and in correction of contractures or bone deformities such as Legg-Calvé-Perthes disease.

Russell traction (Fig. 51-7) uses skin traction on the lower leg and a padded sling under the knee. Two lines of pull, one along the longitudinal line of the lower leg and one perpendicular to the leg, are produced. This combination of pulls allows realignment of the lower extremity and immobilizes the hip and knee in a flexed position. The hip flexion must be kept at the prescribed angle to prevent fracture malalignment, since there is no direct support under the fracture and the skin traction may slip. Special nursing measures include carefully checking the position of the traction so that the amount of desired hip flexion is maintained and damage to the common peroneal nerve under the knee does not produce footdrop. *Split-Russell traction,* in which the lines of pull are modified, is a variation of classic Russell traction.

Ninety-degree–ninety-degree traction is the most common skeletal traction (Fig. 51-8). The lower leg is put in a boot cast and a skeletal Steinmann pin or Kirschner wire is placed in the distal fragment of the femur. From a nursing standpoint this traction facilitates position changes, toileting, and prevention of traction complications.

Balance suspension traction (Fig. 51-9) may be used with or without skin or skeletal traction. Unless used with another traction, the balanced suspension merely suspends the leg in a desired flexed position to relax the hip and hamstring muscles and does not exert any traction directly on a body part. A *Thomas splint* extends from the groin to midair above the foot, and a *Pearson attachment* supports the lower leg. Towels or pieces of felt covered with stockinette are clipped or pinned to the splints for leg support. When the child is lifted off the bed, the traction lifts with the child without loss of alignment. This traction requires very careful checking of splints and ropes to make certain that no slippage or fraying has occurred. The traction is of great value in an older and heavier child when it is essential to lift the patient for care.

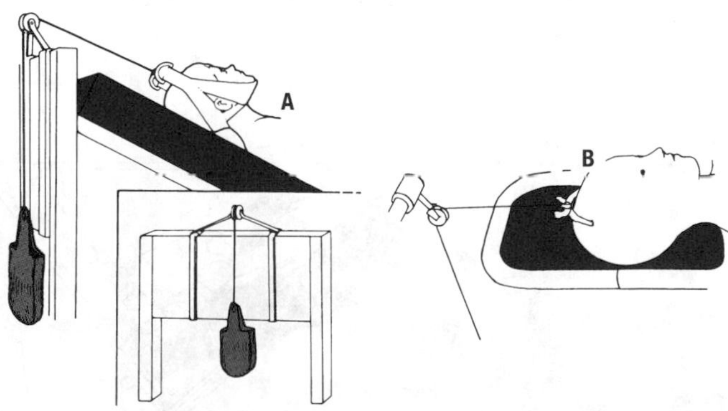

Fig. 51-10 Cervical traction. **A,** With chain strap. **B,** With Crutchfield tongs.

(Figs. 51-5 to 51-10 redrawn from Hilt NE, Schmitt EW: *Pediatric orthopedic nursing,* St Louis, 1975, Mosby.)

Cervical Traction

The cervical area is a vulnerable site for flexion or extension injuries to muscle, vertebrae, and/or the spinal cord. Cervical muscle trauma without other complications is treated with a cervical soft or hard collar to relieve the weight of the head from the fracture site. Intermittent cervical skin traction might be used with a child halter and weight to decrease muscle spasms (Fig. 51-10).

Cervical traction is usually accomplished by the insertion of *Crutchfield* or *Barton tongs* through burr holes in the skull and weights attached to the hyperextended head. As the neck muscles fatigue with constant traction pull, the vertebral bodies gradually separate so that the cord is no longer pinched between the vertebrae. Immobilization until fracture healing can occur is an essential goal of cervical traction. If the injury has been limited to a vertebral fracture without neurologic deficit, a halo cast can be applied to permit earlier ambulation.

Nursing Care Management

Generally the child in traction is hospitalized under the direct care of nurses who develop individualized nursing care plans based on an understanding of correct traction management. Evaluating the therapeutic effects and possible negative consequences is essential to good patient care. Many of the nursing problems associated with a child in traction are related to immobility. However, it is important that nurses understand the basic principles of traction and their role in its maintenance.

Guidelines

TRACTION CARE

Understand therapy

Understand purpose of traction
Understand function of traction in each specific situation

Maintain traction

Check desired line of pull and relationship of distal fragment to proximal fragment
- Check whether fragment is being directed upward, adducted, or abducted

Check function of each component
- Position of bandages, frames, splints
- Ropes: in center tract of pulley, taut, no fraying, knots tied securely
- Pulleys:
  - In original position on attachment bar; have not slid from original site
  - Wheels freely movable
- Weights:
  - Correct amount of weight
  - Hanging freely
  - In safe location

Check bed position—head or foot elevated as directed for desired amount of pull and countertraction
Do not remove skeletal traction or adhesive traction straps on skin traction

Maintain alignment

Observe for correct body alignment with emphasis on alignment of shoulder, hip, and leg
Check after child has moved
Apply restraints when indicated
Maintain correct angles at joints

Skin traction

Replace nonadhesive straps and/or elastic bandage on skin traction *when permitted* and/or absolutely necessary, but make certain that traction on limb is maintained by someone during procedure
Assess bandages to ascertain whether they are correctly applied (diagonal or spiral), neither too loose nor too tightly (which could cause slippage and malalignment of traction)

Skeletal traction

Check pin sites frequently for signs of bleeding, inflammation, or infection
Cleanse and dress pin sites as ordered
Apply topical antiseptic or antibiotic daily as ordered
Cover ends of pins with protective cord or padding to prevent child's being scratched by pin
Note pull of traction on pin; pull should be even
Check pin screws to be certain that screws are tight in metal clamp that attaches traction apparatus to pin

Prevent skin breakdown

Provide sheepskin, waffle mattress, or alternating-pressure mattress underneath hips and back
Make total body skin checks for redness or breakdown, especially over areas that receive greatest pressure; use a small hand mirror to visualize inaccessible skin areas
Wash and dry skin at least daily
Stimulate circulation with gentle massage over pressure areas
Change position at least every 2 hours to relieve pressure

Prevent complications

Check pulse in affected area and compare with pulse in contralateral site
Assess circular dressings for excessive tightness
Assess restraining devices
- Make certain that they are not too loose or too tight
- Remove periodically and check for pressure areas

Encourage deep breathing frequently with maximum inspiratory chest expansion
Note any neurovascular changes, such as:
- Color in skin and nail beds
- Alterations in sensation, increased pain
- Alterations in motor ability

Take immediate action to correct problem or report to practitioner if neurovascular changes are found
Record findings of neurovascular changes
Carry out passive, active, or active-with-resistance exercises of uninvolved joints
Note if any tightness, weakness, or contractures are developing in uninvolved joints and muscles
Take measures to correct and prevent further development of weakness, such as applying foot plate to prevent footdrop

Skeletal traction is never released by the nurse, except under certain circumstances, such as for a child with Legg-Calvé-Perthes disease or scoliosis. The nurse may remove nonadhesive skin traction. In these cases intermittent traction is periodically released and reapplied as ordered. When skin traction must be constantly maintained, as in fractures, nurses may occasionally remove and reapply the elastic bandage if this is approved by the practitioner, provided that *someone manually maintains the traction during the rewrapping process.* It is not uncommon for a child to have several types of traction at one time, and each traction must be assessed separately to prevent problems.

When the child is first placed in traction, an increase in discomfort is common as a result of the traction pull fatiguing the muscle. It has been determined that orthopedic conditions are associated with a higher-than-average number of painful events and a higher percentage of bodily symptoms than other common conditions (Wong and Baker, 1988). Analgesics, including opioids, and muscle relaxants help during this phase of care and should be administered liberally. Children are given an explanation at their level of understanding about what is happening and why they must remain in the device. Children are reassured of the presence of someone who will aid them in adjusting to the traction and coping with the problems of immobilization.

The specific nursing responsibilities for the patient in traction are outlined in the Guidelines box on p. 1719.

DISTRACTION

Unlike traction, which helps bones realign and fuse properly, **distraction** is the process of separating opposing bone to encourage regeneration of new bone in the created space. Distraction can also be used when limbs are of unequal lengths and new bone is needed to elongate the shorter limb.

Ilizarov External Fixator (IEF)

The IEF uses a system of wires, rings, and telescoping rods that permits limb lengthening to occur by manual distraction. In addition to lengthening bones the device can be used to correct angular or rotational defects or to immobilize fractures. The device is attached surgically by securing a series of external full or half rings to the bone with wires. External telescoping rods connect the rings to each other. Manual distraction is accomplished by manipulating the rods to increase the distance between the rings. A percutaneous ostomy is performed when the device is applied to create a "false" growth plate. A special osteotomy or corticotomy involves cutting only the cortex of the bone while preserving its blood supply, bone marrow, endosteum, and periosteum. Capillary blood flow to the transected area is essential for proper bone growth. Cut bone ends typically grow at a rate of 1 cm/month. Use of the IEF can result in up to a 15-cm gain in length (Carlino, 1991).

Nursing Care Management

Success of the IEF depends on the child's and family's cooperation; therefore before surgery they must be fully informed of the appearance of the device, how it accomplishes bone growth, alterations in activities, and home and follow-up care. Children are involved in learning to adjust the device to accomplish distraction. Children who participate actively in their care report less discomfort. Since the device is external, the child and family need to be prepared for the reactions of others and assisted in camouflaging the device with appropriate apparel, such as wide-legged pants that close with self-adhering fasteners around the device (Fig. 51-11). Partial weight bearing is allowed, and the child needs to learn to walk with crutches. Alterations in activity include modifications at school and in physical education. Full weight bearing is not allowed until the distraction is completed and bone consolidation has occurred. Follow-up care is essential to maintaining appropriate distraction until the desired leg length is achieved. The device is removed surgically after the bone has consolidated, and the child may need to use crutches or have a cast for about 1 month after removal.

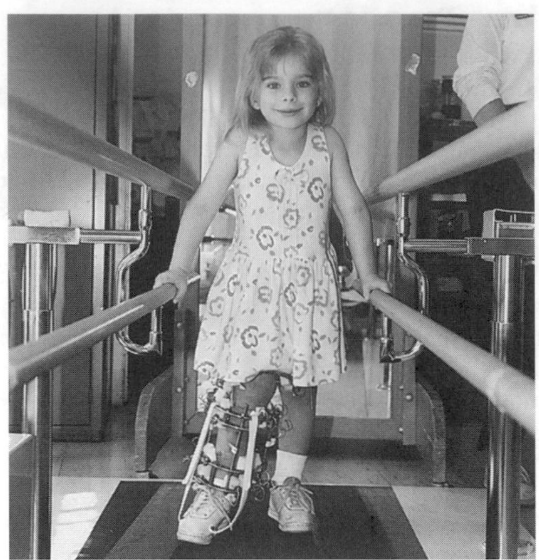

Fig. 51-11 Children with the Ilizarov external fixator must cope with the visible nature of the device.

AMPUTATION

A child may be born with the congenital absence of a body part, have a traumatic loss of an extremity, or need a surgical amputation for a pathologic condition such as osteogenic sarcoma. With today's surgical technology and the quick thinking of bystanders who save a traumatically amputated body part, some children have had fingers and arms reattached with variable degrees of functional use regained. A severed part should be wrapped lightly in a clean cloth or gauze saturated with normal saline solution and sealed in a watertight plastic bag. One should avoid using ice, which might come in contact with the tissue and make implantation impossible. The bag should be labeled with the child's name, the date, and the time and taken to the hospital with the child.

Surgical amputation or the surgical repair of a permanently severed limb focuses on constructing an adequately nourished stump. A smooth, healthy, padded stump, free of nerve endings, is important in prosthesis fitting and subsequent ambulation. In some situations in which there is no vascular or neurologic deficit, a cast is applied to the stump immediately after the procedure, and a pylon, metal extension, and artificial foot are attached so that the patient can walk on the temporary prosthesis within a few hours.

Nursing Care Management

Stump shaping is done postoperatively with special elastic bandaging using a figure-eight bandage, which applies pressure in a cone-shaped fashion. This technique decreases stump edema, controls hemorrhage, and aids in developing desired contours so that the child will bear weight on the posterior aspect of the skin flap rather than on the end of the stump. Stump elevation may be used during the first 24 hours, but after this time the extremity should not be left in this position, because contractures in the proximal joint will develop and seriously hamper ambulation. Monitoring proper body alignment will further decrease the risk of flexion contractures.

For older children and adolescents, arm exercises and bed pushups, as well as parallel bars, which are used in prosthesis-training programs, help build up the arm muscles necessary for walking with crutches. Full range-of-motion exercises of joints above the amputation must be performed several times daily, using active and isotonic exercises. Young children are spontaneously active and require little encouragement.

Depending on the age of the child, the child or parents will need to learn stump hygiene, including careful soap and water washing every day and checking for skin irritation, breakdown, or infection. A tube of stockinette or powder is used to slide the prosthesis on more easily. Skin must be checked carefully every time the prosthesis is removed, and prosthesis tolerance time must be adjusted to prevent skin breakdown.

For children who have had an amputation, *phantom limb sensation* is an expected experience because the nerve-brain connections are still present. Gradually these sensations fade. Preoperative discussion of this phenomenon will aid a child in understanding these "unusual feelings" and not hiding the experiences from others. Limb pain, especially pain that increases with ambulation, should be evaluated for the possibility of a neuroma at the free nerve endings in the stump (see also p. 1736).

Congenital Defects

There are numerous skeletal defects that can be diagnosed at or shortly after birth. The alert nurse is frequently the person who detects the defect and refers the family for correction of the condition. The deviation is often difficult to detect without careful inspection. Therefore it is imperative that nurses become acquainted with signs of these defects and understand the principles of therapy in order to direct others in the care and management of these children.

DEVELOPMENTAL DYSPLASIA OF THE HIP (DDH)

The broad term *developmental dysplasia of the hip* describes a group of disorders related to abnormal development of the hip. A change in terminology from congenital hip dysplasia (CHD) and congenital dislocation of the hip (CDH) to DDH more properly reflects a variety of hip abnormalities in which there is a shallow acetabulum, subluxation, or dislocation. DDH has an incidence of 1 to 2 cases per 1000 live births in the United States. It occurs more commonly in females at a ratio of 6:1 (Bennett and MacEwen, 1989). One fifth of the cases involve both hips; when only one hip is involved, the left hip is affected three times more often than the right.

Pathophysiology

Three degrees of DDH can be identified (Fig. 51-12):

Acetabular dysplasia (or preluxation)—the mildest form, in which there is neither subluxation nor dislocation. The dysplasia reflects an apparent delay in acetabular development evidenced by osseous hypoplasia of the acetabular roof that is oblique and shallow, although the cartilaginous roof is comparatively intact. The femoral head remains in the acetabulum.

Subluxation—accounts for the largest percentage of congenital hip dysplasias. Subluxation implies incomplete dislocation of the hip and is sometimes regarded as an intermediate state in the development from primary dysplasia to complete dislocation. The femoral head remains in contact with the acetabulum, but a stretched capsule and ligamentum teres cause the head of the femur to be partially displaced. Pressure on the cartilaginous roof inhibits ossification and produces a flattening of the socket.

Dislocation—in which the femoral head loses contact with the acetabulum and is displaced posteriorly and superiorly over the fibrocartilaginous rim. The ligamentum teres is elonaged and taut.

Prenatal factors that influence development of hip abnormalities are maternal hormone secretion and mechanical factors of intrauterine posture. The maternal hormone secretion, principally estrogen, that produces laxity of the maternal pelvis toward the end of gestation affects the fetal joints as well. Reliable evidence indicates an association between a higher incidence of developmental hip deformities with breech presentations and cesarean section (often necessitated by abnormal intrauterine position). Legs in frank breech position (i.e., with the hips acutely flexed and knees extended) is an important factor. Other prenatal factors that contribute to hip dysplasia include twinning and large infant size (see the Cultural Considerations box below).

Diagnostic Evaluation

The diagnosis of DDH should be made in the newborn period if possible, since treatment initiated before 2 months of age is most successful (Box 51-4). In the newborn period dysplasia usually appears as hip joint laxity rather than as outright dislocation (Fig. 51-13). Subluxation and the tendency to dislo-

Cultural Considerations 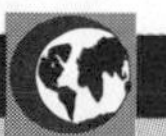

DEVELOPMENTAL DISLOCATION OF THE HIP

A striking relationship exists between the development of the dislocation and methods of handling infants. Among the cultures with the highest incidence of dislocation, newly born infants are tightly wrapped in blankets or other swaddling material or are strapped to cradle boards. In cultures such as the Far East, where mothers traditionally carry infants on their backs or hips in the widely abducted straddle position, the disorder is virtually unknown.

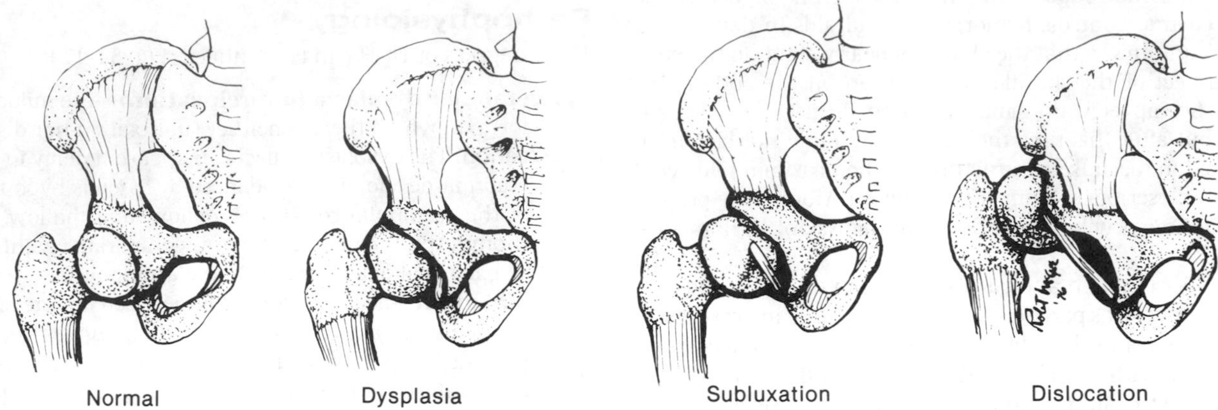

Fig. 51-12 Configuration and relationship of structures in congenital hip deformities.

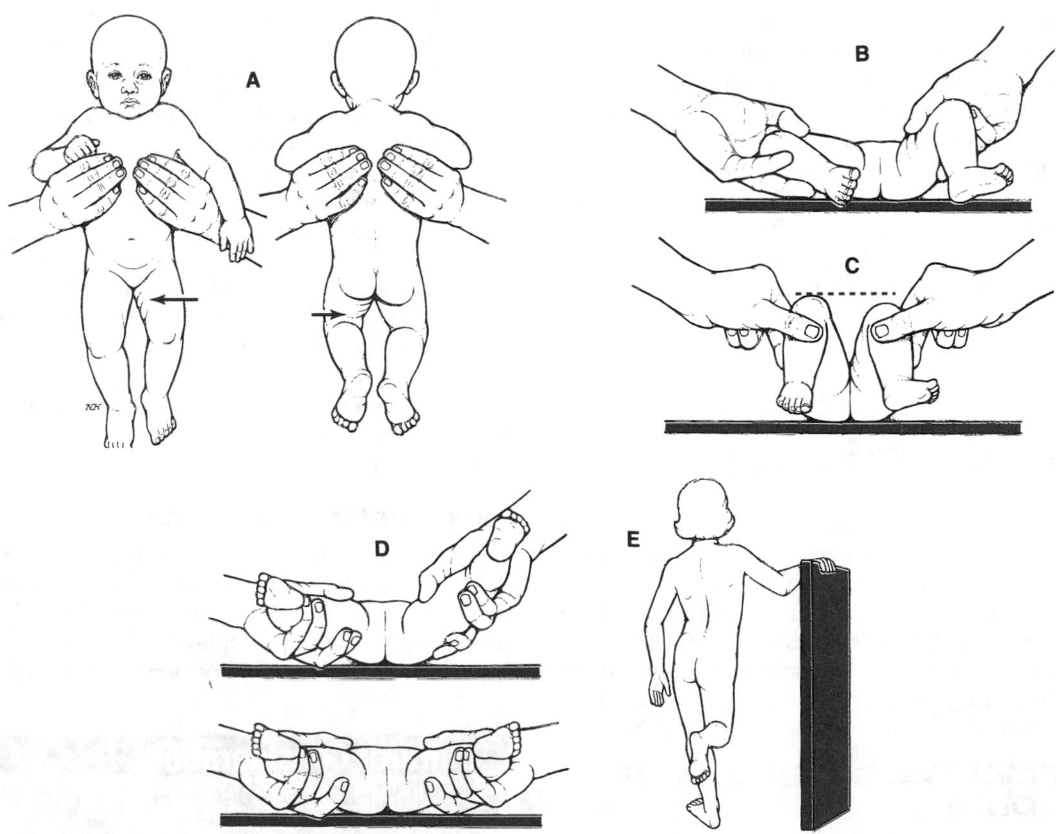

Fig. 51-13 Signs of developmental dysplasia of hip. **A,** Asymmetry of gluteal and thigh folds. **B,** Limited hip abduction, as seen in flexion. **C,** Apparent shortening of femur, as indicated by level of knees in flexion. **D,** Ortolani click (if infant is under 4 weeks of age). **E,** Positive Trendelenburg sign or gain (if child is weight bearing).

BOX 51-4
Clinical Manifestations of Developmental Dysplasia of the Hip

Infant

Shortening of limb on affected side (Galleazzi sign, Allis sign)
Restricted abduction of hip on affected side
Unequal gluteal folds (infant prone)
Positive Ortolani test
Positive Barlow test

Older infant and child

Affected leg shorter than the other
Telescoping or piston mobility of joint
- Head of femur can be felt to move up and down in buttock when extended thigh is pushed first toward child's head and then pulled distally

Trendelenburg sign
- When child stands first on one foot and then on the other (holding onto a chair, rail, or someone's hands) bearing weight on affected hip, pelvis tilts downward on normal side instead of upward, as it would with normal stability

Greater trochanter is prominent and appears above a line from anterior superior iliac spine to tuberosity of ischium
Marked lordosis (bilateral dislocations)
Waddling gait (bilateral dislocations)

cate can be demonstrated by the Ortolani or Barlow test (Fig. 51-13, *B*, *C*, and *D*). There are cases in which dislocation is not diagnosed by these standard tests, and the disorder may not be apparent at birth. Therefore it is recommended that hip examination be included in health supervision until the child begins to walk and the gait is obviously normal.

In older infants and children radiographic examination is useful in confirming the diagnosis. An upward slope in the roof of the acetabulum (the acetabular angle) greater than 40 degrees with upward and outward displacement of the femoral head is a frequent finding in older children. Radiographic examination in early infancy is not reliable, because the bones are largely cartilaginous and difficult to visualize. However, the cartilaginous head can be visualized directly with real-time high-resolution ultrasonography.

Therapeutic Management

Treatment is begun as soon as the condition is recognized, since early intervention is more favorable to the restoration of normal bony architecture and function. The longer treatment is delayed, the more severe the deformity, the more difficult the treatment, and the less favorable the prognosis. The treatment varies with the age of the child and the extent of the dysplasia.

Newborn to age 6 months. The hip joint is maintained by splinting with the proximal femur centered in the acetabulum in an attitude of flexion. Of the numerous devices available, the *Pavlik harness* is the most widely used, and with time, motion, and gravity the hip works into a more abducted, reduced position (Fig. 51-14). The harness is worn continuously until

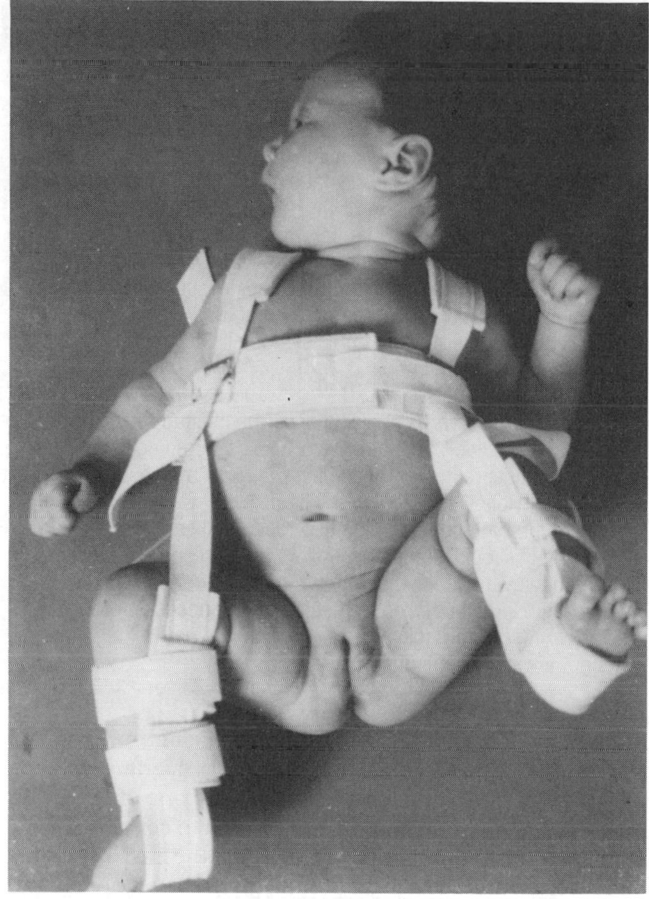

Fig. 51-14 Child in Pavlik harness.

the hip is clinically and radiographically stable, usually in about 3 to 6 months.

When adduction contraction is present, other devices (such as skin traction) are used to stretch the hip slowly and gently to full abduction, after which wide abduction is maintained until stability is attained. When there is difficulty in maintaining stable reduction, a hip spica cast is applied and changed periodically to accommodate the child's growth. After 3 to 6 months, sufficient stability is acquired to allow transfer to a removal protective abduction brace. The duration of treatment depends on development of the acetabulum but is usually accomplished within the first year.

Ages 6 to 18 months. In the 6-to-18-month age group the dislocation is not recognized until the child begins to stand and walk, when attendant shortening of the limb and contractures of the hip adductor and flexor muscles become apparent. Gradual reduction by traction is followed by cast immobilization, which is maintained until radiographic examination confirms a stable joint. Often soft tissue may obstruct and complicate reduction and subsequent joint development. In this case open reduction is performed to remove the obstruction; this is followed by postoperative spica cast immobilization and later replacement with an abduction splint.

Older child. Correction of the hip deformity in older children is inherently more difficult than in younger age groups,

Critical Thinking Q & A

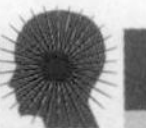

DIAGNOSIS OF DDH

During Kiasha's 4-week well-child visit, her mother comments on a skinfold on the left inner thigh. The history includes a normal pregnancy. A cesarean section was necessitated by breech presentation at 42 weeks' gestation. Given the facts, what intervention should you take, if any?

1. Reassure the mother that her infant has normal vital signs and weight gain and appears very healthy.
2. Explain to the mother that it is adipose tissue, which accumulates rapidly during the first 6 months.
3. Discuss concerns about the "skin fold" with the physician for further examination.
4. Order blood tests.

The correct answer is three. Clinical manifestations of DDH in an infant include unequal gluteal folds, shortening of limb on affected side, restricted abduction of hip on affected side, and positive Ortolani and Barlow test results.

The first intervention is not correct because a thorough assessment should be completed first. The second response is true; however, the key finding is the gluteal fold on the left inner thigh. In general, serum results are not necessary for diagnostic measures. Radiographic examination may be helpful but is not always reliable in infants.

since secondary adaptive changes complicate the condition. Operative reduction, which may involve preoperative traction, tenotomy of contracted muscles, and any one of several innominate osteotomy procedures designed to construct an acetabular roof, is usually required. After the cast is removed and before weight bearing is permitted, range-of-motion exercises help restore movement. Next, rehabilitative measures are instituted. Successful reduction and reconstruction become increasingly difficult after the age of 4 years and are usually impossible or inadvisable to children over 6 years of age because of severe shortening and contracture of muscles and deformity of the femoral and acetabular structures.

Nursing Care Management

Assessment

Nurses are in a unique position to detect DDH in the newborn. During the infant assessment process and routine nurturing activities the hips and extremities are inspected for any deviations from normal. Usually only nurses specially trained in the technique are permitted to perform Ortolani and Barlow tests, but any nurse can be alert to other signs of DDH. These observations are reported to the attending practitioner, and the ambulatory child who displays a limp or an unusual gait should be referred for evaluation. This may indicate an orthopedic or neurologic problem. Nonambulatory children with cerebral palsy should also be assessed for evidence of dislocation (see the Critical Thinking Q & A box above).

Nursing ALERT

Observations during routine care, such as diapering, provide an excellent opportunity to observe the infant for limited movement and a wide perineum, which is an indication to assess for leg shortening, unequal gluteal folds, and limited abduction.

BOX 51-5
Nursing Diagnoses: The Child with Developmental Dysplasia of the Hip

Impaired physical mobility related to correction device
Risk for impaired skin integrity related to presence of corrective device
Altered family processes related to care of a child in a corrective device

Nursing Diagnoses

Nursing diagnoses identified for the child with congenital hip dysplasia are listed in Box 51-5. Other diagnoses will be apparent in specific situations.

Planning

The goals of care for the child in a mechanical device for correction of DDH are as follows:

1. Child will maintain correct position of hip in acetabulum.
2. Child will experience no complications related to wearing corrective device.
3. Family will adapt routine nurturing activities to accommodate corrective device.

Implementation

The major nursing problems in the care of an infant or child in a cast or other device are related to maintenance of the device and adaptation of nurturing activities to meet the needs of the infant or child. Generally treatment and follow-up care of these children are carried out in a clinic, practitioner's office, or outpatient unit. Hospitalization may be necessary for cast application or brace fitting but seldom exceeds 24 to 48 hours. Longer hospitalization is required for open reduction.

The primary nursing goal is teaching parents to apply and maintain the reduction device. The Pavlik harness allows for easy handling of the infant and usually produces less apprehension in the parent than heavy braces and casts. It is important that parents understand the correct use of the appliance, which may or may not allow for its removal during bathing. When the infant has a harness that is not removed, a sponge bath is recommended, and the skin beneath the harness is assessed daily for irritation. Powders and lotions are not used, because they tend to cake or "ball" underneath straps or clothing.

To prevent skin irritation from the straps, long socks and a shirt are worn under the device. Extensions on the shirt that snap at the crotch help keep the shirt in place (Speers and Speers, 1992). Unbuckling or removal of the harness is determined individually on the basis of the family's level of understanding and the degree of deformity in the hip. In general, parents should not adjust the harness without supervision. The child should be examined by the practitioner before any adjustment is attempted to make certain the hips are in correct placement before the harness is resecured.

Casts and orthotic devices ("braces") offer more challenging nursing problems, since they cannot be removed for routine care, although sometimes a brace may be removed for bathing. Care of an infant or small child with a cast requires nursing innovation to reduce irritation and to maintain cleanliness of both the child and the cast, particularly in the diaper area. (See p. 1714 for care of the child in a cast.)

Parents are taught the proper care of the cast (or orthotic device) and are helped to devise means for maintaining cleanliness. A superabsorbent disposable diaper (newborn size) is tucked beneath the entire perineal opening of the cast. A larger (toddler size) diaper can be applied and fastened over the small diaper and cast.

For tightly fitting casts transparent film dressings can be cut into strips as for petaling (see p. 1714), and one edge applied to the cast edge and the other directly to the perineum; this forms a continuous, waterproof bridge between the perineum and the cast to prevent leakage. An additional advantage to the use of this transparent dressing is that it keeps both the skin and the cast dry while allowing for observation of skin beneath the dressing.

Older infants and small children may stuff bits of food, small toys, or other items under the cast; parents should be alerted to this possibility so that suitable preventive measures may be initiated.

Feeding the infant in a hip spica cast offers problems of positioning. Very young infants can be fed in the supine position with the head elevated, and with the infant's hips and legs supported on a pillow at the side, the parent can cuddle the infant in his or her arms during feeding. A somewhat similar position can be used for breastfeeding (i.e., with the infant supported on pillows or held in a "football" hold facing the mother with the legs behind her). An alternate position is to hold the infant upright on the caregiver's lap with the legs of the infant astride the adult's legs.

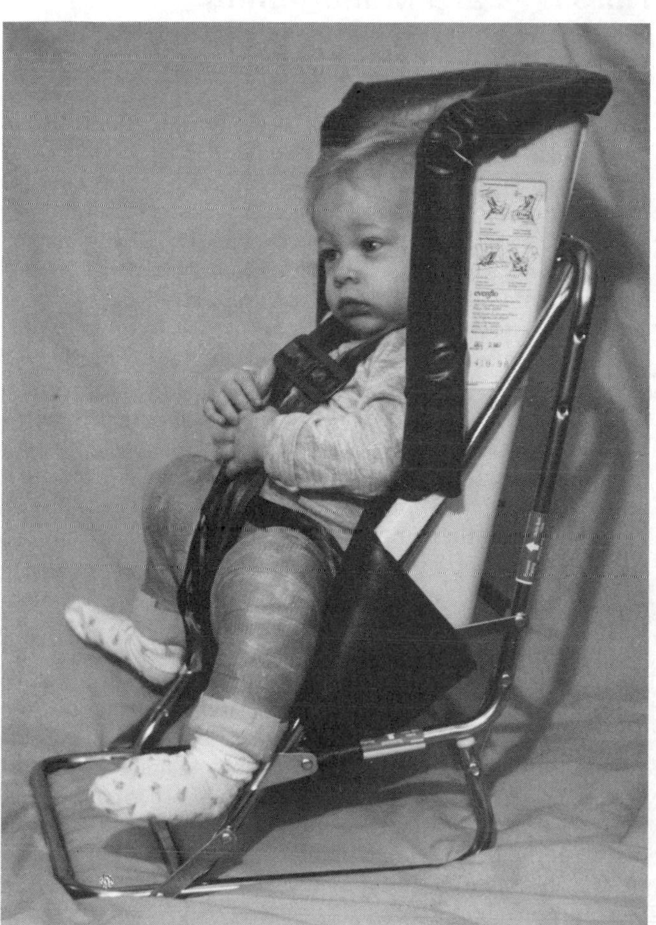

Fig. 51-15 Child in specially designed car restraint (Spelcast).

Infants who are able to sit up can be fed while sitting at a feeding table or in a modified high chair. Parents may be able to fashion a tilt board with a padded seat or an adjustable chair. The table or chair provides an excellent place for the child to play in an upright position. The child's car seat is also a vital consideration. Modifications can be made on several standard, government-approved car seats.* A specially designed car restraint for a young child in a spica cast is shown in Fig. 51-15.

It is important for nurses, parents, and other caregivers to understand that children in corrective devices need to be involved in the same activities as any child in the same age group. Toys that can be used in a prone position on the floor or in the seats devised for feeding and other activities are chosen. Confinement in a cast or appliance should not exclude children from family (or unit) activities. They can be held astride the lap for comfort and transported to areas of activity. The child may be allowed to walk in a cast or orthotic device. An adapted wheelchair, stroller, or scooter can offer mobility to the older infant or child.

Evaluation

The effectiveness of nursing interventions is determined by continual assessment and evaluation of care based on the following observational guidelines and expected outcomes:

1. Inspect corrective device regularly.
2. Inspect child's skin and circulation regularly.
3. Observe family's behavior with child and interview them regarding identified problems and solutions.

Expected outcomes:

1. Hip remains in desired position; corrective device is positioned properly.
2. Skin remains free of irritation; circulation is unimpaired.
3. Family adjusts nurturing activities to accommodate corrective device.

CONGENITAL CLUBFOOT

The general term *clubfoot* is used to describe a common deformity in which the foot is twisted out of its normal shape or position. Any foot deformity involving the ankle is called *talipes*, derived from *talus*, meaning ankle, and *pes*, meaning foot. Deformities of the foot and ankle are described according to the position of the ankle and foot. The more common positions involve the following variations:

Talipes varus—an inversion or a bending inward
Talipes valgus—an eversion or bending outward
Talipes equinus—plantar flexion, in which the toes are lower than the heel
Talipes calcaneus—dorsiflexion, in which the toes are higher than the heel

*For additional information contact the **Automobile Safety for Children Program**, James Whitcomb Riley Hospital for Children, Indiana School of Medicine, 702 Barnhill Dr., Indianapolis, IN 46223; (317) 274-2977 (in Indiana [800] KID-N-CAR).

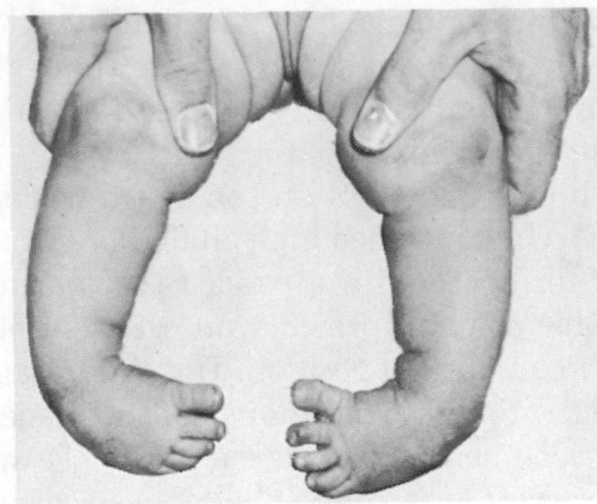

Fig. 51-16 Bilateral congenital talipes equinovarus (congenital clubfoot) in 2-month-old infant. (From Brashear HR Jr, Raney RB: *Handbook of orthopaedic surgery*, ed 10, St Louis, 1986, Mosby.)

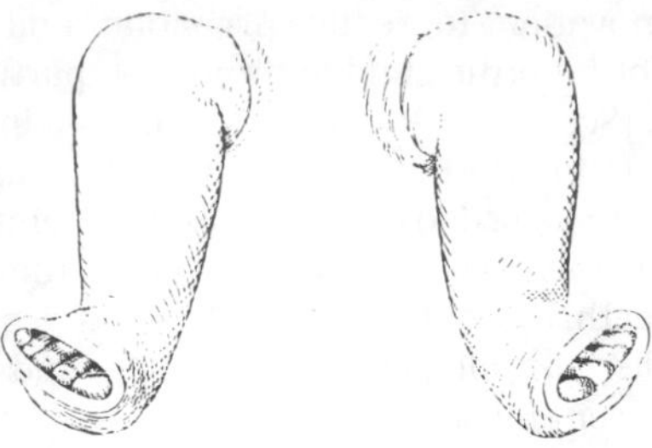

Fig. 51-17 Feet casted for correction of bilateral congenital talipes equinovarus. (From Brashear HR Jr, Raney RB: *Handbook of orthopaedic surgery*, ed 10, St Louis, 1986, Mosby.)

Most clubfeet are a combination of these positions, and the most frequently occurring type (approximately 95%) is the composite deformity *talipes equinovarus* (TEV), in which the foot is pointed downward and inward in varying degrees of severity (Fig. 51-16). Unilateral clubfoot is somewhat more common than bilateral clubfoot and may occur as an isolated defect or in association with other disorders or syndromes, such as chromosomal aberrations, arthrogryposis (a generalized immobility of the joints), cerebral palsy, or spina bifida.

The frequency of clubfoot in the general population is 1:700 to 1:1000 live births, with boys affected twice as often as girls. The 35% concordance in monozygotic twins, as opposed to a 3% concordance in dizygotic twins, indicates a hereditary component.

Pathophysiology

The precise cause of clubfoot is unknown. Some authorities attribute the defect to abnormal positioning and restricted movement in utero, although the evidence is not conclusive. Other experts implicate arrested or abnormal embryonic development. Arrested development during this early stage tends to result in a rigid deformity, whereas mechanical pressures from intrauterine positioning are likely causes of more flexible deformities.

Diagnostic Evaluation

The deformity is readily apparent and easily detected prenatally through ultrasonography or at birth. However, it must be differentiated from some positional deformities that can be passively corrected or overcorrected. The true clubfoot is fixed. Paralytic changes in the lower extremity of children with neuromuscular involvement often produce equinovarus deformity.

Therapeutic Management

Treatment is begun as soon as the deformity is recognized and involves three stages: (1) correction of the deformity, (2) maintenance of the correction until normal muscle balance is regained, and (3) follow-up observation to prevent possible recurrence of the deformity. Some feet respond to treatment readily; some respond only to prolonged, vigorous, and sustained efforts; and the improvement in others remains disappointing even with maximum effort of all concerned.

Correction of TEV is most reliably accomplished by manipulation and the application of a series of casts begun immediately or shortly after birth and continued until marked overcorrection is reached (Fig. 51-17). Successive casts allow for gradual stretching of tight structures on the medial side of the foot and gradual contraction of lax structures on the lateral side. Manipulation and casting are repeated frequently (every few days for 1 to 2 weeks, then at 1- to 2-week intervals) to accommodate the rapid growth of early infancy. The extremity or extremities are casted until the desired result is achieved.

Nursing Care Management

Nursing care of the child with nonsurgical correction of clubfoot is the same as for any child who has a cast (p. 1714). Because the child will spend considerable time in a corrective device, nursing care plans include both long-term and short-term goals. Conscientious observation of the skin and circulation is particularly important in young infants because of their normally rapid growth rate. Since treatment and follow-up care are handled in the orthopedist's office, clinic, or outpatient department, parent education and support are important in nursing care of these children.

Parents need to understand the overall treatment program, the importance of regular cast changes, and the role they play in the long-term effectiveness of the therapy. Reinforcing and clarifying the orthopedist's explanations and instructions; teaching parents about care of the cast or appliance (including vigilant observation for potential problems); and encouraging parents to facilitate normal development within the limitations imposed by the deformity or therapy are all part of nursing responsibilities.

METATARSUS ADDUCTUS (VARUS)

Metatarsus adductus, or metatarsus varus, is probably the most common congenital foot deformity. In most instances it is a result of abnormal intrauterine positioning and is usually detected at birth. The deformity is characterized by medial adduction of the toes and forefoot, frequently in association with inversion, and by convexity of the lateral border of the foot. Unlike TEV, with which it is often confused, the angulation occurs at the tarsometatarsal joint, while the heel and ankle remain in a neutral position. This deformity often causes a pigeon-toed gait in the child.

Management depends on the rigidity of the deformity. Correction can usually be accomplished by gentle manipulation and passive stretching of the foot, which the parent is taught to perform. Repeated and consistent stretching is continued for the first 6 weeks, after which the treatment is based on the flexibility of the foot. Those feet that do not respond to the manipulation require orthopedic therapy. If the child is able to actively overcorrect the deformity voluntarily on stimulation, continued stretching is generally sufficient. If the foot cannot be actively or passively overcorrected, the feet are stretched and manipulated and held with casts and/or orthoses.

Nursing Care Management

The nursing role primarily involves identifying the defect, so that early therapy and instruction of the parents can be initiated. The nurse teaches the parents how to hold the heel firmly and to stretch only the forefoot; otherwise, undue force on the heel may produce a valgus deformity. If casting is needed, the nurse instructs the parents in cast care and observation (see p. 1714).

SKELETAL LIMB DEFICIENCY

Congenital limb deficiencies, or reduction malformations, are manifested by a variety of degrees of loss of functional capacity. They are characterized by underdevelopment of skeletal elements of the extremities. The range of malformation can extend from minor defects of the digits to serious abnormalities, such as *amelia,* absence of an entire extremity, or *meromelia,* partial absence of an extremity, which includes *phocomelia* (seal limbs), an interposed deficiency of long bones with relatively good development of hands and feet attached at or near the shoulder or the hips.

In rare instances prenatal destruction of limbs has been reported, but most reduction deformities are primary defects of development (agenesis, aplasia). Therefore congenital amputations in the literal sense are not amputations, since nonexistent limbs cannot be amputated.

Pathophysiology

Limb deficiencies can be attributed to both heredity and environment and can originate at any stage of limb development. Formation of limbs may be suppressed at the time of limb bud formation, or there may be interference in later stages of differentiation and growth. Heredity appears to play a prominent role, and prenatal environmental insults have been implicated in a number of cases, such as the well-publicized thalidomide tragedy of the 1950s and early 1960s, which demonstrated a clear relationship between the time of exposure of the pregnant woman to the antiemetic drug and the presence and type of limb deformity in the newborn.

Therapeutic Management

Children with congenital limb deficiencies should be fitted with prosthetic devices whenever possible, and such a functional replacement should be applied at the earliest possible stage of development in an attempt to match the motor readiness of the infant. This favors natural progression of prosthetic use. For example a young infant with an upper extremity deficiency is fitted with a simple passive device, such as a mitten prosthesis, to encourage limb exploration, sitting (with the extremities needed for support), and bilateral hand activities.

Lower limb prostheses are applied when the infant is ready to pull to a standing position. In preparation for prosthetic devices, surgical modification is often necessary to ensure the most favorable use of the device, since severe deformity can interfere with its effective use. Phocomelic digits are preserved for controlling switches of externally powered appliances in upper extremities. Digits (in both upper and lower extremities) provide the child with surfaces for tactile exploration and stimulation. Prostheses are replaced to accommodate growth and increasing capabilities of the child.

Nursing Care Management

Prosthetic application training and habilitation are most successfully carried out in a center that specializes in meeting the special needs of these children, especially very young children and those with multiple amputations. It involves a team of health professionals and the parents, who must encourage the child in making age-commensurate adjustments to the environment. Although these children need assistance, excessive overprotection may produce overdependency, with later maladjustment to school and other situations.

OSTEOGENESIS IMPERFECTA (OI)

OI refers to a group of heterogenous inherited disorders of connective tissue characterized by connective tissue and bone defects. The inheritance pattern is autosomal-dominant in the majority of cases, although the most severe form demonstrates autosomal-recessive inheritance.

Persons with OI appear to have abnormal precollagen that prevents the formation of collagen, the major component of connective tissue. At present OI is believed to consist of four different variations (Box 51-6). Type II, the most severe form of OI, is characterized by multiple intrauterine or perinatal fractures, severe deformity, and often, early death. The brittle bones are easily fractured from the slightest trauma.

BOX 51-6
Classification of Osteogenesis Imperfecta

Type		Characteristics
I*	A	Mild bone fragility; blue sclerae; normal teeth; presenile deafness (age 20-30 years); autosomal-dominant inheritance
	B	Same as A except dentinogenesis imperfecta instead of normal teeth
	C	Same as B; no bone fragility
II		Lethal; stillborn or die in early infancy; severe bone fragility, multiple fractures at birth; 10% of OI cases; autosomal-recessive inheritance
III		Severe bone fragility leads to severe progressive deformities; normal sclerae; marked growth failure; most autosomal-recessive; few autosomal-dominant
IV	A	Mild to moderate bone fragility; normal sclerae; short stature, variable deformity; autosomal-dominant
	B	Same as A except dentinogenesis imperfecta instead of normal teeth; approximately 6% of OI cases

*Two thirds of cases are type I.

The diseases of later onset run a milder course. The tendency to fracture appears later (at variable ages) and disappears after puberty. During childhood the shafts of long bones are slender, with reduced cortical thickness resulting from defective periosteal bone formation. In addition to the features already described, the child with OI has thin skin, hyperextensibility of ligaments, a tendency toward recurrent epistaxis, excess diaphoresis, a tendency to bruise easily, and mild hyperpyrexia. The disease shows variable expressivity; that is, the number and extent of pathologic features appear in any individual range, from severe to minimal involvement. The incidence of fractures decreases at puberty, when the body's production of hormones helps strengthen bones.

Therapeutic Management

The treatment is primarily supportive. Several drugs have been tried but appear to be of limited benefit. Light weight braces and splints help support limbs, prevent fractures, and aid in ambulation. Physical therapy helps prevent disuse osteoporosis and strengthens muscles, which in turn improves bone density. Exercises are usually simple ones against light resistance or water exercises with swimming. Patients with milder disease are encouraged to participate in appropriate sports.

Surgery is sometimes used to help treat the manifestations of the disease. Surgical techniques are used to correct deformities that interfere with bracing, standing, or walking. For the child with recurrent fractures, inserting an intermedullary rod provides stability to bones. Unfortunately the rods must be replaced as the child grows; otherwise fractures may occur through the unprotected portion of the bone.

Nursing Care Management

Infants and children with this disorder require careful handling to prevent fractures. They must be supported when they are being turned, positioned, moved, and fondled. Even changing a diaper may cause a fracture in severely affected infants. These children should never be held by the ankles when being diapered but should be gently lifted by the buttocks.

Both parents and the affected child need education regarding the child's limitations and guidelines in planning suitable activities that promote optimum development, as well as protect the child from harm. Realistic occupational planning and genetic counseling are part of the long-term goals of care. Educational materials and information can be obtained from the **Osteogenesis Imperfecta Foundation, Inc.,*** which also has a network that can put a family in contact with other families with a similar problem.

Acquired Defects

LEGG-CALVÉ-PERTHES DISEASE

Legg-Calvé-Perthes disease, sometimes called *coxa plana* or *osteochondritis deformans juvenilis*, is a self-limited disorder in which there is aseptic necrosis of the femoral head. The disease affects children 3 to 12 years of age, but most cases occur in males between ages 4 and 8 years as an isolated event. In approximately 10% to 15% of cases the involvement is bilateral; most of the affected children have a skeletal age significantly below their chronologic age. The male/female ratio is 4:1 or 5:1; white children are affected 10 times more often than black children.

BOX 51-7
Stages of Legg-Calvé-Perthes Disease

Stage I: Aseptic necrosis or infarction of the femoral capital epiphysis with degenerative changes producing flattening of the upper surface of the femoral head—the *avascular stage*

Stage II: Capital bone absorption and revascularization with fragmentation (vascular resorption of the epiphysis) that gives a mottled appearance on radiographs—the *fragmentation*, or *revascularization stage*

Stage III: New bone formation, which is represented on radiographs as calcification and ossification or increased density in the areas of radiolucency; this filling-in process appears to take place from the periphery of the head centrally—the *reparative stage*

Stage IV: Gradual reformation of the head of the femur without radiolucency and, it is hoped, to a spherical form—the *regenerative stage*

Pathophysiology

The cause of the disease is unknown, but there is a disturbance of circulation to the femoral capital epiphysis that produces an ischemic aseptic necrosis of the femoral head. During middle childhood, circulation to the femoral epiphysis is more tenuous than at other ages and can become obstructed by trauma, inflammation, coagulation defects, and a variety of other causes. The pathologic events seem to take place in four stages (Box 51-7). The entire process may encompass as little as 18 months or continue for several years. The reformed femoral head may be severely altered or appear entirely normal.

Diagnostic Evaluation

The diagnosis is suspected from clinical manifestations (Box 51-8) and established by radiographic examination.

Therapeutic Management

Since deformity occurs early in the disease process, the aim of treatment is to keep the head of the femur contained in the acetabulum, which serves as a mold to preserve the spherical shape of the head and to maintain a full range of motion. The initial therapy is rest, which helps reduce inflammation and restore motion. Active motion is encouraged. In some cases traction is applied to stretch tight adductor muscles.

Containment can be accomplished by non–weight-bearing devices, such as an abduction brace, leg casts, or a leather harness sling that prevents weight bearing on the affected limb; by various weight-bearing appliances, such as abduction-ambulation braces or casts, after a period of bed rest and traction; and by surgical reconstructive and containment procedures. Conservative therapy must be continued for 2 to 4

*5005 W. Laurel St., Tampa, FL 33607-3836; (813) 282-1161.

BOX 51-8
Clinical Manifestations of Legg-Calvé-Perthes Disease

Insidious onset
Intermittent appearance of limp on affected side
Pain
- Soreness or aching
- In hip, along entire length of thigh, or in vicinity of knee
- Most evident on rising or at end of a long day
- Usually accompanied by joint dysfunction and limited range of motion

Stiffness
Point tenderness over hip capsule
External hip rotation (late sign)

BOX 51-9
Clinical Manifestations of Slipped Femoral Capital Epiphysis

Obese or tall, lanky youngster
Limp on affected side
Pain in hip
- Continuous or intermittent
- Frequently referred to groin, anteromedial aspect of thigh, or knee

Restricted internal rotation on adduction with external rotation deformity
Loss of abduction and internal rotation as severity increases

years, although braces constructed from lightweight materials allow the child to maintain a nearly normal activity level. Surgical correction returns the child to normal activities within 3 to 4 months.

The disease is self-limited, but the ultimate outcome of therapy depends on early and efficient treatment and the age of onset of the disorder. Younger children, whose epiphyses are more cartilaginous, have the brightest prognosis for complete recovery. The later the diagnosis is made, the more damage has occurred before treatment is implemented. In most cases, with good patient compliance the prognosis is excellent.

Nursing Care Management

Nurses are often the first health professionals to identify affected children and to refer them for medical evaluation. They are also persons on whom the child and the family can rely to help them understand and adjust to the therapeutic measures. Since most of the child's care is conducted on an outpatient basis, the major emphasis of nursing care is teaching the family the care and management of the corrective appliance selected for therapy. The family needs to learn the purpose, function, application, and care of the corrective device and the importance of compliance in order to achieve the desired outcome.

One of the most difficult aspects associated with the disorder is coping with a normally active child who feels well but must remain relatively inactive. Suitable activities must be devised to meet the needs of the child in the process of developing a sense of initiative or industry. Activities that meet the creative urges are well received. This is also an opportune time to encourage the child to begin a hobby, such as collections, model building, or crafts.

SLIPPED FEMORAL CAPITAL EPIPHYSIS

Slipped femoral capital epiphysis, or *coxa vara,* refers to the spontaneous displacement of the proximal femoral epiphysis in a posterior and inferior direction. It develops most frequently shortly before or during accelerated growth and the onset of puberty (children between the ages of 10 and 16 years—median age, 13 for boys, 11 for girls) and is most frequently observed in obese children. Bilateral involvement has been reported as 16% to 40%.

Pathophysiology

The cause of *coxa vara* is unknown, but it occurs most often in "overlarge" youngsters or very tall, thin, rapidly growing children. There has been some evidence to implicate hormonal factors, such as decreased growth hormone and increased sex hormone. It has also been associated with endocrine abnormalities, such as hypothyroidism and renal osteodystrophy, and during growth hormone therapy.

The pathologic processes as seen in radiographs involve first a rarefaction of bone on the lower femoral side of the epiphysis with widening of the growth plate. After trauma or slight injury the femoral portion of the epiphysis slides upward but remains attached by the thick, continuous periosteum. As slipping increases, the epiphyseal displacement becomes posterior and inferior. The slipping produces deformity of the femoral head and stretches the blood vessels to the epiphysis.

Diagnostic Evaluation

The disorder is suspected when an adolescent or preadolescent youngster displays clinical signs or complains of pain (Box 51-9). The diagnosis is confirmed by radiographic examination.

Therapeutic Management

The treatment varies with the degree of displacement but involves surgical stabilization and correction of deformity. In mild cases simple pin fixation is sufficient. More extensive displacement requires skeletal traction followed by pin fixation or osteotomy. The prognosis depends on the degree of deformity and the occurrence of complications, such as avascular necrosis and cartilaginous necrosis. As in other disorders, early diagnosis and implementation of therapy increase the likelihood of a satisfactory cure.

Nursing Care Management

Nursing care is the same as that for a child in a cast or a child in traction, as discussed earlier in this chapter.

KYPHOSIS AND LORDOSIS

Kyphosis is an abnormally increased convex angulation in the curvature of the thoracic spine (Fig. 51-18, *B*). It can occur secondary to disease processes such as tuberculosis, chronic

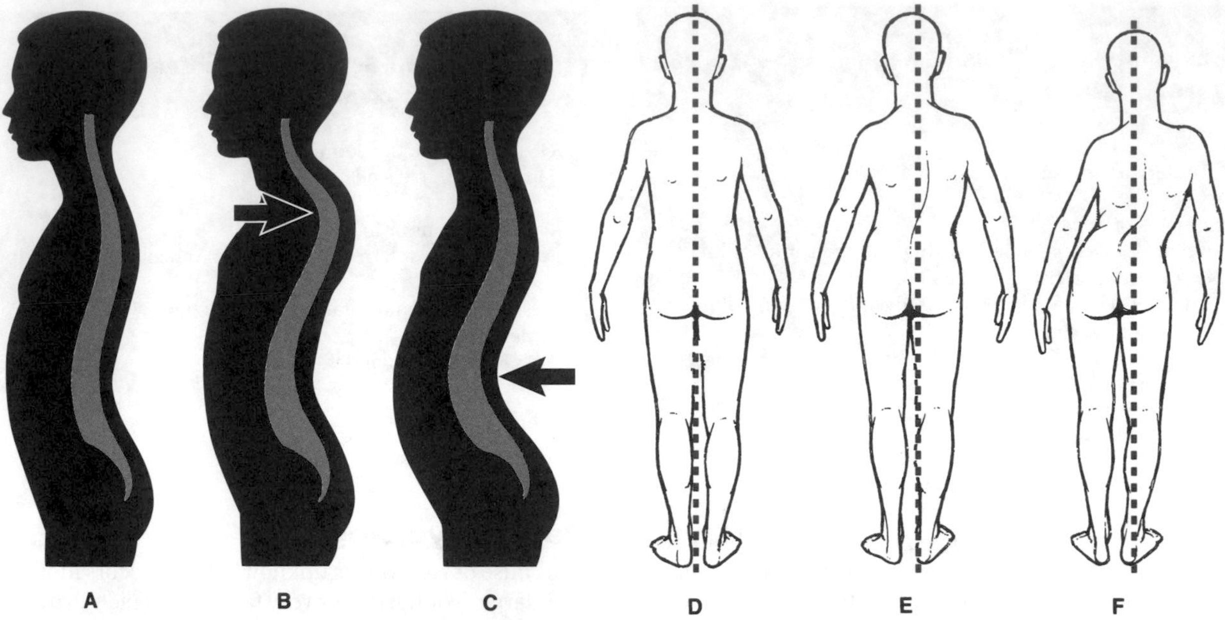

Fig. 51-18 Defects of spinal column. **A,** Normal spine. **B,** Kyphosis. **C,** Lordosis. **D,** Normal spine in balance. **E,** Mild scoliosis in balance. **F,** Severe scoliosis not in balance. **G,** Rib hump and flank asymmetry seen in flexion caused by rotary component. (Redrawn from Hilt NE, Schmitt EW: *Pediatric orthopedic nursing,* St Louis, 1975, Mosby.)

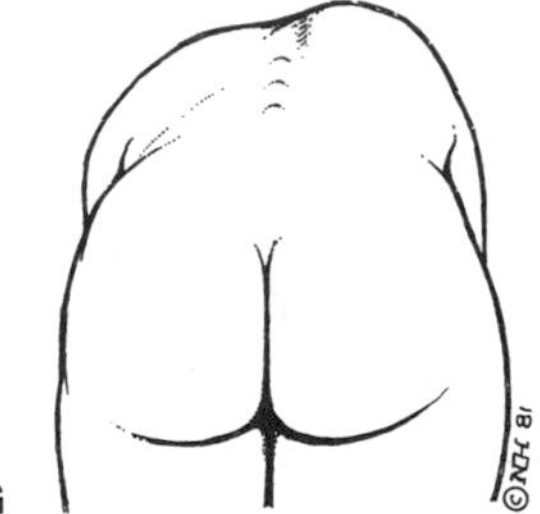

arthritis, osteodystrophy, or compression fractures of the thoracic spine. The most common form of kyphosis is "postural." Children, especially during the time when skeletal growth outpaces growth of muscle, are prone to exaggeration of a tendency toward kyphosis. They assume abnormal sitting and standing positions. This is particularly common in self-conscious adolescent girls who assume a round-shouldered slouching posture in an attempt to hide their developing breasts.

Postural kyphosis is almost always accompanied by a compensatory postural lordosis, an abnormally exaggerated concave lumbar curvature. Treatment consists of postural exercises to strengthen shoulder and abdominal muscles and bracing for more marked deformity. Unfortunately, treatment is difficult; the normal rebellious tendencies of the adolescent, together with continual parental nagging to "stand up straight," often interfere with compliance to a therapeutic regimen. The best approach is to emphasize the cosmetic value of corrective therapy and to place the responsibility on the adolescent for carrying out an exercise program at home with regular visits to and assessments by a therapist. Most adolescents respond well to selected sports as a supplement to regular exercise. Boys prefer weight lifting (preferably performed from a prone or supine position on a bench) and track sports. Girls respond well to dancing classes (ballet or modern dancing). Swimming is excellent and has the added advantages of exercising all muscles, eliminating gravity, and teaching breath control.

Lordosis is an accentuation of the cervical or lumbar curvature beyond physiologic limits (Fig. 51-18, *C*). It may be a secondary complication of a disease process, a result of trauma, or idiopathic. It is often seen in association with flexion contractures of the hip, obesity, congenital dislocated hip, and slipped femoral capital epiphysis. During the pubertal growth spurt lordosis of varying degrees is observed in teenagers, especially girls. In obese children the weight of the abdominal fat alters the center of gravity, causing a compensatory lordosis. Unlike kyphosis, severe lordosis is usually accompanied by pain.

Treatment involves management of the predisposing cause when possible, such as weight loss and correction of deformities. Postural exercises and/or support garments are helpful in relieving symptoms in some cases; however, these do not usually effect a permanent cure.

SCOLIOSIS

Scoliosis, the most common spinal deformity, is a lateral curvature of the spine usually associated with a rotary deformity that eventually causes cosmetic and physiologic alterations in the spine, chest, and pelvis. It can be congenital, or it can develop during infancy and childhood, but it is most common during the growth spurt of early adolescence.

Etiology

Scoliosis can be caused by a number of conditions and may occur alone or in association with other diseases, particularly neuromuscular conditions. In most cases, however, there is no apparent cause, and it is called *idiopathic scoliosis.* There is evidence that it may be genetic and transmitted as an autosomal-dominant trait with incomplete penetrance, and it may be multifactorial.

Diagnostic Evaluation

Diagnosis is made by observation and radiographic examination. Discomfort is rarely present, and there are few outward signs until the deformity is well established. Early detection and treatment are essential to successful management (see also Spine, Chapter 32). The undressed child viewed from the posterior side often reveals primary curvature and a compensatory curvature that places the head in alignment with the gluteal fold (Fig. 51-18, *E*). In uncompensated scoliosis the head and hips are not in alignment (Fig. 51-18, *F*). In advanced cases with rotary deformity, rib hump and flank asymmetry are observed when the child bends from the waist unsupported by the arms (Fig. 51-18, *G*). Radiographs taken in the standing position establish the degree of curvature. Not all spinal curvatures are scoliosis. A curve of less than 10 degrees is considered a postural variation. Curves of under 20 degrees are mild and, if nonprogressive, do not require treatment.

Therapeutic Management

A thorough examination, history, and assessment of the child are carried out to evaluate the status of the deformity, factors contributing to the defect, and factors that may influence the outcome of therapy. Treatment is best undertaken in a center in which a team is available that specializes in management of scoliosis. Current management involves straightening and realignment of the vertebrae by either external (bracing) or internal (surgical) fixation techniques. Bracing is not curative but may slow the progression of the deformity until the spine has reached skeletal maturity.

Bracing and exercise. Exercises alone are rarely of value with scoliosis. However, supplemental exercises are employed daily in and out of the brace to prevent atrophy of spinal and abdominal muscles. Nonoperative treatment by application of a properly constructed and well-fitted external bracing device and close supervision are successful in halting the progression of most curvatures. The two most commonly used types of braces are (1) the *Boston brace,* or underarm orthosis, customized from prefabricated plastic shells, with corrective forces for each patient, using lateral pads and decreasing lumbar lordosis, and (2) the *Milwaukee brace,* an individually adapted plastic and metal brace that includes a neck ring and can be used for curves with an apex of higher than T8 (Fig. 51-19).

The type of brace and wearing schedule (usually between 16 and 23 hours a day) are based on the nature of the curve, the age of the child, and any underlying condition associated with the curve. The underarm brace is usually more cosmetically acceptable to the child, since it is easily hidden under loose-fitting clothing.

Electrical stimulation. Mild to moderate curvatures may be treated with electrical stimulation. An electrical stimulator

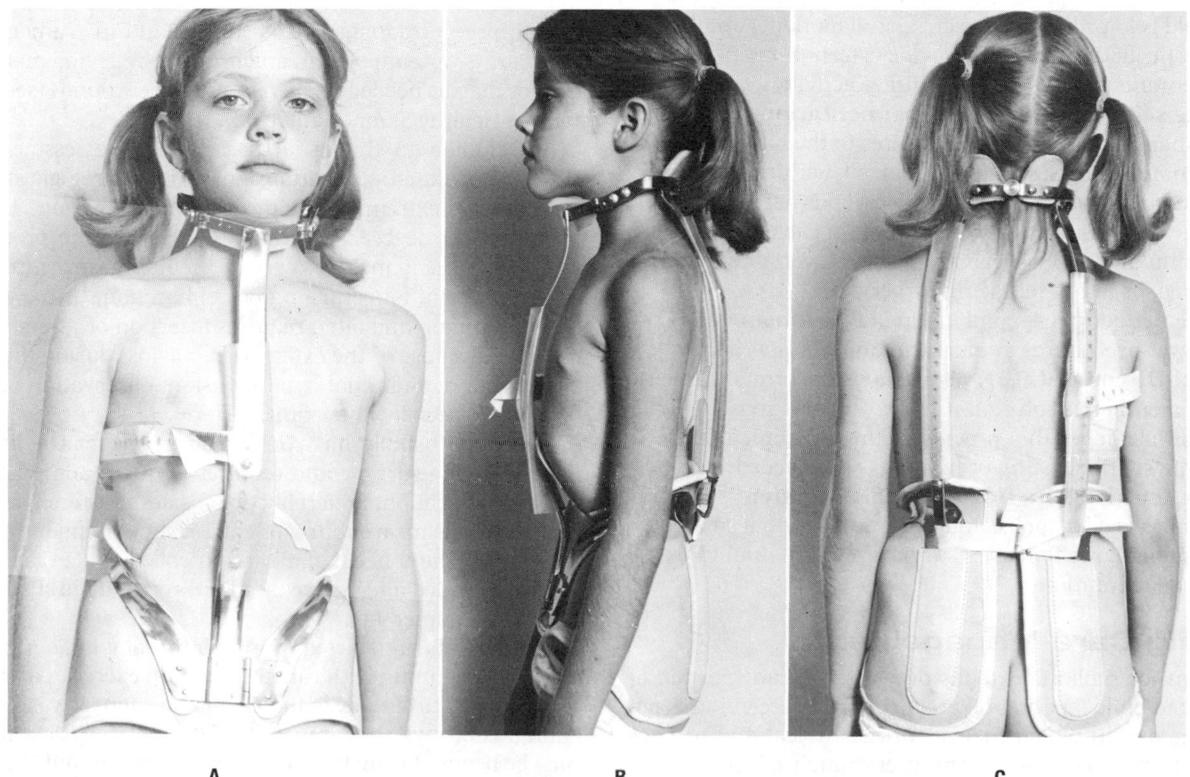

Fig. 51-19 Milwaukee brace. **A,** Front view. **B,** Side view. **C,** Rear view. (From Blount WP, Mueller KH, *Praxis* 8:139-149, 1972.)

generates an electrical pulse that is transmitted to muscles on the convex side of the curvature. This causes the muscles to contract at regular and frequent intervals, possibly straightening the spine. The device is worn at night, allowing unrestricted activity during the waking hours. Not all authorities believe that this therapy is effective.

Surgical correction. Surgical intervention may be required for correction. With few exceptions the techniques consist of spinal realignment and straightening by way of external or internal fixation and instrumentation combined with bony fusion (arthrodesis) of the realigned spine. The age of the child and location of the curvature influence the decision for surgery, and any curve that does not respond to more conservative measures requires surgical correction.

For the most severe scoliotic curvatures, traction is often needed for a time before spinal fusion to provide partial correction and more flexibility. Methods incorporating either continuous or intermittent traction are used. One type consists of a leather head halter and pelvic girdle attached to a system of ropes and pulleys that can be manipulated by the patient. More rigid deformities are best managed by skeletal traction techniques.

When surgical intervention is elected, a variety of spinal fusion techniques may be used. Depending on the surgical procedure, casting or a removable brace may be used for a period of 6 months to a year to produce satisfactory results. The surgical techniques for internal vertebral fixation include:

Harrington instrumentation—implantation of metal rods by way of clips to hold the vertebrae and bone fragments for permanent fusion; postoperatively the child is log-rolled to prevent spinal motion. A molded plastic jacket is used to provide external stabilization of the spine while the child resumes activities.

Luque segmental spinal instrumentation—a flexible L-shaped metal rod fixed by wires to the bases of the spinous processes; patient can walk within a few days, and no postoperative immobilization is necessary

Dwyer instrumentation—a titanium cable through cannulated screws transfixed to each vertebra; child is cared for in bed following surgery

Zielke procedure—combination of Harrington and Dwyer procedures; requires an anterior approach

Cotrel-Dubousset (CD) procedure—a form of bilateral segmental fixation that uses two knurled rods and multiple hooks that provide secure attachment to the spine so that casting or bracing is not needed

Texas Scottish Rite Hospital (TSRH) system—use of bilateral rods, hooks, and cross-link plates; if needed system allows for easier surgical revision than CD instrumentation

Nursing Care Management

Treatment for scoliosis extends over a significant portion of the affected child's period of growth. In adolescents this period is the one in which their identity, physical and psychologic, is formed. For some youngsters much of this time is spent in the hospital setting, immobilized in complex, unattractive appliances. For those treated on an outpatient basis it means having a modified life-style and being "different" from their peers, even though they are usually able to engage in many activities enjoyed by other youngsters.

When a child first faces the prospect of a prolonged period in a brace, cast, or other device, the therapy program and the nature of the device must be explained thoroughly to both the child and the parents so that they will have an understanding of the anticipated results, the way the appliance corrects the defect, the freedoms and constraints imposed by the device, and what they can do to help achieve the desired goal. The management involves the skills and services of a team of specialists, including the orthopedist, physical therapist, orthotist (a specialist in fitting orthopedic braces), nurse, social worker, and sometimes a pulmonary specialist.

It is difficult for the child to be restricted at any phase of development, but the teenager needs continual positive reinforcement, encouragement, and as much independence as can be safely assumed during this time. Guidance and assistance regarding anticipated problems, such as selection of clothing and participation in social activities, are appreciated by adolescents. Socialization with peers is encouraged, and every effort is expended to help the adolescent feel attractive and worthwhile.

Preoperative care. The child hospitalized for surgical management requires preparation for the procedures involved, which are puzzling and often frightening to the young patient. The child needs to know what is going to happen and deserves a full explanation of why the procedure is necessary and the potential outcome of the surgery.

Postoperative care. After surgery, patients are monitored in an intensive care unit and log-rolled when changing position to prevent damage to the fusion and instrumentation. Skin care is very important, and pressure-relieving mattresses or beds may be needed to prevent pressure wounds (see Maintaining Healthy Skin, Chapter 42).

In addition to the usual postoperative assessments—of wound, circulation, and vital signs—the neurologic status of the patient's extremities requires special attention. There is usually some degree of paralytic ileus after the procedure; therefore nursing includes care of the nasogastric intubation and assessment for returning bowel function. Urinary retention is common and often requires insertion of an indwelling catheter. Because of the extensive blood loss during the surgical procedure and renal hypoperfusion, observation of urine output is especially important.

The child usually has considerable pain for the first few days following surgery and requires frequent administration of pain medication, preferably opioids administered on a regular schedule intravenously or epidurally. For children able to understand the concept, patient-controlled analgesia (PCA) is a recommended alternative (see Pain Assessment; Pain Management, Chapter 41).

All patients are started on physiotherapy as soon as they are able, beginning with range-of-motion exercises and many of the activities of daily living. Self-care, such as washing and eating, is always encouraged. Some simple physical therapy may be begun during this acute stage. Throughout the hospitalization, diversional activities and contact with family and friends are important parts of nursing care and planning.

The family is encouraged to become involved with the patient's care to facilitate the transition from hospital to home management. Family members learn to apply and care for the brace or learn cast care. An organization that provides education and services to both families and professionals is the National Scoliosis Foundation, Inc.,* The Scoliosis Research Society,† an organization of physicians and scientists, has published an excellent book, *Scoliosis: A Handbook for Patients.*

See also Nursing Care Plan: The Child with Structural Scoliosis.‡

Infections of Bones and Joints

OSTEOMYELITIS

Osteomyelitis is an infectious process of bone that can occur at any age but that occurs most frequently between 5 and 14 years of age. It is twice as common in boys as in girls.

Pathophysiology

Osteomyelitis can be acquired from exogenous or hematogenous sources. *Exogenous osteomyelitis* is acquired by invasion of the bone by direct extension from the outside as a result of a penetrating wound, open fracture, contamination during surgery, or secondary extension from an overlying abscess or burn. *Hematogenous osteomyelitis* results from spread of organisms from preexisting infectious foci, including furuncles, skin abrasions, impetigo, upper respiratory tract infections, acute otitis media, tonsillitis, abscessed teeth, pyelonephritis, or infected burns.

Any organism can cause osteomyelitis, and there is some relationship between the age of the child and the type of organism responsible. In older children staphylococci are the most common organisms, approximately 80% of which are *Staphylococcus aureus;* in younger children other organisms predominate, especially *Haemophilus influenzae.* In children with sickle cell anemia, *Salmonella* organisms are frequently the responsible agents. Other factors that predispose to development of osteomyelitis are poor physical condition, inadequate nutrition, and surroundings that are not hygienic.

Infective emboli from the focus of infection travel to the small end arteries in the bone metaphysis, where they set up an infectious process that leads to local bone destruction and abscess formation.

Diagnostic Evaluation

The signs and symptoms of *acute hematogenous osteomyelitis* begin abruptly and build up to a maximum intensity during the first few days of the disease, usually less than 1 week (Box 51-10). Symptoms often resemble those observed in other disorders involving bones (e.g., leukemia, arthritis). There are marked leukocytosis and an elevated erythrocyte sedimentation rate. Blood culture findings are usually positive during the early stage, and radiographic findings are often negative or show only soft tissue swelling for 10 to 14 days. After this time the radiographic findings reveal new bone formation. Tomography may reveal bone changes at an early stage (see the Critical Thinking Q & A box on p. 1734).

BOX 51-10
Clinical Manifestations of Acute Osteomyelitis

General manifestations

History of trauma to affected bone (frequent)
Child appears very ill
Irritability
Restlessness
Elevated temperature
Rapid pulse
Dehydration

Local manifestations

Tenderness
Increased warmth
Diffuse swelling over involved bone
Involved extremity painful, especially on movement
Involved extremity held in semiflexion
Surrounding muscles tense and resist passive movement

Most cases involve the femur or tibia and to a lesser extent the humerus and hip. In infants the diagnosis is more difficult because of a lack of systemic symptoms, and the disease may involve multiple bones or joints because of the difficulty in confining an infectious process in children in this age group.

In *subacute hematogenous osteomyelitis* symptoms have been present for a longer period, and the child sometimes has been treated with antibiotics, often for another infection, which modifies the clinical symptoms. In some instances the infection may produce a walled-off abscess rather than a spreading infection.

Therapeutic Management

As soon as blood cultures have been drawn, prompt and vigorous intravenous antibiotic therapy is initiated. The choice of antibiotic is influenced by age, and the dosage determined is sufficient to ensure high blood and tissue levels. The appropriate antibiotic is usually continued for at least 3 to 4 weeks, but the length of therapy is determined by the duration of symptoms, the initial response to treatment, and the sensitivity of the organism in the specific case. Because of prolonged high-dose therapy, it is important to monitor hematologic, renal, hepatic, and other organ systems that may be adversely affected by the drugs (e.g., ototoxic effects).

Antibiotic therapy is accompanied by local treatment. The child is placed on complete bed rest. Immobilization of the affected extremity, which may require a splint or bivalved cast, is continued throughout therapy to limit the spread of infection and, when it is a complication of a fracture, to maintain alignment of bone fragments.

Opinions differ regarding surgical intervention, but many advocate sequestrectomy (removal of dead bone) and surgical

*75 Cabot Place, Stoughton, MA 02072; (617) 341-6333.

†6300 River Rd., Rosemont, IL 60018; (847) 698-1627. The book can be purchased by sending $1.00 to the organization.

‡In Wong DL: *Wong and Whaley's clinical manual of pediatric nursing,* ed 4, St Louis, 1996, Mosby.

Critical Thinking Q & A 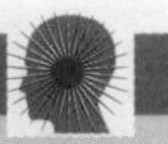

DIAGNOSIS OF OSTEOMYELITIS

Luis, a 12-year-old male, is in the emergency room with a 102° F temperature and a heart rate of 94. He is restless and complains of right leg pain. Laboratory results show an elevated erythrocyte sedimentation rate and leukocytosis. The history includes a recent automobile accident that resulted in hospitalization. During the hospital stay he had acquired a nosocomial *Staphylococcus aureus* infection. What findings would you expect from a thorough assessment?

1. Localized warmth, tenderness, and diffuse swelling above his right knee
2. Ability to extend right leg to full flexion
3. Slight pain with ambulation
4. All of the above

The correct answer is one, which indicates the clinical manifestations of acute osteomyelitis. Other signs would include inability to extend the leg fully and significant pain with ambulation.

drainage to prevent abscess formation. When surgical drainage is carried out, polyethylene tubes are placed in the wound—one tube instills an antibiotic solution directly into the infected area by gravity, and the other, connected to a suction apparatus, provides drainage.

Nursing Care Management

During the acute phase of illness any movement of the affected limb will cause discomfort; therefore the child is positioned comfortably with the affected limb supported. Moving and turning are carried out carefully and gently to minimize pain. Pain medication is administered to provide comfort. Vital signs are taken and recorded frequently, and measures are implemented to reduce a significant temperature elevation.

Antibiotic therapy requires careful observation and monitoring of the intravenous equipment and site. Since more than one antibiotic is usually administered, the compatibility of the drugs is determined, and care is taken to avoid mixing noncompatible drugs. For long-term antibiotic therapy, an intermittent infusion device or peripherally inserted central catheter (PICC) is used (see Venous Access Devices, Chapter 42). Antibiotic therapy is often continued at home.

The child with an open wound may be placed on contact isolation. The wound is managed as prescribed. Antibiotic solution administered directly into the wound is most efficiently accomplished with a regular intravenous infusion setup that is prepared and regulated in the same manner as any other. The drainage tubes are connected to low Gomco or wall suction for continuous removal. Intake and output are measured and recorded, and the character of the wound drainage is noted. The amount and character of drainage on the wound dressing are also noted.

Casts are sometimes used for immobilization, and, if so, routine cast care is carried out. The extremity is examined for sensation, circulation, and pain, and the area over the inflammation is usually left open for observation. The affected area, casted or uncasted, is assessed for color, swelling, heat, and tenderness.

The child usually has a poor appetite at first. Nourishment in the form of high-calorie liquids, such as fruit juices, gelatin, and juice bars, is encouraged until the child begins to feel better. The appetite returns as the acute symptoms subside. During convalescence adequate nutrition must be maintained to aid healing and formation of new bone.

When the acute stage subsides, the child begins to feel better, the appetite improves; the child becomes interested in the surroundings and relationships and may move about in bed. However, bearing weight on the affected limb is not permitted until healing is well under way in order to prevent pathologic fractures. Diversional and constructive activities become important nursing interventions. The child is usually confined to bed for some time after the acute phase but may be allowed to move about in a wheelchair when isolation and bed rest are no longer necessary. As the infection subsides, physical therapy is instituted to ensure restoration of optimal function.

SEPTIC (SUPPURATIVE, PYOGENIC, PURULENT) ARTHRITIS

Infection of the joints, like infection of bone, usually develops through hematogenous dissemination from another focus; occasionally it results from direct extension of a soft tissue infection. Joint infections occur predominantly in males, especially in the adolescent age group. In infancy, however, the incidence in boys and girls is more nearly equal. Any joint may be involved, but the hip, knee, shoulder, and other large joints are more commonly affected. Usually only one joint is involved.

Diagnostic Evaluation

The signs and symptoms of suppurative arthritis, unlike those of osteomyelitis, are usually characteristic (Box 51-11). Fever, leukocytosis, and an increased erythrocyte sedimentation rate are present but may not be demonstrated in affected infants. The most common pathogens are *Staphylococcus aureus,* group A streptococci, and *Haemophilus influenzae.* Diagnosis is made from blood culture, joint fluid aspirate, and radiographs.

Therapeutic Management

Treatment consists of open surgical drainage of hip and shoulder joint disease and repeated needle aspirations of the joint space in other joints. The goals are (1) to cleanse the joint to prevent destruction of articular cartilage, (2) to decompress the joint to prevent interference with the blood supply to the epiphysis, (3) to eradicate the infection with adequate antibiotic therapy, and (4) to prevent secondary bone infection and hematogenous spread. Therapy is similar to that for osteomyelitis; intravenous antibiotic therapy, relief of pain, immobilization of the joint, and prohibition of weight bearing until healing is complete.

Nursing Care Management

Nursing care is the same as that for osteomyelitis.

TUBERCULOSIS

Tubercular infection of the bones is acquired by hematogenous dissemination from a primary tubercular focus. The most common sites in infants and small children are the carpals and phalanges and the corresponding bones of the feet. One or several bones may be involved, with spindle-

BOX 51-11
Clinical Manifestations of Septic Arthritis

History of a traumatic injury to the affected joint (often)
Fever
Involved joint is:
- Warm and tender
- Erythematous
- Swollen
- Painful on even gentle pressure

Superficial involved joints are exquisitely painful
Deep-seated involved joints show little superficial evidence

shaped swelling and tenderness as soft tissues are affected. The process, relatively painless, persists with intermittent symptoms for several months and may leave a permanent deformity. The affected areas are immobilized with a splint or cast.

Tuberculosis of the Spine (Tuberculous Spondylitis)

In older children the infection attacks the body of one or more vertebrae, destroying the bone, and spreads to all the articular tissues, producing a kyphotic deformity. The lower thoracic spine is most frequently affected (Box 51-12 for manifestations).

Treatment consists of immobilization until there is no evidence of active infection, followed by spinal fusion. Antimicrobial therapy and drainage of tubercular abscess are standard therapies. The reparative process is slow, but in most instances recovery takes place with little or no deformity.

Tuberculosis of the Hip

The hip is the most common joint affected by tuberculosis, but the process usually begins in the epiphysis of the femoral head and then erupts into the joint capsule. There is progressive destruction of the femoral head with accompanying symptoms (Box 5-12). There may be abscess formation.

Treatment involves bed rest, traction to reduce muscle spasm, and appropriate drug therapy. Hip fusion may be necessary in severe cases.

BOX 51-12
Clinical Manifestations of Tuberculosis of the Bone

Spinal manifestations

Insidious onset
Irritability
Child complains of persistent or intermittent pain over areas innervated by spinal nerves that arise adjacent to affected vertebrae
Muscle splinting and pain when there is increased pressure applied to head
Child assumes position that best eases weight on diseased vertebrae, such as avoiding bending, walking stiffly and carefully on toes, and resting on abdomen or across a chair or a lap

Hip manifestations

Limp that occurs intermittently
Limp occurs most often on arising in the morning or after exercise
Pain
Thigh gradually becomes fixed and adducted with internal rotation
May be swelling around hip

Bone and Soft Tissue Tumors

GENERAL CONCEPTS: BONE TUMORS

Neoplastic disease can arise from any tissues involved in bone growth. In children the two types that account for 85% of all primary malignant bone tumors are osteogenic sarcoma (osteosarcoma) and Ewing sarcoma.

The peak ages during childhood are 15 to 19 years. The sexes are affected equally until puberty, at which time the ratio approaches 2:1 in favor of males. This propensity for males, with a peak incidence during adolescence, is thought to be related to the accelerated growth rate of osseous tissue. These two bone tumors have several characteristics in common, which are discussed, and then specific information about each tumor is detailed.

Diagnostic Evaluation

A primary objective in diagnosis of bone neoplasm is to rule out causes such as trauma or infection. A history and careful questioning regarding pain help determine the duration and rate of tumor growth (Box 51-13). Physical assessment focuses on the functional status of the affected area, signs of inflammation, size of the mass, involvement of regional lymph nodes, and any systemic indication of generalized malignancy.

Definitive diagnosis is based on radiologic studies (particularly computerized tomography), radioisotope bone scans, and/or surgical bone biopsy to identify the histologic type. Radiologic findings are characteristic for each type of tumor: a "sunburst" appearance produced by needlelike bone projections in osteogenic sarcoma and an "onionskin" appearance caused by layers of new bone in Ewing sarcoma. In both types of bone tumors, soft tissue infiltration may be apparent.

At present there is no reliable biochemical test for bone cancers, although elevated alkaline phosphatase levels may occur in osteoid tumors. Several tests may be performed to rule out metastatic disease from other neoplasms; lung tomography is especially important, since pulmonary metastasis is the most common complication of primary bone tumors. Bone marrow aspiration is helpful in diagnosing Ewing sarcoma in the rare event the child has bone marrow metastasis.

OSTEOGENIC SARCOMA

Osteogenic sarcoma is the most frequently encountered malignant bone cancer in children, with a peak incidence be-

BOX 51-13
Clinical Manifestations of Bone Tumors

Pain localized at affected site
- May be severe or dull
- Often relieved by position of flexion
- Frequently brought to attention when child:
  - Limps
  - Curtails own physical activity
  - Is unable to hold heavy objects

tween 10 and 25 years of age (Link and Eilber, 1993). Most primary tumor sites are in the metaphysis of long bones (wider part of the shaft, next to epiphyseal growth plate), especially in the lower extremities. More than half occur in the femur, particularly the distal portion, with the rest involving the humerus, tibia, pelvis, jaw, and phalanges.

Therapeutic Management

Optimal treatment of osteosarcoma is controversial. The traditional approach has consisted of radical surgery resection or amputation of the affected area. Depending on the tumor site, surgery consists of amputation of the affected extremity at least 7.5 cm (3 inches) above the proximal tumor margin or above the joint proximal to the involved bone (Link and Eilber, 1993). With tumors of the distal femur preservation of the hip joint may be possible. Other procedures include an above-the-knee amputation for tumors of the tibia or fibula, a hemipelvectomy for tumors of the innominate (hip) bone, and a forequarter amputation (removal of arm, scapula, and portion of the clavicle on the affected side) for tumors of the upper humerus. For selected patients *limb salvage procedures* are performed; this involves primary tumor resection with prosthetic replacement of the involved bone. For example, with a tumor in the distal femur a total femur and joint replacement is performed.

Antineoplastic drugs, such as high-dose methotrexate, adriamycin, bleomycin, actinomycin D, cyclophosphamide, ifosfamide, and cisplatin, may be administered in combination or singly both before and after either type of surgery.

Prognosis. With surgery, such as amputation to resect the primary tumor or thoracotomy for pulmonary metastasis, combined with chemotherapy, survival rate is improving. Survival rates depend on the treatment and are influenced by other factors, such as the site of the primary tumor and the presence or absence of metastatic disease at diagnosis. However, approximately 50% of children with osteogenic sarcoma can expect long-term survival, and various cancer centers are reporting higher percentages (Jaffe, 1991).

Nursing Care Management

Nursing care depends on the type of surgical approach, and in either instance preparation of the child and family is critical. Obviously the family may have more difficulty adjusting to an amputation than a limb salvage procedure. Straightforward honesty is essential to gain the cooperation and trust of the child. The diagnosis of cancer should not be disguised with falsehoods such as "infection." To accept the need for radical surgery the child must be aware of the lack of alternatives for treatment. Although the task of informing the child is the responsibility of the physician, the nurse should be present for the discussion or be aware of exactly what is said to the child. The child should be told a few days before surgery, so that he or she has time to think about the diagnosis and consequent treatment and to ask questions.

Sometimes children have many questions about the prosthesis, limitations on physical ability, and prognosis in terms of cure. At other times they react with silence or with a calm manner that masks their concern and fear. Either response is part of the grieving process that accompanies a loss and must be accepted. Children should not be overwhelmed with information. A supportive approach is to answer their questions without offering additional information and to show a willingness to talk, with such expressions as, "Anytime you would like to talk or ask questions about the surgery, tell me." The nurse should not push the topic unless the child initiates the discussion. Silence does not always indicate nonacceptance.

The child is also informed of the need for chemotherapy. Again, caution must be exercised to prevent offering too much information at one time. It is wise to discuss hair loss with emphasis on positive aspects, such as wearing a wig or baseball cap. Since bone tumors affect adolescents and young adults, it is not unusual for them to become angry over all the radical body alterations.

If an amputation is performed, the child may be fitted with a temporary prosthesis immediately after surgery, which permits early functioning and fosters psychologic adjustment. If this is not done, the child requires stump care, which is the same as for any amputee. A permanent prosthesis is usually fitted within 6 to 8 weeks. During hospitalization the child begins physical therapy to become proficient in the use and care of the device.

Phantom limb pain may follow amputation. This symptom is characterized by pain, tingling, itching, burning, and/or cramping in the area of the amputated limb. The child and family need to know that the sensations are real, not imagined. Amitriptyline (Elavil) has been used successfully in children to decrease the pain (Rogers, 1989). However, several pharmacologic and nonpharmacologic interventions, such as transcutaneous electrical nerve stimulation (TENS), may need to be tried to treat phantom limb pain successfully (Rounseville, 1992).

Discharge planning must begin early during the postoperative period. Every effort is made to promote normality and gradual resumption of realistic preamputation activities.* Role playing in anticipation of such experiences is very beneficial in preparing the child for the inevitable confrontation by others. Environmental barriers, such as stairs, are assessed in terms of the accessibility of the school and/or home, especially since the child may need to use crutches or a wheelchair before complete healing and prosthetic competency are achieved.

*Information about special programs for children with amputations, such as "Sunshine Skiers," is available from the **Candlelighters Childhood Cancer Foundation,** 1901 Pennsylvania Ave., N.W., Suite 1001, Washington, DC 20006. Information about prostheses can be obtained from the **National Amputation Foundation, Inc.,** 3840 Church St., Malverne, NY 11565; (516) 887-3600. In Canada: **War Amputations of Canada,** 2827 Riverside Dr., Ottawa, Ontario K1V 0C4; (613) 731-3821.

The family and child need a great deal of support in adjusting not only to a life-threatening diagnosis but also to alteration in body image and function. Since loss of a limb requires a grieving process, those caring for the child need to recognize that anger and depression are normal, necessary reactions. Often parents view the anger as a direct affront to them for allowing the amputation, or they view the depression as rejection. These are not personal attacks but the child's attempts to cope with the loss.

See also the Nursing Care Plan: The Child with Cancer (Chapter 46) and the Nursing Care Plan: The Child with a Bone Tumor.*

EWING SARCOMA

Ewing sarcoma arises in the marrow spaces of the bone rather than from osseous tissue. The principal sites of origin are shafts of long bones (femur, tibia, fibula, humerus, ulna), trunk bones (vertebra, scapula, ribs, pelvis), and skull (Pizzo and Poplack, 1993). The disease occurs almost exclusively in individuals under age 30, with most occurrences in individuals between 4 and 25 years of age.

Therapeutic Management

Surgical amputation is not routinely recommended but may be considered when the results of radiotherapy render the extremity useless or deformed (such as from retarded growth in young children) or the tumor appears resectable. The treatment of choice is intensive irradiation of the involved bone combined with chemotherapy. A widely used drug regimen includes vincristine, actinomycin D, cyclophosphamide, or ifosphamide, VP-16, and adriamycin.

Prognosis. The prognosis is best for children who do not have metastasis at the time of diagnosis. Children with massive tumors or lung or bone marrow metastasis have a much poorer prognosis. Children with distal lesions have the best chance for cure.

Nursing Care Management

The psychologic adjustment to Ewing sarcoma is typically less traumatic than to osteogenic sarcoma because of the preservation of the affected limb. Many families accept the diagnosis with a sense of relief in knowing that this type of bone cancer does not necessitate amputation, and initially they may not be aware of the deleterious effects on the irradiated site, especially severely affected growth, function, and appearance. Consequently they need preparation for the various diagnostic tests, including bone marrow aspiration and surgical biopsy, and adequate explanation of the treatment regimen.

High-dose radiotherapy often causes a skin reaction of dry or moist desquamation followed by hyperpigmentation. The nurse advises the child to wear loose-fitting clothes over the irradiated area to minimize additional skin irritation. Because of increased sensitivity, the area is protected from sunlight and sudden changes in temperature, such as avoiding use of heating pads or ice packs. The child is encouraged to use the extremity as tolerated. Occasionally an active exercise program may be planned by the physical therapist to preserve maximum function.

The child needs the same considerations as any other patient with cancer in adjusting to the effects of chemotherapy, such as hair loss, severe nausea and vomiting, peripheral neuropathy, and possibly cardiotoxicity. Every effort should be made to outline a treatment plan that allows the child maximum resumption of a normal life-style and activities.

See also the Nursing Care Plan: The Child with Cancer (Chapter 46).

RHABDOMYOSARCOMA

Soft tissue sarcomas are malignant neoplasms that originate from undifferentiated mesenchymal cells in muscles, tendons, bursae, and fascia or from such cells as fibrous, connective, lymphatic, or vascular tissue. They are the fourth most common type of solid tumor in children. These disorders derive their name from the specific tissue(s) of origin, such as *myosarcoma* (*myo*—muscle). *Rhabdomyosarcoma* (*rhabdo*—striated) is the most common soft tissue sarcoma in children. Because striated (skeletal) muscle is found almost anywhere in the body, these tumors occur in many sites, the most common of which are the head and neck, especially the orbit. The disease occurs most commonly in children younger than 5 years of age.

Diagnostic Evaluation

The initial signs and symptoms are related to the site of the tumor and compression of adjacent organs (Box 51-14). Some tumor locations, particularly the orbit, produce symptoms early in the course of the illness and contribute to rapid diagnosis and improved prognosis. Other tumors, such as those of the retroperitoneal area, produce no symptoms until they are large, invasive, and widely metastasized. Unfortunately many of the signs and symptoms attributable to rhabdomyosarcoma are vague and frequently suggest a common childhood illness, such as "earache" or "runny nose." In some instances a primary tumor site is never identified.

Diagnosis begins with a careful examination of the head and neck area, particularly palpation of a nontender, firm, hard mass. The nasopharynx and oropharynx are inspected for any evidence of a visible mass. Radiographic studies are performed to isolate a tumor site, accompanied by chest radiographic examinations, lung tomograms, bone surveys, and bone marrow aspiration to rule out metastasis. A lumbar puncture is indicated for head and neck tumors. An excisional biopsy is performed to confirm the histologic type.

Therapeutic Management

Since this tumor is highly malignant, with metastasis frequently occurring at the time of diagnosis, aggressive multimodal therapy is recommended. Complete removal of the primary tumor is advocated whenever possible. However, biopsy is required only in certain tumor locations, such as those of the orbit, when followed by radiation and chemotherapy. This prevents the devastating effects of enucleation, amputation, or pelvic exenteration.

High-dose irradiation to the primary tumor is recommended for most tumors. Radiation usually begins after several chemotherapy courses have been given to shrink the tumor. Drugs that are cytotoxic for rhabdomyosarcoma are

*In Wong DL: *Wong and Whaley's: clinical manual of pediatric nursing*, ed 4, St Louis, 1996, Mosby.

BOX 51-14
Clinical Manifestations of Rhabdomyosarcoma According to Tumor Site

Orbit
Rapidly developing unilateral proptosis
Ecchymosis of conjunctiva
Loss of extraocular movements (strabismus)

Nasopharynx
Stuffy nose (earliest sign)
Nasal obstruction—dysphagia, nasal voice (obstruction of posterior nasal conchae), serous otitis media (obstruction of eustachian tube)
Pain (sore throat and ear)
Epistaxis
Palpable neck nodes
Visible mass in oropharynx (late sign)

Paranasal sinuses
Nasal obstruction
Local pain
Discharge
Sinusitis
Swelling

Middle ear
Signs of chronic serous otitis media
Pain
Sanguinopurulent drainage
Facial nerve palsy

Retroperitoneal area
Usually a "silent" tumor
Abdominal mass
Pain
Signs of intestinal or genitourinary obstruction

Perineum
Visible superficial mass
Bowel or bladder dysfunction (from tumor compression)

vincristine, actinomycin D, and *cyclophosphamide* (collectively known as *VAC*), with or without adriamycin. Other drugs also may be used for more extensive disease.

Prognosis. With current treatment protocols survival rates for children with tumors detected at all clinical stages have increased considerably. Data suggest that children who remain disease-free for 2 years are probably cured; however, if relapse occurs the prognosis for long-term survival is extremely poor (Raney et al, 1993).

Nursing Care Management

The nursing responsibilities are similar to those for other types of cancer, especially the solid tumors when surgery is used. Specific objectives include (1) careful assessment for signs of the tumor, especially during well-child examinations; (2) preparation of the child and family for the multiple diagnostic tests; and (3) supportive care during each stage of multimodal therapy. The reader is urged to review Nursing Considerations under Leukemias in Chapter 46 for physical care of the child, and Chapter 38 for emotional support of the family in the event of a poor prognosis.

Disorders of Joints

JUVENILE RHEUMATOID ARTHRITIS (JRA)

Clinically and pathologically, JRA is an inflammatory disease with an unknown cause. There are two peak ages of onset: between 2 and 5 years of age and between 9 and 12 years of age. Females are affected somewhat more frequently than males. In many instances the disease remains undiagnosed for years.

JRA is not a single disease, but a heterogenous group of diseases. Three major types can be identified. *Systemic-onset disease* is associated with daily temperature spikes (usually in the afternoon) for at least 2 weeks, with or without a maculopapular rash. It accounts for about 30% of all cases. The *polyarticular onset* involves five or more joints and is seen in 25% of cases. The *pauciarticular onset* involves four or fewer joints and is the most common type, accounting for 45% of all cases.

Pathophysiology

The rheumatic process is characterized by a chronic inflammation of the synovium with joint effusion and eventual erosion, destruction, and fibrosis of the articular cartilage. Adhesions between joint surfaces and ankylosis of joints occur if the process persists long enough.

Whether a single joint or multiple joints are involved, the general manifestations (Box 51-15) result from edema, joint effusion, and synovial thickening. The limited motion early in the disease is the result of muscle spasm and joint inflammation; later it is caused by ankylosis or soft tissue contracture. Infections, injuries, or operations often precipitate a flare-up of the arthritis; therefore it is necessary to recognize and treat infections promptly.

Growth may be retarded during periods of active disease, usually with growth spurts during remissions. In severe longstanding cases growth is significantly retarded. Corticosteroid therapy can be a contributing factor.

Diagnostic Evaluation

There are no definitive serologic tests for JRA. The diagnosis is based on criteria established by the American Rheumatism Association (Emery and Miller, 1993). The erythrocyte sedimentation rate may or may not be elevated, depending on the degree of inflammation present. Leukocytosis is generally present in the early stages of classic systemic disease. The result of the latex fixation test, the most common test used to detect the presence of rheumatoid factor (RF) in adults, is negative in 90% of juvenile cases. RFs are found in some children, usually those with disease of later onset. Antinuclear antibodies (ANAs) are found in some types of JRA, especially early-onset pauciarticular disease.

Radiographic findings are variable, but the earliest mani-

BOX 51-15
Clinical Manifestations of Juvenile Rheumatoid Arthritis

Involved joints:
- Stiffness
- Swelling
- Tenderness
- Painful to touch or relatively painless
- Warm to touch (seldom red)
- Loss of motion
- Characteristic morning stiffness or "gelling" on arising in the morning or after activity

festations are widening joint spaces followed by gradual evidence of fusion and articular destruction.

Therapeutic Management

There is no specific cure for JRA. The major goals of therapy are to preserve joint function, prevent physical deformities, and relieve symptoms without causing iatrogenic harm. The child is treated at home under the supervision of the health team, and intermittent treatment by qualified professionals is administered. Hospitalization may be needed during severe exacerbations or when intercurrent illness warrants. Iridiocyclitis, also known as uveitis (inflammation of the iris and ciliary body), is a serious disorder unique to JRA that requires the attention of an ophthalmologist.

Drugs. Several drugs, given alone or in combination, are effective in suppressing the inflammatory process and relieving pain:

Nonsteroidal antiinflammatory drugs (NSAIDs)—(e.g., aspirin, tolmetin sodium, ibuprofen, and naproxen) daily dose usually divided into two or four doses

Slower-acting antirheumatic drugs (SAARDs)—(gold, D-penicillamine, and hydroxychloroquine) may be added to the regimen when one or two NSAIDs have been ineffective

Cytotoxic drugs—(e.g., cyclophosphamide, azathioprine, chlorambucil, and methotrexate) reserved for patients with severe debilitating disease and those who have responded poorly to NSAIDs and SAARDs (White and Ansell, 1992)

Corticosteroids—potent antiinflammatory agents are used for life-threatening disease, incapacitating systemic disease (unresponsive to other antiinflammatory therapy), and iridocyclitis; administered in the lowest effective dose, on alternate days (rather than daily), and for the shortest period possible; undesirable chronic side effects

Physical management. Programs of physical management are individualized for each child and designed to reach the ultimate goal—preserving function and/or preventing deformity. Physical therapy is directed toward specific joints, focusing on strengthening muscles, mobilizing restricted joint motion, and preventing or correcting deformities. Occupational therapy assumes responsibility for generalized mobility and performance of activities of daily living.

General treatment or maintenance programs varies; physiotherapists may be involved several times weekly to monthly in management of a home program, or their visits may be limited to infrequent review of the home program for compliance, effectiveness, and need. Normal activities of daily living and the child's natural tendency to be active are usually sufficient to maintain muscle strength and joint mobility.

Exercising in a pool is excellent therapy, since it allows freedom of movement with support and minimum gravitational pull. When joints are inflamed, heavy resistance aggravates the pain; at such times simple isometric or tensing exercises that do not involve joint movement are generally tolerated and should be encouraged. Range-of-motion exercises are an important aspect of therapy and are continued after evidence of disease has disappeared in order to detect any signs of recurrence.

Most practitioners recommend splinting and positioning during rest to help minimize pain and prevent or reduce flexion deformity. Joints most frequently splinted are the knees, wrists, and hands. Positioning during rest is also important. The child rests on a firm mattress with no pillow or a very low one and has no support under the knee. Loss of extension in the knee, hip, and wrist causes special problems and requires vigilance to detect the earliest signs of involvement and vigorous attention to prevent deformity with specialized passive stretching, positioning, and resting splints.

Prognosis. The course of JRA is highly variable. Thirty percent to 40% of patients have active disease 10 years after the diagnosis, have substantial disability as adults, and require long-term drug therapy. The prognosis is best for children with pauciarticular JRA and worst for children with chronic, polyarticular disease, especially those with positive RF findings (Wallace and Levinson, 1991).

Nursing Care Management

Assessment

Nursing the child with JRA involves assessment of the child's general health, the status of involved joints, and the child's emotional response to all ramifications of the disease—discomfort, physical restrictions, therapies, and self-concept.

Nursing Diagnoses

Nursing diagnoses and management identified for the child with JRA are outlined in Box 51-16. Others will be apparent in individual cases.

Planning

Goals for the child with JRA and family include the following:

1. Child will experience reduction of pain to level acceptable to child.
2. Child will remain healthy.
3. Child will exhibit signs of adequate joint function.
4. Child will perform activities of daily living.
5. Child and family will receive adequate support.

BOX 51-16
Nursing Diagnoses: The Child with Juvenile Rheumatoid Arthritis

Chronic pain related to joint inflammation
Impaired physical mobility related to joint discomfort and stiffness
Bathing/hygiene, dressing/grooming, feeding, or toileting self-care deficit related to impaired joint mobility
Altered family processes related to a situational crisis (child with a chronic illness)

Implementation

The effects of the disease are manifested in every aspect of the child's life—in physical activities, social experiences, and personality development. Much of the children's adjustment to the stresses and demands of the disease and the level of functioning they achieve are directly related to the reaction and support they receive from their family and the health professionals concerned with their care and management.

Relieve pain. The pain of JRA is related to several aspects of the disease—disease severity, functional status, individual pain threshold, family variables, and psychologic adjustment. Although complete pain relief would be highly desirable, it is probably an unrealistic goal. The aim is to provide as much relief as possible with antiinflammatory medication and other therapies to help children tolerate the pain and cope as effectively as possible (Lovell and Walco, 1989). At present opioid administration is not a routine therapy for chronic pain. Nonpharmacologic modalities have proved effective in modifying pain perception (see Pain Management, Chapter 41) and activities that aggravate pain.

Promote general health. The general health of children and their siblings must be considered and is frequently overlooked as parents and health personnel concentrate on the disease. A well-balanced diet and assessment of nutritional status are integral parts of health supervision. The discomfort and increased need for rest may create problems of weight control. Excess weight causes additional strain on inflamed joints, especially those of the lower extremities. Excessive fatigue and overexertion should be prevented by regular periods of rest, especially during acute flare-ups of arthritis. Symptoms may be exacerbated during a viral illness.

Posture and body mechanics are important for children with JRA, both when they are at rest and when they are active. They must have a firm mattress to maintain good alignment of spine, hips, and knees and no pillow or a very thin one. Children who are confined to bed either at home or in the hospital may require supports or splints to maintain positioning. Waterbeds or an electric blanket (or electric sheet) placed under the bottom sheet provides comforting warmth. Lying in the prone position is encouraged to straighten hips and knees; children can do so during rest periods or while watching television. The family is instructed in the principles and purposes of splints so that they can use them judiciously.

Children are encouraged to attend school, even on days when there may be some pain or discomfort. The aid of the school nurse is enlisted so that a child is permitted to take the precribed medication at school and to arrange for rest in the nurse's office during the day. Split days or half days may help a child remain involved in school. Permitting the child to arrive at school late allows time to gain joint movement and reduces the time at school to prevent exhaustion. It is important that the child attend school to learn skills and engage in social interaction, especially if the JRA continues to limit physical skills. Arranging for two sets of textbooks eliminates the need to carry heavy or numerous books to and from school, thus reducing discomfort and difficulty in ambulating.

Facilitate compliance. The child and family are involved in the therapeutic plan. They need to know the purpose and correct use of any splints and appliances and the medication regimen. The family is instructed regarding administration of medications, as well as the value of a regular schedule of administration to maintain a satisfactory drug level in the body. They need to know that aspirin, as well as most NSAIDs, should not be given on an empty stomach and to be alert for signs of aspirin toxicity, which include hyperventilation as a sign of acidosis, bleeding from decreased clotting capacity, tinnitus (ringing in the ears) as a sign of cranial nerve VIII involvement, and undue drowsiness that may indicate central nervous system depression. If evidence of drug toxicity is noted, the family is instructed to stop the medication and notify the health professional.

Encourage heat and exercise. Heat has been shown to be beneficial to children with arthritis. Moist heat is best for relieving pain and stiffness, and the most efficient and practical method is in the bathtub. The temperature and duration of the bath are specified by the therapist but usually do not exceed 10 minutes at 37.8° C. Sometimes a daily whirlpool bath, paraffin bath, or hot packs may be used as needed for temporary relief of acute swelling and pain. Hot packs are easily applied using a bath towel wrung out after being immersed in hot water or heated in a microwave oven, applied to the area and covered with plastic for 20 minutes. Commercial pads that warm in only a few minutes in the microwave are also available. Painful hands or feet can be immersed in a pan of water for 10 minutes two or three times daily in addition to tub baths.

Pool therapy is the easiest method for exercising a large number of joints. Swimming activities strengthen muscles and maintain mobility in larger joints. Children in urban areas have access to a therapy pool, although transportation may be a problem for some families. Very small children who are frightened of the water can carry out their exercises in the bathtub. Small children love to splash, kick, and throw things in the water.

Activities of daily living provide satisfactory exercise for older children to maintain maximum mobility with minimum pain. These children are encouraged in their efforts and patiently allowed to dress and groom themselves, to assume daily tasks, and to care for their belongings. It is often difficult for stiff fingers to manipulate buttons, comb or brush hair, and turn faucets, but parents and other caregivers should not offer assistance to them. In addition, children should learn and understand why others do not help them. Many helpful devices, such as self-adhering fasteners, tongs for manipulating difficult items, and grab bars installed in bathrooms for safety, can be used to facilitate tasks. A raised toilet seat often makes the difference between dependent and independent toileting, since weak quadriceps muscles and sore knees inhibit the ability to raise the body from a low sitting position.

A child's natural affinity for play offers many opportunities for incorporating therapeutic exercises. Throwing or kicking a ball, hanging from monkey bars, and riding a tricycle (with seat raised to achieve maximum leg extension) are excellent moving and stretching exercises for a very young child whose daily living activities are physically limited.

An effective approach to beginning the day's activities is to awaken children early to give them the medication and then to allow them to sleep for an hour. On arising children take a hot bath (or shower) and perform a simple ritual of limbering-up exercises, after which they commence the activities of the day, such as going to school. Exercise, heat, and rest are spaced throughout the remainder of the day according to individual needs and schedules. Parents are instructed in exercises that meet the needs of the child.

Another method of supplying warmth before the child arises is to plug an electric blanket into an appliance timer. Set the blanket to medium or high and adjust the timer to turn on the blanket 1 hour before the child awakens (McIlvain-Simpson and Singsen, 1991).

The Arthritis Foundation and the American Juvenile Arthritis Foundation* provide services for both parents and professionals, and nurses should refer families to these agencies as an added resource.

Support child and family. Rheumatoid arthritis affects every aspect of the child's daily life. The physical pain and limitations interfere with performance of normal tasks and provision of self-care. There may be school difficulties related to transportation to and from school, stairs, and loss of time as a result of exacerbations and hospitalization. Physical limitations interfere with participation in many activities, both curricular and extracurricular, limiting peer contacts and interaction and increasing social isolation. Changes in personality usually accompany JRA, as they do in any child with a chronic illness. They may be temporary, such as demanding, irritable behavior, or they may be manifested in more permanent ways, such as passive hostility, uncommunicativeness, and manipulativeness. Efforts should be made to break through the child's defenses and to identify his or her anxieties, concerns, and conflicts in order to intervene early to prevent the development of permanent personality problems.

Most of the reactions, problems, and concerns of families of a child with JRA are those of any family of a chronically ill and/or disabled child. The problems and needs of these families are discussed in Chapter 38, and the reader is directed to this chapter for guidance in planning care.

Evaluation

The effectiveness of nursing interventions is determined by continual reassessment and evaluation of care based on the following observational guidelines and expected outcomes:

1. Observe child's behavior and use pain assessment techniques.
2. Conduct routine assessment of child's general health.
3. Observe child during planned and unplanned activities, assess mobility of joints, and observe the use of prescribed appliances.
4. Observe child's ability to perform activities of daily living.
5. Observe and interview child and family regarding feelings and concerns.

Expected outcomes:

1. Child is able to move with minimum or no discomfort.
2. Child attains and maintains optimal health status (specify).
3. Child engages in activities suitable to interests, capabilities, and developmental level; joints are mobile, flexible, and free of deformity.
4. Child is involved in self-care activities to maximum capabilities.
5. Child and family demonstrate an understanding of the child's disease and therapies; they verbalize their feelings and concerns.

See also the Nursing Care Plan: The Child with Juvenile Rheumatoid Arthritis.†

SYSTEMIC LUPUS ERYTHEMATOSUS (SLE)

SLE, or lupus erythematosus (LE), is a chronic inflammatory disease of the collagen or supporting tissues of the body. It characteristically follows an unpredictable course of remissions and exacerbations. Because connective tissue is found practically everywhere, almost any organ or structure can be affected.

SLE in childhood consists of two basic types: a transient neonatal disease apparently related to a maternal abnormality and a group of chronic diseases (usually having their onset after infancy) that correspond to the diseases seen in adults. The major portion of the discussion is limited to SLE in childhood.

The cause of SLE is not known, although it is believed that some inciting event, such as stress, infection, extreme fatigue, or exposure to various chemicals, drugs, or excessive sunburn, triggers a reaction that alters the body's immune response to its own tissues. The disease shows a tendency to occur within families.

Diagnostic Evaluation

Because SLE can affect almost any tissue, the clinical manifestations are variable (Box 51-17), and the diagnosis is established by demonstration of any 4 of 11 diagnostic criteria (Box 51-18). However, rapid involvement of vital organs, primarily the kidneys, can herald an accelerated course with minimum or absent involvement of other sites.

*1314 Spring St., N.W., Atlanta, GA 30309; (404) 872-7100 or (800) 283-7800. In Canada: the **Arthritis Society**, 250 Bloor St., E., Suite 401, Toronto, Ontario, Canada M4W 3P2; (416) 967-5679.

†In Wong DL: *Wong and Whaley's clinical manual of pediatric nursing*, ed 4, St Louis, 1996, Mosby.

BOX 51-17
Clinical Manifestations of Systemic Lupus Erythematosus Related to Tissues Involved

Cutaneous lesions—erythematous blush or scaly erythematous patches over bridge of nose and extending to each cheek symmetrically ("butterfly rash"); may extend to scalp, neck, chest, and extremities; sometimes pruritic; resemble severe sunburn or hives or may become bullous
Musculoskeletal system—generalized weakness, usually accompanied by arthritis, myalgia, joint swelling, and stiffness; usually not severe enough to cause deformity; pain may cause temporary disability
Central nervous system—varies from forgetfulness, excitability, and headache to seizures and frank psychosis; seizures may be early sign; any cranial nerves can be affected; paralysis (spinal cord involvement)
Heart and lungs—serous linings may be inflamed; pleurisy (lungs), pericarditis (heart); usually reversible with rest
Kidneys—glomerulus is usual site of destruction; proteinuria; kidney failure
Blood—anemia from decreased erythrocytes is common; amenorrhea secondary to anemia; platelets and plasma proteins may be affected
Lymphoid system—spleen and cervical, axillary, and inguinal lymph nodes are enlarged (sometimes); LE hepatitis may develop
Gastrointestinal tract—nausea, vomiting, diarrhea, and abdominal pain are possible

BOX 51-18
Criteria for Diagnosis of Systemic Lupus Erythematosus

Butterfly rash
Discoid rash
Photosensitivity
Oral ulcers
Arthritis
Serositis
Renal disorder
Neurologic disorder(s) (psychosis, coma, seizures, paresis)
Hematologic disorder(s) (anemia, thrombocytopenia, leukopenia)
Immunologic disorder(s) (anti-DNA, LE prep, anti-SM, STS)
Antinuclear antibody (ANA)

Therapeutic Management

The objectives of medical treatment are (1) to reverse the autoimmune and inflammatory processes and (2) to prevent exacerbations and complications. Therapy involves the use of specific and supportive medications and regulation of activity and diet. The principal drugs used to control inflammation are corticosteroids administered in doses sufficient to suppress symptoms, then tapered to the lowest suppressive dose. Other drugs include the immunosuppressive agents; antimalarial preparations, which are useful against dermatologic, arthritic, and renal symptoms of the disease; and nonsteroidal antiinflammatory agents, which relieve muscle and joint pains and reduce tissue inflammation. Drugs used to control various complications include antiepileptics, antihypertensives, and antibiotics.

The goal of restricted activity is to prevent a recurrence of the disease. An effective schedule must provide for gradual resumption of pre–lupus erythematosus activity and maximum rest periods, usually 8 to 10 hours of sleep a night and one or two rest times during the day. The most frequently prescribed diet modification, if needed, is moderate- or low-salt intake. Low-protein diets may be necessary to prevent elevated nitrogen levels. Weight reduction, if indicated, may help preserve maximum joint function and conserve energy.

Nursing Care Management

The principle nursing goals are to help the child and family adjust to the limitations and treatments of the disease and to prevent exacerbations and complications. Since older female adolescents are the most likely group to be affected, the nurse must be aware of their special needs, such as body image changes, present and future vocational activities, and social relationships. (See Chapter 38 for a discussion of adjusting to a chronic illness.)

Family members need an understanding of the disease process to gain an appreciation of the need for regular, uninterrupted drug administration; moderate activity; and any diet modifications that may be imposed. Usually diagnostic tests are performed during hospitalization, to allow the nurse an opportunity to help the child and parents learn about the disease. Several organizations have been formed to help children and families learn about and adjust to the disease. These groups include the American Lupus Society,* the Lupus Foundation of America Inc.,† and the Arthritis Foundation (see p. 1741).‡

In teaching the child with SLE and the family the nurse stresses the importance of adequate rest and the need to adhere to the medication schedule. Individuals who are sensitive to the sun must avoid exposure. It is important to emphasize that sun filtered through clouds or reflected from snow, water, or white surfaces (such as cement) can cause a severe reaction. Although clothes can protect most areas of the body, sunblocking or sunscreening agents with a high sun protection factor (SPF) are needed on exposed areas such as the face (see Sunburn, Chapter 50). A large-brimmed hat helps in partially shading the face.

Affected persons are advised to maintain regular medical supervision and to seek additional attention during periods of stress, during illness, or before elective surgical procedures, such as dental extraction, because the body may require larger amounts of a drug. People with SLE should carry medical identification emphasizing their dependence on steroids.

---

*P.O. Box 9610, Marina Del Ray, CA 90215; (310) 390-6888.
†4 Research Place, Suite 180, Rockville, MD 20850; (301) 670-9292 or (800) 558-0121.
‡A recommended booklet available from the foundation is *Meeting the Challenge: A Young Person's Guide to Living with Lupus.*

Key Points

- Immobility has a profound effect on all aspects of growth and development.
- The major physical consequences of immobilization are loss of muscle strength, endurance, and muscle mass; bone demineralization; loss of joint mobility; and contractures.
- Features of children's fractures not observed in the adult include presence of growth plate, thicker and stronger periosteum, bone porosity, more rapid healing, and less joint stiffness.
- The goals of fracture management are to regain alignment and length of bony fragments, retain alignment and length, and restore function to injured parts.
- The method of fracture reduction is determined by the age of the child, degree of displacement, amount of overriding, amount of edema, condition of the skin and soft tissues, sensation, and circulation distal to the fracture.
- The primary purposes of traction are to fatigue involved muscles and reduce muscle spasm, position bone ends in desired realignment, and immobilize the fracture site until realignment has been achieved to permit casting or splinting.
- The development of developmental dysplasia of the hip appears to be related to intrauterine, genetic, and cultural factors.
- Treatment of clubfoot consists of manipulation and casting to correct the deformity, maintenance of the correction, and prevention of possible recurrence of the deformity.
- Acquired hip deformities are managed with non–weight-bearing devices (coxa plana) or surgical stabilization (coxa vara).
- Observation for scoliosis is an important part of a routine physical assessment.
- Scoliosis is managed by bracing and exercise or surgical correction.
- Bone infections are managed with vigorous antibiotic therapy, immobilization of the affected part, and (sometimes) surgical drainage.
- Osteosarcoma is a neoplasm of bone-forming tissues; Ewing sarcoma is a neoplasm that arises from bone marrow spaces.
- Rhabdomyosarcoma may occur almost anywhere in the body, but the most common sites are the head and neck.
- Nursing care of the child with juvenile arthritis consists of promoting general health, relieving discomfort, preventing deformity, and preserving function.
- Lupus erythematosus is a chronic autoimmune disorder that affects the collagen tissues of the body.

References

Bennett JT, MacEwen GD: Congenital dislocation of the hip, *Clin Orthop* 247:15-21, 1989.

Bostrom B, McCormick P, Hooke C: Painless procedures with propofol, *J Pediatr Oncol Nurs* 10(2):64-65, 1993.

Carlino HY: The child with an Ilizarov external fixator, *Pediatr Nurs* 17(4):355-358, 1991.

Emery HM, Miller ML: *Ambulatory pediatric care*, ed 2, Philadelphia, 1993, JB Lippincott.

Jaffe N: Osteosarcoma, *Pediatr Rev* 12(11):333-343, 1991.

Link MP, Eilber F: *Osteosarcoma*. In Pizzo PA, Poplack DG: *Principles and practice of pediatric oncology*, ed 2, Philadelphia, 1993, JB Lippincott.

Lovell DJ, Walco GA: Pain associated with juvenile rheumatoid arthritis, *Pediatr Clin North Am* 36:1015-1027, 1989.

McIlvain-Simpson G, Singsen B: Decreasing morning stiffness, *Small Talk* 3(6):8, 1991.

Pizzo PA, Poplack DG: *Principles and practice of pediatric oncology*, ed 2, Philadelphia, 1993, JB Lippincott.

Raney RB et al: *Rhabdomyosarcoma and the undifferentiated sarcomas*. In Pizzo PA, Poplack DG: *Principles and practice of pediatric oncology*, ed 2, Philadelphia, 1993, JB Lippincott.

Rogers AG: Use of amitriptyline (Elavil) for phantom limb pain in younger children, *J Pain Symptom Manage* 4(2):96, 1989.

Rounseville C: Phantom limb pain: the ghost that haunts the amputee, *Orthop Nurs* 11(2):67-71, 1992.

Speers AT, Speers M: Care of the infant in a Pavlik harness, *Pediatr Nurs* 18(3):229-232, 252, 1992.

Tobias JD et al: Oral ketamine premedication to alleviate the distress of invasive procedures in pediatric oncology patients, *Pediatrics* 90(4):537-541, 1992.

Wallace CA, Levinson JE: Juvenile rheumatoid arthritis: outcome and treatment for the 1990s, *Rheum Dis Clin North Am* 17:891-905, 1991.

Wattenmaker I, Kasser JR, McGravey A: Self-administered nitrous oxide for fracture reduction in children in an emergency room setting, *J Orthop Trauma* 4(1):35-38, 1990.

White PH, Ansell BM: Methotrexate for juvenile rheumatoid arthritis, *N Engl J Med* 326(16):1077-1078, 1992.

Wong D, Baker C: Pain in children: comparison of assessment scales, *Pediatr Nurs* 14(1):9-17, 1988.

Bibliography

Immobilization

Brady M, Grey M: Growing pains: a myth or a reality, *J Pediatr Health Care* 3:219-220, 1989.

Bubulka GM, Cipolla F: Preparing for pediatric emergencies, *J Emerg Nurs* 17(4):236-240, 1991.

Mehmert PA, Delaney CW: Validating impaired physical mobility, *Nurs Diagn* 2(4):143-154, 1991.

National Association of Orthopaedic Nurses: Care for orthopaedic patient care: common concerns, *Orthop Nurs* 10(5):73-74, 1991.

Olson EV: The hazards of immobility, *Am J Nurs* 90:43-52, 1990.

Quellet LL, Rush KL: A synthesis of selected literature on mobility: a basis for studying impaired mobility, *Nurs Diagn* 3(2):72-80, 1992.

Sills EM: What's causing the back pain? *Contemp Pediatr* 5(11):85-96, 1988.

Szer IS: Are those limb pains "growing" pains? *Contemp Pediatr* 6(3):143-148, 1989.

Traumatic Injury

Alexander R et al: Serial abuse in children who are shaken, *Am J Dis Child* 144:58-60, 1990.

Campbell LS, Campbell JD: Musculoskeletal trauma in children, *Crit Care Nurs Clin North Am* 3(3):445-456, 1991.

Davis JM, Kuppermann N, Fleisher G: Serious sports injuries requiring hospitalization seen in a pediatric emergency department, *Am J Dis Child* 147(9):1001-1004, 1993.

DuRant RH et al: Findings from the preparticipation athletic examination and athletic injuries, *Am J Dis Child* 146:85-91, 1992.

Dyment PG: How to make the sports physical exciting, *Contemp Pediatr* (10):93-106, 1991.

Feller NG, Stroup K, Christian L: Helping staff nurses become mini-specialists, *Am J Nurs* 89:991-992, 1989.

Hansell MJ: Fractures and the healing process, *Orthop Nurs* 7(1):43-49, 1988.

Hergenroeder AC: Acute shoulder, knee and ankle injuries. I. Diagnosis and Management, *Adolescent Health Update* 8(2):1-8, 1996.

Hergenroeder AC: Acute shoulder, knee, and ankle injuries. II. Rehabilitation, *Adolescent Health Update* 8(3):1-8, 1996.

Kelly JP et al: Concussion in sports, *JAMA* 266(20):2867-2869, 1991.

Leyendecker M et al: Rescuing a multiple trauma victim, *Nursing 89* 19(10):54-61, 1989.

Mansfield MJ, Emans SJ: Growth in female gymnasts: should training decrease during puberty? *J Pediatr* 122(2):237-240, 1993.

Nypaver M, Treloar D: Neutral cervical spine positioning in children, *Ann Emerg Med* 23(2):208-211, 1994.

Reed JL, Keegan MJ: Fat embolism syndrome: a complication of trauma, *Crit Care Nurse* 13(3):33-37, 1993.

Sonzogni JJ, Gross M: Hip and pelvic injuries in the young: fractures and special disorders, part 2, *Emerg Med* 25(8):18-20+, 1993.

Varela CD, Lorfing KC, Schmidt TL: Intravenous sedation for the closed reduction of fractures in children, *J Bone Joint Surg* 77(3):340-345, 1995.

Congenital Defects

Bender LH: Osteogenesis imperfecta, *Orthop Nurs* 10(4):23-32, 1991.

Cmiel PA, Cavanaugh CE: Digital replantation in children, *Am J Nurs* 89:1158-1161, 1989.

McGrath PA, Hillier LM: Phantom limb sensations in adolescents: a case study to illustrate the utility of sensation and pain logs in pediatric clinical practice, *J Pain Symptom Manage* 7:46-53, 1992.

Varni JW et al: Family functioning, temperament, and psychologic adaptation in children with congenital or acquired limb deficiencies, *Pediatrics* 84:323-330, 1989.

Williamson VC: Amputation of the lower extremity: an overview, *Orthop Nurs* 11(2):55-65, 1992.

Musculoskeletal Disorders/Orthopaedic Infections

Bender LH: Osteogenesis imperfecta, *Orthop Nurs* 10(4):23-32, 1991.

Dunst RM: Legg-Calvé-Perthes disease, *Orthop Nurs* 9(2):18-27, 35-36, 1990.

Ekeberg DRE: Promoting a positive attitude in pediatric patients undergoing limb lengthening, *Orthop Nurs* 13(1):41-49, 1994.

Faden H, Grossi M: Acute osteomyelitis in children, *Am J Dis Child* 145(1):65-69, 1991.

Hart K: Using the Ilizarov external fixator in bone transport, *Orthop Nurs* 13(1):35-40, 1994.

Jacobs NM: Pneumococcal osteomyelitis and arthritis in children, *Am J Dis Child* 145(1):70-74, 1991.

Kerrick RC, French C: Torticollis: a head and neck immobilizer, *Am J Occup Ther* 47(1):79-80, 1993.

Ledwith CA, Fleisher GR: Slipped capital femoral epiphysis without hip pain leads to missed diagnosis, *Pediatrics* 89(4):660-662, 1992.

Nance DK, Mardjetko SM: Technical aspects and nursing considerations of limb lengthening, *Orthop Nurs* 13(1):21-33, 1994.

Scoliosis

Brosnan H: Nursing management of the adolescent with idiopathic scoliosis, *Nurs Clin North Am* 26(1):17-31, 1991.

Bunnel WP: Outcome of spinal screening, *Spine* 18(12):1572-1580, 1993.

Cassella M, Hall JE: Current treatment approaches in the nonoperative and operative management of adolescent idiopathic scoliosis, *Phys Ther* 71(12):897-909, 1991.

Cotton LA: Unit rod segmental spinal instrumentation for the treatment of neuromuscular scoliosis, *Orthop Nurs* 10(5):17-23, 1991.

Jacobs-Zacny JM, Horn MJ: Nursing care of adolescents having posterior spinal fusion with Cotrel-Dubousset instrumentation, *Orthop Nurs* 7(1):17-21, 1988.

Johnson JB, Killman-Young J: Adolescence, anxiety, and adaptation: preparing for posterior spine fusion with instrumentation, *J Pediatr Nurs* 3:348-349, 1988.

Murrel GAC et al: An assessment of the reliability of the scoliometer, *Spine* 18(6):709-712, 1993.

National Association of School Nurses Position Paper: Postural screening, *NAS Newsletter* 2:10, 1995.

Rauen KK, Ho M: Children's use of patient-controlled analgesia after spine surgery, *Pediatr Nurs* 15:589-593, 1989.

Richardson A, Taylor M, Murphree B: TSRH instrumentation: evolution of a new system, *Orthop Nurs* 9(6):15-21, 1990.

Scoloveno MA, Yarcheski A, Mahon NE: Scoliosis treatment effects on selected variables among adolescents, *West J Nurs Res* 12(5):616-619, 1990.

Voznak L: My life with scoliosis, *Orthop Nurs* 7(1):22-26, 1988.

Willers U et al: Long-term results of Harrington instrumentation in idiopathic scoliosis, *Spine* 18(6):713-717, 1993.

Bone and Soft Tissue Tumors

Bohm P, Wirth CJ, Jansson V: Limb-preserving operations in the treatment of malignant bone tumors, *Arch Orthop Trauma Surg* 108:218-224, 1989.

Bonilla JA, Healy GB: Management of malignant head and neck tumors in children, *Pediatr Clin North Am* 36(6):1443-1450, 1989.

Hockenberry MJ, Lane B: Limb salvage procedures in children with osteosarcoma, *Cancer Nurs* 11(1):2-8, 1988.

Loughlin KR et al: Genitourinary rhabdomyosarcoma in children, *Cancer* 63:1600-1606, 1989.

Maurer HM, Ragab AH: *Rhabdomyosarcoma.* In Fernbach DJ, Vietti TJ, editors: *Clinical pediatric oncology*, ed 4, St Louis, 1991, Mosby.

Rofary C, Flament F, Donaldson FF: An attempt to use a common staging system in rhabdomyosarcoma: a report of an international work-

shop initiated by the International Society of Pediatric Oncology, *Med Pediatr Oncol* 17:210-215, 1989.
Shochat S: Update on solid tumor management in children, *Pediatr Surg* 72(6):1417-1427, 1992.

Juvenile Rheumatoid Arthritis

Arnett FCL: Revised criteria for the classification on rheumatoid arthritis, *Orthop Nurs* 9(2):58-64, 1990.
Fantini F: Future trends in pediatric rheumatology, *J Rheumatol Suppl* 37:49-53, 1992.
Hughes RB, D'Ambrosia K: Nursing management of a child with juvenile rheumatoid arthritis, *Orthop Nurs* 12(5):17-22, 1993.
Lavigne JV et al: Evaluation of a psychological treatment package for treating pain in juvenile rheumatoid arthritis, *Arthritis Care Res* 5(2):101-110, 1992.
McIlvain-Simpson G: *Juvenile rheumatoid arthritis.* In Jackson PL, Vessey JA, editors: *Primary care of the child with a chronic condition,* ed 2, St Louis, 1996, Mosby.
Page GG: Chronic pain and the child with juvenile rheumatoid arthritis, *J Pediatr Health Care* 5(1):18-23, 1991.
Quirk ME, Young MH: The impact of JRA on children, adolescents, and their families: current research and implications for future studies, *Arthritis Care Res* 3(1):36-43, 1990.
Rose CD: Pharmacological management of juvenile rheumatoid arthritis, *Drugs* 43(6):849-863, 1992.
Sipos DA: M.P. implants for rheumatoid arthritis of the hand, *Orthop Nurs* 12(5):7-14, 1993.
Southwood TR et al: Unconventional remedies used for patients with juvenile arthritis, *Pediatrics* 85:150-154, 1990.
Swann M: The surgery of juvenile chronic arthritis: an overview, *Clin Orthop* (259):70-75, 1990.

Systemic Lupus Erythematosus

Feutren G et al: Effects of cyclosporin in severe systemic lupus erythematosus, *J Pediatr* 111:1063-1068, 1987.
Fuller C, Hartley B: Systemic lupus erythematosus in adolescents, *J Pediatr Nurs* 6(4):251-257, 1991.
Lee LA, Weston WL: Lupus erythematosus in childhood, *Dermatol Clin* 4:151-160, 1986.
Lehman TJA et al: Systemic lupus erythematosus in the first year of life, *Pediatrics* 83:235-239, 1989.
McCurdy DK et al: Lupus nephritis: prognostic factors in children, *Pediatrics* 89(2):240-246, 1992.
Olson NY, Lindsley CB: Neonatal lupus syndrome, *Am J Dis Child* 141:908-910, 1987.
Ramirez-Seijas F, Cepero-Akselrad A: Systemic lupus erythematosus in children, *Int Pediatr* 8(3):334-343, 1993.
Venables PJW: Diagnosis and treatment of systemic lupus erythematosus, *Br Med J* 307:663-666, 1993.

CHAPTER 52

Neuromuscular and Muscular Dysfunction

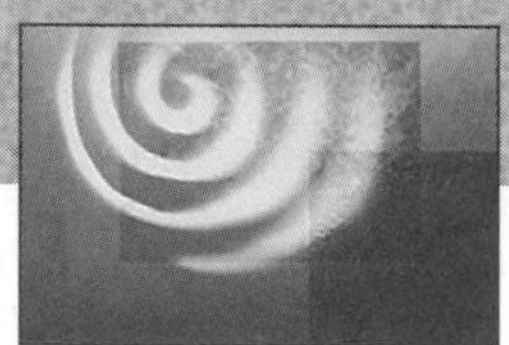

CONGENITAL NEUROMUSCULAR OR MUSCULAR DISORDERS, P. 1746

Cerebral palsy (CP), p. 1746

Spina bifida (myelomeningocele), p. 1751

Progressive infantile spinal muscular atrophy (Werdnig-Hoffmann disease), p. 1759

Juvenile spinal muscular atrophy (Kugelberg-Welander disease), p. 1760

Muscular dystrophies (MDs), p. 1760

Pseudohypertrophic (Duchenne) muscular dystrophy (DMD), p. 1761

ACQUIRED NEUROMUSCULAR DISORDERS, P. 1762

Guillain-Barré syndrome (GBS) (infectious polyneuritis), p. 1762

Tetanus, p. 1763

Botulism, p. 1764

Spinal cord injuries, p. 1765

Congenital Neuromuscular or Muscular Disorders

CEREBRAL PALSY (CP)

CP is a nonspecific term applied to disorders characterized by impaired movement and posture and early onset. It is nonprogressive and may be accompanied by perceptual problems, language deficits, and intellectual involvement. The etiology, clinical features, and course are variable and are characterized by abnormal muscle tone and coordination as the primary disturbances. It is the most common permanent physical disability of childhood, and the incidence is reported as 1.9 to 2.3 in every 1000 live births. A variety of prenatal, perinatal, and postnatal factors contribute to the etiology of CP singly or multifactorially. Although the prevalent hypothesis has been that CP results from perinatal problems, especially birth asphyxia, it is now known that CP results more commonly from existing *prenatal* brain abnormalities. Premature delivery continues to be the single most important determinant of CP; however, in approximately 24% of the cases, no cause is determined.

Pathophysiology

It is difficult to establish a precise location of neurologic lesions based on etiology or clinical signs because there is no characteristic pathologic picture. In some cases there are gross malformations of the brain; in others there may be evidence of vascular occlusion, atrophy, loss of neurons, and degeneration. Anoxia plays the most significant role in the pathologic state of brain damage, which is frequent secondary to other causative mechanisms.

CP has been classified in several ways, but the most useful classification is based on the nature and distribution of neuromuscular dysfunction (Box 52-1).

Diagnostic Evaluation

The neurologic examination and history are the primary modalities for diagnosis. A thorough knowledge of normal variations of motor development is required for detecting abnormal progress, and a careful history is elicited to detect possible etiologic factors. The alert observer may be suspicious when a child demonstrates some of the manifestations outlined in Box 52-2. The child's spontaneous movements and behavior are observed, including posture, attitude, as well as muscle size, function, and tone. Persistence of primitive reflexes may be of value, and two of these aid in the diagnosis: the asymmetric tonic neck reflex and the crossed extensor reflex.

Supplemental diagnostic tests may be employed, such as electroencephalography (EEG), tomography, screening for metabolic defects, and serum electrolyte values. The possibility that the manifestations are those of slowly progressive degenerative disease or early-onset, slowly growing brain tumors must be ruled out.

BOX 52-1
Clinical Classification of Cerebral Palsy

Spastic—May involve one or both sides
- Hypertonicity with poor control of posture, balance, and coordinated motion
- Impairment of fine and gross motor skills
- Active attempts at motion increase abnormal postures and overflow of movement to other parts of the body

Dyskinetic—Abnormal involuntary movement
- Athetosis, characterized by slow, wormlike, writhing movements that usually involve the extremities, trunk, neck, facial muscles, and tongue
- Involvement of the pharyngeal, laryngeal, and oral muscles causes drooling and dysarthria (imperfect speech articulation)
- Involuntary movements may take on choreoid (involuntary, irregular, jerking movements) and dystonic (disordered muscle tone) manifestations that increase in intensity with emotional stress and around adolescence

Ataxic—
- Wide-based gait
- Rapid repetitive movements performed poorly
- Disintegration of movements of the upper extremities when the child reaches for objects

Mixed-type—Combination of spasticity and athetosis

BOX 52-2
Clinical Manifestations of Cerebral Palsy

Delayed gross motor development
- A universal manifestation
- Delay in all motor accomplishments
- Increases as growth advances

Abnormal motor performance
- Very early preferential unilateral hand use
- Abnormal and asymmetric crawl
- Standing or walking on toes
- Uncoordinated or involuntary movements
- Poor sucking
- Feeding difficulties
- Persistent tongue thrust

Alterations of muscle tone
- Increased or decreased resistance to passive movements
- Opisthotonic postures (exaggerated arching of back)
- Feels stiff on handling or dressing
- Difficulty in diapering
- Rigid and unbending at the hip and knee joints when pulled to sitting position (an early sign)

Abnormal postures
- Maintains hips higher than trunk in prone position with legs and arms flexed or drawn under the body
- Scissoring and extension of legs, with the feet plantar flexed in supine position
- Persistent infantile resting and sleeping posture
  - Arms abducted at shoulders
  - Elbows flexed
  - Hands fisted

Reflex abnormalities
- Persistence of primitive infantile reflexes
  - Obligatory tonic neck reflex at any age
  - Nonpersistence beyond 6 months of age
- Persistence or hyperactivity of the Moro, plantar, and palmar grasp reflexes
- Hyperreflexia, ankle clonus, and stretch reflexes elicited in many muscle groups on fast passive movements

Associated disabilities*
- Subnormal learning and reasoning (mental retardation in about two thirds of individuals)
- Seizures
- Impaired behavioral and interpersonal relationships
- Sensory impairment (vision, hearing)

*May or may not be present.

Therapeutic Management

The goals of therapy for children with CP are early recognition and promotion of an optimum developmental course to enable affected children to attain their potential within the limits of their brain dysfunction. The disorder is permanent, and therapy is chiefly symptomatic and preventive.

The broad aims of therapy are (1) to establish locomotion, communication, and self-help; (2) to gain optimum appearance and integration of motor functions; (3) to correct associated defects as effectively as possible; (4) to provide educational opportunities adapted to the individual child's needs and capabilities; and (5) to promote socialization experiences with other affected and unaffected children. Each child is evaluated and managed on an individual basis. The plan of therapy may involve a variety of settings, facilities, and specially trained persons, including the parents.

Ankle-foot orthoses (AFOs) (braces) are worn by many of these children and are used to help prevent or reduce deformity, increase the energy efficiency of gait, and control alignment. Other mobilization devices include wheeled scooter boards that allow children to propel themselves while on the abdomen, wheeled go-carts that provide sitting balance and serve as early "wheelchair" experience for young children, and special devices that leave the upper extremities free (Figs. 52-1 and 52-2).

Nursing ALERT

The use of infant walkers is discouraged. They pose a risk of injury to normal children and are especially hazardous for children with CP. Also, jumping seats, such as those that hang in doorways, should not be used.

Orthopedic surgery may be required to correct contracture or spastic deformities, to provide stability for an uncontrollable joint, and to provide balanced muscle power. This includes tendon-lengthening procedures (especially heel-cord lengthening), release of spastic wrist flexor muscles, and correction of hip and adductor muscle spasticity or contracture to improve locomotion. *Selective dorsal rhizotomy* has provided marked improvement in some children with CP. However, achieving the benefits from the surgery requires intensive physical therapy and family commitment (Brucker, 1990).

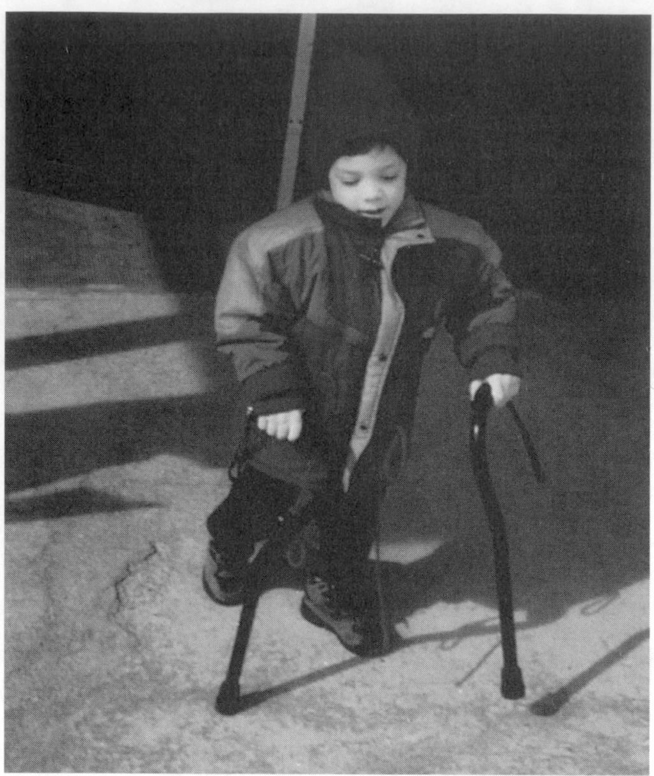

Fig. 52-1 Mobilization device for child.

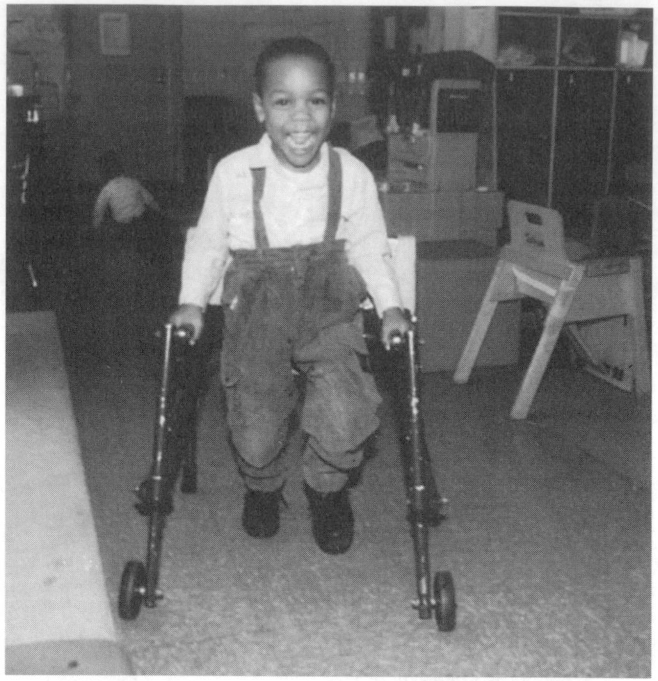

Fig. 52-2 Child ambulating with use of assistive device.

Because the procedure results in flaccid muscles, the child must be retaught to sit, stand, and walk.

Surgical intervention is usually reserved for the child who does not respond to the more conservative measures, but it is also indicated for the child whose spasticity causes progressive deformities. Surgery is primarily used to improve function rather than for cosmetic purposes and is followed by physical therapy. Neurosurgical procedures are used only in selected patients.

Drugs to decrease spasticity have little usefulness in improving function in CP. Antianxiety agents have been used to some extent to relieve excessive motion and tension, particularly in the athetoid child. Skeletal muscle relaxants, such as dantrolene (Dantrium), baclofen, and methocarbamol (Robaxin) may be used on a short-term basis for older children and adolescents. Diazepam (Valium) is often used but should be restricted to older children and adolescents. A local nerve block to motor points of a muscle with a neurolytic agent such as phenol solution reduces spasticity temporarily. Botulinum toxin (Botox) is also being used to paralyze a specific muscle.

Antiepileptic medications (especially phenobarbital and phenytoin) are prescribed routinely for children who have seizures, and hyperactive, dyskinetic children perform better when given dextroamphetamine or other drugs used for the child with attention deficit-hyperactivity disorder (ADHD). Care of visual and auditory deficits requires the attention of appropriate specialists, and speech therapy involves the services of a speech therapist. Dental care is especially important. Regular visits to the dentist and prophylaxis, including brushing, fluoride, and flossing, should be instituted as soon as the teeth erupt. This is especially important for children given phenytoin (Dilantin), who often develop gum hyperplasia.

A wide variety of technical aids are available to improve the functioning of children with CP. These include electromechanical toys that employ the concept of biofeedback and operate from a head unit. The toy is manipulated only when the head and trunk are in correct alignment. Eye-hand coordination can also be enhanced by appropriately designed toys and games. Microcomputers combined with voice synthesizers aid children with speech difficulties to "speak." The computers print messages onto screen monitors and paper. These devices have made it apparent that some children have been erroneously considered to be mentally retarded.

Many other electronic devices allow independent functioning. Sensors can be activated and deactivated by using a headstick, tongue, or other voluntary muscle movement over which the child has control. The application of this technology makes it possible for persons with CP to eventually function in their own residences and can be extended into the workplace.

Physical therapy is one of the most frequently used conservative treatment modalities. It requires the specialized skills of a qualified therapist with an extensive repertoire of exercise methods who can design a program to stimulate each child to achieve his or her functional goals. An active therapy program involves the family, the physical therapist, and often other members of the health team, especially the nurse. The major approach employs traditional types of therapeutic exercises that consist of stretching, passive, active, and resisted movements applied to specific muscle groups or joints to maintain or increase range of motion, strength, or endurance.

Prognosis. Survival rates of children with moderate disability from CP are about the same as for unaffected children for the first 20 years of life. Children with severe disability have a probability of about 50% for surviving 20 or more years (Hutton, Gooke, and Pharaoh, 1994).

Nursing Care Management

Assessment

Early recognition of CP is often a result of alert observation by the nurse. Detection begins at birth, and the nurse should be especially observant for signs in an infant who has a history that includes any of the prenatal or perinatal conditions that predispose to brain dysfunction. Unusual manifestations in a newborn can be signs of various conditions, but an infant who displays poor feeding, rigidity, tenseness, or hypotonia merits closer scrutiny. A history of these unexplained signs is cause for repeated assessment. The disorder is not readily identifiable in the early months of life; often evidence is not apparent until the child begins to walk. Delayed attainment of developmental milestones is one of the most valuable clues to recognizing CP; therefore slow development in a child offers one of the earliest indications of neurologic impairment (Box 52-3).

BOX 52-3
Warning Signs of Cerebral Palsy

Physical signs

Poor head control after 3 months of age
Stiff or rigid arms or legs
Pushing away or arching back
Floppy or limp body posture
Cannot sit up without support by 8 months
Uses only one side of the body, or only the arms to crawl

Behavioral signs

Extreme irritability or crying
Failure to smile by 3 months
Feeding difficulties
  Persistent gagging or choking when fed
  After 6 months of age, tongue pushes soft food out of the mouth

Data from Pathways Awareness Foundation: *Parents . . . if you see any of these warning signs . . . don't delay*, Chicago, 1991, The Foundation.

Nursing Diagnoses

Based on a thorough assessment, several nursing diagnoses identified for the child with CP are primarily related to self-help and to facilitating mobility (see Nursing Care Plan, pp. 1752-1753). Other diagnoses may apply in specific cases.

Planning

The goals of nursing care for the child with CP and the family are as follows:

1. Child will acquire mobility within personal capabilities.
2. Child will acquire communication skills or use appropriate assistive devices.
3. Child will engage in self-help activities.
4. Child will receive appropriate education.
5. Child will develop a positive self-image.
6. Family will receive appropriate education and support in their efforts to meet the child's needs.
7. Child will receive appropriate care if hospitalized.

Implementation

Since children are being treated at an earlier age, parents are participating earlier in treatment programs for their disabled child. They are taught the proper handling and home care of young children with CP and need carefully programmed steps so that their change of role from parent to therapist can be melded into the already-established relationship. Nurses reinforce the therapeutic plan and assist the family in devising and modifying equipment and activities to continue the therapy program in the home.

Therapeutic interventions are those that are most appropriate for the specific problem and that best suit the needs of the individual child at any given time. Passive range-of-motion exercises, stretching, and elongation exercises are valuable at any age, even at early ages when the child is unable to cooperate. They are of particular value for postural abnormalities around various joints.

Training in manual skills and activities of daily living (ADLs) proceeds along developmental lines and according to the child's functional level. Sitting, balancing, crawling, and walking are encouraged at appropriate ages, accompanied by stimulation of protective extension and equilibrium reactions. Hand activities are begun early to improve motor function and provide the child with sensory experiences and information about the environment. As the child progresses from simple feeding and self-care activities, training is extended to include other tasks, such as cooking or typing, that are within the child's developmental and functional capabilities. It should be remembered that a child should not be expected to learn a task until he or she is at the developmental stage at which it would normally be accomplished.

Incorporating play into the therapeutic program often requires a great deal of ingenuity and inventiveness on the part of those involved in the child's care. Objects and toys are chosen to provide needed sensory input, using a variety of shapes, forms, and textures. Nurses can help parents integrate therapy into play activities in natural ways.

The child may need considerable help (and patience) in learning to feed, dress, and care for personal hygiene needs. Children should be fed in the normal eating position. When they have difficulty with sucking and swallowing, it is a temptation to hold them in a semireclining posture to make use of gravity flow. This method does not promote active swallowing, however, and the neck hyperextension may even interfere with swallowing. A more flexed sitting position with arms brought forward to decrease the tendency toward back and neck extension is more natural during bottle- or spoon-feeding and encourages active swallowing.

Because jaw control is compromised, more normal control can be achieved if the feeder provides stability of the oral mechanism from the side or front of the face. When directed

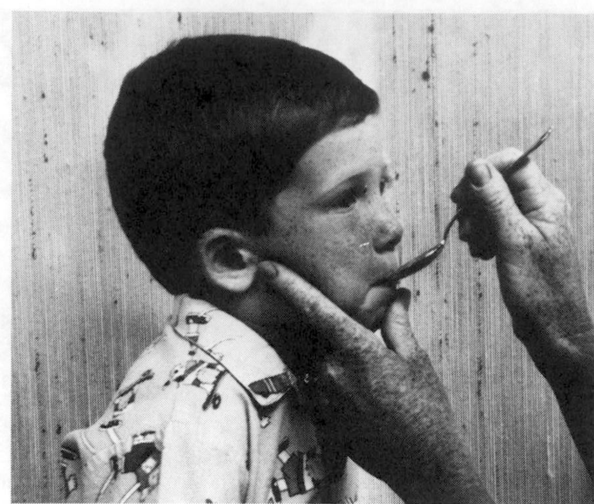

Fig. 52-3 Manual jaw control provided anteriorly.

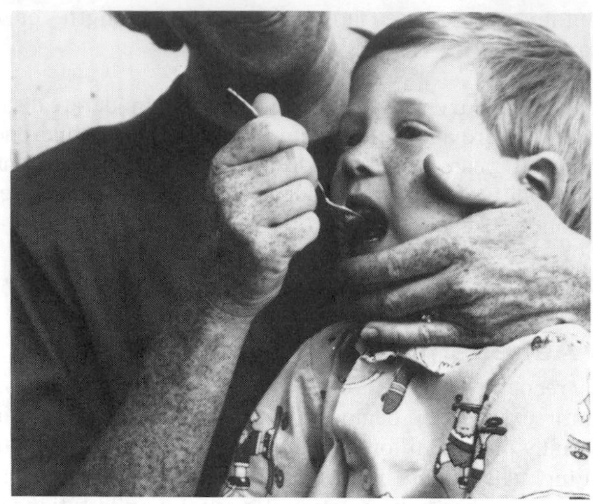

Fig. 52-4 Manual jaw control provided posteriorly.

from the front, the middle finger of the nonfeeding hand is placed posterior to the body portion of the chin, the thumb is placed below the bottom lip, and the index finger is placed parallel to the child's mandible (Fig. 52-3). Manual jaw control from the side assists with head control, correction of neck and trunk hyperextension, and jaw stabilization. The middle finger of the nonfeeding hand is placed posterior to the bony portion of the chin, the index finger is placed on the chin below the lower lip, and the thumb is placed obliquely across the cheek to provide lateral jaw stability (Fig. 52-4).

Speech training under the supervision of a speech therapist is begun early, before the child learns poor habits of communication. Parents and others can help by following the directions of the speech therapist and by talking to the child slowly and using pictures or handling objects about which the adult is speaking. Feeding techniques such as forcing the child to use the lips and tongue in eating help to facilitate speech (e.g., placing food at the side of the tongue, first one side then the other; making the child use the lips to take food from a spoon rather than placing it directly on the tongue; and avoiding using the teeth to remove the food from the utensil). If severe dysarthria prevents articulate speech and the child has reasonable intelligence, nonverbal communication, such as sign language, is taught.

As in all aspects of care, educational requirements are determined by the child's needs and potential. Children with mild to moderate involvement are generally able to participate, for varying amounts of time, in regular classes.

Resource rooms are available in most schools to provide more individualized attention to a child's particular needs. Integration of these children into regular classrooms should be the initial goal. For those who are unable to benefit from formal education, a training program may be appropriate. At adolescence, prevocational and vocational counseling and guidance are arranged. At any phase or in any setting, education is geared toward the child's assets.

Recreational outlets and after-school activities should be considered for the child who is unable to participate in the regular athletic programs and other peer activities. Some children can compete in athletic and artistic endeavors, and there are many games and pasttimes that are suited to their capabilities. Competitive sports are also becoming increasingly available to children with disabilities and offer an added dimension to physical activities. Information on training programs and competition on local, state, regional, and national levels can be obtained from the *National Association of Sports for Cerebral Palsy.**

Recreational activities serve to stimulate children's interest and curiosity, help them adjust to their disability, improve their functional abilities, and build self-esteem. Any accomplishment that helps children approach a "normal" way of life enhances their self-concept.

Family support. Probably the nursing interventions most valuable to the family are support and help in coping with the emotional aspects of the disorder, many of which are discussed in relation to the child with a disability (see Chapter 38). Initially the parents need supportive counseling directed toward understanding the implications of the diagnosis and all the feelings that it engenders. Later they need clarification regarding what they can expect from the child and from health professionals.

Having a child with CP implies numerous problems of daily management and changes in family life (see the Family Focus box on p. 1751).

The nurse needs to support the parents in their frustration, their problem solving, their concerns, their approaches to helping the child, and their lack of gratification, as well as the positive approaches they use. All of these aspects must be explored and discussed. Parents, as well as other members of the family, require much support and counseling. Siblings of a child with a disability are affected and may respond to the presence of the child with overt or less evident behavioral problems. The family needs a relationship with nurses who can provide continued contact, support, and encouragement through the long process of habilitation.

---

*710 Penn Plaza, Suite 804, New York, NY 10001; (800) USA-1UCP. In Canada: *Ontario Federation of Cerebral Palsy*, 1021 Lawrency Ave., W., Suite 303, Toronto, Ontario, M6A 1C8, Canada; (416) 787 1595.

Family Focus

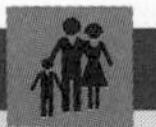

THE REALITY OF ACCEPTANCE OF CEREBRAL PALSY

Acceptance is rarely achieved in the length of time implied in the literature.

In the first place, what is it? To me, it is the end of comparing my son with every other child I see. I focus on *his* gains, not society's expectations.

It is also being able to laugh periodically *at* his "clumsiness." It is "gallows humor" as he achieves adulthood; jokes about CP can be funny now.

The bitterness is gone; I am now happy for people who have children without CP.

I no longer feel sorry for my son, but rather for the people who cannot see him for the great person he is; the CP does *not* come first.

He is now a young man of 25 years and I am learning to accept his independence.

It is a "never-ending story."

Elaine A. Dunham, RN
Shriner's Hospital
Springfield, MA

Parents can also find help and solace from parent groups with whom they can share problems and concerns and from whom they can derive comfort and practical information. Parent support groups are most helpful through sharing experiences and accomplishments. For example, parents can understand from others what it is like to have a child with CP, which is generally not possible from professionals (see the Family Focus box above). The national organization, *United Cerebral Palsy Associations,** has branches in most communities. The address of the nearest branch can be obtained from a local telephone directory, local agency directory, or a local health department or by writing to the national headquarters. The association provides various services for children and families. There are also a number of excellent books available to serve as guides for parents and nurses who work with the child with CP.

The hospitalized child. CP is not a disorder that requires hospitalization; therefore when children with CP are hospitalized, they are usually admitted for another reason or for corrective surgery. Consequently, many nurses are not accustomed to handling these children. Nurses who have never been associated with a child with CP may react in a variety of ways, including fear, revulsion, or overwhelming pity. The basic concept to keep in mind when caring for these children is that they are, first of all, children, who happen to be afflicted with a disorder that limits their capacities in performing some activities of daily living and, for some, in communicating with others.

Children with CP should be approached and treated the same as any child in the hospital. The nurse's actions should convey acceptance, affection, and friendliness and promote a feeling of trust and dependability in the child. This is especially true with older children who have normal intelligence but who may have communication problems. Speech impairment is common in children with CP. All too often, nurses tend to "talk down" to these children and do things for them that they are perfectly capable of doing for themselves, although not as adeptly. This is especially humiliating to teenagers, who value their independence and self-esteem.

To facilitate the care and management of these children, the therapy program should be continued, insofar as their condition allows, during the time they are hospitalized. This should be incorporated into the nursing care plan and every effort expended to make certain that the ground that has been so laboriously gained is not lost. Encouraging the parent to room-in and actively participate in the child's care facilitates a continuation of the home therapy program and helps the child adjust to an unfamiliar environment. However, it is equally important to remember that a hospitalization may be the first time a parent can defer care to a nurse and not be the primary caregiver. This respite may be crucial to the parent's well-being.

Evaluation

The effectiveness of nursing interventions is determined by continual reassessment and evaluation of care based on the following observational guidelines and expected outcomes:

1. Observe child's movements and use of mobilization devices.
2. Observe child's speech and ability to use communication devices.
3. Observe child's activities, especially those related to self-care.
4. Interview family regarding child's activities and school attendance.
5. Observe child's interactions with others and choice of activities; interview child regarding feelings and concerns.
6. Interview family regarding their feelings and concerns and observe family members' interaction with the child.
7. Observe child's behavior and responses during hospitalization.

Expected outcomes:
See the Nursing Care Plan on pp. 1752-1753.

SPINA BIFIDA (MYELOMENINGOCELE)

Abnormalities that are derived from the embryonic neural tube *(neural tube defects [NTDs])* constitute the largest group of congenital anomalies that is consistent with multifactorial inheritance. Normally the spinal cord and cauda equina are encased in a protective sheath of bone and meninges (Fig. 52-5, *A*). Failure of neural tube closure produces defects of varying degrees (Box 52-4). They may involve the entire length of the neural tube or be restricted to a small area.

In the United States, rates of NTDs have declined from 1.3 per 1000 births in 1970 to 0.6 per 1000 births in 1989. A

*710 Penn Plaza, Suite 804, New York, NY 10001; (800) USA-1UCP. In Canada: *Ontario Federation of Cerebral Palsy,* 1021 Lawrency Ave., W., Suite 303, Toronto, Ontario, M6A 1C8, Canada; (416) 787-4595.

Nursing Care Plan

THE CHILD WITH CEREBRAL PALSY

Nursing Diagnosis: Impaired physical mobility related to neuromuscular impairment

Expected Outcome: Child engages in activities appropriate to physical limitations.

• NURSING INTERVENTIONS/*RATIONALES*

Encourage gross and fine motor activities (i.e., sitting, crawling, walking, grasping, throwing) at appropriate ages *to facilitate optimum motor development.*

Refer to therapeutic modalities (physical therapy) that strengthen muscles, relax increased muscle tone, and improve control and balance *to facilitate optimum motor development.*

Balance rest and activity *to provide optimum energy for motor trials.*

Employ aids such as parallel bars, crutches, and orthoses (braces) *to facilitate locomotion.*

Employ passive and active range of motion and stretching exercises *to facilitate muscle development, prevent flexion contractures, and maintain joint flexibility.*

Nursing Diagnosis: Self-care deficit related to physical disability

Expected Outcome: Child engages in self-care activities commensurate with capabilities.

• NURSING INTERVENTIONS/*RATIONALES*

Encourage child to assist in self-care activities as age and capabilities permit, discourage parents from doing it for the child *to foster independence and confidence in abilities.*

Modify environment, introduce use of assistive devices and specialized equipment, devise alternative methods of completing tasks as needed *to facilitate maximum functioning.*

Use therapeutic play and adapted toys *to increase developmental and functional abilities and encourage cooperation of child.*

Emphasize child's abilities, praise effort and accomplishments, promote and reinforce successful endeavors *to foster a sense of self-esteem and competence.*

Refer to therapeutic modalities (e.g., physical therapy [PT], speech therapy, and occupational therapy [OT]) for strengthening of oral motor muscles, development of swallowing control, evaluation and work with adaptive devices *to enhance functional ADLs.*

Nursing Diagnosis: Risk for injury related to physical, perceptual impairment

Expected Outcome: Child exhibits no evidence of injury.

• NURSING INTERVENTIONS/*RATIONALES*

Promote and teach child and family proper use of adaptive and protective devices (i.e., crutches, walkers, braces, helmets, large-handled utensils) *to enhance safety.*

Modify environment as appropriate (i.e., pad furniture; avoid throw rugs, polished floors, deep carpets; put side rails on bed; remove hazards and barriers, clear traffic areas) *to enhance safety.*

Provide adequate rest *to prevent fatigue, which increases injury risk.*

Use feeding techniques and assistive devices (feed in upright position, stroke throat to aid swallowing), which encourage intake and proper swallowing *to minimize choking and aspiration.*

Use restraints in car and when seated *to enhance safety.*

Institute seizure precautions if appropriate and administer seizure medications as ordered *to prevent seizure activity and possible injury.*

Nursing Diagnosis: Impaired verbal communication related to physical, perceptual impairment

Expected Outcome: Child demonstrates ability to communicate needs and wants to caregivers.

• NURSING INTERVENTIONS/*RATIONALES*

Refer to therapeutic modalities (OT, speech therapy) for strengthening of oral motor muscles, evaluation of oral motor abilities, exercises that promote vocalizations/verbalizations, development of verbal and nonverbal communication modalities *to enhance communication.*

Teach caregivers (family, schoolteachers, therapists, nurses) how to use various verbal and nonverbal communication methods and adaptive communications equipment (i.e., communication boards, sign language, computer aids, voice synthesizers) *to enhance communication with others in environment.*

Nursing Diagnosis: Fatigue related to increased energy expenditure

Expected Outcome: Child exhibits signs of adequate rest and optimum nutritional intake.

• NURSING INTERVENTIONS/*RATIONALES*

Balance activity with frequent rest periods; monitor for any signs of tiredness *to reduce fatigue.*

Provide high-calorie, high-protein diet *to meet increased energy expenditure needs.*

Monitor weight *to evaluate adequacy of intake.*

Carry out a regular schedule of health promotion and maintenance (regular checkups with physician, dentist; immunizations; avoidance of people with infections) *to enhance general state of health.*

Nursing Diagnosis: Body image/self-esteem disturbances related to perception of disability, feeling different

Expected Outcome: Child demonstrates acceptance of self, physical appearance, and physical and developmental abilities.

• NURSING INTERVENTIONS/*RATIONALES*

Relate to child on appropriate cognitive level conveying an attitude of caring and acceptance *to encourage positive feelings about self;* serve as role model for others *to foster positive attitudes of acceptance toward child.*

Nursing Care Plan

THE CHILD WITH CEREBRAL PALSY—CONT'D

Relate to child on appropriate cognitive level conveying an attitude of caring and acceptance *to encourage positive feelings about self;* serve as role model for others *to foster positive attitudes of acceptance toward child.*

Encourage child to communicate feelings about the disability (i.e., feelings of differentness, implications of functional limit, difficulty in making friends, views of self) *to facilitate coping.*

Have child identify strengths, assets, things he or she likes about self *to increase positive feelings about self.*

Support positive coping behaviors.

Introduce child to other children who have similar disabilities, arrange for support groups for child and parents *to increase coping skills.*

Refer child for counseling if needed *to enhance adaptation.*

Encourage use of good grooming and age-appropriate dress *to enhance appearance.*

Nursing Diagnosis: Altered family processes related to situational crises (child with lifelong disability)

Expected Outcome: Family will exhibit adaptation of usual roles and functions to accommodate special needs of child, and they will exhibit growth-promoting behaviors.

- **NURSING INTERVENTIONS/*RATIONALES***

Provide opportunity for family to absorb and adjust to diagnosis (i.e., repeat information *to allow time for family to hear and understand;* encourage expression of concerns, fears, and feelings about diagnosis and potential impact *to facilitate adjustment;* identify support systems *to provide resources for coping).*

Assist family to understand expected treatment, rationale, and implications *to provide a sound basis for decision making.*

Explore family reaction to the child; assist them to achieve a realistic view of child's abilities and limitations; encourage family in attempts to promote child growth and development; have family emphasize what child can do; explore ways for family to include child in family activities *to help family increase abilities to cope with and incorporate child into family structure.*

Identify additional resource systems (i.e., relatives, friends, church, health care services, community programs) and strategize with family about making good use of these systems *to develop broad base of support.*

Provide a system of ongoing follow-up and evaluation *to ensure long-term adaptation to challenges presented to family functioning by a child with a chronic disability.*

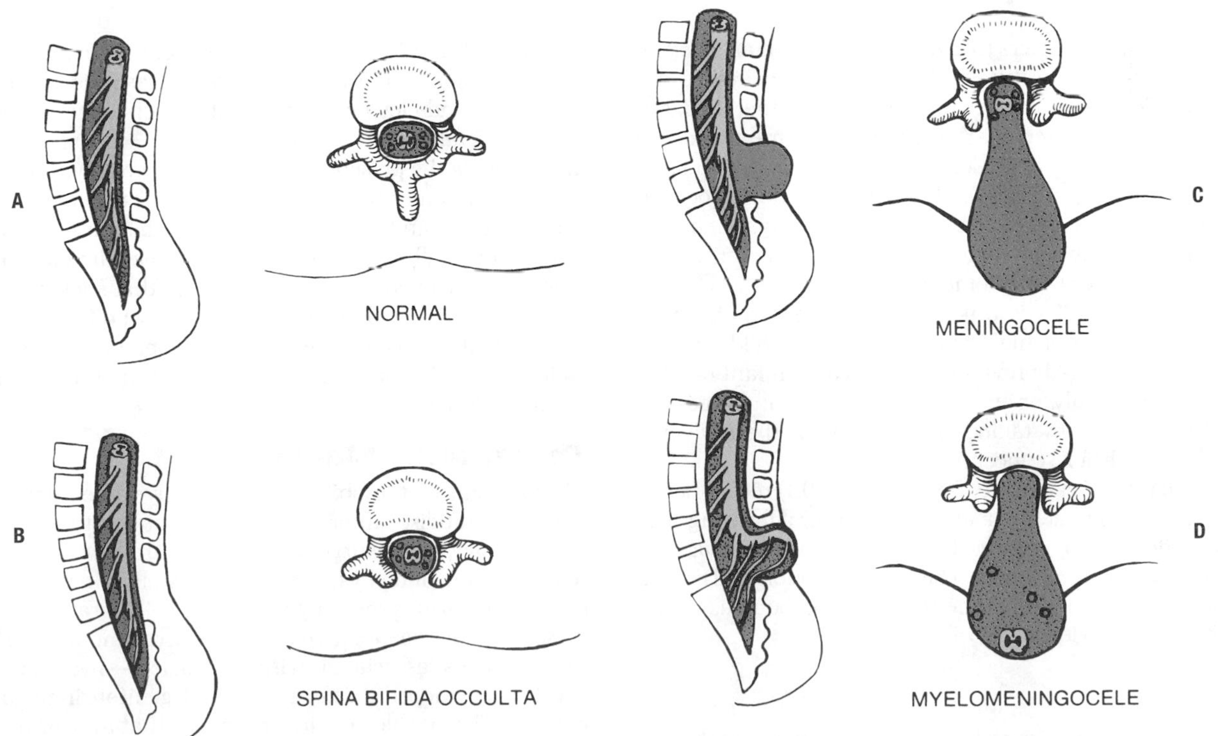

Fig. 52-5 Midline defects of osseous spine with varying degrees of neural herniations.

BOX 52-4
Significant Neural Tube Defects

Craniöschisis—A skull defect through which various tissues protrude
Exancephaly—Brain is totally exposed or extruded through an associated skull defect; fetus usually aborted
Anencephaly—If fetus with exancephaly survives, the brain degenerates to a spongioform mass with no bony covering; incompatible with life usually beyond a few days
Encephalocele—Herniation of brain and meninges through a defect in the skull producing a fluid-filled sac
Rachischisis or spina bifida—Fissure in the spinal column that leaves the meninges and spinal cord exposed
Meningocele—Hernial protrusion of a saclike cyst of meninges filled with spinal fluid (Fig. 51-5, *C*)
Myelomeningocele (meningomyelocele)—Hernial protrusion of a saclike cyst containing meninges, spinal fluid, and a portion of the spinal cord with its nerves (Fig. 51-5, *D*)

partial explanation is the increased use of prenatal diagnostic techniques and termination of pregnancies.

Myelodysplasia refers broadly to any malformation of the spinal canal and cord. Midline defects involving failure of the osseous (bony) spine to close are called **spina bifida (SB),** the most common defect of the central nervous system (CNS). SB is categorized into two types: spina bifida occulta and spina bifida cystica.

Spina bifida occulta refers to a defect that is not visible externally. It occurs most commonly in the lumbosacral area (L5 and S1) (Fig. 52-5, *B*). SB occulta may not be apparent unless there are associated cutaneous manifestations or neuromuscular disturbances.

Spina bifida cystica refers to a visible defect with an external saclike protrusion. The two major forms of SB cystica are **meningocele,** which encases meninges and spinal fluid, but no neural elements (see 52-5, *C*); and **myelomeningocele** (or *meningomyelocele*), which contains meninges, spinal fluid, and nerves (see Fig. 52-5, *D*). Meningocele is not associated with neurologic deficit, which occurs in varying, often serious, degrees in myelomeningocele. Clinically the term *spina bifida* is used to refer to myelomeningocele.

The cause of NTDs is unknown. However, studies have shown that women at high risk for having a child with an NTD because they had previously delivered an infant or fetus with SB, anencephaly, or encephalocele significantly reduced the recurrence rate by taking supplements of the *B vitamin folic acid* (4 mg) before conception.

The American Academy of Pediatrics (1993) recommends daily intake of folic acid for all women of childbearing age. The daily dose of 0.4 mg is the recommended dietary allowance (RDA). Folic acid taken before conception and during early pregnancy can reduce the risk of NTDs, such as SB, by at least 50% (Knowledge, 1995).*

*As of this writing the United States Food and Drug Administration (FDA) has required that folic acid be added to most enriched breads, flours, rice, grits, and other grain products. However, the supplementation may only be 10% of the recommended dietary allowance (RDA).

Nursing ALERT

Educate childbearing adolescent females about the need for folic acid to prevent NTDs. The daily dose of 0.4 mg is most easily obtained from a multivitamin supplement. For women needing a daily dose of 4 mg, special supplements are necessary.

Pathophysiology

The primary defect in NTDs is believed by most authorities to be a failure of neural tube closure during early development of the embryo. However, there is evidence to indicate that the defects are a result of splitting of the already-closed neural tube as a result of an abnormal increase in cerebrospinal fluid pressure during the first trimester. The degree of neurologic dysfunction is directly related to the anatomic level of the defect and thus the nerves involved. Most myelomeningoceles involve the lumbar or lumbosacral area, and hydrocephalus is a frequently associated anomaly (90% of patients).

Diagnostic Evaluation

The diagnosis is made on the basis of clinical manifestations (Box 52-5) and examination of the meningeal sac. Diagnostic measures used to evaluate the brain and spinal cord include magnetic resonance imaging (MRI), ultrasound, computed tomography (CT), and myelography.

Laboratory examinations are used primarily to determine causative organisms in the major complications of myelomeningocele—meningitis and urinary tract infections. Infants with urinary tract incontinence require urinalysis, culture, and evaluation of blood urea nitrogen (BUN) and creatinine clearance.

Prenatal detection. It is possible to determine the presence of some major open NTDs prenatally. Ultrasound scanning of the uterus and elevated concentrations of alpha-fetoprotein (AFP), a fetal-specific gamma-1 globulin, in amniotic fluid may indicate the presence of anencephaly or myelomeningocele. The optimum time for performing these diagnostic tests is between 16 and 18 weeks' gestation, before AFP concentrations normally diminish and in sufficient time to permit a therapeutic abortion. It is recommended that such diagnostic procedures be considered for all mothers who have borne an affected child, and testing is offered to all pregnant women. In addition, elective prelabor cesarean birth may result in less motor dysfunction.

Therapeutic Management

Management of the child who has a myelomeningocele requires a multidisciplinary approach involving the specialties of neurology, neurosurgery, pediatrics, urology, orthopedics, rehabilitation, and physical therapy, as well as intensive nursing care in various specialty areas. The collaborative efforts of these specialists are focused on (1) the myelomeningocele and the problems associated with the defect—hydrocephalus, paralysis, orthopedic deformities, and genitourinary abnormalities; (2) possible acquired problems that may or may not be associated, such as meningitis, hypoxia, and hemorrhage; and (3) other abnormalities, such as cardiac or gastrointestinal malformations.

BOX 52-5
Clinical Manifestations of Spina Bifida

Spina bifida cystica

Sensory disturbances usually parallel motor dysfunction
- Below second lumbar vertebra:
  - Flaccid, are flexic partial paralysis of lower extremities
  - Varying degrees of sensory deficit
  - Overflow incontinence with constant dribbling of urine
  - Lack of bowel control
  - Rectal prolapse (sometimes)
- Below third sacral vertebra:
  - No motor impairment
  - May be saddle anesthesia with bladder and anal sphincter paralysis

Joint deformities (sometimes produced in utero)
- Talipes valgus or varus contractures
- Kyphosis
- Lumbosacral scoliosis
- Hip dislocations

Spina bifida occulta

Frequently no observable manifestations

May be associated with one or more cutaneous manifestations
- Skin depression or dimple
- Port-wine angiomatous nevi
- Dark tufts of hair
- Soft, subcutaneous lipomas

May be neuromuscular disturbances
- Progressive disturbance of gait with foot weakness
- Bowel and bladder sphincter disturbances

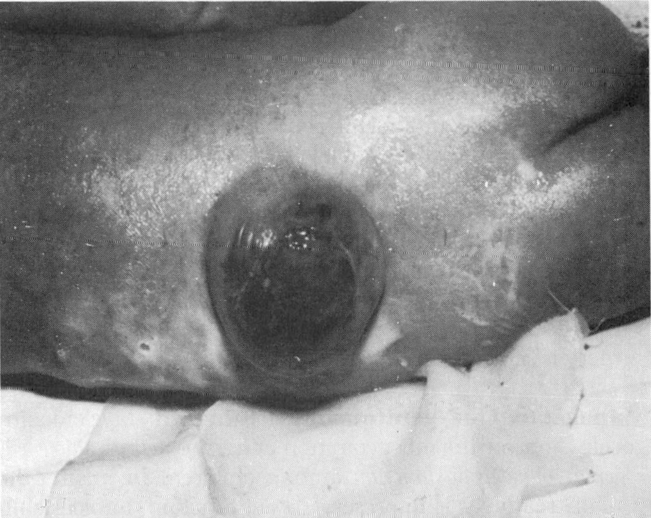

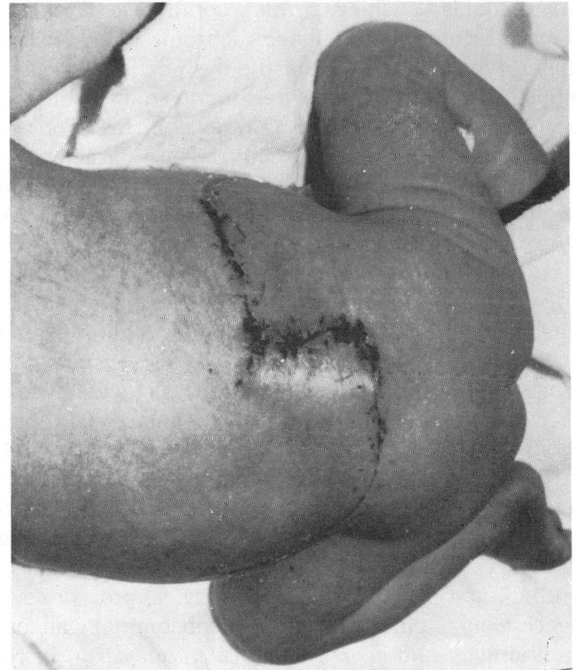

Fig. 52-6 **A,** Myelomeningocele before surgery. **B,** Same patient after surgery. (Courtesy MC Gleason, MD, San Diego, Calif. From Ingalls AJ, Salerno MC: *Maternal and child health nursing*, ed 7, St Louis, 1991, Mosby.)

Infancy. Initial care of the newborn involves prevention of infection; neurologic assessment, including observation for associated anomalies; and dealing with the impact of the anomaly on the family (Fig. 52-6, *A*). Although meningoceles are repaired early, especially if there is danger of rupture of the sac, the philosophy regarding skin closure of myelomeningocele varies. Most authorities believe that early closure, within the first 24 to 72 hours, offers the most favorable outcome. Early closure, preferably in the first 12 to 18 hours, not only prevents local infection and trauma to the exposed tissues, but also avoids stretching of other nerve roots, which may occur as the meningeal sac expands during the first hours after birth, thus preventing further motor impairment.

Other experts contend that surgical repair is best delayed until after further assessment of neurologic function, intellectual potential, and extent of complications. This delay increases the ability of the infant to tolerate the surgical procedure, allows for better epithelialization of the sac (thus reducing the risk of infection), and permits easier mobilization of skin for closure.

Various neurosurgical and plastic surgical procedures can be used for skin closure without disturbing the neural elements or removing any portion of the sac (e.g., Fig. 52-6, *B*). The objective is satisfactory skin coverage of the lesion and meticulous closure. Wide excision of the large membranous covering may damage functioning neural tissue.

Associated problems are assessed and managed by appropriate surgical and supportive measures. Shunt procedures provide relief from imminent or progressive hydrocephalus (see Chapter 48). Meningitis, urinary tract infection, and pneumonia are treated with vigorous antibiotic therapy and supportive measures.

Orthopedic considerations. According to most orthopedists, musculoskeletal problems that will affect later locomotion should be evaluated early, and treatment, where indicated, should be instituted without delay. Neurologic assessment will determine the neurosegmental level of the lesion, recognition of spasticity and progressive paralysis, potential for deformity, and functional expectations. Orthopedic management includes prevention of joint contractures, correction of the deformity, prevention of skin breakdown, and obtaining the best possible locomotor function. The status of the neurologic deficit remains the most important factor in determining the child's ultimate functional abilities.

Various devices are available to provide mobility for children with spinal cord lesions, including lightweight braces, special "walking" devices, and custom-built wheelchairs (see also Chapter 39). Corrective procedures, when indicated, are best initiated at an early age so that the child will not lag significantly behind age-mates in developmental progress. Where there is little hope for lower extremity functioning, surgery is seldom recommended.

Management of genitourinary function. Myelomeningocele is one of the most common causes of *neuropathic (neurogenic) bladder dysfunction* among children. In infants the goal of treatment is to preserve renal function. In older children the goal is to achieve urinary continence (Fernandes et al, 1994). Urinary incontinence, a chronic, often debilitating problem, typically arises from the dysfunctional bladder. In addition, neuropathic bladder dysfunction may predispose the child to *urinary system distress* (infection, ureterohydronephrosis, and vesicoureteral reflux). The characteristics of bladder dysfunction in children vary according to the level of the lesion and the influence of bony growth and development on the spine. Therefore urodynamic testing during infancy and early childhood is important because bladder function changes. The presence of hydrocephalus has the potential to affect bladder function, although spinal influences are predominant.

Treatment of renal problems includes (1) regular urologic care with prompt and vigorous treatment of infections; (2) some type of regular emptying of the bladder, such as clean intermittent catheterization (CIC) taught to and performed by parents and self-catheterization taught to children; (3) medications to improve bladder storage and continence, such as oxybutynin chloride (Ditropan), propantheline (Pro-Banthine), and ephedrine; and (4) surgical procedures such as *vesicostomy* (stoma created on the abdominal wall for urinary drainage) and *augmentation enterocytoplasty* (increases bladder capacity and reduces high bladder pressures).

Infrequently, children with myelodysplasia may develop severe dysfunction of the bladder that compromises renal function or produces debilitating urinary incontinence that is intractable to other means. *Urinary diversion*, typically using a continent neobladder constructed from bowel or stomach, may be required. Whenever feasible, the neobladder is constructed in a way that allows continence, and CIC is used to regularly evacuate urine.

Bowel control. Some degree of fecal continence can usually be achieved in most children with myelomeningocele with diet modification, regular toilet habits, and prevention of constipation and impaction. It is frequently a lengthy process. Fiber supplements, laxatives, suppositories, and/or enemas aid in producing regular evacuation.

Latex allergy. *Latex allergy* has been identified as a serious health hazard occurring in children with SB. These children are at high risk for developing latex allergy because of repeated exposure to latex products during surgery and from numerous bladder catheterizations. Allergic reactions range from urticaria, wheezing, watery eyes, and rashes to anaphylactic shock. More severe reactions tend to occur when latex comes in contact with mucous membranes, wet skin, and the bloodstream and in individuals with atopic disorders. The incidence of latex allergy in children with SB ranges from an estimated 18% to 60%.

Guidelines

IDENTIFYING LATEX ALLERGY

Does your child have any symptoms, such as sneezing, coughing, rashes, or wheezing, when handling rubber products (balloons, tennis or Koosh balls, adhesive bandage strips) or when in contact with rubber hospital products, such as gloves or catheters?
Has your child ever had an allergic reaction during surgery?
Does your child have a history of rashes, asthma, or allergic reactions to medication or foods, especially milk, kiwi, bananas, or chestnuts?
How would you identify or recognize an allergic reaction in your child?
What would you do if an allergic reaction occurred?
Has anyone ever discussed latex or rubber allergy or sensitivity with you?
Has your child had any allergy testing?
When did your child last come in contact with any type of rubber product? Were you present?

Modified from Romanczuk A: Latex use with infants and children: it can cause problems, *Am J Matern Child Nurs* 18(4):208-212, 1993.

The most important goals are prevention of latex allergy and identification of children with a known hypersensitivity (see the Guidelines box above). Allergy testing with the latex extract may be performed with the skin prick test; however, skin testing can cause an allergic reaction. The radioallergosorbent test (RAST) is the most specific test for IgE antibody. Children who are allergic to latex must avoid all latex products and may be given antihistamines and steroids (dexamethasone) before and after surgery to reduce the possibility of a serious reaction.

Prognosis. The early prognosis for the child with myelomeningocele depends on the neurologic deficit present at birth, including motor ability and bladder innervation and the presence of associated cerebral anomalies. Early surgical repair of the spinal defect, antibiotic threapy to reduce the incidence of meningitis and ventriculitis, prevention of urinary system dysfunction, and correction of hydrocephalus have significantly increased the survival rate. Based on current medical knowledge and ethical considerations, aggressive management is favored for the child with meningomyelocele.

With the widespread use of folate supplementation during the childbearing years, the incidence of SB should decrease dramatically. Whether folic acid will lessen the severity of the defect in infants born with SB despite supplementation is unknown.

Nursing Care Management

Assessment

At birth an examination is performed to assess the intactness of the membranous cyst. During transport to the nursery, every effort is made to prevent trauma to this protective covering. In addition to the routine assessment of the newborn (see Chapter 22), the infant is assessed for level of neurologic involvement. Movement of extremities or skin response, especially an anal reflex, that might provide clues to the degree of motor or sensory impairment is noted. It is important to observe the infant's behavior in conjunction with the stimulus, since limb movements can be induced in response to spinal cord reflex activity that has no connection with the higher centers. Observation of urinary output, especially if a diaper remains dry, may indicate urinary retention. The head circumference is measured daily (see Chapter 22), and the fontanels are examined for signs of tension or bulging.

Nursing ALERT

Avoid measuring rectal temperatures on infants with SB. Since bowel sphincter function is often affected, the thermometer can cause irritation and rectal prolapse.

Nursing Diagnoses

Nursing diagnoses identified for the infant with myelomeningocele are listed in Box 52-6. Others will be evident in specific cases and with the child's advancing years.

Planning

The goals for the infant with myelomeningocele and the family include the following:

1. Infant will not experience damage to the myelomeningocele sac.
2. Infant will not experience complications.
3. Family will receive support and education.

Implementation

Care of the myelomeningocele sac. The infant is usually placed in an incubator or warmer so that temperature can be maintained without clothing or covers that might irritate the delicate lesion. When an overhead warmer is used, the dressings over the defect require more frequent moistening because of the dehydrating effect of the radiant heat.

Before surgical closure the myelomeningocele is prevented from drying by the application of a sterile, moist, nonadherent dressing over the defect. The moistening solution is usually sterile normal saline solution. Dressings are changed frequently (every 2 to 4 hours), and the sac is closely inspected for leaks, abrasions, irritation, or any signs of infection. A surgical drape may be used to prevent stool contamination of the SB defect preoperatively. The sac must be carefully cleansed if it becomes soiled or contaminated. Sometimes the sac ruptures during delivery or transport, and any opening in the sac greatly increases the risk of infection to the CNS.

Nursing ALERT

Observe for early signs of infection, such as elevated temperature (axillary), irritability, lethargy, and nuchal rigidity, and for signs of increased intracranial pressure (ICP), which might indicate developing hydrocephalus.

BOX 52-6

Nursing Diagnoses: The Infant With Myelomeningocele

- Risk for infection related to nonepithelialized meningeal sac
- Risk for neurologic trauma related to spinal defect
- Risk for impaired skin integrity related to unprotected meningeal sac; bowel and bladder dysfunction
- Altered family processes related to birth of a child with a congenital defect
- Risk for impaired parent-infant attachment related to birth of a child with a chronic congenital defect

One of the most difficult, important, and challenging aspects in the early care of the infant with myelomeningocele is positioning. Before surgery the infant is kept in the prone position to minimize tension on the sac and the risk of trauma. The prone position allows for optimum positioning of the legs, especially in cases of associated hip dysplasia. The infant is placed flat with the hips only slightly flexed to reduce tension on the defect. The legs are maintained in abduction with a pad between the knees to counteract hip subluxation, and a small roll is placed under the ankles to maintain a neutral foot position. A variety of aids, including diaper rolls, pads, small sandbags, or specially designed frames and appliances, can be used to maintain the desired position.

Prevent complications. The prone position affects other aspects of the infant's care. For example, in this position the infant is more difficult to keep clean, pressure areas are a constant threat, and feeding becomes a problem. The infant's head is turned to one side for feeding. Fortunately, most defects are repaired early, and the infant can be held for feeding as soon as the surgical site is sufficiently healed to permit handling.

Diapering the infant is contraindicated until the defect has been repaired and healing is well advanced or epithelialization has taken place. The padding beneath the diaper area is changed as needed to keep the skin dry and free of irritation. When urinary retention is detected, CIC is employed.* Since the bowel sphincter is often affected, there is continual passage of stool, often misinterpreted as diarrhea, which is a constant irritant to the skin and a source of infection to the spinal lesion.

Areas of sensory and motor impairment are subject to skin breakdown and therefore require meticulous care. Placing the infant on a soft foam or fleece pad reduces pressure on the knees and ankles. Periodic cleansing, application of lotion, and gentle massage aid circulation.

Gentle range-of-motion exercises are sometimes carried out to prevent contractures, and stretching of contractures is performed when indicated. However, these exercises may be restricted to the foot, ankle, and knee joint. Where the hip joints are unstable, stretching against tight hip flexors or ad-

hydrocephalus complication - tx shunt

*Home care instructions on performing clean intermittent self-catheterization are available in Wong: *Wong and Whaley's clinical manual of pediatric nursing*, ed 4, St Louis, 1996, Mosby.

ductor muscles, which act much like bowstrings, may aggravate a tendency toward subluxation. A physical therapy consultation is usually obtained.

Some infants with unrepaired myelomeningocele are unable to be held in the arms and cuddled as unaffected infants are, so their need for tactile stimulation is met by caressing, stroking, and other comfort measures. To facilitate handling and reduce parental anxiety, the infant can recline on a pillow placed in the parent's lap. Black-and-white drawings or geometric shapes can be placed within the infant's view, and other stimulation usually provided for infants is appropriate. All infants respond to pleasant sounds.

Provide postoperative care. Postoperative care of the infant with myelomeningocele involves the same basic care as that of any postsurgical infant—monitoring vital signs, monitoring intake and output, nourishment, observation for signs of infection, and pain management as needed. Wound management is carried out according to the directions of the surgeon and includes close observation for signs of leakage of cerebrospinal fluid. General care is continued as preoperatively.

The prone position is maintained after operative closure, although many neurosurgeons allow a side-lying or partial side-lying position unless it aggravates a coexisting hip dysplasia or permits undesirable hip flexion. This offers an opportunity for position changes, which reduces the risk of pressure sores and facilitates feeding. If permitted, the infant can be held upright against the body, with care taken to avoid pressure on the operative site. Once the effects of anesthesia have subsided and the infant is alert, feedings may be resumed unless there are other anomalies or associated complications.

Since children who have SB are prone to develop an allergy to latex, reducing exposure to latex, from birth on, is hoped to decrease the chance of allergy development. Latex, a natural product derived from the rubber tree, is used in combination with other chemicals to provide elasticity, strength, and durability to many products.

Avoiding latex products is the most important intervention. The establishment of a nonlatex environment is being accomplished in many health care facilities where patients (and health care workers) are at high risk.

Nursing ALERT

Ask *all* patients about allergic reactions to latex, not only those at risk, during the health interview with the parent and/or child. Be sure this is a routine part of all preoperative histories.

Family support and home care. As soon as the parents are able to cope with the infant's condition, they are encouraged to become involved in care. They need to learn how to continue at home the care that has been initiated in the hospital—positioning, feeding, skin care, and range-of-motion exercises when appropriate. They are taught CIC technique when prescribed.* They need to know the signs of complications and how to obtain assistance when needed. When the defect has not been repaired, they are taught to care for the lesion.

The long-range planning with and support of the parents and child begin in the hospital and extend throughout childhood and even beyond. Long-term care of these children is of uncertain length. Nurses assume an important role as a central member of the health team. As a coordinator, the nurse reviews information with the family, takes responsibility for family teaching, and acts as a liaison between inpatient and outpatient services. The child may need numerous hospitalizations over the years, and each one will be a source of stress, to which the younger child is especially vulnerable. (See Chapter 38 for a discussion of care of the child with a disability.)

Habilitation involves not only solving problems of self-help and locomotion, but also solving the most distressing problem of incontinence, which threatens the child's social acceptability. Assistance with preparing the child and the school regarding the special needs of the child helps provide a better initial adjustment to this broader social experience. The Spina Bifida Association of America* is organized to provide services and support for families of children with spinal lesions.

Evaluation

The effectiveness of nursing interventions is determined by continual reassessment and evaluation of care based on the following observational guidelines and expected outcomes:

1. Inspect spinal defect, take appropriate measurements (weight, vital signs, head circumference), observe child's general health status, and check completed care against the preoperative checklist.
2. Take vital signs, inspect operative site (or preoperative lesion), inspect skin (especially dependent areas), measure head circumference, and assess range of motion of lower extremities
3. Observe parent-infant interactions and behavior of family members, and interview family members regarding their feelings and concerns

Expected outcomes:

1. Child is physically prepared for surgical repair of the defect.
2. Child exhibits no evidence of infection (skin, meningeal, or renal), deformities of extremities, or pressure necrosis; signs of complications (e.g., hydrocephalus, hip dysplasia) are detected early, and appropriate interventions initiated.
3. Family members discuss their feelings and concerns and participate in infant's care; family makes contact with appropriate community agencies and facilities.

See also the Nursing Care Plan: The Infant with Myelomeningocele.†

*Home care instructions on performing clean intermittent self-catheterization are available in Wong: *Wong and Whaley's clinical manual of pediatric nursing*, ed 4, St Louis, 1996, Mosby.

*4590 McArthur, N.W., Washington, DC 20007; (202) 944-3285 or (800) 621-3141.

†In Wong DL: *Wong and Whaley's clinical manual of pediatric nursing*, ed 4, St Louis, 1996, Mosby.

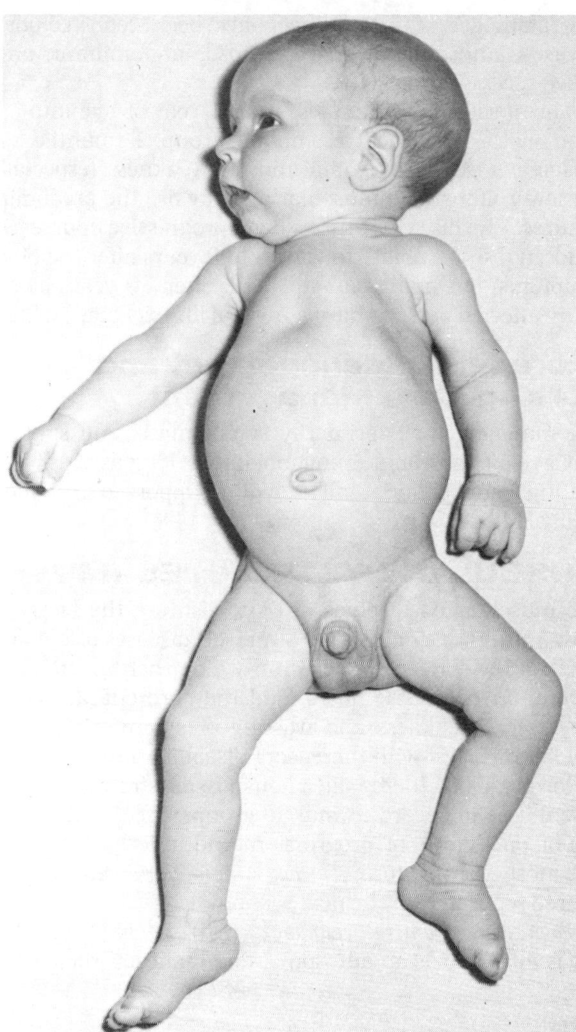

Fig. 52-7 Child with group 1 Werdnig-Hoffmann disease lying in typical posture of abduction of legs at hips and flexion of knees. Arms are flexed slightly with little movement at shoulders. Movements of fingers and toes are present. Pectus excavatum deformity of chest is common and is a result of unopposed diaphragmatic breathing. (From Swaiman KF, Wright FS: *The practice of pediatric neurology*, ed 2, St Louis, 1982, Mosby.)

BOX 52-7

Clinical Manifestations of Werdnig-Hoffmann Disease

Group 1

- Disease acquired in utero or during first 2 months of life
- Inactivity is most prominent feature
- Infant lies in the frog position with legs externally rotated, abducted, and flexed at hips (Fig. 52-7)
- Weakness
- Limited movements of shoulder and arm muscles
- Active movement is usually limited to fingers and toes
- Diaphragmatic breathing with sternal retractions
- Weak cry and cough
- Secretions tend to pool in pharynx
- Alert facies
- Normal sensation and intellect
- Affected infants do not progress to sit alone, roll over, or walk
- Early death (usually by 3 years of age) from respiratory failure or infection

Group 2

- Disease manifested between 2 and 12 months of age
- Early—weakness confined to arms and legs
- Later—becomes generalized
- Legs usually involved to greater extent than arms
- Prominent pectus excavatum
- Movements absent during complete relaxation or sleep
- Some infants able to sit if placed in position
- Life span varies from 7 months to 7 years

Group 3

- Onset of symptoms in second year of life
- Normal head control and can sit unassisted by 6 to 8 months of age
- Thigh and hip muscles weak
- In those who manage to walk:
  - Lumbar lordosis
  - Waddling gait
  - Genu recurvatum
  - Protuberant abdomen
  - Ambulation becomes increasingly difficult
  - Confined to a wheelchair by second decade
- Deep tendon reflexes may be present early but disappear

PROGRESSIVE INFANTILE SPINAL MUSCULAR ATROPHY (WERDNIG-HOFFMANN DISEASE)

Progressive infantile spinal muscular atrophy (Werdnig-Hoffmann disease) is a disorder characterized by progressive weakness and wasting of skeletal muscles caused by degeneration of anterior horn cells. It is inherited as an autosomal-recessive trait and is the most common paralytic form of the "floppy infant syndrome." The site of the pathologic condition is the anterior horn cells of the spinal cord and the motor nuclei of the brainstem, but the primary effect is atrophy of skeletal muscles (Fig. 52-7).

Therapeutic Management

The diagnosis is suspected on the basis of clinical manifestations (Box 52-7). It is established by electromyography demonstrating a denervation pattern and is confirmed by muscle biopsy. Treatment is symptomatic and preventive, primarily preventing infection and treating orthopedic problems, the most serious of which is scoliosis. Many children benefit from powered chairs, lifts, special mattresses, and accessible environmental controls. Vigorous antibiotic therapy and pulmonary physical therapy are implemented during upper respiratory infections.

Prognosis. Prognosis varies according to age of onset or group as described in Box 52-7 above. However, recent observations suggest that the classification is not valid. Individuals with group 1 manifestations had a life span of 4 months to 31 years. Also, some affected persons did not demonstrate progressive loss of strength and function (Russman et al, 1992).

Nursing Care Management

The infant or small child with extensive paralysis requires frequent change of position to prevent physical injury and complications, especially pneumonia. The pharynx requires suctioning to remove secretions, and feeding must be carried out slowly and carefully to prevent aspiration. Since these children are intellectually normal, verbal, tactile, and auditory stimulation are important aspects of care. Supporting them so that they can see the activities around them and transporting them in appropriate conveyances (i.e., carriage, wagon, or wheelchair) for a change of environment provide stimulation and a broader scope of contacts.

Children who are able to sit require proper support and attention to alignment to prevent deformities and other complications. Children who survive beyond infancy will need attention to educational needs and opportunities for social interaction with other children. The parents of a child who is chronically or potentially fatally ill require much support and encouragement (see Chapter 38). The parents of a child with a genetically transmitted disorder also need to be encouraged to seek genetic counseling.

JUVENILE SPINAL MUSCULAR ATROPHY (KUGELBERG-WELANDER DISEASE)

Juvenile spinal muscular atrophy (Kugelberg-Welander disease, juvenile proximal hereditary muscular atrophy) is also the result of anterior horn cell and motor nerve degeneration. The disease is characterized by a pattern of muscular weakness similar to that of infantile spinal muscular atrophy. Several modes of inheritance have been reported for the disease—autosomal-recessive, autosomal-dominant, and X-linked recessive.

The onset occurs from less than 1 year of age into adulthood, with symptoms resembling group 3 infantile spinal muscular atrophy; proximal muscle weakness (especially of the lower limbs) and muscular atrophy are the predominant features. The disease runs a slowly progressive course. Some children lose the ability to walk 8 to 9 years after the onset of symptoms, but many can still walk after 30 years or more. Many affected persons have a normal life expectancy.

Therapeutic Management and Nursing Care Management

The management is primarily symptomatic and supportive and is related to maintaining mobility as long as possible, preventing complications, and providing support to the child and family.

MUSCULAR DYSTROPHIES (MDs)

The muscular dystrophies (MDs) constitute the largest and most important single group of muscle diseases of childhood. They all have a genetic origin in which there is gradual degeneration of muscle fibers, and they are characterized by progressive weakness and wasting of symmetric groups of skeletal muscles, with increasing disability and deformity. In all forms of MD there is insidious loss of strength, but each type differs in regard to muscle groups affected (Fig. 52-8), age of onset, rate of progression, and inheritance patterns. The most common form, *Duchenne muscular dystrophy*, is considered separately in the next section.

Facioscapulohumeral (Landouzy-Déjérine) muscular dystrophy is inherited as an autosomal-dominant disorder with on-

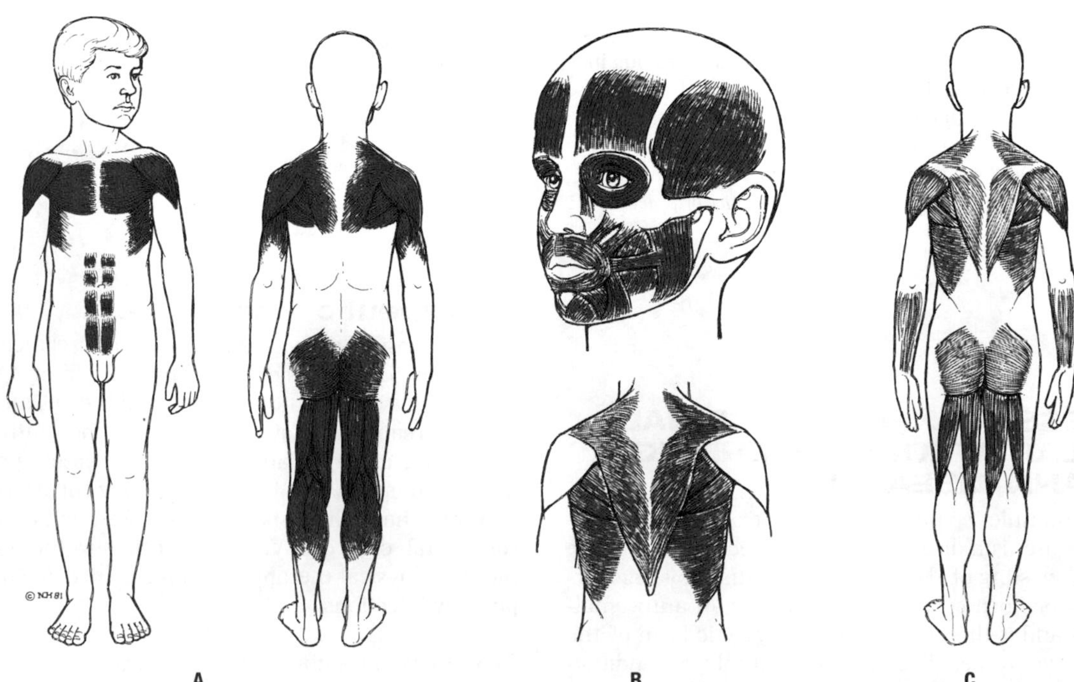

Fig. 52-8 Initial muscle groups involved in muscular dystrophies. **A,** Pseudohypertrophic. **B,** Facioscapulohumeral. **C,** Limb-girdle.

set in early adolescence. It is characterized by difficulty in raising the arms over the head, lack of facial mobility, and a forward slope of the shoulders. The progression is slow.

Limb-girdle muscular dystrophy is an autosomal-recessive disease of later childhood or adolescence with variable but usually slow progression; it is characterized by weakness of proximal muscles of the pelvic and shoulder girdles.

Treatment of the MDs consists mainly of supportive measures, including physical therapy, orthopedic procedures to minimize deformity, and assisting the affected child in meeting the demands of daily living.

PSEUDOHYPERTROPHIC (DUCHENNE) MUSCULAR DYSTROPHY (DMD)

Duchenne muscular dystrophy (DMD) is the most severe and the most common muscular dystrophy of childhood. An X-linked inheritance pattern is identified in most cases; about one third of all cases represent fresh mutations. As in all X-linked disorders, males are affected almost exclusively. The incidence is approximately 1:3500 male births (Multicenter Study Group, 1992). Box 52-8 describes the characteristics of DMD.

Evidence of muscle weakness usually appears during the third year, although there may have been a history of delay in motor development, particularly walking. Difficulties in running, riding a bicycle, and climbing stairs are usually the first symptoms noted. Later abnormal gait on a level surface becomes apparent. In the early years, rapid developmental gains may mask the progression of the disease. Questioning of the parents may reveal that the child has difficulty in rising from a sitting or supine position. Occasionally, enlarged calves are noticed by parents.

The term *pseudohypertrophy* is derived from muscular enlargement caused by fatty infiltration. Profound muscular atrophy occurs in later stages, and as the disease progresses, contractures and deformities involving large and small joints are common complications. Ambulation usually becomes impossible by 12 years of age. Facial, oropharyngeal, and respiratory muscles are spared until the terminal stages of the disease. Ultimately the disease process involves the diaphragm and auxiliary muscles of respiration, and cardiomegaly is common. The cause of death is usually respiratory tract infection or cardiac failure.

BOX 52-8
Characteristics of Duchenne Muscular Dystrophy

Early onset, usually between 3 and 5 years of age
Progressive muscular weakness, wasting, and contractures
Calf muscle hypertrophy in most patients
Loss of independent ambulation by 9 to 11 years of age
Slowly progressive, generalized weakness during teenage years
Relentless progression until death from respiratory or cardiac failure

Diagnostic Evaluation

The disease is suspected on the basis of clinical manifestations (Box 52-9) and confirmed by serum enzyme measurement, muscle biopsy, and electromyography (EMG). The serum creatine phosphokinase, aldolase, and serum glutamic oxaloacetic transaminase (SGOT; more recent term is aspartate aminotransferase, AST) levels are extremely high in the first 2 years of life before the onset of clinical weakness. They diminish with muscle deterioration but do not reach normal levels until severe muscle wasting and incapacitation have occurred. Muscle biopsy reveals degeneration of muscle fibers, with fibrosis and fatty tissue replacement. EMG readings show a decrease in amplitude and duration of motor unit potentials.

Therapeutic Management

No effective treatment exists for childhood MD. Increased muscle bulk and muscle power have been reported after a course of corticosteroids; however, this therapy requires further evaluation before it becomes routine management. Maintaining function in unaffected muscles for as long as possible is the primary goal. It has been found that children who remain as active as possible are able to avoid wheelchair confinement for a longer time. Early recourse to a wheelchair accelerates deconditioning and promotes the development of lower extremity contractures. Maintenance of function often includes range-of-motion exercises, surgery to release contracture deformities, bracing, and performance of activities of daily living. Genetic counseling is recommended for parents, female siblings, and maternal aunts and their female offspring.

Nursing Care Management

The major emphasis of nursing care is to assist the child and family cope with the progressive, incapacitating, and fatal nature of the disease; to help design a program that will afford a greater degree of independence and reduce the predictable and preventable disabilities associated with the disorder; and

BOX 52-9
Clinical Manifestations of Duchenne Muscular Dystrophy

Waddling gait
Lordosis
Frequent falls
Gower sign (child turns onto side or abdomen, flexes knees to assume a kneeling position, then with knees extended gradually pushes torso to an upright position by "walking" the hands up the legs)
Enlarged muscles (especially thighs and upper arms)
  Feel unusually firm or woody on palpation
Later stages: Profound muscular atrophy
Mental deficiency (common)
  Mild (about 20 IQ points below normal)
  Frank mental deficit present in 25% of patients
Complications:
  Contracture deformities of hips, knees, and ankles
  Disuse atrophy
  Obesity

to help the child and family deal constructively with the limitations the disease imposes on their daily lives.

Working closely with other team members, nurses assist the family in developing the child's self-help skills to give the child the satisfaction of being as independent as possible for as long as possible. This requires continual evaluation of the child's capabilities, which are often difficult to assess. It is not always possible to know when children seek parental assistance because they want a little extra attention, when parents are being overprotective, or when the muscles are overtired. Fortunately, most children with MD instinctively recognize this need to become as independent as possible and strive to do so.

Practical difficulties faced by families are physical limitations of housing and mobility. Parents also need assistance in buying and modifying clothing for their child. It is difficult to find clothing and footwear to wear comfortably in a wheelchair, to fit over contracted limbs, and to fit hypertrophied muscles. The parent's social activities are also restricted, and the family's activities must be continually modified to the needs of the affected child.

When the child becomes increasingly helpless, the family may consider a skilled nursing facility or respite care to provide the care needed. Nurses can assist with decision making and support the family in the decision.

No matter how successful the program or how well the family adapts to the disorder, superimposed on the physical and emotional problems associated with a child with a long-term disability is the constant presence of the ultimate outcome of the disease. All of the manifestations seen in the child with a chronic fatal illness are encountered in these families (see Chapter 38). The guilt feelings of the mother may be particularly pronounced in this disorder because of the mother-to-son transmission of the defective gene.

Nurses are especially valuable health professionals as they come to know the family and the family's problems. Nurses can be alert to the problems and needs of the families and make necessary referrals when supplementary services are indicated. The Muscular Dystrophy Association of America, Inc.* has branches in most communities to provide assistance to families in which there is a member with muscular dystrophy.

Acquired Neuromuscular Disorders

GUILLAIN-BARRÉ SYNDROME (GBS) (INFECTIOUS POLYNEURITIS)

GBS, also known as infectious polyneuritis, is an uncommon acute demyelinating polyneuropathy with a progressive, usually ascending flaccid paralysis. Children are less often affected than adults, with children between ages 4 and 10 years having higher susceptibility. Both genders are affected with equal frequency.

Pathophysiology

GBS is an immune-mediated disease often associated with a number of viral or bacterial infections or the administration of vaccines. It has been associated with infectious mononucleosis, measles, mumps, *Borrelia burgdorferi* (Lyme disease), *Helicobacter pylori*, and *Mycoplasma* and *Pneumocystis* infections. Pathologic changes in spinal and cranial nerves consist of inflammation and edema with rapid, segmented demyelination and compression of nerve roots within the dural sheath. Nerve conduction is impaired, producing ascending partial or complete paralysis of muscles innervated by the involved nerves.

Diagnostic Evaluation

Diagnosis of GBS is based on the paralytic manifestations (Box 52-10) and/or EMG findings. Cerebrospinal fluid analysis reveals an increased protein concentration, but other laboratory studies are noncontributory. The symmetric nature of the paralysis helps differentiate this disorder from spinal paralytic poliomyelitis, which usually affects sporadic muscles.

Therapeutic Management

Treatment of GBS is symptomatic. In some reports, corticosteroid therapy has been of benefit in the early stages. Respiratory and pharyngeal involvement requires assisted ventilation, often with tracheostomy. Plasma exchange (plasmapheresis) may be beneficial both in shortening the length of illness and in lessening the long-term disability; intravenous immunoglobulin is also advocated (Vajsar et al, 1994).

Course and prognosis. Better outcomes are associated with younger age, no requirement for respiratory assistance, slower progression of disease, normal peripheral nerve function by electromyograph, and treatment by plasmapheresis.

BOX 52-10

Clinical Manifestations of Guillian Barré Syndrome

Initial symptoms

Muscle tenderness
Paresthesia and cramps (sometimes)
Proximal symmetric muscle weakness

Paralysis

Ascends from lower extremities
Frequently involves muscles of trunk, upper extremities, and those supplied by cranial nerves (especially facial)
Flaccid paralysis with loss of reflexes
May involve facial, extraocular, labial, lingual, pharyngeal, and laryngeal muscles
Intercostal and phrenic nerves:
  Breathlessness in vocalizations
  Shallow, irregular respirations

Other manifestations

Tendon reflexes depressed or absent
Variable degrees of sensory impairment
Muscle tenderness or sensitivity to slight pressure
Urinary incontinence or retention and constipation (frequently)

*10 E. 40th St., Room 4105, New York, NY 10019; (212) 679-6215 or (212) 689-9040. In Canada: *Muscular Dystrophy Association of Canada*, 150 Eglinton Ave, E., Suite 400, Toronto, Ontario M4P 1E8; (416) 488-0030.

Almost all deaths are caused by respiratory failure; therefore early diagnosis and access to respiratory support are especially important. Muscle function begins to return 2 days to 2 weeks after the onset of symptoms, and recovery is complete in most cases. The rate of recovery is usually related to the degree of involvement, which may extend from a few weeks to months. The greater the degree of paralysis, the longer the recovery phase.

Nursing Care Management

Nursing care is essentially supportive and is the same as that required for quadriplegia from any cause. The emphasis of care is on close observation to assess the extent of paralysis and on prevention of complications.

During the acute phase of the disease the child's condition should be carefully observed for possible difficulty in swallowing and respiratory involvement. The child's cardiorespiratory function is monitored, and a respirator, suction apparatus, tracheostomy tray, and vasoconstrictor drugs are kept available at the bedside. Vital signs and level of consciousness are monitored frequently. For the child who develops respiratory dysfunction the care is the same as that for any child with respiratory distress requiring mechanical ventilation.

Throughout the recovery phase, special emphasis is placed on prevention of complications, including proper postural alignment, frequent change of position, and passive range-of-motion exercises. Children with oral and pharyngeal involvement are usually fed via a nasogastric tube to ensure adequate feeding. Bowel and bladder care is needed to avoid constipation and urine retention. Sensory impairment makes the child susceptible to burns and trophic ulcers.

Physical therapy is limited to passive range-of-motion exercises during the evolving phase of the disease. Later, as the disease stabilizes and recovery begins, an active physical therapy program is implemented to prevent contracture deformities and facilitate muscle recovery. This may include active exercise, gait training, and bracing.

Throughout the course of the illness, support of the child and parents is paramount. The usual rapidity of the paralysis and the long period of recovery tax the emotional reserves of all family members greatly. The parents and child benefit from repeated reassurance that recovery is occurring and from realistic information regarding the possibility of permanent disability. In the event of a residual disability, the family needs assistance in accepting and adjusting to the loss of function (see Chapter 38). The Guillain-Barré Syndrome Support Group* is a nonprofit organization devoted to support, education, and research. It provides support to families from recovered persons, publishes informational literature and a newsletter, and maintains a list of practitioners experienced with the disease.

TETANUS

Tetanus, or lockjaw, is an acute, preventable, and often fatal disease caused by an exotoxin produced by the anaerobic spore-forming, gram-positive bacillus *Clostridium tetani.* The disorder is characterized by painful muscular rigidity primarily involving the masseter and neck muscles. There are four requirements for the development of tetanus: (1) presence of tetanus spores or vegetative forms of the bacillus, (2) injury to the tissues, (3) wound conditions that encourage multiplication of the organism, and (4) a susceptible host.

Tetanus spores are found in soil, dust, and the intestinal tracts of humans and animals, especially herbivorous animals. The organisms are more prevalent in rural areas but are readily carried to urban areas by the wind. The organisms are not invasive but enter the body by way of wounds, particularly a puncture wound, burn, or crushed area. They may enter through a very minor, unnoticed break in the skin, such as a thorn or needle prick, bee sting, or scratch. In the newborn, infection may occur through the umbilical cord, usually in situations in which infants are delivered in severely contaminated surroundings. The disease has the greatest incidence in months when persons are more involved in outdoor activities. Substance abusers are especially susceptible from poor injection technique and the use of street heroin, which is often mixed with quinine, a protoplasmic poison that favors the growth of the organism.

Pathophysiology

When conditions are favorable, the organisms proliferate and elaborate a potent exotoxin that affects the central nervous system to produce the clinical manifestations of the disease. The ideal conditions for growth of the organisms are devitalized tissues without access to air, such as wounds that have not been washed or kept clean and those that have crusted over, trapping pus beneath. The exotoxin appears to reach the central nervous system by way of either the neuron axons or the vascular system. The toxin becomes fixed on nerve cells of the anterior horn of the spinal cord and the brainstem. The toxin acts at the myoneural junction to produce muscular stiffness and lower the threshold for reflex excitability.

There are several forms of the disease, but the generalized form is the most common and most dangerous. The incubation period for tetanus varies from 3 days to 3 weeks but generally averages 8 days. The traditional belief that the more extensive the injury, the shorter the incubation period and the more severe the symptoms has not been confirmed in the United States.

The manner of onset varies, but the initial symptoms are usually a progressive stiffness and tenderness of the muscles in the neck and jaw. Eventually all voluntary muscles are affected (Box 52-11). As the child recovers from the disease, the paroxysms become less frequent and gradually subside. Survival beyond 4 days usually indicates recovery, but complete recovery may require weeks.

The mortality rate is about 30%, but the disease is almost invariably fatal in the newborn. The incubation period is short, with the appearance of symptoms 3 to 10 days after exposure. The first symptom is difficulty sucking, which progresses to total inability to suck, excessive crying, irritability, and nuchal rigidity.

Therapeutic Management

Preventive measures are based on the immune status of the affected child and the nature of the injury. Specific prophylactic therapy after trauma is administration of either *tetanus toxoid* or *tetanus antitoxin* (see Immunizations, Chapter 33).

The unprotected or inadequately immunized child sustains a "tetanus-prone" wound (such as, but not limited to, wounds contaminated with dirt, feces, soil, and saliva; puncture

*P.O. Box 262, Wynnewood PA 19096.

BOX 52-11
Clinical Manifestations of Tetanus

Initial symptoms
Progressive stiffness and tenderness of muscles in neck and jaw
Characteristic difficulty in opening the mouth (trismus)
Risus sardonicus (sardonic smile) caused by facial muscle spasm

Progressive involvement
Opisthotonos
Boardlike rigidity of abdominal and limb muscles
Difficulty swallowing
High sensitivity to external stimuli (slight noise, gentle touch, or bright light)
- Trigger paroxysmal muscular contractions that last seconds to minutes
- Contractions recur with increased frequency until almost continuous

Laryngospasm and tetany of respiratory muscles
- Accumulated secretions
- Respiratory arrest
- Atelectasis
- Pneumonia

Other aspects
Mentation unaffected; patient alert
Pain and distress are reflected in:
- Rapid pulse
- Sweating
- Anxious expression

Fever usually absent or only mild

wounds; avulsions; and wounds resulting from missiles, crushing, burns, and frostbite) should receive *tetanus immune globulin (TIG)*. Concurrent administration of both TIG and tetanus toxoid at separate sites is recommended both to provide protection and to initiate the active immune process. Completion of active immunization is carried out according to the usual pattern.

The affected child is best treated in an intensive care facility where close and constant observation and equipment for monitoring and respiratory support are readily available. A quiet environment is preferred to reduce external stimuli. Neonates are placed in an open warmer unit or incubator to maintain a constant environmental temperature and amount of oxygen supplied.

General supportive care, including maintenance of adequate fluid and electrolyte balance and caloric intake, is indicated. Indwelling oral or nasogastric feedings are used whenever possible, but severe laryngospasm may necessitate intravenous parenteral nutrition or gastrostomy feeding. Recurrent laryngospasm or excessive accumulation of secretions may require endotracheal intubation.

TIG therapy to neutralize toxins is the most specific therapy for tetanus. Antibiotics are administered to control the proliferation of the vegetative forms of the organism at the site of infection. Local care of the wound by surgical debridement and cleansing helps reduce the numbers of proliferating organisms at the site of injury. The cleansing should be repeated several times during the first 48 hours, and deep, infected lacerations are usually exposed and debrided.

Sedatives or muscle relaxants are administered to help reduce muscle spasm and prevent convulsions. The most widely used is diazepam (Valium), but phenobarbital, chloral hydrate, the phenothiazines, and paraldehyde may be employed. Patients with severe tetanus and those who do not respond to other sedatives require the administration of a neuromuscular blocking agent, usually pancuronium bromide (Pavulon) or vecuronium. Because of their paralytic effect on respiratory muscles, use of these drugs requires mechanical ventilation with endotracheal intubation or tracheostomy and constant attendance by trained personnel until muscle spasms are controlled. Endotracheal tube insertion or tracheostomy is often indicated and should be performed before severe respiratory distress develops. Administration of corticosteroids has met with success in some instances.

Nursing Care Management

In caring for the child with tetanus, every effort is made to control or eliminate stimulation from sound, light, and touch. Although a darkened room is ideal, sufficient light is essential in order that the child can be carefully observed; light appears to be less irritating than vibratory or auditory stimuli. The infant or child is handled as little as possible, and extra effort is expended to avoid any sudden and/or loud noise.

Medications are administered as prescribed, and vital signs are observed and recorded at frequent intervals. The location and extent of muscle spasms and assessment of their severity are important nursing observations. Respiratory status is carefully evaluated for any signs of distress, and appropriate emergency equipment is kept available at all times. Muscle relaxants and sedatives that may be prescribed can also cause respiratory depression; therefore the child must be assessed for excessive central nervous system depression. Oxygen saturation monitoring and, when needed, blood gases are obtained frequently to evaluate respiratory status. Attention to hydration and nutrition may involve monitoring an intravenous infusion, monitoring nasogastric or gastrostomy feedings, and suctioning oropharyngeal secretions when indicated.

If a potent muscle relaxant such as pancuronium bromide is used, the total paralysis makes oral communication impossible. Therefore all the child's needs must be anticipated and procedures carefully explained beforehand. As the dose of medication is decreased, the child regains movement of the eyelids and facial muscles, which gives the child some opportunity to express emotions and indicate choices through a signal system, for example, blinking the eyelids to indicate "yes" or "no."

Since their mental status is clear, they are aware of what is happening to them and are often in a state of terror. They should not be left alone, and all efforts should be made to reduce anxiety, which can contribute to muscular spasms. A calm and reassuring manner and sympathetic understanding can help immeasurably in getting a child through this crisis situation. Parents are encouraged to stay with the child to offer security and support.

BOTULISM

Botulism is a serious food poisoning that results from ingestion of the preformed toxin produced by the anaerobic bacil-

BOX 52-12
Clinical Manifestations of Botulism

General signs
Weakness
Dizziness
Headache
Difficulty talking and speaking
Diplopia
Vomiting
Progressive, life-threatening respiratory paralysis

Infant botulism
Constipation (a common symptom)
Generalized weakness
Decrease in spontaneous movements
Diminished or absent deep tendon reflexes
Loss of head control
Difficulty feeding
Weak cry
Reduced gag reflex
Progressive respiratory paralysis

lus *Clostridium botulinum*. The most common source of the toxin is improperly sterilized home-canned foods. Central nervous system symptoms appear abruptly about 12 to 36 hours after ingestion of contaminated food and may or may not have been preceded by acute digestive disturbance (Box 52-12).

Treatment consists of intravenous administration of botulism antitoxin and general supportive measures primarily respiratory and nutritional. Toxins vary in protein-binding capacity. Some have a relatively short half-life and do not bind to tissues firmly; therefore therapy is continued until paralysis abates. Other toxins appear to bind irreversibly to nerve endings and are therefore not amenable to neutralization. Respiratory support is often needed and should be available at the bedside, ready for use if indicated.

Infant Botulism

Infant botulism, unlike the disease in older persons, is caused by ingestion of spores or vegetative cells of *C. botulinum* and the subsequent release of the toxin from organisms colonizing the gastrointestinal tract. There appears to be no common food or drug source of the organisms; however, the *C. botulinum* organisms have been found in honey and light or dark corn syrup fed to affected infants (American Academy of Pediatrics, 1994).

There is wide variation in the severity of the disease, from mild constipation to progressive sequential loss of neurologic function and respiratory failure (Box 52-12). The affected infant is usually well before the onset of symptoms. Constipation is a common presenting symptom, and almost all infants exhibit generalized weakness and a decrease in spontaneous movements. Deep tendon reflexes are usually diminished or absent; cranial nerve deficits are common, as evidenced by loss of head control, difficulty in feeding, weak cry, and reduced gag reflex. The most often recognized form of the disease is consistent with the hypotonic infant. Botulism toxin exerts its effect by inhibiting the release of acetylcholine at the myoneural junction, thereby impairing motor activity of muscles innervated by affected nerves.

Diagnosis is made on the basis of the history, physical examination, and laboratory detection of toxin or the organism in the patient or the implicated food. Treatment consists of supportive measures, primarily respiratory and nutritional. Botulism antitoxin, used in adults and older children, is not administered to infants. Evidence indicates that the infants recover without it and that its therapeutic efficacy is lacking. Furthermore, since the antitoxin is made from horse serum, it may cause serum sickness or anaphylaxis and may induce a lifelong hypersensitivity.

The prognosis is generally good if the patient is adequately supported, although recovery may be very slow, requiring weeks to months after severe illness. An infant who is recovering from botulism must avoid contact with other infants for about 3 months or until excretion of organisms has ceased.

Nursing Care Management

Nursing responsibilities include observing for and reporting signs of muscle impairment and providing intensive nursing care when the infant is hospitalized (see Nursing Care of the High-Risk Newborn and Family, Chapter 25). Parental support and reassurance are important. Most infants recover when the disorder is recognized and therapy is implemented. Parents should be aware that during recovery patients tire easily when muscular action is sustained. This has important implications for timing the resumption of feedings because of the risk of aspiration. Parents should also be advised that normal bowel action may not return for several weeks; therefore a stool softener can be beneficial. Cathartics and enemas are not advised.

Home supervision of the outpatient and education regarding possible modes of infection (such as use of honey or corn syrup as a formula sweetener) are nursing responsibilities. Since the prime sources of botulism toxin are inadequately cooked or improperly canned food, families are advised about the danger of home-canned foods, especially vegetables, fruits, fish, and condiments. Boiling is not always adequate, particularly in high altitudes where water boils at a lower temperature, which does not destroy the organisms.

SPINAL CORD INJURIES

Spinal cord injuries with major neurologic involvement are not a common cause of physical disability in childhood. However, there are a sufficient number of children with these injuries who are admitted to major medical centers, and because of the increased survival rate as a result of improved management, nurses are more likely to become involved with such children.

Mechanisms of Injury

In motor vehicle accidents (MVAs), most spinal cord injuries in children are a result of indirect trauma caused by sudden hyperflexion or hyperextension of the neck, often combined with a rotational force. Trauma to the spinal cord without evidence of vertebral fracture or dislocation is particularly apt to occur in an MVA when proper restraints are not used. An unrestrained child becomes a projectile during sudden deceleration and is subject to injury from contact with a variety of objects inside and outside the vehicle. Individuals who use only a lap seat belt restraint are at greater risk of spinal cord injury than those who use a combination lap and shoulder restraint.

Falling from heights occurs less often in children than in adults, but vertebral compression from blows to the head or buttocks can occur in water sports (diving and surfing), falls from horses, or other athletic activities. Birth injuries may occur in breech deliveries from traction force on the spinal cord during delivery of the head and shoulders. An increasing number of teenagers receive spinal cord injuries when they are shot or stabbed in the back.

The injury sustained can affect any of the spinal nerves, and the higher the injury, the more extensive the damage. The child can be left with complete or partial paralysis of the lower extremities *(paraplegia)* or with damage at a higher level and without functional use of any of the four extremities *(quadriplegia)*. A high cervical cord injury that affects the phrenic nerve paralyzes the diaphragm and leaves the child dependent on a respirator.

A mild but equally frightening form of cord trauma is *spinal cord compression*, a temporary neural dysfunction without visible damage to the cord. Complete quadraplegia can result but initially may not be differentiated from serious cord injury.

Therapeutic Management

The management of the child with spinal cord injury is complex and controversial. Initial care begins at the scene of the accident; therefore education and training of rescue personnel in stabilization and transfer techniques to prevent or reduce the severity of injury are of utmost importance. In any situation in which spinal cord injury is suspected or a possibility, the child should be calmed, reassured, and told not to move; no one should be allowed to move the child unless they are able to correctly stabilize the head and trunk to avoid twisting or bending the spine. If conscious, the child is placed supine on a rigid surface to prevent sagging. Infants and small children are removed in their car seats; no attempt should be made to take them out of the seat. Because of the complexity and relative infrequency of these injuries, it is usually recommended that these persons be transferred to a spinal injury center for care by specially trained personnel.

Nursing Care Management

The nursing care of the paraplegic or quadriplegic child is complex and challenging. As a member of the acute care and rehabilitation teams, the nurse is involved in all aspects of care. Ideally, initial care takes place in a special intensive care unit with personnel trained to handle spinal cord injuries. Nursing management is concerned primarily with prevention of complications and maintenance of function.

Once the acute period is over, the lesion is usually static and nonprogressive, regardless of whether the paralysis is secondary to trauma, a congenital defect, infection, a treated tumor, or surgery.

The nurse is a member of a team of specialists, including physicians from a number of specialty areas, physical and occupational therapists, psychologists, social workers, teachers, and vocational counselors. Each team member has a unique contribution to make, and mutual agreement for specific areas of responsibility and evaluation of progress are determined during regularly scheduled team conferences.

To meet the needs of these children, the reader is referred to the extensive discussion in Wong (1995) or to texts devoted to children with spinal cord injuries.

Key Points

- Clinical manifestations of cerebral palsy include delayed gross motor development, abnormal motor performance, alterations of muscle tone, abnormal postures, reflex abnormalities, and associated disabilities such as mental retardation, seizures, attention deficit disorder, and sensory impairment.
- Therapy for cerebral palsy takes into account the nature of the physical disability, defects associated with the disorder, and interpersonal and social influences encountered by the affected child.
- Care of the infant and child with myelomeningocele is directed toward protecting the meningeal sac, preventing infection and skin breakdown, and observing for signs of complications.
- Werdnig-Hoffmann disease is characterized by progressive weakness and wasting of skeletal muscles caused by degeneration of anterior horn cells of the spinal cord.
- Muscular dystrophies are the largest and most important cause of muscular dysfunction of childhood.
- Major complications of Duchenne muscular dystrophy include joint contractures, disuse atrophy, infections, obesity, and cardiopulmonary problems.
- Nursing care of the child with Guillain-Barré syndrome consists of monitoring vital signs, ensuring alignment and positioning, providing physical therapy, and providing support to the child and family.
- Tetanus occurs when tetanus spores or vegetative bacilli enter a wound and multiply in a susceptible host.
- Infant botulism results from the release of toxins from *C. botulinum* colonizing the gastrointestinal tract.
- Therapeutic management of spinal cord injury is directed toward preventing further neuronal damage, avoiding complications, and maintaining vital functions.

References

American Academy of Pediatrics, Committee on Genetics: Folic acid for the prevention of neural tube defects, *Pediatrics* 92(3):493-494, 1993.

American Academy of Pediatrics: *Report of the Committee on Infectious Diseases*, ed 23, Elk Grove Village, Ill, 1994, The Academy.

Brucker JM: Selective dorsal rhizotomy: neurosurgical treatment of cerebral palsy, *J Pediatr Nurs* 5:105-114, 1990.

Fernandes ET et al: Neurogenic bladder dysfunction in children: review of pathophysiology and current management. *J Pediatr* 124(1):1-7, 1994.

Hutton JL, Cooke T, Pharaoh P: Life expectancy in children with cerebral palsy, *Br Med J* 309(6952):431-435, 1994.

Knowledge and use of folic acid by women of childbearing age - United States, 1995, *MMWR* 44(38):716-718, 1995.

Multicenter Study Group: Diagnosis of Duchenne and Becker muscular dystrophies by polymerase chain reaction, *JAMA* 267(19):2609-2615, 1992.

Russman BS et al: Spinal muscular atrophy: new thoughts on the pathogenesis and classification schema, *J Child Neurol* 7(4):347-353, 1992.

Vajsar J et al: Plasmapheresis vs intravenous immunoglobulin treatment in childhood Guillain-Barré syndrome, *Arch Pediatr Adolesc Med* 148(11):1210-1211, 1994.

Wong D: Whaley and Wong's nursing care of infants and children, ed 5, St Louis, 1995, Mosby.

Bibliography

Cerebral Palsy/Spina Bifida

Appleton PL, Minchom PE, Ellis NC: The self-concept of young people with spina bifida, *Dev Med Child Neurol* 36(3):198-215, 1994.

Blasco PA: Primitive reflexes: their contribution to the early detection of cerebral palsy, *Clin Pediatr* 33(7):388-397, 1994.

Dormans JP: Orthopedic management of children with cerebral palsy, *Pediatr Clin North Am* 40(3):645-657, 1993.

Eicher PS, Batshaw ML: Cerebral palsy, *Pediatr Clin North Am* 40(3):537-551, 1993.

Farley JA, Dunleavy MJ: *Myelodysplasia*. In Jackson PL, Vessey JA: *Primary care of the child with a chronic illness*, ed 2, St Louis, 1996, Mosby.

Hobdell EF: Perceptual accuracy and gender-related differences in parents of children with myelomeningocele, *J Neurosci Nurs* 27(4):240-244, 1995.

Knutson LM, Clark DE: Orthotic devices for ambulation in children with cerebral palsy and myelomeningocele, *Phys Ther* 71(12):947-960, 1991.

Kuban KC, Leviton A: Medical progress: cerebral palsy, *N Engl J Med* 330(3):188-195, 1994.

Morrow JD: Temperament of the infant with myelomeningocele, *J Pediatr Nurs* 10(2):99-104, 1995.

Nehring WM, Steele S: *Cerebral palsy*. In Jackson PL, Vessey JA: *Primary care of the child with a chronic condition*, ed 2, St Louis, 1996, Mosby.

Park TS, Owen JH: Surgical management of spastic diplegia in cerebral palsy, *N Engl J Med* 326(11):745-749, 1992.

Peacock WJ, Staudt LA: Management of spasticity in cerebral palsy, *Int Pediatr* 7(2):181-184, 1992.

Peterson PM et al: Spina bifida: the transition into adulthood begins in infancy, *Rehab Nurs* 19(4):229-338, 1994.

Polivka BJ, Nickel JT, Wilkins III Jr: Cerebral palsy: evaluation of a model of risk, *Res Nurs Health* 16(2):113-122, 1993.

Romanczuk AN, Brown JP: Folic acid will reduce risk of neural tube defects, *Am J Matern Child Nurs* 19(6):331-334, 1994.

Sackett CK, Spina bifida, *Urol Nurs* 13(2):58-61, 1993.

Segal ES, Deatrick JA, Hagelgans NA: The determinants of successful self-catheterization programs in children with myelomeningoceles, *J Pediatr Nurs* 10(2):82-88, 1995.

Sprague JB: Surgical management of cerebral palsy, *Orthop Nurs* 11(4):11-19, 1992.

Turnbull JD: Early intervention for children with or at risk of cerebral palsy, *Am J Dis Child* 147(1):54-59, 1993.

Walker MJ: Selective dorsal rhizotomy, reducing spasticity in patients with cerebral palsy, *AORN J* 54(4):759-761, 1991.

Zickler CF, Dodge NN: Office management of the young child with cerebral palsy and difficulty in growing, *J Pediatr Health Care* 8(3):111-120, 1994.

Neuromuscular Dysfunction

Bechler-Karsch A, Berro E: Infant botulism, *Am J Matern Child Nurs* 19(5):275-280, 1994.

Hardy FM, Rittenberry K: Myasthenia gravis: an overview, *Orthopaed Nurs* 13(6):37-42, 1994.

Iannaccone ST et al: Prospective study of spinal muscular atrophy before age 6 years: DCN/SMA Group, *Pediatr Neurol* 9(3):187-193, 1993.

Jansen PW, Perkins RM, Ashwal S: Guillain-Barré syndrome in childhood: natural course and efficacy of plasma pheresis, *Pediatr Neurol* 9(1):16-20, 1993.

Khan MA: Corticosteroid therapy in Duchenne muscular dystrophy, *J Neurol Sci* 120(1):8-14, 1993.

McGhee B, Jarjour IT: Single-dose intravenous immune globulin for treatment of Guillain-Barré syndrome, *Am J Hosp Pharm* 51(1):97-99, 1994.

Mygrant BI et al: Infant botulism, *Heart Lung* 23(2):164-168, 1994.

Pentland B, Donald SM: Pain in the Guillain-Barré syndrome: a clinical review, *Pain* 59(2):159-164, 1994.

Rantala H et al: Epidemiology of Guillain-Barré syndrome in children: relationship of oral polio vaccine administration to occurrence, *J Pediatr* 124(2):220-223, 1994.

Vallee L et al: Intravenous immune globulin is also an efficient therapy of acute Guillain-Barré syndrome in affected children, *Neuropediatrics* 24(4):235-236, 1993.

Wise EJ: Preventing complications in infant botulism, *DCCN* 14(2):86-91, 1995.

Spinal Cord Injury

Ditunno JF, Formal CS: Current concepts: chronic spinal cord injury, *N Engl J Med* 330(8):550-556, 1994.

Joy C: Pediatric spinal cord injury, *Crit Care Nurs Clin North Am* 2(3):415-419, 1990.

Lang SM, Bernardo LM: SCIWORA syndrome: nursing assessment . . . spinal cord injury without radiographic abnormality, *Dimens Crit Care Nurs* 12(5):247-254, 1993.

Mulcahey MJ et al: Outcomes of tendon transfer surgery and occupational therapy in a child with tetraplegia, *Am J Occup Ther* 49(7):607-617, 1995.

Rathbone D et al: Spinal cord concussion in pediatric athletes, *J Pediatr Orthop* 12:616-620, 1992.

Wineman NM, Durand EJ, Steiner R: A comparative analysis of coping behaviors in persons with multiple sclerosis or a spinal cord injury, *Res Nurs Health* 17(3):185-194, 1994.

Yoshimura O et al: Spinal cord injury in a child: a long term follow-up study. Case report, *Paraplegia* 33(6):362-363, 1995.

APPENDIX A

Standards for the Nursing Care of Women and Newborns

I: NURSING PRACTICE

Comprehensive nursing care for women and newborns focuses on helping individuals, families, and communities achieve their optimum health potential. This is best achieved within the framework of the nursing process.

The nurse is responsible for decisions and actions within the domain of the nursing practice, which may include the following:

- Integration of the nursing process components of assessment, planning, implementation, and evaluation in all areas of nursing practice
- Individualization and prioritization of nursing care to meet the physical, psychologic, spiritual, and social needs of patients
- Collaboration with the individual, family, and other members of the health care team
- Promotion of a safe and therapeutic environment for both the recipients and providers of nursing care
- Demonstration and validation of competence in nursing practice
- Acquisition of specialized knowledge and skills and additional formal education to provide specialized care
- Provision for complete and accurate documentation of care

The written or computerized patient record is the documented means of communication among all members of the health care team. It also promotes continuity of care and provides a mechanism for evaluating care. The record should contain accurate and complete recordings of the patient's history and physical examination, as well as the nursing plan of care, including goals, interventions, health education, and evaluation of patient and family responses. Additional documentation may include planned follow-up examinations and appropriate referrals. All information contained in the patient record and related to the care of the patient and family is confidential and should be released only according to institutional policy.

NOTE: **To apply this universal standard to a specific area of gynecologic, obstetric, or neonatal nursing practice, refer directly to the specialty-specific nursing practice standards section.**

Modified from Nurses Association of the American College of Obstetricians and Gynecologists: *Standards for the nursing care of women and newborns*, ed 4, Washington, DC, 1991, NAACOG.

II: HEALTH EDUCATION AND COUNSELING

Health education for the individual, family, and community is an integral part of comprehensive nursing care. Such education encourages participation in, and shared responsibility for, health promotion, maintenance, and restoration.

Comprehensive health education includes the following:

- Identification of the needs and abilities of the learner
- Collaboration with the patient and other health care providers in design, content, and follow-up of the educational plan
- Provision of accurate and current information
- Provision of information based on educationally sound principles of teaching and learning
- Recognition of patient rights, responsibilities, and alternative choices
- Utilization of available educational resources in the practice environment
- Utilization of available educational resources to provide health education information to individuals/families in the community
- Documentation and evaluation of health education including patient response

The nurse participates in and/or coordinates the health education and counseling process. It begins with the initial patient contact or admission to the unit or service and is an ongoing, continuous process.

NOTE: **To apply this universal standard to a specific area of gynecologic, obstetric, or neonatal nursing practice, refer directly to the specialty-specific nursing practice standards section.**

III: POLICIES, PROCEDURES, AND PROTOCOLS

Written policies, procedures, and protocols clarify the scope of nursing practice and delineate the qualifications of personnel authorized to provide care to women and newborns within the health care setting.

The components of policies, procedures, and protocols are based on the following:

- Recognition of the organization's philosophy
- Recognition of the unit's philosophy

- Assessment of the practice setting and determination of types of services to be provided
- Incorporation of a multidisciplinary approach in their development
- Identification of specific areas of practice to be addressed
- Reflection of current practice, standards, and local regulations
- Anticipated use as references for health care providers, orientation of new personnel and students, quality assurance activities, and/or guiding nursing actions in emergency situations

The development of policies, procedures, and protocols should include consideration of staff availability, skill, and licensure; the physical plant and equipment; effects on other departments; and fiscal impact. Policies, procedures, and protocols should be reviewed and revised at least on an annual basis or more frequently as science/technology changes.

NOTE: **To apply this universal standard to a specific area of gynecologic, obstetric, or neonatal nursing practice, refer directly to the specialty-specific nursing practice standards section.**

IV: PROFESSIONAL RESPONSIBILITY AND ACCOUNTABILITY

Comprehensive nursing care for women and newborns is provided by nurses who are clinically competent and accountable for professional actions and legal responsibilities inherent in the nursing role.

Responsibility and accountability for newborns include the following:

- Awareness of changing practices and professional and ethical issues
- Knowledge and clinical skills gained through in-service education, professional continuing education, research data, and professional literature
- Implementation of newly acquired knowledge and skills
- Collaboration through networking and sharing with other professionals
- Participation in the development of standards and policies, procedures, and protocols
- Participation in periodic peer and self-evaluations
- Recognition of certification as one mechanism for the demonstration of special knowledge within a specialty area of practice

Legal accountability extends to the following:

- Nurse practice acts
- Parameters of professional practice established by professional organizations
- Institutional standards
- Legislative changes that affect practice
- Policies, procedures, and protocols within the practice environment

V: UTILIZATION OF NURSING PERSONNEL

Nursing care for women and newborns is conducted in practice settings that have qualified nursing staff in sufficient numbers to meet patient care needs.

Each practice setting should have sufficient nursing personnel to meet patient care requirements. Nursing staff who provide direct care to women and newborns should be supervised by registered nurses who are clinically proficient in the specialty area of practice. The patient care unit or service is managed by a professional nurse who is prepared educationally and clinically to assume a leadership position. In all practice settings, the nurse may practice independently or collaboratively with other health care team members. It is essential that nurses know both the responsibilities and the limitations of professional nursing practice specific to the practice setting.

Many variables are considered in determining both the number and type of nursing staff needed for a practice setting. Among these variables are those related to the patient, practice, organization, and personnel. Patient-related variables may include the following:

- Patient demographics and acuity of patients served
- Length of stay
- Educational needs
- Cultural factors and level of comprehension
- Communication barriers
- Discharge or home care needs

Practice-related variables may include the following:

- Difference in educational and experiential level of nursing staff
- Nursing philosophy
- Type of nursing care delivery system
- Use of assistive personnel
- Use of nurses in expanded roles
- Participation in teaching programs

Organizational variables may include the following:

- Scope of services provided
- Availability of support services
- Patient volume
- Mission or philosophy of the organization
- Risk management concerns
- Quality assurance programs
- Policies, procedures, and protocols
- Physical plant
- Marketing strategies
- Fiscal considerations

Personnel variables relate to the type and number of professional and nonprofessional staff and may include the following:

- Education, skill, and experience of the nursing leadership
- Educational preparation, skill, and experience of staff
- Types and mix of nursing staff
- Availability of qualified alternative staff to deal with emergencies or unanticipated volumes
- Distribution of staff, such as temporary reassignment, floating, on-call, cross-training, and supplemental staffing
- Responsibilities for orientation, precepting, or students
- Turnover rates
- Clinical and technical support

Competency-based job descriptions should be available for each level of nursing staff. Orientation for all personnel should include a general overview of the organization and specific information about the individual practice setting. Performance evaluations for all personnel should be conducted, documented, and discussed on a regular basis with input from the individual, colleagues, and supervisory staff.

VI: ETHICS

Ethical principles guide the process of decision making for nurses caring for women and newborns at all times and especially when personal or professional values conflict with those of the patient, family, colleagues, or practice setting.

The nurses should have the opportunity to participate in the ethical decision-making process. To participate actively, nurses should do the following:

- Clarify their own personal and professional values
- Recognize the difficulty in selecting a course of action that is morally and ethically acceptable to all parties
- Communicate openly and assertively
- Identify options
- Seek consultations

Nurses must carefully examine their own value systems, since values influence the decision-making process. Opportunities should be provided in the practice setting for discussion of potential ethical issues. Each practice setting should have a framework for decision making regarding bioethical dilemmas. Ethical dilemmas generally arise when there is a conflict between loyalties, rights, duties, or values.

For nurses, most ethical dilemmas occur when there is a real or perceived requirement to act in a manner contrary to personal values or when care ordered or provided does not seem compatible with the best interest of the patient. Common areas of concern may include the following:

- Nursing autonomy and decision making
- Maternal interests versus fetal interests
- Issues of duty, obligation, and loyalty (for example, employer to employee, professional to public, professional to professional)
- Patients' rights to resources, privacy, confidentiality, information, participation in decision making, and refusal of therapy
- The right to live or die
- Life cycle concerns, including contraception, sterilization, pregnancy termination, genetic manipulation, infanticide, sexuality and choices of life-style, and euthanasia
- Fetal or neonatal conditions incompatible with life
- Fetal tissue use
- Biomedical intervention

The bioethics literature can provide nurses with strategies to cope with or resolve decisions in situations when conflicts of values occur. For ethical decision-making frameworks to be applied to practice situations, working relationships must be established in which individuals may express their own points of view. All persons potentially affected by an ethical decision have the right to participate in the decision-making process.

VII: RESEARCH

Nurses caring for women and newborns utilize research findings, conduct nursing research, and evaluate nursing practice to improve the outcomes of care.

Knowledge of the research process and participation in scientific inquiry are necessary to do the following:

- Conduct or participate in the conduct of research according to ethical guidelines
- Use research findings to provide appropriate and safe nursing care
- Use research findings as a basis for validating standards of nursing care
- Evaluate the relevance and application of research findings from nursing and related disciplines
- Validate the effect of nursing practice on patient outcomes

VIII: QUALITY ASSURANCE

Quality and appropriateness of patient care are evaluated through a planned assessment program using specific, identified clinical indicators.

Each unit or service should have a written quality assurance plan that reflects a philosophy that is coordinated with the organization's mission and overall quality assurance program. Objectives of the unit-based or service-based quality assurance plan should include the following:

- Assurance of consistent quality patient outcomes
- Identification and correction of potential nursing practice deficiencies
- Promotion of professional nursing practice based on appropriate nursing standards
- Education and participation of staff in quality assurance activities

The unit nurse manager is responsible for developing and implementing the unit-based quality assurance plan. The plan should include the following:

- Responsibilities of all personnel in the quality assurance process
- The scope of service provided
- Important aspects of care or service involving high-risk, high-volume, and problem-prone patients or activities
- Clinical indicators or measurable standards that affect the aspects of care and service that have been identified as important
- Specific criteria and thresholds for use in monitoring clinical indicators
- Methods for the collection and analysis of data, including reference to collection tools, sample size, time frame, and staff responsibility
- Determination of appropriate corrective action, when indicated, that will fall into one of three categories: educational, organizational, or behavioral change
- Follow-up assessment of identified problems
- Documentation of all aspects of the quality assurance program, including results
- A process for communication related to quality assurance activities within the total organization

Nursing Responsibilities in Implementing Intrapartum Fetal Heart Rate Monitoring

The primary goal of perinatal care is to ensure optimal maternal and neonatal outcomes. The intrapartum period represents a time of risk for the mother and the fetus. Assessment of fetal heart rate (FHR) has been recognized as a vital aspect in the evaluation of fetal well-being in response to the stresses of labor and birth.

Auscultation and electronic fetal monitoring (EFM) are the basic techniques used to assess FHR. Each method has its advantages and limitations, necessitating individualized decision making for appropriate use. The method of FHR monitoring selected and the frequency of FHR evaluation should be based on consideration of maternal-fetal risk factors and the availability of nursing personnel who are skilled in the monitoring techniques. The patient's preference regarding the method of FHR monitoring should be taken into consideration.

Nurses who perform FHR monitoring are responsible for their actions and will be held to the established standards of care as defined by their professional organizations, the standards of practice in their institutions, and the scope of practice as defined by their nurse practice act.

METHODOLOGY

Auscultation of the FHR is an auditory assessment procedure that, when properly performed, allows evaluation of FHR both during and immediately after the stress of a uterine contraction. Auscultation between contractions establishes the baseline FHR. Auscultation as a primary technique of FHR surveillance requires a thorough knowledge of the basic principles of the fetal heart and uterine physiology and pathophysiology. Clinical experience in the recognition of and the response to significant FHR changes is required. Validation of competency in the use of this technique must be in accordance with established institutional policy.

Intermittent auscultation of the fetal heart rate with a 1:1 nurse/patient ratio at 15-minute intervals during the active phase of the first stage of labor and at 5-minute intervals during the second stage has been shown to be equivalent to EFM (American Academy of Pediatrics and The American College of Obstetricians and Gynecologists [ACOG], 1992). For low-risk patients, the suggested auscultation frequency is 30-minute intervals in active first-stage labor and 15-minute intervals in second-stage labor (NAACOG,* 1990; ACOG, 1995). For high-risk patients, the suggested auscultation frequency is 15-minute intervals in active first-stage labor and 5-minute intervals in second-stage labor (NAACOG, 1990; ACOG, 1995). Therefore if auscultation is prescribed as the primary technique of FHR surveillance in the second stage of labor, a minimum of a 1:1 nurse/fetus ratio is required.

EFM is an auditory and visual assessment procedure that provides data for the evaluation of uterine activity and fetal heart responses, including baseline heart rate, variability, and FHR change over time. Further, EFM produces a printed record. The use of EFM requires knowledge of its equipment and thorough knowledge of the basic principles of the fetal heart and uterine physiology and pathophysiology. Nurses who use EFM must be able to recognize FHR patterns, variability, and uterine activity.

Fetal monitoring patterns have been given descriptive names, for example, accelerations and early, late, and variable decelerations. Nurses should use these terms in written chart documentation and verbal communication. Deviations from a normal heart rate pattern should be documented. When such changes in a FHR pattern occur, the nurse also should document a subsequent return to a normal pattern.

The patient's medical record should include observations and assessments of FHR and characteristics of uterine activity, as well as specific actions taken when changes in FHR patterns are observed. The monitor tracing is a legal part of the medical record and should include identifying information about the patient, as well as times and events related to the patient's ongoing care.

After identification of a nonreassuring pattern, the nurse is responsible for initiating and documenting appropriate nursing interventions as indicated by the pattern identified and for notifying a physician or certified nurse-midwife. Documentation of such notification should be entered in the patient's medical record. The nurse can expect the physician or certified nurse-midwife to respond after being notified of a nonreassuring pattern. An institutional policy should be established for the nurse to follow in the event that the physician

*Approved by the Executive Board, October 1988. Revised February 1992. Reaffirmed 1994. NAACOG became the Association for Women's Health, Obstetric, and Neonatal Nurses in January 1993.

or certified nurse-midwife is unable to respond in a timely fashion.

Core competencies in FHR monitoring have been published by NAACOG (1991, 1991b). Competency validation of this expertise must be in accordance with established institutional policy (NAACOG, 1988).

EVALUATION AND DOCUMENTATION

The institution should establish policies, procedures, and protocols that define evaluation and documentation of FHR monitoring. In developing policies, procedures, and protocols, the institution should address the following:

- Method(s) for assessment (EFM, auscultation, or a combination of both)
- Maternal-fetal risk factors
- Stage of labor
- Frequency of assessment
- Qualifications of health care providers performing assessments
- Nurse/fetus ratios
- Methods of documentation

Documentation of the evaluation of FHR monitoring information during labor is applicable regardless of the method of monitoring selected and may be accomplished in narrative nurses' notes or by the use of comprehensive flow sheets at the time of assessment. Documentation also may be achieved by the use of abbreviated nurses' notes with follow-up summary nurses' notes at intervals specified by institutional policy. The format for abbreviated notes may include initialing the EFM tracing, annotating the EFM tracing, or annotating basic flow sheets.

Suggested frequencies for interval evaluation of FHR information using auscultation have been addressed. For high-risk patients being monitored with auscultation during the active phase of the first stage and during the second stage of labor, intervals for both the evaluation and recording of FHR information are suggested at 15 and 5 minutes, respectively (NAACOG, 1990). For the same group of patients being monitored electronically, evaluation of the tracing is suggested at the same intervals (ACOG, 1995). For low-risk patients being monitored with auscultation, the suggested intervals for evaluation and recording are at 30 and 15 minutes in the active phase of the first and the second stage of labor, respectively. The standard practice for low-risk patients being monitored electronically is to evaluate and record the FHR at least every 30 minutes in the active phase of the first stage of labor and at least every 15 minutes in the second stage of labor (ACOG, 1995).

Evaluation of FHR information may take place at the intervals suggested above or more frequently as necessitated by the individual patient care situation. Written documentation of these FHR evaluations, however, may occur at longer intervals in narrative, abbreviated, or summary formats in accordance with institutional policy and procedure.

CONFLICT RESOLUTION

The potential for conflict exists in terms of professional judgment and decision making regarding which method of monitoring is best for a particular patient in a given situation. Institutional policies, procedures, and protocols must provide a mechanism that will allow nurses the flexibility to decline to implement the prescribed method of FHR monitoring if any question exists regarding the ability to meet the required staffing ratios or if the methodology is beyond the individual nurse's expertise. Ultimately the responsibility for implementing the prescribed method of FHR monitoring remains with the prescriber. In the event of differences of opinion among professionals regarding the ability to implement the prescribed method, the established institutional policy for resolution of conflict should be followed.

References

American Academy of Pediatrics and American College of Obstetricians and Gynecologists: *Guidelines for perinatal care,* ed 3, Washington, DC, 1992, American Academy of Pediatrics and ACOG.

American College of Obstetricians and Gynecologists: *ACOG technical bulletin: fetal heart rate patterns: monitoring, interpretation, and management,* No 207, Washington, DC, 1995, ACOG.

Nurses Association of the American College of Obstetricians and Gynecologists: *OGN nursing practice resource: fetal heart rate auscultation,* Washington, DC, 1990, NAACOG.

Nurses Association of the American College of Obstetricians and Gynecologists: *Nursing practice competencies and educational guidelines: antepartum fetal surveillance and intrapartum fetal monitoring,* Washington, DC, 1991a, NAACOG.

Nurses Association of the American College of Obstetricians and Gynecologists: *Essentials of electronic fetal monitoring competency validation,* Washington, DC, 1991b, NAACOG.

APPENDIX C

Standard Laboratory Values: Pregnant and Nonpregnant Women

	NONPREGNANT	PREGNANT
Hematologic values		
Complete blood count (CBC)		
Hemoglobin, g/dl	12 to 16*	>11*
Hematocrit, PVC, %	37 to 47	>33
Red blood cell (RBC) volume, ml	1600	1500 to 1900
Plasma volume, ml	2400	3700
RBC count, million/mm³	4 to 5	5 to 6.25
White blood cells, total per mm³	5000 to 10,000	5000 to 15,000
Polymorphonuclear cells, %	55 to 70	60 to 85
Lymphocytes, %	20 to 40	15 to 40
Erythrocyte sedimentation rate, mm/hr	20/hr	Elevated second and third trimesters
MCHC, g/dl packed RBCs (mean corpuscular hemoglobin concentration)	32 to 36	No change
MCH/(mean corpuscular hemoglobin per picogram [less than a nanogram])	27 to 31	No change
MCV μm³ (mean corpuscular volume per cubic micrometer)	80 to 95	No change
Blood coagulation and fibrinolytic activity†		
Factors VII, VIII, IX, X		Increase in pregnancy, return to normal in early puerperium; factor VIII increases during and immediately after birth
Factors XI, XIII		Decrease in pregnancy
Prothrombin time (PT)	12 to 14 sec	Slight decrease in pregnancy
Partial thromboplastin time (PTT)	60 to 70 sec	Slight decrease in pregnancy and again decrease during second and third stage of labor (indicates clotting at placental site)
Bleeding time	1 to 3 min (Duke) 2 to 4 min (Ivy)	No appreciable change
Coagulation time	6 to 10 min (Lee/White)	No appreciable change
Platelets	150,000 to 400,000/mm³	No significant change until 3 to 5 days after birth and then a rapid increase (may predispose woman to thrombosis) and gradual return to normal

*At sea level. Permanent residents of higher levels (for example, Denver) require higher levels of hemoglobin.
†Pregnancy represents a hypercoagulable state.

	NONPREGNANT	PREGNANT
Fibrinolytic activity		Decreases in pregnancy and then abrupt return to normal (protection against thromboembolism)
Fibrinogen	300 mg/dl	600 mg/dl
Mineral/vitamin concentrations		
Vitamin B_{12}, folic acid, ascorbic acid	Normal	Moderate decrease
Serum proteins		
Total, g/dl	6.0 to 8.0	5.5 to 7.5
Albumin, g/dl	3.2 to 4.5	3 to 5
Globulin, total, g/dl	2.3 to 3.4	3 to 4
Blood glucose		
Fasting, mg/dl	115	65
2-hour postprandial, mg/dl	70 to 140	Under 140 after a 100 g carbohydrate meal is considered normal
Cardiovascular determinations		
Blood pressure, mm Hg	90 to 140/60 to 90	Slight decrease during midtrimester and then return to usual value by end of third trimester
Pulse, rate/min	70	80
Stroke volume, ml	45 ± 12	75
Cardiac output, L/min	3.6	6
Circulation time (arm-tongue), sec	15 to 16	12 to 14
Blood volume, ml		
Whole blood	4000	5600
Plasma	2400	3700
RBCs	1600	1500 to 1900
Chest x-ray studies		
Transverse diameter of heart	—	1 to 2 cm increase
Left border of heart	—	Straightened
Cardiac volume	—	70 ml increase
Hepatic values		
Bilirubin total	Not more than 1 mg/dl	Unchanged
Serum cholesterol	150 to 200 mg/dl	↑ 60% from 16 to 32 weeks of pregnancy; remains at this level until after birth
Serum alkaline phosphatase	2 to 4.5 units (Bodansky)	↑ from week 12 of pregnancy to 6 weeks after birth
Serum globulin albumin	2.3 to 3.4 g/dl 3.2 to 4.5 g/dl	↑ slight ↓ 3.0 g by late pregnancy
Renal values		
Bladder capacity	1300 ml	1500 ml
Renal plasma flow (RPF), ml/min	490 to 700	Increase by 25%
Glomerular filtration rate (GFR), ml/min	88 to 128	Increase by 50%
Nonprotein nitrogen (NPN), mg/dl	25 to 40	Decreases
Blood urea nitrogen (BUN), mg/dl	10 to 20	Decreases
Serum creatinine, mg/kg/24 hr	20 to 22	Decreases
Serum uric acid, mg/kg/24 hr	250 to 750	Decreases
Urine glucose	Negative	Present in 20% of pregnant women
Intravenous pyelogram (IVP)	Normal	Slight-to-moderate hydroureter and hydronephrosis; right kidney larger than left kidney

APPENDIX D

Family APGAR Questionnaire

Family APGAR questionnaire

PART I

The following questions have been designed to help us better understand you and your family. You should feel free to ask questions about any item in the questionnaire.

The space for comments should be used when you wish to give additional information or if you wish to discuss the way the question is applied to your family. Please try to answer all questions.

Family is defined as the individual(s) with whom you usually live. If you live alone, your "family" consists of persons with whom you now have the strongest emotional ties.*

For each question, check only one box

A		Almost always	Some of the time	Hardly ever
	I am satisfied that I can turn to my family for help when something is troubling me. Comments: ______	☐	☐	☐
	I am satisfied with the way my family talks over things with me and shares problems with me. Comments: ______	☐	☐	☐
	I am satisfied that my family accepts and supports my wishes to take on new activities or directions. Comments: ______	☐	☐	☐
	I am satisfied with the way my family expresses affection and responds to my emotions, such as anger, sorrow, and love. Comments: ______	☐	☐	☐
	I am satisfied with the way my family and I share time together. Comments: ______	☐	☐	☐

*According to which member of the family is being interviewed the interviewer may substitute for the word "family" either spouse, significant other, parents, or children.

Fig. D-1 Family APGAR questionnaire; may be photocopied for clinical use. **A,** Part I. (Modified from Smilkstein G: The Family APGAR: a proposal for a family function test and its use by physicians, *J Fam Pract* 6(6):1231-1239, 1978.)

Family APGAR questionnaire

PART II

Who lives in your home?* List by relationship (e.g., spouse, significant other,† child, or friend).

Please check below the column that best describes how you now get along with each member of the family listed.

Relationship	Age	Sex	Well	Fairly	Poorly
________	__	__	☐	☐	☐
________	__	__	☐	☐	☐
________	__	__	☐	☐	☐
________	__	__	☐	☐	☐
________	__	__	☐	☐	☐
________	__	__	☐	☐	☐

If you don't live with your own family, please list below the individuals to whom you turn for help most frequently. List by relationship, (e.g., family member, friend, associate at work, or neighbor).

Please check below the column that best describes how you now get along with each person listed.

Relationship	Age	Sex	Well	Fairly	Poorly
________	__	__	☐	☐	☐
________	__	__	☐	☐	☐
________	__	__	☐	☐	☐
________	__	__	☐	☐	☐
________	__	__	☐	☐	☐
________	__	__	☐	☐	☐

*If you have established your own family, consider home to be the place where you live with your spouse, children, or significant other; otherwise, consider home as your place of origin, e.g., the place where your parents or those who raise you live.

†"Significant other" is the partner you live with in a physically and emotionally nurturing relationship, but to whom you are not married.

B

Fig. D-1, cont'd. B, Part II.

APPENDIX E

Developmental/Sensory Assessment

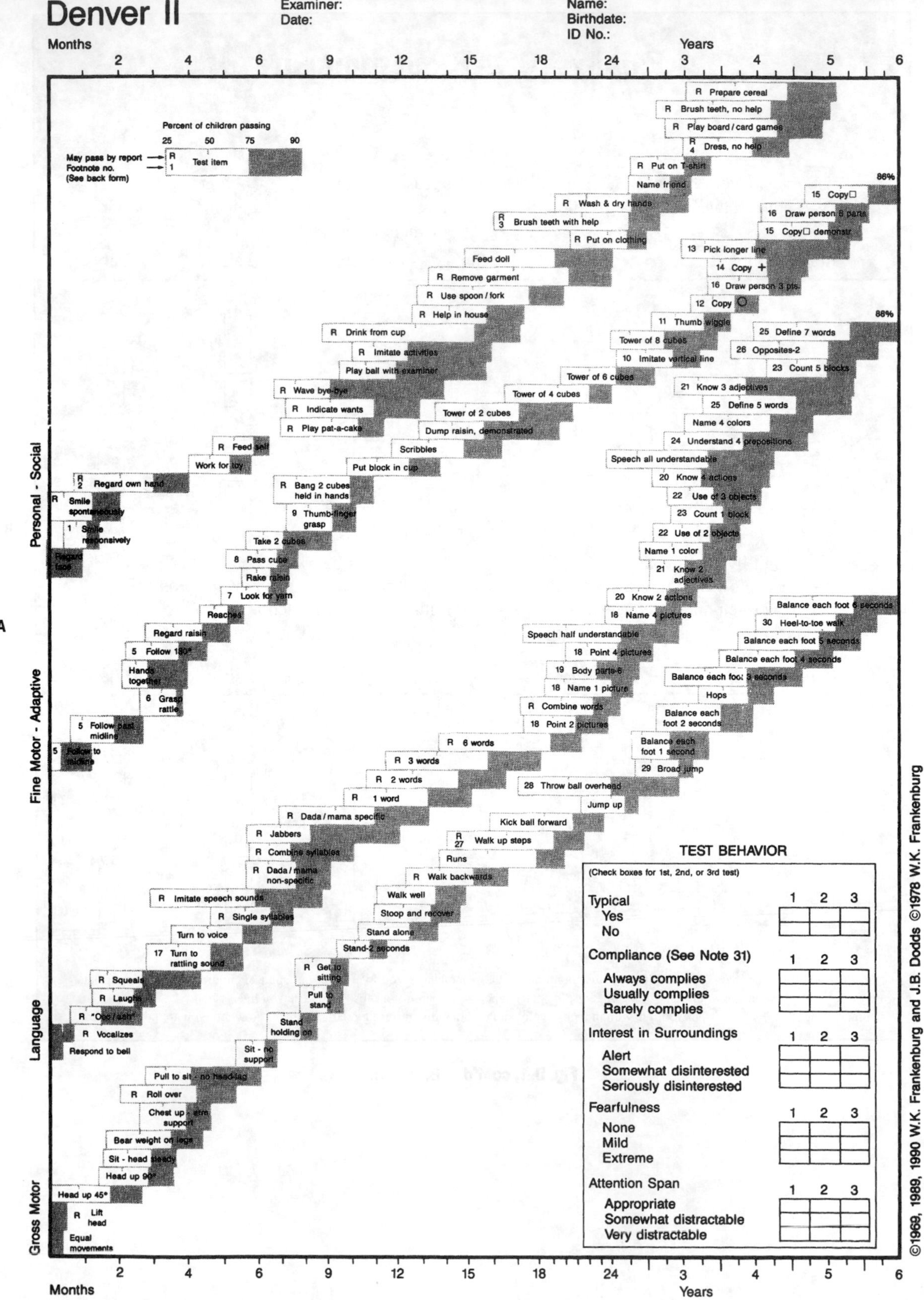

A

DIRECTIONS FOR ADMINISTRATION

1. Try to get child to smile by smiling, talking or waving. Do not touch him/her.
2. Child must stare at hand several seconds.
3. Parent may help guide toothbrush and put toothpaste on brush.
4. Child does not have to be able to tie shoes or button/zip in the back.
5. Move yarn slowly in an arc from one side to the other, about 8" above child's face.
6. Pass if child grasps rattle when it is touched to the backs or tips of fingers.
7. Pass if child tries to see where yarn went. Yarn should be dropped quickly from sight from tester's hand without arm movement.
8. Child must transfer cube from hand to hand without help of body, mouth, or table.
9. Pass if child picks up raisin with any part of thumb and finger.
10. Line can vary only 30 degrees or less from tester's line.
11. Make a fist with thumb pointing upward and wiggle only the thumb. Pass if child imitates and does not move any fingers other than the thumb.

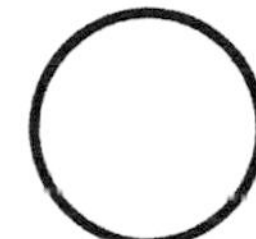

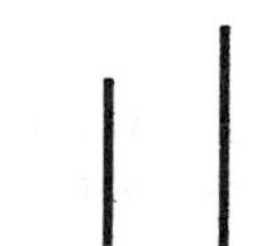

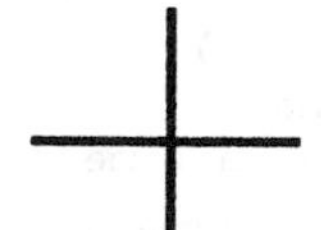

12. Pass any enclosed form. Fail continuous round motions.
13. Which line is longer? (Not bigger.) Turn paper upside down and repeat. (pass 3 of 3 or 5 of 6)
14. Pass any lines crossing near midpoint.
15. Have child copy first. If failed, demonstrate.

When giving items 12, 14, and 15, do not name the forms. Do not demonstrate 12 and 14.

16. When scoring, each pair (2 arms, 2 legs, etc.) counts as one part.
17. Place one cube in cup and shake gently near child's ear, but out of sight. Repeat for other ear.
18. Point to picture and have child name it. (No credit is given for sounds only.) If less than 4 pictures are named correctly, have child point to picture as each is named by tester.

B

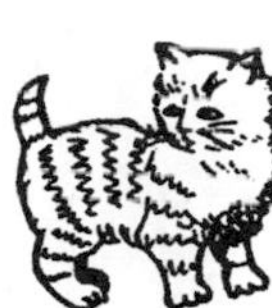

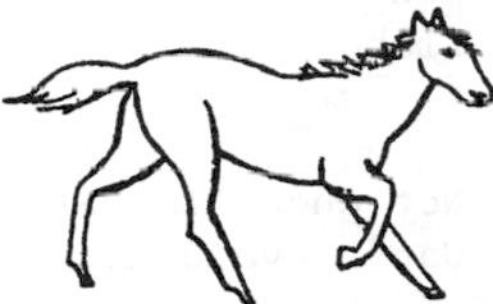

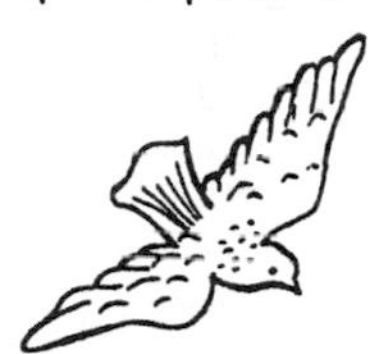

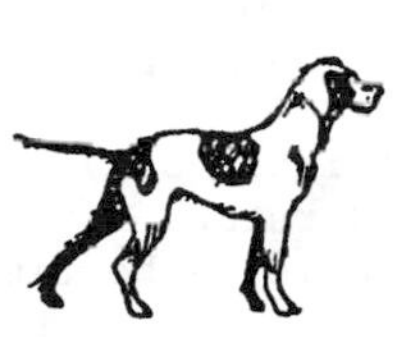

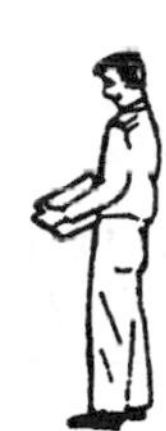

19. Using doll, tell child: Show me the nose, eyes, ears, mouth, hands, feet, tummy, hair. Pass 6 of 8.
20. Using pictures, ask child: Which one flies?... says meow?... talks?... barks?... gallops? Pass 2 of 5, 4 of 5.
21. Ask child: What do you do when you are cold?... tired?... hungry? Pass 2 of 3, 3 of 3.
22. Ask child: What do you do with a cup? What is a chair used for? What is a pencil used for? Action words must be included in answers.
23. Pass if child correctly places and says how many blocks are on paper. (1, 5).
24. Tell child: Put block **on** table; **under** table; **in front of** me, **behind** me. Pass 4 of 4. (Do not help child by pointing, moving head or eyes.)
25. Ask child: What is a ball?... lake?... desk?... house?... banana?... curtain?... fence?... ceiling? Pass if defined in terms of use, shape, what it is made of, or general category (such as banana is fruit, not just yellow). Pass 5 of 8, 7 of 8.
26. Ask child: If a horse is big, a mouse is __? If fire is hot, ice is __? If the sun shines during the day, the moon shines during the __? Pass 2 of 3.
27. Child may use wall or rail only, not person. May not crawl.
28. Child must throw ball overhand 3 feet to within arm's reach of tester.
29. Child must perform standing broad jump over width of test sheet (8 1/2 inches).
30. Tell child to walk forward, → heel within 1 inch of toe. Tester may demonstrate. Child must walk 4 consecutive steps.
31. In the second year, half of normal children are non-compliant.

OBSERVATIONS:

Fig. E-1. **A,** Opposite page—Denver II. **B,** Directions for administration of numbered items on Denver II. (From Frankenburg WK, Dodds JB, 1990.)

DENVER ARTICULATION SCREENING EXAM
for children 2½ to 6 years of age

Instructions: Have child repeat each word after you. Circle the underlined sounds that he pronounces correctly. Total correct sounds is the Raw Score. Use charts on reverse side to score results.

Name:

Hosp. No.:

Address:________________

Date: ________ Child's age: ________ Examiner: ________ Raw score: ____
Percentile: ________ Intelligibility: ________ Result: ________

1. table	6. zipper	11. sock	16. wagon	21. leaf
2. shirt	7. grapes	12. vacuum	17. gum	22. carrot
3. door	8. flag	13. yarn	18. house	
4. trunk	9. thumb	14. mother	19. pencil	
5. jumping	10. toothbrush	15. twinkle	20. fish	

Intelligibility: (circle one)
1. Easy to understand
2. Understandable ½ the time
3. Not understandable
4. Can't evaluate

Comments:

Date: ________ Child's age: ________ Examiner: ________ Raw score: ____
Percentile: ________ Intelligibility: ________ Result: ________

A

1. table	6. zipper	11. sock	16. wagon	21. leaf
2. shirt	7. grapes	12. vacuum	17. gum	22. carrot
3. door	8. flag	13. yarn	18. house	
4. trunk	9. thumb	14. mother	19. pencil	
5. jumping	10. toothbrush	15. twinkle	20. fish	

Intelligibility: (circle one)
1. Easy to understand
2. Understandable ½ the time
3. Not understandable
4. Can't evaluate

Comments:

Date: ________ Child's age: ________ Examiner: ________ Raw score ____
Percentile: ________ Intelligibility: ________ Result: ________

1. table	6. zipper	11. sock	16. wagon	21. leaf
2. shirt	7. grapes	12. vacuum	17. gum	22. carrot
3. door	8. flag	13. yarn	18. house	
4. trunk	9. thumb	14. mother	19. pencil	
5. jumping	10. toothbrush	15. twinkle	20. fish	

Intelligibility: (circle one)
1. Easy to understand
2. Understandable ½ the time
3. Not understandable
4. Can't evaluate

Fig. E-2 **A**, Denver Articulation Screening examination for children 2½ to 6 years of age. (Modified from Drumwright AF, University of Colorado Medical Center, 1971.)

To score DASE words: Note raw score for child's performance. Match raw score line (extreme left of chart) with column representing child's age (to the closest previous age group). Where raw score line and age column meet number in that square denotes percentile rank of child's performance when compared to other children that age. Percentiles above heavy line are ABNORMAL percentiles, below heavy line are NORMAL.

PERCENTILE RANK

Raw Score	2.5 yr.	3.0	3.5	4.0	4.5	5.0	5.5	6 years
2	1							
3	2							
4	5							
5	9							
6	16							
7	23							
8	31	2						
9	37	4	1					
10	42	6	2					
11	48	7	4					
12	54	9	6	1	1			
13	58	12	9	2	3	1	1	
14	62	17	11	5	4	2	2	
15	68	23	15	9	5	3	2	
16	75	31	19	12	5	4	3	
17	79	38	25	15	6	6	4	
18	83	46	31	19	8	7	4	
19	86	51	38	24	10	9	5	1
20	89	58	45	30	12	11	7	3
21	92	65	52	36	15	15	9	4
22	94	72	58	43	18	19	12	5
23	96	77	63	50	22	24	15	7
24	97	82	70	58	29	29	20	15
25	99	87	78	66	36	34	26	17
26	99	91	84	75	46	43	34	24
27		94	89	82	57	54	44	34
28		96	94	88	70	68	59	47
29		98	98	94	84	84	77	68
30		100	100	100	100	100	100	100

To score intelligibility:

	NORMAL	ABNORMAL
2½ years	Understandable ½ the time, or, "easy"	Not understandable
3 years and older	Easy to understand	Understandable ½ time Not understandable

Test result: 1. NORMAL on Dase and Intelligibility = NORMAL

2. ABNORMAL on Dase and/or Intelligibility = ABNORMAL

*If abnormal on initial screening, rescreen within 2 weeks.
If abnormal again, child should be referred for complete speech evaluation.

B

Fig. E-2, cont'd. B, Percentile rank. (From Drumwright AF, University of Colorado Medical Center, 1971.)

SNELLEN SCREENING*

Preparation

1. Hang the Snellen chart on a light-colored wall so that the 20- to 30-foot lines are at eye level when children 6 to 12 years old are tested in the standing position.
2. Secure the chart to the wall with double-stick tape on the back side of all four corners. If the chart must be reversed for use of the letter or E chart, secure it at the top and bottom with tacks. Make sure that the chart does not swing when in place.
3. The illumination intensity on the chart should be 10 to 30 foot candles, without any glare from windows or light fixtures. The illumination should be checked with a light meter.
4. Mark an exact 20-foot distance from the chart. Mark the floor with a piece of tape or "footprints" positioned so that the heels touch the 20-foot line.

Procedure

1. Place child at the 20-foot mark, with the heel edging the line if child is standing or with the back of the chair placed at the marker if child is seated.
2. If the E chart is used, accustom child to identifying which direction the "legs of the E" are pointing. Use a demonstration E card for this purpose.
3. Teach child to use the occluder to cover one eye. Instruct child to keep both eyes open during the test. Provide a clean cover card for each child and then discard after use.
4. If child wears glasses, test only with glasses on.
5. Test both eyes together, then right eye, then left eye.
6. Begin with the 40- or 30-foot line and proceed with test to include the 20-foot line.
7. With child suspected of low vision, begin with the 200-foot line, and proceed until child can no longer correctly read three out of four or four out of six symbols on a line.
8. Use covers on the Snellen chart to expose only one symbol or one line at a time. When screening kindergarten or older children, expose one line but may use a pointer to point to one symbol at a time.

Recording and Referral

1. Record the last line the child read correctly (three out of four or four out of six symbols).
2. Record visual acuity as a fraction. The numerator represents the distance from the chart, and the denominator represents the last line read correctly. For example, 20/30 means that the child read the 30-foot line at a 20-foot distance.
3. Observe the child's eyes during testing and record any evidence of squinting, head tilting, thrusting the head forward, excessive blinking, tearing, or redness.
4. Only make referrals after a second screening has been made on children who are potential candidates for referral.
5. The following children should be referred for a complete eye examination:
   a. Three-year-old children with vision in either eye of 20/50 or less (inability to correctly identify one more than half the symbols on the 40-foot line) *or* a two-line difference in visual acuity between the eyes in the passing range (e.g., 20/20 in one eye and 20/40 in the other)
   b. All other ages and grades with vision in either eye of 20/40 or less (inability to correctly identify one more than half the symbols on the 30-foot line)
   c. All children who consistently show any of the signs of possible visual disturbances, regardless of visual acuity

*Modified from recommendations of the National Society to Prevent Blindness: *Guide to testing distance visual acuity.* Schaumburg, IL, 1988, The Society.

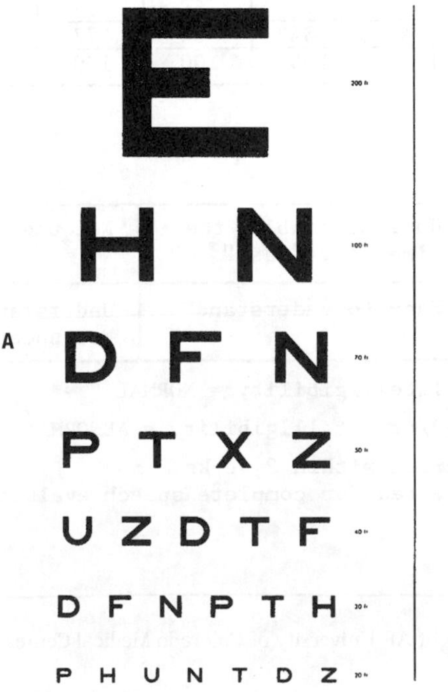

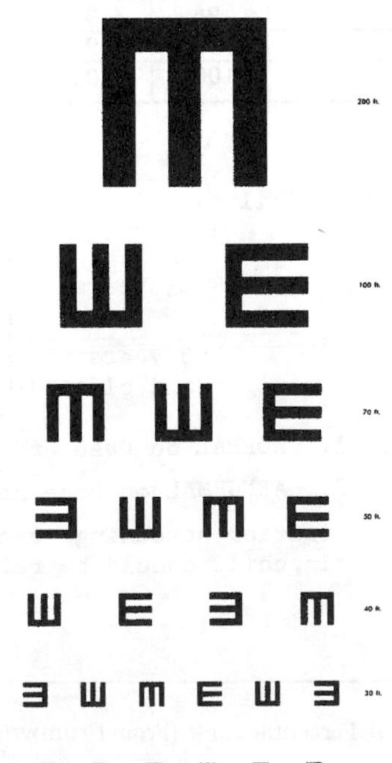

Fig. E-3 Snellen chart. **A,** Letter (alphabet) chart. **B,** Symbol E chart. (From National Society to Prevent Blindness, Schaumburg, IL.)

APPENDIX F

Growth Measurements

HEIGHT AND WEIGHT MEASUREMENTS FOR BOYS

	HEIGHT BY PERCENTILES						WEIGHT BY PERCENTILES					
	5		50		95		5		50		95	
AGE*	cm	INCHES	cm	INCHES	cm	INCHES	kg	lb	kg	lb	kg	lb
Birth	46.4	18¼	50.5	20	54.4	21½	2.54	5½	3.27	7¼	4.15	9¼
3 months	50.7	22¼	61.1	24	65.4	25¾	4.43	9¾	5.98	13¼	7.37	16¼
6 months	63.4	25	67.8	26¾	72.3	28½	6.20	13¾	7.85	17¼	9.46	20¾
9 months	68.0	26¾	72.3	28½	77.1	30¼	7.52	16½	9.18	20¼	10.93	24
1	71.7	28¼	76.1	30	81.2	32	8.43	18½	10.15	22½	11.99	26½
1½	77.5	30½	82.4	32½	88.1	34¾	9.59	21¼	11.47	25¼	13.44	29½
2†	82.5	32½	86.8	34¼	94.4	37¼	10.49	23¼	12.34	27¼	15.50	34¼
2½†	85.4	33½	90.4	35½	97.8	38½	11.27	24¾	13.52	29¾	16.61	36½
3	89.0	35	94.9	37¼	102.0	40¼	12.05	26½	14.62	32¼	17.77	39¼
3½	92.5	36½	99.1	39	106.1	41¾	12.84	28¼	15.68	34½	18.98	41¾
4	95.8	37¾	102.9	40½	109.9	43¼	13.64	30	16.69	36¾	20.27	44¾
4½	98.9	39	106.6	42	113.5	44¾	14.45	31¾	17.69	39	21.63	47¾
5	102.0	40¼	109.9	43¼	117.0	46	15.27	33¾	18.67	41¼	23.09	51
6	107.7	42½	116.1	45¾	123.5	48½	16.93	37¼	20.69	45½	26.34	58
7	113.0	44½	121.7	48	129.7	51	18.64	41	22.85	50¼	30.12	66½
8	118.1	46½	127.0	50	135.7	53½	20.40	45	25.30	55¾	34.51	76
9	122.9	48½	132.2	52	141.8	55¾	22.25	49	28.13	62	39.58	87¼
10	127.7	50¼	137.5	54¼	148.1	58¼	24.33	53¾	31.44	69¼	45.27	99¾
11	132.6	52¼	143.3	56½	154.9	61	26.80	59	35.30	77¾	51.47	113½
12	137.6	54¼	149.7	59	162.3	64	29.85	65¾	39.78	87¾	58.09	128
13	142.9	56¼	156.5	61½	169.8	66¾	33.64	74¼	44.95	99	65.02	143¼
14	148.8	58½	163.1	64¼	176.7	69½	38.22	84¼	50.77	112	72.13	159
15	155.2	61	169.0	66½	181.9	71½	43.11	95	56.71	125	79.12	174½
16	161.1	63½	173.5	68¼	185.4	73	47.74	105¼	62.10	137	85.62	188¾
17	164.9	65	176.2	69¼	187.3	73¾	51.50	113½	66.31	146¼	91.31	201¼
18	165.7	65¼	176.8	69½	187.6	73¾	53.97	119	68.88	151¾	95.76	211

Modified from National Center for Health Statistics (NCHS), Health Resources Administration, Department of Health, Education and Welfare, Hyattsville, MD. Conversion of metric data to approximate inches and pounds by Ross Laboratories, 1977.

*Years unless otherwise indicated

†Height data include some recumbent length measurements, which make values slightly higher than if all measurements had been of stature (standing height).

HEIGHT AND WEIGHT MEASUREMENTS FOR GIRLS

	HEIGHT BY PERCENTILES						WEIGHT BY PERCENTILES					
	5		50		95		5		50		95	
AGE*	cm	INCHES	cm	INCHES	cm	INCHES	kg	lb	kg	lb	kg	lb
Birth	45.4	17¾	49.9	19¾	52.9	20¾	2.36	5¼	3.23	7	3.81	8½
3 months	55.4	21¾	59.5	23½	63.4	25	4.18	9¼	5.4	12	6.74	14¾
6 months	61.8	24¼	65.9	26	70.2	27¾	5.79	12¾	7.21	16	8.73	19¼
9 months	66.1	26	70.4	27¾	75.0	29½	7.0	15½	8.56	18¾	10.17	22½
1	69.8	27½	74.3	29¼	79.1	31¼	7.84	17¼	9.53	21	11.24	24¾
1½	76.0	30	80.9	31¾	86.1	34	8.92	19¾	10.82	23¾	12.76	28¼
2†	81.6	32¼	86.8	34¼	93.6	36¾	9.95	22	11.8	26	14.15	31¼
2½†	84.6	33¼	90.0	35½	96.6	38	10.8	23¾	13.03	28¾	15.76	34¾
3	88.3	34¾	94.1	37	100.6	39½	11.61	25½	14.1	31	17.22	38
3½	91.7	36	97.9	38½	104.5	41¼	12.37	27¼	15.07	33¼	18.59	41
4	95.0	37½	101.6	40	108.3	42¾	13.11	29	15.96	35¼	19.91	44
4½	98.1	38½	105.0	41¼	112.0	44	13.83	30½	16.81	37	21.24	46¾
5	101.1	39¾	108.4	42¾	115.6	45½	14.55	32	17.66	39	22.62	49¾
6	106.6	42	114.6	45	122.7	48¼	16.05	35½	19.52	43	25.75	56¾
7	111.8	44	120.6	47½	129.5	51	17.71	39	21.84	48¼	29.68	65½
8	116.9	46	126.4	49¾	136.2	53½	19.62	43¼	24.84	54¾	34.71	76½
9	122.1	48	132.2	52	142.9	56¼	21.82	48	28.46	62¾	40.64	89½
10	127.5	50¼	138.3	54½	149.5	58¾	24.36	53¾	32.55	71¾	47.17	104
11	133.5	52½	144.8	57	156.2	61½	27.24	60	36.95	81½	54.0	119
12	139.8	55	151.5	59¾	162.7	64	30.52	67¼	41.53	91½	60.81	134
13	145.2	57¼	157.1	61¾	168.1	66¼	34.14	75¼	46.1	101¾	67.3	148¼
14	148.7	58½	160.4	63¼	171.3	67½	37.76	83¼	50.28	110¾	73.08	161
15	150.5	59¼	161.8	63¾	172.8	68	40.99	90¼	53.68	118¼	77.78	171½
16	151.6	59¾	162.4	64	173.3	68¼	43.41	95¾	55.89	123¼	80.99	178½
17	152.7	60	163.1	64¼	173.5	68¼	44.74	98¾	56.69	125	82.46	181¾
18	153.6	60½	163.7	64½	173.6	68¼	45.26	99¾	56.62	124¾	82.47	181¾

Modified from National Center for Health Statistics, Health Resources Administration, Department of Health, Education and Welfare, Hyattsville, MD. Conversion of metric data to approximate inches and pounds by Ross Laboratories.

*Years unless otherwise indicated

†Height data include some recumbent length measurements, which make values slightly higher than if all measurements had been of stature.

GROWTH STANDARDS OF HEALTHY CHINESE CHILDREN

	Weight (kg)		Height (cm)		Head circumference	
Age (months or years)	Boys	Girls	Boys	Girls	Boys	Girls
Birth	3.27	3.17	50.6	50.0	34.3	33.7
1 month	4.97	4.64	56.5	55.5	38.1	37.3
2 months	5.95	5.49	59.6	58.4	39.7	38.7
3 months	6.73	6.23	62.3	60.9	41.0	40.0
4 months	7.32	6.69	64.4	52.9	42.0	41.0
5 months	7.70	7.19	65.9	64.5	42.9	41.9
6 months	8.22	7.62	68.1	66.7	43.9	42.8
8 months	8.71	8.14	70.6	69.0	44.9	43.7
10 months	9.14	8.57	72.9	71.4	45.7	44.5
12 months	9.56	9.04	75.6	74.1	46.3	45.2
15 months	10.15	9.54	78.3	76.9	46.8	45.6
18 months	10.67	10.08	80.7	79.4	47.3	46.2
21 months	11.18	10.56	83.0	81.7	47.8	46.7
24 months	11.95	11.37	86.5	85.3	48.2	47.1
2.5 years	12.84	12.28	90.4	89.3	48.8	47.7
3 years	13.63	13.16	93.8	92.8	49.1	48.1
3.5 years	14.45	14.00	97.2	96.3	49.4	48.5
4 years	15.26	14.89	100.8	100.1	49.7	48.9
4.5 years	16.07	15.63	103.9	103.1	50.0	49.1
5 years	16 88	16.46	107.2	106.5	50.2	49.4
5.5 years	17.65	17.18	110.1	109.2	50.5	49.6
6 years	19.25	18.67	114.7	113.9	50.8	50.0
7 years	21.01	20.35	120.6	119.3	51.1	50.2
8 years	23.08	22.43	125.3	124.6	51.4	50.6
9 years	25.33	24.57	130.6	129.5	51.7	50.9
10 years	27.15	27.05	134.4	134.8	51.9	51.3
11 years	30.13	30.51	139.2	140.6	52.3	51.7
12 years	33.05	34.74	144.2	146.6	52.7	52.3
13 years	36.90	38.52	149.8	150.7	53.0	52.8

Data from Bejing Children's Hospital, 1987, China.

HEAD CIRCUMFERENCE CHARTS

A

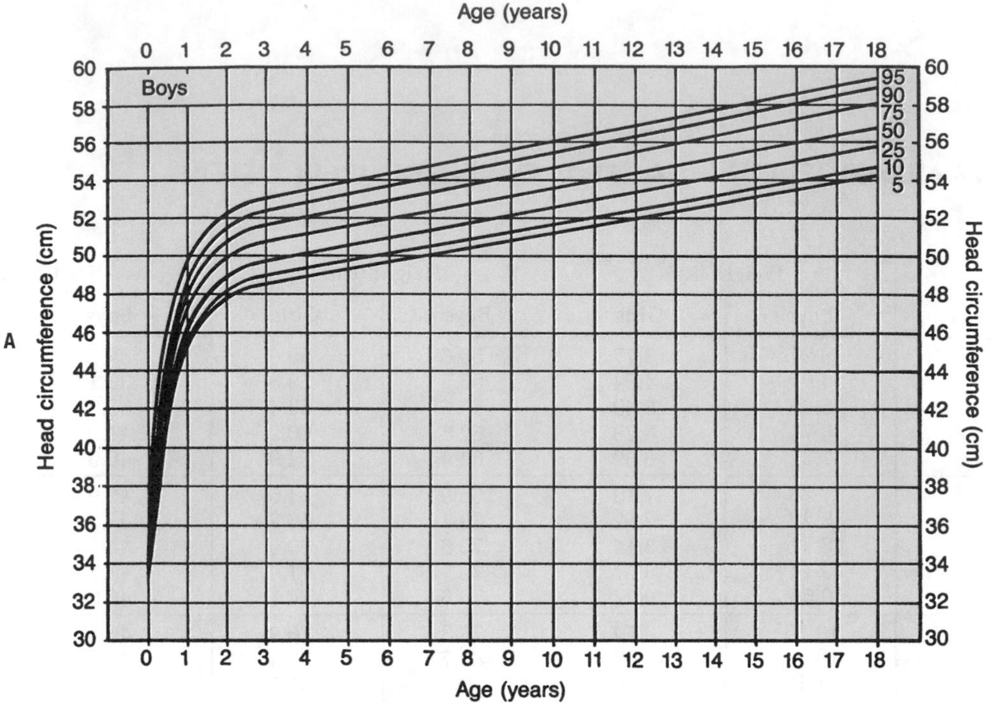

B

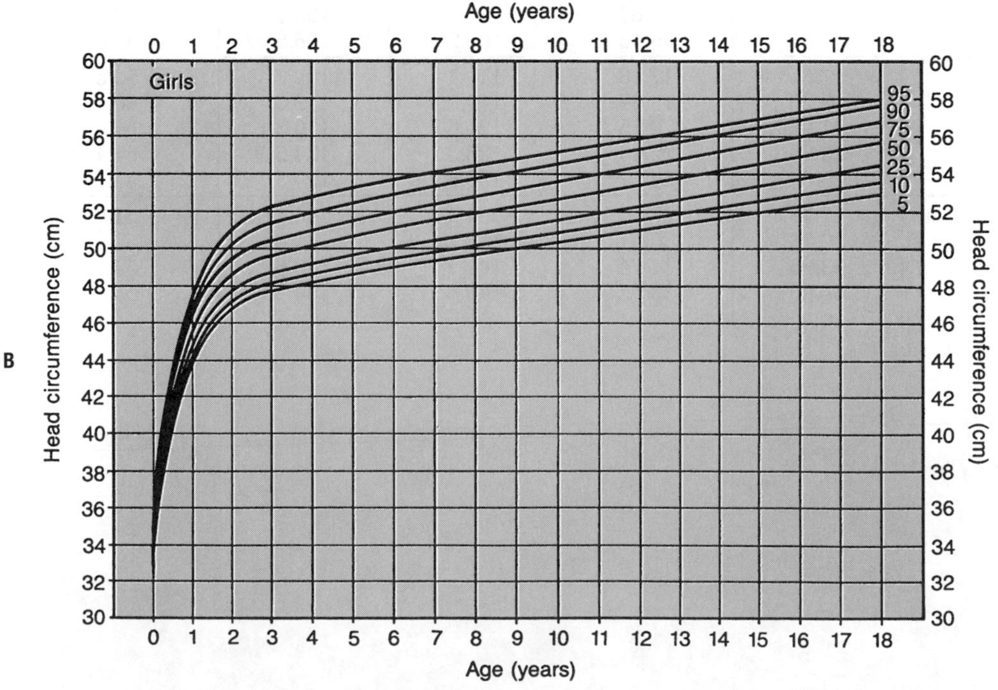

Fig. F-1 Selected percentiles for smoothed head circumference values of children from birth to 18 years. **A,** Boys. **B,** Girls. (From Roche AF et al: Head circumference reference data: birth to 18 years, *Pediatrics* 79(5):706-712, 1987.)

PERCENTILES FOR TRICEPS SKINFOLD

	TRICEPS SKINFOLD PERCENTILES (mm)									
	MALES					FEMALES				
AGE-GROUP (YEARS)	5	25	50	75	95	5	25	50	75	95
1-1.9	6	8	10	12	16	6	8	10	12	16
2-2.9	6	8	10	12	15	6	9	10	12	16
3-3.9	6	8	10	11	15	7	9	11	12	15
4-4.9	6	8	9	11	14	7	8	10	12	16
5-5.9	6	8	9	11	15	6	8	10	12	18
6-6.9	5	7	8	10	16	6	8	10	12	16
7-7.9	5	7	9	12	17	6	9	11	13	18
8-8.9	5	7	8	10	16	6	9	12	15	24
9-9.9	6	7	10	13	18	8	10	13	16	22
10-10.9	6	8	10	14	21	7	10	12	17	27
11-11.9	6	8	11	16	24	7	10	13	18	28
12-12.9	6	8	11	14	28	8	11	14	18	27
13-13.9	5	7	10	14	26	8	12	15	21	30
14-14.9	4	7	9	14	24	9	13	16	21	28
15-15.9	4	6	8	11	24	8	12	17	21	32
16-16.9	4	6	8	12	22	10	15	18	22	31
17-17.9	5	6	8	12	19	10	13	19	24	37
18-18.9	4	6	9	13	24	10	15	18	22	30
19-24.9	4	7	10	15	22	10	14	18	24	34

From Frisancho A: New norms of upper limb fat and muscle areas for assessment of nutritional status, *Am J Clin Nutr* 34:2540-2545, 1981.

PERCENTILES OF UPPER ARM CIRCUMFERENCE

	ARM CIRCUMFERENCE PERCENTILES (mm)									
	MALES					FEMALES				
AGE-GROUP (YEARS)	5	25	50	75	95	5	25	50	75	95
1-1.9	142	150	159	170	183	138	148	156	164	177
2-2.9	141	153	162	170	185	142	152	160	167	184
3-3.9	150	160	167	175	190	143	158	167	175	189
4-4.9	149	162	171	180	192	149	160	169	177	191
5-5.9	153	167	175	185	204	153	165	175	185	211
6-6.9	155	167	179	188	228	156	170	176	187	211
7-7.9	162	177	187	201	230	164	174	183	199	231
8-8.9	162	177	190	202	245	168	183	195	214	261
9-9.9	175	187	200	217	257	178	194	211	224	260
10-10.9	181	196	210	231	274	174	193	210	228	265
11-11.9	186	202	223	244	280	185	208	224	248	303
12-12.9	193	214	232	254	303	194	216	237	256	294
13-13.9	194	228	247	263	301	202	223	243	271	338
14-14.9	220	237	253	283	322	214	237	252	272	322
15-15.9	222	244	264	284	320	208	239	254	279	322
16-16.9	244	262	278	303	343	218	241	258	283	334
17-17.9	246	267	285	308	347	220	241	264	295	350
18-18.9	245	276	297	321	379	222	241	258	281	325
19-24.9	262	288	308	331	372	221	247	265	290	345

From Frisancho A: New norms of upper limb fat and muscle areas for assessment of nutritional status, *Am J Clin Nutr* 34:2540-2545, 1981.

APPENDIX **G**

Translations of FACES Pain Rating Scale

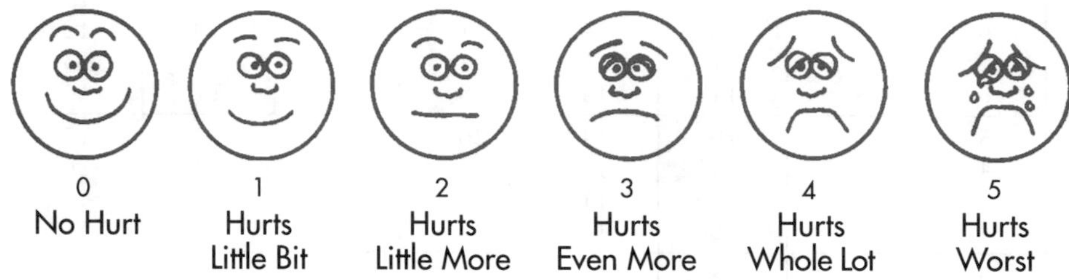

Explain to the person that each face is for a person who feels happy because he has no pain (hurt) or sad because he has some or a lot of pain. **Face 0** is very happy because he doesn't hurt at all. **Face 1** hurts just a little bit. **Face 2** hurts a little more. **Face 3** hurts even more. **Face 4** hurts a whole lot. **Face 5** hurts as much as you can imagine, although you don't have to be crying to feel this bad. Ask the person to choose the face that best describes how he is feeling.

Rating scale is recommended for persons age 3 years and older.

The *brief word instructions* under each face can also be used. Point to each face using the words to describe the pain intensity. Ask the child to choose face that best describes own pain and record the appropriate number. *Note:* In a study of 148 children ages 4 to 5 years, there were no differences in pain scores when children used the original or brief word instructions (In Wong D, Baker C: Reference manual for the Wong-Baker FACES Pain Rating Scale, Durarte, CA, 1996, City of Hope Mayday Pain Resource Center.)

Spanish

Expliquele a la persona que cada cara representa una persona que se siente feliz porque no tiene dolor o triste porque siente un poco o mucho dolor. **Cara 0** se siente muy feliz porque no tiene dolor. **Cara 1** tiene un poco de dolor. **Cara 2** tiene un poquito más de dolor. **Cara 3** tiene más dolor. **Cara 4** tiene mucho dolor. **Cara 5** tiene el dolor más fuerte que usted pueda imaginar, aunque usted no tiene que estar llorando para sentirse asi de mal. Pidale a la persona que escoja la cara que mejor describe su proprio dolor.

Esta escala se puede usar con personas de tres años de edad o más.

French

Expliquez à la personne que chaque visage représent un personne qui est hereux parce qu'elle n'a pas point du mal ou triste parce qu'il a un peu ou beaucoup du mal. **Visage 0** est trés heureux parce qu'elle n'a pas point du mal. **Visage 1** a un petit peu de mal. **Visage 2** a plus du mal. **Visage 3** a encore plus du mal. **Visage 4** a beaucoup du mal. **Visage 5** a autant mal que vous pouvez imaginer, bien que ces mauvais sentiments ne finessent pas nécessairement a vous faire pleurer. Demandez à la personne de choisir le visage qui convient le mieux avec ses sentiments.

Ces evaluations sont recommendés pour des personnes de trois ans et davantage.

Wong-Baker FACES Pain Rating Scale: Available at no charge from The Purdue Frederick Company, 100 Connecticut Ave., Norwalk, CT 06850-3590; (203) 853-0123, ext. 7378. Spanish and Portuguese translations by Ellen Johnsen; French translation by Irene Sherman Liguori and Robert Marino; Italian translation by Madeline Mitchko and Ida DiPietropaolo; Romanian translation by Florin Nicolae; Vietnamese translation by Yen B. Isle; Chinese translation by Hung-Shen Lin; Japanese translation from *After the announcement of cancer,* Tokyo, 1993, Iwanami Shoten, Pub.

Italian

Spiegare a la persona che ogni facien è per una persona che si sente felice perchè non tiene dolore oppure triste perchè ha poco o molto dolore. **Faccia O** è molto felice perchè non tiene dolor. **Faccia 1** tiene poco dolore. **Faccia 2** tiene un po più di dolor. **Faccia 3** tiene più dolore. **Faccia 4** tiene molto dolore. **Faccia 5** tiene molto dolore che non puoi immaginare però non devi piangere per tenere dolore. Domandi ala persona di scegliere quale faccia meglio descrive come si sente.

Grado scale è raccomandata a la person di tre anni in sù.

Portuguese

Explique a pessoa que cada face representa uma pessoa que está feliz porque não têm dor, ou triste por ter um pouco ou muita dor. **Face 0** está muito feliz porque não têm nenhuma dor. **Face 1** tem apenas um pouco de dor. **Face 2** têm um pouco mais de dor. **Face 3** têm ainda mais dor. **Face 4** têm muita dor. **Face 5** têm uma dor máxima, apesar de que nem sempre provoca o choro. Peça a pessoa que escolhe a face que melhor descreve como ele se sente.

Esta escala é aplicável a pessoas de tres anos de idade ou mais.

Romanian

Explică persoanei că fiecare faţă este specifică diferitelor stări fizice; o persoană este ferioita pentru că nu are nici o durere ori tristă pentru că suferă puţin sau mai mult. **Faţa 0** este foarte ferioită pentru că nu are absolut nici o durere. **Faţa 1** are un pic de durere. **Faţa 2** are ceva mai mult. **Faţa 3** suferă şi mai mult. **Faţa 4** suferă foarte mult. **Faţa 5** este greu de imaginat cât de mult suferă, căci nu trebuie neapărat să plângi, oricat de tare te-ar durea. Întreabă persoana să indice figura care-i desorie cel mai bine starea fizică.

Acest **grad de durere** este racomandat pentru persoanele de la 3 ani în sus.

Vietnamese

Xin cắt nghỉa cho mổi người, từng khuôn mặt của một người cãm thấy vui vẽ tại vì không có sự đau đớn hoặc, buồn vì có chút ít hay rất nhiều sự đau đớn.

Cái **mặt** với **số 0** thì rất là vui tại vì mặt ấy không có sự đau đớn. **Mặt số 1** chỉ đau một chút thôi. **Mặt số 2** hơi đau hơn một chút nữa. **Mặt số 3** đau hơn chút nữa. **Mặt số 4** đau thật nhiều. **Mặt số 5** đau không thể tưởng tượng, mặc dù người ta không cần phải khóc mới cảm thấy được sự buồn khổ như thế.

Bạn hỏi từng người tự chọn khuôn mặt nào diển tả được sự đau đớn của chính mình.

Japanese

3歳以上の患者に望ましい。それぞれの顔は、患者の痛み(pain, hurt)がないのでご機嫌な感じ、または、ある程度の痛み・沢山の痛みがあるので悲しい感じを表現していることを説明して下さい。0＝痛みがまったくないから、とても幸せな顔をしている、1＝ほんの少し痛い、2＝もう少し痛い、3＝もっと痛い、4＝とっても痛い、5＝痛くて涙を流す必要はないけれども、これ以上の痛みは考えられないほど痛い。今、どのように感じているか最もよく表わしている顔を選ぶよう、患者に求めて下さい。

Chinese

解釋給人聽用每張臉譜來代表著一個人的感覺是因爲沒有疼痛〔傷痛〕而感快樂或是因爲些許疼痛或者是許多疼痛而感傷心。第零張臉是很快樂的因爲他一點也不覺得疼痛・第一張臉只痛一丁點兒。第二張臉又痛多了一些。第三張臉痛得更多了。第四張臉是非常痛了。第五張臉是爲人們所能想像到的劇痛既使感到這樣難過，卻不一定哭出來。請這人選擇出最能代表他現在感覺的一張臉譜。此量表適用於三歲以上的人。

APPENDIX H

Pediatric Vital Signs and Parameters

TABLE H-1 Normal heart rates for infants and children

AGE	RATE (BEATS/MIN)		
	RESTING (AWAKE)	RESTING (SLEEPING)	EXERCISE (FEVER)
Newborn	100-180	80-160	Up to 220
1 week to 3 months	100-220	80-200	Up to 220
3 months to 2 years	80-150	70-120	Up to 200
2 years to 10 years	70-110	60-90	Up to 200
10 years to adult	55-90	50-90	Up to 200

From Gillette PC: *Dysrhythmias.* In Adams FH, Emmanouilides GC, Riemenschneider TA, editors: *Moss' heart disease in infants, children, and adolescents,* ed 4, Baltimore, 1989, Williams & Wilkins.

TABLE H-2 Normal respiratory rates for children

AGE	RATE (BREATHS/MIN)
Newborn	35
1 to 11 months	30
2 years	25
4 years	23
6 years	21
8 years	20
10 years	19
12 years	19
14 years	18
16 years	17
18 years	16-18

TABLE H-3 Normal blood pressure readings for children—Boys

	SYSTOLIC BLOOD PRESSURE PERCENTILE						DIASTOLIC BLOOD PRESSURE* PERCENTILE				
AGE	5TH	10TH	50TH	90TH	95TH	AGE	5TH	10TH	50TH	90TH	95TH
1 day	54	58	73	87	92	1 day	38	42	55	68	72
3 days	55	59	74	89	93	3 days	38	42	55	68	71
7 days	57	62	76	91	95	7 days	37	41	54	67	71
1 mo	67	71	86	101	105	1 mo	35	39	52	64	68
2 mo	72	76	91	106	110	2 mo	33	37	50	63	66
3 mo	72	76	91	106	110	3 mo	33	37	50	63	66
4 mo	72	76	91	106	110	4 mo	34	37	50	63	67
5 mo	72	76	91	105	110	5 mo	35	39	52	65	68
6 mo	72	76	90	105	109	6 mo	36	40	53	66	70
7 mo	71	76	90	105	109	7 mo	37	41	54	67	71
8 mo	71	75	90	105	109	8 mo	38	42	55	68	72
9 mo	71	75	90	105	109	9 mo	39	43	55	68	72
10 mo	71	75	90	105	109	10 mo	39	43	56	69	73
11 mo	71	76	90	105	109	11 mo	39	43	56	69	73
1 yr	71	76	90	105	109	1 yr	39	43	56	69	73
2 yr	72	76	91	106	110	2 yr	39	43	56	68	72
3 yr	73	77	92	107	111	3 yr	39	42	55	68	72
4 yr	74	79	93	108	112	4 yr	39	43	56	69	72
5 yr	76	80	95	109	113	5 yr	40	43	56	69	73
6 yr	77	81	96	111	115	6 yr	41	44	57	70	74
7 yr	78	83	97	112	116	7 yr	42	45	58	71	75
8 yr	80	84	99	114	118	8 yr	43	47	60	73	76
9 yr	82	86	101	115	120	9 yr	44	48	61	74	78
10 yr	84	88	102	117	121	10 yr	45	49	62	75	79
11 yr	86	90	105	119	123	11 yr	47	50	63	76	80
12 yr	88	92	107	121	126	12 yr	48	51	64	77	81
13 yr	90	94	109	124	128	13 yr	45	49	63	77	81
14 yr	93	97	112	126	131	14 yr	46	50	64	78	82
15 yr	95	99	114	129	133	15 yr	47	51	65	79	83
16 yr	98	102	117	131	136	16 yr	49	53	67	81	85
17 yr	100	104	119	134	138	17 yr	51	55	69	83	87
18 yr	102	106	121	136	140	18 yr	52	56	70	84	88

From the *Second Task Force on Blood Pressure Control in Children,* National Heart, Lung and Blood Institute, Bethesda, Md. Tabular data prepared by Dr. B. Rosner, 1987.

*K4 was used for ages less than 13; K5 was used for ages 13 and over.

TABLE H-4 Normal temperatures in children

AGE	°F	°C
3 months	99.4	37.5
6 months	99.5	37.5
1 year	99.7	37.7
3 years	99.0	37.2
5 years	98.6	37.0
7 years	98.3	36.8
9 years	98.1	36.7
11 years	98.0	36.7
13 years	97.8	36.6

Modified from Lowrey GH: *Growth and development of children*, ed 8, St Louis, 1986, Mosby.

TABLE H-5 Pediatric emergencies

Airway obstruction (choking)	p. 1367
Anaphylaxis	See Shock
Burns	p. 1691
Cardiopulmonary arrest	p. 1363, 1364
Epistaxis	p. 1516
Evulsed tooth	p. 1068
Eye injuries	p. 1175
Fracture	p. 1713
Head injury	p. 1589
Hypoglycemia (insulin reaction)	p. 1649
Poisoning	p. 1438
Seizure	p. 1611
Shock	p. 1491

TABLE H-6 Normal blood pressure readings for children—Girls

	SYSTOLIC BLOOD PRESSURE PERCENTILE						DIASTOLIC BLOOD PRESSURE* PERCENTILE				
AGE	5TH	10TH	50TH	90TH	95TH	AGE	5TH	10TH	50TH	90TH	95TH
1 day	46	50	65	80	84	1 day	38	42	55	68	72
3 days	53	57	72	86	90	3 days	38	42	55	68	71
7 days	60	64	78	93	97	7 days	38	41	54	67	71
1 mo	65	69	84	98	102	1 mo	35	39	52	65	69
2 mo	68	72	87	101	106	2 mo	34	38	51	64	68
3 mo	70	74	89	104	108	3 mo	35	38	51	64	68
4 mo	71	75	90	105	109	4 mo	35	39	52	65	68
5 mo	72	76	91	106	110	5 mo	36	39	52	65	69
6 mo	72	76	91	106	110	6 mo	36	40	53	66	69
7 mo	72	76	91	106	110	7 mo	36	40	53	66	70
8 mo	72	76	91	106	110	8 mo	37	40	53	66	70
9 mo	72	76	91	106	110	9 mo	37	41	54	67	70
10 mo	72	76	91	106	110	10 mo	37	41	54	67	71
11 mo	72	76	91	105	110	11 mo	38	41	54	67	71
1 yr	72	76	91	105	110	1 yr	38	41	54	67	71
2 yr	71	76	90	105	109	2 yr	40	43	56	69	73
3 yr	72	76	91	106	110	3 yr	40	43	56	69	73
4 yr	73	78	92	107	111	4 yr	40	43	56	69	73
5 yr	75	79	94	109	113	5 yr	40	43	56	69	73
6 yr	77	81	96	111	115	6 yr	40	44	57	70	74
7 yr	78	83	97	112	116	7 yr	41	45	58	71	75
8 yr	80	84	99	114	118	8 yr	43	46	59	72	76
9 yr	81	86	100	115	119	9 yr	44	48	61	74	77
10 yr	83	87	102	117	121	10 yr	46	49	62	75	79
11 yr	86	90	105	119	123	11 yr	47	51	64	77	81
12 yr	88	92	107	122	126	12 yr	49	53	66	78	82
13 yr	90	94	109	124	128	13 yr	46	50	64	78	82
14 yr	92	96	110	125	129	14 yr	49	53	67	81	85
15 yr	93	97	111	126	130	15 yr	49	53	67	82	86
16 yr	93	97	112	127	131	16 yr	49	53	67	81	85
17 yr	93	98	112	127	131	17 yr	48	52	66	80	84
18 yr	94	98	112	127	131	18 yr	48	52	66	80	84

From the *Second Task Force on Blood Pressure Control in Children*, National Heart, Lung and Blood Institute, Bethesda, Md.
Tabular data prepared by Dr. B. Rosner, 1987.
*K4 was used for ages less than 13; K5 was used for ages 13 and over.

APPENDIX I

Common Laboratory Tests*

TEST/SPECIMEN	AGE/SEX/REFERENCE	CONVENTIONAL UNITS		INTERNATIONAL UNITS (SI)	
		NORMAL RANGES			
Acetaminophen					
Serum or plasma	Therap. conc.	10-30 µg/ml		66-200 µmol/L	
	Toxic conc.	>200 µg/ml		>1300 µmol/L	
Ammonia nitrogen					
Plasma or serum	Newborn	90-150 µg/dl		64-107 µmol/L	
	0-2 wk	79-129 µg/dl		56-92 µmol/L	
	>1 mo	29-70 µg/dl		21-50 µmol/L	
	Thereafter	15-45 µg/dl		11-32 µmol/L	
Urine, 24 hr		500-1200 mg/d		36-86 mmol/d	
Antistreptolysin O titer (ASO)					
Serum	2-4 yr	<160 Todd units			
	School-age children	170-330 Todd units			
Base excess					
Whole blood	Newborn	(−10) - (−2) mEq/L		(−10) - (−2) mmol/L	
	Infant	(−7) - (−1) mEq/L		(−7) - (−1) mmol/L	
	Child	(−4) - (+2) mEq/L		(−4) - (+2) mmol/L	
	Thereafter	(−3) - (+3) mEq/L		(−3) - (+3) mmol/L	
Bicarbonate (HCO_3)					
Serum	Arterial	21-28 mEq/L		21-28 mmol/L	
	Venous	22-29 mEq/L		22-29 mmol/L	
		Premature (mg/dl)	***Full Term (mg/dl)***	***Premature (µmol/L)***	***Full Term (µmol/L)***
Bilirubin, total					
Serum	Cord	<2.0	<2.0	<34	<34
	0.1 d	8.0	<6.0	<137	<103
	1-2 d	12.0	<8.0	<205	<137
	2-5 d	16.0	<12.0	<274	<205
	Thereafter	2.0	0.2-1.0	<34	3.4-17.1
Bilirubin, direct (conjugated)					
Serum		0.0-0.2 mg/dl		0-3.4 µmol/L	
Bleeding time					
Blood from skin puncture					
Ivy	Normal	2-7 min		2-7 min	
	Borderline	7-11 min		7-11 min	
Simplate (G-D)		2.75-8 min		2.75-8 min	
Blood volume					
Whole blood	Male	52-83 ml/kg		0.052-0.083 L/kg	
	Female	50-75 ml/kg		0.050-0.075 L/kg	

Modified from Behrman RE et al, editors: *Nelson textbook of pediatrics*, ed 14, Philadelphia, 1992, WB Saunders.

*For a description of abbreviations see p. 1802.

TEST/SPECIMEN	AGE/SEX/REFERENCE	CONVENTIONAL UNITS	INTERNATIONAL UNITS (SI)
		NORMAL RANGES	
C-reactive protein (CRP)			
Serum	Cord	52-1330 ng/ml	52-1330 μg/L
	Adult	67-1800 ng/ml	67-1800 μg/L
Calcium, ionized			
Serum, plasma, or whole blood	Cord	50-60 mg/dl	1.25-1.50 mmol/L
	Newborn, 3-24 hr	4.3-5.1 mg/dl	1.07-1.27 mmol/L
	24-48 hr	4.0-4.7 mg/dl	1.00-1.17 mmol/L
	Thereafter	4.8-4.92 mg/dl or 2.24-2.46 mEq/L	1.12-1.23 mmol/L
Calcium, total			
Serum	Cord	9.0-11.5 mg/dl	2.25-2.88 mmol/L
	Newborn, 3-24 hr	9.0-10.6 mg/dl	2.3-2.65 mmol/L
	24-48 hr	7.0-12.0 mg/dl	1.75-3.0 mmol/L
	4-7 d	9.0-10.9 mg/dl	2.25-2.73 mmol/L
	Child	8.8-10.8 mg/dl	2.2-2.70 mmol/L
	Thereafter	8.4-10.2 mg/dl	2.1-2.55 mmol/L
Carbon dioxide, partial pressure (Pco_2)			
Whole blood, arterial	Newborn	27-40 mm Hg	3.6-5.3 kPa
	Infant	27-41 mm Hg	3.6-5.5 kPa
	Thereafter: Male	35-48 mm Hg	4.7-6.4 kPa
	Female	32-45 mm Hg	4.3-6.0 kPa
Carbon dioxide, total (tCO_2)			
Serum or plasma	Cord	14-22 mEq/L	14-22 mmol/L
	Premature (1 wk)	14-27 mEq/L	14-27 mmol/L
	Newborn	13-22 mEq/L	13-22 mmol/L
	Infant, child	20-28 mEq/L	20-28 mmol/L
	Thereafter	23-30 mEq/L	23-30 mmol/L
Cerebrospinal fluid (CSF)			
Pressure		70-180 mm water	70-180 mm water
Volume	Child	60-100 ml	0.06-0.10 L
	Adult	100-160 ml	0.1-0.16 L
Chloride			
Serum or plasma	Cord	96-104 mEq/L	96-104 mmol/L
	Newborn	97-110 mEq/L	97-110 mmol/L
	Thereafter	98-106 mEq/L	98-106 mmol/L
Sweat	Normal (homozygote)	<40 mEq/L	<40 mmol/L
	Marginal (e.g., asthma, Addison) disease, malnutrition	45-60 mEq/L	45-60 mmol/L
	Cystic fibrosis	>60 mmol/L	>60 mmol/L
Cholesterol, total			
Serum or plasma*	Acceptable	<170 mg/dl	<4.4 mmol/L
	Borderline	170-199 mg/dl	4.4-5.1 mmol/L
	High	≥200 mg/dl	≥5.2 mmol/L
Clotting time (Lee-White)			
Whole blood		5-8 min (glass tubes)	5-8 min
		5-15 min (room temp)	5-15 min
		30 min (silicone tube)	30 min

*From National Cholesterol Education Program: Report of the expert panel on blood cholesterol levels in children and adolescents, *Pediatrics* 89 (3, pt 2):527, 1992.

Continued.

COMMON LABORATORY TESTS—cont'd

TEST/SPECIMEN	AGE/SEX/REFERENCE	CONVENTIONAL UNITS	INTERNATIONAL UNITS (SI)
		NORMAL RANGES	
Creatine kinase (CK, CPK)			
Serum	Cord blood	70-380 U/L	70-380 U/L
	5-8 hr	214-1175 U/L	214-1175 U/L
	24-33 hr	130-1200 U/L	130-1200 U/L
	72-100 hr	87-725 U/L	87-725 U/L
	Adult	5-130 U/L	5-130 U/L
Creatinine			
Serum	Cord	0.6-1.2 mg/dl	53-106 μmol/L
	Newborn	0.3-1.0 mg/dl	27-88 μmol/L
	Infant	0.2-0.4 mg/dl	18-35 μmol/L
	Child	0.3-0.7 mg/dl	27-62 μmol/L
	Adolescent	0.5-1.0 mg/dl	44-88 μmol/L
	Adult: Male	0.6-1.2 mg/dl	53-106 μmol/L
	Female	0.5-1.1 mg/dl	44-97 μmol/L
Urine, 24 hr	Premature	8.1-15.0 mg/kg/24 hr	72-133 μmol/kg/24 hr
	Full term	10.4-19.7 mg/kg/24 hr	92-174 μmol/kg/24 hr
	1.5-7 yr	10-15 mg/kg/24 hr	88-133 μmol/kg/24 hr
	7-15 yr	5.2-41 mg/kg/24 hr	46-362 μmol/kg/24 hr
Creatinine clearance (endogenous)			
Serum or plasma and urine	Newborn	40-65 ml/min/1.73 m^2	
	<40 yr: Male	97-137 ml/min/1.73 m^2	
	Female	88-128 ml/min/1.73 m^2	
Digoxin			
Serum, plasma; collect at least 12 hr after dose	Therap. conc.		
	CHF	0.8-1.5 ng/ml	1.0-1.9 nmol/L
	Arrhythmias	1.5-2.0 ng/ml	1.9-2.6 nmol/L
	Toxic conc.		
	Child	>2.5 ng/ml	>3.2 nmol/L
	Adult	>3.0 ng/ml	>3.8 nmol/L
Eosinophil count			
Whole blood, capillary blood		50-350 cells/mm^3 (μl)	50-350 × 10^6 cells/L
Erythrocyte (RBC) count			
Whole blood	Cord	3.9-5.5 million/mm^3	3.9-5.5 × 10^{12} cells/L
	1-3 d	4.0-6.6 million/mm^3	4.0-6.6 × 10^{12} cells/L
	1 wk	3.9-6.3 million/mm^3	3.9-6.3 × 10^{12} cells/L
	2 wk	3.6-6.2 million/mm^3	3.6-6.2 × 10^{12} cells/L
	1 mo	3.0-5.4 million/mm^3	3.0-5.4 × 10^{12} cells/L
	2 mo	2.7-4.9 million/mm^3	2.7-4.5 × 10^{12} cells/L
	3-6 mo	3.1-4.5 million/mm^3	3.1-4.5 × 10^{12} cells/L
	0.5-2.0 yr	3.7-5.3 million/mm^3	3.7-5.3 × 10^{12} cells/L
	2-6 yr	3.9-5.3 million/mm^3	3.9-5.3 × 10^{12} cells/L
	6-12 yr	4.0-5.2 million/mm^3	4.0-5.2 × 10^{12} cells/L
	12-18 yr: Male	4.5-5.3 million/mm^3	4.5-5.3 × 10^{12} cells/L
	Female	4.1-5.1 million/mm^3	4.1-5.1 × 10^{12} cells/L
Erythrocyte sedimentation rate (ESR)			
Whole blood			
Westergren (modified)	Child	0-10 mm/hr	0-10 mm/hr
	<50 yr: Male	0-15 mm/hr	0-15 mm/hr
	Female	0-20 mm/hr	0-20 mm/hr
Wintrobe	Child	0-13 mm/hr	0-13 mm/hr
	Adult: Male	0-9 mm/hr	0-9 mm/hr
	Female	0-20 mm/hr	0-20 mm/hr

TEST/SPECIMEN	AGE/SEX/REFERENCE	CONVENTIONAL UNITS	INTERNATIONAL UNITS (SI)
		NORMAL RANGES	
Fibrinogen			
Plasma	Newborn	125-300 mg/dl	1.25-3.00 g/L
	Thereafter	200-400 mg/dl	2.00-4.00 g/L
Galactose			
Serum	Newborn	0-20 mg/dl	0-1.11 mmol/L
	Thereafter	<5 mg/dl	<0.03 mmol/L
Urine	Newborn	≤60 mg/dl	≤3.33 mmol/L
	Thereafter	<14 mg/dl	<0.08 mmol/L
Glucose			
Serum	Cord	45-96 mg/dl	2.5-5.3 mmol/L
	Newborn, 1 d	40-60 mg/dl	2.2-3.3 mmol/L
	Newborn, >1 d	50-90 mg/dl	2.8-5.0 mmol/L
	Child	60-100 mg/dl	3.3-5.5 mmol/L
	Thereafter	70-105 mg/dl	3.9-5.8 mmol/L
Whole blood	Adult	65-95 mg/dl	3.6-5.3 mmol/L
CSF	Adult	40-70 mg/dl	2.2-3.9 mmol/L
Urine (quantitative)		<0.5 g≠d	<2.8 mmol/d
(Qualitative)		Negative	Negative
Glucose tolerance test (GTT), oral			
Serum			

Dosages		Conventional: *Normal*	Conventional: *Diabetic*	SI: *Normal*	SI: *Diabetic*
Adult: 75 g	Fasting	70-105 mg/dl	>115 mg/dl	3.9-5.8 mmol/L	>6.4 mmol/L
Child: 1.75 g/kg of ideal	60 min	120-170 mg/dl	≥200 mg/dl	6.7-9.4 mmol/L	≥11 mmol/L
weight up to maximum of	90 min	100-140 mg/dl	≥200 mg/dl	5.6-7.8 mmol/L	≥11 mmol/L
75 g	120 min	70-120 mg/dl	≥140 mg/dl	3.9-6.7 mmol/L	≥7.8 mmol/L

TEST/SPECIMEN	AGE/SEX/REFERENCE	CONVENTIONAL UNITS	INTERNATIONAL UNITS (SI)
Growth hormone (hGH, somatotropin)			
Plasma	Cord	10-50 ng/ml	10-50 μg/L
Fasting, at rest	Newborn	10-40 ng/ml	10-40 μg/L
	Child	<5 ng/ml	<5 μg/L
	Adult: Male	<5 ng/ml	<5 μg/L
	Female	<8 ng/ml	<8 μg/L
Hematocrit (HCT, Hct)			
Whole blood	1 d (cap)	48%-69%	0.48-0.69 vol. fraction
	2 d	48%-75%	0.48-0.75 vol. fraction
	3 d	44%-72%	0.44-0.72 vol. fraction
	2 mo	28%-42%	0.28-0.42 vol. fraction
	6-12 yr	35%-45%	0.35-0.45 vol. fraction
	12-18 yr: Male	37%-49%	0.37-0.49 vol. fraction
	Female	36%-46%	0.36-0.46 vol. fraction
Hemoglobin (Hb)			
Whole blood	1-3 d (cap)	14.5-22.5 g/dl	2.25-3.49 mmol/L
	2 mo	9.0-14.0 g/dl	1.40-2.17 mmol/L
	6-12 yr	11.5-15.5 g/dl	1.78-2.40 mmol/L
	12-18 yr: Male	13.0-16.0 g/dl	2.02-2.48 mmol/L
	Female	12.0-16.0 g/dl	1.86-2.48 mmol/L
Hemoglobin A			
Whole blood		>95% of total	0.5 fraction of Hb

Continued.

COMMON LABORATORY TESTS—cont'd

TEST/SPECIMEN	AGE/SEX/REFERENCE	CONVENTIONAL UNITS	INTERNATIONAL UNITS (SI)
		NORMAL RANGES	
Hemoglobin F			
Whole blood	1 d	63%-92% HbF	0.62-0.92 mass fraction HbF
	5 d	65%-88% HbF	0.65-0.88 mass fraction HbF
	3 wk	55%-85% HbF	0.55-0.85 mass fraction HbF
	6-9 wk	31%-75% HbF	0.31-0.75 mass fraction HbF
	3-4 mo	<2%-59% HbF	<0.02-0.59 mass fraction HbF
	6 mo	<2%-9% HbF	<0.02-0.09 mass fraction HbF
	Adult	<2.0% HbF	<0.02 mass fraction HbF
Immunoglobulin A (IgA)			
Serum	Cord blood	1.4-3.6 mg/dl	14-36 mg/L
	1-3 mo	1.3-53 mg/dl	13-530 mg/L
	4-6 mo	4.4-84 mg/dl	44-840 mg/L
	7 mo-1 yr	11-106 mg/dl	110-1060 mg/L
	2-5 yr	14-159 mg/dl	140-1590 mg/L
	6-10 yr	33-236 mg/dl	330-2360 mg/L
	Adult	70-312 mg/dl	700-3130 mg/L
Immunoglobulin D (IgD)			
Serum	Newborn	None detected	None detected
	Thereafter	0-8 mg/dl	0-80 mg/L
Immunoglobulin E (IgE)			
Serum	Male	0-230 IU/ml	0-230 kIU/L
	Female	0-170 IU/ml	0-170 kIU/L
Immunoglobulin G (IgG)			
Serum	Cord blood	636-1606 mg/dl	6.36-16.06 g/L
	1 mo	251-906 mg/dl	2.51-9.06 g/L
	2-4 mo	176-601 mg/dl	1.76-6.01 g/L
	5-12 mo	172-1069 mg/dl	1.72-10.69 g/L
	1-5 yr	345-1236 mg/dl	3.45-12.36 g/L
	6-10 yr	608-1572 mg/dl	6.08-15.72 g/L
	Adult	639-1349 mg/dl	6.39-13.49 g/L
Immunoglobulin M (IgM)			
Serum	Cord blood	6.3-25 mg/dl	63-250 mg/L
	1 mo-4 mo	17-105 mg/dl	170-1050 mg/L
	5 mo-9 mo	33-126 mg/dl	330-1260 mg/L
	10 mo-1 yr	41-173 mg/dl	410-1730 mg/L
	2-8 yr	43-207 mg/dl	430-2070 mg/L
	9-10 yr	52-242 mg/dl	520-2420 mg/L
	Adult	56-352 mg/dl	560-3520 mg/L
Iron			
Serum	Newborn	100-250 μg/dl	17.90-44.75 μmol/L
	Infant	40-100 μg/dl	7.16-1790 μmol/L
	Child	50-120 μg/dl	8.95-21.48 μmol/L
	Thereafter: Male	50-160 μg/dl	8.95-28.64 μmol/L
	Female	40-150 μg/dl	7.16-26.85 μmol/L
	Intoxicated child	280-2550 μg/dl	50.12-456.5 μmol/L
	Fatally poisoned child	>1800 μg/dl	>322.2 μmol/L
Iron-binding capacity, total (TIBC)			
Serum	Infant	100-400 μg/dl	17.90-71.60 μmol/L
	Thereafter	250-400 μg/dl	44.75-71.60 μmol/L

TEST/SPECIMEN	AGE/SEX/REFERENCE	CONVENTIONAL UNITS		INTERNATIONAL UNITS (SI)
		NORMAL RANGES		
Lead				
Whole blood	Child	<10 μg/dl		<0.48 μmol/L
Urine, 24 hr		<80 μg/L		<0.39 μmol/L
		×1000 cells/mm³ (μl)		***×10⁹ cells/L***
Leukocyte count (WBC count)				
Whole blood	Birth	9.0-30.0		9.0-30.0
	24 hr	9.4-34.0		9.4-34.0
	1 mo	5.0-19.5		5.0-19.5
	1-3 yr	6.0-17.5		6.0-17.5
	4-7 yr	5.5-15.5		5.5-15.5
	8-13 yr	4.5-13.5		4.5-13.5
	Adult	4.5-11.0		4.5-11.0
		×1000 cells/mm³ (μl)		***×10⁶ cells/L***
CSE	Premature	0-25 mononuclear		0-25
		0-100 polymorphonuclear		0-100
		1-1000 RBC		0-1000
	Newborn	0-20 mononuclear		0-20
		0-70 polymorphonuclear		0-70
		0-800 RBC		0-800
	Neonate	0-5 mononuclear		0-5
		0-25 polymorphonuclear		0-25
		0-50 RBC		0-50
	Thereafter	0-5 mononuclear		0-5
Leukocyte differential count				
Whole blood	Myelocytes	0%	0 cells/mm³ (μl)	Number fraction 0
	Neutrophils—"bands"	3%-5%	150-400 cells/mm³ (μl)	Number fraction 0.03-0.05
	Neutrophils—"segs"	54%-62%	3000-5800 cells/mm³ (μl)	Number fraction 0.54-0.62
	Lymphocytes	25%-33%	1500-3000 cells/mm³ (μl)	Number fraction 0.25-0.33
	Monocytes	3%-7%	285-500 cells/mm³ (μl)	Number fraction 0.03-0.07
	Eosinophils	1%-3%	50-250 cells/mm³ (μl)	Number fraction 0.01-0.03
	Basophils	0%-0.75%	15-50 cells/mm³ (μl)	Number fraction 0.0-0.0075
Mean corpuscular hemoglobin (MCH)				
Whole blood	Birth	31-37 pg/cell		0.48-0.57 fmol/L
	1-3 d (cap)	31-37 pg/cell		0.48-0.57 fmol/L
	1 wk-1 mo	28-40 pg/cell		0.43-0.62 fmol/L
	2 mo	26-34 pg/cell		0.40-0.53 fmol/L
	3-6 mo	25-35 pg/cell		0.39-0.54 fmol/L
	0.5-2 yr	23-31 pg/cell		0.36-0.48 fmol/L
	2-6 yr	24-30 pg/cell		0.37-0.47 fmol/L
	6-12 yr	25-33 pg/cell		0.39-0.51 fmol/L
	12-18 yr	25-35 pg/cell		0.39-0.54 fmol/L
	18-49 yr	26-34 pg/cell		0.40-0.53 fmol/L

Continued.

COMMON LABORATORY TESTS—cont'd

TEST/SPECIMEN	AGE/SEX/REFERENCE	CONVENTIONAL UNITS	INTERNATIONAL UNITS (SI)
		NORMAL RANGES	
Mean corpuscular hemoglobin concentration (MCHC)			
Whole blood	Birth	30%-36% Hb cell or g Hb/dl RBC	4.65-5.58 mmol or Hb/L RBC
	1-3 d (cap)	29%-37% Hb cell or g Hb/dl RBC	4.50-5.74 mmol or Hb/L RBC
	1-2 wk	28%-38% Hb cell or g Hb/dl RBC	4.34-5.89 mmol or Hb/L RBC
	1-2 mo	29%-37% Hb cell or g Hb/dl RBC	4.50-5.74 mmol or Hb/L RBC
	3 mo-2 yr	30%-36% Hb cell or g Hb/dl RBC	4.65-5.58 mmol or Hb/L RBC
	2-18 yr	31%-37% Hb cell or g Hb/dl RBC	4.81-5.74 mmol or Hb/L RBC
	>18 yr	31%-37% Hb cell or g Hb/dl RBC	4.81-5.74 mmol or Hb/L RBC
Mean corpuscular volume (MCV)			
Whole blood	1-3 d (cap)	95-121 μm^3	95-121 fl
	0.5-2 yr	70-86 μm^3	70-86 fl
	6-12 yr	77-95 μm^3	77-95 fl
	12-18 yr: Male	78-98 μm^3	78-98 fl
	Female	78-102 μm^3	78-102 fl
Osmolality			
Serum	Child, adult:	275-295 mOsmol/kg H_2O	
Urine, random		50-1400 mOsmol/kg H_2O, depending on fluid intake; after 12 hr fluid restriction: >850 mOsmol/kg H_2O	
Urine, 24 hr		≈300-900 mOsmol/kg H_2O	
Oxygen, partial pressure (Po_2)			
Whole blood, arterial	Birth	8-24 mm Hg	1.1-3.2 kPa
	5-10 min	33-75 mm Hg	4.4-10.0 kPa
	30 min	31-85 mm Hg	4.1-11.3 kPa
	>1 hr	55-80 mm Hg	7.3-10.6 kPa
	1 d	54-95 mm Hg	7.2-12.6 kPa
	Thereafter (decreased with age)	83-108 mm Hg	11-14.4 kPa
Oxygen saturation (Sao_2)			
Whole blood, arterial	Newborn	85%-90%	Fraction saturated 0.85-0.90
	Thereafter	95%-99%	Fraction saturated 0.95-0.99
Partial thromboplastin time (PTT)			
Whole blood (Na citrate)			
Nonactivated		60-85 s (Platelin)	60-85 s
Activated		25-35 s (differs with method)	25-35 s
pH			H^+ concentration:
Whole blood, arterial	Premature (48 hr)	7.35-7.50	31-44 nmol/L
	Birth, full term	7.11-7.36	43-77 nmol/L
	5-10 min	7.09-7.30	50-81 nmol/L
	30 min	7.21-7.38	41-61 nmol/L
	>1 hr	7.26-7.49	32-54 nmol/L
	1 d	7.29-7.45	35-51 nmol/L
	Thereafter	7.35-7.45	35-44 nmol/L
	Must be corrected for body temperature		

TEST/SPECIMEN	AGE/SEX/REFERENCE	CONVENTIONAL UNITS	INTERNATIONAL UNITS (SI)
		NORMAL RANGES	
Urine, random	Newborn/neonate	5-7	0.1-10 μmol/L
	Thereafter (average ≈6)	4.5-8	0.01-32 μmol/L (average ≈1.0 μmol/L)
Stool		7.0-7.5	31-100 nmol/L
Phenylalanine			
Serum	Premature	2.0-7.5 mg/dl	120-450 μmol/L
	Newborn	1.2-3.4 mg/dl	70-210 μmol/L
	Thereafter	0.8-1.8 mg/dl	50-110 μmol/L
Urine, 24 hr	10 d-2 wk	1 2 mg/d	6-12 μmol/d
	3-12 yr	4-18 mg/d	24-110 μmol/d
	Thereafter	trace-17 mg/d	trace-103 μmol/d
Plasma volume			
Plasma	Male	25-43 ml/kg	0.025-0.043 L/kg
	Female	28-45 ml/kg	0.028-0.045 L/kg
Platelet count (thrombocyte count)			
Whole blood (EDTA)	Newborn (After 1 wk, same as adult)	$84\text{-}478 \times 10^3/\text{mm}^3$ (μl)	$84\text{-}478 \times 10^9/\text{L}$
	Adult	$150\text{-}400 \times 10^3/\text{mm}^3$ (μl)	$150\text{-}400 \times 10^9/\text{L}$
Potassium†			
Serum	Newborn	3.0-6.0 mEq/L	3.0-6.0 mmol/L
	Thereafter	3.5-5.0 mEq/L	3.5-5.0 mmol/L
Plasma (heparin)		3.4-4.5 mEq/L	3.4-4.5 mmol/L
Urine, 24 hr		2.5-125 mEq/d varies with diet	2.5-125 mmol/L
Protein			
Serum, total	Premature	4.3-7.6 g/dl	43-76 g/L
	Newborn	4.6-7.4 g/dl	46-74 g/L
	1-7 yr	6.1-7.9 g/dl	61-79 g/L
	8-12 yr	6.4-8.1 g/dl	64-81 g/L
	13-19 yr	6.6-8.2 g/dl	66-82 g/L
Total			
Urine, 24 hr		1-14 mg/dl	10-140 mg/L
		50-80 mg/d (at rest)	50-80 mg/d
		<250 mg/d after intense exercise	<250 mg/d after exercise
Total			
CSF		Lumbar: 8-32 mg/dl	80-320 mg/L
Prothrombin time (PT)			
One-stage (Quick)			
Whole blood (Na citrate)	In general	11-15 s (varies with type of thromboplastin)	11-15 s
	Newborn	Prolonged by 2-3 sec	Prolonged by 2-3 sec
Two-stage modified (Ware and Seegers)			
Whole blood (Na citrate)		18-22 sec	18-22 sec
RBC count, see erythrocyte count			
Red blood cell volume			
Whole blood	Male	20-36 ml/kg	0.020-0.036 L/kg
	Female	19-31 ml/kg	0.019-0.031 L/kg

†Potassium ranges are from Johns Hopkins Hospital: *The Harriet Lane handbook*, ed 12, St Louis, 1991, Mosby, p 383.

Continued.

COMMON LABORATORY TESTS—cont'd

TEST/SPECIMEN	AGE/SEX/REFERENCE	CONVENTIONAL UNITS	INTERNATIONAL UNITS (SI)
		NORMAL RANGES	
Reticulocyte count			
Whole blood	Adults	0.5%-1.5% of erythrocytes or 25,000-75,000/mm³ (μl)	0.005-0.015 (number fraction) 25,000-75,000 × 10^6/L
Capillary	1 d	0.4%-6.0%	0.004-0.060 (number fraction)
	7 d	<0.1%-1.3%	<0.001-0.013 (number fraction)
	1-4 wk	<0.1%-1.2%	<0.001-0.012 (number fraction)
	5-6 wk	<0.1%-2.4%	<0.001-0.024 (number fraction)
	7-8 wk	0.1%-2.9%	0.001-0.029 (number fraction)
	9-10 wk	<0.1%-2.6%	<0.001-0.026 (number fraction)
	11-12 wk	0.1%-1.3%	0.001-0.013 (number fraction)
Salicylates			
Serum, plasma	Therap. conc.	15-30 mg/dl	1.1-2.2 mmol/L
	Toxic conc.	>30 mg/dl	>2.2 mmol/L
Sedimentation rate: see erythrocyte sedimentation rate			
Sodium			
Serum or plasma	Newborn	136-146 mEq/L	134-146 mmol/L
	Infant	139-146 mEq/L	139-146 mmol/L
	Child	138-145 mEq/L	138-145 mmol/L
	Thereafter	136-146 mEq/L	136-146 mmol/L
Urine, 24 hr		40-220 mEq/L (diet dependent)	40-220 mmol/L
Sweat	Normal	<40 mEq/L	<40 mmol/L
	Indeterminate	45-60 mEq/L	45-60 mmol/L
	Cystic fibrosis	>60 mEq/L	>60 mmol/L
Specific gravity			
Urine, random	Adult	1.002-1.030	1.002-1.030
	After 12 hr fluid restriction	>1.025	>1.025
Urine, 24 hr		1.015-1.025	
Theophylline			
Serum, plasma	Therap. conc.		
	Bronchodilator	10-20 μg/ml	56-110 μmol/L
	Premature apnea	6-10 μg/ml	28-56 μmol/L
	Toxic conc.	>20	>166 μmol/L
Thrombin time			
Whole blood (Na citrate)		Control time ± 2 sec when control is 9-13 sec	Control time ± 2 sec when control is 9-13 sec
Thyroxine, total (T_3)			
Serum	Cord	8-13 μg/dl	103-168 nmol/L
	Newborn	11.5-24 (lower in low-birth-weight infants)	148-310 nmol/L
	Neonate	9-18 μg/dl	116-232 nmol/L
	Infant	7-15 μg/dl	90-194 nmol/L
	1-5 yr	7.3-15 μg/dl	94-194 nmol/L
	5-10 yr	6.4-13.3 μg/dl	83-172 nmol/L
	Thereafter	5-12 μg/dl	65-155 nmol/L
	Newborn screen (filter paper)	6.2-22 μg/dl	80-284 nmol/L

TEST/SPECIMEN	AGE/SEX/REFERENCE	CONVENTIONAL UNITS		INTERNATIONAL UNITS (SI)	
		NORMAL RANGES			
Tourniquet test (capillary fragility)		<5-10 petechiae in 2.5 cm circle on forearm (halfway between systolic and diastolic); pressure for 5 min; 0-8 petechiae in 6 cm circle (50 torr for 15 min); 10-20 petechiae in 5 cm circle (80 mm Hg)		<5-10 petechiae in 2.5 cm circle on forearm (halfway between systolic and diastolic); pressure for 5 min; 0-8 petechiae in 6 cm circle (50 torr for 15 min); 10-20 petechiae in 5 cm circle (80 mm Hg)	
Triglycerides (TG)					
Serum, after ≥12 hr fast		***mg/dl***		***g/L***	
		M	***F***	***M***	***F***
	Cord blood	10-98	10-98	0.10-0.98	0.10-0.98
	0-5 yr	30-86	32-99	0.30-0.86	0.32-0.99
	6-11 yr	31-108	35-114	0.31-1.08	0.35-1.14
	12-15 yr	36-138	41-138	0.36-1.38	0.41-1.38
	16-19 yr	40-163	40-128	0.40-1.63	0.40-1.28
Triiodothyronine, free					
Serum	Cord	20-240 pg/dl		0.3-3.7 pmol/L	
	1-3 d	200-610 pg/dl		3.1-9.4 pmol/L	
	6 wk	240-560 pg/dl		3.7-8.6 pmol/L	
	Adults (20-50 yr)	230-660 pg/dl		3.5-10.0 pmol/L	
Triiodothyronine, total (T_3-RIA)					
Serum	Cord	30-70 ng/dl		0.46-1.08 nmol/L	
	Newborn	72-260 ng/dl		1.16-4.00 nmol/L	
	1-5 yr	100-260 ng/dl		1.54-4.00 nmol/L	
	5-10 yr	90-240 ng/dl		1.39-3.70 nmol/L	
	10-15 yr	80-210 ng/dl		1.23-3.23 nmol/L	
	Thereafter	115-190 ng/dl		1.77-2.93 nmol/L	
Urea nitrogen					
Serum or plasma	Cord	21-40 mg/dl		7.5-14.3 mmol urea/L	
	Premature (1 wk)	3-25 mg/dl		1.1-9 mmol urea/L	
	Newborn	3-12 mg/dl		1.1-4.3 mmol urea/L	
	Infant/child	5-18 mg/dl		1.8-6.4 mmol urea/L	
	Thereafter	7-18 mg/dl		2.5-6.4 mmol urea/L	
Urine volume					
Urine, 24 hr	Newborn	50-300 ml/d		0.050-0.300 L/d	
	Infant	350-550 ml/d		0.350-0.500 L/d	
	Child	500-1000 ml/d		0.500-1.000 L/d	
	Adolescent	700-1400 ml/d		0.700-1.400 L/d	
	Thereafter: Male	800-1800 ml/d		0.800-1.800 L/d	
	Female	600-1600 ml/d (varies with intake and other factors)		0.600-1.600 L/d	
WBC, see leukocyte					

TABLE I-2 Abbreviations used in laboratory tests

ABBREVIATION	TERM
cap	capillary
CHF	congestive heart failure
conc.	concentration
CSF	cerebrospinal fluid
d	day; diem
EDTA	ethylenediaminetetraacetate
g	gram
m	meter
hr	hour
L, l	liter
mEq	milliequivalent
min	minute
mm	millimeter
mm^3	cubic millimeter
mo	month
mol	mole
mOsmol	milliosmole
s	second
SI	International system of units
Therap.	therapeutic
U	International unit of enzyme activity
vol	volume
wk	week
yr	year
$>$	greater than
$\geq$	greater than or equal to
$<$	less than
$\leq$	less than or equal to
$\pm$	plus/minus
$\approx$	approximately equal to

TABLE I-3 Prefixes denoting decimal factors

PREFIX	SYMBOL	AMOUNT
deci	d	one tenth (10^{-1})
centi	c	one hundredth (10^{-2})
milli	m	one thousandth (10^{-3})
micro	μ	one millionth (10^{-6})
nano	n	one billionth (10^{-9})
pico	p	one trillionth (10^{-12})
femto	f	one quadrillionth (10^{-15})

Index

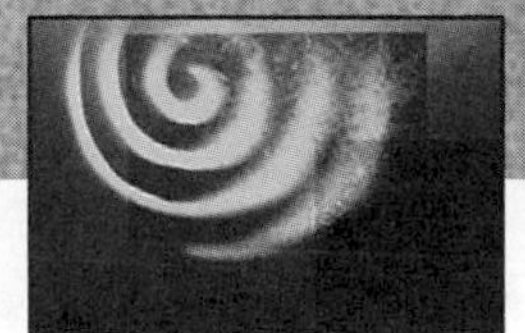

A

AAT; *see* Auscultated acceleration test
Abbreviations used in laboratory tests, 1804
Abdomen
- distention in gastrointestinal dysfunction, 1387
- neuroblastoma, 1599
- newborn, 582, 618, 624
- nutritional status, 889
- physical examination, 924-926
- pregnancy and
  - adaptations during postpartum period, 483
  - first trimester assessment, 129
  - nullipara *versus* multipara, 107
- rhabdomyosarcoma, 1738

Abdominal aorta, 32, 33
Abdominal breathing exercises, 140
Abdominal circumference, 620, 621
Abdominal hernia, 1426
Abdominal hysterotomy, 291
Abdominal orifice of uterine tube, 28
Abdominal pain
- appendicitis, 1408
- gastrointestinal dysfunction, 1387
- respiratory infection, 1322
- school-age child, 1079

Abdominal palpation, 402-406
Abdominal surgery during pregnancy, 285-287
Abducens nerve, 932
Abduction of infant, 495
ABO incompatibility, 768
Abortion
- spontaneous, 216-218
  - after chorionic villus sampling, 94
  - ectopic pregnancy *versus*, 222
  - hydatidiform mole, 223-224
  - hyperthyroidism, 270
- therapeutic and elective, 289-292, 331, 562

Abortus, 2
Abrasion, neonatal birth trauma, 635
Abruptio placentae, 97, 226-228
Absence seizure, 1607
Absolute neutrophil count, 1500
Abstinence, periodic, 515
Abstract communication, 866
Abstract thinking, 1090
Abuse assessment during pregnancy, 311-313
Acceleration injury, 1586
Acceleration of fetal heart rate, 380, 381
Access to care, 4-5
Accessory nerve, 932
Acculturation, 15, 806
Acesulfame K, 184
Acetabular dysplasia, 1721
Acetabulum, 36
Acetaminophen, 1221-1222
- after cardiac surgery, 1479
- equianalgesia, 1225
- fever control, 1270
- for newborn pain, 721
- normal laboratory test ranges, 1794
- pediatric dosage, 1223
- poisoning, 1436

Acetonuria
- diabetes mellitus, 252
- maternal assay, 95

Acetylcholine, 212
Achilles reflex, 931
Achondroplasia, 57
Acid-base balance, 115
Acid-base monitoring, fetal, 385
Acid indigestion, 119, 152
Acid mantle, 647
Acid poisoning, 1436
Acinus, 38
Acme of contraction, 407
Acne, 283, 1684-1687
Acoustic feedback, 1171
Acoustic nerve, 932
Acoustic stimulation test, 98
Acquired immunodeficiency syndrome, 1531-1533
- adolescent, 317-318
- breastfeeding, 156
- hemophilia, 1513
- newborn, 755
- during pregnancy, 234-236

Acrocyanosis, 601, 616
Acrodysesthesia, 118, 153
Acromegaly, 1627
Activated partial thromboplastin time, 231
Active alert state in newborn, 611
Active phase of labor, 394
Activities of daily living
- cerebral palsy, 1749-1750
- postpartum period, 572, 574
- special needs child, 1142

Activity level of newborn, 610, 611
Acute glomerulonephritis, 1556-1558
Acute grief, 1128-1129
Acute laryngotracheobronchitis, 1335-1337
Acute poststreptococcal glomerulonephritis, 1556-1558
Acute renal failure, 1560-1563
Acute spasmodic laryngitis, 1337
Acyclovir, 238-239, 758
Adaptability
- family, 13
- school-age child, 1064

Addiction, 1112
Addison disease, 1635-1636
Adenohypophysis, 1625
Adenoidectomy, 1329
Adenoids, 1328
Adenosine, 1366
ADHD; *see* Attention-deficit hyperactivity disorder
Adipose cell theory, 1107
Adjuvant analgesics, 1222
Admission assessment
- child, 1204-1207
  - emergency, 1242
  - intensive care unit, 1244
- first stage of labor, 395, 397, 398-399

Adnexa, 28
Adolescence, 316, 1084
Adolescent, 1084-1120
- acne, 1684
- anticipatory guidance, 1104
- bereaved, 562
- cognitive development, 317, 1090
- communication with, 874-875
- dental health, 1099
- development of self-concept and body image, 1094-1097
- eating disorders, 1106-1111
- effects of divorce, 838
- epilepsy, 1614
- exercise and activity, 1099
- gender differences in general growth patterns, 1088
- hormonal changes of puberty, 1085
- human immunodeficiency virus infection, 1533
- hypertension, 1487
- immunizations, 1098
- injury prevention, 1102-1104
- insulin-dependent diabetes mellitus, 1650
- mentally retarded, 1162
- moral development, 317, 1090
- nutrition, 1098-1099
- parenthood, 329-331
- personal care, 1099-1100
- physical examination, 895
- physical growth, 1086-1088
- physiologic changes, 316-317, 1088-1089
- pregnancy, 317, 321-329
  - adoption, 329
  - care management, 322-324
  - cultural influences, 322
  - developmental tasks of pregnancy, 321-322
  - under fifteen years of age, 321
  - high risk factor, 81
  - nutrition counseling, 327-328
  - postpartum care, 328-329
  - prenatal care, 325-326
- preparation for procedures, 1255
- psychosocial development, 317, 1089-1090
- rape, 313
- reaction to hospitalization, 1198, 1199-1200

Adolescent—cont'd
  reproductive disorders, 1104-1106
  response to bodily injury and pain, 1203
  sex education and guidance, 318-321, 1101-1102
  sexual maturation, 1085-1086
  sexuality, 515
  sleep and rest, 1099
  smoking, 1111-1112
  social development, 1091-1094
  special needs, 1131, 1145
  spiritual development, 1090-1091
  stress reduction, 1100-1101
  substance abuse, 1112-1115
  suicide, 1115-1117
  understanding and reaction to death, 1134
Adopted child, 835-837
Adoption, 329, 331
Adoptive family, 836-837
Adrenal cortex, 1625, 1634
Adrenal crisis, 1634-1635
Adrenal disorders, 1634-1640
  Addison disease, 1635-1636
  adrenocortical insufficiency, 1634-1636
  congenital adrenogenital hyperplasia, 1637-1639
  Cushing syndrome, 1636-1637
  hyperaldosteronism, 1639
  pheochromocytoma, 1639-1640
Adrenal gland, fetal, 68
Adrenal hyperplasia, congenital, 638
Adrenal medulla, 1625, 1634
Adrenarche, 1085
Adrenocortical insufficiency, 1634-1636
Adrenocorticotropic hormone, 1625
Adrenogenital hyperplasia, 1637-1639
Adult respiratory distress syndrome, 1345
  during pregnancy, 282
  shock, 1489
Advanced life support, 1362
Advanced nurse practitioner, 794
Adventist, 814
Advil; *see* Ibuprofen
Advocacy, family, 793-794
Aerosol therapy, 1304-1305
Affect
  infant development, 944
  pain during delivery, 353
  suicide risk, 1116
Affiliative relationships, 9
Affluence, 803-804
AFP; *see* Alpha-fetoprotein
African-American culture
  adolescent pregnancy, 322
  childbearing and parenting beliefs, 16
  food patterns, 190
  health beliefs and practices, 811, 820-821
Afterbirth pains, 498
Afterpains, 381
AGA; *see* Appropriate-for-gestational-age
Age
  acetaminophen dosage, 1270
  birthrate according to, 3
  classification of hypertension, 1487
  developmental periods, 845
  enema, 1315
  head circumference charts, 1788
  height and weight measurements, 1785-1786
  high risk factor, 81
  parenthood after age 35, 159
  physical examination, 895
  respiratory infections and, 1321-1322
Agency for Health Care Policy and Research, 793
Agenesis, anal, 1431
Agonist-antagonist compounds, 359
Aid to Families with Dependent Children, 321, 790
AIDS; *see* Acquired immunodeficiency syndrome
Airborne precautions, 1272, 1273
Airway
  burn victim, 1692
  cardiopulmonary resuscitation, 1363
  neonatal assessment and maintenance, 630, 631-632
  obstruction, 1365-1368
  unconscious child, 1579
Akinetic seizure, 1606
Alcohol
  adolescent abuse, 1113
  breastfeeding and, 680
  maternal abuse, 759, 760-761
  pregnancy and, 140, 303
    high risk factor, 81
    negative impact on maternal nutrition, 186-187
  psychologic and physiologic signs, 304
Alcohol, Drug Abuse, and Mental Health Block Grant, 790
Aldactone; *see* Spironolactone
Aldomet; *see* Methyldopa
Aldosterone, 1625, 1639
Alertness, 1573
Alfentanil, 721
Alisa Ann Ruch California Burn Foundation, 1699
Alkaline poisoning, 1436
Allele, 52
Allen test, 1283
Allergen, 1349, 1351-1352, 1384
Allergic conjunctivitis, 1181
Allergic reaction to blood transfusion, 1535
Allergy, 1491-1492
Allergy history, 879
Allogenic bone marrow transplantation, 1536
Allograft, burn victim, 1693-1694
Alloimmunization, 1536
Alopecia, 1525, 1680
Alpha cell, 1640
Alpha-fetoprotein, 83, 91, 95
Altered states of consciousness, 1573-1574
Alternate breast massage, 686
Alternative birth center, 172
Alternative family structures, 10-11
Alveolus, mammary, 37
Ambiguous genitalia, 1551
Amblyopia, 1176
Ambulation
  during labor, 414-416
  play activities, 1258
  postpartum, 498-499
Ambulatory setting, 1241-1242
Amelia, 1727
Amenorrhea
  adolescent, 1104-1105
  during pregnancy, 105, 123
American Academy of Pediatrics, 1009
American Alliance for Health, Physical Education, Recreation, and Dance, 1146
American Camping Association, 1146
American Celiac Society, 1433
American Cleft Palate Association, 1422
American Dental Association, 1006
American Diabetes Association, 1645
American Juvenile Arthritis Foundation, 1741
American Lung Association, 1354
American Lupus Society, 1742
American Nurses Association, 5, 796
American Sign Language, 1172
American Society of Dentistry for Children, 1006
American Sudden Infant Death Syndrome Institute, 1148
Amethopterin; *see* Methotrexate
Ammonia nitrogen, 1794
Amnesia during labor, 430
Amniocentesis, 90-93
  injection of urea solution after, 291
  ultrasound adjunct, 85
Amnioinfusion, 383
Amnion, 60, 61
Amniotic fluid, 61
  analysis during first stage of labor, 409-411
  embolism, 437, 477
  meconium-stained, 385-386
  ultrasound assessment, 87-88
Amniotic fluid index, 88
Amniotic fluid volume, 83, 88, 89, 92
Amniotomy, 409-410, 461
Amphetamines, 759, 766
Ampulla, 37-38
  uterine tube, 28, 29

Amputation, 1720-1721
Amylase
  infant, 663, 938
  newborn, 597
ANA; *see* American Nurses Association
Anal membrane atresia, 1431
Anal reflex, 928
Anal sphincter muscle fibers, 36
Anal stage of psychosexual development, 851
Analgesia, 1221
  during labor, 358-373
    administration of medication, 369-373
    anesthesia in obese woman, 366-367
    general anesthesia, 366
    informed consent, 369
    maternal hypothermia after analgesia and anesthesia, 367
    nerve block, 360-365
    systemic analgesia, 358-359
  postpartum, 498
Anaphylaxis, 1491-1492
Androgens, 1085
Android pelvis, 342, 343
Anemia, 1499-1503
  acute renal failure, 1562
  aplastic, 1511-1512
  beta-thalassemia, 1510-1511
  chronic renal failure, 1565
  delayed wound healing, 1660
  infant, 938
  iron deficiency, 1503-1505
  leukemia, 1521
  during pregnancy, 279-281
    iron needs, 184
    laboratory testing, 189
    physiologic, 113-114
  sickle cell, 1505-1510
Anencephaly, 96, 771, 1754
Aneroid sphygmomanometer, 903
Anesthesia
  cesarean birth, 466
  during labor, 358-373
    administration of medication, 369-373
    general anesthesia, 366
    informed consent, 369
    maternal hypothermia, 367
    nerve block, 360-365
    obese woman, 366-367
    recovery following, 489-491
    systemic analgesia, 358-359
  for newborn pain, 721
  skin lesions, 1655
Aneuploidy, 54
Angel dust; *see* Phencyclidine hydrochloride
Angiogenesis, 1658
Angiography, 1451
Angioma, 116-117
Anglican, 815
Animal attack, 977
Animal bite, 1677-1678
Animism, 997
Anisometropia, 1176
Ankle clonus, 206
Ankle edema, 165
Ankyloglossia, 645
Announcement phase, 158
Anorectal malformations, 1431-1432
Anorexia, 1109-1110
  chemotherapy-induced, 1521
  respiratory infection, 1322
Antacids, 1413
Anteflexed uterus, 29
Anterior ligament, 31
Anterior pituitary, 1625
Anteverted uterus, 29
Anthropoid pelvis, 342, 343
Anthropometry, 189, 887
Antibiotics
  hearing loss, 713
  uterine inversion, 541
Anticipatory grief, 552, 717, 1128
Anticipatory guidance, 871
  adolescent, 1104
  infant, 977-979
  preschooler, 1028
  school-age child, 1069-1072
  toddler, 1013
Antidepressants, 299-300
Antidiuretic hormone, 1625
  diabetes insipidus, 1628
  syndrome of inappropriate antidiuretic hormone, 1629
Antidotes, 1439
Antihemophilic factor, 1512
Antimalarial agents, 713
Antipsychotic drugs, 300
Antirheumatic drugs, 1739
Antiseptics, 1660
Antistreptolysin O, 1482, 1557, 1794
Anus, 30
  imperforate, 775
  newborn, 624
  physical examination, 928
  postpartum varicosities, 483
Anxiety during pregnancy, 165
Aorta, 33
Aortic stenosis, 1459
Apgar score, 435, 608-609, 630
Apheresis, 1537
Aphthous stomatitis, 1406
APIB; *see* Assessment of Preterm Infant Behavior
Apical pulse, 593, 616
Aplastic anemia, 1511-1512
Aplastic crisis, 1506
Apnea, 1361
  neonatal, 592, 631
  respiratory distress, 700
Apnea of infancy, 986-988
Appendicitis, 1406-1408
  ectopic pregnancy *versus*, 222
  during pregnancy, 286
Appendix, 119
Appetite
  changes during pregnancy, 118
  hospitalized child, 1268
  postpartum, 484, 493
Appropriate-for-gestational-age infant, 614, 697
Apresoline; *see* Hydralazine
Apt test, 92
Ara-C; *see* Cytosine arabinoside
ARDS; *see* Adult respiratory distress syndrome
Areola, 37
  breast-feeding and, 668
  newborn, 600
ARF; *see* Acute renal failure
Argininosuccinicaciduria, 96
Arm circumference, 899-900
Arm restraint, 1278
Arm strength, 930
Arm traction, 1717
Arousal, 46
Arterial blood gases, 637, 1283, 1795
Arterial hemoglobin saturation, 1800
Arterial switch procedure, 1462
Arteriovenous fistula, 1568
Arthritis
  juvenile rheumatoid, 1738-1741
  during pregnancy, 284-285
  septic, 1734
Arthritis Foundation, 1741, 1742
Arthropod bites and stings, 1674-1677
Articular dysfunction, 1706-1745
  amputation, 1720-1721
  bone and soft tissue tumors, 1735-1738
  cast, 1714-1716
  clubfoot, 1725-1726
  developmental dysplasia of hip, 1721-1725
  distraction, 1720
  fracture, 1711-1714
  immobilization, 1706-1709
  juvenile rheumatoid arthritis, 1738-1741
  kyphosis and lordosis, 1729-1730
  Legg-Calvé-Perthes disease, 1728-1733
  metatarsus adductus, 1726-1727
  osteogenesis imperfecta, 1727-1728
  osteomyelitis, 1733-1734
  scoliosis, 1730-1733
  septic arthritis, 1734
  skeletal limb deficiency, 1727
  slipped femoral capital epiphysis, 1729
  soft tissue injury, 1709-1711
  systemic lupus erythematosus, 1741-1742

Articular dysfunction—cont'd
traction, 1716-1720
tuberculosis, 1734-1735
Artificial airway, 1305
Artificial rupture of membranes, 409-410, 461
Artificial sweeteners, 184
Artificial ventilation, 1362
pediatric nursing interventions, 1305-1311
shock, 1490
Ascariasis, 1404
Ascites, 1552
Ascorbic acid
delayed wound healing, 1660
infant requirements, 664
iron absorption and, 1379
needs during pregnancy, 179, 186
nutritional significance, 1375-1376
ASD; *see* Atrial septal defect
Aseptic meningitis, 1602-1603
Asian-American culture
childbearing and parenting beliefs, 17
health beliefs and practices, 818-819
Aspartame, 184
Asphyxia
fetal responses to, 97
perinatal, 739
Aspiration
bone marrow, 1280
foreign body, 970-973, 1344-1345
meconium, 738
near-drowning, 1593
toddler, 102
Aspiration abortion, 290-291
Aspiration pneumonia, 657, 1345
Aspirin
combination products, 1221
Kawasaki disease, 1488
poisoning, 1436-1437
Assay
alpha-fetoprotein, 95
clotting factor, 231
Assembly of God, 817
Assessment of Preterm Infant Behavior, 713
Assimilation, 15
Association for Care of Children's Health, 1195
Association for Women's Health, Obstetric and Neonatal Nurses, 5, 374, 579
Associative play, 856-857, 1019
Asthma, 281-282, 1347-1356
Asthma and Allergy Foundation of America, 1354
Astigmatism, 1176
Ataractics, 359
Ataxic cerebral palsy, 1747
Athlete's foot, 1669
Atonic seizure, 1606
Atopic dermatitis, 1682-1684
Atraumatic care, 792
Atresia
anal membrane, 1431
biliary, 1417-1418
esophageal, 774, 1422-1425
tricuspid, 1461
Atrial septal defect, 1456
Atrioventricular canal defect, 1457
Atrioventricular heart block, 1485
Atropine sulfate, 1366
Attachment, 506, 507, 567
infant development, 945-946
mentally ill mother, 300-302
newborn, 610-614
postpartum, 506-508
sibling, 585
Attention-deficit hyperactivity disorder, 1075-1077
Attitude, fetal, 337
Atypical pneumonia, 1340
Audiometry, 917
Auditory acuity of newborn, 608
Auditory nerve, 932
Auditory stimulation, 947
Auditory testing, 917, 918
Augmentation enterocytoplasty, 1756
Augmentation of labor, 462
Auscultated acceleration test, 98
Auscultation
abdominal, 925
blood pressure, 903
cardiac, 923-924
fetal heart rate, 1773-1774
newborn heart sounds, 615
pulmonary, 922
Authoritarian parental style, 832-833
Authoritative parenting style, 833
Autism, 988-989
Autism Society of America, 989
Autoimmune disorders, 284-285
Autoimmune hypoparathyroidism, 1633
Autoimmune thrombocytopenic purpura, 231
Autologous bone marrow transplantation, 1536
Autolysis, 484
Autonomic nervous system
Brazelton Neonatal Behavioral Assessment, 610
newborn pain assessment, 719
Autonomy
adolescent, 1091, 1146
Erikson's psychosocial development model, 851-852
ethical decision making, 795
toddler, 995
Autopsy, 557
Autosomal abnormalities, 54
Autosomal dominant inheritance, 57
Autosomal recessive inheritance, 57
Autosome, 51
Avoidance language, 866
AWHONN; *see* Association for Women's Health, Obstetric and Neonatal Nurses
Axillary sensor, 902
Axillary temperature, 616
Azotemia, 1561

B

B cell, 666
B_{12}-binding protein, 666
Babinski reflex, 1576
Babinski sign, 606
Baby blues, 510
Baby powder aspiration, 972-973
Bacille Calmette-Guérin, 1343
Bacitracin, 1694
Back
newborn, 619, 624
physical examination, 928-930
Back transport, 718-719
Backache during pregnancy, 153, 155
Bacteremic shock, 544
Bacterial infection
conjunctivitis, 1181
cutaneous, 1664-1667
diarrhea, 1396-1397
hemolytic-uremic syndrome, 1558
infective endocarditis, 1481-1482
meningitis, 749, 1600-1602
newborn, 758
osteomyelitis, 1733
pneumonia, 1340-1341
short bowel syndrome, 1434
tracheitis, 1337
vaginosis, 241
Bacteriuria, 1546
Bag-and-mask equipment, 699
Bag of waters, 398
Balance suspension traction, 1718
Balanced translocation, 56
Ballard Scale, 713, 732
Ballottement, 109, 110
Bandl ring, 453
Baptist, 814
Barbiturate coma, 1581
Bartholin glands, 27, 928
Barton tongs, 1719
Basal body temperature
contraception, 516, 517
menstrual cycle, 41
Basal layer of endometrium, 29
Basal metabolic rate, 848
changes during pregnancy, 114-115
cold stress in newborn, 596
maternal nutrition, 176
Base excess, 1794
Baseline fetal heart rate, 377
Baseline measurements in newborn, 620-623
Basilar skull fracture, 1587

Basophil count, 1500
Bathing
dead child, 557
hospitalized child, 1266, 1267
newborn, 646-649
during pregnancy, 154
wound care, 1664
Battered woman, 311
Battledore placenta, 229-230
BBT; *see* Basal body temperature
Bearing-down efforts, 344-345, 428-429, 453
Bed rest
preeclampsia, 208
preterm labor, 447, 448
Bed-wetting, 1077
Bee sting, 1675
Behavior
brain tumor, 1595
childhood depression, 1079-1080
cognitive impairment, 1159
maternal, 503-504
newborn, 609-610
newborn pain assessment, 719
suicide risk, 1116
unoccupied, 855-856
Behavior modification, 834
Behavioral contracting, 1220
Behavioral therapy, 1108
Belching, 152
Bell's palsy, 284
Bend fracture, 1712
Beneficence, 795
Benevolent overreaction, 1125
Benzathine penicillin, 234
Bereavement, 551, 1128, 1129
complicated, 562-563
Beta cell, 1640
Beta-thalassemia, 1510-1511
Betadine; *see* Povidone-iodine
Bibliotherapy, 876
Bicarbonate, 1794
Biceps reflex, 206, 930
Biculture, 805
Bicycle safety, 1069, 1071
Bifidus factor, 666
Bile salts, 663
Biliary atresia, 1417-1418
Bililites, 652
Bilingual child, 804-805
Bilirubin, 652
amniocentesis, 91
conjugation, 598
jaundice, 598, 636, 767
kernicterus, 768
neonatal values, 637
normal ranges, 1794
Bilirubinometry, 599
Bill of Rights for Children and Teens, 1219
Billings method of contraception, 515, 516-517
Bimanual compression, 539
Bimanual palpation, 130-131
Binocularity, 909-910, 939
Binuclear family, 9
Biochemical assessment, 90-95
amniocentesis, 90-93
chorionic villus sampling, 94-95
congenital anomalies, 777
maternal assays, 95
percutaneous umbilical blood sampling, 93-94
Biologic skin coverings, 1693
Biomedical model of ethnocentrism, 15
Biophysical assessment, 82-90
daily fetal movement count, 82-83
magnetic resonance imaging, 90
ultrasonography, 83-90
Biophysical profile, 83, 89
maternal diabetes mellitus, 258
ultrasound, 88
Biophysical risks, 80, 81
Biopsy
bone marrow, 1280
heart, 1451
renal, 1543
Biorhythmicity, parent-infant bonding, 508
Biostatistical terminology, 2
Biotin, 1375
Biotinidase deficiency, 638
Biparietal cephalometry, 86
Biparietal diameter, 84, 85, 337, 340
Bipolar disorder, 298
Birth; *see* Childbirth
Birth canal, 338-343
laceration, 538-539
Birth history, 878-879
Birth plan, 128, 141, 147
Birth setting, 172
Birth trauma, 635, 743-744, 746-749
Birthing beds and chairs, 430, 431
Birthing room, 428, 429
Birthrate, 2, 3-4
Birthweight, 614, 616, 620, 724-725
Bishop score, 460
Bite
animal, 1677-1678
arthropod, 1674-1677
human, 1678-1679
rabies, 1605
Biting, infant, 943
Bittersweet grief, 552, 553
Blach test, 636
Black eye, 1175
Black Muslim, 814
Black widow spider, 1675
Blackbird Storybook Home Eye Test, 911, 912, 913
Blackhead, 1684
Bladder, 30, 35
catheterization, 1282
exstrophy, 776, 1551
maternal
changes during pregnancy, 115
distention prevention, 495
home visit assessment, 582
postpartum assessment, 484, 489, 499-501
newborn assessment, 624
pelvic blood supply, 33
ultrasound, 1543
Blanket support, 648
Blastocyst, 60, 62
Blastocyst cavity, 58-60
Blastomere, 58
Blastomycosis, 1670
Bleeding
fourth stage of labor, 495-497
hemophilia, 1514
leukemia, 1518, 1520-1521
Bleeding time, 231, 1794
Blended family, 9-10, 839
Blenoxane; *see* Bleomycin
Bleomycin, 1522
Blighted ovum, 97
Blindism, 1179
Blindness, 1175-1181
Blissymbols, 1161
Bloating, 152
Blood clot, 486, 499
Blood disorders, 1499-1530
disseminated intravascular coagulation, 1516
epistaxis, 1516-1517
hemophilia, 1512-1515
Hodgkin disease, 1528-1530
idiopathic thrombocytopenic purpura, 1515-1516
leukemia, 1517-1528
chemotherapy, 1521-1525
classification, 1517
myelosuppression, 1520-1521
nursing care plan, 1526-1528
pathophysiology, 1517-1518
therapeutic management, 1518-1519
lymphoma, 1528
non-Hodgkin lymphoma, 1530
prenatal diagnosis, 96
red blood cell, 1499-1512
anemia, 1499-1503
aplastic anemia, 1511-1512
beta-thalassemia, 1510-1511
iron deficiency anemia, 1503-1505
sickle cell anemia, 1505-1510
Blood glucose
diabetic mother, 261
newborn, 597
postpartum, 483

Blood loss
during childbirth, 485
postpartum hemorrhage, 482, 495-497, 537
during pregnancy, 216
Blood loss anemia, 1501, 1502
Blood pH, 115
Blood pressure, 903-905
hypertension, 1486-1487
maternal
changes during pregnancy, 112
ectopic pregnancy, 222
postpartum, 485, 489, 492
preeclampsia-eclampsia, 204, 213-214
second trimester, 147
neurologic examination, 1574
newborn, 594
assessment, 615-620
high-risk, 700-701
pediatric, 1792, 1793
Blood specimen, 1282-1284
Blood test
first stage of labor, 409
renal function, 1545
Blood transfusion, 1534-1536
hyperbilirubinemia, 651
hypovolemic shock, 543
respiratory distress syndrome and, 734
Rh incompatibility, 768
Blood typing, 131
Blood urea nitrogen, 1545
Blood vessels, uterine, 32, 33
Blood volume
adaptations during postpartum period, 485
changes during pregnancy, 112-114
maternal nutrition, 176
newborn, 594
normal ranges, 1794
Bloody show, 168, 346, 398
Blue spell, 1472
BMI; *see* Body mass index
BMR; *see* Basal metabolic rate
BNBAS; *see* Brazelton Neonatal Behavioral Assessment
Bodily damage
adolescent, 1103
hospitalized child, 1200-1203, 1219
infant, 976-977
school-age child, 1070
toddler, 1008, 1012-1013
Body fluid loss, 596
Body image
adolescent, 1094-1097
child, 854
infant, 944, 945
preschooler, 1018
school-age child, 1060
toddler, 997
Body mass index, 180, 181
Body mechanics during pregnancy, 154, 155
Body piercing, 1100
Body proportions, 846-847
Body surface area
newborn thermoregulation, 595
water balance, 1387
Body temperature
child, 848-849
near-drowning, 1593
neurologic examination, 1574
normal pediatric values, 1793
physical examination, 900-902
unconscious, 1581-1582
maternal
contraception and, 515, 516, 517
postpartum, 485, 489, 492, 493
puerperal infection, 543-544
newborn, 616, 655
adaptation to extrauterine life, 629-631
assessment, 614-615
bathing, 646-647
home visit assessment, 582
preterm, 726
Body weight
dehydration, 1389
high-risk infant, 707
neonatal assessment, 630
Boil, 1666
Bonding, 567
assessment, 610-614
cultural considerations, 507
infant development, 300
mentally ill mother, 300-302
postpartum, 506-508
sibling, 585
Bone
fracture, 1711-1714
growth and maturation, 847-848
healing and remodeling, 1712-1713
tumor, 1735-1738
Bone age, 847
Bone marrow, leukemia and, 1518, 1519
Bone marrow aspiration, 1280
Bone marrow transplantation, 1519, 1536-1537
Bony pelvis, 36-37
labor, 340-342
Bordetella pertussis, 1034, 1284, 1341
Borrelia burgdorferi, 242, 1678
Boston brace, 1731
Bottle-feeding, 691-693
Botulism, 1764-1765
Bougienage, 1424
Bowel elimination
postpartum, 484, 492, 499-501
spina bifida, 1756
Bowel sounds, 925
Bowleg, 603, 929
BPD; *see* Bronchopulmonary dysplasia
Bra
breastfeeding, 676
maternity, 153
Brachial palsy, 625
Brachycephaly, 1615
Bracing
developmental dysplasia of hip, 1724
scoliosis, 1731
Bradley method of childbirth, 354
Bradycardia
fetal, 378, 379
newborn, 616
Bradydysrhythmia, 1485
Bradypnea, 631
Braille system, 1178, 1179
Brain, 1572-1623
altered states of consciousness, 1573-1584
aseptic meningitis, 1602-1603
bacterial meningitis, 1600-1602
brain tumor, 1594-1599
cranial deformities, 1615
encephalitis, 1603
epilepsy, 1605-1614
febrile seizures, 1614-1615
head injury, 1585-1593
human immunodeficiency virus encephalopathy, 1604
hydrocephalus, 1615-1620
increased intracranial pressure, 1573
near-drowning, 1593-1594
neuroblastoma, 1599
neurologic examination, 1574-1578
rabies, 1604-1605
Reye syndrome, 1603-1604
tumor, 1594-1599
unconscious child, 1578-1585
Brainstem-auditory evoked response, 917
Braun von Fernwald's sign, 109
Braxton-Hicks contractions, 65, 109, 123, 165
Brazelton Neonatal Behavioral Assessment, 331, 610, 713
Breast, 37-39
maternal
adaptations during pregnancy, 111
anatomy, 667
care of, 676, 691
engorgement, 484-485, 498, 501
first trimester assessment, 129
home visit assessment, 582
infection, 544, 684-685
massage, 686
postpartum, 484-485, 492, 493
self-examination, 38, 676-677
newborn, 600, 623-624
pediatric physical examination, 920
pubertal development, 1086
Breast milk
donor milk bank, 688
protein content, 664

Breast milk—cont'd
pumping, 687-688
storage, 678-679
Breast milk jaundice, 599, 682
Breastfeeding, 665-691
adopted baby, 679
breast adaptations during postpartum period, 484
care of mother, 675-677
diabetic mother, 687
drugs and environmental pollutants, 679-680
effects of early discharge, 674
engorgement, 680-681
estrogen levels, 483
expressing, pumping, and storing milk, 677-679
factors affecting breastfeeding practices, 665
failure to thrive, 981
fussy baby, 686-687
infant health, 956-957
jaundiced infant, 599, 681-682
mastitis, 684-685
maternal benefits, 666
maternal substance abuse, 309, 766
milk production, 667-668
monilial infections, 684
nurse role as teacher, 674-675
ovulation suppression, 483
patient teaching, 670-671
plugged milk duct, 684
postpartum analgesia, 498
postpartum promotion, 501
premature or sick infant, 687-688
prenatal support, 665-666
preparation for, 156
promotion, 501
properties of human milk, 666
slow weight gain, 685-686
sore nipples, 683-684
timing and frequency of feedings, 672
twins, 687
weaning, 680
Breath sounds, 922
abnormal breathing, 631
newborn, 592
Breathing
cardiopulmonary resuscitation, 1363
changes during pregnancy, 114
labor techniques, 355-357
neurologic examination, 1575
newborn
abnormal, 631
initial, 591
Breck feeder, 710, 1421
Breech presentation, 337, 412, 455-456
birth trauma, 747
newborn scrotum, 600
spinal cord injury, 749
Brethine; *see* Terbutaline
Bretylium, 1366
British Sign Language, 1172
Broad ligament, 27-29, 28
Bromocriptine
breastfeeding and, 680
lactation suppression, 501
Bronchial asthma, 281-282
Bronchial breath sounds, 922
Bronchial drainage, 1305, 1306-1307
Bronchitis, 1337
Bronchopneumonia, 1339
Bronchopulmonary dysplasia, 735
Bronchospasm, 1352
Bronchovesicular breath sounds, 922
Bronze baby syndrome, 650
Broviac catheter, 1295
Brown fat, 595
Brown recluse spider, 1676
Bruise, 1709-1710
birth trauma, 635, 746, 747
racial differences, 907
skin lesions, 1655
Bryant traction, 1717
Bubble test, 91
Buccal medication administration, 1226
Buck extension traction, 1718
Buckle fracture, 1712
Buckwheat hypersensitivity, 1385
Buddhist Churches of America, 814
Buffered lidocaine, 1229
Bulb syringe, neonatal airway suctioning, 631, 632
Bulbar conjunctiva, 909
Bulbocavernous muscle, 35
Bulbourethral gland, 45
Bulimia, 1110-1111
Bulla, 1657
BUN; *see* Blood urea nitrogen
Burial, 554, 557
Burns, 1687-1703
adolescent, 1103
characteristics, 1687-1690
childhood mortality, 787
emergency care, 1690-1691
infant, 975-976
major, 1692-1700
minor, 1691-1692
pathophysiology, 1690
school-age child, 1070
sunburn, 1700-1703
toddler, 1007, 1010-1011
Burping, 607, 672
Butterfly needle, 640

C

C-reactive protein, 1795
Cabbage leaves for engorgement, 681
Cadaver donor, 1569
Caffeine
breastfeeding and, 680
perinatal risks, 763
Caffeine—cont'd
use during pregnancy, 81, 140, 184, 310
CAGE questionnaire, 306
CAH; *see* Congenital adrenal hyperplasia
Calcaneal nerves, 637
Calcium
hypoparathyroidism, 1633
infant requirements, 664
needs during pregnancy, 178, 185
normal laboratory ranges, 1795
nutritional significance, 1378
placental storage, 65
Calcium channel blockers, 450
Calcium chloride, 1366
Calcium gluconate, 212
Calendar method of contraception, 515, 516
Caloric test, 1576
Calories, 663
breastfeeding and, 675
needs during pregnancy, 178
recommended daily requirements, 848
Campylobacter jejuni, 1397
Canadian Dental Association, 1006
Canadian Hemophilia Society, 1515
Candidiasis, 1669
diaper, 1679
newborn, 758-759
vaginal, 241
Candlelighters Childhood Cancer Foundation, 1736
Canker sore, 1406
Cannula, nasal, 702
Capillary fragility test, 1803
Caput succedaneum, 601, 617, 746
Car safety seat
infant, 974
toddler, 1009
Carbohydrates
energy needs, 663
newborn metabolism, 598
placental storage, 65
Carbon dioxide
lower threshold during pregnancy, 114
normal laboratory ranges, 1795
Carbon dioxide narcosis, 1303
Carbon dioxide partial pressure, 115
Carbon monoxide inhalation, 1345-1347
Carboprost, 494
Carbuncle, 1666
Cardiac catheterization, 1451-1453
Cardiac decompensation, 271
Cardiac dysrhythmia, 1484-1485
Cardiac output
adaptations during postpartum period, 485
changes during pregnancy, 113, 114
noninvasive assessment, 229
Cardinal ligament, 28, 31
Cardinal movements of labor, 347, 348

Cardiogenic shock, 1489
Cardiomyopathy
  infant of diabetic mother, 744
  during pregnancy, 276
Cardiopulmonary resuscitation
  infant, 632, 731
  pediatric, 1362-1365, 1366
  pregnant woman, 278-279
Cardiovascular dysfunction, 1450-1498
  anaphylaxis, 1491-1492
  assessment, 1450-1453
  bacterial endocarditis, 1481-1482
  congestive heart failure, 1465-1472
  defects with decreased pulmonary blood flow, 1457-1465
    aortic stenosis, 1459
    coarctation of aorta, 1458-1459
    hypoplastic left heart syndrome, 1464
    patent ductus arteriosus, 1458
    pulmonary stenosis, 1460
    tetralogy of Fallot, 1460-1461
    total anomalous pulmonary venous connection, 1462-1463
    transposition of great arteries, 1462
    tricuspid atresia, 1461
    truncus arteriosus, 1463-1464
  defects with increased pulmonary blood flow, 1455
  dysrhythmias, 1484-1485
  heart transplantation, 1494
  Henoch-Schönlein purpura, 1493-1494
  hyperlipidemia, 1483-1484
  hypertension, 1486-1487
  hypoxemia, 1472-1474
  Kawasaki disease, 1487-1489
  mixed defects, 1465
  nursing management, 1474-1481
  obstructive defects, 1455-1457
  rheumatic fever, 1482-1483
  shock, 1489-1491
  toxic shock syndrome, 1492-1493
Cardiovascular system
  adaptations during postpartum period, 485
  congenital anomalies, 772
  effects of immobilization, 1707
  newborn, 592-594
  nutritional status, 889
  pregnancy, 270-279
    adaptation in labor, 349
    adaptations during, 111-114, 201
    cardiac disease, 270-276
    cardiopulmonary resuscitation, 278-279
    heart surgery, 276
    nutritional status, 193
    ritodrine-induced complications, 448
  preterm infant, 726
  review of systems, 881
  systemic lupus erythematosus, 1742
Care coordination, 1187
Caries, 1067
Caring, 794
Carotene, 1373
Carpal tunnel syndrome, 118, 153
Carrier, autosomal recessive inheritance, 57
Case management, 792-793
  home care, 1187-1188
Cast
  developmental dysplasia of hip, 1725
  fracture, 1714-1716
Casts, urinary, 1545
Cat-scratch disease, 1679
Cataract, 1177
Catecholamines, 1625
Catheterization, 1282
  hypovolemic shock, 542
  during labor, 415
  postpartum, 495
Cat's eye reflex, 1182
Caudal regression syndrome, 742, 743
Caul, 434
CBC; *see* Complete blood count
Celiac disease, 1432-1433
Celiac Sprue Association, 1433
Cell division, 53-54
Cell-mediated immunity, 1531
Cell-surface immunologic markers, 1517
Cellulitis, 1666
Central access device, 1283
Central auditory imperception, 1168
Central cyanosis, 700
Central nervous system, 1572-1623
  altered states of consciousness, 1573-1584
  aseptic meningitis, 1602-1603
  bacterial meningitis, 1600-1602
  brain tumor, 1594-1599
  cranial deformities, 1615
  encephalitis, 1603
  epilepsy, 1605-1614
  febrile seizures, 1614-1615
  head injury, 1585-1593
  human immunodeficiency virus encephalopathy, 1604
  hydrocephalus, 1615-1620
  increased intracranial pressure, 1573
  lead poisoning, 1441
  leukemia and, 1518, 1519
  near-drowning, 1593-1594
  neuroblastoma, 1599
  neurologic examination, 1574-1578
  newborn
    birth trauma, 749
    congenital anomalies, 770-772
    preterm, 726
  prenatal diagnosis of anomalies, 96
  rabies, 1604-1605
  Reye syndrome, 1603-1604
  shock, 1489
Central nervous system—cont'd
  systemic lupus erythematosus, 1742
  unconscious child, 1578-1585
Central nervous system depressants, 1113
Central nervous system stimulants, 1113
Central venous access device, 1294-1296
Centration, 997
Cephalhematoma, 601, 617, 746
Cephalic presentation, 337
Cephalocaudal development, 66, 602, 845
Cephalometry, biparietal, 86
Cephalopelvic disproportion, 454
Cerebellar functioning, 930
Cerebral dysfunction, 1572-1623
  altered states of consciousness, 1573-1584
  aseptic meningitis, 1602-1603
  bacterial meningitis, 1600-1602
  brain tumor, 1594-1599
  cranial deformities, 1615
  encephalitis, 1603
  epilepsy, 1605-1614
  febrile seizures, 1614-1615
  head injury, 1585-1593
  human immunodeficiency virus encephalopathy, 1604
  hydrocephalus, 1615-1620
  increased intracranial pressure, 1573
  near-drowning, 1593-1594
  neuroblastoma, 1599
  neurologic examination, 1574-1578
  rabies, 1604-1605
  Reye syndrome, 1603-1604
  unconscious child, 1578-1585
Cerebral hyperemia, 1586
Cerebral palsy, 1746-1751, 1752-1753
Cerebrospinal fluid
  hydrocephalus, 1616
  normal laboratory ranges, 1795
Cerebrovascular accident, 277-278
Cerumen, 914
Cervical canal, 32
Cervical cap, 520, 525-528
Cervical mucus
  changes during menstrual cycle, 41, 42
  method of contraception, 516-517
Cervical ripening methods, 460-461
Cervical spine injury, 746
Cervical traction, 1718, 1719
Cervix, 30, 31-32
  adaptations during pregnancy, 110
  changes during menstrual cycle, 41
  incompetent, 219-220
  injury during childbirth, 441
  labor, 343-344, 345
    first stage, 403, 409
    woman's expected responses, 418
  laceration in postpartum hemorrhage, 539
  nullipara *versus* multipara, 107
  postpartum period, 482

Cesarean birth, 465-469
anesthesia, 366
care path, 470-471
CF; *see* Cystic fibrosis
Chadwick's sign, 109
Cheating, 1062
Chelation, 1440, 1442, 1444
Chemical burn, 1175
Chemotherapy
asthma, 1349
bone tumor, 1736
leukemia, 1521-1524
tuberculosis, 1343
Chest
cardiac disease, 1451
newborn assessment, 618, 631
nutritional status, 889
physical examination, 920-921
review of systems, 881
toddler, 993
Chest circumference, 592, 616, 620, 621
Chest compression, 1365
Chest pain, 1323
Chest physiotherapy, 1305, 1308
asthma and, 1350
cystic fibrosis, 1357-1358
Chest radiography, 1451
Chest syndrome, 1506
Chest tubes, 1478
Chickenpox, 242, 1030
Chief complaint, 877-878
Chiggers, 1675
Chilblain, 1703
Child; *see also* Adolescent; Infant; Preschooler; School-age child; Toddler
apheresis, 1537
blood transfusion therapy, 1534-1536
bone marrow transplantation, 1536-1537
cardiovascular dysfunction, 1450-1498
acquired cardiovascular disorders, 1481-1486
assessment, 1450-1453
congenital heart disease, 1453-1455, 1474-1481
congestive heart failure, 1465-1472
defects with decreased pulmonary blood flow, 1457-1465
defects with increased pulmonary blood flow, 1455
heart transplantation, 1494
hypoxemia, 1472-1474
mixed defects, 1464, 1465
obstructive defects, 1455-1457
vascular dysfunction, 1486-1494
cerebral dysfunction, 1572-1623
assessment, 1572-1578
brain tumor, 1594-1599
cerebral malformations, 1615-1620
head injury, 1585-1594
Child—cont'd
cerebral dysfunction—cont'd
intracranial infections, 1600-1605
neuroblastoma, 1599
seizure disorders, 1605-1614
unconscious child, 1578-1585
chronic illness, 1121-1156
changing trends in care, 1121-1123
education about disorder and general health care, 1142-1143
family coping, 1137-1142
impact on child, 1129-1132
impact on family, 1125-1129
impending death, 1132-1135
nurses' reactions to dying child, 1154-1155
planning for future, 1146-1148
promotion of normal development, 1143-1146
reaction of family, 1123-1125
support at time of diagnosis, 1135-1137
terminally ill or dying, 1148-1154
cognitive impairment, 1157-1168
diagnosis and classification, 1157-1158
Down syndrome, 1163-1167
education, 1159-1162
fragile X syndrome, 1167-1168
hospitalization, 1162-1163
endocrine dysfunction, 1624-1653
adrenal disorders, 1634-1640
diabetes mellitus, 1640-1652
pituitary disorders, 1624-1629
thyroid disorders, 1629-1634
gastrointestinal dysfunction, 1386-1403
constipation, 1395-1399
cystic fibrosis, 1356-1357, 1358
dehydration, 1386-1390
diarrhea, 1390-1395
gastroesophageal reflux, 1401-1403
Hirschsprung disease, 1399-1401
vomiting, 1401
genitourinary dysfunction, 1542-1571
acute renal failure, 1560-1563
chronic renal failure, 1563-1568
dialysis, 1568-1569
external defects, 1550-1551
glomerulonephritis, 1556-1558
hemolytic-uremic syndrome, 1558-1559
herpes simplex virus, 1667
kidney transplantation, 1569
myelodysplasia, 1756
nephrotic syndrome, 1551-1556
obstructive uropathy, 1549-1550
renal function assessment, 1542-1545
urinary tract infection, 240-242, 1545-1549
Child—cont'd
genitourinary dysfunction—cont'd
Wilms tumor, 1559-1560
growth and development, 844-865
biologic and physical, 846-848
environmental hazards, 861
heredity, 858-860
interpersonal relationships, 860-861
mass media influence, 862-863
mental, 852-854
nutrition, 860
personality, 850-852
physiologic changes, 848-849
play, 855-858
self-concept, 854-855
socioeconomic level, 861
stages and patterns, 844-846
stress, 861-862
temperament, 849-850
growth measurements, 1785-1789
health promotion, 826-843
adopted child, 835-837
divorce, 837-839
dual-earner families, 840
family roles, relationships, and strengths, 827-831
parenting, 831-835
reconstituted families, 840
single parenting, 839-840
working mothers, 841
hematologic dysfunction, 1499-1530; *see also* Hematologic dysfunction
defects in hemostasis, 1512-1517
neoplastic disorders, 1517-1530
red blood cell disorders, 1499-1512
immunologic deficiency disorders, 1530-1534
integumentary dysfunction, 1654-1705
acne, 1684-1687
burns, 1687-1703; *see also* Burns
dermatitis, 1671-1673
diaper rash, 1679-1682
eczema, 1682-1684
general therapeutic management, 1660-1664
insect and animal contacts, 1673-1679
skin infections, 1664-1671
skin lesions, 1654-1655
wounds, 1655-1660
musculoskeletal and articular dysfunction, 1706-1745
amputation, 1720-1721
bone and soft tissue tumors, 1735-1738
cast, 1714-1716
clubfoot, 1725-1726
developmental dysplasia of hip, 1721-1725
distraction, 1720
fracture, 1711-1714

Child—cont'd
  musculoskeletal and articular dysfunction—cont'd
    immobilization, 1706-1709
    juvenile rheumatoid arthritis, 1738-1741
    kyphosis and lordosis, 1729-1730
    Legg-Calvé-Perthes disease, 1728-1733
    metatarsus adductus, 1726-1727
    osteogenesis imperfecta, 1727-1728
    osteomyelitis, 1733-1734
    scoliosis, 1730-1733
    septic arthritis, 1734
    skeletal limb deficiency, 1727
    slipped femoral capital epiphysis, 1729
    soft tissue injury, 1709-1711
    systemic lupus erythematosus, 1741-1742
    traction, 1716-1720
    tuberculosis, 1734-1735
  neuromuscular dysfunction, 1746-1767
    botulism, 1764-1765
    cerebral palsy, 1746-1751, 1752-1753
    Guillain-Barré syndrome, 1762-1763
    juvenile spinal muscular atrophy, 1760
    muscular dystrophy, 1760-1762
    progressive infantile spinal muscular dystrophy, 1759-1760
    spina bifida, 1751-1758
    spinal cord injuries, 1765-1766
    tetanus, 1763-1764
  nursing interventions; *see* Pediatric nursing interventions
  physical examination, 893-931
    abdomen, 924-926
    anus, 928
    back and extremities, 928-930
    chest, 920-921
    ear, 914-918
    eyes, 908-914
    general appearance, 905-907
    genitalia, 926-928
    growth measurements, 896-900
    head and neck, 907-908
    heart, 922-924
    lungs, 921-922
    lymph nodes, 907
    mouth and throat, 918-920
    neurologic assessment, 930-931
    nose, 918
    physiologic measurements, 900-905
    preparation of child, 893-896
    sequence of examination, 893
    skin, 906-907
  reaction to illness and hospitalization, 1196-1204

Child—cont'd
  reaction to illness and hospitalization,—cont'd
    bodily injury and pain, 1200-1203
    loss of control, 1198-1200
    separation anxiety, 1196-1198
  respiratory dysfunction, 1321-1371; *see also* Respiratory dysfunction
    croup syndromes, 1334-1337
    infection, 1321-1326
    long-term, 1347-1361
    lower airway, 1337-1347
    respiratory emergency, 1361-1368
    upper tract, 1326-1333
  sensory impairment, 1168-1183
    conjunctivitis, 1181-1182
    deaf-blind, 1182
    hearing, 1168-1175
    retinoblastoma, 1182-1183
    visual, 1175-1181
  special needs, 1121-1156
    changing trends in care, 1121-1123
    education about disorder and general health care, 1142-1143
    family coping, 1137-1142
    impact on child, 1129-1132
    impact on family, 1125-1129
    impending death, 1132-1135
    nurses' reactions to dying child, 1154-1155
    planning for future, 1146-1148
    promotion of normal development, 1143-1146
    reaction of family, 1123-1125
    scope of problem, 1121, 1123
    support at time of diagnosis, 1135-1137
    terminally ill or dying, 1148-1154
  vital signs and parameters, 1792-1793
Child care arrangements, 949
Child custody
  adolescent mother, 331
  parenting partnerships, 839
Child neglect, 1039, 1044
Child pornography, 1041
Child prostitution, 1041
Child Welfare Services, 790
Childbearing
  cultural beliefs and practices, 16-17, 18
  practices related to infant temperament, 948
  preconception care, 75-77
Childbed fever, 543
Childbirth, 336-481
  adolescent mother, 328
  changing practices, 2
  complications, 444-481
    amniotic fluid embolism, 477-478
    dystocia, 452-472; *see also* Dystocia
    postdate pregnancy, 472-475
    premature rupture of membranes, 452

Childbirth—cont'd
  complications—cont'd
    preterm, 444-452
    prolapsed umbilical cord, 475
    sequelae of trauma, 546-550
    shoulder dystocia, 475
    uterine rupture, 475-477
  cultural beliefs and practices, 16-17, 18
  diabetic mother, 263
  episiotomy, 439-441
  fetal assessment, 373-393
    basis for, 374-375
    electronic, 376-377
    fetal blood sampling, 385
    fetal heart rate patterns, 377-385
    fetal pulse oximetry, 385-386
    guidelines and standards of nursing care, 387-388
    intermittent auscultation, 375-376
    intrauterine resuscitation, 388-389, 391
    preventive measures, 388
    protocol, 387
    working with monitor, 389-393
  first stage of labor, 394-424
    admission data, 395, 397
    ambulation and positioning, 414-416
    cultural factors, 400-402
    emergency interventions, 411-414
    father/partner role, 418-420
    interview, 398-399
    laboratory tests, 409-411
    physical examination, 402-409
    prenatal data, 395-398
    preparation for giving birth, 421-424
    psychosocial factors, 399-400
    siblings and, 420
    support measures, 416-418
  forceps-assisted birth, 462-464
  lacerations, 440-441
  management of discomfort during labor, 352-374
    administration of medication, 369-373
    anesthesia in obese woman, 366-367
    childbirth preparation methods, 354-355
    expression of pain, 353-354
    general anesthesia, 366
    informed consent, 369
    maternal hypothermia after analgesia and anesthesia, 367
    nerve block analgesia and anesthesia, 360-365
    relaxing and breathing techniques, 355-357
    sedatives, 358
    systemic analgesia, 358-359
  prebirth preparation, 166-168, 170-173

Childbirth—cont'd
preparation methods, 354-355
second stage of labor, 424-436
bearing-down efforts, 428-430
birthing beds and chairs, 430, 431
delivery room, 432-433
duration of, 425
emergency, 435-436
fetal heart rate, 430
maternal position, 427-428
potential problems, 425-427
prebirth considerations, 427, 428
siblings and, 435
vertex presentation, 433-435
as stressor, 14
third stage of labor, 436-441
Children with Special Health Needs, 790
Chilling, 497
Chinese-American culture
factors affecting family care, 19
food patterns, 190
growth standards of healthy children, 1787
health beliefs and practices, 818-819
postpartum care beliefs, 505
Chlamydia trachomatis
conjunctivitis, 1181
newborn infection, 758
during pregnancy, 232-233
respiratory infection, 1321
Chloasma, 116, 283
Chloral hydrate, 1222
Chlorhexidine, 1660
Chloride
normal laboratory ranges, 1795
nutritional significance, 1378
Chlorothiazide, 1467
Choanal atresia, 773
Chocolate hypersensitivity, 1385
Choking, 1008, 1012
Cholecalciferol, 1376-1377
Cholecystitis, 283
Cholelithiasis, 283
Cholera, 1397
Cholestasis, 119
Cholesterol
hypercholesterolemia, 1483-1484
normal laboratory ranges, 1795
Cholestyramine, 1484
Choline magnesium trisalicylate, 1223
Chordee, 619, 1551
Chorioamnionitis, 543
Chorion, 61
Chorionic villus, 60, 61
Chorionic villus sampling, 85, 94-95
Christian Science, 814
Christmas disease, 1512
Chromium, 1378
Chromosomal abnormalities, 54-56
amniocentesis, 91
hydatidiform mole, 222, 223
Chromosomal abnormalities—cont'd
prenatal diagnosis, 96
related risk factors, 82
Chromosomal studies, 1517
Chromosome, 51-53
Chronic hypertension, 201
Chronic illness, 1121-1156
changing trends in care, 1121-1123
education about disorder and general health care, 1142-1143
family coping, 1137-1142
impact on child, 1129-1132
impact on family, 1125-1129
impending death, 1132-1135
nurses' reactions to dying child, 1154-1155
planning for future, 1146-1148
promotion of normal development, 1143-1146
reaction of family, 1123-1125
scope of problem, 1121, 1123
support at time of diagnosis, 1135-1137
terminally ill or dying, 1148-1154
Chronic renal failure, 1563-1568
Chronic sorrow, 1125
Church of Christ Scientist, 814
Church of God, 814
Church of Jesus Christ of Latter Day Saints, 815
Chvostek sign, 1632
Chymotrypsin, 663
Ciliary muscle, 608
Circulation
cardiopulmonary resuscitation, 1363
changes at birth, 1453-1454
changes during pregnancy, 114
delayed wound healing, 1660
fetal, 65-66, 592, 593
human development milestones, 70-72
pulmonary, 592, 594
shock, 1489
Circumcision, 653-655
female, 26
home visit assessment, 582
Cirrhosis, 1416-1417
Citrovorum factor, 1375
Clamping of umbilical cord, 628
Clavicle
neonatal birth trauma, 635, 748
palpation, 623
Clean-catch specimen, 1281
Cleavage, 58, 59
Cleft lip or palate, 710-711, 773-774, 1418-1422
Climacterium, 42
Clinical nurse specialist, 794
Clinical practice guidelines, 793
Clitoris, 25-26, 599
Cloacal exstrophy, 1431
Clonus, 205
Closed captioning, 1172
Closed family, 13
Closed fracture, 1712
Clostridium botulinum, 663, 1397, 1765
Clostridium difficile, 1397
Clostridium perfringens, 1397
Clostridium tetani, 1763
Clothing
first trimester, 145
newborn, 645-646
second trimester, 153-154
Clotting disorders during pregnancy, 230-231
Clotting factors, 114, 486
Clotting time, 1795
Clove hitch restraint, 1278
Clubbing, 1472
Clubfoot, 625, 775, 1725-1726
Co-sleeping, 1027
Coagulation
changes during pregnancy, 114
newborn, 599
tests, 231
Coagulation factors, 114, 486
Coarctation of aorta, 1458-1459
Cobalamin, 1375
Cocaine
adolescent abuse, 1113
breastfeeding and, 766
use during pregnancy, 303-305, 308, 759, 761
Coccidioidomycosis, 1670
Coccygeus muscle, 34
Coccyx, 34, 36-37, 111
Codeine, 1224
Coffee use during pregnancy, 310
Cognitive development, 48
adolescent, 317, 1090, 1096
child, 852-854
function of play, 857-858
infant, 943-944
preschooler, 1017-1018, 1023
school-age child, 1056-1057, 1064-1065
toddler, 995-996
Cognitive impairment, 1157-1168
diagnosis and classification, 1157-1158
Down syndrome, 1163-1167
education, 1159-1162
fragile X syndrome, 1167-1168
hospitalization, 1162-1163
Cognitive power, 1573
Cohabitation, 9
Coining, 812
Coitus interruptus, 515
Cold injury, 1703
Cold sore, 1667
Cold stress, 595-596
Colectomy, 1411
Colestipol, 1484

Colic, 675, 979-980, 981
Collaborative relationships, 1189
Collarbone; *see* Clavicle
Color tool, 1213
Color vision, 913-914
Colostrum, 111, 484, 599, 662, 668
Columnar epithelium, 32
Coma, 1573-1574, 1579
Combined family, 9-10
Combined immunodeficiency disease, 96
Comedone, 1684
Commercial formula, 692
Comminuted fracture, 1712
Common iliac artery, 33
Communal family, 10-11
Communicable diseases, 1028-1039
  chickenpox, 1030
  diphtheria, 1030-1031
  erythema infectiosum, 1032
  exanthema subitum, 1032
  infection control, 1028
  measles, 1032-1033
  mumps, 1034
  nursing care plan, 1038
  pertussis, 1034
  poliomyelitis, 1034-1035
  prevention of complications, 1029
  rubella, 1036
  scarlet fever, 1036-1037
Communication, 866-877
  with child, 872-875, 876-877
  cultural factors, 809-810
  family, 12, 868-875
    health care, 18-19
    special needs child, 1122, 1123
  guidelines for interviewing, 867-868
  high-risk infant, 713
  loss and grief, 554
  mentally retarded child, 1161
  nonverbal, 867
  between parent and child, 506
  parent-professional collaboration in home care, 1189-1190
  parents, 868-872
  techniques, 875, 876-877
  with teenagers, 1091
  verbal, 866-867
Compassionate Friends, 1151-1153
Compensated shock, 1490
Complementary medicine practices, 1207
Complete abortion, 217
Complete blood count
  assessment of hematologic function, 243
  standard laboratory values in women, 1776
Complete breech, 339, 455
Complete fracture, 1712
Complete heart block, 1485
Complex partial seizure, 1606, 1608, 1611
Compliance, 1262-1264
Complicated bereavement, 562-563
Complicated fracture, 1712
Compound fracture, 1712
Compound skull fracture, 1587
Compression
  cerebral, 1586-1587
  chest, 1365
  fetal head, 381
  postpartum hemorrhage, 539
  spinal cord, 1766
  torus fracture, 1712
  umbilical cord, 382
Computed tomography
  cerebral assessment, 1577
  epilepsy, 1608
  genitourinary dysfunction, 1543
  head injury, 1590
Conception, 58-60
Concha, 918
Concrete operations, 853
Concussion, 1586-1587
Condom
  adolescent use, 320
  female, 519, 520
  male, 519-521
Conduction disturbances, 1485
Conduction heat loss, 595
Conduction tests, 917
Conductive hearing loss, 1168
Condylomata acuminata, 239-240
Confidentiality
  adolescent privacy, 331
  interview, 868
Confirming behaviors, 867
Confusion, 1574
Congenital adrenal hyperplasia, 96, 638, 1637-1639
Congenital aganglionic megacolon, 1399-1401
Congenital anal stenosis, 1431
Congenital anomalies, 769-780
  cardiovascular, 772
  central nervous system, 770-772
  cerebral palsy, 1746-1751, 1752-1753
  clubfoot, 1725-1726
  developmental dysplasia of hip, 1721-1725
  diagnosis, 777-779
  family support, 1138
  gastrointestinal, 773-776
  genitourinary, 776-777
  heart; *see* Congenital heart disease
  juvenile spinal muscular atrophy, 1760
  maternal diabetes mellitus, 255, 741-743
  metatarsus adductus, 1726-1727
  muscular dystrophy, 1760-1762
  musculoskeletal, 775-776
  nongenetic factors, 73
  osteogenesis imperfecta, 1727-1728
Congenital anomalies—cont'd
  prenatal diagnosis, 96
  progressive infantile spinal muscular dystrophy, 1759-1760
  respiratory, 772-773
  skeletal limb deficiency, 1727
  spina bifida, 1751-1758
Congenital disability, 1122
Congenital erythropoietic porphyria, 96
Congenital heart disease, 1450, 1453-1455
  congestive heart failure, 1465-1472
  defects with decreased pulmonary blood flow, 1457-1465
    aortic stenosis, 1459
    coarctation of aorta, 1458-1459
    hypoplastic left heart syndrome, 1464
    patent ductus arteriosus, 1458
    pulmonary stenosis, 1460
    tetralogy of Fallot, 1460-1461
    total anomalous pulmonary venous connection, 1462-1463
    transposition of great arteries, 1462
    tricuspid atresia, 1461
    truncus arteriosus, 1463-1464
  defects with increased pulmonary blood flow, 1455
  hypoxemia, 1472-1474
  mixed defects, 1465
  nursing management, 1474-1481
  obstructive defects, 1455-1457
Congenital hypothyroidism, 638
Congenital rubella syndrome, 238, 755-756
Congenital syphilis, 234
Congenital varicella syndrome, 242
Congestive heart failure, 281, 1465-1472
Conjugal family, 9
Conjunctiva, 908
Conjunctivitis, 233, 1181-1182
Connective tissue disorders, 1727-1728
Conscious relaxation, 156
Conscious sedation
  during cerebral assessment, 1577, 1578
  medications for, 1222
  pediatric surgery, 1261
Consciousness, altered states, 1573-1574
Consent
  drugs during labor, 369
  pediatric nursing interventions, 1250-1252
Constipation
  gastrointestinal dysfunction, 1387
  opioid-induced, 1229
  pediatric, 1395-1399
  during pregnancy, 152, 196
Constitutional delay, 1073
Consumer involvement, 4
Contact dermatitis, 1671

Contact lenses, 1181
Contact precautions, 1272-1273
Continuous ambulatory peritoneal dialysis, 1568
Continuous arteriovenous hemodialysis, 1568
Continuous cycling peritoneal dialysis, 1568
Continuous positive airway pressure, 702
Continuous venovenous hemofiltration, 1568
Contraception
  adolescent use, 320, 329, 331
  breastfeeding as, 677
  chemical and mechanical, 517-521
  cultural considerations, 505
  diaphragm, 525, 526-527
  enforced, 524
  intrauterine device, 525-529
  methods, 514
  oral contraceptives, 521-524
  periodic abstinence, 515-517
  postpartum period, 513-515
  predictor test for ovulation, 517
  sterilization, 529-531
  vaginal ring, 524-525
Contraceptive diaphragm, 244, 525, 526-527
Contraction
  first stage of labor, 407-409
  impending labor, 168
  postpartum, 480-481
  primary power in labor, 343-345
  tocolytic suppression, 447-448
Contraction stress test, 95, 97, 98-100
Contusion
  cerebral, 1587
  soft tissue, 1709-1710
Convection heat loss, 595
Conversion reaction, 1079
Cooley anemia, 1510-1511
Coomb's test, 95
Cooper ligaments, 38
Cooperative play, 857
Cooties, 1673-1674
Coping
  adolescent, 1100-1101
  child, 862
  family of special needs child, 1128, 1137-1142
  new families, 510-512
  parenting, 832
  postpartum period, 510-512
  pregnancy, 127, 195
  special needs child, 1131-1132
  suicide, 1116
Copper, 1378
Cord blood testing, 628
Cornea, 909
Cornua, 31
Corpora cavernosa, 43
Corporal punishment, 834-835
Corpus, uterine, 28, 29, 30
Corpus luteum, 107
Corpus spongiosum, 43
Corrosives, 1436
Corticosteroids
  asthma, 1349
  delayed wound healing, 1660
  juvenile rheumatoid arthritis, 1739
  leukemia and lymphoma, 1522
  topical therapy, 1661
Cortisol, 483
Corynebacterium diphtheriae, 1328
Cotrel-Dubousset procedure, 1732
Cotyledon, 64
Cough
  poliomyelitis, 1035
  respiratory infection, 1322, 1323
  whooping, 1034, 1341
Counseling
  genetic, 73-75
  maternal drug abuse, 309
  pregnancy
    diabetes mellitus, 254-255
    iron supplementation, 196
    nutrition, 327-328
    prebirth preparation, 167-168
    TORCH infection, 237
  toddler nutrition, 1003-1004
Countertraction, 1716
Couplet care, 493
Courtesy stigma, 1127
Couvelaire uterus, 228
Cowper's gland, 45
Cow's milk
  as allergen, 663
  allergy, 1385-1386
  unmodified, 695
Coxa plana, 1728-1729
Coxa vara, 1729
Coxsackievirus B, 242
CPAP; *see* Continuous positive airway pressure
CPD; *see* Cephalopelvic disproportion
CPR; *see* Cardiopulmonary resuscitation
CPT; *see* Chest physiotherapy
Crack cocaine, 303-305, 1113
Cradle cap, 1684
Cradling hold, 646, 670
Cramping during pregnancy, 119
Cranial nerves, 746, 931, 932
Craniofacial dysostosis, 1615
Cranioschisis, 1754
Craniosynostosis, 1615
Cranium
  deformities, 1615
  head injury, 1586
  newborn molding, 603
Crawling, 942
Crawling reflex, 605
Cream, contraceptive, 519
Creatine kinase, 1796
Creatinine, 1545
  amniocentesis, 91
  normal laboratory ranges, 1796
Creative expression, 1232-1233
Creativity, 858
Creeping, 942
Creighton method of contraception, 515, 516-517
Cremasteric reflex, 927
Cremation, 554
Crepitus, 635
Creutzfeldt-Jakob disease, 1626
CRF; *see* Chronic renal failure
Cri-du-chat syndrome, 56, 778
Crib-o-gram, 917
Cricoid pressure, 366
Crohn disease, 1409-1412
Crohn's and Colitis Foundation of America, Inc., 1412
Cromolyn sodium, 1349
Cross-eye, 1176
Cross-racial adoption, 837
Crossed extension reflex, 606
Croup syndromes, 1334-1337
Crouzon disease, 1615
Crown-to-heel recumbent length, 898
Crown-to-rump length, 616, 620
Crowning, 433
Crust, 1658
Crutchfield tongs, 1719
Crying, 610, 611, 960, 961
Cryoprecipitate, 1513
Cryotherapy, 239-240
Cryptococcosis, 1670
Cryptorchidism, 1551
CST; *see* Contraction stress test
CTX; *see* Cyclophosphamide
Cuban-American culture, 822-823
Cued speech, 1172
Cul-de-sac of Douglas, 29, 30, 35
Cullen's sign, 221
Cultural considerations, 800-825
  affluence, 803-804
  biculture, 805
  bonding, 507
  circumcision, 653
  communication, 869-870
  customs and folkways, 808-811
  death, 554
  ethnicity, 801-802
  family health, 15-19
  food practices, 190-191, 886
  health beliefs and practices, 811-812
  home care, 1188-1189
  neonates, 643
  peer cultures, 804-805
  postpartum psychosocial assessment, 504, 505
  poverty, 803
  pregnancy

Cultural considerations—cont'd
  pregnancy—cont'd
    adolescent, 322
    antepartum cultural assessment, 80
    beliefs about pain, 367
    birth practices, 400-402
    father participation in childbirth, 419-420
    postpartum period, 504-505
    prenatal care, 143-146
  religion, 804
  schools, 804
  social class, 802-803
  social roles, 801
  susceptibility to health problems, 806-808
Cultural context, 15
Cultural relativism, 15-18, 808
Cultural shock, 806, 809
Culture, defined, 15
Cultured epithelium, 1695
Cupping, 812
Curling ulcer, 1690, 1698
Cushing syndrome, 1636-1637
Customs and folkways, 20, 808-811
Cutaneous stimulation for pain relief, 1220
Cutaneous ureterostomy, 1550
Cutis marmorata, 616
CVS; *see* Chorionic villus sampling
Cyanosis, 1472, 1473
  assessment of respiratory function, 1323
  cardiac disease, 1451
  racial differences, 907
Cyclophosphamide, 680, 1524
Cyclosporine, 680
Cyst, 1657
  ovarian, 286
  prenatal diagnosis, 97
Cystic fibrosis, 58, 1356-1361
  during pregnancy, 282-283
  prenatal diagnosis, 97
Cystic Fibrosis Foundation, 1360
Cystinosis, 96
Cystitis, 1525, 1546
Cystocele, 547
Cystosar; *see* Cytosine arabinoside
Cytabarine; *see* Cytosine arabinoside
Cytochemical markers, 1517
Cytologic studies, 778
Cytomegalovirus
  newborn infection, 756
  during pregnancy, 237, 238
  prenatal diagnosis, 96
Cytosine arabinoside, 1523
Cytotoxic drugs, 1739
Cytotrophoblast, 63
Cytoxan; *see* Cyclophosphamide

D

Dacarbazine, 1524
Daily fetal movement count, 82-83
Daily food guide, pregnancy and lactation, 183, 195
Danazol, 529
Darvocet; *see* Propoxyphene
Darvon; *see* Propoxyphene
DAST; *see* Drug Abuse Screening Test
Data collection process, 19-20
Daunorubicin, 1522
Day care, 949
Deaf, defined, 1168
Deaf-blind child, 1182
Deaf-mute, defined, 1168
Death
  childhood, 1148-1154
    impending, 1132-1135
    reaction of family, 1128-1129
  cultural considerations, 554
  maternal, 562
  newborn, 550-563, 551, 556
    anticipatory grief, 552
    communicating and caring techniques, 554-556
    complicated bereavement, 562-563
    documentation, 558-561
    family issues, 717-718
    grief responses, 551-552
    options for parents, 556-558
    physical comfort, 556
Debridement of burn, 1693
Decannulation, 1310
Deceleration injury, 1586
Deceleration of fetal heart rate, 380-383, 384
Decerebrate posturing, 1576
Decibel, 1168-1169
Decidua basalis, 60
Decidua capsularis, 60, 61
Decision making, 795
Decompensated shock, 1490
Decorticate posturing, 1576
Decrement of contraction, 407
Deep breathing, 1258
Deep dermal burn, 1687, 1689
Deep palpation, 925
Deep sleep state in newborn, 611
Deep tendon reflexes, 605
  physical examination, 930
  preeclampsia-eclampsia, 205
Deformation injury, 1586
Dehydration, 1386-1390
  hospitalized child, 1268
  hypoxemic child, 1473-1474
Delayed hemolytic reaction, 1536
DeLee mucus-trap suction apparatus, 632-633
Delivery room, 431, 432-433
Deltoid injection site, 1291
Demand feeding, 645, 672
Demerol; *see* Meperidine
Democratic parenting style, 833
Denial
  family reaction to child's chronic illness or disability, 1124, 1137
  hospitalized child, 1196-1198
Dental health
  adolescent, 1099
  infant, 961
  during pregnancy, 139
  preschooler, 1027
  school-age child, 1066-1068
  toddler, 1004-1006
Denver Articulation Screening Examination, 1025
Denver Eye Screening Test, 912
Denver II Developmental/Sensory Assessment, 931-934, 1780-1784
Deoxyribonucleic acid, 51, 53-54
Department of Transportation, National Highway Traffic Safety Administration, 1009
Dependent edema, 205
Depressed skull fracture, 1587
Depression
  during and after pregnancy, 296-298
  family reaction to child's chronic illness or disability, 1125
  postpartum, 510
  school-age child, 1079-1080
Dermatitis
  contact, 1671
  diaper, 1679-1682
  eczema, 1682-1684
  pathophysiology, 1655
  seborrheic, 1684
Dermatoglyphics, 778-779, 906-907
Dermatophytoses, 1668, 1669
Dermis, 600
Descent in labor, 347-348, 424, 431
Desensitization, 1025
Desmopressin
  diabetes insipidus, 1628
  enuresis, 1077
  hemophilia, 1513
Desquamation, 601
Detachment, hospitalized child, 1196-1198
Detoxification during pregnancy, 308-309
Deuteranomaly, 913
Development; *see* Growth and development
Developmental delay, 1122
Developmental disability, 1122
Developmental dysplasia of hip, 635-636, 775, 1721-1725
Developmental pace, 846
Developmental/Sensory Assessment, 1780-1784
Developmental task, 844
  of adolescence, 317
  of parenthood, 330-333
  of pregnancy, 321-322

Developmental theory, 13-14
Dextrose, 699
Diabetes insipidus, 1628-1629
Diabetes mellitus, 1640-1652
  breastfeeding, 687
  delayed wound healing, 1660
  etiology, 1640-1641
  infant of diabetic mother, 741-746
  pathophysiology, 1641-1642
  during pregnancy, 251-265
    antepartum care, 259-263
    classification, 252-253
    diet, 195
    fetal and neonatal risks and complications, 255-257
    fetal surveillance, 257-258
    labor and birth, 263
    laboratory tests, 257
    maternal risks and complications, 255
    metabolic changes, 253
    pathogenesis, 252
    postpartum care, 263-265
    preconception counseling, 254-255
    pregestational diabetes, 253-254
  therapeutic management, 1642-1644
Diabetic ketoacidosis, 255, 256, 1644
Diagnosis-related groups, 791
Dialysis, 1565-1567, 1568-1569
Diaper rash, 645, 1679-1682
Diaphoresis
  dehydration, 1389
  postpartum, 484, 486
Diaphragm
  contraceptive, 520, 525, 526-527
  displacement during pregnancy, 108, 114
Diaphragmatic hernia, 96, 773, 1426
Diaphysis, 847
Diarrhea
  gastrointestinal dysfunction, 1387
  malnutrition and, 1384
  pediatric, 1390-1395
  respiratory infection, 1322
Diastasis recti abdominis, 118, 483, 618, 624
Diastatic skull fracture, 1587
Diastolic blood pressure, 594
Diazepam
  conscious sedation, 1222
  eclampsia, 213
Diazoxide, 272
DIC; *see* Disseminated intravascular coagulation
Dick-Read method of childbirth, 354
Dietary history, 188, 879, 886
Dietary intake, 194, 885-886
  adolescent obesity, 1108
  anemia, 1504
  breastfeeding and, 675-677
  chronic renal failure, 1564
Dietary intake—cont'd
  hospitalized child, 1268
  infant dental health, 961
  during pregnancy
    cultural considerations, 146
    diabetic mother, 259-260
    gestational diabetes mellitus, 267
    preeclampsia, 202, 209
  toddler, 1066
Diethylstilbestrol, 529
Differential blood count, 131, 1500
Differentiation, 844, 845-846
Difficult child, 850
Digestion
  infant, 663, 938-939
  newborn, 597
Digestive enzymes, 597
Digital subtraction angiography, 1577
Digital thermometer, 902
Digitalis, 272
Digits, extranumerary, 603
Digoxin
  normal laboratory values, 1796
  toxicity, 1468-1469
Dilation and curettage
  early pregnancy bleeding, 219
  first trimester abortion, 290
  second trimester abortion, 291
Dilation in labor process, 344
Dilaudid; *see* Hydromorphone
Diphtheria, 1030-1031
Diphtheria, tetanus, pertussis immunization, 658, 961-962, 964-965, 968
Dipstick test, 207
Direct bilirubin, 598
Direct-contact transmission, 1272-1273
Disability
  assessment of pregnant woman, 128
  child, 1121-1156
    changing trends in care, 1121-1123
    education about disorder and general health care, 1142-1143
    family coping, 1137-1142
    impact on child, 1129-1132
    impact on family, 1125-1129
    impending death, 1132-1135
    morbidity, 788
    nurses' reactions to dying child, 1154-1155
    planning for future, 1146-1148
    promotion of normal development, 1143-1146
    reaction of family, 1123-1125
    scope of problem, 1121, 1123
    support at time of diagnosis, 1135-1137
    terminally ill or dying, 1148-1154
Disaccharides, 663
Discharge, vaginal
  foul-smelling, 572
Discharge, vaginal—cont'd
  newborn, 599
Discharge planning, 1264
  abdominal surgery during pregnancy, 287
  breastfeeding, 695
  burn victim, 1700
  cardiac surgery, 1479
  child abuse, 1047-1049
  early postpartum, 565-566
  high-risk newborn, 718, 766-767
  home care, 1187, 1188
  hospitalized child, 1237, 1239-1241
  Kawasaki disease, 1488-1489
  newborn, 655-659, 695
  postpartum, 482, 512
  teaching sheet, 573
Discipline
  infant, 949
  mentally retarded child, 1161-1162
  parenting, 833-835
  school-age child, 1062
Disconfirming behaviors, 867
Disease
  growth and development, 861
  prevention, 794
Dislocation, 1710-1711
  hip, 625, 635-636, 1721
Disorientation, 1574
Disseminated intravascular coagulation, 199, 230, 1516
Distancing language, 866-867
Distraction, 1720
Distraction techniques for pain, 1220
Distributive shock, 1489
Diuresis
  magnesium sulfate therapy, 212
  postpartum, 484
Diuretics
  congestive heart failure, 1467
  hearing loss, 713
  use during pregnancy, 115
Diuril; *see* Chlorothiazide
Diverticulum, 1409
Divided custody, 839
Divorce, 837-839
Dizygotic twins, 69, 830
DNA; *see* Deoxyribonucleic acid
Dobutamine, 1366
Documentation
  child abuse, 1046
  during childbirth, 432
  fetal monitoring, 391, 1774
  miscarriage and ectopic pregnancy, 558, 559
  postpartum, 491-492
  stillbirth or newborn death, 560
Doll's head maneuver, 1575
Dolophine; *see* Methadone
Domestic mimicry, 996
Domestic violence, 310-311

Dominant gene, 52
Donor milk bank, 688
Dopamine, 1366
Doppler blood flow analysis, 88
  blood pressure measurement, 903
  preeclampsia-eclampsia, 206
Doppler effect, 88
Doppler ultrasound stethoscope, 133
Dorsogluteal injection site, 1291
Dorsolumbar lordosis, 118
DOT test, 912
Doubt and shame, 995
Douching, 34, 515
Down syndrome, 54-56, 777, 778, 1163-1167
Doxorubicin, 680, 1522
Dramatic play, 856, 1020, 1233
Drawing, communication with child, 877
Dreams, 876
Dressings, 1660, 1661
  topical therapy, 1663-1664
DRGs; *see* Diagnosis-related groups
Drop attack, 1606
Droplet precautions, 1272, 1273
Drowning, 787, 1593-1594
  adolescent, 1103
  infant, 976
  school-age child, 1070
  toddler, 1007, 1010
Drowsiness state in newborn, 611
Drug Abuse Screening Test, 306
Drug tolerance, 1112
Drugs
  administration, 1284-1299
    determination of dosage, 1284-1286
    family teaching and home care, 1298-1299
    intramuscular, 1288-1292
    intravenous, 1293
    nasogastric, orogastric, or gastrostomy, 1296
    optic, otic, and nasal, 1297-1298
    oral, 1286-1288
    peripheral venous access devices, 1294-1296
    rectal, 1296-1297
    subcutaneous and intradermal, 1292-1293
  attention-deficit hyperactivity disorder, 1076
  burn victim, 1692-1693
  cardiopulmonary resuscitation, 1365
  cutaneous reactions, 1672
  effects on breastfeeding, 679-680
  juvenile rheumatoid arthritis, 1739
  during labor, 358-373
    administration of medication, 369-373
    anesthesia in obese woman, 366-367
    general anesthesia, 366
    informed consent, 369
Drugs—cont'd
  during labor,—cont'd
    maternal hypothermia after analgesia and anesthesia, 367
    nerve block, 360-365
    sedatives, 358
    systemic analgesia, 358-359
  during pregnancy, 139-140
    high risk factor, 81
    history during initial assessment interview, 127
    negative impact on maternal nutrition, 186-187
    testing, 303
DTIC-Dome; *see* Dacarbazine
DTP; *see* Diphtheria, tetanus, pertussis immunization
Dual-earner family, 840
Dubowitz scoring system, 614, 713
Duchenne-Erb paralysis, 625, 743, 748
Duchenne muscular dystrophy, 97, 1760, 1761
Ductus arteriosus, 66, 592, 594, 1453
Ductus venosus, 592, 594
Duncan mechanism, 437
Dunlop traction, 1717
Duvall's developmental stages of family, 13
Dwarfism, 1073
Dwyer instrumentation, 1732
Dysfunctional labor, 452-453, 454, 473-474
Dyskinetic cerebral palsy, 1747
Dyslalia, 1025
Dysmature infant, 739-740
Dysmenorrhea, 39, 1105
Dyspareunia
  chlamydial infection, 233
  postpartum, 482
Dysphagia, 1387
Dyspnea during pregnancy, 114, 165
Dysrhythmia, 1484-1485
Dystocia, 452-472
  abnormal labor patterns, 456-458
  alterations of pelvic structure, 453
  augmentation of labor, 462
  cesarean birth, 465-469
  dysfunctional labor, 452-453, 454
  fetal causes, 454-456
  forceps-assisted birth, 462-464
  induction of labor, 460-462
  position of woman, 456
  psychologic response, 456
  shoulder, 475
  vacuum extraction, 464-465
  vaginal birth after cesarean, 469-472
  version, 459-460
Dysuria, 233

E

Ear
  changes during pregnancy, 114
Ear—cont'd
  medication administration, 1297-1298
  newborn, 608
    assessment, 617, 622, 623
    fetal alcohol syndrome, 760
  nutritional status, 888
  otitis media, 1331-1333
  physical examination, 914-918
  review of systems, 881
  rhabdomyosarcoma, 1738
Ear sensor, 902
Early postpartum discharge, 565-566
  effects on breastfeeding, 674
Eastern Orthodox, 815
Eating behavior
  adolescent, 1099
  nutrition questionnaire, 192
Eating disorders, 1106-1111
Ecchymosis, 1709-1710
  birth trauma, 635, 746, 747
  racial differences, 907
  skin lesions, 1655
ECF; *see* Extracellular fluid
Echocardiography, 1451, 1577
Eclampsia, 199, 201, 212-215
ECMO; *see* Extracorporeal membrane oxygenation
Ectocervix, 32, 482
Ectoderm, 62
Ectopic pregnancy, 220-222
  documentation, 558, 559
  prenatal diagnosis, 97
ECV; *see* External cephalic version
Eczema, 1682-1684
Edema
  birth trauma, 635
  burns, 1696
  cerebral, 1588
  delayed wound healing, 1660
  nephrotic syndrome, 1552
  physiologic, 116
  preeclampsia, 200, 201
  pulmonary, 448
Educable mentally retarded, 1158
Education
  cerebral palsied child, 1750
  cognitive impairment, 1159-1162
  preparation for postpartum period, 571-574
Education for All Handicapped Children Act, 790
Education of Handicapped Act Amendments of 1986, 790
Edwards syndrome, 778
EFAs; *see* Essential fatty acids
Effacement, 344, 409
Effleurage, 166, 356
EFM; *see* Electronic fetal monitoring
Eggs
  hypersensitivity, 663, 1385
  needs during pregnancy, 183

Ego, 995, 1059-1060
Egocentrism, 317, 997
EIA test; *see* Enzyme immunoassay
Elastase, 663
Elastic hose, 153
Elbow restraint, 1278
Elective abortion, 289-292
Electrical burn, 976
Electrical stimulation, 1731-1732
Electrocardiography, 1451
Electrode placement in newborn, 701
Electroencephalography, 1577, 1608
Electrolytes
  blood transfusion, 1536
  changes during pregnancy, 115
Electronic fetal monitoring, 95-100, 373, 378-379
  contraction stress test, 98-100
  fetal responses to hypoxia and asphyxia, 97
  guidelines and standards of nursing care, 387-388
  human immunodeficiency virus infected mother, 236
  indications, 95-97
  meconium indication, 93
  nonstress test, 97-98
  nursing responsibilities, 1773-1775
  working with monitor, 389-394
Electronic thermometer, 901
Electrophysiologic studies, 1451, 1452
Elimination
  maternal
    during labor, 415
    postpartum, 492, 493, 495, 499-501
  newborn, 657
    high-risk infant, 708
    home visit assessment, 582
  pediatric nursing interventions, 1315-1316
  unconscious child, 1582
Emancipated minor, 331, 1251
Embalming, 554
Embolism, amniotic fluid, 437, 477
Embryo, 60-65
Emergency admission, 1242
Emergency interventions
  burns, 1690-1691
  eye injury, 1175
  fracture, 1713
  head injury, 1589
  hypoglycemia, 1649
  poisoning, 1435-1439
  pregnancy
    during labor, 411, 412-413
    postpartum hemorrhagic shock, 542
    shoulder dystocia, 475
    vertex presentation, 426, 435-436
  respiratory, 1361-1368
  seizure, 1611
Emergency interventions—cont'd
  shock, 1491
  tracheostomy, 1310
Emergency medical service, 1362
EMLA; *see* Eutectic mixture of local anesthetics
Emotional abuse, 1039, 1043, 1044
Emotional deprivation, 860-861
Emotional neglect, 1039
Emotional support
  after cardiac surgery, 1478-1479
  blind child, 1178
  diabetes mellitus, 1650-1652
  family of special needs child, 1137
  genetic counseling, 75
  during labor, 416-418
  leukemia, 1525
  maternal hemorrhagic disorders, 229
  preeclampsia, 208
  third trimester, 163-164
  unconscious child, 1583
Emotions
  adolescent, 1090
  during and after pediatric procedures, 1256-1257
  cultural factors, 810
  grief, 551, 552
  high risk newborn, 712-713
  pregnancy
    first trimester, 145
    third trimester, 163-164
Empathy, 870
Employment during pregnancy, 136-137
Empowerment, 791
Encephalitis, 1603
Encephalocele, 771, 1754
Encephalopathy
  human immunodeficiency virus, 1604
  lead, 1441
  Reye syndrome, 1603-1604
Encopresis, 1395
  gastrointestinal dysfunction, 1387
  school-age child, 1077-1078
End-stage liver disease, 1417
End-stage renal disease, 1565
Endocarditis, 1481-1482
Endocervical canal, 28, 32
Endocrine dysfunction, 1624-1653
  adrenal disorders, 1634-1640
    Addison disease, 1635-1636
    adrenocortical insufficiency, 1634-1636
    congenital adrenogenital hyperplasia, 1637-1639
    Cushing syndrome, 1636-1637
    hyperaldosteronism, 1639
    pheochromocytoma, 1639-1640
  diabetes mellitus, 1640-1652
    antepartum care, 259-263
    breastfeeding, 687
    classification, 252-253
Endocrine dysfunction—cont'd
  diabetes mellitus—cont'd
    delayed wound healing, 1660
    diet, 195
    etiology, 1640-1641
    fetal and neonatal risks and complications, 255-257
    fetal surveillance, 257-258
    infant of diabetic mother, 741-746
    labor and birth, 263
    laboratory tests, 257
    maternal risks and complications, 255
    metabolic changes, 253
    pathogenesis, 252
    pathophysiology, 1641-1642
    postpartum care, 263-265
    preconception counseling, 254-255
    pregestational diabetes, 253-254
    therapeutic management, 1642-1644
  pituitary disorders, 1624-1629
    diabetes insipidus, 1628-1629
    hyperfunction, 1627
    hypopituitarism, 1624-1627
    precocious puberty, 1627-1628
    syndrome of inappropriate antidiuretic hormone, 1629
  during pregnancy, 251-270
    diabetes mellitus, 251-265; *see also* Diabetes mellitus
    gestational diabetes mellitus, 265-268
    hyperemesis gravidarum, 268
    thyroid disorders, 269-270
  thyroid disorders, 1629-1634
    goiter, 1630
    Graves' disease, 1631-1632
    hyperparathyroidism, 1634
    hypoparathyroidism, 1633-1634
    juvenile hypothyroidism, 1629-1630
    lymphocytic thyroiditis, 1630-1631
    during pregnancy, 269-270
Endocrine system
  adaptations
    during labor, 352
    postpartum, 483
    during pregnancy, 119-120, 201
  fetal, 68
  review of systems, 881
Endoderm, 62
Endometrial cycle, 40, 41
Endometritis, 543
Endometrium, 28, 29
  blastocyst embedded in, 62
  changes during pregnancy, 107
  postpartum, 481
Endorphins, 360
Enema, pediatric, 1315
Energy, 663
  needs during pregnancy, 177-182
  postpartum, 492, 493

Engagement, labor, 338, 347
Engorgement
breast, 484-485, 498, 501, 680-681
splanchnic, 499
Enterobiasis, 1405-1406
Enterocolitis, necrotizing, 736-737
Enterotoxin, 243
Entrainment, 508
Enuresis, 1077
Environmental risks, 80, 81
attention-deficit hyperactivity disorder, 1076
delayed wound healing, 1660
effects on breastfeeding, 679-680
growth and development, 861
high-risk newborn, 714
newborn, 642-643
physical abuse of child, 1040
safety measures in pediatric nursing interventions, 1274
Enzyme immunoassay, 501
Enzyme-linked immunosorbent assay, 105
Enzymes, infant digestion, 597, 663
Eosinophil count, 1500, 1796
Epidermal stripping, 1266
Epidermis
injury, 1655-1656
newborn, 600
Epididymis, 44, 45
Epidural block
during labor, 363-365
pediatric, 1227
Epidural blood patch, 363
Epidural hematoma, 1586-1587
Epidural hemorrhage, 1588
Epiglottis, 1334-1335
Epilepsy, 1605-1614
during pregnancy, 284
Epilepsy Foundation of America, 1613
Epileptogenic focus, 1606
Epinephrine, 1634
for cardiopulmonary resuscitation, 1366
neonatal resuscitation, 699
Epiphyseal cartilage plate, 848
Epiphysis, 847-848
Episcopal, 815
Episiotomy, 433, 434, 439-441, 483
care of, 495, 496
nursing intervention, 498
Epispadias, 619, 776, 1551
Epistaxis, 1516-1517
Epithelial cell, 1656
Epithelial pearls, 619
Epithelium
cultured, 1695
endocervical canal, 32
Epoophoron, 28
Epstein pearls, 597, 617, 623
Epulis, 117, 165
Equianalgesia, 1225
Equipment and supplies
childbirth, 427, 428
neonatal resuscitation, 699
Ergocalciferol, 1376-1377
Ergonovine
dilation and curettage, 219
postpartum hemorrhage, 539
postpartum uterine tone stimulation, 494
uterine subinvolution, 541
Ergot products, 219
Ergotamine, 680
Ergotrate maleate, 494
Erikson's psychosocial development model, 851-852
sense of autonomy, 995
sense of identity, 1089-1090
sense of industry, 1055
sense of initiative, 1017
trust, 943
Erosion, 1659
Erythema
neonatal birth trauma, 635
racial differences, 907
skin lesions, 1655
Erythema chronicum migrans, 1677
Erythema infectiosum, 242-243, 1032
Erythema multiforme, 1681
Erythema toxicum, 616
Erythroblastosis fetalis, 96, 767
Erythrocyte protoporphyrin, 1441
Erythrocyte sedimentation rate, 1796
Erythropoietin, 938
Eschar, 1658-1660
Escherichia coli, 758
Esophagus
atresia, 96, 774, 1422-1425
changes during pregnancy, 119
Esotropia, 1176
Essential fatty acids, 664
Essential hypertension, 1486
Estimated date of birth, 123
Estimated date of confinement, 123
Estriol, 95
Estrogen, 1625
adaptations during pregnancy, 105
breast growth, 37
hormonal changes of puberty, 1085
lactation suppression, 501
oral contraception, 521-522
postpartum, 483
vascular spiders, 117
Ethical considerations, 5
decision making, 795
fetal rights, 95
forced cesarean birth, 465
human immunodeficiency virus screening, 132
pregnant woman with medical complications, 263
screening pregnant women for drug use, 127
Ethical considerations—cont'd
standards of care, 1771-1772
Ethnicity, 800, 801-802
high risk factor, 81
infant behavior, 609
newborn skin color, 601
Ethnocentrism, 15, 802
European-American culture, 17
Eustachian tube, 1332
Eutectic mixture of local anesthetics, 1226, 1228
Evaporated milk, 695
Evaporation in newborn heat loss, 595
Evil eye, 811-812
Evoked otoacoustic emissions, 917
Evolution of child health care, 789-791
Ewing sarcoma, 1737
Exanthema subitum, 1032
Exchange blood transfusion, 651
Excitement phase of sexual response, 47
Excoriation, 1659
Exencephaly, 1754
Exercise
adolescent, 1099, 1108
asthma and, 1350
breastfeeding and, 676
diabetes mellitus, 262, 263, 1643, 1649
juvenile rheumatoid arthritis, 1740-1741
Kegel exercise, 483, 499
menstrual dysfunction, 1104-1105
mentally retarded child, 1160-1161
postpartum, 499, 500
during pregnancy
diabetic mother, 262, 263
first trimester, 138-139, 145-146
maternal nutrition, 187
second trimester, 154
school-age child, 1065-1066
scoliosis, 1731
unconscious child, 1582
Exercise stress test, 1451
Exhibitionism, 1041
Exophthalmos, 1631
Exotropia, 1176
Expectant father, 157-159
Experiential history, 127
Expressive skills, 1161
Exstrophy of bladder, 776, 1551
Extended family, 10, 330
effects of pregnancy, 1127-1128, 1141-1142
Extension in labor, 348
External anal sphincter, 30
External cephalic version, 459
External genitalia, 23-27
External iliac artery, 33
External iliac vessels, 30
External os, 28, 31, 32

Extracellular fluid
infant, 939
newborn, 596
water balance, 1387
Extracorporeal membrane oxygenation, 702
Extrahepatic biliary atresia, 1417-1418
Extrauterine life, 629-632
Extremities
newborn, 603, 625
assessment, 619
birth trauma, 635
nutritional status, 193
physical examination, 928-930
Extremity venipuncture, 1279
Extrusion reflex, 604, 662
Eye
medication administration, 1297-1298
neurologic examination, 1575
newborn, 603-608
assessment, 617, 622
fetal alcohol syndrome, 760
prophylaxis, 630, 632-633
nutritional status, 193, 888
physical examination, 908-914
retinoblastoma, 1182-1183
review of systems, 881
unconscious child, 1582
Eye contact, 507, 810
Eye drops, 1297
Eye patch, 652
Eyebrow, 622

F

Fabry disease, 96
Face and brow presentations, 456
Face of newborn
assessment, 622
birth injury, 746, 748
rash, 645
FACES Pain Rating Scale, 1211, 1790
Facial nerve, 932
Facial paralysis, 743
Facilitative responding, 876
Facioscapulohumeral muscular dystrophy, 1760-1761
Factor VIII, 1512-1513
FAD; *see* Fetal activity determination
Failure of descent, 458
Failure to thrive, 980-984, 1387
Faintness, 152
Fallopian tube, 28, 29
Falls
adolescent, 1103
infant, 974-975
toddler, 1007-1008, 1011-1012
False labor, 394, 395, 399
False Memory Syndrome Foundation, 1042
False pelvis, 37
Family, 8-22
assessment of structure and function, 882-885
child relationships
cerebral palsy, 1750-1751
chronic renal failure, 1567
death, 1148-1154
Down syndrome, 1166-1167
effects of immobilization, 1708
epilepsy, 1613
head injury, 1590
high risk newborn, 719
hydrocephalus, 1619-1620
mental retardation, 1162
special needs child, 1123-1129
communication, 868-875
children, 872-875, 876-877
parents, 868-872
cultural factors, 15-19
defined, 826
extended, 330
function and structure, 8-12
grieving, 555
influence on child health promotion, 826-843
adopted child, 835-837
divorce, 837-839
dual-earner families, 840
family roles, relationships, and strengths, 827-831
parenting, 831-835
reconstituted families, 840
single parenting, 839-840
working mothers, 841
key factors in family health, 14-15
migrant, 803, 807-808
nursing care management, 19-21
postpartum psychosocial assessment, 504
pregnancy and, 122
adolescent, 322
childbirth, 428
violence, 310-311
theories, 12-14, 827
Family advocacy, 793-794
Family and Medical Leave Act, 790
Family APGAR Questionnaire, 884-885, 1778-1779
Family-centered care, 791-792
Family composition, 8-11
Family dynamics, 12
Family history, 880-881
cerebral dysfunction, 1572
pregnancy and, 127
Family life cycle, 11
Family stress theory, 14
Family-to-family support in home care, 1193
Fanconi syndrome, 1511
Fantasy child, 158
Farber disease, 96
Farsightedness, 1176
FAS; *see* Fetal alcohol syndrome
Fat, energy needs, 664
Fat-soluble vitamins, 179, 186
Father
adaptation to newborn, 509-510
adjustment to fatherhood, 509
adolescent, 322, 331-332
relationship with infant, 509-510
role during labor, 418-420
special needs child, 1126
Fatigue
postpartum, 498
during pregnancy, 137
Fatty acids, 666
Faucial tonsil, 1328
Faye Symbol Chart, 912
FBM; *see* Fetal breathing movements
Fears
preschooler, 1025
school-age child, 1062-1063
Febrile seizure, 1614-1615
Feedback
acoustic, 1171
family, 13
relaxation in labor, 355
sexual response, 46
Feeding
cleft lip or palate, 1420-1421
difficulties, 979-984
gavage, 1311-1313
home visit assessment, 582
hospitalized child, 1268, 1269
newborn, 661-695
breastfeeding, 665-691; *see also* Breastfeeding
discharge planning, 695
formula feeding, 691-693
normal development, 661-665
preoperative, 1261
preterm newborn, 731
readiness cues, 662
Feeding tube insertion, 709
Female circumcision, 26, 653
Female condom, 519, 520
Female reproductive system, 23-37
adaptations during postpartum period, 480-483
adaptations during pregnancy, 105-111
adolescent disorders, 1104-1105
bony pelvis, 36-37
breasts, 37-39
external structures, 23-27
fetal, 68
genitalia circumcision, 26, 653
menstrual cycle, 39-42
newborn, 599-600, 618
ovaries, 27-29
pelvic floor and perineum, 34-36
physical examination, 927-928

Female reproductive system—cont'd
 review of systems, 881
 uterine tubes, 29
 uterus, 29-33
 vagina, 33-34
Femoral hernia, 925
Femoral pulse, 618, 926
Femoral thrombophlebitis, 543, 544
Femoral venipuncture, 1279
Femur fracture, 635, 748
Fencing reflex, 604
Fentanyl
 conscious sedation, 1222
 epidural block, 364
 equianalgesia, 1225
 for newborn pain, 721
 pediatric dosages, 1224
 routes and methods of administration, 1226, 1227
Ferguson's reflex, 424-425
Ferning test, 399
Fertility, 3-4
Fertility awareness of contraception, 517
Fertilization, 29, 58-60
Fetal acoustic stimulation, 98
Fetal activity determination, 95, 97-98
Fetal alcohol effect, 303
Fetal alcohol syndrome, 186-187, 303, 760-761
Fetal attitude, 337
Fetal blood sampling, 385
Fetal breathing movements, 87, 88, 89
Fetal circulation, 592, 593
Fetal compromise, 374
Fetal death, 697
Fetal gender determination, 97
Fetal gestational age, 148-149
Fetal heart rate
 biophysical profile, 89
 detection, 133
 eclampsia therapy, 213
 funic souffle, 109
 intermittent auscultation, 375-376
 nursing responsibilities in monitoring, 1773-1775
 patterns, 377-385
  baseline, 377-380
  pattern recognition, 383-385
  periodic changes, 380-383
  prolonged decelerations, 383
 physiologic adaptation to labor, 349, 404-405, 406, 430
 second trimester, 150
 ultrasound, 83
 variability, 97
Fetal hemoglobin, 938
Fetal hemolytic disease, 91-92, 94
Fetal lie, 337
Fetal membranes, 60-61
Fetal monitoring, 373-393
 amniocentesis, 91
Fetal monitoring—cont'd
 basis for, 374-375
 daily fetal movement count, 82-83
 electronic, 95-100, 376-377
  contraction stress test, 98-100
  fetal responses to hypoxia and asphyxia, 97
  human immunodeficiency virus infected mother, 236
  indications, 95-97
  nonstress test, 97-98
 fetal blood sampling, 385
 fetal heart rate patterns, 377-385
 fetal pulse oximetry, 385-386
 guidelines and standards of nursing care, 387-388
 intermittent auscultation, 375-376
 intrauterine resuscitation, 388-389, 391
 maternal diabetes mellitus, 257-258
 nursing responsibilities, 1773-1775
 posttraumatic, 289
 preventive measures, 388
 protocol, 387
 working with monitor, 389-394
Fetal movements, 82-83, 88
 maternal diabetes mellitus, 258
 nonstress test, 97-98
Fetal position, 337-338
Fetal presentation, 337
Fetal pulse oximetry, 385-386
Fetal scalp blood sampling, 93
Fetal scalp stimulation, 385
Fetal tone, biophysical profile, 88, 89
Fetoscope, 133
Fetus, 65-69
 abruptio placentae, 226
 cord insertion and placental variations, 229-230
 development
  first trimester, 132-133
  second trimester, 150-151
  third trimester, 162-163
 diabetic mother, 255-256
 dystocia, 454-456
 head compression, 381
 labor and, 336-338, 349
 maternal infections
  chlamydial, 233
  parvovirus, 242-243
  TORCH, 237, 238
  tuberculosis, 243
  varicella, 242
 preeclamptic mother, 200
 prenatal diagnosis of infection, 96
 response during labor, 374
 risk factor assessment, 80
Fever
 bacteriuria, 1546
 blood transfusion, 1535
 control of, 1268-1271
Fever—cont'd
 gastrointestinal dysfunction, 1387
 as postpartum warning sign, 572
 puerperal infection, 543-544
 respiratory infection, 1322, 1324-1325
 Rocky Mountain spotted fever, 1678
 scarlet fever, 1036-1037
 seizure, 1614
 toxic shock syndrome, 1493
Fever blister, 1667
FHR; *see* Fetal heart rate
Fibrinogen, 1797
Fibrinolytic system, 230
Fibronectin, 666
Fibroplasia, 1658
Fifth disease, 242-243, 1032
Filipino-American culture
 food patterns, 191
 health beliefs and practices, 818-819
Fimbriae, 28
Fine motor development
 infant, 939-940, 950-955
 preschooler, 1016-1017, 1022
 toddler, 994, 1001
Finger-to-nose test, 930
Fire ant sting, 1675
Firearm safety, 1102
First-degree burn, 1687, 1688
First-pass effect, 1225
First stage of labor, 394-424
 admission data, 395, 397
 ambulation and positioning, 414-416
 cultural factors, 400-402
 emergency interventions, 411-414
 father/partner role, 418-420
 interview, 398-399
 laboratory tests, 409-411
 physical examination, 402-409
 prenatal data, 395-398
 preparation for giving birth, 421-424
 psychosocial factors, 399-400
 siblings and, 420
 support measures, 416-418
First trimester, 122-146
 abortion, 290-291
 birth plan, 141
 cultural variations in prenatal care, 143-146
 diagnosis of pregnancy, 123
 education for self-care, 135-141
 expected outcomes, 134
 fetal development, 132-134
 indications for sonography, 84
 laboratory tests, 131-132
 nursing diagnoses, 134
 parent education classes, 141
 pelvic examination, 129-130
 physical examination, 129
 plan of care and implementation, 134-135

First trimester—cont'd
prenatal history form, 124-125
prenatal interview, 126-129
sexual counseling, 141-143
speculum and internal examinations, 130-131
Firstborn child, 829
Fish
hypersensitivity, 1385
needs during pregnancy, 183
Fissure, 1659
Fistula
arteriovenous, 1568
genital, 548, 549
omphalomesenteric, 1409
rectoperitoneal and rectovaginal, 1431
tracheoesophageal, 774, 1422-1425
Flaring of nares, 700
Flatulence, 152
Flea bites and stings, 1675
Flexion in labor, 348
Floppy infant syndrome, 1759-1760
Fluid and electrolyte management
after cardiac surgery, 1478
burn victim, 1692
changes during pregnancy, 115-116
congestive heart failure, 1470
hypovolemic shock, 542-543
hypoxemia, 1473-1474
newborn, 596
pediatric nursing interventions, 1299-1302
unconscious child, 1581
Fluid intake
breastfeeding and, 675-676
infant needs, 664
during labor, 415
play activities, 1258
Fluid loss, neonatal, 707
Fluoride
infant requirements, 664
supplementation, 961, 1005-1006
Fluorine, 1379
Fly bites and stings, 1675
FM; *see* Fetal movements
Foam, contraceptive, 519, 520
Folacin, 1375
Foley catheter, 542
Folic acid
deficiency, 280
needs during pregnancy, 179
nutritional significance, 1375
Folinic acid, 1375
Folk healers, 811
Folk remedies, 811
Folkways and customs, 808-811
Follicle-stimulating hormone, 105, 1625
Follicular phase of menstrual cycle, 39
Folliculitis, 1666
Fontanel, 69, 336
dehydration, 1389
newborn, 617, 622
Food
allergy, 1384
cravings during pregnancy, 152, 187
cultural considerations, 886
customs, 810
high-fiber, 1399
Food frequency record, 887
Food Guide Pyramid, 184, 1382, 1383
Food intolerance, 1384
Food patterns, 190-191
Food poisoning, 1397
Food sensitivity, 1384-1386
Foot
cleansing, 648
clubfoot, 1725-1726
extranumerary, 603
metatarsus adductus, 1726-1727
Football hold, 646, 670
Footling breech, 339
Foramen ovale, 65, 592, 594, 1453
Forced kneeling, 812
Forceps-assisted birth, 462-464
facial paralysis, 743
trauma during, 635, 747
Forebrain, 57
Foreclosure, 317
Foreign body
aspiration, 1344-1345
conjunctivitis, 1181
cutaneous disorders, 1672 1673
delayed wound healing, 1660
visual impairment, 1175
Foreskin, 43
Formal operations, 853
Formula feeding, 691-693
factors affecting, 664
samples given at discharge, 573-574
Fornix of vagina, 28, 30
Four-Square, 817
Fourchette, 27
Fourth stage of labor, 488-512
ambulation, 498-499
bladder and bowel patterns, 499-501
breastfeeding and lactation suppression, 501
comfort, 497-498
coping strategies, 510-512
cultural diversity, 504-505
laboratory tests, 492
maternal adjustment, 508-509
nutrition, 499
parent-infant interactions, 502-504
parental attachment, bonding, and acquaintance, 506-508
paternal adjustment, 509-510
postanesthesia recovery, 489-491
prevention of excessive bleeding, 495-497
Fourth stage of labor—cont'd
prevention of infection, 495
Rh isoimmunization, 501-502
rubella vaccination, 501
transfer from recovery area, 491-492
uterine tone, 494, 495
Fovea centralis, 603
Fracture, 1711-1714
birth trauma, 635, 748
skull, 747, 748, 1587
stress, 1072
Fragile site, 1167
Fragile X syndrome, 57, 1074, 1167-1168
Frank breech, 339, 412, 455
Fraternal twins, 830
Fredt-Ramstedt procedure, 1427
Free-standing birth center, 172
Frenulum, clitoral, 26
Fresh frozen plasma, 543
Freud's psychosexual development, 850-851
Friability, 110
Friction, 1266
delayed wound healing, 1660
Friends, 815
Friendships, adolescent, 1092
Frostbite, 1703
Fruits
hypersensitivity, 1385
needs during pregnancy, 183
Full-term infant, 697
Full-thickness burn, 1688, 1689
Function, term, 8
Functional layer of endometrium, 29
Fundal height, 148
Fundal pressure, 435
Fundus
postpartum assessment, 489
postpartum palpation, 496, 497
uterine, 28, 29
Funduscopic examination, 909, 1576
Fungal infection
cutaneous, 1669-1671
newborn, 749, 758-759
Funic souffle, 109
Furosemide
congestive heart failure, 1467
hearing loss, 713
during pregnancy, 272
Fussy infant, 686-687

G

G-spot, 34
Galactagogue, 676
Galactose, 1797
Galactosemia, 57
neonatal, 637, 638, 778
prenatal diagnosis, 96
Galant reflex, 607

Gallbladder
changes during pregnancy, 119
newborn, 597
Gallstones, 119
Games, 856
Gamete, 53-54
Gametogenesis, 54, 55
Gamma-interferon, 666
Gardnerella vaginalis, 241
Garlic application, 812
Gastric decontamination, 1438-1439
Gastric emptying, newborn, 597
Gastric lavage, 1438
Gastric ulcer, 1412-1414
Gastric washing, 1284
Gastroenteritis, 749, 1393-1395
Gastroesophageal reflux, 1401-1403
Gastrointestinal bleeding, 1387
Gastrointestinal dysfunction, 1386-1403
constipation, 1395-1399
cystic fibrosis, 1356-1357, 1358
dehydration, 1386-1390
diarrhea, 1390-1395
gastroesophageal reflux, 1401-1403
Hirschsprung disease, 1399-1401
during pregnancy, 283
vomiting, 1401
Gastrointestinal system
adaptations
during labor, 352
postpartum period, 484-485
during pregnancy, 118-119
congenital anomalies, 773-776
effects of immobilization, 1707
fetal, 67-68
human development milestones, 70-72
infant, 938-939
newborn, 597
nutritional status, 193
prenatal diagnosis of defects, 96
review of systems, 881
systemic lupus erythematosus, 1742
Gastroschisis, 96, 774, 1426
Gastrostomy, 710
feeding, 1313-1314
medication administration, 1296
Gate-control theory of pain, 353
Gavage feeding, 708-710, 1311-1313
Gay/lesbian family, 11
GBS; *see* Group B streptococci
Gender, differences in general growth patterns, 1088
Gender identity, 47-48
Gene, 51-53
General anesthesia during childbirth, 366
General appearance, 905-907
newborn, 616
nutritional status, 193
General flexion, 337
Generalized seizure, 1608
Genetic counseling, 73-75, 1167
Genetic disorders
amniocentesis, 91
medical interruption of pregnancy, 562
Genetic risk factors, 81, 202
Genetics, 51-58
cell division, 53-54
chromosomal abnormalities, 54-56
cystic fibrosis, 1356
gametogenesis, 54
genes and chromosomes, 51-53
patterns of genetic transmission, 56-58
Genital fistula, 548, 549
Genital gestures and practices, 812
Genital stage of psychosexual development, 851
Genitalia
ambiguous, 776, 1551
cleansing, 648
female, 599, 618
circumcision, 653
external, 23-27
internal, 27-37
human development milestones, 70-72
male, 42-46, 600, 619
newborn, 624-625
physical examination, 926-928
pubertal growth, 1086-1088
Genitourinary dysfunction, 1542-1571
acute renal failure, 1560-1563
chronic renal failure, 1563-1568
dialysis, 1568-1569
external defects, 1550-1551
glomerulonephritis, 1556-1558
hemolytic-uremic syndrome, 1558-1559
herpes simplex virus, 1667
kidney transplantation, 1569
myelodysplasia, 1756
nephrotic syndrome, 1551-1556
obstructive uropathy, 1549-1550
renal function assessment, 1542-1545
urinary tract infection, 240-242, 1545-1549
Wilms tumor, 1559-1560
Genitourinary system
adaptations during postpartum period, 483-484
congenital anomalies, 776-777
effects of immobilization, 1707
review of systems, 881
Genotype, 53
Genu valgum, 929
Genu varum, 929
GER; *see* Gastroesophageal reflux
German measles, 237, 238, 1036
Gestational age, 148-149, 724-725
assessment, 732
birthweight, 724-725
classification, 697
newborn, 612-613, 614
ultrasound confirmation, 83-85
Gestational diabetes mellitus, 252, 265-268
Gestational trophoblastic disease, 83, 85, 222-224
Gestures, cultural factors, 810
GFR; *see* Glomerular filtration rate
Giardiasis, 1403-1405
Gingiva, 919
Gingival granuloma gravidarum, 117
Gingivitis, 165
Glabellar reflex, 604
Glans clitoris, 30
Glans penis, 43
Glaucoma, 1177
Glenn shunt, 1473
Global organization, 997
Glomerular disease, 1551-1558
acute glomerulonephritis, 1556-1558
nephrotic syndrome, 1551-1556
Glomerular filtration rate
changes during pregnancy, 115
newborn, 596
Glomerulonephritis, 1556-1558
Glossopharyngeal nerve, 932
Gloving
infection control, 642
specimen collection, 639
Glucagon, 1625
diabetes mellitus, 1643
pancreatic production, 1640
Glucocorticoids, 1625, 1634
Gluconeogenesis, 939
Glucose
blood
newborn, 597
postpartum, 483
monitoring in diabetes mellitus, 1648
newborn values, 637
normal laboratory values, 1797
urine, 1544
Glucose-6-phosphate dehydrogenase deficiency, 1506
Glucose tolerance, 523
Glucose tolerance test
first trimester, 131
gestational diabetes mellitus, 265-266
normal laboratory values, 1797
Glucosuria, 116
Glue sniffing, 1114
Glutaric acidemia, 96
Gluteal folds, 928
Glycogen, 68
Glycogen storage disease, 96
Glycosuria
diabetes mellitus, 252
maternal assay, 95
Glycosylated hemoglobin, 257, 1643
Gnat bites and stings, 1675
Goiter, 1630
Gonadotropin-releasing hormone, 39
Gonadotropins, 1625

Gonorrhea, 233, 752-753
Goodell's sign, 110
Graft rejection, 1569
Graft-versus-host disease, 1536-1537
Grain products, 183
Grand mal seizure, 1607
Grandparent, 511
  adaptation to pregnancy and birth, 160
  support during labor, 420
Granular casts, 1545
Granulation, 1658
Grasp reflex, 604, 929
Graves' disease, 1631-1632
Gravida, 104
Gravidity, 103-104
Greater vestibular glands, 27
Greek Orthodox, 815
Green-stick fracture, 1712
Grief
  adolescent, 562
  adolescent mother, 329, 562
  bittersweet, 552, 553
  childhood death, 1128-1129, 1153
  complicated bereavement, 562-563
  maternal death, 562
  newborn death, 550-561
    anticipatory grief, 552
    communicating and caring techniques, 554-556
    complicated bereavement, 562-563
    documentation, 558-561
    grief responses, 551-552
    options for parents, 556-558
    physical comfort, 556
  perinatal diagnoses with negative outcome, 561-562
Groshong catheter, 1295
Gross motor development, 940-943, 950-955
  preschooler, 1016-1017, 1022
  toddler, 994, 1000
Group B streptococci
  newborn infection, 758
  upper respiratory tract infection, 1327-1328
  vaginal infection, 241
Group identity, 1089
Growth and development, 60-69, 844-865
  adolescent, 316-317, 1084-1089, 1096
  biologic and physical, 846-848
  blind child, 1178-1179
  chronic renal failure and, 1565
  developmental assessment, 931-934
  embryo, 60-65
  environmental hazards, 861
  fetus, 65-69
    first trimester, 132-133
    second trimester, 150-151
Growth and development—cont'd
  growth measurements, 896-900, 1785-1789
  health history, 880
  heredity, 858-860
  infant, 937-956
    autism, 988-989
    cognitive development, 48, 943-944
    failure to thrive, 980-984
    fine motor behavior, 939-940
    gross motor development, 940-943
    maturation of systems, 938-939
    personality development, 48
    preterm, 727-729
    proportional changes, 937-938
  interpersonal relationships, 860-861
  mass media influence, 862-863
  mental, 852-854
  milestones, 70-72
  newborn
    baseline measurements, 620-623
    high risk, 712-713
    nutrition and feeding, 661-665
    preterm, 727-729
  nongenetic factors, 73
  nutrition, 860, 888
  personality, 850-852
  physiologic changes, 848-849
  physiologic measurements, 900-905
  play, 855-858
  preschooler, 1016-1025
    biologic, 1016-1017
    cognitive, 1017-1018
    preschool and kindergarten experience, 1021-1024
    psychosocial, 1017
    sex education, 1024-1025
    sexuality, 1018
    social, 1018-1021
    special needs, 1130, 1144
    speech problems, 1025
    spiritual, 1018
  school-age child, 1053-1060
  self-concept, 854-855
  socioeconomic level, 861
  special needs child, 1129-1131
  stages and patterns, 844-846
  stress, 861-862
  temperament, 849-850
  toddler, 993-994
Growth factor, 666
Growth hormone, 1625
  deficiency, 1624-1627
  normal laboratory values, 1797
Growth spurts
  breastfeeding requirements, 667
  formula feeding requirements, 692
GTPAL acronym, 104
GTT; *see* Glucose tolerance test
Guided imagery, 1220
Guillain-Barré syndrome, 1762-1763
Guilt, 801, 1137
Gums
  hypertrophy, 117
  physical examination, 919
Gynecoid pelvis, 342, 343
Gynecologic history, 126
Gynecomastia, 1085, 1106

H

Habits, health history, 880
Haemophilus influenzae
  cellulitis, 1666
  epiglottitis, 1335
  osteomyelitis, 1733
  otitis media, 1331
  respiratory infection, 1321
Haemophilus influenzae type b vaccine, 658, 962, 966, 969
Hair
  alopecia, 1680
  changes during pregnancy, 117
  fetal, 69
  hospitalized child, 1267-1268
  lanugo, 601, 621-622
  newborn, 622
  nutritional status, 193, 888
  unconscious child, 1582
Hair follicle, 601-602
Haitian-American culture, 820-821
Hallucinogens, 1114
Hand, neonatal, 648
Hand expression of breast milk, 677, 678
Hand strength, 930
Handicap, 1122
Handwashing, 642-643, 1273
Haploid, term, 53
Hard-of-hearing, 1168
Hardy-Rand-Rittler test, 914
Harlequin color change, 616
Harnessing, 636
Harrington instrumentation, 1732
Harvest mite, 1675
Hashimoto thyroiditis, 270, 1630-1631
Head
  fetal compression, 381, 382
  infant
    control of, 940
    growth, 937
  newborn, 602-603
    assessment, 617, 622-623
    home visit assessment, 582
  nutritional status, 888
  physical examination, 907-908
  review of systems, 881
  toddler, 993
Head circumference, 616, 620, 621, 900, 1788
Head injury, 1585-1593
Head lice, 1673-1674
Head-to-heel length, 616, 621

Headache
after spinal puncture, 361-363
brain tumor, 1595
postpartum, 486
during pregnancy, 118, 153
Health beliefs, 811
Health care
access to, 4-5
changing structure of delivery, 1-2
evolution of pediatric care, 789-791
family socioeconomic characteristics, 14-15
regionalization of services, 80
special needs child, 1121-1122
trends, 4
Health care planning, 796
Health education and counseling, 1769-1770
Health history, 126-127, 875-882
cardiac dysfunction, 1450-1451
chief complaint, 877-878
child abuse, 1044
family medical history, 880-881
hospitalized child, 1204-1207
identifying information, 877
maternal nutrition, 188
neonatal, 634
past history, 878-880
postpartum infection, 545
present illness, 878
psychosocial history, 881-882
review of systems, 880
sexual history, 882
sexually transmitted disease, 244
skin lesions, 1655
Health maintenance organization, 791
Health practices, 811-812
Health promotion, 794
family influences, 826-843
adopted child, 835-837
divorce, 837-839
dual-earner families, 840
family roles, relationships, and strengths, 827-831
parenting, 831-835
reconstituted families, 840
single parenting, 839-840
working mothers, 841
preconception care, 76
Healthy People 2000, 783
Hearing
adolescent, 1100
newborn, 608
unconscious child, 1582
Hearing aid, 1171
Hearing impairment, 713, 1168-1175
Hearing test, 917
Hearing-threshold level, 1169
Heart, 1450-1498
acute renal failure and, 1562
adaptations during postpartum period, 485
Heart—cont'd
anaphylaxis, 1491-1492
assessment, 1450-1453
bacterial endocarditis, 1481-1482
congestive heart failure, 1465-1472
defects with decreased pulmonary blood flow, 1457-1465
aortic stenosis, 1459
coarctation of aorta, 1458-1459
hypoplastic left heart syndrome, 1464
patent ductus arteriosus, 1458
pulmonary stenosis, 1460
tetralogy of Fallot, 1460-1461
total anomalous pulmonary venous connection, 1462-1463
transposition of great arteries, 1462
tricuspid atresia, 1461
truncus arteriosus, 1463-1464
defects with increased pulmonary blood flow, 1455
dysrhythmias, 1484-1485
Henoch-Schönlein purpura, 1493-1494
hyperlipidemia, 1483-1484
hypertension, 1486-1487
hypoxemia, 1472-1474
Kawasaki disease, 1487-1489
mixed defects, 1465
newborn, 592-594
assessment, 618
fetal alcohol syndrome, 760
obstructive defects, 1455-1457
physical examination, 922-924
during pregnancy
adaptations, 111-114
cardiopulmonary resuscitation, 278-279
disease, 270-279
heart surgery, 276
prenatal diagnosis of defects, 96
rheumatic fever, 1482-1483
shock, 1489-1491
systemic lupus erythematosus, 1742
toxic shock syndrome, 1492-1493
transplantation, 1494
Heart block, 1485
Heart murmur, 594, 615, 924
Heart rate
infant, 938
newborn, 592-594, 616
Apgar scoring, 608-609
assessment, 615
home visit assessment, 582
normal child, 1792
Heart sounds, 592-594, 615, 924
Heart surgery, 276
Heartburn, 152, 196
Heat loss
newborn, 595
preterm infant, 739
Heat therapy in juvenile rheumatoid arthritis, 1740-1741
Heavy metal poisoning, 1439-1440
Heel stick, 637-639, 1283
Heel-to-shin test, 930
Hegar's sign, 109
Height, 847, 898
growth measurements, 1785-1786
infant, 937
toddler, 993
Heimlich maneuver
child, 1368
pregnant woman, 278
Helicobacter pylori, 1413
HELLP syndrome, 202-204, 209-214
Hemagglutination inhibition test, 104
Hematemesis, 1387
Hematochezia, 1387
Hematocrit, 1500
first trimester, 131
newborn, 594, 637
normal values, 1797
postpartum, 486
Hematologic dysfunction, 1499-1530
apheresis, 1537
blood transfusion therapy, 1534-1536
bone marrow transplantation, 1536-1537
disseminated intravascular coagulation, 1516
epistaxis, 1516-1517
hemophilia, 1512-1515
Hodgkin disease, 1528-1530
idiopathic thrombocytopenic purpura, 1515-1516
leukemia, 1517-1528
chemotherapy, 1521-1525
classification, 1517
myelosuppression, 1520-1521
nursing care plan, 1526-1528
pathophysiology, 1517-1518
therapeutic management, 1518-1519
lymphoma, 1528
non-Hodgkin lymphoma, 1530
red blood cell disorders, 1499-1512
anemia, 1499-1503
aplastic anemia, 1511-1512
beta-thalassemia, 1510-1511
iron deficiency anemia, 1503-1505
sickle cell anemia, 1505-1510
Hematologic system, 727
Hematoma
epidural, 1586-1587
eye injury, 1175
HELLP syndrome, 204
postpartum hemorrhage, 538-539
Hematopoietic system
fetal, 66
infant, 938
newborn, 594-595
Heme, 1441
Hemimelia, 619

Hemodialysis, 1568
Hemodynamics, 1454
Hemofiltration, 1568
Hemoglobin
  determination, 1500
  first trimester, 131
  newborn, 594-595, 637
  normal values, 1797-1798
  postpartum, 486
Hemolysis, 1501
Hemolytic disease, 682
Hemolytic reaction, 1535
Hemolytic-uremic syndrome, 1558-1559
Hemophilia, 1512-1515
Hemorrhage
  after epidural block, 365
  epidural and subdural, 1588
  intracranial, 749
  leukemia, 1518, 1520-1521
  ocular, 635, 747
  periventricular-intraventricular, 735-736
  postpartum, 482, 495-497, 537-543
  during pregnancy, 216-231
    abruptio placentae, 226-228
    clotting disorders, 230-231
    ectopic pregnancy, 220-222
    hydatidiform mole, 222-224
    incompetent cervix, 219-220
    nursing care management, 228-230
    placenta previa, 224-226
    spontaneous abortion, 216-218
  subarachnoid, 749
  uterine inversion, 539-540
Hemorrhagic cystitis, 1525
Hemorrhagic shock, 542
Hemorrhoids, 119
  nursing intervention, 498
  postpartum, 483, 496
Hemosiderosis, 1511
Hemostasis defects, 1512-1517
Henoch-Schönlein purpura, 1493-1494
Heparin, 272
Heparin lock, 1294
Hepatic disorders
  biliary atresia, 1417-1418
  cirrhosis, 1416-1417
  hepatitis, 1414-1416
Hepatic system
  changes during pregnancy, 119
  fetal, 68
  infant, 939
  leukemia and, 1518
  newborn, 597-599
    assessment, 618, 624
    fetal alcohol syndrome, 760
  palpation, 925-926
  short bowel syndrome and, 1434
Hepatitis, 236-238, 1414-1416
Hepatitis A, 1414
  during pregnancy, 236, 237
  vaccine, 967
Hepatitis B, 1414
  antigen in breast milk, 156
  newborn infection, 754
  during pregnancy, 236-238
  vaccine, 649, 658, 962, 963-964, 969
Hepatitis C, 238, 1414-1415
Hepatitis D, 238, 1415
Hepatitis E, 1415
Heredity, 858-860
  susceptibility to health problems, 806-807
Heritable characteristics, 56
Hernia, 1425, 1426
  diaphragmatic, 773
  inguinal, 625, 1551
  locations, 924
Heroin
  breastfeeding and, 766
  maternal use, 759, 761-762
  psychologic and physiologic signs, 304
  use during pregnancy, 305
Herpes simplex virus infection
  cutaneous, 1667
  newborn, 757-758
  during pregnancy, 237, 238-239
Herpes zoster, 1667
Herpetic gingivostomatitis, 1406
Hertz, 83
Heterosexual relationships, 1092-1093
Heterotopic heart transplantation, 1494
Hiatal hernia, 119, 1426
Hib; *see Haemophilus influenzae* type b vaccine
Hiccups, 607
Hickman catheter, 1295
High density lipoproteins, 1483
High-fiber foods, 1399
High-risk newborn, 696-723
  assessment, 697-699
  classification, 696, 697
  developmental and emotional aspects of care, 712-713
  family care, 719
  neonatal pain, 719-721
  nursing care management, 713-719
  nutrition, 706-712
  respiratory care, 699-704
  thermoregulatory care, 704-706
  transportation, 696-697
High-risk pregnancy, 79
  categories of risk factors, 80-82
  increase in, 4
High-technology care, 4
Hindu, 816
Hip
  developmental dysplasia, 635-636, 775, 1721-1725
  dislocation, 619
  tuberculosis, 1735
Hirschberg test, 910
Hirschsprung disease, 1399-1401
Hirsutism, 117
Hispanic-American culture
  adolescent pregnancy, 322
  childbearing and parenting beliefs, 16
  food patterns, 191
  health beliefs and practices, 820-821
Histoplasmosis, 1670
History taking, 875-882
  cardiac dysfunction, 1450-1451
  chief complaint, 877-878
  child abuse, 1044
  family medical history, 880-881
  hospitalized child, 1204-1207
  identifying information, 877
  neonatal, 634
  past history, 878-880
  postpartum infection, 545
  present illness, 878
  psychosocial history, 881-882
  review of systems, 880
  sexual history, 882
  skin lesions, 1655
HIV; *see* Human immunodeficiency virus
HMO; *see* Health maintenance organization
Hodgkin disease, 1528-1530
Holistic care, 123
Hollister cord clamp, 628
Hollister U-Bag, 640
Holter monitor, 1451
Homans' sign, 499
Home birth, 172-173
Home blood glucose monitoring, 1643
Home care, 4, 1186-1195
  after cardiac surgery, 1479
  after hospitalization of child, 1238-1239
  asthma, 1352, 1353
  burn victim, 1700
  car safety seats, 1009
  case management, 1187-1188
  cast care, 1715
  child abuse, 1047
  child safety home checklist, 978
  child's school experience, 1061
  colic, 980
  cultural diversity, 1188-1189
  cystic fibrosis, 1359-1360
  defined, 1186
  digoxin administration, 1469
  discharge planning and selection of home care agency, 1187, 1188
  family-to-family support, 1193
  fever, 1271
  guidance during adolescence, 1104
  hemophilia, 1514-1515
  lactose intolerance, 1386
  medication administration, 1298-1299
  mother and newborn, 565-590, 658-659

Homecare—cont'd
  mother and newborn—cont'd
    advantages and disadvantages of short-stay maternity care, 566, 567
    early postpartum discharge, 566-571
    home care nursing visits, 574-584
    nursing role in program development, 589
    perinatal coaching, 588-589
    preparatory educational instruction, 571-574
    support groups, 587-588
    telephone follow-up, 584-586
    warm lines/help lines, 586-587
  nursing process, 1190-1191
  parent-professional collaboration, 1189-1190
  during pregnancy
    gestational diabetes mellitus, 267
    incompetent cervix, 220
    postdate pregnancy, 474
    preeclampsia, 208
    preterm labor, 447
    self-administration of insulin, 262
    self-testing of blood glucose level, 261
  preschooler, 1027
  promotion of optimum development, self-care, and education, 1191-1192
  respiratory infection, 1326
  safety issues, 1192
  school-age child, 1071
  skin lesions, 1664
  spina bifida, 1758
  tracheostomy, 1309, 1310-1311
Home pregnancy test, 105
Homelessness, 803, 807
Homocystinuria, 638
Homologues of genitalia, 24, 25
Homosexual family, 11
Homosexuality
  adolescent, 1093
  suicide and, 1115
Honey, 663
Hood therapy, 702
Hookworm disease, 1404
Hormones
  adolescent biologic development, 1084-1085
  breastfeeding benefits, 666
  changes during pregnancy, 119-120
  contraceptive, 521-522, 677
  milk production, 666-667
Hornet sting, 1675
Hospice, 1149, 1186
Hospitalization
  child, 1196-1249
    admission assessment, 1204-1207
    altered family roles, 1236-1237
Hospitalization—cont'd
  child—cont'd
    ambulatory/outpatient setting, 1241-1242
    blind, 1179-1180
    bodily injury and pain, 1200-1203
    cerebral palsy, 1751
    developmentally appropriate activities, 1230
    diabetes mellitus, 1649-1650
    discharge and home care, 1237, 1239-1241
    emergency admission, 1242
    head injury, 1591-1592
    hearing impaired, 1172-1173
    intensive care unit, 1243-1244
    isolation, 1242
    loss of control, 1198-1200, 1218-1219
    mentally retarded, 1162-1163
    minimization of separation, 1216-1218
    nursing care plan, 1235
    pain assessment, 1207-1214
    pain management, 1219-1230; *see also* Pain management
    parent participation, 1237-1238
    parental reactions, 1236
    play, 1230-1233
    preparation for, 1214-1216
    prevention of bodily injury, 1219
    separation anxiety, 1196-1198
    sibling reactions, 1236
  during pregnancy
    diabetes mellitus, 262
    mental disorders, 300
    preeclampsia, 209-211
    preterm labor, 447
Hot lines, warm lines *versus*, 586
hPL; *see* Human placental lactogen
Human bite, 1678-1679
Human chorionic gonadotropin
  placental production, 64
  pregnancy test, 104
  triple marker test, 95
Human development; *see* Growth and development
Human Genome Project, 51, 52
Human Growth Foundation, 1627
Human immunodeficiency virus, 1531-1533
  adolescent, 317-318
  breastfeeding, 132156
  encephalopathy, 1604
  ethical considerations in screening, 132
  hemophilia and, 1513
  newborn, 755
  during pregnancy, 234-236
Human milk, 666, 667-668
Human papillomavirus
  during pregnancy, 239-240
Human papillomavirus—cont'd
  verruca, 1667
Human placental lactogen, 64, 483
Human rabies immune globulin, 1605
Humerus fracture, 635, 748
Humirubin, 650
Humoral immunity, 1531
Hunter syndrome, 96
Huntington's chorea, 57
Hurler syndrome, 96
HUS; *see* Hemolytic-uremic syndrome
Hyaline casts, 1545
Hydatid of Morgagni, 28
Hydatidiform mole, 85, 222-224
Hydralazine, 214
Hydramnios, 61, 255, 410, 777
Hydrocarbons, 1436
Hydrocele, 600, 619, 1551
Hydrocephalus, 96, 771-772, 1579, 1615-1620
Hydrocodone, 1221, 1224
Hydrocolloids, 1661
Hydrogel sheets, 1661
Hydrogen peroxide, 1660
Hydromorphone, 1224
Hydronephrosis, 1549
Hydrops fetalis, 767
Hydrotherapy, 1693
21-Hydroxylase deficiency, 1638
Hygiene
  diabetes mellitus, 1649
  hospitalized child, 1264-1271
  during labor, 415
  physical examination, 905-907
  unconscious child, 1582
Hygroscopic dilators, 461
Hymen, 27, 928
Hymenal tags, 624
Hymenoptera sting, 1675
Hyperactivity, 1075
Hyperalbuminuria, 1552
Hyperaldosteronism, 1639
Hyperbilirubinemia, 598, 767-769, 770
  defined, 652
  infant of diabetic mother, 744-745
  neonatal care, 650-653
  treatment, 681-682
Hypercholesterolemia, 1483-1484
Hypercyanotic spell, 1473
Hyperemesis gravidarum, 195-196, 268
Hyperesthesia, 1655
Hyperglycemia
  diabetes mellitus, 252, 1649
  hypoglycemia *versus*, 256, 1644
Hyperhemolytic crisis, 1506
Hyperinsulinemia, 741
Hyperkalemia, 1561-1562
Hyperlipidemia, 1483-1484
Hyperlipoproteinemia, 96
Hyperopia, 1176

Hyperparathyroidism, 119, 1634
Hyperplasia, prenatal uterine growth, 480
Hypersensitivity, 1384
Hypertension, 1486-1487
acute renal failure, 1562
chronic renal failure, 1565
pregnancy-induced, 187, 199-216
assessment, 204-207
classification, 199-201
control of blood pressure, 213-214
eclampsia, 214-215
HELLP syndrome, 202-204
magnesium sulfate, 211-213
nursing care, 209-210
postpartum care, 215-216
preeclampsia, 201-202, 207-209
Hyperthermia, 1269, 1270-1271
newborn, 596
unconscious child, 1581-1582
Hyperthyroidism, 269-270, 1631-1632
Hypertonic dehydration, 1388, 1389
Hypertonic uterine dysfunction, 452-453, 454
Hypertrophic cardiomyopathy, 276
Hypertrophic pyloric stenosis, 1426-1429
Hypertrophy, prenatal uterine growth, 480
Hyperventilation during labor, 352, 356
Hypervolemia, pregnancy-induced, 485
Hypoalbuminuria, 1552
Hypocalcemia
infant of diabetic mother, 744
neonatal, 636-637
during pregnancy, 118
Hypocapnia, 352
Hypoesthesia, 1655
Hypogastric artery, 32, 33
Hypoglossal nerve, 932
Hypoglycemia, 253
diabetes mellitus, 1643-1644, 1649
hyperglycemia *versus*, 256, 1644
newborn, 636
clinical signs, 707
diabetic mother, 744
preterm, 739
Hypomagnesemia, 744
Hypoparathyroidism, 1633-1634
Hypophosphatasia, 96
Hypophysis, 1624
Hypopituitarism, 1624-1627
Hypoplastic anemia, 1511
Hypoplastic left heart syndrome, 1464
Hyposensitization, 1350
Hypospadias, 619, 776, 1551
Hypotension
after spinal puncture, 361
supine, 112, 404
toxic shock syndrome, 1493
Hypothalamic-pituitary cycle, 39, 40
Hypothalamic-pituitary-ovarian axis, 105
Hypothermia
after analgesia and anesthesia, 367
Hypothermia—cont'd
near-drowning, 1593
neonatal, 629-630
warming techniques, 105
Hypothyroidism, 270
congenital, 638
juvenile, 1629-1630
Hypotonic dehydration, 1388, 1389
Hypotonic uterine dysfunction, 453, 454
Hypovolemia
nephrotic syndrome, 1552
during pregnancy, 115
Hypovolemic shock, 497, 542, 1489
Hypoxemia, 1472-1474
fetal compromise, 374
neonatal, 699-700
Hypoxia
abruptio placentae, 226
fetal compromise, 374
fetal responses to, 97
near-drowning, 1593
sickle cell anemia, 1507
Hysteria, 1079
Hysterotomy, 291

I

I & O; *see* Intake and output
IBD; *see* Inflammatory bowel disease
Ibuprofen, 1223
Ice application, 496, 498
Ice methamphetamine, 304
Ichthyoses, 1679, 1680, 1681
ICP; *see* Intracranial pressure
Icterus neonatorum, 598
IDDM; *see* Insulin-dependent diabetes mellitus
Identical twins, 69, 830
Identifying information, 877
Identity
adolescent development, 1096
Erikson's psychosocial development model, 852
Idiopathic failure to thrive, 980-981
Idiopathic peripartum cardiomyopathy, 276
Idiopathic thrombocytopenic purpura, 1515-1516
IEF; *see* Ilizarov external fixator
Ileal conduit, 1550
Ileocolic intussusception, 1429
Iliac artery, 32, 33
Iliac crest, 36
Iliococcygeus muscle, 34
Ilium, 36
Ilizarov external fixator, 1720
Imaginary playmate, 1020-1021
Imitation
infant development, 944
toddler, 996
Imitative play, 1020
Immobilization, 1706-1709
Immunity, 1530-1531
Immunization
adolescent, 1098
health history, 879
infant, 961-970
meningococcal, 1602
newborn, 658
during pregnancy, 140, 164
Immunoglobulin A
breast-feeding benefits, 666
newborn immune function, 599
Immunoglobulin G, 599
Immunoglobulin M, 599
Immunoglobulins, 1798
Immunologic deficiency disorders, 1530-1534
Immunologic system
breastfeeding benefits, 666
fetal, 68
fetal alcohol syndrome, 760
infant, 939
newborn, 599
during postpartum period, 486
during pregnancy, 164
Immunologic test for pregnancy, 104
Impairment, 1122
Imperforate anus, 775
Impetigo, 1556, 1666
Implantable progestin, 524
Implantation of ovum, 41
Implanted port, 1295
Impulsivity, 1075
In-line skate safety, 1071
Inattention, 1075
Inborn errors of metabolism, 58, 96, 777
Incarcerated hernia, 1425
Incest, 1041
Incision
cesarean birth, 466, 467
episiotomy, 438
home visit assessment, 582
Incompetent cervix, 219-220
Incomplete breech, 455
Incomplete proteins, 1384
Incontinence, postpartum, 547-548
Increased intracranial pressure, 1573
brain tumor, 1595
monitoring, 1579-1581
Increment of contraction, 407
Incubator, 705-706
Indirect bilirubin, 597
Indirect-contact transmission, 1273
Individual Family Service Plan, 1191
Individual identity, 1089-1090
Individuation, 846, 998
Individuation-separation, 1018-1019
Induction of labor, 460-462
Inevitable abortion, 217
Infant, 937-992
abduction, 495
airway obstruction, 1368

Infant—cont'd
- alternate child care arrangements, 949
- anticipatory guidance, 977-979
- apnea of infancy, 986-988
- autism, 988-989
- biologic development, 937-943, 950-955
  - fine motor behavior, 939-940
  - gross motor development, 940-943
  - maturation of systems, 938-939
  - proportional changes, 937-938
- body image, 944, 945
- botulism, 1765
- cognitive development, 48, 943-944
- colic, 979-980
- communication with, 872-873
- constipation, 1398
- dental health, 961
- developmental dysplasia of hip, 1723
- effects of divorce, 838
- failure to thrive, 980-984
- hearing impairment, 1169, 1170
- hydrocephalus, 1617
- hypertension, 1487
- immunizations, 961-970
- increased intracranial pressure, 1573
- infection
  - eczema, 1682
  - human immunodeficiency virus, 1533
  - respiratory, 1322
  - urinary tract, 1547
- injury prevention, 970-977
- limit setting and discipline, 949
- neural tube defects, 1755, 1757
- nutrition, 956-959
- personality development, 48
- physical examination, 895
- postdate, 737-739
- postmature, 737-739
- postpartum risk factors, 83
- preparation for pediatric procedures, 1254
- psychosocial development, 943
- regurgitation, 979
- response to bodily injury and pain, 1200
- separation and stranger fear, 948-949
- shaken baby syndrome, 1042
- shoes, 956
- sleep and activity, 959-961
- social development, 944-948
- special needs, 1130, 1143, 1144
- sudden infant death syndrome, 984-986
- teething, 954-956
- temperament, 948
- thumb-sucking and use of pacifier, 949, 954
- transportation, 1275-1276
- understanding and reaction to death, 1133

Infant—cont'd
- visual acuity testing, 913
- visual impairment, 1178
- vital signs and parameters, 1792-1793
- water balance, 1386-1388

Infant mortality, 2, 3-4, 725

Infantile eczema, 1682

Infantile spasm, 1607

Infection
- blood transfusion-induced, 1536
- bone and joint, 1733-1735
- breast, 544, 684-685
- chronic renal failure and, 1565
- conjunctivitis, 1181-1182
- cutaneous
  - bacterial, 1664-1667
  - fungal, 1669-1671
  - transmitted by arthropods, 1677
  - viral, 1667-1669
- delayed wound healing, 1660
- diarrhea, 1396-1397
- eye, 1177
- intracranial, 1600-1605
- leukemia therapy, 1520
- monilial, 684
- neonatal, 727, 749-759
- postpartum, 495, 543-546
- during pregnancy, 231-247
  - chlamydial, 232-233
  - coxsackievirus B, 242
  - diabetes mellitus-related, 255
  - gonorrhea, 233
  - human immunodeficiency virus, 234-236
  - human papillomavirus, 239-240
  - infection control, 244, 245
  - influenza, 242
  - listeriosis, 242
  - Lyme disease, 242
  - malaria, 242
  - mumps, 242
  - nursing care management, 244-247
  - parvovirus, 242-243
  - rubeola, 243
  - rupture of membranes, 410-411
  - sickle cell anemia-associated, 281
  - syphilis, 233-234
  - TORCH, 236-239
  - toxic shock syndrome, 243-244
  - tuberculosis, 243
  - urinary tract, 241-242
  - vaginal, 240-241
  - varicella, 242
- respiratory, 1321-1344
  - acute laryngotracheobronchitis, 1335-1337
  - acute spasmodic laryngitis, 1337
  - bacterial tracheitis, 1337
  - bronchitis, 1337
  - epiglottis, 1334-1335
  - general aspects, 1321-1326

Infection—cont'd
- respiratory—cont'd
  - infectious mononucleosis, 1330-1331
  - influenza, 1331
  - laryngitis, 1335
  - nasopharyngitis, 1326-1327
  - otitis media, 1331-1333
  - pertussis, 1341
  - pharyngitis, 1327-1328
  - pneumonia, 1339-1341
  - respiratory syncytial virus bronchiolitis, 1337-1339
  - tonsillitis, 1328-1330
  - tuberculosis, 1341-1344
- urinary tract, 1545-1549

Infection control
- communicable disease, 1028
- fourth stage of labor, 495
- high-risk infant, 706
- hospitalized child, 1272-1274
- neonatal, 642-643
- pediatric nursing interventions, 1272-1274
- during pregnancy, 244, 245
- respiratory infection, 1324

Infectious agents, 1321

Infectious mononucleosis, 1330-1331

Infectious polyneuritis, 1762-1763

Infective endocarditis, 1481-1482

Inferior vena cava, 33

Inferior vesical artery, 33

Infertility, 169

Inflammation, 1656-1658

Inflammatory bowel disease, 283, 1409-1412

Inflammatory disorders, 1406-1414
- appendicitis, 1406-1408
- inflammatory bowel disease, 283, 1409-1412
- Meckel diverticulum, 1409
- peptic ulcer, 1412-1414
- stomatitis, 1406

Influenza, 242, 1331

Influenza virus vaccine, 967

Informant, 877

Informed consent
- drugs during labor, 369
- pediatric nursing interventions, 1250-1252

Infrared thermometry, 901

Infratentorial brain tumor, 1594

Infundibulopelvic ligament, 30

Infundibulum of uterine tube, 28, 29

Infus-a-port, 1295

Infusion pump, 1300

Inguinal hernia, 625, 924, 1551

Inhalants, 1114

Inhalation anesthesia, 366

Inhalation injury, 1345-1347

Inhalation therapy, 1227, 1302-1305

Inheritance, 56-58
Initiative, 852, 1017
Injectable progestins, 524
Injection, 1288-1292
 during labor, 370
 newborn, 649-650
 pediatric, 1226
 play activities, 1258
Injury prevention
 adolescent, 1102-1104
 head injury, 1592-1593
 infant, 970-977
 near-drowning, 1594
 newborn, 657
 preschooler, 1027
 school-age child, 1069, 1070-1071
 toddler, 1006-1013
 toy safety, 858, 859
 visually impaired child, 1180-1181
Inlet, pelvic, 37
Inlet contracture, 453
Innervation, uterine, 32-34
Innominate bones, 36
Insect bites and stings, 1674-1677
Insensible water loss, 707-708
Insomnia, 165
Inspiration/expiration ratio, 702
Insulin, 1625, 1640
 diabetes mellitus, 1642-1643, 1646-1648
 pregnancy
  changes during, 120
  hyperglycemia, 252
  needs during, 254
  therapy during, 261
Insulin-dependent diabetes mellitus, 252, 1640, 1650
Insulin pump, 1643
Insulin shock, 256
Insulinase, 483
Intake and output, 1389
 after cardiac surgery, 1478
 measurement of, 1299
Integumentary dysfunction, 1654-1705
 acne, 1684-1687
 animal bites, 1677-1678
 arthropod bites and stings, 1674-1677
 burns, 1687-1703
  adolescent, 1103
  characteristics of burn injury, 1687-1690
  emergency care, 1690-1691
  infant, 975-976
  major, 1692-1700
  minor, 1691-1692
  pathophysiology, 1690
  sunburn, 1700-1703
  toddler, 1007, 1010-1011
 cat-scratch disease, 1679
 cold injury, 1703
 dermatitis
Integumentary dysfunction—cont'd
 dermatitis—cont'd
  contact, 1671
  diaper, 1679-1682
  eczema, 1682-1684
  seborrheic, 1684
 dressings, 1660
 drug reactions, 1672
 foreign bodies, 1672-1673
 human bites, 1678-1679
 infections
  bacterial, 1664-1667
  fungal, 1669-1671
  transmitted by arthropods, 1677
  viral, 1667-1669
 pediculosis capitis, 1673-1674
 poison ivy, oak, and sumac, 1671-1672
 during pregnancy, 283
 relief of symptoms, 1663-1664
 scabies, 1673
 skin lesions, 1654-1655
 systemic therapy, 1662
 topical therapy, 1660-1662, 1663-1664
 wound care, 1662-1663
 wounds, 1655-1660
Integumentary system
 adaptations
  during labor, 352
  postpartum period, 486
  during pregnancy, 116-117
 effects of immobilization, 1707
 fetal, 69
 newborn, 600-602
 review of systems, 881
Intelligence quotient, 1157
Intensive care unit, pediatric, 1243-1244
Intercostal spaces, 920
Intermittent auscultation, 375-376
Internal os, 28, 31
Internal rotation in labor, 348
Internal version, 459-460
International adoption, 837
Interpersonal relationships, 860-861
Interpreter, 871-872
Interstitial cell, 44
Interstitial pneumonia, 1339
Intertrigo, 1680
Interview
 admission during labor, 398-399
 diagnosis of pregnancy, 126
 family assessment, 883-884
 guidelines for interviewing, 867-868
 techniques, 875, 876-877
Intestine
 changes during pregnancy, 119
 infant digestion, 663
 obstruction, 286
 parasitic disease, 1403-1406
Intoxication
 during pregnancy, 309
 psychologic and physiologic signs, 304
Intoxication—cont'd
 water, 664
Intracellular fluid
 newborn, 596
 water balance, 1387
Intracranial birth injury, 746, 749
Intracranial pressure
 brain tumor, 1595
 increased, 1573
 monitoring, 1579-1581
Intradermal medication administration, 1226, 1292-1293
Intramuscular medication administration, 1288-1292
 during labor, 370
 newborn, 649-650
 pediatric, 1226
Intranasal medication administration, 1226, 1642
Intraosseous infusion, 1300
Intrathecal nerve block, 1227
Intrauterine device, 220-221
Intrauterine growth restriction, 697, 725, 739-740
 maternal diabetes mellitus, 254, 256
 maternal nutrition, 176, 177
 related risk factors, 82
 ultrasound indication, 85
Intrauterine pressure catheter, 376, 378, 389, 390
Intrauterine resuscitation, 388-389, 391
Intrauterine transfusion, 768
Intravenous route
 drugs during labor, 370
 medication administration, 1226, 1293
 parenteral fluid therapy, 1299 1302
Introitus, 482-483
Intubation, neonatal resuscitation, 699
Intuitive thought, 1017
Intussusception, 1429-1431
Inversion of uterus, 539-541
Inverted nipple, 156, 157, 668
Involution, 480, 481
Iodine
 needs during pregnancy, 178
 nutritional significance, 1379
IQ, 1157
Iron
 fetal liver storage, 68
 infant requirements, 664
 needs during pregnancy, 178, 184-185, 196, 328
 newborn, 598
 normal laboratory values, 1798
 nutritional significance, 1379-1380
 placental storage, 65
 poisoning, 1437
Iron-binding capacity, 1798
Iron deficiency anemia, 280, 1503-1505
Irreversibility, 997
Irreversible shock, 1490

Ischial spine, 36
Ischial tuberosity, 36
Ischiocavernosus muscle, 35-36
Ischium, 36
Ishihara test, 913-914
Islam, 816
Islands of Langerhans, 1625
Iso-immunization, 767
Isolation, hospitalized child, 1242
Isotonic dehydration, 1388, 1389
Italian food patterns, 191
ITP; *see* Idiopathic thrombocytopenic purpura
IUD; *see* Intrauterine device
IUGR; *see* Intrauterine growth restriction
IWL; *see* Insensible water loss

J

Jacket restraint, 1276
Jacobi, Abraham, 789
Jacquemier's sign, 110
Japanese-American culture
  food patterns, 191
  health beliefs and practices, 818-819
Jargon, 20
Jaundice, 652, 767
  breast milk, 599
  gastrointestinal dysfunction, 1387
  hepatitis, 1415
  hyperbilirubinemia, 598
  newborn, 598-599
  physiologic, 636
  during pregnancy, 119
  racial differences, 907
  treatment, 681-682
Jaw thrust, 1365
Jehovah's Witness, 816
Jet hydrotherapy during labor, 356, 357
Jewish food patterns, 191
Jock itch, 1668
Joint
  disorders, 1738-1742
  pain during pregnancy, 153
  physical examination, 929
Joint custody, 9, 839
Judaism, 816
Jugular venipuncture, 1278-1279
Justice, 795
Juvenile hypothyroidism, 1629-1630
Juvenile rheumatoid arthritis, 1738-1741
Juvenile spinal muscular atrophy, 1760

K

Kangaroo care, 715
Karyotype, 53
Kasai procedure, 1417
Kawasaki disease, 1487-1489
Kegel exercises, 135, 136, 483, 499
Keloid, 1659
Kernicterus, 599, 768-769
Ketamine, 1693
Ketoacidosis, 252, 255, 1641, 1644
Ketone levels, 1544
Ketosuria, 1641
Kidney
  adaptations during labor, 352
  adaptations during pregnancy, 115-116
  dysfunction, 1542-1571
    acute renal failure, 1560-1563
    chronic renal failure, 1563-1568
    dialysis, 1568-1569
    external defects, 1550-1551
    glomerulonephritis, 1556-1558
    hemolytic-uremic syndrome, 1558-1559
    kidney transplantation, 1565, 1569
    nephrotic syndrome, 1551-1556
    obstructive uropathy, 1549-1550
    renal function assessment, 1542-1545
    urinary tract infection, 1545-1549
    Wilms tumor, 1559-1560
  fetal, 66
  gastrointestinal dysfunction and, 1388
  infant, 939
  lead poisoning, 1441
  newborn, 596-597
    assessment, 618, 624
    fetal alcohol syndrome, 760
    nutrition and, 662
  systemic lupus erythematosus, 1742
Kilocalories, 663
  needs during pregnancy, 177-182
Kindergarten experience, 1021-1024
Kinetic stimulation, 947
Kinky-hair disease, 96
Kleihauer-Betke test, 93, 502
Klinefelter syndrome, 56, 1074, 1075
Klumpke's palsy, 748
Knee jerk, 930-931
Knock-knee, 929
Kohlberg moral development, 853, 1018, 1057, 1090
Krabbe disease, 96
Kugelberg-Welander disease, 1760
Kussmaul respirations, 1641
Kwashiorkor, 1384
Kyphosis, 1729-1730

L

Labetalol, 214
Labia, 23-25, 30, 927
  laceration in postpartum hemorrhage, 528
  newborn, 599
Labile cell, 1656
Labor, 336-481
  adolescent mother, 328
  augmentation of, 462
  bearing-down efforts, 344-345
  birth canal, 338-343
  complications, 444-481
    amniotic fluid embolism, 477-478
Labor—cont'd
  complications—cont'd
    dystocia, 452-472; *see also* Dystocia
    postdate pregnancy, 472-475
    premature rupture of membranes, 452
    preterm, 444-452
    prolapsed umbilical cord, 475
    shoulder dystocia, 475
    uterine rupture, 475-477
  cultural beliefs and practices, 16-17
  diabetic mother, 263
  dysfunctional, 452-453, 454
  episiotomy, 439-441
  fetal factors, 336-338
  first stage, 394-424
    admission data, 395, 397
    ambulation and positioning, 414-416
    cultural factors, 400-402
    emergency interventions, 411-414
    father/partner role, 418-420
    interview, 398-399
    laboratory tests, 409-411
    physical examination, 402-409
    prenatal data, 395-398
    preparation for giving birth, 421-424
    psychosocial factors, 399-400
    siblings and, 420
    support measures, 416-418
  fourth stage, 488-512
    ambulation, 498-499
    bladder and bowel patterns, 499-501
    breastfeeding and lactation suppression, 501
    comfort, 497-498
    coping strategies, 510-512
    cultural diversity, 504-505
    laboratory tests, 492
    maternal adjustment, 508-509
    nutrition, 499
    parent-infant interactions, 502-504
    parental attachment, bonding, and acquaintance, 506-508
    paternal adjustment, 509-510
    postanesthesia recovery, 489-491
    prevention of excessive bleeding, 495-497
    prevention of infection, 495
    Rh isoimmunization, 501-502
    rubella vaccination, 501
    transfer from recovery area, 491-492
    uterine tone, 494, 495
  induction of, 460-462
  lacerations, 440-441
  maternal position, 345-346
  normal and abnormal patterns, 458
  pain management, 352-374
    administration of medication, 369-373
    anesthesia in obese woman, 366-367

Labor—cont'd
pain management—cont'd
childbirth preparation methods, 354-355
expression of pain, 353-354
general anesthesia, 366
informed consent, 369
maternal hypothermia after analgesia and anesthesia, 367
nerve block analgesia and anesthesia, 360-365
relaxing and breathing techniques, 355-357
sedatives, 358
systemic analgesia, 358-359
physiologic adaptation, 349-353
process, 346-349
second stage, 424-436
bearing-down efforts, 428-430
birth, 432-435
birthing beds and chairs, 430, 431
duration of, 425
emergency childbirth, 435-436
fetal heart rate, 430
maternal position, 427-428
potential problems, 425-427
prebirth considerations, 427, 428
siblings and, 435
third stage, 436-441
uterine contractions, 343-344
Labor, delivery, recovery, postpartum room, 2, 172, 429, 433
Labor, delivery, recovery room, 2, 172, 429, 433, 491
Laboratory tests, 1794-1804
anemia, 1500, 1502
genitourinary dysfunction, 1542, 1544, 1545
newborn, 637-642
pregnancy
ectopic pregnancy, 222
first stage of labor, 368, 409-411
first trimester, 131-132
fourth stage of labor, 492
high-risk sexual behavior, 319, 324
human immunodeficiency virus, 235
maternal diabetes mellitus, 257
maternal infections, 246
maternal nutrition, 189
preeclampsia-eclampsia, 206-207
second trimester, 147-148
third trimester, 161-162
skin lesions, 1655
standard values in women, 1776-1777
Labored breathing, 1323
Laceration
birth canal, 538-539
care of, 495, 496
cerebral, 1587
during childbirth, 440-441, 635
human bite, 1678
Laceration—cont'd
postpartum hemorrhage, 538-539
wound care, 1663
Lacrimal punctum, 908
Lactation, 665-691
breast engorgement, 680-681
care of mother, 675-677
daily food guide, 183
diabetic mother, 687
drugs and environmental pollutants, 679-680
effects of early discharge, 674
expressing, pumping, and storing milk, 677-679
factors affecting breastfeeding practices, 665
fussy baby, 686-687
jaundice, 681-682
mastitis, 684-685
maternal benefits, 666
milk production, 667-668
monilial infections, 684
nurse role as teacher, 674-675
nutrient needs, 187-188
patient teaching, 670-671
plugged milk duct, 684
postpartum suppression, 501
premature or sick infant, 687-688
prenatal support for breastfeeding, 665-666
properties of human milk, 666
recommended dietary allowances, 178-179
slow weight gain, 685-686
sore nipples, 683-684
suppression, 501
twins, 687
weaning, 680
Lactation consultant, 675
Lactiferous sinus, 37-38, 666
Lactoferrin, 666
Lactogenesis, 666
Lactoovovegetarian diet, 189, 1382
Lactose
in infant diet, 663
intolerance, 185, 1386
Lactovegetarian diet, 189, 1382
Laissez-faire parenting style, 833
Lamaze method of childbirth, 354, 355
Lamb's nipple, 710, 1421
Laminaria tent, 290, 461
Landouzy-Djérine muscular dystrophy, 1760-1761
Language, 20
autism, 988
development, 853
infant, 946
preschooler, 1019, 1022
sign, 1172
toddler, 998, 1001
Lanugo, 69, 601, 621-622
Laparoscopy
hypertrophic pyloric stenosis, 1428
during pregnancy, 285-287
Laparotomy, 285-287
Large-for-gestational-age infant, 614, 697, 724, 740-741
diabetic mother, 256
Laryngeal web, 773
Laryngitis, 1335, 1337
Laryngotracheobronchitis, 1335-1337
Lasix; *see* Furosemide
Last menstrual period, 60, 104, 123
Latch-on, 669, 671
Latchkey children, 1062
Latent phase of labor, 394, 424, 431
Lateral thoracotomy, 1477
Latex agglutination inhibition test, 104
Latex allergy, 1756
Lay midwife, 172
Lazy eye, 1176
LBW; *see* Low-birth-weight infant
Lead
cultural health practices, 812
normal laboratory values, 1799
poisoning, 1440-1444
Learning disability, 1075
Lecithin, 66
Lecithin/sphingomyelin ratio, 66, 90, 91
Left-sided heart failure, 1465
Left-to-right shunt, 1454
Leg
maternal
cramps during third trimester, 165
home visit assessment, 582
postpartum, 492, 493
traction, 1717-1718
varicosities, 499
Leg restraint, 1278
Leg strength, 930
Legal blindness, 1175
Legal considerations
abortion, 289
adolescent issues, 331
pregnancy
cardiac and metabolic emergencies, 273
documentation during childbirth, 432
domestic violence, 311
drugs during labor, 369
early discharge, 512
fetal monitoring standards, 388
home care for preeclamptic patient, 208-209
labor and birth at risk, 459
postdate pregnancy, 474
psychiatric inpatient hospitalization, 300
sexually transmitted disease, 244-245
standards of care for labor, 414

Legal considerations—cont'd
  pregnancy—cont'd
    substance abuse, 302-303
    ultrasound examinations, 89-90
    workplace regulations, 136-137
Legal guardian, 1251
Legg-Calvé-Perthes disease, 1728-1733
Legume hypersensitivity, 1385
Length of newborn, 616, 620, 621, 898
  increased, 661
  measurement, 630
Leopold maneuvers, 402-406
Lesbian couple, 509
Lesch-Nyhan syndrome, 96
Lesion
  chickenpox, 1030
  eczema, 1682
  scabies, 1673
  skin, 1654-1655
Lesser vestibular glands, 27
Let-down reflex, 666, 672
Lethargy, 1574
Letting-go phase of maternal adjustment, 509
Leukemia, 1517-1528
  chemotherapy, 1521-1525
  classification, 1517
  myelosuppression, 1520-1521
  nursing care plan, 1526-1528
  pathophysiology, 1517-1518
  therapeutic management, 1518-1519
Leukocyte differential count, 1799
Leukocyte esterase, 1544
Leukocytes, newborn, 595
Leukocytosis, 486
Leukorrhea
  during pregnancy, 110, 152
  vaginal infection, 240
Levator ani muscle, 30, 34, 35
Level of consciousness, 1573, 1574
  head injury, 1591-1592
Levo-Dromoran; *see* Levorphanol
Levonorgestrel, 522
Levorphanol, 1224
Levothyroxine, 270
Leydig's cell, 44
LGA; *see* Large-for-gestational-age infant
Libido, 47
Lice, 1673-1674
Lichenification, 1658
Lidocaine
  cardiopulmonary resuscitation, 1366
  eutectic mixture of local anesthetics, 1228
  during pregnancy, 272
Lie, fetal, 337
Life-style, nutrition questionnaire, 192
Light sleep state in newborn, 611
Lightening, 109, 346
Lightheadedness, 118, 152
Lighting as neonatal environmental hazard, 714-715
Limit-setting
  infant, 949
  parenting, 833-835
  pediatric nursing interventions, 1275
  school-age child, 1062
Linea alba, 116
Linea nigra, 116
Linear growth, 847
Linear skull fracture, 1587
Lingual tonsil, 1328
Lip, cleft, 1418-1422
Lipase, 597, 663
Lipase hydrolyze, 663
Lipid cell, 91
Lipoproteins, 1483
Lipreading, 1171
Listeriosis
  newborn infection, 758
  during pregnancy, 242
Lithium
  bipolar disorder during pregnancy, 300
  breastfeeding and, 680
Lithotomy position
  childbirth, 432
  pelvic examination, 129-130
Live birth, 697
Liver
  changes during pregnancy, 119
  disorders
    biliary atresia, 1417-1418
    cirrhosis, 1416-1417
    hepatitis, 1414-1416
  fetal, 68
  infant, 939
  leukemia and, 1518
  newborn, 597-599
    assessment, 618, 624
    fetal alcohol syndrome, 760
  palpation, 925-926
  short bowel syndrome, 1434
Living ligature, 31, 32
Living-related donor, 1569
LMP; *see* Last menstrual period
Lobar pneumonia, 1339
Local anesthesia
  eutectic mixture, 1226, 1228
  during labor, 360
  for newborn pain, 719-720
Lochia, 482
  home visit assessment, 582
  postpartum, 489, 492, 493
Lockjaw, 1763
Logical consequences, 834
Lorcet; *see* Hydrocodone
Lordosis, 117, 118, 1729-1730
Lortab; *see* Hydrocodone
Loss and grief
  complicated bereavement, 562-563
  maternal death, 562
Loss and grief—cont'd
  newborn death, 550-561
    anticipatory grief, 552
    communicating and caring techniques, 554-556
    complicated bereavement, 562-563
    documentation, 558-561
    grief responses, 551-552
    options for parents, 556-558
    physical comfort, 556
  perinatal diagnoses with negative outcome, 561-562
Low-birth-weight infant, 3, 80, 697
  maternal nutrition, 176
  skin care, 727
Low-density lipoproteins, 1483
Low income, 81
Low spinal block injection, 361
Lower airway infections, 1337-1341
  bronchitis, 1337
  pneumonias, 1339-1341
  respiratory syncytial virus bronchiolitis, 1337-1339
Lower class, 802-803
Lower esophageal sphincter pressure, 1401
Lower pelvic diaphragm, 34-35
Lumbar puncture, 1279-1280, 1577
Lumbosacral curve during pregnancy, 117, 155
Lung
  adaptations during labor, 352
  adaptations during pregnancy, 114-115
  effects of immobilization, 1707
  fetal, 66
  human development milestones, 70-72
  infant, 938
  newborn, 591-592, 618
  physical examination, 921-922
  review of systems, 881
  systemic lupus erythematosus, 1742
  toddler, 994
  unconscious child, 1579
Lung Association, 1354
Lupron; *see* Luteinizing hormone-releasing hormone
Lupus Foundation of America, Inc., 1742
Luque segmental spinal instrumentation, 1732
Luteal phase of menstrual cycle, 39-41
Luteinizing hormone, 39, 1625
Luteinizing hormone-releasing hormone, 1628
Lutheran, 816
Lying, 1062
Lyme disease, 242, 1677, 1678
Lymph nodes
  leukemia and, 1518
  physical examination, 907
Lymphocyte count, 1500

Lymphocytic thyroiditis, 1630-1631
Lymphoid tissues, 848
Lymphoma, 1528
chemotherapy, 1522-1524
Hodgkin disease, 1528-1530
non-Hodgkin lymphoma, 1530
Lysozyme, 666

M

Mackenrodt's ligament, 28
Macrominerals, 1377
Macrosomia, 256, 743
Macule, 1656
Mafenide acetate, 1694
Magic
communication with children, 877
preoperational thought of toddler, 997
Magical thinking, 1018
Magnesium
needs during pregnancy, 178
nutritional significance, 1380
Magnesium sulfate
preeclampsia, 211-213
suppression of uterine activity, 449-450
Magnet reflex, 607
Magnetic resonance imaging
biophysical assessment, 90
cerebral assessment, 1577
head injury, 1590
Mainstreaming, 1123
Maladaptive behaviors, 503-504
Malaria, 242
Male genitalia
newborn assessment, 619
physical examination, 926-927
Male reproductive system, 42-46
adolescent disorders, 1105-1106
fetal, 68
newborn, 600
Male sterilization, 530-531
Malnutrition
congenital disorders and, 73
malabsorption syndromes, 1432
protein energy, 1384
Malocclusion, 1067
Malposition of fetus, 454
Malpresentation of fetus, 455-456
Maltreatment, 1039-1049
child neglect, 1039, 1044
clinical manifestations, 1043
physical abuse, 1039-1040
prevention, 1047-1049
sexual abuse, 1040-1042, 1044-1045
Mammary gland, 37-39, 111
Mammary papilla, 37
Manganese, 1380
Manic depressive illness, 297
Mantoux test, 1341-1342, 1343
Manual traction, 1717
MAP; *see* Mean arterial pressure
Maple syrup urine disease, 57, 96, 638
Marasmus, 1384
March of Dimes, 1422
Marfan syndrome, 57, 277
Marijuana
breastfeeding and, 766
maternal use, 759, 761
use during pregnancy, 303
Marital status, high risk factor, 81
Mask of pregnancy, 116
Mass media influences, 862-863
Massage
before expressing breast milk, 677, 678
infant, 716-717
Mastitis, 544, 684-685
Masturbation, 997-998
Maternal adaptation, 128, 508-509
after childbirth, 437, 480-487
breastfeeding, 666
distribution of weight gain, 183
first trimester, 132-133
labor, 349-352
multifetal pregnancy, 170
postpartum, 508-509
second trimester, 150-151
third trimester, 161-163, 165
Maternal and Child Health, Crippled Children's Services, 790
Maternal assays, 95
Maternal death, 562
Maternal mortality rate, 2, 4
Maternal nutrition, 176-200
assessment, 188-189, 193
cultural food patterns, 190-191
during lactation, 187-188
during pregnancy
energy needs, 177-182
exercise, 187
minerals and vitamins, 184-186
negative impacts, 186-187
nursing care plan, 199
plan of care and implementation, 194-196
pregnancy-induced hypertension, 187
questionnaire, 192
Maternal-paternal-fetal relationship, 158
Maternal serum alpha-fetoprotein, 95
Maternity bra, 153
Maternity nursing, 1-7
contemporary issues and trends, 1-5
ethical issues in perinatal nursing, 5
family and culture, 8-22
cultural factors, 15-19
function and structure, 8-12
key factors in family health, 14-15
nursing care management, 19-21
theories, 12-14
research into practice, 5
standards of care, 1769-1772
standards of practice, 5
Maternity recovery room record, 489, 490
Matulane; *see* Procarbazine
Maturation, 844
Maturation Index of Colostrum and Milk, 668
Maturational stressor, 14
Maturity-onset diabetes of youth, 1640
McDonald cerclage, 219, 220
McDonald sign, 109
MCH Services Block Grant, 790
McRoberts maneuver, 476
Mean arterial pressure, 112, 903
hypertension, 200
mechanical ventilation, 702
Mean corpuscular hemoglobin, 1500, 1799
Mean corpuscular hemoglobin concentration, 1800
Mean corpuscular volume, 1500, 1800
Measles, 962, 965-966, 969, 1032-1033
Measles-mumps-rubella vaccine, 658
Meat, needs during pregnancy, 183
Mechanical ventilation
neonatal, 702
shock, 1490
Mechanism of labor, 347-349
Mechlorethamine, 1522
Meckel diverticulum, 1409
Meconium, 68, 410, 1398
amniocentesis, 92-93
in newborn stools, 597
prevention of aspiration, 434
Meconium aspiration syndrome, 738
Meconium ileus, 1398
cystic fibrosis, 58, 1356
prenatal diagnosis, 96
Meconium-stained amniotic fluid, 385-386
Median sternotomy, 1477
Medicaid, 790
Medical neglect, 1189
Medication administration, 1284-1299
analgesics, 1226-1227
determination of drug dosage, 1284-1286
family teaching and home care, 1298-1299
intramuscular, 1288-1292
intravenous, 1293
nasogastric, orogastric, or gastrostomy, 1296
optic, otic, and nasal, 1297-1298
oral, 1286-1288
peripheral venous access devices, 1294-1296
rectal, 1296-1297
subcutaneous and intradermal, 1292-1293
unconscious child, 1581
Medication history, 879

Mediport, 1295
Medroxyprogesterone, 522, 524
Megahertz, 83
Meibomian gland, 908
Meiosis, 53, 54
Melanin, 602
Melanocyte-stimulating hormone, 1625
Melanotropin, 116
Melena, 1387
Menarche, 23, 39, 1085
Mendelian inheritance, 56
Meninges, leukemia and, 1518
Meningismus, 1322
Meningitis, 749
Meningocele, 1753, 1754
Meningococcal polysaccharide vaccine, 967
Menkes syndrome, 96
Mennonite, 816
Menopause, 42
Menstrual cycle, 29, 39-42
Menstruation, 39
- breastfeeding and, 677
- ectopic pregnancy, 222
- oral contraception and, 522, 523
- postpartum resumption, 483

Mental health problems
- childhood, 1079-1080
- during pregnancy, 296-317
  - caffeine use, 310
  - emotional complications, 296-302
  - psychoactive substance use, 302-309
  - smoking, 309-310
  - violence against women, 310-313

Mental retardation, 1157-1168
- diagnosis and classification, 1157-1158
- Down syndrome, 1163-1167
- education, 1159-1162
- fragile X syndrome, 1167-1168
- hospitalization, 1162-1163

Menu planning
- diabetes mellitus, 1645-1646
- during pregnancy and lactation, 195, 327
- toddler nutrition, 1004

Meperidine, 1222, 1224
MER; *see* Milk ejection reflex
6-Mercaptopurine, 1523
Mercury, 812, 1439
Mercury glass thermometer, 901
Mercury-gravity sphygmomanometer, 903
Meromelia, 1727
Mesh graft, 1695
Mesoderm, 62
Metabolic acidosis, 1565
Metabolic rate
- fetal, 68
- gastrointestinal dysfunction, 1387-1388
- leukemia and, 1518

Metabolism
- changes associated with pregnancy, 253
- effects of immobilization, 1707
- newborn pain, 719
- physiologic changes in child, 848

Metatarsus adductus, 1726-1727
Metered dose inhaler, 1304-1305
Methadone
- maternal abuse, 762
- for newborn pain, 721
- pediatric dosages, 1224

Methamphetamine, 304, 305, 1113
Methemoglobulin, 1228
Methemoglobulinemia, 1228
Methergine; *see* Methylergonovine
Methodist, 817
Methotrexate, 680, 1523
Methyldopa, 214
Methylergonovine
- postpartum hemorrhage, 539
- postpartum uterine tone stimulation, 494

Methylphenidate, 1076
Methylxanthines, 1350
Mexican-American culture
- food patterns, 191
- health beliefs and practices, 811, 820-821
- postpartum care beliefs, 505

MICAM; *see* Maturation Index of Colostrum and Milk
Microcephaly, 772, 1615
- cri du chat syndrome, 56
- prenatal diagnosis, 96

Microminerals, 1377
Microwave burn, 976
Midazolam
- conscious sedation, 1222
- nasal spray, 1226

Middle child, 829
Middle class, 802
Middle-ear hearing loss, 1168
Middle Eastern food patterns, 190
Midforceps, 464
Midpelvis, 37
Midwife, 172
Mifepristone, 292
Migrant family, 803, 807-808
Milia, 616
Miliaria, 616
Milk
- allergy, 663, 1385-1386
- evaporated, 695
- infant health, 957
- unmodified, 695

Milk banking, 688
Milk duct, plugged, 684
Milk ejection reflex, 666
Milk gland, 666
Milk leg, 543, 544
Milk stool, 597
Milk transfer, 673
Milwaukee brace, 1731
Mimicry, toddler, 996
Mineralocorticoids, 1634
Minerals
- diabetic mother, 260
- infant needs, 664
- needs during pregnancy, 178, 184-186
- nutritional disturbances, 1377-1384
- supplementation in formula feeding, 663

Minilaparotomy approach, 530
Minimal-change nephrotic syndrome, 1551
Minority group, 806
Misbehavior, 833
Miscarriage, 558, 559
Missed abortion, 217
Mitral valve prolapse, 277
Mitral valve stenosis, 277
Mittelschmerz, 42
Mixed conductive-sensorineural hearing loss, 1168
MLBW; *see* Moderately-low-birth-weight infant
MMR; *see* Measles-mumps-rubella vaccine
Moderately-low-birth-weight infant, 697
Modified Blalock-Taussig shunt, 1473
Modified extended family, 9
MODY; *see* Maturity-onset diabetes of youth
Molding of fetal head, 336, 603
Molestation, 1041
Molluscum contagiosum, 1667
Molybdenum, 1380
Mongolian spots, 617
Mongolism, 1163
Moniliasis, 684, 1669
Monitoring
- apnea of infancy, 987
- fetal, 95-100, 373-393
  - amniocentesis, 91
  - basis for, 374-375
  - contraction stress test, 98-100
  - daily fetal movement count, 82-83
  - fetal blood sampling, 385
  - fetal heart rate patterns, 377-385
  - fetal pulse oximetry, 385-386
  - fetal responses to hypoxia and asphyxia, 97
  - guidelines and standards of nursing care, 387-388
  - human immunodeficiency virus infected mother, 236
  - indications, 95-97
  - intermittent auscultation, 375-376
  - intrauterine resuscitation, 388-389, 391
  - maternal diabetes mellitus, 257-258
  - nonstress test, 97-98

Monitoring—cont'd
  fetal—cont'd
    nursing responsibilities, 1773-1775
    posttraumatic, 289
    preventive measures, 388
    protocol, 387
    working with monitor, 389-394
  oxygen therapy, 1303-1304
  patient compliance, 1262-1263
Monitrice, 172
Monoamine oxidase inhibitors, 299
Monocyte count, 1500
Mononucleosis, 1330-1331
Monosomy, 55
Monosomy X, 56
Monozygotic twins, 69, 73, 830
Mons pubis, 927
  female, 23
  male, 43
Montevideo units, 462
Montgomery tubercle, 38, 111
Mood
  disorders during pregnancy, 296-298
  suicide risk, 1116
Mood swings
  chemotherapy-induced, 1525
  during pregnancy, 165
    first trimester, 137
    postpartum blues, 297
Moon face, chemotherapy-induced, 1525
Moral development, 317, 1090
  child, 853
  function of play, 858
  preschooler, 1018
  school-age child, 1057
Morbidity, 787-789
Morgue, 558
Mormon, 815
Morning-after pill, 529
Morning sickness, 123
Moro reflex, 605
Morphine
  conscious sedation, 1222
  epidural block, 365
  for newborn pain, 721
  patient-controlled analgesia, 1227
  pediatric dosages, 1224
Mortality, 783-787
  childhood, 1148-1154
    cultural considerations, 554
    impending, 1132-1135
    maternal, 562
    reaction of family, 1128-1129
  infant, 2, 3-4, 784-785
  newborn, 550-563, 556
    anticipatory grief, 552
    classification, 697
    communicating and caring techniques, 554-556
    complicated bereavement, 562-563
    documentation, 558-561, 560
    family issues, 717-718
Mortality—cont'd
  newborn—cont'd
    gestational age and birthweight, 725
    grief responses, 551-552
    options for parents, 556-558
    physical comfort, 556
Morula, 58, 59
Mosaicism, 55, 1164
Moslem, 816
Mosquito bites and stings, 1675
Mothers Against Drunk Driving, 1148
Motility
  diarrhea, 1390-1393
  postpartum period, 484
Motor function
  Brazelton Neonatal Behavioral Assessment, 610
  neurologic examination, 1576
Motor vehicle injuries
  adolescent, 1102
  childhood mortality, 786-787
  infant safety, 974
  school-age child, 1070
  spinal cord, 1765
  toddler, 1006-1010
Motrin; *see* Ibuprofen
Mourning, 551, 1128, 1129
Mouth
  changes during pregnancy, 119
  newborn
    assessment, 617, 622, 623
    digestion, 663
    fetal alcohol syndrome, 760
  nutritional status, 889
  review of systems, 881
  unconscious child, 1582
Movies influence on child, 862-863
Moxibustion, 812
MRI; *see* Magnetic resonance imaging
MSH; *see* Melanocyte-stimulating hormone
MSUD; *see* Maple syrup urine disease
MTX; *see* Methotrexate
Mucin, 666
Mucocutaneous lymph node syndrome, 1487-1489
Mucopolysaccharidosis, 96
Mucous membranes
  chemotherapy-induced ulceration, 1524
  dehydration, 1389
  physical examination, 919
Mucus-trap suction apparatus, 632-633
Multifactorial inheritance, 56
Multifetal pregnancy, 69-73
  dysfunctional labor, 456
  prenatal care and psychosocial adjustment, 169-170
  prenatal diagnosis, 97
Multigravida, 104
Multipara
  comparison of abdomen, vulva, and cervix, 107
  length of labor, 347
  older woman, 169
Multiple birth, 562, 830
Multiple marker test, 147-148
Multiple sclerosis, 284
Multivitamin-multimineral supplements, 186
Mummy restraint, 1276-1278
Mummy technique, 639, 649
Mumps, 1034
  during pregnancy, 242
  vaccine, 962, 965-966
Munchausen syndrome by proxy, 1039
Muneco, 145
Murmur, 594, 615, 924
Muscular dysfunction, 1746-1767
  botulism, 1764-1765
  cerebral palsy, 1746-1751, 1752-1753
  Guillain-Barré syndrome, 1762-1763
  juvenile spinal muscular atrophy, 1760
  muscular dystrophy, 1760-1762
  progressive infantile spinal muscular dystrophy, 1759-1760
  spina bifida, 1751-1758
  spinal cord injuries, 1765-1766
  tetanus, 1763-1764
Muscular dystrophy, 1760-1762
Musculoskeletal dysfunction, 1706-1745
  amputation, 1720-1721
  bone and soft tissue tumors, 1735-1738
  cast, 1714-1716
  clubfoot, 1725-1726
  developmental dysplasia of hip, 1721-1725
  distraction, 1720
  fracture, 1711-1714
  immobilization, 1706-1709
  juvenile rheumatoid arthritis, 1738-1741
  kyphosis and lordosis, 1729-1730
  Legg-Calvé-Perthes disease, 1728-1733
  metatarsus adductus, 1726-1727
  osteogenesis imperfecta, 1727-1728
  osteomyelitis, 1733-1734
  scoliosis, 1730-1733
  septic arthritis, 1734
  skeletal limb deficiency, 1727
  slipped femoral capital epiphysis, 1729
  soft tissue injury, 1709-1711
  systemic lupus erythematosus, 1741-1742
  traction, 1716-1720
  tuberculosis, 1734-1735
Musculoskeletal system
  adaptations
    during labor, 352
    postpartum period, 486

Musculoskeletal system—cont'd
adaptations—cont'd
during pregnancy, 117-118
effects of immobilization, 1707
fetal, 68-69
human development milestones, 70-72
newborn
Apgar scoring, 608-609
birth trauma, 635-636, 747-748
congenital anomalies, 775-776
fetal alcohol syndrome, 760
nutritional status, 193, 889
physical examination, 929-930
review of systems, 881
Muslim, 814, 816
Mustargen; *see* Nitrogen mustard
Mutation, chromosomal, 57
Myasthenia gravis, 285
Mycobacterium tuberculosis, 758, 1341
Mycoplasma pneumoniae, 1321
bronchitis, 1337
laryngotracheobronchitis, 1335
respiratory infection, 1321
Mycotic infection, 1669-1671
Myelodysplasia, 1754, 1756
Myelomeningocele, 771, 1751-1758
Myelosuppression, 1520
Myerson's reflex, 604
Myoclonic seizure, 1606
Myoepithelium, 37
Myometrium, 28, 31, 32
Myopia, 1176
Myotonia, 46
Myringotomy, 1332

N

Nägele's rule, 60, 123
Nails
changes during pregnancy, 117
physical examination, 906
Naive instrumental orientation, 1018
Name band, 1272
Naprosyn; *see* Naproxen
Naproxen, 1223
Narcotic analgesics
adolescent abuse, 1113
during labor, 359
Narcotic antagonists, 359-360
Nasal blockage
newborn, 592
respiratory infection, 1322
Nasal cannula, 702
Nasal discharge, 1322
Nasal medication administration, 1297-1298
Nasal washing, 1284
Nasogastric medication administration, 1296
Nasogastric tube feeding, 1311-1313
Nasopharyngeal rhabdomyosarcoma, 1738
Nasopharyngitis, 1326-1327
Natal teeth, 617
National Amputation Foundation, Inc., 1736
National Association for Education of Young Children, 1021
National Association for Home Care, 1195
National Association of State Victims of Child Abuse Legislation Organizations, 1042
National Committee for Prevention of Child Abuse, 1049
National Easter Seal Society, 1146
National Father's Network, 1195
National Head Injury Foundation, 1592
National Hemophilia Foundation, 1515
National Hospice Organization, 1149
National Hydrocephalus Foundation, 1620
National Information Center for Children and Youth with Disabilities, 1195
National Information Clearinghouse for Infants with Disabilities and Life-Threatening Conditions, 1195
National Institute of Dental Research, 1006
National Kidney Foundation, 1568
National Organization of Parents of Murdered Children, Inc., 1148
National Sudden Infant Death Syndrome Resource Center, 1148
Native American culture
childbearing and parenting beliefs, 17
food patterns, 190
health beliefs and practices, 822-823
Natural childbirth method, 354
Natural consequences, 834
Natural family planning, 515
Nausea
chemotherapy-induced, 1521
gastrointestinal dysfunction, 1387
during pregnancy, 118
coping, 195-196
ectopic pregnancy, 222
first trimester, 137
Nazarene, 817
NBAS; *see* Brazelton Neonatal Behavioral Assessment
NCAFS; *see* Nursing Child Assessment Feeding Scale
Near-drowning, 1593-1594
Nearsightedness, 1176
Nebulizer, 1304-1305
NEC; *see* Necrotizing enterocolitis
Neck
newborn assessment, 618, 622-623
nutritional status, 888
physical examination, 907-908
review of systems, 881
Necrotizing enterocolitis, 736-737
Nedocromil sodium, 1349
Needle for venipuncture, 639-640
Negative reinforcement, 834
Negativism, toddler, 995, 1002-1003
Negotiation within family, 10
Neisseria gonorrhoeae, 233
Neonatal abstinence syndrome, 763-765
Neonatal death, 697
Neonatal health history, 634
Neonatal intensive care unit, 2
Neonatal mortality, 2, 784
Neonatal narcosis, 360
Neonatal resuscitation, 699
Neonate; *see* Newborn
Neoplastic disorders, 1517-1530
leukemia, 1517-1528
chemotherapy, 1521-1525
classification, 1517
myelosuppression, 1520-1521
nursing care plan, 1526-1528
pathophysiology, 1517-1518
therapeutic management, 1518-1519
Neopresol; *see* Hydralazine
Neosar; *see* Cyclophosphamide
Nephroblastoma, 1559
Nephrotic syndrome, 1551-1556
Nerve block
administration, 370
during labor, 360-365
pediatric, 1227
Nerve deafness, 1168
Neural tube defect, 56, 770-772, 1751-1758
Neuroblastoma, 1599
Neuroendocrine system, 860
Neurofibromatosis, 1681
Neurohypophysis, 1625
Neurolinguistic programming, 870
Neurologic assessment, 1574-1578
child, 930-931
newborn, 625-626
Neurologic system
adaptations
during labor, 352
postpartum, 486
during pregnancy, 118
complications in diabetes mellitus, 254
fetal, 66-67
human development milestones, 70-72
hypoxemia and, 1472
infant growth, 937
maturation, 848
nutritional status, 193, 890
review of systems, 881
Neuromuscular dysfunction, 1746-1767
botulism, 1764-1765
cerebral palsy, 1746-1751, 1752-1753
Guillain-Barré syndrome, 1762-1763
juvenile spinal muscular atrophy, 1760
muscular dystrophy, 1760-1762

Neuromuscular dysfunction—cont'd
progressive infantile spinal muscular dystrophy, 1759-1760
spina bifida, 1751-1758
spinal cord injuries, 1765-1766
tetanus, 1763-1764
Neuromuscular system of newborn, 603-608, 619
Neuropathic bladder dysfunction, 1756
Neuropathy
brain tumor, 1595
chemotherapy-induced, 1525
diabetic, 1641
Neutral thermal environment, 704
Neutrophil count, 1500
Nevus flammeus, 621
Nevus vasculosus, 621
New Ballard Scale, 612-613, 614
Newborn, 591-782
abdomen, 624
adolescent mother, 328
Apgar scoring, 608-609
attachment behaviors, 610-614
back and anus, 624
baseline measurements, 620-623
behavioral assessment, 609-610
birth trauma, 746-749
breastfeeding, 686-687
cardiovascular system, 592-594
clinical gestational age, 612-613, 614
congenital anomalies, 769-780
cardiovascular, 772
central nervous system, 770-772
diagnosis, 777-779
gastrointestinal, 773-776
genitourinary, 776-777
musculoskeletal, 775-776
respiratory, 772-773
constipation, 1398
cultural beliefs and practices, 16-17
death, 550-561, 717
anticipatory grief, 552
communicating and caring techniques, 554-556
complicated bereavement, 562-563
documentation, 558-561
grief responses, 551-552
options for parents, 556-558
physical comfort, 556
developmental dysplasia of hip, 1723
diabetic mother, 741-746
discharge of compromised newborn, 766-767
dysmature, 739-740
effects of epidural block, 365
extremities, 625
fluid and electrolyte balance, 596
gastrointestinal system, 597
genitalia, 624-625
hearing impairment, 1170
hematopoietic system, 594-595
Newborn—con t'd
hepatic system, 597-599
high risk, 696-723
assessment, 697-699
classification, 696, 697
developmental and emotional aspects of care, 712-713
family care, 719
neonatal pain, 719-721
nursing care management, 713-719
nutrition, 706-712
respiratory care, 699-704
thermoregulatory care, 704-706
transportation, 696-697
home care, 565-590
advantages and disadvantages of short-stay maternity care, 566, 567
early postpartum discharge, 566-571
home care nursing visits, 574-584
nursing role in program development, 589
perinatal coaching, 588-589
preparatory educational instruction, 571-574
support groups, 587-588
telephone follow-up, 584-586
warm lines/help lines, 586-587
hyperbilirubinemia, 767-769
hypertension, 1487
immediate assessment and care after birth, 435
immune system, 599
infant mortality and morbidity, 725
infection
bacterial, 758
fungal, 758-759
TORCH, 752-758
urinary tract, 1547
integumentary system, 600-602
intrauterine growth restriction, 739-740
kernicterus, 768-769
large for gestational age, 740-741
massage, 716-717
maternal substance abuse, 759-766
neurologic assessment, 625-626
neuromuscular system, 603-608
nursing care, 627-660
birth through first two hours, 627-629
circumcision, 653-655
discharge planning and teaching, 655-659
eye prophylaxis, 632-633
hyperbilirubinemia, 650-653
intramuscular injection, 649-650
parental support, 643-649
physical injuries, 635-636
physiologic problems, 636-637
protective environment, 642-643
Newborn—cont'd
nursing care—cont'd
restraining infant, 649
specimen collection, 637-642
supporting adaptation to extrauterine life, 629-632
two hours after birth until discharge, 633-635
nutrition and feeding, 645, 661-695
breastfeeding, 665-691; *see also* Breastfeeding
discharge planning, 695
formula feeding, 691-693
normal development, 661-665
pain, 719-721
parent-newborn relationships, 438-439
physical assessment, 616-619
postdate and postmature, 737-739
preterm, 725-737
bronchopulmonary dysplasia, 735
cardiopulmonary resuscitation, 731
feeding, 731
gestational age assessment, 732
growth and development, 727-729
infant stimulation, 730-731
necrotizing enterocolitis, 736-737
parental adaptation, 729
parental support, 731-732
patent ductus arteriosus, 735
periventricular-intraventricular hemorrhage, 735-736
physical care, 730
potential problems, 726-727
respiratory distress syndrome, 732-734
retinopathy of prematurity, 735
reproductive system, 599-600
respiratory system, 591-592
risk factor assessment, 80
skeletal system, 602-603
slow weight gain, 685-686
small for gestational age, 739-740
standards of care, 1769-1772
thermoregulation, 595-596
thorax, 623-624
vital sign, 614-620
NFP; *see* Natural family planning
Niacin
hyperlipidemia, 1484
needs during pregnancy, 179
nutritional significance, 1374
Nicotinamide, 1374
Nicotine, 680, 766
Nicotinic acid
hyperlipidemia, 1484
nutritional significance, 1374
NIDDM; *see* Non-insulin–dependent diabetes mellitus
Niemann-Pick disease, 96
Nifedipine
preeclampsia, 214

Nifedipine—cont'd
  during pregnancy, 272
  suppression of uterine activity, 450
Nightmare, 1026-1027
Nighttime feeding, 960
Ninety-degree-ninety-degree traction, 1718
Nipple
  maternal
    inverted, 668
    sore, 685
  newborn, 600
Nipple confusion, 675
Nipple shield, 685
Nipple-stimulated contraction test, 99-100
Nitrazine test, 399
Nitrogen mustard, 1522
Nitroglycerin, 214
Nitronox, 1693
Nitroprusside, 272
Nits, 1673-1674
Nocturia, 115
Nocturnal emission, 1095
Nodule, 1657
Noise as neonatal environmental hazard, 715
Non-Hodgkin lymphoma, 1530
Non-insulin–dependent diabetes mellitus, 252, 1640
Nondisjunction abnormality, 54
Nonmaleficence, 795
Nonnutritive sucking, 712, 731
Nonopioid analgesics, 1221-1222
Nonorganic failure to thrive, 980, 982-983
Nonoxynol 9, 518
Nonshivering thermogenesis, 595
Nonsteroidal antiinflammatory drugs
  juvenile rheumatoid arthritis, 1739
  pediatric dosages, 1223
Nonstress test, 95
  biophysical profile, 88
  fetal monitoring, 97-98
  indications, 97
  maternal diabetes mellitus, 258
Nontherapeutic relationship, 793
Nonverbal communication, 867
  with child, 877
  family, 12
  mentally retarded child, 1161-1162
Norepinephrine, 1634
Norethindrone, 522, 523
Norgestrel, 522, 523
Normal flora, 597
Normalization, 1122-1123, 1140
  home care, 1191
Normeperidine, 1222
Normodyne; *see* Labetalol
Normoglycemia, 258
Norplant, 524
Norport, 1295
North American blastomycosis, 1670
Norwood procedure, 1464
Nose
  medication administration, 1297-1298
  newborn assessment, 617, 623
  nutritional status, 889
  physical examination, 918
  review of systems, 881
Nosebleed, 1516-1517
NST; *see* Nonshivering thermogenesis, Nonstress test
Nuchal cord, 63, 434
Nuclear brain scan, 1577
Nuclear family, 9
Nulligravida, 104
Nullipara, 104
  comparison of abdomen, vulva, and cervix, 107
  length of labor, 347
  older woman, 169
Numeric pain scale, 1211
Nurse
  liability in fetal monitoring, 388
  reaction to dying child, 1154-1155
  role in contemporary pediatric nursing, 793-796
  role in home care, 1188
  taking baby to morgue, 558
Nursery
  ambient temperature of, 629
  neonatal transfer to, 633
Nursing admission history, 1204-1207
Nursing care plan
  acute respiratory infection, 1325
  anemia, 1504
  asthma, 1355
  burns, 1701-1702
  cerebral palsy, 1752-1753
  child with cancer, 1526-1528
  chronic illness or disability, 1147-1148
  chronic renal failure, 1566-1567
  cleft lip or palate, 1423
  communicable diseases, 1038
  congenital heart disease, 1480
  congestive heart failure, 1471
  diabetes mellitus, 1651
  family of hospitalized child, 1241
  gastroenteritis, 1394
  hearing impairment, 1174
  hospitalized, 1235
  human immunodeficiency virus infection, 1532
  immobilized child, 1710
  maltreatment, 1048
  mental retardation, 1164
  nephrotic syndrome, 1555
  pediatric surgery, 1260-1261
  pregnancy
    active labor, 423
    adolescent, 332
    cocaine abuse, 308
Nursing care plan—cont'd
  pregnancy—cont'd
    dysfunctional labor, 473-474
    electronic fetal monitoring, 391
    first trimester, 144-145
    heart disease, 279
    hyperemesis gravidarum, 269
    lumbar epidural block during labor, 370
    maternal nutrition, 199
    nonpharmacologic management of discomfort during labor, 358
    placenta previa, 227
    postpartum depression, 301
    preeclampsia, 210, 213
    pregestational insulin-dependent diabetes mellitus, 264
    preterm labor, 451
    puerperal infection, 546
    second stage of labor, 436
    second trimester, 149
    third stage of labor, 440
    third trimester, 168
  skin disorder, 1665
  terminally ill or dying, 1152
  unconscious child, 1584-1585
Nursing caries, 1006
Nursing Child Assessment Feeding Scale, 613-614
Nursing diagnoses
  acute respiratory infection, 1325
  anemia, 1504
  asthma, 1355
  burns, 1701-1702
  cerebral palsy, 1752-1753
  child with cancer, 1526-1528
  chronic illness or disability, 1147-1148
  chronic renal failure, 1566-1567
  cleft lip or palate, 1423
  communicable diseases, 1038
  congenital heart disease, 1480
  congestive heart failure, 1471
  diabetes mellitus, 1651
  family health care, 20
  family of hospitalized child, 1241
  gastroenteritis, 1394
  hearing impairment, 1174
  hospitalized, 1235
  human immunodeficiency virus infection, 1532
  immobilized child, 1710
  maltreatment, 1048
  mental retardation, 1164
  nephrotic syndrome, 1555
  pediatric surgery, 1260-1261
  pregnancy
    active labor, 423
    adolescent, 332
    cocaine abuse, 308
    dysfunctional labor, 473-474
    electronic fetal monitoring, 391

Nursing diagnoses—cont'd
  pregnancy—cont'd
    first trimester, 144-145
    heart disease, 279
    hyperemesis gravidarum, 269
    lumbar epidural block during labor, 370
    maternal nutrition, 199
    nonpharmacologic management of discomfort during labor, 358
    placenta previa, 227
    postpartum depression, 301
    preeclampsia, 210, 213
    pregestational insulin-dependent diabetes mellitus, 264
    preterm labor, 451
    puerperal infection, 546
    second stage of labor, 436
    second trimester, 149, 151
    third stage of labor, 440
    third trimester, 168
  skin disorder, 1665
  terminally ill or dying, 1152
  unconscious child, 1584-1585
Nursing practice
  research into, 5
  standards of care, 1769
  trends, 5
Nursing process, 1190-1191
Nursing research, 795-796
Nutrient needs, 663-664
Nutrition
  adolescent, 1098-1099
  anemia, 1504
  assessment, 885-890
  burn victim, 1692, 1697
  child, 860
  diabetes mellitus, 1643
  endocrine system and, 120
  infant, 956-959
  inflammatory bowel disease, 1410-1411
  maternal, 176-200
    assessment, 188-189, 193
    cultural food patterns, 190-191
    during lactation, 187-188
    postpartum, 499
  newborn, 661-695
    breastfeeding, 665-691; *see also* Breastfeeding
    discharge planning, 695
    formula feeding, 691-693
    high risk, 706-712
    normal development, 661-665
    preterm, 726
  during pregnancy
    adolescent, 322-323, 327-328
    energy needs, 177-182
    exercise, 187
    minerals and vitamins, 184-186
    negative impacts, 186-187
    nursing care plan, 199
Nutrition—cont'd
  during pregnancy—cont'd
    plan of care and implementation, 194-196
    preeclampsia, 209
    pregnancy-induced hypertension, 187
  preschooler, 1025-1026
  questionnaire, 192
  respiratory infection, 1326
  school-age child, 1063
  socioeconomic factors, 807
  toddler, 1003-1004
  unconscious child, 1581
Nutritional disturbances, 1372-1449
  delayed wound healing, 1660
  food sensitivity, 1384-1386
  mineral, 1377-1384
  protein energy malnutrition, 1384
  vitamin, 1372-1377
Nutritional history, 127
Nutritional status
  clinical assessment, 888-890
  congestive heart failure, 1470
  physical assessment, 193
  during pregnancy
    assessment, 136
    high risk factors, 81

O

Obesity
  adolescent, 1106-1109
  anesthesia during labor, 366-367
  infant, 959
Object permanence, 943-944
Oblique fracture, 1712
Obstetric admitting record, 396-397
Obstetric history, 126, 395
Obstetric measurements, 342
Obstipation, 1395
Obstructive disorders, 1425-1432
  airway, 1365-1368
  anorectal malformations, 1431-1432
  cardiac, 1455-1457
  hypertrophic pyloric stenosis, 1426-1429
  intussusception, 1429-1431
Obstructive uropathy, 1549-1550
Obtundation, 1574
Obturator artery, 33
Obturator foramen, 36
Occlusive dressings, 1661, 1693
Oculomotor nerve, 932
Oculovestibular response, 1576
Odor, parent-infant bonding, 508
Oil glands, 601-602
Olfactory nerve, 932
Oligohydramnios, 61, 410
  fetal renal dysfunction, 66
  related risk factors, 82
  ultrasound assessment, 87-88
Oligosaccharides, 666
Oliguria, 202
Omphalocele, 67, 96, 774, 775, 1426
Omphalomesenteric fistula, 1409
Oncovin; *see* Vincristine
Onlooker play, 856
Only child, 829
Oogenesis, 54, 55
Open family, 13
Open fracture, 1712
Operculum, 110
Ophthalmia neonatorum, 233, 632
Opioid analgesics, 1221-1222
  for newborn pain, 719-720
  pediatric dosages, 1224
  side effects, 1229
Opportunistic infection, 755
Optic medication administration, 1297-1298
Optic nerve, 932
Optimum state of arousal, 610
OPV; *see* Oral poliovirus vaccine
Oral candidiasis, 758
Oral cavity
  newborn assessment, 622
  nutritional status, 193
Oral contraceptives, 521-523, 524
  adolescent use, 320
  breastfeeding and, 677
  hypertension and, 1487
Oral hygiene
  hospitalized child, 1266-1267, 1299
  unconscious child, 1582
Oral medication administration, 1226, 1286-1288
Oral poliovirus vaccine, 658
Oral rehydration therapy, 1391
Oral stage of psychosexual development, 850-851
Oral temperature, 901
Orbital rhabdomyosarcoma, 1738
Ordinal position, 828-829
Organ donation, 557
Organic failure to thrive, 980
Orgasmic phase of sexual response, 47
Orogastric medication administration, 1296
Orogastric tube, 709
Orthodox Presbyterian, 817
Orthopedics, neural tube defects, 1755-1756
Orthostatic hypotension, 152
Orthotics
  developmental dysplasia of hip, 1724
  scoliosis, 1731
Orthotopic heart transplantation, 1494
Osmolality, 1544, 1800
Ossification, 69
Osteochondritis deformans juvenilis, 1728-1729
Osteodystrophy, renal, 1564

Osteogenesis imperfecta, 96, 1727-1728
Osteogenic sarcoma, 1735-1737
Osteomyelitis, 1733-1734
Ostium primum, 1456
Ostium secundum, 1456
Ostomy, pediatric, 1315-1316
Otic medication administration, 1297-1298
Otitis media, 1331-1333
Otoscopy, 916-918
OTOTEMP, 902
Oucher pain scale, 1211
Outer syncytium, 63
Outlet, pelvic, 37
Outlet contracture, 453
Outpatient setting, 1241-1242
Ovarian artery, 32, 33
Ovarian cycle, 39-41
Ovarian ligaments, 28, 29, 31
Ovary, 27-29, 30
 adaptations during postpartum period, 483
 cyst
  ectopic pregnancy *versus*, 222
  during pregnancy, 286
 newborn, 599
 production of hormones, 1625
Overuse syndromes, 1072
Ovral, 529
Ovulation
 breast-feeding and, 483
 contraception and, 515, 516, 517
 ovarian cycle, 39-41
 ovaries, 29
 postpartum resumption, 483
 predictor test for, 517
 prostaglandin role, 42
Ovum
 conception, 58, 59
 implantation, 41
 uterine tubes, 29
Oximeter sensor, 1303
Oxycephaly, 1615
Oxycodone, 1221
 equianalgesia, 1225
 pediatric dosages, 1224
Oxygen consumption, 596
Oxygen-induced carbon dioxide narcosis, 1303
Oxygen partial pressure, 699, 1800
Oxygen tension, 596
Oxygen therapy
 hypovolemic shock, 542
 newborn, 699, 701-704
 pediatric, 1302-1303
 respiratory distress syndrome, 734
 sickle cell anemia, 1507
Oxygen toxicity, 1303
Oxygenation, 631-632
Oxyhemoglobin dissociation curve, 1304
Oxytocic agents, 541
Oxytocin, 1625
 induction of labor, 461-462, 463
 intrauterine resuscitation, 389
 lactation and, 666, 667
 postpartum contractions, 481
 postpartum hemorrhage, 539
 postpartum uterine tone stimulation, 494
Oxytocin-stimulated contraction test, 100

P

Pacemaker, 1485
Pacifier, 657-658, 949, 954, 970, 973
Packed red blood cells, 543
Pain
 after cesarean birth, 469
 analysis of, 879
 appendicitis, 1408
 assessment in child, 1207-1214
 assessment of respiratory function, 1323
 ectopic pregnancy, 222
 FACES Pain Rating Scale, 1790
 gastrointestinal dysfunction, 1387
 high risk newborn, 719-721
 hospitalized child's reaction, 1200-1203
 postpartum, 497-498
 respiratory infection, 1322
 school-age child, 1079
 undermedication, 1208
Pain assessment record, 1215
Pain management
 after cardiac surgery, 1478-1479
 burn victim, 1692-1693, 1696
 circumcision, 653-654
 fear of addiction, 1509
 fourth stage of labor, 497-498
 hospitalized child, 1219-1230
  nonpharmacologic, 1220-1221
  right dosage, 1223-1225
  right drug, 1221-1222
  right route, 1225-1228
  right time, 1228-1229
  side effects, 1229-1230
 juvenile rheumatoid arthritis, 1739, 1740
 during labor, 352-374
  administration of medication, 369-373
  anesthesia in obese woman, 366-367
  childbirth preparation methods, 354-355
  expression of pain, 353-354
  general anesthesia, 366
  informed consent, 369
  maternal hypothermia after analgesia and anesthesia, 367
  nerve block analgesia and anesthesia, 360-365
Pain management—cont'd
 during labor—cont'd
  relaxing and breathing techniques, 355-357
  sedatives, 358
  sociocultural basis of pain experience, 401
  systemic analgesia, 358-359
 leukemia, 1520
 postpartum, 498
 skin disorders, 1663-1664
Pain rating scale, 1209-1212
Palate, cleft, 1418-1422
Palatine tonsil, 920, 1328
Pallor, 907
Palmar erythema, 117, 152
Palmar grasp, 939
Palmar reflex, 604
Palpation
 abdominal, 600, 925-926
 fundus, 496, 497
 testicular, 600
Palpebral fissure, 908, 909
Palpitations, 152
Palsy, 625
Pancreas
 changes during pregnancy, 119-120
 fetal, 68
 infant digestion, 663
Pancreatic fibrosis, 1356
Pantothenic acid, 1375
Pap smear, 131
Papillomatosis, 240
Papule, 1657
Paracervical block, 365
Parachute reflex, 938
Paralanguage, 867
Parallel play, 856, 999
Paralysis
 Duchenne-Erb, 724, 743, 748
 facial, 748
 forceps delivery, 743
Paralytic ileus, 1425, 1427
Paranasal sinus rhabdomyosarcoma, 1738
Paraplegia, 1766
Parasitic disease, intestinal, 1403-1406
Parathyroid gland
 changes during pregnancy, 119
 disorders, 1633-1634
 functions, 1625
Parathyroid hormone, 1625, 1633
Paraurethral glands, 27
Parenchyma, 37
Parent, 831-835
 adopted child, 835-837
 child abuse, 1040, 1045
 child's school experience, 1061
 communication with, 868-872
 cultural beliefs, 16-17
 divorce, 837-839
 grieving, 556-558

Parent—cont'd
hospitalized child
fostering parent-child relationships, 1233-1234
minimization of separation, 1216-1218
participation in care, 1237-1238
presence during pediatric cardiopulmonary resuscitation, 1362
reactions to, 1236
newborn relationships, 438-439, 502-504, 643-649
presence during neonatal physical examination, 633-634
preterm infant, 729
promotion of skills, 510
relationship with adolescents, 1091-1092, 1096
roles, 827-828
special needs child, 1122, 1123
blind, 1178
coping mechanisms, 1138-1140
death, 1150
impact on, 1125-1126
Parent education classes, 141, 170-171
Parent-professional collaboration, 791-792, 1189-1190
Parenteral fluid therapy
neonatal, 711
pediatric, 1299-1302
Parenthood
adolescent, 329-330
after age 35, 159
Parents Anonymous, 1114
Parents of Murdered Children, 1153
Paresthesia
during pregnancy, 118
skin lesions, 1655
Parity, 103-104
duration of second stage of labor, 425
high risk factor, 81
Parlodel; *see* Bromocriptine
Parotitis, 242, 1035
Paroxysmal abdominal pain, 979-980
Partial mole, 222-223
Partial seizure, 1606, 1607-1608
Partial-thickness burn, 1687, 1689
Partial thromboplastin time, 1800
Partogram, 407, 408, 457
Parvovirus infection, 242-243
Passive smoking, 1346-1347
Past history, 878-880
Patau syndrome, 778
Patch, 1656
Patellar reflex, 206, 930-931
Patent ductus arteriosus, 735, 1458
Paternal adaptation, 158, 509-510
Patient compliance, 1262-1264
Patient-controlled analgesia
pediatric, 1225-1227
sickle cell anemia, 1507
Patient history; *see* Health history
Patient preparation
pediatric procedures, 1252-1257
physical examination, 893-896
Patient teaching
breastfeeding, 670-671
newborn care, 655-659
postoperative complications of cesarean birth, 472
preeclampsia, 208
ultrasound, 90
Pavlik harness, 636, 1723
PCA; *see* Patient-controlled analgesia
PCP; *see* Phencyclidine hydrochloride
PDA; *see* Patent ductus arteriosus
Peak expiratory flow meter, 1352
Peak expiratory flow rate, 1348, 1349
Peak inspiratory pressure, 702
Pearson attachment, 1718
Pectoralis major muscle, 37
Pediatric nurse practitioner, 794
Pediatric nursing interventions, 1250-1320
artificial ventilation, 1305-1311
bathing, 1266, 1267
blood specimens, 1282-1284
bronchial drainage, 1305, 1306-1307
chest physiotherapy, 1305, 1308
control of fever, 1268-1271
enema, 1315
environmental safety measures, 1274
evolution of child health care, 789-791
family teaching and home care, 1271
feeding sick child, 1268
future trends, 796-979
gastrostomy feeding, 1313-1314
gavage feeding, 1311-1313
hair care, 1267-1268
Healthy People 2000, 783
infection control, 1272-1274
informed consent, 1250-1252
inhalation therapy, 1302-1305
limit-setting, 1275
maintenance of skin integrity, 1264-1266
measurement of intake and output, 1299
medication administration, 1284-1299
determination of drug dosage, 1284-1286
family teaching and home care, 1298-1299
intramuscular, 1288-1292
intravenous, 1293
nasogastric, orogastric, or gastrostomy, 1296
optic, otic, and nasal, 1297-1298
oral, 1286-1288
Pediatric nursing interventions—cont'd
medication administration—cont'd
peripheral venous access devices, 1294-1296
rectal, 1296-1297
subcutaneous and intradermal, 1292-1293
morbidity, 787-789
mortality, 783-787
newborn, 649-655
oral hygiene, 1266-1267
ostomy, 1315-1316
parenteral fluid therapy, 1299-1302
patient compliance, 1262-1264
philosophy of care, 791-793
positioning for procedures, 1278-1279
postoperative care, 1261-1262
preoperative care, 1257-1261
preparation for procedures, 1252-1257
reaction of child
bodily injury and pain, 1200-1203
loss of control, 1198-1200
separation anxiety, 1196-1198
restraints, 1276-1278
role of nurse, 793-796
throat specimens, 1284
total parenteral nutrition, 1314
transporting infants and children, 1275-1276
urine specimens, 1280-1282
Pediculosis capitis, 1673-1674
Pedophilia, 1041
PEEP; *see* Positive end-expiratory pressure
Peer cultures, 804-805
Peer group
adolescent, 1092, 1096
school-age child, 1058
Peer pressure, 1115
Pelvic dystocia, 453
Pelvic examination
ectopic pregnancy, 222
first trimester, 129-130
Pelvic floor, 34-35
adaptations during postpartum period, 483
changes during pregnancy, 111
Pelvic relaxation, 483
Pelvic rocking exercise, 140
Pelvic tilt exercise, 155
Pelvis
blood supply, 32, 33
bony, 36-37
dystocia, 453
labor and, 340-342
large-for-gestational-age infant, 740
Penicillin
allergy to, 1492
syphilis, 234
Penis, 43-44
circumcision, 653-655
congenital anomalies, 776

Pentecostal, 817
Pentobarbital, 1222
Peptic ulcer, 1412-1414
Perceptive deafness, 1168
Percocet; *see* Oxycodone
Percodan; *see* Oxycodone
Percussion, chest, 631
Percutaneous umbilical blood sampling, 85, 93-94
Perianal laceration
 care of, 495, 496
 nursing intervention, 498
 postpartum hemorrhage, 538
Perianal pad, 496-497
Perimenopause, 42
Perimetrium, 28
Perinatal asphyxia, 739, 743-744
Perinatal care, 4
Perinatal coaching, 588-589
Perinatal mortality, 2, 697
Perineal body, 35-36
Perineum, 27, 34-35
 adaptations during postpartum period, 482-483
 laceration, 441
 newborn assessment, 624
 postpartum, 489, 492, 493
 rhabdomyosarcoma, 1738
Periodic abstinence, 515
Periodontal disease, 1067
Peripartum heart failure, 276
Peripheral access device, 1283
Peripheral blood smear, 1500
Peripheral venous access devices, 1294-1296
Peripheral vision, 913
Peripherally inserted central catheter, 1294
Peristalsis, 925
Peristaltic waves, 924
Peritoneal dialysis, 1568
Periventricular-intraventricular hemorrhage, 735-736
Permissive parenting style, 833
Persistent fetal circulation, 738
Persistent pulmonary hypertension of newborn, 737-738
Persistent vegetative state, 1574
Personal identity, 1089-1090
Personal space, 19
Personality, 48, 1064-1065
 growth and development, 850-852
 increased intracranial pressure, 1573
Perspiration, changes during pregnancy, 117
Pertussis, 1034, 1341
Pertussis vaccine, 965
Pessary, 549, 550
PET; *see* Positron emission tomography
Petechiae
 neonatal birth trauma, 635, 747
 racial differences, 907
 skin lesions, 1655
Petit mal seizure, 1607
PETT; *see* Positron emission transaxial tomography
pH
 blood, 115
 changes during pregnancy, 110
 normal laboratory values, 1800-1801
 urine, 1544
Phagocytosis, 1658
Phallic stage of psychosexual development, 851
Phantom limb pain, 1736
Pharyngeal tonsil, 1328
Pharyngitis, 1327-1328
Phencyclidine hydrochloride, 761
 breastfeeding and, 766
 psychologic and physiologic signs, 304
 use during pregnancy, 302, 306
Phenindione, 680
Phenobarbital
 hyperbilirubinemia, 651-652
 maternal use, 762
Phenothiazines
 during labor, 359
 during pregnancy, 300
Phenotype, 53
Phenylalanine, 1801
Phenylketonuria, 58, 637, 638, 777-778
Pheochromocytoma, 1639-1640
Pheromone, 26
Phimosis, 653, 1551
Phobia, school, 1078-1079
Phocomelia, 619, 1727
Phosphatidylglycerol, 91, 258
Phospholipids, amniocentesis, 91
Phosphorus
 hypoparathyroidism, 1633
 needs during pregnancy, 178
 nutritional significance, 1380
Photographic pain scale, 1211
Phototherapy
 hyperbilirubinemia, 651-652
 physiologic jaundice, 636
 portable, 583
Phrenic nerve trauma, 749
Physical abuse, 1039-1040, 1043
Physical activity
 adolescent, 1099
 after cardiac surgery, 1478
 hospitalized child, 1230
 infant, 959-961
 newborn, 582
 during pregnancy
  first trimester, 138-139, 145-146
  second trimester, 154
 preschooler, 1026
 school-age child, 1065-1066
Physical activity—cont'd
 toddler, 1004
Physical examination, 893-931
 abdomen, 924-926
 adolescent high-risk sexual behavior and pregnancy, 319, 324
 anus, 928
 back and extremities, 928-930
 cardiac dysfunction, 1450-1451
 cerebral dysfunction, 1572
 chest, 920-921
 child abuse, 1046
 ear, 914-918
 eye, 908-914
 general appearance, 905-907
 genitalia, 926-928
 growth measurements, 896-900
 head and neck, 907-908
 heart, 922-924
 lungs, 921-922
 lymph nodes, 907
 mouth and throat, 918-920
 neurologic assessment, 930-931
 newborn, 579-582, 633-635
 nose, 918
 physiologic measurements, 900-905
 pregnancy
  diabetes mellitus, 257
  first trimester, 129
  during home visit, 579, 580, 582
  during labor, 368
  maternal infections, 245-246
  maternal nutrition, 189
  second trimester, 147
  third trimester, 161
 preparation of child, 893-896
 sequence of examination, 893
 skin, 906-907
Physical neglect, 1039, 1043
Physical therapy, 1748-1749
Physiologic anemia, 113-114, 938
Physiologic changes in child, 848-849
Physiologic edema, 116
Physiologic jaundice, 636, 682
 icterus neonatorum, 598-599
 treatment, 681
Piaget developmental model, 852-853
 abstract thinking, 1090
 concrete operations, 1056-1057
 preconceptual phase, 995-996, 997
 preoperational phase, 1017-1018
 sensorimotor phase, 943-944, 995-996, 997
Pica, 187
Pigeon toe, 929
Pigmentation changes during pregnancy, 116, 152
PIH; *see* Pregnancy-induced hypertension
Pill count, 1263
Pilosebaceous follicle, 1684
Pimple, 1666

Pinard's fetoscope, 133
Pincer grasp, 939
Pinch test, 156, 157
Pinocytosis, 65
Pinworms, 1405-1406
PIP; *see* Peak inspiratory pressure
Piskacek's sign, 109
Pitocin; *see* Oxytocin
Pitting edema, 205
Pituitary disorders, 1624-1629
  diabetes insipidus, 1628-1629
  hyperfunction, 1627
  hypopituitarism, 1624-1627
  precocious puberty, 1627-1628
  syndrome of inappropriate antidiuretic hormone, 1629
  unconscious child, 1581
Pituitary hormones, 483
PKU; *see* Phenylketonuria
Placebo, 1222
Placenta, 63-65
  abruptio placentae, 226-228
  cord insertion variations, 229-230
  placenta previa, 224-226
  prenatal diagnosis of placental conditions, 97
  retained, 539
  separation in third stage of labor, 436-437
  ultrasound assessment, 87
Placenta accreta, 539
Placenta increta, 539
Placenta percreta, 539
Placenta previa, 97, 224-226
Placenta succenturiate, 230
Placental hormones, 483
Plagiocephaly, 1615
Plantar artery, 637
Plantar creases, 625
Plantar nerve, 637
Plantar reflex, 604, 606, 929
Plantar wart, 1667
Plants, poisonous and nonpoisonous, 1435, 1437
Plaque, 1656
Plaque removal, 1004-1005
Plasma glucose, 636
Plasma volume, 1801
Plasmodium falciparum, 242
Plastibell procedure, 653, 655
Plastic strip thermometer, 902
Plateau phase of sexual response, 47
Platelet count, 231, 1500, 1801
Platelet transfusion, 231
Platelets, newborn, 595
Platypelloid pelvis, 342, 343
Play, 855-858
  blind child, 1179
  communication technique, 875, 877
  hospitalized child, 1230-1236
  infant development, 944, 946-948
Play—cont'd
  mentally retarded child, 1160-1161
  during pediatric procedures, 1257, 1258
  preschooler, 1017, 1019-1020
  school-age child, 1059-1060
  toddler, 999
Plugged milk duct, 684
Plumbism, 1440
PMI; *see* Point of maximal impulse
Pneumatic otoscopy, 1332
Pneumococcal polysaccharide vaccine, 967
Pneumocystis carinii pneumonia, 235, 755
Pneumonia, 1339-1341
  aspiration, 657, 1345
  neonatal, 734, 749
  Pneumocystis carinii, 235, 755
Pneumonitis, 1339
Pneumothorax, 1358
Point of maximal impulse, 593
Poison ivy, oak, and sumac, 1671-1672
Poisoning, 789, 1434-1444
  adolescent, 1103
  food, 1397
  heavy metals, 1439-1440
  infant, 975
  lead, 1440-1444
  principles of emergency treatment, 1435-1439
  school-age child, 1070
  toddler, 1007, 1011
Poker chip tool, 1212
Policies, procedures, and protocols, 1770
Polio vaccine, 962, 965, 968
Poliomyelitis, 1034-1035
Poliovirus vaccine, 658
Polish food patterns, 190
Polycystic kidney disease, 57
Polycythemia, 744-745, 1472
Polydactyly, 603, 619, 775-776, 928
Polydipsia, 1628
Polyhydramnios
  maternal diabetes mellitus, 255
  related risk factors, 82
Polyurethane film, 1661
Polyuria
  diabetes insipidus, 1628
  diabetes mellitus, 252
Pompe disease, 96
Pork hypersensitivity, 1385
Pornography, child, 1041
Porphyria, 96
Port-a-cath, 1295
Port-wine stain, 621
Portable phototherapy, 583
Positioning
  childbirth, 427-428
  dystocia and, 456
  ear examination, 914-916
  epidural nerve block, 363-364
Positioning—cont'd
  fetal electronic monitoring, 388
  newborn
    for airway maintenance, 631
    breastfeeding, 669, 670
    burping, 672
    circumcision, 654
    formula feeding, 691
    high-risk infant, 715-716
  pediatric nursing interventions, 1278-1279
  unconscious child, 1582
  woman in labor, 345-346, 414-416, 417
Positive end-expiratory pressure, 702
Positive reinforcement, 834
Positive signs and symptoms of pregnancy, 105, 106, 123
Positron emission tomography, 1577
Positron emission transaxial tomography, 1577
Postanesthesia recovery, 489-491
Postcoital contraception, 529
Postconcussion syndrome, 1590
Postdate birth, 472-475
Postdate infant, 737-739
Postdate pregnancy, 472-475
Posterior pituitary, 1625
Postmature infant, 697, 737-739
Postnatal death, 697
Postneonatal mortality, 784
Postoperative care
  appendicitis, 1408
  brain tumor, 1597
  cardiac disease, 1452-1453
  cesarean birth, 469
  cleft lip or palate, 1421-1422
  congenital heart disease, 1477-1479
  Hirschsprung disease, 1400
  hydrocephalus, 1619
  hypertrophic pyloric stenosis, 1429
  myelomeningocele, 1758
  pediatric nursing interventions, 1261-1262
  scoliosis, 1732-1733
  tracheoesophageal fistula, 1425
  Wilms tumor, 1560
Postpartum blues, 297, 298, 301, 510
Postpartum diuresis, 484
Postpartum period, 480-590
  adolescent mother, 328-329
  cesarean birth, 469
  complications, 537-564
    hemorrhage, 537-543
    mastitis, 544
    sepsis, 543-544
    stillbirth and newborn death, 550-563
    structural disorders of uterus and vagina, 546-550
    urinary tract infection, 543

Postpartum period—cont'd
contraception, 513-515
cultural beliefs and practices, 16-17, 505
diabetic mother, 263-264
discharge teaching, 512
factors placing mother and neonate at high risk, 83
fourth stage of labor, 488-512
ambulation, 498-499
bladder and bowel patterns, 499-501
breastfeeding and lactation suppression, 501
comfort, 497-498
coping strategies, 510-512
cultural diversity, 504-505
laboratory tests, 492
maternal adjustment, 508-509
nutrition, 499
parent-infant interactions, 502-504
parental attachment, bonding, and acquaintance, 506-508
paternal adjustment, 509-510
postanesthesia recovery, 489-491
prevention of excessive bleeding, 495-497
prevention of infection, 495
Rh isoimmunization, 501-502
rubella vaccination, 501
transfer from recovery area, 491-492
uterine tone, 494, 495
gestational diabetes mellitus, 267-268
heart disease, 275
human immunodeficiency virus infected mother, 236
infant risk factors, 83
maternal physiology, 480-487
mother and newborn home care, 565-590
advantages and disadvantages of short-stay maternity care, 566, 567
early postpartum discharge, 566-571
home care nursing visits, 574-584
nursing role in program development, 589
perinatal coaching, 588-589
preparatory educational instruction, 571-574
support groups, 587-588
telephone follow-up, 584-586
warm lines/help lines, 586-587
nutrition, 188, 194-195
preeclampsia-eclampsia, 215
prescribed medications, 513
psychosocial concerns, 504
routine mother and baby checkups, 513
sexual activity, 512-513
thyroid dysfunction, 270
Postterm pregnancy, 82
Posttraumatic stress disorder, 1078
Posttraumatic syndromes, 1590
Postural drainage, 1305-1307
Posture
adolescent, 1100
changes during pregnancy, 117, 154, 155
neurologic examination, 1576
nutritional status, 193
Potassium
normal laboratory values, 1801
nutritional significance, 1381
Poultry
hypersensitivity, 1385
needs during pregnancy, 183
Poverty, 803
failure to thrive, 981
visible *versus* invisible, 803
Povidone iodine, 1660, 1694
Poxvirus, 1667
PPHN; *see* Persistent pulmonary hypertension of newborn
Prebirth education, 170-173
Precipitous labor, 458
Precocious puberty, 1627-1628
Preconception care, 75-77
Preconceptual phase, 995-996, 997
Predictor test for ovulation, 517
Prednisone
leukemia and lymphoma, 1522
nephrotic syndrome, 1553
Preeclampsia, 199, 200-202
home care, 208
hydatidiform mole, 223
maternal diabetes mellitus, 255
Pregestational diabetes, 252, 253-254
Pregnancy, 51-335
adolescent, 317, 321-329
adoption, 329
care management, 322-324
cultural influences, 322
developmental tasks of pregnancy, 321-322
under fifteen years of age, 321
nutrition counseling, 327-328
postpartum care, 328-329
prenatal care, 325-326
anatomy and physiology, 103-121
adaptations to pregnancy, 105, 106
breasts, 111
cardiovascular system, 111-114
endocrine system, 119-120
gastrointestinal system, 118-119
gravidity and parity, 103-104
hypothalamic-pituitary-ovarian axis, 105
integumentary system, 116-117
musculoskeletal system, 117-118
neurologic system, 118
pregnancy tests, 104-105
Pregnancy—cont'd
anatomy and physiology—cont'd
renal system, 115-116
respiratory system, 114-115
uterus, 106-110
vagina and vulva, 110-111
breastfeeding during, 677
cardiovascular disorders
cardiopulmonary resuscitation, 278-279
heart disease, 270-276
heart surgery, 276
cultural beliefs, 16-17
embryo development, 60-65
endocrine disorders, 251-270
diabetes mellitus, 251-265; *see also* Diabetes mellitus
gestational diabetes mellitus, 265-268
hyperemesis gravidarum, 268
thyroid disorders, 269-270
first trimester, 122-146
birth plan, 141
cultural variations in prenatal care, 143-146
diagnosis of pregnancy, 123
education for self-care, 135-141
expected outcomes, 134
fetal development, 132-134
interview, 126-129
laboratory tests, 131-132
nursing diagnoses, 134
parent education classes, 141
pelvic examination, 129-130
physical examination, 129
plan of care and implementation, 134-135
prenatal history form, 124-125
sexual counseling, 141-143
speculum and internal examinations, 130-131
fourth trimester; *see* Postpartum period
genetics, 51-58
cell division, 53-54
chromosomal abnormalities, 54-56
gametogenesis, 54
genes and chromosomes, 51-53
patterns of genetic transmission, 56-58
hemorrhagic disorders, 216-231
abruptio placentae, 226-228
clotting disorders, 230-231
ectopic pregnancy, 220-222
hydatidiform mole, 222-224
incompetent cervix, 219-220
nursing care management, 228-230
placenta previa, 224-226
spontaneous abortion, 216-218
infections, 231-247
chlamydial, 232-233
coxsackievirus B, 242
gonorrhea, 233

Pregnancy—cont'd
infections—cont'd
human immunodeficiency virus, 234-236
human papillomavirus, 239-240
infection control, 244, 245
influenza, 242
listeriosis, 242
Lyme disease, 242
malaria, 242
mumps, 242
nursing care management, 244-247
parvovirus, 242-243
rubeola, 243
syphilis, 233-234
TORCH, 236-239
toxic shock syndrome, 243-244
tuberculosis, 243
urinary tract, 241-242
vaginal, 240-241
varicella, 242
medical disorders, 279-289
abdominal surgery, 285-287
adult respiratory distress syndrome, 282
anemia, 279-281
Bell's palsy, 284
bronchial asthma, 281-282
cholelithiasis and cholecystitis, 283
cystic fibrosis, 282-283
epilepsy, 284
inflammatory bowel disease, 283
integumentary, 283
multiple sclerosis, 284
myasthenia gravis, 285
rheumatoid arthritis, 284-285
systemic lupus erythematosus, 285
trauma, 287-289
medical interruption of, 562
multifetal, 69-73
dysfunctional labor, 456
prenatal care and psychosocial adjustment, 169-170
prenatal diagnosis, 97
nutrition
energy needs, 177-182
exercise, 187
minerals and vitamins, 184-186
negative impacts, 186-187
nursing care plan, 199
plan of care and implementation, 194-196
pregnancy-induced hypertension, 187
postdate, 472-475
pregnancy-induced hypertension, 199-216
assessment, 204-207
classification, 199-201
control of blood pressure, 213-214
eclampsia, 214-215
Pregnancy—cont'd
pregnancy-induced hypertension—cont'd
HELLP syndrome, 202-204
magnesium sulfate, 211-213
nursing care, 209-210
postpartum care, 215-216
preeclampsia, 201-202, 207-209
psychosocial problems, 296-315
caffeine use, 310
emotional complications, 296-302
psychoactive substance use, 302-309
smoking, 309-310
violence against women, 310-313
risk factor assessment, 79-102
amniocentesis, 90-93
categories of risk factors, 80-82
chorionic villus sampling, 94-95
daily fetal movement count, 82-83
electronic fetal monitoring, 95-100
magnetic resonance imaging, 90
maternal assays, 95
percutaneous umbilical blood sampling, 93-94
ultrasonography, 83-90
second trimester, 146-157
assessment, 146-151
discomforts related to maternal adaptation, 152-153
nursing care plan, 149
plan of care and implementation, 153-157
spontaneous abortion, 216-218
after chorionic villus sampling, 94
ectopic pregnancy *versus*, 222
hydatidiform mole, 223-224
hyperthyroidism, 270
standard laboratory values, 1776-1777
therapeutic and elective abortion, 289-292
third trimester, 157-168
expectant fathers, 157-159
fetal assessment, 162
maternal assessment, 161-162
nursing care plan, 168
plan of care and implementation, 163-168
second-time mothers, 157
self-care, 160
Pregnancy-induced hypertension, 187, 199-216
assessment, 204-207
classification, 199-201
eclampsia, 214-215
HELLP syndrome, 202-204
control of blood pressure, 213-214
magnesium sulfate, 211-213
nursing care, 209-210
maternal diabetes mellitus, 255
postpartum care, 215-216
preeclampsia, 201-202, 207-209
Pregnancy tests, 104-105
Preluxation, 1721
Premature dilation of cervix, 219-220
Premature infant; *see* Preterm infant
Premature rupture of membranes, 220, 452, 543
Prenatal care, 5
adolescent pregnancy, 325-326
cultural variations, 143-146
lack of, 81
multifetal pregnancy, 169-170
Prenatal diagnosis, 1754
Prenatal interview
adolescent, 322
first trimester, 126-129
maternal diabetes mellitus, 257
second trimester, 146
Prenatal record
admission during labor, 395-398
history, 124-125
weight gain chart, 182-183
Preoperational thought, 852-853, 996, 997
Preoperative care
brain tumor, 1596-1597
cardiac disease, 1452
cesarean birth, 467
cleft lip or palate, 1421
congenital heart disease, 1476-1477
Hirschsprung disease, 1400
pediatric nursing interventions, 1257-1261
scoliosis, 1732
Wilms tumor, 1560
Prepubescence, 1054-1055
Prepuce
circumcision, 653, 654
clitoral, 26
newborn, 600
penile, 43
Presbyterian, 817
Preschool Vision Screening System, 911
Preschooler, 1016-1052
anticipatory guidance, 1028
biologic development, 1016-1017
cognitive development, 1017-1018
communicable diseases, 1028-1039
chickenpox, 1030
diphtheria, 1030-1031
erythema infectiosum, 1032
exanthema subitum, 1032
infection control, 1028
measles, 1032-1033
mumps, 1034
nursing care plan, 1038
pertussis, 1034
poliomyelitis, 1034-1035
prevention of complications, 1029
rubella, 1036
scarlet fever, 1036-1037
communication with, 873-874

Preschooler—cont'd
- dental health, 1027
- development of body image, 1018
- effects of divorce, 838
- fears, 1025
- injury prevention, 1027
- maltreatment, 1039-1049
  - child neglect, 1039, 1044
  - clinical manifestations, 1043
  - physical abuse, 1039-1040
  - prevention, 1047-1049
  - sexual abuse, 1040-1042, 1044-1045
- mental retardation, 1158
- moral development, 1018
- nutrition, 1025-1026
- physical examination, 895
- preparation for pediatric procedures, 1254-1255
- preschool and kindergarten experience, 1021-1024
- psychosocial development, 1017
- reaction to hospitalization, 1198, 1199
- response to bodily injury and pain, 1201-1202
- sex education, 1024-1025
- sexuality, 1018
- sleep and activity, 1026
- social development, 1018-1021
- special needs, 1130, 1144
- speech problems, 1025
- spiritual development, 1018
- understanding and reaction to death, 1133

Prescription, 143
Present illness, 878
Presenting part, 337
Pressure-equilizing tubes, 1332
Pressure ulcer, 1265-1266
Presumptive signs and symptoms of pregnancy, 105, 106, 123
Pretend play, 856
Preterm, defined, 104
Preterm birth, 444-452
Preterm infant, 3, 697, 725-737
- breastfeeding, 687-688
- bronchopulmonary dysplasia, 735
- cardiopulmonary resuscitation, 731
- difficult temperament, 948
- emergency birth, 436
- feeding, 731
- gestational age assessment, 732
- growth and development, 727-729
- infant stimulation, 730-731
- necrotizing enterocolitis, 736-737
- parental adaptation, 729
- parental support, 731-732
- patent ductus arteriosus, 735
- periventricular-intraventricular hemorrhage, 735-736
- physical care, 730
- potential problems, 726-727

Preterm infant—cont'd
- respiratory distress syndrome, 732-734
- retinopathy of prematurity, 735

Preterm labor, 444-450
- recognition of, 166, 167, 446
- related risk factors, 82
- suppression of uterine activity, 445-448

Preventive care timeline, 896
Priapism, 1507
Prilocaine, 1228
Primary circular reactions, 944
Primary core, 792
Primary germ layers, 62
Primary nursing, 792
Primary sex characteristics, 1085
Primary teeth, 955-956
Primigravida, 104
Primipara, 104
Privacy
- death of child, 557
- interview, 868
- postpartum home visit maternal assessment, 579
- respect for, 1097

Probable signs and symptoms of pregnancy, 105, 106, 123
Problem solving, 12
Procainamide, 272
Procarbazine, 1523
Procardia; *see* Nifedipine
Professional responsibility and accountability, 1770
Progesterone, 1625
- adaptations during pregnancy, 105
- contraceptive, 522
- postpartum levels, 483

Progestin, 521-522, 523-524
Programs for Children with Special Health Needs, 1139
Progressive infantile spinal muscular dystrophy, 1759-1760
Project Copernicus, 1195
Projectile vomiting, 1387
Prolactin, 1625
- changes during pregnancy, 120
- lactation, 666-667
- postpartum levels, 483

Prolapse of umbilical cord, 411, 475
PROM; *see* Premature rupture of membranes
Propionibacterium acnes, 1684
Propoxyphene, 1221, 1225
Propranolol, 272
Propylthiouracil, 270
Proscription, 143
Prostaglandin inhibitors, 450
Prostaglandins, 42
- cervical ripening methods, 460
- second trimester abortion, 291

Prostate gland, 45
Prosthesis
- ocular, 1183

Prosthesis—cont'd
- skeletal limb deficiency, 1727

Prostin/M15; *see* Carboprost
Prostitution, child, 1041
Protective environment, 642-643
Protein, 664
- delayed wound healing, 1660
- diabetic mother, 260
- needs during pregnancy, 178, 182, 183, 184
- normal laboratory values, 1801
- placental storage, 65
- preeclampsia etiology, 202
- recommended daily requirements, 848
- urine, 1544

Protein energy malnutrition, 1384
Proteinuria, 116
- maternal assay, 95
- preeclampsia, 200, 201, 207

Prothrombin time, 231, 1801
Provitamin A, 1373
Proximodistal growth, 845
Pruritus
- during pregnancy, 152
- relief of, 1663
- skin lesions, 1655
- vaginal infection, 240

Pseudohypertrophic muscular dystrophy, 1760, 1761-1762
Pseudohypertrophy, 1761
Pseudohypoparathyroidism, 1633
Pseudomenstruation, newborn, 599, 618
Pseudostrabismus, 910
Psoriasis, 1680
Psychoactive substance use, 302-309
Psychologic response
- dystocia, 456
- grief, 551
- immobilization, 1706-1708
- pediatric procedures, 1252-1256

Psychologic status, 81
Psychomotor retardation, 56
Psychoprophylactic method of childbirth, 354
Psychosexual development, 850-851
Psychosocial adjustment
- adolescent pregnancy, 323
- first stage of labor, 399-400
- multifetal pregnancy, 170

Psychosocial development
- adolescent, 317, 1089-1090, 1096
- child, 851-852
- infant, 943
- preschooler, 1017
- school-age child, 1055-1056
- toddler, 994-995

Psychosocial history, 881-882
Psychosocial problems
- childhood, 1079-1080
- during pregnancy, 296-317
  - caffeine use, 310

Psychosocial problems—cont'd
during pregnancy—cont'd
emotional complications, 296-302
psychoactive substance use, 302-309
smoking, 309-310
violence against women, 310-313
Psychosocial risks, 80, 81
Psychotic features, 296
Psychotropic medications, 299-300
PTSD; *see* Posttraumatic stress disorder
Ptyalin, 938
Ptyalism, 119, 137
Pubarche, 23
Puberty
breast growth, 37
female response, 1095-1097
hormonal changes, 1085
male response, 1095
preadolescence, 1055
precocious, 1627-1628
Pubic bone, 34
Pubic hair, 1087
Pubis, 36
Pubococcygeus muscle, 34
Puborectalis muscle, 34
PUBS; *see* Percutaneous umbilical blood sampling
Pudendal block, 360-361
Pudendum, 927
Puerperal infection, 543-546
Puerperium, 480
Puerto Rican culture
food patterns, 190
health beliefs and practices, 820-821
Pull-to-sit reflex, 607
Pulmonary circulation, changes at birth, 592, 594
Pulmonary disorders; *see* Respiratory dysfunction
Pulmonary edema, ritodrine-induced, 448
Pulmonary function tests, 1348
Pulmonary stenosis, 1460
Pulmonary surfactant, 66
Pulse, 902-903
femoral, 926
location of, 922
neurologic examination, 1574
newborn, 615, 616, 618
postpartum, 485, 489, 492, 493
Pulse oximetry, 701, 1303-1304
Puncture wound, 1663
Punishment and obedience orientation, 1018
Pupil, 909
neurologic examination, 1575
newborn, 608, 622
Purified protein derivative, 243
Purinethol; *see* 6-Mercaptopurine
Purpura
Henoch-Schönlein, 1493-1494
Purpura—cont'd
idiopathic thrombocytopenic, 1515-1516
Purulent arthritis, 1734
Pustule, 1657
PVS; *see* Persistent vegetative state
Pyelonephritis, 1546
Pyloric sphincter, 1426-1431
Pyloromyotomy, 1427
Pyoderma, 1666
Pyogenic arthritis, 1734
Pyridoxine
needs during pregnancy, 179, 186
nutritional significance, 1374
Pyrosis, 119, 196

Q

Quadriceps reflex, 931
Quadriplegia, 1766
Quakers, 815
Quality assurance, 1772
Quickening, 67, 109-110, 123
Quiet alert state in newborn, 611
Quinidine, 272

R

R-PDQ; *see* Revised Prescreening Developmental Questionnaire
Rabies, 1604-1605
Rachischisis, 1754
Radiation, delayed wound healing, 1660
Radiation heat loss, 595
Radiography
cerebral assessment, 1577
fracture, 1713
genitourinary dysfunction, 1543
Radioimmunoassay, 105
Radioreceptor assay, 104
Range of motion, 1258
Range of state, 610
Rape, 313
Rash
Henoch-Schönlein purpura, 1494
measles, 1033
newborn, 645
scarlet fever, 1037
systemic lupus erythematosus, 1742
Rastelli procedure, 1462
RDS; *see* Respiratory distress syndrome
Real-time ultrasonography, 1577
Reasoning, 834
Receptive skills, 1161
Recessive gene, 52-53
Reciprocity, parent-infant bonding, 508
Recommended dietary allowances, 1382
infant, 663
maternal nutrition, 178-179
through adolescence, 848
Reconstituted family, 9-10, 840
Recovery record, 489, 490
Rectal medication administration, 1227, 1296-1297
Rectal temperature, 901
Rectocele, 547, 548
Rectoperitoneal fistula, 1431
Rectovaginal fistula, 548, 549, 1431
Rectovaginal palpation, 131
Rectum, 30, 34
congenital anomalies, 775
newborn assessment, 619
Rectus abdominis, 118
Recumbent length, 897
Recurrent abdominal pain, 1079
Red blood cell count
postpartum, 486
urine test, 1545
Red blood cell disorders, 1499-1512
anemia, 1499-1503
aplastic anemia, 1511-1512
beta-thalassemia, 1510-1511
iron deficiency anemia, 1503-1505
sickle cell anemia, 1505-1510
Red blood cell volume, 1801
Red blood cells
changes during pregnancy, 112-114
newborn, 594-595
normal laboratory values, 1796
Red measles, 243
Red reflex, 622
Red reflex gemini test, 910
Referral form for postpartum home visit, 574, 575
Referred pain, 352
Reflex bradycardia, 275
Reflex irritability, 608-609
Reflexes
Brazelton Neonatal Behavioral Assessment, 610
cognitive development, 944
neurologic examination, 930, 1576
newborn, 603, 604-605, 617, 625
Reflux, vesicoureteral, 1547
Refractive errors, 1175, 1176
Regeneration, 1656
Regression, 1003
Regulation of state, 610
Regurgitation
assessment, 624
gastrointestinal dysfunction, 1387
infant, 979
Rehabilitation, head injury, 1592
Relaxation techniques
hospitalized child, 1220
during pregnancy
labor, 355-357
second trimester, 154-156
Relaxin, 109
Religion, 804
beliefs affecting nursing care, 814-823
customs and folkways, 808-811
health beliefs and practices, 811-812

Religion—cont'd
susceptibility to health problems, 806-808
Remodeling of bone, 1712-1713
Renal biopsy, 1543
Renal failure, 1560-1568
acute, 1560-1563
chronic, 1563-1568
dialysis, 1568-1569
kidney transplantation, 1569
Renal function
assessment, 1542-1545
first trimester, 131
postpartum, 483
Renal osteodystrophy, 1564
Renal plasma flow, 115
Renal system
adaptations during postpartum period, 483-484
adaptations during pregnancy, 115-116
congenital anomalies, 776-777
effects of immobilization, 1707
genitourinary dysfunction, 1542-1571
acute renal failure, 1560-1563
chronic renal failure, 1563-1568
dialysis, 1568-1569
external defects, 1550-1551
glomerulonephritis, 1556-1558
hemolytic-uremic syndrome, 1558-1559
kidney transplantation, 1569
nephrotic syndrome, 1551-1556
obstructive uropathy, 1549-1550
renal function assessment, 1542-1545
urinary tract infection, 1545-1549
Wilms tumor, 1559-1560
infant, 939
preterm newborn, 727
review of systems, 881
systemic lupus erythematosus, 1742
Reproduction, 23-46
female reproductive system, 23-42
adaptations during postpartum period, 480-483
bony pelvis, 36-37
breasts, 37-39
external structures, 23-27
menstrual cycle, 39-42
ovaries, 27-29
pelvic floor and perineum, 34-36
uterine tubes, 29
uterus, 29-33
vagina, 33-34
male reproductive system, 42-46
psychosocial aspects of sexuality, 46-48
sexual response, 46
Research, 795-796
into practice, 5
standards of care, 1772
Residence, high risk factor, 81
Resiliency Model of Family Stress Adjustment and Adaptation, 14
Resolution phase of sexual response, 47
Respirations
assessment of respiratory function, 1323
neurologic examination, 1575
newborn, 615, 616, 657
Apgar scoring, 608-609
home visit assessment, 582
seesaw, 592
physical examination, 903
postpartum, 485
Respiratory alkalosis, 356
Respiratory arrest, 1361
Respiratory distress syndrome, 732-734
early signs, 700
infant of diabetic mother, 744
newborn, 615, 631
phosphatidylglycerol and, 91
promotion of fetal lung maturity, 450
Respiratory dysfunction, 1321-1371
acute laryngotracheobronchitis, 1335-1337
acute spasmodic laryngitis, 1337
adult respiratory distress syndrome, 1345
airway obstruction, 1365-1368
aspiration pneumonia, 1345
asthma, 1347-1356
bacterial tracheitis, 1337
bronchitis, 1337
burns and, 1690, 1692
cardiopulmonary resuscitation, 1362-1365, 1366
congestive heart failure, 1469-1470
cystic fibrosis, 1356-1361
epiglottis, 1334-1335
foreign body aspiration, 1344-1345
infectious mononucleosis, 1330-1331
influenza, 1331
laryngitis, 1335
nasopharyngitis, 1326-1327
opioid-induced, 1230
otitis media, 1331-1333
passive smoking, 1346-1347
pertussis, 1341
pharyngitis, 1327-1328
pneumonia, 1339-1341
during pregnancy, 281-283
respiratory failure, 1361-1362
respiratory syncytial virus bronchiolitis, 1337-1339
smoke and carbon monoxide inhalation, 1345-1347
tonsillitis, 1328-1330
tuberculosis, 1341-1344
Respiratory failure, 1361-1362
Respiratory insufficiency, 1361
Respiratory rate, 1792
Respiratory secretions, 1284
Respiratory syncytial virus bronchiolitis, 1337-1339
Respiratory system
adaptations during labor, 352
adaptations during pregnancy, 114-115
effects of immobilization, 1707
fetal, 66
human development milestones, 70-72
infant, 938
newborn, 591-592
congenital anomalies, 772-773
high risk, 699-704
preterm, 726
review of systems, 881
toddler, 994
unconscious child, 1579
Rest
after cardiac surgery, 1478
child, 849
postpartum, 498
during pregnancy
first trimester, 145-146
hypertonic uterine dysfunction, 453
preeclampsia, 208
preterm labor, 447, 448
second trimester, 154-156
respiratory infection, 1324
school-age child, 1063, 1065
Restitution and external rotation in labor, 348-349
Restraints
neonatal, 639, 649
pediatric, 1276-1278
Resuscitation
infant, 632, 1362-1365, 1366
parent education, 731
preterm, 725
intrauterine, 388-389, 391
neonatal, 699
pregnant woman, 278-279
Retained placenta, 539
Reticulocyte count, 1500, 1802
Retinal hemorrhage, 635, 747
Retinoblastoma, 1182-1183
Retinol, 1373
Retinopathy
diabetic, 1641
of prematurity, 735
Retroflexed uterus, 29
Retroversion, 30, 546
Review of systems, 128, 880, 881
Revised Prescreening Developmental Questionnaire, 934
Reye syndrome, 1603-1604
Rh incompatibility, 767-768
Coomb's test, 95
postpartum Rh isoimmunization, 501-502
Rhabdomyosarcoma, 1737-1738

Rheumatic fever, 1482-1483
Rheumatic heart disease, 277
Rheumatoid arthritis
juvenile, 1738-1741
during pregnancy, 284-285
Rh_o(D) immune globulin, 501-502
Rib cage, 920
Riboflavin
needs during pregnancy, 179
nutritional significance, 1374
RICE regiment, 1711
Richmond screw, 1580
Rickettsial disease, 1677, 1678
Right-sided heart failure, 1465
Right-to-left shunt, 1454
Ringworm, 1669
Rinne test, 917
Risk factor assessment, 79-102
biochemical, 90-95
amniocentesis, 90-93
chorionic villus sampling, 94-95
maternal assays, 95
percutaneous umbilical blood sampling, 93-94
biophysical, 82-90
daily fetal movement count, 82-83
magnetic resonance imaging, 90
ultrasonography, 83-90
categories of risk factors, 80-82
electronic fetal monitoring, 95-100
contraction stress test, 98-100
fetal responses to hypoxia and asphyxia, 97
indications, 95-97
nonstress test, 97-98
fetal and neonatal health problems, 80
hospitalized child, 1204
maternal health problems, 79-80
nursing role, 100
preconception care, 76
preeclampsia-eclampsia, 204
sudden infant death syndrome, 985
Ritalin; *see* Methylphenidate
Ritgen maneuver, 433, 434
Ritodrine, 448
Ritualism
school-age child, 1059
toddler, 995
Rivalry, sibling, 1001-1002
Rocky Mountain spotted fever, 1678
Rogers, Lina, 789
Role clarification, 867
Role confusion, 852
Role learning, 828
Roll-over test, 147
Rolling over, 941
Roman Catholic, 817
Romberg test, 930
Rooting reflex, 604, 623, 662
Roseola, 1032
Round ligament, 30, 31, 33
Round ligament pain, 153
Roundworm, 1404
Roxicodone; *see* Oxycodone
RSV; *see* Respiratory syncytial virus bronchiolitis
RU 486, 292
Rubella, 755-756, 1036
first trimester, 131
postpartum vaccination, 501
during pregnancy, 237, 238
prenatal diagnosis, 96
vaccine, 962, 965-966
Rubeola, 243
Rugae, 34, 482
Rules and rituals, 1059
Rupture
appendix, 1407
uterine, 475-478
Rupture of membranes, 399
Russell traction, 1718
Russian Orthodox, 817

S

Sacral agenesis, 743
Sacral pressure massage during labor, 356
Sacral promontory, 30, 36
Sacroiliac joint, 36
Sacrosciatic notch, 36
Sacrum, 36, 624
Saddle block, 361
Safe passage, 157
Safety
adolescent, 1102-1104
head injury, 1592-1593
home birth, 173
home care, 1192
hospitalized child, 1271-1280
environmental factors, 1274
infection control, 1272-1274
limit-setting, 1275
positioning for procedures, 1278-1280
restraints, 1276-1278
transportation, 1275-1276
infant, 970-977
near-drowning, 1594
nerve block during labor, 370
newborn, 643, 657
nurse during home visit, 579
during pregnancy, 138
preschooler, 1027
school-age child, 1069, 1070-1071
toddler, 1006-1013
toys, 858, 859
ultrasound, 90
visually impaired child, 1180-1181
Saliva, 623
Salmetrol, 1350
Salmonella, 1396
Salpingitis, 222
Same-sex family, 11
Sanfilippo syndrome, 96
Sarcoma, 1735-1737
Sarcoptes scabiei, 1673
SBMC; *see* Single-room maternity care
Scabies, 1673
Scald burn, 976
Scalded skin syndrome, 1666
Scale, 1658
Scalp
assessment, 622
birth injury, 746
caput succedaneum, 601
Scandinavian food patterns, 190
Scaphocephaly, 1615
Scar, 1656, 1659
burn victim, 1698-1699
Scarf sign, 635
Scarlet fever, 1036-1037
Schizophrenia
during pregnancy, 298
school-age child, 1080-1081
School-age child, 1053-1083
altered growth and maturation, 1073-1075
anticipatory guidance, 1069-1072
attention-deficit hyperactivity disorder, 1075-1077
biologic development, 1053-1055
cognitive development, 1056-1057
communication with, 874
conversion reaction, 1079
dental health, 1066-1068
depression, 1079-1080
effects of divorce, 838
encopresis, 1077-1078
enuresis, 1077
exercise and activity, 1065-1066
injury prevention, 1069, 1070-1071
limit setting and discipline, 1062
mental retardation, 1158
moral development, 1057
nutrition, 1063
physical examination, 895
posttraumatic stress disorder, 1078
preparation for pediatric procedures, 1255
psychosocial development, 1055-1056
reaction to hospitalization, 1198, 1199
recurrent abdominal pain, 1079
response to bodily injury and pain, 1202-1203
schizophrenia, 1080-1081
school experience, 1060-1061
school health, 1068-1069
school phobia, 1078-1079
self-concept, 1060
sex education, 1068
sleep and rest, 1063, 1065
social development, 1057-1060
special needs, 1130-1131, 1143-1146
spiritual development, 1057
sports participation, 1072-1073
stress and fears, 1062-1063

School-age child—cont'd
  understanding and reaction to death, 1133-1134
School health, 1068-1069
School phobia, 1078-1079
Schultze mechanism, 437
SCID; *see* Severe combined immunodeficiency disease
Scoliosis, 928, 1730-1733
Scorpion, 1676
Scotoma, 202
Screening
  cystic fibrosis, 1358
  developmental, 934
  human immunodeficiency virus, 132
  vision, 911-914, 1784
Scrotum, 44
  newborn, 600, 619
  ultrasound, 1543
Sebaceous glands
  eyelid, 908
  labial, 25
Seborrheic dermatitis, 1684
Second-degree burn, 1687
Second stage of labor, 424-436
  bearing-down efforts, 428-430
  birthing beds and chairs, 430, 431
  delivery room, 432-433
  duration of, 425
  emergency, 435-436
  fetal heart rate, 430
  maternal position, 427-428
  potential problems, 425-427
  prebirth considerations, 427, 428
  siblings and, 435
  vertex presentation, 433-435
Second-time mother, 157
Second trimester, 146-157
  abortion, 291
  assessment, 146-151
  discomforts related to maternal adaptation, 152-153
  indications for sonography, 84
  nursing care plan, 149
  plan of care and implementation, 153-157
Secondary circular reactions, 944
Secondary sex characteristics, 1085
Secretions, neonatal suctioning, 631-632
Sedatives
  during labor, 358
  pediatric, 1222
Seesaw respirations, 592, 615
Seizure, 1605-1615
  acute renal failure, 1562
  cerebral palsy, 1748
  eclampsia, 199
  epilepsy, 1605-1614
  febrile, 1614
  posttraumatic, 1590
Selenium
  needs during pregnancy, 178
  nutritional significance, 1381
Self-awareness, 858
Self-care
  adolescent, 1099-1100
  diabetes mellitus, 1649
  mentally retarded child, 1160
  during pregnancy, 135-141
  trends, 4
Self-concept
  adolescent, 1094-1097
  child, 854-855
  school-age child, 1060
Self-esteem, 855
Self-image, maternal, 502
Semen, 45-46
Seminal vesicle, 45
Seminiferous tubule, 44
Semivegetarian diet, 189
Sense of industry, 1055
Sense of initiative, 1017
Sense-pleasure play, 855
Sensitization, 1384-1385
Sensorimotor phase, 852, 943-944, 995-996, 997
Sensorineural hearing loss, 1168
Sensory development, 950-955
  function of play, 857
  newborn, 603-608
  toddler, 993-994, 1001
Sensory impairment, 1168-1183
  conjunctivitis, 1181-1182
  deaf-blind children, 1182
  dehydration, 1389
  hearing, 1168-1175
  retinoblastoma, 1182-1183
  visual, 1175-1181
Sentence completion, 876
Separation anxiety, 948-949
  hospitalized child, 1196-1198, 1216-1218
Sepsis
  burns, 1690
  newborn, 749, 751
  postpartum, 543-544
  white blood cell count, 595
Septic abortion, 217
Septic arthritis, 1734
Septic shock, 1491
  newborn, 750
  puerperal shock, 544
Septicemia, 749
Septum, nasal, 918
Sequestration crisis, 1507
Serotonin-selective reuptake inhibitors, 299
Serum bilirubin
  jaundice, 636, 767
  kernicterus, 768
Serum test for pregnancy, 104
Set point, 1107, 1268
Seventh-Day Adventist, 814
Severe combined immunodeficiency disease, 1533-1534
Sex chromosome, 51
Sex chromosome abnormalities, 56, 1074-1075
Sex education, 49, 319-320
  preschooler, 1024-1025
  school-age child, 1068
Sex hormones, 1085, 1625, 1634
Sex role, 47-48
Sex-role identity, 1090
  toddler, 996, 998
Sexual abuse, 1040-1042, 1044-1045
Sexual ambiguity, 776
Sexual counseling
  adolescent, 318-321, 1101-1102
  during pregnancy, 141-143
Sexual desire, 47
Sexual dysfunction, 48
Sexual history, 49, 319, 882
Sexual maturation, 1085-1086
Sexual response, 46, 47
Sexual sensations during breastfeeding, 677
Sexuality
  adolescent, 318-321, 515, 1093, 1096
  mentally retarded child, 1162
  postpartum, 502, 512-513
  during pregnancy
    cultural considerations, 146
    first trimester, 142
    third trimester, 164
  preschooler, 1018
  psychosocial aspects, 46-48
  toddler, 997-998
Sexually transmitted disease
  adolescent, 317-318
  during pregnancy, 234-240, 246
SFD; *see* Small-for-date
SGA; *see* Small-for-gestational age
Shake test, 91
Shaken baby syndrome, 1042
Shame orientation, 801
Shear force, 1266
Sheehan syndrome, 228
Sheet graft, 1694-1695
Shellfish hypersensitivity, 1385
Shigella, 1397
Shingles, 242, 1667
Shirodkar procedure, 219-220
Shivering, postpartum, 497
Shock, 1489-1491
  abruptio placentae, 226
  bacteremic, 544
  childhood death, 1129
  as grief response, 551
  hypovolemic, 497
  postpartum hemorrhagic, 541

Shock—cont'd
reaction of family to child's chronic illness or disability, 1124
uterine inversion hemorrhage, 540
Shock lung, 282
Shoes, infant, 956
Short bowel syndrome, 1433-1434
Short stature, 1073
Shoulder dystocia, 475
Shoulder presentation, 339, 456
Shriners Burn Institutes, 1699
Shunt procedures, 1473
hydrocephalus, 1617-1618
Shut down, 675
SIADH; *see* Syndrome of inappropriate antidiuretic hormone
Sibling Information Network, 1141
Sibling Support Project, 1195
Siblings
adaption to pregnancy and birth, 159, 160
bonding and attachment to newborn, 585
impact of special needs sibling, 1126-1127, 1141
interaction, 829-830
during labor, 420-421, 435
reaction to hospitalized sibling, 1236
rivalry, 511-512, 1001-1002
sexual abuse, 1041
Sick Kids Need Involved People, Inc., 1195
Sickle cell anemia, 57, 96, 280, 281, 1505-1510
Sickle cell hemoglobinopathy, 280
Sickle cell trait, 280
Sickle-turbidity test, 1506
Sickledex, 1506
SIDS; *see* Sudden infant death syndrome
Sign language, 1172
Signs and symptoms of pregnancy, 105, 106
Silver nitrate, 1694
Silver sulfadiazine, 1694
Simian crease, 55, 56
Simple fracture, 1712
Simple partial seizure, 1606, 1608
Sims' position in childbirth, 432, 436
Single-gene inheritance, 56-57
Single-parent family, 9, 839-840
special needs child, 1126
Single-room maternity care, 633
Sinus bradycardia, 1485
Sinus tachycardia, 1485
Sinus venosus defect, 1456
Sitting, infant development, 941, 942
Situational stressor, 14
Sitz bath, 495, 496
Skateboard safety, 1071
Skeletal limb deficiency, 1727
Skeletal system
effects of immobilization, 1707
growth and maturation, 847-848
newborn, 602-603
prenatal diagnosis of deformities, 96
Skeletal traction, 1717
Skene's glands, 27
Skill play, 855
Skin, 1654-1705
acne, 1684-1687
adaptations during labor, 352
adaptations during pregnancy, 116-117
animal bites, 1677-1678
arthropod bites and stings, 1674-1677
burns, 1687-1703
adolescent, 1103
characteristics of burn injury, 1687-1690
emergency care, 1690-1691
infant, 975-976
major, 1692-1700
minor, 1691-1692
pathophysiology, 1690
sunburn, 1700-1703
toddler, 1007, 1010-1011
cat-scratch disease, 1679
chickenpox, 1030
childbirth and, 439-441
cold injury, 1703
dehydration, 1389
dermatitis
contact, 1671
diaper, 1679-1682
eczema, 1682-1684
seborrheic, 1684
dressings, 1660
drug reactions, 1672
effects of immobilization, 1707
fetal, 69
foreign bodies, 1672-1673
human bites, 1678-1679
infections
bacterial, 1664-1667
fungal, 1669-1671
transmitted by arthropods, 1677
viral, 1667-1669
lesions, 1654-1655
maintenance during pediatric nursing interventions, 1264-1266
measles, 1032-1033
neurologic examination, 1575
newborn, 600-602
assessment, 582, 616-617, 621-622
care, 728
fetal alcohol syndrome, 760
preterm, 727
nutritional status, 193, 888
pediculosis capitis, 1673-1674
physical examination, 906-907
poison ivy, oak, and sumac, 1671-1672
Skin—cont'd
postpartum period, 486
relief of symptoms, 1663-1664
scabies, 1673
systemic lupus erythematosus, 1742
systemic therapy, 1662
topical therapy, 1660-1662, 1663-1664
wound care, 1662-1663
wounds, 1655-1660
Skin color of newborn, 601, 621
Apgar scoring, 608-609
home visit assessment, 582
Skin graft, 1694-1695, 1698-1699
Skin test
asthma, 1348, 1349
tuberculin, 658
Skin traction, 1717, 1719
Skinfold thickness, 899-900
Skull
birth injury, 746, 747, 748
cranial deformities, 1615
fracture, 1587
hydrocephalus, 1615-1620
newborn, 602-603
SLE; *see* Systemic lupus erythematosus
Sleep
adolescent, 1099
child, 849
infant, 959-961
newborn, 610, 611
breastfeeding and, 675
home visit assessment, 582
preschooler, 1026
school-age child, 1063, 1065
toddler, 1004
Sleep terror, 1026-1027
Slipped femoral capital epiphysis, 1729
Slow-to-warm-up child, 850
Small-for-date infant, 697
Small-for-gestational age, 614, 697, 724-725, 739-740
Smegma, 26, 600
Smell, newborn, 608
Smoke inhalation, 1345-1347
Smokeless tobacco, 1111
Smoking
adolescent, 1111-1112
breastfeeding and, 680, 766
lactation and, 188
maternal use, 761
passive, 1346-1347
perinatal risk, 759, 761
during pregnancy, 140-141, 309-310
high risk factor, 81
negative impact on maternal nutrition, 186-187
Snacking, 1098
Sneezing, 607
Snellen screening, 1784
Snellen symbol chart, 911, 912

Snuffles, 754
Soak, 1664
  eczema, 1684
  play activities, 1258
Soave endorectal pull-through procedure, 1400
Social-affective play, 855
Social class, 802-803
Social development
  adolescent, 1091-1094
  infant, 944-948
  preschooler, 1018-1021
  school-age child, 1057-1060
  toddler, 998-999
Social history, 127
Social roles, 10, 801
Social Services Block Grant, 790
Socialization, 12, 800
  blind child, 1179
  function of play, 858
  hearing impairment, 1172-1173
  hospitalized child, 1234
  during infancy, 950-955
  mentally retarded child, 1162
  preschooler, 1019, 1023
  school-age child, 1064-1065
  toddler, 998-999, 1001
Sociodemographic risks, 80, 81
Socioeconomic level
  bonding, 507
  growth and development, 861
  susceptibility to health problems, 807-808
Sociogram, 882, 884
Sodium
  needs during pregnancy, 185
  newborn excretion, 596
  normal laboratory values, 1802
  nutritional significance, 1381
Sodium bicarbonate
  for cardiopulmonary resuscitation, 1366
  changes during pregnancy, 115
  neonatal resuscitation, 699
Sodium nitroprusside, 272
Soft tissue dystocia, 453
Soft tissue trauma, 1709-1711
  birth, 635, 746-747
Soft tissue tumor, 1735-1738
Solid food introduction, 662-663, 957-959
Solitary play, 856
Somatic cell, 51
Somatic pain, 352
Somatostatin, 1625
Somatotropin, 1624
Somogyi effect, 1644
Sore throat
  prevention of complications, 1029
  respiratory infection, 1322
Southeast Asian culture
  food patterns, 191
  postpartum care beliefs, 505
Soy hypersensitivity, 1385
Spastic cerebral palsy, 1747
Special needs child, 1121-1156
  changing trends in care, 1121-1123
  education about disorder and general health care, 1142-1143
  family coping, 1137-1142
  impact on child, 1129-1132
  impact on family, 1125-1129
  impending death, 1132-1135
  nurses' reactions to dying child, 1154-1155
  planning for future, 1146-1148
  promotion of normal development, 1143-1146
  reaction of family, 1123-1125
  scope of problem, 1121, 1123
  support at time of diagnosis, 1135-1137
  terminally ill or dying, 1148-1154
Special Olympics, 1146
Specific gravity, 596-597, 1544, 1802
Specimen collection, 637-642, 1280-1284
Spectinomycin, 233
Speculum examination, 130-131
Speech problems, 1025
Speech therapy, 1172
Speed; *see* Methamphetamine
Sperm, 58, 59
Spermatic cord, 44
Spermatogenesis, 44-45, 54, 55
Spermicide, 518, 519, 520, 525
Sphingomyelin, 66
Sphygmomanometer, 903
Spica cast, 1714
Spider angioma, 486
Spider nevus, 152
Spina bifida, 603, 771, 1751-1758
Spina bifida cystica, 96, 1754, 1755
Spina bifida occulta, 1754, 1755
Spinal anesthesia during labor, 361
Spinal cord
  fetal, 67, 68
  membranes and spaces, 362
Spinal cord compression, 1766
Spinal cord injury, 1765-1766
  birth trauma, 746, 749
Spine
  kyphosis and lordosis, 1729-1730
  newborn, 603, 624
  physical examination, 928
  scoliosis, 1730-1733
  tuberculosis, 1735
Spinnbarkeit, 42
Spiral electrode, 376, 378, 389
Spiral fracture, 1712
Spiritual development, 1090-1091
  child, 853-854
  preschooler, 1018
  school-age child, 1057
  toddler, 996-997
Spironolactone, 1467
Spitting up, 979, 1387
Splanchnic engorgement, 499
Spleen
  leukemia and, 1518
  newborn assessment, 618
Splinter, 1672-1673
Split custody, 839
Sponge, vaginal, 519
Sponge bath, 648
Spontaneous abortion, 216-218
  after chorionic villus sampling, 94
  ectopic pregnancy *versus*, 222
  hydatidiform mole, 223-224
  hyperthyroidism, 270
  maternal diabetes mellitus, 255
Spontaneous rupture of membranes, 409
Sports injuries, 1102-1103
Sports participation, 1065-1066, 1072-1073
Sprain, 1711
Sputum, 1323
Squamocolumnar junction, 32
Squamous epithelium, 32
Stammering, 1025
Standard precautions, 1272, 1273
Standards of care, 5, 414, 1769-1772
Standards of practice, 5, 796
Staphylococcus aureus
  food poisoning, 1397
  mastitis, 544
  skin infection, 1666
  toxic shock syndrome, 243, 1492
Startle reflex, 605
State-related behavior, 610
Station in labor, 338, 340
Stature, 897, 1073
Status asthmaticus, 1350
Status epilepticus, 1609
STD; *see* Sexually transmitted disease
Steatorrhea, 1432
Stepfamily, 9-10
Stepping reflex, 605
Sterilization
  contraception, 529-531
  of formula, 692-693
Steroid sex hormones, 29
Steroids, 1634
Stevens-Johnson syndrome, 1681
Stillbirth, 2, 550-563
  anticipatory grief, 552
  communicating and caring techniques, 554-556
  complicated bereavement, 562-563
  documentation, 558-561, 560
  grief responses, 551-552

Stillbirth—cont'd
options for parents, 556-558
physical comfort, 556
Stimulation
newborn
high-risk, 713-714, 715
preterm, 730-731
unconscious child, 1582-1583
Sting, 1674-1677
Stomach
changes during pregnancy, 119
infant digestion, 663
newborn, 597
Stomatitis, 1406
Stool
dehydration, 1389
newborn, 597, 657
specimen, 1282
Stork bite, 617, 621
Storytelling, 876
Strabismus, 910-911, 1176-1177
Strain, 1711
Stranger fear, 945-946, 948-949
Strangulated hernia, 1425
Strawberry as allergen, 663
Strawberry mark, 621
Strep throat, 1327-1328
Streptococci
newborn infection, 758
otitis media, 1331
vaginal infection, 241
Stress
adolescent, 1100-1101
burn care procedures, 1697
child, 861-862
delayed wound healing, 1660
school-age child, 1062-1063
Stress fracture, 1072
Stress ulcer, 1412
Stress urinary incontinence, 548
Stressors
family, 14
hospitalized child, 1196-1204, 1236-1237
bodily injury and pain, 1200-1203
family reactions, 1236-1237
intensive care unit, 1243-1244
loss of control, 1198-1200
separation anxiety, 1196-1198
intensive care unit, 1243-1244
Stretch marks, 116, 486
Stretching, newborn, 607
Striae gravidarum, 116, 486
Stroke during pregnancy, 277-278
Stroma, 37
Strongyloidiasis, 1404
Structural defects, 1418-1425
cleft lip or palate, 1418-1422
esophageal atresia and tracheoesophageal fistula, 1422-1425
hernias, 1425, 1426
Structure, term, 8
Stump care, 1721
Stupor, 1574
Stuttering, 1025
Subarachnoid anesthesia during labor, 361
Subarachnoid bolt, 1580
Subarachnoid hemorrhage, 749
Subconjunctival hemorrhage, 635, 747
Subcultural influences, 801-805
Subculture, 15, 800
Subcutaneous medication administration, 1226, 1292-1293
Subdural hematoma, 1587
Subdural hemorrhage, 1588
Subdural tap, 1577
Subinvolution, 480, 541
Sublimaze; *see* Fentanyl
Sublingual medication administration, 1226
Subluxation, 1721
Suboccipitobregmatic diameter, 337
Substance abuse
adolescent, 1112-1115
during pregnancy, 302-309
Succenturiate placenta, 230
Sucking
newborn, 597
nonnutritive, 712, 731
Sucking reflex, 604
feeding readiness, 662
Suction curettage
first trimester abortion, 290
hydatidiform mole, 224
Suction equipment, 699
Suctioning
neonatal airway, 631-632
tracheostomy, 1308-1309
unconscious child, 1580-1581
Sudamina, 616
Sudden infant death syndrome, 984-986
infant positioning, 645
preterm infant, 731
Sudden Infant Death Syndrome Alliance, 1148
Sufentanil, 721
Suffocation
infant, 973-974
newborn, 657
toddler, 1008, 1012
Suicide, 1115-1117
Sulfamylon; *see* Mafenide acetate
Sulfur, 1381
Sunburn, 976, 1700-1703
Sunscreen, 1700
Suntanning, 1100
Superego, 995
Superficial burn, 1687, 1688
Superior vesical artery, 33
Supine hypotension, 112, 404
first trimester, 130
during labor, 349
second trimester, 152
Supply-meets-demand system, 668
Support systems
adolescent pregnancy, 323, 326
blind child, 1178
brain tumor, 1598
burn victim, 1699
congenital heart disease, 1474-1475
Crohn disease, 1412
cystic fibrosis, 1360
diabetes mellitus, 1645
Down syndrome, 1166
epilepsy, 1613
head injury, 1592
home care, 1193
hospitalized child, 1238-1239
hydrocephalus, 1619-1620
juvenile rheumatoid arthritis, 1741
parenting, 832
postpartum, 587-588
scoliosis, 1733
special needs child, 1128, 1135-1136, 1139-1140
spina bifida, 1758
unconscious child, 1583
Suppository, 1296-1297
contraceptive, 519
Suppurative arthritis, 1734
Supraglottitis, 1334-1335
Suprapubic aspiration, 1282
Suprapubic pressure, 475
Supratentorial brain tumor, 1595
Supraventricular tachycardia, 1485
Surface area, water balance, 1387
Surfactant, 66
administration, 704, 734
newborn, 592
respiratory distress syndrome and, 732-734
Surgery
bone tumor, 1736
genital, 1550-1551
head injury, 1590
pediatric, 1257-1262
during pregnancy, 285-287
scoliosis, 1732
Swaddling for newborn pain, 719
Swallowing reflex, 604, 662, 1387
Sweat glands
labial, 25
newborn, 601-602
Sweating
dehydration, 1389
postpartum, 484, 486
Swimming during pregnancy, 154
Swiss-type lymphopenic agammaglobulinemia, 1533
Sympathy, 870

Symphysis pubis, 30, 36, 111
Symptothermal method of contraception, 517, 518
Synchrony, parent-infant bonding, 508
Syncope, 118, 152
Syndactyly, 603, 619, 928
Syndrome of inappropriate antidiuretic hormone, 1581, 1629
Syngeneic bone marrow transplantation, 1536
Synthetic skin coverings, 1694-1695
Synthroid; *see* Levothyroxine
Syphilis
  congenital, 753-754
  during pregnancy, 233-234
  prenatal diagnosis, 96
Syringe
  intramuscular administration, 1288-1289
  oral administration of medication, 1288
Systemic lupus erythematosus, 285, 1741-1742
Systolic blood pressure, 594

T

T cell, 666
Tachycardia
  fetal, 377-378, 379
  newborn, 616
Tachydysrhythmia, 1485
Tachypnea, 616, 631
Tactile stimulation
  initial newborn breathing, 591
  play during infancy, 947
Tail of Spence, 37
Talipes, 625, 1725-1726
Tall stature, 1073
Tampon, toxic shock syndrome, 244
Tanner stages of puberty, 1085
Tape test, 1405-1406
Taste, newborn, 608
Tay-Sachs disease, 58, 96
TB; *see* Tuberculosis
Tea use during pregnancy, 310
Teacher relationships, 1060-1061
Team play, 1059
Tear gland, 608
Technology-dependent child, 1122
Teeth
  changes during pregnancy, 119
  infant, 939
  newborn assessment, 597, 617
  school-age child, 1066-1068
Teething, 954-956
Telangiectasia, 116-117, 152
Telangiectatic nevus, 617, 621
Telecommunications devices for deaf, 1172
Telegraphic speech, 1019
Telephone follow-up, postpartum, 574, 578, 584-586
Teletypewriter, 1172
Television influence on child, 863
Temper tantrum, 1002
Temperament
  growth and development, 849-850
  infant, 948
Temporary restraint, 648
Tempra-dot, 902
Tenderfoot puncture device, 639
Tension headache, 118
Teratogens, 74
Teratoma, 777
Terbutaline
  asthma, 1349-1350
  suppression of uterine activity, 448-449
Term, defined, 104
Terminal shock, 1490
Tertiary circular reactions, 995-996
Test-tube baby, 5
Testis, 44
  newborn, 600, 619
  self-examination, 1106
  ultrasound, 1543
Testosterone, 45, 1625
  aplastic anemia, 1512
  hormonal changes of puberty, 1085
  lactation suppression, 501
Tet spell, 1472
Tetanus, 965, 1763-1764
Tetany, 1632
Tetracaine, 1226
Tetralogy of Fallot, 1460-1461, 1472, 1473
Texas Scottish Rite Hospital system, 1732
Thalassemia, 1510
  during pregnancy, 280-281
  prenatal diagnosis, 96
Thelarche, 1085
Theophylline, 1802
Therapeutic abortion, 289-292, 562
Therapeutic care, 792
Therapeutic play, 1232
Therapeutic relationship, 793
Thermal injury
  burns, 1687-1703
    adolescent, 1103
    characteristics of burn injury, 1687-1690
    emergency care, 1690-1691
    infant, 975-976
    major, 1692-1700
    minor, 1691-1692
    pathophysiology, 1690
    sunburn, 1700-1703
    toddler, 1007, 1010-1011
  cold, 1703
Thermistor probe, 629
Thermograph, 902
Thermoregulation
  infant, 939
  newborn, 595-596
    high risk, 704-706
    preterm, 726
  unconscious child, 1581-1582
Thiamin
  needs during pregnancy, 179
  nutritional significance, 1373
Thiazides, 272
Third-degree burn, 1688, 1689
Third stage of labor, 436-441
Third trimester, 157-168
  expectant fathers, 157-159
  fetal assessment, 162
  indications for sonography, 84
  maternal assessment, 161-162
  nursing care plan, 168
  plan of care and implementation, 163-168
  second-time mothers, 157
  self-care, 160
Thomas ring splint, 1718
Thoracic cavity, 920
Thoracotomy, 1477
Thorax, newborn, 623-624
Threadworm, 1404
Threatened abortion, 216-217
Throat
  newborn assessment, 617
  physical examination, 918-920
  review of systems, 881
  specimen, 1284
Thrombin time, 231, 1802
Thrombocytopenia, neonatal, 635
Thromboembolism
  postpartum, 486, 499
  sickle cell anemia-associated, 281
Thrombophlebitis, 543, 544
Thrush, 758
Thumb-sucking, 657-658, 949, 954
Thyrocalcitonin, 1625, 1629
Thyroid
  changes during pregnancy, 119
  fetal, 68
  first trimester assessment, 129
  functions, 1625
Thyroid disorders, 1629-1634
  goiter, 1630
  Graves' disease, 1631-1632
  hyperparathyroidism, 1634
  hypoparathyroidism, 1633-1634
  juvenile hypothyroidism, 1629-1630
  lymphocytic thyroiditis, 1630-1631
  during pregnancy, 269-270
Thyroid hormone, 1625, 1629
Thyroid-stimulating hormone, 1625, 1629
Thyroid storm, 270
Thyrotoxicosis, 1631

Thyroxine, 1629
  changes during pregnancy, 119
  normal laboratory values, 1802
Tick, 1676
Tidal volume, 114
Time-out, 834, 835
Time structuring in hospitalization, 1218
Tinea capitis, 1668
Tinea corporis, 1668
Tinea cruris, 1668
Tinea pedis, 1669
Tissue turgor, 906
Title V of Social Security Act, 790
Tobacco
  maternal abuse, 759, 761
  use during pregnancy, 309-310
Tocolytic agents
  incompetent cervix, 220
  magnesium sulfate, 213
  suppression of uterine activity, 447-448
Tocopherol, 1377
Tocotransducer, 376-377, 389, 390
Toddler, 993-1015
  anticipatory guidance, 1013
  biologic development, 993-994
  cognitive development, 995-996
  communication with, 873-874
  dental health, 1004-1006
  development of body image, 997
  injury prevention, 1006-1013
  negativism, 1002-1003
  nutrition, 1003-1004
  physical examination, 895
  preparation for pediatric procedures, 1254
  psychosocial development, 994-995
  reaction to hospitalization, 1198-1199
  regression, 1003
  response to bodily injury and pain, 1200-1201
  sexuality, 997-998
  sibling rivalry, 1001-1002
  sleep and activity, 1004
  social development, 998-999
  special needs, 1130, 1144
  spiritual development, 996-997
  temper tantrums, 1002
  toilet training, 999-1001, 1002
  understanding and reaction to death, 1133
Toeing, 929
Toilet training, 999-1001, 1002
Tolectin; *see* Tolmetin
Tolmetin, 1223
Tongue of newborn
  assessment, 623
  position for breastfeeding, 671
Tonic-clonic seizure, 1607, 1610, 1611
Tonic neck reflex, 604
Tonsillectomy, 1329
Tonsillitis, 1328-1330
Tooth evulsion, 1067, 1068
Toothbrushing, 1004-1005
Topical medication administration, 1226
  burns, 1693
  cutaneous disorders, 1660-1662, 1663-1664
TOPV; *see* Trivalent oral poliovirus vaccine
TORCH infection
  newborn, 752-758
  during pregnancy, 236-239
Torticollis, 618, 908
Torulopsis glabrata, 241
Torus fracture, 1712
Total anomalous pulmonary venous connection, 1462-1463
Total body surface area, 1687
Total colectomy, 1411
Total iron-binding capacity, 1798
Total parenteral nutrition
  neonatal, 711
  pediatric, 1314
Touch
  newborn, 608
  parent-infant bonding, 507-508
Tough Love International, 1114
Tourniquet test, 1803
Toxic shock syndrome, 1492-1493
  contraceptive diaphragm, 525
  during pregnancy, 243-244
Toxocara canis, 1404
Toxoplasmosis
  maternal transmission to newborn, 752
  during pregnancy, 236, 237
Toy safety, 858, 859
TPAL acronym, 104
TPN; *see* Total parenteral nutrition
Tracheitis, 1337
Tracheoesophageal fistula, 774, 1422-1425
Tracheomalacia, 1424
Tracheostomy, 1305-1310
Traction, 1716-1720
Traction reflex, 607
Trainable mentally retarded, 1158
Tranquilizers, 359
Transabdominal intrauterine injection of hypertonic sodium chloride, 291
Transcutaneous bilirubinometry, 599
Transcutaneous electrical nerve stimulation, 356-357
Transcutaneous monitoring, 1303
Transcutaneous oxygen pressure monitoring, 701
Transdermal medication administration, 1226
Transductive thought, 997
Transesophageal echocardiography, 1451
Transfer from recovery area, 491-492
Transferase deficiency, 638
Transfusion therapy, 543
Transillumination, 1577
Transition phase of labor, 356, 394, 424, 431
Translocation of chromosomes, 1164
Transmission-based precautions, 1272
Transmucosal medication administration, 1226
Transpalmar crease, 906
Transplantation
  bone marrow, 1536-1537
  heart, 1494
  renal, 1565
Transportation
  burn victim, 1691-1692
  high risk infant, 696-697
  high-risk infant, 718
  infants and children, 1275-1276
  special needs child, 1142
Transposition of great arteries, 1462
Transvaginal ultrasound, 89
Transverse fracture, 1712
Trauma
  birth, 484, 635, 743-744, 746-749
  cerebral, 1585-1593
  childhood mortality, 786-787
  during pregnancy, 287-289
  soft tissue, 1709-1711
  visual impairment, 1175-1177
Travel during pregnancy, 137-138
Treatment without parental consent, 1251-1252
Tremor
  newborn, 603
  postpartum, 497
Treponema pallidum, 233-234
Trial of labor, 460
Triceps reflex, 930
Triceps skinfold thickness, 899, 1789
Tricholoracetic acid, 240
Trichomonas vaginalis, 241
Trichotillomania, 1680
Trichuriasis, 1404
Tricuspid atresia, 1461
Tricyclic antidepressants, 299
Trigeminal nerve, 932
Triglycerides
  infant requirements, 664
  normal laboratory values, 1803
Triiodothyronine, 1629, 1803
Trilisate; *see* Choline magnesium trisalicylate
Trimesters, 123
Triple marker test, 95
Triple screen test, 147-148
Triple X syndrome, 1074
Triplets, 69-73, 84
Trisomy 12, 778
Trisomy 18, 778
Trisomy 21, 54-55, 56, 778, 1163-1167
Trivalent oral poliovirus vaccine, 658

Trochlear nerve, 932
Trophoblast, 60
Trousseau sign, 1632
True labor, 394, 395
True pelvis, 37
Truncus arteriosus, 1463-1464
Trunk incurvation reflex, 606, 607
Trust
  Erikson's psychosocial development, 851, 943
  hospitalized child, 1198
  preparation for pediatric procedures, 1252
Trypsin, 663
Tub bath, 648
Tubal ligation, 529, 530, 531
Tubal occlusion, 530
Tubal reconstruction, 530, 531
Tubal tonsil, 1328
Tuberculin skin test, 131, 658, 1341-1342, 1343
Tuberculosis, 1341-1344
  bone and soft tissue, 1734-1735
  newborn infection, 758
  during pregnancy, 243
Tuberculous spondylitis, 1735
Tumor
  bone and soft tissue, 1735-1738
  prenatal diagnosis, 97
  retinoblastoma, 1182-1183
  Wilms, 1559-1560
Tunneled catheter, 1295
Turbinates, 918
Turner syndrome, 56, 1074
Twenty-four-hour collection, 1281-1282
Twins, 69, 830
  breastfeeding, 687
  death of one, 562
Tylenol; *see* Acetaminophen
Tylox; *see* Oxycodone
Tympanic membrane compliance tests, 917
Tympanic membrane sensor, 902
Tympanometry, 917, 1332
Tympanostomy, 1332
Typhus, 1678
Typology Model of Adjustment and Adaptation, 14

U

Ulcer, 1659
  chemotherapy-induced, 1524
  Curling, 1690, 1698
Ulcerative colitis, 1409-1412
Ultrasound
  abruptio placentae, 226
  biophysical assessment, 83-90
  congenital adrenogenital hyperplasia, 1638
  ectopic pregnancy, 221
  genitourinary dysfunction, 1543
Ultrasound—cont'd
  percutaneous umbilical blood sampling, 93
Ultrasound transducer, 376, 389, 390
Ultraviolet light, 1175, 1700
Umbilical artery, 33, 594
Umbilical artery velocity wave forms, 88
Umbilical cord, 62-63
  clamping and cutting, 628, 630
  compression, 382
  cross-section, 628
  nuchal cord, 434
  prolapse, 411, 475
  remnant
    assessment, 618, 624, 628
    care of, 645, 648
    home visit assessment, 582
  velamentous insertion, 229-230
Umbilical hernia, 1426
Umbilicus, 924
Unbalanced translocation, 56
Uncompensated shock, 1490
Unconsciousness, 1573
  airway obstruction, 1367
  child, 1578-1585
Uncover test, 910-911
Undermedication of pain, 1208
Unifactorial inheritance, 56-57
Unitarian Universalist, 817
United Nations' Declaration of Rights of Child, 793
United Network for Organ Sharing, 1494
United Ostomy Association, 1412
United States Children's Bureau, 790
Universal precautions, 244, 245
  during childbirth, 402
Unlicensed assistive personnel, 796-797
Unmodified cow milk, 695
Unoccupied behavior, 855-856
Unrelated consequences, 834
UPI; *see* Uteroplacental insufficiency
Upper arm circumference, 1789
Upper class, 802
Upper pelvic diaphragm, 34
Upper respiratory tract infections, 1326-1333
  infectious mononucleosis, 1330-1331
  influenza, 1331
  nasopharyngitis, 1326-1327
  otitis media, 1331-1333
  pharyngitis, 1327-1328
  tonsillitis, 1328-1330
Urachus, 33
Urea nitrogen, 1803
Urea solution injection, 291
Uremia, 1563-1568
Ureter, 28, 30, 115
Urethra
  changes during pregnancy, 115
  female, 30, 34
  laceration during childbirth, 441
Urethra—cont'd
  male, 43, 44
  postpartum, 484
Urethral meatus, 27, 927-928
Urethritis, 1546
Uric acid, 1545
Urinalysis; *see* Urine test
Urinary catheterization
  hypovolemic shock, 542
  postpartum, 495
Urinary frequency during pregnancy, 115, 123
  first trimester, 137
  third trimester, 165
Urinary incontinence, 547-548
Urinary meatus, 27
Urinary stasis, 1546
Urinary system
  adaptations during postpartum period, 483-484
  adaptations during pregnancy, 115-116
  congenital anomalies, 776-777
  effects of immobilization, 1707
  genitourinary dysfunction, 1542-1571
    acute renal failure, 1560-1563
    chronic renal failure, 1563-1568
    dialysis, 1568-1569
    external defects, 1550-1551
    glomerulonephritis, 1556-1558
    hemolytic-uremic syndrome, 1558-1559
    kidney transplantation, 1569
    nephrotic syndrome, 1551-1556
    obstructive uropathy, 1549-1550
    renal function assessment, 1542-1545
    urinary tract infection, 1545-1549
    Wilms tumor, 1559-1560
  infant, 939
  review of systems, 881
Urinary tract infection, 1545-1549
  postpartum, 543
  during pregnancy, 241-242
  prevention, 135
Urine
  creatinine levels, 1796
  dehydration, 1389
  newborn dilution, 596
  normal ranges, 1794, 1803
  postpartum period, 484
Urine collection, 640
Urine culture, 131, 1543
Urine output, 542
  magnesium sulfate therapy, 212
  proteinuria, 207
Urine specimen, 1280-1282
Urine test, 131, 1544-1545
  diabetes mellitus, 1648-1649

Urine test—cont'd
pregnancy, 104
diabetic mother, 261-262
first stage of labor, 409
substance abuse, 303
Urine volume, 1544
Urodynamics, 1543
Urogenital diaphragm, 30
Urosepsis, 1546
Urticaria, 1680
Urushiol, 1671
Uterine artery, 32, 33
Uterine canal, 32
Uterine contraction
first stage of labor, 407-409
impending labor, 168
tocolytic suppression, 447-448
Uterine displacement, 546-547
Uterine-placental-fetal unit
maternal nutrition, 176, 177
preeclampsia-eclampsia, 205
Uterine souffle, 109
Uterine tone, 494, 495
Uterine tube, 28, 29, 30, 31
Uterine wall, 29-31
Uteroplacental insufficiency
electronic fetal monitoring, 382
ultrasound assessment, 88
Uterosacral block, 365
Uterosacral ligament, 28, 30, 31
Uterus
adaptations during pregnancy, 106-110
atony, 538
fourth stage of labor, 494, 495
home visit assessment, 582
hypertonic uterine dysfunction, 452-453
inversion, 539-541
newborn, 599
postpartum, 480-482, 492, 493
prolapse, 546-547
rupture, 475-478
structural disorders, 546-550
subinvolution, 541
UTI; *see* Urinary tract infection
Utilization of nursing personnel, 1770-1771

V

Vaccine
to block pregnancy, 529
diphtheria, tetanus, pertussis, 658, 961-962, 964-965, 968
Haemophilus influenzae type b, 658, 962, 966, 969
hepatitis B, 649
measles-mumps-rubella, 658
varicella zoster virus
infant, 962, 966, 969
during pregnancy, 242
Vacuum abortion, 290
Vacuum extraction in dystocia, 464-465
Vagal maneuvers, 1485
Vagina, 28, 30, 33-34
adaptations during postpartum period, 482-483
adaptations during pregnancy, 110-111
examination during first stage of labor, 409, 410
infection during pregnancy, 240-241
laceration during childbirth, 441, 538
sexually transmitted disease, 246
structural disorders, 546-550
ultrasound, 89-90
Vaginal artery, 33
Vaginal birth
after cesarean, 469-472
nursing care plan, 532-533
Vaginal discharge
foul-smelling, 572
newborn, 599
Vaginal fluid, 34
Vaginal introitus, 27
Vaginal orifice, 30, 928
Vaginal ring, 524-525
Vaginal sheath, 519, 520
Vaginal smear, 131
Vaginal sponge, 519
Vaginal tags, 599
Vaginitis, 240, 1105
Vagotomy, 1414
Vagus nerve, 932
Valium; *see* Diazepam
Valley fever, 1670
Valsalva maneuver
bearing-down efforts and, 429
cardiac disease during pregnancy, 274
fetal heart rate and, 388
during labor, 349
Values, family, 12
Variability of fetal heart rate, 378-380
Varicella zoster virus, 1667
chickenpox, 1030
newborn, 754
during pregnancy, 242
Varicella zoster virus vaccine
infant, 962, 966, 969
during pregnancy, 242
Varicose veins
anal, 483
lower extremity, 499
postpartum period, 486
during pregnancy, 152, 154
Varus, 1726-1727
Vas deferens, 44
Vasa praevia, 229
Vascular dysfunction, 1486-1494
anaphylaxis, 1491-1492
Henoch-Schönlein purpura, 1493-1494
Vascular dysfunction—cont'd
hypertension, 1486-1487
Kawasaki disease, 1487-1489
shock, 1489-1491
toxic shock syndrome, 1492-1493
Vascular spiders, 116-117
Vasectomy, 45, 529, 530-531
Vaso-occlusive crisis, 1505, 1507
Vasopressin
diabetes insipidus, 1628
syndrome of inappropriate antidiuretic hormone, 1629
Vasospasm, preeclamptic, 201
Vastus lateralis injection site, 1290
Vegan diet, 189, 1382
Vegetables, needs during pregnancy, 183
Vegetarian diet, 189, 1382
Velamentous insertion of cord, 229-230
Velban; *see* Vinblastine
Venipuncture, 639-640, 1278-1279
Venous access, 542
Venous access devices, 1294-1296
Venous blood gases, 637
Ventricular peritoneal shunt, 1617-1618
Ventricular septal defect, 1456-1457
Ventrogluteal injection site, 1290
Verapamil, 272
Verbal communication, 866-867
with child, 876-877
family, 12
Vermiform appendix, 1406
Vernix caseosa, 69, 599-600, 601
Verruca, 1667
Version, dystocia and, 459-460
Vertex presentation, 337, 338, 433-435
emergency interventions, 426
Very-low-birth-weight infant, 5, 697, 727
Very-very-low-birth-weight infant, 697
Vesicle, 1657
Vesicotomy, 1756
Vesicoureteral reflux, 1547
Vesicovaginal fistula, 548, 549
Vesicular breath sounds, 922
Vestibule, 27
Vestibulocochlear nerve, 932
Viability, 65, 103
Vibrio cholerae, 1397
Vicodin; *see* Hydrocodone
Video electroencephalography, 1577
Vietnamese-American culture, 818-819
Vinblastine, 1523
Vincristine, 1523
Violence during pregnancy, 310-311
Viral infection
conjunctivitis, 1181
cutaneous, 1667-1669
diarrhea, 1396
laryngitis, 1335
newborn, 749

Viral infection—cont'd
  pneumonia, 1339-1340
  respiratory syncytial virus bronchiolitis, 1337-1339
Visceral larva migrans, 1404
Visceral pain, 352
Vision
  adolescent, 1100
  newborn, 603-608
  testing, 909-914
Visual acuity
  newborn, 608
  testing, 911-913
  toddler, 993-994
Visual analogue scale, 1212
Visual impairment, 1175-1181
Visual stimulation, 947
Vital signs
  adaptations during postpartum period, 485
  brain tumor, 1595
  congenital heart disease, 1477
  dehydration, 1389
  neurologic examination, 1574-1575
  newborn, 614-620
  pediatric values, 1792-1793
Vital statistics, 783
Vitamin A
  needs during pregnancy, 179
  nutritional significance, 1373
Vitamin B_6
  needs during pregnancy, 179, 186
  nutritional significance, 1374
Vitamin B_{12}
  breastfeeding and, 675
  needs during pregnancy, 179
  nutritional significance, 1375
Vitamin C
  delayed wound healing, 1660
  infant requirements, 664
  iron absorption and, 1379
  needs during pregnancy, 179, 186
  nutritional significance, 1375-1376
Vitamin D
  hypoparathyroidism, 1633
  infant requirements, 664
  needs during pregnancy, 179, 186
  nutritional significance, 1376-1377
Vitamin E, 1377
Vitamin K
  infant requirements, 664
  newborn clotting and, 595, 599
  newborn prophylaxis, 633
  nutritional significance, 1377
Vitamins
  diabetic mother, 260
  infant needs, 664
  needs during pregnancy, 179, 184-186
  nutritional disturbances, 1372-1377
  supplementation in formula feeding, 663
VLBW; *see* Very-low-birth-weight infant
Vocalization during infancy, 950-955
Voice
  newborn sensitivity to, 608
  parent-infant bonding, 508
Voiding
  newborn, 596
  postpartum, 492, 495, 499
Vomiting
  brain tumor, 1595
  chemotherapy-induced, 1521
  gastrointestinal dysfunction, 1387
  pediatric, 1401
  during pregnancy
    coping, 195-196
    ectopic pregnancy, 222
    first trimester, 137
  respiratory infection, 1322
von Willebrand disease, 231
Vulva, 927
  adaptations during pregnancy, 110-111
  nullipara *versus* multipara, 107
Vulvovaginal candidiasis, 241
Vulvovaginal glands, 27
VVLBW; *see* Very-very-low-birth-weight infant

W

Wald, Lillian, 789
Waldeyer tonsillar ring, 1328
Walking reflex, 605
War Amputations of Canada, 1736
Warfarin, 272
Warm lines, 586-587
Wart, 1667
Wasp sting, 1675
Water
  balance in infant, 1386-1388
  needs during pregnancy, 182-184
Water intoxication, 664
Water-soluble vitamins, 179, 186
Waterhouse-Friderichsen syndrome, 1634, 1635
Wealth, 803-804
Weaning, 959
  breastfeeding, 680
  formula feeding, 695
Weber test, 917
Weight, 847, 899
  growth measurements, 1785-1786
  infant, 939
  nutritional status, 193
  toddler, 993
Weight gain
  high-risk infant, 707, 708
  neonatal, 685-686
  preeclampsia, 200
  during pregnancy, 180-182, 195, 328
Weight loss
  high-risk infant, 707, 708
  maternal
    breastfeeding and, 676
    postpartum, 484
Werdnig-Hoffmann disease, 1759-1760
West nomogram, 1285
Wet compress, 1663
Wet dream, 1095
Wharton's jelly, 63, 618, 628
Wheal, 1656
Wheat hypersensitivity, 1385
Wheezing, 1323
Whipworm, 1404
Whitaker perfusion test, 1543
White blood cell count, 1500
  changes during pregnancy, 114
  first trimester, 131
  newborn, 595
  postpartum, 486
  urine test, 1545
White blood cells, breast-feeding benefits, 666
White House Conference on Children, 790
Whitehead, 1684
White's classification of diabetes in pregnancy, 253
Whooping cough, 1034, 1341
WIC program, 664, 790
Wilms tumor, 1559-1560
Wiskcott-Aldrich syndrome, 1534
Witch's milk, 68, 600
Withdrawal
  neonatal, 765-766
  during pregnancy, 302
  psychologic and physiologic signs, 304
Withdrawal bleeding, 522, 523
Wolman disease, 96
Women, Infants, and Children's Nutrition Program, 664, 790
Women's liberation movement, 827
Word association game, 876
Word graphic rating scale, 1212
Working class, 802-803
Working mother, 841
Wound, 1655-1660
  burns, 1693-1695, 1697
  care, 1662-1663
  healing and remodeling of bone, 1712-1713
Wristband identification, 493
Wry neck, 618, 908

X

X chromosome, 51-52
X-linked dominant inheritance, 57
X-linked dominant with reduced penetrance inheritance pattern, 1167
X-linked lymphopenic agammaglobulinemia, 1533

X-linked recessive inheritance, 57-58
Xenograft, 1694
XYY male, 1074

Y

Y chromosome, 51-52
Yawn, newborn, 607
Yellen clamp, 653, 654
Yellow jacket sting, 1675
Yersinia enterocolitica, 1397
Yin and yang, 811
Yolk sac, 61
Youngest child, 829
Yutopar; *see* Ritodrine

Z

Zen macrobiotics, 1382
Zielke procedure, 1732
Zinc
  delayed wound healing, 1660
  needs during pregnancy, 178, 186
  nutritional significance, 1382
Zona reaction, 58
Zygote, 54, 58